# Diseases of the Gastrointestinal Tract and Liver

*For Churchill Livingstone*

*Commissioning Editor:* Sheila Khullar
*Project Editor:* Antonia Seymour
*Copy Editor:* Holly Regan-Jones
*Project Controller:* Sarah Lowe
*Indexer:* Monica Trigg

# Diseases of the Gastrointestinal Tract and Liver

Edited by

**David J C Shearman** PhD MBChB FRCP(Ed) FRACP
Mortlock Professor of Medicine, Department of Medicine,
University of Adelaide, Adelaide, Australia

**Niall Finlayson** PhD MBChB FRCP(Lond) FRCP(Ed)
Consultant Physician, Gastrointestinal Liver Service,
Edinburgh Royal Infirmary, Edinburgh, UK

**Michael Camilleri** MD MPhil(Lond) FRCP(Lond) FRCP(Ed) FACP FACG
Professor of Medicine, Gastroenterology Research Unit,
Mayo Foundation, Rochester, Minnesota, USA

Surgical Editor
**Sir David Carter** MD MBChB FRCS(Glas) FRCS(Ed)
Regius Professor of Clinical Surgery, Department of Surgery,
Royal Infirmary, Edinburgh, UK

THIRD EDITION

CHURCHILL LIVINGSTONE
NEW YORK EDINBURGH LONDON MADRID MELBOURNE SAN FRANCISCO AND TOKYO 1997

CHURCHILL LIVINGSTONE
Medical Division of Pearson Professional Limited

Distributed in the United States of America by Churchill Livingstone Inc.,
650 Avenue of the Americas, New York, N.Y. 10011,
and by associated companies, branches and representatives
throughout the world.



First edition 1982
Second edition 1989
Third edition 1997

ISBN 0 443 05147 X



**British Library Cataloguing in Publication Data**
A catalogue record for this book is available from the British Library.

**Library of Congress Cataloging in Publication Data**
A catalog record for this book is available from the Library of Congress.

Medical knowledge is constantly changing. As new information becomes available, changes in treatment, procedures, equipment and the use of drugs become necessary. The editors and contributors and the publishers have, as far as it is possible, taken care to ensure that the information given in this text is accurate and up to date. However, readers are strongly advised to confirm that the information, especially with regard to drug usage, complies with latest legislation and standards of practice.

Printed and bound in Great Britain by
Butler & Tanner Ltd, Frome and London

The publisher's policy is to use paper manufactured from sustainable forests

# Contents

# Contributors

**Graeme J M Alexander** MA MD FRCP
Lecturer, University of Cambridge, School of Clinical Medicine, Cambridge, UK

**David Bartolo** MS FRCS
Consultant Colorectal Surgeon, Royal Infirmary, Edinburgh, UK

**Ian A D Bouchier** CBE MD FRCP FRCPE HonFCP(SAf) FFPHM FRSA FIBiol FRSE
Professor of Medicine, Department of Medicine, University of Edinburgh, Royal Infirmary, Edinburgh, UK

**Ray Brettle** MB ChB MD FRCP(Ed)
Consultant Physician, City Hospital; Reader in Medicine, Department of Medicine, University of Edinburgh, Edinburgh, UK

**Peter Brunt** MD FRCP FRCPE
Consultant Physician and Gastroenterologist, Gastrointestinal and Liver Service, Aberdeen Royal Infirmary; Clinical Professor of Medicine, University of Aberdeen, Aberdeen, UK; Physician to HM The Queen in Scotland

**Michael Camilleri** MD MPhil(Lond) FRCP(Lond) FRCP(Ed) FACP FACG
Professor of Medicine, Gastroenterology Research Unit, Mayo Foundation, Rochester, Minnesota, USA

**Sir David Carter** MD MBChB FRCS(Glas) FRCS(Ed)
Regius Professor of Clinical Surgery, Department of Surgery, Royal Infirmary, Edinburgh

**Albert J Czaja** MD FACP FACG
Professor of Medicine, Mayo Medical School; Consultant in Gastroenterology, Mayo Clinic, Rochester, Minnesota, USA

**G T Davies** MB BCh FRCP(Ed) FRCR FRACR DMRD(Ed)
Consultant Radiologist, Memorial Hospital, North Adelaide, South Australia

**John F Dillon** MB BS MRCP
Consultant Gastroenterologist and Honorary Senior Lecturer, Gastrointestinal Liver Service, Ninewells Hospital and Medical School, Dundee, UK

**Roger Dozois** MD MS FACS FRCS(Glas)(Hon)
Chair, Division of Colon and Rectal Surgery, Mayo Clinic; Professor of Surgery, Mayo Medical School, Rochester, Minnesota, USA

**M G Dunlop** MB ChB FRCS MD
Senior Lecturer in Surgery, MRC Clinician Scientist Fellow and Consultant Surgeon, Institute for Human Gene Therapy, University of Pennsylvania Medical Center, Philadelphia, USA

**Michael J G Farthing** MD FRCP
Professor of Gastroenterology, St Bartholomew's and the Royal London School of Medicine and Dentistry, London, UK

**Niall Finlayson** PhD MBChB FRCP(Lond) FRCP(Ed)
Consultant Physician, Gastrointestinal Liver Service, Edinburgh Royal Infirmary, Edinburgh, UK

**C Richard Fleming** MD
David Murdock Professor of Nutrition Science, Mayo Medical School; Chief of Gastroenterology, Mayo Clinic, Jacksonville, Florida, USA

**M J Ford** MD FRCPE
Consultant Physician, Eastern General Hospital; Honorary Senior Lecturer, University of Edinburgh, Edinburgh, UK

**John A H Forrest** BSc(Hons) MD FRCP
Consultant Physician and Gastroenterologist, Stobhill Hospital, Glasgow, UK

**O James Garden** BSc MD FRCS(Glas & Ed)
Senior Lecturer and Honorary Consultant Hepatobiliary Surgeon, Department of Surgery and Scottish Liver Transplantation Unit, University of Edinburgh, Royal Infirmary, Edinburgh, UK

**A E S Gimson** FRCP
Consultant Physician and Hepatologist, Hepatobiliary and Liver Transplant Unit, Addenbrooke's Hospital, Cambridge, UK

**J B Gross (Jr)** MD
Assistant Professor of Medicine, Mayo School of Medicine; Consultant in Gastroenterology, Mayo Clinic, Rochester, Minnesota, USA

**John P Hanley** MRCP(UK)
Lecturer in Haematology, Department of Haematology, Royal Infirmary, and the University of Edinburgh Medical School, Edinburgh, UK

**Peter C Hayes** BMSc MBChB MD PhD FRCPE
Senior Lecturer and Honorary Consultant Physician, Department of Medicine, Royal Infirmary of Edinburgh, Edinburgh, UK

**Richard M Holloway** BSc(Med) MD FRACP
Senior Consultant Gastroenterologist, Gastrointestinal Medicine, Royal Adelaide Hospital; Clinical Senior Lecturer, Department of Medicine, University of Adelaide, Adelaide, Australia

**Michael Horowitz** MB BS PhD FRACP
Professor of Medicine, Department of Medicine, Royal Adelaide Hospital, Adelaide, Australia

**Peter Katelaris** MB BS FRACP MD
Consultant Gastroenterologist and Clinical Senior Lecturer, Gastroenterology Unit, The University of Sydney, Concord Hospital, Sydney, Australia

**Darlene G Kelly** MD PhD
Assistant Professor of Medicine, Consultant in Gastroenterology and Internal Medicine, Mayo Medical Clinic, Mayo Foundation, Rochester, Minnesota, USA

**Michael J Krowka** MD
Consultant, Division of Pulmonary and Critical Care Medicine, Mayo Clinic, Rochester, Minnesota, USA

**John Lambert** MB BS MMed PhD FRACP FRCP(C)
Associate Professor and Director of Medicine and Gastroenterology, Mornington Peninsula Hospital, Frankston, Melbourne, Australia

**A Lee** BSc MBChB FRCA
Consultant in Anaesthetics and Intensive Care, Department of Anaesthetics, Royal Infirmary, Edinburgh, UK

**Keith D Lindor** MD
Professor of Medicine, Division of Gastroenterology, Mayo Clinic, Rochester, Minnesota, USA

**Christopher A Ludlam** PhD FRCPEdin FRCPath
Consultant Haematologist and Director of the Haemophilia and Haemostasis Centre, Royal Infirmary; Senior Lecturer in Medicine, Department of Medicine, University of Edinburgh Medical School, Edinburgh, UK

**A J MacGilchrist** MD FRCP
Consultant Physician, Scottish Liver Transplant Unit, Royal Infirmary, Edinburgh, UK

**Laurie J Maidl** RN BSN CETN
Certified Enterostomal Therapy Nurse, Mayo Clinic, Rochester, Minnesota, USA

**Janice Main** MB ChB FRCP(Edin & Lond)
Senior Lecturer in Infectious Diseases and General Medicine, Department of Medicine, Imperial College, St Mary's Hospital, London, UK

**Michael N Marsh** DSc DM FRCP
Reader in Medicine, University of Manchester School of Medicine; Consulting Physician, University Department of Medicine, Hope Hospital, Salford, UK

**M V Merrick** MSc BM BCh FRCPE FRCR
Consultant and Head, Department of Nuclear Medicine, Western General Hospital NHS Trust; Consultant in Nuclear Medicine, Royal Infirmary and Royal Hospital for Sick Children, Edinburgh, UK

**David M Nagorney** MD
Professor of Surgery, Mayo Medical School, Mayo Clinic, Rochester, Minnesota, USA

**James Neuberger** DM FRCP
Consultant Physician, Liver and Hepatobiliary Unit, Queen Elizabeth Hospital, Birmingham, UK

**Alan L Ogilvie** MD FRCP(Ed)
Consultant Physician, Northampton General Hospital, Northampton, UK

**Kelvin R Palmer** MD FRCP(Ed)
Consultant Gastroenterologist, Western General Hospital, Edinburgh, UK

**Randall K Pearson** MD
Assistant Professor of Medicine, Mayo Clinic, Rochester, Minnesota, USA

**I W Percy-Robb** MB ChB PhD FRCP FRCPath
Head of Academic Department of Pathological Biochemistry, Western Infirmary, Glasgow, UK

**Eamonn M M Quigley** MD FRCP (Glas, Ed) FACG
Chief, Gastroenterology and Hepatology, University of Nebraska Medical Center, Omaha, Nebraska, USA

**G J Reece** MB BS FRACR FRCR
Senior Visiting Consultant, Department of Radiology, Royal Adelaide Hospital, Adelaide, South Australia

**H Ring-Larsen** MD DSci FRCP(E)
Associate Professor, Division of Hepatology, Rigshospitalet, University of Copenhagen, Copenhagen, Denmark

**Charles B Rosen** MD
Assistant Professor of Surgery, University of Florida College of Medicine, Gainesville, Florida, USA

**Robert Rowland** BSc(Hons,Lon) MBBS(Lon) FRCPath FRCPA
Senior Director and Deputy Head, Division of Tissue Pathology, Institute of Medical and Veterinary Science; Clinical Senior Lecturer, Department of Pathology, University of Adelaide, and Senior Consultant Specialist (Tissue Pathology), Royal Adelaide Hospital, Adelaide, Australia

**Douglas L Seidner** MD
Staff, Department of Gastroenterology, and Co-Director, Nutrition Support Team, Cleveland Clinic Foundation, Nutrition Support Team, Cleveland, Ohio, USA

**David J C Shearman** PhD MBChB FRCP(Ed) FRACP
Mortlock Professor of Medicine, Department of Medicine, University of Adelaide, Adelaide, Australia

**K J Simpson** MD MRCP
Lecturer in Medicine, Department of Medicine, Edinburgh Royal Infirmary, Edinburgh, UK

**Stuart J Spechler** MD
Director, Center for Swallowing Disorders, Beth Israel Deaconess Medical Center; Associate Professor of Medicine, Harvard Medical School, Boston, Massachusetts, USA

**Wei Ming Sun** MB BS PhD
Dr Paul Janssen Senior Lecturer in Medicine, Department of Medicine, Royal Adelaide Hospital, Adelaide, South Australia

**Charles Swainson** MD FRCPE
Consultant Physician, Department of Renal Medicine, Royal Infirmary of Edinburgh; Senior Lecturer, Department of Medicine, University of Edinburgh Medical School, Edinburgh, UK

**William J Tremaine** MD
Associate Professor of Medicine, Mayo Medical School; Director, Inflammatory Bowel Disease Clinic, Mayo Clinic, Rochester, Minnesota, USA

**D Wray** MD BDS MBChB FRSRCPS FDSRCSEd
Professor of Oral Medicine, Glasgow Dental School, Glasgow, UK

# Preface

Fifteen years ago in the preface to this book we described gastroenterology as one of the most exciting of medical specialties. Increasing information about the normal and abnormal functions of the gastrointestinal tract, the hepatobiliary system and the pancreas, better understanding of diseases, and continuing improvements in investigative methods have ensured that this description remains true. Examples of change over these years include better understanding and investigation of gastrointestinal motility disorders, expanding knowledge of viral causes of hepatitis, the transmission of ultrasonic imaging into the gastrointestinal tract and abdomen by endoscopic and laparoscopic ultrasonography, major improvements in therapeutic endoscopy, the appearance of new drugs such as proton-pump inhibitors and a dramatic expansion of liver transplantation. The rate of change inevitably strains the ability of individual doctors to keep abreast of knowledge relating to clinical practice, and in many centres doctors specialise in hollow-organ (gastrointestinal) or solid-organ (hepatobiliary and pancreatic) gastroenterology. Further more, the nature of the changes has ensured that gastroenterology remains a highly clinical specialty dependent on procedures done by clinicians or, particularly, their radiological colleagues.

These changes may raise questions about the wisdom of producing a book covering the two branches of gastroenterology, but our readers remind us that most gastroenterologists in clinical practice look after patients with a wide range of gastrointestinal disease, that general physicians or internists also see such patients, and that even the most highly specialized gastroenterologists can benefit from a broadly-based text. Accordingly, we make no apology for including gastrointestinal, hepatic and pancreatic diseases in one volume and we continue to aim at integrating these diseases into a unified structure using as simple and uniform a style as possible and at producing a balance determined by a clinical approach to the specialty and an extensive but selective referencing. Our aim remains that of providing a clinically orientated text based on an attempt to balance a rapidly expanding and often confusing medical literature with the practical experience of the editors and their contributors. This approach should be of value to physicians in training, to general medical practitioners and to gastroenterologists. Physicians in training are often fascinated by investigations such as endoscopy, but we are aware that about a half of our patients have non-organic or functional disorders which require communication skills as well as technical prowess. We have, therefore, tried to present gastroenterology as a clinical specialty in which investigations serve rather than dominate our patients.

The number of Editors in this edition has increased to four, and the number of contributors to 50. The main reasons for this expansion have been a desire to give this edition an even greater international appeal than previously by the inclusion of Michael Camilleri from the Mayo Clinic so that the editors reflect Australian, United Kingdom and North American practice, and to recognise the integration of medical and surgical gastroenterology by the inclusion of David Carter. The contributors also reflect an international body of opinion and bring their individual expertise to the book. The expansion of our specialty has also led to an expansion of the book in spite of the best efforts of the Editors, and this is reflected in an increase in the number of chapters from 49 to 57, and the inclusion of new or expanded sections on oral diseases, motility disorders, the effects of HIV infection, nutrition, pulmonary aspects of liver disease, the spleen and transplantation. We would like to thank each of our contributors for bringing their skills to this book and providing us with much postgraduate education. Their contributions have brought invaluable improvement but any shortcomings remain the responsibility of the Editors who are still the final common pathway into the text.

We look back in astonishment that we ever agreed to produce a third edition having suffered the traumas of two previous editions. However, it remains as difficult as ever to give up a successful book, and we have been encouraged by the comments of readers and clinical colleagues. Our families have continued to be understanding but equally important they have continued to contribute to the book. Clare Shearman has done extensive work on the gastrointestinal section, Dale Finlayson has done equally extensive work on the hepatobiliary section, and Dr Duncan Finlayson has continued to track down and check all the hepatobiliary references with his insistence for accuracy undiminished by the fact that he is now in his 91st year. We are deeply grateful.

D. J. C. S.
Adelaide and Edinburgh N. D. C. F.

As this is the third and final edition to which I will contribute, I wish to compliment my fellow editors on their hard work, expertise and kindness. Sir David Carter's immense contributions to surgery are evident to all and it has been extremely gratifying that he has had time to continue to contribute to this book. I would also like to thank Michael Camilleri for his contribution and enthusiasm and for bringing to the edition the possibility that this will become a book of worldwide consensus. Those of you who know Niall Finlayson will be aware that he is truly a physician's physician; a careful, diligent, well-read physician to whom you would trust members of your family. In journeying to a new and exciting country in 1975 I suffered the immense loss of the day-to-day friendship I enjoyed with Niall Finlayson. But our friendship remains intact and enhanced despite the tribulations of three editions! I thank Niall for his support, counsel and friendship.

Adelaide David Shearman

# Preface to the second edition

Several important factors contributed to the success of the first edition of *Diseases of the Gastrointestinal Tract and Liver*. Our readers tell us that these were the inclusion of gastrointestinal and liver disease in one volume, the integration of these diseases into a unified structure using as simple and uniform a style as possible, a balance determined by a clinical approach to the specialty and extensive but selective referencing. In the second edition we have aimed to retain these strengths and principles and have sought to build upon them. Our aim, therefore, remains that of providing a clinically oriented text, based on a consensus between a rapidly expanding and often confusing medical literature and the practical experience of the editors and contributors. This approach will be of value to physicians in training, to general medical practitioners and to gastroenterologists. Physicians in training are often fascinated by investigations such as endoscopy but we have tried to present gastroenterology as a clinical specialty in which investigations serve rather than dominate our patients.

The number of contributors in this edition has increased but their contributions mainly embrace sections of several chapters, emphasizing the close coordination which we believe is an essential feature of this book. The importance of surgery to the development of gastroenterology and hepatology and to its clinical implementation is reflected in the appointment of David Carter as surgical editor. Likewise, the increasing impact on our specialty since 1982 of the various forms of imaging has led to an expansion of the chapter on this subject and to the recruitment of two radiologists as contributors. Other changes reflect increasing knowledge of pancreatic diseases, the success of liver transplantation and the need to include paediatric diseases which increasingly impinge on the practice of gastroenterologists and hepatologists. We would like to thank each of our contributors for bringing their individual skills to this book and for providing us with so much instruction. Their contributions have brought major improvements while any shortcomings remain our responsibility, for we are still the final common pathway into the text. Under 'Acknowledgements' we also pay tribute to numerous colleagues who have helped us with the first and the second editions. It is a deep sadness to us that Dr Mike Buist, who was so vital to the first edition, died prematurely in October 1986.

Finally, it has to be questioned why, having survived the rigours of the first edition, we should have subjected ourselves, and particularly our families, to a second edition. Quite simply, it is difficult to part with a successful book. Not only have our families continued to be understanding, they have even continued to contribute; typing and text and reference checking have been carried out by Dale Finlayson, Dr Duncan Finlayson and Clare Shearman, and the last has revised the index. We are deeply grateful.

D.J.C.S.

Adelaide and Edinburgh, 1989 N.D.C.F.

# Preface to the first edition

The last decade has seen the evolution of gastroenterology into one of the most exciting of medical specialties. The impetus for this development has arisen from many sources, but particularly from the development of new endoscopic, radiologic, and ultrasonic methods of diagnosis, a rapid increase of knowledge about liver diseases epitomised by the discoveries regarding the viral causes of acute and chronic hepatitis, and the use of sophisticated methods for elucidating absorptive and secretory mechanisms in the intestines. This has led to the production of many books ranging from highly specialised multiauthor works to monographs on pathological, surgical, biochemical, immunological and other aspects of gastroenterology as well as to works on individual diseases. It is not surprising that many believe the general textbook to be outmoded, as it cannot reflect the latest views on every topic. We subscribe, on the contrary, to the view that a comprehensive text is particularly valuable in this situation as it provides an accessible overview for those training in the specialty and for those in clinical practice.

Our main intention has been to write a textbook which will be of practical value to general physicians, physicians and surgeons with a special interest in gastroenterology and especially to those training in this specialty. The book has been written mainly by two authors, and we have tried to ensure that it is well integrated by working together closely, by cross-referencing the text and by providing an extensive index. Almost all gastroenterologists are consulted on gastrointestinal and hepatological problems, and the book therefore covers gastrointestinal and liver diseases in one volume; few gastroenterologists caring for adult patients are consulted about children, consequently no attempt has been made to cover gastrointestinal and liver diseases in childhood.

The text is designed primarily for clinicians. Such a book obviously needs information from the basic disciplines, but we have tried to restrict such material to that relevant to clinical matters. Radiographs, figures and photomicrographs have been used to illustrate principles as space did not permit that every disease be illustrated. A textbook must also be a stimulus and a source for further exploration of the literature: for this reason we have not stinted on references. We have aimed to include historical, research and clinical papers as well as review articles, monographs and books; our main restrictions have been to refer to articles in English and in the more widely available journals. The order of the text has a specific purpose. The first four chapters describe the important principles of investigational procedures. There are specialised texts on each of these investigations, but we aim to describe their main indications and complications and to relate them to the specialty as a whole. Thereafter, the chapters follow a conventional order, but with close integration of diseases of the liver with those of the pancreas and the biliary tree.

In writing this book we have discovered and benefited from the generosity of innumerable people who have aided our efforts. Most are acknowledged elsewhere, but others we would mention here. It is *de rigeur* for authors to pay tribute to their families to the extent that such tribute may easily ring hollow. However, we know now what demands the writing of a book such as this puts on an author's family; curtailed meals, evaded parental responsibilities, forgotten birthdays and anniversaries, social isolation and that wretched box of papers which even goes on family holidays. The fact is that this book would never have been finished without the generous love and tolerance extended by our wives and children. Family members have also helped directly in our work: Clare Shearman has organised the references for the chapters on gastrointestinal disease, Dale Finlayson has done much emergency typing in what are now called antisocial hours and Dr Duncan Finlayson has organised the references for the chapters on liver disease and has frequently strained family unity by his insistence on accuracy. We have been assisted by contributors who have written chapters on subjects in which they have special expertise. No authors could have had contributors easier to work with and we would pay them all a special tribute here. Our publishers are also due special thanks; Andrew Stevenson, Robert Adam and Claire McLeod have proved patient, helpful and capable of goading in a way which led to tolerable productivity rather than despair.

D.J.C.S.

Adelaide and Edinburgh, 1982 N.D.C.F.

# Acknowledgements

David Shearman would like to acknowledge the work of Dr Robert Rowland and Dr Alan Ogilvie on the pathology sections of this book. He would also like to acknowledge the assistance he has received from Dr Erik Yeoh, Department of Medical Oncology, Royal Adelaide Hospital; Dr David Shaw, Director, Infectious Disease Unit, Royal Adelaide Hospital; Dr Ian Roberts-Thomson, Director of Gastroenterology, The Queen Elizabeth Hospital; Ms Elizabeth English, Clinical Nurse Consultant, Stomal Therapy Department, Royal Adelaide Hospital; and the secretarial assistance of Sue Suter, Department of Medicine, University of Adelaide.

A book such as this cannot be written without reproducing material reported in the medical literature. The origins of all such material are indicated in the captions of the relevant figures and tables, and the names of all the authors, the titles of the publications, the relevant volumes and, in the case of books, the publishers are recorded in the reference lists of individual chapters. We acknowledge here with gratitude the permission granted by individual publishers to reproduce material for which they hold the copyright: Fig. 13.13 is reproduced by permission of Academic Press Inc. (New York) Ltd; Figs 48.7 and 48.8 are reproduced by permission of Acta Chirurgica Scandinavica; Table 38.2 is reproduced by permission of the American Association for the Advancement of Science; Figs 24.7, 36.10, 36.11 and 37.4 and Tables 37.16 and 37.17 are reproduced by permission of the American Association for the Study of Liver Disease; Table 49.1 is reproduced by permission of the American College of Gastroenterology; Figs 36.17 and 36.20 are reproduced by permission of the American Gastroenterological Association and Elsevier Sciences Publishing; Fig. 14.2 is reproduced by permission of the American Gastroenterology Association; Fig. 1.41 is reproduced by permission of the American Journal of Roentgenology; Fig. 11.3 is reproduced by permission of the American Journal of Surgery; Fig. 37.1 is reproduced by permission of the American Journal of the Medical Sciences; Figs 36.6 and 53.8 and Table 37.1 are reproduced by permission of the American Medical Association; Fig. 49.2 is reproduced by permission of the American Physiological Society; Fig. 30.1 is reproduced by permission of the American Society for Biochemistry and Molecular Biology; Fig. 49.8 is reproduced by permission of the American Society for Clinical Investigation; Fig. 13.1 is reproduced by permission of the American Society for Clinical Nutrition; Table 13.1 is reproduced by permission of Annual Reviews Inc.; Fig. 25.7 is reproduced by permission of the Archives of Internal Medicine; Figs 19.3 and 19.6 and Table 31.1 are reproduced by permission of Edward Arnold; Figs 33.3 and 33.6 and Tables 33.3 and 33.9 are reproduced by permission of Australasian Medical Publishing; Figs 9.4, 25.11, 18.4, 47.1, 47.2, 49.1, 54.3 and 55.2 and Tables 23.4 and 23.6 are reproduced by permission of Blackwell Scientific Publications; Fig. 17.1 is reproduced by permission of the BMJ Publishing Group; Table 26.3 is reproduced by permission of the British Journal of Hospital Medicine; Figs 11.18 and 48.2 are reproduced by permission of the British Journal of Surgery; Figs 17.15, 34.3, 50.10 and 53.4 and Tables 17.6, 17.7, 33.5 and 34.8 are reproduced by permission of the British Medical Association and the Editor of Gut; Figs 30.3 and 30.7 and Tables 37.6, 44.1 and 44.2 are reproduced by permission of the British Medical Association and the Editor of the the British Medical Journal; Fig. 30.4 is reproduced by permission of Butterworths; Fig. 31.3 is reproduced by permission of the Canadian Medical Association; Fig. 11.1 is reproduced by permission of Cancer Research; Fig. 49.9 is reproduced by permission of Cell Press; Figs 13.11, 23.2, 24.4, 36.3, 50.1, 50.2, 50.3, 50.12, 50.15, 50.16, 50.17and 56.3 are reproduced by permission of Churchill Livingstone; Figs 9.9, 13.14, 25.2, 25.3, 35.9, 36.4, 37.5, 49.6 and 53.9 and Tables 13.4, 13.5, 23.7, 44.6 and 44.7 are reproduced by permission of Elsevier North Holland; Fig. 30.5 is reproduced by permission of the European Journal of Clinical Pharmacology; Figs 13.10 and 13.15 are reproduced by permission of Federation Proceedings; Figs 10.8 and 16.2 and Table 29.9 are reproduced by permission of Grune &

Stratton; Figs 2.28, 2.29 and 6.2 are reproduced by permission of the Journal of Gastroenterology and Hepatology; Fig. 36.19 is reproduced by permission of S. Karger; Figs 11.4, 23.3, 25.5, 31.10, 51.10, 53.5 and 53.6 and Tables 37.11 and 37.14 are reproduced by permission of the Lancet; Fig. 7.1 and Tables 22.1, 23.9 and 23.10 are reproduced by permission of Lea & Febiger; Fig. 44.4 is reproduced by permission of Lippincott Raven; Table 44.4 is reproduced by permission of Lippincott, Harper & Row; Fig. 2.13 is reproduced by permission of Macmillan Press; Figs 8.2, 15.8 and 15.9 and Tables 22.4 and 29.4 are reproduced by permission of Mayo Clinic Proceedings; Figs 15.7, 15.10, 57.1 and 57.2 are reproduced by permission of the Mayo Foundation for Medical Education and Research; Fig. 49.7 is reproduced by permission of the Medical Journal of Australia; Figs 9.14 and 36.1 are reproduced by permission of C V Mosby; Fig. 11.2 is reproduced by permission of the National Cancer Institute; Figs 13.2, 25.9, 35.5, 36.5 and 43.1 and Tables 25.7, 33.6, 33.7, 34.7, 35.2, 35.3, 35.4, 35.5 and 38.3 are reproduced by permission of the New England Journal of Medicine; 29.13 is reproduced by permission of the New York Academy of Sciences; Fig. 13.6 is reproduced by permission of the Nutrition Society; Figs 10.4 and 31.5 are reproduced by permission of Oxford University Press; Figs 52.3 and 54.2 and Tables 34.10, 34.11 and 34.12 are reproduced by permission of Plenum; Fig. 25.1 is reproduced by permission of Rapid Science Publishers; Fig. 35.8 is reproduced by permission of the Royal College of Physicians; Fig. 36.16 is reproduced by permission of the Royal College of Surgeons of Edinburgh; Figs 13.4, 13.5, 13.7, 13.16, 19.2, 19.7, 25.8, 35.1, 35.6, 36.23 and 52.5 and Tables 24.11, 55.2 and 55.3 are reproduced by permission of W B Saunders; Figs 37.2, 37.3, 49.3, 49.4 and 49.5 are reproduced by permission of Charles B Slack; Figs 43.2 and 50.11 are reproduced by permission of Springer Verlag; Fig. 16.8 is reproduced by permission of Surgery, Gynecology and Obstetrics; Figs 36.18 and 39.1 and Tables 33.8 and 36.3 are reproduced by permission of Technical Publishing; Table 16.8 is reproduced by permission of Charles C Thomas; Tables 9.4, 9.5 and 14.7 are reproduced by permission of Universitetforlaget (Oslo); Fig. 1.8 and Table 55.4 are reproduced by permission of the Editor of Viewpoints on Digestive Diseases and the American Gastroenterological Association; Table 44.3 is reproduced by permission of John Wiley; Figs 31.2, 35.3, 36.22, 43.3 and 53.7 and Tables 25.4, 25.5, 36.10 and 39.1 are reproduced by permission of Williams & Wilkins; Figs 12.5 and 54.1 and Tables 48.4 and 55.1 are reproduced by permission of John Wright.

SECTION 1

# Investigations in gastroenterology and hepatology: general techniques, indications and quality control

# 1. Radiological investigations

*G. J. Reece   G. T. Davies*

PLAIN RADIOGRAPHS (Baker 1990)

The plain radiograph is particularly valuable in the diagnosis of the "acute abdomen" and is sometimes taken prior to other radiological procedures as it shows various soft tissue shadows, demonstrates opacities and is generally regarded as essential before deciding on surgery for small bowel obstruction (Jones 1991). However, with the development of more sophisticated techniques (e.g. ultrasound scanning and computed tomography) to demonstrate individual organs in the abdomen, the value of the plain radiograph is decreasing (Hayward et al 1984, Simeone et al 1985). It is suggested that computed tomography (CT) is the examination of choice in cases of suspected small bowel obstruction when clinical and plain film findings are equivocal (Frager et al 1994). Ultrasound scanning (US) is also more accurate in diagnosing small bowel obstruction, in demonstrating its level and predicting its cause than plain film examinations (Ko et al 1993).

### Indications

A plain radiograph of the abdomen is sometimes required prior to other radiological examinations of the gastrointestinal tract because calculi or calcification in tissues may be obscured by contrast medium. Furthermore, opacities such as tablets, calcification or contrast medium retained after previous investigations may be interpreted as contrast medium introduced in the current examination. An abdominal radiograph is always indicated in patients with acute abdominal pain; in addition, a plain radiograph of the chest is indicated since pain in the abdomen may have a cause in the chest, especially in children. Some abdominal conditions, for example pancreatitis, may cause secondary changes in the chest. The abdominal radiograph is also of value in management, for example in assessing the progress of toxic megacolon or subacute intestinal obstruction. The plain radiograph is insensitive in the detection of ascites (p. 1022). Maximum benefit from the plain abdominal radiograph is obtained when it is reported by a senior radiologist (Lee 1976).

### Procedure

The film should be taken in the radiology department if possible, since portable machines produce films of poorer quality. Films are taken with the patient erect and supine; the former must include both sides of the diaphragm and should be taken 2 min after the patient stands or sits up to allow free gas to accumulate under the diaphragm. A very ill patient may lie on the right and left side alternately and a horizontal X-ray beam is used (lateral decubitus films). It has been suggested that the erect abdominal film should be taken only when the supine film is normal in a patient suspected of having obstruction or when perforation is thought to complicate an obstruction (Simpson et al 1985).

### Interpretation

It is important to examine the radiograph systematically with attention to the following points.

#### *Soft tissue shadows*

The liver, spleen and kidneys can be identified because of their slightly different density to surrounding tissue and in particular to fat in adjacent tissue planes. It is important to define the lateral borders of the psoas muscles (Fig. 1.1) and the layer of extraperitoneal fat in the flank ("flank stripe") because the disappearance of either may indicate an adjacent inflammatory process. Abnormal soft tissue shadows are caused by aneurysms, abscesses, cysts and tumors.

#### *Gas shadows*

The small amount of gas normally present in the small or large intestine has a characteristic pattern which allows the distribution of the bowel within the abdomen to be assessed. Small bowel gas is usually central whereas large

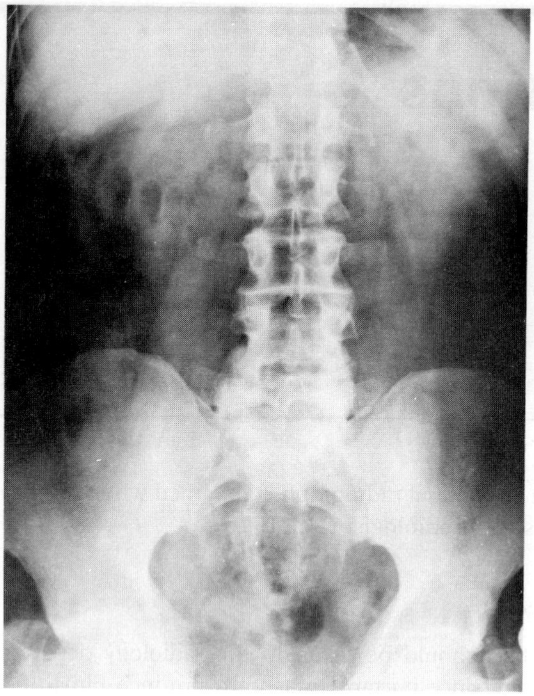

**Fig. 1.1** Normal plain abdominal radiograph. The psoas shadows are seen running obliquely down on either side of the spine. There is a little gas in the stomach and in the colon and rectum but none in the small intestine. The opacity in the right hypochondrium is caused by the liver.

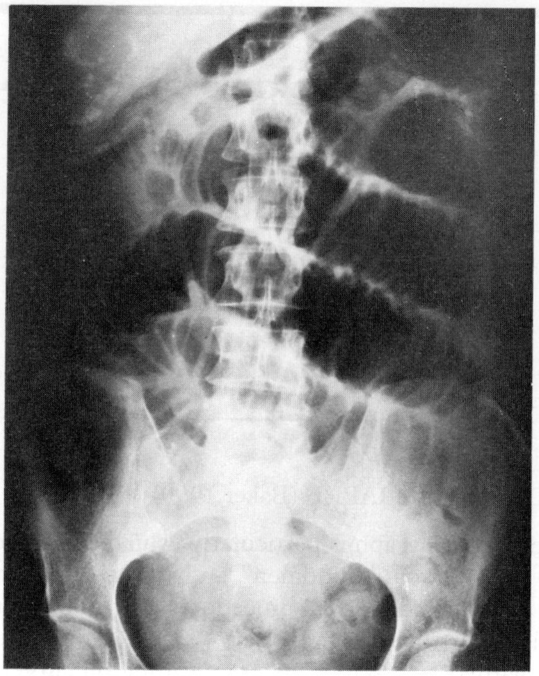

**Fig. 1.2** Obstruction of the small bowel in the ileum. This supine radiograph shows gross distention of bowel proximal to the obstruction with typical cross-hatching. There is practically no gas in the colon. The erect film showed typical fluid levels.

bowel gas tends to be peripheral. Gas is normally seen in the gastric fundus and in the rectum. Gas acts as a contrast medium and occasionally delineates a tumor in the fundus or a strictured or inflamed segment of the bowel (p. 658). Obstruction or paralytic ileus is indicated by fluid levels on the erect film and an excessive amount of gas in the bowel (Figs 1.2 and 1.3). Small bowel fluid levels are arranged in a "step-ladder" pattern centrally in obstruction but tend to be longer and are centrally placed in paralytic ileus. Large bowel fluid levels are longer than those in small bowel disorders and tend to be distributed to the sides of the abdomen or in the pelvis. Complex gas–fluid patterns are to be found in paralytic ileus. There may be a virtual absence of gas in high intestinal obstruction, acute pancreatitis and acute intestinal ischemia.

"Medical" disorders can imitate the abdominal gas patterns of acute surgical disease particularly in infants, children and the elderly, e.g. gastroenteritis, metabolic conditions such as uremia and diabetic ketoacidosis, a history of medication, particularly with ganglion-blocking or anticholinergic drugs, and rare conditions such as lead poisoning, porphyria and some neurological disorders. All physicians ordering abdominal radiographs should be cautious in interpreting appearances in nonsurgical conditions which may simulate an acute surgical emergency and lead to hazardous and unnecessary operations. In cases of doubt consultation with a radiologist and if necessary the performance of more specific investigations should be arranged.

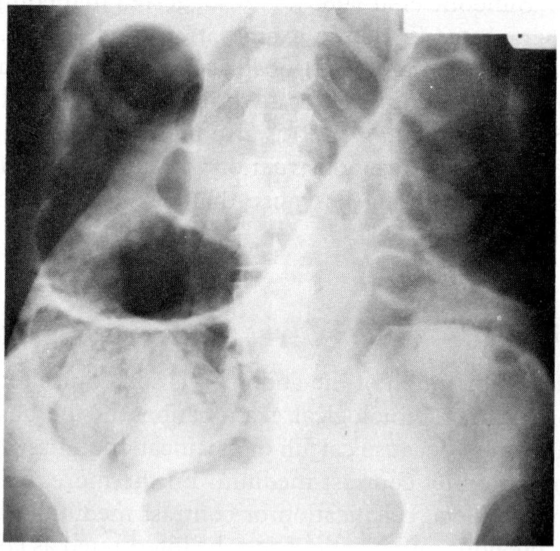

**Fig. 1.3** Gross dilatation of the proximal colon, especially of the cecum, due to obstruction in the descending colon. No "blow-back" into the terminal ileum which could have acted as a safety valve has occurred. In such cases, there is danger of cecal perforation. The obstruction was due to diverticulitis.

Gas may occur in abnormal sites – in the peritoneal cavity as a result of perforation, in a subphrenic abscess, in the bile ducts, gallbladder or portal venous system, in the bowel wall as in pneumatosis intestinalis (p. 1392), or in the colonic wall in colitis or ischemic disease.

*Opacities*

Opacification is usually due to calcium. About 20% of biliary calculi (see Fig. 1.21) and 80% of renal calculi are radio-opaque. Calcification may occur in the liver, gallbladder wall or pancreas (p. 1271), occasionally in cysts and tumors, such as mucoid cancers of stomach or colon, or in the aorta, iliac vessels and aneurysms. Occasionally, confusion may be caused by calcified phleboliths or costochondral calcification and by opaque material, including feces, lying within the lumen of the bowel.

*Bony structures*

The bones should always be inspected for possible causes of abdominal root pain such as degenerative disease of the spine or metastatic deposits.

## GASTROINTESTINAL RADIOLOGY (Gore et al 1994)

### Contrast materials

*Barium sulfate*

Proprietary barium suspensions are of high density and low viscosity (80–90% weight/weight), and are designed to provide maximum adhesion to the gastrointestinal mucosa and to avoid flocculation in the presence of gastric or colonic mucus; these properties are important for producing high-quality radiographs in double-contrast studies. Generators of gas are available commercially mainly in the form of powders or suspensions capable of releasing large volumes of carbon dioxide when in contact with gastric acid.

*Meglumine diatrizoate* (Gastrografin)

This is a water-soluble iodinated contrast medium which is poorly absorbed from the gastrointestinal tract. It is highly osmotic and is rapidly diluted as fluid is pulled into the bowel lumen. This can cause dehydration and its use in children and the elderly must be carefully supervised. Gastrografin is usually given orally in the diagnosis of perforation or obstruction and it can be helpful in demonstrating small intestinal fistulas, provided these are proximal. Gastrografin enemas can be used to investigate known or suspected colonic rupture and when colonic radiographs are required in the presence of a narrow stricture in the distal large bowel. Gastrografin enemas (p. 1240) have been used therapeutically in the management of meconium obstruction in newborn infants, but dehydration must be carefully avoided. Gastrografin must not be used if there is a risk of inhalation or fistula into the lungs, as fatal pulmonary edema can be produced due to its high osmolality. The new, nonionic, water-soluble contrast media such as meglumine and sodium ioxaglate (Hexabrix) and metrizamide (Amipaque) do not harm the lungs in small quantities and do not cause significant reactions in the mediastinum when introduced experimentally (Ginai et al 1985). A new low osmolar compound iohexol (Omnipaque) is a safe alternative to barium or Gastrografin in patients at risk from mediastinitis or pulmonary edema (Brick et al 1988).

### Barium swallow

*Indications*

A barium swallow is regarded by many as the best initial examination for most esophageal disease, especially when dysphagia is present (Caroline 1987). It is also used to demonstrate esophageal varices and to provide information about adjacent abnormalities such as aortic aneurysms, vascular rings and mediastinal lymph node enlargement. Patients with recurrent chest pain in whom coronary artery disease has been excluded may require investigation to identify structural or functional esophageal abnormalities. Barium swallow examination can be most helpful in identifying some of the abnormalities causing such pain (Levine et al 1990).

Recent multidisciplinary approaches to the patient with oropharyngeal dysphagia have been developed utilizing the skills of all medical specialties involved in the care of such patients and, in particular, the close co-operation of the speech therapist (Jones 1992). The development of dynamic recording of the swallowing mechanism utilizing videofluoroscopy and subsequent analysis by the radiologist with the speech therapist and other specialists has enabled the development of criteria for patient management and the design of appropriate therapy (Siebens & Linden 1985).

In patients with suspected gastroesophageal reflux, the examination confirms the presence of a hiatus hernia and/or reflux and can identify sequelae such as reflux esophagitis, peptic strictures, Barrett's esophagus and esophageal adenocarcinoma (Levine & Laufer 1993).

*Contraindications*

Barium is not used if a perforation or leakage from a suture line is suspected. Instead a water-soluble contrast medium is used. If a fistula between the esophagus and the respiratory system is suspected, the newer non-ionic products are indicated.

*Preparation*

The procedure is usually combined with radiological examination of the stomach and duodenum after the patient has been fasted for 12 h. The combined examination is particularly important in disease of the lower esophagus as gastric cancer infiltrating the esophagus may simulate achalasia; furthermore the demonstration of hiatus hernia requires adequate filling of the stomach by barium.

*Procedure*

The details of the procedure, including the dilution of barium, vary with different radiologists; it is essential to provide adequate clinical information so that the radiologist can apply the measures appropriate to the problem. The physiology, radiology and pathology of the oral and pharyngeal phases of swallowing have been reviewed by Dodds et al (1989, 1990). With both the pharynx and the upper esophagus, it is usual to take anteroposterior and lateral radiographs while the esophagus is distended with barium and when cleared, in order to define the mucosal pattern. Oblique radiographs are also helpful in the pharyngeal region and are mandatory in the esophagus to enable views free of the spine.

In general, high-density (80–90% weight/weight) barium is used to examine the pharynx and thoracic esophagus. Initially, each sip is watched by the radiologist so that the stages of relaxation, contraction and resting can be observed. 'Spot' films may be taken during swallowing; mucosal films are taken immediately after the barium has passed through the area. More barium is taken for maximum distention of the esophagus and a mixture of bread and barium or marshmallows of known diameter are sometimes used to demonstrate rings and to investigate dysphagia for solids. More elaborate maneuvers are required for the study of hiatus hernia and gastroesophageal reflux.

The examination should include double-contrast radiographs of the mucosa to assess the morphology, particularly in the diagnosis of esophagitis and early cancer. A dynamic examination, preferably with videofluoroscopy, should be performed to assess function (Levine et al 1990). The patient is asked either to rapidly swallow alternate mouthfuls of barium and water in the prone position or gas-producing granules given in water followed by rapid swallows of barium in the erect position. Intravenous glucagon is helpful in obtaining good double-contrast esophograms, particularly in identifying mucosal changes (Op den Orth 1989).

The pharynx is difficult to examine because the swallowing process is completed quickly. Thus, for the demonstration of neuromuscular problems and webs, rapid sequence filming or videorecording (p. 9) is necessary. However, it is possible to obtain information from the mucosal pattern after thick barium has been swallowed and from the distensibility seen with the patient blowing against closed lips (Valsalva maneuver). A lateral view with a large bolus of barium will demonstrate the posterior wall in the search for vertebral osteophytes and cricopharyngeal hypertrophy.

*Interpretation* (Low & Rubesin 1993)

A radiograph of the pharynx is shown in Figure 1.4 and a diagram in Figure 6.1. When the pharynx and upper esophagus are filled with barium, the posterior wall is straight and runs parallel to the spine; the anterior wall has irregularities at the level of the vallecula, epiglottis and laryngeal vestibule. Contrast films are important to assess the structure and distensibility of the pharynx. A tumor is usually detected visually or by endoscopy, but radiology is used to assess its precise location and extent. As a significant number of tumors in the pharyngeal region are submucosal and are not recognized by palpation, direct laryngoscopy and endoscopy, CT or magnetic resonance imaging (MRI) may be necessary if barium studies are also negative (Harnsberger & Dillon 1994).

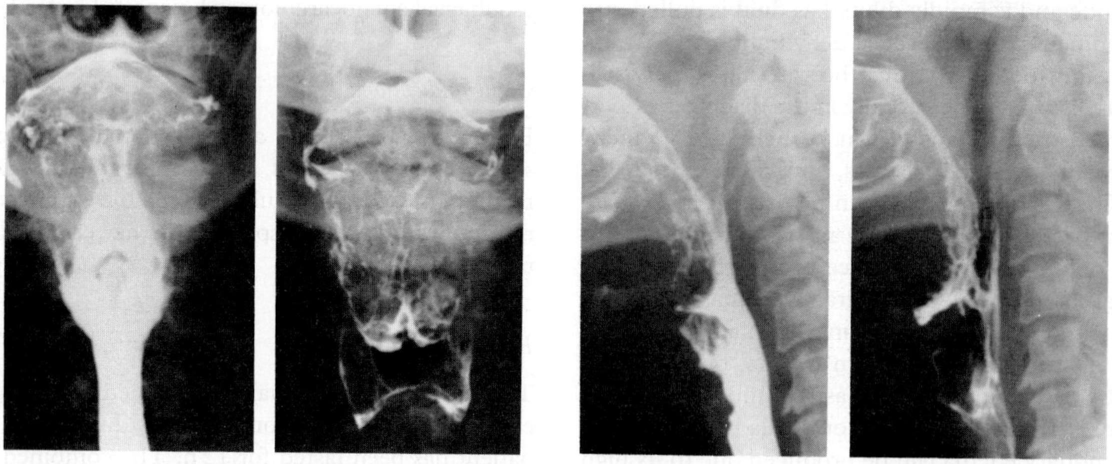

**Fig. 1.4** Radiographs of the normal pharynx during (*left*) and after (*right*) a swallow of barium. Anteroposterior (*left pair*) and lateral (*right pair*) films are shown.

Neuromuscular disorders are often difficult to demonstrate by taking isolated films during the barium swallow examination and thus fluoroscopic observation, rapid-sequence films and videorecording are used. Normally, the bolus is squeezed out of the oral cavity by pressure from the tongue so that it passes through the fauces into the oropharynx. The hyoid and lateral walls of the pharynx are elevated to enclose the bolus and at the same time the posterior part of the tongue obliterates the upper part of the nasopharynx. As the bolus passes further, the epiglottis and the laryngeal musculature prevent entry into the larynx and a rise in pharyngeal pressure accompanied by relaxation of the cricopharyngeus allows the bolus to move into the esophagus. In neuromuscular disturbance barium may enter the larynx or nasopharynx or reenter the mouth. Barium may pool in the pharynx because of inability to contract the pharynx or to relax the cricopharyngeus.

In the examination of the esophagus, the radiologist assesses its position, motility and mucosal features (Figs 1.5 and 1.6). Radiographs are taken in oblique positions in the erect, supine and prone postures. Obstructive lesions are best demonstrated with the patient erect; the recumbent position is used to detect hiatus hernia and motor abnormalities, as the transit of swallowed barium is slower and

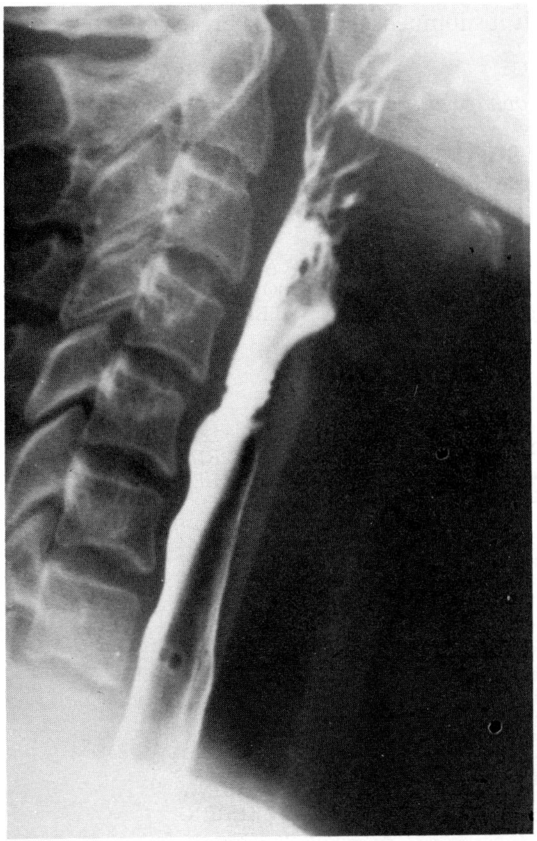

**Fig. 1.5** Normal cervical esophagus. The posterior border of the esophagus is parallel to the cervical spine and separated form it by only a few millimeters.

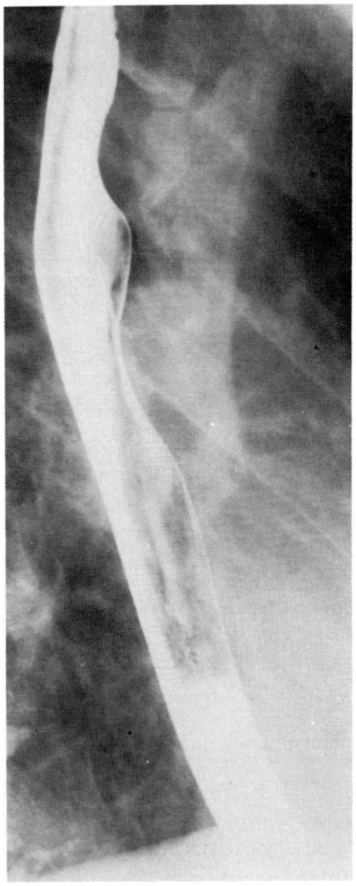

**Fig. 1.6** Normal esophagus. Right anterior oblique view showing extrinsic impressions caused by the aortic arch (*above*) and the left main bronchus (*below*).

hence easier to study and record. The relationship of the esophagus to the great vessels and main bronchi is shown in Figure 1.7. The aortic arch indents the esophagus (Fig. 1.6). Abnormalities are seen with aneurysm of the aorta, aberrant right subclavian artery and right-sided aorta (p. 186). At a slightly lower level, the esophagus is indented by the left main bronchus. Between these two indentations is a small area which is liable to develop pulsion diverticula (p. 181). Below the bronchial indentation, the esophagus is surrounded by lymph nodes and diseases of these nodes may result in traction diverticula (p. 181). Below this, it has close contact with the left atrium.

Under normal circumstances, when liquid barium is swallowed by the erect patient, the esophagus relaxes and the barium momentarily fills its entire length before a primary peristaltic wave empties the esophagus. Relaxation then occurs and any remaining barium is cleared by secondary peristaltic waves. Tertiary contractions are spontaneous nonperistaltic contractions seen in the lower esophagus. They are common in healthy older patients (p. 178). These progressive esophageal movements are best recorded by studying the passage of a single swallow of barium as it proceeds distally. The normal sequence of

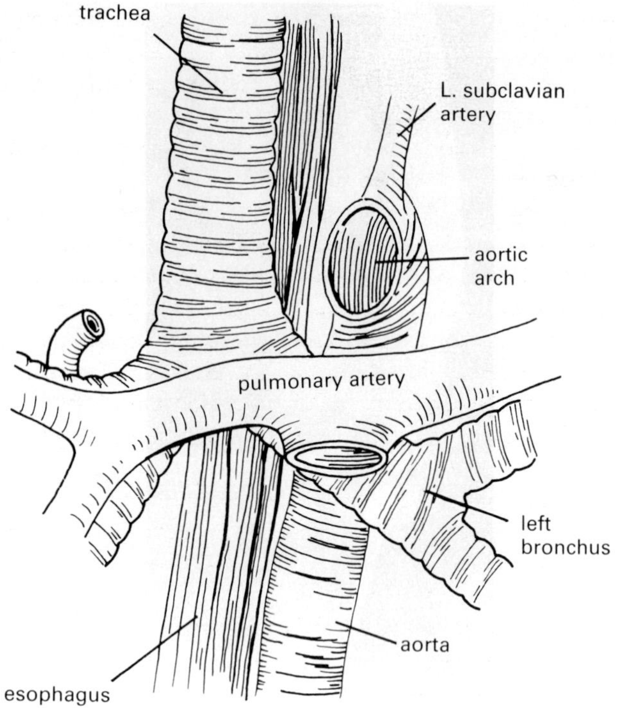


**Fig. 1.7** The relation of the esophagus to the great vessels and main bronchi.

events is nearly always disrupted in the primary motility disorders of diffuse spasm (p. 177) and achalasia (p. 173), and disturbance in motility may also be secondary to organic diseases, such as tumors and peptic esophagitis. Motor disturbances and ring formation (p. 181) may be accentuated by studying the swallowing of solid material.

Tumors are detected by a break in the continuity of the barium column and by the demonstration of a filling defect in the lumen (p. 206). Benign tumors cause a smooth filling defect and do not alter peristalsis; malignant tumors form irregular filling defects and the esophageal walls are rigid. Submucosal infiltration by tumor in the lower part of the esophagus may be difficult to distinguish from achalasia (p. 175) or peptic oesophagitis. In such circumstances computed tomography can be used to study the thickness of the esophageal wall and involvement of neighboring structures.

The normal mucosal pattern consists of parallel longitudinal folds which are best seen after the barium has passed through the esophagus or by utilizing double-contrast techniques. Varices appear as beadlike filling defects (see Fig. 36.6). In the early stages, they occur on the anterolateral wall and thus anterior oblique films are taken, often in deep inspiration, as this lowers the diaphragm and exposes the lowest few centimeters of the esophagus. The demonstration of varices frequently requires multiple films in different positions, particularly supine and prone, and in varying phases of respiration.

Inflammation of the esophagus may thicken or disrupt the longitudinal folds, and there may be motility disturbances. Later, there is narrowing of the esophagus (p. 200), usually due to prolonged spasm but sometimes due to fibrosis if submucosal disease is present.

### *The esophagogastric region*

The normal anatomy (Fig. 1.8) and physiology of this region are difficult to understand because different terms

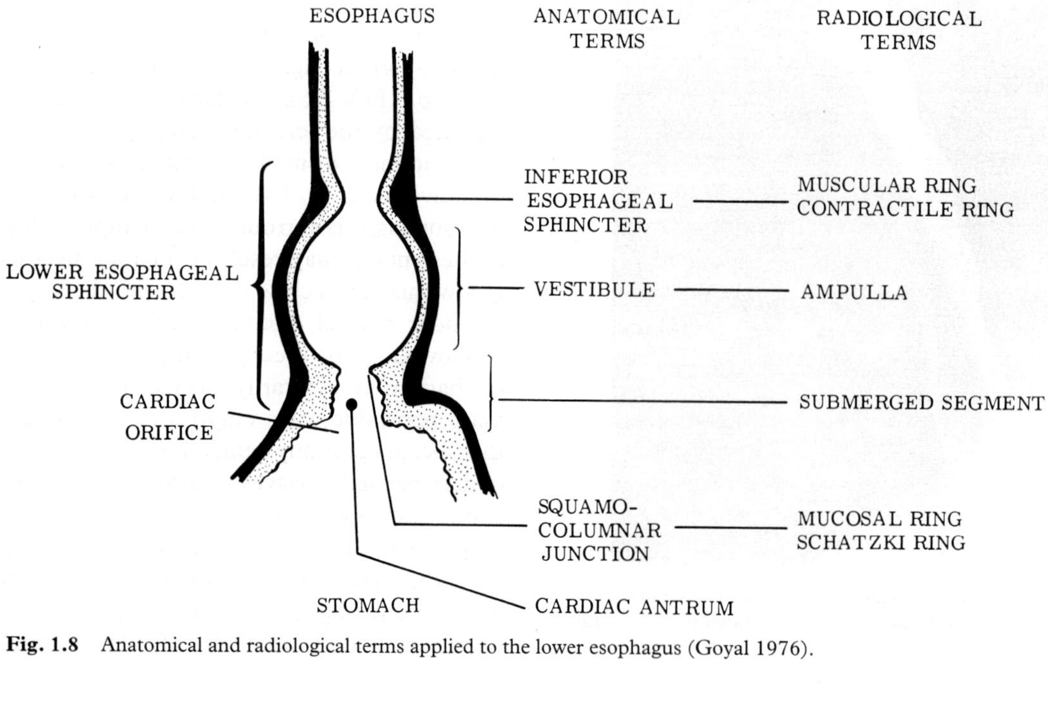


**Fig. 1.8** Anatomical and radiological terms applied to the lower esophagus (Goyal 1976).

have been adopted by radiologists, endoscopists and by those describing the motility of the region. The tubular esophagus joins the (phrenic) ampulla, about 3 cm above the diaphragmatic hiatus. During swallowing, the esophagus closes at its junction with the (phrenic) ampulla, leaving the latter filled with barium which then empties into the stomach. Between the lower limit of the (phrenic) ampulla and the stomach, the esophagus is referred to as the submerged segment because it lies within the abdomen. This segment is narrowed because of the relatively high intra-abdominal pressure. The esophagogastric mucosal junction lies in the submerged segment, but its position cannot be determined radiologically and it cannot be related to the position of the diaphragm. Anatomical terms are also sometimes used. The term "vestibule" denotes the squamous part of the esophagogastric region (Fig. 1.9) and the term "cardiac antrum" denotes the area lined by glandular epithelium. Thus, the stomach includes a short tubular segment of about 1 cm proximal to the cardiac orifice. The high-pressure zone is defined by manometry as the zone of intraluminal pressure which exceeds the pressure within the fundus. It extends above and below the diaphragmatic hiatus for 1–2 cm, the distal margin being the cardiac orifice; the proximal margin is in the region of the junction between esophagus and vestibule which is recognizable at esophagoscopy by the mucosal rosette (p. 104). The term "lower esophageal sphincter" has been used for the high-pressure zone. The term "inferior esophageal sphincter" also requires definition; Wolf (1967) suggests that the term be reserved for the contractile band occasionally seen on radiographs between the esophagus and the vestibule.

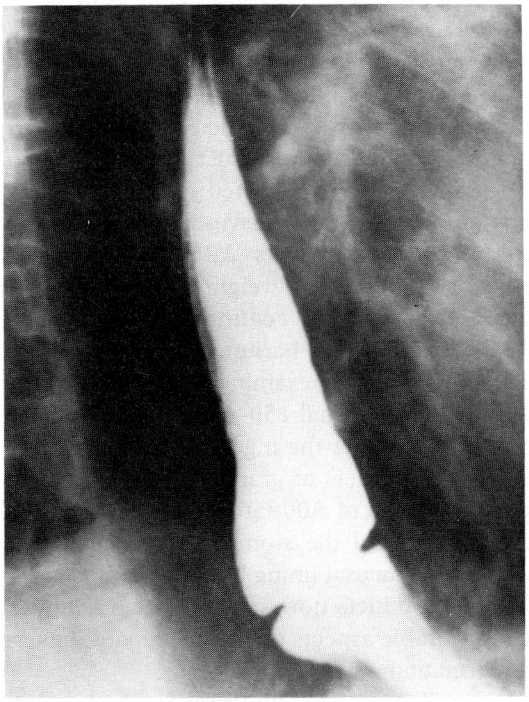

**Fig. 1.9** Normal lower esophagus. The vestibule, a temporary fusiform dilatation at the lower end of the esophagus, is clearly seen. Indentation in the middle of the vestibule is now considered to be due to a prominent ridge of mucosa at the junction between squamous and columnar epithelium.

Radiologically the esophagogastric junction is a complex region and its definition is important in the diagnosis of hiatus hernia and reflux esophagitis. The specific landmark for the squamocolumnar junction is the transition from smooth esophageal to nodular gastric mucosa at the "z" line. The "z" line is normally at the level of the hiatus and can quite frequently be identified on double-contrast films. Upward displacement of this junction is a diagnostic sign of hiatus hernia (Gelfand & Ott 1979). The gastric sling fibers may also notch the lateral aspect of the esophagogastric junction and this may be seen in hiatus hernia (Friedland 1978).

The transverse mucosal fold or B ring may indent the esophagus at the junction (Wolf 1970). It is likely that a Schatzki ring (Schatzki & Gary 1953) is an exaggerated weblike form of the transverse mucosal fold. Another ring indentation can be demonstrated at the proximal end of the vestibule and has been labeled as the muscular ring, the contractile ring or A ring (Wolf 1970).

Radiological definition of a small hiatus hernia can be difficult, firstly because the esophagogastric mucosal junction cannot be seen and secondly because the (phrenic) ampulla may mimic a small hernia by retaining barium which can run back up the esophagus, simulating reflux.

### Videorecording/rapid-sequence filming

(Ott & Pikna 1993)

These provide a detailed and sequential record of the radiological procedures. Videorecording can be repeated slowly or stopped at any point so that interpretation becomes easier and is the optimal method of studying the pharynx and some areas of the esophagus. Videotape systems, which are cheaper and use less radiation, are used to record and display the fluoroscopic image during screening and have largely supplanted cineradiology, though storage is less convenient. Using a photofluorographic camera attached to the image intensifier, up to six frames a second can be recorded on a conveniently stored 100 mm film format.

Videotape studies of the pharynx should always be used to demonstrate neuromuscular disorders (p. 173) and lesions such as small tumors, webs and diverticula. Frontal and lateral views of the pharynx should be recorded routinely and oblique views are sometimes helpful. The technique is also useful in the diagnosis of disorders of motility in the esophagus as it aids the recognition of normal and abnormal contractions. Finally, it has been used to define more precisely abnormalities of motility and rings in the lower esophagus seen on barium swallow (Wolf 1970).

## Barium meal

*Indications*

The barium meal is used to diagnose diseases of the stomach and duodenum and to delineate disorders of the lower esophagus. The radiologist is concerned mainly with the demonstration of the mucosal surfaces, the detection of ulcer craters, filling defects and motility. The use of antispasmodic agents advocated by many for double-contrast examinations precludes observations of peristaltic activity. The barium meal may give information about adjacent masses or viscera, such as the spleen, liver and pancreas, which may displace the stomach and duodenum, though other scanning modalities will give much more accurate information.

Fiberoptic endoscopy has shown that the standard barium meal is inaccurate. However, most studies of the accuracy of double-contrast barium meals indicate a sensitivity of 80–90% (Pyhtinen et al 1982, Gelfand et al 1984). One study (Dooley et al 1984) suggests that the sensitivity of double-contrast barium meal was only 54% against 92% for endoscopy, though specificity was almost as accurate (91–100%).

Realistically, barium examination will not be as sensitive or specific as endoscopy for the evaluation of small mucosal lesions, nor will it compete with computed tomography, ultrasonography or magnetic resonance imaging in evaluating diseases outside the tubular gastrointestinal tract (Maglinte & Miller 1984). However, there is every reason to believe that reproducible, accurate and cost-effective barium examinations will be required for investigation for years to come, remembering that radiology and endoscopy are complementary (Fraser & Earnshaw 1983) and are not mutually exclusive. Whenever there is doubt about the interpretation of the appearance at double-contrast barium meal, an endoscopic opinion should be sought. Similarly the radiologist should be aware of the limitations of endoscopy imposed by observer error and the inadequacy of forceps biopsy.

*Contraindications*

Barium should not be used when gastroduodenal perforation is suspected or when pyloric stenosis is likely, as the examination rarely defines the cause of the stenosis and barium may become inspissated in the stomach. However, preliminary intubation, stomach washouts and aspiration of barium after the procedure may result in a diagnosis, especially when pyloric narrowing prevents diagnostic endoscopy. Rare hypersensitivity reactions have been ascribed to additives, often undisclosed by the manufacturers, in the various barium preparations, the most common being a skin rash (Janower 1986). In patients with suspected gastric or duodenal perforation, Gastrografin and other iodinated compounds may be used if a contrast study is necessary.

*Preparation*

The patient should be fasted for 12 h prior to the procedure. It is essential to inform the radiologist of suspected abnormalities so that a particular search is made for these. Previous radiographs should be made available and precise details of previous gastroduodenal surgery are essential for a satisfactory examination. Some authors have recommended oral metoclopramide, 10 mg, 30 min before the examination to enhance gastric emptying (Hunt & Anderson 1976).

*Procedure*

***Single-contrast barium meal examination.*** Barium sulfate suspension, 250–300 ml, is ingested and radiographs are taken with the patient prone and in varying degrees of rotation to show both stomach and duodenum adequately filled with barium. Some air-contrast films utilizing swallowed air can be obtained by moving the patient from the prone oblique to the supine oblique position or vice versa. The use of compression to disperse the barium and so display the mucosa, either by the examiner's lead-protected hand or by special attachments to the fluoroscopic apparatus, is an essential part of the examination. Fiberoptic endoscopy has shown that the single-contrast examination misses many lesions, particularly in the fundus and upper lesser curvature of the stomach and in the duodenum. Reference to this technique is made as some centers still use it.

***Double-contrast barium meal examination*** (Levine et al 1988). Most radiologists use personal variations of this technique, but the basic principle is to demonstrate all areas in double contrast by the use of a barium pool from which the mucosa can be coated repeatedly, and by the administration of gas to achieve distention and contrast (Scott-Harden 1979, Evers & Kressel 1982). High-density barium (80–90% weight/weight) is essential to maximize the mucosal coating and detail (Gelfand 1978). The quantity of barium suspension varies from 50 ml for the entire examination to 50 ml initially, followed by an additional 150–200 ml. Gas is introduced before, during or after the ingestion of barium by means of gas-releasing tablets or granules or by an effervescent drink. The release of 300–500 ml of carbon dioxide is sufficient to distend the stomach for adequate demonstration of the mucosal lining both in profile and en face. Commercial products now available have removed most of the unfavorable aspects of earlier preparations, such as bubble formation.

There is a difference of opinion as to whether the examination should be performed during gastroduodenal atony induced by pharmacological means; some radiologists always use atony, whilst others prefer motility to continue. Atony can be induced by hyoscine butylbromide

20 mg intravenously, which acts for 15 min, or by glucagon 1–2 mg intravenously, which acts for 10 min. Glucagon does not cause blurring of vision, retention of urine or cardiac arrhythmias, unlike Buscopan, but care is required in diabetic patients as it induces hyperglycemia.

Numerous radiographs in varying degrees of obliquity in supine, prone and erect postures are necessary for a complete display of the mucosal pattern. It is recommended that the radiographic exposures be kept to a moderate level (90–120 kVpeak) to avoid loss of image detail. The use of rare-earth screens in the radiographic cassettes can significantly lower the radiation dosage, allowing exposures in the 70–90 kVpeak range to be used.

Videofluoroscopy may add useful dynamic information and provides a review method for demonstration and teaching.

*Interpretation*

The normal appearance of the stomach is learned by experience. Its position varies widely, ranging from the horizontal to a long J shape; abnormal positions are assessed by anteroposterior, lateral and oblique views with the stomach full of barium. The stomach may be displaced by a pancreatic mass (p. 1257), an enlarged lobe of the liver or an enlarged spleen; the duodenal cap may be indented by a normal gallbladder or common bile duct, though the earlier use of barium examinations to identify masses in adjacent structures has been largely replaced by more specific scanning methods. Normally, peristaltic waves are seen in the body and antrum and their absence, even in a small area, can signify malignant infiltration. With single-contrast radiographs, an ulcer in the stomach or duodenum is diagnosed by the presence of a barium-filled crater seen either in profile or en face, or by disruption of the mucosal pattern with mucosal folds radiating from the ulcer crater. The appearance of the gastric ulcer may indicate whether it is benign or malignant (p. 244). Peptic ulcer disease may be suspected from gastric deformities, such as the "hour-glass" stomach, and from a deformed duodenal cap. The stomach after gastric surgery is difficult to interpret with single-contrast radiographs as distention of the gastric remnant or of the stomach after gastroenterostomy is inadequate because barium rapidly leaves via the anastomosis.

Using the double-contrast barium meal, it is often possible to see the normal, fine, mosaic pattern on the mucosal surface of the stomach, the areae gastricae (Mackintosh & Kreel 1977) (Figs 1.10 and 1.11 and see Fig. 7.14) and of the duodenal cap (Fig. 1.12). Changes in the normal appearances of the gastric rugae and the areae gastricae are sought as evidence of pathological states. Ulcers are shown as craters filled with barium or as ring shadows (p. 244); when an ulcer is benign, straight folds radiate from it, whereas with a malignant ulcer the folds are disorganized

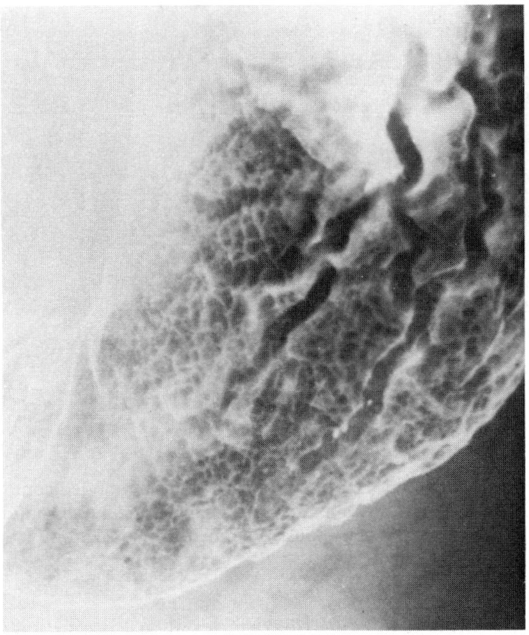

**Fig. 1.10** Normal stomach. Double-contrast technique. Supine view showing the normal mucosal pattern with prominent areae gastricae.

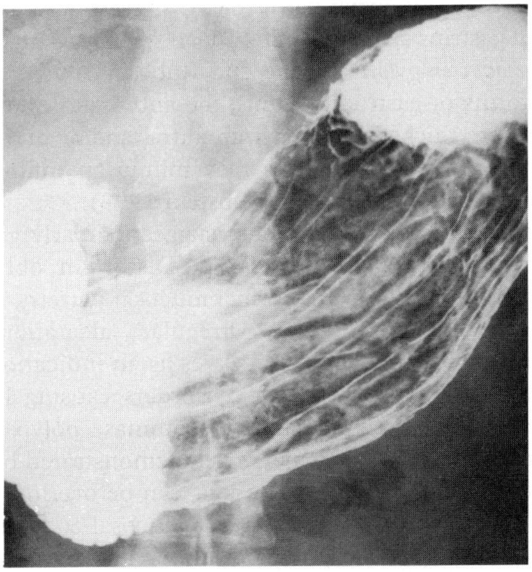

**Fig. 1.11** Normal stomach. Double-contrast technique. The mucosal folds of the anterior wall are seen as thin parallel lines and those of the posterior wall as translucent ridges.

(p. 244). Healed ulcers also retain radiating folds. Duodenal ulcers (p. 241) are recognized by filling of the crater with barium and by radiating folds. The normal duodenal mucosal surface is usually smooth and featureless, though in some patients a fine, lacy reticular pattern is seen in the duodenal cap and rarely in the second part of the duodenum. This is altered by erosive duodenitis, Crohn's disease and celiac disease. The erosive changes in duodenitis are similar to those seen in gastritis, often with

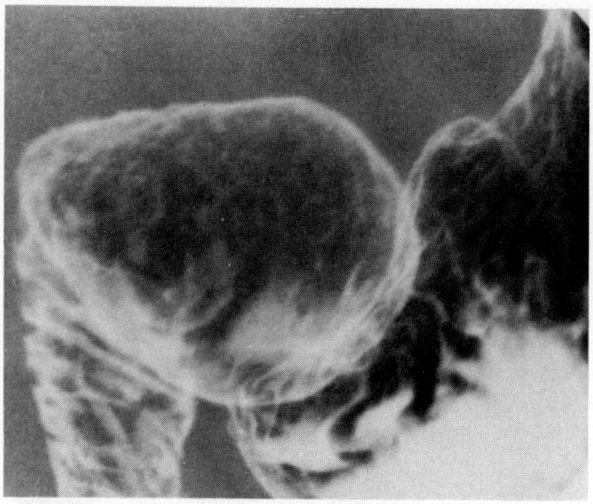

**Fig. 1.12** Normal duodenal cap showing smooth rounded contours and the normal fine mucosal pattern. 20 mg hyoscine butylbromide (Buscopan) was given intravenously to induce duodenal atony.

nodular thickening of the duodenal folds (Glick et al 1984). Gastric erosions are frequently multiple and occur on more than one film as persistent flecks of barium, particularly in the gastric antrum, surrounded by a halo of edema. The radiologist has a role in suggesting the diagnosis of gastritis and duodenitis due to specific agents such as *Helicobacter pylori* (Levine and Rubesin 1995). As in other forms of gastroduodenitis, the antral and duodenal mucosa are thickened, often with antral and/or duodenal ulceration. The appearances may mimic an infiltrating carcinoma or lymphoma (Lichtenstein 1993).

The identification of changes suggesting early gastric cancer (p. 304) requires experience. Distortion, obliteration or irregularity of the normal mucosal pattern, especially if accompanied by irregular ulceration, is suspicious of malignancy and serves as an indication for biopsy of the suspected area. Disorders causing larger filling defects, such as large carcinomas, polyps and benign tumors, are particularly well demonstrated by the double-contrast technique. Lesions can be overlooked if they are situated in an area of poor mucosal coating; gas bubbles may simulate polypoid lesions and barium can flocculate if there is excess mucus in the stomach, leading to opacities which may be interpreted as erosions. Some lesions are too small for resolution, especially minimal mucosal changes.

### Radiology or endoscopy?

Whilst the controversy regarding the decision to utilize endoscopy or barium examinations in patients with upper gastrointestinal symptoms continues, there is no doubt that a fee-for-service environment encourages endoscopists to promote endoscopy (Gelfand et al 1987). Vested interests act as an incentive to burgeoning endoscopic services, especially in the organization of clinical trials. However, the superior accuracy of endoscopy with the access for biopsy must be balanced against the advantages of barium examinations, particularly in esophageal diseases and in showing intramural and extrinsic abnormalities of the upper gastrointestinal tract (Simpkins 1988).

As fewer and fewer upper gastrointestinal examinations are performed, so expertise will diminish and the opportunities for training will decrease. As a consequence, it is becoming increasingly difficult for radiologists in training to acquire sufficient expertise to perform high-quality gastrointestinal studies, with the result that a vicious cycle of events will ultimately lead to a serious reduction in the number of properly trained and experienced experts. Endoscopy remains three to four times more expensive than barium studies and is not without risk (p. 102). As a consequence, radiologists must convince their medical colleagues that the double-contrast upper gastrointestinal technique has a role to play in patients with relevant symptoms and must also ensure the continuation of high-quality diagnostic accuracy in a cost-effective manner (Levine & Laufer 1993).

### Selection of patients for barium studies (Lancet 1980)

Mead et al (1977) found only 24 abnormalities in 100 patients under 50 years undergoing barium meal examinations and in only 11 of these were changes to therapy needed. The authors concluded that the technique was being overused in this age group. Marton et al (1980) considered that the barium meal was being overused and recommended empirical rules, in concert with clinical judgement, to decrease the cost and increase the quality of care. Using any one of four criteria from the history as an indication for a barium study, namely, a previous history of peptic ulcer, age more than 50 years, relief of abdominal pain by food or abdominal pain occurring within an hour of eating, 19% of 483 patients would not have had the examination and the diagnosis would have been missed in six patients: in only one of these would the treatment have changed. Davenport et al (1985) performed a screening interview on 1041 patients with dyspepsia to determine whether they required investigation for organic disease. The patients comprised 496 referred to a hospital dyspepsia/endoscopy clinic, 344 referred for a barium meal and 201 who were interviewed in general practice. The information was analyzed and the patients categorized as high, medium or low risk for organic disease. All patients were followed up until a final diagnosis was reached. Patients predicted to be at low risk had a 10% chance of having ulcer disease and 0.3% chance of having cancer, whereas patients predicted to be at high risk had a 20% chance of ulcer disease and a 10% chance of having cancer. The authors conclude that this form of preliminary screening can separate a group of patients at low risk who will require investigation only if their symptoms do not resolve.

*Selection of patients for endoscopy*

Referral specifically for endoscopy deserves critical appraisal, especially in self-referral situations. An open-access endoscopy service in England (Holdstock et al 1979) showed no rise in the detection of ulcer or cancer following its inception and no decrease in the use of barium meal examinations either. In an attempt to prevent unnecessary endoscopy in an open-access service, Mann et al (1983) investigated factors which best discriminated between patients with major disease and those without. The six factors showing the best discrimination were increasing age, history of vomiting, male sex, smoking and a past history of peptic ulcer or hiatus hernia. Utilizing a scoring system, they showed that it should be possible to reduce the number of endoscopic examinations by 30%, yet still detect 98% of serious disease.

*Direct comparison of radiology and endoscopy*

Holdstock & Bruce (1981) reviewed the radiographic and endoscopic findings in 482 patients with gastric cancer and showed that radiology was almost as successful in diagnosis, although endoscopy was required to confirm the diagnosis. The authors recommended the necessity for endoscopy in those patients with any abnormality of the stomach on barium meal. A report of the endoscopic findings in 140 patients with normal double-contrast barium meal (Salter 1977) showed that in only seven patients were lesions missed and in only three of these was management altered. In the study of Dooley et al (1984) endoscopy was more sensitive (92% versus 54%) and specific (100% versus 91%) than radiology and had a significantly greater effect on management. Commenting on this study, Gelfand et al (1984) defended the use of the barium meal on the grounds of safety, comfort, costs and the ability to diagnose most if not all significant lesions of the upper alimentary tract. It was pointed out that if endoscopy had been performed for decades and radiological examination became available subsequently with its relative cheapness, negligible morbidity and mortality, minimal discomfort and high accuracy then it is likely that radiology would be recommended as the desirable initial examination of the gastrointestinal tract! However, patient acceptability of the double-contrast barium meal is the same as for endoscopy (Dooley et al 1986). This subject is discussed further in relation to peptic ulcer in Chapter 4 and Chapter 9.

*Conclusions*

It is clear that there is little to choose between radiology and endoscopy in terms of diagnostic accuracy for significant lesions which are not confined to the mucosal surface of the stomach and duodenum. Taking this into account, together with the advantages of cost and availability, the double-contrast barium meal has continued in some centers to be the initial investigation in dyspepsia, followed by endoscopy if biopsy is required or if there is doubt about the presence of a lesion. A properly conducted, normal double-contrast barium meal should preclude the necessity for further investigation of the upper gastrointestinal tract and direct attention elsewhere in seeking the cause of symptoms. However, taking into account that many patients then come to endoscopy anyway, there is increasing justification for endoscopy as the initial investigation (p. 102).

The onus for cost-effective use of available resources must rest with the referring clinician and their correct interpretation of the patient's clinical symptoms and signs, together with the likelihood that an undiagnosed lesion will have significant consequences. The choice between radiology and endoscopy as the first line of investigation will largely depend on the availability of resources such as suitable equipment, skilled personnel, appropriate pharmaceutical agents, the comparative safety of the procedure and the acceptability to the patient. In some countries the way in which medical fees are determined may play a significant role, especially where self-referral can occur.

Finally, as recommended by Jones (1985), any diagnostic service which is investigating dyspepsia and is freely available to primary care physicians (and possibly hospital specialists) should reasonably expect to restrict the service to those patients meeting agreed criteria. These criteria, which will include risk factors such as those described by Mann et al (1983), should also encompass the therapeutic and management problems which frequently arise. As Jones (1985) suggests, well-designed prospective trials to better define those patients really in need of investigations are required, so allowing a more cost-effective use of the available resources. One such randomized trial supports the view that endoscopy should be the investigation of choice in patients with persistent dyspepsia, especially those whose age and infirmity may make barium examination suboptimal (Stevenson et al 1991). Cost comparisons and relative complication rates were not recorded.

## **Barium follow-through** (Herlinger & Maglinte 1989)

*Indications* (Dodds & Goldberg 1978)

The diagnostic yield for the barium follow-through study depends upon the reason(s) for which it is performed, based on the history, clinical examination and laboratory findings (Fried et al 1981). The follow-through procedure should not be considered a screening examination for nonspecific abdominal symptoms and signs (Rabe et al

1981). Indications for the procedure likely to produce a high yield include a history of known small bowel disease, symptoms suggestive of small bowel obstruction from whatever cause, inflammatory bowel disease and malabsorption. The origin of gastrointestinal bleeding is rarely demonstrated and arteriography or nuclear isotope scanning is more likely to be diagnostic.

*Procedure*

The patient is prepared as for a barium meal examination. Anticholinergic drugs should be avoided for the previous 24 h since these may cause dilatation (Lumsden & Truelove 1959) and so a double-contrast barium meal using atony cannot be combined with a follow-through study. When the procedure follows an upper gastrointestinal examination, a further 150–250 g of non-flocculating barium is given. However, it should be noted that some of the products used for a double-contrast barium meal are unsuitable for use in follow-through examinations.

Once the duodenal loop has been examined, sequential films are taken at 15 min intervals for 1 h, then at less frequent intervals. Each film is reviewed as it is obtained so that more detailed attention can be focused on any abnormality. The patient is returned to the fluoroscopic screening room for localized films of any abnormality whenever indicated during the procedure. Films are taken until the barium fills the cecum, to ensure adequate films of the ileocecal region. The passage of barium through the small intestine may take up to 5 h in normal subjects and to reduce this metoclopramide 10 mg intravenously is given to increase the rate of gastric emptying, thus delivering barium rapidly to the small intestine.

**Small bowel enteroclysis** (Sellink 1976)

Indications are as for barium follow-through examination.

*Procedure*

The method requires the intubation of the duodenum using a Bilbao or similar tube (Bilbao et al 1967) and the rapid introduction of 150–200 ml of nonflocculating barium sulfate, propelled by a large volume of water (1 L or more) containing methylcellulose or 1 L of iced normal saline. Rapid infusion over 10 minutes is required to preserve the bolus and distend the lumen fully. Frequent fluoroscopic screening and the taking of "spot" radiographs are required to display the whole length of the small intestine. Occasionally metoclopramide 10 mg intravenously is required to facilitate intubation. The patient experiences some discomfort from the intubation and the distention and the radiation dosage is relatively high. However, improvements in the technique have resulted in increased patient comfort and more consistent and reproducible diagnostic examinations (Lappas & Maglinte 1991). A review of 10 years' experience with small bowel enteroclysis indicates a sensitivity of 93.1% and a specificity of 96.9% in 1465 patients in reporting whether the small intestine was normal or whether there was an abnormality to account for the patient's presentation. The correct specific diagnosis was made in 67.5% of examinations which were considered abnormal (Dixon et al 1993).

*Interpretation*

In the normal follow-through examination, the upper jejunum lies in the left upper quadrant and the terminal ileum in the right lower quadrant. The intervening bowel fills the central part of the abdomen (Fig. 1.13). The barium appears as a continuous column and the diameter of barium-filled segments is less than 3 cm. The mucosa in the jejunum is characteristically "feathery", while in the ileum the mucosal folds are more prominent. The width of normal mucosal folds is 2–3 mm. When barium has passed through the small intestine, a stippling of residual barium remains along the intestine.

The most important abnormalities are alterations in the diameter of the lumen which persist throughout the examination, dilution of barium due to excessive secretion, changes in the mucosal fold patterns and the presence of nodules or ulcers in the walls. Fistulae, diverticula, gas in the bowel wall and mesenteric changes may also be observed (Osborn & Friedland 1973).

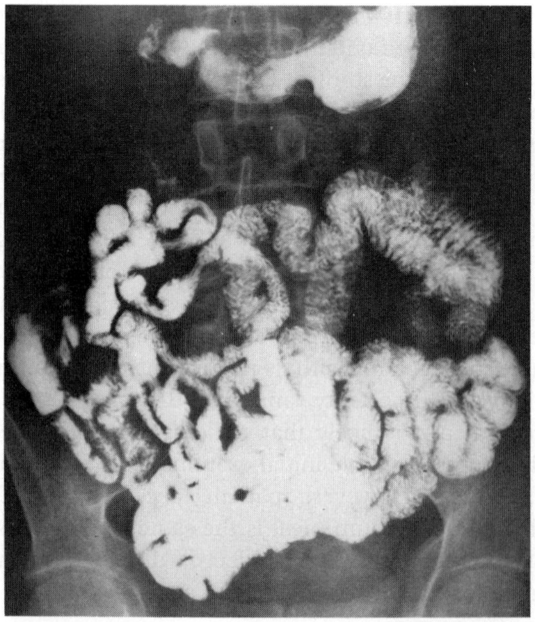

**Fig. 1.13** Normal follow-through radiography of the small intestine 3 h after a barium meal. Note the continuous column of barium from the jejunum to the ileum. Some residual barium is present in the stomach and duodenum.

The follow-through may provide information about an extrinsic mass displacing loops of bowel. Localized structural abnormalities due to Crohn's disease (p. 664), diverticula (p. 464) and tumors (p. 467) often have a characteristic appearance. When there is malabsorption, there is a generalized abnormality of the follow-through, often termed a "sprue or malabsorptive pattern". Formerly, when barium was not prevented from flocculating, flocculation and segmentation were used as signs of malabsorption. Flocculation transformed the homogeneous appearance of the barium into a coarse and granular pattern. Segmentation denotes splitting of the column of barium into short segments. When nonflocculating barium is used, generalized abnormality of the small intestine is denoted by an increase in diameter of the lumen, by dilution of the barium and by changes in the pattern of mucosal folds. Abnormal folds are thickened and may be regular (parallel to each other) or distorted. Distortion of folds may also be caused by mucosal nodules which can produce an abnormal contour of the bowel. In the diagnosis of malabsorption the radiologist's role is to depict changes in the mucosal surface or the bowel outline which may suggest or confirm the cause and demonstrate possible complications (Herlinger 1992). For these reasons, small bowel enteroclysis, with its improved definition and facility to distend the small bowel lumen, is superior to the standard small bowel follow-through examination.

Disease of the ileum is often best defined by a barium enema and some authorities advocate reflux studies of much of the small intestine by the retrograde introduction of contast material from the large bowel, though this technique has been largely replaced by small bowel enteroclysis (Thoeni 1989).

## Peroral pneumocolon

This technique may be employed to demonstrate disease, especially the early lesions of Crohn's disease, in the distal ileum and right half of the colon. Preparation of the colon is as for barium enema and oral barium, accelerated by metocloptamide, is given. Serial films are taken and once the right half of the colon has been outlined with barium, gas is introduced by rectal tube, so distending the colon and distal ileum. Intravenous glucagon may be required to allow passage of the gas through the ileocecal valve. Films are taken in varying positions to show the barium coating of the colonic mucosa through the gas distended lumen without overlap by residual barium in the small bowel (Kressel et al 1982).

## Barium enema

### *Indications*

This is carried out for suspected disease of the large bowel and the terminal ileum; whenever possible a double-contrast enema, which is a reliable method for detecting or excluding the presence of colonic lesions (Fork 1983), should be performed.

### *Contraindications*

The bowel may be perforated during a barium enema when there is active severe ulcerative colitis, acute diverticulitis, a fungating lesion in the rectum or when full-thickness biopsies of the rectum or colon have been performed within the previous week, though not after mucosal biopsy by forceps via the colonoscope (Harned et al 1982); retroperitoneal emphysema has been noted, particularly after a double-contrast enema (Brunton 1960). A barium enema should not be carried out if perforation of the colon is suspected or if there is severe heart disease. The double-contrast enema performed by an experienced examiner takes little more time, is more easily tolerated than the single-contrast method and can be performed in almost all circumstances; exceptions are suspected bowel perforation, suspected intussusception or meconium obstruction in an infant and where there is gross fecal impaction. In these circumstances a water-soluble enema can be utilized and may be therapeutic in some patients. In patients suspected of having large bowel obstruction, the use of a water-soluble contrast enema (Gastrografin) is an accurate and safe method of distinguishing true obstruction of the colon from pseudo-obstruction with a high sensitivity (96%) and specificity (98%) in a series of 140 patients (Chapman et al 1992). A similar technique should always be utilized in patients suspected of having postoperative complications such as a leaking anastomosis. Suspected toxic megacolon is an absolute contraindication to all enemata (p. 669).

A rectal examination and sigmoidoscopy should be carried out prior to a barium enema unless there are good reasons for omitting these.

Some patients experience abdominal pain and/or discomfort during or after the introduction of air as a double-contrast agent and the use of carbon dioxide as the insufflation agent has been shown to significantly reduce the incidence of pain (Robson et al 1993). Twenty-five per cent of patients experience headache after preparation for barium enema, probably as a consequence of dehydration (Kutt et al 1988) induced by the hypertonicity of magnesium citrate solution. This side-effect may be obviated by taking additional fluid (e.g. 500 ml of water) during the preparation period.

### *Preparation*

There is controversy as to how to achieve an adequate preparation and all methods fail in about 10% of patients; the available methods are reviewed by Margulis &

Eisenberg (1979). Constipating drugs such as iron, codeine phosphate and antispasmodics should be stopped 2 days before the enema. Radiologists prefer a potent laxative on the day before the examination, while physicians often prefer less severe laxatives such as bisacodyl or sennosides, e.g. Senokot. Unfortunately, less powerful laxatives do not give adequate results. The regimen recommended by Miller (1976) consists of 60 ml of castor oil at noon and 70 ml "X-prep" (anthraquinoidal glycoside) at 4.00 p.m. on the day before the examination, together with a clear liquid diet and copious oral fluids. On the day of the test, a 2000 ml tap water cleansing enema is given to the patient in the radiology department before the barium enema; all radiology departments must be designed to perform this efficiently. Such methods provide a clean colon in about 95% of patients. Other methods of preparing the colon, for example the oral ingestion of a hypertonic solution such as magnesium citrate, supplemented by bisacodyl tablets and suppository, are used increasingly, as are pharmacological methods to relax the colon which allow a more complete examination and reduce patient discomfort due to spasm. Glucagon is a safe and effective agent for this purpose, though there is no improvement in the sensitivity or specificity of the procedure (Thoeni et al 1984).

Adequate preparation of the colon is exhausting for the patient and those with heart disease should be admitted to hospital and a less vigorous preparation used; a low-roughage diet is given for several days and castor oil must be avoided. Indeed, examination should only be carried out if it is absolutely necessary, because a barium enema may be fatal in patients with pre-existing heart disease (Eastwood 1972). Laxatives should not be given to patients with active ulcerative colitis, ischemic colitis or Crohn's colitis and if contrast examination of the colon is required it should be performed without any preparation. Some centers use the unprepared double-contrast barium enema in monitoring the progress of inflammatory bowel disease – the "instant" enema (Thomas 1979) (see below). An "air enema" may provide a useful, though less precise alternative in patients with severe, acute colitis (Bartram et al 1983).

### *Procedure*

***The conventional enema.*** Barium is introduced into the rectum through a disposable plastic catheter. A retaining balloon can be used for patients who cannot retain barium, but care is required to avoid rupture of the rectum. There should be no evidence of rectal disease on sigmoidoscopy and the balloon should be inflated under radiological control after a small amount of barium has been run into the rectum (Fielding & Lumsden 1973). Barium is introduced under fluoroscopic surpervision until the sigmoid colon is completely filled and "spot" radiographs, if necessary with compression, are taken with varying degrees of rotation to separate visually the loops of sigmoid. A lateral film is taken to assess the retrorectal space. The colon is then filled progressively, with fluoroscopy continuing throughout. Radiographs are taken to show the entire colon and especially the hepatic and splenic flexures, where superimposed loops of bowel are common. Care is taken to see that the cecum is filled completely; this is usually indicated by the filling of the appendix or terminal ileum. The patient is then allowed to empty the bowel and "postevacuation" radiographs are taken (Fig. 1.14).

The conventional enema may fail to show small lesions, especially polyps and tumors, and double-contrast examinations should be performed whenever possible. The conventional enema, nevertheless, remains of value for demonstrating fistulae and in the diagnosis and treatment of intussusception in children. Hydrostatic reduction of intussusception by barium or water-soluble contrast enema has been used for many years but pneumatic reduction of intussusception using introduced gas or air is now performed more frequently (Markowitz & Meyer 1992).

***The double-contrast enema.*** The aim is to coat the colonic mucosa with a thin film of moderately dense and viscous barium sulfate designed to adhere to the mucosa and then to distend the colon with air. The procedure differs from a conventional enema in that the barium is run rapidly into the colon as far as the splenic flexure and "spot" films taken, especially of the rectosigmoid region. The rectosigmoid colon is then drained of barium. Air is introduced in graduated amounts and used to push the

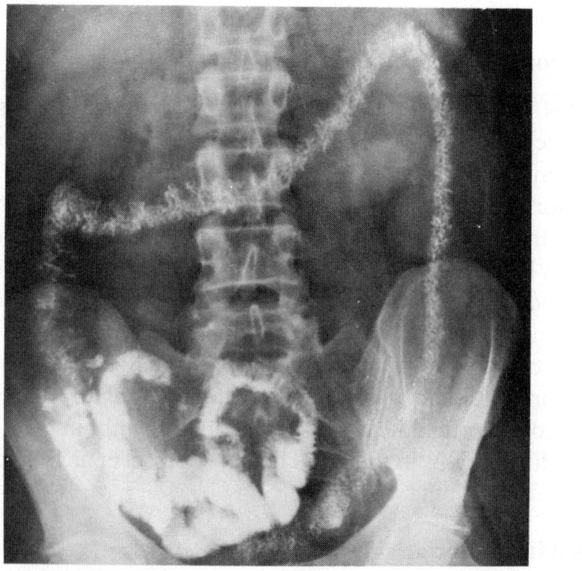

**Fig. 1.14** Normal, conventional postevacuation barium enema radiograph showing the characteristic feathery mucosal pattern. Considerable filling of the terminal ileum is normal.

remaining barium through the colon and distend it. Multiple radiographs are then taken in various postures to display the whole of the colonic mucosa. Difficulty in displaying colonic loops separately occurs when the colon is redundant or if there is excessive reflux into the ileum. Difficulties arise in obtaining a good display of the entire length of the sigmoid colon and in distention and visualization of the cecum.

***The "instant enema"*** (Thomas 1979). This is a limited form of double-contrast barium enema. A preliminary plain abdominal film is obtained to exclude any evidence of toxic dilatation. Then barium is introduced without prior bowel preparation until fecal material is encountered; the barium is then evacuated and insufflation of air is performed, so allowing a limited double-contrast study. In the "air enema" (Bartram et al 1983) air alone is insufflated under fluoroscopic control and radiographs of the air–mucosa pattern assessed.

*Interpretation*

All the evidence suggests that the double-contrast barium enema is more accurate than single contrast in the diagnosis of tumors and inflammatory conditions of the colon (Laufer 1976). Several pitfalls in interpretation occur; adherent fecal residue can simulate polypoid lesions (p. 1349) and fine debris may produce a granular appearance suggesting colitis. Some barium preparations can precipitate, mimicking ulceration, and others cause bubbling of gas but this should be easily distinguished from polyps. The colon is of variable length and when filled with barium to provide single-contrast radiography, it has a smooth outline apart from the presence of haustra. A double contour due to pericolic fat ("fat stripe") may be seen (Fig. 1.15) and should not be mistaken for gas in the bowel wall (p. 670). This outline may be disrupted by diverticula (p. 1384), by filling defects due to cancer (p. 1426), by strictures due to Crohn's disease (p. 664), ulcerative colitis (p. 660) or ischemic colitis (p. 549) or by ulceration extending into the wall of the bowel (p. 661). Occasionally, barium may be seen in a fistula outside the bowel. The retrorectal space may be increased in inflammatory bowel disease; it is measured opposite the fourth sacral vertebra and should not be greater than 2 cm (p. 660).

The double-contrast enema is essential for the definition of mucosal detail and for detecting polyps and small cancers (p. 1405). In ulcerative colitis early radiological changes consist of a granular appearance of the mucosa (p. 659) and mucosal stippling due to the adherence of barium (Margulis & Eisenberg 1979). The earliest mucosal changes of Crohn's disease, small irregular nodules and ulcers, can be identified (p. 664). Polyps and small cancers are best evaluated by the double-contrast (Fig. 1.16) rather than the single-contrast method although, on occasions, the radiographs are difficult to interpret (Fig. 1.17). Lesions may be overlooked because of inadequate cleansing of the colon or because of the superimposition of distended loops of bowel causing confusing shadows. Comparative studies of colonoscopy and double-contrast barium enema have suggested that the latter can detect 98% of lesions greater than 1 cm and 78% of those less than 1 cm (Williams et al 1974). A 92% true positive rate compared with colonoscopy has been reported (Ott et al 1980). Another study (McPherson & Payne 1983) indicated a false positive rate of 34% and a false negative rate of 8% for polyps. Thoeni and Menuck (1977) reported that double-contrast barium enemas and colonoscopy each miss about 12% of polyps; polyps missed radiologically were in areas of colonic redundancy,

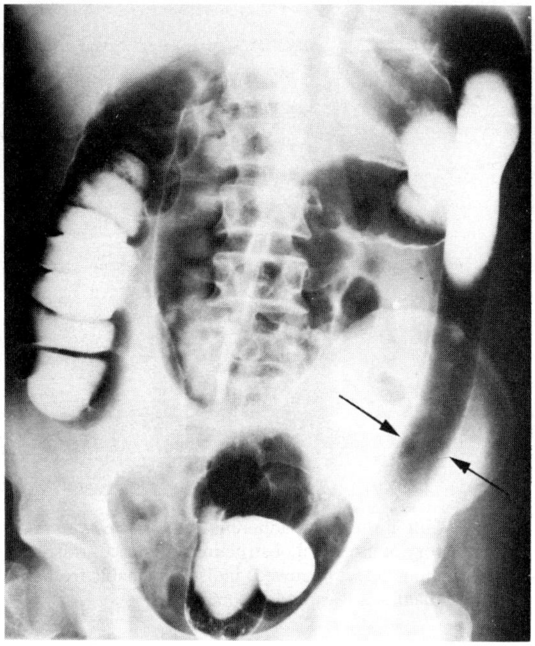

**Fig. 1.15** Air contrast barium enema showing a double contour (arrowed) of the descending colon due to pericolic fat. This must not be mistaken for gas in the bowel wall from a perforation.

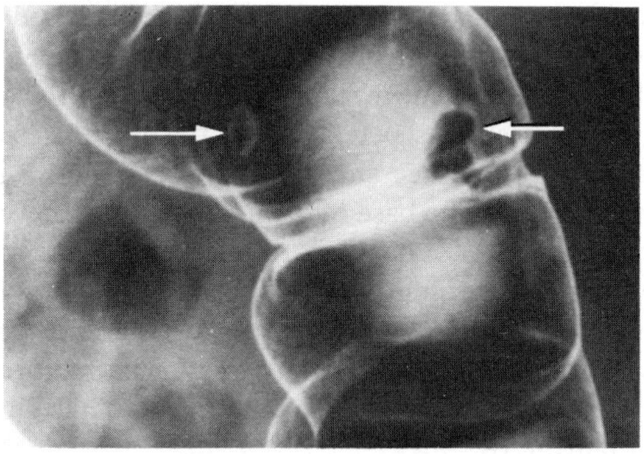

**Fig. 1.16** Two small colonic polyps (arrowed).

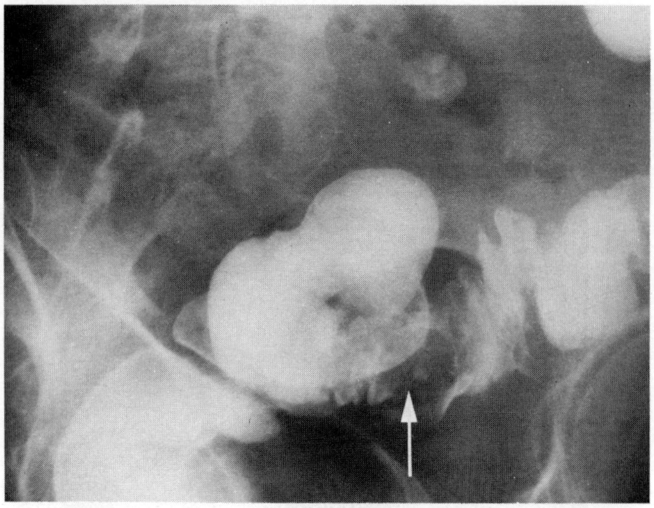

**Fig. 1.17** Fecolith in the pelvis adherent to the bowel wall in a patient with a recent history of intestinal obstruction. Water contrast barium enema shows a filling defect (arrowed) indistinguishable from a carcinoma. The diagnosis was made at operation.

especially in the sigmoid and splenic flexures, their size varying from 2 to 15 mm with an average of 5 mm. The double-contrast enema is particularly valuable in the ascending colon, which is more difficult to reach by colonoscopy, and the examinations are considered to be complementary in many instances. A polyp is seen on the double-contrast enema because barium coats the tumor itself, its base and its pedicle (Fig. 1.16). Sessile polyps appear as rings en face and as the polyp grows, a recess develops between the base of the polyp and the bowel wall which fills with barium. This results in two rings which show varying superimposition depending on the angle of the X-ray beam. When the polyp is pedunculated, the pedicle can be defined in a profile view. The radiographic distinction between a polyp and a diverticulum is illustrated in Figure 1.18.

Patients with diverticular disease tolerate double-contrast barium enema well, particularly if given pharmacological agents such as glucagon. In some patients this is essential to abolish spasm and allow the examination to continue.

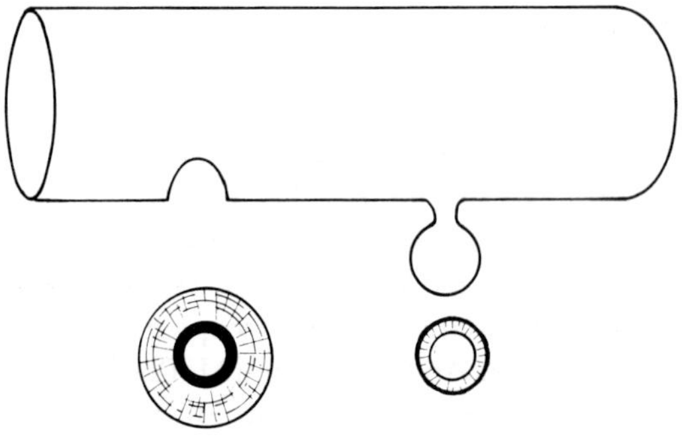


**Fig. 1.18** The radiological appearance of (A) a polyp and (B) a diverticulum. The polyp has a sharp inner border of barium, the diverticulum a sharp outer border.

*Screening for colorectal carcinoma*

Early detection and removal of adenomatous polyps and small carcinomas are very important but large numbers of patients need to be examined by endoscopy complemented by double-contrast barium enema. The role of the barium enema in the detection of colorectal carcinoma has been extensively investigated and a seminal review (Ott 1993) emphasizes the need for high quality and accurate performance by radiologists experienced in the technique. The American College of Radiology has adopted standards for performance and interpretation (Ferrucci 1993). These critical standards include that radiologists should be able to detect 90% of colorectal carcinomas and 80% of polyps of more than 1 cm in diameter. These requirements are essentially identical to those accepted by the American College of Physicians. It is recommended that those patients considered to have a high risk because of family history should attend the first screening at the age of 40, with subsequent colonoscopy or barium enema every 3–5 years and testing for fecal occult blood annually. It has been recommended that other patients should be screened at the age of 50, either by colonoscopy or barium enema, with annual fecal occult blood testing thereafter, but this presents problems (see p. 1422).

**Defecating proctography** (p. 1320)

This is being used increasingly in the investigation of patients with suspected anorectal disorders and constipation (Mezwa et al 1993). The examination is achieved by the introduction of a barium paste plug into the rectum and radiological observation is made as the patient evacuates into a specially constructed commode under fluoroscopic control. "Spot" films and videorecordings are made in the lateral projection with the patient at rest, straining and squeezing. It is vital that the radiologist spends time discussing and explaining the procedure with the patient in private before commencement, to avoid undue embarrassment and to obtain maximum co-operation, particularly with elderly patients.

## BILIARY RADIOLOGY (Bernardino 1991)

Despite significant advances in other imaging techniques such as nuclear medicine (NM), computed tomography (CT) and magnetic resonance imaging (MRI), ultrasound scanning (US) is considered to be the initial investigative technique in the diagnosis of gallbladder diseases and the differential diagnosis of jaundice, particularly as there is no exposure to ionizing radiation, no need for toxic pharmacological agents and it is relatively inexpensive to perform (Meire 1984). Consequently the reduction in usage of contrast biliary radiology has continued apace. Rapid improvements in ultrasound technique and equipment have relegated the role of cholecystography to a secondary one and have virtually replaced intravenous cholangiography. Although oral cholecystography produces good information regarding the presence of gallstones, patency of the cystic duct and abnormalities of the gallbladder mucosa, its role is now secondary in diagnosing conditions such as adenomyomatosis and in patients in whom gallbladder disease is strongly suspected clinically but with negative ultrasound scans (Gelfand et al 1988, Maglinte et al 1991). About 50% of patients with a diagnosis of acalculous cholecystitis on initial ultrasound scanning have gallbladder calculi demonstrated on follow-up examinations which may include further ultrasonography, cholecystography or, rarely, intravenous cholangiography (Ekberg & Weiber 1991). Cholecystography still has an important role to play in the selection of patients for nonsurgical therapy of gallstones such as extracorporeal shockwave lithotripsy (ESWL) and directed dissolution therapy of gallstones with methyl-tert-butyl-ether (MTBE) (vanSonnenberg & Hofmann 1988). In these circumstances oral cholecystography is required to demonstrate gallbladder opacification, the number, size and composition of gallstones, cystic duct patency and the concentrating ability of the gallbladder (Brakel et al 1991).

Oral cholecystography is an accurate investigation at the 92–95% level, comparable to that of ultrasound (de Lacey et al 1984). Most wrong diagnoses occur when gallstones are too small to be visualized even with good technique. Nonvisualization of the gallbladder is a strong indicator of gallstones at about the 92% level (Birch et al 1989).

Despite advocacy of the intravenous cholangiogram as an alternative to routine operative cholangiography (Daly et al 1987) the shortcomings of oral cholecystography, namely ionizing radiation exposure, the use of potentially toxic contrast agents and physiological dependence on normal hepatic function, impose even greater disadvantages on intravenous cholangiography. Even when used widely, it was considered somewhat unreliable and relatively unsafe. The development of laparoscopic cholecystectomy has posed a problem of how best to demonstrate the biliary tree. It can be technically difficult to display the bile ducts via a laparoscope at surgery and it has been suggested that intravenous cholangiography be resurrected for bile duct assessment in association with laparoscopic cholecystectomy. Whilst the introduction of Biliscopin (meglumine iotroxate) 10–15 years ago lessened the incidence of side-effects, these are by no means negligible. The assessment at diagnostic radiography is frequently difficult and always requires conventional tomography for accuracy which significantly increases the radiation dose. Ultrasound scanning is often all that is required for an adequate display of the gallbladder and biliary tree, supplemented wherever possible by operative cholangiography. If there is reason to suspect a bile duct stone on the basis of history, disturbed biochemical tests or suspicious ultrasound findings, then endoscopic retrograde cholangiopancreatography (ERCP) is indicated preoperatively (Dawson et al 1993). For these reasons it is very rarely necessary to advise intravenous cholangiography.

### Contrast materials and contrast toxicity

The contrast materials used for all biliary radiology contain iodine molecules which are excreted almost entirely via the liver into the bile and concentrated in the gallbladder by absorption of water. Iopanoic acid (Telepaque), sodium iopodate (Biloptin) and calcium iopodate (Solubiloptin) are most frequently used for oral cholecystography. Biloptin and Solubiloptin are more soluble in water and less soluble in lipids than Telepaque. Toxicity has been shown to be less with Biloptin (Reiner et al 1980).

For intravenous cholangiography, meglumine iotroxate (Biliscopin) or meglumine iodoxamate (Cholevue) are usually administered by slow intravenous infusion over 30–60 min prior to radiographs being taken. These should include conventional tomography as the degree of opacification is significantly less than that obtained by oral agents.

Common minor side-effects include nausea, vomiting, diarrhea, urticaria and dysuria (Parks 1974). More serious side-effects include hypersensitivity and hypotensive reactions. Renal failure may also be seen in those patients with pre-existing renal disease, diabetes and in dehydrated patients (Heneghan 1978).

Biliary contrast reactions appear to potentiate each other in regard to toxic side-effects and repeat or follow-up examinations should be separated by at least 7 days (Kreel 1973).

### Cholecystography

#### *Indications*

The current role of cholecystography is as an alternative investigation for patients strongly suspected of having biliary disease where the results of other investigations have been unhelpful or dubious. Oral cholecystography is of prime importance in the selection of patients for nonsurgical therapy of gallstones.

#### *Contraindications*

Previous reactions to contrast media or recent exposure to contrast media. Preliminary premedication with prednisolone (20 mg every 8 h for 3 days) may be given to reduce the risks, but alternative methods of investigation are advised.

***Renal disease.*** Oral cholecystography is usually unsuccessful in patients with renal failure (Perrillo et al 1978) but may be successful in patients on renal dialysis.

***Liver disease.*** If the serum bilirubin exceeds 35 μmol/L (2 mg/dL) contrast medium will not enter the biliary tree in sufficient quantity for adequate radiography.

***Recent acute pancreatitis or small bowel diseases.*** Oral contrast is rarely absorbed in sufficient amounts for adequate demonstration of the biliary tree and these are relative contraindications.

*Procedure*

A fractionated dose of 4.5–6 g of either Telepaque or Biloptin given over a 12 h period, with a minimum of 2 L of milk-free fluids and a low-fat diet, usually results in good visualization. Radiographs are taken in varying positions to demonstrate the gallbladder free of overlying bowel gas or fecal material. If no abnormality has been shown on the initial films, a fatty meal is given to induce contraction of the gallbladder and further films taken. Tomography may be helpful if poor opacification has occurred and the extrahepatic bile ducts may sometimes be satisfactorily seen by this method. Contrast may be identified in the bowel and a coarse, granular appearance suggests that the contrast has not been absorbed. If contrast has been absorbed and excreted by the bile, the appearance in the bowel is smooth and homogeneous.

*Interpretation*

***Normal gallbladder.*** This shows as an ovoid or pear-shaped opacity about 10 cm long and 4 cm wide. After a fatty meal, contrast material may enter the cystic and bile ducts and the valves of Heister (p. 1195) may give the former a beaded appearance. Bilateral indentation at the junction of the neck and infundibulum is common and spasm in this region may even result in a complete break in the contrast column. The cystic duct arches to the left, concave superiorly, in its course to the common bile duct, which may show as a smooth tapering column.

Gallbladder anomalies occur in 5–10% of the population. These include the phrygian cap deformity due to a small gallbladder fossa, double gallbladder, bilobed gallbladder and septa. True diverticula and agenesis of the gallbladder are very rare. "Rudimentary" gallbladders in adults are usually due to chronic cholecystitis.

***Failure to visualize the gallbladder.*** Factors other than gallbladder disease should be considered first. They include previous cholecystectomy, failure to ingest the contrast agent, achalasia of the esophagus, pyloric stenosis, diarrhea, intestinal malabsorption and hepatic disease. Cholestyramine has a high affinity for Telepaque and may prevent its absorption (Nelson 1974). Failure to visualize the gallbladder may be due to gallbladder disease, but this cannot be assumed owing to the so-called consecutive dose phenomenon (Berk 1970). This occurs when the gallbladder shows faintly or not at all after a first dose of Telepaque, but shows normally after a second dose. The consecutive dose phenomenon accounts for a third of cases in which the gallbladder shows faintly or not at all on cholecystography. The other two-thirds of patients have gallbladder disease. The use of the fractionated, higher doses of contrast avoids this discrepancy and obviates the need for second dose techniques.

***Abnormalities.*** The plain abdominal radiograph sometimes shows abnormalities such as gallstones (Fig. 1.19). Filling defects in the gallbladder are usually caused by gallstones. They vary greatly in size and may be single or multiple (Figs 1.19, 1.20 and 2.11). Erect films may enhance visualization of multiple stones by showing them layered between the more opaque contrast medium below and the less opaque gallbladder contents above (Fig. 1.21). Only 10–30% of gallstones are radio-opaque. Previously demonstrated gallstones may not be seen on subsequent investigations (MacFarlane & Glenn 1964). This may be due to passage of the gallstones through the biliary tree or through a fistulous communication with the bowel. Air may be seen in the biliary tract when a fistula is present. Other causes of filling defects include adenomas (p. 1211) and adenomyomatosis (Fig. 1.22).

## Infusion cholangiography

*Indications*

The present place of intravenous cholangiography in

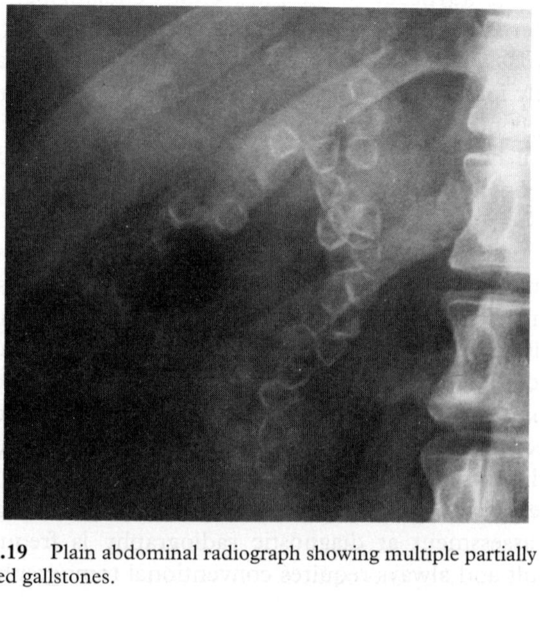

**Fig. 1.19** Plain abdominal radiograph showing multiple partially calcified gallstones.

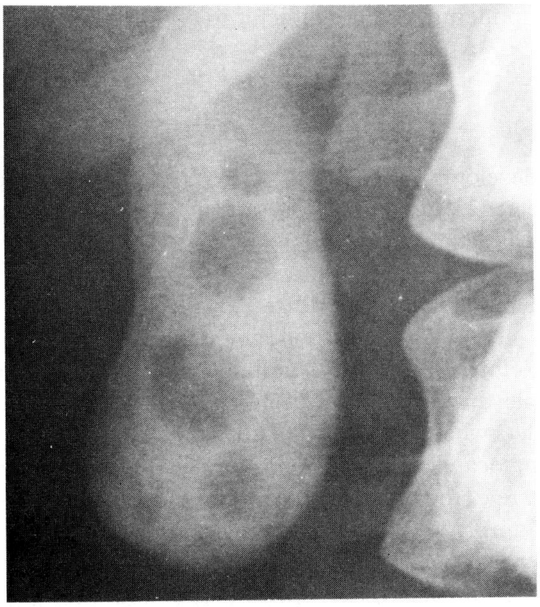

**Fig. 1.20** Cholecystogram showing multiple translucent gallstones.

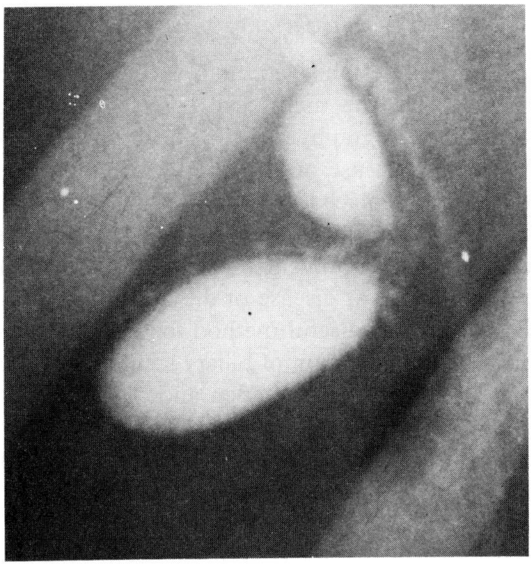

**Fig. 1.22** Cholecystogram showing diffuse adenomyomatosis of the gallbladder. The disease has produced a biloculate gallbladder; contrast has produced a "halo" around the gallbladder by entering the Rokitansky–Aschoff sinuses.

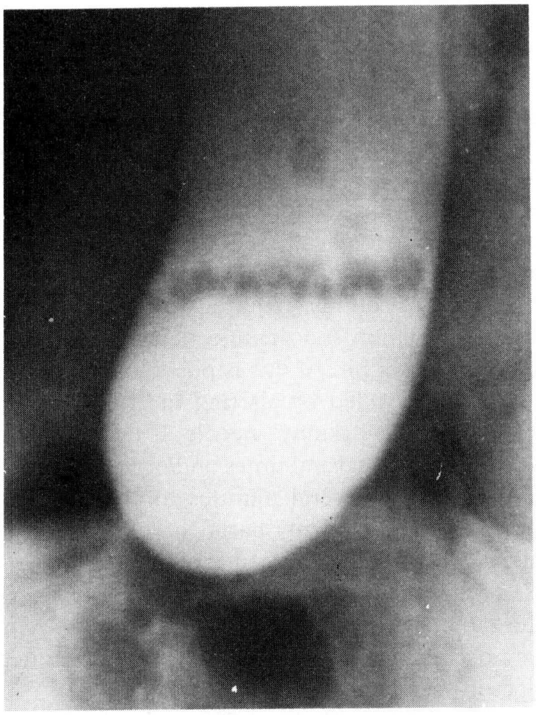

**Fig. 1.21** Cholecystogram showing layering of multiple gallstones in biliary contrast material on a radiograph taken in the erect position.

imaging is now controversial and it is rarely recommended. The preoperative use of intravenous cholangiography as a method of identifying stones in the biliary ducts is much better achieved by alternative methods. Very occasionally, a suspected postoperative common bile duct stone may be visualized by this technique, when ultrasound scanning and/or ERCP are unhelpful or impossible.

*Contraindications*

These are hypersensitivity to iodinated contrast media, impaired liver function, cardiorenal failure and recent oral cholecystography. Dehydration must be corrected before cholangiography.

*Procedure*

Overnight fasting is encouraged and a preliminary laxative is given. Hydration should be maintained with at least 1 L of fluid taken in the period 2–4 h before examination. A preliminary radiograph of the right upper quadrant is taken. An intravenous infusion of Biliscopin is given over 30–45 min. The radiograph of the right upper quadrant is repeated to confirm adequate contrast excretion and then conventional tomography of the biliary tree performed. If the gallbladder is in place, later radiographs may be required, allowing time for filling.

*Interpretation*

The biliary tree is examined for its anatomical appearances, biliary dilatation or stricture, filling defects in the bile ducts, passage of contrast into the duodenum and/or gallbladder and the time density appearance of contrast in the bile ducts (normally this decreases in a nonobstructed bile duct after 1 h). Intrahepatic bile duct visualization before the common bile duct is seen, may be a sign of biliary obstruction (Black & Ferrucci 1978). The visualization of passage of contrast into the duodenum is not necessarily evidence against obstruction.

*Percutaneous transhepatic cholangiography* (PTC)

Although a long-established and successful technique offering an alternative method to endoscopic retrograde cholangiopancreatography (ERCP) for the visualization of the biliary tree, the use of PTC as an imaging technique has been largely replaced by other imaging methods (e.g. US, CT and MRI) (p. 72). However, the technique has enabled dramatic improvements in the management of benign and malignant disease of the liver and biliary system. PTC is a most useful method for percutaneous biliary drainage, the insertion of biliary stents, the dilatation of biliary strictures, the extraction and dissolution of bile duct calculi and for its facility to combine with endoscopic procedures. Percutaneous hepatic puncture by a similar technique allows an approach to portal venous radicles.

*Indications*

PTC can be used to confirm the presence or absence of bile duct obstruction and to define the site and nature of an obstructing lesion. Despite a 95% success rate in defining the site and a 90% success rate in identifying the cause of biliary obstruction, PTC has been largely replaced by ERCP for these purposes. However, if a treatable lesion is suspected, for example an impacted calculus in the common bile duct, and ERCP has failed or is contraindicated, then PTC is an important alternative management method.

If other investigations have suggested a high bile duct problem such as a tumor at the bile duct confluence, then PTC is more likely to define the lesion in detail and gives access for nonoperative drainage of the biliary tree.

*Contraindications and complications*

The high success rate of puncture (95–100%) in the presence of dilated bile ducts and relatively low complication rate (5–15%) can be achieved with careful technique. In a review of 20 006 procedures there was a 3–4% rate of serious complications, including four deaths (Harbin et al 1980).

The major complications include intra-abdominal hemorrhage, biliary peritonitis, bacteremia and septicemia. Therefore a significant increase in the bleeding time poses the major contraindication; the risk may be reduced by the administration of vitamin K and/or fresh frozen plasma.

Broad-spectrum antibiotics (e.g. gentamicin with ampicillin) are given routinely to reduce the risk of infectious complications and are mandatory if infected bile is thought to be present. If infected bile is obtained at puncture, then percutaneous drainage of the biliary tree should be instituted.

End-stage liver disease with cirrhosis, portal hypertension and ascites are relative contraindications, as percutaneous puncture is more difficult to perform in these situations.

*Technique*

The development of a long (15 cm) fine (0.7 mm outer diameter) 22 gauge Chiba or "skinny" needle (Okuda et al 1974) has allowed PTC to be performed successfully with low morbidity and mortality.

The bile ducts, when dilated, are easily punctured and, in the absence of dilatation, there is still a high success rate. Refinements of the technique include the puncture of multiple ducts to demonstrate the complete anatomy in disorders where there may be multiple strictures such as in cholangiocarcinoma and metastatic disease or the selective puncture of the left hepatic duct, particularly in diseases at the hilum.

After preparation with antibiotics and hemostatic agents, if indicated, the patient is given suitable premedication (e.g. diazepam 5–20 mg IV). The skin at the right lateral aspect of the upper abdomen is prepared surgically and the skin and underlying soft tissue are anesthetized (lignocaine 2%) to the depth of the liver capsule with fluoroscopic screening control. The "skinny" needle is advanced into the liver, guided by appropriate skin markers during suspended respiration. Nonionic contrast medium is injected under screening control to confirm the intraductal position of the needle. If there is extravasation of contrast the needle is repositioned until satisfactory duct puncture is obtained. The complication rate is not significantly increased by the number of punctures required.

The volume of contrast required varies with the extent of bile duct dilatation and the injection may be facilitated by the aspiration of bile, if this is possible. Nonopacifying segments may be filled by altering the patient's posture after removal of the "skinny" needle. It may be necessary to rotate the patient several times and/or lie them in a particular position for several minutes to allow contrast to permeate into dependent parts of the biliary tree. Occasionally late films (up to 1 h) may show that contrast has filled previously unfilled segments.

Failure to opacify ducts at a distance from the puncture site may occur, particularly if there is irregular duct narrowing as in sclerosing cholangitis.

After the procedure the patient should be closely observed for 24 h, particularly for signs of hemorrhage or biliary peritonitis.

*Interpretation*

Normal bile ducts have a regular smooth outline and the more distal ducts steadily increase in size (Fig. 1.23). The diameter of the common bile duct should not exceed 10 mm. It may show a notch where its lumen narrows distally (Fig. 1.23) and from that point the duct narrows

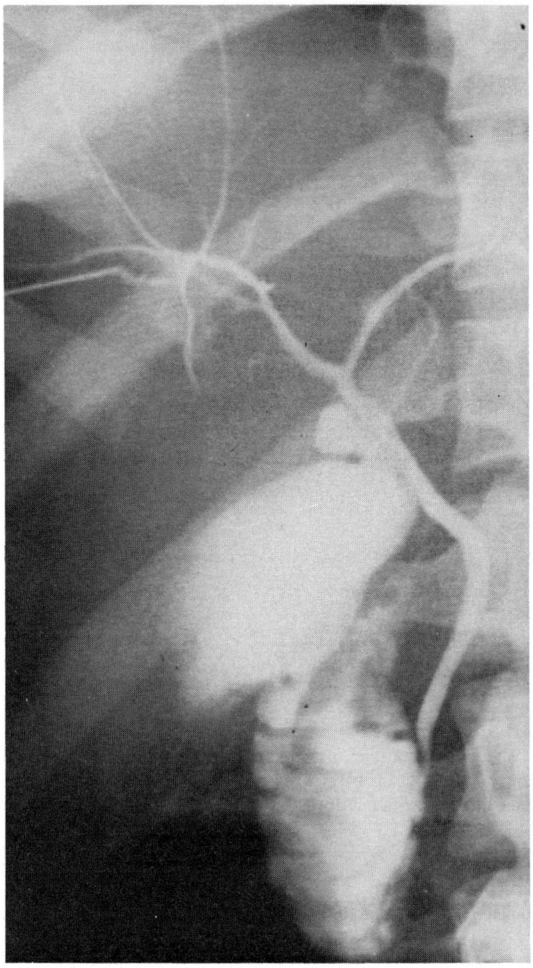

**Fig. 1.23** Transhepatic cholangiogram showing a normal biliary tract in a patient with cholestasis due to viral hepatitis.

markedly and may only be shown as a thread of contrast material. The abnormalities revealed by percutaneous transhepatic cholangiography have been detailed by Fleming et al (1972) and by Kreel (1973). When there has been no previous biliary surgery, an obstructive lesion is generally an impacted stone or a tumor. The convex proximal margin of the former is outlined by the distal end of the contrast column (Fig. 1.24). A tumor at the ampulla of Vater never gives this appearance (Fleming et al 1972). Tumors much more frequently cause a sudden cut-off, with or without distal umbilication, or a distal convexity of the contrast column. The length of the common duct, and whether or not the gallbladder fills, also help to indicate the nature and site of the carcinoma; ampullary cancers are associated with a long common duct and a filled gallbladder (Fig. 1.25), pancreatic cancers give a filled gallbladder with a duct ending at the level of the duodenum (Fig. 1.26) and biliary cancers give a very short duct and cystic duct obstruction prevents gallbladder filling. "Apple-core" or polypoidal lesions in the bile duct are virtually pathognomonic of cancer (Fig. 1.27).

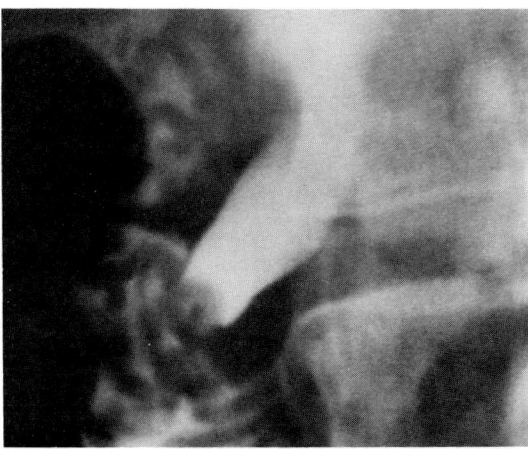

**Fig. 1.24** Transhepatic cholangiogram showing obstruction of the common bile duct by a gallstone. Note the convex proximal margin of the gallstone outlined by contrast medium.

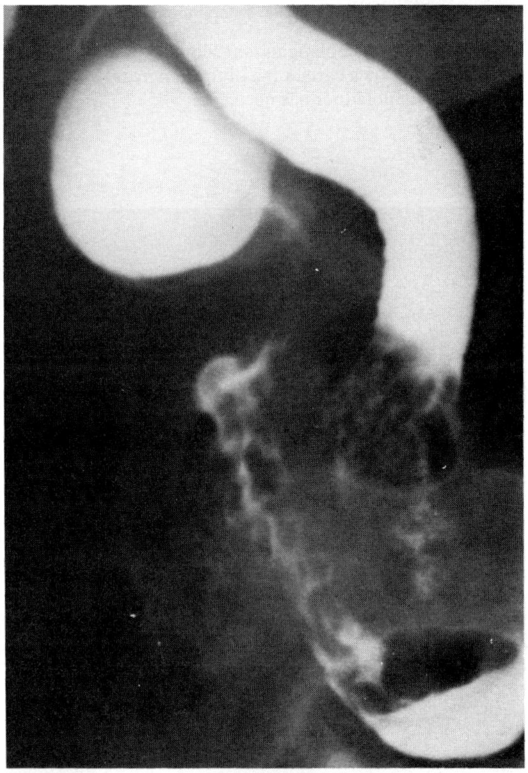

**Fig. 1.25** Transhepatic cholangiogram showing partial obstruction of the common bile duct by a carcinoma of the ampulla of Vater. Contrast outlines the irregular tumor surface at the site of obstruction. The gallbladder has filled.

Intraluminal filling defects may be stones, debris or mucus. Stones cause faceted or rounded translucencies which may move as the patient's position is altered (Fig. 1.28). Translucencies due to mucus often change shape and the debris may give an amorphous appearance. The bile ducts themselves may be abnormal, showing benign strictures (Fig. 31.13) or sclerosing cholangitis

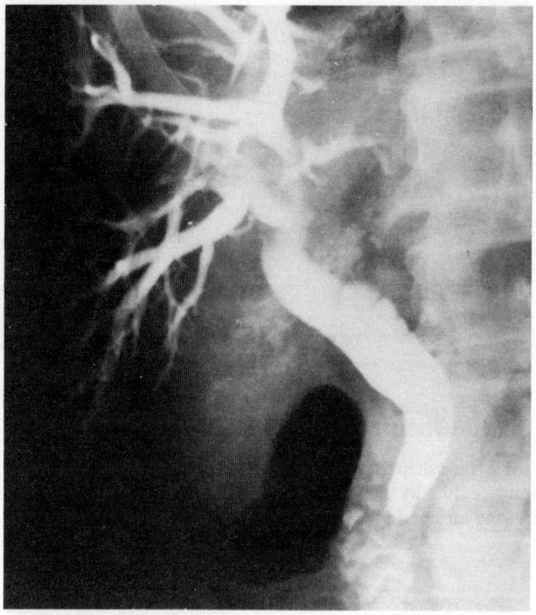

**Fig. 1.26** Transhepatic cholangiogram showing partial obstruction of the common bile duct by a carcinoma of the pancreas. Some filling of the cystic duct and gallbladder has occurred.

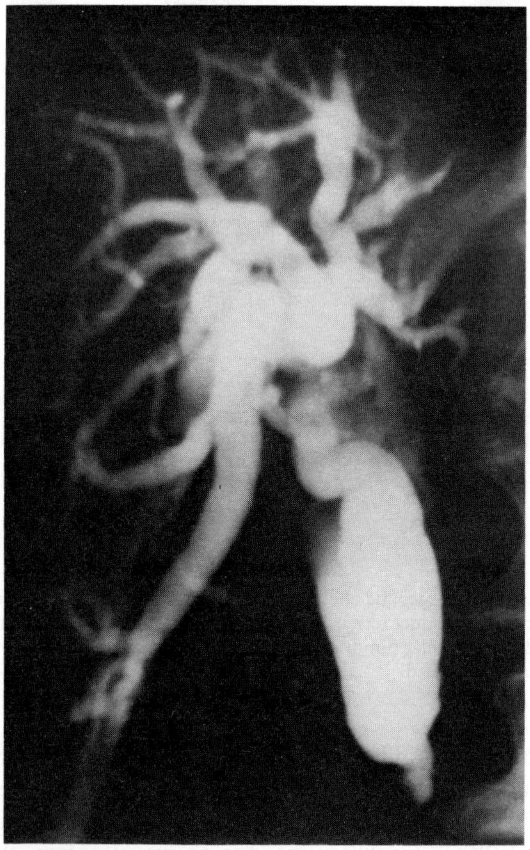

**Fig. 1.27** Transhepatic cholangiogram showing complete obstruction of the common bile duct by a carcinoma of the pancreas. There is an "apple core" appearance and marked dilatation of the bile ducts above the tumor.

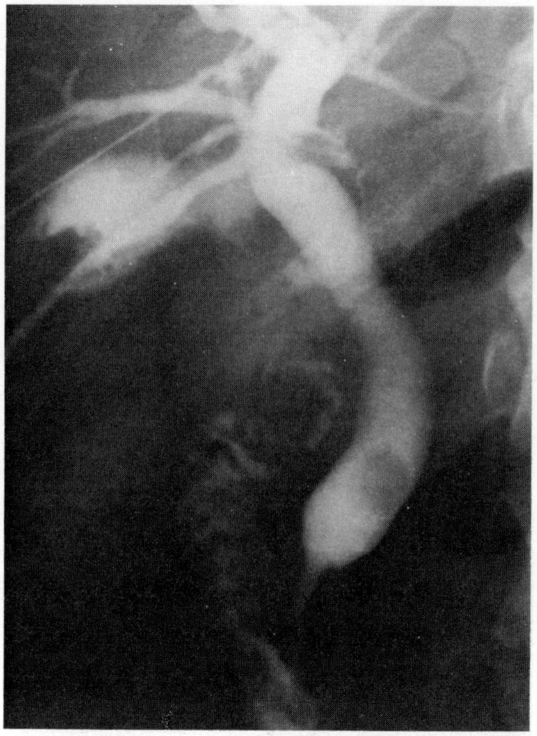

**Fig. 1.28** Transhepatic cholangiogram showing partial obstruction of the common bile duct by a translucent gallstone. There is moderate dilatation of the bile ducts above the gallstone. There are also gallstones in the gallbladder.

(Fig. 48.12). Cystic spaces in communication with the biliary system may be due to Caroli's syndrome (Fig. 24.17), a choledochal cyst (Fig. 24.18) or an abscess. Finally, bile ducts may be compressed or distorted by extrinsic lesions such as tumors or cysts.

*Conclusion*

Whilst a reasonably precise and cost-effective method of investigating patients with cholestatic jaundice, PTC has been initially replaced by other techniques, particularly US and ERCP. However, a progressively modified PTC technique has provided a most important avenue for the nonsurgical interventional management of biliary and liver diseases.

## Operative (peroperative or intraoperative) cholangiography

Operative cholangiography in biliary surgery is well established (Lancet 1970, Kaksos et al 1972, Saltzstein et al 1973, Bremner et al 1974). A review (Doyle et al 1982) has shown a significant reduction in mortality from 3.6% to 1.5% in a cohort study of 4000 consecutive cholecystectomies over 25 years following the introduction of peroperative cholangiography. The reduced mortality was mainly due to the reduced rate of duct exploration necessary once peroperative cholangiography was an established routine. It is used most frequently in patients undergoing cholecystectomy to determine the necessity for common bile duct exploration, but it is also valuable in operations for biliary tumors or strictures. It adds little to operating time, is virtually free of complications with correct technique (p. 1206).

*Procedure*

The operating table should be designed to accommodate the radiographic cassette-holding device and have a radiolucent top. Those personnel required to remain with the patient should wear lead protection to reduce radiation exposure and should wear radiation-monitoring badges. With the patient tilted 15–25° to the right on the operating table, contrast material is injected (25% Hypaque) into the biliary tract via the cystic duct. Initially 3 ml are injected and then further volumes of 5 and 7 ml. Dilated systems may require larger volumes of contrast. A radiograph is taken after each injection. Air must not be injected, as this will form bubbles indistinguishable from stones, and contrast material must not be allowed to extravasate from the biliary tree. Common reasons for poor radiographs include incorrect positioning of the patient on the film cassette, radio-opaque instruments obscuring the radiograph and failure to tilt the operating table to the right so that the biliary tree lies clear of the vertebral column. In the presence of infected bile, which is frequently the case in obstructed systems, intraoperative cholangiography is associated with a high incidence of bacteremia and an increased mortality and morbidity rate (Lygidakis 1982). In these circumstances it is advised that intraoperative cholangiography should be used with extreme care and under manometric control.

*Interpretation*

A satisfactory operative cholangiogram must demonstrate the intrahepatic and extrahepatic ducts. No part of the normal biliary tract is dilated, the common bile duct diameter must not exceed 10 mm and the tapered distal common bile duct must be seen clearly with contrast which has entered the duodenum. The intrahepatic radicles must taper and divide regularly and smoothly. Spasm preventing contrast from entering the duodenum can usually be overcome by an inhalation of amyl nitrate. The appearances of disease are the same as those seen on a percutaneous transhepatic cholangiogram but in addition anatomical variants, particularly the site of insertion of the cystic duct (Hopkinson et al 1983), are of special importance to the surgeon. When a patient with cholestatic jaundice has a normal extrahepatic biliary tree, the intrahepatic ducts need to be examined for a cholangiocarcinoma (p. 1220) at the union of the left and right hepatic ducts. Stones may also be seen in the intrahepatic ducts and in the bile duct (Fig. 1198). Reflux of contrast into the pancreatic duct is an occasional normal finding.

*Conclusions*

Operative cholangiography is safe and adds little to operating time. Its value is illustrated by a review of over 3000 cholecystectomies (Kaksos et al 1972); during the study period, the use of operative cholangiography rose from 2% to 93%, the need for common bile duct exploration fell from 41% to 25% and the frequency of positive findings when exploration was indicated rose from 28% to 62%. The morbidity and mortality of cholecystectomy and choledochotomy were unchanged, but the need for choledochotomy was reduced. Choledochotomy increases morbidity and mortality and is therefore best avoided (Table 1.1). It has to be emphasized that clinical indications for common duct exploration on their own are unreliable and that decisions taken with the help of operative cholangiography give better results (Bremner et al 1974). Operative cholangiography may also reveal anatomical variants, the recognition of which can prevent operative errors which may lead, for example, to strictures. It is therefore mandatory. It is important, however, not to rely solely on operative cholangiography, as stones may not be revealed (Bremner et al 1974) and inadequate films are worse than none at all (Hall et al 1973). The use of the operative choledochoscope (p. 1209) is complementary to operative cholangiography.

Ideally, on completion of a bile duct exploration and insertion of a T drainage tube into the common bile duct, a further cholangiogram is performed. However, frequently during the operative procedure air bubbles are introduced, blood clots and debris are often also present and if procedures such as sphincterotomy have been performed, edema and distortion of the lower end of the common bile duct may be present. Consequently the interpretation of the completion cholangiogram radiographs is often unreliable. Therefore most surgical teams prefer to leave in the T

**Table 1.1** Morbidity and mortality in 3012 patients with gallstone disease undergoing cholecystectomy with or without choledochotomy (Kaksos et al 1972)

| | Cholecystectomy | Cholecystectomy and choledochotomy: All | Abnormal bile duct | Normal bile duct |
|---|---|---|---|---|
| Morbidity* | 16.5% | 27% | — | — |
| Mortality | 0.8% | 1.8%** | 2.5% | 1.1% |

* >85% due to pulmonary, urinary or wound complications, most of which are minor.
** More than half the deaths due to conditions unrelated to the liver or the bile ducts (myocardial infarction, cerebrovascular accident, pulmonary embolism, pancreatitis, renal failure, sepsis, gastrointestinal bleeding).

drainage tube and perform a postoperative study 7–10 days later.

Miniaturized, high-resolution, real-time ultrasonographic equipment is available for use in the operating theatre and a study comparing the accuracy of operative ultrasound scanning and cholangiography in detecting common bile duct stones indicates significant advantages for the former method (Sigel et al 1983).

### Postoperative T-tube cholangiography

If a T drainage tube has been left in place following biliary surgery, it is always advantageous to perform a contrast study through the T-tube at 7–10 days postoperatively as a preliminary to removal of the T-tube. Performed correctly under fluoroscopic control, reliable images of the whole of the extrahepatic and portions of the proximal intrahepatic biliary tree and its drainage should be possible in all cases. The use of dilute contrast medium, fractionated volumes and multiple radiographs should allow the discovery of small retained calculi, complications of surgery and assessment of the rate of drainage in all cases. Attention to detail, the exclusion of air bubbles and the use of varying postures enhance the examination. Excessive filling pressures are to be avoided and a sterile technique should be employed. Occasionally the proximal pancreatic duct will outline but pancreatitis has not been a hazard. If the result of the procedure is in doubt it should be repeated after 24–48 h. Sterile saline solution can be infused for 1 h as a preliminary to flush out persistent air bubbles.

In the event of a retained common bile duct calculus, the T-tube may be left in place for 6 weeks which will allow the T-tube tract to granulate and fibrose, hence allowing a subsequent approach for percutaneous extraction of the retained calculus (p. 38). Similarly, postoperative strictures may be treated by percutaneous balloon dilatation (p. 36).

## VASCULAR RADIOLOGY

From 1960 to 1975 angiography was the most effective radiological method for the investigation of abdominal masses, portal hypertension, some cases of gastrointestinal bleeding and for the confirmation of traumatic rupture of solid viscera. The progress of endoscopy, ultrasound, computed tomography, radionuclide studies and now magnetic resonance imaging has now displaced angiography into a much reduced diagnostic role. The need to display the vascular anatomy usually follows the discovery of an abnormality with "noninvasive" techniques and has an increasing association with therapeutic angiographic procedures (Lang 1979). The uses of pharmacoangiography (Novelline 1982, Cho et al 1989), embolization (Feldman et al 1983, White 1984, Pentecost 1994) and percutaneous angioplasty (Athanasoulis 1980) have also altered the role of the radiologist. As a result of the therapeutic aspects of angiography, the techniques require a high degree of expertise in the manipulation of fine catheters, coaxial catheter systems, embolic material and balloon catheters.

The introduction of intravenous digital subtraction angiography in vascular imaging has not had a major impact in abdominal visceral diagnosis. Intra-arterial digital subtraction angiography (DSA) has application in vascular mapping and the demonstration of portal venous patency prior to hepatic arterial intervention. Due to misregistration artefacts from gut movement DSA has some limitation in defining gut vessels. This movement can be overcome by intra-arterial injections of hyoscine butylbromide (Buscopan) or glucagon. DSA has significant advantages in shortening the procedure time, limiting contrast dose and decreasing film costs. There is also a significantly greater control during interventional vascular procedures using DSA (Rees et al 1989).

### Angiography

*Indications*

***Vascular anatomy.*** The delineation of the often variable upper abdominal visceral blood supply is important prior to many therapeutic considerations. Angiography aids decisions on the surgical management of primary and solitary secondary hepatic tumors and hepatic trauma. Hemobilia from trauma, surgery or previous biopsy is often best managed by embolization techniques at the time of the initial diagnostic angiogram (Perlberger 1977, Fagan et al 1980, Murray 1991).

***Intra-arterial perfusion therapy.*** Chemotherapeutic agents can be delivered either through infusion catheters placed at surgery (Buchwald et al 1980) or via a percutaneous catheter introduced into the hepatic artery by the femoral or axillary route (Kato et al 1981, Patt et al 1981, 1983). Long-term infusion catheters are also placed by percutaneous techniques, with minor surgery to place the pump subcutaneously (Cohen et al 1983). Each of these methods requires a preliminary vascular map to ensure that the therapeutic agent can be delivered via the catheter into the segmental vessel perfusing the tumor and to shorten the operative time if the catheter is to be placed surgically. Portal venous patency should be established prior to catheter placement to ensure hepatic viability if the hepatic artery is inadvertently occluded during therapy (Soo et al 1982). Transcatheter radionuclide studies using $^{99m}$Tc-labeled macroaggregated albumin are of use in assessing both intrahepatic and extrahepatic perfusion (Bledin et al 1982, Ziessman et al 1984).

***Tumor circulation.*** The demonstration of intrahepatic tumor circulation can be useful diagnostically (p. 1122) but its importance in separating primary from secondary tumor has greatly diminished since the introduction of new imaging methods. Primary liver tumors may have some helpful angiographic features, for example arterio-portal shunting and portal vein tumor invasion, but unfortunately these lack a degree of specificity (Freeny 1983).

***Gastrointestinal bleeding.*** Endoscopy and the acceptance of radionuclide studies for the localization of upper and lower intestinal tract bleeding have modified the role of arteriography (Hoare 1975, Alavi & Ring 1981, McKusick et al 1981, Markisz et al 1982). In the upper gastrointestinal tract, angiography is most helpful in patients in whom the bleeding site cannot be identified endoscopically and in those in whom a subsequent therapeutic procedure to control bleeding may avoid surgery. The indications for transcatheter embolization or vasopressin infusion have been reviewed by Athanasoulis (1982), Baum (1982) and Eckstein & Athanasoulis (1984).

Patients with chronic or intermittent gastrointestinal tract hemorrhage and in whom other investigations have been normal also may require angiography. In this instance the procedure aims to demonstrate pathological anatomical abnormalities which may cause bleeding, e.g. arteriovenous malformations, colonic angiodysplasia (Figs 17.10 and 17.11) or sites of diverticular blood loss (Casarella et al 1972). Abnormal tumor circulation can also be demonstrated and identified as a potential site of hemorrhage.

To demonstrate the site of bleeding when there is no anatomical abnormality, the rate of bleeding is the limiting factor (Nusbaum & Baum 1963) (p. 484). The site of bleeding is then indicated by the extravasation of contrast medium into the lumen of the gut. Radionuclide studies have a greater sensitivity (p. 86) (Alavi & Ring 1981) but lack anatomical specificity. In vitro labeled red blood cell techniques have replaced sulfur colloid and should usually be performed prior to angiography. The intermittent nature of gastrointestinal blood loss is always a problem to the angiographer. Pharmacological agents such as vasodilators and anticoagulants have been administered in recurrent massive hemorrhage in patients in whom a site of loss could not be identified by endoscopic, radiological and surgical techniques (Rosch et al 1982). These procedures should only be attempted under closely controlled conditions. Selective studies, particularly of the left gastric artery and the gastroduodenal vessels, may be required in order to show blood loss from gastric or duodenal lesions (Kelemouridis et al 1983). Identification of a bleeding site by superselective arterial studies can be followed by embolization or vasopressin infusion (Gomes et al 1986).

***Intestinal ischemia.*** Angiography is used in the initial investigation of patients suspected of mesenteric ischemia (Boley et al 1978) (p. 546) on the basis that survival is virtually confined to patients in whom a defined vascular occlusion is diagnosed and treated early. The delineation of the blood supply to both small and large bowel by standard arteriographic methods can be of assistance in defining the site and cause of intestinal ischemia. An aggressive approach to the investigation of a patient suspected of having mesenteric ischemia can define whether the arterial disease is occlusive or non-occlusive. "Low flow" states are, however, difficult to diagnose by current methods. Mesenteric venous occlusion is the cause of bowel ischemia in 5%–15% of patients. As an initial investigation CT scanning of the abdomen has proved quite reliable in defining superior mesenteric venous thrombosis rather than proceeding directly to angiography (Alpern et al 1988, Perez et al 1989). Although the patient may be seriously ill, angiography can be performed while supportive and resuscitative therapy is administered. Intra-arterial vasodilators at that time may limit the amount of gut that subsequently needs to be resected. Intra-arterial thrombolysis which is used extensively in other sites of vascular occlusion may eventually be effective in the mesenteric vessels (Flickinger et al 1983). When the cause of abdominal symptoms is shown to be related to stenosis of major mesenteric vessels then percutaneous balloon dilatation or transluminal angioplasty of the appropriate vessel can be performed (Roberts et al 1983, Clark & Gallant 1984, Odurny et al 1988), thus avoiding surgical revascularization.

### *Procedure*

***Angiography.*** Bleeding and clotting studies should be obtained prior to angiography. A prothrombin time of greater than 4 s and a platelet count of $60 \times 10^9$/L or less are relative contraindications. These problems should be corrected by vitamin K injection or platelet infusion before proceeding. Selective catheterization of the celiac axis and the superior and inferior mesenteric arteries can be performed under local anesthesia via either the femoral, axillary or brachial arteries. Access to the lumen of the vessel is performed using the Seldinger technique with five or six French precurved catheters. The catheter shape depends on the vascular configuration and the personal preference of the operator. The techniques are described in detail by Waltman (1982). The volume of contrast and the rate of filming are variable and depend on catheter position, catheter stability, vessel size and the rate of blood flow. Normal volumes and flow rates for hepatic arteriography range from 25 to 80 ml of contrast at a rate of 6–10 ml per second. A high-volume, medium flow rate through a selectively placed catheter into the celiac axis almost always visualizes the portal vein by means of delayed venous phase films.

Firm pressure must be applied to the site of arterial puncture for at least 5 min after the procedure to minimize the risks of bleeding and repeated observations must be made to ensure that this does not occur subsequently. This applies particularly to patients with coagulation abnormalities. Arteriography, for any purpose, has a complication rate of about 2%, usually hypotension or arrhythmia, and a mortality of about 0.03%, most commonly from aortic dissection or rupture of an aneurysm (Hessel et al 1981).

***Normal appearances*** (Fig. 1.29). The anatomy of the mesenteric circulation is variable and celiac or superior mesenteric artery variations occur in almost half of normal persons. The greatest variation occurs in the origin of the hepatic artery (p. 714) (Fig. 1.30). Three vessels usually emanate from the celiac axis: the common hepatic artery, the left gastric artery and the splenic artery. The common hepatic artery gives off the gastroduodenal artery and then divides into the right and left hepatic arteries. These enter the liver and branch into progressively smaller vessels. When the contrast material enters the sinusoids, a "hepatogram" is obtained.

Superselective catheter techniques involve placing the catheter in a second and third order arterial branch and are required for subsequent therapeutic procedures such as infusion of pharmacological agents or the delivery of embolic material. Specific examples are the selection of the left gastric artery from the celiac axis, selection of the gastroduodenal artery from the common hepatic for infusion of vasopressin or embolization in upper gastrointestinal bleeding and selection of the right hepatic artery for embolization of secondary tumor (p. 1124). The procedures can be carried out through the primary angiographic catheter or by coaxial catheter methods, thus enabling the delivery of the therapeutic agent to a specific anatomical site. The coaxial technique involves passing small special-purpose catheters or wires through the lumen of the primary angiographic catheter. For the infusion of chemotherapy, the left axillary approach for the placement of the catheter for angiography is often preferred, since the treatment is usually over a period of 3–5 days and the patient can therefore remain ambulant. The delivery of chemotherapy into the arterial system requires an infusion pump to maintain patency of the catheter.

The newer iso-osmolar, non-ionic contrast agents make the procedure more comfortable for the patient (Schonfeld et al 1984). There is likely to be a reduction in the incidence of renal complications when using high volumes of contrast in patients with pre-existing renal problems, e.g. diabetes. Hypersensitivity responses to contrast medium are significantly decreased with these newer agents (Rapoport et al 1982).

***Digital subtraction arteriography.*** This involves the computed subtraction of images taken during venous or arterial injection of contrast. It is similar in principle to subtraction techniques used in conventional angiography. A preliminary image is taken immediately prior to the injection of contrast and this image is stored within the computer. Following injection of contrast further images are obtained and subtraction of the digitized arteriographic images is carried out by the computer program for display on a television monitor. The technique is very sensitive to differences in the density of contrasts and when injecting into an artery only small volumes of dilute (1:4) arteriographic contrast are used (Harrington et al 1982, Kaufman et al 1984).

For abdominal studies a good map of the major vessels and their branches can be obtained by aortic or selective arterial injection. This mapping technique is useful in planning intra-arterial chemotherapy, embolization and resection of hepatic tumor. Superior detail of the small vessels is obtained using standard film arteriography,

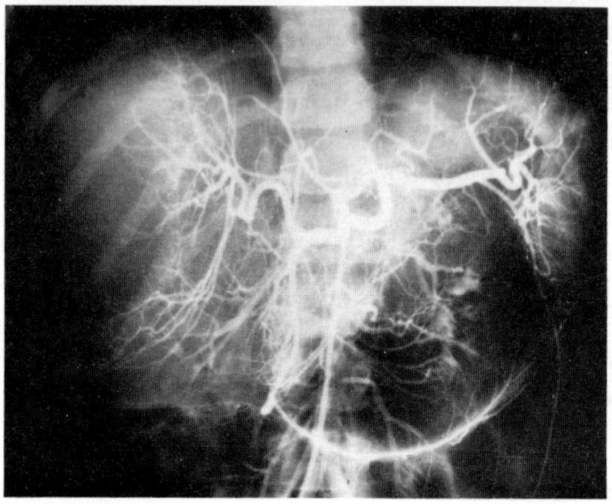

**Fig. 1.29** Hepatic angiogram in a child with an intrahepatic hematoma caused by trauma. The branches of the hepatic artery form an arc around the hematoma.

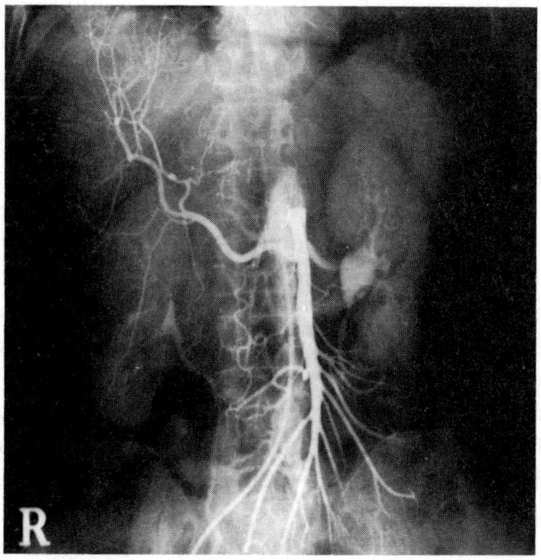


**Fig. 1.30** Common variant of hepatic arterial supply. The right hepatic artery arises from the superior mesenteric artery.

although computed tomography and ultrasound have significantly decreased this requirement in abdominal diagnosis. Portal venous imaging can be performed by this technique but requires a degree of patient co-operation for the delayed venous phase films. The procedure is particularly sensitive to patient movement following injection and therefore respiration during filming significantly reduces the quality of the image (Foley et al 1983).

## Portography

Examination of the portal vein can be elegantly performed using noninvasive methods, with useful information being obtained from ultrasound and bolus injection computed tomography (p. 66). Portal venography, whether by direct or arterial methods, should be reserved for patients in whom the non-invasive methods have not provided sufficient information.

Direct splenoportography is the longest established method and has a major advantage in that portal pressure can be measured directly. Arterioportography following selective splenic and superior mesenteric contrast injection is particularly useful. Transhepatic portography and umbilical vein catheterization will also be described.

### *Indications*

The main indication is the investigation of portal hypertension. This is required most frequently prior to portal systemic shunt surgery and is valuable after surgery if thrombotic occlusion of the shunt is suspected. Following shunt surgery, however, it should be noted that direct access to the portal system is possible through the shunt from the systemic circulation (Redman & Reuter 1969).

Demonstration of the portal venous anatomy is also important prior to embolization or hepatic resection for tumor, since in both of these procedures an adequate portal blood flow may be vital to the viability of the liver. Invasion or obstruction of the portal vein by tumor may be a contraindication to surgical resection of hepatic and pancreatic malignancy. Portal vein invasion is a common finding in hepatocellular carcinoma.

## Arterial portography (Fig. 1.31)

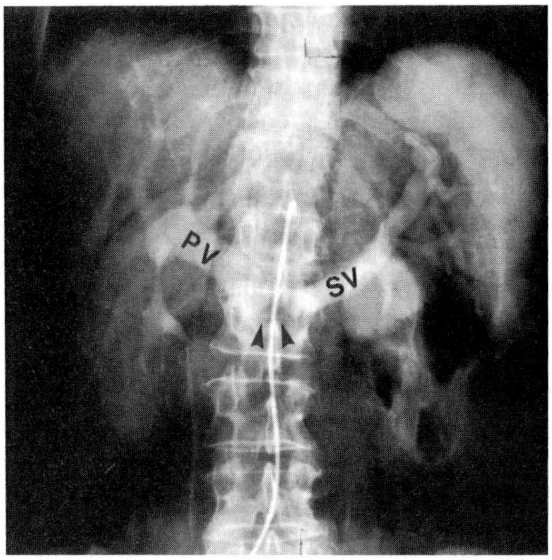


**Fig. 1.31** Arterial portography. Late film following celiac axis injection showing splenic vein (SV) and portal vein (PV). Normal defect (arrows) caused by unopacified blood from superior mesenteric vein.

***Procedure.*** This method is a simple and relatively noninvasive means of demonstrating the portal system and can be performed as part of the angiographic procedure (Viamonte et al 1970 a, b). Large volumes (70–80 ml) of contrast at moderate flow rates (8–10 ml/s) are used in conjunction with delayed venous phase films (10–25 s postinjection) both in the celiac axis and superior mesenteric artery. Tolazoline, an $\alpha$-sympathetic blocking agent, injected into the superior mesenteric artery prior to the contrast improves the flow rate through the mesenteric vascular bed and therefore produces better portal venous opacification (Novelline 1982). Selective splenic artery injection can also be performed with slightly decreased volumes to produce excellent images of the splenic and portal veins. Dilution of contrast by nonopacified mesenteric blood and streamlining of flow is sometimes a problem.

The major disadvantage of arterial portography is the inability to measure portal venous pressure. Furthermore, in low venous flow states, delineation of the system may be inadequate owing to a low density of contrast on the venous side of the splenic or mesenteric vascular bed. In such circumstances, when the demonstration of clinically suspected varices has not been adequate, direct portography may be indicated.

## Direct portography

### *Splenoportography*

In adults, the procedure can be performed under intravenous sedation and local anesthesia. General anesthesia is required in children and in anxious adults. The position of the spleen is determined by palpation, percussion and fluoroscopy. A needle–Teflon sheath combination is inserted into the splenic pulp during mid-respiratory apnea at the ninth intercostal space in the mid-axillary line. The needle is withdrawn and the catheter cleared with 1–2 ml of saline. A pressure measurement can then be taken using an external reference point (usually the mid-axillary line) placed to represent the position of the right atrium. The normal pressure is 3–17 mmHg (p. 997). A test injection of contrast establishes that the catheter is correctly placed and ensures drainage from the splenic pulp into the splenic veins. If the catheter is found to be in a subcapsular position, then it must be repositioned. A pressure injection is then made through the catheter into the splenic pulp using 40–50 ml of contrast medium. Films are taken at one per second over 10–15 s.

***Findings.*** The normal study shows quite dense opacification of the splenic and portal venous systems (Figs 36.4 and 38.8). Major tributaries of these two vessels are not well seen unless there is reversal of normal portal flow and indeed, some dilution of contrast may occur owing to blood entering from the large mesenteric veins. This streaming of contrast should not be mistaken for thrombosis of the portal vein. For gravitational reasons, in the supine patient, the left branch of the portal vein is often less well demonstrated than the right. Some have advocated the prone position to solve this problem and also to demonstrate varices more clearly (Moskowitz et al 1968). Delayed films show a dense hepatogram as the contrast fills the hepatic sinusoids.

Failure to visualize the splenic or portal veins does not necessarily mean that they are occluded. In up to 6% of patients shunting of blood into larger collaterals accounts for the nonvisualization of the patent portal vein (Burchell et al 1965). Ultrasound and computed tomography should help in this group of patients.

***Contraindications and complications.*** Specific contraindications include a nonreversible bleeding diathesis and ascites.

Bleeding is the most important complication. Clinically significant bleeding occurs in about 2% of patients. Usually replacement of blood loss and analgesia is all that is required but about 1% of patients may require splenectomy. Safety can be improved by plugging the needle tract with Gelfoam (Probst et al 1978). Punctures of the left colon, left kidney and lung are also well-documented complications.

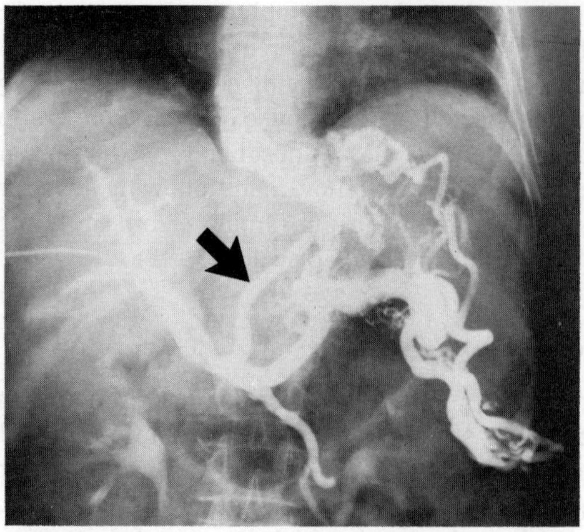

**Fig. 1.32** Transhepatic portogram in a patient with cirrhosis of the liver and portal hypertension. Note the large left gastric vein (arrow) supplying esophageal collateral vessels, and the large collateral vessels from the splenic vein.

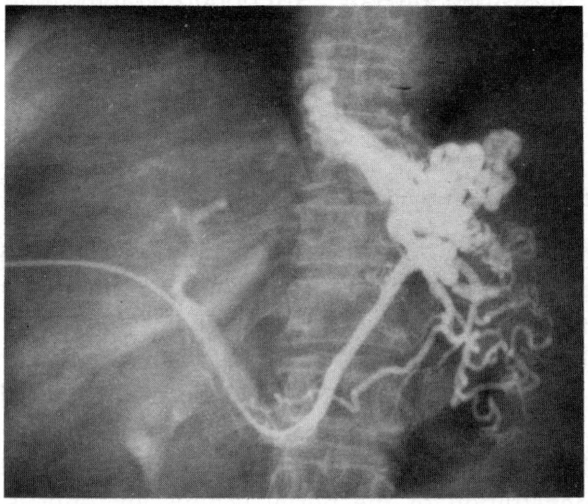

**Fig. 1.33** Transhepatic portogram. The catheter has been placed in the left gastric vein to demonstrate filling of varices from that source.

### *Transhepatic portography*

The percutaneous transhepatic route can be successfully utilized to define portal anatomy or to measure portal venous pressure. Although a difficult technique, it gives direct access to the portal system and allows sclerosis or embolization of varices and venous sampling techniques to be undertaken (Lunderquist & Vang 1974).

Abnormal blood coagulation is a contraindication to the procedure and should be corrected prior to catheter placement. Transhepatic portography can be performed under sedation and local anesthesia. Extended transhepatic embolization procedures may require general anesthesia or neuroleptanesthesia to ensure co-operation of the patient.

Patency of the portal vein should be established by ultrasound, computed tomography or arterial portography before embarking on this technique. A needle–Teflon sheath is inserted into the hepatic parenchyma in a manner similar to catheter placement in biliary drainage procedures. The needle is withdrawn and aspiration through the Teflon sheath confirms the position within a portal venous radicle. A test injection of contrast viewed fluoroscopically shows that the catheter is within the portal vein. Guidewires are then passed into the splenic vein. Portal venous pressure is directly recorded through the catheter. With the catheter tip at the splenic hilum a contrast injection of 40 ml produces excellent opacification of the portal venous system. The catheter is repositioned in the superior mesenteric vein and a second injection made. Excellent definition of varices occurs with delineation of gastric, duodenal, retroperitoneal and mesenteric collaterals (p. 995) (Fig. 1.32). Selective catheterization may then be performed for sclerosant or embolization techniques (Lunderquist et al 1977) (Figs 1.33–1.35). Bleeding may occur at the hepatic puncture site and this can be avoided

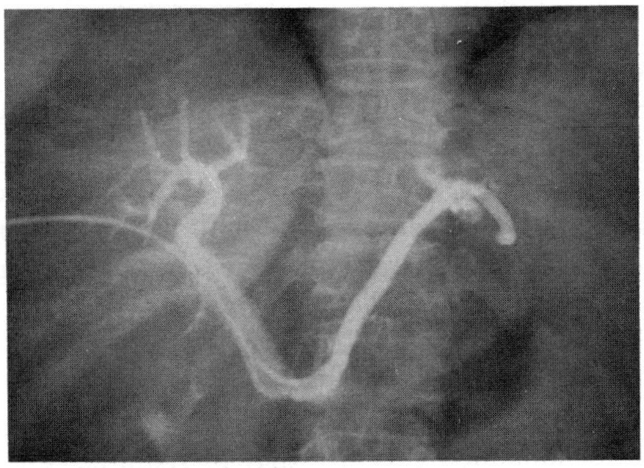

**Fig. 1.34** Transhepatic portogram. Following transcatheter embolization, the collateral vessels shown previously have been occluded.

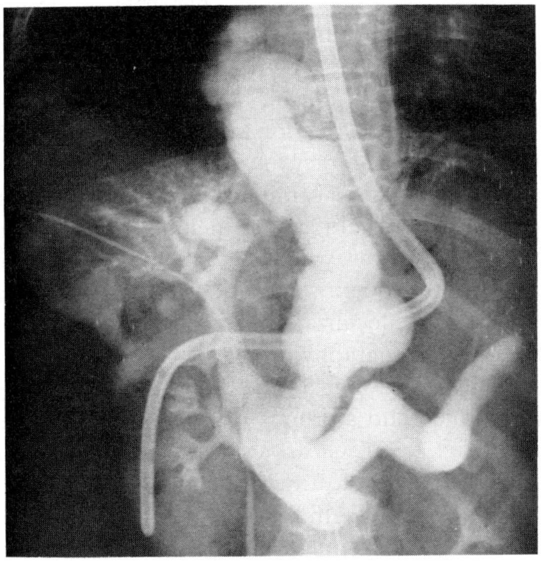

**Fig. 1.35** Transhepatic portogram in a patient with portal hypertension due to hepatic cirrhosis who was bleeding from esophageal varices. The left gastric vein enters an enormous collateral vessel which was shown to pass directly into the vena azygos. Embolization was not performed for fear that emboli would pass into the lungs.

by sealing the needle tract with Gelfoam plugs or a Gianturco spring coil embolus.

***Venous sampling techniques.*** As well as providing access to the portal system, transhepatic portal cannulation allows selective venous sampling and venous mapping of the pancreatic drainage (Ingemansson et al 1975, Roche et al 1982) (p. 1303). The procedure is exacting but localization of insulin-producing tumors has been reported in up to 80% of cases (p. 1303). Only large tumors show displacement of veins and most functioning endocrine tumors are relatively small. It is vital that the techniques of mapping and sampling are methodically performed and documented for the technique to have good correlation with surgical findings.

## Hepatic venography

*Indications*

Hepatic venography is mainly used to diagnose hepatic venous obstruction (Budd–Chiari syndrome, p. 1080). The anatomy of the hepatic venous system can be clearly identified by ultrasound and computed tomography (Sexton & Zeman 1983) and resectability of tumor is better assessed by these methods than by venography. Indirect pressure measurements can also be obtained by either "wedge" techniques or by the balloon occlusion method (p. 996) (Barth & Udoff 1980).

*Procedure*

The veins are catheterized from the right medial antecubital vein or from the femoral vein. Measurement of sinusoidal pressure is obtained by subtracting the intrahepatic caval pressure from the wedged pressure (p. 997). Wedged hepatic venography or free hepatic venography is undertaken by injection of 10–20 ml of contrast at 2–4 ml/s.

*Interpretation*

Injected contrast passes through the sinusoids and is cleared rapidly by other hepatic venous channels (Fig. 1.36). Occasionally portal vein radicles are seen even in normal patients. Hepatic venous occlusion can make entry into the vein difficult and free hepatic injection of contrast may reveal the abnormal collateral vessels and the lace-like pattern that is pathognomonic of venous occlusion (Budd–Chiari syndrome) (Fig. 41.2).

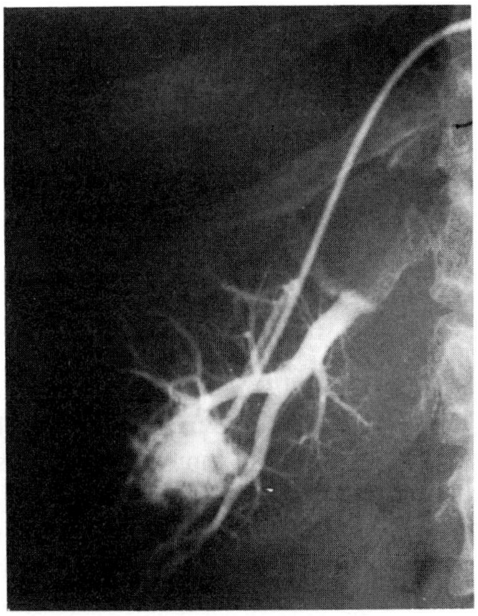

**Fig. 1.36** Normal wedge hepatic venogram showing a patent hepatic vein and contrast medium in the parenchyma.

Cirrhosis produces progressive loss of sinusoidal filling and the hepatic veins become irregular and narrowed owing to fibrosis. Eventually, filling of portal venous branches becomes more prominent as the degree of sinusoidal and hepatic venous obstruction increases. Hepatic venography from the transjugular approach is the starting point for transjugular intrahepatic portosystemic shunt (TIPS) procedure.

## INTERVENTIONAL RADIOLOGY

Developments in the imaging techniques of computed tomography, ultrasound and nuclear medicine have made diagnosis of intra-abdominal masses and fluid collections a precise art. The combination of progress in the field of cytopathology and the use of sophisticated catheter and guidewire techniques has enabled the radiologist to take part in the pathological diagnosis of mass lesions and the management of a variety of intra-abdominal problems.

### Percutaneous biopsy

Percutaneous needle biopsy has been a diagnostic technique since Leyden in 1883 and Menetrier in 1886 introduced the procedure in pulmonary diagnosis (Sargent et al 1974). The current concepts of cytological diagnosis and its recent developments have been reviewed by Koss (1984).

Over the past decade, the parallel development of modern imaging techniques, particularly computed tomography and ultrasound, the refinement of the thin-walled 22 gauge needle (Okuda et al 1974, Ferrucci et al 1976) and the rapid progress in cytological methods have led to the burgeoning increase in diagnosis of fine-needle aspiration. The technique has developed into the most common invasive imaging procedure (Bernardino 1984) and its safety, patient acceptability (Tao et al 1980, Lundquist 1971) and high degree of accuracy are well established (Kline & Neal 1978). The advantages of the technique are its relatively low cost regardless of the imaging modality used and its use on an outpatient basis.

*Indications*

Most abdominal percutaneous biopsies are performed to determine whether a mass that has been found by palpation, ultrasound or computed tomography consists of primary or secondary tumor or inflammatory tissue. Primary tumors of lymphatic origin can be differentiated from lymph node metastasis so that the course of further investigation and therapy can be redirected (Zornoza et al 1977). Staging a tumor or verification of recurrence can also be performed.

*Procedure*

***Biopsy guidance system.*** Superficial or palpable lesions do not require imaging techniques and can be biopsied without concern using fine-gauge needles. If the lesion is impalpable, then the simplest imaging procedure which provides adequate definition of the mass should be employed. Fluoroscopy, ultrasound and computed tomography are the modalities most utilized (Wittenberg et al 1981).

Fluoroscopy is the cheapest and quickest way to biopsy a lesion, but in the abdomen some contrast, for example barium or iodinated contrast, may be required to outline the exact biopsy site (Pereiras et al 1978, Zornoza et al 1977). A surgical clip or biliary drainage tube may also aid fluoroscopic biopsy.

Ultrasound as a guidance system was refined by Holm et al (1975). Since then there has been a progressive improvement in real-time ultrasound images and in special biopsy transducers. The needle tip can now be visualized within the mass during biopsy, thus increasing the yield of appropriate tissue for cytology. Grant et al (1983) reported a 93.4% accuracy in needle placement in 61 consecutive cases using real-time ultrasound guidance alone. Disadvantages with ultrasound include the unpredictable presence of bowel gas, which can preclude visualization of a mass. Small retroperitoneal lesions can also pose a problem for ultrasonic localization.

Computed tomography provides cross-sectional images with excellent anatomical detail (Fig. 8.8). The target is easily identified and a proposed path to the lesion can be outlined (Fig. 1.37). Clear verification of the anatomical accuracy of the needle tip within the mass is an added advantage (Haaga & Alfidi 1976, Ferrucci & Wittenberg 1978). The disadvantages of computed tomography include a longer procedure time than with ultrasound and

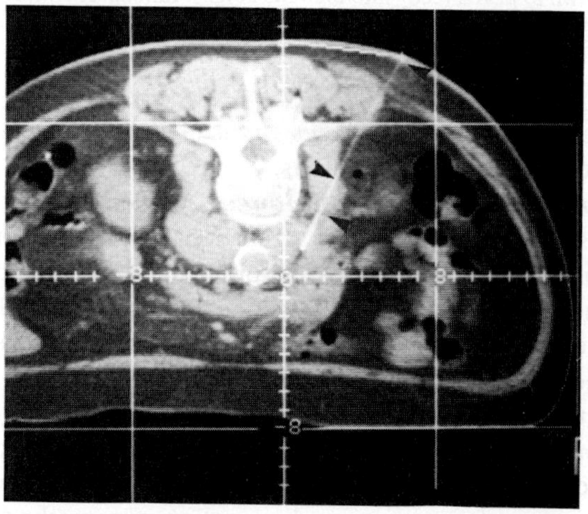

**Fig. 1.37** CT of abdomen showing mensuration guide which allows the operator to identify the area (para-aortic nodes) to be biopsied by means of surface measurements.

the use of ionizing radiation, but with similar expertise and with appropriate patient selection results are comparable (Wittenberg et al 1981).

***Equipment.*** The equipment used is simple, cheap and very effective. It comprises a thin-walled fine needle, a disposable plastic syringe and an aspiration holder which is used to maintain a good vacuum on the syringe during the suction phase of the procedure. There is a large range of needles with varying modifications of the needle tip (Staab et al 1979, Wittenberg et al 1981). Needles fall into two main groups: those for cytological aspirate and those for obtaining histological specimens (Holm et al 1975). The type of needle used depends on the preference of the operator.

Simple 22 gauge needles, usually with a stylet, are used for cytology; for example the 9 cm "spinal" needle or the 15 cm "Chiba" needle. The longer needles have a tendency to bend within the tract. An 18 gauge arterial puncture needle through superficial nonvital tissues can help to give stability and guide the fine needle. A technique to produce a core sample using the fine needle has been described by Isler et al (1981).

As well as the standard "Tru-cut" needles, a range of small gauge needles has been developed to provide a core of tissue for histological section. These include the "Surecut" needle of the Menghini type or the mechanical spring-loaded "Biopty" gun of the Tru-cut style. These needles range from 16 to 22 gauge (Bernardino 1990). A satisfactory tissue core can be obtained routinely (Torp-Pedersen et al 1984).

***Aspiration technique.*** Following the choice of the appropriate guidance system, a local anesthetic (xylocaine, 1%) is infiltrated at the puncture site and through to the peritoneum if a transabdominal approach is used. Premedication is rarely necessary unless the patient is extremely apprehensive.

The fine needle is advanced along the selected tract into the tissue site to be biopsied (Fig. 1.38) and the stylet removed. As soon as the precise position of the needle tip is verified, suction is applied using a 20 ml plastic syringe and the aspiration syringe holder. A connecting tube with a small volume confers flexibility and also gives a better tactile response to the "feel" of the needle in the tissues. Suction is completely released prior to removing the needle from the mass so that the sample cells remain in the needle and are not aspirated into the syringe barrel. The material is deposited on to glass microscope slides and smeared immediately. At this stage expert cytological and pathological support is important so that the small amount of material is handled optimally. Although two to three passes are often necessary to provide good samples, a review of the initial smear can avoid unnecessary further passes. The technique is safe and can be performed on an outpatient basis (Lundquist 1971, Tao et al 1980). Ferrucci et al (1980b) have advocated a 4 h period of observation for outpatients, but as experience has

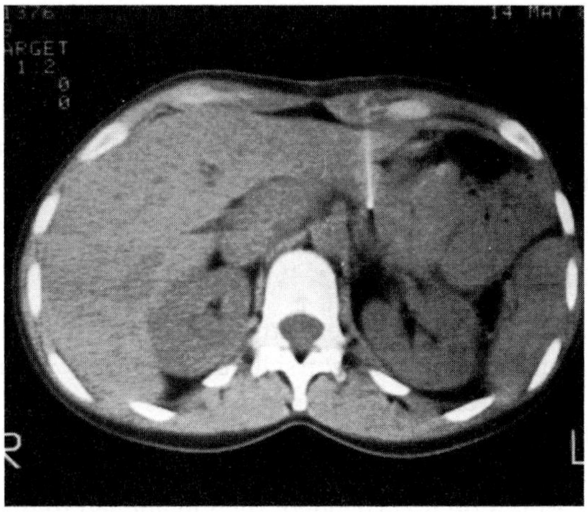

**Fig. 1.38** Patient with secondary gastric carcinoma in a celiac axis node. The needle passes through the liver and pancreas to enter the node. No sequelae.

increased this is probably unnecessary. After Menghini or Tru-cut biopsies for histology the patient must be observed for 4 h unless the biopsy was of a superficial nonvascular mass. In liver biopsy in high-risk patients with a coagulopathy and also with using the larger needles for histology, plugging of the transhepatic needle track with Gelfoam can be helpful in obviating bleeding problems (Zins et al 1992).

***Cytopathology.*** Whilst the techniques of smearing, fixing and staining the material vary between pathologists and institutions, there is merit in having a cytopathologist or technician handle the smears as the biopsies are being performed (Bernardino 1984). A rapid review of each sample can terminate the procedure if it is positive and an adequate specimen has been obtained. Good results depend upon the commitment given by the cytopathological service.

### *Complications*

Complications are rare and are difficult to produce experimentally. Goldstein et al (1977) used transabdominal puncture with fine needles in dogs and were unable to demonstrate significant evidence of bowel perforation or hematoma formation at subsequent laparotomy. Lundquist (1971) performed 2611 fine-needle liver biopsies and reported that only one patient required surgical intervention for hematoma. Livraghi et al (1983) correlated the results of 1700 fine-needle aspiration biopsies and recorded one death, four major and 58 minor complications. Tumor seeding from fine-needle aspiration biopsy was initially reported in a single case by Ferrucci et al (1979). A further four cases have been reported in the literature. The incidence was reviewed by Smith (1985), who concluded that the rate of seeding in the needle track was approximately 1 in 20 000.

## Transjugular hepatic biopsy

Transjugular liver biopsy is an alternative method for obtaining a core sample of liver in patients with a coagulopathy. This technique may also be helpful in patients with ascites.

### *Technique*

Following percutaneous puncture of the internal jugular vein, preferably on the right side, the venotomy is dilated up to 9–10 French and a vascular access sheath is placed into the vein. A modified Ross or Colapinto needle sheath set can then be delivered into a branch of the right hepatic vein. Respiration is suspended, suction applied to the needle and the tip is advanced into the liver parenchyma. The needle is withdrawn and the specimen examined (Velt et al 1984, Gamble et al 1985, Corr et al 1992). A transvenous femoral approach using flexible biopsy forceps is also described and is preferred by some (Lipchik et al 1991). Adequate samples are obtained in 64–100% in reported series (Lebrec et al 1982).

### *Complications*

The major complication is capsular perforation. This occurred in one series in 3.5% of 461 biopsies (Gamble et al 1985). It was clinically significant in only 0.5%. Local neck hematoma, carotid puncture and cardiac arrhythmias are also reported.

## Percutaneous abdominal abscess drainage

During the past 15 years the emphasis has changed from mandatory surgical drainage of abdominal abscesses to percutaneous drainage using imaging techniques. The efficacy of percutaneous drainage was shown by Gerzof et al (1981) and success rates of 80–90% are reported (Haaga & Weinstein 1980, Gerzof et al 1981, Martin et al 1982, vanSonnenberg et al 1984).

### *Diagnosis*

***Plain radiographs.*** For many years the plain radiograph has been the mainstay of diagnosis, although this role is changing (Baker 1993). The presence of abnormal gas shadows, a soft tissue mass or the obliteration of fat planes are all important signs. Often these findings are subtle and are only seen in retrospect. Connell et al (1980) reported finding 71% of upper abdominal abscesses on radiographs, although only 42 out of 82 cases (51%) were reported initially.

***Radionuclide studies.*** Gallium-67 or indium-111 may be used. Intra-abdominal scanning with gallium may produce false positive results owing to excretion of the radionuclide into the colon. Leukocyte-labeling techniques using indium-111 (p. 89) have an accuracy rate of 92% (Knochel et al 1980) and can be used in patients who have no localizing signs and are not critically ill.

***Ultrasound.*** This technique can also be used to demonstrate abscess or fluid collections (p. 59). Usually, these are well-defined echo-free masses with a good through transmission of sound (Fig. 2.9). Septations or gas bubbles may be defined by their ultrasonic characteristics. Multiple locules and fine gas bubbles can produce masses of high echogenicity. An important advantage of ultrasound is its portability, so that it can be taken to the intensive care unit without moving the critically ill patient.

***Computed tomography.*** This has become the primary imaging technique for the diagnosis of intra-abdominal abscess (Aronberg et al 1978, Callen 1979). The classic appearance is of a fluid collection with a well-defined enhancing rim. The presence of small locules of gas within the mass is the most specific sign but is only present in 30% of cases. Diagnostic accuracy rates of 96% (Knochel et al 1980) and 97% (Koehler & Moss 1980) are reported.

### *Indications*

The criteria for percutaneous drainage initially established by Gerzof et al (1981) were: a well-defined unilocular abscess cavity, a safe drainage route, concurring surgical opinion and immediate operative back-up in case of failure or complications. The ability to aspirate pus prior to a formal drainage catheter placement was also considered important (vanSonnenberg et al 1982). As experience has developed, a more aggressive approach has been applied (Gerzof & Johnson 1984, Mueller et al 1984) and indications have broadened, with the inclusion of critically ill patients with complex multilocular abscesses, phlegmons and fistulae (Karlson et al 1982, Papanicolaou et al 1984, vanSonnenberg et al 1984, Lambiase et al 1992). Percutaneous drainage of uninfected cysts, e.g. pseudocysts, can also be accomplished (Fig. 1.39).

### *Contraindications*

The major limitations to percutaneous drainage of an abscess are the inability to provide safe access owing to intervening bowel loops or the risk of traversing sterile cavities, e.g. the pleural space.

### *Procedure* (Gerzof & Johnson 1984)

The procedure must follow basic surgical principles of drainage in that abscesses need to be completely drained without dissemination of infection. Using ultrasound or computed tomographic guidance an appropriate safe route to the abscess is determined. A needle is placed into the collection and a diagnostic aspirate is performed.

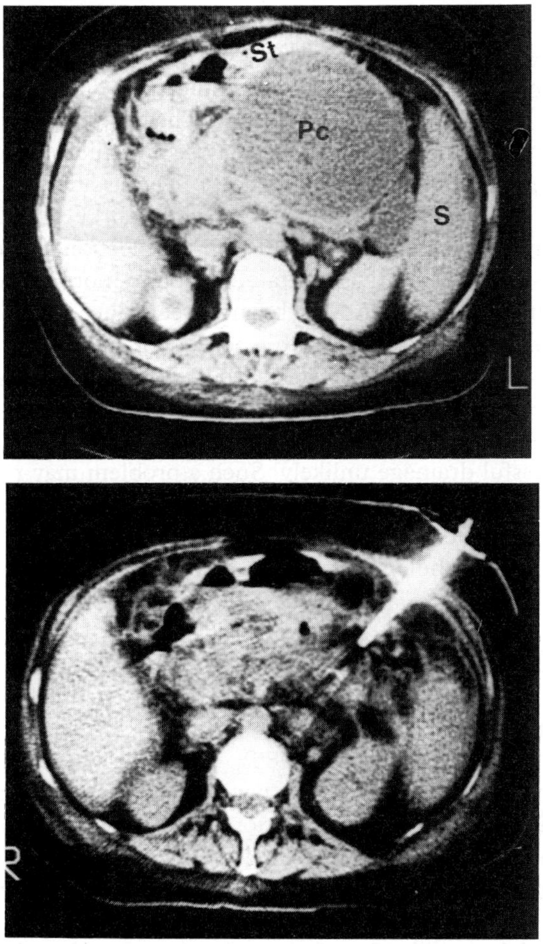


A

B

**Fig. 1.39** Pancreatic pseudocyst. **A** Before drainage, showing stomach (St) displaced by pseudocyst (Pc), spleen (S). **B** After insertion of percutaneous drainage tube. CT has enabled the puncture site to be selected at a point between the spleen and stomach.

Catheter placement and drainage may subsequently be performed using ultrasound, computed tomography or fluoroscopy. The latter is useful particularly in complex collections, after initial CT or ultrasound guided drainage, since catheters can be guided fluoroscopically into specific sites to allow for better drainage of the locules or compartments.

There are two basic methods for catheter placement (vanSonnenberg et al 1981). The first is the Seldinger technique and is based on the principles of arterial access (p. 27). The collection is punctured by a small needle or a needle–sheath combination. A guidewire is passed into the collection through the sheath following removal of the central stylet. A wire is then passed through the sheath and coiled in the abscess cavity. A series of dilators are passed over the wire, up to the size of the drainage catheter. The second technique is the trocar system in which the drainage catheter is mounted over a sharp metal trocar and the whole unit is inserted into the abscess. The latter procedure is more rapid but it can sometimes be difficult to penetrate the thick fibrotic wall that surrounds the longstanding abscess cavity. Irrespective of the method employed, adequate drainage without distention of the cavity is the major aim. If the patient is not on antibiotics prior to the procedure, appropriate antibiotics should be administered following the diagnostic aspirate.

The follow-up of percutaneous abscess drainage and catheter care are particularly important. Routines vary and will depend somewhat on whether adequate drainage is continuing. Very thick pus or necrotic material may require flushing with saline. Mucomyst (*N*-acetylcysteine) has been advocated for thinning non-drainable pus (van Waes et al 1983) but has been doubted by others (Dawson et al 1984).

Drainage times are variable and depend on the complexity of the abscess. Resolution may occur in a few days or may extend to 6 weeks or longer in patients with enteric fistulae (Papanicolaou et al 1984). Johnson et al (1981) reported an average of 17 days. Once the initial period of drainage has occurred, many of the patients can be managed on an outpatient basis until the abscess cavity heals.

### *Results and complications*

In the larger published series (Gerzof et al 1981, Martin et al 1982, vanSonnenberg et al 1982, Lambiase et al 1992) the results are superior to standard surgical drainage. In a comparison of percutaneous with operative drainage the complications (4% vs 16%), inadequate drainage (11% vs 21%), mortality (11% vs 21%), duration of drainage (17 days vs 29 days) and success rates (89% vs 70%) favored percutaneous drainage (Johnson et al 1981). In 250 abscess and fluid collections (vanSonnenberg et al 1984) a success rate of 83.6% was reported. Major complications such as septicemia, hemorrhage and bowel perforation occurred in 2.8% of cases. Minor complications included bacteremia, superficial skin infection, bleeding along the catheter and transgression of the pleural space. Gerzof & Johnson (1984) reviewed 14 series, each of which had more than ten percutaneously drained abscesses, a total of 423 cases. There was a success rate of 78.5%, a complication rate of 10.4% and a recurrence rate of 2.6%.

The method of percutaneous abscess drainage is established as the initial procedure of choice for all intra-abdominal collections because of comparable success rates, technical simplicity and an overall lower complication rate than surgery (vanSonnenberg et al 1992).

## **Percutaneous biliary drainage**

The advent of fine-needle percutaneous transhepatic cholangiography (p. 22) in the 1970s provided a safe method for defining the level and cause of biliary obstruction in jaundiced patients (Okuda et al 1974, Ferrucci et al 1976). Percutaneous transhepatic biliary drainage represents a natural development from this technique. Hoevels et al (1978) reported 15 cases of successful percutaneous biliary drainage. The techniques were further refined by Ring et al (1978) and Ferrucci et al (1980a). Both these groups have progressively improved the techniques and instrumentation (Ferrucci et al 1981, Oleaga et al 1981). Endoscopic techniques and success rates have improved dramatically in recent years and have displaced percutaneous techniques (Summerfield 1988, Ott et al 1992). The indications for percutaneous drainage have not altered but the technique is often reserved for failed or technically impossible endoscopy (e.g. following previous gastric surgery).

*Indications*

Percutaneous biliary drainage is performed in patients with malignant extrahepatic biliary obstruction in order to relieve jaundice and pruritus and treat associated biliary sepsis and hepatic failure. The most common specific indication is in the palliation of malignant biliary obstruction due to carcinoma of the pancreatic head, gallbladder and bile duct and metastatic disease, especially from the colon. Klatskin tumors involving the proximal common hepatic and both right and left hepatic ducts are usually not resectable and percutaneous techniques are effective in their management. Often right and left duct have to be drained separately.

Preoperative decompression of the obstructed biliary tree has been an indication for percutaneous drainage, with some early work suggesting a lowering of peroperative morbidity and mortality (Nakayama et al 1978). This has been supported by some studies (Gundry et al 1984) but not by others (Hatfield et al 1982, Norlander et al 1982). Its use is unresolved.

Biliary sepsis due to acute suppurative cholangitis can be managed initially by percutaneous decompression. In this situation, the high operative mortality of up to 50–75% has been reduced to 17% in a small series of 18 patients (Kadir et al 1982).

Benign biliary strictures are most commonly a direct sequelae of surgical procedures, either at the site of previous biliary enteric anastomosis or due to bile duct injury during cholecystectomy (p. 1215). Balloon dilatation or the insertion of successively larger catheters effectively treat the stricture (Martin et al 1980, Salomonowitz et al 1984, Gallacher et al 1985). Obstruction of biliary enteric anastomoses may also be due to recurrent malignant disease and these strictures need to be managed by an indwelling catheter, plastic stent or by an expandable metal endoprosthesis (Akiyama et al 1990).

*Contraindications*

There are few contraindications to percutaneous transhepatic biliary drainage. Bleeding disorders can be corrected using vitamin K, fresh frozen plasma or platelets. Ascites, although not an absolute contraindication, does add technical and management problems. The fluid gap between the thoracic cage and the liver may be difficult to negotiate owing to buckling of the catheter. The ascitic fluid will tend to leak around the catheter and can be difficult to control (Pogany et al 1985). Bacterial infection in the bile ducts can be a relative contraindication to more aggressive manipulation within the biliary tree, since there is a significant association with subsequent septicemia and shock in these patients, even with antibiotic cover.

Specific contraindications are multiple malignant strictures which sequester parts of the biliary tree and make successful drainage unlikely. Such a problem may require multiple catheters and repeated changes of catheter. The bacterial colonization of the biliary tree may also produce suppurative cholangitis in these segments.

*Procedure*

***Internal/external drainage.*** The techniques are described by Ferrucci et al (1981), Ring & McLean (1981) and Pogany et al (1985).

The patient is placed on parenteral antibiotics (ampicillin and gentamicin) 24 h prior to the procedure. Platelet counts and bleeding times are obtained and if abnormal, vitamin K, platelets or fresh frozen plasma are given. Ferrucci et al (1981) suggest that the prothrombin time should be within 3 s of control value and the platelets should be above $75 \times 10^9$ per liter. Premedication using both sedative and analgesic drugs is required. A general aesthetic is usually not necessary in the adult but the support of an anesthetist to administer further analgesic drugs is often useful during the procedure.

For standard right-sided biliary drainage, the skin of the right lateral chest wall is prepared and draped. A standard 22 gauge fine-needle percutaneous transhepatic cholangiogram is performed and the biliary system opacified. An appropriate right lobe duct is selected and transfixed with an 18 gauge needle–Teflon sheath combination. The needle stylet is removed and bile flow indicates the correct placement of the tip of the sheath within a biliary radicle. A guidewire is then advanced into the biliary system and manipulated down into the duodenum. The sheath is advanced over this guidewire. The hepatic parenchymal tract and stenotic duct are dilated and a multiple side-hole catheter (Ring et al 1979) is placed across the obstruction into the duodenum (Fig. 1.40). If the obstruction cannot be passed, a catheter is left in the proximal biliary tree to drain for 2 or 3 days before a second attempt is made. Cannulation of the duct is often much easier after a period of decompression. Pogany et al (1985) report successful catheter placement in 300 consecutive attempts.

With an obstruction of the bifurcation of the right and

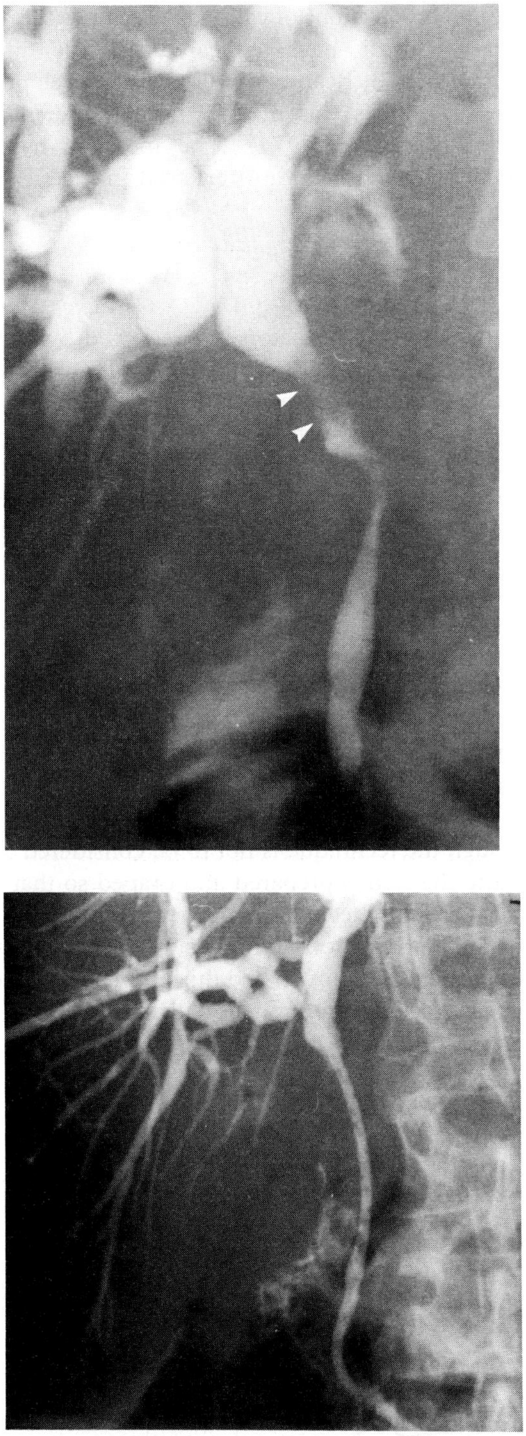
A
B

**Fig. 1.40** Percutaneous biliary drainage. **A** Obstruction of the common hepatic duct (arrows) due to involvement of the lymph nodes in the porta hepatis by secondary carcinoma. **B** Drainage tube in place with its tip in the duodenum.

left hepatic ducts, the left hepatic duct may need to be drained separately. A subxiphoid approach is used for this (Mueller et al 1982a). In contrast to the right-sided biliary drainage for obstruction to the common bile duct, some authors prefer an approach via the subxiphoid and the left hepatic duct (Jaques et al 1982). The procedure is no more difficult but has the disadvantage of a high radiation dose to the operator's hands.

Whether internal or external drainage is achieved, the outer limb of the tube is connected to a drainage bag to allow free decompression of the biliary system. After the procedure, the patient must be observed for 4 h, with half-hourly measurement of pulse and blood pressure and measurement of temperature because of the possibility of septicemia.

***Indwelling stents.*** Completely indwelling stents have been designed and advocated by Ring & McLean (1981), Coons & Carey (1983) and McLean & Burke (1989). Large-bore indwelling 12 French stents have the major advantage of no skin communication and no daily catheter care for the patient. The initial patency rates of 85–95% (Hoevels et al 1980, Coons & Carey 1983) were promising, but there have been problems associated with stent migration and obstruction (Lammer & Neumayer 1986). Mendez et al (1984) had abandoned the technique due to stent blockage, the accessibility of internal/external drainage systems and the high dose of radiation to the operator during stent placement.

The development of self-expanding metallic stents has changed the approach to malignant biliary obstruction by percutaneous techniques (Dawson et al 1991, Lameris et al 1991). The major stents that are deployed are the Wallstent (Schneider, Switzerland) or the Gianturco zigzag stent (Cook, Bloomington, Indiana). With both of these the transhepatic track is smaller and the post-treatment bile duct diameter is larger. In a recent review of the literature median stent patency was 3.6–6.3 months and median survival rates were 3.2–7.5 months (Roddie & Adam 1994). Due to its open nature the Gianturco stent is prone to tumor ingrowth in up to 50% of cases (Irving et al 1989). Tumor ingrowth rate for the finer mesh Wallstent is 6.5% to 11% (Lammer et al 1990). Although there is no clear indication for the use of plastic versus metal stents, it is suggested that plastic stents be used for short-term palliation. They are cheaper, can be removed easily endoscopically and replaced. The metal stents are more permanent, more expensive, but potentially have longer patency rates. Although initial results appear promising (Rossi et al 1990), caution is advised in stenting benign biliary strictures as a primary therapeutic maneuver.

*Complications*

Sepsis is the most frequent complication. In a review (Mueller et al 1982b) severe septicemia occurred in 3.5% of 200 patients and mild transient fever in 10.5%.

Minor bleeding occurs during the procedure and often clot can be identified in the biliary system. However, lysis of the clot occurs in a few days and does not usually present a problem. Intraperitoneal hemorrhage is a major complication and has been reported in 1.5% of 150 cases by Ferrucci et al (1981) and 4.5% of 200 consecutive cases (Mueller et al 1982b). These authors related the increase in bleeding complications to the difficult nature of the cases and a need for multiple needle punctures.

In all, major complications occurred in 8% of 200 patients and the minor complications of fever and hemobilia occurred in 20% (Mueller et al 1982b, Teplick et al 1984). Complications due to catheter blockage, cholangitis and catheter migration are relatively common. Often they can be managed on an outpatient basis by catheter changes to ensure adequate drainage. Fluid and electrolyte problems can occur in patients in whom internal drainage cannot be established. The fluid loss of 500–600 ml per day and the loss of sodium and bicarbonate in this bile can be a problem if external drainage is long term (Ferrucci et al 1981). Extension of tumor along the tube tract in long-term drainage is reported (Oleaga et al 1980) but is rare.

## PERCUTANEOUS BILIARY STONE EXTRACTION

Retained common duct stones following cholecystectomy occur at a rate of 3–4% in spite of the use of operative cholangiography (p. 1208), Fogarty biliary catheters and intraoperative choledochoscopy. Previously, these stones required a second surgical procedure, with its associated increased morbidity and mortality. Percutaneous removal of the stone provides a safe nonoperative method of treatment (Burhenne 1973). In conjunction with endoscopic sphincterotomy (p. 1209) the need for a second operation in this group of patients has diminished.

Although descriptions of various techniques for removal of biliary calculi have appeared in the literature (Mazzariello 1973, Bean et al 1974), the development of modern techniques was mainly through the innovative efforts of Burhenne (1974). The methods have been refined progressively and are reviewed in a series of 661 patients (Burhenne 1980).

### *Procedure*

The detailed technical factors are reviewed by Burhenne (1980) and Ferrucci & Mueller (1981).

Once the diagnosis of a retained stone has been made from the postoperative cholangiogram, a waiting period of 5 weeks must occur to allow the development of a fibrous tract along the tube. The 5-week interval is long enough for a 14 French T-tube tract but an extra 1–2 weeks may be required for smaller T-tubes.

General anesthesia is unnecessary for this procedure and most patients require only mild sedation. Although prophylactic antibiotics are not necessary in all patients, the possibility of bacteremia from manipulation should always be considered when extensive manipulation is required. Patients with previous postoperative pancreatitis or those who have had cholangitis should have antibiotic cover.

Although the technique is not to be considered a sterile procedure the skin is prepared and draped so that principles of surgical cleanliness are employed. A T-tube cholangiogram is performed to ensure that the calculus is still present and has not passed during the interval of 4–5 weeks (Fig. 1.41). If the stone is still present the T-tube is

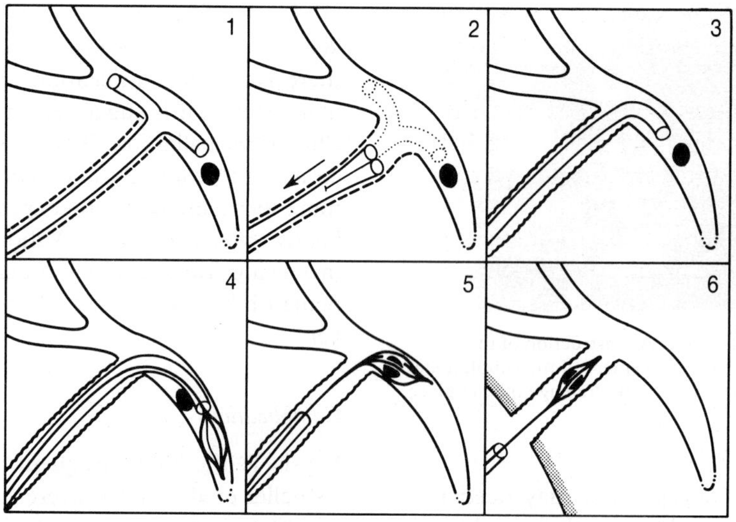


**Fig. 1.41** Transfistula common duct stone extraction. 1. Preliminary cholangiogram confirms presence of stone. 2. T-tube withdrawn. 3. Steerable catheter inserted. 4. Basket placed beyond stone. 5. Stone engaged in basket. 6. Stone, basket and steerable catheter withdrawn as a unit (Burhenne 1973).

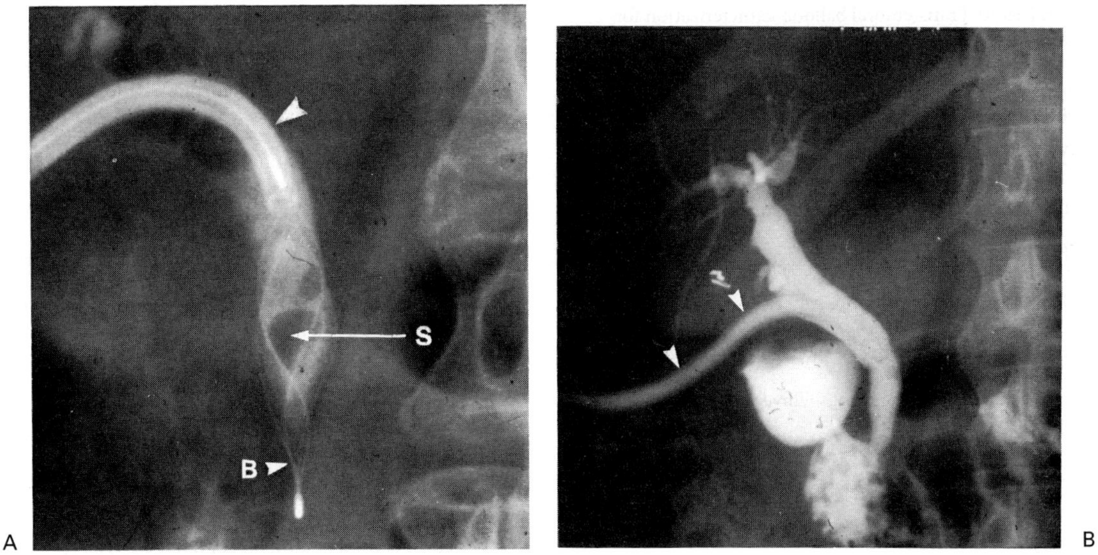


**Fig. 1.42** Percutaneous biliary stone extraction. **A** Steerable catheter (arrow); stone (S); basket (B). **B** Postextraction cholangiogram performed via the tract (arrows). No stone is seen in the common bile duct.

removed. A steerable catheter (Medi-Tech Inc.) is introduced down the tract to a position past the stone. A wire basket can then be introduced through the catheter, which is then gradually withdrawn several centimeters. This allows the basket to open next to the stone, which can often be entrapped by simple rotary or to-and-fro movements. Once the stone is engaged (Fig. 1.42), the basket is withdrawn a little and then the entire system is steadily pulled back through the tract in a single smooth movement. The wire basket and its contents are then examined to see if the stone or stone fragments are present. Fragmentation can occur within the duct or the tract and larger fragments in the duct may have to be removed separately. Smaller fragments will pass spontaneously through the ampulla. If multiple stones are present in the duct the technique is repeated until all calculi have been removed.

After the procedure, contrast is injected into the bile ducts to ensure the system is clear (Fig. 1.42). If air bubbles or blood clot are present, interpretation is difficult; a tube is then reinserted into the duct and the system is gently irrigated with saline prior to being clipped. On the following day, a cholangiogram is performed to define whether all the stones have been removed; if satisfactory, the drainage tube is withdrawn and a small dressing applied.

### *Results*

In Burhenne's review of 661 personal cases, extraction was successful in 95% (Burhenne 1980). Similar results were obtained by Garrow (1977) and Ferrucci & Mueller (1981). The British experience reported from multiple centers showed a success rate of 70% (Mason 1980). This lower success rate was due to the inclusion of centers with fewer than ten extractions, for success increased with operator experience. Burhenne (1980) has suggested that experience with 20 cases is necessary for the radiologist to become proficient.

### *Complications*

Cholangitis is the commonest complication and occurs in 1–2% of patients. The incidence of pancreatitis, false tracts and significant vasovagal reactions amounts to 3% (Burhenne 1976). There were no deaths in 661 patients (Burhenne 1980).

## REFERENCES

Akiyama H, Okazaki T, Takashima I et al 1990 Percutaneous treatment for biliary diseases. Radiology 176: 25–30
Alavi A, Ring E J 1981 Localization of gastrointestinal bleeding: superiority of 99m Tc sulfur colloid compared with angiography. American Journal of Roentgenology 137: 741–748
Alpern M B, Glazer G M, Francis I R 1988 Ischemic or infarcted bowel: CT findings. Radiology 166: 149–152
Aronberg D J, Stanley R J, Levitt R G, Sagel S S 1978 Evaluation of abdominal abscess with computed tomography. Journal of Computer Assisted Tomography 2: 384–387
Athanasoulis C A 1980 Percutaneous transluminal angioplasty: general principles. American Journal of Roentgenology 135: 893–900
Athanasoulis C A 1982 Upper gastrointestinal bleeding of arteriocapillary origin. In: Athanasoulis C A, Pfister R C, Greene R E, Robertson G H (eds) Interventional radiology. W B Saunders, Philadelphia, p 55
Baker S R 1990 The abdominal plain film. Appleton & Lange, East Norwalk
Baker S R 1993 The abdominal plain film. What will be its role in the future? Radiologic Clinics of North America 31: 1335–1344

Barth K H, Udoff E J 1980 Transfemoral balloon catheterization for hepatic wedge pressure measurements. Radiology 135: 779–780
Bartram C I, Preston D M, Lennard-Jones J E 1983 The "air enema" in acute colitis. Gastrointestinal Radiology 8: 61–65
Baum S 1982 Angiography and the gastrointestinal bleeder. Radiology 143: 569–572
Bean W J, Smith S L, Calonje M A 1974 Percutaneous removal of residual biliary tract stones. Problems encountered in a series of 44 cases. Radiology 113: 1–9
Berk R N 1970 The consecutive dose phenomenon in oral cholecystography. American Journal of Roentgenology, Radium Therapy and Nuclear Medicine 110: 230–234
Bernardino M E 1984 Percutaneous biopsy. American Journal of Roentgenology 142: 41–45
Bernardino M E 1990 Editorial: automated biopsy devices: significance and safety. Radiology 176: 615–616
Bernardino M E 1991 Editiorial: imaging of the liver and biliary tree. Radiologic Clinics of North America 29: 11
Bilbao M K, Frische L H, Dotter C T, Rosch J 1967 Hypotonic duodenography. Radiology 89: 438–443
Birch P D, Cook J V, Fletcher C J, Walsh M T 1989 Are multiple examinations of the gall-bladder helpful? Clinical Radiology 40: 262–263
Black E B, Ferrucci J T Jr 1978 New cholangiographic sign of common bile duct obstruction: initial opacification of intrahepatic ducts. American Journal of Roentgenology 130: 61–65
Bledin A G, Kantarjian H M, Kim E E et al 1982 99m Tc-labeled macroaggregated albumin in intrahepatic arterial chemotherapy. American Journal of Roentgenology 139: 711–715
Boley S J, Brandt L J, Veith F J 1978 Ischemic disorders of the intestines. Current Problems in Surgery 15: 1–85
Brakel K, Lameris J S, Nijs H G T, Terpstra O T 1991 The value of ultrasound in predicting non-visualization of the gall-bladder on OCG: implications for imaging strategies in patient selection for non-surgical therapy of gallstones. Clinical Radiology 43: 186–189
Bremner D N, McCormick J StC, Thomson J W W, McNair T J 1974 A study of cholecystectomy. Surgery, Gynecology and Obstetrics 138: 752–754
Brick S H, Caroline D F, Lev-Toaff A S, Friedman A C, Grumbach K, Radecki P D 1988 Esophageal disruption: evaluation with Iohexol esophagography. Radiology 169: 141–143
Brunton F J 1960 Retroperitoneal emphysema as a complication of barium enema. Clinical Radiology 11: 197
Buchwald H, Grage T B, Vassilopoulos P P, Rohde T D, Varco R L, Blackshear P J 1980 Intraarterial infusion chemotherapy for hepatic carcinoma using a totally implantable infusion pump. Cancer 45: 866–869
Burchell A R, Moreno A H, Panke W F, Rousselot L M 1965 Some limitations of splenic portography. I. Incidence, hemodynamics and surgical implications of the nonvisualized portal vein. Annals of Surgery 162: 981–995
Burhenne H J 1973 Nonoperative retained biliary stone extraction. A new roentgenologic technique. American Journal of Roentgenology 117: 388–399
Burhenne H J 1974 The technique of biliary duct stone extraction. Experience with 126 cases. Radiology 113: 567–572
Burhenne H J 1976 Complications of nonoperative extraction of retained common duct stones. American Journal of Surgery 131: 260–262
Burhenne H J 1980 Percutaneous extraction of retained biliary tract stones: 661 patients. American Journal of Roentgenology 134: 888–898
Callen P W 1979 Computed tomographic evaluation of abdominal and pelvic abscesses. Radiology 131: 171–175
Caroline D F 1987 Imaging of the oesophagus – update. Current Opinion in Gastroenterology 3: 812–819
Casarella W J, Kanter I E, Seaman W B 1972 Right-sided colonic diverticula as a cause of acute rectal hemorrhage. New England Journal of Medicine 286: 450–453
Chapman A M, McNamara M, Porter G 1992 The acute contrast enema in suspected large bowel obstruction: value and technique. Clinical Radiology 46: 273–278
Cho K J, Andrews J C, Williams D M, Doenz F, Guy G E 1989 Hepatic arterial chemotherapy: role of angiography. Radiology 173: 783–791
Clark R A, Gallant T E 1984 Acute mesenteric ischemia: angiographic spectrum. American Journal of Roentgenology 142: 555–562
Cohen A M, Greenfield A, Wood W C et al 1983 Treatment of hepatic metastases by transaxillary hepatic artery chemotherapy using an implanted drug pump. Cancer 51: 2013–2019
Connell T R, Stephens D H, Carlson H C, Brown M L 1980 Upper abdominal abscess: a continuing and deadly problem. American Journal of Roentgenology 134: 759–765
Coons H G, Carey P H 1983 Large-bore, long biliary endoprostheses (biliary stents) for improved drainage. Radiology 148: 89–94
Corr P, Beningfield S J, Davey N 1992 Transjugular liver biopsy: a review of 200 cases. Clinical Radiology 45: 238–239
Daly J, Fitzgerald T, Simpson C J 1987 Pre-operative intravenous cholangiography as an alternative to routine operative cholangiography in elective cholocystectomy. Clinical Radiology 38: 161–163
Davenport P M, Morgan A G, Darnborough A, deDombal F T 1985 Can preliminary screening of dyspeptic patients allow more effective use of investigational techniques? British Medical Journal 290: 217–220
Dawson P, Adam A, Benjamin I S 1993 Editorial: intravenous cholangiography revisited. Clinical Radiology 47: 223–225
Dawson S L, Mueller P R, Ferrucci J T Jr 1984 Mucomyst for abscesses: a clinical comment. Radiology 151: 342
Dawson S L, Lee M J, Mueller P R 1991 Metallic endoprosthesis in malignant biliary obstruction. Seminars in Interventional Radiology 8: 242
de Lacey G, Gajjar B, Twomey B, Levi J, Cox A G 1984 Should cholecystography or ultrasound be the primary investigation for gallbladder disease? Lancet 1: 205–207
Dixon P M, Roulston M E, Nolan D J 1993 The small bowel enema: a ten year review. Clinical Radiology 47: 46–48
Dodds W J, Goldberg H I 1978 Roentgen examination of the small bowel using intraluminal contrast media. American Journal of Digestive Diseases 23: 550–552
Dodds W J, Taylor A J, Stewart E T, Kern M K, Logemann J A, Cook I J 1989 Tipper and dipper types of oral swallows. American Journal of Roentgenology 153: 1197–1199
Dodds W J, Logeman J A, Stewart E T 1990 Radiological assessment of abnormal oral and pharyngeal phases of swallowing. American Journal of Roentgenology 154: 965–974
Dooley C P, Larson A W, Stace N H et al 1984 Double-contrast barium meal and upper gastrointestinal endoscopy. A comparative study. Annals of Internal Medicine 101: 538–545
Dooley C P, Weiner J M, Larson A W 1986 Endoscopy or radiography? – the patient's choice. Prospective comparative survey of patient acceptability of upper gastrointestinal endoscopy and radiography. American Journal of Medicine 80: 203–207
Doyle P J, Ward-McQuaid J N, Smith A M 1982 The value of routine peroperative cholangiography – a report of 4000 cholecystectomies. British Journal of Surgery 69: 617–619
Eastwood G L 1972 ECG abnormalities associated with the barium enema. Journal of the American Medical Association 219:719–721
Eckstein M R, Athanasoulis C A 1984 Gastrointestinal bleeding. An angiographic perspective. Surgical Clinics of North America 64: 37–51
Ekberg O, Weiber S 1991 The clinical importance of a thickwalled, tender gall-bladder without stones on ultrasonography. Clinical Radiology 44: 38–41
Evers K, Kressel H Y 1982 Principles of performance and interpretation of double-contrast gastrointestinal studies. Radiologic Clinics of North America 20: 667–685
Fagan E A, Allison D J, Chadwick V S, Hodgson H J F 1980 Treatment of haemobilia by selective arterial embolisation. Gut 21: 541–544
Feldman L, Greenfield A J, Waltman A C et al 1983 Transcatheter vessel occlusion: angiographic results versus clinical success. Radiology 147: 1–5
Ferrucci J T Jr 1993 Screening for colon cancer: controversies and recommendations. Radiologic Clinics of North America 31: 1189–1195
Ferrucci J T Jr, Mueller P R 1981 Post-operative instrumentation of the biliary tract. In: Ferrucci J T Jr, Wittenberg J (eds) Interventional radiology of the abdomen. Williams & Wilkins, Baltimore, p 11–43

Ferrucci J T Jr, Wittenberg J 1978 CT biopsy of abdominal tumors: aids for lesion localization. Radiology 129: 739–744
Ferrucci J T Jr, Wittenberg J, Sarno R A, Dreyfuss J R 1976 Fine needle transhepatic cholangiography: a new approach to obstructive jaundice. American Journal of Roentgenology 127: 403–407
Ferrucci J T Jr, Wittenberg J, Margolies M N, Carey R W 1979 Malignant seeding of the tract after thin-needle aspiration biopsy. Radiology 130: 345–346
Ferrucci J T Jr, Mueller P R, Harbin W P 1980a Percutaneous transhepatic biliary drainage. Technique, results, and applications. Radiology 135: 1–13
Ferrucci J T Jr, Wittenberg J, Mueller P R et al 1980b Diagnosis of abdominal malignancy by radiologic fine-needle aspiration biopsy. American Journal of Roentgenology 134: 323–330
Ferrucci J T Jr, Mueller P R, vanSonnenberg E, Harbin W P 1981 Percutaneous biliary drainage. In: Ferrucci J T Jr, Wittenberg J (eds) Interventional radiology of the abdomen. Williams & Wilkins, Baltimore, p 61–103
Fielding J F, Lumsden K 1973 Large-bowel perforations in patients undergoing sigmoidoscopy and barium enema. British Medical Journal 1: 471–473
Fleming M R, Carlson H C, Adson M A 1972 Percutaneous transhepatic cholangiography. The differential diagnosis of bile duct pathology. American Journal of Roentgenology, Radium Therapy and Nuclear Medicine 116: 327–336
Flickinger E G, Johnsrude I S, Ogburn N L, Weaver M D, Pories W J 1983 Local streptokinase infusion for superior mesenteric artery thromboembolism. American Journal of Roentgenology 140: 771–772
Foley W D, Stewart E T, Milbrath J R, SanDretto M, Milde M 1983 Digital subtraction angiography of the portal venous system. American Journal of Roentgenology 140: 497–499
Fork F-T 1983 Reliability of routine double contrast examination of the large bowel: a prospective study of 2590 patients. Gut 24: 672–677
Frager D, Medwid S W, Baer J W, Mollinelli B, Friedman M 1994 CT of small-bowel obstruction: value in establishing the diagnosis and determining the degree and cause. American Journal of Roentgenology 162: 37–41
Fraser G M, Earnshaw P M 1983 The double-contrast barium meal: a correlation with endoscopy. Clinical Radiology 34: 121–131
Freeny P C 1983 Angiography of hepatic neoplasms. Seminars in Roentgenology 18: 114–122
Fried A M, Poulos A, Hatfield D R 1981 The effectiveness of the incidental small-bowel series. Radiology 140: 45–46
Friedland G W 1978 Historical review of the changing concepts of lower esophageal anatomy: 430 BC–1977. American Journal of Roentgenology 131: 373–388
Gallacher D J, Kadir S, Kaufman S L et al 1985 Nonoperative management of benign postoperative biliary strictures. Radiology 156: 625–629
Gamble P, Colapinto R F, Stronell R D, Colman J C, Blendis L 1985 Transjugular liver biopsy: a review of 461 biopsies. Radiology 157: 589–593
Garrow D G 1977 The removal of retained biliary tract stones: report of 105 cases. British Journal of Radiology 50: 777–782
Gelfand D W 1978 High density, low viscosity barium for fine mucosal detail on double-contrast upper gastrointestinal examinations. American Journal of Roentgenology 130: 831–833
Gelfand D W, Ott D J 1979 Areae gastricae traversing the esophageal hiatus: a sign of hiatus hernia. Gastrointestinal Radiology 4: 127
Gelfand D W, Ott D J, Munitz H A, Chen Y M 1984 Radiology and endoscopy: a radiologic viewpoint. Annals of Internal Medicine 101: 550–551
Gelfand D W, Ott D J, Chen Y M 1987 Primary panendoscopy: a radiologist's response. American Journal of Roentgenology 149: 519–520
Gelfand D W, Wolfman N T, Ott D J, Watson N E Jr, Chen Y M, Dale W J 1988 Oral cholecystography vs gallbladder sonography: a prospective, blinded reappraisal. American Journal of Roentgenology 151: 69–72
Gerzof S G, Johnson W C 1984 Radiologic aspects of diagnosis and treatment of abdominal abscesses. Surgical Clinics of North America 64: 53–65
Gerzof S G, Robbins A H, Johnson W C, Birkett D H, Nabseth D C 1981 Percutaneous catheter drainage of abdominal abscesses. A five-year experience. New England Journal of Medicine 305: 653–657
Ginai A Z, ten Kate F J W, ten Berg R G M, Hoornstra K 1985 Experimental evaluation of various available contrast agents for use in the upper gastrointestinal tract in case of suspected leakage: effects on mediastinum. British Journal of Radiology 58: 585–592
Glick S N, Gohel V K, Laufer I 1984 Mucosal patterns of the duodenal bulb. Subject review. Radiology 150: 317–322
Goldstein H M, Zornoza J, Wallace S et al 1977 Percutaneous fine needle aspiration biopsy of pancreatic and other abdominal masses. Radiology 123: 319–322
Gomes A S, Lois J F, McCoy R D 1986 Angiographic treatment of gastro intestinal haemorrhage. Radiology 146: 1031–1037
Gore R M, Levine M S, Laufer I 1994 Textbook of gastrointestinal radiology (2 vols). W B Saunders, Philadelphia
Goyal R K 1976 The lower esophageal sphincter. Viewpoints on Digestive Diseases 8:
Grant E G, Richardson J D, Smirniotopoulos J G, Jacobs N M 1983 Fine-needle biopsy directed by real-time sonography: technique and accuracy. American Journal of Roentgenology 141: 29–32
Gundry S R, Strodel W E, Knol J A, Eckhauser F E, Thompson N W 1984 Efficacy of preoperative biliary tract decompression in patients with obstructive jaundice. Archives of Surgery 119: 703–708
Haaga J R, Alfidi R J 1976 Precise biopsy localization by computed tomography. Radiology 118: 603–607
Haaga J R, Weinstein A J 1980 CT-guided percutaneous aspiration and drainage of abscesses. American Journal of Roentgenology 135: 1187–1194
Hall R C, Sakiyalak P, Kim S K, Rogers L S, Webb W R 1973 Failure of operative cholangiography to prevent retained common duct stones. American Journal of Surgery 125: 51–63
Harbin W P, Mueller P R, Ferrucci J T Jr 1980 Transhepatic cholangiography: complications and use patterns of the fine-needle technique. A multi-institutional survey. Radiology 135: 15–22
Harned R K, Consigny P M, Cooper N B, Williams S M, Woltjen A J 1982 Barium enema examination following biopsy of the rectum or colon. Radiology 145: 11–16
Harnsberger H R, Dillon W P 1994 The use of imaging in the staging and follow-up of head and neck squamous cell carcinoma. Proceedings of XVIII International Congress of Radiology, Singapore, 581–594
Harrington D P, Boxt L M, Murray P D 1982 Digital subtraction angiography: overview of technical principles. American Journal of Roentgenology 139: 781–786
Hatfield A R W, Terblanche J, Fataar S et al 1982 Preoperative external biliary drainage in obstructive jaundice. A prospective controlled clinical trial. Lancet 2: 896–899
Hayward M W J, Hayward C, Ennis W P, Roberts C J 1984 A pilot evaluation of radiography of the acute abdomen. Clinical Radiology 35: 289–291
Heneghan M 1978 Contrast-induced acute renal failure. American Journal of Roentgenology 131: 1113–1115
Herlinger H 1992 Editorial: radiology in malabsorption. Clinical Radiology 45: 73–78
Herlinger H, Maglinte D D T 1989 Clinical radiology of the small intestine. W B Saunders, Philadelphia
Hessel S J, Adams D F, Abrams H L 1981 Complications of angiography. Radiology 138: 273–281
Hoare A M 1975 Comparative study between endoscopy and radiology in acute upper gastrointestinal haemorrhage. British Medical Journal 1: 27–30
Hoevels J, Lunderquist A, Ihse I 1978 Percutaneous transhepatic intubation of bile ducts for combined internal-external drainage in preoperative and palliative treatment of obstructive jaundice. Gastrointestinal Radiology 3: 23–31
Hoevels J, Lunderquist A, Owman T, Ihse I 1980 A large-bore Teflon endoprosthesis with side holes for nonoperative decompression of the biliary tract in malignant obstructive jaundice. Gastrointestinal Radiology 5: 361–366
Holdstock G, Bruce S 1981 Endoscopy and gastric cancer. Gut 22: 673–676

Holdstock G, Wiseman M, Loehry C A 1979 Open-access endoscopy service for general practitioners. British Medical Journal 1: 457–459

Holm H H, Pedersen J F, Kristensen J K, Rasmussen S N, Hancke S, Jensen F 1975 Ultrasonically guided percutaneous puncture. Radiologic Clinics of North America 13: 493–503

Hopkinson G B, Woodward D A K, Prasad N, Bullen B R 1983 Identification of accessory bile ducts at cholecystectomy. Annals of the Royal College of Surgeons of England 65: 323–324

Hunt J H, Anderson I F 1976 Double contrast upper gastrointestinal studies. Clinical Radiology 27: 87–97

Ingemansson S, Lunderquist A, Lundquist I, Lovdahl R, Tibblin S 1975 Portal and pancreatic vein catheterization with radioimmunologic determination of insulin. Surgery, Gynecology and Obstetrics 141: 705–711

Irving J D, Adam A, Dick R, Dondelinger R F, Lunderquist A, Roche A 1989 Gianturco expandable metallic biliary stents: results of a European clinical trial. Radiology 172: 321–326

Isler R J, Ferrucci J T Jr, Wittenberg J et al 1981 Tissue core biopsy of abdominal tumors with a 22 gauge cutting needle. American Journal of Roentgenology 136: 725–728

Janower M L 1986 Hypersensitivity reactions after barium studies of the upper and lower gastrointestinal tract. Radiology 161: 139–140

Jaques P F, Mandell V S, Delany D J, Nath P H 1982 Percutaneous transhepatic biliary drainage: advantages of the left-lobe subxiphoid approach. Radiology 145: 534–536

Johnson W C, Gerzof S G, Robbins A H, Nabseth D C 1981 Treatment of abdominal abscesses. Comparative evaluation of operative drainage versus percutaneous catheter drainage guided by computed tomography or ultrasound. Annals of Surgery 194: 510–519

Jones G 1992 Editorial: the radiological investigation of oropharyngeal dysphagia. Clinical Radiology 45: 295–297

Jones R 1985 Open access endoscopy. British Medical Journal 291: 424–426

Jones R S 1991 Intestinal obstruction. In: Sarbiston D C (ed) Textbook of surgery. W B Saunders, Philadelphia

Kadir S, Baassiri A, Barth K H, Kaufman S L, Cameron J L, White R I 1982 Percutaneous biliary drainage in the management of biliary sepsis. American Journal of Roentgenology 138: 25–29

Kaksos G S, Tompkins R K, Turnipseed W, Zollinger R M 1972 Operative cholangiography during routine cholecystectomy: a review of 3012 cases. Archives of Surgery 104: 484–488

Karlson K B, Martin E C, Fankuchen E I, Mattern R F, Schultz R W, Casarella W J 1982 Percutaneous drainage of pancreatic pseudocysts and abscesses. Radiology 142: 619–624

Kato T, Nemoto R, Mori H, Takahashi M, Tamakawa Y, Harada M 1981 Arterial chemoembolization with microencapsulated anticancer drug. An approach to selective cancer chemotherapy with sustained effects. Journal of the American Medical Association 245: 1123–1127

Kaufman S L, Chang R, Kadir S, Mitchell S E, White R I Jr 1984 Intraarterial digital subtraction angiography in diagnostic arteriography. Radiology 151: 323–327

Kelemouridis V, Athanasoulis C A, Waltman A C 1983 Gastric bleeding sites: an angiographic study. Radiology 149: 643–648

Kline T S, Neal H S 1978 Needle aspiration biopsy: a critical appraisal. Eight years and 3,267 specimens later. Journal of the American Medical Association 239: 36–39

Knochel J Q, Koehler P R, Lee T G, Welch D M 1980 Diagnosis of abdominal abscesses with computed tomography, ultrasound, and $^{111}$In leukocyte scans. Radiology 137: 425–432

Ko Y T, Lim J H, Lee D H, Lim H W 1993 Small bowel obstruction: sonographic evaluation. Radiology 188: 649–653

Koehler P R, Moss A A 1980 Diagnosis of intra-abdominal and pelvic abscesses by computerized tomography. Journal of the American Medical Association 244: 49–52

Koss L 1984 The thin needle aspiration: an important diagnostic tool. Einstein Quarterly Journal of Biology and Medicine 2: 73

Kreel L 1973 Radiology of the biliary system. Clinics in Gastroenterology 2: 185–212

Kressel H Y, Evers K A, Glick S N, Laufer I, Herlinger H 1982 The peroral pneumocolon examination. Technique and indications. Radiology 144: 414–416

Kutt E, Hall M J, Booth A, Virjee J 1988 Barium enemas are a headache. Clinical Radiology 39: 9–10

Lambiase R E, Deyoe L, Cronan J J, Dorfman G S 1992 Percutaneous drainage of 335 consecutive abscesses: results of primary drainage with 1-year follow-up. Radiology 184: 167–179

Lameris J S, Stoker J, Nijs H G T et al 1991 Malignant biliary obstruction: percutaneous use of self-expandable stents. Radiology 179: 703–707

Lammer J, Neumayer K 1986 Biliary drainage endoprostheses: experience with 201 placements. Radiology 159: 625–629

Lammer J, Klein G E, Kleinert R, Hausegger K, Einspieler R 1990 Obstructive jaundice: use of expandable metal endoprosthesis for biliary drainage. Work in progress. Radiology 177: 789–792

Lancet 1970 Editorial: routine operative cholangiography. Lancet 1: 1379–1380

Lancet 1980 Editorial: Sense and sensitivity about the barium meal. Lancet 1: 1171–1172

Lang E K 1979 Current and future applications of angiography in the abdomen. Radiological Clinics of North America 17: 55–76

Lappas J C, Maglinte D D T 1991 Imaging of the small bowel. Current Opinion in Radiology 3: 414–421

Laufer I 1976a Assessment of the accuracy of double contrast gastroduodenal radiology. Gastroenterology 71: 874–878

Laufer I 1976b The double-contrast enema: myths and misconceptions. Gastrointestinal Radiology 1: 19–31

Lebrec D, Goldfarb G, Degott C, Rueff B, Benhamou J-P 1982 Transvenous liver biopsy. Experience based on 1000 hepatic tissue samplings with this procedure. Gastroenterology 83: 338–340

Lee P W R 1976 The plain X-ray in the acute abdomen: a surgeon's evaluation. British Journal of Surgery 63: 763–766

Levine M S, Laufer I 1993 The upper gastro-intestinal series at the cross-roads. American Journal of Roentgenology 161: 1131–1137

Levine M S, Rubesin S E 1995 The *Helicobacter pylori* revolution: Radiologic perspective. Radiology 195: 593–596

Levine M S, Rubesin S E, Herlinger H, Laufer I 1988 Double-contrast upper gastrointestinal examination: technique and interpretation. Radiology 168: 593–602

Levine M S, Rubesin S E, Ott D J 1990 Update on esophageal radiology. American Journal of Roentgenology 155: 933–941

Lichtenstein J E 1993 Inflammatory conditions of the stomach and duodenum. Radiologic Clinics of North America 31: 1315–1333

Lipchik E O, Cohen E B, Mewissen M W 1991 Transvenous liver biopsy in critically ill patients: adequacy of tissue samples. Radiology 181: 497–499

Livraghi T, Damascelli B, Lombardi C, Spagnoli I 1983 Risk in fine-needle abdominal biopsy. Journal of Clinical Ultrasound 11: 77–81

Low V H S, Rubesin S E 1993 Contrast evaluation of the pharynx and oesophagus. Radiologic Clinics of North America 31: 1285–1291

Lumsden K, Truelove S C 1959 Intravenous pro-banthine in diagnostic radiology of the gastrointestinal tract with special reference to colonic disease. British Journal of Radiology 32: 517–526

Lunderquist A, Vang J 1974 Transhepatic catheterization and obliteration of the coronary vein in patients with portal hypertension and esophageal varices. New England Journal of Medicine 291: 646–649

Lunderquist A, Simert G, Tylen U, Vang J 1977 Follow-up of patients with portal hypertension and esophageal varices treated with percutaneous obliteration of gastric coronary vein. Radiology 122: 59–63

Lundquist A 1971 Fine-needle aspiration biopsy of the liver. Applications in clinical diagnosis and investigation. Acta Medica Scandinavica Supplementum 520: 1–28

Lygidakis N J 1982 Potential hazards in intraoperative cholangiography in patients with infected bile. Gut 23: 1015–1018

MacFarlane J R, Glenn F 1964 The disappearance of demonstrated gallstones. Archives of Surgery 88: 1003–1009

Mackintosh C E, Kreel L 1977 Anatomy and radiology of the areae gastricae. Gut 18: 855–864

McKusick K A, Froelich J, Callahan R J, Winzelberg G G, Strauss H W 1981 99m Tc red blood cells for detection of gastrointestinal bleeding: experience with 80 patients. American Journal of Roentgenology 137: 1113–1118

McLean G K, Burke D R 1989 Role of endoprosthesis in the

management of malignant biliary obstruction. Radiology 170: 961–967
McPherson A, Payne J E 1983 Importance of total colonoscopy in the diagnosis of colonic disorders. Medical Journal of Australia 1: 170–172
Maglinte D D T, Miller R E 1984 Upper gastrointestinal radiology under threat. American Journal of Roentgenology 142: 847–848
Maglinte D D T, Torres W E, Laufer I 1991 Oral cholecystography in contemporary gallstone imaging: a review. Radiology 178: 49–58
Mann J, Holdstock G, Harman M, Machin D, Loehry C A 1983 Scoring system to improve cost effectiveness of open access endoscopy. British Medical Journal 287: 937–940
Margulis A R, Eisenberg R L 1979 The examination of the colon. In: Lodge R, Steiner R E (eds) Recent advances in radiology and medical imaging, Vol 6. Churchill Livingstone, Edinburgh, p 79
Markisz J A, Front D, Royal H D, Sacks B, Parker J A, Kolodny G M 1982 An evaluation of 99m Tc labeled red blood cell scintigraphy for the detection and localization of gastrointestinal bleeding sites. Gastroenterology 83: 394–398
Markowitz R I, Meyer J S 1992 Pneumatic versus hydrostatic reduction of intussusception. Radiology 183: 623–624
Martin E C, Karlson K B, Fankuchen E I, Mattern R F, Casarella W J 1980 Percutaneous transhepatic dilatation of intrahepatic biliary strictures. American Journal of Roentgenology 135: 837–840
Martin E C, Karlson K B, Fankuchen E I, Cooperman A, Casarella W J 1982 Percutaneous drainage of postoperative intraabdominal abscesses. American Journal of Roentgenology 138: 13–15
Marton K I, Sox H C, Wasson J, Duisenberg C E 1980 The clinical value of the upper gastrointestinal tract roentgenogram series. Archives of Internal Medicine 140: 191–195
Mason R 1980 Percutaneous extraction of retained gallstones via the T-tube track – British experience of 131 cases. Clinical Radiology 31: 497–499
Mazzariello R 1973 Review of 220 cases of residual biliary tract calculi treated without reoperation : an eight-year study. Surgery 73: 299–306
Mead G H, Morris A, Webster G K, Langman M J S 1977 Uses of barium meal examination in dyspeptic patients under 50. British Medical Journal 1: 1460–1461
Meire H B 1984 Ultrasound in gastroenterology. Clinics in Gastroenterology 13: 183–203
Mendez G, Russell E, LePage J R, Guerra J J, Posniak R A, Trefler M 1984 Abandonment of endoprosthetic drainage technique in malignant biliary obstruction. American Journal of Roentgenology 143: 617–622
Mezwa D G, Feczko P J, Bosanko C 1993 Radiologic evaluation of constipation and ano-rectal disorders. Radiologic Clinics of North America 31: 1375–1393
Miller R E 1976 The clean colon. Gastroenterology 70: 289–290
Moskowitz H, Chait A, Margulies M, Mellins H Z 1968 Prone splenoportography. Radiology 90: 1132–1135
Mueller P R, Ferrucci J T Jr, vanSonnenberg E et al 1982a Obstruction of the left hepatic duct: diagnosis and treatment by selective fine-needle cholangiography and percutaneous biliary drainage. Radiology 145: 297–302
Mueller P R, vanSonnenberg E, Ferrucci J T Jr 1982b Percutaneous biliary drainage: technical and catheter-related problems in 200 procedures. American Journal of Roentgenology 138: 17–23
Mueller P R, vanSonnenberg E, Ferrucci J T Jr 1984 Percutaneous drainage of 250 abdominal abscesses and fluid collections. Part II: Current procedural concepts. Radiology 151: 343–347
Murray R R 1991 Management of haemobilia by embolotherapy. In: Kadir S (ed) Current practice of interventional radiology. Decker, Philadelphia
Nakayama T, Ikeda A, Okuda K 1978 Percutaneous transhepatic drainage of the biliary tract. Technique and results in 104 cases. Gastroenterology 74: 554–559
Nelson J A 1974 Effect of cholestyramine on telepaque oral cholecystography. American Journal of Roentgenology, Radium Therapy and Nuclear Medicine 122: 333–334
Norlander A, Kalin B, Sundblad R 1982 Effect of percutaneous transhepatic drainage upon liver function and postoperative mortality. Surgery, Gynecology and Obstetrics 155: 161–166
Novelline R A 1982 Pharmacoangiography. In: Athanasoulis C A, Pfister R C, Greene R E, Robertson G H (eds) Interventional Radiology. W B Saunders, Philadelphia
Nusbaum M, Baum S 1963 Radiographic demonstration of unknown sites of gastrointestinal bleeding. Surgical Forum 14: 374–375
Odurny A, Sniderman K W, Colapinto R F 1988 Intestinal angina: percutaneous transluminal angioplasty of the celiac and superior mesenteric arteries. Radiology 167: 59–62
Okuda K, Tanikawa K, Emura T et al 1974 Nonsurgical, percutaneous transhepatic cholangiography – diagnostic significance in medical problems of the liver. American Journal of Digestive Diseases 19: 21–36
Oleaga J A, Ring E J, Freiman D B, McLean G K, Rosen R J 1980 Extension of neoplasm along the tract of a transhepatic tube. American Journal of Roentgenology 135: 841–842
Oleaga J A, McLean G K, Freiman D B, Ring E J 1981 Interventional biliary radiology. In: Ring E J, McLean G K (eds) Interventional radiology, principles and techniques. Little, Brown, Boston, p 369
Op den Orth J O 1989 Use of barium in evaluation of disorders of the upper gastrointestinal tract: current status. Radiology 173: 601–608
Osborn A G, Friedland G W 1973 A radiological approach to the diagnosis of small bowel disease. Clinical Radiology 24: 281–301
Ott D J 1993 Role of the barium enema in colo-rectal carcinoma. Radiologic Clinics of North America 31: 1293–1313
Ott D J, Pikna L A 1993 Review. Clinical and videofluoroscopic evaluation of swallowing disorders. American Journal of Roentgenology 161: 507–513
Ott D J, Gelfand D W, Wu W C, Kerr R M 1980 Sensitivity of double-contrast barium enema: emphasis on polyp detection. American Journal of Roentgenology 135: 327–330
Ott D J, Gilliam J H 3rd, Zagoria R J, Young G P 1992 Interventional endoscopy of the biliary and pancreatic ducts: current indications and methods. American Journal of Roentgenology 158: 243–250
Papanicolaou N, Mueller P R, Ferrucci J T Jr et al 1984 Abscess–fistula association: radiologic recognition and percutaneous management. American Journal of Roentgenology 143: 811–815
Parks R E 1974 Double-blind study of four oral cholecystographic preparations. Radiology 112: 525–528
Patt Y Z, Wallace S, Freireich E J, Chuang V P, Hersh E M, Mavligit G M 1981 The palliative role of hepatic arterial infusion and arterial occlusion in colorectal carcinoma metastatic to the liver. Lancet 1: 349–350
Patt Y Z, Peters R E, Chuang V P, Wallace S, Mavligit G 1983 Effective retreatment of patients with colorectal cancer and liver metastases. American Journal of Medicine 75: 237–240
Pentecost M J 1994 Unresectable hepatic malignancy: regional infusion and embolisation. In: Cope C (ed) Current therapeutics in interventional radiology. Current Medicine, Philadelphia, Ch 6
Pereiras R V, Meiers W, Kunhardt B et al 1978 Fluoroscopically guided thin needle aspiration biopsy of the abdomen and retroperitoneum. American Journal of Roentgenology 131: 197–202
Perez C, Llauger J, Puig J, Plamer J 1989 Computed tomographic findings in bowel ischemia. Gastrointestinal Radiology 14: 241–245
Perlberger R R 1977 Control of hemobilia by angiographic embolization. American Journal of Roentgenology 128: 672–673
Perrillo R P, Zuckerman G R, Koehler R, Stanley R J 1978 Oral cholecystography in chronic renal insufficiency. American Journal of Digestive Diseases 23: 829–832
Pogany A C, Kerlan R K Jr, Ring E J 1985 Percutaneous biliary drainage. Clinics in Gastroenterology 14: 387–402
Probst P, Rysavy J A, Amplatz K 1978 Improved safety of splenoportography by plugging of the needle tract. American Journal of Roentgenology 131: 445–449
Pyhtinen J, Paivansalo M, Myllyla V, Niemela S 1982 Accuracy of single and double contrast barium meal studies. Annals of Clinical Research 14: 177–180
Rabe F E, Becker G J, Besozzi M J, Miller R E 1981 Efficacy study of the small-bowel examination. Radiology 140: 47–50
Rapoport S, Bookstein J J, Higgins C B, Carey P H, Sovak M, Lasser E C 1982 Experience with metrizamide in patients with previous severe anaphylactoid reactions to ionic contrast agents. Radiology 143: 321–325
Redman H C, Reuter S R 1969 Angiographic demonstration of portocaval and other decompressive liver shunts. Radiology 92:

788–792
Rees C R, Palmaz J C, Alvarado R, Tyrrel R, Ciaravino V, Register T 1989 DSA in acute gastrointestinal hemorrhage. Radiology 169: 499–503
Reiner R G, Lawson M J, Davies G T et al 1980 Fractionated dose cholecystography: a comparison between iopanoic acid and sodium ipodate. Clinical Radiology 31: 667–669
Ring E J, McLean G K (eds) 1981 Interventional radiology, principles and techniques. Little, Brown, Boston
Ring E J, Oleaga J A, Freiman D B, Husted J W, Lunderquist A 1978 Therapeutic applications of catheter cholangiography. Radiology 128: 333–338
Ring E J, Husted J W, Oleaga J A, Freiman D B 1979 A multihole catheter for maintaining longterm percutaneous antegrade biliary drainage. Radiology 132: 752–754
Roberts L, Wertman D A Jr, Mills S R, Moore A V, Heaston D K 1983 Transluminal angioplasty of the superior mesenteric artery: an alternative to surgical revascularization. American Journal of Roentgenology 141: 1039–1042
Robson N K, Lloyd M, Regan F 1993 The use of carbon dioxide as an insufflation agent in barium enema – does it have a role? British Journal of Radiology 66: 197–198
Roche A, Raisonnier A, Gillon-Savouret M-C 1982 Pancreatic venous sampling and arteriography in localizing insulinomas and gastrinomas: procedure and results in 55 cases. Radiology 145: 621–627
Roddie M E, Adam A 1994 Self expanding metal stents in the management of bile duct strictures. In: Cope C (ed) Current techniques in interventional radiology. Current Medicine, Philadelphia, Ch 5
Rosch J, Keller F S, Wawrukiewicz A S, Krippaehne W W, Dotter C T 1982 Pharmacoangiography in the diagnosis of recurrent massive lower gastrointestinal bleeding. Radiology 145: 615–619
Rossi P, Bezzi M, Salvatori F M, Maccioni F, Porcaro M L 1990 Recurrent benign biliary strictures: management with self-expanding metallic stents. Radiology 175: 661–665
Salomonowitz E, Castaneda-Zuniga W R, Lund G et al 1984 Balloon dilatation of benign biliary strictures. Radiology 151: 613–616
Salter R H 1977 X-ray negative dyspepsia. British Medical Journal 2: 235–236
Saltzstein E C, Evani S V, Mann R W 1973 Routine operative cholangiography. Archives of Surgery 107: 289–291
Sargent E N, Turner A F, Gordonson J, Schwinn C P, Pashky O 1974 Percutaneous pulmonary needle biopsy. Report of 350 patients. American Journal of Roentgenology 122: 758–768
Schatzki R, Gary J E 1953 Dysphagia due to a diaphragm-like localized narrowing in the lower esophagus ("lower esophageal ring"). American Journal of Roentgenology 70: 911–922
Schonfeld S M, Pinto R S, Schonfeld A R, Berenstein A, Manuell M, Kricheff I I 1984 Iopamidol and Conray 60: comparison in superselective angiography. Radiology 152: 809–811
Scott-Harden W G 1979 The stomach and duodenum. In: Lodge T, Steiner R E (eds) Recent advances in radiology and medical imaging, Vol 6. Churchill Livingstone, Edinburgh, p 65
Sellink J L 1976 Radiological atlas of common diseases of the small bowel. Stenfert Kroese, Leiden
Sexton C C, Zeman R K 1983 Pictorial essay – correlation of computed tomography, sonography, and gross anatomy of the liver. American Journal of Roentgenology 141: 711–718
Siebens A A, Linden P 1985 Dynamic imaging for swallowing reeducation. Gastrointestinal Radiology 10: 251–253
Sigel B, Machi J, Beitler J C et al 1983 Comparative accuracy of operative ultrasonography and cholangiography in detecting common bile duct calculi. Surgery 94: 715–720
Simeone J F, Novelline R A, Ferrucci J T Jr et al 1985 Comparison of sonography and plain films in evaluation of the acute abdomen. American Journal of Roentgenology 144: 49–52
Simpkins K C 1988 Editorial: what use is barium? Clinical Radiology 39: 469–473
Simpson A, Sandeman D, Nixon S J, Goulbourne I A, Grieve D C, McIntyre I M C 1985 The value of an erect abdominal radiograph in the diagnosis of intestinal obstruction. Clinical Radiology 36: 41–42
Smith E H 1985 Fine-needle aspiration biopsy: are there any risks? In: Holm H H, Kristensen J K (eds) Interventional ultrasound. Munksgaard, Copenhagen, p 169
Soo C-S, Wallace S, Chuang V P, Charnsangavej C, Bowers T A 1982 Injury to the intima of the hepatic artery. Results of follow-up in 11 cases. Radiology 143: 373–378
Staab E V, Jaques P F, Partain C L 1979 Percutaneous biopsy in the management of solid intra-abdominal masses of unknown etiology. Radiologic Clinics of North America 17: 435–459
Stevenson G W, Norman G, Frost R, Somers S 1991 Barium meal or endoscopy? A prospective randomized study of patient preference and physician decision making. Clinical Radiology 44: 317–321
Summerfield J A 1988 Biliary obstruction is best managed by endoscopists. Gut 29: 741–745
Tao L C, Pearson F G, Delarue N C, Langer B, Sanders D E 1980 Percutaneous fine-needle aspiration biopsy. 1. Its value to clinical practice. Cancer 45: 1480–1485
Teplick S K, Haskin P H, Matsumoto T, Wolferth C C, Pavlides C A, Gain T 1984 Interventional radiology of the biliary system and pancreas. Surgical Clinics of North America 64: 87–119
Thoeni R F 1989 Small bowel. Current Opinion in Radiology 1: 60–65
Thoeni R F, Menuck L 1977 Comparison of barium enema and colonoscopy in the detection of small colonic polyps. Radiology 124: 631–635
Thoeni R F, Vandeman F, Wall S D 1984 Effect of glucagon on the diagnostic accuracy of double-contrast barium enema examinations. American Journal of Roentgenology 142: 111–114
Thomas B M 1979 The instant enema in inflammatory disease of the colon. Clinical Radiology 30: 165–173
Torp-Pedersen S, Juul N, Vyberg M 1984 Histological sampling with a 23 gauge modified Menghini needle. British Journal of Radiology 57: 151–154
vanSonnenberg E, Hofmann A F 1988 Horizons in gall bladder therapy. American Journal of Roentgenology 150: 43–46
vanSonnenberg E, Wittenberg J, Mueller P R, Simeone J F, Ferrucci J T Jr 1981 Percutaneous abscess drainage. In: Ferrucci J T Jr, Wittenberg J (eds) Interventional radiology of the abdomen. Williams & Wilkins, Baltimore, p 159–191
vanSonnenberg E, Ferrucci J T Jr, Mueller P R, Wittenberg J, Simeone J F 1982 Percutaneous drainage of abscesses and fluid collections: technique, results, and applications. Radiology 142: 1–10
vanSonnenberg E, Mueller P R, Ferrucci J T Jr 1984 Percutaneous drainage of 250 abdominal abscesses and fluid collections. Part I: Results, failures, and complications. Radiology 151: 337–341
vanSonnenberg E, D'Agostino H B, Sanchez R B, Casola G 1992 Percutaneous abscess drainage: editorial comments. Radiology 184: 27–29
van Waes P F G M, Feldberg M A M, Mali W P T H M et al 1983 Management of loculated abscesses that are difficult to drain: a new approach. Radiology 147: 57–63
Velt P M, Choy O G, Shimkin P M, Link R J 1984 Transjugular biopsy in high-risk patients with hepatic disease. Radiology 153: 91–93
Viamonte M Jr, Warren W D, Fomon J J, Martinez L O 1970a Angiographic investigations in portal hypertension. Surgery, Gynecology and Obstetrics 130: 37–53
Viamonte M, Warren W D, Fomon J J 1970b Liver panangiography in the assessment of portal hypertension in liver cirrhosis. Radiologic Clinics of North America 8: 147–167
Waltman A C 1982 Catheter systems used in therapeutic angiography and methods of superselective vessel catheterization. In: Athanasoulis C A, Pfister R C, Greene R E, Robertson G H (eds) Interventional radiology. W B Saunders, Philadelphia, p 14
White R I 1984 Embolotherapy in vascular disease. American Journal of Roentgenology 142: 27–30
Williams C B, Hunt R H, Loose H, Riddell R H, Sakai Y, Swarbrick E T 1974 Colonoscopy in the management of colon polyps. British Journal of Surgery 61: 673–682
Wittenberg J, Mueller P R, vanSonnenberg E, Ferrucci J T Jr 1981 Percutaneous tumor biopsy. In: Ferrucci J T, Jr, Wittenberg J (eds) Interventional radiology of the abdomen. Williams & Wilkins, Baltimore, p 115
Wolf B S 1967 Roentgenology of the esophagogastric junction. In:

Margulis A R, Burhenne H J (eds) Alimentary tract roentgenology. C V Mosby, St Louis, p 371
Wolf B S 1970 The inferior esophageal sphincter – anatomic, roentgenologic and manometric correlation, contradictions, and terminology. American Journal of Roentgenology 110: 260–277
Ziessman H A, Thrall J H, Yang P J et al 1984 Hepatic arterial perfusion scintigraphy with Tc-99m-MAA. Use of a totally implanted drug delivery system. Radiology 152: 167–172
Zins M, Vilgrain V, Gayno S et al 1992 US – guided percutaneous liver biopsy with plugging of the needle tracts: a prospective study in 72 high-risk patients. Radiology 184: 841–843
Zornoza J, Jonsson K, Wallace S, Lukeman J M 1977 Fine needle aspiration biopsy of retroperitoneal lymph nodes and abdominal masses: an updated report. Radiology 125: 87–88

# 2. Transaxial imaging

*G. J. Reece G. T. Davies*

ULTRASONOGRAPHY (Rumack et al 1991)

At the request of the French Navy, Paul Langevin developed an acoustic method for the detection of submarines (Wade et al 1984). He utilized a high-intensity ultrasound beam and pulse-echo technique generated by a piezo-electric transducer, which became popularly known as sonar (sound navigation and ranging). The ultrasound scanners currently used to display abdominal organs utilize the pulse-echo technique to produce echoes and record the intensity of these echoes from different abdominal organs and structures. Major improvements in modern apparatus include the facility to focus and direct an ultrasonic beam using specially designed transducers and the use of sophisticated electronic equipment to time the echoes to a corresponding point on an oscilloscope tube for processing and recording.

Further refinements in electronic focusing allow optimal examination of superficial and deep portions of solid organs such as the liver. The addition of computer technology to scanning apparatus allows storage of enhanced images for editing, copying and reviewing.

Many modern ultrasound scanning systems have duplex Doppler or color Doppler capability, permitting the detection of blood vessels and prograde and retrograde flow patterns in these, the site and sometimes the nature of vascular occlusions and the detection of abnormal vascular channels (Scoutt et al 1990, Taylor & Holland 1990).

A number of substances have been designed as contrast agents for ultrasound scanning. These include free or encapsulated gas bubbles, colloidal suspensions, lipid emulsions and aqueous solutions. These agents are introduced into the vascular system (usually intravenously) to enhance differences between normal or abnormal tissue or to modify a Doppler signal. Alternatively, such agents can be introduced into the lumen of a hollow organ to outline a cavity, define the boundaries better, confirm a persistent stricture or identify a fistula (Ophir & Parker 1989).

Rapid development of rotating ultrasound transducers fitted into fiberoptic endoscopes has allowed good definition of masses in the alimentary tract and adjacent structures. Benign and malignant tumors can be identified, localized and characterized. *Endoscopic ultrasonography* (p. 125) is especially sensitive in the detection of pancreatic neoplasms and patterns of spread (Boyce & Sivak 1990).

**Physical aspects** (Wells 1982)

The spectrum of mechanical vibration contains different frequency bands, including audible sound and ultrasound. The unit of frequency of sound waves is the hertz (Hz) or one cycle per second. Audible sound lies in the range 20–20 000 Hz and ultrasound waves used for diagnostic imaging purposes lie in the 1–10 megahertz (MHz) range. Like audible sound, ultrasound travels through a medium at a definitive speed in a longitudinal waveform. These longitudinal waves interact with structures in a biological medium, especially the soft tissues. The speed ($c$) at which a wave passes through a medium depends on the elasticity ($K$) and the density ($\rho$) of the medium (expressed in the equation $c \sqrt{K/\rho}$. In common with other energy forms, the resoluton of an ultrasound signal is dependent on the wavelength ($\lambda$), which is itself related to the frequency ($f$) and the speed ($c$) of the wave (expressed in the equation $c = f\lambda$). The speed ($c$) is measured in meters per second (m/s) and for soft tissues the speed is about 1540 m/s at a frequency of 1 MHz.

These equations suggest that better resolution of ultrasound images should be anticipated at higher frequencies. However, the attenuation of ultrasound by tissue interaction increases directly with the frequency employed, thus limiting satisfactory demonstration of deeper structures. In practice a compromise is reached between the highest frequency for optimal resolution and that which allows adequate penetration for the deepest structures. Large patients are studied in the 2–3 MHz range and other patients in the 3–5 MHz range.

At the diagnostic frequencies utilized, ultrasound waves are produced and detected by piezo-electric effects. Piezo-electric materials such as quartz crystals provide a coupling between electrical and mechanical energy and are called transducers. When an electrical potential is applied to these materials, changes in the crystal lattice produce a mechanical effect and, conversely, when the crystals are deformed mechanically an electrical field is created. Synthetic materials such as ceramic, lead, zirconate and titanate are used for convenience. A single short pulse of electricity briefly deforms the ceramic transducer, thus setting up a series of mechanical vibrations with alternate compression and rarefaction waves which transmit through the adjacent medium. The return reverberations are received by a transducer and are then amplified, processed and displayed. The circuitry is so designed that whilst up to 1000 pulses or more of ultrasound (each lasting 1 $\mu$s) can be released in 1 second, 99.9% of this second can be utilized for reception of the reflected acoustic signals. Since modern ultrasound apparatus is passively receiving for 99.9% of its operational time the energy transmitted to the tissues is very low, being of the order of a few milliwatts per square centimeter. These levels of intensity are well below those which produce significant effects on mammalian tissues (Nyborg 1982).

As with other forms of energy an ultrasound beam reduces in intensity during transmission through a medium by a process of attenuation. The phenomena occurring during attenuation in biological tissues are incompletely understood and for simplification an assumption is made that the scattering and absorbing properties of tissue are uniform. The attenuation is in part due to a change in direction of the waveform, by divergence, scattering or reflection of the beam, and in part by energy loss in the form of heat production, which is absorbed by the adjacent tissues.

Pulses of ultrasound travel through a medium at a speed ($c$) characteristic of the density ($\rho$) of that medium and this is referred to as the acoustic impedance ($Z$) of the particular medium (expressed in the equation $Z = \rho c$). When the ultrasound beam traverses a substance of varying acoustic impedance there is either a reflection or refraction of the beam at each interface and the echo produced returns through the medium, where it may be detected by the transducer and processed appropriately. The timing and size of these echoes can be expressed in terms of the amplitude of deflection from a baseline and early ultrasound scanners produced this type of "A" mode or amplitude-modulated scan. However, in imaging abdominal structures it is more useful to display the echo as a function of the brightness of the echo – "B" mode or brightness-modulated scan. Using the latter, a single echo is recorded as a single bright spot and with movement on the transducer a whole series of bright spots is obtained, giving a two-dimensional image corresponding to the structures traversed by the ultrasound beam. The signals recorded are then stored on an oscilloscope for analysis and display.

Initially the images produced for display were recorded in black and white and were limited to demonstrations of organ boundaries. However, it became clear that the echo amplitude within organ boundaries contained the most useful diagnostic information and a gray-scale display system was developed. Gray-scale ultrasound imaging has better spatial resolution owing partly to focused and collimated transducers and partly to a better signal-to-noise ratio consequent upon improved technology. As a result, the low-level echoes originating in soft tissues can be amplified to show differences in consistency between normal and abnormal soft tissues.

*Real-time scanners*

The mechanical sector scanners which produced static images have been almost completely replaced by real-time scanners which utilize phased array equipment with no moving parts.

The capability of a computed system to allow observation while a process is being measured or controlled is referred to as 'real-time'. The ultrasound scanners mainly in use now allow rapid production of two-dimensional images so that the motion of an organ can be recorded. The operator has the additional advantage of being able to manipulate the image during observation, unlike the static machines where observation of static events has to be intermittent to allow recording to take place. Ultrasound scans obtained by real-time methods are still two-dimensional "B" mode images, modulated for brightness and hence possessing gray-scale characteristics. The increased speed of data collection and improvements in transducer design produce sequences of images fast enough to follow changes in spatial relationships within the plane of the scan over a period of time. These changes may be due to physiological movements, to movements of the transducer bringing different structures into the scan plane or to combinations of both.

There are many other advantages of real-time systems. The rigid articulated arm used in static systems is absent so the operator is free to carry out scanning movements with the transducer and to display the anatomy to best advantage by continual adjustments to the angles and planes of the scanning sweeps. The technique allows precise measurements with electronic calipers, e.g. the width of the common bile duct. The system has speed, portability and relative economy. Several authors have postulated that pocket-sized real-time scanners will become available for use by physicians at the bedside and in the consulting room (Wells 1982, Margulis 1985). Indeed, even with the current apparatus most experienced ultrasonographers make the diagnosis largely at the time of the scanning procedure, taking appropriate photographic records of the image for archival purposes.

The principal disadvantage of real-time scanners is the relatively small field of view. With such complex technology some unavoidable artefacts will be generated. Some of these are related to assumptions made about the physical uniformity of ultrasound waves and some originate directly in the apparatus. In addition, operator errors can introduce artefactual signals and these are usually due to inexperience. The bodily habitus of the patient, particularly obesity and the inability to co-operate in breath holding, may degrade the image. Additionally, gas, whether in distended bowel or in potential spaces, will totally reflect the ultrasound signal, as will bone. Surgical clips, dressings and open wounds can all prevent the correct application of the transducer to the skin surface.

It is generally accepted that the hand-held real-time system is the most suitable for abdominal ultrasound.

The Doppler effect registers a change in frequency of received echoes due to movement relative to an object, whether towards or away from the object. The most well-known everyday experience of this effect is that of hearing the change in pitch of a railway engine hooter moving towards or away from an observer. In pulsed Doppler equipment, a single transducer is utilized for transmission and reception of the signal and assessed against a time base. In Doppler scanning, the pulsed ultrasound source is kept stationary whilst the receiving, mobile object (usually flow in a blood vessel) modifies the transmitted signal either in a positive or a negative manner. The modified signal is then returned as a Doppler pulse of energy. This can be displayed and analyzed within the apparatus to provide graphical or pictorial display of the underlying moving object. The color coding (red/blue) of positive or negative signals within the instrumentation allows the visual display of the flow pattern and by appropriate manipulation of the equipment and data, flow velocities can be shown and estimated.

### **Procedure** (Taylor 1985)

As with any imaging procedure an abdominal ultrasound scan must be carried out systematically. The application of a transducer probe to the abdominal skin surface requires that the operator, whether ultrasound technician or radiologist, has an accurate knowledge of the underlying three-dimensional anatomy in each section examined. This knowledge is paramount in real-time scanning because the lack of a rigid arm system to define the scanning plane may result in an unsystematic scanning pattern. To meet these requirements the ultrasonographer should have received a thorough and sophisticated training in both the technical and anatomical aspects of ultrasound scanning.

The technique employed should be tailored to the particular clinical indications and examinations are usually organ directed. However, with a systematic approach to the abdominal scan it is usual to perform scans in various defined portions of the abdomen: for example, the right upper quadrant, to include the gallbladder and biliary tree; the left upper quadrant, to include the pancreas; the renal areas; and if indicated, a general examination of the abdominal and pelvic cavities.

### **Gallbladder** (Cohen & Kurtz 1991)

In most centers, ultrasound has replaced oral cholecystography as the procedure of choice in the diagnosis of gallstones, with a sensitivity and specificity as high as cholecystography but with a lower frequency of indeterminate examinations. Ultrasound has also made a most important contribution in the differential diagnosis of jaundice and many authors quote an accuracy of 85–100% in detection of dilated bile ducts (Dewbury et al 1979). Additionally the level of obstruction may be identified in about 50% of patients and in some the cause of the obstruction can be recognized. Dilatation of the biliary tree, even in the absence of clinical jaundice, may give important and accurate anatomical and prognostic information, thus contributing to the speed of diagnosis and comfortable management of the patient.

Developments in the non-surgical treatment of gallstones with extracorporeal shockwave lithotripsy (ESWL) and contact dissolution with methyl-tert-butyl-ether (MTBE) have placed new demands on imaging resources in the diagnosis of gallstones (Simeone et al 1989).

#### *Procedure*

No special preparation is needed, but previous barium examination should be avoided and morning examination of the fasting patient minimizes the amount of intestinal gas and ensures a full gallbladder. Multiple longitudinal and transverse scans of the upper abdomen are made to identify the long axis of the gallbladder. Oblique scans are then made along this axis to show the size of the lumen and to identify any echo-producing structures therein. Sections at small intervals are required to detect the smallest calculi, but if these are less than 2 mm in diameter they are too small to be detected unless they are multiple and aggregate to create echoes. The examination is generally performed in the supine and oblique positions, but sitting and standing may be required. Scanning in different positions will confirm mobile filling defects such as gallstones, which will change position accordingly, whereas fixed filling defects such as polyps or folds will not change position. For the best demonstration of minor echo abnormalities it is important for the patient to be able to hold his or her breath, particularly a deep inspiration. Real-time scanning is particularly helpful in the ease and rapidity of examination, especially in the elderly, the very young and the very sick.

#### *Findings*

***Gallstones.*** The classic appearance of gallstones is a

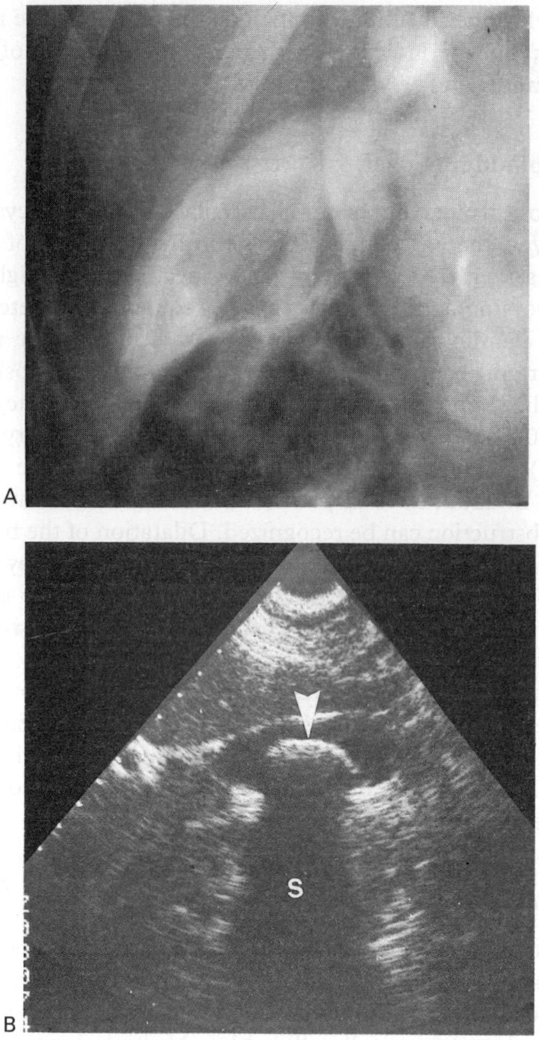


**Fig. 2.1** Cholelithiasis. **A** Cholecystogram showing single stone in the gallbladder; **B** ultrasound of gallbladder in the same patient. Stone (arrow) with acoustic shadow (S).

strong echo-producing area within the gallbladder lumen arising from the interface between bile and the calculus and with an acoustic shadow (echo-free zone) beyond the calculus (Fig. 2.1). The shadow is due to high acoustic reflectivity of the surface of the calculus and its absorption of any remaining ultrasound. The production of a shadow does not depend upon the composition of a stone; any stone will create a shadow if it intersects the majority of the ultrasound beam (Taylor et al 1979). Aggregates of small stones will also form a shadow, though very small individual calculi may not do so. However, the confident diagnosis of a gallstone rests on the demonstration of both echo and shadow together.

***Abnormalities of bile.*** Echogenic bile produces an echo without a shadow. This occurs with bile stasis due, for example, to parenteral feeding. In some patients, "sludge" balls (Fig. 2.2) can be detected in the gallbladder, which may give echoes without shadows. Their nature has not yet been established but they may occur in association with biliary stasis and possibly with lithogenic bile (Filly et al 1980). Occasionally hemorrhage or blood clot in the bile will yield echogenic reflections in the gallbladder and following enterobiliary anastomosis, dense echoes due to gas may be seen in the biliary tree. These are also seen with gas-forming infections in the biliary tract. None of these echogenic abnormalities is associated with significant acoustic shadowing. The selection criteria for ESWL have been strictly defined as the presence of up to three gallstones, none of which exceeds 3 cm in diameter, and they should contain no calcium and the gallbladder should function on oral cholecystography. With such criteria, up to 85% of patients with calculi are excluded from such treatment programs (Ferrucci 1989).

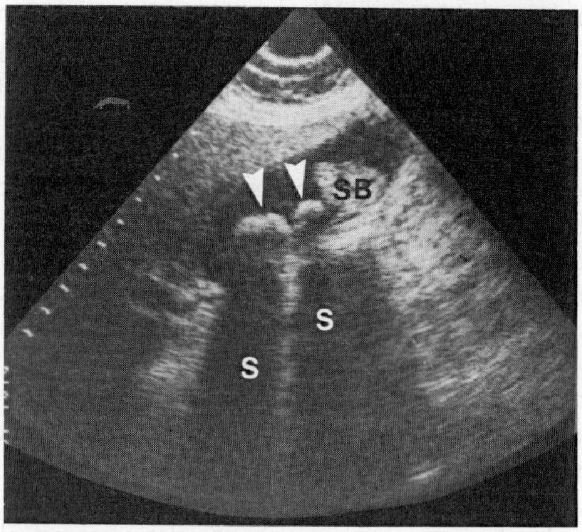


**Fig. 2.2** Stones (arrows) with acoustic shadow (S) and sludge balls (SB), which have no acoustic shadow.

***Acute cholecystitis.*** In the presence of a typical clinical history, tenderness over the gallbladder (ultrasonic "Murphy's sign") on application of the transducer and a thickened gallbladder wall, with or without the presence of gallstones, should suggest the diagnosis of acute cholecystitis. In a series of 427 patients Ralls et al (1982) evaluated the ultrasonic "Murphy's sign". The sensitivity of the sign for the diagnosis of acute cholecystitis was 63%, with a specificity of 93.6%. The authors concluded that whilst relatively insensitive, the sign was a helpful indicator of acute cholecystitis. Other signs indicative of acute cholecystitis include the finding of a gallstone impacted in the cystic duct, fine echoes throughout the lumen due to pus in gallbladder empyema and an adjacent fluid-filled space due to spread of infection from the gallbladder into surrounding tissues creating a pericholecystic abscess. Acutely ill patients with cholecystitis often undergo emergency ultrasound scans and a diagnosis of acalculous cholecystitis is made. In 31 patients with this diagnosis, subsequent examinations showed the presence of gallstones in 21 (Ekberg & Weiber

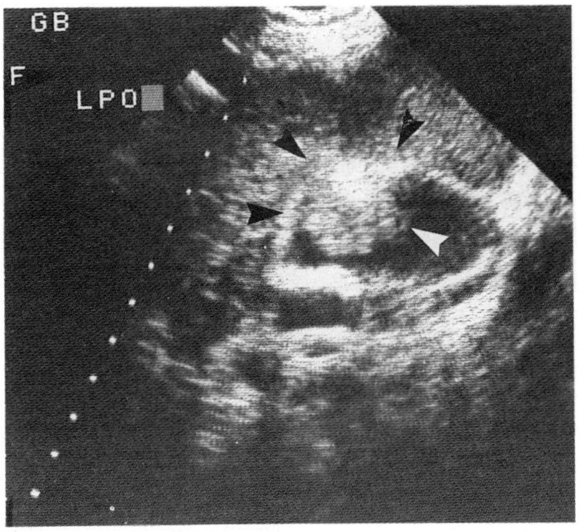


**Fig. 2.3** Carcinoma of the gallbladder. Large focal echogenic filling defect (white arrow) without shadowing and attached to the wall of the gallbladder (black arrows).

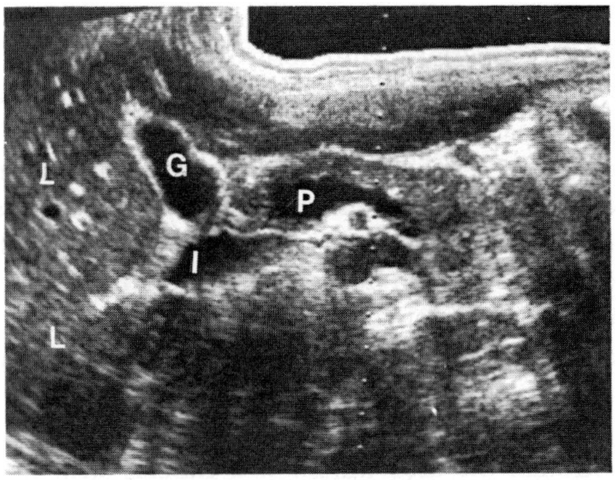


**Fig. 2.4** Section through porta hepatis showing gallbladder (G), portal vein (P), part of right lobe of liver (L) and inferior vena cava (I).

1991). A further five patients were thought to have gallbladder wall thickening secondary to pancreatitis, appendicitis, hepatitis or peptic ulcer. Consequently, a meticulous search for gallstones should be carried out in all patients with ultrasound signs of acute cholecystitis. Localized inflammatory peritoneal fluid collections may also be seen (Kane 1980). When the gallbladder is not demonstrated at ultrasound in the fasting patient, either the gallbladder is absent congenitally (incidence 0.03%) or it is grossly contracted and fibrosed due to cholecystitis. Such gallbladders almost always contain calculi and, instead of the demonstration of a lumen, a highly reflective area is found in the gallbladder fossa with distal acoustic shadows.

***Other abnormalities.*** Other abnormalities may be detected in the gallbladder. Benign tumors (p. 1211) create echoes without acoustic shadows and do not move in relation to gravity. The sinuses of adenomyomatosis (p. 1211) may be visualized as small, fluid-filled spaces in the gallbladder wall. High amplitude periluminal echoes have been described as a constant and prominent feature in adenomyomatosis of the gallbladder (Fowler & Reid 1988). Carcinoma of the gallbladder may be identified as diffuse or focal thickening of the gallbladder wall (Fig. 2.3). More frequently it is seen at an advanced stage as a large mass with low-level echoes in the right upper quadrant, often causing distortion or dilatation of the biliary tree due to direct invasion of the liver (Olken et al 1978).

### **Biliary tree and hepatic blood vessels** (Cohen & Kurtz 1991)

*Anatomy* (Fig. 2.4) (*see also* pp 1195 and 714)

The intrahepatic bile ducts traverse the liver in the portal triads with the intrahepatic arteries and the portal veins. In the porta hepatis the right and left hepatic ducts unite to form the common hepatic duct, which is extrahepatic in position. Normally the intrahepatic ducts are too small to identify but it should be possible to identify the common hepatic duct anterior to the right portal vein in longitudinal scans through the porta hepatis. The right hepatic artery is usually posterior to the common hepatic duct in this plane. Descending through the anterior aspect of the foramen of Winslow (gastrohepatic ligament) the common hepatic duct lies anterior to the main portal vein and lateral to the main hepatic artery. The site of entry of the cystic duct is variable and difficult to define so the exact point at which the common hepatic duct changes to the common bile duct is uncertain, but the convention is that the common bile duct commences at its entry to the head of the pancreas. The common bile duct enters the pancreatic head on the posterolateral aspect, where it lies anterior to the inferior vena cava and posterior to the first part of the duodenum. It terminates at the ampulla of Vater on the medial aspect of the second part of the duodenum.

It is possible to confuse hepatic and portal venous radicles with the biliary tree. However, the three main hepatic veins, namely the right, central and left, pass superiorly through the liver, increasing in width before joining the superior vena cava. The walls of the thinner hepatic veins do not cause the bright echogenic signals which are created by the walls of either biliary ducts or portal veins. The differentiation between portal veins and bile ducts can be more difficult because they show similar orientation and wall signals. This is especially true of the left branch of the portal vein and a thorough knowledge of the normal anatomy and its common variations is required (Marks et al 1979).

The main portal vein is formed by the junction of splenic and superior mesenteric veins posterior to the neck of the pancreas. It runs obliquely to the right and superiorly to the bifurcation in the porta hepatis. The right branch runs a reasonably straight course from the main portal vein through the right lobe of the liver, eventually dividing into anterior and posterior segmental branches. The left branch runs superiorly, anteriorly and to the left from the bifurcation and this in turn divides to give right and left branches to each segment of the left lobe of the liver.

In assessing the biliary ducts the search should begin with the identification of the common hepatic duct, which is recognizable in most patients. It is found most quickly by locating the right portal vein by tracing this from the main portal vein in a longitudinal scan under the costal margin. The right side up or modified Kazam position is particularly helpful for it will often displace overlying bowel and allow better visualization (Behan & Kazam 1978). Sequential scans through the area will show a tubular structure, the common hepatic artery crossing anteriorly, and by altering the obliquity of scan longitudinal sections can then be obtained. Continuation of the scanning in longitudinal and transverse planes should enable the distal portions of the common bile duct to be displayed in about 50% of normal patients (Dewbury 1980), though gas in the duodenum and adjacent hepatic flexure may obscure the whole length of the common bile duct. The duct system is seen by virtue of bright echoes originating in the walls of the bile duct which surround the non-echogenic bile in the lumen.

With the advent of duplex and color Doppler imaging, it is now a relatively straightforward process to distinguish vascular structures from bile ducts in the liver. The recognition of the numerous anatomical variations and intrahepatic bile duct dilatation is thus more readily achieved (Ralls 1990).

*Findings*

***Obstructive jaundice*** (p. 1197). In the jaundiced patient the main use of ultrasound is to identify dilated bile ducts. In severe, long-standing obstructive jaundice, the bile ducts are easily demonstrable by the finding of tortuous, dilated, branching, tubular structures, often referred to as "too many tubes". Laing et al (1978) described five signs in obstructive jaundice with dilated intrahepatic bile ducts: an alteration in the normal anatomy of the porta hepatis, irregular walls of the dilated bile ducts, stellate confluence of the dilated bile ducts, acoustic enhancement behind the dilated bile ducts and the peripheral extension of the dilated bile ducts into the liver substance. When obstruction is less severe, the signs may be less easily recognized and only the main ducts may show changes. In this situation the changes are best seen in the left lobe. The "double-barrelled shotgun" sign described by Weill et al (1978) is the occurrence of two adjacent and parallel structures due to portal vein and bile duct instead of one due to the portal vein alone. The bile ducts lie ventral to the portal vein and its branches. The finding should lead to a search for other evidence of dilated bile ducts.

In early biliary obstruction, there may be extrahepatic bile duct dilatation (Fig. 2.5) without intrahepatic dilatation. Such dilatation may occur before clinical or even laboratory evidence of jaundice (Weinstein & Weinstein 1980, Zeman et al 1980, 1981). There has been considerable controversy in the literature regarding the upper limit of normal for the width of the common bile duct on ultrasound, but there is general acceptance of the opinion of Sample et al (1978) that 6 mm should be considered as the upper limit. In a series of 100 normal patients the largest internal diameter of the common hepatic duct anterior to the portal vein was 4 mm (Cooperberg 1978). Niederau et al (1983) surveyed the size of the common bile duct in 830 healthy blood donors. None had a duct width greater than 7 mm and it was less than 4 mm in 95%. There was a tendency to a slight but significant increase in width as weight and age increased. It has been suggested that 10 mm should be considered as the upper normal value for width of the bile duct in elderly patients (Wu et al 1984).

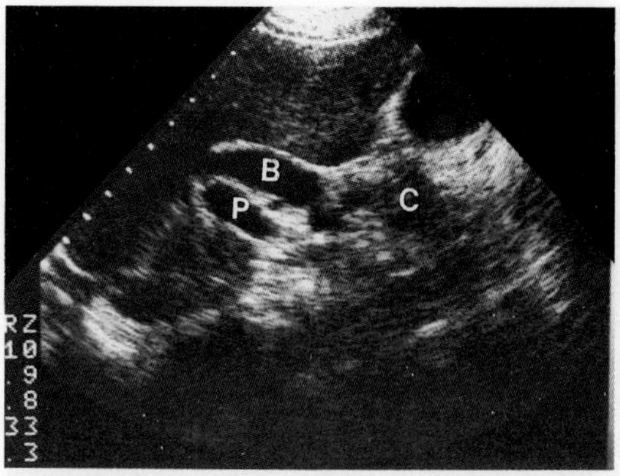


**Fig. 2.5** Carcinoma of the pancreas (C) with dilated common bile duct (B). The portal vein (P) is posterior to the bile duct.

There is conflicting evidence regarding the occurrence of a dilated common duct after cholecystectomy. Graham et al (1980) followed up 67 asymptomatic patients for 16 months after cholecystectomy for gallstones. In 84% of the patients, the width of the common hepatic duct was 4 mm or less and it was concluded that the common hepatic duct is generally not dilated after cholecystectomy. Graham et al (1981) examined 36 symptomatic patients after cholecystectomy who had a common hepatic duct larger than 4 mm and in 64% of these an obstructing cause was found at surgery. In both these series there were patients in whom a dilated common hepatic and/or common bile ducts were shown but no obstructing cause was demonstrated. However, endoscopic retrograde cholangiopancreatography (ERCP) was not used to investigate such cases. Niederau et al (1983) examined 55 patients by ultrasound after cholecystectomy; 58% of these patients had ducts larger than the normal 4 mm, compared to 18% of patients with gallstones in whom operation had not been performed. The authors concluded that the dilatation was not due to previous or persisting obstruction but rather that the common bile duct acted as a reservoir in the postoperative situation. They further believed that after cholecystectomy the finding of a duct size above normal limits requires no further investigation unless there is clinical or laboratory evidence of obstruction. Conversely stones may be found postoperatively in a normal sized common bile duct and therefore in all patients in whom there is good clinical or biochemical evidence of obstruction, ERCP should be performed.

Whilst ultrasound scanning is very accurate in the demonstration of dilated bile ducts, the localization of the level of obstruction and its cause is possible in about 75% of patients. It is usually easy to distinguish a high from a low obstruction but bowel gas frequently obscures the lower common bile duct and so duct stones and pancreatic tumors may be missed. Calculi in the duct may be clearly seen as echo-producing structures and acoustic shadowing in 70–85% of patients (Laing et al 1984, Dong & Chen 1987). The demonstration of calculi in the ducts does not exclude other causes of obstruction. The calculi may be coincidental and when stones are seen in dilated ducts the obstruction may be more distal than the visualized calculi. Other filling defects seen in the bile ducts may cause echoes. For instance, the worms of ascaris infection, which may be revealed as linear, non-shadowing structures, and gas in the bile ducts produce shadows of high echogenicity with relatively little shadowing.

***Other disorders.*** The association of bile duct dilatation on ultrasound with pancreatic and hepatic disorders will be discussed in later sections. From time to time other biliary tract abnormalities will be identified, such as an extrahepatic bile leak or "biloma" following trauma (Gould & Patel 1979), choledochal cyst (Reuter et al 1980) (Fig. 24.11), biliary cystadenomas (Forrest et al 1980) and Caroli's syndrome (p. 727) (Mittelstaedt et al 1980).

### **Liver** (Marn et al 1991)

*Procedure*

The liver is always examined routinely as part of the examination of the gallbladder and biliary tree and vice versa. The right upper quadrant is usually easy to examine because of the acoustic access provided by the liver substance. The patient is examined supine or in the left lateral decubitus position. The flexibility of real-time apparatus allows scanning in the intercostal, subcostal and coronal planes to give an improved demonstration of the portal anatomy and liver parenchyma. Real-time scanning is less hindered by artefacts, though it does not allow the overall liver views which were available on static scanners. Therefore, in assessing liver size and fluid collections around the liver, the sonographer should be fully aware of the anatomy and possible pathological findings. The examination of the right upper quadrant frequently yields additional diagnostic information about the right kidney, pancreas, lymph nodes and great vessels in the superior portion of the retroperitoneum.

Wide variations in size and shape of the liver occur, though the right lobe is usually larger than the left. A large left lobe provides a most useful additional acoustic window for the left upper quadrant and distal pancreas. A Riedel's lobe of the right lobe of the liver is a common normal variant encountered during ultrasound and provides a useful acoustic window for the right kidney and surrounding structures. During scanning the observer notes the liver texture and records are made with different machine settings to identify the presence of diffuse abnormalities.

*Anatomy* (see also pp. 708 and 714)

The portal vein and its branches are characterized by tube-like structures with highly echogenic walls extending outwards from the porta hepatis (Fig. 2.6). The main portal vein approaches the anterior aspect of the inferior vena cava and this is a most important landmark to identify. The posterior wall of the inferior vena cava is normally indented only by the right renal artery and any other impression should lead to suspicion of a retroperitoneal mass. Anteriorly, the inferior vena cava may be indented normally by the pancreas and the caudate lobe of the liver.

As the hepatic veins lie between the various lobes and segments, their recognition is important in defining the segmental anatomy of the liver. This is of particular value for making decisions prior to hepatic resection. Knowledge of segmental anatomy is also of importance in identifying the gallbladder fossa when the gallbladder lumen cannot be identified owing to fibrosis and contraction.

The main hepatic fissure lies between the embryonic right and left lobes and is characterized by a line projected from the gallbladder to the inferior vena cava (Marks et al 1979). The fissure contains the middle hepatic vein and this can be recognized as a sonolucent line on longitudinal

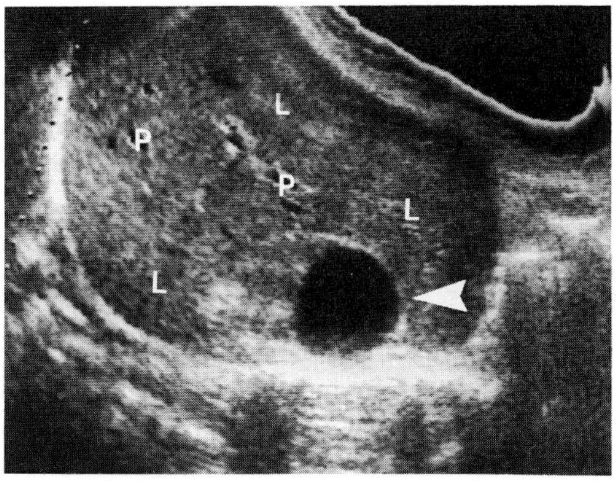


**Fig. 2.6** Simple cyst of liver (arrow). Note normal liver echogenicity (L) and portal vein radicles (P).

scans extending from the portal vein to the gallbladder fossa. This fissure demarcates the anterior portion of the right lobe from the medial segment of the left lobe. Recent surgical advances in hepatic resection, particularly for the removal of secondary colorectal tumors, has meant that the radiologist must be familiar with the hepatic segmental anatomy defined by Couinaud (1957) and amplified by Bismuth et al (1982). The vascular segmental anatomy (Sugarbaker 1990) allows the liver to be theoretically divided by four scissurae – three vertical defined by the left, middle and right hepatic veins and a transverse scissura defined by the right and left portal vein branches. Consequently eight segments may be detailed and numbered (Fig. 24.4). Segment one is the caudate lobe. Segments two and three are the left superior and left inferior lateral segments. Segment four, which is subdivided into subsegments 4a and 4b, is the medial segment of the left lobe. The transverse plane divides the right lobe into segments five and six below the plane and segments seven and eight above the plane. Each segment has its own blood supply (systemic and portal), lymphatics and biliary system. Consequently each segment can be removed individually, the only limitations being the surgeon's ingenuity, the location of the tumor and the percentage of residual hepatic parenchyma after surgery. Whilst ultrasound scanning can identify the major vascular structures defined in the segments, CT portography and MR imaging have been shown to be more sensitive than ultrasound or conventional CT (Nelson et al 1989).

During ultrasound examination of the liver note is made of the upper abdominal aorta and the origins of the celiac axis and superior mesenteric artery. The associated veins also give helpful information. Characteristically the superior mesenteric artery is surrounded by echogenic mesenteric fat and lies between the splenic vein and pancreas anteriorly and the aorta posteriorly. The superior mesenteric vein may also be identified and is a useful landmark as it separates the pancreatic head from the uncinate process. Displacement and involvement of the arteries and veins are of particular value in the diagnosis of pancreatic disease.

As about 80% of the hepatic blood supply is received through the portal vein, the hepatic artery is relatively small. It is, however, possible to define the hepatic artery and its many congenital variations by ultrasound particularly using color Doppler sonography.

### *Findings*

It had been hoped that ultrasound scanning would emerge as an alternative to percutaneous liver biopsy for investigating diffuse parenchymal disease. Whilst there are sometimes specific signs that allow the detection of steatosis from fibrosis, in practice the differential diagnosis is often difficult if not impossible. The reflective "bright" liver signal echogenicity arising in the liver texture in these conditions is often confusing. No quantitative assessment is possible and the determination of echogenicity in the liver remains a subjective assessment (Joseph & Saverymuttu 1991).

In general, focal lesions are more easily identified than diffuse abnormalities.

***Cirrhosis and fatty infiltration.*** A "bright" echo pattern (Fig. 2.7) may be visible, though care must be taken to use appropriate settings on the apparatus. In a series of 66 patients with cirrhosis, brightly echogenic patterns were recorded in 65% and 80% of these had micronodular cirrhosis. However, only 20% of those with macronodular cirrhosis exhibited these changes (Dewbury & Clark 1979). In a series of patients with fatty infiltration a "bright" liver was seen in 60% (Foster et al 1980). The ultrasound differentiation of cirrhosis from fatty changes is not possible, though measurement of attenuation statistics at computed tomography is diagnostic in fatty liver. Of more value is the observation of increased attenuation of the sound beam in conditions like cirrhosis, where there may be difficulty in "penetrating" to the deeper portions of the liver. Sandford et al (1985) studied 125 patients undergoing liver biopsy in whom diffuse parenchymal liver disease had been diagnosed by ultrasound. The diagnosis was correct in 106 patients but ultrasound could not distinguish fat from fibrosis or cirrhosis. The authors concluded that ultrasound is best used in the diagnosis of obstructive jaundice or in the assessment of intrahepatic space-occupying lesions.

Ultrasound scanning may be useful in the detection of cirrhosis because of extrahepatic signs such as splenomegaly, ascites or signs of portal hypertension which may be present. These signs are not specific but when indirect signs are present in the liver, namely enlargement of the liver, hypertrophy of the caudate lobe, increased reflectivity and an irregular liver outline, then the diagnosis of cirrhosis may be made with some confidence (Di Lelio et al 1989).

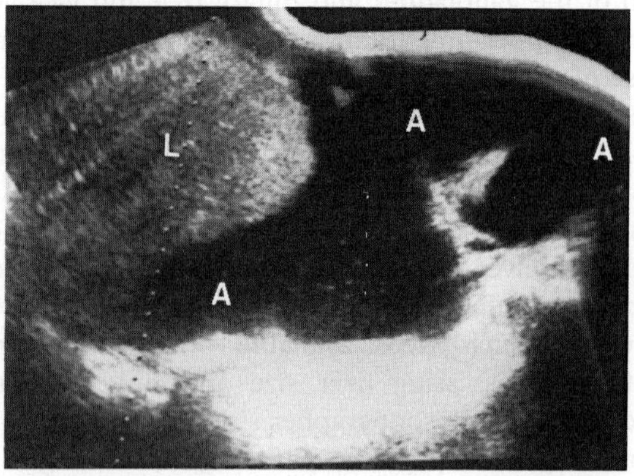


**Fig. 2.7** Cirrhosis in right lobe of liver (L) showing irregular contour increased echogenicity and gross ascites (A).

Occasionally focal fat deposits cause unusual echo patterns and may mimic hepatoma or metastatic disease (Wang et al 1990).

***Metastases.*** Four different ultrasound appearances have been described (Green et al 1977). Discrete echolucent masses were seen in 23%, discrete echogenic masses (Fig. 2.8A) in 30%, echo-free areas in 2% and diffuse alteration in the ultrasound architecture (Fig. 2.8B) in 35%. The variable appearances did not correlate with the findings on histology or arteriography. In another series (Viscomi et al 1981) echolucent masses were described in 38% and purely echogenic masses in 27% of cases. Of the echogenic lesions, 54% were due to colonic cancer and 25% were hepatomas. Of the relatively echolucent masses, 44% were due to lymphoma. Intraoperative ultrasound has also been very helpful in the identification of small deposits not detected by other methods (Parker et al 1989).

***Cysts.*** Simple hepatic cysts may be found in 2.5% of patients examined by ultrasound and are usually coincidental. Occasionally very large hepatic cysts may present with pain, palpable abnormality or biliary obstruction. Echinococcal cysts sometimes have specific ultrasound scanning appearances which can suggest the correct diagnosis. These include the presence of daughter cysts, detachment of the endocyst and densely calcified masses (Lewall & McCorkell 1985). Cystic lesions are identified as clearly defined, often rounded, echolucent structures which may be single (see Fig. 2.6) or multiple. Recognition of cystic disease in the liver should lead to examination for cysts in the kidney and pancreas.

***Benign tumors.*** Hemangiomata are relatively common and are said to be present in 4–7% of the population and most commonly occur in the posterior segment of the right lobe of the liver. They are usually single but may be multiple and most are less than 3 cm in diameter (Nelson & Chezmar 1990). If larger than 4 cm, they are classified as giant hemangiomata. Characteristically hemangioma is diagnosed on ultrasound by virtue of a homogeneous hyperechoic mass with well-defined borders and posterior acoustic enhancement. Unfortunately there is an overlap of these appearances with other tumors such as small hepatocellular carcinomata, particularly in patients likely to develop such malignancies, for example patients with chronic hepatitis from various viral infections, so the differentiation is very important. Each method of differentiation has its own proponents and includes nuclear medicine, CT and MRI.

Focal nodular hyperplasia and liver cell adenomata may also present with the ultrasound scanning appearance of a well-marginated mass, usually with an increased echogenic signal. Complicating features such as hemorrhage and necrosis may cause a complex echo pattern and other investigations are almost always required to make a specific diagnosis (Welch et al 1985).

***Abscesses.*** Single or multiple abscesses are well displayed by ultrasound, which is most useful in monitoring their progress and in the guidance of diagnostic and therapeutic aspiration. Initially abscesses cause an increased echo pattern from the infected area but later there is a more characteristic area of diminished echogenicity, often containing irregular increased echoes due to debris or gas bubbles in the abscess (Meire 1984) (Fig. 2.9). A necrotic liver tumor, whether primary or secondary, may give similar appearances. Hepatosplenic candidiasis is a frequent complication of immune-compromised patients. A number of patterns of abnormality have been described, the most common being of single or multiple uniform hypoechoic or hyperechoic areas (Pastakia et al 1988). *Pneumocystis carinii* infection in AIDS patients can give similar appearances.

***Primary malignant tumors*** (p. 1122). The appearances are similar to those of metastases (Dubbins et al 1981). However, a focal change in echo pattern, especially

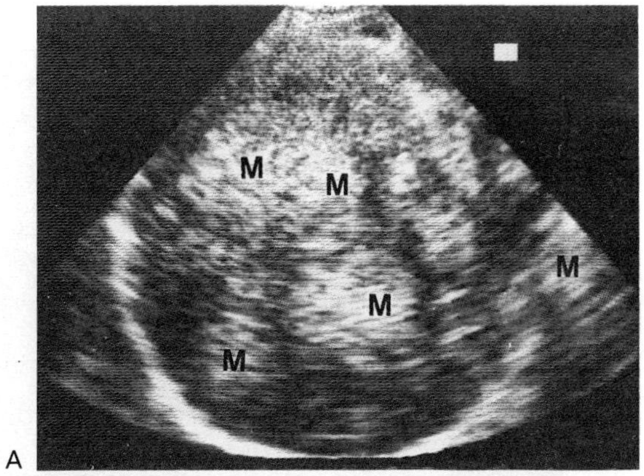


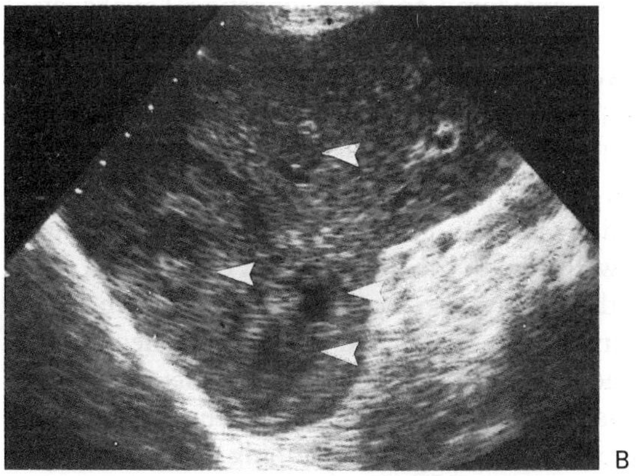


**Fig. 2.8** Secondary tumor of the liver. **A** Large echogenic foci (M) throughout right lobe from metastases from carcinoma of the stomach. **B** Variable echogenicity (arrows) throughout the posterior aspect of the right lobe due to necrotic secondaries from a primary neoplasm of the lung.

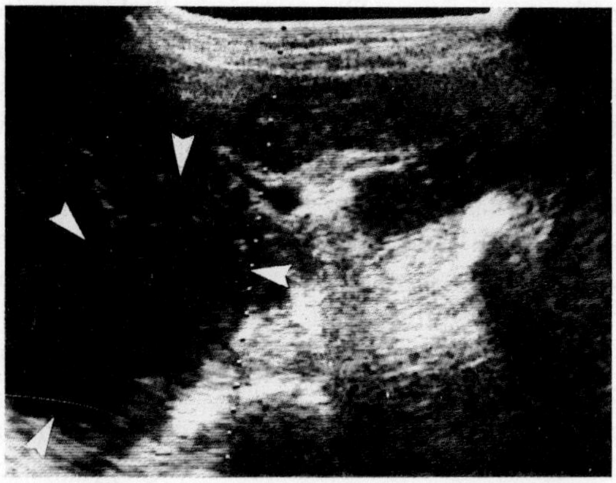

**Fig. 2.9** Pyogenic liver abscess (arrows) due to *Bacteroides*. There is a large irregular echolucent cavity with small irregular echoes within it due to debris.

in a patient known to have cirrhosis, is suspicious of hepatoma. Cholangiocarcinoma may present as a focal echogenic mass with or without evidence of obstructive jaundice and sometimes it will spread widely through the liver with a diffuse echogenic pattern. Occasionally the pattern of bile duct obstruction, especially if there is intrahepatic dilatation with normal extrahepatic ducts, may suggest the diagnosis of a Klatskin-type tumor, particularly if the brunt of obstruction affects the left lobe of the liver. Subtle displacements and distortions of the hepatic veins can lead to the suspicion of a space-occupying lesion in the liver and are most clearly identified with real-time scanning. Ultrasound scanning has advantages in cost and availability and has been suggested as the first screening test for hepatocellular carcinoma, together with alpha-fetoprotein measurement (Curati et al 1988). An overall accuracy of more than 95% has been claimed with modern techniques, including color Doppler flow imaging, in patients with hepatocellular carcinoma. In these patients, a characteristic "basket" pattern due to fine blood flow networks surrounding tumor nodules, together with a specific pulsating pattern on Doppler scanning, is considered to be diagnostic (Tanaka et al 1990).

***Portal hypertension.*** This may be diagnosed by the demonstration of changes in the portal vein or its tributaries and the recognition of portal–systemic anastomoses (Dach et al 1981) (pp. 992 and 995). The porta hepatis may contain multiple echolucent areas with "bright" echogenic walls due to the development of collateral pathways and these may also be identified elsewhere in the abdomen and pelvis. Associated ascites and splenomegaly are easily recognized. In a series of 21 patients with unsuspected portal vein thrombosis (p. 1001), the diagnosis was made by real-time ultrasound scanning (Van Gansbeke et al 1985). An echogenic thrombosis was visible within the lumen of the vein in 67%, collateral circulation was present in 48%, the thrombosed section of portal vein was enlarged in 38% and there was cavernous transformation of the portal vein in 19%. Duplex Doppler ultrasound scanning may provide additional information regarding portal flow rates and direction, though these are affected by physiological changes of posture and respiration. Valuable information regarding the presence of significant portosystemic varices may be obtained.

## Pancreas

Ultrasound scanning of the pancreas is utilized widely because of its availability and lower cost compared to other complex imaging procedures. It is relatively sensitive in identifying the normal from the abnormal pancreas, may assist in discriminating between neoplasm and pancreatitis and is the initial imaging procedure of choice.

*Procedure*

The left upper quadrant is more difficult to examine than the right and various modifications of technique may be required to obtain a suitable "acoustic window". These include scanning through the left lobe of the liver, scanning through the stomach after distention with water, scanning with the patient erect and the use of varying oblique and coronal scanning planes. By utilizing such modifications the pancreas is visualized satisfactorily in 90% of patients (Taylor et al 1981).

*Anatomy* (Figs 2.10, 2.11)

The pancreas, being of a variable size and shape, must be scanned in a variety of transverse and oblique planes. The splenic and left renal veins are excellent guides to the position of the distal body and tail of the pancreas, though gas in the stomach may cause a failure to demonstrate this area and in this circumstance a further scan is indicated

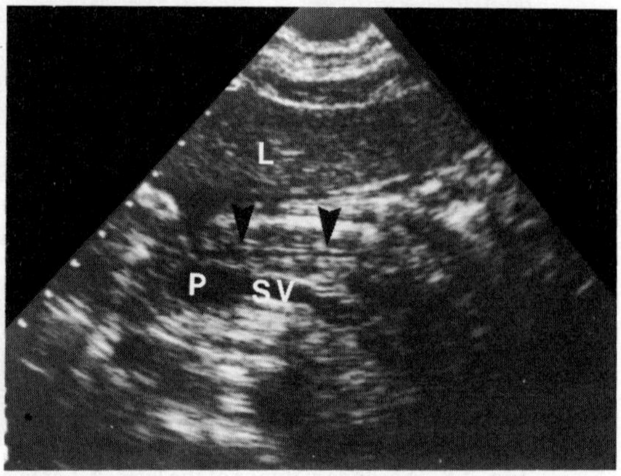


**Fig. 2.10** Transverse section of normal pancreas. Splenic vein (SV), portal vein (P), pancreatic duct (arrows) and left lobe of liver (L).

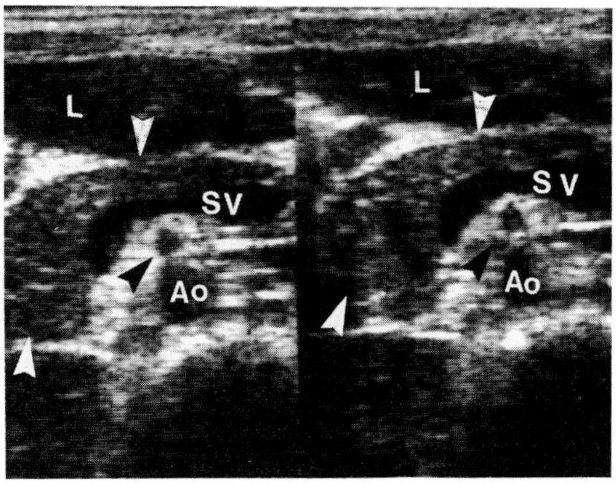


**Fig. 2.11** Transverse sections of normal pancreas. Normal pancreas (white arrows), splenic vein (SV), superior mesenteric artery (black arrows), aorta (Ao), left lobe of liver (L).

after filling the stomach with water. Nevertheless, the tail is often difficult to display and disease in the left lobe of the liver can modify pancreatic echogenicity.

The splenic vein is the most important landmark in the left upper quadrant. It can often be traced from the portosplenic junction towards the splenic hilum. Once the scanning sweep identifies the long axis of the splenic vein, structures crossing through the area should be recognized. These include the left renal vein crossing behind the superior mesenteric artery to join the inferior vena cava, the tortuous splenic artery lying cephalad to the vein, the pancreatic duct (particularly if dilated) lying anterior to the splenic vein within the pancreatic tissue and the common bile duct in its course through the head of the pancreas.

Parasagittal, longitudinal scans in the region of the inferior vena cava are useful to display the head and proximal body of the pancreas. The head lies on the anterior surface of the inferior vena cava just below the crossing of the portal vein. The lower end of the common bile duct passes deep to the head and the gastroduodenal artery lies on its anterior surface. Recognition of changes in the normal relationships of these structures should lead to a search for other signs of pathology, such as changes in the normal contour and echogenicity or significant alterations in the appearance of the pancreatic duct. Current apparatus should allow the demonstration of the pancreatic duct (Fig. 2.10) in many patients and pathological dilatation should be recognizable in most patients with inflammatory or malignant disease (Parulekar 1980).

*Findings*

The width of the normal pancreas falls within a relatively narrow range, generally being larger in the young and reducing in size with age. The head of the pancreas is approximately 2–3 cm in the anteroposterior plane and 3–4 cm in the superoinferior plane. The body is thinner at the pancreatic neck where the great vessels are crossed. Then to the left of the midline the pancreas measures 1.5–2.5 cm in the anteroposterior plane, gradually decreasing in size to 2 cm for the tail (Kreel et al 1977). The mean diameter of the pancreatic duct is 1.6 mm and should not exceed 3 mm in the head and neck or 2 mm elsewhere (Hadidi 1983). The normal echo pattern of the pancreas depends on the amount of interlobular fat and generally it has an echogenicity similar to or greater than that of the liver.

Variations in the size and contour of the gland and pattern of echogenicity, together with variations in duct caliber, comprise the spectrum of ultrasound appearances sought in making the diagnosis of inflammatory or neoplastic disease. About one-half of patients with carcinoma of the pancreas present with obstructive jaundice and ultrasound scanning is an accurate technique in distinguishing obstructive from non-obstructive jaundice. The signs of pancreatic neoplasm may be grouped into those within and those outside the pancreas. Extrapancreatic changes include biliary obstruction, lymph node enlargement, ascites, invasion of vascular structures and hepatic deposits. However, most of these findings are better displayed at CT scanning, which is the most efficient available technique for staging pancreatic carcinoma (Reznek & Stephens 1993).

The main intrapancreatic abnormality in carcinoma is a localized alteration in the echogenicity which is almost always a significant reduction of echogenicity in the affected area. Its borders are usually irregular and quite distinct from the normal echogenic pancreatic tissue. Dilatation of the pancreatic duct is a common finding (Shawker et al 1986). Accompanying pancreatitis modifies these findings and may make the diagnosis of carcinoma difficult or impossible. Cystic neoplasms have no specific features and no differential signs distinguish between benign and malignant cystic tumors. Pseudocysts of the pancreas often show a similar appearance. Thus, the discovery of a cystic lesion almost always requires CT scanning for further differentiation.

Duplex Doppler ultrasound scanning increases the recognition of involvement of the systemic (i.e. superior mesenteric) and portal vessels in pancreatic carcinoma (Campbell & Wilson 1988).

*Endoscopic ultrasound* provides further evaluation and staging of pancreatic neoplasm. The ultrasound source is placed close to pancreatic tissue via the endoscope, so allowing visualization of the pancreas and adjacent structures and allowing access for ultrasound-guided cytological puncture (Tio et al 1990).

*Intraoperative ultrasound* does not replace the preoperative imaging assessment of pancreatic neoplasm but helps to locate a nonpalpable neoplasm and further evaluates the involvement of neighboring structures.

Islet cell tumors are usually difficult to detect with preoperative ultrasound techniques due to their small size and nonspecific echo pattern. However, intraoperative ultrasound scanning has proved an effective means of detecting them when the preoperative assessment has been unhelpful (Galiber et al 1988).

In acute pancreatitis there are technical problems in obtaining good quality scans (Fig. 2.12) because of large volumes of gas in the intestine and the difficulty of applying transducer pressure to the tender abdominal wall. Silverstein et al (1981) found that only 62% of patients with acute pancreatitis had the diagnosis made by ultrasound, compared with 98% by computed tomography. The diagnostic capability of ultrasound scanning may be expected to improve as intestinal ileus resolves, usually 48 h after the onset. Ultrasound findings may be classified by distribution, either focal or diffuse, and by severity, mild, moderate or severe (Freeny 1989a). Complications such as phlegmon, hemorrhage, pseudocyst formation and intra-abdominal fluid collections are well demonstrated. Extrapancreatic complications such as fluid collections in the lesser sac, transverse mesocolon, pararenal spaces or edema of soft-tissue planes and ascites pose a significant challenge in their identification or differentiation (Jeffrey et al 1986) (see also p. 1255).

There has been renewed interest in the ultrasound findings in the difficult diagnosis of chronic pancreatitis and matching these findings with ERCP abnormalities results in a good correlation of the two examinations in the grading of disease severity. These observations form the basis of a revised classification developed by workers in Cambridge, England. Five grades are described – normal, equivocal, mild, moderate and marked – and these depend on the size and shape of the main duct, irregularities of the duct, the presence of calculi or cavities, the overall size of the gland and the echogenic variation within the gland. Contiguous organ involvement is also noted. If less than one-third of the pancreas is involved, the condition is described as focal. These diagnostic features are precise and repeatable.

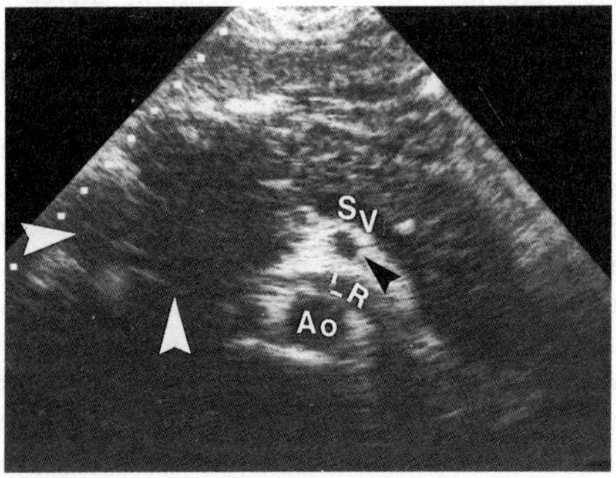


**Fig. 2.12** Acute pancreatitis. Large irregular echolucent area in the head of pancreas (white arrows), superior mesenteric artery (black arrows). Aorta (Ao), splenic vein (SV), left renal vein (LR).

Consequently the diagnosis may be achieved by reference to the simple rules recommended (Jones et al 1988).

## Spleen

The spleen is accessible to ultrasound examination by scanning under the left costal margin and between the ribs. The enlarged spleen provides an "acoustic window" into the left upper quadrant and may be scanned longitudinally in parasagittal sections or obliquely along the subcostal margin.

Cystic structures such as abscess, hematoma and other relatively echolucent lesions such as lymphoma may be demonstrated. Perisplenic collections such as subphrenic abscesses, perisplenic hematoma or localized ascitic collections are easily identified. Echogenic lesions in the spleen may indicate a splenic infarct, granuloma or parasitic infection. Rarely, metastases in the spleen give echogenic foci within the pulp.

## **Bowel** (Carroll 1989)

Despite technical limitations in the use of ultrasound scanning in the investigation of bowel disorders, it has potential advantages. Obstructed bowel loops when full of fluid provide a suitable background for the identification of characteristic patterns of alteration in the valvulae conniventes and haustral markings. The detection of peristaltic activity on real-time scanning helps to distinguish mechanical from paralytic ileus. The recognition of a target-like lesion due to thickened hypoechoic bowel wall surrounding the more echogenic mucosa and submucosa permits the identification and localization of a mass.

In about 20% of patients with acute abdominal pain, ultrasound scanning will change the original clinical diagnosis (McGrath & Keeling 1991). This is particularly so in young females with gynecological disorders where the diagnosis of acute appendicitis may be made clinically in up to 45% (Gaensler et al 1989). Patients with a right iliac fossa mass pose a relatively common diagnostic problem with a wide differential diagnosis ranging from appendix abscess to carcinoma of the cecum and gynecological or urological conditions. Ultrasound scanning is very sensitive (100%) in correctly identifying the presence of such masses with a 97% accuracy in locating the organ of origin (Millard et al 1991).

***Hypertrophic pyloric stenosis.*** Ultrasound scanning is the investigation of choice in infants. Thickening of the pyloric muscle to 4 mm or more, a pyloric diameter of 15 mm or more and a pyloric channel of 17 mm or more in length are diagnostic signs. Prominent gastric peristalsis and retained gastric fluid are additional signs (Blumhagen et al 1988).

***Other conditions.*** Ultrasound examination has been used in childhood atresias and duplications, intussusception of the bowel, congenital hernias and functional obstruction due to meconium. Some intestinal anomalies, as well as meconium ileus and peritonitis, may be recognized in utero.

### Retroperitoneum

Whilst computed tomography is now the mainstay of diagnosis of retroperitoneal disease, ultrasound may give useful information, particularly regarding the abdominal aorta and especially when Doppler scanning is used to estimate aortic size, to detect atherosclerosis and to identify periaortic masses. Technical constraints occur due to the presence of abdominal gas or obesity. Ultrasound scanning is particularly useful in the diagnosis and monitoring of aortic aneurysms. Early diagnosis and surgical treatment with graft replacement improves life expectancy for patients with an aortic aneurysm and no other significant operative risks. In such patients, operations are offered to those in whom an aortic aneurysm is assessed as more than 4 cm in diameter (Crawford & Hess 1989). Whilst the ultrasound examination is very accurate in experienced hands, surgical planning usually requires dynamic contrast-enhanced CT to identify the extent and involvement of arterial branches by the aneurysm.

### Peritoneal space

The facility to identify quickly and painlessly the presence of generalized or localized fluid collections in the peritoneal space gives ultrasound a significant advantage in examining the patient with an acute abdomen (p. 514). Being particularly sensitive to differences between liquid and solid materials, ultrasound can show liquid collections such as abscesses, hematomas and ascites with as little as 100 ml of fluid. With the flexibility and portability of examination by real-time scanners the technique is being used increasingly in emergency and intensive care units and in intraoperative situations. Practical constraints, such as lack of suitably trained staff or up-to-date equipment, have restricted these applications. Ultrasound is also valuable in the patient with postoperative fever in whom an upper abdominal or pelvic abscess or peritonitis is suspected and it has been recommended as the first imaging investigation when an abdominal abscess is suspected (Joseph & McVicar 1990). However, the central portion of the abdomen is always most difficult to examine because of gas-filled bowel, especially in the acute and postoperative situations, and in these circumstances conventional radiological techniques and computed tomography will be necessary.

## COMPUTED TOMOGRAPHY (Moss et al 1992)

Until the advent of computed tomography (CT), X-ray imaging relied on an analog system for the visual display of human anatomy. Various methods were used to display the image, ranging from photographic glass plates to sophisticated photo-electric crystal screens and electronic image intensifiers. Additional assistance was available through the use of administered contrast media and electronic apparatus such as television systems, but basic analog principles prevailed until the early 1970s.

Several technological developments after the Second World War combined to produce a dramatic change. Advances in computer and transistor technology allowed rapid and efficient processing and display of images using digital information. Several mathematical achievements led to methods for computing X-ray information. Radon (1917) developed a mathematical model for reconstructing the location of an object in two dimensions by projecting lines intersecting the object from many angles. In 1955, Cormack independently devised a similar solution using the inhomogeneity of radio-isotope distribution in the body (Cormack 1980). Kuhl & Edwards in 1964 applied similar principles to radio-isotope scanning of the liver and brain and so developed computed emission tomography.

These studies and other observations were virtually neglected until Godfrey Hounsfield developed a prototype CT machine for EMI Ltd which was installed for brain CT at Atkinson Morley's Hospital in London in 1972 (Ambrose 1973, Hounsfield 1973).

Initially, Hounsfield used a gamma ray isotope source which scanned transversely and sensitive radiation detectors measured the emerging attenuated beam, which was digitized and computed. Data collection took 9 days and computer processing 2.5 h (Hounsfield 1980). Because of the extraordinarily long scanning time a conventional X-ray tube was substituted as the X-ray source, so reducing the scanning time to 9 h. After further experimentation the first patient was examined in 1972. So successful has the technique been that more than 5000 CT scanners had been installed by 1982 and many more since. Following the introduction of CT of the brain, development was extremely rapid, with new generations of machines being developed quickly so that examination of other anatomical areas such as the abdomen can now be conducted with speed and precision.

CT is a complex and costly investigation and the judicious selection of patients is paramount. Studies of diagnostic efficacy suggest that CT has had a significant effect on the accuracy of diagnosis, has reduced the need for other investigations, particularly invasive ones, and has altered management in a significant proportion of patients (Fry 1984). In a series of 2619 patients undergoing CT of the body, 53% of examinations provided a unique or substantial contribution to diagnostic understanding and 15% of examinations contributed to a change in treatment. Surgery was reduced by an estimated 14% and angiography by 11% (Fineberg et al 1983). It is anticipated that the major directions of further development will be towards improved spatial resolution and increased speed of scanning. It is likely that the cost of CT will decrease so that it will replace many conventional X-ray procedures (Margulis 1985).

## Principles of computed tomography

The display of human anatomy on radiographic film is the result of a pattern of blackening of the film by an emerging X-ray beam after transmission and attenuation through the body. This blackening is related to the density and thickness of the tissues traversed. During the passage through the subject complex physicochemical interactions occur between the tissues and the X-ray beam, causing variable amounts of attenuation, with bone causing more attenuation than soft tissue. Thus, less radiation emerges from bone, resulting in less blackening of the film image. No quantitative data about the amount of blackening or the physical processes involved are available in such an analog system and the reading of the film is therefore qualitative. The CT scanning process calculates as precisely as possible the attenuation of the transmitted X-ray beam in the particular plane (scan slice) of the subject examined.

When a monochromatic X-ray beam of single energy intensity traverses a homogeneous medium its intensity diminishes due to physicochemical reactions in that medium. When the medium is thin the reduction in intensity is expressed by the equation:

$$\Delta I = -\mu I \Delta X$$

(where I is the incident intensity, $\Delta X$ is the thickness and $\mu$ is the linear attenuation coefficient).

In a slice of the human body the linear attenuation coefficient will vary at different positions so mathematical computations have to be performed to build up the CT image and these would be prohibitively slow without a computer. In carrying out the analysis each scan slice is broken up into a mesh or matrix, each individual component of which is called a picture element or pixel (Fig. 2.13). The third dimension of each pixel, governed by the thickness of the slice, gives a volume to each unit which is then referred to as a voxel. In CT the voxel size is small enough for the assumption of uniform density and atomic number within each voxel. Thus each pixel can be assumed to be uniform. Occasionally a structure or lesion only partly occupies the scanned slice and the average reading, therefore, is an inadequate representation of either tissue. For this reason slice thickness should be no greater than the anticipated size of lesions in the region under study. Usually the slice is broken up into 65 000 or 260 000 pixels by the use of a mesh of 256 × 256 or 512 × 512.

In CT systems, resolution of contrast or the ability to distinguish adjacent areas of differing density is far superior to that in conventional radiography because of the use of special detectors with a very high signal-to-noise ratio. The degree of contrast is also improved by restricting the plane of scan to a narrow width (slice thickness) so that the amount of scattered radiation is reduced.

Conversely spatial resolution, i.e. the ability to distinguish separate objects, is only marginally better than with conventional radiology, because absorption is being measured and two adjacent tissues may exhibit the same absorption.

Spatial resolution can be much improved by using the thin-slice technique, but as the signal-to-noise ratio is inversely proportional to the thickness of the scan plane the degree of noise increases in thin slices.

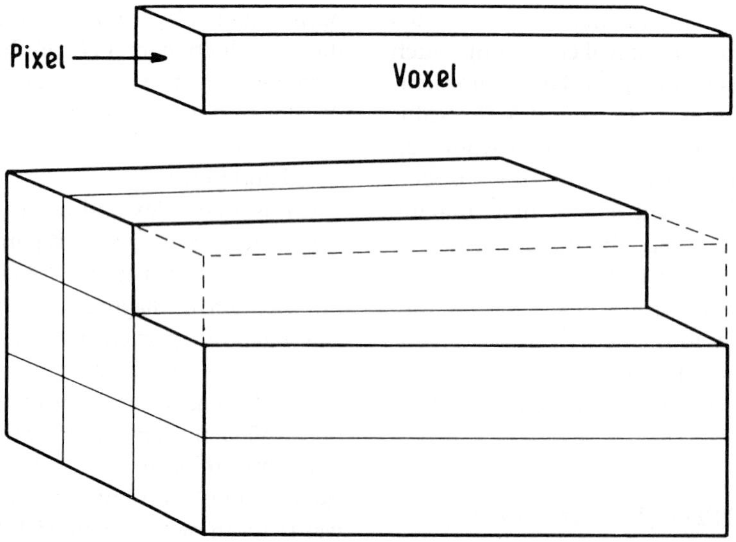


**Fig. 2.13** The configuration of a matrix composed of voxels (Husband & Fry 1981).

The reconstructed CT image is represented in a two-dimensional matrix of CT numbers. The CT numbers are arbitrarily defined utilizing the known linear attenuation coefficients according to the formula:

$$CT = K\,\frac{\mu_{tissue}\,x - 1}{\mu_{water}}$$

where $K = 1000$. On this scale, air is given a value of –1000 and water of zero. Dense bone is in the range +1000 to +2000, fat has a value of –50 to –100 and abdominal soft tissues +20 to +60. The scale is referred to as the Hounsfield scale and the numbers as Hounsfield (H) or CT numbers. CT numbers are a useful guide to the composition of the tissue under examination, but these are not absolute owing to technical factors involving both patient and the apparatus.

## Data recording

Photographic records are usually provided by copying the visual display unit (VDU) image onto film by a multiformat camera. The introduction of laser cameras and films has significantly improved the quality of "hard copy" images.

The VDU image can be manipulated to vary the display and this is essential when interpreting on a scale of shades of gray, of which the human eye can distinguish approximately 16–20. When the gray scale is spread over a wide range or "window" of CT numbers the image lacks contrast but has good detail (spatial resolution). When the shades of gray are distributed more closely over a narrow "window" the image has a sharper black and white quality and has better contrast resolution. Manipulations of the image allow better perception of certain abnormalities, for example liver metastases (Fig. 2.14).

Other software facilities allow the operator to enhance the perception and display of structures. Using different routines the range of CT numbers can be extended, the attenuation of an area can be measured in CT numbers and a lesion may be outlined or subjected to volumetric measurement.

"Dynamic" techniques allow the operator to display graphically attenuation changes occurring in certain tissues over a period of time following the injection of intravenous contrast agents. This provides useful information about certain physical characteristics of a lesion, including its vascularity.

### *Long-term storage*

On completion and recording of an examination the computed data are transferred from the magnetic disk at the operator's console for temporary or permanent storage. Available storage devices include magnetic tape, floppy or optical disks and such records are archived for future reference.

A

B

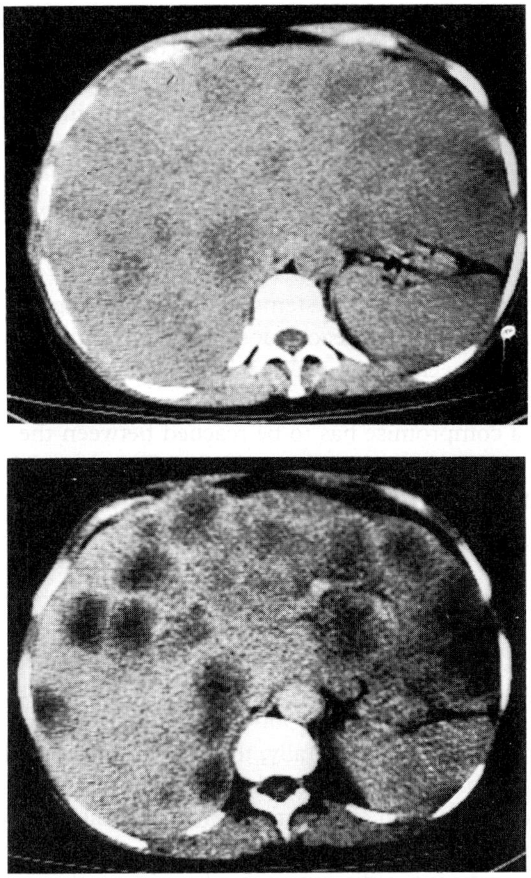

**Fig. 2.14** **A** Axial scan through enlarged liver showing multiple areas of reduced attenuation suspicious of metastases. **B** Same patient after intravenous contrast and different Hounsfield setting confirming multiple metastases.

## Artefacts (Davison 1982)

These may arise because of machine faults, limitations of the reconstruction algorithms, the unwillingness or inability of the patient to be co-operative and involuntary physiological events such as cardiac pulsation and intestinal movements. Streak artefacts may be caused by movement, including breathing, during data collection. Linear and star-shaped artefacts are caused by structures with a high atomic density, such as surgical clips or residual barium in the bowel. Physiological activity is rarely troublesome with modern equipment, but occasionally antiperistaltic agents such as glucagon are necessary to enhance the clarity of an image: for example, with suspected lesions of the head of pancreas duodenal contraction can interfere with data collection. The speed of third and fourth generation scanners has alleviated many problems associated with movement. Helical scanning, with its ability to collect data continuously during the operation of the apparatus, has significantly improved the speed with which data can be collected from a critically ill or unco-operative patient, with marked improvement in the quality of the images. Equipment problems can be minimized by regular calibration checks and servicing.

## Radiation dosage

Owing to the tightly collimated X-ray beam and the great sensitivity of detector systems, CT provides a good diagnostic return from each dose of absorbed radiation. However, because of relationships between spatial and contrast resolution, signal-to-noise ratio and radiation dose, a compromise has to be reached between the image quality and the exposure to radiation. The dose delivered to a patient by a particular CT system will depend on the technical X-ray factors utilized, the condition of the X-ray tube and the patient's position in the scanner circle (Shope et al 1982). The absorbed dose has been calculated as varying from less than 5 mGy to almost 10 mGy for a single CT examination. The overall risk of a CT examination has been expressed as similar to the risks of smoking 600 cigarettes or driving 1500 miles in a motor car (Huda & Sandison 1986). Naturally, the skin receives the highest dose of radiation but the total dose received in CT is usually lower than in conventional radiological procedures because the total volume of tissue exposed is smaller. Some scattered radiation is produced but this may be reduced by lead aprons above and below the patient if circumstances warrant this (McCullough & Payne 1978). Determination of the absorbed radiation dose to various organs is one of the most difficult estimations in radiation physics. However, calculations of fetal and pediatric dosages from phantom experiments have been made and reasonably precise estimates of dosage from CT scanning may be obtained using such experimental data (Fearon & Vucich 1987, Felmlee et al 1989).

## Contrast enhancement

Artificial contrast opacification or enhancement is frequently needed in CT of the abdomen.

***Oral contrast agents.*** The empty or fluid-filled bowel has an attenuation value similar to that of soft tissues and it is necessary to give a substance which will opacify the lumen sufficiently to identify it without causing high-density streak artefacts. A dilute barium preparation such as E-Z Cat, producing a 1% w/w barium sulfate suspension (Megibow & Bosniak 1980) or alternatively an iodinated water-soluble medium such as Gastrografin 1.5–3% (Moss et al 1978) may be used. A volume of 200–300 ml of the selected medium is given 20–30 min before scanning commences to opacify the stomach and small intestine. For investigation of the pancreas, a further dose of 150 ml of oral contrast is given just before commencement of the examination and the patient is placed on the right side for several minutes to ensure good filling of the duodenal loop. If necessary, the pancreas may be scanned in the right lateral decubitus position. If lower abdominal or pelvic structures are to be examined, it is advisable for the initial dose of oral contrast to be administered 1 h before commencement to ensure filling of the distal small bowel and cecum.

***Rectal contrast agents.*** When scanning the pelvis, particularly in the staging of rectal neoplasm or in the search for lymph node enlargement, it is advisable to administer 75–150 ml of dilute contrast medium as an enema on the scanning table to differentiate the rectum and sigmoid colon from other pelvic soft tissue structures.

***Bladder and vaginal contrast agents.*** Occasionally, it is necessary to instil dilute iodinated contrast medium directly into the bladder and the use of a tampon in the vagina can be most helpful in locating the position of the uterine cervix in relation to the vaginal vault (Cohen et al 1977).

***Intravenous contrast agents.*** Iodinated contrast media injected intravenously are used frequently to enhance structures during CT. These are administered either by bolus or infusion or both. The choice of technique depends on the clinical problem under investigation. Each method of enhancement causes different peaks of intensity for varying lengths of time and different examination protocols tend to operate in each department.

A variety of media is available, both ionic, such as meglumine iothalamate (Conray 420), and non-ionic, such as iopamidol (Iopamiro 300). The dosage of iodine received from iodinated contrast medium varies between 40 and 80 g. Injections of contrast medium are valuable in a number of situations, ranging from the opacification of and excretion by normal viscera to the demonstration of abnormal structures by virtue of increased or decreased vascularity, especially in the search for occult lesions. Certain lesions may be better demonstrated after enhancement, for example the differentiation of a cystic from a solid lesion.

When it is necessary to display the detailed vascular structure of solid organs, such as the liver, a dynamic bolus contrast enhancement technique is advised. As intravenous iodinated contrast is given the hepatic attenuation rises in proportion to the volume given and the rate of administration. There is rapid leakage of contrast material from the vascular to the extracellular space and equilibrium is achieved in 2–3 min. Once equilibrium is established there is little or no attenuation difference between liver tumor cells and normal hepatic parenchyma. However, during the critical period before equilibrium it is often possible to display tumors, particularly those which are hypovascular (Nelson 1991).

By rapid delivery of iodinated contrast using a power injector so that 50–60 g of iodine at 1 g/s (120–150 ml

60% iodinated contrast at 2.5 ml/s) and timing the scanning parameters, it is possible to obtain an excellent demonstration of tumor extent and vascularity. The examination is enhanced by the availability of a helical scanning apparatus. By suitable adjustment of the scanning parameters a double-phase examination giving excellent details of the hepatic arterial and portal venous phases may be achieved during the single injection of a bolus of contrast medium (Zeman et al 1993). Such developments avoid the need to perform dynamic CT of the liver following the introduction of an arterial catheter into the celiac axis for contrast delivery. Similar techniques give an accurate visual display of the abdominal aorta and its branches, especially with 3D images.

From time to time the appearances after contrast enhancement may allow a specific diagnosis to be made, such as in cavernous hemangioma of the liver which typically shows delay in contrast enhancement up to 30 min after the commencement of injection.

The normal renal parenchyma will always enhance with intravenous contrast media and this is followed later by filling of the collecting systems, ureters and bladder. Distention of the bladder is usually achieved and this can be helpful in demonstrating pelvic disorders.

Some risks are inherent with intravenous contrast medium (Ansell 1970). However, non-ionic materials appear to be less noxious and should be utilized in patients with a history of allergy, cardiac problems or previous contrast reaction. In addition, systemic contrast medium should be administered with caution to patients with severe renal impairment or diabetes (Hayman et al 1980).

Intra-arterial lipiodol in conjunction with lipophilic chemotherapeutic agents have been used in the treatment of hepatocellular carcinoma. The injection of lipiodol through a catheter in the hepatic artery with subsequent CT has been used very effectively in the detection of small hepatocellular carcinomas. The information derived is also helpful in determining treatment policy, including surgical resection (Choi et al 1989).

*Procedure*

The patient fasts for 4–6 h and a full explanation of the procedure should be given on arrival. As the patient will be required to lie quietly in one position for up to 1 h, they should be encouraged to make themselves comfortable by loosening tight clothing, emptying the bladder and bowel if necessary and instructed in breath holding. The need for and effects of contrast medium administration should also be explained simply. A patient's permission for the procedure should include an understanding of the possible risks of intravenous contrast administration.

The examination is usually made in the supine position, though occasionally other positions are utilized, especially for interventional procedures such as biopsy or abscess drainage. In planning radiotherapy, CT should be performed in the position in which treatment will be given. A satisfactory study requires full co-operation of the patient, who should be able to stay completely still and to breath hold for at least 5 s and preferably to suspend respiration at approximately the same position for each scan slice. It is necessary to obtain the patient's co-operation for breath-holding for up to 30 s when undertaking detailed examinations with helical CT scanning. This applies especially in scanning the upper abdomen. If the patient is unwilling or unable to co-operate a sedative such as Valium 5–10 mg intravenously may be given, though this necessitates careful monitoring. Young children and very old patients need particular care and the help of an anesthetist may be necessary. Very sick patients such as those in intensive care or emergency departments should certainly be under the supervision of the appropriate specialist during CT.

**Abdominal CT** (Gore et al 1994)

Pathological conditions are visible by virtue of either direct changes in attenuation characteristics or indirectly by alteration in the size, shape or position of an organ. CT gives unique information about the margins of abdominal organs and the intervening fat and fascial planes. Abdominal CT relies heavily on the disposition of fat in and around soft tissue structures for the recognition of diseases (Dixon & Nightingale 1984).

Particular problems in the interpretation of abdominal CT include: the lack of specific attenuation characteristics in typing tissue; the difficulty in identifying masses less than 1 cm in size or mucosal lesions of the bowel; the lack of fat in thin or very ill patients; and movement artefacts due to breathing or peristalsis. It has been found that artificial contrast opacification or enhancement of particular structures such as the intestinal lumen or urinary tract can be most helpful.

The addition of helical scanning which allows consistent acquisition of volumetric data has considerable implications for improved diagnosis of abdominal diseases, especially in the liver and pancreas. The use of bolus intravenous contrast injection for dynamic helical scanning of abdominal blood vessels allows excellent visualization including 3D images of the vasculature to third order branches and splenoportal venous structures (Rubin et al 1993).

*Indications*

The indications for abdominal CT are many. A special report was published by the Society for Computed Body Tomography on the indications for body CT in 1979. In this report there were 22 major categories of indication applicable to gastroenterological practice and many further indications have been described since. A close liaison between radiologist and clinician allows the choice of the best diagnostic course in a particular patient (Husband & Golding 1982).

CT and magnetic resonance imaging (MRI) should not be used as screening modalities in patients with non-specific complaints. Kapoor et al (1983) reviewed the indications for abdominal CT scans in 210 patients. Of these, 166 were examined with a specific goal in mind and in 43% of these important new information was revealed: only 16% of the investigations were reported as normal. The other 44 patients were examined without a specific goal (mainly in the evaluation of abdominal pain, fever or weight loss). In only 2% of these was significant new information obtained and in 41% the examination was normal.

In patients with an abdominal mass, CT is excellent for defining the origin and extent of the mass and may be helpful in its characterization. In a series of 101 patients with a palpable or suspected mass a lesion was confirmed in 69 (68%). Of these, the responsible mass or structure was identified in 64 (93%) and the likely nature suggested in 61 (88%) (Williams et al 1984).

Focal disease of the liver, spleen and pancreas is seen well by CT and pathological processes identified in many patients (Foley & Jochem 1991). Because of its facility to localize lesions accurately and so allow precise aspiration biopsy, CT is the method of choice in investigations of such patients (Kreel 1984) (p. 32). Diffuse parenchymal disorders are less well demonstrated and fine-needle aspiration biopsy (under CT or ultrasound monitoring) is more likely to be diagnostic. In obstructive jaundice the site and nature of the cause can be readily identified by CT in up to 95% of patients (Zeman et al 1985) and interventional techniques monitored safely.

Tailored CT scanning of the biliary tree is most helpful in obtaining a precise diagnosis in patients with complex biliary disease (Baron 1991).

CT scanning provides a new perspective for the diagnosis of alimentary tract disease. By virtue of its cross-section facility to demonstrate the bowel lumen, the bowel wall and extraluminal structures, in conditions such as tumors (Thoeni 1989), diverticulitis (Neff & vanSonnenberg 1989) and inflammatory bowel disease (Gore 1989) accurate diagnosis and staging can be achieved promptly and precisely. The need for diagnostic laparotomy has been significantly reduced.

The imaging of retroperitoneal and mesenteric disorders has been revolutionized by modern imaging techniques, especially CT, and the superior image display has considerably increased the ability to manage abscesses and pseudocysts without surgery. Additionally, fine-needle aspiration biopsy of tumors and lymph nodes has become a precise process under CT direction (pp. 32–33).

CT is the most accurate available method for staging malignant disease (p. 207) as a preliminary to surgery and/or radiotherapy (Thompson 1994). Metastatic lesions in distant organs may be detected and this may alter the planned therapeutic approach. The monitoring of progress after surgery or radiotherapy is simple and non-invasive and the recurrence of tumor can be identified at a relatively early stage.

## Risks of CT

As with other radiographic procedures some risk is entailed, whether from radiation exposure (p. 62), the injection of intravenous contrast agents (p. 19) or the use of sedation and anesthetic agents. However, by careful selection of patients and the judicious application of the appropriate technique, such risks are minimized. The need for or withdrawal of other tests and therapy following CT may also reduce or increase the risks for the patient and should be considered in the calculation of net risk (Fineberg 1978).

## Esophagus

As there is often a recognizable amount of fat surrounding the esophagus, it is usually possible to distinguish it from neighboring organs. Normally, the esophageal wall should not exceed 3 mm (Halber et al 1979). Air is normally visible in the esophagus in about half of the patients examined and is seen centrally within the lumen. Dilute contrast medium may be used to enhance the lumen in selected cases.

The soft tissue planes surrounding the esophagus are normally distinct and blurring or distortion of the tissue interfaces is said to be a reliable indicator of disease. Abnormal mediastinal lymph nodes are sought. In a series of 30 patients undergoing CT prior to treatment for proven carcinoma of the esophagus, the extent of spread to the mediastinum was recognized in 27 patients and intra-abdominal metastases were found in 22 patients (Daffner et al 1979). However, Quint et al (1985) found that esophageal cancer was correctly staged in only 13 of 33 patients, the major difficulties being to define individual layers of the esophageal wall and to detect mediastinal invasion. Limitations in staging include difficulty in the detection of aortic invasion, the differentiation of abnormally enlarged lymph nodes due to benign cause and the inability to detect disease in lymph nodes of normal size (Trenkner et al 1994). However, despite continuing controversy over the role of CT in the preoperative staging of esophageal carcinoma, it helps to separate patients into three defined groups: patients with potentially curable disease with no evidence of local invasion or distant metastases, those with obvious unresectable tumor by virtue of local mediastinal invasion and/or distant metastases and a third group with indeterminate results needing other assessment of resectability (Halvorsen & Thompson

1989). The alternative approach to diagnosing local spread of esophageal cancer is endoscopic ultrasonography which is discussed on p. 208.

Abnormalities of the esophagogastric junction can be visualized by CT but care in interpretation is required as normal anatomical structures in this region can be quite prominent, suggesting focal disease (Marks et al 1981). Varices in the lower esophagus and around the esophagogastric junction can be visualized by CT, though contrast enhancement is essential for confirmation. In the study by McCain et al (1985) comparing CT with angiography, there was agreement on the presence or absence of gastroesophageal varices in 70.5% of patients. False negative results were mainly due to technical factors.

## Stomach

If the gastric lumen has been well distended by preliminary oral contrast medium the gastric wall should be readily visible aided by fat in the perigastric tissues. Whilst the gastric wall thickness should not normally exceed 5 mm, the range is quite variable and can be misleading. Only measurements above 1 cm should be considered abnormal (Balfe et al 1981) and then the estimation should be viewed with caution as it is not possible to distinguish between inflammatory and neoplastic disease. All regions of the stomach are examined for alteration of contour, gastric wall thickness, extension of a mass outside the gastric wall and the direct involvement of adjacent or distant organs by metastasis. In the vast majority of carcinomas identified by CT there is a localized thickening of the gastric wall, though in about 10% of cases the thickening is diffuse (Moss et al 1981a).

CT scanning has significant limitations in staging gastric cancer. The assessment of regional lymph nodes and invasion of adjacent organs is unreliable and understaging is frequent. Overstaging also occurs. However, it is a helpful technique in avoiding other than palliative surgery in patients with extensive metastases and in the detection of postoperative recurrence and metastases (Scatarige & DiSantis 1989). Further refinements in technique may enhance diagnostic accuracy but such improvements will hold little reward for patients unless the findings materially alter treatment (Trenkner et al 1994). The CT demonstration of benign gastric tumors is well established (Fig. 2.15) (Megibow et al 1985) and it may be used to identify malignant change.

Occasionally, evidence of the complications of peptic ulcer, particularly penetration by posterior gastric or duodenal ulcers, can be diagnosed by CT (Madrazo et al 1984).

## Small intestine

The small bowel is readily identified when filled by contrast and differentiation of proximal from distal small bowel is possible partly by the position occupied in the abdominal cavity and partly by the more obvious mucosal pattern seen in the jejunum. Under normal circumstances, there should be little separation of adjacent loops and then only by fat in the bowel wall. The suspensory effect of the mesentery with the supplying blood vessels should be seen. Insufficiently or nonopacified bowel loops can pose considerable problems in the interpretation of suspected abdominal masses. In subacute or chronic small bowel obstruction unenhanced bowel loops can simulate cysts or abscesses. With intravenous contrast enhancement the bowel wall may be further enhanced, mimicking a multilocular cyst or even an abscess wall (Kreel 1984). It is of particular importance to distend fully the duodenal loop and proximal jejunum with oral contrast medium in the search for pancreatic abnormalities.

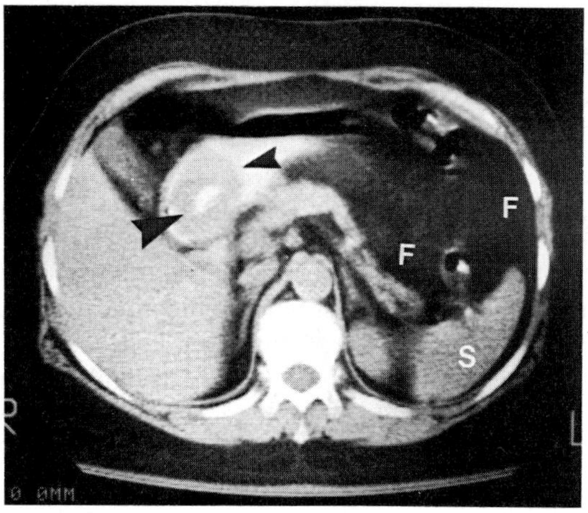


**Fig. 2.15** Leiomyosarcoma of the gastric antrum with surface ulceration (arrows). No evidence of lymph node involvement. Mesenteric fat (F), spleen (S).

Thus, in general, CT is not recommended for the diagnosis of small bowel disease. However, focal disease and its extension to the mesentery can be demonstrated. Lymphoma of the small bowel, which may be symptomatic or occult, can be identified as thickening of the bowel wall and localized dilatation can be used to estimate the extent and staging of the disorder, being shown to correlate well with the Ann Arbor classification (p. 470) of non-Hodgkin's lymphoma (Megibow 1986).

Inflammatory bowel disease may be investigated by CT (p. 665) and, whilst sometimes helpful in the detection of the intrinsic bowel wall disease, it is particularly helpful in the identification of local and widespread complications (Goldberg et al 1983), for example in demonstrating the extent of extracolonic disease and fistulae to structures such as the bladder (Jones 1985). It has been shown that in symptomatic patients with Crohn's disease, CT scanning demonstrates unsuspected findings leading to alteration in medical and surgical treatment in over 25% of cases. CT scanning also enables more accurate and confident assessment of the presence or absence of complications than clinical findings or barium examinations (Fishman et al 1987).

### Large intestine

The colonic wall thickness ranges from 3 to 5 mm and measurements over 5 mm should be the indication for further investigation. Measurements over 1 cm are abnormal if the colon is axial to the slice and is distended normally (Fisher 1982). The colonic lumen is usually smooth when outlined by air or contrast. The outer aspect of the colon is well defined by pericolic fat. Infiltration by tumor and localized inflammatory changes cause loss of normal fat, with increasing soft tissue density. The administration of rectal contrast medium is particularly helpful in examining primary diseases of the distal large bowel and its involvement or otherwise by diseases of other pelvic organs.

Carcinoma of the colon may be identified from the features of the primary mass and the involvement of neighboring or distant structures. As colorectal carcinoma is very common and the prognosis for surgical treatment is related to the stage of disease at the time of diagnosis, CT scanning has been advocated for such staging despite its limitations. CT scanning is particularly good at the detection of local invasion of neighboring structures, liver involvement and distant metastases. The limitations include the inability to determine tumor extension through and along the bowel wall and also the inability to detect involvement of tumor in normal sized lymph nodes (i.e. under 10 mm). Recently the demonstration of perirectal or colonic lymph nodes of any size has been considered to be good evidence of metastases as these are not usually detected on abdominal CT scan in normal patients (Thompson & Trenkner 1994). The detection of such lymph nodes at CT scanning will facilitate more accurate staging.

CT scanning is indicated in patients with suspected recurrent colorectal carcinoma. It can detect abnormalities before the onset of symptoms and when the carcinoembryonic antigen titers are normal (McCarthy et al 1985). The effective demonstration of local tumor recurrence at the site of surgical excision or anastomosis and the detection of isolated hepatic metastases facilitate further management (Moss 1989).

### Liver (Fig. 2.16)

The liver has a complex outline of varying size and configuration. It is seen in the axial tomogram as a relatively homogeneous soft tissue structure occupying most of the right side of the upper abdomen. As described in the ultrasound section (p. 54, see also Fig. 24.4), the segmental anatomy of the liver, described by Couinaud and Bismuth, is now the basis for the correct identification of

A

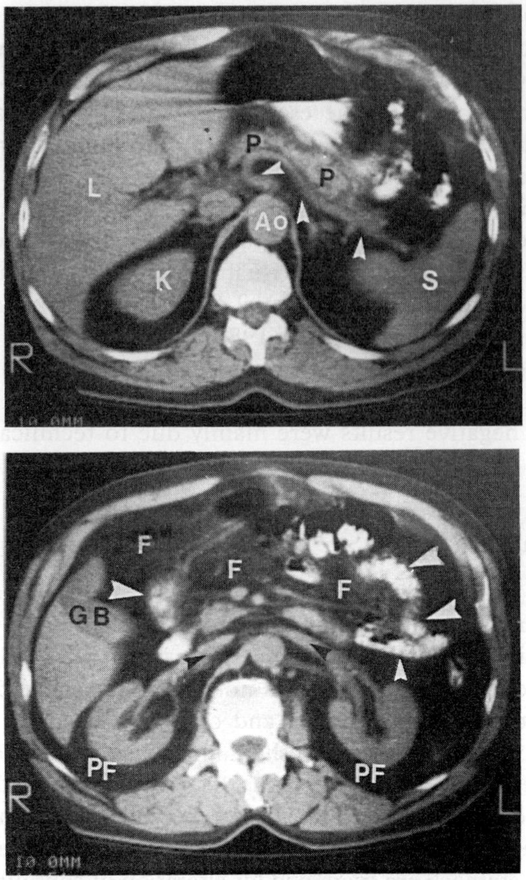


B

**Fig. 2.16** Normal anatomy of the liver. **A** Normal liver (L), spleen (S), kidney (K), pancreas (P), aorta (Ao), celiac axis (arrow), splenic artery (arrows). **B** Gallbladder (GB), contrast medium in small bowel (white arrows), renal veins (black arrow), mesenteric fat (F), perinephric fat (PF).

the internal vascular anatomy of the liver which aids successful surgical resection of a segment or segments of the liver. The liver is divided into eight segments on the basis of the major hepatic veins and four scissurae (Sugarbaker 1990). Consequently surgical planning for partial, single or multiple segmentectomy is facilitated. With this aim, localized lesions of the liver should now be described detailing the segmental position of these as a routine matter when reporting CT scans. The CT examination of the liver has also been significantly improved with the introduction of dynamic contrast enhancement and helical scanning (Bluemke et al 1995).

The CT density of the liver ranges from 54 to 68 Hounsfield units and is generally greater than all other abdominal organs. Owing to this density, the intrahepatic portal and hepatic veins and the bile ducts show up as low density structures. Following contrast enhancement, the blood vessels increase in density and the portal vein can be identified branching from the porta hepatis. The hepatic veins are seen radiating towards the inferior vena cava in the highest slices through the liver. Normally the nondilated intrahepatic bile ducts are not identified. The extrahepatic ducts are seen in one-quarter to one-third of normal patients. The common hepatic duct is 3–5 mm in diameter and is anatomically situated anterior to the portal vein in the porta hepatis. The common bile duct is 3–6 mm in diameter and lies in the lesser omentum behind the duodenal cap, extending downwards to a groove in the head of the pancreas posteriorly, where it unites with the pancreatic duct at the ampulla of Vater. The gallbladder is identified as a thinwalled, circumscribed, oval structure of low attentuation (5–25 Hounsfield units) lying under the liver in the gallbladder fossa.

### *Technique*

Slices through the liver are usually performed both with and without intravenous contrast material, which is given by infusion or bolus techniques (p. 62). Dynamic contrast enhancement is the best method for detecting and differentiating focal lesions of the liver, particularly using the helical scanner (Bluemke & Fishman 1993). Occasionally delayed scanning one or more hours after contrast has been given may help discriminate the hypervascular types of tumor in the liver. Small hepatocellular carcinomas may be detected using lipiodol-enhanced CT. Whilst contrast-enhanced CT is very accurate in the detection and differentiation of liver disease, histological characterization is often complex, requiring both CT and other investigations including fine-needle aspiration biopsy, which may be performed under CT control (Foley & Jochem 1991).

A 10 mm slice thickness with 15–20 mm incrementation is usually sufficient for routine scanning of the liver. Fine cuts of 5 mm or overlapping slices may be required for small lesions or for defining the porta hepatis.

### *Interpretation*

Variations in hepatic density do occur and patients with fatty infiltration (Fig. 2.17) may show a marked decrease in density such that the non-contrasted portal venous radicles may stand out against the low-density hepatic background. Increase in liver density is seen in conditions of increased iron storage; for example, hemochromatosis (Fig. 2.18) or hemosiderosis.

Focal lesions within the hepatic parenchyma are well seen. Cystic disease is usually identified clearly and the most common lesions are simple hepatic cysts and cysts caused by echinococcus. Solid tumors (Fig. 2.14) are differentiated by density differences on the plain scan but can be clarified by contrast enhancement (pp. 61 & 1122). The degree of enhancement varies depending on the vascularity of the tissue and therefore its iodine content during the arterial phase of enhancement. Specific lesions such as cavernous hemangiomata may show progressive enhancement during delayed scans as the contrast-laden blood perfuses slowly through the lesion.

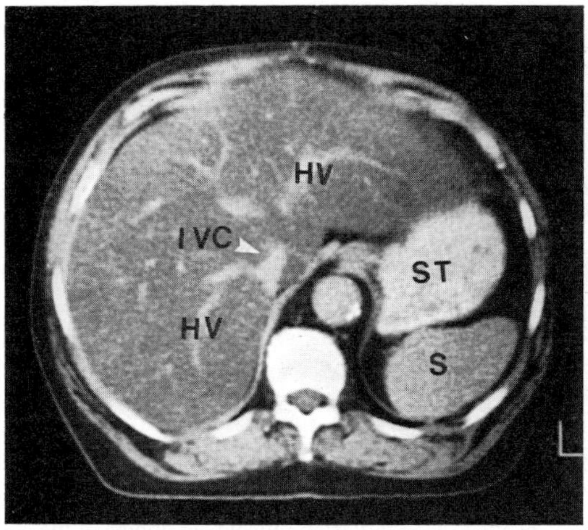


**Fig. 2.17** Fatty infiltration of the liver (alcoholic). Increase in hepatic density. Inferior vena cava (IVC), hepatic veins (HV), stomach (ST), spleen (S).

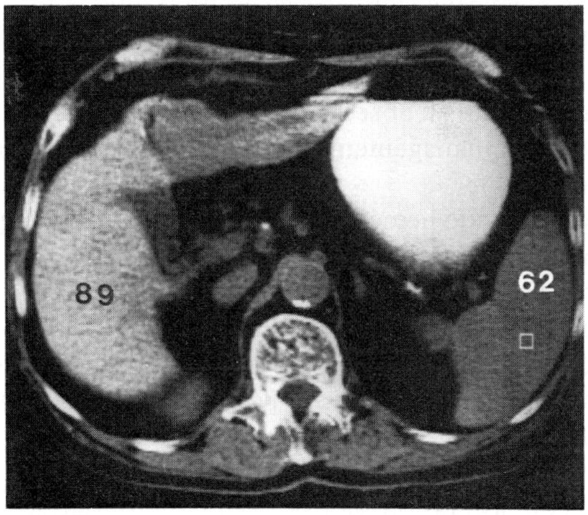


**Fig. 2.18** Hemochromatosis. Axial scan showing dense liver attenuation (89 Hounsfield units) compared with normal splenic density (62 Hounsfield units).

Metastatic disease can be focal (Fig. 2.19) or diffuse (Fig. 2.14). Dynamic hepatic CT has a sensitivity of 85–90% in the detection of metastases in patients with colon cancer and the specificity is more than 95% (Freeny 1988). Hepatic metastases missed at CT are usually less than 1–2 cm in diameter, but it is anticipated that a higher detection rate will be achieved with dynamic helical scanning. Unfortunately the CT characteristics of benign and malignant lesions overlap in nodules smaller than 1 cm and because biopsy of such lesions is often difficult, interval scanning is advised (Ferrucci 1994).

Hepatic abscess may be the result of bacterial, fungal or parasitic organisms, sometimes occurring together. Hematogenous abscesses may complicate arterial or portal venous septic emboli and may be single or multiple. Infections with gas-forming organisms may be identified by the presence of gas in the lesions. Patients with immune

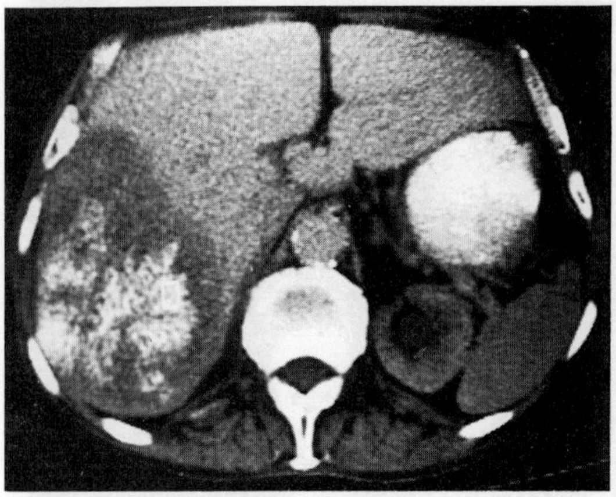

**Fig. 2.19** Calcified secondary from mucoid carcinoma of the colon.

suppression are susceptible to opportunistic viral or fungal infections and hepatic abscess may develop in such patients. Typically such abscesses are multiple and small and there may be similar abscesses in the spleen. CT-guided aspiration biopsy and placement of draining catheters within an abscess are procedures frequently utilized for the management of hepatic abscesses (Foley & Jochem 1991).

Post-traumatic hematoma in the liver and its complications are usually well displayed by CT.

In the evaluation of obstructive jaundice, CT is of particular value in identifying the site and nature of the obstruction and the more distant involvement of other organs (Baron 1991). It is of particular help in resolving the nature of obstruction at the lower end of the common bile duct (Fig. 2.20), especially when combined with fine-needle aspiration biopsy in the appropriate circumstances.

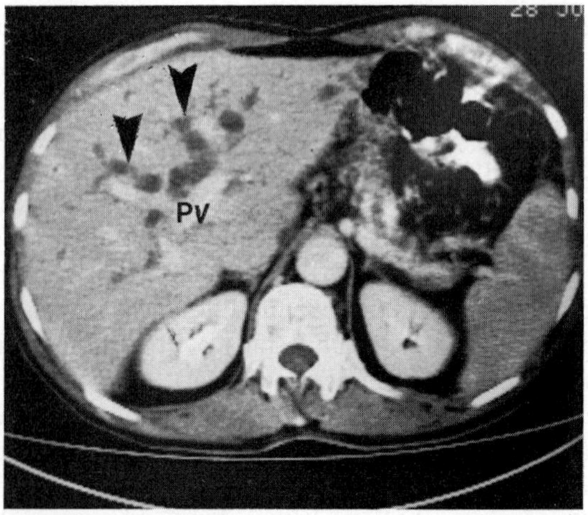


**Fig. 2.20** Obstructive jaundice (secondary to cancer of the pancreas). Dilated intrahepatic ducts (black arrows). Note the relationship to normal portal veins (PV) enhanced with intravenous contrast.

## Spleen

The spleen varies considerably in size and shape but can normally measure up to 14 cm in length. Accessory splenic masses may also be identified. The spleen is homogeneous, with a density of 30–68 Hounsfield units, which is less than that of the liver.

### *Technique*

Scanning is undertaken with 10 mm incremental contiguous slices before and after intravenous contrast given by infusion and by bolus.

### *Interpretation*

Splenic enlargement and volume can be assessed accurately from cross-sectional images taken at 1 cm increments (Moss et al 1981b). In practice, it is usually a subjective opinion considered when the craniocaudal measurement exceeds 14 cm.

In neoplastic disease, CT defines focal abnormalities. Nodules or lymphoma of secondary metastatic disease are identified as regions of lower density against the background of normal splenic tissue (Piekarski et al 1980, Frick et al 1981).

Inflammatory disease is indicated by old calcified granulomas and an abscess by a low-density area similar to abscess in other solid viscera. Pseudocysts associated with pancreatitis in and around the spleen are easily delineated.

CT is currently the best method for assessing blunt abdominal trauma. Dynamic contrast-enhanced CT is very sensitive (95%) for the detection of splenic injury (Taylor et al 1991). The ability to image the organ accurately has supported a conservative approach to splenic trauma and the preservation of splenic tissue.

## Pancreas (Fig. 2.21)

The cross-sectional anatomical display of CT is ideal for the demonstration of the pancreas and its relationships. Generally, it is better displayed in patients with significant adipose tissue in the retroperitoneum and a lack of fat to demarcate tissue planes in thin people and children can make definition difficult. The pancreas lies in a horizontal plane, with the head being slightly caudal to the body and tail. Variations in position dictate how many slices are needed to demonstrate the entire organ. The portal and splenic veins lie behind the head and body of the pancreas such that the contrast-filled splenic vein provides a useful marker of the upper posterior border of the body and tail. Other anatomical features and the size of the pancreas are described on page 56. The texture of the gland varies with age. In the young, it may appear solid and homogeneous, with a smooth margin anteriorly. A lobulated appearance

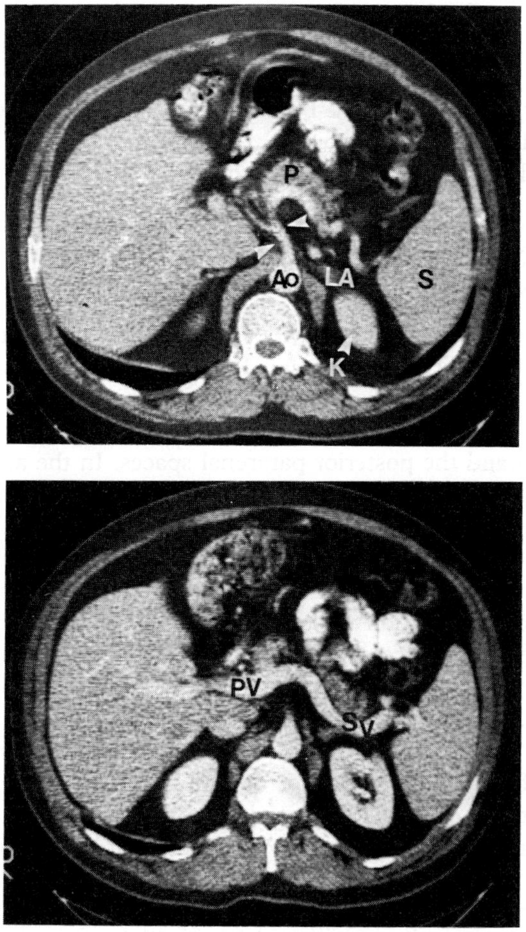


**Fig. 2.21** Normal anatomy of the pancreas. **A** Axial scan through pancreas (P), aorta (Ao), celiac axis (arrows), spleen (S), left adrenal (LA). **B** Section 10 mm below **A** showing splenic vein (SV), portal vein (PV).

is also observed in older or obese patients and this is referred to as fatty replacement or infiltration. It does not usually indicate a compromise of pancreatic function.

*Technique*

The gastric antrum, duodenal loop and proximal small bowel loops can easily be confused with an abnormal mass unless they are well filled with oral contrast. The number of important adjacent vascular structures also requires the liberal use of intravenous contrast by infusion or bolus techniques. The slice thickness used should be 5–10 mm with contiguous or overlapping incrementation.

*Interpretation*

CT is considered to be the most sensitive imaging modality for the diagnosis and staging of acute pancreatitis (Fig. 2.22). Early CT evaluation has allowed the identification of a group of patients at high risk from local

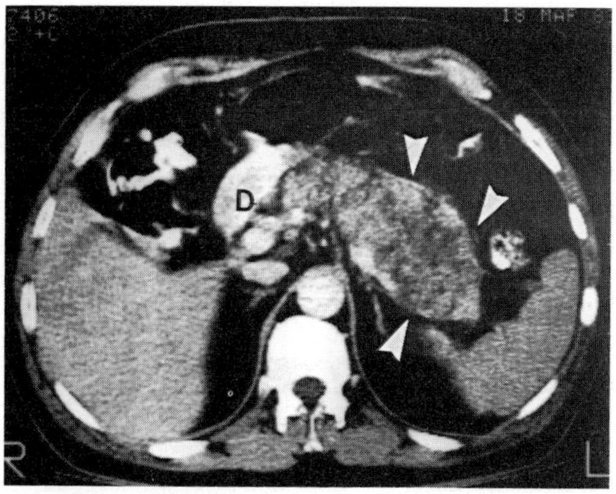


**Fig. 2.22** Acute pancreatitis. Large edematous pancreas, particularly body and tail (arrows). Duodenal loop (D).

complications, particularly those with pancreatic necrosis or extrapancreatic phlegmon (Balthazar 1989). In turn this allows more active clinical monitoring, the early introduction of intensive treatment and further CT monitoring as indicated (p. 1255).

In chronic pancreatitis (Figs 2.23 and 2.24) ultrasound scanning is more effective and economic in the monitoring of progress (p. 1271) though the signs of chronic pancreatitis are well displayed at CT.

CT scanning is the best available method for the detection of tumor spread beyond the margins of the pancreas (p. 1291) or more distantly and therefore identifies those patients unsuitable for curative surgery. Staging of pancreatic carcinoma is likely to be improved with introduction of helical scanning with dynamic contrast enhancement. The CT criteria for resectability include an intrapancreatic neoplasm usually less than 2 cm in diameter, surrounded by normal parenchyma without evidence of local or extracapsular extension, vascular invasion or nodal or hepatic metastases (Freeny 1989b). The pancreatic duct is frequently dilated but is not a specific sign for malignancy or

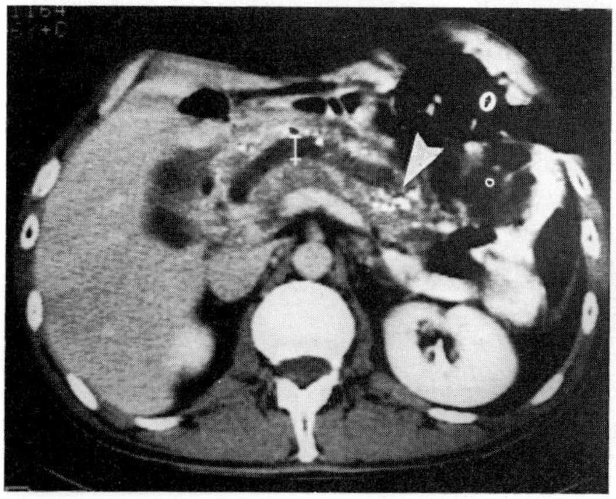

**Fig. 2.23** Chronic pancreatitis. Large dilated duct (1.1 cm), shown by marker. Calcification (arrows).

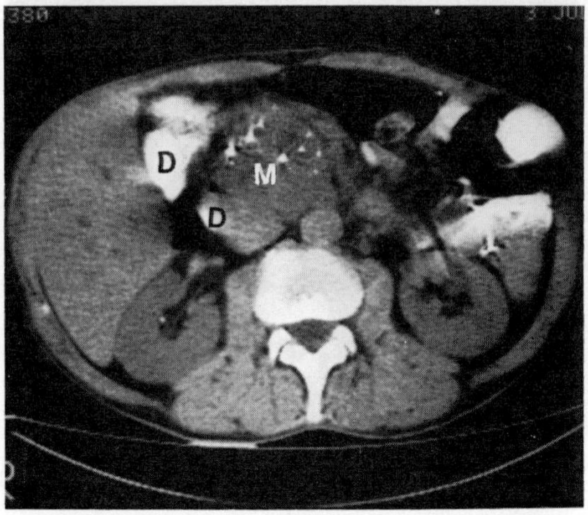


**Fig. 2.24** Acute on chronic pancreatitis. Mass (M) in head of pancreas with calcification but also evidence of acute pancreatitis. There is blurring of the fat plane around the head and displacement of the duodenal loop (D).

chronic pancreatitis (Luetmer et al 1989). Fine-needle aspiration biopsy under CT guidance is often needed to confirm the diagnosis in suspected cases, though sampling may be difficult or misleading, especially in focal inflammatory disease which may accompany carcinoma. Other tumors such as insulinoma and lymphoma can mimic carcinoma on CT scans. The collection of volumetric data by helical scanning, with minimal interference due to patient movement, allows accurate 3D reconstruction of the data and is likely to reveal peripancreatic and vascular involvement in finer detail (Fishman et al 1992).

Cystic neoplasms (Fig. 2.25) can be difficult to distinguish from cystic complications of pancreatitis and there are no characteristic CT findings. However, in suspected cystic lesions fine-needle aspiration biopsy with CT guidance is frequently diagnostic. CT scanning will identify

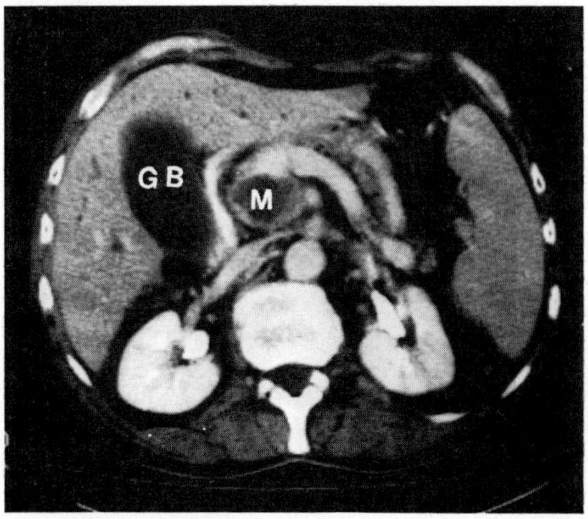


**Fig. 2.25** Cystadenocarcinoma of pancreas (M). Dilated gallbladder (GB).

the site of most endocrine tumors of the pancreas over 2 cm in size and, with attention to technique, many of those between 1 and 2 cm. However, small tumors can rarely be displayed at CT scanning and pancreatic venous sampling and endoscopic (p. 125) or intraoperative ultrasound examination are often required.

### The retroperitoneum and associated structures

(Dodds et al 1986, Rubenstein & Whalen 1986)

The retroperitoneum is divided into several compartments by layers of fascia visible on CT because of the presence of fat along fascial planes. The most important compartments are the anterior pararenal space, the perirenal spaces and the posterior pararenal spaces. In the anterior pararenal space lie the duodenal loop, the pancreas and the ascending and descending colon. This space is the one most commonly affected by retroperitoneal infection. The perirenal spaces contain the kidneys and surrounding fat. No communication exists between the two sides and so perinephric abscesses or fluid collections are usually confined within the posterolateral aspect of the affected space. The posterior pararenal spaces contain a thin layer of fat between the posterior renal fascia and the transversalis fascia. A potential for communication between the two spaces exists via the anterior abdominal wall.

Tumors of the retroperitoneal space are identified by their mass effect and obstruction of the urinary tract. Malignant lesions are associated with obliteration of normal fascial planes, which is often an early sign of malignancy.

Retroperitoneal lymph nodes are recognized by their proximity to normal vascular structures. There are three groups of nodes arranged around the aorta (para-aortic), the inferior vena cava (precaval) and those between these (aortocaval). Typically, the fat plane between the aorta and the inferior vena cava is obscured by lymph node enlargement (Fig. 2.26) and when this is massive, normal contours may be completely lost in an encasing mantle. The outline of neighboring structures such as muscles may also be modified by varying degrees of lymph node enlargement. Retrocrural lymph nodes are visible within the fat contained by the reflections of the diaphragmatic crura and may be distinguished from vascular structures such as the azygos vein by contrast enhancement.

The CT criteria for the size of normal lymph nodes have been difficult to establish. Whilst in the early experience with CT scanning a diameter of 2 cm was taken as the upper limit of normal size for para-aortic lymph nodes, more recently lymph nodes measuring 1 cm or more in diameter have been considered abnormal. Using this criterion the sensitivity for detection of lymph node enlargement with CT ranges from 65% to 95% and the specificity from 80% to 100%. Difficulty remains in detecting disease in lymph nodes less than 1 cm in diameter; lowering the

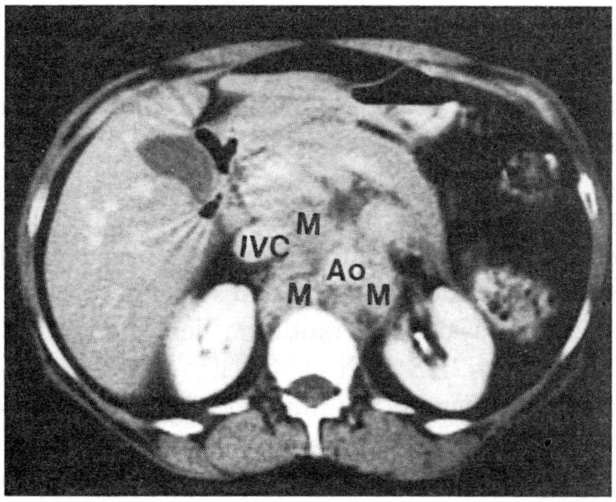


**Fig. 2.26** Retroperitoneal lymphoma (M), aorta (Ao), inferior vena cava (IVC).

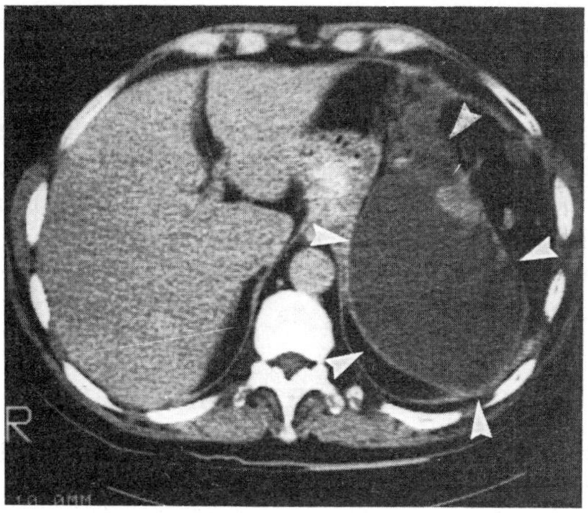


**Fig. 2.27** Large left subphrenic abscess (arrows) following splenectomy for thrombocytopenia.

upper limit of normal lymph node size to 0.5 cm raises the sensitivity to 88% but lowers specificity to 44% (Stomper et al 1987). Whilst combining the use of lymphography with CT improves accuracy, a significant false negative rate persists even after both examinations have been performed.

The normal inferior vena cava lies to the right of the aorta, gradually widening above the union of the common iliac veins. It has a diameter of 2–3 cm and is usually easily seen, though occasionally it is barely discernible. It varies in appearance during differing phases of respiration and may alter in different scan slices in the same patient. Developmental anomalies are not infrequent.

The abdominal aorta has a normal diameter of less than 3 cm and gradually tapers inferiorly to the bifurcation at the L3–4 level. Surrounding fat usually allows good visualization of the aorta and the origins of major branches, particularly with contrast enhancement.

### The peritoneal cavity and mesentery (Meyers 1986)

The peritoneal cavity may be divided into the upper abdomen, the lesser sac and the pelvic cavity. The latter is gravitationally dependent, is frequently the site of abscesses, especially postoperatively, and is a collection area for hematoma or ascites. The paravesical fossae communicate with the upper abdomen via the right and left paracolic gutters. In the upper abdomen, the transverse mesocolon divides the peritoneal cavity into supramesocolic and inframesocolic compartments. In the right upper quadrant the peritoneum reflects over the diaphragm and liver to create right subphrenic and right subhepatic spaces. Peritoneal reflections on the undersurface of the liver form anterior and posterior subhepatic spaces separated by the origin of the transverse mesocolon. The falciform ligament separates the right and left subphrenic spaces, which communicate with each other along the free edges of the ligament. The lesser sac lies behind the lesser omentum, stomach and duodenum, communicating with the peritoneal cavity via the foramen of Winslow. Posteriorly, the lesser sac is bounded by the peritoneum overlying the pancreas and left adrenal gland.

All of these spaces may potentially communicate, allowing the collection and spread of fluids, sterile or infected, throughout the abdominal cavity (Fig. 2.27). CT is an ideal method for the detection of such collections and is of special value in identifying their location and full extent. The nature of the fluid and its source may be documented and CT-guided aspiration and the placement of catheter drainage simplifies therapeutic management (Churchill 1989). CT is particularly helpful when perforation of the bowel has occurred, especially if this has been small, self-sealing or well contained by adjacent structures (Ghahremani 1993). CT scanning is also a very sensitive method of detecting peritoneal metastases in the absence of ascites. Involvement of the bowel wall, omentum or the parietal peritoneum is well displayed (Walkey et al 1988).

The small bowel mesentery reflects from the posterior parietal peritoneum to invest the jejunum and ileum, connecting these viscera to the posterior abdominal wall. The mesenteric attachment extends obliquely downwards across the abdomen from the left upper quadrant to the pelvis in front of the right sacroiliac joint. Within the investing layers of peritoneum may be found fat (especially in obese patients), mesenteric blood vessels, lymphatic channels and nodes.

The transverse mesocolon is a similar structure to the small bowel mesentery, investing the colon especially in its transverse portion. Lymph nodes seen in mesenteric structures should not exceed 1 cm in diameter.

### The pelvic cavity

Ultrasound scanning is the mainstay of imaging the pelvis,

especially in female patients. However, whilst excellent anatomical detail may be seen in the pelvis with CT, magnetic resonance imaging (MRI) is increasingly used for the display of pelvic organs (McCarthy 1992). Optimal results for CT are achieved by ensuring that the bowel loops are well filled with contrast medium. Intravenous contrast material is also given to enhance vascular and urinary structures. Rectal and/or vaginal enhancement may also be needed (p. 62).

## MAGNETIC RESONANCE IMAGING (MRI)

MRI has been heralded as the most exciting current development in diagnostic medicine (Margulis 1985). Although clinical application is recent, MRI scanners have been introduced rapidly in the United States and Europe because the method combines most of the advantages of other diagnostic imaging methods, without many of the disadvantages. Its spectroscopic application will enable biological events to be examined at the molecular level in the living cell (Radda 1985).

MRI techniques evolved in American laboratories in 1946 (Andrew 1984) and the first accounts of successful demonstration of nuclear magnetic resonance (NMR) in matter were published simultaneously (Purcell et al 1946, Bloch et al 1946). In 1973, Lauterbur demonstrated the first image using NMR.

In the application of NMR in human medicine, two distinct approaches have been made. First, large magnets have been used to produce high-resolution NMR spectra from selected tissues particularly for the detection of phosphate ($^{31}$P) and carbon ($^{13}$C) radicals in various biological transformations (Hoult et al 1974, Cady et al 1983). Secondly, and of more immediate clinical application, NMR has been utilized to image organs – magnetic resonance imaging; the word "nuclear" has been conventionally deleted from the title to avoid political and other confrontations (Meaney 1984). Although the sequences of radiofrequency (RF) pulses and magnetic field gradients used to produce MRI are designed primarily to display stationary objects, information can be obtained about motion such as blood flow (Crooks & Kaufman 1984) and MR angiography (MRA) is now well established in the investigation of the portal circulation and of renal vascular disease.

### **Physical principles** (Pykett et al 1982, Rosen & Brady 1983, Baddeley et al 1986)

Atomic nuclei with either an odd number of protons or neutrons (or both) possess the property of spin (intrinsic angular momentum) analogous to the spin of the earth around its axis. Stable atomic nuclei of this type include hydrogen ($^{1}$H), phosphorus ($^{31}$P), carbon ($^{13}$C) and fluorine ($^{19}$F). $^{1}$H and $^{31}$P have been the nuclei most studied in NMR systems. Hydrogen, the most abundant element in living tissues, particularly in body water, consists of a single proton and is the most appropriate element for human study (Mathur-De Vre 1984).

Each nucleus possesses a charge of electrical energy, so that the spinning nucleus creates a magnetic field or moment. The nucleus thus acts as a small magnet dipole. Under the influence of the earth's magnetic field these magnetic charges create a random orientation of the dipolar nuclei (Fig. 2.28). However, if a stronger magnetic field is applied a significant number of dipoles will reorientate themselves to become more aligned along the lines of force of the applied magnetic field. At equilibrium, the magnetic fields of these reorientated nuclei form a macroscopic magnetic moment or vector.

The nuclear resonance phenomenon can be induced by the application of a short radiofrequency (RF) pulse through a coil or antenna surrounding the subject under study. The RF radiation creates a small additional magnetic field rotating around the vector. If an appropriate frequency of rotation is chosen, some of the realigned nuclei experience a force displacing the magnetic moment from the position parallel to the applied magnetic field (Fig. 2.29 a & b). This displacement causes a synchronous rotation of the magnetic moment, termed precession, the motion being analogous to that created in a spinning top under the influence of the earth's gravitational field. The angle of precession between the static field and the magnetization vector is dependent on the amount of energy received from the RF pulse and increases whilst the RF

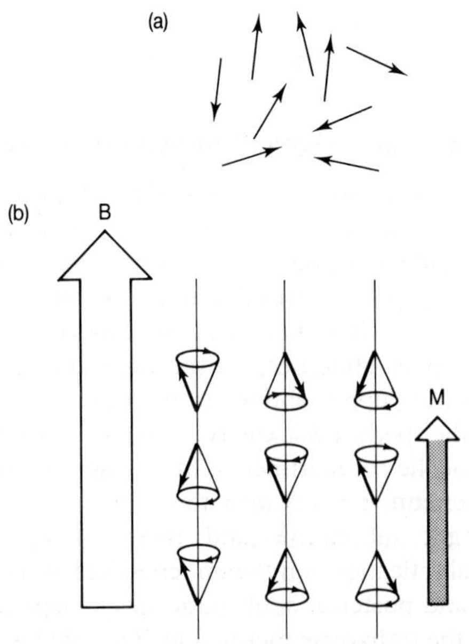


**Fig. 2.28** (a) Protons not exposed to a strong magnetic field are randomly aligned. (b) Protons exposed to a strong magnetic field (B) precess around the axis of the field and have a net longitudinal magnetization (M) (Baddeley et al 1986).

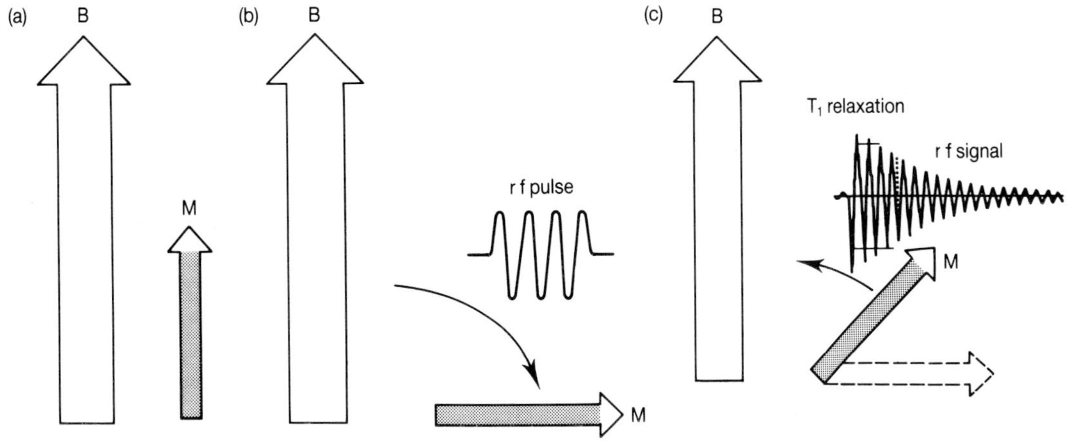


**Fig. 2.29** (a) At rest ($T_1$ longitudinal relaxation) the net proton magnetization (M) is aligned with the main magnetic field. (b) During a 90° excitation RF pulse, net magnetization (M) is rotated into the transverse plane. (c) Following the excitation pulse the magnetization returns towards the longitudinal axis, emitting an RF signal determined by $T_1$ relaxation time.

pulse is switched on. By switching the RF generator on and off, pulses of energy may be transmitted which tip the vector off axis to induce a signal from precessional motion (Fig. 2.29c). Typically values are chosen to rotate nuclear magnetization through 90° and 180° (90° pulse or 180° pulse).

In static magnetic fields, the nuclei of NMR-sensitive elements respond only to stimulation by RF pulses of a particular frequency, termed the resonant or Larmor frequency. The resonant frequency of a subject is directly proportional to the strength of the static magnetic field.

Once precession of the magnetic moment has been induced it is a simple matter to detect this motion. The coil used to transmit the RF pulse can also be used to detect the NMR signal. When the RF pulse is turned off the precessional motion decays and the vector returns to the original position of equilibrium, emitting a fading signal which is referred to as free induction decay (FID). FID can be detected, amplified, encoded and measured.

The physical processes involved are characterized by two species-related time constants: $T_1$ (longitudinal or spin–lattice) and $T_2$ (transverse or spin–spin) relaxation times. These constants account for the excellent contrast obtained in images. Various tissue factors determine $T_1$ and $T_2$ and both are sensitive to the degree of molecular movement. In MRI only the signals from liquids are observed; rigidly bound nuclei do not produce signals, hence proton images from compact bone are 'silent' and appear black on the image. Variations in $T_1$ relaxation time occur according to free water content and inherent differences in tissue relaxation times may therefore be sufficient to distinguish normal from abnormal tissues. The choice of RF pulse sequence utilized for MRI is most important since a number of variables influence the strength of signal obtained in creating an image and the correct choice of parameters for examination is essential for the production of diagnostic images.

*Pulse sequences* (Smith 1985)

The RF pulse sequences which will give optimal information in particular clinical situations depend on intrinsic tissue characteristics and the type of information required. These are determined at the time of examination by the imaging specialist, who aims for optimal tissue contrast.

The physical variables which are utilized in MRI allow the method to be more sensitive and flexible than CT and the promised development of new pulse sequence techniques holds even more favorable possibilities for the future role of magnetic resonance in organ imaging (Glazer et al 1985, Stark et al 1986).

*Image quality*

During MRI a vast amount of information is obtained at each sequence of data collection. The signals measured by the RF coil are converted into a display of relative single intensities. All sequences have a common pathway, starting with spin induction, followed by an excitation phase, an encoding phase, refocusing and then signal collection and display. Each of these phases can be manipulated by control of the scanning parameters to produce the signal best suited to the examination in progress. Modern equipment uses varying signal parameters to enhance $T_1$ and $T_2$ weighting. It is not possible to obtain pure $T_1$ and $T_2$ images because of the mixed signal intensity of both of these physical constants and others such as proton density. However, by suitable manipulation of the scan and protocols, images with emphasis on one or other physical constant (weighting) can be obtained. Factors involved in the quality of the images include the following.

***Contrast resolution.*** The differences in signal intensity from different tissues account for the degree of contrast, which has been assessed as 70 times greater than in CT imaging (Margulis 1985).

***Spatial resolution.*** In all imaging systems there is always some degradation of the signal and in MRI significant impairment of spatial resolution occurs owing to reduced signal-to-noise ratio (SNR). Methods which improve spatial resolution by increasing the signal-to-noise ratio unfortunately increase the time of acquisition of data and a compromise solution is generally sought. One method of reducing the scanning time is to obtain data from many sections of the patient at the same time, a process termed multiple slice acquisition, and all currently produced equipment collects data in this way.

***Magnetic field strength.*** Though spatial resolution in MRI is not yet comparable with CT the use of magnets with high field strength has significantly improved the signal-to-noise ratio obtained and consequently better spatial resolution can be achieved.

***Movement.*** Patient movement, whether voluntary or involuntary, degrades the image. Cardiac and respiratory gating have been utilized to overcome some of the problems.

### *Chemical shift*

The resonant frequency of a nucleus is modified by small changes in the associated magnetic field as a result of the shielding effect of the surrounding molecular electrons. The same nucleus placed in chemically different groups will thus have different resonant frequencies. For example, in ethyl alcohol with three chemical groups, $CH_3$, $CH_2$ and OH, three different resonant frequencies or chemical shifts can be demonstrated and whilst the differences are small, precise information about each chemical group is obtained.

While organic chemists have used the NMR technique for many years, the main medical use for NMR spectroscopy has been in recording the positions and intensities of $^{31}P$ peaks in muscle disorders (Radda et al 1983). However, the distribution of $^{13}C$ (Alger & Shulman 1984) and $^{23}Na$ (Maudsley & Hilal 1984) are under experimental study.

## **Instrumentation** (Pykett 1983, Hanley 1984)

The physically largest component in an MRI system is the magnet, but other items of equipment are equally important. The magnet system provides the means of inducing the static magnetic field whilst the radiofrequency (RF) coils provide the means to "probe" the nuclei and so induce nuclear magnetic resonance.

The RF coils transmit and receive signals which can be coded, stored and processed in systems linked to a computer.

### *Magnets*

The requirements of the magnet include a magnetic field of adequate strength and stability for the duration of study. Whilst organ imaging can be very effective using magnets of relatively low strength from 0.1 to 0.6 tesla (1 tesla (T) = 10 000 gauss (G)), best tissue differentiation is obtained in the 0.5–1.5 T range. The magnetic field strength needed for chemical shift spectroscopy is high, 1.5–2 T. The higher energies employed allow an increase in the signal-to-noise ratio in the system, giving an improvement in sensitivity and therefore better spatial resolution.

Recently, ceramic superconducting materials have been developed and it is likely that cryogenic magnet technology will improve substantially, with significant cost reduction.

The choice of a magnet system is usually determined by the available financial resources. If it is intended to perform NMR chemical spectroscopy in diagnosis, then cryogenic magnet systems are essential.

### *Hazards* (Saunders & Smith 1984)

Some general hazards of high-strength magnetic fields are recognized. These include human injuries and damage which may result from the attraction of magnetic objects to the magnet and interference with surgically implanted devices (e.g. cardiac pacemakers), or cathode ray tubes, magnetic computer tapes and disks and X-ray tubes. Additionally, large moving objects such as motor vehicles and passenger lifts can interfere with the homogeneity of the magnetic field in the diagnostic system and the appropriate shielding of MRI systems may pose considerable design problems.

A number of patients, particularly children, find immersion in the tunnel of the magnet system unbearably claustrophobic. Patient co-operation is a prerequisite for a diagnostic MRI study.

Because of the remote possibility of induced current affecting myocardial muscle contractility, appropriate resuscitation equipment should be available at all installations and a physician trained in resuscitation should always be available.

### *Radiofrequency (RF) coils* (Pykett 1983, Edelman et al 1985)

RF coils are placed around the patient to transmit RF waves for the induction of NMR in the patient and to detect the emitted signal from the resonating nuclei. Various types of coils have been developed, depending on the system in use and the anatomical part of the patient to be examined.

Surface coils are being introduced for specific demonstration of suitable anatomical parts, such as the mastoid process or the orbit. They are designed to demonstrate the particular part of interest to best advantage. Spatial resolution is high with surface coils but the depth of the field examined is limited. Multicoil array development allows the use of more than one surface coil at a time and such arrays have been developed to allow the examination of the entire abdomen and/or pelvis in a short interval of time.

The RF generator with its sophisticated electronic controls and computer provide the measuring system required.

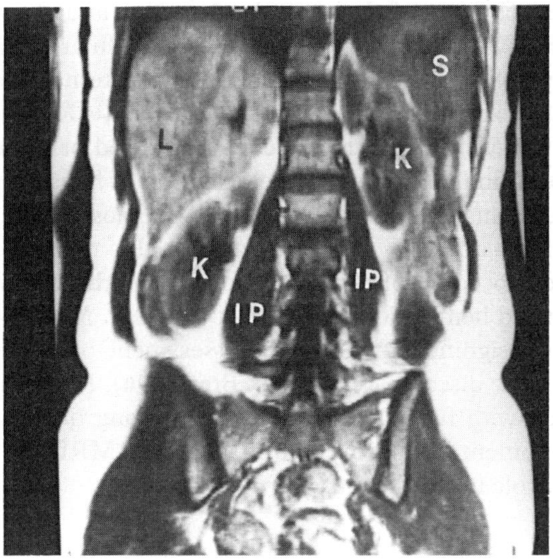


**Fig. 2.30** MRI. Coronal section showing normal anatomy. Liver (L), spleen (S), kidney (K), ileopsoas (IP).

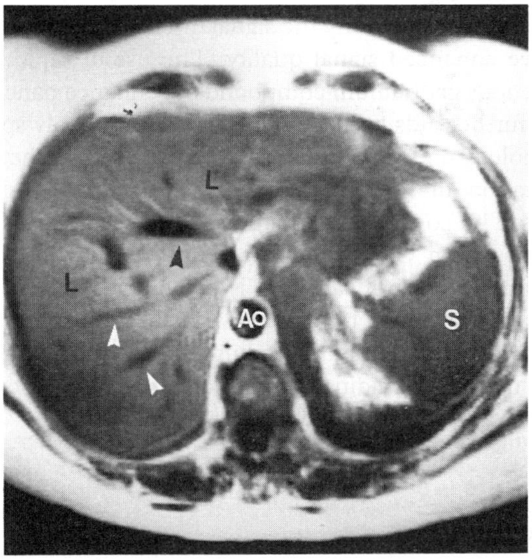


**Fig. 2.31** MRI. Transverse section of upper abdomen. Liver (L), spleen (S), portal vein (black arrow), aorta (Ao), hepatic vein (white arrows).

*Display system*

A dedicated computer is used to control the entire imaging system including display. Because of the relative simplicity of magnetic systems most advances and improvements in MRI will depend on advances in RF coil design and software improvements. Further exploration of the instrumentation, imaging parameters and methods appears to be unlimited (Cho et al 1984). MRI data are displayed on a visual display unit of the type used in CT imaging and similar adjustments to the image through "windowing" can be performed. Images are generally photographed by a multiformat camera. Display of chemical shift spectroscopy is usually graphical.

*Paramagnetic contrast agents* (Carr & Gadian 1985)

The relaxation time ($T_1$ and $T_2$) of nuclei can be altered by the use of paramagnetic compounds. Various agents have been used, particularly iron, manganese, chromium and gadolinium. The action of paramagnetic agents is complex and depends on a number of factors, which include dose, the properties of the agent itself and characteristics of the tissue to be demonstrated and the timing and sequencing of the parameters of investigation.

In the abdominal cavity, iron, especially ferric salts and chelates of gadolinium, are useful in enhancing the gastrointestinal tract, particularly the duodenal loop when imaging the pancreas. Gadolinium chelates enhance liver and pancreatic tumors after intravenous injection. No short-term toxic effects have yet been observed when using gadolinium chelates but long-term toxicity has to be assessed. Disadvantages in using such agents include the need for an intravenous injection and an increase in the time of examination.

## MRI in the abdominal cavity

As yet the application of MRI to diseases of the abdominal cavity is problematic, primarily owing to degradation of image quality due to respiration, cardiac motion and bowel peristalsis (Hricak 1984). Nonetheless, excellent diagnostic images can be achieved, particularly in the pelvic cavity and retroperitoneum. Sections of the normal abdomen are shown in Figures 2.30 and 2.31.

*Liver*

Considerable improvements in scanning methods, especially rapid scanning techniques, motion artefact reduction and improvements in contrast enhancement have resulted in a significant increase in the use of MRI for liver disease (Chezmar 1991). Some authors believe that MRI is the technique of choice in the detection and characterization of liver tumors, especially hepatocellular carcinoma and lymphoma. It is recommended as an alternative or follow-up examination in patients in whom CT scanning with intravenous contrast is contraindicated or where CT has been indeterminate in the detection of hepatic metastases. Hemangioma of the liver is diagnosed with 93% specificity and 89% sensitivity and MRI is recommended as the procedure of choice for confirming the presence of suspected hemangioma (Egglin et al 1990). MRI is developing a significant role in the assessment of biliary and pancreatic disease (Reinhold & Bret 1996). It is anticipated that with further reductions in scanning time and the development of improved contrast agents MRI will play a major role in the diagnosis of liver disease.

### *Pancreas*

Technical advances have improved the results of MRI in pancreatic disease. More rapid scanning techniques which have reduced movement artefact and the development of methods for suppressing the signal intensity obtained from fat have enhanced signal quality. The use of rapid bolus intravenous gadolinium compounds to enhance pancreatic tissue further aids accurate diagnosis. Reasonably specific morphology and signal intensity features permit the characterization of most pancreatic disorders. MRI should therefore be considered in patients with suspicious symptoms in whom CT findings are equivocal or difficult to interpret, where a focal mass is present in patients with chronic pancreatitis, in patients with suspected endocrine tumors and indeterminate findings at CT and in patients with suggestive findings of pancreatitis and uncertain findings at CT (Semelka & Ascher 1993).

### *Abdominal vasculature*

Magnetic resonance (MR) is exceptionally sensitive to movement and this property has been employed to measure blood flow through the vascular system. MR angiography (MRA) identifies blood flowing in blood vessels in terms of velocity and direction. MRA is performed by two different methods: time-of-flight, in which flow-related vascular events are observed, or flow-dependent phase phenomena in which gradients are applied during phase dispersion to identify vascular movement and flow. Two or three-dimensional reconstructions are possible with either technique (Keller et al 1989). MR angiography is an established technique for the noninvasive demonstration of the abdominal aorta and its branches (Edelman 1993). The portal venous system can be displayed reliably and accurately (Hughes et al 1996).

### *Gastrointestinal tract*

MRI remains largely an experimental technique in the diagnosis of disorders of the bowel. Physiological movements are reduced by preliminary fasting, the use of IV glucagon and good breath-holding technique. Faster scanning times and the routine use of paramagnetic contrast agents to enhance the bowel lumen are essential for good signal definition. Optimal small bowel opacification is still difficult to achieve.

With attention to technique and detail, MRI criteria for staging esophageal and colorectal cancer have been determined. However, at present MR does not show any advantage over CT or intraoperative US. It has been proposed as an experimental tool to study gastric emptying as it simultaneously allows measurement of secretion and motor function.

## REFERENCES


Alger J R, Shulman R G 1984 Metabolic applications of high-resolution $^{13}C$ nuclear magnetic resonance spectroscopy. British Medical Bulletin 40: 160–164

Ambrose J 1973 Computerized transverse axial scanning (tomography): Part II. Clinical application. British Journal of Radiology 46: 1023–1047

Andrew E R 1984 A historical review of NMR and its clinical applications. British Medical Bulletin 40: 115–119

Ansell G 1970 Adverse reactions to contrast agents. Scope of problem. Investigative Radiology 5: 374–391

Baddeley H, Doddrell D, Irving M, Brooks W 1986 Magnetic resonance imaging in gastroenterology and hepatology. Journal of Gastroenterology and Hepatology 1: 491–497

Balfe D M, Koehler R E, Karstaedt N, Stanley R J, Sagel S S 1981 Computed tomography of gastric neoplasms. Radiology 140: 431–436

Balthazar E J 1989 CT diagnosis and staging of acute pancreatitis. Radiologic Clinics of North America 27: 19–37

Baron R L 1991 Computed tomography of the biliary tree. Radiologic Clinics of North America 29: 1235–1250

Behan M, Kazam E 1978 Sonography of the common bile duct: value of the right anterior oblique view. American Journal of Roentgenology 130: 701–709

Bismuth H, Houssin D, Castaing D 1982 Major and minor segmentectomies "reglées" in liver surgery. World Journal of Surgery 6: 10–24

Bloch F, Hansen W W, Packard M E 1946 Nuclear induction. Physical Reviews 69: 1–7

Bluemke D A, Fishman E K 1993 Spiral CT of the liver. American Journal of Roentgenology 160: 787–792

Bluemke D A, Soyer P, Fishman E K 1995 Helical (Spiral) C T of the liver. Radiological Clinics of North America 33: 863–886

Blumhagen J D, Maclin L, Krauter D, Rosenbaum D M, Weinberger E 1988 Sonographic diagnosis of hypertrophic pyloric stenosis. American Journal of Roentgenology 150: 1367–1370

Boyce G A, Sivak M V Jr 1990 Endoscopic ultrasonography in the diagnosis of pancreatic tumors. Gastrointestinal Endoscopy 36: S28–S32

Cady E B, Costello A M de L, Dawson M J et al 1983 Non-invasive investigation of cerebral metabolism in newborn infants by phosphorus nuclear magnetic resonance spectroscopy. Lancet 1: 1059–1062

Campbell J P, Wilson S R 1988 Pancreatic neoplasms: how useful is evaluation with US? Radiology 167: 341–344

Carr D H, Gadian D G 1985 Contrast agents in magnetic resonance imaging. Clinical Radiology 36: 561–568

Carroll B A 1989 US of the gastrointestinal tract. Radiology 172: 605–608
Chezmar J L 1991 Magnetic resonance of the liver technique. Radiologic Clinics of North America 29: 1251–1258
Cho Z-H, Kim H S, Oh C H, Park H W, Lee S W 1984 NMR imaging: principles, algorithms and systems. In: Nalcioglu O, Cho Z-H (eds) Selected topics in image science. Lecture notes in medical informatics, Vol 23. Springer-Verlag, Berlin, p 277
Choi B I, Park J H, Kim B H, Kim S H, Han M C, Kim C-W 1989 Small hepatocellular carcinoma: detection with sonography, computed tomography (CT), angiography and Lipiodol-CT. British Journal of Radiology 62: 897–903
Churchill R J 1989 CT of intra-abdominal fluid collections. Radiologic Clinics of North America 27: 653–666
Cohen S M, Kurtz A B 1991 Biliary sonography. Radiologic Clinics of North America 29: 1171–1198
Cohen W N, Seidelmann F E, Bryan P J 1977 Use of a tampon to enhance vaginal localization in computed tomography. American Journal of Roentgenology 128: 1064–1065
Cooperberg P L 1978 High-resolution real-time ultrasound in the evaluation of the normal and obstructed biliary tract. Radiology 129: 477–480
Cormack A M 1980 Early two-dimensional reconstruction and recent topics stemming from it. Science 209: 1482–1486
Couinaud C 1957 Le foie In: Etudes Anatomiques et Chirurgicales. Masson et Cie, Paris
Crawford E S, Hess K R 1989 Abdominal aortic aneurysm. New England Journal of Medicine 321: 1040–1042
Crooks L E, Kaufman L 1984 NMR imaging of blood flow. British Medical Bulletin 40: 167–169
Curati W L, Halevy A, Gibson R N et al 1988 Ultrasound, CT, and MRI comparison in primary and secondary tumors of the liver. Gastrointestinal Radiology 13: 123–128
Dach J L, Hill M C, Pelaez J C, LePage J R, Russell E 1981 Sonography of hypertensive portal venous system: correlation with aterial portography. American Journal of Roentgenology 137: 511–517
Daffner R H, Halber M D, Postlethwait R W, Korobkin M, Thompson W M 1979 CT of the esophagus. II. Carcinoma. American Journal of Roentgenology 133: 1051–1055
Davison M 1982 X-ray computed tomography. In: Scientific Basis of Medical Imaging. Ed: Wells P N T Ch. 2. Churchill Livingstone, Edinburgh
Dewbury K C 1980 Visualization of normal biliary ducts with ultrasound. British Journal of Radiology 53: 774–780
Dewbury K C, Clark B 1979 The accuracy of ultrasound in the detection of cirrhosis of the liver. British Journal of Radiology 52: 945–948
Dewbury K C, Joseph A E A, Hayes S, Murray C 1979 Ultrasound in the evaluation and diagnosis of jaundice. British Journal of Radiology 52: 276–280
Di Lelio A, Cestari C, Lomazzi A, Beretta L 1989 Cirrhosis: diagnosis with sonographic study of the liver surface. Radiology 172: 389–392
Dixon A K, Nightingale R C 1984 Abnormal fat: a useful marker of intra-abdominal disease at computed tomography. Clinical Radiology 35: 469–473
Dodds W J, Darweesh R M A, Lawson T L et al 1986 The retroperitoneal spaces revisited. American Journal of Roentgenology 147: 1155–1161
Dong B, Chen M 1987 Improved sonographic visualization of choledocholithiasis? Journal of Clinical Ultrasound 15: 185–190
Dubbins P A, O'Riordan D, Melia W M 1981 Ultrasound in hepatoma – can specific diagnosis be made? British Journal of Radiology 54: 307–311
Ekberg O, Weiber S 1991 The clinical importance of a thickwalled tender gall-bladder without stones on ultrasonography. Clinical Radiology 44: 38–41
Edelman R R 1993 MR angiography: present and future. American Journal of Roentgenology 161: 1–11
Edelman R R, McFarland E, Stark D D et al 1985 Surface coil MR imaging of abdominal viscera. Part I. Theory, technique, and initial results. Radiology 157: 425–430
Egglin T K, Rummeny E, Stark D D, Wittenberg J, Sanjay S, Ferrucci J 1990 Hepatic tumors: quantitative tissue characteristic with MR imaging. Radiology 178: 107–110
Fearon T, Vucich J 1987 Normalized pediatric organ-absorbed doses from CT examinations. American Journal of Roentgenology 148: 171–174
Felmlee J P, Gray J E, Leetzow M L, Price J C 1989 Estimated fetal radiation dose from multislice CT studies. American Journal of Roentgenology 154: 185–190
Ferrucci J T 1989 Biliary lithotripsy: 1989. American Journal of Roentgenology 153: 15–22
Ferrucci J T 1994 Liver tumor imaging. Current concepts. Radiologic Clinics of North America 32: 39–54
Filly R A, Allen B, Minton M J, Bernhoft R, Way L W 1980 In vitro investigation of the origin of echoes within biliary sludge. Journal of Clinical Ultrasound 8: 193–200
Fineberg H V 1978 Evaluation of computed tomography: achievement and challenge. American Journal of Roentgenology 131: 1–4
Fineberg H V, Wittenberg J, Ferrucci J T Jr, Mueller P R, Simeone J F, Goldman J 1983 The clinical value of body computed tomography over time and technologic change. Roentgenology 141: 1067–1072
Fisher J K 1982 Normal colon wall thickness on CT. Radiology 145: 415–418
Fishman E K, Wolf E J, Jones B Bayless T M, Siegelman S S 1987 CT evaluation of Crohn's disease: effect on patient management. American Journal of Roentgenology 148: 537–540
Fishman E K, Wyatt S H, Ney D R, Kuhlman J E, Siegelman S S 1992 Spiral CT of the pancreas with multiplanar display. American Journal of Roentgenology 159: 1209–1215
Foley W D, Jochem R J 1991 Computed tomography. Focal and diffuse liver disease. Radiologic Clinics of North America 29: 1213–1233
Forrest M E, Cho K J, Shields J J, Wicks J D, Silver T M, McCormick T L 1980 Biliary cystadenomas: sonographic–angiographic–pathologic correlations. American Journal of Roentgenology 135: 723–727
Foster K J, Dewbury K C, Griffith A H, Wright R 1980 The accuracy of ultrasound in the detection of fatty infiltration of the liver. British Journal of Radiology 53: 440–442
Fowler R C, Reid W A 1988 Ultrasound diagnosis of adenomyomatosis of the gall-bladder: ultrasonic and pathological correlation. Clinical Radiology 39: 402–406
Freeny P C 1988 Hepatic CT: state of the art. Radiology 168: 319–323
Freeny P C 1989a Classification of pancreatitis. Radiologic Clinics of North America 27: 1–3
Freeny P C 1989b Radiologic diagnosis and staging of pancreatic ductal adenocarcinoma. Radiologic Clinics of North America 27: 121–128
Frick M P, Feinberg S B, Loken M K 1981 Noninvasive spleen scanning in Hodgkin's disease and non-Hodgkin's lymphoma. Computerized Tomography 5: 73–78
Fry I K 1984 Who needs high technology? British Journal of Radiology 57: 765–772
Gaensler E H L, Jeffrey R B, Laing F C, Townsend R R 1989 Sonography in patients with suspected acute appendicitis: value in establishing alternative diagnoses. American Journal of Roentgenology 152: 49–51
Galiber A K, Reading C C, Charboneau J W et al 1988 Localization of pancreatic insulinoma: comparison of pre- and intraoperative US with CT and angiography. Radiology 166: 405–408
Ghahremani G G 1993 Radiologic evaluation of suspected gastrointestinal perforations. Radiologic Clinics of North America 31: 1219–1234
Glazer G M, Aisen A M, Francis I R, Gyves J W, Lande I, Adler D D 1985 Hepatic cavernous hemangioma: magnetic resonance imaging. Radiology 155: 417–420
Goldberg H I, Gore R M, Margulis A R, Moss A A, Baker E L 1983 Computed tomography in the evaluation of Crohn disease. American Journal of Roentgenology 140: 277–282
Gore R M 1989 CT of inflammatory bowel disease. Radiologic Clinics of North America. 27: 717–729
Gore R M, Levine M S, Laufer I 1994 Textbook of gastrointestinal radiology. W B Saunders, Philadelphia
Gould L, Patel A 1979 Ultrasound detection of extrahepatic encapsulated bile: "biloma". American Journal of Roentgenology 132: 1014–1015
Graham M F, Cooperberg P L, Cohen M M, Burhenne H J 1980 The

size of the normal common hepatic duct following cholecystectomy: an ultrasonographic study. Radiology 135: 137–139

Graham M F, Cooperberg P L, Cohen M M, Burhenne H J 1981 Ultrasonographic screening of the common hepatic duct in symptomatic patients after cholecystectomy. Radiology 138: 137–139

Green B, Bree R L, Goldstein H M, Stanley C 1977 Gray scale ultrasound evaluation of hepatic neoplasms: patterns and correlations. Radiology 124: 203–208

Hadidi A 1983 Pancreatic duct measurements: sonographic measurement in normal subjects. Journal of Clinical Ultrasound 11: 17–22

Halber M D, Daffner R H, Thompson W M 1979 CT of the esophagus: I. Normal appearance. American Journal of Roentgenology 133: 1047–1050

Halvorsen R A Jr, Thompson W M 1989 CT of esophageal neoplasms. Radiologic Clinics of North America 27: 667–685

Hanley P 1984 Magnets for medical applications of NMR. British Medical Bulletin 40: 125–131

Hayman L A, Evans R A, Fahr L M, Hinck V C 1980 Renal consequences of rapid high dose contrast CT. American Journal of Roentgenology 134: 553–555

Hoult D I, Busby S J W, Gadian D G, Radda G K, Richards R E, Seeley P J 1974 Observation of tissue metabolites using $^{31}$P nuclear magnetic resonance. Nature 252: 285–287

Hounsfield G N 1973 Computerized transverse axial scanning (tomography): Part I. Description of system. British Journal of Radiology 46: 1016–1022

Hounsfield G N 1980 Computed medical imaging. Science 210: 22–28

Hricak H 1984 MR imaging of the retroperitoneum and pelvis. British Medical Bulletin 40: 197–201

Huda W, Sandison G A 1986 The use of the effective dose equivalent, HE, as a risk parameter in computed tomography. British Journal of Radiology 59: 1236–1238

Hughes L A, Hartnell G G, Finn J P et al 1996 Time-of slight MR angiography of the portal venous system. Value compared with other imaging procedures. American Journal of Roentgenology 166: 375–378

Husband J E, Fry I K 1981 Computed tomography of the body: a radiological and clinical approach. Macmillan, London

Husband J E, Golding S J 1982 Computed tomography of the body: when should it be used? British Medical Journal 284: 4–8

Jeffrey R B, Laing F C, Wing V W 1986 Extrapancreatic spread of acute pancreatitis: new observations with real-time US. Radiology 159: 707–711

Jones B 1985 Computed tomography and inflammatory diseases of the gastrointestinal tract. In: Margulis A R, Gooding C (eds) Diagnostic radiology. UCSF Printing Department, San Francisco, p 55

Jones S N, Lees W R, Frost R A 1988 Diagnosis and grading of chronic pancreatitis by morphological criteria derived by ultrasound and pancreatography. Clinical Radiology 39: 43–48

Joseph A E A, McVicar D 1990 Editorial: ultrasound in the diagnosis of abdominal abscesses. Clinical Radiology 42: 154–156

Joseph A E, Saverymuttu S H 1991 Editorial: ultrasound in the assessment of diffuse parenchymal liver disease. Clinical Radiology 44: 219–221

Kane R A 1980 Ultrasonographic diagnosis of gangrenous cholecystitis and empyema of the gallbladder. Radiology 134: 191–194

Kapoor W, Hemmer K, Herbert D, Karpf M 1983 Abdominal computed tomography. Comparison of the usefulness of goal-directed vs non-goal-directed studies. Archives of Internal Medicine 143: 249–251

Keller P J, Drayer B P, Fram E K, Williams K D, Dumoulin C L, Souza S P 1989 MR angiography with two-dimensional acquisition and three-dimensional display. Work in progress. Radiology 173: 527–532

Kreel L 1984 Computed tomography in gastroenterology. Clinics in Gastroenterology 13: 235–264

Kreel L, Haertell M, Katz D 1977 Computed tomography of the normal pancreas. Journal of Computer Assisted Tomography 1: 290–299

Kuhl D E, Edwards R Q 1964 Cylindrical and section radioisotope scanning of the liver and brain. Radiology 83: 926

Laing F C, London L A, Filly R A 1978 Ultrasonographic identification of dilated intrahepatic bile ducts and their differentiation from portal venous structures. Journal of Clinical Ultrasound 6: 90–94

Laing F C, Jeffrey R B, Wing V W 1984 Improved visualization of choledocholithiasis by sonography. American Journal of Roentgenology 143: 949–952

Lauterbur P C 1973 Image formation by induced local interactions: examples employing nuclear magnetic resonance. Nature 242: 190–191

Lewall D B, McCorkell S J 1985 Hepatic echinococcal cysts: sonographic appearance and classification. Radiology 155: 773–775

Luetmer P H, Stephens D H, Ward E M 1989 Chronic pancreatitis: reassessment with current CT. Radiology 171: 353–357

McCain A H, Bernardino M E, Sones P J, Berkman W A, Casarella W J 1985 Varices from portal hypertension: correlation of CT and angiography. Radiology 154: 63–69

McCarthy S 1992 Magnetic resonance imaging of the normal female pelvis. Radiologic Clinics of North America 30: 769–775

McCarthy S M, Barnes D, Deveney K, Moss A A, Goldberg H I 1985 Detection of recurrent rectosigmoid carcinoma: prospective evaluation of CT and clinical factors. American Journal of Roentgenology 144: 577–579

McCullough E C, Payne J T 1978 Patient dosage in computed tomography. Radiology 129: 457–463

McGrath F P, Keeling F 1991 The role of early sonography in the management of the acute abdomen. Clinical Radiology 44: 172–174

Madrazo B L, Halpert R D, Sandler M A, Pearlberg J L 1984 Computed tomographic findings in penetrating peptic ulcer. Radiology 153: 751–754

Margulis A R 1985 Future directions of diagnostic imaging. Plenary Session Proceedings. p. 2. XVI International Congress of Radiology, Hawaii

Marks W M, Filly R A, Callen P W 1979 Ultrasonic anatomy of the liver: a review with new applications. Journal of Clinical Ultrasound 7: 137–146

Marks W M, Callen P W, Moss A A 1981 Gastroesophageal region: source of confusion on CT. American Journal of Roentgenology 136: 359–362

Marn C S, Bree R L, Silver T M 1991 Ultrasonography of liver. Technique and focal and diffuse disease. Radiologic Clinics of North America 29: 1151–1170

Mathur-De Vre R 1984 Biomedical implications of the relaxation behaviour of water related to NMR imaging. British Journal of Radiology 57: 955–976

Maudsley A A, Hilal S K 1984 Biological aspects of sodium-23 imaging. British Medical Bulletin 40: 165–166

Meaney T F 1984 Magnetic resonance without nuclear. Radiology 150: 277

Megibow A J 1986 Gastrointestinal lymphoma: the role of CT in diagnosis and management. Seminars in Ultrasound, CT, and MR 7: 43–57

Megibow A J, Bosniak M A 1980 Dilute barium as a contrast agent for abdominal CT. American Journal of Roentgenology 134: 1273–1274

Megibow A J, Balthazar E J, Hulnick D H, Naidich D P, Bosniak M A 1985 CT evaluation of gastrointestinal leiomyomas and leiomyosarcomas. American Journal of Roentgenology 144: 727–731

Meire H B 1984 Ultrasound in gastroenterology. Clinics in Gastroenterology 13: 183–203

Meyers M A (ed) 1986 Computed tomography of the gastrointestinal tract: including the peritoneal cavity and mesentery. Springer-Verlag, New York

Millard F C, Collins M C, Peck R J 1991 Ultrasound in the investigation of the right iliac fossa mass. British Journal of Radiology 64: 17–19

Mittelstaedt C A, Volberg F M, Fischer G J, McCartney W H 1980 Caroli's disease: sonographic findings. American Journal of Roentgenology 134: 585–587

Moss A A 1989 Editorial: imaging of colorectal carcinoma. Radiology 170: 308–310

Moss A A, Kressel H Y, Korobkin M, Goldberg H I, Rohlfing B M, Brasch R C 1978 The effect of Gastrografin and glucagon on CT scanning of the pancreas: a blind clinical trial. Radiology 126: 711–714

Moss A A, Schnyder P, Marks W, Margulis A R 1981a Gastric adenocarcinoma: a comparison of the accuracy and economics of staging by computed tomography and surgery. Gastroenterology 80: 45–50

Moss A A, Friedman M A, Brito A 1981b Determination of liver, kidney, and spleen volumes by computed tomography: an experimental study in dogs. Journal of Computer Assisted Tomography 5: 12

Moss A A, Gamsk G, Genant H K 1992 Computed tomography of the body. W B Saunders, Philadelphia

Neff C C, vanSonnenberg E 1989 CT of diverticulitis, diagnosis and treatment. Radiologic Clinics of North America 27: 743–752

Nelson R C 1991 Techniques for computed tomography of the liver. Radiologic Clinics of North America 29: 1199–1212

Nelson R C, Chezmar J L 1990 Diagnostic approach to hepatic hemangiomas. Radiology 176: 11–13

Nelson R C, Chezmar J L, Sugarbaker P H, Bernardino M E 1989 Hepatic tumors: comparison of CT during arterial portography, delayed CT, and MR imaging for preoperative evaluation. Radiology 172: 27–34

Niederau C, Muller J, Sonnenberg A et al 1983 Extrahepatic bile ducts in healthy subjects, in patients with cholelithiasis, and in postcholecystectomy patients: a prospective ultrasonic study. Journal of Clinical Ultrasound 11: 23–27

Nyborg W L 1982 Ultrasonic intensities generated by real-time devices. In: Winsberg F, Cooperberg P L (eds) Real-time ultrasonography. Churchill Livingstone, New York, Ch 2, p 15

Olken S M, Bledsoe R, Newmark H 1978 The ultrasonic diagnosis of primary carcinoma of the gallbladder. Radiology 129: 481–482

Ophir J, Parker J K 1989 Contrast agents in diagnostic ultrasound. Ultrasound in Medicine and Biology 15: 319–333

Parker G A, Lawrence J Jr, Horsley J S 3rd et al 1989 Intraoperative ultrasound of the liver affects operative decision making. Annals of Surgery 209: 569–577

Parulekar S G 1980 Ultrasonic evaluation of the pancreatic duct. Journal of Clinical Ultrasound 8: 457–463

Pastakia B, Shawker T H, Thaler M, O'Leary T, Pizzo P A 1988 Hepatosplenic candidiasis: wheels within wheels. Radiology 166: 417–421

Piekarski J, Federle M P, Moss A A, London S S 1980 Computed tomography of the spleen. Radiology 135: 683–689

Purcell E M, Torrey H C, Pound R V 1946 Resonance absorption by nuclear magnetic moments in a solid. Physical Review 69: 37–38

Pykett I L 1983 Instrumentation for nuclear magnetic resonance imaging. Seminars in Nuclear Medicine 13: 319–328

Pykett I L, Newhouse J H, Buonanno F S et al 1982 Principles of nuclear magnetic resonance imaging. Radiology 143: 157–168

Quint L E, Glazer G M, Orringer M B, Gross B H 1985 Esophageal carcinoma: CT findings. Radiology 155: 171–175

Radda G K 1985 Magnetic resonance spectroscopy in clinical medicine. Plenary Session Proceedings. p. 5. XVI International Congress of Radiology, Hawaii

Radda G K, Bore P J, Rajagopalan B 1983 Clinical aspects of $^{31}$P NMR spectroscopy. British Medical Bulletin 40: 155–159

Radon J 1917 On the determination of functions from their integrals along certain manifolds. Berichte Sochsische Academic Der Wissenschaften 69: 262

Ralls P W 1990 Color Doppler sonography of the hepatic artery and portal venous system. American Journal of Roentgenology 155: 517–525

Ralls P W, Halls J, Lapin S A, Quinn M F, Morris U L, Boswell W 1982 Prospective evaluation of the sonographic Murphy sign in suspected acute cholecystitis. Journal of Clinical Ultrasound 10: 113–115

Reinhold C, Bret P M 1996 Current status of MR cholangiopancreatography. American Journal of Roentgenology 166: 1285–1295

Reuter K, Raptopoulos V D, Cantelmo N, Fitzpatrick G, Hawes L E 1980 The diagnosis of a choledochal cyst by ultrasound. Radiology 136: 437–438

Reznek R H, Stephens D H 1993 The staging of pancreatic adenocarcinoma. Clinical Radiology 47: 373–381

Rosen B R, Brady T J 1983 Principles of nuclear magnetic resonance for medical application. Seminars in Nuclear Medicine 13: 308–328

Rubenstein W A, Whalen J P 1986 Extraperitoneal spaces. American Journal of Roentgenology 147: 1162–1164

Rubin G D, Dake M D, Napel S A, McDonnell C H, Jeffrey R B Jr 1993 Three-dimensional spiral CT angiography of the abdomen: initial clinical experience. Radiology 186: 147–152

Rumack C M, Wilson S R, Charboneau J W 1991 Diagnostic ultrasound. Mosby Year Book, St Louis

Sample W F, Sarti D A, Goldstein L I, Weiner M, Kadell B M 1978 Gray-scale ultrasonography of the jaundiced patient. Radiology 128: 719–725

Sandford N L, Walsh P, Matis C, Baddeley H, Powell L W 1985 Is ultrasonography useful in the assessment of diffuse parenchymal liver disease? Gastroenterology 89: 186–189

Saunders R D, Smith H 1984 Safety aspects of NMR clinical imaging. British Medical Bulletin 40: 148–154

Scatarige J C, DiSantis D J 1989 CT of the stomach and duodenum. Radiologic Clinics of North America 27: 687–706

Scoutt L M, Zawin M L, Taylor K W J 1990 Doppler US. Part II. Clinical applications. Radiology 174: 309–319

Semelka R C, Ascher S M 1993 MR imaging of the pancreas. Radiology 188: 593–602

Shawker T H, Garra B S, Hill M C 1986 The spectrum of sonographic findings in pancreatic carcinoma. Journal of Ultrasound in Medicine 5: 169

Shope T B, Morgan T J, Showalter C K et al 1982 Radiation dosimetry survey of computed tomography systems from ten manufacturers. British Journal of Radiology 55: 60–69

Silverstein W, Isikoff M B, Hill M C, Barkin J 1981 Diagnostic imaging of acute pancreatitis: prospective study using CT and sonography. American Journal of Roentgenology 137: 497–502

Simeone J F, Mueller P R, Ferrucci J T Jr 1989 Nonsurgical therapy of gallstones: implications for imaging. American Journal of Roentgenology 152: 11–17

Smith M A 1985 The technology of magnetic resonance imaging. Clinical Radiology 36: 553–559

Society for Computed Body Tomography 1979 New indications for computed body tomography. American Journal of Roentgenology 133: 115–119

Stark D D, Wittenberg J, Middleton M S, Ferrucci J T Jr 1986 Liver metastases: detection by phase-contrast MR imaging. Radiology 158: 327–332

Stomper P C, Fung C Y, Socinski M A, Jochelson M S, Garnick M B, Richie J P 1987 Detection of retroperitoneal metastases in early-stage nonseminomatous testicular cancer: analysis of different CT criteria. American Journal of Roentgenology 149: 1187–1190

Sugarbaker P H 1990 Surgical decision making for large bowel cancer metastatic to the liver. Radiology 174: 621–626

Tanaka S, Kitamura T, Fujita M, Nakanishi K, Okuda S 1990 Color Doppler flow imaging of liver tumors. American Journal of Roentgenology 154: 509–514

Taylor A J, Dodds W J, Erickson S J, Stewart E T 1991 CT of acquired abnormalities of the spleen. American Journal of Roentgenology 157: 1213–1219

Taylor K J W (ed) 1985 Atlas of ultrasonography, 2nd edn. Churchill Livingstone, Edinburgh

Taylor K J W, Holland S 1990 Doppler US. Part I. Basic principles, instrumentation and pitfalls. Radiology 174: 297–307

Taylor K J W, Jacobson P, Jaffe C C 1979 Lack of an acoustic shadow on scans of gallstones: a possible artifact. Radiology 131: 463–464

Taylor K J W, Buchin P J, Viscomi G N, Rosenfield A T 1981 Ultrasonographic scanning of the pancreas. Prospective study of clinical results. Radiology 138: 211–213

Thoeni R F 1989 CT evaluation of carcinomas of the colon and rectum. Radiologic Clinics of North America 27: 731–741

Thompson W M 1994 Staging neoplasms. Radiologic Clinics of North America 32: 1

Thompson W M, Trenkner S W 1994 Staging colorectal carcinoma. Radiologic Clinics of North America 32: 25–37

Tio T L, Tytgat G N J, Cikot R J L M, Houthoff H J, Sars P R A 1990 Ampullopancreatic carcinoma: preoperative TNM classification with endosonography. Radiology 175: 445–461

Trenkner S W, Halvorsen R A Jr, Thompson W M 1994 Neoplasms of

the upper gastrointestinal tract. Radiologic Clinics of North America 32: 15–24
Van Gansbeke D, Avni E F, Delcour C, Engelholm L, Struyven J 1985 Sonographic features of portal vein thrombosis. American Journal of Roentgenology 144: 749–752
Viscomi G N, Gonzalez R, Taylor K J W 1981 Histopathological correlation of ultrasound appearances of liver metastases. Journal of Clinical Gastroenterology 3: 395–400
Wade G, Lee H, Schueler C 1984 Acoustical imaging: history, applications, principles and limitations. In: Nalcioglu O, Cho Z-H (eds) Selected topics in image science. Lecture Notes in Medical Informatics, Vol. 23. Springer-Verlag, Berlin, p 221–253
Walkey M M, Friedman A C, Sohotra P, Radecki P D 1988 CT manifestations of peritoneal carcinomatosis. American Journal of Roentgenology 150: 1035–1041
Wang S-S, Chiang J-H, Tsai Y-T et al 1990 Focal hepatic fatty infiltration as a cause of pseudotumors: ultrasonographic patterns and clinical differentiation. Journal of Clinical Ultrasound 18: 401–409
Weill F, Eisencher A, Zeltner F 1978 Ultrasonic study of the normal and dilated biliary tree. The "shotgun" sign. Radiology 127: 221–224
Weinstein B J, Weinstein D P 1980 Biliary tract dilatation in the nonjaundiced patient. American Journal of Roentgenology 134: 899–906
Welch T J, Sheedy P F 2nd, Johnson C M et al 1985 Focal nodular hyperplasia and hepatic adenoma: comparison of angiography, CT, US and scintigraphy. Radiology 156: 593–595
Wells P N T 1982 Ultrasonic imaging. In: Wells P N T (ed) Scientific basis of medical imaging. Churchill Livingstone, Edinburgh, Ch 4, p 4
Williams M P, Scott I H K, Dixon A K 1984 Computed tomography in 101 patients with a palpable abdominal mass. Clinical Radiology 35: 293–296
Wu C-C, Ho Y-H, Chen C-Y 1984 Effect of ageing on common bile duct diameter: a real-time ultrasonographic study. Journal of Clinical Ultrasound 12: 473–478
Zeman R K, Taylor K J W, Burrell M I, Gold J 1980 Ultrasound demonstration of anicteric dilatation of the biliary tree. Radiology 134: 689–692
Zeman R K, Taylor K J W, Rosenfield A T, Schwartz A, Gold J A 1981 Acute experimental biliary obstruction in the dog: sonographic findings and clinical implications. American Journal of Roentgenology 136: 965–967
Zeman R K, Paushter D M, Schiebler M L, Choyke P L, Jaffe M H, Clark L R 1985 Hepatic imaging: current status. Radiologic Clinics of North America 23: 473–487
Zeman R K, Fox S H, Silverman P M et al 1993 Helical (spiral) CT of the abdomen. American Journal of Roentgenology 160: 719–725

# 3. Imaging and other investigations with radionuclides

*M. V. Merrick*

Investigations with radioactive tracers differ from radiological or ultrasound imaging in that they do not in general reveal the appearance of organs but, by selection of an appropriate tracer, permit measurement of the global or local rate and site of specific physiological or biochemical processes; in many cases these processes can, if necessary, be followed noninvasively for hours or days. Interpretation of the findings requires not only a thorough understanding of the constraints imposed by the detecting equipment and the radioactive process, but also of the anatomy, physiology, biochemistry and, in many cases, pharmacology. These investigations in some cases supplement "conventional" imaging techniques and in others provide information otherwise obtainable with difficulty or not at all, but they are rarely direct alternatives. It is important to appreciate that they can often provide direct information of how physiological substances are treated that can otherwise be inferred only from the behavior of unphysiological markers such as barium sulfate.

## GASTROINTESTINAL TRACT

### INTRODUCTION

Radionuclide techniques can be applied to a wide range of clinical problems in the gastrointestinal tract, ranging from the salivary glands to the colon. These techniques have the advantage of being relatively uninvasive and in general they are probably underused.

### SALIVARY GLANDS

The parotid and to a slightly lesser extent the submandibular glands have the ability to take up pertechnetate, iodide and gallium (Mishkin 1981). The sublingual and minor salivary glands cannot be visualized in this way. Perfusion of the salivary glands may be imaged during the first pass of a bolus of any convenient tracer, for example 400–500 MBq (37 MBq = 1 mCi) of sodium pertechnetate. Uptake of pertechnetate reaches a plateau 5–10 min after the first pass of the injection. Stimulation by a sour drink such as lemon juice discharges most of the parotid activity and rather less of the submandibular uptake within a few minutes. This can be demonstrated either by continuous acquisition (Fig. 3.1) or by repeating the original set of projections, using the same duration of acquisition per view, not the same number of counts. Accurate repositioning is essential for quantitative or semi-quantitative studies.

#### Interpretation

Obstructed but still functioning glands have lower uptake than nonobstructed ones and this does not decrease in response to acid stimulation. Stenson's duct may be visualized on the later frames if it is dilated or obstructed, but the normal duct is not visualized. Xerostomia is usually associated with generally poor uptake and failure to respond to acid stimulation. In Sjögren's syndrome, uptake may be normal or reduced, but the response to sialagogues such as lemon juice is usually markedly diminished.

With one important exception, space-occupying lesions are identified as areas of reduced uptake, seen most readily in the lateral oblique projections. The exception is papillary lymphoid cystadenoma (Warthin's tumor), which has greater uptake than normal salivary tissue but does not discharge this activity in response to oral stimulus. Scintigraphy has little application for tumor localization.

#### Clinical application

The principal role of salivary imaging is in patients being assessed for asymmetrical salivary function and in those in whom adequate clinical examination can be impractical, as in cerebral palsy and torticollis. See also p. 142.

### ESOPHAGUS

Functional disorders of swallowing fall into three major

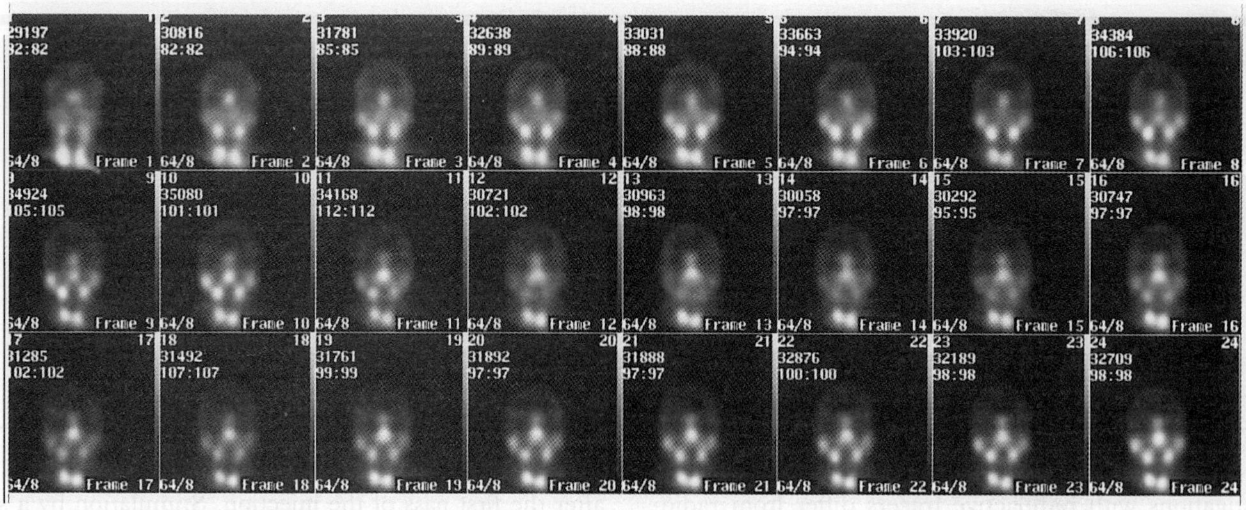


**Fig. 3.1** Consecutive 60-s images starting from the injection of radioactivity. Uptake in the submandibular and parotid glands increases progressively in intensity up to frame 10. A sour drink was given during frame 11 that rapidly discharged the activity in both glands. This subsequently reaccumulates.

categories: oropharyngeal dysphagia, esophageal dysphagia and noncardiac chest pain. Established nuclear medicine methods of assessing esophageal transit and clearance of a liquid, semi-solid or solid bolus offer a simple and reproducible way of investigating esophageal dysphagia and non-cardiac chest pain. Scintigraphic techniques provide better functional but poorer anatomical information than videofluoroscopy with barium for assessment of the progression of a bolus of food or liquid through the esophagus and can more readily be quantitated. Gastroesophageal reflux can also be demonstrated. The clinical value of nuclear medicine techniques is not widely recognized (Datz 1984, Bunker 1992).

### Technique

A gamma camera with a field of view greater than 11 inches (28 cm) diameter, with a general-purpose or high-sensitivity collimator, is suitable for studying the esophagus. The examination should be standardized, that is, always performed with the patient either supine or erect and fasting for 6 h before the test to allow clearance of any residue. The radioactivity is given in a nonabsorbable form; any soluble or stable solution of a technetium-labeled tracer may be used. It is better not to combine esophageal transit with a gastric-emptying study, as the initial requirements of the two are different. The activity may be in plain water, a viscous fluid or a semi-solid bolus. The volume should be small enough to be swallowed comfortably as a single bolus (5–10 ml) and an activity of 10 MBq (0.25 mCi) per swallow is adequate. At least three swallows should be performed, as there is often appreciable variability. A marker (a point source of $^{99m}$Tc or $^{57}$Co) is used to identify the cricoid cartilage and xiphisternum.

### Interpretation

In normal subjects the esophagus clears entirely within the first 60 s, but in patients with achalasia or other motility disorders a prolonged examination is necessary. Time activity curves are drawn for the upper, middle and lower thirds of the esophagus. In addition, time-condensed functional images greatly facilitate interpretation (Figs 3.2 and 3.3). In the normal subject each of the three regional curves shows a transient peak, wider in the distal segment than in the more proximal because of widening of the bolus as it passes down the esophagus and delay at the cardia. In the absence of effective peristalsis, as in achalasia of the cardia or scleroderma, activity in the distal and often in the middle segment rises and may remain constant for an extended period. Diffuse esophageal spasm shows a characteristic pattern of fluctuating activity as the uncoordinated movement causes radioactivity to pass back and forth from one segment to another without emptying the esophagus (Figs 3.4 and 3.5). In these cases, as the count rate falls in one segment there is a corresponding rise in another. Gastroesophageal reflux and aspiration can most readily be detected on time-condensed images following ingestion of a nonabsorbable tracer such as 25–50 MBq (0.5–1.5 mCi) of a technetium-labeled colloid. Its main application is in pediatric practice. Pulmonary aspiration is identified either by inspection of the frames or (preferably) by obtaining time-activity curves from regions over the lungs.

## STOMACH

### Gastric mucosa

Pertechnetate is taken up from the circulation, concentrated and secreted into the lumen by orthotopic or ectopic

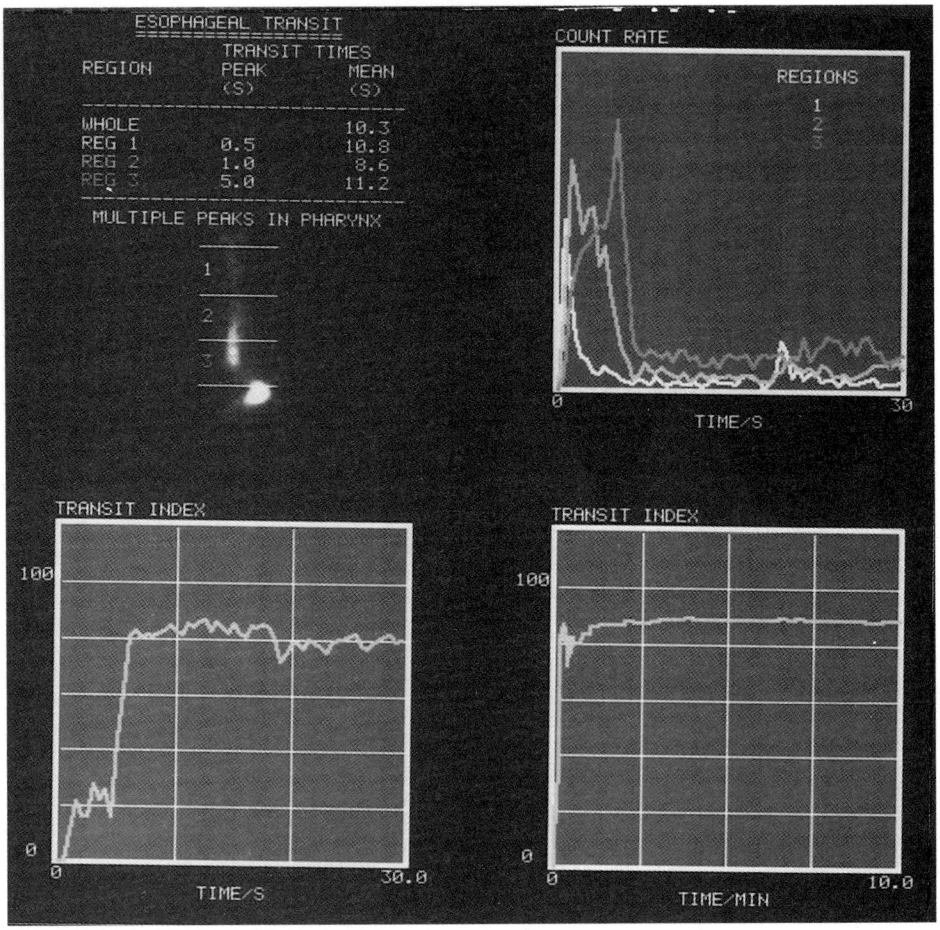


**Fig. 3.2** Normal swallow. *Top right*: time-activity curves from regions enclosing the upper, middle and lower thirds of the esophagus. Note the early peak from the upper region of interest, a slightly later and more delayed peak from the middle region and a still more delayed peak from the distal region. The graph shows (*lower left*) the integral activity over the first 30 s and (*lower right*) over 10 min showing an initial rise followed by a plateau.

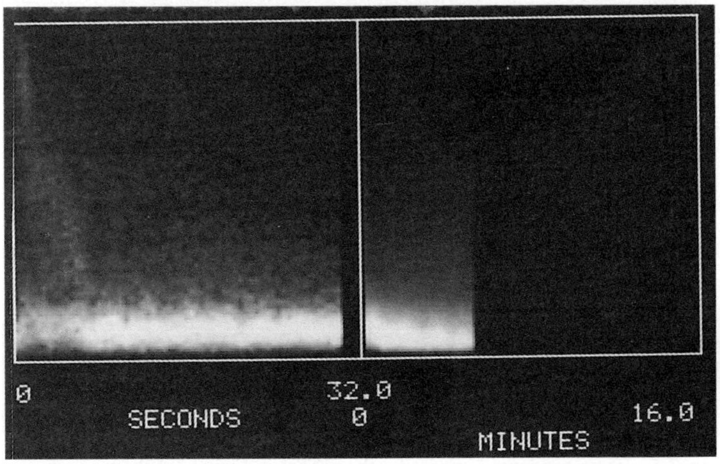


**Fig. 3.3** Time-condensed images from the study shown in Figure 3.2. There is an initial rapid fall on the left-hand side of the first image that represents the first 30 s. The remainder of the study activity remains at or below the cardia.

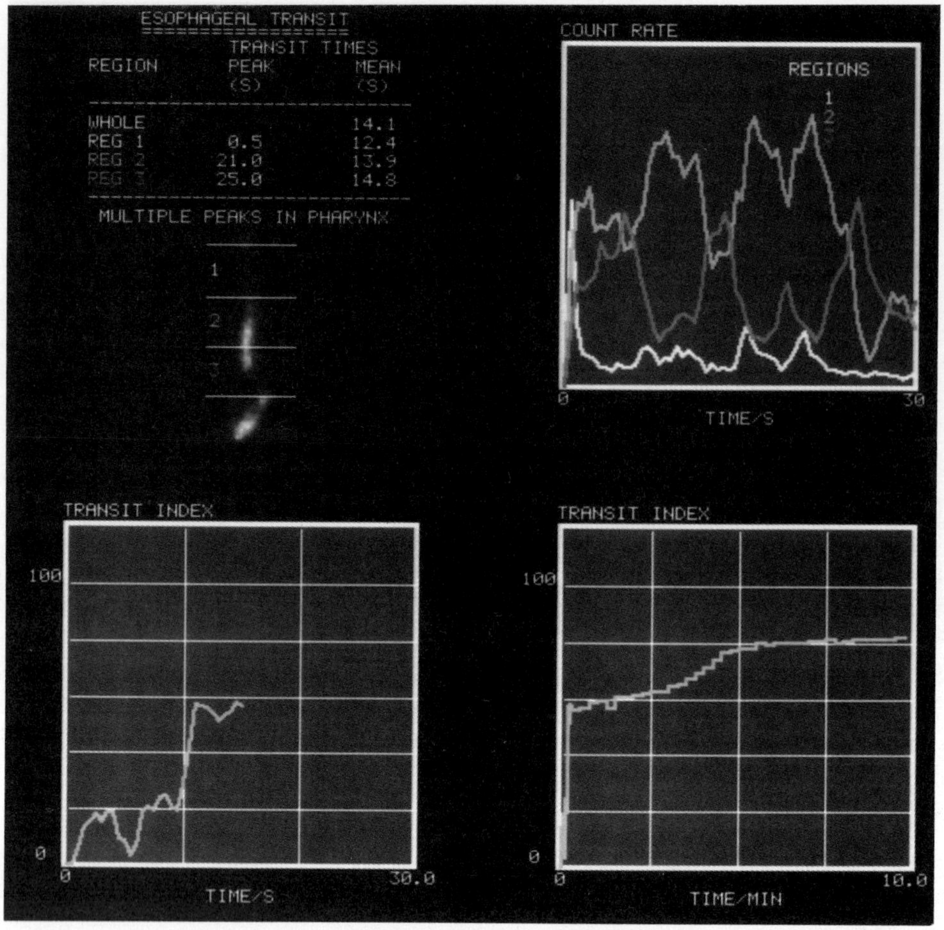


**Fig. 3.4** Time-activity curves from a patient with achalasia. Notice the very disturbed pattern with multiple peaks in all three regions. The integrals (lower two graphs) show a very slow rise to the plateau.

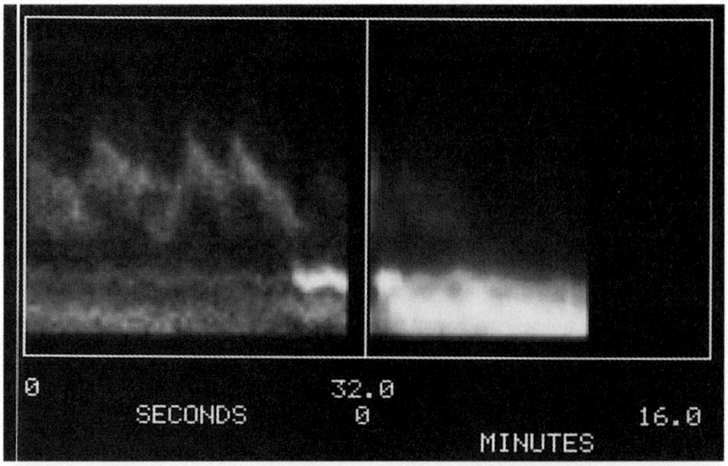


**Fig. 3.5** Time-condensed images for the patient in Figure 3.4 show a very disturbed pattern in the esophagus that persists not only for the first 30 s but continues for some minutes thereafter. Notice the substantial delay before activity reaches the cardia.

gastric mucosa. Uptake probably reflects both mucosal blood flow and the functional state of the mucous cells. It is not a marker of acid production *per se*, although under many circumstances pertechnetate uptake mirrors acid secretion, as both are dependent on blood flow. Gastric mucosa extending above the diaphragm, for example in a hiatus hernia or in Barrett's esophagus, can be visualized if the level of the diaphragm is defined. Ectopic gastric mucosa in other sites, for example Meckel's diverticulum, can be detected with a high degree of accuracy (see below).

### *Helicobacter pylori* infection

*H. pylori* metabolizes urea, with release of carbon dioxide. Measurement of the specific activity (MBq/mMole) in exhaled $CO_2$ 10 min after oral administration of $^{13}C$ or $^{14}C$ labeled urea has been used as a diagnostic test for this infection (p. 224) (Debongnie et al 1991). When urease is present, labeled $CO_2$ is released, absorbed into the circulation and expired in the breath. $^{13}C$ is not radioactive and requires mass spectroscopy for assay. Alternatively $^{14}C$ can be used and measured on a gamma counter.

### Gastric emptying

Radioactive tracers provide a noninvasive and quantitative means of measuring the rate at which the stomach empties its normal contents (Christian et al 1984, Leb & Lipp 1993). The solid and liquid components of a meal leave the stomach at different rates. Solids are stored initially in the fundus and transferred into the antral region for trituration before being expelled into the duodenum (Houghton et al 1988). The overall time-activity curve of a solid meal is initially linear, although there is a delay before emptying starts (the lag phase), while the time-activity curve for a low-nutrient liquid marker is exponential (Collins et al 1983) (Fig. 3.6).

Solid and liquid phase markers are not interchangeable. A solid marker must remain reliably on the solid phase, at least while in the stomach, and there should be no absorption and resecretion subsequently. Pouring a liquid tracer onto a solid meal does not produce a marker of the solid phase; it must be shown that the tracer remains firmly adherent to the solid and that this solid is, or consistently behaves like, a normal constituent of food (Horowitz et al 1985). The most reliable solid-phase marker is $^{99m}Tc$-liver, the $^{99m}Tc$ being incorporated into chicken liver and the latter usually mixed with beef and then cooked. Alternatively technetium-labeled macroaggregate can be added to raw egg and then cooked (into an omelette, scrambled egg, etc.). This remains insoluble in the stomach for long enough (up to 3 h) for the gastric emptying rate to be measured. To date, no preparation suitable for vegans has been validated.

A liquid-phase marker must have a high solubility in aqueous solutions and remain stable at low pH, be resistant to digestion, nonabsorbable, and not exchangeable with any solids present. Chelates of DTPA with either $^{111}In$ or $^{113m}In$ are suitable. $^{111}In$ is relatively expensive and is associated with a substantially higher absorbed radiation dose than $^{113m}In$. $^{113m}In$ now has limited availability and $^{65}Ga$ has been used in some centres. Radioisotopic markers suitable for measurement of gastric emptying of fat, such as $^{99m}Tc(v)$ thiocyanate bound to oil, are also available and likely to be used clinically in the future

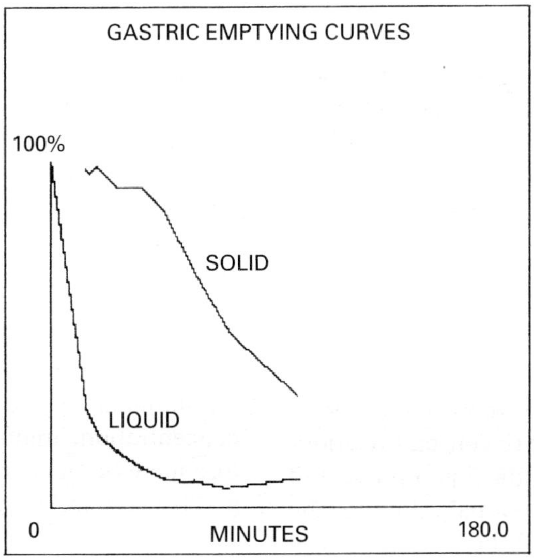


**Fig. 3.6** The normal pattern of simultaneous liquid and solid gastric emptying. The solid phase (the upper right-hand curve) shows an initial lag followed by a linear phase that slows when the stomach is almost empty. The liquid phase emptying is much more rapid and can be fitted by a single exponential function.

(Carney et al 1995). When considering suitable techniques it is necessary to take account of three potential sources of error.

***Scatter and septal penetration.*** The latter is a significant problem only with a high-energy gamma ray such as that of $^{113m}$In or $^{111}$In. Scatter occurs with all radionuclides and results in counts originating from the stomach being ascribed to an extragastric origin. As there is no background correction to be made, the best solution is to draw the region of interest as large as possible, although in practice this is limited in many subjects by overlap of the duodeno-jejunal junction and the stomach. In dual isotope tests, e.g. using $^{99m}$Tc to label solids and $^{113m}$In to label liquids, correction must be made for Compton scatter of photons from the higher energy isotope ($^{113m}$In) into the energy window for the lower energy isotope ($^{99m}$Tc).

***Stomach position.*** The stomach does not lie parallel to the anterior wall and its shape is variable and complex. Therefore, if a single detector is used, changes in count rate may reflect intragastric movement of food from fundus to antrum, rather than gastric emptying. There are a number of techniques which may be used to minimize this error, including calculation of the geometric mean counts, scanning in the left anterior oblique position and the use of correction factors derived from a lateral image of the stomach (Scarpignato 1990). It is often easiest to rotate an erect patient about the vertical axis to obtain anterior and posterior projections. An alternative technique is to acquire all the images in the left anterior oblique position, as this minimizes the differences in depth from the surface of the various parts of the stomach (Scarpignato 1990). The required obliquity is determined by selecting the projection that gives the greatest transverse dimension of the stomach. Once selected, accurate repositioning is crucial. This technique is adequate but may not be accurate in some large subjects with a transverse stomach. There may be difficulty in projecting the antrum clear of the duodenal bulb. As in the straight anterior projection, the duodeno-jejunal junction may be projected over the greater curve.

***Isotope decay.*** Correction is necessary when $^{99m}$Tc or $^{113m}$In is used, particularly in patients with gastric stasis.

#### *Interpretation*

The rate of gastric emptying varies with the population studied, with the composition of the meal and with its calorie content. Liquid meals empty more rapidly than solids (p. 424), but there is no simple or constant relationship between the rate of emptying of the liquid phase and that of the solid phase. The range of normal values for the population under study must be established for a test meal of constant composition that is acceptable to local taste. The volume of the test meal and its fat, carbohydrate and protein content all affect emptying rates. Small meals that do not distend the stomach give smaller attenuation errors than large meals. High calorie, high fat and hyperosmolar meals tend to empty more slowly. Hyperosmolar liquids may exhibit an emptying pattern with an initial lag or retention phase resembling that of solids. The rate of gastric emptying is affected by many extraneous factors, for example smoking or nausea. The changes in solid and liquid phase emptying in gastroparesis and other conditions are discussed on p. 427.

## DUODENOGASTRIC REFLUX

This can be detected and its severity assessed following intravenous administration of any of the hepatobiliary agents by looking for activity that has refluxed into the stomach (Da Costa et al 1992). The technique is principally of value in demonstrating the patency of and the direction of flow in the afferent loop following partial gastrectomy and biliary-enteric and gastro-enteric bypass operations.

## GASTROINTESTINAL BLEEDING

### Meckel's diverticulum

Meckel's diverticulum is a residue of the embryonic omphalomesenteric duct (p. 486). Some diverticula are lined by acid-secreting gastric mucosa instead of normal small intestinal mucosa, the prevalence being variously reported between 20% and 60%. Barium follow-through has a very low sensitivity of detection and cannot differentiate gastric mucosa from small intestinal mucosa in the diverticulum.

Meckel's diverticula are commonly asymptomatic but may present with melena, as anemia due to occult blood loss or as an acute abdomen in consequence of Meckel's diverticulitis. Bleeding occurs only in Meckel's diverticula that contain gastric mucosa and is the commoner presentation in childhood, whereas Meckel's diverticulitis is the more frequent presentation in adults; either may occur at any age. Scintigraphy using pertechnetate is by far the most sensitive and specific test available to detect those Meckel's diverticula that contain gastric mucosa (Cooney et al 1982). The mechanism of uptake of pertechnetate by ectopic gastric mucosa is thought to be identical to that responsible for its uptake in normal gastric mucosa (see above). $H_2$ receptor blockers such as cimetidine inhibit the intraluminal release of pertechnetate, increase the local concentration, minimize small bowel activity and therefore increase the contrast between ectopic gastric mucosa and background (Yeker et al 1984).

#### *Technique*

On the day before the examination an adult patient should

take cimetidine 200 mg early in the morning, before the midday meal and in the evening. Adults should fast from 10.00 p.m. on the evening prior to the examination. In the morning a single dose of cimetidine 400 mg is taken 2 h before the examination. 100–200 MBq (2.5–5 mCi) of $^{99m}$Tc pertechnetate is given intravenously and anterior projections of the abdomen, including both the stomach and the bladder in the field of view, are taken at 5-min intervals for 30 min, acquiring at least 500 000 counts in each. No useful information is obtained from later films. Meckel's diverticula are found most commonly in the right iliac fossa but may occur anywhere in the abdomen Fig. 3.5. If a suspect area is visualized, a lateral projection should be obtained to determine whether the focus is situated anteriorly or posteriorly.

*Interpretation*

The normal structures visualized are the stomach, bladder, kidneys and part or all of the ureters. The uterus may be visualized in adult females. A Meckel's diverticulum should become progressively more clearly identified above background, at the same rate as the stomach itself is visualized. It should be visible in all images, but as gut is commonly freely mobile, it may move between views and can be concealed in some if gut motility is excessive.

The other common causes of false negative examinations are secreted activity entering the small intestine overlying and concealing activity in the Meckel's diverticulum, patient movement, a full bladder, destruction of the gastric mucosa by ulceration and prior administration of drugs such as atropine, which reduces gastric blood flow, and perchlorate, which blocks trapping of iodide and its analogs. The patient should void between films to prevent the bladder becoming prominent. False positives are most commonly due to activity in the ureter, dilatation, stasis or obstruction in the urinary tract, acute inflammatory foci, vascular malformations, rare tumors, local inflammatory disease, intussusception and a normal uterus in adult females. Activity in the renal tract lies posteriorly on a lateral view. Ectopic gastric mucosa concentrates the tracer at the same rate as the stomach; other foci tend to be clearly visualized earlier and remain unchanged. Gastric mucosa can be visualized in other sites such as gastrogenic cysts, enteric duplications, duplication cysts or pockets of gastric mucosa in normal small intestine.

### Bleeding from other sites

It is not necessary to resort to radio-isotope techniques in most patients with gastrointestinal hemorrhage. However, bleeding from the small intestine and occasionally bleeding from the large intestine may be difficult to locate and two radio-isotope techniques may be useful (Robinson 1993).

*Labeled autologous erythrocytes*

Red cells are labeled in vivo by injecting 200–400 MBq (5–10 mCi) of $^{99m}$Tc pertechnetate 10 min after intravenous injection of 1 mg of a stannous ($Sn^{2+}$) salt that "tans" the circulating red blood cells. Anterior and if necessary oblique projections of the abdomen are taken using a large-field gamma camera fitted with a general purpose collimator, at intervals of 15–30 min, starting just after injection of the radioactivity. Imaging should be continued until an abnormal accumulation is identified or for a minimum of 4 h. The chances of detecting an abnormality depend on the duration of the examination and the frequency with which follow-up images are obtained. If no abnormality has been seen by 4 h, further views should be taken at intervals up to 24 h.

Bleeding appears as an area of greater count-rate that subsequently either increases in intensity as more blood loss occurs or becomes less distinct if bleeding stops and the extravasated blood is dispersed within the lumen of the intestine (Fig. 3.7). The site of bleeding cannot be identified with the same precision as angiography, but it is possible to indicate the quadrant that is involved and usually to estimate whether it is in proximal or distal small intestine, large bowel or elsewhere in the gut.

*Intravenous colloid*

If any of the colloidal preparations used for reticulo-endothelial scintigraphy are injected intravenously during hemorrhage, some of the colloid is extravasated at the bleeding site. Because the rest of the colloid is rapidly cleared by the reticulo-endothelial system, any extravasated activity stands out against a comparatively low background. Higher activities (200–400 MBq/5–10 mCi) must be administered than for most other colloid imaging.

*Comparison*

The colloid technique detects lower minimum rates of blood loss, about 0.1 ml/min compared with 5 ml/min for the labeled red cell technique. The disadvantages are the short (<5 min) time-window within which bleeding must occur to be detectable and overlap of activity in the liver and spleen. The two techniques are therefore complementary. The colloid method should be used first if the patient is thought to be bleeding continuously. If negative, it can be followed by the red cell technique not less than 48 h later, to allow activity in the liver and spleen to decay sufficiently for imaging of the upper abdomen to be possible. If bleeding is thought to be intermittent, as is more commonly the case, only the red cell method should be employed.

## GASTROINTESTINAL PROTEIN LOSS

The radioisotope technique is now rarely used as an alter-

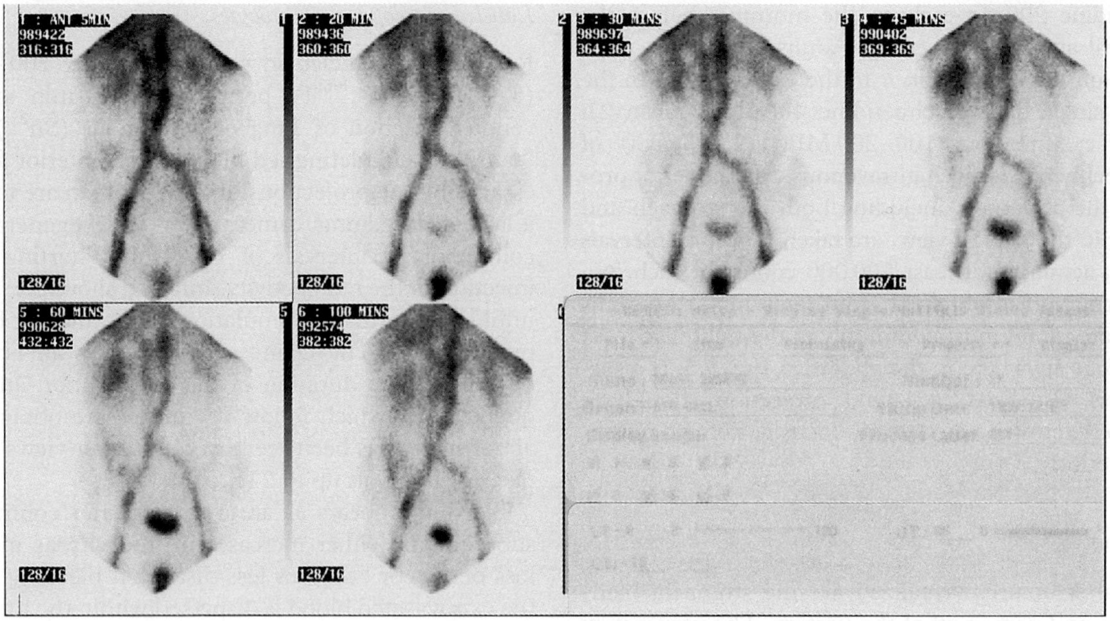

**Fig. 3.7** Consecutive images taken following injection of labeled autologous erythrocytes. There is an initial accumulation of activity in the right iliac fossa that becomes less evident as the activity is dispersed into the colonic contents, but at 60 min (frame 5) there is a further accumulation when a further brisk bleed occurs and this is reinforced in the 100-min image. The upper structures are the aorta, iliac vessels and inferior vena cava. Blood pool in the kidneys is visualized in both hypochondria.

native to stool $\alpha_1$-antitrypsin clearance (p. 348). A test using $^{51}$Cr labeled protein is described on page 348.

## SMALL INTESTINE

A number of substrates may be used to investigate various gastrointestinal transit and absorptive functions; the method of measuring $^{14}CO_2$ output in the breath is similar for all. Exhaled air is passed through a suitable absorber containing a measured quantity (1–2 mmol) of hyamine hydroxide (a basic quaternary amine). A pH indicator shows when the hyamine is fully saturated with carbon dioxide. Provided that the initial concentration of the hyamine is accurately known, the amount of $CO_2$ absorbed can readily be calculated. The absorbent is prepared for beta counting by addition of a suitable scintillation fluor and the $^{14}$C radioactivity content measured. The specific activity of $^{14}$C in the expired air is calculated. Breath samples are collected in this way over a period of 4–8 h, depending on the particular test. Breath tests should be performed with the patient at rest and initially fasting. If a meal is given during the test period, it should be a light meal of a standardized composition, volume and calorie content, formulated according to local taste and custom.

### Fat malabsorption

A number of tests involving radioisotopes (e.g. various $^{14}$C fatty acids) have been described to provide an alternative to fecal fat excretion, although none is universally accepted (King & Toskes 1983). Breath tests to detect fat malabsorption are described on p. 355.

### Carbohydrate malabsorption

Breath tests are described on page 342.

### Other tests

These include $^{14}$C-xylose test (p. 342) and tests of vitamin $B_{12}$ absorption (p. 364).

### Bacterial overgrowth

Small intestinal malabsorption of bile acids produces diarrhea. In the presence of bacterial colonization of the small intestine, deconjugation may occur in the small intestine. This forms the basis of the $^{14}$C glycocholate breath test, which has been used to detect both colonization and bile acid malabsorption (Coates et al 1982).

200 kBq of $^{14}$C glycocholate, the $^{14}$C label being on the glycine moiety, in 50 mg of glycocholate is given orally. Glycocholate is hydrolyzed by many anaerobic bacteria; the $^{14}$C glycine released is oxidized in the host tissues following absorption. $^{14}CO_2$ is measured in the breath over the next 4 h. In the normal subject little $^{14}CO_2$ appears in the breath for 12 h. Each laboratory must establish its own normal range, but as an approximate guide less than 2% of the activity should be recovered in breath within the first 4 h.

Breath output of $^{14}CO_2$ is increased when deconjugating anaerobic bacteria are active in the small intestine. Bile acid malabsorption from any cause, resulting in increased excretion of bile acids into the large intestine, also increases breath $^{14}CO_2$. $^{14}C$ glycocholate is thus a good test for the presence of bile acid deconjugation but does not distinguish between the various possible causes because it does not take account of the rate of bowel transit. It cannot differentiate between accelerated transit into the large bowel, where deconjugation is a normal phenomenon, and colonization of the small bowel. The sensitivity of the test is thus high but the specificity low.

### Bile acid malabsorption

#### *$^{75}$SeHCAT*

Bile acid malabsorption can be detected by stool counting using a labeled bile acid, chemical assay of bile acids in stool and measurement of the whole body retention of a gamma-labeled bile acid analog. The simplest technique in clinical practice is to measure the whole body retention of $^{75}$SeHCAT, the taurine conjugate of the synthetic trihydroxy bile acid, 23-selena-25-homocholic acid (Nyhlin et al 1994). The absorption and excretion of this compound is virtually identical to that of taurocholate and because the label is $^{75}$Se, an efficient gamma ray-emitting isotope, rather than the beta particle-emitting $^{14}$C, it is comparatively simple to measure the percentage of an administered dose remaining in the patient at any time after ingestion. It is thus unnecessary to collect and process stool.

Being the taurine conjugate of a trihydroxy acid, passive diffusion is minimal. Active transport is for practical purposes the only means of absorption and $^{75}$SeHCAT is thus an ideal marker for the active transport mechanism, which is confined to the terminal 1 meter of the ileum. Each bile acid molecule makes on average five circuits of the enterohepatic circulation daily. There is >95% probability of reabsorption on each transit of the circuit and recirculation amplifies the effect of quite small changes in absorption efficiency. After 7 days, assuming no renal excretion (an oversimplification), 17.5% of the original activity will still be in the body if the absorption efficiency of the ileum is 95% but only 8.5% if it is 93%. Bile acid absorption is thus a very sensitive measure of the functional state of the terminal ileum. The test is inaccurate if there is severe hepatic dysfunction.

***Technique.*** The activity is administered absorbed onto an inert carrier in a gelatine capsule. Measurements of retention at 0 and 7 days allow the half-time of excretion to be calculated accurately. The test can be performed using relatively simple equipment, it requires little time from staff or patient and it gives a low radiation dose. Using dedicated whole body counting equipment, as little as 40 kBq is adequate and a second tracer can be used. SeHCAT retention can, for example, be combined with measurement of vitamin $B_{12}$ absorption. Accurate results can also be obtained using a gamma camera either with the collimator removed or fitted with a general-purpose, low-energy collimator. The latter does not significantly attenuate the count-rate for the primary gamma ray emissions of $^{75}$Se but does substantially reduce the background, thus improving signal-to-noise ratio. When using a gamma camera, an administered activity of 400 kBq is required. Because of the relatively poor energy resolution of a gamma camera at these high energies, SeHCAT retention cannot be combined with a second tracer.

***Interpretation.*** Idiopathic bile acid malabsorption is a substantially underdiagnosed cause of intractable diarrhea. SeHCAT retention is by far the most sensitive test of impaired absorptive capacity for bile acid in the terminal ileum. It is specific to the site but not to the nature of the underlying pathology. Diarrhea due to disease affecting the jejunum or colon does not influence the retention of bile acids. Slightly reduced retention values are found in patients with an ileostomy, possibly because the absence of a functioning ileocecal valve reduces the time the intestinal contents spend in the terminal ileum. It is not affected by bacterial overgrowth or colonization and does not require the co-operation of the patient for the collection of excreta nor their processing by technicians. Retention of less than 5% is evidence of bile acid malabsorption. Retention between 5% and 10% is due to malabsorption in half of patients and rapid transit in the other half. Relatively few patients fall into this equivocal range.

#### *7α-hydroxy-4-cholesten-3-one*

There is a strong correlation between the rate of SeHCAT turnover and the plasma concentration of a bile acid precursor 7α-hydroxy-4-cholesten-3-one. Although not currently widely available, assay of this precursor may supercede SeHCAT retention measurement, as it eliminates the need to administer any radioactivity to the patient.

## INFLAMMATORY BOWEL DISEASE

The diagnosis of inflammatory bowel disease is made radiologically and endoscopically (p. 658), but sensitive and noninvasive radionuclide tests can be useful in detecting active or recurrent disease and complications (Rothstein 1991). Autologous leukocytes labeled with $^{111}$In-oxine or tropolone or with $^{99m}$Tc-HMPAO accumulate in areas of inflammation including active Crohn's disease or ulcerative colitis but not where the disease is quiescent. Imaging with $^{99m}$Tc is usually performed at 30 min, 3 h and sometimes 24 h, or at 24 and 48 h when indium is used. Radionuclide tests are particularly useful where active dis-

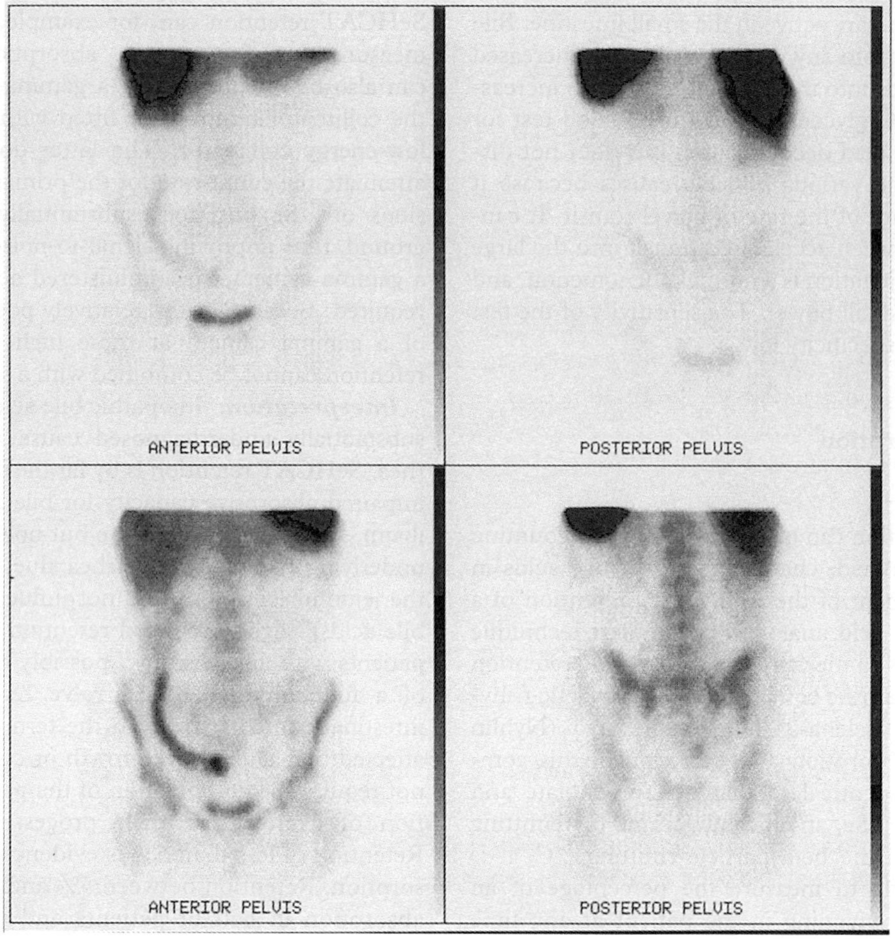


**Fig. 3.8** Labeled white cell images. The upper pair are taken 20 min after injection, the lower at 3 h. There is intense uptake in the right iliac fossa due to active inflammatory bowel disease in the terminal ileum. Uptake is also seen in the spleen, liver and bone marrow. Some activity has been excreted in the bladder. In this patient no biliary excretion is seen at this time.

ease makes radiological or endoscopic investigation hazardous and some regard them as the best tests for assessing disease activity (Fig. 3.8). Extent is demonstrated more readily in the colon, as it is often impossible to unravel the convolutions of the small bowel. A stool collection for 48 h after injection provides an important quantitation of inflammation. Late images allow identification of abscesses and while these should be sought first by computed tomography (CT) or ultrasonography, white cell scintigraphy detects foci in about 10% of patients with clinical evidence of occult infection but normal CT and ultrasound images.

## BOWEL TRANSIT

The various parts of the colon differ morphologically and functionally, while the physical state of the luminal contents varies in different parts of the colon and in the same subject from time to time (Kamm 1992). Study of colonic function is thus complex. Transit through the small intestine is less subject to variability and is less affected by external stimuli, but because of the complexity of its convolutions the only landmarks that can reliably be identified are the pylorus and the cecum.

The standard method for the measurement of gastric, small intestinal and colonic transit uses $^{111}$In and $^{99m}$Tc markers (p. 1348).

# LIVER AND GALLBLADDER

## INTRODUCTION

Radionuclide imaging of the liver and biliary tree can be carried out using radiopharmaceuticals that are taken up by the reticulo-endothelial cells in the hepatic sinusoids or are excreted by the hepatocytes into the biliary tree. The former is used much less than previously, as hepatic imaging by ultrasonography or computed tomography gives better anatomic delineation, but the latter perhaps deserves to be used more often (Watson & Kalff 1991).

## METHODOLOGY

### RADIOPHARMACEUTICALS

*Biliary agents*

The liver and the kidneys are two of the major excretory organs in the body and all substances excreted by one can to some extent be excreted by the other. Biliary excretion plays a major role in the elimination of organic anions and cations and of nonionized molecules that contain polar and lipophilic groups and have a molecular weight in the range 300–1000 daltons. Radiopharmaceuticals excreted in bile are technetium-labeled members of the HIDA (*h*epatic *i*mino *d*i *a*cetic acid) group of compounds and the balance between renal and biliary excretion is determined by the substitution at R (Fig. 3.9). The original HIDA compound is excreted mainly in bile and compounds developed subsequently allow imaging at serum bilirubin concentrations up to 180 mmol/L (10 mg/dl). The mechanism whereby the HIDA compounds enter bile is unknown but is probably carrier moderated.

***Technique.*** Fluids only should be given from the previous evening. Drugs undergoing biliary excretion should be omitted and HIDA excretion can be increased if needed by giving phenobarbitone 5 mg/kg/day for the preceding 5 days. Imaging is carried out with a gamma camera after giving 50 MBq (1–2 mCi) of the HIDA agent intravenously. A normal examination usually takes about 30 min, but occasionally imaging may require up to 24 h.

*Reticulo-endothelial agents*

Colloids given intravenously are rapidly removed by the reticulo-endothelial system, approximately in proportion to blood flow. The distribution is to some extent influenced by particle size. Inorganic tin colloids or denatured albumin millimicrospheres labeled with technetium are given intravenously and 80–90% of a tracer dose is taken up by the liver and spleen, approximately in proportion to the weight of the two organs. The rest accumulates mainly in the bone marrow and very small amounts are retained in the lungs.

***Technique.*** Imaging is carried out with a gamma camera. At least three projections – posterior, anterior and right lateral – are required; supplementary oblique projections occasionally help. Single photon emission computed tomography (SPECT) increases the detection of more deep-seated lesions, but resolution is limited ultimately by respiratory movement.

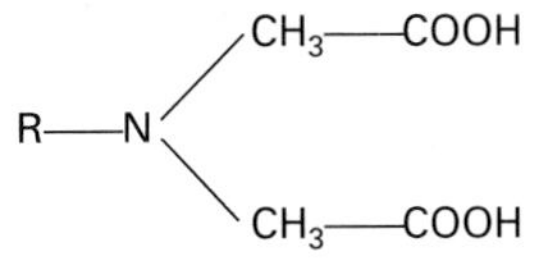


**Fig. 3.9** The general structure of hepatic imino diacetic acid (HIDA) derivatives.

### GALLBLADDER

#### Normal appearance

In the normal subject there is uniform high uptake in the liver within 5 min of injection, intrahepatic bile ducts can be seen by 15 min and the gallbladder, common bile duct and duodenum should always be visualized within 30 min. Small bowel activity can often be identified at 30 min, even in fasting subjects, and by 1 h most of the residual activity is in the small intestine (Fig. 3.10).

#### Acute cholecystitis

Visualization of the gallbladder within 30 min effectively excludes acute cholecystitis, which is associated with cystic duct obstruction in more than 95% of patients. If the gallbladder is not clearly visualized within 30–40 min, morphine sulfate (2 mg) given intravenously may provoke closure of the sphincter of Oddi, enabling visualization of the gallbladder within the following 10–15 min. Morphine should not be administered unless activity has been identified in the small bowel, thereby confirming patency of the common duct. Failure to observe this precaution may lead to perforation of an inflamed, obstructed common bile duct or gallbladder. In patients with a previously normal gallbladder, the sensitivity and specificity of cholescintigraphy are greater than 90%. Nonvisualization of the gallbladder in a patient who does not have acute cholecystitis is associated most commonly with chronic gallbladder disease or previous surgery. The value of cholescintigraphy in cholecystitis therefore depends on the prevalence of chronic gallbladder disease in the population under study.

Indium-labeled white cells accumulate in the gallbladder and its bed in acute cholecystitis. Technetium-labeled cells are more difficult to interpret because of biliary excretion of tracer eluted from the cells. The accumulation of labeled cells in the inflamed gallbladder occurs much earlier than visualization of the gallbladder due to excretion of eluted technetium and is usually more intense. In practice the diagnosis of focal inflammation is usually made clinically and technetium-labeled leukocytes rarely add clinically useful information in the acute phase of the illness. The complexity and cost of white cell labeling can thus rarely be justified, although it is useful in occasional patients postoperatively or where the diagnosis is in doubt.

#### Chronic cholecystitis

Radionuclide imaging is of limited value, as the scintigraphic findings are varied. Appearances may be normal in mild disease; delay in visualizing the gallbladder increases as the severity increases. In some patients it is possible to visualize the gallbladder after cholecystokinin (CCK) administration. Cholescintigraphy is most useful in an acute exacerbation of recurrent upper abdominal pain, as

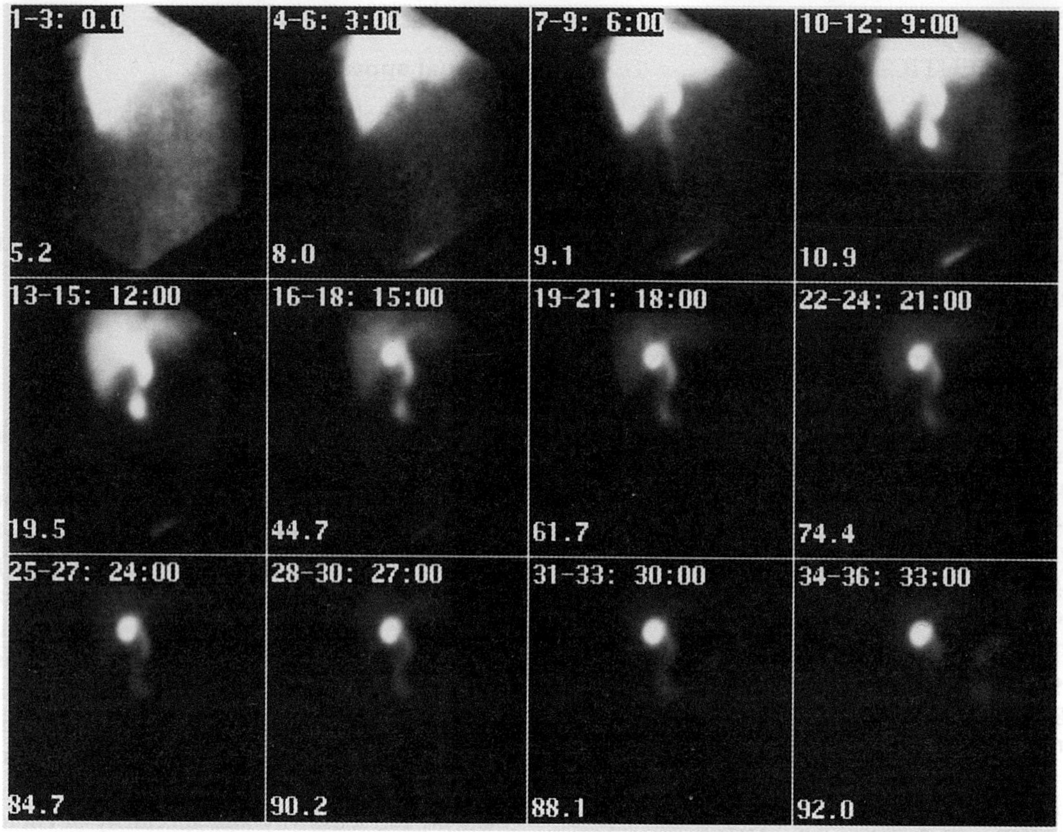


**Fig. 3.10** Normal sequence of images using one of the hepatobiliary agents. In the initial image there is very high uptake in the liver. Within 3 min the common bile duct is seen and this becomes progressively brighter. By 12 min the intrahepatic bile ducts and gallbladder are visualized. By 30 min residual activity is mainly in the gallbladder and bowel activity is visible.

visualization of the gallbladder suggests that this is unlikely to be due to acute or chronic cholecystitis. Unfortunately, the converse is not true.

### Acalculous biliary pain

A gallblader ejection fraction of less than 40% in response to cholecystokinin (CCK8) infusion identifies a group of patients who may obtain symptomatic relief from cholecystectomy despite normal cholecystography or ultrasound of the gallbladder (Krishnamurthy & Krishnamurthy 1992).

## BILE DUCTS

### Sclerosing cholangitis

This condition affects both the intra- and extrahepatic bile ducts, causes multiple sites of obstruction and is often distributed unevenly throughout the liver. A feature of diagnostic importance in sclerosing cholangitis, uncommon in other liver diseases, is that the rate of excretion of imino di acetic acid (IDA) derivatives differs in different parts of the liver, in keeping with the regional differences in disease severity. This causes a typical "beading" pattern due to accumulation of activity between strictures (Buscombe et al 1992). Single photon emission computed tomography of the liver 60–90 min after injection often supplements the planar images and detects lesions in the ducts that are not evident in other images or on contrast cholangiography. Cystic duct obstruction is common and the response to cholecystokinin is poor.

### Choledochal cysts

This uncommon condition, thought to be congenital in origin, may present at any age. The cystic abnormality in the liver or common bile duct can usually be identified by ultrasound or computed tomography, but cholescintigraphy can confirm whether there is communication with the biliary tree (Camponovo et al 1989). Scintigraphically, about a half of cysts show accumulation of hepatobiliary agents within an hour and in half of the remainder the cyst fills if imaging is prolonged up to 24 h. However, in a substantial minority of patients the cyst does not fill. Nonfilling thus cannot be used to exclude a choledochal cyst.

### Postoperative patients

*Cholecystectomy*

Biliary leak is common, especially after laparoscopic cholecystectomy, but is usually of no clinical significance and closes spontaneously. Cholescintigraphy is the simplest method of identifying a leak if one is suspected. It may be necessary to obtain multiple oblique projections to separate the leak from the bile duct and to identify the likely site. Obstruction, for example due to a retained stone, can also be identified, but endoscopic retrograde cholangiopancreatography (ERCP) is the preferred investigation as it allows definitive treatment.

***Biliary-enteric bypass.*** Cholescintigraphy is the best simple technique for determining the patency of biliary-enteric bypass procedures. The anatomy is often difficult to distinguish and multiple projections are necessary.

***Sphincterotomy.*** The normal resting pressure is 15 $cmH_2O$ at the sphincter of Oddi, 12 $cmH_2O$ in the common bile duct and 10 $cmH_2O$ within the gallbladder. Thus, the normal pathway for bile is into the gallbladder. Following sphincterotomy, this gradient is abolished and contrast media may fail to enter the gallbladder.

*Sphincter of Oddi dysfunction*

This condition causes recurrent biliary pain following cholecystectomy. There have been a number of attempts to establish criteria for differential diagnosis using quantitative hepato-biliary scintigraphy, principally by measuring the time to peak uptake or a half-time of washout, under basal conditions and following cholecystokinin (CCK8). Unfortunately, there is appreciable overlap between the normal and abnormal groups (Lisbona 1992). It has been suggested that vasodilators such as amyl nitrite may help to distinguish between dyskinesia and organic stenosis, amyl nitrite increasing the rate of drainage in patients with dyskinesia but not in those with organic stenosis. This interesting development needs to be confirmed.

## LIVER AND SPLEEN

Radionuclide studies of the liver and spleen using agents taken up by the reticulo-endothelial system are used less than previously owing to developments in ultrasound imaging, computed tomography and magnetic resonance imaging. These studies are, however, still used to investigate hepatic disease (Hawkins 1989).

### Normal appearances

There is considerable variation in the shape of the liver and of the spleen. In the anterior projection, the liver appears approximately triangular and the right lobe is substantially larger than the left. A larger left lobe suggests cirrhosis but is occasionally a normal variation. A reduced count-rate may be seen between the left and right lobes due to the porta hepatis and this may be difficult to distinguish from a space-occupying lesion at this site. The female breast or breast prostheses may give rise to a crescentic defect on the diaphragmatic aspect in the anterior projection; a curvilinear area of increased uptake is sometimes seen in the mid or lower third of the liver due to scatter from subcutaneous fat and costal impressions on the right border of the liver may be difficult to distinguish from focal replacement, while the inferior border is often notched by the gallbladder. In the right lateral projection the right and left lobes cannot be distinguished, but a notch on the anterior surface is due to the lower border of the left lobe being projected in front of the right. The diaphragmatic surface is usually a smooth curve but is sometimes unevenly indented by the diaphragm.

In the posterior projection, the peak count-rates from liver and spleen should be approximately equal. There is considerable variation in spleen size between individuals. An impression can usually be identified on the medial aspect of the right lobe of the liver caused by the kidney. The spleen may be identified separately from the liver, but frequently no border can be distinguished. The concentration of radioactivity in the spleen never exceeds that in the normal liver in the anterior projection. When present this indicates displacement or enlargement of the spleen or infiltration of the liver. Nonvisualization of the spleen is always abnormal and may be due to splenectomy, infarction, replacement (for example by tumor), displacement by a space-occupying lesion or suppression of splenic function, for example following a hemolytic crisis. The amount of detail visible in the liver depends on the quality both of the gamma camera and of the display being used. Marrow activity can always be seen with a good display that provides a wide contrast range. However, marrow may not be visualized in normal subjects when using more traditional analog and in poorer quality digital displays.

### Space-occupying lesions

Primary and metastatic tumors, abscesses and benign tumors of the liver do not contain reticulo-endothelial tissue and appear as photon-deficient areas. However, the resolution of both computed tomography and ultrasound is considerably better than that of scintigraphic imaging.

*Hemangioma*

Hemangiomas are identified as photon-deficient areas with both colloid and HIDA imaging of the liver (Middleton et al 1994). A more sensitive and specific method is to demonstrate the increased blood pool in hemangiomas using labeled red cells. They may be visualized immediately after injection if a dynamic study is performed, but most are equally well seen at equilibrium, once mixing of the labeled cells is complete. The pickup rate may be improved by single photon emission computed tomography.

*Hepatocellular carcinoma*

Uptake of HIDA in primary hepatocellular tumors is equal to or greater than that in the surrounding normal liver in two-thirds of patients with well-differentiated and one-third of patients with moderately differentiated tumors. In some this is evident within 30 min but in others the uptake is evident only on delayed scans taken at 3 h. Uptake is not sufficient for visualization in poorly differentiated tumors that appear as nonspecific photon-deficient areas.

### Diffuse liver disease

Cirrhosis, irrespective of the type, is recognized scintigraphically by a number of signs present singly or in any combination (Waxman 1982). They are in general consequent upon fibrosis, which increases vascular resistance in the liver and causes blood to be diverted via collaterals and to the spleen. The earlier signs may be liver enlargement, relative enlargement of the left lobe of the liver and relative increase of uptake of activity in the spleen. Subsequently, as the liver shrinks, the discrepancy between the liver and spleen increases and as more blood is diverted via collaterals into the systemic circulation, the isotope cleared by the marrow increases. Marrow visualization thus becomes progressively more marked. Initially, increased blood flow causes a relative increase in splenic uptake and size and the spleen acquires higher activity than the liver. Subsequently, as fibrosis progresses and collaterals are established, both the size and the relative uptake diminish while the relative uptake in marrow increases.

### Blood flow

*Hepatic perfusion*

Time-activity curves can be drawn over the liver and kidney from the first-pass study and it has been suggested that these can be used to calculate hepatic arterial and portal venous blood flow to the liver (O'Connor et al 1992). However, these claims have been disputed.

*Portasystemic shunting*

The extent of portasystemic shunting can be estimated from measurements following the absorption of tracers administered into the duodenum or the upper rectum. The shunt size can be estimated from time-activity curves over the heart and liver (Urbain et al 1993).

### Tumor-specific uptake

Some tracers are concentrated in tumors to a higher extent than in liver. Many labeled monoclonal antibodies have been investigated, but none is yet clinically useful. High uptake of F-18 fluorodeoxyglucose (FDG) is seen in many deposits, both in the liver and at other sites. Because of the short half-life of F-18 and the high energy of its positron-derived gamma rays, this is currently available only close to a source of production and is not well suited to conventional gamma cameras. It is, however, currently the best means of assessing the metabolic activity of a tumor.

## WILSON'S DISEASE

This rare disorder of copper metabolism can usually be diagnosed fairly readily. However, occasionally diagnosis can be difficult and the blood clearance of a tracer dose of radioactive copper $^{64}$Cu can be useful (Danks et al 1990). In the normal subject given an intravenous tracer dose of $^{64}$Cu, the plasma level at 48 h is higher than that at 2 h, as copper is cleared initially and subsequently returned to the plasma as ceruloplasmin. In Wilson's disease this does not happen and the blood concentration at 48 h is substantially lower than that at 2 h.

## PANCREAS

### Acute pancreatitis

Nonfilling of the gallbladder following the administration of HIDA occurs in over half of patients with acute cholecystitis. This is usually associated with stones in the common bile duct. Visualization of the gallbladder is good evidence that the cystic duct is patent.

## REFERENCES


Bunker C 1992 Esophageal disorders and scintigraphy: one clinician's perspective. Journal of Nuclear Medicine 33: 1301–1303

Buscombe J R, Miller R F, Ell P J 1992 Hepatobiliary scintigraphy in the diagnosis of AIDS-related sclerosing cholangitis. Nuclear Medicine Communications 13: 154–160

Camponovo E, Buck J L, Drane W E 1989 Scintigraphic features of choledochal cyst. Journal of Nuclear Medicine 30: 622–628

Camey B L, Jones K L, Horowitz M, Sun W M, Penagini R, Meyer J H 1995 Gastric emptying of oil and aqueous meal components in pancreatic insufficiency — effects of posture and on appetite. American Journal of Physiology 268: G925–932

Christian P E, Datz F L, Sorenson J A, Taylor A 1984 Technical factors in gastric emptying studies. Journal of Nuclear Medicine 24: 264–268

Coates G, Garnett E S, Webber C E 1982 Detection of deconjugation of bile salts with a $^{14}CO_2$ breath test. Seminars in Nuclear Medicine 12: 99–100

Collins P J, Horowitz M, Cook D J, Harding P E, Shearman D J C 1983 Gastric emptying in normal subjects. A reproducible technique using a single scintillation camera and computer system. Gut 24: 1117–1125

Cooney D R, Duszynski D O, Camboa E, Karp M P, Jewett T C Jr 1982 The abdominal technetium scan (a decade of experience). Journal of Pediatric Surgery 17: 611–619

Da Costa P M, Godinho F, Veiga-Fernandes F 1992 Gastro-oesophageal and bile reflux – simultaneous quantitative assessment with gastric and gallbladder emptying evaluation: clinical applicability of a new computerised gammagraphic method. Nuclear Medicine Communications 13: 817–823

Danks D M, Metz G, Sewell R, Prewett E J 1990 Wilson's disease in adults with cirrhosis but no neurological abnormalities. British Medical Journal 301: 331–332

Datz F L 1984 The role of radionuclide studies in esophageal disease. Journal of Nuclear Medicine 25: 1040–1045

Debongnie J C, Pauwels S, Raat A, de Meeus Y, Haot J, Mainguet P 1991 Quantification of *Helicobacter pylori* infection in gastritis and ulcer disease using a simple and rapid carbon-14-urea breath test. Journal of Nuclear Medicine 32: 1192–1198

Hawkins R A 1989 Radionuclide studies of the liver and hepatobiliary system. Current Opinion in Radiology 1: 499–507

Horowitz M, Collins P J, Shearman D J C 1985 Disorders of gastric emptying in humans and the use of radionuclide techniques. Archives of Internal Medicine 145: 1467–1475

Houghton L, Read N, Heddle R et al 1988 Relationship of the motor activity of the antrum, pylorus, and duodenum to gastric emptying of a solid-liquid mixed meal. Gastroenterology 94: 1285–1291

Kamm M A 1992 The small intestine and colon: scintigraphic quantitation of motility in health and disease. European Journal of Nuclear Medicine 19: 902–912

King C E, Toskes P P 1983 The use of breath tests in the study of malabsorption. Clinics in Gastroenterology 12: 591–610

Krishnamurthy S, Krishnamurthy G T 1992 Gallbladder ejection fraction: a decade of progress and future promise. Journal of Nuclear Medicine 33: 542–544

Leb G, Lipp R W 1993 Criteria for labelled meals for gastric emptying studies in nuclear medicine. European Journal of Nuclear Medicine 20: 185–186

Lisbona R 1992 The scintigraphic evaluation of sphincter of Oddi dysfunction. Journal of Nuclear Medicine 33: 1223–1224

Middleton M L, Milstein D M, Freeman L M 1994 Hepatic mass lesions: scintigraphic update with emphasis on hemangioma detection. In: Freeman L M (ed) Nuclear medicine annual. Raven, New York, p 55–90

Mishkin S 1981 Radionuclide salivary gland imaging. Seminars in Nuclear Medicine 11: 258–265

Nyhlin H, Merrick M V, Eastwood M A 1994 Bile acid malabsorption in Crohn's disease and indications for its assessment using SeHCAT. Gut 35: 90–93

O'Connor M K, Krom R F, Carton E G et al 1992 Ratio of hepatic arterial-to-portal venous blood flow – validation of radionuclide techniques in an animal model. Journal of Nuclear Medicine 33: 239–245

Robinson P 1993 The role of nuclear medicine in acute gastrointestinal bleeding. Nuclear Medicine Communications 14: 849–855

Rothstein R D 1991 The role of scintigraphy in the management of inflammatory bowel disease. Journal of Nuclear Medicine 32: 856–859

Scarpignato C 1990 Gastric emptying measurement in man. In: Scarpignato C, Bianchi Porro G (eds) Clinical investigation of gastric functions, pp 198–246

Smout A, Horowitz M, Armstrong D 1994 Methods to study gastric emptying. Digestive Diseases and Sciences 39: S130–132

Urbain D, Muls V, Dupont M, Jeghers O, Thys O, Ham H R 1993 Physiopathological significance of thallium-201 per rectum scintigraphy in liver cirrhosis. Journal of Nuclear Medicine 34: 1642–1645

Watson A, Kalff V 1991 Hepatobiliary imaging. Current Opinion in Radiology 3: 851–858

Waxman A D 1982 Scintigraphic evaluation of diffuse hepatic disease. Seminars in Nuclear Medicine 12: 75–88

Yeker D, Büyükünal C, Benli M, Büyükünal E, Urgancioglu I 1984 Radionuclide imaging of Meckel's diverticulum: cimetidine versus pentagastrin plus glucagon. European Journal of Nuclear Medicine 9: 316–319

# 4. Endoscopy

*Kelvin R. Palmer* *Peter C. Hayes*

Endoscopy is central to the practice of modern gastroenterology. It is possible to visualize directly and biopsy the entire lumen of the gastrointestinal tract and to examine the biliary tree and pancreas in great detail. The development of therapeutic endoscopy has transformed many aspects of patient management, often avoiding the need for surgical intervention. Endoscopists dilate and stent benign or malignant strictures, arrest life-threatening gastrointestinal hemorrhage, extract gallstones from the biliary tree and destroy or remove tumors. Endoscopy is undertaken by physicians, surgeons and occasionally radiologists. Good results depend upon dexterity, experience and clinical judgment but are impossible without modern, well-maintained equipment and an appropriate environment. Endoscopy is a team effort and expert nursing assistance is vital.

## ENDOSCOPIC NEEDS

It has been estimated that in the United Kingdom the prevalence of gastrointestinal disease is such that 1:100 of the general population require upper endoscopy each year. The corresponding figure for colonoscopy is 1:500 and for endoscopic retrograde cholangiopancreatography (ERCP) 1:1000 (Gastroenterology Services Working Party 1993). For a typical district general hospital serving a population of 250 000, this equals a need for 3500 endoscopic procedures per year.

### Endoscopy unit

A dedicated endoscopy unit is necessary to fulfill these needs. Such a unit is based upon outpatient or day-bed usage and commonly serves both hospital clinical and primary care referral ("open access"). In addition, patients requiring therapeutic endoscopy, who now comprise approximately 20% of all procedures, require inpatient facilities. The endoscopy unit requires a reception area (with appropriate staff and a booking system), a waiting area, an endoscopy suite and a recovery area (Cotton & Williams 1980). In addition, storage space and accommodation are needed. The endoscopy suite ideally comprises at least two rooms, each with a floor area in excess of 30 $m^2$. These rooms should be well ventilated and easily washable, doors should be wide and work surfaces, power points and sinks must be plentiful. Piped oxygen, suction, monitoring devices, resuscitation equipment and endoscopy washing machines are essential. A third room with radiological equipment is necessary for ERCP and other procedures that require radiological screening. An anteroom for the administration of sedation prior to endoscopy is ideal. Patients are endoscoped on trolleys (with brakes), which enable easy transfer to and from the endoscopy suite.

### Nurses

Endoscopy units are dependent upon expert nursing assistants. These individuals are usually trained nurses whose primary role is ensuring the safe practice of endoscopy, but who are often also responsible for much of the administration and day-to-day running of the unit and maintaining the equipment.

During endoscopy, the assistant helps maintain the patency of the airway by removing secretions, ensures optimal patient position and the safety of the instrument by appropriate positioning of the mouthguard and monitors respiration, pulse and oxygen saturation. For routine diagnostic upper intestinal endoscopy at least two assistants are necessary: one to supervise the mouthguard and airway, the other to help with monitoring, biopsy and therapeutic maneuvers. A third assistant is necessary for more complex interventions such as laser photocoagulation. Three assistants are necessary for interventional ERCP, whereas one assistant is sufficient for flexible sigmoidoscopy and colonoscopy. A nursing auxiliary is helpful for a range of less responsible roles and nurses are needed for postendoscopic supervision.

These demands dictate that an active, comprehensive endoscopy service requires one senior nurse-in-charge, three other fully trained nurses and one nursing assistant in addition to day-bed ward staff (British Society of Gastroenterology 1987). Clinical nurse specialists are now being introduced in endoscopy to do diagnostic procedures such as upper gastrointestinal endoscopy and flexible sigmoidoscopy (British Society of Gastroenterology 1994).

### Open access endoscopy

Increasingly, routine diagnostic upper gastrointestinal endoscopy is undertaken on an "open access" basis, without prior consultation from hospital-based physicians or surgeons. This approach has the advantage of increasing the speed with which a diagnosis is made. The diagnostic yield of significant upper gastrointestinal pathology is relatively high and little different from that associated with endoscopy performed after hospital consultation (Gear & Wilkinson 1989). Open access endoscopy reduces pressures upon waiting lists for gastrointestinal outpatient consultations (Bramble 1993). There are moves for routine upper gastrointestinal endoscopy to be done in general practice surgeries (Jones 1995) and this may further reduce pressures upon gastroenterologists.

## EQUIPMENT

### Rigid instruments

The rigid esophagoscope is not usually found in the endoscopy unit, although it remains a useful instrument in otorhinolaryngology and thoracic surgery. It is sometimes necessary for the removal of foreign bodies from the upper gastrointestinal tract and some experts advocate its use for eradication of varices. In both situations, fiberoptic instruments are used first because they are easier to pass, have greater versatility and do not require general anesthesia. Rigid sigmoidoscopy has also largely been replaced by flexible endoscopy. Nevertheless, the proctoscope and rigid sigmoidoscope are still important for examination of the anal canal and rectum, particularly in patients who present with profuse rectal bleeding (Mann et al 1988). The large lumina of these instruments allow easy passage of instruments and blood and colonic fluid can be removed relatively easily. Metal proctoscopes and sigmoidoscopes have been replaced by cheaper, disposable plastic instruments.

### Fiberoptic instruments

The principle of fiberoptics is illustrated in Figure 4.1. Light enters one end of a glass tube and undergoes a series of reflections to exit at the other end. The light is transmitted from a source to illuminate an object via a series of nonaligned fibers. The image is returned along closely aligned fibers – the coherent bundle – to produce an accurate reflection of the object. The resolution of the image depends upon the number of coherent fibers. Modern endoscopes have a wide viewing angle of up to 100°.

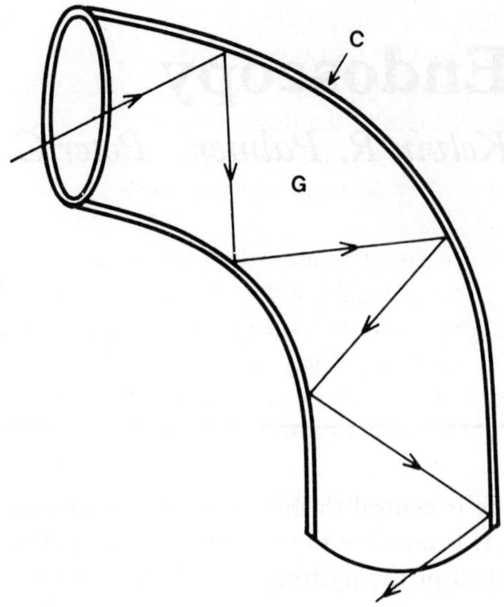


**Fig. 4.1** The principles of fiberoptics. Glass fiber (G), coating on glass fiber (C).

Fiberoptic instruments are extremely flexible, simple to use, easy to pass and extremely maneuverable. They have a distal bending section that can be moved through 360° using an internal pulley system. The distal lens is usually forward-viewing, although side-viewing duodenoscopes are necessary for ERCP and oblique-viewing gastroscopes are sometimes useful for examining the esophagus and duodenal cap. Some instruments have a bridge for adjusting the position of cannulae or forceps. Wheels for moving the bending section and controls for suction, air inflation and cleaning the lens are conveniently situated on the handle of the endoscope. There is a channel for passage of forceps, cannulae or other accessories into the gastrointestinal tract. Endoscopes are fully waterproof, as they need to be immersed for adequate cleaning. The endoscope is connected to a powerful light source which also contains an air pump, necessary for inflating the stomach, and to a suction device for aspiration of gastrointestinal contents.

### Video endoscopes

Fiberoptic endoscopes are being replaced by video endoscopes that are more versatile than their predecessors, more comfortable for the endoscopist and have considerable advantages for training.

The video endoscope is based upon the charged couple device or "chip" (Sivak 1991). This is a silicone-based semiconductive material. Photons of light alter the electrical resistance of the semiconductor by producing an "electron hole" resulting in the production of an electrical current. The surface of the chip is divided by channel stops and electrodes into a grid of numerous photosensitive elements. The channel stops are arranged in parallel rows and act as barriers to the flow of electrons. Parallel rows of electrodes are arranged perpendicular to the channel stops. The chip is thus divided into picture elements known as "pixels".

There is a direct relationship between the number of incident photons reaching the chip and the level of electric charge that is developed: the greater the light intensity, the higher the current. When an image is focused upon the chip using a lens, each pixel stores electrons relative to the number of impinging photons and generates an electronic representation of the image. This is amplified and the image is displayed on a television monitor.

### Cleaning and disinfection

Transmission of infection by endoscopes should not occur if instruments are properly cleaned and disinfected (Axon 1991). Following endoscopy, the instrument is cleaned with soap and water, biopsy channels are brushed and suction and water control buttons are removed. The instrument is then cleaned and soaked in specific disinfectants that have antibacterial, antiviral and antifungal properties. Gluteraldehyde (2%) is the most widely used disinfectant (Bond 1991), but it often causes skin sensitivity and atmospheric pollution may cause respiratory irritation (Working Party of the BSG 1993). Adequate ventilation and automated cleaning machines overcome some of these health and safety problems, although some exposure of staff to the cleaning solution is almost inevitable. Accessories such as biopsy forceps, catheters and snares are cleaned in the same solutions. Alternatives to gluteraldehyde are being sought, but none is currently superior (Babb & Bradley 1995).

Endoscopes are left in cleaning solutions for 20 min. It is wise to perform regular bacteriological culture of equipment and cleaning fluids to ensure that disinfection has been effective. Bacterial and viral infection has been transmitted between patients by inadequately cleaned instruments (Beecham et al 1979, Birnie et al 1983, Allen et al 1987, Safrany 1991), although hepatitis B transmission is very rare and HIV transmission has not been reported.

## SEDATION

Routine intravenous sedation is probably unnecessary for many patients undergoing diagnostic upper gastrointestinal endoscopy. Most patients who have undergone endoscopy without sedation say they would submit themselves to further endoscopy without sedation (Bramble 1993), but the majority of gastrointestinal units continue to use sedative drugs routinely. Intravenous boluses of midazolam or diazepam (Diazemuls) are used most commonly (Quine et al 1995). Care should be employed to give these slowly over a minimum of 2 min and to use the least dose for adequate sedation. The elderly and patients with liver disease are particularly sensitive to midazolam and severe respiratory and cardiac depression will occur if too much is given too quickly. The specific benzodiazepine antagonist flumazenil reverses the central nervous system effects of these drugs and should be available for immediate use in all units. Flumazenil 200 μg is given intravenously over 15 s and then further 100 μg doses are given at 1-min intervals as required to reverse respiratory depression to a total dose of 1 mg (usual dose required 300–600 μg). Where excessive sedation recurs, an infusion of 100–400 μg/h can be used.

Patients undergoing therapeutic procedures such as esophageal dilatation and those undergoing ERCP or colonoscopy usually receive a combination of benzodiazepine and pethidine. This facilitates the examination but increases the degree of cardiorespiratory depression. Patients receiving intravenous sedation should be carefully monitored during and after the endoscopic procedure by continuous measurement of pulse rate and oxygen saturation and an intravenous cannula should be in place. These patients should receive oxygen (3 L/min) through nasal catheters. Equipment for resuscitation should be available.

Gargles or sprays of lignocaine can be used to anesthetize the pharynx. This is probably necessary only for patients not receiving intravenous sedation. Many endoscopists have abandoned its use for routine endoscopy, as the patient is unable to drink for 2 h after the procedure.

## PRECAUTIONS AND COMPLICATIONS

### Consent

Written consent should be obtained by the endoscopist prior to endoscopy. The procedure and its main risks should be explained; information booklets sent to the patient before attending for the procedure are particularly useful.

### Anxiety

It is always sensible to assess the degree of anxiety in each patient. Stoic patients easily swallow endoscopes without needing sedation, while anxious individuals usually need sedative drugs. The endoscopist can learn to identify these two broad groups and appropriate use of intravenous sedation helps make for smooth running of the endoscopy list. Routine diagnostic endoscopy can be performed without the use of intravenous sedation, although pharyngeal anesthesia using lignocaine sprays may be necessary.

### Medications

It is important to obtain an accurate history of drug ingestion. It is generally safe to perform diagnostic endoscopy in patients taking oral anticoagulants, although the prothrombin time should be normalized in those undergoing therapeutic procedures (Choudari et al 1994). This entails stopping warfarin and administering fresh frozen plasma. Vitamin $K_1$ 10 mg intravenously can make reanticoagulation impossible for up to 3 months. Heparinization is necessary before restarting anticoagulants (British National Formulary 1996).

Oral hypoglycemic agents should be omitted on the morning of the procedure in diabetic patients to avoid dangerous falls of blood sugar in the fasted state. Insulin-dependent diabetic patients are best endoscoped at the beginning of a morning endoscopy list; an infusion of dextrose and insulin may be necessary. Patients taking long-term corticosteroids may require intravenous hydrocortisone.

### Emergency endoscopy

This should be undertaken only after the patient has been resuscitated (p. 518). Patients who undergo endoscopy for acute gastrointestinal bleeding while still hypotensive and hypoxic are at high risk of developing cardiac and respiratory complications. Pulmonary aspiration is relatively common, particularly as the endoscopy may be difficult and protracted. Intravenous access through a wide-bore cannula, availability of adequate amounts of blood or colloid and pre-endoscopic oxygenation are mandatory. The highest risk patients are best endoscoped under general anesthetic with an endotracheal tube in place.

### Cardiorespiratory disease

Patients who have severe cardiovascular or respiratory disease may be at risk from life-threatening complications. Those with an unstable myocardium may develop serious arrhythmias (Rostykus et al 1980). Significant falls in arterial oxygen saturation occur during endoscopy (Murray et al 1990) and this assumes particular importance for patients who have chronic obstructive airway disease (Rostykus et al 1980). Those with serious heart disease should be identified prior to endoscopy to ensure that adequate oxygenation is achieved throughout the procedure, heart rhythm is monitored and appropriate antiarrhythmic drugs are available. Tachycardia may be important in producing myocardial ischemia during endoscopy and can be prevented by metoprolol 100 mg as premedication (Rosenberg et al 1996). Patients with poor respiratory function may require pre-endoscopic oxygenation and the smallest possible doses of sedative drugs are used. The fall in arterial $PO_2$ is due to compromise of the upper airway and the respiratory depression of sedative drugs and it is wise to avoid sedatives in patients with severe chronic respiratory disease. It has been recommended that all patients undergoing upper gastrointestinal endoscopy should be monitored by pulse oximetry, receive oxygen supplementation through nasal cannulae and have venous access through an indwelling cannula (Quine et al 1995).

### Bacterial endocarditis

Bacteremia can occur after diagnostic and therapeutic procedures, particularly from the mouth and the genitourinary tract (Durack 1995). Gastrointestinal endoscopic procedures, especially those involving therapeutic manipulation, also cause bacteremia (Botoman & Surawicz 1986, Kohler & Riemann 1987) (Table 4.1) and prophylaxis against bacterial endocarditis may be required in susceptible patients. It is therefore important that heart disease, particularly valvular heart disease, be identified before endoscopy. Bacterial endocarditis can occur in spite of antibiotic prophylaxis and as the frequency of bacteremia during diagnostic endoscopy is low (Table 4.1), the value of prophylaxis during endoscopy has been questioned (Shorvon et al 1983).

The decision regarding the use of antibiotic prophylaxis should be related partly to the risk of bacterial endocarditis associated with particular cardiac lesions (Table 4.2) and partly to the procedure to be carried out and inevitably medicolegal considerations will prompt endoscopists to err on the side of caution and give prophylaxis. At a minimum, all patients who have prosthetic heart valves or who have had bacterial endocarditis previously should be given prophylaxis (Dajani et al 1990, Endocarditis Working Party 1990) and prophylaxis is particularly advisable where therapeutic procedures are to be performed. An appropriate prophylactic regimen for gastrointestinal endoscopy is ampicillin 1 g intravenously and gentamicin 80 mg slowly intravenously over not less than

**Table 4.1** Frequency of bacteremia associated with gastrointestinal events and procedures

| Procedure/event | Frequency (%) | |
|---|---|---|
| | Mean | Range |
| Diagnostic endoscopy | | |
| Upper gastrointestinal | 4 | 0–8 |
| ERCP | 5 | 0–6 |
| Colonoscopy | 5 | 0–5 |
| Rigid sigmoidoscopy | 5 | |
| Proctoscopy | 2 | |
| Therapeutic endoscopy | | |
| Esophageal dilatation | 45 | 8–100 |
| Sclerotherapy | 20 | 5–53 |
| ERCP | 21 | 0–48 |
| Laser therapy | 35 | 30–40 |
| Barium enema | 10 | 5–11 |
| Defecation | 0.6 | |
| Rectal examination | 2 | 0–4 |
| Brushing teeth | 40 | 7–50 |

From: Sontheimer et al 1991, Durack 1995

**Table 4.2** Risk of infective endocarditis associated with pre-existing cardiac disorders (Durack 1995)

| |
|---|
| *Relatively high risk* |
| Prosthetic heart valves |
| Previous infective endocarditis |
| Cyanotic congenital heart disease |
| Patent ductus arteriosus |
| Aortic regurgitation |
| Aortic stenosis |
| Mitral regurgitation |
| Mitral stenosis and regurgitation |
| Ventricular septal defect |
| Coarctation of the aorta |
| Surgically repaired intracardiac lesions with residual hemodynamic abnormality |
| *Intermediate risk* |
| Mitral valve prolapse with regurgitation |
| Pure mitral stenosis |
| Tricuspid valve disease |
| Pulmonary stenosis |
| Asymmetric septal hypertrophy |
| Bicuspid aortic valve or calcific aortic sclerosis with minimal hemodynamic abnormality |
| Degenerative valvular disease in elderly patients |
| Surgically repaired intracardiac lesions with minimal or no hemodynamic abnormality, <6 months after operation |
| *Relatively low risk* |
| Mitral valve prolapse without regurgitation |
| Trivial valvular regurgitation on echocardiography without structural abnormality |
| Isolated atrial septal defect |
| Arteriosclerotic plaques |
| Coronary artery disease |
| Cardiac pacemaker |
| Surgically repaired intracardiac lesions, with minimal or no hemodynamic abnormality, >6 months after operation |

3 min just before the procedure. Vancomycin 1 g infused intravenously over 100 min can be given to patients sensitive to penicillin.

## Other infections

Patients undergoing endoscopy may be at risk of infections other than bacterial endocarditis (Safrany 1991). ERCP in patients with large bile duct obstruction may precipitate cholangitis and those with cholestasis should be given an antibiotic such as ciprofloxacin 750 mg orally 60–90 min before the procedure. Immunocompromised patients such as those with AIDS or who are being given immunosuppressive drugs can also be given antibiotic prophylaxis, particularly when therapeutic manipulations are done. Antibiotic prophylaxis can also be considered to prevent spontaneous bacterial peritonitis (SBP) in ascites due to cirrhosis, particularly where SBP has occurred previously (p. 1033).

## Pyloric stenosis

Patients who have gastric outflow obstruction should be identified before endoscopy. These individuals are at particular risk of aspirating gastric contents into the airway and if pyloric stenosis is likely, it is wise to drain the stomach contents through a nasogastric tube for 24 h before endoscopy.

## Immune deficiency

Immunocompromised patients, particularly those with AIDS, present special problems and should be identified and endoscoped either on a dedicated "high-risk" list or at the end of a routine endoscopy session using endoscopes that have been soaked in glutaraldehyde for at least 60 min (Weller et al 1988). This is because of the importance of destroying mycobacterial organisms that may be relatively resistant to standard disinfection regimens. Mycobacterial organisms have low pathogenicity but may cause severe infection in AIDS patients (Axon et al 1991). Assiduous endoscopic technique, possibly associated with prophylactic antibiotic therapy (p. 100) is necessary. Risks of transmission of infection to the endoscopy staff are minimal providing sensible precautions are taken. These include the use of goggles to prevent conjunctival contamination by vapor, double gloves to minimize risk of transmission through abrasions and plastic aprons, masks and gowns.

## Mortality

Diagnostic upper gastrointestinal endoscopy is extremely safe, with an estimated procedure-related mortality of approximately one per 2000–5000 examinations, and has low morbidity (Arrowsmith et al 1991, Quine et al 1995). Nevertheless, endoscopy carries real risks and these have to be minimized.

## Postendoscopy advice

Patients who have had lignocaine analgesia for the throat should not drink for 2 h. Those who have received sedation for uncomplicated endoscopic procedures should be escorted home and should be advised not to drive or operate machinery for 24 h.

# UPPER GASTROINTESTINAL ENDOSCOPY

## Indications: diagnostic endoscopy

The indications for endoscopy are shown in Table 4.3.

### *Dyspepsia*

The commonest indication for upper gastrointestinal endoscopy is dyspepsia. Anorexia, nausea, fullness or abdominal pain developing after middle age may indicate gastric cancer and these symptoms certainly justify gastroscopy; dyspepsia in younger individuals is rarely due to

**Table 4.3** Indications for diagnostic upper gastrointestinal endoscopy

| |
|---|
| Dyspepsia |
| Heartburn |
| Odynophagia |
| Dysphagia |
| Gastrointestinal bleeding |
| Intestinal bleeding |

malignant disease and many pragmatic clinicians carry out gastroscopy only after failure of response to acid-suppressing drugs. While this does not achieve the ideal of a specific diagnosis, pressure on most endoscopy practices and the low positive yield of endoscopy in young patients make this a reasonable compromise.

Endoscopy is superior to the barium meal in the investigation of the dyspeptic patient. A radiological viewpoint is presented on p. 12. The barium meal is cheaper and visualizes certain abnormalities such as webs, rings and diverticula better than endoscopy; these advantages are offset by difficulties in performing the investigations in immobile, unco-operative patients and by difficulties in interpretation of the postoperative stomach. Endoscopy has the advantages of biopsy and administering therapy. In addition, it is more sensitive and specific in achieving a diagnosis and influencing clinical management (Dooley et al 1984). In one series, patients preferred endoscopy to radiology (Stevenson et al 1991) and the apparent higher costs of endoscopy are at least partly balanced by lower subsequent costs due to improved diagnostic accuracy (Longstreth 1992).

*Heartburn and dysphagia*

Heartburn or painful swallowing (odynophagia) responding poorly to medical therapy are indications for upper gastrointestinal endoscopy. Although most cases are due to acid reflux disease in which treatment is based upon symptoms rather than endoscopic findings, some cases will be associated with Barrett's esophagus or with ulcer, neoplastic disease or infections such as moniliasis. Controversy exists as to the relative merits of a barium swallow or endoscopy as primary investigation for dysphagia. Radiologists and some gastroenterologists (p. 168) argue that a barium swallow should be done first because it shows the site and nature of a stricture, demonstrates a motility disorder and is the investigation of choice for a pharyngeal pouch. Endoscopists argue that the site and nature of a stricture is as well demonstrated endoscopically and that the ability to biopsy and dilate the gullet are considerable advantages. Furthermore, motility is better demonstrated manometrically than by barium radiology and a negative endoscopy in a patient presenting with dysphagia should be followed by esophageal manometry. Although the endoscope may pass into a pharyngeal pouch with the potential for perforation, good endoscopic technique makes this complication rare.

**Table 4.4** Indications for therapeutic upper gastrointestinal endoscopy

| | |
|---|---|
| *Esophageal strictures* | |
| Peptic | Dilatation |
| Malignant | Dilatation plus intubation, laser photocoagulation, alcohol injection |
| Corrosive | Dilatation |
| *Esophageal dysmotility* | |
| Pneumatic balloon dilatation | |
| *Varices* | |
| Injection, banding | |
| *Gastroduodenal bleeding* | |
| Peptic ulcer | Injection, laser, heater probe, diathermy |
| Mallory–Weiss tear | Injection |
| Vascular | Laser photocoagulation |
| *Gastric outflow obstruction* | |
| Balloon dilatation | |
| *Nutritional support* | |
| Gastrostomy tube insertion | |
| *Foreign body removal* | |

*Bleeding*

Upper gastrointestinal endoscopy is the investigation of choice in acute upper gastrointestinal hemorrhage (p. 484). However, endoscopy in actively bleeding patients is potentially hazardous and technically demanding. It should be performed only after adequate resuscitation and by an experienced endoscopist who possesses the ability to apply local hemostatic therapy.

*Intestinal biopsy*

Duodenal biopsy is most conveniently accomplished by endoscopy and the Crosby capsule is now rarely used for investigation of small bowel malabsorption. Wide-bore channels available on certain endoscopes enable multiple large biopsies to be taken.

## Indications: therapeutic endoscopy

The indications for therapeutic upper gastrointestinal endoscopy are shown in Table 4.4.

*Esophageal diseases*

***Strictures*** (p. 200). Esophageal strictures are managed at least in part endoscopically. Benign (peptic) strictures are dilated under direct endoscopic visualization using tapered dilators or balloons (McBride & Ergun 1994). Most patients need repeated dilatations at infrequent intervals but for the great majority, most of whom are elderly, endoscopic dilatation is definitive treatment and operative surgery is rarely performed. Malignant strictures are frequently dilated at the time of diagnosis to effect temporary relief of dysphagia and to facilitate biopsy and cytology. Patients whose tumors are inoperable or unsuitable for radiotherapy are treated endoscopically and operative insertion of endoprostheses is now unnecessary.

Four therapeutic options are commonly available. The best established is intubation using plastic tubes (Ogilvie et al 1982). This is particularly useful for cicatrizing, firm tumors distal to the postcricoid portion of the esophagus. Soft fleshy tumors do not adequately "grip" the prosthesis and tend to migrate; the tube cannot be tolerated in the postcricoid area or pharynx. The advent of expandable, membrane-covered metal stents (Knyrim et al 1993), which are inserted with little morbidity and provide considerable relief of dysphagia, represents a considerable improvement over plastic tubes. Destruction of tumors using Nd:YAG laser energy is particularly suitable for polypoid tumors throughout the gullet (Krasner et al 1987). Long malignant strictures are difficult and tedious to treat by laser and laser vaporization has to be more frequently repeated than intubation (Barr et al 1990). The advent of photodynamic therapy, in which the sensitivity of the tumor to laser energy is increased by prior injection of hematoporphyrin, has the potential to improve the efficacy of the technique (Thomas et al 1987). The cheapest option is perendoscopic injections of absolute alcohol into the tumor (Nwokolo et al 1994). This is done relatively easily and may be particularly applicable to polypoid tumors.

As is often the case in endoscopy, these means for palliating malignant dysphagia are complementary rather than competitive. A patient may require several techniques at different stages of their disease, depending upon the nature of the tumor. For example, a polypoid tumor may respond well initially to laser vaporization, but eventual recurrence may be a hard cicatrizing tumor best treated by intubation. Subsequent tumor overgrowth may require laser vaporization.

***Motility disorders.*** Achalasia of the esophagus can be treated by pneumatic dilatation using a range of balloons (Cox et al 1986, Elta et al 1987). The role of endoscopic dilatation versus surgical myotomy remains controversial; some surgeons do not consider that pneumatic dilatation has any value, while many gastroenterologists refer a patient for myotomy only after failure of endoscopic therapy (Vantrappen & Janssens 1983). Heller's myotomy is an established and effective operation (Csendes et al 1989), but many patients prefer an initial conservative approach. Should laparoscopic myotomy (Shimi et al 1991) prove effective, it is likely that endoscopic therapy will have a lesser role. Neither approach should be undertaken until full endoscopy and manometry have confirmed the diagnosis and excluded "pseudoachalasia" due to infiltration by gastric carcinoma (Tucker et al 1978).

Pneumatic dilatation is occasionally performed for other esophageal motor disorders, including diffuse esophageal spasm (Vantrappen & Hellemans 1980), although its exact value is unclear (see also pp. 176 and 180).

***Varices.*** Bleeding esophageal varices are treated primarily by endoscopic therapy. Currently, evidence dictates that only varices that have bled should be considered for endoscopic treatment (pp. 1009 and 1005); prophylactic sclerotherapy does not improve prognosis and the injections themselves may cause more problems than benefit (Lopes & Grace 1991, Pagliaro et al 1992). The endoscopist plays an important role in the management of actively bleeding esophageal varices. Following resuscitation, endoscopy is performed to confirm the diagnosis and exclude other causes of bleeding. Bleeding peptic ulcer is common in patients with cirrhosis and portal hypertension (Rabinovitz et al 1990). Congestive gastropathy and gastric erosions (Teréz et al 1980) may also cause bleeding in cirrhotic patients, although this is not usually severe.

If esophageal varices are found to be bleeding, they are treated by injection sclerotherapy (Westaby et al 1985, Goff 1993). Bleeding gastric varices are not amenable to injection therapy, except perhaps with tissue glues (Soehendra et al 1987) or thrombin (Williams et al 1994), and are best treated by other means (p. 183). Following initial hemostasis, most gastroenterologists embark upon a course of treatment designed to obliterate residual esophageal varices. This is accomplished either by injection sclerotherapy (Terblanche et al 1983, Copenhagen Esophageal Varices Sclerotherapy Project 1984, Westaby et al 1985) or, particularly if varices are large, by banding (Steigmann et al 1992).

### *Gastroduodenal disease*

A range of endoscopic therapies is available for diseases affecting the stomach and duodenum. Patients who present with bleeding peptic ulcer may be treated by one of several endoscopic therapies (p. 488) including injection of vasoconstricting (Chung et al 1988) or sclerosing agents (Panés et al 1987, Rajgopal & Palmer 1991) and thermal devices including laser photocoagulation (Swain et al 1986), the heater probe (Fullarton et al 1989) and diathermy (Laine 1987). Only patients who at endoscopy are found to be bleeding actively from an ulcer or who have a nonbleeding protuberant vessel within the ulcer base are considered for these treatments, since patients without these endoscopic stigmata stop bleeding spontaneously and do not rebleed in hospital irrespective of specific therapy (Griffiths et al 1979, National Institutes of Health Consensus Conference 1989). Patients who have bled from Mallory–Weiss tears (p. 490) may also respond well to diathermy (Laine 1987) or to injection with dilute adrenaline (Choudari et al 1994), while those who bleed from vascular malformations may be helped by laser photocoagulation (Potomiano et al 1994). A bleeding Dieulafoy malformation (p. 491) is best treated by injection sclerotherapy (Asaki et al 1988). Adenomatous gastric polyps should be removed by snare diathermy, while hyperplastic or hamartomatous polyps are usually left intact unless very large. This is because adenomatous polyps have premalignant potential and also tend to cause anemia (Ming 1977). Leiomyomata are relatively common incidental findings and may also be sources of acute or chronic bleeding. Histological confirmation can be obtained only by surgical resection and the endoscopist can never be certain of the diagnosis despite a classic appearance. These tumors are usually removed surgically, but active bleeding can be managed by endoscopic injection, laser or heater probe therapy.

***Pyloric stenosis.*** When due to peptic ulcer disease, pyloric stenosis is usually treated by gastroenterostomy (p. 285), but elderly or unfit patients may respond to balloon dilatation (Griffin et al 1989). Like many dilatation procedures within the gastrointestinal tract, this may need to be repeated on several occasions and potent acid-suppressing drug therapy should be prescribed to heal active ulceration and minimize scarring.

***Gastrostomy*** (p. 113). Percutaneous endoscopic gastrostomy (PEG) tubes can be used to allow adequate treatment of nutritional disorders. Patients who have chronic bulbar or pseudobulbar palsies may starve and these patients are suitable for nutritional support administered through PEG tubes inserted using a combined percutaneous and endoscopic technique (Panos et al 1994). This approach is far superior to long-term nasogastric feeding (Norton et al 1996).

***Foreign bodies*** (see also p. 184). Foreign bodies, including needles, scalpel or razor blades and batteries, can be removed safely endoscopically (Quinn & Connors 1994). The diagnosis of an ingested foreign body is made by abdominal radiography. Endoscopy is performed through a sheath that allows safe retrieval of potentially damaging sharp objects providing these can be grasped using specialized instruments passed through the biopsy channel of the endoscope. Impacted foreign bodies, for example a dental plate in the esophagus, pose a particular problem, as forceful removal by the endoscopist can be complicated by major hemorrhage. Consultation with thoracic and general surgeons is important before removing impacted foreign bodies.

***Corrosive strictures.*** Patients who ingest corrosives such as household bleach may sustain esophageal perforation and develop extensive fibrosis leading to stricture formation (p. 183) (Kikendall 1991). The decision to endoscope such patients and the timing of endoscopy is difficult. Some studies suggested high perforation rates for dilatation in these patients (Song et al 1992), but others suggest that this procedure is as safe as that performed for peptic strictures (Zargar et al 1989). Corrosive strictures tend to be extensive and rigid and frequent dilatation may be necessary (Broor et al 1993).

## Technique: upper gastrointestinal endoscopy

### *Intubation*

The patient lies in the left lateral position with the neck semiflexed. A mouthguard and nasal catheters are positioned by the assistant. The endoscope is passed to the pharynx, the tip deflected in the midline over the back of the tongue. As the patient swallows, the instrument is advanced across the upper esophageal sphincter into the gullet. The patient is asked to concentrate upon deep respiration and this rapidly relieves gagging and heaving.

Occasionally, intubation using this method fails, usually because the instrument is deflected by the tongue to one side of the pharynx, particularly by elderly patients who may have inco-ordinate swallowing. When this occurs, the endoscopist can guide the instrument into the gullet using the fingers. This should be avoided, as it is unpleasant and is potentially traumatic for the patient, fingers can be bitten and the instrument may be damaged. Once the cricopharyngeus has been passed, the instrument is gently advanced down the gullet under direct vision.

### *The normal esophagus*

The normal mucosa is pale pink in color and is freely mobile. Peristaltic waves are seen. The upper and lower sphincters are tonically contracted, but the lumen of the gullet is easily distended by air and esophagoscopy is easy. Transmitted cardiac and respiratory pulsations are usual and the aortic arch indents the esophagus at a point 23 cm from the incisors. At 38 cm a mucosal rosette is formed by convergence of longitudinal mucosal folds and at 40 cm, the serrated border between the esophagus and stomach ("Z" line) is obvious as the pale esophageal mucosa meets the darker gastric mucosa.

### *The abnormal esophagus*

Esophageal diverticula are common and have no pathological significance. Hiatus hernia is best diagnosed by a barium swallow examination, but it is often recognized by the endoscopist. The endoscopist notes apparent esophageal shortening because the "Z" line between the esophageal and gastric mucosae is less than 40 cm from the incisors and a "sac" is formed by the stomach lying between the "Z" line and the diaphragmatic impression. It is important to examine the hiatus hernia sac carefully, since ulcers or tumors are easily missed.

***Peptic esophagitis.*** The endoscopic recognition of peptic esophagitis is usually straightforward, but the significance of mild abnormalities is unclear. It is well recognized that symptoms of gastroesophageal reflux disease correlate poorly with endoscopic appearances; the most florid examples of erosive esophagitis can be asympto-

**Table 4.5** Endoscopic grading of esophagitis

| | |
|---|---|
| I | Linear nonconfluent erosions |
| II | Longitudinal confluent noncircumferential erosions |
| III | Circumferential erosions |
| IV | Complication: stricture or Barrett's esophagus |

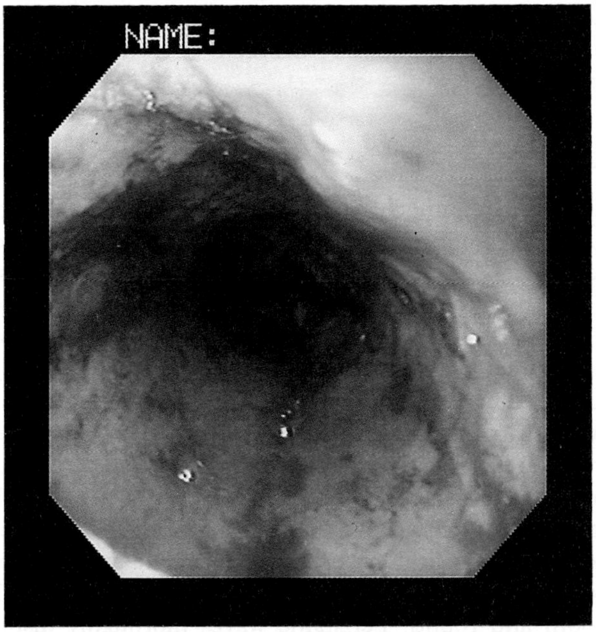


**Fig. 4.2** Distal esophagus showing hemorrhagic linear esophagitis.

matic and the esophagus may appear normal in patients with severe heartburn.

Esophagitis is sometimes graded I–IV (Table 4.5) (Miller 1995). Grade I is characterized by erythema and increased mucosal friability. Grade II is defined as linear streaks of ulceration (Fig. 4.2). Grade III comprises confluent ulceration, while complications such as peptic stricture of Barrett's esophagus define grade IV (Fig. 4.3). Biopsies are performed to exclude other disease. Biopsy evidence of esophagitis does not always correlate with the visual appearance at endoscopy (Ismail-Beigi & Pope 1974).

***Barrett's mucosa.*** Barrett's esophagus is recognized as fingers or confluent areas of gastric mucosa extending from the stomach into the gullet (Fig. 4.4). It is usually associated with hiatus hernia and it is sometimes difficult to differentiate between a hernia sac and Barrett's esophagus. Benign Barrett's ulcer may arise within the abnormal mucosa and has to be differentiated from carcinoma. Barrett's esophagus and ulcer should always be biopsied to seek histological evidence of dysplasia or carcinoma.

***Strictures.*** Esophageal strictures may be obviously malignant with heaped, irregular and friable mucosa. Benign peptic strictures are usually associated with esophagitis and hiatus hernia and they occur in the distal gullet. Rings and webs are covered by normal-looking mucosa. In clinical practice, it is not always possible to be certain of these differences and brush cytology and biopsy is important in all esophageal strictures.

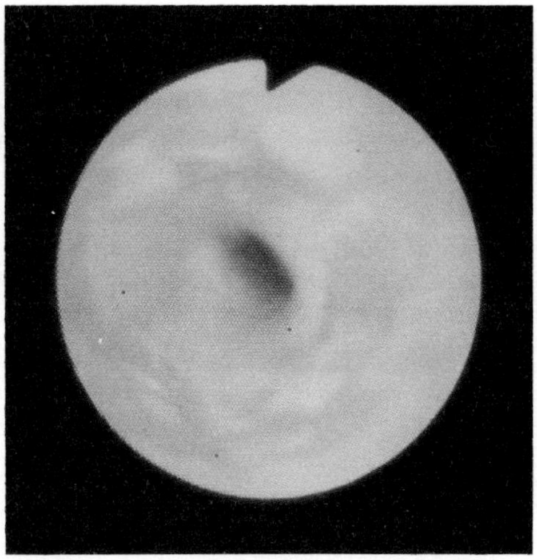

**Fig. 4.3** Distal esophagus showing diffuse circumferential hemorrhagic and ulcerative esophagitis.

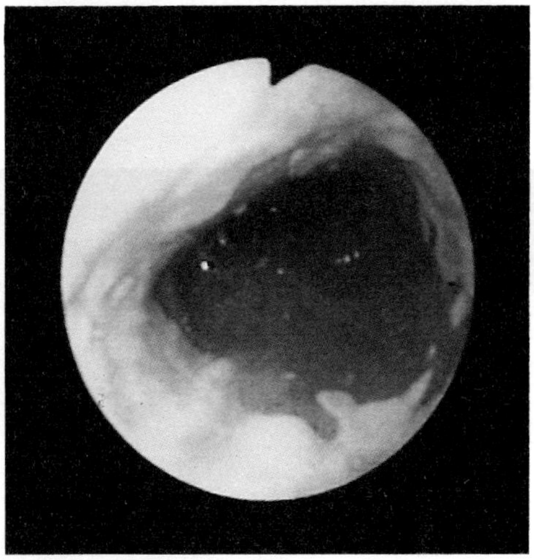

**Fig. 4.4** Distal esophagus showing Barrett's mucosa in the lower esophagus, islands of esophageal mucosa within the Barrett's mucosa and an irregular dentate line between the Barrett's and esophageal mucosae.

***Cancer.*** Esophageal carcinomas present most often as strictures causing dysphagia (above). The tumor usually shows irregular friable mucosa that may protrude into the esophageal lumen (Fig. 4.5) or may be ulcerated. Tumors spreading in the submucosa may not be recognizable at endoscopy and give the appearance of a benign stricture. This occurs most often when a fundal gastric carcinoma seeds up the esophagus.

***Varices.*** Small esophageal varices are sometimes difficult to differentiate from the longitudinal folds that invariably occur in the lower esophagus. Varices, unlike

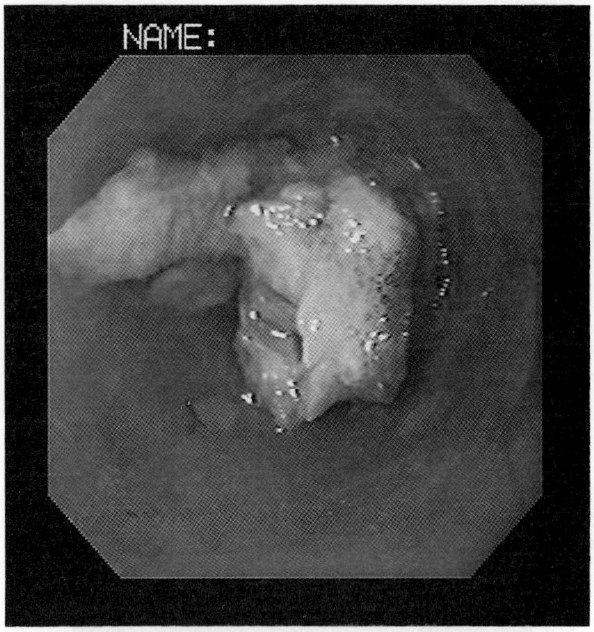


**Fig. 4.5** Fungating esophageal carcinoma obstructing the esophagogastric junction.

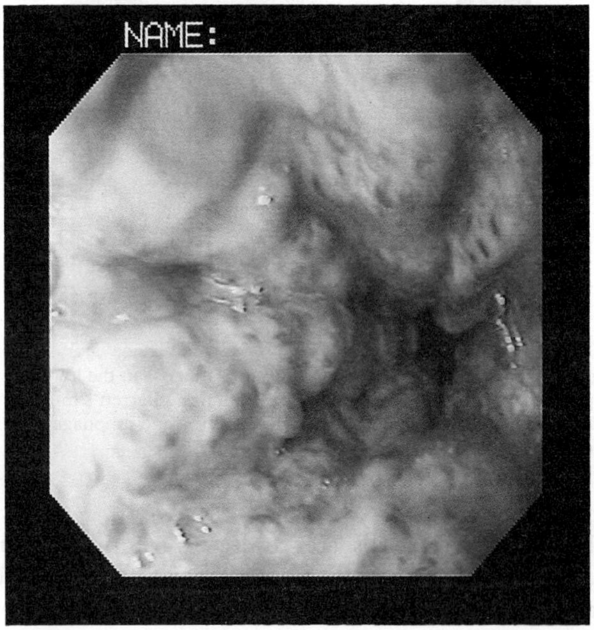


**Fig. 4.6** Large esophageal varices showing multiple red spots indicating a high risk of bleeding.

folds, tend to be tortuous and bluish in color and are not obliterated when the esophagus is distended with air. It is customary to grade variceal size I to IV. Grade I esophageal varices are small (but definite), grade IV varices obliterate the esophageal lumen and grades II and III are intermediate (Fig. 4.6). It is also important to look for blue or red spots or stripes (wales) which indicate an increased risk of bleeding (Fig. 4.6). Esophageal ulcers are often seen following endoscopic sclerotherapy (Schuman et al 1987). Such ulcers develop at the injection site, may be extremely deep and may bleed. They usually heal with or without the use of ulcer-healing drugs.

***Mallory–Weiss tears.*** Mallory–Weiss tears are a relatively common cause of acute gastrointestinal bleeding and are recognized endoscopically as longitudinal ulcers extending across the "Z" line into the gullet. Actively bleeding tears should be considered for endoscopic injection therapy.

*The normal stomach*

The normal stomach may contain some fluid and this should be removed to lessen the possibility of aspiration pneumonia. The endoscope is passed along the lesser curve and the pylorus is intubated without first examining the stomach thoroughly. The gastric antrum, incisura, lesser curve and body are examined as the endoscope is withdrawn through the inflated stomach and the fundus is visualized by retroflexing the endoscope (the "J" maneuver). The mucosa of the stomach is orange-red in color, longitudinal rugae are seen in the body but not in the antrum and the mucosa is sufficiently thick to prevent visualization of the submucosal vessels. The pylorus separates the antrum from the duodenal cap and is normally smooth and round. Peristaltic waves thoroughly display the lining of the stomach.

*The abnormal stomach*

***Gastritis.*** Up to 50% of the asymptomatic population have histological evidence of gastritis (Johnsen et al 1991) and endoscopists often report appearances as "gastritis" (Toukan et al 1985), but the correlation between endoscopic and histological appearances is poor (Khakoo et al 1994). The term "gastritis" should therefore be restricted to a histological diagnosis. The Sydney classification separated endoscopic gastritis into seven categories based on the distribution of mucosal features of edema, erythema, friability, the presence of exudate, erosions, rugal hypertrophy, atrophy, the visibility of vascular pattern, bleeding spots and nodularity (Tytgat 1991). The classification superseded previous methods in which inconsistencies were extremely marked and endoscopic appearance related very poorly to histological findings (p. 224) (Khakoo et al 1994)

There is also a very poor relationship between gastritis (endoscopic and histological) and clinical symptoms (Johnsen et al 1991). The most clinically relevant form of gastritis is that associated with *Helicobacter pylori* and in most endoscopy units it has become routine to biopsy the gastric antrum to diagnose infection by this organism. Biopsies can be examined by a rapid urease slide test (Thillainayagam et al 1991), examined histologically

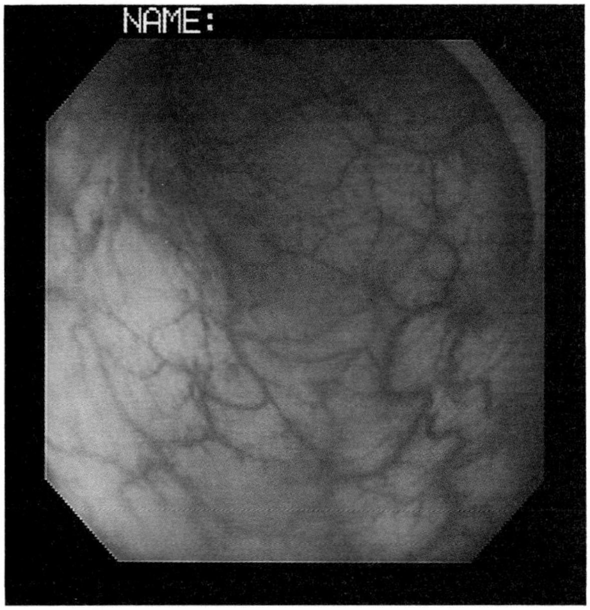


**Fig. 4.7** Gastric mucosal atrophy allowing ready visibility of the submucosal vessels.

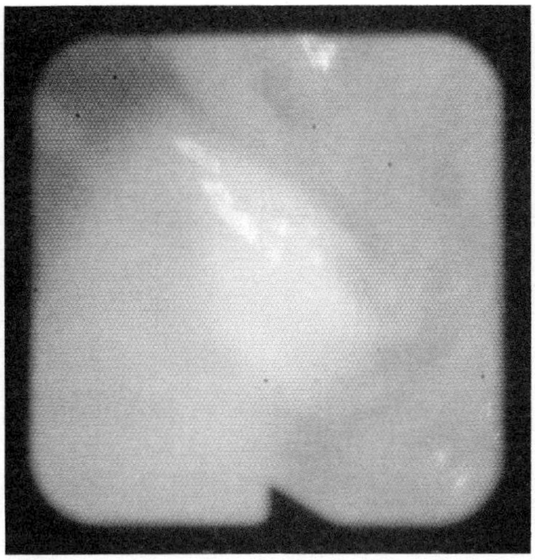

**Fig. 4.8** Benign chronic gastric ulcer showing a regular pale necrotic base and well-defined ulcer margins.

(Gray et al 1986) or occasionally cultured with determination of antibiotic sensitivity (Goodwin et al 1985). Gastritis associated with *H. pylori* tends to involve the antrum and causes erythema, nodularity and superficial erosions (Robert & Weistein 1993). It may be complicated by gastric metaplasia in which a slate gray transformation occurs (Craanen et al 1992). Atrophic gastritis (Fig. 4.7) is recognized by the presence of prominent mucosal blood vessels, as the mucosa is thinned.

***Varioliform gastritis*** (Haot et al 1988). This is a histological entity characterized by the accumulation of small lymphocytes in the surface and foveolar epithelium (p. 326). The endoscopic appearances are nonspecific, although aphthoid nodules and thickened folds within the antrum are common.

***Gastric antral vascular ectasia ("watermelon stomach").*** This is recognized as longitudinal rugal folds traversing the antrum and converging on the pylorus (p. 493), each containing a visible convoluted column of vessels, the aggregates resembling stripes of a watermelon skin (Jabbari et al 1984).

***Congestive (portal hypertension) gastropathy.*** This is a common feature of portal hypertension and is characterized by mosaic-like transformation of the mucosa with acute erosions and friability (p. 1000). The changes tend to be most prominent in the antrum and extend into the duodenum.

***Biliary gastritis*** (p. 271). This is inevitably found following partial gastrectomy or gastroenterostomy. The gastric mucosa is erythematous and erosions are frequent. Some patients also have alkaline gastroesophageal reflux disease.

***Gastric erosions.*** These are commonly seen in the prepyloric regions, including the incisura. They may be associated with erosive duodenitis and duodenal ulcer. These small, shallow mucosal breaches should be differentiated from benign gastric ulcers which are deeper and larger, but differentiation between erosions and ulcers is not always clearcut.

***Ulcers.*** Benign (peptic) gastric ulcers (Fig. 4.8) tend to be situated on the lesser curve of the stomach. Regular mucosal folds radiate from them and, unlike malignant ulcers, their borders are not heaped. Even typically "benign" ulcers may be in fact malignant and all gastric ulcers should be subjected to brushing and biopsies for cytological and histological exclusion of cancer or lymphoma. It is important to record the site and approximate size of an ulcer because repeat endoscopy is undertaken to confirm healing. Duodenal cap examination may show a chronic ulcer (Fig. 4.9), which for practical purposes is always benign, or more or less extensive erosive duodenitis (Fig. 4.10).

***Neoplasia.*** Gastric tumors include a range of benign and malignant diseases and biopsy should be routine for any mucosal lesion. Benign metaplastic polyps are common, tend to occur in the body or fundus and have no malignant potential (Ming 1977). These small, mobile, sessile mucosal lumps are distinguished from adenomata, which often have a pedicle and are purple in color. Adenomata bleed (Fig. 4.11) and may undergo transformation to carcinoma (p. 313); they are removed by snare diathermy, while metaplastic polyps are ignored. Leiomyomata are sessile (Fig. 4.12), clearly submucosal and often have a central, ulcerated "umbilicus". Carcinomas range from malignant ulcers with heaped, irregular walls to polypoid, ulcerated tumors or diffuse infiltration (Fig. 4.13). Linitus plastica causes rigidity of the mucosa, absent peristaltic activity and poor distensibility. Other tumors of the stomach, including lymphoma,

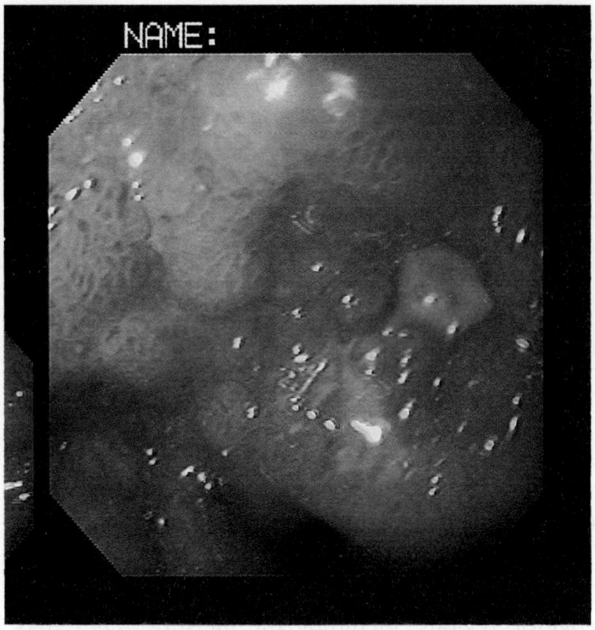


**Fig. 4.9** Chronic duodenal ulcer with surrounding edematous erythemic duodenal cap mucosa.

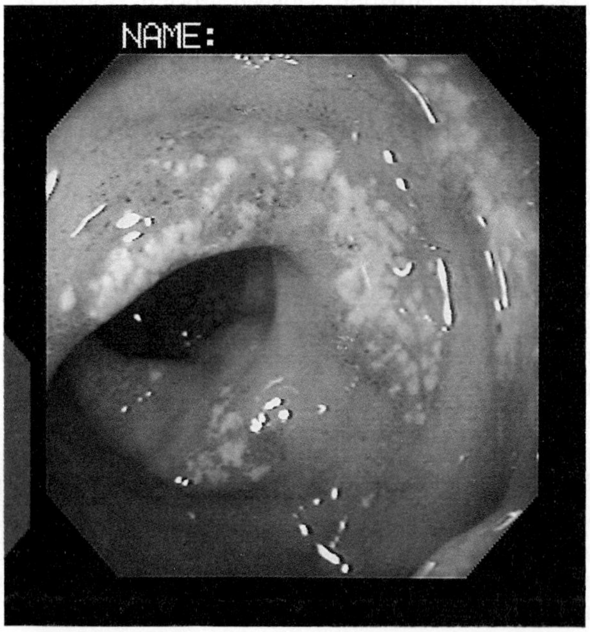


**Fig. 4.10** Erosive duodenitis showing multiple irregular pale and sometimes confluent erosions and associated petechial spots.

sarcoma and carcinoid, are difficult to differentiate from cancer without biopsy.

*Examination of the duodenum*

Most peptic ulcers occur in the first part of the duodenum, but the second part should be examined routinely because postbulbar ulcers or other abnormalities (Fig. 4.14) may

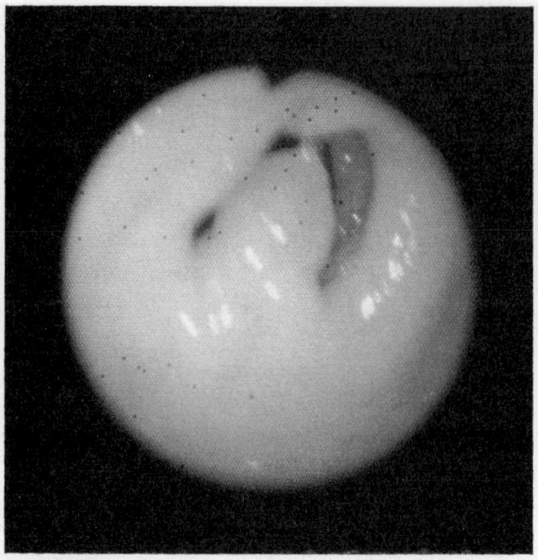

**Fig. 4.11** Benign gastric antral mucosal polyp with a well-defined stalk.

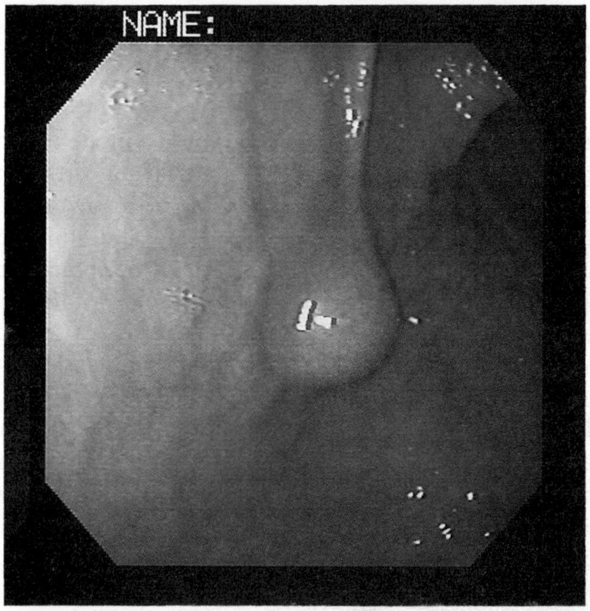


**Fig. 4.12** Benign submucosal polyp covered by normal mucosa in the body of the stomach.

occasionally be found. The duodenum is technically more difficult to examine than the stomach because control over the tip of the instrument is less direct. The duodenum should first be viewed through the pylorus and the instrument is then gently advanced into the bulb. When the instrument is withdrawn, the tip may flick quickly back into the stomach and it may be necessary to advance and withdraw the instrument through the pylorus several times before satisfactory examination of the whole of the duodenal bulb has been achieved. If there is any doubt as to the adequacy of the examination, a side-viewing instrument is used to complete the examination.

The instrument is advanced into the second part of the

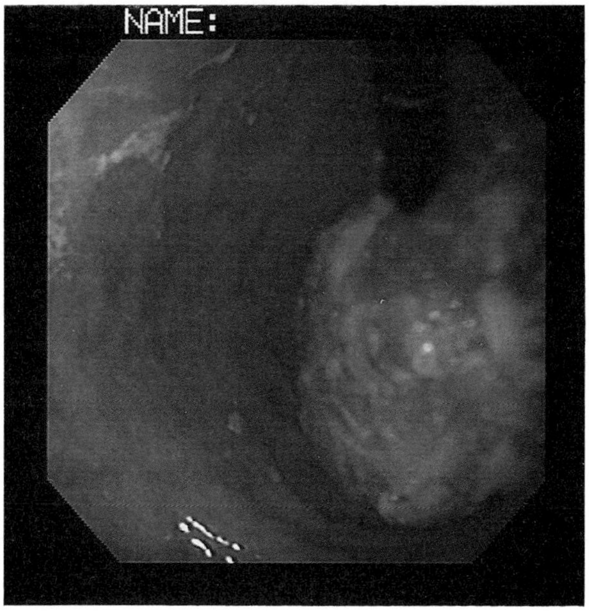


**Fig. 4.13** Irregular fungating carcinoma in the fundus of the stomach viewed with a retroflexed endoscope.

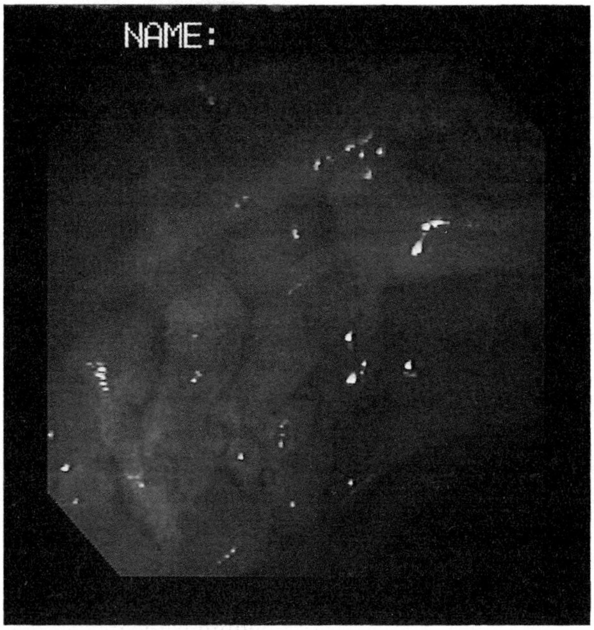


**Fig. 4.14** A villous carcinoma close to the papilla of Vater in the descending duodenum.

duodenum, usually by rotating and deflecting the tip. At this point, air is insufflated to allow the second part of the duodenum with its circular mucosal folds to be seen and withdrawal of the instrument paradoxically causes the tip to advance down the second part because the shaft straightens within the stomach. Further gentle withdrawal at this stage will give adequate views of the second part, although the ampulla of Vater can only be examined adequately using a side-viewing instrument. Patients with celiac disease may lose the circular folds and the mucosa may appear atrophic. The superior duodenal angle itself may be difficult to see, as there is a tendency for the instrument to flick past it quickly.

*Examination of the postoperative stomach*

The postoperative stomach may be difficult to examine completely. Variations in anatomy and in the surgical procedures performed may require the endoscopist to use both end- and side-viewing instruments. The latter may be needed when examining surgically created stomas and deformity produced by pyloroplasty. Other problems with the postoperative stomach include frothing caused by bile reflux and by a small gastric remnant causing difficulty in obtaining gastric distention. Biliary gastritis, a common finding, is usually of little clinical significance.

### Endoscopic biopsy and cytology

One of the particular advantages of endoscopy is the ability to take target biopsies. Close collaboration between the pathologist and the endoscopist is essential, since sensible histological diagnosis often relies upon clinical information. Multiple biopsies should be taken of all suspicious lesions. The initial preparation of the material is carried out by the endoscopic assistant in a way previously agreed with the pathology department. Tissue biopsies are usually mounted on filter paper before being placed in 10% formalin; the larger and deeper the biopsy, the more valuable the information obtained. A selection of biopsy forceps should be available for use in different circumstances. Biopsies should ideally be taken with the forceps perpendicular to the lesion, as this enables the cusps of the forceps to be pressed firmly over the target area; however, it is often the case that a tangential approach is all that can be made. It may sometimes be necessary to use large-channel or side-viewing instruments to obtain suitable material. Particularly larger specimens can be obtained using "hot biopsies" in which diathermy is coupled with large biopsy forceps. Diathermy current is applied at the time of biopsy to lessen the risk of bleeding (Williams 1973).

Cytological examination of abnormal areas is routine. Brushings are usually taken before biopsies to minimize the number of blood cells within the cytology specimen. Specimens are obtained using sleeved brushes; these are smeared onto microscope slides and fixed prior to transfer to the pathology laboratory.

## THERAPEUTIC UPPER GASTROINTESTINAL ENDOSCOPY

### Dilatation of benign esophageal strictures

Benign esophageal strictures are dilated at diagnostic

endoscopy. Many endoscopists use a combination of pethidine and a benzodiazepine for sedation, although care has to be taken since many patients with esophageal stricture are elderly and relatively sensitive to these drugs. Before dilatation, it is important to aspirate esophageal contents to lessen the risks of postendoscopic pneumonia. The stricture is examined carefully, brushed and biopsied to confirm that it is benign. The stricture is dilated either by pushing rigid dilators through its lumen or by using balloons. Although the latter approach may be theoretically more attractive because the force is more appropriately directed, a clinical trial has suggested that the bougie technique is equally safe and has a similar complication rate (Cox et al 1988).

Most techniques involve preliminary passage of a firm metal guidewire with floppy tip through the lumen of the stricture. If possible, the endoscope is first introduced past the stricture to ensure optimal guidewire position. If the stricture is too narrow to allow passage of the endoscope through the stricture, the guidewire is passed under direct vision into the lumen and pushed gently into the distal esophagus and stomach. Radiological screening is useful to confirm passage of the guidewire when strictures are particularly tortuous or following gastric surgery.

After the guidewire has been appropriately positioned the endoscope is withdrawn, taking care to ensure that the guidewire is not withdrawn at the same time. The safety of dilatation depends on making sure that the guidewire does not change position during the procedure. A range of bougies is available. These include spindle-shaped olives (Eder–Puestow dilators), which are screwed onto flexible metal introducers and threaded over the guidewire. These are pushed through the stricture while ensuring that the guidewire is kept in a straight position. Olives of increasing size (to 48 French) are used. These techniques require several "passes" and this is often uncomfortable for the patient. Floppy, graduated plastic olives are more comfortable and easier to use, but the endoscopist appreciates less sensation of obstruction. Celestin dilators are long plastic tubes with a tip graduating from a few millimeters to 16 mm (50 French) (Leichtmann et al 1984). Adequate dilatation is achieved by a single passage, but this approach is used only when the guidewire is positioned well distal to the stricture. It cannot be used for the postoperative stomach because of the risk of gastric perforation.

Balloon dilatation is employed either under direct vision or using radiological screening over a guidewire after the endoscope has been removed (Starck et al 1984). The optimum pressure within the balloon and the duration of the dilatation remain controversial.

Esophageal dilatation is remarkably safe, with low complication rates (Leichtmann et al 1984, Starck et al 1984). Patients who are well following dilatation are given clear fluids after 4 h and allowed home thereafter. Chest or abdominal pain suggests a perforation and subcutaneous emphysema is diagnostic of a perforation of the esophagus. This invariably occurs at the time of the procedure and perforation is confirmed by a chest radiograph. It requires hospital admission for assessment and treatment. The majority of iatrogenic perforations respond well to conservative therapy using antibiotics, parenteral nutrition and management of any pneumothorax (p. 185).

**Table 4.6** Complications following endoscopic treatment for malignant esophageal obstruction

| | | |
|---|---|---|
| Plastic stents | Perforation | |
| | Aspiration pneumonia | |
| | Dysphagia | – bolus obstruction |
| | | – migration |
| | | – tumor growth |
| Metallic stents | Perforation (rare) | |
| | Dysphagia | – bolus obstruction |
| | | – tumor growth |
| Laser | Perforation | |
| | Aspiration pneumonia | |
| | Tracheoesophageal fistula | |
| | Hemorrhage | |
| | Dysphagia | – tumor |
| | | – fibrous stricture |
| Alcohol injection | Pain | |
| | Aspiration pneumonia | |
| | Perforation | |
| | Dysphagia | – tumor |
| | | – fibrous stricture |

## Treatment of malignant strictures

The optimal endoscopic palliative approach is dependent on the nature of the tumor as well as the available equipment and the expertise of the endoscopist. All available methods have complications (Table 4.6).

### *Intubation*

Intubation is performed under intravenous sedation (pethidine and a benzodiazepine) or general anesthesia and requires radiological assistance. The stricture is first dilated and the site and length of the stricture are defined by radiological screening.

### *Plastic prostheses*

The most commonly used stent is that designed by Atkinson (Ogilvie et al 1982). This has a distal flange and a proximal shouldered part to prevent migration. The prosthesis is pushed into position using an introducer and radiological screening is used to judge optimum position. Following intubation, an endoscope is passed to confirm that the tube is placed satisfactorily and to identify possible esophageal tears. If the tube is wrongly placed, the introducer can be reintroduced into the stent and its position adjusted. A modified Atkinson tube with an inflatable cuff has been designed for the palliation of malignant esophagobronchial fistulae (Lux et al 1987). It is introduced by a similar technique.

*Expandable metal stents*

These can be introduced using either endoscopy and radiological screening or under radiological screening alone. A guidewire is passed through the lumen and the stent is then deployed, taking great care to use an appropriately long stent and to position the stent accurately, because the prosthesis shortens when it is fully introduced and its position cannot be adjusted subsequently.

*Complications of intubation*

Intubation using plastic prostheses is complicated by esophageal perforation in up to 10% of cases (Den Hartog Jager et al 1979). Esophageal perforation has a high mortality and rarely responds to conservative therapy. Intubation with expandable metal stents appears much safer (Knyrim et al 1993). Other early complications of intubation include pulmonary aspiration and patients should be nursed in an upright position following the procedure. Late complications include bolus obstruction, tumor overgrowth and displacement of the tube requiring further endoscopic intervention (Loizou et al 1991). Food boluses are usually cleared easily by passing the endoscope or a dilator through the tube. Displacement often requires restenting, although repositioning using the Atkinson introducer or an inflated balloon is possible. Tumor overgrowth is managed by restenting or by laser ablation. Plastic stents will almost certainly be superseded by expandable metal prostheses that have a superimposed membrane designed to limit tumor ingrowth. They are expensive but are easily inserted with little morbidity and achieve excellent palliation of swallowing. Prostheses cannot be tolerated in the postcricoid area and tumors of the upper cervical esophagus are therefore unsuitable for intubation.

*Nd:YAG laser treatment*

A therapeutic endoscope should be used because debris, retained within the obstructed gullet or produced by the procedure, may block the suction channel of standard endoscopes. Many endoscopists prefer an oblique rather than a forward-viewing instrument for laser treatment because of the more appropriate angle of visualization and instrumentation. In addition, the elevator facilitates accurate positioning of the laser fiber. Fiberendoscopes have to be fitted with appropriate filters to prevent damage to the eye of the endoscopist and all individuals in the endoscopy room wear protective goggles.

The flexible laser fiber is passed through the biopsy channel of the endoscope, enabling transmission of light energy to the tumor which is ulcerated by thermal energy. The standard technique avoids preliminary dilatation if at all possible, because bleeding and edema caused by dilating the lumen obscure the view and prevent optimal treatment. The endoscope is passed beyond the stricture and the tumor is treated as the instrument is withdrawn. This is safer than an antegrade approach and difficulties associated with laser-induced edema are avoided. Laser energy is transmitted using a "no touch" technique in which the fiber tip is positioned several millimeters away from the tumor and bursts of energy (50–80 watts for 0.5–1 s) are applied to the mucosa. The amount of energy given is judged by the tissue effect. Low applications leave a small ulcer, higher energy applications cause deep necrotic ulceration, while vaporization occurs with higher and more prolonged settings. It is important to remember that much of the effect of laser therapy is delayed because the mucosa several millimeters below the treated area is damaged by laser energy and these areas necrose within 48 h of a treatment session (Fleischer & Sivak 1985). This and the resolution of local edema caused by photocoagulation account for improving dysphagia 24 h after endoscopy.

The malignant areas are "sprayed" with laser energy in an attempt to produce confluent destruction. Tissue necrosis is associated with acrid smoke formation that irritates the airways, leading to coughing during the procedure. Some endoscopists insert a suction catheter into the esophagus at the time of the procedure to remove this smoke; unfortunately, the catheter often prevents adequate insufflation of air and increases the difficulty of treatment. Frequent aspiration of gas and debris from the stomach and esophagus (best after temporarily removing the laser fiber) through the suction channel is an easier approach but risks blocking the instrument.

If energy is applied when the glass fiber and mucosa are in apposition, the fiber tip is disrupted and the fiber is rendered useless. Unfortunately, it is often difficult to avoid touching the mucosa with the fiber because the lumen is usually narrow and irregular. In this situation, a sapphire laser scalpel can be used to dissect the tumor, but considerable care is necessary because of the high risk of perforation.

Tumor treatment using lasers usually has to be performed on several occasions (median 4) before adequate palliation of dysphagia is achieved (Krasner et al 1987). Repeat therapy is given at weekly intervals and it is then wise to repeat endoscopy with a view to further treatment less frequently (4–6-weekly). The procedure is often prolonged, the obstructed esophagus usually contains food and liquid debris and the patient is invariably frail. These factors predispose to aspiration pneumonia, which is a frequent complication of laser treatment unless endoscopic assistance is of the highest quality. The procedure is also complicated by esophageal perforation in approximately

5% of treatment sessions. This may resolve with conservative approaches but usually requires intubation. Esophagotracheal fistulae may occur after laser treatment. The procedure-related mortality is 1–5%. Late dysphagia is due to tumor recurrence or a fibrous stricture (Table 4.6) (Krasner et al 1987).

The quality of swallowing achieved by laser therapy is at least as good as that following intubation (Loizou et al 1991), lesions in the proximal esophagus are amenable to laser treatment and the risks of immediate complications are lower. This has to be balanced against the need for repeated laser sessions and its higher cost. In clinical practice, laser therapy and intubation must be regarded as complementary rather than competitive and units involved in palliation of esophagogastric tumors should have both options available.

## Pneumatic dilatation of the esophagus

Fibrous or malignant strictures are excluded by endoscopy and biopsy and the diagnosis of achalasia is confirmed manometrically (p. 175). Esophageal contents are removed prior to endoscopy through a wide-bore nasogastric tube and the procedure is performed under pethidine and benzodiazepine sedation, as all patients experience discomfort during the procedure. A guidewire is passed through the biopsy channel of the endoscope into the stomach, the endoscope is removed and an uninflated balloon is passed along the guidewire and positioned using radiological screening. In most units, the Rigiflex balloon system is used (Cox et al 1986). The details of inflation vary widely between units, but most endoscopists inflate the balloon to 4 mmHg for 2 min, then 8 mmHg for 2 min.

The patient is observed overnight and oral fluids are given cautiously after 2–4 h. The risk of perforation is approximately 2–5% (p. 176) (Cox et al 1986). The principal late complication is recurrent dysphagia due to inadequate dilatation. Excessive dilatation causes gastroesophageal reflux, leading to heartburn and regurgitation.

## Esophageal variceal sclerotherapy and banding

These techniques are used to stop active variceal bleeding and to prevent recurrent variceal bleeding thereafter by greatly reducing or obliterating the varices. Sclerotherapy is often more useful in stopping active bleeding, as banding may be difficult or impossible in these circumstances. Banding, on the other hand, is used increasingly to prevent rebleeding (p. 1006) as it is more effective than sclerotherapy, obliterates varices more quickly and has few complications (Hayes 1996).

### *Sclerotherapy*

Flexible endoscopy is performed in the usual manner. The esophageal varices are visualized and hyoscine butylbromide (Buscopan) may then be given to facilitate the injection of sclerosant by paralyzing the esophagus. Each varix should be injected immediately above the esophagogastric junction, as this is the usual site of variceal bleeding (p. 999). Intravariceal injection is probably more effective than paravariceal submucosal injection and may cause fewer complications, but in practice it can be difficult to know whether or not an injection has entered the vein. A long flexible sheathed sclerotherapy needle is passed through the endoscope; the needle is kept retracted in the sheath until the tip of the sheath is applied appropriately to the varix at an acute angle and the needle is then advanced and pushed gently into the varix. The injection proceeds easily and the varix above the needle may fill when the needle is in the varix, whereas when the needle is in the submucosa, ballooning and blanching of the mucosa occurs.

The needle is retracted into the sheath when the injection is complete and some bleeding may then occur from the varix. This is not usually severe. Ethanolamine and sodium tetradecyl sulfate (STD) are the most widely used agents. The authors find that 2 ml of STD (3%) injected into each varix is satisfactory and the injection is reduced to 1 ml if it proves to be extravascular. A Sengstaken tube is passed after injection sclerotherapy only in the unusual event of severe bleeding (p. 501).

### *Banding*

Banding involves the ligation of varices using a rubber band. This is carried out at flexible endoscopy with a device mounted at the end of a forward-viewing endoscope. The device holds an inner cylinder carrying a prestressed rubber band at its distal end and the band can be detached by pulling on a releasing wire running through the biopsy channel to the proximal end of the endoscope. This device makes the passage of the endoscope more difficult, the device itself reduces the endoscopist's field of vision by about a third and the endoscope has to be removed after each banding to allow replacement of the banding device. The procedure is accordingly more time consuming than sclerotherapy, making it less useful in bleeding patients. Repeated passage of the endoscope can be facilitated by using an overtube, but this can cause esophageal damage and is best avoided.

A "speed bander" allowing five variceal bandings is now available but is expensive. Individual varices are drawn into the device on the endoscope using the endoscope suction channel and each varix is then ligated by releasing the rubber band. The ligated varix eventually sloughs off leaving a small ulcer.

### *Complications*

Sclerotherapy and banding give rise to similar complications, but the frequency of complications seems less after banding (Hayes 1996). Significant complications occur after sclerotherapy in about 20% of patients and after banding in about 10%.

Transient chest pain, occasionally severe, dysphagia and fever can occur and a chest radiograph for perforation and blood cultures for bacteremia should be done. Esophageal ulcers are usually asymptomatic but can manifest as bleeding or later as dysphagia due to strictures. Other local complications include esophageal hematomas, infection and perforation and aspiration pneumonia. Bacteremia with distant infections, such as spontaneous bacterial peritonitis or bacterial endocarditis, and portal vein thrombosis can also occur.

## Peptic ulcer bleeding

Duodenal, gastric or stomal ulcers that are bleeding actively or contain a nonbleeding visible vessel are suitable for endoscopic therapy. The same techniques can also be applied to bleeding Mallory–Weiss tears (Laine 1987) and the Dieulafoy malformation (Al-Kawas & O'Keefe 1987, Asaki et al 1988). Gastric contents are removed first. This may be possible by aspiration through the endoscope, although the endoscopist should be careful to avoid blocking the suction channel. It is sometimes necessary to lavage the stomach through an overtube. The source of bleeding is identified and cleaned using a washing tube and nonadherent blood clot is removed from the ulcer base. Hemostasis can be achieved by injection or thermal methods. Other approaches, including application of clips, sprays or sewing machines, are not widely used.

The efficacy of injection and thermal methods are similar and the best results depend upon familiarity and expertise with one technique. Some bleeding lesions may require combination therapy and preliminary injection with adrenaline followed by application of a thermal method may be best for some bleeding lesions. The comparative value of these techniques is discussed on p. 488.

### *Injection*

Most endoscopists inject dilute adrenaline (epinephrine) (4–10 ml 1:10 000 or 1:100 000) in four points around the bleeding point using a 2 m, 23 gauge disposable needle (Chung et al 1988, Rajgopal & Palmer 1991). Adrenaline is particularly useful for stopping active bleeding. Injection is associated with swelling and blanching due to vasoconstriction. Some endoscopists inject sclerosants such as ethanol-amine, ethanol or polidocanol in addition to, or instead of, adrenaline (Panés et al 1987, Rajgopal & Palmer 1991). Complications of injection include perforation and necrosis of the injection site. Further bleeding can be precipitated by the injection, but this usually stops after a second adrenaline injection.

### *Thermal methods*

Nd:YAG lasers have now replaced argon lasers in the treatment of bleeding lesions because of more appropriate physical properties (Swain et al 1986). Relatively low-power laser energy (40 J for 0.5 s) is directed around the bleeding point. A modest tissue effect (a white dot rather than an ulcer) is achieved and the area is progressively encircled. Laser energy is not directed at the bleeding artery itself because this can precipitate bleeding. The laser technique is "nontouch" and it is difficult to treat awkwardly placed ulcers adequately. Consequently, therapy is technically impossible in approximately 10% of cases. Complications are unusual and perforation is the commonest.

Thermocoagulation can also be achieved using the "heater probe" (Fullarton et al 1989). Heat is generated at the Teflon-coated metal tip of a catheter passed through the biopsy channel and positioned adjacent to the bleeding area. Preset units of energy are applied to the tissue on pressing a foot pedal. The area can be washed and adherence of the probe to the bleeding site can be prevented using a powerful integral water jet. The mucosa around the bleeding site is sequentially treated using settings of 20–40 J for 0.5–1 s and the central artery can then be directly treated. The heater probe is attractive because direct or tangential force can be applied to the bleeding area and the washing jet greatly facilitates cleaning and visualization.

### *Diathermy*

The multipolar probe (BICAP) is applied directly to the bleeding area (Laine 1987). Multiple applications are applied around and into the bleeding area. The system is effective, but its greater expense and lack of an integral washing system make it less satisfactory than the heater probe.

## Percutaneous endoscopic gastrostomy (PEG)

Prophylactic intravenous antibiotics (for example, cefotaxime 1 g) and antiseptic mouth washes are given prior to the procedure, which is performed under aseptic conditions (Doyle & Kennedy 1994). Commercially produced sterile kits are available that enable gastrostomy tubes to be inserted easily and safely by an endoscopist with the help of an assistant.

The patient is placed in the supine position and the abdomen washed with antiseptic. The endoscopist passes a standard forward-viewing endoscope into the stomach, inflates it with air and directs the tip toward the anterior gastric wall. The assistant probes the abdomen with a finger and the endoscopist identifies the optimal site for gastrostomy insertion within the distal body of the stomach by observing gastric indentation. Local anesthetic is injected into the chosen site in the abdominal wall and a specialized needle is thrust percutaneously into the stomach. Strong thread is passed through the needle into the stomach, this is grasped by the endoscopist using a snare and endoscope and thread are withdrawn through the mouth. The gastrostomy tube is attached to the thread and pulled through the pharynx into the stomach and across the abdominal wall. The endoscope is then passed into the stomach to ensure adequate positioning of the proximal bulb of the gastrostomy tube. If this is satisfactory, the assistant fixes the tube onto the skin using a plastic flange and connections to a feeding catheter are made. Feeding commences within 24 h.

Gastrostomy tubes may be inserted without endoscopic visualization, but perforation rates are considerably higher and most centers favor the combined percutaneous/endoscopic approach.

Early complications are rare; local sepsis at the gastrostomy site and tube blockage are the major long-term problems. Aspiration of gastric contents into the lungs is unusual. Most patients gain considerable nutritional benefit and the gastrostomy tube is a much more satisfactory approach than long-term nasogastric bleeding (Panos et al 1994).

## ENDOSCOPIC RETROGRADE CHOLANGIOPANCREATOGRAPHY (ERCP)

Diagnostic ERCP involves visualization and cannulation of the ampulla of Vater, then injection of contrast material into the biliary system and pancreatic ducts. The procedure is performed under radiological screening and films are taken. An undercouch table greatly reduces radiation exposure to the nursing and medical personnel. Good radiographic screening is essential during the test to enable appropriate decision making. Magnetic resonance imaging (MRI) may replace much diagnostic ERCP in future (Soto et al 1996), but increasingly ERCP has become a therapeutic tool and successful therapy requires a full range of accessories, expert assistance and an experienced endoscopist.

### Indications: diagnostic ERCP

The general indications for ERCP are shown in Table 4.7.

**Table 4.7** Indications for diagnostic ERCP

| |
|---|
| *Biliary disease* |
| Jaundice or abnormal liver function tests |
| Dilated biliary tree on ultrasound scan |
| *Pancreatic disease* |
| Assessment of chronic pancreatitis |
| Possible pancreatic tumor |
| *Possible ampullary tumor* |

#### *Ampulla of Vater*

ERCP is the investigation of choice for disease affecting the ampulla of Vater. Most patients are referred because ultrasound imaging suggests obstruction to both the pancreatic and bile ducts. The ampulla is visualized directly and can be biopsied at ERCP.

#### *Pancreas*

ERCP is a sensitive method of examining the pancreas and has a role in the assessment of chronic pancreatitis and pancreatic malignancy (Moss et al 1980). The diagnosis and stage of chronic pancreatitis can be confirmed by pancreatography. Radiographic appearances can be graded I–III (Table 4.8). In practice, chronic pancreatitis is usually diagnosed by noninvasive investigations such as ultrasound or computed tomography and ERCP is most useful for planning a surgical operation. ERCP defines strictures, duct size or complications such as biliary disease, calculi, fistulae and pseudocysts and is also useful for defining pancreatic tumors, although operability is best assessed by other means (Warshaw et al 1990).

**Table 4.8** Revised Cambridge classification of the features of chronic pancreatitis on retrograde pancreatography (Jones et al 1988)

| | |
|---|---|
| Normal | Visualization of whole gland with no abnormal features |
| Equivocal (I) | Fewer than 3 abnormal side branches |
| Mild/moderate (II) | More than 3 abnormal side branches |
| | Abnormal main duct and branches |
| Considerable (III) | As above plus one or more of: |
| | Large cavities (>10 mm) |
| | Intraduct calculi |
| | Ductal obstruction with stricture |
| | Grossly irregular main duct |

#### *Jaundice/cholestasis*

ERCP is used in the assessment of jaundice or abnormal liver function and is usually performed following transabdominal ultrasound imaging. Most jaundiced patients undergoing ERCP will require endoscopic sphincterotomy for choledocholithiasis or stenting for malignancy. In other patients, the diagnosis of primary sclerosing cholangitis or congenital biliary disease such as choledochal cyst will be made.

#### *Abdominal pain*

In general, ERCP is not a useful test for the investigation of nonspecific abdominal pain. Diagnostic yield is low unless other biochemical or radiological investigations suggest the possibility of pancreatic disease.

#### *Gastric surgery*

ERCP is difficult following gastric surgery and alternative

**Table 4.9** Indications for therapeutic ERCP

| | |
|---|---|
| *Bile duct stones* | |
| | Endoscopic sphincterotomy or ampullary balloon dilatation |
| | Stone extraction (balloon, basket) |
| | Lithotripsy (mechanical, extracorporeal shockwave, laser) |
| | Drainage (nasobiliary tube, stent) |
| *Acute cholangitis* | |
| | Sphincterotomy and stone extraction, nasobiliary drainage or stent insertion |
| | Replacement of blocked bile duct stent |
| *Acute gallstone pancreatitis* | |
| | In patients with severe acute pancreatitis |
| *Postcholecystectomy syndrome* | |
| | Consider biliary manometry, ampullary dilatation or sphincterotomy |
| *Bile duct injury* | |
| | Consider sphincterotomy and stents for leaks and stenoses |
| *Bile duct strictures* | |
| | Stents for malignancy and in selected benign strictures |
| *Chronic pancreatitis* | |
| | Consider sphincterotomy, stone extraction, stent insertion |
| *Pancreas divisum* | |
| | Accessory stenting in selected patients |

approaches such as MRI should be considered (Forbes & Cotton 1984, Soto et al 1996).

## Indications: therapeutic ERCP

The major therapeutic role of ERCP relates to the biliary tract (Table 4.9). Endoscopic therapy for pancreatic disease is in its infancy.

### *Bile duct stones* (p. 1209)

Biliary sphincterotomy is the treatment of choice for choledocholithiasis. The morbidity and mortality of endoscopic stone removal are lower than those of surgery in elderly patients (Cotton 1984). In young patients the choice is more difficult because bile duct exploration can safely be performed under the age of 60 years, while the complications of biliary sphincterotomy are not age related (Neoptolemos et al 1987). The development of laparoscopic cholecystectomy has complicated this issue further, since it is still not routine to perform laparoscopic cholangiography at the time of cholecystectomy. Patients who have a history of jaundice, acute pancreatitis, abnormal liver function tests or ultrasound evidence of bile duct dilatation should have preoperative ERCP (Perissat et al 1994). If stones are found within the biliary tree, endoscopic sphincterotomy or balloon dilatation of the sphincter of Oddi (Staritz et al 1985) is performed and the bile duct stones are removed. This ensures that most common bile duct stones in patients coming to laparoscopic cholecystectomy are diagnosed and treated, but patients who have silent bile duct stones (up to 10%) will be missed (Southern Surgeons Club 1991). This group either remain asymptomatic or can be treated endoscopically when they develop symptoms.

***Emergency therapy.*** Endoscopic biliary sphincterotomy is usually an elective procedure but is performed urgently in two clinical situations. The first is fulminant cholangitis in which drainage of infected bile from the obstructed bile duct accompanied by appropriate antibiotic therapy achieves rapid resolution of symptoms (Lai et al 1992). The second situation is severe gallstone pancreatitis. Most patients who present with acute pancreatitis respond to conservative therapy and elective ERCP is performed after resolution of the acute event. Patients with jaundice, clinical evidence of cholangitis and abnormal liver function tests and whose condition is poor warrant urgent ERCP with biliary sphincterotomy and gallstone extraction if choledocholithiasis is confirmed (Neoptolemos et al 1988, Fan et al 1993). Complications do not appear to occur more commonly than with elective ERCP and in particular pancreatitis is not exacerbated by the procedure.

***Postcholecystectomy syndrome*** (p. 1210). Biliary sphincterotomy is considered in some cases of postcholecystectomy syndrome. Patients who develop recurrent biliary pain, pancreatitis, abnormal liver function tests or a dilated biliary tree following cholecystectomy are considered for biliary manometry (p. 120). If this confirms ampullary dysfunction or stenosis, it is reasonable to perform endoscopic sphincterotomy, accepting that the symptomatic outlook is uncertain (Geenen et al 1989).

***Ampullary dilatation.*** Dilatation of the ampulla of Vater using small Gruntzig balloons is an alternative to endoscopic sphincterotomy (Staritz et al 1983). Balloon dilatation may be safer than sphincterotomy, although concerns regarding postendoscopic pancreatitis have yet to be resolved. Small and medium-sized calculi can be removed after dilatation and larger stones can be fragmented and extracted using mechanical lithotripsy. The procedure tends to be more difficult, more expensive and more time consuming than sphincterotomy and its exact role is currently unclear.

### *Biliary strictures*

Benign and malignant strictures of the biliary tree are amenable to endoscopic therapy. This may alleviate jaundice prior to surgical resection (p. 1201) or be definitive palliative therapy. Patients with tumors of the ampulla can be treated either by endoscopic sphincterotomy or by stent insertion. In general, sphincterotomy is preferred because it avoids the complications of stenting (principally cholangitis), but the risk of hemorrhage is higher with sphincterotomy than with stenting. Strictures in the common bile duct (usually due to pancreatic cancer or cholangiocarcinoma) are the most suitable for endoscopic stenting and either plastic (Shepherd et al 1988) or expandable metal stents (Davids et al 1992a) are used. Strictures at the confluence of the right and left hepatic ducts or in major intrahepatic biliary radicals are much more difficult to stent and the results are often less satisfactory (Deviere et al 1988).

Benign biliary strictures are best managed jointly by hepatobiliary surgeons and endoscopists. The decision to insert biliary stents in patients with sclerosing cholangitis is often difficult because instrumentation may introduce infection and worsen liver disease. However, jaundice may be relieved by stenting dominant common bile duct strictures and significant remission may follow removal of the stent after a few weeks (Gaing et al 1993). This approach is more successful than balloon dilatation, which achieves only temporary improvement of jaundice. A similar approach is used for anastomotic biliary strictures complicating hepatic transplantation (Van Thiel et al 1993). Most iatrogenic biliary strictures are best managed by choledochojejunostomy (Castrini & Pappalardo 1981), but balloon dilatation or stenting may be useful in selected cases of bile duct injury following laparoscopic cholecystectomy (Davids et al 1992b). Missed retained calculi are extracted after biliary sphincterotomy and bile leaks are managed by temporary insertion of endoscopically placed plastic stents (Davids et al 1992b).

*Pancreas*

Patients who present with benign strictures of the pancreatic duct due to chronic pancreatitis may be considered for stent insertion (Gulliver et al 1992). Pancreatic calculi can be treated by sphincterotomy of the pancreatic orifice followed by stone removal using balloons or baskets or stone destruction by lithotripsy (Delhaye et al 1992). Some enthusiasts advocate stenting or sphincterotomy of the accessory pancreatic ampulla in patients who develop symptoms due to pancreas divisum (Coleman et al 1994). Pancreatic endoscopic therapy is technically demanding, the results remain uncertain and it should be undertaken only after detailed assessment in conjunction with pancreatic surgeons.

## Technique: diagnostic ERCP

Diagnostic ERCP is usually performed on an outpatient basis, although facilities for overnight stay should be available in case of complications or if a therapeutic procedure is undertaken. The procedure requires good radiological facilities, including undercouch screening and the ability to obtain radiographs. Most gastroenterologists use a radiography department and the assistance of a radiographer. A radiologist with a special biliary interest is an advantage, but most institutions consider this a luxury rather than a necessity.

The patient is placed in the left lateral position with the left arm behind the back. Oxygen (3 L/min) is given using nasal catheters and sedation is given through an indwelling cannula in a right forearm vein using a combination of a benzodiazepine and pethidine. Hyoscine is usually also injected at this point to paralyze the duodenum, although some endoscopists prefer to give this only after the duodenum has been entered.

A side-viewing endoscope is passed through the stomach, trying not to overinflate with air, and the pylorus is entered. The patient is turned prone at this point, the endoscope is passed into the descending duodenum, "locked" and then withdrawn. This movement straightens the endoscope within the stomach, paradoxically resulting in forward movement of the tip within the descending duodenum.

*Cannulation*

The instrument is positioned so that the endoscopist is looking directly at the ampulla ("en face") and a contrast-filled plastic cannula is introduced into the duodenal lumen (Fig. 4.15). Pancreatic intubation requires cannulation at about 90° to the ampulla. The bile duct empties above and slightly to the left of the pancreatic duct, therefore biliary cannulation requires upward deflection of the cannula tip toward the 11 o'clock position. It is very important not to be heavy-handed; the ducts will be entered only when the cannula is exactly in line and it then passes easily. Excessive force causes edema and bleeding, increasing the difficulty of the examination.

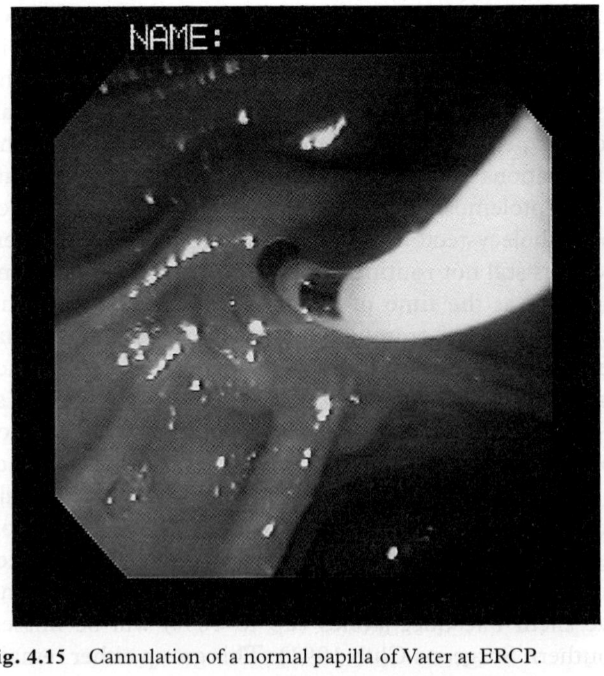


**Fig. 4.15** Cannulation of a normal papilla of Vater at ERCP.

*Pancreas*

Pancreatography includes a preliminary plain radiograph to determine the presence of calcification. Urografin 310 is a suitable contrast medium and it is important to ensure there are no bubbles in the cannula or the syringe. After cannulating the pancreatic duct, contrast is injected carefully. It is important not to overfill the pancreas, since acinar filling predisposes to post-ERCP pancreatitis (Hamilton et al 1983), and the endoscopist may prefer to inject the contrast personally rather than leave this to an assistant. While the pancreatic duct must not be overfilled, it is also important to introduce enough contrast to opacify the pancreatic tail and to demonstrate abnormalities such as pseudocysts. Diagnostic pancreatography should be successful in approximately 95% of cases (Classen & Phillip 1984).

When pancreatography is difficult, two approaches should be considered. The first is to use a fine-tipped (tapered) cannula, although this should be used with some caution because it is easy to inject intramucosally, making subsequent radiography difficult and predisposing to pancreatitis. The second is to consider the possibility of pancreas divisum (p. 1227) (Delhaye et al 1985). The ventral pancreatic duct can be tiny and very difficult to enter even using a fine-tipped cannula. Attempts should be made to cannulate the accessory ampulla. As the endoscopist views it, this lies above and slightly to the right of the main ampulla. In order to obtain an optimum position, it is necessary to produce a "long scope position". The endoscope is first withdrawn into the duodenal cap and the gastric loop is recreated by reintroducing the instrument. This alters the angle of the endoscope tip and reveals the accessory ampulla "en face". Even in this position cannulation is difficult because the punctum is small and the uncomfortable patient may wriggle. A fine-tipped or ball-tipped cannula is necessary to intubate the dorsal pancreatic duct.

*Biliary tract*

Cholangiography is possible in more than 90% of patients (Vaira et al 1989). Some endoscopists prefer to use dilute (1:2 or 1:4) Urografin because small stones may be obscured by full-strength contrast. It is important to screen during cholangiography because this often reveals calculi that are difficult to see on radiographic plates. An early (filling) film should be taken in addition to films of the fully filled biliary system. Difficulty in cannulation may be due to duodenal diverticula which distort the anatomy, making the ampulla of Vater difficult to find. The ampulla usually lies within the left-hand border of a diverticulum. Cannulation is sometimes difficult in the elderly and obese, principally because of difficulties in removing the gastric loop, and cannulation using a "long scope position" is then much more difficult. It is sometimes easier if the patient lies more to the left rather than fully prone. The use of a sphincterotome, which tends to have an upward curve favoring the bile duct, may also help. Once the biliary system has been filled, a final film is obtained after the endoscope has been removed. It is sometimes necessary to turn the patient to a supine position to visualize the distal common bile duct.

*Postgastrectomy ERCP*

ERCP following Polya gastrectomy is difficult. The major problem is that intubation of the afferent jejunal loop is awkward, as the instrument passes preferentially into the efferent loop. Radiological screening helps demonstrate the position of the endoscope and it is easiest to perform the examination while the patient is fully prone. Most endoscopists use a standard duodenoscope, although some advocate forward-viewing instruments. Once the afferent loop has been properly cannulated, and providing it is not excessively long, the ampulla of Vater will eventually be found, but the endoscopist has difficulty because the ampulla is approached from below rather than from the duodenal cap. Manipulations of the cannula essentially have to be reversed, as for example cannulation of the biliary system, which requires a downward rather than upward catheter position. MRI may be preferable to ERCP after Polya gastrectomy.

*Interpretation: pancreas*

***Normal pancreas.*** The normal pancreatogram is characterized by a narrow, regular main duct that crosses the first lumbar vertebra in an oblique and upward direction. Pancreatic radicals are seen throughout the length of the main duct and they divide into tapering secondary ducts. A branch of the main pancreas can often be seen to communicate with the accessory pancreas.

***Pancreas divisum*** (p. 1227). The commonest anatomical variant is pancreas divisum (Sugawa et al 1987). This occurs in approximately 4% of the general population and its association with pancreatic disease is unclear (Delhaye et al 1985). A small ventral pancreas is completely separate from the dorsal duct, which can be opacified only by cannulation of the accessory ampulla.

***Cancer.*** Most commonly, this causes complete obstruction of the main pancreatic duct; there may be corresponding obstruction to the biliary tract ("double duct sign"). Differentiation from benign strictures due to chronic pancreatitis or pancreatic trauma is difficult and relies upon clinical factors (for example, the history and physical findings), pancreatic calcification (suggesting chronic pancreatitis), other abnormalities on the pancreatogram suggesting chronic pancreatitis (below) and the results of other imaging tests. The presence of mucus secretion and cystic changes on the pancreatogram suggest cystadenoma or cystadenocarcinoma (Compagno & Oertel 1978).

***Chronic pancreatitis.*** The Cambridge classification has clarified the endoscopic interpretation of chronic pancreatitis (Jones et al 1988). It is necessary to interpret the radiological report with caution, because there may be a discrepancy between the clinical presentation and the radiographic findings (Bozkurt et al 1994). In addition to aiding diagnosis, the endoscopist has an important role in defining complications of chronic pancreatitis that may be amenable to surgical correction. The site and nature of a stricture, the degree of main duct dilatation, the position of calculi and the presence of a pseudocyst are particularly important. It is also important to visualize the biliary tree in patients with established chronic pancreatitis; this may reveal a distal bile duct stricture (p. 877) and the presence of unsuspected gallstones.

***Trauma.*** ERCP is a useful preoperative test in patients suspected of pancreatic trauma, enabling the site and extent of a leak from the pancreatic duct to be identified prior to surgery.

*Interpretation: biliary system*

***Normal biliary system.*** An adequate cholangiogram demonstrates the common bile and common hepatic ducts and the intrahepatic major bile ducts and their divisions. In addition, the cystic duct and gallbladder should be filled, although caution must be used in interpretation of gallbladder appearances at ERCP as gallbladder pathology is best determined using ultrasound and oral cholecystography. The normal common bile duct is less than 8 mm in diameter and tapers at the ampulla. Screening may reveal peristaltic activity at the ampulla, although this is not an adequate way of defining sphincter function. The bile duct may be dilated in patients who have undergone cholecystectomy, although it is not clear whether this occurs as a consequence of previous choledocholithiasis. The intrahepatic ducts are smooth, tapering and regularly branched.

***Choledocholithiasis.*** Gallstones within the biliary tree have to be distinguished from air bubbles, tumors, blood and parasites. Air bubbles appear as round rather than faceted filling defects and float upwards in the biliary tree. Intraductal tumor is fixed rather than mobile and is often multifocal.

***Hemobilia.*** Hemobilia is diagnosed by observing bloodstained bile at the ampulla.

***Parasites.*** *Ascaris lumbricoides* and other parasites present characteristic radiological appearances.

***Tumors.*** The commonest cause of malignant bile duct obstruction is invasion from pancreatic cancer. When the pancreatic duct is radiologically normal, a cholangiocarcinoma is more likely although pancreatic cancer is still possible. The appearances of cholangiocarcinoma include an apple-core stricture, an eccentric filling defect and multiple strictures indistinguishable from sclerosing cholangitis (Chapman et al 1980).

***Extrinsic obstruction.*** This may be due to compression or invasion by masses, particularly infiltrated lymph nodes.

***Benign strictures.*** Primary sclerosing cholangitis is characterized by multiple strictures of the biliary tree (Chapman et al 1980). The disease may preferentially affect the intrahepatic bile duct. "Pseudodiverticula" of the common bile duct is a characteristic finding. Differentiation from diffuse cholangiocarcinoma may be impossible and some patients present with cholangiocarcinoma complicating established sclerosing cholangitis (LaRusso et al 1984). Rarely, identical radiological appearances can occur following recurrent biliary sepsis due to stone disease, following accidental introduction of formaldehyde into the biliary tree during therapy for hydatid disease, following chemotherapy with floxuridine via the hepatic artery (Doria et al 1986) and in AIDS (Cello 1989).

Benign strictures also occur in biliary trauma, usually complicating laparoscopic cholecystectomy. This may be due to ligation or clipping of the biliary tree or to diathermy-induced ischemia (Zucker et al 1991).

***Congenital disease.*** Jaundice can be due to a range of congenital biliary diseases including choledochal cysts (p. 727), Caroli's disease (p. 727) and biliary atresia in children (p. 730).

## Therapeutic ERCP

Jaundiced patients and those with a history or current evidence of cholangitis should receive prophylactic antibiotics (p. 100). This is not necessary for routine diagnostic ERCP (Lancet 1989). The prothrombin time should be normal and a serum sample saved for crossmatching to allow sphincterotomy to be done safely.

*Biliary sphincterotomy*

A range of sphincterotomes is available, differing according to the position of the cutting wire, length and shape of the distal tip and presence or absence of a guidewire. It is very important to confirm radiologically that the sphincterotome is in the bile duct rather than the pancreatic duct. The cutting wire is positioned under endoscopic control such that only a small portion lies across the sphincter to avoid sudden excessive cutting; the wire is then "bowed" and a combined cutting/coagulation current is applied. The sphincter is cut in a controlled manner in an upward direction until the horizontal mucosal fold which lies proximal to the ampulla is reached. A gush of bile indicates division of the sphincter. Controlled cutting is much more difficult when most of the wire lies within the sphincter; sudden ("zipper") cutting tends to occur in this situation.

It is sometimes impossible to cannulate the bile duct deeply with the sphincterotome and in this situation the endoscopist may resort to using a needle knife. This is used to cut directly into the biliary tree, using the needle tip as a scalpel and making cuts directed from the ampulla toward the bile duct (Tweedle & Martin 1991). The risk of perforation is high and the technique is very much the province of the experienced endoscopist. Once the bile duct has been entered, the sphincterotomy is completed using a standard sphincterotome.

Calculi are removed using extraction balloons that are inflated above the stones or by using Dormia baskets. If possible, the bile duct should be completely cleared at the time of ERCP, since this greatly reduces the risk of post-ERCP cholangitis (Safrany & Cotton 1982). If this proves impossible, check ERCP is necessary to ensure that stones have passed. Patients who have cholangitis and residual calculi should have a stent or a nasobiliary drain passed into the biliary tree to ensure adequate drainage (Cairns et al 1989).

Calculi greater than 2.5 cm in diameter rarely pass through even the largest sphincterotomy. The treatment of choice is mechanical lithotripsy using strong modified Dormia baskets (Sauerbruch et al 1992). Other options include extracorporeal shockwave lithotripsy (Schneider et al 1988), laser lithotripsy (Cotton et al 1990), direct dissolution using methyl tertiary butyl ether (Neoptolemos et al 1990) or a surgical operation.

*Balloon dilatation of the ampulla*

The complications of endoscopic sphincterotomy may be avoided by balloon dilatation of the ampulla (Staritz et al 1983). This is performed using "low profile", Gruntzig-type balloons. Coupled with mechanical lithotripsy, this technique has the potential to remove calculi of all sizes. Small calculi may be removed after relaxation of the ampulla induced by sublingual administration of glyceryl trinitrate (Staritz et al 1985).

*Stent insertion* (see also p. 1294)

The site and length of a stricture is first defined cholangiographically and when possible, brushings and biopsies are taken. Plastic and expandable wire stents are available, both of which require the use of a therapeutic duodenoscope with a wide-bore instrument channel. A preliminary biliary sphincterotomy is usually unnecessary. A guidewire is first passed across the stricture and a plastic stent is then "railroaded" into position using a pusher tube or the metal stent is deployed using standard systems developed by the manufacturers (Fig. 4.16). Plastic stents tend to occlude after 4–6 months but are usually easily replaced. This involves removal of the old stent using "grabbing" forceps or a Dormia basket and restenting using the standard method.

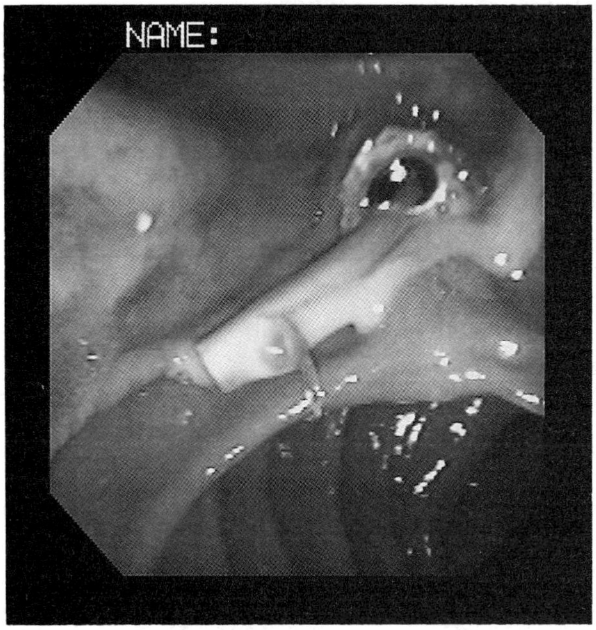


**Fig. 4.16** A biliary stent draining pus into the duodenum in a patient with a biliary stricture and cholangitis.

Deep cannulation of the biliary tree is difficult when the duodenum is infiltrated and distorted by tumor, when a duodenal diverticulum is present and following gastric surgery (Lambert et al 1991). Tight strictures may be overcome only with the use of specialized hydrophilic guidewires and catheters. It is occasionally necessary to use a needle knife to gain entry into the biliary tree. Failed endoscopic stenting is usually an indication for percutaneous insertion of expandable metal prostheses (Nicholson & Royston 1993). These can be introduced into the biliary tree through relatively small tracts and this approach has rendered obsolete the combined percutaneous/endoscopic approach to stenting (Martin 1994).

## Complications of ERCP

ERCP is associated with the complications of any endoscopic procedure including the hazards of sedation and bronchial aspiration (Table 4.10). The need to use combinations of opiates and benzodiazepine drugs in patients who are often elderly makes these complications more likely and careful monitoring and oxygenation are mandatory for ERCP.

The major complication of diagnostic ERCP is acute pancreatitis occurring in 1–4% of procedures (Bilbao et al 1976, Hamilton et al 1983). This is most likely in patients with a history of recurrent pancreatitis. Overfilling of the pancreas with contrast material (and air bubbles) and excessive instrumentation predispose to pancreatitis.

**Table 4.10** Complications of ERCP (%)

| Procedure | Hemorrhage | Pancreatitis | Cholangitis | Perforation | Other |
|---|---|---|---|---|---|
| Diagnostic | 0 | 2–3 | 1–2 | 0 | |
| Biliary sphincterotomy | 2–5 | 2 | 1–4 | 1 | Basket impaction 0.2 |
| Balloon dilatation of ampulla | 0 | 2–6 | 1–2 | 0 | |
| Biliary stent insertion | | | | | |
| – plastic | 2 | 2–4 | 10 early<br>20–50 late | 5 | |
| – metal | 2 | 2–4 | 10 early<br>30 late | 2 | |
| Pancreatic therapy | 4 | 2–20 | 2 | 0 | |

Endoscopic sphincterotomy is complicated by acute pancreatitis (2–4%), hemorrhage (2%), retroperitoneal duodenal perforation (1%), cholangitis (2–3%) and impaction of a Dormia basket within the bile duct (Cairns et al 1989, Freeman et al 1996, Huibregtse 1996). Overall, up to 10% of patients develop a complication and 1% die. Major hemorrhage is due to division of the retroduodenal artery, which usually lies beneath a horizontal fold situated above the ampulla. Local endoscopic therapy such as balloon tamponade and injection of adrenaline is usually ineffective and arterial bleeding often requires surgical correction. Retroperitoneal perforation causes abdominal and back pain and occasionally subcutaneous emphysema of the head and neck. Perforation may be appreciated at ERCP from local extravasation of contrast. Most patients respond to fasting, intravenous fluids and antibiotics. Cholangitis occurs only in the presence of residual calculi. Many endoscopists insert stents or a nasobiliary tube if the duct cannot be cleared to stones. Dormia basket impaction around a calculus which will then not pass through the sphincterotomy should be treated using a mechanical lithotripter.

Endoscopic stenting has a similar range of early complications of which cholangitis is the most important (Speer et al 1987). Patients who have inadequately drained segments of the biliary tree are particularly likely to develop cholangitis and liver abscess. Many endoscopists advocate insertion of multiple stents to prevent this (Deviere et al 1988), although in practice this is technically difficult to achieve. The major late complications of biliary stenting are, for plastic stents, stent occlusion due to infection and biliary debris (Speer et al 1988) and, for metal stents, tumor overgrowth (Adam et al 1991).

### Biliary manometry

Biliary manometry is usually carried out at ERCP, although it can also be done transphepatically or at laparotomy (Geenen et al 1980, Toouli et al 1986, Goff 1988). Pressures can be recorded from the common bile duct and the main pancreatic duct, but the most useful clinical information has come from the measurement of sphincter of Oddi motility (Geenen et al 1980). A triple-lumen Teflon catheter is introduced into the sphincter via the biopsy channel of the endoscope, and pressure is measured with three radially oriented side holes spaced at 2 mm intervals. The catheter is positioned so that all side holes are in the bile duct. Basal sphincter pressure and pattern of motility are recorded using a slow, station pull-through technique. Pressures are referenced to intraduodenal pressure.

The sphincter of Oddi exhibits a basal tone of about 15 mmHg, and superimposed on this basal pressure are phasic contractions occurring at a rate of 2–6 per minute with amplitudes of between 100 and 200 mmHg. Eighty percent of contractions move toward the duodenum, the remainder being simultaneous or retrograde. Sphincter of Oddi dysfunction is associated particularly with high basal pressure (>40 mmHg) and also with high phasic contraction pressure (>240 mmHg) and an increase of simultaneous and retrograde contractions. Associations of sphincter of Oddi dysfunction include transient abnormal liver function tests during biliary-type pain, and a common bile duct of diameter greater than 12 mm and failing to drain over 45 min at ERCP.

Manometry has been used primarily to investigate suspected sphincter of Oddi dysfunction in patients with biliary-type pain, either after cholecystectomy or in patients without evidence of gallstones (p. 1210). Endoscopic sphincterotomy can give prolonged relief from pain when sphincter dysfunction is found (Geenen et al 1989).

## ENTEROSCOPY

Fiberoptic equipment has been designed to examine the whole of the small intestine. However, indications for its use are few and the equipment is expensive and difficult to use.

There are three principal techniques (Classen et al 1976). One is to pass a guidewire through the mouth and thread the endoscope over it once it has appeared at the anus. The second is to use a long, flexible, narrow endoscope that is allowed to pass through the intestine over a number of hours and views are then obtained during withdrawal (Lewis & Waye 1988). The third technique is to pass an enteroscope as one would a duodenoscope and to try and manipulate it through the intestine. This method rarely allows more than the upper part of the jejunum to be visualized. Intraoperative enteroscopy is useful for the detection of bleeding lesions in the small intestine (Lau et al 1986).

## SIGMOIDOSCOPY

### Rigid sigmoidoscopy

The sigmoidoscope is used to examine the rectum and lower sigmoid colon. The distance to which the instrument can be inserted depends upon the skill of the operator, the anatomy of the rectosigmoid junction and the fortitude of the patient. Although a sigmoidoscopy report is usually accompanied by a description of the distance to which the instrument was inserted, this may be erroneous as the rectum may be stretched during the procedure. In a review of several series of cases, Smith (1985) concluded that the average distances reached were 20 cm in males and 18 cm in females.

#### *Indications and contraindications*

Sigmoidoscopy is performed as part of the clinical examination of patients with a wide variety of gastrointestinal disorders, being indicated when there has been a change in bowel habit, rectal bleeding or other anorectal symptoms. In addition to visual diagnosis, rectal biopsy is an important aspect of the procedure. Benign or occasionally malignant tumors can be removed via the sigmoidoscope. There are few contraindications to sigmoidoscopy, the main one being painful conditions of the anus which may mean that the procedure should be carried out under a general anesthetic.

#### *Instruments*

A number of acceptable sigmoidoscopes are available. The provision of a fiberoptic light source has improved their reliability and portable, disposable, prelubricated instruments are available that can be used even in a domiciliary situation.

#### *Technique*

Sigmoidoscopy is usually attempted without bowel preparation, as purgatives may cause mucosal edema and erythema and the appearance of the stool itself may be diagnostically helpful. However, a disposable enema may be needed if stool prevents the examination (Mann et al 1988).

The procedure must be explained to the patient and verbal consent obtained. It is performed with the patient in the left lateral position, lying obliquely with the buttocks over the edge of the couch; the hips should be fully flexed and the legs extended to lie on the opposite side. A small pillow under the left hip increases the room for maneuvering the instrument. Some physicians use the knee–elbow position and this may be more successful because it tends to straighten the rectosigmoid bend; however, the position is uncomfortable and less dignified for the patient. A sigmoidoscopy table is helpful for the aged and those with diarrhea or bleeding, particularly when the procedure is prolonged.

The anal and perianal skin should be examined first. Digital examination must always be carried out, as it dilates the anal sphincter and warns the operator of any condition that precludes the passage of the sigmoidoscope, for example, a painful anal fissure or a tumor just inside the anus. It is also necessary for the assessment of consistency of tumors and to detect abnormalities outside the rectum. Before sigmoidoscopy, the obturator is firmly fixed and the lubricated instrument is passed gently through the anal canal. The tip of the instrument is directed toward the umbilicus until the rectum is entered and then angled toward the sacrum; the obturator is removed, an eyepiece is attached and all subsequent movement of the instrument is made under direct vision. The minimum amount of air is insufflated and relaxation of the patient is encouraged by constant reassurance and by asking the patient to take controlled breaths. Negotiation of the rectosigmoid bend may be difficult for the operator and uncomfortable for the patient. It can be accomplished in about 70% of cases. Pressure should never be used and any pain should lead to termination of the procedure.

After inserting the instrument as far as possible, it is withdrawn slowly and more air is used to obtain distention so that small lesions are not missed. Small amounts of adherent feces can be removed with a swab held in alligator forceps. Rubbing the mucosa with a swab helps to assess the mucosal integrity. As the instrument is withdrawn through the anal canal, the patient is asked to bear down to reveal hemorrhoids. The depth of insertion and the distance from the anus of any lesion or biopsy must be noted.

#### *Interpretation*

Colonic or rectal disease may be revealed by blood, pus or excessive mucus (Fig. 4.17). Normally the rectum is distensible and any areas of rigidity or narrowing should be noted. The normal mucosa glistens, blood vessels can be seen in it and gentle rubbing with a swab does not produce

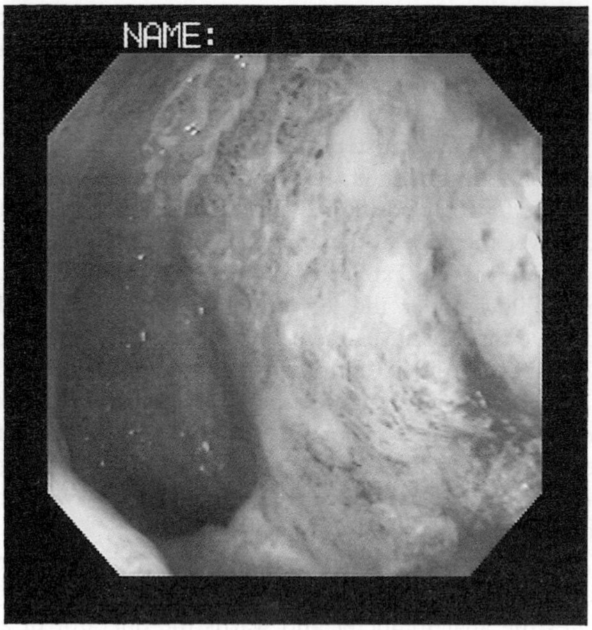


**Fig. 4.17** Diffuse hemorrhagic proctitis in the rectum in ulcerative colitis.

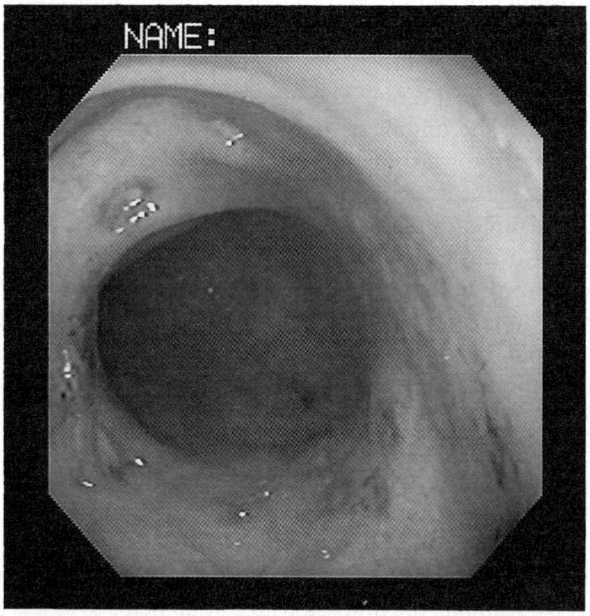


**Fig. 4.18** Aphthous ulceration of the colon in Crohn's disease.

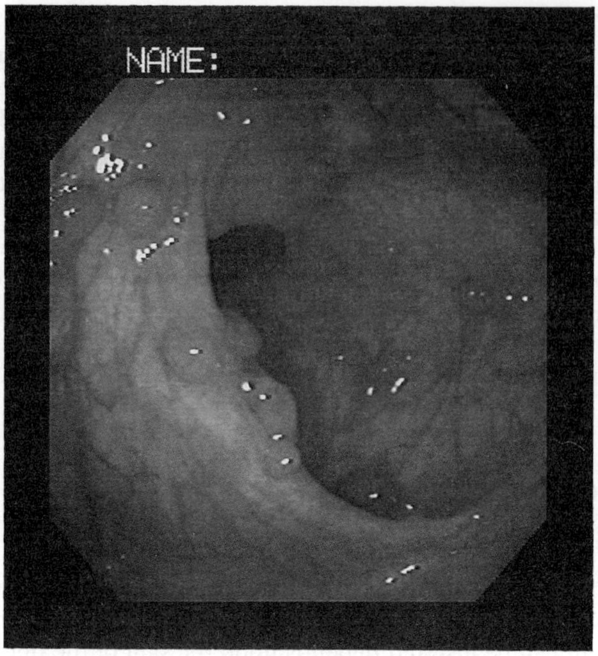


**Fig. 4.19** Multiple benign sessile polyps in the colon.

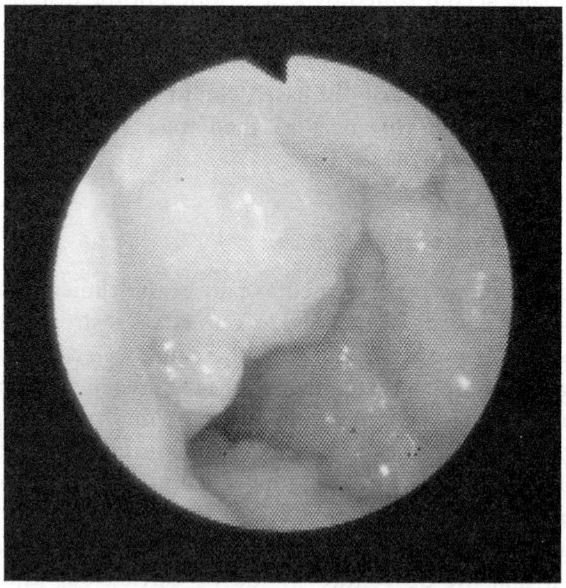

**Fig. 4.20** Pneumatosis coli showing multiple air cysts in the wall of the colon.

bleeding. In proctitis, the vascular pattern is lost as a result of edema and the mucosa is red, granular and loses its light reflex. In some cases, petechiae and bleeding will result from rubbing the mucosa (p. 657). Crohn's disease may reveal changes similar to ulcerative colitis; alternatively, it may have a patchy appearance with discrete ulceration (Fig. 4.18) (p. 667 and Table 23.8). Solitary rectal ulcer appears as a glassy white area and biopsies taken from it may confirm the diagnosis (p. 1330). Other abnormalities that may be seen are tumors, polyps (Fig. 4.19) and the entrances to diverticula. Rare conditions include the cysts of pneumatosis coli (Fig. 4.20) (p. 1393). The stool is worth noting, as it may confirm diarrhea, show pellets as in the irritable bowel syndrome, be pale in malabsorption and can be tested for blood (p. 497) or sent for culture.

### *Biopsy*

Biopsy of the mucosa can be taken at any level, but it

should be remembered that the peritoneal attachment on the anterior rectal wall may be as low as 8 cm from the perineum in the male and 5 cm in the female. Care must be taken to ensure that the biopsy is not too deep and it should be taken under direct vision. The new St Mark's biopsy forceps are safer from this point of view and obtain satisfactory biopsies in the majority of cases. Sigmoidoscopy should be performed prior to barium enema, but if a biopsy is taken, there should if possible be a delay of 10 days between taking the biopsy and performing a barium enema, in view of possible dangers of perforation during the enema examination.

### *Complications*

These are rare. Perforation may result from undue pressure at the rectosigmoid junction, from a large biopsy or in acute ulcerative colitis. It is more likely to occur when the mucosa is thin, but a deep biopsy may perforate normal bowel. Perforation necessitates immediate laparotomy. Occasionally, there may be persistent bleeding after a biopsy; this is treated conservatively with bed rest and sedation. Local cauterization may occasionally be needed. Electrocardiographic abnormality has been noted during sigmoidoscopy and may be responsible for the rare occurrence of sudden death during the procedure.

### *Polyp removal*

Small polyps are often seen in the course of routine rigid sigmoidoscopy and they can be removed conveniently using the biopsy forceps. Larger rectal polyps used to be removed with rigid instruments but since the advent of colonoscopy, this is rarely required. Occasionally, a large polyp can only be treated using the rigid sigmoidoscope if a laparotomy is to be avoided. In these circumstances, the patient is admitted to hospital, the rectum is washed out and the procedure is performed under general anesthesia. A larger operating sigmoidoscope is inserted through the dilated anal sphincter and the polyp is located. Under direct vision, an insulated snare is inserted down the sigmoidoscope and is then opened at the site of the polyp. It is manipulated around the head of the polyp so that it can be closed around its base. Traction is then exerted and a gentle cutting diathermy current is applied to the pedicle. The detached polyp is removed using biopsy forceps, taking care not to crush it. The cut base of the polyp is observed for bleeding and if all is well, the instrument is withdrawn. If the polyp is sessile, removal may have to be piecemeal and great care should be exercised in collecting all the resected pieces so that a complete pathological examination is possible. It must be emphasized that even if a polyp is successfully removed using this technique, the remainder of the colon will still need examination, preferably by colonoscopy, in order to exclude the presence of more proximal polyps.

## Proctoscopy

This procedure is normally performed after sigmoidoscopy. The patient remains in the left lateral position and the instrument and the obturator, both well lubricated, are gently inserted through the anal sphincter into the anal canal up to their hilt. The obturator is then removed and the fiberoptic light source is attached via the appropriate socket to the base of the instrument.

The instrument allows approximately 5–6 cm of anorectum to be visualized. The state of the mucosa is observed with particular reference to the presence of proctitis, tumor, hemorrhoids, fissure or the internal opening of a fistula in ano. Hemorrhoids are best observed at the level of the dentate line and may be exaggerated by asking the patient to bear down. A fissure is often suspected from the outset, as insertion of the instrument may be difficult or impossible owing to anal spasm and pain. In addition, a sentinel pile may be present on first inspection of the anal verge. If proctoscopic examination is allowed to proceed in such patients, the detection of the fissure may be quite difficult as folds of anal mucosa tend to obscure it.

Various therapeutic maneuvers can be carried out, particularly for the treatment of hemorrhoids. These may be injected (p. 1452), banded (p. 1453) or treated by cryoprobe or, more recently, by photocoagulation.

## Flexible sigmoidoscopy

Rigid sigmoidoscopy has been superseded by flexible endoscopy in many institutions. This is because the flexible sigmoidoscope can be used to visualize the rectum, all of the sigmoid colon and in some patients the whole of the descending colon to the splenic flexure. The procedure is performed on an outpatient basis without the need for intravenous sedation and an adequate view can be obtained after use of a single disposable enema. On the other hand, flexible sigmoidoscopy is more expensive than rigid sigmoidoscopy and the instrument requires appropriate maintenance and cleaning. Accordingly, cheap disposable rigid instruments still have an important role in the outpatient assessment of rectal disease and in the management of rectal bleeding.

***Technique.*** A disposable enema is given and the bowel emptied. The examination is performed with the patient in the left lateral position. Digital examination and lubrication of the anal canal are performed and the instrument is introduced into the rectum. The technique of endoscopic visualization is similar to that of colonoscopy.

## COLONOSCOPY

### Indications

Colonoscopy is the best method of examining the colon (Table 4.11) and if resources were adequate, the barium enema would be used only for failures of endoscopy (Leicester 1991). Unfortunately, colonoscopy is more expensive, time consuming and uncomfortable than barium enema and it is likely that both techniques will continue to be employed (p. 17). It has been suggested that barium enema is adequate for patients under the age of 55 years, while colonoscopy is the investigation of choice in older patients (Rex et al 1990).

Colonoscopy is particularly useful for the investigation of colonic bleeding and diarrhea, while barium enema is preferable in the assessment of constipation and colonic pain. The endoscopic approach is more sensitive in disease identification, has the capacity to obtain samples for histological assessment and allows therapy such as polyp removal, hemostasis and stricture dilatation. The barium enema is difficult to interpret in the presence of sigmoid diverticular disease, which may mask filling defects such as polyps or carcinomas (Boulos et al 1984). One approach in these patients is to combine flexible sigmoidoscopy and barium enema (Eckardt et al 1989), but a single colonoscopy seems a more logical approach.

Colonoscopic screening in patients with long-standing colitis (Gyde 1990), adenomatous polyps (Woolfson et al 1990) or a family history of colonic cancer (Mecklin et al 1987) is a controversial area. The risk–benefit and financial implications of these indications are yet to be established.

### Contraindications

The major contraindication is a possible colonic perforation. Discretion is necessary in patients with severe colitis and the procedure can be difficult and onerous in elderly or frail individuals.

### Bowel preparation

A clean colon is required for colonoscopy and a successful procedure depends upon adequate bowel preparation. For the patient, this is often the most unpleasant part of the procedure. One of two approaches is used. The first is based upon avoidance of dietary fiber followed by the use of laxatives such as sodium picosulfate. This regimen works best in mobile outpatients. Immobile inpatients respond less well and bowel washouts, enemas or suppositories may be needed.

The second approach is that of whole-gut lavage using iso-osmolar solutions. Hyperosmolar solutions, such as mannitol, are no longer used since these cause dehydration. The commonest proprietary preparation is Golytely, which is a polyethylene glycol electrolyte solution (Pockros & Foroozan 1985). This is consumed at a rate of 1.5 L/h until 3–5 L have been drunk and the colonic effluent is clear. Nausea and vomiting are minimized by cooling and flavoring the solution, but some patients require nasoenteric infusion.

**Table 4.11** Indications for colonoscopy

| | |
|---|---|
| *Diagnostic* | |
| | Evaluation of abnormal or equivocal barium enema |
| | Rectal bleeding or iron deficiency anemia |
| | Assessment of inflammatory bowel disease |
| *Therapeutic* | |
| | Polypectomy |
| | Laser photocoagulation of vascular lesions |
| | Laser palliation of inoperable colorectal tumors |
| *Surveillance/screening* | |
| | Colonic inflammatory bowel disease |
| | Polyps |
| | Family history of polyps and cancer |

### Technique

Most endoscopists sedate the patient using a combination of a benzodiazepine and pethidine. The patient should be carefully monitored throughout the procedure, as bradycardia is relatively common and is treated by atropine 300–600 μg intravenously or intramuscularly. The examination is usually carried out with the patient in the left lateral position with the buttocks as near the edge of the couch as possible. After visual inspection, a digital examination of the rectum is performed to ensure there is no obstruction or fissure and to relax the anal sphincter. The distal shaft of the colonoscope is lubricated and the tip of the instrument held in the right hand is inserted edgeways into the anus, using gentle pressure with the right index finger. The controls are held in the left hand, which operates the suction button, air flow and up–down angulation. The right hand holds the shaft of the instrument close to the anus and is used to advance, retract and twist. The right hand is also used to control the side-to-side angulation. The length of the colonoscope is allowed to loop downwards over the side of the couch and when the right hand moves from the shaft of the instrument to the controls in order to change side-to-side angulation, the shaft can be prevented from slipping back by pressure of the operator's thigh against the couch, thus trapping the looped instrument.

The tip of the colonoscope is advanced by a series of pushes and pulls, jiggling, twisting and air suction. It is desirable not to allow too much looping to occur within the colon, as this causes difficulty in advancing the instrument and is painful. Overdistention with air tends to cause the colon to elongate and kink, thereby increasing the likelihood of looping. The two areas of greatest difficulty in colonoscopy are passing from the sigmoid colon, which is on a long mesentery, into the relatively fixed descending colon and from the transverse colon, also on a mesentery, into the fixed ascending colon. A number of maneuvers have been described to accomplish these transitions, but in the majority of cases, gentle perseverance, frequent pulling back and the ready use of suction enable total colonoscopy to be performed.

Although the colon is seen as the instrument is advanced, better views are obtained during slow withdrawal, as the tip of the instrument can be kept in the center of the lumen. In spite of this, there may be blind areas where the colon is convoluted and at flexures and it may be necessary to pass the instrument back and forth through a bend several times before an adequate view is obtained. Pancolonoscopy is successful in approximately 75–85% of patients (Lindsay et al 1988). In the remainder, the whole colon is not examined because of extreme tortuosity leading to looping and excessive discomfort. Barium enema is necessary in these failures.

### Complications

Perforations of the colon occur in 1:250–1:500 examinations. They usually respond to fasting, intravenous fluids and antibiotics, but surgical repair is required for large tears (pp. 1394 and 1427) (Macrae et al 1981).

### Polypectomy

The operator must be skilled in colonoscopy before attempting polypectomy and an experienced assistant familiar with the technicalities of the instrument and electrosurgical apparatus should be present. Surgical facilities must be available in case of complications.

Polyps are snared and cut across using diathermy and should then be captured and removed for histology (see p. 109 and Ch. 55). Some polyps are too small for removal in this way but can be destroyed by seizing them in hot biopsy forceps (Williams 1973). The polyp is pulled into the lumen, stretching the mucosa to which it is attached, thus forming a pseudostalk; when diathermy is applied, the current flows through the pseudostalk, which heats up and blanches. The effect of this is to remove the polyp and the hot biopsy forceps are withdrawn containing within them a biopsy of the polyp which has been destroyed. It is not necessary to keep patients in hospital after polyps have been removed, if an experienced colonoscopist performing the procedure is satisfied that there are no complications.

***Complications.*** The main complication of polypectomy is bleeding that may occur at the time of removal and it may then be possible to arrest it by further electrocoagulation of the stalk. Pain immediately following polypectomy suggests a perforation. An abdominal radiograph is taken to look for gas outside the bowel (Webb et al 1985).

### Laser therapy

Nd:YAG laser therapy is used to stop bleeding and to treat tumors.

#### *Hemostatic therapy*

This is used in patients with vascular malformations which are commonly multiple and most frequent in the ascending colon and cecum (Richter et al 1984). Diagnosis requires a perfectly clean colon, good optics and excellent colonoscopic technique. The lesions can be coagulated using low-energy settings (20 watts). Minor bleeding commonly occurs during laser photocoagulation but usually ceases spontaneously or following further laser therapy. The right colon has a relatively thin wall and excessive energy administration can result in perforation.

#### *Neoplastic disease* (p. 1431)

Patients with inoperable cancer, often recurrent disease with metastatic spread, who are unsuitable for further surgery are considered (Krasner 1989). Symptoms of bleeding, mucus discharge, obstruction and diarrhea may respond to laser treatment, but pain does not respond. The principles are similar to those described for ablation of esophagogastric malignancy. Essentially, proximal disease is treated first and relatively high energy settings are used to produce significant tissue effects. The risk of perforation is low, but the procedure may need to be repeated on several occasions. Occasionally, large sessile adenomatous polyps are also treated by Nd:YAG laser (Brunetaud et al 1989) and radiation proctitis may also respond to this therapy (Berken 1985).

## ENDOSCOPIC ULTRASOUND

Endoscopic ultrasound (echoendoscopy) with specially constructed ultrasonic transducers attached to the end of an endoscope provides sonographic images of high resolution. The procedure has become technically easier as more mobile and "user-friendly" systems have been developed, but the procedure remains demanding and requires expertise in both endoscopy and ultrasound. High ultrasound frequencies permit accurate visualization of the various layers within the wall of the gastrointestinal tract and adjacent structures such as the pancreas, biliary tree and lymph nodes are displayed in great detail. The main indication for endoscopic ultrasound is the assessment of tumor spread in relation to the appropriateness of surgical treatment and it has been used successfully for esophageal, gastric, pancreatic, biliary and colorectal tumors.

The most widely used method for staging tumors is the tumor, node, metastasis (TNM) system and endoscopic ultrasound is emerging as superior to computed tomography and magnetic resonance imaging for assessment of local tumor and regional node spread (Lightdale 1991, Ziegler et al 1991, Müller et al 1994).

*Esophagus*

Endoscopic ultrasound is the most sensitive staging method for esophageal cancer. Tumors localized to the mucosa or submucosa or involving all three layers can be identified and resectability, based upon spread of tumor to adjacent structures, can be defined (Lightdale 1991, Ziegler et al 1991, Dittler & Siewert 1993). Direct comparison with other methods suggests that endoscopic ultrasound is superior to computed tomography or magnetic resonance imaging. Benign submucosal tumors, particularly leiomyomata, can be confidently differentiated from carcinoma (Rosch & Dancygier 1990).

*Stomach*

Benign lesions are shown by endoscopic ultrasound to be localized to the stomach wall. It has become the technique of choice for the diagnosis of small submucosal muscle tumors (Yasuda et al 1990). Gastric carcinoma can be accurately staged (Tio et al 1989, Lightdale 1991, Ziegler et al 1991).

*Biliary tract and pancreas*

Endoscopic ultrasound is more accurate than transabdominal ultrasound or computed tomography in the diagnosis of pancreatic cancer and more sensitive in detecting lymph node spread and portal vein invasion (Palazzo et al 1993). Differentiation of pancreatic cancer from chronic pancreatitis can be difficult as with all imaging methods. Endocrine pancreatic tumors are small and often multiple and are best seen by this technique. It may be possible to differentiate between cholangiocarcinoma and pancreatic cancer (Tio & Tytgat 1988) and in the future ultrasound probes capable of passing into the biliary tree may further improve biliary tumor diagnosis (Kuroiwa et al 1994).

*Colon, rectum and anus*

Endorectal ultrasonography using rigid instruments is available for staging rectal tumors and ultrasonography using flexible endoscopes is being developed. Flexible ultrasonography will allow assessment of tumors higher in the bowel, including Dukes C disease (Tio et al 1991). Anal endosonography is discussed on p. 1320.

## LAPAROSCOPY

Laparoscopy (or peritoneoscopy) is primarily used in gastroenterological practice for the investigation of hepatic disorders and may be undertaken under general anesthesia or under sedation with local analgesia. Laparoscopy under local analgesia with modern laparoscopes is a valuable diagnostic tool that deserves wider application. Its advantages include accurate staging of liver disease, recognition of focal lesions, targeted biopsy and high patient acceptance.

### Principles of diagnostic laparoscopy

The principles of diagnostic laparoscopy and the design of laparoscopes have remained relatively unchanged for years, but higher quality lenses, fiberoptic light sources and video endoscopy have improved picture quality greatly.

To provide adequate space in the peritoneal cavity, it is necessary to create a pneumoperitoneum. Insufflation of gas is undertaken using a Veress needle, which consists of an inner blunt needle with lateral holes to transmit the insufflating gas and an outer spring-loaded, sharp-edged sheath. The inner blunt needle protrudes in the resting position. Following insertion, tissue resistance pushes the blunt inner needle into the sheath and the sharp-edged sheath penetrates the abdominal wall. Once the needle has entered the peritoneal cavity, the blunt end protrudes beyond the sheath, reducing the risk of visceral injury. The Veress needle is connected to the insufflator via two plastic tubes, one transmitting the insufflating gas, the other relaying intra-abdominal pressure through the insufflator. Most insufflators have gauges to allow the monitoring of flow rate, intra-abdominal pressure and the total volume of gas administered.

### Choice of gas for insufflation

Three gases may be used for insufflation: air, carbon dioxide and nitrous oxide. Carbon dioxide is absorbed rapidly, is nonflammable (valuable if electrocoagulation is to be used) and gives a clear image, but it is painful if laparoscopy is undertaken under local analgesia. Air is relatively poorly absorbed and is associated with a risk of air embolism. Nitrous oxide is well absorbed, painless and probably the gas of choice for laparoscopy under local anesthesia. Unfortunately, it is relatively combustible and electrocoagulation should therefore be avoided.

### Laparoscope

The laparoscope is a rigid tube with a high-quality lens at one end and a standard or videoendoscopy light system at the other, using glass fibers to transmit cold light. The authors use a 5 mm (pediatric) laparoscope with an oblique-viewing system (50° rotation of the lens) that allows good inspection of the liver. A video camera attached to the eyepiece increases operator comfort, is valuable for teaching and for taking directed biopsies and allows a detailed video record to be kept.

The laparoscope is inserted through a trocar sleeve to the left of and above the umbilicus, as this avoids hypervascular areas, particularly in those patients with portal hypertension. The sleeve incorporates a valve to prevent gas loss and a side arm that is connected to the insufflator enabling automatic replacement of leaking gas. A second trocar may be inserted to allow passage of a palpating probe, which is invaluable for manipulation of bowel and liver and can be used to apply pressure over a biopsy site. Alternatively, a heater probe can be used.

### Patient preparation

The procedure should be explained to the patient beforehand and requires written consent. The prothrombin time and platelet count are used to check adequate coagulation (p. 718), although there is no good relation between the prothrombin time and platelet count and duration of bleeding after laparoscopic liver biopsy (Ewe 1981, Dillon et al 1994). The patient is fasted for at least 6 h and intravenous access is established. In our unit a combination of diamorphine 5–10 mg intravenously followed by diazemuls 5–10 mg intravenously titrated against the level of sedation is used. Both naloxone and flumazenil should be on hand to allow reversal if respiratory depression occurs. Oximetry and supplementary oxygen are used routinely, as mild hypoxia during gas insufflation is common.

Laparoscopy requires a sterile technique and the laparoscopist and assistant should be gowned and gloved. The patient's abdomen is cleaned thoroughly with an antiseptic solution such as chlorhexidine, starting at the umbilicus and working outwards to cover the entire anterior abdominal wall, and the abdomen is covered by sterile drapes exposing only the site of insertion of the laparoscope and biopsy needle.

### Procedure

The site of the Veress needle insertion, usually 1 inch to the left of and above the umbilicus, should be infiltrated with lignocaine. This site is chosen to avoid large collateral vessels that may run in the round ligament on the right side. Bleeding from the insertion site is always a risk, particularly in patients with coagulopathy. Blunt dissection of the muscular and fascial planes should be the rule rather than using a scalpel. As the Veress needle penetrates the anterior fascia and posterior rectus sheath, two distinct "pops" are felt. Once the needle is connected to the insufflator, a free flow of gas at a rate of approximately 1 L/min should be observed without pressure build-up. If high pressure is observed, it is likely the tip of the Veress needle is not free in the peritoneal cavity and it should be withdrawn and repositioned. Once approximately 2 L of nitrous oxide have been insufflated, producing abdominal distention with resonance to percussion over the liver, the needle should be withdrawn and a trocar inserted.

### Inspection of the abdominal cavity and liver

The laparoscope should be inserted carefully through the trocar sheath and moved under direct vision at all times. This is particularly important in patients who have had previous abdominal surgery, as adhesions may interfere with laparoscope movement. The abdominal cavity should be explored carefully by rotating and advancing the instrument until a panoramic view is obtained and then a systematic examination of the liver should be undertaken. The falciform ligament and ligamentum teres should be identified as landmarks and the liver lobes should be inspected thoroughly and an assessment made of their size, shape, surface texture and color and the presence or absence of focal lesions.

The normal liver surface has a faint lobular pattern. In acute hepatitis the liver is usually enlarged, red, smooth and edematous. The normal lobular pattern is exaggerated in chronic hepatitis (Fig. 4.21). The liver is green in cholestasis, rust-brown where there is an excess of iron and yellow in steatosis (Fig. 4.22). The light reflex from the surface of the liver should be circular and bright and fragmentation indicates irregularity of the liver surface. This is common in cirrhosis, where nodularity of varying degrees of severity develops (p. 916). In micronodular cirrhosis the nodules are small, regular in shape, uniform in size and confluent (Fig. 4.23). In macronodular cirrhosis the nodules are large, irregular and variable in size (Fig. 4.24). Portal hypertension is indicated by increased vascularity of the peritoneum and prominence of individual vessels and is often well seen around the fal-

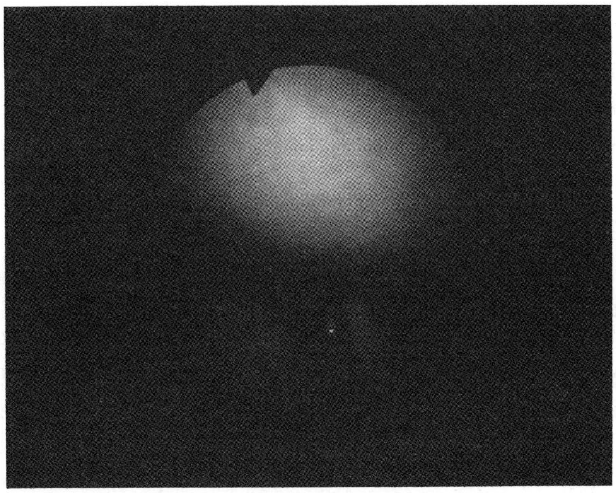

**Fig. 4.21** Chronic hepatitis in an active phase showing an exaggerated ("leopard skin") lobular pattern.

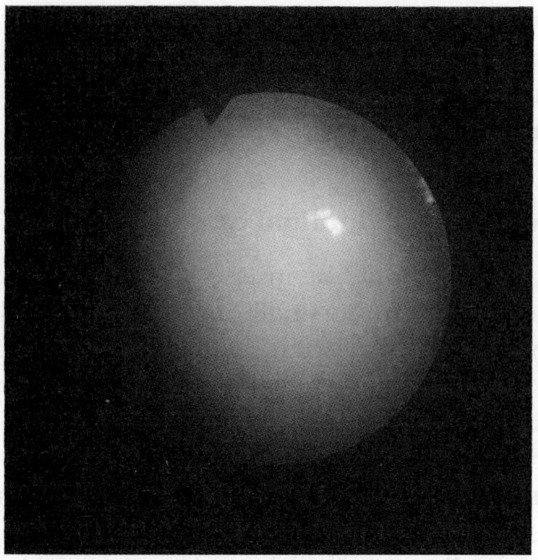

**Fig. 4.22** Severe fatty liver (steatosis) showing a yellow waxy appearance.

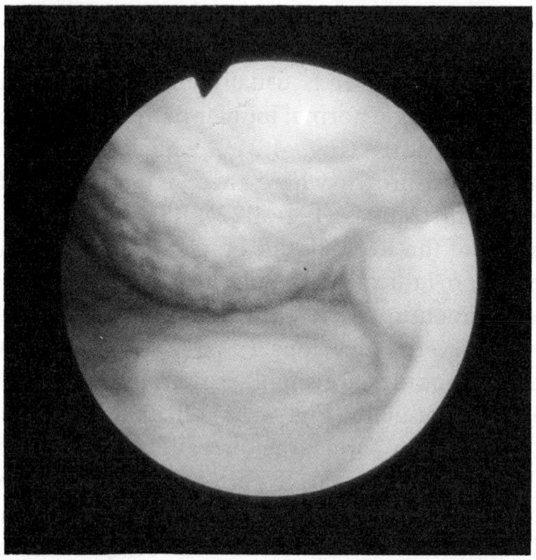

**Fig. 4.23** Alcoholic cirrhosis showing an early diffuse micronodular cirrhosis of the liver.

ciform ligament (Fig. 4.25). It is frequently associated with cirrhosis. Focal lesions such as tumors are usually readily recognized (Fig. 4.26).

## Biopsy

In diffuse liver disease a biopsy is generally undertaken using a Tru-cut needle inserted below the ribs to the left of the xiphisternum. The biopsy should be taken at a 30° angle from the left lobe between segments 2 and 3 (p. 709), which facilitates compression of the biopsy site by a palpating probe or laparoscope to control any bleeding. Different sites of insertion may be required for focal lesions. Transillumination of the abdominal wall with the laparoscope allows large blood vessels to be avoided. The

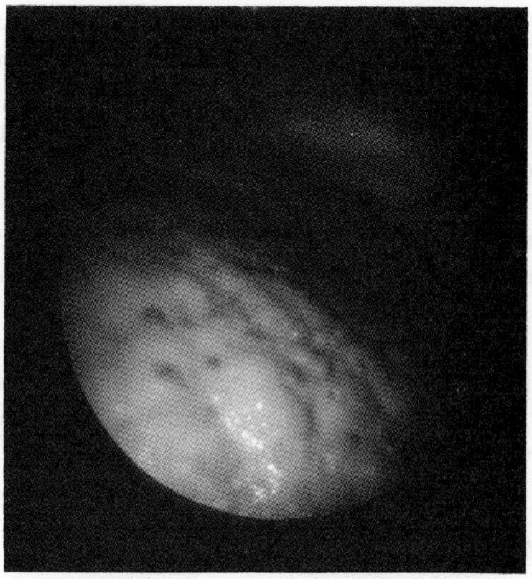

**Fig. 4.24** Primary biliary cirrhosis showing fully established macronodular cirrhosis of the liver.

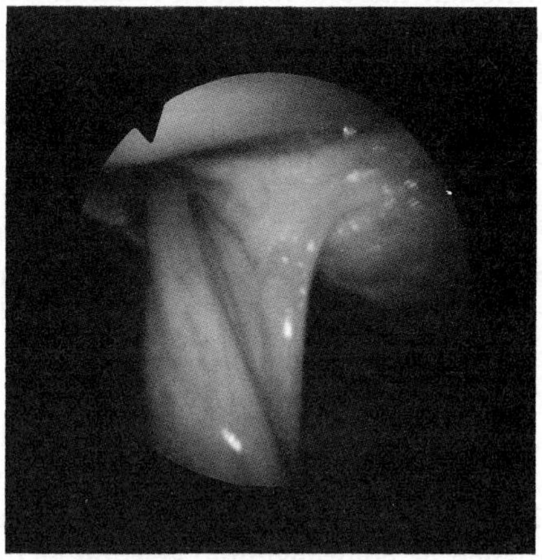

**Fig. 4.25** Prominent vessels around the falciform liver in portal hypertension caused by hepatic cirrhosis.

site of insertion should be visualized as the needle enters the peritoneal cavity. A Menghini needle or pinch biopsies are more suitable than the Tru-cut needle for small surface lesions.

## Postoperative attention

Once the inspection is complete, the laparoscope is withdrawn and the abdomen allowed to deflate before the trocar sleeve is removed and the incision closed with a single silk suture. The blood pressure and heart rate should be monitored for 12 h after the procedure. Occasionally, the patient may require analgesia for left shoulder pain due to diaphragmatic irritation by blood. In patients with ascites, fluid may drain for 24–48 h and should be collected in a colostomy bag. It is important that this should not be allowed to cause hypovolemia. Total paracentesis before

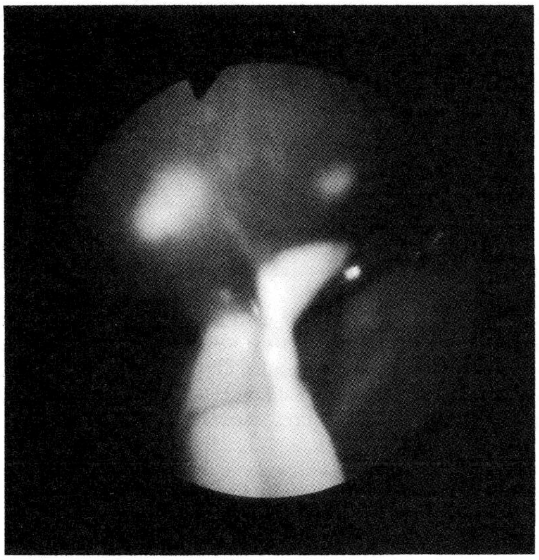

**Fig. 4.26** Metastatic malignant disease in segment 3 (p. 709) of the liver.

**Table 4.12** Indications for laparoscopy

| | |
|---|---|
| *Assessment of liver disease* | |
| | Local lesions (benign and malignant) |
| | Diffuse disease (e.g. cirrhosis) |
| | Presence of portal hypertension |
| | Staging of cirrhosis |
| *Staging for cancer treatment* | |
| | Lymphomas |
| | Hepatocellular carcinoma |
| | Metastases/hepatic tumor resectability |
| *Transplant assessment* | |
| *Ascites of unknown etiology* | |

laparoscopy, if clinically indicated, removes this complication (p. 1029).

## Indications

The main indications for laparoscopy of the liver are listed in Table 4.12 (Plevris & Hayes 1994).

## Focal liver disease

Laparoscopy provides an excellent view of up to two-thirds of the liver surface and it is uncommon for focal liver disease to be missed. Lesions of around 1 mm in diameter can be identified and biopsied (Brady et al 1991). Laparoscopic biopsy has the advantage over scan-directed biopsy, because lesions beyond the resolving power of scanning can be identified. It also identifies lesions of similar echogenicity to the normal liver (Lightdale 1987). Laparoscopy has been found to be at least as accurate as computed tomography and ultrasonography in identifying focal lesions (Mansi et al 1982, Shandall & Johnson 1985, Possik et al 1986, Jeffers et al 1987).

## Chronic liver disease

Liver biopsy can be used to stage chronic liver disease rather than to identify its cause, which is often known. However, biopsy, even at laparoscopy, fails to recognize cirrhosis in approximately 10% of patients, principally in those with macronodular cirrhosis where the tissue is obtained from a single nodule (Boyce 1992). Laparoscopy in these situations is more accurate and, in addition, may identify variations in severity in different segments of the liver. Laparoscopy can also be used prognostically, as more severe disease is typified by well-formed nodules, right lobe atrophy and left lobe hypertrophy (Tameda et al 1990). Portal hypertension may also be recognized as hypervascularity or formation of varices on the falciform ligament.

## Coagulopathy

Pressure or a heater probe can be applied during laparoscopy to control bleeding, allowing biopsies to be undertaken in spite of a degree of coagulopathy. The advantage of being able to undertake liver biopsy safely in cirrhosis with mild to moderate coagulopathy is that sufficient tissue can usually be obtained at laparoscopy for diagnostic purposes, in contrast to transjugular biopsy in which tissue is inadequate in approximately 40% of cases (Lebrec et al 1982). In other cases, where the etiology is known, laparoscopy identifying cirrhosis is sufficient and a biopsy superfluous.

## Contraindications

The main contraindications to laparoscopy are an uncooperative patient, marked obesity, large ventral hernias, abdominal wall sepsis, previous right upper quadrant surgery, coagulopathy (p. 718) and poor cardiorespiratory function.

## Complications

Laparoscopy under local analgesia is safe and has a complication and mortality rate similar to percutaneous biopsy (Henning & Look 1985). The commonest complication, pneumo-omentum and surgical emphysema, is of limited significance and results from incorrect placement of the Veress needle. Abdominal wall bleeding and bleeding from the liver biopsy occur in fewer than 0.25% (Pagliaro et al 1983). Provided a sterile technique is used, infection is not a problem and there is no benefit from performing the procedure in an operating theater rather than an endoscopy suite.

## Conclusion

Laparoscopy can be performed safely under local analgesia and is well tolerated by patients. Visualization of the liver improves diagnostic accuracy and it is cost effective if the need for other procedures such as computed tomography scanning is reduced. It is, however, complementary to other investigations rather than a substitute.

REFERENCES


Adam A, Chetty N, Roddie M, Yeung E, Benjamin I S 1991 Self-expandable stainless steel endoprostheses for treatment of malignant bile duct obstruction. American Journal of Roentgenology 159: 321–325

Al-Kawas F H, O'Keefe J 1987 Nd:Yag laser treatment of a bleeding Dieulafoy's lesion. Gastrointestinal Endoscopy 33: 38–39

Allen J I, Allen M O'C, Olson M M et al 1987 *Pseudomonas* infection of the biliary system resulting from use of a contaminated endoscope. Gastroenterology 92: 759–763

Arrowsmith J B, Gerstman B B, Fleischer D E, Benjamin S B 1991 Results from the American Society for Gastrointestinal Endoscopy/US Food and Drug Administration collaborative study on complication rates and drug use during gastrointestinal endoscopy. Gastrointestinal Endoscopy 37: 421–427

Asaki S, Ohara S, Watanabe Y, Ohara M 1988 Endoscopic diagnosis and treatment of Dieulafoy's ulcer. Tohoku Journal of Experimental Medicine 154: 135–141

Axon A T R 1991 Disinfection of endoscopy equipment. Baillière's Clinical Gastroenterology, Endoscopy update, pp 61–77

Axon A T R, Bond W, Botrill P M 1991 Disinfection and endoscopy: summary and recommendations. Working Party report to the World Congresses of Gastroenterology, Sydney 1990. Journal of Gastroenterology and Hepatology 6: 23–24

Babb J, Bradley C R 1995 A review of gluteraldehyde alternatives. British Journal of Theatre Nursing 5: 20–24

Barr H, Krasner N, Raouf A, Walker R J 1990 Prospective randomised trial of laser therapy only and laser therapy followed by endoscopic intubation for the palliation of malignant dysphagia. Gut 31: 252–258

Beecham H J III, Cohen M L, Parkin W E 1979 *Salmonella typhimurium*. Transmission by fiberoptic upper gastrointestinal endoscopy. Journal of the American Medical Association 241: 1013–1015

Berken C A 1985 Nd:YAG laser therapy for gastrointestinal bleeding due to radiation colitis. American Journal of Gastroenterology 80: 730–731

Bilbao M K, Dotter C T, Lee T G, Katon R M 1976 Complications of endoscopic retrograde cholangiopancreatography (ERCP). A study of 10 000 cases. Gastroenterology 70: 314–320

Birnie G G, Quigley E M, Clements G B, Follet E A C, Watkinson G 1983 Endoscopic transmission of hepatitis B virus. Gut 24: 171–174

Bond W W 1991 Disinfection and endoscopy: microbial considerations. Journal of Gastroenterology and Hepatology 6: 31–36

Botoman V A, Surawicz C M 1986 Bacteremia with gastrointestinal endoscopic procedures. Gastrointestinal Endoscopy 32: 342–346

Boulos P B, Karamanolis D G, Salmon P R, Clark C G 1984 Is colonoscopy necessary in diverticular disease? Lancet 1: 95–96

Boyce H W 1992 Diagnostic laparoscopy in liver and biliary disease. Endoscopy 24: 676–681

Bozkurt T, Braun U, Leferink S, Gilly G, Lux G 1994 Comparison of pancreatic morphology and exocrine functional impairment in patients with chronic pancreatitis. Gut 35: 1132–1136

Brady P G, Peebles M, Goldschmid S 1991 Role of laparoscopy in the evaluation of patients with suspected hepatic or peritoneal malignancy. Gastrointestinal Endoscopy 37: 27–30

Bramble M G 1993 Open access endoscopy – a nationwide survey of current practice. Gut 33: 282–285

British National Formulary 1996 Oral anticoagulants. 31: 106–107

British Society of Gastroenterology 1987 Report of a working party on the staffing of endoscopy units. BSG, London

British Society of Gastroenterology 1994 The nurse endoscopist. Report of the BSG working party. BSG, London

Broor S L, Raju G S, Bose P P et al 1993 Long term results of endoscopic dilatation for corrosive oesophageal strictures. Gut 34: 1498–1501

Brunetaud J M, Maunoury V, Cochelard D, Boniface B, Cortot A, Paris J C 1989 Endoscopic laser treatment for rectosigmoid villous adenoma: factors affecting the results. Gastroenterology 97: 272–277

Cairns S R, Dias L, Cotton P B, Salmon P R, Russell R C G 1989 Additional endoscopic procedures instead of urgent surgery for retained common bile duct stones. Gut 30: 535–540

Castrini G, Pappalardo G 1981 Iatrogenic strictures of the bile ducts: our experience with 66 cases. World Journal of Surgery 5: 763–768

Cello J P 1989 Acquired immune deficiency syndrome cholangiopathy: spectrum of disease. American Journal of Medicine 86: 539–546

Chapman R W G, Arborgh B Å M, Rhodes J M et al 1980 Primary sclerosing cholangitis: a review of its clinical features, cholangiography and hepatic history. Gut 21: 870–877

Choudari C P, Rajgopal C, Palmer K R 1994 Acute gastrointestinal haemorrhage in anticoagulated patients: diagnoses and response to endoscopic treatment. Gut 35: 464–466

Chung S C S, Leung J W C, Steele R J C, Crofts T J, Li A K C 1988 Endoscopic injection of adrenaline for actively bleeding ulcers: a randomised trial. British Medical Journal 296: 1661–1633

Classen M, Phillip J 1984 Endoscopic retrograde cholangiopancreatography (ERCP) and endoscopic therapy in pancreatic disease. Clinical Gastroenterology 13: 819–842

Classen M, Fruhmorgen P, Koch J 1976 Enteroscopy. In: Schiller K F R, Salmon P R (eds) Modern topics in gastrointestinal endoscopy. Heinemann, London, Ch 10, p 139

Coleman S D, Eisen G M, Troughton A B, Cotton P B 1994 Endoscopic treatment in pancreas divisum. American Journal of Gastroenterology 89: 1152–1155

Compagno J, Oertel J E 1978 Mucinous cystic neoplasms of the pancreas with overt and latent malignancy (cystadenocarcinoma and cystadenoma): a clinicopathologic study of 41 cases. American Journal of Clinical Pathology 69: 573–580

Copenhagen Esophageal Varices Sclerotherapy Project 1984 Sclerotherapy after first variceal hemorrhage in cirrhosis. A randomized multicenter trial. New England Journal of Medicine 311: 1594–1600

Cotton P B 1984 Endoscopic management of bile duct stones (apples and oranges). Gut 25: 587–597

Cotton P B, Williams C B 1980 Practical gastrointestinal endoscopy. Blackwell, Oxford

Cotton P B, Kozarek R A, Schapiro R H et al 1990 Endoscopic laser lithotripsy of large bile duct stones. Gastroenterology 99: 1128–1133

Cox J, Buckton G K, Bennett J R 1986 Balloon dilatation in achalasia: a new dilator. Gut 27: 986–989

Cox J G C, Winter R K, Maslin S C et al 1988 Balloon or bougie for dilatation of benign oesophageal stricture? An interim report of a randomised controlled trial. Gut 29: 1741–1747

Craanen M E, Blok P, Dekker W, Ferwerda J, Tytgat G N J 1992 Subtypes of intestinal metaplasia and *Helicobacter pylori*. Gut 33: 597–600

Csendes A, Braghetto I, Henríquez A, Cortés C 1989 Late results of a prospective randomised study comparing forceful dilatation and oesophagomyotomy in patients with achalasia. Gut 30: 299–304

Dajani A S, Bisno A L, Chung K J et al 1990 Prevention of bacterial endocarditis. Recommendations of the American Heart Association. Journal of the American Medical Association 264: 2919–2922

Davids P H P, Groen A, Rauws E A J, Tytgat G N J, Huibregtse K 1992a Randomised trial of self-expanding metal stents versus polyethylene stents for distal malignant biliary obstruction. Lancet 2: 1488–1492

Davids P H P, Rauws E A J, Tytgat G N J, Huibregtse K 1992b Post-operative bile leakage: endoscopic management. Gut 33: 1118–1122

Delhaye M, Engelholm L, Cremer M 1985 Pancreas divisum: congenital anatomic variant or anomaly? Contribution of endoscopic retrograde dorsal pancreatography. Gastroenterology 89: 951–958

Delhaye M, Vandermeeren A, Baize M, Cremer M 1992 Extracorporeal shock-wave lithotripsy of pancreatic calculi. Gastroenterology 102: 610–620

den Hartog Jager F C A, Bartelsman J F W M, Tytgat G N J 1979 Palliative treatment of obstructing esophagogastric malignancy by endoscopic positioning of a plastic prosthesis. Gastroenterology 77: 1008–1014

Deviere J, Baize M, de Toeuf J, Cremer M 1988 Long-term follow-up of patients with hilar malignant stricture treated by internal biliary drainage. Gastrointestinal Endoscopy 34: 95–101

Dillon J F, Simpson K J, Hayes P C 1994 Liver biopsy bleeding time: an unpredictable event. European Journal of Gastroenterology and Hepatology 9: 269–271

Dittler H J, Siewert J R 1993 Role of endoscopic ultrasonography in esophageal carcinoma. Endoscopy 25: 156–161

Dooley C P, Larson A W, Stace N H et al 1984 Double-contrast barium meal and upper gastrointestinal endoscopy: a comparative study. Annals of Internal Medicine 101: 538–545

Doria M I, Shepard K V, Levin B, Riddell R H 1986 Liver pathology following hepatic arterial infusion chemotherapy. Hepatic toxicity with FUDR. Cancer 58: 855–861

Doyle F M, Kennedy N P 1994 Nutritional support via percutaneous endoscopic gastrostomy. Proceedings of the Nutrition Society 53: 473–482

Durack D T 1995 Prevention of infective endocarditis. New England Journal of Medicine 332: 38–44

Eckardt V F, Kanzler G, Willems D 1989 Same-day versus separate-day sigmoidoscopy and double contrast barium enema: a randomized controlled study. Gastrointestinal Endoscopy 35: 512–515

Elta G H, Nostrant T T, Wilson J A P 1987 Treatment of achalasia with the Witzel pneumatic dilator. Gastrointestinal Endoscopy 33: 101–103

Endocarditis Working Party of the British Society for Antimicrobial Chemotherapy 1990 Antibiotic prophylaxis of infective endocarditis. Lancet 335: 88–89

Ewe K 1981 Bleeding after liver biopsy does not correlate with indices of peripheral coagulation. Digestive Diseases and Sciences 26: 388–393

Fan S T, Lai E C S, Mok F P T, Lo C-M, Zheng S S, Wong J 1993 Early treatment of acute biliary pancreatitis by endoscopic papillotomy. New England Journal of Medicine 328: 228–232

Fleischer D, Sivak M V Jr 1985 Endoscopic Nd:YAG laser therapy as palliation for esophagogastric cancer. Parameters affecting initial outcome. Gastroenterology 89: 827–831

Forbes A, Cotton P B 1984 ERCP and sphincterotomy after Billroth II gastrectomy. Gut 25: 971–974

Freeman M L, Nelson D B, Sherman S et al 1996 Complications of endoscopic biliary shpincterotomy. New England Journal of Medicine 335: 909–918

Fullarton G M, Birnie G G, MacDonald A, Murray W R 1989 Controlled trial of heater probe treatment in bleeding peptic ulcers. British Journal of Surgery 76: 541–544

Gaing A A, Geders J M, Cohen S A, Siegel J H 1993 Endoscopic management of primary sclerosing cholangitis: review and report of an open series. American Journal of Gastroenterology 88: 2000–2008

Gastroenterology Services Working Party of the Clinical Services Committee of the British Society of Gastroenterology 1993 Nature and standards of gastrointestinal and liver services in the United Kingdom. Gut 34: 1728–1739

Gear M W L, Wilkinson S P 1989 Open-access upper alimentary endoscopy. British Journal of Hospital Medicine 41: 438–444

Geenen J E, Hogan W J, Dodds W J, Stewart E T, Arndorfer R C 1980 Intraluminal pressure recording from the human sphincter of Oddi. Gastroenterology 78: 317–324

Geenen J E, Hogan W J, Dodds W J, Toouli J, Venu R P 1989 The efficacy of endoscopic sphincterotomy after cholecystectomy in patients with sphincter-of-Oddi dysfunction. New England Journal of Medicine 320: 82–87

Goff J S 1988 The human sphincter of Oddi. Physiology and pathology. Archives of Internal Medicine 148: 2673–2677

Goff J S 1993 Gastroesophageal varices: pathogenesis and therapy of acute bleeding. Gastroenterology Clinics of North America 22: 779–800

Goodwin C S, Blincow E D, Warren J R, Waters T E, Sanderson C R, Easton L 1985 Evaluation of cultural techniques for isolating *Campylobacter pyloridis* from endoscopic biopsies of gastric mucosa. Journal of Clinical Pathology 38: 1127–1131

Gray S F, Wyatt J I, Rathbone B J 1986 Simplified techniques for identifying *Campylobacter pyloridis* from endoscopic biopsies of gastric mucosa. Journal of Clinical Pathology 39: 1279

Griffin S M, Chung S C S, Leung J W C, Li A K C 1989 Peptic pyloric stenosis treated by endoscopic balloon dilatation. British Journal of Surgery 76: 1147–1148

Griffiths W J, Neumann D A, Welsh J D 1979 The visible vessel as an indicator of uncontrolled or recurrent gastrointestinal hemorrhage. New England Journal of Medicine 300: 1411–1413

Gulliver D J, Edmunds S, Baker M E et al 1992 Stent placement for benign pancreatic diseases: correlation between ERCP findings and clinical response. American Journal of Roentgenology 159: 751–755

Gyde S 1990 Screening for colorectal cancer in ulcerative colitis: dubious benefits and high costs. Gut 3: 1089–1092

Hamilton I, Lintott D J, Rothwell J, Axon A T R 1983 Acute pancreatitis following endoscopic retrograde cholangiopancreatography. Clinical Radiology 34: 543–546

Haot J, Hamichi L, Wallez L, Mainguet P 1988 Lymphocytic gastritis: a newly described entity: a retrospective endoscopic and histological study. Gut 29: 1258–1264

Hayes P C 1996 The coming of age of band ligation for oesophageal varices: all the evidence shows it has better outcomes than injection sclerotherapy. British Medical Journal 312: 1111–1112

Henning H, Look D 1985 Laparoskopic atlas und lehrbuch. Thieme, Stuttgart

Huibregtse K 1996 Complications of endoscopic sphincterotomy and their prevention. New England Journal of Medicine 335: 961–963

Ismail-Beigi F, Pope C E II 1974 Distribution of the histological changes of gastroesophageal reflux in the distal esophagus of man. Gastroenterology 66: 1109–1113

Jabbari M, Cherry R, Lough J O, Daly D S, Kinnear D G, Goresky C A 1984 Gastric antral vascular ectasia: the watermelon stomach. Gastroenterology 87: 1165–1170

Jeffers L, Spieglman G, Reddy R et al 1987 Laparoscopically directed fine needle aspiration for the diagnosis of hepatocellular carcinoma: a safe and accurate technique. Gastrointestinal Endoscopy 34: 235–237

Johnsen R, Bernersen B, Straume B, Førde O H, Bostad L, Burhol P G G 1991 Prevalence of endoscopic and histological findings in patients with and without dyspepsia. British Medical Journal 302: 749–752

Jones R 1995 Endoscopy in general practice. British Medical Journal 310: 816–817

Jones S N, Lees W R, Frost R A 1988 Diagnosis and grading of chronic pancreatitis by morphological criteria derived by ultrasound and pancreatography. Clinical Radiology 39: 43–48

Khakoo S I, Lobo A J, Shepherd N A, Wilkinson S P 1994 Histological assessment of the Sydney classification of endoscopic gastritis. Gut 35: 1172–1175

Kikendall J W 1991 Caustic ingestion injuries. Gastroenterology Clinics of North America 20: 847–857

Knyrim K, Wagner H-J, Bethge N, Keymling M, Vakil N 1993 A controlled trial of an expansile metal stent for palliation of esophageal obstruction due to inoperable cancer. New England Journal of Medicine 329: 1302–1307

Kohler B, Riemann J F 1987 Incidence of bacteremia after endoscopic laser treatment of stenosing processes in the upper gastrointestinal tract. American Journal of Gastroenterology 82: 1026–1028

Krasner N 1989 Laser therapy in the management of benign and malignant tumours in the colon and rectum. International Journal of Colorectal Disease 4: 2–5

Krasner N, Barr H, Skidmore C, Morris A I 1987 Palliative laser therapy for malignant dysphagia. Gut 28: 792–798

Kuroiwa M, Tsukamoto Y, Naitoh Y, Hirooka Y, Furukawa T, Katou T 1994 New technique using intraductal ultrasonography for the diagnosis of bile duct cancer. Journal of Ultrasound in Medicine 13: 189–195

Lai E C S, Mok F P T, Tan E S Y et al 1992 Endoscopic biliary drainage for severe acute cholangitis. New England Journal of Medicine 326: 1582–1586

Laine L A 1987 Multipolar electrocoagulation in the treatment of active upper gastrointestinal tract hemorrhage. A prospective controlled trial. New England Journal of Medicine 316: 1613–1617

Lancet 1989 Editorial: antibiotics for cholangitis. Lancet 2: 781–782

LaRusso N F, Wiesner R H, Ludwig J, McCarty R L 1984 Primary sclerosing cholangitis. New England Journal of Medicine 310: 899–903

Lau W Y, Fan S T, Chu K W, Yip W C, Poon G P, Wong S K 1986 Intra-operative fibreoptic enteroscopy for bleeding lesions in the small intestine. British Journal of Surgery 73: 217–218

Lebrec D, Goldfarb G, Degott C, Rueff B, Benhamou J P 1982 Transvenous liver biopsy. An experience based on 1000 hepatic tissue samplings with this procedure. Gastroenterology 83: 338–340

Leicester R J 1991 Primary colonoscopy. Baillière's Clinical Gastroenterology 5: 209–223

Leichtmann G A, Novis B H, Samara M 1984 Dilatation instrumentale des sténoses oesophagiennes et gastrique à l'aide du cathéter de Grüntzig et du dilateur de Celestin. Resultats préliminaires. Gastroenterologie Clinique et Biologique 8: 616–620

Lewis B S, Waye J D 1988 Chronic gastrointestinal bleeding of obscure origin: role of small bowel enteroscopy. Gastroenterology 94: 1117–1120

Lightdale C 1987 Indications, contraindications and complications of laparoscopy. In: Sivak M V (ed) Gastroenterologic endoscopy. W B Saunders, London, pp 1030–1041

Lightdale C J 1991 Endoscopic ultrasonography in the diagnosis, staging and follow-up of esophageal and gastric cancer. Endoscopy 24 (suppl 1): 297–303

Lindsay D C, Freeman J G, Cobden I, Record C O 1988 Should colonoscopy be the first investigation for colonic disease? British Medical Journal 296: 167–169

Loizou L A, Grigg D, Atkinson M, Robertson C, Bown S G 1991 A prospective comparison of laser therapy and intubation in endoscopic palliation for malignant dysphagia. Gastroenterology 100: 1303–1310

Longstreth G F 1992 Long-term costs after gastroenterology consultation with endoscopy versus radiography in dyspepsia. Gastrointestinal Endoscopy 38: 23–27

Lopes G M, Grace N D 1991 Gastroesophageal varices: prevention of bleeding and rebleeding. Gastroenterology Clinics of North America 22: 801–820

Lux G, Wilson D, Wilson J, Demling L 1987 A cuffed tube for the treatment of oesophago-bronchial fistula. Endoscopy 19: 28–30

McBride M A, Ergun G A 1994 The endoscopic management of esophageal strictures. Gastrointestinal Endoscopy Clinics of North America 4: 595–621

Macrae F A, Tan K G, Williams C B 1981 Towards safer colonoscopy: a report on the complications of 5000 diagnostic or therapeutic colonoscopies. Gut 24: 376–383

Mann C V, Gallagher P, Frecker P B 1988 Rigid sigmoidoscopy: an evaluation of three parameters regarding diagnostic accuracy. British Journal of Surgery 75: 425–427

Mansi C, Savarino V, Picciotto A et al 1982 Comparison between laparoscopy, ultrasonography and computed tomography in widespread and localized liver disease. Gastrointestinal Endoscopy 28: 83–85

Martin D F 1994 Combined percutaneous and endoscopic procedures for bile duct obstruction. Gut 35: 1011–1012

Mecklin J P, Järvinen H J, Aukee S, Elomaa J, Karjalainen K 1987 Screening for colorectal carcinoma in cancer family syndrome kindreds. Scandinavian Journal of Gastroenterology 22: 449–453

Miller L S 1995 Endoscopy of the esophagus. In: Castell D O (ed) The esophagus, 2nd edn. Little Brown, Boston. Ch 4, pp 93–132

Ming S C 1977 The classification and significance of gastric polyps. In: Yardley J H, Morgan B C, Abell (eds) The gastrointestinal tract. Williams and Wilkins, Baltimore

Moss A A, Federle M, Shapiro A et al 1980 The combined use of computed tomography and endoscopic retrograde cholangiopancreatography in the assessment of suspected pancreatic neoplasm. Radiology 134: 159–163

Müller M F, Meyenberger C, Bertschinger P, Schaer R, Marincek B 1994 Pancreatic tumours: evaluation with endoscopic US, CT, and MR imaging. Radiology 190: 745–751

Murray A W, Morran C G, Kenny G N C, Anderson J R 1990 Arterial oxygen saturation during upper gastrointestinal endoscopy: the effects of a midazolam/pethidine combination. Gut 31: 270–273

National Institutes of Health Consensus Conference 1989 Therapeutic endoscopy and bleeding ulcers. Journal of the American Medical Association 262: 1369–1372

Neoptolemos J P, Carr-Locke D L, Fossard D P 1987 Prospective randomised study of preoperative endoscopic sphincterotomy versus surgery alone for common bile duct stones. British Medical Journal 294: 470–474

Neoptolemos J P, Carr-Locke D L, London N J, Bailey I A, James D, Fossard D P 1988 Controlled trial of urgent endoscopic retrograde cholangiopancreatography and endoscopic sphincterotomy versus conservative treatment for acute pancreatitis due to gallstones. Lancet 2: 979–983

Neoptolemos J P, Hall C, O'Conner H J, Murray W R, Carr-Locke D L 1990 Methyl-tert-butyl-ether for treating bile duct stones: the British experience. British Journal of Surgery 77: 32–35

Nicholson A A, Royston C M S 1993 Palliation of inoperable biliary obstruction with self-expanding metal endoprostheses: a review of 77 patients. Clinical Radiology 47: 245–250

Norton B, Homer-Ward M, Donnelly M T, Long R G, Holmes G K T 1996 A randomised prospective comparison of percutaneous endoscopic gastrostomy and nasogastric tube feeding after acute dysphagic stroke. British Medical Journal 312: 13–16

Nwokolo C U, Payne-James J J, Silk D B A, Misiewicz J J, Loft D E 1994 Palliation of malignant dysphagia by ethanol induced tumour necrosis. Gut 35: 299–303

Ogilvie A L, Dronfield M W, Ferguson R, Atkinson M 1982 Palliative intubation of oesophagogastric neoplasms at fibreoptic endoscopy. Gut 23: 1060–1067

Pagliaro L, Rinaldi F, Craxi A et al 1983 Percutaneous blind biopsy versus laparoscopy with guided biopsy in diagnosis of cirrhosis. A prospective randomized trial. Digestive Diseases and Sciences 28: 39–43

Pagliaro L, d'Amico G, Sörensen T I A 1992 Prevention of first bleeding in cirrhosis: a meta-analysis of randomized trials of nonsurgical treatment. Annals of Internal Medicine 117: 59–70

Palazzo L, Roseau G, Gayet B et al 1993 Endoscopic ultrasound in the diagnosis and staging of pancreatic adenocarcinoma. Results of a prospective study with comparison to ultrasonograpy and CT scan. Endoscopy 25: 143–150

Panés J, Viver J, Forné M, Garcia-Olivares E, Marco C, Garau J 1987 Controlled trial of endoscopic sclerosis in bleeding peptic ulcers. Lancet 2: 1292–1294

Panos M Z, Reilly H, Moran A et al 1994 Percutaneous endoscopic gastrostomy in a general hospital: prospective evaluation of indications, outcome, and randomised comparison of two tube designs. Gut 35: 1551–1556

Perissat J, Huibregtse K, Keane F B V, Russell R C G, Neoptolemos J P 1994 Management of bile duct stones in the era of laparoscopic cholecystectomy. British Journal of Surgery 81: 799–810

Plevris J N, Hayes P C 1994 Laparoscopy in the investigation of liver disease. Hospital Update 20: 129–138

Pockros P J, Foroozan P 1985 Golytely lavage versus a standard colonoscopy preparation. Effect on normal colonic mucosal histology. Gastroenterology 88: 545–548

Possik R A, Franco E L, Pires D R, Wohnrath D R, Ferre I R A 1986 Sensitivity, specificity and predictive value of laparoscopy for the staging of gastric cancer and for the detection of liver metastases. Cancer 58: 1–6

Potomiano S, Carter C R, Anderson J R 1994 Endoscopic laser treatment of diffuse gastric antral vascular ectasia. Gut 35: 461–463

Quine M A, Bell G D, McCloy R F, Charlton J E, Devlin H B, Hopkins A 1995 Prospective audit of upper gastrointestinal endoscopy in two regions of England: safety, staffing and sedation methods. Gut 36: 462–467

Quinn P G, Connors P J 1994 The role of upper gastrointestinal endoscopy in foreign body removal. Gastrointestinal Endoscopy Clinics of North America 4: 571–593

Rabinovitz M, Yoo Y-K, Schade R R, Dindzans V J, van Thiel D H, Gavaler J S 1990 Prevalence of endoscopic findings in 510

consecutive individuals with cirrhosis evaluated prospectively. Digestive Diseases and Sciences 35: 705–710
Rajgopal C, Palmer K R 1991 Endoscopic injection sclerosis: effective treatment for bleeding peptic ulcer. Gut 37: 727–729
Rex D K, Waddle R A, Lehman G A et al 1990 Flexible sigmoidoscopy plus air contrast barium enema versus colonoscopy for suspected lower gastrointestinal bleeding. Gastroenterology 98: 855–861
Richter J M, Hedberg S E, Athanasoulis C A, Schapiro R H 1984 Angiodysplasia: clinical presentation and colonoscopic diagnosis. Digestive Diseases and Sciences 29: 481–483
Robert M E, Weistein W M 1993 *Helicobacter pylori* – associated gastric pathology. Gastroenterology Clinics of North America 22: 59–72
Rosch T, Dancygier H 1990 Endoskopischer Ultraschall für Diagnostik und Staging von Osophagustumoren. Internist 31: 113–118
Rosenberg J, Overgaard H, Andersen M, Rasmussen V, Schulze S 1996 Double blind randomised controlled trial of effect of metoprolol on myocardial ischaemia during endoscopic cholangiopancreatography. British Medical Journal 313: 258–261
Rostykus P S, McDonald G B, Albert R K 1980 Upper intestinal endoscopy induces hypoxemia in patients with obstructive pulmonary disease. Gastroenterology 78: 488–491
Safrany L 1991 Antibiotic prophylaxis in endoscopy: new round in an old discussion. Endoscopy 23: 91–94
Safrany L, Cotton P B 1982 Endoscopic management of choledocholithiasis. Surgical Clinics of North America 6: 825–836
Sauerbruch T, Holl J, Sackmann M, Paumgartner G 1992 Fragmentation of bile duct stones by extracorporeal shock-wave lithotripsy: a five-year experience. Hepatology 15: 208–214
Schneider M U, Matek W, Bauer R, Domschke W 1988 Mechanical lithotripsy of bile duct stones in 209 patients. Effect of technical advances. Endoscopy 20: 248–253
Schuman B M, Beckman J W, Tedesco F J, Griffin J W, Assad R T 1987 Complications of endoscopic injection sclerotherapy: a review. American Journal of Gastroenterology 82: 823–830
Shandall A, Johnson C 1985 Laparoscopy or scanning in oesophageal and gastric carcinoma? British Journal of Surgery 72: 449–451
Shepherd H A, Royle G, Ross A P R, Diba A, Arthur M, Colin-Jones D 1988 Endoscopic biliary endoprosthesis in the palliation of malignant obstruction of the distal common bile duct: a randomized trial. British Journal of Surgery 75: 1166–1168
Shimi J, Nathanson L K, Cuschieri A 1991 Laparoscopic cardiomyotomy for achalasia. Journal of the Royal College of Surgeons of Edinburgh 36: 152–154
Shorvon P J, Eykyn S J, Cotton P B 1983 Gastrointestinal instrumentation, bacteraemia, and endocarditis. Gut 24: 1078–1093
Sivak M V 1991 Video endoscopy, the electronic endoscopy unit and integrated imaging. Baillière's Clinical Gastroenterology, pp 1–18
Smith L E 1985 Symposium on outpatient anorectal procedures 4. Fibreoptic sigmoidoscopy: an office procedure. Canadian Journal of Surgery 28: 233
Soehendra N, Grimm H, Nam V Ch, Berger B 1987 *N*-butyl-2-cyanoacrylate: a supplement to endoscopic sclerotherapy. Endoscopy 19: 221–224
Song H-Y, Han Y-M, Kim H-N, Choi K-C 1992 Corrosive oesophageal stricture: safety and effectiveness of balloon dilatation. Radiology 184: 373–378
Sontheimer J, Salm R, Friedrich G, von Wahlert J V, Pelz K 1991 Bacteremia following operative endoscopy of the upper gastrointestinal tract. Endoscopy 23: 67–72
Soto J A, Barish M A, Yucel E K, Siegenberg D, Ferrucci J T, Chuttani R 1996 Magnetic resonance cholangiography: comparison with endoscopic retrograde cholangiopancreatography. Gastroenterology 110: 589–597
Southern Surgeons Club 1991 A prospective analysis of 1518 laparoscopic cholecystectomies. New England Journal of Medicine 324: 1073–1078
Speer A G, Cotton P B, Russell R C G 1987 Randomised trial of endoscopic versus percutaneous stent insertion in malignant obstructive jaundice. Lancet 2: 57–62
Speer A G, Cotton P B, Rode J et al 1988 Biliary stent blockage with bacterial biofilm: a light and electron microscopy study. Annals of Internal Medicine 108: 546–553
Starck E, Paolucci V, Herze RM, Crummy A B 1984 Esophageal stenosis: treatment with balloon catheters. Radiology 153: 637–640
Staritz M, Ewe K, Meyer zum Büschenfelde K H 1983 Endoscopic papillary dilatation (EPD) for the treatment of common bile duct stones and papillary stenosis. Endoscopy 15 (suppl): 197–198
Staritz M, Poralla T, Dormeyer H-H, Meyer zum Büschenfelde K-H 1985 Endoscopic removal of common bile duct stones through the intact papilla after medical sphincter dilatation. Gastroenterology 88: 1807–1811
Steigmann G V, Goff J S, Michaletz-Onody P A et al 1992 Endoscopic sclerotherapy as compared with endoscopic ligation for bleeding esophageal varices. New England Journal of Medicine 326: 1527–1532
Stevenson G W, Norman G, Frost R, Somers S 1991 Barium meal or endoscopy? A prospective randomised study of patient preference and physician decision making. Clinical Radiology 44: 317–321
Sugawa C, Walt A J, Nunez D C, Masuyama H 1987 Pancreas divisum: is it a normal anatomic variant? American Journal of Surgery 153: 62–67
Swain C P, Kirkham J S, Salmon P R, Bown S G, Northfield T C 1986 Controlled trial of Nd-Yag laser photocoagulation for bleeding peptic ulcers. Lancet 1: 1113–1116
Tameda Y, Yoshizawa N, Takase K, Nakano T, Kosaka Y 1990 Prognostic value of peritoneoscopic findings in cirrhosis of the liver. Gastrointestinal Endoscopy 36: 34–38
Terblanche J, Bornman P, Kahn D et al 1983 Failure of repeated injection sclerotherapy to improve long-term survival after oesophageal variceal bleeding: a five-year prospective controlled clinical trial. Lancet 2: 1328–1332
Teréz J, Bordas J M, Rimola A, Bru C, Rodés J 1980 Cimetidine in acute gastric mucosal bleeding: results of a double-blind randomized trial. Digestive Diseases and Sciences 25: 92–96
Thillainayagam A V, Arvind A S, Cook R S, Harrison I G, Tabaqchali S, Farthing M J G 1991 Diagnostic efficiency of an ultrarapid endoscopy room test for *Helicobacter pylori*. Gut 32: 467–469
Thomas R J S, Abbot M, Bwathal P S, St John D J, Morstyn G 1987 High-dose photoirradiation of esophageal cancer. Annals of Surgery 206: 193–199
Tio T L, Tytgat G N J 1988 Evaluation of resectability of gastrointestinal tumors. In: Kawai K (ed) Endoscopic ultrasonography in gastroenterology. Igaku Shoin, Tokyo. pp 106–118
Tio T L, Schouwink M H, Cikot R J L M, Tytgat G N J 1989 Preoperative TNM classification of gastric carcinoma by endosonography in comparison with the pathological TNM system: a prospective study of 72 cases. Hepato-Gastroenterology 36: 51–56
Tio T L, Coene P P, van Delden O M, Tytgat G N J 1991 Colorectal carcinoma: preoperative TNM classification with endosonography. Radiology 179: 165–170
Toouli J, Bushell M, Iannos J, Collinson T, Wearne J, Kitchen D 1986 Peroperative sphincter of Oddi manometry: motility disorder in patients with cholelithiasis. Australian and New Zealand Journal of Surgery 56: 625
Toukan A U, Kamal M F, Amr S S, Arnaout M A, Abu-Romiyeh A S 1985 Gastroduodenal inflammation in patients with nonulcer dyspepsia. A controlled endoscopic and morphometric study. Digestive Diseases and Sciences 30: 313–320
Tucker H J, Snape W J Jr, Cohen S 1978 Achalasia secondary to carcinoma: manometric and clinical features. Annals of Internal Medicine 89: 315–318
Tweedle D E F, Martin D F 1991 Needle knife papillotomy for endoscopic sphincterotomy and cholangiography. Gastrointestinal Endoscopy 37: 518–521
Tytgat G N J 1991 The Sydney system: endoscopic division. Endoscopic appearances in gastritis/duodenitis. Journal of Gastroenterology and Hepatology 6: 223–224
Vaira D, D'Anna L, Ainley C et al 1989 Endoscopic sphincterotomy in 1000 consecutive patients. Lancet 2: 431–434
Van Thiel D H, Fagiuoli S, Wright H I, Rodriguez-Rio H, Silverman W 1993 Biliary complications of liver transplantation. Gastrointestinal Endoscopy 39: 455–460
Vantrappen G, Hellemans J 1980 Treatment of achalasia and related motor disorders. Gastroenterology 79: 144–154

Vantrappen G, Janssens J 1983 To dilate or to operate? That is the question. Gut 24: 1013–1019
Warshaw A L, Gu Z, Wittenberg J, Waltman A C 1990 Pre-operative staging and assessment of resectability of pancreatic cancer. Archives of Surgery 125: 230–233
Webb W A, McDaniel L, Jones L 1985 Experience with 1000 colonoscopic polypectomies. Annals of Surgery 201: 626–632
Weller I V D, Williams C B, Jeffries D J et al 1988 Cleaning and disinfection of equipment for gastrointestinal flexible endoscopy: interim recommendations of a working party of the British Society of Gastroenterology. Gut 29: 1134–1151
Westaby D, Macdougall B R, Williams R 1985 Improved survival following injection sclerotherapy for esophageal varices: final analysis of a controlled trial. Hepatology 5: 827–830
Williams C B 1973 Diathermy-biopsy – a technique for the endoscopic management of small polyps. Endoscopy 5: 215–218
Williams S G J, Peters R A, Westaby D 1994 Thrombin – an effective treatment for gastric variceal haemorrhage. Gut 35: 1287–1289
Woolfson I K, Eckholdt G J, Wetzel C R et al 1990 Usefulness of performing colonoscopy one year after endoscopic polypectomy. Diseases of the Colon and Rectum 33: 389–393
Working Party of the British Society of Gastroenterology Endoscopy Committee 1993 Aldehyde disinfectants and health in endoscopy units. Gut 34: 1641–1645
Yasuda K, Cho E, Nakajima M, Kawai K 1990 Diagnosis of submucosal lesions of the upper gastrointestinal tract by endoscopic ultrasonography. Gastrointestinal Endoscopy 36 (suppl 2): S17–S20
Zargar S A, Kochhar R, Nagi B, Mehta S, Mehta S K 1989 Ingestion of corrosive acids: spectrum of injury to upper gastrointestinal tract and natural history. Gastroenterology 97: 702–707
Ziegler K, Sanfe C, Zeitz M et al 1991 Evaluation of endosonography in TN staging of oesophageal cancer. Gut 32: 16–20
Zucker K A, Bailey R W, Gadacz T R, Imbembo A L 1991 Laparoscopic guided cholecystectomy. American Journal of Surgery 161: 36–44

SECTION 2

# Upper gastrointestinal tract

# 5. Common oral disease and oral manifestations of systemic disease

*D. Wray*

The embryonic oral cavity arises from both ectodermal and endodermal origins. The mouth is therefore susceptible to a whole range of gastrointestinal disorders in addition to oral manifestations of cutaneous disease.

The mouth and perioral tissues are extremely sensitive and are frequently a source of symptoms presenting to the general medical practitioner or specialist. Diagnosis of the commoner oral soft tissue diseases allows appropriate identification of those conditions which are purely local and can be managed by local means and those conditions which reflect systemic, particularly gastrointestinal, disease and may indeed be markers of gastrointestinal disease activity.

Oral examination with good illumination is simple to perform and most conditions can be diagnosed on a clinical basis. Where biopsy confirmation is required for a diagnosis, referral to an oral surgeon or oral physician is probably the simplest approach. Physicians examining the mouth should pay particular attention to the lateral borders of the tongue and the floor of the mouth, particularly laterally to the tongue which can be visualized easily with the aid of a tongue spatula. This allows examination of those areas most prone to the development of oral carcinoma, a condition particularly common in those who smoke and drink alcohol but which also occurs in young people without risk factors.

Diseases usually associated with gastrointestinal pathology may affect the mouth directly, such as Crohn's disease or the oral manifestations of ulcerative colitis. Such diseases may also manifest in the mouth indirectly by causing nutritional deficiencies of either iron, folic acid or vitamin $B_{12}$, as a result of gastrointestinal blood loss or malabsorption. The tissue signs of nutritional deficiencies which may manifest in the mouth are shown in Table 5.1. Patients presenting with oral disease that may be a marker of underlying deficiency should have measurement of iron, folic acid and vitamin $B_{12}$ carried out directly in addition to a full blood count as the majority of deficiencies seen in patients with oral disease are latent (Wray & Dagg 1990).

Because of the need to recognize oral conditions and generate a working differential diagnosis the next section on the common oral diseases is presented in a problem-orientated fashion.

## THE PRESENTATION OF ORAL DISEASES

### Bleeding gums/gingivitis

The common causes of bleeding or inflammation of the gums are listed below. The diagnosis and management of these will be discussed in turn.

#### *Plaque-induced gingivitis*

Plaque, which is simply bacterial accumulations, induces inflammation commencing at the margins of the gums with associated redness, puffiness and loss of stippling of the gums. This marginal gingivitis occurs in the presence of inadequate oral hygiene and will occur in all individuals within 3 days of ceasing to brush their teeth. Mild spontaneous hemorrhage may occur and profuse gingival bleeding may occur on brushing. This is due to disturbing pre-existing microulceration around the gingival margins. Bleeding, therefore, is a sign of inadequate oral hygiene rather than excessive brushing. Patients whose gums bleed on brushing should be instructed to brush more vigorously rather than less in order to get the condition to resolve. The prescription of a chlorhexidine mouthwash is an adjunct to successful treatment.

#### *Leukemias*

Spontaneous hemorrhage and gingival swelling occur in the leukemias, especially the acute leukemias, and discreet

**Table 5.1** Oral signs of hematinic deficiency

| |
|---|
| Angular cheilitis |
| Aphthous ulceration |
| Candidiasis |
| Glossitis |
| Paterson–Kelly syndrome |
| Leukoplakia |

gingival swellings may also occur (chloromas). Gingival signs are usually accompanied by more general systemic upset and other obvious signs such as anemia, bruising and lymphadenopathy. Where clinical doubt exists examination of a peripheral blood film is usually diagnostic.

*Acute ulcerative gingivitis* (Vincent's infection)

This is a specific gingival infection particularly common in smokers and the immunocompromised. It is due to a coinfection with *Borrelia vincentii* and *Fusiformis fusiformis*. Clinically there is a characteristic *fetor oris* and ulceration of the gingival papillae between the teeth. The condition responds rapidly to metronidazole or penicillin but patients always require clinical scaling and polishing by a dentist or dental hygienist.

*Gingival hyperplasia*

Hyperplastic overgrowth of the gingivae may occur simply as a fibrous response to inadequate oral hygiene but may also be associated with specific diseases such as Crohn's disease. Several drugs cause gingival hyperplasia including phenytoin, cyclosporin and calcium channel blockers (Scully & Cawson 1993). Gingival overgrowth can be minimized by scrupulous oral hygiene.

*Periodontal disease*

Periodontal disease encompasses a spectrum of gum diseases characterized by loss of the periodontal attachment of the teeth with progressive pocketing, apical migration of the gingival margins and loosening of the teeth. This occurs in some 15% of the adult population and may be aggravated by systemic diseases such as diabetes mellitus or polymorph defects. Prolonged periodontal therapy and scrupulous oral hygiene may inhibit the disease progress. Systemic investigation for patients with periodontal disease is not usually warranted.

*HIV-associated periodontal diseases*

A number of gingival conditions have been specifically associated with HIV disease and may be presenting symptoms. Patients with extremely aggressive or rapidly progressive periodontal destruction should be investigated for evidence of immunodeficiency. Patients with known HIV disease should be referred for periodontal therapy to prevent progression to osteomyelitis which may be significant and life threatening.

*Desquamative gingivitis*

This condition refers to a desquamation of the full thickness of the attached gingivae which is aggravated by tooth brushing. This may be seen in association with vesiculobullous disorders or lichen planus but these diseases may be restricted to the gingival tissues. An intraoral biopsy is necessary to confirm the diagnosis and treatment consists of topical corticosteroid therapy or systemic corticosteroids (Wray & McCord 1987).

### Brown patches

Pigmentation of the oral mucosa is usually asymptomatic and noticed by the patient or as an incidental finding during routine examination. The main causes of pigmented oral lesions are shown in Table 5.2. Amalgam tattoos are due to implantation of filling material during routine dental work and are harmless. Intraoral radiography or mucosal biopsy usually confirms the diagnosis. Addison's disease causes intraoral pigmentation but not in the absence of systemic symptoms. If clinical doubt exists adrenal function should be assessed. Pigmentation may also arise due to an ACTH-producing bronchogenic carcinoma. Several diverse groups of drugs such as anticonvulsants, antimalarials, cytotoxics, hormones and phenothiazines may produce widespread intraoral pigmentation, as will chronic irritation which causes concurrent keratosis. Familial, racial and idiopathic causes of pigmentation are the commonest and are different from the perioral pigmentation seen in Peutz–Jeghers syndrome which is characteristic. Solitary or changing lesions may cause clinical suspicion and malignant melanoma or nevi should be excluded by intraoral biopsy.

### Vesiculobullous disorders

Vesiculobullous disorders are rare but important conditions which traditionally affect the skin, but may first present in the mouth and oral symptoms often dominate the clinical picture (Pisanti et al 1974, Zegarelli & Zegarelli 1977). Even subepithelial bullae, as seen in pemphigoid, are fragile and burst rapidly so that erosions, which may be extensive affecting the oral mucosa, are a more common presenting sign than intact bullae.

The main causes of vesiculobullous disorders are shown

**Table 5.2** Pigmented oral lesions

| |
|---|
| *Exogenous* |
| Amalgam tattoo |
| *Endogenous* |
| Addison's disease |
| Drugs |
| Familial/racial |
| Idiopathic |
| Malignant melanoma |
| Nevi |
| Systemic (Peutz–Jeghers/Albright's syndrome) |
| Trauma (chronic) |

in Table 5.3. The majority of these lesions are clinically indistinguishable and diagnosis relies on direct or indirect immunofluorescent appearances in addition to the histological appearances. Angina bullosa hemorrhagica is the most common and characteristically presents as bloodfilled blisters affecting the soft palate (Fig. 5.1). The direct and indirect immunofluorescence is negative in this condition and the diagnosis relies on the clinical history which is characterized by early healing of bullae once they have ruptured. Erythema multiforme may occasionally be demonstrated to be due to certain drugs or occasionally a reaction to a recurrent herpes infection; usually, however, it is idiopathic. Primary herpetic infections present as a vesicular stomatitis but are self-limiting and are discussed later under the differential diagnosis of oral ulceration.

The mainstay of treatment of noninfective vesiculobullous disorders is systemic steroids with or without steroid-sparing agents such as azathioprine. Dermatitis herpetiformis patients benefit from gluten withdrawal and treatment with either dapsone or sulfamethoxypyridazine.

Patients with angina bullosa hemorrhagica require only reassurance.

## Cheilitis

Cheilitis, or inflammation affecting the lips, may be generalized or affect only the angles. Angular cheilitis is seen particularly in association with intraoral candidal infections in the denture-wearing population or may be associated with *Staphylococcus* or *Streptococcus* infection in younger dentate individuals. In the absence of formal microbiological assessment, patients with angular cheilitis may be treated with miconazole gel which is effective against Gram-positive *Cocci* in addition to *Candida* species. In denture wearers concurrent intraoral candidal infections must be treated. Patients with persistent angular cheilitis should be screened hematologically to exclude nutritional deficiencies. Angular cheilitis is a feature of oral Crohn's disease (p. 149) and HIV disease where it is secondary to infection (p. 601 & 602).

A generalized cheilitis is usually due to allergy or is a feature of orofacial granulomatosis which in turn may be a feature of Crohn's disease. Patients with swollen or inflamed lips should be treated in the first instance with topical steroid creams but persistent cases should be referred for patch testing.

Isolated lip fissures are relatively common, particularly in young people during winter months. Treatment with potent topical steroids such as betamethasone is usually effective although persistent cases may require stretching under local anesthetic. Surgical excision is a last resort.

**Table 5.3** Vesiculobullous disorders

| |
|---|
| Angina bullosa hemorrhagica |
| Benign mucous membrane pemphigoid |
| Bullous pemphigoid |
| Dermatitis herpetiformis |
| Epidermolysis bullosa |
| Erythema multiforme |
| Linear IgA disease |
| Pemphigus vulgaris |
| Viral infections |

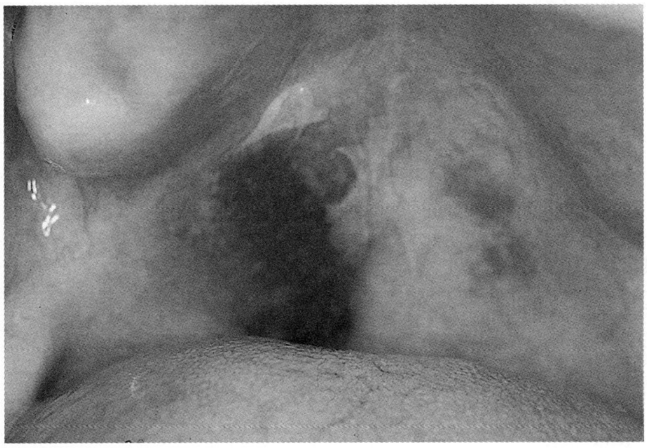

**Fig. 5.1** This 65-year-old woman presented with a large bloodfilled blister of her soft palate which burst on pressure. Healing within 1 week was uneventful. Diagnosis was that of angina bullosa hemorrhagica.

## Glossitis

Glossitis is a common diagnostic problem. It may present as atrophic glossitis with smoothness of the dorsum, pain (glossodynia) or a burning sensation (glossopyrosis). The main causes are:

### *Deficiencies of iron, folic acid or vitamin $B_{12}$*

These deficiencies will produce atrophy of the lingual mucosa leading to a smooth red tongue. Tongue discomfort may precede clinically obvious signs and routine hematological assessment should be carried out on all patients with tongue symptoms. Tongue discomfort or atrophy of the lingual epithelium may precede peripheral blood changes, necessitating individual measurement of iron, folic acid or vitamin $B_{12}$.

### *Geographic tongue*

This is relatively common and is characterized by erythematous areas often surrounded by an incomplete serpiginous periphery (Fig. 5.2). The condition is cyclical and the patches enlarge and migrate across the dorsum of the tongue. The condition may be associated with significant lobulation and fissuring. The condition is usually asymptomatic but is occasionally sensitive to hot or spicy foods. Geographic tongue may be an incidental finding and not responsible for the symptoms of glossitis. If patients pre-

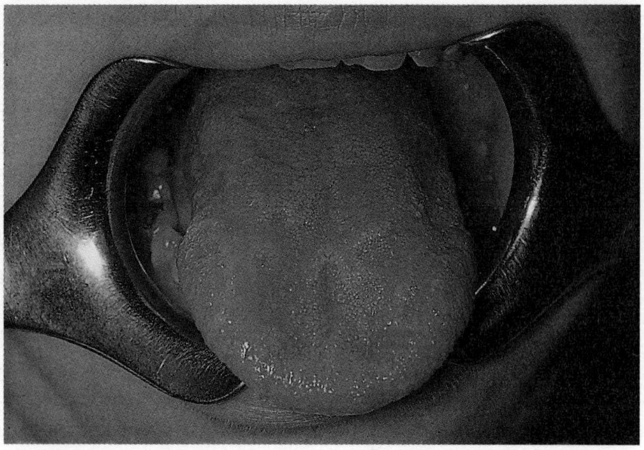

**Fig. 5.2** The characteristic appearance of geographic tongue in a 37-year-old woman with white circles which migrate across the dorsum of her tongue. This patient complained of slight sensitivity to hot and spicy food.

sent with significant discomfort other causes for glossitis should be excluded. Treatment is unsatisfactory but a benzydamine hydrochloride mouthwash may provide symptomatic relief.

*Median rhomboid glossitis* (p. 142)

This form of chronic erythematous candidiasis is common in patients who use steroid inhalers (Walker 1984). It is also more common in HIV disease.

*Hairy leukoplakia*

This presents as white patches on the lateral borders of the tongue but may extend beyond this region. It is a manifestation of HIV disease (p. 602) but is occasionally seen in other immunocompromised groups.

*Coated or black furry tongue*

This is common in dehydrated or debilitated patients but occurs occasionally in otherwise fit and healthy individuals. No specific causes have been identified and treatment consists of mechanical debridement with a toothbrush and the concurrent use of a sodium perborate mouthwash or peroxide mouthwash as a chemical cleansing agent. Patients should be reassured of the benign nature of their condition.

*Glossodynia*

A burning sensation of the tongue (glossodynia) may occasionally be due to nutritional glossitis, candidiasis, diabetes or denture problems. Most commonly, however, this is due to psychogenic oral dysesthesia with or without concurrent anxiety or depression (Harris & Feinmann 1990). Characteristically psychogenic oral dysesthesia presents as a discomfort of the tongue which is constant but shows diurnal variation, being worst in the evenings. It is relieved by eating or drinking but not by analgesics and is commonly associated with symptoms of depression, especially early morning waking and anxiety. Cancer phobia may be a prominent symptom. After organic causes for the oral symptoms have been excluded treatment with psychotropic therapy should be continued for 6 months until symptoms abate or become minimal. Support and reassurance is also essential.

## Halitosis

Patients frequently complain of halitosis which is usually perceived rather than real and is often associated with hypochondriasis (Table 5.4). Other common causes include poor oral hygiene, particularly in association with periodontal disease, dry mouth and ingested products such as food, alcohol or some drugs such as chloral hydrate. Psychogenic causes are by far the most common and present either alone or as part of a spectrum of oral dysesthesia where there may be an associated bad taste (cacogeusia) or a distorted taste sensation (dysgeusia) or there may be a burning sensation in the mouth. Psychogenic causes should be treated in the same way as described under management of burning mouth. Smoking often leaves an unpleasant odor on the breath particularly apparent to nonsmokers and cessation of the smoking habit causes resolution of the problem. Certain systemic diseases such as respiratory infections will cause bad breath, as will regurgitation of stomach contents or gases as a result of obstructive gastrointestinal problems. Renal or liver failure is also associated with characteristic halitosis.

## Pain

Pain is the most common presenting oral symptom.

*Dental pain* (caries, abscess)

Dental pain is by far the most common cause of oral pain since caries is endemic within civilized societies. Dental

**Table 5.4** Halitosis

| |
|---|
| Drugs, e.g. alcohol |
| Dry mouth |
| Food |
| Infection |
| Nasal |
| Oral |
| Psychogenic |
| Smoking |
| Systemic disease, e.g. respiratory, gastrointestinal, diabetes, etc. |

pain may be intense but it is inevitably shortlived and is measured in days rather than weeks. The cause of toothache may be difficult to diagnose on visual examination alone and a dental opinion with or without radiographic investigation is necessary to eliminate dental causes for toothache, especially in an individual with a heavily restored dentition. Dentoalveolar abscess formation may arise due to tooth pulp infection or periodontal disease. Basic surgical principles apply and drainage is a prerequisite to resolution, although antibiotic therapy will cause symptomatic improvement. Dentoalveolar abscesses are usually streptococcal in nature or due to anaerobic Gram-negative bacteria and respond to phenoxymethyl penicillin therapy. In the uncomplicated case broad-spectrum antibiotic therapy is unjustified.

*Chronic facial pain*

This is almost inevitably psychogenic in nature and may manifest itself as temporomandibular disorders, atypical facial pain or oral dysesthesia such as burning mouth (Harris & Feinmann 1990). Temporomandibular disorders may or may not be associated with an audible click of the temporomandibular joint but are inevitably muscular in nature and usually respond to soft diet and reassurance. Dental splint therapy is helpful in the majority of cases although chronic sufferers require psychotropic therapy. An atypical facial pain may be indistinguishable from toothache apart from its duration but inevitably shows a marked diurnal variation with relief in the morning and aggravation in the evening. This is often associated with sleep disturbance and other obvious signs of mild depression. Oral dysesthesias may be bizarre in presentation and have been discussed under the heading of glossitis.

*Periodic migrainous neuralgia*

This pain presents as sporadic episodes of neuralgic type headaches usually focused over one eye in association with nasal stuffiness on one side. The pain characteristically wakes the patient in the early hours of the morning. Patients respond to treatment with indomethacin and prophylaxis with a beta blocker such as propanolol or a calcium channel blocker such as nifedipine.

*Trigeminal neuralgia*

This usually presents with classic lancinating pain in the distribution of one or more branches of the trigeminal nerve. Response to carbemazepine is diagnostic. It should be given in a dose of 300 mg per day in divided doses and increased every 48 h until resolution occurs. Failure of carbemazepine therapy, due to side-effects such as drowsiness, nausea or rash, requires the addition of phenytoin or substitution by phenytoin or baclofen (Sweet 1986). In intractable trigeminal neuralgia surgical intervention may be required: isolated lesions can be treated symptomatically with peripheral nerve block, cryosurgery or nerve ablation using absolute alcohol. Injection of the Gasserian ganglion with absolute alcohol or glycerol is also successful, as is thermal coagulation of the nerve at the point where it exits the foramen ovale (Sharr & Garfield 1977). Morbidity, however, is high with significant areas of facial anesthesia. Microvascular decompression of the nerve in the posterior fossa has a high success rate with no associated analgesia but morbidity is significant and a 1% mortality rate has been reported. Patients with intractable trigeminal neuralgia should be referred for neurosurgical opinion.

### Red patches

Redness of the oral mucosa may arise due to atrophy of the epithelium or mucosal inflammation. Redness may be associated with symptoms of tenderness or frank discomfort or the red patches may be asymptomatic.

*Denture stomatitis*

This is a form of oral candidal infection. Usually it presents asymptomatically as erythema under the fitting surface of a top denture. The inflammation occurs only in that area in contact with the fitting surface of the denture and may be inappropriately diagnosed as acrylic allergy. Treatment consists of improved denture hygiene, especially leaving the denture out at night, and also the use of topical or systemic antifungals. The condition may be associated with angular cheilitis. The dentures are often loose and ill-fitting and may require replacement.

*Erythematous candidiasis* (see also p. 601).

This is also a form of erythematous candidiasis and presents as an erythema which affects any part of the oral mucosa but especially the palate and dorsum of the tongue. It is seen on occasion after the ingestion of broad-spectrum antibiotics but otherwise only occurs in patients who are locally or systemically immunosuppressed. Thus, patients who use steroid inhalers for asthma may develop erythematous candidiasis which may also be a presenting symptom of HIV disease. Patients with persistent or unexplained erythematous candidiasis should be investigated for an underlying disorder, including HIV disease (p. 601).

*Erythroplakia*

This presents as a velvety red patch or a speckled lesion which represents the nonkeratotic presentation of a leukoplakia. Erythroplakias are in general far more sinister and should be biopsied to exclude carcinoma in situ or frank malignancy.

*Lichen planus*

This classically presents as a reticular white patch inside the mouth although atrophic or erosive forms may present as red or eroded patches which are extremely painful. Histopathology confirms the diagnosis. Many lesions of erosive lichen planus occur secondary to drug ingestion, particularly nonsteroidal anti-inflammatory and antihypertensive drugs. Alternative therapeutic agents should be tried since this often causes clinical improvement. Corticosteroid therapy remains the mainstay of treatment which usually consists of topical or systemic corticosteroids with or without steroid-sparing agents (Scully & El-Kom 1985).

*Median rhomboid glossitis*

This is a form of erythematous candidiasis occurring on the central part of the posterior portion of the anterior two-thirds of the tongue. It presents as an amorphous smooth patch which is chronic and asymptomatic. Lesions can be treated with systemic antifungals such as fluconazole 50 mg daily for 2 weeks.

*Iron deficiency anemia or pernicious anemia glossitis*

These classically present as a smooth red tongue. Anemia per se, however, has no influence on the buccal mucosa except to cause pallor when the hemoglobin drops below 8 g/dl. Mucosal atrophy, particularly of the lingual mucosa, occurs secondary to deficiencies of iron, folic acid or vitamin $B_{12}$ and a smooth glossitis or a patchy erythema of the buccal mucosa should be regarded as a tissue sign of deficiencies.

*Trauma*

Trauma from broken teeth, rough fillings or ill-fitting dentures can lead to mucosal erythema and tenderness. The cause is usually obvious and the patient should be referred to their dentist for removal of the traumatic cause.

## Salivary gland disease

Salivary gland disease usually presents as an excess or lack of saliva or salivary gland swelling with or without neurological symptoms of facial palsy. The main causes of salivary gland disease are shown in Table 5.5. Investigation of the salivary glands is carried out by sialography, CT or MRI scanning, the latter having largely superceded radionucleotide scanning (p. 81).

**Table 5.5** Salivary gland disease

| |
|---|
| Drooling |
| Down's syndrome |
| Functional |
| Hemiplegia |
| Dryness |
| Anxiety |
| Drugs |
| Sjögren's |
| Swelling |
| Bacterial sialadenitis |
| Obstruction |
| Sialosis |
| Tumors |
| Viral sialadenitis |

*Drooling or excess saliva*

This is almost inevitably functional in nature. Thus patients with Down's syndrome or hemiplegia may have difficulty in swallowing saliva produced, causing dribbling or drooling of saliva. The salivary glands have a capacity to produce very large quantities of saliva in response to autonomic stimulation. This does not normally cause difficulties in handling saliva. When a patient complains of excessive pooling of saliva or spitting this is almost certainly functional in nature and may be associated with an anxiety or depressive illness. Treatment with tricyclic antidepressants not only corrects the underlying problem but has an anticholinergic effect which reduces salivary flow and causes symptomatic improvement.

*Dryness of the mouth*

Dryness is most commonly caused by drug ingestion, particularly tricyclic antidepressants or diuretics. Chronic anxiety also causes uncomfortable oral dryness which enigmatically may be responsive to tricyclic antidepressant therapy. Sjögren's syndrome occurs in two forms, primary Sjögren's syndrome which presents as dry eyes and dry mouth or secondary Sjögren's syndrome when the symptoms are associated with a connective tissue disorder. Clinical subjective assessment of lacrimal and salivary flow appears to be as accurate as more apparently objective methods of assessment of secretion and antibody assessment which is usually noncontributory. Minor labial salivary gland biopsy performed by an oral surgeon may help the diagnosis if focal lymphocytic sialadenitis is demonstrated histologically. Treatment of oral dryness and Sjögren's syndrome is symptomatic. Patients with some salivary flow can have this stimulated by sialogogues or pilocarpine. Patients with no salivary flow can use saliva substitutes which may be methyl cellulose based or mucin based. It should be remembered that patients with Sjögren's syndrome are 44 times more likely than controls to develop lymphoma (Zulman et al 1978). Unexplained or recent salivary gland enlargement requires investigation to exclude lymphoreticular malignancy.

*Salivary gland swelling* (see also p. 603)

Swelling may arise for the following reasons.

***Bacterial sialadenitis.*** Bacterial sialadenitis, particularly parotitis, occurs in patients who are dehydrated but bacterial sialadenitis may also occur in patients with previously damaged salivary glands or glands obstructed due to mucous plugging or salivary stones, particularly of the submandibular gland. Prompt and prolonged therapy with erythromycin is the treatment of choice and sialography is necessary to assess salivary gland damage after the acute episode has subsided. Sialography in itself may be therapeutic by flushing out the salivary gland concerned.

***Recurrent parotitis of childhood.*** This presents as recurrent bacterial infections of the parotid glands which usually resolve in adolescence.

***Obstructive sialadenitis.*** This occurs either due to mucous plugging or salivary gland calculi. These are most common in the submandibular gland and the majority of calculi are radiolucent. Salivary gland swelling occurs at meal times. Sialography should be undertaken if plain radiographs reveal no calculi.

***Sialosis.*** This is benign enlargement of the salivary glands which is usually idiopathic in nature. It may occur, however, in Sjögren's syndrome, diabetes mellitus, protein malnutrition and alcoholism. The condition may be reversible if the underlying cause is successfully treated.

***Tumors of the salivary glands.*** Tumors of the salivary glands, particularly the parotid glands, are relatively common and usually present as a painless unilateral swelling. Concurrent facial nerve palsies are a sinister sign. The vast majority of salivary gland tumors are pleomorphic salivary adenomas occurring in the superficial part of the parotid gland and superficial parotidectomy is the treatment of choice (Lucas 1984). Salivary tumors may also arise in minor glands, particularly of the soft palate. Biopsy of such lesions is mandatory for satisfactory treatment and to exclude adenoid carcinomas (Seifert 1991).

***Viral sialadenitis.*** Viral sialadenitis due to mumps is relatively common in childhood which presents as bilateral, painful swellings of the salivary glands. Recovery is usually uneventful but may be attended by protracted discomfort.

## Oral swellings

Oral swellings are a common presenting complaint which may be seen in isolation or in association with pain or inflammation. Patients may complain of a diffuse or generalized swelling or they may complain of a specific lump. The commonest causes of swellings and lumps are discussed below.

*Dentoalveolar abscesses*

These commonly arise as a result of neglected teeth or periodontium. When the carious process impeaches upon the dental pulp, infection and acute toothache due to pulpal inflammation rapidly ensue. Continued inflammation of the dental pulp within the hard dental structure leads to pulp necrosis and temporary resolution of symptoms. Subsequently infection spreads through the apex of the tooth causing a periapical abscess which may follow a chronic course but may undergo an acute exacerbation causing expansion of the buccal or palatal alveolus and occasionally gross swelling and cellulitis of the face. As mentioned previously, resolution results from adequate surgical drainage either via root canal therapy or tooth extraction. Antibiotic therapy, usually phenoxymethyl penicillin or metronidazole, will cause improvement in the acute symptoms but surgical drainage is still required. Patients with dentoalveolar swellings should be referred to their dentists for elimination of dental causes.

*Benign tumors*

Several types arise within the oral cavity and may become quite large and interfere with talking or chewing. The commonest lesions are fibrous polyps which are discussed below. Alternatively, benign swellings may be lymphangiomas, fibromas, lipomas, neuromas or squamous papillomas. Simple excision of these lesions under local anesthetic is all that is required, while hemangiomas respond well to cryosurgery.

*Crohn's disease*

This condition may result in generalized lip swelling but, as discussed later, also causes intraoral ulceration and mucosal tags with associated cobblestoning of the buccal mucosa due to lymphedema. Histological confirmation is required for the diagnosis (see below).

*Benign cystic lesions*

These are relatively common and may arise from odontogenic tissue or from nondental tissues. Odontogenic cysts are most common and may be associated with the crown of a buried tooth, as in the case of the dentigerous cyst, or may arise as a result of cyst development in a previous dental abscess. Nonodontogenic cysts are most commonly seen as palatal swellings arising from the incisal canal. Cysts present as expansions of the alveolar bone and radiographically appear as radiolucencies. Enucleation is the treatment of choice when such lesions can be distinguished from cystic neoplasms such as ameloblastomas. The commonest oral soft tissue swellings are simple fibrous polyps or areas of fibroepithelial hyperplasia which may result from previous trauma or from denture irritation. Fibrous polyps or areas of fibroepithelial hyperplasia can become quite large and require surgical removal and elimination of the cause, such as replacement of the denture.

*Malignant tumors*

These most commonly present as ulcers and are discussed in more detail subsequently. Salivary gland tumors, lymphoreticular malignancies and tumor metastases occasionally present as intraoral swellings. All unexplained swellings should be biopsied to exclude malignant causes.

*Viral warts*

Warts occasionally present in the mouth and may be multiple or profuse in immunocompromised individuals. Intraoral warts may arise due to autoinoculation from finger warts or due to sexual contact. Human papilloma virus can be demonstrated in these lesions using in situ hybridization. Cryosurgery or surgical excision usually causes resolution of the lesions.

## Oral ulcers

Oral ulcers are the commonest presenting symptom of oral disease. The main causes for oral ulceration are shown in Table 5.6.

*Recurrent aphthous stomatitis*

This is the commonest oral soft tissue disease. Recurrent aphthae affect some 20% of the population at some time in their lives and have a prevalence of 2% in the general population. Minor aphthous ulcers are the commonest form, affecting 85% of the patient population.

***Etiology.*** This remains unknown but is thought to be mediated by immunological events. A number of host and environmental factors have been shown to be important (Wray 1984a) and these are shown in Table 5.7.

Host factors in recurrent aphthae determine the predisposition of an individual to ulcerate and also the general severity of the ulceration. Family studies have shown a genetic relationship with the majority of first-degree relatives also suffering from oral ulceration. There is a relative risk with the HLA types A2 and B12 although there is no demonstrable Mendelian inheritance pattern. Twenty percent of patients with recurrent aphthae have deficiencies of iron, folic acid or vitamin $B_{12}$, the majority of which are latent in nature (Ferguson et al 1980). Patients with associated nutritional deficiencies often have underlying gastrointestinal disease and those patients with folate deficiencies should be screened for celiac disease (Wray et al 1975). Five percent of women who suffer from recurrent aphthae have premenstrual accentuation of their ulceration. Also 80% of women with recurrent aphthae become ulcer free during pregnancy. Most patients complain that oral ulceration is exacerbated by emotional stress.

**Table 5.6** Oral ulcers

| |
|---|
| Aphthous ulcers |
| Bacterial ulcers |
| Bullous disorders |
| Carcinoma |
| Gastrointestinal diseases |
| Lichen planus |
| Traumatic ulcers |
| Viral stomatitis |

**Table 5.7** Etiological factors in aphthous ulcers

| *Host* | *Environmental* |
|---|---|
| Genetics | Trauma |
| Nutritional | Allergy |
| Hormonal | Infection |
| Psychological | Smoking |

Several environmental factors also influence ulcer incidence. Minor trauma, for example from a dental anesthetic injection or eating sharp foods, may cause inappropriately severe ulceration. A history of trauma therefore does not exclude recurrent aphthous stomatitis as the diagnosis. Food allergy is demonstrable in a third of patients with aphthae using in vitro immunological techniques and patch testing reveals some patients with allergy to cinnamonaldehyde and food additives. Dietary manipulation often causes improvement in the ulceration. Infection with viruses or bacteria has not been shown in patients with recurrent aphthous stomatitis although tetracycline mouthwash often causes a dramatic improvement in recurrent aphthae. Smoking is negatively associated with aphthous ulceration and patients often first complain of oral ulceration on cessation of their smoking habit. Patients with aphthae seem clinically to be less susceptible to intraoral carcinoma and vice versa. Severe aphthous ulceration may occur in HIV disease (p. 602).

***Clinical features.*** Minor ulcers occur singly or in crops and usually last from 5 to 10 days before healing spontaneously without scar formation. They are round or ovoid in nature with a yellow or grey base with an erythematous halo and affect only the moveable nonkeratinized mucosa inside the mouth (Fig. 5.3). The ulcers are usually 2–3 mm in diameter but may be 5–10 mm. Major aphthous ulcers are a more severe variant and are often more than 1 cm in diameter and last for 6 weeks or more before healing with significant scar formation. They are usually single and often affect the fauces but again affect only the moveable nonkeratinized mucosal surfaces. Herpetiform ulcers are so called on the basis of their appearance rather

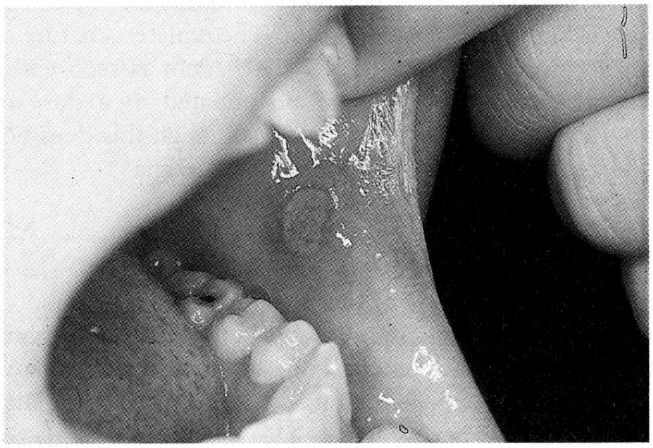

**Fig. 5.3** Four millimeter diameter minor aphthous ulcer on the buccal mucosa of an 18-year-old girl who had had frequent ulceration since the age of 12.

than their etiology. Again, they occur in crops of between 20 and 200 ulcers which are 1–2 mm in diameter and last for up to 3 weeks before healing spontaneously without scar formation. They may be distinguished from primary herpetic gingivostomatitis since they are recurrent and again affect only the moveable mucosal surfaces. The hard palate and the gingival margins are spared. In contrast gingival ulceration may dominate the clinical picture in primary herpetic gingivostomatitis.

The diagnosis of recurrent aphthae rests on the history and clinical examination. Recurrent self-healing ulcers affecting the moveable mucosal surfaces only are inevitably recurrent aphthae.

Patients with recurrent aphthae may occasionally complain of genital ulceration and may therefore be deemed to be suffering from mucocutaneous Behçet's syndrome. Ophthalmic, skeletal, gastrointestinal or neurological complications in Behçet's syndrome are rare in Western civilization, although common in the Middle and Far East.

***Treatment.*** Patients with recurrent aphthae should be screened for nutritional deficiencies before being given empirical therapy. If there is folate deficiency, celiac disease should be considered. Women with recurrent aphthae and premenstrual accentuation of ulceration benefit from depo-progestogens (Ferguson et al 1978). Symptomatic therapy of oral ulcerative conditions is discussed at the end of the section. Patients with severe major aphthae or Behçet's syndrome may require systemic corticosteroids with or without steroid-sparing agents. Thalidomide is also extremely effective in males and in infertile women at a dose of 50 mg daily. Anxiolytic agents are of no benefit.

### *Specific bacterial ulcer*

These are uncommon in the mouth. Ulcers due to mycobacterial infection or syphilis are usually discovered after biopsy examination rather than on clinical grounds.

### *Vesiculobullous disorders*

As discussed above, these usually present as intraoral ulcers which are intransigent and require immunofluorescent examination to confirm the diagnosis.

### *Carcinomas*

These may arise *de novo* from clinically normal mucosa or may arise from pre-existing premalignant conditions such as leukoplakia or lichen planus. Over 90% of carcinomas arise *de novo*. Carcinomas arising in pre-existing lesions will be discussed in the section on white patches (p. 146).

Carcinomas occur on the lateral borders of the tongue or the floor of the mouth in 90% of cases and inspection of these areas as a routine is mandatory for early diagnosis. Thus the majority of carcinomas arise in the lower aspects of the mouth whilst the palate is relatively protected, although carcinomas do occur on the fauces and peritonsillar region. Carcinomas may arise as exophytic growths or intransigent ulcers with rolled edges. Bony involvement is early, as is spread to regional lymph nodes. Pain is often a prominent feature. If an ulcer in the mouth has persisted for more than 2 weeks or there is clinical suspicion a biopsy is required to exclude carcinoma. Early detection is desirable since the prognosis rapidly deteriorates for larger lesions. First line treatment may consist of surgery or radiotherapy and patients should be referred to joint surgical radiotherapy clinics at the earliest possible moment. Smoking and alcohol appear to have a synergistic effect as etiological agents although patients may present without risk factors. In addition, the age at which people develop oral carcinomas appears to have reduced by a decade in the last 20–30 years and patients even in their 20s without risk factors may present with oral carcinoma. Vigilance is therefore necessary in all patients.

### *Ulceration secondary to gastrointestinal disease*

This may present as oral ulceration as a direct result of oral involvement by gastrointestinal disease such as Crohn's disease or ulcerative colitis (p. 149). Gastrointestinal diseases may also cause oral ulceration by creating nutritional deficiencies due to malabsorption or blood loss.

### *Lichen planus*

This is the most common oral soft tissue disease after recurrent aphthous ulceration. It usually presents as a white reticular pattern on the inside of the buccal mucosa but, especially when related to drug ingestion, may be erosive and present as large buccal ulcers. Lichen planus is discussed further under white patches (below).

*Traumatic ulcers*

These may be caused by broken or roughly filled teeth or ill-fitting dentures. The cause is usually evident and removal of the traumatic factor causes rapid resolution of the ulceration without further therapy. Chronic ulcers, however, may be slow to heal because of scar formation and persistent ulcers should be biopsied to exclude malignant change. As mentioned above under recurrent aphthous ulceration, these ulcers may be precipitated by minor trauma and therefore a traumatic etiology does not exclude aphthous ulceration.

*Viral stomatitis*

This appears to be becoming less common within the population, although 50% of 20-year-olds are still seropositive for *Herpes simplex* virus.

**Herpes simplex *virus 1 and 2.*** These are the commonest causes of viral gingivostomatitis and present as an acute infection with a vesicular stomatitis affecting all aspects of the mouth including the hard palate and attached gingivae. The infection is associated with significant pain, fever, malaise and lympadenopathy. Treatment consists of supportive therapy using analgesics, fluids and antiseptic mouthwashes such as chlorhexidine. The patient is acutely ill for 7 days before the ulcers become pain free and start to heal. Resolution is usually complete by 14 days. If the patient is seen within 72 h of the onset of symptoms acyclovir at a dose of 200 mg five times daily should be instituted for 5 days as this is likely to reduce the clinical course of the infection. Regardless of therapeutic intervention the virus becomes sequestered within the trigeminal ganglion or the basal ganglia and 50% of individuals suffer reactivation of the virus with appropriate stimulation such as sunlight, chemical trauma, hormonal variations or emotional stress. Recurrent *Herpes labialis* lesions or cold sores may be controlled at the prodromal stage with 5% acyclovir cream applied five times daily. Routine virological or serological investigation is unnecessary in primary herpetic gingivostomatitis. If this is required, however, virus can be demonstrated by direct immunofluorescence carried out on vesicular fluid, by inoculation of tissue culture or by demonstrating a threefold rise in convalescence serum titers of antibodies against HSV.

***Coxsackie A viruses.*** These may also cause intraoral virus infections in the form of minor epidemics of hand, foot and mouth disease or in isolated cases as herpangina when herpetiform ulcers may be seen predominantly in the soft palate.

**Varicella zoster *virus.*** This may cause shingles in the distribution of the trigeminal nerve and this may be exclusively intraoral in its presentation. The unilateral nature of the ulceration is diagnostic. If the patient is seen early, treatment with acyclovir can be initiated at a dose of 800 mg five times daily for 5 days, although this does not reduce the incidence of postherpetic neuralgia.

## White patches

White patches in general have an increased likelihood of malignant transformation although this varies depending on the nature of the patch. Thus, frictional and smoking keratosis along with hereditary keratosis have no malignant potential whereas leukoplakia has a 5% chance of malignant transformation over a 10-year period. Site is very important in determining malignant potential and the floor of the mouth is particularly susceptible to malignant transformation (Kramer et al 1978). Intraoral leukoplakias do not show progression through the stages of dysplasia to frank malignancy, as is seen in the uterine cervix. Increasing dysplasia, however, implies a greater risk of malignant transformation and all unexplained white patches should be biopsied to assess epithelial dysplasia. Smoking increases the prevalence of white patches although these may resolve on cessation of the smoking habit, thus making leukoplakias in nonsmokers more sinister. Patients with lichen planus are not traditionally regarded as at risk of malignant transformation although the risk is 1–2% over a 10-year period. Erosive lichen planus and lichen planus of the tongue appear particularly susceptible to malignant transformation.

Increased keratosis of the buccal mucosa leads to the clinical presentation of a white patch. There are several disease processes which lead to white patches within the mouth. These are all adherent white patches which cannot be removed by scraping and therefore can be distinguished from pseudomembranous candidiasis which presents as white plaques on the surface of the buccal mucosa which can be wiped away to leave a raw bleeding surface.

*Candidal leukoplakia*

This is a speckled keratosis which occurs usually inside the commissures of the lips and is seen almost exclusively in smokers. Histopathological examination reveals candidal hyphae within the superficial layers of the prickle cells. Systemic antifungals, such as fluconazole, cause dramatic clinical improvements although recurrence is likely if the patient continues to smoke. Candidal leukoplakia has the same premalignant potential as other leukoplakias.

*Carcinomas*

These arise *de novo* although some carcinomas arise in pre-existing leukoplakias or lichen planus. Carcinoma more commonly occurs in speckled or erythroplakic lesions and a change in a white patch or a suspicious area should be biopsied immediately.

*Frictional keratosis*

This is often seen along the buccal mucosa adjacent to the occlusal surfaces of the teeth and may be due to chewing. This is usually merely a habit and the patient may be reassured.

*Hereditary keratoses*

These are seen usually in childhood and other family members may be affected. When clinical doubt exists, histological examination is confirmatory.

*Leukoplakia*

This is defined by the World Health Organization as a white patch that cannot be removed or attributed to any other cause. This is a clinical diagnosis with no histological connotation and is idiopathic although more common among smokers or people who chew betel nut. Leukoplakias which display moderate or severe dysplasia should be excised prophylactically if this is feasible.

*Lichen planus*

This may occur exclusively intraorally or may be associated with skin lichen planus. Lichen planus intraorally may present as a recticular white patch, a red atrophic mucosa or an eroded buccal mucosa (Fig. 5.4). It may appear as a plaque, especially on the dorsum of the tongue in which case it is clinically indistinguishable from leukoplakia. Many cases of clinical lichen planus are a reaction to ingested drugs, particularly nonsteroidal anti-inflammatories or antihypertensives, or may be a reaction to amalgam or metal fillings or crowns. Removal of known causes will allow resolution. In the absence of such improvement the mainstay of therapy is symptomatic, which is discussed later, or the condition may be controlled with systemic corticosteroids with or without the use of steroid-sparing agents such azathioprine.

*Lupus erythematosus*

This presents as a lichen planus-like condition particularly affecting the palate (Fig. 5.5). Diagnosis is usually suggested on the basis of histological features and most cases are localized although systemic lupus erythematosus does occur in the mouth.

*Smoker's keratosis*

This arises as a result of increased keratinization of the buccal mucosa as a result of damage from heat and tobacco products. Classically this occurs on the hard and soft palate as a keratosis with punctate areas of erythema where the minor salivary glands exist. Smoker's palate is a benign condition but in general smoking greatly increases the risk of malignant transformation and patients with smoker's keratosis should be encouraged to stop smoking.

**Symptomatic therapy** (for oral ulcerative and inflammatory conditions)

Ulcerative or inflammatory conditions of the oral mucosa are often extremely painful and intransigent. It is therefore common practice for patients to require symptomatic therapy in the management of these lesions. The most efficacious and useful symptomatic therapies available for intraoral use are discussed below.

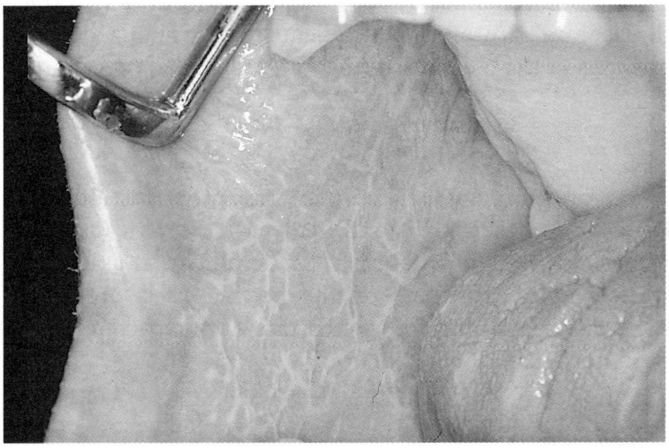

**Fig. 5.4** Reticular lichen planus on the buccal mucosa of a 56-year-old male. The white striations form a lacy pattern over the buccal mucosa on both sides. This patient was asymptomatic.

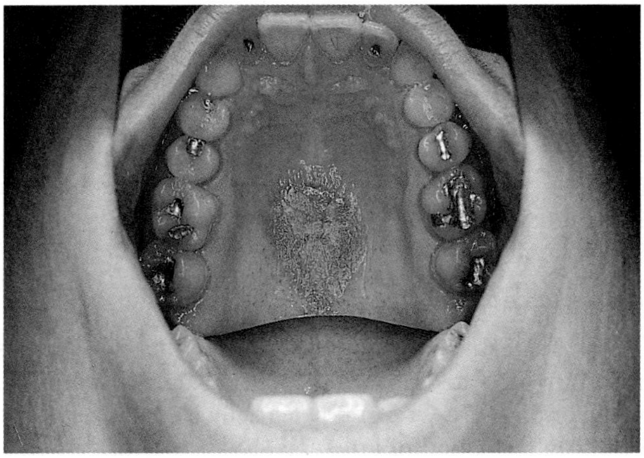

**Fig. 5.5** A chronic eroded and erythematous lesion affecting the hard palate of a 46-year-old woman with systemic lupus erythematosus.

*Xylocaine spray*

This may be very helpful when directed onto painful inflammatory lesions to allow sleep or more comfortable eating. Patients should be warned against overzealous use of the spray in the pharyngeal area so as to prevent inhalation of food.

*Chlorhexidine*

This is the most effective antiseptic mouthwash available and is widely available as a 0.2% mouthwash in the United Kingdom (Corsodyl) and a 0.15% mouthwash in the United States (Peridex). Twice daily mouth rinsing will inhibit oral bacteria, reduce superinfection and cause symptomatic improvement in all patients with inflammatory disorders. It is especially effective in mild forms of lichen planus. 0.2% Chlorhexidine may be too astringent for patients with painful lesions to use and may be diluted to 0.1% in water. Chlorhexidine facilitates the deposition of dark staining foods and drinks on the teeth for several hours after use and patients should be encouraged to avoid such foodstuffs after using the mouthwash. Benzydamine hydrochloride is an anti-inflammatory mouthwash which has mild anesthetic effects on the buccal mucosa, creating a silk-like sensation which most patients appreciate.

*Tetracycline*

This may be used as an antibiotic mouthwash by dissolving capsules in a spoonful of water and washing the mouth with it four times daily. It is particularly effective for some patients with recurrent aphthous ulceration. The mouthwash need only be used when the patient feels the ulcers are developing and may be discontinued when the patient is ulcer free.

*Triamcinolone 0.1% in dental paste*

This is an effective method of covering painful ulcerative lesions and encouraging healing. The preparation must be applied directly to a dried lesion, however, or adhesion will not take place. Patients should be advised to dry the ulcer or lesion with a paper napkin prior to applying the paste, which is particularly effective used last thing at night. It is, however, ineffective for an accessible lesion or lesions on the tongue.

*Beclomethasone spray*

This is as effective as triamcinolone in dental paste but is simpler to use and may be sprayed directly onto the tongue or pharynx. One puff twice daily is usually effective in causing resolution of inflammatory or ulcerative conditions. If the effect is incomplete the dose may be increased or a more potent steroid spray may be used.

*Betamethasone tablets 0.5 mg*

These are available in soluble form and can be used as a mouthwash four times daily. Patients should be instructed to expectorate the mouthwash after use but even so adrenal suppression may occur after using the mouthwash for more than a month. However, there are fewer systemic side-effects than with systemic medication.

*Systemic corticosteroids*

These should be used as a last resort for oral inflammatory or ulcerative conditions but when required, should be prescribed on an initial dose of 40 mg of prednisolone reducing slowly after clinical improvement occurs.

## ORAL MANIFESTATIONS OF SYSTEMIC DISEASE

As discussed above, oral problems may result from localized disease processes or may be oral manifestations of systemic diseases; indeed, oral manifestations of systemic disease may precede other manifestations as seen where glossitis or oral ulceration precedes anemia in nutritionally deficient individuals. The main oral manifestations of systemic disease are, however, gastrointestinal or immunological in nature and these will be discussed in turn.

### Gastrointestinal Disorders

*Paterson–Kelly syndrome (Plummer–Vinson syndrome)*
(see also p. 182)

This encompasses iron deficiency, dysphagia and postcricoid esophageal stricture with ensuing malignant change in the postcricoid area, esophagus or stomach in between 4% and 16% (Kelly 1919, Owen 1950, Shamma-a & Benedict 1958). The condition appears to be less common nowadays with improved early diagnosis of iron deficiency.

Other oral manifestations of upper gastrointestinal tract disease are rare although patients with bulimia develop erosions of the palatal aspects of their maxillary teeth.

*Liver and pancreatic disease*

These are rarely associated with oral problems although both alcoholic cirrhosis and diabetes mellitus cause salivary gland swelling (sialosis). Cystic fibrosis is associated with delayed eruption of the teeth which are often hypoplastic and may be stained due to tetracycline ingestion during childhood.

*Gluten enteropathy*

Recurrent aphthous ulceration, glossitis and angular cheilitis are all seen commonly in gluten-sensitive enteropathy. The ulceration may be a direct result of gluten sensitivity or may manifest secondary to nutritional deficiencies of iron, folic acid or vitamin $B_{12}$. Gluten withdrawal is usually curative.

*Crohn's disease*

Although this disease has a predisposition for the terminal ileum, rectal and oral manifestations are common and indeed oral Crohn's disease may occur in the absence of gastrointestinal manifestations (Tyldesley 1979, Wiesenfeld et al 1985). Thc clinical features of oral Crohn's disease are shown in Table 5.8.

Lip swelling, with a cobblestone appearance or linear ulcers, is the most common feature (Figs 5.6 and 5.7). Lip swelling may fluctuate but never disappears completely. It appears to be caused by lymphedema due to reduced drainage as a result of scarring and granuloma formation. Diagnosis relies on biopsy confirmation demonstrating the presence of noncaseating granulomas but biopsy down to muscle is usually necessary in order to demonstrate these histological features. Similar clinical appearances also occur in patients with sarcoidosis. They may also be seen in association with a fissured tongue and recurrent facial nerve palsy in Melkersson–Rosenthal syndrome or may be seen in isolation. It is becoming increasingly common to group patients with these oral features as suffering from orofacial granulomatosis and in the absence of overt gastrointestinal symptoms, routine gastroenterological investigation is noncontributory. Many patients get acute exacerbations after ingestion of foods, particularly those containing cinnamonaldehydes and benzoates (Patton et al 1985, James et al 1986, Sweatman et al 1986). Patch testing may be helpful. ACE levels should be checked in order to exclude sarcoidosis.

Treatment of orofacial granulomatosis or oral Crohn's disease is unsatisfactory and systemic corticosteroids and sulfasalazine are usually unhelpful. Intralesional triamcinolone may improve the lip swelling and surgical reduction of the lips may provide cosmetic improvement.

**Table 5.8** Oral features of Crohn's disease

| |
|---|
| Angular cheilitis |
| Aphthous ulceration |
| Cobblestoning of buccal mucosa |
| Hyperplastic gingivitis |
| Linear ulcers |
| Lip swelling |
| Localized swelling |
| Mucosal tags |

*Ulcerative colitis*

Patients with ulcerative colitis may develop pyostomatitis vegetans which presents as a vegetative or ulcerative condition with intramucosal abscess formation and a characteristic *fetor oris* (Wray 1984b). Pyostomatitis gangrenosum may also occur as intransigent oral erosions. If oral symptoms warrant it, intraoral biopsy is indicated and histological features are confirmatory. Treatment with corticosteroids and/or sulfasalazine may cause improvement or resolution of the condition.

*Intestinal polyposis* (pp. 1408 & 1413)

This may be associated with a number of intraoral manifestations. Perioral pigmentation is seen in Peutz–Jeghers syndrome and patients with familial polyposis coli (Gardner's syndrome) suffer from jaw osteomas, intraoral fibromas, epidermoid cysts, odontomes and supernumerary teeth. The malignant potential of various intestinal polyps varies but patients with identified syndromes

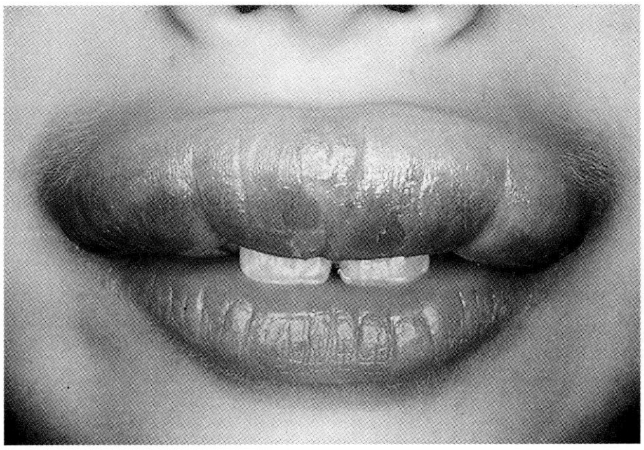

**Fig. 5.6** Gross swelling of the upper lip in an 8-year-old boy with a history of intestinal Crohn's disease.

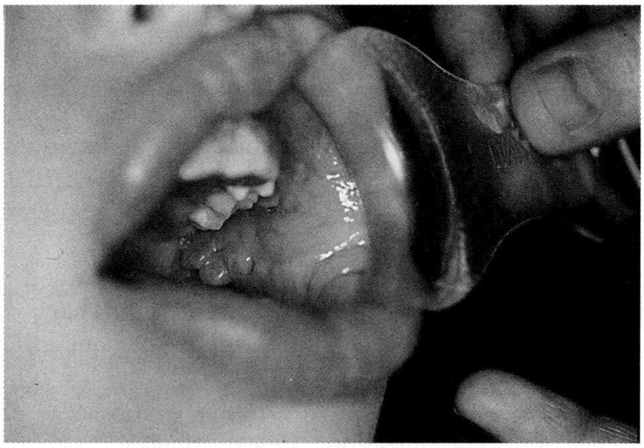

**Fig. 5.7** Buccal cobblestoning and mucosal tag formation with associated lip swelling in a 23-year-old male. There was no evidence of intestinal Crohn's disease or sarcoidosis. This patient was shown to be allergic to cinnamonaldehyde and benzoates on patch testing but was unable to comform to an exclusion diet.

should undergo full gastrointestinal investigation. Patients with colonic polyps have a higher risk of malignant transformation and surgical intervention is usually warranted.

## ORAL MANIFESTATIONS OF IMMUNODEFICIENCY

Primary immunodeficiencies are usually inherited and are uncommon. They may involve cell-mediated immune response, the humoral immune response, the phagocytic system or complement. The oral manifestations of these immunodeficiencies include infections, particularly fungal and viral, and oral ulceration and gum disease. Secondary immunodeficiencies may arise as a result of drug therapy, systemic infection, malnutrition or neoplasia and again viral and fungal infections may arise in the oral cavity in these conditions (Porter et al 1990).

Oral problems are common in HIV disease (p. 601) and indeed oral lesions may dominate the clinical picture. Candidiasis is the most common presenting feature of HIV disease and some conditions such as hairy leukoplakia are almost pathognomonic of this infection. The oral manifestations of HIV infection and AIDS are shown in Table 21.6. These are divided into lesions strongly associated with HIV infection and those lesions less commonly associated with HIV infection (EC Clearinghouse & WHO Collaborating Centre 1993).

Pseudomembranous candidiasis is the most common recognized presenting symptom and sign of HIV infection. Erythematous candidiasis is more difficult to diagnose (Fig. 5.8) but may be more common than pseudomembranous candidiasis. Any form of candidiasis implies progressive immunodeficiency.

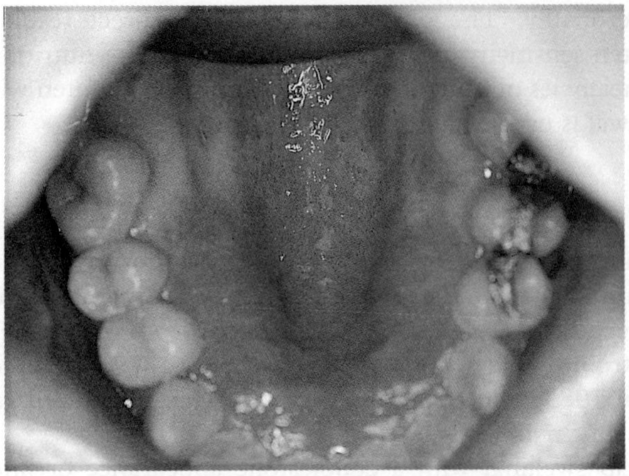

**Fig. 5.8** A red patch of the hard palate due to erythematous candidiasis in an otherwise asymptomatic HIV seropositive 26-year-old male.

Hairy leukoplakia is a keratosis affecting the lateral borders of the tongue and other parts of the mouth may be affected (Fig. 5.9). Definitive diagnosis relies on a demonstration of Epstein–Barr virus within the epithelial cells. Fifty percent of patients with hairy leukoplakia progress to AIDS within 18 months.

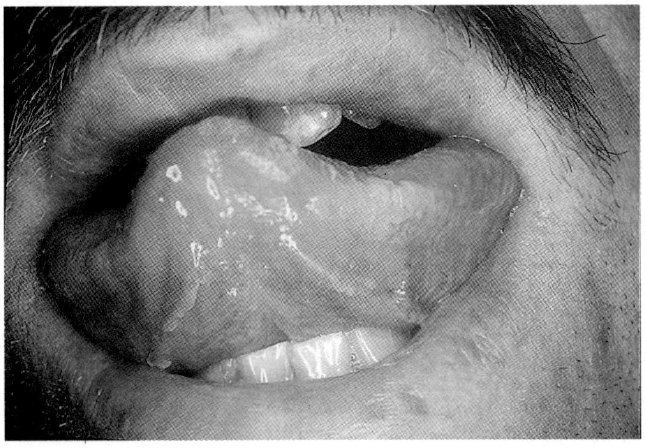

**Fig. 5.9** Hairy leukoplakia in a known HIV seropositive individual showing characteristic vertical corrugations.

The majority of Kaposi's sarcomas arise in the head and neck region and intraoral lesions are common. They present as bluish areas or swellings which may become quite large and interfere with eating or tooth brushing (Fig. 5.10). Kaposi's sarcomas respond to radiotherapy and chemotherapy as well as intralesional cytotoxics (p. 610).

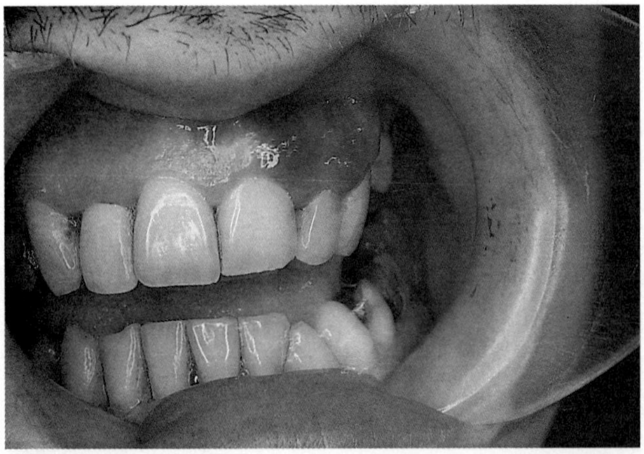

**Fig. 5.10** Gingival Kaposi's sarcoma affecting a 36-year-old male homosexual who was HIV seropositive. The patient had received previous radiotherapy for a Kaposi's sarcoma on his left cheek.

Non-Hodgkin's lymphomas are a late manifestation of HIV infection but may cause severe morbidity. They may present as intraoral swellings when biopsy is required for diagnosis (p. 610).

A number of periodontal conditions appear to be specific for HIV infection. Linear gingival erythema appears to be the result of a candidal infection of the gingival margins and is characterized by a line of erythema around the necks of the teeth. Necrotizing or ulcerative gingivitis involves extensive soft tissue ulceration and

**Table 5.9** Oral disease and side-effects related to drug therapy

| | |
|---|---|
| Angioedema | |
| | Antibiotics |
| | Aspirin |
| | Benzoates |
| | Essential oils |
| Aphthous ulcers | |
| | Vitamin $B_{12}$ deficient, e.g. colchicine |
| | Folic acid deficient, e.g. methotrexate, phenytoin |
| Bullous disorders | |
| | Captopril |
| | Gold salts |
| | Rifampicin |
| Contact stomatitis | |
| | Antibiotics, e.g. penicillin |
| | Antiseptics, e.g. formaldehyde, nitrofurazone |
| | Cosmetics |
| | Dental materials |
| | Food allergy |
| | Toothpaste |
| Drug eruptions | |
| | Barbiturates |
| | Paracetamol (acetaminophen) |
| | Tetracyclines |
| Erythema multiforme | |
| | Barbiturates |
| | Penicillin |
| | Sulfonamides |
| Gingival bleeding | |
| | Drug-induced thrombocytopenia, e.g. antibacterials, anticonvulsants |
| | Anticoagulants, e.g. aspirin, warfarin |
| Gingival hyperplasia | |
| | Calcium channel blockers |
| | Cyclosporin |
| | Oral contraceptives |
| | Phenytoin |
| Halitosis | |
| | Disulfram |
| | Dimethylsulphoxide |
| Infections | |
| | Antibiotics |
| | Corticosteroids |
| | Immunosuppressants |
| | Oral contraceptives |
| Lichenoid eruptions | |
| | Acyclovir |
| | Amalgam |
| | Carbemazepine |
| | Mercury |
| | Penicillamine |
| Neurological disorders | |
| | Parkinsonism, e.g. lithium, methyldopa |
| | Tardive dyskinesia, e.g. phenothiazines |
| | Trigeminal neuropathy, e.g. ergotamine |
| Pigmentation and staining | |
| | Staining, e.g. chlorhexidine, iron |
| | Pigmentation, e.g. anticonvulsants, antimalarials, progestogens, heavy metals, phenothiazines |
| Salivary gland disease | |
| | Enlargement, e.g. insulin, methyldopa, thiouracil |
| | Pain, e.g. clonidine, nitrofurantoin |
| | Ptyalism, e.g. parasympathomimetics |

**Table 5.10** *(cont'd)*

| | |
|---|---|
| Systemic lupus erythematosus | |
| | Carbamazipine |
| | Phenytoin |
| | Methyldopa |
| Taste and smell | |
| | Antihistamines |
| | Antimicrobials, e.g. metronidazole |
| | Antiseptics |
| | Antithyroid drugs |
| | Antihypertensives |
| | Anticonvulsants |
| | Hypoglycemics |
| | Sympathomimetics |
| | Vasodilators |
| Tooth staining | |
| | Extrinsic, e.g. chlorhexidine, iron |
| | Intrinsic, e.g. fluoride, tetracyclines |
| Traumatic ulcers | |
| | Aspirin |
| | Nonsteroidal anti-inflammatories |

necrosis around the necks of the teeth associated with spontaneous gingival hemorrhage. Additionally, necrotizing ulcerative periodontitis involves hard tissues and there is destruction of the supporting tissues of the teeth, leading to tooth loss and bony sequestration in severe cases. All patients found to be HIV seropositive should be referred for prophylactic dental care since established infection of the gums may be difficult to treat.

The lesions less commonly associated with HIV infection are shown in Group 2 of Table 21.6. The herpes infections may be severe and require continuous systemic antiviral therapy to keep them under control. Human papilloma virus infections may cause very extensive wart-like lesions which may require surgical excision or cryotherapy.

## DRUG-ASSOCIATED ORAL DISEASE

A wide variety of drug reactions occur in the mouth (Duxbury 1990). These may manifest in a large number of ways. It is important to identify when drug reactions are involved in the etiology of oral disease since cessation of therapy or switching to an alternative may be associated with marked clinical improvement.

Classification of drug-induced disease is difficult. Table 5.9 lists the common presentations of drug-induced oral disease with examples of drugs typically implicated. Although alteration of therapy may cause clinical improvement in the oral condition, often the underlying disease for which the drug is administered may be severe and warrant continued treatment. In these circumstances the oral disease may be accepted and merely treated symptomatically.

## REFERENCES


Duxbury A J 1990 Systemic pharmacotherapy. In: Jones J H, Mason D K (eds) Oral manifestations of systemic disease, 2nd edn. Baillière Tindall, London, p 411–479

EC Clearinghouse on Oral Problems Related to HIV Infection and WHO Collaborating Centre on Oral Manifestations of the Immunodeficiency Virus 1993 Classification and diagnostic criteria for oral lesions in HIV infection. Journal of Oral Pathology and Medicine 22: 289–291

Ferguson M M, Hart D M, Lindsay R, Stephen K W 1978 Progestogen therapy in menstrually related aphthae. International Journal of Oral Surgery 7: 463–470

Ferguson M M, Wray D, Carmichael H A, Russell R I, Lee F D 1980 Coeliac disease associated with recurrent aphthae. Gut 21: 223–226

Harris M, Feinmann C 1990 Pyschosomatic disorders. In: Jones J H, Mason D K (eds) Oral manifestations of systemic disease, 2nd edn, Baillière Tindall, London, p 30–60

James J, Paton D W, Lewis C J, Kirkwood E M, Ferguson M M 1986 Orofacial granulomatosis and clinical atopy. Journal of Oral Medicine 41: 29–30

Kelly A B 1919 Spasm at entrance to the oesophagus. Journal of Laryngology 34: 285–289

Kramer I R H, El-Labban N, Lee K W 1978 The clinical features and risk of malignant transformation in sublingual keratosis. British Dental Journal 144: 178–180

Lucas R B 1984 Pathology of tumours of the oral tissues. Churchill Livingstone, Edinburgh

Owen R D 1950 The problem of hypopharyngeal carcinoma. Proceedings of the Royal Society of Medicine 43: 157–170

Patton D W, Ferguson M M, Forsyth A, James J 1985 Oro-facial granulomatosis: a possible allergic basis. British Journal of Oral and Maxillofacial Surgery 23(4): 235–242

Pisanti S, Sharav Y, Kaufman E, Posner L N 1974 Pemphigus vulgaris: incidence in Jews of different ethnic groups according to age, sex and initial lesion. Oral Surgery, Oral Medicine, Oral Pathology 38: 382–387

Porter S, Scully C, Greenspan D 1990 Primary and secondary immunodeficiencies. In: Jones J H, Mason D K (eds) Oral manifestations of systemic disease, 2nd edn. Baillière Tindall, London, p 112–182

Scully C, Cawson R A 1993 Medical problems in dentistry, 3rd edn. Wright, Oxford

Scully C, El-Kom M 1985 Lichen planus: review and update on pathogenesis. Journal of Oral Pathology 14: 431–438

Seifert G 1991 Histological typing of salivary gland tumours. Springer-Verlag, Berlin

Shamma-a M H, Benedict E B 1958 Oesophageal webs. A report of 58 cases and an attempt at classification. New England Journal of Medicine 259: 378–384

Sharr M M, Garfield J S 1977 The place of ganglion or root alcohol injection in trigeminal neuralgia. Journal of Neurology, Neurosurgery and Psychiatry 40: 286–290

Sweatman M C, Tasker R, Warner J O, Ferguson M M, Mitchell D N 1986 Orofacial granulomatosis: response to elemental diet and provocation by food additives. Clinical Allergy 16: 331–338

Sweet W H 1986 The treatment of trigeminal neuralgia (tic douloureux). New England Journal of Medicine 315: 174–177

Tyldesley W R 1979 Oral Crohn's and related conditions. British Journal of Oral Surgery 17: 1–9

Walker D M 1984 Infectious diseases with oral manifestations. In: Ivanyi L (ed) Immunological aspects of oral diseases. MTP Press, Lancaster, p 101–123

Wiesenfeld D, Ferguson M M, Mitchell D N et al 1985 Orofacial granulomatosis, a clinical and pathological analysis. Quarterly Journal of Medicine (new series) 54: 101–113

Wray D 1984a Recurrent aphthous stomatitis. Journal of the Royal Society of Medicine 77:1–3

Wray D 1984b Pyostomatitis vegetans. British Dental Journal 157: 316–317

Wray D, Dagg J H 1990 Oral manifestations of diseases of the blood and blood forming organs. In: Jones J H, Mason D K (eds) Oral manifestations of systemic disease, 2nd edn. Baillière Tindall, London, p 660–713

Wray D, McCord J F 1987 Labial veneers in the management of desquamative gingivitis. Oral Surgery, Oral Medicine, Oral Pathology 64: 41–42

Wray D, Ferguson M M, Mason D K, Hutcheon A W, Dagg J H 1975 Recurrent aphthae: treatment with vitamin $B_{12}$, folic acid and iron. British Medical Journal 2: 490–493

Zegarelli D J, Zegarelli E V 1977 Intra-oral pemphigus vulgaris. Oral Surgery, Oral Medicine, Oral Pathology 44: 384–393

Zulman J, Jaffe R, Talal N 1978 Evidence that the malignant lymphoma of Sjögren's syndrome is a monoclonal B-cell neoplasm. New England Journal of Medicine 299: 1215–1220

# 6. Integrative neurohormonal control of gut function

*M. Camilleri   M. J. Ford*

## INTRODUCTION

The integration of gastrointestinal motility is controlled by complex neurohumoral mechanisms involving the extrinsic (central) and intrinsic (enteric) systems, the electrical activity of gut smooth muscle and hormonal systems (enteric, neural and endocrine). The interplay of neural, myogenic and chemical factors in the control of motor function is better understood in the esophagus, stomach and small bowel than in the colon.

The objectives of this chapter are to review the anatomy of the extrinsic and intrinsic neural control and the hormones and peptides involved in the control of gut motor, secretory and absorptive activity, the prime focus being on motor and sensory function. Examples are provided to demonstrate the principle that integrated neurohormonal mechanisms in the control of gut function cannot be meaningfully disassembled into the individual components. The literature on gastrointestinal hormones and peptides is extensive; in contrast, we focus on concepts and examples of relevance to human physiology. Finally, the clinical applications of gut hormone assay are described briefly with particular emphasis on the disorders of motor function.

## EXTRINSIC NERVOUS SYSTEM

### Efferent control

Extrinsic neural control modulates gut function via the parasympathetic and sympathetic nervous systems and their effects on the enteric nervous system and gut smooth muscle. The parasympathetic outflow comprises the cranial and spinal outflows to the gastrointestinal tract. Thus the cervical esophagus receives efferent (motor) fibers from the glossopharyngeal nucleus and the nucleus ambiguus (one of the vagal nuclei).

The parasympathetic innervation of the foregut and midgut originates from the dorsal motor nucleus of the vagus nerve. The hindgut (the anorectum and left hemicolon) receives its parasympathetic efferents from the sacral outflow via the S2–4 roots and the pelvic nerves; the external anal sphincter is supplied by S2–4 and the pudendal nerve.

The sympathetic outflow to the gut arises from the thoracolumbar spinal cord (T5 to L3) and is relayed to the prevertebral ganglia (the celiac, superior mesenteric and inferior mesenteric ganglia). Postganglionic fibers are conveyed via the lumbar colonic, splanchnic and hypogastric nerves and subsequently follow the arterial branches of the mesenteric vasculature. The sympathetic nervous system is particularly important in facilitating the contractile activity of sphincteric muscle and inhibiting the contractile activity of nonsphincteric muscle.

The cerebral cortex and hypothalamus control hunger, satiety and gastrointestinal responses to eating and stress; recent evidence suggests that the effects of stress may be mediated by corticotrophin-releasing factor. The brainstem, spinal cord and prevertebral ganglia modulate enteroenteric reflexes. Thus, extrinsic nerves add a second level of control over and above the intrinsic neural control of sphincteric and nonsphincteric gut motility and gastrointestinal secretion. Visceral sensory pathways also traverse through extrinsic nerves linking the gut to the brain. The motor function of nonsphincteric muscle is stimulated by the vagus nerve and the sacral outflow (pelvic nerves). Inhibition of nonsphincteric muscle contractile activity and gastrointestinal secretion by the sympathetic nervous system provides a "sympathetic brake". In general, sphincteric muscle within the gut is stimulated by alpha sympathetic pathways and inhibited by beta sympathetic pathways. It is also inhibited by nonadrenergic, noncholinergic (NANC) parasympathetic pathways whose neurotransmitters are thought to include VIP, somatostatin, ATP and nitric oxide (Fig. 6.1).

Parasympathetic stimulation increases smooth muscle and secretory activity; parasympathetic ablation has a proportionately greater effect on phasic than tonic contractile activity. When sympathetic innervation is impaired, excessive and unco-ordinated motor and secretory activity are characteristic features (e.g. in diabetic autonomic neuropathy). Disorders such as achalasia and Hirschsprung's

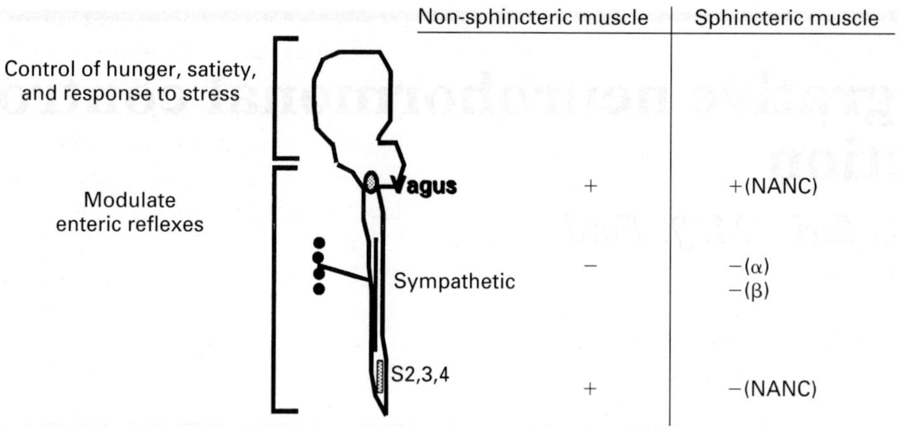


**Fig. 6.1** General organization of the extrinsic neural control of gut motility (NANC = nonadrenergic, noncholinergic pathways).

disease appear to reflect disorders of the enteric nervous system associated with failure of inhibitory neurotransmission (e.g. VIP and NO), resulting in impaired smooth muscle relaxation. The relatively small number of "command" extrinsic nerves modulate function of preprogrammed circuits of hundreds of neurons in the enteric nervous system. This preprogramming of circuits is referred to as "hard-wiring", analogous with the printed circuits in an electronic device. This differs from the classic concept of extrinsic preganglionic vagal fibers synapsing with a small number of enteric neurons.

### Afferent function (see also p. 1345)

Sensory receptors within the gut are responsive to mechanical, chemical, thermal and osmotic stimuli. Most do not exhibit any morphologic specialization and their response characteristics are dependent upon their site within the gut wall. Parasympathetic afferents convey impulses for mucosal and muscle receptors. Mucosal receptors are sensitive to both touch and rapidly changing distention; muscle receptors are sensitive to both isotonic and isometric muscle contraction and to distention, consistent with "in-series" tension receptors. It is thought that C-fibers convey the slowly adapting mechanoreceptor responses which respond to tonic stimuli from the gut. In contrast A-δ fibers convey rapidly adapting mechanoreceptor responses responding to phasic stimuli. Mucosal afferents are activated by non-noxious shearing forces within the lumen. Spinal afferents also supply mechanoreceptors within the mesentery and mesenteric arteries. They produce a slowly adapting response to local pressure and distortion and respond to visceral distention and contraction. Thus, mechanisms are available to respond to different types of distending intestinal stimuli that stimulate specific populations of afferent fibers and respond to stimulation at different depths of distortion of the gut wall.

Sensory receptors in the gut wall and mesenteries are connected to two different types of afferent nerves. Some visceral afferent nerves have their cell bodies within the myenteric and submucosal plexuses; they do not send axonal projections to the central nervous system and do not play a direct role in pain sensation. Spinal and vagal afferent neurons have their cell bodies in spinal and brain-stem ganglia. Visceral sensory fibers account for 75–90% of the vagus nerve and 50% of the pelvic, splanchnic, lumbar colonic and hypogastric nerves. In toto, however, they comprise less than 10% of the sensory inflow to the thoracolumbar spinal cord since the vast majority arise from somatic afferents.

Visceral afferents project to the prevertebral ganglia and are then relayed cephalad to the nucleus of the tractus solitarius, the hypothalamus and higher cortical centers. Afferent nerves travelling within the parasympathetic nerve trunks are principally concerned with the regulatory, sensory functions unassociated with sensation of pain. In contrast, the sympathetic nerves convey information regarding pain sensation; only spinal afferents travelling within sympathetic nerve trunks transmit visceral pain. In this way, cranial (vagal) afferents mediate brain–gut visceral reflexes and spinal afferents mediate viscerovisceral reflexes and pain sensation.

## THE ENTERIC NERVOUS SYSTEM

The intrinsic neural control of gut motor and secretory function is based on the "little brain" located within the gut wall. There are approximately 100 million enteric neurons throughout the gastrointestinal tract, a number that is similar to that found in the spinal cord. The enteric nervous system (ENS) is a network of neurons and fibers located throughout the length of the gut and comprising several ganglionated plexi, each ganglia of which contains up to 100 nerve cell bodies. The ganglionated plexi are concentrated predominantly between the circular and longitudinal muscle layers, the myenteric plexus of Auerbach and in the submucosa of the small and large bowel, the submucosal plexus of Meissner. In addition, there are plexuses deep within the circular muscle layer (Cajal's plexus), in the longitudinal muscle layer and in the lamina propria of the mucosa (Fig. 6.2). Gut smooth muscle receives its innervation almost exclusively from the myenteric plexus; similarly the gut mucosa is innervated almost entirely from the submucosal plexus. The enteric neurons comprise sensory neurons, interneurons (excitatory and inhibitory) and motor neurons.

The characterization of populations of neurons within the ENS is based on their neuronal function and their neurotransmitters. Some neurotransmitters are colocalized, e.g. the excitatory neurotransmitters acetylcholine and substance P may both be present within the same neuron. The enteric nervous system is organized in such a way that it integrates the sensory input from the wall or lumen with the motor input of the autonomic nervous system. The "hard-wiring" of the enteric nervous system can be viewed as multiple integrated circuits programmed to render many of the essential functions of the intestine independent of extrinsic nervous control. The principal functions of the ENS include the control of pacemaking and the migrating motor complex, peristalsis, moment-to-moment regional contractile activity and the processes of sensation and intestinal secretion.

The ENS control of the contractile activity of the gut depends upon the interplay between excitatory and inhibitory motor neurons. Gut smooth muscle is intrinsic-

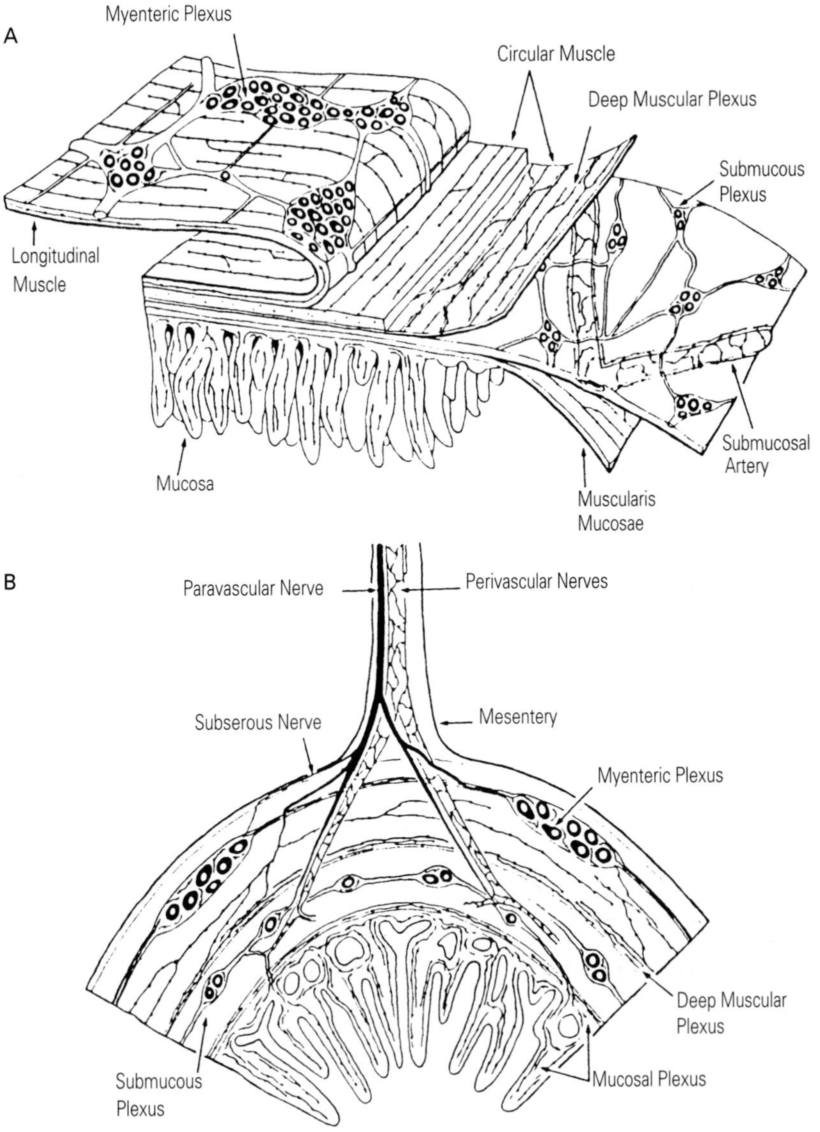


**Fig. 6.2** Diagrammatic representation of the enteric plexuses in whole mounts of intestine **A** and in transverse section **B**. (Reprinted with permission from Furness J B et al 1990. The normal structure of gastrointestinal innervation. *J Gastroenterol Hepatol* 1: 1–9.)

ally active; it is tonically contracted with superimposed, rhythmic, phasic contractions. Individual smooth muscle cells are electrically coupled, enabling pacemaker cells to sequentially activate neighboring cells in both the circular and longitudinal axes. Approximately 40% of myenteric neurons contain VIP and the enzyme nitric oxide synthase and 40% contain acetylcholine and the tachykinins, substance P and substance K. These two populations of motor neurons do not overlap. Of the submucosal neurons, 55% contain acetylcholine and 45% VIP; other transmitters are colocalized in these neurons. In sphincteric muscle, the inhibitory neurons are normally switched off and only switched on as part of a co-ordinated event such as relaxation of a sphincter. In nonsphincteric muscle, inhibitory neuron activation determines the length of the contracting segment by controlling the extent of myogenic excitation.

### The peristaltic reflex

The process of peristalsis, whereby a segment of intestine proximal to a distending stimulus (such as a bolus of food or gas) contracts and the segment below the stimulus relaxes, involves a complex interaction of many neurotransmitters (Fig. 6.3). The ascending wave of contraction that propels the food bolus caudad is mediated by acetylcholine, substance P, substance K and probably serotonin. In contrast, the descending wave of inhibition that induces segmental relaxation to accommodate the oncoming bolus is mediated by VIP, somatostatin, opioids, GABA and probably nitric oxide acting in concert. The initial stimulus, e.g. wall distention by the food bolus, is relayed by sensory neurons and activates somatostatin neurons which in turn stimulate the release of GABA and inhibit the release of opioids. Since GABA stimulates VIP release and opioids inhibit VIP release, both pathways activated by somatostatin produce VIP release which mediates a descending wave of relaxation.

## CHEMICAL AND HORMONAL CONTROL

There is a wide range of chemicals which modulate absorption, secretion, contractile activity and transit either via direct effects on enterocytes or smooth muscle or via effects on the intrinsic and/or extrinsic nervous systems. These chemicals include acetylcholine, amines, peptides and prostaglandins. It is likely that secretory and absorptive processes may also influence transit. Many of the regulatory gut hormones and neuropeptides have major effects on the central nervous system which in turn affects gastrointestinal function, in addition to their direct effects at the enteric level.

### Delivery of regulatory peptides

There are several routes for the delivery of regulatory transmitters to their target site (Fig. 6.4). In the endocrine route, an endocrine cell discharges a transmitter (a hormone such as gastrin) into the bloodstream which transports it to its target site. A more direct route occurs when the transmitter is released by a paracrine cell to diffuse the target cell receptor (e.g. somatostatin D cells in the control of gastrin G cells in stomach). The neurocrine route is similar with neurons discharging a transmitter to the target

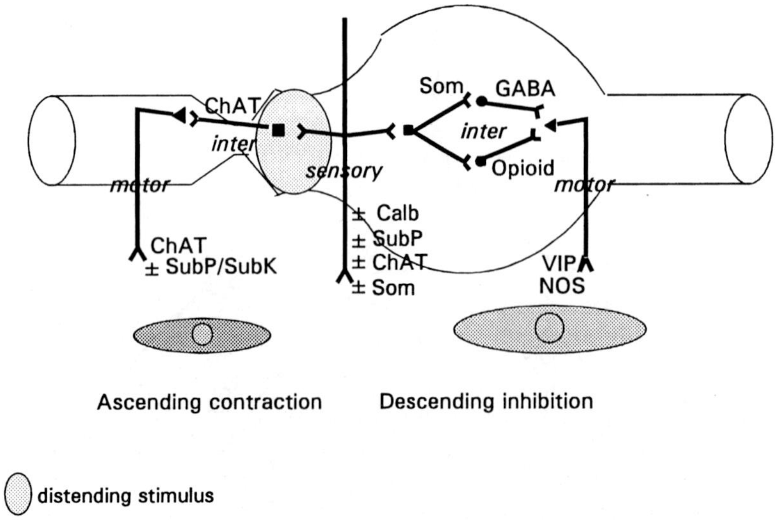


**Fig. 6.3** Neural pathways in the peristaltic reflex. Sensory neurons containing calbindin, substance P, acetylcholine or somatostatin relay information through interneurons to motor neurons that cause contraction orad (through ACh and tachykinins) and dilatation caudad (through VIP and nitric oxide). ChAT = choline acetyl transferase; NOS = nitric oxide synthase.

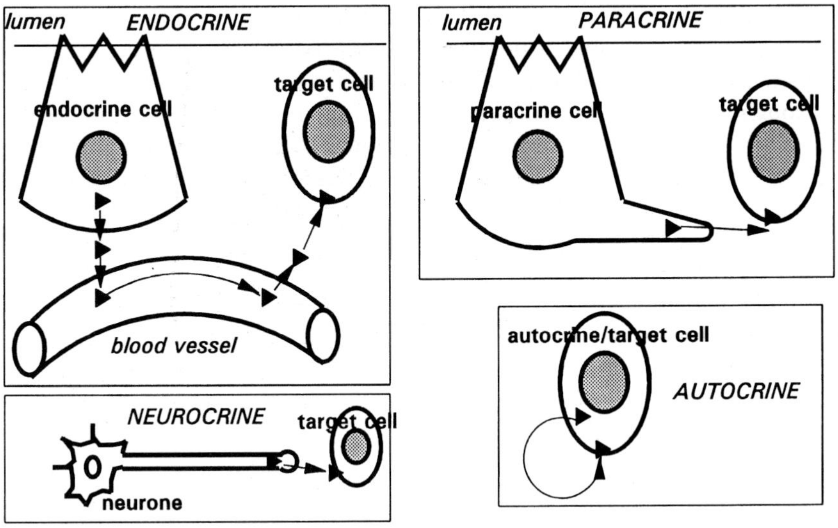


**Fig. 6.4** Delivery of regulatory peptides – endocrine, paracrine, neurocrine or autocrine.

cell. Finally, the transmitter may be released by an autocrine cell, which is itself the target cell, thus regulating its own function.

## Gut neurotransmitters (Table 6.1)

The function of the different populations of enteric neurons is determined by the nature of the transmitters released and by the target receptors. Gut neuropeptides may be colocalized with acetylcholine or norepinephrine in intrinsic nerves, such as substance P and neuropeptide Y respectively. In the guinea pig ileum, almost 30% of neurons are sensory and 60% are either excitatory or inhibitory to the longitudinal and circular muscles. The remaining neurons are either interneurons or secretomotor neurons.

### *Acetylcholine*

Acetylcholine (ACh), released from enteric postsynaptic cholinergic neurons, is the primary stimulant for contraction and acts on smooth muscle muscarinic receptors. It is also the presynaptic mediator of neurons of the extrinsic and intrinsic nervous systems and acts on the nicotinic receptors to stimulate both cholinergic and nonadrenergic noncholinergic (NANC) neurons.

### *Norepinephrine*

Norepinephrine (NE) is released from adrenergic neurons and inhibits the release of acetylcholine by enteric neurons. $\alpha_1$- and $\beta_1$-adrenergic receptors predominate in gut smooth muscle and $\alpha_2$- and $\beta_2$-receptors in enteric neurons. α- and β-adrenergic agonists both induce muscle relaxation but by different routes. $\alpha_1$-agonists reduce smooth muscle activity directly and $\alpha_2$-agonists reduce it indirectly via enteric neurons.

**Table 6.1** Major functions of gut neuropeptides

| Name | Major function |
|---|---|
| VIP | Sphincteric relaxation; peristalsis; descending inhibition; vasodilatation |
| NPY | Vasoconstriction; inhibits ACh release; decreases intestinal secretion |
| Tachykinins | Peristalsis: ascending contraction; sphincteric contraction; vasodilatation; sensory function: nociception |
| Somatostatin | Inhibits GI secretion, peristalsis and sensory function |
| Bombesin | Muscle contraction |
| Gastrin-releasing peptide | Antral gastrin release |
| CGRP | Sensory function; smooth muscle relaxation; vasodilatation |
| μ and δ opioid neuropeptides | Stimulate sphincter contraction; stimulate MMC-like motility; inhibit ACh and VIP release; peristalsis: descending inhibition; inhibit secretion |
| κ opioid neuropeptides | Inhibit visceral sensation; stimulate peristalsis |

In general, $\alpha_2$-agonists have significant effects on gastric and colonic motility and may induce stasis or pseudo-obstruction. An $\alpha_2$-agonist, clonidine, decreases the diarrhea associated with diabetic autonomic neuropathy by virtue of both motor and secretory effects. Other adrenergic agents have less prominent clinical effects on gut motor function. $\beta_2$-adrenergic agonists decrease background or tonic contractility (of the muscle cells) rather than phasic contractions that are typically associated with mixing or peristalsis. β-adrenergic receptor antagonists, unlike α-receptor antagonists, increase upper and lower gastrointestinal contractile activity.

### *Tachykinins*

There are three major tachykinins: substance P, substance

K (which is colocalized and coreleased with substance P) and neuromedin K. There is considerable structural homology and similar bioactivity of these tachykinins. Substance P is present throughout the human gut in similar concentrations in the neurons of the mucosa-submucosal and muscle layers. Receptors for tachykinins are expressed on smooth muscles, enteric neurons and epithelial cells. The neural and myoneural interactions of substance P are complex. It exerts both direct effects and indirect effects via both cholinergic and serotonergic neurons and these effects differ in different parts of the gut. Substance P mediates lower esophageal sphincter contraction when the esophagus is acidified. It is a major component of the peristaltic reflex, splanchnic vasodilatation, pain sensation and the enteric sensory system.

*Serotonin*

Serotonin is released from neurocrine, paracrine and endocrine cells throughout the gastrointestinal tract. It is located predominantly in enterochromaffin cells and in myenteric plexus neurons. Receptors for serotonin are expressed on smooth muscle, enteric neurons and epithelium cells. There are multiple receptor subtypes including 5HT1 and 5HT4 receptors on muscles and neurons, 5HT2 receptors on sphincteric muscle and 5HT3 receptors on cholinergic neurons and sensory afferents. Serotonin has important effects on the peristaltic reflex. Its interactions are complex as different parts of the gut respond in different ways so that some segments exhibit excitation and others inhibition of peristalsis. Experimentally, even within one segment, there may be different pharmacologic actions depending on whether the serotonin originates from the serosal or the mucosal aspect. However, there is no evidence that serotonin from enterochromaffin cells traverses the gut wall to reach targets in the enteric plexus. Hence, motor effects result from local release by serotonergic myenteric neurons. Serotonin has both direct effects on muscle and indirect effects via cholinergic neurons. 5HT4 receptor stimulation results in contraction while 5HT2 stimulation may result in inhibition. Serotonin stimulates the myoelectric activity of the small intestine and is involved in the tonic phase of the gastrocolonic response. It also has important effects on enteric sensory function via 5HT3 receptors.

*VIP, PHI, PHM and neuropeptide Y*

Vasoactive polypeptide (VIP), peptide histidine isoleucine (PHI) and methionine (PHM) are products of the same gene and prohormone and are colocalized in neurons. Neuropeptide Y is colocalized with norepinephrine in sympathetic postganglionic fibers. The motor effects of VIP are predominantly inhibitory; it relaxes the gastric fundus during receptive relaxation and relaxes sphincters such as the lower esophageal sphincter, internal anal sphincter and sphincter of Oddi. VIP is a major mediator in the descending wave of relaxation in the peristaltic reflex. VIP is also an important neurotransmitter mediating vasodilatation in the splanchnic circulation and pancreatic and intestinal secretion. Neuropeptide Y acts like norepinephrine, decreasing the release of acetylcholine, causing vasoconstriction and inhibiting intestinal secretion.

*Endogenous opioids*

Endogenous opioids have both neurocrine and endocrine effects in the gastrointestinal tract. They act on several different receptor subtypes, the mu, delta, kappa opioid, in the gut. β-endorphin, a μ and δ receptor agonist, is released from the hypothalamus during stress and has been shown to have important motor effects on the gastrointestinal tract. The chief endogenous opioid in the myenteric plexus is met-enkephalin which is present at higher concentrations in the colon than in the small intestine.

Endogenous opioids exert their intestinal effects at different levels throughout the nervous system. Central effects include the induction of vomiting, spinal cord effects include mediation of pain sensation and enteric effects include important motor and secretomotor functions. Opioid receptor agonists also inhibit the neuronal release of acetylcholine and VIP, stimulate somatostatin release and play a significant role in the peristaltic reflex.

When administered peripherally, mu opioid agonists stimulate sphincter muscle. μ and δ opioid agonists inhibit nonsphincteric muscle contractions and stimulate MMC-like activity in the small bowel resulting in a net decrease in intestinal transit. μ and δ opioid agonists facilitate intestinal absorption by slowing transit, thereby increasing contact time, and by direct effects on enterocyte function, inhibiting secretion. Opiates and opioid drugs, such as loperamide, delay transit and inhibit secretion. Kappa opioid receptors are also involved in visceral nociception.

*Bombesins and gastrin-releasing peptide* (GRP)

The bombesins, including GRP, are exclusively neuronal in origin and are present in highest concentrations in the nerve endings of the gastric antrum, pancreas and distal ileum. They are released in response to cholinergic stimulation and result in gastrin release and pancreatic exocrine secretion. The bombesins also stimulate lower esophageal sphincter contraction and induce the release of substance P from nerve endings in the colonic mucosa.

*Calcitonin gene-related peptide* (CGRP)

Calcitonin gene-related peptide (CGRP), a 37-amino acid peptide, is produced by the same gene as calcitonin and is expressed in enteric neurons in the submucosal and myenteric plexi. CGRP relaxes contracted gut muscle, causes vasodilatation of the splanchnic circulation and stimulates the release of acetylcholine and somatostatin, thereby inhibiting gastric acid secretion. It is also a major sensory transmitter in the gut.

## Gut regulatory hormones

The regional distribution and localization within endocrine, paracrine and neurocrine cells of the major regulatory hormones are shown in Table 6.2 and Figure 6.5. It is noteworthy that somatostatin is released from endocrine, paracrine and neurocrine cells.

**Table 6.2** Excitatory and inhibitory neurohumoral mediators

| Cell type | Excitatory | Inhibitory |
|---|---|---|
| Endocrine | Gastrin | Pancreatic polypeptide |
| | Secretin | Somatostatin |
| | Cholecystokinin | Gastric inhibitory peptide |
| | Motilin | Neurotensin |
| | Enteroglucagon | Peptide YY |
| | Serotonin | |
| Neurocrine | Acetylcholine | Vasoactive polypeptide |
| | Bombesin (GRP) | Norepinephrine |
| | Tachykinins | Calcitonin-GRP |
| | Serotonin | Somatostatin |
| | | Neuropeptide YY |
| | | Nitric oxide |
| | | Opioids |
| Paracrine | Serotonin | Somatostatin |

## Physiologic functions of the gut hormones

*Gastrin* (see also p. 220)

Gastrin is released by gastric antral G cells in response to stimulation of cholinergic, β-adrenergic, bombesinergic and GABA neurons as well as intraluminal calcium and nutrients such as proteins, peptides and amino acids. Its release is inhibited by somatostatin, secretin, gastric inhibitory peptide (GIP) and luminal acidification. It is a potent stimulus of gastric acid secretion and also exerts a significant trophic effect on peptic mucosa. In addition, the pharmacological effects of gastrin include an increase in the contractility of the lower esophageal sphincter, gastric antrum, small and large bowel. Its role as a physiological mediator of motor responses is unclear.

*Somatostatin*

Somatostatin acts as an endocrine hormone, paracrine agent and neuropeptide. It is secreted mainly by mucosal D cells in the gastric antrum, pancreas and small bowel primarily in response to intraluminal fat, cholinergic and beta-adrenergic stimulation, VIP, GIP, secretin and CCK. It is a potent inhibitor of gastrin and insulin release, biliary, gastric, small and large bowel motility and intestinal absorptive and sensory function. It plays a central role in the descending wave of muscular inhibition during peristalsis. Paradoxically, it induces activity fronts similar to phase III of the MMC.

*Motilin*

Motilin is released by M cells in the duodenum in response to sham feeding, gastric distention, duodenal

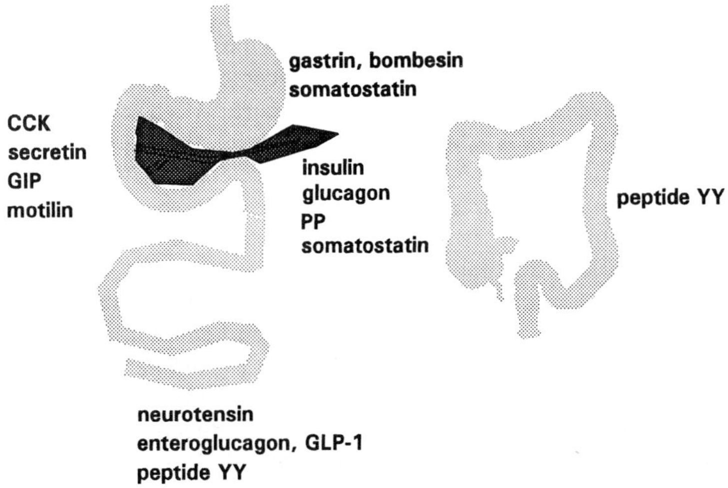


**Fig. 6.5** Regional distribution of endocrine peptides or gut hormones in gastrointestinal mucosa and pancreas. GIP = glucose-stimulated insulinotropic peptide; PP = pancreatic polypeptide; CCK = cholecystokinin; GLP-1 = glucagon-like peptide 1.

exposure to biliary and pancreatic secretions and stimulation by opioid agonists. In the fasted state, the release of motilin is cyclical, being maximal during late phase II and III of the MMC. Motilin stimulates contraction of the lower esophageal sphincter, gastric antrum and duodenum.

*Pancreatic polypeptide*

In the fasted state, the release of pancreatic polypeptide by pancreatic D and F cells has a cyclical pattern like that of motilin. It is released in response to sham feeding, the intake of nutrient, peptides and amino acids, and cholinergic stimulation. It inhibits postprandial pancreatic exocrine secretion.

*Secretin* (see p. 1232)

Secretin is released by the S cells of the duodenum in response to acid or bile in the lumen. Secretin induces pancreatic and duodenal bicarbonate secretion. It also inhibits gastrin release, acid secretion, gastric emptying and lower esophageal sphincter tone.

*Cholecystokinin* (see p. 1233)

Cholecystokinin is released by the I cells of the duodenum in response to nutrient, fat and fatty acids, protein and peptides, and bombesinergic stimulation. It is a potent stimulant of pancreatic exocrine secretion. It produces relaxation of the lower esophageal sphincter, delayed gastric emptying and increased biliary, small and large bowel contractile activity. CCK also stimulates somatostatin and pancreatic polypeptide release and exerts both central and peripheral satiety effects.

*Gastric inhibitory peptide* (GIP)

GIP is released by the K cells of the duodenum in response to nutrient (glucose, fats and amino acids), β-adrenergic and bombesinergic stimulation. GIP is a potent inhibitor of gastric acid secretion and induces intestinal secretion and glucose-dependent insulin release (an "incretin" effect). It may also exert inhibitory effects on the lower esophageal sphincter and gastric antral motility.

*Enteroglucagon*

Enteroglucagon comprises two peptides, glicentin and oxyntomodulin, the products of the same gene which also regulates the production of glucagon-like peptide-1 (GLP-1). They are released by L cells in the distal ileum and proximal colon in response to fats and complex carbohydrates. They are weak physiologic inhibitors of gastric acid and pancreatic secretion and biliary and intestinal motility. As incretins, they enhance insulin release and promote lipolysis, ketogenesis, glycogenolysis and gluconeogenesis.

*Peptide YY*

Peptide YY is colocalized with enteroglucagon within the L cells of the terminal ileum but is present in highest concentration in the rectosigmoid colonic mucosa. It is released in response to intraluminal fat and bile acids in the distal ileum and colon and also following bombesinergic stimulation. It inhibits postprandial gastric acid and pancreatic secretion and delays gastric and small bowel emptying (the "ileal and colonic brake").

*Neurotensin*

Neurotensin is released by N cells in the distal ileum in response to intraluminal fat and bombesinergic stimulation. It inhibits postprandial gastric acid and pancreatic secretion, decreases gastric emptying and increases colonic motility. It is a potent stimulant of pancreatic polypeptide release and also of histamine release from mast cells.

### Neural and hormonal integration

*The brain–gut link*

In the most simplistic of models, the brain–gut interaction is one of parasympathetic stimulation, sympathetic inhibition and hormonal modulation of programmed patterns of activity of the enteric nervous system (Fig. 6.6). The dialogue between these two brains, however, is complex. The cephalic effects on gastrointestinal motility and secretion are most marked in association with psychological stress, eating and excretion. The activities of both brains alter during sleep and during heightened states of arousal and many of the gut hormones and neuropeptides have important receptors within the brain-stem, hypothalamus and higher cortical centers.

In general, there are few responses of the digestive tract that are selectively neural (Fig. 6.7) and most physiologic responses have both neural and hormonal components. Examples of selectively neural responses are receptive gastric relaxation whereby the stomach fundus relaxes in response to deglutition through a reflex mediated by both afferent and efferent fibers of the vagus nerve.

Another example of a selectively neural response is the relaxation of the internal anal sphincter following spontaneous or induced rectal distention, the rectoanal inhibitory reflex. A third example of a selectively neural response is the reflex inhibition of the external anal sphincter following rectal distention mediated by parasympathetic visceral afferent fibers.

However, selective neural responses are the exception

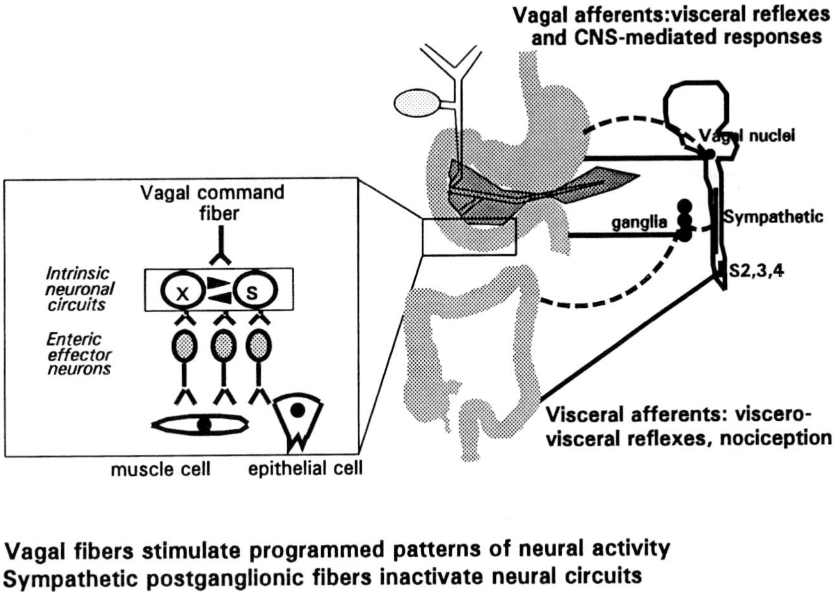


**Fig. 6.6** Integration of extrinsic and enteric neural control. Efferent control by extrinsic fibers modulates "hard-wired" programmed patterns of neural activity, rather than stimulating individual enteric neurons. The functional organization of vagal and visceral afferents is predominantly involved in CNS and nociceptive functions respectively.

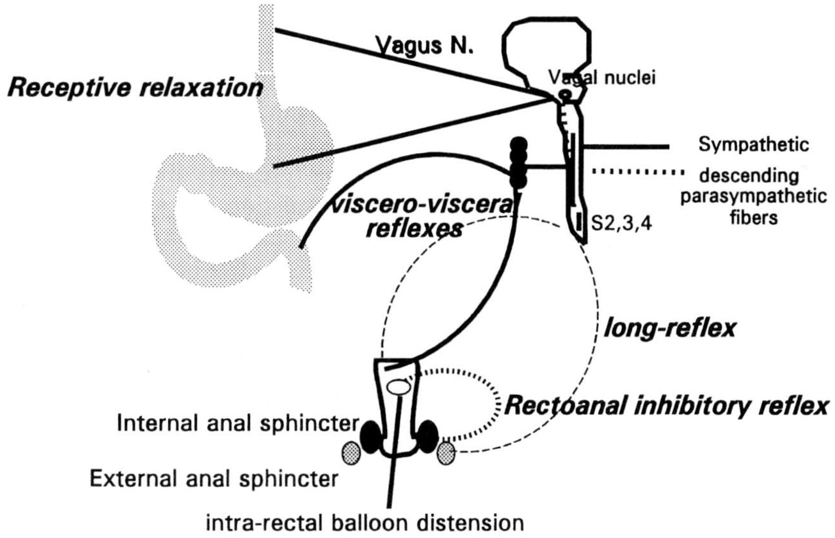


**Fig. 6.7** Examples of the rare phenomenon of selectively neural responses that probably exclude hormonal integration: receptive relaxation during deglutition, the rectoanal inhibitory reflex and a long sacral reflex that results in external anal sphincter contraction during rectal distention.

rather than the rule. In general, physiologic responses are usually integrative neurohormonal phenomena. Consider, for example, the regulation of gastric emptying (Fig. 6.8). Anticipation of feeding evokes a vagally mediated cephalic response stimulating gastric accommodation, the release of gastric antral gastrin, acid secretion and gastric motility. Ingestion of the meal results in gastric distention which produces a vagally mediated, positive feedback stimulating gastric emptying in addition to receptive fundal relaxation. The arrival of nutrient in the duodenum, however, provokes the release of cholecystokinin which mediates negative feedback to inhibit gastric motility and release of motilin which stimulates intestinal motility and may thus enhance the pressure gradient necessary to empty the stomach. Similarly, the arrival of nutrient (unabsorbed complex carbohydrates and fat) in the distal ileum and colon (a rare event in health) stimulates an ileal brake via the release of peptide YY and neurotensin, inhibiting not

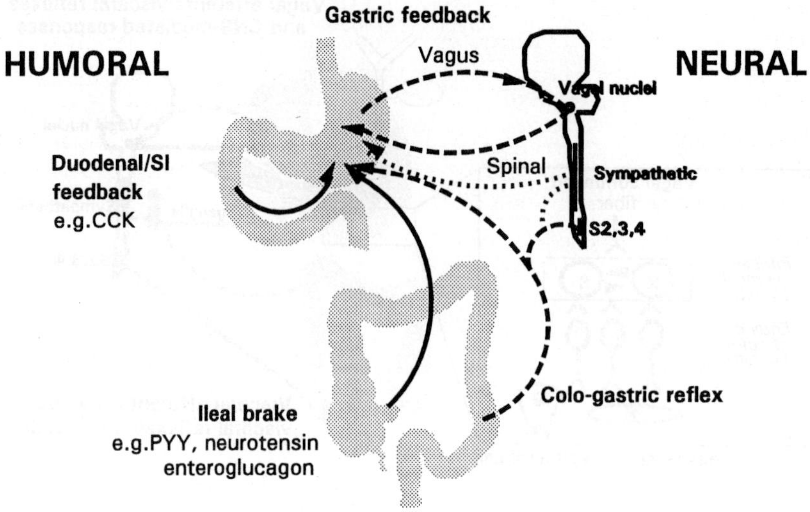


**Fig. 6.8** Examples of integrated neural and humoral responses in the regulation of gastric emptying. Gastric distention stimulates antral contractions through vagal fibers; hormonal feedback from the duodenum generally serves to delay gastric emptying as chemo- or osmoreceptors sense the arrival of chyme from the stomach; complex carbohydrates and fat in the ileum and colon retard gastric emptying through hormonal and possibly neural feedback; distention of the colon or rectum inhibits gastric motility probably by neural reflexes.

only gastric and small bowel motility but also acid and pancreatic secretion and possibly also a colonic brake.

A second example of an integrative physiologic response is the "gastrocolonic" response to food. In this normal reflex, neural and hormonal mechanisms mediate an early and late stimulation of colonic motility in response to a meal. The ensuing movement of colonic residue then elicits a colonogastric reflex, mediated neurally via visceral afferent pathways, to inhibit gastric motility. Examining the gastrocolonic response in more detail reveals the complexity of this integrated neurohormonal response. Pharmacologic studies have implicated a number of neurohumoral mediators which include gastrin, cholecystokinin and prostaglandins, serotonin (5HT3 receptors and opioids). Gastric parasympathetic afferents stimulate the brain-stem vagal nuclei and descending bulbospinal parasympathetic efferents mediate an increase in both gastric and colonic motility respectively.

## Clinical application of gastrointestinal hormones

Gastrointestinal hormones are involved in the production of a number of diarrheal states. Gastrinomas (Zollinger–Ellison syndrome) and VIPomas (Verner–Morrison syndrome) are characterized by secretory diarrheas. Dysmotility-induced diarrheal states attributable to hormonal effects include medullary carcinoma of the thyroid and the carcinoid syndrome. In the carcinoid syndrome, excessive serotonin production results in hyperstimulation of gut motor and secretory function. Increases in jejunal motility and secretion rates provoke a 50% increase in small bowel transit; a six-fold increase in proximal colonic transit is associated with colonic hypermotility in carcinoid diarrhea. Accelerated colonic transit is attributable to the reduction in colonic capacitance associated with increased postprandial colonic tone limiting the absorptive and reservoir functions of the proximal colon.

Manipulation of gastrointestinal hormones provides a useful means of controlling certain gastrointestinal symptoms such as diarrhea and abdominal pain. Typical examples include the use of agents that act on opioid, somatostatin and serotonin receptors.

The mechanisms by which opioid receptor agonists control diarrheal states invoke a complex integration of neurohumoral processes. Mu and δ opioids inhibit the neuronal release of acetylcholine and VIP in both the submucosal and myenteric plexi and stimulate the release of somatostatin. In consequence, gut secretory rates decrease, phase III activity initially is activated before the gut reverts to phasic, nonpropulsive, contractile activity and gastrointestinal transit is markedly slowed.

Somatostatin decreases gastrointestinal secretion and increases small bowel transit time, thereby facilitating intestinal absorption. The somatostatin analog, octreotide, usefully improves symptoms in the short bowel syndrome, postvagotomy diarrhea, small bowel fistulae and carcinoid syndrome.

The use of serotonin receptor agonists and antagonists offers major therapeutic advantages in the management of refractory symptomatology associated with altered visceral afferent function or impaired transit. Therapy with the 5HT3 receptor antagonists, such as ondansetron or tropisetron, has revolutionized the control of cisplatin-induced emesis while 5HT4 agonists, such as cisapride, have clinically significant prokinetic effects that are of value in the treatment of delayed gastric and small bowel emptying and possibly also in colonic inertia.

Finally, the measurement of gastrointestinal regulatory peptides can provide an invaluable diagnostic tool when used in a focused manner. Gut hormone profiles can be pathognomonic of gastrointestinal tumors (e.g. VIPoma, gastrinoma, somatostatinoma and carcinoid syndrome). Measurement of the response of plasma pancreatic polypeptide to modified sham feeding or insulin-induced hypoglycemia is also a simple, safe and robust measure of abdominal vagal function and can be valuable as a test of autonomic function and the completeness of surgical vagotomy.

## FURTHER READING


Adrian T E, Ferri G L, Bacarese-Hamilton A J, Fuessl H S, Polak J M, Bloom S R 1985 Human distribution and release of a putative new gut hormone, peptide Y Y. Gastroenterology 89: 1070–1077

Adrian T E, Ballantyne G H, Longo W E et al 1993 Deoxycholate is an important releaser of peptide YY and enteroglucagon from the human colon. Gut 34: 1219–1224

Anagnostides A A, Christofides N D, Tatemoto K, Chadwick V S, Bloom S R 1984 Peptide histidine isoleucine: a secretagogue in human jejunum. Gut 25: 381–385

Boivin M, Bradette M, Raymond M C, Riberdy-Poitras M, Poitras P 1992 Mechanisms for postprandial release of motilin in humans. Digestive Diseases and Sciences 37: 1562–1568

Camilleri M, von der Ohe M R 1994 Drugs affecting 5HT receptors. In: Hawkey C J (ed), Baillière's clinical gastroenterology: drugs in gastroenterology. Baillière Tindall, London

DeValle J, Yamada J 1990 The gut as an endocrine organ. Annual Review of Medicine 41: 447–455

Fried M, Mayer E A, Jansen J B M J et al 1988 Temporal relationships of cholecystokinin release, pancreatico-biliary secretion and gastric emptying of a mixed meal. Gastroenterology 95: 1344–1350

Furness J B, Costa M 1987 The enteric nervous system. Churchill Livingstone, Edinburgh

Furness J B, Bornstein J C, Smith T K 1990 The normal structure of gastrointestinal innervation. Journal of Gastroenterology and Hepatology 1: 1–9

Holst J J 1983 Gut glucagon, enteroglucagon, gut glucagon-like immunoreactivity, glicentin – current status. Gastroenterology 84: 1602–1613

Kreymann B, Williams G, Ghatei M A, Bloom S R 1987 Glucagon-like peptide-17–36: a physiological incretin in man. Lancet 2: 1300–1303

Kromer W 1988 Endogenous and exogenous opioids in the control of gastrointestinal motility and secretion. Pharmacological Reviews 40: 121–162

Lucey M R 1987 Endogenous somatostatin and the gut. Gut 27: 457–467

Makhlouf G M 1989 Neural and endocrine biology of the gut. In: Handbook of physiology, Vol 11, Section 6. The gastrointestinal tract. Oxford University Press, New York

Maton P N 1993 The management of Zollinger–Ellison syndrome. Alimentary Pharmacology and Therapeutics 7: 467–475

Mayer E A, Raybould H E 1990 Role of visceral afferent mechanisms in functional bowel disorders. Gastroenterology 99: 1688–1704

Sarna S 1985 Cyclic motor activity; migrating motor complex: 1985. Gastroenterology 89: 894–913

Sarna S 1991 Physiology and pathophysiology of colonic motor activity (parts 1 and 2). Digestive Diseases and Sciences 36: 827–862 and 998–1018

Stark M E, Szurszewski J H 1992 Role of nitric oxide in gastrointestinal and hepatic function and disease. Gastroenterology 103: 1928–1949

Sun E A, Snape W J, Cohen S, Renny A 1982 The role of opiate receptors and cholinergic neurons in the gastrocolonic response. Gastroenterology 82: 689–693

Thor K, Rosell S 1986 Neurotensin increases colonic motility. Gastroenterology 90: 27–31

Von der Ohe M R, Camilleri M, Kvols L K, Thomforde G M 1993 Motor dysfunction of the small bowel and colon in patients with the carcinoid syndrome and diarrhea. New England Journal of Medicine 329: 1073–1078

Walsh J H 1987 Gastrointestinal hormones. In: Johnson L R (Ed), Physiology of the gastrointestinal tract. Raven Press, New York, p 181–253

Walsh J H, Grossman M I 1975 Gastrin I and II. New England Journal of Medicine 292: 1324–1334 and 1377–1384

Wood J D 1984 Enteric neurophysiology. American Journal of Physiology 247: G585–G598

Wynick D, Williams S J, Bloom S R 1988 Symptomatic secondary hormone syndromes in patients with established malignant pancreatic endocrine tumors. New England Journal of Medicine 319: 605–607

# 7. The esophagus: physiology, motility and other disorders

*Richard H. Holloway*

The esophagus has one principal function, the controlled movement of solids, liquids and gas between the pharynx and the stomach. This is achieved by co-ordinated activity of the esophageal body and sphincters at its proximal and distal ends which is controlled by central and local neural mechanisms. The primary objective of this chapter is to review normal esophageal motor function and the consequences, symptomatic and functional, of motor dysfunction. Pharyngeal motor function is also included as disturbances of this region share many similarities of symptomatology, investigation and management. The principles of investigation of esophageal disease are discussed, with particular emphasis on esophageal manometry. Details of other diagnostic techniques are included in Chapter 8. This chapter also reviews a number of structural disorders that disturb esophageal transport.

## ANATOMY AND PHYSIOLOGY

### Anatomy

The esophagus consists of a hollow muscular tube about 20–25 cm in length and extends from the cricopharyngeus muscle at the level of the sixth cervical vertebra to the gastroesophageal junction just below the diaphragm. The esophagus is often divided into upper, middle and lower thirds. This is simply a convenience; the upper third extends to the aortic arch, the middle third to the inferior pulmonary vein and the lower third to the gastroesophageal junction. Sometimes these divisions are measured from the incisor teeth; the upper third extends to 18 cm, the middle from 18 to 29 cm and the lower third from 30 cm onward (Pearson 1966), although these measurements take no account of the size of the patient.

It is also necessary to consider the hypopharynx in this chapter because its disorders frequently cause dysphagia. It lies immediately behind the larynx and extends from the epiglottis to the cricopharyngeus. The relationship of the muscles of the pharynx to those of the esophagus is shown in Figure 7.1.

The muscular wall of the esophagus consists of an outer longitudinal and inner circular layer. In the upper third, striated muscle predominates, in the lower third, smooth muscle and in the middle third there is a transition zone containing both striated and smooth muscle. The esophagus is bounded at each end by sphincters which, by maintaining tonic contraction, control the movement of luminal contents. The upper esophageal sphincter (UES) consists mainly of the cricopharyngeus muscle, a small part of the inferior constrictor muscle of the hypopharynx superiorly and some circular muscle fibers of the esophagus inferiorly; together they form a high pressure zone about 3 cm in length (Welch et al 1979). The UES is supplied by pharyngeal branches of the vagus. The lowest 3–5 cm of the esophagus functions as a physiological lower esophageal sphincter (LES) 2–3 cm in length. The circular muscle in this region shows asymmetric thickening and mechanical specialization in comparison to esophageal body muscle (Liebermann-Meffert et al 1979).

The esophagus is lined by squamous epithelium onto the surface of which open numerous mucus-secreting glands of the submucosa. The motor nerves of the esophagus are the vagi; the striated muscle is innervated directly via preganglionic motor fibers whereas the smooth muscle is innervated by postganglionic nerve fibers from Auerbach's plexus.

### Normal esophageal motility (Goyal & Paterson 1989, Cook 1991)

The events during swallowing have been studied by radiological techniques, including fluoroscopic videorecording, (p. 9), and manometry (p. 170). Swallowing can be divided into four phases: preparatory, oral, pharyngeal and esophageal. The oral phase is considered to be largely voluntary whereas the pharyngeal phase, once triggered, is entirely involuntary. The preparatory phase involves the formation of a bolus and lubrication. The tongue pushes the bolus into the pharynx at which time the soft palate rises and seals off the nasopharynx to prevent postnasal regurgitation. As the food is propelled onwards by the

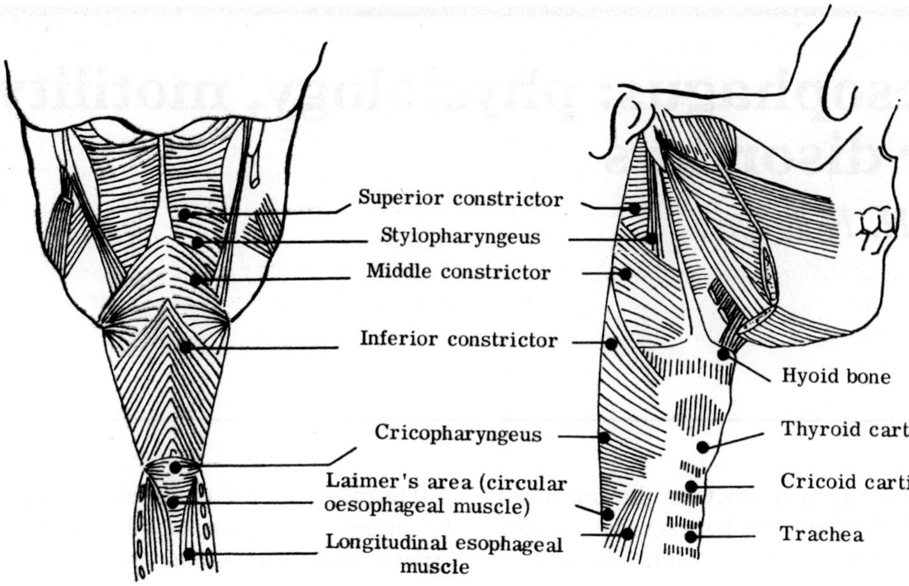


**Fig. 7.1** Posterior and lateral views of pharyngeal constrictors, cricopharyngeus and esophageal musculature. Note that fibers of the cricopharyngeus blend with the lower fibers of the inferior constrictors above, while its lower fibers blend with circular fibers of the esophagus (Payne & Olsen 1974).

sequential contraction of the pharyngeal constrictors, the suprahyoid muscles elevate the larynx and tilt the epiglottis to prevent access to the larynx and thereby aspiration. The most important barrier to aspiration, however, is apposition of the true vocal cords. As the pharyngeal constrictors start to contract, the UES relaxes, allowing food to enter the esophagus, and then immediately contracts so that esophageal contraction does not cause food to regurgitate into the pharynx. In addition to relaxation, UES opening is also a result of external traction on the cricoid cartilage and internal pulsion from the pressure generated within the oncoming bolus.

The swallowed bolus is propelled down the esophagus by primary peristalsis, a propagated wave of contraction initiated by swallowing. Once initiated, the motor responses that follow are relatively stereotyped involuntary ones. The pressure changes and radiological features of esophageal peristalsis are detailed in Chapter 1 and below. Residual material is cleared from the esophagus by secondary peristalsis which is initiated by esophageal distention. Occasionally, a swallow is not followed by a primary peristaltic wave. This happens more frequently in the absence of a bolus (i.e. a dry swallow) and also in the elderly (Khan et al 1977). Relaxation of the LES is also initiated by swallowing and persists until the arrival of the peristaltic wave.

## Control of esophageal motility

*Upper esophageal sphincter* (Miller 1986)

The UES maintains tonic contraction by continuous neural excitation through somatic nerves in the vagus; there is also a small passive component. Relaxation of the UES is controlled by transient inhibition of the tonically active somatic neurons and is followed by hypercontraction. These events are co-ordinated in the swallowing center (see below). The UES prevents reflux of esophageal contents into the pharynx and esophageal distention by air as a result of the decreased intrathoracic pressure induced by respiration. Basal UES pressure in awake subjects who are sitting quietly is relatively stable but falls considerably during sleep (Kahrilas et al 1987). UES pressure increases in response to stress, esophageal acidification (Gerhardt et al 1978) and slow esophageal distention (Kahrilas et al 1987). Sudden esophageal distention, however, as with an air bolus, leads to UES relaxation and belching (Kahrilas et al 1986).

*Esophageal body* (Diamant & El Sharkawy 1977, Christensen 1987)

The excitation of the esophageal muscle is predominantly neurogenic. For esophageal peristalsis initiated by swallowing or by a bolus in the lumen of the upper esophagus, the primary control mechanism resides in a swallowing center in the brain-stem composed of nuclei and reticular formation. From this center a programmed sequence of efferent discharges passes via the trigeminal, facial, vagus and hypoglossal nerves to the oropharynx and to progressively distal segments of esophageal striated muscle. The swallowing center can be influenced by afferent signals from the oropharynx and esophagus; thus the force and velocity of the peristaltic contraction varies with the nature of the swallowed bolus.

Control of the smooth muscle part of the esophagus is initiated in the swallowing center, the nerve supply being via the parasympathetic and sympathetic tracts to the myenteric plexus. However, a peripheral control system exists which can stimulate peristalsis independently from the central nervous system; it is primarily neurogenic and mediated via the myenteric plexus, although mechanisms intrinsic to the smooth muscle may play a role. The mechanism of neuromuscular transmission that produces peristaltic activation of esophageal smooth muscle is complex and poorly understood but is believed to depend on coordination between the stimulation of a noncholinergic nonadrenergic inhibitory mechanism and a cholinergic excitatory mechanism.

### Lower esophageal sphincter

The lowest 3–5 cm of the esophageal body functions as a lower esophageal sphincter (LES). The muscle is thicker and on electron microscopy, in contrast to the esophageal body, the muscle bundles are more widely separated by bands of connective tissue and the circular muscle cells have extensive evaginations of their cell surface (Seelig & Goyal 1978). The LES exhibits different mechanical properties from the esophageal body (Biancani et al 1973); circular muscle strips develop greater active tension that is independent of neural control than do strips from the esophageal body. The mechanisms responsible for maintaining this tone are poorly understood but may involve a lower resting membrane potential than that in the esophageal body, allowing for a slow inward leak of calcium ions (Zelcer & Weisbrodt 1984).

Basal LES pressure also depends on tonic neural input. In humans muscarinic cholinergic blockade with atropine reduces LES pressure by 40%–80% (Dodds et al 1981); alpha-adrenergic mechanisms may also be involved. Experiments in animals suggest that the neural input is predominantly vagal. Evidence that circulating hormones exert significant levels of control on basal LES pressure is at best circumstantial. However, it is possible that the inhibitory effects of fat (Nebel & Castell 1973) and the stimulatory effects of protein (Maher et al 1984) on LES pressure are mediated via hormones. Basal LES pressure often shows considerable variability from minute to minute. In the fasting state, cyclical increases occur during the interdigestive motor cycle. LES pressure is lowest during phase I and increases throughout the cycle. Superimposed on the increase in basal pressure are phasic contractions that occur synchronously with gastric contractions seen during phases II and III (Dent et al 1983). It seems possible that circulating motilin mediates this activity (Holloway et al 1985).

Relaxation of the LES occurs with swallowing, esophageal distention and transiently during belching (Wyman et al 1990). Swallow-induced relaxation is an active process mediated by the vagus nerve via nonadrenergic noncholinergic inhibitory postganglionic motor neurons. Relaxation induced by esophageal distention is mediated by intrinsic nerves. Transient LES relaxation associated with belching or gastroesophageal reflux is currently thought to be a vagal reflex triggered by gastric distention (p. 192) (Holloway & Dent 1990). The neurotransmitters that mediate LES relaxation have yet to be determined; current evidence supports a major role for nitric oxide (Paterson et al 1992) and VIP may also be involved.

## SYMPTOMS

Disturbances of esophageal motility give rise to symptoms because bolus transit is disrupted, contractions are overvigorous or retrograde flow occurs (see Chapter 8). Occasional esophageal symptoms are common, however, and do not always indicate disease. Frequent and persistent dysphagia, odynophagia or chest pain without a cardiac cause point to an esophageal cause that merits further investigation.

### Dysphagia

Dysphagia is defined as a difficulty in swallowing. It always warrants careful and thorough evaluation. True dysphagia should be distinguished from the globus syndrome (see below), aversion to swallowing because of painful pharyngeal or esophageal disorders, odynophagia or painful swallowing and the heightened sensitivity to the normal passage of a bolus, the so-called "tender" esophagus. In an open access dysphagia clinic, of 109 referrals, 90 were judged to have true dysphagia; of these 26% had a malignant stricture, 36% peptic stricture, 13% esophagitis, 7% motility disorder and another 4% had miscellaneous organic disorders. No abnormality was found in 14% (Wilkins et al 1984).

A reliable provisional diagnosis can usually be made on the basis of a careful history. Patients generally present with one of two basic patterns: "high" dysphagia in which the site of hold-up is localized to the neck; and "low" dysphagia in which hold-up is perceived retrosternally. The level at which hold-up is sensed may occasionally be misleading. Whereas dysphagia experienced in the low retrosternal region always indicates a distal esophageal obstruction, hold-up in the mid or proximal esophagus may be localized to the neck or throat, suggesting oropharyngeal dysphagia. Dysphagia solely for solids usually indicates organic obstruction, such as stricture, tumor, ring or web. Bread, meat or potato are frequent offenders. Progressive dysphagia for solids associated with weight loss suggests a malignant stricture. Dysphagia for solids and liquids which may be intermittent suggests a motor disorder. Oropharyngeal dysphagia is usually due to disordered motility and may be accompanied by other symptoms such as coughing or choking during swallowing, difficulty in initiating swallowing, postnasal regurgitation and dysarthria.

When dysphagia is due to a painful condition of the oropharynx, direct inspection will usually reveal the diagnosis. When the history suggests an oropharyngeal cause, neurological examination and visual inspection of the mouth and pharynx are important. A bedside swallow test often yields valuable information. A videoradiographic study of the mouth, pharynx and esophagus should be the initial investigation. As well as outlining structural abnormalities such as pharyngeal pouch, the ability to record multiple swallows and replay them in slow motion provides important information on the nature of the motor dysfunction as well as the presence of unsuspected aspiration.

When the history suggests an esophageal cause, there are two options for investigation. A barium swallow is preferred by most for it is safer. It will diagnose the occasional diverticulum and esophageal displacement and will always indicate the presence of a stricture and its length. When performed as the first test endoscopy may miss an early stricture, fail to adequately assess the length of a stricture and miss webs or diverticula in the proximal esophagus. Endoscopy is insensitive for detecting motor disorders. Endoscopy is always indicated whether the barium swallow is abnormal or not; the mucosa can be inspected and biopsied, the obstructed area can be passed and the stomach and duodenum inspected. Tumors may coexist with achalasia and patients with this disorder should be endoscoped even though the diagnosis may have been made by radiology or manometry. Occasionally other investigations, such as esophageal manometry or radionuclide studies (p. 82), may be required to diagnose the cause of dysphagia.

### *Globus syndrome*

This term describes the sensation of a nonpainful "lump", "tightness", "choking" or "strangling" in the throat which is not related to swallowing. In fact, eating often alleviates the sensation, which is most noticeable between meals. Frequent dry swallowing and emotional stress may aggravate the problem.

## Hiccups (singulus)

In hiccups there is involuntary inspiration against a closed glottis which is mediated by afferent fibers in the phrenic and vagus nerves, brain-stem centers and efferent fibers in the phrenic, vagus, cervical and thoracic nerves. A variety of esophageal lesions may occasionally cause hiccups, including ulcer at the gastroesophageal junction, esophagitis, stricture and bolus obstruction (Kaufmann 1982). Persistent hiccups may itself cause reflux and promote esophagitis (Shay et al 1984). Hiccups may be a sign of diaphragmatic irritation or uremia.

## Esophageal pain

Sensory nerves responding to chemical (e.g. acid), mechanical (e.g. excessive contractions or distention) and thermal stimuli have their endings largely in the submucosa but also in the lamina propria and the basal layers of the squamous epithelium (Christensen 1984). The afferents travel mostly in the vagus nerve but nociceptive sensation travels mostly in the sympathetic nerves. Esophageal pain is felt in dermatomes C8 to T10 which overlap with pain arising in the heart, stomach, liver, pancreas and gallbladder.

### *Heartburn (pyrosis)*

This is a common symptom in the community with about 25% of the adult population experiencing it at least once per month (Smart et al 1986). It is a burning pain located high in the epigastrium or behind the lower end of the sternum, often radiating upwards towards the neck; it characteristically occurs after meals and may be precipitated by bending or stooping. Damage or disruption of the mucosa allows increased access of acid or alkali to nerve endings so that heartburn typically occurs in reflux esophagitis and sometimes in other esophageal mucosal inflammatory disorders.

### *Odynophagia*

This is pain with swallowing. Commonly it occurs when a bolus of food directly irritates an inflamed segment of the mucosa and usually indicates either severe esophagitis or esophageal tumor. Odynophagia may also occur when a bolus of food sticks in the esophagus, particularly when accompanied by excessive contractions.

### *Cardiac-type chest pain* (Holloway 1990)

The esophagus may be a source of pain that is indistinguishable from cardiac pain (Davies et al 1985). Such pain may be described as having a squeezing or burning character and is predominantly retrosternal in location with radiation to the upper chest, neck, jaw and arms. It may be spontaneous but can also be precipitated by swallowing, particularly very hot or cold liquids, meals and emotional stress. Pain episodes may last from a few minutes to several hours and occasionally days. Most patients with esophageal chest pain complain of other esophageal symptoms although about 10% have only chest pain as their presenting complaint.

Chest pain of esophageal origin is often difficult to distinguish from cardiac pain as they share a number of features (Bennett & Atkinson 1966, Davies et al 1985). Nevertheless, helpful clues may be found in the precipitating or relieving factors and the associated symptoms. Features suggestive of an esophageal origin include pain continuing for hours or awakening the patient from sleep, a relationship to swallowing or meals, relief by antacids and the presence of other esophageal symptoms such as heartburn and dysphagia. True angina is more consistently provoked by effort and relieved by rest or nitroglycerine. Both types of pain may be precipitated by emotional stress. Many patients, however, have symptoms of both cardiac and esophageal pain. The prevalence of both cardiac and esophageal disease increases with age and they may therefore coexist. Some patients have what has been termed "linked" angina; that is, they show ECG changes of ischemia when acid is instilled into the esophagus (Davies et al 1985, Anon 1986). The issue is further complicated by the fact that exertional chest pain may result from exercise-induced gastroesophageal reflux (Schofield et al 1987).

### Mechanisms of esophageal pain

Esophageal pain arises by two main mechanisms – stimulation of intramural mechanoreceptors by muscular contraction and/or luminal distention and stimulation of mucosal receptors by the pH, osmolarity or temperature of esophageal contents (Bernstein & Baker 1958, Meyer & Castell 1981, Nasrallah & Hendrix 1987). However, the character of the pain does not necessarily indicate the mechanism of its production. Pain of muscular origin is usually described as gripping or cramping and thus esophageal "spasm" is commonly blamed for all noncardiac chest pain. Mucosal irritation, on the other hand, usually causes a more diffuse retrosternal burning discomfort. However, esophageal distention or excessive contraction may produce a burning discomfort and mucosal irritation may produce angina-like pain (Bernstein et al 1962, Roberts et al 1975). An early notion that esophageal acidification produced pain by triggering esophageal spasm has not been supported by more recent studies (Richter et al 1985). Patients with esophageal chest pain have heightened esophageal sensitivity and experience chest pain at lower distention volumes than normal subjects (Richter et al 1986). Thus altered pain perception may contribute to these patients' reaction to pain stimuli. This may be aggravated by underlying psychological factors (Katon et al 1988).

### Differential diagnosis

A number of esophageal disorders have been identified in patients with cardiac-type chest pain. The actual prevalence of esophageal causes in patients with noncardiac chest pain is unclear because of differences in patient selection and the method of testing among studies and has ranged from 22% to 76% (De Caestecker et al 1985, Katz et al 1987, Richter & Castell 1989, Breumelhof et al 1990, Hewson et al 1990, Lam et al 1992). Ambulatory manometry and pH monitoring have shown that pain is associated with reflux and abnormal motility with about equal frequency. Some patients may experience pain through both acid reflux and dysmotility and the term "irritable" esophagus has been coined to describe this phenomenon.

Other gastrointestinal disorders may cause chest pain, e.g. peptic ulcer, biliary colic, acute cholecystitis and pancreatitis, but these nearly always have other distinguishing features (Long & Cohen 1980).

### Diagnosis

An essential step in the diagnosis of noncardiac chest pain is the exclusion of ischemic heart disease. The extent to which this is done will depend on clinical circumstances. A resting and exercise ECG should be performed. Exercise thallium imaging is often helpful and coronary angiography may be indicated.

Esophageal testing should aim not only to define any underlying esophageal disease but to establish a clear link between the abnormality and chest pain. Endoscopy identifies any erosive or ulcerative esophagitis. Whilst a positive finding does not prove a causal relationship, it is reasonable to give a trial of antireflux therapy before proceeding with further tests. Standard esophageal manometry and Bernstein test may be helpful and are usually performed. The most rewarding investigation, however, is 24-h ambulatory pH monitoring (p. 197). Ambulatory esophageal manometry is also helpful but is not widely available. Prolonged ambulatory tests identify abnormal patterns of motility and reflux and assess the relationship between reflux, motor events and symptoms. Provocative testing with bethanechol or edrophonium is of doubtful value and has largely been abandoned.

### Treatment

Treatment of the causative disorder is undertaken whenever possible. Explanation and reassurance to the patient is of great importance, particularly in relation to negative cardiac investigations, because the outlook for such patients is excellent (Proudfit et al 1966).

Reflux disease should be treated in the usual manner (p. 198). Painful motor disorders may be treated with nitroglycerine 0.6 mg p.r.n., isosorbide 10–20 mg four times a day, nifedipine 10–20 mg three times a day or diltiazem 60–90 mg four times a day. However, there are few controlled clinical trials and the clinical efficacy is variable. If such specific measures fail, or in patients without a definable cause for their pain, low-dose antidepressant therapy, e.g. amitriptyline 25–50 mg at night or trazodone 100–150 mg per day, may be helpful as a pain-modifying approach (Clouse et al 1987).

## ESOPHAGEAL MANOMETRY

Esophageal manometry provides an accurate definition of esophageal motor activity and is the procedure of choice in the diagnosis of esophageal motor disorders. Videofluoroscopy (p. 9) and scintigraphy (p. 82) are complementary techniques. Videofluoroscopy is the diagnostic procedure of first choice for oropharyngeal dysphagia.

### Indications

Esophageal manometry is indicated in patients whose symptoms or other investigations, e.g. radiological studies, suggest a motor disorder. It is particularly useful in the diagnosis of dysphagia. In patients with diffuse spasm, manometry can define the extent of the motor abnormality and thus guide the extent of esophagomyotomy (Pope 1978). Manometry is also useful to define the degree of esophageal motor dysfunction in patients with reflux disease before undergoing antireflux surgery. Normal manometric measurements have been defined by Richter (Richter et al 1987).

### Apparatus

Manometry is usually performed using a perfused manometric assembly about 3–4 mm in diameter containing eight individual lumens. Each lumen terminates in a sidehole orifice. The sideholes are positioned at intervals of 4–5 cm along the assembly to enable pressures to be recorded concurrently from multiple sites along the esophagus. Each lumen is connected to an external pressure transducer and perfused with degassed distilled water at 0.5 ml per min by a low-compliance pneumohydraulic perfusion pump (Arndorfer et al 1977). Occlusion of the sideholes by esophageal contraction results in a rise in pressure within the lumen equal to the pressure exerted on the sidehole. The pressure is sensed by the transducer and converted to an electrical signal that is recorded by either a multichannel chart recorder or a computer. Simultaneous measurement of pressure at several sites permits assessment of co-ordinated motor activity. Recently miniature intraluminal transducers have been developed for recording esophageal motility. However, these are fragile and comparatively very expensive. Such assemblies, therefore, usually incorporate fewer recording sites than standard perfusion manometry and allow only short segments of the esophagus to be evaluated at any one time.

Measurement of pressure in the upper and lower esophageal sphincters entails particular difficulties because of their short length (3–4 cm) and their mobility during swallowing and esophageal peristalsis (Dodds et al 1974). Although sphincter pressure can be sampled for short intervals by drawing a sidehole sensor through the sphincter it is difficult to maintain a sidehole within the sphincter to make prolonged continuous pressure measurements. A sleeve sensor (Dent 1976), 6 cm in length, has been developed which overcomes this problem. It is incorporated into the distal end of the manometric assembly for recording LES pressure and into the middle of the assembly for recording UES pressure (Kahrilas et al 1987). The sleeve accurately records sphincter pressure and relaxation despite axial movement of the sphincter and yields important information about the dynamic sphincter function not possible with sidehole recording.

### Procedure

The assembly is introduced through the nose using topical nasal anesthesia and is passed down the esophagus. If the assembly has a sleeve sensor, it is positioned so that the sleeve straddles the LES. If no sleeve is present, the assembly is passed down so that the distal three radially oriented sideholes are in the stomach. The patient then lies quietly while measurements are made. Manometric assessment of esophageal motor function includes evaluation of the LES, esophageal body and in some instances UES and pharynx. Sphincters are evaluated for their resting pressure and ability to relax. The esophageal body and pharynx are examined for peristaltic and nonperistaltic motor activity.

#### *Lower esophageal sphincter*

***Basal pressure.*** Basal LES pressure can be assessed by three main techniques: station pull-through (or stepwise withdrawal), rapid pull-through (or rapid withdrawal) or using the sleeve sensor. Basal LES pressure is measured at end-expiration and referenced to intragastric pressure. Normal pressures are usually between 10 and 30 mmHg above intragastric pressure and the zone of elevated pressure is usually between 2 and 4 cm in length. Basal pressure may be increased in achalasia (p. 175) and decreased in reflux esophagitis (p. 191) and systemic sclerosis (p. 179).

***Relaxation*** (Fig. 7.2). LES relaxation is evaluated during water swallows of a 5 ml bolus. Normally the LES starts to relax 1–2 s after the initiation of swallowing and relaxes by at least 90% of its resting pressure. Relaxation lasts from 5–10 s and is usually terminated by the oncoming peristaltic wave. Relaxation is impaired in achalasia (p. 175) and Chagas' disease and rarely in diffuse spasm.

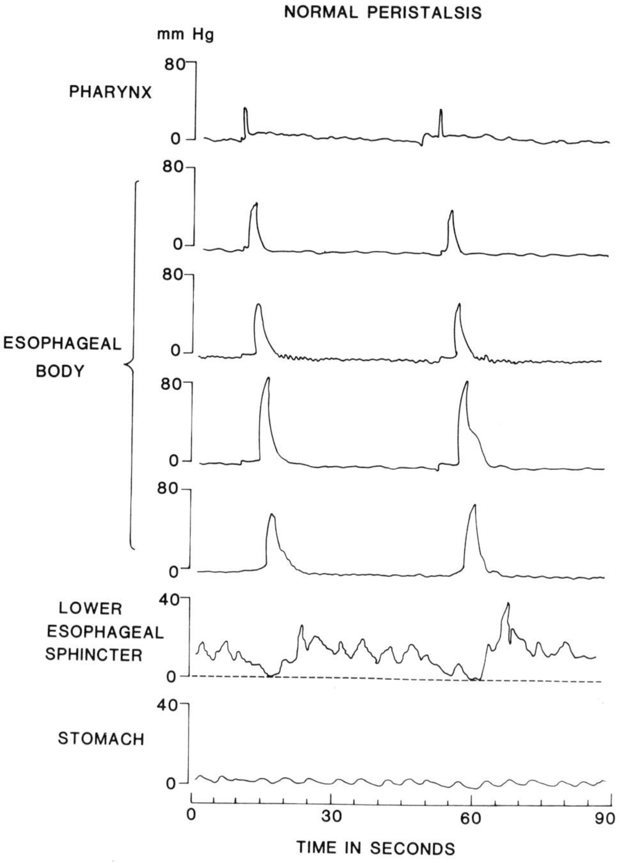


**Fig. 7.2** Esophageal motor response to water swallow. Swallowing, indicated by the brief pharyngeal pressure spike, triggers lower esophageal sphincter relaxation and a complete peristaltic wave that traverses the entire length of the esophagus.

### Esophageal body

Motility of the esophageal body is evaluated best by using a series of sidehole sensors spaced at 3–5 cm intervals which span the entire length of the esophagus (about 20–25 cm). Peristalsis is evaluated using at least ten water swallows of a 5 ml bolus (Richter et al 1987) spaced at least 20 s apart to avoid physiological interference between adjacent esophageal responses (Ask & Tibbling 1980, Vanek & Diamant 1987). Swallowing should be monitored with a pharyngeal sensor and double or multiple swallows discarded from the analysis.

Water swallows usually evoke a propagated contraction that sweeps down the esophagus in a smooth uninterrupted fashion at a speed of 1–5 cm/s (Fig. 7.2). The contraction wave moves fastest in the proximal esophagus and slows distally. Contractions are usually single peaked, although occasionally double-peaked contractions may be seen. Triple-peaked, repetitive or synchronous contractions are abnormal. Contraction amplitude in the distal esophagus is about 80 mmHg (range 70–150 mmHg) and their duration normally <7.5 s (Benjamin et al 1979, Richter et al 1987).

**Pharynx and upper esophageal sphincter** (Orlowski et al 1982, Dodds et al 1987)

Manometric recording of the pharynx and UES places special demands on the recording system. Pharyngeal contractions are of much shorter duration (0.3–0.5 s) and propagate more rapidly (9–25 cm/s) than do esophageal contractions and generally exceed the fidelity of perfusion manometric systems, although the occurrence and timing of the contraction can be recorded adequately. Intraluminal transducers have sufficient fidelity but have limited recording sites. The UES is very short with the zone that yields 50–100% of maximal pressure being less than 1 cm in length (Kahrilas et al 1987) and moves substantially during swallowing, making it difficult to maintain a sidehole sensor within the sphincter. This difficulty has been overcome with a sleeve sensor which is usually incorporated into a special assembly designed to meet the demands of pharyngoesophageal manometry. The sleeve accurately measures basal pressure and the onset and completeness of UES relaxation, although it may underestimate fractionally the duration of relaxation.

***Basal pressure.*** This is measured by the same techniques used to measure LES pressure. Recent studies have shown, however, that the rapid pull-through technique with sidehole sensors may yield falsely high pressures because of stimulation of the sphincter by the assembly. The station pull-through technique, however, yields values comparable to those obtained by sleeve manometry (Kahrilas et al 1987). Basal UES pressures are usually in the range 60–80 mmHg.

***Relaxation*** (Fig. 7.3). The UES relaxes abruptly with the onset of swallowing and pharyngeal peristalsis and usually remains relaxed until the pharyngeal peristaltic wave reaches the sphincter. The duration of relaxation is about 0.5 s and is slightly longer for water than for dry swallows.

## OROPHARYNGEAL DYSPHAGIA

Oropharyngeal dysphagia can be caused by structural or motor disorders (Table 7.1). Structural disorders include the effects of surgery and radiotherapy, tumors, strictures, webs and extrinsic compression of the pharynx or cervical esophagus. Motor disorders are caused by diseases of the central nervous system, peripheral nerve, motor endplate or skeletal muscle. Diseases which involve the pharynx and/or UES have characteristic symptoms. There are repeated attempts to initiate swallowing, coughing whilst eating, food sticking in the throat and nasal regurgitation of liquids whilst trying to swallow.

### Disordered upper esophageal sphincter function

Opening of the UES involves two processes: relaxation of

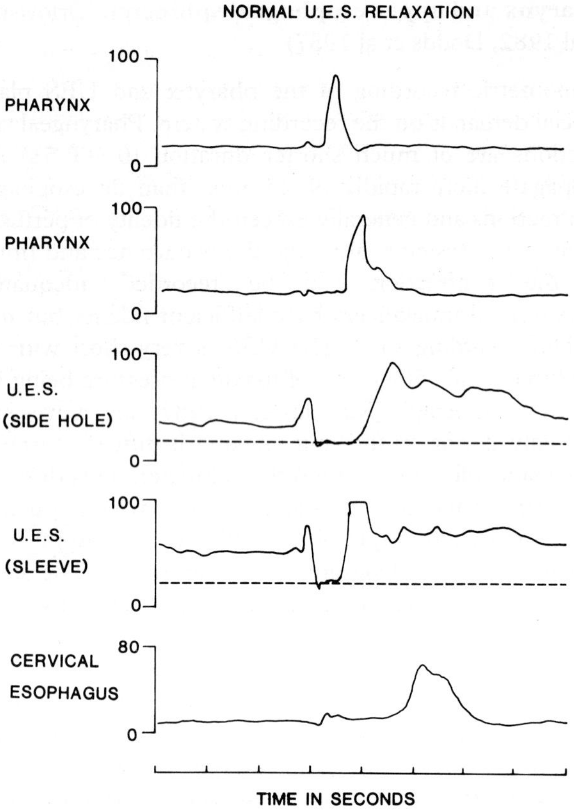


**Fig. 7.3** Normal relaxation of the upper esophageal sphincter (UES).

**Table 7.1** Causes of oropharyngeal dysphagia

| |
|---|
| *Structural lesions* |
| **Intrinsic** |
| Oropharyngeal tumors |
| Inflammatory disorders |
| Surgical resection |
| Radiation fibrosis |
| Cricopharyngeal bar |
| Pharyngeal diverticulum |
| Postcricoid web |
| **Extrinsic** |
| Cervical osteophyte |
| Cervical tumor |
| Thyromegaly |
| *Central nervous system disorders* |
| Cerebrovascular accident |
| Multiple sclerosis |
| Motor neurone disease |
| Extrapyramidal disorders (Parkinson's disease, Wilson's disease, Huntington's chorea) |
| Degenerative diseases (Alzheimer's, Friedreich's ataxia, spinocerebellar degeneration) |
| Familial dysautonomia |
| *Peripheral nervous system disorders* |
| Poliomyelitis |
| Guillain–Barré syndrome |
| Neurotoxins |
| *Neuromuscular junction* |
| Myasthenia gravis |
| Botulism |
| *Muscle disorders* |
| Inflammatory myopathy (polymyositis, dermatomyositis) |
| Muscular dystrophy |
| Thyrotoxic myopathy |

the striated muscle, and mechanical opening by traction from the suprahyoid muscles and pulsion from the oncoming bolus as a result of pharyngeal contraction. Abnormal UES relaxation, or cricopharyngeal "achalasia", is uncommon and rare as an isolated phenomenon. It is seen with lesions affecting the medullary swallow center (e.g. stroke, head trauma) in which impaired sphincter relaxation is accompanied by abnormalities of pharyngeal propulsion. Inco-ordination of UES relaxation has been reported in some cases of dysphagia.

Abnormal UES opening occurs with cricopharyngeal bar (Dantas et al 1990) and Zenker's diverticulum (Cook et al 1992a). Cricopharyngeal bar is often labeled as cricopharyngeal "achalasia" or "spasm". However, when measured manometrically UES relaxation is normal. The abnormal opening in Zenker's diverticulum appears to be a result of decreased muscle compliance because of fibrosis (Cook et al 1992b). Deficient traction can occur in isolation following local muscle damage (e.g. surgery, radiotherapy). More commonly, however, the abnormality has a neurological basis and is accompanied by disordered pharyngeal propulsion.

## Disorders of the nervous system

The commonest cause of oropharyngeal dysphagia is cerebrovascular disease (stroke). Dysphagia occurs particularly when the lesion is in the brain-stem or cerebellum but may also occur with hemisphere lesions. The dysfunction involves both the pharyngeal muscles and the UES. Disordered swallowing is a feature of Parkinson's disease and involves both the oral and pharyngeal phases. The degree of dysfunction apparent radiologically is usually greater than that anticipated on the basis of disease severity or reported symptoms. Dysphagia is common with multiple sclerosis and motor neurone disease (amyotrophic lateral sclerosis) and may be a residual problem after poliomyelitis. In the rare hereditary disorder of dysautonomia (Riley–Day syndrome) there is a widespread derangement of the autonomic nervous system (Margulies et al 1968) which causes pharyngeal dysphagia; decreased esophageal motility and LES pressure and delayed gastric emptying predispose to gastroesophageal reflux disease and recurrent aspiration pneumonia and fundoplication may be necessary to prevent this (Axelrod et al 1987).

### *Disorders of the pharyngeal muscles*

***Polymyositis-dermatomyositis.*** Dysphagia occurs in about 50% of cases. Manometric studies show decreased pharyngeal contractions, decreased UES pressure and decreased contractions in the upper third of the esophagus. There is also dysfunction of the distal esophagus and gastric and esophageal emptying is delayed (Horowitz et al 1986), indicating widespread involvement of smooth muscle. Barium studies show retention of barium in the valleculae, diminished peristaltic activity in the pharynx and nasal reflux of barium during swallowing.

***Myasthenia gravis.*** Occasionally, difficulty in swallowing may be the presenting feature of the disease. The patient swallows normally at the start of the meal but has increasing difficulty as the meal progresses. Pharyngeal motility is diminished.

***Thyrotoxic myopathy.*** Like myasthenia gravis, thyrotoxic myopathy is a treatable myopathy with a predilection for the bulbar muscles.

***Myotonic dystrophy*** (Nowak et al 1982). Characteristically these patients have frontal baldness, cataracts, muscle wasting and myotonia. Dysphagia is common and aspiration pneumonia is the usual cause of death. The muscles of the pharynx, UES and upper third of the esophagus are involved and manometry shows diminished pharyngeal contraction and decreased UES pressure with prolonged relaxation during swallowing. The smooth muscle of the esophagus, stomach and intestines also shows atrophy; there is delay in esophageal and gastric emptying and gastrointestinal symptoms are common (Horowitz et al 1987).

***Oculopharyngeal dystrophy*** (Nowak et al 1982). This autosomal dominant condition occurs predominantly in French Canadians (Duranceau et al 1983) although families in other countries have been reported. Degeneration of facial, extraocular and pharyngeal muscles occurs. Commonly the patient presents with ptosis followed by dysphagia. Pharyngeal and UES pressures are usually decreased. The disorder may be distinguished from myasthenia gravis by the absence of fatiguability and improvement with edrophonium (Tensilon).

***Mixed connective tissue disease*** (Marshall et al 1990). This condition affects predominantly the smooth muscle of the lower esophagus. However, pressures in the UES are also reduced, thus raising the possibility that striated muscle is also involved.

#### *Investigation*

In most instances it is possible to distinguish oropharyngeal from esophageal dysphagia on the basis of a careful history. The most useful and informative test is the video barium swallow which should be the first investigation in most cases. Static radiology is inadequate for resolution of motor abnormalities but may demonstrate important anatomical or structural abnormalities such as strictures, webs, tumors, pouches, bars and external compression. Direct pharyngolaryngoscopy is important for the identification of structural lesions of the larynx, pharynx and cervical esophagus, although it may not be necessary in cases where there is an obvious neurological or myopathic cause. Small tumors in the hypopharynx, postcricoid region or larynx, however, can mimic neuromuscular dysfunction. Manometry can yield additional information and therefore supplements the results of videofluoroscopy. It permits quantification of the strength of pharyngeal contractions and an assessment of the resistance to flow across the UES by measurement of the hypopharyngeal pressure ahead of the pharyngeal wave (Cook et al 1992).

Specific diagnostic tests are necessary to confirm primary muscle disorders such as polymyositis, myasthenia gravis, thyrotoxicosis and connective tissue disease. A CT or MRI scan may be indicated to identify the site and nature of lesions in the central nervous system.

#### *Treatment*

In some patients dysphagia may be improved by treatment of the underlying medical condition, e.g. Parkinsonism and myasthenia gravis; the dysphagia of myotonic dystrophy may respond to procainamide. Cricopharyngeal myotomy is effective for disorders of UES opening or relaxation and may help in other causes of oropharyngeal dysphagia. Dysphagia following a stroke commonly improves with time. Enteral nutrition with a nasogastric tube or percutaneous gastrostomy are established methods for nutritional support.

## MOTILITY DISORDERS OF THE ESOPHAGUS

Motor disorders of the esophagus may be categorized as either primary or secondary to systemic disease. The major primary disorders are achalasia and diffuse spasm.

### Achalasia

The clinical features of this disorder and its treatment by a whalebone bougie were described first in 1674 by Thomas Willis but the term achalasia, meaning "failure to relax", was coined by Sir Arthur Hurst.

#### *Epidemiology*

The disorder has been reported from many countries but there are few studies of its incidence. Investigations in Malmo and Liverpool (Ellis & Olsen 1969) and Edinburgh (Howard et al 1992) suggest an incidence of 1 in 100 000 per year. The sex ratio is approximately equal. It usually occurs between the ages of 40 and 70 years and is uncommon in children. Of 601 patients, only 24 were under the age of 10 when symptoms first developed. The disorder has been reported in twins and siblings.

*Pathology*

The esophagus is dilated above the narrowed cardia, but the muscle wall appears normal, except in long-standing disease when it becomes thin. The epithelium may be ulcerated and there is some predisposition to the development of carcinoma.

On microscopic examination there is degeneration and marked loss of ganglion cells in Auerbach's plexus; this is particularly marked in the dilated segment of the esophagus and in patients with long-standing disease. Other features include variable mononuclear cell inflammation and fibrosis with atrophy and mural scarring. The vagus nerves are normal on light microscopy, but electronmicroscopy has shown both axonal and Schwann cell changes. The dorsal motor nucleus of the vagus shows a decrease in nerve cells. In the lower esophagus there is reduction in the small nerve fibers which contain vasoactive intestinal polypeptide (VIP) (Aggestrup et al 1983) and nitric oxide (Mearin et al 1993). Pharmacological and in vitro studies have shown that there is impairment of the postganglionic inhibitory nerve fibers to the LES with sparing of the cholinergic innervation (Holloway et al 1986, Tottrup et al 1990). The etiology of achalasia is unknown.

*Clinical features*

Dysphagia occurs in almost every case, the patient localizing it to the lower sternum. Initially intermittent, it soon becomes constant. Most patients have more difficulty with solids than with liquids, but when solids stick they can be forced down with large volumes of fluid, particularly fizzy drinks, or by performing a Valsalva maneuver. Regurgitation is very common and occurs particularly soon after eating or at night. The regurgitated material is not sour or bitter to the taste. Dysphagia and regurgitation lead to avoidance of eating in public and at home cold foods and some solid foods are avoided. Respiratory complications are common because of regurgitation and include aspiration pneumonitis, asthma attacks, bronchiectasis or lung abscess. The patient complains of cough at night and dyspnea after meals. Pain occurs in about one-third of cases. It is usually retrosternal, may be referred to the back or shoulders and may be precipitated by cold liquids. It usually occurs early in the disease when there is disordered motility in the body of the esophagus.

Achalasia is a progressive disorder. In the early or mild phase, esophageal dilatation may be absent or only slight. There is motor hyperactivity and occasional pain on swallowing. Regurgitation is not marked. In moderate achalasia the esophagus dilates further, there are simultaneous contractions and retention of food and secretions in the esophagus but food can be forced through the LES by Valsalva maneuver or drinking fizzy drinks. Regurgitation tends to occur immediately after meals. Finally, in severe achalasia, the esophagus is greatly dilated (above 6 cm in diameter) and tortuous and lacks motor activity so that pain no longer occurs. Food cannot be forced through the sphincter, the patient loses weight and regurgitation and pulmonary complications are severe.

Carcinoma may arise secondary to long-standing achalasia (p. 205) and typically occurs in the middle third of the esophagus. Because the esophagus is dilated, the tumor is usually very advanced before additional symptoms are experienced.

*Diagnosis*

***Radiology.*** The chest X-ray characteristically shows a mediastinum widened by the dilated esophagus in which a fluid level may be seen. Gas is usually absent from the gastric fundus.

At barium swallow (p. 5), in the early stages peristalsis is seen to pass normally through the upper third of the esophagus to the level of the aortic arch, but distally there is vigorous and disordered motor activity, sometimes confused with diffuse esophageal spasm. In some patients with early disease these abnormalities are only visible in the prone position with full distention of the esophagus. Later, the esophagus is usually dilated and may be greatly elongated, sometimes assuming a sigmoid shape. The lower end characteristically tapers smoothly like a "bird's beak" over a length of 1–4 cm (Fig. 7.4). Occasionally the esophagus is only slightly dilated, but in almost all estab-

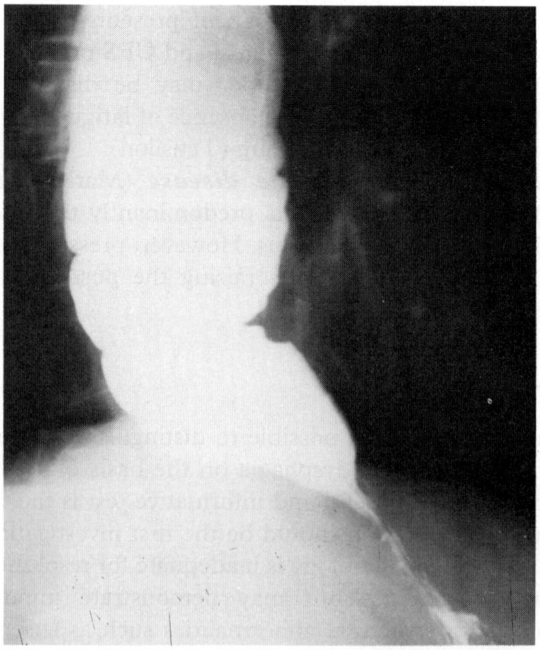

**Fig. 7.4** Achalasia of the esophagus. There is gross dilatation with a large fluid residue, typical "bird beak" narrowing at the lower end, and absence of a gastric air bubble.

lished cases primary peristalsis is absent in the lower two-thirds of the esophagus and the narrowed segment and LES fail to relax after swallowing a bolus. If the double-contrast technique is used, the mucosal folds appear normal, although these are often difficult to display because of food residue. If possible, good views should be obtained of the gastric cardia to look for a tumor as a cause of secondary achalasia.

***Esophageal manometry.*** Although a confident diagnosis can often be made on the basis of a barium swallow, esophageal manometry should be performed in all cases to confirm the diagnosis. The hallmarks of the disease are absent peristalsis and failure of the LES to relax completely with swallowing (Fig. 7.5). With the development of esophageal retention, basal intraesophageal pressure may be higher than intragastric pressure. In about half of the patients basal LES pressure is increased (>30 mmHg). In some patients LES relaxation may be complete but abbreviated (Katz et al 1986). In the early stages simultaneous and repetitive contractions may replace peristalsis. As the esophagus dilates, however, the contractions become feeble and in advanced or classic achalasia there may be no contractions at all. A return of peristalsis has been reported in a minority of patients after treatment (Bianco et al 1986).

A subset of achalasia patients with higher amplitude contractions in the esophageal body have been identified as having vigorous achalasia. Although original reports suggested that chest pain was more common and severe in these patients, more recent studies have shown that they have similar clinical features and response to treatment as patients with typical manometric findings (Goldenberg et al 1991, Todorczuk et al 1991).

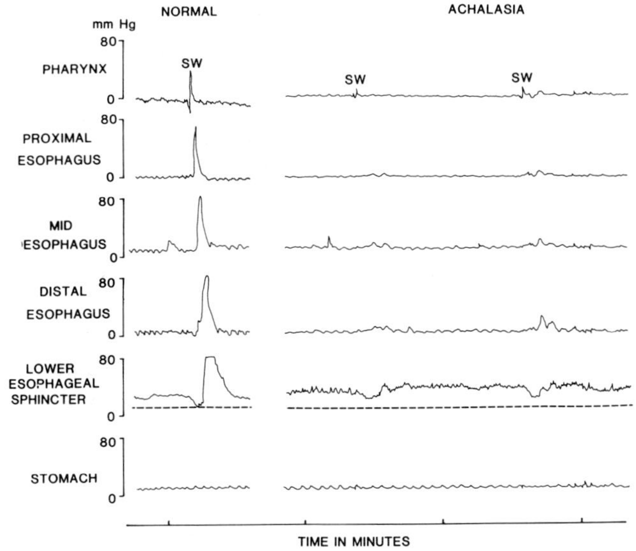


**Fig. 7.5** Esophageal motor response to swallowing in a patient with achalasia (right) and normal subject (left). Note the absence of peristalsis and incomplete lower esophageal sphincter relaxation in achalasia.

***Radionuclide studies*** (see also p. 82). Esophageal emptying is grossly delayed in most patients with achalasia although this is not specific for achalasia (Holloway et al 1983, 1989). The faster emptying after medical or surgical treatment can be used as a measure of success of therapy and correlates with symptomatic improvement.

***Endoscopy.*** This is always required in achalasia in order to exclude a coexistent tumor at the gastroesophageal junction. The esophagus may be dilated and in late stages typically shows little spontaneous activity. It may contain food residue. The gastroesophageal junction does not open spontaneously or with insufflation of air into the stomach but the endoscope passes with no more than gentle pressure.

## Differential diagnosis

The most important differential diagnosis is infiltration of the gastroesophageal junction by tumor (Fig. 7.6). This may produce a secondary or pseudo-achalasia (Tucker et al 1978, Kahrilas et al 1987c). A variety of tumors have

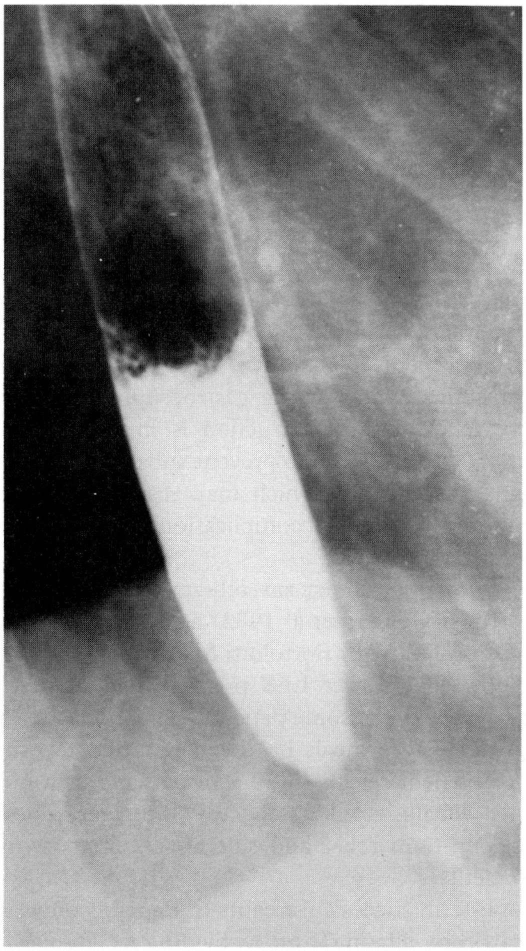

**Fig. 7.6** Carcinoma of the lower end of the esophagus causing obstruction.

**Table 7.2** Tumors associated with secondary or pseudo-achalasia

| |
|---|
| Adenocarcinoma of stomach |
| Squamous cell carcinoma of esophagus |
| Adenocarcinoma of lung |
| Bronchogenic carcinoma |
| Lymphoma |
| Pancreatic carcinoma |
| Hepatoma |
| Prostatic carcinoma |
| Breast carcinoma |
| Neurofibromatosis |

been reported (Table 7.2) and produce their effects by one of two mechanisms: mechanical compression by encirclement of the distal esophagus or infiltration of the esophageal neural plexus. In rare instances tumors may cause an achalasia-like syndrome through a paraneoplastic process. Clinical features suggestive of pseudo-achalasia are a short duration of symptoms (less than 6 months), presentation later in life (over 60 years) and weight loss greater than that expected for achalasia; however, these have relatively poor specificity. Manometry cannot distinguish achalasia from tumor infiltration but the diagnosis can often be suspected by careful radiology and in almost all cases by endoscopy with biopsy of the gastric cardia. Computed tomography and endoscopic ultrasound may reveal tumor not evident at endoscopy.

Chagas' disease affecting the esophagus causes a clinical and manometric picture that closely resembles achalasia (p. 179).

### *Treatment*

The degenerative neural lesion of achalasia cannot be corrected. Treatment is therefore directed at overcoming the obstructive effects at the gastroesophageal junction. Effective relief of this obstruction is important even in early stages of the disease to prevent subsequent dilatation and sigmoid deformity which may result in esophageal retention and pulmonary complications that are resistant to further treatment.

***Drug therapy.*** Direct smooth muscle relaxants such as isosorbide (Gelfand et al 1982) and the calcium channel blocker nifedipine (Bortolotti & Labo 1981, Berger & McCallum 1982) lower LES pressure and may help to alleviate symptoms in some patients. Nifedipine 10–20 mg sublingually before meals has been reported to produce good or excellent results in 72% of patients with mild to moderate achalasia. Drug therapy, however, does not achieve long-term relief and side-effects limit its use in many patients.

All long-term successful treatment depends on weakening the LES by dilating it or by dividing its circular fibers at operation.

***Pneumatic dilatation.*** This procedure is described on page 112. Pneumatic dilatation results in good to excellent relief of symptoms in from 60 to 90% of patients (Vantrappen & Hellemans 1980, McCord et al 1991). The success of dilatation seems to depend on several variables that include the diameter of the bag, the duration of dilatation and the number of dilatations per session although influence of these variables on outcome has not been sufficiently conclusive for standards to have been established. The response rate also appears to be better in older patients with a longer duration of symptoms but without extreme esophageal dilatation (>8 cm) (Vantrappen & Hellemans 1980).

Pain occurs during the dilatation but lasts for only a few seconds. When the pain is prolonged or when fever develops, perforation is suspected. In such instances the patient should have an urgent Gastrograffin swallow. The perforation rate is about 5% and this usually requires emergency operative intervention. Death following pneumatic dilatation has rarely been reported.

***Esophagomyotomy.*** Esophagomyotomy was first performed by Heller. Usually it is carried out by a transthoracic approach. The lower third of the esophagus is exposed and the vagus nerves identified; the myotomy is performed down to the mucosa, the incision extending from a few millimeters distal to the gastroesophageal junction to 7–10 cm proximal to it. Inadvertent incision of the mucosa has been reported in 14–22% of 522 cases collected from the literature and resulted in empyema in 2%. The mortality rate is about 1% (Vantrappen & Hellemans 1980). Good results from myotomy can be expected in over 90% of patients. Myotomy reduces LES pressure more predictably than pneumatic dilatation and this probably explains its higher success rate.

Reflux esophagitis is the most important late complication of the procedure. Its incidence varies considerably in different series of patients, but on average is probably about 10%. The incidence appears to be higher with an abdominal than with a thoracic approach (Andreollo & Earlam 1987). Consequently, many surgeons combine esophagomyotomy with an antireflux procedure, usually a hemifundoplication or Dor technique. Whether this is necessary now that very successful medical therapy for reflux disease is available is controversial (Andreollo & Earlam 1987).

***Choice of treatment.*** Debate continues as to the preferred method of treating achalasia. Pneumatic dilatation tends to be favored by gastroenterologists, largely on the basis of morbidity and cost (Vantrappen & Hellemans 1980, Traube 1991, Parkman et al 1993). Surgery, however, is usually the preferred option for young patients, particularly children. The advent of laparoscopic esophagomyotomy with its attendant lower morbidity and shorter hospital stay may tip the scales in favor of surgery provided that the results are as good as those for open surgery.

**Diffuse esophageal spasm** (Richter & Castell 1984)

This condition is characterized by chest pain, dysphagia and an increased frequency of synchronous contractions in the esophageal body. There is muscular hypertrophy in the lower two-thirds of the esophageal body. Auerbach's plexus is normal, but there are degenerative changes in the vagal nerves (Cassella et al 1965). While diffuse spasm is often regarded as a distinct entity, occasional cases progress to achalasia and it is apparent that a proportion of cases fall into a category between the two diseases (Vantrappen et al 1979).

*Clinical features*

The patients are usually 40–60 years old and the sex ratio is equal. Pain, often severe, is the most common and pronounced symptom. It occurs particularly on eating but also at night and is likely to be precipitated by rapid eating, hot or cold liquids or emotional stress. Pain is retrosternal with radiation to the back, neck or arms. It is sometimes difficult to distinguish from that of myocardial ischemia although it is often more severe. A dull residual discomfort persisting after the severe episode also helps to differentiate the pain from angina (Davies et al 1985a). Pain episodes may last from minutes to hours and swallowing is not generally impaired during the pain.

Dysphagia, present in 30–60% of patients, is intermittent, varying on a daily basis and occurring with solids and liquids. It does not usually coincide with pain, but is often more severe when pain is more severe. In contrast to achalasia, dysphagia is usually not progressive or severe enough to cause weight loss. Rarely patients may experience syncope with swallowing through a vagal reflex mechanism (Bortolotti et al 1982).

Other gastrointestinal symptoms typical of functional bowel disturbance are reported relatively frequently (Clouse & Eckert 1986). Symptoms of psychological dysfunction, especially those of anxiety and depression, are also common (Clouse 1991).

***Radiology.*** The appearances are very different from those of achalasia. Primary peristalsis halts at the aortic arch, often accompanied by slight dilatation of the proximal third of the esophagus. Unco-ordinated contractions occur in the lower two-thirds of the esophagus and may obliterate the lumen, breaking up the barium column into transient sacculations, diffuse segmental narrowing or a spiral corkscrew configuration (Fig. 7.7). These changes result in ineffective transport of the barium bolus and, during episodes of spasm, retrograde passage of barium into the upper third of the esophagus. Minor grades of this condition may be precipitated or exaggerated by giving a solid bolus with the barium, such as a lump of bread or a marshmallow (Davies 1983).

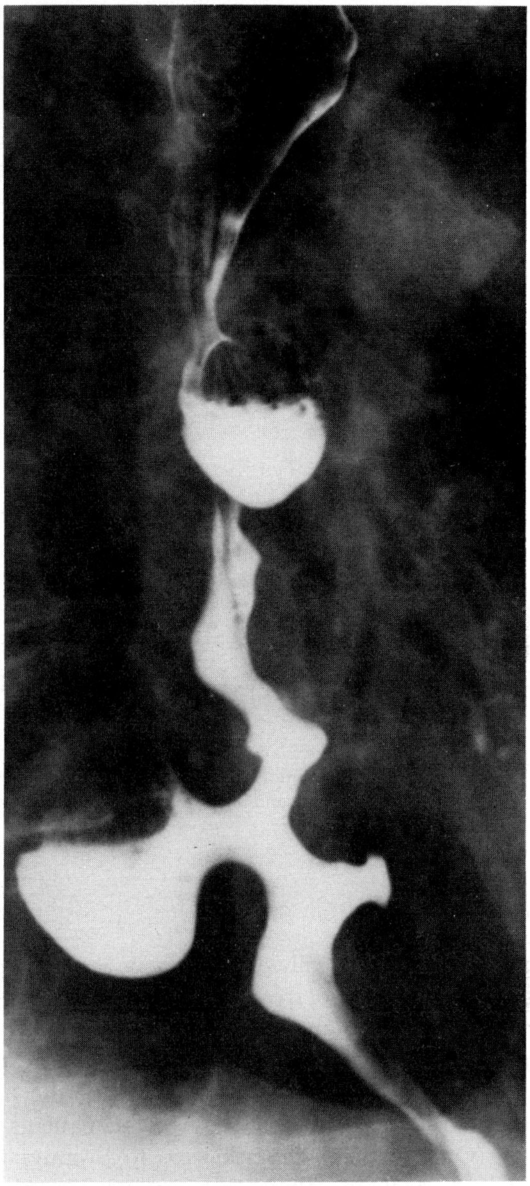

**Fig. 7.7** Corkscrew esophagus associated with diffuse esophageal spasm. Barium swallow shows marked spasm of the lower half of the esophagus with irregular synchronous contractions and formation of large diverticula.

***Esophageal manometry.*** The manometric criteria for the definition of diffuse spasm have been reviewed recently (Richter & Castell 1984, Dalton et al 1991). In contrast to achalasia, primary peristalsis is present. The hallmark of diffuse spasm is an increased prevalence of synchronous contractions in the esophageal body which should occur with at least 10% of water swallows (Fig. 7.8). Contractions are often of high amplitude and may be prolonged and repetitive. Spontaneous activity is often increased and abnormalities of LES function have also been described.

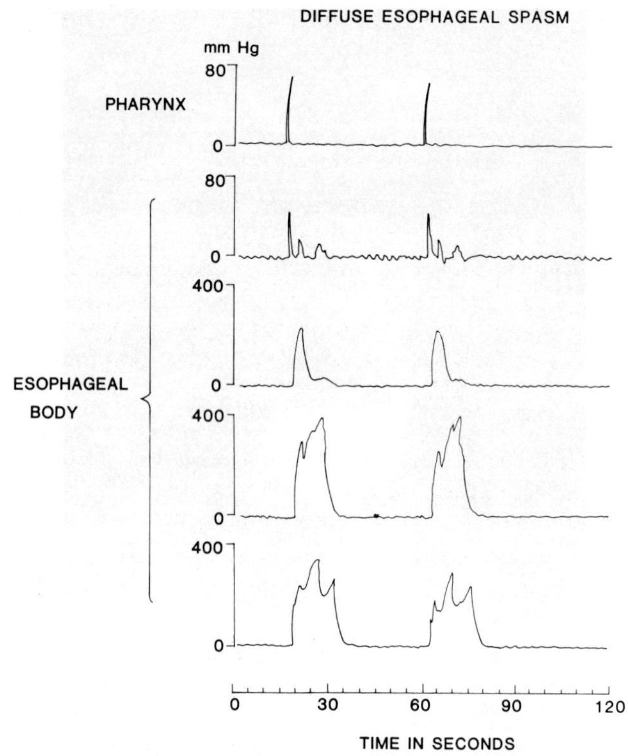


**Fig. 7.8** Pattern of esophageal motility in diffuse esophageal spasm. Note the prolonged, synchronous and high-amplitude contractions in the distal esophagus.

*Treatment* (BMJ 1980)

Diffuse spasm is not usually progressive or associated with major complications so treatment is directed primarily towards relief of symptoms.

***Drug therapy.*** Uncontrolled trials have reported a reduction of symptoms and improvement in the manometric and radiological patterns in some patients with nitrates (Orlando & Bozymski 1973, Swamy 1977, Kikendall & Mellow 1980) and the calcium channel blockers nifedipine (Nasrallah 1982) and diltiazem (Drenth et al 1990). Such agents should be tried in the first instance. Patients should avoid cold foods and should chew all food carefully. Drinking liquids regularly with solids may also be helpful.

***Esophagomyotomy.*** In severe cases, where symptoms are disabling and medical therapy has failed, esophagomyotomy is indicated. In contrast to achalasia, the LES is usually spared and the myotomy extended proximally to the level of the aortic arch. The extent of myotomy may be guided by the manometric findings. A good response has been reported in 70–80% of patients (Ellis et al 1960, Henderson et al 1987). Patients with diffuse spasm and a LES which shows either an elevated basal pressure or incomplete relaxation have been reported to respond well to pneumatic dilatation (Ebert et al 1983).

## Other disorders of esophageal motility

*Tertiary contractions*

These are spontaneous, nonperistaltic contractions in the distal esophagus. They are not of high amplitude and are asymptomatic (Fig. 7.9). On barium swallow, they are manifested by impairment of primary and secondary peristaltic activity in the lower two-thirds of the esophagus and the occurrence of multiple tertiary contractions (Zboralske 1965). As a consequence, delayed emptying and dilatation of the esophagus may occur which are more readily seen in the supine position when the effects of gravity are minimal. Tertiary contractions are common in the elderly, probably due to neuromuscular degeneration. Peristaltic contractions are weaker and progress more slowly with age (Khan et al 1977).

## Hypertensive peristalsis ("nutcracker" esophagus)

This manometric abnormality is characterized by esophageal contractions that are peristaltic but which have an increased amplitude and duration (Benjamin et al 1979). It is more common in patients with noncardiac chest pain. Most patients, however, are asymptomatic during the manometric examination and the relationship of the high-amplitude contractions to the pain has been questioned. The manometric features appear to be vari-

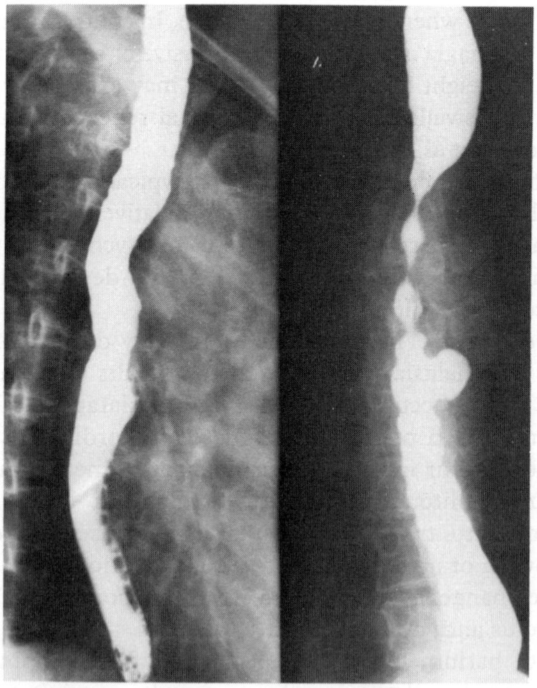

**Fig. 7.9** Symptomless tertiary contractions in the esophagus. (*Left*) Smooth outline. The translucencies in the lower third are due to air bubbles. (*Right*) A few seconds later, showing numerous contractions and a moderately large pulsion diverticulum between two contractions.

able and transition to diffuse esophageal spasm and nonspecific motor disorders has been described (Traube et al 1986, Dalton et al 1988).

### Hypertensive lower esophageal sphincter

An abnormally high resting LES pressure in patients with chest pain and/or dysphagia was first described in 1960 (Code et al 1960). It may be associated with diffuse spasm but may also occur as an isolated abnormality. Its clinical significance, however, remains unclear (Carey 1989).

### Nonspecific motor disorders

The majority of abnormalities on esophageal manometry do not meet the criteria for achalasia or diffuse spasm and are described as nonspecific esophageal motor disorders. They may be found in apparently normal people and in a variety of conditions including gastroesophageal reflux disease and systemic disorders that affect esophageal motility (see below).

## ESOPHAGEAL MOTOR DYSFUNCTION IN SYSTEMIC DISEASES

### **Chagas' disease** (Bettarello & Pinotti 1976, Dantas 1988)

*Etiology and pathology*

Chagas' disease occurs in central Brazil, in Venezuela and in northern Argentina. It is due to infection with *Trypanosoma cruzi*, which lodges in the gastrointestinal tract and heart. There is a progressive destruction of the myenteric plexus and, in addition to megaesophagus, there may be dilatation of the duodenum, colon and rectum. The pathological features in the esophagus are the same as those in achalasia, with marked destruction of the ganglion cells in the smooth muscle portion.

*Clinical features*

The clinical features and progression of the disease are the same as those of achalasia. Initially there is dysphagia, which may commence early in life; later, regurgitation and weight loss are common. Carcinoma of the esophagus occurs in 5–10% of cases. Radiological and motility studies show the same findings as those in achalasia. Chagas' disease can be distinguished from achalasia by a positive serological test and because there is often dilatation elsewhere in the gastrointestinal tract.

*Treatment*

The choice of therapy lies between pneumatic dilatation (p. 112) and esophagomyotomy (p. 176). When these fail, interposition of a jejunal segment between the esophagus and stomach may be required.

### **Scleroderma** (Fulp & Castell 1990)

Esophageal involvement is common in scleroderma. At least 40–50% of patients experience esophageal symptoms such as heartburn and dysphagia, 50–90% of patients will have involvement by manometric or radiological criteria and 74% will have evidence of esophageal involvement at autopsy (Rodman et al 1975). In scleroderma, the smooth muscle of the lower two-thirds of the esophagus undergoes atrophy, leading to failure of peristalsis and incompetence of the lower esophageal sphincter. Erosive peptic esophagitis occurs in 60% of patients with esophageal involvement (Zamost et al 1987).

Patients usually complain initially of heartburn. Dysphagia, especially for solids, develops later and may result from a stricture or from disturbed motility. Occasionally these symptoms may arise before the other manifestations of scleroderma. In advanced cases, a routine chest X-ray may demonstrate air throughout the esophagus. At endoscopy, reflux esophagitis is common. The barium swallow shows dilatation of the esophagus which is less pronounced than in achalasia, retention of barium and lack of peristalsis. Esophageal manometry shows low-amplitude contractions in the distal two-thirds of the esophageal body; in advanced cases peristalsis in this segment may be absent. Peristalsis in the proximal esophagus, however, is normal. Lower esophageal sphincter pressure is reduced and may be absent. As a consequence, gastroesophageal reflux is increased and there is a marked defect of acid clearance causing unusually severe reflux esophagitis in many patients and strictures are common. Gastric emptying of both solids and liquids is delayed (Maddern et al 1984). The findings in scleroderma are not unique to this disorder and may be found in other connective tissue diseases (Clark & Fountain 1967, Turner et al 1973, Tsianos et al 1987).

The problem tends to be progressive and intractable. An aggressive approach should be taken towards the management of reflux disease with acid suppression with acid-pump inhibitors (see p. 199). Antireflux surgery may be necessary in refractory cases but should be performed using a loose fundoplication in order to minimize the risk of postoperative dysphagia.

### **Amyloidosis** (Rubinow et al 1983)

Esophageal deposition of amyloid is common in all forms of generalized amyloidosis. There is decreased amplitude of esophageal contractions and decreased LES pressure which correlate with other evidence of peripheral and/or autonomic neuropathy. Dysphagia and heartburn are common symptoms (Rubinow et al 1983). Radiologically, there is widening of the esophagus which resembles achalasia.

### Diabetes mellitus (Horowitz & Smout 1993)

Abnormalities of esophageal motility are common in diabetes mellitus although they are rarely symptomatic. Manometric abnormalities include a decreased prevalence of peristalsis, increased spontaneous or multi-peaked contractions and reduced LES pressure. Barium swallow may show a dilated esophagus, decrease in the primary peristaltic wave and frequent tertiary contractions. Delayed radionuclide esophageal transit of liquids (Russell et al 1983) and solids (Maddern et al 1985) is also common.

### Alcoholic neuropathy

Abnormalities of esophageal body motility are common in patients with chronic alcohol abuse (Silver et al 1986, Keshavarzian et al 1987, 1992) athough no specific abnormal patterns have been observed. Lower esophageal sphincter pressure may be increased and there may be delayed esophageal transit (Keshavarzian et al 1987). These abnormalities resolve after a period of abstinence.

## DIVERTICULA OF THE PHARYNX AND ESOPHAGUS

A diverticulum is a pouch lined with epithelium. It can cause dysphagia and regurgitation. It is diagnosed by barium swallow and the treatment, if required, is usually resection. Endoscopy requires the greatest caution because of the risk of perforation.

### Posterior pharyngeal (Zenker's) diverticulum

*Etiology, development and pathology*

Ludlow first described the posterior pharyngoesophageal diverticulum in 1764. Zenker & Ziemssen (1878) later proposed that herniation of the pouch proximal to the cricopharyngeus might be caused by high hypopharyngeal pressures, the actual site of herniation being determined by an area of weakness in the posterior hypopharyngeal wall known as Killian's dehiscence. A long-held belief was that high hypopharyngeal pressures arose because of inco-ordination between UES relaxation and pharyngeal peristalsis during swallowing although consistent demonstration of such inco-ordination was lacking. Recent manometric studies have shown that UES relaxation is in fact normal but that UES opening is substantially reduced (Cook et al 1992a), causing an increased pressure in the hypopharynx during swallowing. The impairment of UES opening is caused by fibrosis of the cricopharyngeus (Cook et al 1992b).

*Clinical features*

The condition is much more common in men (Harrington 1945). At first, the patient complains of irritation, excessive mucus in the throat and dysphagia localized to the throat. Later there are gurgling sounds, regurgitation, coughing, fetid breath due to decomposing food and increasing dysphagia. Occasionally, a swelling may occur in the left side of the neck. Complications are chest infections due to regurgitation and aspiration at night and carcinoma in the diverticulum.

The diagnosis is confirmed radiologically. A lateral X-ray of the pharynx may show a fluid level in the sac but a barium swallow is required to confirm its presence and size (Fig. 7.10). Filling defects may be present in the sac owing to retained food and in the later stages, the esophagus is displaced anteriorly and narrowed. Endoscopy is hazardous and so is indicated only if there is esophageal obstruction due to a food bolus or if carcinoma of the diverticulum is suspected.

*Treatment* (Payne & King 1983)

The treatment is surgical, the most favored operation being one-stage excision and primary closure. Cricopharyngeal myotomy is usually performed in addition to excision of the sac and myotomy alone has been

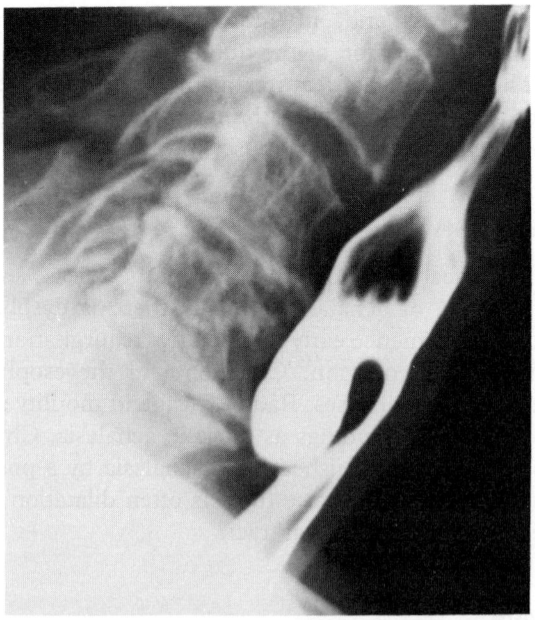

**Fig. 7.10** Large pharyngeal diverticulum in the usual position, posterior to the esophagus. The translucency above the diverticulum is due to a large air bubble.

used for very small diverticula. Some surgeons favor diverticulopexy with myotomy.

### Lateral pharyngeal diverticulum

True lateral pharyngeal diverticula are uncommon and may be congenital. They are derived from the second, third or fourth branchial clefts and arise from the tonsillar fossa or the pyriform recess. Acquired lateral diverticula also arise from the pyriform recess and pierce the thyrohyoid membrane. They are usually found in players of wind instruments or glass blowers and are generally symptomless (Bachman et al 1968).

### Mid-esophageal diverticulum

These arise at the bifurcation of the trachea. The etiology is uncertain. Although they have been attributed to traction from tuberculous mediastinal lymph nodes demonstration of such adhesions is rare at autopsy. A more likely explanation is abnormal motility. Manometric changes consisting of high-amplitude prolonged contractions occur in a high proportion of patients (Allen & Clagett 1965, Kaye 1974). The mouth of the diverticulum is wide and symptoms are rare, but dysphagia and esophageal obstruction can occur. Diagnosis is usually made during barium examination.

### Epiphrenic diverticulum

This diverticulum develops from mechanical or functional obstruction in the lower esophagus. It is usually associated with esophageal motor dysfunction, e.g. diffuse spasm, achalasia and nonspecific abnormalities (Debas et al 1980). The frequency of motor abnormalities increases with the size of the diverticulum (Bruggeman & Seaman 1973). The symptoms are extremely variable, possibly because they are caused by an associated disorder. The most frequent symptoms are dysphagia and regurgitation. The diagnosis is made on barium swallow. Those diverticula causing symptoms require diverticulectomy and correction of any associated condition, such as a myotomy for achalasia or diffuse spasm (Allen & Clagett 1965).

### Intramural pseudodiverticulosis

This is a rare condition in which numerous intramural diverticula develop from dilatation of the excretory ducts of the submucosal glands due to obstruction from a peptic stricture or to chronic submucosal inflammation (Levine et al 1986). Dysphagia is the most common symptom (Sabanthan et al 1985).

## RINGS AND WEBS OF THE ESOPHAGUS

### Mucosal ring (Schatzki ring)

This was first described by Ingelfinger & Kramer (1953) as a "contractile ring of the lower esophagus". When it was shown that it was not muscular the term "contractile" was abandoned. Schatzki & Gary (1953) called them "lower esophageal rings", but to distinguish them from other types of narrowing at the lower end of the esophagus, the term mucosal or Schatzki's ring is now used.

*Pathology*

The ring is a narrowing at the lower end of the esophagus due to an incomplete septum or diaphragm of mucosa. It lies at the junction of squamous and columnar epithelium, with squamous epithelium on its upper surface and columnar epithelium on its lower. The core of the ring consists of fibrous tissue and a few smooth muscle fibers with low-grade inflammation. It may be developmental but some regard it as a peptic stricture (Bremner 1982, Eastridge et al 1984). The inflammatory theory has gained the widest acceptance (Ott et al 1986); it postulates that the ring represents a thin annular stricture just below the squamocolumnar junction and demarcates the lower end of the esophageal vestibule.

*Clinical features*

The condition occurs equally in both sexes, usually after the age of 50 years. Reports on the discovery of Schatzki rings at barium swallow indicate a very variable incidence, from 0 to 32%, but there is an increasing incidence with age (Kaufmann 1979).

Patients describe episodic dysphagia while eating a hurried meal, usually of meat – hence the name "steak-house syndrome". Dysphagia may also be precipitated by emotional stress. It is relieved rapidly by regurgitating the offending bolus and pain is uncommon unless prolonged obstruction occurs. Rarely, such obstruction may lead to esophageal perforation. Attacks tend to occur at intervals of weeks or months and with no symptoms in between. Sometimes, attacks become more frequent and severe.

The diagnosis is confirmed by barium swallow. Motility studies show no diagnostic features and at endoscopy the ring may be missed, as the lower esophagus may not be distended sufficiently to reveal it. Radiological demonstration requires adequate distention of the lower esophagus and gastroesophageal junction and this is best achieved by the patient swallowing barium in the prone position, holding in a deep breath or performing the Valsalva maneuver (Fig. 7.11). The margins of the ring are smooth and usually symmetrical with a fixed maximum internal diameter, occurring a few centimeters above the diaphragm. The appearances should be reproducible with each swallow.

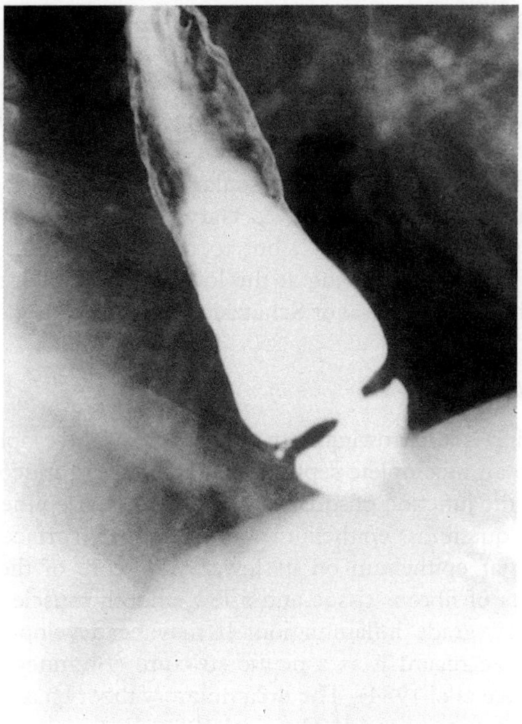

**Fig. 7.11** Schatzki ring.

Schatzki (1963) noted that symptoms occurred only when the ring was less than 13 mm in diameter. Care has to be taken not to mistake a Schatzki ring for the unilateral notch seen on the left side above the hiatus, caused by the insertion of the muscular sling fibers of the stomach (Friedland et al 1966).

*Treatment*

Reassurance and instruction on careful chewing and eating habits may be all that is required. If symptoms continue, bougienage should be performed with a 50 French bougie (Eastridge et al 1984). However, symptoms recur in up to 65% within 6 months to 5 years (Groskreutz & Kim 1990). If symptoms persist, pneumatic dilatation (p. 112) may be tried. Recently, endoscopic therapy in the form of electrosurgical incision with a sphincterotome (Guelrud et al 1987) or Nd:YAG laser (Hubert et al 1990) has led to good short- and long-term results. Surgical removal or dilatation of the ring may eventually be needed in exceptionally severe or resistant cases (Postlethwait & Sealy 1967).

**Other rings and webs in the lower esophagus**

The terminology of these is confused (Goyal et al 1970). In addition to the mucosal ring, a rare mucosal web has been described. This is a fixed structure which, in contradistinction to the mucosal ring, occurs proximal to the squamocolumnar junction so that both surfaces are covered by squamous epithelium. The web is thought to be congenital and may cause symptoms in children and adults.

A muscular or contractile ring is also described. It is caused by hypertrophy of the normal muscle fibers in the sphincteric region of the lower esophagus. Radiologically, it varies in size at different times, depending on the degree of distention of the esophagus. It is a rare cause of dysphagia and is seen most often in children. Some peptic strictures are narrow over a short length and simulate a lower esophageal ring (Ott et al 1984).

**Paterson–Kelly syndrome (Plummer–Vinson syndrome, sideropenic dysphagia)**

This was first described by Paterson & Kelly in 1919. It applies to the association of anemia and glossitis in a patient with dysphagia.

*Epidemiology*

The syndrome has been reported mainly from Sweden, the USA and Great Britain. It occurs over the age of 30 years largely in women (Jacobs & Kilpatrick 1964), but has been reported in boys and girls between the ages of 14 and 19 years (Crawfurd et al 1965).

*Etiology*

The dysphagia is due to changes in the esophageal epithelium, which may include web formation, but it is uncertain whether these result from iron deficiency. Normal serum iron concentrations were found in 68% of women with the Paterson–Kelly syndrome (Wynder & Fryer 1958) and the incidence of iron deficiency in patients with dysphagia, some of whom had a pharyngeal web, was the same as a control group (Elwood et al 1964). Some patients with the syndrome do not have iron deficiency at the time of diagnosis but have had severe iron deficiency previously (Chisolm & Wright 1967). Angular stomatitis, glossitis, atrophy of the tongue mucosa (p. 148) and achlorhydria are common and the latter could predispose to iron deficiency. In other cases, e.g. certain adolescents, these epithelial changes may result from iron deficiency (Crawfurd et al 1965).

*Pathology*

Atrophy of the squamous epithelium occurs in the region of the upper esophageal sphincter. Basal cell hyperplasia and nuclear hyperchromatism may be seen (Entwistle & Jacobs 1965), as well as fibrosis and lymphocytic infiltration. Some patients develop a postcricoid web, which is an epithelial septum lying on a connective tissue stroma with no inflammatory infiltrate. Rare cases of multiple upper esophageal webs have also shown basal cell hyperplasia (Janisch & Eckardt 1982).

### *Clinical features*

The patient complains of sudden dysphagia and choking or of difficulty in initiating swallowing of solids. Commonly there are features of iron deficiency including anemia, atrophy of the tongue mucosa and koilonychia. Occasionally the patient may have pernicious anemia rather than iron deficiency anemia.

### *Investigation*

Barium swallow may reveal a web, best demonstrated by videofluoroscopy in the lateral erect position. A web arises from the anterior and lateral walls in the postcricoid portion of the hypopharynx. The web is usually single, although multiple webs may be seen occasionally. There is often streaming of barium over the shelf-like web and there may be generalized narrowing of the upper esophagus (Fig. 7.12). Sometimes, the postcricoid submucus venous plexus can simulate a web (Pitman & Fraser 1965) but the venous plexus varies in appearance from second to second and may also vary in size with respiration.

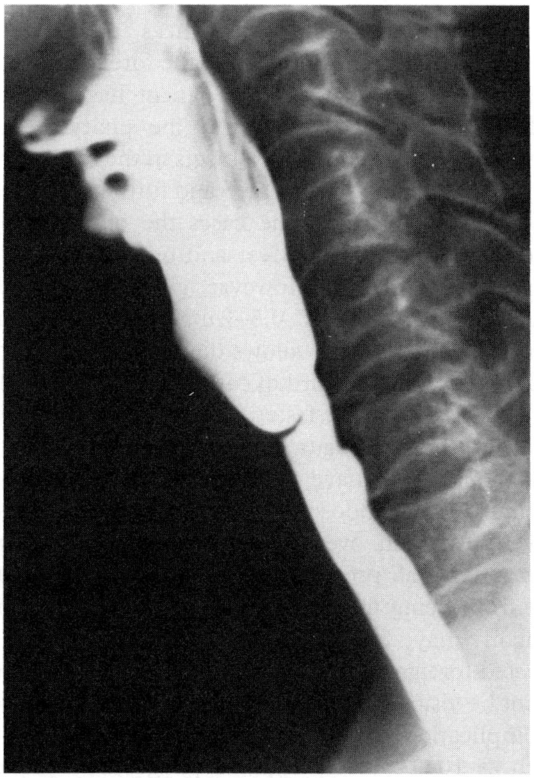

**Fig. 7.12** Postcricoid (sideropenic) web. Typical sharply defined anterolateral filling defect in upper esophagus.

Occasionally, a pharyngeal neoplasm may be present and a careful search for this is necessary.

Endoscopy should be performed because of the high incidence of cancer in this disorder (p. 205). Atrophy of the mucosa may be seen. The web is thin and smooth and is usually ruptured by the instrument before it is seen. The cause of the anemia should be investigated.

### *Treatment*

Anemia should be treated. Dysphagia may be relieved by the endoscopy or by bougies. However, because of the predisposition to carcinoma, surveillance endoscopy with biopsy or brush cytology is recommended.

## **Chemical burns and stricture** (Mellow 1982, Postlethwait 1983)

Burns are usually caused by accidental or deliberate ingestion of strong alkalis present in many cleaning fluids. Clinitest tablets or dental cleaners such as Steradent can cause similar damage if swallowed accidentally. Damage to the lips, mouth, larynx and esophagus is immediate so that there are no "first-aid" measures. Damage to the stomach is relatively uncommon and occurs in only 20% of cases. Ingestion of mineral acid is less common but, in contrast to alkali ingestion, frequently spares the esophagus and causes maximal damage to the distal stomach (Maull et al 1979).

### *Clinical features*

Ingestion is followed within a minute or two by severe mouth, pharyngeal and chest pain. There is dysphagia and retching and the patient spits out mucus and saliva. In severe injury, there may be immediate signs of esophageal perforation. Examination usually shows oral burns but they do not reflect the extent of esophageal damage. If there is shock or evidence of mediastinitis, esophageal perforation is assumed and is confirmed by a Gastrograffin swallow (p. 5). In other patients, endoscopy should be performed to establish the presence of esophageal injury. To avoid perforation, it is preferable to use a small diameter instrument and advance it only as far as the area of severe damage (see also pp. 104 and 329).

Radiological manifestations depend on the nature of the swallowed substance, its concentration and viscosity, the amount swallowed and the length of time the substance is in contact with the esophageal mucosa (Muhletaler et al 1980). In the acute examination, water-soluble contrast medium should be used but later a double-contrast barium examination is likely to be more informative. Early changes (1–4 days) include esophageal mucosal scalloping due to hemorrhage and edema and impaired peristalsis (Donner et al 1981). Painful spasm of the esophagus may occur and sloughing of the mucosa can cause filling defects. Subsequently, the esophagus may become narrowed and atonic with ulceration and irregularity due to persisting edema. Barium swallow is also used to assess stricture formation due to scarring. This is most likely to occur at physiological narrowings such as the upper and lower esophageal sphincters and the levels of the aortic arch and left main bronchus. The strictures may show evidence of proximal dilatation and ulceration may persist.

*Treatment*

All patients in whom burn injury to the esophagus is suspected must be admitted to hospital. Shock is corrected and airway obstruction may demand endotracheal intubation or even tracheostomy. Attempts to dilute or neutralize the damaging agent are of no value and emetics or gastric lavage may aggravate the injury. The patient should receive nothing by mouth. Broad-spectrum antibiotics are given once esophageal injury is diagnosed and are given for only 1 week if the patient remains afebrile. Persistent fever suggests mediastinitis, peritonitis or abscess formation.

Corticosteroids and repeated early dilatation used to be regarded as essential in the prevention of strictures. The role of steroids is controversial and some clinicians consider that their ability to delay healing and mask signs of infection outweigh their benefits (Kirsch et al 1978, Sarfati et al 1987). Similarly, injudicious use of early dilatation may increase the incidence of perforation. Emergency esophagectomy (and gastrectomy) may be needed if alkali ingestion leads to full-thickness necrosis. Gastrointestinal continuity is restored at a later stage by colonic or jejunal interposition. If the esophagus does not perforate but strictures develop, they may respond to dilatation or require subsequent resection. The strictured esophagus may be left in situ if resection is needed, but cancer of the esophagus may develop many years after a caustic burn. Necrosis following acid ingestion is frequently confined to the distal stomach and can be dealt with by subtotal gastrectomy.

## FOREIGN BODIES IN THE ESOPHAGUS (Webb 1992)

Most patients with foreign bodies obstructing the esophagus are children under the age of 10 years or adults past middle age who have dentures or esophageal disease. Children frequently swallow coins and other small metal objects, whereas in adults the obstruction is usually caused by a bolus of meat, fish or chicken bone or swallowed dentures.

*Clinical features*

The symptoms are dysphagia and persistent salivation. Discomfort may be constant when the object is lodged near the cricopharyngeus. Infants regurgitate food or refuse to eat. Sharp objects such as bones, toothpicks and pins may perforate the esophagus with fatal septic or hemorrhagic consequences.

Anyone with a history of swallowing a foreign body should be investigated. X-rays of the chest (posteroanterior and lateral) and cervical spine (lateral) are taken. Foreign bodies tend to lodge in the region of the cricopharyngeus in children and in the lower esophagus in adults. Lodgement in the mid-esophagus is unusual unless the object is pointed. Most objects will be seen on X-ray but some objects such as pull-tabs on aluminum soft-drink cans, small fish bones and wood are radiolucent or nearly so. Air may be seen in the cervical prevertebral space if the upper esophagus has been perforated. Under these circumstances, barium should not be used as it makes endoscopy difficult. A one-mouthful barium swallow is most effective in diagnosing food bolus obstruction. Intravenous glucagon may relax the lower esophageal sphincter and allow the passage of the impacted bolus, which can be monitored fluoroscopically. If associated perforation of the esophagus is suspected, a water-soluble contrast medium should be used, although up to 25% of thoracic esophageal perforations may be missed (Seaman 1981).

*Treatment* (Sanowski 1987)

Treatment is difficult in many instances and considerable experience is required. Removal of the foreign body is not urgent unless it is sharp or the patient has difficulty in breathing. Objects that lodge in the pharynx can be removed at laryngoscopy. For objects in the lower esophagus the patient should be sedated and further X-rays taken after several hours. In some cases the object will have passed into the stomach. Meat and other impacted food often passes with time. However, glucagon given intravenously, in a dose of 0.5–2 mg, relaxes the lower esophageal sphincter and allows the bolus to pass into the stomach in about one-third of cases (Trenkner et al 1983) All patients should be fasted and tubes should not be passed into the esophagus. Food boluses that do not pass spontaneously may have to be dislodged at flexible and sometimes rigid endoscopy. Sharp objects should be removed using an overtube or rigid esophagoscope to facilitate removal, protect the esophagus and prevent the object from being inadvertently dropped into the airway. Glucagon may be helpful to relax the esophagus. Neglected foreign bodies can perforate the esophagus and may not be visible. Esophageal perforation is also a potential complication of removal and has been reported to be as high as 10–12% with rigid esophagoscopy and up to 1–5% with flexible endoscopy.

It is important to perform a barium swallow at a later

stage in all adults who have had a foreign body in the esophagus. This may reveal a ring, stricture, carcinoma, hernia or a motility disorder. Occasionally no lesion is found but focal ulceration secondary to the food impaction may be identified.

## PERFORATION OF THE ESOPHAGUS

The most common causes of esophageal perforation are instrumentation, blunt trauma and forceful vomiting (Boerhaave's syndrome).

### **Instrumental perforation** (Wesdorp et al 1984)

The esophagus may be perforated during endoscopy. The risk is about 1% with rigid endoscopy but only about 0.03% with flexible endoscopy. The risk is increased with difficult intubation, inexperienced endoscopists, uncooperative patients and elderly frail patients with distorted anatomy. Therapeutic endoscopy further increases the risk and the incidence of perforation is almost 1% for dilatation of esophageal strictures, 3–5% for pneumatic dilatation of achalasia (p. 176) and about 10% for palliative intubation in patients with carcinoma.

#### *Clinical features*

Pain is characteristic and occurs immediately after a large perforation. Upper esophageal perforation causes pain in the neck and upper thorax, whilst lower esophageal perforation causes epigastric or thoracic pain which may radiate to the scapular region. Dyspnea, cyanosis, dysphagia and fever may develop. Subcutaneous emphysema may be present and escape of gastric contents leads to mediastinitis. A chest X-ray may reveal air in the mediastinum, mediastinal widening, pleural effusion or even pneumothorax. Contrast X-ray studies should be done either immediately or soon after procedures that carry a high risk of perforation. Perforation should be confirmed radiologically (p. 5).

#### *Treatment*

The objective is to diagnose perforation and institute management before the full-blown clinical picture develops. All patients should be monitored carefully after the endoscopic procedure until fully recovered and pain free. A few sips of water are then allowed and if discomfort is experienced or there are any other symptoms or signs suggesting perforation, investigation is instituted. Perforation of the cervical esophagus may be treated conservatively with broad-spectrum antibiotics, fasting and intravenous feeding. However, patients with significant pain and evidence of local sepsis such as tenderness, fever and tachycardia should be managed surgically. Perforation of the intrathoracic esophagus is more lethal than its cervical counterpart and is usually treated surgically. Conservative management is appropriate in patients with malignant disease and in minor perforations diagnosed early before contamination in patients with nonmalignant disease. Nasoesophageal suction using a tube with multiple sideholes positioned above, at and below the perforation is essential. A Gastrograffin swallow is repeated after 7 days to exclude continuing extravasation. Thoracotomy with primary closure and drainage is indicated if the esophageal tear is large. Subdiaphragmatic perforation of the esophagus should also be treated surgically.

### **Spontaneous perforation (Boerhaave's syndrome)** (Britten-Jones 1988)

Spontaneous perforation may follow a sudden increase in intraesophageal pressure caused by vomiting, straining, convulsions or blunt abdominal trauma. The tear usually occurs on the left posterolateral aspect of the distal thoracic esophagus (Saario et al 1983). Sudden excruciating chest pain starting during an episode of vomiting is the most common feature. The pain is usually retrosternal but may radiate to the upper abdomen and to the interscapular region. Dyspnea, cyanosis and fever are usually present. Subcutaneous emphysema and a pleural effusion may be present.

A plain X-ray in the upright position is the most valuable diagnostic tool. The earliest sign is that of mediastinal air. Later, widening of the mediastinum, pleural effusion with or without pneumothorax develop. Perforation can be confirmed by Gastrograffin swallow.

The differential diagnosis includes perforated peptic ulcer, pulmonary embolism, spontaneous pneumothorax, dissecting aortic aneurysm and pancreatitis.

Treatment is surgical and consists of debridement of the mediastinum, pleural drainage and primary repair of the torn esophagus with reinforcement of the suture line by a flap of diaphragm or pleura. Mortality rises sharply owing to leakage from the suture line if delay exceeds 24 h. For patients coming to surgery beyond this time, pleural and mediastinal drainage are essential. Opinions vary as to the use of additional techniques, but good results have been reported following simple suture and drainage (Finley et al 1980).

## ACQUIRED ESOPHAGEAL FISTULA (Mellow 1982)

### **Broncho- and tracheoesophageal fistulae**

These are commonly secondary to cancer of the lung or esophagus. Occasionally they can result from trauma or chronic inflammatory conditions such as tuberculosis or candidiasis (p. 210).

The patient presents with paroxysmal coughing following the ingestion of liquids but the symptoms can be less dramatic with chronic cough, fever and recurrent pulmonary infection. Fistulae can be localized by nonionic contrast media (p. 5) or barium and the orifice of the fistula biopsied at bronchoscopy or endoscopy.

The treatment of benign fistula is surgical. In general, however, surgery is avoided for malignant fistula. Permanent endoesophageal intubation should be attempted for it allows oral nutrition to continue and reduces cough and pulmonary infection. Lesions must be at least 3 cm below the cricopharyngeus and 3–4 cm above the gastroesophageal junction. The prosthesis is inserted from above after progressive dilatation of the narrowed area.

### Aortoesophageal fistula

The usual cause is foreign body ingestion and slow penetration at the level of the aortic arch. It may also occur secondary to esophageal carcinoma, penetrating Barrett's ulcer and aortic aneurysm, either primary or after repair. Often there is a minor bleed followed after a variable time by a massive bleed. If the condition is suspected because of dysphagia and a "signal" hemorrhage, a chest X-ray should be performed to look for a foreign body. If it cannot be seen, endoscopy is necessary for diagnosis. The treatment is surgical.

A preoperative barium swallow may alert the surgeon to the presence of an aortoesophageal fistula in patients with aneurysm of the thoracic aorta and may save the patient from potentially hazardous endoscopy in this situation (Baron et al 1981).

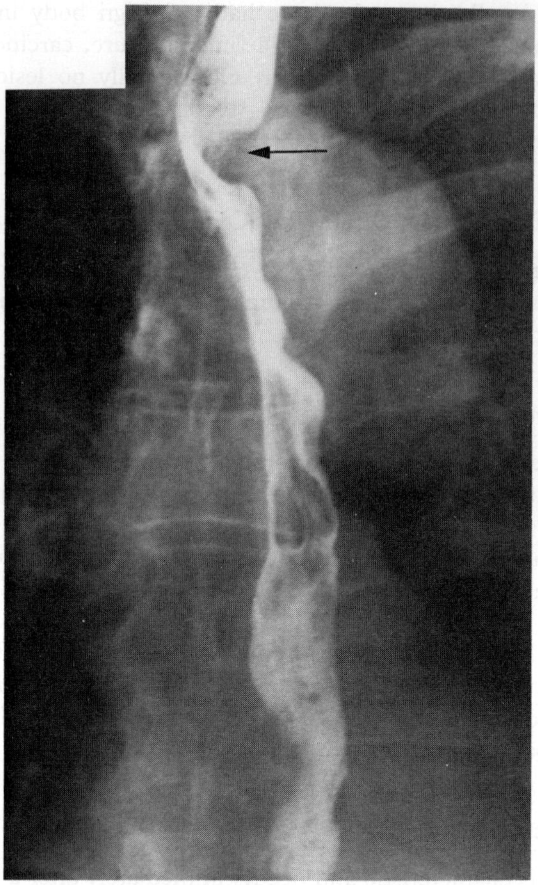

**Fig. 7.13** Aberrant right subclavian artery. Typical smooth indentation (arrow) opposite upper part of aortic arch.

## EXTRINSIC COMPRESSION OF THE ESOPHAGUS

A variety of disorders may compress the esophagus and cause dysphagia. Carcinoma of the bronchus, especially the left main bronchus, can present with dysphagia (Stankey et al 1969). Thyroid enlargement, diseases of lymph nodes (lymphoma or metastatic cancer) and mediastinal cysts (p. 212) can all cause dysphagia. Esophageal compression is described in the ill-defined conditions of mediastinal fibrosis and granuloma (Hache et al 1962, Sakulsky et al 1967).

Aneurysms or aberrant vessels are rare causes of dysphagia (Stewart et al 1964). Obstruction in the lower esophagus can result from aneurysm or tortuousness of the descending thoracic aorta (Mittal et al 1986) and aberrant vessels can form a "vascular ring" which encircles the esophagus and trachea completely or partially. Complete vascular rings may cause severe dysphagia, e.g. a double aortic arch (Wychulis et al 1971) or a right aortic arch with a left ligament arteriosum. "Dysphagia lusoria", described by Bayford in 1794, results from a dilated or tortuous aberrant right subclavian artery (Fig. 7.13).

## REFERENCES


Aggestrup S, Uddmann R, Sundler F 1983 Lack of vasoactive intestinal polypeptide nerves in esophageal achalasia. Gastroenterology 84: 924–927

Allen T H, Clagett O T 1965 Changing concepts in the surgical treatment of pulsion diverticula of the lower esophagus. Journal of Thoracic and Cardiovascular Surgery 50: 455–460

Andreollo N A, Earlam R J 1987 Heller's myotomy for achalasia: is an added anti-reflux procedure necessary ? British Journal of Surgery 74: 765–769

Anon 1986 Angina and esophageal disease. Lancet 1: 191

Arndorfer R C, Stef J J, Dodds W J, Linehan J H, Hogan W J 1977 Improved infusion system for intraluminal esophageal manometry. Gastroenterology 73: 23–27

Ask P, Tibbling L 1980 Effect of time interval between swallows on esophageal peristalsis. American Journal of Physiology 238: G485–G490

Axelrod F B, Maayan C, Hazzi C, Bangaru B S, Shannon D C 1987 Bradycardia associated with hiatal hernia and gastroesophageal reflux relieved by surgery. American Journal of Gastroenterology 82: 159–161

Bachman A, Seaman W, Macken K 1968 Lateral pharyngeal diverticula. Radiology 91: 774—782

Baron R L, Koehler R E, Guttierrez F R, Forrest J V, Weyman P J 1981 Clinical and radiological manifestations of aortesophageal fistulas. Radiology 141: 599–605
Benjamin S B, Gerhardt D C, Castell D O 1979 High amplitude, peristaltic esophageal contractions associated with chest pain and/or dysphagia. Gastroenterology 77: 478–483
Bennett J, Atkinson M 1966 The differentiation between esophageal and cardiac pain. Lancet 2: 1123–1127
Berger K, McCallum R W 1982 Nifedipine in the treatment of achalasia. Annals of Internal Medicine 96: 61–62
Bernstein L M, Baker L A 1958 A clinical test for esophagitis. Gastroenterology 34: 760–781
Bernstein L M, Fruin R C, Pacini R 1962 Differentiation of esophageal pain from angina pectoris: role of the esophageal acid perfusion test. Medicine (Balt) 41: 143–162
Bettarello A, Pinotti H 1976 Esophageal involvement in Chagas' disease. Clinics in Gastroenterology 5: 103–110
Biancani P, Goyal R K, Phillips A, Spiro H M 1973 Mechanics of sphincter action – studies on the lower esophageal sphincter. Journal of Clinical Investigation 52: 2973–2978
Bianco A, Cagossi M, Scrimieri D, Greco A V 1986 Appearance of esophageal peristalsis in treated idiopathic achalasia. Digestive Diseases and Sciences 31: 40–48
BMJ 1980 Leading article. The uneasy esophagus. British Medical Journal 1: 136
Bortolotti M, Labo G 1981 Clinical and manometric effects of nifedipine in patients with esophageal achalasia. Gastroenterology 80: 39–44
Bortolotti M, Cirignotta F, Labo G 1982 Atrioventricular block induced by swallowing in a patient with diffuse esophageal spasm. Journal of the American Medical Association 248: 2297–2299
Bremner C 1982. Benign strictures of the esophagus. Current problems in surgery. Year Book, Chicago
Breumelhof R, Nadorp J H S, Akkermans L M A, Smout A J P M 1990 Analysis of 24-hour esophageal pressure and pH data in unselected patients with noncardiac chest pain. Gastroenterology 99: 1257–1264
Britten-Jones R 1988 Spontaneous injury of the esophagus. (i) Boerhaave's syndrome. In: Jamieson G (ed) Surgery of the esophagus. Churchill Livingstone, Edinburgh, p 397–404
Bruggeman L L, Seaman W B 1973 Epiphrenic diverticula. An analysis of 80 cases. American Journal of Roentgenology 119: 266–272
Carey W D 1989 Hypertensive lower esophageal sphincter. Digestive Diseases and Sciences 34: 1611–1612
Cassella R R, Ellis H, Brown A L 1965 Diffuse spasm of the lower part of the esophagus. Fine structure of esophageal smooth muscle and nerve. Journal of the American Medical Association 191: 379–382
Chisolm M, Wright R 1967 Post-cricoid dysphagia and iron deficiency in men. British Medical Journal 2: 281–283
Christensen J 1984 Origin of sensation in the esophagus. American Journal of Physiology 246: G221–G225
Christensen J 1987 Motor functions of the pharynx and esophagus. In: Johnson L R (ed) Physiology of the gastrointestinal tract, 2nd edn. Raven Press, New York, p 595–612
Clark M, Fountain R B 1967 Esophageal motility in connective tissue disease. British Journal of Dermatology 79: 449–452
Clouse R E 1991 Psychiatric disorders in patients with esophageal disease. Medical Clinics of North America 75: 1081–1090
Clouse R E, Eckert T C 1986 Gastrointestinal symptoms of patients with esophageal contraction abnormalities. Digestive Diseases and Sciences 31: 236–240
Clouse R E, Lustman P J, Eckert T C, Ferney D M, Griffith L S 1987 Low-dose trazodone for symptomatic patients with esophageal contraction abnormalities. A double-blind, placebo-controlled trial. Gastroenterology 92: 1027–1036
Code C F, Schlegel J F, Kelley M L, Olsen A M, Ellis F H J 1960 Hypertensive gastroesophageal sphincter. Mayo Clinic Proceedings 35: 391–399
Cook I J S 1991 Normal and disordered swallowing: new insights. Baillière's Clinical Gastroenterology. 5: 245–280
Cook I J S, Gabb M, Panagopoulos V et al 1992a Pharyngeal (Zenker's) diverticulum is a disorder of upper esophageal sphincter opening. Gastroenterology 103: 1229–1235
Cook I J S, Blumbergs P, Cash K, Jamieson G G, Shearman D J C 1992b Structural abnormalities of the cricopharyngeus muscle in patients with pharyngeal (Zenker's) diverticulum. Journal of Gastroenterology and Hepatology 7: 556–562
Crawfurd M D A, Jacobs A, Murphy B, Peters D K 1965 Paterson–Kelly syndrome in adolescence: a report of 5 cases. British Medical Journal 1: 693–695
Dalton C B, Castell D O, Richter J E 1988 The changing faces of the nutcracker esophagus. American Journal of Gastroenterology 83: 623–628
Dalton C B, Castell D O, Hewson E G, Wu W C, Richter J E 1991 Diffuse esophageal spasm: a rare motility disorder not characterized by high-amplitude contractions. Digestive Diseases and Sciences 36: 1025–1028
Dantas R 1988 Idiopathic achalasia and Chagasic megaesophagus. Journal of Clinical Gastroenterology 10: 13–15
Dantas R, Cook I J S, Dodds W J, Kern M K, Lang I, Brasseur J 1990 Biomechanics of cricopharyngeal bars. Gastroenterology 99: 1269–1274
Davies H A 1983 Diagnostic value of "bread-barium" swallow in patients with esophageal symptoms. Digestive Diseases and Sciences 28: 1094–1100
Davies H A, Jones D B, Rhodes J, Newcombe R G 1985a Angina-like esophageal pain: differentiation from cardiac pain by history. Journal of Clinical Gastroenterology 7: 477–481
Davies H A, Page Z, Rush E M, Brown A L, Lewis M J, Petch M C 1985b Esophageal stimulation lowers exertional angina threshold. Lancet 1: 1011–1013
De Caestecker J S, Brown J, Blackwell J N, Heading R C 1985 The esophagus as a cause of recurrent chest pain: which patients should be investigated and which tests should be used? Lancet 2: 1143–1146
Debas H T, Payne W S, Cameron A J, Carlson H C 1980 Physiopathology of lower esophageal diverticulum and its implications for treatment. Surgery, Gynecology and Obstetrics 151: 593–600
Dent J 1976 A new technique for continuous sphincter pressure measurement. Gastroenterology 71: 263–271
Dent J, Dodds W J, Sekiguchi T, Hogan W J, Arndorfer R C 1983 Interdigestive phasic contractions of the human lower esophageal sphincter. Gastroenterology 84: 453–460
Diamant N E, El Sharkawy T Y 1977 Neural control of esophageal peristalsis: a conceptual analysis. Gastroenterology 72: 546—556
Dodds W J, Stewart E T, Hogan W J, Stef J J, Arndorfer R C 1974 Effect of esophageal movement on intraluminal esophageal pressure recording. Gastroenterology 67: 592–600
Dodds W J, Dent J, Hogan W J, Arndorfer R C 1981 Effect of atropine on esophageal motor functions in humans. American Journal of Physiology 240: G290–G296
Dodds W J, Kahrilas P J, Dent J, Hogan W J 1987 Considerations about pharyngeal manometry. Dysphagia 1: 209–215
Donner M W, Saba G P, Martinez C R 1981 Diffuse diseases of the esophagus: a practical approach. Seminars in Roentgenology 16: 198–205
Drenth J P H, Bos L P, Engels L G J B 1990 Efficacy of diltiazem in the treatment of diffuse esophageal spasm. Alimentary Pharmacology and Therapeutics 4: 411–416
Duranceau A C, Beauchamp G, Jamieson G G, Barbeau A 1983 Oropharyngeal dysphagia and oculopharyngeal muscular dystrophy. Surgical Clinics of North America 63: 825–830
Eastridge C E, Pate J W, Mann J A 1984 Lower esophageal ring: experience in treatment of 88 patients. Annals of Thoracic Surgery 37: 103–107
Ebert E C, Ouyang A, Wright S H, Cohen S, Lipshutz W H 1983 Pneumatic dilatation in patients with symptomatic diffuse esophageal spasm and lower esophageal sphincter dysfunction. Digestive Diseases and Sciences 28: 481–485
Ellis F H, Olsen A M 1969. Achalasia of the esophagus. In: Dunphy J (ed) Major problems in clinical surgery. W B Saunders, Philadelphia
Ellis F H, Code C F, Olsen A M 1960 Long esophagomyotomy for diffuse spasm of the esophagus and hyertensive gastro-esophageal sphincter. Surgery 48: 155–160
Elwood P C, Jacobs A, Pitman R G, Entwistle C C 1964 Epidemiology of the Paterson–Kelly syndrome. Lancet 2: 716–718
Entwistle C C, Jacobs A 1965 Histological findings in the Paterson–Kelly syndrome. Journal of Clinical Pathology 18: 408–415

Finley R J, Pearson F G, Weisel R D, Todd T R, Ilves R, Cooper J 1980 The management of non-malignant intra-thoracic esophageal perforations. Annals of Thoracic Surgery 30: 575–583
Friedland G W, Melcher D H, Berridge F R, Gresham G A 1966 Debatable points in the anatomy of the lower esophagus. Thorax 21: 487–498
Fulp S R, Castell D O 1990 Scleroderma esophagus. Dysphagia 5: 204–210
Gelfand M, Rozen P, Gilat T 1982 Isosorbide dinitrate and nifedipine treatment of achalasia: a clinical manometric and radionuclide evaluation. Gastroenterology 83: 963–969
Gerhardt D C, Shuck T J, Bordeaux R A, Winship D H 1978 Human upper esophageal sphincter. Response to volume, osmotic and acid stimuli. Gastroenterology 75: 268–274
Goldenberg S P, Burrell M, Fette G G, Vos C, Traube M 1991 Classic and vigorous achalasia: a comparison of manometric, radiographic, and clinical findings. Gastroenterology 101: 743–748
Goyal R, Paterson W 1989. Esophageal motility. In: Schultz, S, Wood, J Rauner, B (eds). Handbook of physiology – the gastrointestinal system. Oxford University Press, New York, p 865–908
Goyal R K, Glancy J J, Spiro H M 1970 Lower esophageal ring. New England Journal of Medicine 282: 1298–1305
Groskreutz J L, Kim C H 1990 Schatzki's ring: long-term results following dilation. Gastrointestinal Endoscopy 36: 479–481
Guelrud M, Villasmil L, Mendez R 1987 Late results in patients with Schatzki ring treated by endoscopic electrosurgical incision of the ring. Gastrointestinal Endoscopy 33: 96–98
Hache L, Woolner L B, Bernatz P E 1962 Idiopathic fibrous mediastinitis. Diseases of the Chest 41: 9–14
Harrington S W 1945 Pulsion diverticulum of the hypopharynx at the pharyngo-esophageal junction. Surgery 18: 66–71
Henderson R D, Ryder D, Marryatt G 1987 Extended esophageal myotomy and short total fundoplication hernia repair in diffuse esophageal spasm: five year review in 34 patients. Annals of Thoracic Surgery 43: 25–31
Hewson E G, Dalton C B, Richter J E 1990 Comparison of esophageal manometry, provocative testing, and ambulatory monitoring in patients with unexplained chest pain. Digestive Diseases and Sciences 35: 302–309
Holloway R 1990 Esophageal disease and non-cardiac chest pain. Journal of Gastroenterology and Hepatology 5: 180–193
Holloway R H, Dent J 1990 Pathophysiology of gastroesophageal reflux: lower esophageal sphincter dysfunction in gastroesophageal reflux disease. Gastroenterology Clinics of North America 19: 517–536
Holloway R H, Berger K, Krosin G, Baue A, Lange R, McCallum R W 1983 Radionuclide esophageal emptying of a solid meal to quantitate results of therapy in achalasia. Gastroenterology 84: 771–776
Holloway R H, Blank E L, Takahashi I, Dodds W J, Layman R D 1985 Motilin: a mechanism incorporating the opossum lower esophageal sphincter into the migrating motor complex. Gastroenterology 89: 507–515
Holloway R H, Dodds W J, Helm J F, Hogan W J, Dent J, Arndorfer R C 1986 Integrity of cholinergic innervation to the lower esophageal sphincter in achalasia. Gastroenterology 90: 924–929
Holloway R H, Lange R C, Plankey M, McCallum R W 1989 Detection of esophageal motor disorders by radionuclide transit studies. Digestive Diseases and Sciences 34: 905–912
Horowitz M, Smout A J P M 1993 Disordered esophageal and gastric motility in diabetes mellitus. Advances in Endocrinology and Metabolism 4: 81–114
Horowitz M, McNeil J D, Maddern G J, Collins P J, Shearman D J C 1986 Abnormalities of gastric and esophageal emptying in polymyositis and dermatomyositis. Gastroenterology 90: 434–439
Horowitz M, Maddox A, Maddern G J, Wishart J, Collins P J, Shearman D J C 1987 Gastric and esophageal emptying in dystrophia myotonica. Gastroenterology 92: 570–577
Howard P J, Maher L, Pryde A, Cameron E W J, Heading R C 1992 Five year prospective study of the incidence, clinical features, and diagnosis of achalasia in Edinburgh. Gut 33: 1011–1015
Hubert G, Patrice T, Foultier M-T, Le Bodic L 1990 Dysphagie et anneau de Schatzki: traitment par le laser Nd:YAG chez 14 patients. Gastroenterologie Clinique Biologie 14: 186–190
Ingelfinger F J, Kramer P 1953 Dysphagia produced by a contractile ring in the lower esophagus. Gastroenterology 23: 419–430
Jacobs A, Kilpatrick G S 1964 The Paterson–Kelly syndrome. British Medical Journal 2: 79–82
Janisch H D, Eckardt V F 1982 Histological abnormalities in patients with multiple esophageal webs. Digestive Diseases and Sciences 27: 503–506
Kahrilas P J, Dodds W J, Dent J, Wyman J B, Hogan W J, Arndorfer R C 1986 Upper esophageal sphincter function during belching. Gastroenterology 91: 133–140
Kahrilas P J, Dent J, Dodds W J, Hogan W J, Arndorfer R C 1987a A method for continuous monitoring of upper esophageal sphincter pressure. Digestive Diseases and Sciences 32: 121–128
Kahrilas P J, Dodds W J, Dent J, Haeberle B, Hogan W J, Arndorfer R C 1987b Effect of sleep, spontaneous gastresophageal reflux, and a meal on upper esophageal sphincter pressure in normal human volunteers. Gastroenterology 92: 466–471
Kahrilas P J, Kishk S M, Helm J F, Dodds W J, Harig J M, Hogan W J 1987c Comparison of pseudoachalasia and achalasia. American Journal of Medicine 82: 439–446
Katon W, Hall M L, Russo J et al 1988 Chest pain: relationship of psychiatric illness to coronary arteriographic results. American Journal of Medicine 84: 1–9
Katz P O, Richter J E, Cowan R, Castell D O 1986 Apparent complete lower esophageal sphincter relaxation in achalasia. Gastroenterology 90: 978–983
Katz P O, Dalton C B, Richter J E, Wu W C, Castell D O 1987 Esophageal testing of patients with noncardiac chest pain or dysphagia – results of three years' experience with 1161 patients. Annals of Internal Medicine 106: 593–597
Kaufmann H J 1979 Esophageal roentgenographic "abnormalities" in patients without esophageal symptoms. Journal of Laboratory and Clinical Medicine 83: 1443–1449
Kaufmann H J 1982 Hiccups: an occasional sign of esophageal obstruction. Gastroenterology 82: 1443
Kaye M 1974 Esophageal motor dysfunction in patients with diverticula of the mid-thoracic esophagus. Thorax 29: 666–672
Keshavarzian A, Iber F L, Ferguson Y 1987 Esophageal manometry and radionuclide emptying in chronic alcoholics. Gastroenterology 92: 651–657
Keshavarzian A, Polepalle C, Iber F L, Durkin M 1992 Secondary esophageal contractions are abnormal in chronic alcoholics. Digestive Diseases and Sciences 37: 517–522
Khan A T, Schragge B W, Crispin J S, Lind J F 1977 Effect of aging on the motor function of the esophagus and lower esophageal sphincter. Digestive Diseases and Sciences 22: 1049–1054
Kikendall J W, Mellow M H 1980 Effect of sublingual nitroglycerin and long-acting nitrate preparations on esophageal motility. Gastroenterology 79: 703–706
Kirsch M M, Peterson A, Brown J W, Orringer M B, Ritter F N, Sloan H 1978 Treatment of caustic ingestion of the esophagus: ten years experience. Annals of Surgery 188: 675–678
Lam H G T, Dekker W, Kan G, Breedijk M, Smout A J P M 1992 Acute noncardiac chest pain in a coronary care unit. Gastroenterology 102: 453–460
Levine M S, Moolten D N, Herlinger H, Laufer I 1986 Esophageal intramural pseudodiverticulosis: a reevaluation. American Journal of Roentgenology 147: 1165–1170
Liebermann-Meffert D, Allgower M, Schmid P, Blum A L 1979 Muscular equivalent of the lower esophageal sphincter. Gastroenterology 76: 31–38
Long W B, Cohen S 1980 The digestive tract as a cause of chest pain. American Heart Journal 100: 567–570
Ludlow A 1764 A case of obstructed deglutition from a preternatural dilatation of and bag formed in the pharynx. Medical Observation Inquiries 3: 85–101
McCord G S, Staiano A, Clouse R E 1991 Achalasia, diffuse spasm and non-specific motor disorders. Baillière's Clinical Gastroenterology 5: 307–335
Maddern G J, Horowitz M, Jamieson G G, Chatterton B E, Collins P J, Roberts-Thompson P 1984 Abnormalities of esophageal and gastric emptying in progressive systemic sclerosis. Gastroenterology 87: 922–926

Maddern G J, Horowitz M, Jamieson G G 1985 The effect of domperidone on esophageal emptying in diabetic autonomic neuropathy. British Journal of Clinical Pharmacology 19: 441–444

Maher J W, Olinde A J, McGuigan J E 1984 Suppression of post-prandial lower esophageal sphincter pressure and pancreatic polypeptide by duodenal exclusion. Journal of Surgical Research 37: 467–474

Margulies S I, Brunt P W, Donner M W, Silbiger M L 1968 Familial dysautonomia. Radiology 90: 107–112

Marshall J B, Kretschmar J M, Gerhardt D C et al 1990 Gastrointestinal manifestations of mixed connective tissue disease. Gastroenterology 98: 1232–1238

Maull K I, Scher L A, Greenfield L J 1979 Surgical implications of acid ingestion. Surgery, Gynecology and Obstetrics 148: 895–902

Mearin F, Guarner M F, Salas A, Riveros-Moreno V, Moncada S, Malagelada J-R 1993 Patients with achalasia lack nitric oxide synthase in the gastro-esophageal junction. European Journal of Clinical Investigation 23: 724–728

Mellow M H 1982. Management of esophageal complications. In: Cohen S, Soloway R (eds) Diseases of the esophagus. Churchill Livingstone, Edinburgh, p 215–238

Meyer G, Castell D 1981 Human esophageal response during chest pain induced by swallowing cold liquids. Journal of the American Medical Association 246: 2057–2059

Miller A J 1986 Neurophysiological basis of swallowing. Dysphagia 1: 91–100

Mittal R K, Siskind B N, Hongo M, Flye W, McCallum R W 1986 Dysphagia aortica – clinical, radiological, and manometric findings. Digestive Diseases and Sciences 31: 379–384

Muhletaler C A, Gerlock A J, de Soto L, Halter S A 1980 Gastroduodenal lesions of ingested acids: radiographic findings. American Journal of Roentgenology 134: 1247–1252

Nasrallah S M 1982 Nifedipine in the treatment of diffuse esophageal spasm. Lancet 2: 1285

Nasrallah S M, Hendrix E A 1987 Comparison of hypertonic glucose to other provocative tests in patients with noncardiac chest pain. American Journal of Gastroenterology 82: 406–409

Nebel O T, Castell D O 1973 Inhibition of the lower esophageal sphincter by fat – a mechanism for fatty food intolerance. Gut 14 : 270–274

Nowak T, Ionascescu V, Anuras S 1982 Gastrointestinal manifestations of the muscular dystrophies. Gastroenterology 82: 800–808

Orlando R C, Bozymski E M 1973 Clinical and manometric effects of nitroglycerin in diffuse esophageal spasm. New England Journal of Medicine 289: 23–25

Orlowski J, Dodds W, Linehan J, Dent J, Hogan W, Arndorfer R 1982 Requirements for accurate manometric recording of pharyngeal and esophageal peristaltic pressure waves. Investigative Radiology 17: 567–572

Ott D J, Gelfand D W, Wu W C, Castell D O 1984 Esophagogastric region and its rings. American Journal of Roentgenology 142: 281–287

Ott D J, Chen Y M, Wu W C, Gelfand D W, Munitz H A 1986 Radiographic and endoscopic sensitivity in detecting lower esophageal mucosal ring. American Journal of Roentgenology 147: 261–265

Parkman H P, Reynolds J C, Ouyang A, Rosato E F, Eisenberg J M, Cohen S 1993 Pneumatic dilatation or esophagomyotomy treatment for idiopathic achalasia: clinical outcomes and cost analysis. Digestive Diseases and Sciences 38: 75–85

Paterson W G, Anderson M A B, Anand N 1992 Pharmacological characterization of lower esophageal sphincter relaxation induced by swallowing, vagal efferent nerve stimulation, and esophageal distention. Canadian Journal of Physiology and Pharmacology 70: 1011–1015

Payne W S, King R M 1983 Pharyngesophageal (Zenker's) diverticulum. Surgical Clinics of North America 68: 815–824

Payne W S, Olsen A M 1974 The esophagus. Lea & Febiger, Philadelphia

Pearson J G 1966 The radiotherapy of carcinoma of the esophagus and post cricoid region in southeast Scotland. Clinical Radiology 17: 242–257

Pitman R G, Fraser G M 1965 The post-cricoid impression on the esophagus. Clinical Radiology 16: 34–39

Pope C E II 1978 Esophageal motility – who needs it? Gastroenterology 74: 1337–1338

Postlethwait R W 1983 Chemical burns of the esophagus. Surgical Clinics of North America 63: 915–924

Postlethwait R W, Sealy W C 1967 Experiences with the treatment of 59 patients with lower esophageal web. Annals of Surgery 165: 786–791

Proudfit W L, Shirey E K, Jones F M 1966 Selective cine coronary arteriography. Correlation with clinical findings in 1000 patients. Circulation 331: 901–910

Richter J E, Castell D O 1984 Diffuse esophageal spasm: a reappraisal. Annals of Internal Medicine 100: 242–245

Richter J E, Castell D O 1989 24 hour ambulatory esophageal motility monitoring: how should motility data be analysed? Gut 30: 1040–1047

Richter J E, Johns D N, Wu W C, Castell D O 1985 Are esophageal motility abnormalities produced during the intra-esophageal acid perfusion test? Journal of the American Medical Association 253: 1914–1917

Richter J E, Barish C F, Castell D O 1986 Abnormal sensory perception in patients with esophageal chest pain. Gastroenterology 91: 845–852

Richter J E, Wu W C, Johns D N et al 1987 Esophageal manometry in 95 healthy adult volunteers. Digestive Diseases and Sciences 32: 583–592

Roberts R, Henderson R D, Wigle E D 1975 Esophageal disease as a cause of severe retrosternal chest pain. Chest 67: 523–526

Rodman G P, Medsger T A J, Buckingham R B 1975 Progressive systemic sclerosis-CREST syndrome: observations on natural history and late complications in 90 patients. Arthritis and Rheumatism 18: 423–431

Rubinow A, Burakoff R, Cohen A S, Harris L D 1983 Esophageal manometry in systemic amyloidosis. American Journal of Medicine 75: 951–956

Russell C O H, Gannan R, Coatsworth J et al 1983 Relationship among esophageal dysfunction, diabetic gastroenteropathy and peripheral neuropathy. Digestive Diseases and Sciences 28: 289–293

Saario I, Kostainen S, Salo J, Meurala H, Eerola S 1983 Treatment of spontaneous rupture of the esophagus. Acta Chirugie Scandanavica 149: 771–774

Sabanthan S, Salama F D, Morgan W E 1985 Esophageal intramural pseudodiverticulosis. Thorax 40: 849–857

Sakulsky S B, Harrison E G, Dines D E, Payne W S 1967 Mediastinal granuloma. Journal of Thoracic and Cardiovascular Surgery 54: 279–290

Sanowski R A 1987 Foreign body extraction in the gastrointestinal tract. In: Sivak M (ed) Gastroenterologic endoscopy. W B Saunders, Philadelphia, p 321–331

Sarfati E, Gossot D, Assens P, Celerier M 1987 Management of caustic ingestion in adults. British Journal of Surgery 74: 146–148

Schatzki R 1963 The lower esophageal ring: long-term follow-up of symptomatic and asymptomatic rings. American Journal of Roentgenology 90: 805–810

Schatzki R, Gary J E 1953 Dysphagia due to a diaphragm-like localised narrowing in the lower esophagus ("lower esophageal ring"). American Journal of Roentgenology 70: 911–922

Schofield P M, Bennett D H, Whorwell P J et al 1987 Exertional gastro-esophageal reflux: a mechanism for symptoms in patients with angina pectoris and normal coronary angiograms. British Medical Journal 294: 1459–1461

Seaman W B 1981 Pathophysiology of the esophagus. Seminars in Roentgenology 16: 214–227

Seelig L L, Goyal R K 1978 Morphological evaluation of opossum lower esophageal sphincter. Gastroenterology 75: 51–58

Shay S S, Myers R L, Johnson L F 1984 Hiccups associated with reflux esophagitis. Gastroenterology 87: 205–207

Silver L S, Worner T M, Korsten M A 1986 Esophageal function in chronic alcoholics. American Journal of Gastroenterology 81: 423–427

Smart H L, Nicholson D A, Atkinson M 1986 Gastro-esophageal reflux in the irritable bowel syndrome. Gut 27: 1227–1231

Stankey R M, Roshe J, Sogocio R M 1969 Carcinoma of the lung and dysphagia. Diseases of the Chest 55: 13–17

Stewart J R, Kincaid O W, Edwards J E 1964 An atlas of vascular rings and related malformations of the aortic arch system. Thomas, Springfield

Swamy N 1977 Esophageal spasm: clinical and manometric response to nitroglyceride and long acting nitrites. Gastroenterology 72: 23–27

Todorczuk J R, Aliperti G, Staiano A, Clouse R E 1991 Reevaluation of manometric criteria for vigorous achalasia. Is this a distinct clinical disorder? Digestive Diseases and Sciences 36: 274–278

Tottrup A, Forman A, Funch-Jensen P, Raundahl U, Andersson K-E 1990 Effects of postganglionic nerve stimulation in esophageal achalasia: an in vitro study. Gut 31: 17–20

Traube M 1991 On drugs and dilators for achalasia. Digestive Diseases and Sciences 36: 257–259

Traube M, Aaronson R M, McCallum R W 1986 Transition from peristaltic esophageal contractions to diffuse esophageal spasm. Archives of Internal Medicine 146: 1844–1846

Trenkner S W, Maglinte D T, Lehman G, Chernish S M, Miller R E, Johnson C W 1983 Esophageal food impaction: treatment with glucagon. Radiology 149: 401–403

Tsianos E B, Drosos A A, Chiras C D, Moutsopoulos H M, Kitridou R C 1987 Esophageal manometric findings in autoimmune rheumatic diseases: is scleroderma esophagus a specific entity? Rheumatology International 7: 23–27

Tucker H J, Snape W J, Cohen S 1978 Achalasia secondary to carcinoma: manometric and clinical features. Annals of Internal Medicine 89: 315–318

Turner R, Rittenberg G, Lipshutz W, Schumacher H R, Miller W, Cohen S 1973 Esophageal dysfunction in collagen disease. American Journal of Medical Science 265: 191–203

Vanek A W, Diamant N E 1987 Responses of the human esophagus to paired swallows. Gastroenterology 92: 643–650

Vantrappen G, Hellemans J 1980 Treatment of achalasia and related motor disorders. Gastroenterology 79: 144–154

Vantrappen G, Janssens J, Hellemans J, Coremans G 1979 Achalasia, diffuse spasm and related motility disorders. Gastroenterology 76: 450–457

Webb W A 1992 Foreign bodies in the esophagus. In: Taylor M B (ed) Gastrointestinal emergencies. Williams & Wilkins, Baltimore, p 1–12

Welch R W, Luckmann K, Ricks P M, Drake S T, Gates G A 1979 Manometry of the normal upper esophageal sphincter and its alterations in laryngectomy. Journal of Clinical Investigation 63: 1036–1041

Wesdorp I C E, Bartelsman J F, Huibregtse K, den Hartog Jager F C, Tytgat G N 1984 Treatment of instrumental esophageal perforation. Gut 25: 398–404

Wilkins W E, Walker J, McNulty M R, Britton D G, Gough K R 1984 The organisation and evaluation of an open access dysphagia clinic. Annals of the Royal College of Surgeons of England 66: 115

Wychulis A R, Kincaid O W, Weidman W H, Danielson G K 1971 Congenital vascular ring: surgical considerations and results of operation. Proceedings of the Staff Meetings of the Mayo Clinic 46: 182–189

Wyman J B, Dent J, Heddle R, Dodds W J, Toouli J, Downton J 1990 Control of belching by the lower esophageal sphincter. Gut 31: 639–646

Wynder E L, Fryer J H 1958 Etiologic considerations of Plummer–Vinson (Paterson–Kelly) syndrome. Annals of Internal Medicine 49: 1106–1111

Zamost B J, Hirschberg J, Ippoliti A F, Furst D E, Clements P J, Weinstein W M 1987 Esophagitis in scleroderma. Prevalence and risk factors. Gastroenterology 92: 421–428

Zboralske F F 1965 The esophagus in the geriatric patient. Radiologic Clinics of North America 3: 321–327

Zelcer E, Weisbrodt N W 1984 Electrical and mechanical activity in the lower esophageal sphincter of the cat. American Journal of Physiology 246: G243–G247

Zenker F A, Ziemssen H V 1878. On dilatations of the esophagus. Cyclopaedia of the practice of medicine. Low, Marston, Searle & Rivington, London, p 46–68

# 8. Diseases of the esophageal mucosa

*S. J. Spechler*

GASTROESOPHAGEAL REFLUX DISEASE

Gastroesophageal reflux disease (GERD) can be defined as any symptomatic condition (e.g. heartburn), anatomic alteration (e.g. esophagitis) or both that result from the reflux of noxious material from the stomach into the esophagus. In Western countries, it has been estimated that 20–40% of adults experience heartburn at least occasionally and that endoscopic screening of the general adult population would reveal a 1–2% prevalence of reflux esophagitis (Spechler 1992c). Complications such as esophageal ulceration, stricture and Barrett's esophagus develop in approximately 10–20% of patients who have reflux esophagitis (Spechler 1992b). Clearly, GERD is an extraordinarily common condition in the Western world. The development of GERD is a multifactorial process that often involves dysfunction of a number of normal mechanisms – those that prevent gastroesophageal reflux and those that clear the esophagus of noxious material (Dodds et al 1981, Pope 1994). These mechanisms are reviewed in detail below.

### Antireflux mechanisms

*Lower esophageal sphincter* (LES)

The mean resting pressure in the body of the esophagus is slightly below atmospheric pressure, whereas mean intragastric pressure is slightly higher (Dodds et al 1981). This positive pressure gradient between the abdomen and the thorax promotes gastroesophageal reflux. Indeed, such reflux would occur virtually continuously in the absence of effective antireflux mechanisms (Dodds et al 1981). One of the primary barriers to reflux is the LES, a 1–3.5 cm segment of specialized circular muscle in the distal esophagus (Holloway & Dent 1990) (p. 167). A number of functional characteristics of LES muscle distinguish it from the muscle of the adjacent esophagus and stomach. For example, strips of LES muscle develop spontaneous tension on stretching and relax with transmural electrical stimulation. The LES normally prevents reflux by maintaining a resting pressure 10–30 mmHg higher than that of the stomach (p. 170). Three types of LES dysfunction have been described that can contribute to gastroesophageal reflux:

1. feeble resting LES pressure;
2. inadequate LES response to increased abdominal pressure;
3. transient, inappropriate LES relaxation.

In some individuals, the resting pressure in the LES is so feeble that the sphincter does not pose an effective barrier to reflux. Nearly one-quarter of all episodes of acid reflux in patients with severe GERD are associated with feeble resting LES pressure (Dent et al 1988). Patients who exhibit a feeble resting LES pressure also may have an inadequate LES response to increased abdominal pressure. Normally, increases in abdominal pressure are accompanied by simultaneous increases in LES pressure of similar magnitude. This mechanism ordinarily prevents gastroesophageal reflux during coughing, sneezing, straining and other activities that cause sudden elevations in abdominal pressure. Sometimes, especially in patients whose LES is weak, these sudden increases in abdominal pressure are not accompanied by similar elevations in LES pressure. During these episodes when there is an inadequate LES response to increased abdominal pressure, the resulting pressure gradient can propel gastric material into the esophagus. The precise contribution of this mechanism to GERD is disputed.

The most important LES mechanism for reflux appears to be that of transient, inappropriate LES relaxation (Dent et al 1988). Unlike the brief (3–10 s in duration) appropriate LES relaxations that accompany primary peristalsis, transient LES relaxations are not preceded by a normal peristaltic sequence and last for up to 30 s (Kahrilas et al 1994). In normal individuals, brief episodes of gastroesophageal reflux (called physiologic reflux) occur almost exclusively through the mechanism of transient LES relaxation. Transient LES relaxations can be stimulated by gastric distention and often occur after meals (Kahrilas et al 1994). In patients with GERD, transient LES relaxation is the most frequent, but not necessarily the exclusive cause of reflux. In patients with severe GERD, more than two-thirds of all reflux episodes are associated with transient, inappropriate LES relaxations (Dent et al 1988).

*Crural diaphragm*

The esophagus passes from the thorax into the abdomen through a canal-like opening in the right crus of the diaphragm called the diaphragmatic hiatus. Thus, the crural diaphragm normally encircles a portion of the LES (Mittal 1990). Both the crural and costal portions of the diaphragm contract with inspiration and relax with expiration and both are supplied by the phrenic nerve. However, there appear to be separate neural control mechanisms for each diaphragmatic portion (Mittal 1990). During inspiration, when the abdominothoracic pressure gradient increases so as to favor reflux, the diaphragmatic crurae come together and pinch the distal esophagus. This pinching effect appears to function as an important barrier to reflux during inspiration and during other activities that increase intra-abdominal pressure (Mittal et al 1988). In dogs, gastroesophageal reflux does not occur during transient LES relaxations unless the relaxations are associated with inhibition of the crural diaphragm (Martin et al 1992). This observation suggests that gastroesophageal reflux results only when there is relaxation of both the internal (LES) and external (crural diaphragm) esophageal sphincters. Furthermore, transient LES relaxation with inhibition of the crural diaphragm in dogs is often associated with contraction of the costal diaphragm that further promotes reflux (Martin et al 1992). A similar sequence of events is seen during belching, suggesting that gastroesophageal reflux during transient LES relaxation often occurs through a variant of the belch reflex. In summary, it appears that both the LES and the crural diaphragm contribute importantly to the antireflux barrier. The crural diaphragm buttresses the LES during activities that otherwise might overcome the sphincter's ability to prevent reflux.

Certain anatomic features of the distal esophagus also may contribute to the antireflux barrier. For example, a portion of the distal esophagus ordinarily is located below the diaphragm and is subject to abdominal pressure. Presumably, this external pressure applied to the walls of the intra-abdominal esophagus tends to close the lumen and prevent reflux (O'Sullivan et al 1982).

*Effects of hiatal hernia on the antireflux barrier*

In many patients with GERD, the condition is associated with a sliding hiatal hernia in which both the esophagogastric junction and a portion of the gastric fundus migrate through the diaphragmatic hiatus into the posterior mediastinum. For reasons that are not clear, resting LES pressure is often low in patients who have sliding hiatal hernias. This LES hypotension predisposes to gastroesophageal reflux. Also, hiatal herniation can disrupt the extrasphincteric antireflux mechanisms. With a large hiatal hernia, the distal esophagus is no longer located within the abdomen and, therefore, no longer subject to the external squeeze of abdominal pressure that might prevent reflux. Furthermore, the diaphragmatic crurae no longer pinch the distal esophagus during inspiration. Instead, approximation of the crurae creates an intrathoracic pouch of stomach that may function as a reservoir of material available for reflux. A recent study has shown that the susceptibility to gastroesophageal reflux induced by abrupt elevations of intra-abdominal pressure correlates significantly both with weak LES pressure and with hiatal hernia size (Sloan et al 1992).

Although it appears that hiatal hernia often contributes importantly to GERD, hiatal hernia is neither necessary nor sufficient for the development of reflux esophagitis. Patients who have no hiatal hernia can have GERD and hiatal hernia is not always associated with reflux esophagitis.

## Gastric contents

Refluxed gastric contents must be caustic in order to injure the esophageal mucosa. Acid and pepsin are caustic agents that are normally present in the stomach and readily available for reflux. The dramatic efficacy of potent inhibitors of gastric acid secretion like omeprazole in the treatment of reflux esophagitis underscores the importance of gastric acid in the pathogenesis of reflux esophagitis. However, some patients with severe, ulcerative GERD may not heal completely with acid suppression therapy alone (Hetzel et al 1988). In these patients, substances other than acid and pepsin might contribute to esophagitis. The duodenum contains substances that are potentially harmful to the esophagus including bile acids, lysolecithin and pancreatic digestive enzymes. These noxious substances can reflux into the stomach and from there into the esophagus. The precise contribution of these agents to GERD is disputed, however.

Delayed gastric emptying may play a pathogenetic role in GERD. Using sensitive radionuclide tests, some investigators have found delayed gastric emptying in more than 50% of patients with GERD (McCallum 1990). With delayed gastric emptying, gastric material available for reflux lingers in the stomach and causes gastric distention. Gastric distention has at least two undesirable effects for patients with GERD: it stimulates gastric acid secretion and it triggers transient, inappropriate relaxation of the LES. Prokinetic agents like cisapride that promote gastric motility may be helpful in patients whose GERD is associated with delayed gastric emptying.

## Esophageal clearance mechanisms

Normal individuals experience brief episodes of acid reflux

every day but they do not cause any obvious mucosal injury. To damage the esophagus, refluxed material must have a sufficient duration of contact with the epithelium, which is a function of esophageal clearance mechanisms. There are four important mechanisms for clearing the esophagus of acid: gravity, peristalsis, salivation and intrinsic esophageal bicarbonate production. Most of the material that enters the esophagus is cleared by the effects of gravity and peristalsis (Helm et al 1984) but they are not 100% efficient at clearing the esophagus and even a small quantity of residual acidic material can cause mucosal damage. Fortunately, residual acidic material can be neutralized by swallowed saliva (Helm et al 1984), which is highly alkaline, and by bicarbonate produced by the esophageal mucosa itself (Meyers & Orlando 1992).

GERD can be associated with conditions that interfere with esophageal clearance. Patients who have esophageal motility disorders associated with disordered or absent peristalsis (e.g. scleroderma) frequently have severe GERD. Reflux that occurs during sleep can be particularly damaging to the esophagus for several reasons relating to esophageal clearance. In recumbency, gravity does not facilitate the clearance of material from the esophagus. Swallowing and salivation virtually cease during sleep and, therefore, there is no primary peristalsis and little saliva available to clear acid in the esophageal lumen. Cigarette smoking has been shown to increase esophageal acid exposure by increasing the frequency of acid reflux events and, perhaps, by decreasing salivary flow (Kahrilas 1992). Finally, hiatal hernia has been shown to interfere with esophageal clearance (Sloan & Kahrilas 1991).

## Esophageal mucosal resistance

Three types of defensive factors contribute to esophageal mucosal resistance (Orlando 1991a, 1994):

1. pre-epithelial factors that prevent $H^+$ ions coming into contact with the epithelial cells;
2. epithelial factors that prevent $H^+$ ions in contact with the cell membrane from entering the cells and that buffer or eliminate $H^+$ ions that have penetrated the cells;
3. postepithelial factors that remove $H^+$ ions extruded from the cells and that provide bicarbonate to the epithelium.

Potential components of the pre-epithelial defenses include the surface mucous layer, the unstirred water layer and a layer of bicarbonate ions that line the luminal surface of the epithelial cells. Unlike the stomach and duodenum in which these pre-epithelial factors contribute substantially to mucosal resistance, the pre-epithelial factors in the esophagus are poorly developed and appear to play a minor role in protecting the squamous epithelium from acid-peptic injury. To penetrate the epithelium, $H^+$ ions must pass through the cell membrane or through intercellular spaces where ion movement is restricted by tight junctions and by intercellular material such as lipid and mucin. Both the squamous cell membranes and their intercellular junctional complexes pose formidable barriers to the passage of $H^+$ ions. Nevertheless, exposure to relatively high concentrations of acid can overwhelm these epithelial defenses. $H^+$ ions that enter the epithelial cells can be buffered by intracellular proteins, phosphate and bicarbonate. When the buffers are overwhelmed, squamous cell membranes harbor ion transport systems that can extrude $H^+$ ions out of the cell. These transport systems include a $Na^+/H^+$ exchanger and a $Cl^-/HCO_3^-$ exchange mechanism that appears to have both Na-dependent and Na-independent components. Postepithelial defenses are provided by the esophageal blood supply. The blood delivers the nutrients and oxygen required for normal cell functions and repairs, removes noxious metabolic products such as $CO_2$ and $H^+$ ions and supplies bicarbonate for buffering acid in the intercellular space.

Ambulatory esophageal pH monitoring studies have shown that normal individuals experience brief episodes of acid reflux each day (Orlando 1994). Apparently, the normal esophageal mucosal defenses can resist these brief acid onslaughts. Most patients with reflux esophagitis have an abnormally prolonged duration of esophageal acid exposure. However, some patients have reflux esophagitis despite a normal daily duration of acid reflux as documented by 24-h esophageal pH monitoring studies (Mattioli et al 1989). These patients may have yet uncharacterized defects in esophageal mucosal resistance. It is not clear whether these defects involve the pre-epithelial, epithelial, or postepithelial defense factors.

## NSAIDs and GERD

Circumstantial evidence provided by epidemiologic studies suggests that the ingestion of aspirin and other nonsteroidal anti-inflammatory drugs (NSAIDs) can contribute to GERD (Lanas & Hirschowitz 1991). Patients with esophageal strictures appear to be especially susceptible to NSAID-induced esophageal injury (Wilkins et al 1984). Many NSAID preparations are injurious to the mucosa and severe local injury can result when a stricture impedes passage of the NSAID tablet into the stomach. For patients without strictures, the mechanisms whereby NSAIDS contribute to GERD are not clear.

## Pathology

When the esophagus is examined with the endoscope (see below), a red appearance does not necessarily signify inflammation on histological examination. However, esophagitis can be diagnosed with confidence when the mucosa is ulcerated or when there is a stricture. Longitudinal ridges in the lower esophagus are often seen, the ridges being healing epithelium and the areas between them denuded epithelium.

Early esophagitis is difficult to detect microscopically. Early changes (Fig. 8.1) are thickening of the basal layer of the epithelium and elongation of the papillae (Ismail-Beigi et al 1970) resulting from an increased loss of surface cells and an increased turnover rate of the mucosa. Such changes are found in 85% of patients with symptoms of reflux and in less than 10% of those without symptoms. Only 18% of patients with reflux symptoms have an infiltrate of polymorphonuclear leukocytes in the lamina propria or epithelium, but if patients with severe symptoms are selected, the incidence rises to 40% (Hendrix & Yardley 1976). The presence of lymphocytes does not correlate with symptomatic reflux, but the presence of eosinophils does appear significant (Winter et al 1982). In making histological assessments of reflux damage, it should be emphasized that early changes are common in the distal 2 cm of asymptomatic subjects and therefore biopsies should be obtained more proximally. If the early changes progress, the surface epithelium may be lost, leaving an acutely inflamed submucosa as the esophageal lining. Healing commences with longitudinal epithelial ridges, but continuing damage may prevent this; fibrosis may develop and may be important in shortening the esophagus. With severe ulceration, the inflammatory reaction may extend through the entire wall of the esophagus into the mediastinum.

*Columnar epithelium in the esophagus* (Fig. 8.2)

This is sometimes called Barrett's esophagus after Barrett who first described it; an ulcer in the columnar epithelium is sometimes called a Barrett's ulcer (Fig. 8.3). The columnar epithelium is a metaplastic response to prolonged reflux and esophagitis. Barrett's esophagus was found in 13% of children whose symptoms of reflux were severe enough to lead to esophagoscopy (Dahms & Rothstein 1984), and in adults with reflux between 2% and 12% of patients develop columnar metaplasia (Thompson 1982, Winter et al 1987). In fact, Barrett's metaplasia is a complex and intimate mixture of epithelial cell types. Cell types are gastric-type surface mucous and mucous neck cells, intestinal (Fig. 8.4.), goblet and absorptive cells, chief and parietal cells and neuroendocrine cells (Paull et al 1976). Glands may resemble those of the gastric body, gastric cardia and antral glands or residual esophageal submucosal glands.

The surface epithelium shows all gradations from flat to a normal small intestinal villous pattern (Thompson 1982, Thompson et al 1983). In situ or invasive adenocarcinoma may arise in the columnar mucosa (p. 202).

The macroscopic morphology reveals several important features: the metaplastic mucosa is much deeper red than normal mucosa and the transition between the two is sharp and ulceration is frequent at the junction. The junction usually does not show gross or microscopic evidence of fibrous stricture but focal ulcerations and residual islands of squamous epithelium are frequent (Thompson 1982).

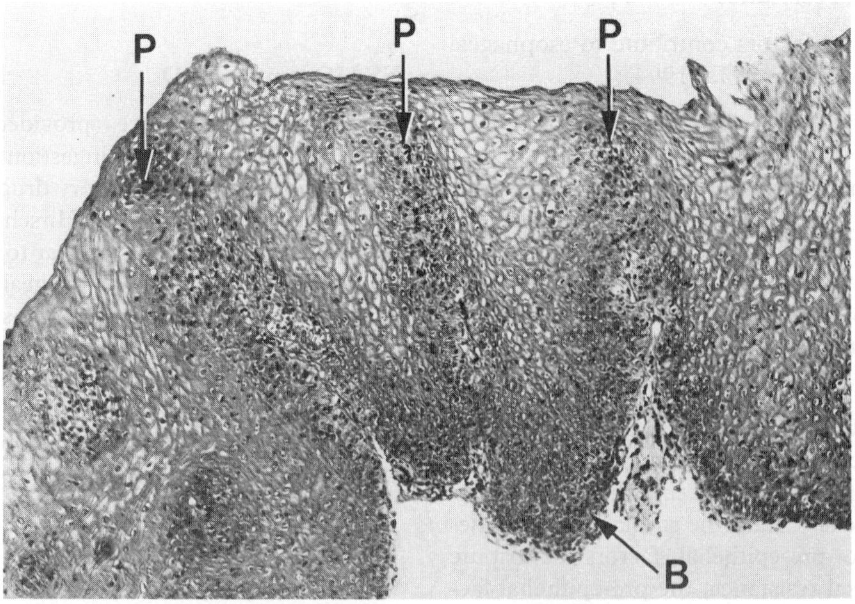


**Fig. 8.1** Preulcerative esophagitis. Esophageal biopsy showing basal cell hyperplasia (B) and increased penetration of papillae (P) towards the surface of the squamous epithelium. (Hematoxylin and eosin ×100.)

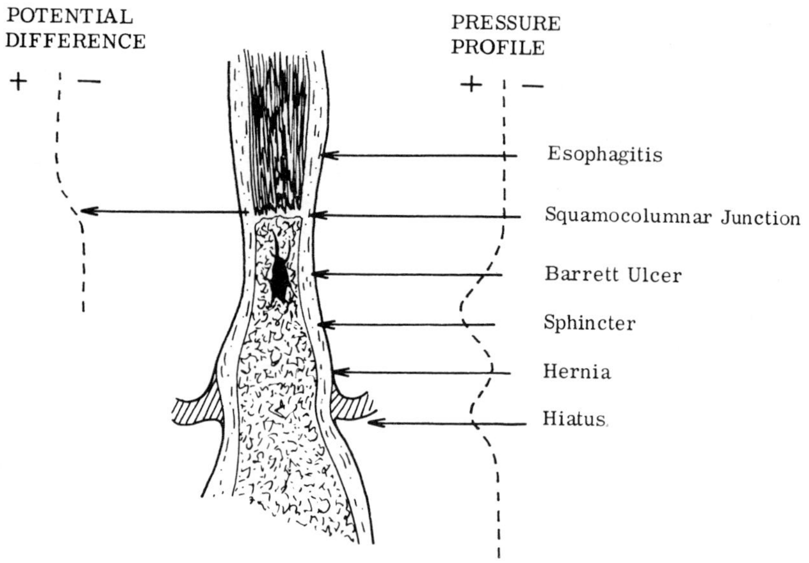


**Fig. 8.2** Barrett's esophagus. Resting pressure and transmucosal potential difference. Potential difference changes abruptly at the squamocolumnar junction, but twin peaks of pressure, marking diaphragmatic hiatus and inferior sphincter, are at a lower level. That portion between mucosal junction and sphincter has typically esophageal motor responses (Burgess et al 1971).

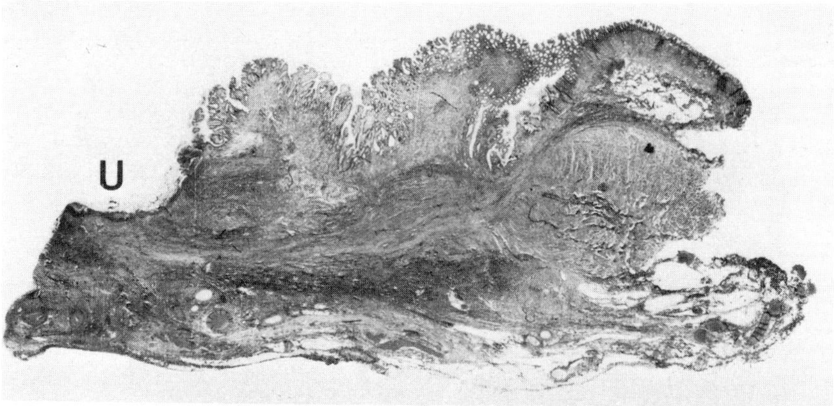


**Fig. 8.3** Peptic ulcer (U) in gastric-type mucosa within the distal esophagus. (Hematoxylin and eosin ×4.)

*Peptic ulcer of the esophagus* (Hendrix & Yardley 1976)

This develops in columnar epithelium close to its junction with squamous epithelium. The ulcer is usually situated on the anterior or posterior wall, is well demarcated and penetrates into the wall of the esophagus. It may result in a localized stricture with eccentric fibrosis, perforation or erosion of an artery.

*Stricture of the esophagus* (Fig. 8.5)

Stricture of the squamous esophagus develops when severe ulceration is prevented from healing by persistent reflux (Bremner 1982). This ulceration may be extensive or localized as a peptic ulcer of the esophagus. Concentric fibrosis commences in the submucosa and then progresses to the muscular coats; the resulting stricture may be several centimeters long. Stricture is most common in patients with Barrett's esophagus, particularly children (Hassall et al 1985). Commonly the stricture is sharply localized and is usually situated just above the squamocolumnar junction, often in the mid-esophagus.

## Clinical features

Symptoms are due to esophagitis and regurgitation and not to hiatus hernia; most patients with hiatus hernia are asymptomatic (Crozier & Jonasson 1964).

Heartburn (p. 168), the cardinal symptom, is a discomfort or burning sensation behind the sternum. It occurs

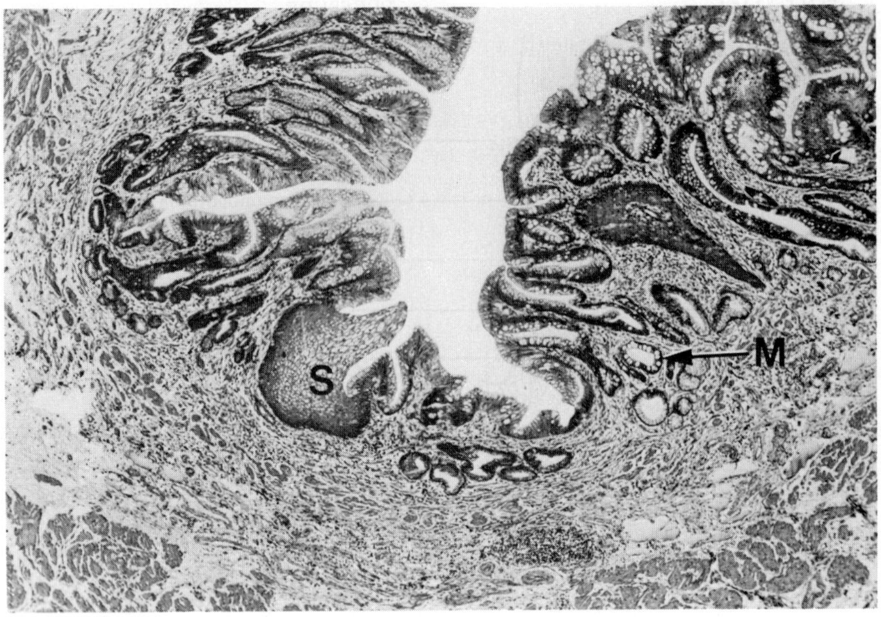


**Fig. 8.4** Metaplasia of squamous epithelium (S) in the distal esophagus to gastric-type mucosa showing intestinal metaplasia (M). (Hematoxylin and eosin ×40.)

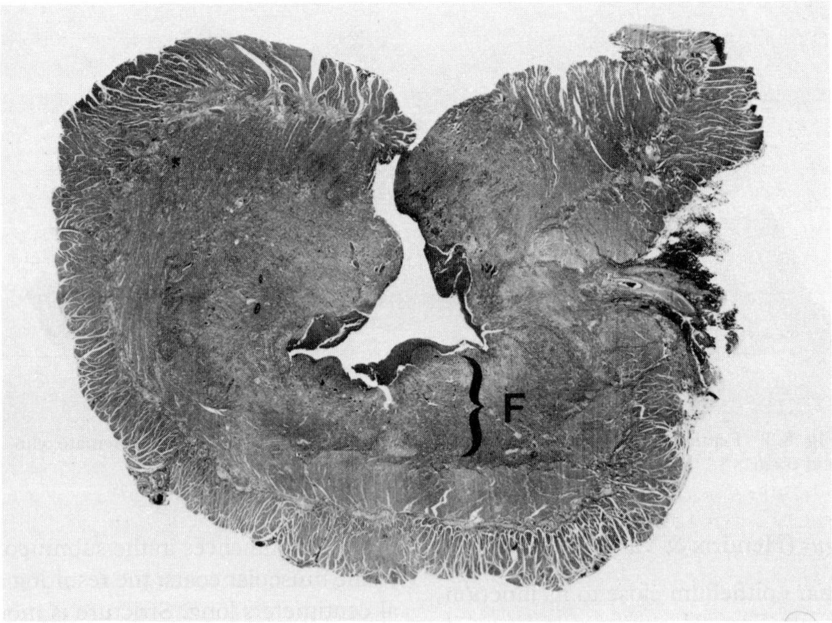


**Fig. 8.5** Peptic stricture. A cross-section of a stricture in the distal esophagus showing ulceration of the epithelium and marked submucosal fibrosis (F). (Hematoxylin and eosin ×3.5.)

one hour or more after food, at night or when bending. It is relieved by antacids within a few minutes and is precipitated by citrus juices. Dysphagia (p. 167) precipitated by solid food may occur but is often transient, occurring characteristically on the first swallow of the meal, and can be relieved by repeated swallowing. It is usually due to dysmotility rather than stricture (p. 200). Persistent dysphagia suggests the development of stricture. Occasionally, swallowing is painful.

Regurgitation of gastric contents into the mouth occurs on bending or during the night and may or may not be accompanied by heartburn. It can result in cough and wheezing due to aspiration pharyngitis and posterior laryngitis. Lung scanning following placement of radio-labeled technetium in the stomach has demonstrated isotope in the lungs (Chernow et al 1979). There is general agreement that this aspiration may contribute to the severity of asthma in some adults and children (Barish et al 1985). Alternatively, reflux may stimulate vagal afferents in the esophagus, leading to bronchoconstriction via vagal efferents in the airways. There is also evidence that gastroesophageal reflux may be contributory in some cases of chronic bronchitis. Adequate therapy for reflux has been shown to improve the respiratory conditions.

Chest pain indistinguishable from angina occurs in 10% of patients with esophagitis (Crozier et al 1972). It can radiate to the neck, jaws and arms, but is not related to exercise (p. 169). Bernstein et al (1962) demonstrated that angina-like substernal chest pain can be induced by acid perfusion of the esophagus in patients with exertional substernal chest pain and no evidence of cardiac disease. This has been confirmed in several studies (Brand 1982, Davies et al 1985). It has been postulated that reflux induces diffuse spasm or high amplitude contractions which cause pain but several groups have failed to demonstrate these during acid perfusion of the esophagus (Burns & Venturatos 1985, Kjellen & Tibbling 1985). The instillation of acid may also act to lower the angina threshold by cardiovascular or neurological mechanisms (p. 169).

Some patients without any other symptoms bleed from the inflamed mucosa. Rarely, this causes a hematemesis and/or melena; more usually, slow bleeding leads to iron deficiency anemia. Very occasionally, an adult with esophagitis may vomit small volumes of gastric content.

Occasionally, the symptomatology may be confusing because another condition is present; this may be cholelithiasis or peptic ulceration, which are commonly associated with peptic esophagitis.

## Diagnostic tests for GERD (Table 8.1)

Barium swallow examination will demonstrate reflux and may define superficial ulceration in the esophageal mucosa (pp. 5 and 8). Endoscopic assessment of severity of esophagitis is discussed in the chapter on endoscopy (p. 105). For patients who have characteristic symptoms of heartburn and regurgitation that respond readily to acid suppression therapy, few diagnostic tests are necessary to confirm the diagnosis of GERD because the characteristic history virtually establishes the presence of the disorder. Nevertheless, an endoscopic examination might be performed to seek evidence of esophagitis that may require more aggressive therapy and evidence of complications such as Barrett's esophagus that cannot be diagnosed on the basis of history alone. Further diagnostic tests may be required for patients with atypical signs or symptoms and for patients with typical signs and symptoms that do not respond well to acid suppression. In such cases, ambulatory monitoring of esophageal pH can be used to document the pattern, frequency and duration of acid reflux and to seek a correlation between reflux episodes and symptoms (Mattioli et al 1989, Mattox & Richter 1990).

*24-h Ambulatory pH monitoring* (Richter & Castell 1982, Atkinson 1987)

Although originally limited by nonportable equipment and the need for hospitalization, the development of portable microprocessors has allowed recordings to be made while the patient is at work or at home.

A pH electrode is positioned 5 cm above the lower esophageal sphincter and is connected to a portable microprocessor, which is carried by the patient on a belt. The microprocessor digitizes the esophageal pH signal and stores the data for subsequent analysis. The microprocessor also contains a signal marker, activated by the patient, to indicate occurrence of symptoms, meals and sleep. The data are decoded by a computer and analyzed for the number of reflux episodes, their duration and the duration of esophageal acid exposure. In most ambulatory systems, an episode of acid reflux is defined (somewhat arbitrarily) as a drop in esophageal pH below 4! Standard 24-h pH monitoring records a number of different variables such as the total number of reflux episodes, the number longer than 5 min in duration, and the duration of the longest episode. The single most clinically applicable variable appears to be the total percentage of the monitoring period that esophageal pH remains below 4 (Mattox & Richter 1990).

The great majority of patients who have both endoscopic signs and symptoms of GERD also have abnormal 24-h esophageal pH monitoring studies, whereas subjects

**Table 8.1** Diagnostic tests for GERD

| | Is there gastro-esophageal reflux? | Is there esophagitis? (inflammation, ulceration) | Is there Barrett's esophagus? | Is there an esophageal stricture? | Are symptoms due to acid reflux? |
|---|---|---|---|---|---|
| UGI series | + | + | + | +++ | – |
| Endoscopy | + | +++ | +++ | ++ | – |
| Esophageal biopsy | – | +++ | +++ | – | – |
| Ambulatory pH monitoring | +++ | – | – | – | +++ |

with no such signs and symptoms usually have normal studies.

*Standard acid reflux test* (Kantrowitz et al 1969)

This test assesses the propensity of reflux to occur under standardized conditions and is usually performed during esophageal manometry. A pH electrode is fastened to the manometric assembly and positioned 5 cm above the manometrically defined lower esophageal sphincter. Three hundred milliliters of 0.1N HCl are instilled into the stomach and esophageal pH is measured basally and during increases in intra-abdominal pressure induced by leg raising, the Valsalva maneuver and coughing. These maneuvers are repeated in the supine and Trendelenburg positions. Reflux is defined as a fall in esophageal pH to 4 or less. The severity of reflux is indicated by the number of reflux episodes and their duration and judged to be significant if reflux occurs basally or with two or more maneuvers.

Although some studies have yielded good discrimination between control subjects and patients with reflux esophagitis, false positive and false negative rates of between 5% and 20% have been reported. A major problem with the test is the highly artificial condition under which it is performed. Because the majority of reflux episodes occur during spontaneous and randomly occurring transient lower esophageal sphincter relaxations, the relevance of the stress maneuvers in such a standardized test is questionable. For this reason pH tests such as ambulatory pH monitoring, which are performed under more physiological conditions, have largely superseded the standard test.

## Management of patients with GERD

The principles of management for patients with GERD emerge from an understanding of the pathophysiologic mechanisms described above (Kitchin & Castell 1991, Katz 1991, deVault & Castell 1994, Pope 1994).

### *Lifestyle modifications*

Management of GERD begins with the lifestyle modifications aimed at reducing acid reflux (Kitchin & Castell 1991, Katz 1991). These modifications include the following:

***Elevate the head of the bed on 4–6 inch blocks.*** This exploits the beneficial effect of gravity on esophageal clearance.

***Advise weight loss for obese patients.*** In theory, obesity may increase abdominal pressure and thereby promote reflux. Studies documenting this effect are not available. Nevertheless, obese patients often report improvement of their GERD symptoms with weight loss. Some authorities attribute this beneficial effect to the elimination of the fatty foods and gastric distention that promote reflux rather than to the weight loss per se. Regardless of the precise mechanism underlying this effect, weight loss seems advisable for obese subjects.

***Avoid bedtime snacks.*** These may stimulate nocturnal acid production by the stomach and stimulate transient LES relaxations, thereby promoting nocturnal reflux. Nocturnal reflux can be especially damaging to the esophagus because recumbency retards esophageal clearance and because the swallowing and salivation that might eliminate refluxed acid cease during sleep.

***Avoid chocolate, fatty foods and carminatives (spearmint, peppermint).*** These foods may decrease LES pressure and delay gastric emptying, thereby promoting acid reflux.

***Avoid cigarettes and alcohol.*** These agents have been found to decrease LES pressure. Cigarette smoking has been shown to increase the frequency of acid reflux events and also may decrease salivation that is important for esophageal acid clearance.

***Avoid drugs that decrease LES pressure and delay gastric emptying if possible.*** These include drugs that have anticholinergic effects and calcium channel blocking agents. Avoid NSAIDs if possible.

### *Drug therapy*

***$H_2$ receptor blocking agents.*** For patients who respond well to the above lifestyle modifications, medications may not be necessary and antacids with or without alginic acid can be used as necessary for occasional episodes of heartburn (Pope 1994). For patients who remain symptomatic, a histamine $H_2$ receptor blocking agent (e.g. cimetidine, famotidine, nizatidine, ranitidine) is a reasonable first medication. When used in conventional doses, relief of GERD symptoms and healing of esophagitis occurs within 12 weeks in approximately one-half to two-thirds of patients (Sontag 1990, Kitchin & Castell 1991, Katz 1991, Pope 1994). If relief is not complete, the dose of the agent can be increased. Although very high doses of histamine $H_2$ receptor blockers (up to eight times the conventional dose) have been used effectively to treat esophagitis in refractory cases (Collen & Johnson 1992), there is little point in prescribing more than a double dose of these agents. When used in very high doses, $H_2$ blockers are expensive and their long-term safety has not been established. For refractory patients, it seems preferable to add another agent or to use a more potent inhibitor of gastric acid secretion such as a proton pump inhibitor (see below).

***Prokinetic agents.*** Prokinetic agents decrease gastroesophageal reflux by elevating LES pressure and by enhancing gastric and esophageal emptying (McCallum 1990). Prokinetic agents include bethanechol, metoclopramide, domperidone and cisapride. Bethanechol is a choline derivative that augments LES pressure. Some authorities do not consider bethanechol a true prokinetic agent because it does not enhance gastric emptying. Bethanechol has been shown to have a therapeutic effect in patients with relatively mild GERD, but the use of this agent is very limited by its frequent side-effects including abdominal cramps, diarrhea, urinary frequency and blurred vision.

Metoclopramide (usual dose 10 mg q.i.d.), a dopamine antagonist and true prokinetic, also has a therapeutic effect in patients with relatively mild GERD. Metoclopramide increases LES pressure and enhances gastric emptying by its effect of co-ordinating motor activity in the stomach, pylorus and duodenum. Like bethanechol, however, the use of metoclopramide often is limited by side-effects such as agitation, restlessness, somnolence and extrapyramidal symptoms that occur in up to 30% of patients.

Domperidone (10 mg q.i.d.) blocks dopamine receptors but it does not have central effects. Cisapride, the newest of these agents, appears to work as a prokinetic by increasing the availability of acetylcholine release from enteric neurons or as an agonist at $5HT_4$ receptors on the smooth muscle cell. It is given in a dose of 10 mg t.d.s. Cisapride has been shown to increase LES pressure, stimulate esophageal peristalsis and enhance gastric emptying. Side-effects are discussed elsewhere. It appears that cisapride may have a therapeutic role primarily in patients with relatively mild GERD where its efficacy appears to be comparable to that of the $H_2$ receptor blockers.

***Sucralfate.*** Sucralfate is an extraordinarily safe medication that has been found to be beneficial in some patients with mild reflux esophagitis (Orlando 1991, Hameeteman 1991). In several studies performed outside the United States, the efficacy of sucralfate in relieving symptoms and healing esophagitis appeared to be similar to that of the $H_2$ receptor blockers. Sucralfate can be administered either in tablet form or as a suspension.

***Proton pump inhibitors.*** The proton pump inhibitors (omeprazole and lansoprazole, daily doses 20 mg and 30 mg respectively) are extremely effective agents for the treatment of GERD (Sontag 1990, Sloan et al 1992, Pope 1994). In patients with mild to moderately severe reflux esophagitis treated with omeprazole 20 mg daily, healing rates of 80% to 100% can be expected within 8 weeks. Very severe (grade 4) esophagitis may persist despite omeprazole therapy administered in conventional dosage in up to 40% of cases; some of these patients will respond to omeprazole 40 mg per day. Two recent studies have shown that aggressive acid suppression with proton pump inhibitors improves dysphagia and decreases the need for esophageal dilatation in patients who have peptic esophageal strictures (Marks et al 1994, Smith et al 1994).

For patients who respond to omeprazole, GERD returns shortly after stopping the drug in the majority of cases. Presently, omeprazole is approved only for the short-term treatment of GERD that is severe or refractory to other forms of therapy (up to 8 weeks). Although the drug is clearly safe for short-term use, there are concerns about the safety of chronic omeprazole therapy, related primarily to the potential carcinogenic effects of profound chronic acid suppression and hypergastrinemia. To date, no such carcinogenicity has been documented in humans. Recent reports suggest that omeprazole is effective in long-term prophylaxis of recurrent esophageal reflux strictures (Hallerbäck et al 1994, Smith et al 1994).

***Antireflux surgery.*** Although there are a number of different antireflux operations (e.g. Nissen fundoplication, Hill posterior gastropexy, Belsey fundoplication), most share several fundamental features (Dunnington & DeMeester 1993). In all these procedures, the surgeon creates an intra-abdominal segment of esophagus, reduces the hiatal hernia and wraps a portion of the gastric fundus around the distal esophagus. The mechanisms whereby these operations prevent reflux are disputed (Jamieson 1987). The surgery narrows the angle of His (the angle formed by the junction of esophagus with stomach), which may create a flap-valve effect, and restoration of the distal esophagus to the positive pressure environment of the abdomen also may prevent reflux. Reduction of the hiatal hernia and approximation of the diaphragmatic crurae may restore the normal antireflux function of the crural diaphragm. The fundoplication may act as a one-way valve and may prevent distention of the gastric fundus that can trigger transient LES relaxations. Finally, LES pressures increase after fundoplication for reasons that are not clear. The importance of the latter mechanism is disputed, because the efficacy of antireflux surgery is not directly proportional to the postoperative increase in LES pressure (Jamieson 1987).

A Department of Veterans Affairs co-operative study compared the efficacy of medical and surgical therapies for 247 veteran patients who had GERD complicated by Barrett's esophagus, esophageal ulceration, esophageal stricture or severe erosive esophagitis (Spechler 1992a). Antireflux lifestyle modifications were prescribed for all study subjects regardless of treatment group. Patients were randomly assigned to receive one of three types of treatment: continuous medical therapy, symptomatic medical therapy or surgical therapy. Continuous medical therapy included antacid tablets and ranitidine taken on a daily basis regardless of symptoms; metoclopramide and sucralfate were added in a stepwise fashion for patients who remained symptomatic. For patients in the symptomatic medical therapy group, drug therapy was used only for control of symptoms. Therapy in these patients began with antacid tablets; ranitidine, metoclopramide and sucralfate were added in a stepwise fashion for symptoms that could not be controlled with antacids alone. Patients in the surgical therapy group had Nissen fundoplications. All three therapies resulted in significant improvements in the symptoms and endoscopic signs of GERD for up to 2 years. However, surgical therapy was significantly better than either medical therapy for the 2-year duration of the study. Overall satisfaction with therapy was also better for patients in the surgical group. Although this study predated the availability of omeprazole, the results are still applicable. The study was prospective and randomized, carefully designed and executed, and clearly demonstrates that surgical therapy is superior to medical therapy without omeprazole.

Presently, antireflux surgery should be considered for patients who have the following indications:

1. esophageal symptoms, ulcerations or strictures due to GERD that are intractable to medical therapy;
2. aspiration pneumonia due to gastroesophageal reflux;
3. patients unwilling to accept lifelong medical therapy;
4. possibly, young patients who require chronic omeprazole or high-dose $H_2$ blocker therapy for control of symptoms and complications.

### Peptic strictures of the esophagus

Most peptic strictures are in the distal 1 or 2 cm of the esophagus. Strictures extending over the lower third of the esophagus have been described and may be caused by prolonged nasogastric intubation or persistent vomiting. Localized peptic strictures can occur higher in the esophagus and the mucosa distal to them is often columnar (p. 195).

The diagnosis of peptic stricture is made by barium swallow and esophagoscopy. While tight esophageal strictures are easily identified at barium swallow, less severe grades of stricture may be missed. It has been shown (Anselm 1979) that the accuracy of barium swallow is inversely related to the diameter of the stricture. However, careful technique will allow the detection of most strictures and the use of the "marshmallow" swallow is very sensitive in the detection of minor strictures and should be utilized in every patient with dysphagia in whom the initial swallow is normal (Stevenson 1984). Barium swallow can overestimate the length of a stricture unless radiographs are taken in a prone, head-down position, so distending the lower esophagus maximally. Endoscopic grading of esophagitis is described on p. 105.

Long strictures of the distal esophagus may be seen in peptic or biliary esophagitis, after persistent vomiting in hyperemesis gravidarum and alcoholism, after nasogastric intubation, rarely in skin disorders such as pemphigus, in moniliasis, following external thoracic trauma or injury caused by instrumentation and after irradiation (Donner et al 1981).

Any elderly patient with esophageal stenosis should always be suspected of having a malignant lesion and investigated appropriately, as from time to time a submucosal infiltrating neoplasm will present as a smooth stricture at barium swallow.

Endoscopic assessment of strictures is mandatory. Endoscopic biopsy and brush cytology should be undertaken to make sure the stricture is not malignant.

#### *Treatment*

Peptic esophageal strictures are managed, at least in part, by direct endoscopic visualization and dilatation using through the scope balloon dilators or tapered dilators (e.g. Savary) passed over an endoscopically placed guidewire. The latter procedure is best performed with the aid of fluoroscopy (p. 109). Most patients require infrequent, repeat dilatations and this can be very effective to avoid surgery. Active ulceration should be treated with standard doses of proton pump inhibitors or $H_2$ blockers (see above). There is good evidence that long-term use of the proton pump inhibitor omeprazole is effective in long-term prophylaxis of recurrent esophageal reflux strictures, thus reducing the number of dilatations needed in follow-up (Hallerbäck et al 1994, Smith et al 1994).

## BARRETT'S ESOPHAGUS

Esophageal squamous cells that are destroyed by gastroesophageal reflux can be replaced either by more squamous cells or, less commonly, by columnar cells through the process of metaplasia. Barrett's esophagus is the condition in which a metaplastic columnar epithelium replaces squamous epithelium in the distal esophagus (Spechler & Goyal 1986). Barrett's esophagus is judged to be a sequel of reflux esophagitis in most cases and the metaplastic mucosa can be recognized in 10–15% of patients who have endoscopic examinations for symptoms of GERD (Winter et al 1987). Barrett's esophagus has clinical importance because it is the major recognized risk factor for adenocarcinoma of the esophagus and gastroesophageal junction (Haggitt 1992).

Up to three different types of columnar epithelia have been described in Barrett's esophagus (Paull et al 1976):

1. *Specialized columnar epithelium* is a form of incomplete intestinal metaplasia that has a villiform surface and intestinal-type crypts lined by mucus-secreting columnar cells and goblet cells. Paneth cells and enteroendocrine cells also can be found in the crypts.

2. *Gastric fundic-type epithelium* has a pitted (foveolar) surface lined by mucus-secreting cells and a deeper glandular layer that contains chief and parietal cells.

3. *Junctional-type epithelium* has a foveolar surface and glands lined almost exclusively by mucus-secreting cells.

The latter two epithelial types cannot be distinguished readily from normal gastric epithelia. The intestinal metaplasia of specialized columnar epithelium, in contrast, is readily distinguished from the mucosa of the normal stomach. Specialized columnar epithelium also is the most common and important of the three epithelial types found in Barrett's esophagus. Dysplasia and carcinoma in this condition are almost invariably associated with intestinal metaplasia (Haggitt & Dean 1985).

## Diagnosis

Barrett's esophagus usually is recognized by its characteristic appearance on endoscopic examination. Columnar epithelium in the esophagus has a red color and velvet-like texture that contrast sharply with the pale, glossy appearance of the adjacent squamous epithelium (Herlihy et al 1984). Barrett's esophagus is recognized readily when long segments of columnar epithelium are seen extending up the esophagus, well above the anatomic junction of esophagus and stomach (Fig. 8.6).

However, diagnostic difficulties arise for patients found to have short segments of columnar lining in the distal esophagus. Although columnar epithelium can be visually distinguished from squamous epithelium in the esophagus, the several types of columnar epithelia cannot be differentiated solely on the basis of endoscopic appearance. The distinction between specialized columnar epithelium and gastric-type columnar epithelia can be made only by histologic examination of biopsy specimens. The finding of gastric-type epithelia in the distal esophagus does not establish a diagnosis of Barrett's esophagus, because gastric mucosa normally can extend at least 2 cm into the distal esophagus (Goyal et al 1970, McClave et al 1987).

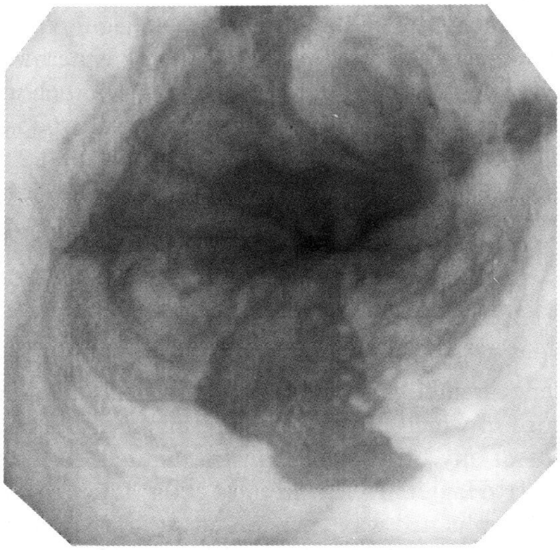

**Fig. 8.6** This endoscopic photograph of the distal esophagus shows long segments of red, columnar epithelium extending well above the esophagogastric junction. This is the characteristic endoscopic appearance of Barrett's esophagus.

Therefore, Barrett's esophagus traditionally has been diagnosed only when columnar lining extends some arbitrary distance (e.g. more than 2–5 cm) up the esophagus (Rothery et al 1986, Spechler & Goyal 1986, Winter et al 1987, McClave et al 1987). Diagnostic criteria based on the extent of esophageal columnar lining clearly are arbitrary and subject to the considerable imprecision both of endoscopic measurement and endoscopic localization of the anatomic esophagogastric junction. To obviate these difficulties, some investigators have contended that the histologic finding of specialized columnar epithelium is so abnormal and distinctive that its presence anywhere in the esophagus establishes the diagnosis of Barrett's esophagus, regardless of extent (Spechler & Goyal 1986, Reid & Weinstein 1987, Hassall 1993). Short segments of specialized columnar epithelium may go unrecognized, however, because endoscopists have been taught that columnar epithelium confined to the distal 2–3 cm of esophagus is a normal finding that does not require biopsy sampling.

Recently, investigators in Boston conducted a prospective study on the frequency, epidemiology and clinical features of patients who had short segments of specialized columnar epithelium at the esophagogastric junction (Spechler et al 1994). All patients scheduled for elective endoscopic examinations in the general endoscopy unit of the Beth Israel Hospital, regardless of indication, had biopsy specimens obtained at the squamocolumnar junction in the distal esophagus irrespective of its appearance and location. Among 142 patients who had columnar epithelium involving $\leq 3$ cm of the distal esophagus, 26 (18%) were found to have specialized columnar epithelium in biopsy specimens of the squamocolumnar junction. Surprisingly, signs and symptoms of esophagitis were not reliable markers for the presence of intestinal metaplasia at the esophagogastric junction. Specific esophageal symptoms (heartburn, regurgitation, dysphagia and odynophagia) were absent in 42% of cases and 69% had few or no endoscopic signs of esophagitis. Indeed, the metaplastic epithelium in these patients would have gone unrecognized if the study protocol had not mandated the acquisition of biopsy specimens from a normal-appearing squamocolumnar junction. Furthermore, for nine of the 26 patients with specialized columnar epithelium, the squamocolumnar junction and the anatomic junction were located at the same level, i.e. columnar epithelium did not extend into the esophagus. For the remaining 17 patients, columnar epithelium extended a variable distance (up to 3 cm) above the esophagogastric junction. A recent report has also highlighted diagnostic inconsistencies in Barrett's esophagus; thus, among patients with specialized columnar epithelium, 20% had this specialized epithelium found on only one of two examinations (Kim et al 1994).

The study of Spechler et al (1994) challenges traditional

concepts on the pathogenesis and diagnosis of Barrett's esophagus. In the meantime, it is important to appreciate that most studies on Barrett's esophagus have included only patients in whom the diagnosis was apparent on endoscopic examination (i.e. columnar epithelium extended well above the esophagogastric junction). It is not clear that conclusions based on these studies are applicable to patients who have short segments of intestinal metaplasia at the esophagogastric junction. The following discussion is based primarily on data obtained from studies on patients for whom the diagnosis of Barrett's esophagus was apparent endoscopically.

## Physiology of GERD in Barrett's esophagus

A number of physiologic abnormalities have been described in these patients that might contribute to the severity of GERD. For example, some patients exhibit hypersecretion of gastric acid and may require extraordinarily high doses of acid-suppressing drugs to facilitate esophageal healing (Collen et al 1990). Some patients also have duodenogastric reflux and, consequently, bile and pancreatic juice may be present in the stomach (Gillen et al 1988). With these abnormalities, the gastric contents available for reflux may be exceptionally injurious, containing high concentrations of acid, bile and pancreatic secretions. Manometric study of the Barrett esophagus often reveals extreme hypotension of the lower esophageal sphincter and therefore these patients are exceptionally predisposed to reflux (Iascone et al 1983). Poor esophageal contractility has also been described and this motility abnormality may interfere with esophageal acid clearance (Zaninotto et al 1989). Some patients have diminished esophageal pain sensitivity and consequently the reflux of noxious material into the Barrett's esophagus may not induce heartburn (Johnson et al 1987). Without heartburn, patients have no warning that they are experiencing gastroesophageal reflux and little incentive to comply with antireflux therapy. Decreased salivary secretion of epidermal growth factor, a peptide that enhances the healing of peptic ulceration, also has been reported in some patients (Gray et al 1991).

In summary, patients who have endoscopically apparent Barrett's mucosa may be exceptionally predisposed to the reflux of unusually caustic gastric material into the esophagus. Such reflux might not elicit pain, the esophagus may be unable to clear the noxious material effectively and healing of the resulting esophageal injury may be delayed by a deficiency of salivary epidermal growth factor. With these abnormalities, it is not surprising that GERD frequently is complicated in patients with Barrett's esophagus.

## Clinical features

Barrett's esophagus has been described in children as young as age 5, but the condition is usually discovered in middle-aged and older adults, with an average age at diagnosis of 55 years. White males predominate in most series and, for unknown reasons, Barrett's esophagus is uncommon in blacks. Most patients are seen initially for symptoms of underlying GERD such as heartburn, regurgitation and dysphagia. The Barrett's epithelium itself causes no symptoms and may even be more resistant to acid-peptic injury than the native squamous mucosa.

Many patients with endoscopically apparent Barrett's esophagus have no symptoms of GERD, however, and recent data suggest that the large majority of patients with Barrett's esophagus do not seek medical attention for esophageal symptoms (Cameron et al 1990). Among patients identified by physicians, the GERD associated with Barrett's esophagus is often severe and associated with esophageal ulceration, stricture and hemorrhage (Spechler & Goyal 1986).

### *Natural history of Barrett's oesophagus*

Given the propensity for severe GERD in patients with Barrett's esophagus, authorities naturally assumed that the metaplasia should progress in extent over the years as more and more columnar epithelium replaced reflux-damaged squamous epithelium. Surprisingly, however, recent data suggest that in most cases Barrett's esophagus develops to its full extent relatively quickly, neither progressing nor regressing substantially with time. Cameron & Lomboy (1992) reviewed the records of 377 patients found to have benign Barrett's esophagus at the Mayo Clinic between 1976 and 1989. When these patients were grouped according to age, the length of esophagus lined by Barrett's epithelium was not found to differ significantly among the various age groups. Twenty-year-old patients had a segment of columnar-lined esophagus similar in length to that of the 80-year-old patients. Furthermore, no significant change in the extent of Barrett's epithelium was found among 101 patients who had follow-up endoscopic examinations performed after a mean interval of 3.2 years. It is not clear why Barrett's esophagus usually does not progress in extent despite ongoing GERD.

## Cancer and dysplasia

Barrett's esophagus is the single most important risk factor for adenocarcinoma of the gastroesophageal junction, the incidence of which has been increasing at a rate exceeding that of any other cancer in the United States (Blot et al 1991, Haggitt 1992). In the 1960s, adenocarcinoma of the esophagus was considered so rare that some authorities questioned its very existence (Raphael et al 1966). Today, adenocarcinomas comprise approximately 50% of all esophageal malignancies in the United States (Blot et al 1993). Adenocarcinomas develop in Barrett's esophagus at the rate of approximately one cancer per 125 patient-years of follow-up (Spechler 1992d). Stated differently, patients with Barrett's esophagus develop esophageal cancer at the rate of approximately 0.8% per year.

As in other tissues, carcinogenesis in Barrett's esophagus appears to involve the activation of proto-oncogenes (e.g. c-erb-B) and the disablement of tumor suppressor genes (e.g. p53) (Blount et al 1993). These changes endow the cells with certain growth advantages. The advantaged cells hyperproliferate and in so doing acquire more genetic alterations that result in neoplasia with autonomous cell growth. Eventually, when enough DNA abnormalities accumulate, a clone of malignant cells emerges – malignant because they have the ability to invade adjacent tissues and to proliferate in unnatural locations. Before the cells acquire enough DNA damage to become frankly malignant, the earlier genetic alterations often cause histologic changes that can be recognized by the pathologist as dysplasia.

Dysplasia in Barrett's epithelium is defined as a neoplastic alteration of columnar cells that remain confined within the basement membranes of the glands from which they arose (Schmidt et al 1985). Dysplasia is widely regarded as the precursor of invasive malignancy and this is what makes dysplasia so interesting for the clinician. The finding of dysplasia provides an opportunity to initiate therapy to interrupt the progression to invasive cancer. Endoscopic surveillance for cancer in Barrett's esophagus is performed primarily to seek high-grade dysplasia, with the rationale that resection of the dysplastic epithelium may prevent the progression to invasive malignancy (Spechler 1987).

In patients found to have high-grade dysplasia in Barrett's esophagus with no apparent esophageal tumor on initial endoscopic examination, a number of reports have suggested that approximately one-third already have invasive cancer (Spechler 1987, Altorki et al 1991). These cancers are missed by the endoscopist because of biopsy sampling error, a problem that can be reduced by increasing the number of biopsy specimens obtained during endoscopic examinations. Recently, Levine et al (1993) reported that they could differentiate high-grade dysplasia from early adenocarcinoma in Barrett's esophagus by adherence to a rigorous endoscopic biopsy protocol wherein the esophagus was sampled extensively. This conclusion was based primarily on findings in seven patients who had esophageal resection for high-grade dysplasia. In all seven cases, only high-grade dysplasia (without invasive cancer) was found in the resected specimens. The biopsy protocol necessary to achieve these results involved obtaining four-quadrant biopsy specimens at 2 cm intervals throughout the columnar-lined esophagus using "jumbo" biopsy forceps. In addition to the four-quadrant biopsies, they obtained specimens from any apparent lesions and took additional samples from sites of known dysplasia. For the seven patients who had esophageal resections for high-grade dysplasia, 29–185 preoperative biopsy specimens were available for review. The one patient who had 185 biopsy specimens had them obtained during five preoperative endoscopies in a period of 10 months. Those 185 specimens came from a segment of Barrett's epithelium that spanned only 3 cm, i.e. more than 60 biopsies per centimeter of metaplastic mucosa! Such a biopsy protocol may be too rigorous to be practical for clinical application.

**Table 8.2** Proposed biomarkers for malignancy in Barrett's epithelium (adapted from Spechler 1994)

| |
|---|
| Ornithine decarboxylase |
| Carcinoembryonic antigen (CEA) |
| Mucus abnormalities |
| Flow cytometry – aneuploidy |
| Flow cytometry – abnormal cellular proliferation |
| Chromosomal abnormalities (trisomy 7, 17p deletions) |
| Oncogenes (c-Ha-ras, c-erb-B) |
| Tumor suppressor genes (p53) |
| Growth regulatory factors (EGF, TGF-α, EGF-R) |
| Proliferating cell nuclear antigen and Ki67 |
| Endosonography – assess invasion |

Another problem with dysplasia as a biomarker for malignancy is the fact that the natural history of dysplasia is not well defined. Available data suggest, however, that high-grade dysplasia progresses to malignancy often and rapidly (Hameeteman et al 1989). For example, in the aforementioned study by Levine et al (1993), seven of 29 patients (24%) with high-grade dysplasia were found to progress to invasive cancer during a follow-up period of 2–46 months. In some cases, however, high-grade dysplasia has persisted for years with no apparent progression to carcinoma (Lee 1985, Altorki et al 1991).

Noting the shortcomings of dysplasia as a biomarker for malignancy, investigators have sought alternatives, as summarized in Table 8.2 (Spechler 1994). For clinical purposes, however, none of these biomarkers has been shown to be superior to the histologic finding of dysplasia for predicting the development of malignancy in Barrett's esophagus. Despite the problems, the finding of dysplasia remains the most appropriate biomarker for the clinical evaluation of patients with Barrett's esophagus.

## Laser ablation of Barrett's epithelium

Recently, investigators have used laser irradiation to obliterate Barrett's epithelium while administering omeprazole to inhibit gastric acid secretion. With no acid reflux to stimulate metaplastic repair, they reason, the damaged esophageal tissue should heal normally, i.e. by regeneration of squamous mucosa. Several recent reports have documented that photoablation of Barrett's epithelium is feasible by this procedure (Brandt & Kauvar 1992,

Berenson et al 1993, Sampliner et al 1993). For example, one report describes the results of argon laser irradiation of Barrett's epithelium in ten patients, all of whom were treated with omeprazole for the duration of the study (6–38 weeks) (Berenson et al 1993). Squamous mucosa was found to replace photoablated columnar epithelium in 38 of 40 treatment locations in these ten patients. Most patients required multiple endoscopic laser treatments to achieve ablation of the irradiated segment. Another recent report describes the use of photodynamic therapy to obliterate dysplasia and early malignancy in Barrett's esophagus with limited success (Overholt et al 1993).

Although these reports document the feasibility of laser ablation of Barrett's epithelium, they do not establish the benefit of the technique. The procedure entails some risk and it is not clear that photoablation reduces the risk of esophageal cancer in these patients. Also, it is not clear whether lifelong, intensive acid suppression will be necessary to prevent return of the columnar epithelium. Further studies addressing these issues are necessary before laser ablation of Barrett's epithelium can be recommended for clinical application (Spechler 1993).

### Management recommendations

There are many unresolved issues regarding the proper management of patients with Barrett's esophagus. For example, the cost-effectiveness of endoscopic surveillance for these patients is disputed because there is no proof that this procedure reduces morbidity and mortality from esophageal cancer. The management of high-grade dysplasia is hotly debated because the natural history of the condition is not clear. Clinicians reviewing the available data on these issues might reasonably arrive at different conclusions regarding management. With minor modifications, the following management approach is that recommended by the 1990 Barrett's Esophagus Working Party of the World Congresses of Gastroenterology (Dent et al 1991).

1. A program of regular endoscopic surveillance for dysplasia and early carcinoma is recommended for patients with Barrett's esophagus unless contraindicated by comorbidity. For patients who have no dysplasia or cancer, endoscopy (with procurement of biopsy and brush cytology specimens from the Barrett's epithelium) is performed every other year.
2. If dysplasia is detected, the finding should be confirmed by at least one other expert pathologist. If any doubt remains, the endoscopic examination is repeated immediately to obtain more biopsy and cytology specimens for analysis.
3. For patients confirmed to have multiple foci of high-grade dysplasia whose operative risk is not inordinate, surgery is advised to resect all of the esophagus lined by columnar epithelium.
4. For patients confirmed to have low-grade dysplasia, intensive medical antireflux therapy (including a proton pump inhibitor) should be given for 8–12 weeks at which time the endoscopic examination is repeated to obtain multiple esophageal biopsy and cytology specimens.
   - For patients whose specimens show histologic improvement, intensive surveillance (e.g. endoscopic examinations every 6 months) is recommended until at least two consecutive examinations reveal no dysplastic epithelium.
   - For patients with persistent low-grade dysplasia, continued intensive treatment and surveillance are recommended.

## HIATAL HERNIAS

### Sliding hiatus hernia

The sliding hiatal hernia is far more common than paraesophageal (periesophageal) hernia. Both the esophagogastric junction and a portion of the proximal stomach migrate through the esophageal hiatus into the posterior mediastinum. Despite the intrathoracic location of the stomach, its anatomic orientation is unaltered. Patients with sliding hiatal hernias may have symptoms of GERD, but the hernias per se rarely cause symptoms. The mechanisms whereby sliding hiatal hernias contribute to GERD are discussed on p. 192.

### Paraesophageal (periesophageal) hernia

The esophagogastric junction is fixed in its normal position within the abdomen and the fundus of the stomach migrates through an enlarged esophageal hiatus into the thorax. Consequently, a portion of the stomach lies within the chest alongside the esophagus. With large periesophageal hernias, the entire stomach can protrude into the chest and assume an upside-down configuration (Fig. 8.7). As the lower esophageal sphincter is competent, reflux is not a feature of paraesophageal hernia. The patient may complain of epigastric fullness, nausea and intermittent dysphagia and distention of the herniated stomach may give rise to dyspnea and severe pain that can simulate angina or cholecystitis. Anemia is common because erosions develop in the congested herniated stomach or a gastric ulcer may occur where the fundus passes through the diaphragm (Windsor & Collis 1967). Most commonly, the hernia is detected when a fluid level is seen on a chest radiograph or during barium meal examination (Fig. 8.7). Twisting (volvulus) of the stomach or progression of the herniation can obstruct the esophagus, the stomach or its blood supply. With a sufficient degree of volvulus, acute vascular compromise can result in gastric infarction and perforation. When surgical intervention is required in this situation, the mortality rate approaches

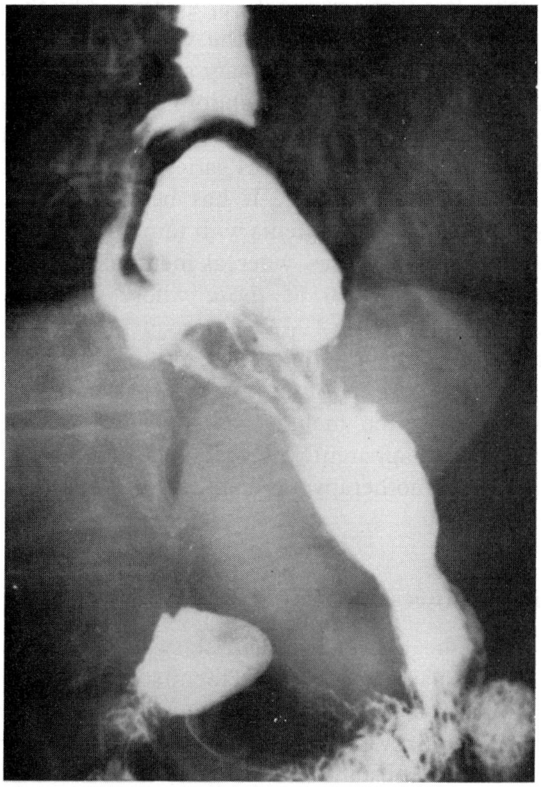

**Fig. 8.7** Large paraesophageal hiatus hernia. The esophagus is of normal length. In spite of its size the hernia was symptomless and was an incidental finding.

50% (p. 328). To prevent the devastating results of acute gastric volvulus, many surgical authorities advise elective repair of periesophageal hernias whenever they are detected. Surgical studies on periesophageal hernias are comprised largely of symptomatic patients, however. It is not clear how often periesophageal hernias are asymptomatic and how often such asymptomatic hernias eventuate in acute gastric volvulus.

## CARCINOMA OF THE ESOPHAGUS

### Epidemiology and pathology

The epidemiology of esophageal cancer is as fascinating as the tumor is lethal (Sons 1987, Moses 1991, Mayer 1993). For squamous cell carcinomas, exceptionally high incidence rates are observed in the Transkei region of South Africa and throughout an esophageal cancer "belt" that extends from the shores of the Caspian Sea (in Iran and the former Soviet Union) across northern China. Interestingly, high-incidence areas are often located near low-incidence areas. Within China itself, for example, incidence rates for esophageal cancer can vary from province to province by a factor of more than 100. Even animals in the high-incidence regions are affected. For example, chickens raised in northern China develop esophageal cancers ten times more frequently than chickens from southern China.

These intriguing epidemiological features have stimulated investigators to identify cultural, dietary and environmental risk factors for esophageal cancer. In the United States and Europe, cigarette smoking and alcoholism are well established as the major recognized risk factors for squamous cell carcinoma of the esophagus (Sons 1987, Moses 1991). However, alcoholism is not a prominent risk factor for esophageal cancer in Moslem Iran where incidence rates for the tumor are exceptionally high. A variety of nutritional deficiencies have also been associated with esophageal cancer including deficiencies in vitamins A and C and in magnesium, selenium and zinc. The esophagus is one of the first organs exposed to ingested carcinogens including N-nitrous compounds that can be formed from the nitrates in pickled vegetables and cured meats. Regional practices such as opium smoking and the ingestion of very hot foods and beverages may play a role in esophageal carcinogenesis and certain high-incidence areas have soils that are poor in certain elements such as molybdenum and zinc.

There has been intense interest recently in the potential role that micro-organisms might play in esophageal carcinogenesis (Chang et al 1992). Indeed, local variations in endemic micro-organisms could explain some of the dramatic regional variations in esophageal cancer incidence rates. The food and water in high-incidence areas frequently are contaminated with fungi and with bacteria that promote the formation of carcinogenic N-nitrous compounds from dietary nitrates. Perhaps even more intriguing is the role that viruses may play in the pathogenesis of esophageal cancer. Human papilloma virus, herpes simplex virus, cytomegalovirus and Epstein–Barr virus can all infect the esophagus and cause alterations in the DNA of the infected cells. These genetic alterations conceivably might promote carcinogenesis by activating cellular oncogenes or by disabling tumor suppressor genes. All of these viruses have been shown to produce tumors in certain animals and all can transform cells in culture. In humans, furthermore, all of these viruses are associated with certain extraesophageal cancers. Researchers recently have found HPV DNA in >20% of human squamous cell carcinomas of the esophagus (Togawa et al 1994). Tumor cells infected with certain HPVs express the genes whose protein products can interact with those of tumor suppressor genes such as the p53 and retinoblastoma genes. Presumably, interference with the normal growth regulatory proteins elaborated by the tumor suppressor genes might lead to hyperproliferation and carcinogenesis. These data suggest that viral infections of the esophagus may play an important role in esophageal carcinogenesis.

A number of medical conditions that predispose to the development of esophageal cancer have also been identified (Sons 1987, Moses 1991, Mayer 1994). For squamous cell carcinoma, these include achalasia, celiac sprue, lye stricture of the esophagus, Plummer–Vinson syndrome and tylosis. There also is a strong association between cancer of the esophagus and malignancies involving the head and neck, perhaps because these tumors share the common risk factors of alcoholism and cigarette smoking (Goldstein & Zornoza 1978). As discussed earlier, the major risk factor for esophageal adenocarcinoma is Barrett's esophagus.

In the United States, there has been a dramatic change in the relative frequency of the different histologic types of esophageal cancer (Hesketh et al 1989, Blot et al 1991, 1993, Mayer 1994). In the 1960s, squamous cell carcinomas comprised more than 90% of all esophageal cancers in this country and adenocarcinomas were considered so uncommon that some authorities questioned whether adenocarcinoma of the esophagus existed at all. For the past two decades, the frequency of adenocarcinoma of the esophagus and the gastroesophageal junction (a similar if not identical tumor) has increased dramatically in the United States and Europe. There are approximately 12 000 new cases of esophageal cancer diagnosed in the United States each year, of which one-half are squamous cell carcinomas and one-half are adenocarcinomas (Blot et al 1993). Both tumors affect men 3–4 times more often than women. Perhaps the most striking epidemiologic difference between the two histologic types of esophageal cancer is the dramatic racial variation in incidence rates. Squamous cell carcinoma affects blacks six times more often than whites, whereas adenocarcinoma is at least four times as common in whites (Blot et al 1991, 1993). Squamous cell cancers clearly are associated with cigarette smoking and alcoholism, whereas the association of these practices with adenocarcinoma is disputed. Although either histologic type of cancer can be found anywhere in the esophagus, squamous cell tumors are located most often in the mid-esophagus, whereas adenocarcinomas are distal tumors that often cross the gastroesophageal junction.

### *The esophageal lymphatic system*

Irrespective of the histologic type, esophageal cancer usually is disseminated at the time of diagnosis. The extensive lymphatic system of the esophagus is the conduit for much of this dissemination (McCort 1952). Small lymphatic vessels in the esophageal mucosa drain into larger submucosal vessels that extend throughout the length of the organ. Similarly, small lymphatics in the muscularis propria drain into larger vessels that traverse the muscular layers and adventitia of the esophagus. These two major groups of esophageal lymphatics intercommunicate with one another and with vessels supplying adjacent lymph nodes, thereby providing the means for both longitudinal and lateral spread of esophageal cancer. Tumor cells often enter these lymphatic channels, as evidenced by the common finding of metastases in the wall of the esophagus widely separated from the primary cancer and by the frequent finding of metastases in abdominal lymph nodes for patients with tumors in the mid- and proximal esophagus.

The prevalence of metastases varies with the size of the primary esophageal cancer. It has been estimated that approximately 50% of patients with tumors less than 5 cm in length have metastases, whereas metastases are present in approximately 90% of those whose tumor length exceeds 5 cm (Fleming 1943). Consequently, simple segmental resection of an esophageal cancer is rarely curative, especially if the primary tumor is large. Attempts at curative treatment often include resection or irradiation of wide margins of apparently normal tissue and the administration of chemotherapy to eradicate distant metastatic deposits.

## Clinical features and diagnosis

There may be dysphagia, painful swallowing or retrosternal chest pain. Dysphagia is the first and most prominent symptom in over 90% of cases. At first, there may be only occasional dysphagia caused by solid foods, but it soon becomes constant and progressive and the patient loses weight. With pharyngeal carcinoma there is pharyngeal dysphagia (p. 171). Cases of mediastinal penetration, hemorrhage and death are recorded (Kikendall et al 1983).

### *Radiology*

Primary pharyngeal carcinoma can be identified by barium swallow and the changes are best recorded by double-contrast barium swallow supplemented by videorecording (p. 9) (Semenkovich et al 1985). As symptoms are usually experienced early the radiographic changes may be very subtle and include minor asymmetry and failure of filling of the valleculae or piriform fossae. The more common abnormalities include a protruding polyp of varying size or shape or an irregular plaque-like filling defect often accompanied by "stiffness" of the pharyngeal walls. The use of the Valsalva or Mueller maneuvers may help to exaggerate the early changes and enhance the double-contrast technique. Sometimes laryngeal carcinomas invade the pharynx directly, giving similar appearances, but the primary site should be recognized by other investigations including computed tomography.

Barium swallow using double contrast may show subtle mucosal changes (Creteur et al 1983) (p. 6). Typically these occur in the upper and mid-esophagus and only occasionally in the lower third. Characteristically, there is a focal collection of multiple, small ulcers often related to the aortic arch impression. Motility is not usually disturbed. Occasionally strictures are seen and, rarely, marked edema accompanying the ulceration may resemble an ulcerating tumor. If the offending agent is withdrawn, a repeat study may show resolution of the changes.

### *Esophageal cytology*

Cytology is an accurate technique which is used in some centers particularly when suspicious lesions have revealed normal biopsies.

Material is now almost always obtained at endoscopy by combining brushing of suspicious lesions with esophageal biopsy (p. 109). Brush cytology can also be performed without endoscopy with very good results (Aste et al 1984) or cells can be obtained by initial aspiration of fasting gastric secretions followed by washings taken from above and below the lesion. Vigorous lavage is performed with 50 ml of isotonic saline at each site and when done rapidly, it is usually possible to recover at least 10–20 ml of saline on each occasion before the rest passes down the esophagus. Usually, a degree of esophageal obstruction enables a good return of fluid to be obtained.

MacDonald et al (1963) correctly diagnosed 94% of 72 malignant tumors involving the esophagus by using a lavage method. As good or better results have been obtained more simply by brush cytology during esophagoscopy (Winawer et al 1976, Hughes et al 1978). Cytology may be more accurate than biopsy and positive results should be investigated carefully before they are regarded as false (Winawer et al 1976).

Cytology is important in regions of high incidence of esophageal cancer. In China a balloon method has been used in more than 500 000 individuals (Shu 1983). The balloon, covered with a mesh net, is swallowed into the stomach, inflated with 25 ml of air and slowly withdrawn. At 18 cm from the teeth, the air is released, the balloon withdrawn and smears prepared from the collected material. The use of the technique showed that 20% of the cases of early cancer were not seen by esophagoscopy. In mass screening surveys, 80% of the defined population in the area were examined and 74% of the lesions detected were early malignant lesions.

### *Endoscopy*

At esophagoscopy, the tumor may appear as a circumscribed ulcer, circumferential ulcer and stricture or a mass lesion. Endoscopy is the standard method to obtain tissue diagnosis of the esophageal malignancy if the less invasive brush cytology without endoscopy (Aste et al 1984) is negative or unavailable. Endoscopic ultrasonography is increasingly utilized in tumor staging (pp. 125 and 208).

## Potential for cure

Most patients with esophageal cancer present with the symptoms of rapidly progressive dysphagia and weight loss. Ordinarily, these symptoms develop only when the tumor has grown to the extent that it has narrowed the lumen of the esophagus substantially or has metastasized. Therefore, the presence of symptoms is usually associated with disseminated disease. This contention is supported by an autopsy study which found evidence of metastases in 85% of patients with squamous cell carcinoma of the esophagus (Anderson & Lad 1982). In the absence of a therapy that reliably eradicates disseminated disease, therefore, cure is not possible for the majority of patients with symptomatic cancer of the esophagus. Furthermore, patients with squamous cell carcinomas are often smokers and drinkers who have severe comorbidity (pulmonary, cardiac, liver disease) that further limits their treatment options. In 1980, a meta-analysis of 122 reported surgical series that included more than 83 000 patients evaluated for surgical treatment of esophageal cancer found that only 58% eventually had an operation and only 39% had their tumors resected (Earlam & Cunha-Melo 1980). Stated differently, surgical cure was deemed impossible because of extensive tumor involvement or severe comorbidity in 61% of cases evaluated for treatment.

The median survival after diagnosis for symptomatic patients with cancer of the esophagus is less than 6 months. However, there are data to suggest that symptomatic patients have in fact harbored their malignancies for years. For example, investigators in China's Henan Province reported the results of a study on mass screening for esophageal cancer (Guanrei et al 1988). Using the technique of exfoliative cytology, these researchers screened 29 235 people and found 125 subjects with asymptomatic esophageal cancer. Ninety of these patients with asymptomatic tumors refused treatment and were followed without intervention. The majority of the patients (58%) remained asymptomatic during a follow-up period ranging from 19 to 78 months. The investigators estimated that esophageal cancers grow for approximately 4.5 years before causing symptoms. Discovery of the neoplasm during an early, asymptomatic phase presumably would improve the chance for cure. Although mass surveillance programs for esophageal cancer are not likely to be cost-effective in Western countries where the incidence of the disease in the general population is low, the Chinese experience supports the concept of surveillance to detect nascent malignancies for certain high-risk groups such as patients with Barrett's esophagus.

## Tumor staging

Accurate tumor staging (Table 8.3) is essential for choosing an appropriate therapy for patients with cancer of the esophagus. Unfortunately, the accuracy of conventional imaging techniques such as computed tomography (Fig. 8.8) for staging esophageal tumors is poor.

**Table 8.3** TNM staging for esophageal cancer

| | |
|---|---|
| Primary tumor (T) | |
| T1 | Invades lamina propria or submucosa |
| T2 | Invades muscularis propria |
| T3 | Invades adventitia |
| T4 | Invades adjacent structures |
| Regional lymph nodes (N) | |
| N0 | No involvement |
| N1 | Involvement |
| Metastases (M) | |
| M0 | None |
| M1 | Present |

Endosonography, which uses high frequency ultrasonic waves to provide exquisitely detailed images of the esophageal wall and its adjacent structures, recently has been used to stage esophageal cancers (Rice et al 1992). A number of studies have shown that endosonography is superior to computed tomography for assessing esophageal wall penetration by the tumor and for detecting regional lymph node involvement. In one recent study of 34 patients with esophageal cancer (Peters et al 1994), endosonography correctly predicted the degree of wall penetration in 26 (76%) and the presence of lymph node involvement in 28 (82%). Furthermore, endosonography correctly predicted tumor stage in 68% of cases. Although endosonography appears to be the best available imaging

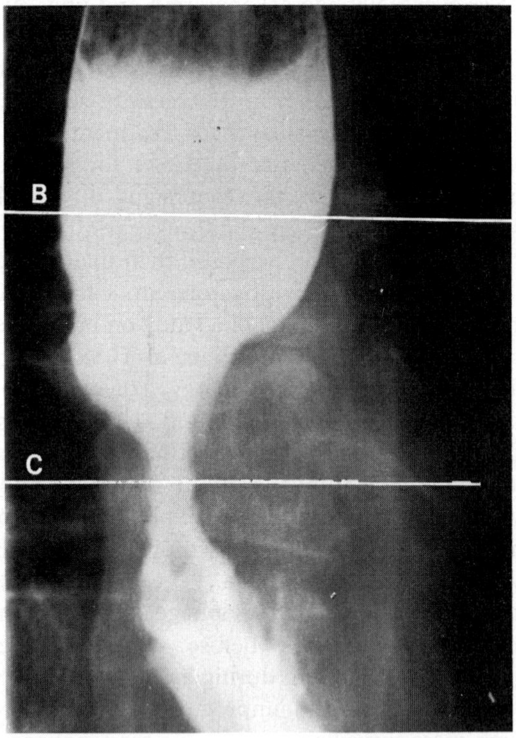


A

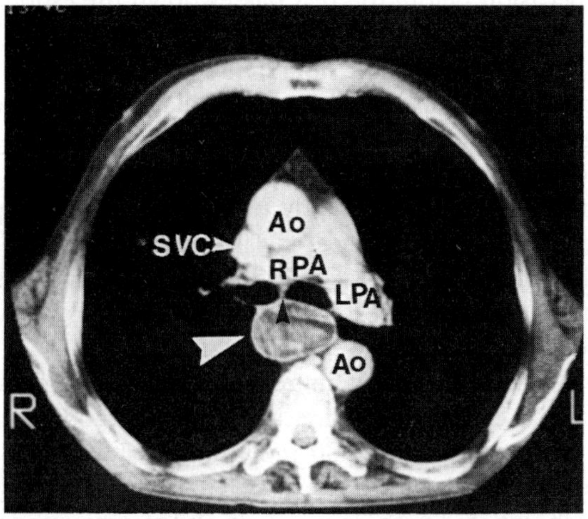


B

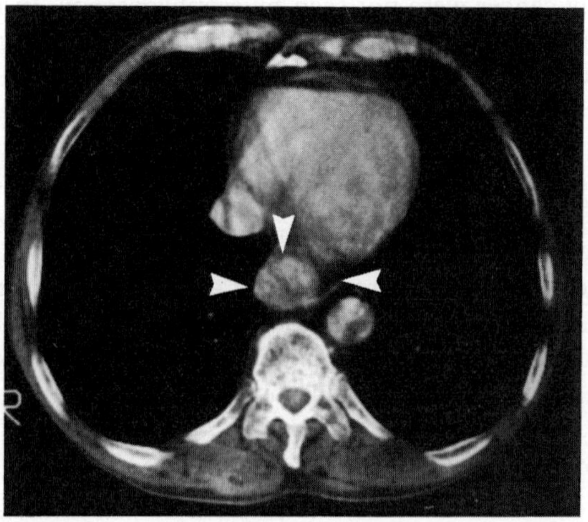

C

**Fig. 8.8** Carcinoma of the esophagus. Use of CT in staging. (a) Barium swallow showing malignant stricture. The horizontal lines indicate the levels of CT in B and C. (b) Dilated esophagus containing fluid (white arrow). The esophageal wall is normal at this point. Aorta (Ao), pulmonary arteries (LPA and RPA), superior vena cava (SVC), carina (arrow). (c) Tumor mass (arrows). No evidence of local invasion.

technique for assessing the depth of tumor invasion and the presence of lymph node involvement by esophageal carcinomas, the accuracy of the technique remains far from ideal. The staging system shown in Table 8.3 was developed by the American Joint Committee on Cancer in conjunction with the International Union Against Cancer in 1987 and is commonly used by endoscopic ultrasonographers (Rice et al 1992).

### Treatment options

Cancer of the esophagus is uniformly fatal without treatment. Unfortunately, overall cure rates for this malignancy remain below 10%. However, treatment can provide substantial palliation for many patients debilitated by dysphagia and aspiration.

Initial treatment usually involves a choice between surgery, radiation therapy and chemotherapy or a combination of these three modalities. Successful surgery provides immediate palliation and is potentially curative. Surgery is associated with substantial morbidity and mortality, however, and the overall cure rate is low. Unlike surgery, the acute mortality of radiation therapy is virtually negligible. Radiation also can cover a wider treatment area than is practical with surgery and radiotherapy is potentially curative. However, radiotherapy usually takes 2–8 weeks to complete, palliation is often delayed for several weeks, there can be substantial damage to surrounding normal tissues and the overall cure rate is low. Chemotherapy is appealing in principle because it has the potential to reach the disseminated disease that usually is present. Unfortunately, it is associated with substantial morbidity and considerable mortality, is often ineffective and the tumor response (if any) is often brief. When used as the sole treatment for esophageal cancer, chemotherapy presently is not curative.

Surgery, radiation and chemotherapy can be used alone or in a variety of combinations and a number of reports have suggested that survival can be improved with combined modality treatments. Much recent interest has focused on the role of chemoradiotherapy, the combination of chemotherapy (usually a regimen of 5-fluorouracil and cisplatin) with radiation therapy for esophageal cancer (Herskovic 1992, Poplin et al 1994). In preliminary studies of patients treated with chemoradiotherapy followed by esophagectomy, complete histologic response (defined as no histologic evidence of tumor in the resected specimen) has been observed in up to 28% of cases. Complete histologic response is not tantamount to cure, however, and the responders frequently succumb eventually to recurrent disease. Furthermore, chemoradiotherapy frequently causes serious toxicity.

*Palliative therapy*

Purely palliative therapies include esophageal dilatation and the placement of intraluminal stents (Tytgat et al 1992, Knyrim et al 1993) (p. 110). There also are palliative techniques designed to ablate the portion of the neoplasm that obstructs the esophageal lumen. These ablative therapies include endoscopic laser irradiation (p. 111), the application of tumor probes that burn the neoplasm directly or the injection of caustic chemicals directly into the tumor body (Murray et al 1988, Jensen et al 1988). Other experimental therapies include the placement of radioactive materials within the esophageal lumen (intraluminal radiotherapy) (Hyden et al 1988), the use of local hyperthermia to enhance the efficacy of radiation and chemotherapy (Matsufuji et al 1988), the use of various radiosensitizing agents to enhance the efficacy of radiation therapy (Schwade et al 1984) and the administration of porphyrins to enhance the efficacy of laser therapy (photodynamic therapy) (Overholt 1992, Overholt et al 1993).

*Management guidelines* (Fig. 8.9)

Presently, the optimal treatment for cancer of the esophagus is unclear and disputed. Pending the results of controlled clinical trials, a strong case can be made for treating newly diagnosed patients according to well-designed, established research protocols whenever possible. This approach eliminates anguish in choosing among treatments of dubious value, provides clear guidelines for patient management and offers an opportunity to evaluate the efficacy of the experimental therapy in a systematic and meaningful fashion.

If the initial use of research protocols is not feasible, an alternative approach is outlined in Figure 8.9. This approach was developed by a panel of experts who participated in a symposium on cancer of the esophagus at the annual meeting of the American Gastroenterological Association in 1994. After the diagnosis of esophageal cancer has been established by barium swallow and endoscopy, the next step is to decide if the patient is fit enough to undergo surgery. If surgery is not a viable option because of advanced age or comorbidity, then primary therapy might include chemoradiation or, preferably, the patient can be enrolled in a clinical trial. If the patient is reasonably fit and a candidate for surgery, then the next step is tumor staging with computed tomography and, if available, endoscopic ultrasonography. In general, surgery is not indicated for patients with T4 tumors that invade adjacent structures or for patients with metastases. Primary therapy for such patients might include chemoradiation or clinical trials.

For tumors that do not invade beyond the muscularis propria and do not involve local lymph nodes, surgery appears to offer the best hope for cure. For lesions that are more advanced due to lymph node involvement or invasion to the adventitia, the choices for primary therapy include chemoradiation with or without surgery or, prefer-

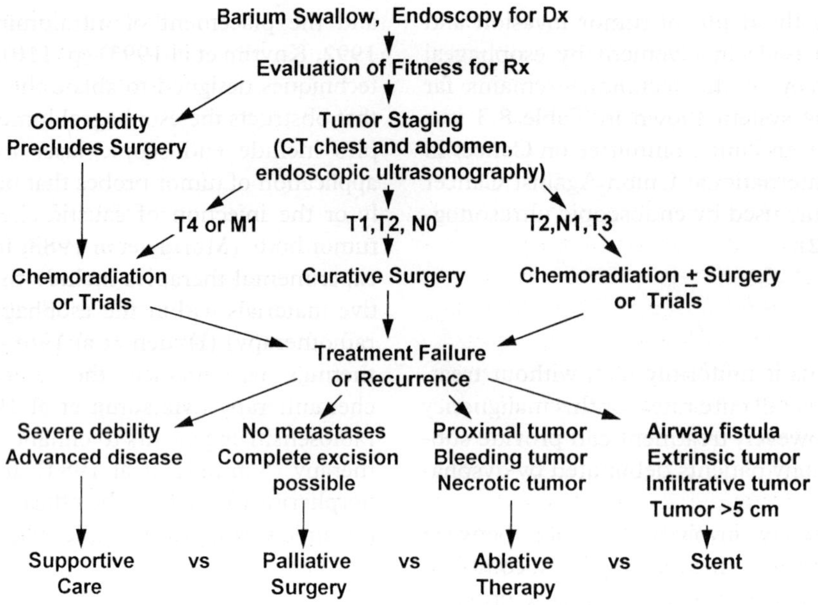


**Fig. 8.9** Management guidelines for cancer of the esophagus, prepared for the 1994 AGA Clinical Practice Section Symposium on Esophageal Cancer by DeMeester TR, Kimmey MB, Kozarek RA, Levin B, Spechler S, Tytgat GNJ.

ably, enrollment in an established clinical trial. If these primary treatments fail or if the tumor recurs, there are a number of treatment options. For a patient who is severely debilitated and who has advanced disease, the most humane option may be only supportive care with careful attention to pain control. If there are no apparent metastases and complete excision of the tumor is possible, then surgery can provide excellent palliation. The other options are ablative therapies or stents. Stents may not provide good palliation for patients with proximal tumors, bleeding tumors and necrotic tumors and ablative therapy may be preferable in these circumstances. Alternatively, ablative therapy has little to offer a patient with an esophagobronchial fistula or a patient with a tumor that is extrinsic or infiltrative. Also, ablative therapy may be difficult and time-consuming for patients with very long tumors and stenting may be preferable in these circumstances.

## INFECTIOUS ESOPHAGITIDES (Baehr & McDonald 1994, Laine 1994)

### Candida esophagitis

Candida esophagitis is common in patients who have impaired immunity due to human immunodeficiency virus (HIV) infection, aggressive chemotherapy, solid organ transplantation and bone marrow transplantation. Other conditions that predispose to candida esophagitis include malignancy, diabetes mellitus, alcoholism, hypochlorhydria, disordered esophageal motility and the administration of antimicrobials, steroids and other immunosuppressive agents. In some cases, candida esophagitis affects otherwise healthy individuals who have no apparent immunodeficiency or other underlying disorder. Although candida infection of the esophagus commonly causes dysphagia and odynophagia, many patients with candida esophagitis are asymptomatic. Oral thrush can be detected on physical examination in most patients with esophageal candidiasis, but thrush is absent in approximately 15% of cases. On endoscopic examination, the esophagus is lined with confluent, raised white plaques that resemble cottage cheese. The plaques cannot be washed away readily and endoscopic attempts to brush them away frequently cause some bleeding. The finding of budding yeast cells, hyphae and pseudohyphae in esophageal biopsy specimens is diagnostic of candida infection.

The infection responds to treatment with a variety of antifungal agents including nystatin, ketoconazole, fluconazole and itraconazole. Unfortunately, recurrent infection is common, particularly in patients with AIDS.

### Herpes simplex virus esophagitis

Primary herpes simplex virus (HSV) infection is commonly acquired in early childhood and takes the form of a self-limiting gingivostomatitis. The acute illness heals, but the virus survives in a latent state in nerve ganglion cells. The latent virus can be reactivated later in life. In the setting of immunodeficiency, the reactivated virus can infect the squamous epithelium of the esophagus. Uncommonly, HSV esophagitis affects otherwise healthy individuals who have no apparent immune disorders.

HSV esophagitis usually is the result of reactivation of the latent virus rather than exogenous infection. In some cases, the esophagitis is severe and can be complicated by bleeding, stricture formation and perforation of the esophagus. The endoscopic appearance of HSV esophagitis varies with the interval between esophageal infection and endoscopic examination. The earliest lesions are small (1–3 mm), rounded vesicles that can be found predominantly in the mid- to distal esophagus. Endoscopy is seldom performed during this early stage of infection and, therefore, these discrete vesicular lesions are not observed commonly. When the vesicles slough, they leave sharply demarcated ulcers that have raised margins and a yellowish base. The mucosa between the ulcerations is often normal in appearance. In more severe cases, the small ulcers coalesce to form larger ulcerations that on rare occasions can cause bleeding, stricture and perforation of the esophagus. Characteristic histologic changes of HSV infection include multinucleated giant cells and intranuclear (Cowdry type A) inclusion bodies. HSV infects squamous cells and therefore biopsy specimens obtained from the ulcer base may yield only nondiagnostic granulation tissue and inflammatory exudate. Biopsy specimens should be taken from the squamous epithelium in the margins of the ulcerated areas. Treatment is discussed on pp. 603 & 610.

### Cytomegalovirus esophagitis

Primary infection with cytomegalovirus (CMV) commonly occurs in preschool children and young adults and therefore most older adults have serologic evidence of CMV infection. After healing of the primary infection, CMV DNA can be found in a latent form in most organs of the body. With the development of immunodeficiency, the latent infection can be reactivated and cause esophagitis. Alternatively, immunocompromised patients can acquire primary CMV disease with esophageal involvement after transfusions of blood products obtained from healthy individuals who have latent CMV infection. Unlike candida and HSV esophagitis that occasionally affect normal individuals, CMV esophagitis virtually is never seen in immunocompetent subjects. The virus often infects extraesophageal organs as well and systemic symptoms are common in patients with CMV esophagitis. Endoscopic examination characteristically reveals very elongated, shallow esophageal ulcerations that can extend for 10–15 cm. The surrounding mucosa often appears normal. These giant ulcerations cannot be distinguished endoscopically from the idiopathic esophageal ulcerations associated with HIV infection. Typical histologic changes of CMV infection include enlarged cells that have amphophilic intranuclear inclusions, a halo surrounding the nucleus and (unlike HSV infection) cytoplasmic inclusion bodies. In contrast to HSV, CMV infects fibroblasts and endothelial cells, but not squamous cells. Therefore, biopsy specimens seeking CMV ideally should be obtained from the base of the esophageal ulceration rather than from its margins. Treatment is discussed on p. 610.

### HIV ulceration

Some patients with HIV infection develop large ulcerations of the esophagus that exhibit no evidence of infection with any micro-organism other than HIV. These idiopathic ulcerations resemble CMV ulcerations in their endoscopic and radiographic appearance. Paradoxically, the idiopathic ulcerations often respond to treatment with corticosteroids or thalidomide (p. 604).

## OTHER CAUSES OF ESOPHAGEAL ULCERATION

**Ulceration due to drugs** (Collins et al 1979, Bonavina et al 1987)

This problem is much more common than previously realized. It is common for tablets to be delayed at the level of the aortic arch, an enlarged left atrium or in the distal esophagus, predisposing factors being recumbency, age and esophageal disease. Capsules, when ingested without water, can remain in the esophagus for up to 2 h (Fisher et al 1982). Tetracycline, doxycycline, emepronium amide, potassium supplements, ferrous sulfate and nonsteroidal anti-inflammatory drugs are most often implicated in the development of ulceration. All patients should take tablets with water while in the sitting position.

*Clinical features*

There may be dysphagia, painful swallowing or retrosternal chest pain. Cases of mediastinal penetration, hemorrhage and death are recorded (Kikendall et al 1983).

Barium swallow using double contrast may show subtle mucosal changes (Creteur et al 1983). Typically these occur in the upper and mid-esophagus and only occasionally in the lower third. Characteristically, there is a focal collection of multiple, small ulcers often related to the aortic arch impression. Motility is not usually disturbed. Occasionally, strictures are seen and, rarely, marked edema accompanying the ulceration may resemble an ulcerating tumor. If the offending agent is withdrawn, a repeat study may show resolution of the changes. Endoscopy shows circumscribed ulceration – sometimes kissing ulcers, focal circumferential esophagitis, erythema and congestion. There can be severe stenosis. Biopsy reveals nonspecific esophagitis and excludes carcinoma.

### Epidermolysis and pemphigoid

These and other disorders of squamous epithelium can involve the esophagus (see Table 5.3).

In the dystrophic form of epidermolysis bullosa, there is involvement of the skin, nails and esophageal mucosa. The latter develops bullae which progress to ulcers and scarring. The patient complains of dysphagia because of strictures. Double-contrast barium swallow examination may show the bullae in these conditions and the later manifestations, namely mucosal lesions progressing to fibrosis and stricture, may also be demonstrated (Tishler et al 1983, Mauro et al 1987).

Conservative therapy consists of systemic corticosteroids (p. 140), semi-liquid foods, dilatation of strictures with balloons and the use of nasogastric feeding when there are tight strictures (Feurle et al 1984). Colonic interposition may be necessary in severe cases.

Bullous lesions, scarring and strictures can occur in pemphigus (Raque et al 1970) and benign mucous membrane pemphigoid (Hardy et al 1971), but this is rare.

### **Graft-versus-host disease** (p. 406)

In those patients with dysphagia, webs or strictures in the upper esophagus are seen on barium swallow (McDonald et al 1984). The strictures are ring-like narrowings or long and tapered. Other patients present with severe esophagitis (Donner et al 1981). At endoscopy, there is desquamation of the epithelium in the upper esophagus and the mucosa is red.

### Crohn's disease

A total of 31 cases of proven or presumed Crohn's disease of the esophagus were reported prior to 1983 (Weterman 1983). In 16 cases, Crohn's disease was present elsewhere in the gastrointestinal tract. A further nine cases were reported by Geboes et al (1986). There is progressive dysphagia which is often painful. Histological features have been reported only rarely but the radiological and endoscopic features may suggest Crohn's disease. The barium swallow and endoscopy show thickened mucosal folds, ulceration or a cobblestone appearance and there may be a tubular or funnel-shaped stenosis. There may be fistulae. The differential diagnosis is from carcinoma, sarcoidosis, tuberculosis and moniliasis. The treatment is that of Crohn's disease (p. 684).

## OTHER ESOPHAGEAL TUMORS

### Leiomyoma and leiomyosarcoma

Leiomyoma occurs in 1 in 20 unselected autopsies (Postlethwait 1983) and accounts for more than 50% of benign esophageal tumors. It originates from smooth muscle and usually projects into the lumen as a lobulated mass which is sometimes ulcerated. It is difficult to distinguish benign and malignant forms histologically. Many are asymptomatic, especially the smaller tumors. Larger ones produce dysphagia and other symptoms similar to a carcinoma (Schmidt et al 1961). At barium swallow, leiomyoma usually presents as a rounded, intramural mass with clear margins. If larger than 5 cm, the possibility of leiomyosarcoma should be considered. Larger tumors may encircle the esophagus and the overlying mucosa may ulcerate. The differential diagnosis of smooth muscle tumors includes duplication and retention cysts. Endoscopy confirms a tumor lying beneath the mucosa. Treatment of symptomatic tumors is surgical.

### **Fibrovascular polyp** (Patel et al 1984)

This polyp, which usually occurs in the upper third of the esophagus, consists of edematous connective tissue covered by squamous epithelium. When it becomes large, the polyp may cause difficulties in swallowing; when it has a long stalk, it may be regurgitated. The polyp should be resected surgically.

### Other benign tumors

Squamous cell papilloma (Javdan & Pitman 1984) is a smooth, round, well-demarcated lesion which usually can be removed at endoscopy, as can granular cell myoblastoma (Subramanyam et al 1984). Benign polyp of the esophagus usually occurs in the cervical region and often has an elongated pedicle.

### Secondary tumors

The esophagus may be invaded by carcinoma of the bronchus (p. 185) or thyroid. At autopsy, eight of 705 cases of lymphoma or leukemia showed esophageal infiltration; five of these had dysphagia (Givler 1970).

### Other malignant tumors of the esophagus

Adenoid cystic carcinoma (Zardawi & Talbot 1983) and malignant melanoma (Takubo et al 1983) may occur as primary esophageal malignancies. Typically they are aggressive neoplasms with a poor prognosis. Lymphoma, which may be primary or secondary, may appear as a polypoid mass with or without ulceration, as irregular strictures, discrete intramural masses, enlarged folds, a tapered lower esophagus or as diffuse nodularity (Levine et al 1985). Kaposi's sarcoma may involve the esophagus (p. 610).

### **Cysts and duplications** (Rhaney & Barclay 1959, Tarnay et al 1970, Postlethwait 1983)

Cysts are lined by ciliated columnar epithelium or occasionally gastric or squamous epithelium and are situated in the outer wall of the esophagus, usually posteriorly. They arise embryologically from diverticula of the foregut. A duplication of the esophagus runs parallel to the esophagus and behaves as a cyst. Cysts and duplications both occur in association with spinal abnormalities. They are asymptomatic or present with pain and dysphagia in adults or respiratory symptoms in children. The treatment is surgical excision.

Congenital fistula without atresia may present in adult life, e.g. a mid-esophageal diverticulum connected by a fistula to the right lower bronchus (Kameya et al 1984).

## REFERENCES


Altorki N K, Sunagawa M, Little A G, Skinner D B 1991 High-grade dysplasia in the columnar-lined esophagus. American Journal of Surgery 161: 97–100

Anderson L L, Lad T E 1982 Autopsy findings in squamous-cell carcinoma of the esophagus. Cancer 50: 1587–1590

Anselm K 1979 Comparison of endoscopy and barium swallow in the diagnosis of esophageal stripture. Gastrointestinal Endoscopy 25: 95

Aste H, Saccomanno S, Munizzi F 1984 Blind pan-esophageal brush cytology. Diagnostic accuracy. Endoscopy 16: 165–167

Atkinson M 1987 Monitoring oesophageal pH. Gut 28: 509–514

Baehr P H, McDonald G B 1994 Esophageal infections: risk factors, presentation, diagnosis, and treatment. Gastroenterology 106: 509–532

Barish C F, Wu W C, Castell D O 1985 Respiratory complications of gastroesophageal reflux. Archives of Internal Medicine 145: 1882–1888

Berenson M M, Johnson T D, Markowitz N R, Buchi K N, Samowitz W S 1993 Restoration of squamous mucosa after ablation of Barrett's esophageal epithelium. Gastroenterology 104: 1686–1691

Bernstein L M, Fruin R C, Pacini R 1962 Differentiation of esophageal pain from angina pectoris: role of the esophageal acid perfusion test. Medicine 41: 143–162

Blot W J, Devesa S S, Kneller R W, Fraumeni J F Jr 1991 Rising incidence of adenocarcinoma of the esophagus and gastric cardia. Journal of the American Medical Association 265: 1287–1289

Blot W J, Devesa S S, Fraumeni J F Jr 1993 Continuing climb in rates of esophageal adenocarcinoma: an update. Journal of the American Medical Association 270: 1320 (letter)

Blount P L, Meltzer S J, Yin J, Huang Y, Krasna M J, Reid B J 1993 Clonal ordering of 17p and 5q allelic losses in Barrett dysplasia and adenocarcinoma. Proceedings of the National Academy of Sciences 90: 3221–3225

Bonavina L, DeMeester T R, McChesney L, Schwizer W, Albertucci M, Bailey R T 1987 Drug induced esophageal strictures. Annals of Surgery 206: 173–183

Brand D L 1982 Chest pain of esophageal origin. In: Cohen S, Soloway R D (eds) Diseases of the esophagus. Churchill Livingstone, Edinburgh, p 137–159

Brandt L J, Kauvar D R 1992 Laser-induced regression of Barrett's epithelium. Gastrointestinal Endoscopy 38: 619–622

Bremner C G 1982 Benign strictures of the oesophagus. Current problems in surgery. Year Book, Chicago

Burgess J N, Payne W S, Andersen H A, Weiland L H, Carlson H C 1971 Barrett esophagus: the columnar-epithelial-lined lower esophagus. Proceedings of the Staff Meetings of the Mayo Clinic 46:725

Burns T W, Venturatos S G 1985 Esophageal motor function and response to acid perfusion in patients with symptomatic reflux esophagitis. Digestive Diseases and Sciences 30: 529–535

Cameron A J, Lomboy C T 1992 Barrett's esophagus: age, prevalence, and extent of columnar epithelium. Gastroenterology 103: 1241–1245

Cameron A J, Zinsmeister A R, Ballard D J, Carney J A 1990 Prevalence of columnar-lined (Barrett's) esophagus. Comparison of population-based clinical and autopsy findings. Gastroenterology 99: 918–922

Carey L C, Darin J C, Worman L W, Wagner K J 1965 Upper gastrointestinal hemorrhage from carcinoma of esophagus. A report of six cases. Archives of Surgery (Chicago) 90: 460–464

Chang F, Syrjänen S, Wang L, Syrjänen K 1992 Infectious agents in the etiology of esophageal cancer. Gastroenterology 103: 1336–1348

Chernow B, Johnson L F, Janowitz W R, Castell D O 1979 Pulmonary aspiration as a consequence of gastroesophageal reflux. A diagnostic approach. Digestive Diseases and Sciences 24: 839–844

Collen M J, Johnson D A 1992 Correlation between basal acid output and daily ranitidine dose required for therapy in Barrett's esophagus. Digestive Diseases and Sciences 37: 570–576

Collen M J, Lewis J H, Benjamin S B 1990 Gastric acid hypersecretion in refractory gastroesophageal reflux disease. Gastroenterology 98: 654–661

Collins F J, Matthews H R, Baker S E, Strakova J M 1979 Drug-induced oesophageal injury. British Medical Journal 1: 1673–1676

Creteur V, Laufer I, Kressel H Y et al 1983 Drug-induced esophagitis detected by double-contrast radiography. Radiology 147: 365–368

Crozier R E, Jonasson H 1964 Symptomatic esophageal hiatus hernias: study of 105 patients. Archives of Internal Medicine 113: 737–743

Crozier R E, Gregg J A, Garabedian M M 1972 Obscure chest pain as a symptom of reflux esophagitis. Medical Clinics of North America 56: 771–780

Dahms B B, Rothstein F C 1984 Barrett's esophagus in children: a consequence of chronic gastroesophageal reflux. Gastroenterology 86: 318–323

Davies H A, Page Z, Rush E M, Brown A L, Lewis M J, Petch M C 1985 Oesophageal stimulation lowers exertional angina threshold. Lancet 1: 1011–1014

Dent J, Holloway R H, Toouli J, Dodds W J 1988 Mechanisms of lower oesophageal sphincter incompetence in patients with symptomatic gastrooesophageal reflux. Gut 29: 1020–1028

Dent J, Bremner C G, Collen M J, Haggitt R C, Spechler S J 1991 Working party report to the World Congresses of Gastroenterology, Sydney 1990: Barrett's oesophagus. Journal of Gastroenterology and Hepatology 6: 1–22

DeVault K R, Castell D O 1994 Current diagnosis and treatment of gastroesophageal reflux disease. Mayo Clinic Proceedings 69: 867–876

Dodds W J, Hogan W J, Helm J F, Dent J F 1981 Pathogenesis of reflux esophagitis. Gastroenterology 81: 376–394

Donner M W, Saba G P, Martinez C R 1981 Diffuse diseases of the esophagus: a practical approach. Seminars in Roentgenology 16: 198–213

Dunnington G L, DeMeester T R 1993 The outcome effect of adherence to operative principles of Nissen fundoplication by multiple surgeons. American Journal of Surgery 166: 654–657

Earlam R, Cunha-Melo J R 1980 Oesophageal squamous cell carcinoma: 1. A critical review of surgery. British Journal of Surgery 67: 381–390

Ellis F H Jr 1990 Diaphragmatic hiatal hernias. Recognizing and treating the major types. Postgraduate Medicine 88: 113–114, 117–120, 123–124

Feurle G E, Weidauer H, Baldauf G, Schulte-Braucks J, Anton-Lamprecht I 1984 Management of esophageal stenosis in recessive dystrophic epidermolysis bullosa. Gastroenterology 87: 1376–1380

Fisher R S, Malmud L S, Applegate G, Rock E, Lorber S H 1982 Effect of bolus composition on esophageal transit: concise communication. Journal of Nuclear Medicine 23: 878–882

Fleming J A C 1943 Carcinoma of the thoracic oesophagus: some notes on its pathology and spread in relation to treatment. British Journal of Radiology 16: 212–216

Geboes K, Janssens J, Rutgeerts P, Vantrappen G 1986 Crohn's disease of the esophagus. Journal of Clinical Gastroenterology 8: 31–37

Gillen P, Keeling P, Byrne P J, Healy M, O'Moore R R, Hennessy T P J 1988 Implication of duodenogastric reflux in the pathogenesis of Barrett's oesophagus. British Journal of Surgery 75: 540–543

Givler R L 1970 Esophageal lesions in leukemia and lymphoma. American Journal of Digestive Diseases 15: 31–36

Goldstein H M, Zornoza J 1978 Association of squamous cell carcinoma of the head and neck with cancer of the esophagus. American Journal of Roentgenology 131: 791–794

Goyal R K, Glancy J J, Spiro H M 1970 Lower esophageal ring. New England Journal of Medicine 282: 1298–1305

Gray M R, Donnelly R J, Kingsnorth A N 1991 Role of salivary epidermal growth factor in the pathogenesis of Barrett's columnar lined oesophagus. British Journal of Surgery 78: 1461–1466

Guanrei Y, Songliang Q, He H, Guizen F 1988 Natural history of early esophageal squamous carcinoma and early adenocarcinoma of the gastric cardia in the People's Republic of China. Endoscopy 20: 95–98

Haggitt R C 1992 Adenocarcinoma in Barrett's esophagus: a new epidemic? Human Pathology 23: 475–476

Haggitt R C, Dean P J 1985 Adenocarcinoma in Barrett's epithelium. In: Spechler S J, Goyal R K (eds) Barrett's esophagus: pathophysiology, diagnosis, and management. Elsevier, New York, p 153–166

Hallerbäck B, Unge P, Carling L et al and the Scandinavian Clinics for United Research Group 1994 Omeprazole or ranitidine in long-term treatment of reflux esophagitis. Gastroenterology 107: 1305–1311

Hameeteman W 1991 Clinical studies of sucralfate in reflux esophagitis. The European experience. Journal of Clinical Gastroenterology 13: S16–S20

Hameeteman W, Tytgat G N J, Houthoff H J, van den Tweel J G 1989 Barrett's esophagus: development of dysplasia and adenocarcinoma. Gastroenterology 96: 1249–1256

Hardy K M, Perry H O, Pingree G C, Kirby T J Jr 1971 Benign mucous membrane pemphigoid. Archives of Dermatology 104: 467–475

Hassall E 1993 Barrett's esophagus: new definitions and approaches in children. Journal of Pediatric Gastroenterology and Nutrition 16: 345–364

Hassall E, Weinstein W M, Ament M E 1985 Barrett's esophagus in childhood. Gastroenterology 89: 1331–1337

Helm J F, Dodds W J, Pele L R et al 1984 Effect of esophageal emptying and saliva on clearance of acid from the esophagus. New England Journal of Medicine 310: 284–288

Hendrix T R, Yardley J H 1976 Consequences of gastroesophageal reflux. Clinics in Gastroenterology 5: 155–174

Herlihy K J, Orlando R C, Bryson J C, Bozymski E M, Carney C N, Powell D W 1984 Barrett's esophagus: clinical, endoscopic, histologic, manometric, and electrical potential difference characteristics. Gastroenterology 86: 436–443

Herskovic A, Martz K, Al-Sarraf M et al 1992 Combined chemotherapy and radiotherapy compared with radiotherapy alone in patients with cancer of the esophagus. New England Journal of Medicine 326: 1593–1598

Hesketh P J, Clapp R W, Doos W G, Spechler S J 1989 The increasing frequency of adenocarcinoma of the esophagus. Cancer 64: 526–530

Hetzel D J, Dent J, Reed W D et al 1988 Healing and relapse of severe peptic esophagitis after treatment with omeprazole. Gastroenterology 95: 903–912

Holloway R H, Dent J 1990 Pathophysiology of gastroesophageal reflux. Lower esophageal sphincter dysfunction in gastroesophageal reflux disease. Gastroenterology Clinics of North America 19: 517–535

Hughes H E, Lee F D, MacKenzie J F 1978 Endoscopic cytology and biopsy in the upper gastrointestinal tract. Clinics in Gastroenterology 7: 375

Hyden E C, Langholz B, Tilden T et al 1988 External beam and intraluminal radiotherapy in the treatment of carcinoma of the esophagus. Journal of Thoracic and Cardiovascular Surgery 96: 237–241

Iascone C, DeMeester T R, Little A G, Skinner D B 1983 Barrett's esophagus. Functional assessment, proposed pathogenesis, and surgical therapy. Archives of Surgery 118: 543–549

Ismail-Beigi F, Horton P F, Pope C E 1970 Histological consequence of gastroesophageal reflux in man. Gastroenterology 58: 163–174

Jamieson G G 1987 Anti-reflux operations: how do they work? British Journal of Surgery 74: 155–156

Javdan P, Pitman E R 1984 Squamous papilloma of esophagus. Digestive Diseases and Sciences 29: 317–320

Jensen D M, Machicado G, Randall G, Tung L A, English-Zych S 1988 Comparison of low-power YAG laser and BICAP tumor probe for palliation of esophageal cancer strictures. Gastroenterology 94: 1263–1270

Johnson D A, Winters C, Spurling T J, Chobanian S J, Cattau E L Jr 1987 Esophageal acid sensitivity in Barrett's esophagus. Journal of Clinical Gastroenterology 9: 23–27

Kahrilas P J 1992 Cigarette smoking and gastroesophageal reflux disease. Digestive Diseases 10: 61–71

Kahrilas P J, Clouse R E, Hogan W J 1994 American Gastroenterological Association technical review on the clinical use of esophageal manometry. Gastroenterology 107: 1865–1884

Kameya S, Umeda Y, Mizuno K, Watanabe T, Kato K, Koike A 1984 Congenital esophagobronchial fistula in the adult. American Journal of Gastroenterology 79: 589–592

Kantrowitz P A, Corson J G, Fleischli D J, Skinner D B 1969 Measurement of gastroesophageal reflux. Gastroenterology 56: 666–674

Katz P O 1991 Pathogenesis and management of gastroesophageal reflux disease. Journal of Clinical Gastroenterology 13: S6–S15

Kikendall J W, Friedman A C, Oyewole M A, Fleischer D, Johnson L F 1983 Pill-induced esophageal injury. Case reports and review of the medical literature. Digestive Diseases and Sciences 28: 174–182

Kim S L, Waring J P, Spechler S J, Sampliner R E, Doos W G et al 1994 Diagnostic inconsistencies in Barrett's esophagus. Gastroenterology 107: 945–949

Kitchin L I, Castell D O 1991 Rationale and efficacy of conservative therapy for gastroesophageal reflux disease. Archives of Internal Medicine 151: 448–454

Kjellén G, Tibbling L 1985 Oesophageal motility during acid-provoked heartburn and chest pain. Scandinavian Journal of Gastroenterology 20: 937–940

Knyrim K, Wagner H J, Bethge N, Keymling M, Vakil N 1993 A controlled trial of an expansile metal stent for palliation of esophageal obstruction due to inoperable cancer. New England Journal of Medicine 329: 1302–1307

Laine L 1994 The natural history of esophageal candidiasis after successful treatment in patients with AIDS. Gastroenterology 107: 744–746

Lanas A, Hirschowitz B I 1991 Significant role of aspirin use in patients with esophagitis. Journal of Clinical Gastroenterology 13: 622–627

Lee R G 1985 Dysplasia in Barrett's esophagus. A clinicopathologic study of six patients. American Journal of Surgical Pathology 9: 845–852

Levine D S, Haggitt R C, Blount P L, Rabinovitch P S, Rusch V W, Reid B J 1993 An endoscopic biopsy protocol can differentiate high-grade dysplasia from early adenocarcinoma in Barrett's esophagus. Gastroenterology 105: 40–50

Levine M S, Sunshine A G, Reynolds J C, Saul S H 1985 Diffuse nodularity in esophageal lymphoma. American Journal of Roentgenology 145: 1218–1220

McCallum R W 1990 Gastric emptying in gastroesophageal reflux and the therapeutic role of prokinetic agents. Gastroenterology Clinics of North America 19: 551–564

McClave S A, Boyce H W Jr, Gottfried M R 1987 Early diagnosis of columnar-lined esophagus: a new endoscopic criterion. Gastrointestinal Endoscopy 33: 413–416

McCort J J 1952 Radiographic identification of lymph node metastases from carcinoma of the esophagus. Radiology 59: 694–711

McDonald G B, Sullivan K M, Plumley T P 1984 Radiographic features of esophageal involvement in chronic graft-vs-host disease. American Journal of Roentgenology 142: 501–506

MacDonald W C, Brandborg L L, Taniguchi L, Rubin C E 1963 Esophageal exfoliative cytology. A neglected procedure. Annals of Internal Medicine 59: 332

Marks R D, Richter J E, Rizzo H, Koehler R E, Spenney J G, Mills T P, Champion G 1994 Omeprazole versus H2-receptor antagonists in treating patients with peptic stricture and esophagitis. Gastroenterology 106: 907–915

Martin C J, Dodds W J, Liem H H, Dantas R O, Layman R D, Dent J 1992 Diaphragmatic contribution to gastroesophageal competence and reflux in dogs. American Journal of Physiology 263: G551–G557

Matsufuji H, Kuwano H, Kai H, Matsuda H, Sugimachi K 1988 Preoperative hyperthermia combined with radiotherapy and chemotherapy for patients with incompletely resected carcinoma of the esophagus. Cancer 62: 889–894
Mattioli S, Pilotti V, Spangaro M et al 1989 Reliability of 24-hour home esophageal pH monitoring in diagnosis of gastroesophageal reflux. Digestive Diseases and Sciences 34: 71–78
Mattox H E III, Richter J E 1990 Prolonged ambulatory esophageal pH monitoring in the evaluation of gastroesophageal reflux disease. American Journal of Medicine 89: 345–356
Mauro M A, Parker L A, Hartley W S, Renner J B, Mauro P M 1987 Epidermolysis bullosa: radiographic findings in 16 cases. American Journal of Radiology 149: 925–927
Mayer R J 1994 The changing nature of esophageal cancer. Chest 103: 404S–405S
Meyers R L, Orlando R C 1992 In vivo bicarbonate secretion by human esophagus. Gastroenterology 103: 1174–1178
Mittal R K 1990 Current concepts of the antireflux barrier. Gastroenterology Clinics of North America 19: 501–516
Mittal R K, Rochester D F, McCallum R W 1988 Electrical and mechanical activity in the human lower esophageal sphincter during diaphragmatic contraction. Journal of Clinical Investigation 81: 1182–1189
Moses F M 1991 Squamous cell carcinoma of the esophagus. Natural history, incidence, etiology, and complications. Gastroenterology Clinics of North America 20: 703–716
Murray F E, Bowers G J, Birkett D H, Cave D R 1988 Palliative laser therapy of advanced esophageal carcinoma: an alternative perspective. American Journal of Gastroenterology 83: 816–819
Orlando R C 1991a Esophageal epithelial defense against acid injury. Journal of Clinical Gastroenterology 13: S1–S5
Orlando R C 1991b Sucralfate therapy and reflux esophagitis: an overview. American Journal of Medicine 91: 123S–124S
Orlando R C 1994 Esophageal epithelial defenses against acid injury. American Journal of Gastroenterology 89: S48–S52
O'Sullivan G C, DeMeester T R, Joelsson B E, Smith R B, Johnson L F, Skinner D B 1982 Interaction of lower esophageal sphincter pressure and length of sphincter in the abdomen as determinants of gastroesophageal competence. American Journal of Surgery 143: 40–46
Overholt B F 1992 Photodynamic therapy and thermal treatment of esophageal cancer. Gastrointestinal Endoscopy Clinics of North America 2: 433–455
Overholt B, Panjehpour M, Tefftellar E, Rose M 1993 Photodynamic therapy for treatment of early adenocarcinoma in Barrett's esophagus. Gastrointestinal Endoscopy 39: 73–76
Patel J, Kieffer R W, Martin M, Avant G R 1984 Giant fibrovascular polyp of the esophagus. Gastroenterology 87: 953–956
Paull A, Trier J S, Dalton M D, Camp R C, Loeb P, Goyal R K 1976 The histologic spectrum of Barrett's esophagus. New England Journal of Medicine 295: 476–480
Peters J H, Hoeft S, Heimbucher J et al 1994 Selection of patients for curative or palliative resection of esophageal cancer based on preoperative endoscopic ultrasonography. Archives of Surgery 129: 534–539
Pope C E II 1994 Acid-reflux disorders. New England Journal of Medicine 331: 656–660
Poplin E A, Khanuja P S, Kraut M J et al 1994 Chemoradiotherapy of esophageal carcinoma. Cancer 74: 1217–1224
Postlethwait R W 1983 Benign tumors and cysts of the esophagus. Surgery Clinics of North America 63: 925–931
Raphael H A, Ellis F H Jr, Dockerty M B 1966 Primary adenocarcinoma of the esophagus: 18-year review and review of literature. Annals of Surgery 164: 785–796
Raque C J, Stein K M, Samitz M H 1970 Pemphigus vulgaris involving the esophagus. Archives of Dermatology 102: 371–373
Reid B J, Weinstein W M 1987 Barrett's esophagus and adenocarcinoma. Annual Review of Medicine 38: 477–492
Rhaney K, Barclay G P 1959 Enterogenous cysts and congenital diverticula of the alimentary canal with abnormalities of the vertebral column and spinal cord. Journal of Pathology and Bacteriology 77: 457–471
Rice T W, Boyce G A, Sivak M V, Adelstein D J, Kirby T J 1992 Esophageal carcinoma: esophageal ultrasound assessment of preoperative chemotherapy. Annals of Thoracic Surgery 53: 972–977
Richter J E, Castell D O 1982 Gastroesophageal reflux. Pathogenesis, diagnosis, and therapy. Annals of Internal Medicine 97: 93–103
Rothery G A, Patterson J E, Stoddard C J, Day D W 1986 Histological and histochemical changes in the columnar lined (Barrett's) oesophagus. Gut 27: 1062–1068
Sampliner R E, Hixson L J, Fennerty B, Garewal H S 1993 Regression of Barrett's esophagus by laser ablation in an anacid environment. Digestive Diseases and Sciences 38: 365–368
Schmidt H G, Riddell R H, Walther B, Skinner D B, Riemann J F 1985 Dysplasia in Barrett's esophagus. Journal of Cancer Research and Clinical Oncology 110: 145–152
Schmidt H W, Glagett O T, Harrison E G 1961 Benign tumors and cysts of the esophagus. Journal of Thoracic and Cardiovascular Surgery 41: 717–732
Schwade J G, Kinsella T J, Kelly B, Rowland J, Johnston M, Glatstein E 1984 Clinical experience with intravenous misonidazole for carcinoma of the esophagus: results in attempting radiosensitization of each fraction of exposure. Cancer Investigation 2: 91–95
Semenkovich J W, Balfe D M, Weyman P J, Heiken J P, Lee J K T 1985 Barium pharyngography: comparison of single and double contrast. American Journal of Roentgenology 144: 715–720
Shu Y-J 1983 Cytopathology of the esophagus. An overview of esophageal cytopathology in China. Acta Cytologica 27: 7–16
Sloan S, Kahrilas P J 1991 Impairment of esophageal emptying with hiatal hernia. Gastroenterology 100: 596–605
Sloan S, Rademaker A W, Kahrilas P J 1992 Determinants of gastroesophageal junction incompetence: hiatal hernia, lower esophageal sphincter, or both? Annals of Internal Medicine 117: 977–982
Smith P M, Kerr G D, Cockel R et al 1994 A comparison of omeprazole and ranitidine in the prevention of recurrence of benign esophageal stricture. Gastroenterology 107: 1312–1318
Sons H U 1987 Etiologic and epidemiologic factors of carcinoma of the esophagus. Surgery, Gynecology and Obstetrics 165: 183–190
Sontag S J 1990 The medical management of reflux esophagitis. Role of antacids and acid inhibition. Gastroenterology Clinics of North America 19: 683–712
Spechler S J 1987 Endoscopic surveillance for patients with Barrett's esophagus: does the cancer risk justify the practice? Annals of Internal Medicine 106: 902–904
Spechler S J 1992a Comparison of medical and surgical therapy for complicated gastroesophageal reflux disease in veterans. The Department of Veterans Affairs Gastroesophageal Reflux Disease Study Group. New England Journal of Medicine 326: 786–792
Spechler S J 1992b Complications of gastroesophageal reflux disease. In: Castell D O (ed) The esophagus. Little, Brown, Boston, p 543–556
Spechler S J 1992c Epidemiology and natural history of gastro-oesophageal reflux disease. Digestion 51: 24–29
Spechler S J 1992d The frequency of esophageal cancer in patients with Barrett's esophagus. Acta Endoscopica 22: 541–544
Spechler S J 1993 Laser photoablation of Barrett's epithelium: burning issues about burning tissues. Gastroenterology 104: 1855–1858
Spechler S J 1994 Barrett's esophagus. Current Opinion in Gastroenterology 10: 448–454
Spechler S J, Goyal R K 1986 Barrett's esophagus. New England Journal of Medicine 315: 362–371
Spechler S J, Zeroogian J M, Antonioli D A, Wang H H, Goyal R K 1994 Prevalence of metaplasia at the gastro-oesophageal junction. Lancet 344: 1533–1536
Stevenson G W 1984 Gastroesophageal reflux. In: Margulis A R, Gooding C A (eds) Diagnostic radiology. University of California Printing Department, San Francisco. p 93
Subramanyam K, Shannon C R, Patterson M, Davis M, Gourley W K 1984 Granular cell myoblastoma of the esophagus. Journal of Clinical Gastroenterology 6: 113–118
Takubo K, Kanda Y, Ishii M, et al 1983 Primary malignant melanoma of the esophagus. Human Pathology 14: 727–730
Tarnay T J, Chang C H, Nugent R G, Warden H E 1970 Esophageal duplication (foregut cyst) with spinal malformation. Journal of Thoracic and Cardiovascular Surgery 59: 293–298
Thompson J J 1982 Esophageal cancer and the premalignant changes of

esophageal diseases. In: Cohen S, Soloway R D (eds) Diseases of the esophagus. Churchill Livingstone, Edinburgh, p 239–276

Thompson J J, Zinsser K R, Enterline H T 1983 Barrett's metaplasia and adenocarcinoma of the esophagus and gastroesophageal junction. Human Pathology 14: 42–61

Tishler J M, Han S Y, Helman C A 1983 Esophageal involvement in epidermolysis bullosa dystrophica. American Journal of Roentgenology 141: 1283–1286

Togawa K, Jaskiewicz K, Takahashi H, Meltzer S J, Rustgi A K 1994 Human papillomavirus DNA sequences in esophagus squamous cell carcinoma. Gastroenterology 107: 128–136

Tytgat G N J, Bartelsman J F W M, Vermeyden J R 1992 Dilatation and prosthesis for obstructing esophagogastric carcinoma. Gastrointestinal Endoscopy Clinics of North America 2: 415–432

Weterman I T 1983 Oral, oesophageal and gastroduodenal Crohn's disease. In: Allan R N, Keighley M R B, Alexander-Williams J, Hawkins C (eds) Inflammatory Bowel Diseases. Churchill Livingstone, Edinburgh, p 299–306

Wilkins W E, Ridley M G, Pozniak A L 1984 Benign stricture of the oesophagus: role of non-steroidal anti-inflammatory drugs. Gut 25: 478–480

Winawer S J, Melamed M, Sherlock P 1976 Potential of endoscopy, biopsy and cytology in the diagnosis and management of patients with cancer. Clinics in Gastroenterology 5: 575–595

Windsor C W O, Collis J L 1967 Anaemia and hiatus hernia: experience in 450 patients. Thorax 22: 73–78

Winter H S, Madara J L, Stafford R J, Grand R J, Quinlan J-E, Goldman H 1982 Intraepithelial eosinophils: a new diagnostic criterion for reflux esophagitis. Gastroenterology 83: 818–823

Winter S C Jr, Spurling T J, Chobanian S J et al 1987 Barrett's esophagus. A prevalent, occult complication of gastroesophageal reflux disease. Gastroenterology 92: 118–124

Zaninotto G, DeMeester T R, Bremner C G, Smyrk T C, Cheng S C 1989 Esophageal function in patients with reflux-induced strictures and its relevance to surgical treatment. Annals of Thoracic Surgery 47: 362–370

Zardawi I M, Talbot I C 1983 Primary adenoid cystic carcinoma of the oesophagus. Diagnostic Histopathology 6: 39–46

# 9. The stomach and duodenum: gastritis, duodenitis and peptic ulceration

*J. R. Lambert*

ANATOMY AND PHYSIOLOGY OF THE STOMACH AND DUODENUM

The stomach lies in the left upper quadrant of the abdomen but is fixed only at the gastroesophageal junction and at the first part of the duodenum, so that its most dependent part may be found as low as the pelvis. Its posterior surface forms part of the wall of the lesser sac and is in contact with the pancreas, kidney and spleen. Its anterior surface is partly covered by the left lobe of the liver and the stomach may be displaced by enlargement of any of these organs. The greater omentum and the transverse colon lie along the greater curve. The duodenum is predominantly retroperitoneal and comprises the cap, descending and distal portions.

The four anatomic regions of the stomach are the cardia, fundus, body and antrum in whose mucosa are varying histologic cell types and secretory products. The anatomical antrum commences at the incisura angularis, an indentation seen on barium meal or endoscopy, two-thirds of the way down the lesser curve (Fig. 9.1).

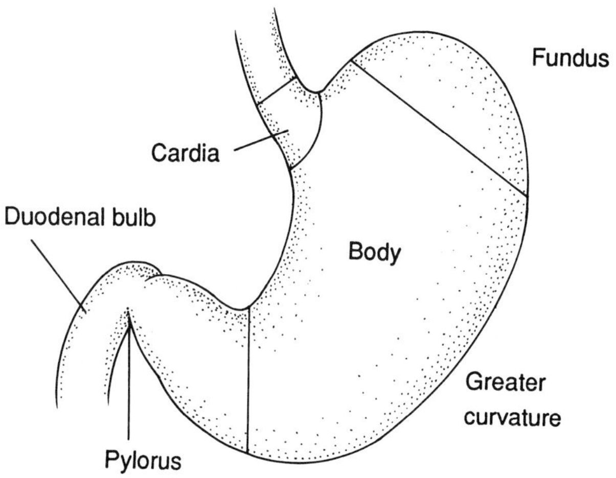


**Fig. 9.1** The anatomical regions of the stomach.

### The anatomical distinction between body and antrum

The body and antrum have distinct secretory and motor functions with no external landmark to separate the two parts. The junction between antral and body mucosa can usually be determined macroscopically, but for an exact demarcation histological studies or measurement in situ of the pH of the secretions are essential. Such studies show that the mucosal junction is variable. Normally the junction occurs 35–44% of the distance on the lesser curve from pylorus to gastroesophageal junction and on the greater curve 11–15% (Landboe-Christensen 1944). Oi & Sakurai (1959) demonstrated that the antral-type mucosa can extend along the lesser curvature to the esophagus and it may also stop short of the pylorus. In Japanese subjects, the studies of Kimura (1972) would suggest that proximal movement of the border occurs with increasing age. Because the border is not static, Grossman (1960) suggested that the term "gastric antrum" should be replaced by the term "pyloric gland area". Gastric ulcers occur predominantly at the junction of the pyloric gland area and the body mucosa.

### The stomach wall

The main muscle layer or muscularis propria consists of inner oblique, middle circular and outer longitudinal layers. The middle circular layer is more concentrated in the antrum. The longitudinal muscle is mainly in continuity with that of the duodenum distally and the esophagus proximally. The pyloric sphincter consists of thickened circular muscle which is partially separated from the duodenal muscle by fibrous tissue. The role of the sphincter and muscle layers in gastric emptying is discussed on p. 423. When the stomach is distended the mucosa is smooth and gastric pits can be seen by the naked eye, but when the stomach is empty the mucosa forms longitudinal folds or rugae. The normal mucosa can also have a cobblestone appearance. A muscularis mucosae is situated between mucosa and the main muscle layer. The function of gastric smooth muscle is controlled jointly by neural and hormonal mechanisms.

## Microscopic appearance of the mucosa

The surface lining of the gastric mucosa consists of tall columnar epithelial cells with basal nuclei and numerous apical granules which contain mucinogen. These surface mucous cells provide the surface mucus, which is an important component of the gastric mucosal barrier. The epithelial cell layer invaginates to form pits or foveolae which occupy one-quarter of the mucosa. Each pit communicates with the gastric glands; there are three specific types of gland: cardiac, oxyntic and pyloric. The proportion of mucosa made up of glands, as well as the cell types (Table 9.1) comprising the various types of glands, differentiate one stomach region from another.

### *Cardiac glands*

These are branched and coiled glands lined by mucous cells that secrete mucus and some pepsinogen. There are relatively few parietal or chief cells in this area.

### *Parietal or oxyntic glands* (Fig. 9.2)

These are present in the fundus and body of the stomach. From three to seven glands empty through the neck region into each gastric pit. The following secretory cells are found within the glands: mucous neck cells, undifferentiated neck cells, parietal (oxyntic) cells, peptic (chief) cells, endocrine cells and mast cells.

The mucous neck cells are interspersed between parietal cells in the neck region of the glands; they are morphologically different from the surface epithelial cells but similar to the mucous cells in the cardiac and pyloric glands. Undifferentiated cells are found at the junction of the gland and pit. They show numerous mitoses and are responsible for the cell renewal of the mucosa. Cells migrate to the surface epithelium, which has a turnover of 1–3 days (Messier & Leblond 1960). By contrast, the migration to form new parietal cells is very slow. While rapid cell turnover of the surface epithelium is a protective mechanism, superficial damage is repaired by restitution within hours. This involves the surviving epithelial cells spreading rapidly over the breached surface to re-establish epithelial continuity.

**Table 9.1** Gastric secretory cells and their products

| Cell type | Secretory products |
|---|---|
| Parietal cells | Hydrochloric acid, intrinsic factor |
| Mucus cells | Mucus, pepsinogen II |
| Chief cells | Pepsinogen I |
| G cells | Gastrin |
| D cells | Somatostatin |
| Mast cells | Histamine |
| Enterochromaffin-like cells | Histamine |

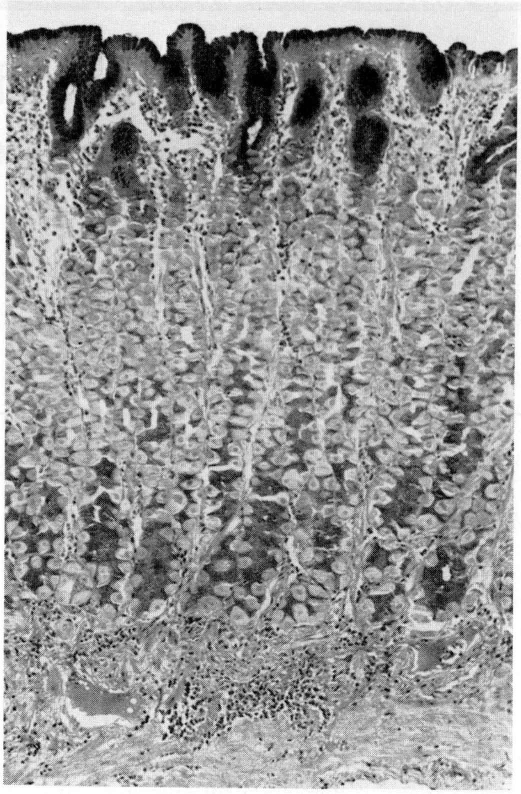

**Fig. 9.2** Normal gastric body mucosa. Short gastric pits, a mid-zone of pale triangular parietal cells and dark chief cells at the gland bases (Maxwell stain, × 110).

The parietal cells are situated predominantly in the upper part of the gland. They are pyramidal in shape, with the base of the pyramid against the basement membrane, and they are eosinophilic. On electronmicroscopy they are seen to contain numerous large mitochondria, intracellular canaliculi which are lined by microvilli, and tubovesicles. In the resting secretory state, tubovesicles predominate and the intracellular canaliculus becomes internalized, distended and devoid of microvilli, but when the cell is stimulated to secrete acid the number of tubovesicles is reduced, microvilli increase and the canalicular system enlarges and opens into the lumen (Rohrer et al 1965). These changes are accomplished by membrane recycling, whereby the tubovesicles fuse with the apical plasma membrane when the cell is stimulated. Return to the resting state involves reincorporation of the surface membrane by endocytosis.

The chief cells are situated mainly in the lower part of the glands, primarily in the corpus but with a few in the cardia. They are columnar or cuboidal and their apical cytoplasm contains numerous zymogen granules; the granules contain pepsinogens.

### *Pyloric glands* (Fig. 9.3)

These are located in the pyloric region of the stomach and

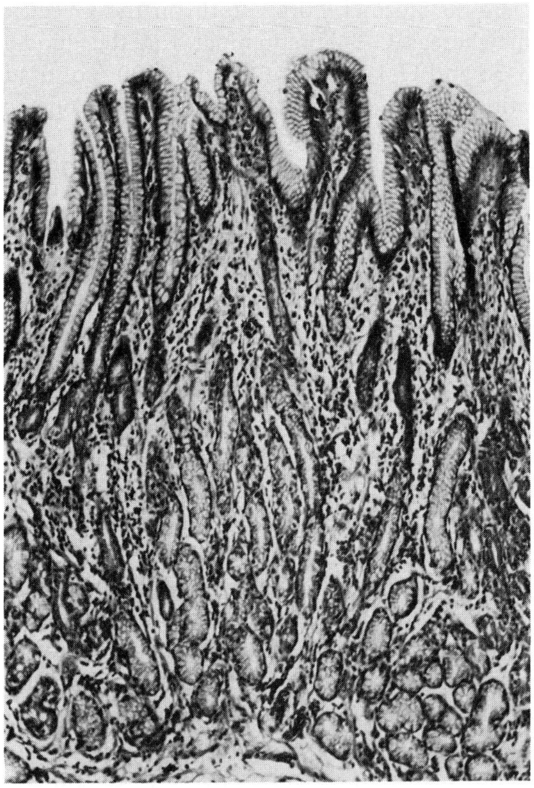

**Fig. 9.3** Normal pyloric antral mucosa. Elongated pits and coiled tubular mucus-secreting glands (hematoxylin and eosin, × 110).

extend into the body for a variable distance, especially along the lesser curvature. They are branched and coiled and are lined by mucus-secreting cells. The glands open into gastric pits which occupy about half the thickness of the mucosa. G cells are found mainly in the mid-portion of the glands (McGuigan 1968). Other endocrine cells are found scattered in the pyloric glands.

At the pylorus, the deeper parts of the pyloric glands become interspersed by muscle fibers and appear to continue into the duodenum as Brunner's glands, which lie deep to the muscularis mucosae.

*Enteroendocrine cells*

Previously characteristics of these cells were based on staining, hence "enterochromaffin", "argentaffin" and "argyrophil" cells. Now these cells are classified by specific immunofluorescence and ultrastructural immunolocalization. The endocrine (EC) cell is also found in the small intestine and the endocrine-like cell (enterochromaffin or ECL cell) is found only in the gastric mucosa. The ECL and mast cells are important sources of histamine which has a central role in the regulation of gastric acid secretion. There are seven other types of endocrine cell in the gastric mucosa, including D cells, which produce somatostatin, and G cells, which produce gastrin (Solcia et al 1987). The hormones and paracrine substances which they produce are involved in the control of gastric secretion and motility and are further discussed on p. 220 and in Chapters 6 and 15.

### The vascular, lymphatic and nervous supply to the stomach

The blood supply to the stomach is mainly via the left gastric, splenic and hepatic branches of the celiac axis. There are widespread anastomoses in the submucosa and an extensive network of capillaries in the mucosa. Gastric mucosal blood flow is proportional to the secretory function of the mucosa (Guth 1982). Mucosal blood flow may be greatly reduced in shock and this reduction is an important factor in the etiology of "stress ulcer". In contrast to the widespread mucosal and submucosal distribution of capillaries, lymphatics are absent from the upper and middle regions of the lamina propria but are found in the deep lamina propria adjacent to the muscularis mucosa. The submucosa has an extensive anastomosing plexus of lymphatics (Lehnert et al 1985). The innervation of the stomach and gastric motility are discussed in Chapter 6.

## THE DUODENUM

The duodenum is approximately 30 cm in length and the second, third and fourth parts are retroperitoneal. The papilla of Vater is situated approximately at the mid-portion of the second or descending part. The structure of the duodenum resembles the rest of the small intestine in having a muscle coat consisting of an inner circular and an outer longitudinal layer and a mucous membrane which is covered with villi. It differs from the rest of the small bowel in having Brunner's glands, a thick layer of glands resembling the pyloric glands of the antral mucosa. These glands lie in the submucosa and their ducts pierce the muscularis mucosae and drain into the base of the crypts. They are most prominent in the first part of the duodenum and diminish in number distal to the papilla of Vater. The alkaline secretion produced may have an important role in protecting the mucosa against gastric acid (Grossman 1958, Isenberg & Flemström 1991).

The mucosa in the first part of the duodenum appears smooth but distally there are crescentic mucosal folds, each of which extends halfway round the wall.

## MOTOR FUNCTION OF THE STOMACH

The stomach is designed to function primarily as a reservoir in which food and liquid are stored, mixed and then expelled by controlled muscle contractions into the duodenum. This complex process is controlled by neurohormonal mechanisms and will be discussed in detail in Chapter 15.

## SECRETORY FUNCTIONS OF THE STOMACH

Gastric juice contains hydrogen ions, pepsin, mucus, bicarbonate, intrinsic factor and water. Parietal cells secrete pure hydrochloric acid at a maximum concentration of 160 mmol/L. When mixed with nonparietal secretions including water, electrolytes and mucus, gastric juice of varying acidity results. Thus the secreted volume of hydrochloric acid is determined by the number of functioning parietal cells, whereas the gastric juice acidity is determined by the relative proportions of parietal and nonparietal secretion.

### Parietal cell secretion

Parietal cell function is modulated by stimulatory and inhibitory substances (Wolfe & Soll 1988). Acid secretion is activated by three, often interacting pathways: the neural, hormonal and paracrine(local) pathways. The major chemical transmitter substances which interact with separate receptors on the parietal cell to activate it are acetylcholine, gastrin and histamine (Fig. 9.24).

At the basolateral parietal cell surface are histamine $H_2$ receptors (Black et al 1972) that bind histamine from local mast cells and ECL cells, gastrin receptors (Baldwin et al 1994) that bind gastrin and muscarinic $M_3$ receptors (Pfeiffer et al 1990) to which acetylcholine binds. A second intracellular messenger is elaborated after binding of each ligand to its receptor.

For histamine, the second messenger is primarily cyclic adenosine monophosphate (cAMP). For gastrin and acetylcholine this messenger is calcium. When histamine binds to the histamine receptor, a stimulatory guanosine triphosphate (GTP) regulatory protein (Gs) activates adenylate cyclase, which generates cAMP. Calcium and cAMP act through protein kinases to activate the proton pump. This pump, or $H^+,K^+$-ATPase, is a membrane-bound enzyme on the apical surface of the parietal cell, which elaborates hydrogen ions in exchange for potassium ions (Sachs 1987). The enzyme $H^+,K^+$-ATPase consists of an α (1030 amino acids) and β subunit (290 amino acids). Omeprazole and other proton pump inhibitors block secretion by blocking the α subunit. The precise function of the β subunit is unknown, but it may protect the enzyme from degradation by pepsin and it is a target antigen in autoimmune gastritis (p. 230).

A number of substances, including prostaglandins and peptides, such as somatostatin, secretin, cholecystokinin, GIP and peptide YY inhibit parietal cell function and suppress acid secretion.

### Gastrin release

Human gastrin exists in many forms based on peptide size. These include G-34, G-17 and G-14. Little gastrin (G-17) is the normal storage form in the G cell of the antrum whereas G-34 predominates in the duodenal G cell. G-34 and G-17 account for about 90% of tissue and circulating gastrin. On a molar basis, G-34 is one-sixth as potent in stimulating acid secretion as G-17 or G-14, but is cleared six times more slowly. Thus G-34, G-17 and G-14 in equimolar doses produce equivalent stimulation of acid secretion. The kidney degrades G-34, G-17 and G-14 whereas smaller fragments and pentagastrin are removed by the liver. Pentagastrin has a similar potency to the C-terminal pentapeptide of gastrin.

Gastrin is released from G cells in the gastric antrum by the presence of food (proteins and amino acids) in the gastric lumen, as well as by the neural release in the antrum of gastrin-releasing peptides (GRP) (Debas 1987). The G cell has microvilli which extend into the lumen of the stomach. The somatostatin D cells are in close proximity to the G cells suggesting that somatostatin acts in a paracrine manner to inhibit gastrin release (Schubert 1991). Hydrogen ions in the gastric lumen may stimulate D cells to further assist in the feedback inhibition of gastrin released by acid. Vagal stimulation with release of acetylcholine also may inhibit the D cell, thus suppressing somatostatin and hence enhancing gastrin release.

Factors which influence the release of gastrin from the G cells are shown in Table 9.2. Gastrin cells also occur in the proximal part of the duodenum and a small number are present in the pancreatic islets. Up to one-third of gastrin release in response to a meal may arise from the duodenum.

### Gastric acid regulation

The overall process of acid secretion is controlled by a complex interaction of a number of pathways discussed below.

#### *Basal acid secretion*

A diurnal pattern of acid secretion occurs in the resting stomach with the rate varying widely among normal indi-

**Table 9.2** Factors regulating the release of gastrin

| | Stimulation | Inhibition |
|---|---|---|
| Luminal | Peptides* and amino acids*<br>Distention* (acting through reflexes) | Acid* |
| Neural | Vagal cholinergic* (initiated from brain or stomach) | |
| Bloodborne | Calcium<br>Adrenaline<br>Bombesin | Secretin, GIP, VIP, glucagon, calcitonin, somatostatin, calcitonin gene-related peptide |

* Factors thought to operate under physiological conditions

viduals. Serum gastrin concentrations correlate poorly with basal acid output (BAO) and vagal tone is probably the important regulatory factor.

*Food-stimulated acid secretion – phases of acid secretion*

The gastric acid secretory response to food occurs in three phases – cephalic, gastric and intestinal (Debas 1987). The cephalic phase of acid secretion occurs in response to sight, taste, smell or thought of food and is mediated centrally by the vagus nerve (Taché 1987). The vagal stimulation may be elicited by sham feeding which directly activates the parietal cell via muscarinic receptors and indirectly stimulates the G cell through GRP with a modest release of gastrin. The vagal stimulation has also been postulated to release histamine from ECL cells as well as inhibiting somatostatin release. Following truncal vagotomy both acid secretion and gastrin release are abolished in response to sham feeding.

The *gastric phase* of acid secretion follows the ingestion of food into the stomach and is mediated by gastric distention and by the specific action of food on gastrin release. Amino acids and other protein digestion products stimulate the G cells to release gastrin. This release accounts for up to 90% of the gastric phase of acid secretion. Distention of the stomach activates mechanoreceptors which stimulate acid secretion via long vagal and short intragastric cholinergic neural reflexes. Gastric distention also releases gastrin. Inhibition of gastrin release occurs with low intragastric pH levels via the local release of somatostatin.

The *intestinal phase* of acid secretion occurs when digested protein enters the small intestine. This is due to the release of gastrin and other stimulatory peptides and to the direct effect on the parietal cell of absorbed amino acids. The intestinal phase accounts, under normal circumstances, for about 5% of acid secretory response to a meal.

Postprandial acid secretion is regulated by a negative feedback mechanism in which antral acidification inhibits the further release of gastrin. As the stomach secretes acid in response to a meal, intragastric pH falls gradually and gastrin release declines. At an intragastric pH of 1.5 gastrin release is completely inhibited. It has been suggested that this inhibition is mediated by intramural cholinergic and noncholinergic neurons (Saffouri et al 1984). In addition protons may directly stimulate somatostatin release which then acts directly on parietal cells to decrease acid secretion (Park et al 1987). Regulatory peptides originating from the small intestine have been shown to inhibit the antral gastrin release with reduction in gastric acid secretion. These agents include gastric inhibitory peptide, secretin, enteroglucagon and peptide YY. The physiological role of other agents which have been shown to inhibit acid secretion, including epidermal growth factor, calcitonin gene-related peptide and vasopressin, is less clear than that of the hormones mentioned above.

## Nonparietal cell secretion

*Pepsinogen secretion* (Konturek 1979, Feldman 1989)

Pepsinogens are present in the mucous cells of cardiac glands, in the chief and mucous neck cells of oxyntic glands, in the mucous cells of pyloric glands and duodenal Brunner's glands. These inactive proenzyme proteases are secreted and activated by acids to the active form pepsin. Although pepsins are important early in life for digestion of milk, their major substrates in later life are meat and other proteins. Only a small amount of digestion occurs in the stomach; however, release of peptides and amino acids by pepsin aids in the release of other hormones, including gastrin and CCK which are important in digestion. There are both cephalic and gastric phases of pepsinogen secretion with the major stimulus being cholinergic.

Two important types of pepsinogen, I and II, are identified by gel electrophoresis and radioimmunoassay (Samloff & Townes 1970). Serum pepsinogen I levels correlate with the acid and pepsin secretory capacity of the stomach. Serum concentrations of pepsinogen I are elevated in subjects with *Helicobacter pylori* gastritis and in patients with duodenal ulcer (Samloff et al 1986, Wagner et al 1991). A decrease occurs when gastric atrophy results in a diminished number of chief cells. Similarly anticholinergic drugs, histamine $H_2$ receptor antagonists and vagotomy decrease pepsinogen secretion. Pepsinogen II is secreted from the entire stomach whereas pepsinogen I is secreted only by chief cells and hence the relative differences in serum concentrations of pepsinogen II to pepsinogen I differ depending on the degree and type of gastritis.

*Intrinsic factor secretion* (Donaldson 1987)

Intrinsic factor is a glycoprotein secreted by parietal cells with a molecular weight of 50 kDa. It contains 351 amino acids and consists of 15% carbohydrate. It is secreted under the same conditions as hydrochloric acid. Its primary role is to facilitate cobalamin (vitamin $B_{12}$) absorption (see p. 363).

Stimulants of acid secretion also stimulate intrinsic factor secretion. $H_2$ receptor antagonists, somatostatin, prostaglandins and epidermal growth factor all inhibit intrinsic factor secretion. Patients with low or absent gastric acid secretion also have reduced intrinsic factor secretion. Rarely intrinsic factor secretion may be absent with normal acid secretion (p. 365). Circulating antibodies to intrinsic factor and parietal cells are found in patients with atrophic gastritis, achlorhydria and pernicious anemia.

*Bicarbonate secretion* (Isenberg & Flemström 1991)

The surface epithelial cells of the stomach and duodenum secrete sodium bicarbonate (Knutson & Flemström 1989). This is an active process dependent on the metabolic integrity of a healthy epithelium. It is stimulated by luminal acid thus protecting the gastroduodenal mucosa from autodigestion by high concentrations of hydrochloric acid. Secretion is also stimulated by acetylcholine, exogenous prostaglandins, glucagon and cyclic GMP and is inhibited by α-adrenergic agonists, GIP, luminal bile acids and prostaglandin inhibitors such as NSAIDs.

Gastrin, secretin, omeprazole and $H_2$ receptor antagonists have no effect on gastric bicarbonate secretion. Sucralfate, colloidal bismuth subcitrate and synthetic prostaglandins enhance bicarbonate secretion (Shorrock et al 1990).

## Gastric mucosal barrier

The gastroduodenal mucosa is able to resist autodigestion by high intraluminal concentrations of hydrochloric acid and pepsin. The protective factors include the integrity of surface epithelial cells, mucus, bicarbonate and mucosal blood flow. Prostaglandins play an important role in mucosal defense.

Hydrophobic phospholipids are incorporated in cell membranes of surface epithelial cells and help to resist digestion (Spychal et al 1989, Hills & Kirkwood 1992).

Gastric mucus consists of about 70% water, glycoproteins, phospholipids, lipids, electrolytes and sloughed cells (Allen 1989). Mucins are the major constituent of mucus and consist of glycoproteins which polymerize and are responsible for its physicochemical properties. The carbohydrate sidechains of the glycoproteins have similar structure to the blood group ABO antigen determinants. The phospholipids in mucus are mainly phosphatidylcholine and phosphatidylethanolamine and may contribute to its protective nature by acting as surfactants. Mucus provides lubrication for food particles and its gel-like nature retains water and bicarbonate close to the surface epithelium. Mucus is secreted by exocytosis, apical expulsion and exfoliation and is formed together with bicarbonate in surface epithelial cells, the mucous neck cells of the body of the stomach, cells in the pyloric glands and by the Brunner's glands of the duodenum.

The mucous layer varies in thickness but averages about 100 μm. Mucus provides a relatively thick hydrophobic, unstirred layer adjacent to the mucosa, which reduces diffusion of $H^+$ ions to four times slower than that through a similar thickness of unstirred water. It also retards the passage of glucose and low molecular weight solutes from the lumen to the cell surface. A hydrogen ion gradient is thus maintained between the gastric lumen and the surface epithelium. When the luminal pH is 2, the pH at the gastric membrane is 6.8–7.

Mucus synthesis and release are inhibited by aspirin and NSAIDs as well as by stress. Cholinergic stimulation and prostaglandins (particularly E type) increase the synthesis of mucus (Allen 1989). Secretion of surface active phospholipids is regulated by both cholinergic and adrenergic mediators, as well as by prostaglandins (Scheiman et al 1991).

Natural prostaglandins, particularly of the E type, probably play an important role in human mucosal defense as evidenced by studies of animal models (Robert 1979). Prevention of the injurious effects of 100% ethanol and boiling water can be prevented by pretreatment of animals with prostaglandins, hence the term "cytoprotection". Rabbits immunized actively or passively against prostaglandins frequently develop gastroduodenal ulcers, thus supporting the role of endogenous prostaglandins in mucosal protection (Redfern & Feldman 1989). In humans the evidence for this role for prostaglandins is indirect. NSAIDs, which block the synthesis of prostaglandin by inhibiting cyclo-oxygenase, predispose to mucosal injury and peptic ulceration (Hawkey 1990). The role of aspirin and NSAIDs in causing damage to the human mucosa will be discussed further on pp. 226, 232 and 485. The actions of prostaglandins which lead to gastroduodenal protection include the maintenance or increase in gastric mucosal blood flow (Konturek 1985), increased secretion of mucus (Jentjens et al 1984), stimulation of bicarbonate secretion (Selling et al 1987) and increased protein synthesis. Prostaglandins also may suppress gastric acid secretion (Chen et al 1988). Prostaglandin E2 prolongs epithelial cell survival time and therefore has a trophic effect (Uribe et al 1986).

The gastric mucosa is perfused by capillary loops arising from arterioles in the submucosa. If mucosal blood flow is compromised, bicarbonate secretion diminishes, juxtamucosal pH falls and ulceration more readily occurs (Frydman et al 1991).

Gastroduodenal mucosal blood flow and the microcirculation are suggested as targets for both ulcerogenic and mucosal protective agents. In response to the application of an irritant to the gastroduodenal mucosa, blood flow increases via mechanisms that are dependent on sensory afferent neurons (capsaicin-sensitive) and the release of mediators such as calcitonin gene-related peptide (CGRP), prostaglandins and nitric oxide (Li et al 1992, Holzer & Lippe 1992). Gastrin and central vagal stimulation increase mucosal blood flow in part via the release of nitric oxide (Pique et al 1992).

Nitric oxide, also known as endothelium-derived relaxing factor, is synthesized in endothelial cells from the precursor amino acid, L-arginine (Palmer et al 1987). Endogenous nitric oxide has been implicated in the regulation of gastric mucosal microcirculation under resting conditions, in response to mucosal irritants and in pentagastrin stimulation of acid secretion (Pique et al 1992).

Inhibition of nitric oxide synthesis results in delayed healing and reduced blood flow of ulcers induced by acetic acid in the rat (Konturek et al 1993).

## ASSESSMENT OF GASTRIC FUNCTION

**Measurement of gastric acid secretion** (Baron 1970)

The stomach secretes a variety of substances but in clinical practice its function is assessed by measuring output of acid and, in certain circumstances, intrinsic factor. The other constituents of gastric juice, including pepsin, bicarbonate and mucus, currently do not provide significant diagnostic information.

*Indications*

Gastric acid output can be measured under basal conditions or in response to stimulation, usually by pentagastrin, or in response to protein stimulus. Clinical indications for gastric analysis are relatively limited. There is little indication for these tests in the diagnosis of gastric or duodenal ulcer, but they remain important in patients suspected of having Zollinger–Ellison syndrome. The adequacy of ulcer surgery in reducing acid secretion can be determined by gastric analysis, especially if postoperative values can be compared with preoperative ones. This is particularly helpful in patients with recurrent ulceration or in patients who have recently had proximal gastric vagotomy and for whom a decision must be made regarding cessation of antisecretory therapy (Baron et al 1975). Gastric analysis also may be important in documenting hypo- or achlorhydria as a cause of hypergastrinemia, particularly in relation to pernicious anemia.

*Technique*

Gastric acid secretion is measured by intubation of the stomach in fasted subjects, followed by sequential aspiration of gastric juice collected in 15 min aliquots from the most dependent part of the stomach. Gastric acidity of each specimen is determined by a pH electrode or by titration to pH 7.0. Acid secretion in mmol per 15 min can then be calculated by multiplying the acidity in mmol/L × the volume in liters per 15 min. All systemic medications to reduce acid secretion should be stopped at least 36 h before gastric analysis and no food or antacid should be ingested for 10 h before the procedure. Proton pump inhibitors should be ceased for 1 week prior to the study. Results are expressed as the amount of acid (mmol or mEq) secreted in the period studied.

Basal acid output (BAO) is the amount of acid secreted in the hour before stimulation. The upper limits of normal for men and women with no *Helicobacter pylori* infection are 15 and 10 mmol per hour respectively. Pentagastrin is the stimulant of choice to determine the ability of the stomach to secrete gastric acid maximally. This is a synthetic pentapeptide and it is given subcutaneously or intramuscularly in a dose of 6 μg/kg. Side-effects are rare unless a higher dose is given and these include nausea, sweating, faintness, weakness of the legs and transient hypotension. Results are expressed in mmol or mEq/h as the maximum acid output (MAO) which is the amount of acid secreted in the first hour following administration of the pentagastrin (sum of the first four 15-min collections). The term "maximum" may be misleading as still greater acid output may be produced in some patients by giving a higher dose of pentagastrin than is usually used. Acid output may also be expressed as peak acid output (PAO) which is the acid output in mmol or mEq/h in the two consecutive highest 15-min outputs after a single injection of the stimulant. The PAO is therefore always greater than the MAO in the same patient as it is calculated as the sum of the two highest consecutive 15-min outputs multiplied by two. The plateau acid output refers to the output during an intravenous infusion of a stimulant. In practice this plateau output is the same as the PAO. The upper limit of PAO for normal men and women is 60 mmol/h and 40 mmol/h respectively.

An alternative method to measure acid secretion uses a homogenized meal at known pH and an in vivo intragastric titration technique (Baron 1978). A continuous 24-h recording of intragastric pH can detect changes in $H^+$ concentration with time (Merki et al 1988). This latter technique does not determine acid output, as secretory volumes are not measured.

Other stimulants including histamine, betazole hydrochloride (Histalog) and insulin-induced hypoglycemia have been used in the past to assess the secretion of acid and pepsin. Histamine causes headache, flushing and changes in pulse rate and blood pressure, as well as pain at the site of injection and thus should not be used unless pentagastrin is unavailable. Betazole is similar to histamine with regards to effects on the gastric mucosa but produces fewer side-effects. Insulin-induced hypoglycemia has been previously advocated to assess the completeness of vagotomy. This is based on the fact that hypoglycemia stimulates vagal centers in the brain, resulting in a vagally mediated increase in the secretion of acid and pepsin. Hypoglycemia induced by the standard insulin test may be severe and cardiac arrhythmias have been reported in up to 50% of patients.

*Sham feeding test* (Mayer et al 1974)

Modified sham feeding has thus replaced the potentially dangerous insulin-induced hypoglycemia as a means of assessing the presence of intact vagus nerve. Subjects during this test will see, smell, taste and chew (but not swallow) an appetizing meal. Gastric acid is collected for

30 min during and 30 min after sham feeding. The total amount of acid collected during this hour is less than 10% of the PAO if an adequate vagotomy has been accomplished. Alternatively, the pancreatic polypeptide response may be measured.

*Normal values*

There is a wide normal range of BAO, PAO and MAO. PAO can be correlated with body weight and calculated lean body mass. The belief that PAO decreases with age has been recently challenged. Elderly persons with no *Helicobacter pylori* infection or atrophic gastritis have acid secretion which is normal or even higher than normal (Goldschmiedt et al 1991).

### Secretin test

The secretin test is used to confirm a diagnosis of gastrinoma (Zollinger–Ellison syndrome) in patients with gastric acid hypersecretion and serum gastrin concentrations above normal, but below 1000 pg/ml (Berg & Wolfe 1991). Patients with acid hypersecretion and gastrin concentrations over 1000 pg/ml do not need further tests to diagnose gastrinoma. Two basal blood samples are initially taken followed by an intravenous bolus of two clinical units per kilogram of body weight of pure porcine secretin. Subsequent blood samples are taken at 2, 5, 10, 15 and 20 min after injection and serum samples assayed for gastrin using radioimmunoassay. A rise in serum gastrin concentrations at least 200 pg/ml above the basal value is considered a positive test.

### Gastric emptying studies

These are discussed in Chapters 3 and 15.

### *Helicobacter pylori* detection (Brown & Peura 1993)

*Helicobacter pylori* (*H. pylori*) is an important factor in the pathogenesis of peptic ulcer disease and gastric malignancy (p. 295). *H. pylori* is detected either by noninvasive tests using a $C^{14}$ or $C^{13}$ urea breath test or detection of serum antibodies to *H. pylori*. Tests requiring endoscopy incorporate assessment of antral biopsy specimens by culture, histology or detection of the presence of urease (rapid urease tests).

### Urease activity

Urease is an enzyme produced in abundance by *H. pylori*. Gastric mucosal biopsies can thus be inoculated on to a urea-containing medium and if urease is present in the mucosal biopsy it splits the urea into ammonia and carbon dioxide. The ammonia results in an elevation of the pH of the medium, with a color change of a pH-sensitive indicator. This test requires several hours to become positive and is neither as sensitive nor as specific as tests that directly assess the presence of *H. pylori*, such as culture (Borromeo et al 1987).

The urea breath test is a noninvasive method of detecting the presence of urease within the stomach (Graham et al 1987, Lin et al 1992) (p. 85). This test is convenient and provides a noninvasive screening test for *H. pylori* in a large number of patients. In addition, it is very useful to monitor patients after eradication therapy.

Tests for gastric urease may be falsely negative if the number of organisms present is small, particularly after recent antimicrobial therapy, or falsely positive in the presence of bacterial overgrowth with other urease-producing organisms.

*Histology*

*H. pylori* causes chronic active inflammation within the gastric mucosa. Organisms can be seen often on routine hematoxylin and eosin stains as well as with special stains including modified Giemsa, Warthin Starry silver stain and acridine orange (Kolts et al 1993).

*Culture* (Hazell 1993)

Culture is considered the gold standard to detect *H. pylori* from gastric mucosal biopsies. The sensitivity of this test is diminished if the number of organisms is small, culture techniques are inadequate or if the patient has recently taken antimicrobial therapy. Cultures should be grown on selective and nonselective media at 35°C in a moist environment with carbon dioxide and hydrogen enrichment. Culture should be maintained for at least 7 days. Culture of the organisms is particularly useful to determine pathogenic strains of *Helicobacter*, including cytotoxin production. In addition, antimicrobial sensitivity testing can be undertaken if the organism is cultured.

*Serum antibodies to* Helicobacter pylori (Schembri et al 1993)

The presence of *H. pylori* can be determined by detecting specific IgG or IgA antibodies in the serum. This test is sensitive for the detection of *H. pylori* infection, but specificity is decreased compared with other tests. Antibody titers may persist for many months after eradication of the organism from the stomach and thus they are not clinically useful for monitoring subjects who have had therapy to eradicate the organism (Hirschl et al 1993).

## GASTRITIS AND DUODENITIS

A number of nonmalignant diseases are limited primarily

to the gastroduodenal mucosa and considerable confusion occurs in relation to nomenclature. In this discussion gastritis will be defined histologically as a diffuse mucosal infiltration of inflammatory cells into mucosa. The Sydney System of classification of gastritis, introduced in 1990 at the World Congress of Gastroenterology in Sydney, Australia, classifies gastritis as acute, chronic and "special forms" (Misiewicz 1991, Fig. 9.4). The system finds common ground between previous classifications. Figure 9.4 is self-explanatory. The etiology and special forms of gastritis are shown in Table 9.3. In Figure 9.4 the nongraded variables are:

**Table 9.3** Etiology or pathogenic associations (special forms) of gastritis (Price 1991)

| |
|---|
| *Helicobacter pylori* |
| Autoimmune associated |
| Idiopathic |
| Drug-associated or other known gastric irritants |
| Infective (excluding *H. Pylori*) |
| Bacterial |
| Viral |
| Parasitic |
| Fungal |
| Special forms |
| Eosinophilic gastritis |
| Lymphocytic gastritis |
| Granulomatous gastritis |
| Crohn's |
| Sarcoid |
| Idiopathic |
| Reactive gastritis |
| Radiation-associated |
| Phlegmonous gastritis |
| Postgastrectomy |

1. nonspecific such as epithelial degeneration, regeneration, mucus depletion, foveolar hyperplasia, edema, erosions, fibrosis, hemorrhage, lymphoid follicles, etc. – they are nonspecific accompaniments to acute, chronic or special forms of gastritis;
2. specific, which are features of the special form of gastritis, e.g. eosinophilic infiltration in eosinophilic gastritis. The latter will be discussed in other sections.

## Acute gastritis

### *Pathology*

In acute gastritis, mucosal changes are generally those of acute inflammation resulting from some form of chemical or other injury. The mucosa is edematous, congested and hemorrhagic with abundant overlying mucus. Dramatic visual damage to the gastroduodenal epithelium generally exists: petechiae, erosions and acute ulcers are commonly present and may all contribute to bleeding. This condition is therefore often called *acute hemorrhagic gastritis*. On

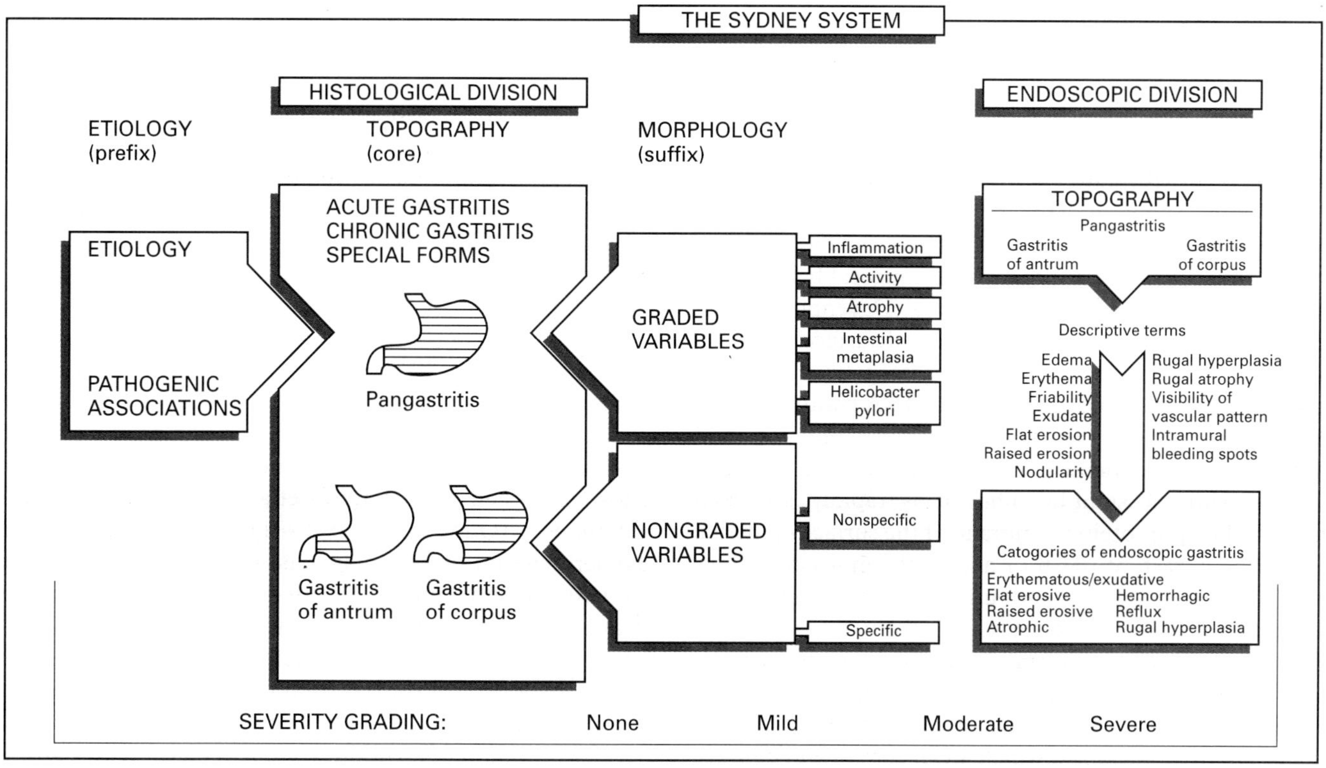


**Fig. 9.4** Main compartments of the histological division of the Sydney System (Misiewicz 1991).

microscopy, there is edema and congestion with variable acute inflammation and reactive changes in the surface epithelial cells. When erosions are present there is necrosis of the epithelium and superficial mucosa. Fibrous exudate and inflammatory slough cover the ulcers so that they appear white at endoscopy. Acute gastritis heals in a few days. A diffuse inflammatory process with abnormal collections of lymphocytes or polymorphonuclear neutrophilic leukocytes is rarely seen. The injury is more correctly considered to be an epithelial burn. Thus it is not truly an acute gastritis as it is not diffuse in nature.

*Etiology*

The etiology of this form of acute inflammation relates to injury induced by aspirin, nonsteroidal anti-inflammatory drugs (NSAIDs), ethanol-induced injury and stress-related mucosal injury. In addition, caustic agents may induce injury and this form of injury is seen after gastrectomy.

*Aspirin and NSAIDs drug injury* (Graham & Smith 1986, Hawkey 1990) (see also pp. 222 and 485)

Two types of mucosal injury may occur after oral aspirin and NSAIDs. The first type relates to ingestion of the agent with the rapid appearance of lesions as a result of suppression of endogenous prostaglandins and the local direct damaging effect on the mucosa. These lesions include hyperemia, erosions and subepithelial hemorrhages (Langman 1970, O'Laughlin et al 1981, Hawkey et al 1991). These acute lesions are probably only of minor consequence. Acute superficial ulceration may, however, develop within a week (Sun et al 1974). There is no relation to symptoms and it rarely produces important bleeding. Resolution frequently occurs with time and a poor correlation exists between the frequency or severity of these acute lesions and the subsequent development of more chronic lesions (Shallcross & Heatley 1990).

Aspirin locally damages the gastric mucosal barrier with back diffusion of acid into the mucosa (Davenport 1964). It causes an increase in the exfoliation of surface epithelial cells from the mucosa, as demonstrated by cytological studies and by measurements on the DNA content of gastric aspirate (Croft 1963). When acetylsalicylic acid (aspirin) is in solution at a pH of less than 3.5, it is undissociated and fat soluble. Thus it is rapidly absorbed through the lipoprotein membrane of the surface epithelial cells. By contrast, at pH 6 or above, the molecule is ionized and water soluble and under these circumstances absorption is slower. In its fat-soluble form, the drug damages the lipoprotein membrane and the intercellular junctions during its absorption. These actions lead to the exfoliation of cells and an increased permeability of the mucosa to hydrogen ions, which are absorbed and damage the deeper layers of the mucosa (Davenport 1967). Dog gastric pouches have been used to demonstrate that aspirin damages the mucosal barrier and that this effect is potentiated by alcohol (Davenport 1967). After injury the surface epithelium is restored by the process of "restitution" within hours (p. 218). Once acid diffuses into the mucosa, mast cells may degranulate with consequent histamine release and this, together with other vasoactive substances, results in microvascular dilatation, edema, hemorrhage and inflammation. NSAIDs damage is induced by local direct damage, inhibition of prostaglandin synthesis and altered mucosal blood flow with increased neutrophil adherence and infiltration into the mucosa (Asako et al 1992). The damaging effects of oxygen radicals and nitric oxide are enhanced by NSAIDs (Vaananen et al 1991).

The second and more important type of lesion is chronic ulceration which will be discussed on p. 232.

*Ethanol-induced injury* (Tarnawski et al 1987)

Ethanol ingestion produces lesions similar to acute NSAID-induced lesions and includes erythema, erosions and epithelial hemorrhages. A poor correlation with symptoms exists and serious bleeding is rare. The importance of such lesions is therefore greatly overemphasized. There is no significant histological inflammation in these subjects and thus the term "alcoholic gastritis" should be abandoned.

*Stress-related mucosal injury, "stress ulcer"* (Durham & Shapiro 1991)

Acute ulcers and erosions of the stomach and duodenum (p. 237) occur in patients with multiple trauma, sepsis, burns (Curling's ulcer), prolonged mechanical ventilation, coagulopathy, multiple organ failure and injury to the central nervous system (Cushing's ulcer) (Lucas et al 1972, Czaja et al 1974). The pathogenesis of these lesions is multifactorial and involves elements of mucosal ischemia in the presence of gastric acid (Kitajima et al 1988). Platelet-activating factor, a vasoconstrictor proinflammatory substance, may have an important role in the mucosal ischemia (Wallace & Whittle 1986). These patients are not usually hypersecretors, but it appears that acid is an essential permissive factor as reduction of gastric acidity in most controlled trials (Lacroix et al 1989) and experimental models (Odonkor et al 1981) prevents the lesions. Hypersecretion of acid may exist in subjects with central nervous system injuries, severe burns or sepsis and this may result in frank peptic ulcers with the appropriate complications of bleeding or perforation (p. 286).

Prophylactic therapy has been primarily used to prevent these lesions with careful attention to support of the subject by ventilation, nutrition, volume replacement, prevention of shock and control of intragastric pH (Shuman et al

1987, Lacroix et al 1989). Antacids and $H_2$ receptor antagonists have been used to control intragastric pH, but major nosocomial pneumonia occurs, presumably caused by aspiration of bacteria from within the hypochlorhydric stomach (Driks et al 1987, Tryba 1987). Several studies have shown that administration of sucralfate in a dose of 1 g every 4–6 h is as effective as either antacid or $H_2$ receptor antagonist prophylaxis and may be associated with a lower incidence of nosocomial pneumonia (Driks et al 1987, Laggner et al 1989). Misoprostol can also be used to prevent stress-related mucosal injury.

*Postgastrectomy injury*

Patients who have had gastric resection, especially associated with surgery to the pylorus, and bile reflux develop histologic and often endoscopic (p. 271) abnormalities of the gastric remnant. Intense hyperemia is often identified on close inspection. Histologically only a minimal inflammatory response exists with more intense epithelial cell and foveolar injury. The pathogenesis of such lesions involves reflux of bile and pancreatic juice. This lesion does not involve *Helicobacter pylori* as the inflammation caused by this bacterium tends to regress after resectional surgery and will recur if biliary diversion is done. *H. pylori* will not grow in bile and the high luminal concentration of bile after resectional surgery may be the mechanism for these observations. (see Alkaline reflux gastritis, biliary gastritis, p. 271)

## Chronic gastritis

Chronic gastritis may be caused by a number of pathogenic or etiologic factors which include *H. pylori* infection, autoimmune disease, lymphocytic gastritis, eosinophilic gastritis and gastritis associated with other systemic diseases. The latter include Crohn's disease, sarcoidosis, syphilis and idiopathic granulomatous gastritis where the etiology is unknown. These latter special forms of gastritis will be discussed in Chapter 12.

### ***Helicobacter pylori*** (Lambert et al 1995)

*Helicobacter pylori* (*H. pylori*) is a microaerophilic Gram-negative spiral bacterium identified only in gastric-type epithelium (Marshall 1983, Warren 1983). Detection and diagnosis is detailed on p. 224. It is found primarily in the stomach and in areas of gastric metaplasia such as in Barrett's oesophagus and in the duodenal bulb. Related organisms have been found in primates and other animals, particularly ferrets and cats. This bacterium is present in a high percentage of the population, increasing in frequency from less than 10% in the young to over 60% in persons of 60 years of age. A high rate of infection occurs among subjects in developing countries, in institutions, among certain population groups and in subjects with peptic ulcer disease and gastric cancer.

*Pathology*

Infection with *H. pylori* causes histologic chronic gastritis involving the antrum and body, with the greatest severity usually within the antrum. The inflammatory cell infiltrate is mixed. However, the hallmark of the inflammatory process is the neutrophil and this is termed "active gastritis" (Fig. 9.5). *H. pylori* causes inflammation as evidenced by human ingestion studies (Marshall et al 1985), animal models, the rapid dissolution of inflammation with bacterial eradication and the systemic antibody responses. The chronic gastritis of *H. pylori* initially starts as an accumulation of chronic inflammatory cells in the lamina propria of the gastric mucosa. Granulocytes often accompany the chronic gastritis and invade the lamina propria and the surface epithelium focally or diffusely (active chronic gastritis). This inflammatory stage of chronic gastritis is commonly referred to as "superficial gastritis" in the former literature (Fig. 9.6). In a number of subjects, gastritis may further progress to atrophy and is termed "*atrophic gastritis*" (Fig. 9.7). This stage of the process is characterized by an increasing loss of normal glands and by a growth of new metaplastic glands with intestinal (Fig. 9.8) or pseudopyloric metaplasias (Fig. 9.7) in the underlying mucosa. Chronic gastritis is generally a stable persistent inflammatory response occurring for life. In some rare instances the chronic gastritis may slow down and even heal, particularly in the antral mucosa. More often it remains stable or progresses to gastritis with atrophy. In the Finnish population the mean annual risk of developing atrophy from chronic gastritis is between 3 and 4% per year (Siurala et al 1985).

*Intestinal metaplasia* (Segura & Montero 1983) has been classified on morphological, immunological and histochemical grounds. Complete intestinal metaplasia consists of mature absorptive small intestinal cells. In incomplete metaplasia the columnar cells secrete mucus

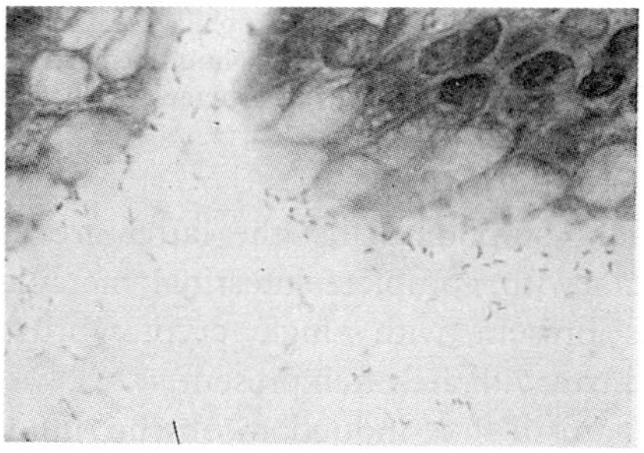

**Fig. 9.5** *H. pylori* infecting gastric epithelium with organisms in gastric gands (Giemsa stain × 100) and activity is shown by the presence of neutrophils and polymorphs within one gastric pit.

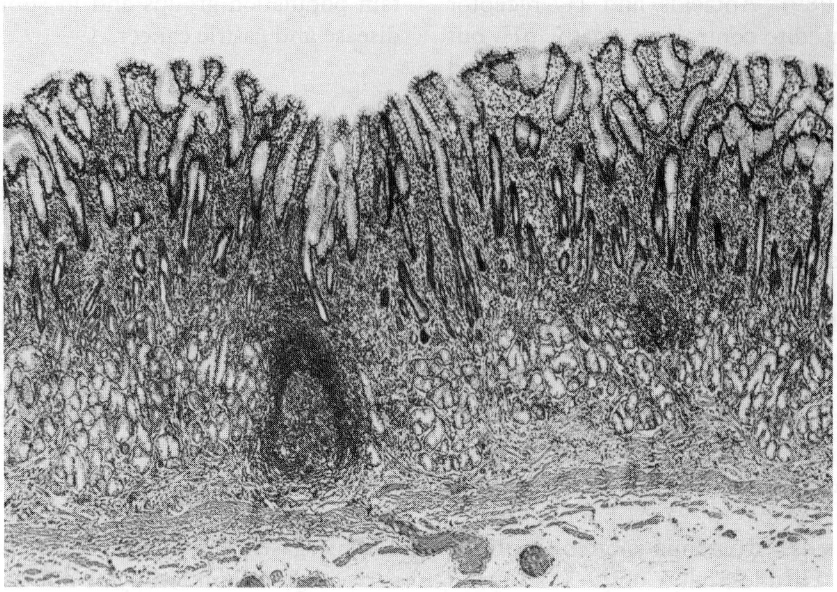

**Fig. 9.6** Chronic active gastritis (pyloric antrum) caused by *H. pylori* with acute and chronic inflammatory cells in the superficial half of the mucosa. A single lymphoid aggregate with germinal center is seen deep in the mucosa (hematoxylin and cosin, × 40).

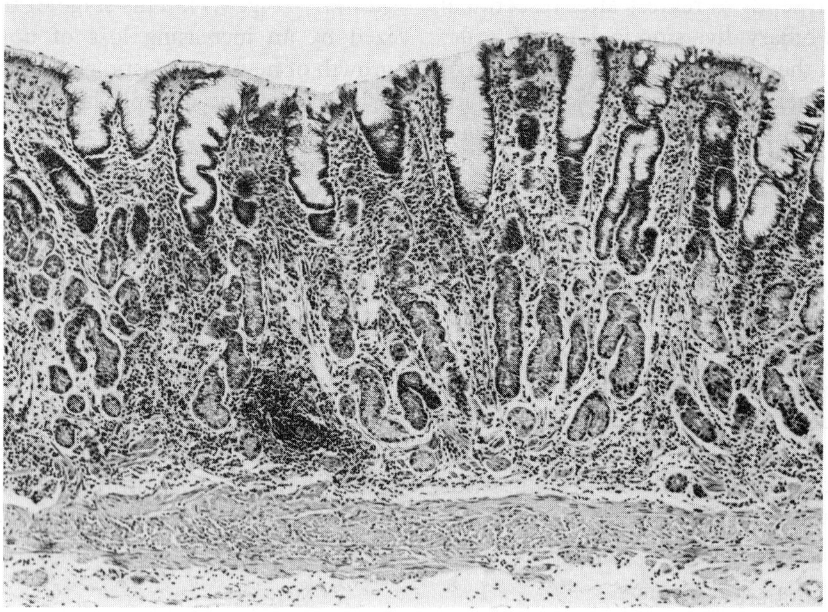

**Fig. 9.7** Atrophic gastritis (body mucosa) with a diffuse chronic inflammatory cell infiltrate throughout the lamina propria with reduction in the number of glands and pseudopyloric metaplasia. Features of activity are absent (hematoxylin and eosin, × 75).

with neutral or sulphomucins; the latter are colonic in type. Subjects with complete intestinal metaplasia have Paneth cells present with single crypts, brush border enzymes and true villi are often present.

The mechanism for induction of the inflammatory response is unknown with a number of potential virulence factors postulated as with other enteric organisms. These factors include bacterial adhesins, cytotoxins, cytotoxin-associated gene protein, enzymes including phospholipases, urease and inflammatory cell products including cytokines (Dunn 1993). These factors permit the organism to avoid destruction by gastric acid, to colonize the gastric epithelium and to damage gastric epithelial cells.

Alteration in the structure and function of gastric mucus, epithelial cell damage, increased mucosal blood flow, decreased secretion of bicarbonate, enhanced serum

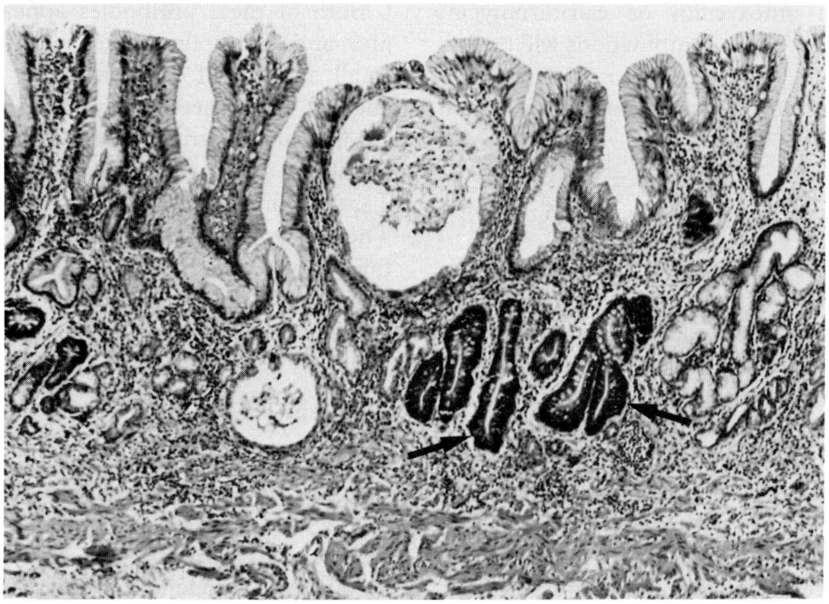

**Fig. 9.8** Severe atrophic gastritis and intestinal metaplasia. A diffuse chronic inflammatory infiltrate is present in the mucosa which shows markedly reduced numbers of glands, some of which are dilated. Prominent foci of intestinal metaplasia (arrows) are present (hematoxylin and eosin, × 70).

gastrin release and probable increased gastric acid secretion occur as a consequence of the inflammation in the distal stomach (McColl et al 1989, Sievert et al 1994). The enhanced gastrin release in response to a protein meal or to gastrin-releasing peptide occurs due to the inflammatory process, most likely as a consequence of the effect of inflammatory products on the antral gastrin and somatostatin cells (Haruma et al 1992). When the organism is eradicated with antimicrobial therapy, there is a diminution in basal and stimulated acid output because the serum gastrin concentration returns to normal (Sievert et al 1994).

*Epidemiology and transmission*

The organism is transmitted from person to person but food, water or animal vectors have not been identified as the source. High levels of infection occur in lower socioeconomic groups and long-residence institutions, as well as within members of the family of an infected individual. The organism may be identified in saliva, gastric and duodenal mucosa, gastric juice, dental plaque and feces, supporting a role for both oral–oral and fecal–oral transmission (Thomas et al 1992, Olsson et al 1993).

*Clinical features*

*H. pylori* gastritis is strongly associated with duodenal and gastric ulcer disease with prevalences of 95% and 75% respectively (Tytgat et al 1993a). The role of *H. pylori* in nonulcer (functional) dyspepsia remains unclear (Lambert 1993). The effect of *H. pylori* eradication in the reduction of ulcer recurrence rate would strongly support a role for this bacteria in the pathogenesis of peptic ulcer disease, and is discussed on p. 231. A poor correlation exists between symptoms, endoscopic findings and *H. pylori* infection (Lambert 1993).

Gastritis caused by *H. pylori* appears to precede the formation of peptic ulcer, suggesting that gastritis is a significant risk factor of ulcer disease (Sipponen et al 1989). Case control studies have suggested that the risk of peptic ulcer is approximately ten times higher in subjects with gastritis compared to those with a normal stomach. The risk of duodenal ulcer is high in males with antral gastritis without coexistent atrophy of the corpus mucosa. This contrasts with the gastric ulcer risk which is high in the presence of gastritis with atrophic antral changes.

Chronic gastritis appears to be a precancerous condition. The prevalence of gastritis with advanced atrophic alterations, with metaplasias and with dysplastic epithelial changes is more common in subjects with gastric carcinoma (p. 295).

The endoscopic appearances of *H. pylori* gastritis are described on p. 107. The diagnosis, made from tests and histology on antral biopsies, is discussed on p. 224.

*Treatment*

*H. pylori* eradication is difficult and requires combination antimicrobial therapy. These therapies include combinations of a bismuth compound, metronidazole and tetracycline or amoxycillin. Other regimens have included proton pump inhibitors, with amoxycillin or clarithromycin, along with metronidazole. These combinations will be further discussed on p. 255. When *H. pylori* is discovered coincidentally, there are no clear guidelines as to which patients should be treated.

### Gastritis associated with gastric antibodies

Two types of atrophic gastritis have been identified previously – type A and type B (Strickland & Mackay 1973). Glass & Pitchumoni (1975) have described a third category – type AB gastritis which is characterized by patchy inflammation and metaplasia of both the antrum and corpus. It is now clear that type B gastritis is caused by *H. pylori* infection in most subjects. Type B gastritis occurs in association with peptic ulcer disease and in the majority of cases of gastric cancer. Type A gastritis is associated with pernicious anemia and tends to involve mainly the body of the stomach with severe atrophy of the corpus mucosa, resulting in achlorhydria and pernicious anemia. Gastrin concentrations are often very high and this may rarely lead to the formation of carcinoid tumors. The pathogenesis of type A gastritis appears to be autoimmune as there are antibodies directed against parietal cells and intrinsic factor. Furthermore, associations exist with other autoimmune diseases such as Addison's disease and Hashimoto's thyroiditis.

#### *Parietal cell antibody*

Parietal cell antibody is detectable by a complement fixation or immunofluorescent techniques and is present in 80–90% of sera from subjects with pernicious anemia and 20–30% of their relatives. It is present in about 2% of the general population over the age of 20 years and in 16% over 60 years of age. Two distinct forms of antigen have been detected (De Aizpurua et al 1983). The first is against the parietal cell surface and the second against microsomes within the parietal cell. The microsomal antibody is inhibitory to the $H^+$, $K^+$-ATPase activity of gastric mucosal tubulovesicular membranes (Burman et al 1989). Thus a number of gastric autoantibodies exist in relation to the parietal cell.

#### *Intrinsic factor antibody* (IFA)

Two types of intrinsic factor antibodies have been described by radioimmunoassay. A blocking (type 1) antibody prevents binding of vitamin $B_{12}$ to intrinsic factor. It occurs in 65–75% of patients with pernicious anemia and occasionally in patients with diabetes mellitus, Addison's disease or thyroid disease. A binding antibody (type 2) has also been identified which binds to intrinsic factor itself or to the intrinsic factor–vitamin $B_{12}$ complex and is present in 30% of patients with pernicious anemia (Strickland 1991).

Both of these antibodies appear in saliva and gastric juice and are responsible for reducing the effectiveness of a small amount of intrinsic factor secreted in pernicious anemia. The mechanism involved in the initiation of autoimmune gastritis remains uncertain, but a genetic susceptibility together with a disturbance of organ-specific T-cell immunoregulation appear to be important factors. There is no evidence that *H. pylori* infection plays a role in this form of chronic gastritis. Autoimmune gastritis results in vitamin $B_{12}$ deficiency, iron deficiency and an increased incidence of gastric neoplasia.

### Duodenitis (Joffe et al 1978)

Inflammatory changes in the duodenal mucosa usually exist in duodenal ulcer disease but may occur less commonly in other conditions such as celiac disease, Crohn's disease and giardiasis. Patchy duodenitis is part of the spectrum of duodenal ulcer disease with areas of gastric-type surface epithelium (gastric metaplasia) infiltrated by polymorphonuclear leukocytes (Noach et al 1993). The morphological changes in duodenal ulcer disease are discussed further on p. 236.

## PEPTIC ULCER

Peptic ulcer is the most important organic gastrointestinal disease and in many Western communities affects approximately 10% of all adult males. In the United States economic studies have suggested the cost of digestive diseases to be $8 \times 10^9$ dollars per annum with peptic ulceration alone amounting to $1 \times 10^9$ dollars (Blumenthal 1968). In England and Wales, 60 000 of 400 000 patients admitted to hospital with digestive diseases had peptic ulcers, with approximately 13 million working days lost in England and Wales as a result of disease of the stomach and duodenum.

### Pathogenesis and etiology

Peptic ulcers occur when the normal balance between acid/pepsin and mucosal defense factors is disrupted. The presence of acid is obligatory for a peptic ulcer to form, but most patients have acid secretion within normal limits. Hypersecretion of gastric acid, moreover, is rarely sufficient by itself to lead to ulceration. The primary event in forming an ulcer is the disruption of normal mucosal defense factors (p. 231). Currently the two most important factors in the pathogenesis of peptic ulcer disease relate to gastric acid secretion and gastroduodenitis caused by *H. pylori.*

#### *Gastric secretion*

The secretion of acid and pepsin is necessary for the development of a peptic ulcer. Benign ulcers do not develop where there is achlorhydria, but will invariably develop in the Zollinger–Ellison syndrome in which there is hypersecretion of acid. Furthermore, most ulcers heal after surgery or during treatment with acid-suppressive drugs.

Many different abnormalities of acid secretion have been described in duodenal ulcer, but the evidence is conflicting (Lam 1984). Patients with duodenal ulcer disease as a group secrete more acid, both basally (Grossman et al 1963, Lam & Sircus 1975) and in response to a variety of stimuli, than do normal subjects. These stimuli include sham feeding (Lam & Sircus 1975, Feldman et al 1980), pentagastrin and histamine. This is due to an increased number of parietal cells which varies between different ethnic groups (Cox 1952). About 30–50% of patients with ulcer have a stimulated acid secretion which exceeds the upper limit for normal subjects (Cheng et al 1977, Lam et al 1980a). However, the majority of patients with duodenal ulcer have an acid secretion which falls within the normal range. Other abnormalities noted in subjects with duodenal ulcer compared to control subjects include an excessive drive to the secretion of gastric acid with elevated serum gastrin (G-17) levels after eating (Fritsch et al 1976, Walsh & Lam 1980); an increased sensitivity of parietal cells to pentagastrin stimulation (Isenberg et al 1975) and to calcium; an abnormal sensitivity of parietal cells to endogenous gastrin released in response to graded doses of a peptone meal (Lam et al 1980b); impaired inhibition of gastric acid secretion by a low intragastric pH (Walsh et al 1975). Additional abnormalities noted in subjects with duodenal ulcer disease include elevated serum pepsinogen I (Samloff et al 1986), and a decrease in epidermal growth factor in saliva, gastric juice and duodenal biopsies (Zandomeneghi et al 1991).

Within the antrum, G cell numbers appear to be normal and the concentration of gastrin elevated, with the somatostatin cell (D cells) numbers and concentration diminished (Moss et al 1992). Thus the ratio of G cells to D cells is elevated. The postprandial hypergastrinemia and antral G and D cell changes are due to concomitant *H. pylori* infection (Haruma et al 1992).

### *Duodenal acid and bicarbonate*

Duodenal ulcer patients as a group have a lower pH in the duodenum for longer periods than control subjects, both in the fasting state and in response to food. This abnormality is a reflection of gastric hypersecretion, since it does not occur in those ulcer patients with a normal acid secretion (Rune & Viskum 1969, Kerrigan et al 1989). Bicarbonate is actively secreted by the human duodenum and patients with duodenal ulcer disease secrete less bicarbonate into the proximal duodenum in response to perfusion with acid than do normal controls.

### *Mucosal blood flow*

Mucosal and submucosal blood flow have been measured in human subjects and it has been suggested that a decrease of flow in certain parts of the duodenum may account for the focal development of mucosal ischemia, leading to chronic duodenal ulceration (Murakami et al 1983). Antral blood flow has also been assessed as being increased in subjects with duodenal ulcer disease whereas in those with active gastric ulcer located at the angulus, blood flow was decreased (Kamada et al 1983).

### *Morphological abnormalities*

A number of morphological abnormalities exist in subjects with peptic ulcer disease. Within the stomach of subjects with both duodenal and gastric ulcer disease chronic histological gastritis (type B) affects the antrum, as well as the body and sometimes the fundus in some individuals. In gastric ulcer the gastritis involves the antrum and commonly the body with progression to atrophic gastritis accompanied by intestinal metaplasia (Maaroos et al 1985). Chronic active antral gastritis due to *H. pylori* infection is found in more than 95% of patients with duodenal ulcer (Kekki et al 1990, Tytgat et al 1993b). Eradication of *H. pylori* results in resolution of this gastritis.

Within the duodenum gastric metaplasia of the surface epithelial cells has been demonstrated in most patients with duodenal ulcer (Patrick et al 1974). The gastric metaplastic areas are due to increased acid entering the duodenum; they develop severe inflammation at the ulcer site. This change may regress upon acid reduction. *H. pylori* can adhere to the duodenal mucosa where there is gastric metaplasia and survive, causing this focal duodenitis (Carrick et al 1989). Controversy exists as to whether the duodenitis represents *H. pylori* infection, the inflammatory reaction of surrounding mucosa to the presence of the ulcer or whether it is part of the pathophysiological spectrum of duodenal ulcer disease.

## Helicobacter pylori (see p. 227)

With the discovery of *H. pylori* in 1983 (Marshall 1983, Warren 1983), considerable interest has been expressed in relation to its role in peptic ulcer disease. *H. pylori* infects the mucosa in 95–100% of patients with duodenal ulcer disease and in 70–80% of patients with gastric ulcer (Graham 1989, Tytgat et al 1993b). The frequency of this infection in a given population increases progressively with age. Neither smoking nor the use of NSAIDs affects the *H. pylori* colonization. Evidence that *H. pylori* causes duodenal and gastric ulcer disease relates to the long-term follow-up of subjects with antral gastritis who are 14 times more likely to develop a peptic ulcer than those with a normal gastric mucosa (Sipponen et al 1990). In addition, *Helicobacter* is closely associated with subjects having duodenal and gastric ulcer disease (Graham 1989). Eradication of *H. pylori* from the antral mucosa induces a prolonged remission and healing of the ulcer disease (Tytgat et al 1993b).

*Mucosal barrier and peptic ulceration*

The mucosal barrier is altered as a consequence of *H. pylori* infection and its impairment may be important in the development of peptic ulceration. In stress ulcer (p. 226), ischemia deprives the epithelial cells of metabolic substrates and oxygen which are needed to maintain the protective mechanisms.

The gastric mucus is more degraded than normal in both gastric and duodenal ulcer patients (Morrissey et al 1983), most likely as a consequence of the production of a number of enzymes including phospholipase and other proteases from *H. pylori* which change its hydrophobicity (Slomiany et al 1989, Spychal et al 1990). The concentration of prostaglandins within the gastric mucosa is reduced in subjects with gastric ulcer (Wright et al 1982) and their synthesis is impaired in duodenal ulcer (Hillier et al 1985). However, measurement of concentrations and synthesis of prostaglandins in mucosal biopsies of the stomach or duodenum is fraught with methodological difficulties and results must be interpreted with caution.

*Mucosal damage due to drugs*

Certain drugs when administered orally or systemically may injure the gastric and duodenal mucosa. These drugs act in various ways by damaging the surface lipoprotein layer of epithelial cells, by reducing bicarbonate secretion and changing the composition of mucus.

The superficial gastric lesions of hyperemia, erosions and subepithelial hemorrhage may result from NSAIDs (see below). Frank ulceration and aggravation of an existing ulcer with bleeding and perforation may also occur.

*Aspirin and NSAIDs*

NSAIDs are associated with approximately a fivefold relative risk of developing a gastric ulcer (McIntosh et al 1985a, Duggan et al 1986). The incidence of new gastric ulcers in patients taking aspirin and NSAIDs is about 10–15% during the first 3 months of use and appears not to vary markedly with the particular NSAIDs used (Piper et al 1981, Duggan et al 1986, Hawkey 1990). Those at risk are usually elderly patients with a history of ulcer disease, multiple NSAIDs and high doses of these agents. Duodenal ulcers also occur as a result of NSAID use, but generally less frequently than gastric ulcers (Gillies & Skyring 1968, Duggan et al 1986). Many subjects with NSAID-induced chronic ulcers are asymptomatic and the problem only becomes important if associated with dyspepsia or with bleeding or perforation (Mellem et al 1985, Skander & Ryan 1988).

The increased incidence of gastric ulcer in young and middle-aged women which occurred in Australia after 1940 was related to regular consumption of compound analgesic powders which contained aspirin, phenacetin and caffeine. An increase in perforated or bleeding gastric ulcer was also described. Studies by the Boston Collaborative Drug Surveillance Program (Levy 1974), from the Mayo Clinic (Cameron 1975) and from Sydney (Piper et al 1981) have confirmed that aspirin abuse is associated with chronic gastric ulcer but not with duodenal ulcer. A case-controlled study of gastric ulcer patients demonstrated that the increased exposure to aspirin occurred before the onset of the ulcer, indicating that the association was causal (McIntosh et al 1985a). The risk of gastric ulcer becomes greater than that in the general population when the weekly dose exceeds 20 tablets (Graham & Smith 1986). Long-term follow-up of patients with rheumatoid arthritis treated with NSAIDs suggests a hazard ratio of gastrointestinal complications requiring hospitalization of 6.5 in NSAIDs users compared with patients not on NSAIDs; the risk is higher in elderly patients with a past history of abdominal pain and peptic ulcer and those on multiple NSAIDs and on corticosteroids (Fries et al 1989). A number of previous small studies of patients with rheumatoid arthritis on long-term NSAIDs have shown prevalence rates of gastric ulcer ranging from 8% to 17% (Sun et al 1974, Gerber et al 1981, Carson et al 1987) and of duodenal ulcer from 1% to 8% (Larkai et al 1987, Gerber et al 1981).

In normal individuals ingestion of aspirin has damaging effects on the gastric and duodenal mucosa. Lesions which resemble duodenal ulcer may result from ingestion of aspirin for one day in normal individuals (Hoftiezer et al 1982). In patients taking eight aspirin tablets daily for more than 3 months endoscopic examination has observed duodenal ulcer in 4%, duodenal erosions in 13% and gastric ulcer in 31% (Lockard et al 1980). Other endoscopic studies have obtained similar results with the risk of an ulcer increasing with the use of combinations of NSAIDs (Caruso & Porro 1980).

The mechanisms of aspirin and NSAID- induced damage to the gastroduodenal mucosa have been discussed (pp. 222, 226 and 485). The synthesis and secretion of mucus is decreased and the secretion of bicarbonate by endogenous prostaglandins is inhibited. Visible damage to the gastric mucosa, including erosions, bleeding and punctate hemorrhages, and ulceration caused by NSAIDs and aspirin is reduced by pretreatment with oral prostaglandin derivatives such as misoprostol (Graham et al 1988). Oral paracetamol (acetaminophen) does not result in gastric and duodenal erosions (Hoftiezer et al 1982).

*Corticosteroids and peptic ulceration in animal studies*

Corticosteroids have been shown to increase gastric secretion, but this does not occur in man (Cooke 1967). Corticosteroids have been implicated in causing gastric ulcer disease in patients with rheumatoid arthritis and other collagen disorders (Cooke 1967). An analysis of 6000 patients from 50 studies failed to show an association between prednisolone or prednisone up to 60 mg/day and peptic ulcer disease (Conn & Blitzer 1976, Piper et al 1991). In patients with renal transplantation who receive very large doses of corticosteroids, there may be a predisposition to complications of ulcer disease. Messer et al (1983) have suggested a higher frequency of peptic ulcer in patients receiving corticosteroids for long periods, those taking high doses and in those with a previous history of ulcer.

*Bile duodenogastric reflux*

The role of bile reflux into the stomach in the causation of gastric ulcer disease is unclear (Heading 1983). In patients with gastric ulcer a high percentage have a higher concentration of bile acids in the stomach and more frequent duodenogastric reflux compared with controls and those with duodenal ulcer disease (Capper et al 1966, Rees & Rhodes 1977). Controversy, however, exists as to the reliability of methods to determine duodenogastric reflux (Muller-Lissner et al 1983). Moreover, the exposure of the gastric mucosa to reflux material also depends on the rate of gastric emptying and Miranda et al (1985) have suggested that patients with gastric ulcer have decreased antral motility and hence an increased concentration of bile acid in the aspirate compared to fasting control subjects.

*Smoking and peptic ulceration*

Peptic ulceration and smoking are strongly associated based on epidemiological and clinical studies (McCarthy 1984a). The frequency of peptic ulcer in both men and women smokers is twice that in nonsmokers with the risk increasing with increased duration and amount of smoking (Friedman et al 1974, Rabkin & Struening 1976, Ainley et al 1986). Cigarette consumption is also associated with ulcer size. Ulcer healing with $H_2$ receptor antagonists is significantly delayed in smokers compared to nonsmokers (Korman et al 1981). With potent acid-suppressing agents including omeprazole and lansoprazole the delay in ulcer healing is less evident (Hui et al 1989). Sucralfate and colloidal bismuth subcitrate, both of which possess cytoprotective properties, as well as the latter having anti-*H. pylori* activity, are able to overcome the adverse effect of cigarette smoking on duodenal ulcer healing (Lambert 1991, Lam 1991). The relapse rate of duodenal ulcer is higher in smokers compared with nonsmokers (Korman et al 1983).

The precise mechanisms whereby smoking causes these effects are not understood. Chronic smoking increases maximal gastric acid secretion (Whitfield & Hobsley 1987) and it also impairs the ability of $H_2$ receptor antagonists to suppress nocturnal acid secretion. Nicotine significantly reduces duodenal, but not gastric mucosal blood flow and in healthy smokers an inhibition of prostaglandin E synthesis has been observed with a reduced concentration of prostaglandin E2 in the gastric juice. Smoking and nicotine administration also adversely affect duodenal neutralizing capacity by inhibiting duodenal and pancreatic bicarbonate secretion (Bynum et al 1972, Ainsworth et al 1993). Therefore these studies suggest that smoking adversely affects both sides of the ulcer equation with an increase in gastric acid secretion and impairment of the defense mechanisms (Kaufmann et al 1990). The prevention of ulcer relapse by the eradication of *H. pylori* is not affected by continued smoking, suggesting that treatment of bacterial infection and a resolution of mucosal inflammation is the more important mechanism (Borody et al 1993).

*Diet and peptic ulceration* (Lin & Lambert 1992)

A number of dietary factors have been implicated in ulcer disease but the role of diet as an independent factor remains unclear. Dietary factors implicated as having a protective effect in prevention of disease include unrefined wheat, vegetables, dietary fiber, essential fatty acid (linoleic) ingestion particularly from fish oil and rice oils. It has been suggested that refined sugars, alcohol, caffeine-containing foods and spices are implicated in causing ulcer disease but the evidence does not support this.

*Stress and psychological factors*

The etiological role of stress in peptic ulcer disease remains unclear. Psychological factors have not been shown conclusively to be important in the etiology of peptic ulcer (Roth 1955, Kessel & Munro 1964, McIntosh et al 1985b). The relationship between personality trait and peptic ulcer disease has also been investigated (Alexander 1934, McIntosh et al 1983). Patients with peptic ulcer have significantly more personality disturbance than controls and a greater tendency to have an excessive number of people dependent upon them, together with overpessimism and hypochondriacal complaints. Considerable difficulty exists in scientifically defining and quantifying an individual's stress. Events giving rise to stress for an individual vary considerably and the perception of stress depends on a large number of factors including intelligence, personality, educational and income level and occupation, as well as age.

Another way of assessing the role of stress is to review the relationship between society stress and peptic ulcer rates. Society stress derives from a stressful event affecting the whole of society or a certain population such as war, periods of migration or urbanization. Rates of complication of peptic ulcer disease have been observed to be increased in London during World War II (Riley 1942), in subjects in Hong Kong during periods of society stress (Hui et al 1990), as well as amongst air traffic controllers in the United States (Rose et al 1987). The incidence of duodenal ulcer in air traffic controllers is estimated to be 2.4 new cases per year per 1000 persons which is higher than that of 1.80 reported by Kurata & Haile (1984) in the general population. In addition, Australian prisoners of war in World War II had a significantly higher incidence of duodenal ulcer than veterans who served in south east Asia but who were not taken prisoner (Goulston et al 1985).

Mechanisms linking psychological factors to ulcer disease are unclear. However, it has been shown that increased gastric acid secretion may be associated with stressful life events. In addition, hard physical exercise with sleep deprivation results in a threefold increase in basal acid secretion (Oktedalen et al 1984).

*Hereditary factors*

Patients with peptic ulcer disease often have a family history of the disease, particularly in subjects who develop the ulcer under the age of 30 (Melrose & Wallace 1965). Two main causes of such a concentration within families relate to a common inheritance and common family environment. The latter may relate to shared dietary habits or shared infection and it is now clear that *H. pylori* infection is more common amongst family members of an infected subject (Drumm et al 1990, Lin et al 1991). Genetic factors may play a role in the etiology of peptic ulcer disease and evidence is based on family studies, twin studies and blood group studies (Rotter & Rimoin 1977). Both genetic and environmental influences exist as identical twins have concordance of less than 100% which is significantly higher than in dizygotic twins.

Blood group O and nonsecretor status are associated with duodenal ulcer, but not with gastric ulcer. Group O nonsecretors are 2.5 times more likely to develop a duodenal ulcer than secretors of Groups A, B and AB (Aird et al 1954, McConnell 1980). The effect of the two genes, O and nonsecretor, on the risk of duodenal ulcer appears to be multiplicative so that individuals who are both O and nonsecretor have a relative risk of approximately 2.5. There is no association between *H. pylori* infection and ABO blood group and secretor status (Hook-Nikanne et al 1990). Group O status has also been shown to be associated with an increased risk of bleeding and perforation (Lam & Ong 1976).

Serum pepsinogen I levels are elevated in subjects with *H. pylori* gastritis (Wagner et al 1991), duodenal ulcer (Samloff et al 1986) and in families with a high prevalence of ulcer (Rotter et al 1979). This was previously considered to be as a consequence of genetic factors but it is clear that serum pepsinogen I levels are elevated as a consequence of *H. pylori*-induced inflammation and are unrelated to specific genetic factors.

Thus, the potential genetic susceptibility to develop peptic ulcer disease may relate in part to the ability to acquire *H. pylori* within families and the levels of gastric acid secreted and entering the duodenum. A reassessment of previous genetic factors must now occur in light of the identification of *H. pylori* as an important etiological factor in ulcer disease.

*Disease association*

There are a number of medical conditions in which peptic ulcer disease occurs at an unexpectedly high frequency. These include patients with chronic obstructive pulmonary disease, cirrhosis and chronic renal failure on hemodialysis or after renal transplantation. Patients with $\alpha_1$-antitrypsin deficiency, hereditary angioedema, cystic fibrosis and certain hematological disorders (leukemias, polycythemia vera and sickle cell disease) are also more prone to ulceration

## EPIDEMIOLOGY

The methods used to assess the epidemiology of ulcers include hospital data (hospitalization rates, ulcer surgery and perforated ulcer rates), mortality statistics, population studies and sickness benefits records. All of these methods have limitations and make comparative studies difficult. In addition, in Australia the number of prescriptions for $H_2$ receptor antagonists has been used to assess the incidence of peptic ulcer as when the drugs were first introduced they could be prescribed only when an ulcer was diagnosed by radiology and endoscopy (Hugh et al 1984).

### Prevalence and incidence of peptic ulcer

Autopsy examination of 13 000 patients in Leeds revealed that chronic duodenal ulcer existed in 7.8% of males and 4% of females dying from causes other than peptic ulcer (Watkinson 1960). Other postmortem studies have suggested that 21–29% of all men and 11–18% of all women have evidence of present or past ulcer disease (Watkinson 1960, Levy & de la Fuente 1963, Lindstrom 1978). Endoscopic surveys have suggested a lifetime prevalence of peptic ulcer of 5.9% and duodenal ulcer alone of 4.2% in a Finnish endoscopic study of 358 control subjects (Ihamaki et al 1979). Bonnevie (1975a, b), in a large study of 500 000 residents of Copenhagen County over 15 years old, revealed an annual incidence of 0.13% for duodenal ulcer, 0.03% for gastric ulcer and 0.02% for combined duodenal and gastric ulcer. These figures are

**Table 9.4** Annual incidence of duodenal ulcer in comparable studies (Bonnevie 1975a). Mean annual incidence rate per 1000 inhabitants aged 15 years and over

| Authors | Period | Area | No. pts | Total | Sex ratio M : F |
|---|---|---|---|---|---|
| Pulvertaft 1959 | 1952–1957 | York, England | 862 | 1.33 | 3.5 : 1 |
| Litton & Murdoch 1963 | 1957–1959 | South west Scotland | 810 | 2.63 | 4.2 : 1 |
| Dunlop 1968 | 1962 | Central Scotland | 259 | 2.70 | 3.4 : 1 |
| Sponheim 1960 | 1950–1952 | Rogaland, Norway | 458 | 1.50 | 4.2 : 1 |
| Bonnevie 1975a, b | 1963–1968 | Copenhagen County | 1475 | 1.32 | 2.2 : 1 |
| Kurata & Haile 1984 | | USA | – | 1.80 | |
| Kuwai 1989 | | Japan | – | 1.00 | |

**Table 9.5** Annual incidence of gastric ulcer in comparable studies (Bonnevie 1975b). Mean annual incidence rate per 1000 inhabitants aged 15 years and over

| Authors | Period | Area | No. pts | Total | Sex ratio M : F |
|---|---|---|---|---|---|
| Pulvertaft 1959 | 1952–1957 | York, England | 257 | 0.40 | 1.7 : 1 |
| Litton & Murdoch 1963 | 1957–1959 | South west Scotland | 134 | 0.34 | 1.2 : 1 |
| Dunlop 1968 | 1962 | Central Scotland | 44 | 0.44 | 1.9 : 1 |
| Sponheim 1960 | 1950–1952 | Rogaland, Norway | 139 | 0.45 | 1.9 : 1 |
| Bonnevie 1975a, b | 1963–1968 | Copenhagen County | 496 | 0.44 | 1.3 : 1 |

similar to the incidence rates for some other European countries (Tables 9.4 and 9.5).

In most European countries, USA and Australia, duodenal ulcer occurs twice as frequently as gastric ulcer, whereas in Finland, Peru, Turkey and Japan, gastric ulcer is more frequent than duodenal ulcer. In Australia the mean annual incidence per 1000 population aged 15 years and over was 3.8% for duodenal ulcer and 0.7% for gastric ulcer, as assessed by prescriptions of cimetidine (Hugh et al 1984). A lifetime prevalence of peptic ulcer of 9% was found in a survey of male physicians from Massachusetts with a mean age of 50 years. In the USA the 1-year point prevalence of self-reported peptic ulcer has been 1.7–1.9% between 1961 and 1981. Therefore about 4 million Americans suffer from active peptic ulcer with 10% developing peptic ulcer during their lifetime (National Center for Health Statistics 1979).

### *Changing trends of peptic ulcer*

Peptic ulcers were rare in the 19th century and became highly prevalent in the 1950s and 1960s. Since then peptic ulcer disease has declined in incidence in some Western countries, as shown by several surveys in Australia, the United Kingdom and United States of America (Wastell 1972, McIntosh et al 1993). Mortality and hospital admission rates for duodenal and gastric ulcers in both sexes fell in England and Wales over the period 1958 to 1977 (Coggon et al 1981) with a decline in the perforation rates for duodenal ulcer and gastric ulcer noted in males. In elderly women, however, an increase in duodenal ulcer mortality has been noted and this has been postulated to be associated with use of NSAIDs (McIntosh et al 1993, Jibril et al 1994). Similar reductions in incidence have been described in West Germany and Switzerland. In the United States of America there was a decline in admissions to hospital for uncomplicated duodenal ulcer by 43% during 1970 to 1978, whereas admissions for gastric ulcer did not change (Elashoff & Grossman 1980); a fall in the death rate and decrease in the male to female ratio was noted in this study. In marked contrast, between 1970 and 1980, hospital admissions for peptic ulcer in Hong Kong increased by 21%. An increased incidence of perforation was also noted during this period with a decline in mortality by 26% (Koo et al 1983).

Susser & Stein (1962) have shown that the annual death rate for duodenal ulcer was greatest in the cohort of population born in the final quarter of the 19th century in Western society. They have interpreted these data as suggesting that some environmental factor operated on this cohort of persons and that the influence of this factor has since declined. A similar birth cohort was demonstrated for peptic ulcer mortality in Switzerland in subjects born between 1870 and 1900 (Sonnenberg 1984). Proposed explanations include early urbanization, economic crisis associated with World War I and social stresses. Another possible explanation of this cohort phenomenon is to incriminate *H. pylori* infection which appears to be decreasing in Western countries (Parsonnet et al 1992).

### *Sex ratio*

The sex ratio of peptic ulcer patients varies in different parts of the world. The male to female ratio for duodenal ulcer varies from 18 : 1 in India (Tovey 1979), 4 : 1 in Hong Kong (Koo et al 1983), 3 : 1 in Scotland (Lam et al 1983), 2 : 1 in Denmark, England and Wales and 1 : 1 in the United States (Kurata et al 1985). The male to female ratio of gastric and duodenal ulcer has fallen considerably in many countries. In Australia the male to female ratio of gastric ulcer has decreased from 2.5 : 1 in 1930 to 0.8 : 1 in 1960 (Billington 1965). The large geographic differences in sex ratios of ulcer disease strongly support the notion that environmental factors play an important etiological role in peptic ulcer.

## Occupational differences and migration

Gastric ulcers occur most frequently in unskilled and manual workers whereas duodenal ulcers occur uniformly in all social groups (Doll et al 1951). However, it has been suggested from the United Kingdom and the United States that there is an increased incidence of duodenal ulcer in the less skilled and unskilled workers (Litton & Murdoch 1963, Pflanz 1971). Thus, reports relating to social class, occupation and urban life have been contradictory and this may reflect differences in data collection, time periods, ethnic grouping and geography. *H. pylori* is more common in the lower socioeconomic groups and this may account for some of the differences noted.

### Geographic and ethnic variations

Considerable variation occurs in the incidence of peptic ulcer within continents and countries. Peptic ulcers are rare among Eskimos in northern Greenland, as well as native Americans in the south west. Similarly ulcers are uncommon amongst Fijians, Indonesians and Australian aborigines. Regional differences in peptic ulcer have been reported from the African continent; it is more prevalent along the west coast of Africa than along the east coast (Tovey & Tunstall 1975). The rural prevalence of ulcer disease in African countries is low with increased frequency of duodenal ulcer in large cities such as Durban, Cape Town and Johannesburg (Shaper & Williams 1959). Marked regional differences have also been identified in India with peptic ulcer more prevalent in southern than in northern India (Tovey 1979). Changes in ulcer prevalence have been attributed to differences in the staple diet with those in the south eating rice compared to wheat, millet and pulses as the staples in northern India.

### Seasonal trends

It is suggested that peptic ulcer and its complications tend to occur or recur during autumn and winter months (Boles & Westerman 1954, Bradley & Bradley 1966, Gibinski et al 1982, Hui & Lam 1988).

## PATHOLOGY

### Chronic peptic ulcer

Chronic gastric ulcer is nearly always single and is usually situated on the lesser curve, adjoining anterior or posterior walls within the antrum or at the junction between body and antral mucosa. Sun & Stempien (1971) found 88% of ulcers along the lesser curvature, 5% on the greater curvature, 6% on the posterior wall and 1% on the anterior wall. In nearly all cases the ulcer is located just distal to the boundary between the body and antral mucosa (Oi et al 1969, Fig. 9.9). Chronic duodenal ulcer is usually in the first part just distal to the junction of pyloric and duodenal mucosa (Oi et al 1969), but occasionally it may be distal to this – postbulbar ulcer (p. 239). In endoscopic terms, the

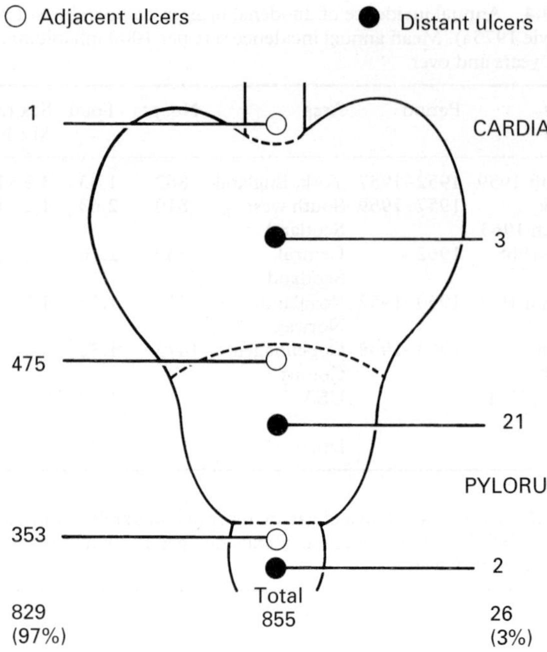


**Fig. 9.9** Location of ulcers in relation to mucosae. Nearly all ulcers are adjacent to mucosal boundaries and on the side of the boundary opposite the fundic gland area (Oi et al 1969).

lesser curvature of the bulb is referred to as the superior wall and the greater curvature as the inferior wall. The following localization of ulcers is found; anterior wall 50%, posterior wall 23%, inferior wall 22% and superior wall 5%. Multiple ulcers are found in 10–15% of cases (Hui & Lam 1987).

Gastric and duodenal ulcers are usually less than 3 cm in diameter, only 8% of duodenal ulcers and 14% of gastric ulcers being larger than this (Niwayama & Terplan 1959). Occasionally, an ulcer can cover a large area of the surface of the mucosa (Lumsden et al 1970) and in the stomach it may be mistaken for carcinoma.

Chronic ulcers are usually circular or oval and have a punched-out appearance. The proximal margin is typically overhanging and the distal sloping. The mucosal folds extend smoothly to the edge of the ulcer. A red zonal gastritis is usually apparent around the ulcer margin. The floor of the active ulcer appears grey or white on endoscopy. The base is rubbery. The serosa overlying an ulcer is red and fibrotic and telangiectatic vessels are a good guide to its location. The adjacent lymph nodes are often enlarged.

Histology of the base shows successive layers of inflammatory and necrotic debris with underlying granulation then fibrous tissue (Fig. 9.10). *Candida* may be seen in the slough. In the chronic ulcer the main muscle coat is destroyed and replaced by fibrous tissue which fuses with the muscularis mucosae at the ulcer margin. Subintimal fibrosis of vessels, neuronal hypertrophy and lymphoid aggregates are present within the wall. The mucosa at the

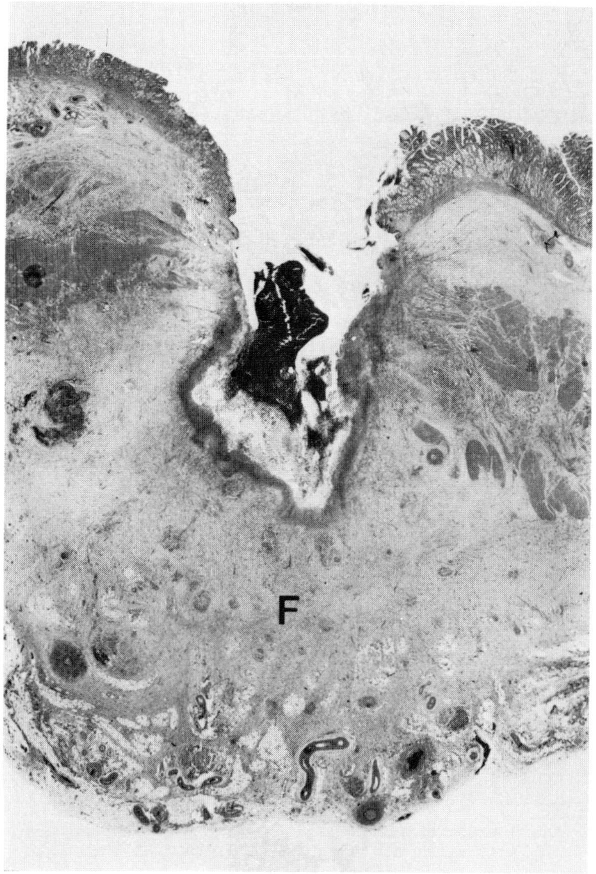


**Fig. 9.10** Chronic penetrating gastric ulcer. Section showing blood clot in the base of a deeply penetrating ulcer. There is much fibrosis in the gastric wall with destruction of all muscle layers (hematoxylin and eosin, × 5).

ulcer margin is hyperplastic and may be polypoid. Misplaced glands may be observed amongst the disturbed muscle fibers. During healing the ulcer becomes smaller and flatter and finally the white slough on the floor is replaced by granulation tissue. Some scarring remains and the main muscle coat is not reconstituted. The site of the healed ulcer is identified by mucosal folds which radiate from the scar.

The ulcer can cause fibrosis, leading to duodenal stenosis or hourglass deformity of the stomach and/or shortening of the lesser curvature of the stomach. Occasionally, a chronic ulcer may perforate or slowly penetrate an adjacent organ, usually the pancreas.

### Acute ulcers and erosions

An erosion (Figs 9.11 and 9.12) is confined to the mucosa, so that its base consists of the gastric glands. Erosions are usually less than 5 mm, shallow, circumscribed and multiple and more common in the stomach than duodenum.

An acute ulcer penetrates the entire thickness of the mucosa and sometimes the muscle coats, which can lead to perforation. Like the erosion, it is more common in the stomach than the duodenum. On histological examination (Fig. 9.13) there is acute inflammation around the ulcer but very little fibrosis.

## CLINICAL FEATURES OF PEPTIC ULCERATION

Dyspepsia is a common symptom caused by peptic ulcer. In only about 20% of subjects presenting with dyspepsia, how-

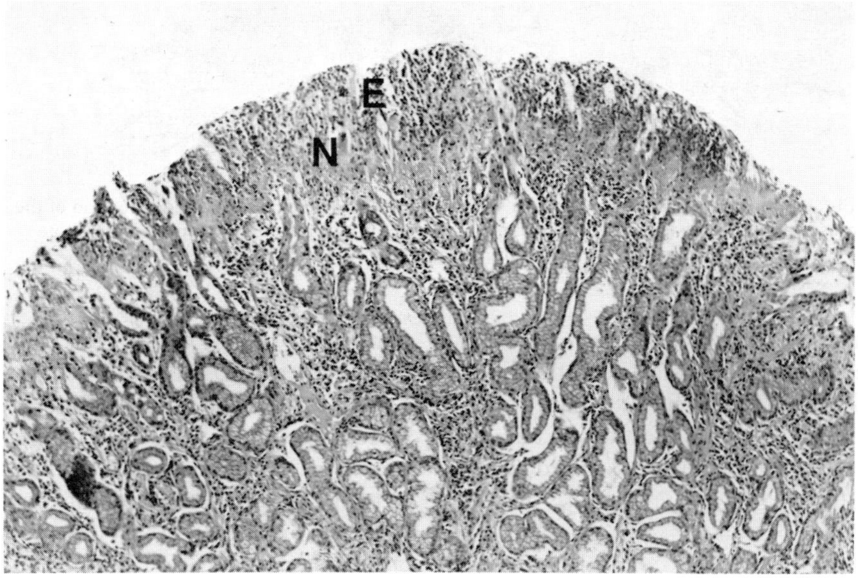


**Fig. 9.11** Gastric erosion. Section showing a prominent superficial zone of necrosis (N) with overlying surface inflammatory exudate (E) (hematoxylin and eosin, × 90).

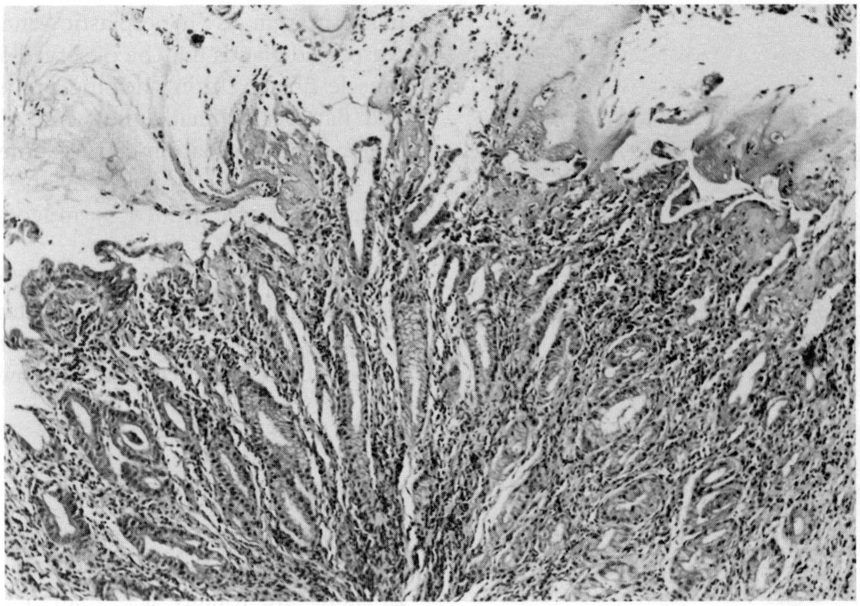

**Fig. 9.12** Section showing a more exudative pattern with a fibrinous exudate arising from the eroded mucosal surface (hematoxylin and eosin, × 90).

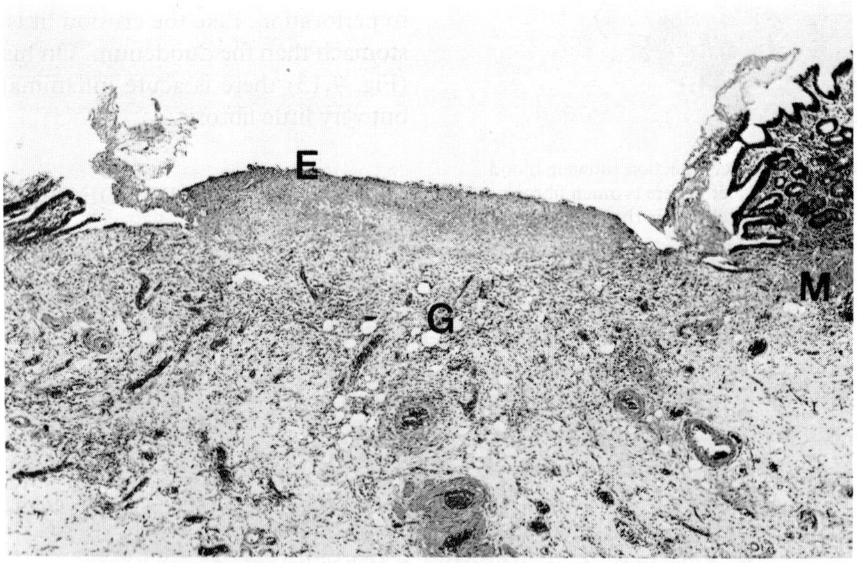


**Fig. 9.13** Acute gastric ulcer. Section showing superficial exudate (E) with destruction of the muscularis mucosae (M) and early granulation tissue (G) formation in the submucosa. Note the lack of mature fibrous tissue (hematoxylin and eosin, × 40).

ever, are the symptoms caused by peptic ulcer, with the majority having no macroscopic abnormalities in the upper gastrointestinal tract (Tibblin 1985). The latter have "functional" dyspepsia (p. 1366). The clinical features of uncomplicated gastric and duodenal ulceration are discussed below.

## Clinical course

The natural history of chronic duodenal and gastric ulcer disease follows a chronic course with frequent relapses and remissions (Boyd et al 1984). In endoscopic studies, relapse rates of 65–80% in 6 months and 80–100% within 1 year have been found for both duodenal and gastric ulcers (Shearman & Hetzel 1979). Asymptomatic recurrences are also common. Presentation with complications of peptic ulcer disease without previous symptoms is also common, particularly in the elderly (Pounder 1989). Overall symptomatic relapse of both gastric and duodenal ulcer occurs on average once every 2 years and there is a lifetime risk of potentially serious complications in 20% of patients. Eradication of *H. pylori* or the use of long-term acid suppression diminishes the risks of complication and lowers the relapse rates.

## Symptoms

### *Pain*

Epigastric pain is the predominant symptom in 60–80% of subjects with duodenal and gastric ulcer disease. With the widespread availability of upper gastrointestinal endoscopy less reliance has now been placed on the symptom pattern, particularly pain, to confirm or refute a diagnosis of peptic ulcer with many subjects with typical "ulcer pain" having no evidence of ulceration at early endoscopy.

Typical pain of duodenal ulcer occurs 1–3 h after meals and frequently awakens the patient at night. This discomfort is relieved by food or antacids and is sometimes described as a burning hunger pain or simply a vague discomfort. The pain is usually episodic with attacks lasting from 0.5 to 2 h. Fleeting pain lasting only seconds or minutes is uncharacteristic of ulcer disease (Edwards & Coghill 1968).

The pain is usually epigastric in site but may be identified in the periumbilical area or right hypochondrium. Radiation to the back is identified in a small percentage of subjects. Ulcer symptoms are typically episodic with relapses lasting up to 2 weeks. This natural history of symptoms is significantly altered by the use of $H_2$ receptor antagonists and failure to respond to these agents makes a diagnosis of simple peptic ulcer unlikely.

The mechanism of abdominal pain is unclear and appears to be multifactorial (Bonney & Pickering 1948, Ruffin 1959). Mechanisms include the action of acid on the ulcer, motility disturbance, serosal irritation and penetration and acid regurgitation into the esophagus. Early studies have attributed an important role to acid in the production of duodenal ulcer pain (Ruffin et al 1953). Pain is relieved by vomiting, by neutralization or by aspiration of gastric contents and is exacerbated by returning contents to the stomach, suggesting acid as an initiator of pain. Study of the precipitation of ulcer pain by nasogastric infusion of acid, however, has shown that there is an inconsistent relationship of pain and acid exposure. Monitoring of the intragastric and intraduodenal pH over a 24-h period along with a symptom diary shows some correlation of periods of high acidity with episodes of pain but most episodes were not associated with increases in duodenal acidity (Fullarton et al 1991). Moreover, it is difficult to understand spontaneous remission of pain when an ulcer crater is still present and recurrence of typical ulcer pain when there is only scarring in the duodenal bulb (Classen 1973, Misiewicz 1978). Thus, acid appears to have a role in the pathogenesis of ulcer pain but other factors must also be important.

### *Vomiting*

Vomiting in peptic ulcer is often self-induced to relieve pain. Nausea and vomiting with minimal or no pain can be the presentation of a pyloric channel ulcer. Vomiting may signify gastric outlet obstruction as a consequence of chronic ulceration or pyloric obstruction associated with a pyloric channel ulcer.

### *Other symptoms*

Weight loss may occur in patients with peptic ulcer, particularly gastric ulcers. Weight gain may occur occasionally in patients who obtain immediate relief of pain by eating.

Complaints of heartburn, regurgitation, excessive salivation, belching and the sensation of epigastric distention are common in peptic ulcer. Heartburn occurs in about 60% of patients with duodenal ulcer (Earlam 1976).

### *Computer-assisted interview system*

Diagnosis of gastric and duodenal ulcer on the basis of the patient's history is difficult and this has led to the use of a standardized interview and examination followed by analyses to determine the value of each symptom or sign (Crean & Holden 1983, Talley et al 1987). Symptoms found to have discriminant value in favor of ulcer are night pain and relief from pain with food, milk or antacids (Talley et al 1987). Other information, including the patient's age, sex, smoking habits and drug use, contributes more to the discrimination between ulcer and nonulcer patients than does the description of dyspepsia itself based on computer-aided analyses of symptoms (Hood et al 1976). These studies suggest that the computer analyses of questionnaire data may increase the precision of diagnosis and hence improve the selection of patients for investigation or treatment.

### *Distinction between gastric and duodenal ulcer*

No specific features differentiate gastric from duodenal ulcer and the problem is made more difficult by the coexistence of gastric and duodenal ulcer in about 7% of patients (Weisberg & Glass 1963). Weight loss, nausea, vomiting and early satiety may be more typical of gastric ulcer but are not diagnostic. The pain of gastric ulcer is not helped by food (2% in one series) and may indeed be precipitated by it (Hood et al 1976). Gastric ulcer is often asymptomatic, particularly in elderly patients taking NSAIDs. Symptoms in gastric ulcer are also less likely to show periodicity (Horrocks & de Dombal 1978).

### *Postbulbar ulcer* (Ramsdell et al 1957, Cooke & Hutton 1958)

This occurs in the first part of the duodenum just distal to the bulb or on the medial wall of the second part proximal to the ampulla. It accounts for less than 5% of duodenal ulcers and may be associated with Zollinger–Ellison syndrome. The pain can be in the right upper quadrant only or in the back, periodicity may be absent and the clinical response to acid reduction is poor. Hemorrhage is more common than with an ulcer in the bulb, occurring in about 40% of cases.

*Pyloric channel and prepyloric ulcers* (Murray et al 1967)

There are problems in definition in that prepyloric ulcer is commonly defined as an ulcer within 2 cm of the pylorus, but often this is difficult to measure. In addition, some studies include pyloric channel ulcers in this definition, while other studies include all ulcers distal to the angulus as prepyloric ulcers.

Vomiting may be a feature in these patients because of pyloric obstruction. Relief of pain by food or antacids may be transient and some develop pain in response to food. Some studies have reported slower healing (Liedberg et al 1985) and more frequent relapse with prepyloric ulcers (Strom et al 1984, 1986) and there is a general opinion that they are more prone to recurrence and complications. In addition, the recurrence rate after highly selective vagotomy may be higher than for other ulcers.

### Peptic ulcer in children

Peptic ulcer in children has been diagnosed more frequently since the introduction of pediatric endoscopy. Acute duodenal ulcers are more likely to occur in children younger than 2 years and are associated with a "viral" illness. These often present with upper gastrointestinal bleeding and a preceding illness with diarrhea, fever or upper respiratory tract infection (Gold et al 1990). Acute ulcers within the stomach and duodenum also are associated with severe burns (Curling ulcer), intracranial lesions (Cushing ulcer), shock, respiratory distress syndrome, sepsis or malignancy. Massive, acute hemorrhage is the usual presentation and mortality is high.

Ulcers in older children are usually chronic with duodenal ulcer six times more common than gastric ulcer in children over 6 years. Symptoms are similar to adults and often a considerable delay in diagnosis occurs, particularly in the younger age group (Murphy et al 1987). A history of duodenal ulcer in family members (20–62%) and nocturnal pain (61%) are important diagnostic pointers. Gastrointestinal bleeding occurs in about 50% of cases while the other complications of perforation, pyloric stenosis and massive bleeding are rare (Chiang et al 1989).

The majority of children with duodenal ulcer have *H. pylori*-associated gastritis with the macroscopic findings of antral nodularity caused by lymphoid hyperplasia (Queiroz et al 1991). Treatment of *H. pylori* gives the same long-term results with a decrease in ulcer relapse, as in adults (Yeung et al 1990).

### Examination of patients with peptic ulcer

A circumscribed area of superficial or deep tenderness in the mid-epigastrium may be found with active peptic ulcer disease; however, it has a poor predictive value (Priebe et al 1982). Some degree of muscle guarding may be felt when there is a penetrating ulcer or when there is a localized perforation.

## INVESTIGATIONS

Peptic ulcer is diagnosed by endoscopic or radiological examination. Both techniques are accurate when carried out by experts (Chs 1 and 4).

### Endoscopy

Most gastroenterologists believe that upper gastrointestinal endoscopy is the procedure of choice in the diagnosis of peptic ulceration. The reasons for its use in preference to double-contrast studies are discussed on pp. 12 and 102. These include the ability of endoscopy to diagnose superficial lesions and ulcer scars and to take multiple biopsies from gastric ulcers and other lesions which may be malignant. In addition, biopsies for *H. pylori* assessment by rapid urease test, culture or histology are important. Endoscopy is preferred in the assessment of a patient with upper gastrointestinal bleeding as it is more accurate and methods of hemostasis may be used. This is not to deny the value of double-contrast studies, rather it reflects the consensus of studies which have used endoscopy after radiology (Cotton & Shorvon 1984). Double-contrast studies carried out by an expert are not quite as accurate as endoscopy and probably even less so in children (Shaw et al 1987).

The endoscopic appearances of gastric and duodenal ulcers are learned by the endoscopist during apprenticeship and subsequent experience (see p. 107). The shape of an ulcer varies considerably: most are round, while the remainder are linear or irregular. They are usually surrounded by edema or reddening; the base appears white, but during healing it develops the color of normal mucosa.

Since most gastroenterologists now perform endoscopy as the first investigation in patients with dyspepsia, under what circumstances should additional investigations be performed if dyspepsia is persistent and it is felt that peptic ulceration might have been overlooked? On occasions endoscopic examination of the first part of the duodenum may be incomplete with an end-viewing instrument and an additional intubation with a side-viewing instrument may be indicated. This also applies to the second part of the duodenum. If it is felt that the initial examination might have been inadequate, then repeat endoscopy is indicated. In other patients, the initial examination might be technically difficult, for example due to scarring in the pyloroduodenal region. Under these circumstances a careful double-contrast study is indicated.

Endoscopy is also the method of choice to assess the response to treatment (Cotton & Shorvon 1984). This should always be carried out in gastric ulcer so that additional biopsies can be obtained to search for malignancy. Repeat endoscopy to assess response to therapy in duodenal ulcer is more debatable. Demonstration of clearance of *H. pylori* by urea breath test and symptom resolution may be all that is required in the future. Endoscopy is indicated when the symptomatic response to therapy is poor, for if the ulcer has healed a search for other causes of the symptoms is indicated.

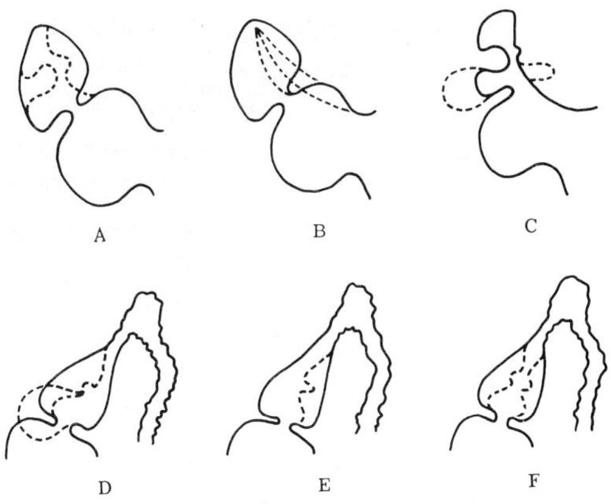


**Fig. 9.14** Variations of duodenal bulb deformities. The top row depicts right anterior oblique position: (A) superior wall ulcer, (B) cicatricial shortening of the lesser curvature aspect of the bulb, (C) pseudodiverticular formation. The bottom row depicts left anterior oblique projection: (D) atypical anterior wall ulcer crater, (E) typical posterior wall crater, (F) "kissing ulcers" (Prevot 1973, after Akerlund 1921).

## Radiology (Cotton & Shorvon 1984)

Acceptable studies of the accuracy of barium meal examination in duodenal ulcer are few (Laufer 1976, Rogers et al 1976, Gelfand et al 1985a). Using the conventional technique, Stein et al (1964) were able to demonstrate craters in only 70% of cases and small craters were commonly overlooked. Using the double-contrast method, agreement with endoscopy was reported in 81% (Rogers et al 1976) and 93% of cases (Laufer 1976). The positive predictive value, i.e. the percentage of positive diagnoses that are correct in double-contrast examination of duodenal ulcer, was 57% (Ott et al 1985). Gelfand et al (1985b) showed that examiner variability (44–80%) and ulcer size (more than 5 mm – 74% sensitivity; less than 5 mm – 69% sensitivity) were the dominant factors in the detection of duodenal ulcers. This study showed no significant difference in the detectability of duodenal ulcer by conventional and the double-contrast method. Others (Op den Orth & Ploem 1977) believe that the double-contrast technique used optimally and supplemented as necessary by views of the duodenal bulb full of barium and with compression provides the best radiographic documentation for detailed analysis.

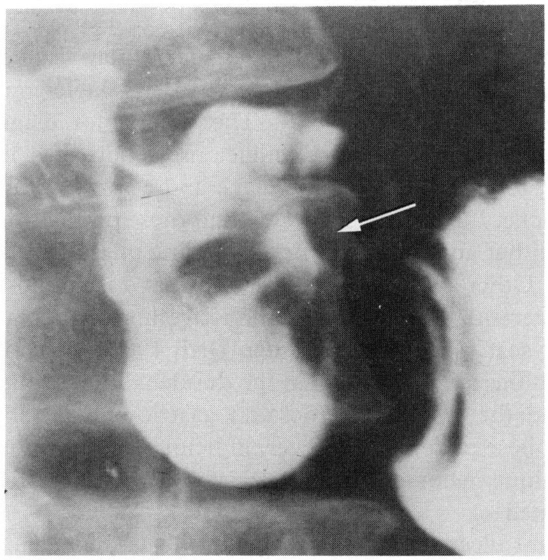

**Fig. 9.15** Large duodenal ulcer (arrow) adjacent to pylorus. Supine film with compression.

### *Radiological signs of duodenal ulceration* (Figs 9.14, 9.15 and 9.16 and p. 11)

Consequent upon improved radiographic techniques it has become apparent that peptic ulcers have a variety of shapes previously only identifiable at endoscopy. In the past, ulcer craters may not have been adequately filled because of spasm; however, the hypotonia induced by hyoscine or glucagon should allow a definitive view of the duodenal mucosa even in the presence of fixed deformity due to fibrosis and scarring, whilst irritative spasm should be completely abolished. Shallow ulcers and erosive changes should be recognized in many instances (Glick et al 1984).

The classic ulcer niche with barium collected in the crater seen en face is no longer the only sign of duodenal ulceration. Whilst this is still a prime sign of ulceration on the posterior wall (the dependent surface with a supine patient), on nondependent surfaces such as the anterior wall barium cannot collect in the crater but will coat the margins of an ulcer and other signs are utilized. If the ulcer edges are sharp a ring shadow may be identified, but it may be necessary to position the patient so that the suspected ulcer comes into profile, often necessitating compression and refilling the crater with barium by repeated turning.

When seen en face, an ulcer crater is usually round or oval, often surrounded by a radiolucent halo of edema and

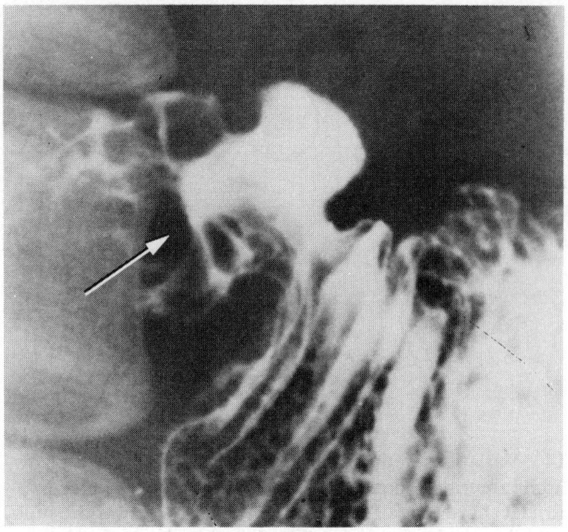

**Fig. 9.16** Duodenal ulcer. Areae gastricae in the gastric antrum.

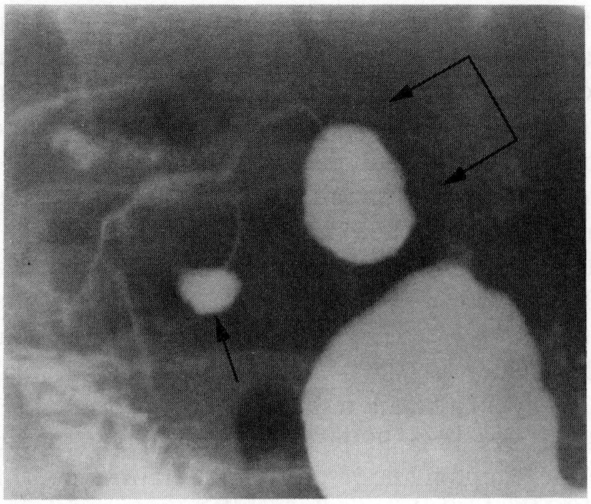

**Fig. 9.17** Two very large duodenal ulcers (arrows). The larger one could be mistaken for the duodenal bulb.

this in turn is surrounded by converging folds, usually signifying chronicity or healing.

Linear and rod-shaped duodenal ulcers may also be visible which were not previously seen by single-contrast studies (Braver et al 1979). The criteria for diagnosis include deformity of the outline, projection of a linear niche, folds radiating to the niche and a fuzzy outline of the niche. It has been suggested that these findings represent either an acute ulcer or the healing phase of a larger ulcer. Other authors have suggested that it is not possible to differentiate between a thin, active linear ulcer and a linear scar (De Roos & Op den Orth 1983). Occasional difficulties are present when the duodenal bulb is hidden behind the pyloric channel and gastric antrum and in very obese patients. However, judicious modifications of technique should enable satisfactory views to be obtained.

Giant ulcers 2–3 cm in diameter in the duodenal bulb (Fig. 9.17) can simulate a normal duodenal bulb. Their major characteristic is constancy of size and shape throughout the procedure and configuration of the ulcer crater which is grossly disorganized. This is detectable with adequate hypotonia and gas distention.

Multiple ulcers may be seen in the duodenal bulb, though these usually occur when there is long-standing disease with gross bulb deformity, making certain detection very difficult. In this situation endoscopy has been shown to have a 25% error rate in detecting multiplicity of ulcers (Shirakabe et al 1975). The presence of large or multiple ulcers in the duodenum, especially if accompanied by hypertrophic mucosa in the stomach and duodenum, with excess resting fluid in the stomach or an abnormal small bowel pattern, should lead to a search for Zollinger–Ellison syndrome (Zboralske & Amberg 1968).

*Secondary signs of ulceration*

Deformity of the duodenal bulb may be due to edema, spasm, fibrosis or combinations of these. Deformity persisting after the induction of hypotonia is almost always due to edema accompanying an acute ulcer or fibrotic scarring from previous ulcer disease and should lead to a careful search for a crater. Scarring can lead to loss of one or both fornices of the bulb, asymmetrical relationship of the pylorus to the base of the bulb, one or more incisura and narrowing of the bulb (see Fig. 9.14). A converging fold pattern can result in the classic "clover-leaf" deformity and with sufficient progression, pseudodiverticula develop. These may mimic ulcer craters but do change size with pressure and peristalsis, unlike ulcer craters. As previously indicated some ulcer craters will heal, leaving a linear cleft in the bulb.

From time to time duodenal bulb deformity results from disease in neighboring organs, especially the pancreas and gallbladder. Occasionally the normal gallbladder or common bile duct will indent the duodenal bulb, although postural changes will usually alter the appearance.

As a consequence of healing, a large duodenal ulcer may give rise to stenosis of the duodenum, leading to obstruction of the gastric outlet.

*Pyloric channel ulcers* (Fig. 9.18)

These are frequently small and shallow and their recognition requires particularly good double-contrast views. Additionally pyloric ulcers on the anterior wall require careful positioning in various prone oblique postures in order to demonstrate the niche. Compression views in the erect barium-filled position are also most helpful. Considerable pyloric spasm and deformity occur with such ulcers and the use of antispasmodics greatly enhances accurate display. Healing of pyloric channel ulcers frequently leads to fibrotic stenosis of the pylorus.

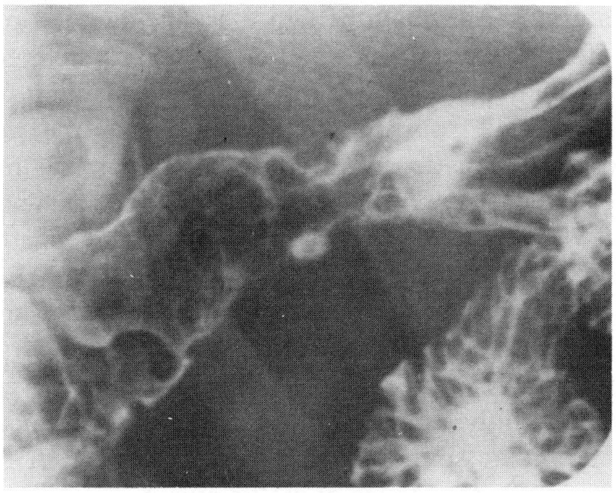

**Fig. 9.18** Pyloric ulcer. Previous pyloroplasty.

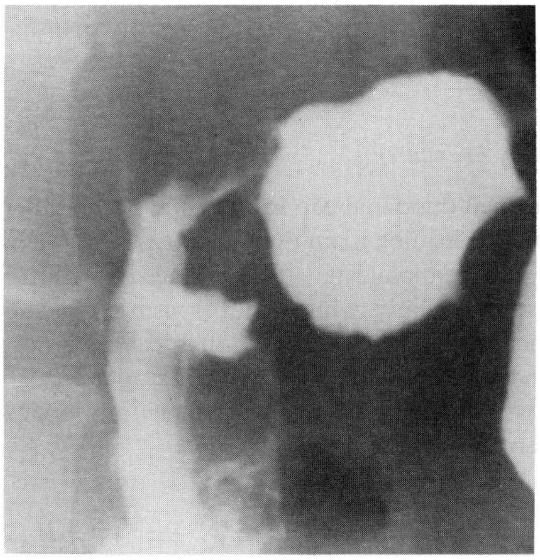

**Fig. 9.19** Large duodenal ulcer arising from second part of duodenum. Some narrowing at the apex of the duodenal bulb due to scarring from a second ulcer.

*Postbulbar ulcers* (Fig. 9.19) (Rodriguez et al 1973)

The ulcer usually occurs in the proximal few centimeters of the second part of duodenum, often on the medial wall. Frequently, there is an incisura opposite the crater and usually there is marked spasm and edema and without adequate hypotonia, the ulcer crater can be very difficult to demonstrate. In healing, a ring stricture may develop proximal to the ampulla (Bilbao et al 1971). If a deeply penetrating ulcer develops, an inflammatory mass may arise in the pancreas, leading to pancreatitis. Difficulties in differential diagnosis occur with carcinoma of the pancreas, acute pancreatitis and Crohn's disease.

*Relationship between the areae gastricae and duodenal ulcer* (see Fig. 9.16)

The appearance of the areae gastricae coated by barium using the double-contrast method is a "cobblestone" mosaic caused by barium lying in the grooves between mounds of mucosal cells (Kreel 1975, Mackintosh & Kreel 1977). The amount of mucus present affects the visibility of the mucosal surface: copious mucus fills the grooves and prevents coating by barium; sparse mucus allows barium to fill the grooves and results in a good demonstration of the areae gastricae. The wide differences in the size of the areae gastricae may be related to variations in parietal cell mass (Mackintosh & Kreel 1977), the areae gastricae being larger in patients with duodenal ulcer (Rose & Stevenson 1981).

*Gastric ulcer* (Figs 9.20, 9.21 and 9.22 and p. 11)

The use of barium studies as opposed to endoscopy in the diagnosis of gastric ulcer is discussed on pp. 12 and 109. The radiological appearances are as follows.

The ulcer crater en face is a round or oval collection of barium or a ring shadow, with barium coating the margins of the crater (Fig. 9.20). In profile, it appears as a conical projection from the lumen. Ulcers may have varying and unusual configurations: linear, rod-shaped or triangular. Most gastric ulcers are situated along the lesser curve and in the distal stomach. There is a preponderance of larger ulcers in the proximal stomach and of smaller ulcers distally (Gelfand et al 1984). Multiple gastric ulcers may occur in up to 23% of patients (Bloom et al 1977) and are frequently small, are often irregular and rarely leave a scar. However, most large benign gastric ulcers heal with a scar and these are seen with a frequency of 1–4% (Gelfand & Ott 1981). Mucosal folds converge towards the scar at the previous ulcer site (Fig. 9.23), which may have a central depression and/or cause gross deformity of the stomach.

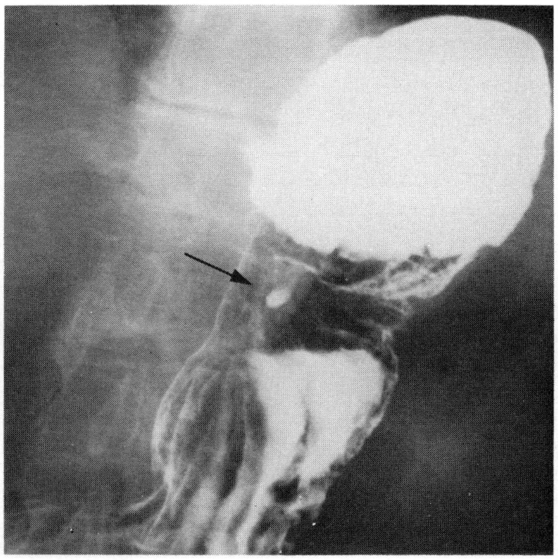

**Fig. 9.20** Gastric ulcer (arrow) high upon the posterior wall of the body of the stomach shown face on. Supine film.

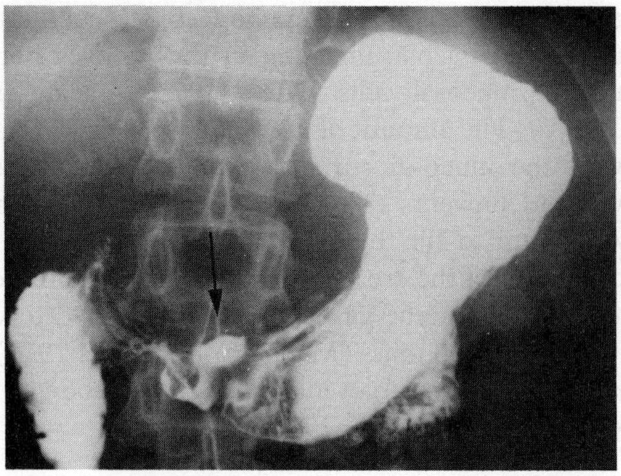

**Fig. 9.21** Simple gastric ulcer (arrow) in the antrum. The filling defect surrounding the ulcer which caused some suspicion of malignancy was due to edema.

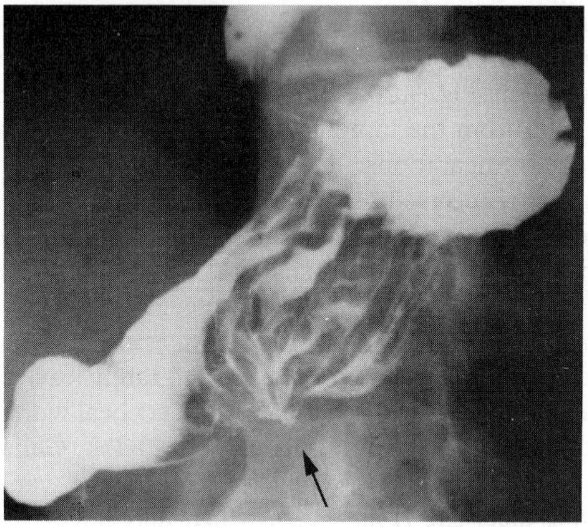

**Fig. 9.22** Simple gastric ulcer (arrow) on greater curvature of stomach in healing phase, with typical radiating folds.

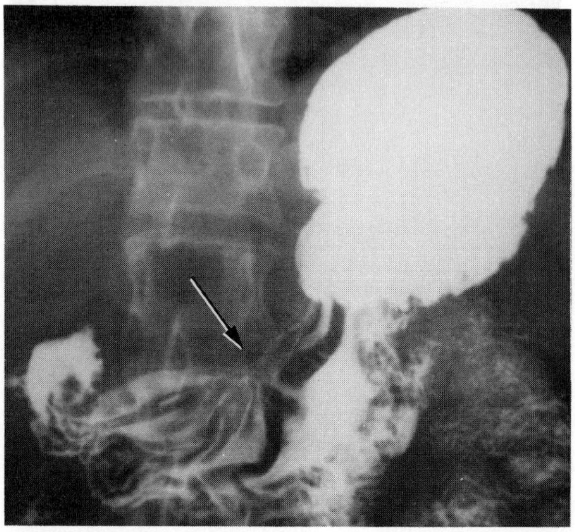

**Fig. 9.23** Scarring (arrow) at the site of a healed gastric ulcer showing typical radiating mucosal folds.

Features suggesting a benign ulcer include: the projection of the crater outside the lumen, sharply defined and smooth margins of the crater, gradual fading of the mound, due to surrounding edema, into the normal mucosa and radiation of the mucosal folds to the margin of the crater (Fig. 9.22) (Ott et al 1985). The areae gastricae, if visible, should be preserved up to the edge of the crater.

In malignant ulceration the crater is mainly intraluminal and its margin may show multiple nodules. The crater is surrounded by an irregular mass often having an abrupt junction with the normal mucosa. Irregular and thickened folds terminate some distance from the crater. A fundal location is often evidence of malignancy but location elsewhere is of little help in decision making. Since malignant ulcers can undergo partial or complete mucosal healing during drug therapy (Sakita et al 1971) we believe that all patients with gastric ulcer diagnosed radiologically should undergo endoscopy and biopsy.

### *Radiology in children*

The normal duodenal cap in the child has a rather irregular contour, leading to an overdiagnosis of duodenal ulceration by radiologists inexperienced with pediatric radiology. Similarly, whilst pylorospasm might suggest the presence of ulceration in an adult it can be a normal feature in children. These features may partly explain the diagnostic disparity between radiology and endoscopy in children (Ament & Christie 1977).

## MEDICAL MANAGEMENT OF PEPTIC ULCER

The medical management of peptic ulceration has advanced markedly over the last two decades with the advent of endoscopy which has allowed accurate diagnosis and assessment of ulcer healing. The introduction of new drugs, assessed rigorously by controlled clinical trials, has demonstrated that medical treatment can speed ulcer healing and provide rapid relief of symptoms as well as delay and decrease the rate of recurrent peptic ulceration. The long-term prevention of relapse and complications of *H. pylori*-associated peptic ulcer by bacterial eradication provides the potential for cure of ulcers.

The efficacy of therapies in preventing relapse of peptic ulcers must take into account the inherent relapse rate of ulcers. Recent clinical trials have provided data on relapse rates in patients receiving placebo preparations which suggest that relapse occurs more rapidly and more frequently than clinical assessment or radiological studies had previously estimated. Relapse rates of 65–80% within 6 months and 80–100% within 1 year have been found in these trials for both duodenal and gastric ulcers. Endoscopy has also shown that one-fifth of ulcers recur in the absence of symptoms.

The remainder of this section will discuss the drugs that are commonly used in the management of peptic ulcer followed by a discussion of their effectiveness in the particular treatment of either duodenal or gastric ulcer.

*Drug therapy for peptic ulceration*

It is now useful to classify the various drugs used in the treatment of peptic ulceration. This enables the physician to select or change therapy on the basis of mechanism of action.

***Receptor-blocking agents.*** The basal and lateral membranes of the parietal cell have three main receptors (Fig. 9.24): for acetylcholine, histamine and gastrin. There may also be an opiate receptor because nalmefine, an opiate receptor antagonist, inhibits acid secretion (Feldman et al 1985). Pirenzepine and $H_2$ receptor antagonists will block the first two, but at present there is no therapeutic agent which blocks the gastrin receptor. In addition there are several hormones which might directly inhibit acid secretion by the parietal cell, including epidermal growth factor, somatostatin and prostaglandins. There are also drugs which will reduce the amount of histamine available at the histamine receptor. For example, the mast cell stabilizer FPL 52694, which is substituted chromone carboxylic acid, will reduce acid secretion by preventing the release of histamine (Reimann et al 1984, Hebnes et al 1986) and histidine decarboxylase inhibitors will reduce the amount of histamine available (Levine et al 1970).

***Inhibitors of secondary messengers.*** Each receptor relays information to its secondary messenger system within the cell (p. 220) and there are several points for potential inhibition of acid secretion. Reduction in the responsiveness of adenylate cyclase may be one of the points of action of endogenous or exogenous prostaglandins but as yet there are no other drugs which act in this way.

***Inhibitors of the proton pump.*** $H^+,K^+$-ATPase, the proton pump, is the final common pathway for the secretion of acid. The inhibition of this pump therefore produces a more reliable and profound inhibition of acid secretion than blockade of any one of the surface receptors.

***Neutralization of acid in the lumen.*** Antacids are designed to effect intragastric neutralization. They continue to be important therapeutically in certain circumstances (stress ulcer).

***Drugs which increase mucosal resistance.*** A variety of drugs enhance mucosal resistance, either generally by influencing the gastric mucosal barrier, e.g. prostaglandins in small doses and sucralfate, or by providing local protection to the ulcer, i.e. site-specific drugs, sucralfate and colloidal bismuth subcitrate.

***Drugs which eradicate*** *H. pylori.* Combination of drugs which reduce acid secretion and antibiotics can effectively treat *H. pylori* infection. These include colloidal bismuth subcitrate or proton pump inhibitors with antibiotics.

***Drugs which act on the central nervous system.***

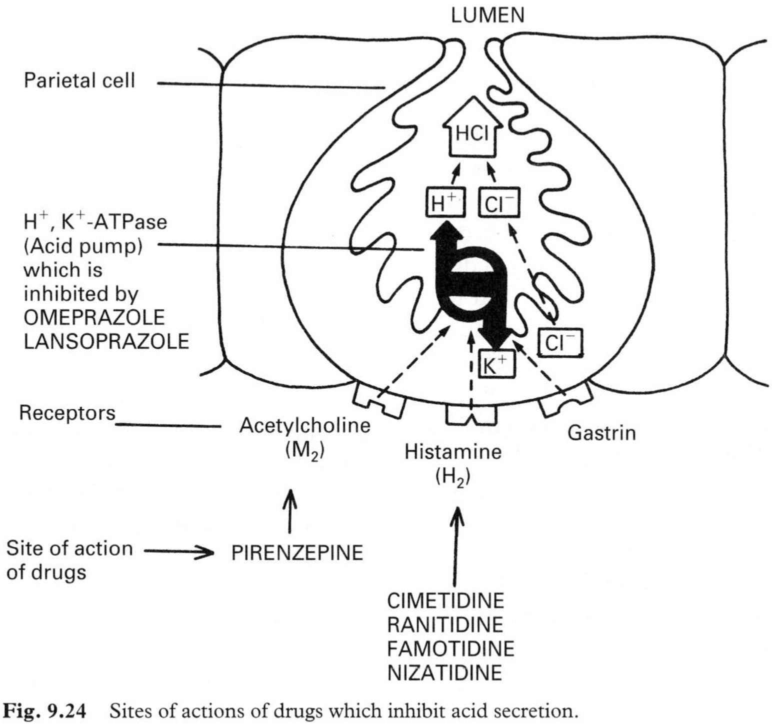


**Fig. 9.24** Sites of actions of drugs which inhibit acid secretion.

Some drugs, e.g. tricyclic antidepressants, probably exert a healing effect on peptic ulceration via central mechanisms.

## Histamine $H_2$ receptor antagonists (Feldman & Burton 1990)

In man there are two distinct types of histamine receptors: $H_1$ and $H_2$ receptors. The actions of histamine on $H_1$ receptors can be blocked by the conventional antihistamines, such as mepyramine, which has no such effect on $H_2$-receptors. Histamine acts on $H_2$ receptors to stimulate gastric acid secretion, to increase the atrial rate of the heart and to inhibit uterine contractions and these effects can be blocked by $H_2$ receptor antagonists (Chand & Eyre 1975). Metiamide and cimetidine have an imidazole ring like histamine. $H_1$ receptor antagonists, which possess a sidechain resembling that in histamine, lack the imidazole ring.

Metiamide was the first $H_2$ receptor antagonist to be used clinically and it inhibited acid secretion in response to a variety of stimulants, histamine, pentagastrin, insulin and food. It also relieved ulcer symptoms and promoted healing of ulcers. However, bone marrow suppression with neutropenia occurred and the drug was withdrawn.

Four $H_2$ receptor antagonists are now available throughout the world: cimetidine, ranitidine, nizatidine and famotidine. Other $H_2$ receptor antagonists include roxatidine (Murdoch & McTavish 1991) and ebrotidine with the latter having gastroprotective and antisecretory properties (Brzozowski et al 1992).

### *Cimetidine*

Cimetidine inhibits the increase in gastric acid secretion in response to histamine, pentagastrin, vagal stimulation and food and inhibits nocturnal acid secretion.

Cimetidine is well absorbed from the small intestine, reaches peak levels in 1–2 h and has a half-life of about 2 h. It is widely distributed throughout the body, apart from the central nervous system. It is given in a dose of 400 mg b.d. It is rapidly excreted by the kidney, mainly as unchanged drug and as the sulfoxide metabolite (Burland et al 1975). It follows that much smaller doses will produce an adequate reduction in acid secretion in patients with renal failure. The following dosages can be used: serum creatinine 0.10–0.20 mmol/L, 200 mg q.i.d; 0.20–0.40 mmol/L, 200 mg t.i.d; greater than 0.40 mmol/L, 200 mg b.d.

### *Ranitidine*

Ranitidine contains a furan ring instead of the imidazole ring of cimetidine. It has the same inhibitory effects on gastric acid secretion as cimetidine. When given intravenously ranitidine is eight times more potent than cimetidine and by mouth it is four times more potent. The increased potency of ranitidine confers a longer duration of action when the drug is used in a dose of 150 mg b.d.

Ranitidine bismuth citrate is a coprecipitate of ranitidine with bismuth citrate providing both gastric acid antisecretory activity and bismuth activity against *H. pylori* (Stables et al 1993).

### *Nizatidine*

This drug is of similar antisecretory potency to ranitidine but it differs in its minimal hepatic clearance after oral administration.

### *Famotidine*

Famotidine contains a thiazole ring instead of the imidazole ring of cimetidine. It has a greater potency and a longer duration of action than either cimetidine or ranitidine (Smith et al 1985), and in a dose of 40 mg once per day, has a healing rate in duodenal ulcer comparable to that of other $H_2$ receptor antagonists (Gitlin et al 1987).

### *Dosages of $H_2$ receptor antagonists*

Similar antisecretory activity of the $H_2$ receptor antagonists is observed with daily doses of cimetidine 800 mg, ranitidine 300 mg, nizatidine 300 mg and famotidine 40 mg (Feldman & Burton 1990). All are absorbed rapidly and apart from nizatidine are subject to extensive first-pass hepatic metabolism. Elimination occurs by a combination of hepatic metabolism, glomerular filtration and renal tubular secretion and thus dosage may need to be adjusted with liver or kidney failure.

The effect of $H_2$ receptor antagonists on intragastric acidity is dose dependent. A sustained decrease of acidity requires dosing four times a day with all agents. Neither gastric emptying or esophageal sphincter function is affected by $H_2$ receptor antagonists. A decrease of intragastric acidity is associated with a rise of plasma gastrin concentration. Chronic dosing with an $H_2$ receptor antagonist is associated with the phenomenon of "tolerance", that is, a small loss of the antisecretory effect. Tolerance develops gradually and reaches a state of equilibrium 1 month after commencement of therapy (Nwokolo et al 1991). The mechanism of this phenomenon is uncertain but may relate to the drug-induced rise of plasma gastrin concentration leading to an increased acid secretory drive.

Sudden withdrawal of $H_2$ receptor antagonist treatment is associated with a transient increase of nocturnal intragastric acidity which resolves within a few days of ceasing treatment (Fullarton et al 1991).

### *Adverse reactions*

$H_2$ receptor antagonists are very well tolerated with a low frequency of nonspecific side-effects including disturbed bowel function, somnolence, headache and fatigue. Idiosyncratic adverse events are rare and include skin rash, anaphylaxis, bone marrow suppression and interstitial nephritis. Mental confusion may develop, particularly in elderly seriously ill patients with multiorgan failure. The binding of dihydrotestosterone to androgen receptors is blocked by cimetidine and its use is associated with gynecomastia in 0.3% of patients (Jones et al 1985) and loss of libido. Gynecomastia is rare with the other $H_2$ receptor antagonists. Cimetidine inhibits the hepatic cytochrome p-450 enzyme system and therefore prolongs the half-life of many drugs including anticoagulants, anticonvulsants and theophylline. These interactions do not occur with ranitidine, famotidine and nizatidine (Sedman 1984).

Cimetidine is secreted by the renal tubules with a 15% increase in the serum creatinine concentration and impaired secretion of theophylline and procainamide. The effect on serum creatinine is due to competition between creatinine and cimetidine for excretion by the renal tubule and is reversed immediately treatment is stopped.

In spite of suggestions that $H_2$ receptor antagonists enhance the absorption of ethanol from the stomach there is no clinically important interaction between $H_2$ receptor antagonists and alcohol (Fraser et al 1992).

### *Potential carcinogenicity of $H_2$ receptor antagonist drugs*

The specter of carcinogenicity in patients receiving $H_2$ receptor antagonist drugs has been raised, particularly in those patients receiving long-term maintenance therapy. Insecurity has been engendered because several developmental $H_2$ receptor antagonist drugs produced gastric tumors or hyperplasia in the stomachs of animals. It should be emphasized that this was not the case with the current $H_2$ receptor antagonists. The potential mechanisms for this occurrence of tumors are (Wormsley 1984): the drug or its metabolite may be a carcinogen; therapeutic inhibition of gastric secretion may allow bacterial colonization of the stomach, with reduction of salivary and dietary nitrate to nitrite which then reacts with secondary and tertiary amines and food proteins to form nitroso compounds; the drug may promote proliferation of components of the gastric mucosa. The 10-year postmarketing surveillance study with cimetidine has been reassuring with only a small, probably unrelated excess of gastric and esophageal malignancy (Colin-Jones et al 1991) (p. 298).

## $H^+$,$K^+$-ATPase inhibitors

Omeprazole, the first of these drugs, acts by irreversible inhibition of $H^+$,$K^+$-ATPase, the gastric proton pump, which is the final step in gastric acid secretion (Maton 1991, Klaassen & de Pont 1994). Omeprazole and the newer similar drugs including lansoprazole (Barradell et al 1992) and pantoprazole (Hannan et al 1992, Classen & della Fave 1994) therefore block acid secretion stimulated by any mechanism.

Omeprazole is degraded by gastric acid and it is formulated in hard gelatin capsules containing enteric-coated granules that release the drug at a pH above 6. Absorption occurs in the small intestine and reaches the gastric parietal cells via the bloodstream. Omeprazole is a weak base, passes through the cell membrane and in the uniquely acidic environment of the intracellular canaliculi of the parietal cell it gains protons and is thus concentrated in this compartment. When protonated, omeprazole changes from an inactive compound to an active form, a sulfonamide, that inhibits $H^+$, $K^+$-ATPase. Acid secretion by the parietal cell resumes when new proton pumps are synthesized.

Omeprazole is rapidly metabolized to inactive forms in blood so that peak plasma concentration occurs 2–4 h after administration and half-life in blood is about 40 min (Anderrson et al 1990). Despite this short half-life, omeprazole 20 mg once daily results in a sustained inhibition of gastric acid secretion with a mean decrease in intragastric acidity of about 80% (Naesdal et al 1984). Almost all duodenal ulcer patients have a profound decrease of intragastric acidity while receiving a morning dose of 40 mg omeprazole, while about one-third respond to 20 mg (Sharma et al 1984).

Adverse events from proton pump inhibitors are uncommon with clinical trials reporting no important side-effects. There is a reduction in vitamin $B_{12}$ absorption (p. 364) but this is not of clinical significance. The pronounced inhibition of gastric acid secretion has been a major source of concern because of development of bacterial overgrowth in the stomach and duodenum, the rise of the plasma gastrin concentration (Clissold & Campoli-Richards 1986) and the theoretical increased susceptibility to enteric infection.

A four-fold rise of the mean 24-h plasma gastrin concentration is observed in duodenal ulcer subjects treated with omeprazole 20 mg daily (Lanzon-Miller et al 1987). Similar changes have been observed with lansoprazole and pantoprazole. Gastrin, a trophic hormone, acts on enterochromaffin-like cells – the ECL cells of the gastric mucosa. Sprague-Dawley rats given high doses of omeprazole for up to 2 years developed, in a dose-dependent manner, gastric carcinoids (Carlsson et al 1986). The same phenomenon has also been demonstrated in the rat with other high-dose, long-term antisecretory drug regimens including ranitidine and lansoprazole (Eason et al 1989, Lee et al 1992). Gastric carcinoids are also a rare complication of patients with pernicious anemia (Borch et al 1985). In the follow-up of patients receiving omeprazole long-term no gastric carcinoids have developed. However, ECL cell hyperplasia is demonstrated often superimposed on a background of accelerated mucosal atrophy (Creutzfeldt & Lamberts 1992).

The $H^+$, $K^+$-ATPase inhibitors have in vitro (Iwahi et al 1991) and in vivo (Sherman et al 1992, Lamouliatte 1993) antibacterial activity against *H. pylori*. Proton pumps are identified in the cell wall of *H. pylori* and may account for the antibacterial action of these agents.

## Colloidal bismuth subcitrate and other bismuth compounds

Colloidal bismuth subcitrate, also termed tripotassium dicitratobismuthate, is a complex bismuth salt of citric acid which precipitates in acid conditions. It has a number of modes of action including cytoprotection of the gastric mucosa and binding to gastric mucus, bile acids and proteins in an ulcer base. In addition, this agent has antibacterial activity against *H. pylori* with the effect of reducing pepsin output and activity, increasing endogenous prostaglandins, improving the duodenal mucosal ultrastructure and increasing binding of epidermal growth factor to ulcer which results in the restitution of gastroduodenal mucosal integrity (Lee 1991).

The action of colloidal bismuth subcitrate and other bismuth compounds is topical with less than 0.042% of ingested bismuth absorbed from colloidal bismuth subcitrate (Dresow et al 1992). Absorption from oral bismuth salicylate nitrate or aluminate is <0.01% of the dose. Colloidal bismuth subcitrate is available as tablet (chew) or coated swallow preparations. One tablet before meals and at night or two tablets twice daily show similar efficacy of ulcer healing. A lower ulcer relapse after initial healing is due to the effect on eradication or suppression of *H. pylori* infection (Lambert 1991).

Side-effects of colloidal bismuth subcitrate include blackening of the tongue (chew preparation) and darkening of the stool, which can be mistaken for melena. No cases of neurotoxicity have been reported with the administration of recommended doses.

Other bismuth preparations including bismuth subsalicylate, bismuth subcitrate and the preparation ranitidine bismuth citrate have been used to treat dyspepsia and peptic ulcer disease. In combination with other antimicrobial agents they are also used to treat *H. pylori* infection. As a single agent colloidal bismuth subcitrate is the most effective of the bismuth compounds in eradicating *H. pylori*.

## Sucralfate

Sucralfate is the aluminum salt of sucrose octasulfate (McCarthy 1991). When taken orally, the tablet forms a viscous paste in the stomach which binds to normal and ulcerated mucosa. The precise mechanism by which sucralfate is beneficial in healing peptic ulcer disease remains unknown. As well as mucosal binding sucralfate has other properties including scavenging oxygen radicals, increasing the production of mucus and gastric and duodenal alkali which in part are mediated via increased prostaglandin production (Hollander et al 1984, 1985). It also adsorbs pepsin and binds bile acids, epidermal growth factor (EGF) and basic fibroblast growth factor (BFGF) (Szabo et al 1991). The EGG and BFGF are thus recruited to the ulcer site.

Sucralfate has a protective effect on drug and alcohol-induced gastric injury in man (Caldwell et al 1987) and animals (Szabo & Brown 1987). After oral administration of sucralfate there is a significant absorption of aluminum with rare reports of aluminum intoxication particularly in patients with kidney failure undergoing dialysis (Marks 1991).

The drug is relatively free of adverse effects except for constipation in up to 15% of patients. Sucralfate, because of its low absorption, decreases the absorption and bioavailability of phenytoin, fluoroquinolone antibiotics, amitriptylline, theophylline, tetracycline, cimetidine and digoxin (McCarthy 1991).

## Prostaglandin analogs

Naturally occurring prostaglandins have a 20-carbon structure and are inactivated at C-15 when given orally. Prostaglandin analogs have been synthesized to contain methyl groups at the C-15 or C-16 position in order to retain activity when orally administered. In spite of the cytoprotective effects of prostaglandin analogs in small doses the clinical benefits are evident at doses that are sufficient to control gastric acid secretion. Misoprostol (15-deoxy, 16-hydroxy, 16-methyl PGE, methyester) and enprostil (dehydro-prostaglandin E2) are the two synthetic agents available (Goa & Monk 1987, Walt 1992).

### *Clinical use of prostaglandins*

Prostaglandins have the theoretical advantage of cytoprotection in the treatment of peptic ulcer. However, their ulcer-healing effect appears to be due to inhibition of acid in that 50 μg misoprostol per day (Brand et al 1985) or 10 μg q.i.d. arbaprostil (Euler et al 1987) is no more effective than placebo. Misoprostol 200 μg four times a day has been shown to be as effective as cimetidine 300 mg four times a day in the healing of gastric and duodenal ulcers (Shield 1985, Nicholson 1985). Prostaglandin probably has an advantage in not increasing serum gastrin levels and in not having a reduced healing effect in smokers. It is not known whether prostaglandin-healed ulcers have a decreased or increased recurrence rate compared to $H_2$ receptor antagonists.

At present there are two unresolved problems with the use of synthetic prostaglandins in peptic ulcer disease. First, diarrhea is a common side-effect; in the trial reported by Vantrappen and colleagues (1982) 34% of patients had this problem. Secondly, prostaglandins can cause hyperplasia of the gastric mucosa but this does not occur in short-term treatment (Herting & Nissen 1986). In the case of misoprostol this is not due to an increase in cellular kinetics (Fich et al 1985). Prostaglandins are contraindicated in pregnancy because of the uterotonic activity.

## Antacids (Halter 1992)

Antacids, chemicals that neutralize gastric hydrochloric acid, are effective in the treatment of peptic ulcers when given in very high doses of over 1000 mmol neutralizing capacity per day (Ippoliti et al 1978). This dose produced diarrhea (magnesium effect) and cimetidine rendered antacids obsolete as primary ulcer therapy. In spite of the studies suggesting low doses of antacids (200 mmol neutralizing capacity per day) are as effective as the original megadoses in primary ulcer therapy (Berstad & Weberg 1986), they are now mainly used for the symptomatic relief of dyspepsia.

### *Side-effects*

Diarrhea due to magnesium salts and constipation caused by aluminum hydroxide are the main side-effects which limit the prolonged use of high doses of antacids, but there are other undesirable effects.

***Acid rebound.*** Calcium antacids produce a rebound increase in acid secretion after their neutralizing effect has subsided; calcium induces the antral mucosa to release gastrin by direct stimulation (Morris & Rhodes 1979). Many physicians feel that because of the hypersecretion induced by calcium antacids these drugs should be excluded from clinical usage; this view is strengthened by studies which suggest that their use delays pain relief.

***The milk alkali syndrome.*** Orwoll (1982) and Burnett et al (1949) used this term to describe a syndrome of severe uremia, hypercalcemia and alkalosis in patients who ingested large amounts of milk and absorbable alkali. The prolonged ingestion of calcium from milk or calcium carbonate leads to hypercalcemia, hypercalciuria and renal impairment. The alkalosis resulting from absorption of sodium or calcium carbonate, together with loss of hydrochloric acid through vomiting, predisposes to nephrocalcinosis since the increased load of calcium phosphate precipitates more readily in alkaline urine. In alkalosis, potassium loss is increased and hypokalemia may result. The patient complains of nocturia, polyuria and polydipsia, together with fatigue, nausea, irritability and dizziness. There is hypercalcemia, alkalosis and renal impairment and hypochloremia, hypokalemia, hyperphosphatemia and hypocalciuria may be present. The syndrome was described particularly in the middle-aged and elderly but it can occur in any individual with predisposing conditions such as renal impairment or diuretic therapy, even when much smaller doses of calcium are consumed.

Treatment involves stopping antacids and milk therapy, rehydration and the provision of a large fluid intake, if necessary with intravenous saline, because of the impaired concentrating ability of the kidneys. Hypokalemia must be corrected. In some cases renal function slowly recovers and in others with either histological or radiological nephrocalcinosis, there is little or no improvement in renal function.

***Interference with other drug therapy*** (Piper 1973). Antacids may affect the absorption of other drugs by adsorbing them or by increasing the intragastric or urinary pH. The absorption of some antibiotics and digoxin is reduced and magnesium hydroxide affects the renal elimination of many drugs by changing urinary pH. Antacids reduce the serum level of salicylates by increasing the pH of the urine, which facilitates their excretion (Levy et al 1975). Antacids do not significantly affect the absorption of $H_2$ receptor antagonist drugs.

***Hypophosphatemia with aluminum antacids.*** Phosphorus depletion, causing weakness, debility and anorexia, has been reported with aluminum antacids; aluminum combines with phosphorus in the intestine and this results in reduced urinary phosphate and raised urinary calcium excretion (Lotz et al 1968). There is increased calcium reabsorption from the bones, leading to osteomalacia (Morris & Rhodes 1979).

***Sodium and edema.*** Most antacids contain enough sodium to cause edema in patients with cardiac failure or hepatic cirrhosis (see also p. 1024). They should not be given to such patients. Low sodium antacids are available.

***Magnesium and aluminum toxicity.*** Small amounts of magnesium and aluminum are absorbed (Kaehny et al 1977) and in patients with renal failure sufficient may be retained to cause magnesium and aluminum toxicity.

### *Antibiotics*

A number of antimicrobial agents with activity against *H. pylori* are now utilized along with proton pump inhibitors and bismuth compounds in subjects with peptic ulcer disease. These include amoxycillin, tetracycline, metronidazole, tinidazole and clarithromycin. These regimens will be discussed below.

## Guidelines to the management of peptic ulcer

Management strategies for peptic ulcer include short-term treatment for relief of symptoms and ulcer healing, as well as long-term prevention of ulcer relapse and complications. In addition some ulcers may be refractory to healing with conventional agents.

General measures include adequate explanation and discussion with ulcer sufferers to alleviate anxiety. This particularly applies to an explanation of *H. pylori* infection. Avoidance of foods which aggrevate symptoms and regular meals are recommended but there is no evidence that other dietary manipulations have any benefit in ulcer healing. Avoidance of smoking, aspirin and NSAIDs in ulcer patients should be recommended. When an analgesic is required paracetamol (acetaminophen) should be recommended.

*Duodenal ulcer*

A wide range of drugs are available for the short-term treatment of duodenal ulcer. Drugs which reduce gastric acid secretion heal duodenal ulcers in relation to the degree of acid suppression (Burget et al 1990). Table 9.6 summarizes duodenal ulcer healing using agents to suppress gastric acid secretion. $H_2$ receptor antagonist drugs are effective in duodenal ulcer healing with cimetidine 400 mg b.i.d. for 4–6 weeks healing the ulcer in 70–80% of patients compared with 30–40% of patients treated with a placebo. Twice daily dosages of cimetidine are comparable to four doses per day or a single high night-time dose. Ranitidine (150 mg b.i.d.), famotidine (20 mg b.i.d.) and nizatidine (150 mg b.i.d.) have similar ulcer healing rates. Relapse occurs when the agents are ceased after initial healing at the same rate as the natural history of the disease.

When patients are receiving other drugs including anticoagulants, anticonvulsants or theophylline preparations, ranitidine, famotidine or nizatidine are recommended.

Ulcer healing rates are almost 100% with more potent acid inhibition from proton pump inhibitors including omeprazole (20 mg once daily)(Wilde & McTavish 1994) and lansoprazole (30 mg once daily). This healing occurs more rapidly and is not influenced by cigarette smoking. When ranitidine 150 mg b.i.d. was compared to omeprazole 20 mg once daily in a double-blind study the latter healed 83% of duodenal ulcers within 2 weeks and 97% within 4 weeks (Bardhan et al 1986); the corresponding figures for ranitidine were 53% and 82%. Similar results can be achieved with lansoprazole.

Sucralfate (4 g/day) (Lam 1991) and colloidal bismuth subcitrate (120 mg × 4/day) result in healing rates similar to those of $H_2$ receptor antagonists. Colloidal bismuth subcitrate and sucralfate achieve ulcer healing in subjects who continue to smoke with cumulative evidence suggesting relapse of 4% per month after colloidal bismuth subcitrate compared to 16% per month after cimetidine (Lambert 1991). This effect is due to the bactericidal effect of the drug on *H. pylori*. Prostaglandin inhibitors achieve ulcer healing primarily due to inhibition of gastric acid with rates of healing similar to those using $H_2$ receptor antagonists (Kollberg & Slezak 1982).

Long-term treatment of duodenal ulcer disease aims to prevent recurrent ulcers as well as complications associated with these recurrences. The ability to diagnose recurrence on symptomatic criteria can be easily achieved without resorting to endoscopy (Hetzel et al 1980). Recurrence of duodenal ulcer can be prevented with long-term $H_2$ receptor antagonists, proton pump inhibitors, eradication of *H. pylori* and surgical procedures to control gastric acid secretion. The rate of ulcer relapse during maintenance treatment with acid-suppressing agents is related to control of nocturnal intragastric acidity (Gough et al 1984). Treatment with ranitidine 300 mg at bedtime results in a low relapse rate compared with rantidine 150 mg at bedtime. Despite prolonged maintenance treatment subjects will relapse at the same rate once treatment is ceased irrespective of how long maintenance therapy has continued (Penston et al 1993). Thus maintenance treatment with an $H_2$ receptor antagonist does not cure duodenal ulcer disease. However, complications such as hemorrhage, perforation or pyloric stenosis appear to be decreased using long-term treatment with low doses of a $H_2$ receptor antagonist (Penston et al 1993). Omeprazole 20 mg daily taken over the long term prevents ulcer recurrence. This is achieved, however, by marked inhibition of gastric acid secretion.

**Table 9.6** Duodenal ulcer healing from published trials meta-analysis

| Drug | Dose | No. patients | Week 4 % healing | Week 8 % healing |
|---|---|---|---|---|
| Cimetidine | 200 mg q.i.d. | 279 | 71 | 90 |
| Cimetidine | 400 mg q.i.d. | 102 | 85 | 100* |
| Cimetidine | 800 mg | 236 | 76 | 92 |
| Enprostil | 35 mg b.i.d. | 134 | 66 | 87† |
| Omeprazole | 20 mg o.m. | 253 | 96 | 97 |
| Ranitidine | 150 mg b.i.d. | 3520 | 81 | 94 |
| Placebo | – | 11 718 | 40 | 49 |

Adapted from Burget et al 1990 * Week 12; † Week 6

## Eradication of *Helicobacter pylori*

A large number of controlled trials and many uncontrolled studies show that eradication of *H. pylori* is associated with prolonged remission or cure of duodenal ulcer disease. Follow-up studies of subjects who had *H. pylori* eradicated reveal a low rate of recurrent ulceration (less than 1%) with no perforation or hemorrhage (Labenz & Borsch 1994, Forbes et al 1994). The coadministration of anti-*Helicobacter pylori* agents along with $H_2$ receptor antagonists or a proton pump inhibitor has been shown to accelerate the healing of duodenal ulcer, as well as markedly eliminating ulcer relapse. The optimal regimen to eradicate *H. pylori* has not yet been established but two alternative regimens have been advocated (Table 9.7). Triple therapy with metronidazole, a bismuth compound (colloidal bismuth subcitrate or bismuth subsalicylate) and either tetracycline or amoxycillin appear to provide

**Table 9.7** Recommended regimens to treat *Helicobacter pylori* infection*

| Drug regimen | Dose | Duration | % eradication |
|---|---|---|---|
| I | | | |
| Bismuth*† | 1 tablet × 4 | 2 weeks | 84 |
| Amoxycillin† | 500 mg × 4 | 2 weeks | |
| Metronidazole | 400 mg × 3 | 2 weeks | |
| II | | | |
| Bismuth* | 1 tablet × 4 | 1 or 2 weeks | 89 |
| Tetracycline* | 500 mg × 4 | 1 or 2 weeks | |
| Metronidazole | 400 mg × 3 | 1 or 2 weeks | |
| III | | | |
| Omeprazole‡ | 20–40 mg b.i.d. | 2 weeks | 73 |
| Amoxycillin | 500 mg × 4 | 2 weeks | |
| IV | | | |
| Omeprazole | 20–40 mg b.i.d. | 2 weeks | 72 |
| Clarithromycin | 500 mg × 3 | 2 weeks | |
| V | | | |
| Omeprazole | 20–40 mg b.i.d. | 1 week | 90 |
| Clarithromycin | 500 mg × 3 | 1 week | |
| Metronidazole | 400 mg × 3 | 1 week | |
| (or amoxycillin) | | | |

* Chiba et al 1992, Tytgat & Noach 1994; † Similar with bismuth subsalicylate, bismuth subnitrate. ‡ Similar with lansoprazole

the best results. The use of proton pump inhibitors (e.g. omeprazole and lansoprazole) along with either amoxycillin or clarithromycin and metronidazole now offer rates of eradication equivalent to that using bismuth triple therapy. The combination of ranitidine bismuth citrate with antibiotics is successful in bacterial eradication in most patients (Wyeth et al 1994). Failure of eradication is associated with poor patient compliance to therapy, metronidazole resistance of the *H. pylori* and predosing with proton pump inhibitors (Tytgat & Noach 1994).

The National Institute of Health consensus statement (NIH 1994) has suggested that *H. pylori* be eradicated in all infected subjects with gastric or duodenal ulcer disease both active and inactive. Follow-up with either endoscopy and antral and body biopsy or the noninvasive tests ($C^{14}$ or $C^{13}$ urea breath tests) is required to ensure that eradication has occurred. These follow-up tests should be undertaken after a minimum of 4 weeks following cessation of therapy. Biopsy of the gastric body is necessary when proton pump inhibitors have been used in the eradication regimen because of migration of the infection into the proximal stomach.

## Refractory duodenal ulcer

Refractory duodenal ulcer is defined as an ulcer that does not respond to medical management and resists healing after 8 weeks of treatment using conventional doses of a $H_2$ receptor antagonist. About 5% of ulcers fail to heal after 8 weeks of treatment (Sonnenberg et al 1981). Others have defined duodenal ulcers as resistant if their size is decreased by less than 25% at 1 month (Lam et al 1984) or as poor responders if they fail to heal with $H_2$ receptor antagonists after treatment for 6 weeks (Gledhill et al 1984). The failure of duodenal ulcers to heal relates to a number of factors including poor compliance to therapy, the continued use of NSAIDs or hypersecretory states such as the Zollinger–Ellison syndrome. Other causes of ulceration in the duodenum not due to peptic ulcer disease include Crohn's disease, tuberculosis, lymphoma, carcinoma or ulceration due to other infections including cytomegalovirus.

Continued dyspepsia after 8 weeks of treatment in a patient with duodenal ulcer disease on full-dose $H_2$ receptor antagonists should lead to repeat endoscopy. Biopsy specimens should be taken from any ulcer site to exclude the rare causes of ulceration (see above). Repeat gastric antral biopsy should be done to determine the *H. pylori* status. If persistent ulceration is evident with no *H. pylori* infection or other etiology observed simple peptic ulceration is an unlikely diagnosis (Nensey et al 1991). A fasting plasma gastrin concentration should be measured to exclude Zollinger–Ellison syndrome. This should be delayed for as long as possible after cessation of therapy commensurate with the patient's symptoms, for the plasma gastrin may be increased by proton pump inhibitors and to a lesser extent by $H_2$ receptor antagonists.

Management strategies for the refractory ulcer include increasing the degree of acid inhibition, the use of site-specific agents, eradication of *H. pylori* and surgical control of gastric acid secretion. High healing rates have been achieved with proton pump inhibitors or high-dose $H_2$ receptor antagonists. If *H. pylori* is present the combination of proton pump inhibitors with antimicrobial agents is appropriate to eradicate the organism. Site-specific agents have been shown to be more effective in refractory ulcer than continuation of $H_2$ receptor antagonists (Lam et al 1984). Patients receiving colloidal bismuth subcitrate one tablet four times a day before meals have achieved 85% healing compared with 40% of patients receiving cimetidine in a dose of 400 mg q.i.d..

It is important to question the patient carefully regarding all other medications including over-the-counter preparations. These may contain aspirin or NSAIDs which will delay healing. Smoking also delays healing and should be discussed with the patient. Patients with resistant duodenal ulcer respond poorly to surgery with a high rate of ulcer recurrence after highly selective vagotomy (Penninckx et al 1990). Truncal vagotomy with antrectomy is the most appropriate procedure in these patients.

## Gastric ulcer – short-term management

Short-term treatment of subjects with gastric ulcer requires an accurate diagnosis based on endoscopy with target biopsy of the edge and/or brushings taken for cytologic examination. Biopsy should also be undertaken after healing has occurred. Attention should be paid to the cessation of smoking and avoidance of aspirin and NSAIDs. Gastric ulcers are often larger than duodenal ulcers and hence take longer to heal. Follow-up endoscopy after 8–12 weeks of treatment is required to confirm complete healing and repeat biopsy and cytologic examination undertaken if malignant change is suspected. $H_2$ receptor antagonists decrease gastric acid secretion in patients with gastric ulcer and result in an increase in the rate of healing at 4 and 8 weeks compared with placebo. The rate of healing is related to the degree of suppression of 24-h intragastric acidity and to the duration of treatment. After 8 weeks of treatment 80–90% of ulcers are healed (Graham et al 1985, Dixon et al 1989). In practice large gastric ulcers may require 12–16 weeks for complete healing. Prepyloric ulcers are often refractory to therapy and may require more prolonged treatment to effect healing (Lauritsen et al 1985, Halter & Eigenmann 1987). Acid suppression using proton pump inhibitors offers little advantage over treatment with conventional doses of an $H_2$ receptor antagonist for patients with benign gastric ulcer (Walan et al 1989). Both sucralfate and colloidal bismuth subcitrate may be used and are as effective an $H_2$ receptor antagonists in ulcer healing. Misoprostol may have a useful role when NSAIDs must be continued but it is not as effective as $H_2$ receptor antagonist therapy in the management of benign gastric ulcer disease.

Recurrence of gastric ulcer after initial healing is probably less common than with duodenal ulcer. Approximately 50% of gastric ulcers relapse within a year of healing with the relapse rate higher in those who smoke, in those using aspirin or NSAIDs and in those with prepyloric ulcers. Eradication of *H. pylori* infection decreases the relapse rate in 12-month follow-up studies. Maintenance therapy with $H_2$ receptor antagonists is recommended for patients with complicated ulcer disease particularly in the elderly who have had hemorrhage and in those with severe concurrent illness.

### Peptic ulcer disease and arthritis

Patients with rheumatoid arthritis or osteoarthritis requiring NSAIDs who develop upper gastrointestinal symptoms or ulceration present considerable management problems. NSAIDs should not be used unless all physical measures and other simple paracetamol (acetaminophen) based analgesics have been tried.

Dyspepsia occurs in 5–25% of aspirin or NSAID users and may simply be due to intolerance to the drug or its formulation. The drug should be taken with meals or another NSAID formulation tried.

When symptoms persist or if subjects have a previous history of peptic ulcer disease endoscopy is indicated. The risk of gastroduodenal complications relates to age, duration, dose and number of NSAIDs, previous history of ulcer disease and concomitant corticosteroid use (Fries et al 1989). The role of *H. pylori* infection in predisposing to mucosal damage from NSAIDs is unclear (Laine et al 1992). If an ulcer or erosions are found a number of measures can be instituted. Reduction or cessation of NSAIDs should be attempted. If necessary suppositories should be used but these do not entirely prevent the development of mucosal lesions. "Second-line" or "disease-modifying" drugs such as gold, chloroquine, methotrexate and sulfasalazine should be used. NSAID-induced dyspepsia often responds to therapy with $H_2$ receptor antagonists (Biljsma 1988). Chronic ulcers diagnosed endoscopically should be treated by the normal measures. Gastric and duodenal ulcers respond to $H_2$ receptor antagonists, proton pump inhibitors, sucralfate and colloidal bismuth subcitrate. More prolonged therapy may be required for complete ulcer healing (Manniche et al 1987).

Prophylaxis with $H_2$ receptor antagonists and proton pump inhibitors is useful in the prevention of duodenal ulcers in those patients taking NSAIDs, but they are not prophylactic for gastric ulceration (Ehsanullah et al 1988). Prophylaxis with misoprostol has been shown to be effective in NSAID-induced gastric ulcer disease (Graham et al 1988).

### Therapy in children

Therapy for peptic ulcer disease is similar to that in adult patients with reduction of gastric acid of primary consideration. $H_2$ receptor antagonists have been recommended in children, including cimetidine and ranitidine (Bradbear et al 1982, Chin et al 1982, Blumer et al 1985). The dose of cimetidine of 20–25 mg/kg per day is recommended (Chin et al 1982) with the side-effects of cerebral toxicity and cholestasis reported (Bale et al 1979). An oral dose of ranitidine of 1.25–1.90 mg/kg orally every 12 h appears to be effective in achieving a greater than 90% suppression of gastric acid output (Blumer et al 1985). Eradication of *H. pylori* is achieved using similar regimens to the adult population. Experience with prostaglandin analogs, colloidal bismuth subcitrate, sucralfate and proton pump inhibitors is more limited in the pediatric age group.

## ZOLLINGER–ELLISON SYNDROME (GASTRINOMA) (Berg & Wolfe 1991)

This syndrome was first reported in 1955 by Zollinger and Ellison and is associated with intractable peptic ulceration, gastric acid hypersecretion, non-β islet cell tumor or hyperplasia or both and diarrhea (40% of patients). The tumor was found to contain gastrin in various molecular forms including small gastrin (G-17) and big gastrin (G-34) and circulating immunoreactive gastrin concentrations were abnormally high (Gregory et al 1967).

## Pathology

The pancreas is the most common site of the tumor (85%) with ectopic tumors found in the duodenum (13%), with 1% in the stomach, upper jejunum and biliary tree (Antonioli et al 1987). Approximately 60% of islet cell tumors are malignant and metastases are found at the time of diagnosis in approximately two-thirds of such cases. The histology and ultrastructure of gastrinomas show variations within and between tumors (Dawson 1976, Creutzfeldt et al 1978). Occasionally a palpable tumor in the pancreas may not be found, instead there is hyperplasia or microadenoma of pancreatic endocrine cells.

Examination of the stomach in Zollinger–Ellison syndrome has shown that the parietal cell mass is increased, reflecting the trophic effects of circulating gastrin. Histological examination of the duodenum and jejunum reveal that the villi are blunted or absent and there may be an infiltrate of polymorphs and eosinophils (Shimoda et al 1968). Gastric metaplasia of the duodenum and hypertrophy of Brunner's glands may be present (Solcia et al 1980).

## Etiology

In about two-thirds of patients gastrinomas are sporadic with no family history (McCarthy 1984b). One-third have features of the multiple endocrine neoplasia syndrome (MEN type I) (see p. 1301). The sporadic gastrinomas occur in the pancreas and also in the walls of the stomach, duodenum and jejunum with malignancy more likely when they occur in the pancreas. By contrast most tumors associated with MEN-I are small, multiple, benign and pancreatic in origin.

## Clinical features

This disorder most commonly occurs in the third or fourth decade and is characterized by a history of peptic ulceration of many years duration before the more florid symptoms of the Zollinger–Ellison syndrome develop. The patient may also present with bleeding, perforation or diarrhea (Ellison & Wilson 1964). Previously this disorder was not recognized until gastric surgery was performed when perforation or bleeding from a recurrent ulcer, often in the postoperative period, ensued. Most patients are now diagnosed when a compatible clinical presentation leads to the ordering of a test to determine serum gastrin concentration which is abnormally high. Resistance to healing with standard ulcer-healing drugs or severe esophagitis in the absence of *H. pylori* in the gastric mucosa suggests the diagnosis of Zollinger–Ellison syndrome. A family history of other endocrine tumors and diarrhea is fairly common. Diarrhea may precede the ulcer symptoms by years and can occur when there is no ulcer (Ellison & Wilson 1964). Diarrhea is caused by high volumes of hydrochloric acid entering the small intestine with resulting damage to the absorptive mucosa and by steatorrhea due to the inactivation of pancreatic lipase and a precipitation of bile acids at a low pH. Formation of micelles is impaired by the low pH. Along with the denaturing of pancreatic lipase, this leads to malabsorption of fat. Endoscopy will demonstrate severe esophagitis, prominent gastric rugal folds with visible hypersecretion, erosive duodenitis, ulcers and erosions in the postbulbar region and occasionally duodenal ulcers.

## Diagnosis

The diagnosis may be suspected from measurements of gastric acid secretion, along with assay of serum gastrin. Basal acid output in most untreated patients with Zollinger–Ellison syndrome will be greater than 15 mmol/h and a ratio of basal to maximal acid secretion greater than 0.6. The 12-h overnight secretion of more than 100 mmol of acid is normally seen. Most patients with gastrinoma have a fasting serum gastrin of greater than 1000 pg/ml, but values of less than 500 pg/ml do occur and normal values have been recorded (Wolfe et al 1985). When the fasting serum gastrin is less than 1000 pg/ml a secretin test should be performed (see p. 224).

### *Localization of tumor* (p. 1302)

Tumor localization may rarely occur following endoscopy or barium studies but in most cases more sophisticated techniques, including ultrasonography (Fig. 51.12), computed tomography and selective arteriography, are required (p. 27). Percutaneous transhepatic portal venous sampling should only be undertaken when computed tomography and selective arteriography have failed to demonstrate the tumor (Lunderquist 1985). A positive result is a large difference in gastrin concentration between the vein and the systemic circulation. Endoscopic ultrasonography (p. 125) is now recognized as a valuable technique. Intraoperative ultrasonography is also of value (p. 1303).

Laparotomy must be regarded as the most important diagnostic procedure in some patients. If the tumor is not found in the pancreas the duodenal wall must be carefully examined along with other upper abdominal organs. Resectable tumors can be found in 40–70% of patients who have surgery, with about 20–30% achieving a cure.

## Treatment

The two goals of management are control of acid hypersecretion and removal of tumors. Adequate pharmacological control of acid secretion with the proton pump inhibitors is now the mainstay of treatment. Gastric acid secretion is generally controlled by omeprazole 60 mg once daily; however, twice daily dosing may be required in a small percentage of patients (Metz et al 1993). Lansoprazole similarly controls gastric acid secretion with a mean dose of 60 mg once or twice each day (Jensen et al 1993). Long-term use of proton pump inhibitors has been effective. The long-acting synthetic octapeptide analog of somatostatin, octreotide acetate, is effective in suppressing gastric acid secretion and results in symptomatic improvement in subjects with gastrinoma (Ahlman & Tisell 1987).

Follow-up and the dosage of drug is determined by acid concentration, i.e. titrate dose to keep acid output to 5–7 mmol/h.

*Surgery*

With the advent of potent antisecretory drugs total gastrectomy is no longer needed routinely for the reduction of acid secretion. The major role of surgery is now to locate and excise the tumor whenever possible. Highly selective vagotomy in patients with disseminated tumor often makes the medical management with antisecretory drugs much easier. The surgical cure rate is still only one in seven of all patients and one in two of those with duodenal wall tumors. Surgery for any MEN-I tumors is controversial as they are often small and multiple and surgical cure is difficult. In patients with MEN-I and primary hyperparathyroidism a parathyroidectomy should be performed as reduction in serum calcium may markedly reduce serum gastrin concentrations and gastric acid output. The 10-year survival rate is 50% in subjects who undergo surgery for Zollinger–Ellison syndrome (Zollinger 1985).

Chemotherapy and other methods of treatment are discussed on p. 1304.

REFERENCES


Ahlman H, Tisell L E 1987 The use of long-acting somatostatin analogue in the treatment of advanced endocrine malignancies with gastrointestinal symptoms. Scandinavian Journal of Gastroenterology 22: 938–942

Ainley C C, Forgacs I C, Keeling P W, Thompson P P 1986 Outpatient endoscopic survey of smoking and peptic ulcer. Gut 27: 648–651

Ainsworth M A, Hogan D L, Koss M A, Isenberg J I 1993 Cigarette smoking inhibits acid-stimulated duodenal mucosal bicarbonate secretion. Annals of Internal Medicine 119: 882–886

Aird I, Bentall H H, Mehigan J A, Roberts J A F 1954 The blood groups in relation to peptic ulceration and carcinoma of colon, rectum, breast, and bronchus. An association between the ABO groups and peptic ulceration. British Medical Journal 2: 315–321

Alexander F 1934 The influence of psychologic factors upon gastro-intestinal disturbances; general principles, objectives, and preliminary results. Psychoanalytical Quarterly 3: 501–539

Allen A 1989 Gastrointestinal mucus. In: Schultz S G, Forte J G (eds) Handbook of physiology. Section 6. The gastrointestinal system. Vol III. Salivary, gastric, pancreatic and hepatobiliary secretion. American Physiological Society, Bethesda, p 359–382

Ament M E, Christie D L 1977 Upper gastrointestinal fibreoptic endoscopy in pediatric patients. Gastroenterology 72: 1244–1248

Andersson T, Andren K, Cederberg C, Lagerstrom P O, Lundborg P, Skanberg I 1990 Pharmacokinetics and bioavailability of omeprazole after single and repeated oral administration in healthy subjects. British Journal of Clinical Pharmacology 29: 557–563

Antonioli D A, Dayal Y, Dvorak A M, Banks PA 1987 Zollinger–Ellison syndrome. Cure by surgical resection of a jejunal gastrinoma containing growth hormone releasing factor. Gastroenterology 92: 814–823

Asako H, Kubes P, Wallace J L, Gaginella T, Wolfe R E, Granger D N 1992 Indomethacin-induced leukocyte adhesion in mesenteric venules: role of lipoxygenase products. American Journal of Physiology 262: G903–908

Baldwin G S, Chandler R, Grego B, Rubira M R, Seet K L, Weinstock J 1994 Isolation and partial amino acid sequence of a 78 kDa porcine gastrin-binding protein. International Journal of Biochemistry 26: 529–538

Bale J F, Roberts C, Book L S 1979 Cimetidine-induced cerebral toxicity in children. Lancet 1: 725–726

Barclay G, Maxwell V, Grossman M I, Solomon T E 1983 Effects of graded amounts of intragastric calcium on acid secretion, gastrin release, and gastric emptying in normal and duodenal ulcer subjects. Digestive Disease and Sciences 28: 385–391

Bardhan K D, Bianchi Porro G, Bose K et al 1986 A comparison of two different doses of omeprazole versus ranitidine in the treatment of duodenal ulcers. Journal of Clinical Gastroenterology 8: 408–413

Baron J H 1970. The clinical use of gastric function tests. Scandanavian Journal of Gastroenterology 5 (suppl 6): 9–46

Baron J H 1978 Clinical tests of gastric secretion: history, methodology and interpretation. Macmillan, London

Baron J H, Griffen W O Jr, Alexander-Williams J 1975 Use and abuse of gastric function tests by British and American gastric surgeons. American Journal of Digestive Diseases 20: 370

Baron J H, Gribble R J N, Rhodes C, Wright P A 1978 Serum carbenoxolone in patients with gastric and duodenal ulcer. Absorption, efficacy and side effects. Gut 19: 330

Barradell L B, Faulds D, McTavish D 1992 Lansoprazole. A review of its pharmacodynamic and pharmacokinetic properties and its therapeutic efficacy in acid-related disorders. Drugs 44: 225–250

Berg C L, Wolfe M M 1991 Zollinger–Ellison syndrome. Medical Clinics of North America 75: 903–921

Berstad A, Weberg R 1986 Antacids in the treatment of gastroduodenal ulcer. Scandanavian Journal of Gastroenterology 21: 385

Bijlsma J W J 1988 Treatment of endoscopy-negative NSAID-induced upper gastrointestinal symptoms with cimetidine: an international collaborative study. Alimentary Pharmacology and Therapeutics 2 (suppl 1): 75–83

Bilbao M K, Frische L H, Rosch J, Benson J A, Dotter C T 1971 Post-bulbar duodenal ulcer and ring stricture. Cause and effect. Radiology 100: 27

Billington B P 1965 Observations from New South Wales on the changing incidence of gastric ulcer in Australia. Gut 6: 121–133

Black J W, Duncan W A, Durant G J et al 1972 Definition and antagonism of histamine $H_2$ receptors. Nature 236: 385–390

Bloom S M, Paul R E, Matsue H, Poplack W E, Goldsmith M R 1977 Improved radiographic detection of multiple gastric ulcers. American Journal of Roentgenology 128: 949

Blumenthal I S 1968 Digestive disease as a national problem. III Social cost of peptic ulcer. Gastroenterology 54: 86

Blumer J L, Rothstein F C, Kaplan B S et al 1985 Pharmacokinetic determination of ranitidine pharmacodynamics in pediatric ulcer disease. Journal of Pediatrics 107: 301

Boles R S, Westerman M P 1954 Seasonal incidence and precipitating causes of hemorrhage from peptic ulcer. Journal of the American Medical Association 156: 1379–1383

Bonnevie O 1975a The incidence of duodenal ulcer in Copenhagen County. Scandinavian Journal of Gastroenterology 10: 385

Bonnevie O 1975b The incidence of gastric ulcer in Copenhagen County. Scandinavian Journal of Gastroenterology 10: 231

Bonney G L W, Pickering G W 1948 Observations on the mechanism of pain in ulcer of the stomach and duodenum. 1. The nature of the stimulus. Clinical Science 6: 63

Borch K, Renvall H, Liedburg G 1985 Gastric endocrine cell hyperplasia and carcinoid tumors in pernicious anaemia. Gastroenterology 88: 638–648

Borody T J, Andrews P, Jankiewicz E, Ferch N, Carroll M 1993 Apparent reversal of early gastric mucosal atrophy after triple therapy for *Helicobacter pylori*. American Journal of Gastroenterology 88: 1266–1268

Borromeo M, Lambert J R, Pinkard K J 1987 Evaluation of "CLO test" to detect *Campylobacter pyloridis* in gastric mucosa. Journal of Clinical Pathology 40: 462–463

Boyd E J, Wilson J A, Wormsley K G 1984 The fate of asymptomatic recurrences of duodenal ulcer. Scandinavian Journal of Gastroenterology 19: 808–812

Bradbear R A, Shepherd R W, Grice J, O'Toole J, Roberts R K 1982 Cimetidine use in children with cystic fibrosis: inhibition of hepatic drug metabolism. Journal of Pediatrics 100: 325

Bradley R L, Bradley E J 1966 Seasonal incidence of perforated ulcer. American Journal of Surgery 111: 656–658

Brand D L, Roufail W M, Thomason A B R, Tapper E J 1985 Misoprostol, a synthetic $PGE_1$ analog, in the treatment of duodenal ulcers. A multicenter double-blind study. Digestive Diseases and Sciences 30: 147S

Braver J M, Paul R E, Philipps E, Bloom S 1979 Roentgen diagnosis of linear ulcers. Radiology 132: 29

Brown K E, Peura D A 1993 Diagnosis of *Helicobacter pylori* infection. Gastroenterology Clinics of North America 22(1): 105–115

Brzozowski T, Majka J, Konturek S J 1992 Gastroprotective and ulcer-healing activities of a new $H_2$-receptor antagonist: ebrotidine. Digestion 51: 27–36

Burget D W, Chiverton S G, Hunt R H 1990 Is there an optimal degree of acid suppression for healing of duodenal ulcers? A model of the relationship between ulcer healing and acid suppression. Gastroenterology 99: 345–351

Burland W L, Sharpe P C, Colin-Jones D G, Turnbull P R G, Bowskill P 1975 Reversal of metiamide-induced agranulocytosis during treatment with cimetidine. Lancet 2: 1085

Burman P, Mardh S, Norberg L, Karlsson F A 1989 Parietal cell antibodies in pernicious anemia inhibit $H^+$, $K^+$-adenosine triphosphatase, the proton pump of the stomach. Gastroenterology 96: 1434–1438

Burnett C H, Commons R R, Albright F, Howard J E 1949 Hypercalcemia without hypercalciuria or hypophosphatemia, calcinosis and renal insufficiency. A syndrome following prolonged intake of milk and alkali. New England Journal of Medicine 240: 787

Bynum T E, Solomon T E, Johnson L R, Jacobson E D 1972 Inhibition of pancreatic function in man by cigarette smoking. Gut 13: 361–365

Caldwell J R, Roth S H, Wu W C et al 1987 Sucralfate treatment of nonsteroidal antiinflammatory drug-induced gastrointestinal symptoms and mucosal damage. American Journal of Medicine 83: 74

Cameron A J 1975 Aspirin and gastric ulcer. Mayo Clinic Proceedings 50: 565

Capper W M, Airth G R, Kilby J O 1966 A test for pyloric regurgitation. Lancet 2: 621–623

Card W I, Marks I N 1960 The relationship between the acid output of the stomach following "maximal" histamine stimulation and the parietal cell mass. Clinical Science 19: 147–163

Carlsson E, Larsson H, Mattsson H, Ryberg B, Sundell C 1986 Pharmacology and toxicology of omeprazole – with special reference to the effects on the gastric mucosa. Scandanavian Journal of Gastroenterology 21 (suppl 118): 31

Carrick J, Lee A, Hazell S, Ralston M, Daskalopoulos G 1989 *Campylobacter pylori*, duodenal ulcer, and gastric metaplasia: possible role of functional heterotopic tissue in ulcerogenesis. Gut 30: 790–797

Carson J L, Strom B L, Soper K A, West S L, Morse M L 1987 The association of nonsteroidal anti-inflammatory drugs with upper gastrointestinal tract bleeding. Archives of Internal Medicine 147: 85–88

Caruso I, Porro B G 1980 Gastroscopic evaluation of anti-inflammatory agents. British Medical Journal 280: 75–78

Chand N, Eyre P 1975 Classification and biological distribution of histamine receptor sub-types. Agents and Actions 5: 277

Chen M C Y, Amirian D A, Toomey M, Sanders M J, Soll A H 1988 Prostanoid inhibition of canine parietal cells: mediation by the inhibitory guanosine triphosphate-binding protein of adenylate cyclase. Gastroenterology 94: 1121–1129

Cheng F C Y, Lam S K, Ong G B 1977 Maximum acid output to graded doses of pentagastrin and its relation to parietal cell mass in Chinese patients with duodenal ulcer. Gut 18: 827–832

Chiang B L, Chang M H, Lin M I, Hsu J Y, Wang C Y, Wang T H 1989 Chronic duodenal ulcer in children: clinical observation and response to treatment. Journal of Pediatric Gastroenterology and Nutrition 8: 161–165

Chiba N, Rao B V, Rademaker J W, Hunt R H 1992 Meta-analysis of the efficacy of antibiotic therapy in eradicating *Helicobacter pylori*. American Journal of Gastroenterology 87: 1716–1727

Chin T W, MacLeod S M, Fenje P, Baltodano A, Edmonds J F, Soldin S J 1982 Pharmacokinetics of cimetidine in critically ill children. Pediatric Pharmacology 2: 285–292

Classen M 1973 Endoscopy in benign peptic ulcer. Clinics in Gastroenterology 2: 315–327

Classen M, della Fave G 1994 Management of acid-related diseases: focus on pantoprazole. Alimentary Pharmacology and Therapeutics 8 (suppl 1): 1–70

Clissold S P, Campoli-Richards D M 1986 Omeprazole, an updated review. Drugs 32: 15–47

Coggon D, Lambert P, Langman M J S 1981 20 years of hospital admissions for peptic ulcer in England and Wales. Lancet 1: 1302–1304

Colin-Jones D G, Langman M J S, Lawson D H, Logan R F, Paterson K R, Vessey M P 1991 Post-cimetidine surveillance for up to ten years: incidence of carcinoma of the stomach and oesophagus. Quarterly Journal of Medicine 78(285): 13–19

Conn H O, Blitzer B L 1976 Nonassociation of adrenocorticosteroid therapy and peptic ulcer. New England Journal of Medicine 294: 473–479

Cooke A R 1967 Corticosteroids and peptic ulcer: is there a relationship? American Journal of Digestive Diseases 12: 323

Cooke L, Hutton C F 1958 Postbulbar duodenal ulceration. Lancet 1: 754–759

Cotton P B, Shorvon P J 1984 Analysis of endoscopy and radiography in the diagnosis, follow-up and treatment of peptic ulcer disease. Clinics in Gastroenterology 13: 383

Cox A J 1952 Stomach size and its relation to chronic peptic ulcer. Archives of Pathology 54: 407–422

Crean G P, Holden R J 1983 Problem areas in diagnosis In: Carter D C (ed) Clinical surgery international (vol 7). Churchill Livingstone, Edinburgh, p 44

Creutzfeldt W, Lamberts R 1992 Inter-relationship between serum gastrin levels, gastric mucosal histology and gastric endocrine cell growth. Digestion 51 (suppl 1): 76–81

Creutzfeldt W, Arnold R, Frerichs H 1978 Insulinomas and gastrinomas. In: Bloom S R (ed) Gut hormones. Churchill Livingstone, Edinburgh, p 589–598

Croft D N 1963 Aspirin and the exfoliation of gastric epithelial cells. Cytological and biochemical observations. British Medical Journal 2: 897

Czaja A J, McAlhany J C, Pruitt B A 1974 Acute gastroduodenal disease after thermal injury. An endoscopic evaluation of incidence and natural history. New England Journal of Medicne 291: 925–929

Davenport H W 1964 Gastric mucosal injury by fatty and acetylsalicylic acids. Gastroenterology 46: 245–253

Davenport H W 1967 Salicylate damage to the gastric mucosal barrier. New England Journal of Medicine 276: 1307

Dawson I M P 1976 The endocrine cells of the gastro-intestinal tract and the neoplasms which arise from them. In: Morson B C (ed) Pathology of the gastro-intestinal tract. Springer-Verlag, Berlin, p 221

De Aizpurua H J, Cosgrove L J, Ungar B, Toh B H 1983 Autoantibodies cytotoxic to gastric parietal cells in serum of patients with pernicious anemia. New England Journal of Medicine 309: 625–629

Debas H T 1987 Peripheral regulation of gastric acid secretion. In: Johnson L R, Christensen J, Jackson M J, Jacobson E D, Walsh J H (eds) Physiology of the gastrointestinal tract, Vol 2, 2nd edn. Raven Press, New York, p 931

De Roos A, Op den Orth J O 1983 Linear niches in the duodenal bulb. American Journal of Roentgenology 140:941
Dixon J S, Worthington P R, Mills J G, Wood J R 1989 Geographical differences of gastric ulcer healing rate in patients treated with ranitidine or placebo. Alimentary Pharmacology and Therapeutics 3: 353–365
Doll R, Jones F A, Bukatzsch M M 1951 Occupational factors in the aetiology of gastric and duodenal ulcers with an estimate of their incidence in the general population. Medical Research Council, Special Report Series No. 276. HMSO, London, p 1–96
Donaldson R M 1987 Intrinsic factor and the transport of cobalamin. In: Johnson L R, Christensen J, Jackson M J, Jacobson E D, Walsh J H (eds) Physiology of the gastrointestinal tract, Vol 2, 2nd edn. Raven Press, New York, p 959
Dresow B, Fischer R, Gabbe E E, Wendel J, Heinrich H C 1992 Bismuth absorption from 205-bi-labelled pharmaceutical bismuth compounds used in the treatment of peptic ulcer disease. Scandinavian Journal of Gastroenterology 27: 333–336
Driks M R, Craven D E, Celli B R et al 1987 Nosocomial pneumonia in intubated patients given sucralfate compared with antacids or histamine type 2 blockers. The role of gastric colonization. New England Journal of Medicine 317: 1376–1382
Drumm B, Perez-Perez G I, Blaser M J, Sherman P M 1990 Intrafamilial clustering of *Helicobacter pylori* infection. New England Journal of Medicine 322: 359–363
Duggan J M, Dobson A J, Johnson H, Fahey P 1986 Peptic ulcer and non-steroidal anti-inflammatory agents. Gut 27: 929–933
Dunn B E 1993 Pathogenic mechanisms of *Helicobacter pylori*. Gastroenterology Clinics of North America 22: 43–57
Durham R M, Shapiro M J 1991 Stress gastritis revisited. Surgical Clinics of North America 71: 791–810
Earlam R 1976 A computerized questionnaire analysis of duodenal ulcer symptoms. Gastroenterology 71: 314
Eason C T, Spencer A J, Pattison A, Bonner F W 1989 The trophic effects of gastrin on fundic neuroendocrine cells of the rat stomach. Alimentary Pharmacology and Therapeutics 3: 245–251
Edwards F C, Coghill N F 1968 Clinical manifestations in patients with chronic atrophic gastritis, gastric ulcer, and duodenal ulcer. Quarterly Journal of Medicine 37: 337
Ehsanullah R S, Page M C, Tildesley G, Wood J R 1988 Prevention of gastroduodenal damage induced by non-steroidal anti-inflammatory drugs: controlled trial of ranitidine. British Medical Journal 297: 1017–1021
Elashoff J D, Grossman M I 1980 Trends in hospital admissions and death rates for peptic ulcer in the United States from 1970 to 1978. Gastroenterology 78: 280–285
Ellison E H, Wilson S D 1964 The Zollinger–Ellison syndrome: reappraisal and evaluation of 260 registered cases. Annals of Surgery 160: 512–530
Euler A R, Tytgat G, Berenguer J et al 1987 Failure of a cytoprotective dose of arbaprostil to heal active duodenal ulcers. Results of a multiclinic trial. Gastroenterology 92: 604
Feldman M 1989 Gastric secretion in health and disease. In: Sleisenger M H, Fordtran J S (eds) Gastrointestinal disease. Pathophysiology, diagnosis, management, 4th edn. W B Saunders, Philadelphia, p 713–734
Feldman M, Burton M E 1990 Histamine$_2$-receptor antagonists. Standard therapy for acid-peptic diseases (two parts). New England Journal of Medicine 323: 1672–1680, 1749–1755
Feldman M, Richardson C T, Fordtran J S 1980 Effect of sham feeding on gastric acid secretion in healthy subjects and duodenal ulcer patients: evidence for increased basal vagal tone in some ulcer patients. Gastroenterology 79: 796–800
Feldman M, Moore L, Walsh J H 1985 Effect of oral nalmefene, an opiate-receptor antagonist, on meal-stimulated gastric acid secretion and serum gastrin concentration in man. Regulatory Peptides 11: 245–250
Fich A, Arber N, Sestieri M, Zajicek G, Rachmilewitz D 1985 Effect of misoprostol and cimetidine on gastric cell labeling index. Gastroenterology 89: 57–61
Forbes G M, Glaser M E Cullen D J E et al 1994 Duodenal ulcer treated with *Helicobacter pylori* eradication: seven-year follow-up. Lancet 343: 258–260
Fraser A G, Hudson M, Sawyer A M, Smith M, Rosalki S B, Pounder R E 1992 Ranitidine, cimetidine, famotidine have no effect on post-prandial absorption of ethanol 0.8 g/kg taken after an evening meal. Alimentary Pharmacology and Therapeutics 6: 693–700
Friedman G D, Siegelaub A B, Seltzer C C 1974 Cigarettes, alcohol, coffee and peptic ulcer. New England Journal of Medicine 290: 469–473
Fries J F, Miller S R, Spitz P W, Williams C A, Hubert H B, Bloch D A 1989 Toward an epidemiology of gastropathy associated with nonsteroidal antiinflammatory drug use. Gastroenterology 96: 647–655
Fritsch W P, Hausamen T U, Rick W 1976 Gastric and extragastric gastrin release in normal subjects, in duodenal ulcer patients, and in patients with partial gastrectomy (Billroth I). Gastroenterology 71: 552–557
Frydman G M, Penney A G, Malcontenti C, O'Brien P E 1991 Inability of cytoprotection to occur during a period of gastric ischemia. Digestive Diseases and Sciences 36: 1353–1360
Fullarton G M, El Nujumi A M, McColl K E 1991 Gastroduodenal pH and duodenal ulcer pain. Gut 33 (abstract T194): S49
Gelfand D W, Ott D J 1981 Gastric ulcer scars. Radiology 140: 37
Gelfand D W, Dale W J, Ott D J 1984 The location and size of gastric ulcer: radiological and endoscopic evaluation. American Journal of Gastroenterology 143: 755
Gelfand D W, Dale W J, Ott D J 1985a Duodenitis: endoscopic-radiologic correlation in 272 patients. Radiology 157: 577–581
Gelfand D W, Dale W J, Ott D J 1985b Effects of examiner variability, ulcer size and technique on duodenal ulcer detection. Proceedings XVI International Congress of Radiology, Hawaii
Gerber L H, Rooney P J, McCarthy D M 1981 Healing of peptic ulcers during continuing anti-inflammatory drug therapy in rheumatoid arthritis. Journal of Clinical Gastroenterology 3: 7–11
Gibinski K, Rybicka J, Nowak A et al 1982 Seasonal occurrence of abdominal pain and endoscopic findings in patients with gastric and duodenal ulcer disease. Scandinavian Journal of Gastroenterology 17: 481–485
Gillies M, Skyring A 1968 Gastric ulcer, duodenal ulcer and gastric carcinoma: a case-control study of certain social and environmental factors. Medical Journal of Australia 2: 1132–1136
Gitlin N, McCullough A J, Smith J L, Mantell G, Berman R 1987 A multicenter, double-blind, randomized, placebo-controlled comparison of nocturnal and twice-a-day famotidine in the treatment of active duodenal ulcer disease. Gastroenterology 92: 48
Glass G B J, Pitchumoni C S 1975 Atrophic gastritis. Structural and ultrastructural alteration, exfoliative cytology and enzyme cytochemistry and histochemistry, proliferation kinetics, immunological derangements and other causes, and clinical associations and sequelae. Human Pathology 6: 219–250
Gledhill T, Buck M, Hunt R H 1984 Effect of no treatment, cimetidine 1 g/day, cimetidine 2 g/day and cimetidine combined with atropine on nocturnal gastric secretion in cimetidine non-responders. Gut 25: 1211
Glick S N, Gohel V K, Laufer I 1984 Mucosal surface patterns of the duodenal bulb. Radiology 150: 317
Goa K L, Monk J P 1987 Enprostil. A preliminary review of its pharmacodynamic and pharmacokinetic properties, and therapeutic efficacy in the treatment of peptic ulcer disease. Drugs 34: 539–559
Gold M S, Hill I D, Bowie M D 1990 Primary peptic ulcer disease in childhood. South African Medical Journal 77: 183–185
Goldschmiedt M, Barnett C C, Schwarz B E, Karnes W E, Redfern J S, Feldman M 1991 Effect of age on gastric acid secretion and serum gastrin concentrations in healthy men and women. Gastroenterology 101: 977–990
Gough K R, Korman M G, Bardhan K D et al 1984 Ranitidine and cimetidine in prevention of duodenal ulcer relapse. A double-blind, randomised, multicentre, comparative trial. Lancet 2: 659–662
Goulston K J, Dent O F, Chapuis P H et al 1985 Gastrointestinal morbidity among Worldwar II prisoners of war: 40 years on. Medical Journal of Australia 143: 6
Graham D Y 1989 *Campylobacter pylori* and peptic ulcer disease. Gastroenterology 96: 615–625
Graham D Y, Smith J L 1986 Aspirin and the stomach. Annals of Internal Medicine 104: 390

Graham D Y, Akdamar K, Dyck W P et al 1985 Healing of benign gastric ulcer: comparison of cimetidine and placebo in the United States. Annals of Internal Medicine 102: 573

Graham D Y, Agrawal N M, Roth S H 1988 Prevention of NSAID-induced gastric ulcer with misoprostol: multicentre, double-blind, placebo-controlled trial. Lancet 2: 1277–1280

Graham D Y, Klein P D, Evans D J et al 1987 *Campylobacter pylori* detected noninvasively by the $^{13}$C-urea breath test. Lancet 1: 1174–1177

Gregory R A, Grossman M I, Tracey H J et al 1967 Nature of the gastric secretagogue in Zollinger–Ellison tumours. Lancet 2: 543–544

Grossman M I 1958 The glands of Brunner. Physiological Reviews 38: 675

Grossman M I 1960 The pyloric gland area of the stomach. A brief survey. Gastroenterology 38: 1

Grossman M I, Kirsner J B, Gillespie I E 1963 Basal and histalog-stimulated gastric secretion in control subjects and in patients with peptic ulcer or gastric cancer. Gastroenterology 45: 14–26

Guth P H 1982 Stomach blood flow and acid secretion. Annual Review of Physiology 44: 3

Halter F 1992 Antacids overview. European Journal of Gastroenterology and Hepatology 4: 947–983

Halter F, Eigenmann F 1987 Is it really more difficult to treat pre-pyloric ulcers? Alimentary Pharamcology and Therapeutics 1 (suppl 1): 433S–438S

Hannan A, Weil J, Broom C, Walt R P 1992 Effects of oral pantoprazole on 24-hour intragastric acidity and plasma gastrin profiles. Alimentary Pharmacology and Therapeutics 6: 373–380

Haruma K, Sumii K, Okamoto S et al 1992 *Helicobacter pylori* infection causes low antral somatostatin content: pathogenesis of inappropriate hypergastrinemia. Gastroenterology 102: A80

Hawkey C J 1990 Non-steriodal anti-inflammatory drugs and peptic ulcers. Fact and figures multiply, but do they add up? British Medical Journal 300: 278–284

Hawkey C J, Hawthorne A B, Hudson N, Cole A T, Mahida Y R, Daneshmend T K 1991 Separation of the impairment of haemostasis by aspirin from mucosal injury in the human stomach. Clinical Science 81: 565–573

Hazell S L 1993 Cultural techniques for the growth and isolation of *Helicobacter pylori*. In: Goodwin C S, Worsley B W (eds) *Helicobacter pylori*. Biology and clincial practice. CRC Press, Boca Raton, p 273

Heading R C 1983 Duodenogastric reflux. Gut 24: 507

Hebnes K, Selbekk B H, Vatn M H 1986 A double-blind crossover study of the effect of a chromone carboxylic acid, FPL 52694, on overnight fasting gastric acid secretion. Scandinavian Journal of Gastroenterology 21: 965

Herting R L, Nissen C H 1986 Overview of misoprostol clinical experience. Digestive Diseases and Sciences 31: S47

Hetzel D J, Hecker R, Shearman D J C 1980 Long term treatment of duodenal ulcer with cimetidine: intermittent or continuous therapy? Medical Journal of Australia 2: 612

Hillier K, Smith C L, Jewell R, Arthur M J P, Ross G 1985 Duodenal mucosa synthesis of prostaglandins in duodenal ulcer disease. Gut 26: 237

Hills B A, Kirkwood C A 1992 Gastric mucosal barrier: barrier to hydrogen ions imparted by gastric surfactant in vitro. Gut 33: 1039–1041

Hirschl A M, Brandstatter G, Dragosics B et al 1993 Kinetics of specific IgG antibodies for monitoring the effect of anti-*Helicobacter pylori* chemotherapy. Journal of Infectious Diseases 168: 763–766

Hoftiezer J W, O'Laughlin J C, Ivey K J 1982 Effects of 24 hours of aspirin. Bufferin, paracetamol and placebo on normal human gastroduodenal mucosa. Gut 23: 692

Hollander D, Tarnawski A, Gergely H, Zipser R D 1984 Sucralfate protection of the gastric mucosa against ethanol-induced injury: a prostaglandin-mediated process? Scandinavian Journal of Gastroenterology 101: 97–102

Hollander D, Tarnawski A, Krause W J, Gergely H 1985 Protective effect of sucralfate against alcohol-induced mucosal injury in the rat. Macroscopic, histologic, ultrastructural, and functional time sequence analysis. Gastroenterology 88: 366

Holzer P, Lippe I T 1992 Gastric mucosal hyperemia due to acid backdiffusion depends on splanchnic nerve activity. American Journal of Physiology 262: G505–509

Hood J M, Spencer E F, MacRae K D, Kennedy T 1976 Predictive value of perioperative gastric acid tests. Gut 17: 998–1000

Hook-Nikanne J, Sistonen P, Kosunen T U 1990 Effect of ABO blood group and secretor status on the frequency of *Helicobacter pylori* antibodies. Scandanavian Journal of Gastroenterology 25: 815–818

Horrocks J C, de Dombal F T 1978 Clinical presentation of patients with "dyspepsia". Detailed symptomatic study of 360 patients. Gut 19: 19

Hugh T B, Coleman M J, McNamara M E, Norman J R, Howell C 1984 Epidemiology of peptic ulcer in Australia. A study based in Government statistics in four states. Medical Journal of Australia 141: 81

Hui W M, Lam S K 1987. Multiple duodenal ulcer: natural history and pathophysiology. Gut 28: 1134–1141

Hui W M, Lam S K 1988 Alimentary tract and pancreas. Monthly variation in frequency of active duodenal ulcer and maximal acid output. Journal of Gastroenterology and Hepatology 3: 457–463

Hui W M, Lam S K, Lau W Y et al 1989 Omeprazole and ranitidine in duodenal ulcer healing and subsequent relapse: a randomized double-blind study with weekly endoscopic assessment. Journal of Gastroenterology and Hepatology 4 (suppl 2): 35–43

Hui W M, Lam S K, Shiu L P, Ng M 1990 A semi-quantitative study of negative social events, stress and incidence of perforated peptic ulcer in Hong Kong over 24 years. Gastroenterology 98(5) Part 2: A61

Ihamaki T, Varis K, Siurala M 1979 Morphological, functional and immunological state of the gastric mucosa in gastric carcinoma families. Comparison with a computer-matched family sample. Scandinavian Journal of Gastroenterology 14(7): 801–812

Ippoliti A F, Sturdevant R A, Isenberg J I et al 1978 Cimetidine versus intensive antacid therapy for duodenal ulcer. A multicenter trial. Gastroenterology 74: 393–395

Isenberg J I, Flemström G 1991 Physiology and pathophysiology of gastroduodenal bicarbonate secretion. Viewpoints of Digestive Disease 23: 27–33

Isenberg J I, Grossman M I, Maxwell V, Walsh J H 1975 Increased sensitivity to stimulation of acid secretion by pentagastrin in duodenal ulcer. Journal of Clinical Investigation 55: 330–337

Iwahi T, Satoh H, Nakao M et al 1991 Lansoprazole, a novel benzimidazole proton pump inhibitor, and its related compounds have selective activity against *Helicobacter pylori*. Antimicrobial Agents and Chemotherapy 35: 490–496

Jensen R T, Metz D C, Koviack P D, Feigenbaum K M 1993 Prospective study of the long-term efficacy and safety of lansoprazole in patients with the Zollinger–Ellison syndrome. Alimentary Pharmacology and Therapeutics 7 (suppl 1): 41–50

Jentjens T, Smits H L, Strous G J 1984 16,16-Dimethyl prostaglandin $E_2$ stimulates galactose and glucosamine but not serine incorporation in rat gastric mucous cells. Gastroenterology 87: 409–416

Jibril J A, Redpath A, MacIntyre I M 1994 Changing pattern of admission and operation for duodenal ulcers in Scotland. British Journal of Surgery 81: 87–89

Joffe S N, Lee F D, Blumgart L H 1978 Duodenitis. Clinics in Gastroenterology 7: 635–650

Jones D G C, Langman M J S, Lawson D H, Vessey M P 1985 Post-marketing surveillance of the safety of cimetidine; twelve-month morbidity report. Quarterly Journal of Medicine 54: 253

Kaehny W D, Hegg A P, Alfrey A C 1977 Gastrointestinal absorption of aluminum from aluminum-containing antacids. New England Journal of Medicine 296: 1389

Kamada T, Kawano S, Sato N, Fukuda M, Fusamoto H, Abe H 1983 Gastric mucosal blood distribution and its changes in the healing process of gastric ulcer. Gastroenterology 84: 1541–1546

Kaufmann D, Wilder-Smith C H, Kempf M et al 1990 Cigarette smoking, gastric acidity and peptic ulceration. What are the relationships? Digestive Diseases and Sciences 35: 1482–1487

Kekki M, Sipponen P, Siurala M, Laszewicz W 1990 Peptic ulcer and chronic gastritis: the relation to age and sex, and to location of ulcer and gastritis. Gastroenterologie Clinique et Biologique (Paris) 14(3): 217–223

Kerrigan D D, Read N W, Taylor M E, Houghton L A, Johnson A G

1989 Duodenal bulb acidity and the natural history of duodenal ulceration. Lancet 2: 61–63
Kessel N, Munro A 1964 Epidemiological studies in psychosomatic medicine. Journal of Psychosomatic Research 8: 67
Kimura K 1972 Chronological transition of the fundicpyloric border determined by stepwise biopsy of the lesser and greater curvatures of the stomach. Gastroenterology 63: 584
Kitajima M, Otsuka S, Shimizu A et al 1988 Impairment of gastric microcirculation in stress. Journal of Clincial Gastroenterology 10 (suppl 1): S120–S128
Klaassen C H W, de Pont J J 1994 Gastric $H^+/K^+$ -ATPase. Cellular Physiology and Biochemistry 4: 115–134
Knutson L, Flemström G 1989 Duodenal mucosal bicarbonate secretion in man. Stimulation by acid and inhibition by the alpha$_2$-adrenoceptor agonist clonidine. Gut 30: 1708–1715
Kollberg B, Slezak P 1982 The effect of prostaglandin E2 on duodenal ulcer healing. Prostaglandins 24(4): 527–536
Kolts B E, Joseph B, Achem S R, Bianchi T, Monteiro C 1993 *Helicobacter pylori* detection; a quality and cost analysis. American Journal of Gastroenterology 88: 650–655
Konturek S J 1979 Gastric secretion: physiological aspects. In: Duthie H L, Wormsley K G (eds) Scientific basis of gastroenterology. Churchill Livingstone, Edinburgh, p 133
Konturek S J 1985 Gastric cytoprotection. Scandanavian Journal of Gastroenterology 20: 543
Konturek S J, Brzozowski T, Majka J, Pytko-Polonczyk J, Stachura J 1993 Inhibition of nitric oxide synthase delays healing of chronic gastric ulcers. European Journal of Pharmacology 239: 215–217
Koo J, Ngan Y K, Lam S K 1983 Trends in hospital admission, perforation and mortality of peptic ulcer in Hong Kong from 1970 to 1980. Gastroenterology 84: 1558–1562
Korman M G, Shaw R G, Hansky J, Schmidt G T, Stern A I 1981 Influence of smoking on healing rate of duodenal ulcer in response to cimetidine or high-dose antacid. Gastroenterology 80: 1451–1453
Korman M G, Hansky J, Eaves E R, Schmidt G T 1983 Influence of cigarette smoking on healing and relapse in duodenal ulcer disease. Gastroenterology 85: 871–874
Kreel L 1975 The surface pattern of the stomach. Proceedings of the Royal Society of Medicine 68: 111
Kurata J H, Haile B M 1984 Epidemiology of peptic ulcer disease. Clinics in Gastroenterology 13: 289–307
Kurata J H, Haile B M, Elashoff J D 1985 Sex differences in peptic ulcer disease. Gastroenterology 88: 96–100
Labenz J, Borsch G 1994 Role of *Helicobacter pylori* eradication in the prevention of peptic ulcer bleeding relapse. Digestion 55: 19–23
Lacroix J, Infante-Rivard C, Jenicek M, Gauthier M 1989 Prophylaxis of upper gastrointestinal bleeding in intensive care units: a meta-analysis. Critical Care Medicine (Baltimore) 17: 862–869
Laggner A N, Lenz K, Base W, Druml W, Schneeweiss B, Grimm G 1989 Prevention of upper gastrointestinal bleeding in long-term ventilated patients. Sucralfate versus ranitidine. American Journal of Medicine 86 (suppl 6A): 81–84
Laine L, Marin-Sorensen M, Weinstein W M 1992 Nonsteroidal antiinflammatory drug-associated gastric ulcers do not require *Helicobacter pylori* for their development. American Journal of Gastroenterology 87: 1398–1402
Lam S K 1984 Pathogenesis and pathophysiology of duodenal ulcer. Clinics in Gastroenterology 13: 447
Lam S K 1991 Treatment of duodenal ulcer with sucralfate. Scandinavian Journal of Gastroenterology 26 (suppl 185): 22–28
Lam S K, Ong G B 1976 Duodenal ulcers: early and late onset. Gut 17: 169–179
Lam S K, Sircus W 1975 Vagal hyperacidity in duodenal ulcer with and without excessive acid secretion. Rendiconti Gastro-enterologia 7: 5–9
Lam S K, Hasan M, Sircus W, Wong J, Ong G B, Prescott R J 1980a Comparison of maximal acid output and gastrin response to meals in Chinese and Scottish normal and duodenal ulcer subjects. Gut 21: 324–328
Lam S K, Isenberg J I, Grossman M I, Lane W H, Walsh J H 1980b Gastric acid secretion is abnormally sensitive to endogenous gastrin released after peptone test meals in duodenal ulcer patients. Journal of Clinical Investigation 65: 555–562
Lam S K, Koo J, Sircus W 1983. Early- and late-onset duodenal ulcers in Chinese and Scots. Scandinavian Journal of Gastroenterology 18: 651–658
Lam S K, Lee N W, Koo J, Hui W M, Fok K H, Ng M 1984 Randomised crossover trial of tripotassium dicitrato bismuthate versus high dose cimetidine for duodenal ulcers resistant to standard dose of cimetidine. Gut 25: 703
Lambert J R 1991 Clinical indications and efficacy of colloidal bismuth subcitrate. Scandinavian Journal of Gastroenterology 185: 13–21
Lambert J R 1993 The role of *Helicobacter pylori* in nonulcer dyspepsia. A debate for. Gastroenterology Clinics of North America 22: 141–151
Lambert J R, Lin S K, Aranda-Michel J 1995 *Helicobacter pylori*. Scandinavian Journal of Gastroenterology 30 (suppl 208): 33–46
Lamouliatte H 1993 Effect of lansoprazole on *Helicobacter pylori*. Clinical Therapy 15 (suppl B): 32–36
Landboe-Christensen E 1944 Extent of the pylorus zone in the human stomach. Acta Pathologica et Microbiologica Scandinavica 54: 671
Langman M J S 1970 Epidemiological evidence for the association of aspirin and acute gastrointestinal bleeding. Gut 11: 627
Lanzon-Miller S, Pounder R E, Hamilton M R et al 1987 Twenty-four hour intragastric acidity and plasma gastrin concentration before and during treatment with either ranitidine or omeprazole. Alimentary Pharmacology and Therapeutics 1: 239–251
Larkai E N, Smith J L, Lidsky M D, Graham D Y 1987 Gastroduodenal mucosa and dyspeptic symptoms in arthritic patients during chronic nonsteroidal anti-inflammatory drug use. American Journal of Gastroenterology 82: 1153–1158
Laufer I 1976 Assessment of the accuracy of double contrast gastroduodenal radiology. Gastroenterology 71: 874
Lauritsen K, Bytzer P, Hansen J, Bekker C, Rask-Madsen J 1985 Comparison of ranitidine and high-dose antacid in the treatment of prepyloric or duodenal ulcer. A double-blind controlled trial. Scandinavian Journal of Gastroenterology 20: 123
Lee H, Hakanson R, Karlsson A, Mattsson H, Sundler F 1992 Lansoprazole and omeprazole have similar effects on plasma gastrin levels, enterochromaffin-like cells, gastrin cells and somatostatin cells in the rat stomach. Digestion 51: 125–132
Lee S P 1991 The mode of action of colloidal bismuth subcitrate. Scandinavian Journal of Gastroenterology 26 (suppl 185): 1–6
Lehnert T, Erlandson R A, Decosse J J 1985 Lymph and blood capillaries of the human gastric mucosa. A morphologic basis for metastasis in early gastric carcinoma. Gastroenterology 89: 939
Levine R J, Vaidya A B, Shearman D J C, Levine S M, Hersh T 1970 Effects of brocresine on Zollinger–Ellison syndrome. Report of 2 cases. American Journal of Digestive Diseases 15(5): 477–484
Levy G, Lampman T, Kamath B L, Garrettson L K 1975 Decreased serum salicylate concentrations in children with rheumatic fever treated with antacid. New England Journal of Medicine 293: 323
Levy I S, de la Fuente A A 1963 A post-mortem study of gastric and duodenal peptic lesions. Gut 4: 349–359
Levy M 1974 Aspirin use in patients with major upper gastrointestinal bleeding and peptic-ulcer disease. A report from the Boston Collaborative Drug Surveillance Program, Boston University Medical Center. New England Journal of Medicine 290: 1158
Li D S, Raybould H E, Quintero G, Guth P H 1992 Calcitonin gene-related peptide mediates the gastric hyperemic response to acid back-diffusion. Gastroenterology 102: 1124–1128
Liedberg G, Davies H J, Enskog L et al 1985 Ulcer healing and relapse prevention by ranitidine in peptic ulcer disease. Scandinavian Journal of Gastroenterology 20: 941
Lin S K, Lambert J R 1992 Nutrition and gastrointestinal disorders. Asia Pacific Journal of Clinical Nutrition 1: 37–42
Lin S K, Lambert J R, Hardikar W, Nicholson L, Schembri M 1991 *Helicobacter pylori* infection in families – evidence for person-to-person transmission. Italian Journal of Gastroenterology 23(suppl 2): 12
Lin S K, Lambert J R, Schembri M et al 1992 A comparison of diagnostic tests to determine *Helicobacter pylori* infection. Journal of Gastroenterology and Hepatology 7: 203–209
Lindstrom C G 1978 Gastric and duodenal peptic ulcer disease in a well-defined population. A prospective necropsy study in Malmö, Sweden. Scandinavian Journal of Gastroenterology 13: 139–143
Litton A, Murdoch W R 1963 Peptic ulcer in south-west Scotland. Gut 4: 360–366

Lockard O O Jr, Ivey K J, Butt J H, Silvoso G R, Sisk C, Holt S 1980 The prevalence of duodenal lesions in patients with rheumatic diseases on chronic aspirin therapy. Gastrointestinal Endoscopy 26(1): 5–7

Lotz M, Zisman E, Bartter F C 1968 Evidence for a phosphorus-depletion syndrome in man. New England Journal of Medicine 278: 409

Lucas C E, Sugawa C, Friend W, Walt A J 1972 Therapeutic implications of disturbed gastric physiology in patients with stress ulcerations. American Journal of Surgery 123: 25–34

Lumsden K, MacLarnon J C, Dawson J 1970 Giant duodenal ulcer. Gut 11: 592–600

Lunderquist A 1985 The pancreas. Clinics in Gastroenterology 14: 255

Maaroos H I, Salupere V, Uibo R, Kekki M, Sipponen P 1985 Seven-year follow-up study of chronic gastritis in gastric ulcer patients. Scandinavian Journal of Gastroenterology 20: 198–204

McCarthy D M 1984a Smoking and ulcers – time to quit. New England Journal of Medecine 311: 726–727

McCarthy D M 1984b The diagnosis and treatment of gastrinoma and Zollinger–Ellison syndrome. In: Santen R J, Manni A (eds) Diagnosis and management of endocrine related tumors. Nijhoff, Boston. p 347–382

McCarthy D M 1991 Sucralfate. New England Journal of Medicine 325: 1017–1025

McColl K E L, Fullarton G M, Nujumi A M, Macdonald A M, Brown I L, Hilditch T E 1989 Lowered gastrin and gastric acidity after eradication of *Campylobacter pylori* in duodenal ulcer. Lancet 2: 499–500

McConnell R B 1980 Peptic ulcer: early genetic evidence – families, twins and markers. In: Rotter J I, Samloff I M, Rimoin D L (eds) Genetics and heterogeneity of common gastrointestinal disorders. Academic Press, New York, p 31

McGuigan J E 1968 Gastric mucosal intracellular localisation of gastrin by immunofluorescence. Gastroenterology 55: 315

McIntosh J H, Nasiry R W, Frydman M, Waller S L, Piper D W 1983 The personality pattern of patients with chronic peptic ulcer. A case-control study. Scandanavian Journal of Gastroenterology 18: 945–950

McIntosh J H, Byth K, Piper D W 1985a Environmental factors in aetiology of chronic gastric ulcer: a case control study of exposure variables before the first symptoms. Gut 26: 789–798

McIntosh J H, Nasiry R W, McNeil D, Coates C, Mitchell H, Piper D W 1985b Perception of life event stress in patients with chronic duodenal ulcer. A comparison of the rating of life events by duodenal ulcer patients and community controls. Scandinavian Journal of Gastroenterology 20: 563–568

McIntosh J H, Byth K, Tsang N, Berman K, Holliday F M, Piper D W 1993 Trends in peptic ulcer mortality in Sydney from 1971 to 1987. Journal of Clinical Gastroenterology 16: 346–353

Mackintosh C E, Kreel L 1977 Anatomy and radiology of the areae gastricae. Gut 18: 855–864

Manniche C, Malchow-Moller A, Andersen J R 1987 Randomised study of the influence of non-steroidal anti-inflammatory drugs on the treatment of peptic ulcer in patients with rheumatic disease. Gut 28: 226

Marks I N 1991 Sucralfate – safety and side effects. Scandinavian Journal of Gastroenterology 26 (suppl 185): 36–42

Marshall B 1983 Unidentified curved bacilli on gastric epithelium in active chronic gastritis. Lancet 1: 1273–1275

Marshall B J, Armstrong J A, McGechie D B, Glancy R J 1985 Attempts to fulfil Koch's postulates for pyloric campylobacter. Medical Journal of Australia 142: 436–439

Maton P N 1991 Omeprazole. New England Journal of Medicine 324: 965–975

Mayer G, Arnold R, Feurle G et al 1974 Influence of feeding and sham feeding upon serum gastrin and gastric acid secretion in control subjects and duodenal ulcer patients. Scandinavian Journal of Gastroenterology 9: 703–710

Mellem H, Stave R, Myren J et al 1985 Symptoms in patients with peptic ulcer and hematemesis and/or melena related to the use of non-steroidal anti-inflammatory drugs. Scandinavian Journal of Gastroenterology 20: 1246–1248

Melrose A G, Wallace J 1965 Multiple cases of duodenal ulcer in one family. Scottish Medical Journal 10: 302

Merki H S, Fimmel C J, Walt R P, Harre K, Rohmel J, Witzel L 1988 Pattern of 24 hour intragastric acidity in active duodenal ulcer disease and in healthy controls. Gut 29: 1583–1587

Messer J, Reitman D, Sacks H S, Smith H Jr, Chalmers T C 1983 Association of adrenocorticosteroid therapy and peptic-ulcer disease. New England Journal of Medicine 309: 21–24

Messier B, Leblond C P 1960 Cell proliferation and migration as revealed by radioautography after injection of thymidine-$H_3$ into male rats and mice. American Journal of Anatomy 106: 247–285

Metz D C, Strader D B, Orbuch M, Koviack P D, Feigenbaum K M, Jensen R T 1993 Use of omeprazole in Zollinger–Ellison syndrome: a prospective nine-year study of efficacy and safety. Alimentary Pharmacology and Therapeutics 7: 597–610

Miranda M, Defilippi C, Valenzuela J E 1985 Abnormalities of interdigestive motility complex and increased duodenogastric reflux in gastric ulcer patients. Digestive Diseases and Sciences 30: 16

Misiewicz J J 1978 Peptic ulceration and its correlation with symptoms. Clinics in Gastroenterology 7: 571

Misiewicz J J 1991 The Sydney System: a new classification of gastritis. Introduction. Journal of Gastroenterology and Hepatology 6: 207–208

Morris T, Rhodes J 1979 Antacids and peptic ulcer – a reappraisal. Gut 20: 538

Morrissey S M, Ward P M, Jayaraj A P, Tovey F I, Clark C G 1983 Histochemical changes in mucus in duodenal ulceration. Gut 24: 909–913

Moss S F, Legon S, Bishop A E, Polak J M, Calam J 1992 Effect of *Helicobacter pylori* on gastric somatostatin in duodenal ulcer disease. Lancet 340: 930–932

Muller-Lissner S A, Fimmel C J, Sonnenberg A et al 1983 Novel approach to quantify duodenogastric reflux in healthy volunteers and in patients with type I gastric ulcer. Gut 24: 510–518

Murakami M, Inada M, Miyake T et al 1983 Regional mucosal blood flow and ulcer healing. In: Koo A, Lam S K, Smaje L H (eds) International symposium on microcirculation of the alimentary tract. World Scientific Publishing, Singapore, p 293–302

Murdoch D, McTavish D 1991 Roxatidine acetate. A review of its pharmacodynamic and pharmacokinetic properties, and its therapeutic potential in peptic ulcer disease and related disorders. Drugs 42: 240–260

Murphy M S, Eastham E J, Jimenez M, Nelson R, Jackson R H 1987 Duodenal ulceration: review of 110 cases. Archives of Disease in Childhood 62(6): 554–558

Murray G F, Ballinger W F, Stafford E S 1967 Ulcers of the pyloric channel. American Journal of Surgery 113: 199

Naesdal J, Bodemar G, Walan A 1984 Effect of omeprazole, a substituted benzimidazole, on 24-h intragastric acidity in patients with peptic ulcer disease. Scandinavian Journal of Gastroenterology 19: 916–922

National Center for Health Statistics 1979 Prevalence of selected chronic digestive conditions, United States 1975. Data from the National Health Interview Survey. Washington, DC: Vital and Health Statistics, p. 14. US Dept of Health, Education and Welfare, p 679–1558

NIH Consensus Development Panel 1994 *Helicobacter pylori* in peptic ulcer disease. Journal of the American Medical Association 272: 65–69

Nensey Y M, Schubert T T, Bologna S D, Ma C K 1991 *Helicobacter pylori*-negative duodenal ulcer. American Journal of Medicine 91: 15–18

Nicholson P A 1985 A multicenter international controlled comparison of two dosage regimes of misoprostol and cimetidine in the treatment of duodenal ulcer in out-patients. Digestive Diseases and Sciences 30: 171S

Niwayama G, Terplan K 1959 A study of peptic ulcer based on necropsy records. Gastroenterology 35: 409

Noach L A, Rolf T M, Bosma N B et al 1993 Gastric metaplasia and *Helicobacter pylori* infection. Gut 34: 1510–1514

Nwokolo C U, Prewett E J, Sawyerr A M, Hudson M, Lim S, Pounder R E 1991 Tolerance during 5 months of dosing with ranitidine, 150 mg nightly: a placebo-controlled, double-blind study. Gastroenterology 101: 948–953

Odonkor P, Mowat C, Himal H S 1981 Prevention of sepsis-induced gastric lesions in dogs by cimetidine via inhibition of gastric secretion and by prostaglandin via cytoprotection. Gastroenterology 80: 375–379

Oi M, Sakurai Y 1959 The location of the duodenal ulcer. Gastroenterology 36: 60

Oi M, Ito Y, Kumagai F et al 1969 A possible dual control mechanism in the origin of peptic ulcer. A study on ulcer location as affected by mucosa and musculature. Gastroenterology 57: 280

Oktedalen O, Guldvog I, Opstad P K, Berstad A, Gedde-Dahl D, Jorde R 1984 The effect of physical stress on gastric secretion and pancreatic polypeptide levels in man. Scandinavian Journal of Gastroenterology 19: 770

O'Laughlin J C, Hoftiezer J W, Ivey K J 1981 Effect of aspirin on the human stomach in normals: endoscopic comparison of damage produced one hour, 24 hours, and two weeks after administration. Scandinavian Journal of Gastroenterology 16 (suppl 67): 211–214

Olsson K, Wadstrom T, Tyszkiewicz T 1993 *H. pylori* in dental plaques (letter). Lancet 341: 956–957

Op den Orth J O, Ploem S 1977 The standard biphasic-contrast gastric series. Radiology 122: 530

Ormand J E, Talley N J, Carpenter H A et al 1990 ($^{14}$C)-urea breath test for diagnosis of *Helicobacter pylori*. Digestive Diseases and Sciences 35: 879–884

Orwoll E S 1982 The milk-alkali syndrome: current concepts. Annals of Internal Medicine 97: 242

Ott D J, Chen Y M, Gelfand D W et al 1985 Positive predictive value and examiner variability in diagnosing duodenal ulcer. American Journal of Radiology 145: 1207

Palmer R M J, Ferrige A G, Moncada S 1987 Nitric oxide release accounts for the biological activity of endothelium-derived relaxing factor. Nature 327: 524–526

Park J, Chiba T, Yamada T 1987 Mechanisms for direct inhibition of canine gastric parietal cells by somatostatin. Journal of Biological Chemistry 262: 14190–14196

Parsonnet J, Blaser M J, Perez-Perez G I, Hargrett-Bean N, Tauxe R V 1992 Symptoms and risk factors of *Helicobacter pylori* infection in a cohort of epidemiologists. Gastroenterology 102: 41–46

Patrick W J A, Denham D, Forrest A P M 1974 Mucous change in the human duodenum: a light and electron microscopic study and correlation with disease and gastric acid secretion. Gut 15: 767–776

Penninckx F, Vuylsteke P, Kerremans R 1990 Recurrences after highly selective vagotomy in refractory and non-refractory duodenal ulcer disease. Acta Chirurgica Belgique 90: 41–45

Penston J G, Dixon J S, Boyd E J, Wormsley K G 1993 A placebo-controlled investigation of duodenal ulcer recurrence after withdrawal of long-term treatment with ranitidine. Alimentary Pharmacology and Therapeutics 7: 259–265

Pfeiffer A, Rochlitz H, Noelke B et al 1990. Muscarinic receptors mediating acid secretion in isolated rat parietal cells are of M3 type. Gastroenterology 98: 218–222

Pflanz M 1971 Epidemiological and sociocultural factors in the etiology of duodenal ulcer. Advances in Psychosomatic Medicine 6: 121–151

Piper D W 1973 Antacid and anticholinergic drug therapy. Clinics in Gastroenterology 2: 361

Piper D W, McIntosh J H, Ariotti D E, Fenton B H, MacLennan R 1981 Analgesic ingestion and chronic peptic ulcer. Gastroenterology 80: 427–435

Piper J M, Ray W A, Daugherty, Griffin M R 1991 Corticosteroid use and peptic ulcer disease: role of nonsteroidal anti-inflammatory drugs. Annals of Internal Medicine 114: 735–740

Pique J M, Esplugues J V, Whittle B J R 1992 Endogenous nitric oxide as a mediator of gastric mucosal vasodilation during acid secretion. Gastroenterology 102: 168–174

Pounder R 1989 Silent peptic ulceration: deadly silence or golden silence? Gastroenterology 96: 626–631

Price A B 1991 The Sydney System: histological division. Journal of Gastroenterology and Hepatology 6: 209–222

Priebe W M, DaCosta L R, Beck I T 1982 Is epigastric tenderness a sign of peptic ulcer disease? Gastroenterology 82: 16

Queiroz D M M, Rocha G A, Mendes E N et al 1991 Differences in distribution and severity of *Helicobacter pylori* gastritis in children and adults with duodenal ulcer disease. Journal of Pediatric Gastroenterology and Nutrition 12(2): 178–181

Rabkin J G, Struening E L 1976 Life events, stress, and illness. Sciences 194: 1013–1020

Ramsdell J A, Bartholomew L G, Cain C R, Davis G D 1957 Postbulbar duodenal ulcer. Annals of Internal Medicine 47: 700–711

Redfern J S, Feldman M 1989 Role of endogenous prostaglandins in preventing gastrointestinal ulceration: induction of ulcers by antibodies to prostaglandins. Gastroenterology 96: 596–605

Rees W, Rhodes J 1977 Bile reflux in gastro-oesophageal disease. Clinics in Gastroenterology 6: 179–188

Reimann H-J, Schmidt U, Ultsch B, Sullivan T J, Wendt P 1984 Action of FPL 52694 on gastric acid secretion in the healthy human stomach. Gut 25: 1221–1224

Riley I D 1942 Perforated peptic ulcer in war-time. Lancet 2: 485

Robert A 1979 Cytoprotection by prostaglandins. Gastroenterology 77: 761–767

Rodriguez H P, Aston J K, Richardson C T 1973 Ulcers in the descending duodenum. Postbulbar ulcers. American Journal of Roentgenology 119: 316

Rogers I M, Sokhi G S, Moule B, Joffe S N, Blumgart L H 1976 Endoscopy and routine double-contrast barium meal in diagnosis of gastric duodenal disorders. Lancet 1: 901

Rohrer G V, Scott J R, Joel W et al 1965 The fine structure of human gastric parietal cells. American Journal of Digestive Diseases 10: 13–21

Rose C, Stevenson G W 1981 Correlation between visualization and size of the areae gastricae and duodenal ulcer. Radiology 139: 371

Rose R M, Jenkins C D, Hurst M W 1987 Air traffic controller health change study. Report to Federal Aviation. Administration under contract FA7 3WA-3211

Roth H P 1955 The peptic ulcer personality. Archives of Internal Medicine 96: 32

Rotter J I, Rimoin D L 1977 Peptic ulcer disease – a heterogeneous group of disorders? Gastroenterology 73: 604

Rotter J I, Petersen G, Samloff I M et al 1979 Genetic heterogeneity of hyperpepsinogenemic I and normopepsinogenemic I duodenal ulcer disease. Annals of Internal Medicine 91(3): 372–377

Ruffin J M 1959 Mechanism of ulcer pain and significance of pain patterns. American Journal of Digestive Diseases 4(11): 871–874

Ruffin J M, Baylin G J, Legerton C W, Texter E C 1953 Mechanism of pain in peptic ulcer. Gastroenterology 23: 252

Rune S J, Viskum K 1969 Duodenal pH values in normal controls and in patients with duodenal ulcer. Gut 10: 569–571

Sachs G 1987 The gastric proton pump: the $H^+$, $K^+$-ATPase. In: Johnson L R, Christensen J, Jackson M J, Jacobson E D, Walsh J H (eds) Physiology of the gastrointestinal tract, Vol 1, 2nd edn. Raven Press, New York, p 865

Saffouri B, DuVal J W, Makhlouf G M 1984 Stimulation of gastrin secretion in vitro by intraluminal chemicals: regulation by intramural cholinergic and noncholinergic neurons. Gastroenterology 87: 557–561

Sakita T, Oguro Y, Takasu S, Fukutomi H, Miwa T, Yoshimori M 1971 Observations on the healing of ulcerations in early gastric cancer. The life cycle of the malignant ulcer. Gastroenterology 60: 835

Samloff I M, Townes P L 1970 Electrophoretic heterogeneity and relationships of pepsinogens in human urine, serum, and gastric mucosa. Gastroenterology 58: 462–469

Samloff I M, Stemmermann G N, Heilbrun L K, Nomura A 1986 Elevated serum pepsinogen I and II levels differ as risk factors for duodenal and gastric ulcer. Gastroenterology 90: 570–576

Scheiman J M, Kraus E R, Bonnville L A, Weinhold P A, Boland C R 1991 Synthesis and prostaglandin $E_2$-induced secretion of surfactant phospholipid by isolated gastric mucous cells. Gastroenterology 100: 1232–1240

Schembri M A, Lin S K, Lambert J R 1993 Comparison of commercial diagnostic tests for *Helicobacter pylori* antibodies. Journal of Clinical Microbiology 31: 2621–2624

Schubert M 1991 Gastric somatostatin. A paracrine regulator of gastrin and acid secretion (letter). Regulatory Peptide 3: 7–11

Sedman A J 1984 Cimetidine-drug interactions. American Journal of Medicine 76: 109

Segura D I, Montero C 1983 Histochemical characterization of different types of intestinal metaplasia in gastric mucosa. Cancer 52: 498–503

Selling J A, Hogan D L, Aly A, Koss M A, Isenberg J I 1987 Indomethacin inhibits duodenal mucosal bicarbonate secretion and endogenous prostaglandin E2 output in human subjects. Annals of Internal Medicine 106(3): 368–371

Shallcross T M, Heatley R V 1990 Effect of non-steroidal anti-inflammatory drugs on dyspeptic symptoms. British Medical Journal 300: 368–369

Shaper A G, Williams A W 1959 Peptic ulcer in Africans. 2: 757–758

Sharma B K, Walt R P, Pounder R E, Gomes M, Wood E C, Logan L H 1984 Optimal dose of oral omeprazole for maximal 24 hour decrease of intragastric acidity. Gut 25: 957–964

Shaw P C, van Romunde L K J, Griffioen G, Janssens A R, Kreuning J, Eilers G A 1987 Peptic ulcer and gastric carcinoma: diagnosis with biphasic radiography compared with fiberoptic endoscopy. Radiology 163(1): 39–42

Shearman D J C, Hetzel D J 1979 The management of peptic ulceration. Annual Review of Medicine 30: 61

Sherman P, Shames B, Loo V, Matlow A, Drumm B, Penner J 1992 Omeprazole therapy for *Helicobacter pylori* infection. Scandinavian Journal of Gastroenterology 27: 1018–1022

Shield M J 1985 Interim results of multicenter international comparison of misoprostol and cimetidine in the treatment of outpatients with benign gastric ulcers. Digestive Diseases and Sciences 30: 178S

Shimoda S S, Saunders D R, Rubin C E 1968 The Zollinger–Ellison syndrome with steatorrhea. II The mechanisms of fat and vitamin $B_{12}$ malabsorption. Gastroenterology 55: 705–723

Shirakabe H, Nishizawa M, Nomoto K, Ariyama J, Hamilton G B 1975 Qualitative comparison of endoscopy and radiology in the diagnosis of duodenal ulcer. Gastroenterology 68: 1031

Shorrock C J, Garner A, Hunter A H, Crampton J R, Rees W D W 1990 Effect of bismuth subcitrate and sucralfate on rat duodenal and human gastric bicarbonate secretion in vivo. Gut 31: 26–31

Shuman R B, Schuster D P, Zuckerman G R 1987 Prophylactic therapy for stress ulcer bleeding: a reappraisal. Annals of Internal Medicine 106(4): 562–567

Sievert W, Allwell L, Lambert J R, Hansky J, Soveny C, Korman M G 1994 Gastrin release and acid secretion are a critical function of *H. pylori* infection. Gastroenterology 106: A180

Sipponen P, Seppala K, Aarynen M, Helske T, Kettunen P 1989 Chronic gastritis and gastroduodenal ulcer: a case control study on risk of coexisting duodenal or gastric ulcer in patients with gastritis. Gut 30: 922–929

Sipponen P, Varis K, Fraki O, Korri U M, Seppela K, Siurala M 1990 Cumulative 10-year risk of symptomatic duodenal and gastric ulcer in patients with or without chronic gastritis. A clinical follow-up study of 454 outpatients. Scandinavian Journal of Gastroenterology 25: 966–973

Siurala M, Sipponen P, Kekki M 1985 Chronic gastritis: dynamic and clinical aspects. Scandinavian Journal of Gastroenterology 109: 69–76

Skander M P, Ryan F P 1988 Non-steroidal anti-inflammatory drugs and pain free peptic ulceration in the elderly. British Medical Journal 297: 833–834

Slomiany B L, Nishikawa H, Piotrowski J, Okazaki K, Slomiany A 1989 Lipolytic activity of *Campylobacter pylori*: effect of sofalcone. Digestion 43: 33–40

Smith J L, Gamal M A, Chremos A N, Graham D Y 1985 Famotidine, a new $H_2$-receptor antagonist. Effect on parietal, nonparietal, and pepsin secretion in man. Digestive Diseases and Sciences 30: 308

Solcia E, Capella C, Buffa R, Frigerio B, Fiocca R 1980 Pathology of the Zollinger–Ellison syndrome. In: Fenoglio C M, Wolff M (eds) Progress in surgical pathology, Vol 1. Masson, New York, p 119–133

Solcia E, Capella C, Buffa R, Usellini L, Fiocca R, Sessa F 1987 Endocrine cells of the digestive system. In: Johnson L R, Christensen J, Jackson M J, Jacobson E D, Walsh J H (eds) Physiology of the gastrointestinal tract, Vol 1, 2nd edn. Raven Press, New York, p 111

Sonnenberg A 1984 Occurrence of a cohort phenomenon in peptic ulcer mortality from Switzerland. Gastroenterology 86: 398

Sonnenberg A, Muller-Lissner S A, Vogel E et al 1981 Predictors of duodenal ulcer healing and relapse. Gastroenterology 81: 1061–1067

Spychal R T, Marrero J M, Saverymuttu S H, Northfield T C 1989 Measurement of the surface hydrophobicity of human gastrointestinal mucosa. Gastroenterology 97: 104–111

Spychal R T, Goggin P M, Marrero J M et al 1990 Surface hydrophobicity of gastric mucosa in peptic ulcer disease. Relationship to gastritis and *Campylobacter pylori* infection. Gastroenterology 98: 1250–1254

Stables R, Campbell C J, Clayton N M et al 1993 Gastric anti-secretory, mucosal protective, anti-pepsin and anti-Helicobacter properties of ranitidine bismuth citrate. Alimentary Pharmacology and Therapeutics 7: 237–246

Stein G N, Martin R D, Roy R H, Finkelstein A K 1964 Evaluation of conventional roentgenographic techniques for demonstration of duodenal ulcer craters. American Journal of Gastroenterology 91: 801

Strickland R G 1991 The Sydney System: auto-immune gastritis. Journal of Gastroenterology and Hepatology 6: 238–243

Strickland R G, Mackay I R 1973 A reappraisal of the nature and significance of chronic atrophic gastritis. American Journal of Digestive Diseases 18(5): 426–440

Strom M, Bodemar G, Lindhagen J, Sjodahl R, Walen A 1984 Cimetidine or parietal-cell vagotomy in patients with juxtapyloric ulcers. Lancet 2: 894

Strom M, Berstad A, Bodemar G, Walen A 1986 Results of short- and long-term cimetidine treatment in patients with juxtapyloric ulcers, with special reference to gastric acid and pepsin secretion. Scandanavian Journal of Gastroenterology 21: 521

Sun D C H, Stempien S J 1971 Site and size of the ulcer as determinants of outcome. Gastroenterology 61: 576

Sun D C H, Roth S H, Mitchell C S, Englund D W 1974 Upper gastrointestinal diseases in rheumatoid arthritis. American Journal of Digestive Diseases 9(5): 405–410

Susser M, Stein Z 1962 Civilization and peptic ulcer. Lancet 1: 115

Szabo S, Brown A 1987 Prevention of ethanol-induced vascular injury and gastric mucosal lesions by sucralfate and its components: possible role of endogenous sulfhydryls. Proceedings of the Society for Experimental Biology and Medicine 185: 493–497

Szabo S, Vattay P, Scarbrough E, Folkman J 1991 Role of vascular factors, including angiogenesis, in the mechanism of action of sucralfate. American Journal of Medicine 91(2A): 158S–160S

Taché Y 1987 Central nervous system regulation of gastric acid secretion. In: Johnson L R, Christensen J, Jackson M J, Jacobson E D, Walsh J H (eds) Physiology of the gastrointestinal tract, Vol 2, 2nd edn. Raven Press, New York, p 911

Talley N J, McNeil D, Piper D W 1987 Discriminant value of dyspeptic symptoms: a study of the clincial presentation of 221 patients with dyspepsia of unknown cause, peptic ulceration, and cholelithiasis. Gut 28: 40–46

Tarnawski A, Hollander D, Stachura J, Klimczyk B, Mach T, Bogdar J 1987 Alcohol injury to the normal human gastric mucosa: endoscopic, histologic and functional assessment. Clinical and Investigative Medicine 10(3): 259–263

Thomas J E, Gibson G R, Darboe M K, Dale A, Weaver L T 1992 Isolation of *Helicobacter pylori* from human faeces. Lancet 340: 1194–1195

Tovey F 1979 Peptic ulcer in India and Bangladesh. Gut 20: 329

Tovey F I, Tunstall M 1975 Duodenal ulcer in black populations in Africa south of the Sahara. The geographical distribution of duodenal ulcer. Gut 16: 564

Tryba M 1987 Risk of acute stress bleeding and nosocomial pneumonia in ventilated intensive care unit patients: sucralfate versus antacids. American Journal of Medicine 83(suppl 3B): 117–124

Tytgat G N J, Noach L A 1994 *Helicobacter pylori* eradication. In: Hunt R H, Tytgat G N (eds) *Helicobacter pylori* – basic mechanisms to clinical cure. Kluwer Academic, Boston, p 350

Tytgat G N, Noach L A, Rauws E A 1993a *Helicobacter pylori* infection and duodenal ulcer disease. Gastroenterology Clinics of North America 22: 127–139

Tytgat G N J, Lee A, Graham D Y, Dixon M F, Rokkas T 1993b The role of infectious agents in peptic ulcer disease. Gastroenterology International 6: 76–89

Uribe A, Rubio C, Johansson C 1986 Cell kinetics of rat gastrointestinal mucosa. Audioradiographic study after treatment with 15(R) 15-methyl-prostaglandin $E_2$. Scandinavian Journal of Gastroenterology 21: 246

Vaananen P M, Meddings J B, Wallace J L 1991 Role of oxygen-derived free radicals in indomethacin-induced gastric injury. American Journal of Physiology 261: G470–475

Vantrappen G, Janssens J, Popiela T et al 1982 Effect of 15(R)-15-methyl prostaglandin $E_2$ (Arbaprostil) on the healing of duodenal ulcer. A double-blind muticenter study. Gastroenterology 83: 357–363

Wagner S M, Varrentrapp M, Haruma D, Gebel M, Schmidt F W 1991 Serum gastrin, pepsinogen I and II in *Helicobacter pylori* positive gastritis and peptic ulcer: effect of bacterial eradication. Gastroenterology 100: A181

Walan A, Bader J-P, Classen M 1989 Effect of omeprazole and ranitidine on ulcer healing and relapse rates in patients with benign gastric ulcer. New England Journal of Medicine 320: 69

Wallace J L, Whittle B J R 1986 Picomole doses of platelet-activating factor pre-dispose the gastric mucosa to damage by topical irritants. Prostaglandins 31: 989–998

Walsh J H, Lam S K 1980 Physiology and pathology of gastrin. Clinics in Gastroenterology 9: 567–591

Walsh J H, Richardson C T, Fordham J S 1975 pH dependence of acid secretion and gastrin release in normal and ulcer patients. Journal of Clinical Investigation 55: 462–468

Walt R P 1992 Misoprostol for the treatment of peptic ulcer and antiinflammatory-drug-induced gastroduodenal ulceration. New England Journal of Medicine 327: 1575–1580

Warren J R 1983 Unidentified curved bacilli on gastric epithelium in acitve chronic gastritis. Lancet 1: 1273

Wastell C 1972 Chronic duodenal ulcer. Butterworths, London

Watkinson G 1960 The incidence of chronic peptic ulcer found at necropsy. A study of 20,000 examinations performed in Leeds in 1930–49 and in England and Scotland in 1956. Gut 1:14

Weisberg H, Glass G B J 1963 Coexisting gastric and duodenal ulcers. A review. American Journal of Digestive Diseases 8: 992

Whitfield P F, Hobsley M 1987 Comparison of maximal gastric secretion in smokers and non-smokers with and without duodenal ulcer. Gut 28: 557

Wilde M I, McTavish D 1994 Omeprazole. An update of its pharmacology and therapeutic use in acid-related disorders. Drugs 48(1): 91–132

Wolfe M M, Soll A H 1988 The physiology of gastric acid secretion. New England Journal of Medicine 319: 1707–1715

Wolfe M M, Jain D K, Edgerton J R 1985 Zollinger–Ellison syndrome associated with persistently normal fasting serum gastrin concentrations. Annals of Internal Medicine 103: 215–217

Wormsley K G 1984 Assessing the safety of drugs for the long-term treatment of peptic ulcers. Gut 25: 1416

Wright J P, Young G O, Klaff L J, Weers L A, Price S K, Marks I N 1982 Gastric mucosal prostaglandin E levels in patients with gastric ulcer disease and carcinoma. Gastroenterology 82: 263

Wyeth J W, Pounder R E, DeKoster E et al 1994 GR122311X (Ranitidine bismuth citrate) with antibiotics for the eradication of *Helicobacter pylori*. Gastroenterology 106: A212

Yeung C K, Fu K H, Yuen K Y et al 1990 *Helicobacter pylori* and associated duodenal ulcer. Archives of Disease in Childhood 65: 1212–1216

Zandomeneghi R, Serra L, Baumgartl U, Poppi M C 1991 The role of epidermal growth factor in the pathogenesis of peptic ulcer disease. American Journal of Gastroenterology 86: 1150–1153

Zboralske F F, Amberg J R 1968 Detection of the Zollinger–Ellison syndrome: the radiologist's responsibility. American Journal of Roentgenology 104: 529

Zollinger R M 1985 Gastrinoma: factors influencing prognosis. Surgery 97(1): 49–54

Zollinger R M, Ellison E H 1955 Primary peptic ulcerations of the jejunum associated with islet cell tumors of the pancreas. Annals of Surgery 142: 709–728

# 10. Surgical treatment of peptic ulcer and its complications

*D. C. Carter*

The incidence of peptic ulceration in Western countries has been declining since about 1960 and with it, the number of elective ulcer operations (Gustavsson et al 1988, Gustavsson 1988). The advent of effective medical therapy undoubtedly accelerated the decline in ulcer surgery. For example, $H_2$ receptor antagonists became widely available in 1977 and in one English region, the proportion of patients admitted with ulcer disease who underwent elective ulcer surgery fell from 74% in 1972–75 to 25% in 1979-84 (Bardhan et al 1989). Elective operations for peptic ulcer are now uncommon in Western centers.

The declining incidence of ulceration and elective surgery has not always been matched by falling rates of admission with ulcer bleeding or perforation (Bardhan et al 1989; see below). For example, in Helsinki between 1977 and 1987, the annual incidence of elective duodenal ulcer operations fell from 15.5 to 6.7 per $10^5$ inhabitants and that of elective gastric ulcer operations from 9.4 to 3.1 per $10^5$ (Paimela et al 1991). The decrease was greatest among men with duodenal ulcer, although the mean age of patients did not change. By contrast, the annual incidence of emergency surgery for ulcer hemorrhage and perforation did not decrease (ranging between 7.2 and 10.2 per $10^5$) and the mean age of the patients rose by approximately 5 years (to 60.4 years for duodenal ulcer and 63.7 years for gastric ulcer). In England and Wales, the number of deaths from peptic ulcer actually increased in the decade after $H_2$ receptor antagonists became available; bleeding and perforation accounted annually for some 4500 deaths and the increase was particularly evident in patients over 65 (Taylor 1989). In the United States some centers have noted a reduced number of admissions for hemorrhage or perforation (Elashoff & Grossman 1980) while others report no change (Gustavsson et al 1988). European centers also show variation (see Bardhan et al 1989) while in Hong Kong, the number of ulcer operations did not fall after introduction of the $H_2$ receptor antagonists and the number of admissions with ulcer perforation increased markedly (Alagaratnam & Wong, 1988)

## ASSESSMENT FOR SURGERY IN UNCOMPLICATED DUODENAL ULCER

A decision to advise surgery is based on the judgement of both the referring physician and surgeon as to whether an ulcer is intractable despite optimal medical treatment and on the risks and benefits of surgery relative to those of continued medical treatment. In patient selection and avoidance of surgical failure the obvious must be emphasized – the patient must have a duodenal ulcer and this must be responsible for the symptoms. It is not sufficient to demonstrate radiological deformity of the duodenal cap; an ulcer crater must be shown radiologically or, preferably, endoscopically.

### Severity of symptoms

The severity of pain and the incapacity it causes are key considerations. The success of surgery does not depend on the duration of symptoms (Small et al 1969, Macintyre et al 1990), although severe pain which persists despite modern medical therapy is now rare and should trigger a search for other causes of pain. Other factors to be considered include the degree to which the ulcer interferes with work (notably shift work), social life and family life.

### Failure of medical treatment

There must have been an adequate trial of medical therapy during which the patient should stop smoking and should moderate alcohol consumption. It is now usually possible to control symptoms rapidly and heal ulcers within weeks of commencing medical treatment, although pyloric channel and postbulbar ulcers may respond less well to medical therapy. The efficacy of modern antisecretory drugs may mean that patients now undergoing elective surgery have a more severe ulcer diathesis (Primrose et al 1988), although all are not agreed that resistance to antisecretory drugs adversely affects the outcome of surgery (Weaver & Temple 1985, Macintyre et al 1990).

The frequency and severity of relapse help to determine

the need for surgery and the patient's ability to comply with long-term medical treatment is critical. It may be unwise to commit a young patient to long-term drug therapy if there are problems of compliance or risks of side-effects, particularly when highly selective vagotomy now offers a safe chance of permanent cure without crippling sequelae. On the other hand, medical treatment has few side-effects and prolonged drug therapy is undoubtedly advisable in the elderly or those in whom surgery carries a higher than usual risk. It must also be recognized that there is some evidence that gastric surgery, or at least gastric resection, may expose patients to an increased risk of gastric cancer in later life (p. 298).

### Secretory status

Acid secretory tests are now rarely used but when they were, patients known to be high secretors (e.g. maximal acid output > 50 mmol/h) were thought less likely to be controlled by long-term medical therapy.

### Previous complications

Stenosis can be an indication for surgery in its own right (p. 283). Even though medical management initially relieved gastric outlet obstruction due to ulceration in 50% of cases in one series, 92% of patients presenting in this way needed surgery within 3 years (Jaffin & Kaye 1985). Previous ulcer bleeding or perforation in patients is usually regarded as strengthening the case for surgery although this has been challenged (Strom et al 1984). While the results of operations such as highly selective vagotomy are no worse in patients who have had previous ulcer complications, the risk of developing such complications falls markedly after surgery (Macintyre et al 1990).

### Other considerations

A strong family history of ulcer disease may be associated with failure to respond to medical therapy, but is also linked with a greater likelihood of ulcer recurrence after operation (Macintyre et al 1990).

## ASSESSMENT FOR SURGERY IN UNCOMPLICATED GASTRIC ULCER

Failure of medical therapy to allow or maintain ulcer healing and alleviate symptoms is the major indication for surgery in gastric ulceration. Anxiety that a gastric ulcer might be malignant has tended to dictate early referral for surgery, particularly when ulceration has recurred or persisted despite medical treatment. If the decision is taken to persist with medical treatment, great care must be taken to exclude malignancy by repeat endoscopy and repeat biopsies and it is well recognized that ulcer healing does not necessarily exclude malignancy. A German study involving 597 patients with gastric ulcers found malignancy in eight patients (1.8%) on repeat endoscopy, four of whom had become asymptomatic (Eckardt et al 1992). Ulcer recurrence does not necessarily mean that a patient is at increased risk of further recurrence or complications (Veterans Administration Cooperative Study on Gastric Ulcer 1971) and as 60% of gastric ulcer patients have major coincidental disease (Mowat et al 1975) there are often cogent reasons for avoiding surgery if at all possible.

## OPERATIONS FOR PEPTIC ULCER (Jamieson 1983, Johnson 1983)

All operations now available (Fig. 10.1) aim to reduce acid-pepsin secretion to levels which allow ulcer healing and prevent recurrence.

### Partial gastrectomy

Between 50% and 70% of the distal stomach is resected

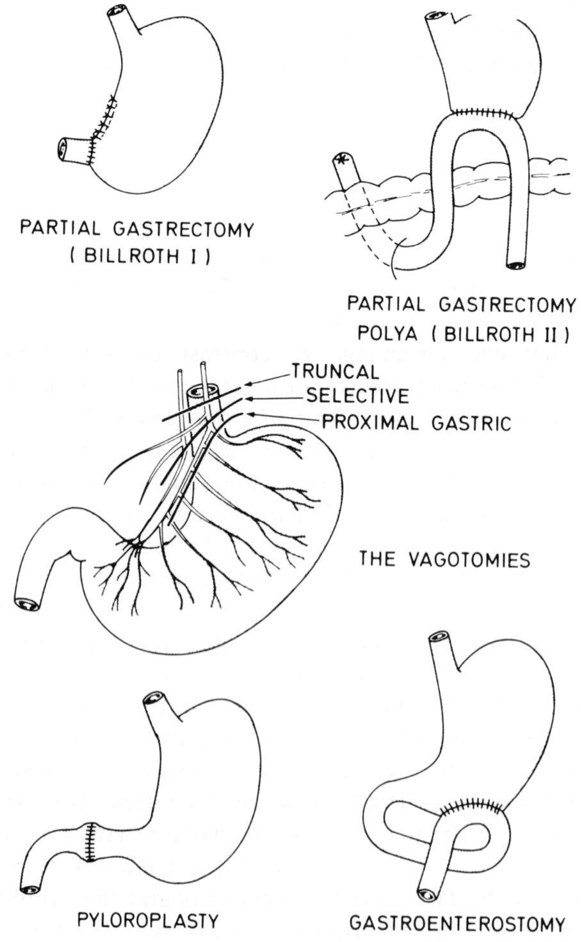


**Fig. 10.1** Operations for peptic ulcer.

and the gastric remnant is anastomosed to the duodenum (Billroth I) or jejunum (Billroth II). Partial gastrectomy removes the gastrin-producing antrum together with a variable amount of the acid-pepsin-secreting corpus and reduces acid secretion by some 70%. Modifications of partial gastrectomy which aim to avoid derangement of gastric emptying include pylorus-preserving gastrectomy (Maki et al 1977) and resection of the distal portion of the acid-secreting corpus combined with removal of the antral mucosa but not the antropyloric musculature (Yan et al 1991).

### Truncal vagotomy and drainage

This operation divides the anterior and posterior vagal trunks just after they enter the abdomen, so denervating the entire stomach, biliary tree, pancreas, small intestine and proximal large intestine. Truncal vagotomy abolishes direct vagal stimulation of acid secretion, reduces vagally mediated release of antral gastrin and desensitizes the parietal cells to humoral stimuli. Up to 40% of patients show evidence of residual vagal innervation on postoperative insulin testing (Smith et al 1972), reflecting the difficulty of identifying and dividing all vagal fibers.

A drainage procedure is normally performed at the same time to overcome the gastric stasis which otherwise follows truncal vagotomy.

#### *Gastroenterostomy (gastrojejunostomy)*

The jejunum is anastomosed to the dependent greater curvature of the stomach, the anastomosis usually being retrocolic (Fig. 10.1). At one time, gastroenterostomy without truncal vagotomy was used in patients with duodenal ulcers and low acid output, although the mechanism of ulcer healing was not understood. When used alone, gastroenterostomy had an unacceptably high ulcer recurrence rate and is no longer used without vagotomy.

#### *Pyloroplasty*

In the Heineke–Mikulicz procedure a 7–10 cm longitudinal incision is made through the distal antrum, pylorus and duodenum and then sewn up transversely. This widens the gastric outlet and disrupts the circular muscle fibers of the antrum and pylorus, so destroying the normal control of gastric emptying. Pyloric dilatation is an alternative to pyloroplasty (Thompson & Galloway 1979). Thoracoscopic or laparoscopic vagotomy has been carried out recently without drainage (McDermott & Murphy 1993); gastric stasis has proved troublesome in 10% of patients but can be dealt with by endoscopic balloon dilatation.

### Selective vagotomy and drainage

Selective vagotomy divided the vagal supply to the stomach, but spared that of the biliary tract, pancreas, small intestine and proximal large bowel. It was hoped that this would ensure complete gastric vagotomy but minimize gastrointestinal side-effects due to vagal denervation of the rest of the foregut and midgut. A drainage procedure was necessary as the antrum and pylorus were also denervated. When compared to truncal vagotomy and drainage, the operation took longer, had the same rate of recurrence and side-effects and is now obsolete.

### Highly selective vagotomy (parietal cell vagotomy, selective proximal vagotomy, parietal gastric vagotomy)

The anterior and posterior vagus nerves run close to the lesser curve of the stomach, giving branches to the corpus and ending in a "crow's foot" of branches which fan out to supply the antrum and pylorus. The aim of highly selective vagotomy is to denervate only the body of the stomach, sparing the vagal supply of the antrum and pylorus (so that a drainage procedure is not required) and other digestive organs. The procedure can be time consuming, especially in obese patients, but is as effective as truncal vagotomy in reducing acid output (Becker & Kelly 1983), does not adversely affect gastric emptying (Mayer et al 1984) and has a low incidence of postprandial side-effects. Provided that the parietal cell mass is denervated completely, the operation appears as effective in patients with high acid outputs as in those with lower outputs (Johnston et al 1975).

Attempts to make the operation easier to perform include lesser curve seromyotomy (Taylor 1979, Taylor et al 1982) and combining anterior highly selective vagotomy with posterior truncal vagotomy (Hill & Barker 1978). In seromyotomy, the vagal fibers supplying the parietal cells are divided by incising the muscle layers only of the body of the stomach, the incision running close to the lesser curve. Laparoscopic posterior truncal vagotomy with lesser curve anterior seromyotomy (Katkhouda & Mouiel 1991) and laparoscopic highly selective vagotomy (Dallemagne et al 1994) have been performed recently. Laparoscopic vagotomy appears to be safe, but as in other areas of minimally invasive surgery, the main advantage is a reduced length of hospital stay and convalescence.

### Truncal vagotomy and antrectomy

The combination of vagal denervation of the parietal cells and removal of the major source of gastrin means that acid secretion is markedly reduced and ulcer recurrence is rare. The operation has been used much more in the USA than in other Western countries.

## SELECTION OF OPERATION FOR DUODENAL ULCER

Each new operation for duodenal ulcer has been claimed as an advance, but enthusiasm has had to be tempered by the emergence of long-term side-effects. Factors influencing the choice of operation are operative mortality, risk of developing side-effects (notably vomiting, dumping, diarrhea and nutritional upsets) and incidence of recurrent ulcer.

### Operative mortality

Procedures involving gastric resection have a greater operative mortality than nonresectional operations. In 1962, Johnson found that the average mortality in the UK for partial gastrectomy was 4.5%, although improved technique and perioperative care brought rates down to 1–2%. The operative mortality after vagotomy and drainage in collected series has fallen below 1% and in one review was only 0.2% (Jamieson 1983). Soon after its introduction, reviews of highly selective vagotomy showed an operative mortality of 0.3% (Johnston 1975) and a number of series now report no mortality (Macintyre & Millar 1991). Vagotomy and antrectomy has approximately the same risks as partial gastrectomy with mortality falling in some series to less than 1% (Postlethwait 1973). As with all ulcer operations, the operative mortality rate is operator dependent and zero mortality rates have been reported from specialist centers even after vagotomy and partial gastric resection (Goligher et al 1968a, Jordan & Condon 1970).

### Recurrent ulceration

The incidence of recurrent ulcer after truncal vagotomy and drainage ranges from 2% to 27% with an overall rate of about 10% (Stabile & Passaro 1983), while after highly selective vagotomy it ranges from 9% to 30% in series followed for at least 5 years (Hoffmann et al 1987, Macintyre et al 1990). The rate is lowest after vagotomy and antrectomy, where it ranges from 0% to 3%, with an overall rate of 1% (Stabile & Passaro 1983). Partial gastrectomy occupies an intermediate position, the recurrence rate being lower when resection is more extensive. Recurrence rates are slightly greater after a Billroth I than a Polya (Billroth II) anastomosis, probably because less stomach is resected in the former operation.

### Other side-effects

Patients who undergo gastric resection are more likely to lose weight and have other nutritional problems, while truncal vagotomy and drainage is more likely to cause diarrhea. In a trial comparing vagotomy and gastroenterostomy, vagotomy and antrectomy, and partial gastrectomy (Polya), the Visick grading (see below) was almost the same for each operation (Goligher et al 1968a). Overall, highly selective vagotomy has fewer side-effects than other operations, but the operation has been blighted by its high recurrent ulcer rate (Stabile & Passaro 1983). While there is some evidence that women are more likely to have sequelae, at least after vagotomy and gastroenterostomy (Goligher et al 1968a), this does not appear to be the case after highly selective vagotomy (Linhardt et al 1982).

### Selection based on acid secretion

Selecting the type of operation on the basis of acid secretion (Bruce et al 1959) was an attractive concept, but the hope that gastroenterostomy alone would suffice when maximal acid output (MAO) was less than 30 mmol/h (Small 1973) has not been sustained. Vagotomy and antrectomy has been advocated in high acid secretors (Robbs et al 1973, Kronborg 1974) although Johnston et al (1975), in their evaluation of highly selective vagotomy, concluded that antrectomy was unnecessary in high secretors as long as the parietal cell mass was completely denervated. Others agree that preoperative acid secretion, duration of symptoms and site of ulceration are not risk factors for recurrence after highly selective vagotomy (Kjaergaard et al 1984).

### Conclusions

As all of the standard operations for duodenal ulcer can produce good results in good hands, the choice of procedure depends on the normal practice of the surgeon and the findings at operation. For example, pyloroplasty is usually contraindicated if the duodenum is grossly deformed and scarred, while highly selective vagotomy alone is inappropriate for patients with obstructing duodenal ulcer (Wang et al 1994). Highly selective vagotomy for uncomplicated duodenal ulcer undoubtedly gives minimal interference with gastrointestinal function, but at the expense of a high recurrence rate (Taylor 1987).

## OPERATIONS FOR GASTRIC ULCER

### Billroth I partial gastrectomy

The overall mortality for elective gastrectomy in collective review is 2% (range 0–6.2%), while recurrent ulceration rates range from zero to 17%, with an overall value of 2.8% (Greenall & Lehnert 1985). There is little difference between the Billroth I and Billroth II operations in terms of operative mortality. Gastrectomy removes the ulcer, allowing complete histological examination, and avoids the risk of leaving a potentially curable neoplasm in situ.

### Vagotomy and drainage

This operation is safer in high-risk patients and when a high gastric ulcer would necessitate extensive and potentially dangerous gastric resection. The collected operative mortality rate is 1.2% (range 0–4.1%) and the recurrent ulcer rate is 9% (range 3–36%) (Greenall & Lehnert 1985). Multiple biopsies (and if possible, cytological examination) are essential before operation and at the time of surgery. Some surgeons prefer to excise the ulcer as part of the operation so as to minimize the risk of leaving a malignant ulcer in situ. Highly selective vagotomy with excision of the ulcer has also been used to treat gastric ulcer (Reid et al 1982) but suffers from the drawbacks of vagotomy and drainage, including a high rate of recurrent ulceration, and is no longer used.

### Conclusions

Although vagotomy with drainage may have a slightly lower operative morbidity and mortality, its long-term results are not sufficiently superior to justify abandoning partial gastrectomy in the treatment of benign gastric ulcer.

## IMMEDIATE POSTOPERATIVE COMPLICATIONS

Complications attributable to any abdominal operation (e.g. chest infection or pulmonary embolus) will not be discussed here but specific complications of gastroduodenal surgery will be considered.

### Leakage of gastrointestinal content

Although leakage from an anastomosis or pyloroplasty is now rare, leakage from the duodenal stump remains a significant cause of death after Billroth II partial gastrectomy. Leakage from the duodenal stump is usually heralded by signs of peritonitis 3–5 days after operation and/or leakage of bile-stained fluid from drains placed down to the duodenal stump at operation. Immediate reoperation is not necessary provided there is adequate external drainage and the patient has no evidence of worsening peritonitis or abscess formation. Nasogastric suction, protection of the skin and intravenous feeding allow the majority of "controlled" fistulae to heal spontaneously provided that there is no distal obstruction of the intestine (Garden et al 1988).

### Lesser curve necrosis

This complication of highly selective vagotomy occurs in about 1 in 500 cases and has a mortality rate of 50%; it results from injury or devascularization of the lesser curve at operation (Johnston 1975). Fundoplication at the time of highly selective vagotomy can be contributory if it entails greater devascularization of the stomach and causes gaseous gastric distention (Kennedy et al 1979). Lesser curve necrosis presents with perforation, usually between the third and seventh postoperative day. Prompt diagnosis and gastrectomy are essential if the patient is to survive.

### Obstruction

Gastric peristalsis recovers slowly after gastric resection or denervation and there is debate as to whether nasogastric suction is advisable. Suction reduces pressure on suture lines but is uncomfortable, predisposes to esophagitis and favors chest infection by inhibiting coughing.

Obstruction can occur after any gastric operation but is particularly common after vagotomy (Bushkin & Woodward 1976c). Edema at the suture line usually resolves on conservative management, but mechanical causes such as internal herniation and intussusception (p. 269) require reoperation. Gastrografin examination is useful in determining the need for reintervention.

### Postoperative bleeding

This occasional complication is usually due to bleeding from the suture line, but an unresected ulcer is occasionally responsible. Suture line bleeding is usually evident within hours of surgery and is initially treated conservatively (p. 482); if bleeding persists the suture line is oversewn. Intraoperative and postoperative bleeding can also result from operative damage to the spleen and, on rare occasions, to the liver.

### Pancreatitis

Potentially lethal pancreatitis occasionally results from pancreatic injury during dissection of a posterior duodenal ulcer. It can also develop after Billroth II partial gastrectomy if afferent loop obstruction leads to raised intraduodenal pressure. Afferent loop obstruction is treated by anastomosing the afferent to the efferent loop.

### Esophageal problems

Perforation of the esophagus during vagotomy occurs in about 0.5% of cases (Koetz & Gewertz 1979) and may prove fatal unless the damage is appreciated at the time and the defect oversewn. Dysphagia occurs after vagotomy in up to 20% of patients but is usually mild and transient.

## ASSESSMENT OF THE RESULTS OF SURGERY (Small 1983)

There are many pitfalls in assessing the success or failure of ulcer surgery. The patient may not wish to appear ungrateful to the surgeon and outcome is best assessed by an independent observer. Grading of symptoms is usually carried out using Visick's classification (Table 10.1). A good or excellent result (grades 1 or 2) is obtained in over 70% of patients and some 5–10% are allocated to the "unsatisfactory" grades 3u or 4 depending on the type of operation. The results in women are often poorer, with more weight loss and a greater incidence of vomiting and dumping (Pulvertaft 1952). The Visick classification is often used to compare results between centers, although lack of preoperative standardization may mean that patient groups are not comparable.

Recurrent ulcer has often been regarded as the main indicator of failure, mainly because the aim of operation was to cure the ulcer. Visick grade 4 includes ulcer recurrence, but it is arguable whether one recurrence, promptly and readily treated, during perhaps 10 years of freedom from symptoms, should be classed as failure. Many now believe that this assignment is inappropriate (Macintyre & Millar 1991) and it is generally agreed that the worst failures of surgery are patients with severe dumping, vomiting, diarrhea and malnutrition, problems which are often unresponsive to treatment.

Success can also be assessed by the ability to work and by the quality of life. The great majority of patients return to normal work. Over 60% of patients have emotional disturbances due to chronic dyspepsia prior to surgery (Small et al 1969), but nearly all return to normal after operation (Philip & Cay 1972).

Despite earlier reports that gastrectomy for peptic ulcer decreased long-term survival, a large Swedish cohort study showed recently that the operation had little effect on life expectancy over the next 20 years, once the patient had survived the first year (Lundergardh et al 1991). The slight but significant decrease in survival thereafter was thought to be attributable to confounding factors (e.g. smoking) linked to the peptic ulcer disease rather than the surgical procedure per se.

There is an association between gastric surgery, particularly partial gastrectomy (Whitlock 1961), and alcoholism. Some patients have been heavy drinkers prior to surgery and alcohol and cigarette smoking may have been contributory factors in their ulcer diathesis. Others become alcoholics after surgery because they can consume alcohol without ulcer pain or because alcohol offsets complications such as dumping. Suicide in males after gastric surgery is three to four times commoner than expected (Westlund 1963) and alcoholism may be an important factor. Some problems, particularly recurrent ulcer, are commoner in patients taking drugs such as salicylates.

In some psychopathic patients, operation is followed by persistent severe symptoms, a state termed the "albatross" syndrome (Johnstone et al 1967). Long-term problems are particularly common when a definitive procedure has been performed in the absence of an ulcer at operation.

**Table 10.1** Visick grading (Visick 1948, Pulvertaft 1952)

| | |
|---|---|
| Grade 1 | No symptoms |
| Grade 2 | Mild symptoms, easily controlled |
| Grade 3s | (s = satisfactory). Mild symptoms, not controlled, but the patient denies that they are causing disability |
| Grade 3u | (u = unsatisfactory). Mild symptoms, not controlled, which are severe enough to restrict the patient's life |
| Grade 4 | Not improved, e.g. recurrence of ulcer after surgery, readmission to hospital because of symptoms or a second definitive operation was necessary |
| Grade 1 plus 2 | = good surgical result |
| Grade 3s | = moderate surgical result |
| Grades 3u plus 4 | = bad surgical result |

## GASTRIC EMPTYING AFTER SURGERY

Epigastric fullness after meals occurs in 30–40% of patients after all forms of gastric surgery, including highly selective vagotomy (Goligher et al 1978). After gastric resection this may reflect the small size of the stomach, but after vagotomy it is due predominantly to abolition of receptive relaxation of the gastric corpus. Vagal denervation of the proximal stomach results in accelerated emptying of liquids, especially during the early phase of gastric emptying, and may contribute to dumping and diarrhea (pp. 272 and 440) (Fig. 15.3c). Postprandial epigastric fullness after all types of vagotomy is usually mild and frequently improves with time and there is evidence that receptive relaxation only remains abnormal in patients who have diarrhea (Hartley & Mackie 1991). Despite its effects on receptive relaxation, highly selective vagotomy usually results in normal gastric emptying after solid meals (Myer et al 1984) and carries a low incidence of dumping and diarrhea.

Denervation of the distal stomach (as occurs in truncal vagotomy) results in delayed emptying of solids due to loss of the antral mill activity. Stasis is normally avoided by a drainage procedure, although this can further accelerate the emptying of liquids. A few patients have delayed emptying of solids after vagotomy despite a drainage procedure and experience nausea and vomiting and even recurrent bezoar formation or gastric mycosis (Rehnberg et al 1982).

Gastric emptying is increased after partial gastrectomy because the antropyloric controlling mechanisms are lost.

## VOMITING

Vomiting may be a problem after vagotomy and drainage or gastric resection (Cox 1968, Cox et al 1969, Goligher 1970), but is rare after highly selective vagotomy (Macintyre et al 1990). It usually amounts to only occasional regurgitation of a mouthful of bile-stained fluid or an occasional small vomit of food.

The term "chronic afferent loop obstruction" implies

vomiting of copious amounts of bile-stained fluid due to mechanical obstruction of an afferent loop. The term "bilious vomiting" is used for all other cases of bile vomiting after food. The term "afferent loop syndrome" should be reserved to describe stasis in the afferent loop in association with bacterial colonization. Biliary gastritis, like bilious vomiting, is caused by reflux of bile into the stomach but is not necessarily accompanied by bilious vomiting. Chronic afferent loop obstruction, bilious vomiting and biliary gastritis are related etiologically and their investigation and management are similar.

### **Gastroparesis** (p. 427)

This is a rare cause of delayed gastric emptying, nausea and vomiting after vagotomy. Radiographic and endoscopic investigations show gastric stasis without organic obstruction or mucosal abnormality. Emptying can be improved by prokinetic agents (p. 433) such as metoclopramide 10–20 mg half an hour before food (Malagelada et al 1980). Bezoar is described on page 327.

### Vomiting caused by organic obstruction

Persistent vomiting of food may be due to duodenal stenosis after pyloroplasty or obstruction of the efferent loop after gastrojejunostomy, usually by edema from recurrent ulcer. Further surgery is required.

### Afferent loop obstruction

This complication of Billroth II partial gastrectomy or gastrojejunostomy can present acutely (usually after gastrectomy) or as chronic intermittent obstruction.

#### *Acute afferent loop obstruction*

This occurs in less than 1% of patients after Billroth II gastrectomy. Two-thirds of cases occur in the first week, but the obstruction can take 5 years to become manifest (Hoffman & Spiro 1961). Causes include herniation of a long afferent loop behind the efferent limb (Dahlgren 1964), volvulus of the afferent loop, sharp angulation of the anastomosis caused by a short afferent loop and retrograde intussusception of jejunal mucosa into the stomach (Robertson & Weder 1968). Retrograde intussusception is recognized radiographically as a filling defect in relation to the stoma (Fig. 10.2).

***Clinical features.*** There is sudden pain in the epigastrium or right hypochondrium, vomiting (without bile) and shock. A mass may be palpable and infarction of the loop may lead to perforation and peritonitis. Jaundice and pancreatitis can develop. A plain abdominal radiograph may show the distended loop and the serum amylase is frequently raised. Early diagnosis and immediate surgery are important as the risk of strangulation and gangrene is high. In one series, 54 of 105 patients died (Dahlgren 1964).

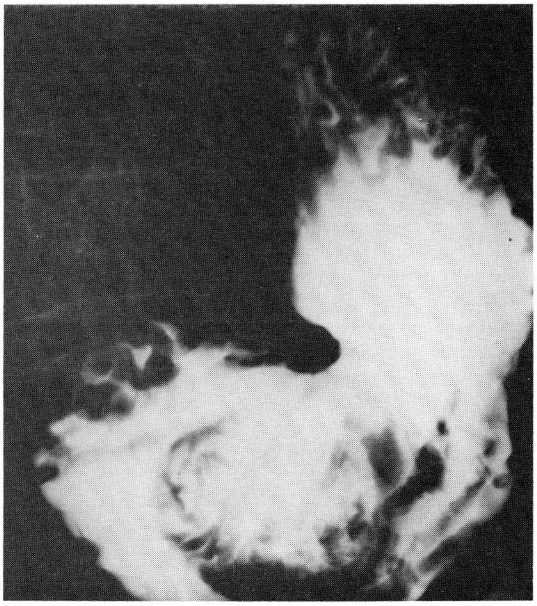

**Fig. 10.2** Retrograde jejunogastric intussusception causing large filling defect in stomach. Patient had a gastroenterostomy several years previously.

#### *Chronic afferent loop obstruction*

Many patients present in the same way as those with bilious vomiting (see below) and the true diagnosis is only made when the obstruction is detected. The condition is rare and most patients thought to have it in the past were probably suffering from bilious vomiting.

Passage of food into the efferent loop stimulates biliary and pancreatic secretion. Pressure rises in the obstructed afferent loop until the obstruction is overcome, the sudden entry of secretions into the stomach leading to vomiting. Causes of chronic obstruction are herniation of the afferent loop, twisting or kinking of the afferent loop and problems at the stoma such as retrograde intussusception, prolapse or inflammation due to ulcer.

***Clinical features.*** Cramping pain in the epigastrium and nausea develop soon after eating and are relieved after about an hour by vomiting a large volume of bile-stained secretion which does not contain food. The straight abdominal radiograph may show air and fluid in a distended loop (see Berenbaum et al 1968). A barium meal using a small volume of barium to avoid obscuring the stomal region may demonstrate a dilated (Fig. 10.3), kinked or unusually long afferent loop. The afferent loop often fails to fill but this is also common in asymptomatic patients. The barium meal may show a left-to-right gastrojejunostomy, which can result in kinking of the efferent loop with afferent loop stasis. This can be demonstrated radiologi-

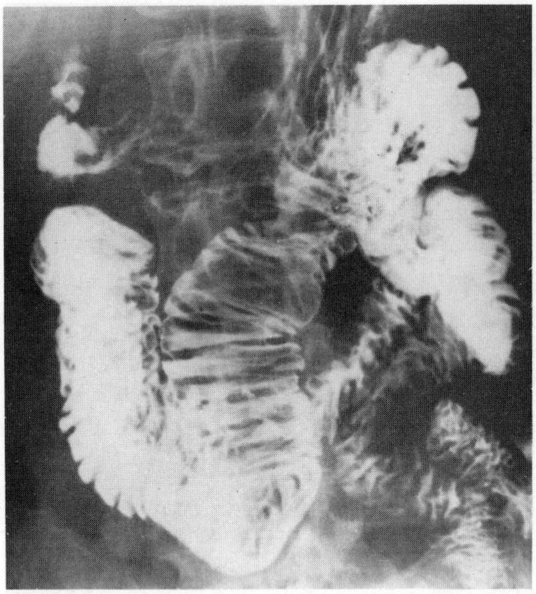

**Fig. 10.3** Dilated afferent loop following gastroenterostomy. History of recurrent attacks of bile vomiting.

cally when the patient is erect, but it is not obvious at operation (Burhenne 1968). Intravenous secretin or cholecystokinin may reproduce the symptoms and cause hyperamylasemia (Bushkin & Woodward 1976a). Surgical treatment is required to relieve the obstruction.

**Bilious vomiting** (Alexander-Williams & Hoare 1979, Meyer 1979)

The mechanism of bile vomiting is unresolved. It was once thought that bile and pancreatic secretions accumulated in the afferent loop, which then emptied and caused vomiting. However, bilious vomiting can occur after pyloroplasty and the stimulus to vomiting is simply the presence of bile in the stomach. It was shown that when a solid meal was mixed with barium, bile appeared on top of the mixture and its presence was related to development of symptoms (Toye & Williams 1965). Gastric emptying studies have confirmed delay in emptying bile and intestinal refluxate from the stomach (Mackie et al 1986) and the amount of bile acids in the fasting stomach correlates with epigastric pain and its relief by vomiting (Alexander-Williams & Hoare 1979, Cabrol et al 1990). However, constituents of upper intestinal content other than bile acids may also cause symptoms (Meshkinpour et al 1980).

Bilious vomiting is more likely after gastrojejunostomy. Goligher et al (1972) found an incidence of 13–14% after operations involving a gastrojejunal anastomosis as opposed to 10% after vagotomy and pyloroplasty. Amdrup et al (1974) found bilious vomiting in 2% of patients after highly selective vagotomy, 8–11% after vagotomy and pyloroplasty, and 16% after truncal vagotomy and gastroenterostomy. Others have reported a low (6%) incidence of bilious vomiting 5 years or more after highly selective vagotomy (Goligher et al 1978).

*Clinical features*

Symptoms develop within 3 months of surgery in two-thirds of cases (Griffiths 1974). Typically, the patient vomits clear, bitter, yellow-green fluid, occasionally mixed with food. Cramping epigastric pain, distention and nausea within an hour of eating are often relieved by vomiting, although vomiting can be unrelated to meals and sometimes occurs at night or on waking in the morning. There may be loss of weight and anorexia. Long periods of freedom can be interspersed with periods when vomiting occurs each day.

*Investigation*

Endoscopy is essential to exclude recurrent ulceration and document the appearances of the gastric mucosa. Alexander-Williams & Hoare (1979) compared asymptomatic patients after gastric surgery with those who had bilious vomiting. There were no endoscopic findings confined to the latter group, although severe erythema affecting the entire stomach, bile staining of adherent mucus and bile reflux throughout the examination were more common. The presence of erosions, edema and contact bleeding were unrelated to symptoms. A "double-barrel stoma" with separate openings for the afferent and efferent loops favors entry of bile into the stomach (Demaret et al 1971) and is associated with a high incidence of pain, vomiting, dumping and diarrhea.

Measurement of intragastric bile acid concentrations and scintigraphy using $^{99m}$Tc-labeled IDA derivatives (p. 86) now allow quantification of duodenogastric reflux (Houghton et al 1986) and patients with bile acid reflux exceeding 80 μmol/h are those likely to benefit from biliary diversion (Cabrol et al 1990).

*Treatment*

Many patients improve with time. Small dry meals, with fluids taken only between meals, may be helpful, as may metoclopramide (10 mg 15 min before meals). Agents which bind bile acids, such as cholestyramine and aluminum hydroxide, give variable results.

If symptoms are severe and intractable, surgery is indicated. Symptoms following truncal vagotomy and gastroenterostomy are best dealt with by closing the gastroenterostomy and, provided that the pyloric canal is patent, pyloroplasty is unnecessary (McMahon et al 1978, Green et al 1978). Patients who have had a Billroth II partial gastrectomy may benefit from conversion to a gastroduodenal anastomosis, but more reliable results are obtained if a 10–15 cm jejunal loop is interposed between stomach and duodenum (Kelly et al 1981). Alternatively, reflux can be prevented by a Roux-en-Y anastomosis, ensuring that duodenal contents enter the jejunum at least 45 cm distal to the gastrojejunal anastomosis (Kennedy & Green 1978, Alexander-Williams & Hoare 1979, Kelly et al 1981, Malagelada et al 1985).

In a review of 111 patients 6–14 years after the onset of vomiting, symptoms had disappeared in 20%, 48% still had occasional vomiting, 9% were disabled and 23% had undergone further surgery (Griffiths 1974).

## ALKALINE REFLUX GASTRITIS (BILIARY GASTRITIS)

### Etiology

Alkaline reflux gastritis is almost inevitable after gastric operations which destroy or remove the antropyloric "gatekeeper" or create a gastrojejunostomy, but is unusual after highly selective vagotomy (Dewar et al 1982). It can also occur after cholecystectomy or sphincteroplasty when there is continuous flow of bile into the duodenum. Predisposing factors are additive and reflux is greater after truncal vagotomy and pyloroplasty plus cholecystectomy than after either procedure alone (Brough et al 1984). Reflux may also occur in individuals who have not had previous gastric or biliary surgery.

Symptomatic biliary gastritis affects less than 5% of patients after gastric surgery and such patients have more reflux than asymptomatic individuals (Cabrol et al 1990). Bile salts cause injury by solubilizing lipids in mucosal membranes and there is debate as to whether deconjugated bile acids, pancreatic enzymes, alkalinity and bacteria add to this toxicity. Gastric emptying in patients with alkaline reflux gastritis may be faster or slower than normal (Pellegrini et al 1985).

### Pathology (see also p. 227)

Given that some degree of gastritis is almost universal after gastric surgery, it is difficult to determine the extent to which this is due to bile reflux (Alexander-Williams & Hoare 1979, Farrands et al 1983). Variable superficial inflammation with focal hemorrhage and ulceration are found, in association with chronic inflammatory infiltration. A degree of atrophic gastritis is common, but the most marked changes are epithelial, especially in the pits (Weinstein et al 1985). The histological apperances do not correlate with endoscopic appearances and have a variable relationship with the presence of symptoms.

### Clinical features (Nath & Warshaw 1984, Ritchie 1984)

Continuous burning epigastric pain is often exacerbated by eating and is sometimes accompanied by nausea, weight loss and anemia. Vomiting of bile may be a feature but many patients with biliary gastritis do not experience bilious vomiting. Symptoms may develop many years after gastric surgery, raising anxiety that gastric cancer is present.

### Investigations

The condition is difficult to diagnose radiologically, even using double-contrast barium meal (Ott et al 1982). Endoscopy is essential and typically reveals erythema, edema, erosions and adherent mucus and sometimes spontaneous mucosal bleeding (which frequently causes iron deficiency anemia). Usually there is a pool of bile-stained fluid in the stomach or gastric remnant. These features are pronounced near the stoma but may be generalized. Biopsy of the gastric mucosa does not add to the information obtained at endoscopy, but is advisable to exclude dysplasia in patients presenting long after gastric surgery.

Some authors have infused upper gastrointestinal contents (Meshkinpour et al 1980) or alkali and gastric contents (Warshaw 1981) into the stomach to reproduce symptoms. Others have used $^{99m}$Tc-HIDA scintigraphy (Tolin et al 1979) or the concentration of bile acids in gastric juice (Cabrol et al 1990) to assess reflux. Transmucosal flux of lithium has also been used to assess the severity of gastritis (Gough et al 1986).

Whichever method of assessment is employed, it is essential to exclude other potential causes of the patient's symptoms, especially biliary and pancreatic disease.

### Treatment

The treatment is the same as that of bilious vomiting. Antacids per se are of no value, but aluminum hydroxide may be used in an attempt to adsorb bile salts. Antibiotics of the type used to treat bacterial overgrowth syndromes (p. 464) are worthy of trial. If surgical treatment is necessary, a Roux-en-Y anastomosis should be created some 45 cm distal to the gastrojejunal anastomosis. While long-term follow-up of 22 patients after Roux-en-Y diversion found that bile reflux gastritis was prevented or treated in all cases, eight patients (36%) were still classified as clinical failures (Visick 3 or 4) (McAlhany et al 1994). The "Roux stasis syndrome" of chronic abdominal pain, nausea and vomiting, particularly after eating (Mathias et al 1985), accounted for six of the failures. Disordered transit in the Roux limb in association with delayed gastric emptying may be responsible for this syndrome and is more likely when a Roux loop is used in revisional as opposed to primary gastric surgery (Britton et al 1987).

## ALKALINE REFLUX ESOPHAGITIS

This is commoner after total gastrectomy or partial gastrectomy, but can occur after other gastric operations and in normal individuals. There is often associated biliary gastritis. Bile acids and proteolytic pancreatic enzymes injure the esophageal mucosa and damage is compounded by acid and pepsin. Indeed, alkaline reflux may play a role in so-called peptic esophagitis (Pellegrini et al 1978) (p. 192).

Severe heartburn aggravated by food is common and swallowing can be painful (Bushkin & Woodward 1976b). There may be waterbrash, vomiting and symptoms related to chronic aspiration. Esophagoscopy reveals severe diffuse inflammation with extreme mucosal friability. "Peptic esophagitis" is excluded in postsurgery patients by demonstrating achlorhydria or marked hypochlorhydria.

The medical measures used to treat biliary gastritis are usually ineffective and Roux loop diversion is indicated (Himal 1977, Alexander-Williams & Hoare 1979).

## CHOLELITHIASIS

The incidence of gallstones increases after gastric resection or vagotomy and drainage surgery for peptic ulcer disease. Gallstones appear to develop within a few years of surgery and cholelithiasis in one recent study of female patients was twice as prevalent as in age- and sex-matched controls (Thompson et al 1994). Vagal denervation is followed by enlargement of the gallbladder, although this may be due to indirect effects such as changes in sphincter of Oddi function or failure to respond to cholecystokinin. The influence of vagotomy on bile composition and lithogenicity is controversial, but bile acid synthesis is now known to be depressed (Thompson et al 1994)

## DUMPING

This complication affects approximately 20% of patients after gastrectomy or vagotomy and gastrojejunostomy and 10% after vagotomy and pyloroplasty (Goligher et al 1972). Fortunately, the symptoms are severe in only 1–3% of patients. After highly selective vagotomy, the incidence after 1 year was 6% in one series (Humphrey et al 1972) and after 5–8 years it was only 0.9% (Goligher et al 1978).

### Clinical features

Weakness, faintness, dizziness, somnolence or drowsiness, sweating, palpitations, pallor and a feeling of abdominal distention develop within half an hour of eating. This is why the condition has been called "early dumping" to distinguish it from the reactive hypoglycemia which can occur 2–3 h after food and which was once called "late dumping" (p. 273). Cramps and diarrhea may develop and all symptoms are helped by lying down. Patients sometimes find that symptoms are worse after fluid meals, such as soups, or after sweet foods. Dumping is most common in the early postoperative period but usually diminishes in frequency and severity over the ensuring months. When it continues, it may lead to food avoidance and weight loss.

### Mechanism of dumping

Dumping is ten times more common after pyloroplasty and vagotomy than after highly selective vagotomy and the most important factor in pathogenesis is loss of control of gastric emptying by the antropyloric region. Creation of a large stoma, reduced gastric reservoir capacity after resection and loss of receptive relaxation after vagotomy are all contributory factors. Dumping may be more common after surgery which markedly reduces acid-secreting capacity (Thomson et al 1974), as acid is one of the factors which slow gastric emptying (p. 424). Although dumping symptoms can occur in individuals with a normal stomach, they are never severe.

If gastric contents empty rapidly into the jejunum, there is no time for them to be rendered isotonic. In 1950, Machella showed that symptoms could be produced in patients and normal subjects by intrajejunal instillation of hypertonic solutions. Entry of such solutions into the jejunum leads to a period of increased jejunal motor activity (Christoffersson et al 1962), spreading the solution along the intestine and evoking an outpouring of fluid into the bowel lumen so that plasma volume is reduced by as much as 20% (Le Quesne et al 1960). This fall in plasma volume, together with abnormal redistribution of blood flow, leads to the feeling of faintness. Mesenteric blood flow is increased (Aldoori et al 1985) with splanchnic pooling and variable effects on peripheral blood flow, including postural hypotension. It is unlikely that the fall in plasma volume is entirely responsible for symptoms since comparable falls induced by venesection do not produce symptoms. Symptoms of dumping have also been produced by distending the jejunum with a balloon (Machella 1950). The feeling of abdominal distention is probably caused by a combination of rapid gastric emptying and profuse secretion of fluid into the jejunum.

The search for a humoral "dumping factor" was triggered by demonstration of such a factor in the portal venous blood of dogs after intrajejunal instillation of hypertonic glucose (Woodward 1976). The release of humoral factor(s) could contribute to postural hypotension by causing peripheral vasodilatation. The rapid transit of hyperosmolar chyme to the distal small intestine results in rapid release of enteroglucagon, neurotensin, vasoactive intestinal polypeptide (VIP) and peptide YY (Adrian et al 1985). The exact significance of these polypeptides is uncertain, although infusion of neurotensin alone does not reproduce symptoms (Pedersen et al 1986). Infusion of somatostatin may block release of these hormones and ameliorate dumping symptoms (see below).

### Treatment

As dumping usually improves with time, reoperation should not be considered until at least 2 years of medical treatment have proved unsuccessful. Two-thirds of 42 patients with dumping in one series were symptom free 3–12 years later and the majority had returned to a normal diet (Chaimoff & Dintsman 1972). Symptoms can often be controlled by eating frequent small dry meals and taking fluids between, rather than with, meals. Sweet foods and soups should be avoided. Symptoms are sometimes alleviated by tolbutamide (250 mg 30 min before food), propantheline, methysergide or propranolol, but their value is uncertain. Somatostatin analogs such as SMS 201–995 (50–100 μg subcutaneously) greatly improve dumping symptoms (Long et al 1985, Hopman et al 1988, Primrose & Johnston 1989) and may act by slowing gastric emptying, delaying intestinal transit and preventing release of other gastrointestinal peptides. A stable fat emulsion (20 g soya bean oil in 100 ml water) given 20 min before food also reduces symptoms of dumping by delaying gastric emptying (Lawaetz et al 1986).

Surgery is considered for patients who are incapacitated despite intensive medical treatment. Incapacity is often equated with inability to work in spite of a previously good work record and the unpredictability of symptoms can pose particular difficulty. Patients with severe dumping frequently have psychiatric or psychological problems (Eldh et al 1974) and/or belong to lower social groups and often cannot come to terms with their symptoms. Such social and psychiatric aspects must be explored fully before embarking on surgery. It is also useful to have objective evidence of dumping. Rapid gastric emptying is inferred if barium reaches the cecum within 30 min (Mattsson & Perman 1962) or there is a rapid initial rise in blood glucose during an oral glucose tolerance test (Stemmer et al 1969). Symptoms may also be produced by a dumping provocation test in which 350 ml of 25% glucose is given orally (Primrose & Johnston 1989). Ralphs et al (1978) used a labeled meal containing hypertonic glucose; gastric emptying was significantly faster and the fall in plasma volume was significantly greater in patients with symptoms of dumping.

Several surgical procedures can be used but overall results are disappointing. Closing a gastroenterostomy without creating a pyloroplasty may be effective (Green et al 1978, McMahon et al 1978) and pyloric reconstruction benefits some patients with dumping after pyloroplasty (Koruth et al 1985). Gastric emptying after surgery is slower in patients who derive symptomatic benefit (Cheadle et al 1985). Billroth II gastrectomy can be converted to a Billroth I anastomosis or an isoperistaltic or retroperistaltic jejunal loop can be interposed between the stomach and duodenum to slow gastric emptying (Mackie et al 1981).

## LATE HYPOGLYCEMIA

Weakness, faintness, anxiety, palpitation, nausea and hunger occurring 90 min or more after a meal and relieved by sweetened drinks can be caused by reactive hypoglycemia. The complication affects about 5% of patients after gastrectomy or vagotomy and drainage and is commoner after gastrojejunal anastomosis (Welbourn et al 1951, Goligher et al 1968b). The symptoms are rarely severe.

### Etiology (Woodward & Neustein 1976)

Partial gastrectomy or truncal vagotomy and drainage disrupt the normal control of gastric emptying, so that a large glucose load enters the small intestine rapidly. The rapid glucose absorption is reflected in an early high peak on the glucose tolerance curve. Simultaneously, excessive release of enteroglucagon sensitizes the β cells of the pancreatic islets, so that the hyperglycemia triggers abnormally large release of insulin.

### Investigation and treatment

An oral glucose tolerance test helps to identify patients prone to develop reactive hypoglycemia. After the oral load, serum insulin concentrations rise to three to four times the levels normally found at 30–60 min and hypoglycemia can be demonstrated at 1.5–3 h.

Late hypoglycemia is managed by carbohydrate restriction (initially to 50 g/day) and by taking frequent dry meals. If symptoms persist, the patient should have a readily available source of carbohydrate, such as sweets.

## DIARRHEA (Cuschieri 1990)

The frequency of bowel movement may increase after any gastric operation and particularly after truncal vagotomy and drainage. The reported frequency of diarrhea after vagotomy varies greatly, some surgeons citing a frequency of up to 20% with severe diarrhea in 0.5–8% of cases (Cuschieri 1990). Much depends on what is meant by "diarrhea". Goligher et al (1968a) defined diarrhea as three or more liquid motions per day and Cuschieri (1990) has emphasized the accompanying urgency and occasional incontinence which may curtail activity and social life. After vagotomy, about one-third of patients notice no change in bowel habit and a third find that instead of being constipated they now have regular formed motions without using laxatives. Johnston et al (1972) found that 25% of 1130 patients had episodic diarrhea after vagotomy with drainage or antrectomy. After vagotomy and gastrojejunostomy, Goligher (1970) reported that 5% of patients have severe diarrhea compared to 1% after partial gastrectomy. Diarrhea after gastrectomy tends to be continuous, whereas after truncal vagotomy it is intermittent and explosive. Diarrhea is more common if truncal vagotomy is combined with cholecystectomy (Taylor et al 1978). After highly selective vagotomy, about 3–4% of patients have mild or moderate diarrhea, but less than half of this number have severe episodic diarrhea (Goligher et al 1978, Macintyre et al 1990).

### Mechanism of diarrhea

Usually, no precise cause can be found. Some patients have marked steatorrhea and others have dumping. The association with dumping suggests that in some cases at least, gastric incontinence exposes the proximal small intestine to a hyperosmolar load. Increased passage of fluid, electrolytes and malabsorbed nutrients into the colon has been demonstrated (Ladas et al 1983) and bile acid diarrhea and impaired pancreatic secretion may also contribute. Fecal excretion of bile acids is certainly excessive in patients with postvagotomy diarrhea who have also had a cholecystectomy (Blake et al 1983).

Rapid intestinal transit is also likely to be important. After truncal vagotomy, intestinal motility is increased (McKelvey 1970) and marked reduction in the feeding pattern of activity allows early resumption of migrating complexes (Thompson et al 1982a). This probably results in a slightly increased fecal fat excretion which is unrelated to bacterial colonization of the upper small intestine (Browning et al 1974). Diarrhea is uncommon after highly selective vagotomy, probably because gastric emptying and pancreatic exocrine function are relatively normal and vagal hepatic fibers are preserved (Ramus et al 1982).

Other potential factors include intolerance to lactose or milk protein as a consequence of rapid gastric emptying (Kern & Struthers 1966) and predisposition to enteric infections because of achlorhydria and/or rapid passage of food into the intestine. Chronic salmonellosis can cause prolonged periods of diarrhea (Waddell & Kunz 1956) and giardiasis may also occur.

### Treatment

If dumping is present, measures to control it (p. 273) should be instituted. It is important to exclude significant steatorrhea and intestinal infection and assess the response to a lactose-free or milk-free diet.

Treatment of episodic diarrhea with urgency is more difficult. The severity of attacks may be limited by regular use of Lomotil (2.5 mg or 5 mg four times a day). In patients not receiving continuous medication, a single dose of Lomotil (5 mg) or codeine phosphate often brings relief within 30 min. An increase in dietary fiber is helpful in some patients. If diarrhea is not controlled by these measures, cholestyramine 4 g/day is worthy of trial (Allan & Russell 1975), particularly in patients who have undergone cholecystectomy. Octreotide can be used (p. 273).

If diarrhea continues to be disabling for at least 2 years despite medical therapy, surgical attempts to slow intestinal transit may be considered, provided that organic gastrointestinal disease has been excluded. When there is marked dumping after vagotomy and drainage, revision of the drainage procedure (see above) may be worthwhile in the first instance. Interposition of an antiperistaltic 10–12 cm jejunal segment at 100 cm beyond the duodenojejunal flexure has been advocated (Herrington et al 1986), but problems with intestinal obstruction and bacterial overgrowth have led others to use an onlay graft of reversed ileum to create a passive nonpropulsive segment some 30 cm from the ileocecal junction (Cuschieri 1990).

## NUTRITIONAL AND ABSORPTIVE DISORDERS

### Weight loss after operation

Postoperative weight should be compared to "ideal" weight according to life assurance tables, since some patients are underweight at the time of operation. Goligher et al (1968a) found insignificant weight loss after vagotomy and drainage but a loss of approximately 10% after vagotomy and antrectomy or subtotal gastrectomy. Other studies (Wastell 1969) show little difference between operations, while Wheldon et al (1970) found that weight loss 15 years after vagotomy and gastroenterostomy was commoner in women. There is no weight loss after highly selective vagotomy.

The cause of weight loss is complex, but most patients with marked loss have reduced food intake (Wheldon et al 1970), usually because of dumping or vomiting. Mild steatorrhea is occasionally contributory. Other causes of weight loss such as gastric cancer and tuberculosis (see below) must be excluded.

*Treatment*

The dietary history, postcibal symptoms and presence of steatorrhea may identify remediable factors. Regular supervision with dietary advice and encouragement to eat more sometimes leads to weight gain.

### Pulmonary tuberculosis and gastric surgery

In male patients with duodenal ulcer, the incidence of pulmonary tuberculosis in general practice was once five times higher than expected (Fry 1964). In England and Wales, 5% of new notifications of tuberculosis used to involve adult males who had undergone partial gastrectomy (Balint 1958) and active tuberculosis can undoubtedly be exacerbated by this operation (Frucht et al 1957). A 7% incidence of tuberculosis has also been reported

15–20 years after vagotomy and gastrojejunostomy (Wheldon et al 1970). Although the situation is now rare, elective ulcer surgery should be avoided in patients with untreated pulmonary tuberculosis.

## Steatorrhea after gastric operations

Weight loss after gastric surgery is usually due to inadequate intake rather than malabsorption (above). Nevertheless, mild steatorrhea is not uncommon and severe malabsorption can occur. Some degree of steatorrhea is present in 10% of patients after Billroth I gastrectomy and in 33–50% after Billroth II gastrectomy (Butler 1961, Clark et al 1964). After vagotomy and drainage, up to 50% of patients have a fecal fat excretion which exceeds 5 g/day, but excretion of more than 8.5 g/day is unusual (Wastell 1972). After highly selective vagotomy, steatorrhea is exceptional (Edwards et al 1974).

### *Mechanism of steatorrhea*

A specific cause for the steatorrhea is found in only a minority of cases.

***Stagnant loop syndrome*** (p. 461). A long afferent loop may act as a blind loop, particularly when there is hypochlorhydria.

***Celiac disease.*** Patients with adult celiac disease can have duodenal ulceration (Finlayson et al 1968) or their symptoms may be misinterpreted as those of duodenal ulcer. Some patients with celiac disease have minimal malabsorption, but severe celiac disease may be precipitated by gastric surgery (Hedberg et al 1966).

***Gastroileostomy.*** The stomach is anastomosed inadvertently to the mid-jejunum or even the ileum. Such technical errors are rare but can lead to severe malabsorption soon after ileal anastomosis or insidious malabsorption if the anastomosis is at a higher level. Malabsorption occurs because the main absorptive area of the bowel has been bypasssed.

***Gastrojejunocolic fistula.*** This leads to a severe loss of fat, protein and other ingested nutrients (see p. 283).

***Pancreatitis.*** Ulcer surgery may unmask pancreatic insufficiency and lead to steatorrhea in patients with chronic pancreatitis.

### *Other etiological factors*

***Mucosal changes in the small intestine.*** Any gross abnormalities in a mucosal biopsy are usually due to preexisting celiac disease (above), as the jejunal mucosa remains normal after gastric surgery.

***Poor mixing of food and digestive secretions.*** Steatorrhea after vagotomy and drainage may involve decreased pancreatic and biliary output (Fields & Duthie 1965) and loss of vagally stimulated release of secretin and cholecystokinin (CCK) (King & Toskes 1976). However, the main cause of steatorrhea after gastric surgery is poor mixing of food and digestive secretions. The problem commences in the stomach with failure to render the meal isotonic and is compounded by uncontrolled gastric emptying. Steatorrhea is more likely after Billroth II than after Billroth I partial gastrectomy (Butler 1961); there is less stimulus to release secretin and CCK if the duodenum has been bypassed and biliary and pancreatic secretions enter the jejunum up to 30 min after food has entered.

Maldigestion of protein can also be a key factor in protein malnutrition after gastric surgery (see below).

### *Investigation and treatment*

In well-nourished patients who are not losing weight, mild steatorrhea has no importance. If there is weight loss, the stagnant loop syndrome should be excluded (p. 463), although jejunal colonization can make results difficult to interpret (Biorneklett et al 1983). Provided there are no other complications arising from the afferent loop, it is treated in the same way as other causes of stagnant loop syndrome (p. 464, King & Toskes 1976).

Celiac disease is diagnosed on jejunal biopsy (p. 387) and responds to a gluten-free diet. Gastroileostomy is diagnosed on a barium follow-through examination and is corrected surgically. Gastrojejunocolic fistula also requires surgical treatment (p. 283).

Patients without a defined cause of steatorrhea and weight loss may benefit from taking regular small meals and pancreatic enzyme supplements.

## Protein malnutrition

A degree of protein malnutrition due to poor intake and absorption is present in any patient with significant weight loss after gastric surgery, but hypoalbuminemia is unusual. Severe protein malnutrition with edema, hypoproteinemia and features of kwashiorkor occasionally follows partial gastrectomy (Neale et al 1967). The problem arises as the result of the stagnant loop syndrome (see p. 462) or pancreatic atrophy. The poor intake provides insufficient amino acids for the synthesis of pancreatic enzymes and this results in further malabsorption and a vicious circle which ends in severe emaciation. Lack of protein also causes partial villous atrophy, which accentuates malabsorption. In one of the patients described by Neale et al (1967), fecal fat excretion fell from 50 g/day to 12 g/day after 150 g albumin was given intravenously. Protein-losing enteropathy can also give rise to hypoalbuminemia after gastric surgery; its cause is not known.

### *Investigation and treatment*

Hypoalbuminemia and severe weight loss after gastric

surgery are investigated by tests to detect blind loop syndrome (p. 463), pancreatic exocrine insufficiency (p. 50.24) and protein loss (p. 348). The stagnant loop is usually corrected surgically, but protein-losing enteropathy is more difficult to manage. Pancreatic insufficiency usually requires permanent treatment with pancreatic enzyme supplements as the atrophy may not recover. Many patients with malnutrition also have dumping or vomiting which reduce food intake.

## **Osteomalacia** (Lancet 1986)

This term denotes impaired calcification of bone and is generally due to vitamin D deficiency.

*Incidence*

Early surveys suggested an incidence of bone disease (principally osteomalacia) after partial gastrectomy of 10–15%, the assessment being based largely on serum alkaline phosphatase and calcium levels. A subsequent comparison of 1228 patients after gastric surgery with peptic ulcer patients (Morgan et al 1965a) found a 5% incidence of postoperative hypocalcemia (which was largely attributable to hypoproteinemia). Serum alkaline phosphatase activity was raised in 8% of patients after vagotomy and drainage and in 12% after Polya gastrectomy, as compared to 6% in the control group. However, bone biopsy in 84 patients did not confirm osteomalacia and alkaline phosphatase activity was not reduced by vitamin D therapy. It was concluded that bone biopsy and response to vitamin D must be tested before the condition can be diagnosed. Of the 1228 patients, only 3% of women and fewer than 1% of men had osteomalacia and all had undergone partial gastrectomy (Morgan et al 1965a). Osteomalacia is not a problem after vagotomy and drainage.

*Etiology*

Since physiological doses of vitamin D cure the condition, poor dietary intake or malabsorption of the vitamin must be implicated (Morgan et al 1965b). Intake of vitamin D after partial gastrectomy tends to be marginal and so any degree of malabsorption can lead to deficiency (Morgan et al 1970). Absorption following a large dose of vitamin D is known to be unaffected in patients with osteomalacia after partial gastrectomy (Thompson et al 1966), but the absorption of physiological doses taken with food has not been fully assessed.

Calcium malabsorption results from the vitamin D deficiency. Patients who had undergone Billroth II partial gastrectomy and did not appear to have vitamin D deficiency showed increased absorption of calcium salts, a finding interpreted as reflecting calcium deficiency consequent upon poor calcium intake (Arman et al 1970).

*Clinical features and treatment*

All 23 patients with osteomalacia after partial gastrectomy in one series had bone pain or muscle weakness, often causing difficulty in walking (Morgan et al 1970). Symptoms usually began 10–14 years after operation. Radiological studies often show Looser's zones and the thickness of the cortex of the metacarpal bones is nearly always reduced. Serum calcium concentration corrected for serum albumin concentration may be low. Bone biopsy reveals an excess of osteoid. Steatorrhea, if present, is rarely severe (Morgan et al 1970).

Vitamin D can be given in the form of calcium and ergocalciferol tablets (1600–2000 units daily for 3 months, reducing to 400 units daily). Parenteral calciferol can also be used (Morgan et al 1965a). Calcitriol can be used in doses of 0.25–3 μg per day. Calcium supplements are advisable during the period of bone recalcification, but as in all patients receiving vitamin D, plasma calcium concentrations should be monitored to avoid hypercalcemia.

## **Osteoporosis**

Osteoporosis is regarded as present when bone density is 2 SD below the normal mean. Osteoporosis is part of the normal process of aging and is more common and more pronounced in women (Morgan et al 1966).

*Etiology*

Osteoporosis may arise because of long-standing negative calcium balance and is correlated with the patient's nutritional state. After gastric surgery, patients with impaired nutrition, as assessed by the ratio of total body fat to total body weight, had an increased incidence of osteoporosis, whereas those in whom nutrition was maintained did not (Morgan & Pulvertaft 1969). The incidence of osteoporosis after gastric surgery rises with age and older patients after partial gastrectomy are most severely affected. Vagotomy and drainage probably increases the risk of osteoporosis slightly in aging patients.

*Clinical features*

Symptoms are due to the collapse of vertebrae or to fractures and the diagnosis is made on routine bone densitometry. Many of the early studies on bone disease after gastric surgery are flawed in that patient groups were not homogeneous, controls were not used and the techniques were inadequate. Klein et al (1987) studied a group of middle-aged men after Billroth II partial gastrectomy and the range of bone abnormalities included decreased mineral content and increase in osteoid and alterations in vitamin D metabolism. A number of treatments are available to prevent bone loss but calcium replacement is essential.

## Anemia after gastric operations

Anemia after partial gastrectomy occurred eventually in 50% of patients in one series (Hines et al 1967) and in 29% of cases in a collective review involving 7222 patients (Chanarin 1969). After partial gastrectomy, the hemoglobin concentration falls progressively with time (Fig. 10.4). Of the 153 anemic patients studied by Hines et al (1967), 135 had predominant iron deficiency, 12 had vitamin $B_{12}$ deficiency and five folate deficiency. Anemia is found in 10–20% of patients after vagotomy and drainage (Pulvertaft & Cox 1969, Kennedy 1977) but does not occur after highly selective vagotomy.

### *Iron deficiency*

After partial gastrectomy, some 20% of patients have a low hemoglobin concentration, while a further 15% have low serum iron concentrations (Deller & Witts 1962). Serum iron levels are frequently low after vagotomy and gastroenterostomy (Pulvertaft & Cox 1969). The etiology has been studied most extensively after partial gastrectomy, but the following discussion probably also applies to vagotomy and drainage.

***Blood loss.*** Iron deficiency anemia within the first year after operation is usually due to preoperative and operative blood loss. There is controversy as to whether subsequent anemia is due to blood loss from the stomach. Using $^{51}$Cr-labeled red cells, Baird et al (1970) failed to show blood loss in the stool but Holt et al (1970), using $^{59}$Fe and whole-body counting, showed that five of 11 male and postmenopausal female patients were losing blood at rates exceeding 150 ml per month. This latter study extended over 3 months and earlier studies may have failed to detect blood loss because of its intermittent nature. Blood is lost occasionally from specific lesions such as stomal ulcer or esophagitis, but gastritis is the usual cause. Increased loss of cells from the gastric mucosa after partial gastrectomy also contributes to the loss of iron from the body (Toskes 1976).

***Deficient intake of iron.*** Reduced iron intake after partial gastrectomy is a major factor in producing anemia (Baird & Wilson 1959) and traditional "ulcer diets" have a low iron content.

***Impaired absorption of iron.*** Malabsorption of food iron is particularly likely after partial gastrectomy (Turnberg 1966). Furthermore, in postgastrectomy patients with iron deficiency, the absorption of food iron remains low (Turnbull 1965), whereas in patients with iron deficiency and an intact stomach, iron absorption increases. Thus, if the iron stores are already depleted before operation, the patient is unable to restore them afterwards. Reasons for poor iron absorption (p. 360) include low secretion of acid-pepsin and iron-binding substances, bypass of the duodenum, intestinal hurry and an inadequate intestinal amino acid concentration because of poor protein intake.

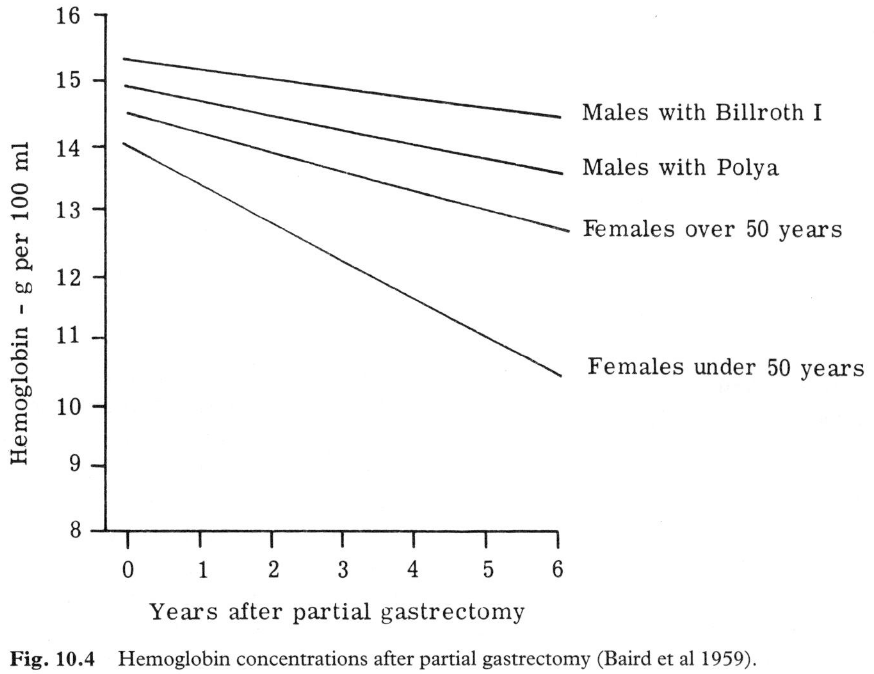


**Fig. 10.4** Hemoglobin concentrations after partial gastrectomy (Baird et al 1959).

*Vitamin $B_{12}$ deficiency*

The incidence of megaloblastic anemia reported after partial gastrectomy varies from 1% to 20% (Hines et al 1967, Toskes 1976) and it is nearly always due to vitamin $B_{12}$ deficiency. Megaloblastic anemia due to vitamin $B_{12}$ deficiency is very rare after vagotomy and gastroenterostomy (Doig & Girdwood 1960, Weir et al 1963).

***Deficiency of intrinsic factor.*** The usual cause of vitamin $B_{12}$ deficiency is inadequate production of gastric intrinsic factor. The collection of gastric secretion for direct measurement of intrinsic factor secretion is difficult after gastric surgery, but deficiency is inferred when malabsorption of vitamin $B_{12}$ can be corrected by oral intrinsic factor. Lous & Schwartz (1959) found that 30% of patients after partial gastrectomy had a $B_{12}$ absorption of less than 10% as assessed by a Schilling test and others have reported a similar or even higher incidence. Care must be exercised when interpreting results of tests in fasting subjects as vitamin $B_{12}$ is absorbed to a greater degree when given with food, as shown by Schilling tests (Turnbull 1967) and whole body counting (Finlayson et al 1969). On the other hand, some studies show that vitamin $B_{12}$ incorporated into eggs is poorly absorbed (Toskes 1976). Vitamin $B_{12}$ malabsorption is more likely after partial gastrectomy for gastric ulcer than for duodenal ulcer, presumably because the stomach of gastric ulcer patients has significant gastritis even before operation. A further factor may be that gastric ulcer patients often lose a greater proportion of the stomach when undergoing partial gastrectomy (Johnson & Hoffbrand 1970).

In the majority of patients with impaired vitamin $B_{12}$ absorption after partial gastrectomy, the impairment is insufficient to cause megaloblastic anemia even though serum vitamin $B_{12}$ levels below 160 pg/ml are found in about 20% of patients (Hines et al 1967). The proportion of patients with low concentrations increases with time because body stores gradually deplete as a result of the slightly reduced absorption. In the series reported by Hines et al (1967), 2% of patients had low serum vitamin $B_{12}$ concentrations after 4 years and 16% after 10 years.

***Intestinal malabsorption.*** This may contribute to $B_{12}$ malabsorption resulting from intrinsic factor deficiency since oral intrinsic factor, while correcting the malabsorption, does not result in a completely normal $B_{12}$ absorption (Lous & Schwartz 1959).

***Stagnant loop syndrome.*** If the afferent loop acts as a "stagnant loop" (p. 461), vitamin $B_{12}$ absorption can only be corrected by giving broad-spectrum antibiotics.

*Folic acid deficiency*

Folic acid deficiency is responsible for one in five cases of megaloblastic anemia following partial gastrectomy (Chanarin 1969), but has not been reported after vagotomy and drainage.

***Etiology.*** Malabsorption of folic acid (p. 362) can be shown in a few patients after partial gastrectomy, but some patients with megaloblastic anemia due to folate deficiency show normal absorption (Gough et al 1965) implying that reduced folate intake is responsible.

*Clinical features and investigation of anemia after gastric surgery*

The onset of anemia is usually insidious. Subacute combined degeneration of the cord or other neurological manifestations are rarely the presenting feature (Williams et al 1969). Features of iron deficiency or megaloblastic anemia are sought on a blood film. When the film is dimorphic, the marrow should be examined. Since the features of megaloblastosis can be concealed by iron deficiency, a serum vitamin $B_{12}$ level is also informative. Anemia should always be treated with iron before marrow examination, which will then be easier to interpret (Hines et al 1967).

***Treatment.*** Established anemia is treated with the appropriate hematinic and it is advisable to continue this for life. The cause of the anemia should be defined and specific lesions treated (e.g. stomal ulcer or stagnant loop syndrome). Anemia is so common, particularly after partial gastrectomy, that a yearly hemoglobin estimation is advisable to detect anemia early and prevent much ill health and debility. It is also advisable to monitor serum iron and vitamin $B_{12}$ concentrations. Falling concentrations signify impending anemia. Low vitamin $B_{12}$ levels are an indication to test vitamin $B_{12}$ absorption and unequivocal malabsorption means that vitamin $B_{12}$ must be given for life.

## RECURRENT ULCER

Recurrent ulceration is classified as jejunal or stomal ulcer (i.e. at an anastomosis between stomach and jejunum), recurrent duodenal ulcer and recurrent gastric ulcer. Suture line ulcer is an additional, and now rare, form of recurrence attributable to the use of nonabsorbable sutures (Small et al 1971).

After surgery for duodenal ulcer (Table 10.2) the ulcer usually recurs in the jejunum or duodenum; gastric ulceration occurs in only 1% of patients but is more common after highly selective vagotomy and to a lesser extent after vagotomy and drainage than afer gastric resection. Inexplicably, operations with the lowest recurrent ulcer rates often fail much earlier than those with higher rates (Stabile & Passaro 1983). For example, most recurrences after vagotomy and antrectomy occur within 3 years, whereas those following gastroenterostomy alone may be deferred for 15 years or more. Recurrence rates after high-

**Table 10.2** Range of incidence of recurrent ulcer after duodenal ulcer surgery

| Type of operation | "Acceptable" incidence (%) | Range in different series (%) | Usual site of ulceration |
|---|---|---|---|
| Vagotomy and antrectomy | 1 | 0–5 | Jejunum or duodenum |
| Billroth II (Polya) partial gastrectomy | 3 | 1–7.5 | Jejunum |
| Vagotomy and gastroenterostomy | 10 | 3–30 | Jejunum |
| Vagotomy and pyloroplasty | 10 | 5–30 | Duodenum |
| Highly selective vagotomy | 15 | 4–30 | Duodenum or stomach |
| Gastroenterostomy alone | 25 | 4–50 | Jejunum |

ly selective vagotomy have continued to rise with time (Macintyre et al 1990, Johnston et al 1991).

After surgery for gastric ulcer, recurrence may be located in the duodenum (after Billroth I gastrectomy or vagotomy and pyloroplasty), jejunum (after Billroth II gastrectomy or vagotomy and gastroenterostomy) or stomach (after any operation).

### Incidence

The incidence of recurrent ulcer varies greatly depending on the selection of patients for surgery, type of operation, skill of the surgeon, thoroughness of the investigation for recurrent ulcer and time elapsed since operation. It must be appreciated that different authors use different definitions of ulcer recurrence, some referring to symptomatic recurrence and others to endoscopically or surgically *proven* recurrent ulcer. It is also important to appreciate that endoscopic or radiological detection of recurrence may be easier after highly selective vagotomy than after operations involving gastric resection or drainage.

***After surgery for duodenal ulcer.*** If gastrectomy alone is used to treat duodenal ulcer, recurrence rates of 36% have been recorded after 30–50% resection, whereas they commonly fall to 12–14% after 50–70% resection and can be as low as 3% (Stabile & Passaro 1976, Postlethwait 1979). This explains why recurrence rates are generally higher after a Billroth I gastrectomy and why limited distal resection (antrectomy) is now combined with truncal vagotomy. One long-term study found a 2.6% recurrence rate 22–30 years after gastrectomy alone (Fisher 1984) but this is exceptional.

If truncal vagotomy and drainage is used, recurrence rates of 10–15% are frequently reported but rates as high as 25–29% are documented when follow-up extends for 10–15 years (Nobles 1966, Stempien et al 1971, Hoffmann et al 1989). Truncal vagotomy and antrectomy has the lowest recurrence rate of all operations with figures of 0–5% reported after follow-up for 4–16 years (see Hoffmann et al 1987).

The incidence of recurrence after highly selective vagotomy is frequently quoted at around 10–15%, but rates of 30% are reported at 5 years by some specialist units (Hoffmann et al 1984). The high rate of recurrence may reflect the fact that the majority of patients now coming to surgery are those with ulcers resistant to modern potent medical management (Primrose et al 1988), although opinions vary as to whether recurrence rates are higher in patients resistant to cimetidine (Hansen & Knigge 1984, Weaver & Temple 1985). In one series with an overall recurrence rate of 13%, there was a 37% recurrence rate in patients with pyloric ulcers (Poppen & Delin 1981) and some surgeons do not use highly selective vagotomy for pyloric or prepyloric ulcers.

***After surgery for gastric ulcer.*** The overall incidence of recurrence after partial gastrectomy in one review was 2.8% and in general there is little difference between Billroth I and Billroth II gastrectomy (Greenall & Lehnert 1984). Reports published in the years 1960–69 have a lower overall incidence (1.5%) than those published a decade later (4.5%), the difference being attributable to longer follow-up in later reports and a more accurate definition of recurrence by endoscopy. The overall recurrence rate after vagotomy and drainage is higher at 9.1% and the difference between decades is much less striking than in the case of gastrectomy. Recurrence rates following highly selective vagotomy ranged from 14.3% to 25.5% in the eight series reviewed by Siewert & Holscher (1986) and the operation is no longer advocated for gastric ulcer.

### Etiology

Recurrence after surgery for duodenal ulcer is usually due to incomplete vagotomy or inadequate partial gastrectomy and consequent failure to reduce acid-pepsin output sufficiently. Truncal vagotomy is incomplete on post-operative insulin testing in up to 40% of cases (Smith et al 1972). The posterior vagal trunk is much more frequently found to be intact at reoperation for ulcer recurrence (Fawcett et al 1969), reflecting its relative inaccessibility. Some surgeons attempt to avoid incomplete vagotomy by using intraoperative pH mapping to detect intact vagal fibers and ensure denervation of the parietal cell area, although unequivocal support for this approach is lacking (Reid et al 1984). When performing highly selective vagotomy, at least 5 cm of esophagus must be cleared of all vagal fibers. Recurrence after highly selective vagotomy is clearly related to surgical technique and in one series, recurrence rates of individual surgeons varied from 5% to 26%, a variation which did not necessarily reflect seniority or experience (Macintyre et al 1990).

Much less frequently, recurrent ulceration is due to causes other than incomplete vagotomy.

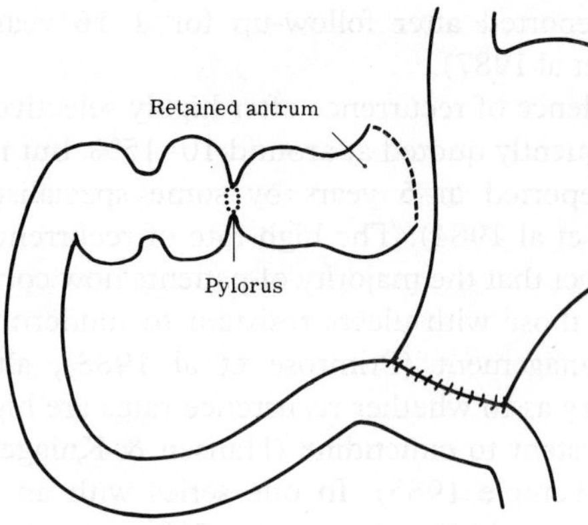


**Fig. 10.5** Retained gastric antrum after Polya partial gastrectomy.

***Retained gastric antrum.*** The antral mucosa may extend 0.5 cm beyond the pylorus and if this mucosa is left behind at Polya partial gastrectomy (Fig. 10.5) it secretes gastrin continuously because there is no acid within the lumen to inhibit the G cells. A similar state of affairs exists if the distal line of surgical resection at Polya gastrectomy passes through the antrum rather than through the first part of the duodenum. "Retained antrum" was once responsible for about 10% of recurrent ulcers after partial gastrectomy (Stabile & Passaro 1976), but is now rare.

***Zollinger–Ellison syndrome, antral G cell hyperplasia and hyperparathyroidism*** (p. 252).

***Long afferent loop following Billroth II gastrectomy.*** This may predispose to recurrent ulceration because the alkaline biliary and pancreatic secretions are delayed in reaching the stoma through which the acid gastric content will pass.

***Unabsorbable sutures.*** Unabsorbable sutures were an occasional cause of ulceration at the anastomosis but are now rarely used in gastric surgery.

***Gastric outlet obstruction.*** Stasis may contribute to recurrent ulceration in that antral distention stimulates gastrin release and so increases acid-pepsin secretion. Recurrence after surgery for gastric ulcer is nearly always due to gastric stasis secondary to inadequate drainage.

***Other factors.*** Continued use of salicylates, smoking and alcohol abuse may favor recurrent ulceration. Recurrence is reported to be more frequent in patients with a strong family history of ulcer disease, giving rise to the suggestion that aggression of the ulcer diathesis could be genetically determined (Macintyre et al 1990).

## Clinical features

Recurrent ulceration can develop at any time following gastric surgery. Recurrence of pain usually heralds its presence but symptoms do not necessarily indicate that ulceration has recurred. Of 250 patients assessed by Macintyre et al (1990) 5–15 years after highly selective vagotomy, 6.9% of those without ulcer recurrence took $H_2$ receptor antagonists daily or on most days. The converse situation where asymptomatic patients harbor ulcer recurrence appears to be much less common (Hoffmann et al 1987). The pain of jejunal ulcer is often severe, persistent and poorly relieved by antacids or food. Its location often differs from that of the original ulcer, being in the left hypochondrium or even the lower abdomen. With recurrent duodenal or gastric ulcer, symptoms are often similar to those of the original ulcer.

All recurrent ulcers may present with bleeding or perforation and a gastrojejunocolic fistula can develop if recurrent ulceration at a gastroenterostomy erodes into the adjacent transverse colon. Hoffmann et al (1987) divided recurrent ulcers into "innocuous" ulcers which respond to a single course of antiulcer medication and do not recur on follow-up and "malevolent" ulcers which do not respond to medical treatment and subsequently require surgery. Of 29 ulcers which recurred after highly selective vagotomy, six were innocuous, while in the experience of Macintyre et al (1990), 19 of their 49 recurrence were "innocuous". It cannot be overemphasized that while recurrent ulceration may appear to represent dramatic and obvious failure of surgery, the relative ease of treatment makes it a less devastating long-term complication than problems such as dumping and diarrhea.

## Investigation

### *Fiberoptic endoscopy*

This is the most reliable means of diagnosing all forms of recurrent ulceration, including suture line ulcer (where nonabsorbable sutures can be seen protruding from the ulcer base).

### *Radiology*

Radiological detection of recurrence is difficult and much less reliable than endoscopy. In detection of gastric ulcer, rapid gastric emptying and folds related to surgery present problems, while ulcers which recur after pyloroplasty often remain hidden in the deformities or pouches created by surgery (Fig. 10.6) or may be mistaken for a pouch. Circumstantial evidence such as delay in the passage of barium through a pyloroplasty should raise suspicion. In some studies the radiological diagnosis was correct in only 50% of cases (Fredens et al 1971) but detection rates improve to 70% if double-contrast techniques are used (Gohel & Laufer 1978, Thompson et al 1982b, Ott et al 1982). Predictive accuracy in one series was only 42% owing to the substantial number of false positive results (Ott et al 1982).

Jejunal ulceration (Fig. 10.7) is missed by contrast radiology in about 50% of cases (Wychulis et al 1966). A small

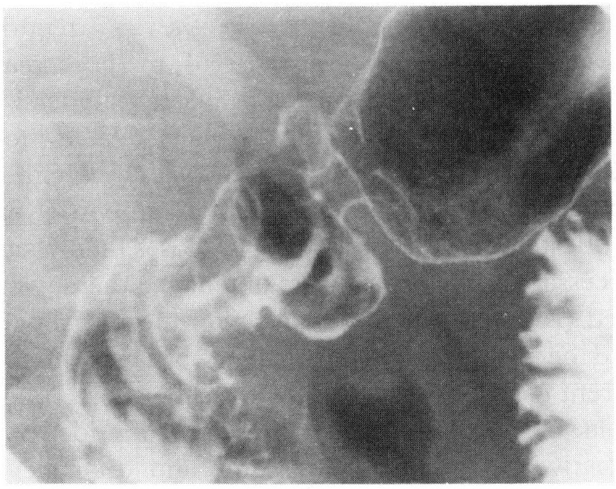

**Fig. 10.6** Typical appearances following pyloroplasty. Some residual deformity of duodenal bulb from the chronic duodenal ulcer. No stenosis.

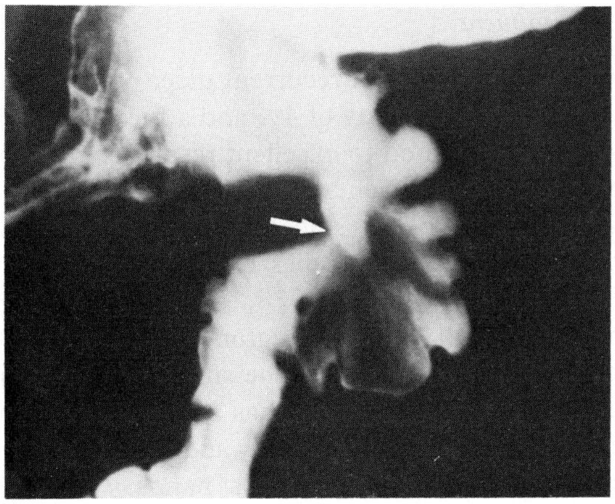

**Fig. 10.7** Stomal ulcer (arrow) complicating gastroenterostomy.

amount of barium must be used so that the anastomosis is not obscured by overlying loops and air is used to distend the stoma region. Superficial ulcers are easily missed, but rigidity of the jejunum should raise suspicion (Schatzki 1968). Even if a crater is not detected, ulceration is almost certain when there is narrowing of the stoma, edema and thickened folds.

A retained antrum can be demonstrated by using a large amount of barium and obstructing the efferent loop manually so as to fill the afferent loop (Burhenne 1967). The retained antrum may not occupy its original position and can be confused with a duodenal diverticulum. Technetium pertechnetate scans now offer a more reliable method of detecting retained antrum (Dunlap et al 1975).

Gastrojejunocolic fistula is best demonstrated by barium enema (Wychulis et al 1966).

### *Tests of gastric secretion*

These tests were once used to audit surgical technique, assess the likelihood of recurrent ulceration and determine whether proven recurrent ulcer was due to failure of vagotomy. In reality, they discriminated poorly between patients with and without recurrent ulcer and their use has diminished greatly with the decline of ulcer surgery and the availability of endoscopy.

Once recurrent ulceration has been diagnosed, secretion tests are occasionally helpful in further management. The acid secretory response to insulin-induced hypoglycemia is the traditional method of evaluating completeness of vagotomy, but the test can be unpleasant and not without dangers if hypoglycemia is profound. A further drawback is the fact that insulin hypoglycemia may have other nonspecific effects, some of which inhibit secretion (Olbe et al 1983) (p. 223).

The "chew and spit" test (see below) and determination of the maximal secretory response to pentagastrin offer alternative means of assessing acid output after gastric surgery (p. 223).

***After vagotomy and drainage.*** Complete vagotomy, as shown by an absence of acid secretory response to insulin, is not associated with recurrent peptic ulcer (Stempien et al 1968). If vagotomy is incomplete, the chance of a recurrent ulcer increases as more of the criteria listed in Fig. 10.8 become positive. In one series, 21 of 25 cases of recurrent ulcer showed an early positive response to insulin and 24 had three or more positive criteria. Patients with five positive criteria had a 77% incidence of recurrent ulcer (Fig. 10.8).

***After vagotomy and antrectomy.*** Antrectomy alone depresses the acid response to vagal stimulation. A positive response to insulin may mean that both the vagotomy and the antrectomy are incomplete, while a negative response cannot be interpreted as proof of satisfactory vagotomy (Ruckley & Sircus 1970).

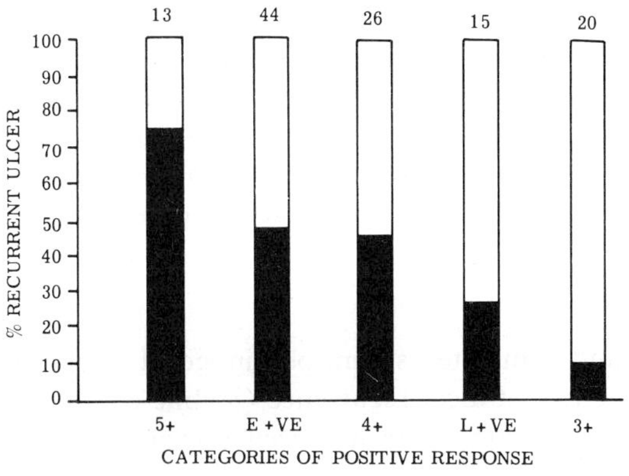


**Fig. 10.8** The incidence of recurrent ulcer in various categories of positive response after vagotomy. Insulin-positive patients have been grouped according to whether they showed 3, 4 or 5 positive criteria and also whether their response occurred in the first post-insulin hour (E +ve) or the second (L +ve). The incidence (%) of recurrent ulcer in each group is shown (shaded). The number of patients in the group is shown above each column (Ruckley & Sircus 1970).

***After partial gastrectomy.*** The pentagastrin test is of limited value after this operation in that it cannot exclude recurrent ulcer, no matter how low the acid output. Conversely a high output (e.g. MAO > 22 mmol/h) is often found with recurrent ulceration and a high basal output suggests excessive gastrin secretion such as occurs with "retained antrum".

***After highly selective vagotomy.*** A positive acid secretory response to insulin in the first week after surgery is followed by a 15% incidence of recurrence, whereas a negative response is associated with a 6% recurrence rate (Blackett & Johnston 1981). Not all agree that the insulin testing at this early stage is a reliable predictor of recurrent ulceration (Johnston et al 1991). The acid secretory response to sham feeding ("chew and spit") in the first 3 months after operation has also been used to predict ulcer recurrence (Stenquist et al 1994). Of 22 patients with incomplete vagotomy on sham feeding, five (23%) had later ulcer recurrence, as opposed to a relapse rate of 8% in those with a secretory response suggesting complete vagotomy. Interestingly, none of the four patients who developed ulcer recurrence more than 5 years after operation had incomplete vagotomy on their sham feeding test, leaving open the possibility of reinnervation as an explanation for late ulcer recurrence.

*Serum gastrin estimations* (see also p. 224 and 253)

Slight increases in circulating gastrin levels are seen after all forms of vagotomy because there is less inhibition of antral G cells by luminal acid. High serum gastrin concentrations are seen in pernicious anemia or atrophic gastritis (when gastric pH is persistently high), in renal failure and after massive small bowel resection. However, the Zollinger–Ellison syndrome is the commonest cause of primary hypergastrinemia (serum gastrin > 500 pg/ml, normal range 20–180 pg/ml) and the syndrome should always be considered in patients with recurrent ulcer. An excluded antrum can lead to comparable increases in gastrin levels, but can be distinguished by a fall in gastrin concentration when secretin is injected (Korman et al 1973). The histology of the gastrectomy specimen should be reviewed to make sure that the distal excision line is clear of antral tissue.

*Serum pepsinogen I estimations*

Basal and stimulated serum pepsinogen I levels correlate with the risk of ulcer recurrence (Stabile et al 1978), but the need for such tests has been obviated by fiberoptic endoscopy.

## Treatment

*Medical management*

Medical management of recurrent ulcer in the pre-cimetidine era was ineffective. In the 297 recurrences reviewed by Stabile & Passaro (1976), medical treatment produced good results in one-third, ulceration persisted or recurred in 42% and there was an ulcer-related mortality of 11%. Modern antisecretory drugs such as cimetidine heal recurrent ulcers in the majority of patients (Kennedy 1978, Festen et al 1979), but higher doses than usual may be necessary and permanent maintenance therapy may be needed (Koo et al 1982). The trial of ulcer-healing drugs should be prolonged in all patients because surgery for recurrent ulcer is often avoidable. Furthermore, long-term sequelae can arise when gastric resection is added to highly selective vagotomy or vagotomy and drainage; some 20–45% of patients remain in Visick grades 3 or 4 and up to 20% of cases require a further operation (Green et al 1978, Muscroft et al 1981, Hoffmann et al 1983).

*Surgical treatment*

The surgical treatment of recurrent ulcer used to carry an overall operative mortality of 4% and a further recurrence rate of 14%, with good to excellent results being achieved in two-thirds of patients (Stable & Passaro 1976). Operative mortality has since fallen appreciably and a number of more recent studies report no mortality after reoperation (Green et al 1978, Muscroft et al 1981, Hoffmann et al 1983, Herrington et al 1984). Much depends on the experience of the surgeon, but reduction in the volume of ulcer surgery has meant that operations for peptic ulceration (both primary and recurrent) are now undertaken increasingly in specialist hands.

The choice of operation is influenced by the nature of the previous operation.

1. Recurrence after vagotomy and drainage or highly selective vagotomy is usually treated by distal gastric resection with or without attempted completion of vagotomy. If a substantial intact vagal trunk(s) is found and divided, antrectomy alone may suffice; if no vagal trunks are found, two-thirds of the distal stomach should be resected. Re-vagotomy alone carried an overall recurrent ulcer rate of 21% (Stabile & Passaro 1976) and attempts to ensure complete vagotomy by using a transthoracic approach have proved disappointing. Recurrence following highly selective vagotomy has been treated by antrectomy with no mortality and a further recurrence rate of only 6% (Hoffmann et al 1983).
2. Recurrence after gastroenterostomy is probably best treated by antral resection combined with vagotomy or by subtotal gastric resection. Vagotomy alone had an overall re-recurrence rate of 24% (Stabile & Passaro 1976)
3. Recurrence after partial gastrectomy is treated by vagotomy unless the initial resection has been limited,

in which case a further resection is combined with vagotomy.

4. Recurrence after vagotomy and resection is an indication to measure serum gastrin levels to exclude retained antrum or Zollinger–Ellison syndrome. At reoperation, any intact vagal trunks are divided. If no intact trunks are found, a 70% distal gastrectomy is advisable.
5. In the case of suture line ulcers, it was sometimes possible to remove the nonabsorbable suture material at endoscopy and allow healing. If ulceration cannot be dealt with in this way or recurs, the anastomosis may have to be reconstructed and additional measures (i.e. completion of vagotomy or gastric resection) taken to reduce acid-pepsin secretion.

## FISTULA SECONDARY TO PEPTIC ULCER

Gastrojejunocolic fistula can complicate ulcer recurrence at a gastrojejunal anastomosis. It presents with severe diarrhea which results from jejunitis rather than from the passage of gastric contents into the colon. The fistula is best demonstrated by barium enema examination. It is dealt with by vagotomy (or completion of previous vagotomy), en bloc resection of the gastric antrum and the fistula and closure of the colonic defect. Gastrocolic fistula may also occur with gastric and colonic cancer and occasionally a benign gastric ulcer is responsible.

Duodenal ulceration and Crohn's disease can each fistulate to the colon on occasions. Duodenal ulcer may also form a fistula to the bile duct or gallbladder (Feller et al 1980), although cholecystoduodenal fistulae are more frequently caused by gallstones eroding into a normal duodenum.

## LATE MORTALITY AFTER GASTRIC SURGERY

Patients who have undergone peptic ulcer surgery may be at risk of premature death, particularly once 20 years have elapsed since operation (Lundegardh et al 1991). In one study of 779 male patients (86% of whom underwent partial gastrectomy) followed for at least 15 years, McLean Ross et al (1982) found an excess mortality relative to the general population and a life expectancy shortened by some 9 years. Smoking-related diseases, notably ischemic heart disease, chronic obstructive airways disease and lung cancer, were the major causes of death and other significant causes of excess mortality were cirrhosis and suicide. Smoking-related diseases also appear to make a major contribution to the excess mortality observed in patients who have undergone vagotomy and drainage procedures (Watt et al 1984).

The link between gastrectomy for peptic ulcer and subsequent gastric cancer is generally accepted (Viste et al 1986, Caygill et al 1986, 1987, Carter 1987), although in Edinburgh, McLean Ross et al (1982) found no increase in incidence. More recent reviews suggest that operations for gastric ulcer largely account for any excess mortality from gastric cancer after ulcer surgery, whereas excess mortality after duodenal ulcer surgery is in the short term the result of the operation itself and in the long-term is largely attributable to cigarette smoking (Macintyre & O'Brien, 1994). The large Balham study found that the risk of developing cancer was greater after Billroth II than Billroth I gastrectomy (Caygill et al 1986, 1987), suggesting the possibility that bile reflux is implicated in carcinogenesis, in addition to factors such as diminished acid secretion, bacterial overgrowth and formation of carcinogenes such as nitrites. As Watt et al (1984) point out, all forms of gastrointestinal cancer are much less frequent causes of death in these patients than smoking-related diseases, notably smoking-related cancers. The link between vagotomy for peptic ulcer and subsequent gastric cancer is much less certain. Despite earlier suggestions from the Aarhus County Vagotomy Trial that mortality from gastric cancer was significantly increased at 8–13 years after vagotomy (Ditlevsen 1989), more recent studies are more cautious, concluding that "longer follow-up is needed before an excess link can be excluded" (Lundergardh et al 1994).

## COMPLICATIONS OF PEPTIC ULCERATION

The complication of hemorrhage is dealt with elsewhere (p. 485) and the remainder of this section is devoted to consideration of pyloric stenosis and ulcer perforation. A number of conditions capable of causing pyloric obstruction which are not complications of peptic ulceration will be dealt with here for convenience.

## PYLORIC STENOSIS

Obstruction in the region of the pylorus may be due to edema and inflammatory reaction around a duodenal or pyloric channel ulcer, to fibrous scarring in the vicinity of a healed ulcer (less common) or to a combination of the two.

In patients referred to hospital with peptic ulcer in Western countries, the incidence of gastric outlet obstruction is 5–10% (Kozoll & Meyer 1964, Jaffin & Kaye 1985). In a series of ulcer patients seen in general practice in the UK only about 1% developed stenosis, whereas 6% suffered perforation and 14% hemorrhage (Fry 1964). Stenosis may be more common and develop more rapidly in developing countries than in Britain or the USA (Tovey & Tunstall 1975).

### Clinical features

*History and examination* (Balint & Spence 1959, Moody et al 1962)

There is nearly always a long history of peptic ulcer disease, but once obstructive symptoms develop the patient usually presents within weeks. Vomiting often occurs two or three times a day and is often more marked later in the day. The vomits are typically of large volume and are free of bile but may contain undigested food such as vegetables which are recognized as having been eaten 12–24 h earlier. Pain tends to be more constant than previously but is relieved by vomiting and sometimes by antacids. There is dehydration, anorexia and weight loss. Constipation is usual but there is occasionally diarrhea. Many cases of pyloric stenosis are now diagnosed at the stage of delayed gastric emptying and before significant vomiting develops.

Examination may reveal evidence of weight loss and dehydration, epigastric distention, a succussion splash and visible peristalsis.

## Investigations

Obstruction is best confirmed by gastric aspiration. A wide-bore nasogastric tube is passed and the stomach emptied. A large volume of gastric contents which contain food residue but no bile confirms obstruction. If aspiration is carried out first thing in the morning, a fasting residue of more than 200 ml indicates obstruction. A barium meal examination is sometimes carried out in an attempt to distinguish between benign and malignant obstruction. This is not essential because in either case surgery is usually necessary; furthermore, differentiation by barium meal is often difficult and unreliable. If the examination is undertaken, as little barium as possible should be used and it should be removed from the stomach by a nasogastric tube after the examination. Sometimes, a barium meal carried out for suspected peptic ulcer may draw attention to early stenosis by showing an atonic stomach which retains a large amount of barium for several hours.

Endoscopy suffers from the same limitations as barium meal examination in that it is usually difficult (or even impossible) to clear the stomach of fasting residue and allow adequate inspection of the lumen.

### *Serum electrolytes* (Howe & Le Quesne 1964)

It is usual to find low serum concentrations of sodium, chloride and potassium, and raised bicarbonate and urea concentrations. In the early stages, loss of chloride ions in vomit leads to their replacement in the plasma by bicarbonate and a resulting metabolic alkalosis. Sodium bicarbonate is excreted in the urine, which is initially alkaline.

Later, the excretion of an alkaline urine entails further loss of sodium and potassium and when the body sodium becomes seriously depleted (usually by about 400 mmol) there is a fall in extracellular fluid and plasma volume. The plasma sodium may be only slightly reduced, but the large sodium deficit is reflected in the fall in plasma volume. This in turn results in a reduced glomerular filtration rate and a rising blood urea. Sodium is ultimately reabsorbed from the tubules in exchange for potassium and hydrogen ions and the urine then becomes acid, the so-called paradoxical aciduria of stenosis. The potassium deficit is usually of the order of 100 mmol, not as large as that of sodium, but deficits of 500 mmol or more can develop in untreated cases. Occasionally, tetany may develop.

## Differential diagnosis

***Organic obstruction.*** Antral or pyloric carcinoma is the major cause of confusion but the history is usually shorter in malignant obstruction. Less common causes of pyloric obstruction include adult hypertrophic pyloric stenosis, congenital diaphragm in the prepyloric region (see below), pancreatic rest in the pylorus (Tonkin et al 1962), annular pancreas, Crohn's disease of the duodenum and duodenal obstruction caused by the superior mesenteric artery, lymphomas, pancreatic carcinoma or adhesions after cholecystectomy.

***Nonorganic obstruction.*** Possible causes of nonorganic obstruction (see Rimer 1966) include inflammation in adjacent organs such as the gallbladder or pancreas, severe infections or electrolyte disturbances and gastroparesis due to diabetic neuropathy, vagotomy and other causes (p. 426). Gastric retention can also be caused by excessive use of anticholinergic drugs.

## Treatment

### *Supportive treatment*

Although a proportion of patients will settle on conservative treatment, more than 90% of those who present with gastric outlet obstruction will ultimately require surgery (Jaffin & Kaye 1985). Pyloric stenosis is not an indication for *urgent* surgery and some days of preparation are advisable with nasogastric suction and intravenous infusion. The wide-bore nasogastric tube inserted for diagnostic purposes is left in situ and the stomach is lavaged with 200 ml volumes of isotonic saline until all food debris is removed. The tube is then replaced with a fine nasogastric tube which is aspirated 2–4-hourly for 3–4 days. If the aspirated volumes decrease markedly during this period it is reasonable to allow oral fluids and assess whether these are being emptied by aspirating a fasting residue. If liquid feeds can be established before surgery this is desirable.

The severity of the metabolic alkalosis is best defined by measuring the standard bicarbonate or calculated base excess. If there is uremia or electrolytic disturbance, some 4 liters of isotonic saline with added potassium are given intravenously in the first 24 h. Subsequently, saline is continued with the addition of 80 mmol of potassium per day until the electrolytic disturbance is corrected. Once the potassium deficit has been corrected intravenous feeding is commenced. These measures are continued for 4–5 days before surgery. Even a severe metabolic alkalosis is usually corrected by giving adequate amounts of saline with appropriate potassium supplements.

*Surgery*

Gastroenterostomy alone is contraindicated because of the high incidence of recurrent ulcer. Vagotomy and antrectomy relieves obstruction and has a low ulcer recurrence rate but may have a higher mortality rate in elderly, frail patients. Vagotomy and drainage (usually gastroenterostomy) is generally recommended as the safest method of relieving obstruction, despite a higher rate of ulcer recurrence (Hoerr & Ward 1972). Fears that vagotomy may produce prolonged stasis have not been realized.

Highly selective vagotomy with dilatation of the stenosis once appeared to offer promise (Dunn et al 1981) but subsequent results proved disappointing, with early recurrent ulcer rates and restenosis rates of around 10% (Blackett et al 1982). Highly selective vagotomy in combination with a drainage procedure has some advocates (Wang et al 1994) but is not used widely.

## ADULT HYPERTROPHIC PYLORIC STENOSIS

Hypertrophic pyloris stenosis affects 5 per 1000 male neonates (Carter 1961). Occasionally presentation is delayed until adult life but some of the cases reported may be secondary to peptic ulcer disease. Families are reported with both adult and infantile forms of the disease.

As in infantile stenosis, the pylorus is enlarged and the circular muscle fibers show uniform hyperplasia and loss of peptide immunoreactivity in nerve fibers (Wellmann et al 1964, Wattchow et al 1987). There is no evidence of ulceration or inflammation of the mucosa.

There is persistent or episodic nausea and vomiting and some patients admit to intermittent symptoms since infancy. Barium meal (Fig. 10.9) shows a narrow elongated pyloric channel, which can be mimicked by carcinoma. Because of this possibility, the narrowed area in adult hypertrophic stenosis is usually resected in preference to pyloromyotomy.

## PREPYLORIC MEMBRANE (ANTRAL WEB) (Banks et al 1967, Woolley et al 1974)

This condition may represent congenital failure of recanalization. While it nearly always presents in neonates, cases have been reported in adult with intermittent pyloric obstruction, although these are probably secondary to gastric ulceration (Huggins et al 1982). Barium examination (Fig. 10.10) shows a "double-bulb" effect, one bulb being the normal duodenal bulb and the other the region between the membrane and the pylorus. Surgical excision of the membrane is indicated.

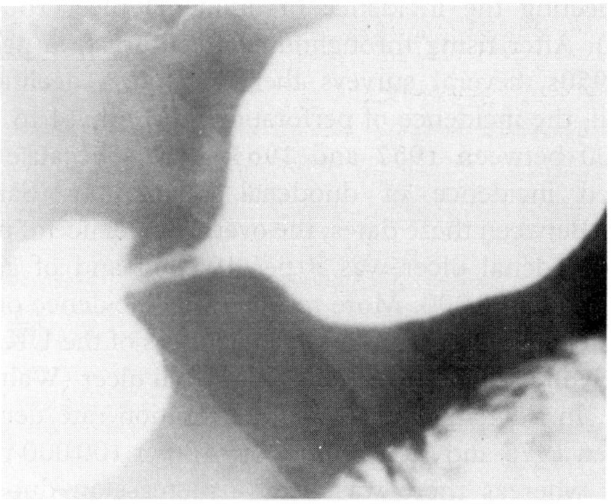

**Fig. 10.9** Adult hypertrophic pyloric stenosis. Smooth narrowed prepyloric segment with lumen of approximately the same caliber as true pylorus. Indentation of base of duodenal bulb by the muscular tumor.

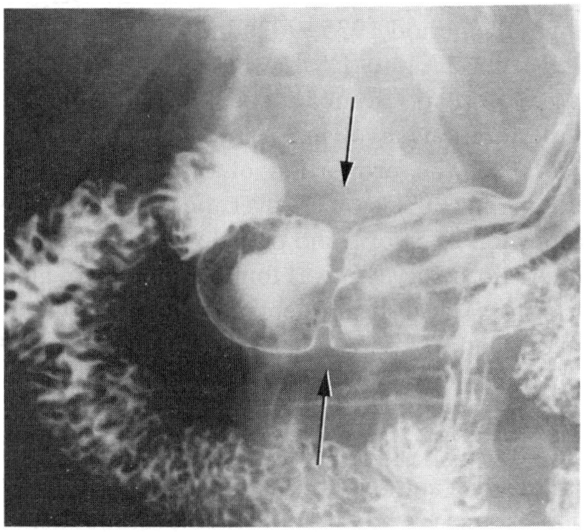

**Fig. 10.10** Congenital diaphragm (arrow) in the antrum causing a typical smooth persistent filling defect, best demonstrated when the antrum is distended.

## DOUBLE PYLORUS (Einhorn et al 1984)

While this may be congenital it usually results from benign fistulous communication between the antrum and duodenal bulb due to peptic ulceration. Barium meal characteristically reveals two channels of barium separated by a relatively smooth radiolucent band of soft tissue. At endoscopy, the fistula is usually clearly visible.

## PERFORATION

### Incidence

The incidence of perforated duodenal ulcer is usually seen

as reflecting the incidence of duodenal ulcer (but see below). After rising throughout the century to a peak in the 1950s, several surveys then showed a decline. In Oxford, the incidence of perforation fell from 14 to 7 per 100 000 between 1957 and 1963, largely because of a reduced incidence of duodenal perforation (Sanders 1967). Between these dates, the overall incidence of perforated duodenal ulcer was 8 per 100 000 and of gastric ulcer, 2 per 100 000. More recently, the incidence of perforation appears to be rising in some areas of the UK, particularly in elderly women with duodenal ulcer (Walt et al 1986). In Scotland, the overall perforation rate declined between 1975 and 1990 from 27 to 15 per 100 000 population, whereas there was a 93% increase in duodenal ulcer perforation in women over 65 years of age (Jibril et al 1994). Whereas there was a male preponderance of some 20:1 in the 1920s in the UK, the ratio decreased to 4:1 in the Oxford series and from 3.7:1 to 1.5:1 in the recent Scottish review. A Norwegian study in the Bergen area examining the period 1935–90 found that the male:female ratio fell from 10:1 to 1.5:1, while the median age rose from 41 to 62 years (Svanes et al 1993). While the proportion of perforations involving gastric ulcers remained constant at 10%, the proportion of duodenal perforations decreased from 80% to 32% over the first 30 years while the proportion of pyloric and prepyloric ulcers rose.

In the Oxford survey it was found that 11% of all peptic ulcers perforated and in a general practice survey over a 15-year period, 6% of ulcers perforated (Fry 1964). Perforation is commoner during the evening than in the early morning and in some series there are peaks in the early summer and early winter (Svanes et al 1993). The reasons for this circadian and seasonal variation are unclear, but the variation is most evident in the case of duodenal and pyloric ulcers.

Some cases are due to perforation of an "*acute ulcer*" (p. 226), but there is some confusion as to what constitutes an acute ulcer. It can be defined histologically by the absence of fibrosis or on the basis of a history of less than 3 months dyspepsia before perforation (Cassell 1969), in which case about 25% of perforated ulcers are acute. This has clinical relevance, since the shorter the duration of symptoms before perforation the less likely the patient is to have further exacerbations of duodenal ulceration after treatment of perforation. Recent evidence indicates that perforation of an acute duodenal ulcer has no association with *H. pylori* infection, suggesting that perforated ulcer may have a different pathogenesis to chronic duodenal ulcer and should not merely be regarded as a complication of it (Reinbach et al 1993).

Nonsteroidal anti-inflammatory drugs (NSAIDs) may play a role in perforation, particularly in the aged (Collier & Pain 1985), and could be implicated in the recent rise in incidence of ulcer perforation in the UK (Walt et al 1986). The prevalence of NSAID use in perforated duodenal ulcer patients ranges from 32% to 82% and steroid use and smoking are other recognized risk factors (Reinbach et al 1993).

## Clinical features

### *History*

There is a sudden onset of severe pain in the upper abdomen which soon becomes generalized and exacerbated by movement. Occasionally, pain is confined to the right side of the abdomen and passage of gastric contents down the right paracolic gutter may produce clinical signs resembling those of acute appendicitis. The symptoms sometimes become slightly less prominent after a few hours, perhaps because peristalsis is inhibited and leakage through the perforation diminishes. However, this "period of illusion" is soon followed by evidence of generalized peritonitis and increasing abdominal pain. In some patients, perforation occurs without a history of peptic ulceration. In about 5% of patients there is hematemesis and/or melena at the time of presentation with perforation.

### *Examination*

The patient usually lies completely still and the abdominal muscles show board-like rigidity with marked rebound tenderness. Respiration is typically shallow and the abdomen does not move on respiration. In some instances the presentation is less dramatic and abdominal pain and tenderness are much less prominent. Such patients may present at a later stage with intra-abdominal abscess formation. Liver dullness may be absent if enough air escapes to produce a substantial pneumoperitoneum. Bowel sounds are usually absent. A plain radiograph of the chest and abdomen with the patient in the erect position confirms the diagnosis in some 70% of cases by demonstrating gas under the diaphragm (Fig. 10.11). Radiology should not be allowed to delay resuscitation and surgery, but contrast studies using the water-soluble medium Gastrografin are valuable when there is diagnostic uncertainty. Acute pancreatitis and acute cholecystitis are the main conditions which can be confused with ulcer perforation.

## Treatment of perforated duodenal ulcer

Initially it is important to relieve pain, correct hypovolemia and establish nasogastric suction. A broad-spectrum antibiotic is usually prescribed.

The choice of operation rests between simple closure and the various definitive ulcer operations. In the era before potent antisecretory drugs were available, some 20% of patients remained asymptomatic after simple closure (Hennessy et al 1976, Griffin & Organ 1976),

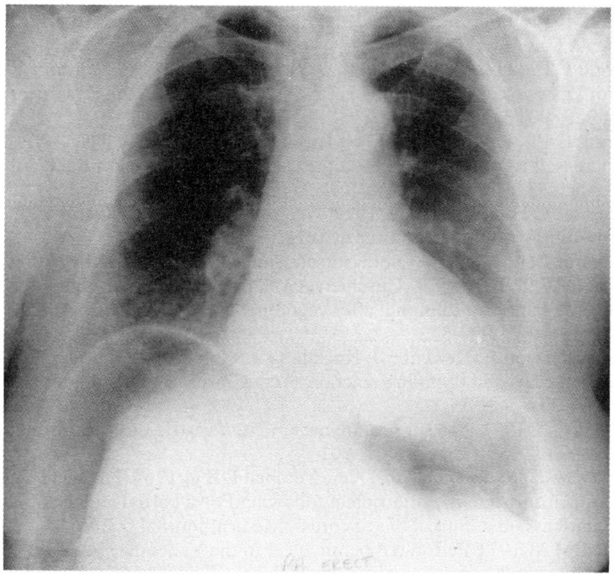

**ßFig. 10.11** Chest radiograph with patient in the upright position showing air under the diaphragm following free perforation of a duodenal ulcer.

although the figure was higher in patients with acute duodenal ulcers who had been asymptomatic before perforation. Simple closure is easy to perform and has a mortality in more recent studies of 5–10% (Morran & Carter 1983). Various laparoscopic methods of closing the perforation or sealing it with an omental patch or sealant have now been described (Darzi et al 1993, Tate et al 1993).

To avoid the need for further surgery, many surgeons used to advocate definitive surgery if the patient had a dyspeptic history of more than 3 months and/or there was chronic scarring at surgery. Truncal vagotomy and pyloroplasty was generally preferred to gastric resection if definitive surgery had to be carried out, although protagonists of highly selective vagotomy reported encouraging results (Jordan 1982). Now that potent antisecretory drugs are available there is a stronger case for simple closure in most patients, given the expectation that healing can be maintained by continued medical therapy and the desirability of avoiding the side-effects of ulcer surgery.

Conservative treatment of ulcer perforation (Taylor 1957) is now seldom undertaken, except in patients who have severe cardiorespiratory disease or who present late when clinical assessment suggests that the perforation has sealed spontaneously and the problem is resolving.

### Mortality

Perforation is a serious complication. In one series of 852 cases (Cohen 1971), there was an overall mortality of 18% and one-third of these deaths were considered to be due to misdiagnosis. In a large Scottish series, perforated duodenal ulcer carried an overall mortality of 11% (MacKay & MacKay 1976) whereas a study from Exeter dealing with the period 1979–86 found that mortality in those under 70 was 13% as opposed to 26% in older patients (Irwin 1989). These figures are probably more representative of the general experience than mortality rates as low as 3% which have been reported in selected patients coming to operation (Booth & Williams 1971). In Bergen in the years 1970–90, perforated duodenal ulcer carried a mortality rate of 7.8%, almost identical to that of perforated pyloric ulcer but half that of perforated gastric ulcer (17.6%) (Svanes et al 1993). Of patients who died in this study, the proportion with intercurrent disease rose throughout the study period from 27% to 85% and it is well recognized that mortality is highest in the elderly, those with cardiorespiratory disease and those in whom diagnosis and treatment are delayed. In view of the increased risk of definitive surgery in the elderly, there is a particularly strong case for simple closure (Irwin 1989).

### Treatment of perforated gastric ulcer

The need for further surgery following simple closure of perforated gastric ulcer exceeds that of duodenal ulcer and may be particularly high in women (Hennessy et al 1976). Furthermore, up to 10% of perforated gastric ulcers prove to be malignant, strengthening the case for definitive surgery (in the form of partial gastrectomy) rather than simple closure. These considerations have to be balanced against the age and general condition of the patient, so that simple closure following excision of the ulcer for histological examination is still often advisable (see Irwin 1989).

Perforation of a gastric ulcer carries a higher mortality than perforated duodenal ulcer, being as high as 27–38% in older series (Sanders 1967, MacKay & MacKay 1976) and remaining high at 17.6% in the more recent Norwegian review (Svanes et al 1993). The high mortality reflects the greater age of gastric ulcer patients and the escape of a large volume of gastric contents into the peritoneal cavity. In Exeter, patients over 70 had a mortality rate of 41% whereas there were no deaths in younger patients (Irwin 1989).

## REFERENCES


Adrian T E, Long R G, Fuessl H S, Bloom S R 1985 Plasma peptide YY (PYY) in dumping syndrome. Digestive Diseases and Sciences 30: 1145–1148

Alagaratnam T T, Wong J 1988 No decrease in duodenal ulcer surgery after cimetidine in Hong Kong. Journal of Clinical Gastroenterology 10: 25–27

Aldoori M I, Qamar M I, Read A E, Williamson R C N 1985 Increased flow in the superior mesenteric artery in dumping syndrome. British Journal of Surgery 72: 389–390

Alexander-Williams J, Hoare A M 1979 Partial gastric resection. Clinics in Gastroenterology 8: 321

Allan J G, Russell R I 1975 Double-blind controlled trial of cholestyramine in the treatment of postvagotomy diarrhoea. Gut 16: 830

Amdrup E, Jensen H E, Johnston D, Walker B E, Goligher J C 1974 Clinical results of parietal cell vagotomy (highly selective vagotomy) two to four years after operation. Annals of Surgery 180: 279–284

Arman E, Nilsson L H, Reizenstein P 1970 Studies in the dumping syndrome. VI. Calcium deficiency after partial gastrectomy. American Journal of Digestive Diseases 15: 455

Baird I M, Wilson G M 1959 The pathogenesis of anaemia after partial gastrectomy. II. Iron absorption after partial gastrectomy. Quarterly Journal of Medicine 28: 35

Baird I M, Blackburn E K, Wilson G M 1959 The pathogenesis of anaemia after partial gastrectomy. I. Development of anaemia in relation to time after operation, blood loss, and diet. Quarterly Journal of Medicine 28: 21

Baird I M, St John D J B, Nasser S S 1970 Role of occult blood loss in anaemia after partial gastrectomy. Gut 11: 55

Balint J A 1958 Pulmonary tuberculosis and partial gastrectomy. Gastroenterologia 90: 65

Balint J A, Spence M P 1959 Pyloric stenosis. British Medical Journal 1: 890

Banks P A, Waye J D, Waitman A M, Cornell A 1967 Mucosal diaphragm of the gastric antrum. Gastroenterology 52: 1003

Bardhan K D, Cust G, Hinchcliffe R F C, Williamson F M, Lyon C, Bose K 1989 Changing pattern of admissions and operations for duodenal ulcer. British Journal of Surgery 76: 230–236

Becker J M, Kelly K A 1983 Implications of vagotomy. In: Carter D C (ed) Peptic ulcer. Churchill Livingstone, Edinburgh, p 77

Berenbaum S L, Lawrence L, Schwartz S 1968 Roentgen exploration of the afferent loop. Radiology 91: 932

Berstad A, Nesland A A 1985 Prepyloric erosions and related changes. Scandinavian Journal of Gastroenterology 20: 779

Biorneklett A, Fausa O, Midtvedt T 1983 Small-bowel bacterial overgrowth in the postgastrectomy syndrome. Scandinavian Journal of Gastroenterology 18: 277

Blackett R L, Johnston D 1981 Recurrent ulceration after highly selective vagotomy for duodenal ulcer. British Journal of Surgery 68: 705–710

Blackett R L, Axon A T R, Barker M C, Pifano E, Baltas D, Johnston D 1982 HSV with pyloric dilatation for pyloric stenosis due to peptic ulcer. British Journal of Surgery 69: 289

Blake G, Kennedy T L, McKelvey S T D 1983 Bile acids and postvagotomy diarrhoea British Journal of Surgery 70: 177

Booth R A D, Williams J A 1971 Mortality of perforated duodenal ulcer treated by simple suture. British Journal of Surgery 58: 42

Britton J P, Johnston D, Ward D C, Axon A T R, Barker M C J 1987 Gastric emptying and clinical outcome after Roux-en-y diversion. British Journal of Surgery 74: 900–904

Brough W A, Taylor T V, Torrance H B 1984 The surgical factors influencing duodenogastric reflux. British Journal of Surgery 71: 770–773

Browning G G, Buchan K A, Mackay C 1974 Clinical and laboratory study of postvagotomy diarrhoea. Gut 15: 644

Bruce J, Card W I, Marks I N, Sircus W 1959 The rationale of selective surgery in the treatment of duodenal ulcer. Journal of the Royal College of Surgeons of Edinburgh 4: 85

Burhenne H J 1967 The retained gastric antrum. Preoperative roentgenologic diagnosis of an iatrogenic syndrome. American Journal of Roentgenology 101: 459

Burhenne H J 1968 The iatrogenic afferent-loop syndrome. Radiology 91: 942

Bushkin F L, Woodward E R 1976a The afferent loop syndrome. Major Problems in Clinical Surgery 20: 34

Bushkin F L, Woodward E R 1976b Alkaline reflux esophagitis. Major Problems in Clinical Surgery 20: 64–71

Bushkin F L, Woodward E R 1976c Delayed gastric emptying. Major Problems in Clinical Surgery 20: 72

Butler T J 1961 The effect of gastrectomy on pancreatic secretion in man. Annals of the Royal College of Surgeons 29: 300

Cabrol J, Navarro X, Sancho J, Simo-Deu J, Segura R 1990 Bile reflux in postoperative alkaline gastritis. Annals of Surgery 211: 239–243

Carter C O 1961 The inheritance of congenital pyloric stenosis. British Medical Bulletin 17: 251

Carter D C 1987 Cancer after peptic ulcer surgery. Gut 28: 921–923

Cassell P 1969 Perforated duodenal ulcer in Reading from 1950 to 1959. Gut 10: 454

Caygill C P J, Hill M J, Kirkham J S, Northfield T C 1986 Mortality from gastric cancer following gastric surgery for peptic ulcer. Lancet 1: 929–931

Caygill C P J, Hill M J, Hall C N, Kirkham J S, Northfield T C 1987 Increased risk of cancer at multiple sites following gastric surgery for peptic ulcer. Gut 28: 924–928

Chaimoff C H, Dinstman M 1972 The long-term fate of patients with dumping syndrome. Archives of Surgery 105: 554

Chanarin I 1969 The megaloblastic anaemias. Blackwell, Oxford, p 622

Cheadle W G, Baker P R, Cuschieri A 1985 Pyloric reconstruction for severe vasomotor dumping after vagotomy and pyloroplasty. Annals of Surgery 202: 568–572

Christoffersson E, Kewenter J, Kock N G 1962 Intestinal motility during provoked dumping reaction. Acta Chirurgica Scandinavica 123: 405

Clagett O T 1971 The surgical management of gastric ulcer. Surgical Clinics of North America 51: 901

Clark C G, Crooks J, Dawson A A, Mitchell P E G 1964 The incidence of malabsorption of radiotriolein following Polya partial gastrectomy in patients on a normal diet. Scottish Medical Journal 9: 365

Cohen M M 1971 Perforated peptic ulcer in the Vancouver area: a survey of 852 cases. Canadian Medical Association Journal 104: 201–205

Collier D St J, Pain J A 1985 Non-steroidal anti-inflammatory drugs and peptic ulcer perforation. Gut 26: 359–363

Cox A G 1968 Comparison of symptoms after vagotomy with gastrojejunostomy and partial gastrectomy. British Medical Journal 1: 288

Cox A G, Spencer J, Tinker J 1969 Clinical results reviewed. In: Williams J A, Cox A G (eds) After vagotomy. Butterworths, London, p 119

Cuschieri A 1986 Surgical management of severe intractable postvagotomy diarrhoea. British Journal of Surgery 73: 981–984

Cuschieri A 1990 Postvagotomy diarrhoea: is there a place for surgical management? Gut 31: 245–246

Dahlgren S 1964 The afferent loop syndrome. Acta Chirurgica Scandinavica (suppl) 327: 1

Dallemagne B, Weerts J M, Jehaes C, Markiewicz S, Lombard R 1994 Laparoscopic highly selective vagotomy. British Journal of Surgery 81: 554–556

Darzi A, Cheshire N J, Somers S S, Super P A, Guillou P J, Monson J R T 1993 Laparoscopic omental patch repair of perforated duodenal ulcer with an automated stapler. British Journal of Surgery 80: 1552

Deller D J, Witts L J 1962 Changes in the blood after partial gastrectomy with special reference to vitamin $B_{12}$. Serum vitamin $B_{12}$, haemoglobin, serum iron, and bone marrow. Quarterly Journal of Medicine 31: 71

Demaret A, Hirschowitz B I, Luketic G C 1971 Double-barrel gastrojejunal stoma and its symptoms and complications in 38 patients. Scandinavian Journal of Gastroenterology 6: 77

Dewar P, King R, Johnston D 1982 Bile acid and lysolecithin concentrations in the stomach in patients with doudenal ulcer before operation and after treatment by highly selective vagotomy, partial gastrectomy, or truncal vagotomy and drainage. Gut 23: 569

Ditlevsen S 1989 Survival after vagotomy: results of the Aarhus county vagotomy trial. World Journal of Surgery 13: 776–781

Doig A, Girdwood R H 1960 The absorption of folic acid and labelled cyanocabolamin in intestinal malabsorption. Quarterly Journal of Medicine 29: 333

Dunlap J A, McLane R C, Roper T J 1975 The retained gastric antrum. A case report. Radiology 117: 371

Dunn D C, Thomas W E G, Hunter J O 1981 Highly selective vagotomy and pyloric dilatation for duodenal ulcer with stenosis. British Journal of Surgery 68: 194

Eckardt V F, Giessler W, Kanzler G, Bernard G 1992 Does endoscopic follow-up improve the outcome of patients with benign gastric ulcers and gastric cancer? Cancer 69: 301–305

Edwards J P, Lyndon P J, Smith R B, Johnston D 1974 Faecal fat excretion after truncal, selective and highly selective vagotomy for duodenal ulcer. Gut 15: 521

Einhorn R I, Grace N D, Banks P A 1984 The clinical significance and

natural history of the double pylorus. Digestive Diseases and Sciences 29: 213
Elashoff J D, Grossman M I 1980 Trends in hospital admissions and death rates for peptic ulcer in the United States from 1970 to 1978. Gastroenterology 78: 280–285
Eldh J, Kewenter J, Kock N G, Olson P 1974 Long-term results of surgical treatment for dumping after partial gastrectomy. British Journal of Surgery 61: 90
Farrands P A, Blake J R S, Ansell I D, Cotton R E, Hardcastle J D 1983 Endoscopic review of patients who have had gastric surgery. British Medical Journal 286: 755
Fawcett A N, Johnston D, Duthie H L 1969 Revagotomy for recurrent ulcer after vagotomy and drainage for duodenal ulcer. British Journal of Surgery 56: 111–116
Feller E R, Warshaw A L, Shapiro R H 1980 Observations on management of choledochoduodenal fistula due to penetrating peptic ulcer. Gastroenterology 78: 126
Festen H P M, Lamers C B H, Driessen W M M, van Tongeren J H M 1979 Cimetidine in anastomotic ulceration after partial gastrectomy. Gastroenterology 77: 83
Fields M, Duthie H L 1965 Effect of vagotomy on intraluminal digestion of fat in man. Gut 6: 301
Finlayson N D C, Shearman D J C, Girdwood R H 1968 A case of coexisting duodenal ulceration and idiopathic steatorrhea. Gastroenterology 55: 626
Finlayson N D C, Simpson J D, Tothill P, Samson R R, Girdwood R H, Shearman D J C 1969 Application of whole body counting to the measurement of vitamin $B_{12}$ absorption with reference to achlorhydria. Scandinavian Journal of Gastroenterology 4: 397
Fisher A B 1984 Twenty-five years after Billroth II gastrectomy for duodenal ulcer. World Journal of Surgery 8: 293–302
Fredens M, Kronborg O, Madsen P, Palbol J 1971 Radiography in the diagnosis of recurrent duodenal ulceration following vagotomy and pyloroplasty. Scandinavian Journal of Gastroenterology 6: 559
Frucht H, Kunkel P, Spiro H M 1957 Pulmonary tuberculosis following gastric resection. Annals of Internal Medicine 46: 696
Fry J 1964 Peptic ulcer: a profile. British Medical Journal 2: 809–
Garden O J, Dykes E H, Carter D C 1988 Surgical and nutritional management of postoperative duodenal fistulas. Digestive Diseases and Sciences 33: 30
Gohel V K, Laufer I 1978 Double-contrast examination of the postoperative stomach. Radiology 129: 601
Goligher J C 1970 The comparative results of different operations in the elective treatment of duodenal ulcer. British Journal of Surgery 57: 780–783
Goligher J C, Pulvertaft C N, de Dombal F T et al 1968a Five- to eight-year results of Leeds/York controlled trial of elective surgery for doudenal ulcer. British Medical Journal 2: 781–787
Goligher J C, Pulvertaft C N, de Dombal F T et al 1968b Clinical comparison of vagotomy and pyloroplasty with other forms of elective surgery for duodenal ulcer. British Medical Journal 2: 787
Goligher J C, Pulvertaft C N, Irvin T T et al 1972 Five- to eight-year results of truncal vagotomy and pyloroplasty for duodenal ulcer. British Medical Journal 1: 7–13
Goligher J C, Hill G L, Kenny T E, Nutter E 1978 Proximal gastric vagotomy without drainage for duodenal ulcer: results after 5–8 years. British Journal of Surgery 65: 145–151
Gough K R, Thirkettle J L, Read A E 1965 Folic acid deficiency in patients after gastric resection. Quarterly Journal of Surgery 34: 1
Gough M J, Woodhouse L, Giles G R 1986 Lithium fluxes across the gastric mucosa after truncal vagotomy and drainage – an objective assessment of mucosal injury. Gut 27: 249
Green R, Spencer A, Kennedy T 1978 Closure of gastrojejunostomy for the relief of post-vagotomy symptoms. British Journal of Surgery 65: 161–163
Greenall M J, Lehnert T 1985 Vagotomy or gastrectomy for elective treatment of benign gastric ulceration? Digestive Diseases and Sciences 30: 353–361
Griffin G E, Organ G H Jr 1976 The natural history of the perforated duodenal ulcer treated by suture plication. Annals of Surgery 183: 382
Griffiths J M T 1974 The features and course of bile vomiting following gastric surgery. British Journal of Surgery 61: 617
Gustavsson S 1988 Peptic ulcer disease – trends in surgical management in Sweden. Scandinavian Journal of Gastroenterology 23 (suppl 155): 152–154
Gustavsson S, Kelly K A, Melton L J, Zinsmeister A R 1988 Trends in peptic ulcer surgery. Gastroenterology 94: 688–694
Hansen J H, Knigge U 1984 Failure of proximal gastric vagotomy for duodenal ulcer resistant to cimetidine. Lancet 2: 84–85
Hartley M N, Mackie C R 1991 Gastric adaptive relaxation and symptoms after vagotomy. British Journal of Surgery 78: 24–27
Hedberg C A, Melnyk C S, Johnson C F 1966 Gluten enteropathy appearing after gastric surgery. Gastroenterology 50: 796
Hennessy E J, Chapman B L, Duggan J M 1976 Perforated peptic ulcer long-term follow-up. Medical Journal of Australia 1: 50
Herrington J L, Scott H W, Sawyers J L 1984 Experience with vagotomy-antrectomy and Roux-en-Y gastrojejunostomy in surgical treatment of duodenal, gastric and stomach ulcers. Annals of Surgery 199: 590–596
Herrington J L Jr, Edwards W H, Carter J H, Sawyers J L 1986 Treatment of severe postvagotomy diarrhoea by reversed jejunal segment. Annals of Surgery 168: 522–541
Hill G L, Barker M C J 1978 Anterior highly selective vagotomy and posterior truncal vagotomy: a simple technique for denervating the parietal cell mass. British Journal of Surgery 65: 702–705
Himal H S 1977 Alkaline gastritis and alkaline esophagitis: a review. Canadian Joumal of Surgery 20: 403
Hines J D, Hoffbrand A V, Mollin D L 1967 The hematologic complications following partial gastrectomy. A study of 292 patients. American Journal of Medicine 43: 555
Hoerr S O, Ward J T 1972 Late results of three operations for chronic duodenal ulcer: vagotomy–gastrojejunostomy, vagotomy–hemogastrectomy, vagotomy–pyloroplasty. Interim report. Annals of Surgery 176: 403
Hoffman W A, Spiro H M, 1961 Afferent loop problems. Gastroenterology 40: 201
Hoffmann J, Jensen H-E, Schulze S, Paulsen P E, Christiansen J 1984 Prospective controlled vagotomy trial for duodenal ulcer: results after five years. British Journal of Surgery 71: 582–585
Hoffmann J, Olesen A, Jensen H-E. 1987 Prospective 14- to 18-year follow-up study after parietal cell vagotomy. British Journal of Surgery 74: 1056–1059
Hoffmann J, Meisner S, Jensen H-E 1983 Antrectomy for recurrent ulcer after parietal cell vagotomy. British Journal of Surgery 70: 120–121
Hoffmann J, Jensen H-E, Christiansen J, Olesen A, Loud F B, Hauch O 1989 Prospective controlled vagotomy trial for duodenal ulcer. Results after 11–15 years. Annals of Surgery 209: 40–45
Holle G E, Frey K W, Thieme Ch, Holle F K 1988 Recurrence of peptic ulcer after selective proximal vagotomy and pyloroplasty in relation to changes in clinical signs and symptoms between 1969 and 1983. Surgery, Gynecology and Obstetrics 167: 271–281
Holt J M, Gear M W L, Warner G T 1970 The role of chronic blood loss in the pathogenesis of postgastrectomy iron-deficiency anaemia. Gut 11: 847
Hopman W P M, Wolberink R G J, Lamers G B H W, van Tongeren J H M 1988 Treatment of the dumping syndrome with the somatostatin analogue SMS 201–995. Annals of Surgery 207: 155–159
Houghton P W J, Mortensen N J McC, Thomas W E G, Cooper M J, Morgan A P, Davies E R 1986 Intragastric bile acids and scintigraphy in the assessment of duodenogastric reflux. British Journal of Surgery 73: 292–294
Howe C T, Le Quesne L P 1964 Pyloric stenosis: the metabolic effects. British Journal of Surgery 51: 923
Huggins M J, Friedman A C, Lichtenstein J E, Bova J G 1982 Adult acquired antral web. Digestive Diseases and Sciences 27: 80
Humphrey C S, Johnston D, Walker B E, Pulvertaft C N, Goligher J C 1972 Incidence of dumping after truncal and selective vagotomy with pyloroplasty and highly selective vagotomy without drainage procedure. British Medical Journal 3: 785–787
Irwin T T 1989 Mortality and perforated peptic ulcer: a case for risk stratification in elderly patients.
Jaffin B W, Kaye M D 1985 The prognosis of gastric outlet obstruction. Annals of Surgery 201: 176–179

Jamieson G G 1983 Operations available for duodenal ulcer: an overview. In: Carter D C (ed) Peptic ulcer. Churchill Livingstone, Edinburgh, p 90

Jibril J A, Redpath A, Macintyre I M C 1994 Changing pattern of admission and operation for duodenal ulcer in Scotland. British Journal of Surgery 81: 87–89

Johnson A G 1983 Operations available for gastric ulcer: an overview. In: Carter D C (ed) Peptic ulcer. Churchill Livingstone, Edinburgh, p 104

Johnson H D 1962 Peptic ulcer in hospital. An analysis of a 10% inpatient enquiry throughout England and Wales. Gut 3: 106

Johnson H D, Hoffbrand A V 1970 The influence of extent of resection, type of anastomosis, and ulcer site on the haematological side-effects of gastrectomy. British Journal of Surgery 57: 33

Johnston D 1975 Operative mortality and postoperative morbidity of highly selective vagotomy. British Medical Journal 4: 545–547

Johnston D, Humphrey C S, Walker B E, Pulvertaft C N, Goligher J C 1972 Vagotomy without diarrhoea. British Medical Journal 3: 788–790

Johnston D, Pickford I R, Walker B E, Goligher I C 1975 Highly selective vagotomy for duodenal ulcer: do hypersecretors need antrectomy? British Medical Journal 1: 716–718

Johnston G W, Spencer E F A, Wilkinson A J, Kennedy T L 1991 Proximal gastric vagotomy: follow-up at 10–20 years. British Journal of Surgery 78: 20–23

Johnstone F R C, Holubitsky I B, Debas H T 1967 Post-gastrectomy problems in patients with personality defects: the "Albatross" syndrome. Canadian Medical Association Journal 96: 1559

Jordan P H 1982 Proximal gastric vagotomy without drainage for treatment of perforated duodenal ulcer. Gastroenterology 83: 179

Jordan P H, Condon R E 1970 A prospective evaluation of vagotomy-pyloroplasty and vagotomy-antrectomy for treatment of duodenal ulcer. Annals of Surgery 172: 547

Katkhouda N, Mouiel J 1991 A new technique of surgical treatment of chronic doudenal ulcer without laparotomy by videocelioscopy. American Journal Surgery 161: 361–364

Kelly K A, Becker J M, van Heerden J A 1981 Reconstructive gastric surgery. British Journal of Surgery 68: 687–691

Kemp D 1967 An evaluation and comparison of the early and late results of standardized Polya gastrectomy. Gut 8: 151

Kennedy T 1977 Which vagotomy? In: Truelove S C, Lee E (eds) Topics in gastroenterology (Vol 5). Blackwell, Oxford, p 263

Kennedy T 1978 Recurrent ulcer after vagotomy or gastrectomy treated with cimetidine. In: Wastell C, Lance P (eds) Cimetidine. The Westminster Hospital Symposium 1978. Churchill Livingstone, Edinburgh, p 79

Kennedy T 1979 A critical appraisal of surgical treatment. In: Truelove S C, Willoughby C P (eds) Topics in gastroenterology (Vol 7). Blackwell, Oxford, p 131

Kennedy T, Green R 1978 Roux diversion for bile reflux following gastric surgery. British Journal of Surgery 65: 323–325

Kennedy T, Magill P, Johnston G W, Parks T G 1979 Proximal gastric vagotomy, fundoplication, and lesser curve necrosis. British Medical Journal 1: 1455–1456

Kern F, Struthers J E 1966 Intestinal lactase deficiency and lactose intolerance in adults. Journal of the American Medical Association 195: 927

King C E, Toskes P P 1976 Malabsorption following gastric resection. Major Problems in Clinical Surgery 20: 129

Kjaergaard J, Esbensen K H, Meisner S, Jensen H-E, Wold S 1984 Ulcer recurrence after parietal cell vagotomy for duodenal ulcer. A multivariate pattern recognition study. Scandinavian Journal of Gastroenterology 19: 255

Klein K B, Orwoll E S, Lieberman D A, Meier D E, McClung M R, Parfitt A M 1987 Metabolic bone disease in asymptomatic men after partial gastrectomy with Billroth II anastomosis. Gastroenterology 92: 608

Koetz H R, Gewertz B L 1979 Vagotomy. Clinics in Gastroenterology 8: 305

Korman M G, Soveny C, Hansky J 1973 Paradoxical effect of secretin on serum immunoreactive gastrin in the Zollinger–Ellison syndrome. Digestion 8: 407

Koo J, Lam S K, Ong G B 1982 Cimetidine versus surgery for recurrent ulcer after gastric surgery. Annals of Surgery 195: 406

Koruth N M, Krukowski Z H, Matheson N A 1985 Pyloric reconstruction. British Journal of Surgery 72: 808–810

Kozoll D D, Meyer K A 1964 Obstructing gastroduodenal ulcers. General factors influencing incidence and mortality. Archives of Surgery 88: 793–799

Kronborg O 1974 Gastric acid secretion and risk of recurrence of duodenal ulcer within 6–8 years after truncal vagotomy and drainage. Gut 15: 714

Ladas S D, Isaacs P E T, Quereshi Y, Sladen G 1983 Role of the small intestine in postvagotomy diarrhea. Gastroenterology 85: 1088–1093

Lancet 1986 Leading article Osteomalacia after gastrectomy. Lancet 1: 77

Lawaetz O, Bloom S R, Stimpel H, Siemssen O J 1986 Effect of soya bean oil on symptoms, gastric emptying and gut hormone release in patients with postvagotomy symptoms. Annales Chirurgiae et Gynaecologie 75: 308

Le Quesne L P, Hobsley M, Hand B H 1960 The dumping syndrome. I. Factors responsible for the symptoms. British Medical Journal 1: 141

Linhardt G E, Stoddard C J, Johnson A G 1982 Do women do worse after proximal gastric vagotomy? British Journal of Surgery 69: 321–322

Long R G, Adrian T E, Bloom S R 1985 Somatostatin and the dumping syndrome. British Medical Journal 290: 886–888

Lous P, Schwartz M 1959 The absorption of vitamin $B_{12}$ following partial gastrectomy. Acta Medica Scandinavica 164: 407

Lundergardh G, Holmberg L, Krusemo U B 1991 Long-term survival in patients operated on for benign peptic ulcer disease. British Journal of Surgery 78: 234–236

Lundergardh G, Ekbom A, McLaughlin J K, Nyren O 1994 Gastric cancer risk after vagotomy. Gut 35: 946–949

Machella T E 1950 Mechanism of the post-gastrectomy dumping syndrome. Gastroenterology 14: 237

McAlhany J C, Hanover T M, Taylor S M, Sticca R P, Ashmore J D 1994 Long-term follow-up of patients with Roux-en-y gastrojejunostomy for gastric disease. Annals of Surgery 219: 451–457

McDermott E W M, Murphy J J 1993 Laparoscopic truncal vagotomy without drainage. British Journal of Surgery 80: 236

Macintyre I M C, Millar A 1991 Highly selective vagotomy – a safe operation for duodenal ulcer. European Journal of Surgery 157: 261–265

Macintyre I M C, O'Brien F 1994 Death from malignant disease after surgery for duodenal ulcer. Gut 35: 451–454

Macintyre I M C, Millar A, Smith A N, Small W P 1990 Highly selective vagotomy 5–15 years on. British Journal of Surgery 77: 65–69

MacKay C, MacKay H P 1976 Perforated peptic ulcer in the West of Scotland 1964–73. British Journal of Surgery 63: 157

McKelvey S T D 1970 Gastric incontinence and past-vagotomy diarrhoea. British Journal of Surgery 57: 741–747

Mackie C R, Hall A W, Clark J, Wisbey M, Baker P R, Cuschieri A 1981 The effect of isoperistaltic jejunal interposition upon gastric emptying. Surgery, Gynecology and Obstetrics 153: 813–819

Mackie C, Hulks G, Cuschieri A 1986 Enterogastric reflux and gastric clearance of refluxate in normal subjects and in patients with and without bile vomiting following peptic ulcer surgery. Annals of Surgery 204: 537

McLean Ross A H, Smith M A, Anderson J R, Small W P 1982 Late mortality after surgery for peptic ulcer. New England Journal of Medicine 307: 519–522

Maki T, Sato T, Shipatori T 1977 Pylorus-preserving procedure in partial and total gastrectomy. Langenbecks Archiv fur Chirurgie 343: 183–193

Malagelada J-R, Rees W D W, Mazzotta L J, Go V L W 1980 Gastric motor abnormalities in diabetic and postvagotomy gastroparesis: effect of metoclopramide and bethanechol. Gastroenterology 78: 286

Malagelada J-R, Phillips S F, Shorter R G et al 1985 Postoperative reflux gastritis: pathophysiology and long-term outcome after Roux-en-Y diversion. Annals of Internal Medicine 103: 178

Mathias J R, Fernandez A, Sninsky C A, Clench M H, Davis R H 1985 Nausea, vomiting and abdominal pain after Roux-en-Y anastomosis: motility of the jejunal limb. Gastroenterology 88: 101–107

Mattsson O, Perman G 1962 Small intestine transit time studied in patients with the dumping syndrome. Acta Chirurgica Scandinavica 124: 326

Mayer E A, Thomson J B, Jehn D et al 1984 Gastric emptying and sieving of solid food and pancreatic and biliary secretions after solid meals in patients with nonresective ulcer surgery. Gastroenterology 87: 1264

Meshkinpour H, Marks J W, Schoenfield L J, Bonnoris G G, Carter S 1980 Reflux gastritis syndrome: mechanism of symptoms. Gastroenterology 79: 1283–1287

Meyer J H 1979 Reflections on reflux gastritis. Gastroenterology 77: 1143

Moody F G, Cornell G N, Beal J M 1962 Pyloric obstruction complicating peptic ulcer. Archives of Surgery 84: 462–466

Morgan D B, Pulvertaft C N 1969 Effects of vagotomy on bone metabolism. In: Williams J A, Cox A G (eds) After vagotomy. Butterworths, London, p 161

Morgan D B, Paterson C R, Woods C G, Pulvertaft C N, Fourman P 1965a Search for osteomalacia in 1228 patients after gastrectomy and other operations on the stomach. Lancet 2: 1085

Morgan D B, Paterson C R, Woods C G, Pulvertaft C N, Fourman P 1965b Osteomalacia after gastrectomy. A response to very small doses of vitamin D. Lancet 2: 1089

Morgan D B, Pulvertaft C N, Fourman P 1966 Effects of age on the loss of bone after gastric surgery. Lancet 2: 772

Morgan D B, Hunt G, Paterson C R 1970 The osteomalacia syndrome after stomach operations. Quarterly Journal of Medicine 39: 395

Morran C G, Carter D C 1983 Complications of peptic ulceration. In: Carter D C (ed) Peptic ulcer. Churchill Livingstone, Edinburgh, p 115

Mowat N A G, Needham C D, Brunt P W 1975 The natural history of gastric ulcer in a community: a four-year study. Quarterly Journal of Medicine 44: 45

Muscroft T J, Taylor E W, Deane S A, Alexander-Williams J 1981 Reoperation for recurrent peptic ulceration. British Journal of Surgery 68: 75

Nath B J, Warshaw A L 1984 Alkaline reflux gastritis and esophagitis. Annual Review of Medicine 35: 383

Neale G, Antcliff A C, Welbourn R B, Mollin D L, Booth C C 1967 Protein malnutrition after partial gastrectomy. Quarterly Journal of Medicine 36: 469

Nobles E R Jr 1966 Vagotomy and gastroenterostomy. 15-year follow-up of 175 patients. American Surgeon 32: 177–182

Olbe L, Forssell H, Stenquist B 1983 The pitfalls in postoperative testing of the completeness of vagotomy. Journal of the Autonomic Nervous System 9: 315–323

Ott D J, Munitz H A, Gelfand D W, Lane T G, Wu W C 1982 The sensitivity of radiography of the postoperative stomach. Radiology 144: 741

Paimela H, Tuompo P K, Perakyla T, Saario I, Hockerstedt K, Kivilaakso E 1991 Peptic ulcer surgery during the $H_2$-receptor antagonist era: a population-based epidemiological study of ulcer surgery in Helsinki from 1972 to 1987. British Journal of Surgery 78: 28–31

Pedersen J H, Beck H, Shokouh-Amiri M, Fischer A 1986 Effect of neurotensin in the dumping syndrome. Scandinavian Journal of Gastroenterology 21: 478

Pellegrini C A, DeMeester T R, Wernly J A, Johnson L F, Skinner D B 1978 Alkaline gastroesophageal reflux. American Journal of Surgery 135: 177

Pellegrini C A, Patti M G, Lewin M, Way L W 1985 Alkaline reflux gastritis and the effect of biliary diversion on gastric emptying of solid food. American Journal of Surgery 150: 166

Philip A E, Cay E L 1972 Psychiatric symptoms and personality traits in patients suffering from gastrointestinal illness. Journal of Psychosomatic Research 16: 47

Poppen B, Delin A 1981 Parietal cell vagotomy for duodenal and pyloric ulcers. I Clinical factors leading to failure of the operation. American Journal of Surgery 141: 323

Postlethwait R W 1973 Five year follow-up results of operations for duodenal ulcer. Surgery, Gynecology and Obstetrics 137: 387–392

Postlethwait R W 1979 Retrospective study of operations for peptic ulcer. Surgery, Gynecology and Obstetrics 149: 703–708

Primrose J N, Johnston D 1989 Somatostatin analogue SMS 201-995 (octreotide) as a possible solution to the dumping syndrome after gastrectomy or vagotomy. British Journal of Surgery 76: 140–144

Primrose J N, Axon A T R, Johnston D 1988 Highly selective vagotomy and ulcers that fail to respond to $H_2$ receptor antagonists. British Medical Journal 296: 1031–1035

Pulvertaft C N 1952 The results of partial gastrectomy for peptic ulcer. Lancet 1: 225

Pulvertaft C N, Cox A G 1969 Effects of vagotomy on haemopoiesis. In: Williams J A, Cox A G (eds) After vagotomy. Butterworths, London, p 150

Ralphs D N L, Thomson J P S, Haynes S, Lawson-Smith C, Hobsley M, LeQuesne L P 1978 The relationship between the rate of gastric emptying and the dumping syndrome. British Journal of Surgery 65: 637

Ramus N I, Williamson R C N, Oliver J M, Johnston D 1982 Effect of highly selective vagotomy on pancreatic exocrine function and on cholecystokinin and gastric release. Gut 23: 553

Rehnberg O, Faxen A, Haglund U, Kewenter J, Stenquist B, Olbe L 1982 Gastric mycosis following gastric resection and vagotomy. Annals of Surgery 196: 21

Reid D A, Duthie, H L, Bransom C J, Johnson A G 1982 Late follow-up of highly selective vagotomy with excision of the ulcer compared to Billroth I gastrectomy for treatment of benign gastric ulcer. British Journal of Surgery 69: 605–

Reid D A, Bird N C, Simms J M, Stoddard C J, Eyre-Brook I, Johnson A G 1984 Controlled trial of the Grassi (pH) intraoperative test for completeness of proximal gastric vagotomy. Surgery, Gynecology and Obstetrics 158: 370–374

Reinbach D H, Cruickshank G, McColl K E L 1993 Acute perforated duodenal ulcer is not associated with *Helicobacter pylori* infection. Gut 34: 1344–1347

Rimer D G 1966 Gastric retention without mechanical obstruction. A review. Archives of Internal Medicine 117: 287

Ritchie W P 1984 Alkaline reflux gastritis: a critical reappraisal. Gut 25: 975

Robbs J V, Bank S, Marks I N, Louse J H 1973 Selection of operation for duodenal ulcer based on acid secretory studies – a reappraisal. British Journal of Surgery 60: 601

Robertson D S, Weder C H 1968 Acute jejunogastric intussusception. Canadian Journal of Surgery 11: 210

Ruckley C V, Sircus W 1970 Tests for gastric secretory function and their clinical applications. In: Glass G B J (ed) Progress in gastroenterology (Vol 11). Grune & Stratton, New York, p 73

Sanders R 1967 Incidence of perforated duodenal and gastric ulcer in Oxford. Gut 8: 58–63

Schatzki R 1968 The significance of rigidity of the jejunum in the diagnosis of postoperative jejunal ulcers. American Journal of Roentgenology 103: 330

Siewert J R, Holscher A H 1986 Billroth I gastrectomy. In: Nyhus L M, Wastell C (eds) Surgery of the stomach and duodenum, 4th edn. Little, Brown, Boston, p 263–290

Small W P 1973 The long-term results of peptic ulcer surgery. Clinics in Gastroenterology 2: 427

Small W P 1983 Reasons for failure. In: Carter D C (ed) Peptic ulcer. Churchill Livingstone, Edinburgh, p 172

Small W P, Cay E L, Dugard P et al 1969 Peptic ulcer surgery: selection for operation by "earning". Gut 10: 996

Small W P, Smith A N, Ruckley C V et al 1971 The continuing problem of jejunal ulcer. American Journal of Surgery 121: 541

Smith I S, Gillespie G, Elder J B, Gillespie I E, Kay A W 1972 Time of conversion of insulin response after vagotomy. Gastroenterology 62: 912

Smithwick R H, Harrower H W, Farmer D A 1961 Hemigastrectomy and vagotomy in the treatment of duodenal ulcer. American Journal of Surgery 101: 325

Stabile B E, Passaro E 1976 Recurrent peptic ulcer. Gastroenterology 70: 124

Stabile B E, Passaro E 1983 Recurrent ulceration. In: Carter D C (ed) Peptic ulcer. Churchill Livingstone, Edinburgh, p 132

Stabile B E, Passaro E, Samloff M, Walsh J H 1978 Serum pepsinogen 1, serum gastrin and gastric acid output in postoperative recurrent peptic ulcer. Archives of Surgery 113: 1136

Stemmer E A, Jones S A, Pearson S C, Connolly J E 1969

Antiperistaltic segments of jejunum in the treatment of the dumping syndrome. Archives of Surgery 98: 396
Stempien S J, Lee E R, Dagradi A E 1968 Clinical appraisal of insulin gastric analysis. American Journal of Digestive Diseases 13: 21
Stempien S J, Dagradi A E, Lee E R, Simonton J H 1971 Status of duodenal ulcer patients ten years or more after vagotomy-pyloroplasty. American Journal of Gastroenterology 56: 99–108
Stenquist B, Forssell H, Olbe L, Lundell L 1994 Role of acid secretory response to sham feeding in predicting recurrent ulceration after proximal gastric vagotomy. British Journal of Surgery 81: 1002–1006
Strom M, Bodemar G, Lindhagen J, Sjodahl R, Walan A 1984 Cimetidine or parietal-cell vagotomy in patients with juxta-pyloric ulcers. Lancet 2: 894–897
Svanes C, Salvesen H, Stangeland L, Svanes K, Soreide O 1993 Perforated peptic ulcer over 56 years. Time trends in patient and disease characteristics. Gut 34: 1666–1671
Tate J J T, Dawson J W, Lau W Y, Li A K C 1993 Sutureless laparoscopic treatment of perforated duodenal ulcer. British Journal of Surgery 80: 235
Taylor H 1957 The non-surgical treatment of perforated peptic ulcer. Gastroenterology 33: 353
Taylor T V 1979 Lesser curve superficial seromyotomy – an operation for chronic duodenal ulcer. British Journal of Surgery 66: 733
Taylor T V 1987 Parietal call vagotomy: long-term follow-up studies. British Journal of Surgery 74: 971–972
Taylor T V 1989 Current indications for elective peptic ulcer surgery. British Journal of Surgery 76: 427–428
Taylor T V, Lambert M E, Quereshi S, Torrance B 1978 Should cholecystectomy be combined with vagotomy and pyloroplasty? Lancet 1: 295–298
Taylor T V, Gunn A A, Macleod D A D, MacLennan I 1982 Anterior lesser curve seromyotomy and posterior truncal vagotomy in the treatment of chronic duodenal ulcer. Lancet 2: 846–848
Thompson D, Wild R, Merrick M V, Brydon G, Macintyre I M C, Eastwood M A 1994 Cholelithiasis and bile acid absorption after truncal vagotomy and gastroenterostomy. British Journal of Surgery 81: 1037–1039
Thompson J D, Galloway J B 1979 Vagotomy and pyloric dilatation in chronic duodenal ulceration. British Medical Journal 1: 1453–1455
Thompson D G, Ritchie H D, Wingate D L 1982a Patterns of small intestinal motility in duodenal ulcer patients before and after vagotomy. Gut 23: 517–523
Thompson G R, Lewis B, Booth C C 1966 Vitamin-D absorption after partial gastrectomy. Lancet 1: 457
Thompson W M, Kelvin F M, Gedgaudas R K, Rice R P 1982b Radiologic investigation of peptic ulcer disease. Radiologic Clinics of North America 20: 701
Thompson J P S, Russell R C G, Hobsley M, LeQuesne L P 1974 The dumping syndrome and the hydrogen ion concentration of the gastric contents. Gut 15: 200
Tolin R D, Malmud L S, Stelzer F et al 1979 Enterogastic reflux in normal subjects and patients with Bilroth II gastroenterostomy. Measurement of enterogastric reflux. Gastroenterology 77: 1027
Tonkin R D, Field T E, Wykes P R 1962 Pancreatic heterotopia as a cause of dyspepsia. Gut 3: 135
Toskes P P 1976 Hematologic abnormalities following gastric resection. Major Problems in Clinical Surgery 20: 119
Tovey F 1979 Peptic ulcer in India and Bangladesh. Gut 20: 329
Tovey F, Tunstall M 1975 Duodenal ulcer in black populations in Africa south of the Sahara. The geographical distribution of duodenal ulcer. Gut: 16: 564
Toye D K M, Williams J A 1965 Post-gastrectomy bile vomiting. Lancet 2: 524
Turnberg L A 1966 The absorption of iron after partial gastrectomy. Quarterly Journal of Medicine 35: 107
Turnbull A L 1965 The absorption of radioiron given with a standard meal after Polya partial gastrectomy. Clinical Science 28: 499
Turnbull A L 1967 Absorption of vitamin $B_{12}$ in patients with anaemia after Polya partial gastrectomy. British Journal of Haematology 13: 752
Veterans Administration Cooperative Study on Gastric Ulcer 1971 Gastroenterology 61: 565
Visick A H 1948 Measured radical gastrectomy. Review of 505 operations for peptic ulcer. Lancet 1: 505, 551
Viste A, Biornestad E, Opheim P et al 1986 Risk of carcinoma following gastric operations for benign disease. A historical cohort study of 3470 patients. Lancet 2: 502
Waddell W R, Kunz L J 1956 Association of salmonella enteritis with operations on the stomach. New England Journal of Medicine 255: 555
Walt R, Logan R, Katschinski B, Ashley J, Langman M 1986 Rising frequency of ulcer perforation in elderly people in the United Kingdom. Lancet 1: 489–492
Wang C-S, Tzen K-Y, Chen P-C, Chen M-F 1994 Effects of highly selective vagotomy and additional procedures on gastric emptying in patients with obstructing duodenal ulcer. World Journal of Surgery 18: 131–138
Warshaw A L 1981 Intragastric alkali infusion. A simple, accurate provocative test for diagnosis of symptomatic alkaline reflux gastritis. Annals of Surgery 194: 297
Wastell C 1969 Long-term clinical and metabolic effects of vagotomy with either gastrojejunostomy or pyloroplasty. Annals of the Royal College of Surgeons 45: 193
Wastell C 1972 Chronic duodenal ulcer. Butterworths, London
Watt P C H, Patterson C C, Kennedy T 1984 Late mortality after vagotomy and drainage for duodenal ulcer. British Medical Journal 288: 1335
Wattchow D A, Cass D T, Furness J B et al 1987 Abnormalities of peptide-containing nerve fibers in infantile hypertrophic pyloric stenosis. Gastroenterology 92: 443
Weaver R M, Temple J G 1985 Proximal gastric vagotomy in patients resistant to cimetidine. British Journal of Surgery 72: 177–178
Weinstein W M, Buch K L, Elashoff J et al 1985 The histology of the stomach in symptomatic patients after gastric surgery: a model to assess selective patterns of gastric mucosal injury. Scandinavian Journal of Gastroenterology 20 (suppl 109): 77
Weir D G, Temperley I J, Gatenby P B B 1963 Anaemia following gastric operations for peptic ulceration in Dublin. II. Deficiency of iron and vitamin $B_{12}$. Irish Journal of Medical Science (Series 6) 448: 151
Welbourn R B, Butler T J, Capper W M 1951 Discussions on postgastrectomy syndromes, Proceedings of the Royal Society of Medicine 44: 773
Wellmann K F, Kagan A, Fang H 1964 Hypertrophic pyloric stenosis in adults. Survey of the literature and report of a case of the localized form (torus hyperplasia). Gastroenterology 46: 601
Westlund K 1963 Mortality of peptic ulcer patients. Acta Medica Scandinavica (suppl) 402: 1
Wheldon E J, Venables C W, Johnston I D A 1970 Late metabolic sequelae of vagotomy and gastroenterostomy. Lancet 1: 437
Whitlock F A 1961 Some psychiatric consequences of gastrectomy. British Medical Journal 1: 1560
Williams J A 1969 Some sequelae of gastric operations including the dumping syndrome and metabolic disorders. In: Maingot R (ed) Abdominal operations, Vol 1, 6th edn. Appleton-Century-Crofts, New York, p 493
Williams J A, Hall G S, Thompson A G, Cooke W T 1969 Neurological disease after partial gastrectomy. British Medical Journal 3: 210
Woodward E R 1976 The early postprandial dumping syndrome: clinical manifestations and pathogenesis. Major Problems in Clinical Surgery 20: 1
Woodward E R, Neustein C L 1976 The late postprandial dumping syndrome. Major Problems in Clinical Surgery 20: 28
Woolley M M, Gwinn J L, Mares A 1974 Congenital partial gastric antral obstruction: an elusive cause of abdominal pain and vomiting. Annals of Surgery 180: 265
Wychulis A R, Priestley J T, Foulk W T 1966 A study of 360 patients with gastrojejunal ulceration. Surgery, Gynecology and Obstetrics 122: 89
Yan C, Zhou H, Ma X, Zhang C 1991 Pylorus and antroseromuscular flap-preserving gastrectomy – a new type of reconstruction after subtotal gastrectomy for treatment of gastroduodenal ulcer: clinical and experimental study. Surgery 109: 756–760

# 11. Carcinoma of the stomach and other tumors

*D. C. Carter*

## CANCER OF THE STOMACH

### EPIDEMIOLOGY AND INCIDENCE

Adenocarcinoma of the stomach accounts for 97% of all gastric malignancies. The incidence of the disease varies markedly between countries (Fig. 11.1) and even within countries. The highest rates have been found in Japan, the Andean areas of Central and South America (Chile and Costa Rica) and northern Europe. The incidence has declined recently in Japan and northern Europe, but Japan still has a high incidence and eastern Europe is now a high incidence area (see Fig. 11.1) (Kurihara et al 1989, Correa 1992). Rates in the white population of the USA are generally low but rates in the north east are some 50% higher than those in the south; such variations may be explained in part by the greater proportion of foreign-born populations in high-incidence areas (Haenszel 1961). In the Netherlands and in Wales, variations in incidence have been related to soil type (BMJ 1965). The incidence is usually higher in lower socioeconomic classes and is linked to poor housing and overcrowding (see below; Barker et al 1990).

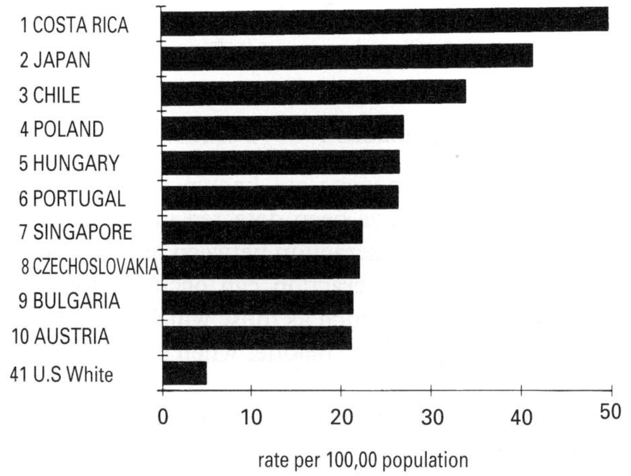


**Fig. 11.1** Annual death rates per 100 000 male population for gastric cancer, 1984–85 in different countries. (Reproduced with permission from Correa 1992.)

The incidence and mortality of gastric cancer has been falling in many countries since before World War II (Fig. 11.2), although in some instances the decline may be more apparent than real as cancer diagnosis has become more accurate (Maartmann-Moe & Hartveit 1985). In Scotland the incidence appeared to be stabilizing (Sedgwick et al 1991) but over the decade to 1990, it fell by 12% in men and 28% in women, whereas relative 5-year survival rates rose from 8% to 10.6% over a similar period (Black et al 1993). The falling incidence reported from most Western countries contrasts with a rising or static incidence of tumors at other sites in the digestive system (Fig. 11.3). There is some evidence (Munoz & Connelly 1971) that the reduced incidence is due to the fall in the number of cases of "intestinal type" cancer. This trend was first shown in Norway (although it is now contested in that country, see below) and now appears to apply to the USA and Japan (Correa & Haenszel 1982).

Conversely, the number of cases of carcinoma of the cardia is increasing significantly in Europe and the USA, both relative to the incidence of gastric cancer at other sites and in absolute terms (Husemann 1989, Hansson et al 1993). The male:female ratio for gastric carcinoma in different countries ranges from 2:1 to 3:2 (Doll 1956). In the age group 25–29 years it is 1:1, rising steadily to 2.2:1 in the 55–59 age group before declining to 1.4:1 in the elderly (Griffith 1968). Tumors of the cardia have a male:female ratio of about 4:1 (Morson & Dawson 1979, Hansson et al 1993).

Despite evidence of declining incidence and mortality in many countries, gastric cancer is still probably the second commonest cause of cancer death worldwide and is the fourth or fifth most common cause of death from cancer in the United Kingdom (Forman 1987, Black et al 1993).

### ETIOLOGY

Gastric cancer is clearly a multifactorial disease, but particular attention is focused on dietary factors and conditions which cause gastritis (notably infection with *H. pylori*).

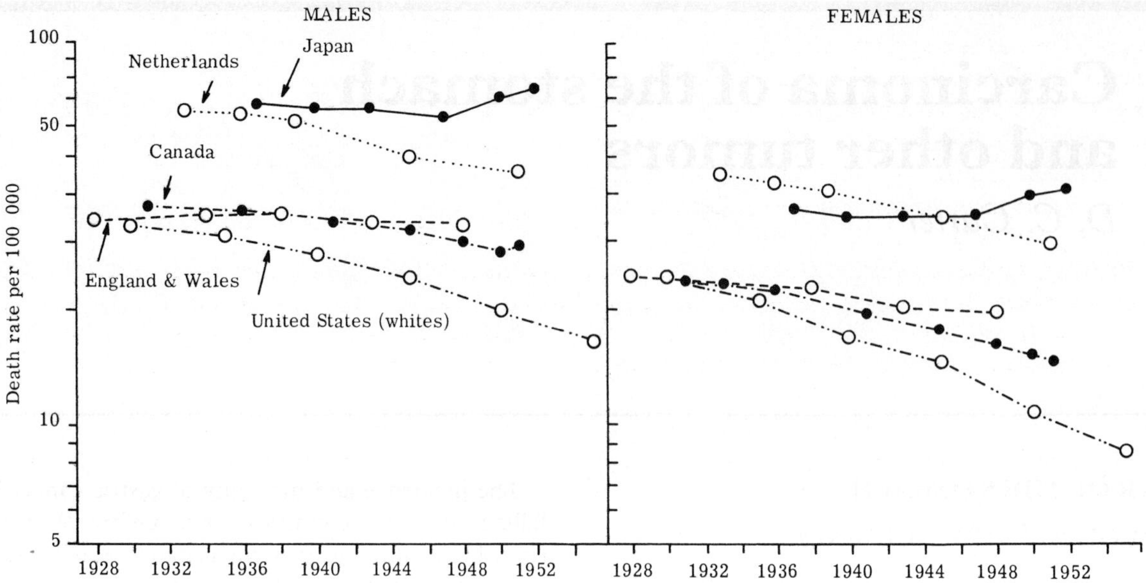


**Fig. 11.2** Trends in age-adjusted mortality per 100 000 population from gastric cancer in five countries. (Reproduced with permission from Haenszel 1958.)

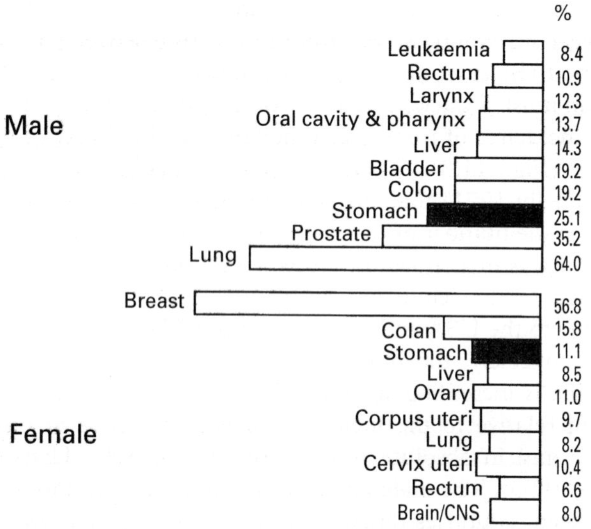


**Fig. 11.3** Estimated incidence of cancer due to various malignancies in the European Community in 1978–82 in males and females (Cancer Research Campaign Scientific Yearbook 1993 p.18)

## Dietary factors

High-risk populations generally consume a diet high in carbohydrate and low in fat, fresh fruit and vegetables (Wynder et al 1976). Carcinogens may be present in foods and additives, produced during cooking or produced by metabolism within the stomach (see below). On the other hand, agents causing atrophic gastritis or intestinal metaplasia may predispose to cancer without themselves being carcinogens.

*Excessive salt intake*

There is strong epidemiological and experimental evidence linking excessive salt intake and gastric cancer (see Correa 1988). Concentrated salt solutions may cause mucosal damage and excessive cell replication and give rise to gastritis and, in time, mucosal atrophy. The incidence of gastric cancer in Japan began to decline some 10 years after a major public health campaign was introduced to reduce salt intake (with the aim of reducing the incidence of cerebrovascular accidents).

*Carcinogens in smoked foods and cigarette smoke*

Cigarette smoking is linked to gastric cancer risk and the relationship between smoked foods and gastric cancer has received particular scrutiny in Iceland and Japan. The carcinogen 3,4-benzopyrene is found in smoked meat and trout and incidence of cancer has declined in areas where singeing and smoking meat has lost popularity (Dungal & Sigurjonsson 1967, Sigurjonsson 1967).

*Nitrosamines* (Tannenbaum 1983, Forman 1987)

These powerful carcinogens are known to cause gastric cancer in rats. They have been detected in smoked foods and can be formed by interaction between nitrites and secondary amines. This interaction can occur in foodstuffs and in acidic conditions such as those which prevail in the human stomach (and in the bladder when bacteria are present).

In the human stomach, nitrate can be converted to nitrite by bacteria when pH is high, but it must be stressed that the rate of formation of N-nitroso compounds is low under these conditions. Nitrates are widely used as a food preservative and are present naturally in green vegetables and drinking water. Secondary amines may form during cooking of protein and during fermentation. Although several epidemiological studies have shown a positive association between nitrate ingestion and gastric cancer (Fraser et al 1980), some populations at high risk of gastric cancer have relatively low exposures to nitrates; furthermore, nitrate concentrations in drinking water in Britain and France do not correlate with gastric cancer incidence (see Forman 1987). A further confounding factor is the presence of inhibitors of N-nitrosation in foods such as vegetables which have a high nitrate content and there is evidence that the antioxidant ascorbic acid may have a key protective role (Correa 1992). Carotenoids such as β-carotene could also counter progression from metaplasia to dysplasia by acting as free radical scavengers.

Japanese who have migrated to a low-incidence area remain at increased risk of gastric cancer although their offspring do not (Haenszel et al 1972). The excess risk persists in those who adopt a Western diet and it may be that diet or gastric infection in early life is important (see below). The decline in gastric cancer in the offspring of migrants is due very largely to a falling incidence of cancer of the intestinal type.

*Rice and its additives*

Some rice is coated with glucose and talc, which is very similar chemically and structurally to asbestos (Merliss 1971). Exposure to asbestos is associated with mesothelioma of the pleura and may also lead to a higher incidence of gastrointestinal cancer (Selikoff et al 1964). In Japan, gastric cancer is commonest where rice is the staple diet (Merliss 1971), but the etiological role of rice additives remains speculative.

## Genetic factors and molecular biology

*Family studies*

Close relatives of patients are at increased risk of gastric cancer (McConnell 1976), particularly in communities with a high incidence of pernicious anemia (see below). Studied in twins have been inconclusive and the genetic basis of inherited susceptibility to gastric cancer is unknown (Wright & Williams 1993).

*ABO blood groups*

Individuals with blood group A have a 20% greater risk of developing gastric cancer (Aird et al 1953, McConnell 1966), further suggesting that hereditary factors are involved. The relationship to blood group A is restricted to the diffuse histological type of cancer (Correa & Haenszel 1982). It can be explained in part by the bias that pernicious anemia also shows to blood group A (Shearman & Finlayson 1967), although group A bias is also found in races such as Negroes and Japanese which have an extremely low incidence of pernicious anemia. Furthermore, most gastric cancers in pernicious anemia are of the intestinal type.

*Molecular biology* (Wright & Williams 1993)

Allele loss has been reported in a number of chromosomes (5q, 18q, and 17p) in gastric cancer. The pattern of loss is similar to that found in colon cancer and could reflect loss of tumor suppressor genes. Mutations in the p53 tumor suppressor gene are common in gastric cancer (Rhyu et al 1994) and overexpression of *ras* oncogenes may also be involved in carcinogenesis and tumor progression.

Gastric cancers contain progesterone receptors and some contain estrogen receptors (Wu et al 1990, 1992), opening the possibility that female sex hormone receptors play a role in cancer growth. To date, attempts to influence outcome by tamoxifen therapy have given conflicting results (see Wu et al 1992), while studies with the gastrin receptor antagonist proglumide have also failed to affect survival (Harrison et al 1990).

Some gastric cancers overexpress epidermal growth factor (EGF) and EGF receptor and there is evidence that tumors which express both EGF and EGF receptor are more likely to be infiltrative (macrodcopically and microscopically), poorly differentiated, scirrhous and deeply invading (Sugiyama et al 1989). It may be that presence of EGF and its receptor identifies tumor cells capable of producing and responding in an autocrine manner to their own growth factor.

## *Helicobacter pylori* and gastric cancer

A recent study involving 17 populations from 13 countries in Europe, North America, North Africa and Japan has confirmed the relationship between seropositivity to *H. pylori* and cumulative rates for both the incidence and mortality of gastric cancer; it has been predicted that mortality from gastric cancer in a population with a 100% prevalence of *H. pylori* infection would be six times that of an uninfected population (Eurogast Study Group 1993) (Fig. 11.4). Chronic gastritis is commonly due to *H. pylori* infection and atrophic gastritis and intestinal metaplasia are recognized precursors of gastric cancer. Furthermore, persistent *H. pylori* infection could induce several mutagenic processes, including cell proliferation, possibly by increased production of epidermal growth factor or DNA damage by neutrophil products released during inflammation (Parsonnet 1993).

Japanese patients with early gastric cancer have a higher prevalence of *H. pylori* infection than asymptomatic controls and the infection in associated with high levels of serum pepsinogen I and II (markers of gastritis and gastric

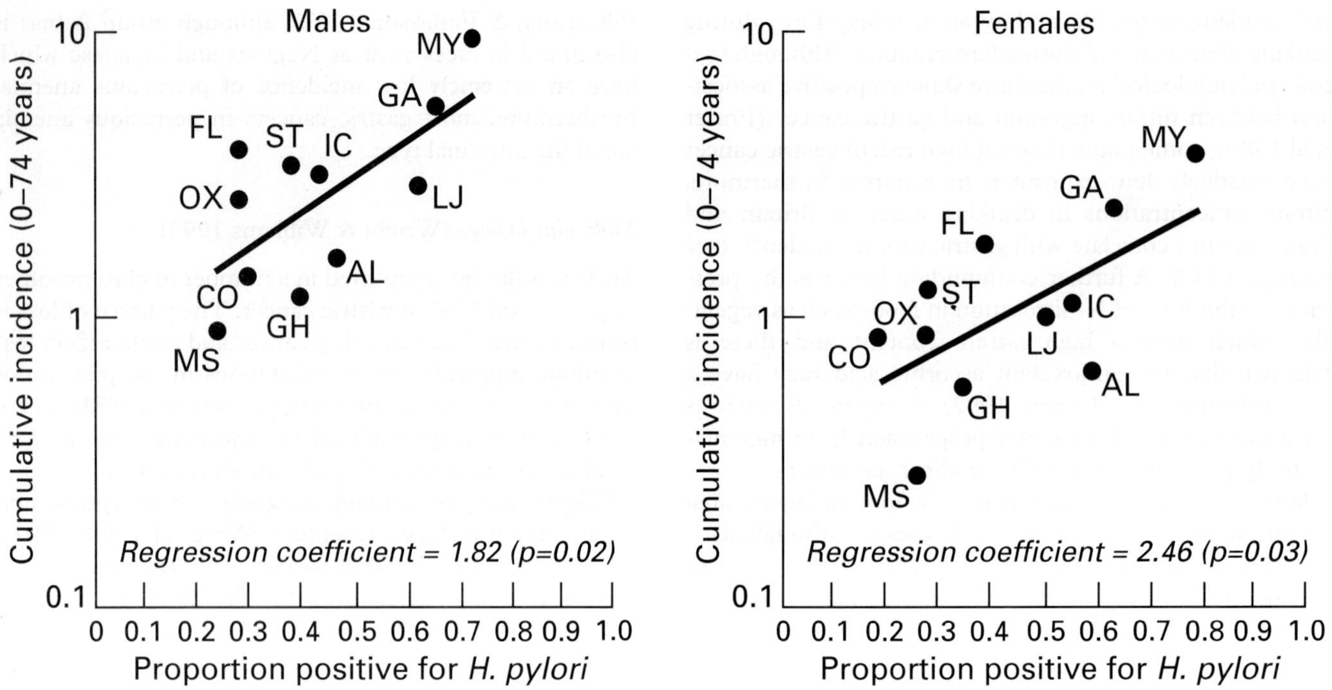


**Fig. 11.4** Incidence rates for gastric cancer in males and females in relation to *H. pylori* seropositivity in various populations (key: Al Algiers, GH Ghent, CO Copenhagen, AU Augsburg, DE Deggendorf, MO Mosbach, CR Crete, IC Iceland, FL Florence, MY Miyagi, YO Yokote, AD Adamowka, GA Gaia, LJ Ljublianja, OX Oxford, ST Stoke, MS Minneapolis-St Paul). (Reproduced with permission from Eurogast Study Group 1993.)

atrophy) in asymptomatic controls (Asaka et al 1992, 1994). For Japanese born after 1950 the frequency of *H. pylori* infection increases at a rate of approximately 1% a year, whereas in those born before 1950 the prevalence is high (70–80%) and relatively constant (Asaka et al 1992). The apparent decrease in prevalence of *H. pylori* infection which has accompanied the Westernization of Japan could well result in a reduction in the frequency of atrophic gastritis and a continuing fall in the incidence of gastric cancer. *H. pylori* infection might also contribute to the link between gastric cancer and socioeconomic status (Barker et al 1990).

Correa (1992) has proposed a multistep and multifactorial etiological hypothesis which explains the progression through chronic gastritis atrophy and intestinal metaplasia to dysplasia. The initial stages of gastritis and atrophy are linked to excessive salt intake and *H. pylori* infection; the intermediate stage is associated with intragastric nitrosation in which the balance between ingestion of nitrate and protective agents such as ascorbic acid may be critical; and the final stage is influenced by the availability of β-carotene and excessive salt intake. As discussed, nitrosating agents are seen as the key carcinogens and could originate in the gastric lumen or in inflammatory infiltrate.

## Pernicious anemia and gastritis

In autopsy series of patients with pernicious anemia, gastric cancer has an overall incidence of 5.2% (range 0.7–12.9%); clinical studies suggest a prevalence of 1–3% (Sjoblom et al 1993) although an increased risk was not found in one study from Minnesota (Schafer et al 1985). Carcinoma of the stomach is also commoner than expected among relatives of patients with pernicious anemia. Atrophic gastritis and gastric atrophy are always present in the stomach in pernicious anemia (type A gastritis, p. 230) and these conditions, or the intestinal metaplasia (p. 227) which usually accompanies them, may predispose to cancer.

Patients with acquired hypogammaglobulinemia (p. 404) also have a greatly increased incidence of gastric cancer (Kinlen et al 1985) and usually have achlorhydria and extensive gastritis.

## Other predisposing factors

### *Gastric ulcer*

Most studies do not support a causal relationship between benign gastric ulcer and gastric cancer (Hirohata 1968). Although both conditions are common in Japan, there is a poor correlation when the incidence of each is matched for each prefecture (Hirohata & Kuratsune 1969).

The term "ulcer cancer" is used when cancer is thought to have developed in a peptic ulcer (Fig. 11.5). The risk of

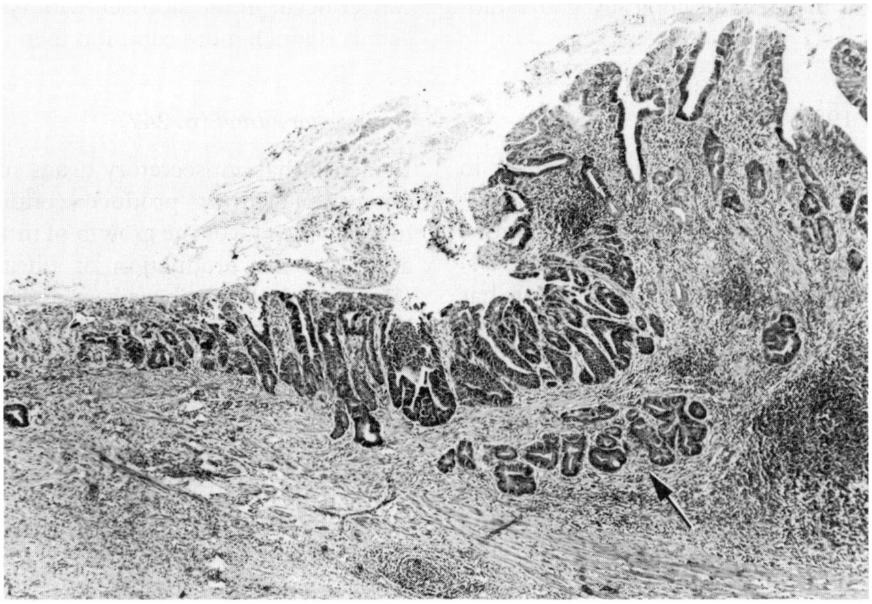

**Fig. 11.5** Ulcer cancer. A focus of malignant glands (arrow) showing early invasion at the edge of what was otherwise a typical benign peptic ulcer in the gastric antrum (hematoxylin and eosin, ×40).

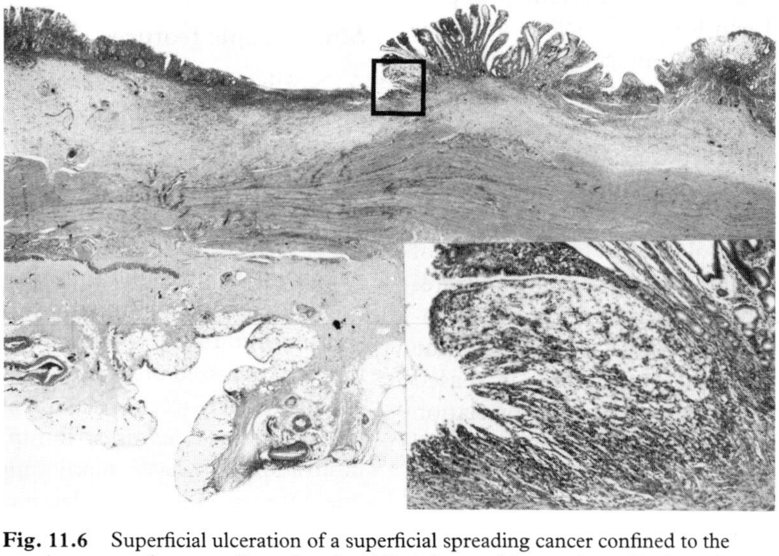

**Fig. 11.6** Superficial ulceration of a superficial spreading cancer confined to the gastric mucosa (hematoxylin and eosin, ×6). A focus of the carcinoma is shown in higher magnification (×35).

such malignant transformation is now thought to be vanishingly small. Japanese workers have found peptic ulceration in up to 70% of patients with gastric cancer (Nakamura et al 1967) and particularly in early gastric cancer (Sano 1971). It is now accepted that early gastric cancers may undergo recurrent cycles of healing and ulceration and so it is virtually impossible to distinguish between peptic ulceration occurring as a result of the breakdown of the abnormal mucosa (Fig. 11.6) and cancer developing at the margin of an ulcer. Microcarcinomas (tumors less than 5 mm diameter) are typically not ulcerated and more recent studies indicate that ulceration is a secondary phenomenon (Sugano et al 1982). In practice, it is important to realize that ulcerated gastric cancers may closely resemble peptic ulcers endoscopically and radiologically.

*Gastric surgery* (Carter 1987)

Most studies report an increased incidence of cancer in the gastric stump after partial gastrectomy. Autopsy studies indicate that 6–15% of patients who have undergone gastric surgery die from gastric cancer (Sonnenberg 1984) and meta-analysis of series of postgastrectomy patients has shown an overall relative risk of stump cancer of 1.66 (95% confidence limits 1.54–1.79)(Tersmette et al 1990). The increased risk is not generally apparent until 15 years have elapsed and in most studies it is greater after surgery for gastric ulcer than for duodenal ulcer (Pickford et al 1984, Tersmette et al 1990). Caygill et al (1986) studied 4466 patients who had gastric surgery between 1940 and 1960. The risk of death from gastric cancer was not increased in the first 20 years after surgery, but duodenal ulcer patients then had a 3.7-fold increase in gastric cancer, the risk in this study being greater after vagotomy than after gastrectomy. Gastric ulcer patients had a 3.0-fold increase in the first 20 years and a 5.5-fold increase thereafter. Patients treated by Billroth II gastrectomy were at higher risk than those undergoing Billroth I gastrectomy. Although most studies report an excess risk of gastric cancer after gastrectomy, it is important to appreciate that not all do (McLean Ross et al 1982) and that the link between vagotomy and drainage operations and gastric cancer is not yet substantiated (Lundergardh et al 1994).

It is assumed that long-term exposure to biliary, pancreatic and intestinal secretions with consequent gastritis contributes to the increased incidence of gastric cancer after gastric surgery (Clark et al 1985). In one study of patients after vagotomy and antrectomy, counts of nitrate-reducing bacteria and nitrite concentrations in the stomach were higher than in control subjects, although the amount of N-nitroso compounds was not increased (Keighley et al 1984). Others report a strong correlation between concentration of nitrite, high gastric pH and moderate or severe mucosal dysplasia in the operated stomach (Watt et al 1984).

*Gastritis* (Correa 1983)

Population studies in countries such as Japan, the USA (Imai et al 1971) and Sweden (Lykke-Olesen 1960) show a correlation between the incidence of gastritis and gastric cancer. The incidence of intestinal metaplasia (p. 227) is related particularly strongly to that of the intestinal type of gastric cancer (Correa & Haenszel 1982). The greater prevalence of gastric cancer in older patients may also reflect the increasing prevalence of gastritis with age (Guiss & Stewart 1943). The majority of cases of gastric cancer occur in the stomach with type B gastritis (p. 230) as this is much more common than type A gastritis.

*Antisecretory drugs* (p. 247)

Evidence that antisecretory drugs such as cimetidine and omeprazole might produce conditions in the gastric lumen which favor the growth of nitrate-reducing bacteria and thus the production of nitrites and nitrosamines (Reed et al 1981, Sharma et al 1984) has given rise to speculation about the risk of gastric cancer in patients on long-term therapy. However, case-control studies and postmarketing surveillance have produced little evidence of long-term risk; any excess incidence of gastric cancer is largely restricted to the first year of treatment where it reflects misdiagnosis of gastric cancer as peptic ulceration (Colin-Jones et al 1982, LaVecchia et al 1990, Moller et al 1992).

*Gastric polyps*

Adenomatous gastric polyps may predispose to the development of cancer but the commoner hyperplastic polyps have no malignant potential (p. 314).

## PATHOLOGY

### Macroscopic features

A North American review found that gastric cancer involved the upper third of the stomach in 30.5% of cases, the middle third in 13.9% and the distal third in 26% of cases (Wanebo et al 1993). The entire stomach was involved in 10% of cases and the site was not defined in 19%. This distribution reflects the increased proportion of patients with proximal tumors and the swing away from a preponderance of tumors in the antropyloric area (Husemann 1989). Tumors of the gastroesophageal junction are discussed on p. 206.

Most macroscopic classifications of tumor type are based on three features: luminal growth, ulceration and infiltration. However, many tumors do not fall clearly into one category and such classifications have limited prognostic value. When a tumor produces a lot of mucin this becomes visible macroscopically as colloid.

*Polypoid tumors*

These grow into the lumen and may ulcerate. They tend to be better differentiated and less infiltrative. They account for about 10% of all gastric cancers.

*Ulcerating tumors*

These account for about half of all gastric cancers. They

may resemble a peptic ulcer or show more extensive ulceration of nodular masses of tumor. There is variable invasion of the muscle coat.

*Diffuse or infiltrating tumors*

***Superficial spreading carcinoma.*** This term describes a tumor which has spread widely within the mucosa and submucosa and is better regarded as a form of early gastric carcinoma (p. 302). Some cases may represent an early stage of diffusely infiltrating carcinoma.

***Diffusely infiltrating carcinoma.*** This common form of cancer invades all layers of the stomach wall. It can involve adjacent organs, commonly metastasizes and has a poor prognosis. The term "linitis plastica" is used when widespread tumor has involved all layers of the stomach wall and given rise to a marked fibrous tissue response which thickens and contracts the stomach. Spread occurs primarily within the submucosa and is facilitated by the rich plexus of submucosal lymphatics. The mucosa often remains intact and appears red, edematous and granular but without visible tumor.

## Microscopic features

The many histological classifications in existence have varied reproducibility and use. Degree of differentiation has long-standing importance and it is held traditionally that well-differentiated adenocarcinomas tend to fungate and metastasize slowly, whereas the poorer prognosis of undifferentiated tumors is related to their invasive nature and tendency to metastasize early (Table 11.1). An alternative explanation for the histological predominance of undifferentiated tumor type in advanced cancer is that the tumor type may alter from differentiated to undifferentiated as the tumor progresses (Ikeda et al 1994).

**Table 11.1** The frequency and prognosis of different histological types of gastric carcinoma in patients treated in the USA in the years 1982 and 1987 (Wanebo et al, 1993)

| Histology | No. of patients | 5-year survival (%) |
|---|---|---|
| Adenocarcinoma | 13 577 (84%) | 12–14 |
| Signet ring cell carcinoma | 1333 (8.3%) | |
| Mucinous adenocarcinoma | 448 (2.8%) | |
| Diffuse type adenocarcinoma | 231 (1.4%) | |
| Intestinal type adenocarcinoma | 208 (1.3%) | 26 |
| Papillary adenocarcinoma | 129 (0.8%) | 16 |
| Undifferentiated carcinoma | 124 (0.8%) | 10 |
| Adenosquamous carcinoma | 40 (0.2%) | 4 |
| Tubular adenocarcinoma | 18 (0.1%) | |

*Note:* The histological evaluation shown in this table did not employ Lauren's classification. When Lauren's classification was used, intestinal cancer had a significantly better 5-year survival rate (23%) than those with diffuse (10%) or mixed lesions (18%).

*The WHO classification* (Oota & Sobin 1977)

This divides adenocarcinomas into papillary, tubular, mucinous and signet ring cell types and also recognizes rarer tumors including adenosquamous and squamous carcinoma, undifferentiated carcinoma and unclassified carcinoma. It has the drawback that the four main histological types do not correlate well with epidemiological data.

*The Lauren classification* (Lauren 1965)

This classification is used widely and although a tumor may show different histological features in different areas, it is usually possible to identify a predominant tumor type. Approximately 50% of tumors are "intestinal", 30% are "diffuse" and the remainder are "mixed". The intestinal type of cancer (Fig. 11.7) has a glandular structure with large and usually well-defined cells, which often have a brush border but usually do not contain secretory products (Table 11.2). The tumor margin is clearly defined and has a marked inflammatory reaction. In contrast, diffuse cancer (Fig. 11.8) is formed by small clusters of solitary cells and brush border formation is rare, although the cells often contain secretory products. Diffuse cancer shows a wider spread within the stomach and has a poorly defined margin with a sparse inflammatory reaction but marked stromal reaction. Macroscopically, some of these tumors are described as "linitis plastica" and some as "superficial spreading cancer".

Lauren found that the intestinal type of cancer had the better prognosis and involved a greater proportion of men and older patients. A recent Japanese study indicated that intestinal-type cancer carried a poorer prognosis, particularly when there was no nodal involvement (10-year survival rates of 70% vs 94%; Iriyama et al 1993), whereas a multicenter Norwegian study found that the Lauren classification did not affect prognosis (Haugstvedt et al 1993).

It seems likely that intestinal and diffuse cancer are etiologically distinct. Earlier reports that a decline in the incidence of gastric cancer in Norway is attributable to a reduced incidence of the intestinal form are now contested (Maartmann-Moe & Hartveit 1985). Other studies suggest that the intestinal form predominates in areas of high incidence, is related to intestinal metaplasia and could be linked to dietary factors (Correa et al 1973). Diffuse cancer predominates in low-risk areas, shows an association with blood group A, but has a less marked association with gastritis and metaplasia than the intestinal type. Etiologically, it may be linked more strongly to host-related factors (Mecklin et al 1988).

*Other classifications*

Other classifications with prognostic relevance include

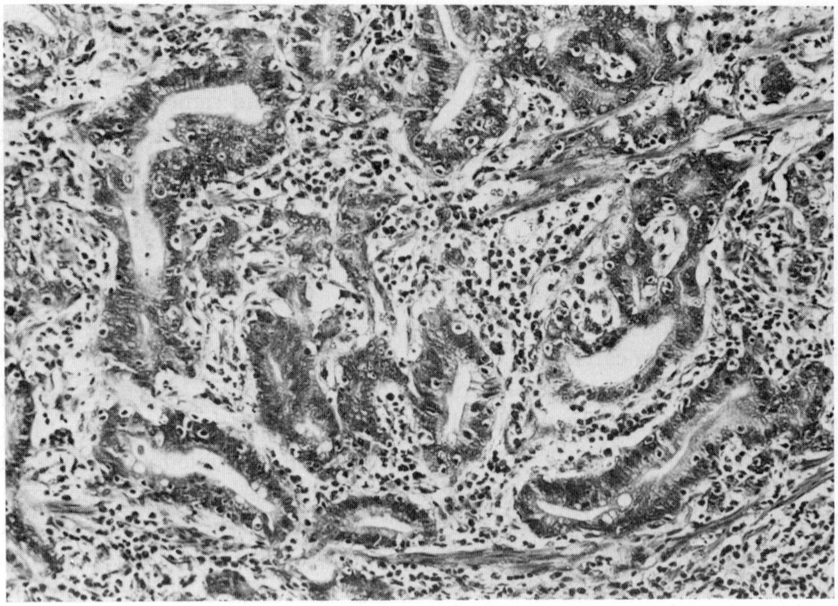

**Fig. 11.7** Gastric cancer. Intestinal type. Irregular glandular acini lined by columnar cells, some of which show a superficial brush border while others show mucus secretion in the form of globlet cells (hematoxylin and eosin, ×165).

**Table 11.2** Implications of the classification of gastric cancer into intestinal and diffuse types according to the Lauren histological classification (after Cunningham 1990).

| | Intestinal | Diffuse |
|---|---|---|
| Histology | Cells resemble intestinal epithelium<br>Little fibrous reaction<br>Inflammatory infiltrate | Cells often single or in "Indian file"<br>Marked stromal reaction<br>Produces signet ring cell tumors |
| Epidemiology | Common in high-incidence areas<br>Male:female 2:1 | Hereditary form of gastric cancer<br>Male:female 1:1<br>linked to blood group A |
| Prognosis | Better than diffuse cancer | Submucosal spread and resection margin involvement more common |

those proposed by Ming (1977), who classified gastric cancer into infiltrative and expanding types, and Goseki et al (1992), who assessed intracellular mucus production and degree of tubular differentiation.

## The Japanese Research Society classification

The Japanese Research Society for Gastric Cancer (1981) has developed detailed guidelines for classifying gastric cancer from both clinical and pathological standpoints. Clinical factors include tumor location, serosal invasion, lymph node invasion, peritoneal dissemination, liver metastases and tumor at resection lines. The macroscopic classification incorporates the classification of early gastric cancer used by the Japanese Gastroenterological Endoscopy Society (p. 302) combined with the gross classification of advanced lesions (p. 298). Lymph node involvement and resection is described according to anatomical groupings (Fig. 11.9). The histological features are handled separately and include epithelial pattern, stromal response, tumor border and depth of invasion into the stomach wall (Japanese Research Society Committee on Histological Classification of Gastric Cancer 1981). The common epithelial patterns are papillary, tubular, well or moderately differentiated, poorly differentiated, mucinous adenocarcinoma and signet ring cell carcinoma. Specific types of tumor include adenosquamous carcinoma, squamous cell carcinoma, carcinoid tumor, undifferentiated carcinoma and miscellaneous.

## The spread of gastric carcinoma

Local spread takes place along the planes of the gastric wall so that both the duodenum and esophagus may be involved and adjacent organs such as pancreas, liver, transverse colon and spleen may be invaded. Malignant cells can disseminate within the peritoneal cavity and form surface deposits on distant organs, including the ovaries where they are one cause of a Krukenberg tumor. Lymph node involvement occurs in about 70% of cases coming to operation (Bollschweiler et al 1992) and nodes in the porta hepatis, celiac axis, mesentery, mediastinum and supraclavicular area may be involved as well as those immediately adjacent to the gastric curvatures. Bloodstream spread frequently involves the liver (50% of cases) and to a lesser extent the lungs (25%) and bones (10%). Pulmonary involvement can result from hematogenous or lymphatic spread.

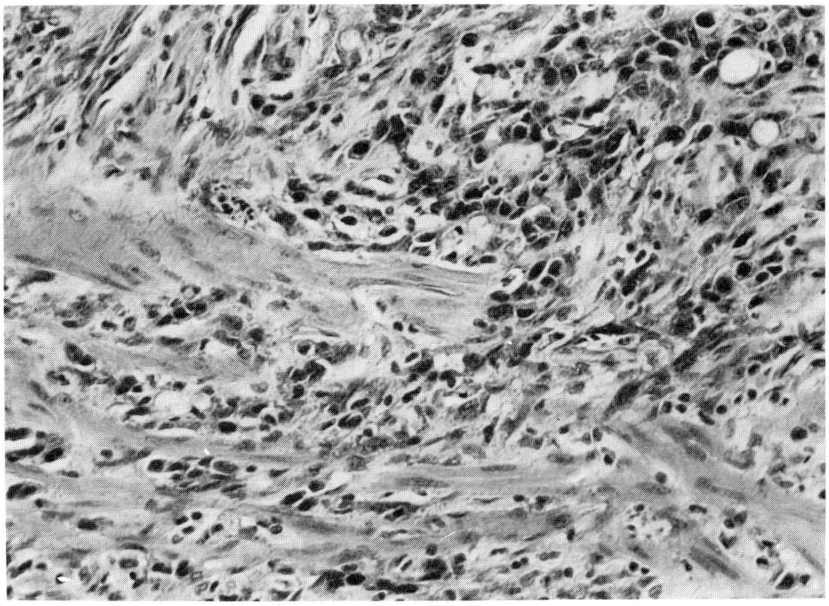

**Fig. 11.8** Gastric cancer. Diffuse type. Pleomorphic cells with irregular, dark-staining nuclei infiltrate muscle fibers. Occasional cells show mucus secretion (hematoxylin and eosin, ×225).

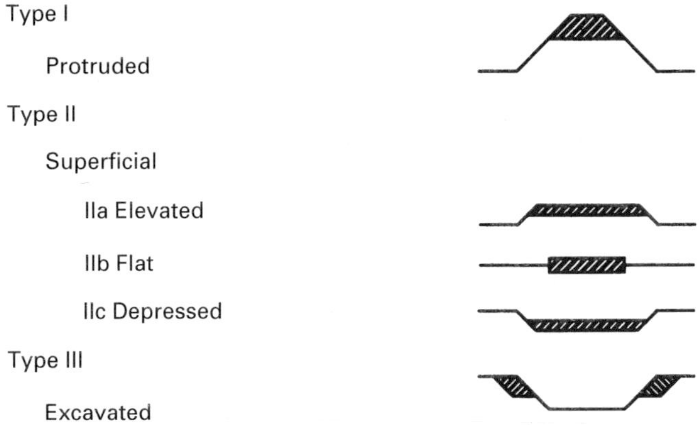


**Fig. 11.9** Macroscopic classification of gastric cancer.

### Prognostic relevance of pathological features

***Histological type.*** As discussed above (Table 11.1) the histological appearances have considerable prognostic significance. For example, the intestinal type of gastric cancer is generally regarded as having a better prognosis than diffuse cancer.

***Depth of invasion.*** Tumor confined to the mucosa and submucosa is called "early gastric cancer". These tumors have a good prognosis because lymphatics are present only in the deepest part of the lamina propria adjacent to the muscularis. Once the lymphatic plexus in the submucosa is infiltrated, the prognosis worsens and it deteriorates further when the main muscle coat and serosa are penetrated. When early gastric cancer recurs, lymph node recurrence is less common than growth of deposits in the liver or bone.

***Lymph node metastasis.*** Survival rates following resection are higher in patients without lymph node metastasis (see below) and the prognosis worsens as more lymph nodes are involved (Adachi et al 1994).

***Local tissue reactions to cancer.*** A marked fibrous and cellular stromal reaction at the tumor margin, lymphoid infiltration of the tumor and sinus histiocytosis within lymph nodes, even if they contain metastases, are thought by some to be favorable prognostic factors (Inokuchi et al 1967, Okamura et al 1983, Oka et al 1992). Not all agree that these appearances confer a favorable prognosis (Martin et al 1994).

All of these prognostic factors are interrelated. For example, the prognosis is more favorable when lymph nodes are not involved, but this is more likely with small tumors and with some microscopic types such as papillary adenocarcinomas. Conversely, lymph node metastasis is common with anaplastic tumors.

### Gastric dysplasia

Gastric dysplasia is regarded as a precancerous lesion (Cuello et al 1979, Morson et al 1980, Watt et al 1983) although even severe dysplasia can regress to normality (Coma del Corral et al 1990). It is important to distinguish dysplasia from "precancerous conditions" such as atrophic gastritis and pernicious anemia. Dysplasia has been observed in association with chronic gastritis and intestinal metaplasia, in the gastric remnant after surgery and in some gastric polyps. Intestinal metaplasia is frequently found adjacent to a gastric cancer and here the expression of intestinal enzymes in the metaplastic cells is

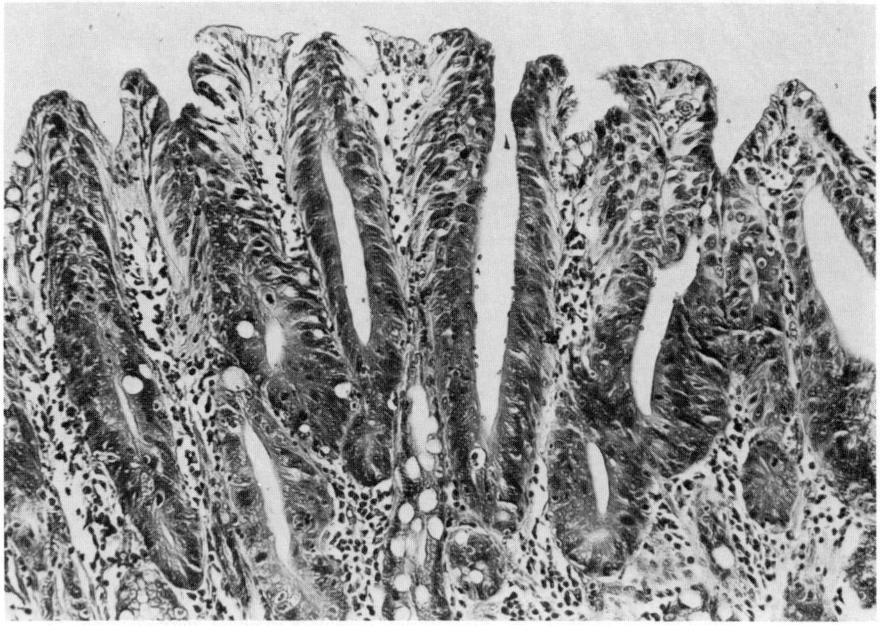

**Fig. 11.10** Gastric carcinoma in situ. There is a marked degree of cellular atypia in the epithelium of the gastric pits. Numerous mitoses and occasional goblet cells are present. The deeper gland in the center shows less pleomorphism of the cells and more obvious intestinal metaplasia (hematoxylin and eosin, ×120).

incomplete. Gastric dysplasia has been divided into adenomatous and intestinal metaplastic types (Jass 1983), each being associated with particular tumor types. Dysplasia is distinguished from carcinoma in situ (Fig. 11.10) by the degree of cytological atypia and the absence of invasion of the lamina propria. It must be distinguished from the inflammatory or regenerative epithelial changes which are often seen at the edge of a benign healing ulcer. Detection of dysplasia is usually seen as an opportunity for early "prophylactic" surgery. At the very least, patients with moderate or severe dysplasia must have frequent endoscopic and biopsy surveillance.

**Early gastric cancer** (Murayami 1971, Hioki et al 1990)

Early gastric cancer is defined as cancer confined to the mucosa, or mucosa and submucosa, regardless of the presence of lymph node metastasis. The definition is not affected by the size of the lesion or the duration of the disease. Many patients have long histories and some have large lesions. In endoscopic studies the proportion of all gastric cancers which are early has varied from one-third in Japan to 6–13% in Europe and the USA (Green et al 1981). Early gastric cancer is multicentric in about 10% of cases. The Japanese classification of early gastric cancer according to endoscopic appearances is widely used (Murayami 1971, see Fig. 11.9).

***Type I (protruded type).*** This is a polypoid carcinoma which may ulcerate and bleed and is sometimes difficult to distinguish from a benign polyp.

***Type II (superficial type).*** This is subdivided into three sybtypes:

- IIa (elevated type) appears as a slight elevation of the gastric mucosa which does not disappear on insufflation. The height of the elevation is less than the thickness of the mucosa.
- IIb (flat type) appears as a discoloration of the mucosa.
- IIc (depressed type) consists of an irregular depressed area with disruption of the mucosal fold pattern, redness of the margins and areas of hemorrhage. The depth of the depression is less than the thickness of the mucosa. This is a common form of early gastric cancer and often occurs with another type, especially type III.

***Type III (excavated type).*** This ulcer would be indistinguishable from a benign ulcer but for its foci of carcinoma.

Early gastric cancer has a variable histological pattern. It ranges from well-differentiated (intestinal type) to poorly differentiated and may include signet ring cell carcinoma (Grundmann 1978). The pattern of histology is related to the macroscopic type of lesion. Types I and IIa lesions are usually well differentiated, type IIb and IIc are variable and type III tumors are often poorly differentiated. There is considerable variation in the pattern of incidence of the different types of early gastric cancer in different countries. Type III lesions are the most common overall, often combined with type IIc. Type I lesions account for up to 22% of cases in Europe and 10–15% in Japan (Bogomoletz 1984).

## CLINICAL FEATURES OF GASTRIC CANCER

### Symptoms

In a series of 18 365 patients presenting with gastric cancer in the USA in 1982 and 1987, 78% of male patients and 82% of female patients were older than 60 years and less than 1% of patients were younger than 30 years (Wanebo et al 1993). The pattern of presenting symptoms is shown in Table 11.3. With the exception of dysphagia, which is said to indicate a poor prognosis, the pattern of symptoms is similar in patients with operable and inoperable gastric cancer (LaDue et al 1950). A large multicenter German study found little difference in the pattern of symptoms between patients with distal and proximal tumors; epigastric pain was slightly more common with distal lesions, while weight loss and dysphagia were more frequent with proximal lesions (Rohde et al 1991).

Weight loss is particularly common and abdominal pain is experienced by more than 50% of patients. The pain sometimes mimics peptic ulcer disease, being located in the epigastrium and relieved by food and antacids. In patients with tumors near the gastroesophageal junction, pain may be continuous or have an unusual distribution suggestive of anginal pain. If the patient complains of a change in bowel habit, either constipation or diarrhea, investigation may be directed initially to the possibility of large bowel cancer. Patients with suspected large bowel cancer and negative investigations should always have investigation of the upper gastrointestinal tract. Hematemesis, usually small in amount, is an occasional presenting feature, but melena is more common. Some patients with advanced disease present with ascites, jaundice or distant metastases. A past history of ulcer disease is common and the patient may be known to have relevant conditions such as pernicious anemia.

**Table 11.3** Pattern of presenting symptoms and previous history at the time of diagnosis in 18 365 patients diagnosed as having gastric cancer in the USA in 1982 and 1987 (Wanebo et al 1993)

| Symptom | Frequency (%) |
|---|---|
| Weight loss | 62 |
| Abdominal pain | 51 |
| Nausea | 34 |
| Anorexia | 32 |
| Dysphagia | 26 |
| Melena | 20 |
| Early satiety | 18 |
| Ulcer-type pain | 17 |
| Edema of lower extremities | 6 |
| *Previous history* | |
| Gastric ulcer | 25 |
| Duodenal ulcer | 7.5 |
| Pernicious anemia | 6 |
| Gastric polyps | 3.5 |
| Large bowel polyps | 3 |
| Achlorhydria | 1.8 |
| Small bowel polyposis | 1.4 |

#### *Early gastric cancer*

The contention that early gastric cancer rarely gives rise to symptoms is not borne out by experience. In many series, the presentation does not differ from that of more advanced disease (Houghton et al 1985, Ballantyne et al 1987). When the cancer ulcerates, the symptoms frequently mimic those of peptic ulceration.

#### *Cancer after gastric surgery*

Cancer arising in the operated stomach produces a similar pattern of symptoms to that arising in an intact stomach and loss of weight, dysphagia and regurgitation are common (Saegesser & James 1972). Gastric cancer should be suspected in any patient who develops symptoms after many years of good health after gastric surgery.

### Physical findings

A mass is palpable in the epigastric region in 30–50% of patients. The only other common finding is evidence of weight loss. About 5% of patients have palpable left supraclavicular lymph nodes. Still fewer patients have palpable hepatic or pelvic metastases. Rectal examination should be carried out to detect Blumer's rectal shelf, i.e. tumor in the peritoneal reflexion, which is present in 1–2% of cases. The tumor can be felt above the prostate, often projecting into the rectum, which it can invade. Pelvic examination may also detect a Krukenberg tumor of the ovary. Gastric cancer can result in metastasis to the skin, including the umbilicus, or may cause acanthosis nigricans.

## INVESTIGATIONS

### Radiology (Sherman 1967, Shirakabe & Maruyama 1983)

Gastric cancer gives rise to morphological and functional radiological signs (Sherman 1967) and the latter are best demonstrated by radiology. Morphologically, the tumor may appear as an ulcer, a mass or an infiltration (Figs 11.11 and 11.12). An infiltrating lesion is suspected when there are changes in the capacity or contour of the stomach. Important functional signs are changes in gastric motility and altered mobility of the stomach when the patient changes position. Double-contrast barium examination diagnosed or suggested malignancy in 92% of 110 patients with advanced cancer in one series and a benign lesion was diagnosed in the other 8%; this compares with figures for

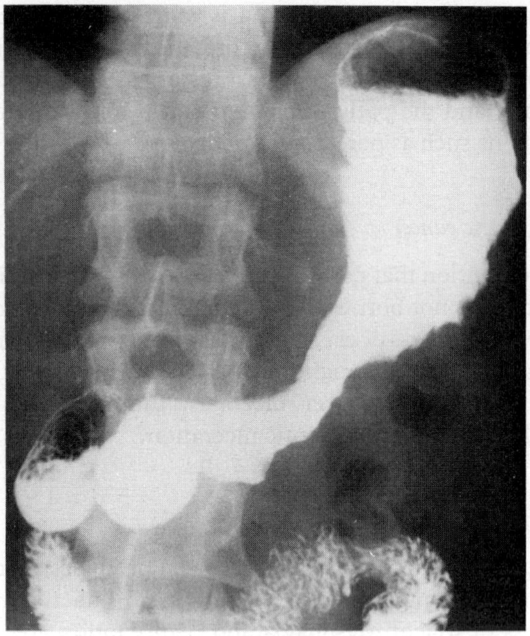

**Fig. 11.11** Carcinoma of body of stomach causing a persistent, irregular filling defect.

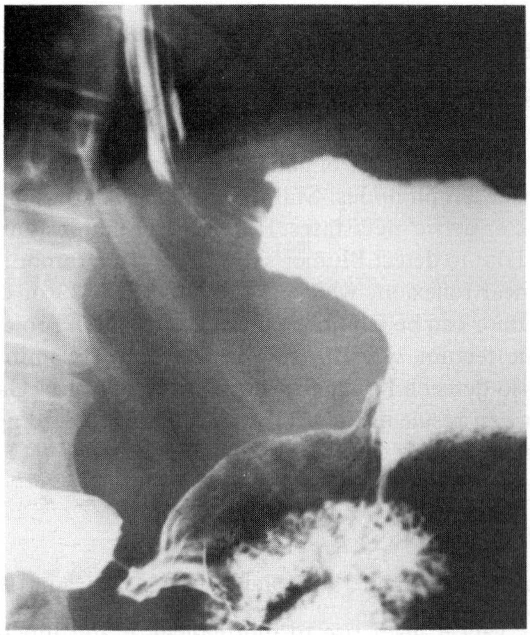

**Fig. 11.12** Carcinoma of fundus of stomach adjacent to the esophagogastric junction causing a filling defect. The tumor has extended into the extreme lower end of the esophagus causing destruction but no significant obstruction.

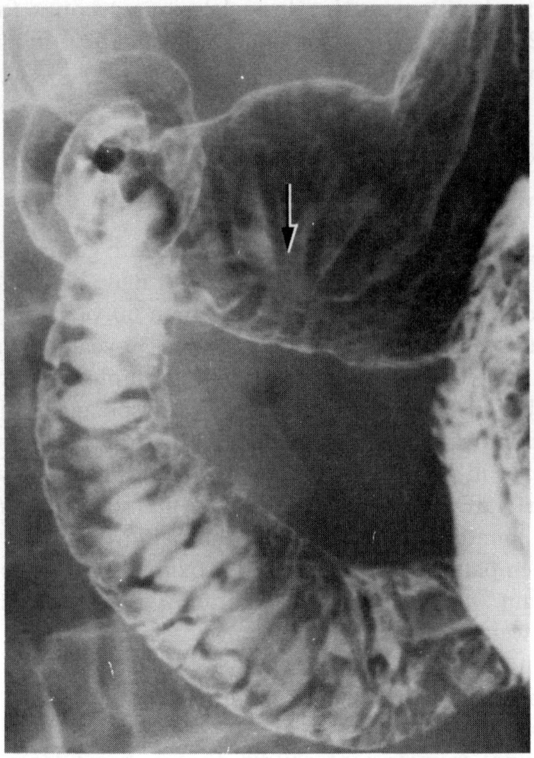

**Fig. 11.13** Early gastric carcinoma. Thickened amputated mucosal folds radiating towards the tumor (arrowed) in the gastric antrum.

endoscopic diagosis of 94% and 6% respectively (Green et al 1981).

*Early gastric cancer*

The double-contrast barium meal is an important means of diagnosing early gastric cancer (Kuru 1966, Shirakabe et al 1982) (Fig. 11.13). In 27 patients with early gastric cancer studied by Green et al (1981), it diagnosed (or suggested) malignancy in 44%, was thought to show a benign lesion in 37% and demonstrated no abnormality in 19%; the corresponding figures for endoscopy were 58%, 38% and 4%. Although endoscopy is regarded as the more accurate method of detecting early gastric cancer in many Western centers, the techniques can be equally accurate (Prolla et al 1969, White et al 1985), particularly if improved photographic methods are used in double-contrast radiology (Hioki et al 1990). With minute early gastric cancers (less than 5 mm in diameter) endoscopy may be more sensitive (Oohara et al 1984).

Detection of early gastric cancer should now be the aim of every radiologist performing upper gastrointestinal examinations, given the much improved prognosis when cancer is detected at this stage. The radiological signs of early gastric cancer reflect those of the pathological changes (Gold et al 1984, White et al 1985). Type I lesions are polypoidal or papillary protrusions and are clearly seen, especially when they extend more than 5 mm into the lumen. Type II lesions are superficial and the most difficult to display. Type III lesions are excavated but their appearances vary considerably; the most common finding is of a depressed, irregular ulcer surrounded by irregular converging folds, often with associated nodularity. It cannot be overemphasized that many early gastric cancers present as ulcerations which may heal with medical therapy (Sakita et al 1971, White et al 1985). If any of the above appearances are seen on radiology, the patient must be referred for endoscopy and biopsy.

*Polypoidal tumors*

The radiographic signs are those of an irregularly contoured mass or masses which project into the lumen and may have surface ulceration (Figs 11.14 and 11.15). There may be an associated large, exophytic soft tissue mass, complete encirclement of the lumen and, if the antrum is involved, gastric outlet obstruction. Differentiation from gastric lymphoma can be difficult (p. 317).

A small polypoidal lesion may be an early gastric cancer and all polyps merit endoscopy to define their nature and detect malignant transformation (Feczko et al 1985). Associated areas of abnormal mucosa suggest that early gastric cancer is present.

*Infiltrative cancer*

This is often suspected from functional findings. Superficial spreading carcinoma is very difficult to detect, the only signs being a reduction in rugal folds and reduced peristalsis. Linitis plastica is easier to detect because the stomach is small and rigid, lacks mucosal folds and peristalsis and empties rapidly. The differential diagnosis of linitis plastica includes corrosive gastritis, Crohn's disease, lymphoma and gastric syphilis. Infiltrative cancer of the prepyloric region cannot be distinguished confidently from the irregularities caused by peptic ulcer or gastritis but the mucosal

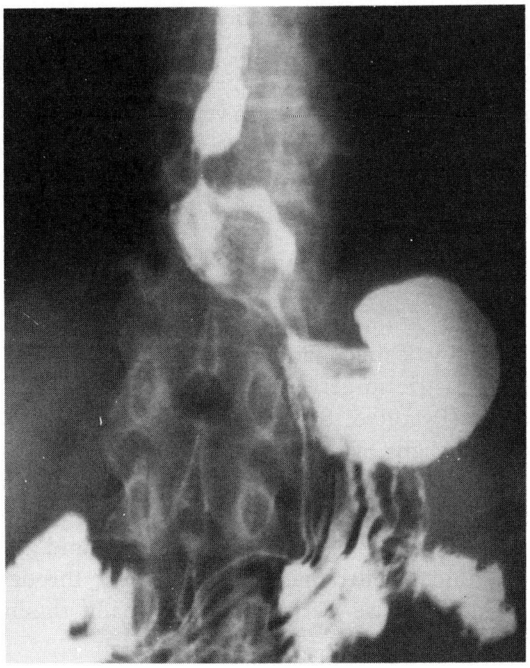

**Fig. 11.15** Gastric carcinoma causing a filling defect in a hiatus hernia and gastric fundus.

surface is often smooth and finely granular. Small infiltrative lesions at the cardia are particularly difficult to detect (Levine et al 1983); they may show as destruction of the mucosal folds or as small changes in the gastric contour. When the esophagus is infiltrated the appearances may resemble those of achalasia.

*Cancer appearing as an ulcer* (Fig. 11.16)

Early gastric cancer may show some central ulceration

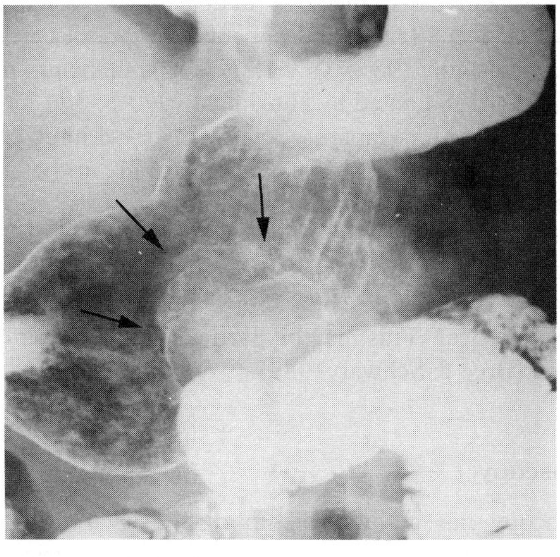

**Fig. 11.14** Large gastric carcinoma. There is clear demarcation between the normal gastric mucosa and the effaced mucosa at the site of the tumor (arrows)

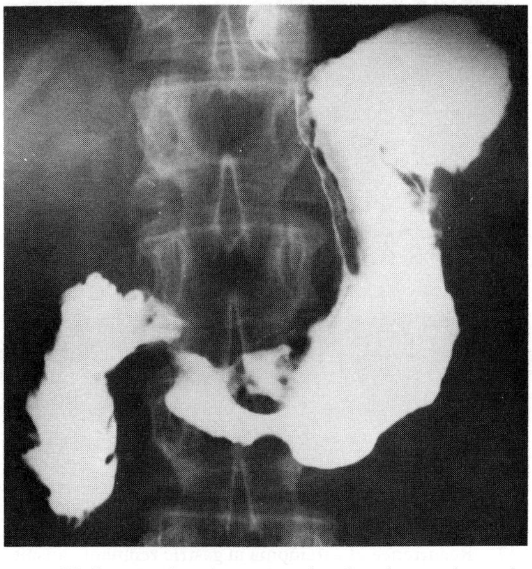

**Fig. 11.16** Malignant ulcer in antrum showing the meniscus sign, i.e. translucency around the crater caused by the rolled margin.

(Type IIc + III) and as ulceration proceeds, the irregular nodularity and mass around the ulcer margins can erode to produce a larger ulcer crater. At this stage, differentiation from a benign ulcer can be very difficult. The size of an ulcer and its location are of no value in differentiation, although ulcers in the fundus are almost certainly malignant (Thompson et al 1982).

*Cancer of the stomach after gastric survery* (Fig. 11.17)

The sensitivity of single- and double-contrast barium meal in the postgastric surgery stomach is poor compared with endoscopy (Pygott & Shah 1968, Ott et al 1982). The radiographic signs of recurrent tumor or "stump cancer" are the same as those of cancer in the intact stomach. However, infiltrating tumors are often missed because of inability to distend the stomach with barium and gas (due to rapid, uncontrolled passage of contrast through the stoma) and because peristalsis is normally diminished after gastric surgery.

*Demonstration of metastases*

In contrast to the frequent demonstration of metastases at pathological examination, metastases are rarely seen on chest radiographs (or skeletel survey) unless computed tomography is employed (Dehn et al 1984). Direct liver infiltration and liver metastases can also be diagnosed by computed tomography (see below).

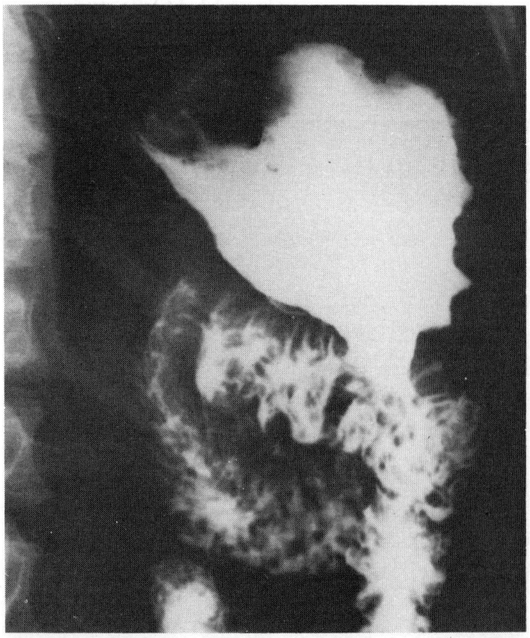

**Fig. 11.17** Recurrence of carcinoma in gastric remnant causing rigidity, irregularity and mucosal destruction. Previous partial gastrectomy for malignant ulcer.

*Staging by computed tomography (CT)*

Approximately one-third of patients present with such advanced disease that resection, whether curative or palliative, is not feasible. It is important to define patients in whom laparotomy should be avoided. Early comparisons of preoperative CT staging with operative findings suggested that CT was useful in defining when curative resection was possible (Moss et al 1981). Features generally regarded as denoting nonresectability include local tumor extension to the posterior abdominal wall, gastrohepatic ligament and diaphragm; spread to the mesocolon and colon; direct and metastatic spread to the liver; and widespread intra-abdominal peritoneal spread with or without ascites. Factors indicating a poor prognosis include spread to the para-aortic lymph nodes, large tumor size and number of other organs involved (Dehn et al 1984).

Ziegler et al (1993) have recently compared computed tomography, endogastric ultrasonography and intraoperative surgical assessment with the findings on histopathological staging in 108 patients treated by total gastrectomy. Depth of invasion (T category) was correctly staged by CT in 43% of cases, by endogastric ultrasonography in 86% and in 56% by intraoperative surgical assessment. Involvement of N1 and N2 lymph nodes (Fig. 11.18) was correctly staged by the three investigations in 51%, 74% and 54% of cases respectively. Whereas computed tomography was accurate for advanced tumors it tended to overstage T category and understage N category. Endogastric ultrasonography was equally accurate for all T stages but tended to understage N categories. The authors conclude that CT scanning and intraoperative surgical assessment "are of little value in staging", and that endogastric ultrasonography should now be used routinely in preoperative assessment.

If computed tomography *is* used, dynamic CT scanning is more sensitive than plain CT in detecting involved lymph nodes (92% vs 88.5%), and nonenhancing nodes are more often metastatic (98% vs 81.5% for enhancing nodes) (Ozaki et al 1984, cited by Hioki et al 1990).

In some centers laparoscopy (with or without laparoscopic ultrasonography) is used increasingly in the evaluation of patients for gastric surgery.

Occasionally, fine-needle aspiration biospy under ultrasound or CT guidance will confirm the diagnosis of gastric carcinoma when endoscopic biopsy has been nondiagnostic or equivocal. This may be particularly helpful in linitis plastica (Bree & Schwab 1985).

## Endoscopy

Endoscopy has a vital role in diagnosis and has contributed to the increase in the proportion of gastric cancer diagnosed at an early stage. It is now frequently used as the primary investigation and has the advantage that biop-

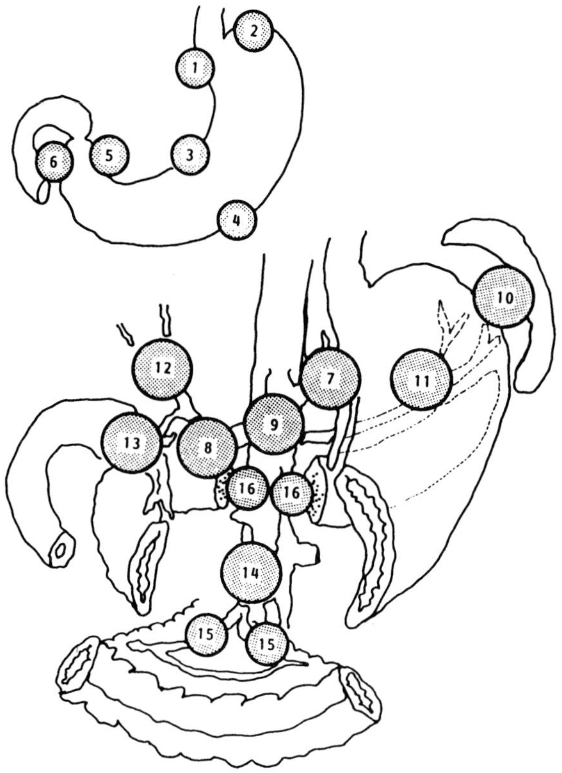


**Fig. 11.18** Lymph node location in gastric cancer according to the general rules of the Japanese Research Committee for Gastric Cancer (1981). Perigastric nodes: 1 (2) right (left) cardiac; 3 (4) lesser (greater) curvature; 5 (6) suprapyloric (subpyloric); Extraperigastric nodes: 7 root left gastric artery; 8 common hepatic artery; 9 coeliac axis; 10 splenic hilus; 11 splenic artery; 12 hepatoduodenal ligament; 13 retropancreatic; 14 mesenteric root; 15 along middle colic vein; 16 along abdominal aorta. (Reproduced with permission of the editors of the British Journal of Surgery, Bollschweiler et al 1992).

sies can be obtained. The visual interpretation of lesions is accurate and in one early series, the gastrocamera interpretation was correct in 93% of cancers and 87% of gastric ulcers, whereas radiography was correct in 83% of cancers and 75% of gastric ulcers (Kato 1966).

As with barium studies, it can be difficult to distinguish benign from malignant. Morrissey & Koizumi (1968) found that of approximately 300 ulcers with a sharply demarcated edge and no evidence of nodularity, only one was malignant. However, in an analysis of 20 benign and 20 malignant ulcers, Gabrielsson (1972) found exceptions to every sign classically held to betoken benignity or malignancy. The most useful endoscopic signs were mucosal folds reaching the edge of the crater in benign ulcer and disruption of folds and blurring of the ulcer edge in malignant ulcer. Two of the malignant ulcers had a sharply demarcated edge. Biospy of all lesions is imperative and at least six biopsies should be taken from the edge of the ulcer so that its entire circumference is examined. The proximal edge of an ulcer can be difficult to biospy with end-viewing instruments and the examination may need to be completed with a side-viewing instrument. It is also important to obtain biopsies from ulcer scars (Sakita et al 1971) and from areas of healing after treatment and to use exfoliative cytology if possible. Because malignant ulcers can heal, it is obligatory to follow all lesions by endoscopy and biopsy; an area of irregularity or nodularity may be seen more easily once the ulcer has healed.

In many Japanese series, biopsy has provided a positive diagnosis in over 90% of cases subsequently shown to be malignant. Technical improvements such as dye spraying, magnified endoscopy, electronic endoscopy and endoscopic ultrasonography may be useful advances, particularly in the case of mucosal, depressed and small (less than 2 mm diameter) tumors (see Hioki et al 1990). Endoscopic ultrasonography offers particular promise in assessing depth of invasion (see above) but fibrosis in the submucosa and muscularis propria can pose problems in early ulcerating gastric cancer. It may also identify involved lymph nodes but, like computed tomography, it cannot discriminate between hyperplasia and neoplasia. Visualization of involved nodes may be improved by endoscopic lymphography (where contrast is injected submucosally near the tumor at endoscopy) or by carrying out endoscopic ultrasonography 2–3 h after oral ingestion of 10% oil-in-water emulsion (see Hioki et al 1990).

Advanced cancers are sometimes missed at endoscopy. An infiltrative tumor may be suspected because of mucosal pallor, decreased peristalsis and an inability to insufflate the stomach, but biopsies may not show any abnormality if the tumor is deep to the mucosa. Infiltrating tumors in the cardia are particularly difficult to detect and biopsy and fine-needle aspiration biopsy under direct vision at endoscopy has been recommended (Iishi et al 1986).

### Gastric cytology

Cytology when added to radiological and endoscopic assessment can increase cancer detection rates to as high as 99.5% (Kato 1966). A study from China suggests that biopsy plus brush cytology is an optimal combination, with an 88% positivity rate (Shanghai Gastrointestinal Endoscopy Cooperative Group 1982). False positive results have been reported and as with all cytological techniques, the skill of the cytologist is paramount.

Endoscopy now allows material to be obtained for cytological examination by brushing or directed lavage and several studies indicate that this can be even more accurate than biopsy (p. 109).

### Other investigations

Acid output in response to histamine or pentagastrin is low in most patients with gastric carcinoma; 20% are achlorhydric (Fischermann & Koster 1962) while a further 45% have a pH in the range 3.3–6.9. As the gastric juice from a few patients with benign ulcer falls within this range, such studies have little diagnostic value. Other analyses of gastric juice, including measurements of lactic dehydrogenase and glucuronidase (Finch et al 1987), have not been used widely.

A moderate normochromic or hypochromic anemia is present in approximately 50% of patients with gastric cancer.

Serum carcinoembryonic antigen (CEA) levels are elevated above 5 ng/ml in almost one-third of patients and can assist staging and assess tumor progression and prognosis after surgery (Nakane et al 1994).

Liver function tests may be abnormal in patients with liver metastases but have poor sensitivity and specificity when used to predict liver involvement.

### Screening for gastric cancer

Screening surveys have allowed the detection of a greater proportion of early gastric cancers. In the USA, early gastric cancer has comprised only 6% of all gastric cancers while in Japan the figure is now as high as 50% in some centers (Sano et al 1992). This discrepancy arises because the high incidence of gastric cancer in Japan led in 1960 to extensive screening programs in which the goal was an annual examination rate of 30% in the population at risk aged 40 years or more (Hisamichi 1989). Double-contrast radiology with standard films was employed, but this is now supplemented by endoscopy and biopsy. Recent comparisons indicate that photofluorography using an image intensifier is almost equivalent to direct radiography and that both of these techniques are superior to screening by photofluorography with a mirror camera, although all three methods have sensitivities and specificities of around 90% (Murakami et al 1990). The number of patients examined has increased steadily so that by 1985, almost 5.2 million individuals were screened and 6240 cases (0.12%) of gastric cancer were detected. The proportion of early gastric cancers detected in one prefecture rose from 13.8% in 1960 to 62.1% in 1985–86 and the mortality rate in patients with screen-detected cancers has been approximately half that of unscreened patients with gastric cancer (Hisamichi 1989). While it is difficult to disentangle the effects of mass screening from the declining incidence of gastric cancer in Japan, the percentage decrease in age-adjusted mortality rate is greater than the decline in the incidence rate (Hisamichi et al 1988).

In general, there has been a low yield of tumors when patients with pernicious anemia have been surveyed using cytology or gastrocamera examinations. The prevalence of gastric cancer probably does not exceed 1–3% in patients with pernicious anemia and only 2% of gastric cancers are associated with the disease (Sjoblom et al 1993). Stockbrugger et al (1983) endoscoped 80 patients with pernicious anemia; 33 had varying degrees of mucosal dysplasia, one patient had a small gastric cancer and 18 had polyps which were often multiple. Borch (1986) gastroscoped 123 patients with pernicious anemia, finding cancer in four (three of whom had early cancer) and carcinoid tumors in five. Others have found that gastric carcinoids are detected as often as carcinomas in patients with pernicious anemia (Sjoblom et al 1993) and the natural history of the carcinoid tumors is uncertain. Despite the low yield of cancer, it still seems sensible to carry out regular endoscopic surveillance in young patients with pernicious anemia.

A theoretical case has been made for a yearly endoscopy to detect early gastric cancer in patients who have undergone gastric surgery (Sonnenberg 1984). However, the strength of the association between gastric surgery and gastric cancer remains controversial (p. 298). Logan & Langman (1983) argue against endoscopic screening after gastric surgery and the risks of further extensive surgery in this aging population should not be underestimated. It is also important to realize that smoking-related diseases are a much more frequent cause of death than gastric cancer in these patients (McLean Ross et al 1982). Although screening after gastric surgery is not generally accepted, regular endoscopy is recommended if severe dysplasia is known to be present (Offerhaus et al 1984).

## TREATMENT

Surgical treatment offers the only hope of cure. Patients who are physically unfit for surgery and most patients with proven metastases to lungs, peritoneum and skin are excluded from consideration. Patients with liver metastases are not necessarily excluded on this criterion alone since surgery may palliate symptoms such as outlet obstruction and bleeding and the metastases are occasionally resectable. Recent American data show that 77% of patients with gastric cancer had treatment which was primarily surgical, but which was complemented by chemotherapy and/or radiotherapy in 35% of cases (Wanebo et al 1993). In patients treated surgically, the rate of gastric resection for upper, middle and distal third lesions was 80%, 83% and 85% respectively, while only 50% of those with involvement of the entire stomach underwent resection.

### Surgery

Subtotal gastrectomy has been the standard operation for gastric cancer, but near-total or total gastrectomy is now often used and extended gastrectomy is employed when other organs have to be resected. Thoracoabdominal esophagogastrectomy is used in extended resection of tumors involving the cardia. The pattern of surgical treatment of patients in the recent North America review is shown in Table 11.4. Distinction is often made between operations which are curative and those which are palliative; in a "curative" procedure the surgeon removes all vis-

**Table 11.4** Types of surgery employed in the treatment of 10 999 patients with gastric cancer in the USA in 1982 and 1987 (Wanebo et al 1993)

| Type of surgery | Anatomical location (%) | | | |
|---|---|---|---|---|
| | Upper third n=3915 | Middle third n=1794 | Lower third n=3923 | Entire stomach n=1362 |
| Extended gastrectomy | 40.7 | 26.9 | 21.1 | 25.3 |
| Subtotal/partial | 29 | 38 | 55 | 8 |
| Total/near total | 4.6 | 14.1 | 6 | 11.3 |
| Exploratory only | 16.9 | 12.3 | 8.6 | 44 |
| Bypass only | 1.4 | 2.3 | 0.8 | 0.8 |
| Other | 8.7 | 8.6 | 9.6 | 10.3 |

ible tumor (see below). It must be emphasized that gastrectomy does not always have to be total to be curative but conversely, many total gastrectomies carried out in the West are noncurative operations (Cuschieri 1986).

A number of systems are used for the surgical staging of gastric cancer (see Cuschieri 1986); the three in most frequent use are those of the Union Internationale Contre le Cancre (UICC), the American Joint Committee and the Japanese Research Society for Gastric Cancer. The stomach is conveniently divided into an upper (C=cardia), middle (M) and lower third (A=antral). In a new TNM classification (Maruyama (1986), the depth of penetration of the stomach wall (T), extent of lymph node involvement (N) and presence or absence of distant metastases is classified, as shown in Table 11.5. Tumor stage (I–IV) can then be defined. The resected specimen is evaluated in detail to identify the histological tumor type, depth of penetration of the stomach wall, freedom of resection margins and involvement of groups or tiers of lymph nodes so that

**Table 11.5** The TNM classification with survival rates according to Maruyama (1986)

| Stage | | | 5-year survival(%) |
|---|---|---|---|
| I | Ia | T1 N0 | |
| | Ib | T1 N0 | 88 |
| | | T2 N0 | |
| II | | T1 N2 | |
| | | T2 N1 | 65 |
| | | T3 N0 | |
| III | IIIa | T2 N2 | |
| | | T3 N1 | 38 |
| | | T4 N0 | |
| IV | | any M1 | 5 |

*T = primary tumor*
T1 tumor limited to mucosa
T2 tumor limited to submucosa
T3 tumor penetrates serosa

*N = regional lymph nodes*
N0 no metastases to regional nodes
N1 involvement of perigastric nodes within 3 cm of tumor
N2 involvement of regional nodes more than 3 cm from tumor

*M = distant metastases*
M0 no evidence of distant metastases
M1 evidence of distant metastases

an accurate pathological TNM (pTNM) classification is possible, the operation then being classified as curative or noncurative. Disease stage emerges consistently as the single most important determinant of prognosis (Maruyama 1986, Haugstvedt et al 1993) and within staging, the total number of involved lymph nodes is a critical prognostic factor (Adachi et al 1994).

The distal margin for gastrectomy should be at the duodenal bulb, while proximal resection margins should be at least 5 cm, although it is possible that a 2 cm margin suffices for early and well-circumscribed cancers (see Cuschieri 1986). Opinions vary as to extent to proximal gastric resection. Some surgeons perform the smallest resection which ensures a tumor-free margin of at least 5 cm and carry out total gastrectomy if need be to achieve this (Brems-Dalgaard & Clausen 1993). Japanese workers advocate total gastrectomy when the tumor is proximal to a line drawn from Demel's point (point between territories of right and left gastroepiploic arteries on the greater curve) and a point 5 cm below the gastroesophageal junction on the lesser curve; tumors distal to this line are dealt with by distal subtotal gastrectomy (Sasako et al 1992).

The lesser and greater omentum (including the anterior layer of the transverse mesocolon) should be removed in all curative resections. Resections are graded R1 when level 1 lymph nodes are removed, as R2 when level 1 and 2 nodes are removed and as R3 when there is additional clearance of the porta hepatis, celiac axis and trifurcation, with splenectomy and pancreatectomy. The extent of lymph node dissection remains a matter of critical concern; anatomical studies indicate that an average of 27 nodes can be expected in the specimen when systematic dissection of level 1 and 2 nodes is performed (Wagner et al 1991).

### *Results of surgery*

***Curative or radical resection.*** Review of surgical results in the English literature dealing with the three decades to 1970, 1980 and 1990 found that operative mortality declined from a median value of 14.9% in the first decade to 4.6% in the last (Macintyre & Akoh 1991). No less than seven series in the decade up to 1990 report no operative mortality, although admittedly none of them comprised more than 60 patients and three were confined to patients with early gastric cancer. In general, Japanese series have the lowest mortality rates and although this undoubtedly reflects technical excellence, contributory factors are the high proportion of patients with early cancer, the relatively young patient population (on average 10 years younger than in Western series), the low incidence of cardiorespiratory disease and the favorable body habitus of Japanese patients. In a large German multicenter series, operative mortality rates were higher following resection of proximal cancers (12%) than after resection of distal cancers (9%) (Rohde et al 1991).

During the period 1961–90 the proportion of patients coming to operation in reported series fell from 92% to 71% while the proportion of operated patients undergoing resection rose from 37% to 48% (Akoh & Macintyre 1992). The 5-year survival rate following all resections rose significantly from 20.7% to 28.4%, while the 5-year survival rate following curative or radical resection also rose significantly, from 37.6% to 55.4%. When Japanese and non-Japanese series are compared, the Japanese resection rate (93.1%) greatly exceeded that of non-Japanese series (35.2%), while the 5-year survival rates after curative or radical resection were 60.5% and 39.4% respectively (Table 11.6). However, there is now evidence that results in Western countries are improving and that stage for stage, they approach those of Japanese centers. In Leeds, Sue-Ling et al (1993) submitted 207 patients to potentially curative gastric resection with R2 lymphadenectomy in the period 1970–89. Operative mortality fell from 9% to 5%, while 5-year survival rates were 60% in patients having curative resection, 98% in those with early gastric cancer and 93%, 69% and 28% in stages I, II and III respectively. The authors emphasize that during this period a significant "shift to the left" was observed in pTNM staging and that the proportion of patients with early gastric cancer increased from 1% to 15%, while the proportion with stage I and II disease rose from 14% to 31%.

Much debate continues to surround the role of extended lymph node dissection during resection for gastric cancer. Japanese surgeons have long advocated extended lymphadenectomy when resecting gastric cancer and 5-year survival rates of 30–50% have been reported in patients with involved level N2 nodes while operative mortality rates have remained below 5% and often below 2% (Thompson et al 1993). In a large multicenter German study (Siewert et al 1993), 1654 patients underwent resection and of these, 558 had a standard lymph node dissection (i.e. fewer than 26 nodes in the specimen) whereas 1096 underwent radical lymphadenectomy (i.e. 26 or more nodes in the specimen). Radical lymphadenectomy significantly improved 5-year survival rates in patients with stage II or IIIA tumors but conferred no advantage on patients with stage I tumors or those with involved $N_2$ nodes or distant metastases. It should be emphasized that the radicality of lymph node dissection had no effect on morbidity or operative mortality (5%) in this series.

**Table 11.6** Comparison of operation rates, resection rates and mean 5-year survival rates in Japanese and non-Japanese series of patients with gastric cancer reported in the English literature in publications from 1970 (Akoh & Macintyre 1992)

| | Japanese series | Non-Japanese series | Total |
|---|---|---|---|
| No. of series | 15 | 85 | 100 |
| Total no. patients | 19 048 | 80 738 | 99 786 |
| Operation rate (%) | 99.8 | 74.1 | 79 |
| Resection rate (%) | 93.1 | 35.2 | 46.3 |
| Curative/radical resection rate (%) | 58.6 | 17.8 | 25.6 |
| Mean 5-yr survival rate (%) after curative/radical resection | 60.5 | 39.4 | 52.2 |

It is a recurring criticism that evaluation of extended lumph node dissection is hampered by a lack of prospective controlled comparison; hopefully this deficiency will now be rectified by the British MRC trial or a Dutch study undertaken with Japanese collaboration to compare R1 (conventional surgery) with R2 (extended node dissection) gastrectomy (Sasako et al 1992).

The role of splenectomy and pancreatectomy in extended gastric resection remains controversial. There are those who resect the spleen as part of an R2 total gastrectomy and who also resect the distal pancreas if there is serosal involvement or a posterior/greater curvature tumor (Sasako et al 1992). Some retrospective studies suggest that adding splenectomy can be beneficial (Noguchi et al 1989) while others do not (Haugstvedt et al 1993). It appears that patients with histologically negative nodes are not benefited (Suehiro et al 1984), whereas involvement of splenic hilar nodes is a poor prognostic sign indicating that resection of spleen and pancreas is unlikely to be therapeutic. This is not to say that organs involved by contiguous spread of otherwise early cancers should not be removed (Korenaga et al 1988).

***Early gastric cancer.*** Ten-year survival rates of 82–97% are reported from Japan when early gastric cancer is resected in the absence of lymph node metastases; when nodes are involved the figure falls to 57–87% (Maehara et al 1992a). Independent risk factors for node positivity in early gastric cancer are tumor size, lymphatic vessel involvement and invasion of the submucosa and some regard these factors as determinants of the need for adjuvant therapy (Maehara et al 1992b).

Recent review of 20 Japanese reports involving 12 785 patients undergoing curative resection of early gastric cancer showed a recurrence rate of 1.9% (range 0.25–4.2%) (Sano et al 1993). The incidence of recurrence was significantly higher in the case of submucosal cancers, cancer of the mixed elevated-depressed type (IIa + IIc), node-positive cancers and differentiated tumors. However, even in node-positive cases the risk of recurrence was only 10% and regarded by the authors as too low to justify routine adjuvant therapy. Bloodstream spread was the prime cause of recurrence in that 59% of patients dying did so with hematogenous metastases. In some cases, recurrence is delayed for more than 5 years after resection and development of a second primary carcinoma after subtotal gastrectomy is a rare but recognized hazard (Sano et al 1993).

Inoue et al (1991) have reported an overall 5-year survival rate of 94% in patients undergoing resection of early gastric cancer, but emphasize that survival in patients with lymph node involvement was only 73% as opposed to 99% in those without. They suggest that R2 gastrectomy is the appropriate operation for early gastric cancer and furthermore, that the term "early gastric cancer" should be confined to carcinomas with invasion confined to mucosa or submucosa and without evidence of lymph node metastases.

Recent experience from Europe and the USA shows encouraging evidence that more gastric cancers are being detected at an early stage and that 5-year survival rates following resection range from 70–98% with 10-year rates of 58–86% (Farley et al 1992, Guadagni et al 1993, Moreaux & Bougaran 1993, Sue-Ling et al 1993). While surgeons outside Japan have shown growing acceptance of the case for extended dissection of the type performed during R2 gastrectomy, anxiety is still expressed about the potential for greater morbidity and operative mortality after this form of surgery (Heesakkers et al 1994). There can be no doubt that technical excellence is demanded and a strong case can be made for confining extended radical gastrectomy to specialist hands.

Sano et al (1992) have recently analyzed the clinical and pathological features of 748 solitary early gastric cancers and defined criteria which make lymph node metastases unlikely and which might be used to identify tumors suitable for endoscopic resection. These criteria are tumor confined to the mucosa, less than 1.5 cm in diameter, macroscopically elevated, macroscopically depressed without intramural ulcers or ulcer scars, and histologically differentiated. The first criterion is the most critical determinant of lymph node involvement and can only be assessed after histological examination of the entire tumor specimen. Modified endoscopic polypectomy is currently being used to resect early gastric cancers in patients with major contraindications to surgery and pilot studies also indicate that intratumoral injection of 5-fluorouracil can cause regression and disappearance of early gastric cancer (Kurayama et al 1984). Although these reports of the use of endoscopic methods are of interest, radical surgery remains the standard and extremely effective treatment of early gastric cancer.

***Palliative gastric surgery.*** In a large retrospective study based on data from 1960–69 in the Birmingham (UK) Cancer Registry, 80% of patients did not have radical surgery (Hallissey et al 1988). Hardly any patients in this group survived for more than 2 years, but operative mortality was significantly lower following palliative resection or bypass than after intubation or laparotomy only. In a report from the Mayo Clinic, in 53 patients who had undergone palliative total gastrectomy, the operative mortality was 8% and six patients required reoperation for complications (Monson et al 1991). The median survival was 19 months and 24% of the patients lived for more than 2 years. The quality of life in survivors was graded as good in 59%, satisfactory in 28% and poor in 13% of cases. Although there is controversy about whether total gastrectomy is an optimal palliative operation, the Norwegian Stomach Cancer Trial found that the mortality (12%) was lower than that of subtotal gastrectomy (18%), while median survival was longer (10 months vs 5.5%) (Haugstvedt et al 1989).

Gastroenterostomy can be used to relieve obstruction in the distal stomach but, in the words of William Mayo, it may only allow the patient "to live and suffer a little longer". When compared to resection, gastroenterostomy provides less palliation without reducing the incidence of postoperative gastrointestinal complications or operative mortality (Ekbom & Gleysteen 1980).

***Resection for stump cancer.*** In a Japanese experience of 52 patients developing gastric cancer after gastrectomy for benign disease, the tumor developed in the anastomostic area, body, cardia and entire stump in descending order of frequency (Sasako et al 1991). Twenty patients were in stage I or II and resection was carried out in 90% of cases and with curative intent in 69%. Five-year survival rates after resection, curative resection and resection when there were metastatic nodes were 43%, 57% and 29% respectively. Radical resection is therefore a viable option and total gastrectomy rather than further partial resection avoids the risk of recurrence (Stael von Holstein et al 1991).

**Chemotherapy** (Wils & Bleiberg 1989, Cunningham 1990)

The chemotherapeutic agent 5-fluorouracil (5-FU) has been used extensively as a single agent in advanced gastric cancer and has an overall response rate of 22% with a response duration of 4–5 months (Comis & Carter 1974). Varying dose schedules have been employed in attempts to improve efficacy and limit toxicity, but use of a weekly intravenous bolus (750–1000 mg/m$^2$) remains the mainstay of treatment. Stomatitis, diarrhea, leukopenia and alopecia have been the most common side-effects. Other single agents used include mitomycin-C, doxorubicin (adriamycin), methyl-CCNU and cisplatin but in general, results have been no better than those achieved with 5-FU.

Many trials of combination therapy have been carried out for advanced gastric cancer. The combination of 5-FU, adriamycin and mitomycin-C (FAM) has emerged as a standard regimen, but 5-FU and adriamycin have also been used in combination with methotrexate (FAMTX) or cisplatin. Randomized studies have failed to show any advantage for the FAM regimen over 5-FU alone (Cullinan et al 1985, Beretta et al 1989). The proportion of patients showing a complete or partial response ranges from about 40% with FAM or FAMTX to about 50% with combinations incorporating cisplatin (Cunningham 1990). The use of cisplatin in combination with adriamycin and etoposide or 5-FU may offer particular promise with 1-year survival rates of some 32% and apparent complete pathological remission in some patients subsequently submitted to surgery (Gastrointestinal Tumor Study Group 1988, Preusser et al 1989). Although chemotherapy now offers more promise, patients with advanced gastric cancer should still not receive this form of treatment on a routine basis outwith prospective controlled clinical trials.

Chemotherapy is frequently used as an adjuvant to surgical resection but convincing objective evidence that it confers benefit is lacking (Cunningham 1990). In Japan, adjuvant chemotherapy, such as oral 5-FU and intravenous mitomycin-C, is employed routinely in many centers, but the lack of controlled comparison with surgery alone in many reports makes evaluation almost impossible. More recently, controlled studies suggest that immunotherapy (using a protein-bound polysaccharide, PSK) in combination with chemotherapy gives significantly better 5-year survival rates than chemotherapy alone after curative gastric resection (73% versus 60%; Nakasato et al 1994). Interest is also being shown in intraoperative hyperthermic peritoneal perfusion of chemotherapeutic agents (Fujimura et al 1994) and intraperitoneal instillation of delayed release forms of mitomycin (Hagiwara et al 1992) in the prevention of peritoneal recurrence.

### **Radiotherapy** (Cunningham 1990)

Radiotherapy has been used alone and in combination with chemotherapy in the preoperative, intraoperative and postoperative management of advanced gastric cancer. Although some studies have used radiotherapy in patients not undergoing surgery, most have concentrated on its use in locally unresectable cancer. There is little convincing evidence that radiotherapy affects survival and toxicity may be increased when it is combined with chemotherapy. The available data do not support the use of radiotherapy as an adjunct to curative resection or in palliation.

### Esophagogastric tubes

Dysphagia due to cancer at the cardia or malignant gastric obstruction can be palliated by endoscopic dilatation and insertion of a prosthesis (p. 110).

### Endoscopic Nd:YAG laser therapy

There is extensive experience in the use of laser therapy to overcome dysphagia caused by oesophageal or gastric cancer (Fleischer 1986). Although a lumen can be re-established in most cases, clinical success is achieved in only 70% and perforation is not infrequent (Lambert 1984, Fleischer 1985, Fleischer & Sivak 1985). The technique has usually been employed in the palliation of patients with advanced and unresectable disease and may be combined with intubation (p. 111).

## PROGNOSIS

Gastric carcinoma remains a grim disease with a fatal outcome in some 90% of patients. However, the past decade has brought some light into what was a picture of unremitting gloom. The incidence of the disease is continuing to decline in most countries and there have been valuable new etiological insights. It must be emphasized that series reported from single surgical centers (many of which have a particular interest in gastric cancer) do not reflect the overall experience of surgical patients or of the entire population of patients with gastric cancer. However, within these limitations, the encouraging results of radical gastrectomy in Japan are now being reflected in improvements in survival following surgery in Western centers. In the decade up to 1990, the overall 5-year survival rate following resection improved to 28% worldwide (Akoh & Macintyre 1992) and after curative or radical resection it rose from 38% to 55%. There has undoubtedly been significant improvement in the selection of patients for surgery and the decline in overall operation rate from 92% to 71% in the period 1961–90 has been accompanied by a fall in operative mortality rates to a median value of 4.6% (Macintyre & Akoh 1991, Akoh & Macintyre 1992). Resection rates and curative/radical resection rates in Japanese series remain higher (93% and 59% respectively) than in non-Japanese series (35% and 18% respectively).

In the American College of Surgeons' review of approved programs, the overall 5-year survival rate of patients with gastric cancer was 14% and it was 19% in those undergoing resection (Wanebo et al 1993). No less than two-thirds of patients in this nationwide review were in stages III and IV and 5-year survival rates of 13.6% and 3% respectively were found following resection (Wanebo et al 1993). In Japan approximately half of the surgical patients are in stages III and IV and 5-year survival rates after resection were 36% and 23% respectively (Table 11.7).

**Table 11.7** Comparison of results of treatment of gastric cancer in the American College of Surgeons study and 56 selected Japanese hospitals (Wanebo et al 1993; Japanese data drawn from Maruyama K. World Journal of Surgery 1987)

| | Incidence (%) | | 5-year survival (%) in resected patients | |
|---|---|---|---|---|
| | Japan | ACS study | Japan | ACS study |
| No. of patients | 15 589 | 18 365 | 12 535 | 10 237 |
| Stage I | 33.7 | 17.1 | 95.6 | 50 |
| Stage II | 14.5 | 16.9 | 70.1 | 29 |
| Stage III | 28.7 | 35.5 | 36.3 | 13 |
| Stage IV | 23.1 | 30.5 | 23.1 | 3 |
| Overall survival | 45.4 | 14 | 56.3 | 19 |

The "earlier" presentation of gastric cancer in Japan has already been discussed (p. 308) and there are encouraging signs that the proportion of patients with early gastric cancer in Western series is beginning to rise, with corresponding improvement in 5-year survival rates into the range 70–98%. There seems little doubt that adoption of the Japanese practice of radical lymphadenectomy is contributing to the improved results of gastrectomy in Western patients.

Factors generally associated with a better prognosis include small tumor size, absence of lymph node metastases, tumor situated in the middle or lower third of the stomach, superficially spreading tumor, fungating rather than infiltrating tumor, well-differentiated tumor (particularly of the intestinal type), marked stromal reaction in the tumor and nodes and absence of distant metastases. There is some evidence that gastric cancer carries a worse prognosis in younger patients and especially in younger women (Maehara et al 1991, 1992b) and the possibility exists that female sex hormone receptors could have a significant role (p. 295; Wu et al 1990, 1992).

## OTHER TUMORS OF THE STOMACH

### POLYPOID LESIONS

Polypoid lesions are usually discovered incidentally on barium meal or endoscopy. While benign polypoid lesions are found in about 0.4% of stomachs at autopsy (Marshak & Feldman 1965), polyps were detected in 1.7% of routine barium examinations (Feczko et al 1985). Lesions which may present as polyps or filling defects include carcinomas, adenomas, regenerative or hyperplastic polyps, intramucosal cysts, leiomyomas, hamartomas or heterotopias (pancreatic rests, p. 1228), carcinoid tumors (p. 315) and inflammatory fibroid polyps (p. 325) (Navas-Palacios et al 1983). A list of rarer tumors of the stomach is shown in Table 11.8.

#### Adenomas

Adenomas are neoplastic polyps of the stomach and must be distinguished from regenerative or hyperplastic polyps. They are usually sessile, but can be pedunculated. They are situated predominantly in the antrum or along the lesser curve. They arise from gastric glands showing intestinal metaplasia or from neck cells and usually adopt a tubulovillous or villous growth pattern (Fig. 11.19) (Oota & Sobin 1977, Morson & Dawson 1979). The epithelium is hyperplastic and pseudostratified and the nuclei show variable atypia. These lesions resemble adenomas of the large bowel and are precancerous, occurring in the same age group as gastric cancer and in some cases in the same stomach. Adenomas have an association with pernicious anemia, but the majority of polyps found in patients with this condition are hyperplastic (Elsborg et al 1977). Adenomas greater than 2 cm in diameter have a 40% risk of malignant change compared to a 1.5% risk in those less than 2 cm (Jamieson & Ludbrook 1971). In one series, long-term follow-up showed that 11% of adenomas underwent malignant change (Kamiya et al 1982).

*Clinical features*

Most adenomas are found coincidentally but some present with epigastric pain or discomfort and occasionally bleeding. A polyp is easily overlooked when the stomach is filled with barium and is best seen on mucosal films (Fig. 11.20). Mobility of a polyp suggests that it is pedunculated and sometimes the stalk can be shown radiologically (Marshak & Lindner 1971). An antral polyp on a stalk can prolapse through the pyloric canal producing a filling detect in the duodenal bulb. Adenomatous polyps look red on endoscopy and may appear ulcerated. Biopsy is difficult and may miss a focus of carcinoma; cytological examination can give valuable additional information.

*Treatment*

Polyps seen on barium examination must be confirmed at

**Table 11.8** Other tumors of the stomach. These are uncommon

| Tumour | Appearance and presentation | Reference |
|---|---|---|
| *Malignant* | | |
| Secondary lymphoid tumors | As for primary lymphoid tumors | |
| Plasmacytoma | As for cancer or ulcer | Scott et al (1978) |
| Leukemia | Nodules or diffuse infiltration | Prolla & Kirsner (1964) |
| Secondary cancer | As primary cancer; rare as the presenting feature | |
| Primary choriocarcinoma | As for cancer | Jindrak et al (1976) Mori et al (1982) |
| *Benign* | | |
| Lipoma | Circumscribed and lobulated; bleeding | Fiddian & Parrish (1960) |
| Neurogenic tumors, neurilemmoma | Similar to leiomyoma, pain and hemorrhage | Rutten (1965) |
| Neurofibroma | Single or multiple; sessile or pedunculated<br>Usually asymptomatic | |
| Glomus tumors | Mass at pylorus; pain and hemorrhage | Appelman & Helwig (1969) |

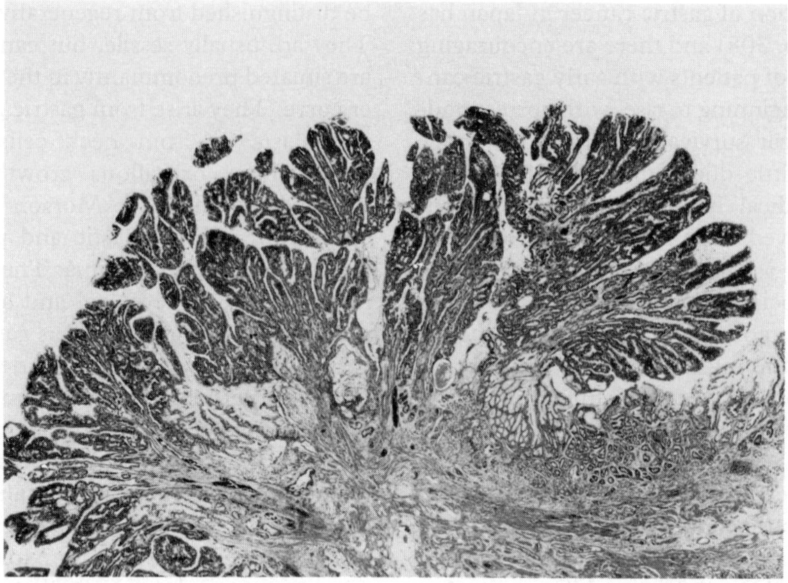

**Fig. 11.19** Gastric adenoma. There is irregular glandular proliferation in the mucosa with production of villous pattern. The adjacent mucosa shows atrophic gastritis with intestinal metaplasia (hematoxylin and eosin ×8).

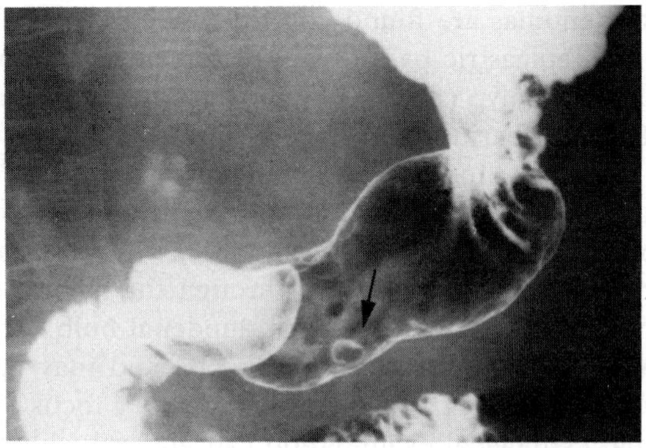

**Fig. 11.20** Small simple tumor (arrow), possibly an adenoma or fibromyoma in the antrum.

endoscopy since the radiological appearances are occasionally due to artefact. Unless they are part of the Peutz–Jeghers syndrome, multiple polyps are nearly always hyperplastic and can be disregarded. Pedunculated polyps should be removed by snaring at endoscopy. If an adenoma is sessile or cannot be snared, it should be removed surgically if it is larger than 2 cm. Polyps less than 2 cm in diameter should be followed by annual gastroscopic or cytological examination.

## Hyperplastic polyps

These result from proliferation of orderly surface and foveolar-type epithelium (Fig. 11.21). When proliferation extends into the glandular region with cyst formation and the presence of muscle fibers, the polyp has been termed hyperplasiogenous (Elster 1976) and has some of the features of a hamartoma. These lesions are unique to the stomach and do not have a large bowel counterpart.

Hyperplastic polyps may be multiple, whereas multiple adenomatous polyposis is rare. Although hyperplastic polyps are not premalignant, an increased incidence of cancer has been noted elsewhere in polyp-containing stomachs (Harju 1986).

## Intramucosal cysts

Intramucosal cysts are benign lesions which appear endoscopically as small nodules or mucosal polyps. The cysts are usually less than 5 mm in diameter and are often multiple. Histologically they may be lined by fundic-type mucosal cells (Sipponen et al 1983) or other gastric mucosal epithelial elements (Kato et al 1983).

## Leiomyoma and leiomyosarcoma

Leiomyomas are probably as common as adenomatous and hyperplastic polyps (Jamieson & Ludbrook 1971). They arise in the main muscle coat and while most are of smooth muscle origin, some appear to be neural (Mazur & Clark 1983). They are circumscribed, project into the lumen (Fig. 11.22) and often aquire a pedicle. It is impossible to distinguish between leiomyoma and leiomyosarcoma using clinical or histological criteria, although leiomyosarcomas are usually larger, have more mitoses and infiltrate surrounding tissues (Ranchod & Kempson

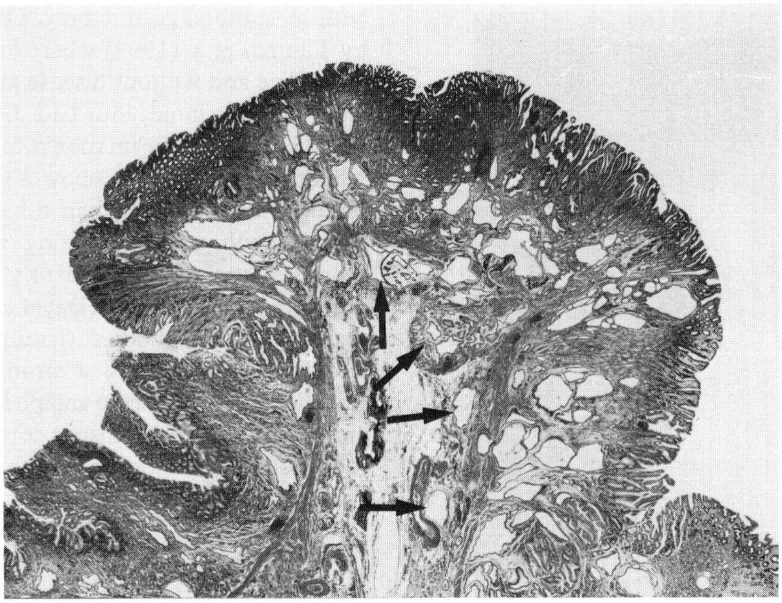

**Fig. 11.21** Gastric hyperplastic polyp. The polyp shows an increase in mucosal thickness with prominent dilatation of the deeper glands which are displaced through the muscularis mucosae (arrows) (hematoxylin and eosin, ×6).

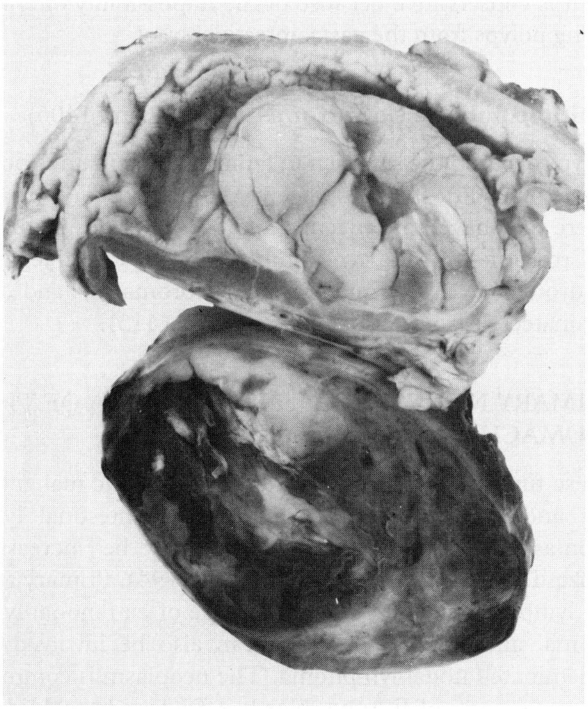

**Fig. 11.22** Gastric leiomyoma. A large dumb-bell shaped tumor with central ulcer crater on the mucosal surface of the intrinsic portion. The extrinsic mass shows central hemorrhagic necrosis.

1977). Conventional indices such as tumor size, grade, cellularity and mitotic index have major limitations in assessing the malignant potential of these tumors and DNA ploidy may have more prognostic value (Suzuki & Sugihira 1993).

*Clinical features*

Tumors larger than 6 cm can produce symptoms, those smaller than 3 cm usually do not (Grafe et al 1960). Pain, anorexia, weight loss and hematemesis and melena are the presenting features. Rarely, the tumor intussuscepts into the duodenum, causing vomiting. Small tumors are difficult to distinguish radiologically from adenomatous polyps. Larger tumors, particularly when intramural, can be distinguished from carcinomas by their smooth, spherical appearance and sharp demarcation from the surrounding mucosa and the tendency to develop central ulceration (Fig. 11.23). Endoscopy may show central ulceration which has not been seen on barium studies, but endoscopic biopsy is of no positive value in diagnosis. Computed tomography may help to identify infiltration in malignant cases (Fig. 2.15) and reveal hematogenous spread to the lungs.

*Treatment*

Leiomyosarcomas are dealt with by gastric resection. Symptomatic leiomyomas and those greater than 2–3 cm in diameter should be resected with a margin of at least 2 cm (Kavlie & White 1972).

**Gastric carcinoids** (Thomas et al 1994)

No more than 2% of all gastrointestinal carcinoids involve the stomach so that this is a less common site for carcinoid tumors than the appendix, small intestine or colon. The tumors have an association with pernicious anemia (p. 230),

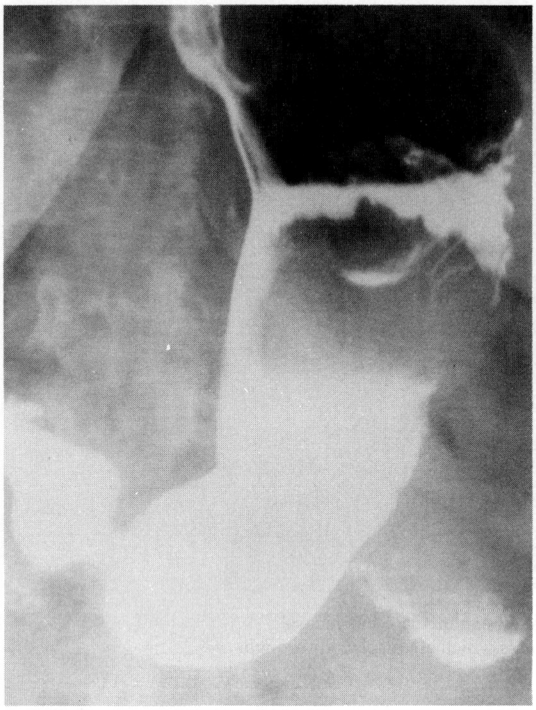

**Fig. 11.23** Leiomyoma of the body of the stomach causing a large, smooth filling defect which projects into the gastric air bubble. A large ulcer crater in the middle of the tumor due to central necrosis shows a barium-fluid level.

chronic gastritis and hypergastrinemia and there is speculation that antisecretory drugs might produce gastric carcinoids by causing hypergastrinemia. Other associations include thyroid disease, hyperplastic gastric polyps and von Recklinghausen's disease. Gastric carcinoids range in size from a few millimeters to as large as 25 cm (in rare cases). Histologically the great majority are argyrophilic but 15% are argentaffin. All stain for chromogranin and secrotonin is detected in about one-third (Thomas et al 1994) (p. 473).

Adult males and females of all age groups are equally affected. Most carcinoids are found incidentally but they can give rise to bleeding, epigastric pain, vomiting and weight loss. Carcinoid syndrome may be present (p. 473).

The tumors are commonest in the proximal stomach and are vascular and yellowish pink lesions which occasionally are polypoid with a wide base. On barium studies, they usually appear as intramural defects simulating leiomyomas, multiple gastric polyps, large gastric ulcers or polypoid intraluminal lesions (Balthazar et al 1982).

Of the 104 patients reviewed by Thomas et al (1994), only one had lymph node metastases at presentation and none has the carcinoid syndrome. Only two patients had transmural invasion and in most cases the lesion was confined to the mucosa and submucosa. In practice, tumors less than 1 cm in diameter are extremely unlikely to have metastasized and are treated by local excision, preferably at endoscopy. Larger gastric tumors are dealt with by subtotal gastrectomy. Of the 62 patients reported by Thomas et al (1994) where follow-up was available, 44 were alive and without disease after 1–10 years, four were alive with carcinoid, four had died from carcinoid and 10 had died from other/unknown causes.

Duodenal carcinoids show a greater similarity to carcinoids of the stomach than other intestinal carcinoids in their growth pattern, setting and serotonin positivity. However, they more frequently stain positive for gastrin/CCK and somatostatin (Dayal et al 1983) and often contain psammoma bodies (laminated calcified basophilic structures). They have a stronger association with von Recklinghausen's disease and pheochromocytoma (Griffiths et al 1984) than their gastric counterparts. Local resection may be possible for small tumors but large ones may require pancreaticoduodenectomy.

### Hamartoma

In the Peutz–Jeghers syndrome, polyps most commonly affect the small intestine (p. 1413) but can occur in the stomach. Gastric polyps may be sessile, but are more often pedunculated and resemble adenomatous polyps. Treatment is conservative because of the impossibility of eradicating polyps from the gastrointestinal tract.

### **Multiple polyposis syndromes** (pp. 468 and 1406)

Polyps occur in the stomach in familial adenomatous polyposis (p. 1406), in multiple juvenile polyposis (p. 1411) where they have both juvenile and adenomatous features, in Cronkhite–Canada syndrome (p. 1413), Peutz–Jeghers syndrome (p. 1413), multiple neurofibromatosis and disseminated gastrointestinal polyposis (p. 1415).

## PRIMARY NON-HODGKINS LYMPHOMA OF THE STOMACH

These tumors account for 1–10% of all gastric malignancies and for 50% of all primary gastrointestinal lymphomas, although their incidence may be increasing (Bozetti et al 1993, Amer & El-Akkad 1994). Primary gastric lymphoma is the commonest type of extranodal lymphoma, although the stomach can also be involved by disseminated nodal lymphoma. The neoplasm is common in certain parts of Europe, North Affrica and the Middle East, but relatively rare in the United States (Amer & El-Akkad 1994). Patients with non-Hodgkins gastric lymphoma are more likely than matched controls to have immunological evidence of prior *H. pylori* infection and a causative role for the organism is plausible but as yet unproven (Parsonnet et al 1994). Gastrointestinal lymphomas affect adults in all age groups, but those with gastric tumors tend to be older than those with intestinal lymphoma. Male preponderance is seen in most series and may be as high as 2.8:1.

**Pathology** (Brooks & Enterline 1983b, Bozzetti et al 1993) (see also p. 468)

The antrum and pylorus are most often involved but any area can be affected. The apperance often resembles that of an infiltrating, polypoid or ulcerating cancer and the tumor frequently arises in an area of chronic inflammation. In contrast to the intestines, multiple lesions are unusual in the stomach. Isaacson et al (1988) have suggested that such extranodal lymphomas arise from lymphoid tissue that developes at extranodal sites in the course of inflammatory disease. Almost all primary gastric lymphomas are B-cell tumors and histologically, they are low- or high-grade lymphomas with features resembling those of mucosa-associated lymphoid tissue (MALT). A number of histological classifications and staging systems exist but those in common current use are shown in Table 11.9. Hodgkins lymphoma and other types of non-Hodgkins lymphoma rarely involve the stomach (Collins et al 1983).

**Clinical features and investigations**

The history is often indistinguishable from that of gastric cancer or peptic ulcer. Abdominal pain and weight loss are common and may be accompanied by anorexia, nausea and vomiting. Hematemesis, melena, obstruction and perforation can occur. On examination, an abdominal mass can sometimes be felt but palpable lymph node enlargement and hepatosplenomegaly are usually absent.

Both radiology and endoscopy may reveal a mass or filling defect; a diffuse infiltrating process with thickened mucosal folds is seen in 20% of cases but ulceration is uncommon. Differentiation from lesions such as carcinoma, Menetrier's disease, chronic gastritis, pseudolymphoma and benign segmental hyperrugosity may be difficult. Biopsy at endoscopy is positive in some 90% of cases but it can show no abnormality or suggest peptic ulcer or cancer (Bozzetti et al 1993). Part of the difficulty stems from the fact that lymphoma grows in the submucosa and may only involve the mucosa at a late stage. Problems may also arise when the stomach is involved secondarily by other forms of lymphoma, as may occur when a para-aortic lymph node mass infiltrates the posterior wall. Computed tomography of the lungs and abdomen should be performed for staging purposes in all patients and a bone marrow aspirate should be examined. Laparotomy is no longer recommended for staging although it is recognized that computed tomography has limited accuracy in assessing lymph node involvement.

Bloodborne metastases from lymphoma elsewhere occasionally give rise to ulcerating mucosal deposits in the stomach and intestine. Such deposits have a "target" appearance if a protruding mound of tumor undergoes central necrosis and ulceration. Target lesions are occasionally seen in other secondary deposits, particularly those of malignant melanoma.

**Table 11.9a** Histopathological classification of primary gastrointestinal lymphoma (see Bozzetti et al 1993)

B cell
- Low-grade B cell lymphoma of MALT*
- High-grade B cell lymphoma of MALT ± evidence of a low-grade, component
- Mediterranean lymphoma (immunoproliferative disease of the small intestine), low, mixed or high grade
- Malignant lymphoma, controcytic (lymphomatous polyposis)
- Burkitt-like lymphoma
- Other types of low- or high-grade lymphoma corresponding to peripheral lymph node equivalents

T cell
- Enteropathy-associated T cell lymphoma
- Other types unassociated with enteropathy

*MALT, mucosa-associated lymphoid tissue

**Table 11.9b** Staging systems for primary gastrointestinal non-Hodgkin's lymphoma (see Bozzetti et al 1993)

| Classification* | | | Description | Relative incidence (%) |
|---|---|---|---|---|
| Ann Arbor | Rao | Musshoff | | |
| IE* | IE | IE | Tumor confined to gastrointestinal tract | 26 |
| IIE | IIE | IIE | Tumor with spread to regional lymph nodes | 26 |
| IIE | IIIE | IIE | Tumor with nodal involvement beyond regional lymph nodes (para-aortic, iliac) | 17 |
| IIIE-IV | IVE | IIIE-IV | Tumor with spread to other intra-abdominal organs (liver, spleen) or beyond abdomen (chest, bone marrow) | 31 |

*E denotes extranodal disease

**Treatment and prognosis** (Bozzetti et al 1993)

There is continuing controversy as to whether gastric lymphomas in stages IE and IIE should be treated by surgery alone (subtotal or total gastrectomy), surgery in combination with chemotherapy and/or radiotherapy, or by chemotherapy or radiotherapy in the first instance. Resectability rates range from 66–88% and 5-year survival rates generally exceed 80% after surgery alone in stage IE; addition of radiotherapy has doubtful value but adding chemotherapy can increase survival rates to virtually 100%. Survival rates in stage IIE are around 40% after surgery alone but improve by some 50% if surgery is followed by adjuvant chemotherapy and/or radiotherapy.

Some have advocated primary chemotherapy with or without radiotherapy as initial treatment in stage IIE, surgery being reserved for nonresponders. This approach has yet to be validated by controlled study and it should not be forgotten that chemotherapy is not without morbidity and in recent reports, treatment-related mortality ranges from 1–10%. Chemotherapy usually involves

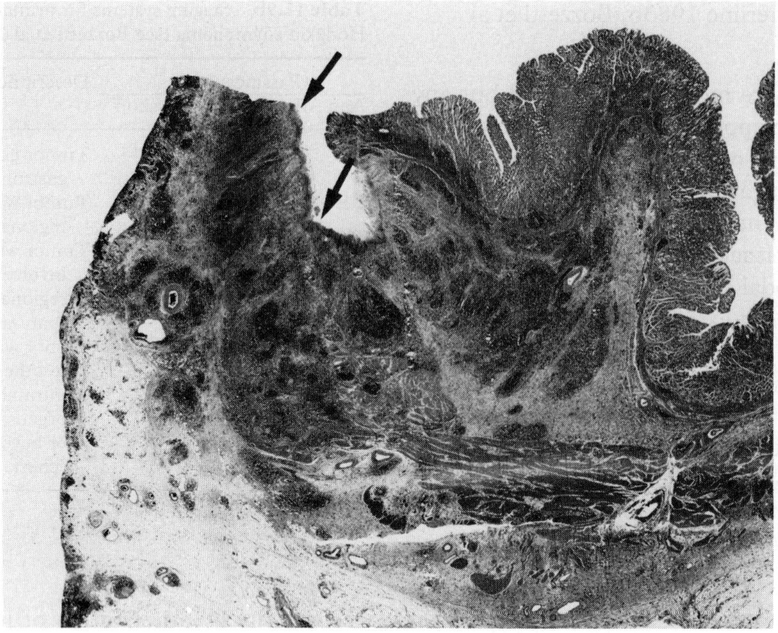

**Fig. 11.24** Gastric pseudolymphoma. There is an area of ulceration (arrows) associated with a very marked focal and nodular lymphatic aggregation in the gastric wall (hematoxylin and eosin, ×5).

administering a combination of cyclophosphamide, vincristine and prednisone with or without agents such as bleomycin and/or procarbazine.

Surgery may have a role in debulking in patients with advanced disease, but combination chemotherapy is the mainstay of therapy if dissemination has been demonstrated.

Emergency surgery is sometimes needed for patients who develop bleeding, obstruction or perforation, either at presentation or when nonsurgical treatment is being employed. Bleeding is the most common problem and affects some 20–30% of patients, although in the experience of Bozzetti et al (1993), emergency surgery was needed for severe bleeding or perforation in 10% of cases.

## BENIGN LYMPHOID HYPERPLASIA (Brooks & Enterline 1983a, Orr et al 1984)

Benign lymphoid hyperplasia or pseudolymphoma of the stomach is an uncommon condition which usually presents with a history of epigastric pain, weight loss and gastrointestinal bleeding and is often misdiagnosed as peptic ulceration or gastric cancer. The lesions form tumor-like thickenings of the mucosa and stomach wall or resemble peptic ulcers, indeed, many cases have coexisting gastric ulceration.

Radiologically and endoscopically, the lesion is often misinterpreted as carcinoma, lymphoma, benign gastric ulcer or thickened rugal folds. Histologically the lesion can be confused with lymphoma and affects the mucosa and submucosa but may involve deeper layers. The lymphoid infiltrate consists mainly of small lymphocytes and follicles with prominent germinal centers (Fig. 11.24). An admixture of plasma cells and eosinophils is usually present and some fibrosis may be seen. Similar lesions may occur in the small bowel or rectum (benign lymphoid polyp of the rectum). The treatment consists of resection and follow-up is advisable as a few cases have progressed to malignant lymphoma (Scoazec et al 1986). The prognosis is otherwise good.

## REFERENCES

Adachi Y, Kanakura T, Mori M, Baba H, Maehara Y, Sugimachi 1994 Prognostic significance of the number of positive lymph nodes in gastric carcinoma. British Journal of Surgery 81: 414–416

Aird I, Bentall H H, Roberts J A F 1953 A relationship between cancer of stomach and A B O blood groups. British Medical Journal 1: 799

Akoh J, Macintyre I M C 1992 Improving survival in gastric cancer: review of 5-year survival rates in English language publications from 1970. British Journal of Surgery 79: 293–299

Amer M H, El-Akkad S 1994 Gastrointestinal lymphoma in adults: clinical features and management of 300 cases. Gastroenterology 106: 846–858

Asaka M, Kimura T, Kudo M et al 1992 Relationship of *Helicobacter pylori* to serum pepsinogens in an asymptomatic Japanese population. Gastroenterology 102: 760–766

Asaka M, Kimura T, Kato M et al 1994 Possible role of *Helicobacter pylori* infection in early gastric cancer development. Cancer 73: 2691–2694

Ballantyne K C, Morris D L, Jones J A, Gregson R H, Hardcastle J D 1987 Accuracy of identification of early gastric cancer. British Journal of Surgery 74: 618–619

Balthazar E J, Megibow A, Bryk D, Cohen T 1982 Gastric carcinoid tumors: radiographic features in eight cases. American Journal of Radiology 139: 1123

Barker D J, Coggon D, Holdsmond C, Wickham C 1990 Poor housing rates and high rates of stomach cancer in England and Wales. British Journal of Cancer 61: 575–578
Beretta G, Arnoldi E, Beretta G D et al 1989 A randomized study of fluorouracil versus FAM polychemotherapy in gastric carcinoma. Proceedings of the EORTC Symposium on Advances in Gastrointestinal Tract Cancer Research and Treatment, p 48
Black R J, Sharp L, Kendrick S W 1993 Trends in cancer survival in Scotland 1968–1990. Information and Statistics Division, Directorate of Information Services, NHS in Scotland, Edinburgh
BMJ 1965 Soil and stomach cancer. British Medical Journal 1: 1
Bogolometz W V 1984 Early gastric cancer. American Journal of Surgical Pathology 8: 381–391
Bollschweiler E, Boettcher K, Hoelscher A H, Sasako M, Kinoshita T, Maruyama K, Siewert J R 1992 Preoperative assessment of lymph node metastases in patients with gastric cancer: evaluation of the Maruyama computer program. British Journal of Surgery 79: 156–160
Borch K 1986 Epidemiologic, clinicopathologic, and economic aspects of gastroscopic screening of patients with pernicious anaemia. Scandinavian Journal of Gastroenterology 21: 21
Bozzetti F, Audiso R A, Giardini R, Gennari L 1993 Role of surgery in patients with primary non-Hodgkins lymphoma of the stomach: an old problem revisited. British Journal of Surgery 80: 1101–1106
Bree R L, Schwab R E 1985 The role of needle aspiration biopsy in the diagnosis of gastric carcinoma. Proceedings of the XVI International Congress of Radiology, Hawaii, p 33
Brems-Dalgaard E, Clausen H V 1993 Survival following microscopically confirmed radical resection of $N_0$ gastric cancer. British Journal of Surgery 80: 1150–1152
Brooks J J, Enterline H T 1983a Gastric pseudolymphoma. Its three subtypes and relation to lymphoma. Cancer 51: 476
Brooks J J, Enterline H T 1983b Primary gastric lymphomas. A clinicopathologic study of 58 cases with long-term follow-up and literature review. Cancer 51: 701
Carter D C 1987 Cancer after peptic ulcer surgery. Gut 28: 921–923
Caygill C P J, Hill M J, Kirkham J S, Northfield T C 1986 Mortality from gastric cancer following gastric surgery for peptic ulcer. Lancet 1: 929–931
Clark C G, Fresini A, Gledhill T 1985 Cancer following gastric surgery. British Journal of Surgery 72: 591
Colin-Jones D G, Longman M J S, Lawson D H, Vessey M P 1982 Cimetidine and gastric cancer: preliminary report from post-marketing surveillance study. British Medical Journal 285: 1311–1313
Collins J, Katon R, Harty-Golder B 1983 Burkitt's lymphoma presenting with gastroduodenal involvement. Endoscopic description and review of the literature. Gastroenterology 85: 425
Coma del Corral M J, Pardo-Mindan F J, Razquin S, Ojeda C 1990 Risk of cancer in patients with gastric dysplasia. Cancer 65: 2078–2085
Comis R L, Carter S K 1974 A review of chemotherapy in gastric cancer. Cancer 34: 1576–1586
Correa P 1983 The gastric pre-cancerous process. Cancer Surveys 2: 437–450
Correa P 1988 A human model of gastric carcinogenesis. Cancer Research 48: 3854–3860
Correa P 1992 Human gastric carcinogenesis: a multistep and multifactorial process – First American Cancer Society Award Lecture on Cancer Epidemiology. Cancer Research 52: 6735–6740
Correa P, Haenszel W 1982 Epidemiology of gastric cancer. In: Correa P, Haenszel W (eds) Epidemiology of cancer of the digestive tract. Martinus Nijhoff, The Hague, p 59
Correa P, Sasano N, Stemmermann G N, Haenszel W 1973 Pathology of gastric carcinoma in Japanese populations: comparisons between Miyagi Prefecture, Japan and Hawaii, Journal of the National Cancer Institute 51: 1449
Cuello C, Correa P, Zarama G, Lopez J, Murray J, Gordillo G 1979 Histopathology of gastric dysplasia. Correlations with gastric juice chemistry. American Journal of Surgical Pathology 3: 491
Cullinan S A, Moertel C G, Fleming T R et al 1985 A comparison of three chemotherapeutic regimens in the treatment of advanced pancreatic and gastric carcinoma. Fluorouracil vs flourouracil and doxorubicin vs fluorouracil, doxorubicin, and mitomycin. Journal of the American Medical Association 253: 2061
Cunningham D 1990 The management of gastric cancer. In: McArdle C S (ed) Surgical oncology. Butterworth, London, p 28–52
Cuschieri A 1986 Gastrectomy for gastric cancer: definitions and objectives. British Journal of Surgery 73: 513–514
Dayal Y, Doos W G, O'Brien M J, Nunnemacher G, DeLellis R A, Wolfe H J 1983 Psammomatous somatostatinomas of the duodenum. American Journal of Surgical Pathology 7: 653
Dehn T C B, Reznek R H, Nockler I B, White F E 1984 The pre-operative assessment of advanced gastric cancer by computed tomography. British Journal of Surgery 71: 413
Doll R 1956 Environmental factors in the aetiology of carcinoma of the stomach. Gastroenterologia 86: 320
Dungal N, Sigurjonsson J 1967 Gastric cancer and diet. A pilot study on dietary habits in two districts differing markedly in respect of mortality from gastric cancer. British Journal of Cancer 21: 270
Ekbom G A, Gleysteen J J 1980 Gastric malignancy: resection for palliation. Surgery 88: 476
Elsborg L, Andersen D, Myhre-Jensen O, Bastrup-Madsen P 1977 Gastric mucosal polyps in pernicious anaemia. Scandinavian Journal of Gastroenterology 12: 49
Elster K 1976 Histologic classification of gastric polyps. In: Morson B C (ed) Pathology of the gastrointestinal tract. Springer-Verlag, New York, p 77
Eurogast Study Group 1993 An international association between *Helicobacter pylori* infection and gastric cancer. Lancet 341: 1359–1362
Farley D R, Donohue J H, Nagorney D M, Carpenter H A, Katzmann J A, IIstrup D M 1992 Early gastric cancer. British Journal of Surgery 79: 539–542
Feczko P J, Halpert R D, Ackerman L V 1985 Gastric polyps: radiological evaluation and clinical significance. Radiology 155: 581
Finch P J, Ryan F P, Rogers K, Holt S 1987 Gastric enzymes as a screening test for gastric cancer. Gut 28: 319
Fischermann K, Koster K H 1962 The augmented histamine test in the differential diagnosis between ulcer and cancer of the stomach. Gut 3: 211
Fleischer D 1985 Washington Laser Symposium: seminar on endoscopic laser therapy. Gastrointestinal Endoscopy 31: 397
Fleischer D 1986 Endoscopic palliative tumour therapy with laser irradiation. Clinics in Gastroenterology 15: 273
Fleischer D, Sivak M V 1985 Endoscopic ND:YAG laser therapy as palliation for esophagogastric cancer. Gastroenterology 89: 827–831
Forman D 1987 Gastric cancer, diet and nitrate exposure. British Medical Journal 294: 528
Fraser P, Chilvers C, Beral V, Hill M J 1980 Nitrate and human cancer: a review of the evidence. International Journal of Epidemiology 9: 3
Fujimura T, Yonemura Y, Muraoka K et al 1994 Continuous hyperthermic peritoneal perfusion for the prevention of peritoneal recurrence of gastric cancer: randomized control study. World Journal of Surgery 18: 150–155
Gabrielsson N 1972 Benign and malignant gastric ulcers. Evaluation of the differential diagnostics in roentgen examination and endoscopy. Endoscopy 4: 73
Gastrointestinal Tumor Study Group (GITSG) 1988 Triazinate and platinum efficacy in combination with 5-fluorouracil and doxorubicin: results of a three-arm randomized trial in metastatic gastric cancer. Journal of the National Cancer Institute 80: 1011–1015
Gold R P, Green P H R, O'Toole K M, Seaman W B 1984 Early gastric cancer: radiographic experience. Radiology 152: 283
Goseki N, Takizawa T, Koike M 1992 Differences in the mode of extension of gastric cancer classified by histological type: new histological classification of gastric carcinoma. Gut 33: 606–612
Grafe W, Thorbjarnarson B, Pearce J M, Beal J M 1960 Benign neoplasms of the stomach. American Journal of Surgery 100: 561
Green P H R, O'Toole K M, Weinberg L M, Goldfarb J P 1981 Early gastric cancer. Gastroenterology 81: 247
Griffith G W 1968 The sex ratio in gastric cancer and hypothetical considerations relative to aetiology. British Journal of Cancer 22: 163
Griffiths D F R, Jasani B, Newman G R, Williams E D, Williams G T 1984 Glandular duodenal carcinoid – a somatostatin rich tumour with neuroendocrine associations. Journal of Clinical Pathology 37: 163

Grundmann E 1978 Early gastric cancer – today. Pathology Research, Practice 162: 347
Guadagni S, Reed P I, Johnson B J et al 1993 Early gastric cancer: follow-up after gastrectomy in 159 patients. British Journal of Surgery 80: 325–328
Guiss L W, Stewart F W 1943 Chronic atrophic gastritis and cancer of the stomach. Archives of Surgery 46: 823
Haenszel W 1958 Variation in incidence and mortality from stomach cancer, with particular reference to the United States. Journal of the National Cancer Institute 21: 213
Haenszel W 1961 Cancer mortality among the foreign-born in the United States. Journal of the National Cancer Institute 26: 37
Haenszel W, Kurihara M, Segi M, Lee R K C 1972 Stomach cancer among Japanese in Hawaii. Journal of the National Cancer Institute 49: 969
Hagiwara A, Takahashi T, Kojima O et al 1992 Prophylaxis with carbon-adsorbed mitomycin against peritoneal recurrence of gastric cancer. Lancet 339: 629–631
Hallissey M, Allum W H, Roginski C, Fielding J W L 1988 Palliative surgery for gastric cancer. Cancer 62: 440–444
Hansson L-E, Sparen P, Nyren O 1993 Increasing incidence of carcinoma of the gastric cardia in Sweden from 1970 to 1985. British Journal of Surgery 80: 374–377
Harju E 1986 Gastric polyposis and malignancy. British Journal of Surgery 73: 532
Harrison D J, Jones J A, Morris D L 1990 The effect of the gastrin receptor antagonist proglumide on survival in gastric carcinoma. Cancer 66: 1449–1452
Haugstved T, Viste A, Edie G E, Soreide O 1989 The survival benefit of resection in patients with advanced stomach cancer. The Norwegian multicentre experience: Norwegian Stomach Cancer Trial. World Journal of Surgery 13: 617–621
Haugstvedt T K, Viste A, Eide G E, Soreide O and Members of the Norwegian Stomach Cancer Trial 1993 Norwegian multicenter study of survival and prognostic factors in patients undergoing curative resection for gastric carcinoma. British Journal of Surgery 80: 475–478
Heesakkers J P F A, Gouma D J, Thunnissen F B J M, Bemelmans M H A, von Meyenfeldt M F 1994 Non-radical therapy for gastric cancer. British Journal of Surgery 81: 551–553
Hioki K, Nakane Y, Yamamoto M 1990 Surgical strategy for early gastric cancer. British Journal of Surgery 77: 1330–1334
Hirohata T 1968 Mortality from gastric cancer and other causes after medical or surgical treatment for gastric ulcer. Journal of the National Cancer Institute 41: 895
Hirohata T, Kuratsune M 1969 The geographical comparison of mortality from cancer of the stomach and ulcer of the stomach in Japan. British Journal of Cancer 23: 465
Hisamichi S 1989 Screening for gastric cancer. World Journal of Surgery 13: 31–37
Hisamichi S, Sugawara N, Fukao A 1988 Effectiveness of gastric mass screening in Japan. Cancer Detection and Prevention 11: 323
Houghton P W J, Mortensen N J McC, Allan A, Williamson R C N, Davies J D 1985 Early gastric cancer: the case for long term surveillance. British Medical Journal 291: 305
Husemann B 1989 Cardia carcinoma considered as a distinct clinical entity. British Journal of Surgery 76: 136–139
Iishi H, Yamamoto R, Iac C T, Tatsuta M, Okuda S 1986 Evaluation of the fine-needle aspiration biopsy under direct vision gastrofiberoscopy in diagnosis of diffusively infiltrative carcinoma of the stomach. Cancer 57: 1365
Ikeda Y, Mori M, Kamakura T, Haraguchi Y, Saku M, Sugimachi K 1994 Increased incidence of undifferentiated type of gastric cancer with tumor progression in 912 patients with early gastric cancer and 1245 with advanced gastric cancer. Cancer 73: 2459–2463
Imai T, Kubo T, Watanabe H 1971 Chronic gastritis in Japanese with reference to high incidence of gastric carcinoma. Journal of the National Cancer Institute 47: 179
Inoue K, Tobe T, Kan N, Nío Y, Sakai M, Takeuchi E, Sugiyama T 1991 Problems in the definition and treatment of early gastric cancer. British Journal of Surgery 78: 818–821
Inokuchi K, Inutsuka S, Furusawa M, Soejima K, Ikeda T 1967 Stromal reaction around tumor and metastasis and prognosis after curative gastrectomy for carcinoma of the stomach. Cancer 20: 1924
Iriyama K, Miki C, Ilunga K, Osawa T, Tsuchibashi T, Suzuki H 1993 Prognostic significance of histological type in gastric carcinoma with invasion confined to the stomach wall. British Journal of Surgery 80: 890–892
Isaacson P G, Spencer J, Wright D H 1988 Classifying primary gut lymphomas. Lancet 1: 1148–1149
Jamieson G G, Ludbrook J 1971 The problems of "benign" polypoid lesions of the stomach. Australian and New Zealand Journal of Surgery 41: 123
Japanese Research Society for Gastric Cancer 1981 The general rules for the gastric cancer study in surgery and pathology. Part I. Clinical classification. Japanese Journal of Surgery 11: 127
Japanese Research Society Committee on Histological Classification of Gastric Cancer 1981 The general rules for the gastric cancer study in surgery and pathology. Part II. Histological classification of gastric cancer. Japanese Journal of Surgery 11: 140
Jass J R 1983 A classification of gastric dysplasia. Histopathology 7: 181–183
Kamiya T, Morishita T, Asakura H, Miura S, Munakata Y, Tsuchiya M 1982 Long-term follow-up study on gastric adenoma and its relation to gastric protruded carcinoma. Cancer 50: 2496
Kato Y 1966 Analysis on the diagnosis of the surgical gastric diseases by gastrocamera – particularly on diagnostic accuracy by combined method with x-ray examination, gastrocamera and exfoliative cytology. Gastroenterological Endoscopy 8: 293
Kato Y, Sugano H, Rubio C A 1983 Classification of intramucosal cysts of the stomach. Histopathology 7: 931
Kavlie H, White T T 1972 Leiomyomas of the upper gastrointestinal tract. Surgery 71: 842
Keighley M R B, Youngs D, Poxon V et al 1984 Intragastric N-nitrosation is unlikely to be responsible for gastric carcinoma developing after operations for duodenal ulcer. Gut 25: 238–245
Kinlen L J, Webster A D B, Bird A G et al 1985 Prospective study of cancer in patients with hypogammaglobulinaemia. Lancet 1: 263
Korenaga D, Haraguchi M, Tsujitani S, Okamura T, Tamada R, Sugimachi K 1986 Clinicopathological features of mucosal carcinoma of the stomach with lymph node metastasis in eleven patients. British Journal of Surgery 73: 431
Korenaga T, Okamura T, Baba H, Saito A, Sugimachi K 1988 Results of resections of gastric cancer extending to adjacent organs. British Journal of Surgery 75: 12–15
Kurayama H, Eastwood G L, Kohashi E, Honda T 1984 Endoscopic local injection of early gastric garcinoma with 5-fluorouracil. Digestive Diseases and Sciences 29: 498–501
Kurihara M, Aoki K, Hisamichi S 1989 Cancer mortality statistics in the world 1950–1985. University of Nagoya Press, Nagoya, Japan
Kuru M 1966 Atlas of early carcinoma of the stomach. NakayamaShoten, Tokyo
LaDue J S, Murison P J, McNeer G, Pack G T 1950 Symptomatology and diagnosis of gastric cancer. Archives of Surgery 60: 305
Lambert R 1984 Laser treatment of colorectal neoplasms. European Laser Workshop, Taunstein
Lauren P 1965 The two histological main types of gastric carcinoma: diffuse and so-called intestinal-type carcinoma. An attempt at a histoclinical classification. Acta Pathologica et Microbiologica Scandinavica 64: 31
LaVecchia C, Negri E, D'Avanzo B, Franceschi S 1990 Histamine-2-receptor anatgonists and gastric cancer risk. Lancet 336: 355–357
Levine M S, Laufer I, Thompson J J 1983 Carcinoma of the gastric cardia in young people. American Journal of Roentgenology 140: 69
Logan R F A, Langman M J S 1983 Screening for gastric cancer after gastric surgery. Lancet 2: 667
Lundergardh G, Ekbom A, McLaughlin J K, Nyren O 1994 Gastric cancer risk after vagotomy. Gut 35: 946–949
Lykke-Olesen O 1960 gastritis in clinically healthy stomachs: a histological study of autopsy material. Munksgaard, Copenhagen
Maartmann-Moe H, Hartveit F 1985 On the reputed decline in gastric carcinoma: necropsy study from Western Norway. British Medical Journal 290: 103
Macintyre I M C, Akoh J A 1991 Improving survival in gastric cancer: review of operative mortality in English language publications from 1970. British Journal of Surgery 78: 773–778

Maehara Y, Orita H, Moriguchi S, Emi Y, Haraguchi M, Sugimachi K 1991 Lower survival rate for patients under 30 years of age and surgically treated for gastric carcinoma. British Journal of Cancer 63: 1015–1017

Maehara Y, Orita H, Okuyama T, Moriguchi S, Tsujitani S, Korenaga D, Sugimachi K 1992a Predictors of lymph node metastasis in early gastric cancer. British Journal of Surgery 79: 245–247

Maehara Y, Orita H, Moriguchi S, Emi Y, Haraguchi M, Sugimachi K 1992b Lower survival rate for patients under 30 years of age and surgically treated for gastric cancer. British Journal of Cancer 63: 1015–1017

Marshak R H, Feldman F 1965 Gastric polyps. American Journal of Digestive Diseases 10: 909

Marshak R H, Lindner A E 1971 Polypoid lesions of the stomach. Seminars in Roentgenology 6: 151

Martin I G, Dixon M F, Sue-Ling H, Axon A T R, Johnston D 1994 Goseki histological grading of gastric cancer is an important predictor of outcome. Gut 35: 758–763

Maruyama K 1986 Results of surgery correlated with staging. In: Cuschieri A, Wellwood J M (eds) Cancer of the stomach. Grune and Stratton, London, p 145–163

Maruyama K 1987 The most important prognostic factors for gastric cancer patients. Scandinavian Journal of Gastroenterology 22: 63

Mazur M T, Clark H B 1983 Gastric stromal tumors. American Journal of Surgical Pathology 7: 507

McConnell R B 1966 The genetics of gastrointestinal disorders. Oxford University Press, London.

McConnell R B 1976 Genetic aspects of gastrointestinal cancer. Clinics in Gastroenterology 5: 483

McLean Ross A H, Smith M A, Anderson J R, Small W P 1982 Late mortality after surgery for peptic ulcer. New England Journal of Medicine 307: 519–522

Mecklin J P, Nordling S, Saario I 1988 Carcinoma of the stomach and its heredity in young patients. Scandinavian Journal of Gastroenterology 23: 307

Merliss R R 1971 Talc-treated rice and Japanese stomach cancer. Science 173: 1141

Ming S 1977 Gastric carcinoma. Cancer 39: 2475

Moller H, Nissen A, Mosbech J 1992 Use of cimetidine and other peptic ulcer drugs in Denmark 1977–1990 with analysis of the risk of gastric cancer among cimetidine users. Gut 33: 1166–1169

Monson J R T, Donohue J H, McIrath D C, Farnell M B, Ilstrup D M 1991 Total gastrectomy for advanced cancer. Cancer 68: 1863–1868

Moreaux J, Bougaran J 1993 Early gastric cancer. A 25-year surgical experience. Annals of Surgery 217: 347–355

Morrissey J F, Koizumi H 1968 The endoscopic diagnosis of gastric cancer. Proceedings of the National Cancer Conference 46: 433

Morson B C, Dawson I M P 1979 Gastrointestinal pathology, 2nd edn. Blackwell, London

Morson B C, Sobin L H, Grundmann E, Johansen A, Nagayo T, Serck-Hanssen A 1980 Precancerous conditions and epithelial dysplasia in the stomach. Journal of Clinical Pathology 33: 711

Moss A A, Schnyder P, Marks W, Margulis A R 1981 Gastric adenocarcinoma: a comparison of the accuracy and economics of staging by computed tomography and surgery. Gastroenterology 80: 45

Munoz N, Connelly R 1971 Time trends of intestinal and diffuse types of gastric cancer in the United States. International Journal of Cancer 8: 158

Murakami R, Tsukuma T, Ubukata T et al 1990 Estimation of validity of mass screening program for gastric cancer in Osaka, Japan. Cancer 65: 1255–1260

Murayami T 1971 Pathomorphological diagnosis, definition and gross classification of early gastric cancer. Gan Monograph on Cancer Research 11: 53–55

Nakamura K, Sugano H, Takagi K, Fuchigami A 1967 Histopathological study on early carcinoma of the stomach: some considerations on the ulcer-cancer by analysis of 144 foci of the superficial spreading carcinomas. Gann 58: 377

Nakane Y, Okamura S, Akehira K, Boku T, Okusa T, Tanaka K, Hioki K 1994 Correlation of preoperative carcinoembryonic antigen levels and prognosis of gastric cancer patients Cancer 73: 2703–2708

Nakasato H, Koike A, Saji S et al 1994 Efficacy of immunochemotherapy as adjuvant treatment for curative resection of gastric cancer. Lancet 343: 1122–1126

Navas-Palacios J J, Colina-Ruizdelgado F, Sanchez-Larrea M D, Cortes-Cansino J 1983 Inflammatory fibroid polyps of the gastrointestinal tract. An immunohistochemical and electron microscopic study. Cancer 51: 1682

Noguchi Y, Imada T, Matsumoto A, Coit D G, Brennan M F 1989 Radical surgery for gastric cancer. A review of the Japanese experience. Cancer 64: 2053–2062

Offerhaus G, Stadt J, Huibregtse K, Tytgat G N J 1984 Endoscopic screening for malignancy in the gastric remnant: the clinical significance of dysplasia in gastric mucosa. Journal of Clinical Pathology 37: 748

Oka M, Yoshino S, Hazama S, Shimoda K, Suzuki M, Suzuki T 1992 Prognostic significance of regional lymph node resection after curative resection of advanced gastric cancer. British Journal of Surgery 79: 1091–1094

Okamura T, Kodama Y, Kamegawa T, Sano C, Kumashiro R, Inokuchi K 1983 Gastric carcinoma with lymphoid stroma: correlation to reactive hyperplasia in regional lymph nodes and prognosis. Japanese Journal of Surgery 13: 177

Oohara T, Aono G, Ukawa S et al 1984 Clinical diagnosis of minute gastric cancer less than 5 mm in diameter. Cancer 53: 162

Oota K, Sobin L H 1977 Histological typing of gastric and oesophageal tumours. International histological classification of tumours No 18. World Health Organization, Geneva, p 37

Orr R K, Lininger J R, Lawrence W 1984 Gastric pseudolymphoma. A challenging clinical problem. Annals of Surgery 200: 185

Ott D J, Munitz H A, Gelfand D W, Lane T G, Wu W C 1982 The sensitivity of radiography of the postoperative stomach. Radiology 144: 741

Parsonnet J 1993 *Helicobacter pylori* and gastric cancer. Gastroenterological Clinics of North American 22: 193–198

Parsonnet J, Hansen S, Rodriguez L et al 1994 *Helicobacter pylori* infection and gastric lymphoma. New England Journal of Medicine 330: 1267–1271

Pickford I R, Craven J L, Hall R, Thomas G, Stone W D 1984 Endoscopic examination of the gastric remnant 31–39 years after subtotal gastrectomy for peptic ulcer. Gut 25: 393

Preusser P, Wilke H, Achterrath W et al 1989 Neoadjuvant chemotherapy with the combination of EAP (etoposide/adriamycin/cisplatin) in locally advanced, non-resectable gastric cancer. Proceedings of the EORTC Symposium on Advances in Gastrointestinal Tract Cancer Research and Treatment, p 42

Prolla J C, Kobayashi S, Kirsner J B 1969 Gastric cancer. Some recent improvements in diagnosis based upon the Japanese experience. Archives of Internal Medicine 124: 238

Pygott F, Shah V L 1968 Gastric cancer associated with gastroenterostomy and partial gastrectomy. Gut 9: 117

Ranchod M, Kempson R L 1977 Smooth muscle tumors of the gastrointestinal tract and retroperitoneum. A pathologic analysis of 100 cases. Cancer 39: 255

Reed P I, Smith P L R, Haines K, House F R, Walters C L 1981 Effect of cimetidine on gastric juice N-nitrosamine concentration. Lancet 2: 553–556

Rhyu M-G, Park W-S, Jung Y-J, Choi S-W, Meltzer S J 1994 Allelic deletions of MCC/APC and p53 are frequent late events in human gastric carcinogenesis. Gastroenterology 106: 1584–1588

Rohde H, Bauer P, Stutzer H, Heitmann K, Gebbensleben B and the German Gastric Cancer TNM Study Group 1991 Proximal compared with distal adenocarcinoma of the stomach: differences and consequences. British Journal of Surgery 78: 1242–1248

Saegesser F, James D 1972 Cancer of the gastric stump after partial gastrectomy (Billroth II principle) for ulcer. Cancer 29: 1150

Sakita T, Oguro Y, Takasu S, Fukutomi H, Miwa T, Yoshimori M 1971 Observations on the healing of ulcerations in early gastric cancer. The life cycle of the malignant ulcer. Gastroenterology 60: 835

Sano R 1971 Pathological analysis of 300 cases of early gastric cancer. With special reference to cancer associated with ulcers. In: Murakami T (ed) Early gastric cancer. Gann Monograph on Cancer Research No. 11. University of Tokyo Press, Tokyo, p 81

Sano T, Kobori O, Muto T 1992 Lymph node metastases from early gastric cancer: endoscopic resection of tumour. British Journal of Surgery 79: 241–244
Sano T, Sasako M, Kinoshita T, Maruyama K 1993 Recurrence of early gastric cancer. Cancer 72: 3174–3178
Sasako M, Maruyama K, Kinoshita T, Okabayashi K 1991 Surgical treatment of carcinoma of the gastric stump. British Journal of Surgery 78: 822–824
Sasako M, Maruyama K, Kinoshita T et al 1992 Quality control of surgical technique in a multicenter prospective randomized controlled study on the surgical treatment of gastric cancer. Japanese Journal of Clinical Oncology 22: 41–48
Schafer L W, Larson D E, Melton L J, Higgins J A, Zinsmeister A R 1985 Risk of development of gastric carcinoma in patients with pernicious anemia: a population-based study in Rochester, Minnesota. Mayo Clinic Proceedings 60: 444
Scoazec J-Y, Brousse N, Potet F, Jeulain J-F 1986 Focal malignant lymphoma in gastric pseudolymphoma. Histologic and immunohistochemical study of a case. Cancer 57: 1330
Sedgwick D M, Akoh J A, Macintyre I M C 1991 Gastric cancer in Scotland: changing epidemiology, unchanging workload. British Medical Journal 302: 1305–1307
Selikoff I J, Churg J, Hammond E C 1964 Asbestos exposure and neoplasia. Journal of the American Medical Association 188: 22
Shanghai Gastrointestinal Endoscopy Cooperative Group 1982 Value of biopsy and brush cytology in the diagnosis of gastric cancer. Gut 23: 774
Sharma B K, Santan I A, Wood E C et al 1984 Intragastric bacterial activity and nitrosation before, during, and after treatment with omeprazole. British Medical Journal 289: 717–719
Shearman D J C, Finlayson N D C 1967 Familial aspects of gastric carcinoma. American Journal of Digestive Diseases 12: 529
Sherman R S 1967 Roentgenologic diagnosis of gastric tumors. In: McNeer G, Pack G T (eds) Neoplasms of the stomach. J B Lippincott, Philadelphia, p 129
Shirakabe H, Maruyama M 1983 Neoplastic diseases of the stomach. In: Margulis A R, Burhenne H J (eds) Alimentary tract radiology, Vol 1, 3rd edn. C V Mosby, St Louis, p 721
Shirakabe H, Nishizawa M, Maruyama M, Kobayashi S 1982 Atlas of X-ray diagnosis of early gastric cancer, 2nd edn. Igaku-Shoin, New York
Siewert J R, Bottcher K, Roder J D et al 1993 Prognostic relevance of systematic lymph node dissection in gastric carcinoma. British Journal of Surgery 80: 1015–1018
Sigurjonsson J 1967 Occupational variations in mortality from gastric cancer in relation to dietary differences. British Journal of Cancer 21: 651
Sipponen P, Laxen F, Seppala K 1983 Cystic "hamartomatous" gastric polyps: a disorder of oxyntic glands. Histopathology 7: 729
Sjoblom S M, Sipponen P, Jarvinen 1993 Gastroscopic follow-up of pernicious anaemia patients. Gut 34: 28–32
Sonnenberg A 1984 Endoscopic screening for gastric stump cancer: would it be beneficial? A hypothetical cohort study. Gastroenterology 87: 489
Stael von Holstein C, Eriksson S, Hammar E 1991 Role of re-resection in early gastric stump carcinoma. British Journal of Surgery 78: 1238–1241
Stockbrugger R W, Menon G G, Beilby J O W, Mason R R, Cotton P B 1983 Gastroscopic screening in 80 patients with pernicious anaemia. Gut 24: 1141–1147
Suehiro S, Nagasue N, Ogawa Y et al 1984 The negative effect of splenectomy on the prognosis of gastric cancer. American Journal of Surgery 148: 645–648
Sue-Ling H M, Johnston D, Martin I G, Dixon M F, Lansdown M R J, McMahon M J, Axon A T R 1993 Gastric cancer: a curable disease in Britain. British Medical Journal 307: 591–596
Sugano H, Nakamura K, Kato Y 1982 Pathological studies of human gastric cancer. Acta Pathologica Japonica 32: 329
Sugiyama K, Yonemura Y, Miyazaki I 1989 Immunohistochemical study of epidermal growth factor and epidermal growth factor receptor in gastric carcinoma. Cancer 63: 1557–1561
Suzuki H, Sugihira N 1993 Prognostic value of DNA ploidy in primary gastric leiomyosarcoma. British Journal of Surgery 80: 1549–1550
Tannenbaum S R 1983 N-Nitroso compounds: a perspective on human exposure. Lancet 1: 629
Tersmette A C, Offerhaus G J A., Tersmette K W F, Giadiello F M, Moore G W, Tytgat G N J, Vandenbroucke J P 1990 Meta-analysis of the risk of gastric stump cancer: detection of high risk patient subsets for stomach cancer after remote partial gastrectomy for benign conditions. Cancer Research 50: 6486–6489
Thomas R M, Baybick J H, Elsayed Al M, Sobin L H 1994 Gastric carcinoids. Cancer 73: 2053–2058
Thompson G B, van Heerden J A, Sarr M G 1993 Adenocarcinoma of the stomach: are we making progress? Lancet 342: 713–718
Thompson W M, Kelvin F M, Gedgaudas R K, Rice R P 1982 Radiologic investigation of peptic ulcer disease. Radiologic Clinics of North America 20: 701
Wagner P K, Ramaswamy A, Ruschoff J, Schmitz-Moorman P, Rothmund M 1991 Lymph node counts in the upper abdomen: anatomical basis for lymphadenectomy in gastric cancer. British Journal of Surgery 78: 825–827
Wanebo H J, Kennedy B J, Chmiel J, Steele G, Winchester D, Osteen R 1993 Cancer of the stomach. Annals of Surgery 218: 583–592
Watt P C H, Sloan J M, Kennedy T L 1983 Changes in gastric mucosa after vagotomy and gastrojejunostomy for duodenal ulcer. British Medical Journal 287: 1407
Watt P C H, Sloan J M, Donaldson J D, Patterson C C, Kennedy T L 1984 Relationship between histology and gastric juice pH and nitrite in the stomach after operation for duodenal ulcer. Gut 25: 246
White R M, Levine M S, Enterline H T, Laufer 1 1985 Early gastric cancer. Recent experience. Radiology 155: 25
Wils J, Bleiberg H 1989 Current status of chemotherapy for gastric cancer. European Journal of Cancer and Clinical Oncology 25: 3–8
Wright P A, Williams G T 1993 Molecular biology and gastric carcinoma. Gut 34: 145–147
Wu C-W, Chi C-W, Chang T-J, Lui W-Y, P'eng F-K 1990 Sex hormone receptors in gastric cancer. Cancer 65: 1396–1400
Wu C-W, Chang H-M, Kao H-L, Lui W-Y, P'eng F-K, Chi C-W 1992 The non-transformed progesterone and estrogen receptors in gastric cancer. Gastroenterology 102: 1639–1646
Wynder E L, Reddy B S, McCoy G D, Weisburger J H, Williams G M 1976 Diet and gastrointestinal cancer. Clinics in Gastroenterology 5: 463
Ziegler K, Sanft C, Zimmer T, Zeitz M et al 1993 Comparison of computed tomography, endosonography, and intraoperative assessment in TN staging of gastric carcinoma. Gut 34: 604–610

# 12. Miscellaneous diseases of the stomach and duodenum

*David Shearman*

## MENETRIER'S DISEASE (HYPERTROPHIC GASTRITIS)

This is a rare disease of unknown cause characterized by protein loss from a hypertrophic gastric mucosa. The histological features are not those of gastritis and therefore the term Menetrier's disease should be used. Menetrier's disease is histologically distinct from hypertrophic lymphocytic gastritis (Wolfsen et al 1993) which is a variant of lymphocytic gastritis (p. 326), though both conditions may result in gastric protein loss.

### **Etiology and pathology** (Scharschmidt 1977, Chouraqui et al 1981)

There is some evidence that the disorder may be caused by the altered expression of TGFα (Dempsey et al 1992). *H. pylori* is not thought to be an etiological factor. Macroscopically, the mucosal folds are greatly enlarged throughout the entire body and fundus or sometimes solely along the greater curvature. The antrum is usually normal. On microscopy (Fig. 12.1), the gastric pits (foveolae) are elongated and tortuous, the glands are also elongated and specialized cells are replaced by mucus-secreting cells. Mucosal cysts develop which contain mucin. The lamina propria is edematous and contains a variable infiltrate of inflammatory cells including eosinophils and strands of smooth muscle extend from the muscularis mucosae towards the surface between the glands.

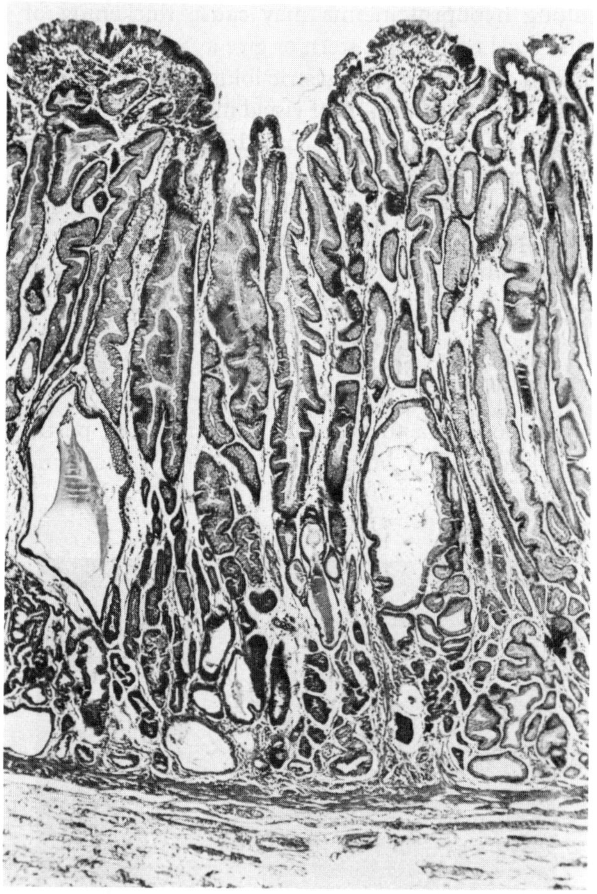

**Fig. 12.1** Menetrier's disease. Section showing thickened gastric mucosa with elongated pits, many of which have a serrated outline and cystic glands (hematoxylin and eosin, ×30).

### **Clinical features** (Searcy & Malagelada 1984, Meuwissen et al 1992)

Most cases occur in middle age, the common presentation being with peripheral edema due to hypoproteinemia. However, some patients have abdominal pain, nausea, vomiting, diarrhea, anorexia or weight loss. The condition is sometimes associated with an increased incidence of severe or recurrent infections, thromboembolic vascular disorders and pulmonary edema. The hypoproteinemia is due to excessive protein loss through widened epithelial tight junctions into the lumen of the stomach. Although this protein is digested and some of the constituent amino acids and peptides are absorbed, the body's capacity to synthesize albumin is exceeded and hypoalbuminemia results. Other serum proteins are lost by the same mechanism. Thus the concentrations of serum albumin and γ-globulins are often reduced. The gastric juice in Menetrier's disease contains 8–9 mg/ml of protein compared to a normal average concentration of 1.7 mg/ml. By contrast, gastric acid secretion is normal, low or absent. Protein loss is best demonstrated by the use of $^{51}$Cr-labeled albumin (p. 348). The use of $\alpha_1$-antitrypsin is not validated as an indicator for gastric protein loss because it is degraded in the stomach (Reinhart et al 1983) (p. 348).

Barium studies (Fig. 12.2) demonstrate tortuous giant rugosal folds predominantly in the proximal stomach and especially along the greater curvature. These folds are flexible in contrast to those caused by lymphoma or carcinoma. The distinction from scirrhous cancer is difficult and may be aided by endoscopic ultrasound (Fujishima et al 1991). Enlarged duodenal folds are common and the resulting hypoproteinemia may cause thickening of the small bowel mucosal pattern or give a "malabsorption pattern". At endoscopy, the gastric folds persist under distention and there are strands of viscid mucus on the surface of the folds. The diagnosis is based on biopsy obtained at endoscopy. The biopsy will not show the full thickness of the mucosa unless forceps with large cusps are used.

In general the course of the disease is protracted but improvement occurs in about half the patients. An increased incidence of gastric cancer is suggested.

### Treatment

There is no satisfactory treatment. Some cases, particularly in childhood (Chouraqui et al 1981), may undergo spontaneous remission. It is thought that the etiology in these children is different from that in adults and may be due to allergy.

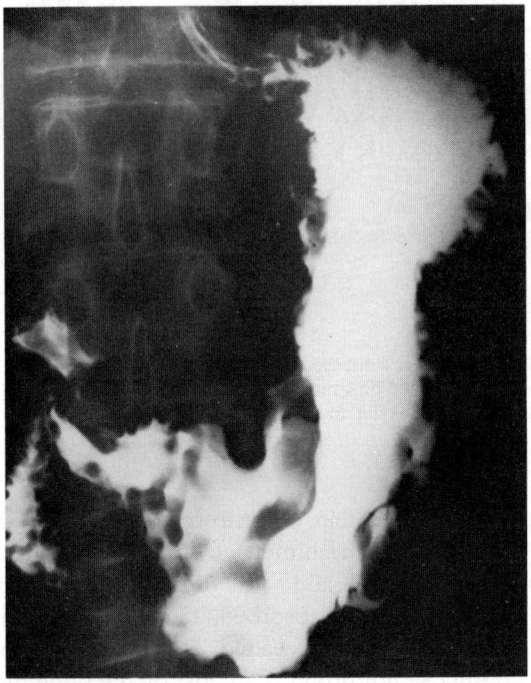

**Fig. 12.2** Menetrier's disease. Giant mucosal folds.

Some patients respond to corticosteroids (Davis et al 1991) but it is possible they have hypertrophic lymphocytic gastritis. Propantheline has been shown to decrease the width of epithelial tight junctions and it reduces protein leakage (Kelly et al 1982). Therapy to reduce acid secretion also reduces protein loss and omeprazole 20 or 40 mg per day has been effective (Bradburn et al 1992). Some cases require partial or subtotal gastrectomy to prevent death from hypoproteinemia.

## EOSINOPHILIC GASTRITIS AND ENTERITIS

### Pathology (Johnstone & Morson 1978a)

Eosinophilic gastroenteritis usually occurs in adults and affects the gastric antrum and pylorus but it may involve the small intestine or very occasionally the large intestine. Macroscopically lesions are typically segmental and appear thickened and indurated. On histology there is edema and a variable eosinophil infiltration of the submucosa (Fig. 12.3). However, in some cases the main muscle coat or subserosa is more affected. This may result in obstruction or ascites with eosinophils in the ascitic fluid. The mucosa is usually spared but may show edema, congestion, eosinophil infiltration, villous abnormality in the small intestine and occasionally ulceration (Katz et al 1977). A band-like infiltrate of eosinophils and mast cells deep in the lamina propria has been observed in some cases associated with connective tissue disorders (DeSchryver-Kecskemeti & Clouse 1984).

### Etiology

The histological features and the peripheral blood eosinophilia support an allergic cause. However, a history of food allergy is usually absent and serum IgE concentrations and other immunological studies are usually normal. Occasional patients with unequivocal allergy to dietary allergens have been described (Caldwell et al 1979). They have raised levels of serum IgE and increased numbers of IgE and IgG cells in the lamina propria of the small intestine. Cases occurring in the tropics may be due to intestinal parasites (Croese 1988), for example the canine hookworm *Ancylostoma caninum* (Croese et al 1994).

### Clinical features

These have been reviewed by Klein et al (1970) and Caldwell et al (1978).

Patients with gastric involvement present with nausea and vomiting and the barium meal may show diffuse ulceration or narrowing of the antrum which is often mis-

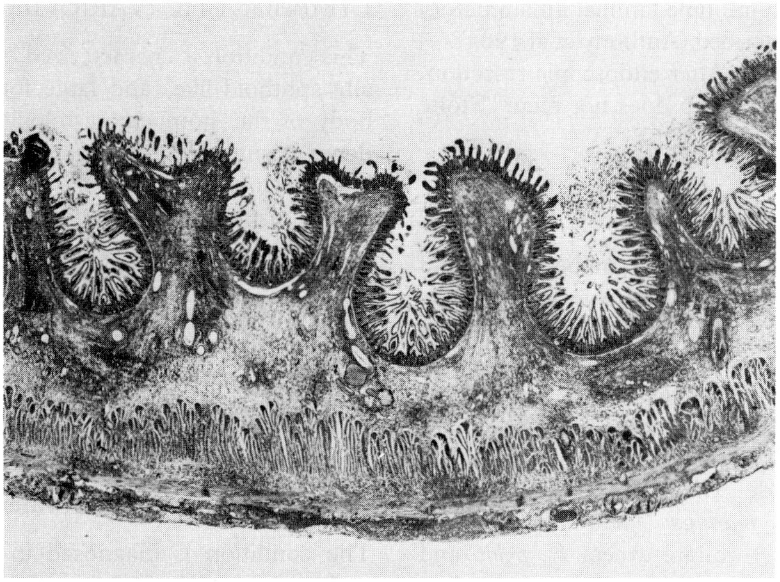

**Fig. 12.3** Esoinophilic enteritis. The wall of the small intestine is thickened by edema and infiltration of the submucosa by eosinophils (hematoxylin and eosin, ×9).

taken for other granulomatous conditions such as tuberculosis, carcinoma, lymphoma or solitary eosinophilic granuloma (see below). Involvement of the intestinal mucosa may cause nausea, vomiting and pain which is often related to the ingestion of specific foods. There may be diarrhea, bleeding and weight loss. However, about half the patients present with symptoms of obstruction. Patients with large bowel involvement present with abdominal pain, diarrhea, nausea, vomiting and weight loss. There may be a palpable mass and rectal bleeding. The cecum and ascending colon are primarily involved (Naylor & Pollet 1985).

The most important findings on investigation are peripheral blood eosinophilia and an increased number of eosinophils in the jejunal biopsy. Biopsies must be obtained from several areas since intestinal involvement is patchy. Occasionally, an eosinophil infiltrate is seen in Crohn's disease or lymphoma. Other common findings are iron deficiency anemia with a positive occult blood test, a decreased serum albumin concentration with evidence of protein-losing enteropathy and abnormal absorption tests. The barium follow-through examination may show solitary or diffuse lesions involving varying lengths of intestine. The combination of irregular fold thickening, ulceration and strictures may simulate the radiological appearances of Crohn's disease. In other patients intestinal lymphoma may be simulated.

Cases caused by *A. caninum* have segmental and/or distal small bowel inflammation with or without ascites and a positive ELISA test against hookworm secretions.

Children with eosinophilic gastritis or enteritis usually present with failure to thrive. Symptoms of vomiting, diarrhea, asthma, rhinitis or urticaria are present in about half of the patients.

### Treatment

Some patients respond well to the elimination of any suspected foodstuff from the diet (Greenberger et al 1967). Most patients respond dramatically to prednisolone 20 mg per day for a week, but sometimes it may be necessary to prolong this therapy or to continue with a reduced dosage for many months. Ulceration secondary to eosinophilic gastritis does not respond to $H_2$ receptor antagonists (Stolte et al 1991). When a parasitic cause is suspected, treatment is with mebendazole (Croese 1988).

## INFLAMMATORY FIBROID POLYP (EOSINOPHILIC GRANULOMA) (Salmon & Paulley 1967, Johnstone & Morson 1978b).

This must be distinguished from eosinophilic gastroenteritis. It consists of a polypoid lesion found most frequently in the stomach or small bowel but occurring also in the large bowel. It is responsible for 5% of all gastric polyps and 87% are in the antrum or at the incisura (Stolte & Finkenzeller 1990). The surface is usually ulcerated and the core is formed by loose vascular connective tissue containing eosinophils. The connective tissue is of variable cellularity and the vessels may be capillary in size or larger, including thickwalled muscular vessels. The deep aspect of the lesion may involve the main muscle coat. Within the stomach, the polyp ulcerates and bleeds or causes pyloric obstruction. Occasionally it appears as an ulcer (Adachi et al 1992).

A polyp in the small intestine or colon may cause abdominal pain, intussusception or bleeding (Shimer & Helwig 1984). There is no history of allergy and no eosinophilia. A family with multiple familial inflammatory fibroid polyps has been described (Anthony et al 1984).

The treatment is resection. After endoscopic resection, gastric inflammatory fibroid polyp does not recur (Stolte & Finkenzeller 1990).

## INFECTIVE GASTRITIS

A number of pathogenic organisms can be found and identified in the gastric mucosa. These include viruses such as cytomegalovirus and *Herpes simplex* virus, bacteria which include *Treponema pallidum, Mycobacterium tuberculosis, Mycobacterium avium-intracellulare* and the most common, *Helicobacter pylori*. Fungi include *Candida albicans, Aspergillus fumigatus*, mucormycosis and *Histoplasma capsulatum*. Parasites include *Giardia intestinalis*, cryptosporidium, *Anasakis marinum* and *Strongyloides stercoralis*. All of the above are rare except *H. pylori* and detection generally should prompt specific antimicrobial therapies. In many instances underlying immunosuppression from diabetes, HIV infection or nutritional deficiencies exists. *H. pylori* can cause an acute gastritis in the acute phase of infection but this is rarely encountered clinically (Morris & Nicholson 1987).

## PHLEGMONOUS GASTRITIS (Miller et al 1975)

This is a rare form of acute gastritis due to intramural infection usually with α-hemolytic streptococci, but sometimes with other organisms. If gas-forming organisms are involved emphysematous gastritis may result (Kussin et al 1982). This condition occurs in subjects with malnutrition, chronic alcoholism and may also follow an upper respiratory tract infection. Endoscopic assessment reveals mucosal edema with an exudate. Microscopy reveals edema of the mucosa and submucosa with an intense inflammatory infiltrate. Bacteria can be identified in the gastric wall. Thrombosis of submucosal vessels and mucosal necrosis and sloughing are also present.

The clinical symptoms are severe acute upper abdominal pain with associated nausea, vomiting, hematemesis and hiccups.

Clinical examination reveals epigastric tenderness and peritonism with occasional epigastric distention. Fever and an elevated white cell count are always present. The provisional diagnosis is often acute appendicitis or pancreatitis and the correct diagnosis is made at laparotomy, when the stomach appears infarcted and there may be peritonitis (Zazzo et al 1992). With emphysematous gastritis the diagnosis may be made on plain radiography of the abdomen with fine, curved collections of gas seen in the wall of the stomach (Meyers & Parker 1967). The mortality is high unless the infected area is resected or drained and large doses of parenteral antibiotics, usually penicillin, are given.

## LYMPHOCYTIC (VARIOLIFORM) GASTRITIS

This condition is characterized by nodules, erosions (usually aphthoid-like) and large folds predominantly in the body of the stomach; histological examination shows a dense accumulation of small lymphocytes in the surface and foveolar epithelium (Haot et al 1988, 1989). Occasionally the large folds may simulate Menetrier's disease (Wolfsen et al 1993) and there may be gastric protein loss. The infiltrate is of mature T-cells and may occur in the stomach in celiac disease (Wolber et al 1990). The condition does not appear to be related to *H. pylori* infection although it may represent a response to a local antigen (Dixon et al 1988).

### Clinical features and treatment

The condition is diagnosed in about 0.1% of patients undergoing upper gastrointestinal endoscopy and in 1% of those with nonulcer dyspepsia (Jaskiewicz et al 1991).

Endoscopic biopsy is vital in making the diagnosis as histological evidence may be found when the characteristic endoscopic appearance is absent (Haot et al 1990). Intraepithelial lymphocytes are increased in number and the epithelium is edematous and infiltrated with lymphocytes. Erosions may be present.

Treatment is symptomatic. In some patients, sodium chromoglycate 200 mg per day has reduced symptoms (André et al 1982).

## OTHER GRANULOMATOUS DISEASES OF THE STOMACH

A variety of other conditions can cause a granulomatous reaction in the stomach, e.g. Crohn's disease (Farman et al 1975) (p. 649), tuberculosis (Balikian et al 1967) (p. 569) and other chronic infections. All present in the same manner with epigastric pain and vomiting, hematemesis or gastric outlet obstruction. When barium studies are performed, the lesion may mimic erosive gastritis (Laufer et al 1976) or linitis plastica (Gonzalez & Kennedy 1974) and if the duodenum is involved in continuity the findings may mimic a previous Billroth I gastroduodenostomy (Nelson 1969).

## BEZOARS

Bezoars are usually composed of hair (trichobezoars) or plant materials (phytobezoars), particularly orange pith and persimmon. In children lactobezoars or food-bolus bezoars, e.g. candy, are reported (Yulevich et al 1993). Bezoars may also form from bulk laxatives (Schneider 1989) or slow-release pharmaceuticals (Prisant et al 1991).

### Etiology and clinical features

Phytobezoars are the more common and usually occur after gastric surgery (Tebar et al 1992) or in conditions with reduced gastric motility (p. 430) such as diabetic gastroparesis.

In bezoar formation after gastric surgery, 80% of patients present with intestinal obstruction (Tebar et al 1992). At laparotomy an attempt is made to fragment the bezoar and milk it to the cecum.

When the bezoar is in the stomach, there is epigastric pain and nausea and gastric ulceration or perforation may occur. On the plain, erect abdominal radiograph, the bezoar may show as a soft tissue mass floating at the air–fluid level and on barium meal examination a movable mass is seen which becomes coated with barium, resulting in a mottled or streaky appearance. Sometimes it has the appearance of a smooth filling defect. Gastroscopy usually shows green or yellow vegetable matter within the mass. Trichobezoars present in the same way but occur most often in young females who have no other gastric disease. Rarely they may cause protein-losing gastropathy.

### Treatment of gastric bezoar

Phytobezoar may resolve spontaneously (Kadian et al 1978) and immediate therapy is necessary only if symptoms are severe. Phytobezoars can be disrupted by lavage or at endoscopy and many can be digested by enzyme (Stanten & Peters 1975). Smaller bezoars may be emptied from the stomach following intravenous erythromycin in a dose of 3 mg/kg by infusion every 8 h. This is particularly useful in patients with diabetic gastroparesis. If these methods fail gastrostomy is indicated. Trichobezoars usually have to be removed surgically.

## GASTRIC DIVERTICULUM (Localio & Stahl 1968)

A gastric diverticulum is found in about 0.1% of upper gastrointestinal studies. It is usually unimportant in itself, but requiring recognition because it may be mistaken for an ulcer.

The most common site is on the posterior wall, a few centimeters below the esophagogastric junction; some 15% occur in the prepyloric region, but they are rarely found elsewhere in the stomach. The prepyloric diverticulum is usually associated with ulceration or another inflammatory process; the juxtacardiac diverticulum, a true diverticulum containing muscularis, probably arises because of a defect in the muscle of the stomach wall. Multiple gastric diverticula are rare (Schweiger & Noonan 1991).

### Clinical features (Palmer 1951, Tillander & Hesselsjo 1968)

Most are diagnosed when barium studies are carried out because of upper gastrointestinal symptoms; when no other lesion is found, the patient's symptoms are attributed to the diverticulum, although it remains in doubt whether or not a diverticulum causes symptoms.

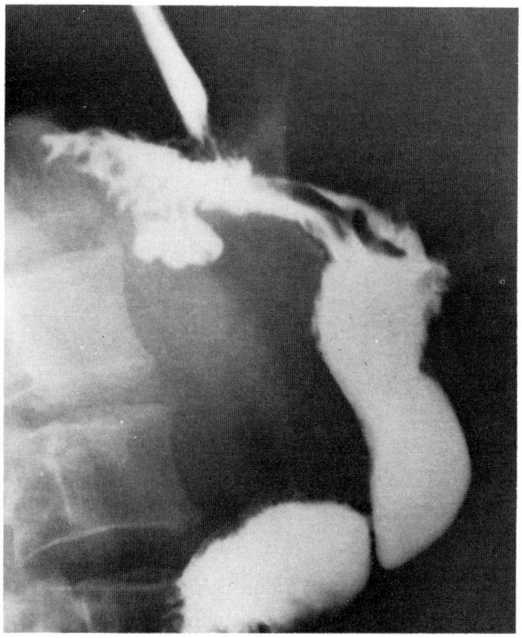

**Fig. 12.4** Gastric diverticulum arising from fundus of stomach – the common site. Note normal mucosal pattern in the diverticulum which differentiates it from gastric ulcer.

The juxtacardiac diverticulum is easy to recognize on barium study: it is smooth, 2–4 cm in diameter with a variable contour and often the gastric folds can be seen to enter the diverticulum (Fig. 12.4). A diverticulum near to the pylorus is more difficult to distinguish from an ulcer, but often it shows the same features as the juxtacardiac type.

### Treatment

Surgery is not indicated unless there is suspicion of mucosal disease within the diverticulum.

## GASTRIC AND DUODENAL DUPLICATION

These are very rare. There is duplication of all layers of the wall of the stomach or duodenum. The lesion usually develops in childhood as a mass; there is pain, vomiting and bleeding (Knight et al 1985). Carcinoma may arise in the duplication (Falk et al 1991).

## GASTRIC VOLVULUS

Volvulus of the stomach is classified according to the axis of twisting (Fig. 12.5). In mixed gastric volvulus, there is

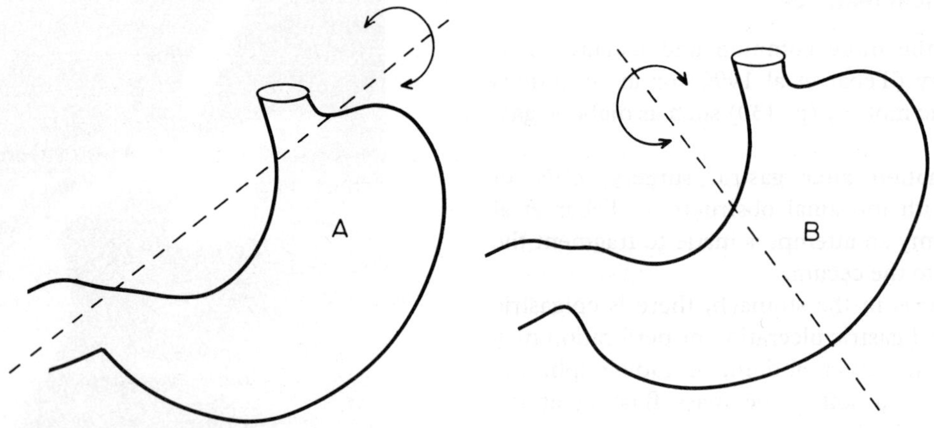


**Fig. 12.5** Types of gastric volvulus. (A) The axis of rotation in an organoaxial volvulus: (B) the axis in a mesenterioaxial volvulus (Wastell & Ellis 1971).

twisting along both axes. Factors predisposing to torsion are weakening of the fibrous attachments or "ligaments" of the stomach and the presence of additional space into which the stomach can rotate, for example a large para-esophageal hiatus (Haas et al 1990) or eventration of the diaphragm (Tanner 1968).

## Clinical features and diagnosis

With acute volvulus, the torsion results in a closed loop obstruction and strangulation. There is severe, continuous epigastric pain, retching but no vomiting and distention of the upper abdomen. Shock supervenes. The diagnosis is made by means of an erect plain radiograph, which shows two distinct fluid levels in the region of the gastric fundus, and by a barium swallow in which barium fails to enter the stomach. The mortality is 50%.

Chronic volvulus is suspected when there is epigastric discomfort or pain, bloating, belching and borborygmi. Symptoms are precipitated by large meals. There may be breathlessness because it is common for part of the stomach to be in the thorax (Fig. 12.6). Barium studies are helpful in that a twisted stomach may be seen (Fig. 12.7), or there may be a paraesophageal hernia or eventration of

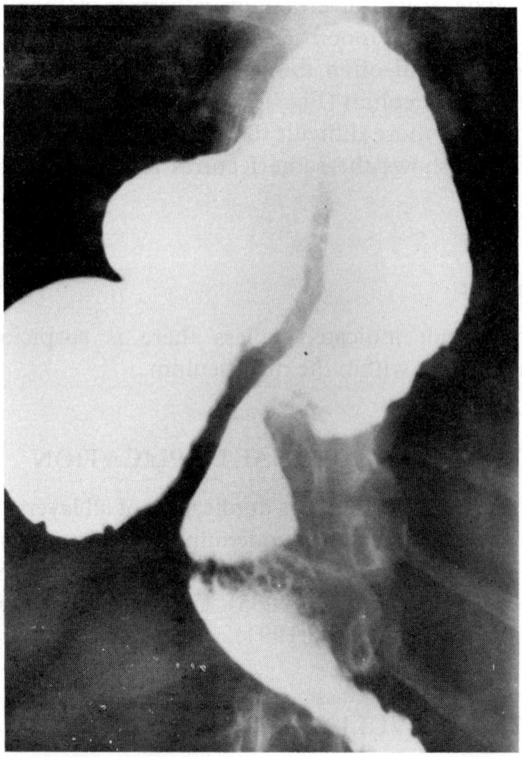

**Fig. 12.6** Intrathoracic stomach. The stomach has rotated and herniated through the esophageal hiatus.

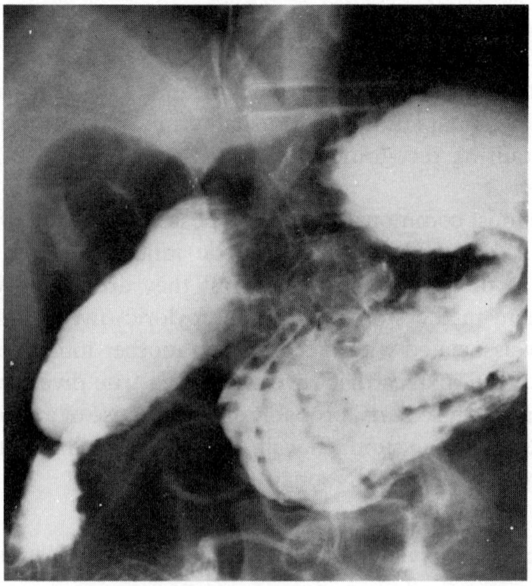

**Fig. 12.7** Volvulus of stomach. The fundus of the stomach is the most dependent part and the greater curvature is uppermost.

the diaphragm which may predispose to intermittent twisting. The mortality is less than 10%.

### Treatment

Both forms of volvulus should be treated surgically regardless of age; in the acute form, the procedure is an emergency. After decompression, gastropexy is performed together with procedures to close a paraesophageal hiatus or eventration (Gosin & Ballinger 1965). In some patients endoscopic correction of the volvulus may be possible (Bhasin et al 1990).

## CHEMICAL DAMAGE TO THE STOMACH

The oesophagus is first in line for injury when acid, alkali or other injurious chemicals are accidentally swallowed (p. 183). When a larger volume is swallowed, injury to the stomach also arises; this tends to occur in adults who are alcoholics or in those attempting suicide.

A wide spectrum of damage occurs, from surface erosion to complete liquefaction of the stomach with perforation. In those patients who survive, antral and pyloric fibrosis and stenosis result because the corrosive agent pools in the antrum.

### Clinical features (Citron et al 1968)

The patient has oral and pharyngeal pain and symptoms of esophageal damage may be present (p. 183). There is immediate severe epigastric pain which can be followed by hematemesis and peritonitis. Patients with less severe injury progress over several months to epigastric pain, vomiting and weight loss as a result of antral stenosis. If the history of ingestion is not obtained, the disease may be mistaken for carcinoma on barium studies, as the radiological appearance is similar (Poteshman 1967); however, endoscopy and biopsy will clearly differentiate the two conditions.

### Treatment (see also p. 184)

There is a case for early fiberoptic endoscopy for the diagnosis of gastric and esophageal injury. With sodium hydroxide burns, early laparotomy to assess gastric damage is recommended followed by adequate gastric resection if necessary (Chung & DenBesten 1975, Meredith et al 1988). Others are treated by nasogastric suction and intravenous fluids. Elective surgery is usually necessary for those who develop antral and pyloric stenosis.

## SPONTANEOUS GASTRIC RUPTURE

Gastric rupture due to blunt abdominal trauma is very rare (Yajko et al 1975). Nontraumatic rupture can result from overeating or drinking, from sodium bicarbonate ingestion (LeDoux et al 1991) or from gastric inflation due to mouth-to-mouth resuscitation or nasal oxygen administration (Demos & Poticha 1964). The patient presents with shock, severe abdominal distention, diffuse peritonitis and sometimes subcutaneous emphysema; it is unusual for the diagnosis to be made before laparotomy and survival is very uncommon.

## INTRALUMINAL DUODENAL DIVERTICULUM
(Karoll et al 1983)

This is rare and probably results from a duodenal diaphragm, although some maintain it is a separate entity because it is attached only to a small segment of the duodenal wall (Mathieu et al 1978). It can therefore be associated with the congenital abnormalities associated with the diaphragm. The diverticulum is a mucosal sac lined on both sides by mucosa and attached to the duodenal wall near to the ampulla of Vater. The diverticulum can be likened to a windsock.

### Clinical features

The patient is nearly always symptomatic; there is abdominal pain and vomiting and gastrointestinal bleeding is common. Pancreatitis occurs when the diverticulum arises near to the ampulla (Willemer et al 1992). There may be obstruction. The diagnosis is made on the radiological appearance of a pear-shaped barium-filled structure commencing in the region of the ampulla and lying entirely within the lumen of the duodenum. However, the sac may not fill with barium and it then has to be recognized by a radiolucent longitudinal streak against the barium-coated duodenal wall.

### Treatment

This is surgical excision or bypass. Alternatively, endoscopic treatment is sometimes successful (Ravi et al 1993). Removal of impacted material from the sac may relieve obstructive symptoms and sometimes the outlet of the diverticulum can be enlarged with a diathermy polypectomy snare.

## DUODENAL DIVERTICULUM (EXTRALUMINAL DIVERTICULUM)

This term is usually reserved for the common form of diverticulum – an outpouching of the duodenal mucosa (Fig. 12.8). The consensus of opinion is that it is acquired and occurs at a point of weakness on the medial duodenal wall. The diverticulum is usually solitary and is seen in 5% of upper gastrointestinal barium or endoscopic studies (Afridi et al 1991). In two-thirds of cases it is on the medial wall of the duodenum near to the ampulla.

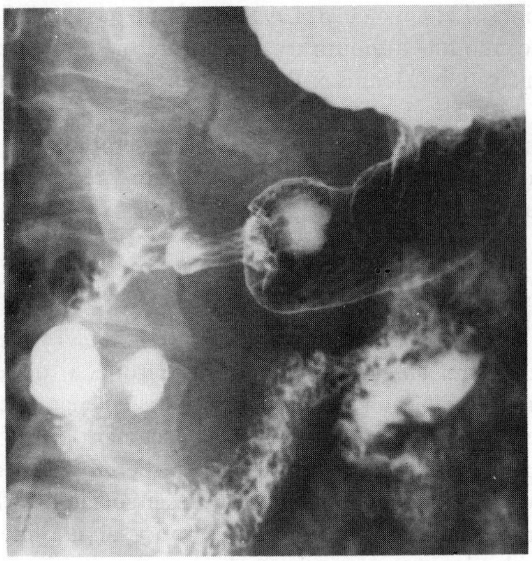

**Fig. 12.8** Two duodenal diverticula opposite the ampulla of Vater – the common site.

### Clinical features

Symptoms are rare; when present, they consist of pain, nausea, vomiting and weight loss. Many are recognized coincidentally during endoscopy or ERCP, when cannulation may be rendered more difficult by the entry of the biliary and pancreatic ducts into or adjacent to a diverticulum of the second part of the duodenum.

*Complications*

When complications arise they are serious and mortality is comman (Munnell & Preston 1966).

***Obstruction to the bile duct or pancreatic duct*** (Afridi et al 1991). The majority of diverticula lie in the region of the ampulla. As the common bile duct often terminates in the diverticulum, where it can be obstructed by kinking or by food or enteroliths, obstructive jaundice or pancreatitis can result. Patients with a diverticulum in the second part of the duodenum have a higher incidence of gallstones than patients with a diverticulum more distally, which suggests that chronic obstruction to the common bile duct may occur. Such patients have higher numbers of bacteria in the duodenum and bile duct than those without diverticula (Skar et al 1989).

***Hemorrhage.*** This is usually severe and results from ulceration of the wall of the diverticulum with erosion of an artery.

***Perforation*** (Duarte et al 1992). This is very uncommon and may be due to the formation of an enterolith which erodes the wall of the diverticulum or to diverticulitis. The perforation is usually retroperitoneal and, at laparotomy, retroperitoneal edema and bile staining are clues to the diagnosis. There is a mortality rate of 13%. A fistula may develop between the diverticulum and the duodenum or other organs.

***Metabolic complications.*** These are rare. Extensive colonization of the diverticulum may occur without malabsorptive problems (Gorbach & Levitan 1970), but in other patients malabsorption has been reported (Breen & Connell 1989).

### **Treatment** (Donald 1979)

Surgical treatment is necessary for hemorrhage, perforation or obstruction to the common duct. Bleeding is localized by endoscopy and arteriography and the diverticulum is excised. Perforated diverticulum is treated by excision, closure and drainage; when the diverticulum is periampullary, the duodenum is mobilized and the common duct exposed before the diverticulum is excised. When there is obstruction to the common duct, it is safer to carry out a choledochoduodenostomy. Patients with pancreaticobiliary disease may be best treated with duodenojejunostomy which avoids the difficulties of resection of the diverticulum (Critchlow et al 1985).

## DUODENAL OBSTRUCTION

A number of congenital abnormalities can produce duodenal obstruction – for example, annular pancreas (p. 1228) and ectopic pancreatic tissue (p. 1228). Nonrotation of the midgut can present in the adult as duodenal obstruction or with chronic abdominal pain (Fukuya et al 1993). Surgery for duodenal atresia may lead to complications in adult life including reduced duodenal peristalsis and duodenal diverticulum (Kokkonen et al 1988).

### Duodenal diaphragm (web)

This is regarded as an incomplete form of *duodenal atresia* and it occurs in association with other anomalies including annular pancreas, midgut malrotation, situs inversus, choledochocele, imperforate anus, Hirschsprung's disease and congenital abnormalities of other systems. The obstruction is periampullary (Madura et al 1991). The proximal duodenum becomes dilated and the obstructing diaphragm may balloon into the distal duodenum to produce an intraluminal duodenal diverticulum (BMJ 1972).

When the condition presents in adulthood, there is vomiting and weight loss. The web is sometimes associated with a peptic ulcer. Surgical treatment consists of excision of the diaphragm or gastrojejunostomy.

### Infiltrative and infective conditions

In Crohn's disease, the duodenum is involved in 1–2% of cases. There is intermittent upper abdominal pain and symptoms of duodenal obstruction (Nugent & Roy 1989).

**Tuberculosis** (Gupta et al 1988)

Duodenal obstruction is common and is due to compression by extrinsic glands or to intrinsic strictures. Ulceration of the duodenum may also occur, leading to symptoms of peptic ulcer.

### Other causes

Duodenal obstruction has occurred in endometriosis (Cuzzo-Kriner 1989), eosinophilic gastroenteritis (Farahvash et al 1990) and Brunner's gland hyperplasia (Peetz & Moseley 1989). The latter may also bleed.

Polyps and tumors may also cause obstruction (p. 466), as may primary malignancy of the duodenum.

Obstruction caused by pancreatic disease is discussed in Chapter 50 and by peptic ulcer in Chapter 10.

The duodenum may be obstructed by a gallstone (Bouveret's syndrome). There is air in the biliary tree (pneumobilia), a large calcified density in the right upper quadrant or a filling defect in the duodenal cap and gastric distention (Crans & Cloney 1991).

### Vascular causes

Superior mesenteric artery syndrome may occur, presenting with chronic (pain and weight loss) or acute obstructive symptoms. Operative treatment may be necessary (Ylinen et al 1989, Marchant et al 1989) but is frequently unsuccessful since there may be an underlying motility disorder of the duodenal loop (p. 440).

Aortic aneurysm may cause direct compression of the duodenum (Sostek et al 1993).

Anomalous (preduodenal) portal vein occurs when the portal vein passes anterior rather than posterior to the duodenum. It may compress the first or second part of the duodenum. It is usually associated with malrotation and other congenital abnormalities.

### Duodenal polyps and tumors

Adenoma, leiomyoma and lipoma account for 90% of benign duodenal tumors (Colborn et al 1989). Duodenal adenomatous polyps develop in nearly all patients with familial adenomatous polyposis coli. They tend to be located close to the duodenal papilla and they become malignant (p. 1408). Duodenal polyps, adenomatous or hamartomatous, also occur in the Peutz–Jeghers syndrome (p. 1413) and are premalignant (Foley et al 1988). Gastric, duodenal and ampullary adenomas occur in the hereditary flat adenoma syndrome (p. 1411) (Lynch et al 1993). (See also Table 55.4 and p. 1411 juvenile polyposis, p. 1413 Cronkhite–Canada syndrome.)

Polyps of the duodenal bulb are commonly due to gastric metaplasia or simple cysts (Matsui & Kitagawa 1993). Commonly they are due to adenoma or Brunner's gland hyperplasia (Kaplan et al 1968) which may be associated with uremia (Paimela et al 1984).

Primary malignancy of the duodenum is usually adenocarcinoma (Colborn et al 1989). These tumors are discussed in conjunction with those of the small intestine (p. 467).

## OTHER ABNORMALITIES OF THE DUODENUM

Other abnormalities may be found when barium studies or endoscopy are performed for upper gastrointestinal symptoms. Duodenitis is discussed on p. 230. Filling defects occur with duodenal varices (Itzchak & Glickman 1977). Duodenal hematoma, resulting from blunt abdominal trauma or due to intramural bleeding as a complication of bleeding diathesis or anticoagulant therapy, is seen on barium study as an intramural mass (Resnicoff & Morton 1969).

## REFERENCES


Adachi Y, Mori M, Iida M, Tsuneyoshi M, Sugimachi K 1992 Inflammatory fibroid polyp of the stomach. Report of three unusual cases. Journal of Clinical Gastroenterology 15: 154–158

Afridi S A, Fichtenbaum C J, Taubin H 1991 Review of duodenal diverticula. American Journal of Gastroenterology 86: 935–938

André C, Gillon J, Moulinier B, Martin A, Fargier M C 1982 Randomised placebo-controlled double-blind trial of two dosages of sodium cromoglycate in treatment of varioliform gastritis: comparison with cimetidine. Gut 23: 348–352

Anthony P P, Morris D S, Vowles K D J 1984 Multiple and recurrent inflammatory fibroid polyps in three generations of a Devon family: a new syndrome. Gut 25: 854–862

Balikian J P, Yenikomshian S M, Jidejian Y D 1967 Tuberculosis of the pyloro-duodenal area. Report of four cases. American Journal of Roentgenology 101: 414–420

Bhasin D K, Nagi B, Kochhar R et al 1990 Endoscopic management of chronic organoaxial volvulus of the stomach. American Journal of Gastroenterology 85: 1486–1488

Bradburn D M, Redwood N F W, Venables C W, Gunn A 1992 Medical therapy of Menetrier's disease with omeprazole. Digestion 52: 204–208

Breen K J, Connell J L 1989 Surgical treatment of duodenal diverticula associated with symptomatic bacterial overgrowth. Australian and New Zealand Journal of Surgery 59: 819–821

British Medical Journal 1972 Editorial: duodenal diaphragm. 2: 482

Caldwell J H, Mekhjian H S, Hurtubise P E, Beman F M 1978 Eosinophilic gastroenteritis with obstruction. Immunological studies of seven patients. Gastroenterology 74: 825–829

Caldwell J H, Sharma H M, Hurtubise P E, Colwell D L 1979 Eosinophilic gastroenteritis in extreme allergy. Immunopathological comparison with nonallergic gastrointestinal disease. Gastroenterology 77: 560–564

Chouraqui J P, Roy C C, Brochu P et al 1981 Menetrier's disease in children: report of a patient and review of sixteen other cases. Gastroenterology 80: 1042–1047

Chung R S K, DenBesten L 1975 Fibreoptic endoscopy in treatment of corrosive injury of the stomach. Archives of Surgery 110: 725–728

Citron B P, Pincus I J, Geokas M C, Haverback B J 1968 Chemical

trauma of the esophagus and stomach. Surgical Clinics of North America 48: 1303–1311
Colborn G L, Gray S W, Pemberton L B, Skandalakis L J, Skandalakis J E 1989 The duodenum. Part 3: Pathology. American Surgeon 55: 469–473
Crans C A, Cloney D J 1991 Bouveret's syndrome: an unusual twist on the classic cause. Southern Medical Journal 84: 1049–1051
Critchlow J F, Shapiro M E, Silen W 1985 Duodenojejunostomy for the pancreaticobiliary complications of duodenal diverticulum. Annals of Surgery 202: 56–58
Croese T J 1988 Eosinophilic enteritis – a recent North Queensland experience. Australian and New Zealand Journal of Medicine 18: 848–853
Croese J, Loukas A, Opdebeeck J, Prociv P 1994 Occult enteric infection by *Ancylostoma caninum*: a previously unrecognized zoonosis. Gastroenterology 106: 3–12
Cuzzo-Kriner M R 1989 Intestinal endometriosis and its complications: case report and review. Mount Sinai Journal of Medicine 56: 334–337
Davis G E, O'Rourke M C, Metz J R, Kindig W V, Sweeney J G, Kane K N 1991 Hypertrophic gastropathy symptoms responsive to prednisone. A case report and a review of the literature. Journal of Clinical Gastroenterology 13: 436–441
Demos N J, Poticha S M 1964 Gastric rupture occurring during external cardiac resuscitation. Surgery 55: 364–366
Dempsey P J, Goldenring J R, Soroka C J et al 1992 Possible role of transforming growth factor $\alpha$ in the pathogenesis of Menetrier's disease: supportive evidence from humans and transgenic mice. Gastroenterology 103: 1950–1963
DeSchryver-Kecskemeti K, Clouse R E 1984 A previously unrecognized subgroup of "eosinophilic gastroenteritis". Association with connective tissue disease. American Journal of Surgical Pathology 8: 171–180
Dixon M F, Wyatt J I, Burke D A, Rathbone B J 1988 Lymphocytic gastritis – relationship to *Campylobacter pylori* infection. Journal of Pathology 154: 125–132
Donald J W 1979 Major complications of small bowel diverticula. Annals of Surgery 190: 183–188
Duarte B, Nagy K K, Cintron J 1992 Perforated duodenal diverticulum. British Journal of Surgery 79: 877–881
Falk G L, Young C J, Parer J 1991 Adenocarcinoma arising in a duodenal duplication cyst: a case report. Australian and New Zealand Journal of Surgery 61: 551–553
Farahvash M J, Bastani B, Farahvash M R, Irvanlou G 1990 Eosinophilic gastroenteritis presenting with biliary and partial duodenal obstruction. American Journal of Gastroenterology 85: 1022–1024
Farman J, Faegenburg D, Dallenmand S, Chen C 1975 Crohn's disease of the stomach: the "ram's horn" sign. American Journal of Roentgenology 123: 242–251
Foley T R, McGarrity T J, Abt A B 1988 Peutz–Jeghers syndrome: a clinicopathologic survey of the "Harrisburg family" with a 49-year follow-up. Gastroenterology 95: 1535–1540
Fujishima H, Misawa T, Chijiiwa Y, Maruoka A, Akahoshi K, Nawata H 1991 Scirrhous carcinoma of the stomach versus hypertrophic gastritis: findings at endoscopic US. Radiology 181: 197–200
Fukuya T, Brown B P, Lu C C 1993 Midgut volvulus as a complication of intestinal malrotation in adults. Digestive Diseases and Sciences 38: 438–444
Gonzalez G, Kennedy T 1974 Crohn's disease of the stomach. Radiology 113: 27–29
Gorbach S L, Levitan R 1970 Intestinal flora in health and in gastrointestinal diseases. In: Glass G B J (Ed) Progress in gastroenterology, Vol II. Grune and Stratton, New York, p 252–275
Gosin S, Ballinger W F 1965 Recurrent volvulus of the stomach. Report of a case with recurrence after simple decompression. American Journal of Surgery 109: 642–646
Greenberger N J, Tennenbaum J I, Ruppert R D 1967 Protein-losing enteropathy associated with gastrointestinal allergy. American Journal of Medicine 43: 777–778
Gupta S K, Jain A K, Gupta J P, Agrawal A K, Berry K 1988 Duodenal tuberculosis. Clinical Radiology 39: 159–161
Haas O, Rat P, Christophe M, Friedman S, Favre J P 1990 Surgical results of intrathoracic gastric volvulus complicating hiatal hernia. British Journal of Surgery 77: 1379–1381
Haot J, Hamichi L, Wallez L, Mainguet P 1988 Lymphocytic gastritis: a newly described entity: a retrospective endoscopic and histological study. Gut 29: 1258–1264
Haot J, Berger F, Andre C, Mouliner B, Mainguet P, Lambert R 1989 Lymphocytic gastritis versus varioliform gastritis. A historical series revisited. Journal of Pathology 158: 19–22
Haot J, Jouret A, Willette M, Gossuin A, Mainguet P 1990 Lymphocytic gastritis – prospective study of its relationship with varioliform gastritis. Gut 31: 282–285
Itzchak Y, Glickman M G 1977 Duodenal varices in extrahepatic portal obstruction. Radiology 124: 619–624
Jaskiewicz K, Price S K, Zak J, Louwrens M D 1991 Lymphocytic gasritis in nonulcer dyspepsia. Digestive Diseases and Sciences 36: 1079–1083
Johnstone J M, Morson B C 1978a Eosinophilic gastroenteritis. Histopathology 2: 335–348
Johnstone J M, Morson B C 1978b Inflammatory fibroid polyp of the gastrointestinal tract. Histopathology 2: 349–361
Kadian R S, Rose J F, Mann N S 1978 Gastric bezoars – spontaneous resolution. American Journal of Gastroenterology 70: 79–80
Kaplan E L, Dyson W L, Fitts W T 1968 Hyperplasia of Brunner's glands of the duodenum. Surgery, Gynecology and Obstetrics 126: 371–375
Karoll M P, Ghahremani G G, Port R B, Rosenberg J L 1983 Diagnosis and management of intraluminal duodenal diverticulum. Digestive Diseases and Sciences 28: 411–416
Katz A J, Goldman H, Grand R J 1977 Gastric mucosal biopsy in eosinophilic (allergic) gastroenteritis. Gastroenterology 73: 705–709
Kelly D G, Miller L J, Malagelada J-R et al 1982 Giant hypertrophic gastropathy (Menetrier's disease): pharmacologic effects on protein leakage and mucosal ultrastructure. Gastroenterology 83: 581–589
Klein N C, Hargrove R L, Sleisenger M H, Jeffries G H 1970 Eosinophilic gastroenteritis. Medicine 49: 299–319
Knight C D, Allen M J, Nagorney D M, Wold L E, DiMagno E P 1985 Duodenal duplication cyst causing massive bleeding in an adult: an unusual complication of a duplication cyst of the digestive tract. Mayo Clinic Proceedings 60: 772–775
Kokkonen M-L, Kalima T, Jaaskelainen J, Louhimo I 1988 Duodenal atresia: late follow-up. Journal of Pediatric Surgery 23: 216–220
Kussin S Z, Henry C, Navarro C, Stenson W, Clain D J 1982 Gas within the wall of the stomach. Report of a case and review of the literature. Digestive Diseases and Sciences 27: 949–954
Laufer I, Trueman T, deSa D 1976 Multiple superficial gastric erosions due to Crohn's disease of the stomach. Radiologic and endoscopic diagnosis. British Journal of Radiology 49: 726–728
LeDoux M S, Sillers M J, Atkins C P 1991 Spontaneous rupture of the stomach in an adult. Southern Medical Journal. 84: 399–401
Localio S A, Stahl W M 1968 Diverticular disease of the alimentary tract. Part II. The esophagus, stomach, duodenum and small intestine. Current Problems in Surgery, January monograph
Lynch H T, Smyrk T C, Lanspa S J et al 1993 Upper gastrointestinal manifestations in families with hereditary flat adenoma syndrome. Cancer 71: 2709–2714
Madura J A, Goulet R J, Wahle D T 1991 Duodenal web in the adult. American Surgeon 57: 607–614
Marchant E A, Alvear D T, Fagelman K M 1989 True clinical entity of vascular compression of the duodenum in adolescence. Surgery, Gynecology and Obstetrics 168: 381–386
Mathieu B, Salducci J, Remacle J-P, Pin G, Monges H 1978 Intraluminal duodenal diverticulum. Report of a case investigated by fiberoptic endoscopy. Digestive Diseases and Sciences 23: 1s–5s
Matsui K, Kitagawa M 1993 Biopsy study of polyps in the duodenal bulb. American Journal of Gastroenterology 88: 253–257
Meredith J W, Kon N D, Thompson J N 1988 Journal of Trauma 28(8): 1173–1180
Meuwissen S G M, Ridwan B U, Hasper H J, Innemee G 1992 Hypertrophic protein-losing gastropathy. A retrospective analysis of 40 cases in The Netherlands. Scandinavian Journal of Gastroenterology 27(suppl 194): 1–7
Meyers H I, Parker J J 1967 Emphysematous gastritis. Radiology 89: 426–431

Miller A I, Smith B, Rogers A I 1975 Phlegmonous gastritis. Gastroenterology 68: 231–238
Morris A, Nicholson G 1987 Ingestion of Campylobacter causes gastritis and raised fasting pH. American Journal of Gastroenterology 82: 192–199
Munnell E R, Preston W J 1966 Complications of duodenal diverticula. Archives of Surgery 92: 152–156
Naylor A R, Pollet J E 1985 Eosinophilic colitis. Diseases of the Colon and Rectum 28: 615–618
Nelson S W 1969 Some interesting and unusual manifestations of Crohn's disease ("regional enteritis") of the stomach, duodenum and small intestine. American Journal of Roentgenology 107: 86–101
Nugent F W, Roy M A 1989 Duodenal Crohn's disease: an analysis of 89 cases. American Journal of Gastroenterology 84: 249–254
Paimela H, Tallgren L G, Stenman S, Numers H V, Scheinin T M 1984 Multiple duodenal polyps in uraemia: a little known clinical entity. Gut 25: 259–263
Palmer E D 1951 Gastric diverticula. Collective review. International Abstracts of Surgery 92: 417–428
Peetz M E, Moseley H S 1989 Brunner's gland hyperplasia. American Surgeon 55: 474–477
Poteshman N L 1967 Corrosive gastritis due to hydrochloric acid ingestion. Report of a case. American Journal of Roentgenology 99: 182–185
Prisant L M, Carr A A, Bottini P B, Kaesemeyer W H 1991 Nifedipine GITS (gastrointestinal therapeutic system) bezoar. Archives of Internal Medicine 151: 1868–1869
Ravi J, Joson P M, Ashok P S 1993 Endoscopic incision of intraluminal duodenal diverticulum. Case report of a new technique. Digestive Diseases and Sciences 38: 762–766
Reinhart W H, Weigand K, Kappeler M et al 1983 Comparison of gastrointestinal loss of alpha-1-antitrypsin and chromium-51-albumin in Menetrier's disease and the influence of ranitidine. Digestion 26: 192–196
Resnicoff S A, Morton J H 1969 Changing concepts concerning intramural duodenal hematomas. Journal of Trauma 9: 561–576
Salmon P R, Paulley J W 1967 Eosinophilic granuloma of the gastro-intestinal tract. Gut 8: 8–14
Scharschmidt B F 1977 The natural history of hypertrophic gastropathy (Menetrier's disease). Report of a case with 16 year follow-up and review of 120 cases from the literature. American Journal of Medicine 63: 644–652
Schneider R P 1989 Perdiem causes esophageal impaction and bezoars. Southern Medical Journal 82: 1449–1450
Schweiger F, Noonan J S 1991 An unusual case of gastric diverticulosis. American Journal of Gastroenterology 86: 1817–1819
Searcy R M, Malagelada J-R 1984 Menetrier's disease and idiopathic hypertrophic gastropathy. Annals of Internal Medicine 100: 565–570
Shimer G R, Helwig E B 1984 Inflammatory fibroid polyps of the intestine. American Journal of Clinical Pathology 81: 708–714
Skar V, Skar A G, Osnes M 1989 The duodenal bacterial flora in the region of papilla of Vater in patients with and without duodenal diverticula. Scandinavian Journal of Gastroenterology 24: 649–656
Sostek M, Fine S N, Harris T L 1993 Duodenal obstruction by abdominal aortic aneurysm. American Journal of Medicine 94: 220–221
Stanten A, Peters H E 1975 Enzymatic dissolution of phytobezoars. American Journal of Surgery 130: 259–261
Stolte M, Finkenzeller G 1990 Inflammatory fibroid polyp of the stomach. Endoscopy 22: 203–207
Stolte M, Gail K, Mihaljevic L 1991 Failure of ranitidine and omeprazole treatment in eosinophilic gastritis with ulceration. Zeitschrift fur Gastroenterologie 29: 426–428
Tanner N C 1968 Chronic and recurrent volvulus of the stomach with late results of "colonic displacement". American Journal of Surgery 115: 505–515
Tebar J C, Campos R R, Paricio P P et al 1992 Gastric surgery and bezoars. Digestive Diseases and Sciences 37: 1694–1696
Tillander H, Hesselsjo R 1968 Juxtacardial gastric diverticula and their surgery. Acta Chirurgica Scandinavica 134: 255–263
Wastell C, Ellis H 1971 Volvulus of the stomach. A review with a report of 8 cases. British Journal of Surgery 58: 557–562
Willemer S, Dombrowski H, Adler G, Bussmann J F, Arnold R 1992 Recurrent acute pancreatitis and intraluminal duodenal diverticulum. Pancreas 7: 257–261
Wolber R, Owen D, DelBuono L, Appelman H, Freeman H 1990 Lymphocytic gastritis in patients with celiac sprue or spruelike intestinal disease. Gastroenterology 98: 310–315
Wolfsen H C, Carpenter H A, Talley N J 1993 Menetrier's disease: a form of hypertrophic gastropathy or gastritis? Gastroenterology 104: 1310–1319
Yajko R D, Seydel F, Trimble C 1975 Rupture of the stomach from blunt abdominal trauma. Journal of Trauma 15: 177–183
Ylinen P, Kinnunen J, Höckerstedt K 1989 Superior mesenteric artery syndrome. A follow-up of 16 operated patients. Journal of Clinical Gastroenterology 11: 386–391
Yulevich A, Finaly R, Mares A J 1993 Candy bezoar: an unusual cause of food bolus bezoar. Journal of Pediatric Gastroenterology and Nutrition 17: 108–110
Zazzo J-F, Troche G, Millat B, Aubert A, Bedossa P, Kéros L 1992 Phlegmonous gastritis associated with HIV-1 seroconversion. Endoscopic and microscopic evolution. Digestive Diseases and Sciences 37: 1454–1459

SECTION 3

# Small intestine and its disorders

# 13. Absorption and its disorders

*Darlene G. Kelly*

## INTRODUCTION

The small intestine extends from the pylorus to the ileocecal valve and consists of the duodenum, jejunum and ileum. Estimates of length of the small intestine of the adult vary (322–717 cm in females, 488–785 cm in males) depending on the circumstances under which the measurement is made (Underhill 1955). The duodenum accounts for the first 30 cm and the jejunum constitutes the proximal two-fifths of the remaining small intestine. The measured length varies depending upon the state of contraction of the muscle and this commonly leads to confusion when estimates are made of the length of resected specimens and of remaining small intestine.

## FUNCTION AND STRUCTURE OF THE SMALL INTESTINE

The function of the small intestine is to digest and absorb the nutrients passed into it from the stomach. Intestinal motility is controlled to maximize exposure of nutrients to the absorptive surface. Nonabsorbable products are delivered by the small intestine to the large intestine for bacterial fermentation.

Four layers make up the wall of the small intestine. The serosa, which is the outer layer, extends from the peritoneum and consists of a single layer of cells associated with loose connective tissue. The muscularis is made up of two layers of smooth muscle, the outer longitudinal layer and the inner circular layer. The submucosa contains lymphatic, venous and nerve plexuses, Brunner's glands (in the duodenum) and small numbers of cells. The mucosa consists of three layers including the muscularis mucosae, a thin smooth muscle sheet, the lamina propria, which is made up of connective tissue, fibroblasts, cells of the immune system, smooth muscle cells, blood and lymph capillaries and lymphatic nodules, and above a thin basement membrane is the epithelial layer, including a single layer of cells which line the crypts and villi and serve the absorptive function of the small intestine.

### The mucosal surface of the small intestine (Fig. 13.1)

The absorptive surface area is magnified by the presence of the valvulae conniventes or folds of Kerckring, crescentic folds of submucosa up to 1 cm in height which increase

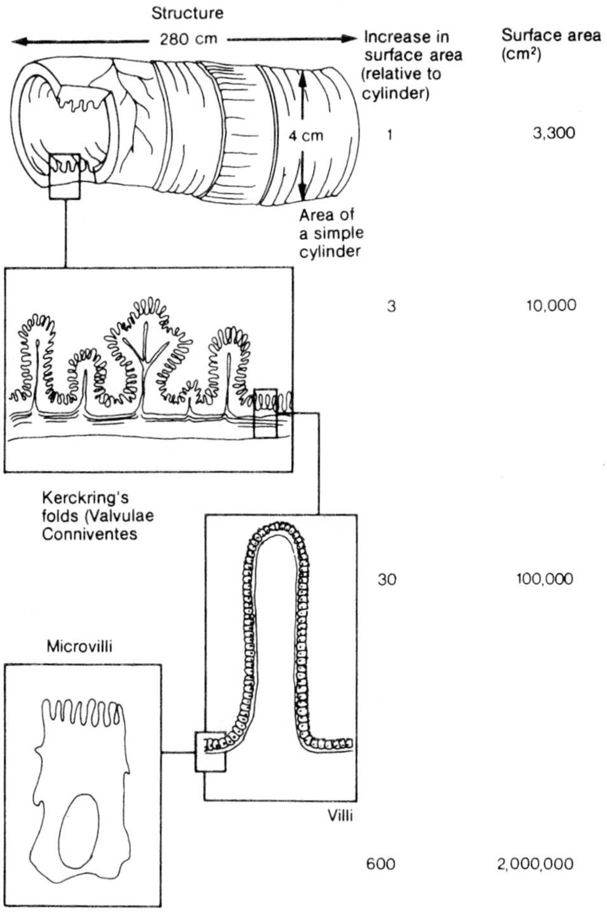


**Fig. 13.1** Morphological structure of the mucosa of the small intestine. The valvulae conniventes, villi, microvilli and brush border provide maximal surface area for contact with food for digestion. (Reproduced with permission from Caspary 1992.)

the surface area by three times, the villi, 0.5–1 mm finger like projections covered by mucosa which further amplify the absorbing surface 10-fold and the microvilli or brush border, a highly specialized structure at the surface of epithelial cells which produces a glycoprotein coat (glycocalyx) containing enzymes for the digestion and absorption of nutrients (Gardner et al 1970). The microvilli and glycocalyx increase the area of membrane by an additional 100 times, thus maximizing contact of intraluminal contents with absorptive surface. The total amplification of surface area which results from these structures is an increase from a hollow tube of 1 $m^2$ to a complex organ of more than 200 $m^2$ (100 times the human body surface area or larger than a doubles tennis court) (Caspary 1992).

Extending into each villus are lymph capillaries (lacteals) and blood vessels, both of which drain the products of digestion and absorption from the villus. The blood vessels ultimately lead to the portal system while the lymphatics drain into the mesenteric lymphatics, the cisterna chyli and finally the thoracic duct. Nerve and smooth muscle fibers, which ascend into the villi, are responsible for control of movement of the villi.

At the base of the villi are pitlike structures, the crypts of Lieberkühn. These contain the mitotic region responsible for cell regeneration and are covered with undifferentiated cells and endocrine cells. The crypts play a specialized role of secretion of fluid and electrolytes.

*The enterocytes*

These tall columnar epithelial cells with nuclei situated near the basement membrane function in absorption of intraluminal nutrients and fluids. Within the cell, histochemical methods have located a variety of enzymes, many of which are concerned with digestion. As cells migrate from crypt to villus, their enzyme content increases and they become fully differentiated and capable of absorption (Fig. 13.2). There is complete development of the microvilli on the villous cells, whereas microvilli are poorly developed in the crypt cells.

*Other epithelial cells*

The undifferentiated cells, produced by mitosis within the crypts, differentiate into goblet cells and enterocytes. The goblet cells, which migrate up the crypts to the villi, appear to have the sole function of producing mucus. The Paneth cells in the basal parts of the crypts contain granules similar to those of the exocrine cells of the pancreas or the salivary glands. The endocrine, argentaffin or enterochromaffin cells are oriented with their secretory granules near the basolateral membrane, suggesting that their products may not be secreted into the lumen. Many immunochemically distinct populations of endocrine cells exist in the crypts.

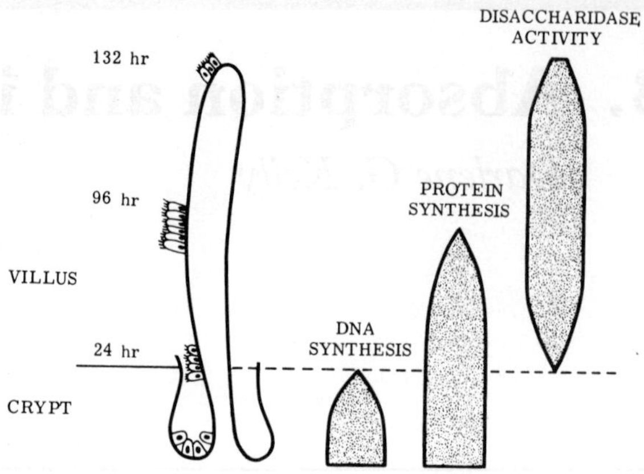


**Fig. 13.2** Correlation of functional activities with location of epithelial cells of the crypt-villus unit. The shaded areas denote the site of the particular activity and the width the relative amount of each functional parameter. Note the tendency for sequential DNA synthesis, protein synthesis and appearance of disaccharidase activity to occur as crypt cells migrate and mature morphologically. (Reproduced with permission from Gray 1975.)

*Cell turnover*

The cells of the small intestine which synthesize DNA are localized to the crypts (Deschner & Lipkin 1976). After division they migrate to the villi, reaching the tip in 2–6 days in humans; they are then shed into the lumen from a small area at the villus tip called the extrusion zone (Eastwood 1977). The basement membrane appears to play an important role in migration of cells along the villi (Timpl 1989, Hahn 1990). The Paneth and endocrine cells are renewed much more slowly. Certain diseases of the small bowel, such as celiac disease and inflammatory disorders, are associated with accelerated cell division, while proliferation is slowed by exposure to ionizing irradiation (Eastwood 1977).

## The ultrastructure of the absorptive cell (Fig. 13.3)

From the point of view of digestion and absorption, the brush border is the most important and complex part of the cell (Gardner et al 1970). The microvilli are about 1 μm in length and 0.1–0.2 μm in width. They are arranged regularly so that the intermicrovillous space varies from only 0.01 to 0.05 μm. The microvilli are enclosed by an extension of the plasma membrane. The microvillous core contains central actin filaments which interact with myosin and other muscle proteins in the region of the cell just subadjacent to the microvilli which is called the terminal web (Mooseker 1985). These filaments allow the microvillus to move in a fanlike manner by means of a circumferential contraction in the region of the

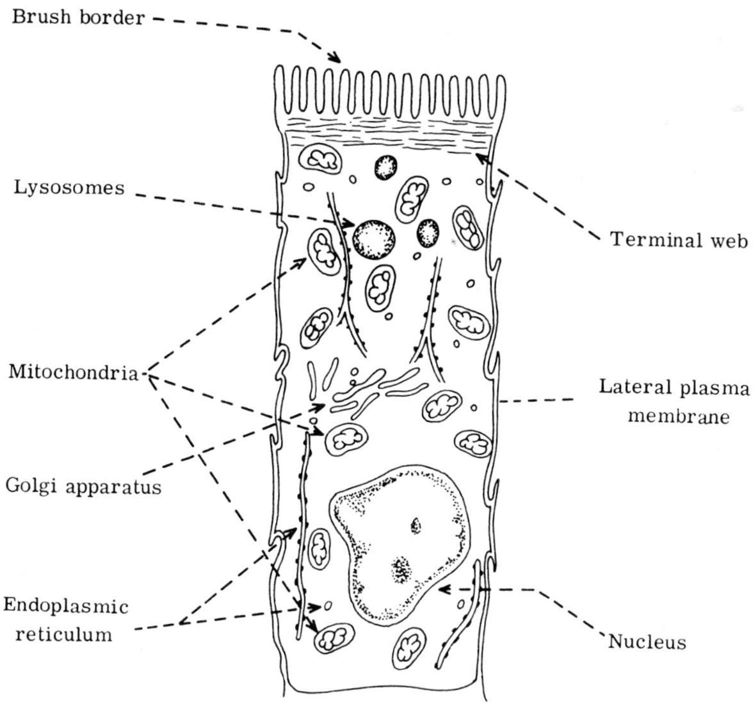


**Fig. 13.3** The ultrastructure of the absorptive cell.

terminal web (Burgess 1982). The surface fuzzy coat, or glycocalyx, is composed of glycoprotein which is manufactured within the cell and extruded from the microvilli as a series of radiating filaments. The glycocalyx is firmly attached to the microvillous membrane. This surface coat and the microvilli contain digestive enzymes (Crane 1975), as well as receptors which selectively bind certain substances which are then available in high concentrations at the cell surface (Bennett 1963). Such a receptor exists in the distal ileum for the intrinsic factor–vitamin $B_{12}$ complex (Mackenzie & Donaldson 1969). The surface coat with its enzymes led Crane (1966) to suggest a "two-layer" hypothesis of membrane function. The concept is of a digestive-absorptive surface in which the elements for both functions are arranged closely together. For example, disaccharides are digested in the glycocalyx and the resulting monosaccharides are then actively absorbed across the plasma membrane.

An unstirred water layer covers the luminal surface of the mucosa and this creates a local milieu which influences both absorptive and defense mechanisms. The thickness of the layer may affect the rate at which solutes, glucose and the products of fat digestion gain access to the absorptive cell. The layer is probably less than 45 μm and should not be rate limiting for the transport of most substances (Levitt et al 1992).

At the upper part of the lateral membrane of the epithelial cell there is a circumferential series of structures which maintain the close apposition of adjacent cells (Farquhar & Palade 1963). From luminal to basal orientation this three-part complex consists of the zonula occludens or tight junction, the zonula adherens or intermediate junction and the desmosome. Although it was originally thought that the tight junctions allow only transport of water and electrolytes via the paracellular route, recent data suggest that this route may be an important nonenergy-requiring pathway for transport of sugars and amino acids (Pappenheimer 1993). The degree of tightness or leakiness of these junctions varies with the crypt junctions being leakier and the villous junctions tighter (Marcial et al 1984). There are also regional differences, with the gastric and rectal junctions being extremely tight and relatively impermeable while the proximal small bowel junctions are quite leaky. The degree of permeability appears to increase postprandially, suggesting a dynamic quality for these structures (Madara 1990). Other organelles present in the absorptive cells are shown in Figure 13.3.

## The lymphatic system

The lymphatic system is responsible for the maintenance of the composition and volume of extracellular fluid and for the absorption of lipids and macromolecules, including serum proteins which escape from the capillaries. In the event of blockage of the lymphatics, the protein molecules are lost into the gut lumen. The lymphatics transport lymphocytes and immunoglobulins, which are produced in the lamina propria, to the general circulation. Lymphocyte counts vary from 900 to 7000/$mm^3$ of lymph.

Lymph flow in the intestinal lacteals is increased by fat

absorption, by increases in intestinal motility and by small increases in intraluminal pressure. Once the lymph has moved into the larger vessels beyond the plexi which are located at the inner surface of the muscularis mucosa, retrograde flow is prevented by a system of valves. Lymphatics play an important role in the absorption of long chain fat and fat-soluble vitamins via chylomicrons which enter the lacteals between gaps in the endothelial cells (Rubin 1966).

The lymphatics in the villi are thin channels. Bank et al (1967) compared small intestinal biopsies from healthy controls and patients with various intestinal disorders and concluded that there is pathological dilatation of lymphatics if lymphatic spaces are seen in more than four out of 50 villi or if the lacteals are dilated beyond 129 μm in length and 64 μm in width. Marked dilatation occurs in lymphangiectasia or in blockage of the lymphatic system.

### Intestinal permeability

This refers to the facility with which various substances can penetrate the intestinal mucosa in a given period of time (Lifschitz 1985). Alterations in permeability may help to explain the pathogenesis of some gastrointestinal disorders, such as celiac disease (Chadwick et al 1977, Bjarnason et al 1985), cystic fibrosis (Leclercq-Foucart et al 1987), food allergy (Du Mont et al 1984), chronic diarrhea (Ford et al 1985) and inflammatory bowel disease (Peled et al 1985). This has been assessed in research settings using inert, water-soluble probe molecules, such as xylose, lactulose, rhamnose, mannitol, $^{51}$Cr-labeled EDTA and polyethylene glycol 400. At present these tests are not in clinical use, but they may have potential for providing useful information on the integrity of the mucosal surface.

## DIGESTION AND ABSORPTION OF CARBOHYDRATE

In the Western diet carbohydrate makes up about 45% of the caloric intake. Of the digestible carbohydrates about 50–65% consists of starch, 25–35% sucrose and 5–10% lactose (Caspary 1992). Fructose is becoming increasingly important as a commercial sweetener, particularly in soft drinks and other beverages. Indigestible complex carbohydrates derived from plant cell walls, gums, mucilages and algal polysaccharides make up dietary fiber. The average American diet is estimated to supply 12 g/day of fiber (Lanza et al 1987).

Carbohydrate digestion begins in the mouth due to action of salivary α-amylase. The enzyme is inactivated at intragastric pH. The degree of hydrolysis by salivary amylase depends on the time that food is chewed and the nature of the food bolus that enters the stomach.

### Intraluminal processes

The glucose polymer starch consists of 20% amylose and 80% amylopectin. Amylose, a straight chain of glucose molecules with α-4 links, is digested at some of these bonds by salivary and pancreatic amylase to form maltose and maltotriose. Amylopectin has α-6 branches in addition to the α-4 bonds. Here too the products of digestion are maltose and maltotriose, but in addition there are residual branched segments termed α-limit dextrins (Fig. 13.4). There is a small amount of glycogen in the diet. Its structure is similar to amylopectin and it is similarly digested.

### Digestion at the brush border

Maltose, maltotriose, α-dextrins, lactose and sucrose are presented to the brush border which contains the di- and trisaccharidases necessary to convert these substances into monosaccharides. A full complement of disaccharidases is present from birth in mature columnar epithelial cells. The highest concentration of sucrase and lactase is in the jejunum, whereas maltase is highest in the ileum (Triadou et al 1983). The ileum also seems to have maximal digestive capacity for more complex oligosaccharides and peptides.

The sequential reactions of hydrolysis and transport are located close together so that the products of hydrolysis become the substrates for transport before there is a chance for them to diffuse away. The rate of hydrolysis is probably limited to some extent by the rate of glucose transport across the cell. Since glucose tends to be present in excess, some moves into the lumen to be absorbed more distally. The unstirred layer may exert control on the rate of absorption of glucose, as the administration of pectin, which increases the thickness of the unstirred layer, reduces the rate of absorption of glucose (Flourié et al 1984). In the case of lactose, however, the slow rate of hydrolysis is probably the limiting step in absorption. Only a very small amount of disaccharide and α-dextrins can enter the mucosa intact and apparently these are not metabolized in the body, as they have been shown to be excreted in the urine.

### Cellular transport of monosaccharides

The above processes result in the presence of glucose and small amounts of fructose and galactose at the cell membrane. Glucose and galactose are absorbed into the cell by active transport. Glucose absorption occurs against a concentration gradient involving the simultaneous translocation of sugar and cation ($Na^+$) with sugar:ion cotransporter proteins functioning as carriers (Crane 1977, Semenza et al 1985). Transport of glucose uphill against a concentration gradient is coupled to the move-

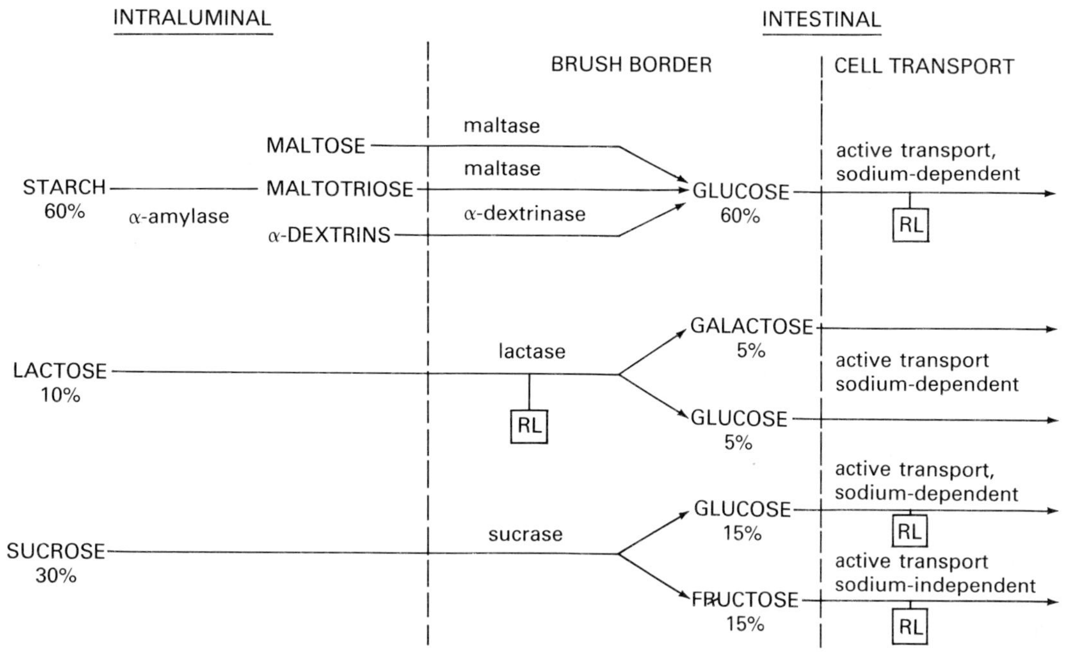


**Fig. 13.4** Carbohydrate digestion and absorption in man. Percentages refer to proportion of total carbohydrate in diet. RL = rate-limiting step in the overall digestive–absorptive process for each carbohydrate. (Modified with permission from Gray 1970.)

ment of sodium ion down its electrochemical gradient. The sodium gradient is maintained by the primary active transport system $Na^+$:$K^+$ ATPase at the basolateral membrane, which pumps sodium out of the cell. The cotransporter contains binding sites for D-glucose and $Na^+$ and these are accessible, through conformational change, from both sides of the membrane. The exit of glucose from the enterocyte occurs along the basolateral membrane as a result of facilitated diffusion using a specific carrier molecule.

Fructose is absorbed at a slower rate than galactose and glucose but more efficiently than passively transported sugars (Rumessen & Gudmand-Hoyer 1986). In humans this takes place by energy-independent facilitated transport using a carrier. Healthy individuals show a large variation in absorption with some incomplete absorption occurring in more than one-third of subjects studied by Ravich et al (1983). Absorption of fructose given as sucrose is faster than when given alone, as glucose stimulates fructose uptake in a dose-dependent fashion. Xylose is probably absorbed partly by passive diffusion and partly by an active process.

## The colon and carbohydrate absorption

Under normal circumstances, 96–98% of an oral load of sucrose is absorbed in the small intestine. Starch in most staple foods is incompletely absorbed by the small intestine in normal individuals. Levitt (1983) estimated that up to 20 g of a 100 g starch load may be metabolized by the colonic flora and as much as 70 g of carbohydrate may reach the colon each day. Wheat, oats, potatoes and corn, but not rice, all cause an increase in breath hydrogen, indicating that they are incompletely absorbed in the small intestine (Levitt et al 1987).

Cellulose, a (1-4)β-linked glucose polymer, also passes unchanged into the colon, where it is fermented and produces short chain fatty acids, hydrogen, carbon dioxide and methane (Cummings 1984). An increased amount of carbohydrate reaches the colon in old age, reflecting reduced absorptive capacity by the small intestine (Feibusch & Holt 1982). Fermentation of unabsorbed carbohydrates and fiber by colonic bacteria is an important salvage mechanism, as the resulting short chain fatty acids are absorbed (Bond et al 1980) and provide a preferred fuel for colonocytes (Roediger 1980).

## Tests of carbohydrate absorption

Absorption of carbohydrate may be tested by giving oral monoglyceride, glucose or xylose, and measuring its concentration in blood or urine or by measuring blood glucose concentrations after an oral load of a disaccharide. In the latter case the test measures hydrolysis of the disaccharide plus absorption of the component monosaccharides. In the assessment of disaccharidase deficiency, it is possible to quantify the disaccharidase in biopsy specimens obtained from the jejunum. Fecal sugar analysis does not provide quantitative information on carbohydrate malabsorption, is unreliable in the newborn period and may give a false negative result.

*Breath tests*

Breath tests are simple, safe and noninvasive methods for the investigation of carbohydrate absorption (Caspary 1978, Newcomer 1984). The principle of these tests is that nonabsorbed carbohydrate is fermented by colonic bacteria, producing hydrogen which appears in the breath within 5 min.

The hydrogen breath test is the most accurate indirect method for detecting lactase deficiency (Newcomer et al 1975). Breath hydrogen is measured at 30–60 min intervals for 2–4 h following a 50 g oral lactose dose. A sustained rise in breath hydrogen of >20 ppm above baseline indicates lactose malabsorption. The test, which has a sensitivity of approximately 95%, is useful in population screening. Sucrose maldigestion may be similarly diagnosed by measurement of breath hydrogen concentrations after an oral sucrose load (Davidson & Robb 1983). Using breath hydrogen determinations, Rumessen & Gudmand-Hoyer (1986) demonstrated that fructose malabsorption occurs in some persons when fructose is given alone but not when presented with glucose or as sucrose.

Rice flour is efficiently absorbed by healthy individuals, with minimal generation of hydrogen. Measurement of breath hydrogen after a rice flour meal has been used to diagnose carbohydrate malabsorption associated with pancreatic insufficiency and small intestinal bacterial overgrowth (Kerlin et al 1984).

The D-xylose hydrogen breath test has been reported to be effective for distinguishing malabsorptive syndromes from irritable bowel syndrome (Casellas & Malagelada 1994). Furthermore, the test may also be useful in following therapeutic response in celiac disease.

Small bowel transit time and bacterial overgrowth of the small intestine can be measured using the nonabsorbable carbohydrate lactulose breath test (Bond & Levitt 1975, Rhodes et al 1979). The $^{14}$C-xylose breath test can also be used to detect bacterial metabolism of carbohydrates. However, the latter test has the disadvantage of using a radioactive tracer.

There are many potential errors associated with measurement of exhaled breath hydrogen. A small proportion (< 5%) of subjects have no hydrogen in the breath after ingesting nonabsorbable carbohydrate due to consumption of hydrogen by colonic bacteria which exceeds production. This can be confirmed by the absence of a breath hydrogen response to a nonabsorbable carbohydrate, e.g. lactulose, or when bowel motility is disturbed. Conditions that influence bowel motility or bacterial flora should be avoided. An early rise in breath hydrogen may result from the passage into the cecum of carbohydrate retained in the ileum from previous meals (Read et al 1985). To ensure a low basal hydrogen excretion nonabsorbable carbohydrates should be avoided for 24 h before the test (Perman et al 1984). Extraintestinal factors, such as hyperventilation, cigarette smoking and hydrogen production by oropharyngeal bacteria, may also adversely affect outcome (Thompson et al 1985). The transient rise in exhaled breath hydrogen from bacteria in the mouth occurs soon after carbohydrate ingestion and is largely abolished by using a bactericidal mouthwash and avoidance of carbohydrate consumption after test meal ingestion (Thompson et al 1986). Breath testing requires end-expiratory collection of breath samples which can be difficult, especially in children. Simultaneous measurement of oxygen, carbon dioxide or nitrogen may be used to normalize data (Newcomer 1984).

*Lactose tolerance test*

Employed in the diagnosis of primary and secondary lactase deficiency, this test uses a dose of 50 g lactose given orally in 400 ml water. Symptoms, e.g. abdominal cramps, bloating and diarrhea, noted over the next few hours occur in >75% of individuals with malabsorption. Samples of blood are taken fasting and at intervals of 20 min for 2 h after the oral load. A rise in blood glucose of less than 1.1 mmol/L (20 mg/100 ml) above baseline indicate lactase deficiency.

An abnormal response to the lactose may be seen in 25% of persons. The glucose peak can be missed for several reasons. The timing may be altered by gastrointestinal dysmotility. Venous blood, rather than capillary samples, also changes the results (McGill & Newcomer 1970). The occurrence of abdominal symptoms during the test is helpful diagnostically. The interpretation of the test is improved by comparing the rise in blood glucose after lactose and after an equivalent amount of the monosaccharides glucose and galactose (Cuatrecasas et al 1965).

This test has limited value in children because it has been shown to have a 25% false positive and false negative rate (Krasilnikoff et al 1975). It is an invasive test requiring multiple blood tests. The breath hydrogen test has largely replaced the lactose tolerance test (Newcomer 1984).

*Mucosal enzyme levels*

It is possible to assay disaccharidase activity in biopsy specimens (Dahlqvist 1968) by preparing a homogenate, incubating it with the appropriate substrate and measuring the yield of glucose. Activity is expressed as units/g of wet weight. It is often important to establish that the normal ratio of disaccharidase activities is altered, for the ratio is usually constant. The ratio of maltase:isomaltase:sucrase: lactase is 6:2:2:1 (Newcomer & McGill 1967). Since there is some variation of enzyme activity along the gut, the biopsy should be obtained from the first 30 cm of jejunum. Many causes of secondary carbohydrate malabsorption can also cause a patchy enteropathy, so activity measured in a single biopsy specimen may be unreliable (Harrison & Walker-Smith 1977).

*D-xylose absorption test*

The pentose D-xylose is absorbed passively and unchanged, mainly from the upper small intestine (Fordtran et al 1962), in contrast to glucose which is absorbed actively over the entire length (Crane 1960). Of the D-xylose which is absorbed, a small proportion is metabolized (Butterworth et al 1959), the remainder being excreted in the urine, where it can be measured. The test can be used to assess the absorptive integrity of the proximal small intestine.

It is performed in a fasting patient who is given an oral dose of D-xylose, 25 g for adults and 5 g for children (Craig & Atkinson 1988). Urine is collected for 5 h after the oral xylose (1 h in children or renal insufficient patients) and the xylose in this specimen is measured. A serum sample may also be collected 1 h after the dose for xylose determination, since this avoids the problems introduced by incomplete urine collections and renal insufficiency.

Normal persons excrete at least 4 g of the xylose in 5 h and the serum level should exceed 25 mg/dl. Subnormal amounts of xylose are excreted in over 90% of patients with celiac disease and tropical sprue, whereas absorption is subnormal in only 7% of patients with pancreatic steatorrhea and no mucosal disease.

The test may be abnormal in renal disease, in ascites because xylose accumulates in the ascitic fluid, after gastric surgery because of rapid intestinal transit, in bacterial overgrowth syndrome and during therapy with aspirin, indomethacin, neomycin and glipizide. In the bacterial overgrowth syndrome about one-third of patients with hypochlorhydria have been shown to have normal 25 g D-xylose tests despite altered $^{14}C$-xylose studies (Saltzman et al 1994), due to bacterial utilization of xylose. Although the D-xylose test is widely used as a screening test for malabsorption, there is disagreement over its reproducibility and usefulness. Furthermore, the ability to obtain biopsies of the proximal small bowel is shifting the approach to suspected malabsorption from functional to morphologic methods of diagnosis.

## Carbohydrate malabsorption

*Disaccharidase deficiencies*

Disaccharidase deficiency may occur as a primary disorder, when the intestinal biopsy is always histologically normal, or secondary to other disorders of the small intestinal mucosa (Enck & Whitehead 1986). Because the disaccharide cannot be hydrolyzed and absorbed, it passes into the colon, where it is split by colonic bacteria into lactic and acetic acids and carbon dioxide. These are osmotically active substances which induce diarrhea.

*Primary lactase deficiency*

***Acquired deficiency.*** Lactase activity in the brush border of the small intestine is high shortly after birth and remains so while the infant continues on a diet with a high milk content. Enzyme levels decline with aging despite continued intake of lactose and other disaccharides (Tadesse 1990). Lactase activity is undetectable in many well-nourished adults who are asymptomatic despite lactose ingestion. The extent of symptoms in those who are lactase deficient may be modified by salvage of short chain fatty acids produced by bacterial fermentation of unabsorbed lactose within the colon (Bond et al 1980). The enzyme present in infantile mucosa crossreacts immunologically with the enzyme found in "persistent" adults (Potter et al 1985, Tsuboi et al 1985).

There are marked racial differences in the prevalence of lactase deficiency (Table 13.1). Races whose ancestors were northern Europeans or residents of the northwestern Indian subcontinent have a high probability of being lactose absorbers in adult life, whereas most blacks, Orientals and South Americans are lactose malabsorbers (Table 13.1).

***Congenital lactase deficiency.*** This is an extremely rare permanent condition which results in severe diarrhea and poor weight gain in the few days after birth (Holzel et al 1959). It is inherited as an autosomal recessive trait. Improvement occurs when milk is withdrawn from the diet.

***Pathology.*** The disorder is due to a deficiency of lactase, which is located in the brush border of the mucosa of the small intestine. There is a gradient of activity along the small bowel in normal and lactase-deficient individuals (Fig. 13.5), hence the necessity for standardization of the biopsy site when enzyme assay is being performed. The histology of the mucosa is normal in primary lactase deficiency.

**Table 13.1** Prevalence of late-onset lactose malabsorption (modified from Büller & Grand 1990)

| Ethnic or racial group | Prevalence (%) |
|---|---|
| Orientals in USA | 100 |
| Native Americans (Oklahoma) | 95 |
| African Americans | 81 |
| Italians | 71 |
| Aborigines (Australia) | 67 |
| Hispanic Americans | 56 |
| Greeks | 53 |
| White Americans | 24 |
| Danes | 3 |
| Dutch | 0 |

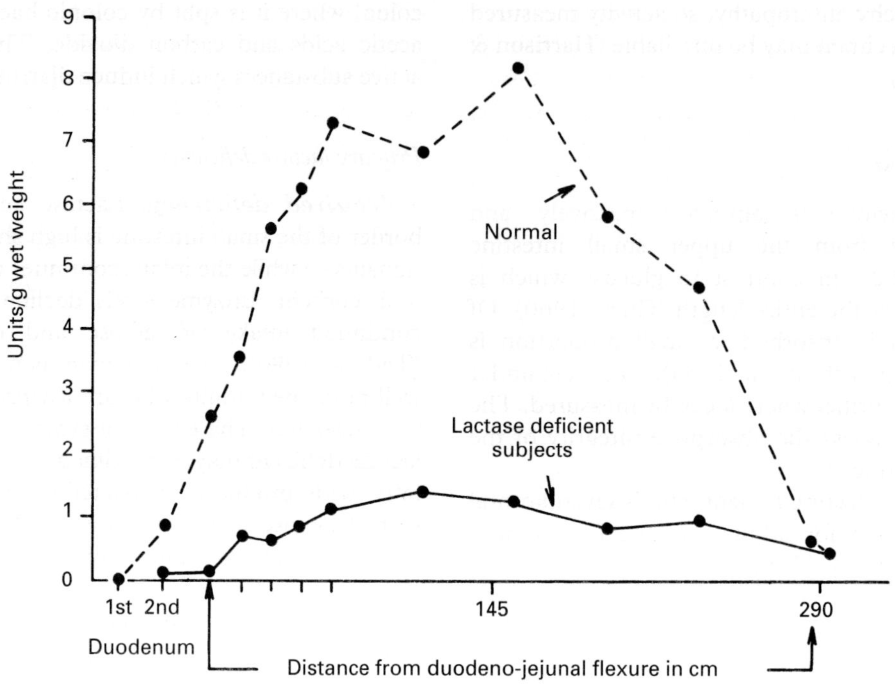


**Fig. 13.5** Distribution of lactase activity in the small intestine of seven normal and seven selected lactase-deficient adults. (Reproduced with permission from Newcomer & McGill 1966.)

***Clinical features.*** Abdominal discomfort occurs after ingesting milk or milk products. This usually takes the form of colic, nausea, a sensation of distention, increased flatus and sometimes watery diarrhea. Malabsorption of lactose does not always lead to lactose intolerance and indeed the range of tolerance is extremely wide among persons with lactase deficiency (Gudmand-Hoyer & Simony 1977). Fifty grams of lactose will produce symptoms in 70–80% of malabsorbers, whereas 10 g lactose (or 200 ml milk) will produce symptoms in only 30–60%. Part of this variability may be explained by the ability of the colonic flora of some individuals to metabolize lactose, the rate of orocecal transit, the dose of lactose ingested, the lactose vehicle and foods consumed at the same time. Some forms of fiber may reduce the breath hydrogen response and symptoms after oral lactose in lactose malabsorbers (Nguyen et al 1982).

A history of intolerance to milk and milk products is much less common than might be expected from the high incidence of lactase deficiency. Often lactase-deficient individuals consciously or unconsciously limit their intakes of lactose, so flatulence and diarrhea are minimized (Bayless et al 1975). Gastric surgery may unmask lactase deficiency because of accelerated gastric emptying. Some symptoms after the ingestion of cow's milk may be due to a milk protein allergy.

***Diagnosis.*** While various diagnostic tests may be used to identify lactase deficiency, the diagnosis is suggested by the ethnic origin, family history and an improvement in symptoms on lactose withdrawal and relapse on its reintroduction.

***Treatment.*** Patients with mild symptoms can be managed only by reducing the amount of milk products consumed. Enzyme (yeast-derived β-galactosidase) in the form of tablets or liquid added to milk or taken prior to ingestion result in hydrolysis of 70–100% of lactose, depending on amount used and incubation time and temperature. Other new food products have been developed which may be used by many persons with lactase deficiency. These include milk substitutes made with soybean protein and milk treated with lactobacillus cultures. When milk is consumed, it should be taken with other foods, resulting in a slower rate of colonic fermentation and thus fewer symptoms (Solomons et al 1985).

Patients with severe symptoms who do not apparently drink an excessive amount of milk should be treated with a lactose-free diet. Since such patients may respond adversely to as little as 5 g of lactose (Gudmand-Hoyer & Simony 1977), the diet must be strict and even medications which contain lactose must be excluded. Careful instruction must be given on the many food products which contain lactose and on the importance of reading labels on convenience foods. Once clinical remission has been achieved, it may be possible in some patients to reintroduce a small amount of milk-containing foods without relapse.

Kolars et al (1984) demonstrated that in patients with lactose intolerance the peak breath hydrogen in response to yoghurt (containing 18 g lactose) is approximately one-third of that in response to 20 g lactose alone and this was associated with a reduced frequency of gastrointestinal symptoms. It appears that yoghurt is digested with fewer symptoms because bacterial lactase remains effective in the product. While these results may not be applicable to all forms of yoghurt, it seems likely that yoghurt will be better tolerated by lactase-deficient subjects than other milk products. Yoghurt-based frozen desserts are also acceptable substitutes for ice cream for some subjects with lactose intolerance.

*Secondary lactase deficiency*

Secondary lactase deficiency is common in conditions with structural abnormalities of the intestinal mucosa, such as celiac disease (Kerlin & Wong 1987), tropical sprue or short bowel syndrome. In these, the brush border is abnormal or there is a decrease in surface area, resulting in an overall deficiency of enzymes. With treatment of celiac disease, lactase activity returns slowly (Plotkin & Isselbacher 1964).

Secondary deficiency of lactase has been reported in many other conditions, such as infectious gastroenteritis, duodenal ulcer, inflammatory bowel disease and after gastric resection, but it is not certain whether the incidence of the deficiency in these disorders is greater than that in a control population. Langman & Rowland (1990) showed that lactase deficiency was seen with peptic duodenitis with the degree of deficiency being proportional to the histologic change. In some of these conditions a lactose-free diet may provide symptomatic relief until the underlying intestinal disorder responds to treatment.

## Malabsorption of other carbohydrates

*Congenital glucose-galactose malabsorption*

This permanent defect in mucosal transport usually presents in the neonatal period with profuse watery diarrhea and abdominal distention when sugar solution or milk is given. Severe dehydration and death can occur in young infants. Some patients are less severely affected and the diagnosis is delayed until adult life. The diagnosis is suggested when there is clinical improvement on withdrawal of dietary glucose and galactose and relapse on reintroduction and when biopsy reveals a structurally normal intestinal mucosa with normal disaccharidase activities. Treatment requires the elimination of glucose- and galactose-containing foods from the diet and the use of fructose as a substitute for glucose and sucrose.

*Sucrase-isomaltase deficiency*

The deficiency of these two enzymes is inherited as an autosomal recessive disease. The prevalence of sucrase-isomaltase deficiency in Western countries is unknown, although a prevalence of 10% has been reported in Eskimos of Greenland (Anonymous 1977). Symptoms occur when sucrose is introduced into the diet, although the initial diagnosis has been reported in adulthood. The decrease in two different enzymes occurs because sucrase-isomaltase is synthesized as a single precursor which is inserted in the plasma membrane. The N-terminal end of the isomaltase moiety acts as an anchor while the sucrase portion projects into the lumen. This is split into its subunits by pancreatic proteases once it has reached the lumen (Hadorn et al 1981). The sucrase-isomaltase complex is a major component of the digestive enzymes in the small intestine, accounting for approximately 80% of the maltase, most of the isomaltase and all the sucrase activity. It appears that most patients with the disease are actually able to synthesize the proenzyme, but subsequent processing intracellularly is defective (Lloyd & Olsen 1987). Since there are other maltases in the mucosa, normal absorption of maltose and maltotriose is maintained despite the deficiency.

Symptoms consist of watery diarrhea, abdominal distention, crampy abdominal pain, excessive gas and excoriation of the buttocks. In young infants severe watery diarrhea is associated with poor weight gain. In older children irritability can be a feature and growth may be retarded or normal (Gudmand-Hoyer & Krasilnikoff 1977).

The sucrose breath hydrogen test is abnormal and sucrase-isomaltase levels are low in a structurally normal small intestinal mucosa. Traditionally treatment has consisted of elimination of sucrose, but not starch, from the diet. However, recent studies indicate that liquid yeast sucrase may offer effective replacement therapy for patients with congenital sucrase-isomaltase deficiency (Treem 1993). Matsuo et al (1992) recently suggested the usefulness of an intestinal sucrase-isomaltase inhibitor in the dietary management of obesity and diabetes mellitus.

*Trehalase deficiency*

Trehalose intolerance occasionally causes diarrhea in adults who eat young mushrooms. These individuals lack trehalase, which hydrolyzes the glycoside to glucose.

*Sorbitol absorption*

Sorbitol is a polyalcohol sugar which cannot be absorbed by humans. When ingested in adequate amounts, it can cause functional gastrointestinal symptoms (Hyams 1983). It is used as a sweetener in diabetic products such as chewing gum and candy and in various medications where it acts as a stabilizer and sweetener in elixirs (Dills 1989). In doses of $\geq 10$ g per day, sorbitol can cause diarrhea (Jain et al 1987). This amount of sorbitol can be reached with typical doses of commonly used medications, such as theophylline or furosemide preparations, given in elixir form. This feature of sorbitol can be used to clinical advantage in cases of constipation, as it is an inexpensive replacement for lactulose and other cathartics (Lederle et al 1990).

*Secondary carbohydrate intolerance*

Temporary defects of monosaccharide absorption and disaccharide digestion may be the result of severe structural damage to the small intestinal mucosa. Causes of secondary carbohydrate intolerance include acute enteritis, giardiasis, celiac disease, protein intolerance (cow's milk, soya, egg) and bacterial overgrowth syndrome. Lactase deficiency is the most common, as lactase is the most labile of the disaccharidases. However, other enzymes and transport systems may be affected as well. Symptoms, including nausea, colicky abdominal pain, abdominal distention, increased flatus, audible borborygmi and watery diarrhea and excoriation of the buttocks, vary with the carbohydrate load. Treatment involves withdrawal of disaccharides and gradual reintroduction as symptoms resolve.

## DIGESTION AND ABSORPTION OF PROTEIN

Most Western diets include 70–100 g protein per day which is in excess of the recommended level of 0.8 g/kg/day (National Research Council 1989). To this are added 17 g protein in secreted juices and 50 g from sloughed cells (Fig. 13.6); this endogenous protein is broken down and absorbed by the same mechanisms as the ingested protein. The fecal nitrogen output, which is equivalent to ≤12.5 g protein per day, represents the end result of all these processes.

There are many analogies between the absorption of proteins and carbohydrates. Protein undergoes initial hydrolysis in the lumen and the resultant short chain peptides are hydrolyzed to their constituent amino acids at the brush border or within the cell. Amino acids and peptides are actively transported across the epithelial cell.

### Absorption of intact protein molecules

Protein can be absorbed as complete molecules in the first few weeks of life in some animals. Antibodies in colostrum are absorbed intact by pinocytosis and are then seen in vacuoles in the cytoplasm (Clark 1959). This mechanism is rapidly lost and is never important nutritionally.

### Intraluminal hydrolysis

Protein undergoes denaturation and partial digestion in the stomach as a result of action of gastric acid and pepsin, respectively. In the small intestine, pancreatic enzymes digest the proteins and the large peptides which remain after peptic digestion. The pancreas produces proenzyme forms of proteases, including trypsinogen, chymotrypsinogen, proelastase and procarboxypeptidase A and B. When the proenzymes reach the small intestinal lumen, the trypsinogen is acted upon by enterokinase, a product of the brush border of intestinal cells, to produce trypsin. Trypsin, in turn, activates the other proenzyme forms.

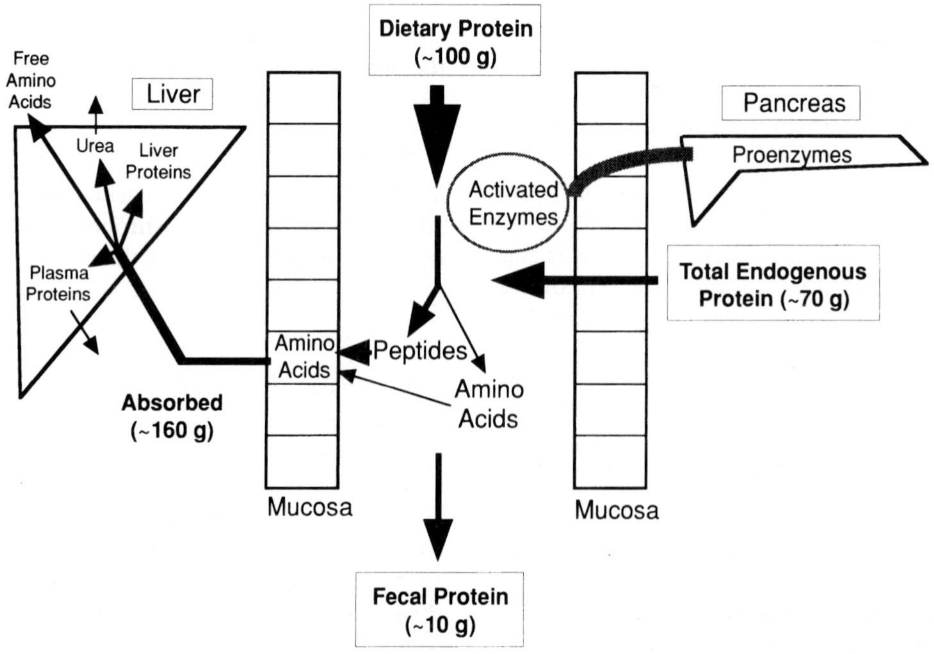


**Fig. 13.6** Digestion, absorption and metabolism of dietary protein and endogenous protein. (Modified with permission from Munro 1976.)

Trypsin, chymotrypsin and elastase are endopeptidases which cleave peptide bonds adjacent to specific amino acids within the protein molecule. By contrast, the carboxypeptidases cleave peptide bonds containing aromatic and aliphatic amino acids at the carboxyl terminals (carboxypeptidase A) or basic amino acids at the carboxyl terminals (carboxypeptidase B). The complementary action of these peptidases yields a mixture of luminal nitrogen substances consisting of about 40% amino acids and 60% oligopeptides of 2–6 amino acids (Erickson & Kim 1990).

### Digestion at the brush border and intracellularly

Peptidases which exist both in the brush border and in the cytosol of the mucosal cells are responsible for further hydrolysis of peptides. Pancreatic proteases, which are adsorbed to the brush border, may assist in this process. Among the brush border peptidases are aminopeptidase A, γ-glutamyl transpeptidase and folate conjugase, each of which has very specific hydrolytic functions. Several types of dipeptidases are present in the brush border and in the cytoplasm of the enterocytes. These enzymes, independent of pancreatic proteases, can initiate hydrolysis of large proteins, such as casein, to yield amino acids and oligopeptides (Erickson & Kim 1990). This may in part be responsible for the delay in protein malabsorption relative to maldigestion of fat in pancreatic insufficiency. In the human small intestine, dipeptidase activities increase distally (Triadou et al 1983).

### Transport into the enterocytes

Amino acids and peptides are actively transported into the mucosa by independent mechanisms. In fact, the enterocyte can transport di- and tripeptides more efficiently than the corresponding free amino acids (Kim & Erickson 1985). In the case of amino acids, transport is stimulated by sodium ions, requires energy and depends on a sodium cotransport mechanism similar to that described for monosaccharides. The L form of amino acids is more readily absorbed than the D form. On the basis of the inherited disorders in amino acid transport, which can involve both intestine and kidney (Milne 1964), and from evidence provided by studies of intestinal transport, four groups of related amino acids have been identified thus far; the members of each group have a similar transport mechanism.

1. the monoamino-monocarboxylic amino acids (alanine, serine, threonine, valine, leucine, isoleucine, phenylalanine, tyrosine, tryptophan, asparagine, histidine, cysteine, methionine and citrulline). Members of this group are involved in Hartnup disease;
2. dibasic amino acids (lysine, arginine, ornithine) and a neutral amino acid, cystine. Members of this group are involved in cystinuria;
3. dicarboxylic amino acids (glutamic and aspartic acids);
4. proline, hydroxyproline and glycine.

There also appears to be an active intestinal transport system for L-carnitine, a trimethylated δ-amino acid which is essential in fatty acid metabolism (Hamilton et al 1986).

Individual peptides compete for transport. It is not yet known whether there is more than one peptide uptake system. A few small peptides cross the intestinal mucosa intact and appear in the peripheral blood. However, most peptides absorbed into the cells are hydrolyzed to amino acids and these are transferred from the mucosal cells to the portal vein. Small peptides are absorbed equally well in the jejunum and ileum, whereas amino acids are absorbed mainly in the jejunum.

The existence of separate absorption mechanisms for amino acids and peptides is of clinical importance. In celiac disease there is a marked reduction in amino acid absorption, but the absorption of dipeptides is affected less. Enteral diets for patients with maldigestion due to intestinal or pancreatic disease should contain peptides in lieu of free amino acids, as this improves absorption and reduces the osmolality of the diet, reducing the risk of diarrhea.

### Hereditary disorders of amino acid transport

In general, these have an autosomal recessive pattern of inheritance and, with the exception of tryptophan malabsorption, they show defective renal tubular transport in addition to the impaired intestinal transport of amino acids. In Hartnup disease and cystinuria the absorption of peptides is normal and so nutrition is maintained.

Hartnup disease is characterized by the onset of pellagra in childhood, as well as episodic cerebellar ataxia and mental retardation in some cases. There is renal aminoaciduria and malabsorption of the monoamino-monocarboxylic amino acids. Unabsorbed tryptophan is degraded by bacteria in the colon to produce an excess of indoles in the stool together with indicanuria.

Cystinuria causes renal calculi in children. The defect in brush border transport involves the dibasic amino acids and cystine.

In tryptophan malabsorption (blue diaper syndrome) there is isolated malabsorption of tryptophan accompanied by hypercalcemia, but no associated renal aminoaciduria. The blue discoloration is due to indigotin, which is formed by the oxidative conjugation of two molecules of indican.

Other defects in amino acid transport which have been reported are methioninc malabsorption, transport defects of the proline, hydroxyproline and glycine group (Joseph's syndrome) and hyperdibasic aminoaciduria due to a defective basolateral membrane transport system (Erickson & Kim 1990).

## Determination of gastrointestinal protein loss

*Radioisotope methods*

Radio-labeled macromolecules which can be given intravenously have been developed to study protein loss into the stool. The ideal labeled protein should be normally metabolized and the label should not be absorbed from or secreted into the gastrointestinal tract unless bound to the protein molecule (Waldmann 1966).

While $^{131}$I- or $^{125}$I-labeled serum proteins behave normally from a metabolic standpoint, free iodine is absorbed from the gastrointestinal tract after digestion of the protein and is secreted by the salivary glands and stomach. Because of these limitations it cannot be used as a quantitative test of fecal loss.

$^{51}$Cr-labeled proteins have the advantage that the chromium label is not absorbed from or secreted into the alimentary tract. The $^{51}$Cr is attached to albumin given intravenously and the stools are collected for a specified number of days. Normal persons excrete 0.1–0.7% of the radioactivity in the stools over 4 days, while those with excessive protein loss excrete 2–40%. False positives and negatives for determination of protein loss into the gut are rare (Waldmann et al 1969). One disadvantage of $^{51}$Cr-labeled albumin is the steady elution of the label and its attachment to other proteins. This precludes its use in the study of albumin synthesis and catabolism. Unfortunately, this radio-labeled protein became unavailable in the USA several years ago.

*Fecal clearance of endogenous $\alpha_1$-antitrypsin ($\alpha_1$-AT)*

$\alpha_1$-AT, a protein which functions as a protease inhibitor, is synthesized by the liver and is present in normal serum in a concentration of 2–5 g/L. It is resistant to proteolysis in the intestines and is therefore excreted into stool undegraded (Durie 1985). $\alpha_1$-AT has a molecular mass similar to albumin, so it would be expected to be lost through the mucosa to the same degree. To determine its clearance, $\alpha_1$-AT is measured by radial immunodiffusion in serum and in a 3-day collection of feces:

$$\text{Fecal } \alpha_1\text{-AT clearance} = \frac{\text{fecal volume} \times \text{fecal } \alpha_1\text{-AT concentration}}{\text{serum } \alpha_1\text{-AT concentration}}$$

The results of fecal $\alpha_1$-AT clearance correlate well with $^{51}$Cr-albumin clearance and provide good separation between controls and patients with protein-losing enteropathy (Hill et al 1981, Karbach et al 1983). However, $\alpha_1$-AT is degraded in the stomach at a pH of less than 3.5. To measure gastric protein loss, the stomach can be continuously aspirated during the intravenous infusion of an $H_2$ receptor antagonist in order to increase gastric pH (Florent et al 1986).

This technique is noninvasive and nonisotopic, making it a much more suitable routine investigative technique in children. Thomas et al (1981) have shown that serial fecal $\alpha_1$-AT concentrations parallel clinical response to therapy in celiac disease, Crohn's disease, intestinal lymphangiectasia and allergic gastroenteropathy. It is possible that random sample collections rather than timed collections may also provide a useful screening test.

## Protein-losing enteropathy

In the normal subject, less than 1% of the total albumin pool is lost into the gastrointestinal tract (Rothschild et al 1970). In some gastrointestinal disorders there is an excessive loss of protein, including albumin, into the lumen; the synthetic capacity of the liver, which at a maximum is twice normal, may be exceeded and hypoproteinemia develops. Equal proportions of the intravascular pool of each protein are lost each day so that the effect is most marked in the case of albumin and immunoglobulins which have a slow turnover, but ceruloplasmin, fibrinogen, transferrin and lipoproteins may also be reduced.

*Mechanisms of protein loss*

Increased cellular turnover, as in celiac disease (p. 382) and atrophic gastritis, results in an increased loss of intracellular protein, but in addition there may be increased loss of serum proteins from the excessive number of extrusion zones. Loss of cells and protein tend to run in parallel (Da Costa et al 1971).

Ulceration occurring in many inflammatory and neoplastic alimentary tract diseases allows direct loss of serum proteins. In active inflammatory bowel disease or graft-versus-host disease, for example, protein loss can be marked. Excessive loss of protein in Menetrier's disease (p. 323) may occur via the mucosal paracellular route (Kelly et al 1982) and from secretions in gastrointestinal tumors and polyps (Gourley et al 1982). In allergic gastroenteropathy protein loss may be secondary to mucosal edema, but the exact mechanism is not understood.

When there is obstruction of the intestinal lymphatic flow, lymph is lost into the gastrointestinal lumen. The loss may occur secondary to increased lymphatic pressure as in congestive cardiac failure, blockage of the lymphatics as in Whipple's disease and lymphoma, or primary disorders of the intestinal lymphatic system such as intestinal lymphangiectasia.

*Clinical features*

In most instances, the clinical features are those of the underlying condition. Protein-losing enteropathy has been demonstrated in a large number of intestinal diseases (Waldmann 1966). However, some conditions present with various degrees of edema (including anasarca) and ascites due to hypoproteinemia.

The etiology of protein-losing enteropathy can be substantiated with endoscopic procedures, gastrointestinal biopsies, radiologic studies and by using radio-labeled serum protein or fecal $\alpha_1$-antitrypsin clearance.

## Intestinal lymphangiectasia

In primary intestinal lymphangiectasia there is congenital malunion of lymphatics resulting in impaired drainage of lacteals and submucosal lymphatics. The lymphatic channels become distended by hydrostatic pressure and then discharge their lymph into the lumen of the small intestine. Most patients have a congenital disorder of the entire lymphatic system, although cases are described where the abnormality is confined to the intestinal lymphatics. The latter may be familial (Shani et al 1974) or sporadic (Waldmann 1966). A minority of patients have congenital hereditary lymphedema (Milroy's disease) which is transmitted as an autosomal dominant trait with incomplete penetrance. Secondary intestinal lymphangiectasia occurs in many neoplastic and infiltrative conditions and also in filariasis.

*Clinical features*

Symptoms usually begin in infancy or childhood. Those presenting soon after birth have marked edema, effusions (often chylous), failure to thrive, diarrhea and steatorrhea. Presentation in childhood or young adulthood is often with asymmetrical edema and mild gastrointestinal symptoms, including intermittent diarrhea. In adulthood, some milder cases have been described, the lymphatic abnormality being confined to the intestine (Roberts & Douglas 1976).

*Diagnostic studies*

Laboratory studies confirm accelerated turnover of albumin (Fig. 13.7), hypoalbuminemia and low serum immunoglobulin concentrations with some reduction in other serum proteins. Lymphocytopenia (500–1000 cells/mm$^3$) is usually present but may not manifest until years after the protein loss appears and this is associated with anergy. Mild to

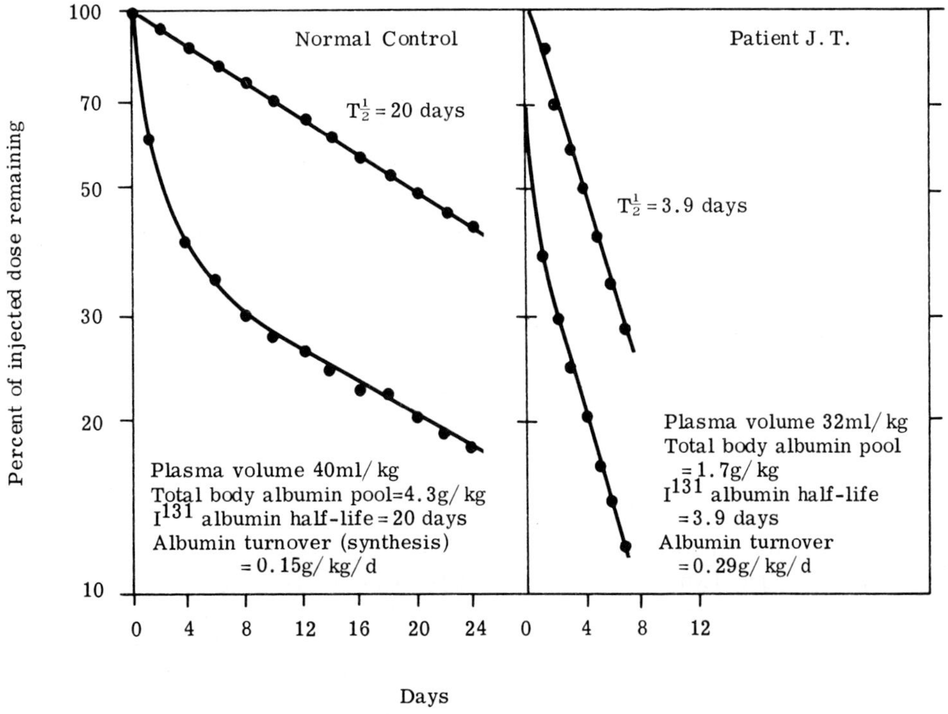


**Fig. 13.7** The turnover of $^{131}$I-labeled albumin in a normal subject and a patient with gastrointestinal protein loss secondary to intestinal lymphangiectasia. The upper curves represent the decline in total body radioactivity with time. The lower curves represent the decline in plasma radioactivity, The total body albumin pool was markedly reduced in patient J.T. The survival half-life of iodinated albumin was markedly shortened and the albumin synthetic rate was slightly greater than normal. (Reproduced with permission from Waldmann 1966.)

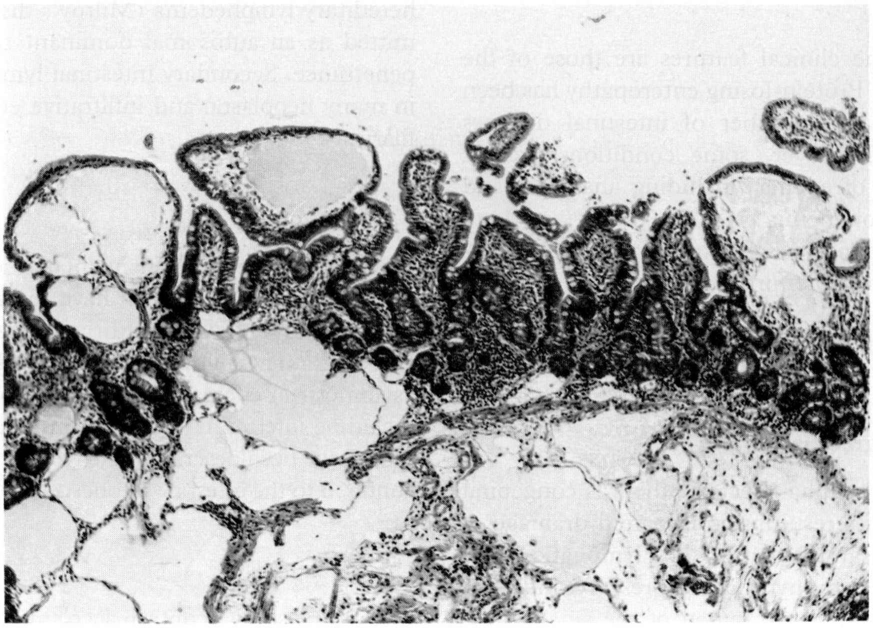

**Fig. 13.8** Lymphangiectasia of small intestine is typified by dilated thinwalled lymphatic channels in the mucosa and superficial submucosa (hematoxylin and eosin, ×75).

moderate steatorrhea is usually present with malabsorption of vitamins D and E as well. Intestinal biopsy after an overnight fast may show gross dilatation of the lymphatic vessels of the submucosa (Fig. 13.8), but this can also occur in lymphatic obstruction caused by Whipple's disease, Crohn's disease and constrictive pericarditis. In some cases, the biopsy may be normal.

The radiological features on barium examination of the small bowel are usually suggestive of the diagnosis, though not specific. In some patients no abnormality is seen, but in most patients there is varying enlargement of the valvulae conniventes, resulting in regular thickening of the small bowel mucosal folds (Fig. 13.9) due to intestinal edema and lymph vessel dilatation. These changes give a serrated outline to the small bowel. In addition there is evidence of increased intestinal secretion but the bowel lumen is rarely dilated (Shimkin et al 1970).

Lymphangiography should be performed in suspected cases. The lower limb lymphatics show either hypoplasia or dilated varicose lymphatics. There may be backflow of contrast into the dermis, reflux into mesenteric lymph nodes and abnormality of the thoracic duct. Lymphangiography occasionally demonstrates localized intestinal disease which can be resected. Enteroscopy may be helpful in making a diagnosis and assessing the extent of the abnormality (Asakura et al 1981). The affected mucosa shows scattered white spots and white tips on the villi.

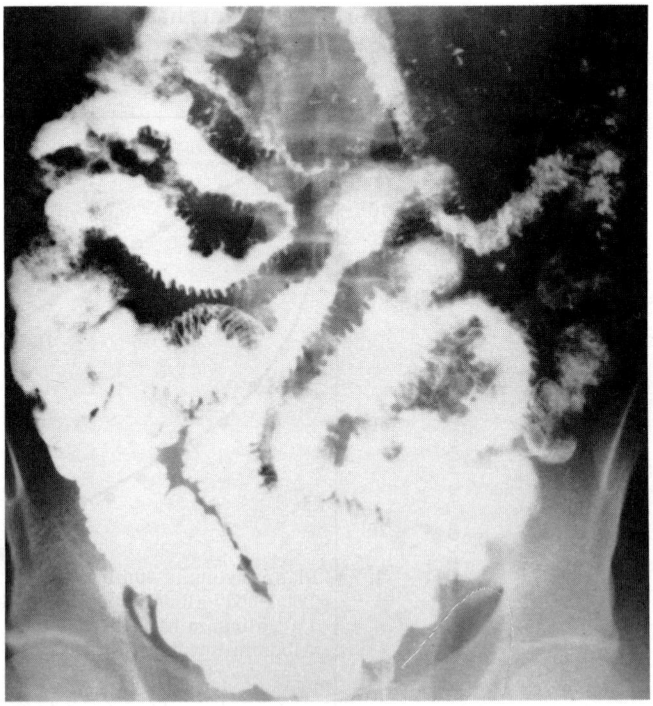

**Fig. 13.9** Congenital lymphangiectasia is depicted by radiologic findings of marked prominence of mucosal folds with regular saw-tooth appearance. Typically there is a history of gross steatorrhea with protein loss resulting in severe hypoproteinemia. Jejunal biopsy shows grossly dilated lymph sacs.

*Differential diagnosis*

The differential diagnosis includes all conditions which cause diffuse enlargement of the intestinal mucosal folds. Among the alternative diagnoses which may cause similar radiologic appearances simulating intestinal lymphangiectasia are Whipple's disease, amyloidosis, systemic mastocytosis, allergic gastroenteritis, Zollinger–Ellison syndrome and constrictive pericarditis with protein-losing enteropathy (Clemett & Marshak 1969).

Lymphoma may develop in patients with long-standing intestinal lymphangiectasia, possibly due to the chronic loss of T-cells into the gut (Broder et al 1981).

#### *Treatment*

It is important to determine if there is an underlying cause which can be treated surgically. In children, malrotation of the gut may cause an increase in lymphatic pressure and lymphangiectasia. Patients with suspected localized involvement of the intestine usually require laparotomy to confirm the diagnosis. Patients who fall into the group without demonstrable underlying cause should receive a trial of corticosteroids (Fleisher et al 1979). In other patients, a low-fat diet or replacement of long chain fatty acids with medium chain triglycerides, which are not transported by the lymphatic system, reduces lymphatic flow and pressure; the loss of protein is thus reduced. Supplements of vitamin D are required to prevent the development of osteomalacia.

## DIGESTION AND ABSORPTION OF LIPIDS

Fat absorption is a complex process with a sequence of steps which converts the hydrophobic long chain triglycerides into a form that can be taken up into the mucosal cells. Once absorbed, the fatty acids themselves become the substrates for re-esterification into triglyceride and incorporation into chylomicrons or they may be delivered directly to the portal bloodstream. A defect in any of the intraluminal, intracellular or lymphatic steps in this sequential interdependent process can lead to malabsorption of fat (see Table 13.2).

### Dietary fat

Lipids provide about 40% of the caloric intake of each individual, amounting to a maximum of 140 g per day in the USA and 60–100 g in the UK. Triglycerides consisting of glycerol esterified to three long chain fatty acids of 16–18 carbon atoms make up >98% of the dietary lipids. A small but variable proportion of lipids contain fatty acids with only 6–10 carbon atoms and are termed medium chain triglycerides (Scheig 1969). In addition, the small intestine is presented with dietary phospholipid, cholesterol and other sterols. Although the diet contains phospholipid, biliary secretion of lecithin provides about 90% of the daily phospholipid load on the intestine, there being 11–12 g of biliary lecithin and 1–2 g of dietary phospholipid.

The absorption of triglyceride is very efficient with more than 95% being absorbed, whereas cholesterol and fat-soluble vitamins are absorbed less efficiently. The absorption of triglyceride is completed in the proximal 100 cm of jejunum, but the more distal bowel can take over this function if the proximal bowel is diseased.

### Intraluminal steps

Several of the processes which occur in the intestinal lumen require the maintenance of a neutral intraluminal pH. When the pH falls below 5, there is inactivation of lipase which reduces lipolysis, precipitation of bile acid which decreases the solubility of fatty acid and monoglyceride, and partitioning of fatty acids into the oil phase. Even in normal subjects, postprandial pH falls below pH 5 intermittently, bringing these mechanisms into action (Zentler-Munro et al 1984).

#### *Emulsification*

This begins in the gastric antrum where the mechanical shearing process produces a coarse emulsion (chyme). In the duodenum the formation of a stable emulsion is enhanced by mechanical mixing and the addition of bile. The detergent-like conjugated bile acids and the lecithin from bile join the phospholipid from the diet in coating the lipid droplets. The emulsification process serves to produce stable lipid particles which have a large lipid:water interfacial surface area.

#### *Hydrolysis*

***Gastric lipase.*** Preduodenal lipase activity in humans is found in the gastric fundic mucosa (Moreau et al 1988). It has a pH optimum of 4.5 (and has some activity at a pH as low as 2.5), so it can digest some of the triglyceride found in food. This enzyme preferentially cleaves the 1α bond of triglycerides, releasing 2,3-diglyceride and one fatty acid molecule. This may be important in assisting with emulsification of lipid and, especially, in digestion of milk fat in the neonate whose pancreatic enzyme function may not be fully developed. The potential activity of gastric lipase is measured to be about 20% of that of pancreatic lipase.

***Pancreatic lipolytic activity.*** Within the duodenum, pancreatic enzyme release is stimulated by fatty acids and amino acids which evoke the release of cholecystokinin (CCK) from the small intestinal mucosa; CCK then causes contraction of the gallbladder and the discharge of pancreatic zymogens. Pancreatic lipase and procolipase are secreted together in a 1:1 molar ratio. Lipase is secreted in its active form but requires activated colipase to participate in hydrolysis of lipid. Procolipase is activated within the small intestinal lumen by trypsin. The peptide sequence of colipase has a hydrophobic moiety which

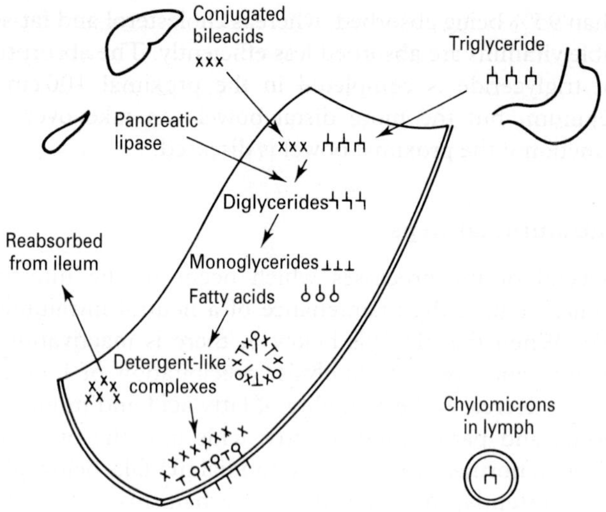


**Fig. 13.10** Scheme depicting the intraluminal events in fat absorption. (Modified with permission from Isselbacher 1967.)

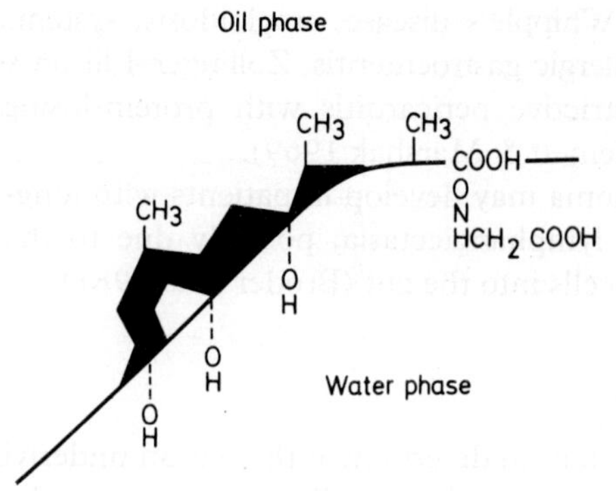


**Fig. 13.11** The alignment of cholic acid conjugate along an oil–water interface. (Reproduced with permission from Eastwood & Mitchell 1979.)

assists its binding to the surface of the lipid emulsion particles, which are also hydrophobic. This process is aided by the conjugated bile acids. It also has a nonhydrophobic moiety which promotes the subsequent binding of the lipase to the surface to bring about the effective hydrolysis of the dietary lipid. Colipase also plays a protective role against inactivation of lipase by bile acids. Pancreatic lipase hydrolyzes the one and three ester bonds of triglyceride to yield 2-monoglyceride and two molecules of fatty acid (Fig. 13.10). These products of lipolysis are removed from the surface of the lipid droplet and solubilized, thus allowing the lipase to continue to act at the oil–water interface of the emulsion. The process of hydrolysis requires pancreatic bicarbonate to maintain an optimal pH for the pancreatic lipase.

### *Solubilization*

Conjugated bile acids play a key role in this process because they have detergent properties. One face of the bile acid molecule with three hydroxyl groups is polar, thus water-soluble, while the other face with two methyl groups is nonpolar and therefore lipid-soluble (Fig. 13.11). The polar carboxyl group on the end of the sidechain contributes to water solubility. Conjugated bile acids are soluble in water when completely ionized at pH 6 in the proximal small intestine.

Conjugated bile acids form polymolecular aggregrates called mixed micelles once their concentration is above a critical concentration of 2 mmol/L (p. 756). Fatty acids and monoglycerides have polar groups which make them highly soluble in the presence of micelles. Nonpolar solutes, e.g. cholesterol, are much less soluble but their solubility increases once polar lipids are included in the micelle.

In the postprandial state bile entering the duodenum is diluted by pancreatic secretions, by the succus entericus and by gastric chyme, the combined effect of this dilution being to reduce the concentration of the conjugated bile acids and hence the stability and numbers of bile acid micelles. At the same time the concentrations of the 2-monoglycerides and fatty acids are rising due to hydrolysis of the dietary triglyceride. Complex interactions occur between these lipids, the conjugated bile acids and phospholipids (mainly lecithin from bile), with the formation of not only mixed micelles but also of much larger disclike phospholipid-conjugated bile acid complexes, resembling liposomes. The composition of these will depend on the proportions of the different lipids present at the stage of digestion reached. Fatty acids are incorporated into the micelle once they are fully ionized and this occurs only at about pH 6.5, induced by pancreatic bicarbonate.

The conversion of an emulsion to micellar particles increases the surface area 10 000-fold, which allows a large amount of monoglyceride and fatty acid to be presented to the intestinal mucosa. The micelles pass through the unstirred layer and since they have a diameter of 4 nm, they are able to pass into the intermicrovillous spaces.

### *Absorption*

Absorption of fat in the normal person occurs predominantly in the duodenum and proximal jejunum. However, when the function of the jejunum is impaired or the jejunum is resected, fat absorption can be taken over by the ileum. A significant proportion of fat, and particularly fatty acids, can be absorbed in the absence of bile as a result of vesicular structures which bud off the emulsion droplets near the brush border membrane and are absorbed immediately unless sufficient bile acids cause their rapid dissolution and uptake into micelles (Rigler et al 1986).

Absorption at the membrane of the absorptive cell does not require energy and probably proceeds merely by passive diffusion. It involves a fatty acid-binding protein in the villi which helps direct fatty acids (especially the unsaturated ones) toward the endoplasmic reticulum for re-esterification (Levy 1992). The high concentrations of lipids solubilized in the micelles acts as a "head" which drives their uptake into the mucosal cells (Fig. 13.10). Recent descriptions of a facilitated diffusion transport mechanism for linoleic acid (Ling et al 1989) and a saturable process for absorption of oleic acid and arachidonic acid indicate that lipid transport may be more complicated than previously thought.

**Intracellular processes** (Fig. 13.12)

*Re-esterification*

Within the small intestinal mucosal cells there are two pathways leading to the resynthesis of triglycerides. These are the monoglyceride pathway and the α-glycerophosphate pathway. Both use absorbed fatty acids which have been bound to coenzyme A as fatty acyl-CoA. This lowers the fatty acid concentration within the mucosal cells, thereby maintaining the gradient for diffusion of fatty acids into the cells and also across the unstirred layer. Both pathways require ATP and are located in the smooth endoplasmic reticulum of the enterocytes.

In the monoglyceride pathway, the 2-monoglyceride is sequentially converted to diglyceride and triglyceride by the addition of fatty acid from acyl-CoA. A closely related group of three enzymes jointly known as triglyceride synthetase is involved. This pathway is used for about 96% of re-esterified triglyceride in the postprandial period.

In the α-glycerophosphate pathway, glycerol which is synthesized de novo from glucose within the mucosal cells is phosphorylated and then acylated by addition of fatty acid residues. A small proportion of the diglyceride formed is used for the synthesis of lecithin. Absorbed lysolecithin is also partly recycled to form lecithin. This pathway functions during fasting.

*Chylomicron formation*

Chylomicrons consist of a hydrophobic core of triglyceride enclosed in a hydrophilic coating of phospholipid, protein and free cholesterol. Lysophosphatidylcholine, which is released from bile-derived phosphatidylcholine in the intestinal lumen as a result of hydrolysis by pancreatic phospholipase $A_2$, acts as the precursor for the mucosal synthesis of phosphatidylcholine, which coats the chylomicrons (Tso et al 1981). The chylomicrons are formed in the smooth endoplasmic reticulum, packaged in vesicles in the Golgi apparatus and secreted into the lymphatic circulation via exocytosis. The lacteals accept the chylomicrons by distending and allowing passage through gaps between the endothelial cells (Sabesin & Frase 1977).

Triglyceride is also converted into very low density lipoproteins (VLDL), which contain less triglyceride and more protein than chylomicrons. In the fasting state, endogenous lipid in the lumen of the intestine is transported as VLDL. Small amounts of dietary fat are also transported in this way, but a large fatty meal is transported by both VLDL and chylomicrons.

Apolipoprotein B, a protein synthesized in the rough endoplasmic reticulum of the enterocyte, is necessary for

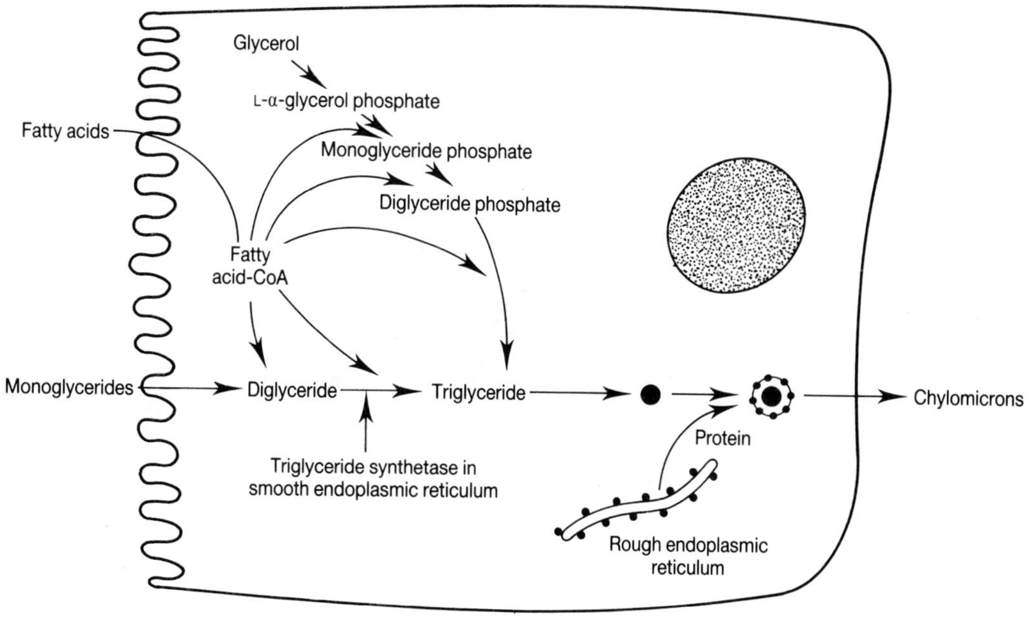


**Fig. 13.12** Major biochemical reactions in the transport of long chain fatty acids and monoglycerides and the production of chylomicrons.

the formation of chylomicrons and VLDL. The lack of apolipoprotein B results in defective formation of chylomicrons and VLDL.

## Absorption of medium chain triglycerides (MCT)

MCT are less hydrophobic than long chain triglycerides (LCT) and, although they form only a small proportion of the dietary intake of fat, they are absorbed more readily than LCT (95.2% absorption of MCT vs 89.9%): this has certain therapeutic advantages (Jensen et al 1986).

The intraluminal hydrolysis of MCT is more rapid and more complete than that of LCT because it presents a greater surface for enzymatic action in any given time (Greenberger & Skillman 1969). The 6–10 carbon fatty acids which are released have greater solubility in water, so bile acids are of less importance for absorption. Furthermore, about 30% of MCT is absorbed intact. Thus, absorption is better than that of LCT when there is a deficiency of pancreatic lipase or bile and when there is a decreased mucosal absorptive area due to intestinal resection. The shorter chain length of the fatty acids derived from MCT allows them to penetrate a diseased mucosal surface more easily. The products are only partly re-esterified within the absorptive cell. Medium chain lipids are largely transported via the portal vein, in contrast to LCT which are transported in the form of chylomicrons via the lymphatic system. A meal of MCT results in a lower concentration of bile acids in the jejunum than a meal of LCT, because gallbladder contraction is weaker. More fluid enters the colon after LCT (Ladas et al 1984). However, patients with pancreatic insufficiency fed MCT-containing formula still require pancreatic enzyme replacement (Durie et al 1980).

## Absorption of fat-soluble vitamins

The major steps in the absorption of the lipid-soluble vitamins A, D, E and K are shown in Figure 13.13. Vitamin esters are hydrolyzed in the intestinal lumen. They are then incorporated into mixed micelles and absorbed by passive diffusion. At this point, vitamin A is re-esterified but this process may not be necessary for the other vitamins. The vitamins are then incorporated into chylomicrons and are absorbed mainly via the lymphatic system, although there is some absorption via the portal vein.

Maximum absorption of fat-soluble vitamins occurs in the proximal jejunum where mixed micelles are formed optimally. β-carotene, a provitamin form of vitamin A, is also absorbed in the proximal small bowel and it is cleaved to form active vitamin A within the enterocytes. Because of the need for incorporation specifically into mixed micelles, absorption is not as efficient as for triglycerides and severe malabsorption can occur when there is defi-

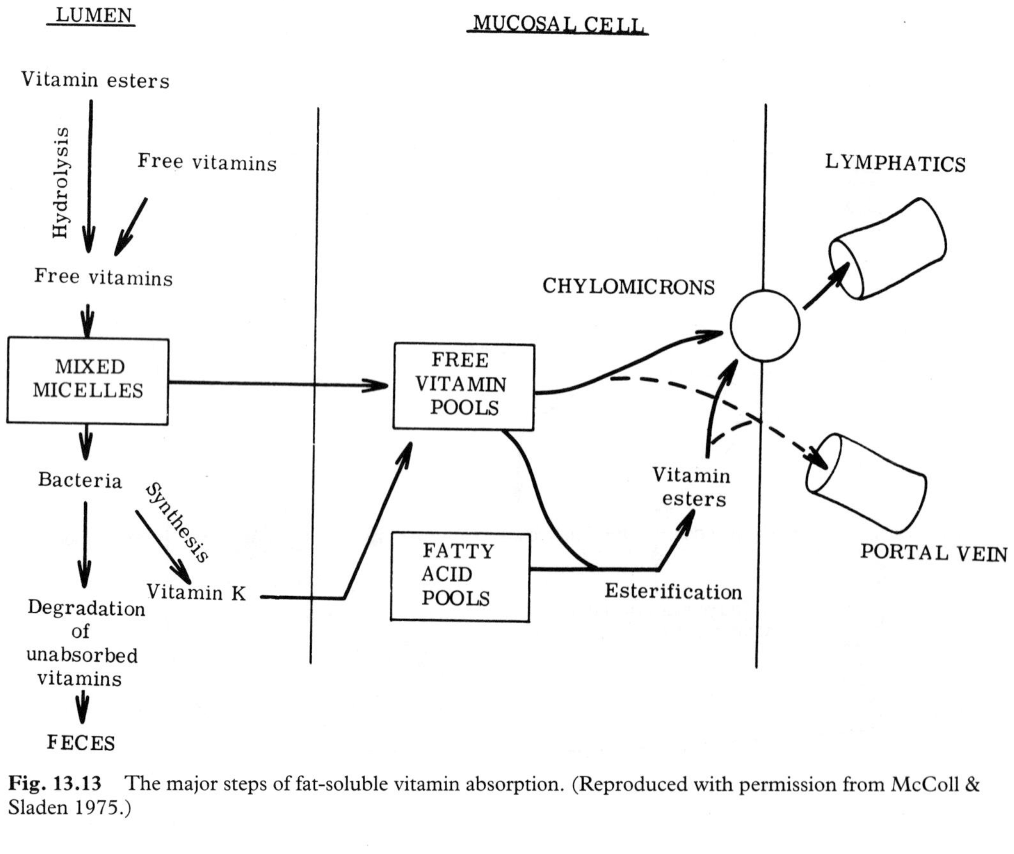


**Fig. 13.13** The major steps of fat-soluble vitamin absorption. (Reproduced with permission from McColl & Sladen 1975.)

ciency of bile acids and when there is damage to mucosal cells, as in celiac disease.

## Cholesterol absorption

Cholesterol in the intestinal lumen is both endogenous (derived from bile, from cholesterol synthesized in intestinal mucosal cells and indirectly from serum cholesterol) and dietary. Cholesterol ester is hydrolyzed to free cholesterol by pancreatic carboxylester lipase (or cholesterol esterase). The unesterified cholesterol is then solubilized in mixed micelles. It is absorbed by passive diffusion and incorporated into chylomicrons before passing into the lymphatic circulation. Its absorption is markedly dependent upon conjugated bile acids. In this respect, the different bile acids have varying effects on absorption, with the therapeutic agent ursodeoxycholic acid (p. 1204) being least effective (Fromm 1984).

## Tests of fat absorption

An estimate of fat absorption can be made directly by qualitatively or quantitatively analyzing the stool or indirectly using alternate methods.

### *Origin of fecal fat*

Studies on fasting subjects suggest that 0.5–2 g/day of fat in the feces is endogenous, arising from fat secreted through the intestinal wall and from fat in desquamated cells and bacteria. The remainder of the fecal fat is derived from unabsorbed dietary fat.

### *Measurement of fecal fat*

The "gold standard" for measurement of fat malabsorption is the quantitative assay using the method of Van de Kamer et al (1949). The fatty acids are liberated from the triglyceride and measured. Fatty acids of a chain length of less than 10 carbon atoms are not measured satisfactorily; thus for patients receiving MCT, the unabsorbed MCT in the stool are not measured without modification of the method. In that case, the method of Jeejeebhoy et al (1970) should be used.

Wollaeger et al (1947) found fecal fat excretion of 4.1 ± 0.5 g/day on an intake of 102 g/day and 8.7 ± 0.7 g/day on an intake of 208 g/day. Other studies support the concept of higher excretion of fat in both normal individuals and patients with steatorrhea when dietary intake of triglyceride is increased. When a 48–72 h stool collection is obtained from a patient receiving a diet of 100 g fat per day, the upper limit of normal is accepted to be 7 g/day. Because fecal fat excretion is nearly linear, the result can be expressed as a percentage of consumed fat, in which case 7% represents the upper limit of normal. Fat absorption and excretion may be better expressed as a coefficient of absorption or the percentage of dietary fat absorbed:

$$\text{Coefficient of absorption} = \frac{\text{dietary fat} - \text{fecal fat}}{\text{dietary fat}} \times 100$$

The coefficient of fat absorption varies with age, premature infants excreting more fat than full-term infants. Adult levels of fat excretion occur by 3 years of age (St Louis et al 1991). Fine & Fordtran (1992) demonstrated that fecal fat levels of up to 14 g per day occurred when diarrhea was induced in normal subjects by cathartic administration.

Complete collection of feces is essential for this test. The difficulty of obtaining a complete collection can be a serious limitation of fecal fat studies.

### *Visual examination of feces*

Gross fecal observation and microscopic examination using Sudan red stain on the feces is thought to be reasonably reliable when there is moderate or severe steatorrhea. With mild steatorrhea the stool looks normal and microscopic examination is also unreliable.

### *Serum carotene*

Serum carotene has been used as a screening test for steatorrhea, assuming an inverse relationship between carotene levels and fecal fat excretion. Its primary function was as an indicator of mucosal disease causing generalized malabsorption. This test is quite insensitive and apart from steatorrhea, low concentrations are found in patients with poor dietary intake of carotene and with liver disease.

### *Tests with isotopically labeled fat*

Tests using $^{131}$I-labeled trioleate have the potential advantage of avoiding fecal fat estimations, but after extensive studies it has to be concluded that blood radioactivity correlates poorly with fat absorption. Measurement of fecal radioactivity is unreliable when compared to fat estimation by the chemical method.

### *Breath tests to detect fat malabsorption*

Metabolism of absorbed fat produces carbon dioxide, which is exhaled in the breath. These techniques use $^{14}$C-trioctanoate, which is an MCT with the advantage of rapid hydrolysis and absorption, or $^{14}$C-trioleate or $^{14}$C-tripalmitate, which are long chain triglycerides requiring a longer period of breath collection. After ingestion of the labeled fat, $^{14}CO_2$ is measured in the expired air. In initial studies with these techniques, there was a wide overlap of results in patients with and without steatorrhea, but subsequently the results of the $^{14}C$-trioleate test have been shown to correlate with the presence of steatorrhea (West et al 1981). However, in patients with altered metabolism of oleic acid due to thyroid disease, obesity, diabetes, chronic liver disorders or hyperlipidemia or with lung disease and altered $CO_2$ release, the test is likely to be inaccurate. The sensitivity may be insufficient for detection of early pancreatic insufficiency.

## Classification of steatorrhea

A physiological abnormality at any of the intraluminal or intracellular stages may result in steatorrhea (Table 13.2). Emulsification is interrupted by lack of mechanical forces in the stomach and by decreased bile secretion. Hydrolysis is incomplete when secretion of lipolytic enzymes is insufficient or the enzymes are inactivated by acid in the intestinal lumen. Solubilization is affected by inadequate bile acid concentration in the lumen. Absorption is suboptimal when contact with the mucosal surface area is reduced by resection, mucosal disease or rapid transit. The re-esterification step is limited if enzymes are decreased, such as in celiac disease or Addison's disease (McBrien et al 1963). Impaired transport of chylomicrons results from altered lymph flow. Impaired lipoprotein synthesis results from genetic disease and drug effect.

### *Steatorrhea in HIV infection*

While fat malabsorption is common in AIDS, Kapembwa et al (1990) demonstrated that exocrine pancreatic insufficiency is unusual and, when present, mild. The villous atrophy identified in the jejunum and intestinal infections are more likely causes of malabsorption of fat and other nutrients in these patients.

### *Abetalipoproteinemia*

The normal human intestine synthesizes the major apolipoproteins, apo-B, apo-A-I and apo-A-IV (Green et al 1982). Abetalipoproteinemia is a rare disease, inherited in an autosomal recessive manner, characterized by steatorrhea and central nervous system abnormalities. There is a lack of apolipoprotein B-containing lipoprotein in the plasma, possibly due to increased degradation rather than lack of synthesis, with the result that chylomicrons and very low density lipoproteins cannot be produced. This leads to fat retention in the enterocyte (Glickman et al 1979, 1991).

The appearance of the small intestinal mucosa on biopsy may be diagnostic. In the fasting state the mucosa is structurally normal except that the enterocytes are engorged with large lipid droplets. Low serum cholesterol and triglyceride concentrations often occur. The diagnosis is confirmed by the absence of serum β-lipoprotein.

The disease usually presents in infancy with failure to thrive, often accompanied by features of intestinal malabsorption. Later in childhood cerebellar ataxia and retinitis pigmentosa may develop, primarily as a result of vitamin E deficiency (Rader & Brewer 1993). Steatorrhea can be mild or absent in older children.

The steatorrhea is effectively controlled by the dietary substitution of MCT for LCT. A vitamin E supplement in a water-miscible form (d-α-tocopherol polyethylene glycol 1000 succinate) may prevent the development or arrest the progression of the neurological complications (Muller et al 1983). The other fat-soluble vitamins should be given in a water-miscible form.

### *Homozygous hypobetalipoproteinemia*

Familial hypobetalipoproteinemia is a rare genetic disorder distinct from classic abetalipoproteinemia (Kane & Havel 1989). Low density lipoprotein and apolipoprotein B are reduced but patients remain asymptomatic.

### *Chylomicron retention disease*

This is a recessively transmitted disorder in children which

**Table 13.2** Classification of steatorrhea

| Stage of fat absorption | Abnormality occurs in |
|---|---|
| Emulsification | Gastric surgery, deficiency of bile |
| Intraluminal hydrolysis | Pancreatic disease – deficiency of lipase |
| | Zollinger–Ellison syndrome — low pH which inactivates lipase |
| | Pancreatic disease |
| Solubilization | Bile acid deficiency |
| | Biliary obstruction |
| | Interrupted enterohepatic circulation |
| | Blind loop syndrome |
| Absorption | Resection – reduction in number of absorptive cells |
| | Damage to mucosal cells, e.g. celiac disease |
| | Decreased transit time, e.g. thyrotoxicosis |
| Re-esterification | Lack of mucosal enzymes – celiac disease, Addison's disease |
| Impaired lipoprotein synthesis | Abetalipoproteinemia |
| leading to impaired chylomicron formation | Puromycin-induced steatorrhea |
| Impaired transport of chylomicrons | Intestinal lymphangiectasia, Whipple's disease, lymphoma |

differs from the above conditions in that the enterocytes are filled with fat which has the morphological appearance of chylomicrons (Roy et al 1987).

## CALCIUM ABSORPTION

### Dietary calcium

The majority of calcium in the diet is found in milk and milk products. It is present primarily in a bound form, for example as calcium caseinate, but some is in the form of ionized calcium. The daily dietary calcium requirement in adults is uncertain, with estimates varying from 500 mg to 1200 mg of elemental calcium per day. Increased calcium requirements occur with pubertal growth, lactation and pregnancy and after menopause. In postmenopausal women the dietary requirement of calcium is likely to be at least 1000 mg of elemental calcium per day.

In addition to the dietary calcium, 600–700 mg enter the intestinal lumen in intestinal secretions (Norman 1990). Of the approximate total of 1600 mg calcium presented to the small intestine, about 700 mg is absorbed or reabsorbed, representing a net gain of 100 mg. This would be matched by a urinary and sweat output of about 100 mg, if calcium balance is achieved. About 900 mg calcium is excreted in stool. There is also an obligatory urinary loss of calcium.

### Absorption

Calcium is absorbed in its ionized form. Absorption from the intestinal lumen and transfer into blood may take place by both a saturable active transcellular route, which is found primarily in the duodenum, and a passive paracellular route which occurs in all parts of the small intestine. Quantitatively, the passive route is more important due to the short mucosal contact time for chyme in the duodenum relative to the remainder of the small intestine. The overall passive transfer of calcium depends on the relative concentrations of calcium ions in the lumen and in blood. The rate of calcium movement through the tight junction and into the paracellular space is slower than expected on the basis of simple diffusion, so the junction itself must specifically inhibit calcium and fluid transport (Bronner 1992). Active transfer becomes more important when the gradient between lumen and blood is unfavorable for diffusion of calcium.

Three phases of transcellular calcium absorption are recognized. At the brush border of the mucosal cells uptake is based on a steep downhill electropotential gradient for calcium and probably occurs via a calcium channel in the apical membrane (Bronner 1992). Transit through the cellular cytosol involves calbindin, a vitamin D-inducible calcium-binding protein (Staun et al 1986), the concentrations of which correlate directly with the rate of calcium transport. At the basolateral membrane of the mucosal cells a $Ca^{++}$-dependent ATPase transports calcium ions out of the cell against a concentration gradient.

Calcium absorption is stimulated by vitamin D and its metabolites, the most active of which is 1,25-dihydroxyvitamin $D_3[1,25(OH)_2D_3]$, by increasing transport at every step of the transcellular pathway, including increased synthesis of calbindin intracellularly (Karbach 1991) and stimulation of $Ca^{++}$ pump units in the basolateral membrane (Wasserman et al 1992). There is also some evidence for stimulation of both the brush border and basolateral membrane phases of calcium uptake by $1,25(OH)_2D_3$ (Nemere & Norman 1986). Parathyroid hormone increases the concentration of $1,25(OH)_2D_3$, thereby increasing calcium absorption, but parathyroid hormone probably also has a direct effect on calcium transport (Nemere & Norman 1986).

The absorption of calcium (and magnesium and zinc) may be increased by the presence of certain dietary sugars such as glucose (Bei et al 1986) and lactose (Cochet et al 1983) by an unknown mechanism. Net intestinal absorption of calcium is subject to metabolic regulation. Long-term adaptations are determined by alterations in vitamin D metabolism and intestinal responsiveness to vitamin D metabolites. Deficiency of either calcium or phosphorus leads to increased production of $1,25(OH)_2D_3$. Bile acids and prolactin have also been shown to stimulate calcium and/or phosphorus absorption, but this effect appears to be via vitamin D-independent mechanisms (Lee et al 1990). The transport of calcium is depicted in Figure 13.14.

### Tests of calcium absorption

Many techniques have been proposed for measurement of calcium absorption in humans during the last 20 years. The better ones have proved useful as research methods, but to date none has found clinical acceptance. In clinical

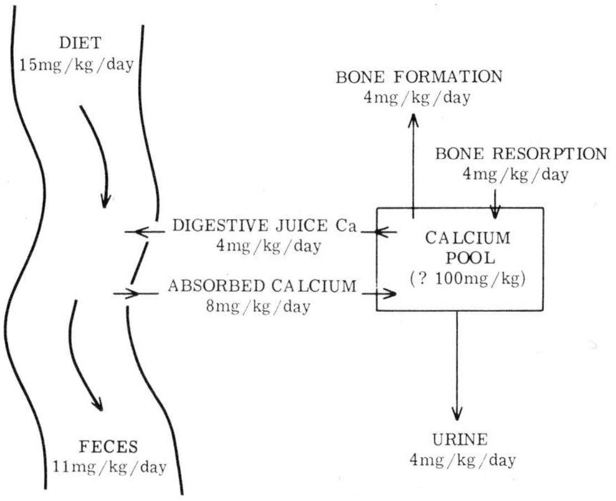


**Fig. 13.14** Calcium absorption in man.

practice, malabsorption of calcium may be inferred from a low serum calcium level. Prolonged vitamin D deficiency may lead to osteomalacia, which can be suggested by radiological study of the bones or inferred from a reduced but sometimes measurable 25-hydroxyvitamin D concentration and raised plasma alkaline phosphatase activity.

Calcium balance can be measured by conventional balance techniques, but these are difficult and time consuming. The isotopes $^{45}Ca$ and $^{47}Ca$ can be used to obtain more information about calcium absorption. While these isotopes can be diagnostically helpful in particularly difficult cases of bone disease, their use is rarely necessary in the clinical setting.

*Serum calcium*

Less than 2% of the body content of calcium is in the plasma and extracellular fluid, yet its concentration is controlled within narrow limits. Calcium is present in the serum in both ionized and protein-bound forms, a small proportion (5–10%) being complexed with anions such as bicarbonate, phosphate and citrate. The normal range for total calcium is 9–10.5 mg/dl (2.2–2.6 mmol/L). In vitamin D deficiency, the serum calcium may fall below 9 mg/dl, but before attaching significance to a low value the concentration of serum proteins must be known. If these are low, total calcium may be reduced while the ionized component remains normal. A simple correction for this effect is to add total serum calcium concentration +0.8 mg/dl for each 1 g/dl reduction of albumin concentrations below normal.

*Alkaline phosphatase activity* (Warnes 1972)

Vitamin D deficiency leads to increased osteoblastic activity and a rise in alkaline phosphatase activity in blood. A raised enzyme activity in a patient with bowel disease or after gastric surgery may be indicative of osteomalacia due to malabsorption of calcium, provided liver disease and other bone disorders such as Paget's disease can be excluded. The problem of the origin of the alkaline phosphatase can be solved by the use of electrophoresis which separates the liver, bone and intestinal alkaline phosphatases.

## Vitamin D deficiency

Vitamin D deficiency may cause two types of bone disease, firstly hyperparathyroidism leading to accelerated bone loss and secondly osteomalacia. The presence of osteomalacia is suggested by radiological study of the bones or inferred from a reduced but sometimes measurable 25-hydroxyvitamin D concentration associated with elevations in plasma concentrations of parathyroid hormone and alkaline phosphatase activity. Also in osteomalacia fasting (24 h) urinary calcium is low and hydroxyproline is high.

## Malabsorption

*Small intestinal disease*

Absorption of calcium is often normal in adult celiac disease. It may be abnormal when there is steatorrhea, perhaps because of the formation of calcium soaps with the unabsorbed fat but also because of vitamin D deficiency. Vitamin D malabsorption occurs frequently and there may be endogenous loss of 25-hydroxyvitamin D in the bile.

Malabsorption of calcium has also been reported in patients after jejunoileal bypass surgery or small intestinal resections. In these the malabsorption may be reversed by administration of $1,25(OH)_2D_3$ (Nunan et al 1986).

*Gastric surgery* (see also p. 276)

Malabsorption in this setting may be due to various factors, including vitamin D malabsorption and deficiency, anatomical changes, more rapid small intestinal transit and interference with the preparation of the ionic forms for absorption. Contrary to earlier speculation the hypochlorhydria resulting from some forms of gastric surgery is unlikely to play a major role in the malabsorption of dietary calcium (Bo-Linn et al 1984, Recker 1985). Malabsorption of calcium due to altered vitamin D metabolism is likely to be a significant factor contributing to the development of metabolic bone disease after gastric surgery (Klein et al 1987).

*Liver disease*

There is vitamin D malabsorption and deficiency in chronic liver disease, particularly that associated with cholestasis, and this leads to calcium malabsorption. It is unlikely that liver disease affects the hydroxylation of vitamin D into the more active form 25-hydroxyvitamin D.

*Corticosteroids*

The administration of glucocorticoids may be associated with a reduction in the intestinal absorption of calcium. There are two major hypotheses to explain this. One is that corticosteroids have an effect on vitamin D metabolism and the other is that they have a direct effect on mucosal cell function, impairing the calcium transport mechanism. Malabsorption of calcium is probably an important etiological factor in the development of corticosteroid-associated osteoporosis. In addition, bone formation is decreased and renal calcium excretion is increased.

*Malabsorption in the elderly*

The absorption of calcium has been shown to decrease after the age of 60 years with decreased absorption in all persons over 80 years (Bullamore et al 1970). In addition, calcium absorption declines marginally in the menopause. Dietary vitamin D deficiency and impaired renal function are likely to be more important factors than a general decline in gastrointestinal function. Malabsorption of calcium is certainly a risk factor for osteoporosis and occurs in 50% of patients with post menopausal osteoporosis. This malabsorption of calcium responds to oral calcium. Nordin et al (1985) have suggested that osteoporosis results from resorption of calcium from the bone in an attempt to hold serum calcium levels stable in the face of calcium malabsorption. It has been attributed by some workers to low plasma levels of $1,25(OH)_2D_3$ but is likely to be multifactorial in origin (Nordin et al 1985).

*Chronic renal failure*

One of the earliest manifestations of renal insufficiency is a fall in calcium absorption. This is such a sensitive expression of renal failure that it may become apparent before the renal impairment has any other physiological effect, i.e. when the glomerular filtration rate is about 60 ml per min or plasma creatinine concentrations are above 150 μmol/L (Juttmann et al 1981). Malabsorption is due to a reduced 1α-hydroxylation of $25(OH)_2D_3$ by the kidney, leading to decreased production of $1,25(OH)_2D_3$, the plasma level of which is a very sensitive indicator of renal function. It follows that there is a correlation between calcium absorption and plasma $1,25(OH)_2D_3$ in subjects with varying degrees of renal insufficiency. Malabsorption of calcium in renal failure is immediately responsive to treatment with $1,25(OH)_2D_3$ or 1α-dihydroxyvitamin D. Because 24,25-dihydroxyvitamin D is also produced in the kidney, the plasma level of this less active metabolite is reduced in renal failure, but the clinical significance of this is uncertain.

*Hyperthyroidism*

Intestinal calcium transport, particularly its active component, is reversibly decreased in hyperthyroidism, probably due to rapid intestinal transit. This decrease is likely to result from calcium-regulating mechanisms as a consequence of the net calcium efflux from bone in this disease (Peerenboom et al 1984). Overtreatment of hypothyroidism with replacement hormone is likely to be important clinically with respect to bone loss as well.

## MAGNESIUM ABSORPTION

Magnesium is the fourth most abundant cation in the body. The proportional distribution of magnesium in serum as ionized, protein bound and complexed is similar to that of calcium. It is absorbed predominantly in the distal small intestine (Kayne & Lee 1993) and descending colon (Hardwick et al 1991), primarily by passive diffusion via the paracellular pathway, although saturable active absorption transcellularly may occur during times of physiological stress (Hardwick et al 1990). Within the physiological range, net absorption of magnesium and phosphate varies linearly with dietary supply. Thus the intestine plays a greater role in the adaptation to changes in exogenous availability of calcium than magnesium. Vitamin D in pharmacological doses increases magnesium absorption, but it also increases urinary excretion of magnesium (Hardwick et al 1991)

Magnesium depletion most commonly occurs in gastrointestinal disorders associated with malabsorption and diarrhea, such as celiac disease, short bowel syndrome, radiation enteritis or inflammatory bowel disease. In borderline short bowel syndrome that is adequate for most nutrient absorption, hypomagnesemia, often accompanied by nephrolithiasis, can sometimes be the factor which necessitates the use of prolonged parenteral nutrition.

### Neonatal hypomagnesemia

This is a selective defect of magnesium absorption which presents in the neonatal period and is characterized by repeated convulsions. A defect in carrier-mediated transport of magnesium has been postulated (Milla et al 1979). Hypocalcemia and hyperphosphatemia as well as hypomagnesemia are noted. Calcium absorption is normal. Treatment of the acute situation is with parenteral magnesium chloride or sulfate. Long-term treatment with oral magnesium gluconate (1 g q.i.d.) will prevent symptoms and normalize serum calcium, but magnesium levels remain low.

## IRON ABSORPTION

The total complement of iron in the adult is ~4 g with about 2.5 g present in red blood cells, 1 g in storage, 300 mg in myoglobin and respiratory chain enzymes and 4 mg in the plasma (Conrad 1987). The iron status of the body is closely controlled through the mechanisms of iron absorption. Dietary iron is prepared for absorption in the upper alimentary tract and the proportion absorbed depends indirectly upon the state of the body stores.

### Dietary iron

The diet of a Western adult (nonvegetarian) contains about 6 mg/1000 kcal or 10–20 mg iron, of which most is inorganic or nonheme iron (85–90%). The amount of iron absorbed varies depending on the chemical form of iron, other dietary factors and various other physiological determinants, but on average 0.5–1.0 mg is absorbed. With an increase in iron stores or a depression of erythropoiesis a smaller amount may be absorbed and in iron deficiency anemia absorption may increase to 3 or 4 mg. Only a small proportion of the iron in food is available for absorption and the availability in different foods varies considerably.

The route and efficiency of absorption depend upon the proportion of heme iron and the ability to keep inorganic iron in an absorbable form. Even when iron is present in a soluble form, other dietary constituents may act as binding or chelating agents. For example, phytate from bran, phosphate and oxalate reduce absorption due to precipitation of the iron. Tea decreases iron absorption as a result of the formation of insoluble iron tannate complexes. The eating of clay, as in geophagia, impairs absorption by cation exchange, with the formation of insoluble complexes in the gut lumen (Minnich et al 1968). Some dietary substances, such as citric acid, lactic acid and ascorbic acid, enhance the absorption of iron. Of these organic acids, ascorbic acid is the most potent promoter of nonheme iron absorption (Baynes & Bothwell 1990) The effect of ascorbic acid is dose related and also affected by the degree of iron deficiency, with doses of 500 mg of ascorbate maximizing iron absorption in subjects with deficient or marginal iron nutriture (Bendich & Cohen 1990).

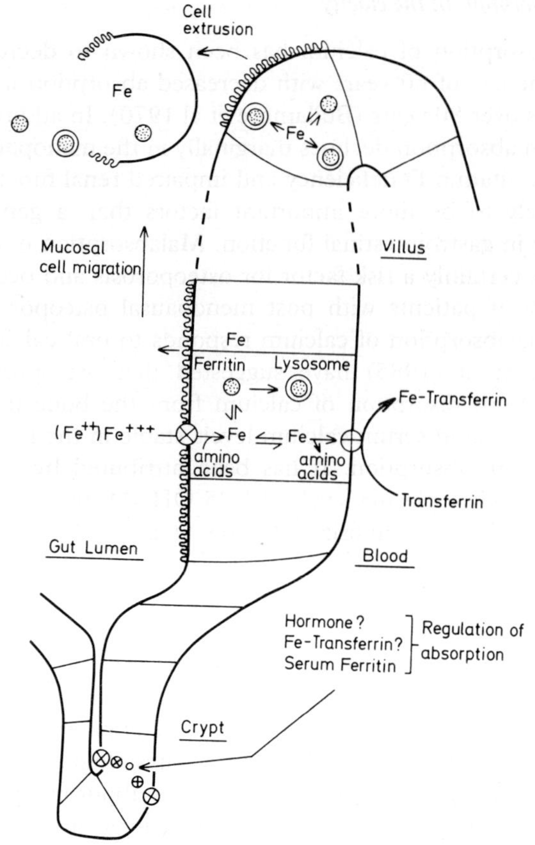


**Fig. 13.15** The mechanism and regulation of iron absorption in the intestinal mucosa. (Reproduced with permission from Linder & Munro 1977.)

### Intraluminal factors affecting absorption

Gastric acid is important in maintaining nonheme iron in the ferrous state rather than the ferric form which is insoluble in aqueous solutions with a pH >3. The ferrous iron is more available for chelation with substances that increase its absorption at the higher pH of the small intestine. Some sugars, amines and amino acids improve absorption by decreasing precipitation and polymerization of iron in solution.

In contrast to inorganic iron, heme iron is most soluble at a neutral pH and is absorbed more efficiently (5–10 fold greater absorption). The heme proteins are digested in the small intestine and the heme fragments are absorbed as metalloporphyrin without release of the iron. Then iron is released within the cell by the action of mucosal heme oxygenase. The absorption of heme iron is unaffected by such factors as alkalinity, ascorbic acid and chelating agents, because the porphyrin part of the molecule protects the iron.

### Mechanism and regulation of iron absorption
(Fig. 13.15)

The small intestine proximal to the jejunum is more efficient in iron absorption than the distal portion and most iron is absorbed from the duodenum and upper jejunum. Nonheme iron is primarily absorbed by an energy-dependent controlled pathway, but it may also be transported via the paracellular route as a result of diffusion and by a transcellular route which is accelerated by lipid. Ferrous iron is oxidized to the ferric form at the brush border before it can interact with its carrier. It is then transferred to the cytoplasm by an active process. Within the cytoplasm nonheme iron and that released from heme is taken up by binding proteins. It is delivered to the basolateral membrane where it is transported out of the cell and becomes attached to transferrin. Most of the iron in this form is transported through the mesenteric circulation.

Iron which is not transported into the plasma is retained in the cell as ferritin and is lost into the lumen when the cell is extruded from the tip of the villus. Ferritin is thought to protect the enterocyte from oxidative damage by free iron. One hypothesis for the control of iron absorption suggests that ferritin was the critical molecule which regulates iron uptake (the mucosal block theory). While there are data relating intestinal concentrations of ferritin and absorption of nonheme iron, it is still unknown whether ferritin plays an active or passive role (Cook 1990).

Iron absorption is stimulated by hypoxemia, decreased iron stores and increased erythropoiesis. These stimuli increase uptake of nonheme and heme iron. By contrast, when iron stores are high, the mucosa is believed to block excessive absorption.

### Tests of iron absorption

These tests are difficult to carry out and are usually used for research purposes rather than as diagnostic tests. Most studies have compared absorption of iron from different iron compounds or foods and for this purpose the isotopes $^{55}Fe$ and $^{59}Fe$ can be used. Day-to-day variations in absorption are overcome by performing multiple absorption tests on the same subject. The absorption is measured by the incorporation of radioactivity into red blood cells or by whole body counting.

### Malabsorption and loss of iron in gastrointestinal disorders

Iron deficiency is common after gastric resections because of failure to reduce iron to the more easily absorbed ferrous form due to the reduced acid output. Bypass of the duodenum and rapid transit through the upper jejunum also decrease transport of iron. Atrophic gastritis with achlorhydria in the intact stomach may be a factor in the development of iron deficiency in some patients (Shearman et al 1966). In the small intestine, disorders which affect the absorptive cell such as celiac disease and tropical sprue result in reduced iron absorption and iron deficiency may develop.

Excessive loss of iron may also result from increased turnover of intestinal cells, which leads to extrusion into the lumen of the cell and its content of iron. This has been called "free iron loss", i.e. nonheme iron (Baird 1973), and it occurs in atrophic gastritis, celiac disease and after partial gastrectomy.

## ZINC ABSORPTION

The majority of dietary zinc is from animal products, especially meat. The zinc that is derived from plants is found mainly in cereals. The zinc in animal products is most bioavailable, while that in cereal grains may be bound by phytates and unavailable.

Zinc is absorbed throughout the small intestine, but the highest capacity for absorption in humans appears to be in the jejunum (Sandström 1992). Recent studies in pigs have identified a saturable carrier-mediated process as well as an unsaturable transport process for zinc in the apical membrane (Tacnet et al 1990). Intraluminal glucose enhances zinc absorption, suggesting a common carrier in the brush border (Sandström 1992). Transport across the cell to the serosal surface is by a low molecular mass zinc-binding protein.

Zinc undergoes enterohepatic circulation, so that zinc excreted in bile is reabsorbed in the distal small intestine. The major losses of zinc occur via the gastrointestinal tract, particularly in association with enterocutaneous and biliary fistulae and inflammatory disease. Zinc absorption and balance are regulated by zinc uptake. One to two mg/day are absorbed from an average zinc intake of 15 mg.

### Acrodermatitis enteropathica

Acrodermatitis enteropathica is a rare autosomal recessive disorder of zinc absorption leading to chronic diarrhea and characteristic acral and orofacial skin lesions (Hambidge & Walravens 1982). A similar clinical picture can occur in any acquired zinc deficiency state. Diseases that lead to increased enteric zinc loss or dietary zinc deficiency can cause an acquired acrodermatitis enteropathica, including patients on total parenteral nutrition devoid of zinc (McClain et al 1980a), Crohn's disease (McClain et al 1980b) and some patients with ileostomy and jejunoileal bypass (Atkinson et al 1978).

#### *Pathogenesis*

Moynahan (1974) first recognized that all the manifestations of acrodermatitis enteropathica could be reversed by giving oral zinc supplements. Atherton et al (1979) have shown that patients have a markedly reduced zinc accumulation in jejunal mucosal biopsy specimens compared with controls. The location and identification of the inherited molecular defect remains undetermined.

#### *Clinical features*

The most typical clinical feature is severe dermatitis consisting of erythematous, pustular, vesiculobullous or eczematoid lesions in an acral and orofacial distribution. Other lesions include nail dystrophy, alopecia, loss of eyebrows, conjunctivitis, photophobia and corneal opacities. The rash first occurs in early infancy except in breastfed infants, in whom it develops after weaning. The zinc concentration in breast milk is similar to cow's milk but is more bioavailable.

Chronic diarrhea, anorexia, failure to thrive and neuropsychiatric manifestations such as irritability, lethargy and depression are common as the disease progresses. Increased susceptibility to infections and hypogonadism in adolescence is reported.

#### *Diagnosis*

This should be suspected on clinical grounds, especially

on the characteristic distribution of the rash. A plasma or serum zinc of less than 6 μmol/L (40 μg/dl) is the most helpful confirmatory test. When severe zinc deficiency is found it is necessary to distinguish acrodermatitis enteropathica from other causes of acquired severe zinc deficiency. The clinical features of acrodermatitis enteropathica have recently been described in a few breastfed premature infants due to a defect of zinc secretion by the mammary gland.

*Treatment and prognosis*

Oral zinc therapy leads to rapid clinical and biochemical remission and in the inborn disorder has to be continued indefinitely. The quantity of elemental zinc required for replacement varies from 30 to 45 mg daily, unrelated to age or weight. It can be given as zinc sulfate or acetate.

## FOLIC ACID ABSORPTION

### Dietary folate

Folic acid is present in many foods, particularly green vegetables, liver and legumes, and this is found primarily in the polyglutamate conjugate of methyl or formyl folate. Because it is easily destroyed, with up to 50% loss during storage, processing and cooking, the recommended intake for adults is 180–200 μg, as compared to the estimated requirement of 50 μg (National Research Council 1989).

### Absorption

Some dietary folate is bound to protein; this must be released within the intestinal lumen but little is known about the process. Only the monoglutamate form is absorbed, therefore for efficient absorption, polyglutamates must be deconjugated by folylpolyglutamate hydrolase which is synthesized in the intestine. Two enzymes are present: one in the brush border which is a carboxypeptidase that cleaves one glutamate residue at a time and one which is an intracellular microsomal endopeptidase (Halsted et al 1986).

Absorption is by a saturable, sodium-dependent, pH-sensitive process throughout the length of the small intestine, although it is most efficient proximally. However, pharmacological amounts of folic acid are probably absorbed passively along the whole length of the small intestine. Daily fecal excretion of folate in healthy humans is about 200 μg (Herbert et al 1984).

The monoglutamates are absorbed via the portal vein to be distributed to the liver and peripheral tissues. Both nonspecific and specific binding proteins are involved in this distribution. The preferential uptake by hepatocytes, erythrocytes, renal tubular cells and enterocytes is executed by binding sites on these cells.

Monoglutamate in the liver is released for distribution to the peripheral tissues by an enterohepatic cycle. Thus the liver exerts a regulatory control in folate metabolism by means of the enterohepatic circulation and by receiving and redistributing folate from tissue turnover.

### Tests of folic acid absorption

A low red cell folate concentration is usually taken to indicate deficiency of folic acid. Serum folate concentrations of less than 2 ng/ml (4.5 nmol/L) are considered abnormal. They do, however, occur in many conditions and do not necessarily signify malabsorption. Folate deficiency may be due to insufficient intake, malabsorption, drug effects or alcoholism.

Folic acid absorption tests are available but are not often used. In these tests, the patient's stores are saturated by a daily intramuscular injection of 15 mg folic acid for 3 days. A standard oral dose of folate is then given and any subsequent rise in serum folate is measured. Other tests measure the absorption of $^{3}$H-folic acid. The amount of radioactivity excreted in the feces subtracted from the total dose used gives a quantitative measurement of the amount absorbed. Normally, less than 35% of the oral dose is excreted (Anderson et al 1960). This method suffers from the disadvantage of requiring a complete collection of feces over 5 or 7 days. In addition, $^{3}$H is difficult to count in fecal samples, requiring combustion of samples for accurate counts. A urinary excretion test has been described as an alternative (Freedman et al 1973).

### Malabsorption

This occurs particularly in disorders which affect the absorptive cells, such as celiac disease and tropical sprue. It is thought that mucosal disease impairs absorption by decreasing the transport of the monoglutamate, probably due to decreased brush border enzyme for deconjugation of folate polyglutamate. Malabsorption also occurs after reduction of the absorptive area of the intestine following resection. Folate deficiency is common in alcoholism, as alcohol reduces folate absorption and also causes increased renal excretion (Weir et al 1985). Drug-induced folate malabsorption results with diphenylhydantoin and sulfasalazine. Although methotrexate alters folate metabolism, it does not decrease absorption (Freedman et al 1973).

Dietary folic acid deficiency in childhood can lead to a megaloblastic anemia, chronic diarrhea and failure to thrive, associated with significant small intestinal mucosal injury. In addition to the megaloblastic erythrocytes, megaloblasts are found in the intestinal mucosa, a change which is reversible with folate supplementation (Davidson & Townley 1977).

A genetic condition which presents with megaloblastic

anemia, diarrhea, stomatitis, failure to thrive, mental retardation and convulsions in the first few months of life has been shown to be due to folic acid malabsorption. It is likely that there is a defect in the specific transport process for monoglutamate (Halsted 1980). These children are able to maintain normal serum folate levels when given large oral doses of folic acid (40 mg/day) or 100–200 μg of folic acid intramuscularly daily.

## VITAMIN $B_{12}$ ABSORPTION

### Dietary vitamin $B_{12}$

Vitamin $B_{12}$ is synthesized by bacteria and fungi, but cannot be produced by plants and animals. While it is obtained from animal products, including eggs and milk, the source is ultimately bacterial synthesis. Fruits and vegetables are essentially devoid of the vitamin. The recommended daily intake for adults is 2 μg, an amount which is contained in most mixed diets but not in a strict vegetarian diet (National Research Council 1989). The total body store of vitamin $B_{12}$ is 2–3 mg which resides mainly in the liver. This is a sufficient supply for 2–5 years, the length of time before megaloblastic anemia develops after total gastrectomy.

Vitamin $B_{12}$ in physiological doses is absorbed only after it has formed a complex with intrinsic factor. By contrast, pharmacological doses in the form of free cyanocobalamin given orally are absorbed across the intestinal mucosa by a process of diffusion (Herbert & Colman 1988).

Although vitamin $B_{12}$ is attached to dietary protein and is in the coenzyme form, most is available for absorption (Okuda et al 1968). Pretreatment of egg with acid and pepsin does not improve the absorption of its vitamin $B_{12}$ when given together with intrinsic factor to patients with pernicious anemia (Schade & Schilling 1967). However, some achlorhydric patients do have malabsorption of vitamin $B_{12}$ incorporated into food, whereas their absorption of cyanocobalamin is normal (Doscherholmen et al 1983). This is likely the result of passive diffusion of the pharmacologic form rather than a requirement for gastric acid or pepsin.

### Absorption

*Intraluminal processes*

Although it was previously believed that dietary vitamin $B_{12}$ was immediately bound to gastric intrinsic factor (produced by parietal cells of the gastric fundic gland region), it is now known that vitamin $B_{12}$ is freed from food proteins by acid and pepsin is then bound to salivary R protein at the low pH in the stomach (Donaldson 1985). This interaction may be important in avoiding destruction of the vitamin at the low pH of the stomach or perhaps as a protection against excess or useless, possibly harmful metabolites. In the alkaline environment of duodenum, the R protein–vitamin $B_{12}$ complex is cleaved by pancreatic protease, allowing the free vitamin to bind with intrinsic factor in the chyme. The vitamin $B_{12}$–intrinsic factor complex proceeds along the intestine to the terminal ileum, where it is absorbed. It is probable that an adequate concentration of calcium ions and a narrow pH range are necessary conditions for absorption (Seetharam & Alpers 1982).

*Site of absorption*

The ileum is the only site of active vitamin $B_{12}$ absorption in humans. If the distal ileum is resected there is total failure of absorption of the vitamin (Cornell et al 1961). Absorption is reduced with resection of more than 120–180 cm of ileum.

*Mechanism of absorption*

***Apical membrane transport.*** The vitamin $B_{12}$–intrinsic factor complex attaches to the brush border of the terminal ileum by a specific mechanism in which the intestinal receptor reacts with intrinsic factor. Antibodies prepared against microvillous membranes of the distal small intestine (but not from proximal small intestine) block the attachment of the complex to brush borders from the distal small intestine (Mackenzie et al 1968). The attachment of the complex to receptors in the intermicrovillous pits requires divalent cations, especially calcium, which probably induce the appropriate configuration of the receptor (Donaldson 1987). Whether vitamin $B_{12}$ is released from intrinsic factor before entering the cell has been debated, but there is now evidence that intrinsic factor may enter the cell as well (Kapadia et al 1983).

With regard to the mechanism of entry into the cell, Donaldson (1985) suggests that the process is probably receptor-mediated endocytosis. The fact that only a limited amount of vitamin $B_{12}$ can be taken up at any one time is in keeping with a specific absorptive mechanism in the ileum. The average maximum daily uptake is about 1.5 μg irrespective of the size of the oral dose (Chanarin 1969); for example, about 75% of an oral dose of 0.5 μg is absorbed and about 50% of a 1 μg dose.

***Intracellular transport.*** Within the ileal cell vitamin $B_{12}$ is released from intrinsic factor and then is bound to transcobalamin II either in the cell or at the basal surface of the ileal enterocyte. It then carries vitamin $B_{12}$ via the portal vein into the circulation and stimulates its uptake by the reticulocyte and liver cell. By contrast, in the fasting state, most of the circulating vitamin $B_{12}$ is bound to transcobalamin I.

The whole process of attachment and transport is slow and when labeled vitamin $B_{12}$ is used, radioactivity appears in the plasma after 4 h and reaches a maximum only after 8–12 h. The receptor sites in the ileum become free to receive further vitamin after 4 h (Schade & Schilling 1967). In part, this may be explained by gastrointestinal transit time from ingestion to distal ileum.

## Tests of vitamin $B_{12}$ absorption

*Serum vitamin $B_{12}$ analysis*

This is measured to detect vitamin $B_{12}$ deficiency. The assay used may be microbiological or radiodilutional. The latter gives higher values and may miss some cases of vitamin $B_{12}$ deficiency (Cohen & Donaldson 1980).

*Absorption of radio-labeled vitamin $B_{12}$*

Vitamin $B_{12}$ absorption tests depend upon the labeling of the vitamin with $^{57}Co$ or $^{58}Co$. After an oral dose of vitamin $B_{12}$, the following methods can be used (Chanarin 1969).

***Urinary excretion method (Schilling test).*** $^{57}Co$- or $^{58}Co$-labeled vitamin $B_{12}$ in a dose of 0.5–2.0 µg is given orally to the fasting patient; 100–200 ml of water are used and the container is carefully rinsed so that the patient receives all of the dose. One or two hours later 1000 µg of nonradioactive vitamin $B_{12}$ is given intramuscularly as a flushing dose. Urine is collected for 24 h following the oral dose and is counted for radioactivity.

The injected vitamin $B_{12}$ saturates the plasma and tissue vitamin $B_{12}$ binders and the absorbed radio-labeled vitamin is excreted in the urine. The free vitamin is filtered by the glomerulus and there is no tubular absorption or excretion. About one-third of the oral dose which has been absorbed is excreted in the urine. The normal excretion of the radio-labeled dose is >8% in 24 h.

The test can be used to distinguish the various causes of vitamin $B_{12}$ deficiency by using several steps: the baseline use of oral free vitamin is followed by a separate study using oral intrinsic factor bound vitamin; an additional study uses free vitamin following an oral course of antibiotics; finally oral pancreatic enzymes are given with the free vitamin. The respective steps can then determine the etiology of malabsorption (Table 13.3).

False positive tests may occur in renal insufficiency. The test depends upon a complete 24-h collection of urine, which may be difficult to obtain in elderly patients or in young children.

***Hepatic uptake method.*** Counting over the liver with a gamma camera allows an estimate to be made of the amount of $^{57}Co$- or $^{58}Co$-labeled vitamin absorbed and deposited in the liver. Difficulties arise because the patient must be in exactly the same position for subsequent counts and, furthermore, the test is unreliable in the presence of liver disease.

***Assessment of plasma radioactivity.*** The radioactivity is measured in a blood sample 8–12 h after the oral dose.

**Table 13.3** Diagnosis of vitamin $B_{12}$ deficiency with the Schilling test

| Cause of deficiency | Free $B_{12}$ | $B_{12}$-IF | Antibiotics | Pancreatic |
|---|---|---|---|---|
| Normal | Normal | – | – | – |
| Pernicious anemia (lack of intrinsic factor) | Abnormal | Corrected | – | – |
| Bacterial overgrowth syndrome | Abnormal | Abnormal | Corrected | – |
| Pancreatic insufficiency | Abnormal | Abnormal | Abnormal | Corrected |
| Ileal disease or resection | Abnormal | Abnormal | Abnormal | Abnormal |

***Whole body counting methods.*** The patient is counted immediately after ingesting the oral dose and again 7–10 days later to determine the proportion of the oral dose which has been retained. Care must be taken to ensure that the patient's bowels have moved regularly during the period of the test because unabsorbed radioactivity retained within the bowel lumen will be interpreted as absorbed radioactivity. The test is accurate and reproducible (Finlayson et al 1969).

Of these tests, the hepatic uptake and plasma radioactivity tests are only semiquantitative. The fecal excretion method is not used clinically because of difficulties of stool collection. In practice, the urinary excretion method (Schilling test) is used for routine clinical assessments and the whole body counting method is used for research studies. All tests using radioactive vitamin $B_{12}$ occasionally suffer from the problem of normal absorption in achlorhydric subjects who nevertheless malabsorb protein-bound cobalamin and who are cobalamin-deficient (King et al 1979).

## Malabsorption of vitamin $B_{12}$

*Lack of intrinsic factor*

***Pernicious anemia.*** This is megaloblastic anemia which occurs in the setting of achlorhydria. Intrinsic factor output is greatly depressed by atrophic gastritis which alters the ability of parietal cells to secrete. In some patients antibodies to intrinsic factor and/or parietal cells can be detected in the plasma (p. 230). In the absence of intrinsic factor vitamin $B_{12}$ must be given parenterally.

***Gastric surgery.*** While the intrinsic factor output may be greatly reduced in partial gastric resection, other factors may contribute to malabsorption, such as bacterial overgrowth syndrome. Total gastrectomy results in complete lack of absorption of vitamin $B_{12}$ (p. 278).

***Acid secretory inhibitors.*** Inhibitors of acid secretion block parietal cell release of acid either through antagonism of the histamine-2 receptor or in the case of omeprazole, by inhibiting $H^+/K^+$ATPase. There is evidence that the $H_2$ blockers (Steinberg et al 1980) and omeprazole (Marcuard et al 1994) decrease absorption of vitamin $B_{12}$. It is likely that the mechanism for this involves inhibition of intrinsic factor production by the parietal cell.

*Abnormalities in the intestinal lumen*

***Bacterial overgrowth syndrome*** (p. 461). In this condition, bacteria in the lumen of the small intestine are able to take up free vitamin $B_{12}$ or, less commonly, the vitamin $B_{12}$–intrinsic factor complex. Giardiasis may cause vitamin $B_{12}$ malabsorption, probably by similar mechanisms (Cowan & Campbell 1973).

***Fish tapeworm*** (Diphyllobothrium latum) (p. 587). The tapeworm acts by taking up free vitamin $B_{12}$ and by releasing the vitamin from vitamin $B_{12}$–intrinsic factor complex (Schjönsby 1973). The diagnosis is made by finding ova or segments in the stool. Treatment is with niclosamide or paromycin.

***Other conditions.*** In pancreatic exocrine insufficiency, tests of vitamin $B_{12}$ absorption may show malabsorption, probably due to lack of protease to release the vitamin from R protein. Deficiency of vitamin $B_{12}$ is unusual in pancreatic disease, but this may not be surprising as decreased protease production is a late manifestation in pancreatic insufficiency.

Malabsorption of vitamin $B_{12}$ may occur in Zollinger–Ellison syndrome. This is often explained on the basis of a low pH in the small intestine, but this is not proven.

*Disorders of the terminal ileum*

Malabsorption of vitamin $B_{12}$ can result from extensive ileal resection (p. 453) or disease, such as Crohn's disease (p. 646), celiac disease or tropical sprue (p. 399). There is some evidence that deficiency of either vitamin $B_{12}$ or folic acid may affect the vitamin $B_{12}$ absorptive mechanism of the ileal cells; thus correction of the deficiency leads to recovery of absorption.

*Vitamin $B_{12}$ deficiency in infancy*

This is rare. While it may be due to juvenile pernicious anemia, familial selective vitamin $B_{12}$ malabsorption or transcobalamin II deficiency, most reported cases are dietary in origin. This may occur in breastfed infants of mothers who are deficient in vitamin $B_{12}$, usually on the basis of inadequate maternal diet or undiagnosed maternal pernicious anemia. Infants of vitamin $B_{12}$-deficient mothers can present with profound hematological, neurological and metabolic abnormalities (Lampkin et al 1966, Higginbottom et al 1978).

***Juvenile pernicious anemia.*** These patients have absent or very low levels of intrinsic factor in their gastric secretions but they do not have achlorhydria or gastric atrophy. They absorb vitamin $B_{12}$ when it is given with exogenous intrinsic factor (Levine & Allen 1985). This disorder is transmitted as an autosomal recessive and hematological and neurological signs of vitamin $B_{12}$ deficiency become apparent within the first 3 years of life (Hall 1973).

***Familial selective vitamin $B_{12}$ malabsorption (Immerslund-Grasbeck syndrome).*** Like congenital absence of intrinsic factor, this is an autosomal recessive disorder. It presents in the first 2 years of life with pallor, weakness, anorexia, growth retardation and neurological and hematological signs of vitamin $B_{12}$ deficiency. It is accompanied by proteinuria without other renal abnormalities. There is a defect in the ileal receptors for intrinsic factor-bound vitamin $B_{12}$ (Burman et al 1985). Gastric and small intestinal structure and function are normal. The Schilling test with and without intrinsic factor is abnormal and serum vitamin $B_{12}$ is low.

***Transcobalamin II deficiency.*** This is a rare disorder in which vitamin $B_{12}$ deficiency manifests itself in the first month of life, because transcobalamin II is necessary for the delivery of vitamin $B_{12}$ to the bone marrow. Severe megaloblastic anemia, vomiting, diarrhea, oral ulceration and atrophy of the mucosa of the tongue develop in the first few weeks after birth. The condition does not arise in utero because transcobalamin II is obtained from the maternal circulation (Hall 1973). The disease is transmitted in an autosomal recessive manner and usually responds well to frequent large doses of vitamin $B_{12}$.

## WATER AND ELECTROLYTE ABSORPTION AND SECRETION IN THE GASTROINTESTINAL TRACT

Large amounts of water and electrolytes enter the lumen of the gastrointestinal tract in the form of secretions necessary for the processes of digestion and absorption. About 9 L of water and 800 mmol of sodium enter each day (Table 13.4) and are subsequently almost completely reabsorbed from the jejunum, ileum and colon (Table 13.5).

The regional variations in this reabsorptive process have been reviewed by Phillips (1972). It can be calculated that the daily volume in the duodenum is 9000 ml, in the jejunum 5000 ml and in the ileum 1500 ml. Ultimately, 150 ml of water are excreted in the stool. Thus, the efficiency of water absorption is approximately 44% in the jejunum, 70% in the ileum and 93% in the colon, although, of course, the greatest volume is absorbed in the jejunum.

### The role of the duodenum and small intestine

The gastric mucosa acts as a barrier to the free movement of water and ions. Thus, the gastric chyme is not isosmolar

**Table 13.4** Volume and composition of fluids entering the gut per 24 h (Phillips 1972)

| | Volume (ml) | Sodium (mmol) | Potassium (mmol) | Chloride (mmol) |
|---|---|---|---|---|
| Diet | 2000 | 150 | 50 | 200 |
| Saliva | 1000 | 50 | 20 | 40 |
| Gastric juice | 2000 | 100 | 15 | 280 |
| Bile | 1000 | 200 | 5 | 40 |
| Pancreatic juice | 2000 | 150 | 5 | 40 |
| Succus entericus | 1000 | 150 | 5 | 100 |
| Total | 9000 | 800 | 100 | 700 |

**Table 13.5** Efficiency of water and sodium absorption in the intestine (Phillips 1972)

| Segment | Volume leaving ml/24 h | Na leaving mmol/24 h | % of Duodenal load absorbed | | % of Segmental load absorbed | |
|---|---|---|---|---|---|---|
| | | | Water | Na | Water | Na |
| Duodenum | 9000 | 800 | – | – | – | – |
| Jejunum | 5000 | 700 | 44 | 13 | 44 | 13 |
| Ileum | 1500 | 200 | 39 | 62 | 70 | 72 |
| Colon | 100 | 3 | 16 | 25 | 93 | 99 |
| Entire gut | 100 | 3 | 99 | 99+ | – | – |

with plasma when it enters the duodenum and various feedback mechanisms influence the rate of gastric emptying so that the chyme can be rendered isosmotic and neutral in the duodenum (p. 423). This involves the secretion of bicarbonate into the pancreatic juice, bile and succus entericus and the movement of water or ions out of or into the lumen, depending on whether the meal is hypo-osmolar or hyperosmolar, respectively. By the time the chyme reaches the major absorptive region, the jejunum, it has been rendered isosmotic and it remains so throughout the jejunum, ileum and proximal colon. Therefore, a major role of the duodenum is to osmotically equilibrate its contents rapidly with plasma.

## Electrolyte and water absorption

There are three proposed routes by which sodium can enter the absorbing enterocyte from the intestinal lumen. A sodium–potassium ATPase pump in the basolateral membrane of the enterocyte exchanges intracellular sodium for extracellular potassium and is essential to the maintenance of a downhill gradient which favors sodium absorption. This electrochemical gradient, thus the pump, is essential to all three sodium routes.

Sodium may enter by an apical membrane sodium channel, the driving force for sodium entry being a downhill electrochemical gradient between the lumen and cytoplasm of the enterocyte. This pathway does not involve simultaneous transport of other ions, so there is net transfer of charge; thus it is electrogenic. In the small intestine this is a minor route but it may represent the major route for sodium entry in the colon.

Sodium can also enter the small intestinal mucosa coupled to the absorption of organic solutes such as amino acids and glucose. Here too the driving force for the coupled entry of sodium with organic solute is an inward electrochemical gradient for sodium. This transport mechanism is the basis for oral rehydration solution replacement of fluids in cholera and infantile diarrheas.

Thirdly, there exists a $Na^+$ and $Cl^-$ cotransport system in the brush border. This is probably the main route for the entry of both ions, on a one-to-one basis, in the small intestine. Electroneutrality is maintained by concomitant entry of chloride ions or exchange of luminal sodium for intracellular hydrogen ion.

Water accompanies the movement of sodium regardless of the mechanism of sodium transport. In the jejunum water is also absorbed with organic solutes by the process of solvent drag.

In addition to the cotransport with sodium, a $Cl^-$ absorption mechanism is recognized in the ileum. This transport which involves exchange with $HCO_3^-$ is driven by an electrochemical gradient which favors bicarbonate secretion. The jejunum absorbs $HCO_3^-$ as a result of sodium absorption coupled with secretion of hydrogen derived from cellular water (the $OH^-$ ion remains in the cell). The hydrogen ion interacts with luminal $HCO_3^-$ to form carbonic acid which dissociates to carbon dioxide and water. The $CO_2$ is absorbed and forms $HCO_3^-$ within the enterocyte when it interacts with hydroxyl ion left behind in the cell.

Potassium is absorbed passively from both jejunum and ileum. There is net absorption in the proximal small bowel and distal colon. In the distal small intestine and proximal colon net potassium secretion occurs. Potassium is the cation which is normally present at the highest concentration in the stool.

## Secretion by crypt cells of the small intestine

There is strong evidence that, whereas villous cells have an absorptive role, the undifferentiated crypt cells are an important site of secretion. In the crypt cells there is a $Na^+$-dependent $Cl^-$ secretion. $Cl^-$ enters the mucosal cell at the basolateral membrane coupled to entry of $Na^+$ down its electrochemical gradient. $Cl^-$ then exits via the chloride permeable apical membrane. It appears that $Ca^{++}$, cyclic AMP and cyclic GMP can act as intracellular modifiers of this $Cl^-$ secretion process with stimulation of $Cl^-$ secretion being mediated through activation of intracellular protein kinases (Donowitz & Welch 1987). There is evidence for regulation of chloride secretion by a neurohumoral regulatory pathway (Sjövall et al 1986) which is affected by cholera endotoxin and the heat-stable enterotoxin from *E. coli*.

Under physiological conditions, several hormones are secretagogues for the small intestinal mucosa. Among these are VIP, secretin, neurotensin, substance P, acetylcholine and peptide histidine-isoleucine (Anagnostides et al 1984).

### The effect of drugs on diarrhea

Opiates such as codeine, diphenoxylate and loperamide reduce cathartic-induced diarrhea and decrease ileostomy fluid excretion. There are two potential points of action for these opiate drugs. They slow intestinal transit (thus allowing more time for absorption) by increasing non-propulsive muscle activity, particularly in the circular muscle. There is evidence (p. 1363) that loperamide acts to delay small bowel transit by increasing its capacitance (Schiller et al 1984) and increasing transit time predominantly in the jejunum but not in the ileum or colon (Kachel et al 1986). The effect of loperamide is mediated through $\mu$-opioid receptors since it is antagonized by naloxone (Basilisco et al 1985). The increase in non-propulsive muscular activity by opiates can increase intracolonic pressure, which can be dangerous in severe colitis or diverticular disease. However, others have demonstrated marked effects of loperamide on colonic transit (Ewe et al 1993) and it may also significantly enhance anal sphincter function (Hallgren et al 1994).

Opiates also have effects on the water and electrolyte transport in the intestine. The latter is via peripheral mechanisms rather than through the central nervous system and consists of stimulation of absorption and/or the inhibition of secretion via opiate receptors in the intestinal mucosa (McKay et al 1981, 1982). Additionally, loperamide may act by reducing intestinal secretion in response to secretagogues but does not alter absorption under basal conditions (Hughes et al 1984).

It is possible that diarrhea can be alleviated by other drugs. Clonidine, an $\alpha_2$-adrenergic agonist, slows small intestinal transit and increases absorption. It may act on $\alpha_2$ receptors both in the intestinal musculature and on the enterocyte membranes (Schiller et al 1985). Lidamidine hydrochloride may also act as an $\alpha_2$ agonist to enhance absorption or inhibit secretion of fluid and electrolytes. It has no effect on small intestinal transit (Sninsky et al 1986) and is not superior to placebo in functional diarrhea (p. 1363). $\beta_2$-adrenergic agonists have been shown to decrease rectosigmoid motility (Lyrenäs et al 1985). Lithium carbonate, which inhibits cyclic AMP synthesis, has been reported to ameliorate secretory diarrhea (Owyang 1984).

### Water and electrolyte absorption from the colon

The primary function of the colon is the conversion of the fluid ileal contents into semisolid feces for excretion, with consequent conservation of sodium and water. While an established ileostomy discharges on average a daily volume ≤500 ml, intubation studies suggest that ileum in the intact gut delivers into the colon ~1500 ml per day (fasting flow rates of 0.3–1.6 ml/min and postprandial flow rates of 4–8 ml/min). All but 100–150 ml water are absorbed together with 95% of the 200 mmol of sodium. About 60 mmol of bicarbonate and 5 mmol of potassium are absorbed. Most of the sodium and water absorption occurs in the ascending colon. Perfusion with isotonic saline has shown that the colon has the capacity to absorb up to 5.7 liters of water, 816 mmol of sodium and 44 mmol of potassium each day (Debongnie & Phillips 1978). Thus, under normal circumstances, the colon has a reserve capacity for absorption which can compensate for impaired absorption by the small intestine.

### Mechanisms of absorption from the colon

Sodium is absorbed across the apical membrane of the cell down an electrochemical potential gradient which is maintained by the action of the $Na^+/K^+$ATPase situated in the basolateral membrane. This pathway is electrogenic. There is also an electroneutral cotransport mechanism for chloride with sodium, the process probably being linked to the $Na^+/H^+$ and $Cl^-/HCO_3^-$ (chloride absorbed) exchange across the colonic mucosa. The colon has the ability to actively secrete chloride from the crypt cells. The potassium concentration in stool water is much higher than in plasma and this results from the absorption of water along the colon and from the secretion of potassium in the proximal colon. Mucus from both the diseased (Crane 1965) and normal (Giller & Phillips 1972) colon contains a high concentration of dialyzable potassium and may account for the increased loss of potassium in diarrhea. The electrogenic sodium absorptive mechanism is stimulated in the colon by aldosterone and its analogs. Aldosterone also stimulates potassium secretion by the colon. This may be important in the response to dehydration and in Addison's disease.

Since water movement is secondary to net solute movement, the capacity of the epithelium to absorb fluid will be indirectly affected by the ease with which water can cross the mucosa. As in the small intestine, absorption of water from the majority of the colon is passive and closely follows the osmotic pressure gradient created by sodium absorption. Thus in the proximal colon the absorbed fluid is nearly isotonic with luminal fluid and a transmural osmotic pressure difference is not maintained. By contrast, the distal colon can absorb hypertonic fluid and maintain a transmural osmotic pressure difference. Typically diarrheal stool water is isosmotic with plasma, as transit through the distal colon is too rapid to establish a hypertonic stool.

## Short chain fatty acids

The major anions in the colonic contents are short chain fatty acids (SCFAs) (Hoverstad 1986). These are present in low concentration in the terminal ileum but rise significantly in the ascending colon as the result of carbohydrate fermentation by colonic anaerobic bacterial flora (Mitchell et al 1985). Plant polysaccharides are the main precursors of these organic acids, but up to 20% of ingested starch and simple sugars which have escaped small intestinal digestion and mucus are also potential precursors. The pKa values of SCFAs are close to 4.8, so that at the near neutral pH of the large intestine they are ionized. Production of organic acid in the large bowel accounts for the disappearance of most of the bicarbonate which is secreted by the intestinal mucosa. The following reaction accounts for the high $PCO_2$ of the colonic lumen:

$$CH_3COOH + Na^+ + HCO_3^- = CH_3COONa + H_2O + CO_2$$

Concentrations of SCFAs fall again in the distal colon owing to absorption and metabolism. Acetate is the principal SCFA, contributing 60% of the total, with the other two major acids propionate and butyrate at almost 20% each.

Roediger (1980) has shown that SCFAs are substantially metabolized by isolated colonic epithelial cells and when present can suppress glucose oxidation, suggesting they are the preferred metabolic fuel for the colonic mucosal cells. Dependence on butyrate as a fuel appears to be greater in the distal bowel. SCFAs have been shown to inhibit bacterial proliferation. When dissociated, these acids can enter the bacterial cell and inhibit bacterial metabolism.

Absorption of SCFA from the colonic lumen coincides with bicarbonate secretion and sodium and water reabsorption. Stool output in various diarrheal states correlates with SCFA output and it was once thought that SCFAs caused fluid retention in the colon by an osmotic effect. However, as fecal SCFA levels remain more or less constant despite dietary changes, any factor increasing stool weight will increase output of these acids, even laxatives. The change in stool output in diarrhea caused by carbohydrate malabsorption is now thought to be partly due to the osmotic effect of malabsorbed sugars (Saunders & Wiggins 1981).

Evidence for diminished oxidation of SCFAs has been provided in ulcerative colitis (Roediger et al 1984). This effect may be secondary to the disease process rather than causative.

## Regulation of ion transport

### *Hormonal mechanisms*

Mineralocorticoids increase the absorption of sodium and water and probably exert an overall control on their transport. They appear to act primarily by increasing apical membrane permeability to sodium. Loss of sodium stimulates secretion of the hormone, which in turn acts on the colon to retain sodium but with an increased potassium loss. Such changes have been demonstrated in normal subjects given mineralocorticoids and in patients with hyperaldosteronism. Under normal circumstances, the fecal loss of potassium amounts to 20% of the total daily loss, but this can be increased fivefold in primary aldosteronism (Shields et al 1968). It is also relevant to note that secondary hyperaldosteronism can occur in patients addicted to laxatives.

### *Neuronal mechanisms*

Although there is broad understanding of the role of the enteric nervous system in the motor activity of the intestine, its role in the regulation of ion transport is not well understood. It is accepted, however, that the enteric nervous system may have the main responsibility for ion transport (Bridges & Rummel 1986). Neurotransmitters which act at the postsynaptic neural receptors in the enteric ganglia stimulate secretion (acetylcholine, CCK, 5-hydroxytryptamine, TRH and VIP) and absorption (enkephalin, galanin, norepinephrine and somatostatin) (Cooke 1994). Neurotransmitters also control water and electrolyte transport directly at the epithelial cells. Excitatory substances cause secretion at this level (acetylcholine, CGRP, 5-hydroxytryptamine, substance P and VIP) while inhibitory substances increase absorption (neuropeptide Y, norepinephrine, peptide YY and somatostatin) (Cooke 1994).

### *Intracellular mechanisms*

As a result of the application of cloning techniques to cell membranes, there is now an increased understanding of the interaction of ligands with their specific receptors and of the intermediary couplers involved, such as G proteins (Holenberg 1991). Cyclic AMP, cyclic GMP, tyrosine kinase, inositol 1,4,5-triphosphate (Berridge 1993) and $Ca^{++}$ are among the intracellular mediators of various neuronal and hormonal stimuli. Inositol triphosphate controls many cellular processes by generating inositol calcium signals. It operates through receptors that closely resemble the calcium-mobilizing ryanodine receptors of muscle. Tyrosine kinase protein has been localized to the plasma membrane and to the membrane of secretory vesicles in secretory cells, suggesting that tyrosine phosphorylations may be associated with the process of secretion.

Cyclic AMP or agents which increase cyclic AMP, such as VIP, prostaglandins, cholera toxin and theophylline, inhibit the absorption of sodium and chloride and stimulate the secretion of chloride. Furthermore, adenylate cyclase-coupled receptors for VIP and the active moiety of cholera toxin have been demonstrated in isolated membranes from the enterocytes (Sharp et al 1977). When the ileum is diseased or resected (p. 452), bile acids enter the colon, where the dihydroxy bile acids inhibit water and sodium absorption and may also stimulate secretion by increasing mucosal cyclic AMP. Hydroxy fatty acids (p. 462) and castor oil (p. 462) also act by stimulating colonic secretion.

## Congenital chloridorrhea

This is a rare disorder which is inherited in an autosomal recessive manner manifested from birth. It is characterized by severe watery diarrhea associated with hypochloremia, hypokalemia and metabolic alkalosis (in contrast to the usual acidosis in severe diarrhea). The excessive loss of chloride in the stool reaches as high as 150 mmol/L and always exceeds the sum of the $Na^+$ and $K^+$ concentrations. The condition is associated with maternal hydramnios and all affected infants are born prematurely. The primary defect in this condition lies in the anion exchange mechanism in both ileum and colon, with a reversal of the normal chloride/bicarbonate exchange (Turnberg 1971).

Treatment consists of intravenous replacement therapy initially and oral electrolyte replacement later. In order to prevent renal and arteriovascular changes, replacement solutions should contain both NaCl and KCI (Holmberg et al 1977).

## Fecal weight and composition

As a result of the physiological processes described above, the mean daily fecal weight is about 120 g and 60–85% of this is water. When the stool weight exceeds 200 g/day in Western communities, diarrhea is usually present. In the normal stool there is a daily loss of ~4 mmol of sodium and 9–12 mmol of potassium. In diarrhea, the concentration of sodium in the stool increases with the severity of the diarrhea and at stool flow rates of 3 L or more per 24 h the electrolyte content approaches that of plasma (Fig. 13.16).

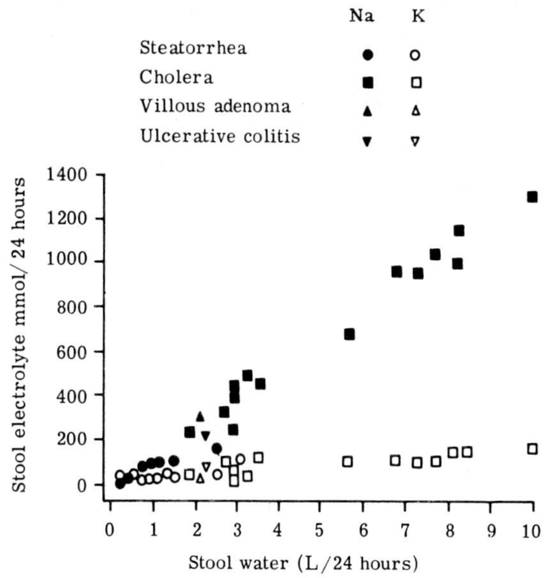


**Fig. 13.16** Relation of stool water to sodium and potassium loss in diarrhea. The points of cholera, ulcerative colitis and villous adenoma refer to single patients. The points for steatorrhea represent the average of 3–5 patients. (Reproduced with permission from Fordtran & Dietschy 1966.)

## Mechanisms of diarrhea

### *Definition of diarrhea*

Diarrhea is an increase in fluidity, volume or frequency of bowel movement. This involves a change in bowel habits or characteristics. Diarrhea can occur without an increase in stool volume, called "small volume" diarrhea. This often occurs with disease or dysfunction of the distal colon or rectum and the stool often consists of blood or mucus.

## Classification of diarrhea

Diarrhea may be caused by a variety of mechanisms. In any one disease more than one mechanism may be in operation.

***Osmotic diarrhea.*** An excess of water-soluble molecules in the gut lumen results in the osmotic retention of water within the lumen of the colon. Osmotic diarrhea occurs with many laxatives and in carbohydrate malabsorption (p. 344). When there is diffuse disease of the small intestine, a variety of other substances may contribute to the osmotic load, e.g. amino acids.

***Secretory diarrhea.*** This can be defined as diarrhea resulting from a net movement of fluid into the gut lumen despite fasting. The stool osmolality in adults is accounted for by total stool electrolytes.

Secretory diarrhea results from the stimulation of active ion secretion by the small intestine or colon. This is mediated by an increase in intracellular cyclic AMP or calcium which allows $Cl^-$ to enter the lumen, followed by $Na^+$ and water. The absorption of NaCl via the NaCl cotransport mechanism (p. 367) is also inhibited by cyclic AMP, but $Na^+$ absorption by the glucose and amino acid carrier mechanism remains intact. Thus absorption can continue if stimulated by glucose. This forms the basis for the treatment of cholera (p. 564) and other diarrheas by glucose-electrolyte oral rehydration solutions. Cholera, some *E. coli* and salmonella infections act via stimulation of intracellular cyclic AMP (pp. 558 and 564), as do prostaglandins, VIP and dihydroxy bile acids in the colon (p. 452). A variety of other agents suspected to act through the cyclic AMP cause diarrhea, e.g. ricinoleic acid or castor oil and some other gastrointestinal hormones. Other pathological processes can lead to secretory diarrhea, e.g. mucosal injury, inflammatory processes and the excessive secretion from villous adenomas.

***Diarrhea due to inhibition of ion absorption.*** Several agents, for example bile acids and hydroxylated fatty acids (pp. 452 and 462), may act by preventing ion absorption as well as by stimulating colonic secretion.

***Motility disorders.*** Often, the disordered motility which accompanies diarrhea is secondary to an inflammatory process or an increase in intraluminal contents. However, some diarrheal disorders may be due primarily to disturbed motility, e.g. irritable bowel syndrome and diabetic diarrhea (p. 445). In some cases, markedly slowed motility, as in scleroderma or radiation fibrosis of the muscularis, can cause bacterial overgrowth syndrome (p. 442) with resulting diarrhea.

*Clinical distinction between secretory and osmotic diarrhea*

***The effect of fasting.*** When the patient is fasted for 48–72 h (with fluid and electrolytes given by intravenous infusion), osmotic diarrhea stops unless osmotic laxatives are taken surreptitiously (p. 1337). By contrast, secretory diarrhea usually continues during fasting, unless it has been induced by bile acids in the colon, in which case it stops with fasting.

***Investigation of the stool.*** Stool osmotic gap may be estimated based on the premise that stool is isosmotic to plasma, particularly when stool is not allowed to remain in the rectum (as would be expected in diarrhea). Therefore, plasma osmolality can be determined or a typical plasma osmolality of 290 mOsm/kg can be assumed. Stool sodium and potassium concentrations are then measured, added and multiplied by two (to account for anions as well as the measured cations). When this number is subtracted from the plasma osmolality or 290, the resulting value is the osmotic gap. In patients with secretory diarrhea the gap should be $\leq 50$. In osmotic diarrhea, the stool osmotic gap is $>50$ and usually 100 or more, owing to the presence of other unabsorbed solutes.

Measurements of the actual osmolality of fecal fluid must be used with caution, as bacterial fermentation of unabsorbed solutes can artificially elevate the osmolality and thus the osmotic gap (Fine et al 1993).

**Oral rehydration solution** (p. 282)

Fluid and electrolyte imbalances resulting from cholera, infantile diarrhea, especially in Third World countries, and short bowel syndrome have been treated effectively using oral rehydration solutions which draw upon basic physiologic concepts of water and electrolyte transport (Ghisan 1988). These solutions base their success on principles of cotransport of sodium and glucose with resulting water absorption and on minimization of osmotic activity within the bowel lumen. In some cases of short bowel syndrome this approach to therapy may eliminate the need for home parenteral nutrition (Camilleri et al 1992). This example of applied physiology demonstrates how an understanding of the basic physiologic mechanisms of absorption may be beneficial to effective therapy of gut dysfunction.

REFERENCES

Anagnostides A A, Christofides N D, Tatemoto K, Chadwick V S, Bloom S R 1984 Peptide histidine isoleucine: a secretagogue in human jejunum. Gut 25: 381–385

Anonymous 1977 Sucrose malabsorption. British Medical Journal 1: 1558–1559

Anderson B, Belcher E H, Chanarin I, Mollin D L 1960 The urinary and fecal excretion of radioactivity after oral doses of H3-folic acid. British Journal of Haematology 6: 439–459

Asakura H, Miura S, Morishita T et al 1981 Endoscopic and histopathological study on primary and secondary intestinal lymphangiectasia. Digestive Diseases and Sciences 26: 312–320

Atherton D J, Muller D P R, Aggett P J, Harries J T 1979 A defect in zinc uptake by jejunal biopsies in acrodermatitis enteropathica. Clinical Science 56: 505–507

Atkinson R L, Dahms W T, Bray G A, Jacob R, Sandstead H H 1978 Plasma zinc and copper in obesity and after intestinal bypass. Annals of Internal Medicine 89: 491–493

Baird I M 1973 Gastrointestinal causes of iron deficiency. Clinics in Haematology 2: 291–302

Bank S, Fisher G, Marks I N, Groll A 1967 The lymphatics of the intestinal mucosa. A clinical and experimental study. American Journal of Digestive Diseases 12: 619–632

Basilisco G, Bozzani A, Camboni G et al 1985 Effect of loperamide and naloxone on mouth-to-cecum transit time evaluated by lactulose hydrogen breath test. Gut 26: 700–703

Bayless T M, Rothfeld B, Massa C, Wise L, Paige D, Bedine M S 1975 Lactose and milk intolerance: clinical implications. New England Journal of Medicine 292: 1156–1159

Baynes R D, Bothwell T H 1990 Iron deficiency. Annual Reviews of Nutrition 10:133–148

Bei L, Wood R J, Rosenberg I H 1986 Glucose polymer increases jejunal calcium, magnesium, and zinc absorption in humans. American Journal of Clinical Nutrition 44: 244–247

Bendich A, Cohen M 1990 Ascorbic acid safety: analysis of factors affecting iron absorption. Toxicology Letters 51: 189–201

Bennett H S 1963 Morphological aspects of extracellular polysaccharides. Journal of Histochemistry and Cytochemistry 11: 14–23

Berridge M J 1993 Inositol triphosphate and calcium signaling. Nature 361: 315–325

Bjarnason I, Marsh M N, Price A, Levi A J, Peters T J 1985 Intestinal permeability in patients with coeliac disease and dermatitis herpetiformis. Gut 26: 1214–1219

Bo-Linn G W, Davis G R, Buddrus D J, Morawski S G, Santa Ana C, Fordtran J S 1984 An evaluation of the importance of gastric acid secretion in the absorption of dietary calcium. Journal of Clinical Investigation 73: 640–647

Bond J H, Levitt M D 1975 Investigation of small bowel transit time in man utilizing pulmonary hydrogen (H2) measurements. Journal of Laboratory and Clinical Medicine 85: 546–555

Bond J H, Currier B E, Buchwald H, Levitt M D 1980 Colonic conservation of malabsorbed carbohydrate. Gastroenterology 78: 444–447

Bridges R J, Rummel W 1986 Mechanistic basis of alterations in mucosal water and electrolyte transport. Clinics in Gastroenterology 15: 491–506

Broder S, Callihan T R, Jaffe E S et al 1981 Resolution of longstanding protein-losing enteropathy in a patient with intestinal lymphangiectasia after treatment for malignant lymphoma. Gastroenterology 80: 166–168
Bronner F 1992 Current concepts of calcium absorption: an overview. Journal of Nutrition 122: 641–643
Bullamore J R, Gallagher J C, Wilkinson R, Nordin B E C, Marshall D H 1970 Effect of age on calcium absorption. Lancet 2: 535–537
Büller H A, Grand R J 1990 Lactose intolerance. Annual Review of Medicine 41: 141–148
Burgess D H 1982 Reactivation of intestinal epithelial cell brush border motility. ATP-dependent contraction via a terminal web contractile ring. Journal of Cell Biology 95: 853–863
Burman J F, Jenkins W J, Walker-Smith J A et al 1985 Absent ileal uptake of IF-bound vitamin $B_{12}$ in vivo in the Imerslund-Grasbeck syndrome (familial Vitamin $B_{12}$ malabsorption with proteinuria). Gut 26: 311–314
Butterworth C W, Perez-Santiago E, Martinez J J, Santini R 1959 Studies on the oral and parenteral administration of *d* (+) xylose. New England Journal of Medicine 261: 157–164
Camilleri M, Prather C M, Evans M A, Andresen-Reid M L 1992 Balance studies and polymeric glucose solution to optimize therapy after massive intestinal resection. Mayo Clinic Proceedings 67: 755–760
Casellas F, Malagelada J R 1994 Clinical applicability of shortened D-xylose breath test for diagnosis of intestinal malabsorption. Digestive Diseases and Sciences 39: 2320–2326
Caspary W F 1978 Breath tests. Clinics in Gastroenterology 7: 351–374
Caspary W F 1992 Physiology and pathophysiology of intestinal absorption. American Journal of Clinical Nutrition 55: 299S–308S
Chadwick V S, Phillips S F, Hofmann A F 1977 Measurements of intestinal permeability using low molecular weight polyethylene glycols (PEG 400). II Application to normal and abnormal permeability states in man and animals. Gastroenterology 73: 247–251
Chanarin I 1969 The megaloblastic anaemias. Blackwell, Oxford
Clark S L Jr 1959 The ingestion of proteins and colloidal materials by columnar absorptive cells of the small intestine in suckling rats and mice. Journal of Biophysical and Biochemical Cytology 5: 41–49
Clemett A R, Marshak R H 1969 Whipple's disease. Roentgen features and differential diagnosis. Radiologic Clinics of North America 7: 105–111
Cochet B, Jung A, Griessen M, Bartholdi P, Schaller P, Donath A 1983 Effects of lactose on intestinal calcium absorption in normal and lactase-deficient subjects. Gastroenterology 84: 935–940
Cohen K L, Donaldson R M Jr 1980 Unreliability of radiodilution assays as screening tests for cobalamin (Vitamin $B_{12}$) deficiency. Journal of the American Medical Association 244: 1942–1945
Conrad M E 1987 Iron absorption. In: Johnson L R (ed) Physiology of the gastrointestinal tract, 2nd edn. Raven Press, New York, p 1437–1453
Cook J D 1990 Adaptation in iron metabolism. American Journal of Clinical Nutrition 51: 301–308
Cooke H J 1994 Intestinal salt and water transport. In: Walsh J H, Dockray G J (eds) Gut peptides: biochemistry and physiology. Raven Press, New York, p 749–763
Cornell G N, Gilder H, Moody F, Frey C, Beal J M 1961 The pattern of absorption following surgical shortening of the bowel. Bulletin of the New York Academy of Medicine 37: 675–688
Cowan A E, Campbell C B 1973 Giardiasis – a cause of vitamin $B_{12}$ malabsorption. American Journal of Digestive Diseases 18: 384–390
Craig R M, Atkinson A J 1988 D-xylose testing: a review. Gastroenterology 95: 223–231
Crane C W 1965 Observations on the sodium and potassium content of mucus from the large intestine Gut 6: 439–443
Crane R K 1960 Intestinal absorption of sugar. Physiological Reviews 40: 789–825
Crane R K 1966 Enzymes and malabsorption: a concept of brush border membrane disease. Gastroenterology 50: 254–262
Crane R K 1975 A digestive-absorptive surface as illustrated by the intestinal cell brush border. Transactions of the American Microscopical Society 94: 529–544
Crane R K 1977 The gradient hypothesis and other models of carrier-mediated active transport. Reviews of Physiology, Biochemistry and Pharmacology 78: 99–159
Cuatrecasas P, Lockwood D H, Caldwell J R 1965 Lactase deficiency in the adult. A common occurrence. Lancet 1: 14–18
Cummings J H 1984 Cellulose and the human gut. Gut 25: 805–810
Da Costa L R, Croft D N, Creamer B 1971 Protein loss and cell loss from the small-intestinal mucosa. Gut 12: 179–183
Dahlqvist A 1968 Assay of intestinal disaccharidases. Analytical Biochemistry 22: 99–107
Davidson G P, Robb T A 1983 Detection of primary and secondary sucrose malabsorption in children by means of the breath hydrogen technique. Medical Journal of Australia 2: 29–32
Davidson G P, Townley R R W 1977 Structural and functional abnormalities of the small intestine due to nutritional folic acid deficiency in infancy. Journal of Pediatrics 90: 590–594
Debongnie J C, Phillips S F 1978 Capacity of the human colon to absorb fluid. Gastroenterology 74: 698–703
Deschner E E, Lipkin M 1976 Cell proliferation in normal, preneoplastic and neoplastic gastrointestinal cells. Clinics in Gastroenterology 5: 543–561
Dills W L 1989 Sugar alcohols as bulk sweeteners. Annual Reviews of Nutrition 9: 161–186
Donaldson R M 1985 How does cobalamin (Vitamin $B_{12}$) enter and traverse the ileal cell? Gastroenterology 88: 1069–1071
Donaldson R M 1987 Intrinsic factor and the transport of cobalamin. In: Johnson L R (ed) Physiology of the gastrointestinal tract, 2nd edn. Raven Press, New York, p 959–973
Donowitz M, Welch M J 1987 Regulation of mammalian small intestinal electrolyte secretion. In: Johnson L R (ed) Physiology of the gastrointestinal tract, 2nd edn. Raven Press, New York, p 1351–1388
Doscherholmen A, Silvis S, McMahon J 1983 Dual isotope Schilling test for measuring absorption of food-bound and free Vitamin $B_{12}$ simultaneously. American Journal of Clinical Pathology 80: 490–495
Du Mont G C L, Beach R C, Menzies I S 1984 Gastrointestinal permeability in food-allergic eczematous children. Clinical Allergy 14: 55–59
Durie P R 1985 Intestinal protein loss and fecal $\alpha$1-antitrypsin. Journal of Pediatric Gastroenterology and Nutrition 4: 345–347
Durie P R, Newth C J, Forstner G G, Gall D G 1980 Malabsorption of medium-chain triglycerides in infants with cystic fibrosis: correction with pancreatic enzyme supplements. Journal of Pediatrics 96: 862–864
Eastwood G L 1977 Gastrointestinal epithelial renewal. Gastroenterology 72: 962–975
Eastwood M A, Mitchell W D 1979 Biliary excretion by the liver. In: Duthie H L, Wormsley K G (eds) Scientific basis of gastroenterology. Churchill Livingstone, Edinburgh, p 288–305
Enck P, Whitehead W E 1986 Lactase deficiency and lactose malabsorption. A review. Zeitschrift fur Gastroenterologie 24: 125–134
Erickson R H, Kim Y S 1990 Digestion and absorption of dietary protein. Annual Reviews of Medicine 41: 133–139
Ewe K, Ueberschaer B, Press A G 1993 Influence of senna, fibre, and fibre + senna on colonic transit in loperamide-induced constipation. Pharmacology 47: 242–248
Farquhar M F, Palade G E 1963 Junctional complexes in various epithelia. Journal of Cell Biology 17: 375–412
Feibusch J M, Holt P R 1982 Impaired absorptive capacity for carbohydrate in the aging human. Digestive Diseases and Sciences 27: 1095–1100
Fine K D, Fordtran J S 1992 The effect of diarrhea on fecal fat excretion. Gastroenterology 102: 1936–1939
Fine K D, Krejs G J, Fordtran J S 1993 Diarrhea. In: Fordtran M H, Fordtran J S (eds) Gastrointestinal disease pathophysiology, diagnosis, management, 5th edn. W B Saunders, Philadelphia, p 1043–1072
Finlayson N D C, Simpson J D, Tothill P, Samson R R, Girdwood R H, Shearman D J C 1969 Application of whole body counting to the measurement of Vitamin $B_{12}$ absorption with reference to achlorhydria. Scandinavian Journal of Gastroenterology 4: 397–405
Fleisher T A, Strober W, Muchmore A V, Broder S, Krawitt E L,

Waldmann T A 1979 Corticosteroid-responsive intestinal lymphangiectasia secondary to an inflammatory process. New England Journal of Medicine 300: 605–606

Florent C, Vidon N, Flourié B et al 1986 Gastric clearance of alpha-1-antitrypsin under cimetidine perfusion. New test to detect protein losing gastropathy? Digestive Diseases and Sciences 31: 12–15

Flourié B, Vidon N, Florent C H, Bernier J 1984 Effect of pectin on jejunal glucose absorption and unstirred layer thickness in normal man. Gut 25: 936–941

Ford R P K, Menzies I S, Phillips A D, Walker-Smith J A, Turner M W 1985 Intestinal sugar permeability: relationship to diarrheal disease and small bowel morphology. Journal of Pediatric Gastroenterology and Nutrition 4: 568–574

Fordtran J S, Dietschy J M 1966 Water and electrolyte movement in the intestine. Gastroenterology 50: 263–285

Fordtran J S, Clodi P H, Soergel K H, Ingelfinger F J 1962 Sugar absorption tests, with special reference to 3-O-methyl-d-glucose and d-xylose. Annals of Internal Medicine 57: 883–891

Freedman D S, Brown J P, Weir D G, Scott J M 1973 The reproducibility and use of the tritiated folic acid urinary excretion test as a measure of folate absorption in clinical practice; effect of methotrexate on absorption of folic acid. Journal of Clinical Pathology 26: 261–267

Fromm H 1984 Gallstone dissolution and the cholesterol-bile acid lipoprotein axis. Propitious effects of ursodeoxycholic acid. Gastroenterology 87: 229–233

Gardner J D, Brown M S, Laster L 1970 The columnar epithelial cell of the small intestine: digestion and transport. New England Journal of Medicine 283: 1196–1201, 1264–1271, 1317–1324

Ghisan F K 1988 The transport of electrolytes in the gut and the use of oral rehydration solutions. Pediatric Clinics of North America 35: 35–51

Giller J, Phillips S F 1972 Electrolyte absorption and secretion in the human colon. American Journal of Digestive Diseases 17: 1003–1011

Glickman R M, Green P H R, Lees R S, Lux S E, Kilgore A 1979 Immunofluorescence studies of apolipoprotein B in intestinal mucosa. Absence in abetalipoproteinemia. Gastroenterology 76: 288–292

Glickman R M, Glickman J N, Magun A, Brin M 1991 Apolipoprotein synthesis in normal and abetalipoproteinemic intestinal mucosa. Gastroenterology 101: 749–755

Gourley G R, Odell G B, Selkurt J, Morrissey J, Gilbert E 1982 Juvenile polyps associated with protein-losing enteropathy. Digestive Diseases and Sciences 27: 941–945

Gray G M 1970 Carbohydrate digestion and absorption. Gastroenterology 58: 96–107

Gray G M 1975 Carbohydrate digestion and absorption. Role of the small intestine. New England Journal of Medicine 292: 1225–1230

Green P H R, Lefkowitch J H, Glickman R M, Riley J W, Quinet E, Blum C B 1982 Apolipoprotein localization and quantitation in the human intestine. Gastroenterology 83: 1223–1230

Greenberger N J, Skillman T G 1969 Medium-chain triglycerides. Physiologic considerations and clinical implications. New England Journal of Medicine 280: 1045–1058

Gudmand-Hoyer E, Krasilnikoff P A 1977 The effect of sucrose malabsorption on the growth pattern in children. Scandinavian Journal of Gastroenterology 12: 103–107

Gudmand-Hoyer E, Simony K 1977 Individual sensitivity to lactose in lactose malabsorption. American Journal of Digestive Diseases 22: 177–181

Hadorn B, Green J R, Sterchi E E, Hauri H P 1981 Biochemical mechanisms in congenital enzyme deficiencies of the small intestine. Clinics in Gastroenterology 10: 671–690

Hahn U 1990 Facts and problems of the intestinal basement membranes. Digestion 46 (suppl 2): 40–48

Hall C A 1973 Congenital disorders of Vitamin $B_{12}$ transport and their contribution to concepts. Gastroenterology 65: 684–686

Hallgren T, Fasth S, Delbro D S, Nordgren S, Oresland T, Hulten L 1994 Loperamide improves anal sphincter function and continence after restorative proctocolectomy. Digestive Diseases and Sciences 39: 2612–2618

Halsted C H 1980 Intestinal absorption and malabsorption of folates. Annual Review of Medicine 31: 79–87

Halsted C H, Beer W H, Chandler C J et al 1986 Clinical studies of intestinal folate conjugases. Journal of Laboratory and Clinical Medicine 107: 228–232

Hambidge K M, Walravens P A 1982 Disorders of mineral metabolism. Clinics in Gastroenterology 11: 87–117

Hamilton J W, Li B U K, Shug A L, Olsen W A 1986 Carnitine transport in human intestinal biopsy specimens. Gastroenterology 91: 10–16

Hardwick L L, Jones M R, Brautbar N, Lee D B N 1990 Site and mechanism of intestinal magnesium absorption. Mineral and Electrolyte Metabolism 16: 174–180

Hardwick L L, Jones M R, Brautbar N, Lee D B N 1991 Magnesium absorption: mechanisms and the influence of vitamin D, calcium and phosphate. Journal of Nutrition 121: 13–23

Harrison M, Walker-Smith J A 1977 Reinvestigation of lactose intolerant children: lack of correlation between continuing lactose intolerance and small intestinal morphology, disaccharidase activity, and lactose tolerance tests. Gut 18: 48–52

Herbert V, Colman N 1988 Folic acid and Vitamin $B_{12}$. In: Shils M E, Young V R (eds) Modern nutrition in health and disease, 7th edn. Lea & Febiger, Philadelphia, p 388–416

Herbert V, Drivas G, Manusselis C, Mackler B, Eng J, Schwartz E 1984 Are colon bacteria a major source of cobalamin analogues in human tissues? 24-h human stools contain only about 5 μg cobalamin but about 100 μg apparent analogues (and 200 μg folate). Transactions of the Association of American Physicians 97: 161–171

Higginbottom M C, Sweetman L, Nyhan W L 1978 A syndrome of methylmalonic aciduria, homocystinuria, megaloblastic anemia and neurologic abnormalities in a Vitamin $B_{12}$ deficient breast-fed infant of a strict vegetarian. New England Journal of Medicine 299: 317–323

Hill R E, Hercz A, Corey M L, Gilday D L, Hamilton J R 1981 Fecal clearance of α-1-antitrypsin: a reliable measure of enteric protein loss in children. Journal of Pediatrics 99: 416–418

Holenberg M D 1991 Structure-activity relationships for transmembrane signaling: the receptor's turn. FASEB Journal 5: 178–186

Holmberg C, Perheentupa J, Pasternack A 1977 The renal lesion in congenital chloride diarrhea. Journal of Pediatrics 91: 738–743

Holzel A, Schwarz V, Sutcliffe K W 1959 Defective lactose absorption causing malnutrition in infancy. Lancet 1: 1126–1128

Hoverstad T 1986 Studies of short-chain fatty acid absorption in man. Scandinavian Journal of Gastroenterology 21: 257–260

Hughes S, Higgs N B, Turnberg L A 1984 Loperamide has antisecretory activity in the human jejunum in vivo. Gut 25: 931–935

Hyams J S 1983 Sorbitol intolerance: an unappreciated cause of functional gastrointestinal complaints. Gastroenterology 84: 30–33

Isselbacher K J 1967 Biochemical aspects of lipid malabsorption. Federation Proceedings 26: 1420–1425

Jain N K, Patel V P, Pichumoni C S 1987 Sorbitol intolerance in adults. Journal of Clinical Gastroenterology 9: 317–319

Jeejeebhoy K N, Ahmad S, Kozak G 1970 Determination of fecal fats containing both medium and long chain triglycerides and fatty acids. Clinical Biochemistry 3: 157–163

Jensen C, Buist N R M, Wilson T 1986 Absorption of individual fatty acids from long chain or medium chain triglycerides in very small infants. American Journal of Clinical Nutrition 43: 745–751

Juttman J R, Buurman C J, de Kam E, Visser T J, Birkenhager J C 1981 Serum concentrations of metabolites of vitamin D in patients with chronic renal failure (CRF). Consequences for the treatment with 1-α-hydroxy derivatives. Clinical Endocrinology 14: 225–236

Kachel G, Ruppin H, Hagel J, Barina W, Meinhardt M, Domschke W 1986 Human intestinal motor activity and transport: effects of a synthetic opiate. Gastroenterology 90: 85–93

Kane J P, Havel R J 1989 Disorders of the biogenesis and secretion of lipoproteins containing the B apolipoproteins. In: Scriver C R, Beaudet A C, Sly W S, Valle D (eds) The metabolic basis of inherited disease, 6th edn. McGraw-Hill, New York, p 1139–1164

Kapadia C R, Serfilippi D, Voloshin K, Donaldson R M Jr 1983 Intrinsic factor mediated absorption of cobalamin by guinea pig ileal cells. Journal of Clinical Investigation 71: 440–448

Kapembwa M S, Fleming S C, Griffin G E, Caun K, Pinching A J, Harris J R W 1990 Fat absorption and exocrine pancreatic function in human immunodeficiency virus infection. Quarterly Journal of Medicine 273: 49–56

Karbach U 1991 Segmental heterogeneity of cellular and paracellular calcium transport across the rat duodenum and jejunum. Gastroenterology 100: 47–58

Karbach U, Ewe K, Bodenstein H 1983 $Alpha_1$-antitrypsin, a reliable endogenous marker for intestinal protein loss and its application in patients with Crohn's disease. Gut 24: 718–723

Kayne L H, Lee D B N 1993 Intestinal magnesium absorption. Mineral and Electrolyte Metabolism 19: 210–217

Kelly D G, Miller L J, Malagelada J-R, Huizenga K A, Markowitz H 1982 Giant hypertrophic gastropathy (Ménétrier's disease): pharmacologic effects on protein leakage and mucosal ultrastructure. Gastroenterology 83: 581–589

Kerlin P, Wong L 1987 Lactose tolerance despite hypolactasia in adult coeliac disease. Journal of Gastroenterology and Hepatology 2: 233–237

Kerlin P, Wong L, Harris B, Capra S 1984 Rice flour, breath hydrogen, and malabsorption. Gastroenterology 87: 578–585

Kim Y S, Erickson R H 1985 Role of peptidases of the human small intestine in protein digestion. Gastroenterology 88: 1071–1073

King C E, Leibach J, Toskes P P 1979 Clinically significant Vitamin $B_{12}$ deficiency secondary to malabsorption of protein-bound Vitamin $B_{12}$. Digestive Diseases and Sciences 24: 397–402

Klein K B, Orwoll E S, Lieberman D A, Meier D E, McClung M R, Parfitt A M 1987 Metabolic bone disease in asymptomatic men after partial gastrectomy with Billroth II anastomosis. Gastroenterology 92: 608–616

Kolars J C, Levitt M D, Aouji M, Savaiano D A 1984 Yogurt – an autodigesting source of lactose. New England Journal of Medicine 310: 1–3

Krasilnikoff P A, Gudmand-Hoyer E, Moltke H H 1975 Diagnostic value of disaccharide tolerance tests in children. Acta Paediatrica Scandinavica 64: 693–698

Ladas S D, Isaacs P E T, Murphy G M, Sladen G E 1984 Comparison of the effects of medium and long chain triglyceride containing liquid meals on gall bladder and small intestinal function in normal man. Gut 25: 405–411

Lampkin B C, Shore N A, Chadwick D 1966 Megaloblastic anemia of infancy secondary to maternal pernicious anemia. New England Journal of Medicine 274: 1168–1171

Langman J M, Rowland R 1990 Activity of duodenal disaccharidases in relation to normal and abnormal mucosal morphology. Journal of Clinical Pathology 43: 537–540

Lanza E, Jones D Y, Block G, Kessler L 1987 Dietary fiber intake in the USA population. American Journal of Clinical Nutrition 46: 790–797

Leclercq-Foucart J, Forget P P, van Cutsem J L 1987 Lactulose-rhaminose intestinal permeability in children with cystic fibrosis. Journal of Pediatric Gastroenterology and Nutrition 6: 66–70

Lederle F A, Busch D L, Mattox K M et al 1990 Cost-effective treatment of constipation in the elderly: a randomized double-blind comparison of sorbitol and lactulose. American Journal of Medicine 89: 597–601

Lee D B N, Hardwick L L, Hu M-S, Jamgotchian N 1990 Vitamin D-independent regulation of calcium and phosphate absorption. Mineral and Electrolyte Metabolism 16: 167–173

Levine J S, Allen R H 1985 Intrinsic factor within parietal cells of patients with juvenile pernicious anemia. A retrospective immunohistochemical study. Gastroenterology 88: 1132–1136

Levitt M D 1983 Malabsorption of starch: a normal phenomenon. Gastroenterology 85: 769–770

Levitt M D, Hirsh P, Fetzer A, Sheahan M, Levine A S 1987 H2 excretion after ingestion of complex carbohydrates. Gastroenterology 92: 383–389

Levitt M D, Strocchi A, Levitt D F 1992 Human jejunal unstirred layer: evidence for extremely efficient luminal stirring. American Journal of Physiology 262: G593–G596

Levy E 1992 Selected aspects of intraluminal and intracellular phases of intestinal fat absorption. Canadian Journal of Physiology and Pharmacology 70: 413–419

Lifschitz C 1985 Intestinal permeability. Journal of Pediatric Gastroenterology and Nutrition 4: 520–522

Linder M C, Munro H N 1977 The mechanism of iron absorption and its regulation. Federation Proceedings 36: 2017–2023

Ling K Y, Lee H Y, Hollander D 1989 Mechanisms of linoleic acid uptake by rabbit small intestinal brush border membrane vesicles. Lipids 24: 51–55

Lloyd M L, Olsen W A 1987 A study of the molecular pathology of sucrase-isomaltase deficiency A defect in the intracellular processing of the enzyme. New England Journal of Medicine 316: 438–442

Lyrenäs E, Abrahamsson H, Doteval G 1985 Rectosigmoid motility response to beta-adrenoreceptor stimulation in patients with the irritable bowel syndrome. Scandinavian Journal of Gastroenterology 20: 1163–1174

Mackenzie I L, Donaldson R M 1969 Vitamin $B_{12}$ absorption and the intestinal surface. Federation Proceedings 28: 41–45

Mackenzie I L, Donaldson R M, Kopp W L, Trier J S 1968 Antibodies to intestinal microvillous membranes. II. Inhibition of intrinsic factor-mediated attachment of Vitamin $B_{12}$ to hamster brush borders. Journal of Experimental Medicine 128: 375–386

Madara J L 1990 Pathobiology of the intestinal epithelial barrier. American Journal of Pathology 137: 1273–1281

Marcial M A, Carlson S L, Madara J L 1984 Partitioning of paracellular conductance along the crypt-villus axis: a hypothesis based on structural analysis with detailed consideration of tight junction structure-function relationships. Journal of Membrane Biology 80: 59–70

Marcuard S P, Albernaz L, Khazanie P B 1994 Omeprazole therapy causes malabsorption of cyanocobalamin (Vitamin $B_{12}$). Annals of Internal Medicine 120: 211–215

Matsuo T, Odaka H, Ikeda H 1992 Effect of an intestinal disaccharidase inhibitor (AO-128) on obesity and diabetes. American Journal of Clinical Nutrition 55: 314S–317S

McBrien D J, Jones R V, Creamer B 1963 Steatorrhea in Addison's disease. Lancet i: 25–26

McClain C J, Soutor C, Steele N, Levine A S, Silvis S E 1980a Severe zinc deficiency presenting with acrodermatitis during hyperalimentation: diagnosis, pathogenesis, and treatment. Journal of Clinical Gastroenterology 2: 125–131

McClain C, Soutor C, Zieve L 1980b Zinc deficiency: a complication of Crohn's disease. Gastroenterology 78: 272–279

McColl I, Sladen G E 1975 Intestinal absorption in man. Academic Press, London

McGill D B, Newcomer A D 1970 Primary and secondary disaccharidase deficiencies. In: Glass G B J (ed) Progress in gastroenterology, Vol 11. Grune & Stratton, New York, p 392–408

McKay J S, Linaker B D, Turnberg L A 1981 Influence of opiates on ion transport across rabbit ileal mucosa. Gastroenterology 80: 279–284

McKay J S, Linaker B D, Higgs N B, Turnberg L A 1982 Studies of the antisecretory activity of morphine in rabbit ileum in vitro. Gastroenterology 82: 243–247

Milla P J, Aggett P J, Wolff O H, Harries J T 1979 Studies in primary hypomagnesaemia: evidence for defective carrier-mediated small intestinal transport of magnesium. Gut 20: 1028–1033

Milne M D 1964 Disorders of amino-acid transport. British Medical Journal 1: 327–336

Minnich V, Okcuoglu A, Tarcon Y et al 1968 Pica in Turkey. II Effect of clay upon iron absorption. American Journal of Clinical Nutrition 21: 78–86

Mitchell B L, Lawson M J, Davies M et al 1985 Volatile fatty acids in the human intestine: studies in surgical patients. Nutrition Research 5: 1089–1092

Mooseker M S 1985 Organization, chemistry and assembly of the cytoskeletal apparatus of the intestinal brush border. Annual Review of Cell Biology 1: 209–241

Moreau H, Laugier R, Gargouri Y, Ferrato F, Verger R 1988 Human preduodenal lipase is entirely of gastric fundic origin. Gastroenterology 95: 1221–1226

Moynahan E J 1974 Acrodermatitis enteropathica: a lethal inherited human zinc-deficiency disorder. Lancet 2: 399–400

Muller D P R, Lloyd J K, Wolff O H 1983 Vitamin E and neurological function. Lancet 1: 225–227

Munro H N 1976 Regulation of body protein metabolism in relation to diet. Proceedings of the Nutrition Society 35: 297–308

National Research Council 1989 Recommended dietary allowances, 10th edn. National Academy Press, Washington, D C

Nemere I, Norman A W 1986 Parathyroid hormone stimulates calcium

transport in perfused duodena of normal chicks: comparison with the rapid (transcaltachic) effect of 1,25-dihydroxyvitamin D3. Endocrinology 119: 1406–1408
Newcomer A D 1984 Screening tests for carbohydrate malabsorption. Journal of Pediatric Gastroenterology and Nutrition 3: 6–8
Newcomer A D, McGill D B 1966 Distribution of disaccharidase activity in the small bowel of normal and lactase-deficient subjects. Gastroenterology 51: 481–488
Newcomer A D, McGill D B 1967 Disaccharidase activity in the small intestine: prevalence of lactase deficiency in 100 healthy subjects. Gastroenterology 53: 881–889
Newcomer A D, McGill D B, Thomas P J, Hofmann A F 1975 Prospective comparison of indirect methods for detecting lactase deficiency. New England Journal of Medicine 293: 1232–1236
Nguyen K N, Welch J D, Manion C V, Ficken V J 1982 Effect of fiber on breath hydrogen response and symptoms after oral lactose in lactose malabsorbers. American Journal of Clinical Nutrition 35: 1347–1351
Nordin B E C, Robertson A, Seamark R F et al 1985 The relation between calcium absorption, serum dehydroepiandrosterone, and vertebral mineral density in postmenopausal women. Journal of Clinical Endocrinology and Metabolism 60: 651–657
Norman A W 1990 Intestinal calcium absorption: a vitamin D-hormone-mediated adaptive response. American Journal of Clinical Nutrition 51: 290–300
Nunan T O, Compston J E, Tonge C 1986 Intestinal calcium absorption in patients after jejuno-ileal bypass or small intestinal resection and the effect of vitamin D. Digestion 34: 9–14
Okuda K, Takara I, Fujii T 1968 Absorption of liver-bound Vitamin $B_{12}$ in relation to intrinsic factor. Blood 32: 313–323
Owyang C 1984 Treatment of chronic secretory diarrhea of unknown origin by lithium carbonate. Gastroenterology 87: 714–718
Pappenheimer J R 1993 On the coupling of membrane digestion with intestinal absorption of sugars and amino acids. American Journal of Physiology 265: G409–G417
Peerenboom H, Keck E, Kruskemper H L, Strohmeyer G 1984 The defect in intestinal calcium transport in hyperthyroidism and its response to therapy. Journal of Clinical Endocrinology and Metabolism 59: 936–940
Peled Y, Watz C, Gilat T 1985 Measurement of intestinal permeability using $^{51}$Cr-EDTA. American Journal of Gastroenterology 80: 770–773
Perman J A, Modler S, Barr R G, Rosenthal P 1984 Fasting breath hydrogen concentration: normal values and clinical application. Gastroenterology 87: 1358–1363
Phillips S F 1972 Diarrhea: a current view of the pathophysiology. Gastroenterology 63: 495–518
Plotkin G R, Isselbacher K J 1964 Secondary disaccharidase deficiency in adult celiac disease (nontropical sprue) and other malabsorption states. New England Journal of Medicine 271: 1033–1037
Potter J, Ho M-W, Bolton H, Furth A J, Swallow D M, Griffiths B 1985 Human lactase and the molecular basis of lactase persistence. Biochemical Genetics 23: 423–439
Rader D J, Brewer H B 1993 Abetalipoproteinemia. New insights into lipoprotein assembly and vitamin E metabolism from a rare genetic disease. Journal of the American Medical Association 270: 865–869
Ravich W J, Bayless T M, Thomas M 1983 Fructose: incomplete intestinal absorption in humans. Gastroenterology 84: 26–29
Read N W, Al-Janabi M N, Bates T E et al 1985 Interpretation of the breath hydrogen profile obtained after ingesting a solid meal containing unabsorbable carbohydrate. Gut 26: 834–842
Recker R R 1985 Calcium absorption and achlorhydria. New England Journal of Medicine 313: 70–73
Rhodes J M, Middleton P, Jewell D P 1979 The lactulose hydrogen breath test as a diagnostic test for small bowel bacterial overgrowth. Scandinavian Journal of Gastroenterology 14: 333–336
Rigler M W, Honkanen R E, Patton J S 1986 Visualisation by freeze fracture, in vitro and in vivo, of the products of fat digestion. Journal of Lipid Research 27: 836–857
Roberts S H, Douglas A P 1976 Intestinal lymphangiectasia: the variability of presentation. A study of five cases. Quarterly Journal of Medicine 45: 39–48
Roediger W E W 1980 Role of anaerobic bacteria in the metabolic welfare of the colonic mucosa in man. Gut 21: 793–798
Roediger W E W, Lawson M J, Kwok V, Kerr Grant A, Pannall P R 1984 Colonic bicarbonate output as a test of disease activity in ulcerative colitis. Journal of Clinical Pathology 37: 704–707
Rothschild M A, Oratz M, Schreiber S S 1970 Current concepts of albumin metabolism. A review. Gastroenterology 58: 402
Roy C C, Levy E, Green P H R et al 1987 Malabsorption, hypocholesterolemia, and fat-filled enterocytes with increased intestinal apoprotein B. Chylomicron retention disease. Gastroenterology 92: 390–399
Rubin C E 1966 Electron microscopic studies of triglyceride absorption in man. Gastroenterology 50: 65–77
Rumessen J J, Gudmand-Hoyer E 1986 Absorption capacity of fructose in healthy adults. Comparison with sucrose and its constituent monosaccharides. Gut 27: 1161–1168
Sabesin S M, Frase S 1977 Electron microscopic studies of the assembly, intracellular transport, and secretion of chylomicrons by rat intestine. Journal of Lipid Research 18: 496–511
St Louis P J, Freedman M H, Richardson S E, Petrie M, Karmale M A 1991 Laboratory studies. In: Walker W A, Durie P R, Hamilton J R, Walker-Smith J A, Watkins J B (eds) Pediatric gastrointestinal disease, Vol 2. B C Decker, Philadelphia, p 1363–1395
Saltzman J R, Kowdley K V, Pedrosa M C et al 1994 Bacterial overgrowth without clinical malabsorption in elderly hypochlorhydric subjects. Gastroenterology 106: 615–623
Sandström B 1992 Dose dependence of zinc and manganese absorption in man. Proceedings of the Nutrition Society 51: 211–218
Saunders D R, Wiggins H S 1981 Conservation of mannitol, lactulose, and raffinose by the human colon. American Journal of Physiology 241: G397–G402
Schade S G, Schilling R F 1967 Effect of pepsin on the absorption of food Vitamin $B_{12}$ and iron. American Journal of Clinical Nutrition 20: 636–640
Scheig R 1969 What is dietary fat? American Journal of Clinical Nutrition 22: 651–653
Schiller L R, Santa Ana C A, Morawski S G, Fordtran J S 1984 Mechanism of the antidiarrheal effect of loperamide. Gastroenterology 86: 1475–1480
Schiller L R, Santa Ana C A, Morawski S G, Fordtran J S 1985 Studies of the antidiarrheal action of clonidine. Effects on motility and intestinal absorption. Gastroenterology 89: 982–988
Schjönsby H 1973 The mechanism of Vitamin $B_{12}$ malabsorption in blind-loop syndrome. Scandinavian Journal of Gastroenterology 8: 97–99
Seetharam B, Alpers, D H 1982 Absorption and transport of cobalamin. Annual Review of Nutrition 2: 343–369
Semenza G, Kessler M, Schmidt U, Venter J C, Fraser C M 1985 The small-intestinal sodium-glucose cotransporter(s). Annals of the New York Academy of Science 456: 83–96
Shani M, Theodor E, Frand M, Goldman B 1974 A family with protein-losing enteropathy. Gastroenterology 66: 433–445
Sharp G W G, Fischer J, Lipson L G et al 1977 Time course studies on the mechanism of action of cholera toxin. In: Bonfils S, Fromageot P, Rosselon G (eds) Hormonal receptors in digestive tract physiology. Elsevier, Amsterdam, p 447–454
Shearman D J C, Delamore I W, Gardner D L 1966 Gastric function and structure in iron deficiency. Lancet 1: 845
Shields R, Miles J B, Gilbertson C 1968 Absorption and secretion of water and electrolytes by the intact colon in a patient with primary aldosteronism. British Medical Journal 1: 93–96
Shimkin P M, Waldmann T A, Krugman R L 1970 Intestinal lymphangiectasia. American Journal of Roentgenology 110: 827–841
Sjövall H, Abrahamsson H, Westlander G et al 1986 Intestinal fluid and electrolyte transport in man during reduced circulatory blood volume. Gut 27: 913–918
Sninsky C A, Davis R H, Clench M H, Thomas K D, Mathias J R 1986 Effect of lidamidine hydrochloride and loperamide on gastric emptying and transit of the small intestine. A double-blind study. Gastroenterology 90: 68–73
Solomons N W, Guerrero A-M, Torun B 1985 Dietary manipulation of postprandial colonic lactose fermentation. 1. Effect of solid foods in a meal. American Journal of Clinical Nutrition 41: 199–208

Staun M, Sjoström H, Noren O 1986 Calcium-binding protein from human small intestine. Purification and characterization of a 10 000 molecular weight protein. European Journal of Clinical Investigation 16: 468–472

Steinberg W M, King C E, Toskes P P 1980 Malabsorption of protein-bound cobalamin but not unbound cobalamin during cimetidine administration. Digestive Diseases and Sciences 25: 188–191

Tacnet F, Watkins D W, Ripoche P 1990 Studies of zinc transport into brush border membrane vesicles isolated from pig small intestine. Biochimica et Biophysica Acta 1024: 323–330

Tadesse K 1990 The effect of continued feeding of physiological amounts of lactose on the level of intestinal lactase and other disaccharidase enzyme activities in the rat. Experimental Physiology 75: 231–238

Thomas D W, Sinatra F R, Merritt R J 1981 Random fecal alpha-1 antitrypsin concentration in children with gastrointestinal disease. Gastroenterology 80: 776–782

Thompson D G, Binfield P, De Belder A, O'Brien J, Warren S, Wilson M 1985 Extra intestinal influences on exhaled breath hydrogen measurements during the investigation of gastrointestinal disease. Gut 26: 1349–1352

Thompson D G, O'Brien J D, Hardie J M 1986 Influence of the oropharyngeal microflora on the measurement of exhaled breath hydrogen. Gastroenterology 91: 853–860

Timpl R 1989 Structure and biological activity of basement membrane proteins. European Journal of Biochemistry 180: 487–502

Treem W R, Ahsan N, Sullivan B et al 1993 Evaluation of liquid yeast-derived sucrase enzyme replacement in patients with sucrase-isomaltase deficiency. Gastroenterology 105: 1061–1068

Triadou N, Bataille J, Schmitz J 1983 Longitudinal study of the human intestinal brush border membrane proteins. Distribution of the disaccharidases and peptidases. Gastroenterology 85: 1326–1332

Tso P, Kendrick H, Balint J A, Simmonds W J 1981 Role of biliary phosphatidylcholine in the absorption and transport of dietary triolein in the rat. Gastroenterology 80: 60–65

Tsuboi K K, Kwong L K, d'Harlingue A E, Stevenson D K, Kerner J A, Sunshine P 1985 The nature of maturation decline of intestinal lactase activity. Biochimica et Biophysica Acta 840: 69–78

Turnberg L A 1971 Abnormalities in intestinal electrolyte transport in congenital chloridorrhoea. Gut 12: 544–551

Underhill B M L 1955 Intestinal length in man. British Medical Journal 2: 1243–1246

Van de Kamer J H, ten Bokkel Huinink H, Weyers H A 1949 Rapid method for determination of fat in feces. Journal of Biological Chemistry 177: 347–355

Waldmann T A 1966 Protein-losing enteropathy. Gastroenterology 50: 422–443

Waldmann T A, Wochner R D, Strober W 1969 The role of the gastrointestinal tract in plasma protein metabolism. American Journal of Medicine 46: 275–285

Warnes T W 1972 Alkaline phosphatase. Gut 13: 926–937

Wasserman R H, Chandler J S, Meyer S A et al 1992 Intestinal calcium transport and calcium extrusion processes at the basolateral membrane. Journal of Nutrition 122: 662–671

Weir D G, McGing P G, Scott J M 1985 Folate metabolism, the enterohepatic circulation and alcohol. Biochemical Pharmacology 34: 1–7

West P S, Levin G E, Griffin G E, Maxwell J D 1981 Comparison of simple screening tests for fat malabsorption. British Medical Journal 282: 1501–1504

Wollaeger E E, Comfort M W, Osterberg A E 1947 Total solids, fat and nitrogen in the feces. III. A study of normal persons taking a test diet containing a moderate amount of fat; comparison with results obtained with normal persons taking a test diet containing a large amount of fat. Gastroenterology 9: 272–283

Zentler-Munro P L, Fine D R, Fitzpatrick W J F, Northfield T C 1984 Effect of intrajejunal acidity on lipid digestion and aqueous solubilisation of bile acids and lipids in health, using a new simple method of lipase inactivation. Gut 25: 491–499

# 14. Celiac disease and other mucosal disorders of the small intestine

*M. N. Marsh*

GLUTEN SENSITIVITY (Celiac sprue disease)

Initially, celiac disease was viewed as a gross malabsorption syndrome of children (Gee 1888) while malabsorption in adults was invariably termed idiopathic steatorrhea, even though there were hints of an association in certain patients who complained of recurrent disease since childhood (Low 1928, Holmes & Starr 1929, Bennett et al 1932, Haynes & McBryde 1936).

The introduction of the peroral intubation technique for obtaining specimens of unautolysed jejunal mucosa (c1960 onwards) provided evidence of severe mucosal lesions both in children and adults, thus showing for the first time that celiac disease persists into adult life and is therefore a lifelong condition (Doniach & Shiner 1957, Shiner & Doniach 1960, Rubin et al 1960, Anderson 1960).

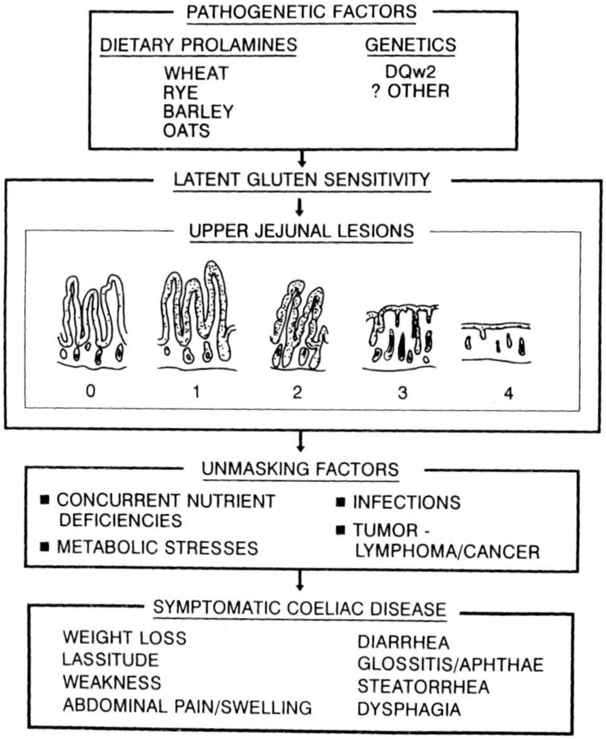


**Fig. 14.1** The pathogenesis of gluten sensitivity. Although most patients will be latent (asymptomatic) irrespective of proximal mucosal pathology, symptomatology, if unmasked, will tend to mirror the predisposing environmental factor.

## Definition

Nowadays it is preferable to use the term "gluten sensitivity" to describe those people who, through inheritance of specific Class 2 MHC D sublocus genes, are predisposed to develop some aspect of this protean condition. Evidence to date suggests that only 30–40% of sensitized people are symptomatic, i.e. develop an overt symptomatic "celiac" malabsorption syndrome usually in response to environmental stress or other stimuli (Fig. 14.1): the remainder exhibit either atypical (Table 14.1) or other non-gastrointestinal symptoms or signs or remain asymptomatic: to these latter individuals, the term "latent" gluten sensitivity is applied even though some will have a severe proximal jejunal lesion (Marsh 1992a).

## Prevalence

Figures for prevalence probably give only a very crude estimate of all gluten-sensitized individuals. Estimates have invariably been based solely on symptomatic cases with malabsorption and flat mucosae derived from hospital series (and hence national celiac society records): such populations are likely to be biased because of selective hospital referral patterns (Logan 1992).

Overall the prevalence is 1 per 1000 or 2000 of the population, although in West Ireland the figure is 1 in 500. These data raise questions as to the diagnostic criteria employed and the proportion of sensitized cases which remain undetected because of latency. Viewed in this context, there are few accurate data and 1:300 may be somewhat nearer the truth (Auricchio et al 1990).

Similar criticisms apply to the numerous family studies

**Table 14.1** Presenting features in gluten sensitivity

| Typical | Atypical |
|---|---|
| Weakness, fatigue, lethargy | Pigmentation, hypotension (?Addisons) |
| Weight loss | Rapid weight loss ± diarrhea |
| Diarrhea | Hair loss |
| Abdominal distention | Unusual skin rashes |
| Nausea, vomiting, anorexia | Arthropathy, "rheumatism" |
| Cramps, tetany | (vit D deficiency) |
| Skin bleeding | Arthropathy (mono/poly) |
| Edema | (small/large joint inflammation) |
| Glossitis | Peripheral neuropathy |
| | Abdominal pain |
| | Dental hyperplasia |
| | Infertility |
| | Growth defect |
| | Abnormal "liver function tests" |
| | Obesity |

which have indicated that 10–20% of relatives may be affected, depending on analyses of siblings, parents or more widely dispersed members of a kindred. Invariably these are individuals who agree to jejunal biopsy and have significant mucosal lesions. The future identification of all gluten-sensitized individuals will require use of far more stringent tests or demonstrations of sensitization to gluten. Such tests will probably reveal a far greater percentage of relatives with the condition than was hitherto suspected.

The same considerations apply to studies of discordance/concordance rates for the condition in identical twin pairs. It is not at all certain whether all the *discordant* identical twin pairs are valid either because mucosal lesions were not characteristic or not present at the particular time of sampling (Polanco et at 1981). The value of twin studies is further hampered by the effects of environmental factors on subsequent (somatic) programming of the immune system. Nevertheless, as with insulin-dependent diabetes mellitus, other genes in addition to the MHC Class 2 background are more than likely to be involved in determining both susceptibility, as well as degree of sensitivity, to gliadin. These concepts require revision based on more stringent tests of gluten sensitivity.

## Etiology

Gluten sensitivity arises in genetically susceptible individuals because of interactions between cereal proteins (wheat, rye, barley and oats prolamins) and T-lymphocytes, resulting in mucosal damage. There are strong grounds for supposing that sensitization of mesenteric T-lymphocytes, rather than humoral immunity, is a basic prerequisite of the disease process as well as for the induction of mucosal pathology, both spontaneously or by gluten challenge (Kagnoff et al 1982, Marsh 1992b). This view is strengthened by the knowledge that gluten sensitivity occurs frequently with IgA deficiency (Crabbe & Heremans 1967) and even rarely in severer forms of immunodeficiency (e.g. common variable immunodeficiency) (Webster et al 1981). Thus although antibodies to gluten (often in high titer) abound in the intestinal tissues and blood, and the presence of breakdown products of activated complement (Halstensen et al 1992) is demonstrable within the mucosa, such mechanisms have never been shown to selectively induce the *range* of mucosal lesions (Fig. 14.2) which typify gluten sensitivity or other allied forms of enteropathy (Marsh 1992b). Nevertheless, the mechanism(s) whereby T-lymphocytes in the presence of gluten bring about the characteristic alterations in mucosal architecture have yet to be defined, although there is no doubt that as with other immunological models of T-cell activation or sensitization, the mucosa is subject to analogous patterns of cellular change or morphologic injury (Mowat & Ferguson 1982, Ferguson 1987, MacDonald & Spencer 1988, Mowat & Felstein 1991, Macdonald 1992, Marsh 1992b, Marsh & Cummins 1993).

## Genetic background

Gluten sensitivity is very strongly associated with genes which are encoded at the MHC Class 2 D subloci on the short arm of chromosome 6 (Kagnoff 1992).

Although an association with certain Class 1 genes (A1,B8) was observed almost two decades ago and later with DR3, these genes are now recognized to comprise an "extended haplotype" of which the allotype DQw2 (defined serologically) is the major gene product, being present in 95–96% gluten-sensitized individuals (Roep et al 1988, Sollid et al 1989, Kagnoff et al 1989, Sollid & Thorsby 1993): the remaining 4–5% are DR4. Both Class 1 and 2 MHC gene products are concerned in the binding of endogenous or exogenous peptides respectively and their subsequent presentation to T-cells. While Class 1 antigens are ubiquitously expressed, Class 2 alloantigens are only expressed on certain cells, such as T- and B-lymphocytes and antigen-presenting dendritic cells.

The Class 2 D subloci comprise three sets of alleles: DR, DQ and DP lie nearer the centromere than Class 1 B, C and A loci which are distributed at the distal end of the short arm. Between the A and B Class 1 loci lie the Class 3 genes, which code for complement system proteins, and other proteins like HSP 70 and TNF α, β (Fig. 14.3). These genes are all highly polymorphic (express certain variable amino acids at particular positions) and exhibit a high degree of linkage disequilibrium, resulting in the inheritance of a specific cluster of genes (or "haplotype"). Despite such marked polymorphism, only a limited number of haplotypes is expressed throughout the population, in general.

The Class 2 molecule is a heterodimer comprising an α chain (Mr ~ 33 kDa) encoded by an A gene and a β chain

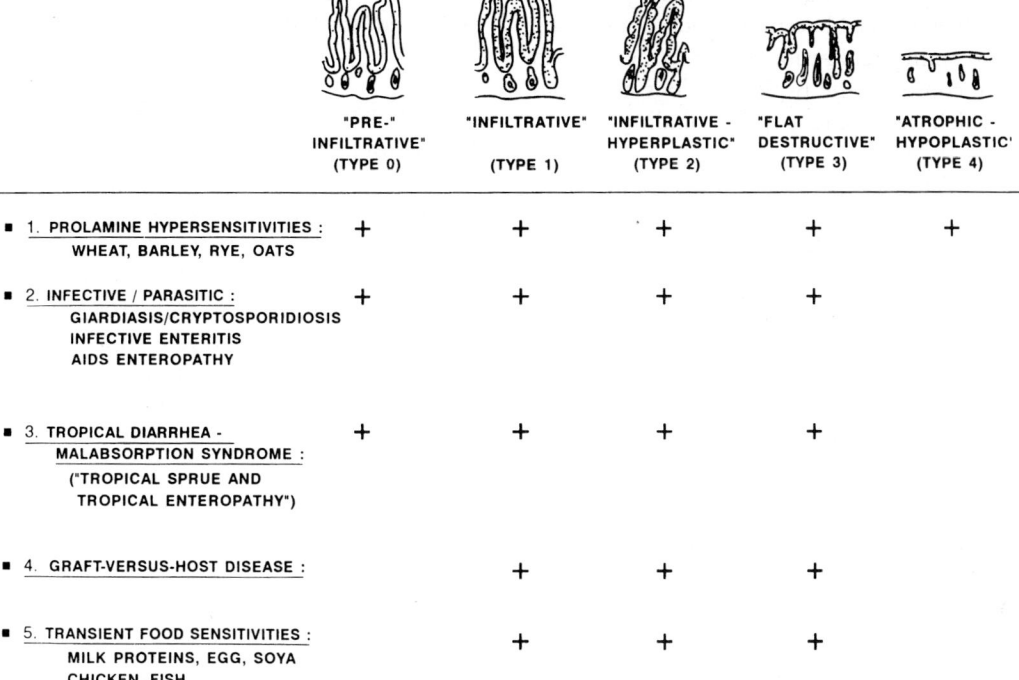

| | "PRE-" INFILTRATIVE" (TYPE 0) | "INFILTRATIVE" (TYPE 1) | "INFILTRATIVE - HYPERPLASTIC" (TYPE 2) | "FLAT DESTRUCTIVE" (TYPE 3) | "ATROPHIC - HYPOPLASTIC" (TYPE 4) |
|---|---|---|---|---|---|
| ▪ 1. PROLAMINE HYPERSENSITIVITIES : WHEAT, BARLEY, RYE, OATS | + | + | + | + | + |
| ▪ 2. INFECTIVE / PARASITIC : GIARDIASIS/CRYPTOSPORIDIOSIS, INFECTIVE ENTERITIS, AIDS ENTEROPATHY | + | + | + | + | |
| ▪ 3. TROPICAL DIARRHEA - MALABSORPTION SYNDROME : ("TROPICAL SPRUE AND TROPICAL ENTEROPATHY") | + | + | + | + | |
| ▪ 4. GRAFT-VERSUS-HOST DISEASE : | | + | + | + | |
| ▪ 5. TRANSIENT FOOD SENSITIVITIES : MILK PROTEINS, EGG, SOYA, CHICKEN, FISH | | + | + | + | |

**Fig. 14.2** The major structural alterations in gluten sensitivity consist arbitrarily of the infiltrative (type 1) infiltrative-hyperplastic (type 2) and classic flat-destructive (type 3) lesions. The preinfiltrative (type 0) lesion is associated with florid antibody production only, while rarely the truly atrophic and irreversible lesion (type 4) is uniquely associated with tumor development in a minority of gluten-sensitive patients only. The literature fully attests to the development of a similar range of mucosal lesions in the other categories listed. These are all evidently T-cell-mediated, host-driven responses to each type of environmental antigen at local mucosal level. (After Marsh 1992c, copyright American Gastroenterological Association.)

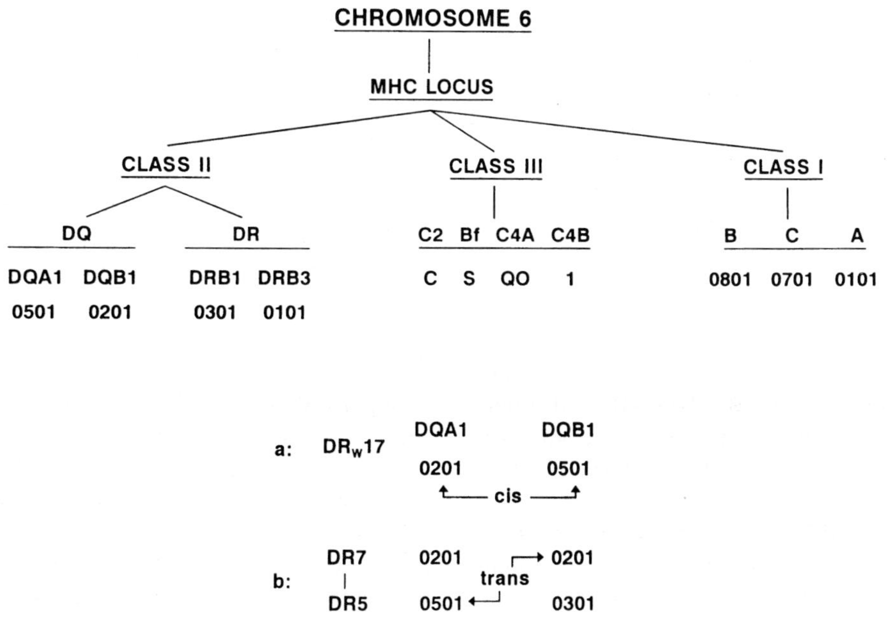


**Fig. 14.3** The upper part of the diagram illustrates a typical extended haplotype for a gluten-sensitive individual. The serological DQw2 specificity can either be assembled in cis (a) or in trans (b) in DR5/7 heterozygotes.

(Mr ~ 29 kDa) encoded by a B gene. The most polymorphic regions are their distal N termini, each comprising approximately 100 amino acid residues and termed $\alpha_1$ and $\beta_1$ domains: these comprise the β-pleated floor and adjacent α-helices which form the peptide-binding groove (Brown et al 1988, 1993).

Class 2 positive cells are able to express a variety of alloantigens with either DR, DQ and DP specificity, although the density of DR expression per cell is greatest, in comparison with the other two sublocus products: usually more than one DR gene product is expressed (e.g. DRA1 and DRB2, and DRA1, DRB3/4 or 5). Furthermore, because there are two chromosomes, a mixed molecule may be produced, a process termed *trans* as opposed to *cis*, by gene combinations along the same chromosome (Fig. 14.3): therefore, any cell may express a variety of DR, DQ and DP alloantigens. Class 2 molecules, in general, bind exogenous peptides as fragments produced by endocytosis and re-expression by macrophages, epithelial cells and dendritic cells while Class 1 molecules usually express endogenous cell products, including those of viral pathogens. Class 1 peptides are presented in the context of $CD8^+$ cell surface markers, usually resulting in cytolysis, while Class 2 peptides react preferentially with $CD4^+$ cells resulting in lymphokine release (IFN-γ IL2, IL4, IL5, etc.) which modulate, and amplify, the immune response.

The earliest reported association of gluten sensitivity to the Class 1 B8 specificity was subsequently found to be due to its linkage disequilibrium with the Class 2 serological marker DRw17 (previously known as DR3). However, DRw17 is, in turn, very tightly associated with DQw2 and this combination has been found in 90–100% of all northern European patients of Caucasian extraction, the background expression of DQw2 in nongluten-sensitized subjects being ~20–25%.

However, particularly in southern European patients, there is heterozygosity involving DR5/7 (Mearin et al 1983, Morellini et al 1988). Both DR7 and DRw17 type serologically as DQw2 (because they have identical β chains (DQB1*0201) while their α chains are different (DRB1*0701 and DRB1*0301 respectively): this results in the expression of different αβ heterodimers at the cell surface. Likewise, DRw17 and DR5 share the same α chain (DQA1*0501), so that DR5/7 heterozygotes are able to express the same αβ (A1*0501/DRB1*0201) heterodimer as DRw17 individuals, each derived from DR5 and DR7, respectively, in trans (Fig. 14.3) (Kagnoff 1992).

Further work has identified genes in the DP sublocus which contribute to the susceptibility to gluten protein (Bugawan et al 1989, Rosenberg et al 1989, Hall et al 1990). These are DPB1 0301 and 0101 in northern Europeans and northern Italians: DPB*0301 appears independent, while DPB1*0101 is linked to DRw17. In southern Europeans DPB1*0301 or DPB1*0402 are expressed, the latter being related to DR5/7 heterozygotes.

## Gluten chemistry and immunogenicity

That gluten protein, in contradistinction to gluten (starch) carbohydrate, plays a major role in the pathogenesis of gluten sensitivity was first demonstrated by Dicke (c1950). Studies by Dicke, Weijers and van de Kamer (Dicke et al 1953, van de Kamer et al 1953) and by followers such as Anderson et al (1952) led to the confirmation of this important observation, as well as laying the foundations for the clinical introduction and adoption of the gluten-free diet as a key therapeutic advance. Another extension of these early studies was that barley and rye were also shown to exacerbate the condition, while the pivotal role of oats is still undecided (Shewry et al 1992): maize ("corn flour") and rice are not implicated (Fig. 14.4).

In all grasses which exacerbate the condition and thus bring about variable changes in upper jejunal mucosal pathology, their relevant immunogenic proteins are termed "prolamins" due to a high proportion of prolamine and amine residues, particularly glutamine. The relevant active proteins are gliadins (wheat), hordeins (barley), secalins (rye) and avenins (oats) (Fig. 14.5) with molecular weights 30–100 kDa.

The immunogenic sequences which could be presented by MHC Class 2 molecules to T-cell receptor(s) are not yet known. However, studies in vitro appear to have demonstrated activity in the N-terminus of a gliadin which, in common with other disease-active prolamins, comprise, in part, the common amino acid sequences or motifs SPQQ, PQQP (De Ritis et al 1984) (Fig. 14.4). In vitro studies have produced some confusing results regarding the sequence of homology between α-gliadin (residues 211–217) and the adenovirus 12 E1B protein (Kagnoff 1992). Since mucosae from gluten-sensitive individuals in subsequent studies have failed to demonstrate the presence of adenovirus 12 DNA, the validity of this hypothesis and the role of crossreacting sensitivities between virus and gluten are still somewhat uncertain.

## Mucosal pathology

The peroral biopsy technique was a major breakthrough in the assessment of malabsorption disorders, not only because it provided fresh, unautolysed mucosal tissue from unanesthetized subjects, but also because it paved the way for the discovery, description and investigation of many other disorders of the small bowel which hitherto were either unknown and unrecognized or inaccessible to further study (Booth 1970).

In the early days, particularly in Britain, it became customary to examine the mucosal appearance of jejunal

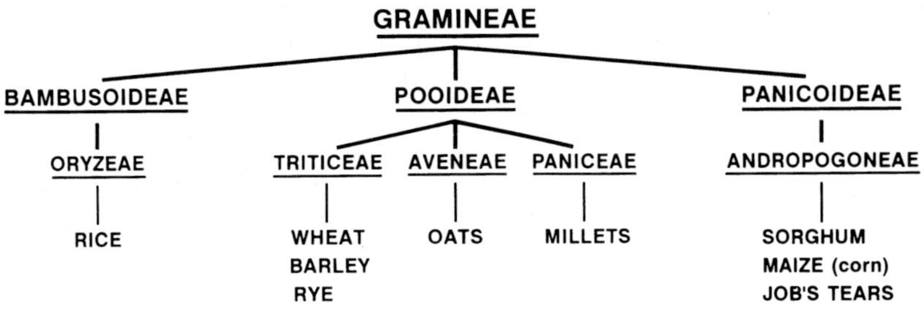


CONSENSUS SEQUENCES OF POOIDEAE:

1. WHEAT
(N) V R V P V P Q L Q P Q N P S Q Q Q P Q E Q V P L V Q Q Q Q F L G Q Q Q P F P P Q Q P

2. BARLEY
Q Q Q P F P Q Q P I P Q Q P Q P Y P Q Q P Q P Y P Q Q P F P Q Q P F P Q Q P

3. RYE
N M Q V N P G G Q V Q W P Q Q Q P P P Q S Q Q P F . . Q P Q . Q F P Q

4. OATS
T T T V Q Y N P S E Q Y Q P Y P E Q Q E P F V

5. MILLET
Y I S P V S A V A A T A S P L F W P Q A T S I A A T H P F V

**Fig. 14.4** Classification of the edible grasses, including the Triticeae and Aveneae (Pooideae), that exacerbate gluten sensitivity. Note that oats prolamins contain sequence motifs (underlined) similar to wheat, barley and rye prolamins. Millet clearly lacks such homology, while rice (oryzeae) is safe, as is maize (corn or Zea). Note single letter code for amino acids: P, proline; Q, glutamine; S, serine; F, phenylalanine; E, glutamic acid.

| | WHEAT | BARLEY | RYE |
|---|---|---|---|
| 1. SULFUR-RICH | | | |
| (a) monomeric | | | |
| γ TYPE | γ-GLIADIN | γ-HORDEIN | γ-SECALINS |
| α TYPE | αβ-GLIADIN (30-45kDa) | — | — |
| (b) polymeric aggregated | LMW GLUTENIN | B-HORDEIN | — |
| 2. SULFUR-POOR | ω-GLIADIN (60kDa) | C-HORDEIN | ω-SECALINS |
| 3. HMW PROLAMINS | HMW GLUTENIN (65-90kDa) | D-HORDEIN | HMW-SECALINS |

**Fig. 14.5** Molecular species involved in disease pathogenesis are the sulfur-rich and sulfur-poor prolamins (MW 30–60 kDa). The aggregated or polymeric high molecular weight (HMW) glutenins (MW > 65 kDa) are not pathogenic.

biopsies through the low-powered dissecting (binocular) microscope. Various descriptive terms such as flat, flat-mosaic and convoluted evolved together with a further vocabulary directed to variations in villous shape evident both within a single biopsy and, comparatively, in biopsies obtained from various parts of the world. That all these changes are part of a continuously evolving spectrum, from finger-shaped villi to a flat mucosa, became evident with the use of the scanning electron microscope whose high resolving power provided far greater revelations about mucosal surface detail than was possible with its optical equivalent (Marsh 1972). Nowadays, the examination of biopsies in this way is essentially historical and of passing interest only: in addition, the endless arguments as to the significance of leafy, or fused, villi are now outdated.

The histological appearances of the superficial intestinal mucosa have become established as the major characteristic of the gluten-induced lesion. It should be pointed out that earlier information (Paulley 1954) of a transmural lesion was eclipsed by peroral biopsies which provided only superficial mucosal tissues. This new technique thus helped to give undue emphasis to Frazer's view (Frazer et al 1959, Frazer 1960) of a congenital (cellular) "peptidase" deficiency by focusing on the damaged enterocytes that now came under scrutiny by various techniques such as light and transmission electron microscopy and histochemistry. Thus early research tended to concentrate solely on attempts to demonstrate the intracellular defect considered responsible for the disease.

The fully established, classic flat mucosal lesion of gluten sensitivity is extremely complicated (Watson & Wright 1974, Cooke & Holmes 1984, Marsh 1992b). The major architectural features comprise the flat, avillous surface which consists of irregularly arranged, unhealthy-looking surface cells which have a cuboidal appearance in sectioned profile: their volumes are also decreased

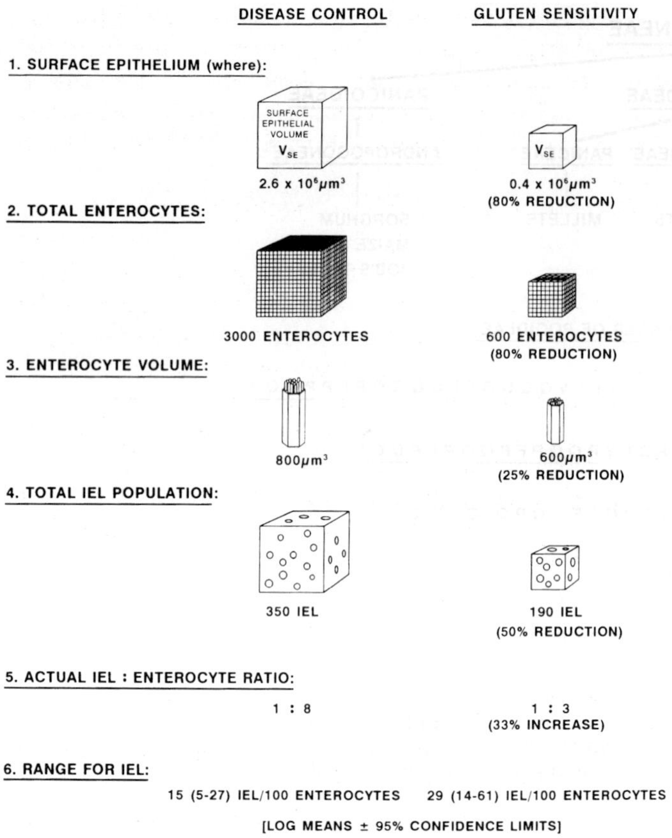


**Fig. 14.6** This diagram is based on computerized morphometry of representative groups of disease-control and flat (type 3) gluten-sensitive mucosae. In the latter surface enterocytes are reduced by 80%, while their mean volume is reduced by 25% compared with control mucosae. The total population of IEL is reduced by 50%, although in relative terms, their ratio to enterocyte is raised to 1:3 (control mucosae have density ratios of 1:10). New log-transformed data for IEL populations are 15 (95% confidence limits 5–27) per 100 enterocytes for disease-control mucosae and 29 (14–61) per 100 enterocytes for flat (type 3) gluten-induced lesions. (Based on Crowe & Marsh, 1993, 1994.)

(Fig. 14.6), although the mechanism whereby these cells become small is still uncertain (Crowe & Marsh 1993). The crypts, on the other hand, are hypertrophied both lengthwise and in diameter. Cell turnover and production by these crypts is increased at least sixfold over control mucosae, a phenomenon accomplished by an increased population of mitotic cells ("growth fraction"), a reduced duration of mitosis (40 min compared with 1 h for controls) and a reduction in the intermitotic interval (Watson & Wright 1974). In other words, newly formed daughter crypt cells re-enter mitosis at a faster rate than those of control mucosae: in addition, the interval taken to complete cell division is reduced by 30%.

This vastly increased output of cells per crypt is accompanied by an increased rate of migration upwards towards the luminal surface (Trier & Browning 1970) and matched by a similar rate of loss of cells from the surface epithelium. Despite this heightened turnover by the epithelium, the histological appearances do not immediately give any hint of such prodigious cell production and turnover, except for the increase in mitotic figures within crypt epithelium.

The lamina propria is also involved in the process: its volume is doubled over control mucosae, due to edema resulting from microvascular dilatation and increased permeability, and from the influx of cells of all types – lymphocytes, plasma cells, eosinophils, neutrophils, mast cells and basophils. It is thought that these, and their products, are secondarily recruited into the lesion and triggered by the presence of gluten in the predisposed host, probably resulting in a secretory and hyperpermeable mucosa, as demonstrated by $^{51}$Cr EDTA and double-sugar "absorption" (urinary) ratios (Marsh 1983, 1992b).

During the 1960s other advances drew attention to the importance of the small bowel as an organ of major immunologic importance. At first the mucosal IgA system was described, but following that the presence of the intraepithelial lymphocyte (IEL) pool was discovered. This was to become a subject of considerable interest since IEL are present in the interface between the internal and external milieu. However, their functions are still poorly understood. In the early phases of this "immunological" era, enterocyte damage in gluten sensitivity came to be attributed to a wide variety of possible immunologic phenomena, such as T-cell cytotoxicity, NK cell targeting and antibody-dependent cell-mediated cytotoxicity. Even the subclass of IEL cells termed $\gamma\delta$, which are usually increased in the majority of gluten-sensitive lesions, is not an exclusive marker for this condition: furthermore, since the local functions of this subset of lymphocytes are virtually unknown, its contribution to the immunopathology of gluten sensitivity is far from clear. Thus, none of these speculative views has stood the test of time: furthermore, their underlying basis has become questionable since it is now certain that the target of gluten-induced intestinal damage is not the enterocyte at all (Marsh 1983); instead, it is evident that the lamina propria is the prime seat of initiation of immune events which ultimately leads to mucosal inflammation, its architectural remodelling and the secondary surface enterocyte damage with its corresponding impairment of digestive–absorptive function (Marsh 1983, 1988, 1992b&c, Marsh & Cummins 1993).

### *The immunopathology of the gluten-associated mucosal lesion*

A more acceptable explanation of the mucosal lesions in gluten sensitivity is that they are due to T-lymphocyte activity (Figs14.2 and 14.7). Such a view is based on parallels drawn between the lesions in gluten-sensitized individuals and those in immunologic models of intestinal mucosal damage in experimental animals, such as allograft rejection, graft-versus-host reactions and the effects of worm and parasite infestations (trichiniasis, nippostrongyliasis and giardiasis). It is through these latter

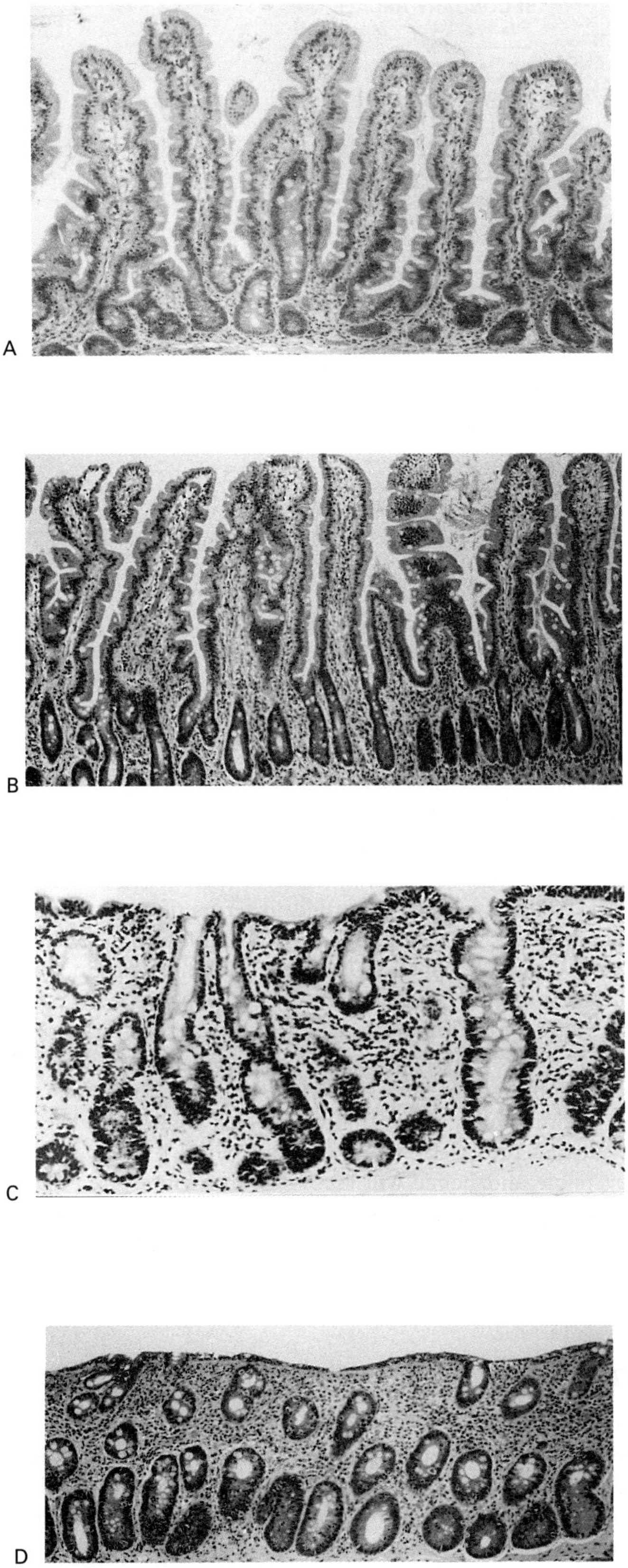


**Fig. 14.7** Histological appearance of **A** apparently normal mucosa (dermatitis herpetiformis), **B** hyperplastic mucosa (large crypts), **C** typical flat lesion and **D** unresponsive, atrophic lesion.

studies that our knowledge and understanding of the varied, although stereotyped, ways in which the intestinal mucosa responds to or is altered by local T-cell-mediated influences has been enhanced (Ferguson 1987, Mowat & Felstein 1991, MacDonald 1992, Marsh 1992b&c, Marsh & Cummins 1993).

Competent T-lymphocytes, probably acting through lymphokine secretion, are necessary for the evolution of such tissue reactions, including changes in the established villous architecture. Furthermore, the maturation of the fetal/neonatal intestine at or around the time of weaning is likewise a T-cell-dependent phenomenon, associated with evidence of mast cell discharge, release of circulating IL2-R antigen and a rapid increase in the population of IEL (Marsh & Cummins 1993).

Experimental approaches to GVH demonstrate less florid changes than villous effacement, like the infiltrative-hyperplastic lesion in the neonatal model (Mowat & Ferguson 1982); these have revealed more varied and subtle effects of T-cell-mediated influences on mucosal architecture resembling milder human lesions seen after low-dose gluten challenge (Leigh et al 1985), in dermatitis herpetiformis (Marsh 1989a), in relatives of known celiac patients (Marsh et al 1990) and in other enteropathies such as giardiasis, tropical enteric syndromes and sensitivities to various food antigens seen predominantly in children below 2–3 years of age (Fig. 14.2).

It should also be remembered that gluten reactivity has been demonstrated from upper jejunum to terminal rectum (Rubin et al 1960, 1962, Dobbins & Rubin 1964) (Fig. 14.8). Since undigested (immunogenic) gluten is only "seen" by the upper intestine, how are these phenomena best interpreted? It is suggested the answer lies in earlier experiments which elucidated the potential of mesenteric T- and B-lymphocytes and immunoblasts to recirculate and relocate within the gastrointestinal tract and showed that secondary antigen recall responses, which could be elicited at sites distant from the original site of priming, are restricted to areas in contact with that antigen.

Like the mild infiltrative lesion seen in dermatitis herpetiformis and first-degree family members, the rectal mucosa of untreated celiac patients is infiltrated by $CD3^+$ and $\alpha\delta^+$ receptor-bearing lymphocytes: gluten restriction causes a prompt fall in $CD3^+$, but a much slower reduction in $\alpha\delta^+$ cells (Ensari et al 1993a), a response that exactly mirrors the jejunal response to a gluten-free diet (Kutlu et al 1993). Conversely, rectal gluten challenge evokes very specific responses (Loft et al 1989, 1990) which are even evident by 4 h (Ensari et al 1994): discriminant analysis permits calculation of a diagnostic score for accurate identification of gluten-sensitized individuals, based on information on $CD3^+$ and $\alpha\delta^+$ lymphocyte populations in a postchallenge biopsy (Ensari et al 1994).

The exquisite sensitivity of rectal mucosa to gluten challenge is very striking and based on recruitment and activa-

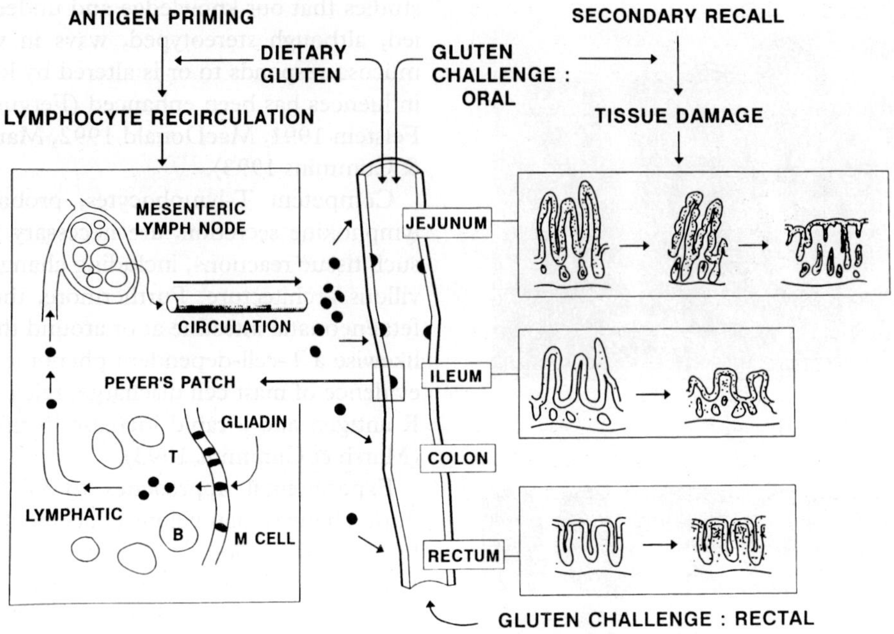


**Fig. 14.8** Initial priming of mucosal T-cells for gluten sensitivity will occur via M cells in follicle-associated epithelium of Peyer's patches, followed by their expansion in local mesenteric lymph nodes. After passing through the circulation, T-cells home to the intestine and migrate within lamina propria and epithelium from upper duodenum/jejunum to distal rectum (*left*). Continued exposure to gluten (until diagnosis) leads to typical lesion pathology (*right*) which affects a variable length of upper small intestine. On the same basis, secondary recall responses of sensitized T-cells may be elicited at any point along the bowel, as demonstrated clinically, or experimentally by (a) peroral or (b) rectal challenge. Since Peyer's patches are presumed to be a source of B blasts in humans, similar circuitry for gluten-induced humoral responses throughout the gastrointestinal tract is also assumed (see Fig. 14.13).

tion of gluten-specific memory T-cells (Fig. 14.8) within the mesenteric pool (Loft et al 1989), acting via addressins expressed on the local microvasculature (Ensari et al 1993b). These data therefore indicate that the rectal response to gluten is (immunologically) identical to that evoked in jejunum by either the presence or removal of gluten in the luminal contents, but without architectural disturbance. Indeed, within the diagnostic armamentarium for gluten sensitivity, rectal challenge is the only test which dynamically elicits specific T-cell sensitization to gluten (Loft et al 1990, Ensari et al 1994).

Thus, it is important for the clinician to understand the basis of the lesions in gluten sensitivity and to recognize that a spectrum of mucosal patterns varying from mild to severe is possible (Marsh 1992c). Moreover, it has been shown that these varied patterns are interrelated and progressively become more severe spontaneously (Marsh 1989b) or during gluten challenge when the dose of gluten is progressively increased per challenge (Marsh et al 1992). Therefore, the amount of gluten ingested, together with the underlying extended genetic haplotype, are sufficient causes to explain any degree of mucosal damage.

The descriptive terms applied to this series of lesions are ad hoc (Figs 14.2 and 14.7), but they are consistent with the nomenclature evolved in the field of experimental GVH. They are best construed in terms of architectural change (Marsh 1992c), patterns of IEL infiltration (Marsh 1980, Crowe & Marsh 1994) or of antibody production (O'Mahony et al 1990, Arranz & Ferguson 1993) for purposes of recognition, or for clinical practice.

It is necessary to appreciate that these mucosal lesions are manifestations of T-cell-mediated, *host* responses to environmental antigens that are operative at the mucosal level, that these lesions are not "atrophic" but invariably reversible and hence will recover with a gluten-free diet. Thus, they are not "autoimmune" phenomena: neither is gluten sensitivity an "autoimmune" disorder since it improves once the offending environmental antigen is removed from the diet.

### *The irreversible (atrophic) lesion*

In a small minority of patients, the intestinal mucosa is progressively destroyed, despite use of a gluten-free diet (Fig. 14.7d), a process somewhat analogous to the autoimmune lesion, in which infiltrating lymphocytes seem to be the agents of tissue destruction.

The "unresponsiveness" which attends this small group of gluten-sensitive patients may result from the development of suppressor T-lymphocyte clones. This is evident in other chronic T-cell-mediated conditions which may be MHC Class 2 related. Alternatively the development of tumor may lead to a condition analogous to chronic GVH, resulting in wasting, cachexia, lymphoid hypoplasia and immunosuppression (Mowat & Felstein, 1991). Nevertheless, it does seem probable that this tiny facet of the natural history of gluten sensitivity most likely arises from multifocal clones of malignant T-cells. These either directly invade and irreparably destroy the entire intestinal mucosa or by some other mechanism render the patient (who may, at some earlier time, have demonstrated a typical response to dietary treatment) unresponsive to further gluten withdrawal. Nevertheless the evolution of this very unusual syndrome requires recognition of a presumptive T-cell-mediated, end-stage lesion (Fig. 14.2, Table 14.2) which causes complete atrophy of the intestinal mucous membrane in some people with undoubted gluten sensitivity (Marsh 1992c).

## Clinical features

The presenting complaints of gluten sensitivity are protean (Table 14.1) and there is no specific characteristic group of symptoms (Dawson & Kumar 1985, Howdle & Losowsky 1992). Thus a high degree of suspicion is always required if the diagnosis is not to be missed, because the presentation is often based on very few symptoms or atypical features which may not immediately indicate a cause in the small intestine (Table 14.1). The frequently observed delay in diagnosis suggests that clinical awareness of the condition is not as acute as it might be, even though approximately one-third of adults give a history of childhood disorder. Features at this younger age include recurrent diarrhea after weaning, failure to thrive, vomiting and even constipation and reduced height and weight achievement.

Although symptoms may begin at any time, figures obtained through 1980–90 by the British Celiac Society show bimodal (diagnostic) peaks, the first for children (0–10 years) and the second for adults with females outnumbering males (2:1) and presenting a decade earlier (40–50) than males.

### *Constitutional symptoms*

Lassitude, weakness, malaise and lack of energy are frequent. In the absence of specific symptoms, such patients are unlikely to achieve rapid diagnosis: conversely once diagnosis is made and treatment instituted, a patient is much more able to perceive the degree of malaise suffered beforehand, a state of affairs which he or she came to believe was "normal". Weight loss is a more variable complaint, while a normal weight or even obesity do not exclude diagnosis.

### *Gastrointestinal symptoms*

Diarrhea is still the commonest gastrointestinal complaint but may not be characterized by features of severe steatorrhea. Although diarrhea may be continuous, it is more likely to be recurrent or precipitated by foreign travel (Marsh 1993a). The diarrhea may be associated with weight loss, although this may be variable or regained during periods of remission. There may also be lower abdominal colicky discomfort which may be interpreted as

**Table 14.2** Principal causes of mucosal lesions of small bowel mucosa

| Infiltrative/infiltrative-hyperplastic lesions | Flat | Atrophic-irreversible |
|---|---|---|
| Gluten sensitivity | Gluten sensitivity | Unresponsive gluten sensitivity (lymphoma) ? other |
| Tropical enteric diseases | Tropical enteric diseases | Protracted diarrhea of infancy |
| Giardiasis, cryptosporidiosis | AIDS complex | Scleroderma |
| AIDS enteropathy | Parasites | Chronic radiation |
| Crohn's disease | Giardiasis | Diffuse lymphoma |
| Acute enteritis | Cryptosporidiosis | Ischemia |
| Food-protein hypersensitivity | Immunodeficiency | Inflammatory (Crohn's) |
| Graft-versus-host disease | Lymphoma (Eastern/Western) | |
| | Protracted diarrhea of infancy | |
| | Drugs | |
| | Colchicine | |
| | Antimetabolites | |
| | Nonsteroidal anti-inflammatory | |
| | Zollinger–Ellison syndrome | |
| | Dietary protein hypersensitivity – milk, egg, fish, soya | |
| | Mucosal transplantation | |
| | Allograft | |
| | Ileal conduit | |
| | Gastroenterostomy | |
| | Graft-versus-host disease | |

irritable bowel syndrome. If nocturnal diarrhea occurs, this should always be regarded with suspicion and followed by a full diagnostic evaluation. The presence of severe abdominal colic, with or without diarrhea, should suggest intestinal obstruction either from small bowel carcinoma, lymphoma or stricture: such complications may further cause hemorrhage or perforation, even in well-treated patients.

Nausea, anorexia or vomiting are also relevant symptoms in about one-third of patients, with or without diarrhea. Given that so many patients now come to upper gastroduodenoscopy, even on an "open access" basis, endoscopists should be aware of this presentation and be careful to evaluate the duodenal mucosa for loss of folds and take a routine biopsy for histological analysis.

Aphthous ulceration (pp. 144 and 148) of the buccal mucosa is a presenting feature of gluten sensitivity in ~10% patients: thus any patient presenting with this complaint should be carefully reviewed with this diagnosis in mind. Likewise a presentation with glossitis, especially in the presence of an atrophic tongue, due to iron deficiency, should prompt the appropriate investigations.

*Other symptoms*

Gluten sensitivity may present with a variety of other non-gastrointestinal symptoms, such as peripheral edema or spontaneous bleeding. Joint pains may be due either to mono/polyarthropathy or osteomalacia with accompanying proximal girdle weakness, waddling gait and difficulty in climbing stairs, rising from a chair or lifting the arms. Backache and weakness from severe osteoporosis are occasionally striking and unexpected presentations. In these patients, it is important to note that diarrhea, and in particular the features of steatorrhea, are often absent. Although there may be cramps, paresthesiae or spontaneous tetany, osteomalacia usually develops insidiously, so that the bone pain is more likely to be interpreted as rheumatism, fibrositis or osteoarthritis and thus dismissed as the inevitable scourge of increasing age.

A true peripheral neuropathy with numbness, tingling, unsteadiness and weakness may include the legs. Men appear to be involved more often and there may be more complex neurological syndromes, involving brain and spinal cord, that are not responsive to gluten restriction.

As part of the presentation some patients, knowingly or unknowingly, may suffer periods of irritability and depression or may simply be very difficult to relate to or work with. This kind of negativism is often experienced by the physician when performing a biopsy or other investigative procedure: the difference in temperament once dietary gluten exclusion has commenced is very noticeable and may even become apparent to the patient once treatment has been established.

In addition to nocturnal diarrhea, nocturnal diuresis may be a troublesome complaint that may not be related to the urinary tract. Although water absorption may be delayed from the gastrointestinal tract, this is not the simplistic explanation for the phenomenon, which does respond to gluten restriction.

Untreated (and particularly unsuspected) gluten sensitivity may be associated with infertility, oligospermia, and end-organ unresponsiveness to testosterone. In females, menstruation may be delayed in onset and irregular, while difficulty in conceiving is occasionally encountered. Gluten sensitivity may relapse during pregnancy with anemia, malnutrition, diarrhea or tetany, particularly if prenatal care is not optimal. Although described but not widely appreciated, celiac disease can present in the puerperium with diarrhea and weight loss: this type of presentation needs to be recognized (Pauzner et al 1992).

*Other disease associations*

Gluten sensitivity may be associated with, or masked by, other coexisting disorders. There is an association with insulin dependent diabetes and difficulty in maintaining euglycemia may be due to underlying gluten sensitivity, while conversely the latter may not favorably respond until the need for insulin has been recognized.

The occurrence of rapid weight loss and diarrhea may suggest hyperthyroidism. There appears to be an increased risk of thyroid disease in gluten sensitivity, including goiter, myxedema and thyroidism (Cooke & Holmes 1984). The association of weakness, lethargy and skin pigmentation, with or without hypotension, may suggest hypoadrenalism, but gluten sensitivity (and Whipple's disease) should be considered.

The presence of disturbed circulating liver enzymes may be the only feature of underlying gluten sensitivity: these abnormalities revert to normal on treatment (Hagander et al 1977, Ledingham & More 1978, Lindberg et al 1978, Maggiore et al 1986). There may be a possible association with primary biliary cirrhosis.

There is an increased risk of ulcerative colitis, both in patients and family members, and a rare association with Crohn's disease. Thus diarrhea may arise from both small intestine and colon and thus require sigmoidoscopy or colonoscopy with biopsies (Marsh 1993a). Other reported associations with polymyositis, Sjögren's syndrome, rheumatoid and systemic lupus erythematosus may be by chance alone. Similarly associated pulmonary disorders such as sarcoidosis and pulmonary fibrosis may not have a single etiology. The occurrence of bird fancier's lung due not to sensitization to albumin, as commonly occurs throughout the normal population, but to avian β-globulin is seen in gluten-sensitized patients. The latter may also suffer other pulmonary infectious complications, including lung abscess.

## Diagnosis

Suspicions are raised in the presence of diarrhea and steatorrhea, weight loss and anemia. The anemia is microcytic, hypochromic if due to iron deficiency, or macrocytic if due to folate deficiency. However, the features of iron deficiency may obscure coexisting folate deficiency: thus, measurement of appropriate factors in the blood will clarify the issue. Splenic atrophy occurs in ~30% of patients and may be manifest as Howell–Jolly bodies (damaged red cell remnants) in the blood film. Additional diagnostic corroboration may include a history of similar complaints in childhood (perhaps 30%), a family history of the disorder or Irish ancestry. However, the diagnosis of gluten sensitivity may be more difficult particularly if symptoms are mild, if the complaints are of tiredness or vague ill health or if presenting features do not immediately suggest a gastrointestinal cause.

Diagnosis is most commonly established, or confirmed, by mucosal biopsies of duodenum or upper jejunum.

### *Jejunal biopsy*

A single biopsy of the small intestinal mucosa can be obtained with the Crosby–Kugler capsule and multiple biopsies with the Rubin or Quinton tubes.

***Indications.*** Biopsy of the small intestine is indicated when there is reason to suspect malabsorption. Some disorders display characteristic histologic/diagnostic features (Table 14.2): repeat biopsies are sometimes necessary to assess response to therapy, as in celiac disease and in Whipple's disease. Biopsies should not be performed on patients with a bleeding diathesis: thus prothrombin time and platelet counts should be checked.

***Crosby–Kugler capsule.*** The instrument consists of a metal capsule attached to a stiff radio-opaque catheter: if further stiffening is required a Seldinger wire can be passed down the catheter. There is a small port in the side of the capsule, so that suction via the catheter draws in mucosa and acts on a rubber diaphragm to trigger a knife which separates the indrawn fragment from the bowel. A screw is required to keep the cap in place. The Watson capsule is a modification of the Crosby–Kugler capsule.

The patient is fasted overnight and the throat sprayed with local anesthetic before the capsule is swallowed. It is then pushed into the pylorus under radiological control, for which the Seldinger wire may be needed. If intubation through the pylorus proves difficult, an outer polythene sleeve, for example Portex PP 325 tubing, may be used: an intravenous injection of metoclopramide (10 mg) is also helpful in facilitating its progress. When the capsule is in the duodenum the Seldinger wire is withdrawn, for its removal may become impossible once the capsule has passed round the duodenal loop. Once through the pylorus, the capsule invariably moves on quickly to the biopsy site at or beyond the duodenojejunal flexure. Fluoroscopy is necessary to obtain correct positioning of the capsule. Once in the jejunum, the capsule is cleared of secretions or mucus by injection of a small amount of air down the tube. Firing is achieved by two or three pulls with a 20 ml syringe attached to the distal end of the tubing. Slow suction should not be applied since this may draw too much mucosa into the port of the capsule. If the capsule has been fired correctly there is resistance to the passage of further air down the catheter. The capsule is then removed by steady, upward traction on the catheter. Resistance to removal should be investigated by fluoroscopy; if the knife has not severed the mucosa, the capsule will spring back to its previous position, once traction is stopped. Under these circumstances it is dangerous to apply further traction and 24–48 h must be allowed for the biopsy to slough off.

***The multipurpose suction biopsy tube (Rubin tube).*** This was developed by Brandborg et al (1959) for suction biopsy of the stomach or small bowel. Two intestinal biopsies can be obtained on each intubation, but two operators are required. The tube is passed and positioned in the same way as the Crosby–Kugler capsule and with the knife pulled closed, air is injected through the tube to confirm patency. A manometer is attached and a measured negative pressure of 4–10 mmHg is applied rapidly for 1–2 s by one operator, while the second operator excises the biopsy specimen by closing the knife rapidly. The instrument is withdrawn 1–2 cm under radiological control and a second biopsy is performed in the same manner. This apparatus may be used to obtain gastric biopsies in such conditions as Menetrier's disease and gastritis. The distribution of gastritis may be patchy and consequently multiple biopsies have to be taken.

***Directable suction biopsy tube*** (Linscheer & Abele 1976). This is a modification of a Rubin tube which uses wires to guide the tube quickly through the pylorus and duodenum.

***The Quinton hydraulic multiple biopsy tube*** (Flick et al 1961, Quinton et al 1962). This instrument has the great advantage that multiple biopsies can be taken. This is important because the abnormalities in various enteropathies may be patchy. It utilizes a hydraulic system which activates the knife and transports the biopsy specimens to the exterior. The tube is stiff and it can be pushed into the correct position in the jejunum. Local anesthesia of the throat and sedation with intravenous diazepam are necessary preliminaries. Two operators are needed, one to check that the correct pressure is maintained in the system and the other to fire the knife and withdraw the tube 1–2 cm after each biopsy. The procedure fails in only 3% of patients (Scott & Losowsky 1976) in comparison with a higher failure rate with other methods (Sheehy 1964).

***Biopsy of the jejunum in infants.*** This can be carried out with a pediatric version of the Crosby–Kugler capsule which is two-thirds the size of the adult capsule. It is attached to radio-opaque polyvinylchloride tubing (Portex R/1 SH 90): an outer polythene (Portex PP 260) tube can be used for stiffening. A pediatric version of the Watson biopsy capsule is also available. The technique is similar to that in the adult (Anderson & Burke 1975). Biopsies can be performed more rapidly with a directable Medi-Tech instrument (Ferry & Bendig 1981).

***Small bowel biopsy at endoscopy.*** The ease of endoscopy has led to a trend for endoscopic biopsy of the duodenum in preference to capsule biopsy in the diagnosis of celiac disease and other diffuse lesions of the small intestine. Mee and colleagues (1985) compared endoscopic and capsule biopsies and concluded that endoscopic biopsy of the second part of the duodenum is a reliable method for detecting mucosal abnormalities provided at least four specimens are obtained with standard-size forceps. However, because duodenal histological changes are more variable than those in the jejunum, doubt remains regarding the reliability of duodenal biopsy. Certainly, unless the duodenum biopsies are unequivocally normal or abnormal, it is advisable to perform jejunal biopsy: this is particularly important if the small endoscopic biopsy is poorly orientated, for then sensible interpretation is impossible.

We are still a long way from developing an easy test (preferably based on a blood sample) which will identify all gluten-sensitized subjects. Since endoscopic gastroduodenoscopies are performed so widely, a greater awareness of the flattening and scalloping of mucosal folds and readiness to take duodenal biopsies as a routine on all patients will provide another route to higher rates of diagnosis (Maurino et al 1993, van Bergeijk et al 1993a).

***Complications of intestinal biopsy.*** These are relatively rare, but are slightly more common when hydraulic instruments are used and when biopsies are obtained from infants. Bleeding occurs in about 0.1% of cases (Tytgat 1976). Perforation is much rarer and usually involves very young malnourished children and/or adults with very thin mucosae: the ileum is also more prone to perforation than jejunum. Perforation is also liable to occur from failure to withdraw the multiple (Quinton) biopsy tube by 2 cm between successive attempts at biopsy. Perforation should not occur if the recommended pressures are adhered to when using multiple biopsy tubes and if sudden suction is applied to fire the knife when using the Crosby–Kugler capsule.

Retention of the capsule occurred in 1.3% of 700 patients (Sheehy 1964) and was due to incomplete section of the mucosa so that the capsule remained attached to the bowel wall. This situation can be identified readily at screening (above) and is avoided by maintaining a sharp knife and avoiding excessive suction or pressure.

Damage to other parts of the upper gastrointestinal tract can occur in children when relatively large tubes are being manipulated.

***Care of instruments.*** All instruments are delicate. The instructions of the manufacturers should be followed carefully and the instrument scrupulously cleaned with any commercial disinfecting agent after individual use. The cutting parts of each instrument should then be immersed in 25% glutaraldehyde solution for 30 min to minimize the possibility of transmitting hepatitis.

### *Preparation of biopsies and interpretation*

Biopsies are rapidly retrieved from the capsule and gently spread on card, dental wax or a sliver of cucumber: the mucosal surface must be uppermost. Use of a low-power binocular microscope will aid correct orientation of the biopsy. The biopsy is then cut into smaller fragments if further studies other than routine histology are anticipated (determination of brush border membrane hydrolase levels, for example). Furthermore, more complex microscopic analyses (immunopathology or cytochemistry) will require either freezing in liquid nitrogen or immersion in special fixatives. However, for routine, diagnostic use, the orientated specimen is embedded to ensure sectioning that is perpendicular to the mucosal (luminal) surface: most usually, hemotoxylin and eosin or the periodic acid/Schiff stains are most helpful for interpretation. If correct processing has been achieved, the villi will appear uninterrupted along their entire length, while the crypts should not appear as circular cross-sections (see Figs 14.2 and 14.7).

### *Immunohistological techniques*

Although diagnosis, hitherto, has rested on the "gold standard" of a flat, proximal jejunal lesion, this is no longer an adequate criterion (Fig. 14.7): in addition the significance of milder lesions may not be appreciated or dismissed as nonspecific. In this regard, a further adjunct to tissue diagnosis is to determine whether the number of $\gamma\delta^+$ mucosal lymphocytes (especially IEL) are raised, preferably as a ratio of $\gamma\delta^+$/CD3$^+$ cells. In our hands, this has a specificity of 90–95% even when the villi appear histologically normal (Table 14.3). Alternatively, rectal challenge is another option, which is based on quantitative analysis (Loft et al 1990, Ensari et al 1994).

**Table 14.3** Diagnostic options in gluten sensitivity

| | |
|---|---|
| 1. Jejunal biopsy : | a) morphologic spectrum |
| | b) high $\gamma\delta^+$CD3 IEL ratio |
| 2. Gluten challenge: | a) oral deterioration |
| | b) rectal discriminant score influx $\gamma\delta^+$CD3cells |
| 3. Antibody screen: | a) antigliadin |
| | b) antiendomysial |
| 4. Intestinal antibody: | "CIA" pattern (see Arranz & Ferguson 1993) |

*Antigliadin and antiendomysial antibodies*

Diagnosis can be helped by screening for antigliadin and antiendomysial antibodies (Ferreira et al 1992, Uibo et al 1993), particularly in younger patients, but it should be noted that antigliadin (IgA) antibodies lose specificity with advancing age. Endomysial antibodies will also fail to identify gluten-sensitized individuals in the presence of milder jejunal lesions.

*Intestinal permeability tests* (p. 340)

While various types of "intestinal permeability" tests have been advocated in diagnosis, especially those which assay the urinary ratio of two ingested sugars (e.g. lactulose/mannitol), the prospective specificity of such procedures is unknown and unlikely to be high. They do have a potential role in assessing responses to dietary gluten restriction, although because of cost it is likely that periodic checks on antigliadin antibody titers which fall to control levels within 3–6 months of treatment will provide a simpler and probably more financially attractive test.

*Absorption tests*

The most commonly encountered abnormality is an increase in fecal fat excretion (p. 355). A mean daily output exceeding 7 g fat per day is indicative of steatorrhea and will thus initiate a search for small intestinal pathology.

The 25 g oral xylose test shows an excretion in a 5-h urine sample of less than 4 g of the ingested dose (p. 343). There may be impaired excretion of urinary xylose in the elderly: thus test results must be carefully interpreted in such individuals.

Hypoalbuminemia, due to protein-losing enteropathy, can occur with gluten sensitivity. The excess intestinal loss is confirmed with the use of the intravenous $^{51}CrCl_3$ test (p. 348). There is excretion of more than 2%. Alternatively the fecal clearance of $\alpha_1$-antitrypsin can be measured (p. 348).

## Latent gluten sensitivity

Twenty to thirty years ago, the diagnosis of celiac disease came to depend on the presence of severe villous flattening of upper jejunal mucosa associated with diarrhea, steatorrhea or some demonstrable form or consequence of malnutrition. Subsequent mucosal regeneration following institution of a strict gluten-free diet provided a further valuable diagnostic criterion.

*Definition*

Nowadays, such a simplistic view of "celiac disease" is inappropriate to current clinical or diagnostic needs (Marsh 1993b). This is due to the fact that many patients are either symptomless or have borderline features that are either dismissed or not interpreted within this context. In addition, it has become evident that other patients, adult or juvenile, may present with a variety of atypical symptoms which do not directly point to a gastrointestinal etiology (Table 14.1). The most convenient way to define asymptomatic subjects is by the term "latent" which is defined in the dictionary as "present, but not manifest".

Nevertheless, there is much confusion regarding the use and hence meaning of the word "latent". It was first used by Weinstein (1974) when he showed that by feeding gluten to some patients with dermatitis herpetiformis, a mild type 1 or type 2 lesion could be converted to a more severe lesion, such as type 3. This description of "mucosal latency" was, of course, a rather narrow use of the word, which does not have relevance to the important concept of *clinical* latency. The literature demonstrates that many individuals who are sensitized to gluten may have any lesion (type 0–4) on proximal jejunal biopsy and *yet be asymptomatic* (Fig. 14.1) (Marsh 1992a,c).

*Latency in "celiac" patients*

Latent gluten sensitivity is discovered:

1. by performing a jejunal biopsy in suspicious clinical circumstances, such as the presence of ill health, weakness, exhaustion, loss of weight, growth deficiency, unexplained osteomalacia or osteopenia or other nutritional deficiency, especially chronic, unresponsive iron deficiency (Egan-Mitchell et al 1981);
2. in systematic studies of family members of a known or recently diagnosed patient with classic symptomatic celiac disease; here it should be noted that as many as 50% immediate family members may have a proximal flat (type 3) lesion and yet be virtually asymptomatic (Table 14.4);
3. when acute complications arise such as diffuse jejunoileitis with or without ulceration and perforation, bleeding or obstruction due to a coexisting intestinal cancer or lymphoma;
4. when intestinal symptoms are unmasked by intercurrent infection (Marsh 1993a) (Table 14.5, Fig. 14.9).

*Latency in dermatitis herpetiformis*

This condition is characterized by intensely itchy "water blisters" that develop symmetrically over elbows, buttocks, knees, face or other exposed surfaces. The rash is gluten driven and is therefore an external marker for gluten sensitivity. The diagnosis is confirmed by the demonstration of IgA deposits along the dermoepidermal junction by immunofluorescence in *uninvolved* skin (Fry 1992).

**Table 14.4** Mucosal disease in latent compensated family members with gluten sensitivity

| Source | Region | Prevalence of celiac disease (flat mucosa) among first-degree relatives | Percentage of asymptomatic celiac patients (with flat mucosae) among first-degree relatives | Percentage of families affected |
|---|---|---|---|---|
| MacDonald et al (1965) | Seattle, N. America | 10 | 50 | 35 |
| Mylotte et al (1974) | Galway, Ireland | 10 | 50 | 25 |
| David & Adjukiewicz (1975) | Bristol, UK | 10 | – | – |
| Stokes et al (1976a) | Birmingham, UK | 20 | 50 | – |
| Shipman et al (1975) | Melbourne, Australia | 10 | 45 | 25 |
| Rolles et al (1974) | Birmingham, UK | 6 | 55 | 20 |
| Sagaro & Jiminez (1981) | Cuba, C. America | 5 | – | – |
| Mean values(%): | | 10 | 50 | 30 |

Note: (a) In the larger series, about 10% of all relatives were found to have a flat-destructive proximal jejunal lesion, of which at least half were latent or asymptomatic. (b) Of all families surveyed, only 30% appeared to reveal additional cases with mucosal lesions, whether symptomatic or not.

**Table 14.5** Common factors involved in unmasking latent gluten sensitivity (irrespective of proximal mucosal pathology)

| | |
|---|---|
| 1. *Gastrointestinal infections* | 3. *Metabolic stress* |
| Enteric bacteria/toxins (*Escherichia coli, Salmonella, Yersinia, Campylobacter, Aeromonas*) | Surgery of stomach/gallbladder/appendix |
| Viral (rotavirus/astrovirus/adenovirus) | Acute pancreatitis/trauma |
| Parasitic (*Giardia*/cryptosporidium) | Pregnancy/postpartum period |
| 2. *Coexisting nutritional deficiencies* | Acute febrile illness (influenza/pneumonia) |
| Iron deficiency | |
| poor dietary intake (low iron-content food) | 4. *Malignancies* |
| excessive losses (pregnancy/menstruation) | Diffuse lymphoma (unresponsive end-stage disease ± inflammatory jejunoileitis) |
| Folate deficiency | Mass lesions (intestinal obstruction/pain/ hemorrhage/perforation) |
| poor dietary intake (vegetables) | Esophagus (dysphagia) |
| increased utilisation (pregnancy/skin disease/ increased enterocyte turnover) | Stomach (anorexia) |
| Vitamin D | Other? |
| diet low in fish/fish oil/dairy products | |
| low exposure to sunlight | |

Only 50% of patients with dermatitis herpetiformis have a severe proximal lesion: the remainder have lesser degrees of change, characterized by infiltrative or infiltrative-hyperplastic lesions (Marsh 1989a). Nevertheless, only a few patients develop intestinal symptoms, but a jejunal biopsy should be performed in order to assess the degree of proximal mucosal damage or involvement and a gluten-free diet instituted in all cases. Parenthetically, it should be appreciated that because dermatitis herpetiformis acts as a skin marker for gluten sensitivity we have, through proximal jejunal biopsies in these patients, obtained a firm grasp of the spectrum of mucosal changes in gluten sensitivity (Marsh 1989a, O'Mahony et al 1990, Fry 1992).

*Diagnosis of latent gluten sensitivity*

The term "gluten sensitivity" should be employed in order to embrace all patients with typical or atypical symptoms of celiac disease, dermatitis herpetiformis and the remaining and largest proportion of individuals who are latent or asymptomatic. Gluten sensitivity may then be defined as a state of heightened immunologic responsiveness (cell mediated and humoral) to gluten protein in a genetically predisposed (DQw2 positive) individual. Note that this definition makes no implication (i) about the nature of the proximal jejunal mucosa nor (ii) mucosal response, since the latter *may not be demonstrable* with either a type 0 or irreversible flat-atrophic (type 4) lesion (Fig. 14.2).

Clearly a patient is either sensitized or not. Given a state of hypersensitivity to gluten, any type of mucosal lesion may be present (as demonstrable by proximal jejunal biopsy) *but irrespective of type of lesion present* that individual would either be symptomatic (i.e. present with a celiac malabsorption syndrome, whatever the lesion) or subclinical and latent (whatever the lesion) (Marsh 1992a).

Thus the recognition and diagnosis of gluten sensitivity (as opposed to celiac malabsorption of previous decades and centuries) has become a difficult problem and is based often on very subtle hints or the physician's high degree of awareness. In this respect it should be recalled that cases have been reported when the initial jejunal biopsy was apparently normal and only shown to be abnormal a few or several years later, despite absence of major symptomatology or severe nutritional deficiency (Challacombe et al 1975, McConnell & Whitwell 1975, Scott & Losowsky 1977, Egan-Mitchell et al 1981, Marsh 1989b, Mäki et al 1990). *A normal biopsy can no longer be relied on to exclude gluten sensitivity*, particularly in family relatives or in other patients with atypical presentations or vague ill health.

Celiac disease is not simply malabsorption accompanied

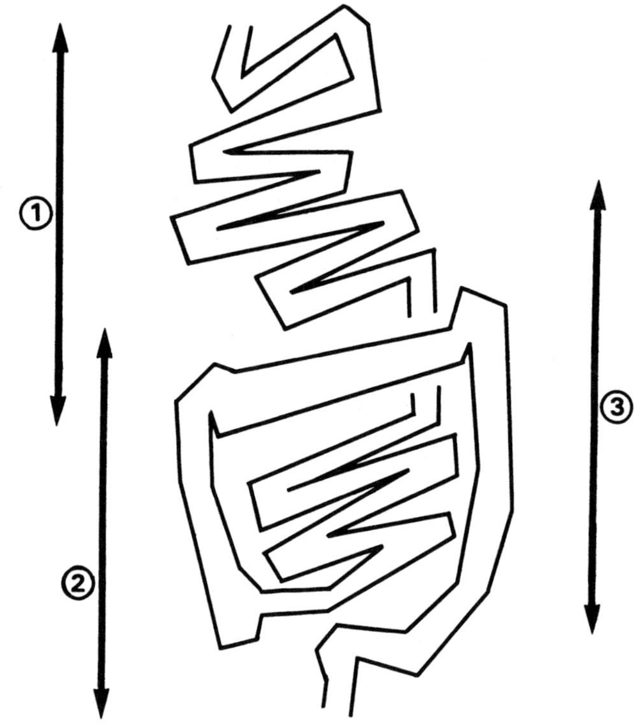


**Fig. 14.9** Occurrence of symptoms is dependent on the length of jejunum involved (1). The commonest precipitant of symptoms, at any age, must be infection, either directly or via toxic or cytopathic effects: these effects may impair the hindgut (2) which invariably compensates the proximal defect, thereby preventing diarrhea in most patients. Once this area is compromised the distal colon (3) will be overloaded (see Marsh 1993a for extended discussion). Note that infection does not necessarily drive the proximal lesion to a more severe form in order to produce symptomatic diarrhea or malabsorption.

by a flat jejunal mucosa. The possibilities of an atypical presentation or of latency must always be kept in mind, especially if there is a positive family history. Commonly borderline symptoms are dismissed and minor mucosal abnormalities interpreted as nonspecific.

This raises the question as to how to diagnose gluten sensitivity, what technique or approach is most likely to fulfill that task and whether mucosal biopsy is still necessary or the most desirable option (Table 14.3). The answers can only come with further study, but in pursuing such studies the value of any diagnostic test must be evaluated in terms of the entire mucosal spectrum and not confined to the minority of patients with the typical flat-destructive proximal lesion.

## Treatment

*The gluten-free diet*

This is the mainstay of treatment. Commonly the newly diagnosed patient is given a list of foods which cannot or must not be eaten. This practice should continue but should be accompanied by positive information about a core diet which can be adopted immediately. This diet is based around rice, soya and cornflour products, together with meat (unprocessed) and fresh fish, vegetables and fruit which provides a reasonably "healthy" diet. This may then be gradually supplemented by other safe gluten-free foods, as experience is gained with the diet: in this way the confidence of the patient is maintained. An early appointment is given with an experienced dietitian who should also be trained to stress the positive aspects of what can be eaten and arrange membership of the local celiac society so that updated food lists are received. With this approach the patient can be encouraged to embark on the diet with confidence, if not enthusiasm.

It is important to avoid making the patient confused or even afraid to eat anything. This can be monitored by frequent follow-up appointments so that body weight can be checked: while not every patient responds to the diet by an increase in weight, there should certainly be no loss. If this does occur, then rapid steps must be taken to ensure an increased caloric intake.

Many patients find that gluten-free products are unpalatable or difficult to handle. However, there is now a wide variety of products available and it is important that the newly diagnosed patient is advised to try as many as possible in order to find the most compatible products. Most celiac groups run cookery demonstrations which provide considerable support in the early days of the diet. The patient must always be on the lookout for changes in the specification of "safe" food products, as some manufacturers may add gluten without notification. All processed types of food should be carefully watched, especially if symptoms consistently arise after their use.

Restrictions must apply to wheat, barley, rye and oats-derived products. The risks of contamination in alcoholic beverages with gluten is extremely small (Shewry et al 1992) and therefore some physicians believe that beer or malt whisky is not contraindicated, but understandably, some patients prefer not to take the risk.

*Supplements*

Some supplemental medicine may be necessary during the first 6–12 months of treatment.

***Hematinics.*** It is vital that body stores of iron are totally replaced until serum ferritin levels become normal: this can be done either by oral or intramuscular iron or a total (intravenous) body infusion. Similarly, folate stores may require replenishment and careful monitoring to ensure they remain stable. Use of folate to correct a megaloblastic anemia may rapidly exhaust borderline iron stores as hemopoiesis is stimulated: thus iron status should be regularly checked for masked iron deficiency when folate supplements are initially given alone.

***Calcium and vitamin D.*** Metabolic bone disease (osteomalacia) may either be treated with vitamin D injections (50–100 000 units IM) or oral calcium/cholecalciferol tablets, provided serum calcium levels are regularly checked. Studies of bone mineralization ("osteoporosis") in gluten-sensitive patients indicate the possibility of considerably low bone-mass densities in children and adults, in the absence of steatorrhea, skeletal symptoms, biochemical abnormalities and when on treatment with a gluten-free diet (Caraceni et al 1988, Molteni et al 1990, Mazure et al 1994). While female patients diagnosed and commenced on treatment during childhood (Molteni et al 1990, Mora et al 1993) appear to gain a normal bone marrow density when adult, a female patient diagnosed in adult life is still very likely to have a reduced bone marrow density. However, this state of affairs is unlikely to affect final height attainment, which normalizes within 1.8–3 years treatment with a gluten-free diet (Bosio et al 1990, Bode et al 1991, Mora et al 1993). However, there is a particular need to maintain a careful watch on bone density in adult (female) celiacs as they continue to age and hence lose total bone mass (Melton et al 1990). Furthermore, there is evidence that in normal women peak bone mass may never be achieved and that dietary calcium intake may be far below that necessary for positive calcium balance (Haeney et al 1977), the latter requiring different levels of calcium intake, especially during periods of adolescent growth and beyond the menopause (Haeney 1991). The average fractional absorption is ~30% of intake (Haeney & Recker 1985). Thus supplementation with 0.5–1.5 g calcium per day together with milk (if tolerated) may be vital (Dawson-Hughes et al 1990, Haeney 1991) in females in order to achieve peak bone mass and to protect against inevitable bone attrition associated with aging and the menopause. Screening is now rapid, cheap and noninvasive (Melton et al 1990): the responsibility lies with the physician.

## Response to a gluten-free diet

As Rubin showed over 30 years ago the intestinal mucosa heals from below, so that the proximal jejunal lesion is the last event to normalize. Provided nutrition is maintained and serum antigliadin levels fall, there is little need for repeated jejunal biopsies. More telling evidence of a response can be gleaned from clinical and other observations (especially falling titers of antigliadin antibody) than by further mucosal sampling. Maintenance of nutritional indices without supplements provides evidence of improved intestinal function and absorption and hence response to diet.

In children, diagnosis is based on symptoms, suspicions or family history and confirmed by a proximal jejunal biopsy. A response to diet is manifested by significant weight gain or relief of symptoms (Walker-Smith 1988).

The original diagnostic criteria from the European Society of Pediatric Gastroenterology and Nutrition are no longer applied. However, it is advisable to rechallenge a child who never had a biopsy before commencing the diet or who was diagnosed before the age of 2 years. With a gluten challenge, relapse either histological or clinical usually occurs within 2 years. If not, the gluten containing diet may be continued, with close surveillance and further repeat biopsies: in such cases, it is difficult to be dogmatic as relapse, if it occurs, may take several years. Thus the rule is careful follow-up if diagnosis is in doubt. It may be necessary to refer the patient, at a later date, to a gastroenterologist to maintain surveillance.

### *Failure of response*

For reasons that are not evident, a few patients fail to improve immediately once the diagnosis is made and dietary treatment has been commenced. This picture is unlikely to occur in a patient with a mild or minimal type of proximal lesion. Therefore, the physician must be certain that a severe lesion is due to gluten sensitivity and not due to other causes of a flat mucosa (Table 14.2). It is also important to be sure that there have been no dietary lapses, particularly during the early months of treatment, when dietary adherence must be most strict. Indiscretions may be due to deliberate noncompliance, unwitting departures, inability to grasp the implications of the diet or use of a product which the manufacturer has altered or is unsuspected to contain gluten (tablets, sweets, confections). Hyperthyroidism, hypothyroidism, coexisting diabetes mellitus or even alcoholism should also be considered.

***Prednisolone.*** Once the above options have been considered, corticosteroids may be useful, commencing with 20 mg prednisolone daily and slowly reducing over 3–6 months. This often brings about an improvement in clinical well-being. However, such treatment should be used with caution: it is not uncommon for aching joints to follow in the wake of such treatment, so that some preliminary warning of the after-effects might be given. There is always the possibility of repeating the course if progress is not maintained or the response appears to slow.

***Other causes of non-response.*** Very rarely, secondary complications of gluten sensitivity may blunt the response and these possibilities must be excluded, such as pancreatic dysfunction or bacterial overgrowth (Marsh 1993a). Other abdominal symptoms with bloating or diarrhea may be due to symptomatic lactose intolerance. Therefore, a trial of a milk-free diet may be useful. However, it is very difficult for the patient to maintain both a strict gluten- and milk-free diet, so careful follow-up is necessary in these circumstances.

Although patients are frequently referred as "?unresponsive celiac syndrome, ?lymphoma", the reasons for a slow response are usually more obvious, as outlined above.

True unresponsiveness is usually a different phenomenon, with progressive weight loss, continued diarrhea,

**Table 14.6** Ulceration of the small intestine

| | |
|---|---|
| 1. *Nonspecific ulcerative jejunoileitis* | 4. *Infective* |
| (a) Unresponsive gluten sensitivity | Typhoid |
| (b) Gluten-induced lymphoma | *Campylobacter jejuni* |
| (c) Idiopathic: solitary | Tuberculosis |
| diffuse | Actinomycosis |
| | *Yersinia* |
| 2. *Malignant* | Cytomegalovirus |
| Carcinoma | *Candida* |
| Lymphoma (primary) | Mucormycosis |
| Leiomyosarcoma | |
| (Metastatic) | 5. *Vascular* |
| | Polyarteritis |
| 3. *Drug-induced* | Behçet's syndrome |
| Potassium salts (enteric-coated) | Ischemia |
| Nonsteroidal anti-inflammatory agents | |
| Iron sulfate | 6. *Chronic radiation damage* |
| Phenylbutazone | |
| Salicylates | |
| Indomethacin | 7. *Meckel's diverticula* (ectopic gastric mucosa) |

onset of a gradual fall in serum albumin and progressive inanition which invariably but slowly results in death. Usually mucosal atrophy is the cause. For a while, a plateau can be maintained with use of steroids, additional nutritional support including parenteral nutrition and even immunosuppressive drugs. These cases are usually due to lymphoma although its objective diagnosis may be extremely difficult, even at postmortem.

## True (unresponsive) mucosal atrophy

### *Etiology*

The nature of this clinical syndrome with its attendant irreversible mucosal atrophy is unclear, although it undoubtedly includes cases of gluten sensitivity because of associated splenic atrophy, a typical proximal (type 3) flat-destructive lesion, a history of childhood disorder or a family relative with the same disorder and appropriate HLA (DQw2) genetic background (Holmes & Thompson 1992). It is not evident whether such patients become antigen insensitive or anergic or whether a separate process evolves which progressively destroys the intestinal mucosa and the patient with it. Sometimes there is associated *diffuse jejunoileitis*, with or without mucosal ulceration, or frank lymphoma.

### *Clinical features and treatment*

Ill health or continued diarrhea may persist for several years, in the presence of a flat mucosa, and where a postulated failure to adhere to the diet is an insufficient and indeed naive explanation for the phenomenon. This type of presentation usually appears in the middle-aged or beyond, with a malabsorption syndrome that is unresponsive to gluten withdrawal. It may be ameliorated by the use of steroids, azathioprine, cyclosporin or FK506. Even then, there may still be a downhill course, with continuing weight loss, cachexia, a lowering of the serum albumin or hemoglobin levels, despite use of parenteral alimentation and other maneuvers, such as milk-free diet. Alternatively, the presentation may be abrupt with onset of diarrhea, pain and abdominal masses in a well-treated patient or with bleeding, perforation and obstruction resulting from tumor masses or mucosal fissuring, ulceration or stricture formation. In this setting the ulcers, which are probably microfoci of lymphoma, seem distinct from the other solitary or multiple punched-out ulcers that may be associated with gluten sensitivity (or drug usage (p. 395)) (Table 14.6).

## The malignant complications of gluten sensitivity

The relationship between gluten sensitivity, lymphoma and carcinoma of the gastrointestinal tract is now well defined and is a tribute to the continued surveillance by the Birmingham, England, physicians in studies initiated by the late Dr W T Cooke. Their most recent publication draws attention to the apparent role of a strict gluten-free diet in reducing the risk of developing either a lymphoma or carcinoma (Holmes et al 1976, 1989, Holmes & Thompson 1992).

The concept of protection against a malignant outcome by adherence to a reasonably strict gluten-free diet is relevant to those with minimal or clinically inapparent disease, that is, patients with latent disease. Since the highest number of latent gluten-sensitive patients is likely to be found among the relatives of known patients, our attentions should naturally fall on this group of individuals.

Note should therefore be taken of the 10-fold increase in deaths from malignancy, in comparison with age- and sex-matched controls, in a study of 1400 relatives of known gluten-sensitive patients from Birmingham, UK (Stokes et al 1976b). The risk was for esophageal, bladder and cerebral malignancy in male relatives and for breast cancer in females. There were also some deaths from lymphoma, although figures were too small for any statistical significance to be drawn: nevertheless, the information obtained is highly suggestive, indicating that the physician should be aware of these increased cancer rates and therefore try to identify those at risk (having latent gluten sensitivity) within these kindreds (Holmes & Thompson 1992).

There can be little doubt that chronic gluten exposure in susceptible individuals leads to malignancy (Holmes & Thompson 1992). It appears that the more severe the (proximal) lesion, the greater the risk (Holmes et al 1989). It should be remembered that ~50% latent family relatives have a severe (type 3) flat-destructive lesion (MacDonald et al 1965, Mylotte et al 1974, Stokes et al 1976a) and are therefore most at risk (Table 14.4).

However, malignancy has also been described in patients whose jejunal mucosal lesions were of minimal degree (Gjone & Nordoy 1970, Mansson 1971, Freeman & Chiu 1986) so that they could have been easily overlooked and hence missed. The density of IEL counts either may not be elevated (Leonard et al 1983) or become reduced, this latter phenomenon predating onset of lymphoma by 5 years (Ferguson et al 1974).

Malignancy is also a complication of dermatitis herpetiformis. It is important that all these patients, irrespective of proximal jejunal lesional pathology, be offered and advised to adhere to a strict gluten-free diet. There still appears to be a misconception that dermatitis herpetiformis, if either unaccompanied by symptomatic gastrointestinal disease or a significantly abnormal proximal jejunal biopsy, does not require dietary restriction as an adjunct to oral dapsone treatment (Fry 1992).

### *Lymphomas*

The background historical evidence, which largely suggested that malabsorption is a complication of intestinal malignancy (lymphoma), has been reviewed (Cooke & Holmes 1984, Isaacson 1987, Wright & Isaacson 1989). It was work from Bristol (Gough et al 1962, Austad et al 1967, subsequently supported by very extensive data from Birmingham, UK (Harris et al 1967), which firmly established the malignant potential of gluten sensitivity and, later, of dermatitis herpetiformis (Freeman et al 1977).

***Pathology*** (p. 459)

***Clinical features.*** The presentation of lymphoma is varied and affects males and females equally. It is not necessarily confined to the elderly since it has been recognized in patients in their third decade, but it has never been reported in children. The disease may arise rapidly in an apparently healthy, well-treated patient with onset of abdominal pain, recurrence of diarrhea and presence of abdominal masses. It may even occur as an acute surgical emergency with intestinal obstruction, perforation or hemorrhage arising from ulceration, tumor mass or stricturing of the bowel: often the cause is only discovered in these cases at laparotomy. Furthermore, the relationship to gluten sensitivity may then not be determined unless a proximal jejunal biopsy is subsequently performed. In other patients the onset may be more chronic and insidious, with diarrhea, slow and continued weight loss, falling serum albumin and a poor or transient response to steroids, azathioprine or cyclosporin.

The common presenting symptoms of lymphoma are weakness, weight loss and diarrhea: these are also the major features of typical celiac disease, although response to a conventional dietary regimen may be poor in the presence of lymphoma. Muscle weakness, in the absence of neuropathy or vitamin D deficiency, has also been identified as an important discriminatory symptom in this setting, as is the occurrence of a pyrexia: over 60% cases in one series presented with fever (Holmes & Thompson 1992). Early symptoms of vague ill health, lethargy and inanition may not always suggest the underlying diagnosis or prompt a particular search for features of gluten sensitivity. Patients over the age of 50 years need careful follow-up, since their chances of malignancy are high (Cooper et al 1982).

***Investigations.*** There are no useful laboratory, histologic or radiologic features which prospectively aid diagnosis. The radiological presence of strictures, narrowed segments or a nodular mucosal pattern are indications of suspicious pathology which probably require operative resection for correct diagnosis. Gastroduodenoscopy may, of course, identify upper gastrointestinal malignancies, if biopsies are taken.

The use of abdominal ultrasound and computed tomography provides a further useful means of searching for tumor deposits and assessing the longer term effects of treatment on established tumor masses.

***Treatment.*** Treatment options are variable. A localized mass may be resectable and given postoperative radiotherapy and chemotherapy, a tolerable lifestyle may be possible for some additional years. In others, the downhill course is so rapid that diagnosis (by biopsy or laparotomy) may not be possible, while others may already have features of widespread dissemination. In general, the prognosis is extremely gloomy.

### *Carcinoma*

Carcinoma of the small bowel is the second most common malignant complication of gluten sensitivity (Swinson et al 1983, Holmes & Thompson 1992). There is a marked male predominance for this type of neoplasm, occurring in 21 of 29 reported cases (Holmes & Thompson 1992). Occult blood loss leads to anemia and weakness or obstruction occurs with vomiting, abdominal pain and distention and a palpable mass may be present. Radiology is helpful in defining narrowed segments or apple-core lesions of small bowel: features of intestinal obstruction in the known setting of gluten sensitivity may suggest a carcinoma. Surgery is the preferred option, with reasonable optimism (Holmes & Thompson 1992). In addition to carcinoma of the jejunum, malignancies of the mouth, pharynx and esophagus are statistically more common in individuals with gluten sensitivity.

## ULCERATION OF THE SMALL INTESTINE

Ulceration of the small intestine occurs in many conditions (Table 14.6) but particularly occurs as a result of infective (tuberculosis and typhoid) inflammatory (Crohn's disease), vascular and neoplastic diseases (especially lymphoma) (Wayte & Helwig 1968, Booth & Neale 1985).

## Chronic ulcerative nongranulomatous jejunoileitis

Patients with celiac disease only rarely develop extensive ulceration of the small intestine; the consensus of opinion is that ulcerative jejunoileitis is a distinct disorder. It is also called idiopathic mucosal enteropathy or idiopathic chronic ulcerative enteritis. Some patients with associated hypogammaglobulinemia have a deficiency of T-cells and a failure of B-cells to produce normal amounts of immunoglobulin (Saxon et al 1977).

*Pathology*

The ulcerative lesion and severe mucosal atrophy is patchy but usually extends throughout the small intestine. No specific features of the ulceration have been identified. Strictures may develop secondary to ulceration. A subepithelial layer of collagen may be seen but is not specific for it may occur in celiac disease. It has been suggested that the epithelium is hyporegenerative, in contrast to the hyperregenerative mucosa of celiac disease, because the crypts are hypoplastic or even absent. This hypoplasia leads to loss of villi and to ulceration. The condition is often difficult to distinguish from malignant histiocytosis (Robertson et al 1983).

*Clinical features* (Jeffries et al 1968, Modigliani et al 1979)

There is severe intractable diarrhea, abdominal pain, fever and weight loss. The ulceration may lead to hemorrhage, perforation or obstruction due to strictures. There may be abdominal distention and peripheral edema. Steatorrhea is severe and other tests of absorption are usually abnormal; there is hypoproteinemia due to protein-losing enteropathy, anemia due to iron and folate deficiency and intermittent leukocytosis. Zinc deficiency may occur. Intestinal biopsy may show normal mucosa, partial or total villous atrophy, because the mucosal lesion is patchy (see above). Biopsy rarely shows ulceration, which is usually only seen at enteroscopy or laparotomy. In early disease the barium follow-through examination shows changes of malabsorption, whilst later there are strictures and proximal dilatation. Ulcers are rarely demonstrated (Lamont et al 1982).

*Treatment*

The prognosis is poor, whatever treatment is carried out. In one series of 13 patients, nine (69%) died within 1–5 years of the onset of abdominal symptoms (Jeffries et al 1968). A gluten-free diet should be tried; a response indicates that the patient has celiac disease. By definition, patients with chronic ulcerative nongraulomatous jejunoileitis do not respond. Prednisolone, in an initial dosage of 40–80 mg/day gradually reducing to 10–20 mg/day, may be of temporary benefit.

## Behçet's syndrome

Small intestinal ulceration is rare in patients from Western countries but is common in Japan (p. 145).

*Pathology*

The ulcers occur predominantly in the ileum and cecum. They are nonspecific in appearance but the inflammation is transmural and perforation may occur at more than one site. There may be thrombosis of the vessels around the ulcer, together with perivascular infiltration (Booth & Neale 1985).

*Clinical features*

The condition is chronic and intermittent with attacks of anorexia, nausea, vomiting, abdominal pain, distention and diarrhea. Radiological examination shows dilated loops of small intestine and ulceration of the ileum may be seen. Malabsorption may occur.

## Nonspecific ulceration (primary ulcer)

*Etiology*

Many patients with nonspecific ulceration of the small intestine give a history of therapy with enteric-coated potassium tablets (Watson 1963, Wayte & Helwig 1968), nonsteroidal anti-inflammatory drugs (Madhok et al 1986) or diuretics and it is assumed that these drugs, and possibly others as well, cause damage to the mucosa at the location where they dissolve. Ulceration also occurs in patients with vascular diseases and in these instances the ulceration may have a vascular etiology.

*Pathology*

The ulcer (Fig. 14.10) is usually solitary and situated in the ileum. Characteristically, the ulcer produces a "napkin ring" constriction and there is proximal dilatation of the bowel. On histological examination, the mucosal ulceration overlies submucosal fibrosis.

*Clinical features*

The ulcer presents with partial small intestinal obstruction or, less commonly, with perforation or hemorrhage. The symptoms of obstruction are often of short duration, but in some patients they arise slowly over several months. On investigation, the findings are those of intestinal obstruction and on barium examination of the small intestine a short narrow annular stricture with proximal dilatation may be seen (Carlson 1969). The precise diagnosis is only made at surgery. The ulcerated area is resected and the small bowel should be inspected for additional areas of ulceration.

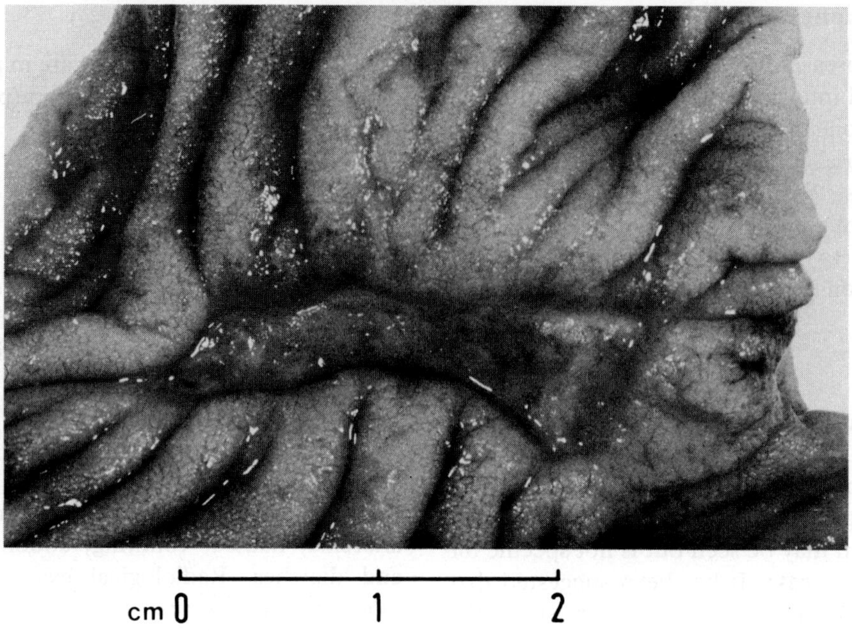

**Fig. 14.10** Nonspecific ileal ulcer. The ulcer is shallow and flat-based. There is no abnormality of the adjacent mucosa.

## TROPICAL SPRUE (TROPICAL DIARRHEAL MALABSORPTION SYNDROME)

The importance of this condition grew out of its effects on civilian and military personnel involved in British, Dutch, French and American interests in the Far East, as witnessed over a period of about three centuries (c1650 onwards). Indeed, the word "sprue" is an anglicized version of the Dutch word (sprouw) for the association of oral aphthous ulceration and diarrhea and reflects the involvement of the Dutch East India Company in the economic trade between India and Europe. Nevertheless, all descriptions of so-called "tropical sprue" made before the advent of peroral biopsy techniques are beyond interpretation, since certain "epidemics" of this condition could have been due to waterborne giardiasis (Cooke 1985). Furthermore, the term itself is inappropriate and inaccurate and its etiology never satisfactorily explained.

### Definition

Tropical sprue is a malabsorption syndrome peculiar to tropical and subtropical areas of the world. It affects the indigenous populations as well as those who come to inhabit these areas on a more temporary basis. Classically sprue was seen in India, south east Asia and in certain parts of the Hispanic Caribbean, such as Haiti and Puerto Rico, but it seems more likely that it involves a large number of underprivileged peoples across the world between the tropics of Cancer and Capricorn, including central and southern Africa and central and southern America.

### Mucosal pathology and immunopathology

Following the use of the peroral biopsy technique from 1960 onwards, it became apparent that mucosal lesions similar to those recently demonstrated in children and adults with gluten sensitivity were present in this disease (Chacko et al 1961, Baker et al 1962a, Schenk et al 1965, 1968, Swanson & Thomassen 1965). However, there were three major distinctions: patients with symptomatic, full-blown sprue rarely seemed to have as severe a lesion as the characteristic flat-destructive (type 3) lesion of gluten sensitivity. Observations from India and the Caribbean indicated that only 5% of patients develop a flat mucosa. Furthermore, another 5% of mucosal biopsies were apparently indistinguishable from biopsies from the local population. In most patients, there was an "inflamed" mucosa (increased lymphocytes, plasma cells, etc) on an architectural background of mild to moderate abnormality, ranging from blunting of villous tips to a more severe reduction in villous height with prominent hypertrophic crypts. The surface epithelial cells were often damaged, being cuboidal in section like celiac cells and infiltrated by small lymphocytes (Fig. 14.11).

Secondly, although the proximal lesion was generally less severe than that encountered in gluten sensitivity, the lesion in sprue patients was far more extensive and tended to involve the entire small bowel mucosa, including ileum: this was invariably manifested by impaired vitamin $B_{12}$ absorption.

Finally, a most important observation was that the majority of so-called normal individuals demonstrated minor abnormalities in intestinal structure and function,

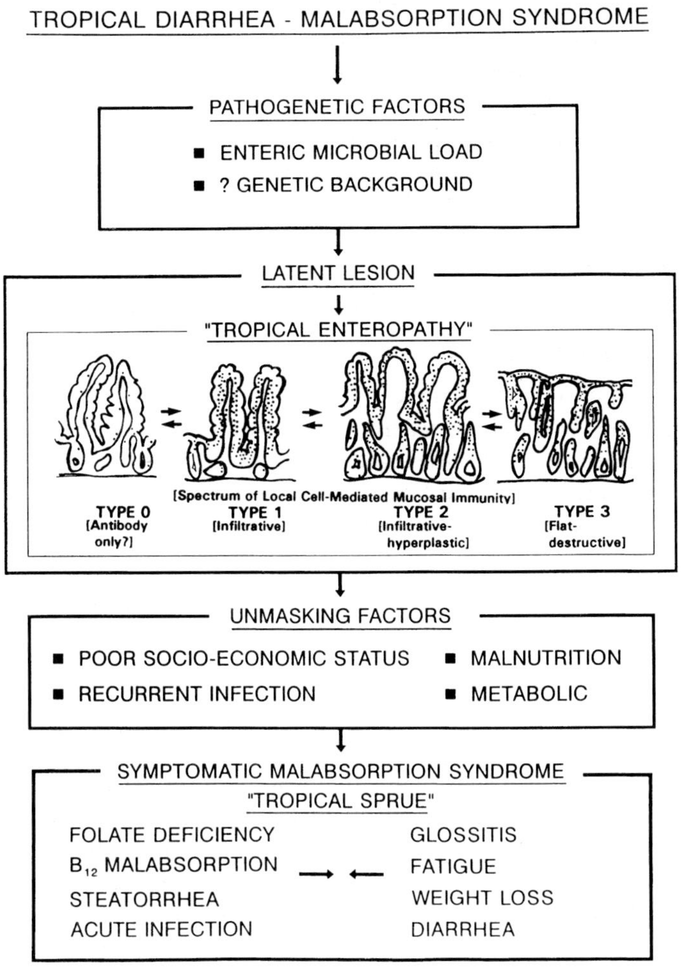


**Fig. 14.11** The pathogenesis of the tropical diarrhea malabsorption syndrome (tropical enteropathy, tropical sprue) is largely based on continued exposure to a heavy microbial intestinal load: variations in response may be genetically determined. This leads to a "latent" tropical enteropathy, which may become symptomatic by a variety of environmental factors, but especially acute enteric infections. Compare with Fig. 14.1.

although diarrhea, weight loss or constitutional upset were never a major problem. This mild, albeit demonstrable, abnormality gained the term "tropical enteropathy" to distinguish it from the symptomatic and generally more severe malabsorption picture termed "tropical sprue". Importantly, in terms of etiopathology, it was shown that a similarly mild derangement of small bowel structure and function invariably affected Westerners who took up residence in tropical and subtropical areas. The changes were more marked in individuals adopting rural habitats, such as peace corps volunteers (Lindenbaum et al 1966), than their compatriots living under more sanitized urban conditions. These intestinal changes invariably and rapidly reverted to normal after repatriation to a Western style of living (Baker 1982).

Many studies showed that this mild, asymptomatic form of intestinal derangement was invariably associated with xylose or $B_{12}$ malabsorption, mild steatorrhea or increased fecal nitrogen losses. The lesional pathology, comprising mild blunting of villi, tongue or ridged shaped villi and moderate infiltration of epithelium and lamina propria, was acquired early in childhood and persisted throughout adulthood. It can be concluded that the majority of the indigenous and expatriate populations of the periequatorial regions of the world have a *latent* form of environmentally induced, cell-mediated enteropathy that is distinct, and quantitatively different, when compared with the "control" Western intestinal tract.

The overlap between the mucosal pathology of clinically apparent "sprue" and that of latent tropical enteropathy deserves further comment. Although symptomatic sprue patients might have severe folate deficiency and significant $B_{12}$ deficiency resulting in weakness, lack of energy, weight loss and severe exhaustion, replacement therapy by oral or parenteral exogenous folate (Spies et al 1946) or $B_{12}$ injections could reverse symptoms, but not mucosal morphology. Indeed, despite successful clinical responses, persisting abnormalities in vitamin absorption, together with mild steatorrhea, persistent xylose and $B_{12}$ malabsorption, were still evident. Neither did mucosal morphology always return to normal (Sheehy et al 1962, Baker 1982). In other words, treatment of acute deficiency states by appropriate nutrients, and diarrhea by antibiotics, merely returned the patient to the previous state of latent tropical enteropathy.

## Etiology – immunopathology

This has never been satisfactorily resolved. No "sprue agent" has ever been identified which effectively explains the nature of the disease, its characteristic territorial distribution or its spectrum of mucosal pathologies. During the last 150 years, yeasts, fungi, algae, bacteria, viruses, parasites and even amebae have been implicated as etiological agents. Klipstein (1981) has suggested that toxigenic *E.coli* is the pathogenic agent, but this is more likely to be a superadded infection or colonizer which precipitates, rather than causes, the condition. Furthermore, it is not at all clear that a microbial toxin, of itself, could result in the spectrum of mucosal pathology (Figs 14.2 and 14.11) which characterizes "tropical enteropathy/sprue".

It has been suggested that there is no specific condition of tropical sprue caused by one particular organism and this is why a specific "sprue agent" has never been, or cannot be, found (Marsh 1992d). Indeed, the key to any rational interpretation of the etiology and pathogenesis of the two arbitrary conditions of tropical enteropathy and tropical sprue must surely lie in the interpretation of the mucosal lesion.

A ready source of published micrographs of jejunal and ileal morphology is to be found in the Wellcome Trust Collaborative Study (1971). A critical examination of the varied lesions shows that they fulfill the criteria of type 1 (infiltrative), type 2 (infiltrative-hyperplastic) and type 3 (flat-destructive) pathology which characterizes the fully developed spectrum of mucosal lesions in gluten sensitivity (Fig. 14.2). In "sprue" of either Indian or Caribbean type, the mucosal lesion invariably spans the infiltrative/infiltrative-hyperplastic part of the spectrum, with 5% demonstrating severe (type 3) lesions and ~10% apparently having normal biopsies (Fig. 14.11). This latter statement must be cautiously received, since lesion pathologies, like that in gluten sensitivity, may be locally patchy and because (as is clearly evident in the Wellcome Symposium) mucosae that obviously show a type 1 or type 2 appearance were often described as "normal".

Despite such shortcomings, reflective of an age in which mucosal immunology was not a considered option, the mucosal changes described represent a pathological spectrum consistent with an environmentally produced, but *host-directed* response of cell-mediated immune type, operative at mucosal level to the heavy microbial intestinal load experienced in these parts of the world. For such reasons, it seems quite unwarranted to regard tropical sprue and enteropathy as two distinct, nosologic conditions: indeed, avoidance of such terminologies in favor of the less specific "tropical diarrhea malabsorption syndrome" is to be preferred.

It must be appreciated that there is a widespread, latent form of bowel pathology, comprising cell-mediated "inflammatory" changes induced by environmental conditions imposed by living in tropical and subtropical areas of the world. This picture is little different from the high proportion of gluten-sensitized individuals with latent disease and mucosal pathology: indeed, it may be difficult to differentiate between them (Van Bergeijk et al 1993b). Furthermore, as a full-blown symptomatic celiac syndrome can arise in a latent subject in response to a variety of nonspecific environmental stimuli (Table 14.5: Fig. 14.1) (Marsh 1993a) so, likewise, symptomatic tropical sprue can develop on the common background of mild enteropathy given similar types of environmental stimuli (Fig. 14.11).

In the tropics, such predisposing factors may include poor socioeconomic status, borderline or frank undernutrition, concurrent parasitism, metabolic stress and, particularly, recurrent intestinal infections. As in gluten sensitivity (Marsh 1993a), acute enteric infections must be, by far, the most common factor to precipitate acute malabsorption. Thus, so-called acute or "epidemic" sprue (with time–space clustering) is accounted for by community-acquired/spreading infections (Baker & Mathan 1961, Baker et al 1962b): abrupt onset with fever and bloodflecked watery diarrhea suggests dysenteric episodes. In other cases, the syndrome develops more insidiously (as in adult gluten sensitivity) with marked steatorrheic stools, weight loss, profound weakness and anergy and marked nutritional deficiencies, especially of folate and iron, together with reduced $B_{12}$ stores. Careful inquiry reveals that these patients may give a history of preceding episodes of acute diarrhea, frequently over many years, suggesting that recurrent infection, the cumulative effects of postinfectious enteropathy, and progressive malabsorption combined with poor socioeconomic conditions create a downward spiral resulting in severe intestinal deficiency, malabsorption and further impaired immune responsiveness.

## Epidemiology

It is clear that "tropical diarrhea malabsorption syndrome" is widely prevalent, especially among the growing numbers of underprivileged and starving populations of the world, including South America, East Africa and the Far East. Although masked by overlying malnutrition and recurrent, high infection rates, it still represents a problem of major importance and gravity.

This condition widely affects children (Santiago-Borrero et al 1970), although the classic literature is not extensive. In a recent study of malnourished, infected infants in the Gambia, intestinal mucosal histology was interpreted to be consistent with local cell-mediated changes, which were highly reminiscent of the spectrum of changes seen in gluten sensitivity (Sullivan et al 1991).

Importantly, follow-up study of this cohort at 1 month, following intense in-hospital rehabilitation and antibiotic therapy, revealed no alteration in mucosal architecture, while in some it deteriorated, as had also been noted previously in "sprue" patients (Sheehy et al 1962). Moreover, the jejunal mucosal morphology remained unchanged at a year after discharge, when these individuals had returned to their natural habitat (Sullivan et al 1992). This experience again underlines the view that treatment can improve symptoms, and perhaps nutritional status, but is unlikely ever to improve mucosal morphology, since the antigenic exposure remains the same. One of the problems relating to all similar studies is that the state of the intestinal mucosa, before clinical illness began, has never been adequately documented in the patients studied. Treatment invariably returns the patient to the pre-existing clinical state: clearly, only removal to a more sanitized environment will reduce the risk of further nutritional impairment, recurrent infection and long-term malabsorption. Apart from its clinical effects on the patients, the disease importantly has a devastating impact on the economic fitness and performance of the society and country of the affected individual.

## Clinical features

These are varied and may be related to the duration of the disease. Initially, there is fatigue, anorexia, diarrhea, abdominal distention and some weight loss. If the disorder continues, weight loss becomes severe and eventually the continued malabsorption of vitamins, especially folic acid, results in megaloblastic anemia. Anorexia and weight loss are caused partly by vitamin deficiency (Klipstein & Corcino 1977).

In the visitor to the tropics the disease is usually heralded by an explosive episode of watery, non-bloody diarrhea, often with malaise, fever and weakness. After a week or so, the diarrhea may become chronic. There is intolerance of milk. Disease contracted by the visitor may persist for up to 20 years after return to temperate climates. Furthermore, it may commence for the first time many years after leaving the tropics (Mollin & Booth 1970). Exacerbations in expatriates would be similar to a gluten challenge, that is, due to antigenic recall by mucosal T-cells in response to infection previously encountered abroad.

Features on examination include abdominal distention, hyperpigmentation, especially on the back of the hands, edema, glossitis and stomatitis. The diagnosis depends upon a history of appropriate travel, the demonstration of malabsorption of fat, xylose and vitamin $B_{12}$, and the response to broad-spectrum antibiotics.

Table 14.7 shows some of the abnormalities present in several series of patients with tropical sprue in different areas of the world. Generally, there is malabsorption of more than one substance, but the effect is variable (Jeejeebhoy et al 1966). When the disorder occurs in individuals who have returned from a short visit to the tropics, giardiasis needs to be excluded (Klipstein 1981).

## Diagnosis

### *Radiology*

While abnormalities may be demonstrable, radiology is used to exclude a structural cause for malabsorption. The findings in tropical sprue are identical to those in celiac disease.

### *Tests of absorption*

Steatorrhea is not always present. It may be caused by secondary abnormalities of the absorptive cell, as in celiac disease, or by deconjugation of conjugated bile acids by bacteria (Banwell & Gorbach 1969). Malabsorption of xylose is extremely common; mucosal disaccharidase activity is reduced but may improve with treatment. Malabsorption of vitamin $B_{12}$ is common and is not corrected by the administration of intrinsic factor. In most cases, bacterial proliferation is the precipitant of the malabsorption with some resolution provided by broad-spectrum antibiotics.

### *Folic acid malabsorption*

Malabsorption of a pharmacological dose of pteroylmonoglutamate is common, whereas a physiological dose is better absorbed (Klipstein 1970). The polyglutamate is commonly malabsorbed (p. 362) and, since it forms the major component of dietary folate, folate deficiency results. Folate deficiency which is not due to poor dietary intake can occur in patients with normal absorption of physiological doses of folic acid (Hoffbrand et al 1969). Furthermore, patients receiving a hospital diet may show a favorable hematological response only when treated with a physiological dose of folic acid, implying that dietary folate is not available for absorption (Klipstein 1970).

### *Hematological abnormalities*

Malabsorption of vitamin $B_{12}$ and polyglutamate usually leads to deficiency of one or both of these vitamins and megaloblastic anemia occurs in about two-thirds of cases. The anemia is invariably due to folate deficiency, but vitamin $B_{12}$ deficiency is seen in those with long-standing disease: folate deficiency occurs earlier because tissue stores are exhausted within 2–3 months of onset (Klipstein 1970).

### *Hypoalbuminemia and edema* (Klipstein 1970)

This occurs in about 25% of cases. Several factors are responsible: poor diet, malabsorption of amino acids, protein loss from the bowel and reduced synthesis of albumin.

### *Other deficiencies*

Low serum calcium concentrations may occur in about

**Table 14.7** Frequent abnormalities in patients with tropical sprue (figures amalgamated from several series listed by Klipstein 1970)

| Location | Number of subjects | Megaloblastic anemia (%) | Malabsorption (%) | | | Abnormal jejunal morphology (%) |
|---|---|---|---|---|---|---|
| | | | Fat | Xylose | $B_{12}$ | |
| Northern and western India | 158 | 27 | 71 | 28 | 21 | 79 |
| Southern India | 300 | 64 | 97 | 90 | 50 | 100 |
| Puerto Rico | 189 | 24 | 94 | 91 | 15 | 98 |
| New York City* | 40 | 88 | 85 | 100 | 96 | 97 |

* Expatriates from the West Indies

half the patients, due to malabsorption and deficiency of vitamin D. Signs of deficiency of B vitamins are seen and there may be iron deficiency, although this may be exacerbated by other factors, including hookworm infestation. Deficiency of vitamin K may also occur. When diarrhea is severe, there is an increased loss of fluid and electrolytes in the stool, with resultant dehydration, hyponatremia and hypokalemia.

### Differential diagnosis

Enteric bacterial pathogens and parasites must be excluded, including *Yersinia, Giardia intestinalis, Strongyloides stercoralis, coccidia* and *Isospora*. Thereafter, deficiency of folate, vitamin $B_{12}$, albumin and calcium, and the presence of macrocytic anemia, should be sought. Malabsorption is established by xylose and vitamin $B_{12}$ absorption tests and a 3-day stool collection for daily fecal fat output. Radiology is used to exclude other disorders. Jejunal biopsy establishes the presence of morphological abnormalities and will exclude other small bowel disorders. Confirmation of the diagnosis rests with a response, within 2 weeks, to folic acid and tetracycline.

### Treatment

In general, this consists of correcting nutritional deficiencies and prescription of long-term antibiotics.

#### *Fluid and electrolytes*

The correction of abnormalities is extremely important in the severely ill patient and a great reduction in mortality is effected by early treatment (Baker & Mathan 1970).

#### *Vitamin $B_{12}$ and folic acid*

Vitamin $B_{12}$ given intramuscularly and folic acid given orally in a dosage of 5 mg four times a day will bring about a hematological response. Often, gastrointestinal symptoms improve and weight gain commences.

#### *Antibiotics*

Tetracycline or oxytetracycline 1 g/day for 1 month and 500 mg/day for 5 months is the preferred treatment (Guerra et al 1965); poorly absorbed sulfonamides are also effective (Maldonado et al 1969). Treatment usually results in an improvement in absorption and intestinal histology, although some degree of steatorrhea may persist. Antibiotics are said to produce a more rapid response in the jejunal mucosa than folic acid (England 1968). In expatriates Klipstein (1981) recommends oral folic acid 5 mg per day and tetracycline 250 mg four times a day for several months or until evidence is obtained for normalization of intestinal function.

## THE INTESTINAL IMMUNE SYSTEM

The intestinal tract provides a large surface for the entry of many substances or agents capable of sensitizing the host to result in local or systemic disease (Marsh & Ensari 1994). Various factors confer protection at the mucosal surface (Udall & Walker 1987), such as nonimmune secretions (gastric acid, mucus, lactoferrin, lysozyme), a normal resident microflora, other factors such as peristalsis and motility and specific immune mechanisms subserved by B-cells (IgA secretion) (Brandtzaeg et al 1985), T-cells (cytolysis, memory) and other effector mechanisms (MacDermott & Elson 1991).

Mucosal defense, however, is not only concerned with protective events operative at the mucosal surface or within the intestinal lumen. Cells located both within epithelium and lamina propria are concerned with the control and elaboration of antibody and also fulfil cell-mediated activities against foreign antigen or allergens, in association and through the recruitment of ancillary cells such as neutrophils, mast cells and basophils (Mowat 1987). Finally the Kupffer cells (comprising 30% of total hepatic mass) provide a further hepatobiliary tier of defense which sequesters antigens present in portal venous blood and helps to return antigen–antibody complexes from the circulation to the intestinal lumen.

### The local immune system

This comprises T-lymphocytes diffusely distributed throughout epithelium and lamina propria and localized within the organized milieu of mesenteric lymph nodes and Peyer's patches. In addition, there is a major contribution by B-lymphocytes and their terminally formed cell elements, the immunoglobulin-secreting plasma cells. Dendritic (antigen-presenting) cells also play an important role in controlling local immune responses (Bland & Kambarage 1991) and influencing the activation and cell–cell interactions between T-cells or T- and B-lymphocytes. Other effector agents comprise cells (such as eosinophils, mast cells, neutrophils) whose secretions may amplify the immune response and cause tissue damage, while a wide and very complex system of cell surface "addressins" provides the molecular basis for regulating cell traffic within the intestinal tissues and focusing responses to the site of entry of foreign material.

#### *The receptor system*

Much of our information concerning the function and integration of the local intestinal immune system is derived from experimental work in laboratory animals. Peyer's patches (Carlson & Owen 1987) are the major site for receipt of antigen via the specialized M ("membrane") cells within their follicle-associated epithelium. M cells transfer antigen to the subjacent dome area (Fig. 14.12) which leads to antigen priming for subsequent T- or B-cell responses. The dome regions comprise diffuse T-dependent areas and organized primary and secondary follicles which represent B-cell territory. The patches are a major source of the predominant intestinal secretory IgA through B-cells that are influenced by specific T-cells (Elson 1985). These primed B-cells, through gene rearrangements, emigrate via local lymphatics to mesenteric lymph nodes, where further development and expansion occur. Having first circulated, they then return to the lamina propria where they mature into plasma cells elaborating antibody to the original antigen encountered via follicle-associated epithelium (Fig. 14.13). Presumably T-cells (and T immunoblasts) follow a similar priming/expansion/recirculatory pathway (Fig. 14.8), although this is less well documented.

*The effector system*

This comprises the local immunoglobulin secretory system. IgA is invariably secreted as dimers, or higher polymers, that are bound by a J piece, a molecule also synthesized by plasma cells (Underdown & Schiff 1986).

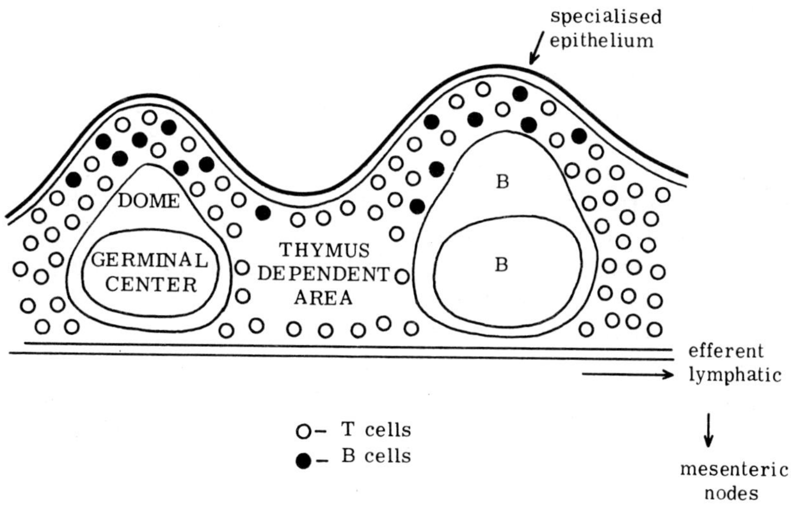


**Fig. 14.12** The structure of Peyer's patch.

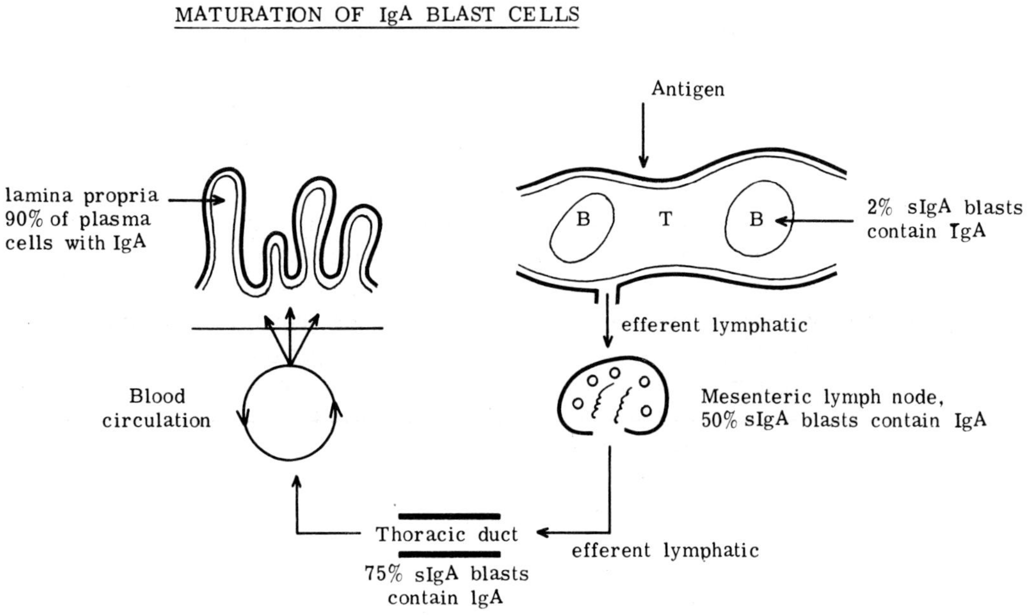


**Fig. 14.13** The maturation and circulation of IgA cells.

The secretory form of IgA is then transported to the mucosal surface via epithelium and the polyclonal receptor, "secretory component". Secretory IgA provides various surface protective functions, including neutralization of viruses, toxins and enzymes, interference with bacterial adherence, opsonization of bacteria, reduction of antigen penetration through epithelium and enhancement of other antibacterial substances like lactoperoxidase and lactoferrin.

While most IgA is destined for the mucosal surface, about 10% of circulating (polymeric) IgA is intestinally derived, the remainder (monomeric) arising from the bone marrow. Secretory component, unlike in many animals, is not expressed on human hepatic sinusoidal cell membranes and transport of polymeric IgA into bile is presumably dependent on secretory component expression by biliary epithelial cells. Serum levels of polymeric IgA are known to rise in patients with chronic liver disease.

Other specific effectors are the intraepithelial lymphocytes (Marsh 1985) and additional lymphocyte populations within the lamina propria. The latter comprise CD4 ("helper") cells (Elson 1985) that mediate immune cellular events via MHC Class 2-expressing cells (other T-lymphocytes, B-cells, macrophages). Despite extensive investigation, convincing roles for IEL have yet to be assigned: these are an extensively heterogeneous set of cells derived both from thymic and nonthymic (bone marrow) sources. The role of T-cell receptor expression ($\alpha\beta$ or $\gamma\delta$) (Viney et al 1990) is not yet clarified. The role of effector T-cells in the intestinal mucosa awaits further clarification.

## IMMUNODEFICIENCY SYNDROMES

The consequence most commonly encountered in any patient with a defect in the intestinal immune system is infection or infestation. There are many conditions within this category, most of which are either excessively rare and hence unlikely to be encountered by the average physician during a working lifetime or will require the help of a regional center specifically devoted to the diagnosis and aftercare of such individuals. Although recent and very detailed accounts are available for reference (Ross 1987), conditions of some practical importance are listed (Table 14.8) and briefly described below.

### Common variable immune deficiency (common variable hypogammaglobulinemia)

*Etiology*

This is unknown, but results in panhypogammaglobulinemia and recurrent infections, particularly of chest and intestinal tract.

*Pathology*

The basic defects are heterogeneous and include absence of plasma cell precursors, failure of B-cells to mature and absence of plasma cells within the lamina propria or failure of synthesis of immunoglobulin or its release. Overactive "suppressor" T-cells have also been involved in some cases, their removal allowing B-cells to function in an apparently normal fashion: other patients demonstrate lymphopenia. Common variable hypogammaglobulinemia is characterized by low levels of IgG (level less than 200 mg/100 ml) and undetectable levels of M and A. Disease is usually thought to have started from the onset of clinical symptoms which usually present in adult life. However, this leaves open the question as to when the defect started or for how long it may have lain dormant. In some instances the condition is familial.

Nodular lymphoid hyperplasia is a pathological variant seen in 20–50% of patients with common variable hypogammaglobulinemia. The nodules comprise hypertrophied lymphoid tissue, particularly in the small bowel mucosa, but are also seen in colon and stomach (Fig. 14.14). These nodules are also seen in patients with selective IgA deficiency, suggesting they may be uncontrolled hyperplasias of B-cells as a result, possibly, of bacterial stimuli within the lumen. Despite claims and counterclaims, it is likely that nodular lymphoid hyperplasia is not especially associated with chronic giardiasis.

*Clinical features*

A childhood form normally occurs between ages 2–16 and thus may include unrecognized cases of X-linked agammaglobulinemia or Bruton's disease. The median age of onset is 5 in children, and 30 in adults. Sinopulmonary infections are due to pneumococci and *H. influenzae* while mycoplasmas may cause urinary

**Table 14.8** Immunodeficiency and allied syndromes

| | |
|---|---|
| 1. *Antibody (B cell) defects* | 3. *T and B cell defects* |
| Common variable immune deficiency (CVID) | Severe combined immune deficiency (SCID) |
| X-linked agammaglobulinemia (Bruton) | Ataxia-telangiectasia |
| Selective IgA deficiency | Wiskott–Aldrich syndrome |
| 2. *T cell defects* | 4. *Miscellaneous disorders* |
| Thymic aplasia (DiGeorge) | Chronic granulomatous |
| Mucocutaneous candidiasis | Deficiency of complement proteins |
| | Secondary immunodeficiencies |

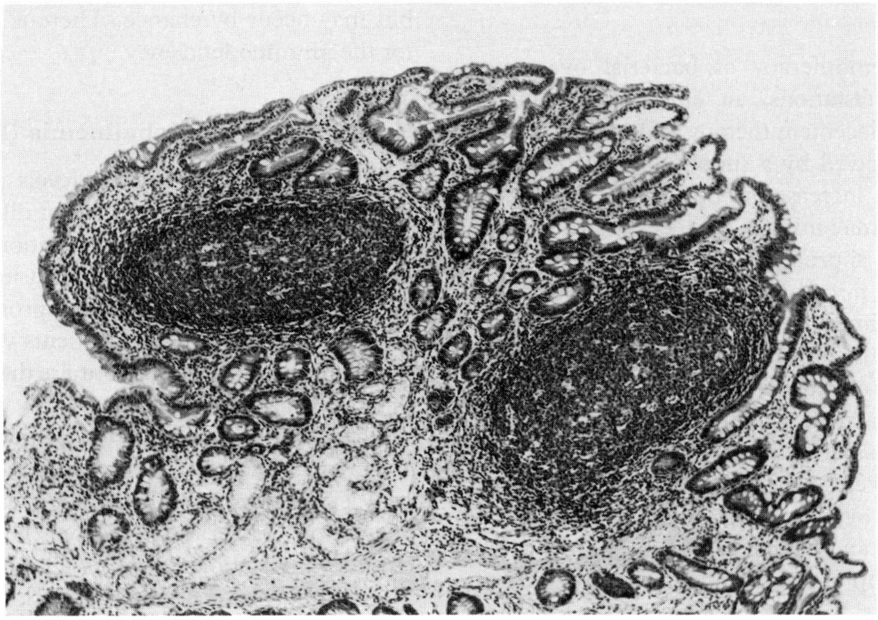

**Fig. 14.14** Nodular lymphoid hyperplasia of the small intestine. The lymphoid follicles lie within the mucosa and produce a surface nodule (hematoxylin and eosin, ×75).

infection and joint problems: intestinal infections are seen in 30–65% of patients. The patient will present with multiple, recurrent infections, diarrhea or a sprue-like malabsorption syndrome. In children, there may be growth deficiency and infantilism.

*Diagnosis*

The history of recurrent infections and the finding of low or absent circulating immunoglobulin concentrations will point to the diagnosis. In the context of diarrhea or malabsorption, a broader based investigative schema will be necessary, but should include estimation of serum immunoglobulins as well as an assessment of nutritional deficiency and the presence of specific deficits, like iron, calcium or vitamin D. Once the cause is known, a detailed and intensive search for intestinal pathogens will be undertaken.

Bacterial overgrowth with aerobic and anaerobic (*Bacteroides*, lactobacillus and *Clostridia* spp.) organisms does occur but the $^{14}$C-glycocholate breath test may occasionally be normal (Ament et al 1973). In vitro, bile acid deconjugation has been demonstrated and hence cholestyramine may have some practical use in the control of diarrhea (Gleich & Hofmann 1971). Other sporadic infections may occur and *Campylobacter* diarrhea may last for several weeks (Melamed et al 1983).

The major problem involves chronic giardiasis and its control. It is likely that T- and B-cell defects contribute in common variable hypogammaglobulinemia patients who suffer with chronic giardiasis (Ross 1987, Webster 1980). This is based on the view that in normal individuals, evidence of an immune response to this parasite has been demonstrated by (i) an increase in intraepithelial lymphocytes, (ii) an increase in mucosal plasma cells, (iii) the production of local and circulating antibodies, (iv) a requirement for competent T ($CD4^+$) cells, and (v) prompt and spontaneous resolution within 1–4 weeks. Clearly, both arms of the immune system (T- and B-cells) are necessary for adequate protection and resolution of infection with *Giardia trophozoites*. Other common protozoal infections are cryptosporidiosis and coccidiosis (*Isospora belli*) which may, occasionally, be prolonged and life-threatening. Diagnosis is difficult because the organism may not be seen in biopsy material, or in feces, unless special techniques are employed for their identification (Brandborg et al 1970, Sloper et al 1982).

The variable forms of malabsorption seen in common variable hypogammaglobulinemia, accompanied by equally variable changes in proximal jejunal mucosal morphology, have given rise to the term "hypogammaglobulinemic sprue". Although such cases rarely may coexist with tropical sprue (Ross & Mathan 1981) or gluten sensitivity (Webster et al 1981), the basis for the malabsorption is likely to be due to giardiasis, bacterial overgrowth or undiagnosed coccidiosis infestation. Inflammatory bowel disease is a recently documented problem (Hermaszewski & Webster 1993). Nongranulomatous jejunoileitis and protein-losing enteropathy are also occasionally encountered (Ament & Ochs 1973). Cholelithiasis, either reflecting ileal mucosal involvement or the chronic effects of bile acid deconjugation secondary to bacterial overgrowth, is seen in approximately 30% of patients in some series (Heremans et al 1976).

*Treatment*

This comprises chemotherapy of bacterial overgrowth and/or protozoal infestations, an effective schedule of immunoglobulin replacement therapy and adequate nutritional repletion, followed by a supply of calories to promote growth and an increase in body weight: short-term parenteral nutrition may initially be necessary to rehabilitate the patient. This approach requires good co-operation between clinician, microbiologist, immunologist and dietitian. Such a regimen, pursued aggressively, will considerably improve the clinical status, nutritional competence and well-being of such patients.

There is no treatment for nodular lymphoid hyperplasia, which is not considered to be a pregmalignant condition. There is, however, an increased risk for neoplasia in common variable hypogammaglobulinemia including intestinal lymphoma and gastric carcinoma (Spector et al 1978, Scientific Group on Immunodeficiency 1983).

Specific treatments for giardiasis are given elsewhere (p. 577) but may have to be prolonged. *Campylobacter jejuni* infection is treated with erythromycin 500 mg four times daily and this may have to be continued for several weeks. Eradication may still be difficult, so it is essential that good nutrition and adequate attention to immunoglobulin replacement therapy are secured: antibiotics alone will achieve little success.

## Selective IgA deficiency

This is defined by a concentration of less than 1 mg/100 ml serum and has an estimated prevalence of 1 in 700 (Holt et al 1977). Like its more global counterpart, common variable hypogammaglobulinemia, selective IgA deficiency is probably a heterogeneous collection of defects, including T-cell subset deficiency to varying failures of development of pre-B-cells to mature IgA-secreting plasma cells. Its frequent occurrence in gluten sensitivity may thus reflect a more profound disturbance in T-cell function, while in those who are asymptomatic, the deficiency may be due to a heavy chain gene malexpression or some other regulatory/environmental factor, as with drug-induced IgA deficiency due to antiepilepsy therapy.

In the majority of patients, there is no "disease complex" or symptomatology. Small intestinal structure is normal, although circulating high-titer antibodies to food are present in serum. Secretory IgM probably compensates and accounts for the increased population of IgM-secreting plasma cells in the lamina propria. It should be noted that anti-IgA antibodies may give rise to anaphylactic reactions in such individuals during the administration of plasma or blood. Nodular lymphoid hyperplasia may be seen, but in general giardiasis is not a particular complication. Various other "associations" have been documented, but may occur by chance. There is no specific treatment for the immunodeficiency.

## X-linked agammaglobulinemia (Bruton)

There are undetectable levels of all circulating immunoglobulins and a failure of differentiation of pre-B-cells to B-cells. The presentation is with recurrent episodes of upper respiratory tract infections, otitis media or meningitis. Gastrointestinal problems are much less common or severe than in patients with common variable hypogammaglobulinemia, but are diagnosed and managed as in these latter patients.

The majority of infections are viral, with the enterovirus group particularly troublesome (Ross 1987). Echovirus may cause myositis, ligneous edema of the legs and meningitis. Bacterial overgrowth has been recorded and chronic infestations with *Giardia*, *Campylobacter* and rotavirus may be encountered: a Whipple's-type syndrome has also been recorded. Most have responded to appropriate antibiotic therapy (Ament et al 1973, Rhee et al 1975, Saulsbury et al 1980, Melamed et al 1983). Patients may be at risk from either leukemia or generalized lymphoma (Kirkpatrick 1976, Hermaszewski & Webster 1993).

## T-cell-mediated defects

These are more rare than the antibody deficiency syndromes described above. They also tend to occur in young infants and hence are less well portrayed in pathologic terms. There may be an associated defect in B-cell maturation with hypogammaglobulinemia, otherwise known as severe combined immune deficiency.

## Thymic hypoplasia

A defect in the development of the embryonic third and fourth branchial arches leads to a congenital absence of the thymus and parathyroid glands, congenital heart disease and loss of the right side of the aortic arch. While heart failure and tetany (due to hypoparathyroidism) are the common presenting features, there may also be severe oroesophageal and gastrointestinal candidiasis, diarrhea and malabsorption: the esophagus may be atretic. Surprisingly there is no lack of immunoglobulins although their production is T-cell dependent. Survival occurs only in those with a partial thymic deficiency.

## Severe combined immune deficiency

The features of this comprise a severe deficit of both T- and/or B-cell systems associated with diarrhea, malabsorption and mucocutaneous candidiasis. Jejunal morphology is often abnormal and contains PAS-positive macrophages. Bone marrow transplantation is now the treatment of choice (Horowitz et al 1974, Stephan et al 1993).

### Wiskott–Aldrich syndrome

These patients present soon after birth with eczema, thrombocytopenia and recurrent infections. Inherited as an X-linked recessive trait, it comprises elevated IgE levels with allergic phenomena, failure of the T-cell system, increased catabolism of immunoglobulins, with bloody diarrhea or protein-losing enteropathy. The latter may reflect acute allergic reactions to environmental proteins. Treatment is most effectively accomplished by bone marrow transplantation (Huntley & Dees 1957, Ament et al 1973, Gryboski & Walker 1983).

## OTHER MISCELLANEOUS DISORDERS

### Chronic granulomatous disease

Resulting from a defect in the intracellular killing of phagocytosed pathogens by neutrophils and monocytes, the diagnosis is made by a failure of these cells to reduce the dye nitroblue tetrazolium. Other tests for intracellular killing capacity are also available. The usual presentation is in infancy with recurrent infections, abscesses and lymphadenopathy. There may be widespread (granulomatous) involvement of the gastrointestinal tract with recurrent oral ulceration, gastric outlet obstruction and Crohn's-like inflammatory disease of small and large bowel, with perianal involvement. This granulomatous reaction is caused by the ability of catalase-negative organisms such as staphylococci and *Serratia marcescens* to survive within the defective tissue macrophages. Bone marrow transplantation is essential before ineradicable fungal infection and tissue destruction renders this treatment option useless (Ament & Ochs 1973).

### $C_1$-esterase deficiency

This is the only defect in complement metabolism which affects the gastrointestinal tract. Deficiency of $C_1$-esterase is inherited as an autosomal dominant, most commonly causing low levels and more rarely, a functionless molecule (Frank 1982). It may also be secondarily acquired by patients with lymphoid malignancy, paraproteinemias and autoimmune diseases, due to consumption of the enzyme by activation by autoantibody, a cryoglobulin or other form of paraprotein (Gelfand et al 1979) or by antigen–antibody complexes giving angioedema as part of a more generalized lupus-type syndrome (Sissons et al 1974).

Affected patients suffer recurring attacks of localized swellings of face, lips, tongue and pharynx, this latter being a potentially life-threatening event. Alternatively, gastrointestinal symptoms occur, comprising recurrent attacks of colicky abdominal pain, vomiting or watery diarrhea. An edematous segment of bowel may induce intussusception.

Attacks are precipitated by oral trauma, for example at the dentist, exercise or menstruation. Pregnancy seems to lead to a temporary respite. The absence of $C_1$-esterase is determined in the laboratory. Treatment is with low-dose danazole (200 mg daily) or stanozolol (5 mg biweekly) which is effective in reducing attacks (Warin et al 1980).

### Secondary immunodeficiencies

Intestinal lymphangiectasia, whether primary (p. 349) or secondary, may lead to a generalized reduction in circulating immunoglobulin concentrations, sometimes with a depressed lymphocyte count. However, these patients do not usually have a coexisting reduction in serum albumin concentration, which helps to distinguish them from "hypogammaglobulinemic sprue". Further investigations involve demonstrating either normal recall to standard B-cell antigens (tetanus toxoid or pneumococcal polysaccharide) or showing a normal complement of Ig-secreting plasma cells in intestinal mucosa, for example by rectal biopsy. None of these patients is predisposed to recurrent bacterial, fungal or protozoal infection.

There is a growing population of individuals which is therapeutically immunosuppressed, either as a result of transplantation surgery (kidney, heart, lungs, bone marrow, etc), or from long-term chemotherapy for lymphoma, myeloproliferative disease and other malignancies and for collagen-vascular diseases. Such patients are especially predisposed to gastrointestinal infections like candidiasis and particularly cytomegalovirus, the latter being capable of mimicking a wide range of disorders from mouth to rectum (Goodgame 1993). These patients may, from time to time, present to a general physician, who must therefore be aware of the growing numbers of immunocompromised individuals that now survive for prolonged periods in the population.

Since these individuals may have variable defects of B- and T-cell function, any type of opportunistic infection may be seen, while chronic candidiasis of mouth, pharynx or esophagus should always raise the possibility of an acquired type of immunodeficiency.

Note should also be made of "super-infection" by parasites, especially *Strongyloides stercoralis* (Boyd & Bachman 1982) (p. 583). In immunocompromised hosts, the larvae develop into filariform species which invade the intestinal wall leading to an endless cycle of local reinfection and septicemia. Thus, in the presence of an unexplained acute gastrointestinal episode of vomiting, abdominal pain or diarrhea in such patients, an active search for worm larvae in the stools should be made (Lima & Delgado 1961).

### Graft-versus-host disease

This is common when bone marrow is transplanted into patients with cellular immunodeficiency or into patients who are irradiated and receive chemotherapy to prevent graft rejection. Donor T-cells are then responsible for tissue damage which is mediated by cytokines (Rowe et al 1994).

The condition is separated into acute and chronic forms. The acute form is graded histologically and clinically into four grades according to the involvement of skin, liver and gastrointestinal tract. The grading has prognostic significance in that grade 1 has a long-term survival of 88% compared to 45% for grades 2–4. The chronic form is graded on the basis of the overall extent of this disease for it involves multiple organs. Intestinal and hepatic graft-versus-host disease is discussed further on p. 1167, Chapter 46.

## AIDS-RELATED MALABSORPTION (see p. 610)

## ADVERSE REACTIONS TO FOOD

### Etiological mechanisms

There is nothing so uncertain, confused or emotive as the subject of food allergy and of adverse reactions to food. While some of the relevant anecdotes are fairly impressive, the underlying science and understanding of the pathophysiology of these conditions is still very weak, while the absence of universally acceptable diagnostic criteria, as well as diagnostic tests, creates an air of uncertainty and of distrust between doctors and the public. Matters have not been made any better by attempts to relate the "chronic fatigue syndrome" and other ill-understood clinical entities to food-induced allergic mechanisms.

It is recognized, however, that not all adverse food reactions are the result of immune-mediated mechanisms (Table 14.9). Some reactions may be due to nonspecific histamine release or to the unpleasant side-effects of food additives, such as sodium metabisulfite, sodium benzoate or tartrazine dyes. Other reactions may be biochemical, due to lactase, trehalase or other mucosal enzyme deficiencies.

**Table 14.9** Nonallergic causes of food intolerances

| | |
|---|---|
| *Chemical* | *Toxins* |
| Caffeine | Ethanol |
| Salicylates | Quinine |
| Tartrazine dyes | Fava beans |
| Sodium metabisulfite | Aflatoxins |
| Monosodium glutamate | Pesticides (cholinesterase inhibitors) |
| Nitrites, nitrates | |
| Tyramine | |
| Hexachlorobenzene | |
| *Irritants* | *Psychological* |
| Onions | Phobias |
| Phenylethylamine | Anxiety state |
| Spices | Hysterical |
| Curries | Food fads |

### Prevalence

It is difficult to be certain of the numerical extent of true allergic food reactions: figures given by various authors often reflect particular interests and are meaningless for constructing useful generalizations. It is clear that these syndromes affect youngsters far more than adults and in this regard, it is noteworthy that experimentally induced intestinal anaphylaxis can only be induced in relatively young, as opposed to adult, animals. What is less certain is whether any particular genetic background predisposes to food allergic disease and, more importantly, whether and to what extent any alterations in intestinal permeability are involved in initiating or perpetuating the state of sensitization.

### Diagnosis

True food allergies are much more common in young children than adults, by far the commonest offenders being milk, eggs, nuts and fish. The symptoms most commonly attributed to food allergic reactions are gastrointestinal, cutaneous and respiratory. The reactions should be reproducible on challenge and in order to obtain firm evidence for this, challenges should be performed with a defined protocol, on a strictly double-blind basis. If challenges cannot be performed in this manner, there is little hope of producing a firm, reliable diagnosis. Clearly, appropriate clinical arrangements need to be at hand in order to achieve this ideal. This implies the presence of dedicated centers and the need for staff who are trained in this kind of work and who can perform individual challenges in the appropriate manner, without hurry or mistakes. Detection of the offending agent will therefore require much time and often repeated sessions, unless the patient has already made some incisive observations, and this rarely happens. Once the offending agent is identified, an appropriate diet should be given.

### Pathology and molecular basis

Although much has been written about "intestinal permeability" and the entry of antigens to the mucosa, it is equally accepted that under normal physiologic conditions sufficient undigested antigen gains access to the mucosa to stimulate antibodies (IgE/$IgG_4$) which may either arm mast cells for subsequent discharge once these antibodies are bridged by specific allergen or cause other forms of damage (?antigen–antibody complex mediated) following repeated ingestion of the offending, sensitizing antigen.

Some intestinal lesions associated with milk, egg, soya and other sensitivities resemble the spectrum of presumptive T-cell-mediated lesions which have now been recognized in gluten sensitivity, giardiasis and the tropical diarrhea malabsorption syndrome (Figs 14.2 and 14.11). This suggests that there is a range of immunological reactions to a variety of food antigens which, in some individuals, may be mixed.

Another difficulty with the literature pertaining to human studies is the lack of a well-defined molecular approach to the problem. Of the most frequent offenders (milk, eggs and fish) the sequences of their major constituent proteins are now known, such as α-lactalbumin, β-lactoglobulin and casein. One of the most interesting approaches to this area has been the delineation of the epitopes of the M allergen of cod muscle protein (Aas 1966). It may be relevant to the pathophysiology of all these conditions that the relative molecular mass of these proteins is 10–20 000 kDa, similar to that for gluten sensitivity.

## Cow's milk protein intolerance

*Etiological factors*

The most widely and intensively researched syndrome has been cow's milk protein intolerance. The almost universal decrease in breastfeeding in most developed countries has made this reaction an important cause of infant morbidity (Salvilahti 1981) with an incidence of about 2% (Jakobsson & Lindberg 1979). Since most infants develop antibodies to milk proteins without adverse effect, diagnosis is dependent on the clinical response to cow's milk ingestion or challenge. Of those affected 80–90% will react within the first few months of life (Hill et al 1984). Symptoms due to lactose intolerance should be excluded by giving breast milk which has a high content of lactose.

The role of concurrent infection is unclear, since all neonates and young children are subject to these as they slowly mature and respond to environmental microbial challenge. Some clinicians argue that milk allergy is precipitated by a specific infective event, whereas others indicate that removal of cow's milk from the feed permits resolution of infection and diarrhea. However, this train of events is reminiscent of latent gluten sensitivity and tropical enteropathies, both of which may become clinically apparent as a result of acute infection: thus, in terms of individuals predestined to develop intestinal cell-mediated immune responses, recurrent episodes of diarrhea may awaken a latent susceptibility and result in the onset of clinical symptoms. Thus, where milk sensitivity appears to follow an acute gastrointestinal illness, its diagnosis is only valid after exclusion of persistent bacterial gastroenteritis, giardiasis or secondary lactase deficiency by intestinal biopsy and enzyme assay (Hill et al 1984).

*Clinical features*

There is acute diarrhea, colic, vomiting, acidosis and dehydration, which may simulate an infective entity in young infants, or chronic diarrhea with vomiting and failure to thrive in older infants. These may also be associated with fecal blood loss, failure of weight gain, abdominal protuberance and hypotonia.

In a computerized analysis of symptoms developing after application of a strict challenge protocol, Hill and colleagues (1984) divided their 100 patients into three cohorts.

1. Twenty-six infants reacted within 45 min of challenge. A large proportion developed circumoral or other cutaneous eruptions, while 1 in 3 developed respiratory symptoms like wheezing, coughing or rhinitis. Rarely stridor occurred. The mean age of this group of infants was 15 months and all had positive skin reactions to cow's milk proteins.
2. Fifty-seven patients (mean age 12 months) developed symptoms within 20 h of challenge which were largely confined to the gastrointestinal tract, with skin pallor, vomiting and diarrhea. Review of these individuals revealed evidence of instability and failure to thrive and their skin reactivity was negligible.
3. The remaining 17 patients developed symptoms >20 h after challenge, of which >50% developed diarrhea or respiratory symptoms. Eczema was also more common to this reactive group, whose mean age was 30 months. Patients with eczema had positive skin tests.

***Immunopathogenesis.*** Although mechanisms for reactivity in each of the three groups identified were not addressed in this study, it seems likely that the group 1 response which occurred within an hour of challenges was due to IgE-mediated allergic sensitization, as has been noted by previous investigators (Goldman et al 1963, Dannaeus & Johansson 1979, Hill et al 1979, Savilahti 1981).

In contrast, in group 2 reaginic antibody levels are low or absent (Dannaeus et al 1977, 1978, Hill et al 1979). This suggests that the slower, evolving reactions are due to other mechanisms and are probably associated with the cellular and architectural changes characteristic of local T-cell-mediated reactivity (Kuitenen et al 1973, Iyngkaran & Yadav 1987). These could also lie dormant and be awakened by infection, the infective process being associated with enterocyte damage, reductions in membrane hydrolase activity and involvement of other parts of the intestine beyond that damaged directly by the milk protein sensitivity.

Clearly there is a possible analogy to latent gluten sensitivity (Fig. 14.1) and the paradox (Fig. 14.11) of differentiating latent "tropical enteropathy" from clinically apparent "tropical sprue". In relationship to cow's milk protein intolerance, the possibility of a *latent* infiltrative or flat lesion existing before the acute event (?infection) brought the child to hospital cannot be excluded. In this regard it is noteworthy that Walker-Smith (1988) has suggested the occurrence of a primary (immunologic) and secondary (postinfectious/mucosal damage) forms of cow's milk protein intolerance. The other possibility is that the infective insult merely awakened a pre-existing though latent condition. After all, if several children with lifelong gluten sensitivity can escape detection in early life because their lesion remains latent, why not those with cow's milk hypersensitivity as well? Indeed, the symptomatic children may merely represent the small tip of yet another intestinal hypersensitivity iceberg induced by milk protein.

The evidence for complement activation (Yadav & Iyngkaran 1981) and consumption is least convincing and not well represented in the literature regarding cow's milk allergy. Such a mechanism could, however, underlie the morbilliform and eczematous skin reactions observed in reactions of intermediate/late timing (groups 2 and 3 above).

### *Diagnosis*

The diagnosis cannot be effected by any single test, but only by reproducible responses to milk challenge under suitably controlled conditions, as indicated by the studies of Goldman and colleagues (1963) or Davidson and colleagues (1976).

The problems with these criteria include reluctance to submit children to more than one potentially dangerous challenge, the fact that some children take more than 48 h to relapse and that intercurrent illnesses can completely mimic challenge symptoms.

The exclusion of common nonimmune causes of gastrointestinal milk intolerance is very important and this can be done by following the protocol of Davidson et al (1976). Stool microscopy, culture and electronmicroscopy exclude most infectious causes. The initial small bowel biopsy further excludes giardiasis and sucrase-isomaltase deficiency and provides a basis for interpreting postchallenge mucosal changes. Because lactose intolerance, the commonest cause of milk intolerance, can be secondary to cow's milk protein intolerance as well as many other conditions, it may be difficult to distinguish from cow's milk protein intolerance. The distinction can be made at the time of milk challenge by a prior lactose tolerance test, using the breath hydrogen test. Serial small intestinal biopsies at initial presentation, after a clinical response to milk withdrawal and after symptomatic response to milk challenge, may be useful in excluding conditions such as gluten sensitivity, but are generally not required. The gastrointestinal mucosal response is quite variable and may remain normal even in the face of gastrointestinal symptoms (Berg et al 1979).

#### *Cow's milk challenge*

The following procedure is adopted. Following symptomatic response to milk withdrawal the child is admitted to hospital. A prechallenge small bowel biopsy is carried out to show that the mucosa has returned to normal; if so, a lactose tolerance test is performed the next day. If the child remains asymptomatic, a cow's milk challenge is performed 24 h later. The volume of milk used varies according to the severity of the child's previous symptoms. If severe, the amount of milk given should be small (0.5 ml). In most children 15 ml is a safe amount and this is doubled every half hour until a diet containing a normal volume of cow's milk for the child's weight is established or a positive response elicited. When clearcut symptoms develop within 48 h of milk challenge, repeat small bowel biopsy appears to add little to the management. However, if the response is doubtful, if there is a suspicion of an intercurrent hospital-acquired illness or if symptoms occur more than 48 h after challenge, a repeat biopsy is the only way to diagnose relapse. The failure of symptoms to reappear more than 48 h after challenge makes a diagnosis of cow's milk protein intolerance unlikely. Having established the diagnosis a further milk challenge will be required to determine the return of milk tolerance. Usually this can be delayed until the age of 2 years and should be done in hospital; a small bowel biopsy is not necessary at this time.

If access to investigative facilities are not readily available a trial of a milk-free diet is acceptable. A symptomatic response is suggestive of the diagnosis and the child should then be referred to a pediatric center for evaluation and milk challenge under controlled conditions. This differs from celiac disease, where there is never any indication for a trial of a gluten-free diet without prior intestinal biopsy.

The diagnosis of cow's milk protein-induced colitis can be confirmed by sigmoidoscopy and rectal biopsy.

True cow's milk protein intolerance is uncommon and is unfortunately overdiagnosed, leading to a great degree of parental anxiety, overuse of elimination diets and excessive expenditure on costly milk substitutes. The most misdiagnosed child is the one who presents with chronic diarrhea, but no evidence of growth disturbance. These children usually fall into the group variously labeled "toddler's diarrhea", "irritable colon syndrome of infancy" or "chronic nonspecific diarrhea" (Walker-Smith 1980). Diarrhea usually starts around 6–12 months of age and disappears by 2–3 years. The motions are sloppy, often contain undigested food and occur 4–6 times a day. Elimination diets in the majority of these children will only lead to guilt and anxiety in the mother who, despite adhering to rigid dietary restriction, will still have a child with intermittent sloppy stools who may begin to fail to grow because of the restricted diet (Lloyd-Still 1979).

In conclusion, the diagnosis of cow's milk protein intolerance depends on the demonstration of a *reproducible* response to cow's milk challenge under controlled clinical conditions and is greatly aided by the use of serial small intestinal biopsies. When in doubt, and particularly if the child is thriving, it is better to observe the child rather than restrict dietary intake.

*Management*

The majority of children with cow's milk protein intolerance can be managed using a casein hydrolysate formula. Occasionally it is necessary to use an elemental formula. Soy formula should probably be avoided as 30–50% of infants with cow's milk protein intolerance are also soy protein intolerant (Hill et al 1984). Goat's milk is not satisfactory as there is crossreactivity between some goat's milk and cow's milk proteins. Goat's milk is also grossly deficient in folic acid and if used as the major source of nutrients, can cause chronic diarrhea and growth failure. It is also extremely important to remember that all foods containing cow's milk protein must be removed from the diet.

Most children with cow's milk protein intolerance tolerate milk satisfactorily by 3 years of age, but a small number continue to have symptoms beyond this age and require continued milk restriction. When elimination diets are used in children it is vitally important that the diet is nutritionally adequate for the growing child. Elimination diets can be hazardous (David et al 1984) and it is essential that they are regularly supervised by a pediatrician and/or dietitian.

It is noteworthy that sensitivity to soy protein, which also causes cell-mediated-type mucosal lesions of the intestinal tract (Ament & Rubin 1972), is often associated with cow's milk hypersensitivity (Jakobsson & Lindberg 1979). Although it is usual for these syndromes to spontaneously revert by the age of 2 or 3 years, it is reasonable to recommend avoidance of all foods that may give rise to similar forms of short-term sensitization including gluten, fish, eggs and soya. Since these conditions recover spontaneously, they are clearly different from the lifelong, genetically determined form of gluten sensitivity: their origin may be thus related to a transient failure of the intestinal immune system to tolerize the individual to these dietary proteins (Marsh & Cummins 1993). What that defect is, and what puts it right, is still far from understood.

## RADIATION DAMAGE TO THE INTESTINAL TRACT (Yeoh & Horowitz 1987)

Radiation treatment for abdominal or pelvic malignancy often results in damage to the gastrointestinal tract, although this may not always be clinically evident. In general, fixed parts of the bowel such as terminal ileum, duodenojejunal flexure, ascending and descending colon and rectum are most prone to damage: in planning courses of radiotherapy, thought should be given to avoid excessive exposure to these areas. Other parts of bowel may become fixed following surgery through adhesions or associated pathology such as pelvic inflammatory disease.

### Prevalence

It is generally agreed that acute radiation damage (arbitrarily occurring within 3 months of treatment) characterized by diarrhea with or without abdominal pain is an inevitable consequence of therapeutic pelvic irradiation. The prevalence of chronic radiation damage is, however, uncertain and figures based on retrospective studies of patients treated for gynecological neoplasms will be skewed because of cumulated deaths due to malignancy and because the patient may be able to put up with the problem or, if symptoms develop several years after treatment, may be misinterpreted and not ascribed to a previous episode of radiation treatment.

The risk of developing obvious chronic complications (strictures, fistula, bowel perforation, severe enteritis or proctitis) depends both on total radiation dose received and daily incremental dose: thus, a minimal tolerance dose estimated to create a 5% risk at 5 years is 45 Gy for small bowel, 55 Gy for sigmoid colon and rectum for a daily incremental dose of 1.50–2.00 Gy (Roswit et al 1972) (1 Gy = 100 Rads). Addition of a further 15 and 25 Gy to each category respectively increases the 5-year risk to 50%. Other factors may compound the cumulative risk, such as the effects of previous surgery, use of chemotherapy with radiotherapy and undernutrition at the time when treatment is given (Van Nagell et al 1974). Finally, the likelihood of chronic radiation damage may be higher if acute radiation damage is more severe: alternatively the absence of an acute syndrome by no means excludes the occurrence of chronic radiation damage (Bourne et al 1983). It is also important to realize that radiation damage may present symptomatically several decades after treatment was given and this kind of past medical history must always be sought when dealing with any new case with severe intestinal damage which is initially suggestive of diffuse Crohn's disease or lymphoma.

### Pathology

That radiation directly damages the intestines, leading to clinical symptoms of anorexia, weight loss, vomiting or diarrhea and acute pathological changes or chronic strictures, was established in early studies in experimental animals (Warren & Whipple 1922, Martin & Rogers 1924) and in hospital-based series (Desjardins 1931, Jones 1939, Warren & Friedman 1942).

In acute radiation damage, the crypt stem cell is highly

vulnerable: ensuing intestinal damage is related both to the rate of absorption and cumulative dose of radiation in these highly mitotic cells (Trier & Browning 1966, Wiernik 1966). The range of lesions observed varies from moderate changes, such as focal cellular death and degeneration, to a wider effect on mucosa, with edema, villous effacement and related functional disturbances. Up to four single doses of abdominal irradiation of approximately 10 Gy weekly over 4 weeks is biologically equivalent to at least 33 daily doses of abdominal irradiation of approximately 2 Gy weekly over 6.5 weeks. There may also be mucosal denudation, leading to hemorrhage and extensive loss of fluid, with microvascular necrosis, infarction and blockage. The lamina propria is disorganized and infiltrated by neutrophils and other inflammatory cells (Fig. 14.15).

Recovery may be rapid and complete with smaller insults, although with heavier dosage regimens, damage may persist resulting in (localized) areas of true mucosal atrophy with hypoplastic crypts and variable degrees of villous flattening. Persisting damage may be severe enough to induce permanent alterations in bowel habit (Newman et al 1973, Kinsella & Bloomer 1980).

Whether structural recovery of the mucosa occurs or not during the acute stage, it is during this period that the stage is set for further long-term, chronic effects of radiation. This latter phenomenon depends on two key factors, chronic vascular endarteritis and ischemia and submucosal fibrosis.

The gross appearances of the bowel are thickening, with a dull, grayish looking serosa which displays extensive telangiectasia. Stenotic areas or perforations may also be present. Histologically the major change is seen in the submucosa where there is prominent fibrosis, above which is an atrophic mucous membrane with small, shrunken crypts, atrophic villi with small, cuboid-shaped enterocytes. Affected vessels are located within the submucosa and mesentery. There is myointimal proliferation with or without the presence of foamy macrophages and medial fibrosis: thrombosis may be present where these changes are most severe and hence may underlie areas of necrosis, frank ulceration or fistula formation. Lymphatic dilatation is also a prominent feature. Microradiological studies have emphasized the severe degree of vascular ischemia and its consequent reduced tissue perfusion (Carr et al 1984) (Figs 14.16, 14.17, 14.18).

## Clinical features

Acute features are invariably confined to the anorectum, with small volume diarrhea, bleeding and tenesmus being common in elderly men irradiated for prostatic cancer. Watery diarrhea with or without abdominal pain is also common when the irradiated area includes the distal small intestine, especially the terminal ileum. Middle-aged women are obvious candidates because of gynecological neoplasms, but these symptoms may arise in young men following irradiation for testicular tumors with the addition of nausea and vomiting since part of the stomach is also irradiated. It is important to recognize that symptoms may be due to irradiation and thus thought of and considered, in addition to weighing whether tumor or even Crohn's disease is responsible for recurrent complaints or onset of "new" ones (Fig. 14.19).

If the acute radiation phase is mild, symptoms will abate

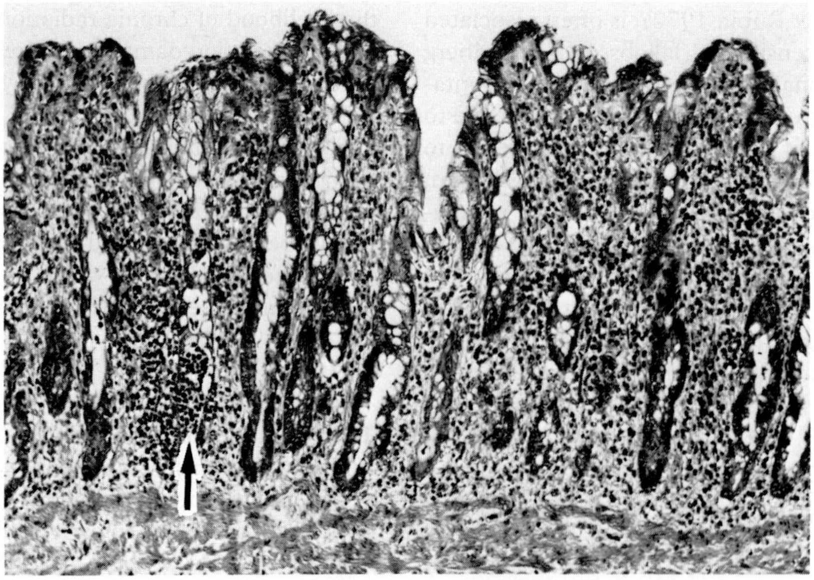

**Fig. 14.15** Acute radiation proctitis. There is acute inflammation of the mucosa with crypt abscess formation (arrow) and regenerative hyperplasia of crypt epithelium (hematoxylin and eosin, ×100),

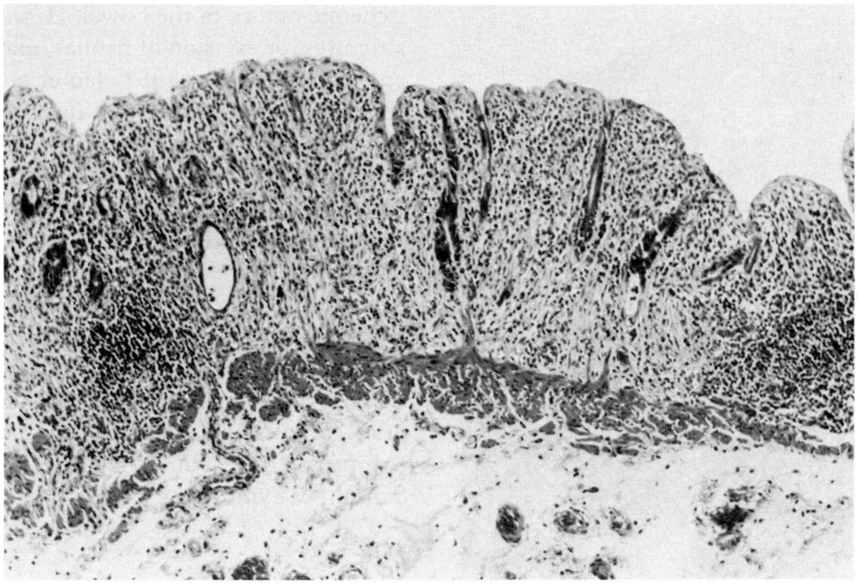

**Fig. 14.16** Subacute radiation proctitis. The crypts are atrophic and there is continuing inflammation of the mucosa (hematoxylin and eosin, ×100).

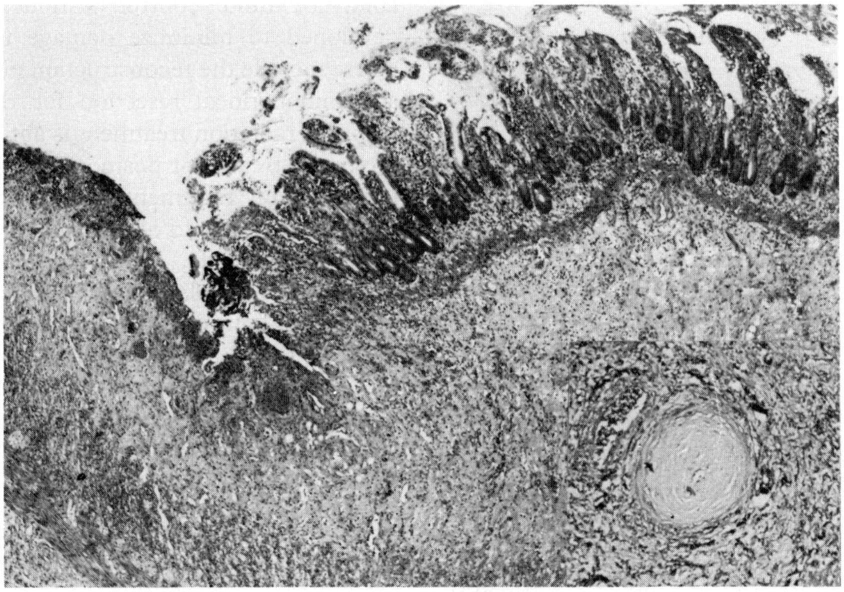

**Fig. 14.17** Chronic radiation enteritis. There is erosion and ulceration of the mucosa, with associated inflammation and submucosal fibrosis (hematoxylin and eosin, ×35).

without further trouble. Occasionally more severe reactions may extend, without interruption, to a chronic syndrome. Most commonly there is a period, often of several years, between the acute and chronic phase. The latter usually takes the form of recurrent small bowel obstruction, but there may also be evidence of malabsorption (impaired $B_{12}$ absorption, steatorrhea) or disturbed motility with bacterial overgrowth. Other possibilities are segmental infarction, perforation or fistula formation and sometimes hemorrhage. This may be due to mucosal ulceration or to a solitary rectal ulcer that lies adjacent to the tip of the cervix.

## Treatment

Treatment of acute radiation syndrome is directed to relief of symptoms, with attention paid to fluid and electrolyte replacement, especially of potassium. Corticosteroids, antibiotics or bile-acid binding agents may provide additional help. The chronic phase will often involve the differential diagnosis of diffuse disease, such as Crohn's disease, lymphoma or amyloidosis: a proper history will indicate the past exposure to ionizing radiation. Thus treatment will be determined by the abnormalities demonstrated by

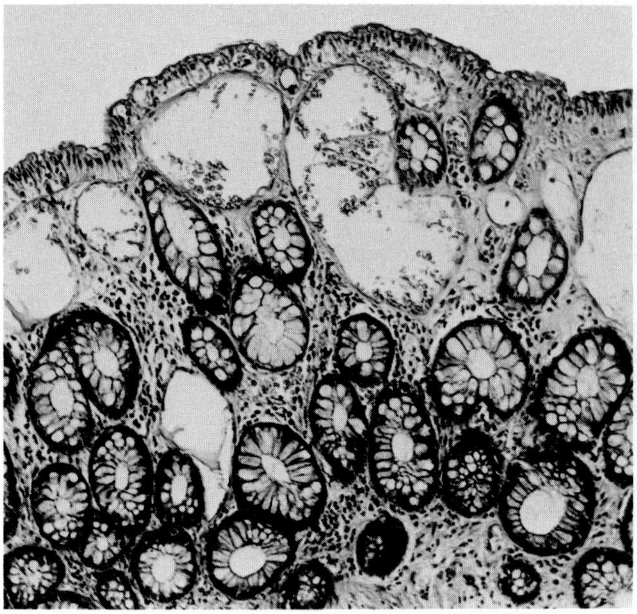

**Fig. 14.18** Postirradiation telangiectatic vessels in the mucosa (hematoxylin and eosin, ×100).

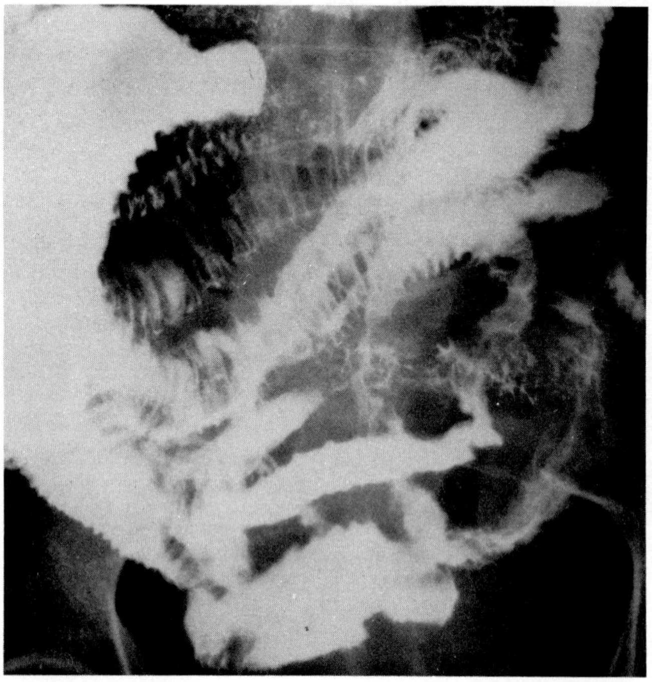

**Fig. 14.19** Radiation enteritis. Barium follow-through showing generalized changes with narrowing, irregularity and mucosal swelling.

the investigations and will involve use of steroids, antibiotics, antidiarrheals or dietary manipulations to reduce bulk or fat intake: parenteral nutrition may also be required in the most severe cases, usually when single or multiple strictures are present.

Surgery is fraught with difficulties because of the ischemic nature of the bowel. However, operative relief of strictures, or excision of fistulas, may have to be undertaken (Cochrane et al 1981, Jao et al 1986). The approach should be conservative and directed towards the specific problem: no attempt to excise all involved bowel should ever be contemplated or undertaken. Before operation is carried out, the patient should receive intense nutritional support in order to maximize success and reduce the risk of postoperative failures or additional complications. Emergency procedures should tackle the immediate precipitating cause, leaving the definitive procedure to a later date, once proper control of nutrition has been secured. If these well-established principles are followed, surgically induced disasters will be reduced to the minimum (Morgenstern et al 1977, 1985, Localio et al 1979, Schmitt & Symmonds 1981).

### Prevention

In recommending radiotherapy a risk of injury to normal tissues has to be accepted in order to achieve a good probability of tumor control. Various techniques have been developed to minimize damage to the small intestine. These include the reconstruction of the pelvic floor during abdominoperineal resection for rectal carcinoma when adjuvant radiation treatment is anticipated, and the use of the prone treatment position and bladder distention during radiation treatment. Methods of removal of small bowel from the field of radiation, such as by a mesh sling inserted surgically, are being developed (Rodier et al 1991). It is possible to identify those patients who are at a greater risk of small bowel injury by identifying areas of small bowel fixation on barium follow-through examination. Radiation dosimetry and positioning are then modified accordingly. Careful planning and co-ordination of external beam and intracavitary radiotherapy are very important.

## WHIPPLE'S DISEASE

This condition was first distinguished and described by Whipple in 1907. The patient was affected by weight loss, arthritis, diarrhea, malabsorption and cough. Whipple initially called the condition "intestinal lipodystrophy" on account of the large number of lipid-filled, foamy macrophages present within the lamina propria and the enlarged mesenteric lymph nodes. Although after silver impregnation, rod-shaped bacteria, approximately 2 μm in length, were abundant in one node, he still concluded that a disorder in lipid metabolism was the most likely cause of the illness.

Extraintestinal manifestations are common and subsequent studies identified similar foamy macrophages in liver, adrenals, heart valves and other tissues (Hendrix et

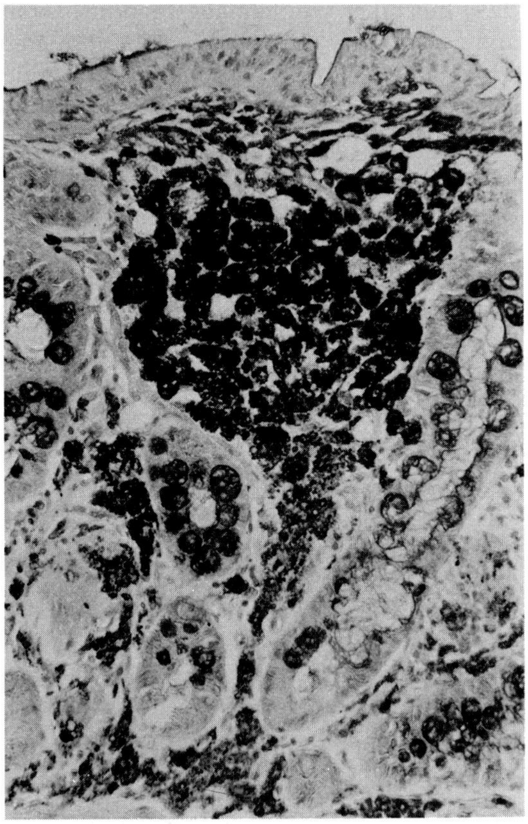

**Fig. 14.20** Whipple's disease. Section of small intestine showing the positive granules within the macrophges (PAS, ×270).

al 1950, Upton 1952, Sieracki & Fine 1959). However, the infectious nature and curability of the condition was first demonstrated by Paulley in 1952 who achieved a spectacular, long-lived remission in his patient with long-term chloramphenicol treatment.

## Pathology

The characteristic lesion is invariably present within the jejunum (Fig. 14.20) in which typically there is blunting of villi by the massive accumulation of PAS-positive macrophages within the lamina propria. There is also infiltration by neutrophils and dilatation of lymphatics by fat-filled material. Similar accumulations of macrophages are seen within involved lymph nodes and other extraintestinal tissues. Studies with the electronmicroscope have demonstrated the presence of rod-shaped bacilli within macrophages and lying freely in the tissues. The PAS-positive glycolipid probably represents remains of cell walls of phagocytosed bacteria.

Note should be taken of the vegetations which occur on heart valves, as a result of infiltration by macrophages: importantly secondary subacute streptococcal bacterial endocarditis can involve the damaged valves.

## Etiology (see also p. 568)

DNA technology has recently permitted identification of the organism responsible for this infection: nucleotide sequences were similar to *Rhodococcus*, *Arthrobacter* and *Streptomyces* species (Wilson et al 1991): the bacterium was named *Tropheryma whippelii* (Relman et al 1992) and identified in extraintestinal tissue. However, it seems that infection is related to an intrinsic defect in macrophage/monocyte degradation of bacterial protein and other components, although why this leads to a specific infection with only one particular organism has yet to be determined. One possibility is of an enzyme defect necessary for degradation of cell wall material from this particular agent (Bjerknes et al 1985, 1988). Nevertheless the histological similarity between Whipple's disease and *M. avium-intracellulare* infections in AIDS enteropathy is intriguing, particularly as both organisms share homologies in their 16s ribosomal DNA (Wilson et al 1991).

## Clinical features

The disease typically affects males in the fourth of fifth decades. Gastrointestinal symptoms predominate with diarrhea occurring in over 75% of patients. Stools are watery, steatorrheic and malodorous and are accompanied by abdominal distention and cramping pains. Bleeding may sometimes occur. Other important features are skin pigmentation, lymphadenopathy, a low-grade fever and arthropathy.

Symptoms of joint involvement occur in 80% of patients and in about one-third of cases antedate onset of diarrhea by up to 5 years (Fleming et al 1988). Usually the peripheral joints are involved, often in a transient, flitting manner. Use of nonsteroidal anti-inflammatory drugs may lead to mucosal ulceration, anemia or frank hemorrhage. Pleuritic pain or cough is another characteristic feature, while heart murmurs suggest endocardial involvement. Large masses in the abdomen indicate mesenteric lymphadenopathy: hepatosplenomegaly is another feature.

Central nervous involvement occurs in 10% of patients and sometimes is manifest only when antibiotics are withdrawn after treatment of gastrointestinal symptoms. Neural involvement is widespread, leading to various syndromes – peripheral neuropathy, cranial nerve lesions, cortical defects and visual or brain-stem impairment. Thus, the patient will present with dementia, confusion, ataxia, cranial nerve lesions or sensory-motor signs in limbs.

## Diagnosis and treatment

Whipple's disease is still rare, so that diagnosis may be delayed on account of the varied forms of presentation. Classically, the presence of fever, skin pigmentation, lym-

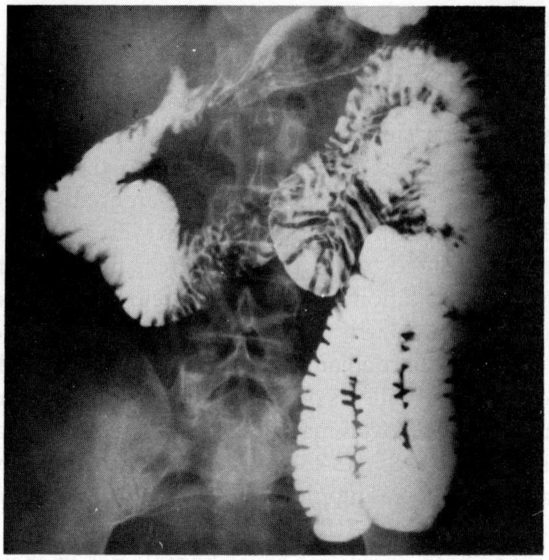

**Fig. 14.21** Whipple's disease. Some dilatation of the jejunum with coarsening of mucosal pattern and moderate atrophy.

phadenopathy, arthritis and wasting should suggest the diagnosis and prompt an intestinal biopsy. On barium follow-through examination there is marked thickening of the mucosal folds in the duodenum and jejunum (Fig. 14.21).

Until the advent of chemotherapy, Whipple's disease was uniformly fatal. Successful treatment has been achieved with various regimens, such as penicillin, trimethoprim-sulfa-methoxazole or erythromycin. Treatment should be continued for at least 1 year, until all evidence of jejunal bacteria has disappeared (Trier et al 1965). The occurrence of cerebral/neural symptoms requires combinations which cross the blood–brain barrier and agents such as ceftriaxone usefully fulfill this role: moreover, drug side-effects are minimal (Adler & Galetta 1990, Zighelboim et al 1993).

## SYSTEMIC MASTOCYTOSIS

Abnormal proliferations of mast cells result in (i) infiltration of skin (urticaria pigmentosa), (ii) infiltration of the gastrointestinal tract or (iii) diffuse involvement of several organs or tissues (systemic mastocytosis). Involvement of the gastrointestinal tract may give rise to vomiting or dyspeptic symptoms due to gastric involvement or diarrhea from diffuse infiltration of the bowel wall. The characteristic radiologic features are increased size of rugal folds or nodular filling defects in the jejunum (Clemett et al 1968). Jejunal biopsy may reveal the mucosal infiltrates (Scott et al 1975). The diarrhea associated with bowel mast cell infiltrates is copious and watery. Whether malabsorption is a feature is unknown, since the case reported by Broitman et al (1970) probably had gluten sensitivity, with villous effacement of the mucosa. Treatment with cromoglycate may be effective (Soter et al 1979) but other symptomatic support may also be necessary: occasionally the disease can be extremely persistent (Mahood et al 1982). Other patients may develop malignancies such as lymphoma or a myeloproliferative disorder.

## MACROGLOBULINEMIA

Steatorrhea has been reported in this condition (Khilnani et al 1969), but the mechanism is unknown. Barium follow-through examination of the small intestine shows dilatation and thickened folds.

## PNEUMATOSIS INTESTINALIS (p. 1392)

When this condition occurs in the small intestine it is usually secondary to other diseases. Occasionally, when the pneumatosis is extensive, it may result in steatorrhea (Hughes et al 1966).

## LIVER DISEASE AND STEATORRHEA (pp. 922 & 934)

Steatorrhea occurs in liver disease, particularly that associated with cholestasis (p. 934). Several factors contribute to this.

## MALABSORPTION INDUCED BY DRUGS (George & Holdstock 1985)

Drugs may act by: direct morphological damage to the mucosa (neomycin, colchicine, cytotoxics, alcohol, mefenamic acid); inhibition of mucosal enzymes (laxatives, PAS, biguanides); interference with micelle formation (cholestyramine); chelation (tetracycline will chelate iron, calcium and magnesium); influencing motility.

### Neomycin

This is an aminoglycoside which inhibits protein synthesis within the bacterial lysosomes. It can produce steatorrhea and malabsorption of many other substances. The degree of malabsorption is dose dependent and is reversible on withdrawal of the drug. It causes moderate villous effacement, edema and changes in the morphology of the mucosal cells and acts at several points in the intraluminal digestive and absorptive processes; in particular, it precipitates bile acids and also causes disaccharidase deficiency.

### Colchicine

This binds to microtubular protein to cause metaphase arrest, which can lead to variable degrees of mucosal flattening. It can cause nausea, vomiting, colicky abdominal pain and diarrhea. If used as a long-term treatment for gout it causes steatorrhea and there is malabsorption of vitamin $B_{12}$.

### Cytotoxic agents

Alkylating agents have the potential to damage the intestinal mucosa but diarrhea is a rare complication because nitrogen mustard is given intravenously and cyclophosphamide requires metabolic activation within the microsomes of the liver.

By contrast, antimetabolites affect the gastrointestinal tract more frequently. Methotrexate, a folate antagonist, can induce villous flattening. 5-Fluorouracil acts on the synthesis of DNA and may also produce mucosal abnormalities. It causes stomatitis, nausea, vomiting and diarrhea. The vinca alkaloid vincristine can cause intestinal ulceration and adynamic ileus due to a neuropathic process.

### Alcohol

With chronic use, alcohol damages the lipoprotein membranes of the enterocyte, leading to ultrastructural changes. The activity of the brush border enzymes is reduced, so that there is malabsorption of many nutrients. In vitro studies with intestinal biopsies indicate that alcohol inhibits triglyceride synthesis and secretion (Zimmerman et al 1986).

### Mefanamic acid

This is a nonsteroidal anti-inflammatory agent which acts by inhibition of prostaglandin synthetase. It has produced steatorrhea by direct damage to the intestinal mucosa.

### Para-amino salicylic acid (PAS)

This antitubercular drug is still used in developing countries. It causes steatorrhea without affecting the histology of the jejunum.

### Biguanides

The oral hypoglycemic drugs metformin and phenformin reduce glucose absorption by a direct action on active transport mechanisms. There is also a reduced absorption of amino acids and vitamin $B_{12}$.

### Other drugs

Folic acid deficiency occurs in up to two-thirds of patients who take diphenylhydantoin regularly; the drug reduces the absorption of folic acid by an unknown mechanism. Sulfasalazine also reduces the absorption of folic acid (Halsted 1980). Aluminum hydroxide reduces phosphate absorption (p. 249).

## AMYLOIDOSIS (Neale & Booth 1985)

Amyloid protein is discussed on p. 979. The following forms of amyloidosis are described.

***Primary.*** This is rare. Amyloid is deposited in the heart, kidneys, gastrointestinal tract, liver and spleen, mainly in the outer walls of the muscular layers of the intestine. A similar distribution of deposition occurs in multiple myeloma.

***Secondary.*** This occurs in Crohn's disease, ulcerative colitis and in other chronic inflammatory disorders. In the small intestine, amyloid is deposited in the inner wall of small bowel vessels and in the mucosa, often just beneath the surface epithelium, and may cause malabsorption.

***Heredofamilial amyloidosis.*** The small intestine is frequently involved in types I and III, particularly the muscularis mucosae, muscle layers and enteric nerve plexuses (Ikeda et al 1982).

***Senile or localized amyloidosis.*** Local deposition of amyloid is common in the aged and occurs in heart, pancreas, aorta and brain, but not in the small intestine. However, local deposition of amyloid has been found in the small intestine in some healthy subjects (Griffel et al 1975).

### Clinical features

Motility disorders, including pseudo-obstruction of the small intestine (p. 441), develop in heredofamilial amyloidosis type I and in primary amyloidosis (Monteiro 1968).

Malabsorption occurs in 5–10% of patients with diffuse amyloidosis (Kyle & Bayrd 1975). Sometimes this results in diarrhea. The causes of malabsorption are deposition of amyloid in the mucosa, vascular insufficiency (Herskovic et al 1964), pancreatic infiltration (Casad & Bocian 1965) or bacterial overgrowth secondary to disordered motility.

The barium follow-through examination shows nonspecific changes. The most significant abnormality is the demonstration of motor dysfunction in the esophagus, with gastroesophageal reflux, delayed gastric emptying, dilatation of the small bowel and a prolonged transit time (Legge et al 1970). Additionally, deposition of amyloid tissue in the small intestine can cause thickening or effacement of the valvulae conniventes, but these changes are nonspecific (Seliger et al 1971).

Ischemia may result in infarction or ulceration with perforation, bleeding or protein-losing enteropathy.

The diagnosis is obtained on rectal biopsy when there is generalized disease. Occasionally, the diagnosis can be made by a biopsy of small intestine.

**Treatment**

There is no specific therapy. In secondary amyloidosis, successful treatment of the underlying cause may result in regression of amyloid deposits. In other patients, treatment is supportive and, depending on the cause of diarrhea, broad-spectrum antibiotics or pancreatic replacements may be of value.

REFERENCES


Aas K 1966 Studies of hypersensitivity to fish. Internal Archives of Allergy and Applied Immunology 29: 453–469

Adler C H, Galetta S L 1990 Oculo-facial-skeletal myorhythmia in Whipple disease: treatment with ceftriaxone. Annals of Internal Medicine 112: 467–469

Ament M E, Ochs H D 1973 Gastrointestinal manifestations of chronic granulmatous disease. New England Journal of Medicine 288: 382–387

Ament M E, Rubin C E 1972 Soy protein – another cause of the flat intestinal lesion. Gastroenterology 62: 216–226

Ament M E, Ochs H D, Davis S D 1973 Structure and function of the gastrointestinal tract in primary immunodeficiency syndromes: a study of 39 patients. Medicine 53: 227–248

Anderson C M 1960 Histological changes in the duodenal mucosa in coeliac disease. Reversibility during treatment with a wheat gluten free diet. Archives of Disease in Childhood 35: 419–427

Anderson C M, Burke V 1975 Paediatric gastroenterology. Blackwell, London

Anderson C M, Frazer A C, French J M, Gerrard J W, Sammons H G, Smellie J G 1952 Coeliac disease. Gastrointestinal studies and the effect of dietary wheat flour. Lancet 1: 836–842

Arranz E, Ferguson A 1993 Intestinal antibody pattern of celiac disease: occurrence in patients with normal jejunal biopsy histology. Gastroenterology 104: 1263–1272

Auricchio S, Greco L, Troncone R 1990 What is the true prevalence of coeliac disease? Gastroenterology International 3: 140–142

Austad W I, Cornes J S, Gough K R, McCarthy C F, Read A E A 1967 Steatorrhea and malignant lymphoma. The relationship of malignant tumors of lymphoid tissue and celiac disease. American Journal of Digestive Diseases 12: 475–490

Baker S J 1982 Idiopathic small intestinal diseases in the Tropics. Critical Reviews in Tropical Medicine 1: 197–245

Baker S J, Mathan V I 1961 Syndrome of tropical sprue in South India. American Journal of Clinical Nutrition 21: 984–993

Baker S J, Mathan V I 1970 Tropical sprue. In: Card W I, Creamer B (eds) Modern trends in gastro-enterology, Vol 4. Butterworths, London, p 198

Baker S J, Ignatius M, Mathan V I, Vaish S K, Chacko C C 1962a Intestinal biopsy in tropical sprue. In: Wolstenholme G E W, Cameron M P (eds) Intestinal biopsy (Ciba Foundation Study Group No. 14). Churchill Livingstone, London, p 84

Baker S J, Mathan V I, Joseph I 1962b Epidemic tropical sprue. American Journal of Digestive Diseases 7: 959–964

Banwell J G, Gorbach S L 1969 Tropical sprue. Gut 10: 328–333

Bennett T I, Hunter D, Vaughan J M 1932 Idiopathic steatorrhoea. A nutritional disturbance associated with tetany, osteomalacia, and anaemia. Quarterly Journal of Medicine 1: 653–667

Berg N O, Jakobsson I, Lindberg T 1979 Do pre- and post-challenge small intestinal biopsies help to diagnose cow's milk protein intolerance? Acta Paediatrica Scandinavica 68: 657–661

Bjerknes R, Laerum O D, Ødegaard S 1985 Impaired bacterial degradation by monocytes and macrophages from a patient with treated Whipple's disease. Gastroenterology 89: 1139–1146

Bjerknes R, Ødegaard S, Bjerkvig R, Børkje B, Laerum O D 1988 Whipple's disease. Demonstration of a persisting monocyte and macrophage dysfunction. Scandinavian Journal of Gastroenterology 23: 611–619

Bland P W, Kambarage D M 1991 Antigen handling by the epithelium and lamina propria macrophages. Gastroenterological Clinics of North America 20: 577–596

Bode S H, Bachmann E H Gudmund-Hoyer E, Jensen G 1991 Stature of adult coeliac patients: no evidence for decreased attained height. European Journal of Clinical Nutrition 45: 145–149

Booth C C 1970 Enterocyte in coeliac disease. British Medical Journal 3: 725–731

Booth C C, Neale G 1985 Ulcerative lesions. In: Booth C C, Neale G (eds) Disorders of the small intestine. Blackwell, Oxford, p 209

Bosio L, Barera G, Mistura L, Sassi G, Bianchi C 1990 Growth acceleration and final height after treatment for delayed diagnosis of celiac disease. Journal of Pediatric Gastroenterology and Nutrition 11: 324–329

Bourne R G, Kearsley J H, Grove W D, Roberts S J 1983 The relationship between early and late gastrointestinal complications of radiation therapy for carcinoma of the cervix. International Journal of Radiation Oncology, Biology and Physics 9: 1445–1550

Boyd W P, Bachman B A 1982 Gastrointestinal infections in the compromised host. Medical Clinics of North America 66: 743–753

Brandborg L L, Rubin C E, Quinton W E 1959 A multipurpose instrument for suction biopsy of the esophagus, stomach, small bowel and colon. Gastroenterology 37: 1–16

Brandborg L, Goldberg S, Breidenbach W C 1970 Human coccidiosis – a possible cause of malabsorption. The life-cycle in small-bowel mucosal biopsies as a diagnostic feature. New England Journal of Medicine 283: 1306–1313

Brandtzaeg P, Valnes K, Scott H, Rognum T O, Bjerke K, Baklien K 1985 The human gastrointestinal secretory immune system in health and disease. Scandinavian Journal of Gastroenterology 20 (suppl 114): 17–38

Broitman S A, McGray R S, May J C et al 1970 Mastocytosis and intestinal malabsorption. American Journal of Medicine 48: 382–389

Brown J H, Jardetzky T, Saper M A, Samraoui B, Bjorkman P, Wiley D C 1988 A hypothetical model of the foreign antigen binding site of class II histocompatibility molecules. Nature 332: 845–850

Brown J H, Jardetzky T S, Gorga J C et al 1993 Three-dimensional structure of the human class II histocompatibility antigen HLA-DR1. Nature 364: 33–39

Bugawan T L, Angelini G, Larrick H, Auricchio S, Ferrara G, Erlich H A 1989 A combination of a particular HLA-DP beta allele and an HLA-DQ heterodimer confers susceptibility to coeliac disease. Nature 339: 470–473

Caraceni M P, Molteni N, Bardella M, Ortalani S, Nogara A, Bianchi P 1988 Bone and mineral metabolism in adult celiac disease. American Journal of Gastroenterology 83: 274–277

Carlson H C 1969 Localized nonspecific ulceration of the small intestine. Radiologic Clinics of North America 7: 97–103

Carlson J R, Owen R L 1987 Structure and functional role of Peyer's patches. In: Marsh M N (ed) Immunopathology of the small intestine. Wiley, Chichester, p 21–40

Carr N D, Pullen B R, Hasleton P S, Schofield P F 1984 Microvascular studies in human radiation bowel disease. Gut 25: 448–454

Casad D E, Bocian J J 1965 Primary systemic amyloidosis simulating acute idiopathic ulcerative colitis. Report of a case. American Journal of Digestive Diseases 10: 63–74

Chacko C, Job C, Johnson S 1961 Histopathological changes in upper jejunum in tropical malabsorption syndrome studied by transoral jejunal biopsy. Indian Journal of Pathology and Bacteriology 4: 203–213

Challacombe D, Hawkins P, Baylis J, Robertson K 1975 Small intestinal histology in coeliac disease. Lancet 1: 1345–1346

Clemett A R, Fishbone G, Levine R J, James A E, Janower M 1968 Gastrointestinal lesions in mastocytosis. American Journal of Roentgenology 103: 405–412

Cochrane J P S, Yarnold J R, Slack W W 1981 The surgical treatment of radiation injuries after radiotherapy for uterine carcinoma. British Journal of Surgery 68: 25–28

Cooke G C 1985 Parasitic infection. In: Booth C C, Neale G (eds) Disorders of the small intestine. Blackwell, Oxford, p 283

Cooke W T, Holmes G K T 1984 Coeliac disease. Churchill Livingstone, Edinburgh

Cooper B T, Holmes G K T, Cooke W T 1982 Lymphoma risk in coeliac disease of later life. Digestion 22: 89–92

Crabbe P A, Heremans J F 1967 Selective IgA deficiency and steatorrhea. A new syndrome. American Journal of Medicine 42: 319–326

Crowe P T, Marsh M N 1993 Morphometric analysis of small intestinal mucosa. IV Measuring epithelial cell volumes. Virchows Archiv; A: Pathological Anatomy and Histology 422: 459–466

Crowe P T, Marsh M N 1994 Morphometric analysis of intestinal mucosa. VI Principles in enumerating intra-epithelial lymphocytes. Virchows Archiv; A: Pathological Anatomy and Histology 424: 301–306

Dannaeus A, Johansson S G O 1979 A follow-up study of infants with adverse reactions to cow's milk. I. Serum IgE, skin test reactions and RAST in relation to clinical course. Acta Paediatrica Scandinavica 68: 377–382

Dannaeus A, Johansson S G O, Foucard T, Ohman S 1977 Clinical and immunological aspects of food allergy in childhood. I. Estimation of IgG, IgA and IgE antibodies to food antigens in children with food allergy and atopic dermatitis. Acta Paediatrica Scandinavica 66: 31–37

Dannaeus A, Johansson S G O, Foucard T 1978 Clinical and immunological aspects of food allergy in childhood. II. Development of allergic symptoms and humoral immune response to foods in infants of atopic mothers during the first 24 months of life. Acta Paediatrica Scandinavica 67: 497–504

David T J, Ajdukiewicz A B 1975 A family study of coeliac disease. Journal of Medical Genetics 12: 79–82

David T J, Waddington E, Stanton R H J 1984 Nutritional hazards of elimination diets in children with atopic eczema. Archives of Disease in Childhood 59: 323–325

Davidson G P, Hill D J, Townley R R W 1976 Gastrointestinal milk allergy in childhood: a rational approach. Medical Journal of Australia 1: 945–947

Dawson A M, Kumar P 1985 Coeliac disease. In: Booth C C, Neale G (eds) Disorders of the small intestine. Blackwell, Oxford, p 153–178

Dawson-Hughes B, Dallal G E, Krall E A, Sadowski L, Sahyoun N, Tannenbaum S 1990 A controlled trial of the effect of calcium supplementation on bone density in postmenopausal women. New England Journal of Medicine 323: 878–883

De Ritis G, Auricchio S, Jones H W, Lew E, Bernardin J E, Kasarda D D 1984 In vitro (organ culture) studies of the toxicity of specific A-gliadin peptides in celiac disease. Gastroenterology 94: 41–49

Desjardins A U 1931 Action of Roentgen rays and radium on the gastrointestinal tract. American Journal of Roentgenology 26: 337–370

Dicke W K, Weijers H W, van de Kamer J H 1953 Coeliac disease. II The presence in wheat of a factor having a deleterious effect in cases of coeliac disease. Acta Paediatrica Scandinavica 42: 34–42

Dobbins W O, Rubin C E 1964 Studies of the rectal mucosa in celiac sprue. Gastroenterology 47: 471–479

Doniach I, Shiner M 1957 Duodenal and jejunal biopsies. Gastroenterology 33: 71–86

Egan-Mitchell B, Fottrell P F, McNicholl B F 1981 Early or pre-coeliac mucosa: development of gluten enteropathy. Gut 22: 65–69

Elson C O 1985 Induction and control of the gastrointestinal immune system. Scandinavian Journal of Gastroenterology 20 (suppl 114): 1–15

England N W J 1968 Intestinal pathology of tropical sprue. American Journal of Clinical Nutrition 21: 962–975

Ensari A, Marsh M N, Loft D E, Morgan S, Moriarty K J 1993a Morphometric analysis of intestinal mucosa. V. Quantitative histological and immunocytochemical studies of rectal mucosae in gluten sensitivity. Gut 34: 1225–1229

Ensari A, Ager A, Marsh M N, Morgan S, Moriarty K J 1993b Time-course of adhesion molecule expression in rectal mucosa of gluten-sensitive subjects after gluten challenge. Clinical and Experimental Immunology 93: 303–307

Ensari A, Marsh M N, Morgan S, Moriarty K J, Lobley R, Unsworth D J 1994 A comparative, prospective study of rectal gluten challenge in the diagnosis of gluten-sensitivity. Gut 35 (suppl 2): Abst S29

Ferguson A 1987 Models of immunologically-driven small intestinal damage. In: Marsh M N (ed) The immunopathology of the small intestine. Wiley, Chichester, p 225–252

Ferguson R, Asquith P, Cooke W T 1974 The jejunal cellular infiltrate in coeliac disease complicated by lymphoma. Gut 15: 458–461

Ferreira M, Lloyd Davies S, Butler M, Scott D, Clark M, Kumar P 1992 Endomysial antibody: is it the best screening test for coeliac disease? Gut 33: 1633–1637

Ferry G D, Bendig D W 1981 Peroral small-bowel biopsies in infants and children using a directable biopsy instrument. Digestive Diseases and Sciences 26: 142–145

Fleming J L, Wiesner R H, Shorter R G 1988 Whipple's disease: clinical, biochemical, and histopathologic features and assessment of treatment in 29 patients. Mayo Clinic Proceedings 63: 539–551

Flick A L, Quinton W E, Rubin C E 1961 A peroral hydraulic biopsy tube for multiple sampling at any level of the gastrointestinal tract. Gastroenterology 40: 120–126

Frank M M 1982 The $C_1$ esterase inhibitor and hereditary angioedema. Journal of Clinical Immunology 2: 65–68

Frazer A C 1960 Pathogenetic concepts of the malabsorption syndrome. Gastroenterology 38: 389–398

Frazer A C, Fletcher R F, Ross C A, Shaw B, Sammons H G, Schneider R 1959 Gluten-induced enteropathy. The effect of partially-digested gluten. Lancet 2: 252–255

Freeman H J, Chiu B K 1986 Multifocal small bowel lymphoma and latent celiac sprue. Gastroenterology 90: 1992–1997

Freeman H J, Weinstein W M, Shnitka T K, Piercy J R A, Wensel R H 1977 Primary abdominal lymphoma. Presenting manifestations of celiac sprue, or complicating dermatitis herpetiformis. American Journal of Medicine 63: 585–594

Fry L 1992 Dermatitis herpetiformis. In: Marsh M N (ed) Coeliac disease. Blackwell, Oxford, p 81

Gee S 1888 On the coeliac affection. St Bartholomew's Hospital Reports 24: 17–20

Gelfand J, Boss G, Conley C, Reinhart R, Frank M M 1979 Acquired C1 esterase inhibitor deficiency and angioedema: a review. Medicine 58: 321

George C F, Holdstock G E 1985 Drug-induced disorders. In: Booth C C, Neale G (eds) Disorders of the small intestine. Blackwell, Oxford, p 398

Gjone E, Nordoy A 1970 Dermatitis herpetiformis, steatorrhoea and malignancy. British Medical Journal 1: 610

Gleich G J, Hofmann A F 1971 Use of cholestyramine to control diarrhea associated with acquired hypogammaglobulinemia. American Journal of Medicine 51: 281–286

Goldman A S, Anderson D W, Sellers W A et al 1963 Milk allergy. I Oral challenge with milk and isolated milk proteins in allergic children. Pediatrics 32: 425–443

Goodgame R W 1993 Gastrointestinal cytomegalovirus disease. Annals of Internal Medicine 119: 924–935

Gough K R, Read A E, Naish J M 1962 Intestinal reticulosis as a complication of idiopathic steatorrhoea. Gut 3: 232–239

Griffel B, Man B, Kraus L 1975 Selective massive amyloidosis of small intestine. Archives of Surgery 110: 215–217

Gryboski J, Walker A W 1983 Gastrointestinal problems in the infant. W B Saunders, Philadelphia, p 642

Guerra R, Wheby M, Bayless T M 1965 Long-term antibiotic therapy in tropical sprue. Annals of Internal Medicine 63: 619–634

Haeney R P 1991 Lifelong calcium intake and prevention of bone fragility in the aged. Calcified Tissue International (suppl 49) 49: S42–S45

Haeney R P, Recker R R 1985 Estimation of true calcium absorption. Annals of Internal Medicine 103: 516–521

Haeney R P, Recker R R, Saville P D 1977 Calcium balance and calcium requirements in middle-aged women. American Journal of Clinical Nutrition 30: 1603–1611

Hagander B, Brandt L, Sjölund K, Berg N, Norden A, Stenstam M 1977 Hepatic injury in adult coeliac disease. Lancet 2: 270–272

Hall M A, Lanchbury J S S, Bolsover W J, Welsh K, Ciclitira P 1990 Celiac disease is associated with an extended HLA-DR3 haplotype which includes HLA-DPw1. Human Immunology 27: 220–228

Halsted C H 1980 Intestinal absorption and malabsorption of folates. Annual Review of Medicine 31: 79–87

Halstensen T S, Hvatum M, Scott H, Brandtzaeg P 1992 Association of subepithelial deposition of activated complement and immunoglobulin G and M response to gluten in celiac disease. Gastroenterology 102: 751–759

Harris O D, Cooke W T, Thompson H, Waterhouse J A H 1967 Malignancy in adult coeliac disease and idiopathic steatorrhoea. American Journal of Medicine 42: 899–912

Haynes F M, McBryde A 1936 Identity of sprue, non-tropical sprue and celiac disease. Archives of Internal Medicine 58: 1–16

Hendrix J P, Black-Schaffer B, Withers R W, Handler P 1950 Whipple's intestinal lipodystrophy. Archives of Internal Medicine 85: 91–131

Heremans P E, Diaz-Buxo J A, Stobo J D 1976 Idiopathic late-onset immunoglobulin deficiency. American Journal of Medicine 61: 221–237

Hermaszewski R A, Webster A D B 1993 Primary hypogammaglobulinaemia: a survey of clinical manifestations and complications. Quarterly Journal of Medicine 86: 31–42

Herskovic T, Bartholomew L G, Green P A 1964 Amyloidosis and malabsorption syndrome. Archives of Internal Medicine 114: 629–633

Hill D J, Davidson G P, Cameron D J, Barnes G L 1979 The spectrum of cow's milk allergy in childhood. Acta Paediatrica Scandinavica 68: 847–852

Hill D J, Ford R P K, Shelton M J, Hosking C S 1984 A study of 100 infants and young children with cow's milk allergy. Clinical Reviews of Allergy 2: 125–142

Hoffbrand A V, Necheles T F, Maldonado N, Horta E, Santini R 1969 Malabsorption of folate polyglutamates in tropical sprue. British Medical Journal 2: 543–547

Holmes G K T, Thompson H 1992 Malignancy as a complication of coeliac disease. In: Marsh M N (ed) Coeliac disease. Blackwell, Oxford, p 105

Holmes G K T, Stokes P L, Sorahan T M, Prior P, Waterhouse J A H, Cooke W T 1976 Coeliac disease, gluten-free diet, and malignancy. Gut 17: 612–619

Holmes G K T, Prior P, Lane M R, Pope R N, Allan R N 1989 Malignancy in coeliac disease – effect of a gluten free diet. Gut 30: 333–338

Holmes W H, Starr P 1929 A nutritional disturbance in adults resembling celiac disease and sprue: emaciation, anemia, tetany, chronic diarrhea and malabsorption of fat. Journal of the American Medical Association 92: 975–980

Holt P D, Tandy N, Anstee D J 1977 Screening of blood donors for IgA deficiency: a study of the donor population of south-west England. Journal of Clnical Pathology 30: 1007–1010

Horowitz S, Lorenzsohn V W, Olsen W A 1974 Small intestinal disease in T cell deficiency. Journal of Pediatrics 85: 457–462

Howdle P D, Losowsky M S 1992 Coeliac disease in adults. In: Marsh M N (ed) Coeliac disease. Blackwell, Oxford, p 49

Hughes D T D, Gordon K C D, Swann J C, Bolt G L 1966 Pneumatosis cystoides intestinalis. Gut 7: 553

Huntley C C, Dees S C 1957 Eczema associated with thrombocytopenic purpura and purulent otitis media. Report of five fatal cases. Pediatrics 19: 351–354

Ikeda S-I, Makishita H, Oguchi K, Yanagisawa N, Nagata T 1982 Gastrointestinal amyloid deposition in familial amyloid polyneuropathy. Neurology 32: 1364–1368

Isaacson P G 1987 The association between coeliac disease and malignant lymphoma. In: Marsh M N (ed) Immunopathology of the small intestine. Wiley, Chichester, p 401

Iyngkaran N, Yadav M 1987 Food allergy. In: Marsh M N (ed) Immunopathology of the small intestine. Wiley, Chichester, p 415

Jakobsson I, Lindberg T 1979 A prospective study of cow's milk protein intolerance in Swedish infants. Acta Paediatrica Scandinavica 68: 853–858

Jao S W, Beart R W, Gunderson L L 1986 Surgical treatment of radiation injuries of the colon and rectum. American Journal of Surgery 151: 272–277

Jeejeebhoy K N, Desai H G, Noronha J M, Antia F P, Parekh D V 1966 Idiopathic tropical diarrhea with or without steatorrhea (tropical malabsorption syndrome). Gastroenterology 51: 333–344

Jeffries G H, Steinberg H, Sleisenger M H 1968 Chronic ulcerative (nongranulomatous) jejunitis. American Journal of Medicine 44: 47–59

Jones T E 1939 Benign strictures of the intestine due to irradiation. Surgical Clinics of North America 19: 1185–1194

Kagnoff M F 1992 Genetic basis of coeliac disease: role of HLA genes. In: Marsh M N (ed) Coeliac disease. Blackwell, Oxford, p 215

Kagnoff M F, Austin R K, Johnson H C, Bernardin J E, Dietler M D, Kasarda D D 1982 Celiac sprue: correlation with murine T cell responses to wheat gliadin components. Journal of Immunology 129: 2693–2697

Kagnoff M F, Harwood J, Bugawan T, Erlich H A 1989 Structural analysis of the HLA-DR, -DQ and -DP alleles on the celiac disease-associated HLA-DR3 (DRw17) haplotype. Proceedings of the National Academy of Sciences USA 86: 6274–6278

Khilnani M T, Keller R J, Cuttner J 1969 Macroglobulinemia and steatorrhea: roentgen and pathologic findings in the intestinal tract. Radiological Clinics of North America 7: 43–55

Kinsella T J, Bloomer W D 1980 Tolerance of the intestine to radiation therapy. Surgery, Gynecology and Obstetrics 151: 273–284

Kirkpatrick C H 1976 Cancer and immunodeficiency diseases. Birth Defects 12: 61–78

Klipstein F A 1970 Recent advances in tropical malabsorption. Scandinavian Journal of Gastroenterology (suppl) 6: 93–114

Klipstein F A 1981 Tropical sprue in travelers and expatriates living abroad. Gastroenterology 80: 590–600

Klipstein F A, Corcino J J 1977 Factors responsible for weight loss in tropical sprue. American Journal of Clinical Nutrition 30: 1703–1708

Kuitenen P, Rapola J, Savilahti E, Visakorpi J K 1973 Response of the jejunal mucosa to cow's milk in the malabsorption syndrome with cow's milk intolerance. Acta Paediatrica Scandinavica 62: 585–595

Kutlu T, Brousse N, Rambaud C, Le Deist F, Schmitz J, Cerf-Bensussan N 1993 Numbers of T cell receptor (TCR) $\alpha\beta^+$ but not TCR $\gamma\delta^+$ intraepithelial lymphocytes correlate with the grade of villous atrophy in coeliac patients on a long term normal diet. Gut 34: 208–214

Kyle R A, Bayrd E D 1975 Amyloidosis: review of 236 cases. Medicine 54: 271–299

Lamont C M, Adams F G, Mills P R 1982 Radiology in idiopathic chronic ulcerative enteritis. Clinical Radiology 33: 283–287

Ledingham I, More J G 1978 Liver damage in coeliac disease. Lancet 2: 390

Legge D A, Carlson H C, Wollaeger E E 1970 Roentgenologic appearances of systemic amyloidosis involving the gastrointestinal tract. American Journal of Roentgenology 110: 406–412

Leigh R J, Marsh M N, Crowe P, Kelly C, Garner V, Gordon D 1985 Studies of intestinal lymphoid tissue. IX. Dose-dependent, gluten-induced lymphoid infiltration of coeliac jejunal epithelium. Scandinavian Journal of Gastroenterology 20: 715–719

Leonard J N, Tucker W F, Fry J S et al 1983 Increased incidence of malignancy in dermatitis herpetiformis. British Medical Journal 286: 16–18

Lima J P, Delgado P G 1961 Diagnosis of strongyloidiasis: importance of Baerman's method. American Journal of Digestive Diseases 6: 899–904

Lindberg T, Berg N O, Borulf S, Jacobsson I 1978 Liver damage in coeliac disease or other food intolerance in childhood. Lancet 1: 390–391

Lindenbaum J, Kent T, Sprinz H 1966 Malabsorption and jejunitis in American Peace Corps volunteers in Pakistan. Annals of Internal Medicine 65: 1201–1209

Linscheer W G, Abele J E 1976 A new directable small bowel biopsy device. Gastroenterology 71: 575–576

Lloyd-Still J D 1979 Chronic diarrhea of childhood and the misuse of elimination diets. Journal of Pediatrics 95: 10–13

Localio S A, Pachter H L, Gouge T H 1979 The radiation-injured bowel. Surgery Annual 11: 181–205

Loft D E, Marsh M N, Sandle G I et al 1989 Studies of intestinal lymphoid tissue. XII. Epithelial lymphocyte and mucosal responses to rectal gluten challenge in celiac sprue. Gastroenterology 97: 29–37

Loft D E, Marsh M N, Crowe P 1990 A prospective study of rectal gluten challenge: a new diagnostic test for coeliac disease. Lancet 335: 1293–1295

Logan R F A 1992 Epidemiology of coeliac disease. In: Marsh M N (ed) Coeliac disease. Blackwell, Oxford, p 192
Low G C 1928 Sprue. Quarterly Journal of Medicine 21: 523–534
MacDermott R P, Elson C O 1991 Mucosal immunology. W B Saunders, Philadelphia
MacDonald T T 1992 T cell-mediated intestinal injury. In: Marsh M N (ed) Coeliac disease. Blackwell, Oxford, p 283
MacDonald T T, Spencer J 1988 Evidence that activated mucosal T cells play a role in the pathogenesis of enteropathy in human small intestine. Journal of Experimental Medicine 167: 1341–1349
MacDonald W C, Dobbins W O, Rubin C E 1965 Studies of the familial nature of celiac sprue using biopsy of the small intestine. New England Journal of Medicine 272: 448–456
Madhok R, MacKenzie J A, Lee F D, Bruckner F E, Terry T R, Sturrock R D 1986 Small bowel ulceration in patients receiving non-steroidal anti-flammatory drugs for rheumatoid arthritis. Quarterly Journal of Medicine 58: 53–55
Maggiore G, de Giacomo C, Scotta M, Sessa F 1986 Celiac disease presenting as chronic hepatitis in a girl. Journal of Pediatric Gastroenterology and Nutrition 5: 501–503
Mahood J M, Harrington C L, Slater D N, Corbett C L 1982 Forty years of diarrhoea in a patient with urticaria pigmentosa. Acta Dermato-Venereologica 62: 264–265
Mäki M, Holm K, Koskimies S, Hällström O, Visakorpi J K 1990 Normal small bowel biopsy followed by coeliac disease. Archives of Disease in Childhood 65: 1137–1141
Maldonado N, Horta E, Guerra R, Perez-Santiago E 1969 Poorly absorbed sulfonamides in the treatment of tropical sprue. Gastroenterology 57: 559–568
Mansson T 1971 Malignant disease in dermatitis herpetiformis. Acta Dermato-Venereologica 51: 379–382
Marsh M N 1972 The scanning electron microscope and its application to the investigation of intestinal structure. In: Badenoch J, Brooke B N (eds) Recent advances in gastroenterology, 2nd edn. Churchill Livingstone, Edinburgh, p 81
Marsh M N 1980 Studies of intestinal lymphoid tissue. III. Quantitative analyses of epithelial lymphocytes in the small intestine of human control subjects and of patients with celiac sprue. Gastroenterology 79: 481–492
Marsh M N 1983 Immunocytes, enterocytes and the lamina propria: an immunopathological framework of coeliac disease. Journal of the Royal College of Physicians (London) 17: 205–212
Marsh M N 1985 Functional and structural aspects of the epithelial lymphocyte, with implications for coeliac disease and tropical sprue. Scandinavian Journal of Gastroenterology 20 (suppl 114): 55–75
Marsh M N 1988 Studies of intestinal lymphoid tissue. XI The immunopathology of cell-mediated reactions in gluten sensitivity and other enteropathies. Scanning Microscopy 2: 1663–1684
Marsh M N 1989a Studies of intestinal lymphoid tissue. XV Histopathologic features suggestive of cell-mediated reactivity in jejunal mucosae of patients with dermatitis herpetiformis. Virchows Archiv; A: Pathological Anatomy and Histology 416: 125–132
Marsh M N 1989b Studies of intestinal lymphoid tissue. XIII. Immunopathology of the evolving celiac sprue lesion. Pathology, Research and Practice (Stuttgart) 185: 774–777
Marsh M N 1992a Gluten sensitivity and latency: the histological background. In: Auricchio S, Visakorpi J K (eds) Dynamic nutrition research, Vol 2. Common food intolerances: 1. Epidemiology of coeliac disease. Karger, Basel, p 142
Marsh M N 1992b The mucosal pathology of gluten-sensitivity. In: Marsh M N (ed) Coeliac disease. Blackwell, Oxford, p 136
Marsh M N 1992c Gluten, major histocompatibility complex, and the small intestine. A molecular and immunobiologic approach to the spectrum of gluten sensitivity ("celiac sprue"). Gastroenterology 102: 330–354
Marsh M N 1992d Celiac and allied sprue syndromes. In: Turnberg L A (ed) Absorption and malabsorption. Seminars in Gastrointestinal Disease 4: 214–223
Marsh M N 1993a Mechanisms of diarrhoea and malabsorption in gluten-sensitive enteropathy. European Journal of Gastroenterology and Hepatology 5: 796–807
Marsh M N 1993b Editorial: gluten sensitivity and latency: can patterns of intestinal antibody secretion define the great "silent majority"? Gastroenterology 104: 1550–1553
Marsh M N, Cummins A G 1993 The interactive role of mucosal T lymphocytes in intestinal growth, development and enteropathy. Journal of Gastroenterology and Hepatology 8: 270–278
Marsh M N, Ensari A 1994 The gut associated lymphoid tissue and immune system. In: Whitehead R (ed) Oesophageal and gastrointestinal pathology. Churchill, Edinburgh pp 201–225
Marsh M N, Bjarnason I, Shaw J, Ellis A, Baker R, Peters T J 1990 Studies of intestinal lymphoid tissue. XIV. HLA status, mucosal morphology, permeability and epithelial lymphocyte populations in first degree relatives of patients with coeliac disease. Gut 31: 32–36
Marsh M N, Loft D E, Garner V G, Gordon D 1992 Time/dose responses of coeliac mucosae to graded oral challenges with Frazer's fraction III of gliadin. European Journal of Gastroenterology and Hepatology 4: 667–674
Martin C L, Rogers F T 1924 Roentgen-ray cachexia. American Journal of Roentgenology 11: 280–286
Maurino E, Capizzano H, Niveloni S et al 1993 Value of endoscopic markers in celiac disease. Digestive Diseases and Sciences 38: 2028–2033
Mazure R, Vazquez H, Gonzalez D, Mautalen C, Boerr L, Bai J C 1994 Bone mineral density in asymptomatic adult patients with celiac sprue. American Journal of Gastroenterology 89: 2130–2134
McConnell R B, Whitwell F 1975 Small intestinal histology in coeliac disease. Lancet 2: 418
Mearin M L, Biemond I, Pena A S et al 1983 HLA-DR phenotypes in Spanish coeliac children: their contribution to the understanding of the genetics of the disease. Gut 24: 532–537
Mee A S, Burke M, Vallon A G, Newman J, Cotton P B 1985 Small bowel biopsy for malabsorption: comparison of the diagnostic adequacy of endoscopic forceps and capsule biopsy specimens. British Medical Journal 291: 769–772
Melamed I, Bujanover Y, Siegman Y, Schwartz D, Zakuth V, Spirer Z 1983 Campylobacter enteritis in normal and immunodeficient children. American Journal of Diseases of Children 137: 752–753
Melton L, Eddy D, Johnson C 1990 Screening for osteoporosis. Annals of Internal Medicine 112: 516–528
Modigliani R, Poitras P, Galian A et al 1979 Chronic non-specific ulcerative duodenojejunoileitis: report of four cases. Gut 20: 318–328
Mollin D L, Booth C C 1970 Chronic tropical sprue in London. In: Tropical sprue. Wellcome Trust. Churchill, London, p 61–127
Molteni N, Caraceni M P, Bardella M T, Ortalani S, Gandolini G G, Bianchi P 1990 Bone mineral density in adult celiac patients and the effect of gluten-free diet from childhood. American Journal of Gastroenterology 85: 51–53
Monteiro J G 1968 Familial amyloidosis with gastrointestinal neuropathy. Gut 9: 353–354
Mora S, Weber G, Barera G et al 1993 Effect of gluten-free diet on bone mineral content in growing patients with celiac disease. American Journal of Clinical Nutrition 57: 224–228
Morellini M, Trabace S, Mazzilli M et al 1988 A study of HLA class II antigens in an Italian paediatric population with coeliac disease. Disease Markers 6: 23–28
Morgenstern L, Thompson R, Friedman N B 1977 The modern enigma of radiation enteropathy: sequelae and solutions. American Journal of Surgery 134: 166–172
Morgenstern L, Hart M, Lugo D, Friedman N B 1985 Changing aspects of radiation enteropathy. Archives of Surgery 120: 1225–1228
Mowat A McI 1987 The cellular basis of gastrointestinal immunity. In: Marsh M N (ed) Immunopathology of the small intestine. Wiley, Chichester, p 41
Mowat A McI, Felstein M 1991 Intestinal graft-versus-host reactions in experimental animals. In: Burakoff S J, Ferrar H (eds) Graft-versus-host disease. Dekker, New York, p 205
Mowat A McI, Ferguson A 1982 Intraepithelial lymphocyte count and crypt hyperplasia measure the mucosal component of the graft-versus-host reaction in mouse small intestine. Gastroenterology 83: 417–423
Mylotte M, Egan-Mitchell B, Fottrell P F, McNichol B, McCarthy C F 1974 Family studies in coeliac disease. Quarterly Journal of Medicine 171: 359–369

Neale G, Booth C C 1985 Infiltrative lesions. In: Booth C C, Neale G (eds) Disorders of the small intestine. Blackwell, Oxford, p 128

Newman A, Katsaris J, Blendis L M, Charlesworth M, Walter L H 1973 Small-intestinal injury in women who have had pelvic radiotherapy. Lancet 2: 1471–1473

O'Mahony S, Vestey J P, Ferguson A 1990 Similarities in intestinal humoral immunity in dermatitis herpetiformis without enteropathy and in coeliac disease. Lancet 335: 1487–1490

Paulley J W 1952 A case of Whipple's disease (intestinal lipodystrophy). Gastroenterology 22: 128–133

Paulley J W 1954 Observations on the aetiology of idiopathic steatorrhoea. Jejunal and lymph-node biopsies. British Medical Journal 2: 1318–1321

Pauzner R, Rothman P, Schwartz E, Neumann G, Farfel Z 1992 Acute onset of celiac disease in the puerperium. American Journal of Gastroenterology 87: 1037–1039

Polanco I, Biemond I, van Leeuwen A 1981 Gluten sensitive enteropathy in Spain: genetic and environmental factors In: McConnell R B (ed) Genetics of coeliac disease. MTP, Lancaster, p 211

Quinton W E, Flick A L, Rubin C E 1962 The design of a hydraulic suction tube for peroral biopsy of the human gastrointestinal tract. Gastroenterology 42: 281–284

Relman D A, Schmidt T M, MacDermott R P, Falkow S 1992 Identification of the uncultured bacillus of Whipple's disease. New England Journal of Medicine 327: 293–301

Rhee J W, Gryboski J D, Sheaham D G, Dolan T, Dwyer J M 1975 Reversible enteritis and lymphopenia in infantile X-linked agammaglobulinaemia. American Journal of Digestive Diseases 20: 1071–1075

Robertson D A F, Dixon M F, Scott B B, Simpson F G, Losowsky M S 1983 Small intestinal ulceration: diagnostic difficulties in relation to coeliac disease. Gut 24: 565–574

Rodier J-F, Jansen J-C, Rodier D et al 1991 Prevention of radiation enteritis by an absorbable polyglycolic acid mesh sling. A 60-case multicentric study. Cancer 68: 2545–2549

Roep B O, Bontrop R E, Pena A S, van Eggermond M C, van Rood J, Giphart M J 1988 An HLA-DQ alpha allele identified at DNA and protein level is strongly associated with celiac disease. Human Immunology 23: 271–279

Rolles C J, Myint T D, Sin W K, Anderson C M 1974 Family study of coeliac disease. Gut 15: A827

Rosenberg W M, Wordsworth B P, Jewell D, Bell J 1989 A locus telomeric to HLA-DPß encodes susceptibility to coeliac disease. Immunogenetics 30: 307–310

Ross I 1987 Primary immunodeficiency and the small intestine. In: Marsh M N (ed) Immunopathology of the small intestine. Wiley, Chichester, p 283–332

Ross I, Mathan V I 1981 Immunological changes in tropical sprue. Quarterly Journal of Medicine 50: 435–460

Roswit B, Malsky S J, Reid C B 1972 Severe radiation injuries of the stomach, small intestine, colon and rectum. American Journal of Roentgenology 114: 460–475

Rowe J M, Ciobanu N, Ascensao J et al 1994 Recommended guidelines for the management of autologous and allogeneic bone marrow transplantation. A report from the Eastern Cooperative Oncology Group (ECOG). Annals of Internal Medicine 120: 143–158

Rubin C E, Brandborg L L, Phelps P C, Taylor H C Jr 1960 Studies of celiac disease. I. The apparent identical and specific nature of the duodenal and proximal jejunal lesion in celiac disease and idiopathic sprue. Gastroenterology 38: 28–49

Rubin C E, Brandborg L L, Flick A L, Phelps P C, Parmentier C, van Neil S 1962 Studies of celiac sprue. III The effect of repeated wheat instillation into the proximal ileum of patients on a gluten-free diet. Gastroenterology 43: 621–641

Sagaro E, Jiminez N 1981 Family studies of coeliac disease in Cuba. Archives of Disease in Childhood 56: 132–133

Santiago-Borrero P J, Maldonado N, Horta E 1970 Tropical sprue in children. Journal of Pediatrics 76: 470–479

Saulsbury E T, Winkelstein J A, Yolken R 1980 Chronic rotavirus infection in immunodeficiency. Journal of Pediatrics 97: 61–65

Savilahti E 1981 Cow's milk allergy. Allergy 36: 73–88

Saxon A, Stevens R H, Ashman R F, Parker N H 1977 Dual immune defects in nongranulomatous ulcerative jejunoileitis with hypogammaglobulinemia. Clinical Immunology and Immunopathology 8: 272–279

Schenk E, Samloff I, Klipstein F 1965 Morphologic characteristics of jejunal biopsy in celiac disease and tropical sprue. American Journal of Pathology 47: 765–781

Schenk E, Samloff I, Klipstein F 1968 Morphology of small bowel biopsies. American Journal of Clinical Nutrition 21: 944–961

Schmitt E H, Symmonds R E 1981 Surgical treatment of radiation induced injuries of the intestine. Surgery, Gynecology and Obstetrics 153: 896–900

Scientific Group on Immunodeficiency 1983 Primary immunodeficiency diseases. Clinical Immunology and Immunopathology 28: 450–475

Scott B B, Losowsky M S 1976 Peroral small-intestinal biopsy: experience with the hydraulic multiple biopsy instrument in routine clinical practice. Gut 17: 740–743

Scott B B, Losowsky M S 1977 Coeliac disease with mild mucosal abnormalities: a report of four patients. Postgraduate Medical Journal 53: 134–138

Scott B B, Hardy G J, Losowsky M S 1975 Involvement of the small intestine in systemic mast cell disease. Gut 16: 918–924

Seliger G, Krassner R L, Beranbaum E R, Miller F 1971 The spectrum of roentgen appearance in amyloidosis of the small and large bowel: radiologic-pathologic correlation. Radiology 100: 63

Sheehy T 1964 Intestinal biopsy. Lancet 1: 959–962

Sheehy T W, Baggs B, Perez-Santiago E, Floch M H 1962 Prognosis of tropical sprue. A study of the effect of folic acid on the intestinal aspects of acute and chronic sprue. Annals of Internal Medicine 57: 892–908

Shewry P R, Tatham A S, Kasarda D D 1992 Cereal proteins and coeliac disease. In: Marsh M N (ed) Coeliac disease. Blackwell, Oxford, p 305

Shiner M, Doniach I 1960 Histopathologic studies in steatorrhea. Gastroenterology 38: 419–440

Shipman R T, Williams A L, Day R, Townley R R W 1975 A family study of coeliac disease. Australian and New Zealand Journal of Medicine 5: 250–255

Sieracki J C, Fine G 1959 Whipple's disease – observations on systemic involvement. II. Gross and histologic observations. Archives of Pathology 67: 81–93

Sissons J G P, Peters D K, Williams D G, Boulton-Jones J M, Goldsmith H J 1974 Skin lesions, angioedema and hypocomplement-aemia. Lancet 2: 1350

Sloper K S, Dourmashkin R R, Bird R B, Slavin G, Webster A D B 1982 Chronic malabsorption due to cryptosporidiosis in a child with immunoglobulin deficiency. Gut 23: 80–82

Sollid L M, Thorsby E 1993 HLA susceptibility genes in celiac disease: genetic mapping and role in pathogenesis. Gastroenterology 105: 910–922

Sollid L M, Markussen G, Ek J, Gjerde H, Vartdal F, Thorsby E 1989 Evidence for a primary association of celiac disease to a particular HLA-DQ alpha/beta heterodimer. Journal of Experimental Medicine 169: 345–350

Soter N A, Austin K F, Wasserman S I 1979 Oral disodium cromoglycate in the treatment of systemic mastocytosis. New England Journal of Medicine 301: 465–468

Spector B D, Perry G S, Kersey J H 1978 Genetically-determined immunodeficiency diseases (GDID) and malignancy. Clinical and Immunological Immunopathology 11: 12–29

Spies T, Milanes F, Menendez A 1946 Observations on treatment of tropical sprue with folic acid. Journal of Laboratory and Clinical Medicine 31: 227–241

Stephan J, Vlekova V, Le Deist F et al 1993 Severe combined immunodeficiency: A retrospective single-center study of clinical presentation and outcome in 117 patients. Journal of Pediatrics 123: 564–572

Stokes P L, Ferguson R, Holmes G K T, Cooke W T 1976a Familial aspects of coeliac disease. Quarterly Journal of Medicine 180: 567–582

Stokes P L, Prior P, Sorahan T M, McWalter R J, Waterhouse J A H, Cooke W T 1976b Malignancy in relatives of patients with coeliac disease. British Journal of Preventative Social Medicine 30: 17–21

Sullivan P B, Marsh M N, Mirakian R, Hill S M, Milla P J, Neale G 1991 Chronic diarrhea and malnutrition – histology of the small intestinal lesion. Journal of Pediatric Gastroenterology and Nutrition 12: 195–203

Sullivan P B, Lunn P G, Northrop-Clewes C, Crowe P T, Marsh M N, Neale G 1992 Persistent diarrhea and malnutrition – the impact of treatment on small bowel structure and permeability. Journal of Pediatric Gastroenterology and Nutrition 14: 205–215

Swanson V, Thomassen R 1965 Pathology of the jejunal mucosa in tropical sprue. American Journal of Pathology 46: 511–551

Swinson C M, Slavin G, Coles E C, Booth C C 1983 Coeliac disease and malignancy. Lancet 1: 111–115

Trier J S, Browning T H 1966 Morphologic response of the mucosa of human small intestine to X-ray exposure. Journal of Clinical Investigation 45: 194–204

Trier J S, Browning T H 1970 Epithelial-cell renewal in cultured duodenal biopsies in celiac sprue. New England Journal of Medicine 283: 1245–1364

Trier J S, Phelps P C, Eidelman S, Rubin C E 1965 Whipple's disease: light and electron microscope correlation of jejunal mucosal histology with antibiotic treatment and clinical status. Gastroenterology 48: 384–407

Tytgat G 1976 Risks of small bowel biopsy techniques. Scandinavian Journal of Gastroenterology 12 (suppl 47): 18–24

Udall J N, Walker W A 1987 Mucosal defence mechanisms. In: Marsh M N (ed) Immunopathology of the small intestine. Wiley, Chichester, p 3

Uibo O, Uibo R, Kleimola V, Jogi T, Mäki M 1993 Serum IgA anti-gliadin antibodies in an adult population sample. High prevalence without celiac disease. Digestive Diseases and Sciences 38: 2034–2037

Underdown B, Schiff J 1986 Immunoglobulin A: strategic defense initiative at the mucosal surface. Annual Reviews in Immunology 4: 389–417

Upton A C 1952 Histochemical investigation of the mesenchymal lesions in Whipple's disease. American Journal of Clinical Pathology 22: 755–764

Van Bergeijk J D, Meijer J W R, Mulder C C 1993a Endoscopic abnormalities in patients screened for coeliac disease. Journal of Clinical Nutrition and Gastroenterology 8: 136–139

Van Bergeijk J, Mulder C, Thies J 1993b Coeliac disease. Three cases delayed after a sojourn in the tropics. Netherlands Journal of Medicine 43: 222–226

Van de Kamer J H, Weijers H A, Dicke W K 1953 Coeliac disease. IV An investigation into the injurious constituents of wheat in connection with their actions on patients with coeliac disease. Acta Paediatrica Scandinavica 42: 223–231

Van Nagell J R, Maruyama Y, Parker J C, Dalton W L 1974 Small bowel injury following radiation therapy for cervical cancer. American Journal of Obstetrics and Gynecology 118: 163–167

Viney J, MacDonald T T, Spencer J 1990 Gamma/delta T cells in gut epithelium. Gut 31: 841–844

Walker-Smith J 1980 Toddler's diarrhoea. Archives of Disease in Childhood 55: 329

Walker-Smith J 1988 Diseases of the small intestine in childhood, 3rd edn. Butterworth, London

Warin A P, Greaves M W, Gatecliff M, Williamson D, Warin R P 1980 Treatment of hereditary angioedema by low dose attenuated androgens. British Journal of Dermatology 103: 405–409

Warren S, Friedman N B 1942 Pathology and pathological diagnosis of radiation lesions in the gastrointestinal tract. American Journal of Pathology 18: 499–513

Warren S L, Whipple G H 1922 Roentgen ray intoxication. Journal of Experimental Medicine 35: 187–202

Watson M R 1963 Primary nonspecific ulceration of the small bowel. Archives of Surgery 87: 600

Watson A J, Wright N A 1974 Morphology and cell kinetics of the jejunal mucosa in untreated patients. Clinics in Gastroenterology 3: 11–31

Wayte D M, Helwig E B 1968 Small-bowel ulceration – iatrogenic or multifactorial origin? American Journal of Clinical Pathology 49: 26–40

Webster A D B 1980 Giardiasis and immunodeficiency disease. Transactions of the Royal Society of Tropical Medicine and Hygiene 74: 440–443

Webster A D B, Slavin G, Shiner M, Platts-Mills T A E, Asherson G L 1981 Coeliac disease with severe hypogammaglobulinaemia. Gut 22: 153–157

Weinstein W M 1974 Latent celiac sprue. Gastroenterology 66: 489–493

Wellcome Trust Collaborative Study (1961–1969) 1971 Tropical sprue and megaloblastic anaemia. Churchill Livingstone, Edinburgh

Whipple G H 1907 A hitherto undescribed disease characterized anatomically by deposits of fat and fatty acids in the intestinal and mesenteric lymphatic tissues. Bulletin of the Johns Hopkins Hospital 18: 382–391

Wiernik G 1966 Radiation damage and repair in the human jejunal mucosa. Journal of Pathology 91: 389–393

Wilson K H, Blitchington R, Frothingham R, Wilson J A P 1991 Phylogeny of the Whipple's-disease-associated bacterium. Lancet 338: 474–475

Wright D H, Isaacson P G 1989 Gut associated lymphoid tumours. In: Whitehead R (ed) Gastrointestinal and oesophageal pathology, Churchill Livingstone, Edinburgh, p 643

Yadav M, Iyngkaran N 1981 Immunological studies in cow's milk protein sensitive enteropathy. Archives of Disease in Childhood 56: 24–30

Yeoh E K, Horowitz M 1987 Radiation enteritis. Surgery, Gynecology and Obstetrics 165: 373–379

Zighelboim J, Carpenter H A, Talley N J 1993 A patient with diarrhea, arthralgias, and fever. Gastroenterology 105: 923–930

Zimmerman J, Gati I, Eisenberg S, Rachmilewitz D 1986 Ethanol inhibits triglyceride synthesis and secretion by human small intestinal mucosa. Journal of Laboratory and Clinical Medicine 107: 498–501

# 15. Gastric and intestinal motility disorders

*M. Horowitz    M. Camilleri*

## GASTRIC MOTILITY DISORDERS

The application of novel techniques to evaluate gastric motor function in humans has demonstrated that abnormal gastric motility is a frequent and clinically important problem. Abnormal gastroduodenal motility may result in delayed or, less frequently, excessively rapid emptying of the stomach. Gastroparesis can be defined as delayed gastric emptying resulting from disordered motility, rather than gastric outlet or proximal small intestinal obstruction; 30–50% of those patients who have chronic unexplained upper abdominal symptoms or long-standing diabetes mellitus have gastric stasis. Disordered gastroduodenal motility may be associated with upper gastrointestinal symptoms, altered oral drug absorption and, in patients with diabetes mellitus, poor control of blood glucose concentrations. However, there is a poor correlation between the presence of symptoms such as nausea and early satiety and abnormal gastric emptying. The mechanism(s) by which disordered motility causes symptoms are still poorly understood. In this chapter current knowledge of the etiology, pathophysiology, investigation and treatment of disordered gastric and intestinal motor function in humans is discussed.

### NORMAL GASTRIC MOTOR FUNCTION

Gastric emptying is a complex process which involves storage of ingesta, mixing with gastric secretions, grinding of solid food into small particles and delivery of chyme into the small intestine at a rate designed to optimize digestion and absorption. The mechanical factors by which the stomach moves its contents into the small intestine are incompletely understood, largely because of the technical difficulties associated with the investigation of human gastric motility; many studies have attempted to define the role of individual motor components, such as the antrum, in an integrated system, whereas few studies have related patterns of gastroduodenal motility to simultaneously measured gastric emptying or transpyloric flow (Horowitz & Dent 1994). Most liquified chyme is propelled into the duodenum as a series of small gushes (Fig. 15.1); that is, gastric emptying is predominantly pulsatile, rather than continuous (King et al 1984, Malbert & Ruckebusch 1991). The duration and volume of individual flow pulses vary considerably from one cycle to the next – forward, interrupted and reverse flow may all occur. Furthermore, no motor component should be considered to exert the dominant control over normal gastric emptying (Heddle et al 1993).

#### The proximal stomach

During swallowing there is a transient receptive relaxation of the proximal region of the stomach (comprising the fundus and upper body), followed by a prolonged relaxation known as accommodation, so that meal ingestion is not usually associated with a substantial rise in intragastric pressure. Proximal gastric tone is neurally modulated with cholinergic stimuli causing increased tone and nonadren-

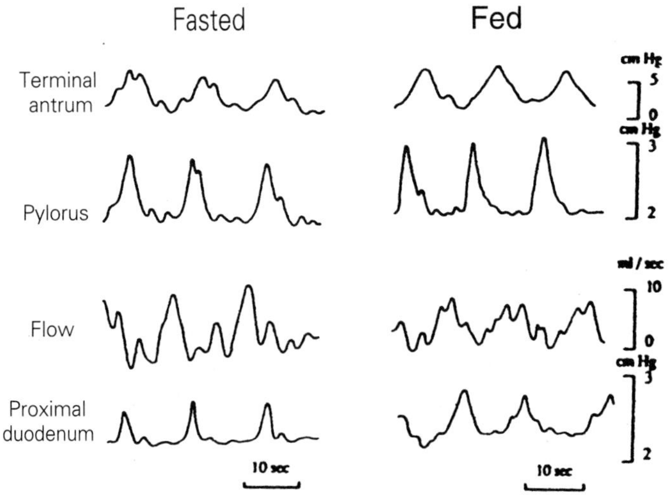


**Fig. 15.1** Antroduodenal pressures and transpyloric flow in the dog measured in the fasted and fed states. Flow, recorded with an electromagnetic flow-meter probe positioned in the duodenal bulb, is predominantly pulsatile rather than continuous (from Malbert & Ruckebusch 1991).

ergic, noncholinergic stimuli inducing relaxation (Azpiroz & Malagelada 1987). During emptying of a meal from the stomach there is a gradual increase in proximal stomach tone, which favors the delivery of ingesta into the distal stomach. Following ingestion of a solid–liquid meal solid food is retained predominantly in the proximal stomach until the majority (~80%) of the liquid has emptied (Houghton et al 1988). This storage contributes to the lag phase of up to 60 min before solids begin to empty from the stomach.

### The distal stomach

The contractions of the distal stomach, consisting of the lower body, antrum and pylorus, are controlled by electrical signals generated by a pacemaker region located on the greater curvature. The gastric pacemaker discharges at a rate of about 3 per min (Kelly 1980) and these electrical potentials are propagated towards the pylorus. Whether this electrical activity results in a contraction or not is determined by the interaction of neural and, possibly, hormonal inputs. While the onset of the majority of contractions follows a peristaltic pattern, the onset of contraction-induced lumen occlusion is rarely peristaltic, unlike the esophagus. Patterns of lumen occlusion are of major importance in determining flow, because when the lumen is occluded neither antegrade nor retrograde flow can occur. The characteristics of both fasting and fed lumen-occlusive antral pressure waves – extent, amplitude and timing of onset – are extremely variable (Sun et al 1993).

Normal fasting antral motility consists of three phases which have a cycle time of about 100 min: phase 1 – motor quiescence, phase 2 – irregular contractions, and phase 3 – regular high amplitude contractions at the maximal rate of about 3 per min for about 5 min (Wingate 1981). The latter move towards the distal small intestine to reach the terminal ileum in about 3 h. About 20% of phase 3 episodes commence in the small intestine and do not involve the stomach. Fasting antral motor activity is not interrupted by the intake of small volumes (<150 ml) of nonnutrient liquids (including tablets and capsules) (Oberle et al 1990). Gastric emptying of larger (>5 mm) nondigestible solids occurs predominantly during phase 3. Antral contractions play the major role in grinding digestible solids into small particles (<1 mm in size). Contractions localized to the pylorus occur over a narrow zone (~4 mm) and regulate transpyloric flow by acting as a brake (Heddle et al 1988, Tougas et al 1992).

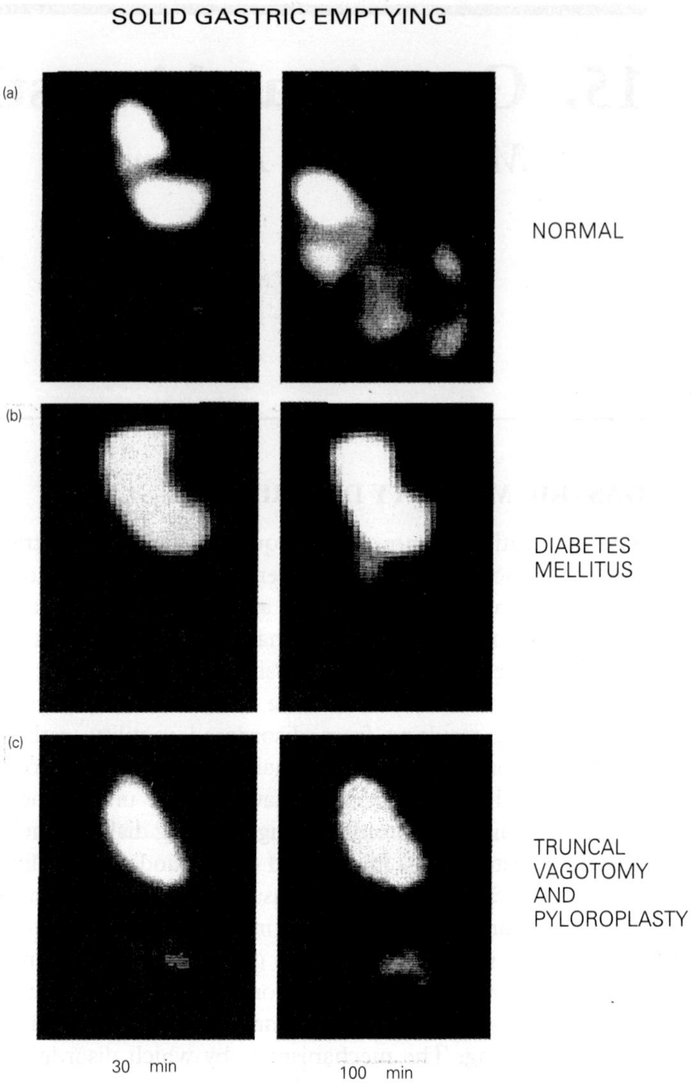


**Fig. 15.2** Scintiphotographs showing the abdominal distribution of radioactivity after ingestion of a mixed solid (100 g minced beef containing chicken liver labeled with $^{99m}$Tc sulfur colloid) and liquid (150 ml of 10% dextrose labeled with $^{113m}$In DTPA) meal in the seated position in (a) a normal volunteer, (b) a diabetic patient with symptoms of nausea and vomiting who had a normal barium meal study and (c) a patient with symptoms of "dumping" 2 years after truncal vagotomy and pyloroplasty. For commentary on findings refer to Fig. 15.3 (from Horowitz & Dent 1991).

### Patterns of gastric emptying of solids and liquids

Solids, nutrient-liquids and nonnutrient liquids empty from the stomach at different rates and patterns (Fig. 15.2). The overall gastric emptying rate of digestible solids is characterized by a lag phase before emptying commences, when food moves from the proximal into the distal stomach and is ground into small particles, followed by an emptying phase that approximates a linear pattern (Fig. 15.2 and 15.3) (Collins et al 1983, Lin et al 1992). A major factor controlling gastric emptying of nutrient liquids and "liquified" solids is feedback from receptors in the small intestinal lumen (Horowitz & Dent 1991, Edelbroek et al 1994). There are "specific" small intestinal chemoreceptors for carbohydrate, fatty acids, amino acids and $H^+$ (Cooke 1977, Lin et al 1989, 1990a & b), with substantial variations in receptor number and type between the duodenum, jejunum and ileum. The extent of

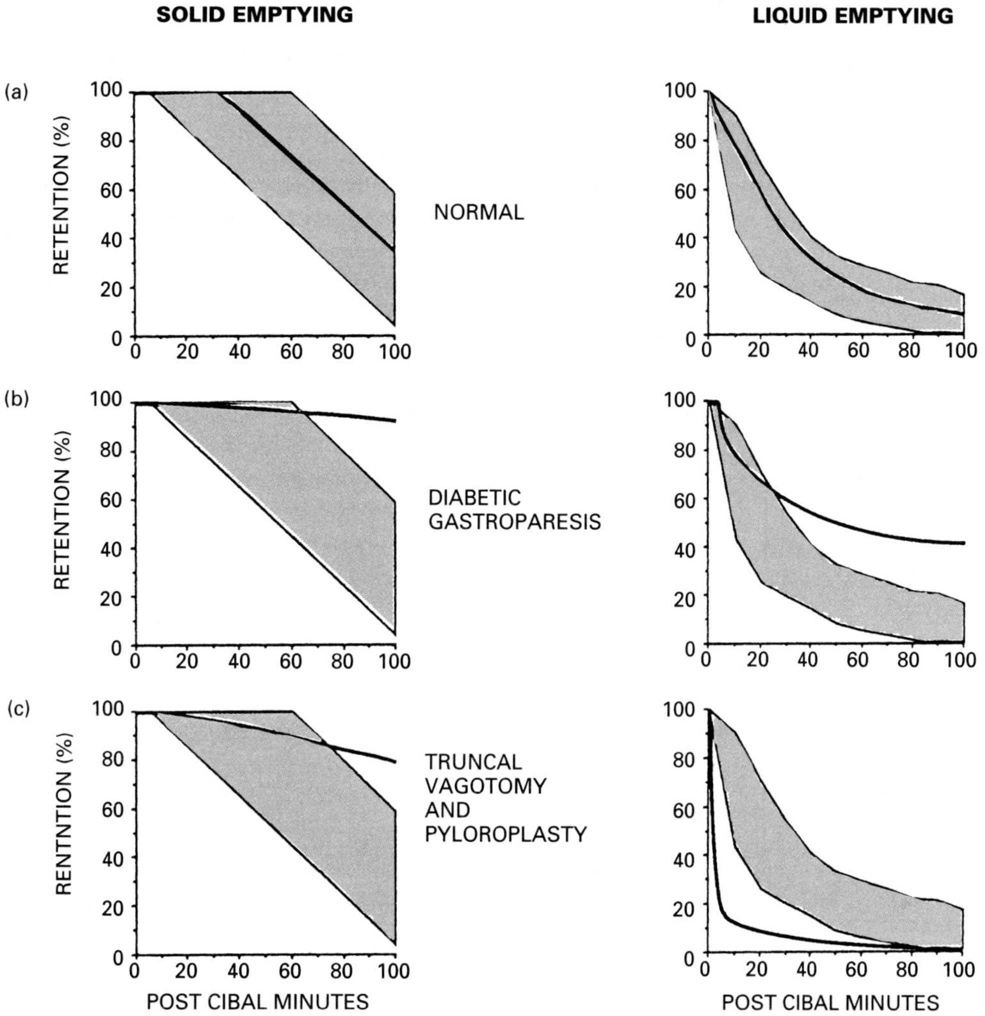


**Fig. 15.3** Gastric emptying curves for a mixed solid (100 g minced beef) and liquid (150 ml 10% dextrose) meal consumed in the sitting position in a (a) a normal subject, (b) a diabetic patient with gastroparesis and (c) a patient after truncal vagotomy with pyloroplasty. The normal range for gastric emptying (mean ± 2 SD) is shown in the shaded areas. In the normal subject gastric emptying of minced beef is characterized by a lag phase, followed by a linear emptying phase, while emptying of dextrose is faster than minced beef and in a nonlinear pattern. There is a marked delay of solid and liquid emptying in the diabetic patient. After truncal vagotomy and pyloroplasty, the initial emptying rate of liquid is very rapid, while there is an overall delay in solid emptying (from Horowitz & Dent 1991).

small intestinal feedback inhibition is dependent on both the number and site of the receptors which are exposed (Lin et al 1989, 1990a & b) and mediated by both neural and hormonal (such as cholecystokinin) mechanisms. Nutrient liquids normally empty from the stomach at an overall linear rate of about 2 kcal/min (Brener et al 1983). Feedback from small intestinal chemoreceptors can be influenced by patterns of prior nutrient intake. For example, dietary supplementation with glucose or fat is associated with more rapid gastric emptying of glucose (Cunningham et al 1991a) and fat (Cunningham et al 1991b) respectively. Volume and gravity are the major determinants of emptying of low nutrient liquids which empty from the stomach in a monoexponential pattern.

### Motor mechanisms controlling gastric emptying

The motor mechanisms which regulate gastric emptying are complex. Pulses of transpyloric flow appear to be generated primarily by antropyloric and body contractions (Malbert et al 1992). Variability of transpyloric flow patterns appears to result from changes in the temporal and spatial patterning of tone and active lumen occlusion, as well as the strength of contractions, in different regions of the stomach and small intestine. In most cases stimuli which influence gastric emptying act on multiple motor components. For example, infusion of nutrients into the small intestine is associated with a decrease in fundic tone (Azpiroz & Malagelada 1985), suppression of phasic antral pressure waves and stimulation of pressure waves which are localized to the pylorus (Heddle et al 1989) (Fig. 15.4). Gastric emptying is most rapid when contractions in the antrum, pylorus and duodenum produce sequential lumen occlusion (Fraser et al 1992, Tack et al 1992). Nonlumen occlusive gastric wall movements may also have a major impact on gastric emptying (Horowitz & Dent 1994). The stomach is capable of considerable compensation before the overall rate of emptying, as opposed to the characteristics of individual flow pulses, is modified substantially (Malbert & Mathis 1994). In general, provided that small intestinal feedback is intact, the elimination of individual motor components does not prevent the slowing of emptying by nutrients.

## PREVALENCE AND ETIOLOGY OF DISORDERED GASTRIC MOTILITY

Abnormally slow stomach emptying may result from impaired myogenic, intrinsic or extrinsic neural (including gastric electrical activity) or hormonal control mechanisms or increased small intestinal feedback. While defective motor control could result in weak pumping, delay in gastric emptying could also reflect an increased resistance to

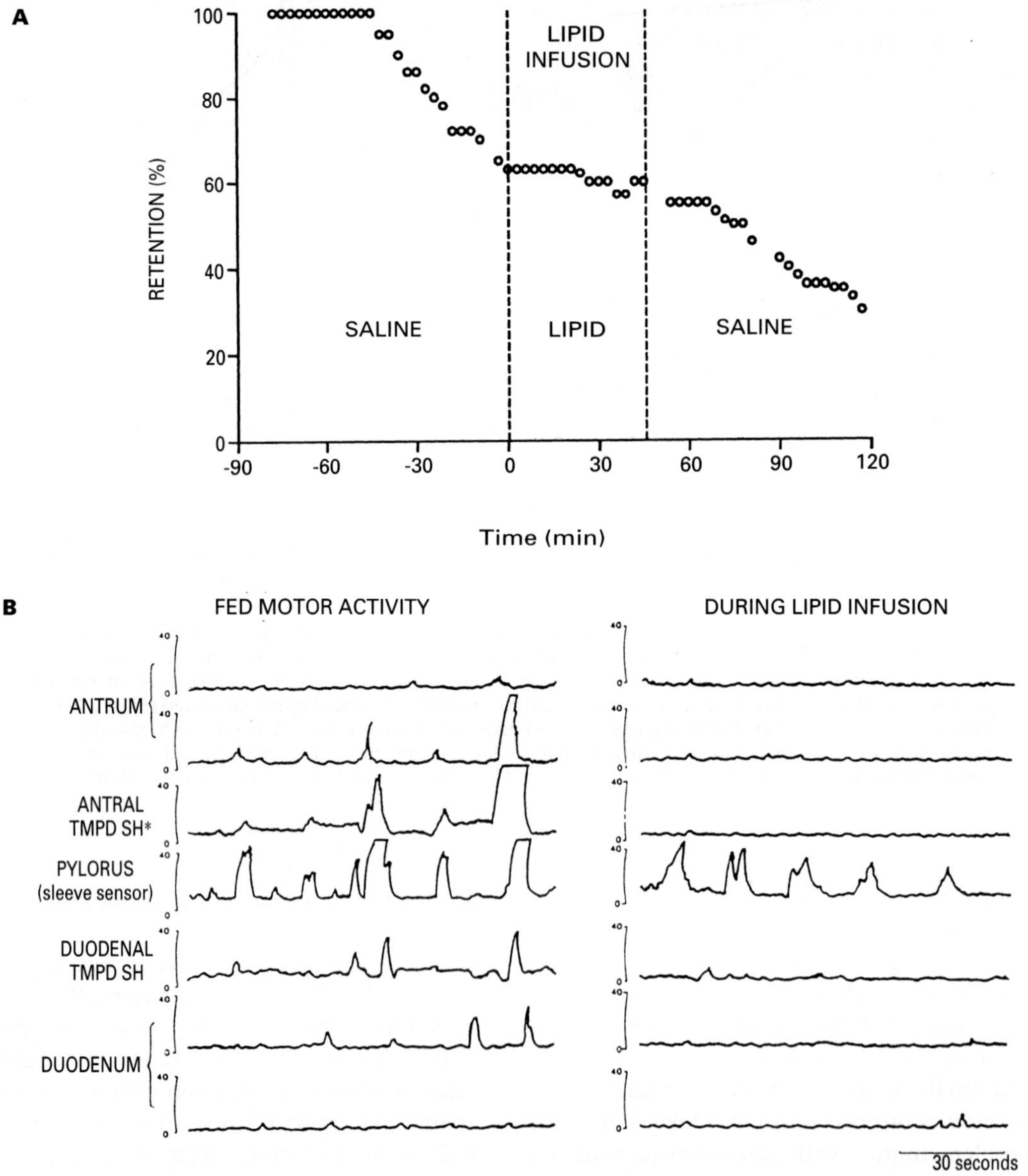


**Fig. 15.4** Effects of an intraduodenal triglyceride infusion (Intralipid 10%, 1 ml/min for 45 min) on **A** gastric emptying of a solid meal and **B** antropyloroduodenal motility in a normal subject. The lipid infusion slows gastric emptying and this retardation is associated with stimulation of pressure waves localized to the pylorus and suppression of antral pressure waves. Pyloric pressures are recorded with a sleeve sensor. The position of the sleeve sensor is monitored by measurement of the antroduodenal transmucosal potential difference (TMPD) gradient (from Heddle et al 1989).

outflow, i.e. contractions which display a disordered organization. Disordered gastric motility is usually diagnosed by measurement of gastric emptying. The prevalence of abnormal gastric emptying presumably represents an underestimate of the prevalence of disordered gastroduodenal motility.

## Causes of gastroparesis

Gastroparesis may be acute or chronic (arbitrarily defined as lasting more than 3 months) and there may sometimes be a combination of acute and chronic dysfunctions. There are many causes of gastric stasis (Table 15.1). Common causes of acute gastroparesis include drugs and electrolyte disturbances. Cigarette smoking slows gastric emptying (Johnson et al 1991). In patients with diabetes mellitus gastric emptying is slower during hyperglycemia (~15 mmol/L) when compared to euglycemia (Fraser et al 1990) and accelerated during hypoglycemia (Schvarcz et al 1993). The most common causes of chronic gastroparesis are idiopathic (often presenting as "nonulcer" or "functional" dyspepsia (Waldron et al 1991, Scott et al 1993)) and associated with diabetes mellitus (Horowitz et al 1991) where there is a prevalence of 30–50% (Fig. 15.5). Idiopathic gastroparesis occurs most frequently in young (<40 yr) females (Tucci et al 1992). There is little evidence of acid secretory abnormalities in patients with "nonulcer" dyspepsia (Waldron et al 1991). Delay in gastric emptying, like cardiovascular autonomic impairment, is not inevitably a "late" complication of diabetes (Horowitz & Fraser 1994). Chronic gastroparesis is a frequent accompaniment of diseases which cause motor dysfunction throughout the gastrointestinal tract, such as progressive systemic sclerosis. It is therefore not uncommon for patients with gastroparesis to have abnormal

**Table 15.1** Etiology of gastroparesis

| |
|---|
| *Transient delayed gastric emptying* |
| Postoperative ileus |
| Acute viral gastroenteritis |
| Hyperglycemia |
| Hypokalemia |
| Hypothyroidism |
| Drugs: morphine, anticholinergics, levodopa, β-adrenergic agonists, nicotine |
| Stress: labrynthine stimulation, cold pain |
| *Chronic gastric stasis* |
| Idiopathic ("nonulcer" or "functional" dyspepsia) |
| Diabetes mellitus |
| Postsurgical: postvagotomy |
| Gastroesophageal reflux disease |
| Anorexia nervosa |
| Progressive systemic sclerosis |
| Chronic idiopathic intestinal pseudo-obstruction |
| Amyloidosis |
| Myotonia dystrophica |
| Dermatomyositis |
| Autonomic degeneration |
| Brain-stem tumor |
| Spinal cord injury |
| Tumor associated (carcinoma lung, pancreas) |
| Postirradiation |
| Porphyria |
| Neurofibromatosis |
| Ischemic |

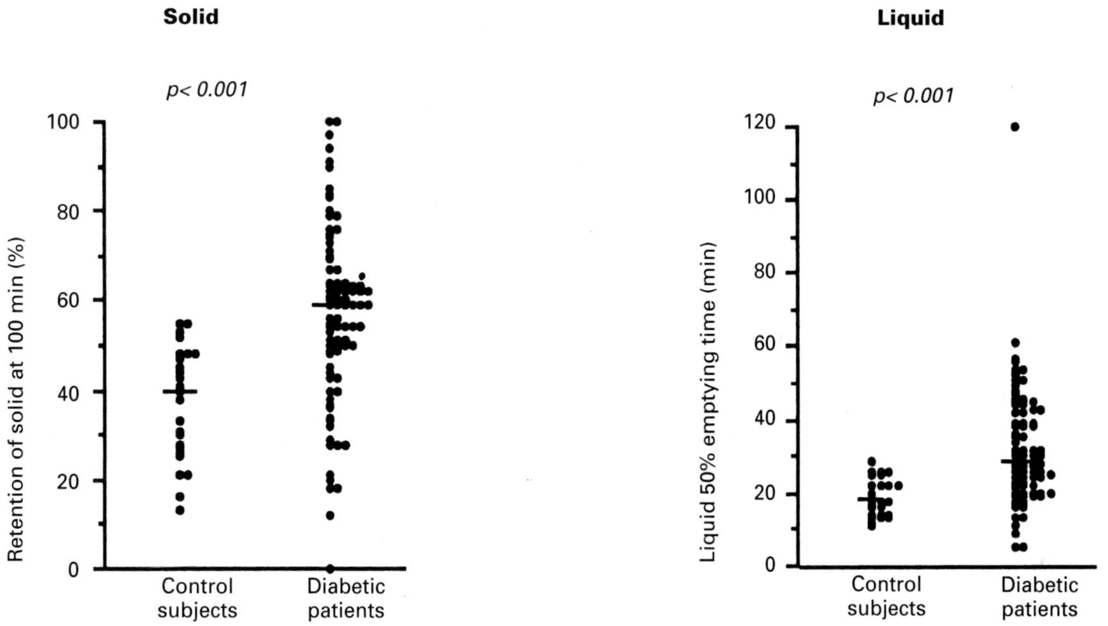


**Fig. 15.5** Gastric emptying expressed as the amount of solid (100 g minced beef) remaining in the stomach at 100 min after meal completion and the 50% emptying time for liquid (150 ml 10% dextrose) in 87 randomly selected outpatients with diabetes mellitus (67 insulin-dependent; 20 noninsulin-dependent) and 25 normal volunteers. Horizontal lines represent median values (from Horowitz et al 1991).

motility in the esophagus, small intestine, colon or anorectum (Camilleri et al 1986a). Gastroparesis occurs in about 40% of patients with gastroesophageal reflux disease, but the delay in gastric emptying is usually not marked and its significance is uncertain (Cunningham et al 1991c). Infection with *Helicobacter pylori* does not cause delayed gastric emptying and patients with dyspepsia who are *H. pylori*-positive may be less likely to have gastroparesis (Tucci et al 1992). Gastric emptying is delayed in many patients with primary anorexia nervosa (Stacher et al 1987). Gastroparesis may be a complication of malignancy, i.e. in the absence of gastric or intestinal obstruction. Tumor-associated gastroparesis occurs frequently in association with carcinomas of the pancreas and lung.

### Causes of rapid gastric emptying

For practical purposes abnormally rapid gastric emptying is usually only important following gastric surgery (Table 15.2). In patients with duodenal ulceration or the Zollinger–Ellison syndrome, gastric emptying is often rapid, but there is considerable overlap with normal values. "Early" noninsulin-dependent diabetes may be associated with more rapid emptying of nutrient liquids (Phillips et al 1992). Exocrine pancreatic insufficiency is associated with faster gastric emptying of fat which may contribute to malabsorption (Carney et al 1995). Because fats must be hydrolyzed to fatty acids in order to slow gastric emptying, this acceleration is likely to reflect a reduction in small intestinal feedback regulation.

### Pathophysiology of gastroparesis

#### *Neural and myogenic abnormalities*

Many gastric motility disorders result from defects in intrinsic (myenteric) or extrinsic (parasympathetic and sympathetic) neural innervation, although in many cases a neurological disorder is not obvious (Bharucha et al 1993). For example, patients with functional (nonulcer) dyspepsia (Greydanus et al 1991) and gastroesophageal reflux disease (Cunningham et al 1991c) often have evidence of autonomic nerve dysfunction on specific testing. Although diabetic gastroparesis has been attributed to vagal damage, earlier descriptions of vagal segmental demyelination (Smith 1974) have not been confirmed in more recent studies (Yoshida et al 1988). Because the blood glucose concentration influences gastric motor function in diabetes, in some cases of diabetic gastroparesis delay in gastric emptying may be due to hyperglycemia and, hence, be reversible (Horowitz & Fraser 1994). Abnormalities of the myenteric plexus have been demonstrated in some patients with intestinal pseudo-obstruction (Krishnamurthy & Schuffler 1987). In most patients with gastroparesis presumed to result from viral infections the pathogenesis has not been defined, but intranuclear inclusion bodies have been demonstrated after cytomegalovirus infection (Sonsino et al 1984). A lymphocytic infiltration of the myenteric plexus is often evident in gastroparesis associated with paraneoplastic syndromes (Schuffler et al 1983) and in some trials a specific antibody directed against neural components of the myenteric plexus can be demonstrated (Lennon et al 1991). In some patients with gastroparesis, gastric pacemaker activity is abnormal (You et al 1981).

**Table 15.2** Etiology of rapid gastric emptying

| |
|---|
| Postgastric surgery |
| Pancreatic exocrine insufficiency |
| Zollinger–Ellison syndrome |
| Duodenal ulcer disease |
| Diabetes mellitus |

Myogenic abnormalities are important in only a minority of patients with gastroparesis. In Duchenne muscular dystrophy and myotonic dystrophy, there is replacement of smooth muscle by connective tissue (Bahron et al 1988). In polymyositis and dermatomyositis, gastric smooth muscle dysfunction appears to be due to lymphocytic infiltration, atrophy and, ultimately, fibrosis of muscle fibers (Horowitz et al 1986). Infiltration of smooth muscle and autonomic nerves by amyloid is well recognized in systemic amyloidosis. Replacement of smooth muscle fibers with collagen occurs in patients with progressive systemic sclerosis, but the motility disturbances in this condition may also reflect neuropathic changes (Greydanus & Camilleri 1989).

#### *Hormones*

Hypothyroidism is associated with delayed gastric emptying. Otherwise it is uncertain whether hormonal changes contribute to abnormal gastric motility. For example, an increase in plasma motilin has been reported in patients with gastroparesis (Achem-Karam et al 1985), but this has not been a consistent observation (Tack et al 1992).

#### *Sensory dysfunction*

Gastroparesis has been traditionally considered to reflect "pump" failure. However, slow gastric emptying could result from sensory dysfunction – in particular, a defect in the signalling process from small intestinal receptors leading to inappropriate retardation of gastric emptying (Read & Houghton 1989). This hypothesis, whilst interesting, remains unproven. In many patients with anorexia nervosa delayed gastric emptying improves with the commencement of oral renutrition (Rigaud et al 1988) and may therefore reflect excessive small intestinal feedback as an adaptive response to nutrient deprivation.

*Motor dysfunctions*

Gastroparesis may theoretically result from defective mechanical breakdown of food, ineffective propulsion of intragastric content or an abnormally high resistance to emptying. In view of the incomplete understanding of the mechanisms which underlie normal gastric emptying, it is not surprising that knowledge of the dysfunctions responsible for delayed gastric emptying is even more limited. In particular, there is considerable uncertainty about the relative contribution of regional abnormalities of motor function to disordered emptying. The emphasis of most studies has been on antral motor function. Most investigators have assumed that gastroparesis reflects reduced motility. The possibility that delay in gastric emptying could result from disordered sequencing of contractions has largely been ignored because the technologies required to evaluate the organization of contractions have only recently become available. Furthermore, many studies have been performed in patients who were assumed to have gastroparesis on the basis of symptoms, but in whom measurement of gastric emptying was not performed. It now appears that gastroparesis arises from a heterogeneous mix of motor dysfunctions, which is not surprising given the diverse etiologies of delayed gastric emptying, and that abnormal organization of gastropyloroduodenal motility is important in some cases (Horowitz & Dent 1994).

There is little information about proximal stomach motor function in patients with gastroparesis. Patients with postsurgical gastroparesis often have a dilated gastric remnant with a reduced contractile response to distention (Azpiroz & Malagelada 1987). Proximal gastric tone is abnormal in some patients with nonulcer dyspepsia (Scott et al 1993, Troncon et al 1994) and diabetes mellitus (Oliveira et al 1984). Both fasting and postprandial antral hypomotility occur frequently in gastroparesis, being reported in nonulcer dyspepsia (Labo et al 1986), as well as gastroparesis associated with truncal vagotomy (Malagelada et al 1980), gastroesophageal reflux disease (Behar & Ramsby 1978), progressive systemic sclerosis (Bortolotti et al 1991), anorexia nervosa (Stacher et al 1987) and diabetes mellitus (Camilleri & Malagelada 1984) (Fig. 15.6). In the fasted state antral phase 3 activity is absent or diminished in frequency in many patients with gastroparesis (Labo et al 1986) and suppressed dur-

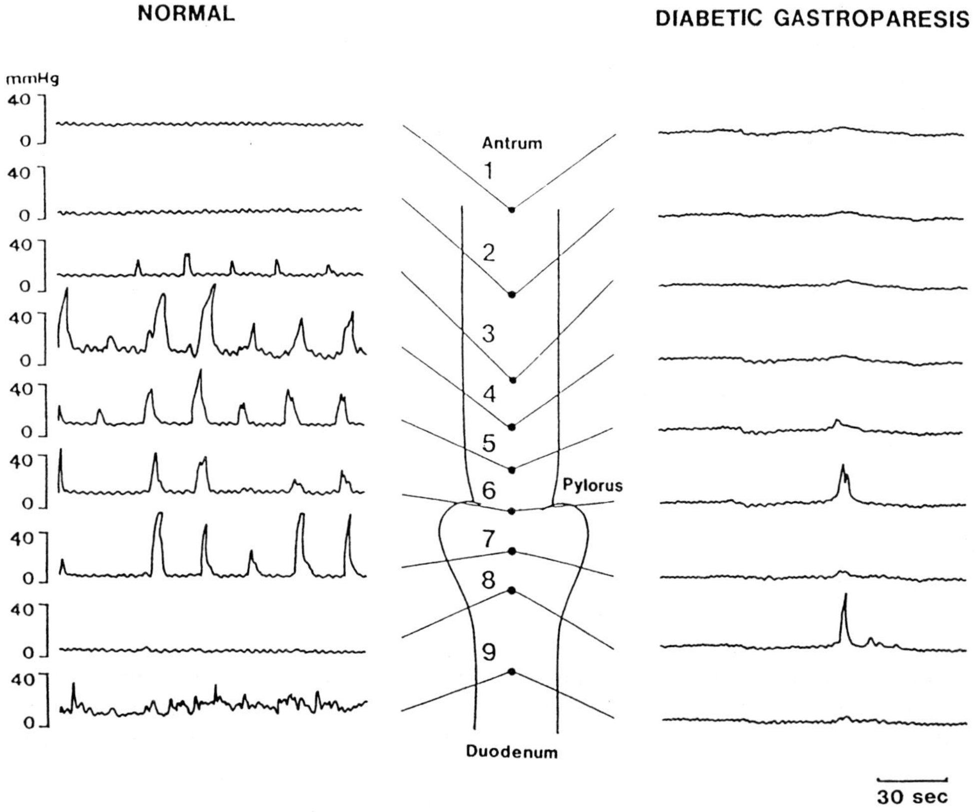


**Fig. 15.6** Manometric recording of pressures in the antrum, pylorus and duodenum after ingestion of a solid (minced beef) meal in a normal volunteer (*left*) and a diabetic patient with gastroparesis (*right*). In the normal volunteer there are a number of antral pressure waves. In the diabetic patient there is antral hypomotility. The position of the manometric sideholds (spaced at 1–2 cm intervals) used to record antral, pyloric and duodenal pressures is shown (from Horowitz & Dent 1991).

ing hyperglycemia (Barnett & Owyang 1988). As antral phase 3 activity is associated with expulsion of nondigestible food residues into the small intestine, a reduction in this activity may contribute to bezoar formation and delayed absorption of tablets or capsules which are not degraded in the stomach.

In some patients, the frequency of postprandial antral contractions is normal, but there is a reduction in the number of antral pressure waves which are temporally associated with duodenal pressure waves (Fraser et al 1993). Ultrasonographic studies have shown that, as a group, patients with nonulcer dyspepsia have a wider antrum, both fasting and postprandially, than healthy subjects (Hausken et al 1994), suggesting that antral tone is reduced in these patients. An increased frequency of phasic and tonic pressure waves localized to the pylorus has been reported in diabetic patients with nausea and vomiting (Mearin et al 1986), but pyloric pressures were evaluated by a suboptimal technique. Furthermore hyperglycemia, per se, stimulates pyloric motility (Fraser et al 1991) and blood glucose concentrations were not monitored in this study. A recent report suggests that an increased frequency of pyloric contractions is not a major factor contributing to retardation of transpyloric flow in diabetic patients (at least during euglycemia) and in other forms of gastroparesis (Fraser et al 1993). A number of motor abnormalities of the proximal small intestine occur in patients with gastroparesis which may contribute to delayed emptying. It has been suggested that disordered small intestinal motility retards the emptying phase, rather than the lag phase, of a solid meal (Camilleri et al 1986b).

## Clinical features

The potential clinical consequences of disordered gastric motility are upper gastrointestinal symptoms, impaired control of blood glucose concentrations and altered oral drug absorption.

### *Gastrointestinal symptoms*

Although some patients with gastric stasis are asymptomatic, many suffer from severe symptoms including nausea, vomiting, abdominal pain, bloating and early satiety. Symptoms are usually most marked postprandially. Vomiting of large volumes many hours after eating is strongly suggestive of gastroparesis. Physical examination is usually unremarkable. The cause of symptoms in patients with gastroparesis is poorly understood. There is a poor correlation between symptoms and delay in gastric emptying (Horowitz et al 1991), so that some patients with grossly delayed emptying have few or no symptoms. Delayed and rapid gastric emptying, which frequently coexist after gastric drainage procedures, may be associated with similar symptoms (Smout et al 1987). Furthermore, while treatment of gastroparesis with prokinetic drugs often relieves symptoms, in some patients normalization of emptying appears to have no clinical effect and there is only a weak correlation between the change in gastric emptying and the magnitude of symptomatic improvement. Delay in gastric emptying should, therefore, be regarded as a marker of gastric and/or proximal small intestinal motor abnormality, rather than the direct cause of symptoms.

Symptoms, which are presumed to result primarily from disordered motility, are likely to be multifactorial in origin. For example, symptoms may reflect disordered esophageal, small intestinal or colonic motility; in other patients psychiatric dysfunction may be important (Clouse et al 1989). The role of abnormal gastric pacemaker function is unclear (Koch et al 1989). In patients with diabetes, hyperglycemia induces abnormal gastric myoelectrical activity (Jebbink et al 1994). Recent studies support the concept that abnormal feedback from mucosal afferent sensory receptors in the stomach or small intestine may cause symptoms (Lemann et al 1991, Coffin et al 1994). For example, patients with nonulcer dyspepsia have an increased sensitivity to gastric, but not duodenal, distention and an impaired gastric motor response to duodenal distention (Coffin et al 1994).

Patients with rapid gastric emptying may complain of similar symptoms to those with delayed gastric emptying, i.e. nausea, vomiting, abdominal pain and bloating, which may reflect excessive feedback from small intestinal receptors. In a minority of patients vasomotor symptoms, such as palpitations and faintness, are present and reflect the rapid delivery of hyperosmolar gastric contents into the jejunum. Symptoms of "dumping" occur most frequently (5–30% of cases) after a gastric drainage procedure, such as a Billroth II gastrectomy or vagotomy with pyloroplasty (Smout et al 1987).

### *Glycemic control*

In normal subjects and patients with diabetes mellitus, the rate of gastric emptying is a significant factor in blood glucose homeostasis by controlling the delivery of carbohydrate to the small intestine (Horowitz et al 1993a, Jones et al 1995). For example, in normal subjects gastric emptying accounts for about 34% of the variance in peak plasma glucose after a 75 g oral glucose load, so that the latter is greater if gastric emptying is faster (Horowitz et al 1993a). It seems likely that abnormal gastric emptying contributes to poor glycemic control in diabetic patients, particularly those with insulin-dependent diabetes, by causing a mismatch between the action of exogenously administered insulin or oral hypoglycemic drug and the absorption of nutrients from the small intestine (Horowitz & Fraser 1994). Such a relationship, if established, would have major implications for the management of patients with poorly controlled diabetes, particularly in view of the convincing evidence that optimal control of blood glucose concentrations reduces the risk of long-term diabetic complications substantially. However, it should also be recognized that delayed gastric emptying could be an advantage, particularly in noninsulin-dependent diabetes, because carbohydrate may be absorbed more slowly in coordination with the delayed insulin release characteristic of this disorder (Horowitz & Fraser 1994). The beneficial effects of high glycemic-index foods and certain forms of fiber on blood glucose control in noninsulin-dependent diabetes are likely to reflect retardation of gastric emptying, as well as slower intestinal carbohydrate absorption.

*Oral drug absorption*

Most drugs are absorbed from the small intestine more rapidly than the stomach because the small intestine has a much greater surface area. The rate of gastric emptying is therefore an important determinant of oral drug absorption (Nimmo 1976, Horowitz et al 1989, Hebbard et al 1995) and gastric stasis may lead to abnormalities in the serum concentrations of orally administered drugs. As examples, after some forms of gastric surgery the rate of alcohol absorption is faster and the absorption of oral hypoglycemic agents may be delayed during hyperglycemia (Hebbard et al 1995). When oral pharmaceuticals are given on a chronic basis changes in gastric emptying, in the absence of vomiting, would not be expected to have a major influence on the steady-state concentrations of drugs that have a relatively long half-life.

## Diagnosis

The nonspecific nature of symptoms means that objective measurement is required for the diagnosis of gastric motor dysfunction. Evaluation of autonomic nerve function, usually by standardized cardiovascular reflex tests, may be useful in some cases, particularly when other methods are unavailable. A number of approaches have been devised to assess gastroduodenal motility (Table 15.3). These methods fall into three categories: measurements of gastric emptying, intraluminal pressure measurements and recording of gastric electrical activity. No single technique measures flow, pressure and wall motion concurrently and in research studies most information is therefore obtained by the simultaneous use of a combination of techniques. The lack of standardization of methods has hindered comparison of the results of studies between different centers. Routine tests such as endoscopy and barium meal and follow-through are usually normal, although endoscopy may reveal retained food after an overnight fast. Although other techniques used to measure gastric emptying, such as ultrasound and radioisotopic breath tests, show considerable promise, scintigraphy is at present the most accurate and arguably the only clinically applicable method. At present the use of manometry is in general limited to a research setting, but it is likely to gain acceptance of clinical procedure.

**Table 15.3** Techniques for measurement of gastroduodenal motility in humans

| |
|---|
| *Invasive techniques* |
| Intubation/aspiration of gastric contents |
| Endoscopy |
| Manometry |
| *Noninvasive techniques* |
| Scintigraphy |
| Radiology |
| Ultrasound |
| Radioisotopic breath testing |
| Applied potential tomography |
| Impedance epigastrography |
| Absorption kinetics of orally administered drugs |
| Magnetic resonance imaging |
| Electrogastrography |

### Measurement of gastric emptying

***Scintigraphy.*** Scintigraphic measurement of gastric emptying, by incorporating radioisotopes into meal components, is the most convenient and physiological measure of gastric emptying currently available. The procedure is noninvasive and requires a relatively low exposure to ionizing radiation so that, except in pregnancy, several studies can be performed in each patient to evaluate clinical progress or the effect of therapeutic agents. Radioisotopic markers, most frequently $^{99m}Tc$, are incorporated into solid, liquid or mixed solid and liquid meals and a gamma camera is used to measure the abdominal distribution of radioactivity over the next 2–6 h. For individual studies gastric emptying is best expressed as a curve showing the amount of isotope remaining in the stomach against time, superimposed on a normal range (Fig. 15.3 & 3.6).

There is considerable variation in the performance of scintigraphic tests, particularly the nature of the isotope and the meal (Horowitz et al 1985a, Scarpignato 1990). As discussed on p. 81, a technique which measures both solid and nutrient liquid emptying should ideally be used, since the pattern of emptying of one of these does not predict emptying of the other. In particular, delayed emptying of solid food may be associated with accelerated emptying of liquid. This is characteristic of gastric emptying after gastric drainage procedures (Smout et al 1987). There is little information about the appropriate test meal for the optimum detection of differences between health and disease, but it is generally accepted that it should be representative of an ordinary meal (usually 250–500 ml in volume) (Moore et al 1988, Christian et al 1980). There is a strong temptation to use small-volume, bland meals because these are less likely to lead to vomiting during the test and, in normal subjects, the majority of the meal empties from the stomach in a relatively short time period, but nonnutrient liquids, such as water, which do not stimulate mechanisms which retard gastric emptying should not be used. If it is only possible for a single isotope to be used a marker for the solid components of a meal is probably preferable. There is some evidence that the use of test meals designed to provoke symptoms, such as fatty meals (Houghton et al 1993, Horowitz et al 1993b) and evaluation of the intragastric distribution of meals (Mangnall et al 1994, Troncon et al 1994), show a higher prevalence of abnormality. A number of methodological variables such as patient movement, radionuclide decay and attenuation of $\gamma$ rays due to intragastric redistribution of the test meal also need to be taken into account during a scintigraphic study (Scarpignato 1990). In patients with diabetes mellitus blood glucose concentrations should be measured during the test and taken into account in the interpretation of results.

Although the high cost of equipment sometimes limits the availability of scintigraphy, in most clinical studies continuous monitoring of gastric emptying is not required (Camilleri et al 1991). Scintigraphic techniques may also be used to evaluate contractions in the distal stomach by monitoring changes in isotope activity within small regions of interest drawn over the antrum (Urbain et al 1993). Current scintigraphic techniques do not have sufficient temporal resolution to quantify transpyloric flow on a short-term basis.

*Radiological techniques*

Radiological techniques, such as fluoroscopy, are insensitive and associated with a high radiation burden. X-ray tracking of radio-opaque markers has been used to measure emptying of nondigestible solids (Feldman et al 1984). The passage of markers out of the stomach is almost certainly related to the occurrence of phase 3 of the interdigestive migrating motor complex in the antrum and is therefore not a reflection of gastric emptying per se.

*Radioisotopic breath testing*

The indirect measurement of solid and liquid gastric emptying by detection of radio-labeled $CO_2$ has recently been reported and shows considerable promise (Ghoos et al 1993, Maes et al 1994). This technique is relatively simple and yields gastric emptying times which correlate well with those obtained by scintigraphy. For example, $^{14}C$ octanoic acid bound to egg is hydrolyzed in the duodenum, rapidly absorbed and oxidized in the liver to yield $^{14}CO_2$. The radiation dose is only about 1% of conventional scintigraphic techniques.

*Ultrasound*

Percutaneous, high-resolution, real-time ultrasonography is a promising technique to evaluate gastric emptying, wall motion in the distal stomach and transpyloric flow (King et al 1984, Bolondi et al 1985, Marzio et al 1989, Hausken et al 1991, 1994). Ultrasound techniques are noninvasive, not associated with exposure to radiation and use equipment which is usually readily available. In most cases gastric emptying is calculated from the changes in antral area (or diameter) which occur after ingestion of a meal (Bolondi et al 1985). Gastric emptying of liquids (~300 ml) is usually measured; ultrasound is less suited to measurement of gastric emptying of solids and cannot discriminate between solids and liquids. The quality of ultrasound images is dependent on anatomical factors such as body weight and the location of the antrum. With further development ultrasound is likely to be used clinically, but it will be necessary to demonstrate that the close concordance between ultrasound and scintigraphic measurements in normal subjects also applies to patients with disordered gastric emptying. Doppler techniques also enable the relationship between antropyloroduodenal contractions and transpyloric flow to be evaluated (Hausken et al 1991).

*Applied potential tomography and impedance epigastrography*

These techniques use portable and relatively inexpensive equipment to quantify changes in electrical resistivity or impedance to measure gastric emptying of liquids (Avill et al 1987). The clinical role of these methods remains to be established. Gastric emptying of solid meals cannot be evaluated reliably and pharmacological inhibition of gastric acid secretion is required.

*Absorption kinetics of orally administered drugs*

Determination of the rate of gastric emptying by measurement of blood or salivary concentrations of orally administered drugs, such as paracetamol and alcohol, is simple and relatively inexpensive (Horowitz et al 1989), but not sufficiently accurate for the use of this technique to be recommended for clinical purposes.

*Intubation/aspiration methods*

Although considerable knowledge of gastric emptying has been derived from techniques utilizing intubation and aspiration of gastric contents, their use for both research and clinical purposes has essentially been rendered obsolete because of the availability of other methods.

*Magnetic resonance imaging*

By incorporating a gadolinium complex in a liquid meal magnetic resonance imaging can be used to measure gastric emptying and gastric secretion (Schwizer et al 1992).

A three-dimensional image of the stomach and its contents is obtained by performing multiple transaxial T1-weighted images. Magnetic resonance imaging is expensive and requires equipment with limited availability but is a promising research technique. The use of high-speed magnetic resonance imaging enables gastric contractile activity to be evaluated.

*Manometry*

The use of manometry to measure pressures in the antrum, pylorus and duodenum has provided substantial insights into the physiology of normal gastric emptying and the dysfunctions associated with disordered gastric emptying, but remains a highly specialized technique (Horowitz & Dent 1991). Diagnostic manometry is at present performed in only a few centers, partly because considerable experience is required to perform and interpret studies, but also because the clinical utility of the test has not been clearly established. It is, however, probable that manometry will gain increased acceptance as a clinical procedure because of the capacity to characterize the motor dysfunctions responsible for disordered gastric emptying and also demonstrate whether the motor disturbance involves the small intestine or the stomach alone. Manometry may also be useful to define whether the underlying pathophysiological process is myopathic or neuropathic and to exclude small intestinal obstruction (Camilleri 1993). At present manometry is clinically indicated in patients with disabling symptoms, associated with poor nutritional status, who do not respond to conventional therapies. Such studies should be performed in specialized centers.

Pressures can be measured with miniature intraluminal transducers or by external transducers linked to multiple lumen manometric catheters (Fig. 15.6). Computerized methods are used increasingly in data analysis. Because of the variation in luminal pressures over short distances in the antrum and pylorus, optimal measurement in this region requires an array of closely spaced (1–1.5 cm apart) sensors. Because the pylorus is highly mobile and its zone of contraction narrow, pyloric pressures are optimally measured with a sleeve sensor, an adaptation of the sensor originally developed for manometry of the lower esophageal sphincter (Horowitz & Dent 1991). Manometry cannot indicate the timing of gastric wall motion reliably and will not usually recognize this event when it does not result in lumen occlusion. This is especially important in the fundus where nonlumen occlusive contractions are common (Vassallo et al 1992a). In research studies proximal stomach tone is most effectively measured with a barostat technique (Azpiroz & Malagelada 1987) in which a large capacity thin-walled bag is placed in the proximal stomach and intrabag pressure is set and then made constant by the barostat through fractional inflation and deflation of the bag. The volume of gas delivered or removed by the barostat unit gives a direct indication of changes in proximal gastric tone.

*Electrogastrography*

Gastric electrical activity can be recorded using cutaneous electrodes, a technique known as external electrogastrography (Smout et al 1980). While this is a promising technique to diagnose abnormal gastric pacemaker function, it does not have the ability to monitor gastric contractile activity accurately (Sun et al 1995).

## Treatment

*Gastroparesis*

The major rationale for treatment of disordered gastric motility associated with gastric stasis is the occurrence of gastrointestinal symptoms. All patients with symptoms suggestive of abnormal gastric motility should have an endoscopy to exclude gastric outlet obstruction secondary to peptic ulcer disease or malignancy. Patients with disordered gastric motility may, not infrequently, have their symptoms ascribed to psychological problems (Stacher et al 1986). Symptoms due to gastroparesis must be differentiated from rumination.

Reversible causes of gastroparesis, such as a drug side-effect and electrolyte abnormalities, must always be excluded. In patients with diabetes blood glucose control should be optimized. Although the effect of dietary modifications (e.g. low-fat, frequent meals and avoidance of nondigestible solids) on symptoms is often disappointing, the use of liquid supplements may help optimize nutritional status. The outcome of present surgical treatments for gastroparesis is frequently unsatisfactory and may be associated with deterioration. Surgery should only be performed in specialized centers when the patient has failed to respond to all other treatments. While electrical pacing of gastric muscle is technically possible, experience with this approach is too limited for it to be considered (Karlstrom & Kelly 1989a).

Antiemetic agents, such as prochlorperazine, are usually relatively ineffective, although they may provide some relief of nausea and vomiting. While cholinomimetic agents, such as bethanechol, stimulate smooth muscle contraction they do not usually induce a contraction pattern that favors aboral transit of chyme and therefore should not be used. Moreover, their lack of specificity is associated with multiple cholinergic side-effects.

*Prokinetic drugs*

Drug therapy with prokinetic agents forms the mainstay of treatment. The currently available drugs include metoclopramide (Albibi & McCallum 1983), domperidone (Brogden et al 1982), cisapride (Wiseman & Faulds 1994) and erythromycin (Peeters 1993). These agents usually accelerate gastric emptying, in dose-related fashion, when the latter is delayed and, with the possible exception of erythromycin, have been shown to improve symptoms better than placebo. Their pharmacological properties which lead to improvement in gastric emptying are poorly understood, but involve dopamine receptor blockade (domperidone and metoclopramide), stimulation of motilin receptors and cholinergic pathways (erythromycin) and stimulation of 5-hydroxytryptamine receptors (metoclopramide and cisapride). The majority of the motor-stimulating properties of cisapride result from $5HT_4$-mediated increased release of acetylcholine from the myenteric plexus (Wiseman & Faulds 1994).

The heterogeneous nature of both the pathogenesis and motor dysfunctions in gastroparesis implies that it may be impossible to achieve correction of all motor/sensory abnormalities with one drug. The symptomatic and gastrokinetic response to prokinetic therapy is variable (Horowitz et al 1987); there is some evidence that myopathic disorders (Hyman et al 1993) and neuropathic disorders due to defective extrinsic neural innervation (Camilleri et al 1994) may respond less well. Although there have been few formal comparisons between drugs, cisapride (usual dose 10 mg t.d.s. or q.i.d.) is probably the drug of first choice, as its prokinetic effect is sustained during long-term administration and it has virtually no adverse effects (Wiseman & Faulds 1994). Loose stools and abdominal cramps may occur, but are usually transient. Cisapride may also affect bladder function. The beneficial effects of cisapride on motility in other regions of the gastrointestinal tract may be therapeutically useful. Cisapride is not available as a parenteral formulation. Metoclopramide (usual dose 10 mg q.i.d.) and domperidone (usual dose 10 mg q.i.d.) are useful alternatives, particularly for initial control of nausea, although there is some evidence that their beneficial effects on gastric emptying are not sustained (Schade et al 1985, Horowitz et al 1985b). Metoclopramide has central antiemetic properties, but central nervous system side-effects, which occur in up to 20% of patients, limit its use. Because of the absence of antidopaminergic properties, cisapride does not have central nervous system side-effects when given in therapeutic doses. The antibiotic erythromycin has recently been shown to have potent motor effects on gastrointestinal motility. When given intravenously, in doses less than required for antimicrobial effects, erythromycin is the most potent of the prokinetic drugs. For example, in patients with diabetic gastroparesis erythromycin in a dose of about 3 mg/kg IV accelerates gastric emptying to a rate faster than normal (Janssens et al 1990). This may not be totally desirable as grinding of solids is impaired and larger particles enter the small intestine (Lin et al 1994). Parenteral erythromycin may, however, be of particular value in the initial management of patients with severe nausea and vomiting and in facilitating the passage of transpyloric tubes (DiLorenzo et al 1990). Oral erythromycin (usual dose 250 mg t.d.s.) is less potent and there are uncertainties about its long-term efficacy (Richards et al 1993, Fiorucci et al 1994). The probability that certain drug combinations will be synergistic, particularly domperidone and cisapride, has not been adequately addressed (Tatsuta et al 1992).

There is relatively little information about the mechanical effects which are responsible for faster gastric emptying. Cisapride and erythromycin increase the number of antral, pyloric and duodenal pressure waves which are temporally related and suppress those pressure waves which are localized to the pylorus, i.e. change the organization of gastric contractions to an expulsive pattern (Fraser et al 1992, 1994). The effects of erythromycin on gastric motility are dependent on dosage (Catnach & Fairclough 1992).

Ideally gastric emptying should be measured before the commencement of prokinetic therapy, but this is often impractical. It is therefore reasonable to give a trial of therapy, for perhaps 4 weeks. Gastric emptying should be measured if symptoms fail to improve or relapse after the cessation of therapy and in all patients with symptoms after gastric surgery. There is a high placebo response, so a positive therapeutic result does not equate with a definitive diagnosis. Therefore, although many patients with severe gastroparesis will require prolonged therapy with prokinetic agents, a favorable effect on symptoms does not in itself justify the use of long-term therapy. It is also recognized that in some patients with gastroparesis symptoms improve spontaneously, so that medical therapy can be withdrawn.

Despite improvements in pharmacotherapy, treatment of symptoms presumed to result from disordered gastroduodenal motility is not uniformly satisfactory and there is a need for new therapeutic approaches. Where drug treatment fails it may be necessary to resort to enteral feeding either via a nasoenteric tube or via an endoscopically placed jejunostomy tube. Pharmacological modification of sensory feedback from the stomach and small intestine, rather than prokinetic therapy, may provide useful agents for treatment of symptoms. A number of novel agents, including $5HT_3$ receptor antagonists, $\kappa$ opiate agonists, somatostatin analogs and motilin agonists devoid of antibiotic activity, are currently being evaluated.

### *Rapid gastric emptying*

Symptoms of the "early" dumping syndrome related to rapid emptying frequently improve with minor dietary modifications and time (p. 273). Patients should eat frequent small solid meals, avoid simple carbohydrates and not drink soon after eating. Lying down after a meal may also improve symptoms. The addition of guar gum has been reported to be beneficial. Octreotide (50–100 μg s.c. before meals) may also be helpful in some patients, perhaps by slowing gastric emptying and inhibiting the release of gastrointestinal hormones. Ingestion of a small amount of liquid nutrient (e.g. oil) before a meal may be of benefit by slowing small intestinal transit of the remainder of the meal. Definition of the type of emptying abnormality can be used to tailor dietary advice and drug treatment of postoperative gastric motor disorders, e.g. if gastric emptying of liquids is accelerated patients should be advised to consume liquids after solid food.

## VOMITING

### Physiology

The motor mechanisms responsible for vomiting are reasonably well characterized (Thompson & Malagelada 1982, Lang et al 1993). Vomiting is associated with an initial reduction in the tone of the antrum, fundus and lower esophageal sphincter, followed by retrograde contractions involving the small intestine, duodenum and stomach which are accompanied by strong contractions of the abdominal muscle. The cricopharyngeus muscle contracts and then relaxes immediately before the ejection of gastric content. Following vomiting, the fundus and lower esophageal sphincter remain relaxed for some time. Retching encompasses the same motor events, with the exception that the glottis remains closed and gastric contents are therefore not ejected. Vomiting is often accompanied by salivation, sweating, tachycardia or bradycardia and, sometimes, by defecation. Nausea usually precedes vomiting and is associated with a reduction in vagal tone, increased release of catecholamines and vasopressin, abnormalities of gastric pacemaker function (particularly tachyarrhythmias) and slowing of gastric emptying (Koch et al 1990). It is uncertain whether changes in gastric motility contribute directly to nausea or represent epiphenomena (Reid et al 1995).

The act of vomiting is co-ordinated by a vomiting center located in the dorsal medulla which receives input from the alimentary tract and a number of other sites (Borison & Wang 1953). Thus, there are receptors in the pharynx, pyloric region, the entire bowel, the biliary ducts and, probably, in the mesenteric vessels, heart and vestibular system. Afferent impulses travel in the vagus to the vagal nuclei and in sympathetic nerves to the nucleus tractus solitarius; these nuclei are near the vomiting center and the chemoreceptor trigger zone. The latter is located in the area postrema in the floor of the fourth ventricle. A number of drugs (digoxin, opioid narcotics and some chemotherapeutic agents) and metabolic disturbances (diabetic ketoacidosis, uremia) which induce vomiting act via the chemoreceptor trigger zone which stimulates the vomiting center. Some other brain centers may be sensitive to emetic drugs and metabolic disturbances. The efferent control of vomiting is via the vagi and sympathetic systems and via the phrenic and other nerves which supply the pharynx, diaphragm and abdominal muscles.

### Clinical approach to the patient with vomiting
(Hanson & McCallum 1985)

Vomiting occurs in a wide variety of causes and algorithms for the evaluation of patients with vomiting have been suggested. However, history and routine examination will usually indicate the cause. Vomiting must be distinguished from regurgitation and rumination (p. 436). It may be useful to classify causes according to the duration of vomiting as acute (<48 h) or chronic (>48 h) (Table 15.4) (Schoen & Brandt 1993).

Extragastrointestinal causes such as myocardial infarction, uremia, drugs and migraine should become obvious. The timing and nature of the vomiting may provide indications as to its cause. For example, the presence of food eaten many hours before in the vomitus is strongly suggestive of gastric outlet obstruction or gastroparesis, while vomiting immediately after meals is characteristic of psychogenic vomiting or sometimes a pyloric channel ulcer. Epigastric pain relieved by vomiting occurs in peptic ulcer and early morning vomiting before food is eaten is characteristic of pregnancy, alcohol intoxication and uremia. Neurological causes may be associated with projectile vomiting.

When the cause is not obvious from initial history and examination it is wise to re-examine the cranial nerves and fundi thoroughly and look for signs of autonomic neuropathy, including evaluation of cardiovascular reflexes. A

**Table 15.4** Differential diagnosis of nausea and vomiting (modified from Schoen & Brandt 1993)

| |
|---|
| *Acute symptoms* (<48 h) |
| Viral gastroenteritis, e.g. Norwalk virus |
| Toxins, e.g. staphylococcus enterotoxin |
| Visceral pain, e.g. appendicitis, cholecystitis, pancreatitis, hepatitis, renal colic, biliary colic, myocardial infarction |
| Vestibular: motion sickness, labyrinthitis |
| Acute mechanical obstruction of the gastrointestinal tract |
| Drugs, e.g. alcohol, opiate analgesics, chemotherapeutic agents, digoxin |
| Central nervous system disorders, e.g. meningitis, migraine |
| *Chronic symptoms* (>48 h) |
| Mechanical obstruction, e.g. gastric outlet, small or large bowel obstruction |
| Metabolic: diabetic ketoacidosis, pregnancy, uremia, Addison's disease, hypercalcemia |
| Psychiatric disease: anorexia nervosa, bulimia nervosa, psychogenic |
| Central nervous system disorders: increased intracranial pressure, brainstem lesions |
| Peritoneal irritation, e.g. peritonitis, irradiation |
| Peptic ulcer disease |
| Other disorders affecting gastrointestinal motility (see Table 15.1) |
| Idiopathic |

thorough drug history must be taken and consideration given to endocrine disorders. Endoscopy of the upper gastrointestinal tract is essential in most cases of chronic vomiting to search for relevant lesions. Psychiatric assessment may be helpful. Psychogenic vomiting can be a response to depression, anxiety or acute stress, particularly conflict or bereavement. While in many cases this may be shortlived, in other individuals a conversion reaction may result in chronic vomiting (Fitzgerald & Walsh 1977).

When all these investigations are negative further investigation is indicated to search for gastroparesis and disorders of intestinal motility (p. 441). Central nervous system disorders, such as brain-stem tumors, may cause vomiting by affecting intestinal motility (Wood et al 1985). Abnormal gastrointestinal motility may also be the cause of cyclical vomiting (Abell et al 1988). In up to 50% of cases of unexplained chronic vomiting gastric emptying is delayed and abnormal gastric pacemaker activity also occurs frequently.

### Treatment

Pharmacological or surgical treatment should be ideally directed towards the correction of a specific disorder, but in many cases a nonspecific approach is necessary. As discussed on, hospitalization may be required for management of dehydration and severe nutritional impairment. Phenothiazines, such as prochlorperazine, represent the first choice, nonspecific therapy for vomiting and act by antagonizing dopaminergic input to the chemoreceptor trigger zone. As discussed on p. 433 these drugs do not stimulate gastric emptying and their use is frequently associated with extrapyramidal symptoms and anticholinergic effects. Transdermal scopolamine is effective in the treatment of motion sickness. Therapy with prokinetic agents (cisapride, metoclopramide, domperidone and erythromycin) is indicated when vomiting is associated with gastroparesis (p. 433). The use of serotonin ($5HT_3$) antagonists such as ondansetron, particularly when combined with dexamethasone, represents a major advance in the treatment of vomiting induced by chemotherapeutic agents, such as cisplatin and radiation (Cubeddu et al 1990, De Mulder et al 1990, Perez 1995). These agents act as antagonists of $5HT_3$ receptors located in the area postrema, the gastrointestinal mucosa and on vagal efferent nerves. $5HT_3$ antagonists are relatively expensive and their use is associated with few side-effects. At present there is little information about the effect of ondansetron in the treatment of nausea and vomiting due to gastrointestinal causes.

## RUMINATION SYNDROME IN ADULTS

Rumination, which may be defined as the voluntary, repetitive, regurgitation of gastric contents, is a relatively frequent condition in infants and adults of subnormal intelligence. In adults of normal intelligence rumination has been considered to occur only rarely, but the prevalence has probably been underestimated due to a lack of awareness of the condition (O'Brien et al 1995). A detailed history is pivotal to diagnosis, particularly as the rumination syndrome may easily be confused with other disorders, including vomiting and gastroesophageal reflux. Regurgitation of gastric contents usually commences within 10 min after a meal and persists for 1–2 h. The undigested or partly digested food which is regurgitated lacks an acidic taste and is usually swallowed, but may be expectorated. Significant nutritional disturbances are unusual. Rumination occurs most frequently in young women and a history of psychiatric disturbance is not uncommon (O'Brien et al 1995).

While the mechanisms responsible for regurgitation are incompletely understood, manometric studies have demonstrated that episodes of regurgitation are often preceded by abdominal muscle contraction (Amarnath et al 1986) and it has been suggested that repetitive increases in abdominal pressure may induce relaxation of the lower esophageal sphincter (Smout & Breumelhof 1990). While the characteristic history is usually sufficient for diagnosis, combined esophageal manometric and pH studies may be useful in some cases (Weusten & Smout 1994). Rumination often persists for many years, although there is little information about the natural history (O'Brien et al 1995). Treatment consists primarily of reassurance to clarify the benign nature of the condition. There is some evidence that behavioral therapy may be useful.

## BULIMIA NERVOSA (Herzog & Copeland 1985)

Bulimia is a syndrome distinct from anorexia nervosa characterized by compulsive episodes of secretive binge-eating, often of high caloric "junk" foods, followed by acts to prevent weight gain, including self-induced vomiting, laxative or diuretic abuse, fasting and excessive physical activity. Unlike anorexia nervosa body size is normal, although bulimic symptoms can occur in anorexia nervosa.

### Prevalence and etiology

In women less than 30 years of age the prevalence of bulimia is greater than 1% and this group accounts for about 95% of cases. As with anorexia nervosa, cultural, psychological and biological factors appear to be important. In particular, abnormal regulation of several neurotransmitters including serotonin, catecholamines, opioids and cholecystokinin (Geracioti & Liddle 1988) have been demonstrated which gives additional rationale to pharmacological treatment with drugs such as imipramine. As in anorexia nervosa, gastric emptying is frequently delayed (Kiss et al 1990).

### Clinical features

The criteria for diagnosis given in the American Psychiatric Association's *Diagnostic and Statistical Manual of Mental Disorders* include:

1. recurrent episodes of binge-eating;
2. recurrent inappropriate compensatory behavior in order to prevent weight gain;
3. both binge-eating and inappropriate compensatory behaviors occur at least twice a week for 3 months;
4. self-evaluation is unduly influenced by body shape and weight;
5. the disturbance does not occur exclusively during episodes of anorexia nervosa.

Only a minority (perhaps 10%) of patients with bulimia seek medical attention. Patients may have menstrual irregularities. Organic gastrointestinal disease must always be excluded (Kiss et al 1990). Gastrointestinal abnormalities include acute gastric dilatation and rupture, parotid enlargement due to repeated vomiting, erosion of dental enamel, esophagitis, Mallory–Weiss tears and esophageal rupture. Laxative abuse and vomiting may cause electrolyte abnormalities. Other features are aspiration pneumonia and ipecac poisoning leading to fatal myocardial dysfunction.

### Treatment

Behavioral therapy is frequently successful as bulimics generally have greater insight into psychosocial issues than patients with anorexia nervosa. Antidepressant medications are effective in reducing the number of binges and improving body image.

## ANOREXIA NERVOSA (Stonehill 1986)

Patients with anorexia nervosa are frequently referred to the gastroenterologist for evaluation of gastrointestinal symptoms such as vomiting, abdominal pain and constipation, or when severe weight loss and malnutrition suggest malabsorption or Crohn's enteritis.

### Incidence and etiology

The incidence (number of new cases each year) of anorexia nervosa in most Western societies is about 0.6 per 100 000 and appears to be increasing. The prevalence has been estimated at about 1% in the UK and USA. Caucasian females account for 90–95% of cases and characteristically these come from affluent families. In most cases the onset of the disorder is within 8 years of the menarche. Social, psychological and biological factors have all been implicated in the etiology of anorexia nervosa. The cultural value currently placed on thinness and family dysfunction, including sexual abuse, may be particularly important. The prevalence of anorexia nervosa is higher in monozygotic than dizygotic twins and it is possible that there is a primary neurochemical abnormality. In 20% of cases the menstrual periods cease before there is substantial weight loss and these patients have evidence of increased endogenous opioid activity.

### Clinical features

The use of standardized criteria for diagnostic purposes is recommended, particularly as the severity of the disorder varies considerably. Furthermore, attitudes and behavior consistent with anorexia nervosa but without substantial weight loss are very common in young women in Western society. The current criteria for diagnosis detailed in the fourth edition of the American Psychiatric Association's *Diagnostic and Statistical Manual of Mental Disorders* (DSM-IV) are:

1. refusal to maintain body weight over a minimal normal weight for age and height;
2. intense fear of gaining weight or becoming fat, even though underweight;
3. disturbance in the way in which body weight, size or shape is experienced;
4. absence of at least three consecutive menstrual cycles (in postmenarchal females).

While in most cases weight loss occurs primarily as a result of dietary restriction and exercise, about 50% of patients with anorexia nervosa induce vomiting or take purgatives and the DSM criteria now subdivide patients into "restricting" or "bulimic" types.

The features of anorexia nervosa in males and females are similar. The patient may insist that a normal diet is eaten and the marked disturbance of body image is often apparent when "fatness" is commented on by the wasted patient. Self-induced vomiting and purgation may be concealed. The findings on examination correlate with nutritional status but there may be emaciation, hypotension, bradycardia, arrhythmias, hypothermia, acrocyanosis, carotenemia, dry skin, a diffuse growth of lanugo hair and ankle edema. In contrast to patients who are emaciated from organic disease, energy and activity are usually unimpaired. There may be dehydration and hypokalemia due to laxative and diuretic abuse, and vomiting. Endocrine abnormalities relating to gonadotrophin, thyroid hormone and cortisol secretion occur frequently and are reversible with weight gain. Estrogen deficiency predisposes to osteoporosis.

The gastrointestinal symptoms, including vomiting, abdominal bloating and constipation, which occur frequently in patients with anorexia nervosa, accentuate weight loss and are probably the result of disordered gastrointestinal motility (Stacher et al 1986, Abell et al 1987,

Kamal et al 1991). Gastric emptying is delayed in about 50% of patients and this is associated with postprandial antral hypomotility (Stacher et al 1986, Abell et al 1987). Gastric pacemaker function may also be abnormal (Abell et al 1987). Whole gut transit is frequently delayed (Kamal et al 1991). Many of these abnormalities are likely to be secondary to dietary restriction. For example, the delay in gastric emptying frequently improves with the commencement of oral renutrition (Rigaud et al 1988) and therefore probably reflects excess small intestinal feedback by arrival of nutrients into the small intestine at times when the patient's intake is diminished (Corvilain et al 1995).

Anorexia nervosa may easily be confused with organic gastrointestinal disease. In particular, achalasia and other esophageal motility disorders have been described in patients classified as having anorexia nervosa (Stacher et al 1986). Thus a patient with features of anorexia nervosa who has dysphagia or chest pain should have a full esophageal investigation. The gastroenterologist may be worried that an emaciated patient has malabsorption or Crohn's enteritis. In most cases a psychiatric opinion should be sought before embarking upon investigations for these possibilities.

### Treatment

Treatment is difficult and a multidisciplinary approach focusing on nutritional status, medical complications and psychological issues is essential. Hospitalization is necessary when there is severe malnutrition (weight <65% of ideal) and enteral (jejunal) feeding is required when oral intake is inadequate. Prokinetic drugs may increase the tolerance to enteral feeding (Stacher et al 1993). While refeeding is usually associated with resolution of gastrointestinal symptoms, excessively rapid refeeding may cause acute gastric or duodenal dilatation, diarrhea and pancreatitis. Although psychotropic medications are frequently used, none has clearly been shown to be effective. While the short-term prognosis is usually favorable, relapse requiring hospitalization occurs in about 50% of cases and the long-term mortality is about 10%, 2–5% being due to suicide. The degree of social integration provides a guide to long-term prognosis.

## SMALL BOWEL MOTILITY DISORDERS

Motility disorders of the small intestine are increasingly recognized as clinical syndromes characterized by acute, recurrent or chronic episodes suggestive of mechanical obstruction of the small bowel. However, such episodes are unassociated with any physical obstruction of the gut lumen. Impairment of motor function may be intrinsic to the gut's neuromuscular apparatus, associated with disturbances of extrinsic neural control, accompany systemic diseases or may result from the effects of medications. Small intestinal motor disorders may be associated with motor disorders of the esophagus, stomach, colon and urinary bladder. Acute gastroparesis or pseudo-obstruction syndromes tend to be associated with severe or catastrophic extraintestinal conditions including myocardial infarction or total hip arthroplasty and the mechanisms resulting in disturbed gut motility are still largely unexplained. In contrast, chronic disturbances of the neuromuscular apparatus of the gut, whether familial or sporadic, are somewhat better understood and usually result in recurrent or chronic intestinal pseudo-obstruction.

The pathophysiology of disorders primarily affecting small intestinal motility and the underlying diseases are discussed briefly (Table 15.5).

## PHYSIOLOGY

### Normal small intestinal motor function

Normal intestinal motor function is characterized by the occurrence of cyclical motor activity during the fasting state (Kellow et al 1986); postprandially, triturating, mixing and propulsive activity result in the aboral movement of chyme (Fig. 15.7).

### Small bowel motility: integrative physiology in health and disease

Motor activity of the small intestine is organised into a recurrent pattern of different phases known as the migrat-

**Table 15.5** Diseases associated with abnormal small intestinal motility

| Type | Comment |
|---|---|
| *Structural disorders* | |
| Crohn's disease | Identifiable by contrast |
| Radiation enteritis | X-ray; component of secondary |
| Infiltrative disorders | neuromuscular dysfunction |
| Postgastric surgery | (e.g. radiation plexus damage; |
| Small bowel surgery | amyloid neuropathy or myopathy) |
| Jejunal diverticulosis | |
| *Irritable bowel syndrome* | |
| *Mucosal disease* | |
| Celiac sprue | Rarely associated with motility disturbance |
| *Pseudo-obstruction* | See Table 15.1 |
| Myopathic, neuropathic | |
| Acute, chronic | |
| *Neurologic disorders* | See Table 15.1 |
| *Endocrine/metabolic disorders* | |
| Thyrotoxicosis | Direct hormonal effects on |
| Myxedema | neuromuscular apparatus; |
| Hypercalcemia | secretory effects may alter |
| Carcinoid | transit; rarely associated |
| Zollinger–Ellison syndrome | with neuropathy (e.g. porphyria) |
| VIPoma | |
| Somatostatinoma | |
| Porphyrias | |

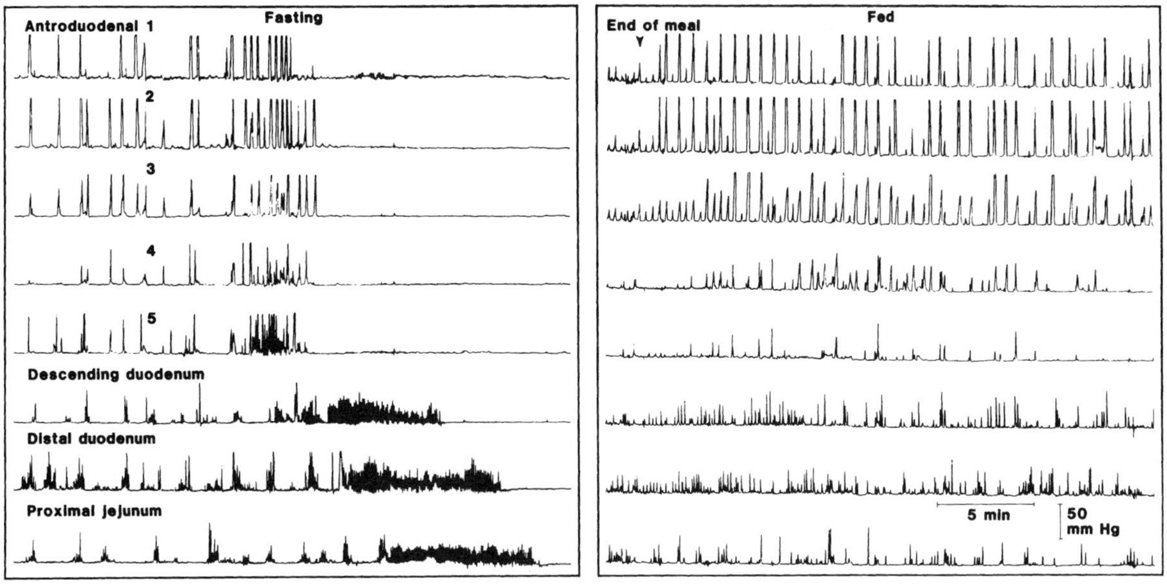


**Fig. 15.7** Normal manometric profile of the stomach and small bowel (fasting and postprandial). The migrating motor complex characteristic of the fasting state is demonstrated by presence of quiescence (phase I), intermittent activity (phase II) and an activity front (phase III). The postprandial pattern features high amplitude, irregular, but persistent phasic pressure activity at all levels. (Reproduced with permission from Malagelada et al 1986.)

ing motor complex. The fasting phase is characterized by the interdigestive motor complex, which commences in the gastroduodenal region and propagates down the small bowel (Kellow et al 1986), but only infrequently reaches the distal ileum or traverses the ileocecal junction. This cyclic activity consists of a period of quiescence (phase I); phase II exhibits intermittent phasic pressure activity (contractile activity that is unassociated with alterations in muscle tone); during the "activity front", or phase III, there are regular, repetitive contractions at the maximal frequency typical for that locus (3 per minute in the human antrum, up to 12 per minute in the human small bowel, with a gradient ranging from 12 per minute in duodenum to about 9 per minute in the ileum). The interdigestive motor complex serves the role of a "housekeeper", sweeping products of digestion and debris towards the colon. Postprandially, cyclical motor activity disappears and gastric and small bowel contractions of variable amplitude occur fairly consistently, although irregularly. These contractions propagate for shorter distances and propel the contents less rapidly than the organized "activity front" or phase III that occurs during fasting. Postprandial small intestinal contractions mix and propel triturated solids and liquids through the small bowel. The duration of the "fed" pattern depends on the size and nutrient content of the meal. The arrival of nutrients such as complex carbohydrates and fats in the distal ileum stimulates an ileal brake mechanism which serves to delay gastric emptying and proximal small intestinal motility. The precise mechanism that results in this inhibitory response in the upper gut following the arrival of nutrients in the ileum is unclear, but putative mediators include neurotensin, PYY, and glucagon-like peptide-1. There is also evidence of a neural reflex inhibiting gastric function in response to the arrival of nutrients in the ileum.

Some of the effects of deranged small bowel motility can be predicted from a simple understanding of flow dynamics in a hydraulic system. Thus, the propulsive function of the proximal small intestine is an important determinant of gastric emptying (Camilleri et al 1986a). Other characteristics of normal and/or abnormal motility reflect specific functions of certain regions. The major roles of the jejunum are the mixing of digestive biliopancreatic juices with incoming, partially digested chyme, the transfer of chyme between relatively low pressure systems and aboral movement that is slow enough to allow for maximal absorption of nutrients. Hence, most contractions are of relatively low amplitude, but on average exceed 15 mmHg in health and may be organized in short clusters. This is in sharp contrast to the ileum, which is a region of relative storage where chyme accumulates before being propelled into the colon in sudden or relatively rapid bolus movements.

The ileocolonic sphincter (Phillips et al 1988) serves as a watershed between the high bacterial counts of the colon and the ileum (see p. 459), with its specialized regional functions for absorption of vitamin $B_{12}$ and bile acids (see Chapter 16), and its role in the salvage of nutrients not absorbed more proximally. In the ileum, "power" or prolonged propagated contractions (Quigley et al 1984) sweep across the ileocecal junction. However, the precise motor mechanisms that result in the bolus transfer of chyme are unclear (Hammer et al 1993). Reflux of colonic contents, such as short chain fatty acids, into the ileum likely results in the generation of powerful contractions

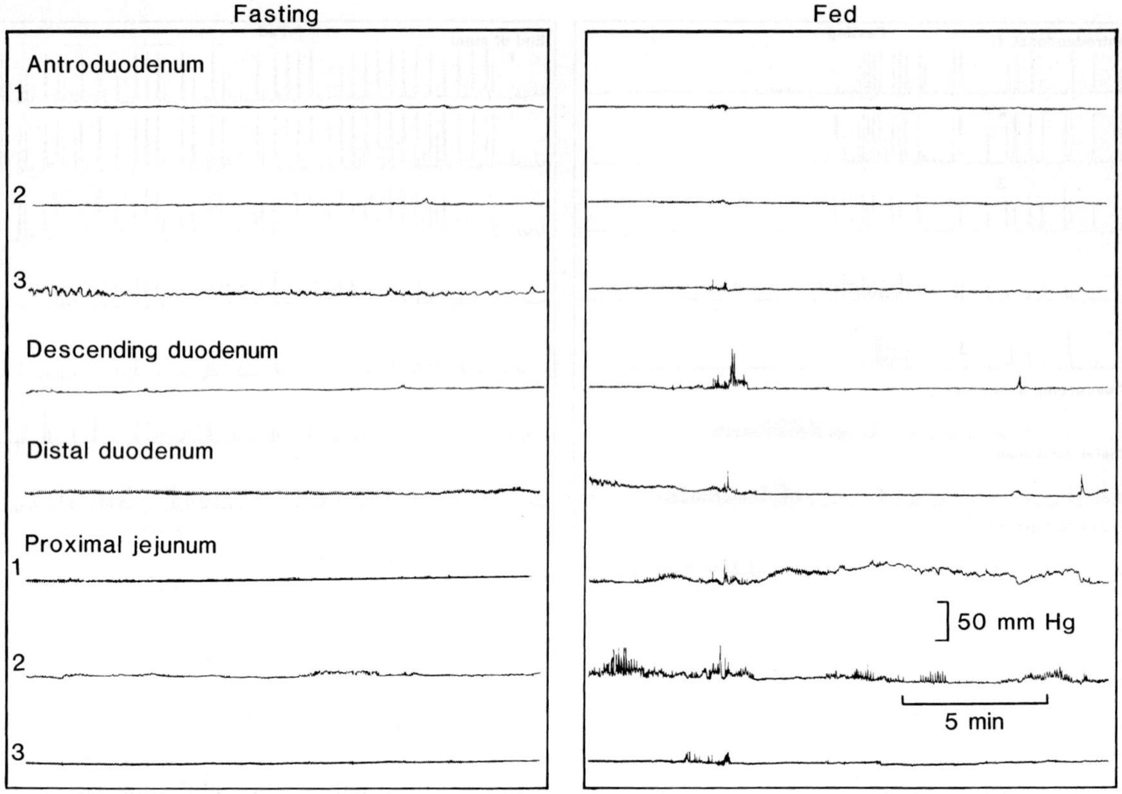


**Fig. 15.8** Manometric profile (fasting and postprandial) showing pronounced hypomotility in a 30-year-old man with hollow visceral myopathy. Eating causes no change in the featureless record. (Reproduced with permission from Colemont & Camilleri 1989.)

(Kamath et al 1987) that effectively clear the small bowel of digestive residues and of any colonic contents that had refluxed into the small bowel.

### Control of gastrointestinal motor function

Motility of the gut is dependent upon the contraction of smooth muscle cells; ion fluxes alter the cell membrane potential and the contractile state of the cell. Contractions are integrated and modulated by intrinsic nerves in the gut wall or by extrinsic nerves (see Chapter 6). The key extrinsic inputs to the enteric neuromuscular apparatus are cranial (vagal) and sacral (S2,3,4) parasympathetic nerves and the thoracolumbar sympathetic outflow. Prevertebral sympathetic ganglia are important in the integration of afferent impulses from the gut and in modulating supraspinal facilitatory and inhibitory control. Derangements at any of these levels of control may result in abnormal bowel motility.

## ACUTE INTESTINAL PSEUDO-OBSTRUCTION

Acute intestinal pseudo-obstruction is most frequently encountered as an isolated colonic disturbance, usually arising in hospitalized patients as a complication of another, often major illness such as cardiac ischemia, major surgery, hip or knee replacements and trauma (Anuras & Baker 1986). Hence, it will not be discussed further.

## CHRONIC MOTILITY DISORDERS OF THE SMALL BOWEL

### Structural diseases and their effect on small bowel motility

Disturbances of proximal small bowel motility are frequently observed following gastric surgery. Mathias et al (1985) demonstrated inco-ordinated phasic pressure waves in the Roux limb after Roux-en-Y gastrectomy and postulated that these were responsible for the nausea, vomiting and gastric stasis. Similar contractile patterns were observed in asymptomatic Roux-en-Y patients (Miedema et al 1992). Dysfunction in the vagotomized gastric remnant may also play a role in the etiology of symptoms since contractile activity of the gastric remnant is deranged after vagotomy and partial gastric resection (Azpiroz & Malagelada 1987); in practice, further resection of the gastric remnant relieves the symptoms of upper gut stasis in about two-thirds of patients in one series (Karlstrom & Kelly 1989b), and hence the role of further resective surgery is unclear.

Subacute mechanical intestinal obstruction often shows one of two contractile patterns of motility: (1) rhythmic,

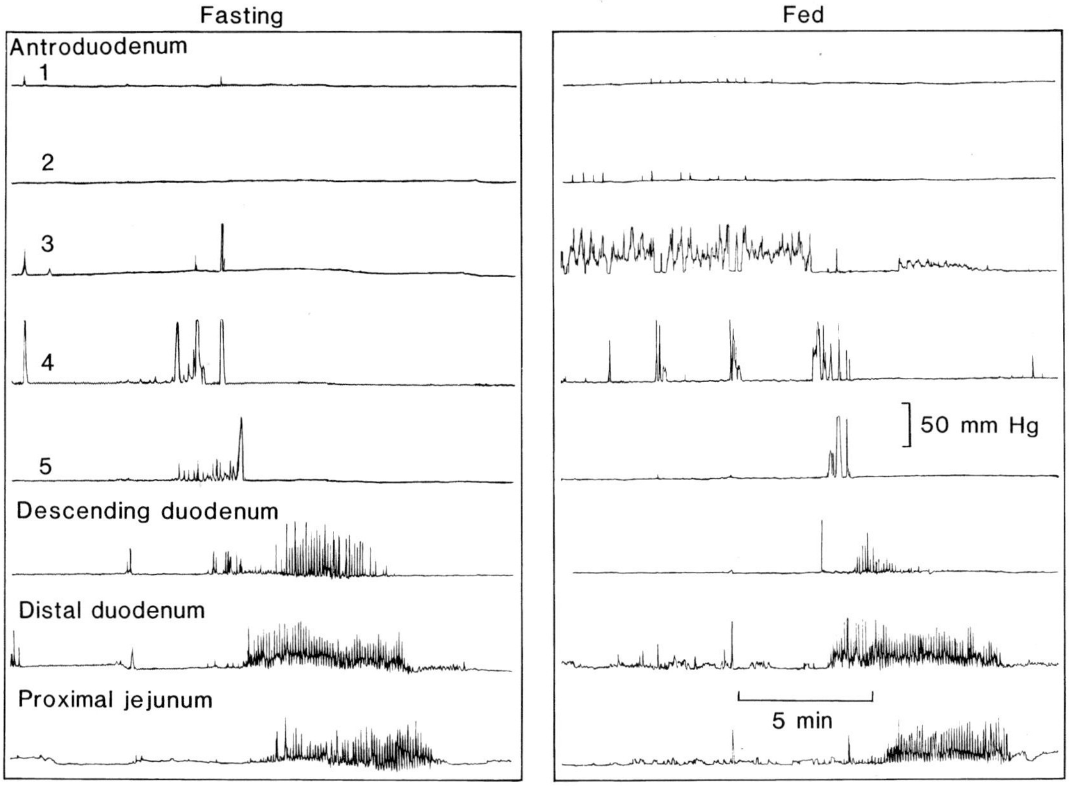


**Fig. 15.9** Neuropathic intestinal pseudo-obstruction due to diabetic autonomic neuropathy. Note the lack of distal antral contractions (fasting and postprandial), abnormal propagation of phase III of the interdigestive migrating motor complex (*left*) and the failure of the solid–liquid meal to induce a fed pattern. (Reproduced with permission from Colemont & Camilleri 1989.)

clustered contractions (Summers et al 1983, Camilleri 1989), which may also be observed in patients with chronic intestinal pseudo-obstruction (Summers et al 1983) and after ileal pouch–anal anastomosis (Stryker et al 1985); and (2) simultaneous prolonged contractions (Fig. 15.9) separated by periods of motor quiescence (Camilleri 1989, Frank et al 1994). This pattern has a positive predictive value for obstruction of 80% in a tertiary referral clinical practice (Frank et al 1994).

Small bowel fistulae, diverticula and postsurgical blind loops are all associated with bacterial overgrowth, but whether bacteria are responsible for the motility disorders or vice versa is not always clear. Bacterial toxins induce migrating action potential complexes in the rabbit ileum (Mathias et al 1976). Multiple jejunal diverticulosis may result from abnormal neuromuscular function (Krishnamurthy et al 1983).

### "Superior mesenteric artery syndrome"

This symptom complex, characterized by nausea, vomiting, early satiety, postprandial bloating and epigastric discomfort, is associated with dilatation of the duodenal loop with an apparent narrowing of the lumen of the third portion of the duodenum by the superior mesenteric artery.

It occurs in two clinical settings. The first is in patients immobilized because of spinal injury who suffer pronounced weight loss. Such patients are thought to have true mechanical obstruction by the superior mesenteric artery (SMA). The second clinical scenario is in ambulant, usually young women with recurrent vomiting and abdominal pain associated with dilatation of the proximal duodenum; the SMA appears to be responsible for partial mechanical obstruction, but the radiological "obstruction" of the duodenum is more likely due to dilatation that results from hypomotility or unco-ordinated contractions of the duodenal loop.

### Chronic intestinal pseudo-obstruction

Chronic intestinal pseudo-obstruction (CIP) is a rare syndrome characterized by recurrent episodes of symptoms and signs of intestinal obstruction (Faulk et al 1978, Schuffler 1981, Schuffler et al 1981, Stanghellini et al 1988). These symptoms occur in the absence of mechanical obstruction in any of the organs affected and result from impaired gut motility. The characteristic symptoms in this syndrome (Stanghellini et al 1987) are nausea, vomiting, abdominal distention, bloating, abdominal pain and an alteration in bowel movements (most typically, constipation). Weight loss and malnutrition may become prominent features in the more advanced stages of the disorder.

This syndrome is sometimes associated with involvement of extraintestinal smooth muscle organs, such as the urinary bladder, particularly in patients with myopathic processes. As the motility disturbances in CIP are not restricted to the small intestine, the clinical manifestations may also include dysphagia, heartburn, distention and constipation. Almost half the young female patients with severe idiopathic constipation (or chronic colonic pseudo-obstruction) in several series had evidence of esophageal, gastric or small bowel dysmotility, either at the time of colectomy or subsequently (Preston et al 1984, Leon et al 1987). Other localized variants of CIP include megaduodenum (Cohen et al 1985) and selective left colonic pseudo-obstruction (Suzuki et al 1987) or selective left colonic transit disorders (Chaussade et al 1989, Stivland et al 1991, Kamm et al 1991).

### *Pathophysiologic types*

Chronic intestinal pseudo-obstruction may be due to a variety of underlying diseases, as shown in Table 15.1. In clinical practice, identification of the underlying disease process, such as scleroderma or diabetes mellitus, in the history may be all that is necessary to attribute classic symptoms of gastric or intestinal stasis to its associated gut dysmotility. In eliciting the history, symptoms suggesting an underlying disease process should be sought: for example, postural dizziness, visual disturbances and sweating abnormalities are indicative of an autonomic neuropathy and urinary symptoms suggest genitourinary involvement by a generalized visceral neuromyopathic disorder. The family history is particularly relevant in myopathic pseudo-obstruction and suggests a congenital disorder. Patients should also be questioned about the use of anticholinergic drugs, phenothiazines, antihypertensive agents such as clonidine and tricyclic antidepressants. Physical examination should include a neurological, including pupillary, examination, measurement of blood pressure with the patient both in supine and standing positions and a search for abdominal distention or a succussion splash.

For those patients in whom the etiology is not immediately apparent, the most practical approach (Colemont & Camilleri 1989, Camilleri & Phillips 1989) starts with a noninvasive transit test (e.g. gastric emptying and/or small bowel transit) and goes on to address the pathophysiology of the motility disturbance, which can be broadly subdivided into: 1. a myopathic variety (e.g. scleroderma, amyloidosis, hollow visceral myopathy); and 2. a neuropathic variety (including the "idiopathic" variant which is thought to result from a disorder of the myenteric plexus). Patterns of gastric and small bowel motility in health (Fig. 15.7) are well established and provide the basis for assessing the pathophysiologic type of chronic pseudo-obstruction. The myopathic variant is characterized by low amplitude (average small bowel amplitude <15 mmHg), but normally co-ordinated pressure activity in the affected segments (Fig. 15.5); the neuropathic type produces excessive or unco-ordinated manometric profiles of the small bowel (Fig. 15.9) (Malagelada et al 1986). Some conditions, such as amyloidosis and, less commonly, scleroderma (Greydanus & Camilleri 1989), are initially associated with a neuropathic pattern and later, a myopathic one.

Identification of the neuropathic variant of pseudo-obstruction necessitates a more detailed search for the underlying cause (Camilleri 1990), a disturbance in the extrinsic neural supply (for example, a brain-stem tumor or, more commonly, autonomic neuropathy) or a disorder of the intrinsic nervous system (for example, idiopathic or paraneoplastic chronic intestinal pseudo-obstruction). The extrinsic neural supply may be assessed by structural examinations (such as computed tomographic scanning or magnetic resonance imaging of the brain) or noninvasive tests of sympathetic and parasympathetic function. These include pharmacologic tests of the pupils, autonomic reflexes such as sweating in response to acetylcholine and cardiovascular responses to Valsalva maneuver and deep breathing, the plasma pancreatic polypeptide response to hypoglycemia or sham feeding, and plasma norepinephrine levels after intravenous edrophonium (Camilleri 1990). This information may lead to the identification of a potentially treatable lesion, for example, a tumor of the posterior cranial fossa (Wood et al 1985).

Identification of a myopathic pseudo-obstruction should lead to a more thorough family history, fat or rectal biopsy for amyloidosis, serologic tests for infiltrative disorders such as scleroderma or a generalized muscle disease (Camilleri 1990).

Disorders of the enteric nervous system are suspected when patients with chronic intestinal pseudo-obstruction associated with inco-ordinated excessive small bowel contractility or antral hypomotility have normal autonomic tests, suggesting that the extrinsic neural control is normal. Indirect evidence of abnormal myoelectric activity can be obtained by measurements under baseline conditions and in response to neostigmine (Sullivan et al 1977); however, there are no current methods to evaluate adequately the function of the myenteric plexus before resection of a full-thickness segment of the affected bowel. Histologic studies of the myenteric plexus have been predominantly based on light microscopy or silver staining (see below).

### *Diagnosis of chronic intestinal pseudo-obstruction*

The greatest diagnostic difficulties presented by chronic

intestinal pseudo-obstruction are first, the lack of specificity of the clinical features and the absence of diagnostic radiologic features; and second, overlap with the symptoms and signs of other "functional syndromes", such as nonulcer dyspepsia, irritable bowel syndrome and chronic idiopathic constipation. The diagnosis requires recognition of the nonspecific clinical syndrome, exclusion of mechanical obstruction or mucosal disease of the gastrointestinal tract and confirmation of a disorder of small intestinal motor function. In a referral practice, the patient has often undergone exploratory laparotomy before the diagnosis is considered.

***Radiologic studies.*** The most important role of radiology is to exclude mechanical obstruction. The radiologic findings depend on the anatomic regions affected; visceral myopathy is typified by pronounced duodenal enlargement, lack of haustration, increased colonic caliber and poor to absent contractions (Rohrmann et al 1984). On the other hand, visceral neuropathy is mainly characterized by disordered smooth muscle contractility, which is best appreciated on fluoroscopy. The radiologic features of progressive systemic sclerosis, which results in close approximation of the valvulae conniventes in the small bowel and wide-mouthed sacculations in the colon, are the most specific findings in patients with pseudo-obstruction. More frequently, dilatation of the small intestine is a nonspecific feature of all types of chronic intestinal pseudo-obstruction.

Other radiologic studies may be indicated to discover the etiology of the CIP. These include brain CT or MRI in patients with neuropathic CIP in whom autonomic function tests suggest an extrinsic autonomic neuropathy (Camilleri 1990) or chest X-rays and computed tomographic scans in heavy smokers or others with risk factors for lung cancer (Sodhi et al 1989).

***Histologic analysis.*** A full-thickness biopsy specimen of the small bowel obtained during laparotomy or laparoscopy would ideally be part of the diagnostic work-up of patients with chronic intestinal pseudo-obstruction.

Krishnamurthy & Schuffler (1987) extensively reviewed the histopathologic findings in full-thickness biopsy sections of the small intestine and colon in patients with a large variety of neuromuscular disorders and showed either neuronal intranuclear inclusions, reductions in the number of ganglion cells and replacement by glial cells, inflammatory cell infiltration of the enteric plexus ganglia or abnormalities in the neuronal processes (dendritic or axonal). Immunohistochemical studies of gut neuropeptides and other transmitters are in progress. In other studies (Jayachandar et al 1988, Venizelos et al 1988), histologic evaluation of full-thickness biopsies has not provided a clear cut diagnosis of the disorder of motor function, particularly in distinguishing systemic sclerosis from visceral myopathy; the histologic changes in familial visceral myopathy can be quite variable (Fitzgibbons & Chandrasoma 1987). In a number of tissue specimens from adults (Loening-Baucke et al 1987) and children, a significant number show no specific neural or muscular histologic abnormality. Rectal biopsy may be of value when the diagnosis of intestinal neuronal dysplasia is considered (Achem et al 1987).

***Motility studies.*** Findings at the Mayo Clinic suggested that qualitative analysis of small bowel manometric studies (Stanghellini et al 1987, Colemont & Camilleri 1989) may provide complementary evidence of a motility disorder in the small bowel. Esophageal motility and anorectal sphincter responses to rectal distention (Schuffler 1981, Schuffler et al 1981) may also be abnormal. In myopathic processes, the amplitude of contractions and the frequency of MMCs are decreased (Vantrappen et al 1977).

***Gastrointestinal transit.*** Noninvasive tests of small bowel motor function facilitate the diagnosis of chronic intestinal pseudo-obstruction. Mouth-to-cecum transit of solids and liquids and transit of solid radio-label ($^{131}$I-labeled fiber or $^{111}$In resin pellets) through the small bowel are significantly prolonged. Gastric emptying of solids is also delayed (Camilleri et al 1986a & b, Mayer et al 1988).

Ileocolonic transfer of radio-labeled solid 1 mm resin pellets occurs less frequently and less efficiently in patients with myopathic pseudo-obstruction than in those with neuropathic disorders and healthy controls (Greydanus et al 1990).

## Treatment of chronic intestinal pseudo-obstruction

The goals of treatment of chronic intestinal pseudo-obstruction are the restoration of normal intestinal propulsion and adequate nutrition and treatment of complications such as bacterial overgrowth.

### *Nutritional support*

The physical nature of food can be important in the delivery of oral nutrients for the absorption by the intestine, especially if gastric emptying is impaired; thus, blenderized or liquid food is tolerated better. Other dietary measures include the use of a low lactose, low fiber, polypeptide or hydrolyzed protein diet with multivitamins and specific supplementation with iron, folate, calcium and vitamins D, K and $B_{12}$. A minority of patients with mild to moderate symptoms will be controlled adequately with nutritional supplements and dietary modifications. Supplementation of oral or enteral nutrition with liquid caloric and protein-rich formula is necessary in more severe cases. Elemental diets confer no advantage. If oral supplementation is not tolerated, a trial of nasoenteric feeding with volumes of at least 60 ml iso-osmolar nutrient per hour should be performed before placing a feeding jejunostomy. If the patient tolerates nasoenteric feeding, enteral feeding can usually be continued long term through a feeding jejunostomy tube. The more severe forms of myopathic pseudo-obstruction can only seldom have their nutritional supplements by enteral routes and often require parenteral nutrition, which is successful in maintaining the patient's weight and reversing trace element and vitamin deficiencies (Warner & Jeejeebhoy 1985, Kadowaki et al 1987). However, this treatment is associated with significant morbidity and mortality and is costly. Among ten adults receiving home parenteral nutrition with a maximal follow-up of 5 years, four required reinsertion of their lines, three for catheter sepsis and septicemia; one developed immune complex glomerulonephritis and another thrombosed the superior vena cava preterminally (Warner & Jeejeebhoy 1985).

*Bacterial overgrowth*

Treatment of bacterial overgrowth and secondary fat malabsorption with broad-spectrum antibiotics has been successful in only a small number of patients (Keshavarzian et al 1983). In patients with demonstrated steatorrhea, antibiotics are given on a rotational basis for 7–10 days each month. Commonly used antibiotics are doxycycline, metronidazole, co-trimoxazole, amoxycillin or ciprofloxacin.

*Pharmacological agents*

Cholinergic agents, including metoclopramide and neostigmine, have been ineffective in the treatment of patients with CIP. Metoclopramide has been used in the treatment of familial visceral myopathy, idiopathic CIP (Maldonado et al 1970, Lipton & Knauer 1977, Lewis et al 1978) and scleroderma (Schuffler et al 1981), but its overall efficacy has been disappointing. Its main use is intravenously in acute presentations. Erythromycin is an alternative for IV use (3 mg/kg, every 8 h), but long-term effects are disappointing (Miller et al 1990).

Cisapride, a serotonin type 4 receptor agonist, enhances the release of acetylcholine from the myenteric nerve endings in the digestive tract (Schuurkes et al 1985). In patients with CIP, cisapride reduced the delayed intestinal transit time (Camilleri et al 1986b) to normal (Fig. 15.10). In single-day studies or for up to 6 weeks (Camilleri et al 1989), oral cisapride has been shown to correct impaired propulsion in the stomach and small bowel of patients with CIP. Medium-term efficacy is less in patients with extrinsic vagal neuropathy (Camilleri et al 1994). Long-term relief of symptoms is best achieved with 20 mg t.i.d. (Camilleri et al 1995) rather than 10 mg t.i.d. (Abell et al 1991).

The analog of somatostatin, octreotide, induces migrating motor complexes in patients with progressive systemic sclerosis of the small bowel and in an uncontrolled, short study, it improved symptoms in these patients (Soudah et al 1991). However, more recent studies show that it also inhibits antral motility (Haruma et al 1994) and significantly delays small bowel transit time; in healthy subjects, small bowel transit is prolonged (Von der Ohe et al 1995) to levels observed in patients with small bowel neuropathies or myopathies (Greydanus et al 1990).

*Surgical treatment*

Surgical bypass of affected segments might be beneficial in highly selected patients. In a review of 73 operations performed on 12 patients with CIP, Schuffler & Deitch (1980) found that some procedures were not helpful (e.g. gastrojejunostomy and resection of the small bowel), whereas others were beneficial when a short segment of the bowel was involved (e.g. side-to-side duodenojejunostomy for megaduodenum or colectomy for colonic pseudo-obstruction). In planning surgery, it is important to remember that chronic intestinal pseudo-obstruction may be a generalized process (Leon et al 1987). In patients with familial visceral myopathy, Anuras et al (1979) reported variable results from duodenojejunostomy for megaduodenum. They recommended preoperative treatment of bacterial overgrowth. Sometimes, intractable and incapacitating symptoms may necessitate radical resection of the small bowel (Schuffler et al 1985, Mughal & Irving 1988). However, the principal surgical treatments are resection of localized disease or providing access for venting or enteral feeding (Murr et al 1995), usually by laparoscopy.

*Venting*

A venting enterostomy relieves gaseous distention and bloating and reduces, by a factor of 6, the need for nasogastric intubation and repetitive hospitalization for the "obstructive" episodes commonly encountered in these patients (Pitt et al 1985, Murr et al 1995). Double-lumen tubes facilitate decompression and enteral feeding.

*Experimental treatments*

Small bowel transplantation has been performed in patients with CIP; however, the indications, complications and risk–benefit ratio are still unclear.

## RAPID TRANSIT DYSMOTILITIES OF SMALL BOWEL

Rapid transit through the small bowel may constitute a minor component of an illness, such as that observed in

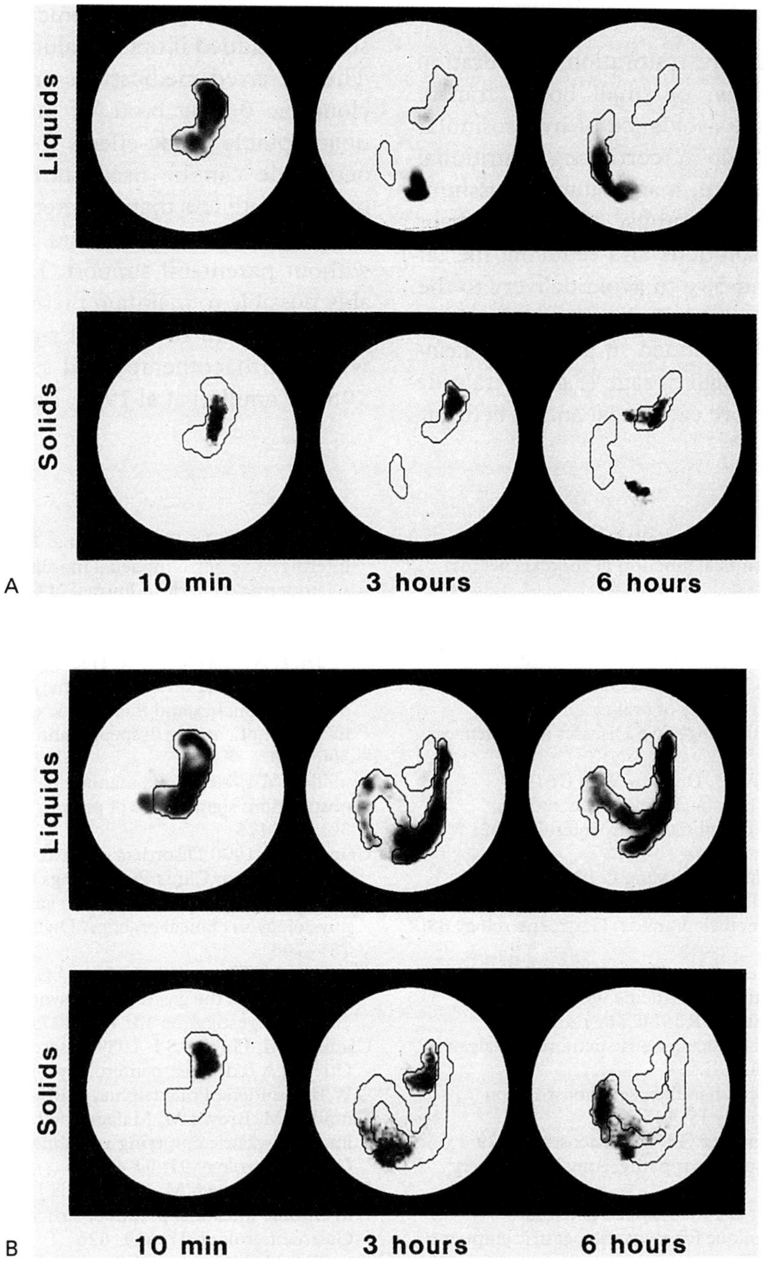


**Fig. 15.10** Effect of a prokinetic agent, cisapride, on gastric emptying and small bowel transit in a diabetic patient with antral hypomotility as shown by radioscintigrams. (a) Note delayed emptying, particularly of solids. (b) Acceleration of emptying by cisapride. (Reproduced with permission from Malagelada et al 1986.)

irritable bowel syndrome (Cann et al 1983, Vassallo et al 1992b). However, it is a major component of other diseases and results in a significant loss of fluid and osmotically active solutes that overwhelm colonic capacitance and reabsorptive capacity, resulting in severe diarrhea. Examples include *postvagotomy diarrhea* (O'Brien et al 1988), *short bowel syndrome*, *diabetic diarrhea* and *carcinoid diarrhea* (Von der Ohe et al 1993). These disturbances of small bowel transit are typically identified by scintigraphic (optimally) or by lactulose-hydrogen breath test. Manometrically, the small bowel sometimes shows prolonged duration, high amplitude and very rapidly propagated contractions (Camilleri, unpublished observations) or rapidly propagated spike bursts by intraluminal electromyography (Coremans et al 1987). Similar myoelectric activity has been noted in a series of bacterial or toxic diarrheas induced in experimental animals by Mathias et al (1976).

## Treatment

The objectives of treatment are restoration of hydration and nutrition and retardation of small bowel transit. Dietary interventions include avoidance of hyperosmolar drinks (e.g. virtually all "pop"), correcting nutritional deficiencies (commonly calcium, magnesium, potassium, water- and fat-soluble vitamins) and use of iso-osmolar or hypo-osmolar rehydration solutions and reducing the fat content in the diet to around 50 g to avoid delivery to the colon of unabsorbed fat whose metabolites are cathartic.

Pharmacotherapy should be added in a stepwise fashion: first, an opioid agent in high dosage (e.g. loperamide 4 mg q.i.d.) half an hour before each meal and at bedtime to suppress the gastrocolonic response; second-line measures are added if opioids alone do not control symptoms. The preferred medications are verapamil 40 mg b.i.d. or clonidine 0.1 mg b.i.d.; if ineffective or associated with unacceptable side-effects (e.g. postural dizziness), octreotide can be used starting at 50 µg t.i.d. Clearly, patients with less than 1 meter of residual small bowel may be unable to maintain fluid and electrolyte homeostasis without parenteral support. However, it is almost invariably possible to maintain these parameters in patients with more than 1 m of residual small bowel on oral nutrition with pharmacotherapy and supplements (Rodrigues et al 1989, Camilleri et al 1992, Farthing 1993).

REFERENCES

Abell T L, Malagelada J R, Lucas A R et al 1987 Gastric electromechanical and neurohormonal function in anorexia nervosa. Gastroenterology 93: 958–965

Abell T L, Kim C H, Malagelada J-R 1988 Idiopathic cyclic nausea and vomiting – a disorder of gastrointestinal motility. Mayo Clinic Proceedings 63: 1169–1175

Abell T L, Camilleri M, DiMagno E P, Hench V S, Zinsmeister A R, Malagelada J-R 1991 Long-term efficacy of oral cisapride in symptomatic upper gut dysmotility. Digestive Diseases and Sciences 36: 616–620

Achem S R, Owyang C, Schuffler M D, Dobbins W O III 1987 Neuronal dysplasia and chronic intestinal pseudo-obstruction: rectal biopsy as a possible aid to diagnosis. Gastroenterology 92: 805–809

Achem-Karam S, Funakoshi A, Vinik A, Owyang C 1985 Plasma motilin concentration and interdigestive migrating motor complex in diabetic gastroparesis: effect of metoclopramide. Gastroenterology 88: 492–499

Albibi R, McCallum R W 1983 Metoclopramide: pharmacology and clinical application. Annals of Internal Medicine 98: 86–95

Amarnath R P, Abell T L, Malagelada J-R 1986 The rumination syndrome in adults. A characteristic manometric pattern. Annals of Internal Medicine 105: 513–518

Anuras S, Baker C R Jr 1986 The colon in the pseudoobstruction syndrome. Clinical Gastroenterology 15: 745–762

Anuras S, Shirazi S, Faulk D L, Gardner G D, Christensen J 1979 Surgical treatment in familial visceral myopathy. Annals of Surgery 189: 306–310

Avill R, Mangnall Y F, Bird N C et al 1987 Applied potential tomography: a non invasive technique for measuring gastric emptying. Gastroenterology 92: 1019–1026

Azpiroz F, Malagelada J-R 1985 Intestinal control of gastric tone. American Journal of Physiology 249: G501–G509

Azpiroz F, Malagelada J-R 1987 Gastric tone measured by an electronic barostat in health and post surgical gastroparesis. Gastroenterology 92: 934–943

Bahron R, Levine E, Olson J, Mendell J 1988 Gastric hypomotility in Duchenne's muscular dystrophy. New England Journal of Medicine 319: 15–18

Barnett J L, Owyang C 1988 Serum glucose concentration as a modulator of interdigestive gastric motility. Gastroenterology 94: 739–744

Behar J, Ramsby G 1978 Gastric emptying and antral motility in reflux oesophagitis. Gastroenterology 74: 253–256

Bharucha A E, Camilleri M, Low P A, Zinsmeister A R 1993 Autonomic dysfunction in gastrointestinal motility disorders. Gut 34: 397–401

Bolondi L, Bortolotti M, Santi V, Salletti T, Gaiani S, Labo G 1985 Measurement of gastric emptying time by real-time ultrasonography. Gastroenterology 89: 752–759

Borison H L, Wang S C 1953 Physiology and pharmacology of vomiting. Pharmacological Reviews 5: 193

Bortolotti M, Turba E, Tosti A et al 1991 Gastric emptying and interdigestive antroduodenal motility in patients with esophageal scleroderma. American Journal of Gastroenterology 86: 743–747

Brener W, Hendrix T, McHugh P R 1983 Regulation of the gastric emptying of glucose. Gastroenterology 85: 76–82

Brogden R N, Carmine A A, Heel R C, Speight T M, Avery G S 1982 Domperidone. A review of its pharmacological activity, pharmacokinetics and therapeutic efficacy in the symptomatic treatment of chronic dyspepsia and as an antiemetic. Drugs 24: 360–400

Camilleri M 1989 Jejunal manometry in distal subacute mechanical obstruction: significance of prolonged simultaneous contractions. Gut 30: 468–475

Camilleri M 1990 Disorders of gastrointestinal motility in neurologic diseases. Mayo Clinic Proceedings 65: 825–846

Camilleri M 1993 Study of human gastrojejunal motility: applied physiology in clinical practice. Digestive Diseases and Sciences 38: 785–794

Camilleri M, Malagelada J 1984 Abnormal intestinal motility in diabetics with the gastroparesis syndrome. European Journal of Clinical Investigation 14: 420–427

Camilleri M, Phillips S F 1989 Disorders of small intestinal motility. In: Ouyang A (ed) Gastroenterology clinics of North America. W B Saunders, Philadelphia, p 405–424

Camilleri M, Brown M, Malagelada J 1986a Relationship between impaired gastric emptying and abnormal gastrointestinal motility. Gastroenterology 91: 94–99

Camilleri M, Brown M, Malagelada J 1986b Impaired transit of chyme in chronic intestinal pseudoobstruction. Correction by cisapride. Gastroenterology 91: 619–626

Camilleri M, Malagelada J-R, Abell T L, Brown M L, Hench V, Zinsmeister A R 1989 Effect of six weeks of treatment with cisapride in gastroparesis and intestinal pseudoobstruction. Gastroenterology 96: 704–712

Camilleri M, Zinsmeister A R, Greydanus M P, Brown M L, Proano M 1991 Towards a less costly but accurate test of gastric emptying and small bowel transit. Digestive Diseases and Sciences 36: 609–615

Camilleri M, Prather C M, Evans M A, Andresen-Reid M L 1992 Balance studies and polymeric glucose solution to optimize therapy after massive intestinal resection. Mayo Clinic Proceedings 67: 755–760

Camilleri M, Balm R K, Zinsmeister A R 1994 Determinants of response to a prokinetic agent in neuropathic chronic intestinal motility disorder. Gastroenterology 106: 916–923

Camilleri M, Balm R K, Zinsmeister A R 1995 Continued symptomatic improvement during one-year treatment of neuropathic chronic intestinal dysmotility with cisapride. Gastroenterology 108: A578 (abstract)

Cann P A, Read N W, Brown C, Hobson N, Holdsworth C D 1983 Irritable bowel syndrome: relationship of disorders in the transit of a single solid meal to symptom patterns. Gut 24: 405–411

Carney B L, Jones K L, Horowitz M, Sun W-M, Penagini R, Meyer J H 1995 Gastric emptying of oil and aqueous meal components in pancreatic insufficiency – effects of posture and on appetite. American Journal of Physiology 268: G925–932
Catnach S M, Fairclough P D 1992 Erythromycin and the gut. Gut 33: 397–401
Chaussade S, Khyari A, Roche H, Garret M, Gaudric M, Couturier D, Guerre J 1989 Determination of total and segmental colonic transit time in constipated patients. Digestive Diseases and Sciences 34: 1168–1172
Christian P, Moore J, Sorenson J, Coleman R, Weich D 1980 Effects of meal size and correction technique on gastric emptying time: studies with two tracers and opposed detectors. Journal of Nuclear Medicine 21: 883–885
Clouse R E, Lustman P J 1989 Gastrointestinal symptoms in diabetic patients: lack of association with neuropathy. American Journal of Gastroenterology 84: 868–872
Coffin B, Azpiroz F, Guarner F, Malagelada J-R 1994 Selective gastric hypersensitivity and reflex hyporeactivity in functional dyspepsia. Gastroenterology 107: 1345–1351
Cohen L B, Field S P, Sachar D B 1985 The superior mesenteric artery syndrome. The disease that isn't, or is it? Journal of Clinical Gastroenterology 7: 113–116
Colemont L, Camilleri M 1989 Chronic intestinal pseudoobstruction: diagnosis and treatment. Mayo Clinic Proceedings 64: 60–70
Collins P J, Horowitz M, Cook D J, Harding P E, Shearman D J C 1983 Gastric emptying in normal subjects. A reproducible technique using a single scintillation camera and computer system. Gut 24: 1117–1125
Cooke A 1977 Localisation of receptors inhibiting gastric emptying in the gut. Gastroenterology 72: 875–880
Coremans G, Janssens J, Vantrappen G, Chaussade S, Ceccatelli P 1987 Migrating action potential complexes in a patient with secretory diarrhea. Digestive Diseases and Sciences 32: 1201–1206
Corvilain B, Abramowicz M, Fery F et al 1995 Effect of short term starvation on gastric emptying in normal and obese subjects – relationship to oral glucose tolerance. American Journal of Physiology 269: G512–517
Cubeddu L X, Hoffmann I S, Fuenmayor N T, Finn A L 1990 Efficacy of ondansetron (GR38032F) and the role of serotonin in cisplatin-induced nausea and vomiting. New England Journal of Medicine 322: 810
Cunningham K, Horowitz M, Read N 1991a The effect of short-term dietary supplementation with glucose on gastric emptying in humans. British Journal of Nutrition 65: 15–19
Cunningham K, Daly J, Horowitz M, Read N 1991b Gastrointestinal adaptation to diets of differing fat composition in human volunteers. Gut 32: 483–486
Cunningham K, Horowitz M, Riddell P et al 1991c Relationships among autonomic nerve dysfunction, oesophageal motility and gastric emptying in gastrooesophageal reflux disease. Gut 32: 1436–1440
De Mulder P H M, Seynaeve C, Vermorken J B et al 1990 Ondansetron compared with high dose metoclopramide in prophylaxis of acute and delayed cisplatin-induced nausea and vomiting. Annals of Internal Medicine 113: 834–840
DiLorenzo C, Lachman R, Hyman P E 1990 Intravenous erythromycin for postpyloric intubation. Journal of Paediatric and Gastroenterological Nutrition 11: 45–47
Edelbroek M, Horowitz M, Dent J et al 1994 Effect of duodenal distension on fasting and postprandial antropyloroduodenal motility in humans. Gastroenterology 106: 583–592
Farthing M J 1993 Octreotide in dumping and short bowel syndromes. Digestion 54: 47–52
Faulk D L, Anuras S, Christensen J 1978 Chronic intestinal pseudoobstruction. Gastroenterology 74: 922–931
Feldman M, Smith H, Simon T 1984 Gastric emptying of solid radiopaque markers: studies in healthy subjects and diabetic patients. Gastroenterology 87: 895–902
Fiorucci S, Distrutti E, Gerli R, Morelli A 1994 Effect of erythromycin on gastric and gallbladder emptying and gastrointestinal symptoms in scleroderma patients is maintained medium term. American Journal of Gastroenterology 89: 550–555
Fitzgerald O, Walsh N 1977 Functional dysphagia and vomiting (including anorexia nervosa). Clinics in Gastroenterology 6: 557
Fitzgibbons P L, Chandrasoma P T 1987 Familial visceral myopathy. Evidence of diffuse involvement of intestinal smooth muscle. American Journal of Surgical Pathology 11: 846–854
Frank J W, Sarr M G, Camilleri M 1994 Use of gastroduodenal manometry to differentiate mechanical and functional intestinal obstruction: an analysis of clinical outcome. American Journal of Gastroenterology 89: 339–344
Fraser R, Horowitz M, Maddox A et al 1990 Hyperglycaemia slows gastric emptying in type I diabetes mellitus. Diabetologia 33: 675–680
Fraser R, Horowitz M, Dent J 1991 Hyperglycaemia stimulates pyloric motility in normal subjects. Gut 32: 475–478
Fraser R, Shearer T, Fuller J et al 1992 Intravenous erythromycin overcomes small intestinal feedback in antral, pyloric and duodenal motility. Gastroenterology 103: 114–119
Fraser R, Maddox A, Horowitz M, Dent J 1993 Organization of antral, pyloric and duodenal motility in patients with gastroparesis. Journal of Gastrointestinal Motility 5: 167–175
Fraser R, Horowitz M, Maddox A, Dent J 1994 Postprandial motility and gastric emptying in gastroparesis – the effect of cisapride. Gut 35: 172–178
Geracioti T D Jr, Liddle R A 1988 Impaired cholecystokinin secretion in bulimia nervosa. New England Journal of Medicine 319: 683–688
Ghoos Y, Maes B, Geypens B et al 1993 Measurement of gastric emptying rate of solids by means of carbon-labeled octanoic breath test. Gastroenterology 104: 1640–1647
Greydanus M P, Camilleri M 1989 Abnormal postcibal antral and small bowel motility due to neuropathy or myopathy in systemic sclerosis. Gastroenterology 96: 110–115
Greydanus M P, Camilleri M, Colemont L J, Phillips S F, Brown M L, Thomforde G M 1990 Ileocolonic transfer of solid chyme in small intestinal neuropathies and myopathies. Gastroenterology 99: 158–164
Greydanus M P, Vassallo M, Camilleri M et al 1991 Neurohormonal factors in functional dyspepsia: insights on pathophysiological mechanisms. Gastroenterology 100: 1311–1318
Hammer J, Camilleri M, Phillips S F, Aggarwal A, Haddad A M 1993 Does the ileocolonic junction differentiate between solids and liquids? Gut 34: 222–226
Hanson J S, McCallum R W 1985 The diagnosis and management of nausea and vomiting: a review. American Journal of Gastroenterology 80: 210–218
Haruma K, Wiste J A, Camilleri M 1994 Effect of octreotide on gastrointestinal pressure profiles in health, functional and organic gastrointestinal disorders. Gut 35: 1064–1069
Hausken T, Odegaard S, Berstad A 1991 Antroduodenal motility studied by real-time ultrasonography. Effect of enprostil. Gastroenterology 100: 59–63
Hausken T, Thune N, Matre K et al 1994 Volume estimation of the gastric antrum and the gallbladder in patients with non-ulcer dyspepsia and erosive prepyloric changes, using three-dimensional ultrasonography. Neurogastroenterology and Motility 6: 263–270
Hebbard G S, Sun W-M, Bochner F, Horowitz M 1995 Pharmacokinetic considerations in gastrointestinal motility disorders. Clinical Pharmacokinetics 28: 41–66
Heddle R, Dent J, Read N et al 1988 Antropyloroduodenal motor responses to intraduodenal lipid infusion in healthy volunteers. American Journal of Physiology 254: G671–G679
Heddle R, Collins P, Dent J et al 1989 Motor mechanisms associated with slowing of the gastric emptying of a solid meal by an intraduodenal lipid infusion. Journal of Gastroenterology and Hepatology 4: 437–447
Heddle R, Miedema B W, Kelly K A 1993 Integration of canine proximal gastric, antral, pyloric and proximal duodenal motility during fasting and after a liquid meal. Digestive Diseases and Sciences 38: 856–869
Herzog D B, Copeland P M 1985 Eating disorders. New England Journal of Medicine 313: 295–303
Horowitz M, Dent J 1991 Disordered gastric emptying: mechanical basis, assessment and treatment. Bailliere's Clinical Gastroenterology 5: 371–407
Horowitz M, Dent J 1994 The study of gastic mechanics and flow: a

Mad Hatter's tea party starting to make sense. Gastroenterology 107: 302–306
Horowitz M, Fraser R 1994 Disordered gastric motility in diabetes mellitus. Diabetologia 37: 543–551
Horowitz M, Collins P J, Shearman D J C 1985a Disorders of gastric emptying in humans and the use of radionuclide techniques. Archives of Internal Medicine 145: 1467–1475
Horowitz M, Harding P E, Chatterton B E, Collins P J, Shearman D J C 1985b Acute and chronic effects of domperidone on gastric emptying in diabetic autonomic neuropathy. Digestive Diseases and Sciences 30: 1–9
Horowitz M, McNeil J D, Maddern G J et al 1986 Abnormalities of gastric and oesophageal emptying in polymysitis/dermatomyositis. Gastroenterology 90: 434–439
Horowitz M, Maddox A, Harding P E et al 1987 Effect of cisapride on gastric and esophageal emptying in insulin-dependent diabetes mellitus. Gastroenterology 92: 1899–1907
Horowitz M, Maddox A, Bochner M et al 1989 Relationships between gastric emptying of solid and caloric liquid meals and alcohol absorption. American Journal of Physiology 257: G291–G298
Horowitz M, Maddox A F, Wishart J M et al 1991 Relationships between oesophageal transit and solid and liquid gastric emptying in diabetes mellitus. European Journal of Nuclear Medicine 18: 229–234
Horowitz M, Edelbroek M A L, Wishart J, Straathof J 1993a Relationship between oral glucose tolerance and gastric emptying in normal healthy subjects. Diabetologia 36: 857–862
Horowitz M, Jones K, Edelbroek M, Smout A, Read N W 1993b The effect of posture on gastric emptying and intragastric distribution of oil and aqueous meal components and appetite. Gastroenterology 105: 382–390
Houghton L, Read N, Heddle R et al 1988 Relationship of the motor activity of the antrum, pylorus, and duodenum to gastric emptying of a solid–liquid mixed meal. Gastroenterology 94: 1285–1291
Houghton L A, Mangnall Y F, Dwivedi A, Read N W 1993 Sensitivity to nutrients in patients with non-ulcer dyspepsia. European Journal of Gastroenterology and Hepatology 5: 109–113
Hyman P E, Di Lorenzo C, McAdams L et al 1993 Predicting the clinical response to cisapride in children with chronic intestinal pseudoobstruction. American Journal of Gastroenterology 88: 832–836
Janssens J, Peeters T, Vantrappen G et al 1990 Improvement of gastric emptying in diabetic gastroparesis by erythromycin. Preliminary studies. New England Journal of Medicine 322: 1028–1031
Jayachandar J, Frank J L, Jonas M M 1988 Isolated intestinal myopathy resembling progressive systemic sclerosis in a child. Gastroenterology 95: 1114–1118
Jebbink R J A, Samson M, Bruijs P P M et al 1994 Hyperglycaemia induces abnormalities of gastric myoelectrical activity in patients with Type 1 diabetes mellitus. Gastroenterology 107: 1390–1397
Johnson R D, Horowitz M, Maddox A et al 1991 Cigarette smoking and rate of gastric emptying – effect on alcohol absorption. British Medical Journal 302: 20–23
Jones K L, Horowitz M, Wishart J M et al 1995 Gastric emptying and intragastric meal distribution in diabetes mellitus – relationship between gastric emptying and blood glucose concentrations. Journal of Nuclear Medicine 36: 2220–2228
Kadowaki H, Ouchi M, Kaga M et al 1987 Problems of trace elements and vitamins during long-term total parenteral nutrition: a case report of idiopathic intestinal pseudo-obstruction. Journal of Parenteral and Enteral Nutrition 11: 322–325
Kamal N, Chami T, Andersen A, Rusell F A, Schuster M M, Whitehead W E 1991 Delayed gastrointestinal transit times in anorexia nervosa and bulimia nervosa. Gastroenterology 101: 1320–1324
Kamath P S, Hoepfner M T, Phillips S F 1987 Short-chain fatty acids stimulate motility of the canine ileum. American Journal of Physiology 253: G427–G433
Kamm M A, van der Sijp J R, Hawley P R, Phillips R K, Lennard-Jones J E 1991 Left hemicolectomy with rectal excision for severe idiopathic constipation. International Journal of Colorectal Disease 6: 49–51
Karlstrom L, Kelly K A 1989a Ectopic jejunal pacemaker and gastric emptying after Roux gastrectomy: effect of intestinal pacing. Surgery 106: 867–871
Karlstrom L, Kelly K A 1989b Roux-Y gastrectomy for chronic gastric atony. American Journal of Surgery 157: 44–49
Kellow J E, Borody T J, Phillips S F, Tucker R L, Haddad A C 1986 Human interdigestive motility: variations in patterns from esophagus to colon. Gastroenterology 91: 386–395
Kelly K A 1980 Gastric emptying of liquids and solids: roles of proximal and distal stomach. American Journal of Physiology 239: G71–G76
Keshavarzian A, Isaacs P, McColl I, Sladen G E 1983 Idiopathic intestinal pseudo-obstruction and contaminated small bowel syndrome – treatment with metronidazole, ileostomy, and indomethacin. American Journal of Gastroenterology 78: 562–565
King P M, Adam R D, Pryde A et al 1984 Relationships of human antroduodenal motility and transpyloric fluid movement : non-invasive observations with real-time ultrasound. Gut 25: 1384–1391
Kiss A, Bergmann H, Abatzi T A et al 1990 Oesophageal and gastric motor activity in patients with bulimia nervosa. Gut 31: 259–265
Koch K L, Stern R M, Stewart W R, Vasey M W 1989 Gastric emptying and gastric myoelectrical activity in patients with diabetic gastroparesis: effect of long-term domperidone. American Journal of Gastroenterology 84: 69–75
Koch K L, Summy-Long J, Bingaman S et al 1990 Vasopressin and oxytocin responds to illusory self-motion and nausea in man. Journal of Clinical Endocrinology and Metabolism 71: 1269–1275
Krishnamurthy S, Schuffler M 1987 Pathology of neuromuscular disorders of the small intestine and colon. Gastroenterology 93: 610–639
Krishnamurthy S, Kelly M M, Rohrmann C A, Schuffler M D 1983 Jejunal diverticulosis: a heterogenous disorder caused by a variety of abnormalities of smooth muscle or myenteric plexus. Gastroenterology 85: 538–547
Labo G, Bortolotti M, Vezzadini P et al 1986 Interdigestive gastroduodenal motility and serum motilin levels in patients with idiopathic delay in gastric emptying. Gastroenterology 90: 20–26
Lang J M, Sarna S K, Dodds W J 1993 The pharyngeal, esophageal and proximal gastric responses associated with vomiting. American Journal of Physiology 265: G963
Lemann M, Dederding J P, Flourie B et al 1991 Abnormal perception of visceral pain in response to gastric distension in chronic idiopathic dyspepsia. The irritable stomach syndrome. Digestive Diseases and Sciences 36: 1249–1254
Lennon V, Sas D, Busk M et al 1991 Enteric neuronal autoantibodies in pseudoobstruction with small-cell lung carcinoma. Gastroenterology 100: 137–142
Leon S H, Krishnamurthy S, Schuffler M D 1987 Subtotal colectomy for severe idiopathic constipation: a follow-up study of 13 patients. Digestive Diseases and Sciences 32: 1249–1254
Lewis T D, Daniel E E, Sarna S K, Waterfall W E, Marzio L 1978 Idiopathic intestinal pseudoobstruction: report of a case, with intraluminal studies of mechanical and electrical activity, and response to drugs. Gastroenterology 74: 107–111
Lin H, Doty J, Reedy T, Meyer J 1989 Inhibition of gastric emptying by glucose depends on length of intestine exposed to nutrient. American Journal of Physiology 256: G404–G411
Lin H, Doty J, Reedy T, Meyer J 1990a Inhibition of gastric emptying by acids depends on pH, titratable acidity, and length of intestine exposed to acid. American Journal of Physiology 259: G1025–1030
Lin H, Doty J, Reedy T, Meyer J 1990b Inhibition of gastric emptying by sodium oleate depends on length of intestine exposed to nutrient. American Journal of Physiology 259: G1031–G1036
Lin H, Elashoff J D, Go Y-G, Meyer J H 1992 Effect of meal volume on gastric emptying. Journal of Gastrointestinal Motility 4: 157–163
Lin H, Sanders S L, Gu Y-G, Doty T E 1994 Erythromycin accelerates solid emptying at the expense of gastric sieving. Digestive Diseases and Sciences 39: 124–128
Lipton A B, Knauer C M 1977 Pseudo-obstruction of the bowel: therapeutic trial of metoclopramide. American Journal of Digestive Diseases 22: 263–265
Loening-Baucke V A, Anuras S, Mitros F A 1987 Changes in colorectal function in patients with chronic colonic pseudoobstruction. Digestive Diseases and Sciences 32: 1104–1112
Maes B D, Hiele M I, Geypens B J et al 1994 Pharmacological modulation of gastric emptying rate of solids as measured by the

carbon labelled octanoic acid breath test: influence of erythromycin and propantheline. Gut 35: 333–337
Malagelada J, Rees W, Mazzotta L, Go V 1980 Gastric motor abnormalities in diabetic and post-vagotomy gastroparesis: effect of metoclopramide and bethanecol. Gastroenterology 78: 286–293
Malagelada J-R, Camilleri M, Stanghellini V 1986 Manometric diagnosis of gastrointestinal motility disorders. Thieme, New York
Malbert C, Mathis C 1994 Antropyloric modulation of transpyloric flow of liquids in pigs. Gastroenterology 107: 37–46
Malbert C, Ruckebusch Y 1991 Relationship between pressure and flow across the gastroduodenal junction in dogs. American Journal of Physiology 260: G653–G657
Malbert C, Serthelon J P, Dent J 1992 Changes in antroduodenal resistance induced by cisapride in conscious dogs. American Journal of Physiology 263: G202–G208
Maldonado J E, Gregg J A, Green P A, Brown A L Jr 1970 Chronic idiopathic intestinal pseudo-obstruction. American Journal of Medicine 49: 203–212
Mangnall Y F, Houghton L A, Johnson A G, Read N W 1994 Abnormal distribution of a fatty liquid test meal within the stomach of patients with non-ulcer dyspepsia. European Journal of Gastroenterology and Hepatology 6: 323–327
Marzio L, Giacobbe A, Conoscitore P et al 1989 Evaluation of the use of ultrasonography in the study of liquid gastric emptying. American Journal of Gastroenterology 84: 496–500
Mathias J R, Carlson G M, DiMarino A J, Bertiger G, Morton H E, Cohen S 1976 Intestinal myoelectric activity in response to live *Vibrio cholerae* and Cholera enterotoxin. Journal of Clinical Investigation 58: 91–96
Mathias J R, Fernandez A, Sninsky C A, Clench M H, Davis R H 1985 Nausea, vomiting and abdominal pain after Roux-en-Y anastomosis: motility of the jejunal limb. Gastroenterology 88: 101–107
Mayer E A, Elashoff J, Hawkins R, Berquist W, Taylor I L 1988 Gastric emptying of mixed solid–liquid meal in patients with intestinal pseudo-obstruction. Digestive Diseases and Sciences 33: 10–18
Mearin F, Camilleri M, Malagelada J 1986 Pyloric dysfunction in diabetics with recurrent nausea and vomiting. Gastroenterology 90: 1919–1925
Miedema B W, Kelly K A, Camilleri M, Hanson R B, Zinsmeister A R, O'Connor M K, Brown M L 1992 Human gastric and jejunal transit and motility after Roux gastrojejunostomy. Gastroenterology 103: 1133–1143
Miller S M, O'Dorisio T M, Thomas F B, Mekhjian H S 1990 Erythromycin exerts a prokinetic effect in patients with chronic idiopathic intestinal pseudo-obstruction. Gastroenterology 98: A375
Moore J, Datz F, Christian P et al 1988 Effect of body posture on radionuclide measurements of gastric emptying. Digestive Diseases and Sciences 33: 1592–1595
Mughal M M, Irving M H 1988 Treatment of endstage chronic intestinal pseudoobstruction by subtotal enterectomy and home parenteral nutrition. Gut 29: 1613–1617
Murr M M, Sarr M G, Camilleri M 1995 The surgeon's role in the treatment of chronic intestinal pseudo-obstruction. American Journal of Gastroenterology 90: 2147–2151
Nimmo W S 1976 Drugs, diseases and altered gastric emptying. Clinical Pharmacokinetics 1: 189–203
O'Brien J D, Thompson D G, McIntyre A, Burnham W R, Walker E 1988 Effect of codeine and loperamide on upper intestinal transit and absorption in normal subjects and patients with postvagotomy diarrhoea. Gut 29: 312–318
O'Brien M D, Bruce B K, Camilleri M 1995 The rumination syndrome: clinical features rather than manometric diagnosis. Gastroenterology 108: 1024–1029
Oberle R L, Chen T S, Lloyd C et al 1990 The influence of the interdigestive migrating myoelectric complex on the gastric emptying of liquids. Gastroenterology 99: 1275–1282
Oliveira R B, Troncon L E A, Meneghelli U G et al 1984 Gastric accommodation to distention and early gastric emptying in diabetics with neuropathy. Brazilian Journal of Medical & Biological Research 17: 49–53
Peeters T L 1993 Erythromycin and other macrolides as prokinetic agents. Gastroenterology 105: 1886–1899
Perez E A 1995 Review of the preclinical pharmacology and comparative efficacy of 5-hydroxytryptamine-3 receptor antagonists for chemotherapy-induced emesis. Journal of Clinical Oncology 13: 1036–1043
Phillips S F, Quigley E M M, Kumar D, Kamath P S 1988 Motility of the ileo-colonic junction. Gut 29: 390–406
Phillips W T, Schwartz J G, McMahan C A 1992 Rapid gastric emptying of an oral glucose solution in Type 2 diabetic patients. Journal of Nuclear Medicine 33: 1496–1500
Pitt H A, Mann L L, Berquist W E, Ament M E, Fonkalsrud E W, DenBesten L 1985 Chronic intestinal pseudo-obstruction: management with total parenteral nutrition and a venting enterostomy. Archives of Surgery 120: 614–618
Preston D M, Hawley P R, Lennard-Jones J E, Todd I P 1984 Results of colectomy for severe idiopathic constipation in women (Arbuthnot Lane's disease). British Journal of Surgery 71: 547–552
Quigley E M M, Borody T J, Phillips S F, Wienbeck M, Tucker R L, Haddad A 1984 Motility of the terminal ileum and ileocecal sphincter in healthy humans. Gastroenterology 87: 857–866
Read N, Houghton L 1989 Physiology of gastric emptying and pathophysiology of gastroparesis. Gastroenterological Clinics of North America 18: 359–373
Reid K, Grundy D, Khan M I, Read N W 1995 Gastric emptying and symptoms of vection-induced nausea. European Journal of Gastroenterology and Hepatology 7: 103–108
Richards R D, Davenport K, McCallum R W 1993 The treatment of idiopathic and diabetic gastroparesis with acute intravenous and chronic oral erythromycin. American Journal of Gastroenterology 88: 203–207
Rigaud D, Bedig G, Merrouche M et al 1988 Delayed gastric emptying in anorexia nervosa is improved by completion of a renutrition program. Digestive Diseases and Sciences 33: 919–925
Rodrigues C A, Lennard-Jones J E, Thompson D G, Farthing M J 1989 The effects of octreotide, soy polysaccharide, codeine and loperamide on nutrient, fluid and electrolyte absorption in the short-bowel syndrome. Alimentary Pharmacology and Therapeutics 3: 159–169
Rohrmann C A Jr, Ricci M T, Krishnamurthy S, Schuffler M D 1984 Radiologic and histologic differentiation of neuromuscular disorders of the gastrointestinal tract: visceral myopathies, visceral neuropathies, and progressive systemic sclerosis. American Journal of Roentgenology 143: 933–941
Scarpignato C 1990 Gastric emptying measurement in man. In: Scarpignato C, Bianchi Porro G (eds) Clinical investigation of gastric functions. Karger, Basel, Switzerland p 198–246
Schade R R, Dugas M C, Chotsky D M et al 1985 Effect of metoclopramide on gastric liquid emptying in patients with diabetic gastroparesis. Digestive Diseases and Sciences 30: 10–15
Schoen R E, Brandt L J 1993 A 19 year old woman with unexplained vomiting. Gastroenterology 104: 302–309
Schuffler M D 1981 Chronic intestinal pseudo-obstruction syndromes. Medical Clinics of North America 65: 1331–1358
Schuffler M D, Deitch E A 1980 Chronic idiopathic intestinal pseudo-obstruction: a surgical approach. Annals of Surgery 192: 752–761
Schuffler M D, Rohrmann C A, Chaffee R G, Brand D L, Delaney J H, Young J H 1981 Chronic intestinal pseudo-obstruction: a report of 27 cases and review of the literature. Medicine 60: 173–196
Schuffler M, Baird H, Fleming C et al 1983 Intestinal pseudo-obstruction as the presenting manifestation of small-cell carcinoma of the lung. A paraneoplastic neuropathy of the gastrointestinal tract. Annals of Internal Medicine 98: 129–134
Schuffler M D, Leon S H, Krishnamurthy S 1985 Intestinal pseudoobstruction caused by a new form of visceral neuropathy: palliation by radical small bowel resection. Gastroenterology 89: 1152–1156
Schuffler M D, Pagon R A, Schwartz R, Bill A H 1988 Visceral myopathy of the gastrointestinal and genitourinary tracts in infants. Gastroenterology 94: 892–898
Schuurkes J A J, van Nueten J M, van Daele P G H, Reyntjens A J, Janssen P A J 1985 Motor-stimulating properties of cisapride on isolated gastrointestinal preparations of the guinea pig. Journal of Pharmacology and Experimental Therapeutics 234: 775–783
Schvarcz E, Palmer M, Aman J et al 1993 Hypoglycaemia increases gastric emptying rate in patients with insulin-dependent diabetes mellitus. Diabetic Medicine 10: 660–663

Schwizer W, Maecke H, Fried M 1992 Measurement of gastric emptying by magnetic resonance imaging in humans. Gastroenterology 103: 369–376

Scott A M, Kellow J E, Shuter B et al 1993 Intragastric distribution and gastric emptying of solids and liquids in functional dyspepsia. Digestive Diseases and Sciences 38: 2247–2254

Smith B 1974 Neuropathology of the oesophagus in diabetes mellitus. Journal of Neurology, Neurosurgery and Psychiatry 37: 1151–1154

Smout A J P M, Breumelhof R 1990 Voluntary induction of transient lower esophageal sphincter relaxations in an adult patient with the rumination syndrome. American Journal of Gastroenterology 85: 1621–1625

Smout A J P M, van der Schee E J, Grashius J L 1980 What is measured in electrogastrography? Digestive Diseases and Sciences 25: 179–187

Smout A J P M, Akkermans L M A, Roelofs J M M et al 1987 Gastric emptying and postprandial symptoms after Billroth II resection. Surgery 101: 27–34

Sodhi N, Camilleri M, Camoriano J K, Low P A, Fealey R D, Perry M C 1989 Autonomic function and motility in intestinal pseudoobstruction caused by paraneoplastic syndrome. Digestive Diseases and Sciences 34: 1937–1942

Sonsino E, Mouy R, Foucard P et al 1984 Intestinal pseudoobstruction related to cytomegalovirus infection of myenteric plexus. New England Journal of Medicine 311: 196–197

Soudah H C, Hasler W L, Owyang C 1991 Effect of octreotide on intestinal motility and bacterial overgrowth in scleroderma. New England Journal of Medicine 325: 1461–1469

Stacher G, Kiss A, Wiesnagrotzki S et al 1986 Oesophageal and gastric motility disorders in patients categorised as having primary anorexia nervosa. Gut 27: 1120–1126

Stacher G, Bergmann H, Wiesnagrotzki S et al 1987 Intravenous cisapride accelerates delayed gastric emptying and increases antral contraction amplitude in patients with primary anorexia nervosa. Gastroenterology 92: 1000–1006

Stacher G, Peeters T L, Bergmann H et al 1993 Erythromycin effects on gastric emptying, antral motility and plasma motilin and pancreatic polypeptide concentrations in anorexia nervosa. Gut 34:166–172

Stanghellini V, Camilleri M, Malagelada J-R 1987 Chronic idiopathic intestinal pseudo-obstruction: clinical and intestinal manometric findings. Gut 28: 5–12

Stanghellini V, Corinaldesi R, Barbara L 1988 Pseudoobstruction syndromes. Baillière's Clinical Gastroenterology 2: 225–254

Stivland T A, Camilleri M, Vassallo M et al 1991 Regional gut transit in scintigraphic measurement of idiopathic constipation. Gastroenterology 101: 107–115

Stonehill E 1986 Keep on taking the weed killer? Gut 27: 1115

Stryker S J, Borody T J, Phillips S F, Kelly K A, Dozois R R, Beart R W Jr 1985 Motility of the small intestine after proctocolectomy and ileal pouch–anal anastomosis. Annals of Surgery 201: 351–356

Sullivan M A, Snape W J Jr, Matarazzo S A, Petrokubi R J, Jeffries G, Cohen S 1977 Gastrointestinal myoelectrical activity in idiopathic intestinal pseudo-obstruction. New England Journal of Medicine 297: 233–238

Summers R W, Anuras S, Green J 1983 Jejunal manometry patterns in health, partial intestinal obstruction and pseudoobstruction. Gastroenterology 85: 1290–1300

Sun W M, Malbert C, Jones K et al 1993 Variation in spatial patterns of antropyloric pressure waves – a determinant of gastric mechanics. Gastroenterology 104: A589

Sun W M, Smout A, Malbert C et al 1995 Relationship between surface electrogastrography and antropyloric pressures. American Journal of Physiology 268: G424–430

Suzuki H, Amano S, Matsumoto K, Kitagawa T, Masuda T 1987 Chronic idiopathic intestinal pseudo-obstruction caused by acquired visceral neuropathy localized in the left colon: report of two cases. Japanese Journal of Surgery 17: 302–306

Tache Y, Garrick T, Raybould H 1990 Central nervous system action of peptides to influence gastrointestinal motor function. Gastroenterology 98: 517–528

Tack J, Janssens J, Vantrappen G et al 1992 Effect of erythromycin on gastric motility in controls and in diabetic gastroparesis. Gastroenterology 103: 72–79

Tatsuta M, Iishi H, Nakaizumi A, Okuda S 1992 Effect of treatment with cisapride alone or in combination with domperidone on gastric emptying and gastrointestinal symptoms in dyspeptic patients. Alimentary Pharmacology and Therapeutics 6: 221–228

Thompson D G, Malagelada J-R 1982 Vomiting and the small intestine. Digestive Diseases and Sciences 27: 1121–1125

Tougas G, Anvari M, Dent J et al 1992 Relation of pyloric motility to pyloric opening and closure in healthy subjects. Gut 33: 466–471

Troncon L E A, Bennett R J M, Ahluwalia N K, Thompson D G 1994 Abnormal intragastric distribution of food during gastric emptying in functional dyspepsia patients. Gut 35: 327–332

Tucci A, Corinaldesi R, Stanghellini V et al 1992 *Helicobacter pylori* infection and gastric function in patients with chronic idiopathic dyspepsia. Gastroenterology 103: 768–774

Urbain J L, Vekemans M C, Bouillon R et al 1993 Characterization of gastric antral motility disturbances in diabetes using a scintigraphic technique. Journal of Nuclear Medicine 34: 576–581

Vantrappen G, Janssens J, Hellemans J, Ghoos Y 1977 The interdigestive motor complex of normal subjects and patients with bacterial overgrowth of the small intestine. Journal of Clinical Investigation 59: 1158–1166

Vassallo M J, Camilleri M, Prather C M et al 1992a Measurement of axial forces during emptying from the human stomach. American Journal of Physiology 263: G230–G239

Vassallo M, Camilleri M, Phillips S F, Brown M L, Chapman N J, Thomforde G M 1992b Transit through the proximal colon influences stool weight in the irritable bowel syndrome. Gastroenterology 102: 102–108

Venizelos I O, Shousha S, Bull T B, Parkins R A 1988 Chronic intestinal pseudoobstruction in two patients. Overlap of features of systemic sclerosis and visceral myopathy. Histopathology 12: 533–540

Von der Ohe M, Camilleri M, Kvols L K, Thomforde G M 1993 Motor dysfunction of the small bowel and colon in patients with the carcinoid syndrome and diarrhea. New England Journal of Medicine 329: 1073–1078

Von der Ohe M R, Camilleri M, Thomforde G M, Klee G G 1995 Differential regional effects of octreotide on human gastrointestinal motor function. Gut 36: 743–748

Waldron B, Cullen P T, Kumar R et al 1991 Evidence for hypomotility in non-ulcer dyspepsia: a prospective multifactorial study. Gut 32: 246–251

Warner E, Jeejeebhoy K N 1985 Successful management of chronic intestinal pseudo-obstruction with home parenteral nutrition. Journal of Parenteral and Enteral Nutrition 9: 173–178

Weusten B L A M, Smout A J P M 1994 The secondary rumination syndrome. European Journal of Gastroenterology and Hepatology 6: 1171–1176

Wingate D L 1981 Backwards and forwards with the migrating complex. Digestive Diseases and Sciences 26: 641–666

Wiseman L R, Faulds D 1994 Cisapride: An updated review of its pharmacology and therapeutic efficacy as a prokinetic agent in gastrointestinal motility disorders. Drugs 47: 116–152

Wood J R, Camilleri M, Low P A, Malagelada J R 1985 Brainstem tumour presenting as an upper gut motility disorder. Gastroenterology 89: 1411–1414

Yoshida M, Schuffler M, Sumi S 1988 There are no morphological abnormalities of the gastric wall or abdominal vagus in patients with diabetic gastroparesis. Gastroenterology 94: 907–914

You C H, Chey W Y, Lee K Y et al 1981 Gastric and small intestinal myoelectric dysrhythmia associated with chronic intractable nausea and vomiting. Annals of Internal Medicine 95: 449–451

# 16. Structural disorders of the small intestine

*David Shearman*

The physiology of the bile acid circulation is discussed on p. 755.

## INTESTINAL RESECTION

Resection of large amounts of the terminal ileum due to Crohn's disease or vascular insufficiency with gangrene may lead to diarrhea and severe malabsorption. Extensive resection also occurs in patients with radiation enteritis, intestinal pseudo-obstruction and with volvulus leading to infarction in the neonatal period. It is often difficult to relate the expected degree of malabsorption to the length of bowel removed at operation and in the case of an extensive resection, it is more important for the surgeon to estimate the length of viable bowel which remains. This is because the normal length of the small intestine shows a wide variation (p. 337). Resection of a short length (even 20–30 cm) of terminal ileum can cause derangement of the absorptive processes, whereas up to 50% of the mid small intestine can be resected without significant problems. Survival is recorded when only 15–46 cm of small bowel remain in addition to the duodenum. In children, survival with normal growth is recorded when only 11 cm of jejunoileum together with an intact ileocecal valve or 25 cm without the valve remain (Dorney et al 1985).

Ileal resection or disease reduces the surface area of intestine capable of absorbing bile acids. Experiments using controlled interruption of the enterohepatic circulation in the Rhesus monkey have shown that when more than 20% of the bile flow is diverted, the bile acid pool decreases (Dowling 1973). Interruption of the enterohepatic circulation by resection of less than 100 cm of ileum has the following effects on bile acid metabolism. Fecal concentration and daily excretion of bile acids are increased, the primary bile acids, cholic acid and chenodeoxycholic acid being dehydroxylated to deoxycholic and lithocholic acid. In some patients, dehydroxylation is inhibited, resulting in a persistence of primary bile acids. The concentration of bile acids may be maintained in the duodenum by increased hepatic synthesis. There is diarrhea because increased amounts of bile acids enter the colon, but steatorrhea is absent or mild. With resections of more than 100 cm, duodenal bile acid concentrations may only be adequate for the first meal of the day because of overnight synthesis and storage in the gallbladder, but they are inadequate for fat absorption during later meals and steatorrhea results.

### Results of intestinal resection

*Fluid and electrolyte depletion*

The diarrhea associated with the short bowel syndrome (p. 454) arises predominantly from endogenous secretions which amount to 8 liters per 24 h (p. 627). Normally 80% of endogenous secretions are reabsorbed in the small intestine, the remainder being absorbed by the colon.

*Gastric hypersecretion*

This may occur after massive small bowel resection. Animal experiments suggest that the degree of hypersecretion increases with the degree of resection. Hypergastrinemia has been demonstrated in some patients and it is likely that inhibitors of gastrin such as gastric-inhibiting polypeptide and vasoactive intestinal polypeptide are removed with the resected bowel. The hypersecretion is often an initial, transient event but it can persist, thereby lowering intestinal pH sufficiently to affect absorptive processes. In particular the low jejunal pH may precipitate bile acids thus reducing their effective jejunal concentration (Fitzpatrick et al 1986). Furthermore, the low jejunal pH is promoted by more rapid gastric emptying of acid because of removal of the ileal brake mechanism (Williams et al 1985) and feedback mechanisms in the colon (Nightingale et al 1993) that normally retard upper gastrointestinal transit.

*Adaptation (compensation) by the residual bowel* (Weser 1976, Dowling 1982a & b)

Much of our knowledge is derived from studies in laboratory animals, but there are sufficient data to confirm a similar pattern of responses in man (Williamson 1978).

Adaptation for the loss of bowel involves the colon as well as the remaining proximal and distal small intestine; colectomy also stimulates ileal adaptation (Williamson 1982). Hyperplasia of the enterocytes resulting in enlargement of the villi is detectable within 1–2 days and becomes maximal 1–2 weeks after resection; subsequently, there may be some elongation of the residual bowel. The response of the ileum to proximal resection is much greater than the response of the jejunum to ileal resection.

Several factors influence adaptation (Lentze 1989).

Intraluminal nutrients promote adaptation whereas parenteral nutrients generally do not. Long chain triglycerides and in particular their free fatty acids, oleic and linoleic acids are the most effective inducers of adaptation and may act independently or through the release of enteroglucagon. Medium chain triglycerides are less effective than long chain trigycerides. Undigested proteins and pectin or water-soluble fiber polysaccharide also stimulate adaptation. The latter is fermented to short chain fatty acids in the colon; these are absorbed and have a trophic effect on intestinal mucosa, which also occurs when they are given in parenteral nutrition (Koruda et al 1988).

Humoral factors are important in adaptation as illustrated by crosscirculation experiments. Enteroglucagon is the most important of these (Bloom & Polak 1982, Buchan et al 1985). A possible role for cholecystokinin, secretin and pancreaticobiliary secretions is controversial. Various growth factors including epidermal growth factor and prostaglandins may also play a role.

Some or all of the factors responsible for adaptation are likely to act through ornithine decarboxylase within the epithelial cell (Dowling 1990). This is the rate-limiting enzyme for polyamine synthesis, which in turn is necessary for rapid growth. The polyamines concerned are spermine, spermidine and putrescine and they promote synthesis of deoxyribonucleic acid.

*Catharsis due to bile acids in the colon*

Bile acids which are unabsorbed because of ileal resection or disease pass into the colon. They are deconjugated by anaerobic bacteria; thereafter, they inhibit water and electrolyte absorption and may even cause a net secretion (Mekhjian et al 1971), resulting in watery diarrhea. The secretory effects may be mediated by stimulation of the enzyme adenylate cyclase, by activating reflexes in the enteric nervous system (Karlström 1986) or by altering mucosal permeability (Chadwick et al 1979). The rate of fecal bile acid excretion correlates with the fecal excretion of water and some studies show that unconjugated dihydroxy bile acids exert most of this purgative effect. Bile acids may exert a further diarrheal effect by increasing colonic motility by stimulating the enteric nervous system (Karlström 1986). Fecal pH is also an important factor in that high concentrations of dihydroxy bile acids are found with an alkaline fecal pH whereas with severe steatorrhea, fecal pH is acidic and the concentration of dihydroxy bile acids is low (McJunkin et al 1981).

It is important to realize that diarrhea due to an excessive loss of bile acids into the colon need not be associated with steatorrhea if the jejunal concentration of conjugated bile acid is maintained by increased hepatic synthesis. This is often the case when the ileal resection is less than 100 cm. The severity of diarrhea is influenced not only by the length of the ileal resection but also by the length of colonic resection. The relation between colonic resection and the severity of diarrhea applies to patients with ileal resection of both less and greater than 100 cm (Mitchell et al 1980).

*Malabsorption*

The absorption of fat and fat-soluble vitamins is partly dependent on an adequate concentration of conjugated bile acids in the jejunum (p. 352). Steatorrhea is common if more than 100 cm of ileum are resected (Fromm et al 1973). Other factors may add to the severity of steatorrhea; the rapid transit time after large resections leaves insufficient time for digestion and absorption and bacterial colonization of the shortened bowel is common, particularly if the ileocecal valve has been removed. This leads to excessive deconjugation of the bile acids and an increase in steatorrhea. However, an important cause of diarrhea in these patients is the malabsorption of fatty acids which causes colonic secretion (p. 462). Steatorrhea also increases the absorption of oxalate and this has been noted particularly after ileal resection. The rapid transit through the small intestine is due to more frequent migrating motor complexes which are propulsive (phase III) and a reduction in phase II activity which is segmenting (Remington et al 1983).

Carbohydrate malabsorption is another major cause of watery diarrhea in patients with short bowel syndrome. Usually intestinal lactase activity is decreased and unhydrolyzed lactose is fermented by intestinal bacteria. In some patients up to 65% of dietary carbohydrate is excreted in the stool (Ameen et al 1987).

*Oxalate nephrolithiasis*

An increased incidence of renal oxalate stones has been reported after ileal resection and after jejunoileal bypass; they result from an increased absorption of oxalate (Chadwick et al 1973). Under normal circumstances, calcium in the intestinal lumen binds oxalate to form insoluble calcium oxalate. When there is steatorrhea, calcium soaps are formed and there is an increased concentration of oxalate in the aqueous phase of intestinal fluid with increased absorption and ultimately renal excretion. Thus both ileal disease and steatorrhea are necessary for oxalate nephrolithiasis; neither is a risk factor when it occurs alone (Dharmsathaphorn et al 1982). Oxalate absorption through the colonic mucosa is also favored by the greater permeability due to effects of unabsorbed fatty acids and bile acids which are present in increased amounts after ileal resection. A reduction in dietary oxalate does not reduce the urinary excretion of oxalate in all patients because protein-rich foods can be oxalogenic (Hofmann et al 1983).

*Cholesterol gallstones*

Resection or disease of the terminal ileum is associated with a fourfold increase in the incidence of gallstones (Heaton & Read 1969, Cohen et al 1971). In ileal dysfunction, the bile is usually supersaturated with cholesterol (Dowling et al 1972) and this may be due in part to a diminished bile acid pool.

## Ileal resection or dysfunction

*Clinical features*

In ileal resection or disease due to radiation enteropathy or Crohn's disease, the patient has painless diarrhea, the severity of which depends on the extent of the affected bowel. The diarrhea is usually watery, regardless of the presence of steatorrhea, and occurs only after meals. It is often most severe after breakfast, when bile acid secretion is at its greatest.

*Diagnosis*

***Stool weight.*** Significant bile acid malabsorption is excluded by the finding of a normal daily stool weight.

***Vitamin $B_{12}$ absorption.*** If the measurement of vitamin $B_{12}$ absorption shows malabsorption in the presence of ileal resection, interruption of the bile acid circulation is also likely (Fromm et al 1973). However, interruption of the enterohepatic circulation, as indicated by $^{75}$SeHCAT, may exist when vitamin $B_{12}$ absorption is normal.

***Bile acid absorption.*** This can be assessed by the oral administration of $^{14}$C glycocholate and the measurement of radioactivity in stool, blood or breath. It is not common for nonlabeled bile acids to be measured in feces because of the difficulties of fecal analysis. The stool radioactivity is assessed (Roda et al 1977) over several days or over 24 h if a stool marker is used (Thaysen 1977). Stool radioactivity is increased in contrast to patients with bacterial overgrowth or stagnant loop syndrome; such patients show normal or decreased radioactivity. The $^{14}$C-glycocholic acid breath test (ch. 3) is of occasional value although it is an insensitive way of detecting malabsorption of bile acids in comparison to the direct measurement of radioactivity in feces (Lauterburg et al 1978). For example, it has been shown that normal breath tests may occur with severe bile acid malabsorption. In addition, it is not possible to distinguish bacterial overgrowth from malabsorption of bile acid in the ileum.

***$^{75}$SeHCAT absorption.*** Bile acid absorption is best measured by $^{75}$SeHCAT retention using whole body counting (p. 89).

***Other investigations.*** Other investigations which have implications for therapy and management are a stool fat estimation (p. 355), serum calcium concentration and prothrombin time and an assessment of urinary oxalate output.

*Treatment*

A combination of cholestyramine, dietary fat restriction and antidiarrheal agents will render most patients asymptomatic. Measures to reduce oxalate absorption may also be necessary.

***Cholestyramine*** (Beher 1976). This is an anion-binding resin which is not absorbed and which binds conjugated bile acids and other anions in the jejunum. It is administered as the chloride salt; chloride ions exchange with bile acid anions in the small intestine and hyperchloremic acidosis may therefore occur in patients with renal failure. It is used to treat diarrhea after ileal resection (Rowe 1967), being effective when the resection is less than 100 cm. It is given orally at meal times in a dose of 4 g one to four times per day. One sachet (4 g of cholestyramine) is placed on the surface of a glass of water or fruit juice, allowed to stand for 2 min and then stirred just prior to drinking. It can also be mixed with liquid foods, but should not be taken dry. Other drugs should not be administered at the same time since these may be bound to the resin and hence malabsorbed. Therapy should be commenced with 4 g at breakfast and the dosage increased over several days until the minimum dose effective in controlling the diarrhea is established. For example, some patients with only a small degree of interruption of the enterohepatic circulation often obtain control with a 4 g dose at breakfast. This treatment may increase the amount of fecal fat excreted and it is important to give supplements of vitamins A, D and K. Serum calcium concentration and alkaline phosphatase activity should be checked regularly.

The response to cholestyramine is often poor in patients with marked steatorrhea (Hofmann & Poley 1969), as the diarrhea in these cases is often related to steatorrhea rather than bile acid catharsis and responds to dietary restriction of long chain triglycerides. Such patients usually have an ileal resection greater than 100 cm. Cholestyramine is also said to bind ingested oxalate (Stauffer et al 1973), but whether this is sufficient to prevent the excessive absorption of dietary oxalate is not known.

In one patient, cholestyramine was absorbed and deposited in various body tissues; the portal of entry was probably an ulcerated distal esophagus (McDonald & Vracko 1984).

***Treatment of hyperoxaluria.*** This occurs particularly after ileal resection. With the patient on a normal diet, the 24-h urinary oxalate should be assessed. If it is elevated, dietary restriction of oxalate, a high fluid intake and oral calcium supplements should be instituted. Dietary fat restriction is also of value. The important high oxalate foods are mainly fruits and vegetables, but tea, coffee, cocoa and malt drinks should be remembered (Stauffer 1977). Many other drinks, particularly beer and cola, also have a high oxalate content (Earnest 1977).

## SHORT BOWEL SYNDROME

This cannot be defined by the specific length of residual intestine. Rather, it is a combination of clinical signs and symptoms characterized by intractable diarrhea, steatorrhea and malabsorption of other nutrients and vitamins, weight loss, dehydration and malnutrition (Dudrick et al 1991). Factors which determine the severity and features of the presentation are shown in Table 16.1.

Usually short bowel syndrome is present when 75% or more of the small intestine is resected, leaving the patient with 70–100 cm of intestine. The problem is likely to be severe if the terminal ileum and ileocecal valve are lost. In addition, preservation of the colon is important for the maintenance of sodium and water balance and for the absorption of calcium (Hylander et al 1990).

### Clinical features (p. 627)

The patient has intractable high volume diarrhea, loss of weight, dehydration and malnutrition. Additional symptoms arise from hypovolemia, hypoalbuminemia, loss of potassium, calcium and magnesium, vitamin deficiencies and metabolic acidosis.

### Treatment

This is conveniently discussed under the following headings.

**Table 16.1** Short bowel syndrome. Factors which determine the severity and features of presentation

| |
|---|
| Extent of resection |
| Site of resection |
| Presence or absence of the ileocecal valve |
| Presence or absence of the colon |
| Residual function of small bowel, stomach, pancreas and biliary tract |
| Adaptive capacity of residual small intestine |
| Primary disease that caused the problem |
| Extent and activity of residual disease |

1. Measures which should be undertaken in the preoperative period if surgery is not an emergency.
2. The immediate preoperative period – this is defined as the first 2 months by Dudrick et al (1991).
3. The bowel adaptation period – 2 months to 2 years (Dudrick et al 1991).
4. Long-term management.

A summary of management options is shown in Table 16.2.

#### *Preoperative management* (Shaffer et al 1976)

Preoperative nutritional support in patients about to undergo intestinal resection for inflammatory bowel disease should be considered if their weight is 10% below ideal body weight or if the serum albumin concentration is less than 25 g/L. Usually, 10–14 days of nutritional support is indicated; positive nitrogen balance may be achieved after 1–2 days with a daily nitrogen intake of about 14 g along with carbohydrate and lipid contributing 150–200 kcal/g nitrogen, 150 kcal/g being used in parenteral nutrition and 200 kcal/g when nutrition is by the enteral route. Higher rates of carbohydrate and fat may be appropriate in patients with sepsis or those taking corticosteroids. Nutrition can be given both intravenously and orally as an enteral diet, the proportion of each depending on the presence of intestinal obstruction or diarrhea.

At the initial resection the surgeon must make every attempt to preserve the maximum amount of intestine. If possible, the ileocecal valve should be retained and also the right colon because of its capacity to absorb water and electrolytes (Mitchell et al 1980).

#### *Immediate postoperative management*

Initially, fluid and electrolytes are given intravenously. On the second or third postoperative day parenteral nutrition with 3000–4000 kcal/g/day is given. The intravenous regimen consists of amino acids for the replacement of protein losses and a nonprotein calorie source such as glucose, often together with lipid, which contributes essential fatty acids and prevents excess insulin secretion which accompanies the use of glucose as the sole source of calories. The selection of appropriate intravenous regimens has been reviewed (Gilder 1986). The inevitable large fluid, sodium and potassium losses must be replaced intravenously as the fluid loss can be up to 10 L/day (Bochenek et al 1970); calcium, magnesium and phosphate deficiency and hypoprothrombinemia must be watched for. Oral diphenoxylate, codeine or loperamide may be used to treat diarrhea. The somatostatin analog octreotide may also be of value at doses of 100–300 μg t.i.d. With very large resections, gastric hypersecretion may be assumed and an $H_2$

**Table 16.2** Management of short bowel syndrome (modified from Dudrick et al 1991)

| Immediate postoperative period (first 2 months) | Bowel adaptation period (first 2 years) | Long-term management (after 2 years) |
|---|---|---|
| Fluid and electrolyte replacement<br>Lactated Ringer's solution<br>Dextrose 5% in water<br>Human serum albumin<br>$K^+$, $Ca^{2+}$, $Mg^{2+}$ supplementation<br>Strict intake and output monitoring<br>Daily body weight<br>Graduated metabolic monitoring | Progression of oral diet<br>Water, tea, broth<br>Simple salt solutions<br>Simple sugar solutions<br>Complex salt/sugar solution<br>Dilute chemically defined diets<br>High carbohydrate, high protein<br>Near-normal, normal diet | Apply previous principles<br>as indicated individually<br><br>Ambulatory home TPN<br>Supplemental or total<br>Continuous, cyclic or intermittent |
| Antacid therapy<br>Liquid antacid (30–60 ml via nasogastric tube) or 2-hourly<br>Carafate 1 g p.o. 6-hourly | Enteral supplementation<br>Coconut oil 30 ml p.o. t.i.d.<br>Safflower oil 30 ml p.o. t.i.d.<br>Multiple vitamins 1 ml b.i.d.<br>Iron 1 ml t.i.d.<br>Ca gluconate 6–8 g/day<br>Na bicarbonate 8–12 g/day | Surgical managment<br>Treat operative complications<br>Drain abscesses<br>Resect fistulae<br>Lyse adhesions<br>Reduce obstructions<br>Restore bowel continuity<br>Cholecystectomy for symptomatic gallstones |
| Antisecretory-antimotility therapy<br>Cimetidine 300 mg IV q 6 h<br>Ranitidine 150 mg IV q 12 h<br>Famotidine 20 mg IV q 12 h<br>Codeine 60 mg IM q 4 h<br>Loperamide 4–16 mg p.o. daily<br>Lomotil 20 mg p.o. q 6 h<br>Octreotide 50–150 μg SC q 6 h<br>Cholestyramine 4 g p.o. q 8 h | Parenteral supplementation<br>Electrolytes<br>Divalent cations<br>Trace elements<br>Albumin<br>Packed erythrocytes<br>Lipid emulsion | |
| TPN<br>1 L on second postop day<br>Gradually increase dosage as tolerated<br>Supplement fluids, electrolytes and colloids as needed | Antisecretory<br>Famotidine 20 mg p.o. q 12 h<br>(or other $H_2$ antagonist)<br>Omeprazole 20 mg p.o. q day | |
| Oral and enteral supplementation<br>Introduction of small amounts as soon as possible | Antimotility<br>as in column 1 | |

receptor antagonist should be given as a parenteral infusion. This has been shown to reduce the output from a jejunostomy (Jacobsen et al 1986). Antacid therapy or sucralfate is given to reduce the tendency for acute ulceration or erosions.

Oral nutrition is started 1–3 weeks after surgery while intravenous nutrition is being given. An elemental diet (p. 630) which will promote compensatory adaptation whilst supplying some nutritional requirements with minimum stimulation of digestive secretions is given. Initially, 1 liter of quarter strength solution is given daily through a small-bore nasogastric tube and the concentration and volume are increased gradually until several liters are given each day.

Periods of up to 21 days on an elemental diet are followed by a gradual introduction of a low-lactose, low-fat, high-protein and high-carbohydrate diet. Milk is avoided because of lactase deficiency (although yoghurt may be taken) and supplements of medium chain triglycerides (MCT) are given. However, the use of a low-fat diet means that more carbohydrate has to be given and it has been debated whether such diets are advantageous (Woolf et al 1983, Young 1983); there is no difference in loss of water and electrolytes between high-fat and high-carbohydrate diets (Jeejeebhoy 1983).

*Bowel adaptation period*

This is the period of adaption to the gradual introduction of the above diet, whilst support from parenteral nutrition is gradually decreased. Initially oral sodium bicarbonate for metabolic alkalosis and calcium gluconate for hypocalcemia are nearly always required and may need to be continued indefinitely after extensive resections. Other supplementations are listed in Table 16.2.

*Long-term management*

A minority of patients require supplemental parenteral nutrition continuously or intermittently for life. However, the majority will manage with a modified oral diet, an enteral diet, total or supplementary, or an oral or enteral diet supplemented with intravenous fluid and electrolytes. The outcome depends on the degree of intestinal adaptation. Recent studies suggest that in patients with at least 75 cm of small bowel, fluid needs can be supplemented with hyperosmolar glucose-electrolyte solutions.

Subsequent surgical treatment is indicated for gallstones which are common (p. 1202). A variety of surgical procedures which slow intestinal flow are described (Dudrick et al 1991) but none is recommended.

## GASTROINTESTINAL SURGERY FOR MORBID OBESITY (Adibi & Stanko 1984, O'Brien 1994) (Fig. 16.1)

Severe obesity is unequivocally associated with significant medical morbidity and given the ineffectiveness of conservative therapy, surgery may offer an approach to treatment. The American Society for Clinical Nutrition has published guidelines for surgery for obesity. The indications for surgery include the criterion that prospective patients should be morbidly obese – at least 100% or 45 kg above ideal body weight.

Initially, small intestinal bypass procedures were used to achieve weight loss by creating malabsorption but because of side-effects, these have been largely superseded by gastric reduction operations. However biliopancreatic bypass and ileal bypass are occasionally used and are described below. In addition, jejunoileal bypass is described because the side-effects must be recognized and treated in previous recipients of the operation. Most reports of gastric reduction operations have described a low incidence of complications, large mean weight losses (associated with improvements in medical disorders such as diabetes mellitus, lipid abnormalities and hypertension) and psychological benefits (Stunkard et al 1986). During the first year after operation the magnitude of weight loss is extremely variable, but averages at approximately 50% of excess weight and is similar with all procedures. There are few long-term studies, but weight loss appears to plateau after the first year. Nevertheless, previous experience with jejunoileal bypass dictates that any gastrointestinal operation for treatment of obesity should be subjected to comprehensive eval-

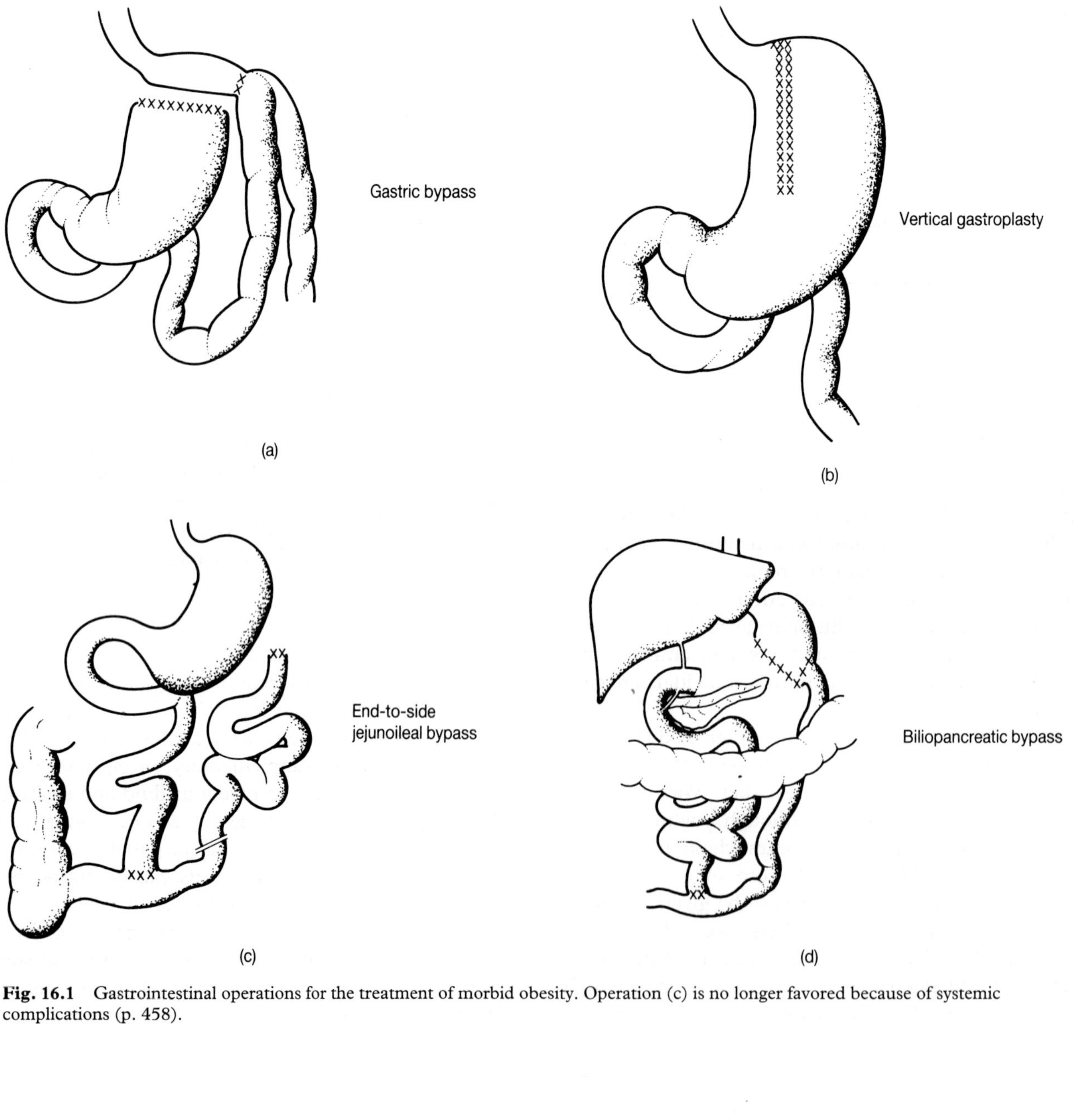


**Fig. 16.1** Gastrointestinal operations for the treatment of morbid obesity. Operation (c) is no longer favored because of systemic complications (p. 458).

uation and assessment before being widely used and at this time surgery for obesity should not be performed for cosmetic reasons or for obesity of less than great severity.

### Gastric partitioning procedures

These procedures have become the most widely performed surgical treatment for obesity. The basic principles of these operations are to produce a small gastric reservoir of 30–50 ml and a small stoma (1 cm diameter) to communicate with the remainder of the gastrointestinal tract. They markedly reduce the volume of food which can be consumed at any one time and thus differ radically from intestinal bypass, which permits unlimited consumption subject only to the discomfort of the subsequent diarrhea. In some gastric restriction procedures, the gastric reservoir may empty food more slowly, resulting in a prolonged sense of fullness (Horowitz et al 1984). Failure of these procedures, which may necessitate revision, may be caused by dilatation of the gastric reservoir or outlet. Weight loss is also likely to be unsatisfactory if the patient eats frequent small meals or consumes high-calorie liquids. Unlike jejunoileal bypass there appears to be minimal loss of lean body mass with these procedures and hepatic complications have not been reported.

*Gastric bypass* (Griffen et al 1981)

Gastric bypass, the first gastric restriction procedure, was introduced in 1967 by Mason & Ito. It involves the construction of a fundic pouch of approximately 50 ml volume which is connected to the jejunum by a gastroenterostomy (approximately 1 cm diameter) and a distal bypassed stomach, which remains as a blind pouch that empties into the duodenum. Gastric bypass is technically more difficult to perform than jejunoileal bypass and is associated with a significant risk of immediate postoperative complications, such as anastomotic leaks, stomal obstruction and peritonitis. The long-term complications of gastric bypass are far fewer and less severe than those following intestinal bypass. In general, depending on the patient's ability to cope with the small pouch, excessive nausea and vomiting do not persist for more than 3 weeks postoperatively. Liver disease has been documented only in a small number of patients (Rucker et al 1982) and nephrolithiasis is also uncommon. Vitamin $B_{12}$ malabsorption may also occur (Behrns et al 1994). Since these patients rarely have diarrhea, electrolyte imbalances are uncommon.

*Gastroplasty* (Gomez 1981a & b)

The technical difficulties of gastric bypass are greatly reduced by gastroplasty procedures. Vertical banded gastroplasty is widely considered as the operation of choice for morbid obesity, as it is simpler and easier to perform than other gastric restriction procedures and preserves a normal sequence in the passage of food. The operative technique involves the production of a stapled pouch 20–60 ml in volume, orientated along the lesser curvature of the stomach, and an outlet at the lower end of the pouch measuring approximately 12 mm in diameter. To provide additional support for the outlet, a Marlex mesh collar may be sewn around the outside of the stomach wall, where it is rapidly enveloped by connective tissue. Location of the pouch along the lesser curvature takes advantage of the greater muscle strength of this region and decreases the tendency towards distention that has plagued traditional pouches located in the fundus. Reinforcement of the stoma with a plastic collar eliminates the stomal dilatation that has occurred with other gastric restriction procedures.

*Adjustable silicone gastric banding*

At laparoscopy the band is placed around the upper stomach to create a small pouch and small stoma. Subsequently the size of the stoma can be adjusted to increase or decrease weight loss.

*Biliopancreatic bypass* (Scopinaro et al 1981)

This procedure creates a maldigestion which results in a selective malabsorption for main foodstuffs with caloric value, with no interruption of the bile acid enterohepatic circulation and no blind loop. A distal gastrectomy is performed, with closure of the duodenal stump. A Roux-en-Y reconstruction is made, the enterostomy being placed at a distal ileal level. In the new anatomic situation, three intestinal tracts can be recognized: the alimentary tact where only foods not requiring digestion can be absorbed; the biliopancreatic tract, conducting pancreatic and biliary juices to the distal ileum; and the common tract of terminal ileum, which is necessary for complete bile acid absorption and where digestion and absorption of fats, starch and proteins begin.

### Ileal bypass for familial hypercholesterolemia

Familial hypercholesterolemia usually causes premature ischemic heart disease. Ileal bypass which excludes the distal one-third of the small intestine reduces plasma cholesterol, especially the low density lipoproteins, more efficiently than alternative treatments such as neomycin or cholestyramine. The operation results in an increase of bile acids in the stool and there is diarrhea and slight steatorrhea (Faergeman et al 1982). The malabsorption of cholesterol after operation slowly returns to normal over a period of 8 years due to intestinal adaptation, whereas malabsorption of bile acid continues (Koivisto & Miettinen 1986). The florid side-effects of the more radical bypass operations have not been reported but there is an increase in the renal excretion of oxalate, a decrease in calcium absorption and minor rises in serum alanine aminotransferase (Faergeman et al 1982).

## Jejunoileal bypass

This invariably induces initial weight loss, diarrhea and a variety of beneficial and undesirable side-effects (Juhl et al 1979, Joffe 1981, Adibi & Stanko 1984).

The usual operation was a jejunoileostomy in which the proximal 35 cm of jejunum was anastomosed end-to-side or end-to-end to the last 10 cm of the ileum and the proximal end of the defunctioned jejunum was closed. With the end-to-end bypass the excluded intestinal segment was anastomosed to the colon. Thus 90% of the small intestine was bypassed. The operative mortality was around 3%. There is a 30% incidence of postoperative complications.

A large proportion of patients lose 35–50 kg of their body weight in the first year after operation; thereafter weight loss levels off due to intestinal adaptation. Weight loss is due mainly to reduced intake. The metabolic benefits of this weight reduction are an increase in glucose tolerance so that those patients requiring insulin or oral hypoglycemic agents may be able to discontinue them, a decline in serum cholesterol and triglyceride, a reduction in hypertension and an improvement in psychological features related to the obesity.

Diarrhea and steatorrhea result (Iber & Cooper 1977) because of a shortened transit time and malabsorption of bile acids (Faloon et al 1977) and osmotic diarrhea because of malabsorption of sugars. The diarrhea is most severe in the first year after surgery during which weight loss is most pronounced; depletion of calcium, potassium and magnesium is common. However, a prospective study of patients undergoing jejunoileal bypass suggests that the initial abnormalities in mineral metabolism tend to correct themselves after 2 years (Sellin et al 1984).

### *Liver disease*

Progressive liver disease may develop during this period and is sometimes fatal (p. 976). The etiological factors are thought to be protein malnutrition and bacterial overgrowth.

### *Stagnant loop syndrome*

A stagnant loop syndrome may develop from bacterial overgrowth in the defunctioned jejunum and treatment with metronidazole retards the development of hepatic steatosis (Drenick et al 1982).

### *D-Lactic acidosis*

D-Lactic acidosis associated with neurological dysfunction has been reported in patients with extensive small bowel resection. This problem is caused by an increase in fecal Gram-positive anaerobes such as *Bifidobacterium, Eubacterium* and *Lactobacillus* and a reduction in Gram-negative anaerobes such as *Bacteroides* (Stolberg et al 1982). The former organisms produce D-lactic acid.

The patient complains of dizziness, ataxia, dysarthria, disorientation, confusion, somnolence, loss of memory, headache, behavioral changes, weakness, inco-ordination of the arms and blurring of vision. Symptoms usually develop 5 years after bypass.

There is a hyperchloremic metabolic acidosis and in most patients there are D-lactate levels of greater than 0.5 mmol/L (Thurn et al 1985).

Treatment with neomycin, neomycin plus ampicillin or vancomycin has corrected the clinical, biochemical and microbiological abnormalities.

### *Enteropathy of excluded bowel*

Enteropathy of the excluded bowel has been described (Drenick et al 1977). Microscopy shows a nonspecific inflammatory process and there is often marked proliferation of enteric bacteria within the lumen. Symptoms, which include persistent diarrhea with abdominal distention sometimes giving rise to the features of pseudo-obstruction (p. 441), respond to broad-spectrum antibiotics or metronidazole.

It is likely that the excluded loop is responsible for many of the abdominal symptoms after bypass operations. Pneumatosis intestinalis occurs in about 10% of patients. The appearance of arthritis and skin lesions resembling erythema nodosum is due to circulating immune complexes arising in the wall of the excluded bowel (Duncan 1977) (see below).

### *Protein malnutrition*

When protein nutrition is assessed by the profile of amino acids in venous blood, alterations typical of kwashiorkor are found in the period 12–36 months after operation. There is speculation that these deficiencies are a contributory factor in the development of liver disease.

### *Renal disease*

This results from oxalate nephropathy (p. 452). There is also deposition of immune complexes which leads to mesangial injury.

### *Arthritis and dermatitis*

These result from bacterial overgrowth in the excluded

jejunum and are usually accompanied by the symptoms of enteropathy. The absorption of bacterial antigen leads to the formation of cryoglobulin immune complexes which are deposited in the skin and joints. The joint symptoms which occur in 35% of patients vary from episodic polyarthralgia to a persistent polyarthritis (Delamere et al 1983) which is negative for rheumatoid factor. The skin lesions include urticaria and pustular necrosis.

### Other surgical methods in the treatment of obesity

*Jaw wiring* (Kark 1980)

Jaw wiring, or maxillomandibular fixation, is a standard treatment for jaw fractures. In the treatment of severe obesity, jaw wiring has been used to restrict the intake of solid food while permitting the ingestion of liquid foods. Typically, weight loss averages 35 kg over a 9-month period. Because patients who have lost weight by jaw wiring usually regain the lost weight when the wires are removed, it should not be accepted as a treatment by itself. It has a place as a preparation for surgery but has not gained acceptance.

*Vagotomy* (Kral & Görtz 1981)

A rationale for this procedure is provided by the fact that vagotomy reduces the food intake and body weight of a variety of species, although it has little effect on the genetic forms of obesity. Humans treated by vagotomy for duodenal ulcer may report little or no feeling of hunger. Kral & Görtz (1981) performed truncal vagotomy on 21 severely obese patients. At 1 year, mean weight loss was $20 \pm 4$ kg with a range of 0 to 52 kg and patients reported less hunger and a greater ease of adherence to a traditional weight reduction program. This procedure must still be considered experimental.

*Intragastric balloons*

Intragastric balloons (free floating or attached to a nasal cannula) were introduced in an effort to achieve gastric restriction by noninvasive means. This idea is plausible as gastric distention has been recognized as a satiety mechanism in the experimental animal for many years and bezoars can present as weight loss in otherwise healthy subjects. These procedures have not gained acceptance because of complications including balloon deflation and have been prohibited by the FDA.

## BACTERIAL OVERGROWTH IN THE SMALL INTESTINE – THE STAGNANT LOOP SYNDROME

Bacterial overgrowth in the small intestine occurs in structural abnormalities and motility disorders and occasionally in immunological deficiency diseases. The overgrowth may result in steatorrhea, malabsorption of vitamin $B_{12}$ and other absorptive problems (Tabaqchali & Booth 1970).

As early as 1890, White suspected a relationship between small bowel strictures and an anemia which resembled pernicious anemia and in 1924, Seyderhelm et al showed that removal of a stricture cured the anemia (see Donaldson 1970). Today, the terms "blind loop" or "stagnant loop" syndromes are used to describe absorptive disorders resulting from bacterial overgrowth. Because the syndrome can arise without a structural blind loop, the term "contaminated small bowel syndrome" is also used (Gracey 1971, 1983).

### Bacteria in the normal intestine (Finegold et al 1983, Simon & Gorbach 1984)

The normal intestinal flora in the adult is represented in Figure 16.2 (Gorbach & Levitan 1970). The microflora of the stomach is mainly Gram-positive and aerobic with $<10^3$ colony-forming units/ml, the common organisms being streptococci, staphylococci, lactobacilli and fungi with occasional oral anaerobes. The duodenum and jejunum have low concentrations ($10^1$–$10^4$) of these organisms, although these counts are higher in residents of developing countries. Such organisms are probably derived from the saliva (Hamilton et al 1982). Coliforms are seen occasionally, but counts do not exceed $10^3$/ml. In the ileum, there is a greater number of bacteria ($10^3$–$10^8$/ml) and coliforms and anaerobes are found regularly. The ileocecal valve tends to separate the flora into two types (Gorbach 1967). In the ileum, there is a preponderance of the Gram-positive aerobes, whereas in the cecum ($10^8$–$10^{12}$ organisms/ml) the flora consists mainly of anaerobes, including large numbers of *Bacteroides*, *Bifidobacterium*, *Eubacterium*, coliforms, enterococci and *Clostridia*.

### Bacteria in the small intestine in stagnant loop syndromes

The population tends to resemble that of the large intestine and counts as high as $10^8$–$10^{10}$ organisms/ml are obtained. Many different organisms are present (Drasar & Hill 1974) and the abnormal proliferation of bacteria may be generalized or localized (Gorbach & Tabaqchali 1969). Diagnostic criteria are discussed on p. 463.

### Mechanisms controlling the normal bacterial flora (Drasar & Hill 1974)

***Gastric acidity.*** This plays an important part in controlling the number of bacteria in the upper small intestine. Most oral bacteria are killed by acid and pepsin

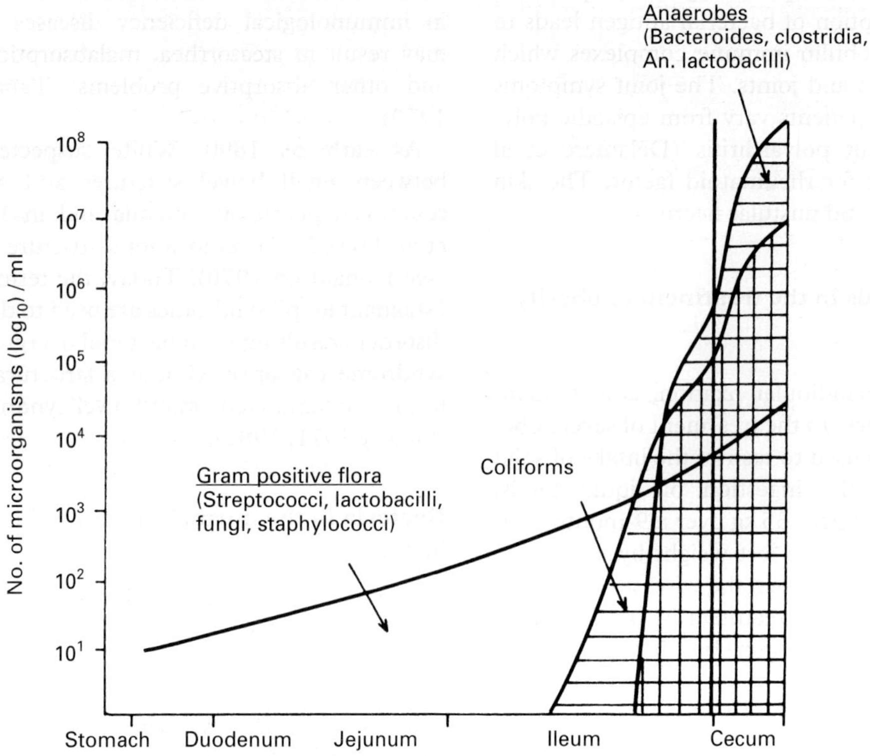


**Fig. 16.2** The normal bacterial flora (Gorbach & Levitan 1970).

(Gray & Shiner 1967), but a small number of acid-resistant forms are passed into the duodenum during eating. When there is achlorhydria due to atrophic gastritis or proton pump inhibitors, bacterial counts in the stomach and upper small intestine are increased. Gastric acid is a major defense mechanism against infection with enteric pathogens, e.g. cholera (p. 563).

***Intestinal motility.*** Animal studies have shown that bacteria placed in the small intestine can be recovered quantitatively from the large bowel. Thus small intestinal motility, particularly in the fasting state, is probably responsible for the generally low bacterial counts in the upper small intestine. The slow progression of residue in the large intestine is one of the factors which allows proliferation of bacteria there.

***Other factors.*** Other secretions, such as bile or saliva, may inhibit certain organisms, but there is no evidence that they play a major role in the control of the flora. Although intestinal motility ensures that organisms in the lumen do not proliferate unduly, it has been shown by repeated washings that large numbers of bacteria cannot be dislodged from the small bowel surface (Dubos et al 1965) because they are within the mucus which is adherent to the mucosa (Savage 1983). The relative importance of epithelial cell turnover, surface mucus and secretory immunoglobulins in the defense against commensal bacteria is not known (Shearman et al 1972). A minor role for immunoglobulin is suggested by the finding that bacterial overgrowth is not always a problem in patients with hypogammaglobulinemia (Parkin et al 1972a). However, specific antibody does have a role in the control of pathogens (LaBrooy & Shearman 1979); parasites and unusual organisms proliferate in the intestine of patients with immunological deficiency. Specific antibody to pathogenic bacteria prevents their adherence to the mucosa, reduces their motility and agglutinates them. Agglutinated organisms are more susceptible to clearance by peristalsis (p. 400). Within the colon, organisms are regulated by microbial interactions. Some organisms produce colicins which are bactericidal while the production of short chain fatty acids inhibits bacterial proliferation. Alterations in the normal gut flora affect the metabolism of many drugs; for example, in a minority of patients antibiotics, by altering the flora, can greatly increase the absorption of digoxin (Lindenbaum et al 1981).

## Abnormalities of the stomach and small intestine which result in an abnormal bacterial flora

Bacterial overgrowth may occur because of failure of one of the above mechanisms which control proliferation. The common cause of proliferation is stasis due to a mechanical cause or a motility disorder such as scleroderma (Stellaard et al 1987) but achlorhydria, immunological

**Table 16.3** Causes of the "stagnant loop syndrome"

| | |
|---|---|
| Failure of gastric secretion | Pernicious anemia[1]<br>Gastric operations[2]<br>Treatment with $H_2$ receptor antagonist or proton pump inhibitor[3] |
| Stasis (1) due to localized mechanical causes | Chronic afferent loop obstruction<br>Strictures and surgical blind loops<br>Single duodenal diverticulum[4]<br>Multiple jejunal diverticula<br>Enteroanastomosis |
| Stasis (2) due to abnormal motility | Intestinal pseudo-obstruction<br>Scleroderma<br>Diabetic neuropathy<br>Biguanide drugs[5] |
| Communication with a heavily colonized area | Extensive bowel resection<br>Enterocolic or gastrocolic fistula<br>Chronic biliary infections |
| Immune deficiency | Hypogammaglobulinemia<br>Leukemia[6] |
| Other conditions | Cirrhosis[7]<br>Chronic malnutrition<br>Irradiation |

[1]Dellipiani & Girdwood (1964), Sherwood et al 1964; [2]Goldstein et al (1961), Wirts & Goldstein (1963); [3]Ruddell & Losowsky (1980); [4]Goldstein et al (1961); [5]Caspary et al (1977); [6]Smith et al (1990); [7]Martini et al (1957)

deficiency and other factors may play a role in some patients. The inhibition of acid secretion by $H_2$ receptor antagonists can increase the intragastric bacterial count to $10^6$/ml (Deane et al 1980). The causes of the stagnant loop syndrome are summarized in Table 16.3. It must be realized that overgrowth of bacteria in the stomach and small intestine does not always result in malabsorption. In general, it is the presence of anaerobes which leads to metabolic disturbances.

Many of the responsible disorders can be classified, but the cause of proliferation in others is not so clear, for example in cirrhosis (Martini et al 1957) and hypogammaglobulinemia (Parkin et al 1972a).

## The effects of bacterial overgrowth

### *Steatorrhea*

Studies in the experimental animal and in the human favor the concept that the steatorrhea is due to malabsorption of dietary fat rather than an increased loss of endogenous lipid. Firstly, fecal fat excretion is not raised when fat is excluded from the diet of patients with the stagnant loop syndrome. Secondly, when $^{14}$C-labeled triolein or oleic acid is fed to rats or patients with bacterial overgrowth the fecal radioactivity correlates with the total fat excretion (Donaldson 1965).

It is established that high bacterial counts in the human small intestine may lead to deconjugation and dehydroxylation of conjugated bile acids; both processes normally occur predominantly in the colon. Thus unconjugated bile acids are present in the jejunum and this is reflected in increased levels in the serum (Tabaqchali & Booth 1985, Stellaard et al 1987). Steatorrhea may occur and broad-spectrum antibiotics reverse these features (Donaldson 1965, Tabaqchali & Booth 1966). There are two possible mechanisms for the production of steatorrhea. Firstly, the unconjugated bile acids may be toxic to the intestinal mucosa or, secondly, the deconjugation of bile acids may reduce the levels of the conjugated bile acids below the concentration required for fat absorption. These two mechanisms have been reviewed in detail (Heaton 1976, 1977).

Unconjugated bile acids can be demonstrated in jejunal aspirates. Patients usually, but not always, have an abnormal $^{14}$C-glycocholic acid breath test and anaerobes capable of deconjugating bile acids can be cultured from jejunal aspirates. Studies in vitro (Aries & Hill 1970) show that *Clostridium*, *Veillonella*, enterococci, *Streptococcus fecalis*, *Bifidobacterium* and particularly *Bacteroides* spp. (Gorbach & Tabaqchali 1969) are capable of carrying out deconjugation and that it is likely that $10^4$ organisms per ml are necessary. Most strains of coliforms do not have this activity.

***Damage to the jejunal mucosa.*** Patchy abnormalities of the jejunal mucosa are present on light microscopy (Ament et al 1972) and electronmicroscopy shows a reduced number of fat particles in the damaged absorptive cells. There is evidence from animal studies that these appearances are due to the direct toxic effects of deconjugated bile acids (Heaton 1976, 1977) and because the brush border is damaged, malabsorption of other substances also occurs. However, in humans with stagnant loop syndrome, Schjønsby et al (1983) have measured a large number of epithelial cell enzymes and have not found any abnormalities.

***Jejunal concentrations of bile acids.*** There is good evidence that the steatorrhea is related to the reduction in the concentration of bile acids. In dogs with experimental blind loop syndrome and steatorrhea, the steatorrhea was abolished simply by feeding bile acids (Kim et al 1966) and humans with steatorrhea due to the stagnant loop syndrome have reduced concentrations of bile acids (Tabaqchali et al 1968). Postprandial samples of jejunal juice contained only 3.4 mmol/L of bile acids compared with 7.4 mmol/L in controls (Northfield 1973).

Other changes in bile acid metabolism can be demonstrated; it is probable that the deconjugated bile acids are effectively absorbed by passive diffusion throughout the small intestine and therefore, the enterohepatic circulation of bile acids remains intact though short circuited. However, these events have two other consequences: firstly, there are high concentrations of unconjugated bile acids in the serum and, secondly, the glycine:taurine ratio is high in bile and serum because of the relative unavailability of taurine as a result of increased bile acid conjugation.

*Vitamin $B_{12}$ malabsorption*

Enteric bacteria bind dietary vitamin $B_{12}$ and, once bound, the vitamin $B_{12}$ is unavailable for absorption and passes into the large intestine with the bacteria (Schjønsby 1973).

Studies examining this process have shown that some bacteria can take up vitamin $B_{12}$ bound to intrinsic factor. The uptake of intrinsic factor-bound vitamin $B_{12}$ has been demonstrated in vivo in rats (Donaldson 1962) and in humans with the stagnant loop syndrome. In the latter study, the centrifuged deposit from ileal aspirate of patients who were fed radioactive vitamin $B_{12}$ bound to intrinsic factor showed a much higher radioactivity than the centrifuged deposit from control patients. In addition, antibiotic treatment decreased the amount of radioactivity in the centrifuged deposit and vitamin $B_{12}$ absorption became normal. Stasis may be an important condition for bacterial uptake because in studies in vitro, several hours are required (Donaldson 1962).

*Protein absorption*

Although hypoproteinemia is common in the stagnant loop syndrome (Badenoch et al 1955, Cooke et al 1963), its exact cause is not known. Possible causes are protein-losing enteropathy, bacterial degradation of dietary protein and inhibition of amino acid absorption by deconjugated bile acids.

Protein-losing enteropathy occurs in the rat with stagnant loop syndrome (Nygaard & Rootwelt 1968) but has been reported in only a few patients (Jeejeebhoy & Coghill 1961, King & Toskes 1979).

Organisms such as *E.coli*, *Bacteroides* and some strains of *Klebsiella* possess the enzyme tryptophanase which converts tryptophan to indole. This is absorbed and carried to the liver where it is hydroxylated and conjugated with sulfate to form indoxylsulfate (indican). An excessive amount of indican then appears in the urine (Greenberger et al 1968). Other amino acids are degraded and are no longer available for absorption but it is not yet known whether this is the main cause of hypoproteinemia.

In vitro studies on rat intestine have suggested that amino acid transport is inhibited by deconjugated bile acids (Pope et al 1966) and this is one further way in which protein malnutrition might occur in the blind loop syndrome.

*Carbohydrate absorption*

Carbohydrate absorption may be impaired in the stagnant loop syndrome (p. 463). Three mechanisms have been suggested. Firstly, aerobic intestinal bacteria have been shown to utilize D-xylose in vitro (Goldstein et al 1970) and they may therefore utilize other sugars. Secondly, intestinal monosaccharide uptake can be inhibited by deoxycholic acid which is the product of bacterial action (Gracey 1971) and thirdly, direct mucosal injury can cause lactase deficiency and lactose malabsorption (King & Toskes 1979). Volatile fatty acids resulting from bacterial metabolism of carbohydrate can be found in the jejunum (Chernov et al 1972).

*The mechanisms of other absorptive problems*

In addition to their possible effect on monosaccharide and amino acid absorption, it has been shown that deconjugated bile acids can impair water, sodium and potassium transport in the jejunum in vitro (Gracey 1971). Malabsorption of folate resulting in a deficiency is rarely reported (Cooke et al 1963); more often, the serum folate concentration is high (Hoffbrand et al 1966) because of the synthesis of folate by the proliferating bacteria. Similarly, deficiency of other vitamins is uncommon, presumably because most of them, apart from vitamin D, are synthesized by bacteria.

*Diarrhea and the stagnant loop syndrome*

Diarrhea is usually due to several causes. It can be associated with steatorrhea. Enteric bacteria are capable of hydroxylating fatty acids (Asselineau & Lederer 1960) and an increased quantity of hydroxylated fatty acid appears in the stool in a variety of intestinal disorders (Kim & Spritz 1968a); in the dog with induced bacterial overgrowth, this increase in hydroxylated fatty acids has been demonstrated in the small intestine (Kim & Spritz 1968b). Hydroxylated fatty acids may be responsible for diarrhea by the same mechanisms as ricinoleic acid, a hydroxylated fatty acid which is a constituent of castor oil. Furthermore, whilst steatorrhea and increased hydroxylated fatty acid excretion usually coexist, the experiments on the dog (Kim & Spritz 1968b) show that increased fatty acid excretion can occur without steatorrhea. This may provide one explanation for the diarrhea in patients with stagnant loop syndrome who do not have steatorrhea.

It is not known whether the deconjugated bile acids play a direct role in the production of diarrhea. Since there is no increase in the fecal excretion of bile acids (Heaton 1977), deconjugates would have to exert their effect on secretory mechanisms in the small intestine.

## Clinical features

The term "stagnant loop syndrome" has been used for an intestinal abnormality associated with bacterial overgrowth in the small intestine resulting in steatorrhea and vitamin $B_{12}$ malabsorption, both of which are improved by oral broad-spectrum antibiotics. The term should also be used for other metabolic complications of bacterial proliferation.

The most common presentation is with anemia; this is nearly always due to vitamin $B_{12}$ deficiency. More rarely, it is due to folate deficiency (above) or to bone marrow depression secondary to the overgrowth of bacteria (Hines et al 1967). Anemia often occurs independently of steatorrhea, which is present in about one-third of cases. The patient may present with diarrhea, deficiency of minerals and vitamins and edema due to hypoproteinemia. Severe malnutrition occurs on occasions, as described in three patients after partial gastrectomy (Neale et al 1967). Occasionally, vitamin $B_{12}$ deficiency leads to subacute combined degeneration of the spinal cord (Richmond & Davidson 1958). In the child, malnutrition may result in failure to grow (Bayes & Hamilton 1969).

The patient may also have symptoms due to underlying causes, such as diverticula or strictures.

## Diagnosis

This is based on the following criteria:

1. The reversal of malabsorption by oral broad-spectrum antibiotics. Vitamin $B_{12}$ malabsorption should be corrected (Table 13.3) and fecal fat excretion returned to normal.
2. The demonstration of a causative lesion or disease (Table 16.3). Most lesions will be diagnosed on a barium follow-through examination but a duodenocolic or enterocolic fistula usually requires a barium enema for its demonstration.
3. A positive breath test or culture of small bowel aspirate.

### *Glycocholic acid breath test*

This is a test of bile acid deconjugation which was devised by Sherr et al (1971) and by Fromm & Hofmann (1971). It is usually abnormal in stagnant loop syndrome. Occasionally, the test is normal in patients who have other clear evidence of bacterial overgrowth (Parkin et al 1972b, Lauterburg et al 1978). In addition, a small number of patients may have an abnormal test without evidence of significant bacterial overgrowth or malabsorption.

The test is described on p. 88.

### *Breath tests for carbohydrate malabsorption*

There may be a significant elevation in breath hydrogen after absorbable carbohydrates such as glucose (King & Toskes 1986) or rice flour. An early peak in hydrogen followed by a normal, higher, sustained colon peak may be observed after oral administration of the nonabsorbable carbohydrate lactulose but this test is probably less sensitive than using glucose because peaks resulting from small bowel metabolism or arrival in the colon may fuse. Bacterial overgrowth may be associated with an elevated fasting breath hydrogen level, possibly because glycoproteins of endogenous origin may act as substrates for hydrogen production by enteric flora.

### *$^{14}$C-xylose breath test*

Measurement of breath $^{14}CO_2$ after $^{14}$C-xylose is probably the most appropriate breath test for the diagnosis of bacterial overgrowth (King et al 1980, King & Toskes 1986) for it has the advantage of the substrate being absorbed from the upper small intestine, thus avoiding problems of interpretation due to colonic metabolism.

***Procedure.*** 10 μCi $^{14}$C-D-xylose is given with 1 g unlabeled D-xylose in 250 ml water followed by a further 250 ml water. The concentration of $^{14}CO_2$ in the breath is measured after trapping 2 mmol $CO_2$ in a 1:1 (vol/vol) 95% ethanol/hyamine hydroxide solution with 1% phenolphthalein indicator. The result is abnormal if the $^{14}CO_2$ concentration at 30 min exceeds 0.0013% of the administered dose per mmol $CO_2$.

### *Jejunal intubation for aspiration*

This enables bacterial counts to be carried out and unconjugated bile acids to be detected. An assessment of the jejunal concentration of bile acids may be of value. The results of bacteriological studies need to be interpreted cautiously because *Bacteroides* species, which can deconjugate bile acids in vitro, have been cultured from the intestine when malabsorption has not been present. Furthermore, local lesions may cause local bacterial proliferation and deconjugation without steatorrhea because the proliferation does not extend along a sufficient length of bowel (Tabaqchali et al 1968).

***Procedure.*** Intubation is carried out with a sterile radio-opaque double-lumen tube (internal diameter 1.8 mm). No antibiotics should be given for a week before the test and the patient is fasted overnight prior to the test. The proximal end of the tube is clamped and the tube is then passed orally and screened with the aid of fluoroscopy into the upper jejunum. Rapid passage through the small intestine is ensured by attaching a mercury bag to the tip or by a small balloon which can be inflated once the tip has passed through the pylorus. Once the tube is in position, 5 ml of intestinal content are aspirated and discarded and a further 2–5 ml are then aspirated and inoculated immediately on to media for aerobic and anaerobic culture. Samples are taken from multiple sites in the small intestine and on each occasion the exact position of the tube is checked radiologically. About 300 cm of tubing is required to reach the terminal ileum. Simultaneous sampling at different levels in the small intestine can be performed with a triple-lumen tube with the orifices 50 cm apart.

***Interpretation.*** Methods have been described (Shiner

et al 1963) using a capsule for the collection of intestinal secretion in order to avoid the contamination of samples from higher levels which was thought to result from the long tube method. However, the validity of the long tube method has been established (Gorbach et al 1967) and furthermore, it has become apparent that samples must be obtained from different levels of the small intestine (Gorbach & Tabaqchali 1969), whereas a capsule allows only one sample to be taken.

In the normal small bowel, there are few organisms proximally although some increase occurs distally (Kalser et al 1966, Gorbach 1967). Bacterial counts of less than $10^4$ occur in the upper jejunum (Gorbach & Levitan 1970) although higher counts can occur without metabolic consequences in achlorhydric patients (Parkin et al 1972b) (Fig. 16.2).

Since there are many different types of bacteria in the small intestine, a large number of selective culture media must be used. However, culture by such media introduces several possible errors (Gorbach & Levitan 1970). The culture of intestinal anaerobes presents particular difficulties and various methods of attempting to ensure anaerobic conditions are in use. The number of bacteria of a given species is determined from culture, but because of the exacting growth requirements of some organisms, underestimates are likely. For example, direct microscopic counts of fecal bacteria may be 10 to 100 times as high as those determined from culture (Van Houte & Gibbons 1966). In conclusion, bacteriological studies have been used to elucidate the metabolic role of bacteria in the syndrome, but they are used for diagnosis infrequently. In the upper jejunum, counts of aerobes of $10^5$/ml or greater and of anaerobes of $10^3$/ml or greater indicate that blind loop syndrome may be present.

*Screening tests for bacterial overgrowth*

The measurement of indicanuria has been suggested, but an increased excretion rate of indican occurs in other gastrointestinal diseases (Hamilton et al 1970, Dyer & Hawkins 1972).

## Treatment

*Antibiotics*

It is usual for vitamin $B_{12}$ malabsorption and steatorrhea to be corrected within 3–4 days of starting treatment. The antibiotics of choice are tetracycline or chlortetracycline 1–2 g per day in divided dosage. Any antibiotic which affects the anaerobic flora is likely to be effective, for example lincomycin (Polter et al 1968, Donaldson 1970). Neomycin is said to be ineffective, probably because the drug itself can cause malabsorption (p. 415), but since it can reverse the abnormal Schilling test (Murray-Lyon et al 1968) it must have an antibacterial effect in some patients. Unless there is a nutritional deficiency the aim of treatment is to alleviate symptoms, usually diarrhea, and to this end antibiotics may be given for as few as 7–10 days every 6 weeks (King & Toskes 1979) or for several months during which antibiotics such as co-trimoxazole, metronidazole and ciprofloxacin should be alternated. In cases where vitamin $B_{12}$ deficiency is the only manifestation of stagnant loop syndrome, antibiotics should not be given.

*Dietary measures and supplements* (Banwell et al 1981)

Diarrhea can often be relieved by reducing dietary long chain triglycerides. A supplement of vitamin $B_{12}$, 1000 μg hydroxycobalamin once monthly is necessary if there is a reduced absorption of the vitamin. If there is steatorrhea, supplements of fat-soluble vitamins should be given. Persistent lactase deficiency may require a lactose-free diet.

*Surgery*

Single or localized abnormalities are best treated surgically. Strictures and fistulae, for example, can be dealt with by local resection. The more extensive diseases, such as jejunal diverticulosis and motility disorders, cannot be corrected.

# JEJUNAL AND ILEAL DIVERTICULA

## Etiology and incidence

Jejunal diverticula, which are seen in about 1% of barium follow-through studies (Cooke et al 1963), are thought to be acquired (Edwards 1954), arise from the mesenteric

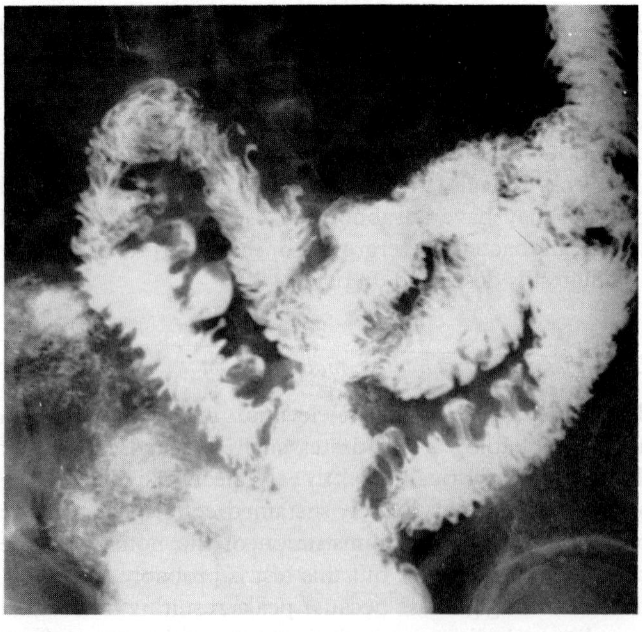

**Fig. 16.3** Multiple jejunal diverticula. Such diverticular may show air-fluid levels on erect radiograph.

border of the small intestine and extend into the mesentery. They are usually multiple (Fig. 16.3). They are pseudodiverticula with a wall consisting of mucosa and submucosa. Abnormal jejunal motility is undoubtedly an etiological factor for some patients also have pseudo-obstruction with underlying scleroderma, visceral myopathy of unknown cause or visceral neuropathy (Krishnamurthy et al 1983). Jejunal diverticulosis is also reported in Fabry's disease in which the neurones of the myenteric plexus are damaged (Friedman et al 1984) and in amyloidosis of the intestine (Patel et al 1993). Ileal diverticulum is less frequent than jejunal diverticulum and is usually solitary (Longo & Vernava 1992).

### Clinical features

Most patients are over the age of 50 years and nearly all are asymptomatic. Occasionally, there may be abdominal pain, obstructive symptoms, perforation, volvulus, severe hemorrhage or malabsorption (Donald 1979). Intestinal obstruction may occur secondary to volvulus, adhesions, enterolith formation (Yang & Fondacaro 1992) or compression from a large diverticulum (Longo & Vernava 1992). In other patients abdominal pain may be chronic or intermittent and colicky and may be due to disordered motility in the affected segments of the bowel (Altemeier et al 1963). The combination of colicky abdominal pain, borborygmi and abdominal distention sometimes leads to a plain radiograph of the abdomen, whereby the presence of fluid levels in the diverticula is mistaken for obstruction. This may lead to unnecessary laparotomy (Krishnamurthy et al 1983). Malabsorption is due to the stagnant loop syndrome (p. 459), but the reasons for its development in only a minority of patients are not well understood. Achlorhydria may facilitate jejunal colonization in some patients (Murray-Lyon et al 1968) and in others the type of organism present may determine whether deconjugation of bile acids occurs. Deconjugation has to occur over a significant length of intestine before steatorrhea results. Malabsorption of vitamin $B_{12}$ may occur with or without steatorrhea.

The diagnosis of diverticulosis of the jejunum or ileum is usually made by barium follow-through examination but enteroclysis is a more reliable technique because it distends the bowel (Maglinte et al 1986).

Bleeding may be acute or chronic (Shackelford & Marcus 1960). Acute bleeding is usually severe with the passage of red blood per rectum and occurs in a patient with no previous abdominal complaints (Thomas et al 1967); chronic bleeding tends to be associated with a history of abdominal complaints. The diagnosis of bleeding diverticulum should be suspected when diverticulosis is seen on a barium follow-through study but upper gastrointestinal endoscopy fails to locate a bleeding lesion. A precise diagnosis can be made by angiography (p. 27) during active bleeding if the contrast material pools in a diverticulum in sufficient quantity to be visualized.

Other complications include intestinal obstruction, volvulus, acute diverticulitis, pneumoperitoneum and peritonitis.

### Treatment

Resection and primary anastomosis is the treatment of choice for perforation, bleeding or obstruction (Donald 1979) otherwise surgery is best avoided.

Patients with diarrhea and malabsorption may require repeated courses of antibiotics and when there is malnutrition and pseudo-obstruction, parenteral feeding may be required.

## DISTURBANCE OF BILE ACID CIRCULATION IN OTHER DISEASES

This is reviewed by Heaton (1977).

In Crohn's disease of the small intestine (p. 676), features resembling those of terminal ileal resection or stagnant loop syndrome, or both, can occur. Similar features may arise after radiotherapy (p. 412) with damage to the terminal ileum.

In celiac disease (p. 377), there is no evidence of deconjugation or malabsorption of bile acid, but there may be an increased pool size of bile acids due to stasis in the gallbladder. This stasis leads to a poor bile acid output into the duodenum in the initial stages of digestion and this is compounded by increased intraluminal dilution as a result of the increased volume of jejunal juice in celiac disease; thus, bile acid concentrations below the critical micellar concentration occur in some patients. It is concluded that bile acid deficiency may contribute to malabsorption in some patients.

In tropical sprue (p. 399), the evidence for disturbance of bile acid metabolism is conflicting. Reduced concentrations of bile acid are found in the jejunum; the causes may be the same as in celiac disease.

Diarrhea after truncal vagotomy and drainage (p. 274) may be due to intestinal hurry and bile acid malabsorption. Similarly diabetic autonomic neuropathy may be associated with bile acid catharsis (Scarpello et al 1976).

## TUMORS OF THE SMALL INTESTINE

The distribution of benign and malignant tumors is shown in Tables 16.4 and 16.5.

### **Benign tumors** (River et al 1956, Braasch & Denbo 1964)

Most commonly, these are adenomas (papillomas), leiomyomas or lipomas. Of the adenomas, islet cell adenoma is considered on p. 1301 and Brunner's gland adenoma is

**Table 16.4** Benign tumors of the small intestine: Combined results of 11 series (from Mason 1986)

| | Duodenum | Jejunum | Ileum | Total | (%) |
|---|---|---|---|---|---|
| Leiomyoma | 31 | 84 | 61 | 176 | (31) |
| Adenoma | 42 | 42 | 41 | 125 | (22) |
| Lipoma | 25 | 17 | 48 | 90 | (16) |
| Miscellaneous | 40 | 73 | 58 | 171 | (31) |
| | 138 (25) | 216 (38) | 208 (37) | 562 | (100) |

**Table 16.5** Malignant tumors of the small intestine: Combined results of 11 series (from Mason 1986)

| | Duodenum | Jejunum | Ileum | Total | (%) |
|---|---|---|---|---|---|
| Carcinoid | 15 | 19 | 229 | 263 | (35) |
| Adenocarcinoma | 97 | 99 | 34 | 230 | (32) |
| Lymphoma | 6 | 64 | 85 | 155 | (21) |
| Sarcoma | 15 | 29 | 37 | 81 | (11) |
| Miscellaneous | 1 | 4 | 4 | 9 | (1) |
| | 134 (18) | 215 (29) | 389 (53) | 738 | (100) |

a localized hyperplasia. The common adenomas or papillomas (Fig. 16.4) have the same histological features as those in the large intestine and may be sessile or pedunculated. Villous adenomas are usually sessile and occur in the duodenum (Cooperman et al 1978, Ryan et al 1986) or upper jejunum and, like colonic villous tumors, are prone to malignancy (Mir-Madjlessi et al 1973). They are commonly found in patients with familial adenomatous polyposis. Leiomyomas have the same features as those described elsewhere in the gastrointestinal tract (pp. 212 and 314) and occur most frequently in the jejunum. As with leiomyoma elsewhere, there is a problem in defining malignancy. Lipomas are found most frequently in the distal ileum; they arise from submucosal fat and protrude into the lumen as small yellow nodules. They may ulcerate but malignancy is rare.

Also included under the classification of benign tumors is heterotopic gastric mucosa, which occurs in the first part of the duodenum (p. 230) and heterotopic pancreas, which occurs in the duodenum and jejunum as a nodular lesion (p. 1228). Inflammatory fibroid polyp (p. 325) also occurs in the small intestine, especially the ileum. In children and young adults lymphoid hyperplasia may form polypoid lesions.

### *Clinical features*

Benign tumors occur most commonly in the elderly. Adenomatous polyps and lipomas are usually asymptomatic but occasionally cause bleeding or obstruction. Brunner's gland adenomas cause these symptoms even more rarely whereas the rare villous adenoma commonly causes these symptoms. Leiomyoma presents with bleeding in two-thirds of cases and the remainder present with obstruction.

Tumors in the upper jejunum or terminal ileum may be diagnosed with contrast studies of the small bowel or barium enema respectively. Those between these levels are commonly missed by radiography and are diagnosed at laparotomy (Aubrey et al 1971). Bleeding benign tumors may be diagnosed by angiography or by enteroscopy.

Symptomatic tumors should be treated surgically.

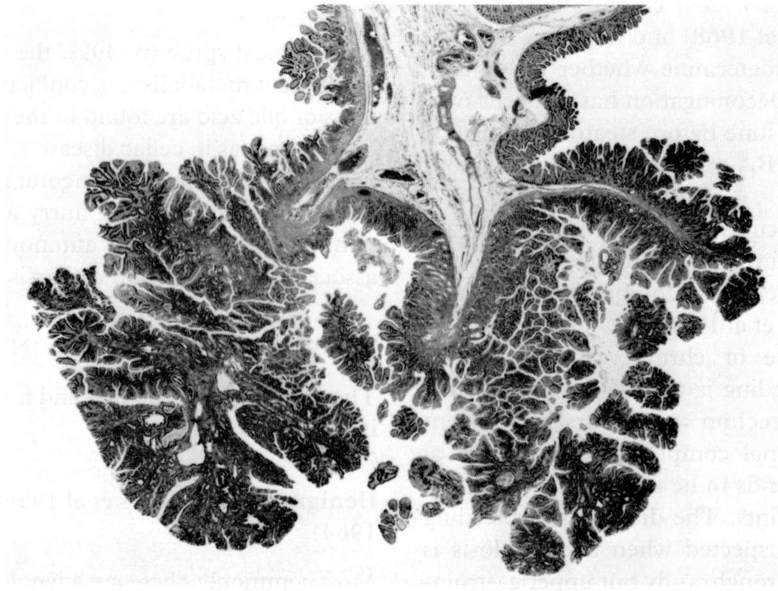

**Fig. 16.4** Villous adenoma originating in the duodenum (hematoxylin and eosin × 2.5).

### Neurogenic tumors (Slavin 1985)

Neurilemmoma (schwannoma) may arise de novo or as part of von Recklinghausen's syndrome. The lesions commence in a nerve plexus but may ulcerate the mucosa. Malignant schwannomas and ganglioneuromas also occur.

Gangliocytic paraganglioma, which is benign, occurs in the second part of the duodenum near to the ampulla. It presents as a polyp which ulcerates.

### Vascular tumors (Slavin 1985)

Hemangiomas of the small bowel occur at any age and may be single or multiple. They may be circumscribed vascular polyps or they may infiltrate. They present most commonly with bleeding but they may cause obstruction or intussusception. Malignant vascular tumors are rare.

### Malignant tumors

Malignant tumors of the small intestine amount to 1–2% of all gastrointestinal malignancies with an age adjusted annual incidence rate per 100 000 varying from 0.1 in Poland to 2.8 in Switzerland (Stemmermann et al 1992). The more common ones are adenocarcinoma, lymphoma and leiomyosarcoma. Lymphoma is discussed on p. 468. Kaposi's sarcoma may involve the gastrointestinal tract, particularly in patients with AIDS (p. 610).

Adenocarcinoma occurs predominantly in the duodenum, proximal jejunum and distal ileum. It may arise from a pre-existing polyp (Johansen & Larsen 1969). It may be associated with Crohn's disease (Thompson et al 1983), celiac disease (p. 394), the Peutz–Jeghers syndrome (p. 1413), familial adenomatous polyposis (p. 1409) neurofibromatosis and juvenile familial polyposis. In addition hereditary non-polyposis colon cancer or Lynch syndrome is associated with adenocarcinoma of the distal jejunum and the ileum. A study of small intestinal adenocarcinoma in Hawaiian Japanese men demonstrated a relationship to multicentric large bowel cancer and the first-degree relatives had stomach and colon cancer.

The peak incidence of adenocarcinoma is in the seventh decade. By contrast, lymphoma occurs predominantly in the distal jejunum and ileum in younger patients (p. 468). Leiomyosarcomas (Starr & Dockerty 1955) occur at all levels in the small intestine. Small intestinal carcinoids are most common in the ileum and appendix and the malignant ones present with metastases as well as with local symptoms (p. 472).

Adenocarcinoma usually ulcerates and infiltrates to produce a ring stricture but polypoid lesions also occur. At diagnosis it is usual for there to be invasion through the bowel wall and an enterocolic fistula may develop.

*Clinical features* (Dorman et al 1967, Ashley & Wells 1988)

All malignant tumors of the small intestine cause abdominal pain, weight loss and usually a palpable mass. Obstruction, intussusception, change in bowel habit and perforation also occur. Duodenal carcinoma (Fig. 16.5) presents with obstruction, pain and bleeding, leading to anemia (Kibbey et al 1976, Alwmark et al 1980). Initially, the symptoms may be mistaken for duodenal ulceration. Jaundice may occur. Leiomyosarcoma presents with recurrent melena but pain and a palpable abdominal mass are also common.

Duodenal tumors are easily detected by barium studies (Joesting et al 1981) or endoscopy. The diagnosis is difficult to establish at more distal sites (Termansen & Linde 1971), when small bowel enema, a follow-through examination (Fig. 16.6) or barium enema has to be used.

Usually a preoperative diagnosis is made in only 20–50% of patients who are symptomatic.

*Treatment and prognosis*

Surgery is usually necessary to confirm the diagnosis; the tumour should be resected. Radiotherapy is effective in lymphoma (p. 470). The 5-year survival rate is about 20% for adenocarcinoma, 55% for lymphoma (p. 470) and 40–50% for leiomyosarcoma and carcinoids. In one series (Ouriel & Adams 1984) 65% of patients underwent resection and the overall 5-year survival was 30%. When nodes were negative survival was 70%, but with positive nodes, survival was 13%.

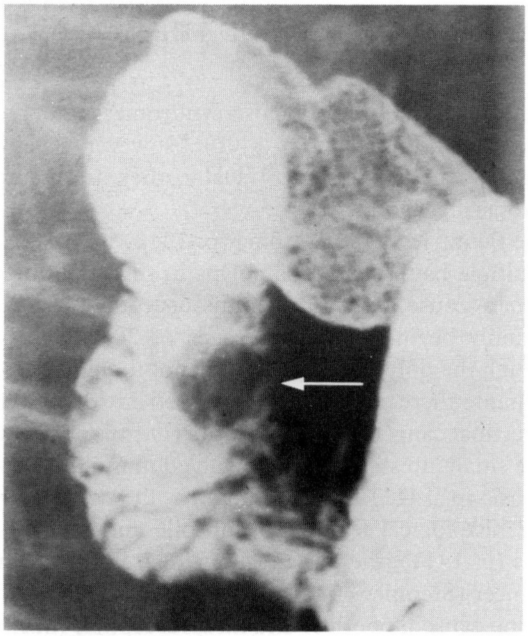

**Fig. 16.5** Carcinoma of the duodenum adjacent to papilla of Vater causing an irregular defect (arrow).

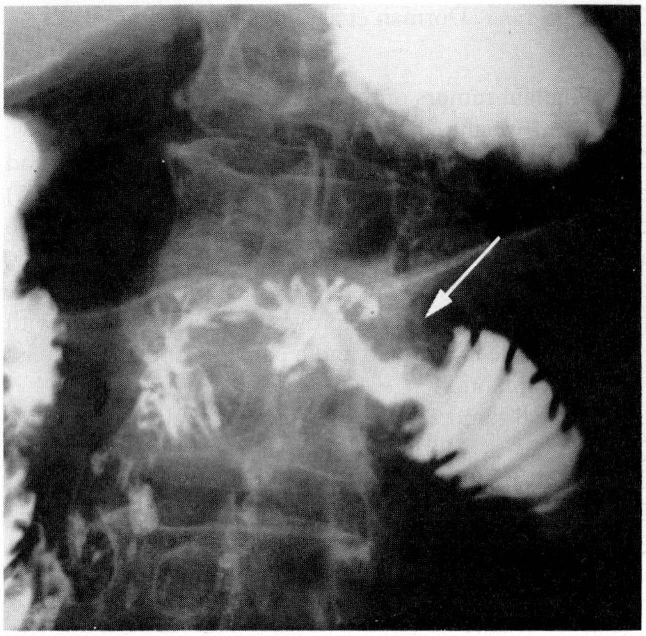

**Fig. 16.6** Carcinoma of jejunum. Typical irregular filling defect (arrow) with mucosal destruction.

### Secondary carcinoma

The small intestine may be involved in direct or metastatic spread. Secondary spread is from melanoma of the skin, carcinoma of lung, kidney, adrenal, ovary, uterus, stomach and large intestine (De Castro et al 1957). The metastasis may simulate a primary tumor but metastasis from malignant melanoma may produce characteristic polypoidal lesions (Fraser-Moodie et al 1976).

## MULTIPLE POLYPOSIS AND THE SMALL INTESTINE

The inherited multiple polyposis syndromes are of greatest importance in the colon (p. 1406). However, several also involve the small intestine. Usually, they are recognized radiologically (Dodds 1976).

The Peutz–Jeghers syndrome (p. 1413) is characterized by multiple hamartomatous polyps in the small intestine; they can cause anemia or intussusception. Symptoms commonly begin between the ages of 20 and 30 years. Although the polyps themselves are not thought to be premalignant, there may be an increased incidence of gastrointestinal cancer in these patients (Dozois et al 1969).

The small intestine may be involved in multiple juvenile polyposis (p. 1411). In some patients, the polyps have the mixed histological features of juvenile and adenomatous polyps (p. 1411); there is a high incidence of gastrointestinal cancer (Stemper et al 1975). Such polyps in the small intestine cause blood loss and intussusception (Sachatello et al 1970). The Cronkhite–Canada syndrome (p. 1413) also consists of generalized juvenile polyposis; the polyps in the small intestine may cause malabsorption and protein-losing enteropathy (Johnson et al 1972).

Occasionally, small intestinal polyps occur in familial polyposis of the colon (p. 1409), in Gardner's syndrome (p. 1409), in disseminated gastrointestinal polyposis (p. 1415) and in multiple neurofibromatosis (p. 1415).

## LYMPHOMA OF THE SMALL INTESTINE
(Rambaud 1983) (see Table 11.9a)

Malignant lymphoma of the gastrointestinal tract may be primary or secondary. Primary malignant lymphomas of the gastrointestinal tract are defined as those tumors in which the lesion has arisen in the lymphoid tissue of mucosa or submucosa. They are most common in the stomach (p. 316), followed by the small intestine and colon (p. 1436). By contrast, in secondary malignant lymphoma the intestinal involvement is only one manifestation of more generalized disease originating elsewhere, e.g. in regional lymph nodes. Primary malignant lymphoma of the gastrointestinal tract has three main disease patterns: namely, the Western type of lesion, which is sporadic and typically forms ileal masses; lymphoma developing in association with celiac disease; and the Mediterranean type of lymphoma (immunoproliferative small intestine disease), in which the lesion is diffuse and incomplete $\alpha$ chains may be produced. The latter is sometimes called Eastern lymphoma (Khojasteh 1987).

A number of different classifications of malignant lymphomas have been developed. Various series of gastrointestinal tract lymphoma have used different classifications and so are not readily comparable. Earlier classifications were purely morphological but those developed more recently have a functional basis and depend on marker studies and immunocytochemical techniques which can identify distinctive T- and B-lymphocyte-associated antigens as well as others related to the histiocytes (Knowles 1985). There are two broad categories of primary gut lymphoma: (i) B-cell which includes the Western type lymphoma, immunoproliferative small intestinal disease, malignant lymphomatous polyposis and Burkitt-like lymphoma; (ii) T-cell lymphoma which occurs in celiac disease.

The Working Formulation is valuable in that it compares the various classifications and indicates as far as possible equivalent lesions described under different names (National Cancer Institute 1982). The full range of cell types of malignant lymphomas occur in the gastrointestinal tract.

### Primary lymphoma of the small intestine

These tumors are defined above.

*Pathology* (Lewin et al 1978, Morson & Dawson 1979)

Lymphoma which occurs in the West is sporadic and there

is no underlying mucosal or serum protein abnormality. The lesions most commonly occur in the distal small intestine (Table 16.5), forming malignant ulcers or nodular masses, and in Lewin et al's series (1978) averaged 70 mm in diameter at the time of diagnosis. Other tumors may be stenotic or form plaques. The lymphomatous tissue is usually soft and gray with areas of necrosis and hemorrhage. The local lymph nodes may be enlarged owing to reactive or secondary neoplastic involvement. At operation, the tumor may have already spread directly through the full thickness of the bowel wall into the mesentery or adjacent organs. Histologically low, intermediate and high grades of tumor account for 7.6%, 53% and 39.4% respectively (Rambaud 1983). Alternatively, 59% of tumors are the diffuse "histiocytic" type of Rappaport (42% diffuse large cell, 17% immunoblastic of the National Cancer Institute 1982). The most recent classification defines low grade and high grade B-cell lymphomas (Lancet 1991). Western-type lymphomas, which occur most commonly in the stomach, have been termed MALTomas by Isaacson & Wright (1983), indicating that they arise from mucosa-associated lymphoid tissue. The tumor comprises parafollicular centrocyte-like B-cells. The centrocyte-like cell has a propensity to invade epithelial glandular structures, thus giving rise to the hallmark of this type of tumor – the "lymphoepithelial" lesion. That gastric MALTomas may arise because of chronic *H. pylori* infection and regress on chemotherapy is a recently advanced, provocative claim. Intestinal tumors are of similar type and tend to remain localized to the intestinal tissues so that spread beyond the confines of the local nodes is very late in disease evolution. Thus, in their very early stages, tumor resection can be very effective, when followed by radiotherapy (Gray et al 1982). By contrast, the childhood lesions are indifferentiated Burkitt and non-Burkitt type tumors of Rappaport (small noncleaved cell lymphomas of the National Cancer Institute 1982).

Typically, all tumors spread to the local lymph nodes before becoming disseminated.

***Malignant lymphoma complicating celiac disease.*** Celiac disease is complicated by the development of malignant T-cell lymphoma in a significant number of cases (p. 394). Initially, it was shown that the lymphoma associated with celiac disease had macrophage or true histiocyte markers such as cytoplasmic $\alpha_1$-antitrypsin, $\alpha_1$-chymotrypsin or erythrophagocytosis. It is now recognized that the cells in celiac disease lymphoma carry T-cell markers, particularly the IEL marker HML-1. Histological examination of the intestine shows pleomorphic large cells and frequent eosinophilic infiltration.

The lymphomas in celiac disease most commonly occur in the upper small intestine where the mucosal lesion is most severe and are sometimes associated with severe small intestinal ulceration and perforation. The lesion is usually a localized or circumferential ulcer or solitary or multiple nodules. Another feature is that macroscopic examination of the intestine sometimes fails to show evidence of involvement. Chronic ulcerative jejunitis may be an early stage of T-cell lymphoma.

*Incidence of primary lymphoma*

The incidence is 5 per million in northeast Scotland (Green et al 1979) and comprises 12% of all small intestinal malignancies in specialist referral hospitals (Mittal & Bodzin 1980), being exceeded by adenocarcinoma and carcinoid tumors (Table 16.5). The series from Scotland comprised 45 cases of gastrointestinal lymphoma, of which 15 were primary. The male to female ratio for primary tumors is 2 or 3:1 and they occur in the fifth or sixth decades.

*Clinical features*

The patient complains of abdominal pain, which may be periumbilical and colicky, and nausea and vomiting due to intestinal obstruction. There may be perforation, intestinal bleeding, anemia and loss of weight. In fact, approximately half of all patients present with acute symptoms requiring surgical intervention (Green et al 1979). Less common modes of presentation are malaise, fatigue, fever, night sweats or intussusception. On examination, an abdominal mass is present in about one-third of cases, but in contrast to patients with carcinomas of a similar size, marked emaciation is unusual. Finger clubbing is uncommon except in 'Mediterranean-type' lymphoma. Rarely, the lymphoma may present with malabsorption (p. 472). Primary T-cell lymphoma of the small intestine may also occur in patients with celiac disease (p. 394).

*Investigations* (Bush & Ash 1969, Craig & Gregson 1981)

The specific radiological diagnosis of small bowel lymphoma is made difficult by the overlap of signs with those seen in Crohn's disease. Sartoris et al (1984) examined retrospectively the radiographs of 27 patients with lymphoma and 23 patients with Crohn's disease with reference to 10 radiological findings. In about one-half of the patients in each group a confident radiological diagnosis could not be made. Craig & Gregson (1981) also had difficulty distinguishing lymphoma from Crohn's disease and from tuberculosis. Most studies have used single contrast but double-contrast studies give better definition of the tumor (Iida et al 1991).

The most frequent radiological abnormalities in lymphoma are segments of irregular, mucosal thickening of the small bowel which can be associated with ulceration, nodularity and mass effect. In addition, localized perforations with fistulae and abscesses are relatively frequent. Many patients show more than one of these signs and multiple sites of involvement can occur. The terminal ileum may be the only site of involvement in primary lymphoma and the cecum may be deformed. There may be a malabsorption pattern. Stricture and aneurysmal dilatation of the small bowel, said to be highly suggestive of lymphoma (Cupps et al 1969), are seen in both Crohn's disease and lymphoma (Sartoris et al 1984). Ultrasound examination is useful in defining the tumors when the presentation is with an abdominal mass (Goerg et al 1990).

### *Staging of lymphoma*

The Ann Arbor system of staging has been recommended (Gray et al 1982) (Table 16.6). Under this system lymphoma of the gastrointestinal tract, being an extralymphatic site, will carry the subscript "E". Thus $I_E$ = tumor limited to a single site within the stomach or bowel. $II_E$ = as $I_E$, plus limited regional node involvement in the mesentery, celiac or para-aortic lymph nodes. $III_E$ = limited intestinal involvement plus widespread lymph node disease. IV = multiple sites of involvement of the gastrointestinal tract, either alone or with other extranodal disease, with or without lymph node involvement; this is the most common stage when lymphoma affects the gastrointestinal tract. The staging system also acknowledges the poor prognostic significance of the systemic symptoms of fever, night sweats or weight loss by designating the stage as A = without and B = with systemic symptoms (see also Table 11.9b).

Staging is accomplished by routine radiological procedures followed by a lymphangiogram, computed tomography (p. 24), an assessment of the renal collecting system and bone marrow biopsy.

**Table 16.6** Ann Arbor staging classification of the lymphomas

| | |
|---|---|
| *Stage I* | Involvement of a single lymph node region (I) or of a single extralymphatic organ or site ($I_E$) |
| *Stage II* | Involvement of two or more lymph node regions on the same side of the diaphragm alone (II) or with involvement of limited, contiguous extralymphatic organ or tissue ($II_E$) |
| *Stage III* | Involvement of lymph node regions on both sides of the diaphragm (III), which may include the spleen ($III_E$) or both ($III_{ES}$) |
| *Stage IV* | Multiple or disseminated foci of involvement of one or more extralymphatic organs or tissues, with or without lymphatic involvement |

All cases are subclassified to indicate the absence (A) or presence (B) of the systemic symptoms of significant fever, night sweats and unexplained weight loss exceeding 10% of normal body weight. The clinical stage (CS) denotes the stage as determined by all diagnostic examinations and a single diagnostic biopsy only. If a second biopsy of any kind has been obtained, whether negative or positive, the term "pathologic stage" (PS) will be used and the results of the additional biopsies shown by an agreed-upon designation.

### *Treatment*

For a stage $I_E$ gastric lesion, limited surgery is followed by irradiation of the upper abdomen to 4000 rads, including 2500 rads to the liver. For stage $I_E$ intestinal, limited surgery is followed by whole abdominal irradiation to a dose of 3500–4000 rads, with 2500 rads to the liver. For $II_E$, limited surgery can be followed by chemotherapy and radiotherapy. Patients with $III_E$ or IV are managed primarily with combination chemotherapy. Chemotherapy regimens usually consist of CHOP (cyclophosphamide, adriamycin, vincristine and prednisolone) or C-MOPP (cyclophosphamide, vincristine, procarbazine and prednisolone).

### *Prognosis*

It is difficult to identify those factors which have bearing on prognosis in gastrointestinal tract lymphomas because even large series consist of only 100–150 patients and are retrospective. In addition, not all patients have been fully staged and treatment regimens have varied (Appelman et al 1985).

Prognosis is related to site, with gastric lymphoma having the best prognosis, small intestinal cases intermediate and colonic the poorest. The actuarial survival of gastrointestinal lymphomas in all sites and stages showed a progressive decrease to 44% at 4 years in one large series (Lewin et al 1978).

The stage of the disease is the single most important factor in predicting prognosis (Weingrad et al 1982). Thus when the tumor is confined to the viscus the prognosis is better than when it has spread to lymph nodes or become disseminated. In one series of gastric lymphomas the 5-year survival for lesions without lymph node metastasis was 86% compared with 55% for those with lymph node metastasis (Brooks & Enterline 1983). Gray et al (1982) quote a 75% cure of stage $I_E$ disease. Depth of penetration of the lesion into the viscus wall has been shown to affect prognosis, with best results being found in superficial lesions (Saraga et al 1981). Another factor possibly related to depth of penetration is that tumors less than 7 cm in diameter carried a better prognosis than larger ones (Brooks & Enterline 1983).

Histological subtype also appears to affect prognosis, with low-grade tumors doing better than intermediate or high-grade lesions (Appelman et al 1985).

## Secondary lymphoma

This is involvement of the intestine in a generalized lymphomatous process which began elsewhere in the body. It occurs clinically in 10% and at postmortem in approximately 50% of patients with generalized lymphoma (Rosenberg et al 1961, Herrmann et al 1980).

*Clinical features*

The age of the patient, the site of the tumor and its histology are like those of primary lymphoma (p. 468). The presentation is also similar but there is often lymphadenopathy, splenomegaly and a raised white cell count, none of which is present in primary lymphoma. There is weight loss, diarrhea and sometimes steatorrhea. The management is of the intestinal aspect of the tumor and is similar to primary lymphoma (p. 470) but the prognosis is much worse.

## Immunoproliferative small intestinal disease ($\alpha$-heavy chain disease)

This form of lymphoma evolves from a premalignant plasmacytoid infiltration of the small intestine and is relatively common in the Mediterranean region and the Middle East, although it is reported sporadically from countries elsewhere. Because the condition occurs in socially disadvantaged populations, there has been speculation that ingested micro-organisms may provide a stimulus to its development, but as yet there is no evidence for this.

The majority of patients have incomplete $\alpha$-heavy chains in the serum, urine and jejunal secretions. This protein consists of Fc fragment and part of the Fd fragment of IgA subclass 1.

*Pathology* (Khojasteh et al 1983)

This typically affects the duodenum and upper jejunum but can involve the entire small bowel. The mucosa is diffusely thickened owing to a massive lymphoplasmacytic infiltration (Nassar et al 1978). This infiltration leads to widening and shortening of villi and an apparent loss of crypts, causing partial or subtotal villous atrophy. The surface epithelium may show transepithelial lymphocyte migration and erosion. The lymphoplasmacytic infiltration consists of an admixture of mature plasma cells and larger lymphoid cells, including immunoblasts. Transition forms are typical. When malignant lymphoma supervenes the infiltration becomes cytologically malignant and extension occurs locally through the bowel wall and to the intra-abdominal lymph nodes and viscera. There is also spread to the postnasal space, bone marrow and blood (Doe 1985).

Khojasteh (1987) has defined three stages of the disease. Stage A is a dense plasmacytic infiltrate associated with a high percentage of abnormal $\alpha_1$-heavy chain fragments. In stage B, the infiltrate extends outside the lamina propria to invade the submucosa and is associated with additional lymphoid infiltrates and lymphoid nodules. In stage C solid tumor masses appear, although spread outside the gastrointestinal tract is late. At this stage $\alpha_1$-chain production is lost.

*Clinical features*

These have been extensively reviewed by Khojasteh (1987). The disease appears to arise on a chronic background of poor socioeconomic status, low levels of hygiene, high parasitism rates and frequent attacks of intestinal infections throughout early life.

Clinically, the presentation is fairly uniform, typically involving young adults who present with intermittent diarrhea and malabsorption, progressing to more severe disease with edema and ascites due to hypoalbuminemia, finger clubbing and diffuse abdominal pain. In advanced cases, tumor masses with surgical complications of obstruction, perforation, intussusception and bleeding may arise or there may be fever, extra-abdominal nodal enlargement, hepatosplenomegaly and cachexia. There may also be development of a secondary neoplasm, extensive skin warts or mycosis fungoides. Heavy infestations with *Giardia* parasites may occur.

*Investigation*

Commonly, features of malabsorption are present and there is often a marked increase in serum alkaline phosphatase activity of intestinal origin (Doe 1985).

The radiological changes seen on the barium follow-through examination are those of lymphoma (Vessal et al 1980).

In 100 cases of primary intestinal lymphoma from Iran examined by Vessal et al (1980), 38 patients had evidence of generalized lymphoma, particularly infiltrative and nodular lesions, while 62 fulfilled the criteria of primary small bowel lymphoma. In 46 patients lymphomatous changes were confined to the duodenum and jejunum and all had evidence of immunoproliferative small intestinal disease. In addition a sprue pattern was present in non-lymphomatous segments of the gut. By contrast, primary lymphomatous changes confined to the ileum occurred in 14 patients, none of whom had evidence of immunoproliferative small intestinal disease. Whilst Crohn's disease must be considered in the differential diagnosis, it is extremely rare in developing countries (Vessal et al 1980).

Intestinal biopsy shows extensive infiltration of the lamina propria, but in contrast to celiac disease the surface epithelial cells are relatively normal.

Evidence of parasitic or protozoan infection is common and usually there is overgrowth of bacteria in the upper small intestine, so that a stagnant loop syndrome may contribute to the steatorrhea.

Diagnosis is made by the detection of the abnormal $\alpha$-chain in serum, secretions or urine. As the disease progresses, evidence for the abnormal $\alpha$-chain fragment disappears and it cannot be detected in serum. In 5% of cases serum protein electrophoresis is abnormal, showing an abnormally broad band in the $\alpha_2$ or $\beta$ region.

Immunoelectrophoresis using antisera monospecific for IgA usually reveals an abnormal precipitin arc extending from the $\alpha_1$ to the $\beta_2$ region. An immunoselection technique is the most sensitive for detecting $\alpha$-chain disease polypeptide (Doe & Spiegelberg 1979).

*Treatment*

The prognosis is relatively good since most patients are stage $I_E$ when they present. In the premalignant phase, when the plasma cell infiltrate is confined to the lamina propria, remission of clinical, histological and immunological features has been reported, often after prolonged treatment with tetracycline and removal of the patient to a less infected environment. If the infiltrate is less differentiated, a 6-month trial of tetracycline 1 g daily will determine the reversibility. This regimen also produces occasional remission in more advanced disease. With lymphoma confined to the intestine, total abdominal irradiation with or without chemotherapy is recommended treatment. With chemotherapy, multiple drug regimens have been shown to be useful. CHOP is probably best (Rambaud et al 1983) and comparable with the effects of irradiation, although both are poorly tolerated by extremely debilitated patients. The effects of surgical debulking on survival, and also subsequent responses to ancillary treatment schedules, are unknown.

*Nonsecretory immunoproliferative small intestinal disease*

Patients are described with diffuse malignant B-cell infiltration of the small intestine but without the secretion of $\alpha$-chains (Matuchansky et al 1989, Cammoun et al 1989).

## Multiple lymphomatous polyposis

This is characterized by polypoid accumulations of malignant centrocytic lymphoid cells of B-cell origin and is associated with a high frequency of dissemination beyond the gastrointestinal tract and a poor outlook. It predominantly involves the ileocecal region. Some of these cases can be classified as follicular lymphomas (LeBrun et al 1992).

## Malabsorption and lymphoma

Lymphoma is occasionally associated with a malabsorption syndrome and it is thus important to consider it in the differential diagnosis of celiac disease. Table 16.7 depicts the various relationships between lymphoma and malabsorption. Lymphoma may result in malabsorption by involvement of the lymphatic channels and by mucosal damage. In patients with a primary intestinal lymphoma, malabsorption may be a major feature of clinical presentation (Sleisenger et al 1953). Often, the malabsorption precedes other symptoms of lymphoma by a few months and there may be a transient response to a gluten-free diet, but the underlying lymphoma soon results in abdominal pain and fever and clinical deterioration. The association with immunoproliferative small intestinal disease is much more common.

**Table 16.7** Lymphoma and malabsorption

| | | Malabsorption |
|---|---|---|
| Primary lymphoma: | (a) "Western" lymphoma | Unusual |
| | (b) $\alpha$-Heavy chain disease | Common |
| Primary lymphoma: associated with celiac disease | | Already present |
| Secondary involvement of the intestine by systemic lymphoma | | Very rare |

## Solitary plasmacytoma of intestine (Asselah et al 1982)

The majority of solitary plasmacytomas occur in the oral cavity and upper respiratory tract and only about 10% have been in the gastrointestinal tract, including stomach, small and large intestine (Asselah et al 1982). Rarely, there is a paraprotein in the serum and association with multiple myeloma is uncommon. The tumors consist of sheets of well-differentiated and monoclonal plasma cells. Although lymph node metastases are often present these do not appear to affect prognosis.

# CARCINOID TUMORS

After the appendix, the small intestine is the second most common site of gastrointestinal carcinoid tumors (Godwin 1975). The most common site in the small intestine is the ileum. The pathology is discussed below.

## Clinical features

Most patients are in the fifth to seventh decades. The presenting features are abdominal pain, diarrhea, loss of weight and rectal bleeding or symptoms of the carcinoid syndrome (see below). Obstruction may be due to the dense fibrotic reaction to the tumor. About 30% of patients present with the carcinoid syndrome (p. 473). Many carcinoids, however, are asymptomatic and are found incidentially during operations.

The principles of surgical treatment include a wide excision of the tumor including adjacent mesentery, resection of all visible metastases and a search for multiple tumors. An ileo-right colectomy is the usual procedure. Hepatic metastases which cannot be resected are treated with hepatic artery ligation, embolization or infusion with chemotherapeutic agents (Martin et al 1983). The overall 5-year survival rate is 54% (Godwin 1975).

## Carcinoid syndrome

Carcinoid tumors arise in many different organs (Table 16.8) and represent 1.5% of all gastrointestinal neoplasms. They are most common in the appendix (30–40%), the small intestine and then the rectum (p. 1435). These tumors are discussed under site. The carcinoid syndrome occurs with only about 4% of all tumors and is most frequent with tumors of the ileum and jejunum (30%) and with teratomas of the ovary. More rarely, the syndrome has been reported with cancer of the thyroid, cervix and testis.

The term "carcinoid syndrome" refers to the systemic symptoms produced when the secretory products of neoplastic enterochromaffin cells are released into the systemic circulation. The precise biochemical mechanisms of the syndrome have not been clearly defined, although an increase in serotonin production is almost always observed. Overproduction and excessive urinary excretion of its metabolite 5-HIAA is the diagnostic hallmark of the syndrome and serotonin is a cause of diarrhea in these patients. The flushing is probably caused by the release of tachykinins (such as neuropeptide K, neurokinin A), rather than 5HT, in the case of small intestinal carcinoids and histamine in the case of gastric carcinoids (Oates 1986). Many other biologically active substances, e.g. bradykinin, prostaglandins, substance P, gastrin, insulin, calcitonin, VIP, ACTH, corticotrophin-releasing factor, growth hormone-releasing factor and neuropeptide Y, may be released (Connell et al 1987).

Carcinoid tumors also produce local symptoms at the site of the origin (pp. 315, 524 and 1436).

## Pathology

Carcinoid tumor occurs at many sites in the gastrointestinal tract (Table 16.8). In the appendix typical carcinoids are almost always benign but adenocarcinoids in which mucin production is seen may behave aggressively (p. 524). Warkel et al's study (1978) of 39 cases showed six instances of metastasis. Glandular carcinoids have also been reported in the duodenum, some associated with von Recklinghausen's disease (Griffiths et al 1984). Carcinoids in the small bowel are usually in the ileum and should be thought of as carcinomas of low-grade malignancy (Morson & Dawson 1979).

The tumors are usually less than 1.5 cm in diameter and are multiple in about 20% of cases. The lesions are usually well demarcated, growing towards the lumen and into the submucosa and deeper tissues. Commonly there is a surrounding fibrotic reaction which may extend to the mesentery. They appear yellow to the naked eye and may ulcerate. There may be evidence of ischemia, with elastosis of vessels and smooth muscle hyperplasia in adjacent tissues. Gastrointestinal carcinoids metastasize to the abdominal lymph nodes and particularly to the liver so that only 40% are localized at the time of diagnosis; even tumours of 1 cm or less have lymphatic invasion in 19% of cases (Strodel et al 1983). The microscopic features of ileal tumors are clusters, cords or acini of small polygonal or round cells (Fig. 16.7) with prominent round or oval basophilic nuclei. The cytoplasm is weakly eosinophilic

**Table 16.8** Prevalence of the carcinoid syndrome in carcinoid tumors in the alimentary tract (Sanders 1973)

| Site of tumor | Number of patients | Number with the carcinoid syndrome |
|---|---|---|
| Esophagus | 1 | 0 |
| Stomach | 98 | 7 |
| Duodenum | 80 | 1 |
| Small bowel | 992 | 39 (4%) |
| Meckel's diverticulum | 46 | 6 |
| Appendiceal | 1609 | 2 |
| Cecum and ascending colon | 59 | 3 |
| Left colon | 35 | 0 |
| Rectum | 706 | 0 |
| Gallbladder | 7 | 0 |

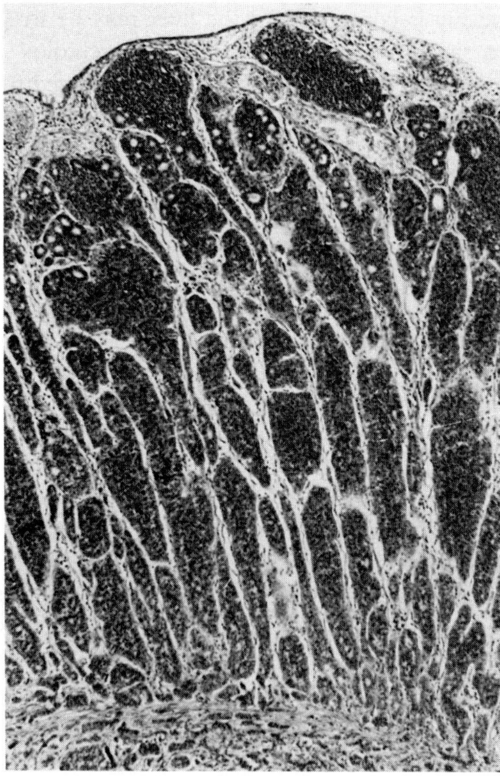

**Fig. 16.7** Carcinoid tumor of the ileum showing uniform small cells which form aggregates in which occasional acini are seen. There is some invasion through the musculanis mucosae (hematoxylin and eosin, × 60).

and finely granular. Various histological patterns of carcinoid have been identified and these bear some relation to prognosis (Johnson et al 1983). However, a mixed pattern is the commonest.

## Clinical features (Davis et al 1973, Walsh & Roth 1976, Grahame-Smith 1977)

Flushing is common and various patterns have been described; it may be diffuse and transient, affecting the face, neck and upper chest, or it can last for an hour or more, with watery eyes and conjunctival redness. Flushing may last for 2–3 days, especially with bronchial carcinoids; generalized flushing with weal formation, especially just after meals, occurs with gastric carcinoids, which produce histamine. Wheezing may accompany flushing attacks. Diarrhea is a common symptom; it is periodic, accompanied by colic and is due to increased motility (Von der Ohe et al 1993); attacks are usually independent of vasomotor features. Attacks of flushing or diarrhea may be precipitated by alcohol, food or exercise. Other features include edema and high-output cardiac failure with lesions of the valves of the right side of the heart. Symptoms may arise from the release of other hormones.

The carcinoid syndrome occurs when the humoral products of the tumor are not inactivated by the liver and therefore enter the systemic circulation. This occurs when there are extensive liver metastases; on examination, hepatomegaly is common and the liver may be irregular. However, as ovarian and bronchial carcinoids drain directly into the systemic venous circulation, features of the syndrome can occur without liver metastases. Occasional patients with jejunal and ileal carcinoid are described who develop the syndrome but have no hepatic metastases; instead they have intra-abdominal metastases which drain into the systemic circulation (Feldman & Jones 1982). About one-third of patients with the syndrome develop facial telangiectasia and the skin may become permanently plethoric.

## Diagnosis

The various tumor products are summarized in Table 16.9. The 5-hydroxytryptamine (5-HT or serotonin) elaborated by the tumor is metabolized within the tumor and circulation to 5-hydroxyindoleacetic acid (5-HIAA). Urinary excretion of >7 mg/24 h (37 mmol) 5-HIAA is abnormal, provided foods containing serotonin (mainly bananas and tomatoes) and certain drugs (phenothiazines, reserpine) are not ingested. However, other substances, especially bradykinin and histamine, are released by the tumor and these are mainly responsible for the flushing attacks. Bronchial, pancreatic and gastric (i.e. foregut) carcinoids release 5-HTP and 5-HT and the urine contains 5-HTP, 5-HT and 5-HIAA; these finding are useful diagnostically.

**Table 16.9** Characteristics of carcinoid tumors derived from different embryonic divisions of the gut (Williams & Sandler 1963, Grahame-Smith 1977)

| | Foregut | Midgut |
|---|---|---|
| Histological structure | Tendency to be trabecular; may differ widely form classic pattern | Characterisitc (see text) |
| Argentaffin and diazo reactions | Usually negatice | Positive |
| Association with the carcinoid syndrome | Frequent | Frequent |
| Tumor 5-HT content | Low | High |
| Urinary 5-HIAA | High | High |
| 5-HTP secretion | Frequent | Rare |
| Metastases to bone (usually osteoblastic) and skin | Common | Unusual |
| Associated with other endocrine secretion | Frequent | Not described |

Intravenous pentagastrin 0.06 μg/kg body weight given by intravenous injection induces a flush in carcinoid patients who have liver metastases (Richter et al 1986). The plasma concentration of tachykinin has been proposed as a useful tumor marker for the diagnosis and follow-up of patients with carcinoid tumors of midgut origin (Norheim et al 1986). For these tumors, the measurement of both urinary 5-HIAA and plasma tachykinins may be appropriate.

Localization of the tumors is assisted by magnetic resonance imaging and whole body scintigraphy with radiolabeled analogs of somatostatin (Kvols & Reubi 1993, Kwekkeboom et al 1993).

## Treatment

### *Surgery*

Surgery is palliative rather than curative in most patients with carcinoid syndrome because hepatic metastases have already occurred. Surgical treatment is also important because of the generally poor response of these tumors to chemotherapy and radiotherapy. Reduction of the tumor mass by removal of the primary and if possible by partial hepatectomy (p. 1132) will relieve symptoms, often for long periods of time, and it is also possible that the development of cardiac valvular lesions will be delayed. Since noncarcinoid malignancies, especially adenocarcinoma of the colon, accompany carcinoid tumors in many instances these should be sought by investigation and during surgical treatment (Peck et al 1983). Anesthesia presents special problems because of the release of vasoactive substances. Promethazine may be given preoperatively and aprotonin, E-aminocaproic acid and the somatostatin analog, octreotide (see below) have been used during induction of anesthesia (Haller 1985).

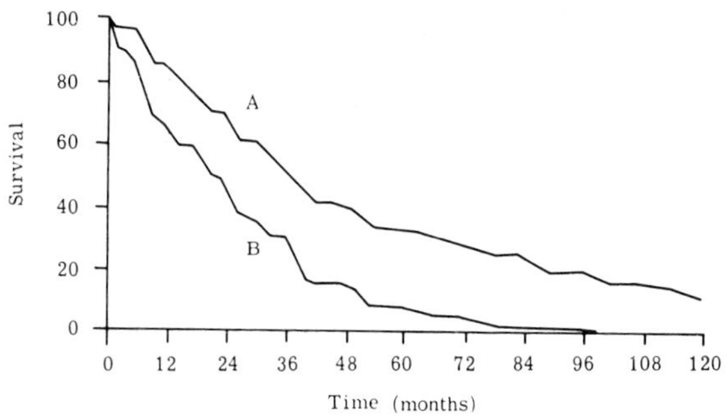


**Fig. 16.8** Survival of patients with malignant carcinoid syndrome. (A) Survival of 60 patients measured from the onset of flushing. (B) Survival of 91 patients measured from the first determination of elevated urinary 5-hydroxyindoleacetic acid (Davis et al 1973).

### *Pharmacological therapy*

A variety of pharmacological agents have been used to control symptoms (Grahame-Smith 1977). These include $H_1$ and $H_2$ blockers, serotonin antagonists (methysergide, cyproheptadine) bradykinin antagonists and corticosteroids (Moertel 1983), but these agents have only occasionally and partly suppressed the endocrine effects of the tumor, and usually only the diarrhea, and without any changes in serotonin production. Parachlorophenylalanine has been shown to relieve both flushing and diarrhea and to reduce urinary excretion of 5-HIAA, but the side-effects of this agent usually make it intolerable for long-term use.

The synthetic, long-acting somatostatin analog octreotide acetate, given by subcutaneous injection in a dose of 150 μg three times a day, relieves flushing and diarrhea in 85% of patients, associated with a reduction in the urinary excretion of 5-HIAA and few side-effects (Maton 1993). Therapy with somatostatin analogs has also been used successfully to treat a carcinoid crisis associated with the induction of anesthesia (Kvols et al 1985). Octreotide may also control tumor growth for a short period of time (Arnold et al 1993). Recombinant interferon α-2a will also control symptoms in 80% of patients and can be used in combination with octreotide or after octreotide has failed (Janson & Oberg 1993).

### *Chemotherapy*

A decision to give chemotherapy with its entailed hazards must be balanced against the slow progression of the malignancy (Fig. 16.8). The median lifespan from the date of the first episode of flushing is 38 months. Streptozotocin, which is effective in some other hormone-producing adenomas, is unlikely to produce improvement and other agents used alone also produce a low response rate with a short duration. Combination therapy is being assessed (Haller 1985) and for hepatic secondary tumors 5-fluorouracil has been infused into the hepatic artery prior to ligation and thereafter into a tributary of the portal vein to act on any areas of surviving carcinoid tissue (see also p. 1304).

The most promising treatment of hepatic secondary tumor is with hepatic artery chemoembolization which controls the symptoms and produces some regression of the tumor (Ruszniewski et al 1993).

## REFERENCES


Adibi S A, Stanko R T 1984 Perspectives on gastrointestinal surgery for treatment of morbid obesity: the lesson learned. Gastroenterology 87: 1381–1391

Altemeier W A, Bryant L R, Wulsin J H 1963 The surgical significance of jejunal diverticulosis. Archives of Surgery 86: 732

Alwmark A, Andersson A, Lasson A 1980 Primary carcinoma of the duodenum. Annals of Surgery 191: 13–18

Ameen V Z, Powell G K, Jones L A 1987 Quantitation of fecal carbohydrate excretion in patients with short bowel syndrome. Gastroenterology 92: 493–500

Ament M E, Shimoda S S, Saunders D R, Rubin C E 1972 Pathogenesis of steatorrhea in three cases of small intestinal stasis syndrome. Gastroenterology 63(5): 728–747

Appelman H D, Schnitzer B, Hirsch S D, Coon W W 1985 Clinicopathologic overview of gastrointestinal lymphomas. American Journal of Surgical Pathology 9: 71

Aries V, Hill M J 1970 Degradation of steroids by intestinal bacteria. I. Deconjugation of bile salts. Biochimica et Biophysica Acta 202: 526–534

Arnold R, Benning R, Neuhaus C, Rolwage M, Trautmann M E 1993 Gastroenteropancreatic endocrine tumours: effect of Sandostatin on tumour growth. German Sandostatin Study Group. Digestion 54 (suppl 1): 72–75

Ashley S W, Wells S A Jr 1988 Tumors of the small intestine. Seminars in Oncology 15: 116–128

Asselah F, Crow J, Slavin G, Sowter G, Sheldon C, Asselah H 1982 Solitary plasmacytoma of the intestine. Histopathology 6: 631–645

Asselineau F, Lederer E 1960 Chemistry and metabolism of bacterial lipides. In: Bloch K (ed) Lipide metabolism. Wiley, New York, p 337

Aubrey D A, Blumgart L H, Davies G T, Gravelle I H 1971 Occult small-bowel tumours: their diagnostic features and management. British Journal of Surgery 58: 678–684

Badenoch J, Bedford P D, Evans J R 1955 Massive diverticulosis of the small intestine with steatorrhoea and megaloblastic anaemia. Quarterly Journal of Medicine 24: 321

Banwell J G, Kistler L A, Giannella R A, Weber F L, Lieber A, Powell D E 1981 Small intestinal bacterial overgrowth syndrome. Gastroenterology 80: 834–845

Bayes B J, Hamilton J R 1969 Blind loop syndrome in children. Malabsorption secondary to intestinal stasis. Archives of Disease in Childhood 44: 76–81

Beher W T 1976 Bile acids: chemistry and physiology of bile acids and their influence on atherosclerosis. Karger, Basel

Behrns K E, Smith C D, Sarr M G 1994 Prospective evaluation of gastric acid secretion and cobalamin absorption following gastric bypass for clinically severe obesity. Digestive Diseases and Sciences 39: 315–320

Bloom S R, Polak J M 1982 The hormonal pattern of intestinal adaptation. A major role for enteroglucagon. In: Polak J M, Bloom S R, Wright N A, Daly M J (eds) Adaptation pathophysiology of intestinal response to disease. Proceedings of the third symposium in a series on basic science in gastroenterology. Scandinavain Journal of Gastroenterology 17 (suppl 74): 93–103

Bochenek W, Rodgers J B, Balint J A 1970 Effects of changes in dietary lipids on intestinal fluid loss in the short-bowel syndrome. Annals of Internal Medicine 72: 205–213

Braasch J W, Denbo H E 1964 Tumors of the small intestine. Surgical Clinics of North America 44: 791–809

Brooks J J, Enterline H T 1983 Primary gastric lymphomas. A clinicopathologic study of 58 cases with long-term follow-up and literature review. Cancer 51: 701–711

Buchan A M J, Griffiths C J, Morris J F, Polak J M 1985 Enteroglucagon cell hyperfunction in rat small intestine after gut resection. Gastroenterology 88: 8–12

Bush R S, Ash C L 1969 Primary lymphoma of the gastrointestinal tract. Radiology 92: 1349–1354

Cammoun M, Jaafoura H, Tabbane F, Halphen M, TUFRALI Group 1989 Immunoproliferative small intestinal disease without α-chain disease: a pathological study. Gastroenterology 96: 750–763

Caspary W F, Zavada I, Reimold W V, Emrich D, Willms B 1977 Increased deconjugation of bile acids and vitamin $B_{12}$ malabsorption in diabetics on treatment with biguanides. In: Paumgartner G, Stiehl A (eds) Bile acid metabolism in health and disease. MTP Press, Lancaster, p 271–284

Chadwick V S, Modha K, Dowling R H 1973 Mechanism for hyperoxaluria in patients with ileal dysfunction. New England Journal of Medicine 289: 172–176

Chadwick V S, Gaginella T S, Carlson G L, Debongnie J C, Phillips S F, Hofmann A F 1979 Effect of molecular structure on bile acid-induced alterations in absorptive function, permeability, and morphology in the perfused rabbit colon. Journal of Laboratory and Clinical Medicine 94: 661–674

Chernov A J, Doe W F, Gompertz D 1972 Intrajejunal volatile fatty acids in the stagnant loop syndrome. Gut 13: 103–106

Cohen S, Kaplan M, Gottlieb L, Patterson J 1971 Liver disease and gallstones in regional enteritis. Gastroenterology 60: 237–245

Connell J M, Corder R, Asbury J et al 1987 Neuropeptide Y in multiple endocrine neoplasia: release during surgery for phaeochromocytoma. Clinical Endocrinology 26: 75–84

Cooke W T, Cox E V, Fone D J, Meynell M J, Gaddie R 1963 The clinical and metabolic significance of jejunal diverticula. Gut 4: 115–131

Cooperman M, Clausen K P, Hecht C, Lucas J G, Keith L M 1978 Villous adenomas of the duodenum. Gastroenterology 74: 1295–1297

Craig O, Gregson R 1981 Primary lymphoma of the gastrointestinal tract. Clinical Radiology 32: 63–72

Cupps R E, Hodgson J R, Dockerty M, Adson M A 1969 Primary lymphoma in the small intestine: problems of roentgenologic diagnosis. Radiology 92: 1354–1362

Davis Z, Moertel C G, McIlrath D C 1973 The malignant carcinoid syndrome. Surgery, Gynecology and Obstetrics 137: 637–644

De Castro C A, Dockerty M B, Mayo C W 1957 Metastatic tumors of the small intestines. Surgery, Gynecology and Obstetrics 105: 159–165

Deane S, Youngs D, Poxon V, Keighley M R B, Alexander-Williams J, Burdon D W 1980 Cimetidine and gastric microflora. British Journal of Surgery 67: 371

Delamere J P, Baddeley R M,Walton K W 1983 Jejuno-ileal bypass arthropathy: its clincial features and associations. Annals of the Rheumatic Diseases 42: 553–557

Dellipiani A W, Girdwood R H 1964 Bacterial changes in the small intestine in malabsorptive states and in pernicious anaemia. Clinical Science 26: 359

Dharmsathaphorn K, Freeman D H, Binder H J, Dobbins J W 1982 Increased risk of nephrolithiasis in patients with steatorrhea. Digestive Diseases and Sciences 27: 401–405

Dodds W J 1976 Clinical and roentgen features of the intestinal polyposis syndromes. Gastrointestinal Radiology 1: 127–142

Doe W F 1985 Lymphoma and alpha-chain disease. In: Booth C C, Neale G (eds) Disorders of the small intestine. Blackwell, Oxford, p 179–194

Doe W F, Spiegelberg H L 1979 Characterization of an antiserum specific for the Fabalpha fragment. Its use for detection of alpha-heavy chain disease protein by immunoselection. Journal of Immunology 122: 19–23

Donald J W 1979 Major complications of small bowel diverticula. Annals of Surgery 190: 183–188

Donaldson R M Jr 1962 Malabsorption of $CO^{60}$ labelled cyanocobalamin in rats with intestinal diverticula. I. Evaluation of possible mechanisms. Gastroenterology 43: 271–281

Donaldson R M Jr 1965 Studies on the pathogenesis of steatorrhea in the blind loop syndrome. Journal of Clinical Investigation 44: 1815

Donaldson R M Jr 1970 Small bowel bacterial overgrowth. In: Stollerman G H (ed) Advances in internal medicine, Vol 16. Year Book Medical Publishers, New York, p 191–212

Dorman J E, Floyd C E, Cohn I Jr 1967 Malignant neoplasms of the small bowel. American Journal of Surgery 113: 131–136

Dorney S F, Ament M E, Berquist W E, Vargas J H, Hassal E 1985 Improved survival in very short small bowel of infancy with use of long-term parenteral nutrition. Journal of Pediatrics 107: 521–525

Dowling R H 1973 Bile acids and the intestine. In: Truelove S C, Jewell D P (eds) Topics in gastroenterology, Vol. 1 Blackwell, Oxford, p 139–154

Dowling R H 1982a Small bowel adaptation and its regulation. In: Polak J M, Bloom S R, Wright N A, Daly M J (eds) Adaptation pathophysiology of intestinal response to disease. Proceedings of the third symposium in a series on basic science in gastroenterology. Scandinavian Journal of Gastroenterology 17 (suppl 74): 53–74

Dowling R H 1982b Intestinal adaptation and its mechanisms. In: Jewell D P, Selby W S (eds) Topics in gastroenterology, Vol. 10. Blackwell, Oxford, p 135–156

Dowling R H 1990 Polyamines in intestinal adaptation and disease. Digestion 46 (suppl 2): 331–344

Dowling R H, Bell G D, White J 1972 Lithogenic bile in patients with ileal dysfunction. Gut 13: 415–420

Dozois R R, Judd E S, Dahlin D C, Bartholomew L G 1969 The Peutz–Jehgers syndrome: is there a predisposition to the development of intestinal malignancy? Archives of Surgery 98: 509–517

Drasar B S, Hill M J 1974 Human intestinal flora. Academic Press, London

Drenick E J, Ament M E, Finegold S M, Passaro E Jr 1977 Bypass enteropathy: an inflammatory process in the excluded segment with systemic complications. American Journal of Clinical Nutrition 30: 76–89

Drenick E J, Fisler J, Johnson D 1982 Hepatic steatosis after intestinal bypass – prevention and reversal by metronidazole, irrespective of protein-calorie malnutrition. Gastroenterology 82: 535–548

Dubos R, Schaedler R W, Costello R, Hoet P 1965 Indigenous, normal, and autochthonous flora of the gastrointestinal tract. Journal of Experimental Medicine 122: 67–76

Dudrick S J, Latifi R, Fosnocht D E 1991 Management of the short-bowel syndrome. Surgical Clinics of North America 71: 625–643

Duncan H 1977 Arthropathy and the intestinal bypass operation for obesity. Journal of Rheumatology 4: 115–117

Dyer N H, Hawkins C 1972 Blind loop syndrome. In: Badenoch J, Brooke B N (eds) Recent advances in gastroenterology, 2nd edn Churchill Livingstone, Edinburgh, p 250–275

Earnest D L 1977 Perspectives on incidence, etiology and treatment of enteric hyperoxaluria. American Journal of Clinical Nutrition 30: 72–75

Edwards H C 1954 Intestinal diverticulosis and diverticulitis. Annals of the Royal College of Surgeons 14: 371–388

Faergeman O, Meinertz H, Hylander E, Fischerman K, Jarnum S, Nielsen O V 1982 Effects and side-effects of partial ileal by-pass surgery for familial hypercholesterolaemia. Gut 23: 558–563

Faloon W W, Rubulis A, Knipp J, Sherman C D, Flood M S 1977 Fecal fat, bile acid and sterol excretion and biliary lipid changes in jejunoileostomy patients. American Journal of Clinical Nutrition 30: 21–31

Feldman J M, Jones R S 1982 Carcinoid syndrome from gastrointestinal carcinoids without liver metastasis. Annals of Surgery 196: 33–37

Finegold S M, Sutter V L, Mathisen G E 1983 Normal indigenous intestinal flora. In: Hentges D J (ed) Human intestinal microflora in health and disease. Academic Press, New York, p 3–31

Fitzpatrick W J F, Zentler-Munro P L, Northfield T C 1986 Ileal resection: effect of cimetidine and taurine on intrajejunal bile acid precipitation and lipid solubilisation. Gut 27: 66–72

Fraser-Moodie A, Hughes R G, Jones S M, Shorey B A, Snape L 1976

Malignant melanoma metastases to the alimentary tract. Gut 17: 206–209
Friedman L S, Kirkham S E, Thistlethwaite J R, Platika D, Kolodny E H, Schuffler M D 1984 Jejunal diverticulosis with perforation as a complication of Fabry's disease. Gastroenterology 86: 558–563
Fromm H, Hofmann A F 1971 Breath test for altered bile-acid metabolism. Lancet 2: 621–625
Fromm H, Thomas P J, Hofmann A F 1973 Sensitivity and specificity in tests of distal ileal function: prospective comparison of bile acid and vitamin $B_{12}$ absorption in ileal resection patients. Gastroenterology 64: 1077–1090
Gilder H 1986 Parenteral nourishment of patients undergoing surgical or traumatic stress. Journal of Parenteral and Enteral Nutrition 10: 88–99
Godwin J D 1975 Carcinoid tumors. An analysis of 2837 cases. Cancer 36: 560–569
Goerg C, Schwerk W B, Goerg K 1990 Gastrointestinal lymphoma: sonographic findings in 54 patients. American Journal of Roentgenology 155: 795–798
Goldstein F, Wirts C W, Kramer S 1961 The relationship of afferent limb stasis and bacterial flora to the production of post-gastrectomy steatorrhea. Gastroenterology 40: 47–55
Goldstein F, Cozzolino H J, Wirts C W 1963 Diarrhea and steatorrhea due to a large solitary duodenal diverticulum. American Journal of Digestive Diseases 8: 937
Goldstein F, Karacadag S, Wirts C W, Kowlessar O D 1970 Intraluminal small-intestinal utilization of *d*-xylose by bacteria. A limitation of the *d*-xylose absorption test. Gastroenterology 59: 380–386
Gomez C A 1981a Gastroplasty in intractable obesity. International Journal of Obesity 5: 413–420
Gomez C A 1981b Gastroplasty in morbid obesity: a progress report. World Journal of Surgery 5: 823–828
Gorbach S L 1967 Population control in the small bowel. Gut 8: 530–532
Gorbach S L, Levitan R 1970 Intestinal flora in health and in gastrointestinal diseases. In: Glass G B J (ed) Progress in gastroenterology, Vol. II Grune & Stratton, New York, p 252–275
Gorbach S L, Tabaqchali S 1969 Bacteria, bile and the small bowel. Gut 10: 963–972
Gorbach S L, Plaut A G, Nahas L, Weinstein L, Spanknebel G, Levitan R 1967 Studies of intestinal microflora. II. Microorganisms of the small intestine and their relations to oral and fecal flora. Gastroenterology 53: 856–867
Gracey M 1971 Intestinal absorption in the 'contaminated small-bowel syndrome'. Gut 12: 403–410
Gracey M 1983 The contaminated small bowel syndrome. In: Hentges D J (ed) Human intestinal microflora in health and disease. Academic Press, New York, p 495–515
Grahame-Smith D G 1977 The carcinoid syndrome. In: Truelove S C, Lee E (eds) Topics in Gastroenterology, Vol. 5. Blackwell, Oxford, p 285–312
Gray G M, Rosenberg S A, Cooper A D, Gregory P B, Stein D T, Herzenberg H 1982 Lymphomas involving the gastrointestinal tract. Gastroenterology 82: 143–152
Gray J D A, Shiner M 1967 Influence of gastric pH on gastric and jejunal flora. Gut 8: 574–581
Green J A, Dawson A A, Jones P F, Brunt P W 1979 The presentation of gastrointestinal lymphoma: study of a population. British Journal of Surgery 66: 798-801
Greenberger N J, Saegh S, Ruppert R D 1968 Urine indican excretion in malabsorptive disorders. Gastroenterology 55: 204–211
Griffen W O, Bivins B A, Bell R M, Jackson K A 1981 Gastric bypass for morbid obesity. World Journal of Surgery 5: 817–822
Griffiths D F R, Jasani B, Newman G R, Williams E D, Williams G T 1984 Glandular duodenal carcinoid – a somatostatin rich tumour with neuroendocrine associations. Journal of Clinical Pathology 37: 163–169
Haller D G 1985 Chemotherapeutic management of endocrine-producing tumors of the gastrointestinal tract. In: Cohen S, Soloway R D (eds). Hormone-producing tumors of the gastrointestinal tract. Churchill Livingstone, New York, p 129–157
Hamilton I, Worsley B W, Cobden I, Cooke E M, Shoesmith J G, Axon A T R 1982 Simultaneous culture of saliva and jejunal aspirate in the investigation of small bowel bacterial overgrowth. Gut 23: 847–853
Hamilton J D, Dyer N H, Dawson A M et al 1970 Assessment and significance of bacterial overgrowth in the small bowel. Quarterly Journal of Medicine 39: 265–285
Heaton K W 1976 Clinical aspects of bile acid metabolism. In: Bouchier I A D (ed) Recent advances in gastroenterology, Vol. 3 Churchill Livingstone, Edinburgh, p 199–230
Heaton K W 1977 Disturbances of bile acid metabolism in intestinal disease. Clinics in Gastroenterology 6: 69–89
Heaton K W, Read A E 1969 Gall stones in patients with disorders of the terminal ileum and disturbed bile salt metabolism. British Medical Journal 3: 494–496
Herrmann R, Panahon A M, Barcos M P, Walsh D, Stutzman L 1980 Gastrointestinal involvement in non-Hodgkin's lymphoma. Cancer 46: 215–222
Hines J D, Hoffbrand A V, Mollin D L 1967 The hematologic complications following partial gastrectomy. A study of 292 patients. American Journal of Medicine 43: 555–569
Hoffbrand A V, Tabaqchali S, Mollin D L 1966 High serum-folate levels in intestinal blind-loop syndrome. Lancet 1: 1339–1342
Hofmann A F, Poley J R 1969 Cholestyramine treatment of diarrhea associated with ileal resection. New England Journal of Medicine 281: 397–402
Hofmann A F, Laker M F, Dharmsathaphorn K, Sherr H P, Lorenzo D 1983 Complex pathogenesis of hyperoxaluria after jejunoileal bypass surgery. Oxalogenic substances in diet contribute to urinary oxalate. Gastroenterology 84: 293–300
Horowitz M, Collins P J, Chatterton B E, Harding P E, Watts J McK, Shearman D J C 1984 Gastric emptying after gastroplasty for morbid obesity. British Journal of Surgery 71: 435–437
Hylander E, Lakefoged K, Jarnum S 1990 Calcium absorption after intestinal resection. The importance of a preserved colon. Scandinavian Journal of Gastroenterology 25: 705–710
Iber F L, Cooper M 1977 Jejunoileal bypass for the treatment of massive obesity. Prevalence, morbidity and short- and long-term consequences. American Journal of Clinical Nutrition 30: 4–15
Iida M, Suekane H, Tada S et al 1991 Double-contrast radiographic features in primary small intestinal lymphoma of the 'Western' type: correlation with pathological findings. Clinical Radiology 44: 322–326
Isaacson P G, Wright D H 1983 Malignant lymphoma of mucosa-associated lymphoid tissue. Cancer 52: 1410–1416
Jacobsen O, Ladefoged K, Stage J G, Jarnum S 1986 Effects of cimetidine on jejunostomy effluents in patients with severe short-bowel syndrome. Scandinavian Journal of Gastroenterology 21: 824–828
Janson E T, Oberg K 1993 Long-term management of the carcinoid syndrome. Treatment with octreotide alone and in combination with alpha-interferon. Acta Oncologica 32: 225–229
Jeejeebhoy K N 1983 Therapy of the short-gut syndrome. Lancet 1: 1427–1430
Jeejeebhoy K N, Coghill N F 1961 The measurement of gastrointestinal protein loss by a new method. Gut 2: 123–130
Joesting D R, Beart R W, van Heerden J A, Weiland L H 1981 Improving survival in adenocarcinoma of the duodenum. American Journal of Surgery 141: 228–231
Joffe S N 1981 Surgical management of morbid obesity. Gut 22: 242–254
Johansen A, Larsen E 1969 Adenomas of the small intestine. A report of four cases with special reference to their relation to carcinomas. Acta Pathologica Microbiologica Scandinavica 75: 247–256
Johnson G K, Soergel K H, Hensley G T, Dodds W J, Hogan W J 1972 Cronkite Canada syndrome: gastrointestinal pathophysiology and morphology. Gastroenterology 63: 140–152
Johnson L A, Lavin P, Moertel C G et al 1983 Carcinoids: the association of histologic growth pattern and survival. Cancer 51: 882–889
Juhl E, Dano P, Quaade F 1979 The small bowel. Part II. Shunt operations for obesity. Clinics in Gastroenterology 8: 386–397
Kalser M H, Cohen R, Arteaga I et al 1966 Normal viral and bacterial flora of the human small and large intestine. New England Journal of Medicine 274: 500–505, 558–563

Kark A E 1980 Jaw wiring. American Journal of Clinical Nutrition 33: 420–424

Karlström L 1986 Evidence of involvement of the enteric nervous system in the effects of sodium deoxycholate on small-intestinal transepithelial fluid transport and motility. Scandinavian Journal of Gastroenterology 21: 321–330

Khojasteh A 1987 Immunoproliferative small intestinal disease (IPSID) in Third World countries. In: Marsh M N (ed) Immunopathology of the small intestine. Wiley, Chichester, p 121–150

Khojasteh A, Haghshenass M, Haghighi P 1983 Immunoproliferative small intestinal disease. A 'third-world lesion'. New England Journal of Medicine 308: 1401–1405

Kibbey W E, Sirinek K R, Pace W G, Thomford N R 1976 Primary duodenal tumors. A diagnostic and therapeutic dilemma. Archives of Surgery 111: 377–380

Kim Y S, Spritz N 1968a Hydroxy acid excretion in steatorrhea of pancreatic and nonpancreatic origin. New England Journal of Medicine 279: 1424–1426

Kim Y S, Spritz N 1968b Metabolism of hydroxy fatty acids in dogs with steatorrhea secondary to experimentally produced intestinal blind loops. Journal of Lipid Research 9: 487–491

Kim Y S, Spritz N, Blum M, Terz J, Sherlock P 1966 The role of altered bile acid metabolism in the steatorrhea of experimental blind loop. Journal of Clinical Investigation 45: 956–962

King C E, Toskes P P 1979 Small intestine bacterial overgrowth. Gastroenterology 76: 1035–1055

King C E, Toskes P P 1986 Comparison of the 1-gram [$^{14}$C] xylose, 10-gram lactulose-$H_2$, and 80-gram glucose-$H_2$ breath tests in patients with small intestine bacterial overgrowth. Gastroenterology 91: 1447–1451

King C E, Toskes P P, Guilarte T R, Lorenz E, Welkos S L 1980 Comparison of the one-gram *d*-[$^{14}$C] xylose breath test to the [$^{14}$C] bile acid breath test in patients with small-intestine bacterial overgrowth. Digestive Diseases and Sciences 25: 53–58

Knowles D M II 1985 Lymphoid cell markers. Their distribution and usefulness in the immunophenotypic analysis of lymphoid neoplasms. American Journal of Surgical Pathology 9 (suppl 3): 85

Koivisto P, Miettinen T A 1986 Adaptation of cholesterol and bile acid metabolism and vitamin $B_{12}$ absorption in the long-term follow-up after partial ileal bypass. Gastroenterology 90: 984–990

Koruda M J, Rolandelli R H, Settle R G, Zimmaro D M, Rombeau J L 1988 Effect of parenteral nutrition supplemented with short-chain fatty acids on adaptation to massive small bowel resection. Gastroenterology 95: 715–720

Kral J G, Görtz L 1981 Truncal vagotomy in morbid obesity. International Journal of Obesity 5: 431–435

Krishnamurthy S, Kelly M M, Rohrmann C A, Schuffler M D 1983 Jejunal diverticulosis. A heterogeneous disorder caused by a variety of abnormalities of smooth muscle or myenteric plexus. Gastroenterology 85: 538–547

Kvols L K, Reubi J C 1993 Metastatic carcinoid tumors and the malignant carcinoid syndrome. Acta Oncologica 32: 197–201

Kvols L K, Martin J K, Marsh H M, Moertel C G 1985 Rapid reversal of carcinoid crisis with a somatostatin analogue. New England Journal of Medicine 313: 1229–1230

Kwekkeboom D J, Krenning E P, Bakker W H, Oei H Y, Kooij P P, Lamberts S W 1993 Somatostatin analogue scintigraphy in carcinoid tumours. European Journal of Nuclear Medicine 20: 283–292

LaBrooy J T, Shearman D J C 1979 Antibody in the defences of the gut. In: Truelove S C, Willoughby C P (eds) Topics in gastroenterology, Vol. 7. Blackwell, Oxford, p 177–203

Lancet 1991 Leading article: primary gut lymphomas. Lancet 337: 1384–1385

Lauterburg B H, Newcomer A D, Hofmann A F 1978 Clinical value of the bile acid breath test. Evaluation of the Mayo Clinic experience. Mayo Clinic Proceedings 53: 227–233

LeBrun D P, Kamel O W, Cleary M L, Dorfman R F, Warnke R A 1992 Follicular lymphomas of the gastrointestinal tract. Pathologic features in 31 cases and bcl-2 oncogenic protein expression. American Journal of Pathology 140: 1327–1335

Lentze M J 1989 Intestinal adaptation in short-bowel syndrome. European Journal of Pediatrics 148: 294–299

Lewin K J, Ranchod M, Dorfman R F 1978 Lymphomas of the gastrointestinal tract. A study of 117 cases presenting with gastrointestinal disease. Cancer 42: 693–707

Lindenbaum J, Rund D G, Butler V P Jr, Tse-Eng D, Saha J R 1981 Inactivation of digoxin by the gut flora: reversal by antibiotic therapy. New England Journal of Medicine 305: 789–794

Longo W E, Vernava A M III 1992 Clinical implications of jejunoileal diverticular disease. Diseases of the Colon and Rectum 35: 381–388

Maglinte D D T, Chernish S M, DeWeese R, Kelvin F M, Brunelle R L 1986 Acquired jejunoileal diverticular disease: subject review. Radiology 158: 577–580

Martin J K, Moertel C G, Adson M A, Schutt A J 1983 Surgical treatment of functioning metastatic carcinoid tumors. Archives of Surgery 118: 537–542

Martini G A, Phear E A, Ruebner B, Sherlock S 1957 The bacterial content of small intestine in normal and cirrhotic subjects: relation to methionine toxicity. Clinical Science 16: 35

Mason G R 1986 Tumors of the duodenum and small intestine. In: Sabiston D C Jr (ed) Textbook of surgery, 13th edn. W B Saunders, Philadelphia, p 868–873

Mason E E, Ito C 1967 Gastric bypass in obesity. Surgical Clinics of North America 47: 1345–1351

Maton P N 1993 Use of octreotide acetate for control of symptoms in patients with islet cell tumors. World Journal of Surgery 17: 504–510

Matuchansky C, Cogné M, Lemaire M et al 1989 Nonsecretory a-chain disease with immunoproliferative small-intestinal disease. New England Journal of Medicine 320: 1534–1539

McDonald G B, Vracko R 1984 Systemic absorption of oral cholestyramine. Gastroenterology 87: 213–215

McJunkin B, Fromm H, Sarva R P, Amin P 1981 Factors in the mechanism of diarrhea in bile acid malabsorption: fecal pH – a key determinant. Gastroenterology 80: 1454–1464

Mekhjian H S, Phillips S F, Hofmann A F 1971 Colonic secretion of water and electrolytes induced by bile acids: perfusion studies in man. Journal of Clinical Investigation 50: 1569–1577

Mir-Madjlessi S-H, Farmer R G, Hawk W A 1973 Villous tumors of the duodenum and jejunum: report of 4 cases and review of the literature. American Journal of Digestive Diseases 18: 467-476

Mitchell J E, Breuer R I, Zuckerman L, Berlin J, Schilli R, Dunn J K 1980 The colon influences ileal resection diarrhea. Digestive Diseases and Sciences 25: 33–41

Mittal V K, Bodzin J H 1980 Primary malignant tumors of the small bowel. American Journal of Surgery 140: 396–399

Moertel C G 1983 Treatment of the carcinoid tumor and the malignant carcinoid syndrome. Journal of Clinical Oncology 1: 727–740

Morson B C, Dawson I M P 1979 Gastrointestinal pathology. Blackwell, Oxford

Murray-Lyon I M, Finlayson N D C, Shearman D J C 1968 Studies on two patients with concomitant intrinsic factor secretory defect and jejunal diverticulosis. Scandinavian Journal of Haematology 5: 383–389

Nassar V H, Salem P A, Shahid M J et al 1978 'Mediterranean abdominal lymphoma' or immunoproliferative small intestinal disease. Part II: pathological aspects. Cancer 41: 1340–1354

National Cancer Institute Sponsored Study of Classifications of Non-Hodgkin's Lymphomas 1982 Summary and description of a working formulation for clinical usage. Cancer 49: 2112–2135

Neale G, Antcliff A C, Welbourn R B, Mollin D L, Booth C C 1967 Protein malnutrition after partial gastrectomy. Quarterly Journal of Medicine 36: 469–494

Nightingale J M D, Kamm M A, van der Sijp J R M et al 1993 Disturbed gastric emptying in the short bowel syndrome. Evidence for a 'colonic brake'. Gut 34: 1171–1176

Norheim I, Theodorsson-Norheim E, Brodin E, Oberg K 1986 Tachykinins in carcinoid tumors: their use as a tumor marker and possible role in the carcinoid flush. Journal of Clinical Endocrinology and Metabolism 63: 605–612

Northfield T C 1973 Intraluminal precipitation of bile acids in stagnant loop syndrome. British Medical Journal 2: 743–745

Nygaard K, Rootwelt K 1968 Intestinal protein loss in rats with blind segments on the small bowel. Gastroenterology 54: 52–55

Oates J A 1986 The carcinoid syndrome. New England Journal of Medicine 315: 702–703

O'Brien P E 1994 The surgical treatment of morbid obesity: current status and prospects. Medical Journal of Australia 160: 741–742
Ouriel K, Adams J T 1984 Adenocarcinoma of the small intestine. American Journal of Surgery 147: 66–71
Parkin D M, McClelland D B L, O'Moore R R, Percy-Robb I W, Grant I W B, Shearman D J C 1972a Intestinal bacterial flora and bile salt studies in hypogammaglobulinaemia. Gut 13: 182–188
Parkin D M, O'Moore R R, Cussons D J et al 1972b Evaluation of the 'breath test' in the detection of bacterial colonisation of the upper gastrointestinal tract. Lancet 2: 777–780
Patel S A, Al-Haddadin D, Schopp J, Cantave I, Duarte B, Watkins J L 1993 Gastrointestinal manifestations of amyloidosis: a case of diverticular perforation. American Journal of Gastroenterology 88: 578–582
Peck J J, Shields A B, Boyden A M, Dworkin L A, Nadal J W 1983 Carcinoid tumors of the ileum. American Journal of Surgery 146: 124–132
Polter D E, Boyle J D, Miller L G, Finegold S M 1968 Anaerobic bacteria as cause of the blind loop syndrome. A case report with observations on response to antibacterial agents. Gastroenterology 54: 1148–1154
Pope J L, Parkinson T M, Olson J A 1966 Action of bile salts on the metabolism and transport of water-soluble nutrients by perfused rat jejunum in vitro. Biochimica et Biophysica Acta 130: 218–232
Rambaud J-C 1983 Small intestinal lymphomas and alpha-chain disease. Clinics in Gastroenterology 12: 743–766
Rambaud J-C, Galian A, Danon F G et al 1983 Alpha-chain disease without qualitative serum IgA abnormality. Report of two cases, including a 'non-secretory' form. Cancer 51: 686–693
Remington M, Malagelada J-R, Zinsmeister A, Fleming C R 1983 Abnormalities in gastrointestinal motor activity in patients with short bowels: effect of a synthetic opiate. Gastroenterology 85: 629–636
Richmond J, Davidson S 1958 Subacute combined degeneration of the spinal cord in non-Addisonian megaloblastic anaemia. Quarterly Journal of Medicine 27: 517
Richter G, Stöckmann F, Conlon J M, Creutzfeldt W 1986 Serotonin release into blood after food and pentagastrin. Studies in healthy subjects and in patients with metastatic carcinoid tumours. Gastroenterology 91: 612–618
River L, Silverstein J, Tope J W 1956 Benign neoplasms of the small intestine. A critical comprehensive review with reports of 20 new cases. International Abstracts of Surgery 102: 1–38
Roda A, Roda E, Aldini R et al 1977 Determination of $^{14}CO_2$ in breath and $^{14}C$ in stool after oral administration of cholyl-l-[$^{14}C$]glycine: clinical application. Clinical Chemistry 23: 2127–2132
Rosenberg S A, Diamond H D, Jaslowitz B, Craver L F 1961 Lymphosarcoma: a review of 1269 cases. Medicine 40: 31–84
Rowe G G 1967 Control of tenesmus and diarrhea by cholestyramine administration. Gastroenterology 53: 1006
Rucker R D, Horstmann J, Schneider P D, Varco R L, Buchwald H 1982 Comparisons between jejunoileal and gastric bypass operations for morbid obesity. Surgery 92: 241–249
Ruddell W S J, Losowsky M S 1980 Severe diarrhoea due to small intestinal colonisation during cimetidine treatment. British Medical Journal 281: 273
Ruszniewski P, Rougier P, Roche A et al 1993 Hepatic arterial chemoembolization in patients with liver metastases of endocrine tumors. A prospective phase II study in 24 patients. Cancer 71: 2624–2630
Ryan D P, Schapiro R H, Warshaw A L 1986 Villous tumors of the duodenum. Annals of Surgery 203: 301–306
Sachatello C R, Pickren J W, Grace J T 1970 Generalized juvenile gastrointestinal polyposis. A hereditary syndrome. Gastroenterology 58: 699–708
Sanders R J 1973 Carcinoids of the gastrointestinal tract. Thomas, Illinois
Saraga P, Hurlimann J, Ozzello L 1981 Lymphomas and pseudolymphomas of the alimentary tract. An immunohistochemical study with clinicopathologic correlations. Human Pathology 12: 713–723
Sartoris D J, Harell G S, Anderson M F, Zboralske F F 1984 Small-bowel lymphoma and regional enteritis: radiographic similarities. Radiology 152: 291–296
Savage D C 1983 Associations of indigenous microorganisms with gastrointestinal epithelial surfaces In: Hentges D J (ed) Human intestinal microflora in health and disease. Academic Press, New York, p 55–78
Scarpello J H B, Hague R V, Cullen D R, Sladen G E 1976 The $^{14}C$-glycocholate test in diabetic diarrhoea. British Medical Journal 2: 673–675
Schønsby H 1973 The mechanism of vitamin $B_{12}$ malabsorption in blind-loop syndrome. Scandinavian Journal of Gastroenterology 8: 97
Schjønsby H, Andersen K-J, Nordgard K, Skagen D W 1983 Enzymatic activities in jejunal biopsy specimens from patients with the stagnant-loop syndrome. Scandinavian Journal of Gastroenterology 18: 599–602
Scopinaro N, Gianetta E, Civalleri D, Bonalumi U, Friedman D, Bachi V 1981 Partial and total biliopancreatic bypass in the surgical treatment of obesity. International Journal of Obesity 5: 421–429
Sellin J H, Meredith S C, Kelly S, Schneir H, Rosenberg I H 1984 Prospective evaluation of metabolic bone disease after jejunoileal bypass. Gastroenterology 87: 123–129
Shackelford R T, Marcus W Y 1960 Jejunal diverticula – a cause of gastrointestinal hemorrhage: a report of three cases and review of the literature. Annals of Surgery 151: 930–938
Shaffer E A, Brown R A, Dutton J W 1976 The effects of massive small bowel resection. In: Bouchier I A D (ed) Recent advances in gastroenterology, 3rd edition. Churchill Livingstone, London, p 73
Shearman D J C, Parkin D M, McClelland D B L 1972 The demonstration of function of antibodies in the gastrointestinal tract. Gut 13: 483–499
Sherr H P, Sasaki Y, Newman A, Banwell J G, Wagner H N, Hendrix T R 1971 Detection of bacterial deconjugation of bile salts by a convenient breath-analysis technic. New England Journal of Medicine 285: 656–661
Sherwood W C, Goldstein F, Haurani F I, Wirts C W 1964 Studies of the small-intestinal bacterial flora and of intestinal absorption in pernicious anemia. American Journal of Digestive Diseases 9: 416–425
Shiner M, Waters T E, Allan J D, Gray J D A, Lambert R A 1963 Culture studies of the gastrointestinal tract with a newly devised capsule. Results of tests in vitro and in vivo. Gastroenterology 45: 625
Simon G L, Gorbach S L 1984 Intestinal flora in health and disease. Gastroenterology 86: 174–193
Slavin G 1985 Tumours and tumour-like conditions. In: Booth C C, Neale G (eds) Disorders of the small intestine. Blackwell, Oxford, p 363–375
Sleisenger M H, Almy T P, Barr D P 1953 The sprue syndrome secondary to lymphoma of the small bowel. American Journal of Medicine 15: 666
Smith G M, Chesner I M, Asquith P, Leyland M J 1990 Small intestinal bacterial overgrowth in patients with chronic lymphocytic leukaemia. Clinical Pathology 43: 57–59
Starr G F, Dockerty M B 1955 Leiomyomas and leiomyosarcomas of the small intestine. Cancer 8: 101–111
Stauffer J Q 1977 Hyperoxaluria and calcium oxalate nephrolithiasis after jejunoileal bypass. American Journal of Clinical Nutrition 30: 64–71
Stauffer J Q, Humphreys M H, Weir G J 1973 Acquired hyperoxaluria with regional enteritis after ileal resection. Role of dietary oxalate. Annals of Internal Medicine 79: 383–391
Stellaard F, Sauerbruch T, Luderschmidt C H, Leisner B, Paumgartner G 1987 Intestinal involvement in progressive systemic sclerosis detected by increased unconjugated serum bile acids. Gut 28: 446–450
Stemmermann G N, Goodman M T, Nomura A M Y 1992 Adenocarcinoma of the proximal small intestine. A marker for familial and multicentric cancer? Cancer 70: 2766–2771
Stemper T J, Kent T H, Summers R W 1975 Juvenile polyposis and gastrointestinal carcinoma. A study of a kindred. Annals of Internal Medicine 83: 639–646
Stolberg L, Rolfe R, Gitlin N et al 1982 D-Lactic acidosis due to abnormal gut flora. Diagnosis and treatment of two cases. New England Journal of Medicine 306: 1344–1348
Strodel W E, Talpos G, Eckhauser F, Thompson N 1983 Surgical therapy for small-bowel carcinoid tumors. Archives of Surgery 118: 391–397

Stunkard A J, Stinnett J L, Smoller J W 1986 Psychological and social aspects of the surgical treatment of obesity. American Journal of Psychiatry 143: 417–429

Tabaqchali S, Booth C C 1966 Jejunal bacteriology and bile-salt metabolism in patients with intestinal malabsorption. Lancet 2: 12–15

Tabaqchali S, Booth C C 1970 Bacteria and the small intestine. In: Card W I, Creamer B (eds) Modern trends in gastroenterology, Vol. 4. Butterworths, London, p 143–172

Tabaqchali S, Booth C C 1985 Bacterial overgrowth. In: Booth C C, Neale G (eds) Disorders of the small intestine. Blackwell, Oxford, p 249–269

Tabaqchali S, Hatzioannou J, Booth C C 1968 Bile-salt deconjugation and steatorrhoea in patients with the stagnant-loop syndrome. Lancet 2: 12–16

Termansen N B, Linde N C 1971 Primary tumours of the small intestine. Scandinavian Journal of Gastroenterology 9 (suppl): 119–126

Thaysen E H 1977 Diagnostic value of the $^{14}$C-cholylglycine breath test. Clinics in Gastroenterology 6: 227–245

Thomas C S Jr, Tinsley E A, Brockman S K 1967 Jejunal diverticula as a source of massive upper gastrointestinal bleeding. Archives of Surgery 95: 89–92

Thompson E M, Clayden G, Price A B 1983 Cancer in Crohn's disease – an 'occult' malignancy. Histopathology 7: 365–376

Thurn J R, Pierpont G L, Ludvigsen C W, Eckfeldt J H 1985 D-Lactate encephalopathy. American Journal of Medicine 79: 717–721

Van Houte J, Gibbons R J 1966 Studies of the cultivable flora of normal human feces. Antonie Van Leeuwenhoek Journal of Microbiology and Serology 32: 212–222

Vessal K, Dutz W, Kohout E, Rezvani L 1980 Immunoproliferative small intestinal disease with duodenojejunal lymphoma: radiologic changes. American Journal of Roentgenology 135: 491–497

Von der Ohe M R, Camilleri M, Kvols L K, Thomforde G M 1993 Motor dysfunction of the small bowel and colon in patients with the carcinoid syndrome and diarrhea. New England Journal of Medicine 329: 1073–1078

Walsh J H, Roth B E 1976 Hormone-secreting tumours of the gastrointestinal tract. In: Bouchier I A D (ed) Recent advances in gastroenterology, Vol. 3. Churchill Livingstone, Edinburgh, p 49

Warkel R L, Cooper P H, Helwig E B 1978 Adenocarcinoid, a mucin-producing carcinoid tumor of the appendix. A study of 39 cases. Cancer 42: 2781–2793

Weingrad D N, Decosse J J, Sherlock P, Straus D, Lieberman P H, Filippa D A 1982 Primary gastrointestinal lymphoma: a 30-year review. Cancer 49: 1258–1265

Weser E 1976 The management of patients after small bowel resection. Gastroenterology 71: 146–150

Williams E D, Sandler M 1963 The classification of carcinoid tumours. Lancet 1: 238–239

Williams N S, Evans P, King R F G J 1985 Gastric acid secretion and gastrin production in the short bowel syndrome. Gut 26: 914–919

Williamson R C N 1978 Intestinal adaptation. New England Journal of Medicine 298: 1393–1402, 1444–1450

Williamson R C N 1982 Intestinal adaptation: factors that influence morphology. Scandinavaian Journal of Gastroenterology 17 (suppl 74): 21–29

Wirts C W, Goldstein F 1963 Studies of the mechanism of postgastrectomy steatorrhea. Annals of Internal Medicine 58: 25–36

Woolf G M, Miller C, Kurian R, Jeejeebhoy K N 1983 Diet for patients with a short bowel: high fat or high carbohydrate? Gastroenterology 84: 823–828

Yang H K, Fondacaro P F 1992 Enterolith ileus: a rare complication of duodenal diverticula. American Journal of Gastroenterology 87: 1846–1848

Young E A 1983 Short bowel syndrome: high-fat versus high-carbohydrate diet. Gastroenterology 84: 872–875

SECTION 4

# Generalized alimentary problems

# 17. Gastrointestinal bleeding

*Kelvin R. Palmer   Peter C. Hayes   J. A. H. Forrest*

## DEFINITIONS

Acute gastrointestinal bleeding is defined as the development of sudden blood loss from the gastrointestinal tract leading to melena or hematemesis. *Melena* is the passage of black, tarry stools due to the presence of altered blood and 95% of cases originate from the upper gastrointestinal tact. *Hematemesis* is the vomiting of blood. This may be fresh and red or black ("coffee grounds") due to the action of acid upon hematin. It is almost invariably due to bleeding from sources proximal to the duodenojejunal flexure. *Rectal bleeding* is the passage of bright or dark red blood. It usually originates from the colon, although massive upper gastrointestinal blood loss can cause bright red bleeding rather than melena. *Occult bleeding* is the presence of blood in the stool detected only by biochemical testing.

## UPPER GASTROINTESTINAL BLEEDING

### Incidence and epidemiology

In the years 1960–1980 the annual incidence of acute gastrointestinal bleeding was estimated to be 48–144 episodes per 100 000 population (Herner et al 1965, Schiller et al 1970, Cutler & Mendeloff 1981). These figures are very similar to those reported more recently (Laine & Peterson 1994, Rockall et al 1995). It is estimated that acute gastrointestinal bleeding is responsible for 8% of admissions to hospitals in the United Kingdom.

The epidemiology of acute gastrointestinal bleeding is nevertheless changing. The most striking change has been the increasing age of patients in industrialized countries, where the proportion over 60 years had reached a half by 1975 and two-thirds by 1993 (Logan & Finlayson 1976, Rockall et al 1995). It has also been observed that admissions for bleeding ulcer rise in winter and fall in summer (Bendahan et al 1992) and over a 10-year period in the United States the incidence of bleeding gastric ulcer rose by 100%, probably because of increased consumption of nonsteroidal anti-inflammatory drugs (NSAIDs) (Laine & Peterson 1994).

### Mortality

The mortality of patients admitted to hospital because of gastrointestinal hemorrhage is approximately 10%, although this varies widely between hospitals (Rockall et al 1995). There is no evidence that mortality has fallen over the last few decades (Allan & Dykes 1976, Silverstein et al 1981, Rockall et al 1995). Furthermore, gastrointestinal bleeding occurring in hospital in patients with unrelated diseases continues to have particularly high mortality (Clason et al 1986, Branicki et al 1990, Rockall et al 1995). This disappointing situation has occurred despite reduction in the incidence and virulence of peptic ulcer over the past 30 years (Hollander & Tarnawski 1986) and in spite of undoubted improvements in diagnosis, intensive care and nonoperative and surgical treatments. The explanations are complex, but several factors may be responsible for continuing high hospital mortality.

Firstly, the average age of patients admitted to hospital because of gastrointestinal bleeding continues to rise and advanced age is an important adverse risk factor (Logan & Finlayson 1976, Rockall et al 1995). Mortality rises steadily and appreciably with age (Fig. 17.1) and serious associated disease is much commoner in older patients. Most patients do not die of exsanguination but from medical complications associated with blood lost and from postoperative complications. Secondly, gastrointestinal bleeding is a common accompaniment of many life-threatening diseases such as cancer, renal failure and sepsis. About a third of patients die when gastrointestinal bleeding complicates another illness in hospital (Rockall et al 1995). Thirdly, admission to hospital for bleeding frequently leads to the discovery of serious underlying disease unrelated to the gastrointestinal tract. For these reasons, it is likely that the mortality of patients entering hospital with a diagnosis of gastrointestinal bleeding will

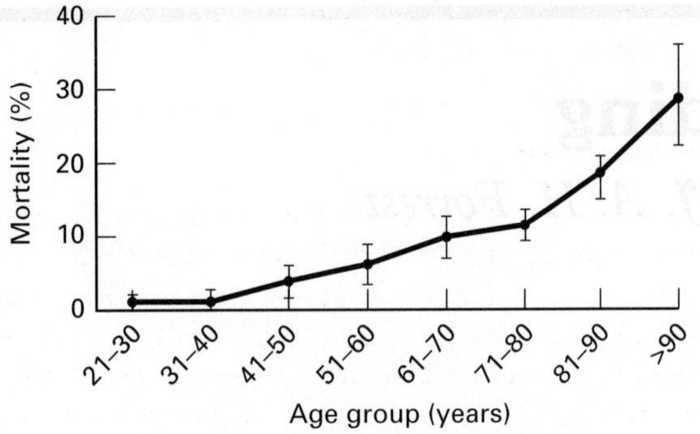


**Fig. 17.1** Mortality following emergency hospital admission for acute upper gastrointestinal hemorrhage related to age and showing 95% confidence intervals (Rockall et al 1995).

remain significant. The challenge is to improve prognosis in patients with remedial gastrointestinal disease.

## MANAGEMENT OF ACUTE GASTROINTESTINAL BLEEDING

The important initial steps are to assess the severity of bleeding and to resuscitate the patient by restoring hemodynamic stability. Thereafter, the source of the bleeding must be located and treated.

### Assessment of severity

*History and examination*

The combination of hematemesis and melena suggests more severe bleeding than either hematemesis or melena alone (Schiller et al 1970). The normal adult blood volume is approximately 4–5 L (70 ml/kg) and healthy adults suffer no symptoms when blood loss is less than 500 ml. Loss of 1–1.5 L leads to syncope, dizziness, palpitations, sweating and postural hypotension. Older patients tend to withstand bleeding less well than younger subjects because their vasomotor control is less effective and they frequently have coexisting vascular disease.

The patient is pale with cool, sweaty extremities. The important features on examination include assessment of pulse, blood pressure and skin perfusion. A resting pulse rate greater than 100 beats/minute and systolic blood pressure less than 100 mmHg indicate blood loss in excess of 1.2 L and are associated with high risk of uncontrolled hemorrhage and rebleeding (Bornman et al 1985). Postural hypotension (a fall in arterial systolic pressure of at least 20 mmHg) occurs with less severe bleeding. Renal hypoperfusion leads to oliguria and cerebral hypoperfusion can cause confusion, particularly in elderly subjects. History and examination should also be directed to the detection of factors influencing management and prognosis, including cardiac and respiratory disease. Assessment for possible liver disease is particularly important, since specific management is indicated for patients who bleed from varices in conditions such as cirrhosis (p. 499).

*Pulse and blood pressure*

Unfortunately, physical examination cannot predict accurately the amount of blood loss and it is therefore very important to assess carefully and monitor all patients with gastrointestinal bleeding. The pulse and blood pressure are recorded immediately and then half-hourly until bleeding is judged to have stopped and the pulse and blood pressure have returned to normal, indicating reasonable restoration of the blood volume. Thereafter, the pulse and blood pressure should be recorded hourly for 12 h, 2-hourly to 24 h and 4-hourly to 72 h.

*Investigations*

A blood sample is taken for measurement of hemoglobin concentration, platelet count, urea, creatinine and electrolytes. A sample is taken for urgent crossmatching and a minimum of 2 units of red blood cell concentrate should be made available. In patients suspected of liver disease, the prothrombin time and serum liver function tests (p. 735) are also measured. The hemoglobin concentration (and hematocrit) may provide useful information regarding blood loss. A hemoglobin less than 10 g/dl on admission is an adverse risk factor (Bornman et al 1985). However, measurement of hemoglobin and hematocrit may not always reflect magnitude of blood loss. Hemodilution is relatively slow and severe acute blood loss can be associated with normal values; only after 24–72 h will they reflect the degree of blood loss. A low hemoglobin concentration at the time of admission may be due to chronic blood loss, which can be confirmed by a blood film that shows evidence of iron deficiency and low plasma ferritin concentration. A blood urea concentration in excess of 8.5 mmol/L with a normal serum creatinine concentration indicates significant blood loss in excess of 1 L (Pumphrey & Beck 1980). This is because of breakdown of blood in the gastrointestinal tract. The serum creatinine reflects renal function.

### Resuscitation

Resuscitation is the essential first step in the management of acute gastrointestinal bleeding.

*Transfusion*

At the time of initial assessment, a wide-bore indwelling intravenous catheter is inserted into a large vein. Patients who are shocked are given oxygen via a face mask and a catheter is passed into the urinary bladder if there is any doubt about the ability of the patient to pass urine spontaneously. An intravenous infusion should be started at the time of entry to hospital. Initially, 1 L of 0.9% sodium chloride is given at a rate dictated by the clinical state. If the patient is shocked (pulse >100 beats/min or systolic blood pressure <100 mmHg), this can be given over a few minutes followed by infusion of a colloid to expand the blood volume. The most suitable volume expanders are gelatin solutions such as Hemaccel or plasma protein solution (PPS) (p. 518). After 2 L of crystalloid or colloid, a red cell concentrate or red cell concentrate supplement is infused. The supplemented form (containing red cells suspended in saline, adenine, glucose, mannitol or an alternative nutrient) has a better flow rate than the concentrate alone. Infusions given at a rate faster than 50 ml/kg/h should be administered through a warmer.

### *Observations during transfusion*

During infusion of colloid and blood, the following clinical measurements are made.

***Pulse and blood pressure.*** These are taken every 15 min initially, reducing in frequency according to the clinical state (p. 515).

***Central venous pressure.*** This is not necessary in all patients but is wise in the elderly, in those with severe bleeding and in those with a history of cardiorespiratory disease because it facilitates appropriate fluid replacement and reduces the risk of cardiac failure by overtransfusion.

***Urine output.*** This gives a useful measure of the adequacy of transfusion therapy and of renal function. A urinary catheter should be passed when patients cannot pass urine spontaneously.

***Nasogastric aspiration.*** This has little value in the management of bleeding patients. Endoscopy is a far superior method of determining that bleeding originates in the upper gastrointestinal tract and the nasogastric tube is uncomfortable and irritating with the potential to cause complications.

***Hemoglobin.*** The frequency of determination of the hemoglobin depends on the severity of bleeding and its continuation or recurrence but even when bleeding seems to have stopped, measurements should be made at least daily for several days to ensure the hemoglobin concentration remains stable. Fit younger patients maintain adequate cardiovascular function down to a hemoglobin of 70 g/L, but concentrations of about 100 g/L are safer in older patients (>60 years), in those with arterial disease or where oxygen requirement is increased, for example by infection (Lundsgaard-Hansen 1992).

***Creatinine.*** The blood creatinine concentration should be measured daily to check the adequacy of renal function. The blood urea concentration rises above 8.5 mmol/L when blood loss into the proximal gut has exceeded 1 L and does not in those circumstances reflect renal function (Pumphrey & Beck 1980).

### *Massive transfusion*

This is defined as the replacement of the patient's total blood volume by stored homologous bank blood in less than 24 h (Hewitt & Machin 1990). In general, it can be avoided in gastrointestinal bleeding by attempts to stop the bleeding at a relatively early stage. These procedures include endoscopic or radiological interventions or a surgical operation. Indeed, it is extremely important to define, in any one patient, the amount of blood transfusion to be allowed before such intervention. This is because the morbidity and mortality of massive transfusion are high, partly due to the complications of transfusion and partly because of the underlying cause of the bleeding (Donaldson et al 1992, Lundsgaard-Hansen 1992).

***Complications.*** The major complications of massive blood transfusion are the adult respiratory distress syndrome (ARDS), defective hemostasis, hypothermia, reduced oxygen-carrying capacity, metabolic disturbances and reduced plasma colloid osmotic pressure.

ARDS (p. 518) is due principally to pulmonary microemboli from white cell and platelet fragments. The incidence is reduced by using blood filters with a pore size of 170 μm. Although micropore filters (20–40 μm) are more effective in preventing microemboli, they greatly reduce blood flow. Treatment is discussed on p. 518. Abnormal coagulation can occur during massive transfusion and it cannot be prevented by prophylactic administration of fresh frozen plasma or platelets. Accordingly, coagulation tests and platelet counts should be measured frequently during massive transfusion and specific replacements are given as appropriate. Microvascular bleeding manifesting as oozing from the mucosae and skin puncture sites is the usual clinical manifestation of coagulopathy and is usually due to thrombocytopenia due to dilution or platelet consumption with or without deficiency of soluble coagulation factors. Disseminated intravascular coagulation may also occur. In general, significant thrombocytopenia develops when about twice the blood volume has been lost and platelets are needed when the count falls below $50 \times 10^9$/L. Fresh frozen plasma should only be given if coagulopathy develops. The plasma fibrinogen, prothrombin time (PT), activated partial thromboplastin time (APTT) and measurement of fibrin degradation products are used to guide therapy. Clinical features of coagulopathy, a PT or APTT prolonged more than one and a half times and a fibrinogen <0.8 g/L indicate the need for fresh frozen plasma and 4 units are usually given initially. Specialist advice is desirable for further therapy or the use of cryoprecipitate.

Hypothermia is avoided by using bloodwarming devices

whenever infusion rates above 50 ml/kg/h are used. Hypothermia increases the oxygen affinity of hemoglobin, reduces citrate metabolism and increases the risks of cardiac arrhythmias due to hyperkalemia and hypocalcemia. Modern anticoagulant red cell preservative solutions ensure adequate concentrations of 2,3-diphosphoglycerate and therefore of oxygen-carrying capacity for up to 14 days after collection of blood. Consequently, defective oxygen-carrying capacity following transfusion is rare unless blood stored for long periods of time is used.

Metabolic disturbances are usually clinically insignificant but are sometimes important when large amounts of blood are transfused. Hypocalcemia is rarely significant and prophylactic infusions are not recommended as complications from giving calcium are likely to be more harmful than hypocalcemia itself. If hypocalcemia does develop, 20 ml of 10% calcium gluconate is infused, with electrocardiogram monitoring. Supernatant plasma potassium concentrations in stored red blood cells may reach 30 mmol/L, but hyperkalemia is usually transient and unimportant. A combination of hypocalcemia and hyperkalemia caused by rapid transfusion of blood stored at 4°C can cause cardiac arrhythmias. Citrate toxicity does not occur unless liver disease is present. Although stored blood has a reduced pH due to accumulation of lactic acid, acidosis in recipients of massive transfusion does not occur because citrate metabolism causes alkalosis.

Reduced plasma colloid oncotic pressure follows replacement of blood loss with large volumes of crystalloids and synthetic colloids. This may contribute to development of adult respiratory distress syndrome and transfusion of albumin may be necessary.

Resuscitation in patients who have bled in association with severe liver disease is a special case and is discussed elsewhere (p. 499).

## Diagnosis of the cause of bleeding

### *History and examination*

These are not usually helpful in identifying the cause of bleeding. It is nevertheless important to inquire about a history of indigestion, known peptic ulcer (including peptic ulcer surgery) and ingestion of NSAIDs. Features of liver disease are important (p. 991), as variceal bleeding requires specific therapy (p. 499). A history of anticoagulant drug consumption is important because these drugs increase the amount of bleeding from gastrointestinal sources.

### *Endoscopy*

Upper gastrointestinal endoscopy is undertaken after the patient has been resuscitated. The procedure is performed on the next available elective endoscopy list, usually on the day after admission. Patients who continue to bleed, who rebleed or who are suspected of having varices should be endoscoped as soon as is feasible. Studies in the 1970s suggested that early endoscopy had no effect upon hospital mortality in bleeding patients (Logan & Finlayson 1976, Dronfield et al 1977). This was not surprising, since these studies merely observed the natural history of the bleeding episodes and specific therapy was not undertaken in response to the endoscopic findings. Logical treatment requires accurate diagnosis and the prognosis of certain diseases is undoubtedly improved by specific therapies such as sclerotherapy of ulcers and sclerotherapy or banding of varices. In addition, endoscopy provides prognostic information. For example, active peptic ulcer hemorrhage in a shocked patient is associated with uncontrolled bleeding or rebleeding in 80% of cases and 50% of patients found to have a nonbleeding visible vessel in the ulcer base rebleed in hospital. In contrast, patients who present with peptic ulcer bleeding without these endoscopic stigmata rarely rebleed and have an excellent prognosis (Foster et al 1978, Bornman et al 1985, Wara 1985).

Several studies have shown that endoscopy should be done as soon as is practicable after bleeding has occurred. If carried out within 12–24 h of admission, endoscopy will find the site of bleeding in 80–90% of cases (Zambartas et al 1982), whereas if there is a delay of 36–48 h the bleeding source is detected in only about 30% of cases (Forrest et al 1974).

### *Angiography*

This should be considered when endoscopy fails to reveal a cause in a patient with continuing or recurrent bleeding (p. 27). Prior barium examinations preclude satisfactory definition for several days. Relative contraindications to angiography include severe coagulation disorders and advanced atherosclerosis which may cause arterial embolization. Angiography is likely to be positive only if the patient is bleeding at a rate of 1–2 ml/min (Balint et al 1977). A diagnosis is achieved in 33–100% (Baum et al 1965, Frey et al 1967, Koehler & Salmon 1967, Allison et al 1982). Angiography may show a likely source of bleeding even if acute bleeding is not found and diagnoses include aneurysms, angiomas, arteriovenous malformations and angiodysplasia (Tarin et al 1978, Allison et al 1982). Thompson et al (1987) reviewed 131 patients with obscure gastrointestinal bleeding. The responsible lesions were angiodysplasia (52), smooth muscle tumors in the small intestine (7) and gastric vascular anomalies (4). In 69 (53%) patients the lesion was first demonstrated by angiography, in 23 (18%) the diagnosis was made at laparotomy and in 11 (8%) at endoscopy.

### *Radionuclide techniques*

$^{99m}$Tc-labeled red blood cells circulate continuously, permitting monitoring for as long as 24 h so that foci that bleed slowly or intermittently can be identified (p. 87). This technique may occasionally be useful but is used infrequently.

*Laparotomy*

In some patients bleeding is so profuse that diagnosis and treatment require a laparotomy associated with on-table endoscopy

## Treatment

The treatment of acute upper gastrointestinal bleeding is directed largely at the specific cause. Medical treatment is often instigated for patients who present with bleeding, but trials of medical treatments aimed at reducing mortality and morbidity from upper gastrointestinal bleeding have largely been unrewarding. Large trials have shown no clear effect in reducing mortality from all causes with various ulcer-healing drugs. These drugs include $H_2$ receptor antagonists (Collins & Langman 1985) and proton pump inhibitors (Daneshmend et al 1992), although these agents tend to improve blood clot stability by increasing intragastric pH (Patchett et al 1989) and may reduce rates of rebleeding and operation (Collins & Langman 1985). The fibrinolytic inhibitor tranexamic acid (Henry & O'Connell 1989) and somatostatin, which reduces splanchnic blood flow (Christiansen et al 1989), also confer no clear benefit.

*Units to manage hematemesis and melena*

There is increasing evidence that the best outcome is achieved by units specially devoted to patients admitted to hospital because of gastrointestinal bleeding (Bramley et al 1993). These units are run jointly by physicians and surgeons and have full facilities for resuscitation and endoscopy. One of the earliest units, in Melbourne, Australia, reported an overall reduction in hospital mortality from 8.5% to 5.8% following development of the unit (Hunt et al 1979). This contrasted with an unchanged mortality of 12% in a similar, adjacent hospital with no bleeding unit (Hunt 1984).

Similar results have been achieved in other special units throughout the world (Sanderson et al 1990, Clements et al 1991, Jeans et al 1991, Masson et al 1996). Reasons for improved prognosis within this setting are multifactorial and include appropriate and early resuscitation, awareness of specific disease entities that demand particular approaches, including liver disease, and appropriate timing of diagnostic and therapeutic endoscopy and surgery.

# SPECIFIC CAUSES OF ACUTE UPPER GASTROINTESTINAL BLEEDING

The common causes of acute upper gastrointestinal bleeding and their approximate frequencies are shown in Table 17.1.

**Table 17.1** Common causes of upper gastrointestinal hemorrhage

| Cause | Approximate frequency (%) |
|---|---|
| Peptic ulcer | 40–55 |
| Gastroduodenal erosions | 20–30 |
| Esophagitis | 10 |
| Esophageal/gastric varices | 2–7 |
| Mallory–Weiss tear | 5 |
| Tumors | 2 |
| Vascular anomalies | 4 |

# PEPTIC ULCER

Peptic ulcer is the commonest cause of acute upper gastrointestinal bleeding, accounting for approximately 50% of cases (Silverstein et al 1981, Gilbert 1990, Rockall et al 1995). Bleeding ulcer is responsible for approximately 150 000 admissions to hospital annually in the United States (Laine & Peterson 1994). Although hospitalization and elective surgery for uncomplicated ulcers have fallen dramatically in the US and Europe over the past 30 years, the number of admissions for ulcer bleeding (and perforation) has been unchanged over this period (Mäkelä et al 1992).

## Etiology

Significant ulcer bleeding is due to erosion of an artery. In most cases the diameter of the artery is small (0.1–1.8 mm) (Swain et al 1986a). The severity of bleeding and the hospital mortality increase when larger arteries are eroded; for arteries 1.5–3.4 mm in diameter, mortality approaches 25% (Swain et al 1993). Bleeding from ulcers in the posterior wall of the duodenal cap may be particularly severe because of erosion of the posterior duodenal artery (Swain et al 1986a).

*NSAIDs and aspirin* (see also pp. 222, 226 & 232)

The use of NSAIDs and aspirin is an important risk factor for bleeding ulcers. Case control and cohort studies show that the risk of peptic ulcer bleeding and perforation is higher for patients who consume NSAIDs compared with those who do not (Somerville et al 1986, Griffin et al 1991, Laporte et al 1991) and this is confirmed by meta-analysis (Gabriel et al 1991). All NSAIDs and aspirin are associated with an increased risk of peptic ulcer bleeding (Table 17.2). It is likely that NSAIDs precipitate dose-related bleeding from both gastric and duodenal ulcers. In a study of aspirin prophylaxis for transient ischemic attacks, patients receiving 300 mg of aspirin daily had a significant increase in bleeding risk compared to placebo (relative risk 7.7), while for patients receiving 1200 mg

**Table 17.2** Liability of nonsteroidal anti-inflammatory drugs to cause acute gastrointestinal bleeding shown in decreasing order of risk (Langman et al 1994)

| |
|---|
| Azapropazone |
| Ketoprofen |
| Piroxicam |
| Indomethacin |
| Naproxen |
| Diclofenac |
| Ibuprofen |

daily the relative risk of bleeding was twice that for patients receiving 300 mg a day (Shorrock et al 1992).

***Mechanism of damage.*** The means whereby aspirin and NSAIDs produce anti-inflammatory effects and unwanted side-effects is poorly understood (Hayllar & Bjarnason 1995). An important advance in understanding was the recognition that these drugs inhibit cyclo-oxygenase (Cox), an enzyme that exists in two distinct forms (Cox-1 and Cox-2). Cox-1 is found in most tissues and is important in cell homeostasis, including the production of prostaglandins from arachidonic acid, which maintains microvascular integrity, regulates cell division and promotes mucus production in the gastrointestinal tract. Cox-2 is not found normally in most tissues but is present in inflammatory cells and is inducible at sites of inflammation where the prostaglandins produced may be important in pain mediation. Cox-1 inhibition may therefore contribute to producing side-effects, while Cox-2 inhibition causes therapeutically useful effects. Study of Cox-1 and Cox-2 inhibiting capacity of different NSAIDs related to gastrointestinal toxicity gives some support to this view but does not explain fully differences between NSAIDs. NSAIDs also uncouple oxidative phosphorylation in mitochondria, leading to a deficiency of ATP in the cells. This and Cox-1 inhibition may be important in increasing intestinal permeability, allowing back-diffusion of acid and other toxic agents leading to local inflammation and ulceration. Future development of specific Cox-2 inhibitors may give the benefits of NSAIDs without their undesirable effects.

***Prophylactic treatment.*** Unfortunately, measures to prevent gastrointestinal damage have been only partly successful. These include "pro-drugs" which are absorbed from the gastrointestinal tract and are then metabolized to the active agent. The use of NSAID suppositories is associated with gastrointestinal side-effects including peptic ulcer bleeding. Combination of an NSAID with a synthetic prostaglandin analog does not reliably protect the gastrointestinal tract. The most promising approach may be the development of drugs affecting the activity of enzymes mediating the undesirable effects of NSAIDs (above).

#### *Corticosteroids*

When prescribed alone, these do not increase the risk of ulcer formation or of ulcer bleeding, but the combination of corticosteroids and NSAIDs is associated with a tenfold increased risk of bleeding (Piper et al 1991).

#### *Helicobacter pylori*

Although most peptic ulcers are associated with *Helicobacter pylori*, the prevalence of this organism is 15–20% lower than in patients with nonbleeding ulcers (Hosking et al 1992, Jensen et al 1992).

#### *Anticoagulant drugs*

Bleeding tends to be worse in anticoagulated patients, but anticoagulant drugs do not themselves cause bleeding.

### Clinical features

Many patients have symptoms suggesting peptic ulcer, but bleeding often occurs in previously asymptomatic patients (Forrest & Finlayson 1974). This is particularly the case in elderly patients taking NSAIDs. Twenty percent of patients present with melena, 30% with hematemesis and 50% with both (Wara & Stødkilde 1985). Those with bleeding in excess of 1 L (approximately 5%) present with bright red rectal bleeding (Schiff et al 1942). In 80% of cases, bleeding stops spontaneously, while mortality occurs almost exclusively in the remaining 20% who continue to bleed or rebleed in hospital (Bornman et al 1985, Clason et al 1986).

### Prognostic factors

The mortality of patients admitted with acute peptic ulcer bleeding is 6–7% in most centers and has not improved significantly over several decades (Avery-Jones 1956, Silverstein et al 1981, Dronfield et al 1982, Rockall et al 1995). However, in centers with a special interest better results have been reported with mortalities of 1–3% (Jeans et al 1991, Rajgopal & Palmer 1991, Bramley et al 1993, Masson et al 1996). These figures may not reflect the full mortality, however, as some studies do not include bleeding occurring in hospital and others are relatively small. Rockall et al (1995) reviewed virtually all patients in 74 English hospitals over a 4-month period (4185 patients), where 84% had been admitted with bleeding, 14% bled while in hospital and 2% had been transferred from other hospitals, and found an overall mortality of 14% (emergency admissions 11%, hemorrhage in inpatients 33%).

The major factors influencing outcome are the magnitude of the initial bleeding episode, whether bleeding persists or recurs, age and comorbid conditions (Table 17.3). Clinical markers indicating severe bleeding include shock (pulse rate >100 beats/min, systolic blood pressure <100 mmHg), repeated hematemesis of red blood and/or

**Table 17.3** Risk factors for death following peptic ulcer bleeding

| |
|---|
| Shock (pulse >100/min; systolic BP <100 mmHg) |
| Anemia (hemoglobin <10 g/dl) |
| Comorbid disease |
| Advanced age |
| Endoscopic stigmata (active bleeding or nonbleeding visible vessel) |

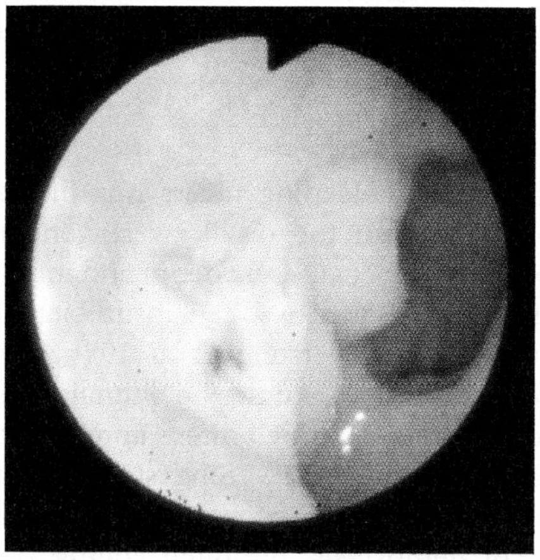

**Fig. 17.2** Benign gastric ulcer showing flat red and black spots related to previous acute gastrointestinal bleeding.

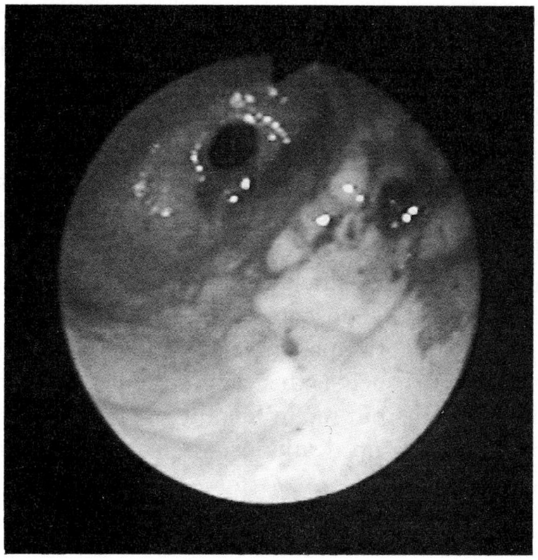

**Fig. 17.3** Malignant gastric ulcer showing a prominent visible vessel related to previous acute gastrointestinal bleeding.

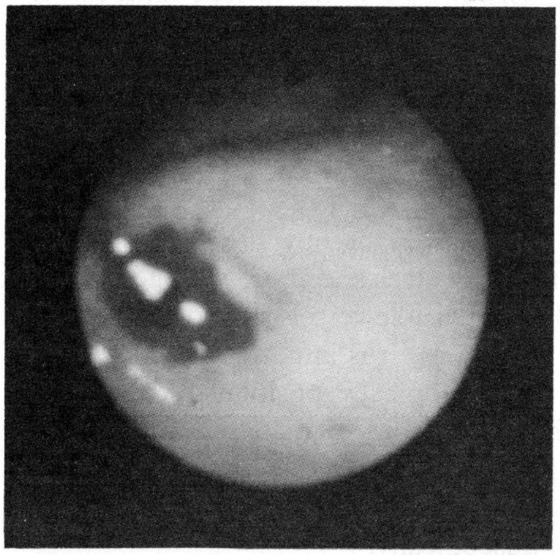

**Fig. 17.4** Duodenal ulcer showing steady oozing of blood after washing related to previous acute gastrointestinal bleeding.

rectal bleeding (Schiller et al 1970, Wara & Stødkilde 1985, Branicki et al 1990). Rebleeding in hospital is associated with tenfold increase in mortality (Bornman et al 1985). Advanced age (Fig. 17.1) and the presence of serious underlying medical illness are important predictive factors. Death in the elderly is mainly due to postoperative complications following emergency surgery (Logan & Finlayson 1976), whereas the outcome in elderly patients treated endoscopically is similar to that of younger patients (Choudari & Palmer 1995). Rockall et al (1995) showed the importance of associated disease in patients admitted with acute gastrointestinal bleeding. The overall mortality in the absence of comorbidity was 5% by comparison with 16% where another disease was present. Malignancy, respiratory disease, and cardiac, renal, or hepatic failure carried the worst prognoses.

Although clinical characteristics are valuable, the endoscopic appearances of the ulcer provide the most helpful prognostic information in respect of rebleeding. The ulcer may have a clean base or have one of several stigmata of hemorrhage: a flat red or black spot (Fig. 17.2), adherent clot, a visible nonbleeding vessel (Fig. 17.3) or active bleeding (spurting or oozing) (Fig. 17.4). A clear ulcer base and spots are rarely associated with further bleeding and carry insignificant mortality. Adherent clots are associated with rebleeding in approximately 20% of patients, with a 10% surgical operation rate and mortality of 7%. Nonbleeding visible vessels, in reality a pseudoaneurysm of the artery or a thrombin plug (Swain et al 1986a), carry a 40% risk of further bleeding, 34% chance of requiring emergency surgery and 11% mortality. At least 55% of patients who present with active bleeding at endoscopy continue to bleed or rebleed in hospital, 35% require an urgent surgical operation and 11% die during that admission (Laine & Peterson 1994). Patients who present with shock and spurting hemorrhage have the worst prognosis; up to 80% of these continue to bleed in hospital and require urgent intervention (Bornman et al 1985).

Larger ulcers have a poorer prognosis than small ones (Branicki et al 1990); "giant" duodenal ulcers often have multiple protuberant visible vessels and fare particularly badly (Branicki et al 1990). It has also been suggested that clear or translucent visible vessels do worse than opaque vessels, but endoscopic impressions are not always reliable or reproducible.

Some enthusiasts advocate the use of Doppler probes, which are passed endoscopically and positioned at the ulcer base, but these are not widely available. Rebleeding is said to be rare in the absence of a Doppler signal (Beckley & Casebow 1986).

Prognostic factors such as those discussed above (Table 17.3) have been used to construct risk-scoring systems. Rockall et al (1996) devised a numerical risk-scoring system based on age, shock, associated disease, the cause of the bleeding and endoscopic stigmata of recent bleeding which could categorize patients into groups related to risk of death. Systems such as this cannot predict outcome for individual patients but might identify patients suitable for early discharge, as no deaths occurred in the lowest risk groups.

## Treatment

The first important steps are resuscitation followed by endoscopy. Drug therapy of peptic ulcer does not improve the prognosis of a bleeding episode although it is clearly sensible to start ulcer therapy at an early stage (p. 485).

### Endoscopic therapy (see also p. 113)

*Selection of patients*

Patients who at endoscopy are found to be bleeding actively from an ulcer and those with adherent blood clot or nonbleeding visible vessels should be treated endoscopically (Table 17.4). It is important to clean the ulcer base using an endoscopically positioned washing catheter to define the endoscopic stigmata and to facilitate accurate localization of endoscopic therapy. This may itself precipitate active bleeding, although bleeding can usually be controlled endoscopically.

It is important to recognize the limitations of endoscopy. Massive bleeding from a major artery does not respond to endoscopic treatment and patients presenting in this way require early emergency surgery; their operation should not be delayed by endoscopic therapy that has little chance of success. Endoscopic treatments have their main application in managing moderately severe bleeding and this treatment can avoid the need for a surgical operation and may reduce transfusion requirements. However, as endoscopic therapy has limited value in the more profusely bleeding patient, its impact upon reducing hospital mortality is modest. Minor bleeding usually settles with supportive therapy.

**Table 17.4** Endoscopic therapy for nonvariceal upper gastrointestinal bleeding

| |
|---|
| *Thermal methods* |
| Argon laser |
| Nd:YAG laser |
| Monopolar electrocoagulation |
| Multipolar electrocoagulation |
| Heater probe |
| *Injection therapy* |
| Adrenaline |
| Sclerosants |
| Alcohol |
| Thrombin |
| *Other therapy* |
| Clips |
| Sprays |

*Lasers*

Photocoagulation of bleeding ulcers was first attempted using argon lasers, but the results were generally disappointing, principally because the depth and intensity of tissue damage they produce is often insufficient to induce arterial thrombosis (Silverstein et al 1976, Swain et al 1981, Vallon et al 1981). Studies on animals subsequently showed Nd:YAG lasers to be a more appropriate thermal agent (Dixon et al 1979, Silverstein et al 1979). Obliterative coagulation is probably the most important mechanism of hemostasis, although edema surrounding the vessel may be an additional factor (Dixon et al 1979, Rutgeerts et al 1981).

Most controlled trials performed in the 1980s showed significant benefit from treatment with Nd:YAG lasers (Rutgeerts et al 1982, Swain et al 1986b, Matthewson et al 1990). Rebleeding, transfusion requirements, operation rates and mortality were reduced. Laser therapy for bleeding has proved safe, with low perforation rates, and although bleeding can be precipitated by the treatment itself, this either stops spontaneously or can be arrested by further photocoagulation. However, laser treatment is technically difficult and about 10% of bleeding ulcers cannot be treated. This occurs when ulcers are in awkward sites, as in a deformed duodenal cap, or when continuing bleeding prevents circumferential treatment of the bleeding site. Criticisms of laser therapy include its high capital and running costs, inability to tamponade the bleeding point and lack of portability.

*Electrocoagulation*

Electrocoagulation devices cause arterial thrombosis by passing an electric current through the bleeding area. Monopolar units apply current using a ball-tipped probe, and the circuit is completed through a plate attached to the patient. This technique has the drawbacks of tissue adherence, unpredictable tissue damage and the frequent need to clear the tip of the instrument. An electrical conducting fluid can be used to transmit the current to the mucosa (liquid monopolar coagulation) and this largely overcomes the problem of tissue adherence. Three controlled trials have shown that bleeding can be arrested and rebleeding rates reduced by monopolar electrocoagulation

(Papp 1982, Freitas et al 1985, Moretó et al 1987), but because it is unpredictable, the device has been superseded by other contact methods.

Bipolar coagulation works by completing an electrical circuit between probes applied to the mucosa. The multipolar electrocoagulation pulse, known as BICAP, has three pairs of electrodes on its side and tip and electrocoagulation can be performed if any pair of electrodes are in tissue contact, thus allowing tangential treatment. The amount of energy applied to the area and the degree of tissue damage is much more predictable than with monopolar units. Early clinical trials with the BICAP were disappointing, but two subsequent prospective controlled studies showed the device to be effective in bleeding ulcer. One small clinical study showed a significant hemostatic effect in actively bleeding patients (Laine 1987) and the other showed reduction of rebleeding in patients with nonbleeding visible vessels (Laine 1989). Both studies showed reduced need for emergency surgery and reduction in blood transfusion and duration of hospital admission.

Perforation is unusual with BICAP. Bleeding is precipitated by treatment in up to a third of cases but usually stops with repeated applications. A particular advantage of contact probes is the ability to stop bleeding by tamponade and the best results with BICAP are associated with forceful application of the larger (3.2 mm) probe using a low-frequency (coagulation) current at the midrange power settings. The commercially available systems are portable, have irrigation systems that are helpful in managing active bleeding and have a low failure of access to the ulcer.

*Heater probe*

The heater probe transmits predetermined amounts of energy to the mucosa through a Teflon-coated tip. The probe may be applied tangentially and almost all lesions are accessible. Several early uncontrolled studies showed the heater probe to be safe and effective and subsequent randomized controlled trials in high-risk patients confirmed that treatment reduced rebleeding rates and the need for emergency surgery (Lin et al 1990, Chung et al 1991, Choudari et al 1992). Repeated application after 24–48 h is thought to be safe and effective.

Optimum therapy is best administered using the 3.2 mm probe. A twin-channelled therapeutic endoscope is useful to keep the treated area free of debris. Firm tamponade is possible by pressing the probe against the mucosa. At least 120 joules are applied to the bleeding area before the probe position is changed. The heater probe is attractive because it is relatively cheap and portable. The ability to apply tamponade at a bleeding area, the capacity to apply the probe tangentially in the emergency situation and a powerful water jet that cleans and irrigates the area are particular advantages.

*Injection therapy*

Endoscopic injection into bleeding ulcers has received considerable attention. Early uncontrolled studies showed that dilute adrenaline stopped active bleeding and other workers subsequently examined the effects of combinations of injection therapies comprising dilute adrenaline and a range of sclerosants (polidocanol, STD, ethanolamine) (Chung et al 1988, Rajgopal & Palmer 1991, Lin et al 1993, Choudari & Palmer 1994). The rationale is that adrenaline causes vasoconstriction and stops active bleeding and sclerosants lead to a vigorous inflammatory response around the ulcer, causing endarteritis and arterial thrombosis that prevents rebleeding. Whether this actually occurs in practice is unknown. In experimental mucosal ulcers in animals, neither adrenaline nor sclerosants cause arterial damage but only adrenaline reduces rebleeding and consequently the combination approach may have little basis in fact (Rajgopal et al 1992). In reality, it is difficult to study the effects of injected materials around a bleeding ulcer in humans because histology is rarely available and the inflammatory response associated with the ulcer itself makes interpretation of the effects of injection impossible.

Several groups have shown that the prognosis of bleeding peptic ulcer is improved by injection treatment. The most convincing data relate to rebleeding rates, but meta-analysis has revealed a significant reduction of hospital mortality (Cook et al 1992). The best regimen is unclear. Most endoscopists first inject 1–2 ml of 1:10 000 adrenaline at four sites around the periphery of the ulcer. This results in blanching and active bleeding usually stops. Smaller volumes of sclerosants may then be injected around and into the bleeding point. Some endoscopists use adrenaline alone and others use sclerosants without adrenaline. All the regimens appear effective and safe. Complications are unusual, with a low incidence of perforation and no evidence of impaired ulcer healing. Nevertheless, successful therapy demands careful technique and excessive injection of sclerosants can cause catastrophic perforation.

Treatment failures occur because of torrential bleeding or inaccessibility. Torrential bleeding usually arises from a large breach in a major artery and no endoscopic therapy is successful in this situation. Adrenaline injection is probably the most effective initial hemostatic approach in such cases; laser photocoagulation is difficult when the mucosa is obscured by blood and contact thermal methods are difficult because of adherence to coagulum. Approximately 10% of ulcers are inaccessible to injection treatment; these are almost invariably duodenal ulcers within deformed duodenal caps. Retroflection and other manipulations of the endoscope usually allow successful injection of gastric ulcers.

Endoscopic therapy is carried out at the initial diagnostic endoscopy. Many endoscopists now reinject 24–48 h after the first treatment. This is particularly useful for patients with active bleeding, because it is often difficult to be sure that adequate treatment has been given. Repeat endoscopy up to 48 h after injection usually shows that protuberant vessels are little changed by the first treatment.

## Surgery

*Indications*

Surgery is indicated when endoscopic therapy has been unsuccessful. This occurs when therapeutic endoscopy is impossible because of severe bleeding or when patients rebleed after endoscopic treatment. Continuing uncontrolled bleeding is the major reason for surgical intervention. Surgery is indicated when hemodynamic instability recurs and when blood transfusion exceeds about 4–6 units of blood, particularly in patients over 60 years of age. It is very important to resuscitate the patient prior to surgery and assessment by anesthetic and intensive care colleagues is appropriate.

In general, a single rebleed in a high-risk patient (over 60 years of age or with significant comorbid disease) is an indication for surgery. An aggressive, early surgical approach in elderly patients is associated with a better outcome than that which follows more conservative therapy (Morris et al 1984). In patients aged less than 60 years who do not have coexisting cardiorespiratory disease, it may be safe to permit two rebleeds before embarking upon a surgical operation. Repeated endoscopic therapy may be attempted in this group.

The operation performed is dependent upon the site and size of the ulcer. When possible, the most conservative approach is taken with the aim of arresting active bleeding and preventing rebleeding. Modern drug therapy almost invariably heals ulcers and surgery to cure the ulcer is not needed. Undersewing the bleeding point is often sufficient. Large ulcers sometimes require more radical operations such as partial gastrectomy for gastric ulcers or giant duodenal ulcers, but these operations are associated with high risk of postoperative complications and death.

# OTHER NONVARICEAL CAUSES OF ACUTE BLEEDING

## Gastric erosions (p. 225)

Gastroduodenal erosions are a common cause of bleeding (Sugawa et al 1973, Forrest & Finlayson 1974), accounting for 36–41% of cases (Table 17.1). Erosions are frequently associated with NSAID consumption. They are superficial and rarely cause major blood loss. When extensive, the appearance is called *acute hemorrhagic gastritis* (Fig. 17.5). Occasionally massive bleeding occurs, usually

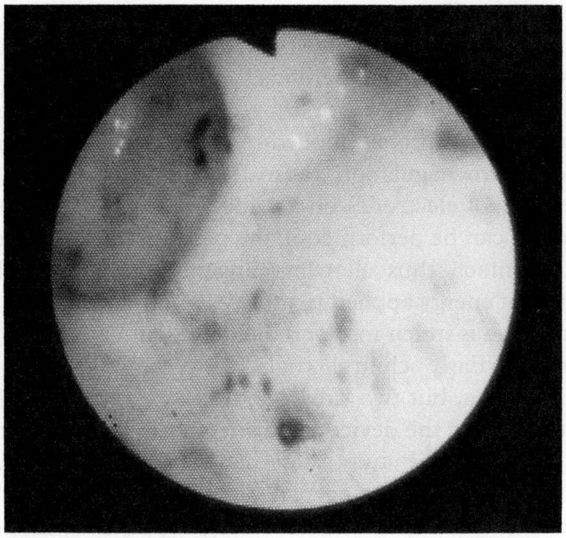

**Fig. 17.5** Multiple hemorrhagic gastric erosions related to previous acute gastrointestinal bleeding.

in patients who are ill because of other diseases and particularly where renal failure or respiratory failure is present. In this situation, an emergency gastrectomy may be necessary, but mortality is high.

## Stress ulcers

Stress ulcers are defined on p. 226. They develop in patients suffering from severe systemic illness. Although these gastroduodenal lesions were once thought common in intensive care patients, recent evidence suggests that clinically important bleeding from stress ulcers is relatively uncommon. Approximately 1–2% of such patients develop bleeding from stress ulcers, respiratory failure and coagulopathy being the most important risk factors (Cook et al 1994). Perforation of stress ulcers is even less common. The cause of stress ulcers is multifactorial (p. 226). Although prophylaxis is often given (p. 226), there is debate as to whether this improves mortality. It is important to reduce the risk of stress ulcers by the assiduous correction of hypoxia and acid base balance in critically ill patients (Peterson 1994).

## Mallory–Weiss syndrome

The Mallory–Weiss tear, described in 1929 (Mallory & Weiss 1929), is defined as a mucosal laceration of the cardia or gastroesophageal junction induced by retching or vomiting. In the cardia the tears are often circumferential, while in the esophagus they are longitudinal (Fig. 17.6). In most series, Mallory–Weiss tears account for 5% of cases of upper gastrointestinal bleeding (Katz & Salas 1993).

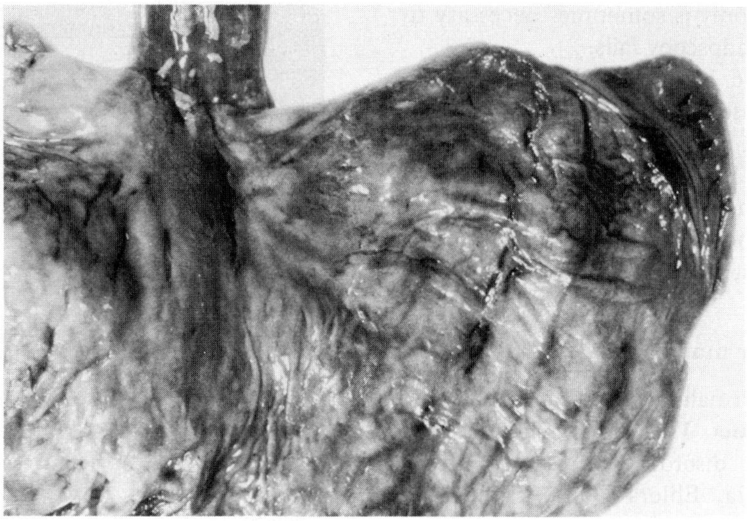

**Fig. 17.6** Mallory–Weiss syndrome. Linear mucosal tears in the gastric cardia and fundus.

*Etiology*

The mucosal tear results from transient large pressure gradients between the intrathoracic and intragastric compartments, leading to sudden dilatation of the gastroesophageal junction. This occurs most frequently during retching and vomiting. Hiatus hernia may be a predisposing factor because of pressure generated by the hernia (Watts 1976).

*Clinical features*

Bleeding usually occurs at the time of retching but occasionally is delayed. Thirty to 80% of patients present with repeated violent retching and vomiting following an alcoholic binge and culminating in hematemesis. In the remainder antecedent retching may be absent. Hematemesis is found in 80%, but 10% of patients present with melena alone (Sugawa et al 1983).

Almost all patients have an underlying predisposing cause. The commonest is alcohol abuse, but other include blunt trauma, straining at stool, coughing, heavy lifting, seizures, cardiopulmonary resuscitation and raised intracranial pressure. Some have coexisting gastrointestinal disease such as peptic ulcer or gastric outflow obstruction.

*Diagnosis and treatment*

The diagnosis is made at endoscopy. Most tears are found in the region of the gastroesophageal junction, but they are occasionally seen within the body of the stomach. Although more than 95% of cases stop bleeding spontaneously and transfusion requirements are usually modest, a few patients require intervention. Active bleeding found at endoscopy should be treated by injection with dilute adrenaline (pp. 113 & 489) or a thermal probe (pp. 113 & 489). Compression of the bleeding point can be attempted using the Minnesota tube, although this is potentially dangerous in the presence of a hiatus hernia (Welch et al 1987). Other approaches, including the use of intra-arterial infusion of vasoconstricting agents and embolization, cannot be recommended and if endoscopic therapy is unsuccessful, surgical oversewing of the bleeding point is necessary.

## Dieulafoy abnormality

This has been considered a rare cause of upper gastrointestinal bleeding, accounting for 0.3–6.7% of patients admitted to hospital because of bleeding (Broberg et al 1982, Strong 1984, Lin et al 1989). This may be an underestimate, because diagnosis is often difficult or impossible unless the patient is endoscoped at the time of bleeding.

The Dieulafoy abnormality is a large, tortuous submucosal artery that ruptures through the mucosa, resulting in profuse hemorrhage. The involved artery is 1–3 mm in diameter and is histologically normal, without evidence of vasculitis or atheromatous change. The majority of lesions are found in the body of the stomach. Approximately 75–95% are within 6 cm of the gastroesophageal junction on the lesser curvature of the stomach, but they have been reported at other sites including the duodenum and colon. The average age of presentation is 55 years (range 20 months to 93 years) and males outnumber females by 2:1 (Reilly & Al-Kawas 1991). There is sudden, profuse upper gastrointestinal bleeding without warning and without dyspeptic symptoms or a history of NSAID ingestion.

Diagnosis is made at endoscopy but is often missed unless active bleeding is present at examination. At other times a small, raised, purple lesion may be identified; ulceration is not a feature. Angiography (Durham et al

1990) or a surgical gastrotomy is sometimes necessary to make the diagnosis when endoscopy fails.

The treatment of choice is endoscopic therapy with electrocautery, Nd:YAG laser, the heater probe or injection therapy (Hoffmann et al 1984, Boron & Mobarhan 1987, Pointer et al 1988, Lin et al 1989, Reilley & Al-Kawas 1991). The best treatment is unclear, as controlled trials have not been performed. Surgical resection is necessary if endoscopic treatment proves impossible.

## Gastroduodenal vascular malformations

A range of vascular abnormalities may cause bleeding from the gastrointestinal tract. These lesions may be part of a generalized inherited disorder such as hereditary hemorrhagic telangiectasia, Ehlers–Danlos syndrome or pseudoxanthoma elasticum. More commonly, vascular malformations occur sporadically, usually in older patients.

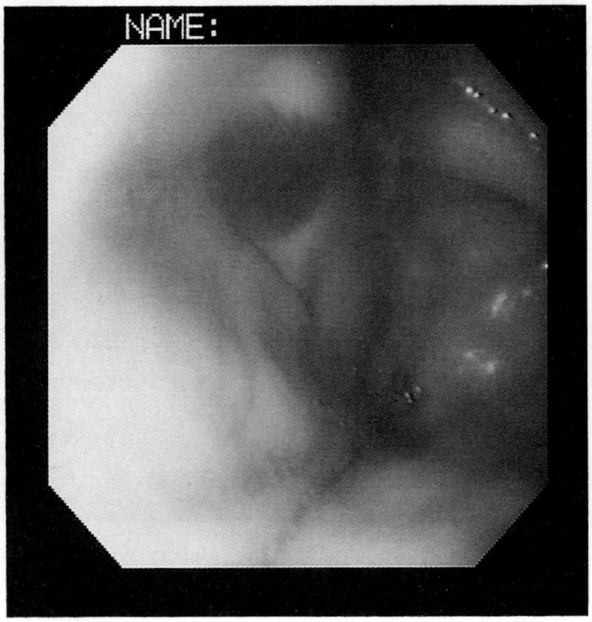


**Fig. 17.7** Arteriovenous malformation in the proximal stomach causing acute gastrointestinal bleeding in a patient with ischemic heart disease on warfarin therapy.

## Arteriovenous malformations

These are commonly found in elderly subjects and rarely cause massive bleeding. More often they cause anemia due to chronic blood loss. They are associated with other medical conditions including chronic renal failure, systemic sclerosis (Rosekrans et al 1980) and cor pulmonale (Rogers 1980). Arteriovenous malformations account for approximately 1–5% of bleeding episodes (Clouse et al 1985), but this rises to 24% in patients with chronic renal failure (Zuckerman et al 1985).

At endoscopy, lesions appear as flat or raised bright red spots that can occur anywhere in the gastrointestinal tract (Fig. 17.7); enteroscopy reveals many otherwise undiagnosed lesions in the small intestine (Gostout et al 1988). Large simple lesions are amenable to therapy by Nd:YAG laser photocoagulation (Cello et al 1986), but many patients present with multiple lesions and endoscopic therapy is impractical. In these patients, oral ethinyl estrodiol 0.05 mg daily may reduce transfusion requirements (Van Cutsem et al 1990).

### *Angiodysplasia*

Angiodysplasia is considered in relation to colonic bleeding (p. 495).

### *Hereditary hemorrhagic telangiectasia*

Inherited as an autosomal dominant condition, this disease is due to an inborn error of vascular structure. Patients present at any age, although many are diagnosed in childhood. Characteristic small red or purple spots are found around the lips, palmar surfaces of the hands, nail beds, ears and mucous membranes of the mouth. A history of recurrent epistaxis is characteristic. Twenty percent of patients present with gastrointestinal bleeding from malformations that can occur anywhere in the gastrointestinal tract. Other patients present with complications due to vascular malformation in the lungs or central nervous system and these should be borne in mind when dealing with patients who have gastrointestinal bleeding in association with the disease. Rarely, hepatic malformations can cause portal hypertension and variceal bleeding (p. 1086). Diagnosis and management of the gastrointestinal lesions is identical to that of spontaneous arteriovenous malformations.

### *Pseudoxanthoma elasticum*

Gastrointestinal hemorrhage may be the presenting feature in this disorder, which is inherited as an autosomal recessive condition. Degeneration of connective tissue is responsible for the characteristic coarse, leathery skin with yellowish modules around the neck and in the anticubital fossae and angoid streaks in the optic fundus. The collagen defect is probably also responsible for the gastrointestinal manifestations of the disease. These include bleeding from mucosal or submucosal lesions and intestinal ischemia and infarction (Cocco et al 1969).

### *Ehlers–Danlos syndrome*

This rare condition is caused by a generalized defect of the vascular wall associated with a coagulation defect. It presents with lax skin and joints and with scarring over bony prominences. Approximately 5% present with gastrointestinal complications including gastrointestinal bleeding from lesions such as ulcers, arteriovenous malformations and retroperitoneal hemorrhage. Other gastrointestinal disorders include motility defects, particularly megaesophagus, gastroparesis, rectal prolapse and megacolon. Surgery is avoided whenever possible because wound healing is poor.

*Aortoduodenal fistula*

Aortoduodenal fistulae are responsible for 80% of all enteroaortic fistulae. Most fistulae occur in patients with a synthetic aortic graft, although they can occur rarely with aortic aneurysms due to atherosclerosis (p. 532) or to infections with syphilis, salmonella or tuberculosis. Bleeding is characteristically intermittent. An initial "herald" bleed is brief and stops spontaneously. Massive hemorrhage follows hours to days later and leads to exsanguination. Many patients have a history of back pain prior to bleeding and some have evidence of sepsis in the aortic graft. Emergency endoscopy rarely identifies the bleeding point because profuse hemorrhage prevents adequate visualization. Bleeding originating from the second or third part of the duodenum, particularly in patients with a history of aortic surgery, suggests the diagnosis. The investigation of choice is abdominal computed tomography. This will visualize the aneurysm and may identify extraluminal gas associated with the aorta (Ibrahim et al 1989). Frequently, patients are too ill for investigations and emergency laparotomy is performed by vascular and gastrointestinal surgeons.

*Gastric antral vascular ectasia*

Gastric antral vascular ectasia is also known as the "watermelon stomach". It presents with acute gastrointestinal bleeding or insidious blood loss leading to chronic anemia. It tends to be a disease of elderly women (sex ratio 9:1, median age 70 years). It usually occurs sporadically but has been associated with atrophic gastritis, cirrhosis and systemic sclerosis (Jabbari et al 1984).

At endoscopy, friable, raised red stripes of gastric mucosa emanate from the pylorus into the gastric antrum (Fig. 17.8). Biopsy reveals foveolar hyperplasia, fibromuscular spindle cell hyperplasia of the lamina propria and dilated mucosal capillaries with focal thrombosis and dilated submucosal channels (Gilliam et al 1989).

Treatment is by Nd:YAG laser photocoagulation, which ablates the abnormal submucosal blood vessels. Multiple sessions are sometimes necessary, but success is achieved in the majority of cases (Gostout et al 1989). Failure of this treatment requires surgical antrectomy.

*Hemobilia*

Hemobilia is defined as bleeding through the ampulla of Vater, originating from the liver, biliary tree or pancreas. Forty percent of cases are complications of percutaneous transhepatic radiological or drainage procedures or of liver biopsy (Yoshida et al 1987, Czerniak et al 1988). Other causes include trauma, systemic infection, gallstones, and aneurysms of the hepatic artery (p. 1081) and tumor.

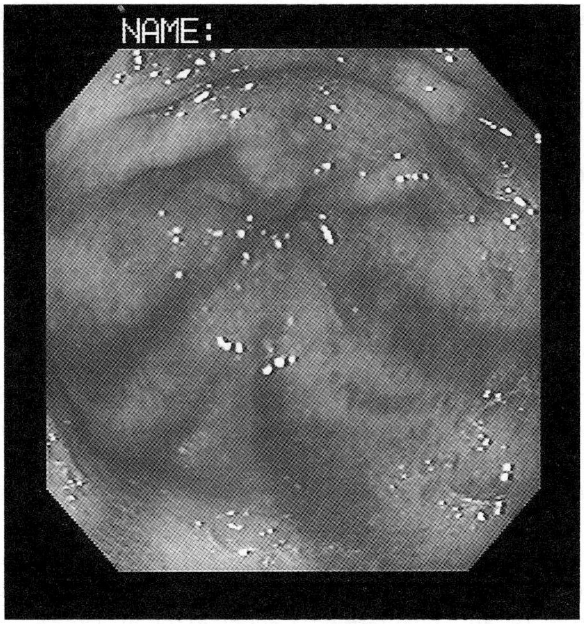


**Fig. 17.8** Linear erythemic areas of friable hemorrhagic antral gastric mucosa ("watermelon stomach") in a patient with recurrent iron deficiency anemia.

The classic presentation is a triad of right upper quadrant abdominal pain, jaundice and gastrointestinal bleeding, although this is present in only 40% of cases. The majority of patients present approximately 4 weeks after injury. Diagnosis is suggested by the appearance of blood (particularly clots) coming from the ampulla. It is confirmed by angiography, which demonstrates arteriovenous fistulation and/or aneurysm formation (Blackstone 1984). The treatment of choice is transcatheter embolization with gelfoam and coils (Uflacker et al 1989). Surgical therapy, principally ligation of the hepatic artery, is necessary in some cases.

## Other causes of bleeding

Tumors can cause acute gastrointestinal hemorrhage, but they account for only 3–4% of cases; most are gastric cancers (Schiller et al 1970, Forrest & Finlayson 1974). Leiomyoma of the stomach or intestine can present with recurrent hemorrhage. Those in the intestine are best diagnosed by radionuclide techniques, angiography or careful palpation of the bowel at operation. Pancreatic rests, gastric lymphoma and other gastric tumors can also present with hematemesis or melena. Carcinomas of the head of the pancreas, duodenum, papilla of Vater or jejunum and polypoid conditions such as the Peutz–Jeghers syndrome rarely cause hematemesis and/or melena. Meckel's diverticulum (p. 486), a range of inflammatory and malignant pancreatic diseases and ulcers of the small bowel are causes of bleeding described elsewhere. Systemic diseases affecting the gut such as polyarteritis nodosa (p. 227), systemic lupus erythematosus (p. 227), Henoch–Schönlein purpura (p. 536) and amyloidosis may also cause bleeding. Bleeding in HIV infection is discussed on p. 604.

### Gastrointestinal bleeding and anticoagulants

Patients who bleed while taking anticoagulant drugs pose a difficult clinical dilemma. They are usually anticoagulated for good reason and to stop treatment risks thromboembolism, while continuation of therapy risks exsanguination. Bleeding usually occurs in anticoagulated patients from underlying coexisting gastrointestinal disease, although the risk of hemorrhage increases with the degree of anticoagulation (Landefeld et al 1989). The commonest cause of upper gastrointestinal bleeding is peptic ulcer, accounting for approximately 50% of cases. The treatment of bleeding in anticoagulated patients is to stop the anticoagulant, normalize the prothrombin time using fresh frozen plasma and then perform endoscopy. It is generally unwise to give vitamin K because its effect is delayed by hours and subsequent reanticoagulation may be impossible for several weeks. If vitamin K is used, the dose should be restricted to 1 mg intravenously to allow reanticoagulation. Upper gastrointestinal endoscopy may reveal the bleeding source and if endoscopic stigmata are found, local hemostatic therapy using injection or a thermal method is performed. The results are similar to those found in bleeding patients not receiving anticoagulants (Choudari & Palmer 1995). If upper gastrointestinal endoscopy is negative and bleeding is severe, immediate colonoscopy or visceral angiography may be necessary. Reanticoagulation may be considered if there is a strong indication once an ulcer has been healed and *H. pylori* eradicated. In this situation, lifelong maintenance ulcer treatment should be recommended.

## BLEEDING FROM THE LOWER GASTROINTESTINAL TRACT

Rectal bleeding is common (Fig. 17.9) and when a patient presents with fresh rectal bleeding, anal examination may show hemorrhoids or a fissure to account for the bleeding. However, in patients who have colonic symptoms and in those aged 45 years or more, more serious diseases including colorectal neoplasia should be suspected.

### Causes

The common important diagnoses are colorectal neoplasia, diverticular disease and angiodysplasia (Table 17.5). Acute, life-threatening rectal bleeding can occur in Crohn's disease and ulcerative colitis because of erosion of a major artery, but much more commonly these diseases cause chronic blood loss and are considered in detail elsewhere (Ch. 23). Rectal bleeding is a common feature of infective colitides (p. 560) but is rarely a diagnostic dilemma or in itself of clinical importance.

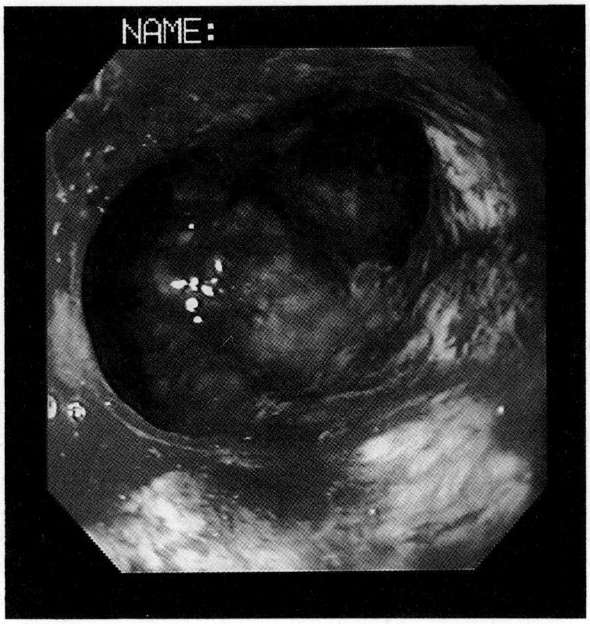


**Fig. 17.9** Fresh blood in the rectum in a patient with acute rectal bleeding due to ulcerative colitis.

**Table 17.5** Causes of acute rectal bleeding in adults

| |
|---|
| Anal disease: |
| hemorrhoids (p. 1451) |
| anal fissure (p. 1456) |
| Diverticular disease (p. 1388) |
| Colorectal neoplasia: |
| cancer (p. 1423) |
| adenomatous polyps (p. 1404) |
| Vascular malformations: |
| angiodysplasia |
| arteriovenous anomalies |
| Inflammatory bowel disease (Ch. 23) |
| Infective: |
| bacterial dysentery (p. 560) |
| amebiasis (p. 573) |
| Ischemic colitis (p. 547) |
| Solitary rectal ulcer (p. 1329) |
| Meckel's diverticulum (p. 496) |
| Radiation enterocolitis (p. 410) |

### Diverticular disease

Diverticular disease is the commonest cause of profuse rectal bleeding and this is described elsewhere (p. 1388). In elderly patients, diverticular disease and angiodysplasia together account for approximately two-thirds of admissions to hospital for acute rectal bleeding (Boley et al 1979). Diverticular disease is very common in Western populations (Parks 1969) and it is wise to be sure that other bleeding sources have been excluded even in the presence of severe diverticular disease. Colonoscopy and barium enema may be technically difficult in severe sigmoid diverticular disease and polyps or carcinoma can be missed.

## Angiodysplasia

Angiodysplasia is a degenerative vascular ectasia of previously normal blood vessels which is distinct from congenital vascular lesions such as hereditary hemorrhagic telangiectasia, hemangiomata and other vascular disorders that affect the gastrointestinal tract (Boley et al 1977a, 1981).

### *Etiology and pathology*

Angiodysplasia is found in more than 25% of asymptomatic patients over the age of 60 years and occurs only rarely in young patients. The lesions occur almost exclusively in the cecum and ascending colon and appear as bright red spots on endoscopy. Histological identification is impossible using standard techniques, but casts of the vessels can be made by injecting polymers into the blood vessels of resected specimens (Boley et al 1977b). When this is done, the lesions are found to be ectatic, distorted, thinwalled venules and veins with minimal amounts of smooth muscle within the wall (Fig. 17.10). The lesions drain into dilated veins in adjacent submucosa. In the most severe cases, a mass of dilated and distorted channels develop.

It is thought that angiodysplasia arises from repeated episodes of colonic distention. This leads to increases in tension of the bowel wall and obstruction to the veins as they pass through the muscle layers. Eventually this results in dilatation of the submucosal veins, disruption of valves within those vessels and the development of arteriovenous fistulae.

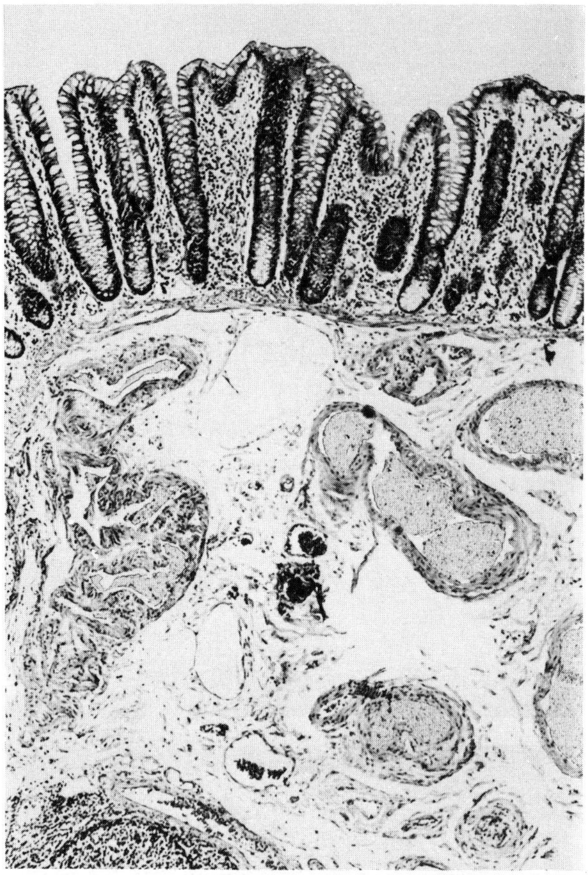

**Fig. 17.10** Angiodysplasia in the ascending colon showing numerous abnormal dilated vessels in the submucosa.

### *Clinical features and investigation*

Patients bleed without warning. Bleeding is often relatively mild but is life-threatening in up to 15% of cases. A similar proportion of patients present with anemia due to chronic low-grade bleeding (Boley et al 1979). There is a close association with aortic valve disease, particularly aortic stenosis, although the explanation for this is unknown (Imperale & Ransohoff 1988). Patients with angiodysplasia and those with aortic valve disease have low circulating levels of von Willebrand's factor. Angiography is the diagnostic test of choice during a bleeding episode and may show active bleeding into the lumen of the cecum or ascending colon. The characteristic findings are a densely opacified, slowly emptying, tortuous vein, a vascular tuft and a vein that fills early (Fig. 17.11). In patients who are not actively bleeding, colonoscopy is indicated. Excellent bowel preparation is required and angiodysplasia must be differentiated from suction artefact, hereditary telangiectasia and radiation injury.

### *Treatment*

The treatment of angiodysplasia includes therapeutic endoscopy, surgical resection and drugs. Argon and Nd:YAG laser photocoagulation, endoscopic injection and electrocoagulation all stop active bleeding and prevent recurrent bleeding, but the lesions themselves are frequently multiple and tend to recur (Rutgeerts et al 1985). Should bleeding continue despite these approaches, a right hemicolectomy is indicated. The use of embolization at the time of angiography cannot be advocated because of the risk of colonic infarction and delayed stricture formation (Sniderman et al 1978). Oral ethinyl estrodiol 0.05 mg daily may be of value.

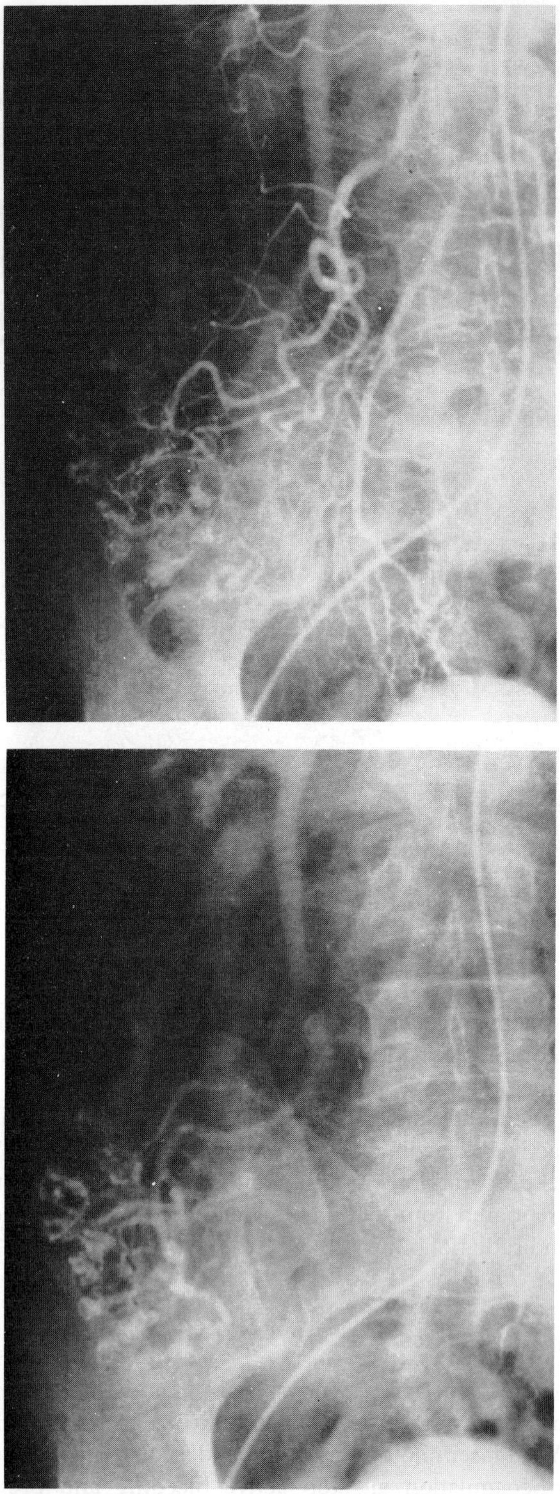

**Fig. 17.11** Arterial (*above*) and venous (*below*) phases of a mesenteric angiogram showing early filling and late pooling of contrast in abnormal vessels (angiodysplasia) in the cecum.

### Other causes of lower gastrointestinal bleeding

Other causes of lower gastrointestinal bleeding are described elsewhere and are listed in Table 17.5.

## BLEEDING FROM THE SMALL INTESTINE

Bleeding from the small intestine is responsible for 3–5% of admissions to hospital for gastrointestinal hemorrhage (Netterville et al 1968). Diagnosis is difficult because radiological techniques are relatively insensitive and enteroscopy is not widely available. The commonest causes of acute small bowel hemorrhage are vascular malformations, leiomyoma, Crohn's disease, Meckel's diverticulum and NSAID-associated enteropathy. Vascular malformations, including angiodysplasia, account for approximately 80% of cases (Lewis 1994). Leiomyomas and leiomyosarcoma are responsible for 5–10% of cases (Ashley & Wells 1988).

### Meckel's diverticulum

This is a remnant of the vitelline duct and is found in 2% of the population (p. 486). It is located about 100 cm from the ileocecal valve. In approximately one-quarter of patients, the tip of the diverticulum is attached by a fibrous cord to the abdominal wall at the umbilicus. Intestinal obstruction can be caused by intussusception or by volvulus around the fibrous cord. The diverticulum can become inflamed and present like acute appendicitis (p. 525) or it can perforate. Neoplasms may arise from heterotopic or normal mucosal elements in the diverticulum. Ileal ulceration occurs when the diverticulum contains acid-secreting gastric epithelium or pancreatic tissue and this may cause brisk arterial bleeding (Ghahremani 1986). Bleeding usually occurs in childhood or adolescence and may be severe. Occasionally, bleeding is the consequence of intussusception of the diverticulum (Ponka 1956). Diagnosis is made by radioisotope scanning using technetium ($^{99m}$Tc) pertechnetate which accumulates in the mucin-secreting cells of gastric mucosa (p. 86) (Duszynski et al 1971). Meckel's scans are most often positive in children, but false positive and false negative scans are common in adults (Dixon & Nolan 1987).

### Diagnosis of small intestinal hemorrhage

The inaccessibility of the small bowel is reflected in the wide range of methods used in the investigation of small bowel bleeding. The initial diagnostic step is to exclude bleeding from the upper gastrointestinal tract or colon. Small bowel contrast studies using barium or enteroclysis are rarely useful unless additional symptoms suggest small bowel disease (Rabe et al 1981). Radionuclide scans involving injection of $^{99m}$Tc-labeled autologous red cells (p. 87) may demonstrate that bleeding originates in the small bowel, but this test does not identify the cause (Markisz et al 1982). A Meckel's scan is useful in young adults and children. Angiography is the investigation of choice for brisk, active bleeding but will not be helpful when bleeding occurs at a rate less than 0.5 ml/min (Browder et al 1986).

The small bowel can be examined endoscopically (p. 120) using enteroscopy in which a particularly long, narrow, flexible instrument with a balloon at its tip is allowed to pass through the small bowel into the ileum; the small bowel is examined as the instrument is withdrawn through the bowel. The procedure is extremely time consuming and operator dependent and neither biopsy nor therapy is possible. Push enteroscopy with a long gastroscope will visualize much of the jejunum (80–120 cm beyond the ligament of Treitz), but the ileum is inaccessible. Biopsy and heater probe therapy can be used (Morris et al 1992).

In some patients, the diagnosis is made at laparotomy. This involves intubation of the gastrointestinal tract by an endoscope which is passed orally or through a cecotomy. The bowel is inflated with air and in the darkened theater the bowel wall is transilluminated in an attempt to visualize mucosal vascular lesions. This approach will establish a diagnosis in almost all cases of bleeding and enables the surgeon to resect the abnormal segment (Whelan et al 1989, Desa et al 1991).

## OCCULT GASTROINTESTINAL BLEEDING

Blood loss into the gastrointestinal tract is normally 0.5–1.5 ml/day (Ahlquist et al 1984) and does not increase with age. Occult gastrointestinal bleeding is defined as abnormal loss of blood into the digestive tract that is not apparent to the patient. It presents as iron deficiency anemia with constant or intermittent positive tests for blood in the stool. The importance of occult bleeding is that it can indicate colonic cancer, although a range of alternative gastrointestinal diseases may be responsible.

***Iron deficiency unassociated with gastrointestinal bleeding.*** When a patient presents with iron deficiency anemia, confirmed by a hypochromic microcytic blood film and low serum ferritin concentration, gastrointestinal bleeding is one of several possible causes. Others include bleeding from other sites including menorrhagia and even recurrent epistaxis, poor dietary iron intake and malabsorption of iron (p. 361). The assessment of iron deficiency anemia therefore includes a dietary and menstrual history, inquiry about recurrent bleeding from other sites and consideration of malabsorption (particularly celiac disease). Once the alternatives have been excluded, bleeding from the gastrointestinal tract is likely.

***Anticoagulants and gastrointestinal bleeding.*** Physiological bleeding is not increased by anticoagulant therapy (Choudari & Palmer 1995). Patients who bleed while taking warfarin require investigation of the gastrointestinal tract.

***Exercise-related gastrointestinal bleeding.*** Long-distance running (but not long-distance walking) causes a slight but significant increase in fecal blood loss (Robertson et al 1987). Some long-distance runners suffer abdominal pain, diarrhea or occasionally overt bleeding during or soon after running, although such bleeding may be less marked in well-trained athletes (Fogoros 1980). The exact cause is unknown, but intestinal ischemia due to alterations in splanchnic blood flow has been proposed. Panendoscopy performed shortly after marathon runs has shown hyperemia and mucosal erosions in the stomach and at the splenic flexure which heal rapidly (Schwartz et al 1990). Ultrasonic measurements show reductions in mesenteric arterial blood flow of up to 80% during vigorous exercise (Clausen 1977). Aggravation of pre-existing lesions such as hemorrhoids may also cause bleeding.

### Fecal occult blood tests

These are most useful in screening asymptomatic populations at risk of colorectal cancer rather than in the assessment of patients with iron deficiency anemia or symptoms of gastrointestinal disease, who need investigation irrespective of the results of tests for occult blood.

#### *Hemoccult test*

This is the most widely used test for detecting occult blood in feces. It is based upon a color change of a guaiac-based colorless dye caused by the peroxidase activity of hemoglobin. The test is positive in 80–90% of cases when fecal blood loss exceeds 20 ml/day and sensitivity is increased by testing on three separate days. False positive results occur in 7–12% of cases. Certain foods high in peroxidase activity, such as raw fruits and vegetables and rare meat, should be eliminated from the diet prior to testing, since they may produce false positive results. Aspirin and NSAIDs, which invariably increase gastrointestinal bleeding in normal subjects, should be stopped, although this may be impractical in patients taking these drugs because of painful arthritis. Few patients with positive tests have upper gastrointestinal bleeding and about one-third of such patients have colorectal neoplasia. Most false positive tests are due to technical reasons rather than hemorrhoids or other benign gastrointestinal lesions (Johnson 1989).

***Cancer screening.*** The Hemoccult test has been used in screening programs for colonic cancer detection, but the impact of these programs remains ill defined (p. 1422). The predictive value of a positive Hemoccult test is 4–10% (Barry et al 1987, Ahlquist et al 1989).

#### *Labeled red blood cells*

Gastrointestinal bleeding can be quantified using autologous $Cr^{51}$-labeled red blood cells (p. 87).

### Causes

The causes of occult and clinically apparent gastrointestinal bleeding are similar. The commonest cause worldwide is infestation with hookworm (p. 581), involving millions of individuals in the tropics and subtropics (Roche & Layrisse 1966) and leading to enormous morbidity. In industrialized countries, the most important cause is lower gastrointestinal cancer but, as shown in Table 17.5, a great range of diseases may be responsible.

### Investigations

Patients who describe specific gastrointestinal symptoms in association with anemia are investigated first in relation to those symptoms. Gastroscopy will be appropriate in those with dyspepsia, while colonoscopy will be undertaken in patients who present with altered bowel habit. When patients have no gastrointestinal symptoms, the first investigations should be directed at excluding colonic disease by colonoscopy. If this proves normal, gastroscopy can be done at the same endoscopic session (Rockey & Cello 1993). Patients who have certain upper gastrointestinal pathology may require additional colonoscopy. For example, esophagitis can cause anemia, but because esophagitis is an extremely common entity in the general population, it is wise to exclude a coexisting colonic cancer. How far any one patient should be investigated following discovery of upper gastrointestinal pathology is a matter of clinical judgment but in general, anemic patients with esophagitis, hiatus hernia, gastritis and duodenitis also require colonoscopy. Those who present with anemia in association with previous gastric surgery or peptic ulcer rarely have additional colonic pathology (Rockey & Cello 1993). In patients with negative gastroscopy and colonoscopy, small bowel disease should be considered although the yield of barium follow-through, enteroclysis and enteroscopy is low (Rockey & Cello 1993).

In up to one-third of patients, diagnostic tests are negative. Some of these patients are subjected to repeated radiological and endoscopic investigations, only some of which are necessary to ensure the validity of previously negative tests. The prognosis for these patients, who are presumably bleeding repeatedly from small vascular anomalies, is generally very good.

## BLEEDING DUE TO PORTAL HYPERTENSION

Overt bleeding due to portal hypertension is almost always from varices. Variceal hemorrhage is an uncommon cause of such bleeding, but it is important because it is often severe, carries a high mortality and requires early and specific treatment if the best results are to be obtained. Bleeding also occurs from the congested mucosa in portal gastropathy, but this usually causes iron deficiency anemia and overt bleeding is uncommon (p. 1000).

### Sites and causes of varices

Portal hypertension leads to the formation of varices in the esophagus (Figs 4.6 & 36.6); bleeding from these varices is common (Fig. 36.5) and usually occurs within 2–3 cm of the esophagogastric junction due to rupture or erosion of a varix (Fig. 17.12). Varices can also form elsewhere in the gastrointestinal tract, but bleeding from them is uncommon (p. 1000). The structure of the varices in the distal 5 cm of the esophagus is a major contributory factor to an increased risk of bleeding, as the vessels within the esophageal mucosal folds are more numerous and superficial (Fig. 36.12) than elsewhere and are therefore more likely to bleed than gastric varices or varices higher up the esophagus (Spence 1984). Portal hypertension is usually caused by intrahepatic portal venous obstruction and cirrhosis is the usual cause in most countries (p. 990). Schistosomiasis is the main cause in countries where this disease is endemic. Extrahepatic portal venous obstruction also causes portal hypertension and since these patients have a relatively good prognosis, it is important to establish the cause of portal hypertension (p. 1082). Transient portal hypertension can occur in acute viral hepatitis or alcoholic hepatitis but this is not usually a cause of bleeding.

Mortality is high, no matter the form of treatment, and it is highest in those with severe cirrhosis (p. 505). Approximately a third of patients die of their initial bleed, a further third bleed again within the following 6 weeks and only a third survive 1 year.

### Etiology of variceal bleeding

The underlying cause of varices can usually be determined (p. 992), but the factors that predispose to bleeding are much more obscure (p. 998). Larger varices (Lebrec et al 1980), red spots, red ridges (wales) and red stripes on the varices (Fig. 4.6), a portal venous pressure above 12 mmHg and advanced liver disease seem to be the most important predisposing factors (p. 999). Clinical experience suggests that salicylates, other nonsteroidal anti-inflammatory drugs, alcohol and perhaps corticosteroids can induce variceal bleeding, but gastroesophageal acid reflux is probably not important. Continuous bleeding and early rebleeding are also common and may be a result of portal hemodynamics in portal hypertension (McCormick et al 1995).

### Incidence

In the UK, bleeding varices account for 2.5–5% of patients admitted to hospital with hematemesis and

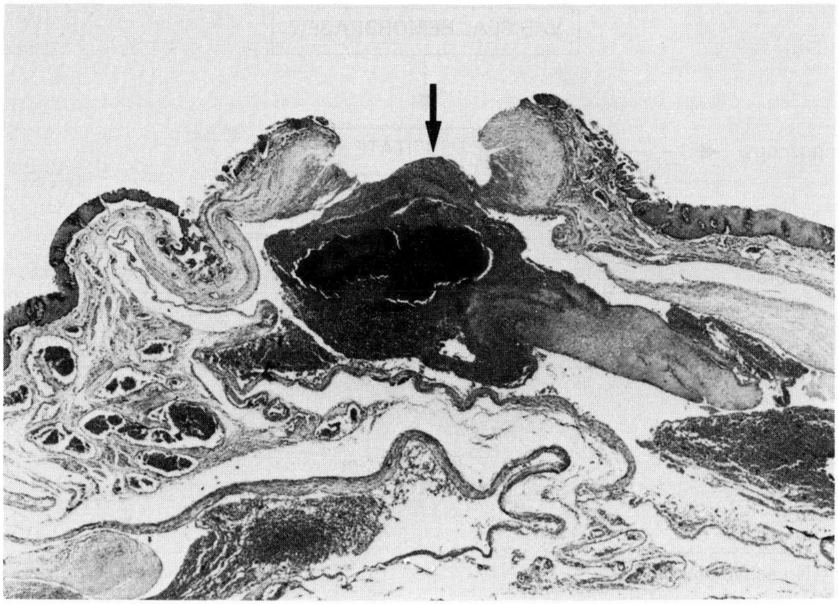

**Fig. 17.12** Esophageal varices. A small punctate ulcer has penetrated through the squamous epithelium into an underlying submucosal varix. A small plug of thrombus (arrow) is occluding the defect in the vein wall (hematoxylin and eosin, × 13).

melena (Jones 1956, Schiller et al 1970, Forrest et al 1974, Rockall et al 1995). In other countries bleeding varices are more common and in the United States they account for 10–15% of patients with acute gastrointestinal hemorrhage.

## Clinical features

The diagnosis should be suspected in any patient with a history of alcoholism or liver disease. Examination will usually reveal one or more of the external signs of liver disease (pp. 918 & 991), but this is not always the case. Complications of liver disease, such as encephalopathy or ascites, should be sought.

## Investigations

### *Endoscopy*

Endoscopy is important in gastrointestinal bleeding possibly due to portal hypertension, as sites of bleeding other than varices, such as erosions, portal hypertensive gastropathy or peptic ulceration, may be responsible. The proportion of patients with portal hypertension with non-variceal bleeding may be as high as 30% (Waldram et al 1974), but in the authors' experience this is probably an overestimate. Sometimes, particularly when endoscopy is delayed, the variceal source of bleeding may be missed and gastric erosions, which may develop after upper gastrointestinal bleeding, presumed to be the source of blood loss. Accordingly, and because treatment by injection sclerotherapy or band ligation of varices can be started, endoscopy should be undertaken as soon as possible after resuscitation in patients with known or suspected portal hypertension. This usually distinguishes reliably between variceal and other bleeding lesions and when varices are found but no source of bleeding can be identified, the varices can justifiably be regarded as the source and treated (Mitchell et al 1978).

### *Other investigations*

Investigations that raise the possibility of liver disease in portal hypertension include abnormal liver function tests, although these are frequently not available at the time of bleeding. A full blood count is valuable since thrombocytopenia and/or leukopenia suggest hypersplenism consequent on portal hypertension, a prothrombin time gives warning of coagulation abnormality and the blood urea and creatinine give a measure of renal function. A disproportionately high blood urea concentration points to a severe bleed (p. 482).

## Treatment

The treatment of active variceal hemorrhage is discussed below (see Fig. 17.13). Prevention of rebleeding from varices and prophylactic treatment in patients with varices that have not bled are considered elsewhere (p. 1005).

### *Resuscitation*

Resuscitation has been discussed previously (p. 482) and its principles are as in other causes of acute gastrointestinal

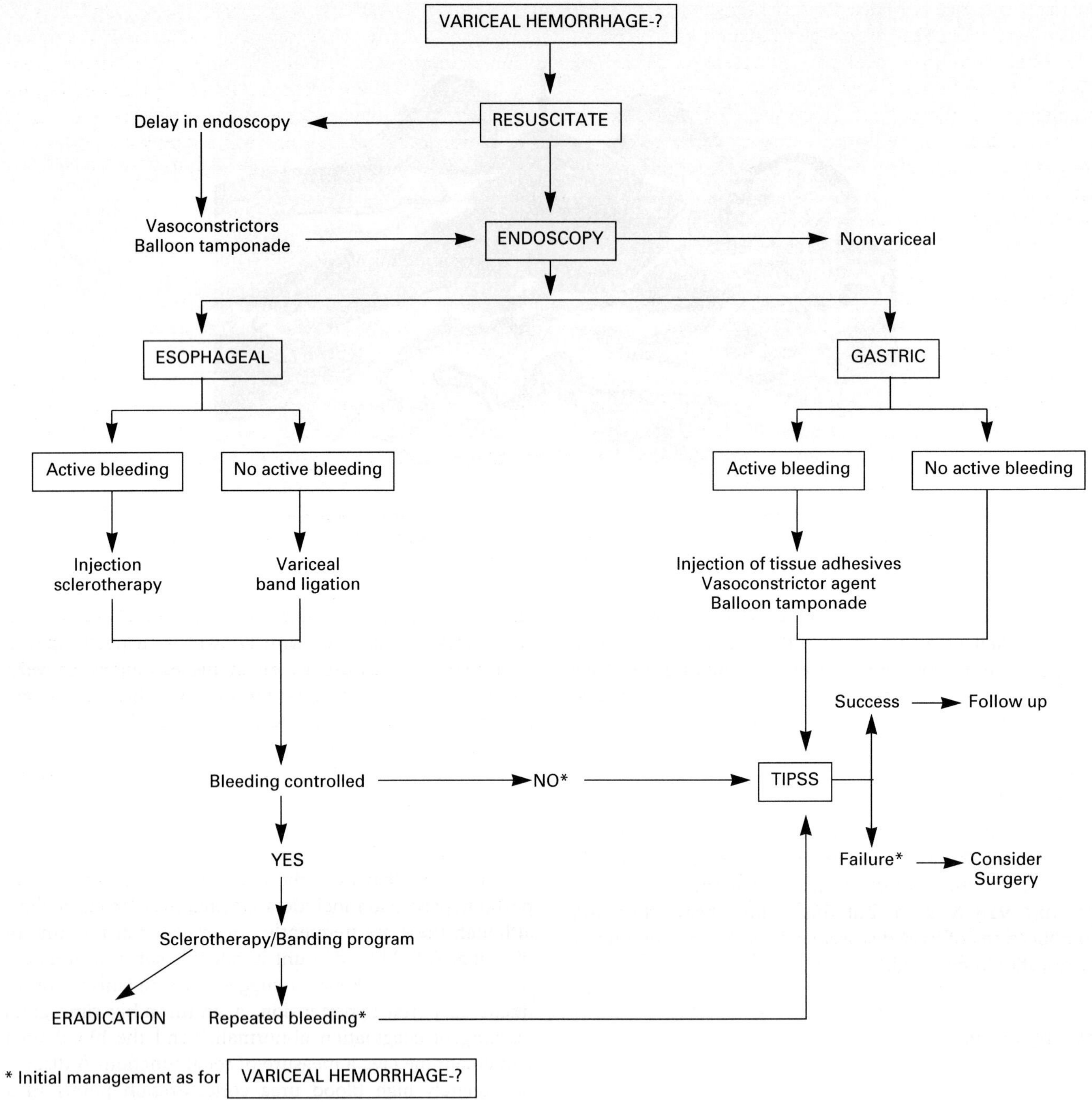


**Fig. 17.13** Schematic plan for the management of acute variceal bleeding in portal hypertension.

bleeding. Particular care should be taken to avoid overtransfusion, as this may precipitate rebleeding (McCormick et al 1995). Patients with cirrhosis have impaired hemodynamic responses to blood loss, presumably due to their systemic vasodilatation (p. 920) and autonomic neuropathy (p. 923). A recent study showed that venesection of 15% of the circulating blood volume in patients with portal hypertension caused no compensatory tachycardia or increase in systemic vascular resistance in spite of a significant decrease in cardiac output and blood pressure (Gimson & Vlavianos 1992). Such patients also show covert tissue hypoxia that may result in critical reductions in oxygen supply and consumption when bleeding occurs (Moreau et al 1989). For this reason it is important that patients be given supplementary oxygen (3–4 L/min) to maximize tissue oxygen supply, particularly when they are anemic. Pulmonary aspiration occurs readily in encephalopathic patients and expert nursing care is needed to avoid its occurrence.

Fluid replacement should be with colloid initially,

preferably using gelatin-based solutions such as Hemaccel as they have less effect on platelet function and bleeding time compared with dextran or hydroxyethyl starch (Tschirren et al 1974). Blood transfusion should be with a combination of packed red blood cells and fresh frozen plasma (5:1) to restore oxygen-carrying capacity and to minimize coagulopathy. Some recommend the slow administration of fresh frozen plasma (one unit per 6 h) once bleeding has been controlled, but this should be used cautiously in patients with ascites or edema as the sodium in plasma promotes fluid retention. Vitamin K (phytomenadione 10 mg) is usually administered parenterally for three successive days when the prothrombin time is prolonged, but its value is questionable. Vitamin K deficiency is rarely the cause of prolongation of the prothrombin time other than in chronic cholestatic liver disease and deficiency is adequately corrected by a single 10 mg dose given intravenously over not less than 5 min. Thrombocytopenia is rarely important in continued bleeding and platelet transfusions do not raise the platelet count in patients with a palpable spleen. Platelets need only be given where the count is below $50 \times 10^9$/L and are best administered at the time of a hemostatic treatment such as sclerotherapy.

*Hepatic encephalopathy*

It should be assumed that bleeding will precipitate hepatic encephalopathy in patients with portal hypertension and treatment should be given to prevent this. Blood should be removed from the stomach by aspiration and lavage if a Sengstaken tube has been passed and from the colon by lactulose 15–30 ml (Duphalac) 8-hourly, magnesium sulfate (30 ml of 25%) given orally on one or two occasions or colonic washouts. Dietary protein intake should not exceed 20 g/day, sedation should be avoided unless an uncomfortable treatment such as balloon tamponade is being performed and a poorly absorbed antibiotic such as neomycin may reduce infections as well as alleviate encephalopathy provided there is no renal failure (p. 1053).

*Sedation*

If sedation is required, the smallest dose of midazolam (p. 99) needed to produce drowsiness can be given by a slow intravenous injection (0.5 mg/min). Flumazenil (p. 99), the benzodiazepine antagonist, should be available to reverse excessive sedation, to which these patients are particularly prone.

## Control of bleeding

Many treatments are available to control active variceal hemorrhage and depend on local availability and expertise. Certain treatments, such as vasopressin, are less used now than formerly, while new approaches such as variceal banding and transjugular intrahepatic portasystemic stent shunting (TIPSS) are becoming more popular but require longer term evaluation. The treatments discussed below are not mutually exclusive and it is not uncommon for two or more to be required during an episode of active variceal hemorrhage.

*Variceal sclerotherapy*

Endoscopic injection sclerotherapy is probably the best initial treatment in controlling active variceal bleeding (p. 112). It is done at diagnostic endoscopy and controls hemorrhage in around 90% of patients (Westaby et al 1989). To obtain such success, sclerotherapy may have to be repeated on more than one occasion during the first 48 h. When bleeding at endoscopy has stopped or is minor, sclerotherapy is relatively straightforward, as visibility is good. However, when more active hemorrhage makes visualization of the varices difficult, small-volume injections (STD 3% 0.5–1 ml) paravariceally 2–3 cm above the gastroesophageal junction will often stop bleeding and allow intravariceal injections to be undertaken. If bleeding is severe, perseverance in trying to control bleeding may be harmful, particularly in causing pulmonary aspiration, and it is then best to apply balloon tamponade to control hemorrhage. Sclerotherapy can then be repeated some hours later with a blood-free field.

It is sometimes uncertain whether hemostasis has been obtained after sclerotherapy and it has been advocated that balloon tamponade be used after the procedure to localize the sclerosant around the lower esophagus. There is no good evidence to support this practice and balloon tamponade after sclerotherapy is recommended only when bleeding is clearly continuing.

*Variceal ligation*

Endoscopic band ligation of varices is effective in controlling active variceal hemorrhage but is more difficult to carry out than sclerotherapy (p. 112). This technique has advantages over endoscopic injection sclerotherapy in the prevention of rebleeding, as complications are less common (p. 113), eradication of varices more rapid and rebleeding less frequent (Hayes 1996). A combination of small-volume sclerotherapy injections to control active bleeding followed by band ligation may be the most effective approach.

*Balloon tamponade*

Sengstaken & Blakemore (1950) developed balloon tamponade for the control of bleeding from esophageal and gastric fundal varices and a four-lumen modification of the original Sengstaken tube (Minnesota tube) is now the most widely used means of achieving balloon tamponade (Boyce 1962). The distal balloon, by virtue of its size, serves as an anchor in the stomach, while the proximal balloon compresses the varices in the esophageal wall. The distal end of the esophageal balloon is reinforced to prevent its sliding into the stomach. The large central lumen is used to aspirate the stomach and to administer foods or drugs and the fourth lumen is used to aspirate secretions lying above the esophageal balloon. An alternative is the Linton–Nachlas tube, which has a single large gastric balloon.

***Use.*** Endoscopic injection sclerotherapy should be undertaken if variceal bleeding is identified at endoscopy, but if this is not available or if bleeding persists despite sclerotherapy, a Sengstaken tube should be passed without delay. Although uncomfortable, balloon tamponade is more effective than vasoconstrictor therapy and is the best second-line treatment for active variceal hemorrhage.

***Procedure.*** A new tube should be used for each patient and the balloons must be tested for leaks prior to insertion. Storing the tubes in a refrigerator (not a freezer) keeps them cold, which increases rigidity and eases insertion. The procedure should be explained to the patient, who should be lightly sedated before the balloon is passed. The lubricated tube should be passed via the mouth and, if active bleeding is present, the patient rolled onto the left side to help prevent aspiration. The patient should be encouraged to swallow as the tube is advanced to at least the 50 cm mark, so that its tip passes well into the stomach. Blood frequently emerges spontaneously from the gastric aspiration port and should be aspirated. Auscultation over the upper abdomen while air is injected into the gastric aspiration port checks that this port is in the stomach.

Air (150 ml) is then inflated slowly into the gastric balloon and if pain occurs, the balloon should be deflated immediately, as pain implies that the balloon is still in the esophagus. Particular care is required in patients after gastric resection, as the gastric balloon may pass into the jejunum and inflation there will cause a rupture (Goff et al 1982). Once inflation of the balloon can be achieved painlessly, the tube should be withdrawn until the balloon impacts in the cardia, which usually occurs with the 35–40 cm mark at the teeth. The balloon should then be taped in place and an X-ray taken of the upper abdomen and lower chest to ensure satisfactory position. Thereafter the volume of air in the gastric balloon should be increased to 400 ml, the tube doubly clamped and steady traction applied to maintain impaction of the balloon in the cardia. This is essential, as impaction in the cardia and partial herniation of the balloon into the lower esophagus is the mechanism whereby hemorrhage is controlled. The best means we have found of maintaining traction is to tape two wooden tongue-depressors across the tube where it leaves the mouth. This traps the tube effectively and stops slippage, but it is important to apply sufficient sponge and/or swabs around the wood to prevent damage to the skin. It is essential that a note is made of the calibrated marking on the tube at the teeth and this should be checked regularly to confirm that traction is maintained. A common cause of failure to control bleeding is slippage of the tube either because the gastric balloon is deflated, in which case the tube calibration marks are lower than originally noted, or because traction has been lost, in which case the marks at the teeth will be higher.

***Management.*** The patient needs continuous supervision by a personal nurse who has immediate access to medical help. Aspiration is a major complication and accordingly the patient should be nursed on the side, the head of the bed should be elevated 15–20 cm to prevent reflux of gastric content and some use atropine (0.6–1.2 mg) to reduce secretion of saliva. The risk of aspiration is related to encephalopathy and patients in grade III or IV (p. 1045) should be considered for ventilation before the tube is passed. The esophagus, the stomach and the pharynx should be aspirated and the tube traction checked at least every half hour and the site of traction pressure on the lips should be changed regularly to avoid ulceration. Further sedation may be needed during therapy but before this is given, the need for pharyngeal aspiration should be checked and pain due to a complication of therapy should be considered. Bleeding can usually be arrested with the gastric balloon alone but if not, the esophageal balloon should be inflated to 30–40 mmHg using a sphygmomanometer connected to the tube via a Y-connection. If the esophageal balloon has been used, pressure should be checked regularly and the balloon deflated for 5 min every 6 h to prevent esophageal mucosal damage. Airway obstruction due to upward migration of the esophageal tube is rapidly fatal and the supervising nurse should have no hesitation in transecting the tube with heavy scissors and removing it if respiratory distress cannot be relieved by pharyngeal aspiration.

The balloon is usually kept in place for around 12 h after control of hemorrhage, when endoscopy and sclerotherapy can be undertaken in a bloodless field. If bleeding has not been controlled after an hour or so, consideration should be given to an alternative site of bleeding or alternative treatments (see below) should be instituted. Continuing bleeding can usually be identified by aspiration of fresh blood from the gastric or esophageal aspiration ports. Occasionally, however, blood cannot be aspirated despite ongoing bleeding recognized by persistent tachycardia, hypotension, a falling central venous pressure and ongoing transfusion requirement.

***Complications.*** Approximately 30% of patients experience complications related to balloon tamponade. Aspiration pneumonia occurs in at least 10% and is more likely in patients with hepatic encephalopathy. The most

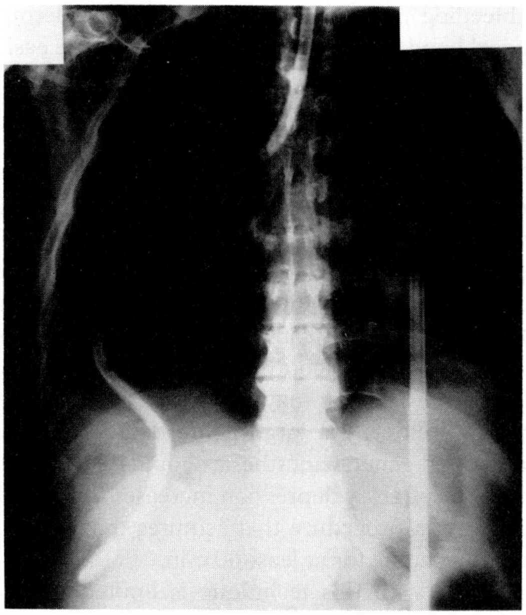

**Fig. 17.14** Chest radiograph in a patient with hepatic cirrhosis and bleeding esophageal varices. The Sengstaken tube has perforated the esophagus and lies in the pleural cavity. The proximal part of the Sengstaken tube seen on the right is lying on the anterior chest wall.

life-threatening complication is obstruction of the airway by the esophageal balloon and other serious complications include esophageal rupture and mucosal ulceration (Fig. 17.14).

***Results.*** Balloon tamponade is highly effective in controlling variceal bleeding and experienced users obtain hemostasis in around 90% of patients (Panés et al 1988). The Sengstaken tube is probably more effective in controlling bleeding from esophageal varices, while the Linton tube may be better for bleeding gastric varices (Terés et al 1978). Esophageal tamponade is not a definitive treatment but allows temporary control of bleeding to be achieved. Without further definitive treatment a quarter of patients will bleed within 24 h of deflating the balloon and a further quarter within the next 10 days (Panés et al 1988).

*Vasoconstrictor therapy*

Vasoconstrictor therapy has been used for over 30 years in the treatment of variceal bleeding. Vasopressin was the drug used originally and more recently vasopressin analogs, combination treatments and somatostatin or octreotide have been advocated.

The place of vasoconstrictor therapy is controversial. It is less effective than sclerotherapy, variceal banding or balloon tamponade and it is now used most often as an adjuvant therapy in continuing bleeding. Whether this is appropriate when treatments such as TIPSS are so effective is debatable. Some use vasoconstrictor therapy rather than emergency sclerotherapy in patients suspected of a variceal hemorrhage, but we believe that urgent diagnostic endoscopy should be performed, as there seems little logic in delaying sclerotherapy where expertise is available. Where this is not the case, vasoconstrictor drugs may be useful in controlling bleeding while the patient is transferred to another hospital.

*Vasopressin*

Vasopressin (antidiuretic hormone) is an endogenous vasoconstrictor that at pharmacological doses reduces splanchnic blood flow and consequently portal blood flow and portal pressure (Bosch 1985). More recently, it has been shown to reduce azygos blood flow by approximately 35% (Bosch et al 1985) and this is a measure of portasystemic collateral blood flow and variceal pressure (Bosch et al 1988). It has been used for many years in variceal hemorrhage and has an efficacy of 30–70% (Bosch & Terés 1992). It is usually administered by continuous intravenous infusion starting at a dose of 0.4 units/min increasing to 0.8 units/min if required. Regional infusions into the superior mesenteric artery have been attempted but have not been shown to be superior to intravenous administration (Mallory et al 1980). Unfortunately, it has significant adverse effects because of its widespread vasoconstrictor action. Injection sclerotherapy or band ligation should be undertaken within 24 h of control of bleeding.

*Vasopressin and nitroglycerine*

Nitroglycerine given with vasopressin can prevent the adverse vasoactive effects of vasopressin, which include cardiac arrhythmias, cardiac ischemia and even myocardial infarction. Nitroglycerine reduces portal pressure in its own right (Hayes et al 1988); when it is combined with vasopressin, the portal pressure is reduced even further (Fig. 17.15). Three studies have shown that vasopressin and nitroglycerine are more effective in controlling bleeding than vasopressin alone (Gimson et al 1986, Tsai et al 1986, Bosch et al 1989). Nitroglycerine can be administered sublingually or transdermally, but impaired peripheral blood flow due to bleeding or vasopressin may reduce the efficacy of nitroglycerine given by this route. We therefore recommend that it be given by intravenous infusion (single dose of 1000 μg followed by 200 μg/min), generally after the vasopressin infusion has been started as this tends to raise arterial pressure and avoids hypotension. The dose can then be gradually increased until the systolic blood pressure falls to around 100 mmHg.

*Glypressin*

Glypressin (terlipressin or triglycyl lysine vasopressin) is a synthetic vasopressin analog from which vasopressin is released gradually into the circulation following endoge-

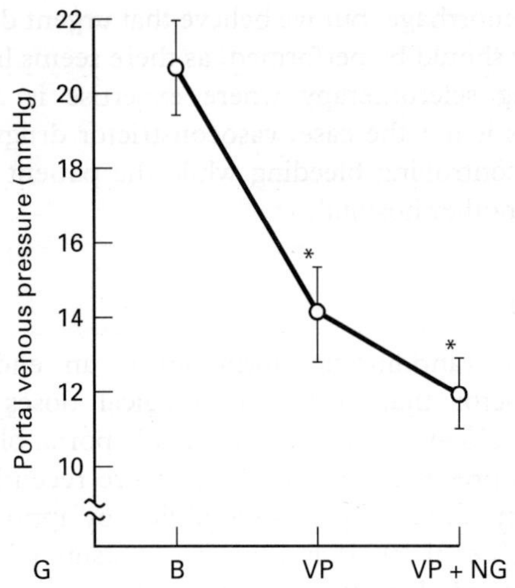


**Fig. 17.15** Portal venous pressure before (B) and after vasopressin (VP) and vasopressin and nitroglycerine (VP+NG) therapy (Westaby et al 1988).

nous removal of glycyl residues. It can be administered by bolus injection (2 mg/4 h) continued until bleeding has ceased for 24 h. Two controlled trials have demonstrated its effectiveness in controlling variceal hemorrhage (Freeman et al 1989, Söderlund et al 1990).

Glypressin seems to produce fewer side-effects than vasopressin, but the reason for this is unclear as its primary action is dependent upon endogenous vasopressin release. The effect of concurrent nitroglycerine administration is unclear (Fort et al 1990).

*Somatostatin and octreotide*

Both these drugs have minor and variable effects on wedged hepatic venous pressure, but they consistently reduce azygos venous blood flow, which is a measure of collateral blood flow. The variable effect on portal pressure may be less important than orginally supposed, as the actions of vasoconstrictive drugs in patients bleeding actively may be different from those in hemodynamically stable persons.

The effectiveness of these drugs in stopping acute variceal bleeding is debatable. One large recent controlled study found it effective (Burroughs et al 1990), but a second found it less effective than placebo (Valenzuela et al 1989). Several studies have compared the effectiveness of somatostatin and octreotide relative to vasopressin, vasopressin and nitroglycerine, balloon tamponade and sclerotherapy and the results have been variable. Thus, somatostatin and octreotide, although popular because of freedom from side-effects, probably have limited ability to control variceal bleeding. Somatostatin can be used as an initial dose of 250 μg intravenously followed by 250 μg/h and octreotide as an initial dose of 50 μg followed by 50 μg/h. They may have some place in reducing the severity of bleeding prior to endoscopy to allow sclerotherapy or variceal band ligation to be undertaken more easily.

*Transjugular intrahepatic portasystemic stent shunting (TIPSS)* (p. 1007)

This relatively new approach in the management of bleeding varices has been used most in the prevention of rebleeding (p. 1008) and it has also been very successful in treating active bleeding (LaBerge et al 1993, Simpson et al 1994). When TIPSS can be undertaken successfully (approximately 90%), control of bleeding is almost universal but liver function may deteriorate in a few patients, particularly following a large hemorrhage. Endotracheal intubation and general anesthesia should be used, because associated respiratory depression increases the risk of aspiration during a procedure that requires the patient to be sedated and supine for at least 60 min.

Experience with this technique is limited and further assessment is required, but it looks promising as a method of controlling variceal hemorrhage where others have failed. When available, it deserves consideration before surgical intervention in patients with a patent portal vein (McCormick et al 1994, Jalan et al 1994).

*Surgery*

Surgery is indicated when bleeding cannot be controlled by any of the methods outlined above. Patients are usually poor surgical risks and it is questionable whether operation is justified in patients with obvious ascites and encephalopathy. There are two types of surgical procedure: direct interruption of the varices and portasystemic shunts (Marks 1976).

***Portalazygos disconnection operations.*** A variety of operations to arrest and prevent variceal bleeding by interrupting the flow of blood from the portal venous system to the azygos venous system (portalazygos disconnection) have been devised. All involve combinations of esophageal transection and esophagogastric devascularization, with or without splenectomy, and they have been developed to stop continuing bleeding, to prevent rebleeding and to preserve portal blood flow to the liver, thereby minimizing postoperative encephalopathy. They do stop continuing variceal bleeding and varices can disappear postoperatively (Umeyama et al 1983), but they do not alter the underlying portal hypertension and subsequent rebleeding occurs in 20–50% of patients (Keagy et al 1986). Acceptably low overall operative mortality rates have been achieved in large series, but these have included elective operations on patients with good liver function; the operative mortality for bleeding patients with poor liver function (grade C) is high at around 30–50%.

Operations are now generally undertaken abdominally using a staple gun to transect the esophagus, with or without additional devascularization procedures (Johnston 1982). Complications of the stapling gun operation include leakage from the transection line and dysphagia from esophageal narrowing. The latter usually resolves spontaneously but may need esophageal dilatation. Hepatic encephalopathy is not a particular problem, in contrast to portasystemic shunt operations. Japanese surgeons have achieved good results using much more radical operations, including esophageal transection, extensive gastric devascularization and splenectomy as the preferred surgical therapy for the prophylaxis and the prevention of rebleeding (Sugiura & Futagawa 1977, Koyama et al 1980). However, such operations have little role in the emergency treatment of acute variceal bleeding and surgeons in other countries have not been able to reproduce the Japanese results (Gouge & Ranson 1986, Keagy et al 1986). The authors use esophageal transection to stop variceal bleeding when other treatments, including TIPSS, have been unsuccessful but do not advocate its use electively where variceal bleeding has stopped.

*Portasystemic shunts*

Although there is still debate about portasystemic shunt surgery in the prevention of rebleeding from varices, there is little doubt that it now has almost no place in the treatment of acute hemorrhage. Even in the most experienced hands, the mortality of an emergency portacaval shunt is about 50% (Orloff et al 1977) and no patient with a combination of ascites, jaundice, encephalopathy and muscle wasting has survived a year postoperatively. Shunt surgery should only be considered to control active bleeding in those with good liver function where TIPSS is not available or where there is portal vein thrombosis.

## Prognosis

Mortality from bleeding esophageal varices in patients with cirrhosis is related closely to the severity of bleeding and to underlying hepatocellular function (Novis et al 1976, Graham & Smith 1981, Burroughs & McCormick 1992). Severity of bleeding, as evidenced by active bleeding at endoscopy and by blood transfusion requirement, is particularly important at an early stage, as bleeding accounts for two-thirds of deaths in the first week. Other important factors include deteriorating liver function evidenced by ascites or encephalopathy, renal failure, infections such as pneumonia and complications related to treatment. Graham & Smith (1981) found that only a third of patients suffering a complication of treatment survived and only a half of those suffering any complication. Novis et al (1976) emphasized the importance of hepatocellular function in survival to leave hospital by relating this to simple clinical measures of liver function (Tables 17.6 and 17.7) and Burroughs & McCormick (1992) showed that mortality was related clearly to the Child grade with mortalities of 5% for grade A, 25% for grade B and 50% or more for grade C. Other factors related to early rebleeding and increased mortality include laboratory measures of poor liver function such as hypoalbuminemia and a prolonged prothrombin time, uremia and a hepatic venous pressure gradient greater than 16 mmHg (Garden et al 1985, Vinel et al 1986, Ready et al 1991).

**Table 17.6** Prognosis in cirrhosis with bleeding varices related to clinical features of hepatic failure (Novis et al 1976)

| Indices of liver function: jaundice, ascites, encephalopathy | Survival (%) To leave hospital | 1 year | 2 years |
|---|---|---|---|
| None present | 92 | 62 | 31 |
| One present | 53 | 12 | 12 |
| Two present | 38 | 15 | 9 |
| Three present | 23 | 0 | 0 |

**Table 17.7** Prognosis in cirrhosis with bleeding varices related to serum albumin concentration (Novis et al 1976)

| Serum albumin (g/L) | Survival to leave hospital (%) |
|---|---|
| >30 | 69 |
| 25–30 | 53 |
| <25 | 9 |

REFERENCES


Ahlquist D A, McGill D B, Schwartz S, Taylor W F, Ellefson M, Owen R A 1984 HemoQuant, a new quantitative assay for fecal hemoglobin. Annals of Internal Medicine 101: 297–302

Ahlquist D A, McGill D B, Fleming J L 1989 Patterns of occult bleeding in asymptomatic colorectal cancer. Cancer 63: 1826–1830

Allan R, Dykes P 1976 A study of the factors influencing mortality rates from gastrointestinal haemorrhage. Quarterly Journal of Medicine 45: 533–550

Allison D J, Hemingway A P, Cunningham D A 1982 Angiography in gastrointestinal bleeding. Lancet 2: 30–33

Ashley S, Wells S A Jr 1988 Tumors of the small intestine. Seminars in Oncology 15: 116–128

Avery-Jones F 1956 Hematemesis and melena: with special reference to causation and to the factors influencing the mortality from bleeding peptic ulcers. Gastroenterology 30: 166–190

Balint J A, Sarfeh I J, Fried M B 1977 Gastrointestinal bleeding – diagnosis and management. Clinical Gastroenterology Monograph Series. Wiley, New York

Barry M J, Mulley A G, Richter J M 1987 Effect of workup strategy on the cost-effectiveness of fecal occult blood screening for colorectal cancer. Gastroenterology 93: 301–310

Baum S, Roy R, Finkelstein A K, Blakemore W S 1965 Clinical application of selective celiac and superior mesenteric arteriography. Radiology 84: 279–295

Beckley D E, Casebow M P 1986 Prediction of rebleeding from peptic ulcer: experience with an endoscopic Doppler device. Gut 27: 96–99

Bendahan J, Gilboa S, Parem H et al 1992 Seasonal pattern in the

incidence of bleeding caused by peptic ulcer in Israel. American Journal of Gastroenterology 87: 733–735
Blackstone M O 1984 Endoscopic interpretation. Raven Press, New York, pp 392–393
Boley S J, Sammartano R, Adams A, DiBiase A, Kleinhaus S, Sprayregen S 1977a On the nature and etiology of vascular ectasias of the colon: degenerative lesions of aging. Gastroenterology 72: 650–660
Boley S J, Sprayregen S, Sammartano R J, Adams A, Kleinhaus S 1977b The pathophysiologic basis for the angiographic signs of vascular ectasias of the colon. Radiology 125: 615–621
Boley S J, DiBiase A, Brandt L J, Sammartano R J 1979 Lower intestinal bleeding in the elderly. American Journal of Surgery 137: 57–64
Boley S J, Brandt L J, Frank M S 1981 Severe lower intestinal bleeding: diagnosis and treatment. Clinics in Gastroenterology 10: 65–91
Bornman P C, Theodorou N A, Shuttleworth R D, Essel H P, Marks I N 1985 Importance of hypovolaemic shock and endoscopic signs in predicting recurrent haemorrhage from peptic ulceration: a prospective evaluation. British Medical Journal 291: 245–247
Boron B, Mobarhan S 1987 Endoscopic treatment of Dieulafoy hemorrhage. Journal of Clinical Gastroenterology 9: 518–520
Bosch J 1985 Effect of pharmacological agents on portal hypertension: a haemodynamic appraisal. Clinics in Gastroenterology 14: 169–184
Bosch J, Terés J 1992 Immediate management of variceal hemorrhage. Gastrointestinal Endoscopy Clinics of North America 2: 43–58
Bosch J, Mastai R, Kravetz D, Bruix J, Rigau J, Rodés J 1985 Measurement of azygos venous blood flow in the evaluation of portal hypertension in patients with cirrhosis. Clinical and haemodynamic correlations in 100 patients. Journal of Hepatology 1: 125–139
Bosch J, Bordas J M, Mastai R et al 1988 Effects of vasopressin on the intravariceal pressure in patients with cirrhosis: comparison with the effects on portal pressure. Hepatology 8: 861–865
Bosch J, Groszmann R J, García-Pagán J C et al 1989 Association of transdermal nitroglycerin to vasopressin infusion in the treatment of variceal hemorrhage. A placebo-controlled clinical trial. Hepatology 10: 962–968
Boyce H W 1962 Modification of the Sengstaken–Blakemore balloon tube. New England Journal of Medicine 267: 195–196
Bramley P N, Masson J, Walshe D et al 1993 The impact of a specialised bleeding unit serving Grampian region: the way forward? Gut 34 (S60): F236
Branicki F J, Coleman S Y, Fok P J 1990 Bleeding peptic ulcer: a prospective evaluation of risk factors for rebleeding and mortality. World Journal of Surgery 14: 262–270
Broberg A, Ihre T, Pyke E, Raaschou-Nielson T 1982 Exulceratio simplex as a conceivable cause of massive gastric hemorrhage. Surgery, Gynecology and Obstetrics 154: 186–188
Browder W, Cerise E J, Litwin M S 1986 Impact of emergency angiography in massive lower gastrointestinal bleeding. Annals of Surgery 204: 530–536
Burroughs A K, McCormick P A 1992 Natural history and prognosis of variceal bleeding. Baillière's Clinical Gastroenterology 6: 437–450
Burroughs A K, McCormick P A, Hughes M D, Sprengers D, D'Heygere F, McIntyre N 1990 Randomized, double-blind, placebo-controlled trial of somatostatin for variceal bleeding. Emergency control and prevention of early variceal bleeding. Gastroenterology 99: 1388–1395
Cello J P, Grendell J A 1986 Endoscopic laser treatment for gastrointestinal vascular ectasias. Annals of Internal Medicine 104: 352–354
Choudari C P, Palmer K R 1994 Endoscopic injection therapy for bleeding peptic ulcer: a comparison of adrenaline alone with adrenaline plus ethanolamine oleate. Gut 35: 608–610
Choudari C P, Palmer K R 1995 Acute gastrointestinal haemorrhage in patients treated with anticoagulant drugs. Gut 36: 483–484
Choudari C P, Rajgopal C, Palmer K R 1992 Comparison of endoscopic injection therapy versus the heater probe in major peptic ulcer haemorrhage. Gut 33: 1159–1161
Christiansen J, Ottenjann R, von Arx F 1989 Placebo-controlled trial with the somatostatin analogue SMS 201-995 in peptic ulcer bleeding. Gastroenterology 97: 567–574
Chung S C S, Leung J W C, Steele J R C, Croft T J, Li A K C 1988 Endoscopic injection of adrenaline for actively bleeding ulcers: a randomised trial. British Medical Journal 296: 1631–1633
Chung S C S, Leung J W C, Sung J Y, Lo K K, Li A K C 1991 Injection or heater probe for bleeding ulcer. Gastroenterology 100: 33–37
Clason A E, MacLeod D A D, Elton R A 1986 Clinical factors in the prediction of further haemorrhage or mortality in acute upper gastrointestinal haemorrhage. British Journal of Surgery 73: 985–987
Clausen J P 1977 Effect of physical training on cardiovascular adjustments to exercise in man. Physiological Reviews 51: 779–815
Clements D, Aslan S, Foster D, Stamatakis J, Wilkins W E, Morris J S 1991 Acute upper gastrointestinal haemorrhage in a district general hospital: audit of an agreed management policy. Journal of the Royal College of Physicians of London 25: 27–30
Clouse R E, Costigan D J, Mills B A, Zuckerman G R 1985 Angiodysplasia as a cause of upper gastrointestinal bleeding. Archives of Internal Medicine 145: 458–461
Cocco A E, Grayer D I, Walker B A, Martyn L J 1969 The stomach in pseudoxanthoma elasticum. Journal of the American Medical Association 210: 2381–2382
Collins R, Langman M 1985 Treatment with histamine $H_2$ antagonists in acute upper gastrointestinal hemorrhage: implications of randomized trials. New England Journal of Medicine 313: 660–666
Cook D J, Guyatt G H, Salena B J, Laine L A 1992 Endoscopic therapy for acute nonvariceal upper gastrointestinal hemorrhage: a meta-analysis. Gastroenterology 102: 139–148
Cook D J, Fuller H D, Guyatt G H et al 1994 Risk factors for gastrointestinal bleeding in critically ill patients. New England Journal of Medicine 330: 377–381
Cutler J A, Mendeloff A I 1981 Upper gastrointestinal bleeding: nature and magnitude of the problem in the U.S. Digestive Diseases and Sciences 76 (suppl): 90S–96S
Czerniak A, Thompson J N, Hemingway A P et al 1988 Hemobilia. A disease of evolution. Archives of Surgery 123: 718–721
Daneshmend T K, Hawkey C J, Langman M J S, Logan R F A, Long R G, Walt R P 1992 Omeprazole versus placebo for acute upper gastrointestinal bleeding: randomised double blind controlled trial. British Medical Journal 304: 143–147
Desa L A, Ohri S K, Hutton K A P 1991 Role of intraoperative enteroscopy in obscure gastrointestinal bleeding of small bowel origin. British Journal of Surgery 78: 192–195
Dixon P M, Nolan D J 1987 The diagnosis of Meckel's diverticulum: a continuing challenge. Clinical Radiology 38: 615–619
Dixon J A, Berenson M M, McCloskey D W 1979 Neodymium-Yag laser treatment of experimental canine gastric bleeding: acute and chronic studies of photocoagulation, penetration, and perforation. Gastroenterology 77: 647–651
Donaldson M D J, Seaman M J, Park G R 1992 Massive blood transfusion. British Journal of Anaesthesia 69: 621–630
Dronfield M W, McIllmurray M B, Ferguson R et al 1977 A prospective randomised study of endoscopy and radiology in acute upper-gastrointestinal-tract bleeding. Lancet 1: 1147–1169
Dronfield M W, McIllmurray M B, Ferguson R, Atkinson M, Langman M J S 1982 A prospective randomised study of endoscopy and radiology in acute gastrointestinal tract bleeding. Lancet 1: 1167–1169
Durham J D, Kumpe D A, Rothbarth L J, van Steigmann G 1990 Dieulafoy disease: arteriographic findings and treatment. Radiology 174: 937–941
Duszynski D O, Jewett T C, Allen J E 1971 $Tc^{99m}$Na pertechnetate scanning of the abdomen with particular reference to small bowel pathology. American Journal of Roentgenology 113: 258–262
Eddy D M, Nugent F W, Eddy J F et al 1987 Screening for colorectal cancer in a high-risk population. Results of a mathematical model. Gastroenterology 92: 682–692
Fogoros R N 1980 "Runner's trots": gastrointestinal disturbances in runners. Journal of the American Medical Association 243: 1743–1744
Forrest J A H, Finlayson N D C 1974 The investigation of acute upper gastrointestinal haemorrhage. British Journal of Hospital Medicine 12: 160–165
Forrest J A H, Finlayson N D C, Shearman D J C 1974 Endoscopy in gastrointestinal bleeding. Lancet 2: 394–397

Fort E, Sautereau D, Silvain C, Ingrand P, Pillegand B, Beauchant M 1990 A randomized trial of terlipressin plus nitroglycerin vs balloon tamponade in the control of acute variceal hemorrhage. Hepatology 11: 678–681
Foster D N, Miloszewski K J A, Losowsky M S 1978 Stigmata of recent haemorrhage in diagnosis and prognosis of upper gastrointestinal bleeding. British Medical Journal 1: 1173–1177
Freeman J G, Cobden I, Record C O 1989 Placebo-controlled trial of terlipressin (Glypressin) in the management of acute variceal bleeding. Journal of Clinical Gastroenterology 11: 58–60
Freitas D, Donato A, Monteiro J G 1985 Controlled trial of liquid monopolar electrocoagulation in bleeding peptic ulcers. American Journal of Gastroenterology 80: 853–857
Frey C F, Ernst C, Lindenauer S M, Bartlett J, Bookstein J 1967 Use of arteriography in the diagnosis of occult gastrointestinal and traumatic intra-abdominal hemorrhage. American Journal of Surgery 113: 137–148
Gabriel S E, Jaakkimainen L, Bombardier C 1991 Risk for serious gastrointestinal complications related to use of nonsteroidal anti-inflammatory drugs: a meta-analysis. Annals of Internal Medicine 115: 787–796
Garden O J, Motyl H, Gilmour W H, Utley R J, Carter D C 1985 Prediction of outcome following acute variceal haemorrhage. British Journal of Surgery 72: 91–95
Ghahremani G G 1986 Radiology of Meckel's diverticulum. Critical Review of Diagnostic Imaging 26: 1–43
Gilbert D A 1990 Epidemiology of upper gastrointestinal bleeding. Gastrointestinal Endoscopy 36 (suppl): S8–S13
Gilliam J H III, Geisinger K R, Wu W C, Weidner N, Richter J E 1989 Endoscopic biopsy is diagnostic in gastric antral vascular ectasia: the "watermelon stomach". Digestive Diseases and Sciences 34: 885–888
Gimson A E S, Vlavianos T 1992 Resuscitative measures in acute variceal haemorrhage. Gastrointestinal Endoscopy Clinics of North America 2: 31–41
Gimson A E S, Westaby D, Hegarty J, Watson A, Williams R 1986 A randomized trial of vasopressin and vasopressin plus nitroglycerin in the control of acute variceal hemorrhage. Hepatology 6: 410–413
Goff J S, Thompson J S, Pratt C S, Tomasso G I, Penn I 1982 Jejunal rupture caused by a Sengstaken–Blakemore tube. Gastroenterology 82: 573–575
Gostout C J 1988 Acute gastrointestinal bleeding. A common problem revisited. Mayo Clinic Proceedings 63: 596–604
Gostout C J, Ahlquist D A, Radford C M, Bowyer B A, Viggiano T R, Balm R K 1989 Endoscopic laser therapy for watermelon stomach. Gastroenterology 96: 1462–1465
Gouge T H, Ranson J H C 1986 Esophageal transection and paraesophagogastric devascularization for bleeding esophageal varices. American Journal of Surgery 151: 47–54
Graham D Y, Smith J L 1981 The course of patients after variceal hemorrhage. Gastroenterology 80: 800–809
Griffin M R, Piper J M, Daugherty J R, Snowden M, Ray W A 1991 Nonsteroidal anti-inflammatory drug use and increased risk for peptic ulcer disease in elderly persons. Annals of Internal Medicine 114: 257–263
Hayes P C 1996 The coming of age of band ligation for oesophageal varices. All the evidence shows it has better outcomes than injection sclerotherapy. British Medical Journal 312: 1111–1113
Hayes P C, Westaby D, Williams R 1988 Effect and mechanism of action of Isosorbide-5-mononitrate. Gut 29: 752–755
Hayllar J, Bjarnason I 1995 NSAIDs, Cox-2 inhibitors, and the gut. Lancet 346: 521–522
Henry D A, O'Connell D L 1989 Effects of fibrinolytic inhibitors on mortality from upper gastrointestinal haemorrhage. British Medical Journal 298: 1142–1146
Herner B, Källgärd B, Lauritzen G 1965 Haematemesis and melaena from a limited reception area during a 5 year period. Acta Medica Scandinavica 177: 483–492
Hewitt P E, Machin S J 1990 Massive blood transfusion. British Medical Journal 300: 107–109
Hoffmann J, Beck H, Jensen H-E 1984 Dieulafoy's lesion. Surgery, Gynecology and Obstetrics 159: 537–540
Hollander D, Tarnawski A 1986 Dietary essential fatty acids and the decline in peptic ulcer disease – a hypothesis. Gut 27: 239–242
Hosking S W, Yung M Y, Chung S C, Li A K C 1992 Differing prevalence of Helicobacter in bleeding and nonbleeding ulcers. Gastroenterology 102 (suppl): A85
Hunt P S 1984 Surgical management of bleeding chronic peptic ulcer. A 10-year prospective study. Annals of Surgery 199: 44–50
Hunt P S, Korman M G, Hansky J, Marshall R D, Peck G S, McCann W J 1979 Bleeding duodenal ulcer: reduction in mortality with a planned approach. British Journal of Surgery 66: 633–635
Ibrahim I M, Raccuia J S, Micale J, Zafar A 1989 Primary aortoduodenal fistula. Diagnosis by computed tomography. Archives of Surgery 124: 870–871
Imperale T F, Ransohoff D F 1988 Aortic stenosis, idiopathic gastrointestinal bleeding and angiodysplasia: is there an association? A methodologic critique of the literature. Gastroenterology 95: 1670–1676
Jabbari M, Cherry R, Lough J O, Daly D S, Kinnear D G, Goresky C A 1984 Gastric antral vascular ectasia: the watermelon stomach. Gastroenterology 87: 1165–1170
Jalan R, John T G, Redhead D N, Garden O J, Finlayson N D C, Hayes P C 1994 A comparative study of TIPSS and oesophageal transection in the management of uncontrolled variceal haemorrhage. Gut 35: W43
Jeans P L, Padbury R T A, Toouli J 1991 A prospective evaluation of the management of bleeding peptic ulcer. Australian and New Zealand Journal of Surgery 61: 187–193
Jensen D M, You S, Pelayo E, Jensen M E 1992 The prevalence of *Helicobacter pylori* and NSAID use in patients with severe UGI hemorrhage and their potential role in recurrence of ulcer bleeding. Gastroenterology 102 (suppl): A90
Johnson D A 1989 Fecal occult blood testing: problems, pitfalls and diagnostic concerns. Postgraduate Medicine 85: 287–288, 293–299
Johnston G W 1982 Six years' experience of oesophageal transection for oesophageal varices, using a circular stapling gun. Gut 23: 770–773
Jones F A 1956 Hematemesis and melena: with special reference to causation and to the factors influencing the mortality from bleeding peptic ulcers. Gastroenterology 30: 166–190
Katz P O, Salas L 1993 Less frequent causes of upper gastrointestinal bleeding. Gastroenterology Clinics of North America 22: 875—889
Keagy B A, Schwartz J A, Johnson G Jr 1986 Should ablative operations be used for bleeding esophageal varices? Annals of Surgery 203: 463–469
Koehler P R, Salmon R B 1967 Angiographic localization of unknown acute gastrointestinal bleeding sites. Radiology 89: 244–249
Koyama K, Takagi Y, Ouchi K, Sato T 1980 Results of esophageal transection for esophageal varices. Experience of 100 cases. American Journal of Surgery 139: 204–209
LaBerge J M, Ring E J, Gordon J L et al 1993 Creation of transjugular intrahepatic portosystemic shunts with the Wallstent endoprosthesis: results in 100 patients. Radiology 187: 413–420
Laine L 1987 Multipolar electrocoagulation in the treatment of active upper gastrointestinal tract hemorrhage. New England Journal of Medicine 316: 1613–1617
Laine L A 1989 Multipolar electrocoagulation in the treatment of peptic ulcers with nonbleeding visible vessels: a prospective controlled trial. Annals of Internal Medicine 110: 510–514
Laine L, Peterson W L 1994 Bleeding peptic ulcer. New England Journal of Medicine 331: 717–727
Landefeld C S, Rosenblatt M V, Goldman L 1989 Bleeding in outpatients treated with Warfarin: relation to the prothrombin time and important remediable lesions. American Journal of Medicine 87: 153–159
Langman M J S, Weil J, Wainwright P et al 1994 Risks of bleeding peptic ulcer associated with individual non-steroidal anti-inflammatory drugs. Lancet 343: 1075–1078
Laporte J-R, Carné X, Vidal X, Moreno V, Juan J 1991 Upper gastrointestinal bleeding in relation to previous use of analgesics and non-steroidal anti-inflammatory drugs. Catalan Countries Study on Upper Gastrointestinal Bleeding. Lancet 337: 85–89
Lebrec D, De Fleury P, Rueff B, Nahum H, Benhamou J-P 1980 Portal hypertension, size of esophageal varices and risk of gastrointestinal bleeding in alcoholic cirrhosis. Gastroenterology 79: 1139–1144
Lewis B S 1994 Small intestinal bleeding. Gastroenterology Clinics of North America 23: 67–91

Lin H J, Lee F Y, Tsai Y T, Lee S D, Lee C H, Kang W M 1989 Therapeutic endoscopy for Dieulafoy's disease. Journal of Clinical Gastroenterology 11: 507–510

Lin H J, Lee F Y, Kang W M, Tsai Y T, Lee S D, Lee C H 1990 Heat probe thermocoagulation and pure alcohol injection in massive peptic ulcer haemorrhage: a prospective randomised controlled trial. Gut 31: 753–757

Lin H J, Perng C L, Lee F Y et al 1993 Endoscopic injection for the arrest of peptic ulcer hemorrhage: final results of a prospective, randomized comparative trial. Gastrointestinal Endoscopy 39: 15–19

Logan R F A, Finlayson N D C 1976 Death in acute upper gastrointestinal bleeding. Can endoscopy reduce mortality? Lancet 1: 1173–1175

Lundsgaard-Hansen P 1992 Treatment of acute blood loss. Vox Sanguinis 63: 241–246

Mäkelä J, Laitinen S, Kairaluoma M I 1992 Complications of peptic ulcer disease before and after the introduction of H2-receptor antagonists. Hepato-Gastroenterology 39: 144–148

Mallory A, Schaefer J W, Cohen J R, Holt S A, Norton L W 1980 Selective intra-arterial vasopressin infusion for upper gastrointestinal tract hemorrhage. Archives of Surgery 115: 30–32

Mallory G K, Weiss S 1929 Hemorrhages from lacerations of the cardia orifice of the stomach due to vomiting. American Journal of the Medical Sciences 178: 506–515

Markisz J A, Front D, Royal H D, Sacks B, Parker J A, Kolodny G M 1982 An evaluation of $99^{m}$-Tc labeled red blood cell scintigraphy for the detection and localization of gastrointestinal bleeding sites. Gastroenterology 83: 394–398

Marks C 1976 The anatomical basis for portal decompressive surgery. Annals of the Royal College of Surgeons of England 58: 293–299

Masson J, Bramley P N, Herd K et al 1996 Upper gastrointestinal bleeding in an open-access dedicated unit. Journal of the Royal College of Physicians of London 30: 436–442

Matthewson K, Swain C P, Bland M, Kirkham J S, Bown S G, Northfield T C 1990 Randomized comparison of Nd-Yag laser, heater probe and no endoscopic therapy for bleeding peptic ulcers. Gastroenterology 98: 1239–1244

McCormick P A, Dick R, Panagou E B et al 1994 Emergency transjugular intrahepatic portasystemic stent shunting as salvage treatment for uncontrolled variceal bleeding. British Journal of Surgery 81: 1324–1327

McCormick P A, Jenkins S A, McIntyre N, Burroughs A K 1995 Why portal hypertensive varices bleed and bleed: a hypothesis. Gut 36: 100–103

Mitchell K J, Macdougall B R D, Silk D B A, Williams R 1978 Importance of repeated endoscopy in determining the source of haemorrhage in portal hypertension. Gut 19: A955

Moreau R, Lee S, Hadengue A, Ozier Y, Sicot C, Lebrec D 1989 Relationship between oxygen transport and oxygen uptake in patients with cirrhosis: effects of vasoactive drugs. Hepatology 9: 427–432

Moretó M, Zaballa M, Ibañez S, Setién F, Figa M 1987 Efficacy of monopolar electrocoagulation in the treatment of bleeding gastric ulcer: a controlled trial. Endoscopy 19: 54–56

Morris A J, Wasson L A, MacKenzie J F 1992 Small bowel enteroscopy in undiagnosed gastrointestinal blood loss. Gut 33: 887–889

Morris D L, Hawker P C, Brearley S, Simms M, Dykes P W, Keighley M R B 1984 Optimal timing of operation for bleeding peptic ulcer: a prospective randomised trial. British Medical Journal 288: 1277–1280

Netterville R E, Hardy J D, Martin R S Jr 1968 Small bowel hemorrhage. Annals of Surgery 167: 949–957

Novis B H, Duys P, Barbezat G O, Clain J, Bank S, Terblanche J 1976 Fibreoptic endoscopy and the use of the Sengstaken tube in acute gastrointestinal haemorrhage in patients with portal hypertension and varices. Gut 17: 258–263

Orloff M J, Duguay L R, Kosta L D 1977 Criteria for selection of patients for emergency portacaval shunt. American Journal of Surgery 134: 146–152

Panés J, Terés J, Bosch A, Rodés J 1988 Efficacy of balloon tamponade in treatment of bleeding gastric and esophageal varices. Results in 151 consecutive episodes. Digestive Diseases and Sciences 33: 454–459

Papp J P 1982 Endoscopic electrocoagulation in the management of upper gastrointestinal tract bleeding. Surgical Clinics of North America 62: 797–806

Parks T G 1969 Natural history of diverticular disease of the colon: a review of 521 cases. British Medical Journal 4: 639–642

Patchett S E, Enright H, Afdhal N, O'Connell W, O'Donoghue D P 1989 Clot lysis by gastric juice: an in vitro study. Gut 30: 1704–1707

Peterson W L 1994 Prevention of upper gastrointestinal bleeding. New England Journal of Medicine 330: 428–429

Piper J M, Ray W A, Daugherty J R, Griffin M R 1991 Corticosteroid use and peptic ulcer disease: role of nonsteroidal anti-inflammatory drugs. Annals of Internal Medicine 114: 735–740

Pointer R, Schwab G, Königsrainer A, Dietze O 1988 Endoscopic treatment of Dieulafoy's disease. Gastroenterology 94: 563–566

Ponka J L 1956 Intussusception due to invaginated Meckel's diverticulum. American Journal of Surgery 92: 545–557

Pumphrey C W, Beck E R 1980 Raised blood urea concentration indicates considerable blood loss in acute upper gastrointestinal haemorrhage. British Medical Journal 1: 527–528

Rabe F E, Becker G J, Besgozzi M, Miller R E 1981 Efficacy study of the small bowel examination. Radiology 140: 47–50

Rajgopal C, Palmer K R 1991 Endoscopic injection sclerosis: effective treatment for bleeding peptic ulcer. Gut 32: 727–729

Rajgopal C, Lessels A M, Palmer K R 1992 Mechanisms of action of injection therapy for bleeding peptic ulcer. British Journal of Surgery 79: 782–784

Ready J B, Robertson A D, Goff J S, Rector W G Jr 1991 Assessment of the risk of bleeding from esophageal varices by continuous monitoring of portal pressure. Gastroenterology 100: 1403–1410

Reilly H F III, Al-Kawas F H 1991 Dieulafoy's lesion: diagnosis and management. Digestive Diseases and Sciences 36: 1702–1707

Robertson J D, Maughan R J, Davidson R J L 1987 Faecal blood loss in response to exercise. British Medical Journal 295: 303–305

Roche M, Layrisse M 1966 The nature and causes of "hookworm anemia". American Journal of Tropical Medicine and Hygiene 15: 1029–1100

Rockall T A, Logan R F A, Devlin H B, Northfield T C 1995 Incidence of and mortality from acute upper gastrointestinal haemorrhage in the United Kingdom. British Medical Journal 311: 222–226

Rockall T A, Logan R F A, Devlin H B, Northfield T C 1996 Risk assessment after upper gastrointestinal haemorrhage. Gut 38: 316–321

Rockey D C, Cello J P 1993 Evaluation of the gastrointestinal tract in patients with iron deficient anemia. New England Journal of Medicine 329: 1691–1695

Rogers B H 1980 Endoscopic diagnosis and therapy of mucosal vascular abnormalities of the gastrointestinal tract occurring in elderly patients and associated with cardiac, vascular and pulmonary disease. Gastrointestinal Endoscopy 26: 134–138

Rosekrans P C, deRooy D J, Bosman F T, Eulderink F, Cats A 1980 Gastrointestinal telangiectasia as a cause of severe blood loss in systemic sclerosis. Endoscopy 12: 200–204

Rutgeerts P, Vantrappen G, Geboes K, Broeckaert L 1981 Safety and efficacy of Neodymium-Yag laser photocoagulation: an experimental study in dogs. Gut 22: 38–44

Rutgeerts P, Vantrappen G, Broeckaert L et al 1982 Controlled trial of YAG laser treatment of upper digestive hemorrhage. Gastroenterology 83: 410–416

Rutgeerts P, Van Gompel F, Geboes K, Vantrappen G, Broeckaert L, Coremans G 1985 Long term results of treatment of vascular malformations of the gastrointestinal tract by Neodymium Yag laser photocoagulation. Gut 26: 586–593

Sanderson J D, Taylor R F H, Pugh S, Vicary F R 1990 Specialized gastrointestinal units for the management of upper gastrointestinal haemorrhage. Postgraduate Medical Journal 66: 654–656

Schiff L, Stevens R J, Shapiro N, Goodman S 1942 Observations on the oral administration of citrated blood in man. II. The effect on the stools. American Journal of the Medical Sciences 203: 409–412

Schiller K F R, Truelove S C, Williams D G 1970 Haematemesis and melaena, with special reference to factors influencing the outcome. British Medical Journal 2: 7–14

Schwartz A E, Vanagunas A, Kamel P L 1990 Endoscopy to evaluate gastrointestinal bleeding in marathon runners. Annals of Internal Medicine 113: 632–633

Sengstaken R W, Blakemore A H 1950 Balloon Tamponade for the control of hemorrhage from esophageal varices. Annals of Surgery 131: 781–789

Shorrock C J, Langman M J S, Warlow C 1992 Risks of upper GI bleeding during TIA prophylaxis with aspirin. Gastroenterology 102 (suppl): A165

Silverstein F E, Auth D C, Rubin C E, Protell R L 1976 High power argon laser treatment via standard endoscopes. 1. A preliminary study of efficacy in control of experimental erosive bleeding. Gastroenterology 71: 558–563

Silverstein F E, Protell R L, Gilbert D A et al 1979 Argon vs. neodymium YAG laser photocoagulation of experimental canine gastric ulcers. Gastroenterology 77: 491–496

Silverstein F E, Gilbert D A, Tedesco F J, Buenger N K, Persing J 1981 The national ASGE survey on upper gastrointestinal bleeding. II. Clinical prognostic factors. Gastrointestinal Endoscopy 27: 80–93

Simpson K J, Chalmers N, Redhead D N, Dillon J F, Finlayson N D C, Hayes P C 1994 Emergency transjugular intrahepatic portasystemic stent shunts to control acute variceal haemorrhage resistant to sclerotherapy. European Journal of Gastroenterology and Hepatology 6: 423–428

Sniderman K W, Franklin J Jr, Sos T A 1978 Successful transcatheter gelfoam embolization of a bleeding cecal vascular ectasia. American Journal of Roentgenology 131: 157–159

Söderlund C, Magnusson I, Törngren S, Lundell L 1990 Terlipressin (triglycyl-lysine vasopressin) controls acute bleeding oesophageal varices. A double-blind, randomized, placebo-controlled trial. Scandinavian Journal of Gastroenterology 25: 622–630

Somerville K, Faulkner G, Langman M 1986 Non-steroidal anti-inflammatory drugs and bleeding peptic ulcer. Lancet 1: 462–464

Spence R A J 1984 The venous anatomy of the lower oesophagus in normal subjects and in patients with varices: an image analysis study. British Journal of Surgery 71: 739–744

Strong R W 1984 Dieulafoy's disease: a distinct clinical entity. Australian and New Zealand Journal of Surgery 54: 337–339

Sugawa C, Werner M H, Hayes N F, Lucas C E, Walt A J 1973 Early endoscopy. A guide to therapy for acute hemorrhage in the upper gastrointestinal tract. Archives of Surgery 107: 133–137

Sugawa C, Benishek D, Walt A J 1983 Mallory Weiss syndrome. A study of 224 patients. American Journal of Surgery 145: 30–33

Sugiura M, Futagawa S 1977 Further evaluation of the Sugiura procedure in the treatment of esophageal varices. Archives of Surgery 112: 1317–1321

Swain C P, Bown S G, Storey D W, Kirkham J S, Northfield T C, Salmon P R 1981 Controlled trial of argon laser photocoagulation in bleeding peptic ulcers. Lancet 2: 1313–1316

Swain C P, Storey D W, Bown S G et al 1986a Nature of the bleeding vessel in recurrently bleeding gastric ulcers. Gastroenterology 90: 595–608

Swain C P, Kirkham J S, Salmon P R, Bown S G, Northfield T C 1986b Controlled trial of Nd-Yag laser photocoagulation for bleeding peptic ulcers. Lancet 1: 1113–1116

Swain C P, Lai K C, Kalabakas A, Grandison A, Pollock D 1993 A comparison of size and the pathology of vessel and ulcer in patients dying from bleeding gastric and duodenal ulcers. Gastroenterology 104 (suppl): A202

Tarin D, Allison D J, Modlin I M, Neale G 1978 Diagnosis and management of obscure gastrointestinal bleeding. British Medical Journal 2: 751–754

Terés J, Cecilia A, Bordas J M, Rimola A, Bru C, Rodés J 1978 Esophageal tamponade for bleeding varices. Control trial between the Sengstaken–Blakemore tube and the Linton–Nachlas tube. Gastroenterology 75: 566–569

Thompson J N, Selem P R, Hemingway A P et al 1987 Specialist investigation of obscure gastrointestinal bleeding. Gut 28: 47–51

Tsai Y T, Lay C S, Lai K H et al 1986 Controlled trial of vasopressin plus nitroglycerin vs vasopressin alone in the treatment of bleeding esophageal varices. Hepatology 6: 406–409

Tschirren B, Affolter U, Elsasser R et al 1974 Der klinische plasmaersatz mit gelatin: zwolf jahre erfahrungen mit 3932. Einheiten Physiogel Infusionstherapie 1: 651–662

Uflacker R, Mourao G S, Piske R L 1989 Hemobilia: transcatheter occlusive therapy and longterm follow-up. Cardiovascular Intervention Radiology 12: 136–141

Umeyama K, Yoshikawa K, Yamashita T, Todo T, Satake K 1983 Transabdominal oesophageal transection for oesophageal varices: experience in 101 patients. British Journal of Surgery 70: 419–422

Valenzuela J E, Schubert T, Fogel M R et al 1989 A multicenter, randomized, double-blind trial of somatostatin in the management of acute hemorrhage from esophageal varices. Hepatology 10: 958–961

Vallon A G, Cotton P B, Laurence B H, Armengol Miro J R, Oses J C S 1981 Randomised trial of endoscopic argon laser photocoagulation in bleeding peptic ulcers. Gut 22: 228–233

Van Cutsem E, Rutgeerts P, Vantrappen G 1990 Treatment of bleeding gastrointestinal vascular malformations with oestrogen-progesterone. Lancet 335: 953–955

Vinel J P, Cassigneul J, Levade M, Voigt J J, Pascal J P 1986 Assessment of short-term prognosis after variceal bleeding in patients with alcoholic cirrhosis by early measurement of portohepatic gradient. Hepatology 6: 116–117

Waldram R, Davis M, Nunnerley H, Williams R 1974 Emergency endoscopy after gastrointestinal haemorrhage in 50 patients with portal hypertension. British Medical Journal 4: 94–96

Wara P 1985 Endoscopic prediction of major rebleeding – a prospective study of stigmata of hemorrhage in bleeding ulcer. Gastroenterology 88: 1209–1214

Wara P, Stødkilde H 1985 Bleeding pattern before admission as guideline for emergency endoscopy. Scandinavian Journal of Gastroenterology 20: 72–78

Watts H D 1976 Lesions brought on by vomiting: the effect of hiatus hernia on the site of bleeding. Gastroenterology 71: 683–688

Welch G H, McArdle C S, Anderson J R 1987 Balloon tamponade for the control of Mallory–Weiss haemorrhage in patients with coagulation defects. British Journal of Surgery 74: 610–611

Westaby D, Gimson A, Hayes P C, Williams R 1988 Haemodynamic response to intravenous vasopressin and nitroglycerin in portal hypertension. Gut 29: 372–377

Westaby D, Hayes P C, Gimson A E S, Polson R J, Williams R 1989 Controlled clinical trial of injection sclerotherapy for active variceal bleeding. Hepatology 9: 274–277

Whelan R L, Buls J G, Goldberg S M 1989 Intra-operative endoscopy: University of Minnesota experience. American Surgeon 55: 281–286

Yoshida J, Donohue P E, Nyhus L M 1987 Hemobilia: review of recent experience with a worldwide problem. American Journal of Gastroenterology 82: 448–453

Zambartas C, Cregeen R J, Forrest J A H, Finlayson N D C 1982 Accuracy of early endoscopy in acute upper gastrointestinal bleeding. British Medical Journal 285: 1540

Zuckerman G R, Cornette G L, Clouse E, Harler H R 1985 Upper gastrointestinal bleeding in patients with chronic renal failure. Annals of Internal Medicine 102: 588–592

# 18. The acute abdomen

*D. C. Carter*

In this chapter, the principles of assessment and management of the acute abdomen are defined and specific problems considered in detail. Common causes of acute abdominal pain are shown in Table 18.1. Some specific causes such as perforated peptic ulcer, cholecystitis, acute pancreatitis and diverticular disease are considered separately elsewhere and are only mentioned here in terms of the differential diagnosis of abdominal pain.

## PRINCIPLES OF ASSESSMENT

### History and examination

A full history and thorough physical examination are the basis of diagnosis and successful management. Pain and tenderness are of central importance and their origin and significance will be discussed.

*Abdominal pain*

The perception of abdominal pain is subserved by both the autonomic (visceral pain) and somatic nervous systems (parietal pain).

***Visceral abdominal pain*** is evoked by distention of hollow viscera and excessive contraction of their muscle wall. Inflammation and stretching of the peritoneum, ischemia and traction on the mesentery can also produce pain. In some conditions such as peptic ulceration, the mechanism of pain production is uncertain.

Colic is produced when a hollow organ such as the gut, gallbladder or ureter undergoes waves of excessive smooth muscle contraction, usually as a consequence of obstruction and distention. Pain is experienced in the region of the abdomen which reflects the embryonic development of the viscus. For example, colic originating in organs derived from the embryonic foregut is appreciated in the epigastrium, midgut colic is felt in the periumbilical region and hindgut colic is appreciated in the hypogastrium (Fig. 18.1). This explains why the initial pain of acute appendicitis is felt typically in the perium-

**Table 18.1** Common causes of acute abdominal pain (data drawn from series of 1204 patients reported by Dixon et al 1991)

| Diagnosis | No. of patients |
|---|---|
| Nonspecific abdominal pain | 463 |
| Acute appendicitis | 449 |
| Renal colic | 61 |
| Gynecological disorders | 44 |
| Intestinal obstruction | 32 |
| Urinary tract infection | 30 |
| Gallbladder disease | 12 |
| Perforated ulcer/dyspepsia | 10 |
| Diverticular disease | 6 |
| Other diagnoses | 58 |
| No diagnosis established | 39 |

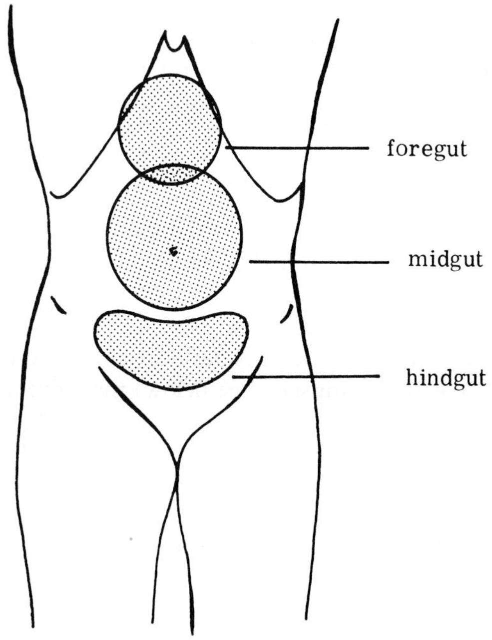


**Fig. 18.1** Site of appreciation of abdominal colic according to the area of gut involved.

bilical region despite the fact that the appendix lies in the right iliac fossa or pelvis. Visceral pain is dull, deepseated and poorly localized. The sympathetic nerves responsible for its mediation are derived from segments T5 to L2 of the spinal cord and their nerve endings lie in visceral muscle. The vagus nerve has no role in the appreciation of visceral pain.

***Parietal abdominal pain*** results from inflammation of the parietal peritoneum. The parietal peritoneum is innervated by the spinal nerves which supply the overlying abdominal wall and parietal pain is localized to the area affected. The eventual development of pain and tenderness in the right iliac fossa in acute appendicitis reflects the onset of inflammation of the parietal peritoneum.

### *Abdominal tenderness*

Abdominal tenderness and associated muscle guarding are the most reliable signs of peritonitis. The need to examine the patient before an analgesic is given has been overemphasized and on no account should a patient be left in pain while awaiting examination. Effective analgesia usually makes evaluation easier, particularly in children.

Inflammation of the peritoneum lining the anterior abdominal wall is readily detectable because tenderness and guarding are elicited so readily. Detection of peritonitis in "nondemonstrative" areas is more difficult. For example, pelvic peritonitis may produce little or no tenderness or guarding on abdominal examination (although tenderness may be elicited on digital rectal examination). Inflammation of the diaphragmatic peritoneum may not give rise to abdominal tenderness or guarding but is suggested by shoulder-tip pain and hyperesthesia and by clinical or radiological evidence of restriction of diaphragmatic movement. The referral of pain to the shoulder tip is explained by the common segmental origin (C3, 4 and 5) of nerves supplying the diaphragm and shoulder area.

Peritonitis involving the posterior parietal peritoneum may also produce few signs on abdominal examination (e.g. inflammation confined to the lesser sac in acute pancreatitis). Inflammation of the posterolateral parietal peritoneum (e.g. in retrocecal appendicitis) may also give rise to little abdominal tenderness but restriction of movement of the psoas major muscle (see below) may give a clue to its presence.

While guarding and rigidity of the anterior abdominal wall usually denote peritonitis, they are also present in some cases of renal colic, neurological disorders, hysterical overlay and malingering. The muscle spasm of renal colic defies ready explanation but is usually confined to the rectus muscle of the affected side.

***Murphy's sign*** is positive when tenderness in the right hypochondrium is elicited as the patient breathes in and the inflamed gallbladder moves down into contact with the examiner's hand. About 85% of patients with acute cholecystitis are tender in the right hypochondrium, although only 60% have tenderness confined to this area (Staniland et al 1972). Localized tenderness in the right hypochondrium is unusual in any other condition.

***Rebound tenderness*** denotes parietal peritonitis but its value is controversial and some surgeons believe that sharp localized pain on coughing (a "positive cough test") may be at least as reliable a sign (Jeddy et al 1994). Staniland et al (1972) elicited rebound tenderness in only 39% of patients with a perforated peptic ulcer, while Dixon et al (1991) found rebound tenderness in only 53% of patients with acute appendicitis and in 25% of those without appendicitis. On the other hand, Jones (1969) elicited rebound tenderness in 80% of children with acute appendicitis, but in only 1% of those with nonspecific causes for abdominal pain, suggesting that the sign can be of value if carefully elicited and interpreted.

***Rovsing's sign*** is positive when deep palpation of the left iliac fossa produces pain in the right iliac fossa in patients with acute appendicitis. In practice the sign is inconstant and unreliable.

***The iliopsoas test*** can be used to detect inflammation which restricts movement of the iliopsoas muscle. The patient lies on the unaffected side and the contralateral iliopsoas is stretched by fully extending the thigh. Pain is elicited in some cases of retrocecal appendicitis and perinephric abscess and the patient may even lie with the hip flexed on the affected side to avoid stretching the inflamed iliopsoas muscle.

***Carnett's test*** can help to determine whether abdominal tenderness is of parietal or visceral origin, although it is of more value in patients with chronic abdominal pain (Thomson et al 1991). The site of maximum tenderness is defined and the patient is then asked to cross his arms and sit halfway forwards. If further palpation elicits greater tenderness the sign is positive and the problem is likely to lie in the abdominal wall; if there is less tenderness once the abdominal wall muscles are tensed, the problem is more likely to lie within the peritoneal cavity.

### *Pitfalls in assessment of the acute abdomen*

***Misinterpretation of vital signs.*** The temperature is frequently normal in the early stages of peritonitis and in shocked patients may be normal or even subnormal. Tachycardia is a relatively late sign of peritonitis and a normal pulse rate does not exclude infection. Infection usually causes leukocytosis, but a normal white cell count does not exclude early peritonitis. Lee (1973) found that 18% of patients with acute appendicitis had leukocyte counts of less than $10 \times 10^9$ L (10 000/mm$^3$) at the time of admission.

***Failure to distinguish between intrathoracic and***

***intra-abdominal disease.*** Pleurisy, pneumonia and myocardial disease, especially myocardial infarction, may produce abdominal pain. The true source of pain is reflected in associated symptoms such as dyspnea, cough and production of purulent sputum or by finding a pleural rub, crepitations, consolidation or a triple rhythm. However, these clues may be absent and a chest radiograph should be obtained in all patients presenting with acute abdominal pain. An electrocardiogram is indicated if diagnostic doubt remains.

***Failure to examine the mouth, throat and ears.*** Abdominal pain and vomiting are not infrequent early features of otitis media, influenza and pharyngitis in children and cervical lymphadenopathy should be sought routinely.

***Inadequate auscultation.*** Repeated auscultation may be needed to assess changes in peristaltic activity. Peristalsis is increased in mechanical intestinal obstruction and gastroenteritis and when there is blood in the gut. Activity ceases in paralytic ileus, but movement of the patient can cause fluid to spill from one distended loop to another, producing a sound not unlike that of peristaltic activity.

***Failure to examine the groin.*** Groin herniae are easily overlooked and the patient may not be aware that they have a small femoral hernia. A small groin lump is easily missed on examination when the clinical picture is dominated by the central abdominal colic of small bowel obstruction.

Tuberculous pus tracking down the psoas sheath into the groin is now exceptionally rare, but colonic neoplasms occasionally perforate retroperitoneally, producing crepitus and erythema in the groin. The external genitalia must be examined routinely and the presence of both testes in the scrotum confirmed. Femoral artery pulsation should be recorded, noting any asymmetry between the two sides.

***Failure to carry out digital rectal examination.*** Dixon and colleagues (1991) found that in patients with right lower quadrant pain, digital rectal examination added little to their ability to diagnose acute appendicitis once rebound tenderness had been assessed. However, most would argue that rectal examination is still essential in all patients presenting with acute abdominal pain. Rectal tenderness can be decisive in diagnosing pelvic appendicitis, cervical tenderness may indicate salpingitis and pelvic masses may be palpable. Fecal impaction can be excluded, the state of the prostate can be assessed and a specimen of stool can be obtained for occult blood testing. The need for proctoscopy and sigmoidoscopy can also be determined following digital rectal examination.

***Failure to carry out vaginal examination.*** A full menstrual history and vaginal examination are essential when abdominal symptoms are thought to arise from disease of the uterus, fallopian tubes or ovaries. Insertion of a vaginal speculum, Gram staining of any vaginal discharge and subsequent culture and sensitivity determinations allow prompt diagnosis and management of pelvic inflammatory disease.

***Failure to reassess the patient.*** If the diagnosis and need for surgery are at first uncertain, signs and symptoms should be reassessed periodically. Jones (1976) demonstrated the value of "active observation" in 363 children admitted with acute abdominal pain; 106 had a probable surgical cause for their pain and were operated on without delay, 20 developed such evidence over 6 h of active observation and came to surgery and 237 did not require an operation. Of those operated upon, 90% had a surgical cause for abdominal pain and perforation of the appendix was found in only one patient where operation was delayed.

## Establishing a diagnosis

Once the history has been taken and the physical examination completed, an attempt should be made to define the nature of the disease process responsible and the organ or system involved. A differential diagnosis is constructed and a working diagnosis made pending the results of appropriate investigations. The need for operation can then be determined.

## Laboratory investigations

The hemoglobin concentration, hematocrit and white cell count are determined routinely. Urea and electrolyte concentrations are seldom of diagnostic significance but are useful when managing fluid and electrolyte derangements. Liver function tests are seldom available in time to influence initial management but are helpful in the subsequent evaluation of hepatobiliary and pancreatic disease. The serum amylase activity should be determined in all patients with abdominal pain of uncertain origin.

The urine must be tested routinely for glucose, acetone, protein, bilirubin and urobilinogen and for porphobilinogen if porphyria is suspected. Microscopy may reveal pus cells and bacteria in urinary tract infection and red blood cells in ureteric colic.

A specimen of stool should be tested for occult blood and stool culture for bacterial pathogens such as *Campylobacter* and *Salmonella* is indicated when diarrhoea is present.

### *Radiology*

While a chest radiograph is always advisable on admission, the value of routine abdominal films is debatable as only 10% of abdominal radiographs in unselected patients with abdominal symptoms show an abnormality. Restricting abdominal radiography to those with moderate to severe tenderness or clinical suspicion of bowel obstruction, renal or ureteric calculi, trauma, ischemia or gallbladder disease will avoid 50% of unnecessary radiographs (Eisenberg et al 1983). Erect abdominal radiographs add little to the information available on the supine view (Field et al 1985). Contrast studies are helpful if intestinal obstruction or perforation is suspected and water-soluble contrast medium such as Gastrografin is used where the gastrointestinal tract may have perforated (p. 5).

Ultrasound scanning has an established role in the diagnosis of obstetric and gynecological disorders and can provide diagnostic information not available on the plain abdominal radiograph in patients with abdominal pain (p. 59). Ultrasonography can be particularly useful in the diagnosis of acute appendicitis (Schwerk et al 1989), pancreatitis and biliary disease. Intravenous pyelography or ultrasonography may also be indicated in patients thought to have urinary tract obstruction. Angiography has been superseded by ultrasonography in the diagnosis of aortic aneurysm, but may still be indicated in the diagnosis of mesenteric vascular occlusion.

### *Fiberoptic endoscopy*

Upper gastrointestinal endoscopy is invaluable when abdominal pain is thought to be due to the peptic ulcer diathesis and may be indicated in the diagnosis and treatment of gallstone disease, including gallstone pancreatitis (p. 1265). Sigmoidoscopy and colonoscopy may be helpful in the diagnosis and management of some colorectal disorders responsible for acute abdominal pain (p. 531).

### *Computer-assisted diagnosis*

Only two-thirds of patients with acute abdominal pain present with "typical" features of their disease (Staniland et al 1972) and using a computerized database was shown to increase diagnostic accuracy from 72–80% to 92% in patients with acute abdominal pain (De Dombal et al 1972). In acute appendicitis, computer-assisted diagnosis was correct in 97% of 145 cases and reduced the rate of appendix perforation and gangrene from 40% to 5% and the negative laparotomy rate from 25% to 7% (De Dombal et al 1974). Structured history and data collection sheets may be the most important element in the success of computer-aided diagnosis (Paterson-Brown 1991), particularly when used in conjunction with a computerized teaching package (De Dombal et al 1991).

### *Other aids to diagnosis*

***Peritoneal lavage*** is an established means of assessing blunt abdominal trauma. It has not been used widely as a means of defining the cause of acute abdominal pain and is contraindicated in patients with gross distention or multiple abdominal scars.

Fine catheter aspiration is an alternative to lavage in which a small umbilical catheter is inserted under local anesthesia so that a peritoneal aspirate can be examined microscopically. An increased proportion of polymorphonuclear cells is a reliable index of acute intra-abdominal inflammation (Stewart et al 1986) and can be used to determine the need for laparotomy or laparoscopy (Paterson-Brown 1991). In one recent study, peritoneal aspiration cytology had a sensitivity of 91% and specificity of 94% in acute appendicitis and the negative appendicectomy rate was reduced to 10% overall and to 11% in women of reproductive age (Caldwell & Watson 1994).

***Laparoscopy*** (p. 126) is used increasingly in patients with acute abdominal pain. It can be carried out under local anesthesia, but is generally performed under general anesthesia. The reported complication rate for gynecological laparoscopy is about 3% with a procedure-related mortality rate of eight per 100 000 cases (Chamberlain & Carron Brown 1978) and the recent widespread adoption of laparoscopic cholecystectomy has made the technique increasingly familiar to general surgeons.

Laparoscopy undoubtedly reduces the incidence of unnecessary laparotomy (Sugarbaker et al 1975). In one early series of 32 patients in whom the diagnosis of appendicitis was uncertain, laparoscopy confirmed the diagnosis in 17 cases, revealed another disease in eight and avoided unnecessary operation in 12 patients so that the negative appendicectomy rate was reduced to 1% (Leape & Ramenofsky 1980). In patients with abdominal pain when the decision to operate is in doubt, laparoscopy can reduce management error rates to zero (Paterson-Brown et al 1986a) and is of particular value in females with suspected appendicitis (Olsen et al 1993). The normal appendix is not visible at laparoscopy in one in four cases (Paterson-Brown et al 1986b) and nonvisualization does not necessarily mean that the appendix is inflamed and has to be removed. However, even if the appendix cannot be seen, laparoscopy may reveal signs of inflammation in the right iliac fossa or detect alternative causes for abdominal pain (Paterson-Brown 1991).

## Treatment

All patients admitted with acute abdominal pain are confined to bed, given nothing by mouth and observed "actively" if urgent operation is not thought necessary. Vomiting patients may benefit from a nasogastric tube so that the stomach can be kept empty by regular aspiration. An intravenous infusion is established when there is blood loss, dehydration, electrolyte disturbance or shock and a fluid balance chart is maintained. The bladder is catheterized in shocked patients and when there is doubt about urine retention. Pulse, blood pressure, temperature and hourly urine output are recorded regularly in all shocked patients and central venous pressure (CVP) monitoring may be needed.

Antibiotics are not prescribed routinely but are reserved for specific indications. For example, they are essential in patients with acute cholecystitis (p. 1207) or perforated diverticular disease (p. 1390) but unnecessary in cases of nonspecific abdominal pain. Antibiotic therapy is commenced prior to surgery when infection is considered life-threatening, but only after blood samples have been obtained for bacteriological culture. Specimens of infected material are taken at the time of surgery so that therapy can be modified as appropriate. The use of antibiotics in the prevention of wound infection will be considered below.

Assessment of the need for laparotomy must not become the sole objective of examination; an attempt must be made to define the nature and severity of the underlying disease process. However, surgeons have to balance the desire for precise preoperative diagnosis against the penalties for delaying operation in the face of worsening intra-abdominal disease. For example, the risks of unnecessary laparotomy in mesenteric adenitis are outweighed by the dangers of gangrene and perforation when removal of an acutely inflamed appendix is unduly delayed.

The timing of operation is dictated by the nature of the disease process, by the general condition of the patient and by the need for preoperative resuscitation. Considerable delay may have occurred before the patient reaches hospital and in general, conditions requiring surgery do deteriorate with time. Delay can be disastrous following rupture of an aortic aneurysm, whereas adequate preoperative fluid and electrolyte replacement may be lifesaving for the patient with gross dehydration due to mechanical intestinal obstruction.

It cannot be overemphasized that an initial period of active observation is advisable in the large group of patients in whom the diagnosis and need for surgery are uncertain at the time of presentation. The term "nonspecific abdominal pain" is used when a cause for abdominal pain cannot be defined. Over one-third of patients presenting to hospital with abdominal pain are so classified (Adams et al 1986, Dixon et al 1991, Gunn 1991) and in many series, nonspecific abdominal pain rivals or outstrips acute appendicitis as the commonest cause of the acute abdomen.

## THE SHOCKED PATIENT

Shock can be defined as an acute alteration in the circulation leading to a state of inadequate tissue perfusion and is a common complication of acute abdominal disease. Despite the variety of mechanisms involved (Table 18.2), assessment and resuscitation are based on common principles. The aim of resuscitation is to restore the circulation to normal or acceptable levels as quickly as possible and so permit treatment of the underlying cause.

**Table 18.2** Factors contributing to shock in acute abdominal disease

1. Low flow states

*Hypovolaemia – loss of blood, plasma or water and electrolytes*

- External loss (including loss into the gut lumen)
- Sequestration
- Extravascular pooling, e.g. ruptured aneurysm, peritonitis, pancreatitis
- Intravascular pooling
- Septicemia
- Endotoxemia

*Cardiogenic factors*

- Primary myocardial failure (as a cause of nonocclusive intestinal infarction)
- Secondary myocardial failure (as a complication of shock due to hypovolemia or sepsis)

2. High flow states

*Septic shock – primary impairment of cellular oxygen uptake or utilization, with compensatory hyperdynamic circulation*

Earlier definitions of shock stressed the failure of the cardiovascular system to maintain blood flow, leading to poor tissue oxygenation and impaired organ function. This definition still applies to hypovolemic and cardiogenic shock, but septic shock may involve primary impairment of tissue oxygen uptake or utilization. The circulation in septic shock is characteristically hyperdynamic and cardiac output increases while peripheral vascular resistance falls. When sepsis complicates pre-existing hypovolemic shock, the circulation may remain hypodynamic despite the adverse effect of sepsis on tissue oxygen utilization.

### Assessment of the shocked patient

The severity of shock and response to treatment can only be assessed by regular examination of the circulation (Table 18.3).

#### *Clinical examination of the circulation*

Valuable information is obtained by inspection and palpa-

**Table 18.3** Important measurements in shocked patients

| | Normal value |
|---|---|
| Regular clinical assessment | |
| Pulse rate | 60–90 beats/min |
| Arterial blood pressure | Systolic 110–140 mmHg<br>Diastolic 60–95 mmHg |
| Central venous pressure | 5–10 $cmH_2O$ |
| Hourly urine output | 30–50 ml/h |
| Hematocrit | 40–54% |
| Arterial blood | |
| Hydrogen ion | 36–44 nmol/L |
| pH | 7.37–7.43 |
| $PO_2$ | 12–15 kPa (90–113 mmHg) |
| $PCO_2$ | 4.4–5.6 kPa (33–42 mmHg) |
| Base excess | +2.3 mmol/L (mEq/L) |

tion. Blood loss produces pallor and all forms of hypovolemia result in peripheral vasoconstriction with poor capillary and venous filling and cold clammy extremities. This picture contrasts with the warm dry extremities and bounding pulse of the hyperdynamic circulation of early septic shock.

Serial pulse rate and blood pressure measurements are essential and an arterial line allows continuous monitoring as well as repeated sampling for arterial blood gas analysis. Pulse rate and blood pressure must not be interpreted in isolation; blood pressure can sometimes be maintained despite critical reduction in tissue perfusion and a fall in urine output.

*Central venous pressure*

Central venous pressure (CVP) is determined by the volume of blood arriving in the great veins and the ability of the right ventricle to propel that blood into the pulmonary circulation. Trends in CVP are a valuable adjunct to management; low readings reflect hypovolemia, while a high or rapidly rising CVP denotes overtransfusion and/or impaired right ventricular function.

CVP is not a sensitive index of left ventricular function and does not give early warning of left ventricular overload. It is recognized that pulmonary venous pressure can rise until pulmonary edema occurs without increased CVP. Pulmonary capillary wedge pressure, as measured by a Swan–Ganz catheter (pulmonary artery flotation catheter), is a more reliable index of left heart function than CVP and correlates more closely with radiological signs of pulmonary congestion. A Swan–Ganz catheter also allows measurement of parameters such as right atrial pressure and cardiac output and permits calculation of pulmonary and systemic vascular resistance.

Insertion of a CVP or Swan–Ganz catheter requires meticulous aseptic technique. The tip of a CVP catheter should lie in the superior vena cava just short of the right atrium. The catheter can be introduced via the cephalic vein, but sometimes fails to pass through the clavipectoral fascia and access by the basilic, subclavian or internal jugular veins is usually preferred. Care must be taken to avoid causing pneumothorax and/or hemothorax when cannulating the subclavian vein. A chest radiograph is obtained routinely to check catheter position and detect complications. The length of catheter introduced is a useful guide to correct placement while awaiting the radiograph and the fluid level within the manometer tubing should swing freely when the patient coughs or inspires deeply.

CVP measurements are made from the level of the right atrium and the mid-axillary line is the reference point in the supine patient. An intravenous giving set attached to a three-way tap maintains catheter patency between readings. Hypovolemia is associated with a CVP of less than 5 $cmH_2O$, while circulatory overload produces pressures above 12 $cmH_2O$.

A Swan–Ganz catheter is inserted in a similar manner to a CVP catheter and has two monitoring/sampling channels. When the opening in the catheter tip lies in the pulmonary artery, the opening of the other channel lies 30 cm back in the right atrium or superior vena cava. Inflation of a balloon in the catheter tip causes it to move forwards into a "wedged" position so that pulmonary capillary wedge pressure can be measured as an index of left atrial filling pressure.

*Hourly urine output*

The value of measuring hourly urine output in shock far outweighs the hazard of introducing infection by bladder catheterization. The kidney is one of the vital organs which is deprived of blood as the body attempts to maintain perfusion of the heart and brain. An inadequate urine output can reflect hypovolemia or inadequate cardiac output (with resulting impairment of renal blood flow) or intrinsic renal failure. Oliguria is present when output falls below that required to maintain a normal blood urea or creatinine concentration. As a clinical rule of thumb, an output of less than 30 ml/h (or approximately 0.5 ml/kg/h) represents oliguria. A high urine osmolality in such circumstances indicates good renal tubular function but inadequate renal perfusion. Failure of the urine osmolality to rise in patients with oliguria points to intrinsic renal failure.

*Hematocrit*

The hematocrit is a guide to the type of fluid required rather than the volume or rate of administration. It falls after blood loss because extracellular fluid (ECF) crosses the capillaries to restore plasma volume. This process is relatively slow so that the hematocrit takes some hours to fall after acute hemorrhage (p. 482). The hematocrit rises following plasma or ECF loss, reflecting the need for crystalloid or plasma rather than blood transfusion.

Resistance to hypovolemic shock in experimental models is greatest if the animal commences with a hematocrit of 42% (Baue et al 1967). With higher hematocrits, perfusion may be impaired by red cell aggregation, while blood oxygen-carrying power is reduced when the hematocrit is low. However, recent evidence indicates that oxygen delivery to peripheral tissues is greatest with a hematocrit of 30% and isovolemic hemodilution with agents such as dextran 60 may prove valuable in conditions such as acute pancreatitis (Klar et al 1993). In practice, one should probably aim for a hematocrit of 30–35%.

*Arterial blood gases and pH*

The partial pressure of oxygen ($PaO_2$) in arterial blood is a key measurement in shock and can be monitored by a pulse oximeter attached to a finger or ear lobe. The amount of oxygen available to the tissues can be calculated as the product of cardiac output, arterial blood oxygen saturation and oxygen-carrying capacity (Nunn & Freeman 1964). The "available oxygen" is normally about 1000 ml oxygen/min:

Available oxygen = cardiac output (5.25 L/min) × arterial oxygen saturation (95/100) × hemoglobin concentration (150 g/L) × 1.34 ml/g = 1000 ml oxygen/min

The overall resting requirements for the body are only 250 ml/min, but certain tissues, notably the heart, have above average oxygen requirements. A reduction in all three parameters causes a profound fall in available oxygen, although the reduction in each parameter may not appear striking in isolation. For example, if all three are reduced by one-third, available oxygen falls to only 300 ml/min.

Inadequate tissue perfusion and oxygenation lead to anaerobic metabolism, increased lactate production and metabolic acidosis. Acid–base status is determined by measurement of arterial pH, $PCO_2$ and base excess. Blood lactate concentrations also reflect tissue oxygen debt and a high lactate may be present in sepsis despite high cardiac output and oxygen delivery.

*Core and peripheral temperature measurements*

Assessment of skin temperature by hand is a useful guide to peripheral perfusion and core and peripheral temperature measurements (by thermistor) provide an accurate index of tissue perfusion.

## Treatment of shock

Guidelines for the treatment of shock are summarized in Table 18.4. The time available for resuscitation depends on the underlying disease. Massive continuing blood loss is the most urgent indication for surgery and in the case of ruptured aortic aneurysm, stabilization of the circulation may only be possible once the aorta has been cross-clamped. Time is also vital if the blood supply is to be restored to strangulated but still viable bowel and vigorous resuscitation is essential if early surgery is to prevent continuing contamination of the peritoneum after bowel perforation. Resuscitation must never be dilatory and even in simple mechanical intestinal obstruction there is the danger that strangulation will supervene. Delayed or inadequate resuscitation exposes the shocked patient to the dangers of secondary organ failure from prolonged underperfusion and deficient oxygenation.

**Table 18.4** Guidelines for assessment and management of the shocked patient

| | |
|---|---|
| 1. | Initial clinical assessment and diagnosis |
| 2. | Establish oxygen therapy (6 L/min) |
| 3. | Establish an intravenous infusion (isotonic saline or Ringer lactate)<br>Withdraw blood for hemoglobin, hematocrit, crossmatching<br>Urea and electrolytes (sodium, potassium and bicarbonate)<br>Blood gases (if required)<br>Blood culture (except in shock due to bleeding)<br>Measurements – pulse, blood pressure, respiration rate |
| 4. | Establish a CVP line – assess response to initial rapid infusion<br>Measurement – CVP |
| 5. | Insert indwelling urinary catheter<br>Measurement – hourly urine output |
| 6. | Pass nasogastric tube<br>Measurement – fluid balance chart |
| 7. | Review:<br>General clinical state and diagnosis<br>Trends in clinical observations<br>Available laboratory data |
| 8. | Adjust management if required<br>More data needed on:<br>blood gases<br>biochemical data<br>pulmonary wedge venous pressure (Swan–Ganz catheter)<br>Alter fluid therapy<br>Institute ventilatory support |
| 9. | Consider the need for antibiotics, diuretics, digitalis, vasoactive drugs, corticosteroids |
| 10. | Undertake surgery at the optimal time determined by the balance between the urgency of the underlying disease and needs of resuscitation |

*Position of the patient*

The Trendelenburg (head-down) position improves venous return transiently but embarrasses ventilation and increases the risk of aspiration of gastric contents. The patient is best nursed supine. The stomach should be kept empty by a nasogastric tube in obstructed patients and those with persistent vomiting.

*Oxygen therapy*

Oxygen is administered continuously through a close-fitting mask. A flow rate of 4–6 L/min provides an inspired oxygen concentration of 40–60%, while flow rates of 15 L/min give an inspired oxygen concentration of 70%. Positive pressure ventilation with endotracheal intubation is needed if the $PaO_2$ remains below 8.6 kPa (65 mmHg) despite high flow oxygen therapy. Patients with chronic obstructive airway disease can be given oxygen-enriched air, but care must be taken to avoid carbon dioxide retention.

*Establishing intravenous infusion*

At least one free-flowing line other than a CVP line is established. Venoconstriction may dictate the use of central veins and more than one line may be needed to contend with major continuing blood loss.

### *Choice of fluid replacement*

Blood is taken on admission for grouping and crossmatching and measurement of blood urea and electrolyte concentrations and blood gases. The hematocrit can help to determine the need for blood transfusion, bearing in mind the timescale of compensatory hemodilution (p. 482).

The objective of resuscitation in hypovolemic shock is to replace the type of fluid lost and the problem is simplified if the nature of the underlying abdominal disease is known. For example, blood is needed following rupture of an ectopic pregnancy, plasma and crystalloid are usually needed in acute pancreatitis (p. 1263), while crystalloid alone will replace ECF losses in mechanical intestinal obstruction. In septic shock, crystalloid and colloid (and on occasions, blood) may be needed to maintain the compensatory hyperdynamic state.

The intravenous infusion is established with isotonic saline or Ringer lactate solution. The priorities are to ensure an adequate venous return and maintain cardiac output. Provided that the initial CVP reading is not high, 500–1000 ml of crystalloid is infused over 30 min while CVP is monitored. A persistently low CVP indicates a continuing volume deficit, a rise into the normal range indicates that venous return is adequate, for the moment at least, while an abnormally high or rising CVP is a warning of overtransfusion or cardiac failure which may require diuretics and inotropic agents.

***Blood transfusion*** is indicated if there are signs of major blood loss and a low hematocrit. Packed red blood cells given after an intravenous dose of a diuretic (frusemide 40 mg) are advisable for patients with impaired cardiac function. Storage of blood reduces oxygen-carrying power and the freshest blood available is preferred. If massive transfusion is needed, a filter helps to prevent the adult respiratory distress syndrome (ARDS) by trapping microemboli.

***Plasma*** does not replenish oxygen-carrying capacity and is only a temporary substitute for blood following major hemorrhage. Infused plasma may not remain in the vascular compartment and is distributed throughout the extracellular fluid compartment if capillary permeability is increased. Nevertheless, plasma or albumin is of great value when given with crystalloid when plasma losses are a dominant feature, as in acute pancreatitis (p. 1263).

***Plasma substitutes*** such as dextran (molecular mass 70 000) can maintain plasma volume for up to 48 h but may cause clotting defects when over 1 L is infused and can interfere with subsequent crossmatching. Low molecular mass dextran (molecular mass 40 000) leaves the vascular compartment even more rapidly, but may improve tissue perfusion by nonspecific volume expansion and possibly by preventing red blood cell aggregation.

***Crystalloid solutions*** such as Ringer lactate and isotonic saline are the mainstay of resuscitation in all forms of shock and even in patients with blood loss, there is significant loss of extravascular ECF. Ringer lactate resembles ECF in its electrolyte content once its lactate has been metabolized to bicarbonate. The theoretical danger of compounding lactic acidosis is more than compensated for by the benefits of improved tissue perfusion. Overinfusion of crystalloids induces pulmonary congestion and must be avoided.

***Dextrose solutions*** provide water without electrolytes and can induce a hypo-osmolar state with cellular edema. They should be avoided in shock.

### *Acid–base imbalance*

Metabolic acidosis is treated by improving tissue perfusion rather than by giving bicarbonate. Bicarbonate becomes available in any event from metabolism of lactate in Ringer lactate solution and from metabolism of citrate in stored blood. Further bicarbonate administration may precipitate metabolic alkalosis and can only be justified in situations such as cardiac arrest when acidosis is profound (pH $<7.2$). In these circumstances, sodium bicarbonate is best given as a small volume of concentrated solution (i.e. 50 ml of 8.4% solution) while plasma pH is monitored.

### *Specific organ failure*

***Cardiac failure*** is a common accompaniment of the acute abdomen in the elderly and those with pre-existing cardiac disease. Electrocardiography and insertion of a Swan–Ganz catheter provide essential information while cardiac failure and arrhythmias are treated in the usual way.

***Pulmonary insufficiency (adult respiratory distress syndrome, ARDS)*** can complicate all forms of shock and especially septic shock. No single cause is responsible and fluid overload, disseminated intravascular coagulation, transfusion, microemboli, endotoxemia, oxygen toxicity, aspiration pneumonitis and secondary infection have all been implicated. Abnormal capillary permeability is responsible for pulmonary edema and a generalized permeability abnormality. Shunting of blood through underventilated lung can also contribute to the persistently low arterial oxygen tension and saturation. Circulatory overload must be avoided at all costs in patients who develop pulmonary insufficiency and measurement of pulmonary capillary wedge pressure (p. 516) helps to exclude primary pump failure. Oxygen is administered by mask or nasal catheter, but endotracheal intubation with positive pressure ventilation is necessary if there is continuing hypoxia. A diuretic is prescribed to reduce interstitial edema and inotropic support is indicated if pulmonary edema remains. Sequential chest radiographs are used to monitor progress (see also p. 1259).

***Renal failure*** reflects inadequate organ perfusion and oxygenation. Oliguria demands restoration of circulating blood volume in the first instance, but if the patient remains oliguric once the circulation has been restored, a diuretic is given (e.g. frusemide 40 mg intravenously). Doses of 250–500 mg may eventually be required to produce a diuresis. Failure to induce a diuresis indicates renal damage and the need for fluid restriction and dialysis, with or without ultrafiltration.

***Hepatic dysfunction*** with jaundice may occur (p. 1099) and ischemic-hypoxic injury in the gut may critically impair the gut mucosal barrier to endotoxin absorption.

*Vasoactive drugs*

Vasoconstrictor drugs are contraindicated. It is futile to raise arterial pressure by inducing further peripheral vasoconstriction and so cause a further deterioration in tissue perfusion. Vasodilator drugs, notably dopamine or dobutamine, may be of benefit as they increase cardiac output and improve tissue perfusion and renal function. Dopamine is given by intravenous infusion (2–5 μg/kg/min), the dose being titrated by assessing blood pressure, urine flow and general tissue perfusion. Higher doses (5–20 μg/kg/min) have a predominantly inotropic effect, while even higher doses cause predominantly α-adrenergic effects with vasoconstriction. Dobutamine acts directly on $\beta_1$-adrenergic receptors and achieves its inotropic effects with a less marked effect on heart rate.

*Antibiotics*

Antibiotics are essential in septic shock. Until the results of culture are available, a combination of penicillin, gentamicin and metronidazole is usually appropriate (p. 520) when shock complicates acute abdominal disease.

*Other measures*

Corticosteroid therapy in septic shock (using massive intravenous doses) remains empirical and uncertain in its effect and is no longer advocated. A variety of measures to combat the effects of endotoxin and other mediators in septic shock (e.g. monoclonal antibodies against endotoxin) have not yet established a place in management.

## PERITONITIS

Peritonitis is such a frequent complication of acute abdominal disease that it deserves special consideration. Peritoneal inflammation may be bacterial or chemical.

*Bacterial peritonitis*

Bacteria gain access to the peritoneal cavity from inflamed or perforated viscera and occasionally through penetrating wounds. In the rare primary or spontaneous bacterial peritonitis (p. 521), infection is bloodborne or enters by the ostia of the fallopian tubes.

In most cases, the organisms responsible are members of the normal gut flora. Gastric contents are normally sterile, but pathogenic bacteria such as *E. coli* or *Strep. fecalis* may colonize the stomach of achlorhydric patients and contaminate the peritoneum following perforation. The organisms most often present in infected bile include *E. coli*, *Klebsiella aerogenes* and *Strep. fecalis*, but anaerobic streptococci and clostridia may be present. Peritonitis arising from the bowel and appendix is due to anaerobes (*Bacteroides*) in combination with aerobic coliform bacilli. Peritonitis is only occasionally due to infection with nonalimentary organisms such as pneumococci, gonococci and *Mycobacterium tuberculosis*.

The severity of peritonitis depends on the type, number and virulence of infecting organisms, the rapidity of onset and the ability of the patient's defenses to contain and overcome infection. Bacteria are removed from the peritoneal cavity by lymphatic drainage, killed by the action of complement or phagocytosis or trapped by fibrin and omentum. Adhesions help to prevent generalized peritonitis, but elderly or debilitated patients and those on corticosteroid therapy are often unable to prevent dissemination. Bacteria leaving the peritoneal cavity are cleared rapidly by the reticuloendothelial system and this may trigger a systemic response to sepsis. Macrophages normally resident within the peritoneal cavity have considerable capacity to engulf bacteria and within 4–6 h of bacterial invasion of the peritoneal cavity, their defensive role is reinforced by the influx of large numbers of activated polymorphonuclear leukocytes. Unfortunately, bacterial opsonization in peritoneal exudate is poor and complement components and immunoglobulins are destroyed by proteases, giving rise to the suggestion that restoration of opsonization by intra-abdominal administration of normal serum may be beneficial (Billing et al 1994).

*Chemical peritonitis*

Chemical peritonitis is caused by irritants such as gastric contents, bile, pancreatic enzymes, blood or meconium. It is frequently followed by secondary bacterial infection. Bile peritonitis has an evil reputation, but large quantities of sterile bile can accumulate before dramatic physical signs are produced. Blood can be surprisingly irritant, giving rise to abdominal and rectal tenderness and to shoulder-tip pain due to diaphragmatic irritation.

Granulomatous peritonitis caused by starch granules

introduced at the time of surgery can be regarded as a form of chemical peritonitis.

## Clinical presentation of peritonitis

Abdominal pain and tenderness are prominent and become diffuse as peritonitis disseminates, although they may remain maximal in the area initially involved. Reflex guarding and muscle rigidity are found when a "demonstrative" area of peritoneum is inflamed (p. 512) and pelvic peritonitis is associated with tenderness on rectal examination. Physical signs may be unimpressive or absent in elderly, obese or debilitated patients and in those receiving corticosteroid therapy.

Vomiting is common initially but often diminishes in frequency and severity, only to return with the onset of toxemia and paralytic ileus. Rigidity wanes as toxemia increases and abdominal distention can embarrass breathing and interfere with venous return. Fever and tachycardia reflect progressing infection and the patient becomes dehydrated, shocked and confused. The classic Hippocratic facies is a late manifestation of peritonitis.

## Principles of management

*Resuscitation prior to surgery*

This may not be necessary in patients presenting with early localized peritonitis but is essential in shocked patients presenting with advanced diffuse peritonitis. Hypovolemia develops as extracellular fluid is lost by peritoneal exudation, vomiting and accumulation in the lumen of the paralysed obstructed gut. Systemic absorption of bacteria and their products from the peritoneum compounds the problem and leads to circulatory collapse.

The assessment and resuscitation of shocked patients is described on p. 515. Failure to replace fluid losses before surgery is a major avoidable factor in mortality and considerable clinical judgement is often needed to select the optimal time for surgery. Infection progresses with time and there is often a critical period beyond which continuing attempts at resuscitation produce diminishing returns.

*Antibiotic therapy*

The choice of antibiotic is dictated by past experience of the spectrum of organisms responsible for the disease in question, by culture and sensitivity determinations on samples obtained at operation or on blood culture and by immediate Gram staining of infected material. Blood cultures should be taken prior to commencing antibiotic therapy in the resuscitation of patients with major sepsis.

The commonest organisms present in intra-abdominal sepsis are *E. coli* and *Bacteroides fragilis* (see Table 18.5).

**Table 18.5** Bacterial species identified in intra-abdominal sepsis (Solomkin 1988)

| Bacterial species | % of cases |
|---|---|
| Aerobes | |
| *Eschercichia coli* | 62 |
| *Klebsiella* spp. | 15 |
| *Proteus* spp. | 15 |
| *Pseudomonas* spp. | 8 |
| *Enterobacter* spp. | 5 |
| Other Gram negative bacteria | 16 |
| Enterococci | 22 |
| *Staphylococcus aureus* | 9 |
| Other *Staphylococcus/Streptococcus* spp. | 19 |
| Anaerobes | |
| *Bacteroides fragilis* | 46 |
| *Bacteroides* spp. | 38 |
| *Clostridium* spp. | 23 |
| Other anaerobes | 43 |

The majority of biliary tract bacteria are sensitive to gentamicin or cephalosporins (e.g. cefuroxime 750 mg every 6–8 h intravenously or intramuscularly), but amoxycillin (500 mg every 8 h intravenously) is recommended if Gram staining reveals Gram-positive bacteria in the infected bile. Metronidazole (500 mg 8-hourly by intravenous infusion) combined with gentamicin (2–5 mg/kg daily in divided doses every 6–8 h by injection) is effective against fecal anaerobes and aerobic coliform bacteria and is recommended for use in peritonitis associated with bowel organisms. Triple therapy with gentamicin, metronidazole and penicillin is used when broad-spectrum cover is needed, although single broad-spectrum agents such as the newer cephalosporins offer a viable alternative which avoids the potential toxicity of gentamicin (Solomkin 1988). In one recent study, patients treated with a single broad-spectrum antibiotic (in the majority of cases a cephalosporin) fared better than those treated with multiple antibiotics and predictably, patients given empiric treatment with inappropriate antibiotics did particularly badly (Mosdell et al 1991).

The choice of antibiotics is modified in the light of subsequent culture and sensitivity determinations, although it must be admitted that in reality, this may not influence outcome; in one recent review less than 10% of patients had an appropriate change in antibiotic therapy once the results of culture became available (Mosdell et al 1991). The duration of treatment depends on the severity of infection, but a minimum of 5 days is recommended.

*Operative management*

The first aim of laparotomy is to prevent further contamination of the peritoneal cavity by dealing effectively with the primary focus of disease. Perforation of a viscus can be controlled temporarily by occlusion clamps while a sample is taken for culture and sensitivity determination and all infected material is evacuated from the peritoneum. Failure to clear all peritoneal recesses increases the risk of residual abscess formation. On the other hand, if it is obvious that peritonitis has been contained prior to laparotomy, it is unwise to risk spreading infection by needless exploration.

Lavage with saline containing tetracycline (1 g/L) is used in some centers as a means of reducing peritoneal and wound infection after operation for peritonitis. In one series of 276 emergency "dirty" operations where tetracycline lavage was employed, the sepsis-associated mortality rate was 4% (Krukowski et al 1986). If lavage is used, all fluid should be aspirated prior to wound closure so as to avoid dilution of natural defense mechanisms.

***Wound closure.*** Leaving drains in the peritoneal cavity does not prevent postoperative sepsis. The deep layers of the wound are closed with continuous monofilament material such as nylon, taking large tissue bites and employing a suture length to wound length ratio greater than 4:1 to avoid undue tension. Deep tension sutures may be harmful and are no longer used to prevent wound dehiscence.

The high incidence of wound infection after laparotomy in the presence of peritonitis can be reduced by systemic antibiotics. For example, in acute appendicitis, a single intravenous dose of metronidazole or a metronidazole suppository (1 g) can be used to reduce the incidence of wound sepsis.

In the presence of gross contamination, the risks of wound infection can be reduced if only the deeper layers are closed and the skin is left open to await delayed primary suture when the wound is clean. Alternatively, the entire wound may be packed and left open to heal by granulation ("laparostomy"), an approach which also allows easy and repeated access to deal with intraperitoneal sepsis in conditions such as necrotising pancreatitis (Mughal et al 1986). Marlex mesh (with or without a zipper) can be used to reduce fluid loss, prevent evisceration and reduce the risk of fistula formation if laparostomy is employed (Walsh et al 1988).

It should be stressed that most wounds are closed conventionally after dealing with intra-abdominal infection and its underlying cause. It is arguable whether closed peritoneal lavage is of benefit (Leiboff & Soroff 1987) but in some centers, the problem of continuing necrosis and infection after pancreatic necrosectomy is dealt with by leaving multiple catheters for continuing peritoneal lavage (p. 1266).

## Uncommon forms of peritonitis

The common specific causes of peritonitis are dealt with elsewhere and tuberculous peritonitis is discussed on p. 569, but two uncommon forms of peritonitis will be considered here.

*Primary (spontaneous) bacterial peritonitis* (p. 1033)

The terms "primary" and "spontaneous" denote that there is no recognizable source of infection. Gram-negative bacteria, pneumococci and hemolytic streptococci are the organisms chiefly responsible, but gonococci are occasionally to blame. There is debate regarding the way in which organisms reach the peritoneum. The condition was once common among young girls, suggesting that bacteria can gain access from the genital tract. Patients with ascites (usually due to cirrhosis or the nephrotic syndrome) and immune-deficient patients are especially prone to the disease.

***Clinical features and management.*** The onset is typically abrupt, with abdominal pain, fever and vomiting. Toxicity is marked, occurs early and is out of all proportion to the abdominal signs. Pain and tenderness are maximal in the lower abdomen, but rigidity is uncommon. If there is no obvious associated cause such as cirrhosis, laparotomy is indicated to confirm the diagnosis and exclude conditions requiring surgery and deal with any abscesses. Diffuse peritonitis is usually found and is often most severe in the pelvis. Peritoneal lavage is advisable and the peritoneum is closed without drainage. Antibiotic therapy (p. 520) is commenced immediately after Gram staining.

*Granulomatous peritonitis*

The incidence of granulomatous peritoneal reaction has been reduced by using starch rather than talc as surgical glove powder. Starch was thought originally to be nonirritant and easily absorbed, but widespread granulomas and adhesions can be produced experimentally and sporadic cases of granulomatous peritonitis are reported (Cox 1970).

***Clinical features.*** Abdominal pain, low-grade fever, anorexia, nausea and vomiting usually begin within weeks of operation. The abdomen is tender and may contain a palpable mass or becomes distended from adhesion obstruction or ascites. Occasionally, the presentation is delayed for years after surgery.

***Diagnosis.*** The clinical picture often resembles that of intestinal obstruction or peritonitis due to more common causes. Laparotomy can be avoided if diagnostic paracentesis yields sterile amber fluid in which starch granules are detected. If laparotomy is undertaken, the multiple white pinhead nodules can mimic disseminated malignancy or tuberculosis. Biopsy reveals vacuolated granules, 10–70 μm in size, surrounded by a chronic granulomatous reaction. The granules are birefrigent under polarized light and have a characteristic Maltese cross appearance.

***Prevention and treatment.*** Surgeons should avoid using glove powder or wash off excess powder before surgery. If granulomas do develop, they tend to resolve spontaneously and it is doubtful whether corticosteroids reduce the risk of adhesion obstruction. Laparotomy is indicated only to exclude other causes of peritonitis or deal with persisting adhesion obstruction.

## ACUTE APPENDICITIS

### Incidence

Acute appendicitis is predominantly a disease of Western civilization, but after a steep rise at the beginning of this century, the incidence in countries such as the UK has declined continuously in the second half of the century (Barker 1988). Approximately one in seven individuals is still affected and highest incidence is in the age group 10–14 in boys and 15–19 in girls (West & Carey 1978). Appendicitis remains the commonest abdominal emergency in childhood, adolescence and young adult life. Less than 2% of cases occur in infants under 2 years but diagnosis is notoriously difficult in this group, a fact reflected in a perforation rate of around 80% (Wilkinson et al 1969). The incidence of appendicitis diminishes with age and less than 5% of cases occur in patients over 60 years of age (Peltokallio & Jauhiainen 1970).

### Etiology and pathogenesis

A combination of bacteria and obstruction are needed to produce appendicitis experimentally and the initial abdominal colic suggests that obstruction is also important in man. Obstruction causes accumulation of secretion and distention, leading to pressure necrosis of the mucosa with invasion by luminal bacteria. The peak incidence of appendicitis coincides with the period of maximal development of lymphoid tissue and it is conceivable that lymphoid hyperplasia obstructs the lumen. Fecoliths are also a potential cause of obstruction; kinks, adhesions and neoplasia are occasionally responsible.

The "hygiene hypothesis" attributes the rise in appendicitis in Britain during the first half of this century and the fall that followed to improvements in hygiene (Barker 1985). The hypothesis is based on the postulate that the response to certain infections is different in early childhood and later life. Young children begin to escape infection as household hygiene improves, but this renders them vulnerable to appendicitis when exposed to infection in adolescence and early adulthood. This initial increase in susceptibility with improving hygiene is supported by the steep rise in the incidence of appendicitis in Hong Kong when housing, sanitation and water supplies improved after World War II (Donnan 1986). The association between appendicitis and overcrowding and the clustering of cases suggests that organisms responsible for respiratory and enteric infections may cause appendicitis (Barker 1988). With continued improvement in hygiene, exposure to infection eventually declines and with it the incidence of acute appendicitis. The rate of acute appendicitis in the British Isles in 1979–82 was correlated with the percentage of households still lacking amenities, in particular fixed baths and hot water systems (Barker 1988).

*Yersinia* infection was implicated serologically in almost one-third of cases with histologically proven appendicitis in one Irish study (Attwood et al 1987). It is conceivable that many patients with acute abdominal pain have *Yersinia* infection in lymphoid tissue and that this may resolve spontaneously, progress to mesenteric adenitis or to acute appendicitis.

Dietary factors are also implicated in that a low consumption of vegetables other than potatoes is associated with a high incidence of appendicitis, while green vegetables and tomatoes may actually protect against appendicitis by an effect on the gut flora (Barker 1988). Appendicitis has a high incidence in some communities with high cereal or sugar consumption, but the suggestion that lack of dietary fiber may be contributory is now largely discounted (Heaton 1987).

Threadworm infestation occasionally causes discomfort in the right iliac fossa, but it is doubtful whether it causes acute appendicitis.

Once appendicitis develops, progressive obstruction and infection may lead to impairment of the blood supply. The antimesenteric border is most vulnerable and small patches of gangrene appear first in its mid-portion. Morbidity rises sharply as bacteria pass through the devitalized areas into the peritoneum, even before frank perforation occurs. The outcome then depends on containment of infection by the peritoneal defenses. Gangrene and perforation are five times as common in patients over the age of 60 years for a given duration of symptoms (Peltokallio & Jauhiainen 1970), and in one series from the English Midlands no less than 37% of patients with appendicitis over the age of 60 were found to have perforation of the appendix at operation (Sherlock 1985). A recent report from Sweden offers the intriguing suggestions that perforating and nonperforating appendicitis may be separate entities and that spontaneous resolution of appendicitis may be common (Andersson et al 1994). In this study, the incidence of perforation in the period 1984–89 was constant, independent of age and uninfluenced by the rate of laparotomy, whereas nonperforating appendicitis was age dependent, decreasing over time, and related to diagnostic accuracy and rate of removal of a normal appendix.

In infancy, localization is inadequate because the greater omentum is not fully developed, but delay in diagnosis is the major cause of the high incidence of gangrene and perforation. The average delay between onset and diagnosis was 4 days in the 40 infants reviewed by Bartlett et al (1970), while Williams (1947) reported that of a series of 42 infants under 3 years, only six had not developed an appendix mass or generalized peritonitis before operation. Although the number of deaths from appendicitis in childhood has fallen, a third of these deaths still occur in children younger than 4 years, giving a death rate of one in 320 cases in this age group as opposed to one in 4760 cases in children aged 5–14 years (Pledger et al 1987).

### Clinical features

Delay is the most important determinant of morbidity and mortality of acute appendicitis. It must be clearly understood that the "typical" signs and symptoms may not be present or only appear in the later stages of the disease.

Periumbilical colic is usually the first symptom and can be severe or amount to no more than aching discomfort. Children often appear well between bouts of pain. It is easy to attribute this central colic to intestinal obstruction, especially when vomiting occurs, but tenderness and guarding in the right iliac fossa should suggest the true diagnosis.

In the majority of cases, pain remains periumbilical for some hours before shifting to the right iliac fossa with the development of parietal peritonitis. In approximately 30% of patients, pain commences and remains in the right iliac fossa (Winsey & Jones 1967).

Anorexia is almost invariable. Vomiting is seldom marked in adults but can be prominent in children, particularly when diagnosis is delayed. Alteration in bowel habit is uncommon, but diarrhea in children can simulate gastroenteritis when pain is not severe.

Fever and tachycardia are not features of early appendicitis and the pulse may not rise significantly before perforation. Fetor is a frequent but nonspecific accompaniment.

Right iliac fossa tenderness and guarding are the most constant and reliable signs but initially they can be masked by colic. Peritonitis arising in the pelvis may not produce abdominal guarding or rigidity until late in the disease. In retrocecal appendicitis, signs are more marked in the right flank and loin, while in pelvic appendicitis tenderness is often elicited on rectal examination.

Advanced disease with diffuse peritonitis leads to generalized tenderness, guarding and rigidity and eventually to the silent abdomen of paralytic ileus. Even at this stage, tenderness is usually still maximal in the right iliac fossa.

### Investigation

Leukocytosis is present in the majority of cases on admission (Lee 1973) but a fall in lymphocyte count may be associated with gangrenous appendicitis (Jahangiri & Wyllie 1990). The urine is examined to exclude urinary tract infection and renal colic, remembering that a few pus cells may be present in acute appendicitis.

There are no specific radiological signs of appendicitis and signs said to be associated with it are in fact present with roughly the same frequency in patients who do not have the disease (Jenkins & Lee 1970). The presence of positive radiographic signs in 80% of infants with appendicitis reflects the high incidence of perforation in this age group (Wilkinson et al 1969). A radio-opaque fecolith in a patient with clinical signs in the right iliac fossa strongly suggests appendicitis and such patients have a higher incidence of perforation and abscess.

Ultrasound scanning can distinguish between various types of mass in the right iliac fossa and pelvis (p. 59) and in one study had an overall accuracy of 95.7% in the diagnosis of appendicitis while reducing the negative laparotomy rate from 23% to 13% (Schwerk et al 1989). Criteria for the ultrasound diagnosis of appendicitis include a "target-like" appearance of the appendix in cross-section (hypoechoic fluid-filled lumen, hyperechoic inner ring of mucosa and submucosa and hypoechoic outer ring of muscle), noncompressibility, lack of peristalsis and a diameter exceeding 7 mm.

### Diagnosis

Many of the conditions which can be confused with appendicitis do in any case require laparotomy, but it is important to exclude causes of the acute abdomen, such as basal pneumonia and myocardial infarction (p. 537), in which operation is contraindicated.

In patients with central abdominal colic, appendicitis is easily confused with intestinal obstruction and gastroenteritis. Mesenteric adenitis, irritable bowel syndrome (p. 1358), mesenteric vascular occlusion (p. 546) and acute pancreatitis (p. 1253) are among the many conditions which can be simulated in patients with central abdominal pain.

With the shift of pain and tenderness which follows the development of parietal peritonitis, the differential diagnosis is influenced by the position of the appendix. Right iliac fossa tenderness can suggest mesenteric adenitis, acute terminal ileitis (p. 205), Meckel's diverticulitis (p. 205), ovarian disease (p. 534) and salpingitis, although the tenderness in salpingitis is often bilateral and lower in the abdomen (p. 535). Ureteric colic can be associated with pain and tenderness on deep palpation over the ureter, but is seldom difficult to distinguish from appendicitis. Pelvic appendicitis may mimic salpingitis, ovarian disease and urinary tract infection. Retrocecal appendicitis causes pain and tenderness in the right flank and can mimic perinephric abscess, acute pyelitis and acute cholecystitis.

Once a mass develops in the right iliac fossa the differential diagnosis includes intussusception in young children; mesenteric adenitis, acute terminal ileitis (p. 525) and Crohn's disease (p. 656) in older children and adults; ovarian cysts in women; and neoplasia in older patients.

Once diffuse peritonitis develops, it is difficult clinically to determine the original site of infection. However, tenderness usually remains maximal in the right iliac fossa, although spread of infected material down the right paracolic gutter can produce confusing right iliac fossa signs in perforated peptic ulcer.

## Treatment and problem areas

The aim of treatment is to carry out appendicectomy before gangrene and perforation supervene. While undue delay should be avoided, recent studies have shown that patients who present between midnight and 6.00 a.m. have higher rates of unnecessary appendicectomy and that in most cases, the decision to operate and the operation itself can be safely postponed until the following morning (McLean et al 1993, Surana et al 1993).

There is some evidence that laparoscopic appendicectomy may have advantages over conventional open appendicectomy in terms of hospital stay and return to normal activity (Attwood et al 1992, Tate et al 1993, Vallina et al 1993).

### *Uninflamed appendix*

It was once commonplace for an uninflamed appendix to be removed in at least one in four patients undergoing emergency appendicectomy and it was accepted that to await signs allowing certain clinical diagnosis resulted in an increased morbidity and mortality from gangrene and perforation (Berry & Malt 1984). Improved diagnosis and the use of ultrasonography can virtually halve the negative laparotomy rate without incurring any increase in perforation rates, which at 20% remain well within the reported range of 17–39% (Schwerk et al 1989). Selective use of laparoscopy in patients where the need for operation was uncertain also reduced the incidence of unnecessary appendicectomy from 28% to 16% in one recent report (Paterson-Brown et al 1988).

Other pathology must be excluded before removing a normal appendix. Peritoneal fluid is clear yellow in mesenteric adenitis, bile-stained following perforation of peptic ulceration or an inflamed gall bladder, fecal in colonic perforation and blood-stained after infarction of gut. Free blood denotes rupture of a vessel, solid organ or ectopic pregnancy.

If there is no apparent pathology, the distal ileum is inspected to exclude a Meckel's diverticulum, terminal ileitis and mesenteric adenitis. The right tube and ovary are inspected in the female. Once surgical pathology has been excluded most surgeons would remove a normal appendix, although this becomes increasingly questionable in older adults (Berry & Malt 1984) and is contraindicated in the elderly and immunocompromised.

### *Difficult appendicectomy*

If difficulty is encountered during emergency appendicectomy, the incision is extended if necessary and it is often useful to divide the appendix base to allow retrograde removal. If continuing manipulation is considered hazardous, the area should be drained and interval appendicectomy considered (p. 526).

An excessively long appendix stump can cause subsequent "stump appendicitis", while portions of necrotic tip can be overlooked during retrograde removal. Free fecoliths which have eroded through a necrotic appendix are a rare cause of residual infection and abscess formation.

### *Pregnancy*

The reported rate of appendicectomy varies between 1:1000 and 1:5529 deliveries (DeVore 1980, Horowitz et al 1985) but there is general agreement that pregnancy does not affect the incidence of appendicitis. Early diagnosis is vital but difficult. Upward displacement of the appendix produces pain and tenderness which is higher in the abdomen than usual and lessens the value of rectal and vaginal examination. The white cell count is normally elevated in pregnancy and has to be interpreted with caution. In the series reported by Horowitz et al (1985), up to 9 days elapsed between the onset of symptoms and appendicectomy and perforation had occurred in no less than six of the 10 cases, resulting in one maternal death and the loss of three fetuses. Ultrasound scanning is particularly helpful in diagnosis and in excluding complications of pregnancy.

Delay is so harmful to mother and child that one should operate on reasonable clinical suspicion once urinary tract infection has been excluded. Death results not from appendicectomy but from delaying operation until perforation and peritonitis supervene. Hinshaw (1963) reported an overall maternal mortality of 5% and a fetal loss of 20%; in uncomplicated appendicitis the fetal mortality was only 3% whereas it was 30% following perforation.

### *Appendiceal neoplasms*

***Carcinoid tumors.*** The appendix is the commonest site for carcinoid tumors (Table 16.8). Carcinoids account for 85% of appendiceal neoplasms and are found in some 0.3% of appendices (Moertel et al 1968). The tumors are usually found incidentally and are small gray-yellow lesions located near the tip of the appendix. Muscle infiltration and spread into the mesoappendix is common, metastatic spread is relatively rare although it has been reported even with small tumors (MacGillivray et al 1992), and the carcinoid syndrome is virtually unknown. In a long-term study of 150 cases, there were no metastases in the 127 patients with tumors less than 2 cm in diameter, whereas seven of the 23 patients with larger tumors had metastatic spread (Moertel et al 1987). Larger tumors and metastases were more common in younger patients. The patient with an appendiceal carcinoid can present with acute appendicitis or chronic right lower quadrant pain and should be treated by appendicectomy in the first instance unless the tumor is larger than 2 cm and metastases are obvious. In doubtful cases, the appendix is removed and suspicious lesions are biopsied. Larger tumors are probably best treated by right hemicolectomy.

***Adenocarcinoids*** are tumors in which mucin production is present in addition to the carcinoid component. They can be identified by immunocytochemical localization of serotonin and CEA (Klappenbach et al 1985). These tumors behave more aggressively than carcinoids but less so than adenocarcinoma. In one series of 10 cases, one patient had died and two had persistent disease 1–5 years after surgery (Edmonds et al 1984). Other names applied to these tumors are argentaffin cell adenocarcinoma, argyrophil mucus-secreting adenocarcinoma, goblet cell carcinoid and neuroendocrine carcinoma.

***Carcinomas*** of the appendix are much less common than carcinoid tumors. It may be difficult to distinguish between primary lesions of the cecum and appendix, but right hemicolectomy is the treatment of choice in either case. Inflammation of a solitary cecal diverticulum can mimic the clinical presentation of appendicitis and the operative appearance of carcinoma. The diverticulum, which is probably congenital, occurs close to the ileocecal valve and may cause problems in young adults. Although there is debate about the desirability of local excision, right hemicolectomy is generally regarded as the treatment of choice (Riseman & Wichterman 1989).

### *Terminal ileitis* (p. 561)

Acute terminal ileitis is usually a self-limiting infection with *Yersinia* organisms (*Y. enterocolitica* and *Y. pseudotuberculosis*) which can mimic appendicitis and which was once confused with Crohn's disease. Preceding gastrointestinal upset with malaise and diarrhea is common. At laparotomy the terminal ileum is red and thickened, mesenteric adenitis is obvious and the rest of the bowel, including the appendix, is normal. Histology of nodes and appendix shows nonspecific inflammatory changes.

When faced with terminal ileitis at laparotomy, appendicectomy should be carried out to avoid any confusion caused by a subsequent attack of appendicitis (Gurry 1974). Serological tests for *Yersinia* are available if diagnostic confirmation is needed and are preferred to culture of enlarged lymph nodes or appendiceal luminal content. Even when one is faced at laparotomy with true ileal Crohn's disease, appendicectomy is still indicated to prevent subsequent appendicitis and confusion if right iliac fossa pain recurs. Fistula formation in such cases involves the diseased ileum rather than appendix stump and is a consequence of the laparotomy rather than the appendicectomy.

If right iliac fossa pain persists in patients with confirmed *Yersinia* infection, tetracycline (in adults only) or co-trimoxazole is the antibiotic of choice (Attwood et al 1989).

### *Meckel's diverticulum*

Inflammation of Meckel's diverticulum (p. 496) cannot be distinguished clinically from acute appendicitis. Excision is indicated for diverticula giving rise to problems and a V-shaped rim of ileum is included to ensure removal of any ectopic gastric mucosa (Fig. 18.2). Opinions differ regarding management when a Meckel's diverticulum is discovered as an incidental finding. The risk of late complications developing has been reported at 4.2% when the diverticulum was found in infancy, 3% when found in adults and zero when discovered at the age of 75 years (Soltero & Bill 1976).

The following guidelines have been suggested (Leijonmarck et al 1986, Lancet 1983):

1. In the presence of acute appendicitis no search should be made for a Meckel's diverticulum.
2. If during an operation for abdominal pain a normal appendix is found, a diverticulum should be sought and removed with the appendix.
3. If a diverticulum is found in a child or young adult during nonacute surgery, it should be removed (particularly if narrow-necked), provided that the patient's general condition and nature of the primary operation are appropriate.
4. The finding of a band between diverticulum and umbilicus at any age is an indication to divide the band between ligatures and resect the diverticulum if appropriate.
5. In a patient over 40 years, an incidental nonadherent Meckel's diverticulum should be left alone.

### *Mass and abscess*

Patients occasionally present with a history extending over some days, a palpable mass in the right iliac fossa and a soft abdomen which is only tender in the region of the mass. Provided that the general condition is good, an expectant attitude can be adopted to allow the inflammation to resolve with disappearance of the mass. Oral intake is stopped, fluids are given parenterally and progress is followed by 4-hourly pulse and temperature readings and by twice-daily delineation of the mass. A CT scan or ultrasonography is advisable and if a phlegmon or small abscess is shown, conservative treatment should continue (Nitecki et al 1993). Conservative treatment is abandoned if the general condition deteriorates, fever fails to settle or the mass does not diminish in size. Percutaneous drainage now offers an alternative to surgical drainage if intervention is needed (Haaga 1990) (p. 32). Larger abscesses

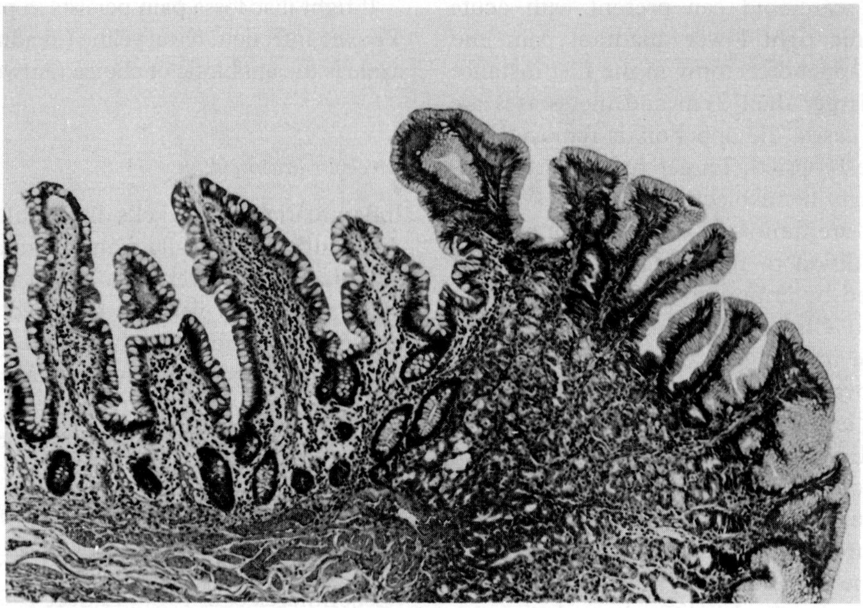

**Fig. 18.2** Meckel's diverticulum. Ectopic gastric mucosa is seen on the right and normal ileal villi on the left (hematoxylin and eosin, ×60).

are probably best treated by percutaneous drainage while complex multilocular abscesses are probably best managed by open surgery using an extraperitoneal approach if possible. Adequate drainage is the main objective if surgery has to be undertaken, but the appendix is removed if possible.

If the mass subsides without surgery, appendicectomy at a later date was once advised routinely in order to avoid recurrent inflammation and exclude other causes of mass formation. However, recent reviews advise against routine interval appendicectomy (Nitecki et al 1993). Radiological studies must be undertaken to exclude malignancy in patients older than 40 years of age for as many as 3% of patients with appendicitis in this age group prove to have an obstructing neoplasm (Peltokallio 1966).

The distinction between appendix mass and appendix abscess is a little artificial in that both result from localization of inflammation. Patients with an appendix abscess have a definite collection of pus and usually have more serious systemic upset. Both conditions are dangerous. The risks of expectant treatment are greatest in young children, pregnant women and the elderly, and conservative treatment of an appendix mass or abscess is usually contraindicated in such patients.

*Intraperitoneal abscess*

Prevention of intraperitoneal abscess by early diagnosis and treatment of appendicitis cannot be overemphasized. Pelvic abscesses are the commonest problem and follow gravitation of pus from a pelvic appendix. A pelvic abscess usually takes 4–5 days to become manifest and the clinical condition gradually deteriorates with tachycardia, a fluctuating temperature and leukocytosis. There are few abdominal signs at first, but a mass is palpable rectally and often causes diarrhea with tenesmus and passage of mucus. Frequency and dysuria are sometimes present. Deep suprapubic palpation may elicit tenderness. Ultrasound or CT scanning have proved of immense value in localization of intra-abdominal abscesses and transvaginal ultrasonography is particularly useful in examining the pelvis (Adam & Page 1991).

In the past, a number of abscesses pointed into the rectum and discharged spontaneously or were encouraged to do so with a finger or sinus forceps. Percutaneous drainage is now a valuable alternative to surgery in the treatment of these difficult abscesses and drainage can be undertaken transabdominally or transvaginally as appropriate (Adam & Page 1991). Intraperitoneal sepsis at best means a prolonged illness and subsequent adhesions may cause intestinal obstruction, while sterility may follow occlusion of the ostia of fallopian tubes.

*Portal pyemia*

This complication is now rare. Suppurative thrombophlebitis can give rise to multiple hepatic abscesses (Table 29.1) which typically become manifest between the sixth and 10th postoperative days. Septicemia is controlled by antibiotic therapy and operations such as portal vein ligation are no longer indicated. The prognosis remains grave. Portal vein thrombosis can give rise to portal hypertension which becomes manifest after a prolonged interval.

*Appendicectomy wounds*

Peritoneal drainage is not indicated, even after removal of a perforated appendix (Greenall et al 1978). At one time, one-third of appendicectomy wounds became infected but this problem has been reduced greatly by giving a single dose of a prophylactic antibiotic such as metronidazole (500–1000 mg) at the time of premedication. Some surgeons prescribe additional cover against aerobic organisms if the appendix is found to be perforated at operation. The incidence of wound infection in recent trials of laparoscopic and conventional appendicectomy has ranged from zero to 14%; in general, lower rates have been recorded following laparoscopic appendicectomy (Attwood et al 1992, Tate et al 1993, Vallina et al 1993).

## Prognosis

The overall mortality rate of acute appendicitis has declined markedly. A comparison of the periods 1929–39 and 1974–78 showed that overall mortality fell from 3.1% to 0.8% at the Massachusetts General Hospital (Berry & Malt 1984) and the mortality from uncomplicated appendicitis should now be less than 0.1%. Gangrene and perforation increase morbidity and mortality, especially in infancy, pregnancy and old age.

# INTESTINAL OBSTRUCTION

Intestinal obstruction can be classified according to the level of obstruction, rate of progression (acute, subacute, chronic or acute-on-chronic), site of the obstructing process (luminal, mural or extramural) or pathological process responsible (mechanical obstruction, paralytic ileus, strangulation) (Table 18.6). The pathological classification of "true" intestinal obstruction has great clinical importance in that strangulation worsens the prognosis and necessitates urgent surgical intervention. The types of obstruction shown in Table 18.6 are not mutually exclusive. For example, an inguinal hernia initially produces simple mechanical obstruction but strangulation may supervene, while obstruction due to colonic carcinoma may be complicated by perforation and the development of paralytic ileus.

The relative frequency of the causes of intestinal obstruction is affected by age and by geographical and racial factors. Intussusception and inguinal hernia are common in infancy, while neoplastic obstruction is the major problem in the elderly. In the UK, external hernia accounts for 35%, large bowel cancer for 30% and bands and adhesions for 25% of all adult admissions with intestinal obstruction (Jones 1974). When small bowel obstruction in adults is considered in isolation, adhesions account for up to 80% of cases, the remainder being due to carcinomatous obstruction, previous abdominal irradiation, Crohn's disease and hernias (Riveron et al 1989). Colorectal cancer is the commonest cause of large bowel obstruction in adults and up to one-third of large bowel cancers present in this way (Lothian Surgical Audit). The risk of obstruction varies according to the site of the tumor; as shown in Table 18.7, cancers at the splenic flexure are relatively uncommon but 50% present with obstruction, whereas cancers of the right and left colon obstruct in less than one in four cases (Phillips et al 1985). Sigmoid volvulus is relatively uncommon in most Western countries, but in some parts of Africa ranks second only to external hernia as a cause for obstruction in adults.

**Table 18.6** Classification and common causes of intestinal obstruction

| |
|---|
| *Mechanical obstruction* |
| Luminal obstruction (obturation) |
| Fecal impaction |
| Gallstone ileus (p. 1217) |
| Foreign bodies (p. 1394) |
| Worms (p. 580) |
| Intrinsic lesions of bowel wall |
| Tumor |
| Strictures |
| Crohn's disease (p. 671) |
| Ischemia (p. 549) |
| Potassium chloride (p. 395) |
| Intussusception |
| Extrinsic compression |
| Hernias |
| Adhesions |
| Volvulus |
| *Strangulation obstruction* |
| *Paralytic (adynamic) ileus* |
| Postoperative (post-traumatic) |
| Peritonitis |
| Vascular occlusion (p. 545) |
| Hypokalemia |
| Uremia |
| *Intestinal pseudo-obstruction* (pp. 441 & 531) |

**Table 18.7** Risk of large bowel obstruction according to site of cancer (Phillips et al 1985)

| Tumour site | Non-obstructing (n) | Obstructing (n) | Risk of obstruction (%) |
|---|---|---|---|
| Right colon | 857 | 242 | 22 |
| Splenic flexure | 84 | 80 | 49 |
| Left colon | 784 | 236 | 23 |
| Rectum/ rectosigmoid | 1881 | 128 | 6 |
| Other (e.g. multiple) | 267 | 27 | 9 |

## Pathophysiology

*Consequences of simple mechanical obstruction*

***Intestinal distention.*** Fluid and gas distend the bowel above the obstructing lesion and this stimulates marked peristalsis and colic. The gas which accumulates is mainly nitrogen from swallowed air, with a small contribution from gases such as hydrogen and methane produced by putrefaction within the bowel lumen. Ileal obstruction seldom produces pressures in excess of 8 cm $H_2O$, but colonic obstruction can produce pressures as high as 50 cm$H_2O$ if the ileocecal valve prevents backflow (Sperling 1938). Experimental obstruction of the colon doubles the blood flow to the distended large bowel and increases flow to the ileum (Papanicolaou et al 1989). Distention offsets the increases in intraluminal pressure, but capillary filling is eventually impaired as tension rises in the bowel wall and mucosal ischemia may result.

***Extracellular fluid depletion.*** Altered mucosal function in the obstructed bowel leads to net accumulation of water and electrolytes in the lumen (Shields 1965). Some of this fluid may be lost overtly by vomiting and substantial "hidden" losses are inevitable as fluid accumulates in the gut. The fluid lost is isotonic and has a relatively high potassium concentration. Pyloric stenosis leads to loss of acid and a resultant metabolic alkalosis (p. 284). Obstruction lower in the gut leads to loss of slightly alkaline fluid, but significant acid–base imbalance is exceptional in the absence of shock.

***Shock.*** Shock is a relatively late event in simple mechanical obstruction and is due initially to progressive extracellular fluid depletion. The patient becomes increasingly dehydrated and develops tachycardia, hypotension and oliguria. The CVP is low. Intestinal distention elevates the diaphragm and may embarrass breathing. The luminal bacterial content increases and bacteria and endotoxin may translocate into the portal circulation from obstructed and distended bowel, even before strangulation supervenes. Activation of submucosal leukocytes and hepatic Kupffer cells may have a key role by releasing the cytokines and other mediators implicated in the pathogenesis of multiple organ failure (Deitch 1992, Border 1992).

### *Consequences of strangulation obstruction*

Venous drainage from the obstructed bowel is occluded initially. Arterial blood continues to enter until no more blood can be forced into the infarcted gut. The attendant losses of plasma and blood are substantial and usually overshadow the losses of extracellular fluid incurred by preceding mechanical obstruction. Blood and plasma losses are particularly marked in strangulated sigmoid volvulus and it has been shown experimentally that up to 70% of blood volume can be sequestered (Ya et al 1957).

The development of shock is accelerated as bacteria and their toxins pass through the ischemic bowel wall into the peritoneum and are absorbed into the bloodstream. Thorough peritoneal lavage is essential at the time of surgery to prevent continued absorption of bacteria and their toxins from the peritoneal cavity.

## Clinical features

### *Mechanical obstruction*

***Abdominal colic*** is the cardinal symptom and its distribution depends on the region of gut obstructed. The bouts of colic may last for up to a minute and are often associated with marked restlessness. The clinical picture contrasts with that of peritonitis where the patient is afraid to move for fear of exacerbating the pain. Auscultation during attacks of colic reveals runs of bowel sounds which become high-pitched and tinkling if obstruction is unrelieved. Peristalsis is occasionally visible and in infants with intussusception the mass hardens as the child begins to scream at the onset of colic.

***Vomiting*** is a marked early feature of high obstruction but is often a late development in the course of colonic obstruction.

***Abdominal distention*** is inversely related to vomiting and is particularly marked in low intestinal obstruction. Ascites and gross obesity can confuse, but the gaseous distention of intestinal obstruction produces a resonant note on percussion.

***Constipation*** follows complete obstruction, but patients may pass flatus and even some feces in the early stages as waves of peristalsis carry on past the obstruction to empty the distal bowel.

***Examination*** may reveal the cause of obstruction. Abdominal scars raise the possibility of adhesion obstruction and may be the result of previous surgery for a disease liable to cause recurring obstruction (e.g. Crohn's disease). The dangers of overlooking a small hernia in the groin cannot be overemphasized. A femoral hernia is readily overlooked in that there may be little local pain or tenderness, while central abdominal colic tends to focus attention away from the causal lesion.

Digital rectal examination is essential and frequently reveals an empty rectum when obstruction is due to large bowel cancer. In some cases, the obstructing cancer is palpable. Fecal impaction is a frequent cause of obstruction in the elderly .

***Proctoscopy and sigmoidoscopy*** are carried out when low intestinal obstruction is suspected. Sigmoidoscopy may allow relief of obstruction in some cases of sigmoid volvulus (see p. 531).

### *Strangulation obstruction*

Strangulation is notoriously difficult to detect clinically in its early stages and can never be excluded confidently without laparotomy. Silen et al (1962) found that 41% of their patients with strangulation obstruction had only one or none of the four "classic findings" (fever, leukocytosis, localized pain and absent bowel sounds) said to be associated with strangulation. Others consider that absence of all four "classic findings" can allow a period of conservative observation with a low risk of missing strangulation (Stewardson et al 1978, Riveron et al 1989). The danger of strangulation lends urgency to surgical intervention in all patients with mechanical intestinal obstruction. Severe constant localized pain with tenderness and guarding is suggestive of strangulation with local peritonitis. The suspicion is increased if the patient appears more ill than might be expected from the length of history and when signs of shock develop early.

## Investigation

***Abdominal radiographs*** reveal gaseous distention with fluid levels in the erect or lateral decubitus views (Fig. 18.3). High intestinal obstruction is exceptional in that little or no intestinal gas is seen, although gastric distention and a gastric fluid level may be detected. The diagnosis of intestinal obstruction cannot always be made by plain radiograph of the abdomen and as many as 20% of patients will have no radiological evidence of obstruction (Tiblin 1969). Erect films seldom provide significant additional information to that obtained from supine films (Hayward et al 1984, Simpson et al 1985).

The site of obstruction can often be inferred. Small bowel occupies the center of the abdomen, shows markings which extend across the whole diameter of the bowel (valvulae conniventes) and does not attain the diameter of distended colon (Fig. 1.2). The large bowel occupies a peripheral position, has haustral indentations and may become grossly distended, particularly in closed loop obstruction. The lowest point in the bowel at which gas can be seen indicates the level of the obstructing lesion.

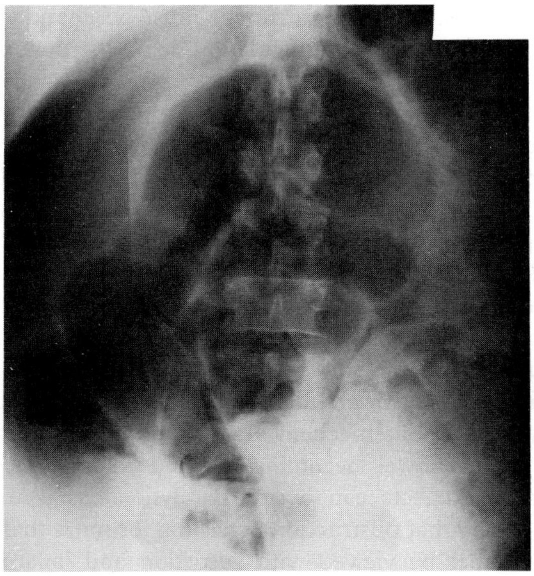

**Fig. 18.3** Sigmoid volvulus of the pelvic colon. The plain radiograph shows considerable distention of the pelvic colon with tapering and approximation of its extremities.

Contrast examination is indicated if the diagnosis remains in doubt or more specific information is required. In a retrospective review of 229 patients with a final diagnosis of small bowel obstruction, 145 had an upper gastrointestinal series, barium enema or both investigations because the findings on clinical examination and abdominal plain films remained equivocal (Riveron et al 1989). Useful information (complete obstruction, unobstructed passage of contrast or diagnosis other than adhesion obstruction) was obtained from 86% of the contrast studies and it was concluded that contrast radiology is a safe and effective means of increasing diagnostic accuracy when small bowel obstruction is suspected.

Barium is the most effective contrast agent and is used unless there is any suggestion of perforation of the gastrointestinal tract, in which case water-soluble media such as Gastrografin should be used. Water-soluble contrast media are progressively diluted in the small intestine when given orally and are usually of little value in identifying the site or nature of the obstruction. Barium should not be given orally until large bowel obstruction has been excluded by a contrast enema, because barium and feces compact proximal to the obstructive lesion to compound the obstruction. In large bowel obstruction, contrast enemas or fiberoptic endoscopy may be of value.

When giving barium from above, a small volume (100–150 ml) is instilled by mouth or by a duodenal tube. As the barium advances, the site and, in some cases, the nature of the obstructing lesion will be revealed by sequential radiographs. The large volume of intestinal fluid proximal to the obstruction prevents the barium from hardening.

## Management

Prompt diagnosis is essential to reduce the risk of strangulation and the old adage that "the sun must not be allowed to set on a bowel obstruction" remains essentially correct. However, conservative management may be appropriate in certain circumstances (see below).

### *Resuscitation*

Resuscitation is essential before operation (p. 515), though it may be impossible to normalize the circulatory state and fluid and electrolyte balance, particularly in the presence of strangulation. The benefits of delaying operation to allow resuscitation must be balanced against the risk of progressive circulatory impairment in the obstructed bowel.

### *Principles of surgery*

***Small bowel obstruction.*** Obturation is managed by

milking the obstructing agent into the large bowel or by removing it through an enterotomy. Lesions in the bowel wall require resection of the involved segment with end-to-end anastomosis. Extrinsic causes of obstruction such as bands, adhesion and hernial rings are divided.

Strangulation of small bowel demands resection of dead gut. An end-to-end anastomosis is usually performed after small bowel resection but in cases of mesenteric ischemia it may be advisable to re-explore the abdomen 24 h later to check bowel viability or to exteriorize both ends of the intestine.

***Large bowel obstruction.*** Obstructing lesions of the right colon are usually managed by right hemicolectomy with immediate ileocolic anastomosis. Palliative bypass without resection is only used in patients with unresectable carcinoma (p. 1430).

Obstructing lesions of the left colon are more difficult to manage, as emergency resection with immediate anastomosis carries a higher risk of anastomotic leakage. A staged approach is usually employed. In the classic three-stage approach, emergency transverse colostomy was performed to relieve obstruction. The patient was then prepared for elective resection of the affected bowel 3–4 weeks later. Although bowel preparation for this elective procedure reduced the risk of anastomotic leakage, the transverse colostomy was usually retained to divert the fecal stream until anastomotic healing had been confirmed by instilling barium into the distal loop. The third stage consisted of colostomy closure about 8 weeks later.

The classic three-stage approach to left-sided large bowel obstruction is now obsolete. Emergency resection with immediate end-to-end anastomosis can be undertaken in selected cases following on-table lavage of the obstructed bowel (Dudley et al 1980), but resection without immediate restoration of continuity is a more frequent option. If continuity is not restored immediately, the cut proximal and distal ends of bowel can both be exteriorized or the distal bowel can be oversewn with only the proximal cut end of colon being brought to the surface as a colostomy (Hartmann's procedure). Intestinal continuity is restored at a second elective operation after full bowel preparation.

Strangulated or perforated large bowel must always be resected. Right-sided lesions are dealt with by right hemicolectomy with ileocolic anastomosis or exteriorization of both bowel ends. Immediate anastomosis is not recommended after resection of strangulated or perforated left colon or rectum. Both ends of bowel can be exteriorized or a Hartmann's procedure can be performed.

Rarely, a patient with large bowel obstruction is not fit for laparotomy and "blind" cecostomy (i.e. undertaken through a small incision without exploration of the peritoneal cavity), performed if necessary under local anesthesia, may prove life-saving as a temporary measure.

*Nonoperative treatment*

Conservative management may be the appropriate in the following situations.

***Paralytic ileus.*** Paralytic ileus may complicate long-standing mechanical obstruction or result from peritonitis, retroperitoneal bleeding or acute pancreatitis (p. 1259). Paralysis probably results from interference with splanchnic nerve function, but a direct toxic effect on the bowel wall may be involved in peritonitis. Gross electrolyte disturbances, notably potassium and magnesium deficiency, can also cause ileus.

The abdomen is distended, tenderness is minimal or absent and there is little guarding on palpation. Bowel sounds are absent. Vomiting is often copious, as fluid spills back into the stomach from the distended gut. Plain abdominal radiographs show gaseous distention and multiple fluid levels throughout the gut and contrast radiography is frequently helpful (Riveron et al 1989).

Conservative treatment consists of nasogastric aspiration and intravenous fluid and electrolyte replacement. Surgery is only required for a surgically correctable lesion, but the patient must be reviewed twice daily and a positive decision taken to persist with conservative therapy. Mechanical intestinal obstruction or strangulation must not be allowed to escape notice.

***Mechanical obstruction.*** Conservative treatment for mechanical obstruction is only indicated in specific circumstances.

***Adhesion obstruction*** is treated conservatively, particularly if the patient has already undergone multiple operations. Further surgery carries little prospect of avoiding further episodes of obstruction and there is considerable risk that the bowel lumen will be entered inadvertently. Conservative treatment must be abandoned if there are any signs of strangulation or if obstruction persists.

***Intra-abdominal malignancy*** in patients known to have carcinomatosis may be a contraindication to surgery.

***Crohn's disease*** is often complicated by bouts of subacute obstruction which frequently resolve on conservative management (pp. 656 & 695).

***Pyloric stenosis*** usually requires operation, but surgery is best deferred for 4–5 days to allow rehydration, correction of electrolyte and acid–base disturbances and adequate gastric decompression (p. 284).

***Postoperative obstruction*** is generally attributable to paralytic ileus but mechanical obstruction due to adhesions or to bowel becoming trapped in peritoneal or mesenteric defects can occur. Paralytic ileus is usually transient, so that obstruction persisting for more than 2 or 3 days must be viewed with suspicion and laparotomy should be undertaken if mechanical causes cannot be excluded.

***Ileocecal intussusception*** in infants can be treated by the hydrostatic method of Ravitch (Ravitch 1958), provided that there is no risk of ischemia, facilities for operation are available and there is free reflux of barium into the ileum. Adult intussusception requires operation because there is often an underlying cause which requires surgery.

***Sigmoid volvulus*** accounts for some 5% of large bowel obstructions in Western communities; it is at least four times more common than cecal volvulus and infinitely more common than volvulus of the transverse colon. Sigmoid volvulus is the most frequent cause of large bowel obstruction in regions such as East Africa, where a high-residue diet is consumed. Elongation of the sigmoid mesocolon is a major predisposing factor. Over half the patients in Western countries are over 70 years and the condition is often encountered in the bedridden and mentally ill who fail to evacuate the bowel regularly. Chagas' disease is a cause in parts of South America and high altitude (with expansion of gas in the colonic lumen) and constipation caused by chewing coca leaves may be contributory in some areas.

The bowel usually twists in an anticlockwise direction about its mesentery and a closed loop obstruction occurs when it has rotated through 180°. Further rotation leads to impaired venous drainage and strangulation.

The patient presents with abdominal colic, complete constipation and gross asymmetrical abdominal distention. Plain abdominal radiographs show characteristic appearances in about two-thirds of patients. Classically there is an inverted U-shaped loop due to the massively distended sigmoid colon which is usually devoid of haustra, extends high in the abdominal cavity and sometimes reaches the diaphragm (Fig. 18.3). Proximal large bowel obstruction is also present, usually with gaseous distention, and there may be small bowel distention if the ileocecal valve is incontinent. If diagnostic difficulty persists, a contrast enema will show the typical smooth, tapered narrowing likened to a "bird's beak" appearance at the point of twisting.

Sigmoid volvulus is treated by passing a soft lubricated rubber tube into the twisted loop at rigid sigmoidoscopy or by introducing a flexible sigmoidoscope. The maneuver succeeds in 80–90% of cases (Arigbabu et al 1985) and expulsion of flatus and liquid feces with immediate disappearance of abdominal distention denotes satisfactory decompression. Residual tenderness in the left iliac fossa suggests strangulation and is an indication for laparotomy, as is failure to deflate the bowel. Elective sigmoid colectomy is usually recommended, as volvulus otherwise recurs in up to half of the patients.

***Acute colonic pseudo-obstruction.*** In 1948, Ogilvie described two patients with constipation, abdominal distention and colicky pain who did not have colonic obstruction at laparotomy but in whom the diaphragmatic crura and celiac axis were infiltrated by malignancy. It is now recognized that a clinical picture mimicking mechanical obstruction may develop in patients who do not have a mechanical cause and that while the large or small bowel can be affected, acute colonic "pseudo-obstruction" is particularly common (Dudley et al 1958).

The pathogenesis of pseudo-obstruction is unknown but in more than 80% of cases, it complicates other clinical conditions (Dorudi et al 1992) (see Table 18.8). One explanation offered is that surgery, retroperitoneal bleeding or neoplasia causes dysfunction of the parasympathetic nerves supplying the distal colon and rectum (S2 to S4), leading to atony or spasticity and a functional obstruction. The transition between collapsed and distended bowel is often near the splenic flexure and abnormal balance between the inhibitory sympathetic and excitatory parasympathetic nerves has been implicated, attention centering on reflex sympathetic-induced inhibition (Dorudi et al 1992). In dogs, reflex relaxation of the colon can be produced by ileal distention and multiple mechanisms are involved (Basilisco & Phillips 1994). The association of pseudo-obstruction with pregnancy, pelvic surgery and trauma suggests reflex stimulation from the uterus could block the efferent parasympathetic nerve supply from S2 to S4 (Spira et al 1976) or that the distal sigmoid colon could be obstructed by the uterus falling backwards (Munro & Jones 1975).

The patient presents with rapid and progressive abdominal distention which mimics acute large bowel obstruction. The plain radiograph of the abdomen shows a gas-filled cecum, ascending colon and transverse colon with a cut-off at the splenic flexure, rectosigmoid junction or hepatic flexure. If the diagnosis is in doubt, a barium enema is invaluable to exclude organic obstruction.

Acute colonic pseudo-obstruction can be treated conservatively for up to 72 h provided there is no right iliac fossa tenderness and the cecum is not grossly distended. Sequential measurement of cecal diameter is helpful in that cecal perforation is unlikely when its diameter is less than 12 cm but the risk increases markedly once the diameter exceeds 14 cm (Dorudi et al 1992).

Colonic decompression succeeds in about 80% of cases but is often difficult and time consuming and has a mortality rate of up to 5% (Dorudi et al 1992). Laparotomy may still be needed when the diagnosis is in doubt or when gross distention raises fears of cecal perforation. Tube cecostomy is then the treatment of choice in the absence of gross cecal necrosis and can be carried out under local or general anesthesia. A large Foley catheter is usually left in the cecum for some 2–3 weeks. It is now possible to insert cecostomy tubes percutaneously with the assistance of the colonoscope. The incidence of cecal perforation varies from 14% to 40% and in its presence, mortality rates rise to some 50%; in general the mortality rate of patients requiring surgery (30%) is twice as high as in patients managed by nonoperative means (Dorudi et al 1992).

**Table 18.8** Conditions associated with acute colonic pseudo-obstruction (from Dorudi et al 1992)

| | |
|---|---|
| Idiopathic | |
| Cardiovascular | |
| | Myocardial infarction |
| | Congestive cardiac failure |
| | Cerebrovascular accident |
| | Subarachnoid haemorrhage |
| | Pulmonary embolus |
| | Mesenteric ischaemia |
| | Peripheral vascular disease |
| After trauma | |
| | Intra-abdominal |
| | Pelvic fractures |
| | Spinal fractures/retroperitoneal haematoma |
| | Femoral fractures |
| | Burn injury |
| After operation | |
| | Abdominal surgery |
| | Pelvic/gynaecological surgery |
| | Postpartum |
| | Caesarean section |
| | Renal transplantation |
| | Cardiothoracic surgery |
| | Hip surgery |
| | Spinal surgery |
| | Neurosurgery |
| Malignant | |
| | Retroperitoneal |
| | Disseminated |
| | Leukaemia |
| | Pelvic radiotherapy |
| | Phenol ablation of renal tumour |
| Infective/inflammatory | |
| | Intra-abdominal/pelvic abscess |
| | Acute appendicitis |
| | Acute cholecystitis |
| | Acute pancreatitis |
| | Systemic sepsis |
| | Herpes zoster infection |
| Respiratory | |
| | Pneumonia |
| | Mechanical ventilation |
| Metabolic | |
| | Electrolyte disturbances |
| | Renal failure |
| | Liver failure |
| | Alcohol abuse |
| | Thyroid dysfunction |
| | Diabetes |
| | Parkinson's disease |
| Drugs | |
| | Antidepressants |
| | Phenothiazines |
| | Antiparkinsonian |
| | Opiates/narcotic addiction |
| | Neurological |
| | Nerve root compression |
| | Multiple sclerosis |
| | Low spinal cord disease |

The obstructive features of chronic colonic pseudo-obstruction and small intestinal pseudo-obstruction are discussed on p. 441.

## VASCULAR DISEASE AND THE ACUTE ABDOMEN

Ruptured abdominal aortic aneurysm and primary disease of the mesenteric blood vessels are important causes of the acute abdomen. Mesenteric vascular disease is considered elsewhere (p. 544).

### Ruptured aortic aneurysm

*Incidence*

The vast majority of aortic aneurysms occur in older men and approximately 5% of men aged 55–74 years harbor an asymptomatic aneurysm (Collin et al 1988). Rupture accounts for 1.7% of all deaths in men aged 64–75 years (Collin 1985). The risk of rupture of an asymptomatic aneurysm is approximately 25% per annum and doubles if the aneurysm is symptomatic. If rupture occurs, as many as two-thirds of patients may fail to reach hospital alive (Hopkins 1979) although more recent estimates suggest that this figure has fallen beneath 20% (Jenkins et al 1986).

*Pathology*

Atherosclerotic degeneration is the commonest cause. Occlusion of the nutritive vasa vasorum leads to reduced tensile strength, aneurysmal dilatation and ultimately to rupture.

*Clinical features*

The classic triad of abdominal pain, a pulsatile mass and shock is not always present or not always appreciated. Pain is the outstanding clinical feature and is severe, central or low and may ease only to return with renewed severity. Hemorrhage is usually retroperitoneal at first and shock may confuse the diagnosis. Back pain can simulate acute pancreatitis (p. 1253) and loin pain may mimic renal colic. The acute episode is preceded by up to 3 weeks of mild backache in as many as one-third of cases and slow leakage of blood can cause bruising of the abdominal wall, flank or perineum or produce a tender mass simulating inflammation.

Gastrointestinal bleeding can occur if the mesenteric circulation is compromised or if the aneurysm ruptures into the duodenum (p. 493). Aortocaval fistulae have also been reported.

*Treatment*

Survival depends on prompt diagnosis and immediate surgery. A lateral plain abdominal radiograph shows an expanded calcified vessel in some 80–90% of cases. While the urgency of the situation usually precludes refined investigations, portable real-time ultrasound scanning does allow rapid confirmation of the diagnosis. Computed tomography scanning in fast mode can also give valuable information while resuscitative and preanesthetic preparations are being carried out. However, diagnosis is essentially clinical; the correct place to investigate a ruptured aneurysm is in the operating theatre.

The patient's blood must be crossmatched immediately, two intravenous lines established, a catheter inserted into the bladder and operation commenced. Hemorrhage is arrested by crossclamping the aorta and the aneurysm is treated by insertion of a synthetic graft. Involvement of the renal arteries was once regarded as a contraindication to resection but occurs in only 1% of cases (Jenkins et al 1986) and may be overcome by transplanting a kidney to the iliac vessels or reimplanting the renal arteries .

Elective surgery for nonruptured aneurysm carries a mortality rate of 2–15% as opposed to 30–60% after emergency repair following rupture. If the patient survives the repair, there is no significant difference in long-term survival between the two patient groups and 8-year survival rates of 41–45% have been reported recently (Stonebridge et al 1993).

## OBSTETRIC AND GYNECOLOGICAL CAUSES OF THE ACUTE ABDOMEN

### Ruptured ectopic pregnancy

The fertilized ovum implants outside the uterus approximately once in every 200–300 pregnancies and there were an estimated 88 400 ectopic pregnancies in the United States in 1989 (Carson & Buster 1993). The fallopian tube is the commonest site of implantation (Fig. 18.4) and implantation in the cervix, ovary or peritoneal cavity is exceptional. Delayed or impaired transit of the ovum to the uterus is the major cause and may result from previous tubal infection (notably gonococcal salpingitis), use of an intrauterine contraceptive device, use of progestogens as a sole contraceptive agent (possibly) and conception following tubal surgery, tubal ligation or in vitro fertilization (Setchell & Cass 1990). The decidual reaction in the fallopian tube is inadequate for the needs of the developing conceptus and the erosive trophoblast penetrates the wall, leading to rupture. The conceptus may also be extruded from the fimbrial end of the tube. Interstitial pregnancy may continue for 16 weeks, but embryos implanting in the isthmus do not often survive beyond 6 weeks.

#### *Clinical features*

Delayed diagnosis is the major cause of morbidity and mortality in ectopic pregnancy (Report 1989). Most patients present with recurrent abominal pain, often associated with fainting and vaginal bleeding. Abdominal pain almost always occurs and begins suddenly as a cramping pain in one or other iliac fossa. Sudden rupture is much less common and produces more generalized pain with rebound tenderness and rigidity and shock due to intra-abdominal bleeding. Shoulder-tip pain occurs in about 10% of patients.

Amenorrhea and/or abnormal vaginal bleeding is noted by some 75% of patients. The menstrual history may mislead in that rupture can occur before the next period would have been expected or bleeding at the start of rupture may be mistaken for a period. Vaginal bleeding associated with rupture is dark ("prune juice"), scanty and follows the pain, in contrast to the profuse, bright red bleeding of abortion which precedes the pain.

Signs of pregnancy, such as enlargement of the breasts and uterus, are not usually obvious, but cervical softening and tenderness are apparent on gentle pelvic examination. The pregnancy may rupture between the layers of the broad ligament, producing a tender hematoma and an

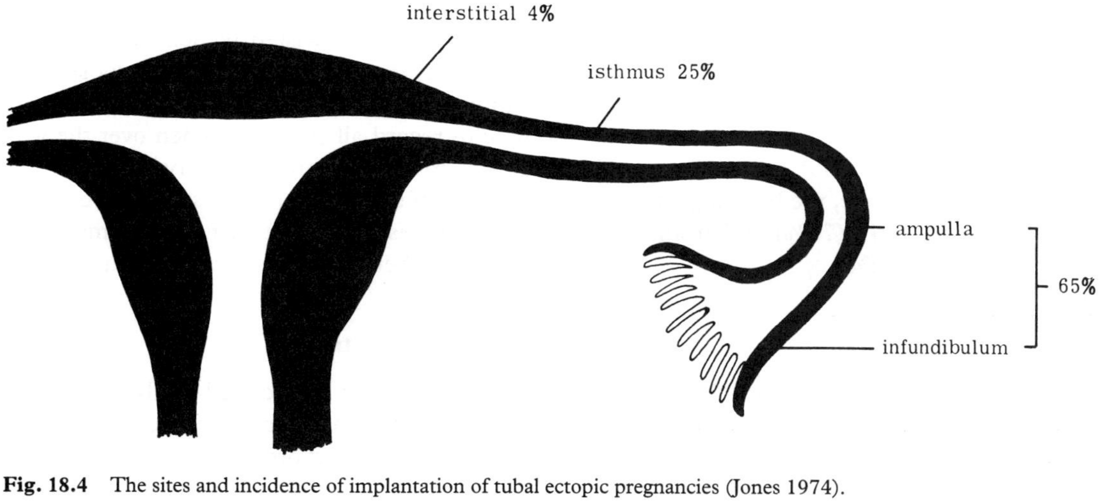


**Fig. 18.4** The sites and incidence of implantation of tubal ectopic pregnancies (Jones 1974).

adnexal mass is palpable through the vaginal wall in up to 50% of cases.

Presymptomatic diagnosis is now possible as early as 4.5 weeks after gestation (Carson & Buster 1993). Serum progesterone levels reflect stimulation of the corpus luteum by a viable pregnancy. Failure of the pregnancy causes serum levels to fall so that progesterone levels can be used to exclude ectopic pregnancy and identify nonviable pregnancies. Utrasensitive assays for the β subunit of human chorionic gonadotrophin (β-hCG) are also useful; a negative β-hCG virtually discounts pregnancy whereas a positive test confirms pregnancy but does not indicate whether it is ectopic. In normal pregnancy the serum concentration of β-hCG doubles every 2 days and patients with ectopic pregnancy have reduced production with prolonged doubling times.

Once pregnancy is confirmed, abdominal ultrasonography can confirm whether it is intrauterine and transvaginal ultrasonography may be particularly useful. Laparoscopy can prove useful when the diagnosis remains in doubt and given the advent of laparoscopic salpingostomy or salpingectomy, laparotomy is now needed less frequently. Medical treatment with agents such as systemic methotrexate can now be used in some women to abort the ectopic pregnancy and avoid narrowing of the fallopian tube involved (Carson et al 1993).

*Treatment*

Rupture with massive intraperitoneal bleeding demands urgent surgery. It may be impossible to keep up with the blood loss until the affected tube has been clamped at operation and resuscitation should be regarded as part of the operation rather than a preliminary measure. Tubal pregnancy is usually treated by removing the involved tube but in some cases it may be possible to conserve the tube by performing a linear salpingostomy.

**Rupture of "functional" ovarian cysts**

Ovulation with rupture of a Graafian follicle normally occurs 14 days after the onset of menstruation. The follicle then becomes a corpus luteum and this degenerates before the start of the next menstrual period unless conception occurs. Hoyt & Meigs (1936) reported that in 58 operations for ovarian hemorrhage, the bleeding was coming from a corpus luteum in 45 (78%) and from a ruptured Graafian follicle in 13 (22%).

*Clinical features*

The patient is usually in the age group 15–25 years and complains of sudden iliac fossa pain. Nausea and vomiting may be present, but the patient remains afebrile and the pain usually settles within hours. Tenderness and guarding in the right iliac fossa can mimic acute appendicitis and in a minority of cases there is sufficient bleeding to suggest rupture of an ectopic pregnancy. Rectal examination often reveals tenderness in the rectovaginal pouch and ultrasound scanning may confirm the diagnosis.

*Treatment*

Observation is indicated in young females complaining of iliac fossa pain in the middle of a menstrual cycle ("Mittelschmerz"). The pain usually settles spontaneously and laparoscopy can be undertaken to exclude acute appendicitis or ruptured ectopic pregnancy.

**Torsion or rupture of ovarian cysts**

Over 90% of ovarian neoplasms in women under the age of 30 years are benign. Between the ages of 30 and 50 years this figure falls to 80% and in women over 50 years of age about half are malignant. Many of these neoplasms are cystic and difficult to evaluate at laparoscopy.

Dermoid cysts make up less than 10% of ovarian cysts, but are liable to torsion because of their long pedicles. They account for half the twisted ovarian cysts in young women.

*Clinical features*

Cramping lower abdominal pain is present and a smooth rounded mass is often palpable higher in the abdomen than might be expected. Tenderness and guarding are elicited over the mass and peritonism becomes marked if the cyst ruptures. A fallopian tube and pedunculated uterine fibroids may also undergo torsion and present with a similar clinical picture. Ultrasound scanning may reveal free fluid but laparoscopy or laparotomy may be needed to confirm the diagnosis.

*Treatment*

At operation the twisted pedicle is transfixed and ligated and the ovary removed. Adequate exposure is essential, as rupture of the cyst can disseminate malignant cells. It is wise to regard all cysts in women over the age of 30 years as malignant until proved otherwise. Pelvic clearance with removal of both tubes, ovaries and uterus may be required if the cyst is malignant and surgery may need to be followed by chemotherapy or radiotherapy.

**Acute salpingitis**

Most cases are associated with sexually transmitted infection and gonococci are the organsims most often responsible. Other organisms, such as streptococci and *Mycobacterium tuberculosis*, may be responsible and the risk of salpingitis is increased by use of an intrauterine contraceptive device and by recent pregnancy. Three to six days after gonococcal infection there is urethritis, cervicitis and vaginal discharge. Tubal involvement is unusual at this stage and tends to follow a menstrual period as organisms spread from the endocervix to the lining of the uterus and tube. Both tubes are commonly involved and edema and adhesions may close off the fimbriated ends, leading to pyosalpinx.

*Clinical features*

The pain and tenderness of salpingitis are commonly bilateral and low in the abdomen, often just above the pubis and inguinal ligaments. Urinary frequency is common but dysuria is rare. An irregular menstrual history is often obtained. The temperature rises early to 39° or 40°C, and leukocytosis is common.

Vaginal examination reveals unusual vaginal warmth, cervical tenderness and a purulent discharge. In closed pyosalpinx there may be no discharge and vaginal, cervical and urethral swabs may not reveal the causal organism. Ultrasound scanning is often diagnostic.

*Treatment*

Aggressive antibiotic therapy is essential to reduce the risk of permanent tubal damage and sterility. Erythromycin or tetracycline with metronidazole can be used until the results of cultures are available, but ampicillin may be preferred if gonococcal infection is confirmed (Setchell & Cass 1990). Laparotomy is undertaken if acute appendicitis or an ectopic pregnancy cannot be excluded, but the affected tube is removed only if it contains a closed pyosalpinx. Otherwise, a specimen of pus is obtained for culture (including anaerobic and *Chlamydia*) and the abdomen closed without drainage and without removing the appendix.

## MEDICAL CAUSES OF THE ACUTE ABDOMEN

Acute abdominal pain can be produced by a number of medical conditions and surgery may have to be undertaken if the diagnosis cannot be established.

### Endocrine or metabolic diseases

*Diabetes mellitus*

Severe abdominal pain and tenderness can occur in diabetic ketoacidosis. Campbell et al (1975) reported this in 46 of 211 (21%) episodes of diabetic ketoacidosis. A cause for ketoacidosis was found in three-quarters of the 46 episodes and in 17 cases (37%) could have accounted for the pain. In the remaining episodes, the cause of the pain was unknown. Although hyperamylasemia may be associated with diabetic ketoacidosis, pancreatitis is rarely responsible for the abdominal pain. The abdominal pain of diabetic ketoacidosis should resolve rapidly once treatment is started; if it does not, a cause such as acute appendicitis, which may itself have caused the ketoacidosis, should be sought. Ketoacidosis requires vigorous treatment if surgery is required.

*Hereditary hepatic porphyria (acute porphyria)* (p. 35.24)

Acute porphyria is commoner in women but rare before puberty; in some women there are monthly attacks of pain which occur in the late luteal phase of the menstrual cycle (Bonkovsky 1993). The abdominal pain is severe and resembles small bowel colic, but with less marked tenderness. Vomiting and obstipation are common and motor and sensory neurological deficits can develop. The diagnosis rests on finding increased levels of porphobilinogen and/or 5-aminolevulinate (ALA) in the urine, but it must be remembered that some patients with intermittent abdominal pain due to other causes can show marginal increases in urinary porphyrins. Surgery is contraindicated in acute porphyria; the patient is advised to avoid porphyrogenic drugs and alcohol and can be treated with agents such as intravenous heme.

*Hemochromatosis* (p. 954)

Abdominal pain occurs in approximately one-third of patients with hemochromatosis. The pain is dull and boring, but may be severe and simulate acute appendicitis or acute cholecystitis.

*Lead poisoning*

The clinical features resemble acute porphyria and the diagnosis is suggested by a history of exposure to lead, muscle palsy, a blue line on the gums and punctate basophilia of the red blood cells.

### Diseases of the blood and blood vessels

*Hereditary spherocytosis*

Attacks of abdominal pain, nausea, vomiting, tenderness and guarding may coincide with episodes of hemolysis in which anemia worsens and jaundice may deepen. Emergency laparotomy is seldom indicated, but cholelithiasis occurs in half of these patients and cholecystitis should always be considered.

*Hemophilia and other bleeding disorders*

Bleeding disorders such as thrombocytopenic purpura,

hemophilia, leukemia and overanticoagulation can cause abdominal pain due to bleeding into the gut wall, mesentery or retroperitoneum. Such patients may get diseases such as appendicitis, but abdominal pain is more commonly due to bleeding. Anscombe (1970) reviewed 100 patients admitted to a hemophilia center with acute abdominal pain; only five required surgery, four for acute appendicitis and one for intestinal strangulation. Extraperitoneal bleeding is common and hemorrhage into the psoas sheath can simulate appendicitis. Hematoma in the gut wall can cause intussusception.

Collections of blood in the mesentery or muscle compartments such as the psoas or anterior rectus sheaths can be easily identified by ultrasound scanning or computed tomography, allowing conservative management. Hematological advice is essential to ensure or restore normal coagulation, prevent further bleeding and permit surgery if required.

*Anaphylactoid purpura*

Henoch–Schönlein purpura occurs predominantly in children and usually presents with purpura followed by polyarthritis and abdominal symptoms. Other features include proteinuria and hematuria due to glomerulonephritis and cutaneous edema, pleurisy and pericarditis. Over half of the patients have gastrointestinal symptoms with severe abdominal colic, vomiting and occasionally hematemesis and melena. The pain can precede the purpura and children may present only with abdominal pain and undergo unnecessary laparotomy. The abdominal pain is due to intestinal obstruction, but only edema and hemorrhage are found at laparotomy. Intussusception or perforation are uncommon in adults but can occur in children.

Barium studies of the small bowel usually confirm the presence of hemorrhage into the bowel wall or edema and should prevent unnecessary surgery. Follow-through studies may be used to monitor the response to medical therapy, but it must be borne in mind that the appearances can simulate nonhemorrhagic conditions such as Crohn's disease or lymphoma (Glasier et al 1981).

Corticosteroids relieve abdominal pain within 24 h and may reduce bleeding. They have no beneficial effect on outcome and can mask signs of perforation. Intussusception and perforation require surgical treatment. Chronic nephritis is the major cause of mortality and morbidity in the children and does not respond to corticosteroids.

*Sickle cell disease* (p. 1103)

This hereditary disease is virtually confined to blacks, particularly those originating from West Africa. Hemoglobin-S crystallizes when oxygen tension is reduced, causing rigidity and deformity of red cells and increased blood viscosity. Small blood vessels become blocked, leading to painful skeletal and abdominal crises. Abdominal pain, which is usually severe, is felt in the upper abdomen and may be due to splenic infarction. Nausea, vomiting and leukocytosis are usual and potentially confusing. The crisis may last from hours to days. The true diagnosis is suggested by associated anemia, leg ulcers and characteristic bony changes and can be confirmed by blood film examination. Gallstones occur in a third of patients.

Surgery is contraindicated unless a surgical disease requiring laparotomy cannot be excluded. Particular care is needed to avoid hypoxia during anesthesia or dehydration, as these worsen the crisis.

*Polycythemia rubra vera*

Spontaneous thrombosis occasionally causes splenic and mesenteric infarction.

*Polyarteritis nodosa* (p. 551)

Polyarteritis nodosa often affects the small and medium-sized arteries of the gut leading to ischemia and fibrinoid necrosis. The resulting gangrene and ulceration is usually located in the small intestine and presents with bleeding or perforation. Abdominal pain is very common; it is usually colicky and situated in the right upper quadrant or epigastrium. Anorexia, nausea and vomiting are also common and peptic ulcer, cholecystitis or appendicitis may be suspected. Peritoneal or retroperitoneal hemorrhage are also reported. When the small vessels of the colon are involved, the presentation can resemble ulcerative colitis. Selective mesenteric angiography may reveal the presence of multiple small aneurysms.

When a patient with polyarteritis nodosa presents with acute abdominal pain, a trial of corticosteroids is justified if there are no signs of perforation or peritonitis.

*Systemic lupus erythematosus* (p. 551)

Abdominal pain due to arteritis may also occur in this disease.

## Infections

*Acute mesenteric adenitis*

The etiology is uncertain, but viral infection is probably responsible. The mesenteric nodes are large, discrete, soft and fleshy. Microscopy reveals nonspecific hyperplasia and edema and culture is negative.

The patients are usually between 5 and 15 years old and give a history of central colicky abdominal pain, anorexia, nausea and vomiting. There may have been previous attacks or a recent upper respiratory tract infection. The patient is frequently flushed and pyrexial, with injection of the fauces and cervical lymphadenopathy. Abdominal tenderness is found higher than is usual in appendicitis, varies in severity on repeated examination and shifts when the child changes position. Guarding and rebound tenderness are unusual and a mass of glands is sometimes palpable in the right iliac fossa.

Jones (1969) reported that of 462 children undergoing emergency laparotomy for suspected appendicitis, 42 (9%) had mesenteric adenitis. However, as bedside diagnosis of adenitis was rarely feasible because typical features were frequently missing, there should be no hesitation in carrying out laparotomy if acute appendicitis cannot be excluded confidently after a period of observation.

*Acute terminal ileitis*

This is discussed on p. 525.

*Other infections*

Generalized abdominal pain may be a feature of acute tonsillitis, pharyngitis, otitis media and influenza. Gastroenteritis can simulate retroileal and pelvic appendicitis, but vomiting and diarrhea are usually prominent. Prodromal or anicteric acute viral hepatitis can produce nausea, vomiting and pain in the right hypochondrium. Coxsackie viral infections cause fever with intercostal and abdominal pain, but a pleural rub and thoracic muscle tenderness are usually diagnostic.

### Neurological and psychiatric diseases

*Herpes zoster* affecting the lower thoracic nerve roots can cause pain in the anterolateral abdominal wall before herpetic vesicles appear. Careful examination usually reveals that pain is confined to the distribution of a nerve root and seldom crosses the mid-line. Bilateral *Herpes zoster* is rare. Abdominal pain with tenderness and guarding may appear before headache and neck stiffness in meningitis and can cause confusion in diagnosis. Tabes dorsalis with gastric crises is now exceedingly rare. The severe lightning pains are associated with vomiting, but rigidity is absent.

The Munchausen syndrome is a recurring diagnostic problem. Careful objective examination is essential, as these patients do occasionally suffer from conditions needing surgery. The temptation to "beat the patient at his own game" must be resisted and emphasis should be placed on vital signs and on abdominal findings when the patient's attention is distracted.

### Intrathoracic disease

Respiration is typically rapid and shallow in patients with severe acute abdominal pain. Even though pulmonary or cardiac disease can also produce abdominal pain, tachypnea, dyspnea, fever, cough, purulent sputum or cyanosis usually indicate the true source of the problem. In acute respiratory disease, such as pneumonia, the alae nasi may move with respiration.

In almost all instances a plain chest radiograph will confirm the clinical signs and reveal the underlying abnormality.

*Pleurisy and pneumonia*

Abdominal pain and guarding frequently appear before obvious chest signs (p. 512). Unilateral pain of abdominal origin is often associated with tenderness when the opposite side of the abdomen is pressed, whereas pain referred from the chest is not associated with such tenderness.

*Myocardial infarction*

The pain of myocardial infarction is occasionally maximal in the epigastrium, but in such cases retrosternal pain is usually also present. The pain is unaffected by abdominal examination and signs of left ventricular failure or arrhythmia may be found. The diagnosis is confirmed by an electrocardiograph and by serum enzyme measurements. The electrocardiogram can be normal in the early stages of a myocardial infarct and it needs to be repeated in a few hours if an infarct is to be diagnosed electrocardiographically. Acute abdominal diseases, on the other hand, may sometimes be associated with electrocardiographic changes, though rarely those typical of myocardial infarction. Fortunately, abdominal signs are marked, or soon become so, in abdominal diseases requiring emergency surgery and there is then seldom doubt as to the source of the primary illness.

### Genitourinary diseases

Pain in the loin or iliac fossa can be caused by acute pyelitis and is a particular problem during infancy, childhood and pregnancy. Dysuria and frequency are usual in pyelitis and there is gross contamination of the urine by pus cells and bacteria. Pus cells are also found in the urine of some patients with acute appendicitis, but contamination is seldom gross. Uremia is often complicated by vomiting and abdominal distention.

Renal colic is sudden in onset, radiating from the loin down to the iliac fossa and groin. The patient is pale, restless and complains of nausea and vomiting. Abdominal tenderness and guarding are not as marked as in peritonitis. The diagnosis is confirmed by finding red blood cells in the urine and plain abdominal radiographs may show a calcified stone in the urinary tract in about 80% of patients. Subsequent ultrasound scanning or intravenous pyelography will reveal the site and possibly the nature of the obstruction.

Dysuria and frequency usually denote lower urinary tract infection. Acute retention causes severe lower abdominal pain and tenderness and assessment is impossible until the bladder has been decompressed. Chronic retention with overflow incontinence causes painless bladder distention.

Torsion of an undescended testis may simulate strangulation of an inguinal hernia, a pitfall which is avoided by always examining the testes and scrotum.

## Nonspecific abdominal pain

De Dombal et al (1974) found that about half of 552 patients admitted to hospital with abdominal pain had no detectable disease. Many recovered spontaneously, some had no abnormality at laparotomy and a few had urinary tract infection of doubtful significance. Nonspecific pain may be due to mesenteric adenitis, urinary tract infection, gastroenteritis, irritable bowel syndrome, cyclical ovarian changes and emotional problems. There is a relationship between the onset of pain and life events such as the break-up of close relationships (Creed 1981) and psychosocial problems are significantly more common in patients with nonspecific pain (Fraser et al 1992). Psychological factors in some patients may explain why the "closed eyes sign" (i.e. the patient keeps their eyes closed during abdominal examination to elicit tenderness) is present in one-third of patients with nonspecific abdominal pain as opposed to only 4% of those with appendicitis (Gray et al 1988).

Acute appendicitis is the most frequent cause for concern, as tenderness is often present in the right iliac fossa. Jones (1969) reported that 40% of children admitted with suspected acute appendicitis recovered after a day or two without treatment.

A period of active observation (p. 514) is essential and if pain and tenderness persist laparotomy is usually undertaken to exclude conditions requiring surgery.

REFERENCES


Adams I D, Chan M, Clifford P C et al 1986 Computer aided diagnosis of acute abdominal pain: a multicentre study. British Medical Journal 293: 800–804

Adam E J, Page J E 1991 Intra-abdominal sepsis: the role of radiology. In: Williamson R C N & Thompson J N (eds) Gastrointestinal Emergencies: Part I. Baillière Tindall, London, pp 587–610

Andersson R, Hugander A, Thulin A, Nystrom P O, Olaison G 1994 Indications for operation in suspected appendicitis and incidence of perforation. British Medical Journal 308: 107–110

Anscombe A R 1970 Surgery in haemophilia and allied disorders. Annals of the Royal College of Surgeons of England 47: 125

Arigbabu A O, Badejo O A, Akinola D O 1985 Colonoscopy in the emergency treatment of colonic volvulus. Diseases of the Colon and Rectum 28: 795–798

Attwood S E A, Cafferkey M T, West A B et al 1987 Yersinia infection and acute abdominal pain. Lancet 1: 529–533

Attwood S E A, Cafferkey M T, Keane F B 1989 Yersinia infection in surgical practice. British Journal of Surgery 76: 499–504

Attwood S E A, Hill A D K, Murphy P G, Thornton J, Stephens R B 1992 A prospective randomized trial of laparoscopic versus open appendectomy. Surgery 112: 497–501

Barker D J P 1985 Acute appendicitis and dietary fibre: an alternative hypothesis. British Medical Journal 290: 1125–1127

Barker D J P, Morris J 1988 Acute appendicitis, bathrooms, and diet in Britain and Ireland. British Medical Journal 296: 953–955

Barker D J P, Osmond C, Golding J, Wadworth M E J 1988 Acute appendicitis and bathrooms in three samples of British children. British Medical Journal 296: 956–958

Bartlett R H, Eraklis A J, Wilkinson R H 1970 Appendicitis in infancy. Surgery Gynecology and Obstetrics 130: 99

Basilisco G, Phillips S F 1994 Ileal distension relaxes the canine colon: a model of megacolon? Gastroenterology 106: 606–614

Baue A E, Tragus E T, Wolfson S K, Cary A L, Parkins W M 1967 Hemodynamic and metabolic effects of Ringer's lactate solution in hemorrhagic shock. Annals of Surgery 166: 29

Berry J, Malt R A 1984 Appendicitis near its centenary. Annals of Surgery 200: 567–575

Billing A G, Frohlic D, Konecny G et al 1994 Local serum applications: restoration of sufficient host defence in human peritonitis. European Journal of Clinical Investigation 24: 28–35

Bonkovsky H L 1993 Advances in understanding and treating "the little imitator", acute porphyria. Gastroenterology 105: 590–594

Border J R 1992 Multiple systems organ failure. Annals of Surgery 216: 111–116

Caldwell M T P, Watson R G K 1994 Peritoneal aspiration cytology as a diagnostic aid in acute appendicitis. British Journal of Surgery 81: 276–278

Campbell I W, Duncan L J P, Innes J A, MacCuish A C, Munro J F 1975 Abdominal pain in diabetic metabolic decompensation. Journal of the American Medical Association 233: 166–168

Carson S A, Buster J E 1993 Ectopic pregnancy. New England Journal of Medicine 329: 1174–1181

Chamberlain G V P, Carron Brown J A 1978 Report of the working party of the confidential enquiry into gynaecological laparoscopy. In: Royal College of Obstetricians and Gynaecologists, London.

Collin J 1985 The incidence of abdominal aortic aneurysm. British Journal of Surgery 72: 499

Collin J, Araujo L, Walton J, Lindsell D 1988 Oxford screening programme for abdominal aortic aneurysm in men aged 65 to 74 years. Lancet 2: 613–615

Cox K R 1970 Starch granuloma—pseudomalignant seedlings. British Journal of Surgery

Creed F 1981 Life events and appendicectomy. Lancet 1: 1381–1385

de Dombal F T, Leaper D J, Staniland J R, McCann A P, Horrocks J C 1972 Computer-aided diagnosis of acute abdominal pain. British Medical Journal 2: 9–13

de Dombal F T, Leaper D J, Horrocks J C, Staniland J R, McCann A P 1974 Human and computer-aided diagnosis of abdominal pain: further report with emphasis on performance of clinicians. British Medical Journal 1: 376–380

de Dombal F T, Dallos V, McAdam W A F 1991 Can computer aided teaching packages improve clinical care in patients with acute abdominal pain? British Medical Journal 302: 1495–1497

Deitch E A 1992 Multiple organ failure. Pathophysiology and potential future therapy. Annals of Surgery 216: 117–134

DeVore G R 1980 Acute abdominal pain in the pregnant patient due to pancreatitis, acute appendicitis, cholecystitis, or peptic ulcer disease. Clinical Perinatology 7: 349–369

Dixon J M, Elton R A, Rainey J B, Macleod D A D 1991 Rectal examination in patients with pain in the right lower quadrant of the abdomen. British Medical Journal 302: 386–388

Donnan S P B 1986 Appendicitis in Hong Kong. In: (ed) The aetiology of acute appendicitis. (Scientific Report No. 7). MRC Environmental Epidemiology Unit, Southampton, pp 16–19

Dorudi S, Berry A R, Kettlewell M G W 1992 Acute colonic pseudo-obstruction. British Journal of Surgery 79: 99–103
Dudley H A F, Sinclair I S, McLaren I F, McNair T J, Newsam J E 1958 Intestinal pseudo-obstruction. Journal of the Royal College of Surgeons of Edinburgh 3: 206–217
Dudley H A F, Radcliffe A G, McGeehan D 1980 Intraoperative irrigation of the colon to permit primary anastomosis. British Journal of Surgery 67: 80–81
Edmonds P, Merino M J, LiVolsi V A, Duray P H 1984 Adenocarcinoid (mucinous carcinoid) of the appendix. Gastroenterology 86: 302–308
Eisenberg R L, Heineken P, Hedgcock M W, Federle M, Goldberg H I 1983 Evaluation of plain abdominal radiographs in the diagnosis of abdominal pain. Annals of Surgery 197: 464–469
Field S, Guy P J, Upsdell S M, Scourfield A E 1985 The erect abdominal radiograph in the acute abdomen: should its routine use be abandoned? British Medical Journal 290: 1934–1936
Fraser S C A, Smith K, Agarwal M, Bates T 1992 Psychological screening for non-specific abdominal pain. British Journal of Surgery 79: 1369–1371
Glasier C M, Siegel M J, McAlister W H, Shackelford G D 1981 Henoch–Schonlein syndrome in children: gastrointestinal manifestations. American Journal of Roentgenology 136: 1081
Gray D W, Dixon J M, Collin J 1988 The closed eyes sign: an aid to diagnosing non-specific abdominal pain. British Medical Journal 297: 837
Greenall M J, Evans M, Pollock A V 1978 Should you drain a perforated appendix? British Journal of Surgery 65: 880–882
Gunn A A 1991 The acute abdomen: the role of computer-assisted diagnosis. In: Williamson R C N & Thompson J N (eds) Gastrointestinal emergencies: part 1. Ballière Tindall, London, pp 639–665
Gurry J F 1974 Acute terminal ileitis and Yersinia infection. British Medical Journal 1: 264–266
Haaga J R 1990 Imaging intra abdominal abscesses and non-operative drainage procedures. World Journal of Surgery 14: 204–209
Hayward M W J, Hayward C, Ennis W P, Roberts C J 1984 A pilot evaluation of radiography of the acute abdomen. Clinical Radiology 35: 289
Heaton K W 1987 Aetiology of acute appendicitis. British Medical Journal 294: 1632–1633
Hinshaw J R 1963 The acute abdomen complicating pregnancy. Journal of the Oklahoma Medical Association 56: 4–10
Hopkins N F G 1979 Abdominal aortic aneurysm. British Medical Journal 294: 790–791
Horowitz M D, Gomex G A, Satniesteban R, Burkett G 1985 Acute appendicitis during pregnancy: diagnosis and management. Archives of Surgery 120: 1362–1367
Hoyt W F, Meigs J V 1936 Rupture of the Graafian follicle and corpus luteum. Surgery Gynecology and Obstetrics 62: 114–119
Jahangiri M, Wyllie J H 1990 Peripheral blood lymphopenia in gangrenous appendicitis. British Medical Journal 301: 215
Jeddy T A, Vowles R H, Southam J A 1994 "Cough sign": a reliable test in the diagnosis of intra-abdominal inflammation. British Journal of Surgery 81: 279
Jenkins D, Lee P W R 1970 Radiology in acute appendicitis. Journal of the Royal College of Surgeons of Edinburgh 15: 34–37
Jenkins A M, Ruckley C V, Nolan B 1986 Ruptured aortic aneurysm. British Journal of Surgery 73: 395–398
Jones P F 1969 Acute abdominal pain in childhood with special reference to cases not due to acute appendicitis. British Medical Journal 2: 551–554
Jones P F 1974 Emergency abdominal surgery. Blackwell, Oxford.
Jones P F 1976 Active observation in management of acute abdominal pain in childhood. British Medical Journal 2: 551–553
Klappenback R S, Kurman R J, Sinclair C F, James L P 1985 Composite carcinoma – carcinoid tumors of the gastrointestinal tract. A morphologic, histochemical, and immunocytochemical study. American Journal of Clinical Pathology 84: 137
Klar E, Foitzik T, Buhr H, Messmer K, Herfarth C 1993 Isovolemic hemodilution with dextran 60 as treatment of pancreatic ischaemia in acute pancreatitis. Annals of Surgery 217: 369–374
Krukowski Z H, Koruth N H, Matheson N A 1986 Antibiotic lavage in emergency surgery for peritoneal sepsis. Journal of the Royal College of Surgeons of Edinburgh 31: 1–6
Lancet 1983 Leading article. Meckel's diverticulum: surgical guidelines at last? Lancet 2: 438–439
Leape L L, Ramenofsky M L 1980 Laparoscopy for questionable appendicitis—can it reduce the negative laparoscopy rate? Annals of Surgery 191: 410–413
Lee P W R 1973 The leucocyte count in acute appendicitis. British Journal of Surgery 60: 618
Leiboff A R, Soroff H S 1987 The treatment of generalized peritonitis by closed postoperative peritoneal lavage. Archives of Surgery 122: 1005–1100
Leijonmarck C-E, Bonman-Sandelin K, Frisell J, Raf L 1986 Meckel's diverticulum in the adult. British Journal of Surgery 73: 146–149
MacGillivray D C, Heaton R B, Rushin J M, Cruess D F 1992 Distant metastasis from a carcinoid tumor of the appendix less than one centimeter in size. Surgery 111: 466–471
McLean A D, Stonebridge P A, Bradbury A W, Rainey J B, Macleod D A D 1993 Time of presentation, time of operation, and unnecessary appendicectomy. British Medical Journal 306: 307
Moertel C G, Dockerty M B Judd E S 1968 Carcinoid tumours of the vermiform appendix. Cancer 21: 270–278
Moertel C G, Weiland L H, Nagorney D M, Dockerty M B 1987 Carcinoid tumor of the appendix: treatment and prognosis. New England Journal of Medicine 317: 1699–1701
Mosdell D M, Morris D M, Voltura A et al 1991 Antibiotic treatment for surgical peritonitis. Annals of Surgery 214: 543–549
Mughal M M, Bancewicz J, Irving M H 1986 "Laparostomy": a technique for the management of intractable intra-abdominal sepsis. British Journal of Surgery 73: 253
Munro A, Jones P F 1975 Abdominal surgical emergencies in the puerperium. British Medical Journal 4: 691–694
Nitecki S, Assalia A, Schein M 1993 Contemporary management of appendiceal mass. British Journal of Surgery 80: 18–20
Nunn J F, Freeman J 1964 Problems of oxygenation and oxygen transport during haemorrhage. Anaesthesia 19: 206
Ogilvie H 1948 Large intestine colic due to sympathetic deprivation. A new clinical syndrome. British Medical Journal 2: 671–673
Olsen J B, Myren C J, Haahr P E 1993 Randomized study of the value of laparoscopy before appendicectomy. British Journal of Surgery 80: 922–923
Papanicolaou G, Ahn Y K, Nikas D J, Fielding L P 1989 Effect of large bowel obstruction on colonic blood flow: an experimental study. Diseases of the Colon and Rectum 32: 673–679
Paterson-Brown S 1991 Strategies for reducing inappropriate laparotomy rate in the acute abdomen. British Medical Journal 303: 1115–1118
Paterson-Brown S, Eckersley J R T, Sim A J W, Dudley H A F 1986(a) Laparoscopy as an adjunct to decision making in the acute abdomen. British Journal of Surgery 73: 1022–1024
Paterson-Brown S, Olunfunwa S A, Galazka N, Simmons S C 1986(b) Visualisation of the normal appendix at laparoscopy. Journal of the Royal College of Surgeons of Edinburgh 31: 106–107
Paterson-Brown S, Thompson J N, Eckersley J R T, Ponting G A, Dudley H A F 1988 Which patients with suspected appendicitis should undergo laparoscopy? British Medical Journal 296: 1363–1364
Peltokallio P 1966 Acute appendicitis associated with carcinoma of the colon. Diseases of the Colon and Rectum 9: 453–456
Peltokallio P, Jauhiainen K 1970 Acute appendicitis in the aged patient. Archives of Surgery 100: 140
Phillips R K S, Hittinger R, Fry J S, Fielding L P 1985 Malignant large bowel obstruction. British Journal of Surgery 72: 296–302
Pledger H G, Fahy L T, van Mourik G A, Bush G H 1987 Deaths in children with a diagnosis of acute appendicitis in England and Wales 1980–4. British Medical Journal 295: 1233–1235
Ravitch M M 1958 Intussusception in infancy and childhood. New England Journal of Medicine 259: 1058
Report 1989 Report on confidential enquiries into maternal deaths in England and Wales 1982–1984. HMSO, London.
Riseman J A, Wichterman K 1989 Evaluation of right hemicolectomy for unexpected cecal mass. Archives of Surgery 124: 1043–1044
Riveron F A, Obeid F N, Horst M, Sorensen V J, Bivins B A 1989 The

role of contrast radiography in presumed bowel obstruction. Surgery 106: 496–501
Schwerk W B, Wichtrup B, Rothmund M, Ruschoff J 1989 Ultrasonography in the diagnosis of acute appendicitis: a prospective study. Gastroenterology 97: 630–639
Setchell M E, Cass P L 1990 Gynaecological causes of the acute abdomen. In: Williamson R C N & Cooper M J (eds) Emergency abdominal surgery. Clinical Surgery International (17). Chuchill Livingstone, Edinburgh, pp 233–241
Sherlock D J 1985 Acute appendicitis in the over-sixty age group. British Journal of Surgery 72: 245–246
Shields R 1965 The absorption and secretion of fluid and electrolytes by the obstructed bowel. British Journal of Surgery 52: 774–779
Silen W, Hein M F, Goldman L 1962 Strangulation obstruction of the small intestine. Archives of Surgery 85: 137–145
Simpson A, Sandeman D, Nixon S J, Goulbourne I A, Grieve D C, MacIntyre I M C 1985 The value of an erect abdominal radiograph in the diagnosis of intestinal obstruction. Clinical Radiology 36: 41
Solomkin J S 1988 Use of new beta-lactam antibiotics for surgical infection. Surgical Clinics of North America 68: 1–24
Soltero M J, Bill A H 1976 The natural history of Meckel's diverticulum and its relation to incidental removal. American Journal of Surgery 132: 168–173
Sperling L 1938 Mechanics of simple intestinal obstruction. Archives of Surgery 36: 778
Spira I A, Rodrigues R, Wolff W I 1976 Pseudo-obstruction of the colon. American Journal of Gastroenterology 65: 397–408
Staniland J R, Ditchburn J, de Dombal F T 1972 Clinical presentation of acute abdomen: study of 600 patients. British Medical Journal 3: 393–398
Stewardson R H, Bombeck C T, Nyhus L M 1978 Critical operative management of small bowel obstruction. Annals of Surgery 187: 189–193
Stewart R J, Gupta R K, Purdie G L, Isbister W H 1986 Fine-catheter aspiration cytology of peritoneal cavity improves decision-making about difficult cases of acute abdominal pain. Lancet 2: 146–149
Stonebridge P A, Callam M J, Bradbury A W, Murie J A, Jenkins A M, Ruckley C V 1993 Comparison of long-term survival after successful repair of ruptured and non-ruptured abdominal aortic aneurysm. British Journal of Surgery 80: 585–586
Sugarbaker P H, Bloom B S, Sanders J H, Wilson R E 1975 Preoperative laparoscopy in diagnosis of acute abdominal pain. Lancet 1: 442–445
Surana R, Quinn F, Puri P 1993 Is it necessary to perform appendicectomy in the middle of the night in children? British Medical Journal 306: 1168
Tate J J T, Chung S C S, Dawson J et al 1993 Conventional versus laparoscopic surgery for acute appendicitis. British Journal of Surgery 80: 761–764
Thomson W H F, Dawes R F H, Carter S S C 1991 Abdominal wall tenderness: a useful sign in chronic abdominal pain. British Journal of Surgery 78: 223–225
Tiblin S 1969 Diagnosis of intestinal obstruction with special regard to plain roentgen examination of the abdomen. Acta Chirurgica Scandinavica 135: 249
Vallina V L, Velasco J M, McCulloch C S 1993 Laparoscopic versus conventional appendectomy. Annals of Surgery 218: 685–692
Walsh G L, Chiasson P, Hedderich G, Wexler M J, Meakins J L 1988 The open abdomen. The marlex mesh and Zipper technique. Surgical Clinics of North America 68: 25–40
West R R, Carey M J 1978 Variation in rates of hospital admission for appendicitis in Wales. British Medical Journal 1: 1662–1664
Wilkinson R H, Bartlett R H, Eraklis A J 1969 Diagnosis of appendicitis in infancy. American Journal of Diseases of Chidren 118: 687–692
Williams H 1947 Appendicitis in the young child. British Medical Journal 2: 730
Winsey H S, Jones P F 1967 Acute abdominal pain in childhood: analysis of a year's admissions. British Medical Journal 1: 653–655
Ya P M, Perry J F, Thein M S, Wangensteen O H 1957 Measurement of sequestration of red cell mass in strangulating intestinal obstruction utilising radioactive Cr51. Surgical Forum 7: 411

# 19. Intestinal ischemia and vasculitis

*D. C. Carter M. Camilleri*

## INTESTINAL ISCHEMIA

The term "intestinal ischemia" embraces a spectrum of clinical conditions. Increased awareness of its varied manifestations, improved radiological techniques and clear separation of ischemic bowel disease from inflammatory bowel diseases have combined to allow a more rational approach to the problem. There are four clinical syndromes (Marston 1977) namely, acute intestinal failure with threatened or complete ischemia in the distribution of the superior mesenteric artery (SMA); ischemic colitis which can range from transient colitis with complete recovery to stricture formation; chronic intestinal ischemia, otherwise known as intestinal angina; and focal ischemia of the small intestine with development of a stricture.

## ANATOMY OF THE INTESTINAL CIRCULATION

The celiac axis supplies the foregut and has a collateral supply from esophageal vessels, from the phrenic branches of the aorta and from the anastomosis between the superior and inferior pancreaticoduodenal arteries (Fig. 19.1). Ischemia in the distribution of the celiac artery is exceptional, due in part to this plentiful collateral supply.

The superior mesenteric artery (SMA) supplies the midgut and is functionally an end artery in that its collateral supply is usually inadequate after acute occlusion of the main trunk. The anastomosis between the pancreaticoduodenal arteries is the only major source of collateral supply, but the inferior pancreaticoduodenal artery begins close to the origin of the SMA and is usually occluded by the thrombosis or embolus which blocks the parent vessel. There is a tenuous anastomosis with the inferior mesenteric artery at the splenic flexure (Fig. 19.1), but this is seldom able to nourish significant lengths of midgut after SMA occlusion and the colon is particularly susceptible to ischemia at the splenic flexure. The small bowel is nourished by a series of arterial arcades, whereas the proximal colon depends on the marginal artery formed by connections between the ileocolic, right and middle colic branches of the SMA. It was once thought that the SMA was totally or partially occluded in two-thirds of individuals over the age of 55 years (Derrick et al 1959), but more recent autopsy studies have shown that while mild stenosis is common, critical stenosis (i.e. 50% reduction in vessel diameter) is rare, affecting less than 5% of celiac and superior mesenteric arteries and 11% of inferior mesenteric arteries (Croft et al 1981). Gradual occlusion allows collateral flow to develop which can nourish the intestine, but abrupt occlusion of the SMA is disastrous; only 25–30 cm of proximal jejunum may survive while the rest of the midgut becomes necrotic.

The inferior mesenteric artery (IMA) supplies the hindgut and its terminal superior rectal branch ends in a profuse anastomosis with the middle and inferior rectal branches of the internal iliac arteries. Ischemic proctitis is rare but can occur, particularly in patients with occlusive disease affecting the internal iliac arteries (Parks et al 1972) and IMA occlusion may occur without clinical effects. Dick et al (1967) failed to visualize the IMA in 40 of 100 lateral lumbar aortograms and drew attention to its relatively small caliber. The ratio of the diameter of the celiac to the superior mesenteric and to the inferior mesenteric arteries is normally 4 : 4.5 : 1. In terms of cross-sectional area, these ratios become 64 : 81 : 4 and it is not surprising that IMA occlusion may pass unnoticed. However, such occlusion may prove critical if flow through the SMA is already impaired.

## PATHOGENESIS OF ACUTE INTESTINAL ISCHEMIA

Ischemia results from occlusion of arterial inflow, occlusion of venous outflow or failure of perfusion; these factors may act singly or in combination.

### Arterial inflow occlusion

*Atheroma* is the commonest cause of mesenteric vascular

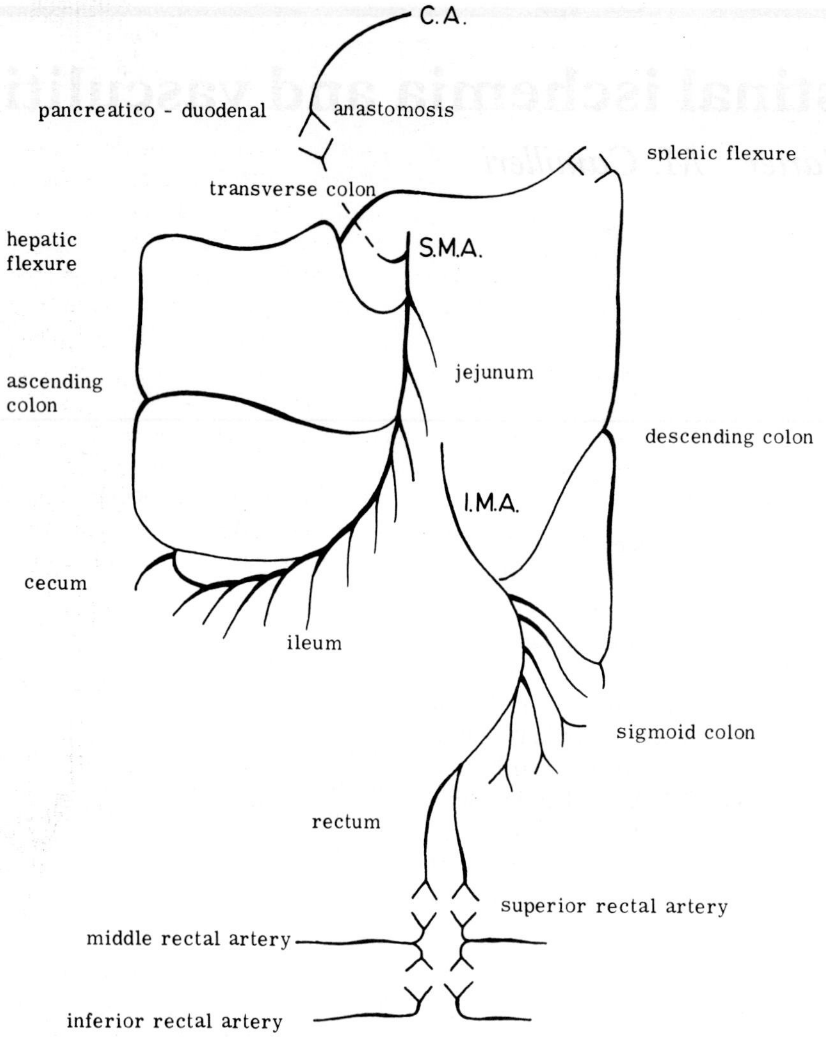


**Fig. 19.1** Diagrammatic representation of the blood supply of the gastrointestinal tract from the celiac axis (CA), superior mesenteric artery (SMA) and inferior mesenteric artery (IMA).

disease. It is most severe at the ostia and start of the mesenteric arteries, sparing the more peripheral vessels. Ischemia is unlikely until the cross-sectional area of the main arteries is reduced to less than two-thirds of normal (Dick et al 1967), but any narrowing may prove critical during episodes of hypotension or if thrombosis supervenes.

*Thrombosis* is commonly the final event in atheromatous narrowing and SMA thrombosis accounts for up to two-thirds of cases of acute intestinal ischemia (Mosley & Marston 1989, Storey & Cunningham 1993). Thrombosis may also be associated with trauma, polycythemia, sickle cell disease, disseminated intravascular coagulation from any cause and amyloid disease.

*Embolus* blocking the SMA was once responsible for approximately 50% of cases of acute mesenteric ischemia, but has become less common with the falling incidence of rheumatic heart disease and improved control of arrhythmias and acute myocardial ischemia. In one Scottish series, 33% of cases of acute superior mesenteric ischemia were due to embolus (Wilson et al 1987). The angle of emergence of the SMA from the aorta means that it readily accepts emboli whereas the IMA is seldom occluded in this way. Most emboli originate from thrombi in the left side of the heart; paradoxical emboli, emboli from aneurysmal thrombus and embolism from ulcerated atheromatous plaque are rare alternative sources.

*Aortic disease* can occlude the ostia of mesenteric vessels by atheroma, aneurysmal thrombosis or dissection of an aneurysm. Ligation of the inferior mesenteric artery is unavoidable during resection of aortic aneurysms, but subsequent colonic ischemia is rare.

*Arteritis* is rare and may be due to polyarteritis nodosa, "necrotizing enteritis", thromboangiitis obliterans, Takayasu's disease or radiation angiitis (p. 409).

*Neoplasia* is a rare cause of inflow occlusion. Vessels can be occluded or invaded by retroperitoneal tumors and occasionally vasoconstriction due to circulating catecholamines can be a manifestation of pheochromocytoma.

*Iatrogenic* causes include operative damage to vessels and rare complications of angiography.

### Venous outflow occlusion

Mesenteric venous thrombosis in the absence of arterial thrombosis or mechanical intestinal obstruction is rare, accounting for no more than 0.1% of emergency surgical admissions and some 5–15% of all cases of ischemia in the absence of gut obstruction (Grendell & Ockner, 1982).

Conditions associated with mesenteric venous thrombosis are shown in Table 19.1. Intra-abdominal infection, neoplasia, previous abdominal surgery and portal cirrhosis with congestive splenomegaly are the more common causes (Johnson & Baggenstoss 1949, Grendell & Ockner 1982). Hypercoagulability from any cause is a predisposing factor. Sporadic cases have been reported in pregnancy, in the puerperium and in young women taking oral contraceptives (Hoyle et al 1977), but the mechanism by which estrogens could cause thrombogenesis is uncertain and the association is still in doubt. Given the enormous number of women taking oral contraception, any increase in the risk of mesenteric venous thrombosis must be very small.

### Infarction without occlusion

Approximately one-third of patients dying with acute ischemic necrosis of the midgut have no demonstrable occlusion of a major vessel, although in some series 50% of cases of mesenteric ischemia are due to this cause (Ottinger & Austen 1967). Nonocclusive infarction occurs when intestinal blood flow is greatly reduced (Renton 1972) and reduced cardiac output due to ventricular failure or arrhythmia is responsible for at least 75% of cases. Aortic insufficiency with a high pulse pressure and heart surgery are occasional causes. Hypotension due to hypovolemia or septicemia can also cause this form of intestinal infarction.

**Table 19.1** Associated diseases in ischemic colitis in 98 patients over 50 years of age (Marcuson & Farman 1971)

| Associated disease | Number of patients |
|---|---|
| Atheroma | 24 |
| Colon surgery or disease | 12 |
| Cardiac disease | 9 |
| Diabetes mellitus | 8 |
| Aortic aneurysm | 7 |
| Hypotensive episode | 7 |
| Hypertension | 7 |
| Arrhythmia | 5 |
| Superior mesenteric artery occlusion | 5 |
| Collagen disease | 2 |
| Blood dyscrasia | 1 |
| None found | 42 |

The splanchnic bed has a low priority in shock and is denied its normal 20% of cardiac ouput in an attempt to maintain perfusion of more vital areas. The sympathetic nervous system and catecholamines constrict splanchnic arteriolar sphincters, causing selective reduction of intestinal flow. The combination of increased splanchnic resistance and systemic hypotension leads readily to intestinal ischemia and mucosal hypoxia may be amplified during low-flow states by a countercurrent exchange of oxygen at the villous base (Lundgren & Haglund 1978, Haglund & Lundgren 1979). Once the tips of villi become anoxic, tissue damage may release toxic substances which adversely affect the cardiovascular system and impairment of the intestinal mucosal barrier may allow absorption of bacteria and their toxins from the gut lumen.

## PATHOLOGY

### Functional consequences of ischemia

The severity of injury is inversely related to the rate of blood flow during the ischemic period. In canine jejunal loops, substantial transmucosal leakage of albumin is only seen when blood flow is reduced to a level where oxygen consumption falls by at least 50% (Bulkley et al 1985) (Fig 19.2). Cellular oxidative metabolism becomes compromised with depletion of intracellular energy stores, increasing functional impairment and cell death. The importance of mucosal hypoxia is emphasized by experiments showing that intraluminal perfusion with oxygenated saline can greatly reduce the severity of mucosal injury during ischemia (Haglund et al 1976). The mucosa is much more susceptible to ischemia than the muscle layers

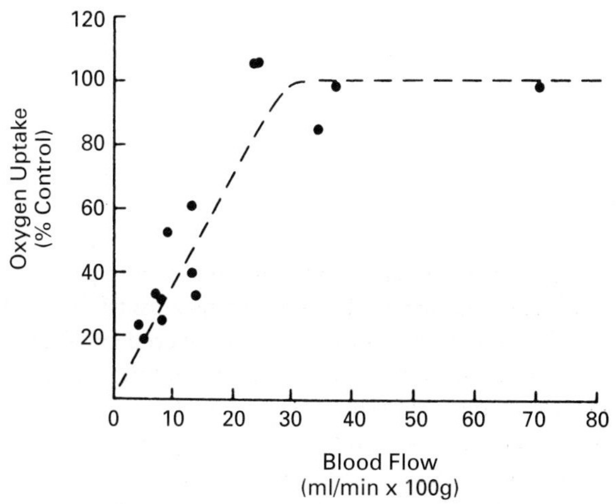


**Fig. 19.2** Relationship between blood flow and oxygen uptake in the canine small intestine. (Reproduced with permission from Bulkley et al 1985.)

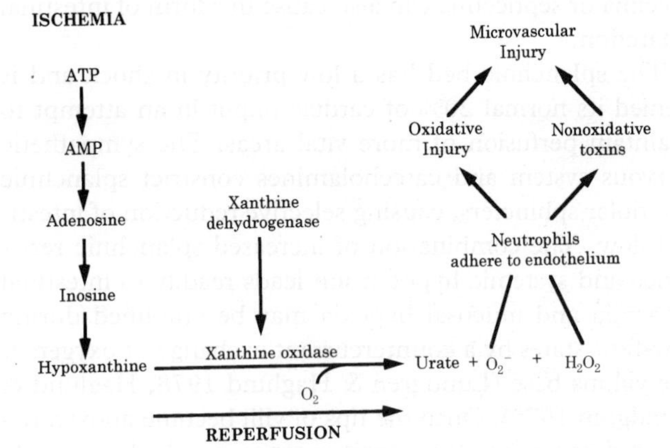


**Fig. 19.3** Potential relationships between xanthine oxidase generated superoxide ($O_2$), neutrophil infiltration and microvascular injury in intestinal ischemia. (Reproduced with permission from Grisham & Granger 1989).

and although small intestinal mucosa is more susceptible to damage, it can recover more rapidly than ischemic colonic mucosa (Robinson et al 1981).

There is abundant evidence that injury sustained during intestinal ischemia is exacerbated during reperfusion if the blood supply is restored (Parks & Granger 1986). Reperfusion injury appears to be mediated by cytotoxic free radicals derived from oxygen such as superoxide radicals, hydrogen peroxide and hydroxyl radicals. It has been proposed that mucosal xanthine oxidase is the prime source of reactive metabolites (Fig. 19.3) and that neutrophils then adhere to vascular endothelium with secondary microvascular damage (Grisham & Granger 1989). Mechanisms by which neutrophils might cause damage include release of further reactive oxygen metabolites and secretion of myeloperoxidase. Myeloperoxidase could act on hydrogen peroxide and chloride ions to yield hypocholorous acid (a potent cytotoxin which is the active ingredient of bleach) and may also promote proteolysis by inactivating local protease inhibitors (Grisham & Granger 1989).

### Macroscopic changes in ischemic necrosis

The bowel initially appears pale and spastic but gradually dilates, becomes flaccid and reddens as blood enters from collateral vessels. Its color darkens in severe ischemia, it loses its sheen and after 24–48 h it turns a mottled purple-green, becomes friable and thin and covered by flecks of fibrin. Gas bubbles appear in the mesenteric veins and frank perforation is then not long delayed.

The lumen fills with bloodstained fluid and submucosal congestion produces a pseudopolypoid appearance of the mucosa in the early stages. The mucosa ulcerates, becomes covered by greenish-white patches of slough and ultimately turns gangrenous.

The distribution and severity of these changes depend on the cause of the ischemia. Major vessel occlusion causes segmental infarction, while nonocclusive infarction is characteristically patchy.

### Microscopic changes in ischemic necrosis

Necrosis of the superficial epithelium is apparent within minutes of infarction. Submucosal hemorrhages follow and an inflammatory polymorphonuclear response becomes marked within 12–24 h (Fig. 19.4), demarcating the dead inner zone. Bacterial invasion from the lumen accentuates this response and pus may form beneath the dead superficial tissue. Clostridia and other fecal organisms are often found within the bowel wall. The muscle layers are remarkably resistant to ischemia but develop similar histological changes if severe ischemia persists.

### Sequelae of ischemic necrosis

*Gangrene*

Unrelieved ischemia usually causes necrosis of all layers of the bowel with gangrene and perforation. Death is inevitable unless the gangrenous bowel is resected.

*Transient ischemia*

Temporary occlusion of a mesenteric artery is compatible with full structural and functional recovery. Muscle withstands approximately 6 h of ischemia and restoration of flow within this period may allow full recovery. Repair after transient ischemia involves replacement of dead tissue by granulation and fibrous tissue and reconstitution of the epithelium. Macrophages laden with hemosiderin are conspicuous (Fig. 19.5). The mucosa may appear hyperemic, edematous, ulcerated or nodular.

*Ischemic stricture*

Ischemia of a short segment of bowel may be compatible with survival even though damage extends deeply into the submucosa and underlying circular muscle. Healing is slow, fibrosis is pronounced and a concentric stricture results. Ischemic strictures of the large bowel are not uncommon (p. 549), but ischemic small bowel strictures are rare.

## ACUTE INTESTINAL FAILURE

The term "acute intestinal failure" was introduced by Marston (1977) to replace the numerous terms used to describe necrosis of bowel supplied by the SMA. The condition appears to have increased in frequency and is predominantly a disease of the elderly (Fig. 19.6). Current

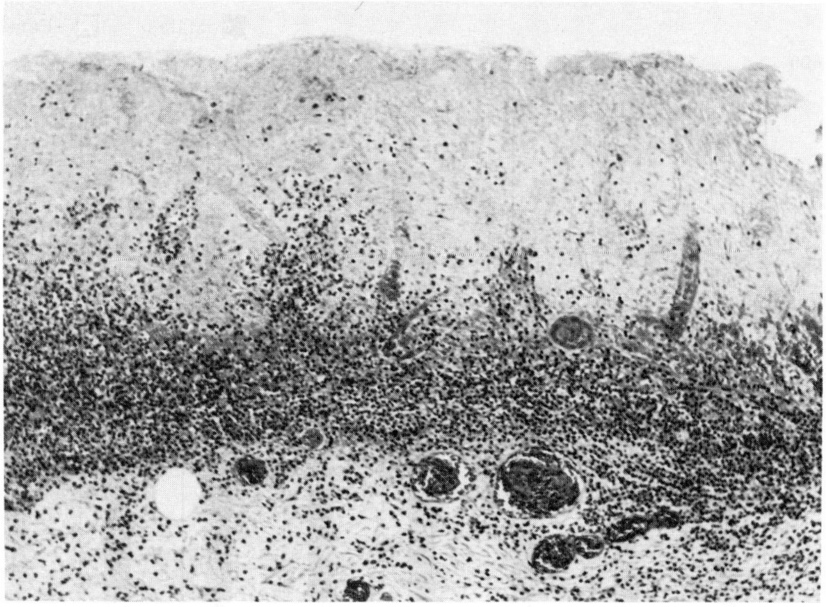

**Fig. 19.4** Acute ischemic colitis. The mucosa is necrotic with an inflammatory infiltrate replacing the muscularis mucosae. There is marked capillary congestion (hematoxylin and eosin, × 100).

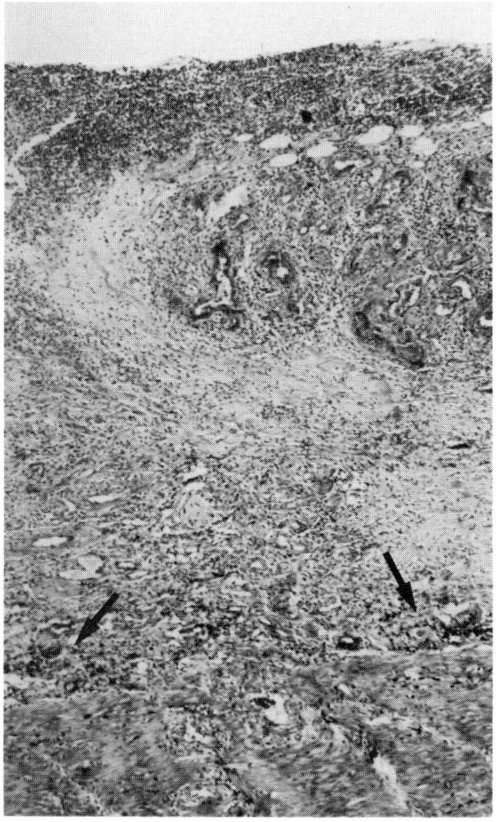

**Fig. 19.5** Chronic ischemic colitis. The mucosa is ulcerated and the submucosa is fibrotic. Groups of macrophages containing hemosiderin are present (arrows) (hematoxylin and eosin, × 60).

estimates suggest that a district hospital draining a catchment area of 250 000 individuals will see about one case a month, but the true incidence may still be underestimated as up to 50% of cases are diagnosed for the first time at autopsy (Wilson et al 1987).

Acute occlusion of the SMA leads to complete necrosis and gangrene of most of the midgut unless blood flow can be restored surgically. Failure to restore flow within 6 h makes massive midgut resection necessary and even if the patient survives, the nutritional problems which follow can jeopardize survival (p. 454). Acute superior mesenteric artery occlusion is a vascular emergency and early diagnosis is essential if the mortality rate is to be brought beneath 90% (Mavor 1972, Wilson et al 1987).

It cannot be overemphasized that about one-third of patients with acute intestinal failure have nonocclusive infarction in which the major intestinal arteries remain patent.

## Presentation and early diagnosis

Early diagnosis of acute intestinal failure is difficult. In the experience of Mavor et al (1962), 70% of patients had abdominal pain for at least 12 h before admission and in 54% there was a delay of more than 12 h between admission and laparotomy. More recently, Wilson et al (1987) found that in the 49 of their 102 cases where the diagnosis was made in life, 53% were admitted within 24 h of the onset of symptoms and 47% had laparotomy on the day of admission. Of the 53 patients diagnosed at

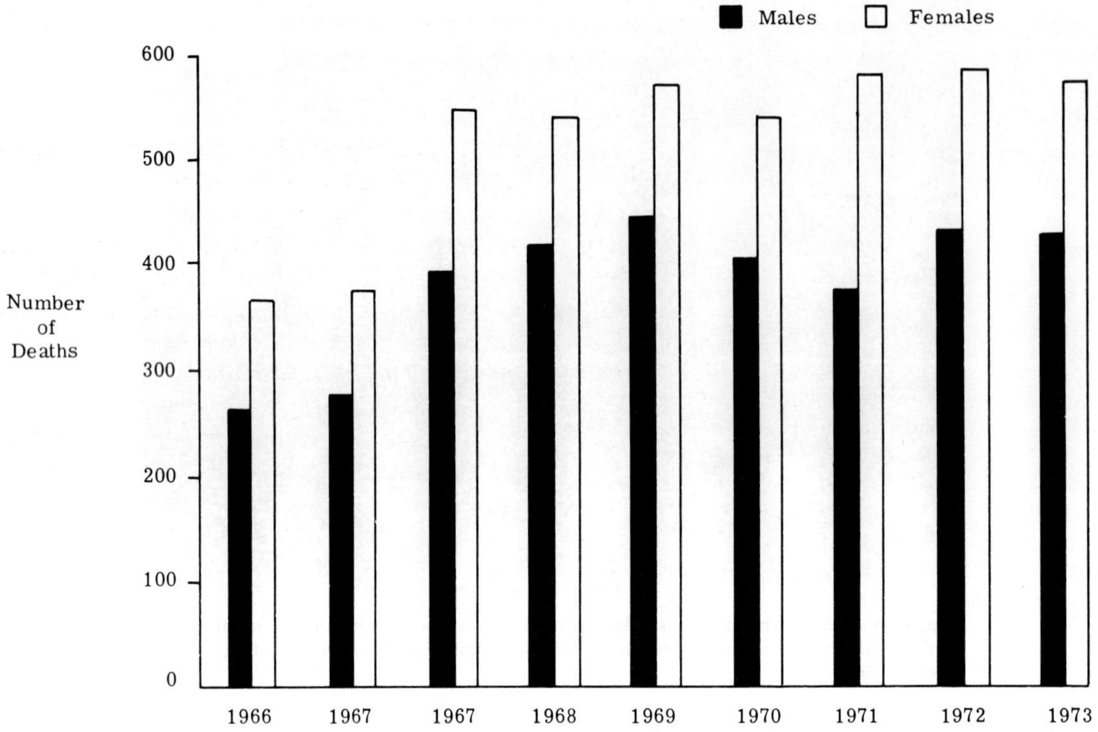


**Fig. 19.6** Deaths from arterial embolism and thrombosis of the mesenteric artery in England and Wales from 1966 to 1973 (Marston 1977). Note: 1967 International Classification of Disease Index (ICD) No. 7th Revision 570.2, 8th Revision 444.2.

postmortem, the diagnosis had been "suspected" in life in 60% of cases but the patient's condition precluded operation.

A prodrome of chronic or episodic abdominal pain, often related to meals, with diarrhea and weight loss is a valuable pointer to the diagnosis. Patients with thrombosis tend to have more insidious onset of symptoms than those with embolism where the onset is typically abrupt. Concomitant or previous vascular disease such as cerebrovascular accident, myocardial infarction and acute limb ischemia is common. Abdominal pain is invariably present on admission but varies greatly in severity and distribution. It may be central or epigastric, constant or colicky, episodic or continuous. The pain eventually becomes agonizing, constant and diffuse. Vomiting is common at the onset of pain; watery and later bloody diarrhea occurs in up to one-third of cases.

In the early stages the patient typically appears more ill and in more pain than the lack of physical signs would suggest. A high index of suspicion is essential, particularly in patients with pre-existing vascular disease and cardiac diseases associated with production of emboli. Abdominal signs are a late feature and tenderness, guarding, rigidity and gross abdominal distention denote peritonitis following full-thickness necrosis. Fetor, confusion and cyanosis may develop and multiorgan failure supervenes.

## Investigations

Plain abdominal radiographs usually show no intestinal abnormality in the critical early period, although aortic calcification and sometimes an aneurysm may denote atherosclerosis. Common findings on the plain abdominal radiograph include gas-filled and edematous loops of small bowel and fluid-filled small bowel loops which have a "gasless" appearance (Field 1984). Linear streaks of gas indicating gangrenous changes and gas in the portal vein secondary to bowel necrosis are grave, but not inevitably fatal, prognostic signs (Krankendonk et al., 1983). The diagnosis can be confirmed by percutaneous transfemoral arteriography, but time usually does not permit this investigation. If arteriography can be undertaken adequate hydration must be maintained as an integral part of resuscitation and the procedure may prove therapeutic as well as diagnostic (see below). It must be remembered that a patent arterial tree does not exclude nonocclusive infarction.

Hemoconcentration is usual and a leukocytosis of 20–30 $\times$ $10^9$/L (20 000–30 000 cells/$mm^3$) is often an early finding which suggests intestinal ischemia in a patient with unimpressive abdominal signs. A metabolic acidosis and base deficit is common. The serum amylase levels are normal in more than 50% of patients with acute mesenteric infarction, but on occasions may rise to levels normally associated with acute pancreatitis (Wilson & Imrie 1986). A raised serum inorganic phosphate follows experimental SMA occlusion (Jamieson et al 1982) but initial clinical studies suggest that phosphate levels rise in mesenteric ischemia only when the entire small bowel is infarcted (Mosley & Marston 1989)

## Treatment

*Resuscitation* (p. 517)

Delay in diagnosis increases the need for vigorous resuscitation before operation and large volumes of blood, plasma and crystalloid may be required. Full monitoring is required and oxygen is essential.

*Operation*

The presence and extent of obvious gut necrosis is determined and the mesenteric vessels are inspected carefully to determine whether they are pulsatile and filled or nonpulsatile and collapsed. Lack of pulsation and collapsed vessels signify occlusion of the SMA and attempts should be made to remove embolus or thrombus from the vessel with a Fogarty catheter. Boley et al (1981) advocate early angiography, not only as an aid to diagnosis but as a means of infusing vasodilators such as papaverine (30–60 mg/h) intra-arterially to overcome spasm before and after surgery in patients with superior mesenteric emboli. Attempts to achieve clot lysis by infusing streptokinase are of uncertain value. Alternatively, mesenteric arterial flow may be supplemented by anastomosis of the ileocolic artery to the right common iliac artery (Marston 1977).

Gangrenous bowel requires resection, but resection of the whole midgut is futile in elderly patients. When ischemia is present but gangrene is not obvious, an attempt should be made to restore blood flow in the hope that resection will be minimized. There is considerable merit in a "second look" operation when bowel of questionable viability is left in situ (Shaw & Rutledge 1957, Shaw & Maynard 1958). This operation is undertaken 24 h later, the decision to reoperate being made at the time of the first laparotomy. If resection is undertaken, there is a strong case for avoiding immediate end-to-end anastomosis of bowel of doubtful viability and electing to exteriorize both bowel ends as a temporary expedient. Continuity can be restored after approximately 2 weeks (Mosley & Marston 1989).

If the mesenteric vessels are pulsating despite gut necrosis, it must be assumed that there is no occlusion of the superior mesenteric artery and that there is no purpose in attempting revascularization. Conservatism is recommended for infarction without occlusion (Marston 1977) and gut resection is only undertaken when there is obviously necrotic bowel. A second look operation is also recommended in such patients.

## Postoperative care

Restoration of blood flow to ischemic bowel is followed by the loss of blood, plasma and fluid into the bowel wall and lumen; vasoactive substances and bacteria and their toxins enter the bloodstream; blood pressure and blood volume fall as the splanchnic bed reopens and metabolic acidosis is common. Intensive care is essential and therapy must include oxygen and intravenous heparin (20 000 i.u. followed by 10–15 000 i.u. 6-hourly according to the thromboplastin time) to prevent extension of thrombus and counter disseminated intravascular coagulation. Antibiotics are given once blood has been taken for culture and a combination of gentamicin, metronidazole and crystalline penicillin (p. 520) is used in the first instance. Despite its ability to constrict mesenteric vessels (Bynum & Hanley 1982), digitalis may be beneficial in controlling atrial fibrillation and so increasing cardiac output and inotropic agents such as dopamine may help to increase mesenteric blood flow.

## Prognosis

Patients suffering from acute intestinal failure are usually elderly and frequently have diseases of the heart, kidneys and lungs. Survival is virtually confined to patients in whom a defined vascular occlusion is diagnosed and treated early. Acute intestinal failure has carried a mortality rate of 90% in most hospitals for some 50 years and although more aggressive treatment including arteriography may lower mortality to the order of 50% in some centers (Veith & Boley 1986, Levy et al 1990), it will be difficult to improve survival prospects for the vast majority of patients (Wilson et al 1987). The ready availability of long-term parenteral nutrition now means that selected patients with the "short bowel syndrome" can be nourished effectively after massive resection (Mughal & Irving 1986).

# ISCHEMIC COLITIS

In addition to its involvement in superior mesenteric artery occlusion, the colon may become ischemic without involvement of the small bowel. It is recognized that necrosis of the left colon may follow ligation of the IMA during resection of an aortic aneurysm or in the course of colonic surgery. The adequacy of anastomosis between the middle colic artery, which is derived from the SMA, and the left colic artery, which is a branch of the IMA, at the splenic flexure (Fig. 19.1) and the integrity of the marginal artery of the colon are important determinants of bowel survival following such ligation. Reversible or irre-

**Table 19.2** Associated diseases in ischemic colitis in 24 patients under 50 years of age (Marcuson & Farman 1971)

| Associated disease | Number of patients |
|---|---|
| Oral contraceptives | 6 |
| Diabetes mellitus | 3 |
| Mesocolon hematoma | 2 |
| Rectal carcinoma | 1 |
| Abdominoperineal resection | 1 |
| Buerger's disease | 1 |
| Mesenteric embolism | 1 |
| Rheumatoid arthritis | 1 |
| Thrombophlebitis | 1 |
| Postpartum | 1 |
| None found | 6 |

versible ischemia of the left colon may follow spontaneous IMA occlusion and many patients previously considered to have atypical forms of inflammatory bowel disease are now known to be suffering from colonic ischemia (Boley et al 1963, Marston et al 1966). Marcuson & Farman (1971) collected 122 cases of ischemic colitis and the associated factors are shown in Tables 19.1 and 19.2.

Ischemic colitis may be transient and followed by complete healing, lead to ischemic stricture formation or progress to gangrene. In practice, the important distinction is between gangrenous colitis (which is part of the spectrum of acute intestinal failure as discussed on p. 544) and the nongangrenous forms. The term "ischemic colitis" is now restricted to the nongangrenous forms of the disease and has been defined as an inflammatory disorder, caused by a vascular accident, but which does not involve complete death of tissue (Marston 1989a).

## Gangrenous colitis

Only 12% of the patients with colonic ischemia reported by Marcuson & Farman (1971) presented with gangrenous colitis. The presentation is similar to that described for SMA occlusion except that the pain often begins in the left lower quadrant. Diagnosis is frequently not made until generalized abdominal pain and shock indicate generalized peritonitis. Laparotomy is undertaken after resuscitation and gangrenous bowel is resected with exteriorization of both ends of the remaining viable colon.

## Ischemic colitis

Transient colitis accounted for 40% of Marcuson & Farman's cases. It occurs when ischemic damage is confined to the mucosa and innermost submucosa and full recovery is usual. Often the diagnosis is only certain in retrospect. Almost half the patients described by Marcuson & Farman (1971) developed ischemic strictures (Fig. 19.7). Progression of ischemic colitis to gangrene is rare, occurring in only two of 180 cases dealt with by Marston (1989a).

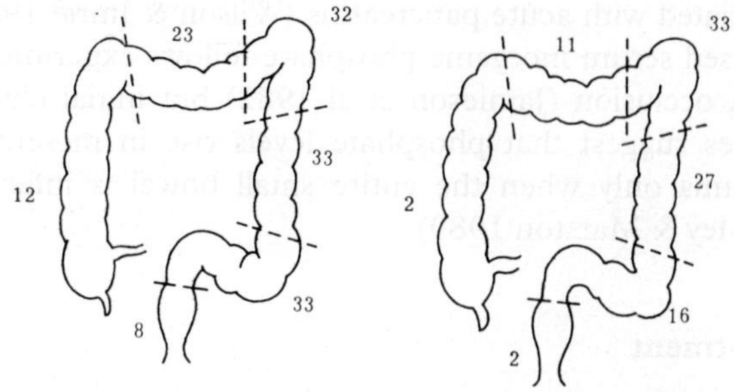


**Fig. 19.7** Distribution of lesions in 73 patients with ischemic colitis (*left*) and 58 patients with ischemic strictures of the colon (*right*). The figures indicate the number of patients with damage in the sites shown; long lesions count at two or more adjacent sites (Marcuson 1972).

*Clinical features*

The patient is usually middle-aged or elderly and often has a history of cardiovascular or cerebrovascular disease. The presentation varies from a severe acute illness to a mild upset which may not require hospital admission. Colicky lower abdominal pain, nausea, vomiting and diarrhea with the passage of blood and mucus are typical. There may have been similar preceding attacks or abdominal angina following meals. Tachycardia and fever are common. Abdominal examination reveals tenderness and guarding in the left lower quadrant. A palpable mass is unusual. Bowel sounds are usually present. Persistent bleeding suggests that a stricture may be forming. The differential diagnosis often includes other bowel diseases such as ulcerative colitis, Crohn's disease, acute diverticular disease, carcinoma and bacillary dysentery.

*Investigations*

Leukocytosis is usually present.

Sigmoidoscopy is usually normal in ischemic colitis unless blood is seen coming down from the proximal bowel or ischemic change extends to the rectum. Rectal biopsy may help to exclude other forms of inflammatory bowel disease but should be deferred if barium enema will be performed. Colonoscopy is being used increasingly in diagnosis and may reveal an irregular edematous mucosa which appears bluish-purple and bleeds on contact. If carried out at a later stage, colonoscopy may reveal ulceration or a smooth stricture.

The plain radiograph shows characteristic 'thumbprinting' of the bowel wall caused by submucosal hemorrhage and edema in about 20% of patients (Fig. 19.8). The involved segment may cause obstruction with distention of the proximal bowel (Field 1984).

Double-contrast barium enema is usually diagnostic and, until the advent of colonoscopy, was the mainstay of diagnosis. As a result of submucosal bleeding, separation of the mucosa occurs and mucous sloughing and thumbprinting may be present (Fig. 19.9). Ulceration is

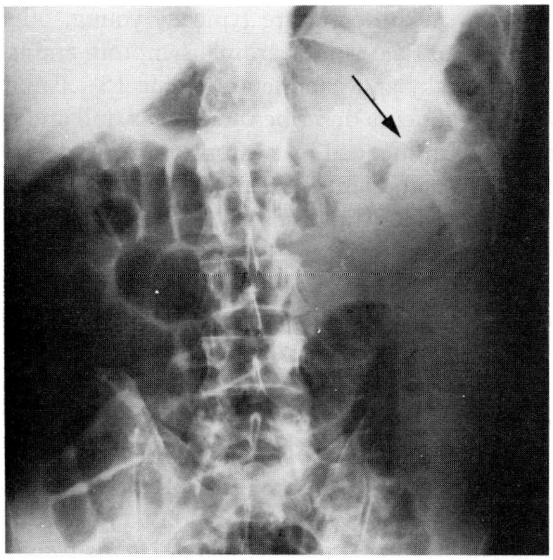

**Fig. 19.8** Acute ischemic colitis affecting the splenic flexure and adjacent transverse colon. Plain radiograph showing narrowing with a soft-tissue shadow due to edema of the bowel wall (arrow). The lumen of the bowel is depicted by gas and is narrowed.

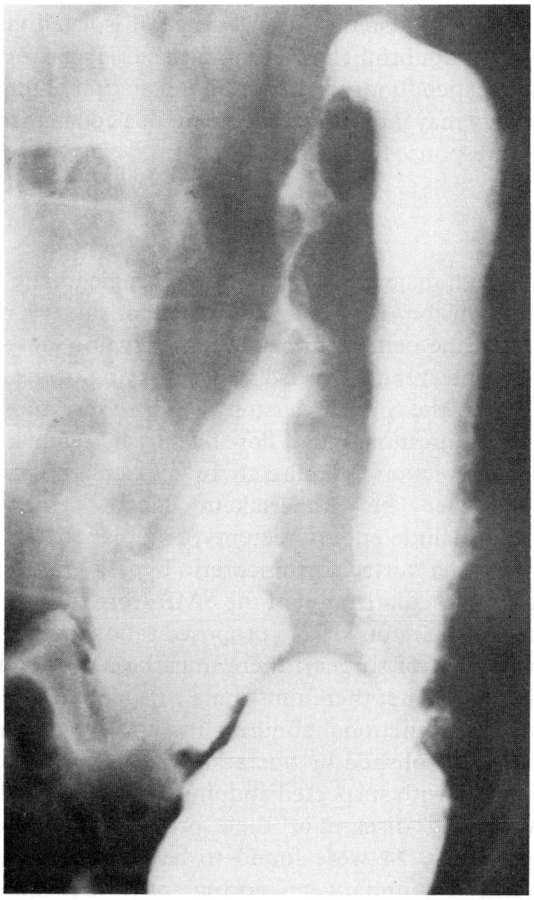

**Fig. 19.9** Ischemic colitis of the splenic flexure in the acute phase. Considerable narrowing with characteristic "thumbprinting".

maximal 5–10 days from the onset. The ulcers may be of variable size and depth and can even mimic the appearances of ulcerative colitis or Crohn's disease in some patients. Varying lengths of colon may be affected by these radiological changes with the splenic flexure and descending colon most commonly involved, though the rectum is almost always spared (Simpkins 1984).

These changes develop early and persist for up to 10 days after the onset of symptoms. Serial barium enemas show gradual resolution of thumbprinting and ulceration (Fig. 19.10), but in patients who progress to stricture formation, the narrowed area of bowel shortens, becomes smooth and develops a funnelled appearance at either end. In a few patients an annular constricting lesion results which can be difficult to distinguish from carcinoma of the colon. It should be remembered that ischemic colitis can occasionally develop proximal to a carcinoma.

Angiography is unnecessary for the diagnosis of ischemic colitis and its routine use in this context cannot be justified.

*Treatment*

With conservative treatment, pain and bloody diarrhea should settle rapidly in 2–3 days. Intravenous fluids are used until abdominal signs settle and antibiotics (e.g. gentamicin and metronidazole) may be prescribed although there is no objective evidence that they are of benefit. A barium enema is repeated after 1 week to confirm resolution. Deterioration with signs of spreading peritonitis are indications to abandon conservative therapy in favor of

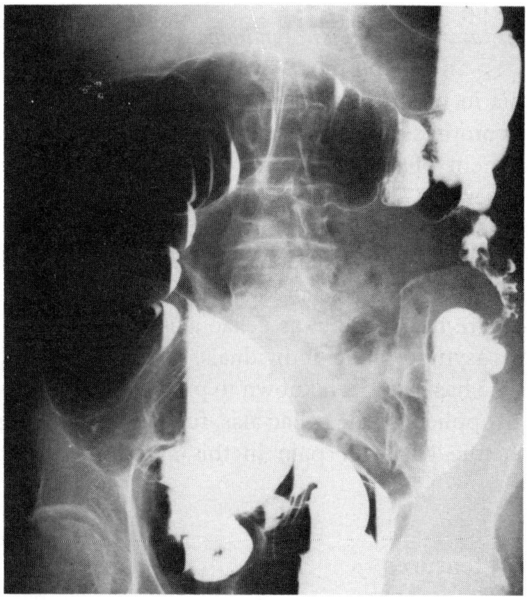

**Fig. 19.10** Localized ischemic colitis of mid-descending colon causing some obstruction. The affected area shows considerable narrowing with irregularity. Healing phase.

laparotomy. Persistent bleeding and continued pain and tenderness due to stricture formation may also lead to early laparotomy and resection of the narrowed segment. However, some patients with radiological stricture formation improve spontaneously and surgery should not be undertaken unless absolutely essential. Forty-nine of the 58 patients with ischemic strictures reported by Marcuson (1972) required resection. There were few deaths in the group undergoing resection and one death in the nine patients treated conservatively.

Occasionally, patients present with subacute intestinal obstruction due to a stricture without a preceding acute illness. In such patients, a barium enema and a colonoscopy are required to exclude Crohn's disease and carcinoma.

## CHRONIC INTESTINAL ISCHEMIA

Interest in intestinal ischemia as a cause of abdominal pain was stimulated by Dunphy's (1936) observation that seven of 12 patients dying with mesenteric vascular occlusion had experienced prodromal abdominal pain for up to 2 years. Mavor et al (1962) found that almost half of their patients with acute mesenteric infarction had a history of pain consistent with chronic intestinal ischemia. However, the concept of "abdominal angina" remains controversial. While stenosis of the visceral arteries is common, intestinal angina is rare and there is no relationship between the degree of occlusion and presence of symptoms (Croft et al 1981). If symptoms are present, they are usually ascribed to ischemia of the gut muscles, although recent evidence suggests that in some patients there may be "steal" of blood into the gastric mucosa in response to a meal (Poole et al 1987).

*Celiac axis compression syndrome* (Abu-Nema & Eklof 1984) is an uncommon variant of chronic intestinal ischemia in which recurrent abdominal pain is said to be due to compression of the celiac axis by the median arcuate ligament of the diaphragm or by the celiac ganglion (Sleisenger 1977, Brandt & Boley 1978). The diagnosis is entertained only after careful search for other causes of abdominal pain and the existence of the condition is by no means universally accepted. Even the arteriographic findings are not specific, as celiac axis narrowing is common in asymptomatic individuals. No patient with the syndrome has ever been known to progress to infarction of viscera supplied by the celiac axis, further evidence against an ischemic basis for pain in this syndrome (Jamieson 1986).

### Clinical features

The patient is often elderly and may have pre-existing coronary artery disease, hypertension or peripheral vascular disease. The celiac compression syndrome is exceptional in that its sufferers are typically young, otherwise healthy women. Pain is the cardinal symptom and is often epigastric, colicky and experienced some 15–20 min after meals. Some patients describe the pain as dull and aching and it may be influenced by posture or exercise or radiate to the back. The patient is often afraid to eat and weight loss is common. Constipation may occur as a consequence of diminished intake, but occasional patients have diarrhea and steatorrhea due to malabsorption. Manifestations of generalized vascular disease and a systolic bruit over the upper abdomen support the diagnosis of chronic intestinal ischemia, although Edwards et al (1970) detected such bruits in 13 of a series of 200 healthy young adults.

### Investigations

Most patients have been investigated exhaustively before the diagnosis of intestinal ischemia is entertained. Arteriography with selective catheterization of the visceral arteries is the key investigation. Arterial narrowing is sought, bearing in mind that ischemia is unlikely unless the cross-sectional area of the main trunks is reduced by at least one-third (Dick et al 1967) and that symptoms are unlikely until at least two of the three visceral arteries have become compromised. As indicated above, radiological demonstration of stenosis or blockage of isolated visceral arteries has doubtful clinical significance. Hypertrophy of the pancreaticoduodenal arcade and dilatation of the marginal artery may indicate development of a collateral circulation in response to ischemia.

### Treatment

Patients with major vessel occlusion on angiography and a suggestive history should be considered for surgery, recognizing that the pendulum has probably swung away from operative intervention for isolated narrowing of the celiac axis or even the SMA (Marston 1989b). Operation aims to improve intestinal blood flow directly by removing the arterial obstruction or indirectly by revascularization and should never be undertaken lightly. Operations described include endarterectomy, reimplantation of the SMA into the aorta, aortomenteric bypass grafting and retrograde vascularization of the SMA from the common iliac artery. Marston (1977) proposed rational criteria for the evaluation of surgery: there must be a constant and definite syndrome; there must be a constant and definite structural or functional abnormality; and the abnormality must be abolished by operation. In his experience of 100 patients with suspected abdominal angina, 37 clearly had unrelated disease or their problems disappeared spontaneously, 14 were found to have other causes of pain and 58 underwent aortography. Of these 58 patients, 21 had no arterial lesion, and of the 37 with arterial lesions, 31 were subjected to reconstruction

(Marston 1989b). Three of the patients undergoing surgery died in the postoperative period and there were five late deaths from a variety of vascular causes. Of the 23 survivors, two were unchanged or worse, two were lost to follow-up and 19 were asymptomatic over periods ranging from 6 to 160 months.

Treatment of the celiac axis compression syndrome by division of constricting bands has given variable results. Most patients are relieved of pain immediately after the operation, but less than half remain free of symptoms for more than 3 years. It is difficult to exclude a "placebo effect" of surgery and any success attributable to the operation may result from interruption of afferent pain fibers rather than an effect on blood flow.

## FOCAL ISCHEMIA OF THE SMALL INTESTINE

Focal ischemia of the small bowel with stricture formation may result from strangulation by bands and external herniae, abdominal trauma with mesenteric hematoma formation, radiation enteritis, other forms of vasculitis and from ischemia induced by drugs such as enteric coated potassium tablets (p. 395). The presentation is one of subacute small bowel obstruction and resection of the stricture with end-to-end anastomosis is indicated.

## SYSTEMIC VASCULITIS

Vasculitis is characterized by inflammation and necrosis of blood vessels. It is a relatively common phenomenon when it occurs as part of the pathological process of infection or allergy. In these situations it is characterized by mild, often transient symptoms confined to the skin. Infrequently, extensive vasculitis affects many organs and may cause life-threatening illness.

### Etiology and classification

Systemic vasculitis may be a primary disorder or complicate an underlying disorder. Table 19.3 shows a classification that is based on the size of vessels affected, the presence of granulomas histologically and the coexistence of an underlying disease (Camilleri et al 1983). The etiology of primary systemic vasculitis can only rarely be ascertained with certainty. One cause is a rare response to hepatitis B virus infection, often when complicated by cryoglobulinemia. Cytomegalovirus infection in patients with acquired immunodeficiency syndrome (Kyriziakis & Mitra 1992) or those receiving immunosuppressive treatment (Sackier et al 1991) may also result in vasculitic ulcers that may perforate. More often, vasculitis is secondary to an underlying collagen-vascular disease (Helliwell et al 1985, Marshall et al 1990) or inflammatory myositis (Schullinger et al 1985).

**Table 19.3** Classification of systemic vasculitis

| Size of vessel | Granulomas absent | Granulomas present |
|---|---|---|
| Arteries: | | |
| Large | Takayasu's<br>Kawasaki | Giant cell arteritis |
| Medium | Polyarteritis nodosa | Churg–Strauss syndrome |
| Small | Microscopic polyarteritis or leukocytoclastic angitis | Wegener's granulomatosis |
| Venules | Henoch–Schönlein syndrome | |

Associated diseases cause a small vessel vasculitis: SLE, rheumatoid disease, essential mixed cryoglobulinemia, malignancy (leukemia, lymphoma, cancer), Behçet's, endocarditis, childhood dermatomyositis

### Pathology

Vasculitis involves one of several pathogenetic mechanisms: immune complex deposition, antibody-mediated injury or cytotoxic T-cell-induced injury. The pathology of affected organs demonstrates inflammation of the blood vessel wall with fibrin deposition ("fibrinoid necrosis") and neutrophil phagocytosis of nuclear debris of other inflammatory cells or leukocytoclasis. Some types are associated with granulomas and giant cells; the inflammatory cells are usually neutrophils and mononuclear cells, except in Churg–Strauss angiitis where eosinophils predominate.

### Gastrointestinal and systemic features

Vasculitis results in hemorrhage, inflammation or perforation of the gut. Rarely, inflammation may result in the necrotic "casts" of the segment of affected colon being passed per rectum. The spectrum of gut manifestations also depends on the size of the vessels affected by the specific type of vasculitis (Table 19.4). Vasculitis of the gut is almost invariably associated with evidence of systemic involvement: palpable purpura in the skin, peripher-

**Table 19.4** Spectrum of gastrointestinal manifestations in systemic vasculitis

| Arteries | GI manifestations/complications |
|---|---|
| *Large* | |
| Takayasu (pulseless disease) | Ischemia, aneurysm |
| Kawasaki (mucocutaneous lymph node syndrome) | Obstructions, perforation |
| Giant cell arteritis | Ischemia, aneurysm |
| *Medium* | |
| PAN | Ulceration, pancreatitis, cholecystitis, perforation, hemorrhage |
| Churg–Strauss (allergic angiitis) | Perforation, focal on regional inflammation, cholecystitis |
| *Small* | |
| Wegener's | Focal inflammation, ulcer, stricture |
| Henoch–Schönlein | Hemorrhage, intussusception |
| SLE | Pancreatitis, focal inflammation, protein-losing enteropathy |

al neuropathy, glomerulitis or hypertension. In one series (Camilleri et al 1983), the gastrointestinal tract was affected in 27% of patients with a variety of "primary" vasculitides. The diagnosis depends on a high index of suspicion in the setting of the systemic disorder and further investigations are dictated by the accompanying features. Thus, in the presence of hypertension, but an inactive sediment on microscopy of the urine, selective visceral angiography is most useful to identify medium-sized vessel vasculitis. Conversely, in the presence of clinical and laboratory evidence of glomerulonephritis, a percutaneous renal biopsy is indicated since a small vessel vasculitis is most likely (Camilleri et al 1983).

The digestive tract involvement is usually apparent by endoscopy or barium contrast radiology; endoscopic findings include erythema, edema, petechiae, hemorrhage, erosions or ulcers (Shepherd et al 1983, Kato et al 1992). Thickening of bowel loops may be identified ultrasonographically (Kagimoto 1993). Visceral angiography will also document medium-sized vessel aneurysms in the territory of the superior mesenteric artery or organ infarcts (Cohen et al 1980). Gastrointestinal and laparoscopic peritoneal biopsies have, on occasion, shown diagnostic features of an arteritis and eosinophilic infiltration suggests an allergic angiitis such as Churg–Strauss syndrome.

Circulating liver enzymes are sometimes deranged during the process of a systemic vasculitis; however, significant hypoalbuminemia is more suggestive of an associated glomerulonephritis or nephrotic syndrome since the hepatic derangement rarely results in significant synthetic dysfunction.

## Management

The principles of management are to treat the underlying systemic vasculitis (initially with oral cyclophosphamide 3 mg/kg daily, with or without prednisone 60 mg/day) and support the patients through the gastrointestinal manifestations. Some authors prefer using azathioprine 1.5–2.0 mg/kg because of the risks of bladder and gonadal toxicity and oncogenesis with cyclophosphamide. Close follow-up is essential to detect complications that may require surgical treatment, such as massive hemorrhage, obstruction (Murphy et al 1987) or perforation; the latter may be clinically silent, particularly in those patients treated with corticosteroids (McCauley et al 1985).

Maintenance treatment is aimed at controlling the underlying systemic vasculitis. Gastrointestinal and renal involvement are indicative of a worse prognosis, particularly when bowel infarction or severe gastrointestinal bleeding occur or when renal failure supervenes.

REFERENCES

Abu-Nema T, Eklof B 1984 Evaluation of coeliac artery reconstruction. In: Bergan J T (ed) Arterial surgery. Clinical surgery international, Vol 8. Churchill Livingstone, Edinburgh, p 109

Boley S J, Schwartz S, Lash J, Sternhill V 1963 Reversible vascular occlusion of the colon. Surgery, Gynecology and Obstetrics 116: 53

Boley S J, Feinstein F R, Sammartano R, Brandt L J, Sprayregen S 1981 New concepts in the management of emboli of the superior mesenteric artery. Surgery, Gynecology and Obstetrics 153: 561–569

Brandt L J, Boley S J 1978 Celiac axis compression syndrome. A critical review. American Journal of Digestive Diseases 23: 633

Bulkley G B, Kvietys P R, Parks D A, Perry M A, Granger D N 1985 Relationship of blood flow and oxygen consumption to ischemic injury in the canine small intestine. Gastroenterology 89: 852–857

Bynum T E, Hanley H G 1982 Effect of digitalis on estimated splanchnic blood flow. Journal of Clinical Medicine 99: 84–91

Camilleri M, Pusey C D, Chadwick V S, Rees A J 1983 Gastrointestinal manifestations of systemic vasculitis. Quarterly Journal of Medicine 52: 141–149

Cohen R D, Conn D L Ilstrup D M 1980 Clinical features, prognosis, and response to treatment in polyarteritis. Mayo Clinic Proceedings 55: 146–155

Croft R J, Menon G P, Marston A 1981 Does "intestinal angina" exist? A critical study of obstructed visceral arteries. British Journal of Surgery 68: 316–318

Derrick J R, Pollard H S, Moore R M 1959 The patterns of arteriosclerotic narrowing of the celiac and superior mesenteric arteries. Annals of Surgery 149: 684–689

Dick A P, Graff R, Gregg D McC, Peters N, Sarner M 1967 An arteriographic study of mesenteric arterial disease. Gut 8: 206

Dunphy J A 1936 Abdominal pain of vascular origin. American Journal of the Medical Sciences 192: 109–112

Edwards A J, Hamilton J D, Nichol W D, Taylor G W, Dawson A M 1970 Experience with the coeliac axis compression syndrome. British Medical Journal 1: 342

Field S 1984 Plain films: the acute abdomen. Clinics in Gastroenterology 13: 3

Grendell J H, Ockner, R K 1982 Mesenteric venous thrombosis. Gastroenterology 82: 358–372

Grisham M B, Granger D N 1989 Free radicals: reactive metabolites of oxygen as mediators of postischemic reperfusion injury. In: Marston A, Bulkley G B, Fiddian-Green R G, Haglund U (eds) Splanchnic ischemia and multiple organ failure. Edward Arnold, London, p 135–144

Haglund U, Lundgren O 1979 Non-occlusive acute intestinal vascular failure. British Journal of Surgery 66: 155–158

Haglund U, Abe T, Ahren C, Braide I, Lundgren O 1976 The intestinal mucosal lesions in shock. I. Studies on the pathogenesis. European Journal of Surgical Research 8: 435–447

Helliwell T R, Flook D, Whitworth J, Day D W 1985 Arteritis and venulitis in systemic lupus erythematosus resulting in massive lower intestinal haemorrhage. Histopathology 9: 1103–1113

Hoyle M, Kennedy A, Prior A L, Thomas G E 1977 Small bowel ischaemia and infarction in young women taking oral contraceptives and progestational agents. British Journal of Surgery 64: 533–537

Jamieson C W 1986 Coeliac axis compression syndrome. British Medical Journal 293: 159–160

Jamieson W G, Marchik S, Rowson J, Durand D 1982 The early diagnosis of massive acute intestinal ischaemia. British Journal of Surgery 69: 552–553

Johnson C C, Baggenstoss A H 1949 Mesenteric vascular occlusion. I. Study of 79 cases of occlusion of veins. Proceedings of the Staff Meetings of the Mayo Clinic 24: 628–636

Kagimoto S 1993 Duodenal findings on ultrasound in children with Schönlein–Henoch purpura and gastrointestinal symptoms. Journal of Pediatric Gastroenterology and Nutrition 16: 178–182

Kato S, Shibuya H, Naganuma H, Nakagawa H 1992 Gastrointestinal endoscopy in Henoch–Schönlein purpura. European Journal of Pediatrics 151: 482–484

Krankendonk S E, Bruining H A, van Urk H 1983 Survival after portal venous gas due to mesenteric vascular occlusion British Journal of Surgery 70: 183–184
Kyriziakis A P, Mitra S K 1992 Multiple cytomegalovirus-related intestinal perforations in patients with acquired immunodeficiency syndrome. Report of two cases and review of the literature. Archives of Pathology and Laboratory Medicine 116: 495–499
Levy P J, Krausz M M, Manny J 1990 Acute mesenteric ischemia: improved results – a retrospective analysis of ninety-two patients. Surgery 107: 372–380
Lundgren O, Haglund U 1978 The pathophysiology of the intestinal countercurrent exchanger. Life Science 23: 1411–1422
Marcuson R W 1972 Ischaemic colitis. Clinics in Gastroenterology 1: 745–763
Marcuson R W, Farman J 1971 Ischaemic disease of the colon. Proceedings of the Royal Society of Medicine 64: 1080
Marshall J B, Kretschmar J M, Gerhardt D C et al 1990 Gastrointestinal manifestations of mixed connective tissue disease. Gastroenterology 98: 1232–1238
Marston A 1977 Intestinal ischaemia. Edward Arnold, London
Marston A 1989a Ischemic colitis. In: Marston A, Bulkley G B, Fiddian-Green R G, Haglund U (eds) Splanchnic ischemia and multiple organ failure. Edward Arnold, London, p 301–322
Marston A 1989b Chronic intestinal ischemia: intestinal angina. In: Marston A, Bulkley G B, Fiddian-Green R G, Haglund U (eds) Splanchnic ischemia and multiple organ failure. Edward Arnold, London, p 323–336
Marston A, Pheils M T, Thomas M L, Morson B C 1966 Ischaemic colitis. Gut 7: 1
Mavor G E 1972 Acute occlusion of the superior mesenteric artery. Clinics in Gastroenterology 1: 639
Mavor G E, Lyall A D, Chrystal K M R, Tsapogas M 1962 Mesenteric infarction as vascular emergency – the clinical problems. British Journal of Surgery 50: 219–225
McCauley R L, Johnston M R, Fauci A S 1985 Surgical aspects of systemic necrotizing vasculitis. Surgery 97: 104–110
Mosley J G, Marston A 1989 Acute intestinal ischemia: embolus, thrombosis and non-occlusive infarction. In: Marston A, Bulkley G B, Fiddian-Green R G, Haglund U (eds) Splanchnic ischemia and multiple organ failure. Edward Arnold, London, p 279–289
Mughal M, Irving M 1986 Home parenteral nutrition in the United Kingdom and Ireland. Lancet 2: 383
Murphy D J Jr, Morrow W R, Harberg F J, Hawkins E P 1987 Small bowel obstruction as a complication of Kawasaki disease. Clinical Pediatrics 26: 193–196
Ottinger L W, Austen W G 1967 A study of 136 patients with mesenteric infarction. Surgery, Gynecology and Obstetrics 124: 251–261
Parks D A, Granger D N 1986 Contributions of ischemia and reperfusion to mucosal lesion formation. American Journal of Physiology 250: G749–G753
Parks T G, Johnston C W, Kenedy T L, Gough A D 1972 Spontaneous ischaemic proctocolitis. Scandinavian Journal of Gastroenterology 7: 241–246
Poole J W, Sammartano R J, Boley S J 1987 Hemodynamic basis of the pain in chronic mesenteric ischemia. American Journal of Surgery 153: 171–176
Renton C J C 1972 Non-occlusive intestinal ischaemia. Clinics in Gastroenterology 1: 655–673
Robinson J W L, Mirkovitch V, Winistorfer B, Saegesser F 1981 Response of the intestinal mucosa to ischaemia. Gut 22: 512–527
Sackier J M, Kelly S B, Clarke D, Rees A J, Wood C B 1991 Small bowel haemorrhage due to cytomegalovirus vasculitis. Gut 32: 1419–1420
Schullinger J N, Jacobs J C, Berdon W E 1985 Diagnosis and management of gastrointestinal perforations in childhood dermatomyositis with particular reference to perforations of the duodenum. Journal of Pediatric Surgery 20: 521–524
Shaw R S, Maynard E P 1958 Acute and chronic thrombosis of the mesenteric arteries associated with malabsorption. New England Journal of Medicine 258: 874
Shaw R S, Rutledge R H 1957 Superior-mesenteric-artery embolectomy in the treatment of massive mesenteric infarction. New England Journal of Medicine 257: 595–598
Shepherd H A, Patel C, Bamforth J, Isaacson P 1983 Upper gastrointestinal endoscopy in systemic vasculitis presenting as an acute abdomen. Endoscopy 15: 307–311
Simpkins K C 1984 Double-contrast examination. Part III: Colon. Clinics in Gastroenterology 13: 99
Sleisenger M H 1977 The celiac artery syndrome – again? Annals of Internal Medicine 86: 355
Storey R J, Cunningham C G 1993 Acute mesenteric ischemia Surgery 114: 489–490
Veith F J, Boley S J 1986 Mesenteric ischaemia. In: Cameron J L (ed) Current surgical therapy, 1986–1987. C V Mosby, St Louis, p 399
Wilson C, Imrie C W 1986 Amylase and gut infarction. British Journal of Surgery 73: 219–221
Wilson C, Gupta R, Gilmour D G, Imrie C W 1987 Acute superior mesenteric ischaemia. British Journal of Surgery 74: 279–281

# 20. Tropical and infective diseases of the gastrointestinal tract and liver

*Peter Katelaris    Michael J. G. Farthing*

Infectious diseases of the gastrointestinal tract are perhaps the commonest infections of mankind. The heaviest burden of these diseases falls on the majority of the world's population that live in developing countries. Children in these regions still suffer unacceptably high morbidity and mortality from intestinal infections. Acute viral and bacterial diarrheal disease remains a major killer of preschool children. Parasites, particularly the geohelminths, are increasingly recognized as important contributors to childhood malnutrition and growth impairment. Many bacterial and parasitic intestinal infections are endemic in developed countries although the prevalence of these infections is generally much lower than in developing countries. With increasing numbers of travelers and immigrants, tropical infectious diseases must be considered in the differential diagnosis of many clinical presentations in nonendemic regions. This chapter details the epidemiology, pathophysiology, clinical features, diagnosis, treatment and prevention of the major tropical infections of the gastrointestinal tract and liver.

## DIARRHEAL DISEASE

Infections of the gastrointestinal tract are the most common intestinal disorders. Intestinal infections have their major impact in the developing world and are still responsible for the deaths of up to 4 million preschool children each year. Acute diarrheal disease in children is most commonly due to rotavirus and enterotoxigenic *Escherichia coli* infections although other types of pathogenic *E. coli*, *Shigella* spp., *Salmonella* spp. and *Campylobacter jejuni* are also important bacterial enteropathogens. Intestinal protozoa are important causes of *persistent* diarrhea particularly *Giardia intestinalis* (formerly *lamblia*), *Entamoeba histolytica*, *Cryptosporidium parvum* and the more recently recognized organisms of the *Microsporidium* spp. Diarrheal illness in children is almost inextricably linked to undernutrition and retardation of linear growth. Thus, the dangerous cycle of recurrent intestinal infection and undernutrition is never more obvious than in acute and persistent diarrheal disease. Despite the life-saving intervention of oral rehydration therapy, diarrheal disease attack rates remain largely unchanged because of the continuing high prevalence of bacterial, viral and protozoal enteropathogens. Until there is widespread provision of high-quality drinking water and adequate disposal of sewage and other waste, it is unlikely that there will be major changes in the prevalence of diarrheal disease in the poorer countries of the world.

Epidemiological studies indicate that intestinal infection is increasing even in developed countries. This relates to a number of factors which include food contamination during production (for example, poultry colonized with *Salmonella* spp. and *Campylobacter* spp.), the use of raw or partially cooked foods such as eggs and the adoption of other food cultures such as eating raw fish. Gastrointestinal infection affects 30–50% of travelers from Western countries to the developing world and is now well described in association with swimming in the sea, fresh inland waters and swimming pools. Other high-risk groups include the extremes of age, particularly those in daycare centers and residential institutions, and the immunocompromised, notably those with HIV/AIDS.

The science of intestinal infection continues to develop apace. New developments have occurred in our understanding of the epidemiology of these infections, new organisms have been discovered and new mechanisms of diarrhea elucidated. The techniques of molecular genetics have permitted the development of new diagnostic approaches and through our appreciation of the pathogenesis and pathophysiology of infective diarrhea, new treatments have emerged. The sophistication and efficacy of vaccines for enteric infection continue to improve such that these should be available for the majority of important gut infections early in the next millennium.

## BACTERIAL INFECTIONS

### Travelers' diarrhea

Diarrheal illness is the most common ailment associated

with travel and usually has an infective origin. Attack rates of 30–50% are common among travelers from developed countries who visit developing countries (Steffen & Boppart 1987). Travelers' diarrhea is usually defined as the passage of three or more unformed stools per 24 h occurring during or shortly after travel or any number of loose stools when associated with fever, abdominal pain or vomiting. Passage of any number of dysenteric stools (diarrhea with blood) associated with travel is also included in the definition of travelers' diarrhea.

### *Etiology and epidemiology*

High-risk destinations include most parts of Asia, Africa and South and Central America. The enteropathogens responsible are mostly transmitted via contaminated food and drink (Table 20.1). Bacterial pathogens are by far the most frequent causes, of which enterotoxigenic *Escherichia coli* (ETEC) is undoubtedly the single most common. It should be noted that cholera is rare in travelers. Enteric viruses may be responsible for a significant minority of cases. Protozoa and helminths may cause acute diarrhea but make up a greater proportion of cases presenting with prolonged diarrhea on return from abroad. *Giardia intestinalis* is the most common protozoal infection of travelers. *Entamoeba histolytica* is not common in travelers and when present, is usually not associated with invasive disease.

**Table 20.1** Spectrum and prevalence of pathogens that may cause diarrhea in travelers

| | Estimated proportion of total (%)* |
|---|---|
| **Bacteria** | |
| Enterotoxigenic *E. coli* (ETEC) | >40 |
| *Shigella* spp. | 8 |
| *Campylobacter jejuni* | >5 |
| *Salmonella* spp. | 3 |
| *Vibrio parahaemolyticus* | 1 |
| *Aeromonas* spp. | 3 |
| *Plesiomonas* spp. | 2 |
| Enteroinvasive *E. coli* | 2 |
| **Viruses** | |
| Rotavirus } | |
| Norwalk } | 10 |
| **Protozoa** | |
| *Giardia intestinalis* | 2 |
| *Entamoeba histolytica* | <1 |
| *Cryptosporidium parvum* | 1 |
| *Blastocystis hominis* | <1 |
| **Helminths** | 1–2 |
| **No pathogen identified** | 20–50 |
| **Multiple pathogens** | 20 |

*Estimates from many sources including Steffen & Boppart 1987. Regional and seasonal variation exists

### *Clinical features*

Symptoms may begin at any time during travel or shortly after return but the peak onset is on the third day after arrival abroad. The clinical features are an unreliable guide to the particular pathogen responsible. Most cases are mild episodes of acute watery diarrhea which are self-limiting and more inconvenient than medically hazardous but in a minority of travelers the illness may be a serious problem. There may be a prodrome of constitutional symptoms. Untreated, most episodes last only a few days (a median of 2 days) but occasionally may be protracted (Steffen & Boppart 1987). Dehydration is rarely marked and systemic symptoms are usually mild or absent. Associated symptoms may include anorexia, nausea, vomiting, abdominal cramps, bloating or low-grade fever. Dysentery occurs in less than 10% of cases and may be associated with abdominal pain, tenesmus and fever. Probably less than 1% of travelers suffer prolonged diarrhea. This is often due to nonbacterial causes, particularly *Giardia intestinalis*, other protozoa and occasionally helminths. Salmonellosis and *Campylobacter* colitis are occasionally protracted, causing symptoms for 2–3 months, or may relapse after initial improvement. Travelers with reduced host defenses, such as the very young, the elderly, those with achlorhydria or those who are specifically immunocompromised, are at increased risk for infection.

### *Diagnosis*

As most cases of travelers' diarrhea are mild and self-limiting they do not usually require laboratory investigation. However, when symptoms are protracted or severe or there is dysentery, investigations are warranted. Initially fresh stool (ideally three specimens) should be sent for microscopy, culture and drug sensitivity testing. If stool tests are negative, sigmoidoscopy or colonoscopy with biopsies may aid diagnosis and exclude noninfective diseases such as idiopathic inflammatory bowel disease. Serology for dysentery is usually unhelpful with the exception of amebic colitis in which at least 75% of infected individuals have specific anti-*Entamoeba. histolytica* IgG antibodies (Arvind et al 1988). In patients with chronic diarrhea investigations should begin with thorough microscopy of multiple fresh stool specimens to search for *Giardia intestinalis*, *E. histolytica*, *Cryptosporidium parvum* and *Isospora belli* and cultures also done to identify bacterial pathogens. Parasites may prove elusive to identify in feces, particularly in laboratories which do not examine positive specimens regularly. If stool examination is negative, endoscopy, aspiration of duodenal fluid and small intestinal biopsy may be helpful in identifying *G. intestinalis* or other protozoa or for the diagnosis of tropical sprue.

*Treatment*

Prior to travel the principles of self-treatment while abroad should be explained to patients. The mainstay of therapy is the maintenance of hydration and electrolyte balance. For adults this can usually be achieved by increasing the intake of fluids and by ensuring adequate sodium intake by adding salt to food or eating salty foods. There is no reason to fast during an attack. For diarrhea in young children, the aged or infirm it is sensible to have oral rehydration sachets on hand to use during attacks. In healthy adults with acute watery diarrhea, self-therapy with loperamide may be used in the short term but is not a substitute for adequate fluid intake. The usual dose for adults is 4 mg initially followed by 2 mg after each loose stool to a maximum of 16 mg/day. The usual daily dose is 6–8 mg/day. It should not be used in infants or young children or in those with dysentery. Bismuth subsalicylate has also been used to decrease stool frequency but is not as convenient or effective as loperamide.

A 3–5 day course of an antibiotic can reduce the duration of an acute diarrheal episode in travelers, irrespective of whether investigations are done to identify the causative enteropathogen. Doxycycline (100 mg daily), trimethoprim (TMP) alone or in combination with sulfamethoxazole (SMX) in a dose of TMP/SMX 160 mg/800 mg twice daily and the 4-fluoroquinolone drugs, ciprofloxacin 500 mg twice daily, norfloxacin 400 mg twice daily and ofloxacin 300 mg twice daily have all demonstrated efficacy (DuPont et al 1982, Taylor et al 1991). Even shorter courses of quinolones are effective. A single dose of ciprofloxacin 500 mg can markedly reduce the duration and severity of traveler's diarrhea (Salam et al 1994). The possibility of side-effects and the risk of drug resistance emerging should discourage indiscriminate use of antimicrobials for what is mostly mild self-limiting illness. Antibiotic resistance in bacterial enteropathogens is common, particularly in the developing world. Antibiotics should be avoided unless diarrhea is moderate or severe (>6 stools/day) or there is dysentery. Empirical therapy with a quinolone is reasonable in cases of dysentery as they are effective against many of the causative bacteria.

*Prevention*

For the traveler to a high-risk area, the motto "Cook it, peel it, boil it or forget it" is sound advice with regard to choice of food and drink but the ubiquitous distribution of enteropathogens means that even the most careful often succumb. Prophylactic use of antibiotics markedly decreases the risk of travelers' diarrhea with efficacy rates up to 80–90% (DuPont et al 1983, Scott et al 1990) but is not generally recommended because of the problems of increasing drug resistance, poor compliance, cost and side-effects. More important is careful attention to hygiene and appropriate intervention for an acute attack, as self-treatment of the acute episode may limit illness to less than 1 day. For short-term travelers (generally less than 3 weeks) to high-risk areas who are at increased risk of infection or in whom a diarrheal illness would greatly reduce the benefit of the trip, prophylactic antibiotics may be given. Doxycycline 100 mg, TMP/SMX 160 mg/800 mg, ciprofloxacin 500 mg or norfloxacin 400 mg all once daily may be used. Nonantibiotic prophylaxis using bismuth preparations is relatively effective but has never been popular. At present there is no effective vaccine for the prevention of travelers' diarrhea although various oral vaccines are being developed.

## *Escherichia coli* infections

*E. coli* is the major contributor to the aerobic bacterial flora of the human intestinal tract. It was initially thought that because of their ubiquitous nature these organisms did not cause disease, although by the 1940s the link between certain serotypes and diarrheal disease had become apparent. Since then at least five major categories of pathogenic *E. coli* have been described, each with defined epidemiology, clinical syndromes and differing pathogenesis (Levine 1987). The major groups include enterotoxigenic *E. coli* (ETEC), enteroinvasive *E. coli* (EIEC), enteropathogenic *E. coli* (EPEC), enterohemorrhagic *E. coli* (EHEC) and enteroadherent *E. coli* (EAEC) of which a subgroup, the enteroaggregative *E. coli* (EAggEC), is emerging as a clinically important group of organisms.

Traditionally, *E. coli* have been distinguished by serotyping using somatic (O) and flagella (H) antigens although with the identification of specific virulence factors such as enterotoxins, cytotoxins, invasins and adhesins, these earlier typing systems have become less important.

*Enterotoxigenic* E. coli

ETEC is one of the most prevalent bacterial enteropathogens in the developing world and thus, a common cause of acute diarrhea in infants and young children and in travelers (Sack 1975). The illness is characterized by acute watery diarrhea, which on average lasts 3–5 days and in young children may be associated with severe dehydration and in some cases acidosis. Virulence of ETEC depends on expression of two factors, namely (i) adhesins which mediate attachment of the organism to the intestinal epithelium, and (ii) the elaboration of secretory enterotoxins which are either heat labile (LT), which are now known to be a family of related toxins (LT-I, LT-IIa and LT-IIb), or the low molecular weight heat-stable toxin (ST). A variety of adhesins are now recognized including colonization factor antigens (CFA) and coli sur-

**Table 20.2** Properties of cholera toxin (CT) and *Escherichia coli* heat-labile (LT) and heat-stable (STa) toxins

| Property | LT/CT | STa |
|---|---|---|
| Onset | 1 h | Minutes |
| Duration | Prolonged | Shortlived |
| Molecular weight | 86 kDa | ~2 kDa |
| Toxin internalized | Yes | No |
| Cyclase dependency | Adenylate – cAMP | Guanylate – cGMP |

face (CS) fimbriae. The genes encoding both adhesins and enterotoxins are present in the organism as extra-chromosomal plasmid DNA. LT and ST differ in their molecular weight, enterocyte receptors and onset and duration of action (Table 20.2). Both ST and LT produce intestinal secretion by increasing intracellular concentrations of cyclic nucleotides, with LT stimulating adenylate cyclase, resulting in increase in cAMP levels, whereas ST activates guanylate cyclase, increasing cGMP. Although bioassays were initially used to identify these toxins, their presence can now be detected using specific DNA probes and molecular genetic analysis.

Infection with ETEC is usually self-limiting and thus antibiotic treatment is not routinely required. However, travelers may opt for a short course of a broad-spectrum antibiotic which can reduce both the severity and duration of the illness. Suitable antibiotics include TMP/SMX (co-trimoxazole), doxycycline or one of the 4-fluoroquinolones, as for travelers' diarrhea.

### *Enteroinvasive* E. coli

EIEC are similar to *Shigella* spp. with respect to both the clinical illness and pathogenesis of disease (Echeverria et al 1991). EIEC produce a dysenteric illness as a result of direct invasion of the distal ileum and colon. An important virulence factor of this group of organisms is the presence of invasins, surface proteins which mediate entry into the host epithelial cell. These proteins are encoded by genes contained in a large 120–140 MDa plasmid. In addition to their ability to invade the intestinal epithelium there is also evidence that EIEC may produce an enterotoxic factor which can produce intestinal secretion in a bioassay system. The classic test for demonstrating EIEC is the Sereny test in which a keratoconjunctivitis is produced in guinea pigs following inoculation into the conjunctivae.

### *Enteropathogenic* E. coli

EPEC were one of the first *E. coli* subtypes to be recognized as a human enteropathogen (Donnenberg & Kaper 1992). Their major impact is in children in whom they cause outbreaks of diarrhea in nurseries and daycare centers, which may be persistent. EPEC are noninvasive and do not produce classic enterotoxins but induce a characteristic attaching and effacing lesion with marked disruption of the intestinal microvilli. The organism attaches intimately to the epithelial cell surface membrane which is associated with high concentrations of filamentous actin at the adherence site. The ability to produce this lesion is encoded in the chromosome by the *eae* gene, the gene product being the protein intimin (Jerse & Kaper 1991). In addition to the ultrastructural changes to the host cell, EPEC induce an elevation in intracellular calcium and phosphorylation of a host cell protein. It has been suggested that this process may also be involved in an intestinal secretory response and thus the production of diarrhea.

### *Enterohemorrhagic* E. coli

EHEC typically produce outbreaks of self-limiting bloody diarrhea, which may be preceded by watery diarrhea and is usually associated with severe abdominal pain. Infection may be complicated by the hemolytic uremic syndrome or thrombocytopenic purpura which have a substantial morbidity and mortality in young children and the elderly. Transmission is usually through food with major outbreaks originating from hamburgers and milk. Outbreaks have been described in nursing homes and daycare centers and a recent study indicates that infection may also be transmitted by swimming in natural fresh waters.

EHEC are noninvasive but produce a similar attaching and effacing lesion as EPEC and possess the same *eae* gene thought to be responsible for this attachment mechanism. In addition, EHEC produce two antigenically distinct toxins called verocytotoxin (VT-I and VT-II), also known as Shiga-like toxin (SLT-I and SLT-II). These toxins are potent inhibitors of protein synthesis and have been implicated in the pathogenesis of the hemolytic uremic syndrome, possibly by damaging the renal microvasculature.

### *Enteroadherent* E. coli

EAEC is a heterogeneous group of *E. coli*, not all of which are thought to cause diarrhea. They can be differentiated from other adherent *E. coli* by the pattern of adherence to the HEp-2 cell line in which the localized adherence pattern of EPEC is not seen, adherence being diffuse across the cell surface. Although some studies have shown an association between this organism and acute diarrhea, human challenge studies failed to confirm this.

### *Enteroaggregative* E. coli

EAggEC have a classic "stacked brick" lattice pattern of adherence to epithelial cells and cells in tissue culture. There is now a consistent relationship between the presence of this organism and acute diarrhea and thus it is considered to be an enteropathogen (Yamamoto et al

1992). About 10% of cases associated with this organism have bloody diarrhea and hemorrhagic lesions have been produced when inoculated into animal models. EAggEC produce a heat-stable enterotoxin (EAST-1) which shows some sequence homology to *E. coli* STa. Further work is required to determine the precise role of this organism in persistent diarrhea in children.

## Campylobacter infection

### *Etiology*

Campylobacters are now recognized as one of the most common bacterial diarrheal pathogens of man. They are fastidious, spiral or curved nonsporulating Gram-negative rods. *Campylobacter jejuni* is the most common species responsible for human diarrheal disease. *C. fetus* has been isolated in immunocompromised individuals in whom it is associated with septicemia (Blaser & Reller 1981). There are occasional reports of diarrhea with *C. coli*, *C. laridis*, *C. upsaliensis* and *C. hyointestinalis*.

### *Epidemiology*

Contamination of animal food sources is probably the major mode of transmission although waterborne transmission also occurs. *Campylobacter* spp. can frequently be isolated from domestic and farm animals although poultry probably form the most important human reservoir of disease. At least 60% of chickens in the United Kingdom carry the organism and a similar proportion of carcasses remain contaminated as supplied to retailers. Infections are more common in summer months. In developed countries there is a peak of infection in children less than 1 year old and a second peak in adolescents and young adults.

### *Pathogenesis and pathology*

*Campylobacter jejuni* produces an enterocolitis with a marked inflammatory response in the mucosa (Bukholm & Kapperud 1987). The organism is known to produce two toxins: an enterotoxin which is similar to cholera toxin and activates adenylate cyclase and a cytotoxin which is presumed to be responsible for epithelial cell death and the associated acute inflammatory response (Guerrant et al 1987). The precise role of these toxins in the pathogenesis of Campylobacter colitis remains to be established.

### *Clinical features*

The spectrum of the clinical presentation is broad, ranging from mild watery diarrhea to severe dysentery (Black et al 1988). The incubation period is usually 24–72 h although it may be as long as 10 days. In 50% of cases a prodromal illness characterized by fever, headache, myalgia and malaise precedes the onset of diarrhea and sometimes overshadows the enteric symptoms. Fever, severe cramping, lower abdominal pain, anorexia and vomiting are often present with diarrhea. The disease is usually self-limiting with recovery occurring in 7–10 days. Persistent infection may occur in patients with HIV (Perlman et al 1988). Other nonenteric manifestations include arthralgia and the Guillain–Barré syndrome.

### *Diagnosis*

As *C. jejuni* infection is common and often closely linked to the ingestion of chicken, a presumptive clinical diagnosis can often be made in a patient with bloody diarrhea and severe lower abdominal pain. The presence of the organism can be confirmed by dark-field or phase-contrast microscopy in which the highly motile organisms can be seen in a saline wet mount of feces. Infection can be confirmed by culture on selective media, incubated at 42°C under microaerophilic conditions. As Campylobacters are relatively small in size, they may also be isolated by selective filtration from stool specimens followed by culture.

### *Treatment*

The primary goal in therapy of *Campylobacter* spp. infection is to restore water and electrolyte homeostasis and then to consider whether additional therapy is necessary. Antidiarrheal medication is not advised in patients with overt dysentery. The role of antibiotics remains controversial. If the individual presents late in the course of the illness and dysentery is absent or mild, then it is probably reasonable to withhold specific antimicrobial chemotherapy. There is little evidence to suggest that the late administration of antibiotics significantly alters the natural history of the illness. However, in patients who present early with severe dysentery then an antibiotic is recommended, such as erythromycin 250–500 mg four times daily for 5–7 days or a fluoroquinolone antibiotic such as ciprofloxacin 500 mg twice daily for a similar period. Ciprofloxacin reduces fecal excretion of the organism and appears effective in reducing the duration of symptoms. It is probably the drug of choice in confirmed *Campylobacter* enterocolitis in adults. Even without specific antimicrobial chemotherapy, recovery is usually rapid and complete although there is now an established link between *Campylobacter* spp. infection and Guillain–Barré syndrome (polyneuropathy) which may persist for weeks or months.

### *Prevention*

Reduction in the animal reservoirs of *Campylobacter* spp. must be a major goal for the future. In the meantime all chicken products should be considered to be potentially contaminated and therefore cooked thoroughly. Food preparers should also be aware that it is possible to contaminate other foods such as salads after handling an uncooked carcass. Thus great care must be taken in handling foodstuffs that will not eventually be subjected to high temperature cooking.

## Shigellosis

### *Etiology*

*Shigella* spp. produce a broad spectrum of clinical disease ranging from watery diarrhea to dysentery (Formal et al 1982, Keusch & Bennish 1989). Shigellosis is a disease that can rapidly rise to epidemic proportions because it is spread easily from person to person by transfer of a small number of organisms. *Shigella* spp. are members of the Enterobacteriaceae, are Gram-negative and closely resemble *E. coli*, although they are nonmotile. A variety of species are recognized, namely, *Shigella dysenteriae*, *S. flexneri*, *S. boydii* and *S. sonnei*. All species can produce dysentery, although *S. dysenteriae* produces the most serious disease.

### *Epidemiology*

*Shigella* spp. are found worldwide although *S. dysenteriae* is most commonly found in the tropics. It was responsible for many thousands of deaths in the Central American pandemic which raged from 1969 to 1972. Further outbreaks in Central America and other areas in the tropics have continued to occur. In the developed world, *S. sonnei* is found most commonly and often exhibits seasonality, with infections occurring most frequently in the winter. Humans constitute the only natural host for *Shigella* spp. and thus are the only important clinical reservoir of infection. The organism is transmitted usually by person-to-person contact but foodborne epidemics have been described.

### *Pathogenesis and pathology*

*Shigella* spp. produce several virulence factors which are thought to be important in the pathogenesis of infection (Sansonetti 1991). The ability of *Shigella* spp. to invade the host epithelial cell appears to be a central feature of pathogenesis and is known to be mediated by the ability to produce specific outer membrane proteins such as invasion plasmid antigens (*IPA*), invasion factors (inv) and virulence regulation factors (vir). Isolates with invasive potential always contain a large plasmid 120–140 MDa which closely resembles that found in EIEC (Maurelli et al 1985). The invasion process relies on complicity by the host cell which is an energy-dependent, active process.

A second important virulence factor is thought to be the production of Shiga toxin which is produced in large amounts by *S. dysenteriae* and to a lesser extent by other *Shigella* spp. (Acheson et al 1991). Shiga toxin is a potent inhibitor of protein synthesis and acts by irreversibly inactivating the 60S ribosomal subunits. It is thus directly cytotoxic but has also been shown to have enterotoxic and neurotoxic activity.

Although the precise role of Shiga toxin in the pathogenesis of shigellosis is not fully defined the resultant effects of infection are clear. Shigellosis produces a severe inflammatory colitis usually associated with large numbers of polymorphonuclear leukocytes, microabscess formation, goblet cell depletion and often frank mucosal ulceration. It is likely that neutrophil products such as prostaglandins, leukotrienes and reactive oxygen metabolites are involved in continuing the inflammatory cascade and possibly inducing intestinal secretion.

### *Clinical features*

Shigellosis is characteristically described as a two-phase illness, the first beginning with watery diarrhea and abdominal pain sometimes associated with fever. In the primate model of infection, it has been suggested that this might be the small intestinal phase of infection. The second phase usually begins 3–5 days after the initial illness when stool volume decreases and tends to be mainly blood and mucus, often associated with severe tenesmus and, in children, rectal prolapse. This is considered to be the colonic phase of the illness when colitis predominates. If severe, the colitis can progress to toxic megacolon and occasionally surgery is required because of colonic perforation. Other serious complications, which are generally associated with *S. dysenteriae* infection in children, include the hemolytic uremic syndrome and seizures.

### *Diagnosis*

Shigellosis cannot be reliably diagnosed clinically although a high index of suspicion is helpful, particularly during epidemics. Clinically the infection cannot be easily distinguished from other causes of bacillary dysentery. Sigmoidoscopy will often reveal the presence of a colitis but again there are no specific features which will distinguish this from other infective colitides or nonspecific inflammatory bowel disease. Culture of feces or a rectal swab is required to confirm the diagnosis microbiologically. An ELISA has been developed for the detection of Shiga toxin in feces although this is not widely available as a routine laboratory test.

### *Treatment*

General supportive measures are required as in all acute diarrheal disease and antidiarrheal preparations should be avoided, as in other forms of dysentery. In its mildest form, shigellosis is a self-limiting illness and no specific antimicrobial chemotherapy is required. However, in infection with *S. dysenteriae* and in other forms of shigellosis in which there are severe systemic symptoms, antibiotic therapy is indicated. Although ampicillin and co-trimoxazole have in the past been effective, safe and economic treatments for shigellosis, resistance to these antibiotics is now common. Knowledge of the origin of the *Shigella* spp. may be helpful in determining the likelihood of antibiotic resistance prior to sensitivity data being available. Nalidixic acid (1 g three times daily for 5 days) continues to be the treatment of choice in southern Asia for the treatment of *S. dysenteriae* although the newer fluoroquinolone drugs (such as ciprofloxacin 500 mg twice daily for 3–5 days) are emerging as first-line treatment, their superiority to other standard therapies having been clearly shown in clinical trials.

*Prevention*

The key to preventing shigellosis is to interrupt the transmission pathway from person to person. When infections are isolated in the community, strictest instructions must be given with regard to personal hygiene to avoid the high secondary attack rate that will inevitably follow if such precautions are not taken. Vaccine development is under way but it seems unlikely that this will reduce the size of the human reservoir for many years to come.

## Yersiniosis

*Yersinia enterocolitica* is the organism responsible for the majority of human intestinal infections with this genus. Other *Yersinia* species can be isolated from domestic and farm animals. The organism multiplies and is motile at low temperatures (22–29°C) which almost certainly contributes to its ability to survive in the environment outside its mammalian hosts.

*Epidemiology*

The reservoirs of *Y. enterocolitica* include humans, a variety of domestic and farm mammalian species and foods including milk, ice cream and other milk products. In certain parts of the world, notably Europe, isolation rates in humans closely parallel those in pigs. The organism is mostly found in temperate climates such as northern Europe, particularly Scandinavia, and also in Canada. Seasonality is described in some geographic locations, notably in Europe, where isolations are at their peak in autumn and early winter. In most series in Europe and USA, preschool children are the most commonly affected.

*Pathogenesis and pathology*

*Y. enterocolitica* is an invasive organism and depends on the presence of a 103 kDa invasin which appears to be vital to mediate the invasion process. The organism has a predilection for the epithelium overlying Peyer's patches and proliferates within the lymph follicles. The organisms then migrate into the lamina propria and are taken up by macrophages. The organism also produces an enterotoxin in vitro when cultured at 25°C but not at 37°C. The role of this toxin in the pathogenesis of diarrhea is unclear. Additional virulence factors include a chromosomal gene, the *AIL* locus which is involved in attachment and invasion and other plasmid encoded factors which control autoagglutination, and factors which enable *Y. entercolitica* to resist the bactericidal effects of serum and phagocytosis. As a result of the invasion process there is marked hyperemia, neutrophil infiltration and often overt epithelial ulceration. There is generally associated lymphoid hyperplasia with resulting mesenteric adenitis.

*Clinical features*

The illness is characterized by diarrhea, fever and lower abdominal pain, often in the right iliac fossa (Simmonds et al 1987). Diarrhea is more pronounced in young children. The illness may mimic appendicitis. The illness is usually self-limiting with recovery occurring on average within 14–17 days. Chronic abdominal symptoms have been associated with yersiniosis although whether this relates strictly to continuing infection or a postinfective functional disturbance is unclear. Occasionally terminal ileitis (Fig. 20.1) may be so severe as to require surgical resection.

Extraintestinal manifestations include polyarthritis which may be associated with inflammatory skin lesions such as erythema nodosum and erythema multiforme, indicative of Reiter's syndrome. Arthritis may occur in up to 2% of infected individuals and is more common in those with HLA-B27.

*Diagnosis*

It is difficult to distinguish yersiniosis from other intestinal infections. Diagnosis can be confirmed in the early stages of the illness by culture of feces, blood or mesenteric lymph nodes if surgery is performed for appendicitis. Selective media with culture at 25°C are required to isolate the organism. Serological testing can be used to demonstrate whether infection has occurred although the results are usually only available after the illness has resolved (Bottone & Sheehan 1983).

*Treatment*

There is no clearcut evidence that treatment with antibi-

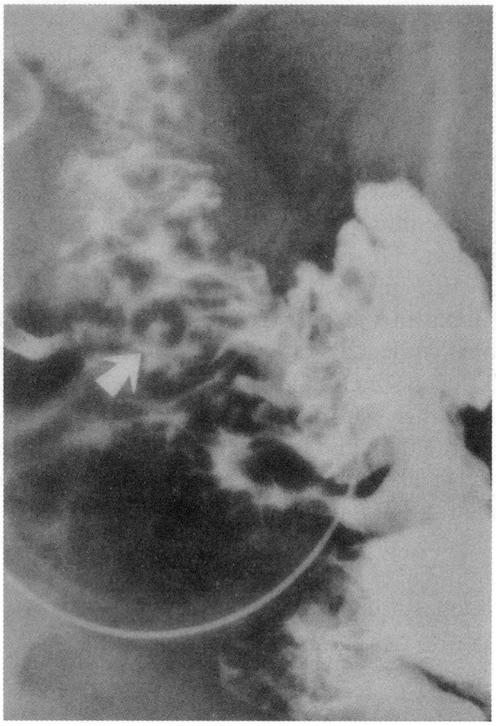

**Fig. 20.1** Barium follow-through examination showing ileal ulceration (arrow) due to yersiniosis.

otics alters the natural history of this infection (Hoogkampe-Korstanje 1987). However, the organism is usually sensitive to co-trimoxazole, tetracyclines and the fluoroquinolones. Antibiotics, however, are indicated when there are severe systemic symptoms and when there is obvious metastatic spread in bones, joints, lungs, the central nervous system and other tissues.

## Salmonellosis

Infection with *Salmonella* spp. occurs as five major clinical syndromes:

1. gastroenteritis
2. bacteremia
3. localized infection
4. enteric fever (typhoid)
5. the asymptomatic carrier state.

*Salmonella* is a genus of the family Enterobacteriaceae and possesses somatic (O) and flagella (H) antigens that are used for serotyping related organisms. Vi is an additional virulence antigen and in some strains, particularly *S. typhi*, it prevents agglutination with O antisera. There are approximately 1700 serotypes known to cause disease in humans, although 90% of genotypes fall into groups A–E which contain 40 serotypes.

### *Epidemiology*

*Salmonella* spp. colonize the gastrointestinal tract of many vertebrates and some invertebrates. The organisms are also found in fresh and seawater, in sewage and certain foods, particularly chicken and eggs. There is a close similarity between the serotypes isolated from animals and human feces and it is estimated that at least 50% of human infections are derived from contaminated animal products (Sharp 1988, Rampling et al 1989). The peak incidence of salmonella infection is in the summer months, with the highest attack rates in children and the elderly. The immunocompromised, particularly individuals with HIV/AIDS, are at increased risk of salmonellosis.

### *Pathogenesis and pathology*

*Salmonella* spp. infects the ileum and colon producing an inflammatory ileocolitis with mucosal inflammation. There is marked mucosal edema and polymorphonuclear leukocyte infiltration. Salmonellae are invasive enteropathogens and contain a plasmid that encodes for the invasive characteristics (Jones et al 1982). Other virulence factors enable the organism to survive within macrophages following phagocytosis. Salmonellae have the ability to penetrate lymphatic and blood vessels within the gut wall and thus disseminate to other parts of the body including bones, joints, the heart and many other soft tissues.

### *Clinical features*

The clinical presentations of salmonellosis are variable and depend on the group and serotype of the organism involved and the extent to which the disease is disseminated throughout the body (Saphra & Winter 1957).

***Gastroenteritis.*** This accounts for approximately 75% of infections and usually follows the ingestion of contaminated foods. Early symptoms include nausea and vomiting which are followed by diarrhea and cramping abdominal pain. Fever occurs in approximately 50% of infected patients; the illness is usually short lived (2–5 days) and self-limiting. Diarrhea varies from watery to overt dysentery.

***Bacteremia.*** Salmonellae can be detected in blood and bone marrow in approximately 10% of infected individuals. It may be transient and occurs in some patients with otherwise uncomplicated gastroenteritis, but may be persistent in patients with AIDS.

***Localized infection.*** This form of the disease occurs in individuals with severe and prolonged bacteremia and may be present in as many as 5% of cases seen by clinicians. Common complications include osteomyelitis, septic arthritis, endocarditis and local abscesses in soft tissues. Disseminated salmonellosis occurs more commonly in individuals with sickle cell anemia, malaria and other hemolytic anemias.

***Asymptomatic carriage.*** Less than 1% of individuals with symptomatic infection with *Salmonella* spp. go on to develop the asymptomatic carrier state. Carriage may be higher in individuals infected with typhoidal strains and is most commonly found in the elderly, in women and in the presence of gallstones. The gallbladder is still considered to be an important reservoir of infection. If carriage persists for more than 1 year, it is unlikely that spontaneous clearance of the organism will occur.

***Typhoid (enteric fever).*** *S. typhi* and *S. paratyphi* strains are responsible for the majority of cases although occasionally other Salmonellae can produce this clinical form of the disease. Typhoid is predominantly a systemic infection and not a major intestinal disease. The incubation period is approximately 7–14 days. This is followed by the first stage of the illness which is characterized by high fever, headache and abdominal discomfort which is either diffuse or localized to the right iliac fossa; 50% of patients are constipated during the first week of the illness. During the second phase, which again lasts approximately 1 week, the patient becomes increasingly unwell with a continuous fever. The typical "rose spots" usually develop at this time, often associated with splenomegaly. During the third week, the illness increases in severity with severe toxemia and disorientation. Diarrhea may develop at this stage and be complicated by hemorrhage and perforation from intestinal ulceration, usually the ileum. Other complications result from metastatic spread of infection and include pneumonia, pyelonephritis, brain abscess, osteomyelitis and septic arthritis. Acute hepatic infection associated with cholestasis also occurs. During the fourth week of the illness the fever usually subsides and clinical recovery ensues.

*Diagnosis*

Diagnosis of nontyphoidal gastroenteritis is generally made by stool culture. In severely ill patients the organism may also be detected in blood and synovial fluid. In typhoidal salmonellosis, blood culture is positive in 90% of patients during the first week and for several following weeks if antimicrobial chemotherapy is not given. Bone marrow cultures remain positive for several weeks, despite antibiotic treatment. Stool cultures are only positive during the later stage of the illness as Peyer's patches ulcerate in the distal ileum. The organism may also be recovered from duodenal fluid and urine.

Serological testing in the form of the Widal test which relies on the detection of anti-O and anti-H antibody has been used in the past. However, this test lacks precision and thus vigorous attempts must be made to isolate the organism by culture.

*Treatment*

For uncomplicated nontyphoidal gastroenteritis, antibiotic therapy is not indicated. There are still concerns that inappropriate use of antibiotics can increase the chances of developing a chronic carrier state (Keusch 1988). Antibiotics are, however, indicated in immunocompromised individuals such as those with HIV infection, those with malignant disease and patients who have recently undergone organ transplantation. Treatment is also recommended for individuals with prosthetic heart valves or prostheses elsewhere in the body, those with hemolytic anemia and those at the extremes of age. Antibiotics may also be given when there is evidence of serious systemic involvement. There is now widespread resistance to ampicillin and co-trimoxazole but if the strain is sensitive there is no reason why these antibiotics cannot be used, (ampicillin 0.25–1 g four times daily, TMP/SMX 160 mg/800 mg twice daily, each for 5 days). Alternatives include fluoroquinolones such as ciprofloxacin 500 mg or norfloxacin 400 mg twice daily for 5 days. Chloramphenicol is less used now but may be appropriate in cases of multiple drug resistance.

For typhoid, chloramphenicol is the classic therapy, usually 2 g/day for adults given orally in four divided doses. In the severely ill it may be administered intravenously (in the same dosage). Alternatives include oral amoxycillin 1 g four times daily or intravenous ampicillin 6 g/day in divided doses. Co-trimoxazole (in the dosages above) and the third-generation cephalosporins have also been used. The fluoroquinolones are active against *S. typhi* although resistance has been described. Antibacterial therapy should be continued for 10–14 days. Fluoroquinolones have been used successfully to eradicate the carrier state and this is thought to be related to the high drug concentrations that are achieved in the gallbladder.

## Cholera

Cholera is one of the most devastating human diarrheal diseases. It produces severe, high-volume watery diarrhea which may exceed 20 L per day which without treatment results in a high mortality from dehydration and acidosis. The disease was recognized by Hippocrates but the modern history of cholera dates from 1817 when "Asiatic cholera", previously restricted to India and beyond, came to Europe and North America. Between 1817 and 1889, there were six cholera pandemics which resulted in approximately 400 000 deaths in the UK and USA. The seventh pandemic began in south east Asia in the early 1960s and has spread throughout the tropics and subtropics through Africa and more recently into Central and South America.

*Etiology*

*Vibrio cholerae* O1 is the classic organism responsible for cholera. The organism may be subdivided into serotypes Ogawa and Inaba on the basis of agglutination tests with type-specific antisera for the lipopolysaccharide, heat-stable somatic O-antigen. In addition two biotypes have been identified. The classic biotype was responsible for the first six world pandemics while the El Tor biotype is responsible for the current seventh pandemic. El Tor produces a milder form of the disease than the classic biotype and may be carried asymptomatically. The ratio of infection to clinical disease is approximately 100:1 with the El Tor biotype compared to 10:1 with the classic vibrio.

Non-O1 V. *cholerae* are found in the same geographic areas as *V. cholerae* O1. The former organisms may account for up to 3% of patients with diarrhea in cholera areas. Towards the end of 1993 a new organism responsible for outbreaks of cholera-like diarrheal disease was found and has been designated *V. cholerae* O139 (Cholera Working Group 1993). This organism differs genetically from El Tor and classic *V. cholerae* but produces cholera toxin and other virulence factors and it has been suggested that *V. cholerae* O139 is a mutant of the El Tor biotype.

*V. parahaemolyticus* is another non-O group organism and is responsible for a relatively mild diarrheal illness usually associated with the ingestion of uncooked fish and seafood.

### *Epidemiology*

*V. cholerae* O1 is transmitted by contaminated water, shellfish and other seafood and by person-to-person contact (Feachem 1982). The infective dose is around $10^9$ vibrios but may fall to as low as $10^3$ in situations of low gastric acidity. In endemic areas, children are at greatest risk with age-specific prevalence falling with increasing age due to acquired immunity. Infants, however, have a reduced risk of infection presumably as a result of less exposure to vibrios combined with the protective effects of breastfeeding. There is seasonality of cholera in endemic areas, being more common in the warmer, wetter months of the year.

### *Pathogenesis and pathology*

Following ingestion of *V. cholerae* the highly motile vibrios colonize the proximal small intestine by penetrating the mucus coat and multiplying in close proximity to the intestinal epithelium. The organism does not cause light microscopic or ultrastructural damage to the epithelial cells but releases cholera toxin which activates the enzyme adenylate cyclase, causing a marked increase in the concentration of intracellular cyclic AMP (Farthing 1993). This leads to stimulation of protein kinase A which results in phosphorylation of a membrane protein related to the chloride channel in the apical membrane of the enterocyte. This results in chloride ion secretion which is then followed by sodium ions and water. Recently, two other toxins have been identified in *V. cholerae.* Zonular occludens toxin (ZOT) has been shown to enhance the secretory state by disrupting the zonular occludens (tight junction) and accessory cholera enterotoxin (ACE) also produces electrogenic secretion although the precise mechanism has not been fully elucidated (Fasano et al 1991, Trucksis et al 1993).

In addition, recent studies suggest that neurohumoral pathways may be involved in cholera-toxin induced intestinal fluid secretion. There is increasing evidence to suggest that cholera-toxin is able to release 5HT from enterochromaffin cells in the small intestine, possibly by activation of the adenylate cyclase-cAMP system in these cells. The release of 5HT is then thought to activate prostaglandin $E_2$ formation via $5HT_2$ receptors which will further enhance the secretory response. It has also been proposed that 5HT may also act via $5HT_3$ receptors on enteric nerves which, via interneurones in the myenteric plexus, activate submucosal nerves (possibly VIPergic) that terminate close to the basolateral membrane of the enterocyte (Farthing 1991).

### *Clinical features*

Mild cholera in adults and children may be indistinguishable from diarrhea due to other infective agents. This form of the disease occurs in the majority of infected individuals. However, severe cholera begins abruptly, often at night, with severe diarrhea up to 1 L/h in the first 24 h. Fever is usually absent but vomiting is common in the early stages of the illness. Stools take on the typical "rice water" character due to the presence of mucus particles in the watery stool. Dehydration, acidosis and hypotension follow rapidly. When the fluid deficit is >8% there is usually evidence of cardiovascular collapse and oliguria. Ultimately, the patient loses consciousness and death follows when fluid losses exceed 12%. Untreated cholera has a mortality rate of 20–50% but with adequate rehydration therapy, no patient should die.

### *Diagnosis*

In endemic and epidemic cholera, diagnosis is usually made on clinical criteria, namely the extremely high-volume watery diarrhea with profound dehydration and acidosis. Microbiological diagnosis can be achieved by dark-field examination of the stool revealing the highly motile cholera vibrio and confirmed by the immobilizing effect of specific antisera. The presence of *V. cholerae* can be confirmed by culture.

### *Treatment*

The most important aspects of the treatment of cholera

are (i) rapid rehydration and correction of acidosis and (ii) reduction of bacterial colonization and eradication of vibrios with antibiotics. Tetracycline 250 mg four times daily for 3–5 days decreases both the duration and severity of diarrhea. *V. cholerae* O1 is also sensitive to ampicillin, chloramphenicol, co-trimoxazole, doxycycline and furazolidone. A single dose of doxycycline (200–300 mg) has recently been shown to be as effective as the standard multiple dose tetracyline regimen (Alam et al 1990).

In the late 1960s the World Health Organization recommended the use of an oral rehydration solution (sodium 90, glucose 111, potassium 20, citrate 10 mmol/L) for the treatment of cholera. Providing there is no evidence of marked hypovolemia and severe hypotension, fluid and electrolytes may be administered orally or by nasogastric tube. This solution has been widely used in the treatment of epidemic cholera and has dramatically reduced mortality. Simple glucose electrolyte solutions, while being effective for rehydration, do not reduce stool output. However, the use of complex carbohydrate oral rehydration solutions, particularly those containing rice powder, do reduce stool output and total requirements for oral rehydration solutions in cholera. In the presence of cardiovascular collapse and severe acidosis intravenous rehydration is mandatory.

#### *Prevention*

Administration of tetracycline to family members of patients with cholera can substantially decrease the secondary attack rate (e.g. doxycycline 300 mg as a single dose for adults). Even mass treatment has been used to limit the spread during epidemics although this adds to the development of multiple antibiotic-resistant strains of *V. cholerae* O1. Mass treatment is not economically viable and should be restricted to immediate family members.

Cholera vaccines have been available for many decades but the early parenteral vaccines are generally of low efficacy. More recently, live oral vaccine strains have been developed, particularly the genetically manipulated strains of *V. cholerae* O1 in which the genes encoding cholera toxin, ACE and ZOT have been deleted. These vaccine strains produce little or no diarrhea, are immunogenic and produce impressive protection in challenge studies. Large field studies are currently under way to assess their efficacy (Levine et al 1988, Clemens et al 1990).

### ***Aeromonas* spp. and *Plesiomonas shigelloides***

*Aeromonas* spp. and *Plesiomonas shigelloides* are ubiquitous micro-organisms which are found in fresh and salt waters and particularly river estuaries. *Aeromonas* spp. have been known to be pathogens to fish for many years but there is increasing evidence to suggest an association with human diarrheal disease (Taylor et al 1985). *Aeromonas* can also cause extraintestinal disease including bacteremia, endocarditis, septic arthritis and skin infections. Both *Aeromonas* and *Plesiomonas* can be contracted from shellfish.

*Aeromonas* spp. are known to produce a variety of enterotoxins, cytotoxins and hemolysins. The organism is not invasive and as yet the relative importance of these potential virulence factors has not been determined with respect to pathogenesis (Pitarangsi et al 1982). The mechanisms involved in the pathogenesis of *Plesiomonas* infection have not been established. *Aeromonas* infection can present as watery diarrhea, acute bloody diarrhea which can closely resemble acute ulcerative colitis or as persistent diarrhea which may continue for many weeks.

Treatment is generally supportive and the role of antibiotics not clearly established. However, the organism is usually sensitive to co-trimoxazole and also to tetracyclines, chloramphenicol, third-generation cephalosporins and the fluoroquinolones. Antibiotics are usually advised for systemic infection.

### **Foodborne diarrheal disease**

Foodborne diarrheal disease is most commonly due to enteropathogenic bacteria which either colonize and truly infect the intestinal tract or are consumed in food in which there is preformed enterotoxin. The most common forms of "infective" food poisoning are due to *Salmonella* spp., *Shigella* spp., *Campylobacter jejuni* and ETEC for which there is usually an incubation period of 24–48 h. The second variety of food poisoning is when preformed toxins are ingested in the contaminated food and thus, the symptoms of vomiting and diarrhea usually occur within a few hours. This type of food poisoning is most commonly associated with *Staphylococcus aureus*, *Clostridium perfringens* and *Bacillus cereus* (Table 20.3).

#### Staphylococcus aureus

This organism produces a variety of enterotoxins which are heat stable. Between 1–6 h after ingestion of toxin, nausea, vomiting and eventually diarrhea occur (Tranter 1990). The illness is usually shortlived with complete recovery within 24 h. Fever is not usually present. Food is usually contaminated by a food handler who is a carrier and commonly implicated foods include cold dishes such as milk-containing desserts, mayonnaise, ice cream and coleslaw. Enterotoxin can be detected directly in food or following culture of *S. aureus*.

#### Clostridium perfringens

This organism survives in the environment by production of heat-resistant spores; these spores are responsible for food poisoning (Lund 1990). Spores can be detected in

**Table 20.3** Bacterial causes of food poisoning

| Organism | Source | Incubation period | Symptoms | Diagnosis | Recovery |
|---|---|---|---|---|---|
| *Staphylococcus aureus* | Contaminated food, usually by humans | 2–6 h | Diarrhea, vomiting and dehydration | Culture organism in vomitus or remaining food | Rapid (few hours) |
| *Bacillus cereus* | Spores in food (often rice) survive boiling | 1–6 h | Diarrhea, vomiting and dehydration | Culture organism in feces and food | Rapid |
| *Clostridium perfringens* | Spores in food survive boiling | 8-22 h | Watery diarrhea and cramping pain | Culture organism in feces and food | 2–3 days |
| *Clostridium botulinum* | Spores survive cooking but only germinate in anaerobic conditions, e.g. canned or bottled food | 18–36 h | Brief diarrhea and paralysis due to neuromuscular blockade | Demonstrate toxin in food or feces | 10–14 days |
| *Salmonella enteritidis* | Bowels of animals, especially fowl | 12–24 h | Abrupt diarrhea, fever and vomiting | Culture organism in stool | Usually 2–5 days, but may be up to 2 weeks |
| *Campylobacter jejuni* | Bowels of animals, especially fowl; also milk | 48–96 h | Diarrhea ± blood, fever, malaise and abdominal pain | Culture organism in stool | 3–5 days |

raw meat and animal and human feces. Diarrhea and cramping abdominal pain begins 10–24 h following ingestion of contaminated food but the illness is self-limiting and usually resolves within 24 h. An extremely severe form of the disease is caused by *C. perfringens* type C which causes enteritis necroticans (pig-bel disease) which in the past was common in Papua New Guinea.

### *Clostridium botulinum*

This is another potentially serious form of clostridial food poisoning and is again due to the ingestion of preformed toxins in bacterial spores (Lund 1990). This illness has been associated with the bottling and canning industry. Nausea and vomiting occur only in the early phases of the disease prior to the development of the neurological complications which include flaccid paralysis which may require ventilation.

### *Bacillus cereus*

This organism is responsible for two food poisoning syndromes namely (i) diarrhea and abdominal pain which occur 8–16 h after eating contaminated foods and (ii) isolated vomiting 1–5 h after ingestion of reheated rice. The diarrhea and abdominal pain are thought to be due to ingestion of preformed enterotoxins although the etiology in the second is unclear. It is presumed, however, that it relates to ingestion of a heat-stable, preformed toxin.

## ANTIBIOTIC-ASSOCIATED DIARRHEA

This is common and occurs in 10–20% of patients treated with lincomycin or clindamycin and 5–10% treated with ampicillin. It is also common with amoxycillin and cephalosporins but can occur with any antibiotic. In about 25% of patients with antibiotic-associated diarrhea, infection with *C. difficile* is responsible. The remainder have osmotic diarrhea. The antibiotic alters the colonic microflora, thereby impairing the fermentation of carbohydrate which reaches the colon (Rao et al 1988); this results in an osmotic diarrhea which is probably accentuated by a diet high in complex carbohydrate.

Diarrhea usually begins a few days after antibiotic is commenced; there is abdominal discomfort and several loose stools per day but these are negative for pathogens and leukocytes. Sigmoidoscopy shows a normal mucosa and the patient has no fever or leukocytosis.

## *C. difficile* infection and pseudomembranous colitis

*C. difficile* produces toxins which are responsible for virtually all cases of pseudomembranous colitis and for up to 25% of cases of antibiotic-associated diarrhea without colitis (Kelly et al 1994).

### *Epidemiology*

Children born in hospital frequently acquire the organism at birth but rarely develop symptoms or colitis because toxin receptors are absent from their mucosal cells; they then become colonized with commensal organisms which inhibit the growth of *C. difficile*.

By contrast a colonization at the rate of 21% was found when adults are admitted to hospital (McFarland et al 1989) in contrast to a carriage rate of 3% in healthy adults in the community. The spores of *C. difficile*, which are heat resistant, are widely distributed in hospitals, in bathrooms, on linen and on commonly handled objects. The spores are carried from room to room on the hands or instruments of healthcare workers. When ingested, if the spores pass through the barrier of gastric acid, they may colonize the large intestine. The overwhelming predisposing factor is the use of antibiotics which alter colonic flora. Antibiotics most frequently involved are clindamycin, lincomycin, ampicillin, amoxycillin and cephalosporins: less frequently involved are the penicillins, quinolones, erythromycin, sulfamethoxazole and trimethoprim. Antibiotics rarely involved are parenteral aminoglycosides, vancomycin, metronidazole and bacitracin. Additional predisposing factors are age, reduction in gastric acidity due to $H_2$ receptor antagonists or proton pump inhibitors and immune deficiency including AIDS (Cappell & Philogene 1993). The organism may also be acquired in the community from pet droppings.

*Pathology and pathogenesis*

Within the human colon, two large protein exotoxins are produced. Toxin A (308 kDa) is an enterotoxin and toxin B (250–270 kDa) is a cytotoxin. Both have the potential to cause colonic inflammation. These toxic effects follow their binding to receptors on the membranes of enterocytes.

In pseudomembranous colitis, the membrane usually appears as adherent plaques covering areas of superficial ulceration. The mucosal change is focal and the mucosa between the plaques is normal (Price & Davies 1977). Occasionally, the membrane covers the entire mucosa as a result of coalescence of plaques. The histological features are graded into three types. Type I, the early lesion, has patchy epithelial necrosis and an exudate of fibrin and neutrophils. Type II has a more prominent exudate that erupts as "volcanoes" from foci of epithelial ulceration, but the surrounding mucosa remains intact. The type III lesion shows more diffuse epithelial necrosis and ulceration with a pseudomembrane of mucin, fibrin, leukocytes and cellular debris. The mucosa itself is infiltrated with lymphocytes and polymorphs (Sumner & Tedesco 1975) and the glands are distended with mucin. Focal areas of inflammation can be seen in the mucosa in the absence of a membrane. In some instances, the histological features are difficult to distinguish from ulcerative colitis or amebiasis; there is no membrane formation and mucosal changes are general rather than focal. Finally, the rectum is normal or shows only edema in some cases.

*Clinical features and investigation*

The symptoms commence during or after oral or parenteral antibiotic therapy (Hoberman et al 1976) with diarrhea which is accompanied by blood only in severe cases. Occasionally development of symptoms may be delayed until after antibiotic therapy. Most cases are mild with little systemic response and last for 2–3 weeks. Fever and leukocytosis may only when colitis is severe. To make the diagnosis a stool cytotoxin test for the B toxin is the most sensitive and specific assay but requires overnight incubation. Enzyme immunoassays are available which detect toxins A and B in stool samples. The diagnosis is usually confirmed on sigmoidoscopy and biopsy of the mucosa; a pseudomembrane is often present, but if the colitis has been active for some time a hemorrhagic and friable mucosa may be seen and the differential diagnosis from ulcerative colitis is more difficult. Some patients have a normal rectosigmoid colon with more proximal pseudomembranous colitis (Tedesco 1979). A plain radiograph of the abdomen may show an increase in thickness of the colonic wall, thumb printing and mucosal irregularity due to the presence of plaques (Tedesco 1977). In severe cases electrolyte imbalance, hypoproteinemia and toxic dilatation may develop.

*Treatment*

Antibiotic therapy should be discontinued if possible. In patients with mild diarrhea this and supportive treatment may be all that is required. When symptoms are persistent or severe or when antibiotic therapy cannot be ceased, metronidazole is the drug of choice, with vancomycin reserved for the minority of patients with the most severe disease. Both are equally effective in treating diarrhoea caused by *C. difficile* infection (Wenisch et al 1996). Symptomatic improvement should occur within 3 days with complete resolution of the illness in most patients within 10 days (Bartlett 1985, Kelly et al 1994). The usual dose of metronidazole is 250–500 mg 3–4 times per day orally for 10 days (Teasley et al 1983). It is widely available, inexpensive, generally reasonably well tolerated and resistance is uncommon. However, it is readily absorbed in the upper gastrointestinal tract and in severe disease, particularly when there is ileus, it may not reach the colonic lumen in sufficient concentration (Bolton & Culshaw 1986). Therefore vancomycin is often used in patients with severe disease; the dose is 125 mg orally four times daily for 10 days but it is expensive and not readily available in all parts of the world. Moreover, the recent rise in the prevalence of vancomycin-resistant enterococci, particularly in hospitals, may be due in part to its increased use. As this is plasmid mediated, the risk of other organisms acquiring vancomycin resistance should restrict its use. Both drugs can be given via a naso-gastric tube if necessary. When the oral route cannot be used, intravenous metronidazole can be given, however reliance on this alone is not recommended and if possible oral vancomycin should be given as well. Intravenous vancomycin does not reliably produce adequate stool concentrations although it has been used in conjuction with metronidazole parenterally in severe cases. When vancomycin is given both orally and parenterally serum concentration should be monitored. Occasionally emergency colectomy for toxic dilatation is necessary as a life saving measure (p. 23.43).

Relapse is common in the 4 weeks after discontinuation of therapy. In one series 46 of 189 patients (24%) had one relapse and of these 46 patients, 21 (46%) had a further relapse (Bartlett 1984). Relapse may therefore be due to failure to eradicate the organism because of sporulation. Relapses are more prone to occur in the elderly and in those who have undergone abdominal surgery (Young et al 1986). Often the relapse is mild and does not require further treatment, but in more severe cases a further course of metronidazole or vancomycin is given. Administration of the yeast *Saccharomyces boulardii* has been reported to reduce the risk of relapsing infection (McFarland et al 1994).

## NEW AND EMERGING GUT PATHOGENS

### *Cyclospora cayetanensis*

In 1988 a previously unidentified organism was found in the stools of 55 immunocompetent foreign visitors in Nepal (Taylor et al 1988). The new organism had characteristics of both *Coccidia* and *Cyanobacteria* species and was associated with a prolonged diarrheal illness with anorexia, fatigue and weight loss. A similar organism was identified in Peruvian children during the same period and a further case-controlled study has confirmed the association between chronic diarrhea and detection of coccidian-like or cyanobacterium-like bodies in the feces (Ortega et al 1993). The organism has been tentatively designated *Cyclospora cayetanensis* and has recently been identified in an intracellular location in the jejunal epithelium of humans (Bendall et al 1993). Exposure to potassium dichromate induces sporulation of fecal sporocysts within 5–13 days, following which complete excystation occurs, liberating two sporozoites. Electronmicroscopy has confirmed that the intracellular organelles are characteristic of coccidian parasites. Infection with *Cyclospora* produces shortening of villi and results in increased numbers of intraepithelial lymphocytes in the small intestine. Diagnosis relies on microscopic identification of the parasite in feces or small intestinal aspirates. Co-trimoxazole in standard doses for 7 days will cure infection in about 95% of cases.

### *Tropheryma whippelii*

Whipple's disease (p. 412) has been recognized to have an infective etiology for more than eight decades. Bacilli have been identified in macrophages and extracellular locations in the intestine but characterization has been impossible because of the inability to culture the organism. Using genetic analysis of the 16S-like ribosomal RNA (rRNA) it has been possible to classify this organism and relate it to other bacterial species since the 16S rRNA sequence mutates and makes it useful as an evolutionary clock. According to this phylogenetic analysis the organism is a Gram-positive actinomycete and is not closely related to any known genus. It has been given the name *Tropheryma whippelii* (Wilson et al 1991, Relman et al 1992). This work is not only of interest because of its contribution to the classification of the Whipple's bacillus but it has inevitably lead to the development of highly specific primers which can be used in a DNA-based polymerase chain reaction assay for detecting the organism in blood and bone marrow. This is an important advance since it may now be possible to screen for this disease without the necessity of obtaining biopsy material from small intestine or brain.

### Toxic phytoplankton

Algal blooms now constitute an important health risk worldwide (Epstein et al 1993). Toxic phytoplankton blooms are associated with paralytic, diarrheal and amnesic shellfish poisoning and with histamine (scromboid), puffer fish and ciguatera fish poisoning. Algal blooms (red, green, gold, brown, bioluminescent) are widely distributed in marine, estuarine and inland waters in the Americas, Japan, south east Asia and Australia. Increase in algal blooms has been attributed to a variety of environmental factors, including a rise in sea temperatures, pollution and overharvesting of fish and shellfish. The seasonality of cholera has been related to coastal algal blooms but this reservoir of cholera vibrios remained undetected until recently. However, a viable nonculturable form of *Vibrio cholerae* has been found associated with certain varieties of surface marine life. Under the conditions which favor algal blooms, *V. cholerae* reverts to its culturable and infectious state. The algal bloom "red-tide" has been associated with the deaths of humpback whales in the Cape Cod area of Massachusetts.

### *Helicobacter pylori*

This important pathogen infects gastric mucosa and causes active chronic gastritis. It is central to the pathogenesis of peptic ulcer disease and is implicated in the etiology of gastric cancer. It is perhaps the commonest bacterial infection of humans with up to half the world's population harboring the organism. Despite its ubiquitous distribution the organism was only recognized in 1983. Although it is common in developed countries, the prevalence of infection is highest in developing countries as infection has been linked to poor standards of hygiene and sanitation. The organism is discussed in detail on p. 227.

## INTESTINAL TUBERCULOSIS

Abdominal tuberculosis has been recognized since the time of Hippocrates. Tuberculosis is one of the most common human infections with estimates of 8 million new infections each year worldwide and an annual mortality approaching 3 million. Abdominal tuberculosis is an important clinical entity in immigrant populations in industralized countries and needs to be clearly distinguished from idiopathic inflammatory bowel disease such as Crohn's disease and intra-abdominal malignancy.

## Etiology

Although *Mycobacterium bovis* has for many years been regarded as the organism responsible for abdominal tuberculosis, the importance of this organism has diminished dramatically; *M. tuberculosis* accounts for more than 90% of cases of abdominal tuberculosis in patients presenting in the developed world. This is largely due to the fact that the majority of dairy herds are tuberculosis free and because milk consumed by humans is now generally pasteurized.

## Epidemiology

Abdominal tuberculosis is found worldwide although prevalence rates are still highest in the developing world. Due to immigration, however, abdominal tuberculosis is increasing in some developed countries (Palmer et al 1985, Schofield 1985, Cook 1985). During the past 10 years there has been an increasing number of cases of abdominal tuberculosis in patients with AIDS (Rosengart & Coppa 1990) (see pp. 605 & 607). In these individuals, the infection is often more severe with complications requiring surgery.

## Pathogenesis

Tubercle bacilli probably infect the abdominal cavity and its organs either directly by being swallowed or by hematogenous spread during a primary pulmonary infection. It is thought that the bacilli cross the epithelium and enter Peyer's patches most commonly in the distal ileum and then spread into mesenteric lymph nodes to cause hyperplasia and subsequent caseation and necrosis. Retrograde spread of bacilli may occur from these lymph nodes to the bowel wall where it is thought that an inflammatory endarteritis leads to transmural inflammation, ulceration and sometimes perforation. Hematogenous spread of bacilli can occur from a primary pulmonary infection, possibly accounting for disseminated peritoneal infection. Mycobacteria do not produce any known classic virulence factors such as toxins, proteolytic enzymes or hemolysins but their pathogenicity appears to rest on their capacity to multiply and survive within macrophages. The presence of bacilli in tissue initiates an inflammatory cellular immune response leading to a local necrotising allergic reaction.

## Clinical features

Abdominal tuberculosis has three major categories of clinical presentation, (i) gastrointestinal disease, (ii) mesenteric lymphadenopathy and (iii) peritonitis.

### *Abdominal disease*

***Ileocecal disease.*** This is found both in the tropics and in immigrants to industrialized countries where it probably accounts for 40–60% of patients with abdominal tuberculosis. Abdominal pain is a prominent feature of infection in this region of the intestinal tract and may be either obstructive in character or localized to the right iliac fossa as a result of transmural focal inflammation. A mass may be palpable and there is often fever, diarrhea and general malaise. Perforation is unusual. Tuberculosis may also involve the anal canal where it produces a painless ulcer sometimes associated with fistula formation and ischiorectal abscess.

***Esophageal and gastroduodenal disease.*** Dysphagia is the most common presentation of esophageal involvement, either as a result of extrinsic compression from enlarged mediastinal lymph nodes or from a mass lesion within the esophagus itself. Discrete tuberculous ulcers occur in the esophagus which can penetrate to produce a bronchoesophageal fistula. Ulceration in the stomach and duodenum may occur and be indistinguishable from typical peptic ulcers. An inflammatory mass in the prepyloric region may mimic Crohn's disease or neoplasia.

***Mesenteric lymphadenopathy.*** This is the most common variety of tuberculosis found in the tropics and may be associated with lymphadenopathy in other locations although a pulmonary lesion is notable by its absence. The illness begins insidiously with weight loss, intermittent low-grade fever and general malaise. As the disease progresses, abdominal swelling occurs as a result of ascites and massive lymph node enlargement. Anemia, hypoalbuminemia and peripheral edema become apparent as the disease progresses. Massive caseation of mesenteric lymph nodes occurs and the major complication of this form of abdominal tuberculosis is node rupture with dissemination of bacilli throughout the abdominal cavity.

***Peritonitis.*** This appears to be a common presentation of disease in immigrants from developing countries. Onset is usually insidious over several months (Bastani et al 1985). Symptoms include fever, weight loss, anorexia and lethargy. In the "wet" form of the disease there is progressive ascites (straw colored) and the peritoneal surface of the bowel and omentum is covered with fine white tubercles. In the more advanced "dry" form, bowel loops and omentum are matted together and give rise to abdominal pain and tenderness, moderate distention, a mass in approximately 25% and a doughy feel to the abdomen. Such patients occasionally present with obstructive features secondary to tuberculous adhesions. Peritonitis may begin abruptly following bowel perforation or massive rupture of caseating abdominal lymph nodes but is most commonly due to reactivation of latent peritoneal disease following hematogenous spread from a primary focus.

*Diagnosis*

In all cases of suspected abdominal tuberculosis attempts should be made to achieve a microbiological diagnosis by the identification of *M. tuberculosis* or *M. bovis* in tissue or secretions or by the identification of caseating granulomas in tissues. In gastrointestinal tuberculosis, tissue may be obtained at endoscopy which should then be submitted to histopathological examination and microbiological culture (Morgante et al 1989). The macroscopic appearances of intestinal disease either at endoscopy or by contrast radiology are generally not diagnostic although the combination of ulceration and stricturing of the terminal ileum, obliteration of the ileocecal angle and shortening of the ascending colon and cecum are highly suggestive (Fig. 20.2). Tissue diagnosis can be obtained in mesenteric lymphadenopathy by guided biopsy or lymph node aspiration. If this is technically impossible or considered hazardous, laparotomy may be required, particularly if there is concern about the possibility of lymphoma. In tuberculous peritonitis, ascites if present should be removed and examined microscopically and submitted to microbiological culture. Peritoneal fluid has a relatively high protein content (greater than 2.5 g/100 ml) (p. 1021) and characteristically has a high lymphocyte count. Acid-fast bacilli are only seen occasionally. Sometimes peritoneal biopsy can provide the diagnosis although laparoscopy may be required to enable peritoneal tubercles to be directly visualized and biopsied.

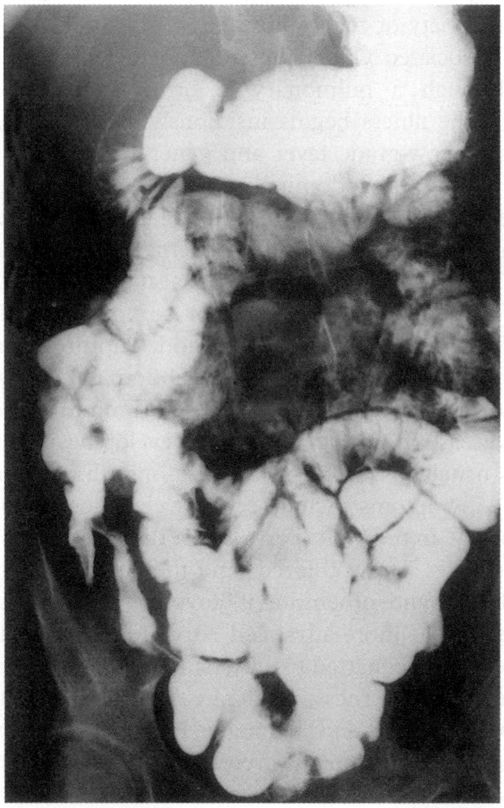

**Fig. 20.2** Barium follow-through examinations showing ileocecal tuberculosis.

*Treatment*

It is currently recommended that extrapulmonary tuberculosis should be treated with triple therapy, namely, isoniazid and rifampicin for 6 months with pyrazinamide included for the first 2 months (Ormerod 1990). A fourth drug such as streptomycin or ethambutol should be added initially if drug resistance is suspected, particularly in patients who may have imported the disease from a developing country. Major adverse reactions are not common but liver biochemistry should be assessed before treatment starts.

## VIRAL GASTROENTERITIS

It is only during the past 20 years that some of the causes of viral gastroenteritis have been identified and the clinical features that distinguish them described. Although there are a number of viruses that can be isolated from the gastrointestinal tract, only four major groups are recognized to cause gastroenteritis in humans: rotavirus, enteritic adenovirus, calicivirus and astrovirus (Cukor & Blacklow 1984). All of these infections are relatively mild and self-limiting and as yet there is no specific therapy or widely available vaccine. *Cytomegalovirus* is discussed on p. 600.

### Rotaviruses

This is the most common cause of gastroenteritis in infants and young children worldwide (Fig. 20.3). The vast majority of children in both the industrialized and developing worlds are infected either clinically or sub-clinically during the pre-school years, which probably accounts for the reason why clinical illness is rare in adults (Haffejee 1991).

The rotavirus genome contains 11 segments of double-stranded RNA, each of which encodes a single protein. The two major surface proteins, VP4 and VP7, are the major determinants of protective antibody-mediated immunity. Rotaviruses are classified serologically into groups A–G, although only A, B and C have been found in humans and animals. Rotavirus group A is the predominant cause of severe gastroenteritis in children. Rotavirus has a distinct seasonal pattern with peak prevalence occurring in the winter months. The incubation period is between 2–4 days and there is a wide spectrum of disease ranging from subclinical infection to severe dehydrating diarrheal disease with acidosis. In addition to diarrhea there may be fever and marked vomiting, usually early in the illness. Infection is self-limited with recovery usually occurring within a few days although occasionally symp-

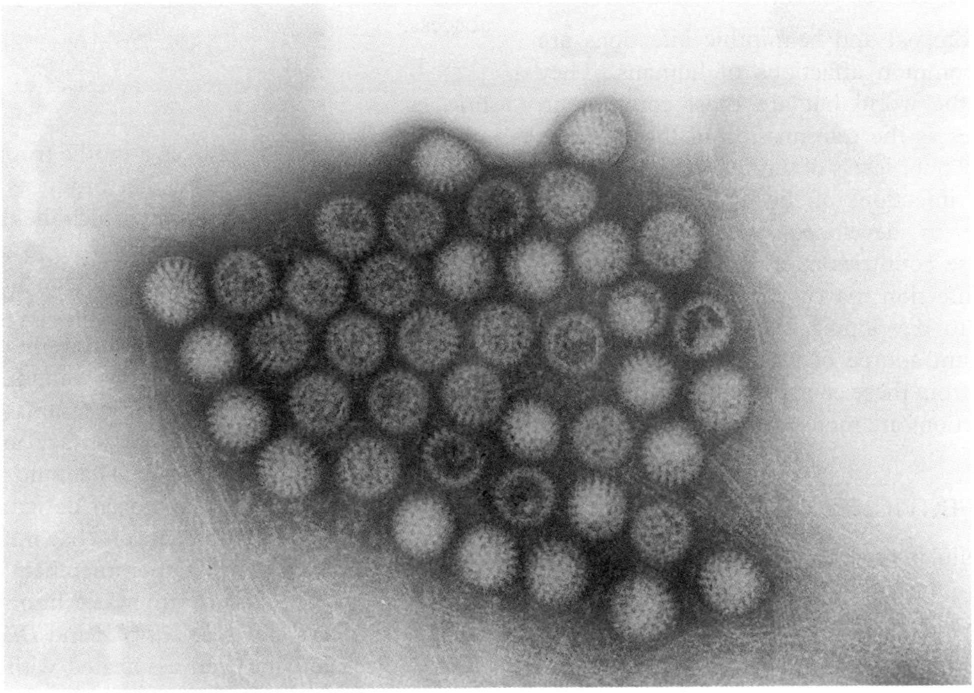

**Fig. 20.3** Electronmicrograph showing rotavirus particles (× 180 000).

toms may persist for up to 2 weeks. Treatment is supportive with replacement of fluid and electrolyte losses by oral rehydration therapy being of most importance. Live oral rotavirus vaccines have been developed and submitted to field trials. A bovine rotavirus has been shown to protect infants and young children in the industrialized world but results have been disappointing in developing countries. Other approaches using rhesus rotaviruses, human-rhesus rotavirus reassortants and the relatively avirulent neonatal rotavirus strains are currently under evaluation. It seems likely that an oral live rotavirus vaccine will be widely available within the next 5 years.

A recent study using probiotics (harmless commensal bacteria) in formula milk has been shown to protect infants from rotavirus infection and reduce the severity of disease in those infected. This may be a reasonable alternative approach to prevention but further clinical studies are required to confirm these preliminary observations.

### Enteric adenoviruses types 40 and 41

Adenoviruses are DNA viruses and are the second most common cause of viral gastroenteritis in infants and young children (Uhnoo et al 1984, Richmond et al 1988). The clinical features are similar to rotavirus although the incubation period is longer at 8–10 days and like rotavirus, transmission is by the fecal–oral route. While the diarrheal illness may be of greater duration than rotavirus infection, lasting up to 12 days, dehydration is usually less severe. Unlike rotavirus there is no obvious seasonality in infection.

### Caliciviruses

Norwalk and the Norwalk-like family viruses tend to affect older children and adults (Kapikian et al 1972). Caliciviruses are small, round structured RNA viruses containing a single structural protein. Infection classically occurs in outbreaks of diarrhea in families, schools, on cruise ships and in other closed communities (Iversen et al 1987, Reid et al 1988). Epidemics are characterized by the extremely high secondary attack rate. The virus is spread by the fecal–oral route with a short incubation period of 12–48 h. The illness tends to be mild and of short duration with diarrhea and vomiting being the predominant features. Associated symptoms may include fever, myalgia and headaches.

### Astroviruses

Astroviruses are single-stranded RNA viruses with a stellate configuration apparent on electronmicroscopy. Five human serotypes have been identified. Astrovirus predominantly affects infants and preschool children and has been associated with outbreaks in residential institutions. The incubation period is 24–36 h but the illness is generally of short duration, lasting up to 4 days. Infection rates, as with rotavirus, are greatest during the winter months. Diarrhea is the predominant symptom although vomiting and fever occur in approximately 30% of patients. Recovery occurs without any specific therapeutic interventions although supportive therapy with oral rehydration solutions may be required if dehydration is a problem.

## PARASITIC INFECTIONS

Gastrointestinal protozoal and helminthic infections are among the most common afflictions of humans. They occur throughout the world but are most common in developing countries as the transmission of these organisms is facilitated by poor levels of sanitation and hygiene. However, parasitic infections of the gut do occur with varying prevalence in developed countries (Farthing et al 1993). In these countries many parasitic infections are endemic and infection may occur sporadically or in outbreaks. Travel to developing and tropical countries remains an important source of imported parasitic diseases and migrants from these countries are another group in whom these infections are more commonly seen.

## PROTOZOAL INFECTIONS

Protozoa are unicellular organisms that can multiply in their hosts and are found in blood and tissue as well as the gastrointestinal tract (Table 20.4). Amebiasis, giardiasis and cryptosporidiosis are the commonest gastrointestinal protozoal infections. Uncommon infections occur with *Balantidium coli* and *Coccidia* and occasionally disease is associated with species that are usually nonpathogenic. Although more common in tropical countries, protozoa are cosmopolitan organisms that are found worldwide (Katelaris 1992). They have an increased prevalence in particular high-risk groups including children, residents of institutions, the immunocompromised, travelers, homosexuals and wherever personal hygiene is poor. The increasing incidence of HIV infection has been associated with particular gut protozoal infections which are often manifest as severe and chronic diarrhea.

### Amebiasis

Amebiasis is one of the most important parasitic diseases of the gastrointestinal tract, affecting approximately 480 million individuals. The majority are asymptomatic carriers with the organism existing in the intestine as a commensal. Approximately 10% develop clinical disease in the colon with a relatively smaller proportion suffering extraintestinal manifestations such as hepatitis and liver abscess.

**Table 20.4** Intestinal protozoal infections

| **Pathogenic** | **Nonpathogenic** |
|---|---|
| *Entamoeba histolytica* | *Entamoeba dispar* |
| *Giardia intestinalis* | *Entamoeba coli* |
| *Cryptosporidium parvum* | *Entamoeba hartmani* |
| *Isospora belli* | *Entamoeba polecki* |
| *Sarcocystis* spp. | *Endolimax nana* |
| *Balantidium coli* | *Iodamoeba butschlii* |
| *Blastocystis hominis* | |
| *Dientamoeba fragilis* | |
| *Microsporidium* spp. | |
| *Cyclospora cayetariensis* | |

#### *Etiology*

*Entamoeba histolytica* exists as a motile trophozoite, which is the form of the organism that produces intestinal and hepatic disease, and as a cyst by which the disease is transmitted and which enables the parasite to survive outside the human host. It is now accepted that there are distinct strains of *E. histolytica*. Pathogenic strains are responsible for human disease while nonpathogenic strains reside within the colon but are noninvasive and not associated with clinical disease states. These strains can be distinguished by isoenzyme analysis, surface antigen profiles and DNA analysis (Clark & Diamond 1991). Nonpathogenic *E. histolytica* have been designated *E. dispar*. Other species of nonpathogenic amebae include *E. coli*, *E. hartmani* and *E. polecki*. Other members of the family Entamoebidae are known to infect humans. Of these, *Endolimax nana*, *Iodamoeba butschlii* and *Dientamoeba fragilis* have occasionally been associated with diarrheal disease and colitis.

#### *Epidemiology*

It is estimated that 12% of the world's population are infected with *E. histolytica* resulting in an annual mortality of 40 000–110 000 individuals. Prevalence varies widely from about 1% in industrialized countries to 50–80% in certain areas in the tropics. *E. histolytica* is also commonly found in homosexual men although this is almost invariably with nonpathogenic strains. AIDS patients do not have an increased risk of severe infections.

Infection is transmitted by the fecal–oral route with food and drink being the major vehicles. Infection is also spread by person-to-person contact with asymptomatic cyst carriers being the main reservoir of infection. Epidemics occur when raw sewage contaminates water supplies. Infection may also be transmitted during sexual contact.

#### *Pathogenesis and pathology*

*E. histolytica* produces dysentery by destruction of the intestinal epithelium with subsequent ulceration and inflammation (Fig. 20.4). The cellular and molecular mechanisms involved in this process are beginning to be characterized. Several virulence factors have been identified including adhesion molecules, toxins, contact-dependent cytolysis, proteases and phagocytic activity (Ravdin 1990). Following excystation in the large intestine, *E. histolytica* trophozoites adhere to the surface epithelium via a surface membrane galactose-binding lectin (Petri et al 1987). This lectin is a 260 kDa heterodimeric glycoprotein which consists of 170 and 35 kDa

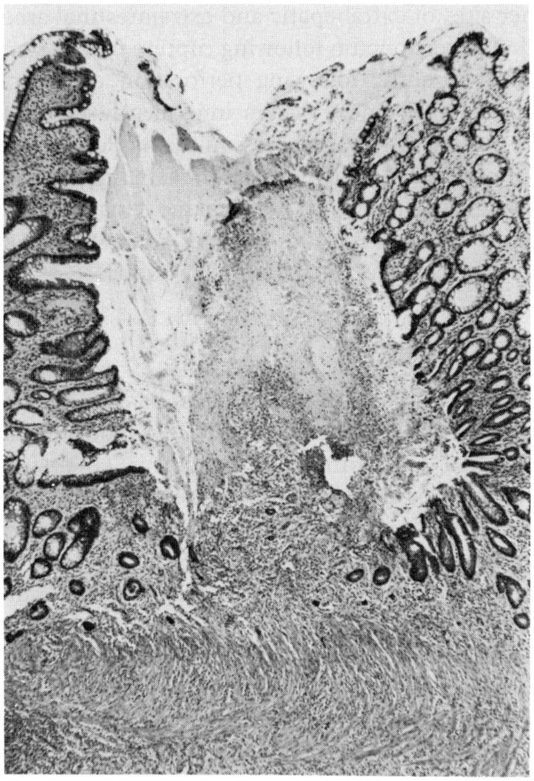

**Fig. 20.4** An amebic ulcer in the colon. The ulcer is superficial and appears cup-shaped owing to the shouldering of the adjacent mucosa.

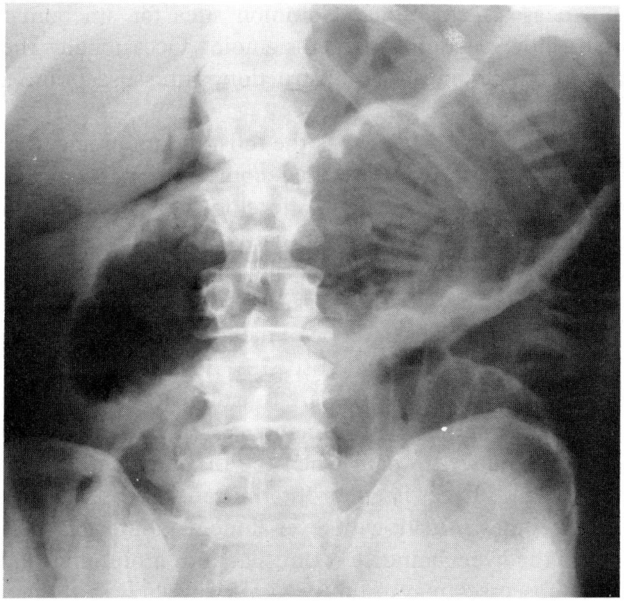

**Fig. 20.5** Dilatation of the colon in fulminating amebic colitis.

subunits. This galactose-specific lectin mediates adherence of amebae to human colonic mucus and epithelial cells.

Following contact with the host epithelial cell, cytolysis of the colonocyte occurs rapidly. Cytolysis is dependent on parasite microfilament function and on phospholipase A enzyme activity. Cytolysis is calcium dependent which relates at least in part to its interaction with phospholipase A. Although target cell death is associated with a substantial rise in intracellular calcium, amebic calcium does not appear to be a second messenger for amebic cytolysis. However, *E. histolytica* does contain a pore-forming peptide of 4–5 kDa known as amebapore. This protein is capable of forming pores in artificial lipid bilayers and target cell membranes and has recently been purified. The N-terminal amino acid sequence has marked structural similarities to melittin, the membranolytic polypeptide of bee venom. It is thought that this protein forms ion-channel pores spanning the membrane of the target cell which leads to ion disequilibrium across the cell membrane. Proteolytic and hydrolytic enzymes are also released at this time which may facilitate the invasion process. *E. histolytica* is able to phagocytose dead or dying cells, allowing deeper penetration into the intestinal wall.

Amebae probably spread from the intestine to the liver through the portal circulation. In the early stages of hepatic amebic invasion, intrahepatic trophozoites produce foci of neutrophil accumulation which is followed by necrosis and granulomatous infiltration. The size of the granulomas gradually increases and finally the lesions coalesce to produce necrotic lesions which eventually develop into abscesses.

*Clinical features*

Amebiasis may present as a variety of clinical syndromes including: (i) asymptomatic infection, (ii) intestinal amebiasis, (iii) amebic liver abscess, and (iv) extrahepatic and extraintestinal amebiasis.

***Asymptomatic infection*** is the most common clinical situation, accounting for at least 80–90% of infections. In carriers the parasite remains within the gut lumen without invasion. *E. histolytica* isolates from asymptomatic individuals differ genetically from those that produce invasive disease.

***Intestinal amebiasis*** usually has an insidious onset and is characterized by abdominal discomfort, bloody diarrhea and tenesmus (Lewis & Antia 1969). The colitis may be fulminant with toxemia and colonic dilatation (Fig. 20.5). This form of the disease is more prevalent in pregnancy, in the puerperium and in undernourished infants and young children. Complications include intestinal perforation with amebic peritonitis or localized perforation with a paracolic abscess. Chronic intestinal amebiasis also has an insidious onset with intermittent rather than continuous symptoms. It is often associated with headache, anorexia, nausea and low-grade fever. Complications include stricture formation in the colon or the development of an annular mass of granulation tissue, known as an ameboma. Common sites for amebomata include the cecum and rectosigmoid. Occasionally they may produce intestinal obstruction, intussusception or severe hemorrhage.

***Amebic liver abscess*** is the most common and clinically significant extraintestinal complication of amebic infection. Liver abscess may develop within days of the onset of amebic colitis, but in half of the cases of amebic liver abscess there is no clear clinical history of intestinal disease. Liver abscesses are usually single and most commonly found in the right lobe of the liver. In advanced disease, however, multiple abscesses do occur. In acute fulminant amebic abscess there is usually localized pain in the right upper quadrant, sometimes associated with pleuritic or shoulder-tip pain when the diaphragmatic pleura are involved. Fever is either intermittent or absent. Deep abscesses may present with fever alone without signs referable to the liver. Jaundice is unusual and, if present, mild. Large abscesses may produce visible swelling in the epigastrium or between the intercostal spaces. The liver is usually enlarged and tender. Chronic amebic abscess may be present for months or even years; the abscess is usually large, single and located in the right lobe. Evidence of liver abscess may be present on a chest radiograph (raised right hemidiaphragm, pleural effusion, right basal pneumonia), but diagnosis is usually confirmed by abdominal ultrasound or CT scan. "Acute amebic hepatitis" is an outmoded concept that should be discarded. The liver remote from an amebic abscess is histologically normal and there is therefore no evidence for a diffuse process occurring in the liver in amebic infection.

Other sites of extrahepatic and extraintestinal amebiasis include the peritoneum following rupture of a liver abscess or, less frequently, following perforation of the cecum. Pericardial involvement occurs infrequently but generally follows perforation of an abscess in the left lobe of the liver into the pericardial cavity. Similarly, there may be spread of disease into the pleura or lung parenchyma. Occasionally amebiasis can spread to the brain or genitourinary system and may even develop in abdominal wounds.

### *Diagnosis*

*E. histolytica* trophozoites or cysts can be demonstrated by light microscopy in feces. *E. histolytica* trophozoites can be distinguished from other nonpathogenic amebae as the former are erythrophagic or contain red blood cells. Multiple stool specimens may be required to confirm the diagnosis. Fecal specimens need to be taken rapidly to the laboratory and examined with a saline wet mount on a heated microscope stage, as trophozoites rapidly die and disintegrate once they leave the host. Fecal leukocytes are usually absent in amebic colitis, which helps distinguish it from bacterial dysentery. Sigmoidoscopy may reveal small, shallow amebic ulcers with undermined edges covered with yellow exudate. The intervening mucosa is usually normal. Mucosal exudate from ulcers may show the presence of trophozoites. Rectal mucosal biopsy from the edge of an ulcer may also reveal trophozoites together with associated inflammatory changes (Fig. 20.6). Fecal antigen ELISA is being developed as an alternative approach to diagnosis. Specific anti-*E. histolytica* antibodies can be

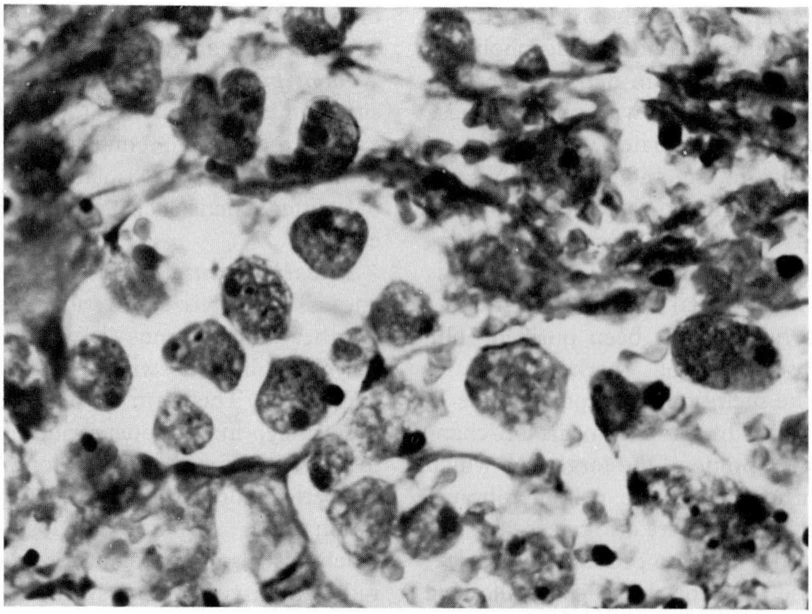

**Fig. 20.6** Irregularly rounded *Entamoeba histolytica* with single dark nuclei and foamy cytoplasm in which an occasional erythrocyte can be seen (hemotoxylin and eosin, × 700).

**Table 20.5** Drug therapy for amebiasis

| Drug | Adult dose |
|---|---|
| **Intestinal infection/ liver abscess** | |
| Metronidazole followed by | 750–800 mg three times daily for 10 days |
| Diloxanide furoate | 500 mg three times daily for 10 days |
| **Asymptomatic carrier** | |
| Diloxanide furoate or | 500 mg three times daily for 10 days |
| Paramomycin | 25–30 mg/kg in three doses, for 7–10 days |

detected in serum in more than 90% of patients with amebic liver abscess and 70–80% of patients with amebic colitis (Arvind et al 1988).

*Treatment*

Medical treatment for intestinal and hepatic amebiasis is summarized in Table 20.5. Surgery should rarely be required providing antimicrobial chemotherapy is started promptly. However, certain complications will require surgical management including toxic dilatation, perforation, severe hemorrhage and colonic strictures. In acute severe colitis, subtotal colectomy and ileostomy is the procedure of choice. Aspiration of liver abscess may sometimes be necessary but is usually reserved for large abscesses in the left lobe of the liver in which there is concern about rupture into the pericardium, pleura or peritoneal cavity.

## Giardiasis

*Giardia* is the commonest gut protozoan infection of humans. The World Health Organization lists it among the top 10 parasitic diseases with more than 200 million new cases estimated to occur annually, a number that would appear to be a gross underestimate.

*Etiology*

*Giardia intestinalis* is ingested in the cyst form and excysts in the upper small intestine. The motile trophozoites (Fig. 20.7) are pear-shaped, 15 μm in length and 4 μm wide and contain a pair of nuclei situated anteriorly and four pairs of flagella. On the ventral surface is a "sucker" disk which is important for attachment to the small intestinal mucosa. Cysts are shed in the stool and may remain viable for many months on the surface of cool water. Infection may occur by the fecal–oral route, by waterborne transmission or as a zoonosis.

*Epidemiology*

Infection occurs worldwide, in tropical, temperate and arctic regions and affects children as well as adults. The frequency of infection is highest in developing countries in association with poor standards of hygiene and sanitation. In these situations the prevalence has been reported to be between 20–50%, with infection being ubiquitous in young children (Miotti et al 1986).

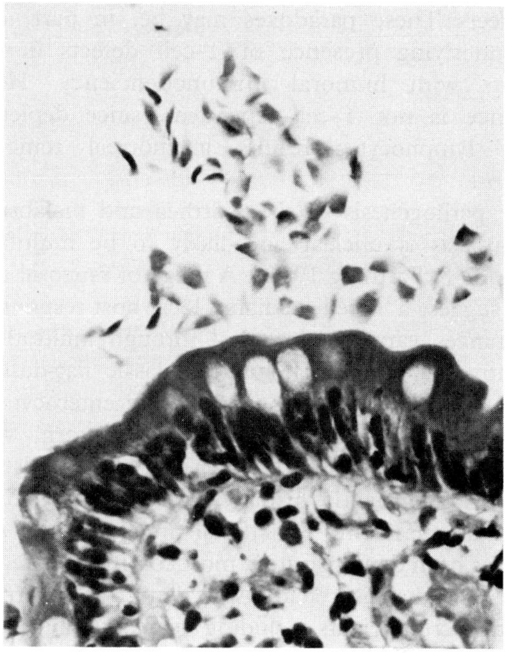

**Fig. 20.7** Biopsy of the small intestine showing numerous *Giardia intestinalis* seen in profile and en face above the epithelium, (hemotoxylin and eosin, × 700).

In developed countries, the prevalence in the general population varies between 2% and 12% (Boreham & Phillips 1986) with a peak in preschool children, particularly those in childcare facilities in whom very high rates of infection (>20%) have been documented (Pickering & Engelkirk 1990). In developed countries several high-risk groups have been identified. These include travelers, male homosexuals and the immunocompromised, particularly those with hypogammaglobulinemia (Hartong et al 1979). Giardiasis occurs in HIV-infected subjects but not with the greatly enhanced frequency of some other infections.

*Pathogenesis and pathology*

Humoral and cell-mediated responses both appear necessary for the adequate clearance of *Giardia*. Patients with variable combined immunodeficiency are prone to giardiasis, whereas those with primary immunodeficiency (antibody) syndromes are not. Furthermore, giardiasis is not a complication of selective IgA deficiency, suggesting that control of infection is taken over by other compensatory mechanisms, probably local IgM production. Infection leads to systemic IgG, IgA and IgM responses and local IgA is produced following deliberate infection in human volunteers These paradoxes may be, in part, due to the underlying presence of T-cell defects in certain patients with humoral immunodeficiency. However clearance is not T-cell-dependent, since depletion of $CD8^+$ lymphocytes results in normal removal of *G. muris*.

The pathogenesis of the diarrhea and malabsorption in giardiasis is unclear and likely to be multifactorial (Katelaris & Farthing 1992). A range of mucosal appearances suggest a T-cell-mediated local host response. The appearances vary from normal through infiltrative and infiltrative-hyperplastic lesions to classic flat-destructive lesions with flattened, cuboidal surface enterocytes. The commonest lesion is the infiltrative pattern, while a preinfiltrative (high antibody titer only) state is also likely. Mucosal abnormalities usually recover quickly following successful treatment. Functional impairment of enterocytes has been demonstrated, most commonly a reduction of brush border disaccharidase activity. Malabsorption of fat and micronutrients including folate, vitamin $B_{12}$, vitamin A and carotene may occur. As the morphological abnormalities are often minor and not invariably present despite diarrhea and malabsorption it has been suggested that derangements to luminal components of digestion may also be important. Possible mechanisms include consumption of bile acids by *Giardia*, inhibition of pancreatic lipase and proteolytic enzymes (Katelaris et al 1991) and increased intestinal transit.

**Table 20.6** Symptoms in acute and chronic giardiasis

| Clinical features | Acute giardiasis* (%) | Chronic giardiasis* (%) |
|---|---|---|
| Diarrhea | 96 | 62.9 |
| Weakness/ fatigue | 72 | 28.6 |
| Weight loss | 62 | 18.1 |
| Abdominal pain | 61 | 32.4 |
| Nausea/anorexia | 60 | 40.0 |
| Steatorrhea | 57 | 52.9 |
| Flatulence | 35 | 46.7 |
| Vomiting | 29 | 4.8 |
| Fever | 17 | 3.8 |

*Data derived from 324 subjects with acute giardiasis (Moore et al 1969) and 105 subjects with chronic giardiasis of undetermined duration (Wolfe 1990).

### *Clinical features*

Infection with *Giardia* results in a variable and broad clinical spectrum ranging from asymptomatic cyst passage (probably most cases) to acute or chronic diarrhea with malabsorption. The incubation period is typically 1 week but may range from 1 to 45 days. Acute giardiasis may result in a wide variety of symptoms (Moore et al 1969). Nonspecific constitutional and upper abdominal symptoms may precede or accompany the onset of diarrhea (Table 20.6). These commonly include nausea, anorexia, dyspepsia, malaise and sometimes low-grade fever. Distasteful belching often occurs ("sulfur burps"). Occasionally the upper abdominal symptoms may mimic peptic ulcer disease. There is often a sudden onset of diarrhea which may be explosive and watery but more often comprises loose, foul-smelling, bulky stools associated with flatulence, abdominal distention, borborygmi and cramps.

Chronic giardiasis is characterized by ongoing diarrhea with evidence of malabsorption of fat, carbohydrate and micronutrients (Hartong et al 1979, Wolfe 1990). Anorexia and steatorrhea may cause significant weight loss. Typical symptoms of chronic giardiasis are shown in Table 20.6. Other occasional findings are $B_{12}$ malabsorption or folate deficiency, protein-losing enteropathy (Korman et al 1990) or severe hypokalemia with secondary myopathy. Rarely there may be eosinophilia, urticaria, uveitis, arthropathy or coughing: in some volunteer infections, fever seems to be associated with elevations of hepatic transaminase levels while cholangitis with granulomas has also been recorded. Further symptoms after recovery may represent recrudescence, reinfection or postinfectious irritable bowel. Some persistent symptoms may be due to secondary lactase deficiency.

Acute giardiasis may not be distinguishable from other acute infections but is suggested by a typical history. The presence of blood or mucus in the stool or a high fever strongly suggests a different diagnosis. Chronic giardiasis must be distinguished from other chronic intestinal infections including amebiasis, cryptosporidiosis, isosporiasis or strongyloidiasis. Tropical sprue and tropical enteropathy must also be considered along with noninfectious disorders of the gut including inflammatory bowel disease, celiac disease and irritable bowel syndrome.

### *Diagnosis*

Investigations are necessary for a definitive diagnosis. However, when symptoms are typical, it is sometimes justifiable to treat empirically with an appropriate agent and reserve investigations for when this approach is not successful. Diagnosis is usually made by identification of cysts in stool by light microscopic examination of an iodine-stained wet preparation or a concentrated specimen. The sensitivity of light microscopy is operator dependent. A single wet smear examination may diagnose only 30–70% of cases. As cysts and trophozoites are shed erratically, it may be necessary to examine up to three stools on separate occasions. In experienced hands this raises the diagnostic sensitivity to more than 90%. When stool microscopy is negative, *Giardia* may be identified histologically by examination of a jejunal biopsy taken with a Crosby capsule or, more conveniently, from an endoscopic distal duodenal biopsy (Fig. 20.7). Duodenal fluid may be aspirated and concentrated for direct microscopic examination for trophozoites. A mucosal biopsy may also be examined by a smear impression technique. The string test (Enterotest) involves swallowing a gelatine capsule on a string and sampling duodenal fluid for examination in this way but it has a low sensitivity. Diagnosis by stool or duodenal examination should be considered complementary rather than competing methods, as one test may be positive while the other is negative (Goka et al 1990a). Immunofluorescent and ELISA methods for stool diagnosis are available but not widely used routinely. Serological tests have also been employed but are neither sensitive nor specific enough for diagnosis of acute infection in individual patients. Hematological and other tests may document the presence and degree of malabsorption but are not helpful diagnostically. Eosinophilia is rare.

*Treatment*

The nitroimidazoles, metronidazole (400 mg three times daily for 5 days or 2 g daily for 3 days) or tinidazole (2 g as a single dose) are the drugs of choice with a cure rate of 90% or better (Jokipii & Jokipii 1990). Side-effects include nausea and vomiting, metallic taste and a disulfiram-like effect with alcohol. An alternative drug is furazolidone, a nitrofuran. This is used in children but the dosage regimen is lengthy and cumbersome (100 mg four times daily for 7–10 days) and may also cause nausea and vomiting. Mepacrine (100 mg three times daily for 7 days) is commonly used in the USA but this agent may cause yellowing of the skin, is poorly tolerated by children and has potentially serious side-effects, including exfoliative dermatitis, blood dyscrasias and toxic psychosis. Albendazole, a benzimidazole which is widely used for helminthiasis, is being evaluated for use in giardiasis.

Treatment failure occurs for a variety of reasons including patient noncompliance or intolerance. Nitroimidazole resistance is not a major problem. Treatment failures most often occur in compromised hosts where host defenses do not aid clearance of the organism. Several strategies for the management of first-line treatment failures may be tried. Initially, after metronidazole or tinidazole failure, treatment may be repeated for longer, the other nitroimidazole substituted or furazolidone or mepacrine substituted. Combinations of different agents may be tried simultaneously or serially.

In children with diarrhea malnutrition, giardiasis is very common and may be facilitated by the high prevalence rates for *Helicobacter pylori*-induced gastritis hypochlorhydria, in addition to depressed immune responsiveness and generalized T-cell anergy. In these circumstances, eradication of the parasite is more difficult and requires a multipronged attack comprising improving caloric intake, nutritional replacement and use of antibiotics to eradicate the *H. pylori* infection.

*Prognosis and prevention*

Acute giardiasis often resolves spontaneously. In adults it is usually a mild to moderately severe illness but in children chronic infection or repeated reinfection may contribute to failure to thrive. In patients with hypogammaglobulinemia giardiasis may be severe and protracted. *Giardia* is widely distributed geographically and it is unlikely that the organism will ever be eliminated either from the environment or from human or animal reservoirs. Strenuous public health measures are clearly required to ensure that water supplies are *Giardia* free. Similarly, attention to personal hygiene should minimize person-to-person transmission, particularly in high-risk situations such as daycare centers and residential institutions.

## Enteric coccidial infections

*Coccidia* parasitizing the human intestine are recognized as important causes of chronic diarrhea in immunocompromised patients but they also cause disease in immunocompetent individuals. They are characterized by a sexual cycle of reproduction that occurs within epithelial cells of the small intestine that leads to the excretion of oocysts in the feces.

## Cryptosporidiosis

*Etiology and epidemiology*

Human infection is due to C. parvum and is well recognized as a cause of acute self-limiting diarrhea in healthy individuals, especially young children, and of a debilitating chronic diarrhea in immunodeficient patients, particularly those with AIDS (p. 609). Infection occurs in both developed and developing countries. Transmission may be sporadic, by person-to-person spread or in association with travel or animal contact, such as with cattle or domestic pets (Wolfson et al 1985, Public Health Laboratory Service Study 1990). Food and waterborne outbreaks also occur.

*Cryptosporidium* infection is initiated by ingestion of oocysts. Sporozoites localize onto the microvillus membrane of the small intestine and become intracellular, but extracytoplasmic, lying just beneath the enterocyte luminal membrane. Here they develop through either asexual or sexual stages to produce new oocysts which may release sporozoites to maintain the infection or sporulate to be excreted in an infective form. *Cryptosporidia* do not destroy host cells but blunting of villi, loss of microvilli and an inflammatory response are seen in small bowel biopsies in immunocompetent patients. However, the precise mechanism involved in the pathogenesis of diarrhea is still unclear.

*Clinical features*

The symptoms of cryptosporidiosis are variable and cannot be distinguished from those caused by other enteropathogens, particularly Giardia intestinalis. Typically, in immunocompetent patients the incubation period is about a week (5–14 days) followed by the onset of diarrhea. This is usually profuse, offensive, watery or mucoid and lasts 1–2 weeks before resolving spontaneously. Anorexia, nausea and vomiting and cramping abdominal pain are common and a low-grade fever may be present (Table 20.7). In children especially, excessive fluid losses may lead to dehydration. Some patients may excrete infective oocysts for up to 2 months after clinical resolution. A carrier state has been described although most cases are probably symptomatic. While in most immunocompetent subjects infection is self-limiting, prolonged symptoms may occur in a few. In contrast to this, in immunodeficient patients, particularly those with AIDS, Cryptosporidium infection is often a catastrophic debilitating chronic illness associated with copious cholera-like fluid losses which contributes to cachexia and death in many cases (p. 609).

*Diagnosis*

Although the clinical features may be suggestive, they are nonspecific and Cryptosporidium must be considered in the appropriate clinical context. The diagnosis is most readily made by identification of oocysts in fecal samples but needs to be specifically sought as routine stains used for other parasites are not useful. An Auramine stain or a modified Ziehl–Neelsen staining method on direct smears or formalin-ether concentrations is most routinely used (Casemore et al 1984). In experienced hands the diagnosis can be made on a single specimen in nearly all cases but as stools from infected subjects may occasionally be intermittently negative, further samples may be necessary. A stool immunofluorescence test is also available though not widely used. Diagnosis may also be made from histological examination of intestinal mucosal biopsies. Since the advent of reliable methods of diagnosis by stool examination this method is seldom required. Serodiagnostic methods using either immunofluorescence or ELISA methods are available but not in general use.

**Table 20.7** Clinical features of cryptosporidiosis in immunocompetent patients

| | Fayer & Ungar 1986 (n=586) (%) | Public Health Laboratory Service Study 1990 (n=62 421) (%) |
|---|---|---|
| Diarrhea | 92 | 98 |
| Abdominal pain | 45 | 60 |
| Anorexia | nr | 51 |
| Nausea | 51 | 35 |
| Vomiting | 51 | 49 |
| Low-grade fever | 63 | 36 |

nr=not reported

*Treatment and prevention*

In most immunocompetent patients the illness is self-limiting and treatment is supportive. Oral and occasionally parenteral rehydration therapy may be required when fluid losses are marked, especially in young children with severe diarrhea. In immunodeficient subjects, unless the source of immunosuppression can be removed, the infection is often life-threatening with dehydration and cachexia despite intensive parenteral fluid replacement and nutritional support. No antimicrobial agent of the many tested has been shown to be an effective or specific treatment for cryptosporidiosis. The macrolide antibiotic spiramycin did show some initial promise which does not seem to have been fulfilled.

No specific prophylactic therapy is available for *Cryptosporidium* and the usual care with food, water and personal hygiene is prudent advice for the traveler. Unfortunately, oocysts may be found in "clean" water supplies as standard chlorination is ineffective and filtration unreliable (Smith 1990). Oocytes, however, are unable to survive heating for 30 min to temperatures above 65°C (Tzipori 1983).

## Isosporiasis

Oocytes of *Isospora belli* are ingested with fecally contaminated food. Asexual and sexual reproduction occurs within enterocytes and unsporulated oocysts are shed in the stool. Autoinfection may occur as oocysts are also capable of sporulation within the gut. It appears very uncommon in healthy subjects in developed countries, although it may be underdiagnosed. It occasionally infects travelers but is more commonly recognized to infect AIDS patients (p. 609). *Isospora* may damage enterocytes resulting in diarrhea and malabsorption. Morphological damage to the small intestine ranges from mild to subtotal villous atrophy in association with an inflammatory infiltrate. Unlike most protozoal infections there may be an eosinophilia. In healthy hosts, infection is usually acute and self-limiting with fever and abdominal pain in association with diarrhea. Occasionally it causes a chronic illness which may persist for years associated with malabsorption and weight loss. In AIDS patients the profuse watery diarrhea is often severe and protracted and accompanied by wasting. Diagnosis is usually made by identifying oocysts using an acid-fast staining technique on a stool sample or duodenal aspirate. Parasites may also be identified on small intestinal biopsies. Co-trimoxazole (TMP/SMX 160 mg/800 mg four times daily for 10 days) has demonstrated efficacy. Pyrimethamine is a useful alternative treatment where there is sulfur allergy. Therapy may need to be maintained in AIDS patients to prevent relapses. Sulfadoxine/pyrimethamine 500 mg/25 mg once weekly or TMP/SMX 160 mg/800 mg three times weekly are effective for ongoing prophylaxis (Pape et al 1989).

### *Sarcocystis* spp.

Unlike *I. belli* which appears specific for man, this coccidian alternates between intermediate hosts, such as pigs and cattle, and a definitive primate host. Infection occurs following ingestion of cysts in contaminated undercooked beef or pork. Epidemiological data regarding this organism are sparse but a 2% prevalence in diagnostic stool samples has been reported from a hospital for tropical diseases in Paris (Deluol et al 1980). *Sarcocystis*, like *Isospora*, is an intracellular parasite and may cause mucosal morphological damage including a segmental eosinophilic necrotizing enteritis (Bunyaratvej et al 1982). Symptoms may occur hours to days following infection with nausea, abdominal pain and an abrupt onset of diarrhea which may mimic food poisoning. Eosinophilia may be present. The illness is usually self-limiting. The diagnosis may be made by identification of the parasite in concentrated stool specimens. Treatment with metronidazole, tinidazole and paromomycin have been tried.

### Other protozoal parasites

#### *Blastocystis hominis*

The epidemiology of *B. hominis* is ill defined but the fecal–oral route, including contamination of food and water, appears important to transmission (Zierdt 1991). The pathogenicity of this organism has been controversial. As it has been isolated in association with other known pathogens and asymptomatic carriage is often noted, its causal role in producing diarrheal illness has been questioned. However, there is growing evidence for its role in producing disease in humans. In one report (Doyle et al 1990), the commonest symptoms in patients in whom *Blastocystis* infection was the likely cause of illness were diarrhea (74%), abdominal pain (58%) and gas (42%). Infection in AIDS patients may cause chronic diarrhea, although even in this group it may not always be associated with intestinal symptoms. The organism may be identified in stool by examination of wet preparations or concentrated trichrome-stained smears. Therapy for asymptomatic excretion has not been recommended. Treatment of symptomatic infection with metronidazole (250–750 mg three times daily for 7–10 days) is the drug of choice and has been associated with clinical and parasitological cure; furazolidone, dehydroemetine and co-trimoxazole have been suggested as alternative treatments.

#### Microsporidium *sp.* (Enterocytozoon bieneusi)

These tiny intracellular spore-forming organisms are associated primarily with AIDS patients (pp. 606 & 609). The organism infects enterocytes and may be found in nearly all enterocytes in severe cases. Diagnosis has relied on demonstration of the organism in small intestinal biopsy specimens using light and/or electronmicroscopy. However, spores of *E. bieneusi* have been identified in stool and duodenal fluid samples using standard concentration methods and Giemsa or toluidine blue staining (Orenstein et al 1990). Microsporidiosis responds to albendazole 400–800 mg twice daily but only infection with a recently described microsporidium *Septafa intestinalis* is completely cured by albendazole.

#### Balantidium coli

*Balantidium* spp. may be found in primates, rats and pigs. It is a motile ciliate and the largest human protozoal parasite. It occurs most commonly in tropical regions, particularly in communities that raise and live in close proximity to pigs. Transmission may occur by direct person-to-person contact, by ingestion of contaminated food and in occasional waterborne epidemics (Walzer et al 1973). It is often found in asymptomatic subjects where it is a non-invasive and self-limiting infection, but it may invade the colonic mucosa and produce deep ulceration and necrosis resulting in acute dysentery associated with sudden onset of abdominal pain, tenesmus and nausea. Perforation occurs occasionally in severe cases. Infection may also manifest as a chronic diarrheal illness. The large motile trophozoites can be identified in fresh saline suspensions of feces or from mucosal ulcer exudates or mucosal biopsies taken at sigmoidoscopy. Amebic dysentery is the main differential diagnosis, particularly when discrete areas of ulceration are seen at endoscopy. The parasite is best treated with tetracycline (500 mg four times daily for 10 days). If this fails, metronidazole (250–500 mg four times daily for 7 days) may be tried. Surgery may be required for severe fulminant colonic infection.

## HELMINTH INFECTIONS

Helminthic parasites may be found in the gut, tissues or blood and disease may be due to adult or immature (lar-

**Table 20.8** Intestinal helminthic infections

| Nematodes | Cestodes | Trematodes |
|---|---|---|
| *Ascaris lumbricoides* | *Taenia saginata* | *Schistosoma* spp. |
| *Ancylostoma duodenale* | *Taenia solium* | *Fasciolopsis buski* |
| *Necator americanus* | *Diphyllobothrium latum* | *Heterophyes heterophyes* |
| *Trichuris trichiura* | *Hymenolepsis nana* | *Metagonimus yokogawai* |
| *Strongyloides stercoralis* | *Echinococcus* spp. | *Clonorchis sinensis* |
| *Enterobius vermicularis* | | *Opisthorchis* spp. |
| *Toxocara* spp. | | *Fasciola hepatica* |
| *Trichinella spiralis* | | |
| *Capillaria philippinensis* | | |
| *Trichostrongylus* spp. | | |
| *Angiostrongylus costaricensis* | | |
| *Anisaksis* spp. | | |

val) forms of these worms. Infestation with helminths are among the most common infections of humans worldwide (Table 20.8). They occur throughout the developing world and especially in the poorest countries. Estimates vary but the major geohelminths, *Ascaris lumbricoides*, *Trichuris trichiura* and hookworm, may each infect about 1 billion people (Bundy 1994). As infection with helminths is ubiquitous in many areas, their impact on health has been consistently underestimated. While many infections appear asymptomatic it has become apparent that considerable morbidity and mortality may result. For example, while the mortality rate directly related to ascariasis is low the absolute number of deaths is relatively high because of the high prevalence of infection. Furthermore, it is now unequivocally established that intestinal helminthiasis may have adverse developmental consequences for children due to physical growth stunting and impaired cognition and educational achievement (Stephenson et al 1989, Nokes et al 1992). In developed countries helminthic infections may occur in small endemic foci as well as being commonly recognized in returned travelers or immigrants.

The manifestations of helminthic infections depend on the pathogenicity of the parasite, the host immune response and the worm burden. Subjects with light infection are often asymptomatic although occasionally even a single worm can produce significant disease such as when an adult *Ascaris* migrates into the biliary tree or pancreatic duct. Some parasites, such as the beef tapeworm *Taenia saginata*, appear relatively benign. Other parasites may cause significant tissue injury, eliciting damaging immune responses or having direct toxic effects.

With few exceptions helminths do not usually multiply within the definitive host. Therefore the infective parasite load is important as it affects the intensity of infection which in turn is an important determinant of disease expression. Most helminths develop in soil or require one or more intermediate hosts and are dependent on environmental conditions. Only *Strongyloides* and *Capillaria* are able to multiply in man. *Enterobius* is the only helminth commonly transmitted directly from person to person. Helminths survive in the host for a variable time which may be several years. The intensity of infection with the commonest helminths, *Ascaris lumbricoides* and *Trichuris trichiura*, is heaviest in children whereas the prevalence and intensity of hookworm infection rises throughout childhood and adolescence to peak in early adulthood (Bundy et al 1992). Acquired immunity may influence and limit the parasite burden but does not generally clear the infection. Intestinal helminths are neither uniformly nor randomly distributed among individuals. It is now established that more intense infections are highly aggregated so that most individuals have light infections whereas a small proportion of the population harbor disproportionally large worm burdens. This minority of heavily infected people not only comprises the individuals most likely to suffer disease but also is the major source of infection within a community. Control of intestinal helminths at a population level is dependent in the long term on improvements in economic conditions which lead to better education, sanitation and water supply. Meanwhile, morbidity and transmission can be reduced by mass treatment of populations by either targeting those who are most heavily infected or by treating whole sections of the community. In recent years selective targeting of school age children, who typically harbor the most intense infections with *Ascaris* and *Trichuris*, has shown to be of benefit not only for the physical and cognitive development of the children but also for reducing the intensity and prevalence of infections in a community as a whole (Stephenson et al 1989, 1993, Hall 1993).

## NEMATODES

Nematodes are nonsegmented worms with a surface cuticle enclosing longitudinal muscle which gives them mobility. The sexes are differentiated. Fertilized ova are passed in the stool or they release larvae in the gut. Infection occurs following ingestion or cutaneous invasion. After infection some nematodes reach the gut by way of the lungs and other viscera. Disease is due to larval and adult forms in the case of natural human parasites or due to the larval forms of some nonhuman parasites.

### Ascariasis

*Ascaris lumbricoides* (roundworm) is probably the most common worm that infects humans. The adult worm may grow to 30 cm in length and resides in the lumen of the small bowel. Ova are shed in the stool and develop in soil. Infection occurs when contaminated food or water is ingested. Larvae penetrate the small intestinal mucosa and travel in the bloodstream through the liver to the lungs. Larvae are then coughed up and swallowed. Maturation and fertilization takes place in the small intestine. A gravid female may produce 200 000 eggs per day. *Ascaris* has a global prevalence but is found most commonly in tropical and developing countries. In some of these communities infection of children may be virtually ubiquitous (Pawlowski 1987).

*Pathophysiology*

During passage through the lung, hypersensitivity to larval antigens may cause transient pulmonary eosinophilic infiltrates. In the intestine there may be an inflammatory infiltration of the lamina propria and some mild villous abnormalities but these are usually not marked. Worms may migrate into the biliary tree or the pancreas and cause obstructive problems or result in secondary bacterial infection. The direct impact of *Ascaris* on small intestinal function has been difficult to determine as infected subjects are often infected with multiple other parasites and/or bacteria. However, there is strong evidence that with intense infection they contribute significantly to growth retardation in children and may contribute to protein calorie malnutrition and vitamin A deficiency. In addition, in heavy infections a bolus of worms may cause intestinal obstruction and perforation, which is the leading cause of death due to *Ascaris* (Blumenthal & Schultz 1975). Appendicitis, volvulus, intussusception, perforation and peritonitis have all been described.

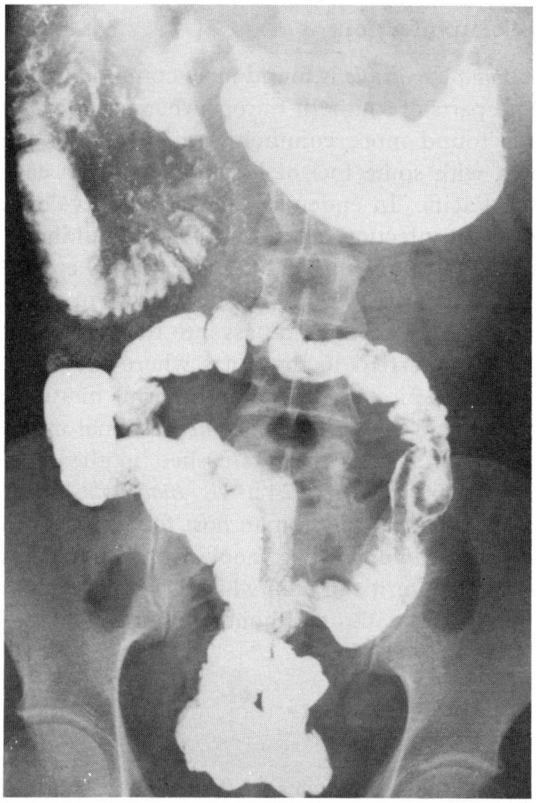

**Fig. 20.8** *Ascaris lumbricoides* in the jejunum causing filling defects about 25 cm long. They were found incidentally in a patient with a chronic duodenal ulcer.

*Clinical features*

During the pulmonary phase patients may present with cough, fever and dyspnea which usually subsides spontaneously after about a week. Most infections are of light intensity and probably asymptomatic but nonspecific abdominal pain and anorexia have been ascribed even to light infection. Some patients present initially following passage of an adult worm in stool or vomitus. The migration of a worm into the biliary tree may cause a clinical picture indistinguishable from calculus disease with biliary colic or cholangitis. Similarly, passage into the pancreatic duct may result in pancreatitis (Khuroo et al 1990). In children with heavy infection the initial presentation may be with intestinal obstruction or perforation in which case a worm mass may often be visible or palpable.

Travelers or expatriates returning from developing countries are sometimes found to have eggs of *Ascaris* in their stool. These infections are almost always light and usually asymptomatic. When symptoms are present they are not distinguishable from symptoms in other uninfected travelers.

*Diagnosis*

The diagnosis is most easily made by demonstration of *Ascaris* eggs in a wet preparation or concentrated stool specimen. Worms are occasionally demonstrated on barium radiology of the gut (Fig. 20.8) and can be demonstrated in the pancreas or biliary tree using ERCP. Identification of an adult worm in vomitus or stool also may establish the diagnosis. To date no clinically useful serological test is available.

*Treatment*

Several different compounds may be used to treat ascariasis. Mebendazole is a safe broad-spectrum benzimidazole anthelmintic with established efficacy. The usual dose is 100 mg twice daily for 3 days although single dose regimens are also used. As it is also effective against *Trichuris trichiura*, hookworm and pinworm infection it is particularly useful in areas where polyparasitism is common. It should be avoided in pregnancy and in children less than 2 years of age. Albendazole, a similar agent, is very effective as a single 400 mg dose and is increasingly used. Piperazine may be used and several dose regimens are available. A single dose (75 mg/kg) or two consecutive doses over 2 days are effective. This drug appears safe in pregnancy. Pyrantel (10 mg/kg) as a single dose is also highly effective. Levamisole is often used as a cheap therapy for mass treatment of whole communities. Intestinal obstruction can often be managed conservatively but may require surgery. Worms in the biliary tree may be removed endoscopically.

## Hookworm infection

*Ancylostoma duodenale* is found most commonly in Africa, Asia and parts of southern Europe whereas *Necator americanus* is found more commonly in Central and South America with some foci of infection in south east Asia and the Pacific. In endemic regions the prevalence and intensity of infection rises throughout childhood and reaches a plateau in early adulthood (Bundy et al 1992). Man is the major reservoir. Infective larvae in soil invade through the intact skin and pass into the venous circulation and are carried to the lungs where they are swallowed with respiratory secretions. Worms mature in the duodenum and attach to the small intestinal mucosa by their buccal capsules. Eggs are shed in the feces and hatch into larvae within 24 h. *A. duodenale* larvae may remain dormant in the human host for up to 8 months. *Ancylostoma caninum* (dog hookworm) may cause an eosinophilic enteritis in man which is usually manifest as abdominal pain with or without a peripheral eosinophilia (Croese et al 1994).

### *Pathophysiology*

Hookworm may cause localized dermatitis at the site of skin penetration and pneumonitis during passage through the lung. At the site of attachment to the intestinal mucosa there is an inflammatory reaction. Suction by the hookworm pulls mucosa cells free of the lamina propria, villous capillaries burst and blood flows into the lumen of the worm. Plugs of mucosal tissue are ingested along with blood which together may result in iron deficiency anemia and protein loss which contribute to malnutrition, particularly in those with heavy infections. There is no evidence of generalized malabsorption.

### *Clinical features*

Light infection is frequently asymptomatic. Localized skin irritation, so-called "ground itch", may occur at the site of entry through the skin. A transient fever and cough associated with eosinophilia and pulmonary infiltrates may occur during passage of larvae through the lungs. There may also be transient mild diarrhea and associated abdominal discomfort. Nonspecific dyspepsia is sometimes attributed to hookworm and may cause confusion with peptic ulcer disease.

The major clinical manifestations are those that result from iron deficiency anemia due to chronic blood loss and include fatigue and lassitude, breathlessness, palpitations and syncope (Maxwell et al 1987). In adults the ability to work is impaired. In severe cases congestive cardiac failure may ensue. Hypoproteinemia with edema may accompany heavy infections with marked protein loss from the gut (Gilman 1982). In children with heavy infection physical growth may be stunted and cognitive function impaired with adverse effect on education as well as health (Stephenson et al 1993). In women in their reproductive years hookworm infection may be one of many factors, including poor oral intake of iron, menstrual losses and blood loss in childbirth, that all contribute to iron deficiency.

### *Diagnosis*

The diagnosis is made by the detection of eggs in feces. An iodine-stained wet preparation may yield the diagnosis but a concentration technique is often needed, particularly in light infections. When stools are not examined for some time larvae may hatch in stool in a warm environment and be observed by microscopy. Diagnostic sensitivity can be increased by the use of Harada and agar plate culture methods which enhance the hatching of eggs into filariform larvae. Diagnosis may also be made by examination of duodenal fluid where stool tests are negative.

### *Treatment*

Mebendazole 100 mg twice a day for 3 days is effective treatment with minimal side-effects. Albendazole in a single oral dose of 400 mg is also very effective. As these benzimidazoles are effective against the major geohelminths they are very useful in the common situation where hookworm infection coexists with *Ascaris* and *Trichuris* infection. Other effective agents include pyrantel, bephenium and in some developing countries tetrachlorethylene. The choice depends on the presence of other parasites, availability and cost. Oral iron supplements are needed to treat the iron deficiency and careful blood transfusion may be needed in severe cases. Nutritional supplementation may be needed for severe protein deficiency. Personal prevention of reinfection includes the wearing of footwear and improved sanitation and personal hygiene.

## Trichuriasis

*Trichuris trichiura* (whipworm) is probably the third most common intestinal worm after *Ascaris* and hookworm. Adult worms are 2.5–5 cm in length with a whiplike anterior portion. *Trichuris* infection is distributed globally with similar epidemiology and population dynamics as *Ascaris* (Booth & Bundy 1992). The prevalence and intensity of infection are similarly greatest in school-age children. Eggs are shed in feces and embryonation occurs in the soil. Eggs are ingested and larvae are released in the stomach and pass into the intestine. These larvae penetrate and anchor into the colonic mucosa, particularly in the cecum where maturation to adult worms occurs.

*Pathophysiology*

There may be superficial localized inflammation at the site of worm penetration of the colonic mucosa. There is generally no increase in intraepithelial lymphocytes, but an increase in mucosal macrophage numbers and an IgE-mediated mast cell response has been identified, suggesting local anaphylaxis may have a role in producing diarrhea and protein loss from the gut (Cooper et al 1991, MacDonald et al 1991). In heavy infections worms are seen in a progressively distal distribution and there may be a diffuse colitis and proctitis. Rectal prolapse may occur with heavy infections in children. A large number of worms may occlude the appendix and cause appendicitis.

*Clinical features*

Most light infections are asymptomatic. Heavy infections may result in the Trichuris-dysentery syndrome characterised by small frequent diarrheal stools with blood and mucus, although stools can be watery. Passage of blood and mucus may predominate without diarrhea. There may be accompanying abdominal pain, tenesmus and rectal prolapse associated with anorexia and weight loss. Anemia and finger clubbing are associated with severe infection. Growth stunting in heavily infected children is common and well documented (Gilman et al 1983). There is increasing evidence that less intense infection may also have a deleterious effect on physical growth and cognitive performance (Nokes et al 1992). This may or may not be associated with chronic diarrhea. Population-based intervention studies have demonstrated improved growth velocity in children in whom the infection has been eradicated or the intensity of infection lowered.

*Investigation*

Diagnosis depends on identifying the characteristic barrel-shaped ova in the stool by light microscopic examination of a wet preparation or concentrated stool specimen. Endoscopic examination of the rectum and colon may enable adult worms to be directly visualized.

*Treatment and prevention*

*Trichuris* is less susceptible to anthelmintic agents than *Ascaris*. Mebendazole and albendazole are the most effective agents but need to be given in multiple dosage regimens to ensure eradication of the parasite. Albendazole 400 mg daily for 3 days or mebendazole 100 mg twice daily for 3 days are usually used. Oxantel has also reported efficacy. Risk of personal infection can be lowered by scrupulous personal hygiene and sanitary disposal of feces, as with other soil-transmitted helminths.

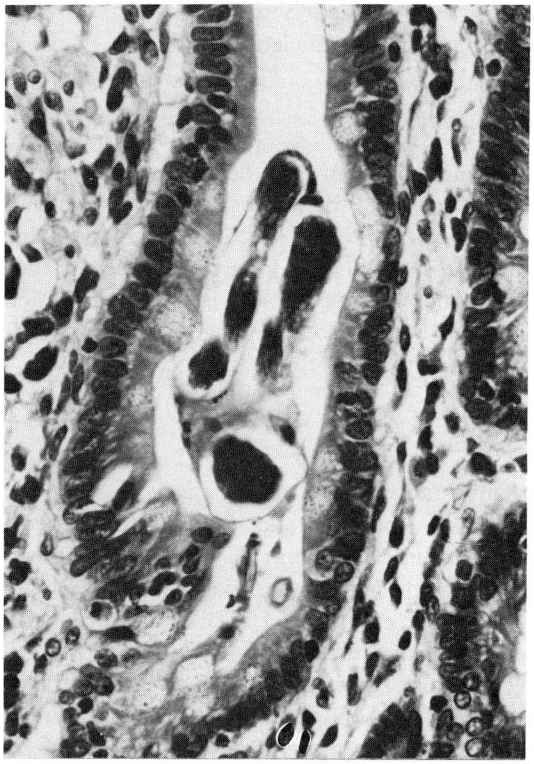

**Fig. 20.9** Adult forms of *Strongyloides stercoralis* in a small intestinal crypt (hematoxylin and eosin, × 250).

## Strongyloidiasis

*Strongyloides stercoralis* differs from most other intestinal nematodes as it can complete its lifecycle within the definitive host. Adult worms reside in the upper small intestine where the female worm burrows into the mucosa to lay eggs (Fig. 20.9). Rhabditiform larvae hatch and pass into the stool. In warm, humid soil they may either molt into infective filariform larvae or develop into free-living adults. The filariform larvae penetrate the skin or the mucosa on contact and are carried to the lungs via the venous system. Here they mature and migrate up the respiratory tree and are then swallowed and so reach the intestine where full adult maturation is completed and egg production begins. Some rhabditiform larvae develop into filariform larvae within the host and may penetrate the colonic mucosa or perianal skin, resulting in auto-infection. This may lead to prolonged infection over many years without the need for reinfection to maintain survival in the host. In studies of British and Australian ex-prisoners of war in south east Asia infection has been found in some more than 30 years after their return from endemic areas (Grove 1980). Although the distribution of *S. stercoralis* is most prevalent in tropical countries and is similar to that of hookworm, pockets of endemic infection have been found in some temperate regions including parts of Europe and the USA (Genta et al 1988). Infection may be asymptomatic or associated with chronic intermittent symptoms. Hyperinfection with systemic dissemination may occur in immunodeficiency.

*Pathology*

Adult female worms invade the proximal small intestine and directly damage the mucosa, causing mild or partial villous atrophy and an accompanying inflammatory infiltrate of eosinophils and mononuclear cells. Thickening of the intestinal wall may be seen in chronic infection. The colonic mucosa may also be damaged during autoinfection by filariform larvae.

*Clinical features*

The manifestations of strongyloidiasis may be chronic, nonspecific and periodic and must be considered in the appropriate clinical setting. Asymptomatic infection is common. Symptomatic cases may have many manifestations. There may be a brief local reaction consisting of itch, erythema and urticaria following penetration of the skin by filariform larvae. About a week later as the parasite passes through the lungs there may be transient cough, wheeze and pulmonary infiltrates associated with eosinophilia. Abdominal fullness, bloating, postprandial discomfort or severe epigastric or abdominal pain may follow. Bowel habit may vary between episodic mild diarrhea and constipation. Malabsorption may occur in heavy infection. Larva currens is highly suggestive of strongyloidiasis. This is a pruritic, migratory, linear cutaneous eruption that mostly appears on the back, chest, abdomen, buttocks and thighs. It is thought to be associated with cutaneous migration of filariform larvae during autoinfection and may be an allergic reaction to parasite antigens as it is observed more often in Caucasians with long-standing infection rather than in subjects living in endemic areas who are continually exposed to reinfection. Less common manifestations may include colitis or granulomatous hepatitis.

Hyperinfection may occur in patients immunocompromised by HIV infection, malnutrition, malignancy (particularly lymphoma) and immunosuppressive drugs such as corticosteroids and chemotherapy (Morgan et al 1986). The infection becomes heavy as the autoinfection cycle is enhanced. Small intestinal and colonic ulceration and hemorrhage occur because of the heavier parasite burden resulting in severe abdominal pain, vomiting and bloody diarrhea. The infection may then disseminate, resulting in large numbers of larvae and adult worms reaching other organs. Parasites have been found in virtually all tissues. Disseminated strongyloidiasis has a high mortality rate. Bacterial septicemia due to enteric organisms is a common cause of death in this syndrome. Bacteria are thought to be carried across the colon with migrating larvae.

*Diagnosis*

The diagnosis may be made by identification of larvae, eggs or adult females in specimens including feces, duodenal fluid, sputum or tissue samples. Stool examination is a relatively insensitive diagnostic method as the concentration of larvae in stool is often very low. Examination of multiple specimens using concentration techniques may increase the sensitivity but may still result in the diagnosis being overlooked. Use of culture techniques such as Harada or agar plate culture may increase the diagnostic yield. Microscopy of duodenal aspirates is more sensitive than stool examination and may be useful when fecal examination is negative (Goka et al 1990b). Inflammation and ulceration of the colon may be evident endoscopically. Serological diagnosis using an ELISA is available as a screening test and is reasonably sensitive.

*Treatment and prevention*

Thiabendazole in a dose of 25 mg/kg twice daily for 3 days orally is moderately effective, but is associated with side-effects including anorexia, vomiting, nausea and dizziness. Longer or repeated courses may be given if there is initial therapeutic failure. Mebendazole 100 mg or albendazole 400 mg twice daily for 3 days are less toxic than thiabendazole and have been used, but are probably less efficacious. Repeated stool examination at intervals over several months may be necessary to detect treatment failure. Individual prevention of infection is dependent on the avoidance of skin contact with contaminated soil.

## Enterobiasis

Infection with the small nematode *Enterobius vermicularis* (pinworm) is extremely common and is found in tropical and temperate locations in developing and affluent communities. Infection is most common in young schoolchildren and is acquired by ingestion of eggs from contaminated hands, food or, less commonly, water. While usually considered a nocturnal nuisance, it may cause significant morbidity in children. Transmission within families of infected children is common (Cook 1994).

After ingestion, eggs hatch in the upper gut and larvae migrate to the ileum, cecum and appendix. Gravid worms migrate from the colon through the anus and traverse the perianal or perineal skin, where eggs are layed. Transmission may therefore be by direct autoinfection or by exposure to soiled and contaminated night clothes or bedding. Pruritus ani is the most common symptom, although many infections are asymptomatic. Other symptoms in children ascribed to infection include insomnia, tiredness, anorexia and irritability but these have not been definitively proven to be due to infection. There may be local skin trauma and excoriation with secondary infection.

Diagnosis may be made presumptively on history but only definitively by accurate identification of adult worms or eggs. These may be visualized in the perianal region, particularly after use of the sellotape method to identify the parasite. Fecal examination is insensitive. Adult worms are occasionally visualized during colonoscopy. Single dose treatment with mebendazole 100 mg, albendazole 200–400 mg or pyrantel 10 mg/kg are each effective. The benzimidazoles are the drugs of choice because of the excellent safety profile and low incidence of side-effects but are not recommended for pregnant patients or children under 2 years of age. In these cases piperazine in a 7-day course is an alternative and single dose preparations are available, but this drug is associated with more adverse reactions (Cook 1994). Close attention to personal hygiene and living conditions is important to prevent re-infection. It is wise to treat the whole family of an infected child. Reinfection is frequent and repeated treatment of individuals and whole families may be required.

### Visceral larva migrans

This is a syndrome characterized by eosinophilia, tender hepatomegaly and occasional involvement of other organs and is due to tissue migration of larval nematodes in a nondefinitive host. In humans this is most commonly due to infection with *Toxocara canis* (dog roundworm) or *T. catis* (cat roundworm) and occasionally with larvae of other nematodes.

### Toxocariasis

Infection with *T. canis* and *T. catis* occur by ingestion of eggs in contaminated soil. Infection is commonest in young children who often have a history of pica. Larvae hatch in the small bowel and penetrate the mucosa to enter the portal circulation and reach the liver, lungs and occasionally other sites including the brain. Ocular lesions are seldom associated with the visceral syndrome and tend to occur in older children. Adult worms do not develop. Manifestations of visceral larva migrans relate to the intensity of infection, prior exposure and the host immune response. Dead larvae excite a granulomatous reaction with prominent eosinophils and sometimes fibrosis. Infection is often asymptomatic. Symptomatic cases may have fever, nausea, vomiting, abdominal pain and bronchospasm with hepatosplenomegaly, leukocytosis and persistent eosinophilia.

The diagnosis is suggested by the clinical picture. Serology using an ELISA technique is sensitive (Ogilvie & de Savigny 1982). Larvae surrounded by tissue destruction with eosinophilic granulomas may be seen on liver biopsy. The illness is usually self-limiting. Treatment with diethylcarbamazine 3 mg/kg three times daily for 10–20 days has been recommended, particularly for ocular or cerebral involvement. A role for corticosteroids in the acute phase is controversial. Prevention relies on control of infection in pets and of their feces in public areas.

### Trichinosis

*Trichinella spiralis* causes a disease primarily of skeletal muscle but acute gastrointestinal symptoms may occur early in infection. It is found worldwide and is transmitted to humans following ingestion of inadequately cooked meat containing larvae. Ingested larvae invade the intestinal mucosa where they mature, mate and discharge a new generation of larvae which are carried to skeletal muscle via the circulation. Intestinal symptoms develop after 1–7 days. Diarrhea is usually shortlived. Abdominal cramps, nausea, anorexia and diarrhea are accompanied by fever, malaise and eosinophilia. The acute myositis develops from 9–28 days after infection and the illness may be complicated by encephalitis or myocarditis. The diagnosis is often unsuspected until myositis develops and is confirmed on muscle biopsy. Adult worms or larvae are rarely seen in feces. Serological tests become positive after about 2 weeks of infection. Treatment is aimed at eradicating adult worms from the intestine, but there is no effective treatment for larvae in muscle. Mebendazole 200 mg twice daily, pyrantel 10 mg/kg/day and albendazole 200–400 mg twice daily, each for 5 days, are used. Prevention depends on adequate cooking of pork and of preventing infection in pigs, although other animals from wild or domestic sources may also harbor this parasite (Kociecka 1987).

### Capillariasis

*Capillaria philippinensis* is a small nematode found predominantly in the Philippines and Thailand. Infection occurs by ingestion of inadequately cooked fish infected with this parasite (Cross 1992). Adult worms invade the small intestinal mucosa causing mucosal damage sometimes associated with protein-losing enteropathy. Ova and larvae are released and internal autoinfection occurs. Infection can cause severe diarrhea with malabsorption associated with copious steatorrhea which may be associated with profound weight loss and even death over a period of a few months if untreated. Ova, larvae or adult worms may be identified in feces or small intestinal biopsies. Treatment is with mebendazole 200 mg twice daily which needs to be given for 20–30 days. Prevention rests on the adequate cooking of fish in endemic areas. A related parasite, *Capillaria hepatica*, is a zoonosis and human infection has been described. It infrequently causes visceral larva migrans.

### Trichostrongyliasis

*Trichostrongylus* spp. are common intestinal parasites of

herbivores. Human infection is incidental. Infection is found in parts of the Middle East, Asia and South America and follows consumption of vegetables contaminated with infected animal feces (Wolfe 1978). This parasite attaches to the small intestinal mucosa and sucks blood. Epigastric pain, anemia and diarrhea occur with heavy infection. Ova are found in the stool and larvae can be cultured. The ova resemble hookworm ova and must be distinguished from these. Thiabendazole 25 mg/kg twice daily for 3 days or pyrantel 10 mg/kg as a single dose are effective treatments.

### Angiostrongyliasis

Human infection with the rodent nematode *Angiostrongylus costaricensis* occurs when the larval stage is ingested in the slug intermediate host. Larvae penetrate the gut wall in the ileocecal region and clinically the illness may resemble intestinal obstruction or appendicitis for which surgery is performed (Hulbert et al 1992). No effective treatment is known and the illness usually regresses within weeks.

### Anisakiasis

Human anisakiasis is caused by larval stages of anisakid nematodes (Bier et al 1987). Infection occurs by eating raw, salted or pickled fish or shellfish containing larvae. The parasite does not mature in man and larvae are not found in stools. Most cases have been reported from Japan and The Netherlands, although increasing cases have been found worldwide with the increasing popularity of sushi (Hubert et al 1989). Larvae penetrate the stomach, small intestine and rarely the colon, causing eosinophilic granulomas with edema and induration which is thought to be due to a hypersensitivity reaction. Occasionally intestinal perforation with peritonitis occurs.

Anisakiasis can be asymptomatic or cause acute or chronic illness. In the acute gastric syndrome, epigastric pain, nausea and vomiting may occur as early as 1 h after the ingestion of raw fish. At endoscopy worms may be seen and can be physically removed using biopsy forceps. In small intestinal anisakiasis symptoms do not usually appear until 1–2 weeks after ingestion of the parasite. There may be constant or intermittent abdominal pain, fever and vomiting sometimes mimicking an acute abdomen. Eosinophilia is inconstant. Diagnostic ova or larval stages are not seen in feces or blood and serology is not yet widely available so that the diagnosis is usually made by demonstration of larvae in tissue. The disease usually subsides spontaneously but occasionally a chronic illness develops which may require surgery. No specific anthelmintic treatment has proven to be effective. Prevention of the disease rests with the avoidance of eating potentially contaminated raw seafoods.

## CESTODES

Infection with cestodes (tapeworms or flatworms) is common and widespread throughout the world (Pawlowski 1984). Man is the definitive host to several intestinal cestodes, most commonly *Taenia saginata* (beef tapeworm), *T. solium* (pork tapeworm), *Diphyllobothrium latum* (fish tapeworm) and *Hymenolepis nana* (dwarf tapeworm). *Echinococcus granulosus* and *E. multilocularis* are other species of tapeworms which infect humans in the larval stage and in whom humans are an intermediate host. With these parasites, larvae enter the circulation and lodge in the liver, lungs and occasionally other organs and develop into hydatid cysts.

### Taeniasis

Mature adult *Taenia* live in the intestinal tract of humans, the definitive host, where they may reside for many years. Worms attach by a scolex (head) which has four strong hemispherical suckers. The neck and body of the worms consist of several segments (proglottids). Each proglottid has male and female reproductive organs. Both intact proglottids or the eggs released from proglottids are passed in the stool. The larval form may live in a wide range of intermediate hosts where they penetrate the intestinal mucosa to become encysted in tissues. These fluid-filled sacs are called cysticerci. Humans are infected with cysticerci by consuming raw infected beef (*T. saginatum*) or pork (*T. solium*). Highly endemic regions include much of central and east Africa and the Middle East. Light to moderate infection rates occur in many European countries, south east Asia and South America. Although found in many developed countries, the prevalence is very low.

The pathophysiology of taeniasis is not well studied. There may be some morphological derangement to the small intestinal mucosa with deformed villi and a cellular infiltrate. Most infections are with a single tapeworm and do not produce significant malabsorption. Whether infection with large numbers of worms produces malabsorption is not definitively known. The vast majority of infections are asymptomatic and come to notice only when a patient becomes aware of passing proglottids in the stool. Nonspecific symptoms including abdominal discomfort or pain, hunger sensations and nausea have been ascribed to infection. Occasionally, proglottids may crawl through the anus and cause much distress to a host. *T. solium* may undergo larval development in human tissue to cause cysticercosis (Despommier 1992). It is thought this results from the ingestion of eggs and subsequent development of the larval stage. Cysticerci may develop in subcutaneous tissue, muscles or viscera but most importantly in the eye and brain (Fig. 20.10). Inflammatory changes provoked by dead ova may cause raised intracranial pressure and fitting or simulate many neurological disorders.

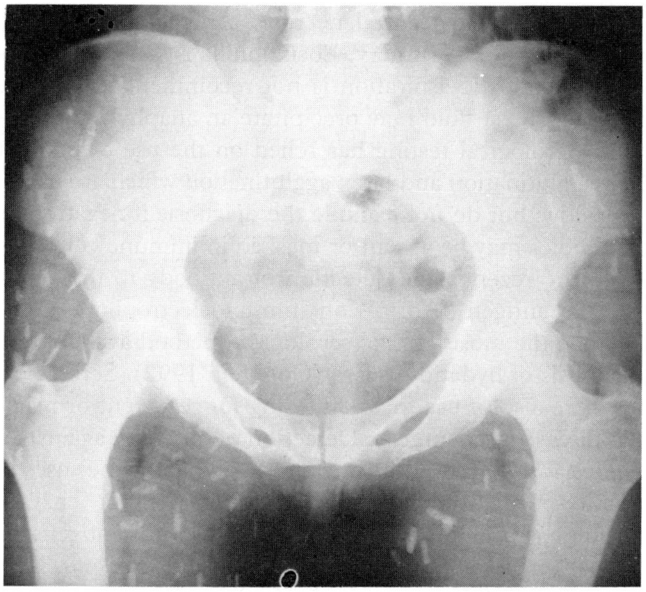

**Fig. 20.10** Radiograph showing tissue calcification due to cysticercosis.

Diagnosis is usually made by the identification of proglottids or eggs in stools. Eggs may also be found by applying adhesive tape to the perianal region as for pinworm infection. Examination of proglottids is necessary for species identification as egg morphology is not diagnostic. Occasionally adult worms may be identified on radiological studies done for a variety of reasons. At present immunologically based diagnosis is not routinely available.

Niclosamide (2 g as a single dose chewed) is the drug of choice and is highly effective. Praziquantel 10–20 mg/kg as a single dose is also effective. Cerebral cysticercosis may improve with praziquantel but surgical intervention may sometimes be required. The disease can be controlled by measures aimed at reducing animal infection. For personal protection, eating inadequately cooked meat in endemic areas should be avoided.

## Diphyllobothriasis

*Diphyllobothrium latum*, a tapeworm of fish, is found in populations that consume raw fish and is commonest in temperate and subarctic Europe and America. The lifecycle includes two intermediate hosts, small freshwater crustaceans and then fish. Human infection is acquired by the ingestion of live encysted larvae in infected fish. The adult worms are the longest that infect man and may grow as long as 15 m. The adult worm attaches to the ileal mucosa. Most infection is asymptomatic or causes mild nonspecific symptoms. The worm is able to compete successfully with its host for vitamin $B_{12}$ and many infected subjects have low serum vitamin $B_{12}$ levels although only a small minority develop megaloblastic anemia or neurological sequelae (Pawlowski 1984). Diagnosis is made by detection of eggs, which are typically plentiful in stool. Proglottids are not usually seen as they disintegrate in the human intestine. Infection responds well to either niclosamide or praziquantel. Disease can be prevented by avoidance of ingestion of raw freshwater fish.

## Hymenolepiasis

*Hymenolepis nana*, the dwarf tapeworm, infects humans and rodents and has a widespread distribution. Children and those in institutions are most commonly affected. Infection may occur directly by person-to-person spread or by the fecal–oral route. It differs from other tapeworms as both the larval stages and adult phases occur in the same host. Gravid proglottids disintegrate in the bowel and eggs, which are immediately infective, are passed in the feces. Ingested eggs hatch, penetrate the intestinal mucosa and develop into the next larval stage, the cysticercoid. These larvae migrate back into the lumen, attach and mature into adult worms. *H. nana* may cause minor damage at the site of attachment. Heavier infection may be associated with anorexia, nausea, diarrhea or weight loss. Diagnosis is made by identification of eggs in stool. Treatment with niclosamide 2 g daily for 1 week (which may be repeated in 2 weeks in heavy infection) or praziquantel 25 mg/kg as a single dose is effective (Groll 1980). Personal hygiene is the most important preventive measure. In institutions screening of newcomers may avoid epidemics.

## Echinococcosis

*Etiology and epidemiology*

Echinococcosis is a tissue infection caused by *Echinococcus granulosus* and the less common *E. multilocularis*. Canines are the definitive hosts for *E. granulosus* (dog tapeworm). Intermediate hosts are most commonly sheep and cattle. Humans serve as an intermediate host following accidental ingestion of eggs from the feces of infected canines. Rodents are the usual natural intermediate host for *E. multilocularis* and various carnivores including wolves and foxes as well as domestic dogs and cats are the definitive hosts. The lifecycle for both species is similar. Gravid proglottids release eggs either before or just after passage in the stool. Following ingestion by a human, the oncospheres (embryos) are released from the ova, penetrate the intestinal mucosa and enter the portal circulation. Most lodge in the liver (60%) with a lesser proportion reaching the lung (20–30%). A minority may reach the systemic circulation and localize to the brain, kidney, bones, heart or other tissues. Larvae develop into hydatid cysts. In the case of *E. granulosus* these are unilocular with an external laminated cuticula and an inner germinal layer and are normally fluid filled. Brood capsules and daughter cysts develop from the germinal layer. So-called "hydatid sand" within cysts consists of scolices liberated from ruptured brood capsules. The hydatid cyst of *E. multilocularis* differs in that the larval form remains in the proliferative phase and the cyst is multilocular (alveolar). The lesion infiltrates adjacent tissue by extension from the germinal layer. When a hydatid cyst is ingested by a definitive host, such as when offal from sheep or cattle is fed to farm dogs, the cycle is completed. Hydatid cysts due to *E. granulosus* are found frequently in many parts of the Middle East and also occur in South Africa, South America, central and eastern Europe, Australia and New Zealand. *E. multilocularis* infections are generally confined to colder regions of the northern hemisphere including Alaska, Siberia and Switzerland.

### *Clinical features*

Echinococcosis is often acquired in childhood and several decades may pass before clinical manifestations occur as cysts grow slowly over a period of many years. Some cysts may be detected in asymptomatic individuals undergoing imaging investigations for other reasons. Hydatid cysts of *E. granulosus* may become very large. Enlarging cysts usually produce tissue damage by mechanical means and symptoms depend on the site and rate of growth of the lesions. Patients with hepatic disease may present with abdominal pain and hepatomegaly and a mass may be palpable. Cysts may rupture into the bile duct, peritoneal cavity or pleural space and this may produce fever, pruritus, rash or an anaphylactic reaction which may be fatal. Numerous scolices are released which leads to disseminated infection. In a minority of patients, calcified cysts are extruded via the biliary tract causing symptoms indistinguishable from cholecystitis. Biliary obstruction may result in jaundice and pain. The alveolar cyst of *E. multilocularis* usually presents as a slowly growing mass in the liver and is commonly fatal if untreated due to progressive destruction of the liver with erosion into vital structures.

### *Diagnosis*

On plain abdominal radiograph hepatic hydatid cysts of *E. granulosus* show a smooth rim of calcification in about half of cases and the diaphragm may be elevated. CT scanning or ultrasonography are invaluable in demonstrating the morphology of a cyst. However, in some cases a simple fluid-filled cyst may be indistinguishable from other benign hepatic cysts. The finding of daughter cysts and hydatid sand strongly suggests infection. Egg shell calcification may indicate active disease. With alveolar hydatids CT scan may demonstrate an indistinct mass lesion, often with central necrosis. Angiography may be necessary prior to surgery. Eosinophilia is sometimes present. Diagnostic aspiration is not recommended because leakage of cyst fluid may precipitate an anaphylactic reaction. Serological testing has relied on the use of indirect hemagglutination and latex agglutination which are useful if positive but do not exclude the diagnosis if negative, as antibodies may be absent or masked in immune complexes. More recently the detection of antibody to the genus specific antigen "Arc 5" on immunoelectrophoresis has become the most specific serological method available for diagnosis of hydatid disease (Gottstein 1992). Serological tests are also of use for monitoring for recurrent or residual disease after surgery. Detection of antibody against *E. multilocularis* has improved markedly with the use of affinity-purified and recombinant antigen in enzyme immunoassays (Gottstein 1992). However, antigens of similar quality are not yet available for *E. granulosus*. New diagnostic molecular methods involving DNA probes are currently being studied.

### *Treatment and prevention*

Surgery remains the mainstay of treatment. However, asymptomatic patients with small cysts found incidentally may not need intervention if no symptoms develop and there is no enlargement observed over time. Various surgical methods have been described. With a large cyst the contents should be sterilized with hypertonic saline before the cyst is opened. The entire endocyst should then be removed and the residual space obliterated. Care is needed to prevent seeding of daughter cysts into the peritoneal cavity. Medical therapy with high-dose mebendazole (40–200 mg/kg) has been used, particularly in subjects medically unfit for surgery or where there is extensive disease rendering surgical cure impossible (Bryceson et al 1982). Results are variable and blood levels should be monitored. Albendazole may be more effective as it appears to achieve higher concentrations in cysts. These drugs have also been used at the time of surgery to reduce the risk of intraoperative metastatic spread. Successful percutaneous drainage of hepatic hydatid cysts has been reported although in general this should be avoided because of the risk of leakage of cyst fluid. Transmission of the disease can be interrupted by controlling the infection in dogs by reducing their access to offal and by regular deworming. Where there is no cycle in wild animals these procedures may be very effective, as evidenced by the successful control of the disease in several areas of endemic infection.

## TREMATODES

Trematodes or flukes include species that are found in blood (*Schistosoma*), the intestine (*Fasciolopsis*) and the liver (*Clonorchis and Fasciola*). Infection with trematodes is usually associated with water contact, consumption of aquatic intermediate hosts or water plants.

### Schistosomiasis

The major schistosome species *S. mansoni*, *S. japonicum* and *S. haematobium* and a number of less common species such as *S. mekongi* and *S. intercalatum* probably infect more than 200 million people. Schistosomiasis (also known as bilharziasis) is a chronic life-threatening infection which may cause hepatic fibrosis and portal hypertension, intestinal lesions, bladder lesions and obstructive renal disease. Disease arises from granulomatous and fibrous reaction to retained *Schistosoma* ova. Clinical features vary with the site of predilection of the ova, which is mainly the intestine and liver in *S. mansoni* and *S. japonicum* infections and the bladder for *S. haematobium*.

#### *Epidemiology and lifecycle*

*S. mansoni* is found in Africa, south west Asia, the Caribbean and South America. *S. japonicum* is limited to China, the Philippines, Japan and parts of south east Asia while *S. haematobium* occurs only in Africa. In all countries the distribution is focal. All ages and both sexes are infected, with the highest prevalence in children. Morbidity is largely related to the intensity of infection. Serious disease occurs in only a small proportion of infected individuals. Schistosomiasis only occurs as an imported disease in developed countries, in travelers and immigrants. Man is the definitive host of the three major schistosome species and is the sole reservoir of importance except for *S. japonicum*, which is also found in domestic and wild animals. Nonhuman schistosomes may cause dermatitis ("swimmer's itch") but no other disease.

Intestinal and hepatosplenic schistosomiasis are caused by *S. mansoni* and *S. japonicum*. Adult worms live in the portal vessels and migrate down the inferior and superior mesenteric veins, reaching terminal vessels where they deposit ova which penetrate the intestinal wall (Fig. 20.11). Most ova are carried to the liver but a proportion reach the bowel lumen and are excreted. If ova reach water, miracidia hatch, penetrate the snail intermediate host, develop over 4–6 weeks and leave the snail as cercariae to reinfect the definitive host through the skin. After penetrating the skin, cercariae undergo further morphological change to schistosomula and travel from subcutaneous tissue through the lymphatics and peripheral circulation to the lungs to reach their final destination in the portal vasculature after approximately 1 week. After a further 4 or 5 weeks they are fully mature and egg laying commences, but a further 1–2 weeks elapse before ova are found in the stool. The intermediate hosts of *S. mansoni* are freshwater *Biomphalaria* snails and of *S. japonicum* amphibious

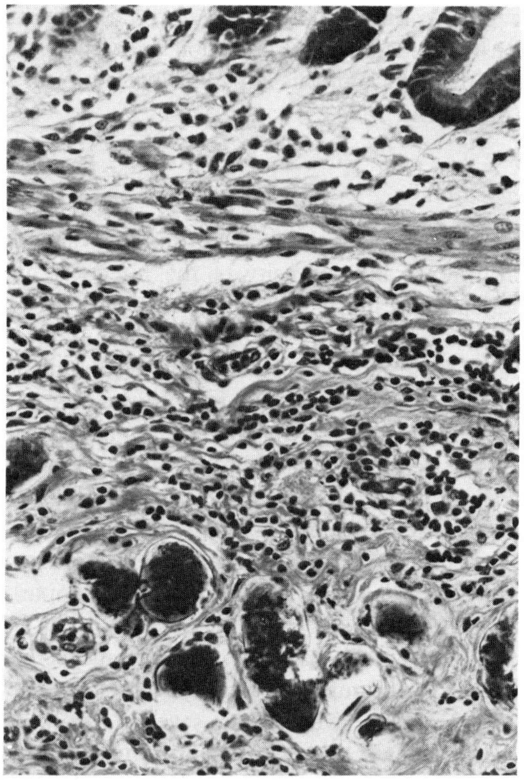

**Fig. 20.11** Numerous *Schistosoma* ova present in the submucosa of the appendix (hematoxylin and eosin, × 150).

*Oncomelania* snails. Dam construction and irrigation schemes have extended the range of schistosomiasis.

#### *Pathology and immunology*

Most pathological changes of schistosomiasis are mediated by the immune response, which is also partly protective. Immediately following cutaneous penetration hypersensitivity may cause transient focal cutaneous edema and eosinophilic infiltration. Dead ova in tissues provoke a granulomatous reaction dependent on cell-mediated immunity. Early granulomata are diffuse, with a predominance of mononuclear cells and some eosinophils. Later they become smaller and infiltrated with macrophages, lymphocytes and fibroblasts. Collagen deposition is followed by fibrosis. Extensive fibrosis of the liver is seen in end-stage disease (Symmers clay pipe-stem fibrosis), being greatest around portal areas. Portal hypertension is due to obstruction of presinusoidal vessels. The collateral circulation enables ova to reach the lungs, nervous tissue and other organs and for immune complexes to cause glomerulonephritis. Focal dense deposits of eggs in the colon elicit a granulomatous response. Usually the involvement is slight, but extensive areas may be involved with large hemorrhagic granulomata, ulcers, polyps and fibrosis. Prolonged *Salmonella* infection may occur that only responds to treatment after schistosomal chemotherapy is given. There also appears to be a relationship between hepatitis B and C infection and schistosomiasis, although the nature of this apparent interaction is not yet clear (Strickland 1994).

*Clinical features*

Clinical manifestations of schistosomiasis vary with the stage, duration and intensity of the infection, with the infecting species and with the host response. In endemic areas many infections go unrecognized. Acute symptoms are mainly limited to visitors. A localized allergic dermatitis (cercarial dermatitis) develops within a day or two of cercarial penetration and may become more generalized in highly sensitized individuals. The symptoms are self-limiting and resolve within 2 weeks. Katayama fever develops 4–6 weeks after infection and is characterized by fever, cutaneous and respiratory allergic manifestations, enlargement of the liver and spleen, lymphadenopathy and peripheral eosinophilia.

Established hepatic disease may be suspected when hepatomegaly or features of portal hypertension are evident. The left lobe of the liver is more severely involved. Portal hypertension may present with gastrointestinal bleeding, splenomegaly, ascites or anemia. Features of liver failure such as gynecomastia and spider nevi are uncommon except terminally or following portocaval shunt. Transient ascites and peripheral edema may develop after hemorrhage. The schistosomal cause is confirmed by detecting the parasite but in endemic areas schistosomiasis may be coincidental to cirrhosis or other causes of portal hypertension. Ova reaching the lungs, the brain and the spinal cord can cause severe symptoms but pulmonary fibrosis is unusual in the absence of extensive hepatic disease.

Established intestinal schistosomiasis may present, or be found incidentally, months or years after infection. The major symptoms are of colitis with diarrhea, which may contain blood, and nonspecific abdominal pain. Patients may also complain of tiredness, anorexia and weight loss. Physical examination may be normal or the liver and spleen may be palpable. In severe infections protein-losing enteropathy and anemia occur.

*Diagnosis*

Detection of ova in the stool is the simplest way to confirm the diagnosis but even using concentration methods stool examination is insensitive and likely to miss light infections. Stool examination is particularly insensitive in acute syndromes occurring during the prepatent period (the time between infection and the appearance of ova) and in long-standing infections. Tissue biopsy is more sensitive and rectal mucosal biopsy is a sensitive method to detect ova in active infections. The diagnosis may be suspected by the macroscopic appearances at colonoscopy (Mohamed et al 1990) which may vary from pinpoint hemorrhages and mucosal granularity to marked polypoid change with ulceration. Stricture formation is rare. A serum ELISA is now available and can be used as a screening test for acute infection. Ultrasonography is increasingly used to evaluate schistosomal morbidity. It can assess liver and spleen size and grade periportal fibrosis and portal vein diameter (Strickland & Abdel-Wahab 1993). Confirmation of schistosomal hepatic fibrosis requires demonstration of ova and histological changes in the liver and may need open liver biopsy, as needle biopsy may fail to detect focal lesions.

*Treatment*

Treatment of schistosomiasis has altered considerably with the advent of relatively nontoxic drugs which have simplified treatment of individual patients and facilitated community chemotherapy. In addition to lower toxicity, the newer drugs facilitate some regression of established disease (Davis 1986, Strickland & Abdel-Wahab 1993). Chemotherapy is seldom contraindicated in advanced disease and may improve the prognosis. Praziquantel and oxamniquine have replaced older drugs such as the triantimonials and niridazole. Praziquantel is effective against all human schistosomes and a range of other parasite infections and represents a major advance in parasite chemotherapy. Praziquantel 40 mg/kg is given orally as a single dose for *S. mansoni* infection and 60 mg/kg in three divided doses over 24 h for *S. japonicum*. Oxamniquine is reasonably effective against *S. mansoni* and has been used in population-based chemotherapy. The complications of portal hypertension are treated in the standard ways.

*Prevention and control*

In endemic areas control relies on strategies directed at reducing morbidity and the human reservoir through chemotherapy, improving sanitation and water supplies and attempting to reduce the prevalence of the intermediate host. Praziquantel is probably the best drug available for community or selective chemotherapy, but cost limits its use in many places. In spite of considerable research an effective vaccine is not yet available. In the individual, prevention is only possible by avoiding exposure. Swimming and other water activities in endemic areas are the major causes of infection and should be avoided.

**Intestinal flukes**

Many species of intestinal flukes have been found to infect humans but the pathogenicity of most of these remains unknown. Approximately 50 million people are estimated to be infected with one or more species of intestinal fluke.

### Fasciolopsis buski

*F. buski*, the giant intestinal fluke, is the largest intestinal fluke, varying in length between 20 and 75 mm. Certain freshwater snails are the intermediate hosts after which cercariae encyst on water plants. Infection follows ingestion of these plants raw. Pigs are the main nonhuman reservoir. *F. buski* is endemic in parts of India and south east Asia. The flukes attach to the duodenal and jejunal mucosa. Attachment causes local inflammation and may cause abscesses or hemorrhage at the site of deep ulceration. Most infections are light and asymptomatic. Symptoms may include abdominal pains which mimic peptic ulcer, anorexia, nausea and vomiting. Diarrhea may alternate with constipation initially but diarrhea usually becomes persistent. Malabsorption may occur with foul-smelling stools that contain undigested food. Protein-losing enteropathy secondary to mucosal damage may result in ascites and edema of the face and trunk. In heavy infection the presentation may be with acute ileus or bowel obstruction.

The diagnosis is made by identifying the eggs in stool samples. These must be distinguished from eggs of *Echinostoma* spp. and also *Fasciola* spp. Flukes are occasionally seen in vomitus or feces. Nonspecific laboratory findings may include a leukocytosis with eosinophilia. Praziquantel is very effective and is the drug of choice, in a single dose of 15 mg/kg (Harinasuta et al 1987). The organism is killed by immersion of infected water plants in boiling water for a few seconds. Cessation of the use of human night soil and preventing pig excrement from contaminating pond water may reduce the prevalence of infection.

### Heterophyes heterophyes *and* Metagonimus yokogawai

The lifecycle of these minute heterophyids includes two intermediate hosts, freshwater snails then fish. Man becomes infected by eating parasitized raw fish. *H. heterophyes* is found in parts of the Middle East, particularly along the Nile delta, with foci of infection also found in Asia. *M. yokogawai* is probably the most common intestinal fluke in Asia with endemic foci of infection particularly in Japan and Korea. Attachment to the small intestinal mucosa results in inflammation and superficial necrosis. Mild intermittent diarrhea with mucus, colicky abdominal pain and dyspepsia may result. With *M. yokagawai* severe abdominal pain, watery diarrhea and prostration may follow ingestion of a single parasitized raw fish in a previously uninfected individual. Eggs of either parasite may enter the systemic circulation and cause serious systemic sequelae, particularly in the heart and central nervous system, probably due to embolic occlusion of blood vessels. Diagnosis is based on the identification of eggs in stools but as these are virtually indistinguishable and resemble other heterophyids, the definitive diagnosis may only be made by identification of adult flukes recovered after antihelminthic therapy (Harinasuta et al 1987). Praziquantel is effective in a single dose of 15–25 mg/kg. Avoidance of the consumption of raw fish will prevent infection.

## Liver flukes

### *Clonorchiasis and opisthorchiasis*

*Clonorchis sinensis* and *Opisthorchis* spp. are trematodes that infect the biliary tree. The former occurs mostly in China, Japan and parts of south east Asia whereas the latter is also found in parts of eastern Europe and Siberia. Many mammals may serve as reservoirs. The adult flukes live in the bile ducts and are acquired by eating inadequately cooked infected fish, including pickled and salted fish. Flukes are hermaphrodite and fertilized ova are passed in the stool. Further development takes place in freshwater molluscs and then fish.

After ingestion of infected fish, larvae are released in the upper gut and immature flukes ascend the biliary tree and grow to maturity. Adults generally have heaviest infections. In nonendemic countries cases occur in immigrants or travelers or following consumption of infected imported fish products. Infection may be asymptomatic or associated with acute or chronic symptoms. During migration of the larvae an acute febrile illness occurs associated with hepatosplenomegaly, jaundice and eosinophilia. In heavy chronic infections the flukes cause inflammation in the biliary tree with pericholangitis followed by periductal fibrosis, focal obstruction and intrahepatic biliary calculi. Secondary pyogenic cholangitis and hepatic abscess formation may follow biliary obstruction with dead flukes, with or without intrahepatic choledocholithiasis. Late in the disease there may be biliary cirrhosis and portal hypertension. The risk of cholangiocarcinoma is enhanced after long periods of infection (Chan & Lam 1987).

The diagnosis is often suggested by the clinical and epidemiological setting. The organism can be detected by finding eggs in the stool. Eggs may also be found on examination of duodenal aspirates. There may be eosinophilia or neutrophilia when pyogenic sepsis supervenes. An elevated serum alkaline phosphatase concentration is usual when there is biliary obstruction. Endoscopic retrograde cholangiography may show the typical uniform size slender filling defects in dilated intrahepatic ducts with wall irregularities and tortuosities (Choi et al 1984). Biliary calculi may also be evident. A variety of imaging procedures may be necessary to delineate the complications of infection, particularly hepatic abscess.

Praziquantel 75 mg/kg in three divided doses on a single day effectively kills the flukes. Calculous biliary disease and hepatobiliary sepsis are treated in the usual fashion. Thorough cooking of freshwater fish will prevent infection.

*Fascioliasis*

Adult *Fasciola hepatica* infect sheep in many tropical and temperate countries. The adult worm is found in the biliary ducts of the definitive host and eggs are passed in the stool. Further development occurs in freshwater molluscs and released cercariae encyst on water vegetation to be ingested by sheep. Infection occurs sporadically in humans after eating infected uncooked water plants, especially watercress. From the duodenum the parasite migrates through the intestinal wall to the peritoneal cavity and from there through the liver capsule to enter the liver parenchyma and so to reach the bile ducts. Clinical manifestations during the invasive stage include fever, painful hepatomegaly, jaundice, urticaria, diarrhea and eosinophilia (Chan & Lam 1987). Eggs appear in the stool about 4 months after infection.

In the bile ducts *F. hepatica* may cause biliary obstruction with hyperplasia of the ductal epithelium and periportal fibrosis. Cholangitis and jaundice may occur and stones may also form. Cirrhosis and cholangiocarcinoma do not usually occur. Leukocytosis and eosinophilia are common in the acute phase and eosinophilia is chronically present. Liver enzymes may reflect biliary obstruction. Diagnosis depends on recognition of eggs (which closely resemble *F. buski*) in the stool or duodenal aspirates. Serological tests have been developed but their role is uncertain. The differential diagnosis of fever, hepatomegaly and eosinophilia due to liver flukes includes visceral larva migrans and tropical eosinophilia of filarial origin. Bithional has been used for treatment and praziquantel has been used more recently, as described for clonorchiasis. Infection can be prevented by avoiding uncooked water plants in endemic regions.

REFERENCES


Acheson D W K, Donohue-Rolfe A, Keusch G T 1991 The family of Shiga and Shiga-like toxins In: Alouf J E, Freer J H (eds) Sourcebook of bacterial protein toxins. Academic Press, London, p 415–534

Alam A N, Alam N H, Ahmed T, Sack D A 1990 Randomised double-blind trial of single dose doxycycline for treating cholera in adults. British Medical Journal 300: 1619–1621

Alp M H, Hislop I G 1969 The effect of *Giardia lamblia* infestation on the gastro-intestinal tract. Australian Annals of Medicine 18: 232–237

Ambrose N S, Hutchison S, Tejan J 1989 Folate deficiency due to giardiasis. Journal of the Royal Society of Medicine 82(1): 48–49

Ament M E, Ochs H D, Davis S D 1973 Structure and function of the gastrointestinal tract in primary immunodeficiency syndromes: a study of 39 patients. Medicine 52: 227–248

Arvind A S, Shetty N, Farthing M J G 1988 Serodiagnosis of amoebiasis. Serodiagnosis and Immunotherapy 2: 79–84

Bartlett J G 1984 Treatment of antibiotic-associated pseudomembranous colitis. Reviews of Infectious Diseases 6: S235

Bartlett J G 1985 Treatment of Clostridium difficile colitis. Gastroenterology 89: 1192

Bastani B, Shariatzdeh M R, Dehdashti F 1985 Tuberculous peritonitis – report of 30 cases and review of the literature. Quarterly Journal of Medicine 56: 549–557

Bendall R P, Lucas S, Moody A, Tovey G, Chiodini P L 1993 Diarrhoea associated with cyanobacterium-like bodies: a new coccidian enteritis of man. Lancet 341: 590–592

Bier J W, Deardorff T L, Jackson G J, Raybourne R B 1987 Human anisakiasis. In: Pawlowski Z S (ed) Baillière's clinical tropical medicine and communicable diseases. Intestinal helminthic infections. Baillière Tindall, London, p 723–733

Black R E, Levine M M, Clements M L, Hughes T P, Blaser M J 1988 Experimental *Campylobacter jejuni* infections in humans. Journal of Infectious Diseases 157: 472–479

Blaser M J, Reller L B 1981 *Campylobacter enteritis*. New England Journal of Medicine 305: 1444–1452

Blenkinsopp W K, Gibdon J A, Haffenden G P 1978 Giardiasis and severe jejunal abnormality. Lancet 1: 994

Blumenthal D S, Schultz M G 1975 Incidence of intestinal obstruction in children infected with *Ascaris lumbricoides*. American Journal of Tropical Medicine and Hygiene 24: 801–805

Bolton R P, Culshaw M A 1986 Faecal metronidazole concentrations during oral and intravenous therapy for antibiotic associated colitis due to *Clostridium difficile*. Gut 27: 1169

Booth M, Bundy D A P 1992 Comparative prevalences of *Ascaris lumbricoides*, *Trichuris trichiura* and hookworm infections and the prospects for combined control. Parasitology 105: 151–157

Boreham P F, Phillips R E 1986 Giardiasis in Mt Isa, north west Queensland. Medical Journal of Australia 144: 524–528

Bottone E J, Sheehan D J 1983 *Yersinia enterocolitica*: guidelines for serologic diagnosis of human infections. Reviews of Infectious Diseases 5: 898–906

Buckley A 1986 Severe megaloblastic anaemia due to giardiasis. British Medical Journal 292: 992

Bukholm G, Kapperud G 1987 Expression of *Campylobacter jejuni* invasiveness in cell cultures co-infected with other bacteria. Infection and Immunity 55: 2816–2821

Bundy D A P 1994 The global burden of intestinal nematode disease. Transactions of the Royal Society of Tropical Medicine and Hygiene 88: 259–261

Bundy D A P, Hall A, Medley G F, Savioli L 1992 Evaluating measures to control intestinal parasite infections. World Health Statistics Quarterly 45: 168–179

Bunyaratvej S, Bunyawongwiroj P, Nitiyanant P 1982 Human intestinal sarcosporidiosis: report of six cases. American Journal of Tropical Medicine and Hygiene 31: 36–41

Bryceson ADM, Woestenborghs R, Michiels M, van den Bossche H 1982. Bioavailability and tolerability of mebendazole in patients with inoperable hydatid disease. Transactions of the Royal Society of Tropical Medicine and Hygiene 76: 563–564

Cappell M S, Philogene C 1993 *Clostridium difficile* infection is a treatable cause of diarrhea in patients with advanced human immunodeficiency virus infection: a study of seven consecutive patients admitted from 1986 to 1992 to a university teaching hospital. American Journal of Gastroenterology 88: 891–897

Casemore D P, Armstrong M, Jackson F B 1984 Screening for cryptosporidium in stools. Lancet 2: 734–735

Cervello A, Alfaro A, Chumillas M J 1993 Hypokalemic myopathy induced by *Giardia lamblia*. New England Journal of Medicine 329: 210–211

Chan C W, Lam S K 1987 Diseases caused by liver flukes and cholangiocarcinoma. In: Gyr K E (ed) Baillière's clinical gastroenterology. Tropical gastroenterology. Baillière Tindall, London 1: 297–318

Choi T K, Wong K P, Wong J 1984 Cholangiographic appearance in clonorchiasis. British Journal of Radiology 37: 681–684

Cholera Working Group ICDDR 1993 Large epidemics of cholera-like disease in Bangladesh caused by *Vibrio cholerae* O139 synonym Bengal. Lancet 342: 387–390

Clark C G, Diamond L S 1991 Ribosomal RNA genes of "pathogenic" and "non-pathogenic" *Entamoeba histolytica* are distinct. Molecular and Biochemical Parastiology 49: 297–302

Clemens J D, Sack DA, Harris J R 1990 Field trial of oral cholera vaccines in Bangladesh: results from longterm follow-up. Lancet 335: 270–273

Cook G C 1985 Tuberculosis – certainly not a disease of the past. Quarterly Journal of Medicine 56: 519–521

Cook G C 1994 *Enterobius vermicularis* infection. Gut 35: 1159–1162
Cooper E S, Spencer J, Whyte-Alleng C A M et al 1991 Immediate hypersensitivity in the colon of children with chronic *Trichuris trichiura* dysentery. Lancet 338: 1104–1107
Cowen A E, Campbell C B 1973 Giardiasis – cause of vitamin $B_{12}$ malabsorption. American Journal of Digestive Diseases 18(5): 384–390
Croese J, Loukas A, Opdebeeck J, Prociv P 1994 Occult enteric infection by *Ancylostoma caninum*: a previously unrecognised zoonosis. Gastroenterology 106: 3–12
Cross J H 1992 Intestinal capillariasis. Clinical Microbiological Reviews 5: 120
Cukor G, Blacklow NR 1984 Human viral gastroenteritis. Microbiological Reviews 48: 157–159
Davis A 1986 Recent advances in schistosomiasis. Quarterly Journal of Medicine 58: 95–110
Deluol A M, Mechali D, Cenac J, Savel J, Coulaud JP 1980 Incidence and clinical aspects of intestinal coccidioses in a tropical medicine practice. Bulletin de la Societe de Pathologie Exotique 73: 259–265
Desai H I, Chandra R K 1982 Giardiasis. In: Chandra R K (ed) Critical reviews in tropical medicine, vol 1. Plenum Press, New York, p 109
Despommier D D 1992 Tapeworm infection – the long and the short of it. New England Journal of Medicine 327: 727–728
Donnenberg M S, Kaper J B 1992 Enteropathogenic *Escherichia coli*. Infection and Immunity 60: 3953–3961
Doyle P W, Helgason M M, Mathias R G, Proctor E M 1990 Epidemiology and pathogenicity of *Blastocystis hominis*. Journal of Clinical Microbiology 28: 116–121
Duncombe V M, Bolin T D, Davis A E, Cummins A G, Crouch R L 1978 Histopathology in giardiasis: a correlation with diarrhoea. Australian and New Zealand Journal of Medicine 8: 392–396
DuPont H L, Reves R R, Galindo E, Sullivan P S, Wood L V, Mendiola J G 1982 Treatment of travelers' diarrhoea with trimethoprim/sulfamethoxazole and with trimethoprim alone. New England Journal of Medicine 307: 841–844
DuPont H L, Galindo E, Evans D G, Cabada F J, Sullivan P, Evans D J 1983 Prevention of travelers' diarrhea with trimethoprim-sulfamethoxazole and trimethoprim alone. Gastroenterology 84: 75–80
Echeverria P, Sethabutr O, Pitarangsi C 1991 Microbiology and diagnosis of infections with *Shigella* and enteroinvasive *Escherichia coli*. Reviews of Infectious Diseases 13 (S4): S220–225
Epstein P R, Ford TE, Colwell R R 1993 Marine ecosystems. Lancet 342: 1216–1219
Farthing M J G 1991 5-hydroxytryptamine and 5-hydroxytryptamine-3 receptor antagonists. Scandinavian Journal of Gastroenterology 26 (suppl 188): 92–100
Farthing M J G 1993 Pathophysiology of infective diarrhoea. European Journal of Gastroenterology and Hepatology 5: 796–807
Farthing M J G, Katelaris P H, Dias J, Munzer D, Popovic O 1993 Bacterial and parasitic infections in Europe. Gastroenterology International 6: 149–166
Fasano A, Kay B A, Russell R G et al 1991 *Vibrio cholerae* produces a second enterotoxin which affects intestinal tight junctions. Proceedings of the National Academy of Science 88: 5242–5246
Fayer R, Ungar B L P 1986 *Cryptosporidium* spp. and cryptosporidiosis. Microbiology Reviews 50: 458–483
Feachem R G 1982 Environmental aspects of cholera epidemiology: III Transmission and control. Tropical Diseases Bulletin 79: 1–47
Formal S B, Hale T L, Sansonetti P 1982 Invasive enteric pathogens. Reviews of Infectious Diseases 5: S702–S707
Genta R M, Gatti S, Linke M J, Cevini C, Scaglia M 1988 Endemic *Strongyloides* in Northern Italy: clinical and immunological aspects. Quarterly Journal of Medicine 68: 679–690
Gilman R H 1982 Hookworm disease: host-pathogen biology. Reviews of Infectious Diseases 4: 824–829
Gilman R H, Chong T H, David C, Greenberg B, Virik H K, Dixon H B 1983 The adverse consequences of heavy *Trichuris* infection. Transactions of the Royal Society of Tropical Medicine and Hygiene 77: 432–438
Goka A K J, Rolston D D, Mathan V I, Farthing M J G 1990a The relative merits of faecal and duodenal juice microscopy in the diagnosis of giardiasis. Transactions of the Royal Society of Tropical Medicine and Hygiene 84: 66–67
Goka A K J, Rolston D D K, Mathan V I, Farthing M J G 1990b Diagnosis of *Strongyloides* and hookworm infections: comparison of faecal and duodenal fluid microscopy. Transactions of the Royal Society of Tropical Medicine and Hygiene 84: 829–831
Gottstein B 1992 Molecular and immunological diagnosis of echinococcosis. Clinical Microbiological Reviews 5: 248–261
Groll E 1980 Praziquantel for cestode infections in man. Acta Tropica 37: 393–396
Grove D I 1980 Strongyloidiasis in allied ex-prisoners of war in south-east Asia. British Medical Journal I: 598–601
Guerrant R L, Wanke C A, Pennie R A, Barrett L J, Lima A, O'Brien A D 1987 Production of a unique cytotoxin by *Campylobacter jejuni*. Infection and Immunity 55: 2526–2530
Haffejee I E 1991 The pathophysiology, clinical features and management of rotavirus diarrhoea. Quarterly Journal of Medicine 79: 289–299
Hall A 1993 Intestinal parasitic worms and the growth of children. Transactions of the Royal Society of Tropical Medicine and Hygiene 87: 241–242
Harinasuta T, Bunnag D, Radomyos P 1987 Intestinal fluke infections. In: Pawlowski Z S (ed) Baillière's clinical tropical medicine and communicable diseases. Intestinal helminthic infections. Baillière Tindall, London 2: 695–721
Hartong W A, Gourley W K, Arvanitakis C 1979 Giardiasis: clinical spectrum and functional-structural abnormalities of the small intestinal mucosa. Gastroenterology 77: 61–69
Heyworth M F 1989 Intestinal IgA responses to *Giardia muris* in mice depleted of helper T lymphocytes and in immunocompetent mice. Journal of Parasitology 75(2): 246–251
Hoberman L J, Eigenbrodt E H, Kilman W J et al 1976 Colitis associated with oral clindamycin therapy: a clinical study of 16 patients. American Journal of Digestive Diseases 21: 1
Hoogkampe-Korstanje A 1987 Antibiotics in *Yersinia enterocolitica* infections. Journal of Antimicrobial Chemotherapy 20: 123–131
Hoskins L C, Winawer S J, Broitman S A, Gottleib L S, Zamchek N 1967 Clinical giardiasis and intestinal malabsorption. Gastroenterology 53: 265–279
Hubert B, Bacou J, Belveze H 1989 Epidemiology of human anisakiasis: incidence and sources in France. American Journal of Tropical Medicine and Hygiene 40: 301–303
Hulbert T V, Larsen R A, Chandrasoma P T 1992 Abdominal angiostrongyliasis mimicking acute appendicitis and Meckel's diverticulum: report of a case in the United States and review. Clinical Infectious Diseases 14: 836–840
Iversen A M, Gill M, Bartlett C L R 1987 Two outbreaks of foodborne gastroenteritis caused by a small round structured virus: evidence of prolonged infectivity in a food handler. Lancet 2: 556–558
Jerse A E, Kaper J B 1991 The *eae* gene of enteropathogenic *Escherichia coli* encodes a 94 kilodalton membrane protein, the expression of which is influenced by the EAF plasmid. Infection and Immunity 59: 4302–4309
Jokipii L, Jokipii A M M 1990 Nitroimidazole treatment of giardiasis. In: Meyer E A (ed) Giardiasis. Human parasitic diseases, Vol 3. Elsevier, Amsterdam, p 315–323
Jones G W, Rabert D K, Svinarich D M, Whitfield H J 1982 Association of adhesive, invasive and virulent phenotypes of *Salmonella typhimurium* with autonomous 66-megadalton plasmids. Infection and Immunity 38: 476–486
Kapikian A Z, Wyatt R G, Dolin R, Thornhill T S, Kalica A R, Chanock R M 1972 Visualization by immune electron microscopy of a 27-nm particle associated with acute infectious non-bacterial gastroenteritis. Journal of Virology 10: 1075–1081
Katelaris P H 1992 Intestinal parasitoses in Europe. European Journal of Gastroenterology and Hepatology 4: 771–777
Katelaris P H, Seow F, Ngu M C 1991 The effect of *Giardia lamblia* trophozoites on lipolysis *in vitro*. Parasitology 103: 35–39
Katelaris P H, Farthing M J G 1992 Diarrhoea and malabsorption in giardiasis: a multifactorial process. Gut 33: 295–297
Kelly C P, Pothoulakis C, LaMont J T 1994 *Clostridium difficile* colitis. New England Journal of Medicine 330: 257–262
Keusch G T 1988 Antimicrobial therapy for enteric infections and typhoid fever: state of the art. Reviews of Infectious Diseases 10: S199–S205

Keusch G T, Bennish M L 1989 Shigellosis: recent progress, persisting problems and research issues. Pediatric Infectious Diseases Journal 8: 713–719

Khuroo M S, Zaregar S A, Mahajan R 1990 Hepatobiliary and pancreatic ascariasis in India. Lancet 335: 1503–1506

Kociecka W 1987 Intestinal trichinellosis. In: Pawlowski Z S (ed) Baillière's clinical tropical medicine and communicable diseases. Intestinal helminthic infections. Baillière Tindall, London 2: 755–764

Korman S H, Bar-Oz B, Mandelberg A, Mototh I 1990 Giardiasis with protein-losing enteropathy: diagnosis by fecal $\alpha_1$-antitrypsin determination. Journal of Pediatric Gastroenterology and Nutrition 10: 249

Levine M M 1987 *Escherichia coli* that cause diarrhea: enterotoxigenic, enteropathogenic, enteroinvasive, enterhemorrhagic and enteroadherent. Journal of Infectious Diseases 155: 377–389

Levine M M, Kaper J B, Herrington D 1988 Safety, immunogenicity and efficacy in man of recombinant live oral cholera vaccines, CVD 103 and CVD 103-HgR. Lancet ii: 467–470

Levinson J D, Nastro L J 1978 Giardiasis with total villous strophy. Gastroenterology 74(2): 271–275

Lewis E A, Antia A U 1969 Amoebic colitis: review of 295 cases. Transactions of the Royal Society of Tropical Medicine and Hygiene 63: 633–638

Lund B M 1990 Foodborne disease due to *Bacillus* and *Clostridium* species. Lancet 336: 982–986

MacDonald T T, Choy M Y, Spencer J et al 1991 Histopathology and immunohistochemistry of the caecum in children with *Trichuris* dysentery syndrome. Journal of Clinical Pathology 44: 191–199

McFarland L V, Mulligan M R, Kwok R Y Y, Stamm W E 1989 Nosocomial acquisition of *Clostridium difficile* infection. New England Journal of Medicine 320: 204–210

McFarland L V, Surawicz C M, Greenberg R N et al 1994 A randomized placebo-controlled trial of Saccharomyces boulardii in combination with standard antibiotics for Clostridium difficile disease Journal of the American Medical Association 271: 1913–1918

Maurelli A T, Baudry B, d'Hauteville II, Hale T L, Sansonetti P J 1985 Cloning of plasmid DNA sequences involved in invasion of HeLa cells by *Shigella flexneri*. Infection and Immunity 49: 164–171

Maxwell C, Hussain R, Nutman T B et al 1987 The clinical and immunological responses of normal human volunteers to a low dose hookworm (*Necator americanus*) infection. American Journal of Tropical Medicine and Hygiene 37: 126–134

Miotti P G, Gilman R H, Santosham M, Ryder R W, Yolken R H 1986 Age-related rate of seropositivity and antibody to *Giardia lamblia* in four diverse populations. Journal of Clinical Microbiology 24: 972–975

Mohamed A E, Karawi M A, Yasawy M I 1990 Schistosomal colonic disease. Gut 31: 439–442

Moore G T, Cross W M, McGuire D et al 1969 Epidemic giardiasis at a ski resort. New England Journal of Medicine 281: 402–407

Morgan J S, Schaffner W, Stone W J 1986 Opportunistic strongyloidiasis in renal transplant recipients. Transplantation 42: 518–524

Morgante P E, Gandara M A, Sterle E 1989 The endoscopic diagnosis of colonic tuberculosis. Gastrointestinal Endoscopy 35: 115–118

Nash T E, Herrington D A, Losonsky G A, Levine M M 1987 Experimental human infections with *Giardia lamblia*. Journal of Infectious Diseases 156(6): 974–984

Nokes C, Grantham-McGregor S M, Sawyer A W, Cooper E S, Robinson B A, Bundy D A P 1992 Moderate to heavy infections of *Trichuris trichiura* affect cognitive function in Jamaican schoolchildren. Parasitology 104: 539–547

Ochs H D, Ament M E, Davis S D 1972 Giardiasis with malabsorption in X-linked agammaglobulinemia. New England Journal of Medicine 287: 342–342

Olgivie B M, de Savigny D 1982 Immune response to nematodes. In: Cohen S, Warren K S (eds) Immunology of parasitic infections, 2nd edn. Blackwell, Oxford, p 715–

Orenstein J M, Zierdt C W, Zierdt C, Kotler D P 1990 Identification of spores of *Enterocytozoon bieneusi* in stool and duodenal fluid from AIDS patients. Lancet 336: 1127–1128

Ormerod J P 1990 Chemotherapy and management of tuberculosis in the United Kingdom: Recommendations of the Joint Tuberculosis Committee of the British Thoracic Society. Thorax 45: 403–408

Ortega Y R, Sterling C R, Gilman R H, Cama V A, Diaz F 1993 Cyclospora species – a new protozoan pathogen of humans. New England Journal of Medicine 328: 1308–1312

Palmer K R, Patil D H, Basran G S, Riordan J F, Silk D B A 1985 Abdominal tuberculosis in urban Britain – a common disease. Gut 26: 1296–1305

Pape J W, Verdier R-I, Johnson Jr W D 1989 Treatment and prophylaxis of *Isospora belli* infection in patients with the acquired immunodeficiency syndrome. New England Journal of Medicine 320: 1044–1047

Pawlowski Z S 1984 Cestodiasis: taeniasis, diphyllobothriasis, hymenolipiasis and others. In: Warren K S, Mahmoud A A F (eds) Tropical and geographic medicine. McGraw Hill, New York, p 471–486

Pawlowski Z S 1987 Ascariasis. In: Pawlowski Z S (ed) Baillière's clinical tropical medicine and communicable diseases. Intestinal helminthic infections. Baillière Tindall, London 2: 595–616

Perlman D M, Ampel N M, Schifman R B et al 1988 Persistent *Campylobacter jejuni* infections in patients infected with human immunodeficiency virus (HIV). Annals of Internal Medicine 108: 540–545

Petri W A, Smith R D, Schlesinger P H, Murphy C F, Ravdin J I 1987 Isolation of the galactose-binding lectin that mediates the *in vitro* adherence of *Entamoeba histolytica*. Journal of Clinical Investigation 80: 1238–1244

Pickering L K, Engelkirk P G 1990 *Giardia* among children in day care. In: Meyer E A (ed) Giardiasis. Human parasitic diseases, Vol 3. Elsevier, Amsterdam, p 295–303

Pitarangsi C, Echeverria P, Whitmire R et al 1982 Enteropathogenicity of *Aeromonas hydrophila* and *Plesiomonas shigelloides*: prevalence among individuals with and without diarrhea in Thailand. Infection and Immunity 35: 666–673

Price A B, Davies D R 1977 Pseudomembranous colitis. Journal of Clinical Pathology 30: 1

Public Health Laboratory Service Study 1990 Cryptosporidiosis in England and Wales: prevalence and clinical and epidemiological features. British Medical Journal 300: 774–777

Rampling A, Upson R, Ward LR, Anderson JR, Peters E, Rowe B 1989 *Salmonella enteritidis* phase type 4 infection of broiler chickens: a hazard to public health. Lancet ii: 436–438

Rao S S C, Edwards C A, Austen C J, Bruce C, Read N W 1988 Impaired colonic fermentation of carbohydrate after ampicillin. Gastroenterology 94: 928–932

Ravdin J E 1990 Cell biology of *Entamoeba histolytica* and immunology of amebiasis. In: Wyler D J (ed) Modern parasite biology. W H Freeman, New York, p 126–150

Reid J A, Caul E O, White D G, Palmer S R 1988 Role of infected food handler in hotel outbreak of Norwalk-like viral gastroenteritis: implications for control. Lancet ii: 321–323

Relman D A, Schmidt T M, MacDermott R P, Falkow S 1992 Identification of the uncultured bacillus of Whipple's disease. New England Journal of Medicine 327: 293–301

Richmond S J, Wood D J, Bailey A S 1988 Recent respiratory and enteric adenovirus infection in children in the Manchester area. Journal of the Royal Society of Medicine 8: 15–18

Roberts-Thomson I C 1987 Giardiasis: the role of immunological mechanisms to host-parasite relationships. In: Marsh M N (ed) Immunopathology of the small intestine. Wiley, Chichester, p 209

Rosengart T K, Coppa G F 1990 Abdominal mycobacterial infections in immunocompromised patients. American Journal of Surgery 159: 125–131

Sack R B 1975 Human diarrheal disease caused by enterotoxigenic *Escherichia coli*. Annual Reviews of Microbiology 29: 333–353

Salam I, Katalaris P, Leigh-Smith S, Farthing M J G 1994 A randomised placebo-controlled trial of single dose ciprofloxacin in treatment of travellers' diarrhoea. Lancet 344: 1537–1539

Sansonetti P J 1991 Genetic and molecular basis of epithelial cell invasion by *Shigella* spp. Reviews of Infectious Disease 13 (suppl 4): 285–292

Saphra I, Winter J W 1957 Clinical manifestations of salmonellosis in man. New England Journal of Medicine 256: 1128–1134

Schofield P F 1985 Abdominal tuberculosis. Gut 26: 1275–1278

Scott D A, Haberberger R L, Thornton S A, Hyam K C 1990 Norfloxacin for the prophylaxis of travelers' diarrhea in US military personnel. American Journal of Tropical Medicine and Hygiene 42: 160–164

Sharp J C M 1988 Salmonellosis and eggs. British Journal of Medicine 297: 1557–1558

Simmonds S D, Noble MA, Freeman HJ 1987 Gastrointestinal features of culture-positive *Yersinia enterocolitica* infection. Gastroenterology 92: 112–117

Smith H V 1990 Environmental aspects of *Cryptosporidium* species: a review. Journal of the Royal Society of Medicine 83: 629–631

Steffen R, Boppart I 1987 Travellers' diarrhoea. In: Gyr K E (ed). Tropical Gastroenterology. Baillière's clinical gastroenterology. Baillière Tindall, London 1: 361–376

Stephenson L S, Latham M C, Kurz K M, Kinoti S N, Brigham H 1989 Treatment with a single dose of albendazole improves growth of Kenyan schoolchildren with hookworm, *Trichuris trichiura*, and *Ascaris lumbricoides* infections. American Journal of Tropical Medicine and Hygiene 41: 78–87

Stephenson L S, Latham M C, Adams E J, Kinoti S N, Pertet A 1993 Weight gain of Kenyan schoolchildren infected with hookworm, *Trichuris trichiura*, and *Ascaris lumbricoides* is improved following once- or twice-yearly treatment with albendazole. Journal of Nutrition 123: 656–665

Strickland G T 1994 Gastrointestinal manifestations of schistosomiasis. Gut 35: 1334–1337

Strickland G T, Abdel-Wahab M F 1993 Abdominal ultrasonography for assessing morbidity from schistosomiasis. 1. Community studies. Transactions of the Royal Society of Tropical Medicine and Hygiene 87: 132-134.

Sumner H W, Tedesco F J 1975 Rectal biopsy in clindamycin-associated colitis. Archives of Pathology 99: 237

Taylor D N, Blaser MJ, Blacklow N, Echeverria P, Pitarangsi C, Cross J, Weniger B G 1985 Polymicrobial aetiology of travellers' diarrhoea. Lancet i: 381–383

Taylor D N, Houston R, Shlim D R, Bhaibulaya M, Ungar B L P, Echeverria P 1988 Etiology of diarrhea among travelers and foreign residents in Nepal. Journal of the American Medical Association 260: 1245–1248

Taylor D N, Sanchez J L, Candler W, Thornton S, McQueen C, Echeverria P 1991 Treatment of travelers' diarrhea: ciprofloxacin plus loperamide compared with ciprofloxacin alone. A placebo-controlled, randomized trial. Annals of Internal Medicine 114: 731–734

Teasley D G, Gerding D N, Olson M M et al 1983 Prospective randomised trial of metronidazole vs vancomycin for *Clostridium difficile*-associated diarrhoea and colitis. Lancet 2: 1043

Tedesco F J 1977 Clindamycin and colitis: a review. Journal of Infectious Diseases 135 (suppl 95):

Tedesco F J 1979 Antibiotic associated pseudomembranous colitis with negative proctosigmoidoscopy examination. Gastroenterology 77: 295

Tranter H S 1990 Foodborne staphylococcal illness. Lancet 336: 1044–1046

Trucksis M, Galen J E, Michalski J, Fasano A, Kaper J B 1993 Accessory cholera enterotoxin (ACE), the third toxin of *Vibrio cholerae* virulence cassette. Proceedings of the National Academy of Science 90: 5267–5271

Tzipori S 1983. Cryptosporidiosis in animals and humans. Microbiological Reviews 47: 84–96

Uhnoo I, Wadell G, Svensson L, Johansson M E 1984 Importance of enteric adenoviruses 40 and 41 in acute gastroenteritis in infants and young children. Journal of Clinical Microbiology 20: 365–372

Walzer P D, Judson F N, Murphy K B, Healey G R, English D K, Schultz M G 1973 Balantidiasis outbreak in Truk. American Journal of Tropical Medicine and Hygiene 22: 33–41

Wenisch C, Parschalk B, Hasenhundl M, Hirschl A M, Graninger W 1996 Comparison of vancomycin, teicoplanin, metronidazole and fusidic acid for treatment of *Clostridium difficile*-associated diarrhoea. Clinical Infectious Diseases 22: 813–818

Wilson K H, Blitchington R, Frothingham R, Wilson J A P 1991 Phylogeny of the Whipple's disease associated bacterium. Lancet 338: 474–475

Wolfe M S 1978 *Oxyuris*, *Trichostrongylus* and *Trichuris*. Clinical Gastroenterology 7: 201–217

Wolfe M S 1990 Clinical symptoms and diagnosis by traditional methods. In: Meyer E A (ed) Giardiasis. Human parasitic diseases, Vol 3. Elsevier, Amsterdam, p 175–185

Wolfson J S, Richter J M, Waldron M A, Weber D J, McCarthy D M, Hopkins C C 1985 Cryptosporidiosis in immunocompetent patients. New England Journal of Medicine 312: 1278–1282

Wright S G, Tomkins A M, Ridley D S 1977 Giardiasis: clinical and therapeutic aspects. Gut 18(4): 343–350

Yamamoto T, Koyama Y, Matsunoto M et al 1992 Localized aggregative and diffuse adherence to HeLa cells, plastic and human small intestines by *Escherichia coli* isolated from patients with diarrhea. Journal of Infectious Diseases 166: 1295–1310

Yardley J H, Takano J, Hendrix T R 1964 Epithelial and other mucosal lesions of the jejunum giardiasis. Jejunal biopsy studies. Bulletin of the Johns Hopkins Hospital 115: 389–406

Young G P, Bayley N, Ward P et al 1986 Antibiotic-associated colitis caused by *Clostridium difficile*: relapse and risk factors. Medical Journal of Australia 144: 303

Zierdt C H 1991 *Blastocystis hominis* – past and future. Clinical Microbiological Reviews 4: 61–79

# 21. HIV, AIDS and the gastrointestinal tract and liver

*R. P. Brettle*

## HIV RETROVIRUS

The original description of the acquired immune deficiency syndrome (AIDS) appeared in 1981 and since then cases have been noted in most parts of the world (Centers for Disease Control 1982). The causative virus involved in AIDS was isolated first in 1983 by Montagnier and propagated in a cell line by Gallo in 1984 (Barré-Sinoussi et al 1983, Gallo et al 1984). A variety of names was used for the virus, including LAV, ARV and HTLV-III, but these have all now been replaced by the term human immunodeficiency virus or HIV (Coffin et al 1986). HIV is an RNA retrovirus; it utilizes an enzyme known as DNA polymerase or reverse transcriptase to produce a DNA provirus that is able to insert itself into host DNA.

HIV preferentially infects lymphocytes that function as T helper cells. These cells are characterized by a specific receptor molecule known as CD4 after the monoclonal antibodies that specifically recognize the molecule. In addition to helper lymphocytes, this receptor molecule is found on 10–20% of monocytes or macrophages, Langerhans cells in the dermis and microglial cells in the central nervous system (Weber & Weiss 1988). The various viral proteins produced by HIV infection stimulate an immune response, although in many individuals this antibody immune response does not neutralize or protect against the virus.

HIV infection results in depletion of CD4 cells. Initially there is a balance between a huge production and clearance of the virus and the destruction and degeneration of CD4 cells (Ho et al 1995). Eventually, the numbers of CD4 cells are reduced due to their destruction. This suggests that antiviral therapy should be given early in the infection rather than be delayed until CD4 cells are reduced in number. It is also recognized that the spread of HIV outside the cells of the immune system occurs late in HIV infection and may lead to the presentation of disease in specific organs (Donaldson et al 1994).

AIDS is at present a fatal condition; at any one time, approximately 50% of the cumulative number of AIDS cases reported have died (Anonymous 1988a). Survival times vary with the type of presentation; the initial median survival time for patients with Kaposi's sarcoma in the absence of opportunistic infections was between 4 and 11 months (Moss et al 1984, Rivin et al 1984). This differential remains for some conditions but not others; for instance, the median survival of patients with Kaposi's sarcoma in Europe was 21 months between 1979 and 1989 compared to 28 months for tuberculosis, 20 months for *Pneumocystis carinii* pneumonia, 19 months for esophageal candidiasis, but only 15 months for toxoplasma encephalitis (Lundgren et al 1994). However, for any other condition the median survival was not more than 13 months (Lundgren et al 1994).

## CLASSIFICATION

The Centers for Disease Control (CDC) developed a descriptive classification system for HIV infection (Centers for Disease Control 1987) which essentially details four mutually exclusive categories or groups of HIV infection, as shown in Table 21.1. It includes a number of medical conditions such as thrombocytopenia, neuropathies, myopathy, dementia, wasting syndrome, recurrent bacter-

**Table 21.1** Classification of the effects of HIV infection

| CDC stage | Clinical description |
|---|---|
| I | Acute infection with seroconversion |
| II | Asymptomatic infection |
| III | Persistent generalized lymphadenopathy |
| IV | Symptomatic HIV disease |
| IVA | Constitutional symptoms and disease |
| IVB | Neurological disease |
| IVC | Immunodeficiency |
| IVC1 | 1982 CDC definition of AIDS |
| IVC2 | Infections outwith AIDS definition |
| IVD | Tumors in CDC definition of AIDS |
| IVE | Other, e.g. Hodgkin's disease, carcinoma, lymphoid interstitial pneumonia, symptomatic thrombocytopenia |

Note: CDC = Centers for Disease Control

ial infections, shingles, etc. related to HIV infection other than AIDS itself.

The CDC classification of HIV is not meant to describe the natural history of HIV infection, nor to suggest that every individual has to progress through all stages. It is hierarchical, however, in that staging progresses from II to IV and patients do not revert to earlier stages if the signs or symptoms settle. By contrast, CDC stage IV is subdivided into five subgroups (A–E) that are not mutually exclusive and patients may be included in one or more of the subgroups. The conditions detailed in stage IV contain all those conditions currently used for the definition of AIDS as well as others that indicate clinically significant HIV infection.

With the increasing availability of CD4 counts, a new World Health Organization/CDC classification system is increasingly being utilized (World Health Organization 1990, Centers for Disease Control 1992). It consists of three broad clinical stages: well or asymptomatic, HIV-related disease and AIDS combined with three stages of immunodeficiency as measured by either CD4 counts (≥500, 200–500 and ≤200 cells/mm$^3$) or lymphocyte counts (Table 21.2). When combined in a three-way table, there are thus nine possible stages.

In the United States, in addition to the clinical definition of AIDS (C1–C3), everyone with a CD4 count below 200 (A3, B3) is also to be classified as having AIDS. At present this laboratory definition of AIDS has not been adopted by Europe (Centers for Disease Control 1992). The CDC also proposed that three new clinical problems be added to the 1987 definition of AIDS (Centers for Disease Control 1992). These are invasive cervical cancer, two episodes of bacterial pneumonia in a 12-month period and pulmonary tuberculosis. These new clinical definitions of AIDS have recently been added to the UK and Australian definitions of AIDS.

**Table 21.2** WHO/CDC classification system for human immunodeficiency virus (HIV) infection

| Laboratory classification | | | Clinical category* | | |
|---|---|---|---|---|---|
| | Absolute CD4 *or* count | Total lymphocyte count (TLC) | A | B | C |
| 1 | ≥500/mm$^3$ | ≥2000/mm$^3$ | A1 | B1 | C1 |
| 2 | 201–499/mm$^3$ | 1001–1999/mm$^3$ | A2 | B2 | C2 |
| 3 | ≤200/mm$^3$ | ≤1000/mm$^3$ | A3 | B3 | C3 |

Clinical category A (asymptomatic disease): Acute infection with HIV; persistent generalized lymphadenopathy; asymptomatic. Conditions in groups B and C must be absent.
Clinical category B (symptomatic disease): Any symptomatic conditions not included in category C. Examples are bacterial infections, candidiasis (oral or vulvovaginal) for more than 1 month, cervical dysplasia or carcinoma, constitutional symptoms, oral hairy leukoplakia. Two distinct episodes of herpes zoster or involving more than one dermatome, idiopathic thrombocytopenic purpura, mycobacterium tuberculosis, peripheral neuropathy.
Clinical category C: Any condition that meets the 1987 CDC/WHO case definition for AIDS.

## EPIDEMIOLOGY OF HIV AND AIDS

The initial pattern of the epidemic was characteristic of a bloodborne or blood-associated virus, since transmission occurred via direct blood contact, via penetrative sexual intercourse in either sex and perinatally. Consequently, particular groups of individuals were most likely to be affected (Table 21.3).

The majority of HIV transmission in the US and Europe has involved homosexuals or bisexuals and injecting drug users, whereas in Africa it has always appeared to be a heterosexually transmitted disease (Clumeck 1989). In other areas of the world, HIV is seen as a sexually transmitted disease in individuals traveling to and from areas of high seroprevalence. Alternatively, HIV occurs because of the importation of infected blood products from areas of high seroprevalence. These patterns of spread have been designated types I, II and III respectively by the WHO (Chin 1988). In the United States, 70% of AIDS cases are associated with homosexual intercourse, 24% with drug use with or without homosexual intercourse, 2% with heterosexual intercourse, 2% with receiving blood transfusions and 1% with hemophilia (Anonymous 1993a). In Europe, however, injecting drug use is a commoner risk factor for AIDS than in the US and accounts for 34% of reported AIDS cases (Anonymous 1993b). Some 87% of these injection-related cases have been reported by just three countries (France, Italy and Spain). There is a small but increasing number of pediatric cases, the majority of which are associated with HIV infection in the mother (Anonymous 1993b). In the UK, 74% of AIDS cases have been associated with homosexual or bisexual intercourse, 11% with heterosexual intercourse, 4% with injecting drug use and 6% with blood products (Anonymous 1993c). The number of HIV reports by risk activity also shows a predominance of homosexual and bisexual transmission.

There appears to be little variation between the risk groups with regard to the clinical presentation of AIDS. In the US, figures available on the first 30 000 cases of AIDS notified to the CDC show that conditions such as Kaposi's sarcoma are unusual in the absence of homosexuality or bisexuality (Selik et al 1987). In drug users, Kaposi's sarcoma, cytomegalovirus and chronic cryptosporidiosis are all significantly less common than for all other risk groups notified with AIDS, while *Pneumocystis carinii* pneumonia, tuberculosis, esophageal candidiasis and extrapulmonary

**Table 21.3** Risk categories associated with human immunodeficiency virus (HIV) infection

| |
|---|
| Homosexuals or bisexuals |
| Heterosexual contacts of infected individuals |
| Injection drug users |
| Children of infected females |
| Blood product transfusion (e.g. coagulation factor*) |

*Particularly prior to availability of HIV tests in 1985.

cryptococcosis are all more common. However, in drug users the number of AIDS cases has been found to greatly under-represent the extent of serious HIV disease. For instance, in New York by 1986, for every AIDS-related death in a drug user there was one other as a consequence of such conditions as tuberculosis, endocarditis and bacterial pneumonia. Similar data have appeared from Europe. This problem may in part be overcome by the additional clinical conditions contained in the new AIDS definition (Centers for Disease Control 1992).

## CLINICAL FEATURES OF EARLY HIV INFECTION

### Primary HIV infection

***CDC stage I.*** During seroconversion to HIV a self-limiting illness frequently occurs, manifested as a "glandular fever"-like condition, meningoencephalitis or peripheral neuropathy. However, many seroconversions are subclinical. The incubation period (time from exposure to clinical symptoms of acute HIV infection) ranges from a few days to a few months. Seroconversion time, defined as time from infection to the detection of specific antibodies, may be from 8 days to 10 weeks after the onset of acute illness. Severe immunosuppression occurs during acute HIV infection and esophageal candidiasis has been reported during acute HIV infection, while other opportunistic infections such as tuberculous meningitis have been reported only 8 weeks after acute HIV infection.

### Early manifestations of HIV infection

***CDC stage II.*** These are individuals who are well or asymptomatic.

***CDC stage III.*** This stage shows enlarged lymph nodes (>1 cm) at two or more nonadjacent sites for longer than 3 months in the absence of any other illness to explain the findings (persistent generalized lymphadenopathy). Massive enlargement can occur and there may be other symptoms such as tiredness, lethargy, excessive sweating, aches and pains in muscles or joints.

### Late manifestations of HIV infection

***CDC stage IV* (subsections A–E).** This stage is usually more serious, although individuals may be relatively well. The symptoms and signs of AIDS-related complex (ARC), a term now no longer used, are all included in stage IV disease.

*CDC stage IVA* – constitutional symptoms of stage III and/or unexplained diarrhea, fever (>38°C) for longer than 1 month or unexplained weight loss of more than 10% of body weight.

*CDC stage IVB* – neurological problems (other than during stage I) such as neuropathy and myelopathy. In addition, cognitive and/or motor dysfunction, loss of memory and loss of skills such as mental arithmetic or decision making may occur. Relatives may notice changes in personality, frank mental illness, dementia or loss of consciousness. If no other pathogens are found, it is assumed to result from HIV encephalopathy, which is now considered to be a feature of AIDS.

*CDC stage IVC* – infection secondary to immunodeficiency divided into two subgroups, IVC1 and IVC2:

CDC stage IVC1 – one or more of 12 infections that formed the basis of the original CDC definition of AIDS.

CDC stage IVC2 – infections commonly associated with serious HIV but not in the original description of AIDS, such as recurrent salmonella bacteremia, extensive herpes zoster, recurrent oral candidiasis, oral hairy leukoplakia and tuberculosis.

*CDC stage IVD* – cancers associated with HIV. As with IVC1, some of these conditions also fulfill the CDC definition of AIDS, e.g. Kaposi's sarcoma. Also cancers of the lymph nodes such as non-Hodgkin's lymphoma or primary lymphoma of the brain.

*CDC stage IVE* – conditions not yet described or not yet understood such as chronic lymphoid interstitial pneumonitis.

## LONG-TERM CONSEQUENCES OF HIV INFECTION

The major effect of HIV appears to be damage to cell-mediated immunity resulting in susceptibility to opportunistic infections. This deficiency is usually associated with infections due to intracellular organisms or the appearance of tumors, with depletion of peripheral blood CD4 lymphocytes, and in adults with reasonable B-cell immunity although recurrent bacterial infections do occur in some individuals. In children, where, depending upon age, B-cell immunity may be immature, the patient may be rendered effectively hypogammaglobulinemic. Particular immunological defects noted in patients with HIV infection include leukopenia and lymphopenia, loss of CD4 lymphocytes from the peripheral blood, hypergammaglobulinemia, skin anergy, decreased in vitro lymphocyte proliferation, cytotoxic T-cell response and antibody production to new antigens, and elevated levels of immune complexes, acid labile $\alpha$-interferon and $\beta_2$-microglobulin.

## LABORATORY MARKERS OF DISEASE PROGRESSION FROM HIV TO AIDS

Laboratory and clinical markers predicting rapid progression to AIDS may appear very early in HIV infection. In one study, patients who had an acute seroconversion illness lasting longer than 14 days had a progression rate of

78% in 3 years compared to those who were symptom free or who had minor symptoms. Primary humoral responses to HIV proteins may also be associated with clinical outcome of infection, as patients with high and persistent antibody responses to core viral proteins seem to progress to AIDS more slowly.

### Lymphocyte subsets estimations

The CD4 lymphocyte seems to be the main target cell for HIV and the primary immunological defect in patients with AIDS is severe depletion of CD4 lymphocytes. As HIV infection progresses, there is a progressive decline in the percentage and number of CD4 cells. Patients with an absolute CD4 count below 200 cells/mm$^3$ or a rapidly falling CD4 count have a greater chance of progression, while patients with CD4 counts higher than 500 have a much lower probability of progression. This correlation between low and/or declining CD4 counts and disease progression is well established in the various risk groups.

The number of CD8 cells declines shortly before the development of AIDS. In some studies, high numbers of CD8 cells predicted a rapid decline in CD4 cells and it is possible that CD4/CD8 ratio may be a better predictor of rapid progression to AIDS than the absolute number of CD4 cells.

### HIV serological markers

Low titers or absence of antibodies to core viral proteins correlate strongly with rapid disease progression, as does the appearance of these viral proteins in serum.

### Other immunological markers

A variety of immunological parameters have been associated with HIV disease progression, but most of them are impractical for everyday clinical practice and are also expensive. However, elevated serum IgA and $\beta_2$-microglobulin concentrations are predictive of clinical progression.

## PROGRESSION FROM HIV TO AIDS

The explanation for progression from early HIV to AIDS is unknown, but the rate of progression to AIDS may be described reasonably accurately for groups of patients and is detailed in Table 21.4 for different durations of infection. The median time for progression from infection to AIDS has now risen to 11 years. Another way to look at progression is to consider the risk for individual patients, which seems on average to be around 8% per year. A number of factors could be involved including genetic susceptibility, gender, pregnancy, risk activity, coinfection with other viruses and age. A number of markers of progression have been described including age of the patient, low numbers of CD4 lymphocytes, immune thrombocytopenic purpura, the presence of HIV antigen in serum and rising levels of $\beta_2$-microglobulin. The risk of progression can be predicted approximately according to CD4 counts (Table 21.5).

**Table 21.4** Rates of progression to AIDS after infection with HIV

| Time from infection (years) | Percentage progressing to AIDS |
|---|---|
| 2 | 0–2 |
| 4 | 5–10 |
| 6 | 10–25 |
| 8 | 30–40 |
| 10 | 51 |

**Table 21.5** Annual risk of progression to AIDS according to CD4 count

| CD4 lymphocytes (cells/mm$^3$) | Percentage progression to AIDS per year |
|---|---|
| >500 | 1 |
| 350–500 | 3 |
| 200–350 | 10–12 |
| <200 | 20 |

## SURVIVAL AFTER AIDS

While survival has improved from around 6 months, only about 50% of patients with AIDS survive 1 year, 25–40% 2 years and 5–20% 3–4 years. In the author's experience, the median survival from fulfilling the 1987 definition of AIDS is 20 months; survival is 40 months when the CD4 count falls to 200 cells/mm$^3$ (Brettle et al 1993). A patient with the 1992 definition of AIDS (one CD4 count <200) has a median survival of 50 months. Survival rates at 2 years are respectively 42% (1987 AIDS), 71% (CD4 count of <200 cells/mm$^3$ $\times$ 2) and 80% (CD4 count of <200/mm$^3$ $\times$ 1).

## GASTROINTESTINAL CLINICAL PROBLEMS OF HIV

The clinical problems of HIV and AIDS may be conveniently classified in relation to the various anatomical systems such as pulmonary, gastrointestinal, skin or neurological. However, many HIV complications such as infections or tumors are multisystem, although they may have a predominant presentation in one system. *Pneumocystis carinii* pneumonia, for example, generally presents with respiratory symptoms but pneumocystis abscesses may develop elsewhere, for instance in the eye, brain or liver. This is a problem to be aware of, particularly in those on aerosolized prophylaxis. As a consequence, all physicians need to be aware of the potential multisystem presentation of a variety of pathogens.

### Frequency of gastrointestinal problems in HIV and AIDS

Although risk activity overall seems not to affect presentation, the author's experience has been that gastrointestinal problems such as diarrhea are uncommon in drug users either because they have had relatively little exposure to gut pathogens prior to acquiring HIV or because self-administered opiates suppress the symptoms. In Edinburgh, Scotland, the cumulative frequency of early clinical manifestations over a period of 7 years in a cohort of over 600 individuals (70% drug-related) were: minor skin problems (9%), minor bacterial infections (4%), major bacterial problems (6.5%), oral thrush (16%), oral hairy leukoplakia (12%), significant weight loss of >10% (8.5%) and HIV-related thrombocytopenia (4%). Thus, while overall the gastrointestinal manifestations accounted for around one-third of the non-AIDS clinical problems, diarrhea itself was an uncommon early clinical problem.

Particular conditions at the time of diagnosis of AIDS included multiple index events and single events. Eleven percent had multiple index conditions at presentation, the commonest of which was *Pneumocystis carinii* pneumonia in conjunction with other opportunistic infections and this occurred in 7% of the index diagnoses. In the remainder, AIDS was diagnosed via a single event: *Pneumocystis carinii* pneumonia alone (51%), esophageal candidiasis (15%), Kaposi's sarcoma (5.5%), HIV dementia (4%), atypical mycobacteria (4%), cerebral toxoplasmosis (2.5%), lymphoma (2%), cytomegalovirus disease (1.5%) and extrapulmonary tuberculosis (1.5%). Thus, *Pneumocystis carinii* pneumonia was involved in 58% of the AIDS index conditions. In Edinburgh, esophageal candidiasis was commoner in drug users than in homosexuals, although this has not been reported by others.

In the author's practice in Edinburgh, the cumulative chance of an individual patient developing AIDS-related conditions were as follows: *Pneumocystis carinii* pneumonia (91%), esophageal candidiasis (28%), Kaposi's sarcoma (11%), disseminated *Mycobacterium avium intracellulare* (29%), HIV dementia (10%), cytomegalovirus disease (21%), extrapulmonary tuberculosis (2%). Expressed as a rate per 100 person-years of AIDS, the morbidity was as follows: *Pneumocystis carinii* pneumonia (69.4), esophageal candidiasis (21.6), Kaposi's sarcoma (8.5), disseminated *Mycobacterium avium intracellulare* (22.4), HIV dementia (7.3), cytomegalovirus disease (15.8), extrapulmonary tuberculosis (1.5). Gastrointestinal cryptosporidiosis occurred at a rate of 3.1 and recurrent salmonella septicemia at a rate of 0.8. Thus, if all cases of *Mycobacterium avium intracellulare* are included, gastrointestinal manifestations occur at a rate of at least 48 per 100 person-years or one event every 2 years for each patient with AIDS.

**Table 21.6** Oral lesions associated with HIV infection

| |
|---|
| *Lesions strongly associated with HIV infection* |
| Candidiasis |
| Erythematous |
| Pseudomembranous |
| Angular cheilitis |
| Aphthous ulceration |
| Hairy leukoplakia |
| Kaposi's sarcoma |
| Non-Hodgkin's lymphoma |
| Periodontal disease |
| Linear gingival erythema |
| Necrotizing (ulcerative) gingivitis |
| Necrotizing (ulcerative) periodontitis |
| *Lesions less commonly associated with HIV infection* |
| Melanotic hyperpigmentation |
| Salivary gland disease |
| Thrombocytopenic purpura |
| Viral infections |
| Herpes simplex virus |
| Human papillomavirus |
| Varicella zoster virus |

## ORAL DISEASE

The mouth is a common area for a variety of problems seen in HIV/AIDS. The commonest infection is thrush or oral candidiasis, but malignancies such as Kaposi's sarcoma or malignant lymphoma may also present in the mouth, as they can throughout the rest of the gastrointestinal tract. The oral problems to be considered in patients with HIV are shown in Table 21.6.

### Candidiasis or thrush (see also p. 150)

This fungal infection, an important clinical marker of immunodeficiency, is often asymptomatic in the early stages but can also cause burning discomfort in the mouth. Four varieties are recognized: the commonest is pseudomembranous candidiasis (white lesions over the mucosal surface or classic thrush) and the others are erythematous/atrophic, hyperplastic and angular cheilitis (Anonymous 1989a). The erythematous variety is probably also common but is often missed by inexperienced observers (Anonymous 1989a) (Fig. 5.8). Characteristically, candidiasis involves the palate, tongue and buccal mucosa. In a San Francisco cohort of gay men, the prevalence of pseudomembranous candidiasis in any year was 5.8% while that of erythematous candidiasis was 1.1% and the likelihood of developing candidiasis was significantly related to low CD4 counts (Feigal et al 1991). Recurrent fungal infection of mucous membranes of the mouth or vagina herald progression from the asymptomatic stage of HIV to CDC stage IVC2.

The importance of recurrent thrush lies in the fact that

it is a clinical predictor of progression to AIDS (see above). Without the use of specific antiretroviral therapy or prophylactic agents, as many as 80% of individuals with oral thrush progress to AIDS within 2 years. If candidiasis spreads to the esophagus, trachea or lungs, then this becomes an index diagnosis for AIDS.

*Treatment*

Initial therapy for mild oral thrush is topical with chlorhexidine mouth washes, amphotericin B lozenges, nystatin solutions or pastilles and miconazole gels. The efficacy and safety of the new oral azoles such as fluconazole (100–400 mg/day for 1–3 days) have led to their widespread use as first-line therapy in more severe or recalcitrant disease. Fluconazole has been used as secondary prophylaxis and even as primary prophylaxis in patients with advancing immunodeficiency to prevent the initial development of oral thrush (50–200 mg/day). Ketoconazole (200 mg/day) is cheaper and has the advantage of good skin and nail penetration but has the disadvantages of hepatotoxicity, nausea, variable absorption and drug interaction. Itraconazole (200–400 mg/day) is a newer azole that has a different spectrum of activity and is often of use in patients not responding to fluconazole. It has variable absorption, is hepatotoxic and costly.

While systemic antifungal prophylaxis is convenient and attractive, caution is required in view of reports of failures of oral systemic antifungal agents after prophylaxis which may represent de novo resistance or overgrowth with resistant candida species. Susceptibility to oral candidiasis is reduced by antiretroviral agents such as zidovudine and this avoids continuous prophylaxis.

**Oral hairy leukoplakia**

This condition was originally thought to be pathognomonic of HIV immunodeficiency (Fig. 5.8) with probable progression to AIDS within 2 years (Greenspan 1984). The underlying cause seems to be advancing immunodeficiency and an opportunistic infection rather than direct infection with HIV. Epstein–Barr virus is present in the lesions of oral hairy leukoplakia and is thought to be the underlying cause. Similar lesions have now been reported in other immunosuppressed states, as after transplantation, and they seem more a characteristic of chronic advanced immunosuppression than of HIV infection itself.

*Pathology*

The histological features are characteristic and include hyperparakeratosis, hyperplasia, ballooning of prickle cells, depletion of Langerhans cells and only a sparse inflammatory infiltrate in the lamina propria (Anonymous 1989b).

*Clinical features*

The lesions are usually found on the lateral margins of the tongue and have a white corrugated or shaggy appearance. The condition is usually asymptomatic, but occasionally burning discomfort may be experienced along the edge of the tongue, particularly with spicy or acidic substances. Candidiasis may also be present, but confusion can be resolved by antifungal agents which do not benefit hairy leukoplakia. In clinical practice, it is unnecessary to biopsy the lesions to establish the diagnosis.

*Treatment*

No therapy is required in the vast majority of cases. Antiviral agents such as acyclovir and ganciclovir can cause regression of oral hairy leukoplakia, although this is not a consistent response. Symptoms can usually be controlled by antiretroviral therapy or by locally applied podophyllin which usually produces resolution of symptoms in 4–5 days.

*Aphthous ulceration*

This is a painful ulcerative condition of the mouth (or esophagus, p. 604) of unknown cause. Initially it does not differ from the condition seen in the non-HIV patient (p. 144), but it is generally more persistent with larger and more numerous ulcers. It can be extremely distressing for the patient and treatment is unsatisfactory. Local corticosteroids and analgesics are the mainstays of therapy, although some success has been reported with the use of thalidomide (below).

**Oral herpes simplex infections**

In normal individuals, this condition resolves within about 14 days (p. 146). Chronic mucocutaneous ulceration for more than 1 month is indicative of AIDS, although this is now unusual in Europe or the United States in view of the widespread availability of acyclovir. The ulceration is particularly deep and investigation of ulcerated lesions for herpes simplex is mandatory. Diagnosis can be made by isolation from surface swabs transported in viral medium or from biopsy tissue. The histologic appearance of inclusion bodies is characteristic but not diagnostic. Acyclovir is highly effective. Continuous prophylaxis may be required if recurrent. Resistance to acyclovir may develop and other antiviral agents such as phosphonoformic acid (Foscarnet) may be required (below).

**Angular cheilitis**

Angular cheilitis (p. 139) may be a manifestation of candidiasis or herpes simplex infection and produces erythema, cracks and fissures at the corners of the mouth. Topical antifungal treatment or systemic acyclovir results in improvement. It is worth trying systemic acyclovir if antifungal treatment fails to bring about improvement.

### Parotitis

Parotid enlargement, particularly in children, has been noted without any yet identified cause other than association with Didanosine. Diagnosis of an HIV-related salivary gland disease may require labial salivary gland biopsy or other major salivary gland fine needle aspiration (Schiodt et al 1989).

### Gingivitis and periodontitis

A number of specific abnormalities have been noted to be associated with HIV (pp. 137, 150). These include an HIV-associated gingivitis manifesting as a fiery red marginal line along the gingiva, acute necrotizing gingivitis, rapidly progressive periodontitis and necrotizing stomatitis. As a consequence, teeth may loosen and fall out and bone may be exposed or sequestrated. Referral to a dentist specializing in the oral manifestations of chronic immunosuppression is required, since standard therapy often fails. Treatment consists of combinations of topical antiseptics such as chlorhexidine or povidone iodine with prolonged systemic agents such as metronidazole and broad-spectrum antibiotics.

## ESOPHAGEAL DISEASE

Approximately 50% of esophagitis is due to candidiasis and one-third is a result of viral infections such as herpes simplex or cytomegalovirus (Bonacini et al 1991). Approximately 25% of patients have multiple etiologies. Over 40% of patients with esophagitis do not have oral candidiasis (Bonacini et al 1991). In addition to infective causes of dysphagia, it is necessary to consider peptic ulceration, idiopathic ulceration and malignant disease. In one-third of cases of esophagitis, no cause can be found even after an abnormal endoscopy (Bonacini et al 1991). Bonacini et al (1991) reported idiopathic ulceration in 5% of cases; other studies have reported rates over 50%. The differences are likely to be due to selection and sensitivity of viral studies (Wilcox & Schwartz 1992).

### *Clinical features and diagnosis*

The majority of conditions occurring in the mouth also affect the esophagus. The classic symptom of esophagitis is retrosternal pain on swallowing (odynophagia), possibly exacerbated by hot or cold liquids, with or without actual difficulty in swallowing (dysphagia). The diagnosis of esophagitis can often be made from symptoms, but the etiology cannot. Dysphagia is unusual in patients with AIDS and suggests malignant disease such as Kaposi's sarcoma or lymphoma of the esophagus.

### *Treatment*

All patients who are significantly immuno-compromised (CD4 <200) are treated empirically with fluconazole or other systemically active antifungal agents (Porro et al 1989). If symptoms are relieved within 3–4 days, a presumptive diagnosis of candidal esophagitis may be made. If symptoms continue, endoscopy is advisable (p. 101).

***Candidiasis.*** Despite gastric hypochlorhydria in the late stages of HIV (Lake-Bakaar et al 1988), additional symptomatic relief may be obtained by the use of $H_2$ receptor antagonists to reduce the damaging effect of reflux in patients with severe discomfort from infective esophagitis.

The treatment of choice for candidal esophagitis is oral fluconazole 200 mg/day for 7 days. Occasionally, courses of up to 2 weeks may be required. Possible causes of failure of fluconazole therapy include concurrent drugs known to induce liver enzymes (p. 839). If increased metabolism or malabsorption is suspected, higher doses may be required (800 mg/day). Fluconazole may occasionally be required intravenously. Other systemic agents for candidal esophagitis are ketoconazole, which is cheaper than fluconazole but may cause liver dysfunction, and itraconazole. Both have poorer bioavailability and higher rates of adverse events. Intravenous amphotericin (0.5 mg/kg/day) with or without 5-flucytosine (200 mg/kg/day) is the alternative in the clinically resistant case. Unfortunately, in some patients resistance may develop to the azole antifungal drugs. This may be due to the stepwise development of resistant species of *Candida albicans* or to the selection of other fungal species such as *C. kruzei* or *C. (Torulopsis) glabrata* that have intrinsic resistance to the azole compounds. These events are more likely to occur in patients with low CD4 counts, prolonged survival and maintenance therapy with azoles.

When systemic agents are not available, topical therapies such as chlorhexidine mouth washes, amphotericin B lozenges, nystatin solution or pastilles, miconazole gel or clotrimazole (available in the UK only as pessaries that can be given orally; in the US oral troches, effervescent tablets similar to pessaries, are available) may be considered.

***Viral esophagitis.*** The initial therapy for herpes simplex esophagitis is acyclovir, 200 mg five times/day orally or 5 mg/kg three times/day by intravenous infusion. Alternatives are newer agents such as valciclovir (2000 mg four times/day for 7 days) or famciclovir (250 mg three times/day for 7 days). Considerable use of acyclovir may lead to resistance and this requires the use of agents prescribed for cytomegalovirus (see below). If cytomegalovirus is implicated, then induction therapy and maintenance will be required (p. 610).

***Idiopathic ulceration.*** Idiopathic ulceration of the mouth and/or esophagus is thought to be related to aphthous ulceration and responds to oral corticosteroids and thalidomide (Youle et al 1989, Youle et al 1990, Ryan et al 1992, Wilcox & Schwartz 1992). Systemic corticosteroids may be effective, but there is concern over further immunosuppression. Success has been reported with prednisolone 40 mg/day tapering to 10 mg/day over 1 month. Dexamethasone 0.5 mg combined with sucralfate 1 g four times/day and tapered on control of symptoms was also thought to be effective (the sucralfate is thought to bind preferentially to ulcers allowing delivery of the corticosteroid to the surface of the ulcer). Thalidomide 100–200 mg/day has been found to be helpful, although the duration of treatment is not clear since relapse may occur. It is available in the UK on a named patient basis, but it is not recommended for treatment in women except under the most stringent conditions. The major limiting toxicity is a painful, nonreversible neuropathy and it is strongly recommended that regular assessments are undertaken for this complication, if possible using serial sensory nerve action potential measurements.

**Table 21.7** Classification of hepatic disorders in AIDS

| | | |
|---|---|---|
| **Infection** | | |
| | Bacterial | *M. avium intracellulare* |
| | | *M. tuberculosis* |
| | | *K. pneumoniae* |
| | | *Staph. aureus* |
| | | *R. quintana* |
| | Viral | Hepatitis A, B, C, D |
| | | Cytomegalovirus |
| | | Herpes virus |
| | Fungal | *C. albicans* |
| | | Coccidiodes |
| | | Cryptococcus |
| | | Histoplasmosis |
| | Protozoan | *P. carinii* |
| | | Cryptosporidium |
| | | Toxoplasmosis |
| **Neoplasia** | | |
| | Kaposi's sarcoma | |
| | B-cell lymphoma | |
| **Vascular** | | |
| | Sinusoidal congestion/dilatation | |
| | Peliosis hepatis | |
| **Miscellaneous** | | |
| | Steatosis | |
| | Granulomas | |
| | Portal/periportal inflammation | |
| | Focal necrosis | |
| | Fibrosis/cirrhosis | |

## GASTROINTESTINAL BLEEDING

The principles of diagnosis and management are broadly the same as those discussed elsewhere (p. 482). However, in addition to the usual causes of bleeding such as peptic ulcer, some are particular to HIV-infected patients. Cytomegalovirus can cause bleeding from the esophagus, stomach or colon, because it infects vascular endothelium leading to mucosal ulceration. Common colonic bacterial pathogens are more likely to cause severe bloody diarrhea than in normal individuals. Kaposi's sarcoma and non-Hodgkin's lymphoma, particularly of the stomach and duodenum, are liable to acute hemorrhage (Parente et al 1991). Mortality in patients with gastrointestinal hemorrhage is high (Cappell & Geller 1992).

## HEPATIC DISEASE

Hepatic involvement becomes common as AIDS advances and disease is found in a third to three-quarters of patients at autopsy (Schneiderman et al 1987). A classification of hepatic disease in AIDS in shown in Table 21.7. The main clinical features are upper abdominal pain, weight loss, fever and hepatomegaly. Jaundice may also occur, but splenomegaly may reflect extrahepatic effects of AIDS rather than portal hypertension. Abnormal liver function tests in asymptomatic patients and in those with extrahepatic disease are common and these abnormalities are not good predictors of intrahepatic pathology. However, dominant increases of alanine aminotransferase activity suggest viral or drug hepatitis, while significant elevation of alkaline phosphatase activity suggests mycobacterial infection or lymphoma (Schneiderman et al 1987). Computed tomography and ultrasound imaging are most useful for detecting intrahepatic tumor masses and biliary disease.

### Infections

Infections are common causes of hepatic disease in AIDS and the organisms involved and the manifestations of disease are often different from those encountered in immunocompetent patients.

#### *Viruses*

Hepatitis virus infections are common and have accounted for 18% of deaths in drug users with AIDS in Edinburgh, Scotland. Hepatitis B infection is common in intravenous drug users and in male homosexuals (p. 784) and is particularly common in those with HIV infection. In the UK, 91% of drug users with HIV infection have serological evidence of past or current hepatitis B infection compared with 51% who do not have HIV infection. Hepatitis D infection is not common in male homosexuals in Europe and North America but is common in intravenous drug users (Novick et al 1988). One study has reported an adverse effect of hepatitis B infection on the progression of HIV disease, as the relative risk of progression of AIDS for those with antibodies to hepatitis B compared with those without antibodies was 3.6 (Eskild et al 1992).

Coincident HIV and hepatitis B virus infection alters the natural history of the hepatitis B virus infection in that markers of infection such as HBV-DNA are present at higher concentration and rates of clearance of HBV-DNA are lower (Krogsgaard et al 1987). At the same time, plasma transaminase activity and histological evidence of liver damage is less in coincident HIV and hepatitis B virus infection, reflecting the likely importance of immune mechanisms in hepatitis B virus liver damage (p. 783). Conversely, combined hepatitis B and D infection in HIV-infected patients is associated with higher trans-aminase activity and more severe liver disease, reflecting the more direct effect of hepatitis D on the liver (Novick et al 1988). Reactivation of hepatitis B and D infections during HIV infection has also been described (Shattock et al 1987, Maeland et al 1989). Patients lose antibodies against the hepatitis B and D viruses (Hadler et al 1986, Biggar et al 1987) and the δ antigen and HBsAg may reappear subsequently. Furthermore, HBsAg and δ antigen have been found to be more common in AIDS patients than in asymptomatic patients with HIV (Kreek et al 1990, Outtra et al 1990). This liability to reactivation of infectivity has implications for infection control practices and staff caring for HIV-infected patients should be vaccinated against hepatitis B. With the onset of immunodeficiency (CD4 cells <200 cells/mm$^3$), regular monitoring of HBsAg and δ antigen should be undertaken in those with evidence of past infection and they should always be checked before invasive procedures are carried out.

Hepatitis C is also common in patients with AIDS. This is particularly the case in intravenous drug users (p. 788), where serological markers of hepatitis C virus infection can be found in 80% of such patients (Chamot et al 1992). HIV infection may also affect the course of chronic hepatitis C virus infection, but this is still poorly understood. Hepatitis A virus infection is more common in homosexual men (Corey & Holmes 1980) and in intravenous drug users (Anonymous 1988b) and is therefore also common in HIV-infected patients. Other hepatic viral infections encountered in HIV-infected patients include cytomegalovirus and herpes simplex virus.

***Treatment.*** Interferon can be used for hepatitis B and hepatitis C virus infections (pp. 902 & 903) but is less effective than in patients without HIV infection (McDonald et al 1987, Brook et al 1989). Ganciclovir (above) for 14–21 days may be useful in cytomegalovirus infection (Bach et al 1985).

### *Bacteria*

Mycobacteria, particularly *Mycobacterium avium intracellulare* (MAI), are the most common bacterial infections of the liver in AIDS. An interesting more recently reported infection is related to bacillary angiomatosis.

***Mycobacteria.*** Mycobacterial infection is common in AIDS and is due to *M. tuberculosis* or MAI. The frequency of *M. tuberculosis* is related to the frequency of latent tuberculosis in the community, but MAI infection seems to be due mainly to new environmental exposure and has been found in 59% of AIDS patients at autopsy in a US study (Hawkins et al 1986). Both organisms can affect the liver in AIDS, but MAI is the most commonly diagnosed hepatic infection in this disease (Schneiderman et al 1987). Liver involvement may take the form of well-formed granulomas with or without caseation that is almost always due to *M. tuberculosis* or aggregates of foamy macrophages, plasma cells and lymphocytes usually due to MAI. Granulomas are often atypical in HIV infection and even when the granulomas look characteristic, they frequently show immunohistological abnormalities (Shen et al 1988). No reaction may occur in liver infection but either organism may be revealed on liver smears or culture, which should always be done when AIDS patients are biopsied. Antituberculous therapy may be effective for *M. tuberculosis* but is rarely effective for MAI (above). MAI usually persists despite therapy and disseminated disease is generally found at autopsy (Hawkins et al 1986).

***Bacillary peliosis hepatis.*** This condition is caused by bacilli similar to those seen in bacillary angiomatosis and is another cause for abnormal liver function tests. Bacillary angiomatosis is a chronic bacterial infection most commonly involving the skin. The bacterium appears to be caused by a rickettsia-like organism related closely to *Rochalimaea quintana* (Relman et al 1991) and is distinct from the related agent (*Afipia felis*) involved in cat scratch disease (Koehler et al 1992). The skin lesions usually look like granulation tissue or slowly healing sores. Visceral disease with or without skin disease is possible involving the liver, spleen or bones. The condition should be considered in patients with hepatosplenomegaly, abdominal pain and abnormal liver function tests. Diagnosis is made from the histopathological appearances and by specific staining techniques. Treatment is usually with erythromycin or doxycycline for 6–8 weeks in the case of skin lesions or 3–4 months for visceral lesions.

### *Other organisms*

Many other organisms, including fungi and protozoans, can cause liver disease in patients with AIDS (Table 21.7). They account for less than half of liver infections in such patients and liver function tests are not helpful in identifying specific organisms.

## Neoplasms

Kaposi's sarcoma forms purple-brown nodular areas of

vascular endothelial cells and pleomorphic spindle cells in the liver. Hepatic involvement is rarely diagnosed from liver biopsy during life but is a common finding at autopsy (Schneiderman et al 1987). Extrahepatic disease leads to diagnosis in life in most patients. Lymphomas in AIDS patients are usually B-cell lymphomas and can be diagnosed by imaging and biopsy. They may occasionally arise in the liver (Caccamo et al 1986).

### Vascular lesions

Vascular hepatic lesions in AIDS include sinusoidal dilatation and congestion and peliosis hepatis (Scoazec et al 1988).

### Drugs

Patients with AIDS receive many drugs in the course of their disease. These should be considered possible causes of hepatic abnormality and such drugs include sulfonamides, antituberculous drugs and zidovudine (Table 30.7). Multiple pathology in AIDS often makes the attribution of hepatic abnormality to drugs difficult, but the range of hepatic pathology caused by drugs is wide (Chapter 30) and includes granulomas that are common in AIDS.

### Other lesions

Liver histology in patients requiring liver biopsy or coming to autopsy is almost always abnormal (Schneiderman et al 1987). Fatty change (steatosis) is common and may be related primarily to weight loss and cachexia. Deaths associated with massive fatty change have been reported and may be related to drugs such as zidovudine (Freiman et al 1993). Portal and periportal tract inflammation is also common and occasionally aggressive hepatitis or cirrhosis of unknown cause may be present.

## BILIARY DISEASE

Acalculous cholecystitis and sclerosing cholangitis occur in patients with AIDS (Cello 1989, Bouche et al 1993, Forbes et al 1993). Presentation is usually with upper abdominal pain, fevers and elevated serum alkaline phosphatase activity. Diagnosis may be delayed in patients on large doses of opiates and drug users may present late with empyema of the gallbladder. Jaundice is uncommon, but many patients have diarrhea. Hepatomegaly may be present and most patients have lost weight. Ultrasound imaging may show biliary dilatation and thickening of the bile ducts or gallbladder wall. Endoscopic retrograde cholangiopancreatography (ERCP) is diagnostic and disease patterns include sclerosing cholangitis and papillary stenosis (38%), papillary stenosis alone (12%), sclerosing cholangitis alone (15%) and long extrahepatic bile duct strictures (12%) (Cello 1989).

The commonest pathogens have been cytomegalovirus and cryptosporidia (15%), which can be found in ampullary or small intestinal biopsies or in the stool. Several pathogens may be present. Cytomegalovirus may also affect the gallbladder and can result in acalculous cholecystitis. More recently, it has been suggested that the microsporidia *Enterocytozoon bieneusi*, an obligate intracellular protozoan, can also cause cholangitis (Pol et al 1993) (p. 579). The pathogens involved in the biliary tract may vary with the risk activity involved in the acquisition of HIV. In drug users, classic gallbladder disease due to stones or enteric bacteria is as frequent as cryptosporidiosis or cytomegalovirus.

Treatment has not proved effective but includes opiates for pain relief, antibiotics and possibly ganciclovir (p. 610) or foscarnet (p. 610) for those with cytomegalovirus infection. Endoscopic sphincterotomy may relieve severe recurrent pain. Patients with AIDS-related sclerosing cholangitis tend to have relatively advanced AIDS and a half or more are dead within a year of diagnosis.

## PANCREATIC DISEASE

The frequency of acute pancreatitis in different series varies from uncommon to as high as 46%. Usually, it is associated with drugs used in AIDS such as co-trimoxazole and pentamidine as well as a nucleoside analog DDI (Table 21.8). Its presentation is not changed by HIV or AIDS but may be masked in those on large doses of opiates. It should certainly be considered in anyone on maintenance opiates with abdominal pain. The diagnosis is made as in non-HIV patients, but it is important that HIV infection itself is associated with plasma amylase activities up to twice normal. Therapy is as for pancreatitis unassociated with HIV.

## ENTEROPATHIC DISEASE

Patients with advancing HIV immunodeficiency are susceptible to the gastrointestinal tract infections seen in immunocompetent individuals, although they are often more prolonged and may be complicated by systemic infection. Gastric hypoacidity also increases susceptibility to gut pathogens such as salmonella and there is a significant association between diarrhea, bacterial overgrowth of the upper gastrointestinal tract and gastric hypoacidity (Belitsos et al 1992). While infection with salmonella species was not in the original definition of AIDS, recurrent infection with these bacteria has been a particular problem in patients with AIDS (Jacobs et al 1985). Treatment is difficult and even prolonged antibiotic therapy may fail to eliminate the organisms. In addition, there is a variety of more unusual pathogens, usually protozoa,

**Table 21.8** Drugs causing pancreatitis in AIDS

| |
|---|
| *Drugs commonly used in the treatment of HIV disease* |
| Alcohol |
| Cimetidine |
| Corticosteroids (prednisolone) |
| Diphenoxylate |
| Dideoxyinosine (DDI or didanosine) |
| Dideoxycytidine (DDC or Zalcitabine) |
| Metronidazole |
| Nitrofurantoin |
| Opiates |
| Paracetamol |
| Pentamidine |
| Ranitidine |
| Sulfonamides |
| Tetracycline |
| Thiazide diuretics |
| Valproic acid |
| *Drugs occasionally used in the treatment of HIV disease* |
| L-Asparginase |
| Azathioprine |
| Cytosine arabinose |
| Estrogens |
| 6-Mercaptopurine |
| Methyldopa |
| Phenformin |
| Piroxicam |
| Procainamide |
| Vitamin D |
| Sulfasalazine |

which can colonize the gastrointestinal tract and cause illness with the onset of HIV-related immunodeficiency.

Diarrhea is very common in patients with HIV, but the risk group is an important co-factor. Drug users with a high consumption of opiates are much less likely to present with diarrhea unless opiate withdrawal occurs. In these patients, abdominal pain and constipation are much commoner than intractable diarrhea. Large doses of opiates also make it more difficult to diagnose serious intra-abdominal diseases such as appendicitis, cholecystitis, spontaneous peritonitis and large bowel perforations that may go unrecognized for a number of days in those on methadone or other long-term opiates. To a certain extent, previous microbiological exposure is important in determining the spectrum of pathology seen in HIV-related gastrointestinal disorders. Thus certain sexual practices, particularly oral–anal contact, dramatically increase the likelihood of colonization with gut pathogens such as ameba, cryptosporidium and giardia and such patients are therefore much more likely to present with diarrhea.

The frequency of causes of diarrhea varies in different populations, but one survey from the United States revealed that protozoa accounted for 33% and bacteria for 21% of cases of diarrhea (Smith et al 1988). The single commonest agent identified was cytomegalovirus. *Clostridium difficile* has also been associated with AIDS and in one study was responsible for 4% of admissions. It was particularly associated with clindamycin therapy (used in the treatment of both *Pneumocystis carinii* pneumonia and toxoplasmosis) and with prolonged hospitalization (Hutin et al 1993). More recently, diarrhea has also been associated with rifabutin therapy for the treatment of disseminated *Mycobacterium avium intracellulare* (McBride et al 1994).

**Table 21.9** Common pathogens causing diarrhea in HIV infection (AIDS)

| Pathogens | Small intestine (duodenum/jejunum) | Large intestine (colon/terminal ileum) |
|---|---|---|
| Bacteria | *Mycobacterium avium intracellulare*<br>Salmonella | Campylobacter<br>Shigella<br>Yersinia<br>Aeromonas<br>*C. difficile* |
| Protozoa | Cryptosporidium<br>Isosporiasis<br>Microsporidium<br>Cyclospora<br>*Giardia intestinalis* | |
| Viruses | Rotavirus<br>Astrovirus<br>Calavirus<br>Picornavirus<br>HIV | Cytomegalovirus<br>Adenovirus<br>Herpes simplex virus |

Table 21.9 lists the bacterial, protozoal, and viral infections found in HIV infection. In the history it is useful to distinguish between small and large bowel symptoms, to review all medication and to document previous opportunistic illnesses. Figure 21.1 provides guidance for investigation. The recommendations need to be implemented in the context of the stage of disease. For example, in late-stage patients, endoscopy may be done only if symptomatic therapy fails.

## Mycobacterium tuberculosis

Extrapulmonary or disseminated *M. tuberculosis* (cultured from the blood, bone marrow or other normally sterile sites) indicates AIDS in those who are HIV positive. This infection may be a recurrence because of lowered immunity or may be acquired from an external source, as HIV patients are more likely to be reinfected. Not surprisingly, there is a high incidence in Africa, southern Europe and New York because the background rate of tuberculosis infection in the communities at risk of HIV is very high.

## Atypical mycobacteriosis

*Etiology*

*Mycobacterium avium intracellulare* (MAI or MAC) infection tends to occur in the course of AIDS with a CD4 count <50 cells/mm$^3$, although it can occasionally be the first manifestation of AIDS. Infection probably occurs from the environment, where these organisms are very common.

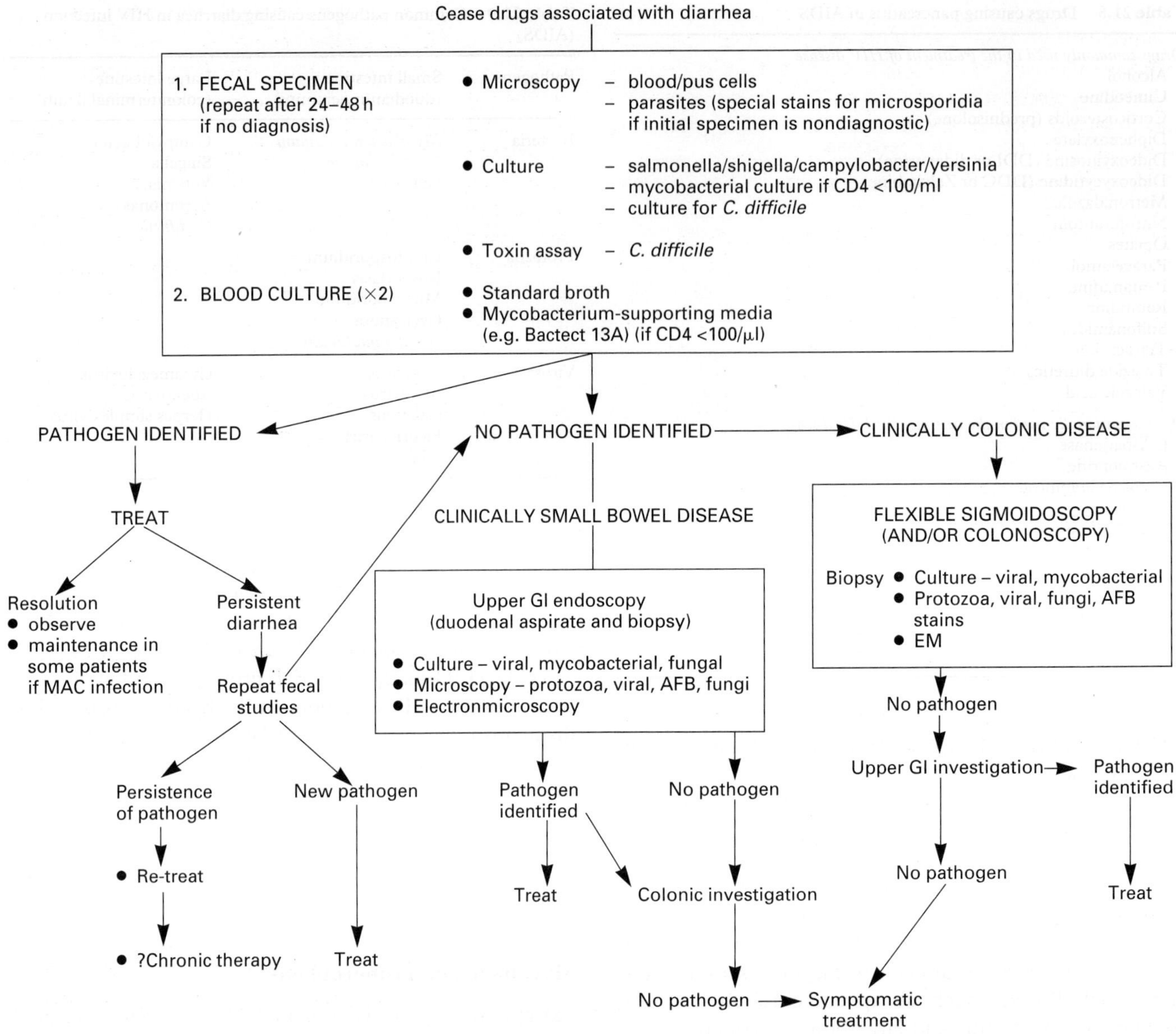


**Fig. 21.1** Algorithm for management of HIV-infected patients with diarrhea

Initially, there is colonization at a nonsterile site such as the gut or the respiratory tract, followed by a phase of localized infection, again often at a nonsterile site such as the gastrointestinal or respiratory tract, and finally the infection disseminates and spreads to other sterile sites such as the liver, blood and lymph nodes (Benson 1994). Isolation of MAI from two sterile sites is required to define disseminated MAI infection. This is because isolation at one sterile site only such as urine might indicate simply local infection.

*Clinical features*

Gastrointestinal presentations include weight loss, abdominal pain and/or fever with a rising alkaline phosphatase. Patients may also present with jaundice from compression of the bile ducts by enlarged lymph nodes. The histology of MAI in the bowel closely resembles Whipple's disease (Roth et al 1983). There is little in the way of a cellular response such as granulomata and the macrophages are full of organisms. Gastrointestinal MAI infection may be identified by finding acid-fast bacilli in the stools, blood cultures, bone marrow cultures or liver biopsy. With the advent of BACTEC technology, bone marrow culture seems to have no advantage over blood cultures that yield a result in 1–2 weeks.

*Treatment*

Treatment for MAI is usually difficult, as the majority of

strains are resistant to conventional tuberculous chemotherapy (isoniazid, rifampicin, ethambutol and pyrazinamide). Ethambutol seems to assist penetration of other drugs into the organism and it therefore seems sensible to include it in most treatment regimens. Possible drug regimens include ciprofloxacin, clarithromycin, azithromycin, rifabutin and amikacin. There is no generally accepted regimen, but recently the National Institutes of Health in Washington have published guidelines suggesting at least two drugs (one being clarithromycin or azithromycin) (Masur 1993, Benson 1994). Additional drugs such as ethambutol, clofazamine, rifabutin, ciprofloxacin or amikacin may be considered. Prophylaxis against MAI infection with rifabutin in the US, Canada, Australia and New Zealand should be considered for all patients with a CD4 count below 100 cells/mm$^3$ (Masur 1993, Benson 1994).

Fluconazole increases bioavailability of rifabutin and dosage adjustments may be necessary since iritis appears more frequently with higher doses. If the patient is taking ketoconazole, it is advisable to change to fluconazole and regular liver function tests should be performed. Patients should be warned that their urine might turn red with the use of rifampicin or rifabutin and soft contact lenses become permanently discolored. The use of rifampicin in any patient on long-term opiates will lead to increased turnover of opiates and subsequent withdrawals after around 3–7 days. Experience has shown that increases in opiate doses of 2–3 times the daily dose may be needed. Care is also required when rifampicin is discontinued. Patients taking oral contraceptives should be warned of possible "contraceptive pill failure" with rifampicin or rifabutin.

Although MAI is commoner as a late presentation of HIV, tuberculosis can mimic MAI. Patients with weight loss and positive blood cultures for acid-fast bacilli may in fact have tuberculosis. Those patients not responding to MAI treatment may respond to routine antituberculous treatment. It may be 4–6 weeks before the exact type of mycobacterial infection can be determined unless genetic probes are used.

## Protozoal infections of the gastrointestinal tract

A number of protozoa that infect the gastrointestinal tract cause prolonged primary infections or may recur. The most frequent protozoal causes of diarrhea in the US are cryptosporidiosis (11%), amebiasis (11%), giardiasis (5%), isosporiasis (3%) and strongyloidiasis (3%) (Smith et al 1988). *Isospora belli* is found in at least 15% of patients with AIDS in Haiti (DeHovitz et al 1986).

### *Cryptosporidiosis* (p. 577)

Cryptosporidia predominantly invade the columnar epithelium of the small bowel and ultimately lead to villous atrophy. In the immunocompetent host, the infection is transient and after about 5–14 days the organism is eliminated (Current et al 1983). However, in the presence of immunodeficiency, failure of elimination of the organism occurs with persistent infection, diffuse abdominal pain, symptoms of voluminous diarrhea of up to 15 L/day and rapid weight loss. The diagnosis is usually made by requesting an acid-alcohol-fast stain of the stools (p. 578).

There is no universally accepted successful therapy for cryptosporidiosis. Some success has been achieved with paromomycin, a nonabsorbed aminoglycoside, but symptomatic relief with opiates is often the only successful therapy. Rarely, octreotide may be of use in alleviating the symptoms of high volume, secretory diarrhea, although a recent study did not show any particular benefit (Simon et al 1995).

### *Isosporiasis*

Infection with *Isospora belli* is associated with chronic watery diarrhea and weight loss and is indistinguishable from cryptosporidiosis (DeHovitz et al 1986). Therapy with co-trimoxazole (p. 609) is effective and long-term prophylaxis with the standard dose three times a week is also possible (DeHovitz et al 1986, Pape et al 1989). The wider scale use of co-trimoxazole for *Pneumocystis carinii* pneumonia prophylaxis may explain the low frequency of disease in the United States.

### *Strongyloidiasis*

This may present with abdominal pain (p. 584). Dissemination of strongyloidiasis to extragastrointestinal sites such as the central nervous system has been noted in those exposed to this protozoal infestation. Treatment is discussed on p. 584.

### *Enterocytozoon bieneusi*

*Enterocytozoon bieneusi* is an obligate intracellular protozoan (p. 579). It was detected in 27% of AIDS patients with unexplained diarrhea for more than 1 month compared with only 2.5% in matched patients without diarrhea (Eeftinck Schattenkerk et al 1991). Some success in treatment has been noted with metronidazole (Eeftinck Schattenkerk et al 1991).

## Viral infections

Severe anal and oral disease secondary to herpes simplex virus may be an early presentation of AIDS, but gastrointestinal involvement with viral pathogens tends to be a late complication. At any time in the course of HIV infection, patients may develop enteric infection with viruses such as rotavirus and adenovirus. Such infections are usually transient and require only symptomatic therapy. There are, however, some particular viral syndromes that are more common in the immunodeficient patient. These are cytomegalovirus, herpes simplex and HIV enteropathy.

*Cytomegalovirus infection*

The commonest presentation of this recurrent herpetic viral infection is cytomegalovirus (CMV) retinitis, which presents as visual disturbance or visual loss. However, it can also present as esophageal ulceration (pp. 211 & 603), colitis, acalculous cholecystitis, adrenalitis (dehydration and hypotension) and pneumonitis. Colitis causes abdominal pain and diarrhea with blood and mucus and appearances suggest ulcerative colitis but inflammation of the terminal ileum may also occur. Abdominal radiology may show colonic dilatation and the virus may be isolated from stools. Sigmoidoscopy reveals diffuse submucosal hemorrhages and ulceration. A near-normal appearance occurs in about 10% of patients with histological CMV colitis. Colonic biopsies are the definitive method of diagnosis and show vasculitis, neutrophilic infiltration, nonspecific inflammation and viral inclusions. Episodes of colonic dilatation often resolve spontaneously over a few days, but necrosis of the bowel wall and perforation may occur unless antiviral therapy is commenced.

***Treatment.*** Treatment usually commences with ganciclovir, initially in a dose of 10 mg/kg/day in two divided doses each as a 1-h infusion in dextrose or saline, for 2–3 weeks, followed by maintenance therapy in a dose of 5 mg/kg/day, 5–7 days a week. Ganciclovir is myelotoxic and there is a need for frequent full blood counts. Myelotoxicity is more likely when the patient is also on zidovudine and this drug should be discontinued and an alternative retroviral considered.

An alternative but more toxic drug is foscarnet, available in a solution of 24 mg/ml. The solution may be administered undiluted via a central vein after fluid loading or, if diluted, via a peripheral vein. It is given as an initial test dose of 20 mg/kg infused in 5% dextrose over 30 min. The daily dose is usually in the region of 100–200 mg/kg/day for 3 weeks and is dependent on renal function. This is usually given as a continuous intravenous infusion of 60 mg/kg every 8 h. Renal toxicity is less likely if 2.5 L of normal saline can be given per day. This treatment is followed by maintenance therapy of 100 mg/kg/day. Foscarnet causes abnormalities in serum calcium, renal impairment fits and genital ulcers. If the patient is also taking pentamidine, caution is required because of the possibility of intractable hypocalcemia. The dose of foscarnet will depend on the renal function and serum creatinine and creatinine clearance must be known before commencement.

*HIV enteropathy*

HIV itself was detected in epithelial cells from two out of four bowel biopsy specimens from patients with AIDS and chronic diarrhea of unknown cause (Nelson et al 1988). Consequently, it has been suggested that an HIV enteropathy could account for cases of chronic diarrhea or slim disease (Anonymous 1989c).

*Other enteric viruses*

Patients with HIV and AIDS are just as likely as the rest of the population to be affected by enteric viruses circulating in the population. However, persistent infection is also possible with prolonged symptoms. One study found enteric viruses in the stools of 35% of patients with diarrhea compared to 12% for patients without diarrhea. Viruses such as astroviruses, picobirnaviruses, calciviruses and adenoviruses were all more common in patients with diarrhea, suggesting a possible etiological relationship (Grohmann et al 1993). These viruses may be of more importance in the causation of diarrhea than HIV enteropathy.

## MALABSORPTION

The clinical triad of diarrhea, weight loss and malabsorption may occur as a result of many different pathogens in HIV/AIDS (Anonymous 1989c). Even when all of the known pathogens have been excluded, there are patients with malabsorption and partial villous atrophy on small intestinal biopsy (Anonymous 1989c). Substantial deficiency of lactase activity has been reported, suggesting that treatment for lactose intolerance may improve patients' well-being even if no other enteropathy can be diagnosed (Anonymous 1989a).

## MALIGNANT DISEASE

Malignant disease may affect any portion of the gastrointestinal tract from the mouth to the anus. Obstruction of the esophagus, stomach, small bowel, large bowel or anal canal can be a presentation. The two main malignant diseases are Kaposi's sarcoma and non-Hodgkin's lymphoma. Both malignancies tend to be multicentric in origin rather than metastatic.

The commonest neoplasm in AIDS is Kaposi's sarcoma, which has occurred in 15% of reported cases of AIDS although this is associated mainly with homosexuals and is reported in only around 3% of drug users (Beral et al 1990). Its appearance is discussed elsewhere (p. 438, Fig. 5.9). By comparison, the commonest malignancy associated with drug use appears to be malignant lymphoma or non-Hodgkin's lymphoma, which has been reported in 8% of surgical specimens from drug users (Vazquez et al 1989).

Postmortem studies reveal that most patients with Kaposi's sarcoma of the skin have gastrointestinal lesions (77%) and these occur even in the absence of skin lesions (Friedman et al 1985). The lesions may coalesce or ulcerate, causing obstruction, diarrhea, bleeding or perforation. Similar problems may occur with non-Hodgkin's lymphoma, which may also present with malabsorption, weight loss, abdominal pain or an abdominal mass.

Therapy for Kaposi's sarcoma should be reserved for those with symptoms. In general, local treatment of Kaposi's sarcoma lesions by infiltration under the lesion is useful only for oral, esophageal or rectal lesions. A variety of agents have been injected under Kaposi's sarcoma lesions including sterile water, α-interferon, vinblastine and vincristine and all seem to be successful in local control of lesions. Local radiotherapy is useful for particular problems such as lymphedema of limbs. Chemotherapy is usually reserved for patients with widespread cutaneous disease and/or those with major organ involvement, but it is important not to worsen the patient's lot with aggressive therapy, as treatment is palliative only. Vincristine or bleomycin has until recently formed the mainstay of chemotherapy. However, more recently reasonable success has been achieved with adriamycin or liposomal daunorubicin. Interferon treatment for Kaposi's sarcoma is reserved for patients with well-preserved immunity (CD4 count >350 cells/mm$^3$) but is usually ineffective.

Therapy for non-Hodgkin's lymphoma depends upon the presentation. Obstruction, for instance, may require resection, although this treatment is not curative because of the multicentric origin of the lymphoma. Aggressive chemotherapy, which usually results in a good but short-lived response, is useful especially in those with well-preserved immunity. Those with end-stage disease tolerate chemotherapy poorly and palliative chemotherapy with corticosteroids alone is all that can be given without worsening their quality of life. In patients receiving chemotherapy, it is important to commence prophylaxis for conditions such as *Pneumocystis carinii* pneumonia or toxoplasmosis, since the immunosuppression of chemotherapy increases the occurrence of these infections.

## ANORECTAL DISORDERS

### Etiology

The anus and rectum, like the mouth, are common sources of problems for patients with HIV/AIDS. The possible HIV-related manifestations include viral infections such as herpes simplex or cytomegalovirus as well as malignant disease including squamous cell carcinoma, Kaposi's sarcoma and non-Hodgkin's lymphoma. In homosexuals and some heterosexuals, sexually transmitted diseases also need to be considered including *Neisseria gonorrhoea*, *Chlamydia trachomatis*, *Treponema pallidum* and herpes simplex virus, which may all cause a proctitis or anal ulceration. Proctocolitis may occur with traditional sexually transmitted diseases such as *Neisseria gonorrhoea* or *Chlamydia trachomatis* as well as with enteric organisms such as shigella or campylobacter species acquired sexually. The causes of anorectal problems in 148 HIV patients included 30% due to condylomata and 28% to ulceration, of which 61% were secondary to herpes simplex virus and 21% to cytomegalovirus, while 12% were idiopathic; bacterial sepsis accounted for 11%, hemorrhoids for 12% and fissures for 6% (Schmitt & Wexner 1994). Thirteen of the 148 patients with HIV had malignant lesions (Kaposi's sarcoma or non-Hodgkin's lymphoma). Cancer of the anus in HIV patients is discussed on p. 1437.

### Clinical features and diagnosis

Early in the natural history of HIV, patients often suffer from recurrent herpes simplex alone, while later persistent ulceration and malignancies are more common. Chronic perineal herpes simplex virus is in fact an indicator disease of AIDS if present for more than 1 month. Acyclovir has made this diagnosis relatively less common. Patients often present with severe anorectal pain, perianal ulceration, tenesmus, constipation and sacral plexus dysfunction causing a neurogenic bladder or impotence. Proctoscopy, which may be impossible initially, reveals a friable mucosa, diffuse ulceration or possibly vesicles. Recurrent anal herpes is also possible without extensive rectal involvement and causes only perianal pain and pruritus.

Patients presenting with rectal or anal ulceration require a thorough evaluation in order to pinpoint treatable conditions (Schmitt & Wexner 1994). Failure to undertake such an evaluation may lead to a purely surgical approach with disappointing results. For instance, in the mid-1980s a study of surgical treatment for anorectal problems in 73 patients revealed poor healing with 13% of patients having failed to heal by 6 months, 43% were dead by 6 months and the 30-day mortality rate was 18%. In addition, patients undergoing any form of sphincterotomy all experienced a degree of incontinence after the operation. It is now appreciated that results depend in part upon the stage of HIV. As an example, 100% of patients in CDC stage II healed at 6 weeks compared with 11% in CDC stages III and IV. It is likely that the poor results from earlier studies were a result of misdiagnosing ulcerative lesions as fissures with subsequent poor healing. Consequently, extensive and thorough evaluation is vital to successful management. In a recent study, delayed healing at 3 months occurred in only 12% of 74 operations (Schmitt & Wexner 1994).

The correct evaluation of anorectal problems requires a history for specific details relating to anal intercourse and diarrhea as well as staging of the HIV disease with CD4 counts. External examination of any lesion is required as well as proctoscopy and sigmoidoscopy if the lesions are not tender. If there is significant tenderness, then a general anesthetic is required both for patient comfort and for operator safety. All ulcerating lesions need to be biopsied and cultures sent for herpes simplex, cytomegalovirus, acid-fast bacilli and fungi and other enteric pathogens, since these may exacerbate anal problems.

At any time seborrheic dermatitis, bacterial infections and/or abscess formation can be troublesome. The majority of conditions already described for oral, esophageal and enteropathic disease can also affect the rectal area. Particularly troublesome may be malignancies (Kaposi's sarcoma and non-Hodgkin's lymphoma) which can mimic fistulae or infection early on. A recent analysis of the risks of squamous cell carcinoma of the anus suggests an increased risk both before and after onset of AIDS (Melbye et al 1994).

### Treatment

Specific therapy should be started once the results of cultures are available, although empiric therapy with broad-spectrum antibiotics and acyclovir can be considered. All patients require fiber supplements and possibly local anesthetics. An assessment of anal tone and anal manometry is required before sphincterotomy to determine if surgical intervention is appropriate. Recent reports suggest that incontinence can be avoided with such an approach. Occasionally, a diversionary colostomy is required for extensive ulceration. In the case of inflammatory bowel disease, the decision to use immunosuppressive treatment should be based on the level of underlying immunodeficiency and a frank discussion with the patient over the possible disadvantages and advantages of such therapy. For instance, many patients are willing to take the risks of further immunosuppression and a shortening of life in order to achieve better quality of life. Sulfasalazine and related drugs may also be used.

## REFERENCES


Anonymous 1988a Statistics from the World Health Organization and the Centers for Disease control. AIDS 2: 145–149

Anonymous 1988b Hepatitis A among drug abusers. Morbidity and Mortality Weekly Reports 37: 297–305

Anonymous 1989a Oral candidiasis in HIV infection. Lancet 2: 1491–1492

Anonymous 1989b Oral hairy leucoplakia. Lancet 2: 1194

Anonymous 1989c HIV associated enteropathy. Lancet 2: 777–778

Anonymous 1993a Statistics from the World Health Organization and the Centers for Disease Control. AIDS 7: 297–298

Anonymous 1993b AIDS surveillance in Europe: quarterly report to 31st June 1990. Communicable Diseases (Scotland) Unit 93/26 (A302): 1–5

Anonymous 1993c AIDS and HIV-1 infection: United Kingdom. Communicable Disease Report 3: 197–200

Bach M C, Bagwell S P, Knapp N P, Davis K M, Hedstrom P S 1985 9-(1,3-dihydroxy-2-propoxymethyl) guanine for cytomegalovirus infections in patients with the acquired immunodeficiency syndrome. Annals of Internal Medicine 103: 381–384

Barré-Sinoussi F, Chermann J C, Rey F et al 1983 Isolation of a T-lymphotropic retrovirus from a patient at risk for acquired immune deficiency syndrome (AIDS). Science 220: 868–871

Belitsos P C, Greenson J K, Yardley J H, Sisler J R, Bartlett J G 1992 Association of gastric hypoacidity with opportunistic enteric infections in patients with AIDS. Journal of Infectious Diseases 166: 277–284

Benson C 1994 *Mycobacterium tuberculosis* and *Mycobacterium avium* complex disease in patients with HIV infection. AIDS 7: 95–107

Beral V, Peterman T A, Berkelman R L, Jaffe H W 1990 Kaposi's sarcoma among persons with AIDS: a sexually transmitted infection? Lancet 335: 123–128

Biggar R J, Goedert J J, Hoofnagle J 1987 Accelerated loss of antibody to hepatitis B surface antigen among immunodeficient homosexual men infected with HIV. New England Journal of Medicine 316: 630–631

Bonacini M, Young T, Laine L 1991 The causes of esophageal symptoms in human immunodeficiency virus infection. A prospective study of 110 patients. Archives of Internal Medicine 151: 1567–1572

Bouche H, Housset C, Dumont J-L et al 1993 AIDS-related cholangitis: diagnostic features and course in 15 patients. Journal of Hepatology 17: 34–39

Brettle R P, Gore S M, Bird A G, McNeil A J 1993 Clinical and epidemiological implications of the Centers for Disease Control/World Health Organization reclassification of AIDS cases. AIDS 7: 531–539

Brook M G, McDonald J A, Karayiannis P et al 1989 Randomised controlled trial of interferon alfa 2A (rbe) (Roferon-A) for the treatment of chronic hepatitis B virus (HBV) infection: factors that influence response. Gut 30: 1116–1122

Caccamo D, Pervez N K, Marchevsky A 1986 Primary lymphoma of the liver in the acquired immunodeficiency syndrome. Archives of Pathology and Laboratory Medicine 110: 553–555

Cappell M S, Geller A J 1992 The high mortality of gastrointestinal bleeding in HIV-seropositive patients: a multivariate analysis of risk factors and warning signs of mortality in 50 consecutive patients. American Journal of Gastroenterology 87: 815–824

Cello J P 1989 Acquired immune deficiency syndrome cholangiopathy: spectrum of disease. American Journal of Medicine 86: 539–546

Centers for Disease Control 1982 Update on Kaposi's sarcoma and opportunistic infections in previously healthy persons – United States. Mortality and Morbidity Weekly Report 31: 294

Centers for Disease Control 1987 Revision of the CDC surveillance case definition for acquired immunodeficiency syndrome. Mortality and Morbidity Weekly Report 36 (1S)

Centers for Disease Control 1992 1993 revised classification system for HIV infection and expanded surveillance case definition for AIDS among adolescents and adults. Mortality and Morbidity Weekly Report 41 (RR-17): 1–19

Chamot E, de Saussure Ph, Hirschel B, Deglon J J, Perrin L H 1992 Incidence of hepatitis C, hepatitis B, and HIV infection among drug users in a methadone maintenance programme. AIDS 6: 430–431

Chin J 1988 The global epidemiology and projected impacts of AIDS. WKPL/GPA/5E, Geneva, 27–28 June

Clumeck N 1989 Aids in Africa. In: J A Levy (ed) Aids pathogenesis and treatment. Marcel Dekker, New York, pp 37–63

Coffin J, Haase A, Levy J A et al 1986 What to call the AIDS virus. Nature 321: 10

Corey L, Holmes K K 1980 Sexual transmission of hepatitis A in homosexual men. Incidence and mechanism. New England Journal of Medicine 302: 435–438

Current W L, Reese N C, Ernst J V, Bailey W S, Heyman M B, Weinstein W M 1983 Human cryptosporidiosis in immunocompetent and immunodeficient persons. Studies of an outbreak and experimental transmission. New England Journal of Medicine 308: 1252–1257

DeHovitz J A, Pape J W, Boncy M, Johnston W D Jr 1986 Clinical manifestations and therapy of *Isospora belli* infection in patients with the acquired immune deficiency syndrome. New England Journal of Medicine 315: 87–90

Donaldson Y K, Bell J E, Ironside J W et al 1994 Redistribution of HIV outside the lymphoid system with onset of AIDS. Lancet 343: 382–385

Eeftinck Schattenkerk J K M, van Gool T et al 1991 Clinical significance of small intestinal microsporidiosis in HIV-1-infected individuals. Lancet 337: 895–898

Eskild A, Magnus P, Peterson G et al 1992 Hepatitis B antibodies in HIV-infected homosexual men are associated with more rapid progression to AIDS. AIDS 6: 571–574

Feigal D W, Katz M H, Greenspan D et al 1991 The prevalence of oral lesions in HIV infected homosexual and bisexual men: three San Francisco epidemiological cohorts. AIDS 5: 519–525

Forbes A, Blanshard C, Gazzard B 1993 Natural history of AIDS related sclerosing cholangitis: a study of 20 cases. Gut 34: 116–121

Freiman J P, Helfert K E, Hamrell M R, Stein D S 1993 Hepatomegaly with severe steatosis in HIV seropositive patients. AIDS 7: 379–385

Friedman S L, Wright T L, Altman D F 1985 Gastrointestinal Kaposi's sarcoma in patients with acquired immune deficiency syndrome. Gastroenterology 89: 102–108

Gallo R C, Salahuddin S Z, Popovic M et al 1984 Frequent detection and isolation of cytopathic retroviruses (HTLV-III) from patients with AIDS and at risk for AIDS. Science 224: 500–503

Greenspan D, Greenspan J S, Conant M, Petersen V, Silverman S Jr, de Souza Y 1984 Oral "hairy" leucoplakia in male homosexuals: evidence of association with both papillomavirus and a herpes-group virus. Lancet 2: 831–834

Grohmann G S, Glass R I, Pereira H G et al 1993 Enteric viruses and diarrhea in HIV-infected patients. New England Journal of Medicine 329: 14–20

Hadler S C, Francis D P, Maynard J E et al 1986 Long term immunogenicity and efficacy of hepatitis B vaccine in homosexual men. New England Journal of Medicine 315: 209–214

Hawkins C C, Gold J W M, Whimbey E et al 1986 *Mycobacterium avium* complex infections in patients with acquired imunodeficiency syndrome. Annals of Internal Medicine 105: 184–188

Ho D D, Neumann A U, Perelson A S, Chen W, Leonard J M, Markowitz M 1995 Rapid turnover of plasma virions and CD4 lymphocytes in HIV-1 infection. Nature 373: 123–126

Hutin Y, Molina J M, Casin I et al 1993 Risk factors for *Clostridium difficile*-associated diarrhoea in HIV-infected patients. AIDS 7: 1441–1447

Jacobs J L, Gold J W M, Murray H W, Roberts R B, Armstrong D 1985 Salmonella infections in patients with acquired immune deficiency syndrome. Annals of Internal Medicine 102: 186–188

Koehler J E, Quinn F D, Berger T G, LeBoit P E, Tappero J W 1992 Isolation of Rochalimaea species from cutaneous and osseous lesions of bacillary angiomatosis. New England Journal of Medicine 327: 1625–1631

Kreek M J, des Jarlais D C, Trepo C L, Novick D M, Abdul-Quader A, Raghunath J 1990 Contrasting prevalence of delta hepatitis markers in parenteral drug abusers with and without AIDS. Journal of Infectious Diseases 162: 538–541

Krogsgaard K, Lindhardt B O, Nielsen J O et al 1987 The influence of HTLV-III infection on the natural history of hepatitis B virus infection in male homosexual HBsAg carriers. Hepatology 7: 37–41

Lake-Bakaar G, Quadros E, Beidas S et al 1988 Gastric secretory failure in patients with the acquired immune deficiency syndrome. Annals of Internal Medicine 109: 502–504

Lundgren J D, Pedersen C, Clumeck N et al 1994 Survival differences in European patients with AIDS, 1979–89. British Medical Journal 308: 1068–1073

Maeland A, Skaug K, Stofvold G, Kittleson P 1989 Reactivation of hepatitis B. Lancet 1: 1083

Masur H and the Public Health Service Task Force on Prophylaxis and Therapy for *Mycobacterium Avium* Complex 1993 Recommendations on prophylaxis and therapy for disseminated *Mycobacterium avium* complex disease in patients infected with the human immunodeficiency virus. New England Journal of Medicine 329: 898–904

McBride M O, Coker R J, Horner P J, Weston R, Weber J N 1994 Diarrhoea associated with *Clostridium difficile* in AIDS patients receiving rifabutin. Lancet 343: 417

McDonald J A, Caruso L, Karayiannis P et al 1987 Diminished responsiveness of male homosexual chronic hepatitis B virus carriers with HTLV-III antibodies to recombinant α-interferon. Hepatology 7: 719–723

Melbye M, Coté T R, Kessler L, Gail M, Biggar R J and the AIDS/Cancer Working Group 1994 High incidence of anal cancer among AIDS patients. Lancet 343: 636–639

Moss A R, McCallum G, Volberding P A, Bacchetti P, Dritz S 1984 Mortality associated with mode of presentation in the acquired immune deficiency syndrome. Journal of the National Cancer Institute 73: 1281–1284

Nelson J A, Wiley C A, Reynolds-Kohler C, Reese C E, Margaretten M, Levy J A 1988 Human immunodeficiency virus detected in bowel epithelium from patients with gastrointestinal symptoms. Lancet 1: 259–262

Novick D M, Farci P, Croxson T S et al 1988 Hepatitis D virus and human immunodeficiency virus antibodies in parenteral drug abusers who are hepatitis B surface antigen positive. Journal of Infectious Diseases 158: 795–803

Outtra S A, Meite M, Aron Y, Akran V, Gody M, de Manlan L K 1990 The G. Increase of the prevalence of hepatitis B virus surface antigen related immunodeficiency inherent in AIDS. Journal of Acquired Immune Deficiency Syndromes 3: 282–286

Pape J W, Verdier R-I, Johnson W D Jr 1989 Treatment and prophylaxis of *Isospora belli* infection in patients with the acquired immune deficiency syndrome. New England Journal of Medicine 320: 1044–1047

Parente F, Cernuschi M, Valsecchi L et al 1991 Acute upper gastrointestinal bleeding in patients with AIDS: a relatively uncommon condition associated with reduced survival. Gut 32: 987–990

Pol S, Romana C A, Richard S et al 1993 Microsporidia infection in patients with the human immunodeficiency virus and unexplained cholangitis. New England Journal of Medicine 328: 95–99

Porro G B, Parente F, Cernuschi M 1989 The diagnosis of esophageal candidiasis in patients with acquired immune deficiency syndrome: is endoscopy always necessary? American Journal of Gastroenterology 84: 143–146

Relman D A, Falkow S, LeBoit P E et al 1991 The organism causing bacillary angiomatosis, peliosis hepatis, and fever and bacteremia in immunocompromised patients. New England Journal of Medicine 324: 1514

Rivin B E, Monroe J M, Hubschman B P, Thomas P A 1984 AIDS outcome: a first follow-up. New England Journal of Medicine 311: 857

Roth R I, Owen R L, Keren D F 1983 AIDS with *Mycobacterium avium-intracellulare* lesions resembling those of Whipple's disease. New England Journal of Medicine 309: 1324–1325

Ryan J, Colman J, Pedersen J, Benson E 1992 Thalidomide to treat esophageal ulcer in AIDS. New England Journal of Medicine 327: 208–209

Schiodt M, Greenspan D, Daniels T E et al 1989 Parotid gland enlargement and xerostomia associated with labial sialadenitis in HIV-infected patients. Journal of Autoimmunity 2: 415–425

Schmitt S L, Wexner S D 1994 Treatment of anorectal manifestations of AIDS: past and present. International Journal of STD and AIDS 5: 8–10

Schneiderman D J, Arenson D M, Cello J P, Margaretten W, Weber T E 1987 Hepatic disease in patients with the acquired immune deficiency syndrome (AIDS). Hepatology 7: 925–930

Scoazec J-Y, Marche C, Girard P-M et al 1988 Peliosis hepatis and sinusoidal dilatation during infection by the human immunodeficiency virus (HIV). An ultrastructural study. American Journal of Pathology 131: 38–47

Selik R M, Starcher E T, Curran J W 1987 Opportunistic diseases reported in AIDS patients: frequencies, associations, and trends. AIDS 1: 175–182

Shattock A G, Finlay H, Hillary I B 1987 Possible reactivation of hepatitis D with chronic δ antigenaemia by human immunodeficiency virus. British Medical Journal 294: 1656–1657

Shen J-Y, Barnes P F, Rea T H, Meyer P R 1988 Immunohistology of

tuberculous adenitis in symptomatic HIV infection. Clinical and Experimental Immunology 72: 186–189
Simon D M, Cello J P, Valenzuela J et al 1995 Multicenter trial of octreotide in patients with refractory acquired immunodeficiency syndrome-associated diarrhea. Gastroenterology 108: 1753–1760
Smith P D, Lane H C, Gill V J et al 1988 Intestinal infections in patients with acquired immune deficiency syndrome. Annals of Internal Medicine 108: 328
Vazquez M, Rotterdam H, Sidu G 1989 Malignant neoplasms in surgical specimens of different AIDS risk groups. V International Conference on AIDS: 4–9 June 1989, Montreal, Canada. Abstract MBP 293
Weber J N, Weiss R A 1988 The virology of human immunodeficiency viruses. British Medical Bulletin 44: 20–37
Wilcox C M, Schwartz D A 1992 A pilot study of oral corticosteroid therapy for idiopathic esophageal ulcerations associated with human immunodeficiency virus infection. American Journal of Medicine 93: 131–134
World Health Organization 1990 Acquired immune deficiency syndrome (AIDS): interim proposal for a WHO staging system for HIV infection and disease. Weekly Epidemiological Research 65: 221–224
Youle M, Clarbour J, Farthing C et al 1989 Treatment of resistant aphthous ulceration with thalidomide in patients positive for HIV antibody. British Medical Journal 298: 432
Youle M, Hawkins D, Gazzard B 1990 Thalidomide in hyperalgic pharyngeal ulceration of AIDS. Lancet 335: 1591

# 22. Nutrition

*Douglas L. Seidner C. Richard Fleming*

The primary role of the gastrointestinal tract is to digest and absorb nutrients in sufficient quantities so that normal body composition and function are maintained throughout life. Gastrointestinal diseases result in significant impairment of normal digestive function and often lead to the development of malnutrition. This is obvious in patients with severe Crohn's disease, postgastrectomy syndrome and upper gastrointestinal malignancy where malnutrition is quite commonly seen. Nutritive factors may also be responsible for gastrointestinal disease as is the case with conditions such as celiac sprue, alcoholic liver disease and pancreatitis. It is therefore important for gastroenterologists to have a strong working knowledge of the interaction between nutrition and digestive health so that optimal patient care can be provided.

In this chapter, we will cover several fundamental aspects of malnutrition including prevalence, pathogenesis and diagnosis as well as determination of nutritional requirements. Specific considerations for the management of patients with acute pancreatitis, chronic liver disease, inflammatory bowel disease and short bowel syndrome will be discussed. Lastly, methods for the safe and effective delivery of enteral and parental nutrition will be reviewed.

## FUNDAMENTALS OF NUTRITION SUPPORT

### Definition of malnutrition

Malnutrition is the end result of any condition which leads to an alteration in either body composition or function. Malnutrition may result from either an excess or deficit in calories, protein, vitamins and minerals. In general, digestive diseases are more likely to result in undernutrition, especially where disease is severe and/or prolonged.

Protein calorie malnutrition is the most common form of undernutrition seen in clinical practice. Protein calorie malnutrition is not just one disease; rather, it is a set of afflictions which span the pathophysiologic consequences of starvation and injury (McMahon & Bistrian 1990). Marasmus is at one end of this continuum and develops when there is a reduction in the availability of all nutrients resulting in a diminution in protein and fat stores. Voluntary starvation in the form of anorexia nervosa represents the purest form of marasmus. More commonly, the marasmic form of protein calorie malnutrition occurs because of decreased intake or malabsorption associated with illnesses such as short bowel syndrome, severe cardiac disease (e.g. cardiac cachexia) or advanced malignancy. Clinical characteristics of marasmus include reductions in weight, visceral and skeletal muscle and fat stores in the presence of a normal serum albumin. At the other end of the spectrum is kwashiorkor or hypoalbuminemic protein calorie malnutrition. Clinical findings include depressed serum albumin values, fluid overload, hepatic steatosis and abnormalities in cellular immunity and muscle function. Features of kwashiorkor are commonly seen in the intensive care setting where it is commonly associated with trauma, surgery and sepsis (Wilmore 1991).

### Prevalence of malnutrition

The prevalence of protein calorie malnutrition in hospitalized patients ranges from 30% to 50% whether one surveys a community or teaching hospital or medical or surgical ward (Bistrian et al 1974, 1976, Hill et al 1977, Weinsier et al 1979). In patients with Crohn's disease and alcoholic liver disease, the likelihood of developing a nutritionally associated abnormality may approach 80% (Driscoll & Rosenberg 1978, McCullough et al 1989). The importance of recognizing this problem is that patients with significant protein calorie malnutrition are at increased risk for infections, poor wound healing, respiratory failure and death (Buzby et al 1980). Other less serious morbidity associated with malnutrition, such as fatigue and muscle weakness, has a more pernicious impact on the patient's health.

### Pathogenesis of malnutrition

The mechanisms responsible for the development of malnutrition can be broadly categorized into four main groups: inadequate intake, malabsorption, excessive losses and altered metabolism. In most patients, more than one of these factors is operational. For example, a patient with Crohn's disease may have diminished intake because of the presence of abdominal pain and diarrhea, malabsorption secondary to mucosal inflammation, bacterial overgrowth or previous intestinal resection (Rosenberg et al 1985) and increased catabolism. Malnutrition is almost always secondary to an underlying disease and management of the primary illness is necessary to optimize nutritional therapies.

*Diminished intake*

Inadequate intake of food, whether it is due to anorexia, inability to eat, voluntary starvation or poor dietary habits, is the most common cause of undernutrition. The pathogenesis of anorexia is complex but is in part mediated through the elaboration of cytokines such as interleukin 1 and tumor necrosis factor that are released in response to infection and/or inflammation (Sternberg et al 1992). Patients with gastrointestinal diseases often avoid food to minimize symptoms such as abdominal pain, diarrhea, nausea and vomiting. Patients with eating disorders may also become malnourished by following self-imposed restrictive diets. Occasionally, therapeutic diets that are not closely followed can lead to inadvertent removal of a required nutrient from the diet. Lastly, patients with alcoholism frequently consume approximately 35% of their calories as alcohol (Neville et al 1986).

*Maldigestion and malabsorption*

Maldigestion and malabsorption can result from defects in the intraluminal, intestinal or lymphatic transport stages. The intraluminal stage is responsible for the bulk of digestion of protein (p. 346), carbohydrate (p. 340) and fat (p. 351). Pancreatic insufficiency, postgastrectomy syndrome and the Zollinger–Ellison syndrome are examples of conditions that can adversely affect intraluminal digestion. The intestinal or mucosal stage is responsible for the terminal digestion and transport of small peptides and monosaccharides. Since the length of the small bowel is considerable (p. 337), intestinal surface area is usually not an issue unless mucosal disease is diffuse and severe or large lengths of small bowel have been resected (p. 454). Since certain nutrients are absorbed in specific segments of the bowel, the site of disease or resection is important. The distal portion of the ileum is responsible for absorption of vitamin $B_{12}$ (Gerson et al 1973) and bile acids (Hofmann & Poley 1972). When the terminal ileum is resected (p. 453), as in the management of Crohn's disease, vitamin $B_{12}$ deficiency is likely to occur; however, hepatic reserves are usually so great that 2 or 3 years may pass before biochemical evidence of vitamin $B_{12}$ deficiency occurs. Receptors for bile acids are most concentrated in the distal 100 cm of the ileum; severe inflammation or surgical resection of this segment results in depletion of the bile acid pool (p. 452) with maldigestion of fat and fat-soluble vitamins. Optimal absorption of iron, calcium and folate occurs within the duodenum so mucosal disease which predominantly affects this portion of the bowel, such as celiac sprue, can lead to deficiencies of these and many other nutrients. Conditions that affect the lymphatic stage of absorption include lymphoma, intestinal lymphangiectasia and transmural diseases such as Crohn's disease. Excessive pressure within the intestinal lymphatics leads to leakage of lymph fluid into the small bowel lumen and losses of proteins and white blood cells.

*Excessive losses*

Normal gastrointestinal function involves the secretion of fluid, electrolytes, minerals and digestive enzymes. When the secretory function of the intestinal tract exceeds its absorptive capacity, large amounts of fluids and electrolytes may be lost. Large volume diarrhea and fistula losses can lead to depletion of sodium, potassium, magnesium and zinc (Wolman et al 1979). Divalent cations such as calcium, magnesium and zinc are poorly solubilized at the alkaline pH of the small intestine. Under normal circumstances, 30–40% of these cations are absorbed; however, with steatorrhea they form insoluble precipitates with intraluminal fatty acids and become less available for absorption. Hence, these cations may be depleted when steatorrhea is significant, as in pancreatic insufficiency and the short bowel syndrome (p. 454). Since intestinal secretions are also rich in protein, depletion of this nutrient also occurs in the short bowel syndrome. More commonly, excessive protein losses occur with inflammatory conditions of the mucosa such as protein-losing enteropathies (p. 348). Iron deficiency often results from chronic blood loss associated with gut diseases.

*Altered metabolism*

Altered metabolism may be the result of the underlying disease or the therapies used to treat it. Energy requirements may be transiently increased in patients with fever or infection (Long et al 1979). Inflammation associated with the primary disease, such as alcoholic hepatitis (John et al 1989) and inflammatory bowel disease (Chan et al 1986), often does not significantly increase energy requirements. Medications, especially those used to treat inflammatory bowel disease, can directly impact on nutrient absorption. Sulfasalazine competitively inhibits the absorption of folic acid (Franklin & Rosenberg 1973). Corticosteroids diminish the absorption of calcium and often contribute to the osteopenia seen in patients on long-term corticosteroids (Reid 1989). The mineralocorticoid effect of corticosteroids may increase potassium and phosphate losses in the urine. Bile acid-binding resins such as cholestyramine used in the management of cholerrheic diarrhea can increase steatorrhea minimally and accelerate the loss of fat-soluble vitamins (Compston & Horton 1978).

## Patient assessment and monitoring

A comprehensive nutritional assessment includes a thorough history, a physical examination that includes anthropometric measurements and laboratory studies. A complete evaluation should also help determine the severity and cause of the malnutrition so that the timing of nutritional support can be determined and the etiologic factors can be managed. Finally, these techniques can also be used to determine the response to nutritional therapy.

### *Body composition*

An understanding of body composition helps define the available stores of fat, glucose and protein that are utilized during periods of starvation and injury. Knowledge of body composition is also useful in interpreting the results of a nutrition assessment. Fat stores normally constitute 20–25% of the body weight or 12–16 kg and are the major repository of energy, containing 25 000–37 500 kJ (105 000–157 500 kcal) (Moore et al 1963, Bistrian 1977a). Nearly all of the body fat can be used during prolonged periods of negative energy balance. Glucose is stored as glycogen in the liver and muscle and is used as a source of fuel during the immediate postprandial period. Unfortunately, of the 1 kg which is stored, only one quarter or 5000 kJ (21 000 kcal) is available as fuel. After this portion of glycogen is used glucose is produced by the liver and to a lesser degree by the kidney through gluconeogenesis.

The remaining tissues are referred to as the fat-free mass (FFM) which comprises skeletal and visceral muscle, plasma and extracellular protein and bone. The metabolically active portion of the FFM is referred to as the body cell mass which includes skeletal and visceral muscle. Though the body cell mass can provide 7000 kJ (30 000 kcal) through the conversion of amino acids to glucose, the body spares protein, especially that in visceral muscle (Cahill 1970, Young & Scrimshaw 1971).

### *Clinical history*

The magnitude and pattern of weight loss compared to the usual weight are crucial components of the history. A recent loss of 5–10%, 10–20% and more than 20% body weight signifies mild, moderate and severe protein calorie malnutrition, respectively. The pattern of weight loss is also important. For example, a patient with a 7 kg loss over a 3-month period is at greater risk than one who loses 9 kg and then gains 2 kg over the same time. Severe weight loss has been shown to markedly increase the risk of postoperative complications, nosocomial infection and mortality (Harvey et al 1981).

Medical, social, drug and dietary information are also important components of the nutritional history. Conditions such as diabetes mellitus, thyroid disease and previous gastrointestinal surgery may impact on the development and management of undernutrition. Increased metabolic needs are often associated with sepsis, trauma, open wounds, abscesses and fistulae. A history of alcohol or chemical dependence should also be elicited. Unusual dietary habits, social setting and the effect of presenting symptoms on oral intake are all important factors which will affect nutritional health.

### *Physical examination*

The signs of nutritional deficiencies (Table 22.1), including muscle wasting, edema, thinning of the hair, dry scaling skin, stomatitis and cheilosis, can be easily detected on physical examination. Unfortunately, most of these findings appear only after a moderate to severe deficiency occurs and are not specific for malnutrition. Whenever possible, patients should be treated before these signs develop.

Anthropometry of the upper arm is a simple, inexpensive and noninvasive method to indirectly measure body composition (Heymsfield et al 1982). Two metabolically distinct body compartments, fat and skeletal muscle, are estimated with these techniques. Triceps skinfolds (TSF) measure fat stores while both triceps skinfolds and mid-arm circumference are used to calculate mid-upper arm muscle circumference (MUAMC) which is an estimate of skeletal muscle stores. Diminished fat stores do not correlate directly with outcome since a marked reduction can be well tolerated in the setting of pure starvation (Bistrian 1977a). Serum albumin and weight loss correlate with MUAMC and have been shown to predict operative morbidity in patients undergoing a variety of operative procedures (Young & Hill 1979). Values below the fifth percentile of population standards are indicative of severe protein calorie malnutrition (Heymsfield et al 1982). The limitation of upper arm anthropometry is the expertise required to obtain reproducible measurements.

Body weight is a composite of total body energy stores with changes coinciding with energy and nitrogen balance. The accurate determination of body weight and comparison with premorbid or desirable body weight are important. A simple equation proposed by Hamwi (1964) can be used to calculate ideal body weight: for women 45.5 kg is allowed for the first 5 feet and 2.3 kg are added for each inch thereafter; for men 48.2 kg are allowed for the first

**Table 22.1** Signs of specific vitamin and nutritional deficiencies

| Organ system | Signs | Deficiencies |
|---|---|---|
| Hair | Coiled, corkscrew | Vitamins A, C |
| | Dry | Vitamins E, A |
| | Color change | Zinc |
| | Brittle | Biotin |
| | Easy pluckability | Protein, biotin, zinc |
| | Loss | Protein, $B_{12}$, folate |
| Skin | Petechiae | Vitamins A, C |
| | Pigmentation, cracking, crusting | Niacin |
| | Desquamation | Riboflavin |
| | Perifollicular hemorrhage | Vitamin C |
| | Purpura | Vitamins C, K |
| | Xerosis | Essential fatty acid |
| | Edema | Protein, thiamine, vitamin E |
| Oral | Swollen, spongy, bleeding gums | Vitamin C |
| | Gingivitis, loosening of teeth | Vitamin C |
| | Large, swollen tongue | Iodine, niacin |
| | Fissure, raw tongue | Niacin |
| | Cheilosis, angular stomatitis | B-complex, iron, protein |
| | Ulcers | Folate |
| Extremities | Weakness | Thiamine |
| | Paresthesiae | Thiamine, $B_{12}$, biotin |
| | Numbness, tingling | $B_{12}$ |
| | Arthralgias | Vitamin C |
| | Muscle wasting | Protein |
| | Pain in calves | Thiamine |
| Central nervous system | Ophthalmoplegia, foot drop | Thiamine |
| | Depressed sensation – vibratory, position | $B_{12}$, Vitamin E |
| | Anxiety, depression, hallucinations | Niacin |
| | Memory disturbance | $B_{12}$ |
| | Hyporeflexia | Thiamine, $B_{12}$ |
| General | Anorexia | Thiamine, vitamin C, folate, $B_{12}$, biotin |
| | Hypotension, hypothermia | Thiamine |
| | Thrombocytopenia | Folate, vitamin C |
| | Parotid enlargement | Protein |
| | Thyroid enlargement | Iodine |

Adapted from Shils & Young 1988

5 feet and 2.7 kg are added for each additional inch. Interpretation of body weight becomes difficult with sodium and fluid retention secondary to hepatic, renal and cardiac disease. Body weight is a good measure of long-term nutritional status. Increases in weight in physically active individuals usually represents an equal gain in skeletal muscle and fat stores. Rapid changes in weight are more likely to represent changes in body water.

While weight loss is important, one must not lose sight of the consequences of excessive body weight. Obesity is clearly a risk factor for hypertension, atherosclerosis, diabetes, cancer and premature death. A simple measurement of obesity is known as the Body Mass Index (BMI) which compares weight and height in the following relationship:

$$\text{BMI} = \frac{\text{weight (kg)}}{\text{height}^2\ \text{(m)}}$$

An individual with a BMI greater than 29.5 is clearly obese and at high risk for its detrimental effects, while those over 23.5 for men and 24.5 for women are above the normal range and are at modest health risk.

A variety of other nutrition assessment techniques have been used to study body composition and response to therapy (Lukaski 1987). They are mentioned for completeness but are used for the most part as research tools. They include computed tomography, ultrasonography, magnetic resonance imaging, bioelectrical impedance, isotope dilution measurements and neutron activation. In most cases, these techniques have been used to validate the more readily available assessment methods.

*Laboratory assessment*

Serum proteins, including albumin, transferrin and prealbumin, are commonly measured to assess the visceral protein compartment. Malnutrition, especially injury-associated protein calorie malnutrition, leads to diminished hepatocellular biosynthesis and a reduction in the serum concentrations of these proteins. Other factors which affect their concentrations include altered plasma volume, catabolism and excretion.

Albumin is the most commonly measured marker of visceral protein status. It is normally synthesized at a rate of 120–270 mg/kg/24 h, is distributed between the intravascular (40%) and extravascular (60%) spaces, transports many small molecules and helps maintain plasma oncotic pressure (Doweiko & Nompleggi 1991a). As part of the metabolic response to injury, serum albumin levels decrease because synthesis is decreased, a greater fraction is distributed into the extravascular space and its catabolism is increased (Doweiko & Nompleggi 1991b). This is contrasted with the preservation of normal albumin levels in patients with marasmus, such as anorexia nervosa, even in its most severe form. Because of these apparent discrepancies, albumin is often a better marker of severity of illness than it is of nutrition status; however, it has been clearly shown that albumin concentrations correlate with overall morbidity and mortality and thus identify patients who might benefit from nutritional support (Studley 1936, Cannon et al 1944, Reinhardt et al 1980, McClave et al 1992). The long serum half-life of albumin (18–21 days), changes in distribution and frequent exogenous administration make it a poor marker of short-term nutritional repletion.

Liver secretory proteins of shorter half-life are more sensitive than albumin in assessing response to adequate nutritional support. Transferrin, which transports iron from the plasma to the bone marrow, has a half-life of 7–8 days and has been shown to reflect the severity of protein calorie malnutrition (Reeds & Laditan 1976). Concentrations may be falsely elevated in iron deficiency, blood transfusion, estrogen therapy and acute hepatitis.

Prealbumin transports thyroxine in the blood and has a half-life of 2–3 days. Its rapid turnover and relationship to protein depletion and injury make it a very sensitive marker of protein intake. Levels may be falsely elevated with renal failure, its chief site of catabolism.

Urinary creatinine excretion, which reflects creatine turnover within muscle, can be used as a measure of body cell mass as long as dietary protein intake and renal function are stable (Heymsfield et al 1983). It can be used to assess the amount of metabolically active tissue and is especially useful in patients where anthropometric measurement of skeletal muscle may be inaccurate (i.e. fluid overload). The creatinine height index (CHI) is the comparison of the measured 24-h creatinine excretion and the expected urinary creatinine excretion (Bistrian et al 1975). The expected creatinine excretion per day can be calculated by multiplying the patient's ideal weight by 18 mg for women and 23 mg for men. The CHI is expressed as a percentage by dividing the observed by the expected creatinine excretion and multiplying this number by 100. A CHI between 60% and 80% indicates moderate depletion of muscle mass while a value less than 60% suggests severe depletion.

### *Nitrogen balance*

Nitrogen balance is the difference between nitrogen ingested and nitrogen lost (MacKenzie et al 1974). Since protein has an average nitrogen content of 16%, dietary protein is multiplied by 0.16 or divided by 6.25 to be converted to grams of nitrogen. Nitrogen losses equal urinary urea nitrogen (UUN) measured in a 24-h collection plus 4 g to account for skin, stool and nonurea urinary nitrogen losses. All values are expressed in grams and results are calculated as follows:

$$N_{balance} = N_{in} - N_{out}$$

$$N_{in} = \text{protein intake} \div 6.25$$

$$N_{out} = \text{UUN} + 4\text{g}$$

Nitrogen balance studies are best performed in patients with stable renal function and after the patient has been maintained on a stable diet for at least 4 days. This test is indicated in patients requiring prolonged nutrition support to assure that adequate amounts of protein and energy are being provided.

### *Functional assessment*

Nutrition is known to affect immune function and muscle strength; therefore, the function of each can be used as indirect measures of nutrition. Immune function is the easiest to assess with total lymphocyte count and delayed hypersensitivity skin testing (DHST). Lymphocyte counts below 1500, 1200, and 800 $mm^{-3}$ are considered mild, moderate and severely depressed, respectively, with changes being seen with injury-associated protein calorie malnutrition and not starvation (Blackburn et al 1977). DHST is performed by placing at least three recall antigens intradermally on the forearm and reading the results at 24 and 48 h. Induration of 5 mm or more is considered positive. Anergy to DHST can be seen with either severe starvation or injury (Bistrian 1977b). The frequency of postoperative sepsis and death can be as high as 52% and 36% respectively in patients with anergy, whereas the frequency of these complications is 7% and 2% when reactivity to these tests is preserved. Both of these measures show improvement following nutritional repletion with a reduction in associated morbidity and mortality (Harvey et al 1981).

Muscle weakness is a common complaint in malnourished patients. Hand grip dynamometry and measurement of inspiratory force have been used to quantify muscle strength and both have been shown to correlate with nutrition-associated complications (Fraser et al 1984, Kalfarentzos et al 1989). Supramaximal nerve stimulation is a more objective way to study the force, relaxation and endurance characteristics of various skeletal muscles. Rapid functional changes in muscle function have been demonstrated with nutrient deprivation prior to any compositional changes in body protein stores (Russell et al 1983). In addition, muscle function has been shown to be a more accurate measure of surgical risk than anthropometric changes in muscle and protein compartments (Windsor & Hill 1988). Sepsis, trauma and corticosteroid administration do not appear to affect these measurements and nutritional repletion results in normalization within 4 days (Brough et al 1986).

### *Predictive equations*

In an attempt to stratify patients more reliably according to hospital morbidity and mortality, several predictive models have been developed. These include the Hospital Prognostic Index (HPI) (Harvey et al 1981) and the Prognostic Nutritional Index (PNI) (Buzby et al 1980), each of which requires the measurement of various nutritional and functional parameters. Bedside assessments by experienced clinicians may provide equally useful information. The subjective global assessment (Detsky et al 1987) combines historical features, such as amount and pattern of weight loss, change in dietary intake, the presence of gastrointestinal symptoms and functional capacity, and signs of malnutrition to determine the degree of malnutrition.

### *Patient selection and route of administration*

Patient selection focuses on the proper identification of those who require specialized nutrition support and the decision as to when this therapy should be provided. In addition, the question as to which route, enteral or parenteral, is more appropriate is often answered at this juncture of the patient's assessment.

Any patient with moderate to severe malnutrition or catabolism who is unable to eat for 5 or more days should receive nutritional support. Three important variables, the presence of protein calorie malnutrition, the degree of the injury response and the absence of adequate oral consumption, determine the urgency with which nutritional support should be given.

Specialized nutritional support is usually not required when weight loss is less than 10% of usual body weight, when the degree of injury or inflammation is mild and when an oral diet is expected to resume within 1 week. Patients with mild to moderate degrees of weight loss and/or stress may be supported with peripheral vein intravenous fluids until their clinical course can be more adequately predicted. This intermediate group may require specialized nutritional support within the first or second week of hospitalization. Lastly, certain clinical conditions require prompt intervention, even if weight loss has not occurred. These include patients with a severe closed head injury, trauma or third-degree burns. A scheme which can be used in deciding when to provide nutrition support is presented in Table 22.2.

Specialized nutrition support is given by the enteral or parenteral route. A brief list of indications for each mode of therapy is outlined in Table 22.3.

***Tube enteral nutrition.*** This is the preferred method for providing support. The advantages of enteral compared with parenteral nutrition are that nutrients are more efficiently utilized, gut integrity is maintained (Dominioni et al 1984, Mochizuki et al 1984), complications are less severe (Cataldi-Betcher et al 1983) and expense is only one-tenth that of total parenteral nutrition. Tube feeding should be considered in patients who are unable to meet their nutritional requirements through the consumption of an oral diet plus supplements and have functioning gastrointestinal tracts. Patients with dysphagia because of a neurologic disease or head and neck cancers are ideal candidates for tube feeding. Critically ill patients are far more challenging to tube feed but may have enhanced recovery through the use of early enteral feeding. Early enteral feeding in the intensive care unit may have additional benefits of decreasing bacterial translocation across the gut barrier and diminishing the catabolic response to injury (Deitch 1990). Even patients with inflammatory conditions of the gastrointestinal tract can be tube fed with standard formulas. In the case of Crohn's disease, enteral nutrition has been successfully used as primary therapy (p. 629) (see below).

Tube feeding should not be used in patients with mechanical bowel obstruction, acute severe pancreatitis, acute bowel ischemia, intractable vomiting and diarrhea, active gastrointestinal bleeding and a high output gastrointestinal fistula arising from the proximal small bowel. Some patients with severe malabsorption and intestinal pseudo-obstruction also may not be suitable candidates for this therapy.

***The parenteral route.*** This is the preferred method for patients requiring nutritional support whose gastrointestinal tract is nonfunctional. The contraindications for enteral nutrition are often the indications for parenteral nutrition. Contraindications for parenteral nutrition include treatment anticipated for less than 7–10 days, a functioning gastrointestinal tract and inability to obtain or maintain central venous access. Peripheral vein parenteral nutrition can avoid many of the more serious complications associated with central vein cannulation; however, these solutions are just as expensive as the more calorically dense formulae delivered via a central vein and require similar monitoring. Thus, it is suggested that these formulae be used for the same indications as total parenteral nutrition. Since it can be difficult to provide full nutritional support with peripheral solutions, they are mainly used when therapy is required for less than 7 days in patients who are not hypermetabolic or when central vein cannulation is not practical.

**Table 22.2** Degree of malnutrition and initiation of nutrition support

| Weight loss (%) | Level of stress* | Intervention† |
|---|---|---|
| < 10 | Mild or moderate | Fluid and electrolytes |
| 10–20 | Mild | Fluid and electrolytes |
| | Moderate or severe | Nutrition |
| > 20 | Any | Nutrition |
| Any | Severe | Nutrition |

*Clinical markers of stress: fever, leukocytosis, depressed visceral proteins
†See text for timing of intervention

**Table 22.3** Indications for nutritional support

| Category | Examples |
|---|---|
| Hypermetabolism | Sepsis, trauma, burns, major surgery |
| Organ system failure | Cardiac, hepatic, respiratory, renal |
| Neurologic | Cerebral vascular accident, head trauma, dementia |
| Gastrointestinal | Esophageal obstruction, inflammatory bowel disease, pancreatitis |
| Oncologic | Chemotherapy, radiotherapy, surgery |

Enteral nutrition is preferred with the following exceptions: mechanical bowel obstruction; ileus; severe vomiting, diarrhea, GI bleeding; high output fistula (>200 ml/d); and early phase of acute pancreatitis

## Metabolic response to starvation and injury

The physiologic changes that accompany starvation and injury are predictable. The metabolic response to starvation leads to adaptive changes which help preserve the body cell mass, the compartment that includes skeletal and smooth muscle and visceral proteins (Cahill et al 1966). This assures survival by preserving organ function in the face of diminished substrate availability. On the other hand, injury results in a prioritization of energy, protein and micronutrients for recovery (Powanda 1977). This response to injury is well tolerated for a short duration in the well nourished, but in a poorly nourished patient or with prolonged injury, a critical loss of body cell mass can result in multisystem organ failure and death. The metabolic response to injury depends on both the severity and duration of the underlying illness. Since most diseases lead to a mixed picture, it is best to view protein calorie malnutrition as a continuum between starvation and injury.

*Metabolic response to starvation*

The neurohumoral response to starvation includes a depression in sympathetic nervous system and thyroid function (Cahill et al 1966). These changes plus a decrease in physical activity contribute to reduced energy expenditure (Young & Scrimshaw 1971). Energy requirements are initially met through glycogenolysis but this store of fuel is usually depleted in 24–48 h, after which protein catabolism supplies substrate for gluconeogenesis. Over time this would result in a profound loss of muscle stores if it were not for the shift in substrate utilization from glucose to fat. The average adult requires 125 g of glucose each day for metabolic function of the central nervous system, renal medulla and red and white blood cells (Cahill 1970). The adaptive response to starvation diminishes this obligatory need for glucose to 40 g per day. This shift in substrate utilization occurs as a result of decreased insulin secretion and insulin to glucagon ratio which favor lipolysis and ketogenesis. Ketone bodies can be utilized by the brain during starvation. The adaptive response to starvation takes several weeks to be fully realized and helps preserve protein, as demonstrated by a decreasing urinary nitrogen excretion.

*Metabolic response to injury*

The neurohumoral response to injury is contrasted with the response to starvation in Table 22.4. There is an increase in insulin and the counter-regulatory hormones glucagon, epinephrine, cortisol and growth hormone. In addition, interleukin 1 and tumor necrosis factor, along with other cytokines, orchestrate the flow of substrate which is necessary for the synthesis of acute phase proteins, polymorphonuclear leukocytes, collagen formation and other processes that allow recovery (Wilmore 1991). Where the response to starvation helps conserve protein, injury results in an outpouring of protein to provide ample quantities of amino acids for synthetic function and gluconeogenesis. This is manifest as a markedly negative nitrogen balance. Gluconeogenesis in the liver and lipolysis of adipose stores to provide fatty acids supply the necessary fuel to drive the injury response.

**Table 22.4** Protein calorie malnutrition: comparison of chemical mediators and metabolic response in starvation and injury

| | Starvation | Injury |
|---|---|---|
| Mediators | | |
| Insulin | ↓ | ↑ |
| Counter regulatory hormones* | ↑ | ↑↑ |
| Sympathetic nervous system | ↓ | ↑↑ |
| Cytokines† | ø | ↑↑ |
| Metabolic | | |
| Energy expenditure | ↓ | ↑ |
| Proteolysis | ↑ early<br>↓ late | ↑↑ |
| Glycogenolysis | ↑ early<br>ø late | ø |
| Gluconeogenesis | ↑ | ↑ |
| Lipolysis | ↑ late | ↑ |
| Ketogenesis | ↑ | ø |
| Body cell mass | ↓ gradual | ↓↓ rapid |

*Counter-regulatory hormones — glucagon, epinephrine, cortisol, growth hormone
†Cytokines — tumor necrosis factor, interleukin-1, -2, -6
ø = None

*Gut barrier function and the injury response*

The gastrointestinal tract serves as a protective barrier which prevents a variety of infectious pathogens and their toxins from gaining entrance into the bloodstream (Deitch 1990). This barrier is maintained by direct stimulation and the neurohumoral response to intraluminal food (Levine et al 1974, Eastwood 1977). A wide array of clinical conditions, including burns, trauma, pancreatitis and intestinal obstruction (Fink 1991), have been shown to disrupt this barrier and make the intestine more permeable to micro-organisms and microbial products. This process, known as bacterial translocation, is believed to sustain the systemic response to injury in some critically ill patients who appear septic but have no apparent source of fever. Early enteral feeding has been shown to maintain gut integrity and decrease the metabolic response to injury in laboratory animals (Dominioni et al 1984, Mochizuki et al 1984). Though it has been difficult to directly demonstrate this process in humans, several lines of evidence support this concept including intestinal permeability studies in septic patients (Ziegler et al 1988) and subjects given low-dose endotoxin (O'Dwyer et al 1988) and in clinical trials comparing enteral to parenteral nutrition in trauma patients where lower rates of pneumonia and intra-abdominal abscesses have been found in the patients on tube enteral feeding (Moore et al 1989, Kudsk et al 1992). Glutamine, which is the primary fuel of the gastrointestinal tract, has been shown to prevent TPN-induced mucosal atrophy and bacterial translocation in laboratory animals (Fox et al 1988) and to improve nitrogen retention, decrease the incidence of bacterial infections and shorten the length of stay in patients undergoing bone marrow transplantation (Ziegler et al 1992).

## Substrate utilization

### *Protein and nitrogen balance*

The major objective of nutrition support is to maintain or replace protein stores. This can only be done if protein of high biologic value is provided in an adequate amount. There are important relationships between protein, energy and the metabolic state that determine the success of any nutritional program.

Under normal conditions, nitrogen balance is tightly regulated by the body to be zero (Edens et al 1986). When nitrogen is provided in excess of these quantities it is oxidized and when there is an insufficient amount of nitrogen provided, negative nitrogen balance ensues. In the latter case nitrogen losses are modest but with time, the body adapts to help conserve protein and thus minimize these losses and in some cases nitrogen balance is again reached. Patients who display an injury response are by definition hypercatabolic and are unable to conserve protein as previously mentioned because of the body's need to provide a sufficient amount of protein to fuel the injury response. Under these circumstances, protein must be provided in sufficient amount to meet this added demand.

In health, protein breakdown and synthesis are closely matched, with synthesis being quite efficient relative to the amount of new dietary protein taken. On the other hand, the injury response markedly increases protein breakdown and synthesis with the former being greater than the latter. This results in an increase in urinary urea nitrogen loss which parallels the severity of the injury (Bistrian 1979).

Nitrogen balance can usually be obtained in patients with mild stress; however, this goal cannot be reached when stress is more severe. Streat and colleagues (1987) studied eight septic postoperative patients who were given TPN for 10 days (mean of 11 550 kJ and 127 g protein). Despite a substantial increase in fat stores, which suggested adequacy of the TPN formula, the patients lost a significant amount of lean tissue. These results underscore the importance of treating the primary illness while providing reasonable amounts of nutrients to minimize nitrogen losses. The temptation to escalate the nutritional formula in this setting should be avoided as it will often lead to intolerance and possibly complications of overfeeding (Meguid et al 1984).

### *Glucose and energy balance*

Glucose is the major oxidative fuel of most diets and nutrition support formulas. When there is an energy deficit, negative nitrogen balance will occur even when protein intake is near normal. With complete starvation in unstressed subjects, 12 g of nitrogen are lost on the first day (Cahill et al 1966) and it declines to only 3 g per day after 5 weeks (Owen et al 1967). The addition of only 120 g of glucose (1680 kJ/24 h) reduces the nitrogen loss by one half whereas 700 g glucose (10 000 kJ/24 h will only reduce the amount of nitrogen lost by half again (Wolfe et al 1977). The relatively small amount of glucose which is required to markedly reduce protein breakdown reflects the basal amount needed to meet the demands of tissues that require glucose for fuel (brain, renal medulla, leukocytes, red blood cells) which has previously been mentioned. This is the pivotal feature in the synergistic relationship between energy and nitrogen balance.

This endogenous production of glucose is incompletely suppressed by glucose infusion with injury (Shaw & Wolfe 1986). The hormonal milieu which occurs with injury favors protein catabolism despite glucose infusion. In addition, the stress response impairs the rate of glucose oxidation with more severe injury leading to a greater degree of impairment. These patients should be given no more than 5–6 mg/kg/min or 105–126 kJ/kg/24 h in parenteral solutions (Wolfe et al 1979). Glucose given beyond this rate favors fatty acid synthesis which can result in hepatic steatosis, liver dysfunction, excessive carbon dioxide production and hyperglycemia. These problems are generally avoided when fat is used as a portion of the nonprotein calories; however, careful calculation of nutritional requirements is still advised so that overfeeding is avoided.

### *Fat*

Fat is given with TPN as a lipid emulsion of long chain triglycerides (LCTs) to provide a source of energy and essential fatty acids. As long as 125–150 g/24 h of glucose is supplied, intravenous fat is able to spare nitrogen to the same degree as glucose. It appears that most of the nitrogen-sparing effect of fat is derived from the glycerol used to prepare the lipid emulsion and the glycerol moiety of the triglyceride molecule, both of which lead to the production of glucose. Fat oxidation is not suppressed with the infusion of excess glucose (Stoner et al 1983) and it is a major fuel in patients with moderate to severe injury (Nordenstrom et al 1982). A three-in-one formula which supplies 20–40% of the calories as fat can help minimize the development of hepatic steatosis, maintain the respiratory quotient in a normal range for patients with lung disease and help control blood sugars more easily in diabetics as opposed to a glucose-based parenteral solution. Fat is also the major energy source of peripheral parenteral nutrition formulae.

Essential fatty acids (EFA) should make up 2–4% of total calories to avoid deficiency (Burr & Burr 1930). Linoleic acid, an n-6 polyunsaturated fatty acid (PUFA), is a precursor of arachidonic acid which is necessary for normal wound healing, skin and hair growth and platelet and immune function. Deficiency of this fat results in a characteristic diffuse, scaly rash. α-Linolenic acid is an n-3 PUFA which is important in the neurologic development of neonates (Holman et al 1982) and may be important in adults (Bjerve et al 1987). Both of these fatty acids are abundant in parenteral lipid emulsions that are derived from soybean or safflower oil. Enteral products consist of either corn, soybean or other vegetable oil which also contain sufficient n-6 PUFA to meet EFA requirements.

Long chain triglycerides (LCTs) are calorically dense nutrients; however, there are several concerns regarding their clinical application. The digestion and absorption of LCTs require an efficient level of gastrointestinal function (p. 354) which may be compromised in patients with digestive diseases. Lipoprotein lipase is inhibited by the cytokines released during severe injury and may lead to impaired fat clearance and oxidation (Kinsella et al 1990). Lipid emulsions contain moderate amounts of linoleic acid and may lead to an exaggerated production of eicosanoids during the stress response which may adversely affect immune competence and vascular integrity. Excessive amounts of fat may therefore be detrimental in certain settings. In a study of severely burned patients being given enteral products with a variety of lipid-based formulae, the solution high in linoleic acid was associated with the greatest mortality (Gottschlich et al 1990). In addition, parenteral LCT emulsions have been shown to impair reticuloendothelial function if they are infused too rapidly (i.e. >110 mg/kg/h) (Seidner et al 1989).

Medium chain triglycerides (p. 354) are available for enteral use as a readily absorbed and oxidized source of fat calories and are added to many tube feeding formulae. Unfortunately, they do not provide EFAs for normal eicosanoid production.

## Determination of nutrient requirements

Protein, carbohydrate and fat must be given in every nutritional prescription so that essential metabolic processes can occur. These requirements are most often established by using predictive equations, but on occasion direct measurement of substrate use is determined by gas exchange techniques. Electrolyte requirements depend on fluid status, renal function, the presence of extrarenal electrolyte losses and current blood values. Vitamins and minerals for enteral feeding are usually provided in accordance with requirements as determined by the Food and Nutrition Board of the National Academy of Sciences (National Research Council 1989). The Nutrition Advisory Group of the American Medical Association Department of Foods and Nutrition has established guidelines for vitamins and trace elements which should be provided in parenteral solutions (Nutrition Advisory Group 1979).

*Energy requirements*

Three descriptive terms are commonly used to describe energy requirements. The first is basal energy expenditure (BEE) which accounts for the energy required to maintain basal body temperature in a thermoneutral environment and to perform essential body functions such as respiratory and cardiac function. It is the minimal heat production measured 12–18 h postprandially at complete muscular rest. Resting energy expenditure (REE) is the energy expenditure obtained at rest in a supine position and includes physical stress and variations in ambient or body temperature. Measured REE is approximately 10% higher than BEE. Total energy expenditure (TEE) is comprised of BEE and the clinical factors which affect REE, plus diet-induced thermogenesis, shivering and nonshivering thermogenesis (the energy to maintain body temperature above ambient temperature) and physical activity. REE represents the major component of TEE in the hospitalized patient while diet-induced thermogenesis, shivering and nonshivering thermogenesis account for approximately 10% of TEE.

The Harris–Benedict equation is used to calculate the BEE and was derived from indirect calorimetric data obtained from 239 healthy subjects (Harris & Benedict 1919). Two formulae were developed from regression analysis of four independent variables: age, gender, height and current weight. These four factors reflect the relationship between body weight and body cell mass, the metabolically active tissue of the body. The calculated BEE is then adjusted for physical activity and stress hypermetabolism to determine the TEE (Long et al 1979). It should be noted that even patients with severe hypermetabolism, such as those with extensive third-degree burns, rarely will exceed 200% of their BEE. Calculation of TEE in hospitalized patients is summarized in Table 22.5.

The accuracy of predictive methods to estimate energy needs is dependent on a valid assessment of weight and stress level. The Harris–Benedict equation may overestimate energy requirements for starved patients who have

**Table 22.5** Calculation of adult energy requirements

*Harris–Benedict equations*

Men: BEE (kcal/d) = 66.47 + 13.57 (W) + 5.0 (H) − 6.76 (A)

Women: BEE (kcal/d) = 655.1 + 9.56 (W) + 1.85 (H) − 4.68 (A)

W = weight in kg; H = Height in cm; A = Age in years

| *Stress factor* | |
|---|---|
| Mild starvation | 0.85–1.0 |
| Postoperative | 1.00–1.05 |
| Peritonitis | 1.05–1.25 |
| Severe infection | 1.30–1.55 |
| Cancer | 1.10–1.45 |

*Activity factor* = 1.25 if ambulatory

*Total energy expenditure (TEE)*

TEE = BEE × stress factor × activity factor

undergone an adaptive decrease in BEE and for obese patients who tend to have a disproportionate increase in body fat stores to lean tissue (Paauw et al 1984, Hunter et al 1988). Most patients who are less than 120% of their ideal body weight (IBW) will need 120–170 kJ/kg/24 h. This estimate can be used to check the estimates established by other predictive equations. An adjusted body weight (ABW) is calculated for obese patients who are more than 120% of their IBW as follows:

$$\text{ABW} = (\text{current weight} - \text{IBW}) \times 0.25 + \text{IBW}.$$

This assumes that excess body fat has only one-quarter the metabolic activity of lean tissue.

Energy expenditure can be measured either by direct calorimetry, which measures the amount of heat released to the environment, or indirect calorimetry, which measures oxygen consumption and carbon dioxide production. Because direct calorimetry is too cumbersome for clinical practice, portable metabolic carts made it possible to measure REE by indirect calorimetry in hospitalized patients (Feurer & Mullen 1986). These instruments use sensitive gas analyzers along with a microcomputer to calculate REE using the Weir (1949) formula. TEE approximates 130% of the measured REE. Indirect calorimetry can also be used to measure the respiratory quotient (RQ), thus providing valuable information on substrate utilization. Ideally, the RQ should range from 0.85 to 0.95. Values greater than 1.0 indicate fat synthesis and overfeeding and suggest a need to reduce total calories, while an RQ less than 0.82 suggests that total calories need to be increased.

While there has been some concern that predictive equations may lead to over- and underestimation of energy needs for individual patients, most will not suffer any ill effects while using these equations along with close monitoring of the response to nutritional therapy. Since performing indirect calorimetry can be time consuming and costly, its use is often reserved for the critical care setting. Indirect calorimetry is most beneficial in patients who are severely stressed (e.g. closed head injury, major burns, multiple trauma), markedly volume overloaded where dry weight estimates are uncertain, difficult to wean from mechanical ventilation because of severe lung disease and are at the extremes of normal body composition (morbidly obese, severely malnourished) where predictive equations are most inaccurate (McMahon & Bistrian 1990). Patients who do not fit into one of these categories yet need prolonged nutritional support may also benefit from measurement of REE, especially if improved nutritional status, as measured by visceral proteins, immune function and nitrogen balance, is not seen. Indirect calorimetry is only a component of a complete nutritional assessment, providing a small but important bit of information regarding the overall nutritional status and needs of a patient.

*Protein requirements*

The source of nitrogen should contain a mixture of essential and nonessential amino acids to meet requirements which might be "essential" during periods of physical stress. This concept of conditionally essential nutrients has been best described with the amino acids arginine and glutamine which appear to play important roles in maintaining immune function and intestinal integrity, respectively, in the critically ill (Wilmore 1991).

The dose of protein which is needed depends on body weight, nonprotein calorie intake and level of stress. Requirements range from 0.8 to 1.5 g/kg/24 h (Shaw et al 1987). Patients with marasmic-type malnutrition can easily achieve nitrogen balance with the lower end of this range. When renal disease results in significant uremia (BUN>100 mg/dl) and liver disease causes hepatic encephalopathy (HE), protein restriction or specialized formulae may need to be considered. If protein restriction is required it should not be much below 0.8 g/kg/24 h and under no circumstance should large amounts of nonprotein calories be given without nitrogen. Patients with excessive losses of protein from enteric fistulae, inflammatory bowel diseases, short bowel syndrome, hemo- or peritoneal dialysis losses and open wounds may require greater amounts of protein relative to their level of stress.

Parenteral amino acids are available as standard crystalline amino acid solutions which contain the nine essential and six to eight nonessential amino acids. A 10% solution is equivalent to 10 g of amino acid per 100 ml and provides 1 kJ of energy and 0.16 g of nitrogen per gram (6.25 g of protein = 1 g of nitrogen). Specialized amino acid solutions for renal failure contain essential amino acids only and formulae for patients with hepatic encephalopathy from chronic liver disease are enriched with branched chain amino acids and low in aromatic amino acids. These specialized formulae are far more costly than the standard solutions and have not been shown to improve patient outcome. We recommend the use of the renal formulations for uremic patients who cannot be dialyzed to a blood urea nitrogen of less than 17–20 mmol/L (Seidner et al 1994); hepatic formulae are advised when standard amino acids cannot be tolerated in patients with spontaneous hepatic encephalopathy.

Enteral nutrition products provide whole or partially hydrolyzed protein of high biologic grade and are suitable for the majority of patients. A few formulae are available with crystalline amino acids; however, it is not clear if they are superior to hydrolyzed products for patients with malabsorption.

*Nonprotein substrate requirement*

Nonprotein calories are usually given as 60–80% carbohydrate and 20–40% fat.

***Parenteral nutrition formulae.*** These are prepared from standard concentrations of glucose monohydrate and long chain triglycerides. Parenteral formulae can be made to meet the exact metabolic demands of each patient since base solutions are used. The total amount to be given depends on the energy requirements as determined by predictive equations or direct measurement of substrate utilization. Substrate tolerance is usually acceptable as long as nutrient requirements are determined and these ranges provided.

***Tube feeding products.*** These are prepared with fixed amounts of carbohydrate and fat. They are prepared from modified corn starch, glucose polymers, maltodextrins and a variety of vegetable oils. A formula is chosen for a patient depending on the underlying medical condition and the digestive capacity of the gut. If a patient's nutritional requirements are not met by an existing formula then modular forms of protein, carbohydrate and fat can be added to tailor the best available product to meet these needs.

*Fluid requirements*

Fluid requirements should be divided into three components: maintenance fluids which are needed for normal renal function, stool and insensible fluid losses; fluids required for any excessive losses; and fluids for the correction of any imbalances in volume status. Maintenance fluids for an adult approximate 35 ml/kg/24 h where weight is usually based on current body weight. Excessive fluid losses can be added to maintenance requirements and can be categorized as being renal (e.g. recovery from acute tubular necrosis, osmotic diuresis, salt-losing nephropathy) or extrarenal (e.g. diarrhea, vomiting or nasogastric decompression and insensible losses). Daily fluid losses can be determined by keeping strict intake and output records. Insensible losses, resulting from fever, large burns and open wounds, can be approximated by predictive equations. Less fluid should be provided to patients with fluid overload. Fluid overload, which may be manifested as pedal edema, ascites, jugular venous distention and pulmonary edema, is commonly seen in patients with cardiac, renal and liver diseases. Dilutional hyponatremia, hypoalbuminemia, anemia and low blood urea nitrogen may also be present as additional signs of fluid excess. Extra fluid is needed for patients with signs of dehydration that include poor skin turgor, dry mucus membranes, an orthostatic drop in blood pressure, an elevated ratio of blood urea nitrogen to creatinine and possibly hypernatremia (depending on the sodium content of the fluids which are lost). Most adults will receive 1.5–3.0 L/24 h of fluids. Regardless of the fluid status, if a patient has severe intravascular depletion a sufficient amount of fluid must be given within the first 24–48 h to ensure hemodynamic stability.

*Electrolyte requirements*

Electrolyte requirements depend on renal function, fluid status and extrarenal fluid losses. Patients receiving TPN will have higher electrolyte requirements than patients receiving standard intravenous fluids. Proteolysis during administration of 5% glucose solutions is associated with release of intracellular fluids which are rich in potassium, magnesium, sulfate and phosphate. Infusion of TPN reduces proteolysis and results in anabolism that requires additional amounts of electrolytes and minerals. Table 22.6 lists the usual adult requirements for TPN electrolytes. Excessive losses of gastric, pancreatic, small bowel secretions and other extrarenal fluids can lead to severe electrolyte and acid–base disturbances. Table 22.7 lists the electrolyte concentrations of various body fluids so losses from these sources can be replaced and then maintained.

*Vitamin and trace element requirements*

Vitamins are an essential component of all forms of nutritional therapy and must be provided every day. Adequate quantities of fat- and water-soluble vitamins are needed for the effective utilization of protein, carbohydrate and fat. This is especially true with parenteral feedings where deficiencies of water-soluble vitamins can rapidly develop when these vitamins are not supplied.

In the United States, the Food and Nutrition Board of the National Academy of Sciences has established recommended dietary allowances (RDAs) for vitamins and some minerals. The recommended allowances are set two standard deviations above the estimated mean requirements of normal individuals to ensure that all patients

**Table 22.6** Daily electrolyte and mineral IV requirements in patients with adequate renal function

| Electrolyte and minerals | Usual adult daily dose |
|---|---|
| Sodium | 100–150 mEq |
| Potassium | 60–120 mEq |
| Chloride | 100–150 mEq |
| Calcium | 9–22 mEq |
| Magnesium | 8–24 mEq |
| Phosphate | 15–30 mM |

**Table 22.7** Approximate electrolyte composition of various body fluids

| Source | Volume (ml/d) | Electrolytes (mEq/L) $Na^+$ | $K^+$ | $HCO_3^-$ | $Cl^-$ |
|---|---|---|---|---|---|
| Gastric | 2000–2500 pH <4 | 60 | 10 | — | 90 |
| | pH >4 | 100 | 10 | — | 100 |
| Pancreatic | 1000 | 140 | 5 | 90 | 75 |
| Bile | 1500 | 140 | 5 | 35 | 100 |
| Small bowel | 3500 | 100 | 15 | 25 | 100 |
| Diarrhea | 1000–4000 | 60 | 30 | 45 | 45 |
| Urine | 1500 | 40 | 40 | — | 20 |
| Sweat | | 50 | 5 | — | 55 |

receive an adequate amount of these nutrients. Similar standards have been established in the United Kingdom and Canada (Health and Welfare Canada 1990, Panel on Dietary Reference Value 1991). The Nutrition Advisory Group of the American Medical Association (1979) recommended guidelines for the intravenous dosing of fat- and water-soluble vitamins based on the RDAs. It should be noted that water-soluble vitamins are rapidly excreted when provided in this fashion and so the AMA guidelines are two to three times greater than the RDAs. The RDAs for oral vitamins are compared to the AMA guidelines for intravenous vitamins in Table 22.8. Vitamin K is not present in intravenous vitamin preparations. It may be given intramuscularly as 10 mg every week or as 1 mg/24 h in the parenteral solution.

Trace elements are essential cofactors in numerous metalloenzymes involved in various metabolic processes. Clinical deficiencies have been recognized for chromium, copper, iron, iodine, selenium and zinc. The five trace elements which are given with TPN are listed in Table 22.9 along with dose adjustments which should be considered in patients with large volume diarrhea or ostomy losses. Tube feeding formulae provide a sufficient amount of vitamins and trace elements when caloric requirements are met. Patients with malabsorption may require supplementation of individual vitamins and minerals. Table 22.10

**Table 22.8** Recommended daily vitamin dosing for adults

| Vitamin | RDA adult range | Intravenous multivitamin formulation |
|---|---|---|
| Vitamin A | 4000–5000 i.u. | 3300 i.u. |
| Vitamin D | 400 i.u. | 200 i.u. |
| Vitamin E | 12–15 i.u. | 10 i.u. |
| Ascorbic acid (vitamin C) | 45 mg | 100 mg |
| Folic acid | 400 μg | 400 μg |
| Niacin | 12–20 mg | 40 mg |
| Riboflavin (vitamin $B_2$) | 1.1–1.8 mg | 3.6 mg |
| Thiamin (vitamin $B_1$) | 1.1–1.5 mg | 3 mg |
| Pyridoxine (vitamin $B_6$) | 1.6–2.0 mg | 4 mg |
| Cyanocobalamin (vitamin $B_{12}$) | 3 μg | 5 μg |
| Pantothenic acid | 5–10 mg | 15 mg |
| Biotin | 150–300 μg | 60 μg |

**Table 22.9** Daily intravenous trace element requirements

| | Stable adult | Adult with intestinal losses |
|---|---|---|
| Chromium | 10–15 μg | 20 μg |
| Copper | 0.5–1.5 mg | same |
| Manganese | 0.15–0.8 mg | same |
| Selenium | 50–120 μg | up to 200 μg |
| Zinc | 2.5–4.0 mg<br>+2 mg if catabolic | 12 mg/kg small bowel fluid lost;<br>17 mg/kg of stool or ileostomy output |

**Table 22.10** Oral vitamin and mineral supplements in gastrointestinal disease

| Name | Form | Strength | Regimen |
|---|---|---|---|
| *Vitamins* | | | |
| Vitamin A | cap | 25 000 i.u., 50 000 i.u. | 5000–10 000 i.u./d |
| | liq | 50 000 i.u./ml | |
| Vitamin D: calcitriol | cap | 0.25 μg | 0.25–1 μg qd |
| Vitamin D: ergocalciferol | cap | 50 000 i.u. | 50 000 i.u. 2–3 times/week<br>Rickets: 12 000–500 000 i.u./d |
| | liq | 8000 i.u., 200 i.u./drop | |
| Vitamin E: D-α-tocopherol | cap | 100 i.u. | 100–200 i.u./d |
| | liq | 50 i.u./ml | |
| Vitamin K: phytonadione | tab | 5 mg | 5–10 mg/d |
| *Minerals** | | | |
| Calcium carbonate | tab | 1.25 g (500 mg Ca) | 1000–3000 mg/d (Ca) |
| | ch tab | 500 mg (200 mg Ca) | |
| | susp | 500 mg/5 ml | |
| Ca glubionate | syr | 5.4 g/15 ml (345 mg Ca) | |
| Calcium gluconate | ch tab | 500 mg (46 mg Ca), 1 g | |
| Calcium lactate | tab | 300 mg, 600 mg (84 mg Ca) | |
| Magnesium oxide | cap | 400 mg (240 mg Mg) | 400–1200 mg/d |
| Magnesium lactate | tab | 700 mg (84 mgMg) | 2100–6300 mg/d |
| Zinc sulfate | cap | 220 mg (50 mgZn) | 50–150 mg/d |
| Potassium chloride | tab | 10 mEq, 20 mEq | As needed to replace potassium deficit |
| | liq | 20 mEq K/15 ml | |
| Potassium and sodium phosphate | cap | 250 mg (8 mM) $PO_4$<br>(7.125 mEq Na & 7.125 mEq K) | 250–2000 mg/d |
| Sodium bicarbonate | tab | 650 mg | 1300–5200 mg/d |
| Bicitra | liq | Each ml = Na 1 mEq, $HCO_3$ 1 mEq | As needed |
| Polycitra | liq | Each ml = Na 1 mEq, K 1 mEq, $HCO_3$ 2 mEq | |

cap=capsule, liq=liquid, tab=tablet, syr=syrup
*In divided doses 2–4 times each day

outlines the strength and dosing of some of these micronutrients which may be given orally or by tube feeding.

## MANAGEMENT OF SELECTED GASTROINTESTINAL CONDITIONS

### Short bowel syndrome

*Pathophysiology*

The short bowel syndrome typically occurs following extensive resection of small bowel (pp. 451 & 454) (Greenberger 1978). Resection of more than 75% of the small intestine will almost certainly require some means of specialized nutritional care (Weser 1983). In terms of the length of bowel required to survive on oral intake alone, it is generally regarded that 60–80 cm of small bowel distal to the ligament of Treitz is needed when it is in continuity with the colon, while 150 cm of small bowel is needed when it ends in a stoma, provided that the intact bowel is normal.

The severity of diarrhea which develops following intestinal resection depends on the absorption by the remaining bowel. Protein, carbohydrate and water-soluble vitamins are for the most part absorbed within the first 200 cm of jejunum. Fat absorption is proportional to the quantity that is ingested; however, when moderate degrees of steatorrhea occur, the unabsorbed fat can result in a secretory diarrhea from the colon. Sodium absorption in the jejunum, which is coupled to the absorption of glucose and certain amino acids, can only occur over a small concentration gradient since moderate amounts of sodium normally diffuse back from the interstitial space between the enterocytes into the lumen. Perfusion studies using isotonic, glucose-containing solutions in patients with a proximal jejunostomy have shown positive sodium balance (absorption > secretion) when test solutions contain at least 90 mmol/L of sodium. Below this concentration sodium balance is negative, placing the patient at risk for sodium and extracellular fluid depletion without the provision of oral rehydration solutions. Sodium balance in patients with an intact ileum and/or colon is not as difficult to maintain because, even though sodium absorption is not as efficient as that which occurs in the jejunum, the back diffusion into the lumen is very low. Therefore, patients who have an intact ileum and/or colon usually do not require oral rehydration solutions.

The diarrhea associated with the short bowel syndrome comes predominantly from endogenous gastrointestinal secretions that amount to 8–9 L/24 h. Resection of the proximal small bowel is unlikely to result in massive diarrhea because of the ability of the ileum and colon to compensate. However, if equal lengths of ileum and colon are resected, diarrhea is likely to develop. The ileum also plays an important role in bile acid reabsorption and resection of more than 100 cm will result in steatorrhea from bile acid depletion (Hofmann & Poley 1972) (p. 451). Hypergastrinemia and gastric hypersecretion may result (p. 451) and cause inactivation of pancreatic enzymes.

The remaining small intestine undergoes morphologic and physiologic adaptation (p. 451). Although there are no practical tests to see how much a patient has adapted to intestinal resection, the response to an oral meal can be used to judge whether they will require parenteral nutrition or not (Nightingale et al 1990). Patients who are given an appropriate diet and who are found to have diarrheal losses that exceed oral intake will require drugs that slow transit or enhance absorption or parenteral nutrition (or both).

*Management of short bowel syndrome* (p. 454)

The initial consequences of extensive small bowel resection include marked depletion of fluid, sodium, potassium and the divalent cations (calcium, magnesium and zinc). A severe metabolic acidosis may occur through the loss of bicarbonate. The immediate postoperative management is discussed on p. 454, including the use of antidiarrheal agents. The somatostatin analog, octreotide, when given at 100 μg every 8 h subcutaneously, has decreased gut losses of fluid and electrolytes. Balance studies by O'Keefe et al (1994a) performed in 10 stable patients with end-jejunostomy syndrome demonstrated significant reductions in stomal outputs of fluid and electrolytes (sodium, potassium and chloride) that permitted reductions in intravenous fluid requirements. There was no significant change in the absorption of nitrogen, fat and calories. While octreotide may help manage the fluid and electrolyte problems experienced by these patients, it inhibits amino acid uptake by the small bowel and may suppress adaptation (O'Keefe et al 1994b).

Dietary requirements need to be modified for each patient's digestive defects. Oral rehydration solutions can be tried first. It has been suggested that the fluid contains (in mmol/L): glucose 200; sodium 85–90; potassium 12; bicarbonate 9; and chloride 80–90 (Fleming & Jeejeebhoy 1994). Others have suggested the use of a hypo-osmolar (240 mOsm/kg vs 330 mOsm/kg) solution which contains a rice-based glucose polymer as opposed to monomeric glucose (Thillainayagam et al 1993). This latter solution has been shown to improve water absorption while maintaining a positive sodium balance. Some patients may benefit from tube feeding with a hydrolyzed feeding formula (Cosnes et al 1992). Finally an attempt should be made to provide a normal diet for most patients. Though some patients with intact colons may need fat restriction, those with jejunostomy tolerate additional dietary fats well (McIntyre et al 1986). Patients tend to compensate for the severe malabsorption by consuming a hypercaloric, hyperprotein diet (Messing et al 1991).

TPN is tapered in response to weight gain and fluid and electrolyte balance. If this occurs, it is usually within the first 1–2 years following resection during the adaptive phase. Oral supplementation with calcium, zinc, iron, bicarbonate, magnesium and phosphate salts may be needed for some patients. Whereas many of these patients require TPN for the rest of their lives, recent evidence suggests that by using growth hormone, oral glutamine and fiber, some can reduce or eliminate their need for parenteral nutrition (Byrne et al 1992).

## Acute pancreatitis

### *Energy and substrate requirements*

Energy expenditure, as measured by indirect calorimetry, has not been shown to be significantly increased in a group of patients with acute pancreatitis and ongoing sepsis (Bouffard et al 1989). Acute pancreatitis leads to impaired clearance of both glucose (Mizuma et al 1978, Shaw & Wolfe 1986) and lipids (Cameron et al 1974) and it may be necessary to provide a mixed fuel system to meet energy expenditure. A report of fat emulsion-induced pancreatitis (Lashner et al 1986) initially raised concern over its use; however, it appears that most patients tolerate glucose and lipid-based formulae well (Silberman et al 1982, Grant et al 1984, Van Gossum et al 1988, Sitzmann et al 1989). Severely catabolic patients may remain in negative nitrogen balance despite the provision of adequate caloric intake (Streat et al 1987).

At times metabolic constraints may not permit infusion of the desired amount of macronutrients. Patients with hyperglycemia should only receive 150–200 g of glucose initially to meet essential requirements (Cahill 1970) and thereafter increase the amount infused to keep blood glucose levels below 10 mmol/L. Insulin usually is required to control blood glucose (Van Gossum et al 1988) and may be added in increasing amounts to the TPN as glucose is increased. Lipid emulsions should be withheld in patients with hypertriglyceridemia-induced acute pancreatitis. Lipid emulsions should also be limited when triglycerides are greater than 4.5 mmol/L either prior to or during lipid administration.

### *Parenteral nutrition*

Total parenteral nutrition has been advocated for patients with severe acute pancreatitis within the first 72 h of hospitalization (Corcoy et al 1988) because of the anticipated requirements for prolonged bowel rest and the hypermetabolic state (Bouffard et al 1989). Parenteral nutrition does not appear to affect pancreatic secretions to a significant degree in animals (Stabile & Debas 1981) or humans (Grundfest et al 1980, Edelman & Valenzuela 1983, Bivins et al 1984). Retrospective studies suggest a favorable effect of TPN on clinical outcome (Feller et al 1974, Blackburn et al 1976); however, others failed to confirm this (Goodgame & Fischer 1977, Grant et al 1984). One prospective controlled trial of TPN in acute mild pancreatitis did not show any advantage (Sax et al 1987). Despite the lack of evidence to support the use of TPN in acute pancreatitis, late complications, especially those which require surgical intervention, might be expected to have an improved outcome based on prospective studies examining the effect of preoperative TPN in severely malnourished patients (Mullen et al 1980, Muller et al 1986, Veterans Affairs Total Parenteral Nutrition Co-operative Study Group 1991).

### *Enteral nutrition*

Transition to enteral feeding should be considered when ileus subsides or a jejunostomy can be placed in patients who undergo abdominal surgery. Distal duodenal or jejunal feeding is preferred over the intragastric route (Raggins et al 1973, Kelly & Nahrwold 1976), to minimize neurohumoral stimulation of the pancreas. Most studies using elemental formulae have shown less stimulation of the pancreas compared with polymeric ones (Cassim & Allardyce 1974, Vidon et al 1978). We therefore suggest that patients recovering from acute pancreatitis receive enteral tube feeding delivered at or beyond the ligament of Trietz and that the formula be composed of free amino acids and low in fat. If this is well tolerated, it may be transitioned to a conventional polymeric formula.

## Inflammatory bowel disease

Nutrient deficiencies are commonly seen in patients with inflammatory bowel disease (IBD), especially Crohn's disease of the small bowel (Driscoll & Rosenberg 1978). The extent, location and activity of disease are important determinants that contribute to malnutrition. Previous intestinal resection and medications used to treat IBD are also important considerations (see p. 676).

### *Oral diet*

The control of disease activity can often replete individuals with mild nutrient deficiencies. Every effort should be made to ensure that patients consume a nutritionally adequate diet. This can usually be done with a regular diet; however, patients with mild malabsorption may require supplementation with vitamins and minerals that exceed the recommended dietary allowances.

Dietary modification should be instituted in only a few settings. While lactose intolerance has been reported to be common in patients with IBD (p. 676), evidence suggests that lactase deficiency may actually parallel the prevalence in healthy ethnic group controls (Kirschner et al 1981). Since dairy products are an important source of protein and calcium it would seem prudent in some situations to document the presence of lactose malabsorption prior to suggesting that lactose-containing foods be avoided. Dietary fiber should be restricted in patients with symptomatic partial bowel obstruction secondary to strictures of the bowel and in some patients with enteroenteric fistulae. Steatorrhea occurs infrequently and when present can usually be managed with a modest fat restriction (i.e. 70–80 g/day). Steatorrhea can be associated with hyperoxaluria and calcium oxalate kidney stones (p. 452). Patients with hyperoxaluria should restrict their consumption of dietary fat and oxalate, increase calcium intake (p. 454) and if necessary, take bile acid-binding resins that also bind intraluminal oxalate (Dobbins & Binder 1976).

*Enteral and parenteral nutrition*

Enteral and parenteral nutrition are usually used as adjuncts in the management of patients with IBD. Since intraluminal antigens derived from dietary protein and bacterial components may be implicated in the pathogenesis of IBD, alteration of intraluminal proteins has been investigated as primary treatment for Crohn's disease.

Trials comparing hydrolyzed enteral formula to corticosteroids have generally shown that steroids result in clinical remission more commonly and faster. In two large studies from the European Co-operative Crohn's Disease Study, clinical remission rates of 41–53% in patients on hydrolyzed enteral formulae were not as favorable as the response to steroids which ranged from 73% to 79% (Malchow et al 1990, Lochs et al 1991). In addition, nutritional therapy required a mean of 4 weeks to achieve remission whereas the response time to steroids was a mean of 8 days. One caveat from these trials is that patients with Crohn's colitis and perianal disease respond poorly to enteral nutrition and relapse rates are high after a regular diet is resumed. Enteral nutrition should be considered as primary or adjunctive therapy for malnourished patients with long-standing Crohn's disease involving the small bowel who are refractory to or have major complications from corticosteroid therapy or are poor surgical candidates.

Controlled trials using hydrolyzed "elemental" diets (i.e. all nitrogen as free amino acids) have reported short-term clinical remissions of 60–82% (O'Morain et al 1984, Saverymuttu et al 1985). Unfortunately these formulae are quite unpalatable and appear to show no benefit when compared to hydrolyzed (Malchow et al 1990, Lochs et al 1991, Lindor et al 1992) and polymeric (Gonzalez-Huix et al 1993) formulae. Patients with proximal small bowel obstruction and fistulae should be excluded from this form of treatment. A standard polymeric formula should be tried first. Many sick Crohn's patients will not drink enough to meet their needs so it may need to be given by a continuous drip through a nasogastric tube.

Parenteral nutrition in patients with Crohn's disease has been associated with short-term remission rates of up to 71%; however, this was not significantly better than enteral nutrition (58%) (Greenberg et al 1988). The main role of parenteral nutrition in IBD is as preoperative support for patients with moderate to severe malnutrition, for postoperative fistulae due to anastomotic leaks and as home parenteral nutrition for patients with gut failure from either short bowel or extensive small bowel Crohn's disease.

## Liver disease

The liver plays a central role in the metabolism of nitrogen, carbohydrate and lipids. Protein calorie malnutrition occurs in 20–80% of patients with alcoholic liver disease admitted to tertiary care hospitals (McCullough et al 1989). In patients with established cirrhosis, it approaches 100%. A reduction in dietary intake is the primary cause and is most often due to anorexia and encephalopathy (Munro et al 1975). Exocrine pancreatic insufficiency and malabsorption have also been demonstrated (Mezey 1975). The synthesis and activation of certain nutrients, such as choline and vitamin D, can also be impaired in patients with liver disease (Chawla et al 1989). An impaired ability to store adequate quantities of glycogen in the liver results in a rapid transition from the fed to the fasted state and therefore a greater reliance on amino acids for gluconeogenesis (Swart et al 1989). This observation stresses the importance of providing an adequate amount of protein in patients with chronic liver disease. A bedtime snack has been proposed because of the adverse effects of prolonged fasting on protein metabolism.

*Nutrition assessment in liver disease*

Identifying patients with malnutrition may be difficult because of the progressive retention of sodium and water in chronic liver disease. Weight loss may not be a sensitive indicator of malnutrition because of fluid retention. Upper arm anthropometry may be used in many patients since edema tends to accumulate in the lower extremities. Measurement of visceral proteins may be helpful; however, caution must be exercised in interpreting the results. Hypoalbuminemia has often been attributed to decreased synthesis by the liver; however, it has been shown that synthetic rates are at the lower end of the normal range in advanced liver disease (Hehir et al 1985). More often, low albumin concentrations reflect a dilutional effect associated with intravascular volume expansion along with an increased protein catabolic rate. A compensatory increase in albumin synthesis does not occur because of inadequate protein intake, inadequate synthetic reserve or both.

*Nutrition therapy in chronic liver disease*

Dietary counseling is advised in all ambulatory patients with advanced liver disease to ensure that an adequate amount of protein and a properly balanced diet are consumed. Protein restriction should only be imposed when hepatic encephalopathy cannot be managed with conventional medications. In general, a protein intake of 1.0–1.2 g/kg/24 h is tolerated well.

Patients who are unable to eat, as may occur in hospital, may require supplementation with either enteral or parenteral nutrition. Though both enteral and parenteral nutrition have been shown to improve hepatocellular function, these therapies should be directed toward repleting patients with moderate to severe malnutrition. Enteral nutrition is preferred since it is more physiologic, safer and is less expensive than the parenteral route. Standard amino acid formulae should be used in most patients except when encephalopathy cannot be controlled with conventional medical therapy. When it appears that standard amino acid formulae cannot be tolerated, even at a restricted dose, then branched chain amino acids may be used so that further deterioration in mental status can be prevented while providing adequate quantities of amino acids to meet nitrogen requirements.

***Enteral nutrition in chronic liver disease.*** Two recent randomized controlled trials comparing supplemental tube feeding with a standard diet have shown improvement in hepatocellular function as measured by serum albumin, bilirubin, antipyrine clearance and Child's score (Cabre et al 1990, Kearns et al 1992). In one of these trials encephalopathy improved even though the formula was casein-based (Kearns et al 1992). Other randomized controlled trials comparing branched chain amino acids to casein-based formulae provided as a diet supplement have shown no clear advantage for the branched chain amino acids group (McGhee et al 1983, Christie et al 1985, Marchesini et al 1991). In general, these trials were performed in patients with latent hepatic encephalopathy.

***Peripheral parenteral nutrition in alcoholic liver disease.*** Several randomized studies have investigated the use of peripheral parenteral nutrition (PPN) as a part of the treatment for patients with alcoholic hepatitis. Nasrallah & Galambos (1980) were the first to demonstrate significant improvement in serum albumin, bilirubin and survival in patients who received PPN compared with controls who were given a regular diet. Though several subsequent studies have shown improvement in liver enzymes, hepatocellular function and histology, none has been able to duplicate the improvement in clinical outcome (Diehl et al 1985, Achord 1987, Simon & Galambos 1988, Bonkovsky et al 1991). Despite the greater amount of protein received by the supplemented patients, none developed hepatic encephalopathy.

***Branched chain amino acid for hepatic encephalopathy.*** In some patients with chronic liver disease, the normal ratio of the branched chain amino acids to aromatic amino acids is decreased. This change is believed to play a role in the development of encephalopathy secondary to the accumulation of aromatic amino acids in the brain and the production of false neurotransmitters which interfere with normal neural function (Fischer & Baldessarini 1971). Though this theory has been superseded by several others, it led to the development of a branched chain amino acids enriched/aromatic amino acids restricted parenteral solution for the treatment of encephalopathy in patients with chronic liver disease (Fischer et al 1975). Several randomized controlled trials have investigated these solutions (Rossi-Fanelli et al 1982, Wahren et al 1983, Michel et al 1984, Cerra et al 1985, Fiaccadori et al 1985). Three of these studies demonstrated branched chain amino acids to be superior (Cerra et al 1985, Fiaccadori et al 1985) or equivalent (Rossi-Fanelli et al 1982) to conventional treatment while in one trial the treatment group fared worse than controls (Wahren et al 1983). In one study (Cerra et al 1985), overall mortality was also improved. The only study that compared branched chain amino acids to standard amino acids showed no advantage in the patients who received branched chain amino acids (Michel et al 1984). Unfortunately, all of the other trials used lactulose or neomycin along with IV solutions containing high concentrations of dextrose in the control arm. The dextrose solution may have had a negative impact on the control groups by interfering with normal nitrogen utilization that occurs during fasting.

## PROVISION OF NUTRITION SUPPORT

### Enteral nutrition

*Tube selection and placement*

***Nasogastric tubes.*** The optimal tube feeding route depends on the anticipated duration of therapy, the adequacy of gastric function and competence of the lower esophageal sphincter. Most hospitalized patients should be fed through nasogastric tubes. Patients at high risk for aspiration of gastric contents, such as those who are mentally obtunded, have an incompetent lower esophageal sphincter with gastroesophageal reflux or gastroparesis, should have feeding instilled into the third portion of the duodenum or beyond. Patients who require tube feedings for more than 30 days should undergo endoscopic or surgical placement of gastrostomy or jejunostomy tubes.

Small-bore pliable tubes made of biologically inert materials are preferred for nasoenteric feeding. Adult patients will tolerate a tube diameter of 10 French. This size tube easily accepts standard or viscous fiber-containing formulae without difficulty, whether administered by pump, gravity or bolus administration. Tubes which are 8 French in size or smaller are usually reserved for pediatric use and often require an infusion pump to reliably deliver the enteral formula. A standard tube length of 110 cm is sufficient for nasogastric and transpyloric placement.

The distal ends of nasal tubes may be placed into the stomach, duodenum or proximal jejunum. Nasogastric feeding tubes are easy to place and have the advantage that tube feeding products can be instilled by bolus, intermittent gravity or continuous drip. Adequate length of insertion can be estimated by adding the distances from the tip of the nose to the ear and from the ear to the xiphoid process (Hanson 1979). Great care must be taken while inserting feeding tubes to avoid inadvertent placement into the trachea where lung and pleural injury can occur. Patients who are obtunded or comatose are at a greater risk for tube malposition. Contrary to popular belief, a cuffed endotracheal tube does not prevent this complication. Nasoduodenal or jejunal tube placement is far more challenging. An active bedside technique for placing tubes into the small bowel has been described by Zaloga (1991) and involves careful advancement of the tube while rotating it around its long axis. This author was able to successfully place feeding tubes beyond the pylorus in 213 of 231 consecutive patients (92%). Prokinetic agents may also be used to assist in the transpyloric placement of feeding tubes. In a series of consecutive patients, Kalfarentzos and colleagues (1987) achieved nasoduodenal tube placement within 4 h in nine of 10 patients (90%) when 10 mg of metoclopramide was given intravenously before nasogastric placement of the tube. When metaclopramide was given after nasogastric tube placement only one of 10 patients (10%) had successful transpyloric passage at 24 h. In a randomized placebo-controlled trial Kittinger and colleagues (1987) confirmed that metoclopramide is ineffective when given after tube placement except in a subgroup of patients with diabetes mellitus. In a study comparing weighted versus unweighted feeding tubes in critically ill patients, Lord and colleagues (1993) gave metoclopramide before tube passage and demonstrated spontaneous transpyloric tube placement in 84%, 86% and 92% for unweighted and 36%, 48%, and 56% for weighted tubes on radiographs obtained at 4 h, 1 day and 2 days. Erythromycin has also been used to facilitate duodenal placement of feeding tubes. In a randomized controlled study, six of eight tubes were successfully positioned into the duodenum when an elixir of erythromycin was administered through the feeding tube (Stern & Wolf 1994). In the nine control patients none had transpyloric tube placement. Fluoroscopic and endoscopic tube placement allows proper tube placement in 86% of patients but is much more costly because of the need for expensive equipment and properly trained personnel (Gutierrez & Balfe 1991).

None of these methods, except fluoroscopy, can guarantee proper tube placement prior to the start of tube feeding and thus still require radiographic confirmation of tube position. Lastly, for critically ill patients at risk for gastroparesis, a sump drain can be placed in the stomach to collect gastric secretions during transpyloric feeding and to monitor the possibility of retrograde flow of feedings or dislodgement of the feeding tube (Montecalvo et al 1992).

***Gastrostomy tubes.*** These may be used for tube feeding or gastric decompression. When placed for feeding, gastric emptying should be normal and gastroesophageal reflux minimal. Percutaneous endoscopic gastrostomy (PEG) is the most frequently used method for long-term access (Kirby et al 1986, Larson et al 1987). A skin level PEG, referred to as a "button", is popular with ambulatory patients (Ferguson et al 1993). The procedure is simple and well tolerated even in debilitated patients. An experienced operator can place a tube in a patient with previous abdominal and/or gastric surgery. Surgical gastrostomy should be considered when access to the stomach is anticipated during a major abdominal procedure or when PEG cannot be done safely. Surgical gastrostomies are of three types: the Stamm type is simple to perform; the Witzel type adds a seromuscular tunnel to minimize gastrocutaneous reflux of gastric contents; and the Janeway type creates a permanent stoma and allows periodic intubation for feeding.

***Jejunostomy tubes.*** These are reserved for patients with abnormal gastric emptying or severe gastroesophageal reflux that increases the risk for aspiration (Weltz et al 1992). Endoscopy or fluoroscopy can be used to position a small-bore feeding tube through a PEG tube resulting in a combination of two tubes, often referred to as a jejunal extension tube with percutaneous endoscopic gastrostomy (JET-PEG) (Ponsky et al 1984). JET-PEG can offer simultaneous gastric decompression with small bowel feedings through a single enterogastric stoma. Unfortunately the JET is technically difficult to place and migration back into the stomach is common (Kaplan et al 1989, Wolfsen et al 1990, DiSario et al 1990). True percutaneous endoscopic jejunostomy (PEJ) has been described but is rarely performed (Shike et al 1987). Surgical jejunostomy is the favored method for prolonged tube placement into the small bowel. The procedure may be done as an open or laparoscopic procedure.

### *Enteral formulae*

Enteral formulae are available for a wide range of clinical conditions. The choice of the most appropriate formula will depend on the integrity of the gastrointestinal tract and the desired metabolic effect. These formulae can be divided into three major categories: polymeric, hydrolyzed and modular. Most commercial products from the first two categories are nutritionally complete and provide the daily requirements of nitrogen, energy, essential fatty acids and micronutrients when given in sufficient amount. Modular products are used to augment protein, carbohydrate and fat content of existing commercial formulae and, under certain circumstances, to enhance the efficacy of an oral diet. Products can be subcategorized according to several other attributes including composition and quality of protein and fat, caloric density and presence of fiber.

Polymeric formulae contain intact protein most commonly derived from casein and soy protein isolates, polysaccharides and glucose polymers and a mixture of long and medium chain triglycerides in proportions which are similar to a regular diet. Standard polymeric formulae are isotonic, provide 0.24 kJ/ml and are relatively inexpensive. High nitrogen polymeric formulae share many of the features of standard polymeric formulae except that the protein content is higher. If more protein is required a modular protein product may be added to an existing formula. High calorie or concentrated polymeric formulae have a caloric density of 0.36–0.48 kJ/ml and are useful when fluid restriction is indicated. The osmolalities of these formulae can range from 450 to 600 mOsm/kg of water depending on the product. These hypertonic formulae are well tolerated in most patients. High nitrogen–high calorie polymeric formulae are also available and should be considered in severely malnourished patients who require fluid restriction.

Partially hydrolyzed formulae combine macronutrients which have been partially or completely hydrolyzed. Various quantities of oligopeptides, short peptides and glucose oligosaccharides are combined to permit optimal absorption when intraluminal digestion or intestinal surface area is compromised by disease. Some of these formulae have free amino acids as their nitrogen source and have been called "elemental diets", though this is something of a misnomer since their glucose and fat sources are not elemental. Elemental diets are more properly considered as partially hydrolyzed formulae. Even though they have free amino acids, they contain glucose polymers and a mixture of triglycerides. These solutions are very low in fat content (1–15% of calories). These products are four to five times more expensive than polymeric formulae and are hypertonic with osmolalities that range from 450 to 700 mOsm/kg of water.

Disease-specific products for renal, liver and lung disease, trauma and diabetes mellitus are also available. Renal formulae are low in protein yet enriched in essential amino acids, are concentrated and may be restricted in their content of electrolytes and fat-soluble vitamins. Liver formulae are high in branched chain amino acids and low in aromatic amino acids. Trauma formulae may be enriched in branched chain amino acids, low in polyunsaturated fatty acids, moderately concentrated and supplemented with conditionally essential amino acids (glutamine, arginine). Pulmonary formulae provide a majority of the calories as fat. Lastly, formulae for glucose-intolerant patients are low in carbohydrate, high in fat, isotonic and supplemented with fiber.

### *Administration of tube feeding*

The method selected for the delivery of tube feeding depends on several factors which include the location of the feeding tube, the ability of the stomach to empty, the risk of gastroesophageal reflux, the digestive function of the gastrointestinal tract and the mobility of the patient. Tube feedings can be instilled by continuous or intermittent technique. The continuous method provides feeding with an infusion pump or by gravity drip and is often used for small bowel feeding or when gastric emptying is impaired. Intermittent feeding may be given by syringe as a bolus, by infusion pump or gravity drip over several minutes or it may be cycled with an infusion pump over a portion of the day. Intermittent feeding is more convenient than continuous feeding and is favored in ambulatory patients who are at home or in rehabilitation.

### *Complications of tube feeding*

Complications of tube feeding can be divided into mechanical, infectious, gastrointestinal and metabolic (Cataldi-Betcher et al 1983). These complications are quite frequent but fortunately most are easily managed. Most of these problems can be avoided by using the proper technique during tube placement, by paying strict attention to the details of tube care and formula administration and by monitoring the patient's tolerance and response to the feeding formula.

The frequency of mechanical complications, such as nasal injury, sinusitis, otitis media, esophageal erosion, ulceration and stricture, has markedly decreased with the development of small pliable feeding tubes (Silk et al 1987). These tubes should always be favored over large polyvinylchloride tubes which are used for gastric decompression. Tube misplacement is perhaps the most serious complication of small-bore feeding tube insertion. This problem is most common in patients who are either uncooperative, obtunded or seriously ill (Bohnker et al 1987). The presence of an endotracheal tube does not prevent its occurrence. Since tube misplacement can lead to esophageal or pleural perforation and the inadvertent administration of feeding into the mediastinum or lung, a chest radiograph is mandatory after tube placement and prior to the start of feeding. Inadvertent tube removal is another common problem, occurring in up to 60% of patients (Silk et al 1987). This often results in the provision of inadequate amounts of formula. The solution to this problem is often unsatisfactory; restraining the patient or the application of a nasal bridle can lead to significant injury and is only advised in exceptional circumstances. If tube misplacement becomes a major problem then alternative means of feeding, such as gastrostomy tubes, should be considered. The use of preoperative antibiotics (Jain et al 1987) minimizes the risk of infection.

The development of aspiration pneumonia is a serious complication of tube feeding. It is important to differentiate the aspiration of tube feeding from the aspiration of oropharyngeal secretions since patients with the latter problem will aspirate while receiving any form of nutrition support (Hassett et al 1988, Fay et al 1991, Shailesh et al 1992). A decrease in the rate of gastric emptying is the most common risk factor for aspiration and is due to a wide variety of medical conditions including sepsis, trauma, head injury, electrolyte abnormalities and anticholinergic and narcotic drugs. Gastroesophageal reflux can occur when a tube is placed across the lower esophageal sphincter; however, this risk is greatest when the patient is supine (Singh & Richter 1992). In addition, rapid bolus feeding can lead to transient relaxation of the lower esophageal sphincter (Coben et al 1994). Intragastric feeding should be given with the patient's head raised 30° or more and if intermittent feeding is administered the patient should remain in this position for at least 1 h (Ibanez et al 1992). If mild gastroparesis is suspected, feeding should be given by continuous drip. Early enteral feeding in the intensive care setting should be administered transpylorically (with simultaneous nasogastric decompression) (Montecalvo et al 1992). JET-PEG and needle catheter jejunostomy may also be used to feed critically ill patients soon after injury (Kirby et al 1991). As these patients recover, they may be cautiously fed into the stomach.

***Bacterial contamination of enteral formulae.*** This has been reported to cause colonization of the respiratory tree, enterotoxin-induced diarrhea, gastroenteritis and sepsis (De-Leeuw & Vandewoude 1986). This problem is lessened if there is proper formula preparation and storage, use of the "no touch" technique while transferring the formula to the delivery system, limiting infusion time to 12 h or less while administering the feeding by pump or gravity drip and keeping the delivery system clean by rinsing it with water every 8 h. If these precautions cannot be followed, consideration should be given to the use of a closed delivery system for tube feeding.

***Gastrointestinal intolerance.*** This is the most common complication of tube feeding (Cataldi-Betcher et al 1983). Symptoms include nausea, vomiting, diarrhea, constipation, abdominal pain and distention. In many cases, the patient's disease or medications used to manage it contribute to these symptoms. If nausea and vomiting are due to gastric distention or gastroesophageal reflux, a slow continuous infusion of the diet may reduce these symptoms. A prokinetic agent, such as metoclopramide or cisapride, may also be used. A similar approach should be taken for patients with abdominal distention and pain believed to be due to altered gastrointestinal motility.

Diarrhea is perhaps the most common gastrointestinal complication of tube feeding, occurring in up to 30% of all patients; the causes include concomitant use of antibiotics, *Clostridium difficile* toxin with or without pseudomembranous colitis, the use of sorbitol-based liquid medications, hypoalbuminemia and magnesium in the formula (Keohane et al 1984). Prior to investigation and treatment, the presence of diarrhea should be confirmed since some patients may have only small volume, frequent stools which are less than 200 g/24 h (Benya et al 1991). When causes of diarrhea other than those associated with tube feeding are excluded, the formula can be manipulated to help manage this problem. Decreasing the rate of infusion is often helpful but will result in diminished efficacy of feeding. Antidiarrheal agents (e.g. loperamide and diphenoxylate/atropine) and/or kaopectate are often adequate for most patients and can permit the provision of the required amount of feeding. Fiber-containing formulae may help some patients with diarrhea by increasing intestinal transit time and by supplying the colon with fermentable fiber which produces short chain fatty acids, the primary fuel of the colon.

Confusion still exists regarding the dilution of hypertonic formula and the development of diarrhea. Water enters the lumen from the interstitial space when a hypertonic meal enters the proximal small bowel in order to make the intestinal contents isotonic. This physiologic response to a hypertonic meal is the basis for the dumping symptoms following gastric surgery. It is, however, doubtful that this occurs to a significant degree when tube feeding is instilled into the stomach. Since studies have shown that dilute and full-strength formulae are tolerated equally when infused into the stomach in patients with normal and diseased gastrointestinal tracts, we generally start all patients on full-strength formulae (Keohane et al 1984, Rees et al 1986). On the other hand, small bowel feeding should be started slowly with an isotonic formula and advanced as tolerated.

The relationship between hypoalbuminemia and diarrhea is still unsettled. Though several studies suggest that an albumin of less than 25 g/L is associated with diarrhea, it is unclear if this is related to the low albumin with intestinal edema or is just another severity of illness marker in this extremely ill group of patients (Brinson & Pitts 1989). Some investigators have suggested that albumin infusion can diminish the severity of diarrhea while others have shown good tolerance in patients with low albumin to polymeric and hydrolyzed formulae (Mowatt-Larssen et al 1992). We find that most critically ill patients tolerate high-nitrogen polymeric formulae well and only rarely require the use of a hydrolyzed product or parenteral albumin administration. Many commercially available formulae are low in dietary residue and result in a diminished stool frequency and volume. For patients who are uncomfortable because of a decrease in the number of bowel movements, an enteral formula which is enriched with fiber may be used. Alternatively, a liquid preparation of kaolin and pectin may be added to the feeding formula or given directly via the feeding tube.

***Metabolic complications.*** These are also common in patients receiving tube feeding. Glucose intolerance, hyperkalemia, hypokalemia, hyponatremia, hypernatremia, hypophosphatemia and dehydration are some of the problems that can be encountered. Usually the patient's underlying disease, such as diabetes mellitus, renal insufficiency, starvation with refeeding, and the medications used to treat them account for most of these difficulties. Generally, these complications can be avoided by reviewing the patient's medications and by examining the contents of their enteral product. Electrolytes can be replaced by supplementing the tube feeding or by providing them parenterally. Oral potassium salts can cause gastrointestinal upset while magnesium and phosphate salts can result in diarrhea. Restriction of electrolytes can be achieved by using a renal-specific product or by diluting a concentrated formula. Rarely, a modular formula must be devised to provide a safe diet.

## Parenteral nutrition

### *Venous access*

Infraclavicular subclavian vein cannulation is the most common approach for the administration of TPN. Relative contraindications to this approach are conditions which distort the normal anatomy including radical neck dissection, radical mastectomy and clavicular fracture. Under these circumstances and when the development of pneumothorax would be disastrous, such as in patients with severe pulmonary disease, congestive heart failure and pneumonia, cannulation of the internal jugular vein is preferred. Catheters may also be placed in the femoral vein; however, the exit site of these catheters is difficult to keep clean and may predispose the patient to a higher rate of catheter sepsis. Swan–Ganz and hemodialysis catheters and arteriovenous fistulae and shunts have also been used to deliver TPN, although these routes are subject to a greater risk of infection and venous thrombosis. As a last resort cannulation of the right atrium via open thoracotomy may be necessary. Peripherally inserted central catheters (PICC lines) have been used recently to gain access to the deep venous system via the basilic vein and their use is clearly associated with a decreased incidence of pulmonary complications which occur with infraclavicular line placement. Unfortunately there is little information regarding the frequency of complications associated with these lines and they must be removed when catheter sepsis is suspected.

Central venous catherization is usually performed using the Seldinger technique. Whenever possible, catheter placement should be performed electively in a co-operative patient who is adequately hydrated. The patient should be placed in the Trendelenburg position for cannulation of the subclavian or internal jugular vein to promote venous distention and prevent air embolization. Strict aseptic technique should be followed to minimize the risk of catheter sepsis.

Catheters are made of silastic or polyurethane materials which are both durable and of low thrombogenicity. Single-lumen catheters are preferred because they have the lowest incidence of catheter-associated infection; however, double- and triple-lumen catheters may be required in the critical care setting or in patients who require antibiotics or other medications which are incompatible with TPN solutions (Hilton et al 1988). Once the catheter is in position it should be converted to a standard intravenous solution and a sterile occlusive dressing should be placed over the exit site. A plain radiograph of the chest should be obtained to confirm that the tip is in the proper position within the superior vena cava and to exclude the presence of pneumothorax. Hypertonic TPN solutions should not be administered through the catheter until its proper placement is confirmed.

Changing a previously placed central venous catheter over a guidewire is useful under several circumstances. The first is in the management of a patient in whom catheter sepsis is suspected (Pettigrew et al 1985). Since most patients, especially those in the intensive care unit, who develop a fever or leukocytosis are likely to have a source for sepsis other than their central line, this procedure is a means whereby the suspected catheter can be surveyed by removing it and the patient is not subject to the complications of a catheter replacement. Blood cultures are usually obtained from a peripheral vein and through the central line prior to catheter exchange. The catheter tip can also be cultured. This information can be used to determine if the catheter is the source of the fever and whether catheter removal is warranted (see below).

### *Formula preparation and delivery*

TPN solutions are mixed in the pharmacy under sterile conditions in a laminar flow hood. A high-speed computerized compounder allows easy data entry, calculation, label preparation and rapid, accurate mixing. Stock solutions which are typically attached to the compounder include 10% amino acids, 70% dextrose and 20% lipid emulsion. A precise quantity of each solution is mixed to provide the desired amount of protein, carbohydrate and fat and sterile water is added to bring the solution to its final volume. Electrolytes, vitamins and trace elements are added to the solution to provide the necessary micronutrients. As clinically indicated, other additives such as heparin, insulin, and $H_2$ blockers are added to diminish the risk of venous thrombosis, control blood sugar concentrations and reduce gastric secretion and possibly the risk of gastric ulceration, respectively.

Classically, TPN solutions are given as a mixture of amino acid and dextrose, referred to as two-in-one solutions, with fat emulsions being given separately on 2–3 days each week. For many years, two-in-one solutions were provided in 1 L bottles with most patients receiving 2–3 bottles each day. Bags for TPN fluid ranging in size from 1 to 4 L now make it possible to provide one bag for most patients each day. This system decreases the workload on the departments of nursing and pharmacy. The advantage of two-in-one TPN is that it is physically stable over a broad range of electrolyte concentrations and is compatible with numerous medications. Total nutrient admixtures (TNAs), also called three-in-one formulae, contain all three macronutrients in a single 24-h container and are even more convenient since they require one less infusion pump. Since TNAs provide fat emulsion every day there is a tendency to give less carbohydrate with this system compared to a two-in-one formula. TNAs may be more desirable in patients with diabetes mellitus, severe pulmonary disease and hepatic steatosis. Since the fat emulsion is administered over 24 h it is more effectively cleared from the systemic circulation and does not lead to impairment of the reticuloendothelial system (Seidner et al 1989). The major disadvantage of TNAs is that they may limit the number of medications which can be given in the TPN and modest amounts of divalent cations can lead to cracking of the lipid emulsion.

Protein requirements for hospitalized patients typically provide 15–20% of total calories. The nonprotein calories are usually given as 60–80% carbohydrate and 20–40% fat. A typical TPN formula for a 70 kg patient is illustrated in Table 22.11. Our TPN order form provides an easy way to express the desired formula for each patient by requesting that only the grams of protein, total calories, nonprotein calorie ratios, total volume and rate be given.

TPN should provide glucose at 42–63 kJ/kg (200–300 g/24 h for a 70 kg man) the first day to assess glucose tolerance and should only be advanced when blood sugar is adequately controlled. To prevent this, blood glucose monitoring is done every 6 h, usually by capillary sampling. Protein, fluid and lipid can be given in the desired amount on the first day. If glycemic levels are acceptable the formula can be advanced to provide the target goals. If blood sugars are greater than 10 mmol/L then insulin should be added to the formula. We usually start with 0.1 units of regular insulin per gram of dextrose per day (i.e. 20 units of insulin per 200 g of glucose).

**Table 22.11** Parenteral nutrition orders

| Base solutions | |
|---|---|
| Standard amino acids* | 105 g |
| Total calories* | 10 300 kJ |
| Nonprotein calorie distribution† | Dextrose 70%<br>Fat 30% |
| Total volume‡ | 2450 ml |
| Infusion rate | 102 ml/h |

*Based on weight of 70 kg providing protein 1.5 g/kg/24 h, calories 150 kJ/kg/24 h
†Calorie distribution just equals 100%: for this example true calorie distribution equals protein 1760 kJ (17%), dextrose 5980 kJ (58%), fat 2560 kJ (25%)
‡Maintenance fluid requirements 35 ml/kg/24 h

## Complications of parenteral nutrition

Complications of parenteral nutrition can be divided into three categories: mechanical, infectious and metabolic. These complications have been well described and emphasize why proper patient selection is so important in the provision of this therapy. Patients who are well nourished or who are going to be fed within a few days should not be subjected to the risks which accompany the provision of TPN. If possible, this therapy should be provided by a multidisciplinary team, including physicians, dietitians, nurses and pharmacists, since nutrition support teams have been shown to decrease complications and improve cost effectiveness.

### *Mechanical complications*

The mechanical complications of central venous catheters include pneumothorax that occurs in 1–8% of patients. The patient should be examined and a chest radiograph checked after the procedure. A small pneumothorax can often be observed with serial films; however, larger ones require chest tube placement. Air embolus is much less common but can be life-threatening. It can be prevented by placing the patient in the Trendelenburg position while placing the catheter. This complication should be suspected if hypotension and cyanosis develop during or immediately after line insertion. A harsh murmur can be auscultated over the precordium. If an air embolism is suspected, the patient should immediately be placed in the head-down position, lying on the left side. This will help displace the air bubbles into the right atrium where they can be aspirated with a long catheter. Hemothorax is more often associated with difficult vein cannulation and occurs when the subclavian artery is inadvertently punctured. The needle should be removed and pressure should be applied over the insertion site. If continued bleeding is evident, angiography to identify the site of bleeding and thoracotomy to control bleeding are necessary. Malpositioned catheters which are identified soon after initial placement can sometimes be manipulated into proper position through fluoroscopic guidance. Venous thrombosis is a late complication and is suspected when edema of the upper extremity, chest and neck on the side of the catheter develops with or without superficial venous distention.

Inability to withdraw blood or infuse intravenous fluids may also suggest thrombosis. Duplex ultrasound or venography can be used to confirm this diagnosis. If diagnosed early, thrombolytic therapy can be given followed by full anticoagulation with heparin and then coumadin. This is to minimize the risk of pulmonary embolization which has been reported to occur with a frequency of 15% for upper extremity deep venous thrombosis. If patency of the vein is re-established the catheter may be left in position if it is still required.

*Infectious complications*

Catheter-associated infection should be suspected when fever, leukocytosis or sudden glucose intolerance develops. Examination and ancillary studies to identify the site of infection should be performed. Since hospitalized patients on parenteral nutrition often have many potential causes for their fever, including the central venous catheter, it is prudent to perform a guidewire change (described above) as a means of surveying the catheter.

Catheter-associated sepsis is a serious complication of parenteral nutrition if it is not promptly diagnosed and treated. The pathogenesis of this problem includes touch contamination of the catheter hub with migration of micro-organisms down the lumen of the catheter, transcutaneous passage of micro-organisms at the site of catheter insertion, colonization of the fibrin sheath which coats the catheter from a distant hematogenous source and contamination of parenteral solutions. The results of culture from blood obtained from the central line, peripheral vein and the tip of the catheter can be used to differentiate catheter sepsis, catheter infection and a distant focus of infection (Bozzetti et al 1983, Porter et al 1988). A positive catheter tip and peripheral blood culture with or without a central culture is considered to be catheter sepsis and warrants catheter removal. A positive tip and/or central blood culture with a negative peripheral culture is considered a catheter infection and may be managed with repeat catheter exchange. A positive peripheral, with or without a positive central vein culture, and a negative tip suggests a distant source of infection and requires catheter exchanges weekly if the patient remains febrile. *Staphylococcus epidermidis*, *S. aureus*, *Enterococcus*, *Enterobacteriaceae* spp. and *Candida albicans* are the most common micro-organisms encountered with parenteral nutrition-associated catheter sepsis. Guidewire exchange is not indicated for patients with septic shock, documented catheter sepsis, fungemia and a purulent catheter exit site. Since methicillin resistance is quite common for *S. epidermidis* and *S. aureus*, empiric treatment should include intravenous vancomycin and, for Gram-negative bacilli, gentamicin. Other antibiotics are acceptable and should be tailored to the sensitivity profile for the micro-organisms in a given community. Fungal bacteremia requires special mention. Patients with documented fungemia should undergo a thorough examination including a fundoscopic examination to exclude *Candida* endophthalmitis since this complication necessitates prolongation of therapy.

Quantitative blood cultures have become helpful in assessing patients with permanent venous access devices where surveillance is not possible by guidewire exchange (Mosca et al 1987). When these cultures reveal a greater growth of bacteria through a permanent catheter compared to the peripheral culture, it is strongly suggestive of an infected vascular device that should be treated with long-term antibiotics. If the bloodstream infection is not controlled as demonstrated by continued sepsis or positive cultures, the device needs to be removed.

*Metabolic complications*

Severely malnourished patients who have been without food for an extended length of time are at risk for the development of acute confusion, seizures, cardiac arrhythmias, profound muscle weakness and respiratory failure soon after nutrition support is instituted, even when calories are provided in a normal amount. These symptoms, whether they occur together or separately, have been referred to as the refeeding syndrome and are the result of rapid and profound decreases in serum potassium, phosphate and magnesium. Acute vitamin deficiencies have also been implicated as the etiology of this condition. Since it is difficult to predict which patients will develop this problem it has been suggested that all patients at risk for the refeeding syndrome should be started on nutrition support at total energy intakes of 105 kJ/kg (25 kcal/kg) of actual BW per day and with glucose provisions being initially limited to 2.9 g/kg/day (41.4 kJ based on 14.3 kJ/g of parenteral dextrose). If electrolyte levels remain stable or are easy to maintain the formula can be advanced over a 5–7-day period. Hyperglycemia can result in neutrophil dysfunction, an osmotic diuresis with dehydration and electrolyte abnormalities and is due to the infusion of glucose coupled with insulin resistance which is often seen in ill patients. Patients at risk for hyperglycemia include those with diabetes or sepsis/stress or who are receiving corticosteroids. Blood sugars should be kept below 11.2 mmol/L and if they rise above 19.5 mmol/L the TPN solution should be stopped. Guidelines to minimize this problem have already been discussed. Hyperglycemia in a patient who had previously been stable suggests an added metabolic stress, such as an infection, and should prompt appropriate investigation.

***Hypoglycemia.*** This is seen when excess insulin is given relative to the patient's level of stress. It occurs most often during recovery and can be prevented by avoiding too stringent blood glucose control. Low blood glucose also occurs when TPN solutions are abruptly discontinued. Intravenous fluid with 10% dextrose should be given if TPN must be immediately discontinued or the TPN should be given at half the usual rate for 1–2 h before discontinuation. Both of these maneuvers permit the rate of endogenous insulin secretion to return to a more normal level.

A significant and sometimes life-threatening decrease in serum potassium, phosphate and magnesium can occur with the institution of TPN. In fact, low concentrations of these electrolytes may develop with any type of nutrition support; however, they are more likely to occur with the administration of large amounts of parenteral glucose that stimulates insulin secretion and tissue anabolism. During the first 3–4 days of TPN, as total glucose calories are increased, these electrolytes must be closely monitored.

***Hypokalemia.*** This occurs with tissue anabolism or increased renal and intestinal losses. Diuretics, corticosteroids, some antibiotics (especially amphotericin), cisplatin and alkalosis lead to excessive renal excretion of potassium while diarrhea and upper gastrointestinal fistulae result in increased intestinal losses of potassium. Vomiting and nasogastric suction lead to alkalosis that increases renal losses. Lethargy, mental status changes, weakness, myalgias, nausea, vomiting, diarrhea and ileus are some of the symptoms of hypokalemia. Estimates of total body deficits based on serum levels have been suggested as follows: serum 3.0–3.5 mmol/L = deficit of 100–200 mEq, serum 2.5–3.0 mmol/L = deficit of 200–400 mEq, and 2.0–2.5 mmol/L = deficit of 400–800 mEq. Oral replacement is favored if the gastrointestinal tract is intact and deficiency is mild to moderate (2.5–3.5 mmol/L). Otherwise, the parenteral route is advised. Systemic alkalemia and hypomagnesemia should be corrected since these disturbances can impair successful potassium repletion.

***Hypophosphatemia.*** Patients at greatest risk are those with severe marasmus, alcoholism and hyperglycemia. Decreased intestinal absorption and increased urinary losses can also contribute to this problem and can be due to phosphate-binding antacids, corticosteroids, diuretics, vitamin D deficiency and hyperparathyroidism. Signs and symptoms include encephalopathy, seizures, paresthesias, muscle weakness, rhabdomyolysis and hemolytic anemia. Serum concentrations of phosphorus between 0.32 and 0.81 mmol/L are moderately depressed while those below 0.32 mmol/L are severely depressed. Sodium or potassium phosphate salts are used to replete low serum levels. Oral supplements are preferred for patients on enteral tube feeding but they may cause diarrhea. Parenteral replacement is used for patients with severely low serum concentrations and who are unable to tolerate enteral repletion. Dosing typically ranges from 0.08 to 0.16 mmol/kg which must be infused over 6 h to avoid hypocalcemia and calcium phosphate precipitates in the renal tubules and other body tissues.

***Magnesium depletion.*** Magnesium is essential for proper neuromuscular and cardiac function and the activity of many enzymes. In addition, the secretion of parathyroid hormone in response to hypocalcemia and the renal response to parathyroid hormone are dependent on normal levels of serum magnesium. Intestinal absorption is poor due to its relative insolubility; magnesium levels are maintained by the ability of the kidneys to retain and excrete magnesium over a very broad range. Renal tubular dysfunction, diabetes, alcoholism (p. 876), hyperparathyroidism, hypercalcemia, hypophosphatemia and various medications including diuretics, antibiotics (aminoglycosides, amphotericin, ticarcillin), cisplatin and digitalis can all contribute to magnesium depletion. Just as with phosphorus repletion, oral administration of magnesium is favored for mild depletion when the gut is intact although diarrhea is a common side-effect. Intravenous magnesium sulfate can be given empirically until serum levels return to normal. Each gram of this salt provides 8 mEq of magnesium.

### *Elevation of liver-associated enzymes*

This is one of the most commonly observed abnormalities seen in patients who receive TPN. Lindor and colleagues (1979) described a pattern of liver enzyme elevations in hospitalized adult patients who received fat-free TPN for 2 weeks or longer. Transaminase, alkaline phosphatase and bilirubin concentrations increased 3.0-, 1.9- and 0.25-fold respectively and peaked between days 9 and 12 after starting TPN. TPN should not cause jaundice in adults and if it occurs, other causes should be considered including sepsis, drugs, viral hepatitis and extrahepatic obstruction. The most frequent pathology is hepatic steatosis followed by nonspecific triaditis and intrahepatic cholestasis (Sheldon et al 1978). Infusion of excessive calories, especially glucose, with an elevated portal vein insulin to glucagon ratio is believed to be responsible for the hepatic steatosis (Hall et al 1984, Li et al 1989). Other factors that have been implicated in the development of steatosis include sepsis/cytokines (Matsui et al 1993) and amino acid and essential fatty acid deficiencies. TPN rarely needs to be stopped for increased liver enzymes. Calories should be reduced to meet basal energy requirements and the carbohydrate to fat calories should be given in a ratio of 70 to 30. Occasionally, TPN needs to be infused in a cyclic fashion. Normalization of liver enzymes usually occurs within 2–3 weeks after the discontinuation of TPN. Steatohepatitis has been described in adults on long-term home TPN; its cause is not completely understood (Bowyer et al 1985). Approximately 15% will develop persistent elevations in their liver tests, biopsies usually find steatohepatitis and 5% have progressed to fibrotic–cirrhotic stages.

### *Monitoring*

Careful monitoring is essential to avoid many of the complications associated with TPN. Patients should be weighed and examined daily and strict intake and output records need to be maintained. A complete serum electrolyte profile should be obtained on the first 3 days of therapy and weekly thereafter. A complete blood count and coagulation profile is needed before central line placement. Capillary blood glucose determination should be done twice times daily. This can be decreased to once daily for nondiabetics when their blood sugars are under good control. Liver enzymes are measured periodically in stable patients. Subsequent laboratory determinations must be individualized for the patient's active medical problems. Though hyperkalemia, hyperphosphatemia and hypermagnesemia were not discussed in detail, patients with moderate to severe renal dysfunction or those receiving medications which affect renal acid–base and electrolyte status require monitoring of these and other electrolytes 2–3 times per week.

REFERENCES


Achord J L 1987 A prospective randomized clinical trial of peripheral amino acid-glucose supplementation in acute alcoholic hepatitis. American Journal of Gastroenterology 82: 871–875

Benya R, Layden T J, Mobarhan S 1991 Diarrhea associated with tube feeding: the importance of using objective criteria. Journal of Clinical Gastroenterology 13: 162–172

Bistrian B R 1977a Nutritional assessment and therapy of protein-calorie malnutrition in the hospital. Journal of the American Dietetic Association 71: 393–397

Bistrian B R 1977b Interaction of nutrition and infection in the hospital setting. American Journal of Clinical Nutrition 30: 1228–1235

Bistrian B R 1979 A simple technique to estimate severity of stress. Surgery, Gynecology and Obstetrics 148: 675–678

Bistrian B R, Blackburn G L, Hallowell E, Heddle R 1974 Protein status of general surgical patients. Journal of the American Medical Association 230: 858–860

Bistrian B R, Blackburn G L, Sherman M, Scrimshaw N S 1975 Therapeutic index of nutritional depletion in hospitalized patients. Surgery, Gynecology and Obstetrics 141: 512–516

Bistrian B R, Blackburn G L, Vitale J, Cochran D, Naylor J 1976 Prevalence of malnutrition in general medical patients. Journal of the American Medical Association 235: 1567–1570

Bivins B A, Bell R M, Rapp R P, Toedebusch W H 1984 Pancreatic exocrine response to parenteral nutrition. Journal of Parenteral and Enteral Nutrition 8: 34–36

Bjerve K S, Mostad L, Thoresen L 1987 Alpha-linolenic acid deficiency in patients on long-term gastric-tube feeding: estimation of linolenic acid and long-chain unsaturated n–3 fatty acid requirement in man. American Journal of Clinical Nutrition 15: 66–77

Blackburn G L, Williams L F, Bistrian B R et al 1976 New approaches to the management of severe acute pancreatitis. American Journal of Surgery 131: 114–124

Blackburn G L, Bistrian B R, Maini B S, Schlamm H T, Smith M F 1977 Nutritional and metabolic assessment of the hospitalized patient. Journal of Parenteral and Enteral Nutrition 1: 11–22

Bohnker B K, Artman L E, Hoskins W J 1987 Narrow bore nasogastric feeding tube complications. A literature review. Nutrition in Clinical Practice 2: 203–209

Bonkovsky H L, Fiellin D A, Smith G S, Slaker D P, Simon D, Galambos J T 1991 A randomized, controlled trial of treatment of alcoholic hepatitis with parenteral nutrition and oxandrolone. I. Short-term effects on liver function. American Journal of Gastroenterology 86: 1200–1208

Bouffard Y H, Delafosse B X, Annat G J, Viale J P, Bertrand O M, Motin J P 1989 Energy expenditure during severe acute pancreatitis. Journal of Parenteral and Enteral Nutrition 13: 26–29

Bowyer B A, Fleming C R, Ludwig J, Petz J, McGill D B 1985 Does long-term home parenteral nutrition in adult patients cause chronic liver disease? Journal of Parenteral and Enteral Nutrition 9: 11–17

Bozzetti F, Terno G, Bonfanti G et al 1983 Prevention and treatment of central venous catheter sepsis by exchange via a guidewire. A prospective controlled trial. Annals of Surgery 198: 48–52

Brinson R R, Pitts W M 1989 Enteral nutrition in the critically ill patient: role of hypoalbuminemia. Critical Care Medicine 17: 367–370

Brough W, Horne G, Blount A, Irving M H, Jeejeebhoy K N 1986 Effects of nutrient intake, surgery, sepsis, and long term administration of steroids on muscle function. British Medical Journal 293: 983–988

Burr G O, Burr M M 1930 On the nature and role of the fatty acids essential in nutrition. Biological Chemistry 86: 587–621

Buzby G P, Mullen J L, Matthews D C, Hobbs C L, Rosato E F 1980 Prognostic nutritional index in gastrointestinal surgery. American Journal of Surgery 139: 160–167

Byrne T A, Morrissey T B, Ziegler T R, Gatzen C, Young L S, Wilmore D W 1992 Growth hormone, glutamine, and fiber enhance adaptation of remnant bowel following massive intestinal resection. Surgical Forum 43: 151–153

Cabre E, Gonzalez-Huix F, Abad-Lacruz A et al 1990 Effect of total enteral nutrition on the short-term outcome of severely malnourished cirrhotics. A randomized controlled trial. Gastroenterology 98: 715–720

Cahill G F Jr 1970 Starvation in man. New England Journal of Medicine 282: 668–675

Cahill G F Jr, Herrera M G, Morgan A P et al 1966 Hormone–fuel interrelationships during fasting. Journal of Clinical Investigation 45: 1751–1769

Cameron J L, Capuzzi D M, Zuidema G D, Margolis S 1974 Acute pancreatitis with hyperlipemia. Evidence for a persistent defect in lipid metabolism. American Journal of Medicine 56: 482–487

Cannon P R, Wissler R W, Woolridge R L, Benditt E P 1944 The relationship of protein deficiency to surgical infection. Annals of Surgery 120: 514–525

Cassim M M, Allardyce D B 1974 Pancreatic secretion in response to jejunal feeding of elemental diet. Annals of Surgery 180: 228–231

Cataldi-Betcher E L, Seltzer M H, Slocum B A, Jones K W 1983 Complications occurring during enteral nutrition support: a prospective study. Journal of Parenteral and Enteral Nutrition 7: 546–552

Cerra F B, Cheung N K, Fischer J E et al 1985 Disease-specific amino acid infusion (F080) in hepatic encephalopathy: a prospective, randomized, double-blind, controlled trial. Journal of Parenteral and Enteral Nutrition 9: 288–295

Chan A T H, Fleming C R, O'Fallon W M, Huizenga K A 1986 Estimated versus measured basal energy requirements in patients with Crohn's disease. Gastroenterology 91: 75–78

Chawla R K, Wolf D C, Kutner M H, Bonkovsky H L 1989 Choline may be an essential nutrient in malnourished patients with cirrhosis. Gastroenterology 97: 1514–1520

Christie M L, Sack D M, Pomposelli J, Horst D 1985 Enriched branched-chain amino acid formula versus a casein-based supplement in the treatment of cirrhosis. Journal of Parenteral and Enteral Nutrition 9: 671–678

Coben R M, Weintraub A, DiMarino A J Jr, Cohen S 1994 Gastroesophageal reflux during gastrostomy feeding. Gastroenterology 106: 13–18

Compston J E, Horton L W L 1978 Oral 25-hydroxyvitamin $D_3$ in treatment of osteomalacia associated with ileal resection and cholestyramine therapy. Gastroenterology 74: 900–902

Corcoy R, Sanchez J M, Domingo P, Net A 1988 Nutrition in the patient with severe acute pancreatitis. Nutrition 4: 269–275

Cosnes J, Evard D, Beaugerie L, Gendre J P, Le Quintrec Y Le 1992 Improvement in protein absorption with a small-peptide-based diet in patients with high jejunostomy. Nutrition 8: 406–411

Deitch E A 1990 The role of intestinal barrier failure and bacterial

translocation in the development of systemic infection and multiple organ failure. Archives of Surgery 125: 403–404
De-Leeuw I H, Vandewoude M F 1986 Bacterial contamination of enteral diets. Gut 27(suppl 1): 56–57
Detsky A S, McLaughlin J R, Baker J P et al 1987 What is subjective global assessment of nutritional status? Journal of Parenteral and Enteral Nutrition 11: 8–13
Diehl A M, Boitnott J K, Herlong H F et al 1985 Effect of parenteral amino acid supplementation in alcoholic hepatitis. Hepatology 5: 57–63
DiSario J A, Foutch P G, Sanowski R A 1990 Poor results with percutaneous endoscopic jejunostomy. Gastrointestinal Endoscopy 36: 257–260
Dobbins J W, Binder H J 1976 Effect of bile salts and fatty acids on the colonic absorption of oxalate. Gastroenterology 70: 1096–1100
Dominioni G, Trocki O, Mochizuki H et al 1984 Prevention of severe postburn hypermetabolism and catabolism by immediate gastric feeding. Journal of Burn Care and Rehabilitation 5: 106–112
Doweiko J P, Nompleggi D J 1991a Role of albumin in human physiology and pathophysiology. Journal of Parenteral and Enteral Nutrition 15: 207–211
Doweiko J P, Nompleggi D J 1991b The role of albumin in human physiology and pathophysiology, part III: albumin and disease states. Journal of Parenteral and Enteral Nutrition 15: 476–483
Driscoll R H Jr, Rosenberg I H 1978 Total parenteral nutrition in inflammatory bowel disease. Medical Clinics of North America 62: 185–201
Eastwood G L 1977 Small bowel morphology and epithelial proliferation in intravenously alimented rabbits. Surgery 82: 613–620
Edelman K, Valenzuela J E 1983 Effect of intravenous lipid on human pancreatic secretion. Gastroenterology 85: 1063–1066
Edens N K, Gil K M, Elwyn D H 1986 The effects of varing energy and nitrogen intake on nitrogen balance, body composition, and metabolic rate. Clinics in Chest Medicine 7: 3–17
Fay D E, Poplausky M, Gruber M, Lance P 1991 Long-term enteral feeding: a retrospective comparison of delivery via percutaneous endoscopic gastrostomy and nasoenteric tubes. American Journal of Gastroenterology 86: 1604–1609
Feller J H, Brown R A, Toussaint G P, Thompson A G 1974 Changing methods in the treatment of severe pancreatitis. American Journal of Surgery 127: 196–201
Ferguson D R, Harig J M, Kozarek R A, Kelsey P B, Picha G J 1993 Placement of a feeding button ("one-step button") as the initial procedure. American Journal of Gastroenterology 88: 501–504
Feurer I M, Mullen J L 1986 Bedside measurement of resting energy expenditure and respiratory quotient via indirect calorimetry. Nutrition in Clinical Practice 1: 43–49
Fiaccadori F, Ghinelli F, Pedretti G et al 1985 Branched-chain amino acid solutions in the treatment of hepatic encephalopathy: a controlled trial. Italian Journal of Gastroenterology 17: 5–10
Fink M P 1991 Gastrointestinal mucosal injury in experimental models of shock, trauma, and sepsis. Critical Care Medicine 19: 627–641
Fischer J E, Baldessarini R J 1971 False neurotransmitters and hepatic failure. Lancet 2: 75–80
Fischer J E, Funovics J M, Aguirre A et al 1975 The role of plasma amino acids in hepatic encephalopathy. Surgery 78: 276–290
Fleming C R, Jeejeebhoy K N 1994 Advances in clinical nutrition. Gastroenterology 106: 1365–1373
Fox A D, Kripke S A, de Paula J, Berman J M, Settle R G, Rombeau J L 1988 Effect of a glutamine-supplemented enteral diet on methotrexate-induced enterocolitis. Journal of Parenteral and Enteral Nutrition 12: 325–331
Franklin J L, Rosenberg I H 1973 Impaired folic acid absorption in inflammatory bowel disease; effects of salicylazosulfapyridine (Azulfidine). Gastroenterology 64: 517–525
Fraser I M, Russell D M C R, Whittaker S et al 1984 Skeletal and diaphragmatic muscle function in malnourished chronic obstructive lung disease. American Review of Respiratory Disease 129: A269
Gerson C D, Cohen N, Janowitz H D 1973 Small intestinal absorptive function in regional enteritis. Gastroenterology 64: 907–912
Gonzalez-Huix F, de Leon R, Fernandez-Banares F et al 1993 Polymeric enteral diets as primary treatment of active Crohn's disease: a prospective steroid controlled trial. Gut 34: 778–782
Goodgame J T, Fischer J E 1977 Parenteral nutrition in the treatment of acute pancreatitis: effect on complications and mortality. Annals of Surgery 186: 651–658
Gottschlich M M, Jenkins M, Warden G D et al 1990 Differential effects of three enteral dietary regimens on selected outcome variables in burn patients. Journal of Parenteral and Enteral Nutrition 14: 225–236
Grant J P, James S, Grabowski V, Trexler K M 1984 Total parenteral nutrition in pancreatic disease. Annals of Surgery 200: 627–631
Greenberg G R, Fleming C R, Jeejeebhoy K N, Rosenberg I H, Sales D, Tremaine W J 1988 Controlled trial of bowel rest and nutritional support in the management of Crohn's disease. Gut 29: 1309–1315
Greenberger N J 1978 State of the art: the management of patients with short bowel syndrome. American Journal of Gastroenterology 70: 528–540
Grundfest S, Steiger E, Selinkoff P, Fletcher J 1980 The effect of intravenous fat emulsions in patients with pancreatic fistula. Journal of Parenteral and Enteral Nutrition 4: 27–31
Gutierrez E D, Balfe D M 1991 Fluoroscopically guided nasoenteric feeding tube placement: results of a 1-year study. Radiology 178: 759–762
Hall R I, Grant J P, Ross L H, Coleman R A, Bozovic M G, Quartfordt S H 1984 Pathogenesis of hepatic steatosis in the parenterally fed rat. Journal of Clinical Investigation 74: 1658–1668
Hamwi G J 1964 Changing dietary concepts in diabetes mellitus: diagnosis and treatment. American Diabetes Association, New York
Hanson R L 1979 Predictive criteria for length of nasogastric tube insertion for tube feeding. Journal of Parenteral and Enteral Nutrition 3: 160–163
Harris J A, Benedict F G 1919 Biometric study of basal metabolism in man (publication no. 279). Carnegie Institute, Washington
Harvey K B, Moldawer L L, Bistrian B R, Blackburn G L 1981 Biological measures for the formulation of a hospital prognostic index. American Journal of Clinical Nutrition 34: 2013–2022
Hassett J M, Sunby C, Flint L M 1988 No elimination of aspiration pneumonia in neurologically disabled patients with feeding gastrostomy. Surgery, Gynecology and Obstetrics 167: 383–388
Health and Welfare Canada 1990. Nutrition recommendations. Report of the Scientific Review Committee. Supply and Services Canada, Ottawa, Canada
Hehir D J, Jenkins R L, Bistrian B R, Blackburn G L 1985 Nutrition in patients undergoing orthotopic liver transplantation. Journal of Parenteral and Enteral Nutrition 9: 695–700
Heymsfield S B, Stevens V, Noel R, McManus C, Smith J, Nixon D 1982 Biochemical composition of muscle in normal and semistarved human subjects: relevance to anthropometric measurements. American Journal of Clinical Nutrition 36: 131–142
Heymsfield S B, Arteaga C, McManus C, Smith J, Moffitt S 1983 Measurement of muscle mass in humans: validity of the 24-hour urinary creatinine method. American Journal of Clinical Nutrition 37: 478–494
Hill G L, Blackett R L, Pickford I et al 1977 Malnutrition in surgical patients. An unrecognized problem. Lancet 1: 689–692
Hilton E, Haslett T M, Borenstein M T, Tucci V, Isenberg H D, Singer C 1988 Central catheter infections: single- versus triple-lumen catheters. Influence of guide wires on infection rates when used for replacement of cathetes. American Journal of Medicine 84: 667–672
Hofmann A F, Poley J R 1972 Role of bile acid malabsorption in the pathogenesis of diarrhea and steatorrhea in patients with ileal resection. I. Response to cholestyramine or replacement of dietary long chain triglyceride by medium chain triglyceride. Gastroenterology 62: 918–934
Holman R T, Johnson S B, Hatch T F 1982 A case of human linolenic acid deficiency involving neurological abnormalities. American Journal of Clinical Nutrition 35: 617–623
Hunter D C, Jaksic T, Lewis D, Benotti P N, Blackburn G L, Bistrian B R 1988 Resting energy expenditure in the critically ill: estimations versus measurement. British Journal of Surgery 75: 875–878
Ibanez J, Penafiel A, Raurich J M, Marse P, Jorda R, Mata F 1992 Gastroesophageal reflux in intubated patients receiving enteral nutrition: effect of supine and semirecumbent positions. Journal of Parenteral and Enteral Nutrition 16: 419–422

Jain N K, Larson D E, Schroeder K W et al 1987 Antibiotic prophylaxis for percutaneous endoscopic gastrostomy. Annals of Internal Medicine 107: 824–828

John W J, Phillips R, Ott L, Adams L J, McClain C J 1989 Resting energy expenditure in patients with alcoholic hepatitis. Journal of Parenteral and Enteral Nutrition 13: 124–127

Kalfarentzos F, Alivizatos V, Panagopoulos K, Androulakis J 1987 Nasoduodenal intubation with the use of metoclopramide. Nutritional Support Services 7: 33–34

Kalfarentzos F, Spiliotis J, Velimezis G, Dougenis D, Androulakis J 1989 Comparison of forearm muscle dynamometry with nutritional prognostic index as a preoperative indicator in cancer patients. Journal of Parenteral and Enteral Nutrition 13: 34–36

Kaplan D S, Murthy U K, Linscheer W G 1989 Percutaneous endoscopic jejunostomy: long-term follow-up of 23 patients. Gastrointestinal Endoscopy 35: 403–406

Kearns P J, Young H, Garcia G et al 1992 Accelerated improvement of alcoholic liver disease with enteral nutrition. Gastroenterology 102: 200–205

Kelly G A, Nahrwold D L 1976 Pancreatic secretion in response to an elemental diet and intravenous hyperalimentation. Surgery, Gynecology and Obstetrics 143: 87–91

Keohane P P, Attrill H, Love M, Frost P, Silk D B A 1984 Relation between osmolality of diet and gastrointestinal side effects in enteral nutrition. British Medical Journal 288: 678–680

Kinsella J E, Lokesh B, Broughton S, Whelan J 1990 Dietary polyunsaturated fatty acids and eicosanoids: potential effects on the modulation of inflammatory and immune cells: an overview. Nutrition 6: 24–44

Kirby D F, Craig R M, Tsang T et al 1986 Percutaneous endoscopic gastrostomies: a prospective evaluation and review of the literature. Journal of Parenteral and Enteral Nutrition 10: 155–159

Kirby D F, Clifton G L, Turner H, Marion D W, Barrett J, Gruemer H D F 1991 Early enteral nutrition after brain injury by percutaneous endoscopic gastrojejunostomy. Journal of Parenteral and Enteral Nutrition 15: 298–302

Kirschner B S, DeFavaro M V, Jensen W 1981 Lactose malabsorption in children and adolescents with inflammatory bowel disease. Gastroenterology 81: 829–832

Kittinger J W, Sandler R S, Heizer W D 1987 Efficacy of metoclopramide as an adjunct to duodenal placement of small-bore feeding tubes: a randomized, placebo-controlled double-blind study. Journal of Parenteral and Enteral Nutrition 11: 33–37

Kudsk K A, Croce M A, Fabian T C et al 1992 Enteral versus parenteral feeding. Annals of Surgery 215: 503–513

Larson D E, Burton D D, Schroeder K W, DiMagno E P 1987 Percutaneous endoscopic gastrostomy. Gastroenterology 93: 48–52

Lashner B A, Kirsner J B, Hanauer S B 1986 Acute panceatitis associated with high-concentration lipid emulsion during total parenteral nutrition therapy for Crohn's disease. Gastroenterology 90: 1039–1041

Levine G M, Deren J J, Steiger E, Zinno R 1974 Role of oral intake in maintenance of gut mass and disaccharide activity. Gastroenterology 67: 975–982

Li S, Nussbaum M S, McFadden D W, Dayal R, Fischer J E 1989 Reversal of hepatic steatosis in rats by addition of glucagon to total parenteral nutrition (TPN). Journal of Surgical Research 46: 557–566

Lindor K D, Fleming C R, Abrams A, Hirschkorn M A 1979 Liver function values in adults receiving total parenteral nutrition. Journal of the American Medical Association 241: 2391–2400

Lindor K D, Fleming C R, Burnes J U, Nelson J K, Ilstrup D M 1992 A randomized prospective trial comparing a defined formula diet, corticosteroids, and a defined formula diet plus corticosteroids in active Crohn's disease. Mayo Clinic Proceedings 67: 328–333

Lochs H, Steinhardt H J, Klaus-Wentz B et al 1991 Comparison of enteral nutrition and drug treatment in active Crohn's disease. Results of the European Co-operative Crohn's Disease Study IV. Gastroenterology 101: 881–888

Long C L, Schaffel N, Geiger J W, Schiller W R, Blakemore W S 1979 Metabolic response to injury and illness: estimation of energy and protein needs from indirect calorimetry and nitrogen balance. Journal of Parenteral and Enteral Nutrition 3: 452–456

Lord L M, Weiser-Maimone A, Pulhamus M, Sax H C 1993 Comparison of weighted vs unweighted enteral feeding tubes for efficacy of transpyloric intubation. Journal of Parenteral and Enteral Nutrition 17: 271–273

Lukaski H C 1987 Methods for the assessment of human body composition: traditional and new. American Journal of Clinical Nutrition 46: 537–556

MacKenzie T A, Blackburn G L, Flatt J P 1974 Clinical assessment of nutritional status using nitrogen balance. Federation Proceedings 33: 683 (abstract)

Malchow H, Steinhardt H J, Lorenz-Meyer H et al 1990 Feasibility and effectiveness of a defined-formula diet regimen in treating active Crohn's disease. European Co-operative Crohn's Disease Study III. Scandinavian Journal of Gastroenterology 25: 235–244

Marchesini G, Dioguardi F S, Bianchi G P et al 1991 Long-term branched-chain amino acid treatment in chronic hepatic encephalopathy. A randomized double-blind casein-controlled trial. The Italian Multicenter Study Group. Journal of Hepatology 11: 92–101

Matsui J, Cameron R G, Kurian R, Kuo G C, Jeejeebhoy K N 1993 Nutritional, hepatic, and metabolic effects of cachectin/tumor necrosis factor in rats receiving total parenteral nutritrion. Gastroenterology 104: 235–243

McClave S A, Mitoraj T E, Thielmeier K A, Greenburg R A 1992 Differentiating subtypes (hypoalbuminemic vs marasmic) of protein-calorie malnutrition: incidence and clinical significance in a university hospital setting. Journal of Parenteral and Enteral Nutrition 16: 337–342

McCullough A J, Mullen K D, Smanik E J, Tabbaa M, Szauter K 1989 Nutritional therapy and liver disease. Gastroenterology Clinics of North America 18: 619–643

McGhee A, Henderson J M, Millikan W J Jr et al 1983 Comparison of the effects of Hepatic-Aid and a casein modular diet on encephalopathy, plasma amino acids and nitrogen balance in cirrhotic patients. Annals of Surgery 197: 288–293

McIntyre P B, Fitchew M, Lennard-Jones J E 1986 Patients with a high jejunostomy do not need a special diet. Gastroenterology 91: 25–33

McMahon M M, Bistrian B R 1990 The physiology of nutritional assessment and therapy in protein-calorie malnutrition. Disease-a-Month 36: 375–417

Meguid M M, Akahoshi M P, Jeffers S, Hayashi R J, Hammond W G 1984 Amelioration of metabolic complications of conventional total parenteral nutrition: a prospective randomized study. Archives of Surgery 119: 1294–1298

Messing B, Pigot F, Rongier M, Morin M C, Ndeïndoum U, Rambaud J C 1991 Intestinal absorption of free oral hyperalimentation in the very short bowel syndrome. Gastroenterology 100: 1502–1508

Mezey G 1975 Intestinal function in chronic alcoholism. Annals of the New York Academy of Sciences 252: 215–227

Michel H, Pomier-Layrargues G, Aubin J P et al 1984 Treatment of hepatic encephalopathy by infusion of a modified amino-acid solution: results of a controlled study in 47 cirrhotic patients. In: Capocaccia L, Fischer J E, Rossi-Fanelli F (eds) Hepatic encephalopathy in chronic liver failure. New York, Plenum, p 323–333

Mizuma K, DeLamater P V, Lee P C, Appert H E, Howard J M 1978 Changing circulating levels of lipids, insulin and glucagon during experimental acute pancreatitis. Surgery, Gynecology and Obstetrics 147: 577–582

Mochizuki H, Trocki O, Dominioni L, Brackett K A, Joffe S N, Alexander J W 1984 Mechanism of prevention of postburn hypermetabolism and catabolism by early enteral feeding. Annals of Surgery 200: 297–308

Montecalvo M A, Steger K A, Farber H W et al 1992 Nutritional outcome and pneumonia in critical care patients randomized to gastric versus jejunal tube feedings. Critical Care Medicine 20: 1377–1387

Moore F A, Moore E E, Jones T N, McCroskey B L, Peterson V M 1989 TEN versus TPN following major abdominal trauma – reduced septic morbidity. Journal of Trauma 29: 916–922

Moore F D, Olesen K H, McMurrey J D et al 1963 The body cell mass and its supporting environment: body composition in health and disease. W B Saunders, Philadelphia

Mosca R, Curtas S, Forbes B, Meguid M M 1987 The benefits of

isolator cultures in the management of suspected catheter sepsis. Surgery 102: 718–723
Mowatt-Larssen C A, Brown R O, Wojtysiak S L, Kudsk K A 1992 Comparison of tolerance and nutritional outcome between a peptide and a standard enteral formula in critically ill, hypoalbuminemic patients. Journal of Parenteral and Enteral Nutrition 16: 20–24
Mullen J L, Buzby G P, Matthews D C, Smale B F, Rosato E F 1980 Reduction of operative morbidity and mortality by combined preoperative and postoperative nutritional support. Annals of Surgery 192: 604–613
Muller J M, Keller H W, Brenner U, Walter M, Holzmuller W 1986 Indications and effects of preoperative parenteral nutrition. World Journal of Surgery 10: 53–63
Munro H N, Fernstrom J D, Wurtman R J 1975 Insulin, plasma amino acid imbalance, and hepatic coma. Lancet 1: 722–724
Nasrallah S M, Galambos J T 1980 Amino acid therapy of alcoholic hepatitis. Lancet 2: 1276–1277
National Research Council 1989 Recommended dietary allowances, 10th edn. National Academy Press, Washington
Neville J N, Eagles J A, Samson G, Olson R E 1986 Nutritional status of alcoholics. American Journal of Clinical Nutrition 21: 1329–1340
Nightingale J M D, Lennard-Jones J E, Walker E R, Farthing M J G 1990 Jejunal efflux in short bowel syndrome. Lancet 336: 765–768
Nordenstrom J, Carpentier Y A, Askanazi J et al 1982 Metabolic utilization of intravenous fat emulsion during total parenteral nutrition. Annals of Surgery 196: 221–231
Nutrition Advisory Group, American Medical Association 1979 Multivitamin preparations for parenteral use. Journal of Parenteral and Enteral Nutrition 3: 258–262
O'Dwyer S T, Michie H R, Ziegler T R, Revhang A, Smith R J, Wilmore D W 1988 A single dose of endotoxin increases intestinal permeability in healthy humans. Archives of Surgery 123: 1459–1464
O'Keefe S J D, Peterson M E, Fleming C R 1994a Octreotide as an adjunct to home parenteral nutrition in the managememnt of permanent end-jejunostomy syndrome. Journal of Parenteral and Enteral Nutrition 18: 26–34
O'Keefe S J D, Haymond M W, Bennet W M, Oswald B, Nelson D K, Shorter R G 1994b Long-acting somatostatin analogue therapy and protein metabolism in patients with jejunostomies. Gastroenterology 107: 379–388
O'Morain C, Segal A W, Levi A J 1984 Elemental diet as primary treatment of acute Crohn's disease: a controlled trial. British Medical Journal 288: 1859–1862
Owen O E, Morgan A P, Kemp H G, Sullivan J M, Herrera M G, Cahill G F Jr 1967 Brain metabolism during fasting. Journal of Clinical Investigation 46: 1589–1595
Paauw J D, McCamish M A, Dean R E, Ouellette T R 1984 Assessment of caloric needs in stressed patients. Journal of the American College of Nutrition 3: 51–59
Panel on Dietary Reference Values 1991 Dietary reference values for food energy and nutrients for the United Kingdom. Report of the Panel on Dietary Reference Values of the Committee on Medical Aspects of Food Policy. HMSO, London
Pettigrew R A, Lang S D R, Haydock D A, Parry B R, Bremmer D A, Hill G L 1985 Catheter-related sepsis in patients on intravenous nutrition: a prospective study of quantitative catheter cultures and guidewire changes for suspected sepsis. British Journal of Surgery 72: 52–55
Ponsky J L, Gauderer M W L, Stellato T A, Aszodi A 1984 Percutaneous approaches to enteral alimentation. American Journal of Surgery 149: 102–105
Porter K A, Bistrian B R, Blackburn G L 1988 Guidewire catheter exchange with triple culture technique in the management of catheter sepsis. Journal of Parenteral and Enteral Nutrition 12: 628–632
Powanda M C 1977 Changes in body balances of nitrogen and other key nutrients: description and underlying mechanisms. American Journal of Clinical Nutrition 30: 1254–1268
Raggins H, Levenson S M, Singer R A, Stamford W, Seifter E 1973 Intrajejunal administration of an elemental diet at neutral pH avoids pancreatic stimulation. American Journal of Surgery 126: 606–614
Reeds P J, Laditan A A O 1976 Serum albumin and transferrin in protein-energy malnutrition. Their use in the assessment of marginal undernutrition and the prognosis in severe undernutrition. British Journal of Nutrition 36: 255–263
Rees R G P, Keohane P P, Grimble G K et al 1986 Elemental diet administered nasogastrically without starter regimens to patients with inflammatory bowel disease. Journal of Parenteral and Enteral Nutrition 10: 258–262
Reid I R 1989 Pathogenesis and treatment of steroid osteoporosis. Clinical Endocrinology 30: 83–103
Reinhardt G F, Myscofski J W, Wilkens D B, Dobrin P B, Mangan J E Jr, Stannard R T 1980 Incidence and mortality of hypoalbuminemic patients in hospitalized veterans. Journal of Parenteral and Enteral Nutrition 49: 357–359
Rosenberg I H, Bengoa J M, Sitrin M D 1985 Nutritional aspects of inflammatory bowel disease. Annual Review of Nutrition 5: 463–484
Rossi-Fanelli F, Riggio O, Cangiano C et al 1982 Branched-chain amino acids vs lactulose in the treatment of hepatic coma. A controlled study. Digestive Diseases and Sciences 27: 929–935
Russell D M C R, Leiter L A, Whitwell J, Marliss E B, Jeejeebhoy K N 1983 Skeletal muscle function during hypocaloric diets and fasting: a comparison with standard nutritional assessment parameters. American Journal of Clinical Nutrition 37: 133–138
Saverymuttu S, Hodgson H J F, Chadwick V S 1985 Controlled trial comparing prednisolone with an elemental diet plus non-absorbable antibiotics in active Crohn's disease. Gut 26: 994–998
Sax H C, Warner B W, Talamini M A et al 1987 Early total parenteral nutrition in acute pancreatitis: lack of beneficial effects. American Journal of Surgery 153: 117–124
Seidner D L, Mascioli E A, Istfan N W et al 1989 Effects of long-chain triglyceride emulsions on reticuloendothelial system function in humans. Journal of Parenteral and Enteral Nutrition 13: 614–619
Seidner D L, Matarese L E, Steiger E 1994 Nutritional care of the critically ill patient with renal disease. Seminars in Nephrology 14: 53–63
Shailesh L T C, Kadakia S C, Sullivan H O, Starnes E 1992 Percutaneous endoscopic gastrostomy or jejunostomy and the incidence of aspiration in 79 patients. American Journal of Surgery 164: 114–118
Shaw J H F, Wolfe R R 1986 Glucose, fatty acid, and urea kinetics in patients with severe pancreatitis. Annals of Surgery 204: 665–672
Shaw J H F, Wildbore M, Wolfe R R 1987 Whole body protein kinetics in severely septic patients: the response to glucose infusion and total parenteral nutrition. Annals of Surgery 205: 288–294
Sheldon G F, Petersen S R, Sanders R 1978 Hepatic dysfunction during hyperalimentation. Archives of Surgery 113: 504–508
Shike M, Schroy P, Ritchie M A, Lightdale, C J, Morse R 1987 Percutaneous endoscopic jejunostomy in cancer patients with previous gastric resection. Gastrointestinal Endoscopy 33: 372–374
Shils N E, Young V R 1988 Modern nutrition in health and disease, 7th edn. Lea and Febiger, Philadelphia, p 843–845
Silberman H, Dixon N P, Eisenberg D 1982 The safety and efficacy of a lipid-based system of parenteral nutrition in acute pancreatitis. American Journal of Gastroenterology 77: 494–497
Silk D B A, Rees R G P, Keohane P P, Attrill H 1987 Clinical efficacy and design changes of "fine-bore" nasogastric feeding tubes: a seven-year experience involving 809 intubations in 403 patients. Journal of Parenteral and Enteral Nutrition 11: 378–383
Simon D, Galambos J T 1988 A randomized controlled trial of peripheral parenteral nutrition in moderate and severe alcoholic hepatitis. Journal of Hepatology 7: 200–207
Singh S, Richter J E 1992 Effects of a pH electrode across the lower esophageal sphincter. Digestive Diseases and Sciences 37: 667–672
Sitzmann J V, Steinborn P A, Zinner M J, Cameron J L 1989 Total parenteral nutrition and alternate energy substrates in treatment of severe acute pancreatitis. Surgery, Gynecology and Obstetrics 168: 311–317
Stabile B E, Debas H T 1981 Intravenous versus intraduodenal amino acids, fats, and glucose as stimulants of pancreatic secretion. Surgical Forum 32: 224–226
Stern M A, Wolf D C 1994 Erythromycin as a prokinetic agent: a prospective, randomized, controlled study of the efficacy in nasoenteric tube placement. American Journal of Gastroenterology 89: 2011–2013

Sternberg E M, Chrousos, G P, Wilder R L, Gold P W 1992 The stress response and regulation of inflammatory disease. Annals of Internal Medicine 117: 854–866

Stoner H B, Little R A, Frayn K N, Elebute A E, Tresadern J, Gross E 1983 The effect of sepsis on the oxidation of carbohydrate and fat. British Journal of Surgery 70: 32–35

Streat S J, Beddoe A H, Hill G L 1987 Aggressive nutritional support does not prevent protein loss despite fat gain in septic intensive care patients. Journal of Trauma 27: 262–266

Studley H O 1936 Percentage of weight loss: a basic indicator of surgical risk in patients with chronic peptic ulcer. Journal of the American Medical Association 106: 458–460

Swart G R, Zillikens M C, van Vuure J K, van den Berg J W O 1989 Effect of a late evening meal on nitrogen balance in patients with cirrhosis of the liver. British Medical Journal 299: 1202–1203

Thillainayagam A V, Carnaby S, Dias J A, Clark M L, Farthing M J G 1993 Evidence of a dominant role for low osmolality in the efficacy of cereal based oral rehydration solutions: studies in a model of secretory diarrhoea. Gut 34: 920–925

Van Gossum A V, Lemoyne M, Greig P D, Jeejeebhoy K N 1988 Lipid-associated total parenteral nutrition in patients with severe acute pancreatitis. Journal of Parenteral and Enteral Nutrition 12: 250–255

Veterans Affairs Total Parenteral Nutrition Co-operative Study Group 1991 Perioperative total parenteral nutrition in surgical patients. New England Journal of Medicine 325: 525–532

Vidon N, Hecketsweiler P, Butel J, Bernier J J 1978 Effect of continuous jejunal perfusion of elemental and complex nutritional solutions on pancreatic enzyme secretion in human subjects. Gut 19: 194–198

Wahren J, Denis J, Desurmont P et al 1983 Is intravenous administration of branched chain amino acids effective in the treatment of hepatic encephalopathy? A multicenter study. Hepatology 3: 475–480

Weinsier R L, Hunker E M, Krumdieck C L, Butterworth C E Jr 1979 Hospital malnutrition. A prospective evaluation of general medical patients during the course of hospitalization. American Journal of Clinical Nutrition 32: 418–426

Weir J B de V 1949 New methods for calculating metabolic rate with special reference to protein metabolism. Journal of Physiology 109: 1–9

Weltz C R, Morris J B, Mullen J L 1992 Surgical jejunostomy in aspiration risk patients. Annals of Surgery 215: 140–145

Weser E 1983 Nutritional aspects of malabsorption: short gut adaptation. Clinics in Gastroenterology 12: 443–461

Wilmore D W 1991 Catabolic illness: strategies for enhancing recovery. New England Journal of Medicine 325: 695–702

Windsor J A, Hill G L 1988 Weight loss with physiologic impairment: a basic indicator of surgical risk. Annals of Surgery 207: 290–296

Wolfe B M, Culebras J M, Sim A J W, Ball M R, Moore F D 1977 Substrate interaction in intravenous feeding: comparative effects of carbohydrate and fat on amino acid utilization in fasting man. Annals of Surgery 186: 518–540

Wolfe R R, Allsop J R, Burke J F 1979 Glucose metabolism in man: responses to intravenous glucose infusion. Metabolism 28: 210–220

Wolfsen H C, Kozarek R A, Ball T J, Patterson D J, Botoman V A 1990 Tube dysfunction following percutaneous endoscopic gastrostomy and jejunostomy. Gastrointestinal Endoscopy 36: 261–263

Wolman G M, Anderson G H, Marliss E B, Jeejeebhoy K N 1979 Zinc in total parenteral nutrition: requirements and metabolic effects. Gastroenterology 76: 458–467

Young G A, Hill G L 1979 Assessment of protein-calorie malnutrition in surgical patients from plasma proteins and anthropometric measurements. American Journal of Clinical Nutrition 31: 429–435

Young V R, Scrimshaw N S 1971 The physiology of starvation. Scientific American 225: 14–21

Zaloga G P 1991 Bedside method for placing small bowel feeding tubes in critically ill patients: a prospective study. Chest 100: 1643–1646

Ziegler T R, Smith R J, O'Dwyer S T, Demling R H, Wilmore D W 1988 Increased intestinal permeability associated with infection in burn patients. Archives of Surgery 123: 1313–1319

Ziegler T R, Young L S, Benfell K et al 1992 Clinical and metabolic efficacy of glutamine-supplemented parenteral nutrition after bone marrow transplantation. A randomized, double-blind, controlled study. Annals of Internal Medicine 116: 821–828

# 23. Inflammatory bowel disease

*W. J. Tremaine   R. R. Dozois*

The idiopathic inflammatory bowel diseases include Crohn's disease and ulcerative colitis, which account for nearly all of the cases, and collagenous colitis and microscopic colitis, which are uncommon. The causes of the inflammatory bowel diseases remain unknown and there are no known cures. Crohn's disease and ulcerative colitis share a number of similarities in their epidemiology and also in clinical features. Indeed, Crohn's colitis and ulcerative colitis cannot be distinguished on the basis of histology (p. 654) and clinical data in up to 20% of patients (Kirsner 1975). The medical treatment of inflammatory bowel disease has improved during the past 10 years because of the availability of new agents. The surgical treatment of inflammatory bowel disease is also evolving.

**Table 23.1** Selected reports of incidence (per 100 000) of inflammatory bowel disease

| Location | Year | Ulcerative colitis incidence | Crohn's disease incidence |
|---|---|---|---|
| North Tees, UK | 1971 | 15.1 | 5.3 |
| Northern Norway | 1983–86 | 12.8 | 5.8 |
| Copenhagen, Denmark | 1962–78 | 8.1 | |
| | 1970–78 | | 2.7 |
| Olmsted Co., MN, USA | 1960–79 | 5.0 | |
| | 1943–82 | | 4.3 |
| South Africa | 1980–84 | 5.0 | 2.6 |
| Tel Aviv, Israel | 1961–70 | 3.7 | |
| | 1970–76 | | 1.3 |

Modified from Sandler (1994)

## EPIDEMIOLOGY

Ulcerative colitis and Crohn's disease are considered together in most epidemiological studies.

### Incidence, prevalence and mortality

Information is available on the annual incidence rate, i.e. the rate of occurrence per 100 000 persons at risk per year, or the prevalence, i.e. the total number of persons afflicted at any one point in time. The data are subject to error because of problems in diagnosis and interpretation, for example whether acute Crohn's disease represents a separate disease entity. Furthermore, many figures are based on hospital experience of inflammatory bowel diseases rather than on community studies.

Incidence rates of ulcerative colitis and Crohn's disease are shown in Table 23.1. In general, prevalence rates for ulcerative colitis in Western communities are 12 times the annual incidence rates and the prevalence of Crohn's disease is about 15–20 times the incidence. The prevalence rate for ulcerative colitis in Oxford was 80 per 100 000 for the year 1960 and the mortality was 0.7 per 100 000 (Evans & Acheson 1965). In Rochester, Minnesota, the prevalence rate was 225 per 100 000 in 1980 (Stonnington et al 1987). In the same study, the prevalence rate for Crohn's disease was nine per 100 000. The prevalence rate for Crohn's disease is much higher in some other countries, for example 33 and 56 per 100 000 in parts of the UK and 54 and 75 per 100 000 in Stockholm and Malmo (Mayberry & Rhodes 1984). Mortality rates for ulcerative colitis in the USA, UK and Scandinavia vary between 0.5 and 1.0 per 100 000 (Kristensen & Mosbech 1977). In general the incidence of both diseases runs in parallel and are highest in northern Europe and North America and lowest in southern and eastern Europe, Africa, Asia, South America and Japan.

### Race and ethnicity

In the United States inflammatory bowel disease appears to be much more common among whites than nonwhites. The differences may be in part socioeconomic, because with increased urbanization and Westernization the incidence appears to rise in nonwhites, in some cases to equal the rates in whites in the same location. The apparent racial differences may also be due to a lower rate of identification of the diseases among nonwhites due to a difference in access to healthcare. The incidence of ulcerative colitis in the Maori population of New Zealand is much lower than that in white New Zealanders (Wigley & MacLaurin 1962). Among Medicare recipients with inflammatory bowel disease in the United States, hospital discharge rates were twice as high for whites as blacks and there were also lower rates for Asians, native Americans and Hispanics as compared to whites (Sonnenberg et al 1991). There is a higher incidence and prevalence of inflammatory bowel disease among Jews, particularly in Europe and North America where the risk is 2–3 times higher than for non-Jews.

### Age and gender

Both ulcerative colitis and Crohn's disease have a peak age of onset between 15–25 years. Most studies show a bimodal age distribution with a second peak between ages 50 and 80. Men are slightly more likely than women to develop ulcerative colitis and women are at a 20–30% greater risk than men to develop Crohn's disease (Sandler 1994).

### Changes in incidence

There is a general impression that inflammatory bowel disease is becoming more common in Western society. This increase is probably due to both a true increase and to an increased awareness of the disease. The incidence of Crohn's disease increased dramatically until the 1970s and now appears to have stabilized. The incidence of ulcerative colitis has remained unchanged for decades.

## ETIOLOGY

The causes of inflammatory bowel disease are unknown. There is increasing evidence that some individuals have a genetic predisposition to one of these disorders and that there are specific immunologic derangements that occur. From the current data available, the inflammatory bowel diseases appear to be either an excessive response to a normal stimulus (such as an autoimmune disorder) or a normal response to a chronic abnormal stimulus (such as a chronic infection) (Podolsky 1991).

### Immunological features

The immunology of inflammatory bowel disease is an area of intense research that holds promise for defining the underlying pathogenesis of these disorders.

#### *Immunoglobulins*

In the normal intestine, the IgA immunoglobulins are predominant. These mucosal-based molecules are able to bind and inactivate gut antigens without activating the complement system and causing an inflammatory reaction. In patients with inflammatory bowel disease, there is a marked increase in the intestinal production of IgG, up to 30 times normal. Unlike IgA, IgG can bind complement and activate other inflammatory cells that may cause local tissue injury. In ulcerative colitis there is an increased expression of IgG1 and in Crohn's disease there is increased expression of IgG2 in both the serum and in dispersed intestinal mononuclear cells (Fantry & James 1993). These differences in the production of IgG subclasses appear to be in part genetically determined, as healthy monozygotic twins of patients with ulcerative colitis also have increased IgG1-producing cells (Helgeland et al 1992). In contrast, the healthy monozygotic twins of patients with Crohn's disease do not necessarily have the same immunoglobulin production pattern. Differences also exist between ulcerative colitis and Crohn's disease with regard to mucosal complement fixation and the potential role of autoantibodies in tissue injury. In both diseases, there is deposition of C3b and terminal complex components on the luminal surface, but only in ulcerative colitis is there also colocalizing IgG, C1q and C4c, suggesting that complement deposition is less likely to have been initiated by IgG deposition in Crohn's disease (Halstensen et al 1992). The colonic biopsies of some patients show an increase in eosinophils in the mucosa. Their presence, together with increased numbers of IgE-containing cells and mast cells, suggests that immediate hypersensitivity reactions may play a part in the local inflammation.

Circulating autoantibodies to colonic epithelium, present in 13–73% of patients with ulcerative colitis (Snook et al 1991), are directed against lipopolysaccharide in goblet cells or on colonic cell membranes. They are rare in normal subjects and uncommon in patients with Crohn's disease. In ulcerative colitis, both colonic and circulating IgG reacts with a 40 kDa molecular weight antigen (Das et al 1987), but the relevance of this antigen and antibody response to the pathogenesis of inflammatory bowel disease has not been established.

#### *Antineutrophil cytoplasmic antibody*

Antineutrophil cytoplasmic antibodies (ANCA) are found in the sera of patients with several diseases, including Wegener's granulomatosis, glomerulonephritis and ulcerative colitis. In ulcerative colitis, the ANCA is perinuclear (p-ANCA), nongranular and it does not react with myeloperoxidase as does the p-ANCA found in glomerulonephritis (Saxon et al 1990). The ANCA is useful in distinguishing ulcerative colitis from Crohn's colitis as it is present in about 70% of patients with ulcerative colitis, in about 6% of patients with other types of colitis (including Crohn's colitis and infectious colitis) and in about 3% of healthy controls (Duerr et al 1991a). The ANCA is found in about 16% of healthy relatives of patients with ulcerative colitis as compared to 3% in unrelated healthy controls (Shanahan et al 1992). The presence of the ANCA is not influenced by the duration, activity or location of the disease in ulcerative colitis. The ANCA is found with an even higher frequency in patients with ulcerative colitis who have primary sclerosing cholangitis (Duerr et al 1991b) and in patients who have undergone colectomy for ulcerative colitis and who have pouchitis following ileal pouch placement (Sandborn et al 1993). The ANCA does not appear to be pathogenic in ulcerative colitis and probably is a result of the underlying immune-mediated disorder.

### *Cytokines*

Cytokines are activated immune cell-derived peptides that mediate activity, particularly in the immune system (Fiocchi 1994). They are key components in the pathogenesis of inflammatory bowel disease, but the factors that trigger their release and activation are still unknown (Sartor 1994). These inflammatory mediators include interleukins 1–10, tumor necrosis factor α, and a number of others (Table 23.2). Among this bewildering array of cell products (Cominelli & Kam 1993), interleukin 1 and tumor necrosis factor α exert key influences on the tissue inflammatory response in inflammatory bowel disease.

### *Adhesion molecules*

Adhesion molecules control the localization of circulating lymphoid cells and thus control the local inflammatory response. Adhesion molecule levels are markedly increased in patients with inflammatory bowel disease, including levels of endothelial leukocyte adhesion molecule (ELAM), intercellular adhesion molecules (ICAMS) and vascular adhesion molecules (VCAMS).

**Table 23.2** Inflammatory mediators in the intestine in patients with inflammatory bowel disease

| Mediator | Ulcerative colitis | Crohn's disease |
|---|---|---|
| Interleukin 1 | Increased | Increased |
| Interleukin 1 receptor antagonist | Increased | Stable/decreased |
| Interleukin 2 | Decreased | Increased (mRNA only) |
| Interleukin 2 receptor | Increased | Increased |
| Interleukin 6 | Increased | Increased |
| Interleukin 8 | Increased | Comparable |
| Prostaglandin E | Increased | Increased |
| Leukotriene B4 | Increased | Increased |
| Tumor necrosis factor α | Comparable | Comparable |
| Interferon γ | Decreased | Decreased |
| Transforming growth factor β | Comparable | Comparable |
| Substance P | Increased | Increased |
| Somatostatin | Decreased | Decreased |

Modified from Cominelli & Kam 1993

## **Inflammatory bowel disease and arachidonic acid metabolism** (Donowitz 1985)

There are two potential pathways for the metabolism of arachidonic acid in the colon: in the cyclo-oxygenase pathway there is an increased production of prostaglandins, thromboxanes and prostacyclin and all of these metabolites are increased in active colitis. The second pathway is via lipoxygenase metabolism to hydroperoxyeicosatetraenoic acids (HPETEs), hydroxyeicosatetraenoic acids (HETEs) and leukotrienes; these products are also increased in inflammatory bowel disease (Nielsen et al 1987). At present, the cells responsible for these increases are unknown. However, the lipoxygenase pathway is predominant in mucosal leukocytes which are markedly increased in colitis. Some metabolites, e.g. prostaglandin $E_2$, from both pathways act to stimulate diarrhea by increasing active chloride secretion and decreasing active sodium and chloride absorption. While the nature of the stimulants to arachidonic metabolism in inflammatory bowel disease is not yet understood, an appreciation of the pathways is relevant to drug therapy. Glucocorticoids prevent the formation of free arachidonic acid from membrane-bound arachidonic acid and thus they block both the cyclo-oxygenase and lipoxygenase pathways. Sulfasalazine and 5-aminosalicylic acid inhibit both pathways. Sulfapyridine, which is not effective in colitis, inhibits the synthesis and release of $PGE_2$ to the same degree as sulfasalazine. It can be concluded, therefore, that the lipoxygenase pathway is of more importance in colitis, particularly since cyclo-oxygenase inhibitors such as indomethacin are not effective in treatment. Within the lipoxygenase pathway, both sulfasalazine and 5-ASA inhibit synthesis of both 5-HETE and leukotriene B4, whereas 5-aminosalicylic acid does not significantly inhibit the synthesis of 5-HETE but inhibits the formation of leukotriene B4.

## **Animal and experimental models**

There are no animal models that are identical to inflammatory bowel disease in humans. There are a number of animal models currently in use in research, each with some features of inflammatory bowel disease.

### *Spontaneous disease in animals*

In the cotton-topped tamarin, a monkey from the jungles of Colombia, colitis develops in 50% of animals in captivity (Madara et al 1985). As in humans, the colitis is chronic and can progress to adenocarcinoma. These animals do not have serum antineutrophil cytoplasmic antibodies (ANCA) as found in humans, although neutrophils from the animals are recognized by antigen-positive sera of humans with ulcerative colitis (Stenson 1994).

*Toxin-induced colitis*

The two animal models that have been used most commonly in experimental trials have been in rats. In one, 5% acetic acid is injected into the lumen of the colon and in the other, trinitrobenzenesulfonic acid (TNBS) is administered with 30% ethanol as an enema. These models cause an acute colitis that is primarily toxin induced, although the TNBS model may also be in part immune mediated. Both preparations are easily delivered and reproducible and are suitable for studying the inflammatory response in colitis.

*Carrageenan-induced colitis*

Carrageenan is a sulfated polysaccharide of high molecular weight which induces colonic ulceration or granuloma formation when fed orally to animals such as guinea pigs and rabbits. The ulceration is confined largely to the mucosa and there is pseudopolyp formation and the occasional crypt abscess. However, in contrast to man, the disease occurs predominantly in the cecum and there is also a pronounced macrophage response.

*Immune complex colitis*

Lesions similar to colitis have been produced in animals by the Arthus, Schwartzman, and Auer reactions and by direct antigen–antibody reactions (MacPherson & Pfeiffer 1976). It is also possible to produce colonic inflammation by delayed hypersensitivity reactions; rabbits or guinea pigs are sensitized to dinitrochlorobenzene (DNCB) by skin painting, and this is followed by rectal instillation of DNCB 10 days later; alternatively successive rectal instillations of DNCB can be employed (Streilein 1978). Persistence of colitis has been induced in the rabbit following the injection of soluble immune complexes after immunization with common enterobacterial antigen plus irritation of the rectum with dilute formalin (Mee et al 1979). Although immune-mediated experimental colitis may appear to be more akin to inflammatory bowel disease than toxin-induced colitis, there is no evidence that immune complexes cause idiopathic inflammatory bowel disease and no convincing data that the immune complex model is superior.

## Psychological factors

It is now generally accepted that psychological disorders in individuals with inflammatory bowel disease are a result, not a cause of the underlying illness. Earlier studies that proposed a classic psychosomatic etiology for inflammatory bowel disease were flawed by selection bias and the lack of appropriate control groups. Depression and anxiety occur commonly in patients with inflammatory bowel disease. Helzer et al (1984) studied 50 subjects with Crohn's disease and 50 control subjects with other chronic medical illness. A significantly greater number of patients with Crohn's disease had depression and other psychiatric disorders. In contrast, patients with ulcerative colitis were no more likely than control patients with other chronic medical illnesses to have depression (Helzer et al 1982). Currently, the main focus for psychosocial investigation in inflammatory bowel disease is the effect on the overall quality of life. Mendeloff et al (1970) assessed various life stresses in patients with ulcerative colitis, with irritable bowel syndrome and in a group of normal subjects. Those with irritable bowel syndrome gave a history of more stressful situations than the other two groups, both of which showed a similar history. Patients with inflammatory bowel disease readily discuss symptoms that concern bowel function, pain and energy level, but only a minority volunteer information about emotional problems or social stresses unless prompted to do so (Mitchell et al 1988). The most frequently mentioned fears and concerns listed by inflammatory bowel disease patients on a self-reporting form were concerns about sexual intimacy, loss of bowel control, pain and suffering, feeling alone and being unable to achieve full potential (Drossman et al 1989). Most patients with inflammatory bowel disease who undergo surgery adapt well postoperatively. As an example, in a follow-up of 51 patients with Crohn's disease, 92% noted improvement in their quality of life and would choose surgery again, despite the recurrence of disease or the need for a permanent ileostomy in some (Meyers et al 1980). Social support, both from family and peer groups in lay organizations such as the Crohn's and Colitis Foundation of America and similar support groups in other countries, is now recognized as an important factor in maintaining or improving the quality of life of such patients.

## Cigarette smoking

Many environmental factors have been assessed as possible etiologies in inflammatory bowel disease. The most striking and widely observed association has been with cigarette smoking. Former smokers are 1.7 times as likely as never-smokers to develop ulcerative colitis. The risk of developing ulcerative colitis among current smokers is only 40% that of nonsmokers (Calkins 1989). In contrast to ulcerative colitis, smokers are more than twice as likely to develop Crohn's disease as nonsmokers and smoking may also increase the risk of recurrent disease. Studies in children from North Carolina (Sandler et al 1992) indicate that passive smoking among children in households with smokers has the same effects on the future development of inflammatory bowel disease as active smoking in adults.

## GENETIC FACTORS

There are abundant data that the development of inflammatory bowel disease is at least partly determined by genetic influences. The precise role of inheritance has not been determined.

### Family studies

There is approximately a 30-fold increase in disease prevalence among siblings compared to the prevalence in the community (Fielding 1986). Ulcerative colitis is more likely to occur among family members of a proband with the disease and Crohn's disease occurs more commonly among family members of a proband with Crohn's disease. However, the disorders also may occur in the family member of a proband who has a different disease, either ulcerative colitis or Crohn's disease. A positive family history is more common in patients with Crohn's disease than with ulcerative colitis (Table 23.3) (Yang et al 1993). Individuals in whom inflammatory bowel disease developed at less than 20 years of age have an increased risk of having affected family members as compared to a group of such patients of more varied ages (Farmer 1989).

### Twin studies

There is a higher concordance for monozygotic twins than for dizygotic twins for both Crohn's disease and ulcerative colitis (Sirlin et al 1986, Monsen et al 1987). When data from selected and unselected series are pooled, there is a 67% vs 5% concordance for monozygotic vs dizygotic twin Crohn's disease patients and a lower concordance for ulcerative colitis patients (20% vs 0) comparing monzygotic and dizygotic twins (Yang & Rotter 1994). These data add strong support for a genetic role in these disorders. The risk of inflammatory bowel disease in the children of parents who are both affected with the disease is as high as 36% (Bennett et al 1991).

### Association with other disorders

Inflammatory bowel disease is associated with at least three other genetic disorders: Turner's syndrome, the Hermansky–Pudlak syndrome (a form of oculocutaneous albinism) and glycogen storage disease type Ib (Price 1979, Schinella et al 1980, Roe et al 1986).

In approximately 3 000 patients with inflammatory bowel disease reviewed by Kirsner (1973), 3% had ankylosing spondylitis. McBride et al (1963) studied 870 patients with ankylosing spondylitis and found 16 with ulcerative colitis and four with Crohn's disease. Jayson et al (1970) investigated 47 patients with ankylosing spondylitis and found eight with evidence of colitis. Either the bowel disease or the spondylitis may occur first, which implies that one is not a complication of the other. Ankylosing spondylitis is a familial disease and is associated with the HLA-B27 histocompatibility antigen in over 90% of cases. Of those patients with inflammatory bowel disease who also have spondylitis, about 80% with ulcerative colitis and a smaller proportion of those with Crohn's disease have the HLA-B27 antigen. This indicates that inflammatory bowel disease is a potent initiating or potentiating factor in the development of ankylosing spondylitis.

Primary sclerosing cholangitis occurs in about 5% of patients with ulcerative colitis and in less than 1% of patients with Crohn's disease. Other disorders that are rarely found in association with inflammatory bowel disease include psoriasis, multiple sclerosis and celiac disease.

**Table 23.3** Positive family history of inflammatory bowel disease in ulcerative colitis (UC) and Crohn's disease (CD) probands

| Disease in probands | Number of probands | Disease in relatives UC (%) | CD (%) | Mixed (%) | Total (%) |
|---|---|---|---|---|---|
| UC | 269 | 37 (13.8) | 6 (2.2) | 4 (1.5) | 47 (17.5) |
| CD | 258 | 19 (7.4) | 32 (12.4) | 9 (3.5) | 60 (23.3) |
| Total | 527 | 56 (10.6) | 38 (7.2) | 13 (2.5) | 107 (20.3) |

From Yang et al (1993)

## PATHOLOGY

### Macroscopic appearances of ulcerative colitis

The disease always involves the rectum and it may spread proximally to involve a portion of or the entire colon. Although the inflammation is usually most severe in the rectum, in some patients there may appear to be rectal sparing on endoscopic or radiographic examination, but microscopically the disease is always in continuity with the rectum (Table 23.4).

The mucous membrane has a hemorrhagic, granular or velvety appearance and ulceration may be superficial or deep. Polyps, often termed pseudopolyps or inflammatory

**Table 23.4** Macroscopic pathology of the large intestine in ulcerative colitis and Crohn's disease (adapted from Morson & Dawson 1979)

| Ulcerative colitis | Crohn's disease |
|---|---|
| Disease in continuity | Disease discontinuous |
| Rectum always involved | Rectum involved in 50% |
| Terminal ileum involved in 10% | Terminal ileum involved in 30% |
| Mucosa granular and ulcerated but not fissured | Mucosa discretely ulcerated, with cobblestones and fissures |
| Vascular | Not vascular |
| Serosa normal | Serosa inflamed |
| Colon shortened because of muscle changes, fibrous strictures rare | Colon shortened because of fibrosis, fibrous strictures common |
| Inflammatory polyposis common | Inflammatory polyposis uncommon |
| Anal lesions in 25%: fissures, excoriations and occasonal fistulae | Anal lesions in 75%: fistulae in 10%; fistulas, fissure and ulceration severe |

polyps (Fig. 23.1), are present in 20% of patients with colonic involvement (De Dombal et al 1966b) and they represent the residual mucosa after ulceration and healing of the entire depth of the mucosa (Fig. 23.2). The mucosa of the distal 5–25 cm of ileum is inflamed in about 10% of colectomy specimens (Morson & Dawson 1979), commonly termed "backwash ileitis", and in these cases the ileocecal valve is rigid and incompetent. In chronic cases the involved colon is usually grossly shortened as a result of muscle thickening and contracture and the diameter is also reduced. Except in fulminant disease, the serosa is intact but often shows vascular congestion. Strictures may occur and these are usually mild and rarely cause obstruction of the lumen. In general, anal lesions are acute and superficial.

## Microscopic appearances of ulcerative colitis

Except in the case of fulminating colitis, histological changes are confined mainly to the mucosa, although the submucosa may be involved to a lesser degree. The mucosal inflammatory changes are diffuse. In active colitis, there is congestion of the vessels, intramucosal hemorrhage and edema. Goblet cells are reduced or absent (Fig. 23.3).

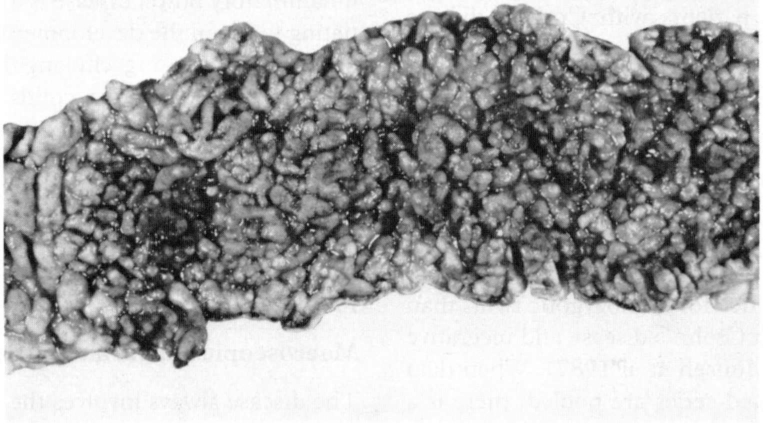

**Fig. 23.1** Ulcerative colitis. Marked inflammatory polyposis with intervening ulceration.

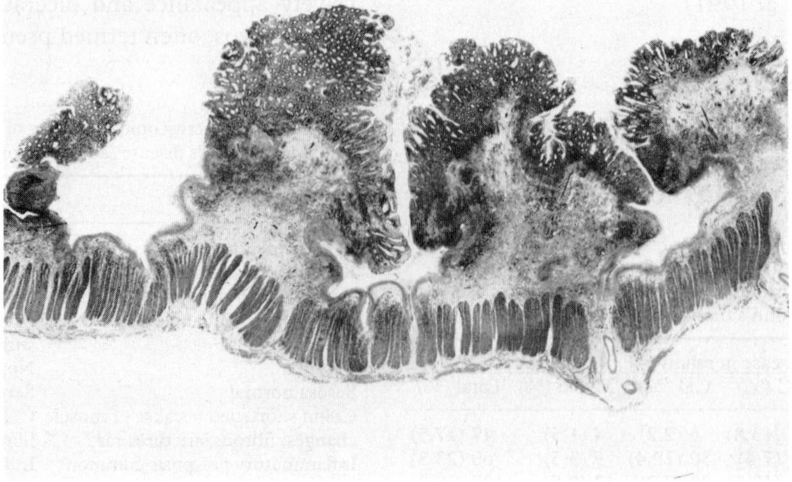

**Fig. 23.2** Ulcerative colitis, inflammatory polyps (pseudopolyps) and intervening ulcers (hematoxylin and eosin, ×5).

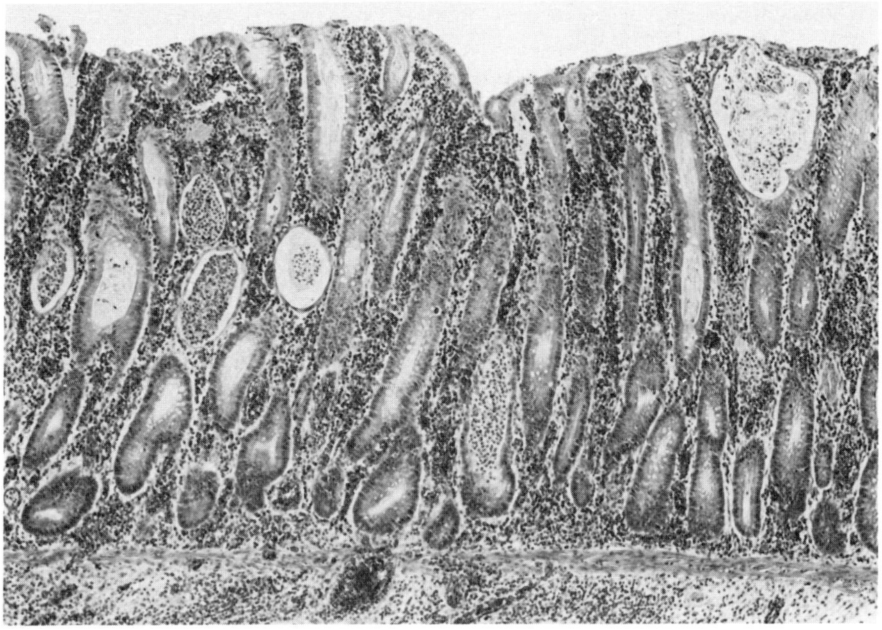

**Fig. 23.3** Active ulcerative colitis (with predominantly acute inflammatory changes). There are no erosions or ulcers, the crypts show goblet cell depletion and crypt abscess formation. The lamina propria is congested and shows an inflammatory cell infiltrate (hematoxylin and eosin, ×60).

The lamina propria is infiltrated by lymphocytes, plasma cells, eosinophils and foci of polymorphs and some lymphoid follicles may be enlarged. In some patients, eosinophil infiltration in the mucosa is pronounced (Wright & Truelove 1966a). Crypt abscesses occur and consist of a collection of polymorphonuclear leukocytes and organisms in the crypts of Lieberkuhn. The spread of crypt abscesses may play a role in the production of ulceration. These inflammatory changes are associated with disturbance of the mucosal architecture. Although crypt abscesses are often present in active ulcerative colitis, it must be stressed that they occur in other inflammatory disorders of the colon, e.g. Crohn's disease (Table 23.5), amebiasis (Madanagopalan et al 1968), shigellosis (Gonzalez-Licea & Yardley 1966) and radiation enteritis (Gelfand et al 1968). The process of resolution is accompanied by a reduction in crypt abscesses and inflammatory cells and a gradual restoration of goblet cells. However, even when all evidence of active inflammation has disappeared, histological evidence of the attack remains. The crypts are reduced in number, irregular and branched, and often fail to extend to the muscularis (Fig. 23.4); there is Paneth cell metaplasia at the base of the crypts; there may be some permanent loss of goblet cells; and there may be a chronic inflammatory infiltrate (Fig. 23.5).

## Macroscopic appearances of Crohn's disease

Crohn's disease can affect any region of the gastrointestinal canal, including the mouth, esophagus and gastroduodenum, but in all areas similar macroscopic and histological features are seen. These have been reviewed by Morson (1972). The term "metastatic" Crohn's disease has been used to denote Crohn's disease of the perineum, abdominal wall, penis or elsewhere (Slaney et al 1986) which is separated from the gut by normal skin.

From several series, disease limited to the small intestine occurs in 40–80% (Kyle 1971, Fielding 1972, De Dombal et al 1974, Farmer et al 1975) and in the remainder of patients the disease involves either the colon alone or the colon and small bowel together. When the small

**Table 23.5** Site and macroscopic appearance of Crohn's disease

| Site | Macroscopic appearance |
|---|---|
| Mouth | Aphthous-like ulceration (a) |
| Esophagus | Thickened folds in the lower esophagus simulating stricture (b) (see also p. 212) |
| Stomach | Thickening and rigidity of the antrum simulating carcinoma (c); thickened folds with ulceration |
| Duodenum | Thickening of the mucosal folds with ulceration, narrowing or stricture (d) |
| Small intestine | Narrowing and ulceration of the terminal ileum; cobblestone appearance of the terminal ileum; strictures in the jejunum and ileum |
| Appendix | Inflamed appendix |
| Large intestine | Total diffuse involvement, strictures or proctitis (e) |
| Anus | Chronic fissure, anal fistula or ulceration (f) |
| Skin | Ulceration in the perineum, genitalia or abdominal wall (g) |

(a) Croft & Wilkinson (1972), (b) Dyer et al (1969), (c) Johnson et al (1966), (d) Farmer et al (1972), (d) Goldberg et al (1979), (e) Ewen et al (1971), (f) p. 672 (g) this page

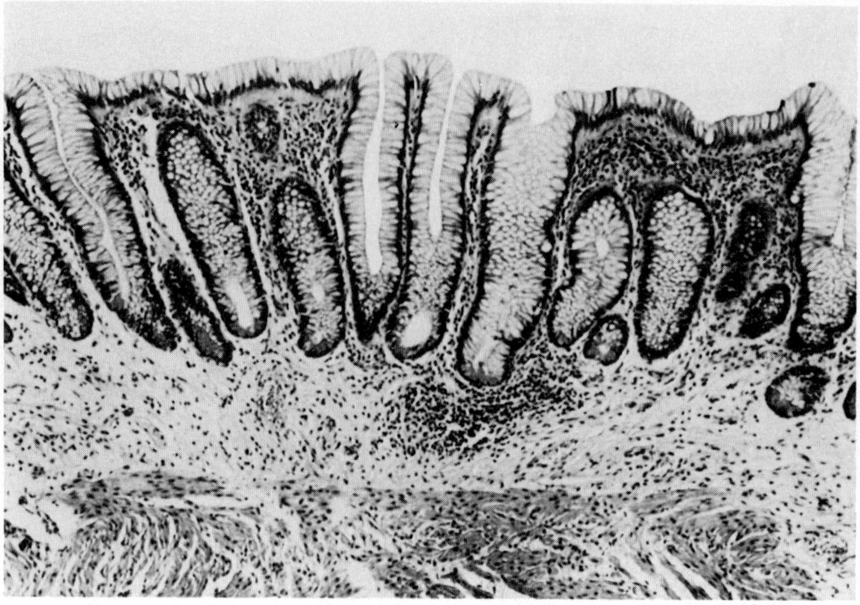

**Fig. 23.4** Quiescent ulcerative colitis. There is a very mild chronic inflammatory infiltrate in the lamina propria. The crypts are slightly irregular and markedly shortened (hematoxylin and eosin, ×85).

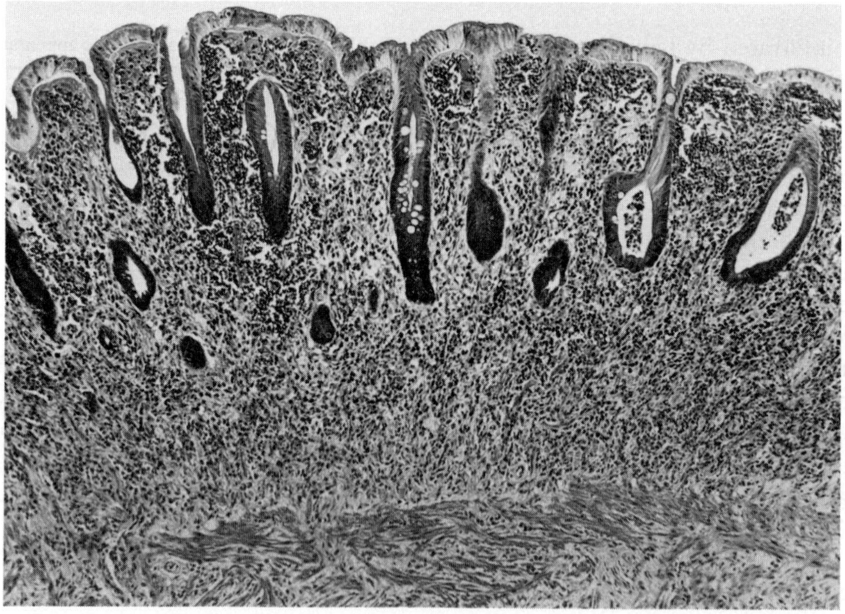

**Fig. 23.5** Active ulcerative colitis (with predominantly chronic inflammatory features). The crypts are shortened and separated by an infiltrate of chronic inflammatory cells which forms a band-like zone between the crypt bases and the muscularis mucosa. There is still goblet cell depletion and occasional crypt abscesses indicating continuing activity (hematoxylin and eosin, ×90).

bowel is involved, the terminal ileum is the site in over 90% of patients. Four to five percent of patients have gastroduodenal disease and this is usually associated with more distal disease (Fielding et al 1970, Weterman 1983). In the National Co-operative Crohn's Disease Study (NCCDS), disease was confined to the small intestine in 31% of patients and to the colon in 11%; ileocolitis occurred in 58% of patients (Mekhjian et al 1979). In general, series from the UK show a higher incidence of involvement of the colon alone than series from the USA. In UK studies, anal disease occurs in approximately 75% of colonic Crohn's disease and in up to 25% of small intestinal disease. In the NCCDS, anal disease occurred in 36% of all patients and in 47% of those with disease of the colon alone.

In Crohn's disease the inflammation is typically segmental and transmural. Mucosal involvement is characterized by inflammation and ulceration. The ulcers are of two main types: superficial and fissuring.

Small ulcers in Crohn's disease, called aphthous ulcers (McGovern & Goulston 1968), develop in the mucosa overlying lymphoid aggregates and have a white base with a surrounding congested margin. Microerosions – less than 1 mm diameter ulcers – are also described (Poulsen et al 1984). Larger superficial ulcers are serpiginous and are separated by normal-looking mucosa (Fig. 23.6).

When an area is extensively involved by linear ulceration the nodular edematous mucosa between ulcers produces the so-called cobblestone pattern (Fig. 23.7). The wall of the affected segment is thickened from edema and later fibrosis. The serosa is red, the mesenteric fat extends around the bowel and the lymph nodes are enlarged. The fissures lead to abscesses and fistulae, the mural inflammation to strictures and the serosal inflammation to adhesions. A typical affected segment of small intestine is shown in Figure 23.8.

The usual macroscopic appearance of Crohn's disease at different sites in the gastrointestinal tract is shown in Table 23.5.

Crohn's disease of the colon is often discontinuous, the

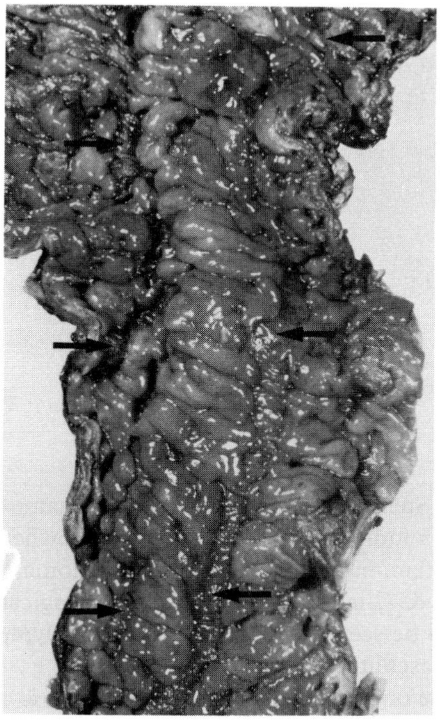

**Fig. 23.6** Crohn's disease of the colon showing numerous irregular serpiginous ulcers (arrows). The intervening mucosa is edematous but not inflamed and granular as in ulcerative colitis.

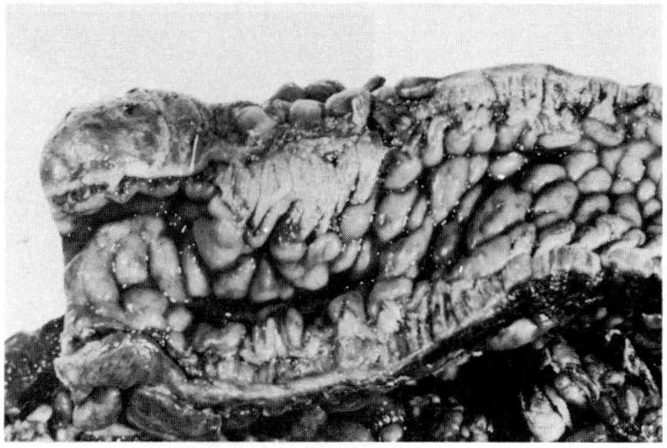

**Fig. 23.7** Crohn's colitis with cobblestoning and mural thickening.

involved areas being separated by normal tissue, but it can also present as a diffuse, continuous, colonic inflammation. The wall of the colon is thickened, the serosa is inflamed, fibrous strictures are often present and the mucosa is edematous but not unduly vascular. Fistulae, abscess formation and severe perianal lesions are common. In the chronic phase the bowel is thickened and in contrast to ulcerative colitis, it is fibrous and the serosa can be covered by granulations.

### Macroscopic differentiation of Crohn's and ulcerative colitis

The major macroscopic differences between ulcerative colitis and Crohn's disease of the colon are summarized in Table 23.4. However, it is not always possible to differentiate one form from the other.

Cook & Dixon (1973) reviewed the various criteria which have been used to separate the two disorders and studied 50 cases of their own. In Crohn's disease, confluent linear ulcers along the axis of the bowel and deep fissures were the most characteristic features, whereas in ulcerative colitis fissures were absent and there was a loss of mucosal folds indicative of areas of healed mucosa.

### Microscopic features of Crohn's disease

The inflammation in Crohn's disease is aggregated, lymphocytic and transmural (Fig. 23.9), but the single most valuable aid to diagnosis is the presence of noncaseating granulomas (Fig. 23.10) (sarcoid or tuberculoid granulomas). Granulomas are focal aggregates of epithelioid histiocytes. They may have a surrounding rim of lymphocytes and contain giant cells. Granulomas are seen in 50–70% of cases and in 40–50% of rectal biopsies (Schmitz-Moormann et al 1984) and in about a quarter of these they are also found in the regional lymph nodes. Attention has been drawn to the importance of microgranulomas (Rotterdam et al 1977). These are very small collections of histiocytes not quite amounting to granulomas.

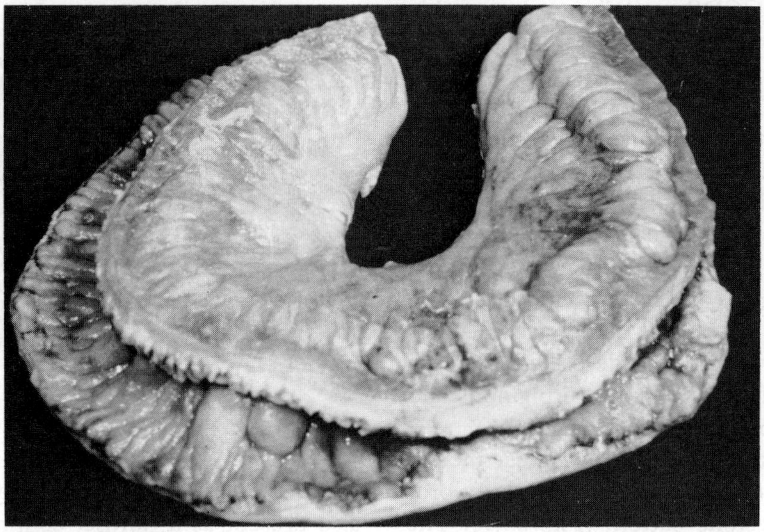

**Fig. 23.8** Crohn's of the small intestine. There is a central stricture with associated linear ulceration, an irregular poorly developed cobblestone area to the left of the stricture and an overlying serositis.

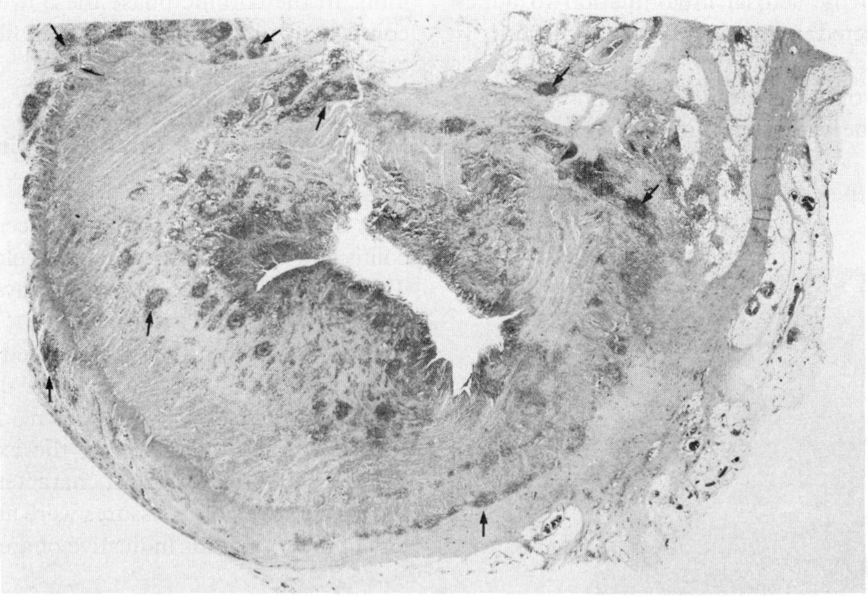

**Fig. 23.9** Crohn's ileitis. The lumen is narrowed due to the transmural involvement. Numerous lymphoid aggregates (arrows), many associated with granulomas, are seen throughout the wall of the ileum (hematoxylin and eosin, ×4.5).

Microerosions and aphthous ulcers (Fig. 23.11) develop as shallow ulcers over the lymphoid aggregates of the mucosa. Biopsy of these lesions shows marked inflammatory changes and granulomas (Makiyama et al 1984). Fissures (Fig. 23.12) are lined by granulation tissue and histiocytes. The mucosal inflammation is typically patchy and mononuclear in type and in large bowel is associated with less architectural disturbance and fewer crypt abscesses than ulcerative colitis. Duodenal involvement is probably more common than was previously recognized (Nyhlin & Stenling 1984) and includes the same histological features indicative of the diagnosis elsewhere, that is marked inflammation usually with granuloma formation (Schuffler & Chaffee 1979). Other histological features which may be seen are neural hypertrophy, lymphangiectasia and vasculitis.

No single one of these histological changes is characteristic of Crohn's disease; it is the spectrum of findings which confirms the diagnosis. The pathological differentiation from tuberculosis of the small intestine is usually

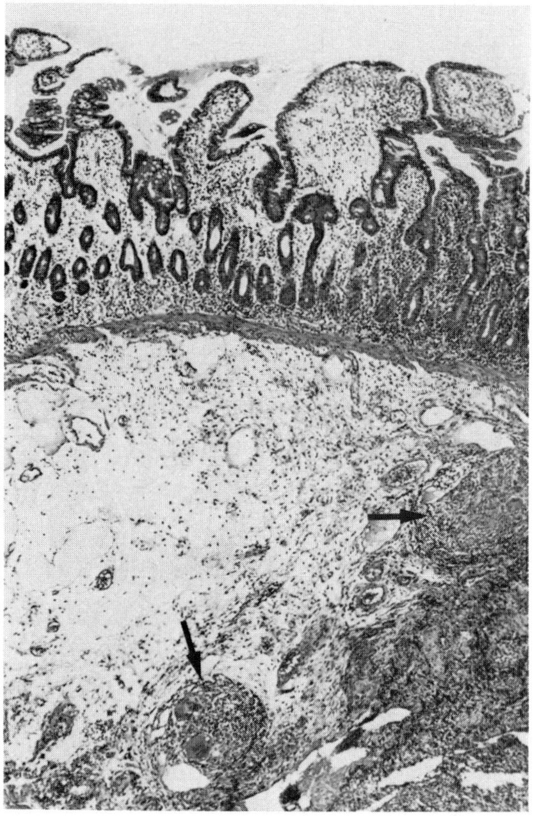

**Fig. 23.10** Crohn's disease. Patchy chronic inflammatory cell infiltrate in the small intestinal mucosa with submucosal edema and focal submucosal granulomas (arrow) (hematoxylin and eosin, ×45).

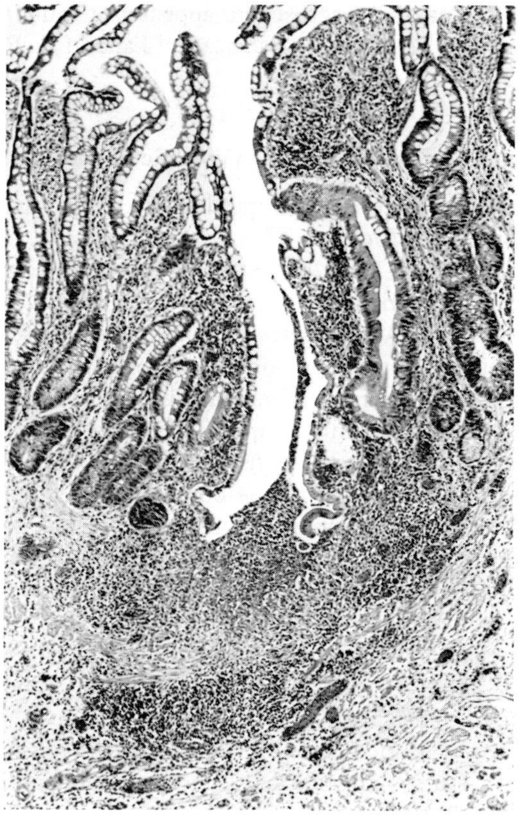

**Fig. 23.11** Crohn's disease. Early lesion showing ulceration at the base of a crypt overlying a lymphoid aggregate with early inflammatory cell response (hematoxylin and eosin, ×60).

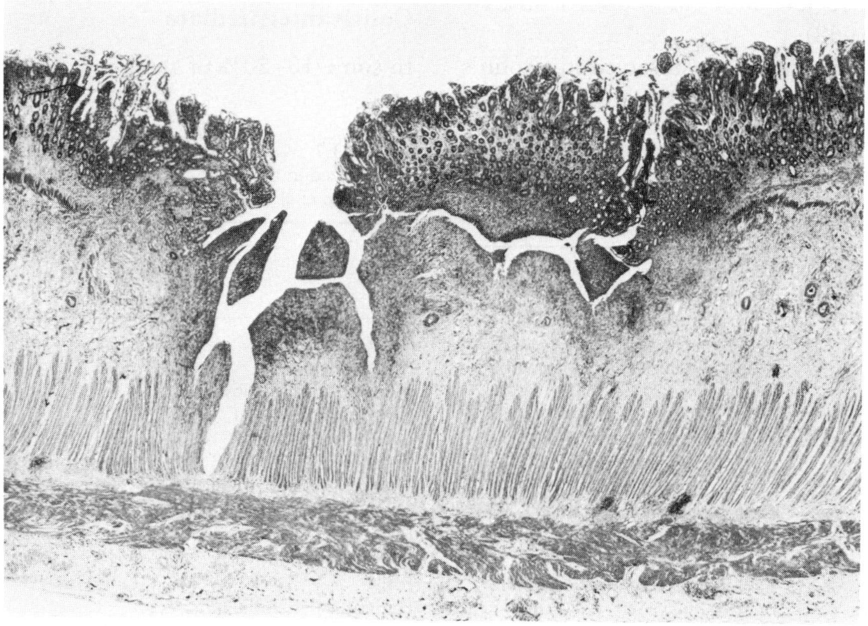

**Fig. 23.12** Crohn's disease. Extensive fissuring and ulceration penetrating the circular muscle coat (hematoxylin and eosin, ×8).

impossible on the macroscopic appearance, but the distinction can be made histologically (Tandon & Prakash 1972).

### Microscopic appearances of colonic Crohn's disease

The essential differences from ulcerative colitis are listed in Table 23.6. However, it is not always possible to make this distinction. The acute stage is characterized by edema, lymphatic dilatation and a generalized scant infiltration with lymphocytes and plasma cells. Essentially, the crypts and their population of goblet cells remain normal in areas away from ulceration. The aphthous-like ulcer is due to ulceration in a lymphoid aggregate (Fig. 23.11). Ulceration in the form of fissures (Fig. 23.12) at right angles to the long axis of the bowel is also present; the ulcers are lined by granulation tissue, histiocytes and sometimes foreign body giant cells. Fibrosis occurs secondary to inflammation and also as a generalized process in the submucosa.

Aggregates of inflammatory cells and sarcoid-like granulomas (Fig. 23.13) are characteristic features in the histological diagnosis of Crohn's disease (Cook & Dixon 1973). Fully formed granulomata may occur, consisting of focal aggregates of histiocytes, sometimes containing giant cells and showing a surrounding rim of lymphocytes. Necrosis is not a feature of the granulomas, which may occur in any layer of the bowel wall or be located in the draining lymph nodes. Microgranulomas are also useful diagnostic features (Rotterdam et al 1977). The more sections cut, the more granulomas will be found.

Histological evidence of fissuring (Table 23.7) in the form of linear ulcers lined by necrotic inflammatory cells provides firm evidence in favor of Crohn's disease (Lennard-Jones et al 1968).

Various vascular lesions have been observed in Crohn's disease, including thromboembolic disease, polyarteritis, giant cell arteritis (Teja et al 1980) and Takayasu's arteritis (Owyang et al 1979).

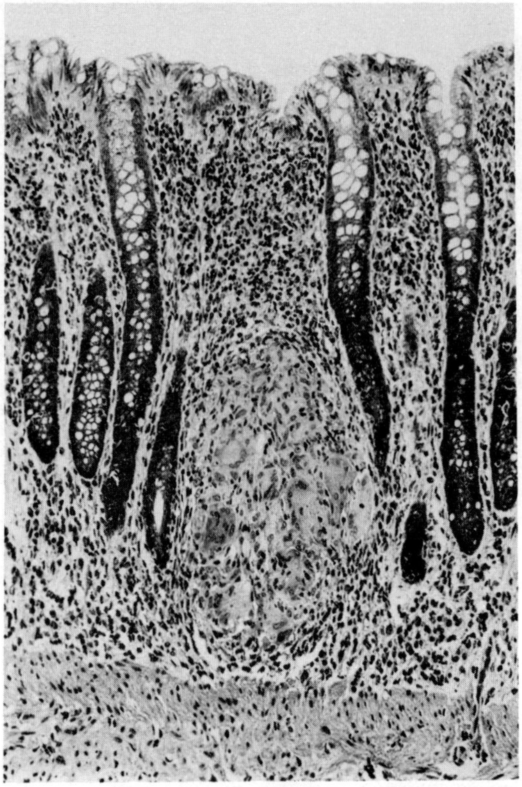

**Fig. 23.13** Crohn's disease. Rectal biopsy. A well-formed granuloma in the lamina propria. The crypt epithelium is hyperplastic and there is an excess of inflammatory cells in the lamina propria (hematoxylin and eosin, ×165).

### Colitis intermediate

In some 10–20% of cases it is not possible to make a dis-

**Table 23.6** Microscopic pathology of the large intestine in ulcerative colitis and Crohn's disease (Morson & Dawson 1979)

| Ulcerative colitis | Crohn's disease |
|---|---|
| Mucosal and submucosal inflammation only | Transmural inflammation |
| Width of submucosa normal or reduced | Width of submucosa normal or increased |
| Increased vascularity | Marked edema |
| Focal lymphoid hyperplasia limited to mucosa and superficial submucosa | Focal lymphoid hyperplasia in all layers of the bowel wall |
| Crypt abscesses common | Crypt abscess infrequent |
| Loss of goblet cells | Normal population of goblet cells |
| Paneth cell metaplasia common | Paneth cell metaplasia rare |
| Granulomas absent | Granulomas in bowel and nodes in 70% |
| Anal lesions show nonspecific inflammation | Anal lesions often show granulomas |

**Table 23.7** Clinical manifestations in Crohn's disease in patients randomized in the National Cooperative Crohn's Disease Study (Mekhjian et al 1979)

| | All patients with Crohn's disease (569) | Patients with disease of the colon alone (60) |
|---|---|---|
| Diarrhea | 92 | 92 |
| Abdominal pain | 95 | 93 |
| Bleeding from the lower gastrointestinal tract | 41 | 62 |
| Weight loss (>5 lbs) | 85 | 88 |
| Fever | 56 | 72 |
| Anal fissure, abscess or fistula | 36 | 47 |
| Other internal fistula | 16 | 9 |
| Enterocutaneous fistula | 5 | 3 |
| Arthritis or spondylitis | 19 | 22 |
| Iritis | 4 | 7 |
| Hepatitis, pericholangitis | 4 | 5 |
| Erythema nodosum/ pyoderma gangrenosum | 5 | 8 |

tinction between ulcerative colitis and Crohn's disease (Price 1978). In children, Chong et al (1985) also found that 15% could not be categorized after clinical, radiological and endoscopic assessment, including colonic biopsy. Diagnostic difficulties are sometimes resolved when biopsy material becomes available during the follow-up or when patients develop clear evidence of Crohn's disease such as small intestinal or perianal disease.

### Rectal biopsy

The rectal biopsy is important for the detection of microscopic mucosal abnormalities when sigmoidoscopy and barium studies are normal or of doubtful significance (Goodman et al 1977). A common problem is hyperemia of the rectal mucosa, which may be due either to mild chronic idiopathic proctitis or acute infectious or nonspecific causes; biopsies may help resolve the problem. Features indicative of inflammatory bowel disease are distorted crypt architecture, increased numbers of both round cells and neutrophils in the lamina propria, a villous surface, epithelioid granuloma, crypt atrophy, basal lymphoid aggregates and basally located isolated giant cells. The diagnosis of acute self-limited colitis is based on the absence of these features (Surawicz & Belic 1984). Evidence of previous attacks of inflammation can be inferred if there is crypt atrophy, which suggests colitis, or if there are foci of lymphocytes or increased cellularity, which suggest Crohn's disease. When the diagnosis of Crohn's disease seems possible because of radiological abnormalities in the terminal ileum or elsewhere in the bowel, a rectal biopsy that shows granulomas supports the diagnosis. For Crohn's disease, granulomas may be found in up to 14% of cases even when the appearance of the rectum is normal (Rotterdam 1982). Nostrant et al (1987) found that plasmacytosis extending through to the base of the mucosa and mucosal distortion were always present in ulcerative colitis but absent in acute self-limited colitis, provided the biopsy was taken within 4 days of the onset of symptoms.

Biopsy is often helpful in distinguishing Crohn's disease from ulcerative colitis, particularly if many colonoscopic biopsies can be taken (Chong et al 1985). Although not always found, epithelioid granulomata are highly specific for Crohn's disease (Surawicz et al 1981). It is also important in the exclusion of other forms of colitis, particularly amebic colitis, pseudomembranous colitis and ischemic colitis.

The rectal biopsy in homosexual men requires special consideration. Surawicz et al (1986) found that acute inflammation was common in both symptomatic and asymptomatic homosexuals and was associated with a variety of pathogens including *C. jejuni* or *C. intestinalis*, *Herpes simplex*, *N. gonorrhoeae*, *C. trachomatis* and *T. pallidum*. However, when chronic inflammation was present it was significantly associated with syphilis, *Herpes simplex* virus type II and *C. trachomatis* infection. The conclusions from this study were that rectal biopsy is not generally helpful in homosexuals because the histological abnormalities are usually nonspecific. Biopsy is recommended for specific lesions and as an aid to diagnose syphilis, *Chlamydia* and tuberculosis.

## CLINICAL FEATURES

### Symptoms

*Ulcerative colitis*

The onset may be insidious with a gradual increase in rectal bleeding or sudden with an increase in the number of bowel movements that may be bloody, as well as fecal urgency, cramping abdominal pains and fever. The course of the disease varies; some patients have only a single attack, while in others the first attack may be so severe that colectomy is necessary. Most patients experience exacerbations and remissions of the disease, which has been called "chronic intermittent colitis", while in a small proportion the disease becomes chronic and continuous.

The symptoms depend partly on the severity and extent of the disease. In most series, distal colitis, left-sided colitis and pancolitis each account for one-third of cases. However, data from population-based studies rather than referral centers indicate that 50% of patients have proctitis alone. Severe attacks occur in 20–50% of cases in referral center series and in 10% of patients overall. Patients with colitis confined to the rectum and lower sigmoid colon were studied by Farmer & Brown (1967). Of 124 patients, all but one had rectal bleeding, but in some cases this was mild and led to a diagnosis of hemorrhoids. Diarrhea occurred in 107 patients, abdominal pain was present in one half and weight loss was uncommon. In a large series of men with ulcerative colitis, 79% had diarrhea, 71% abdominal pain and 55% rectal bleeding. Other symptoms found at the onset of the illness were tenesmus (16%), fever (11%), weight loss (18%) and vomiting (14%) (Nefzger & Acheson 1963). These systemic symptoms usually occur when there is severe proctocolitis rather than proctitis alone.

Diarrhea may vary from one to two up to 20 or more loose or liquid stools a day, often with urgency and sometimes fecal incontinence; diarrhea is worse in the morning, owing to the accumulation of blood, mucus and secretions overnight, and immediately after meals. Patients with moderately or severely active disease may have nocturnal stools.

Constipation is a presenting symptom in 5% (Nefzger & Acheson 1963) to 15% (Sim & Brooke 1958) of all patients with ulcerative colitis and in 25% of patients when the disease is confined to the rectum (Jalan et al 1970a). The constipation usually resolves when the inflammation subsides.

Rectal bleeding is usually characterized by blood mixed with a liquid stool; on rare occasions bleeding may be severe (pp. 671 & 685) and lead to hypotension. In proctitis, the blood may streak a formed stool and resemble hemorrhoidal bleeding.

Pain may take the form of tenesmus due to rectal involvement or cramping lower abdominal pain that is worse after meals or bowel movements. Sometimes the abdominal pain is constant during an exacerbation. Anorexia, nausea and vomiting in the absence of bowel obstruction are common when the disease is severely active and extensive. Patients with extensive and severely active colitis may lose weight because of anorexia, fear of eating and loss of protein in the stool.

Less overt presentations may occur at the extremes of life. In the elderly, colitis can present as an intermittent obstruction of the large bowel (Diethelm et al 1968). In children, urgency, incontinence and upper gastrointestinal symptoms are more frequent and growth failure is common (Davidson 1975).

Rarely, patients may present with extraintestinal manifestations, such as ankylosing spondylitis, arthritis or liver disease, before the bowel disease becomes apparent.

*Severity of colitis*

The severe attack of ulcerative colitis was defined by the following criteria (Truelove & Witts 1955): severe diarrhea with six or more motions per day; macroscopic blood in the stools; fever with an evening temperature of 37.2°C (99°F) or more; tachycardia of 90 beats/min or over; anemia with a hemoglobin of 75% or less; ESR of 30 mm/h or more. In the first instance, it is safer to regard any attack with six or more stools per day as severe, particularly if there is evidence of systemic disturbance, such as fever.

A mild attack of ulcerative colitis is characterized by four or less motions per day and only a small amount of blood in the stool. The criteria for a moderate attack lie between severe and mild.

*Crohn's disease of the colon*

The clinical manifestations in 60 patients admitted to the NCCD study are shown in Table 23.7. It is almost impossible to distinguish Crohn's colitis from ulcerative colitis on the basis of symptoms. It is often stated that bleeding is less common in Crohn's colitis, but it occurs in nearly 50% of cases (Farmer et al 1975). Rarely it may be severe (Mellor et al 1982). The only important distinguishing clinical feature is the presence of rectal fistulae, present in 20% of Crohn's colitis either at the time of diagnosis or later during the illness.

*Small intestinal Crohn's disease*

Most commonly, the patient has abdominal pain, diarrhea and fever. Because of the predilection for the terminal ileum, the pain is colicky and in the mid or lower abdomen; a more persistent pain may be felt in the right iliac fossa. However, the pain may resemble that of acute appendicitis or it can be due to intestinal obstruction.

The severity of diarrhea is variable and it may be accompanied by pain; the stool can be watery or soft and sometimes contains blood or mucus. In the case of terminal ileal disease, there are usually fewer than six stools per day, but with diffuse small intestinal disease the diarrhea is frequent and profuse. A persistent, low-grade fever is usual with active disease and, indeed, this was the sole presenting symptom in 11 of 542 cases reviewed by Crohn & Yarnis (1958). Nonspecific constitutional symptoms such as malaise, poor appetite and loss of weight are common. In patients with Crohn's disease in remission, recurrent symptoms may be due to intercurrent viral (Gorbach 1982) or bacterial infection rather than to reactivation of the Crohn's disease.

Other presentations include anal or perianal disease, small bowel obstruction in up to 30% of patients (Banks et al 1969).

*Gastroduodenal Crohn's disease*

Crohn's disease of the stomach or duodenum usually presents as upper abdominal pain and vomiting or symptoms of peptic ulcer disease (Farmer et al 1972, Haggitt & Meissner 1973). Rarely, Crohn's disease may present as an isolated disease of the stomach (Cary et al 1989). Symptomatic gastroduodenal involvement occurs in up to 4% of cases of Crohn's disease and the gastric involvement is almost always confined to the antrum (Fielding et al 1970). Radiographically, the lesions of gastric Crohn's disease are similar to those seen in patients with erosive gastritis. Endoscopic examination usually shows mucosal nodularity and strictures. Discrete ulcers without other mucosal disease are unusual in Crohn's gastroduodenal disease. Biopsies may show granulomas, but these are not invariably present. The diagnosis is made on the basis of the combination of endoscopic, radiographic and histologic features. In some cases, it is difficult to differentiate Crohn's gastroduodenal disease from peptic disease, particularly in patients who are taking ulcerogenic medications such as nonsteroidal anti-inflammatory drugs. In some cases, the response to a therapeutic trial of an $H_2$ blocker or omeprazole in combination with prednisolone is helpful in differentiating the Crohn's disease from peptic ulcer.

*Other presentations*

Complaints may also relate to the many possible complications of inflammatory bowel disease: anemia due to malabsorption or chronic gastrointestinal blood loss, malnutrition, iritis, arthritis and spondylitis; liver disease; skin abnormalities including erythema nodosum and pyoderma gangrenosum, and growth failure in children.

Some patients present suddenly with symptoms indistinguishable from those of acute appendicitis. At laparotomy, the diagnosis of acute ileitis is made when an inflamed, edematous terminal ileum is found. Some of these presentations are probably due to *Yersinia* or other infective agents, as only the minority eventually develop Crohn's disease. In one series, 15 out of 54 patients presenting as acute ileitis developed chronic Crohn's disease after a follow-up period of 25 years (De Dombal et al 1974).

### Examination

In patients with severely active or long-standing active disease, there may be signs of weight loss, dehydration and anemia. Patients with proctosigmoiditis and more extensive colonic involvement may have mild generalized or left lower abdominal tenderness and patients with proctitis alone usually have normal findings on abdominal examination. With more severely active disease, there may be localized abdominal tenderness, guarding and rigidity. Patients with colonic dilatation may have abdominal distention.

A mass in the abdomen or severe anal lesions (see below) indicate a high probability of Crohn's disease, although anal lesions that are less severe can occur in ulcerative colitis. Findings on examination of the anal region in Crohn's disease are perianal edema, fissures which are often deep and lateral to the anus in contrast to the usual midline fissure, and perianal or ischiorectal abscesses that lead to fistula formation. Occasionally in Crohn's disease, some perianal ulceration may spread over a wide area and there may be "metastatic" ulceration of the skin elsewhere (Mountain 1970).

Examination of the abdomen in patients with terminal ileal Crohn's disease often demonstrates tenderness and fullness in the right iliac fossa. If there is a mass, it can vary from diffuse and ill defined to circumscribed and from tender and soft to hard and irregular, resembling a tumor. There may be features of abdominal abscess, fistula or anal lesions and any of the associated disorders of inflammatory bowel disease in the skin, joints, eyes or liver may be present.

## INVESTIGATION

### Clinical activity indices

Several combinations of clinical symptoms and signs have been proposed over the years (Bartholomeusz & Shearman 1989); the most widely used are the Truelove & Witts criteria (1955) for ulcerative colitis and either the Crohn's Disease Activity Index (Best et al 1976) or adaptation of the Harvey & Bradshaw Index for Crohn's Disease (1980).

### Laboratory studies

Iron deficiency anemia due to blood loss is common and losses of up to 150 ml/week can occur without any visible blood in the stool (Ormerod 1967, Stack et al 1969). The erythrocyte sedimentation rate and other acute phase reactants (e.g. C-reactive protein, orosomucoid) may be raised, with leukocytosis and thrombocytosis. Hypoproteinemia results from protein exudation from the inflamed mucosa. During a severe attack, hyponatremia, hypokalemia and hypomagnesemia can occur due to losses in the stool. In patients with small bowel Crohn's disease, there may be malabsorption of vitamin $B_{12}$ from the terminal ileum, and folate and fat malabsorption. However, on their own, these laboratory indices have relatively low sensitivity and specificity for activity and severity of inflammatory bowel disease (Camilleri & Proano 1989).

### Flexible sigmoidoscopy and colonoscopy

These procedures provide more diagnostic information than radiology, although total colonoscopy may be impossible in about 5% of adults due to tortuosity of the bowel or partial obstruction (Waye 1982, Axon & Dickinson 1983, Williams 1983). Radiology usually underestimates the extent of disease, compared to colonoscopy and biopsy. In particular, mild extensive disease can be missed by double-contrast barium enema and even by visual inspection at colonoscopy, but is detected from biopsies.

In assessing changes in the mucosa and the degree of abnormality, there are observer variations and the reader is referred to the studies by Baron et al (1964) and Watts et al (1966b). The reliable features in the diagnosis are the vascular pattern, which is not seen in proctitis, bleeding on contact with the instrument or swab, edema and ulceration. However, ulceration is not a prominent feature. Often, the appearance of the mucosa returns to normal once healing has taken place. If the disease becomes chronic, some evidence of inflammation remains and the lumen of the rectum may become narrowed. Rectal biopsy should always be taken. For the purposes of assessment and comparison, the rectal changes have been graded (Goligher et al 1968).

1. **Normal.** The vessel pattern is normal and there is no contact bleeding.
2. **Mild.** The vessel pattern is absent, but there are no other abnormalities.
3. **Moderate.** Rectal changes in this category are between grades 2 and 4.
4. **Severe.** The vessel pattern is absent, there is contact bleeding and edema and there may be other features such as inflammatory polyps, stricture or ulceration.

A Crohn's disease endoscopic index of severity has also been used extensively but it correlates poorly with the

Crohn's Disease Activity Index (Mary & Modigliani 1989).

*Differential diagnosis at colonoscopy*

Colonoscopy is important in distinguishing Crohn's disease from ulcerative colitis. For example, rectal sparing, which is common in Crohn's disease, can occur in ulcerative colitis, particularly following treatment, and in this regard biopsies from the normal-appearing rectum will show histological changes of chronic colitis. Sometimes a typical visual appearance of Crohn's disease is seen, for example, aphthous ulcers, discontinuity of the inflammation and cobblestone appearance of the mucosa. Other differentiating features between Crohn's disease and ulcerative colitis are shown in Table 23.8. Pera et al (1987) found that the most discriminating features were discontinuous involvement and cobblestoning in Crohn's disease and small ulcers and granularity in ulcerative colitis. On occasion, colonoscopy and biopsy are also of value in the diagnosis of the many other infective and non-infective causes of colitis (see below).

In patients with Crohn's disease, recurrent disease is found in about three-quarters of patients by colonoscopy 1 year after resection of all identifiable disease (Rutgeerts et al 1984). A scoring system to quantitate the severity of Crohn's disease was developed by the French study group GETAID (Anonymous 1987).

## Stool culture

The sigmoidoscopic appearance of inflammatory bowel disease, and particularly ulcerative colitis, is difficult to distinguish from infections such as salmonellosis, shigellosis, gonorrhoea, amebiasis (p. 572), *Campylobacter* colitis (p. 559) and on occasions solitary rectal ulcer. Thus, three specimens of stool (p. 556), mucosal swabs and rectal biopsies must be taken for culture and to examine for amebae. It is also wise to repeat culture of the stool at each exacerbation since ulcerative colitis and salmonellosis may coexist (Dronfield et al 1974).

**Table 23.8** Endoscopic differentiation between Crohn's disease and ulcerative colitis (derived from Waye 1977, 1978, Axon & Dickinson 1983)

| Crohn's disease | Ulcerative colitis |
|---|---|
| Rectum often normal | Rectum usually involved |
| Walls may be asymmetrically involved | Loss of vessel pattern – usually diffuse and symmetrical |
| Mucosal involvement may be discontinuous | Discontinuous involvement unusual |
| Cobblestone appearances frequently seen | Granularity common |
| Friability unusual | Friability usual |
| Ulcers may occur in otherwise normal mucosa | Ulcers occur in inflamed mucosa |
| Ulcers well circumscribed or deep and longitudinal | Ulcers small, diffuse and superficial |

## Upper gastrointestinal endoscopy (Ariyama et al 1980, Rutgeerts et al 1980)

Upper gastrointestinal endoscopy in Crohn's disease usually reveals thickening and stiffening of the gastric mucosal folds, a cobblestone appearance, ulceration or erosions. The mucosa may be friable and bleed easily. All these findings may also be seen in the duodenum. The lumen may be narrowed in the antrum or the first and second parts of the duodenum.

## Radiology (Gardiner & Stevenson 1982)

Because the colon can react to injury in only limited ways, there is marked overlap in the clinical, radiological and pathological findings in the various form of colitis. While it is possible to differentiate ulcerative colitis from Crohn's colitis in a majority of cases, some radiological features are common to both diseases and differentiation may be impossible by radiological and even pathological criteria. The radiographic differentiation is based on differences of mucosal pattern, the distribution of involvement and the presence of complicating features.

*The plain radiograph*

***Colitis.*** This is of the greatest importance in the diagnosis of toxic dilatation, which is usually due to ulcerative colitis but can also occur in Crohn's disease. It also provides valuable information in less severe cases. For example, the absence of haustra usually correlates with an area of disease, whereas haustration and feces in a segment of bowel indicate a healthy mucosa in that segment (Halls & Young 1964). However, lack of haustra in the absence of other features of colitis is of no diagnostic value. In distal proctocolitis, the involved area is commonly devoid of feces whilst the unaffected proximal colon is filled with feces. Sometimes, there is fecal stasis in the proximal colon. A variety of other features may be seen on the straight radiograph, such as shortening of the colon and the presence of inflammatory polyps, which may appear as thumbprinting.

***Small intestinal Crohn's disease.*** The plain film may show changes of intestinal obstruction or, rarely, perforation of the small bowel may be present. An enterolith can develop proximal to an obstructing lesion and this may calcify and hence become visible on the abdominal radiograph (Nelson 1969). Extraluminal gas may be seen in the soft tissues if fistulae or sinuses are present and also in localized abscess cavities. Some patients will develop renal calculi which are usually visible on the plain abdominal radiograph. Gallstones may be seen, being more frequent in patients with terminal ileal disease than in normal individuals.

*Barium studies*

Seriously ill patients with suspected inflammatory bowel disease should always be examined first with a plain abdominal radiograph, together with sigmoidoscopy, rectal biopsy and stool culture. In general, barium studies and all other enemas should not be performed in the acute stage of colitis because they can precipitate toxic dilatation.

A single-contrast barium enema will demonstrate some of the features of inflammatory bowel disease, although mucosal features are best demonstrated by the double-contrast enema and this has generally superseded the single-contrast enema (p. 16). Margulis et al (1971), using the single-contrast barium enema, retrospectively diagnosed 70% of patients with Crohn's disease and 79% of patients with ulcerative colitis. Kelvin et al (1978), using the double-contrast enema, diagnosed 98% of patients with Crohn's colitis and 83% of patients with ulcerative colitis. Winthrop et al (1985), in reviewing the barium enema examinations of patients with suspected inflammatory bowel disease, correctly categorized Crohn's colitis or ulcerative colitis in 93% when the double-contrast method was used, compared to 86% with the single-contrast method. However, in patients with early disease the double-contrast enema detected 91% of cases compared with only 70% of single-contrast method, whereas both methods detected all cases of advanced disease.

*Radiological features of ulcerative colitis* (Figs 23.14–17)

These are produced by edema and ulceration of the mucosa, by changes in the motility of the colon and by the presence of secretions.

The characteristic normal fine reticular pattern of the mucosa is altered in various ways; it may be lost completely so that the mucosa is entirely covered by a thin film of barium (effacement) or it may show granularity or frank ulceration. A diffuse granular mucosal pattern is the earliest radiographic abnormality and when ulceration supervenes this is nearly always imposed on this background of diffuse granularity (Bartram 1977).

The granularity seen in early ulcerative colitis (p. 17) is strikingly different from the early findings of Crohn's disease. The granularity is due to fine punctate lesions and closely matches the findings of edema, hyperemia and loss of vascularity seen on endoscopy and the erosive changes seen pathologically.

The ulceration of the colonic mucosa is at first superficial, rarely more than 3 mm in depth, giving rise to a stippling of the mucosal surface, but as the mucosa is

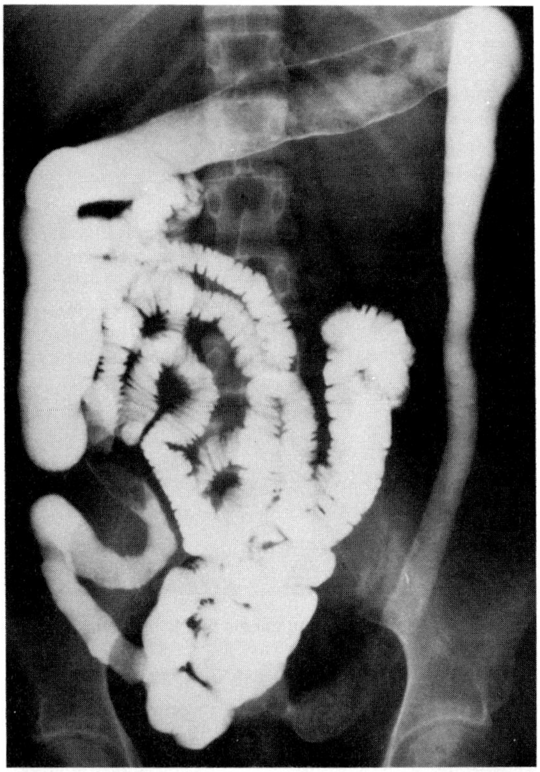

**Fig. 23.14** Ulcerative colitis of many years' duration with a shortened colon that has a smooth outline. The stricture at the hepatic flexure is smooth due to extensive mucosal destruction. A long segment of ileum has been filled with barium.

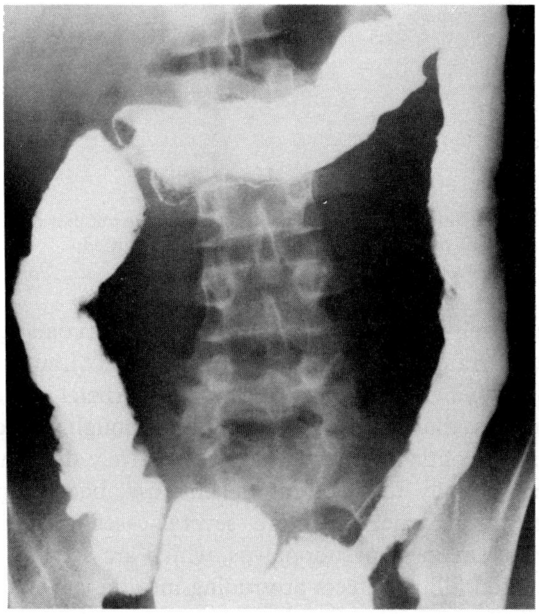

**Fig. 23.15** Chronic ulcerative colitis with a narrow rigid shortened colon and a smooth outline. Stricture at the hepatic flexure which proved to be benign, but radiologically a carcinoma could not be excluded.

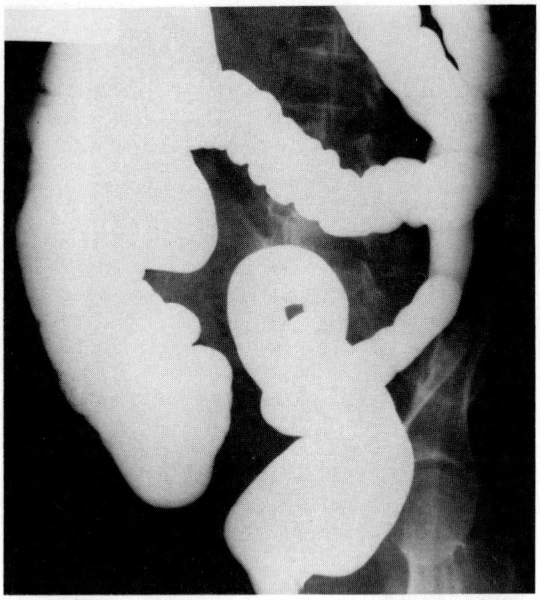

**Fig. 23.16** Conventional barium enema that is normal.

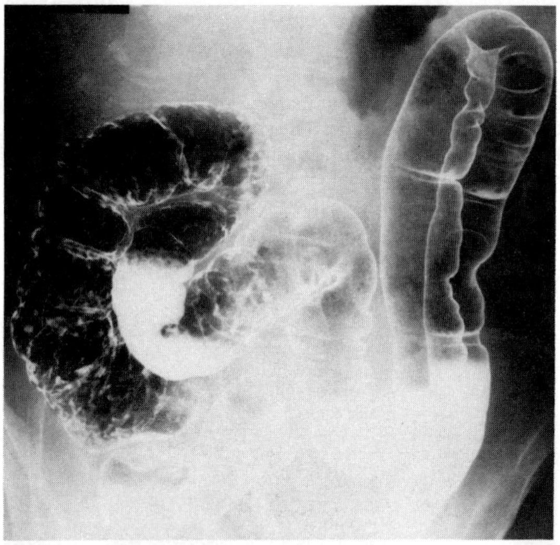

**Fig. 23.17** Contrast barium enema showing a large number of ulcers in the right side of the colon. The distal colon is narrowed.

progressively denuded the more characteristic coarse granular or serrated appearance becomes evident (Laufer et al 1976). In general, the ulcers are more superficial in ulcerative colitis than in Crohn's colitis, although in severe ulcerative colitis the ulcers may progressively deepen and extend laterally to undercut the mucosa, becoming the collar-button type. In more severe cases, islands of mucosa remain as pseudopolyps, which are seen as barium-coated filling defects protruding into the gas-distended lumen. Such pseudopolyps may also create a thumbprinting appearance on plain abdominal radiographs. When pseudopolyps are few in number, they may be difficult to distinguish from neoplastic polyps. Masses of postinflammatory polyps can develop, giving the appearance of multiple branching worm-like filling defects known as filiform polyposis (Zegel & Laufer 1978). These changes can also sometimes be seen in patients recovering from Crohn's colitis.

In the chronic stage of colitis, the bowel is shortened and narrowed; haustra are lost and the bowel has the appearance of a smooth tube. Widening of the retrorectal space on a lateral radiograph is a well-documented feature of chronic ulcerative colitis and is due to perirectal inflammation and a reduced caliber of the rectum. The space is usually measured opposite S4 where the rectum is running parallel to the sacrum; its upper normal limit is 2 cm (Chrispin & Fry 1963). Tapered benign fibrous strictures are usually benign but the possibility of malignancy should be considered. In some patients radiological abnormalities may be seen in areas subsequently shown to contain dysplasia (Frank et al 1978), although barium studies are not sensitive enough to use routinely in the surveillance for dysplasia.

Ulcerative colitis almost always affects the rectal mucosa and spreads proximally in a continuous fashion to a relatively well-defined zone of demarcation within the colon or it may involve the entire colon. Backwash ileitis may occur with a dilated and fixed ileocecal valve and granular mucosal changes in the distal ileum, sometimes up to 20 cm in length.

Using predetermined signs, Kelvin et al (1978) identified ulcerative colitis in 83% of patients on the basis of continuous distal involvement (86%), granular mucosa (79%) and diffuse rectal disease (79%). In a series of 41 children with inflammatory bowel disease reviewed by Winthrop et al (1985), the most informative signs of ulcerative colitis were symmetrical or continuous involvement (73%), mucosal granularity (87%) and superficial ulceration (67%).

*Radiological changes with time*

Barium enema studies have demonstrated extension of the ulcerative proctocolitis in a minority of patients. In the series reported by Edwards & Truelove (1963), five of 50 patients with involvement of the rectum and rectosigmoid region and 12 of 84 patients with substantial involvement beyond the rectum showed extension of the disease subsequently. Goligher et al (1968) studied 50 patients with rectal involvement and found that seven developed total involvement and 17 substantial involvement beyond the rectum.

Ulceration is the most common finding in early ulcerative colitis (De Dombal et al 1968), but other radiological features may appear rapidly and major radiological changes can sometimes be seen after only a short history. This may be explained by the muscular contraction which arises rapidly during the acute attack and results in a loss of haustration and narrowing of the colon. Such changes are to some extent reversed during remission. However, eventually, contraction of the muscle and foreshortening of the colon becomes permanent.

The role of the double-contrast enema in a symptomatic patient thought to have ulcerative colitis is initially that of making a specific diagnosis, assessing the extent and severity of the disease and then the identification of complicating features. In quiescent disease the double-contrast enema is much less accurate and considerably underestimates the degree of involvement (see below).

*Correlation between radiology, endoscopy and pathology*

Barium enemas underestimate the severity of the mucosal changes, which tended to be masked by debris in the colon (Dick et al 1959). Biopsy at colonoscopy showed that the double-contrast enema underestimated the extent or severity of the disease in eight out of 11 patients with proctocolitis (Warwick et al 1973). This applies particularly to quiescent disease (Gabrielsson et al 1979).

Both sigmoidoscopy (Dick et al 1966, Wright & Truelove 1966b) and colonoscopy (Warwick et al 1973) can show a visually normal mucosa and yet the histology shows evidence of inflammation. The same applies to Crohn's disease, in which histological abnormalities may be found in spite of normal endoscopic appearances.

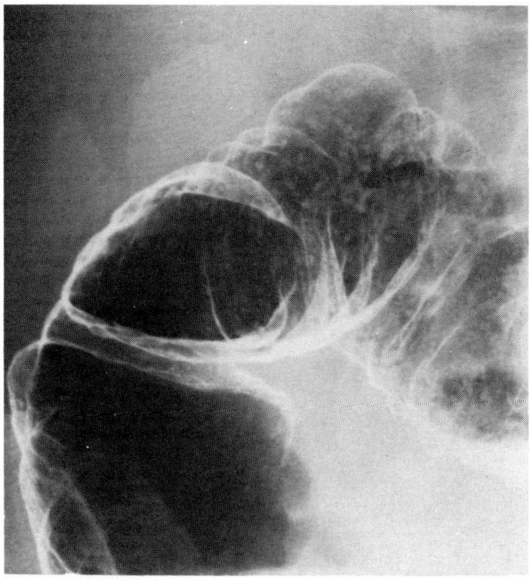

**Fig. 23.18** Crohn's disease of colon with aphthoid ulcers at the hepatic flexure seen as multiple discrete pits or dots of barium with a surrounding translucent halo.

*Radiological features of colonic Crohn's disease*
(Figs 23.18–22)

The radiological appearance of the colon in Crohn's disease differs from ulcerative colitis in three main ways.

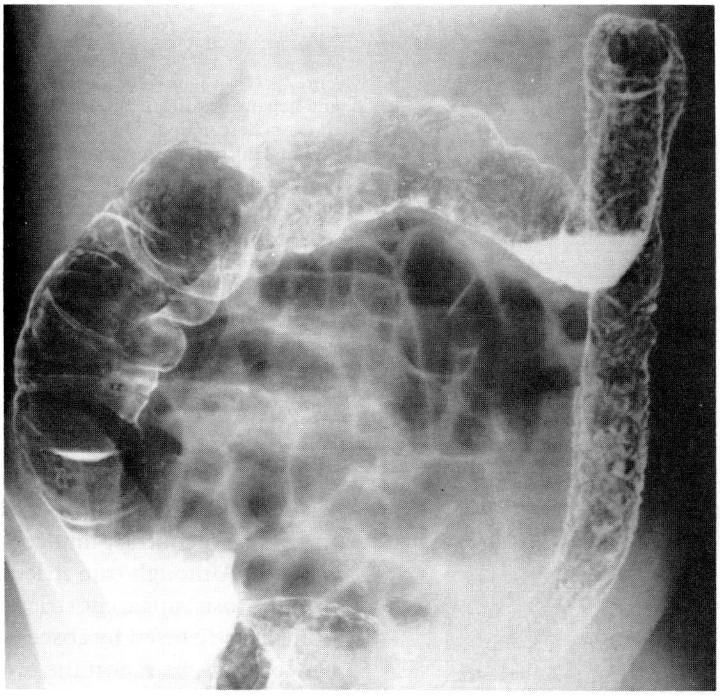

**Fig. 23.19** Crohn's disease of colon with extensive ulceration of the left side of the colon and multiple discrete aphthoid ulcers in the ascending colon and at the hepatic flexure.

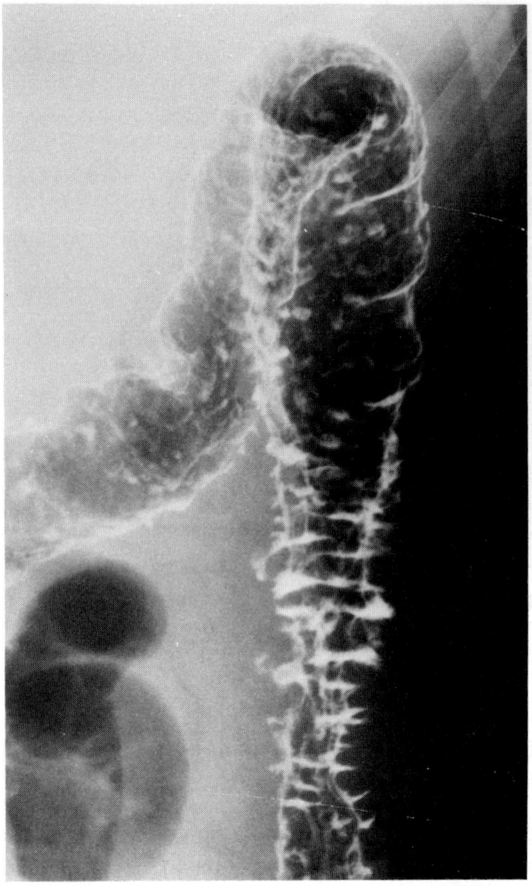

**Fig. 23.20** Severe Crohn's disease of colon showing both discrete aphthoid ulcers and deep penetrating ulcers.

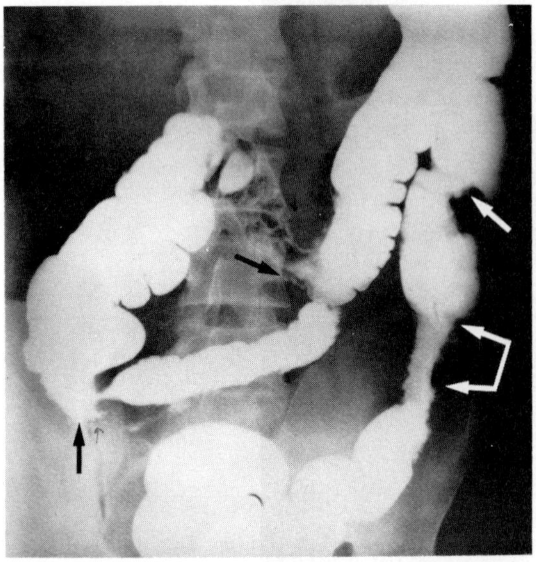

**Fig. 23.21** Crohn's disease of colon with segmental distribution – a common finding. The affected areas (arrows) show narrowing with irregularity due to ulceration.

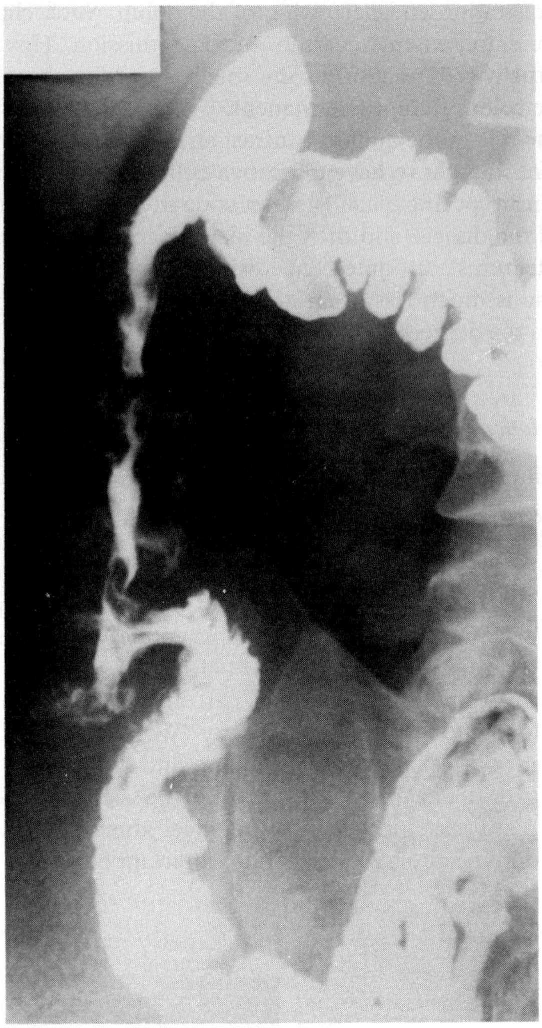

**Fig. 23.22** Right-sided Crohn's colitis. The cecum, ascending colon and hepatic flexure are affected with irregularity, shortening and mucosal destruction. The terminal ileum is also involved and there is minimal dilatation proximally, indicative of partial obstruction.

First, the disease is often discontinuous and although strictures may lead to narrowing of the bowel as in ulcerative colitis, the narrowing is not symmetrical. Secondly, ulceration is much more marked and penetrating, with deep collar-button ulcers and fissures. The mucosal pattern may show linear ulcers or a cobblestone appearance. As a consequence of the deep ulceration, there may be evidence of intramural abscesses and fistulae. Thirdly, the terminal ileum in Crohn's disease may be narrow and irregular, in contrast to ulcerative colitis in which it is featureless. Although true strictures in Crohn's disease result from fibrosis, apparent strictures at the rectosigmoid junction can be caused by abscesses arising from the ileum.

Most authors report the presence of ulcers as the earliest sign of Crohn's disease (Laufer et al 1976, Kelvin et al 1978). Simpkins (1977) described the radiographic appearances of aphthous ulceration as a small fleck of barium of varying size (a target lesion) surrounded by a translucent halo due to granulomatous inflammation amidst a pattern of normal mucosa. Nolan (1981) suggested that in a small number of cases of Crohn's disease of the terminal ileum, aphthoid ulceration is the only demonstrable abnormality, hence it is the earliest change. Others claim that the superficial ulceration does not develop in an otherwise normal mucosa (Ekberg et al 1980) and that the search for early disease should start with the identification of an edematous segment followed by careful scrutiny of those segments for ulceration. The course of aphthous ulcers is unpredictable; some remain unchanged for years, some disappear completely and others progress to large ulcers and consequent loss of the aphthous changes (Ni & Goldberg 1986). Aphthous ulcers were demonstrated in 40 of 91 patients with Crohn's colitis. In Simpkins' view aphthous ulceration is a strong indication and the earliest sign of Crohn's colitis. However, aphthous ulceration is not pathognomonic of Crohn's colitis and is also seen in colitis due to ameba, shigella, tuberculosis, *Yersinia*, herpes virus, Behçet's disease and oral contraceptives (Max & Kelvin 1980). Rarely, aphthous ulcers occur in idiopathic ulcerative colitis and in diversion colitis.

Although a normal variant, extensive lymphoid hyperplasia, especially if the follicles are of variable size and are larger than 3.5–4 mm diameter, should be regarded as suspicious of Crohn's colitis (Jones 1985).

Deep fissures are common and may become confluent to form longitudinal or transverse fissures which are not seen in ulcerative colitis. Severe edema of the mucosa and submucosa leads to the cobblestone appearance. As in ulcerative colitis, some cases show radiographic improvement during remission, with healing of ulcers and the return of haustra (Jones et al 1969).

One of the hallmarks of Crohn's disease of the colon is its discontinuous nature along the length of the bowel and often of a more localized asymmetrical involvement of the circumference of one area of the bowel. As a consequence, sacculations or pseudodiverticula may occur on the opposite wall of the colon. Strictures which are asymmetrical may occur anywhere in the colon, often with fissured ulcers on the antimesenteric border in the same section of bowel. The distribution of abnormalities may be helpful; involvement of the right half of the colon, especially disease of the cecum when the terminal ileum is almost invariably involved, indicates Crohn's colitis. The rectum is often spared.

The double-contrast barium enema is of value in detecting the anorectal features of inflammatory bowel disease. In a series of 74 patients with Crohn's disease and 32 with ulcerative colitis, half the patients with Crohn's colitis had fissures, fistulae or abscesses in relation to the anal canal, in comparison to 13% with small bowel Crohn's disease and 6% with ulcerative colitis. It was also evident that extensive perianal disease may be seen radiographically before it presents clinically (DuBrow & Frank 1983).

Kelvin et al (1978) found the most useful signs in diagnosing Crohn's colitis were discontinuous or eccentric involvement (88%) and aphthous (discrete) ulcers (67%). Winthrop et al (1985) studied 41 children with inflammatory bowel disease in whom the most informative signs were asymmetrical or discontinuous involvement (64%), aphthous ulcers (71%), deep mucosal ulceration (57%) and disease confined to the right side of the colon (64%).

***Differential diagnosis: radiology.*** The barium enema is sensitive and fairly specific in Crohn's disease, but other conditions such as amebic colitis, *Yersini* enterocolitis, tuberculosis and ischemic colitis can mimic the findings. Infiltration by lymphoma and secondary deposits or pelvic infection and endometriosis can also cause similar and sometimes identical appearances. However, in assessing the extent of the disease and in the demonstration of complications such as fistulae and obstructive lesions the double-contrast enema is essential. It is also helpful in assessing postoperative recurrences.

### *Barium examination of the small intestine in Crohn's disease*

The indications for barium examination of the small bowel are: to establish the diagnosis; to determine the extent of disease; and to search for complications such as strictures with obstruction or abscess formation in patient exacerbations.

***Methodology.*** The barium small intestinal follow-through examination is the most widely used procedure, though increasingly duodenal intubation techniques for small bowel enteroclysis are being used (Nolan 1981, Herlinger 1982). The peroral pneumocolon examination is a refinement of the follow-through study of the small intestine which enables detailed display of the ileocecal region (p. 15). Ekberg (1977) showed that the small bowel enema technique was far superior to the follow-through examination in demonstrating the proximal extent, the diameter and length of a stricture and in showing early changes of the disease. The main advantage in this technique seems to be related to the full distention of the small bowel lumen which can be achieved. However, the barium follow-through study may be favored because of time saving, lower radiation dose and better acceptance (Ott et al 1985). These authors compared the accuracy of the follow-through technique with the intubation method. Overall the sensitivity of the follow-through was 92% and the specificity 94%, compared with a sensitivity of 94% and specificity of 89% for the intubation technique. There was no difference in the sensitivity of diagnosis of Crohn's disease between the methods.

The small intestinal barium study has considerable false positive and false negative rates in the diagnosis of inflammatory bowel disease. In the NCCDS (Goldberg et al 1979) many of the radiographic examinations were inadequate and the available data on the nature and extent of the disease were likely to have underestimated these factors. Admans et al (1980) studied 140 patients with Crohn's disease. In only 13% of patients with small bowel disease and in only 21% of the group as a whole was the diagnosis correctly made after initial investigations. Many misdiagnoses were made and in patients with small bowel disease 19% were first thought to be suffering from psychiatric disorders.

Dyer et al (1970) reported a study of retrospective observer error using the barium follow-through technique in 50 patients with known Crohn's disease. The most reliable radiographic signs were persistent and fixed narrowing of the bowel lumen. Ulceration, fissures and irregularity of the mucosal surface were also frequent and reliable signs. Other radiographic abnormalities were less reliable. Ekberg et al (1980), in a retrospective study using the intubation small bowel enema in 53 patients previously operated on for Crohn's disease, reported a close correlation of the severity of radiographic features and subsequent clinical recurrence. The authors paid particular attention to early signs such as submucosal edema and superficial ulceration and 27% of patients with these findings had signs of recurrence. When transmural disease was demonstrated radiographically 87% of patients had a clinical recurrence.

***Early manifestations.*** The earliest manifestation of Crohn's disease in the small bowel is generally thought to be blunting, thickening, flattening and distortion of the valvulae conniventes (Marshak & Lindner 1976). These changes are due to hyperplasia of the lymphoid tissue and nodules may develop (Herlinger 1982). Although these changes are probably the earliest detectable radiological signs and may be the only change (Nolan 1981), the appearances are not specific and similar abnormalities are found in radiation enteritis, ischemia, lymphoma and conditions associated with hypoalbuminemia (Nolan & Gourtsoyiannis 1980). Glick & Teplick (1985), using a peroral pneumocolon technique in a group of 43 consecutive patients with Crohn's disease, recognized a diffuse granular pattern occupying all of the mucosal surface of the involved segment of bowel. At resection the pattern represented lymphocytic infiltration of the villi, which were widened and blunted. The authors claim that the granular appearance is the earliest manifestation of Crohn's disease. However, most authors believe that the demonstration of aphthous ulceration is the earliest specific radiological sign of Crohn's disease in the bowel (Laufer & Costopoulos 1978) (p. 662).

***Other radiological findings.*** In addition to discrete aphthous ulcers, fissures are common and best seen in profile. Frequently these are not deep but some may penetrate the intestinal wall for 5 mm or more and these can develop into small abscess cavities below the muscularis. These may progress to sinuses and fistulae. The combination of discrete and fissure ulcers is highly suggestive of Crohn's disease, though tuberculosis and *Yersinia* enteritis may give identical appearances. A combination of longitudinal and transverse fissures separating islands of intact mucosa creates a cobblestone appearance.

Asymmetric involvement of the bowel wall, particularly the mesenteric border, with straightening, shortening and more extensive ulceration with nodularity is seen frequently. It is characteristic of Crohn's disease. Pseudodiverticula (Fig. 23.23) may be seen along the shortened mesenteric border (Nolan & Gourtsoyiannis 1980). Skip lesions with intervening areas of normal small intestine are seen in about 10% of patients. Strictures affect about 40% of patients. These may be single or multiple, short or long. In the absence of other evidence an isolated stricture is not diagnostic of Crohn's disease and other conditions such as ischemia, malignant infiltration, adhesions from previous surgery, previous radiotherapy or abdominal trauma should be considered in the differential diagnosis. Dilatation of bowel loops with stasis of contents proximal to strictures is a frequent finding. However, the well-known "string" sign (Fig. 23.24) described by Kantor (1934) is now thought to be due to spasm and irritability of the bowel wall and does not always indicate stenosis. Occasionally small rounded filling defects may protrude into the bowel lumen and are described by Marshak & Lindner (1976) as pseudopolyps.

In about half of patients with Crohn's disease there will be clear evidence of irregular thickening of mucosal folds in the affected segment, often with thickening of the bowel wall, and in some there will be a soft tissue mass around or adjacent to the involved loops of small bowel, especially in the region of the terminal ileum and cecum (Fig. 23.25). In most instances patients with abnormalities of the terminal ileum have continuous disease in the cecum and right colon.

The ileocecal valve is a common site of sinus and fistula formation in Crohn's disease (Goldberg & Jeffrey 1980) and careful examination of this structure is necessary.

Fistulae can be identified, particularly to the sigmoid colon, which fills with barium during the follow-through examination before the remainder of the colon.

Jejunal involvement (Fig. 23.26) is characterized by dilated and chronically obstructed loops and gastric involvement may appear like antral carcinoma (Legge et al 1970) or there may be erosions detected by double-contrast radiography (Ariyama et al 1980) or a cobblestone appearance.

Duodenal abnormalities were seen in one-fifth of the patients in the NCCDS and in one-third of these the features were considered typical of Crohn's disease. There was narrowing of the duodenal bulb and loop (Fig. 23.27), with stiffening and flattening of the wall, thickened irregular folds and shallow ulceration. In the other two-thirds of patients the findings were considered nonspecific (Goldberg et al 1979).

Recurrent Crohn's disease after surgical resection usually

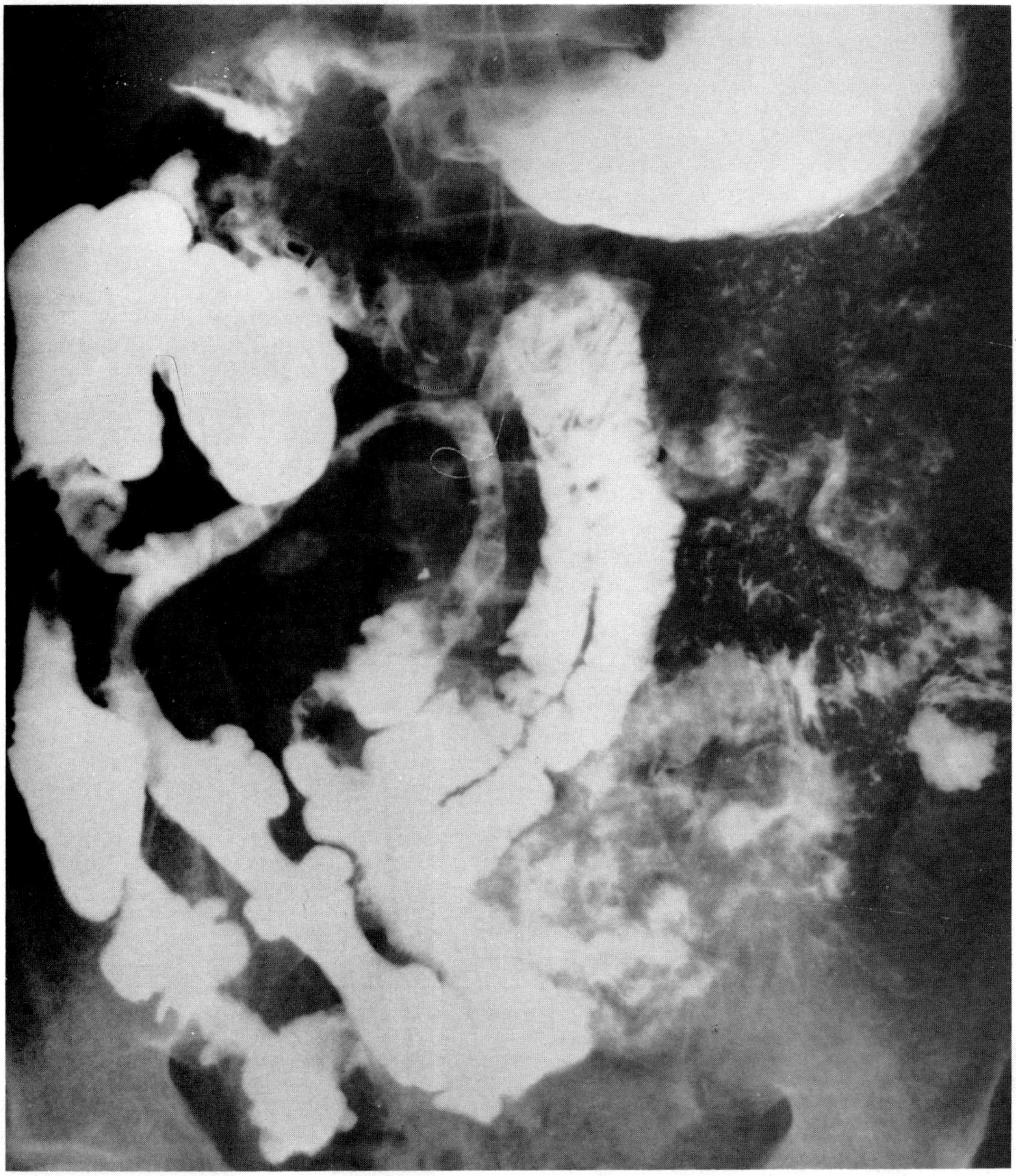

**Fig. 23.23** Diffuse Crohn's disease of small bowel with narrowing, mucosal destruction and ulceration. Numerous sacculations are also present.

occurs in continuity with the operative site. Jejunal involvement is also more common in patients who have had resection (Nolan 1981). The radiographic signs include ulceration, mucosal nodularity and stricture formation.

The differential diagnosis of small intestinal Crohn's disease includes: tuberculosis, *Yersinia* enteritis and small bowel lymphoma (Sartoris et al 1984).

*Computed tomography*

This examination is particularly useful in demonstrating some of the intra-abdominal complications of Crohn's disease (p. 65). In studying the cause of an abdominal mass or the separation of bowel loops seen on the small bowel series, CT can differentiate an abscess cavity from necrotic or fibrofatty tissue and enlarged lymph nodes. CT is also of value in the detection of perirectal and psoas abscesses (Gore et al 1985, Fishman et al 1987).

*Leukocyte scans*

Radionuclide scans ($^{111}$indium, $^{67}$gallium, $^{99m}$technetium) are useful in identifying active areas of inflammation, particularly in the small intestine (Froelich 1987) (p. 89). These techniques allow both the identification of the site of disease and also quantitation of the severity.

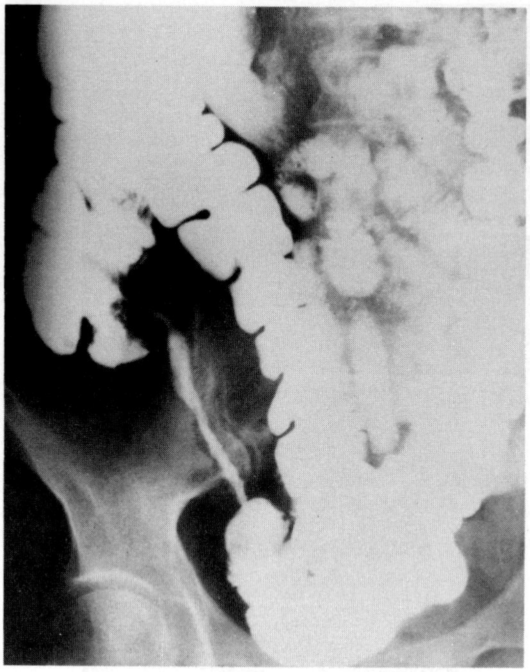

**Fig. 23.24** Crohn's disease of terminal ileum and cecum. Follow-through of barium meal shows rigidity, narrowing and mucosal destruction of the terminal ileum – the "string sign".

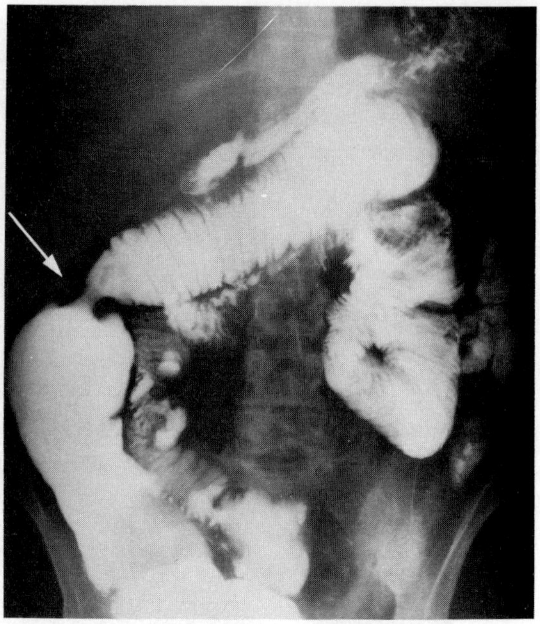

**Fig. 23.26** Stricture in the jejunum (arrow) due to Crohn's disease, with dilatation proximally. There is also gross dilatation distal to the stricture due to a second stricture not demonstrated on this radiograph.

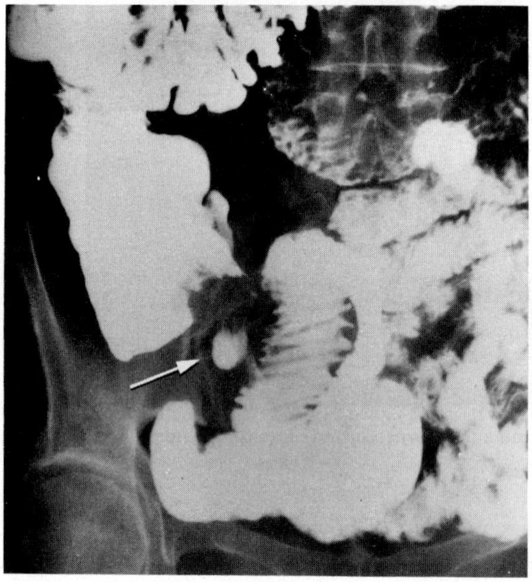

**Fig. 23.25** Crohn's disease of terminal ileum. Large ulcer (arrow) in the middle of a large inflammatory mass which displaces the ileum and cecum.

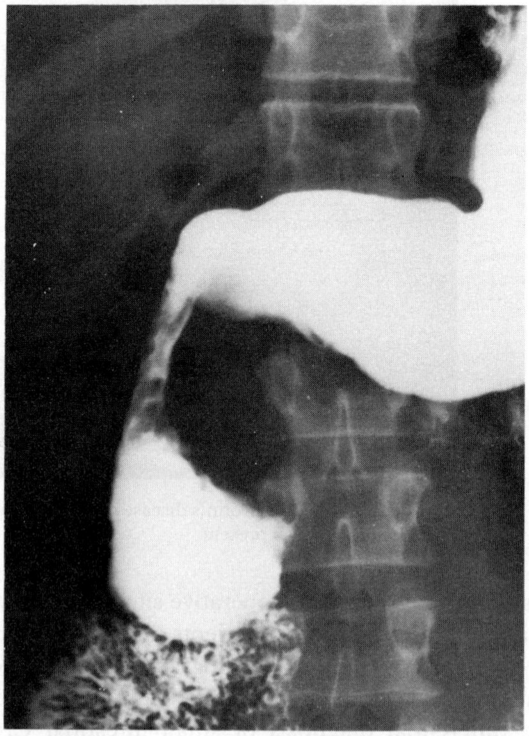

**Fig. 23.27** Crohn's disease of the duodenum causing obstruction at the junction of the second and third parts. In addition there is persistent narrowing in the middle of the second part due to another lesion.

They may be of most value in clinical trials to assess efficacy.

## Choice of investigations for diagnosis of inflammatory bowel disease: best practice

The diagnosis of inflammatory bowel disease is made with a combination of clinical, endoscopic, radiologic and histologic information and no one single modality is solely diagnostic. For a patient with ulcerative colitis, or Crohn's disease with colonic involvement, a flexible sigmoidoscopic examination often provides sufficient confirmatory information, particularly if used in combination with an air contrast barium enema. Colonoscopy is being used with increasing frequency in the diagnosis of inflammatory bowel disease for several reasons: it permits inspection of the entire colon and in the majority of instances, inspection of the terminal ileum as well; biopsies can be obtained from multiple levels in the colon and in the ileum, for confirmation of a segmental distribution of disease in the case of Crohn's; abnormal lesions such as dysplastic areas or polyps can be biopsied; the number of tests can be reduced, with colonoscopy as a single test rather than a flexible sigmoidoscopic examination, barium enema, and small intestinal barium study to examine the terminal ileum; many patients find colonoscopy with sedation much more comfortable than an air contrast barium enema.

Colonoscopy is important in distinguishing Crohn's disease from ulcerative colitis, e.g. rectal sparing, which is common in Crohn's disease, can occur in ulcerative colitis and thus multiple biopsies of the entire colon are often necessary to make the diagnosis – in this regard, it is the biopsies from areas which appear normal or are only mildly diseased which most often provide important information. Sometimes a typical visual appearance of Crohn's disease is seen, e.g. aphthous ulcers, discontinuity of the inflammation and cobblestone appearance of the mucosa. Other differentiating features between Crohn's disease and ulcerative colitis are shown in Table 23.8. Pera et al (1987) found that the most discriminating features were discontinuous involvement and cobblestoning in Crohn's disease and small ulcers and granularity in ulcerative colitis. On occasions, colonoscopy and biopsy are also of value in the diagnosis of the many other infective and non-infective causes of colitis (see below).

The distinction of pseudopolyp from adenomatous polyp can be made by the removal of the polyp at colonoscopy. Strictures must be investigated with biopsy and cytology brushings to determine whether they are fibrous or malignant or indeed whether they are due to other conditions such as ischemic colitis.

## DIFFERENTIAL DIAGNOSIS

At the onset of symptoms it is not always apparent whether the diagnosis is idiopathic inflammatory bowel disease or whether another colonic condition is present. Conditions which should be considered are listed in Table 23.9. Rectal infections in HIV patients are discussed on p. 611.

### Salmonellosis and shigellosis

The clinical and endoscopic features at the onset of these disorders are often indistinguishable from ulcerative colitis. For this reason, stool cultures are always necessary.

### *Campylobacter* gastroenteritis

This can be difficult to distinguish clinically and histologically from ulcerative colitis.

**Table 23.9** Conditions simulating nonspecific inflammatory bowel disease (Johnson & Roth 1975)

| |
|---|
| *Specific infections* |
| Bacterial |
| Salmonellosis |
| Shigellosis |
| Tuberculous enterocolitis |
| Gonorrheal proctitis |
| Staphylococcal enterocolitis |
| Fungal |
| Histoplasmosis |
| Parasitic |
| Amebic dysentery |
| Schistosomiasis |
| *Other specific diseases* |
| Radiation proctitis |
| Diverticulitis |
| Ischemic colitis |
| *Neoplasms and premalignant diseases* |
| Lymphoma |
| Familial polyposis |
| *Miscellaneous disorders* |
| Pseudomembranous enterocolitis |
| Behçet's syndrome |
| Polyarteritis |
| Solitary ulcer of the rectum |
| Cathartic colon |
| Soap colitis |
| Irritable bowel syndrome |
| Hemorrhoids |

### Hemorrhagic colitis due to Enterohemorrhagic *E. coli* (p. 558)

### Gonorrhea and other venereal infections

In gonorrheal proctitis, the symptoms and endoscopic features are indistinguishable from ulcerative proctitis; however, gonorrheal infection does not spread beyond the rectum and causes only mild mucosal abnormalities. The presence of proctitis should lead to questioning about sexual preferences and habits and if condyloma acuminata are found on examination, cultures for gonococcus should be obtained. Other sexually transmitted infections, amebiasis and shigellosis, should also be considered.

Other infections are: syphilis, which may cause solitary or multiple erosions and ulcers at the anal verge or in the canal; anorectal *Herpes simplex*, which causes severe rectal pain, urinary and fecal retention; chlamydial proctitis; lymphogranuloma venereum, which may cause a proctocolitis with the development of fistulae and perianal abscesses. Narrowing of the lumen of the rectum is a characteristic feature.

### Amebiasis

Amebic dysentery can mimic ulcerative colitis both at its onset and during long phases of remissions and exacerbations. In many instances, the endoscopic appearance cannot be distinguished from ulcerative colitis or Crohn's proctitis, but features which suggest amebic colitis are fine, punctate mucosal changes without friability of the mucosa, which occur in mild cases, and raised ulcers or irregular penetrating ulcers in more severe cases. The diagnosis is made by three separate examinations of the stool for *E. histolytica* or by obtaining mucus and debris from the ulcers at sigmoidoscopy (p. 574).

### Other parasitic infections

Parasitic infections which can cause a colitis are schistosomiasis, balantidiasis, *Strongyloides stercoralis* and anisakiasis.

### Pseudomembranous colitis (p. 566)

This commences with profuse watery diarrhea and, depending on the severity, it may simulate ulcerative colitis and may progress to toxic dilatation. Most patients have a history of recent antibiotic use, but *C. difficile*, the causative organism, is contagious and not all patients have a history of prior antibiotic use.

The endoscopic appearance is of value in making the diagnosis because there is often a yellowish, adherent membrane and even when this is not obvious the rectal biopsy is usually characteristic. However, in some cases, the endoscopic features are indistinguishable from ulcerative colitis.

### Tuberculosis (p. 568)

Tuberculosis of the ileocecal region must be considered in the differential diagnosis of Crohn's disease. Tuberculosis may also involve the colon and rectum. Histoplasmosis can also involve the ileocecal region.

### Radiation proctitis/colitis (p. 409)

This can usually be inferred from the history of radiotherapy up to 30 years previously. However, patients who have had radiotherapy could also develop ulcerative colitis or Crohn's disease as the cause of rectal symptoms. Endoscopy in the acute stage shows redness, friability and edema; the chronic phase is characterized by atrophic mucosa with scattered telangiectasias, often extensive.

### Ischemic colitis

The differentiating features from ulcerative and Crohn's colitis are shown in Table 23.10. The most important are the occurrence of ischemic colitis in older patients with generalized vascular disease (although it has been reported in young women taking oral contraceptives), thumbprinting on the barium enema and a normal rectum at sigmoidoscopy. Ischemic proctitis occurs occasionally but involves the lower rectum only rarely; the mucosa is dark and there is an abrupt demarcation to normal mucosa.

**Table 23.10** Differential diagnosis of ischemic colitis (Johnson & Roth 1975)

| Feature | Ischemic colitis | Chronic ulcerative colitis | Crohn's disease of the colon |
|---|---|---|---|
| Onset | Very rapid | Gradual; occasionally rapid | Gradual |
| >50 years | 80% | <10% | <5% |
| Rectal bleeding | Once | Every stool | Uncommon |
| Stricture formation | Common | Uncommon | Common |
| Prior cardiovascular disease | Common | Rare | Rare |
| Progress of disease | Acute; rapidly changing | Chronic | Chronic |
| Segmental involvement | Common | Rare | Common |
| Thumbprinting on barium enema | Common | Rare | Uncommon |
| Most common involvement | Splenic flexure; descending colon; transverse colon | Rectum, sigmoid and descending colon in continuity; entire colon | Terminal ileum and right colon; entire colon |

### Microscopic colitis

In this condition the radiological and endoscopic appearance of the colon is usually normal or there may be nonspecific erythema, but biopsy of the colon shows a mild uniform, diffuse inflammation of the lamina propria.

The patient has severe watery diarrhea with a stool volume usually greater than 500 ml/day. This volume is greatly reduced on fasting. The diarrhea is probably due to a reduction in colonic water absorption (Bo-Linn et al 1985). There may be anemia, a raised ESR, hypokalemia and hypoalbuminemia. Some patients respond to sulfasalazine.

This condition is distinct from ulcerative colitis and Crohn's disease and there is no evidence that microscopic colitis evolves into one of these other diseases. Microscopic colitis should be considered in the differential diagnosis of irritable bowel syndrome and diarrhea-producing tumors.

### Collagenous colitis

The clinical features of collagenous colitis and microscopic colitis are usually indistinguishable and these may in fact be different manifestations of the same entity (Carpenter et al 1992). This is a rare cause of abdominal pain and watery diarrhea, usually in middle-aged women. The stool volume can range from normal up to 5 L/day. There may be vomiting, nocturnal diarrhea, urgency and incontinence. The disorder shows exacerbations and remissions. Some patients may have rheumatoid arthritis or related disorders (Fausa et al 1985, Kingham et al 1986, Palmer et al 1986).

On investigation, the colon may be normal or have nonspecific abnormalities such as erythema and granularity at endoscopy and the barium is typically normal (Steadman et al 1987). Biopsy of the rectum shows that the subepithelial collagen band is greater than 15 μm compared to a normal thickness of 10–15 μm.

There have not been any controlled trials for the treatment of collagenous or microscopic colitis. In general, medications that are effective for the treatment of mildly to moderately active ulcerative colitis also appear effective for the treatment of these conditions, such as sulfasalazine and other aminosalicylates and prednisolone.

### Gold-induced enterocolitis

This is probably a hypersensitivity reaction to gold. It presents with acute diarrhea, predominantly in women, within 3 months of starting therapy (Jackson et al 1986). Both the small intestine and colon may be involved, with an infiltration of plasma cells and eosinophils. There may also be some crypt abscesses and surface ulceration. Other features are peripheral blood eosinophilia and a petechial appearance of the mucosa on endoscopy. Treatment with corticosteroids is probably of no benefit. Gold therapy must be stopped and if the colitis is severe, surgery may be necessary.

The gold preparation Auranofin can cause diarrhea by increasing intestinal permeability, which results in an increased fecal loss of sodium and water. In these patients the rectal biopsy is normal (Behrens et al 1986).

### Other conditions

A number of other conditions may occasionally be confused with ulcerative or Crohn's colitis. Diffuse lymphoma and Kaposi's sarcoma of the colon may simulate ulcerative colitis (Friedman et al 1968, Weber et al 1985), cytomegalovirus colitis occurs in acquired immune deficiency syndrome (Meiselman et al 1985), colitis may occur in Behçet's syndrome (O'Duffy et al 1971) and involvement of the gastrointestinal tract in polyarteritis nodosa (Goldgraber & Kirsner 1957) and other vasculitides including Wegener's granulomatosis (Sokol et al 1984) may cause ulceration, infarction and proctitis. Chronic granulomatous disease can result in a colitis similar to Crohn's disease (Werlin et al 1982) and eosinophilic gastroenteritis can present as colitis (Naylor & Pollet 1985). In the hemolytic uremic syndrome, in which there is acute microangiopathic hemolytic anemia, thrombocytopenia and oliguric renal failure, thrombosis of small submucosal vessels in the colon can lead to a colitis similar to ulcerative or pseudomembranous colitis (Whitington et al 1979). Colitis occurs in severe neutropenia (Mulholland & Delaney 1983) and in 2.6% of patients with acute leukemia (Mower et al 1986) and is termed neutropenic colitis or typhlitis (Kunkel & Rosenthal 1986). Secondary amyloidosis may also cause proctitis. The radiological features of cathartic colon can be indistinguishable from those of ulcerative colitis. Diverticular disease localized to the sigmoid colon may be difficult to distinguish from Crohn's disease and the conditions may coexist; at sigmoidoscopy, the mucosa at the rectosigmoid junction may be pale and edematous in both conditions. Ulcerative proctitis must also be distinguished from a rectal prolapse with inflammatory distal proctitis; in this situation, inflammation is commonly localized to the anterior wall of the rectum, indicating the solitary ulcer syndrome.

## LOCAL COMPLICATIONS

### Toxic dilatation (acute colonic dilatation)

This medical emergency can lead rapidly to colonic perforation and death. The condition occurs because of the severity of the colitis and not because of some identifiable endogenous or exogenous toxin, as the name may suggest, and some prefer the terms "acute colonic dilatation" or "megacolon in colitis". Toxic dilatation may also occur in pseudomembranous colitis, ischemic colitis, amebic colitis and salmonellosis.

#### *Incidence*

The incidence varies in different centers; it was 1.6% in Oxford (Edwards & Truelove 1964), 3% at the Mayo Clinic (McInerney et al 1962), 14% in Edinburgh (Jalan et al 1969) and 6% in Chicago (Greenstein et al 1985) but its incidence would appear to be decreasing. This variation is probably related to the severity of colitis in referred patients. There is much less information about the incidence of the complication in Crohn's colitis, but it probably occurs in about 6% of cases (Grieco et al 1980). In another series, toxic dilatation occurred in 10% of patients with ulcerative colitis, compared to 2.2% of patients with Crohn's colitis or ileocolitis (Greenstein & Aufses 1985).

#### *Etiology and pathology*

The affected colon is usually dilated and intensely congested. There is extensive mucosal sloughing present and the wall is thinned and may be necrotic in places. On histology the inflammation is transmural and the ulcers extend down into the main muscle coat, which shows myocytolysis (Rowland & Pounder 1982). There is transmural extension of the inflammatory process (Lumb et al 1955, Jalan et al 1969). Dilatation in colonic Crohn's disease occurs more often early in the course of the disease before the colon has become thickened and fibrotic.

While it is accepted that dilatation is the final stage of severe inflammation, certain factors are suspected of precipitating the event. Hypokalemia may contribute. In one series, 17 of 36 patients had received opiates a short time previously (Garrett et al 1967). Anticholinergics are also suspected (Smith et al 1962). Performing a barium enema in a patient with severe colitis may precipitate dilatation (Jalan et al 1969). Goligher et al (1968) postulated that mechanical obstruction distally may play a role in the dilatation of the transverse colon, the obstruction being due, presumably, to inflammation and edema of the pelvic colon. There is no evidence that corticosteroids predispose to dilatation.

*Clinical features*

Dilatation can occur either during the initial attack of colitis or during a relapse. It is more common in patients with total colonic involvement; in one series of 55 cases, only nine developed dilatation associated with partial involvement of the colon (Jalan et al 1969). The patient with a severe attack of colitis is ill, with fever, tachycardia and leukocytosis, and commonly the hemoglobin and serum albumin are reduced. Impending dilatation may be heralded by a reduction in the number of stools or occasionally by increased rectal bleeding (Marshak et al 1960). On examination of the abdomen, bowel sounds may be reduced and there may be distention with tenderness. Jalan et al (1969) found distention or tenderness in only 24 of 55 patients and radiological diagnosis is therefore all-important. Perforations usually occur in the transverse or pelvic colon and are often multiple. Prompt diagnosis is essential because of the likelihood of perforation if immediate treatment is not instituted. Once perforation has occurred, the surgical mortality is greatly increased. Whether dilatation of the colon is always the precursor of perforation is controversial. Goligher et al (1968) maintain that perforation can occur without dilatation, whereas others (Jalan et al 1969) think that this is rare. Massive hemorrhage and septicemia are other serious complications of dilatation.

*Radiological features*

An anteroposterior film is taken with the patient supine. Usually, the transverse colon is distended (Fig. 23.28); less frequently, there is distention of the descending and sigmoid colon. A lateral decubitus or an erect film should be taken to exclude free air. Dilatation is diagnosed when the diameter of the transverse colon is greater than 5.5 cm (Jones & Chapman 1969) or 6 cm (Neschis et al 1968). Recognition is aided by the observation that, under normal circumstances, the diameter of the transverse colon should not exceed that of the cecum or ascending colon. The haustral pattern is completely absent from the involved area and it is usual to see mucosal irregularities; these are mucosal islands indicating that the full thickness of the surrounding mucosa has been denuded.

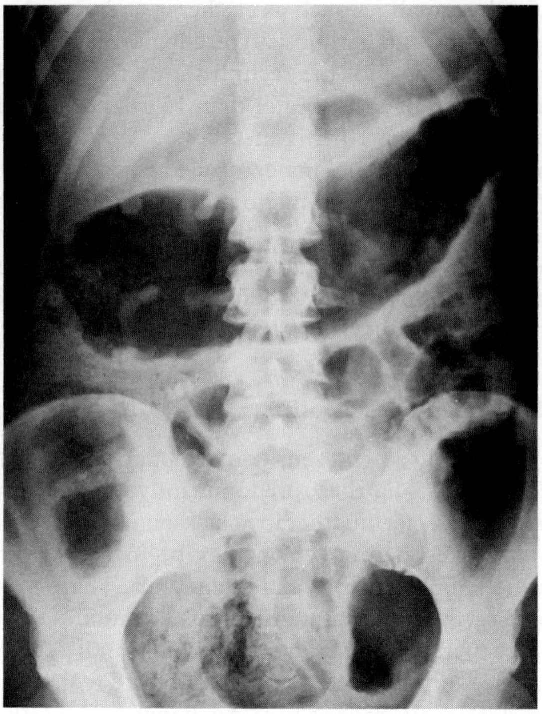

**Fig. 23.28** Ulcerative colitis with toxic dilatation. The transverse colon – the most common site – is particularly involved. Numerous inflammatory polyps cause filling defects when seen en face and marginal thumbprinting when seen in profile.

Other findings are subserosal radiolucent lines and dilatation of the small intestine. The radiolucent lines may represent submucosal accumulations of gas and they must be distinguished from the normal pericolic fat stripe, which is thinner, longer and more regular (Simon et al 1962). Marked distention of some areas of the colon associated with narrowed or normal areas elsewhere in the colon distinguishes this condition from mechanical obstruction in which the colon is uniformly distended proximal to the obstruction (Marshak et al 1960).

**Perforation without dilatation**

Perforation can occur without preceding acute colonic dilatation and in one series only 38% of patients with perforation had evidence of dilatation (Goligher et al 1968). However, others believe that perforation without previous dilatation is rare (Jalan et al 1969).

The incidence of perforation varies from 29% in patients with colonic dilatation to 3% in patients without dilatation (De Dombal et al 1965). In the Oxford series (Edwards & Truelove 1964) the incidence of perforation was 3.2% and of dilatation 1.6%. In the absence of toxic dilatation, the incidence of colonic perforation is similar in ulcerative colitis and Crohn's colitis (Greenstein & Aufses 1985). From their own data, Goligher et al (1968) estimate that a patient with a severe first attack of colitis has a

10% risk of perforation and a patient with total involvement has a 15% risk. The risk was 30% with severe total involvement. There is no evidence that corticosteroid therapy contributes to perforation.

*Clinical features*

Perforation occurs in severe and sometimes in moderate attacks of colitis, especially first attacks, but is less common in Crohn's disease. Perforation is difficult to recognize clinically with or without colonic dilatation. Because patients are usually on high doses of corticosteroids, symptoms and signs of perforation may be insidious and the diagnosis not suspected until several hours after it has taken place. The sudden appearance of tachycardia may be its only indication, although a few patients will complain of an increased abdominal or referred shoulder pain and signs of peritonitis. Sepsis may lead to shock. A high index of suspicion is therefore critical when managing patients with severe colitis with or without toxic megacolon, especially if the patient is undergoing steroid therapy, and any change in the patient's clinical status should alert the physician to the possibility of perforation. Plain radiographs of the abdomen often help in making the diagnosis; erect, supine and lateral decubitus views are taken.

## Hemorrhage

Massive hemorrhage, defined as bleeding requiring repeated transfusion, occurs in less than 4% of patients with ulcerative colitis and is often associated with toxic megacolon. Most bleeding abates during treatment but if it continues, surgery must be considered (p. 685).

## Stricture of the colon or rectum

Colonic strictures occur in Crohn's disease, ulcerative colitis and in ischemic colitis. Stricture may be defined as a constant, localized narrowing of the colon or rectum, often only a few centimeters in length but occasionally much longer.

*Incidence*

In ulcerative colitis, the incidence is about 11% (De Dombal et al 1966b), whereas in Crohn's disease stricture formation is extremely common.

*Pathology*

The pathogenesis of strictures in ulcerative colitis is controversial. There is some evidence that strictures are due to fibrosis of the submucosa, with muscular and mucosal hypertrophy (De Dombal et al 1966b). However, other data suggest that the problem is primarily muscular thickening and contraction, with hypertrophy of both the inner circular layer and the outer longitudinal layer of the muscularis (Goulston & McGovern 1969).

In Crohn's colitis, strictures result from fibrosis following transmural inflammation and they tend to be longer than those in ulcerative colitis.

In small intestinal Crohn's disease, partial obstruction is common and it may be due to either edema from inflammatory disease or stricture due to fibrostenotic disease.

*Clinical features*

Strictures may be single or multiple and occur at any site in the colon or rectum. Strictures in ulcerative colitis are more common in extensive disease and while they have been regarded as a feature of long-standing colitis, they can occur after one severe attack (De Dombal et al 1966b); in one series, one-third of strictures occurred within 5 years of the onset of the colitis (Edwards & Truelove 1964).

Often, the stricture does not add to the symptomatology of the colitis but is found on examining the rectum or at barium enema. In some patients, however, the stricture may be responsible for obstructive symptoms. While the vast majority of strictures are benign, it is difficult to determine when cancer is present. By barium enema, the stricture in ulcerative colitis is usually concentric with smooth contours and tapering margins, but it can also be eccentric with an irregular contour (Marshak & Lindner 1966).

*Management of strictures*

In patients with ulcerative colitis, a colonic stricture should raise concern for a possible underlying malignancy, even if colonoscopic biopsies do not show malignant or dysplastic changes. As the strictures in ulcerative colitis are usually mild, they are asymptomatic and do not require treatment on a symptomatic basis.

For patients with Crohn's disease, strictures are often symptomatic. A fibrotic, anastomotic stricture may be amenable to colonoscopic balloon dilatation (Blomberg et al 1991). However, dilatation of inflammatory strictures should not be attempted because of the risk of perforation. A surgical approach can be taken for small intestinal strictures with strictureplasty and for resection of anastomotic strictures.

## Anal fissure, abscess and fistula

*Incidence*

These complications are uncommon in ulcerative colitis (Table 23.11). Fistulae-in-ano were found in 4% of patients with ulcerative colitis (Edwards & Truelove 1964).

**Table 23.11** Incidence of fissure, abscess and fistula in ulcerative colitis

| Series | Patients | Incidence % | | |
|---|---|---|---|---|
| | | Fissure | Abscess | Fistula |
| Hightower et al 1958 | 220 | 0.5 | 2.0 | 3.0 |
| Edwards & Truelove 1964 | 624 | – | 4.2 | 7.7 |
| De Dombal et al 1966a | 465 | 12.3 | 6.0 | 7.6* |

*Including rectovaginal fistula

In contrast, anal lesions can occur in up to 82% of Crohn's disease (Baker & Milton-Thompson 1974); they occur in 50% or more of patients with diffuse colonic and rectal disease, but are less common in disease of the terminal ileum (Williams et al 1981).

*Clinical features*

In ulcerative colitis, the anorectal complications are often mild and usually occur in relation to an exacerbation.

The anal complication is the presenting feature in 25% of cases of Crohn's disease, often preceding colonic and small intestinal symptoms by months or years; fissure-in-ano is usually indolent, multiple and surrounded by edema and it is often difficult to tell if a fistula is present. Perianal abscess usually presents during an exacerbation of the disease; in contrast to ulcerative colitis, it occurs at some time in 25% of patients with Crohn's colitis and the abscess is likely to extend into the ischiorectal fossa. An abscess is suspected when there is pain aggravated by sitting and by defecation; ulceration and redness are seen close to the anus; digital examination is painful and an indurated area is felt external to the anal canal. Fistula-in-ano arises either as a result of a perianal abscess or as an insidious process. The patient complains of a discharge; on inspection, the opening of the fistula is near to the anus and on digital examination or proctoscopy, the internal opening is usually near to the anal valves. Multiple fistulae or a fistula at some distance from the anus suggest Crohn's disease.

### Enteric fistulae

Excluding perianal fistulae, enteric fistulae occur in 20–40% of cases, equally divided between internal and external fistulae (Williams 1972). Internal fistulae vary with the site of Crohn's disease; they occurred in 34% of patients with ileocolic disease, 16% with small intestinal and 17% with colonic disease (Farmer et al 1975). Fistulae are usually multiple. Internal fistulae occur between loops of bowel and between bowel and bladder, vagina or uterus. Less commonly, a fistula may develop between the ileum and the sigmoid colon, the ileum and the duodenum or the colon and the stomach or duodenum (Jacobson et al 1985). More usual causes of coloduodenal fistula are duodenal ulcer, appendix abscess, duodenal diverticulitis, foreign body perforation and trauma (Korelitz 1977, Ferguson & Moncure 1985). External fistulae usually occur after surgery for Crohn's disease. It is thought that the serosa of the inflamed gut adheres more easily to the incised parietal peritoneum and as a result the fistula develops through the scar. In a study of 47 fistulae occurring after surgery for Crohn's disease, Steinberg et al (1973) found a 5% incidence after resection, 13% after a bypass procedure, 11% after diagnostic laparotomy and 24% after appendicectomy. External fistulae to the abdominal wall may arise spontaneously but are much less common than fistulae arising after surgery.

### Intra-abdominal and pelvic abscess

An abscess develops from slow penetrating ulceration of the bowel wall. It may resolve by discharging into the lumen of the bowel or into another organ, resulting in a fistula. Occasionally, it points to the skin and requires drainage; an external fistula usually results.

Preoperative abscess occurred in 10% of all consecutive patients with Crohn's disease (Keighley et al 1982). Most were solitary and occurred in those with small bowel disease. Psoas abscess is also reported (Burul et al 1980). Usually the abscess is small and is not detected by investigations such as CT, gallium scan, leukocyte imaging or ultrasonography. Usually the white cell count is normal. Some patients have high serum alkaline phosphatase. In a majority of cases the abscess is unsuspected. In the same series of patients postoperative abscess occurred in 14%. Postoperative abscesses occur soon after operation or a few months later. The early ones are usually due to anastomotic dehiscence, fecal fistula or an infected hematoma. Late abscesses are often recurrent. The organisms usually isolated are *Escherichia coli, Bacteroides fragilis*, enterococci and *Streptococcus viridans*.

Treatment is resection of the diseased bowel in continuity with the abscess.

Liver abscess is a rare complication of Crohn's disease (Valero et al 1985, Mir-Madjlessi et al 1986).

## CARCINOMA ASSOCIATED WITH ULCERATIVE COLITIS

Patients with ulcerative colitis of more than 8–10 years duration and particularly those with extensive disease are at an increased risk of developing colorectal cancer (Kewenter et al 1978, Prior et al 1982, Ekbom et al 1990). The magnitude of the increased risk and the appropriate management are controversial. Patients who are at risk often have minimal if any symptoms of colitis, because patients with persistent active symptoms usually have undergone colectomy before the disease has been present for 8–10 years. It has been pointed out that only "interval" cancers should be included, i.e. those identified at review or at operation at least 1 year after the date first seen (Prior et al 1982). In adults, the overall mortality is about 11 times the expected rate in a sample of the general population matched for age and sex (De Dombal et al 1966b, Prior et al 1982). When only "interval" cancers were considered, there was a sixfold risk after 15 years from the diagnosis of ulcerative colitis (Prior et al 1982). Initial studies in referral centers report an increased risk of 10–20% per decade once the disease has lasted 10 years (Devroede 1980). Most recent estimates indicate a cumulative risk of cancer to be less – about 5% after 20 years of disease and 12% at 25 years (Prior et al 1982, Hendriksen et al 1985, Brostrom et al 1987, Gilat et al 1988, Ekbom et al 1990).

The cancer risk in left-sided colitis (not extending more proximal than the splenic flexure) is probably less than with more extensive disease, but more than in the general population (Dixon et al 1988).

### Cancer in the rectum following colectomy

After surgery, either colectomy with ileorectal anastomosis or total colectomy leaving a blind rectal pouch, an increased incidence of rectal cancer remains. Five rectal cancers occurred in 237 cases of ileorectal anastomosis (MacDougall 1964), an incidence 65 times greater than would be expected, and this increased incidence has been confirmed in other series (Aylett 1971, Hulten et al 1971, Baker et al 1978). In a review of the literature, Slaney & Brooke (1959) found that 34 of 304 cases of cancer in patients with ulcerative colitis had occurred after surgery.

### Site and multiplicity of cancers

In patients without colitis the majority of tumors occur in the rectum, whereas cancer of the colon in ulcerative colitis is evenly distributed. In figures prepared by Langman (1966) from several series, 76% of tumors occurred in the rectum and sigmoid in patients without colitis, whereas in patients with colitis only 47% occurred in the rectum and sigmoid. Cancer in patients with ulcerative colitis is often multiple, 20–25% in various series having more than one tumor.

### Pathology of cancer in ulcerative colitis

The carcinoma is sometimes flat and difficult to recognize macroscopically and may be associated with a stricture (Sommers 1985). Earlier reports indicated that carcinoma associated with ulcerative colitis is more aggressive than in noncolitic colon cancer. However, data from a prospective study indicated that colon cancer in patients with ulcerative colitis had a similar distribution of histologic grades, of clinical stages and prognosis as in patients with colon cancer without colitis (Lennard-Jones et al 1983).

### Dysplasia in ulcerative colitis

Dysplasia is the unequivocal neoplastic alteration of the colonic epithelium that remains confined within the basement membrane of the gland within which it arose (Riddell 1983) (Fig. 23.29). Early on, there is no macroscopic abnormality of the mucosa, but as dysplasia progresses the mucosa may become granular, nodular, even

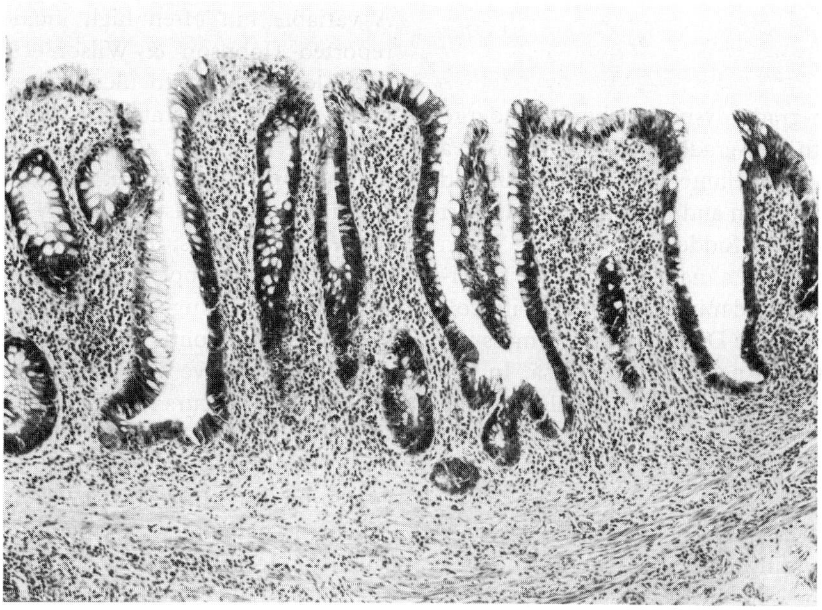

**Fig. 23.29** Dysplasia in ulcerative colitis. The mucosa shows abnormal crypts of villous configuration with marked atypia of the lining epithelial cells (hematoxylin and eosin, ×75).

polypoid and may develop plaques. The histology of a benign colorectal adenoma is histologically indistinct from dysplasia in ulcerative colitis and in some cases it is difficult for a pathologist to distinguish between the two. A dysplasia-associated lesion or mass (DALM) in the setting of ulcerative colitis is a marker for a high risk of malignancy.

There is a strong association between dysplasia and cancer in ulcerative colitis. When colectomy is performed in patients who had dysplasia alone on biopsies, 30–70% have a clinically unsuspected colon carcinoma (Rosenstock et al 1985). It may take up to 13 years or more for patients in whom dysplasia has been found to develop a colon cancer (Yardley & Keren 1974). Mapping studies using flow cytometry have shown that single or multiple aneuploid cell populations are often present in colons resected for ulcerative colitis with dysplasia or cancer and each population probably represents a clone of cells derived from an original abnormal cell (Levine et al 1991).

*Surveillance for dysplasia*

Several centers conducting surveillance programs recommend colonoscopy with multiple biopsies at 10 cm intervals throughout the colon, at 1–2 year intervals in patients who have had ulcerative colitis for more than 8 years. However, the current data do not permit a firm conclusion as to how often surveillance should be done and how many biopsies should be taken. Since left-sided colitis has a lesser risk of cancer, it may be reasonable to defer regular surveillance until after 12–15 years of disease. At colonoscopy, pseudopolyps should be avoided for surveillance biopsies. Strictures should be carefully evaluated with extensive biopsies, but cancer in a stricture should be suspected even if the biopsies do not show malignancy.

*Management of dysplasia*

Patients who have high-grade dysplasia should undergo colectomy. Patients with low-grade dysplasia without a mass or biopsies that are indefinite for dysplasia should undergo follow-up examination and biopsies after a short interval, less than 6 months (Riddell et al 1983). When low-grade dysplasia is found in a mass, it should be determined if the mass is located and mucosa involved with colitis (in which case the lesion is a DALM) or if the mass is a sporadic adenoma arising in non-colitic mucosa. In the latter case, the lesion is considered an incidental adenoma and not a DALM.

*Surgery versus surveillance for dysplasia*

A patient with long-standing ulcerative colitis who is a risk for cancer should be counseled about the options – colectomy (p. 687) or colonoscopic surveillance. It should be pointed out that surveillance is not an entirely safe approach (pp. 685 & 691) and it is possible that colon cancer may develop despite regular surveillance, with biopsies that show no evidence of dysplasia. The surgical option should be revisited periodically with patients who choose to enter a surveillance program.

## COLONIC CANCER IN CROHN'S COLITIS

Patients with long-standing Crohn's colitis are also at an increased risk of colon cancer (Hamilton 1985) pp. 696 & 1419, but probably at a much lower risk than patients with ulcerative colitis. In contrast to ulcerative colitis, there does not appear to be a correlation between the extent of disease and the risk of malignancy. Dysplasia occurs in Crohn's colitis. However, whether surveillance programs with colonosopic biopsies for dysplasia are indicated in long-standing Crohn's colitis is controversial.

## SYSTEMIC COMPLICATIONS

A wide variety of systemic manifestations have been described in ulcerative colitis and it is becoming apparent that most also occur in Crohn's disease of the colon. Many, such as those in the eyes, joints and skin, may be due to immune reactions. Occasionally, the "complication" or associated disease manifests itself before the bowel disease; six cases of undiagnosed ulcerative colitis were found in a study of 77 cases of ankylosing spondylitis (Jayson & Bouchier 1968). Thus, inflammatory bowel disease may already exist in an early form in patients who first present with symptoms of the complication.

### Skin lesions

A variable but often high incidence of skin lesions is reported (Johnson & Wilson 1969). Characteristically, these lesions tend to ulcerate, even erythema nodosum which does not ulcerate when associated with other conditions.

***Erythema nodosum.*** This occurs in about 2% of patients with colitis, especially women, and consists of tender red nodules, usually on the anterior tibial surfaces and also on the upper limbs (Edwards & Truelove 1964). They occur during exacerbations of colitis and usually subside as the colitis improves (Du Boulay & Whorwell 1982); they resolve with corticosteroid treatment and after colectomy. It occurs less frequently in Crohn's disease. In Crohn's disease, some lesions resembling erythema nodosum have been called nodular necrobiosis.

***Pyoderma gangrenosum.*** This is a rare condition except in patients with inflammatory bowel disease, in whom it occurs in 1–5% and in patients with arthritis (Kirsner 1979, Powell et al 1985). The lesion starts as a raised, red, tender area on the anterior aspect of the legs, bullae develop and ulcerate and the lesions spread, becoming extensive and chronic. They may occur elsewhere, such as the chest and face. The onset and course of pyoderma is not related to the onset or the activity of the colitis. The lesions may improve with systemic corticosteroids. Healing does not necessarily occur following colectomy.

***Papulonecrotic lesions.*** These are small scattered erythematous papules which suppurate to form small ulcers.

***Ulcerating erythematous plaques.*** These flat lesions, often 7–8 cm in diameter, occur on the shins and break down to produce a group of small ulcers.

***Psoriasis.*** Yates et al (1982) found that the prevalence of psoriasis was 11% in Crohn's disease and 6% in ulcerative colitis, compared to 1.5% in a control group.

## Joint complications

### *Arthritis*

This is common in both ulcerative colitis and Crohn's disease; its incidence is about 10% in colitis and up to 20% in Crohn's disease. The inflammatory process affects the synovium and can be distinguished from rheumatoid arthritis by the radiological findings which show soft tissue swelling without joint destruction and clinically, nodules and tendonitis are absent. The ESR is usually increased, but specific serologic markers for rheumatoid arthritis are absent. The synovial fluid is turbid, with a white count raised to 10 000–15 000/$mm^3$.

There is asymmetric large joint arthritis, with acutely painful and swollen joints, particularly knees, ankles and wrists; the arthritis is transient and recurrent. Exacerbations may last for 6–12 weeks and are often associated with the activity of the colitis. The joint symptoms usually improve with treatment of the colitis. However, in some patients the joint symptoms are the most disabling aspect of the illness, with continued symptoms despite improvement in the colitis. These patients may require nonsteroidal anti-inflammatory agents or prednisolone for control. The joint symptoms usually resolve following colectomy.

### *Ankylosing spondylitis*

This occurs in about 3% of patients with ulcerative colitis or Crohn's disease. Sacroiliitis is present in 20% of patients (Wright & Watkinson 1965, Haslock & Wright 1973), but usually this does not progress to ankylosing spondylitis. Ninety percent of patients with primary ankylosing spondylitis are males, whereas in ankylosing spondylitis associated with colitis, only 60% are male (Russell 1977).

Spondylitis and sacroiliitis are not related to the extent, severity or duration of the bowel disease and may precede the onset of colitis. Colectomy has no influence on their progression.

## Eye lesions

These are conjunctivitis, iritis and episcleritis (Korelitz & Coles 1967, Billson et al 1967). They are prone to occur early in the course of the disease, particularly during a severe attack. The iritis occurs in 0.5–3% of patients and is strongly associated with arthritis and sacroiliitis and also with erythema nodosum and aphthous ulceration. There is pain in the eyes, with blurred vision and headaches. The diagnosis is confirmed by slit-lamp examination which shows perilimbic erythema, conjunctival injection and cells in the anterior chamber. The condition resolves during remissions of colitis and is usually cured by colectomy. Episcleritis occurs in 3–4% of patients with inflammatory bowel disease, especially in Crohn's disease (Greenstein et al 1976). It is associated with disease activity and presents with burning and itching.

## Oral manifestations

### *Aphthous ulceration* (see also p. 144)

This is especially common during the acute attack of colitis and is usually eradicated by colectomy. Oral ulceration is common in Crohn's disease and Croft & Wilkinson (1972) reported an incidence of 6.1% in 332 cases. Sometimes, biopsy of the ulcer reveals histological evidence of Crohn's disease.

*Angular cheilitis and swelling of the lips* occurs in Crohn's disease (pp. 139 and 143).

*Other oral features of Crohn's disease* (p. 149 and Table 5.8).

*Pyostomatitis occurs in ulcerative colitis* (p. 149).

## Finger clubbing (Young 1966, Jalan et al 1970b, Kirschner et al 1978)

This occurs in 5–15% of patients with ulcerative colitis and in about half of patients with Crohn's disease (Fielding & Cooke 1971). It is associated with severe and extensive disease and regresses after surgical treatment.

## Nephrolithiasis and other urinary tract problems

Urinary calculi are more prone to occur in patients with ulcerative colitis (2–3%) and Crohn's disease (6–10%), both before and after colectomy, than in the general population (Fleckenstein et al 1977). Amyloid occurred in 1% of patients with inflammatory bowel disease, particularly those with Crohn's disease (Greenstein et al 1976), but is less frequent than this in other series (Lowdell et al 1986).

Kyle (1983) studied 90 patients with urinary tract symptoms in 429 patients with Crohn's disease during the period 1955–80. Of these, 70 had cystitis, nine had renal or ureteric calculi, nine had hydronephrosis, nine had ileovesical fistulae, three had a retroperitoneal abscess, one female had retention of urine and one male had a rectourethral fistula.

Cystitis occurred especially in females with long-established Crohn's disease. The predisposing factor may be the presence of inflamed bowel lying close to the bladder. Of the nine patients with renal or ureteric calculi, seven had had previous intestinal resection and oxalate stones (p. 452). Radionuclide renography suggests that minor degrees of ureteral stasis are common in Crohn's disease (Schofield et al 1968). Hydronephrosis can occur in either kidney and is most likely to develop when Crohn's disease recurs after resection (Kyle 1983).

Crohn's disease is the commonest cause of ileovesical fistula. The problem often presents with a minor attack of cystitis followed by a sudden increase in frequency, strangury and pneumaturia.

## Malnutrition

Malnutrition in Crohn's disease usually results from a combination of malabsorption, poor appetite and food intake, increased catabolism and loss of protein and secretions from the bowel and fistulae (Heatley 1984). The growth retardation, which occurs in one-fifth of children with Crohn's disease, is due largely to poor caloric intake superimposed on a deficiency of protein, vitamins and minerals (Kirschner et al 1978).

In patients with chronic diarrhea, sodium, potassium and water depletion are common; the serum potassium level is a poor indication of intracellular potassium and it is reasonable to assume potassium depletion. Magnesium and zinc (Sturniolo et al 1980) deficiency may also occur. The absorption of vitamin D may be impaired and there may be evidence of osteomalacia (Sitrin et al 1980). Plasma 25-hydroxycholecalciferol is reduced in patients who have active disease and are undernourished (Harries et al 1985) and osteoporosis is very common in patients with small intestinal disease when resections have been performed (Compston et al 1987). Anemia is common (Beeken 1975) and is due to iron, folic acid or vitamin $B_{12}$ deficiency or a combination of these. Folic acid absorption is impaired by mucosal disease and by sulfasalazine.

The judicious use of absorption tests may define the absorptive abnormalities. With extensive involvement of the jejunum, folic acid absorption (Cox et al 1958) and D-xylose absorption can be abnormal, although they remain unaffected in most patients (Gerson et al 1973). With ileal disease, vitamin $B_{12}$ malabsorption depends upon the extent of involvement, 60–90 cm needing to be resected or diseased for malabsorption to occur (Gerson et al 1973), but D-xylose absorption is normal (Dotevall & Kock 1968). The status of the enterohepatic circulation of bile acids can be tested by $^{75}$SeHCAT.

## Lactase deficiency

Many series before 1969 reported that 50% of patients with colitis suffered from this form of malabsorption, but the studies of Gudmand-Hoyer & Jarnum (1970) and Newcomer & McGill (1967) found an incidence not much greater than in the population at large. There is also disagreement as to whether the malabsorption is transient during the acute stage of the disease, when the histological changes in the small intestine are most marked, or whether it can be a chronic feature. Pena & Truelove (1973) found that some patients with ulcerative colitis had permanent hypolactasia, but the number was no greater than would be expected in the general population. However, other patients had hypolactasia only during a moderate to severe attack of colitis. Whatever the incidence or mechanism of the deficiency, a milk-free diet is beneficial in some patients with ulcerative colitis. Wright & Truelove (1965) showed that in comparison to patients on a control diet, those on a milk-free diet had fewer relapses and symptoms and that one in five patients benefited from the diet; nevertheless, it is possible that the beneficial effect in some patients is due to mechanisms other than lactase deficiency since Gudmand-Hoyer & Jarnum (1970) demonstrated a clinical improvement in patients receiving a milk-free diet who did not have lactose malabsorption.

## Thrombosis and embolism

Venous thrombosis occurs in 5% of patients during the first attack of colitis (Edwards & Truelove 1964) and in 1.3% of 7199 patients with ulcerative colitis or Crohn's disease (Talbot et al 1986); this is usually in the leg veins but may be widespread and rarely includes the cerebral veins (Borda et al 1973) and the hepatic veins, thus causing the Budd–Chiari syndrome (Chesner et al 1986). Embolism and arterial thrombosis occur occasionally, particularly after surgery (Talbot et al 1986). Abnormalities of the coagulation mechanism may offer an explanation for these phenomena. Thrombocytosis occurs frequently (Morowitz et al 1968, Talstad et al 1973). In their study, Talstad et al (1973) showed that the thrombocytosis is proportional to the activity of the disease and that there is a reduced half-life and an increased turnover of platelets. Thrombocytosis occurs in both ulcerative colitis and Crohn's disease of the small bowel. There is an increase in factor VIII deficiency, which results in accelerated thromboplastin generation, and there is also an increase in fibrinogen. These abnormalities are related to the activity and the extent of the disease (Lee et al 1968). At the same time, other patients can show a coagulation defect, a prolonged one-stage prothrombin time due to decreases in factors VII and X as a result of vitamin K deficiency.

### Hepatobiliary disease

Hepatic enzyme abnormalities are not uncommon in patients with inflammatory bowel disease. Some of the abnormalities are due to medications, malnutrition and viral hepatitis related to blood transfusions. Primary sclerosing cholangitis is the main hepatic disorder associated with ulcerative colitis and Crohn's disease. A mean of 77% of patients with primary sclerosing cholangitis have inflammatory bowel disease and most have ulcerative colitis and a small minority have Crohn's disease. In most patients the onset of inflammatory bowel disease precedes the development of the primary sclerosing cholangitis, but in some the reverse is the case. Primary sclerosing cholangitis can develop years after proctocolectomy for ulcerative colitis (Cangemi et al 1989). Patients with inflammatory bowel disease are also at a greater risk for cholangiocarcinoma, which usually develops in the setting of primary sclerosing cholangitis. This is discussed further on p. 1101.

### Other complications

Cutaneous vasculitis (Ball & Goldman 1976), pulmonary vasculitis (Forrest & Shearman 1975) and autoimmune hemolytic anemia (Altman et al 1979) have been described. There is an increased risk of ulcerative colitis.

### Pregnancy and inflammatory bowel disease

Because inflammatory bowel disease commonly occurs in young adults, it is not unusual for a clinician to encounter women with inflammatory bowel disease who are pregnant or who are contemplating pregnancy. In the pregnant patient, the potential of adverse effects that tests and treatment may have on the fetus must be considered. Likewise, the effects of pregnancy and delivery on the course of the disease must be addressed.

#### *Fertility*

Recent reports indicate that women with ulcerative colitis and Crohn's disease have normal fertility. However, most large series include twice as many women with inflammatory bowel disease in remission at the onset of pregnancy as compared to those with active disease, so there may actually be a decreased fertility rate in patients with active disease (Donaldson 1985, Mayberry & Weterman 1986).

#### *Effect of inflammatory disease on the course of pregnancy*

For both ulcerative colitis and Crohn's disease, pregnancy is at least twice as likely to end in spontaneous abortion if the bowel disease is active at the time of conception than if the disease is quiescent. Cesarean sections are needed mainly for obstetric indications and are usually indicated for patients with active perineal Crohn's disease as well. Vaginal deliveries are reported in women who have previously undergone proctocolectomy with ileal reservoir–anal anastomosis for ulcerative colitis. Emergency surgery for fulminant colitis or for intestinal obstruction can be undertaken during pregnancy without ill effects to the fetus (Anderson et al 1987).

The stool and blood studies, sigmoidoscopic examination and rectal biopsies that are done in most patients to diagnose inflammatory bowel disease can be performed safely in the pregnant patient. More invasive studies such as colonoscopy or barium enema should be avoided unless they are essential in the management of a patient (Korelitz 1992).

#### *Medications during pregnancy*

Sulfasalazine and corticosteroids appear safe during pregnancy. However, sulfasalazine may temporarily impair male fertility due to effects on spermatogenesis. Other aminosalicylates do not affect male fertility. Although azathioprine and 6-mercaptopurine have been used in patients with inflammatory bowel disease at the time of conception and during pregnancy without apparent ill-effects (Alstead et al 1990), most physicians recommend discontinuing these drugs 3 months before proceeding with conception. Metronidazole and methotrexate should be avoided during pregnancy. Cyclosporin has been taken during pregnancy, primarily in organ transplant recipients, with the only consistent abnormalities of prematurity and low birth weights. Nutritional therapy should be prompt and aggressive in the malnourished pregnant patient with inflammatory bowel disease (Teahon et al 1991).

#### *Effect of pregnancy on the activity of inflammatory bowel disease*

About 30% of women with quiescent inflammatory bowel disease who become pregnant have exacerbations of the disease during pregnancy, which is about the same risk in nonpregnant patients over a 9 month period. Exacerbations of colitis during pregnancy occur most often during the first trimester and during the immediate postpartum period. Pregnancy does not appear to have any consistent effect on the activity of Crohn's disease, except that women with active disease at conception are likely to have continued activity of the disease throughout the pregnancy.

## MEDICAL TREATMENT OF ULCERATIVE AND CROHN'S COLITIS

In this section, treatment options for ulcerative colitis and Crohn's disease are reviewed and strategies are presented for the management of disease ranging from mild limited involvement to severe extensive activity.

## Aminosalicylates

*Sulfasalazine* (Peppercorn 1984)

Sulfasalazine (Salazopyrin, Azulfidine) is a diazo compound of salicylic acid and sulfapyridine and is of value in the acute stage of ulcerative colitis and also prevents exacerbations. It is effective in active Crohn's disease but does not prevent relapse in quiescent Crohn's disease or after surgical treatment (Lennard-Jones & Powell-Tuck 1979). It is usually given orally but can be used in enema or suppository form.

***Metabolism and mode of action*** (Azad Khan & Truelove 1976). After ingestion, 10–30% of the drug is absorbed from the small intestine and the remainder passes into the colon, where the azo link is split by colonic bacteria to produce sulfapyridine and 5-aminosalicylic acid (5-ASA). Most of the former is absorbed and about 80% appears in the urine as metabolites of sulfapyridine. 5-ASA is excreted mainly in the feces as Ac-5-ASA, the acetylation occurring in the bowel wall and in the lumen by the action of colonic bacteria. This sequence of events has been confirmed in two ways: firstly, in germ-free rats most of the sulfasalazine is recovered unchanged in the feces; secondly, in ileostomy patients there is a marked decrease in the concentration of sulfapyridine in the serum and urine (Das et al 1974). The peak serum level of sulfasalazine occurs 3–5 h after a single dose whereas the sulfapyridine peak is reached at 12–24 h. During treatment a steady state of serum sulfapyridine is achieved in about 5 days.

Its mode of action is not understood. Studies on mice (Hanngren et al 1963) suggest that both sulfasalazine and 5-aminosalicylic acid may have an affinity for the connective tissue of the colon and their increased concentration might be important for their therapeutic effect. 5-aminosalicylic acid is the effective part of the molecule because it or sulfasalazine given rectally results in improvement in proctitis, whereas sulfapyridine does not (Azad Khan et al 1977, Van Hees et al 1980). Both sulfasalazine and 5-aminosalicylic acid act on the metabolism of arachidonic acid and may also have the ability to remove oxygen radicals (Miyachi et al 1987).

***Dosage.*** The drug should be given after food in a dosage of 1 g 2–4 times a day. Treatment is started with 500 mg or 1 g the first day and gradually increased in similar increments to the final dose, to avoid dose-related side-effects. Enteric-coated tablets may be given to patients who experience nausea or abdominal discomfort.

***Clinical effects.*** Several controlled trials have demonstrated that remission or improvement in the acute phase of colitis occurs in about two-thirds of patients, whereas only one-third respond to a placebo. There is improvement in the systemic symptoms and the appearance of the rectal mucosa. However, improvement is not as dramatic as that produced by corticosteroid therapy.

The main value of the drug is in preventing exacerbations. Misiewicz et al (1965) studied two comparable groups of patients with ulcerative colitis. In the treated group of 34 patients who received 2 g/day, 24 were still in remission after 1 year whereas in the placebo group only seven of 33 were still in remission (Fig. 23.30). Maintenance therapy for periods of longer than 1 year has been studied in two trials. In one trial, a continuation of the therapy beyond 1 year provided no additional benefit. In the other trial, it was found that patients who were changed to placebo after 1 year's therapy had more than four times the relapse rate of those who continued to receive sulfasalazine (Lennard-Jones & Powell-Tuck 1979).

The NCCDS showed that sulfasalazine was effective in Crohn's colitis and ileocolitis, but in contrast to its effect in ulcerative colitis, it does not prevent relapse or recurrence (Summers et al 1979). A benefit in Crohn's ileitis has not been demonstrated.

Sulfasalazine suppositories which contain 1 g sulfasalazine can be used for mild proctitis. In a controlled trial, suppositories were used for 28 days (Watkinson 1967); 15 of 18 receiving the drug improved, compared to five of 18 who received a placebo suppository. No side-effects were reported, but the drug stains clothing and is unpopular with patients. Enemas which contain 3 g sulfasalazine in 100 ml spread throughout the colon and are also effective (Palmer et al 1981, Kruis et al 1982). Sulfasalazine suppository and enema preparations are not approved for use in the US.

***Side-effects.*** In various studies, side-effects occur in 20–40% of patients who receive 2–4 g/day of sul-

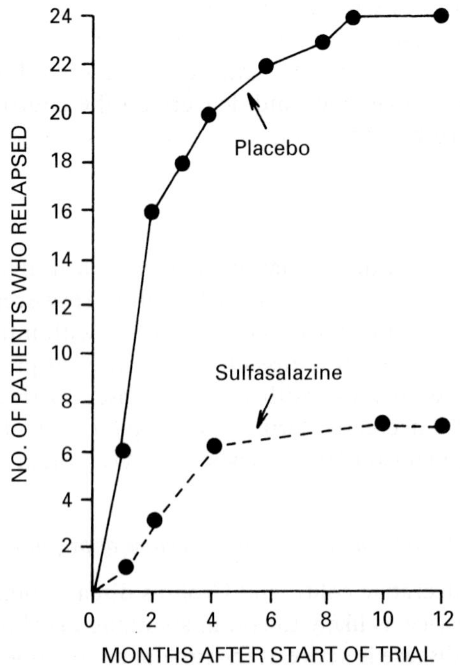


**Fig. 23.30** Relapse in 33 patients receiving placebo or 34 patients receiving sulfasalazine (Misiewicz et al 1965).

fasalazine. Side-effects increase with increasing dosage of the drug and with any given dosage, they are more likely to occur in patients who are slow acetylators of the drug.

Nausea and epigastric discomfort are the most common complaints. They usually occur soon after starting treatment, they have been attributed to gastric irritation and may be avoided by the use of enteric-coated tablets. Nausea may occasionally develop after many months of treatment and this is usually due to a high level of sulfapyridine; stopping the drug for a week and restarting with a lower dose is a remedy. Some patients complain of headache and dizziness, particularly with exercise.

A variety of hematological disorders may occur. Leukopenia, agranulocytosis and aplastic anemia are rare but serious complications which contraindicate further use of the drug. Hemolytic anemia, usually of the Heinz body type, often starts within a few weeks of starting treatment. The drug should be stopped but can often be reintroduced at a lower dose after a few weeks. In other patients, there may be transient reticulocytosis without evidence of hemolysis. Sulfasalazine may interfere with the absorption of folic acid and deficiency may occur; supplements should be given to patients on maintenance therapy. Pancytopenia due to acute megaloblastic arrest secondary to severe folate deficiency has been described (Logan et al 1986). Cyanosis can occur due to methemoglobinemia and/or sulfhemoglobulinemia.

Other side-effects are drug fever, lymphadenopathy, arthralgia and rash which are often due to hypersensitivity and usually preclude further use of the drug. The scarlatiniform rash usually begins during the first 2 weeks of treatment. Patients with these reactions can be desensitized by giving sulfasalazine 1 mg/day, which is gradually increased (Holdsworth 1981). Rarely, a form of fibrosing alveolitis may occur, particularly in the early months of treatment, and cause dyspnea, cough, weight loss and fever; opacities are seen on the chest radiograph. Cholestatic hepatitis may occur. Rarely sulfasalazine may be responsible for an exacerbation of colitis (Schwartz et al 1982, Chakraborty et al 1987) and this is probably due to salicylate sensitivity.

Sulfasalazine causes oligospermia, reduced sperm motility and an increased proportion of abnormal sperm. The resulting infertility is reversible when the drug is stopped (O'Morain et al 1984b).

The incidence of nausea, vomiting, anorexia, headache, arthritis and arthralgia caused by sulfasalazine in patients with Crohn's disease in the NCCDS was no greater than in patients receiving placebo (Singleton et al 1979a).

### *5-Aminosalicylic acid derivatives* (5-ASA)

The side-effects of sulfasalazine are due largely to the sulfapyridine moiety. 5-ASA is effective when given topically but is unstable in aqueous solution. Thus, several pharmaceutical preparations have been developed to deliver 5-ASA to the colon without the use of sulfapyridine. These use another carrier molecule or join two molecules of 5-ASA together.

#### *Azodisalicylate*

This consists of two molecules of 5-ASA joined together by an azo bond. The drug is given orally in a dose of 250 mg four times daily after food. There is very little absorption of the parent drug. Bacteria in the colon split the bond, releasing the two molecules of 5-ASA (Lauritsen et al 1984). The 5-ASA is excreted in the feces mainly as Ac-5-ASA. When a trial of azodisalicylate or placebo was carried out in 160 patients who were intolerant to sulfasalazine for a variety of reasons, most could tolerate it and the relapse rate was less than on placebo (Sandberg-Gertzen et al 1986b). However, azodisalicylate does cause diarrhea in some patients. When given to patients with ileostomy, it increases ileostomy fluid output (Sandberg-Gertzen et al 1986a) and its side-effect of diarrhea may therefore be due to an increased flow of fluid into the colon. The diarrhea usually occurs soon after starting therapy. Adaptation occurs in some patients and so the drug should be stopped and then restarted in a small dose which is slowly increased over 1 week. Alternatively, the drug can be started in a small dose and increased every 2–3 days.

#### *Mesalazine*

This is single molecule 5-ASA with delayed release or controlled release coatings so that the drug is delivered to specific sites in the gut. Asacol® contains 400 mg of 5-ASA coated with an acrylic, eudragit-S, that releases the drug when the pH rises to greater than 7, usually in the region of the ileocecal valve. It is effective in the treatment of active ulcerative colitis in doses up to 4.8 g/d (Schroeder et al 1987) and in the maintenance of remission (Dew et al 1982, Riley et al 1988). Claversal®, not available in the US, has a different coating, eudragit-L, that dissolves more proximally in the gut at pH >6. Pentasa® contains 5-ASA microencapsulated in ethylcellulose and is gradually released throughout the small intestine and colon and has been shown to be effective in the treatment of ulcerative colitis (Hanauer et al 1993).

Other preparations involve the linking of 5-ASA to a carrier molecule to form ipsalazide or balsalazide (Chan et al 1983) and these are not approved for use in the US. To date, efficacy of oral 5-ASA preparations in the treatment of active Crohn's disease has not been published.

#### *5-ASA enemas* (Campieri et al 1985, Sutherland et al 1987)

These are poorly absorbed and so probably exert a local

effect. They are as effective as 100 mg hydrocortisone enemas and are available in a 4 g preparation in the US.

*5-ASA suppositories*

These are effective in the treatment of proctitis with demonstrated coating to 15 cm above the anal verge (Williams 1990). They are available in a 500 mg form and can be used 1–3 times daily.

## Corticosteroids

Corticosteroids are effective in the treatment of both ulcerative colitis and Crohn's disease and induce remissions in up to 80% of cases. Oral, intravenous, enema and suppository preparations are available.

*Pharmacology*

Oral prednisolone is absorbed from the small intestine with peak blood levels after 3 h and a plasma half-life of 200 min, partly bound to albumin and $\alpha_1$-globulin transcortin. The biological half-life is much longer, probably 18–36 h. The free prednisolone is the metabolically active form. Plasma levels of prednisolone after rectal administration of prednisolone-21-phosphate are similar to those after the same oral dose (Powell-Tuck et al 1976). ACTH acts by releasing endogenous cortisol from the adrenal glands, but has more mineralocorticoid and androgenic side-effects than prednisolone. Corticosteroids have an anti-inflammatory effect, probably by acting at several different points in the inflammatory process. Furthermore, they stimulate water and sodium absorption in the distal colon, which reduces diarrhea (Sandle et al 1986).

*New corticosteroids*

Two strategies have been used in the development of new formulations to deliver corticosteroids to the site of disease without suppression of the pituitary adrenal axis. In one approach, prednisolone metasulfobenzoate, a poorly absorbed steroid, has been coated with the pH-dependent acrylic polymer eudragit-S to deliver the drug to the colon for treatment of ulcerative colitis (Ford et al 1992). Use of this preparation in Crohn's colitis has not been reported. The second strategy is use of rapidly metabolized steroids that have limited systemic bioavailability. Although several compounds have been tested in clinical trials, of primary clinical interest at present is budesonide, a nonhalogenated glucocorticosteroid that is currently used in inhaled and intranasal forms for the treatment of asthma and allergic rhinitis. Budesonide enemas, suppositories and coated controlled ileal release tablets have been used in clinical trials in inflammatory bowel disease and appear promising (Löfberg et al 1993).

*Systemic corticosteroids*

Controlled trials have shown that corticosteroids are more effective than placebo in acute ulcerative colitis. In the first trial (Truelove & Witts 1955), cortisone 100 mg day induced remission in 40% of patients, compared to 16% in the placebo group. For first attacks, 42% achieved remission, whereas only 26% of relapsing cases responded, whatever the degree of severity of the colitis. Similar results have been obtained in subsequent controlled trials. Initial doses of prednisolone 40–60 mg per day are more effective than 20 mg per day (Baron et al 1962). Maintenance treatment of ulcerative colitis with corticosteroids is not recommended because of the risk of side-effects. Controlled trials (Truelove & Witts 1959, Lennard-Jones et al 1965) showed that cortisone 50 mg/day or prednisolone 15 mg/day failed to prevent relapse of ulcerative colitis.

Corticosteroids are used for moderate to severe Crohn's colitis and mild to severe Crohn's ileitis. Systemic steroids are particularly helpful for extraintestinal manifestations of inflammatory bowel disease including polyarthritis, iritis, oral aphthous ulcers and erythema nodosum.

For systemic therapy, the alternatives are ACTH 40 units/day by continuous intravenous infusion (or 40 units of corticotrophin gel by intramuscular injection twice daily), hydrocortisone 300–400 mg/day by slow intravenous infusion or prednisolone 40–60 mg/day orally in divided doses for initial treatment. The physician should be aware that absorption of oral prednisolone can be variable, particularly with small intestinal Crohn's disease (Shaffer et al 1983). The NCCD study confirmed the value of corticosteroids in active Crohn's ileocolitis, but efficacy in active Crohn's colitis could not be determined because of the small number of patients (Summers et al 1979). Corticosteroids can also be used in cases of subacute obstruction, particularly in patients with a short history of Crohn's disease, since these symptoms may be due to edema and inflammation rather than fibrosis. Corticosteroids should be avoided if there is clinical or radiological evidence of chronic stenosis or abscess formation and they must be used cautiously when there is an abdominal mass since this may actually be an abscess; the presence of a fistula is not a contraindication when corticosteroids are indicated for active or extensive disease. Maintenance treatment with retention enemas on two successive nights each week also failed to prevent relapses (Truelove 1958). In patients with Crohn's ileocolitis or colitis, both before and after surgery, maintenance corticosteroids failed to prevent recurrence (Summers et al 1979).

*Adverse effects of corticosteroids*

Side-effects from systemic steroid therapy depend on the dose and duration of therapy and are a common source of morbidity. In a group of patients with ulcerative colitis (Goligher et al 1968), 42 of 296 patients (15%) developed side-effects: 25 had moon face, seven had severe mental disturbance, four had severe electrolyte imbalance, three had severe osteoporosis and two had gross obesity. In the NCCDS (Summers et al 1979) minor side-effects were noted, including moon face, acne, striae, hirsutism, easy bruising and petechiae. Joint disease due to aseptic necrosis is an uncommon, disabling complication. Ocular side-effects include cataracts and increased intraocular pressure. Other adverse effects are suppurative perianal or skin conditions, moniliasis (Truelove & Witts 1959) and other fungal infections. The development of hypercortisonism (fluid retention, hypertension, glycosuria, mooning and hirsutism) was more common with ACTH than with cortisone (Truelove & Witts 1959).

Corticosteroids do not appear to have an adverse effect on the outcome of subsequent surgery. In a retrospective study of 140 patients, Jalan et al (1970c) found no difference in operative results, complications and healing of the perineal wound between those treated and those not treated with corticosteroids, provided the comparison was between patients with the same severity of colitis. However, Watts et al (1966a) found that 50% of patients who had received corticosteroids had an unhealed perineal wound at 6 months, whereas only 19% of those not treated with corticosteroids remained unhealed.

Corticosteroids do not increase risk of bowel perforation or mask the presence of a pre-existing perforation. Goldgraber et al (1957) showed that perforation occurred twice as often in a period before corticosteroid therapy than in a 7-year period when corticosteroids were used. In patients with toxic dilatation, corticosteroids did not increase the risk of perforation (Jalan et al 1969).

*Topical corticosteroids*

In patients with distal ulcerative colitis, 100 mg hydrocortisone enemas daily for 1 week resulted in improvement in 60% of patients and after 3 weeks of daily treatment there was apparent remission in 72% (Truelove 1958). Similar results have been obtained with prednisolone-21-phosphate (20 mg). A foam base (Cortifoam®) may be used in those patients who find liquid enemas difficult to retain. Corticosteroid enema preparations produce some adrenal suppression: Farmer & Schumacher (1970) found that 30–50% of a hydrocortisone enema was absorbed in patients with ulcerative colitis and that there was temporary adrenal suppression in some patients. The clinical response to treatment was more rapid than after oral therapy and enemas appear to exert an effect locally rather than systemically. Hydrocortisone enemas are distributed in the left colon as high as the splenic flexure, as demonstrated by radio-opaque marker studies (Matts & Gaskell 1961) and foam preparations reach the sigmoid colon (Farthing et al 1979). Budesonide enemas appear to have better efficacy than prednisolone enemas, with less suppression of the pituitary adrenal axis (Danielsson et al 1987). Budesonide enemas are not approved for use in the United States.

Topical corticosteroids are indicated for the treatment of colitis of mild to moderate severity. However, the patient with severe colitis is usually unable to retain the enema for a sufficient time and insertion of the rigid enema tip could injure markedly inflamed mucosa.

*Corticosteroid suppositories*

These contain prednisolone-21-phosphate and are used for distal proctitis. In one trial (Lennard-Jones et al 1962), 14 of 16 patients treated in this way improved symptomatically, whereas only nine of 23 patients treated with an inert suppository improved. In proctocolitis, as would be expected, the suppository is not as effective as the corticosteroid enema (Watkinson 1961). These are not approved for use in the United States.

*Azathioprine and 6-mercaptopurine*

Azathioprine and 6-mercaptopurine are both purine analogs that disrupt several steps in purine ribonucleotide synthesis and in the DNA synthesis phase of the cell cycle (Hawthorne & Hawkey 1989). Azathioprine differs from 6-mercaptopurine only in that it contains a methylnitroimidazole side group that is removed by hepatic enzymatic action, yielding 6-mercaptopurine. Therefore, the mechanisms of action and pharmacologic effects of the two compounds are thought to be identical. There are clinical trials that have addressed the question of whether one of the agents has therapeutic advantages over the other. These agents are further metabolized by multiple enzymatic pathways including xanthine oxidase. Thus, when the xanthine oxidase inhibitor allopurinol is given, the dose of azathioprine must be reduced. Another pathway for catabolism is via the red cell enzyme, thiopurine methyltransferase (TPMT). Levels of TPMT are controlled by genetic factors and one in 300 people has very low levels and is at increased risk for toxicity from these drugs (Lennard et al 1989). The blood TPMT level can be measured in patients for whom therapy is contemplated. The mechanism of action of these drugs in the treatment of inflammatory bowel disease is unknown, although in Crohn's disease the effect may be to suppress natural killer (NK) cell cytotoxicity (Shih et al 1982).

The most common side-effect of these purine analogs is bone marrow suppression with cytopenias, either leukopenia, anemia or pancytopenia, and these complications are rare if the dose is kept below 2.5 mg/kg body weight per day. The blood counts should be monitored regularly as long as patients remain on therapy (Connell et al 1992).

Other side-effects are headache, nausea, fever, skin rashes, arthralgias and hepatitis. Pancreatitis occurs in up to 15% of patients and is usually mild and typically resolves within a few days of withdrawing therapy (Present et al 1989). Experience with the drug in patients with renal transplants suggests that its use increases the risk of malignant tumors, although an increased risk in patients treated for inflammatory bowel disease has not been demonstrated (Present et al 1989).

These drugs have not been shown in a placebo-controlled trial to be efficacious in the treatment of active ulcerative colitis, although a steroid-sparing effect has been demonstrated (Rosenberg et al 1975). A recent trial showed benefit of azathioprine in maintaining remission in ulcerative colitis (Hawthorne et al 1992).

In Crohn's disease, multiple controlled trials during the 1970s gave conflicting results regarding efficacy of azathioprine and 6-mercaptopurine, but the negative studies may have been a result of an inadequate length of treatment (Present et al 1980). The mean time to clinical response with 6-mercaptopurine is 3 months, with a range of 2 weeks to 9 months, and 20% of patients do not respond until after 4 months of therapy. The purine analogs are indicated for patients with chronic active Crohn's disease who are steroid dependent or steroid resistant and for patients with fistulous disease. A starting dose of 50 mg/day can be used and if no response is seen in 3–4 months then the dose can gradually be increased in 25 mg/day increments each month up to as high as 1.5 mg/kg/day. Because of the delay in the onset of action, corticosteroids should be continued for 2 months then slowly tapered.

### *Cyclosporin*

Cyclosporin, a cyclic oligopeptide, inhibits immune responses mediated by T-lymphocytes. It has been shown in a 3-month controlled trial to be effective when used orally in the treatment of steroid-unresponsive Crohn's disease (Brynskov et al 1989) although the long-term benefit (for 6 months) could not be established in a follow-up study by the same group (Brynskov et al 1991). The addition of low-dose (2.5 mg/kg/day) cyclosporin to conventional therapy does not provide any benefit in the treatment of Crohn's disease (Feagan et al 1994). In several uncontrolled trials, intravenous cyclosporin has healed Crohn's fistulae in a matter of a few days or 1–2 weeks (Sandborn & Tremaine 1992, Hanauer & Smith 1993).

In patients with severe ulcerative colitis unresponsive to high-dose steroids, intravenous cyclosporin in a dose of 4 mg/kg/day was effective in a placebo-controlled trial in avoiding the need for urgent surgery (Lichtiger et al 1994) although the toxicity and unproven benefit are drawbacks to this approach. Cyclosporin enemas are not effective in the treatment of distal ulcerative colitis (Sandborn et al 1994).

Cyclosporin therapy has numerous potential side-effects including a reversible decrease in the glomerular filtration rate of about 20%, neurological symptoms in about 20% of patients, including a risk of seizures in patients with a total cholesterol level below 120 mg/dl, hypertrichosis, nausea, vomiting, gingival hyperplasia and hyperglycemia, among others.

### *Methotrexate*

Methotrexate, a folic acid antagonist, has been reported in open trials to be beneficial in patients with steroid-resistant Crohn's disease (Kozarek et al 1989), and it also has steroid-sparing effects (Baron et al 1993). There is no evidence for a long-term benefit in Crohn's disease and its usefulness in ulcerative colitis has not been established.

### *Metronidazole*

Metronidazole produced clinical improvement in patients with chronic perineal Crohn's disease (Brant et al 1982). Pain, tenderness, erythema and swelling all improved and in some patients the perineal wound healed completely. The dose used in this study was 20 mg/kg/day divided into 3–5 doses. A reduction in dosage was followed by relapse. A comparative study of metronidazole 0.4 g b.d. and sulfasalazine 1.5 g b.d. in active Crohn's disease indicated that metronidazole was slightly more effective (Ursing et al 1982), but in other studies it conferred no additional advantage to sulfasalazine and corticosteroids (Blichfeldt et al 1978). The side-effects are a metallic taste, dark urine and occasional nausea and vomiting. Peripheral neuropathy occurs especially with higher doses and in children (Duffy et al 1985) but is usually reversible.

### *Other therapies*

A variety of other treatments for inflammatory bowel disease have been tested in recent years. Nicotine patches were effective in patients with ulcerative colitis (Pullan et al 1994). Bismuth foam enemas were as effective as 5-ASA enemas (Pullan et al 1993). Disodium cromoglycate showed conflicting results when used in trials of patients with ulcerative colitis (Binder et al 1981). Leukotriene B4 antagonists such as fish oil preparations and Zileuton were not effective in controlled trials for the treatment of ulcerative colitis. The use of enteral and parenteral nutrition to induce remission is discussed on p. 629.

### *Treatment of severe ulcerative colitis*

Patients with severely active ulcerative colitis have more than six stools a day with visible blood, fever, tachycardia, anemia and an increased sedimentation rate (Truelove & Witts 1955) (p. 656). These patients should be hospitalized, enteric infection should be excluded with stool examinations for ova and parasites, a stool culture for enteric pathogens, and a stool *C. difficile* toxin assay. Supine and upright abdominal films should be done to rule out colonic dilatation or free air. Oral fluid and food should be stopped, intravenous fluids should be given and electrolyte disturbances should be corrected. Severe anemia may require red cell transfusions. Anticholinergics, narcotics and antidiarrheal medications should not be given because of the possibility of precipitating colonic dilatation. In a patient in whom the diagnosis has not been previously established, a careful and limited proctoscopic examination should be performed, with insertion of the instrument only as far as necessary to make a diagnosis of colitis. Corticosteroids are administered intravenously with divided doses in the range of hydrocortisone 300 mg/day, prednisolone 60 mg/day or methylprednisolone 40–60 mg/day. For the patient who has not been on corticosteroids, intravenous ACTH 80–120 units per day is a consideration (Meyers et al 1983). Patients who respond will improve within 7 days. Thereafter, oral nutrition may be reintroduced gradually and oral steroids in doses equivalent to the intravenous dose can be started. For the patient who does not improve on steroids after 1 week of hospitalization and intravenous steroids, then surgical resection or cyclosporin treatment should be considered.

If the patient has toxic megacolon as manifested by dilatation of the transverse colon to more than 6 cm, then additional measures are necessary. These patients are at risk for perforation and the condition is a medical emergency. Broad-spectrum antibiotic coverage for enteric organisms should be given, such as metronidazole and an aminoglycoside or a second- or third-generation cephalosporin. Nasogastric suction and rolling the patient from side to side and to the prone position to help evacuate intestinal gas can be done (Present et al 1981). Twice daily or daily abdominal films to look for worsening of the dilatation or signs of perforation should be performed. The patient should be followed closely by a surgeon and if there is no improvement in 48 h or if there is deterioration, then colectomy should be done.

### *Mild and moderate active ulcerative colitis*

Patients with mildly to moderately active disease may be managed as outpatients. Stool studies to exclude infection, including a stool examination for ova and parasites, a culture for enteric pathogens and a stool *C. difficile* toxin assay should be done. Sigmoidoscopy following a small volume enema or without any preparation establishes the extent (proctosigmoiditis or more extensive disease), whether the abnormalities are diffuse, patchy or segmental and the severity of the abnormalities. Biopsies are supportive of the diagnosis of ulcerative colitis but not diagnostic and can help identify specific infection such as amebiasis, pseudomembranous colitis or cytomegalovirus infection in at-risk patients. The finding of granulomas supports a diagnosis of Crohn's disease.

If symptoms are mild, oral therapy with sulfasalazine – the least expensive 5-ASA preparation – could be started in a dose of 500 mg twice daily and increased by 1 g daily up to 3 or 4 g per day total. Folate 1 mg may be given daily along with the sulfasalazine. In patients who develop side-effects with sulfasalazine, another oral aminosalicylate such as Asacol or Pentasa may be used. Patients with disease that extends proximal to the splenic flexure need oral treatment with aminosalicylates. Patients with disease limited to the distal 20 cm of the rectosigmoid may be treated with 5-ASA suppositories or with 5-ASA or cortisone enemas. For disease that extends more proximally in the left colon, 5-ASA enemas or cortisone enemas may be used; 5-ASA enemas have been demonstrated to give coverage to the splenic flexure (Chapman et al 1992). For patients with more troublesome symptoms, the 5-ASA enemas or hydrocortisone enemas are a good choice, with one enema nightly for 2–3 weeks.

Patients with moderate symptoms may require the addition of oral prednisolone 40–60 mg per day to aminosalicylate treatment. Once the patient responds, the prednisolone may be tapered rapidly, usually over 4–6 weeks, and then discontinued.

Symptomatic therapy with antispasmodic or antidiarrheal medications can be used as needed along with anti-inflammatory therapy, but in general these agents should not be used as primary treatments.

The diet should be individualized for the patient. If there is constipation, as occurs in some patients with proctitis, then fiber supplements are helpful. Patients should evaluate the effect on their symptoms of milk products, fresh fruit and vegetables and spicy foods and if symptoms worsen within 1–2 h after meals, the offending food should be avoided. However, most patients do not need any specific food restriction.

### *Maintenance of remission*

The benefit of maintenance therapy in ulcerative colitis has been demonstrated in several controlled clinical trials. Sulfasalazine in a dose of 2–4 g/day, Dipentum 1 g/day, Asacol 0.8–2.4 g/day and Pentasa 1.5–4 g/day all have been shown to be of benefit in maintaining clinical remission. Patients with ulcerative proctitis or proctosigmoiditis who have frequent exacerbations – more than one or two a year – may also be placed on maintenance oral therapy. However, some patients with distal disease have a better response to topical treatment and can be maintained on suppositories or enemas used every other day or every third day. There are other patients with distal disease in whom remission is best maintained with a combination of oral and topical aminosalicylates. In summary, maintenance treatment with aminosalicylates should be individualized with attention to the effectiveness, the cost and the least cumbersome form of therapy.

Prednisolone and corticosteroid enemas are not effective for maintenance of remission in ulcerative colitis and should be tapered and discontinued as soon as possible. Azathioprine is effective in maintaining remission (Hawthorne et al 1992) and is most often used in patients who have previously been steroid dependent.

## Treatment of Crohn' diseases

Enteral and parenteral nutrition is considered on p. 629.

### *The initial episode*

For patients with Crohn's colitis or ileocolitis, sulfasalazine is effective (Summers et al 1979). The initial dose is 500 mg twice a day increased by 1 g/day up to 3–4 g/day. Folic acid 1 mg/day is given along with sulfasalazine. For patients who are intolerant to sulfasalazine, Pentasa in doses of 2–4 g/day or Asacol may be used. Sulfasalazine should not be given at the same time as corticosteroids (Singleton et al 1979b) and it is unlikely to be effective if corticosteroids have proved ineffective. In patients with colitis or ileocolitis who do not respond to aminosalicylates, there are several options. Metronidazole is as effective as sulfasalazine (Ursing et al 1982) and can be used in divided doses of 10–20 mg/kg/day. Prednisolone in an initial dose of 40–60 mg/day is often chosen for use because of the prompt response in many patients, within 1–3 weeks of starting treatment. An elemental diet has been advocated as being as effective as corticosteroids for Crohn's disease (O'Morain et al 1984a), although the effectiveness of this approach has not been confirmed in some trials (see also p. 629).

For patients with Crohn's ileitis, initial therapy with prednisolone 40–60 mg/day is the most immediately effective. Some clinicians advocate the use of broad-spectrum antibiotics in this setting, but there are no controlled data to support this strategy.

### *Chronic steroid-dependent disease*

Some patients achieve symptomatic remission while on prednisolone but have recurrent symptoms when the dose is tapered or discontinued and are considered steroid dependent. These patients are excellent candidates for immunomodulatory therapy with 6-mercaptopurine or azathioprine. As it takes a mean of 3 months for patients to respond to oral therapy with these immunomodulators, an effective dose of prednisolone can be continued to maintain remission during this time and then it can be gradually tapered thereafter. The starting dose is usually 50 mg/day. If symptoms deteriorate as the prednisolone is tapered, the immunomodulator dose can be increased gradually up to 1.5 mg/kg/day while maintaining a therapeutic dose of prednisolone, with reductions in the dose after each increase in the dose of the 6-MP or azathioprine. These agents are effective in at least two-thirds of patients and the success rate may be even higher in this subset who are steroid responsive. For patients who are intolerant to 6-MP or azathioprine or in whom these drugs are ineffective, methotrexate is an option. In uncontrolled trials, methotrexate 15–25 mg/week intramuscularly appeared effective as a steroid-sparing agent.

### *Steroid-resistant Crohn's disease*

If a patient fails to respond to treatment with corticosteroids, the possibility of partial bowel obstruction or of a fistula with abscess should be considered. For patients without these complications who do not achieve remission with aminosalicylates and prednisolone, 6-MP or azathioprine is effective in about two-thirds, in doses as discussed above. Cyclosporin was effective in steroid-resistant patients over a 3-month period, although it has not been shown to have long-term benefit (Brynskov et al 1989). Methotrexate also appears effective in the short-term, although long-term treatment has not been shown to be effective.

### *Maintenance of remission*

In contrast to patients with ulcerative colitis, sulfasalazine has not been shown in controlled trials to be effective in maintaining remission in Crohn's disease, probably because the dose of 5-ASA is too low (Tremaine 1992). Other aminosalicylates, Asacol and Pentasa, do appear effective in maintaining remission and are used in doses of 2–4 g/day. Because of the serious potential side-effects of long-term use, prednisolone is not a good agent for maintaining remission. Azathioprine and 6-MP are appropriate maintenance drugs when an aminosalicylate is not effective and some patients have been maintained on therapy for more than 10 years.

# SURGERY FOR INFLAMMATORY BOWEL DISEASE

## Ulcerative colitis

While the treatment of ulcerative colitis remains primarily medical, surgery continues to have a central role in its management because it may save the patient's life, it is curative and it eliminates the long-term risk of cancer. The advent of novel sphincter-saving procedures that preserve physiological functions additionally improve the overall quality of life of patients after proctocolectomy. Finally, further understanding of the role and timing of surgery and better care of stomas have all contributed to improved surgical management of this disease.

*Indications for surgery*

Surgery in ulcerative colitis is indicated either because of failure of medical treatment or because of complications of the disease (Table 23.12).

*Failure of medical management*

The response to current medical therapies is generally good but varies depending on the severity of the disease and the patient's ability to tolerate the medication. For mild and moderate disease, the remission rate is 92% and 87% respectively (Jarnerot et al 1985). The remission rate for severe disease, however, is much less favorable, either because of the severity of the attack itself for which the medication has minimal or no effect and the patient continues to have disabling symptoms, or because the response is satisfactory but the steroid requirements are excessive or cannot be reduced. Some patients have deleterious side-effects, allergic reactions or cannot tolerate the medication. Finally, some patients are noncompliant.

*Complications of ulcerative colitis*

***Fulminant colitis.*** Severe fulminant colitis should be treated aggressively with medication and nutritional support. If the clinical status does not show any significant improvement or if continued deterioration is witnessed, surgery should be undertaken. In the past, severe colitis was associated with high morbidity but with current and effective medical management and earlier operative approach, if necessary, mortality has decreased to less than 3% (Hawley 1988).

**Table 23.12** Indications for surgery in ulcerative colitis

| |
|---|
| *Failure of medical treatment* |
| Fulminant/unresponsive nature of first attack |
| Incomplete response |
| Excessive steroid dose required |
| Side-effects/intolerance/complications related to medications |
| Noncompliance with medication |
| *Complications of the disease* |
| Acute: fulminant colitis |
| Acute toxic megacolon |
| Perforation |
| Hemorrhage |
| Chronic: |
| Recurrent hemorrhage |
| Obstruction |
| Risk of carcinoma |
| Growth retardation in children |
| Extraintestinal manifestations of ulcerative colitis |
| Perianal disease |

Derived from Juhasz et al (1995)

***Toxic megacolon.*** The clinical features and diagnosis are defined on p. 669. Because the risk of perforation tends to increase with a more prolonged toxicity and the higher mortality seems to be related to the presence of perforation (up to 40% with perforation compared to 4% with no perforation) (Heppell et al 1986), surgery should be contemplated early rather than late. Urgent colectomy with rectal preservation is indicated if vigorous medical treatment is not associated with definite improvement of the patient's condition within 24–48 h or if deterioration manifested by persistent tachycardia, lowered blood pressure and increasing abdominal pain and tenderness are witnessed. It is well to remember that even patients who do respond to medical treatment frequently have a second attack of fulminant colitis or toxic megacolon (29%) and many eventually need colonic resection (47%), not uncommonly as an emergency (Grant & Dozois 1984).

***Perforation.*** The clinical features and diagnosis are described on p. 670. The mortality associated with perforation is high, ranging between 20% and 40% (Greenstein et al 1985, Heppel et al 1986), and the importance of early surgical intervention to prevent perforation in patients with fulminant disease or toxic megacolon cannot be overemphasized.

***Hemorrhage.*** Massive hemorrhage (p. 671) accounts for approximately 10% of emergency colectomies. Since rectal hemorrhage after colectomy may continue in as many as 12% of patients (Korelitz et al 1969), the surgeon must decide whether abdominal colectomy with rectal preservation will be sufficient or whether proctectomy should be added. The proctoscopic appearance of the rectum at the time of surgery, the perseverance of rectal stump bleeding and other considerations that make the future possibility of restorative surgery less likely may make immediate proctectomy preferable (Robert et al 1990).

***Obstruction.*** Obstruction in a patient with long-standing ulcerative colitis is almost invariably a result of malignancy. Benign colonic or rectal strictures (p. 671) are seen infrequently and are rarely obstructive. Despite the appearance on barium enema or colonoscopy or even the histologic suggestion that a stricture is benign, one must remain suspicious of underlying malignancy. Once a stricture is documented, colectomy is indicated.

***Risk of cancer.*** There is general agreement that after patients have had extensive disease for 8–10 years they should enter a close surveillance program or be offered prophylactic proctocolectomy. With the more acceptable alternative of the ileal pouch–anal anastomosis as opposed to proctocolectomy and ileostomy, surgery is becoming more attractive when compared to the pitfalls of surveillance (Collins et al 1987, Jones et al 1988). Surveillance, while useful, has many limitations. When patients have quiescent or mild disease, it may be difficult to convince them to undergo annual or biannual colonoscopy. If colonoscopy is performed, areas of abnormalities may not be recognized. Moreover, dysplasia does not always precede carcinoma and is not evenly distributed (Ransohoff et al 1985) and the carcinoma may be flat or submucosal and escape detection. Most importantly, carcinoma is already present in many patients with severe dysplasia (Lennard-Jones et al 1983). Finally, patients have continued to develop carcinoma while on surveillance programs and these carcinomas are not uncommonly advanced. If a surveyed patient develops dysplasia or a dysplasia-associated lesion or mass (DALM), surgery becomes necessary since the latter is associated with a greater than 50% chance of invasive cancer (Blackstone et al 1981).

***Growth retardation.*** Ulcerative colitis may retard children's growth at times even before the onset of typical bowel symptoms. The chronic illness, the nutritional deficiency and the use of steroids all may contribute to growth retardation. Within 12 months of surgery eliminating the disease, children often experience a growth spurt several times normal. It is of interest to note that improvement in growth may be less after rectal anastomosis than after proctocolectomy, possibly due to residual disease. Surgery to reverse growth retardation should take place before puberty when fusion of the epiphysis occurs (Berger et al 1975, Kirschner et al 1978).

***Perianal disease.*** Perianal abscesses, fissures and simple fistulae do occur in ulcerative colitis, although with less frequency and complexity than in Crohn's disease. Abscesses should be drained and fissures and fistulae should be treated as warranted. The presence of perianal disease should always raise suspicion of Crohn's disease, especially when contemplating restorative proctocolectomy.

***Extraintestinal manifestations.*** Approximately 30% of patients with ulcerative colitis will have one or more extraintestinal manifestations of their colonic disease (Danzi 1988). The cutaneous, eye, joint and vascular manifestations (p. 674) often regress and do not recur after resection of the entire colonic and rectal disease. The exceptions include ankylosing spondylitis and rheumatoid arthritis, which are probably separate disease processes with a common genetic predisposition (Gravallese & Kantrowitz 1988), pyoderma gangrenosum and primary sclerosing cholangitis, which may continue to evolve to cirrhosis, portal hypertension, and liver failure even after a proctocolectomy (Cangemi et al 1989). While most of these manifestations will improve as the disease severity declines, proctocolectomy should still be considered if troublesome symptoms persist, especially when other indications for surgery are present.

## Preoperative preparation

Adequate preparation for surgery is most important. In trying to tailor the operation to the patient's needs, type of disease and lifestyle, it is critical for the surgeon to discuss frankly with the patient the various surgical alternatives available and their respective advantages and disadvantages. In this respect, the assistance of a stomal therapist is essential, not only to again review the various surgical alternatives but also to include a psychological preparation using modern educational tools, particularly if a stoma is planned. Nutritional requirements are also important, especially if a period of medical management with total parenteral nutrition is contemplated. For those patients who require urgent surgery, postoperative nutritional support may be beneficial in the malnourished patient to prevent further protein depletion during the period of recovery. The severity of the disease and continued blood loss may lead to significant anemia and perioperative blood transfusion may be necessary. This is particularly so in older patients and in those with low iron stores.

A half-day mechanical bowel preparation with polyethylene glycol (GoLytely®) lavage combined with antibiotics is adequate and well tolerated by most patients. Patients requiring emergency surgery usually cannot undergo mechanical bowel preparation and should receive broad-spectrum systemic antibiotics perioperatively. Correction of electrolyte abnormalities is important and may be accomplished during the 12–18 h preceding the surgery. Some patients may also benefit from respiratory therapy preoperatively. A stoma site should be marked by an enterostomal therapist, who also has a crucial role in counseling these patients about the future care of the stoma and expectations. Support hose and intermittent pneumatic calf compression devices are routinely used to prevent thromboembolic complications. Heparin may be needed in patients at higher risk of such accidents. It is imperative that patients who have taken steroids within the 12 months prior to surgery be given steroids preoperatively and the medication should be continued postoperatively and tapered over a period of 4–6 weeks.

## Choice of operative procedures

Numerous surgical alternatives are now available to patients with ulcerative colitis. There is little question that in recent years the ileal pouch–anal anastomosis has become the more acceptable alternative for most colitic patients. However, it is important to remember that the other alternatives still have a role and a place. Thus, the choice of operation should be based on an individual patient's needs and include: proctocolectomy with Brooke ileostomy, continent ileostomy of Kock and colectomy with ileorectal anastomosis. More recently, a modification of the conventional ileal pouch–anal anastomosis has been developed whereby no mucosectomy is carried out and the ileal reservoir is anastomosed to the distal rectum or upper anal canal (ileal pouch–distal rectal anastomosis), most often with a stapling device.

Ileal pouch–anal anastomosis may sometimes be carried

out as a three-stage procedure with abdominal colectomy, total rectal preservation and Brooke ileostomy being performed as the first operation. This approach may be advantageous when a patient requires emergency life-saving surgery, when Crohn's disease cannot be ruled out or when a patient is extremely malnourished as a result of chronic illness and/or steroid use (Nicholls et al 1989). A temporary ileostomy is not without problems (Metcalf et al 1986a) but thus far, a one-stage procedure without ileostomy has been advocated by very few surgeons (Parks & Nicholls 1978). In highly selected patients (those who are not taking steroids or are well nourished and have a technically perfect operation with a tension-free anastomosis), a one-stage operation is safe (Galandiuk et al 1991) and indeed may have a broader application.

### Ileal pouch–anal anastomosis

Currently, the ileal pouch–anal anastomosis (Fig. 23.31) is the operation of choice for the majority of patients suffering from ulcerative colitis because it avoids a permanent stoma, restores physiological functions and cures the disease (Kelly et al 1992). In nearly all of our patients, the operation is done in two stages. In the first stage, the cecum, colon and proximal two-thirds of the rectum are removed, the mucosa of the distal rectum and anal canal is excised endoanally starting at the dentate line and the ileal reservoir is anastomosed to the anal canal at the dentate line. In most instances, 30–40 cm of ileum are used to construct the reservoir. Whenever possible, we have preferred the J-shaped reservoir because of its ease of construction and the fact that it empties readily. Other designs, such as an S-shaped or W-shaped reservoir, have also been chosen, usually for anatomical reasons, in 4% of our patients. A temporary protective loop ileostomy is established in the right lower quadrant area to help reduce the risk of sepsis. At the second stage, usually 2–3 months later, the ileostomy is removed and ileal continuity is restored.

In the emergency setting, a three-stage procedure may prove necessary, with abdominal colectomy and preservation of the entire rectum with an end ileostomy only being done as the first stage. When the patient has fully recovered and the nature of the colitis is clearly established, an ileal pouch–anal anastomosis may be carried out if this is the desire of the patient. A one-stage procedure without ileostomy is not widely practiced for ulcerative colitis, although it can be safely performed in very carefully selected patients under optimal conditions, i.e. mild or inactive disease, absence of steroids for more than 1 year and a technically easier operation.

#### *Indications*

Ileal pouch–anal anastomosis is suitable for most patients

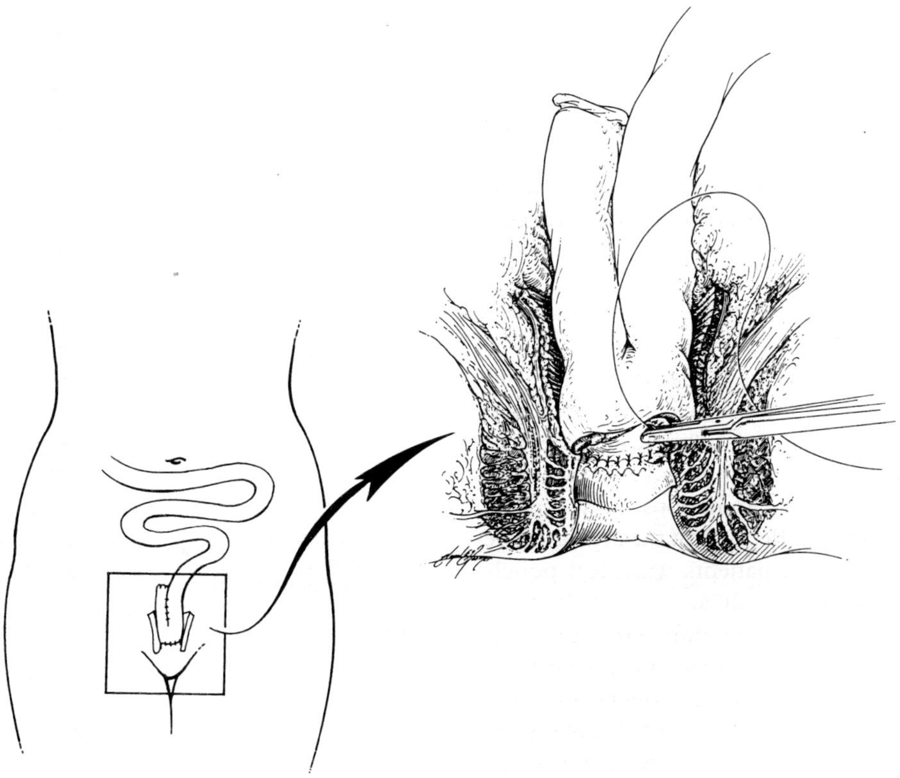

**Fig. 23.31** Ileal pouch–anal anastomosis.

who have ulcerative colitis and are younger than 65 years of age provided they have effective anal sphincter function. Patients older than 65 years are unlikely to be good candidates because of impaired anal sphincter function, as are those with previously damaged sphincters or those with some degree of existing incontinence and oftentimes associated medical problems which make the risk of this complex operation greater. While we do not subscribe to routine manometric studies of anal sphincter competency in all patients preoperatively, we do for patients who are older than 50 years of age and for those who are suspected of anorectal incompetency by history and physical examination. It is also important to inform older patients that their functional results may not be quite as good as those of younger patients. Patients who may not be suitable candidates for the operation because of anticipated technical difficulties should be forewarned preoperatively. Other patients who are not suitable are those with cancer of the rectum and those in whom Crohn's disease is strongly suspected.

A number of other pouch designs have been championed by various authors and the results of the various designs are fairly similar. The S-pouch was initially associated with significant functional difficulties with emptying (Parks et al 1980), mostly because of the long, tortuous efferent limb. With shortening of the latter, these functional problems would appear to have been largely overcome (McHugh et al 1987). The S-pouch may at times be easier to anastomose to the anal area and should be used preferentially when the J-shaped design does not allow this. The S and W designs also provide a larger reservoir, at least initially, theoretically leading to less frequent bowel movements (Nicholls & Pezim 1985), but little difference has been noted. The choice of the reservoir design should be individualized, based primarily on personal experience and technical considerations in any particular patient.

### *Advantages and disadvantages*

The operation is advantageous because it not only removes all of the diseased mucosa while preserving the anal route of defecation, but also because it restores patients to their previous way of life with very few restrictions. The operation does have limitations, however, and is not suitable for all patients. Because of the increased frequency of bowel movements, patients with ileal pouch–anal anastomosis may require ready access to toilet facilities and this situation may cause difficulties for some workers whose occupation takes them away from such facilities. Some patients may also experience problems with imperfect continence, especially at night. Finally, the time required away from normal activity with the staging of this procedure may be a disadvantage for younger patients, especially students.

### *Results*

***Mortality.*** The operation is safe and very few deaths have been reported in the literature. In our own experience with 1600 such operations, two patients (less than 0.1%) have died in the immediate postoperative period, one patient after a massive pulmonary embolism and another after perforation of a large steroid-induced gastric ulcer.

***Indications, demographics, complications in Mayo series.*** In the most recent evaluation of our experience with 1193 ileal pouch–anal operations performed at the Mayo Medical Center in Rochester, Minnesota, 89% of the procedures were done for ulcerative colitis. The most commonly used design of reservoir was the J-pouch, initially described by Utsunomiya (Utsunomiya et al 1980). In 4% of the patients another design of reservoir was employed, namely the W-shaped or the S-shaped reservoir, most often for technical reasons, especially in tall or obese patients in whom reaching the dentate line area proved to be nearly impossible with the J-shaped reservoir. The mean age of the patients was 32 years and there was an equal number of men and women. The overall complication rate was 30% (Table 23.13) compared with a 13–54% incidence reported by others (Kelly et al 1992). The most frequent complication was small bowel obstruction, occurring in 13% of patients, half requiring reoperation. This incidence of intestinal obstruction does not differ greatly from that reported by others with proctocolectomy and ileostomy or with colectomy and ileorectostomy (Francois et al 1989).

Perhaps the most feared complication of ileal pouch–anal anastomosis, pelvic sepsis, has occurred in 5% of

**Table 23.13** Postoperative morbidity after ileal pouch–anal anastomosis and after closure of the ileostomy in 390 patients

| Complication | % of patients with complication |
|---|---|
| *After ileal pouch–anal anastomosis* | |
| Small bowel obstruction | 13 |
| Transient | 8 |
| Required reoperation | 5 |
| Pelvic sepsis | 5 |
| Antibiotics alone | 3 |
| Required reoperation | 2 |
| Wound infection | 3 |
| Urinary retention | 7 |
| Transient | 5 |
| Required catheterization | 2 |
| *After closure of ileostomy* | |
| Small bowel obstruction | 9 |
| Transient | 4 |
| Required reoperation | 5 |
| Anastomotic leakage | 2 |
| *Longer term* | |
| Anastomotic stricture | 5 |
| Pouchitis | 31 |

Derived from Pemberton (1991)

patients overall. This incidence, however, has decreased from 8% in our early experience to 4% in our latest experience. Others have reported a similar decreasing risk with increasing experience (Dozois 1988). Antibiotics or CT-guided drainage or both have been successful for well-encapsulated abscesses (Dozois 1988). In about one-third of the patients, however, abdominal surgical intervention was necessary; of those, only 29% ultimately had a satisfactorily functioning pouch (Galandiuk et al 1990). Wound infection occurred in 3% of patients and urinary retention occurred in 5%. No long-term urinary dysfunction ensued and impotence and retrograde ejaculation occurred in 1.5% and 2%, respectively (Kelly et al 1992).

Long-term complications after ileostomy closure included small bowel obstruction in 9% of patients, half of whom required operations.

Patients usually pass six stools during the day and one stool at night. The frequency of bowel movements changes little with time, but the need for medication to slow intestinal transit or increase bulk and stool consistency decreases with time (Table 23.14) (Pemberton et al 1987). In contrast, night-time spotting has occurred in 20–30% of patients more than 12 months after the operation, but frank soiling is rare (Pemberton et al 1987). With time, night-time continence does seem to improve and reliance on medication diminishes (Pemberton et al 1987). Older patients, women and those patients with a greater preoperative stool frequency are more likely to be incapacitated by imperfect continence at night than younger patients, men and those with less diarrhea preoperatively (Pemberton et al 1987). The ability to discriminate gas from stool and to defer bowel movements also improves considerably with time.

An anastomotic stricture (5%), which may occur as a result of ischemia, undue anastomotic tension, sepsis or a combination thereof, may require single or repeated dilatation or even surgical revision (Galandiuk et al 1990). Long, dense and nonpliable strictures are difficult to manage and may require advancement of anoderm and pouch mucosa after excision of the strictured fibrotic segment (Galandiuk et al 1990). Pouch–perineal fistulae (5%) and pouch–vaginal fistulae (4%) can often be managed successfully by proximal diversion and/or repair of the fistula (Dozois 1988).

**Table 23.14** Functional results of ileal pouch–anal anastomosis from 6 months to 5 years postoperatively in 389 patients

| Parameter | Follow-up | | | | | |
|---|---|---|---|---|---|---|
| | 6 mo. | 1 yr. | 2 yr. | 3 yr. | 4 yr. | 5 yr. |
| Number of stools (mean ± SD) | | | | | | |
| Day | 5 ± 2 | 5 ± 3 | 6 ± 3 | 6 ± 2 | 6 ± 3 | 6 ± 2 |
| Night | 1 ± 1 | 1 ± 1 | 2 ± 2 | 2 ± 1 | 1 ± 1 | 2 ± 1 |
| Able to discriminate gas from stool (% of pts) | 69 | 77 | 73 | 84 | 77 | 86 |
| Lomotil (% of pts) | 26 | 19 | 17 | 25 | 5 | 4 |
| Metamucil (% of pts) | 43 | 36 | 40 | 38 | 30 | 27 |

Derived from Pemberton (1991)

***Pouchitis.*** Nonspecific inflammation of the reservoir, or pouchitis, is clinically characterized by the sudden onset of diarrhea, bleeding, fever and, at times, exacerbation of extracolonic manifestations. While the etiology of this entity remains unknown, numerous contributing factors have been implicated, including bacterial overgrowth, poor pouch emptying and the presence or absence of extracolonic manifestations preoperatively (Lohmuller et al 1990). The incidence has steadily risen as follow-up has increased, although some authors report a lesser incidence. In a recent survey, we found that 31% of patients had experienced at least one episode of pouchitis with almost two-thirds having had more than one episode (Kelly et al 1992). While this may at first appear somewhat distressing, it is important to remember that most patients readily respond to antibiotics and that the clinical syndrome is infrequently a serious problem. Indeed, only two patients have had to have their pouch excised because of this condition and even in these instances there was some serious concern about the possibility of Crohn's disease. Finally, because it occurs very rarely in patients with polyposis, the cause of pouchitis may in some way be related to the cause of colitis. More recently, we have found that the risk of pouchitis in patients with ulcerative colitis and primary sclerosing cholangitis far exceeds that of patients with ulcerative colitis alone (64% vs 32%, respectively) (Penna et al 1994). Moreover, the presence of p-ANCA positive testing in those patients with pouchitis as opposed to negative testing in those patients without pouchitis (Sandborn et al 1993) not only points to a common etiology for primary sclerosing cholangitis and pouchitis, but also suggests some type of immunologic incompetence.

Failure of the operation, that is, the patient requiring pouch excision or permanent ileostomy, has occurred in 6% of our patients because of poor functional results, later appearance of Crohn's disease or insurmountable sepsis (Kelly et al 1992). With time, however, the failure rate would seem to rise slowly. In a recent evaluation of our first 1000 patients with this operation for colitis, a cumulative risk of failure at 10 years was 10%. Others have reported a failure rate of 12% (Gemlo et al 1992).

## Ileal pouch–distal rectal anastomosis

In order to improve night-time continence, some surgeons have advocated avoiding the mucosectomy portion of the operation and stapling the reservoir to the lower rectal or upper anal canal mucosa. In two separate controlled trials conducted thus far (Choen et al 1991, Luukonen & Jarvinen 1992) the double-stapled technique without mucosectomy would not appear to provide superior night-time continence. Although there are yet no clearcut benefits to this technique, the risks associated with residual diseased mucosa should remain a concern. These may include recurrent exacerbations of the residual ulcerated and bleeding mucosa, potential exacerbation of extracolonic manifestations and a long-term risk of cancer (Tsunoda et al 1990). A further objective evaluation by randomization is needed in a larger number of patients followed for a longer time. In our view, the double-stapled technique without mucosectomy should not be performed in those patients with severe distal rectal disease, in those with extracolonic manifestation or in those with colitis associated with dysplasia or carcinoma elsewhere in the large bowel (Dozois & Juhasz 1993).

Finally, both the conventional ileal pouch–anal anastomosis and the double-stapled ileal pouch–distal rectal anastomosis offer patients a quality of life better than that expected with the alternative operations, but certainly the limitations of postoperative complications, frequency of stool passage and pouchitis persist for both operations.

## Quality of life

Assessment of the benefits of surgery is a difficult task. Not only do the tangible benefits such as eradication of the disease and return to normal lifestyle need to be perceived, but other less tangible benefits or disadvantages also need to be assessed. These include return to work, social and sporting activities and general lifestyle activities, as well as changes in sexuality and self-esteem.

Regardless of the type of surgery performed, patients return to normal health and enjoy a better quality of life after a complete removal of their disease. Several studies have compared the quality of life of patients undergoing Brooke ileostomy, Kock pouch or ileal pouch–anal anastomosis. After Brooke ileostomy, most patients have a normal lifestyle and are able to return to work. Restrictions in activity appear to be less common among patients with the Kock pouch than those with the Brooke ileostomy (Table 23.15) (McLeod & Fazio 1984, McLeod et al 1986, 1991, Pemberton et al 1989, Kohler et al 1991). The results would appear to be even better after ileal pouch–anal anastomosis (Kohler et al 1991) (96% pleased, 94% having returned to work or school). Sporting and sexual activity have been higher in patients with an ileal pouch–anal anastomosis than those with a Brooke ileostomy or a Kock pouch, suggesting that the presence of a stoma, whether continent or not, has some limiting effect on some physical activities (Tables 23.15 and 23.16).

The majority of women who develop ulcerative colitis are in their reproductive years, and the impact of ileal pouch–anal anastomosis on their sexual functions and ability to conceive has considerable importance. Women with ulcerative colitis have normal fertility rates (Miller 1986). If they have active ulcerative colitis after becoming pregnant, they should be treated in much the same way as nonpregnant women, preferably with medication. If surgery becomes necessary, especially if urgent, the risk of spontaneous abortion may be expected to increase.

Various surgical options appear to affect sexual function differently. After proctocolectomy and Brooke ileostomy, painful intercourse may occur in 7%, a problem substantially less common than after ileorectostomy (53%)

**Table 23.15** Patient satisfaction after creation of Brooke ileostomy, Kock pouch or ileal pouch–anal anastomosis

| Categories | % Responding | | |
|---|---|---|---|
| | Brooke ileostomy (n=406) | Kock pouch (n=313) | Ileal pouch–anal anastomosis (n=298) |
| Diet restricted | 28 | 46 | 22 |
| Satisfied with diet | 97 | 96 | 95 |
| Returned to work or school | 98 | 96 | 94 |
| Desired change but satisfied | 33 | 11 | 3 |
| Definitely desired change | 6 | 3 | 1 |
| Overall satisfaction | 93 | 98 | 96 |
| Attitude since operation | | | |
| Improved | 60 | 60 | 62 |
| No change | 35 | 36 | 34 |
| Deteriorated | 5 | 4 | 4 |

Derived from Kohler et al (1991)

**Table 23.16** Patient performance responses after creation of Brooke ileostomy, Kock pouch or ileal pouch–anal anastomosis

| Categories and responses | % Responding | | |
|---|---|---|---|
| | Brooke ileostomy (n=406) | Kock pouch (n=313) | Ileal pouch–anal anastomosis (n=298) |
| Social activity | | | |
| Restricted | 21 | 22 | 14 |
| No change | 51 | 41 | 42 |
| Improved | 28 | 38 | 44 |
| Sports | | | |
| Restricted | 42 | 30 | 17 |
| No change | 42 | 44 | 43 |
| Improved | 15 | 26 | 40 |
| Housework | | | |
| Restricted | 14 | 8 | 9 |
| No change | 68 | 70 | 52 |
| Improved | 19 | 22 | 39 |
| Recreation | | | |
| Restricted | 30 | 24 | 17 |
| No change | 42 | 43 | 42 |
| Improved | 22 | 33 | 41 |
| Family relationships | | | |
| Restricted | 8 | 6 | 8 |
| No change | 68 | 64 | 51 |
| Improved | 24 | 30 | 41 |
| Sexual activity | | | |
| Restricted | 29 | 17 | 14 |
| No change | 56 | 52 | 42 |
| Improved | 15 | 30 | 45 |
| Travel | | | |
| Restricted | 26 | 32 | 20 |
| No change | 48 | 35 | 37 |
| Improved | 26 | 33 | 42 |

Derived from Kohler et al (1991)

(Penna et al 1994). Postoperative dyspareunia also ensues more often after proctocolectomy and continent ileostomy than after ileal pouch–anal anastomosis (38% vs 18%, respectively) (Metcalf et al 1986b). Also, some women with a Kock pouch have episodic vaginal discharge (18%), a problem not reported by women with ileal pouch–anal anastomosis (Metcalf et al 1986b). It would thus appear that the presence of an ileal reservoir interposed between the vagina and sacrum and less pelvic floor disruption after endorectal mucosectomy and ileoanal anastomosis may be beneficial. We have also found that ileal pouch–anal anastomosis allows for safe pregnancy and delivery. Delivery does not adversely affect bowel function except for a modest increase in nocturnal stool passage during the last trimester of the pregnancy and the initial 3 months after delivery (Nelson et al 1989). Similarly, the type of delivery, whether vaginal or by cesarean section, does not seem to influence bowel movement frequency or continence (Dozois et al 1993). The decision to perform cesarean section should be based on obstetric indications. Whether multiparity will affect pudendal nerve integrity or continence in the long term is unknown.

## INTRAOPERATIVE MANAGEMENT OF UNUSUAL SITUATIONS

### Indeterminate colitis

At the time of colectomy, it may be difficult to distinguish between ulcerative colitis and granulomatous colitis and the nature of the colitis may remain "indeterminate". In the past, it has been our practice to proceed with ileal pouch–anal anastomosis and our initial results would suggest that there is no major difference in the complication rate and long-term functional results of these patients (Pezim et al 1989). More recently, however, we have observed that patients who have so-called indeterminate colitis who have had previous perianal complications of their colitis are more likely to have failure of their ileal pouch–anal anastomosis in the long term. Also, when Crohn's disease is clinically suspected preoperatively and the pathologist remains uncertain about the exact nature of the disease at the time of the colectomy, more of these patients will ultimately prove to have Crohn's disease and are more likely to fail the ileal pouch–anal anastomosis (McIntyre et al 1993). In instances where the nature of the colitis is indeterminate, it is important to review the dilemma and risks posed by the construction of an ileal reservoir with the patient's relatives so that they clearly understand before the surgeon embarks on the construction of the reservoir.

### Cancer

The exact magnitude of the risk of colorectal cancer in ulcerative colitis remains debated, but all surveys indicate that such a risk is increased (p. 672). The malignancies are at times difficult to diagnose preoperatively and the process may be advanced when discovered intraoperatively. Indeed, these tumors are often flat, ulcerated and of a higher grade than the usual colon or rectal tumors and are not easily detectable radiographically or even endoscopically. The advent of restorative proctocolectomy has added a new dimension to this problem. Young patients with a long life expectancy are at a higher risk of developing cancer but, the feasibility of performing an ileal pouch–anal anastomosis is also higher and its risks of postoperative mortality and morbidity are lower. In contrast, older patients with a shorter life expectancy have a lesser risk of cancer and restorative proctocolectomy carries a greater risk of both short- and long-term complications and may not be advisable. Such factors should be discussed carefully when reviewing alternatives with patients. Moreover, the finding of carcinoma at surgery may not necessarily preclude the possibility of constructing an ileal pouch–anal anastomosis. If the carcinoma is located in the colon and diagnosed at an early stage (Dukes' A or B1), an ileal pouch–anal anastomosis is still a reasonable option. When the colon cancer is more advanced and adjuvant therapy will be required, it may be preferable to avoid the ileal pouch–anal anastomosis because of the much greater risk of complications in such patients. In these patients an ileorectostomy may be considered at least until there is fair certainty that the malignant process will not recur. If rectal carcinoma is diagnosed early, an ileal pouch–anal anastomosis should be considered only if the tumor is located in the upper rectum. In such instances, the proctectomy should be done in the more radical fashion to reduce the risk of recurrence. For carcinomas of the mid and lower rectum, a more conventional radical proctectomy should be combined with a Brooke ileostomy.

### Primary sclerosing cholangitis, portal hypertension and peristomal varices

It is now quite clear that proctocolectomy has no beneficial effect on primary sclerosing cholangitis complicating ulcerative colitis (Cangemi et al 1989). Also, if a Brooke ileostomy is established after proctocolectomy in patients with ulcerative colitis and primary sclerosing cholangitis, the risk of peristomal varices is quite high (43% within 4 years) (Wiesner et al 1986) and the varices may pose very difficult management problems. In such patients, we now prefer to construct an ileal pouch–anal anastomosis, an operation that has proven to be safe and not associated with the development of perianal varices (Kartheuser et al 1993). More recently, we have found that the long-term risk of pouchitis is quite significant (Kartheuser et al 1993) and that the pouchitis seems to have a more intractable clinical course and be more difficult to manage (Penna et al 1994). If at the time of surgery, colectomy proves to be unduly difficult due to severe bleeding, an ileorectostomy should be preferred to a Brooke ileostomy if the extent of the disease in the rectum is such that reasonable results can be anticipated.

## Proctocolectomy and Brooke ileostomy

Since the advent of better appliances and improved surgical techniques, most of the initial problems encountered early after the end ileostomy have been avoidable and proctocolectomy and Brooke ileostomy (Daly & Brooke 1967) continues to be an acceptable procedure for patients with ulcerative colitis (Fig. 23.32). Indeed, the procedure has been the established standard for many years. While its role is now more limited, it still has a place in certain categories of patients.

### *Indications*

This may be the operation of choice for patients who are not suitable for sphincter-preserving procedures because of age, inadequacy of the anal sphincter apparatus or advanced malignancy, especially in the rectum, or if other medical problems would make the more technically demanding ileal pouch–anal anastomosis a more risky operation in medically handicapped patients. The operation may also be better suited for those patients whose work make it easier for them to handle an appliance.

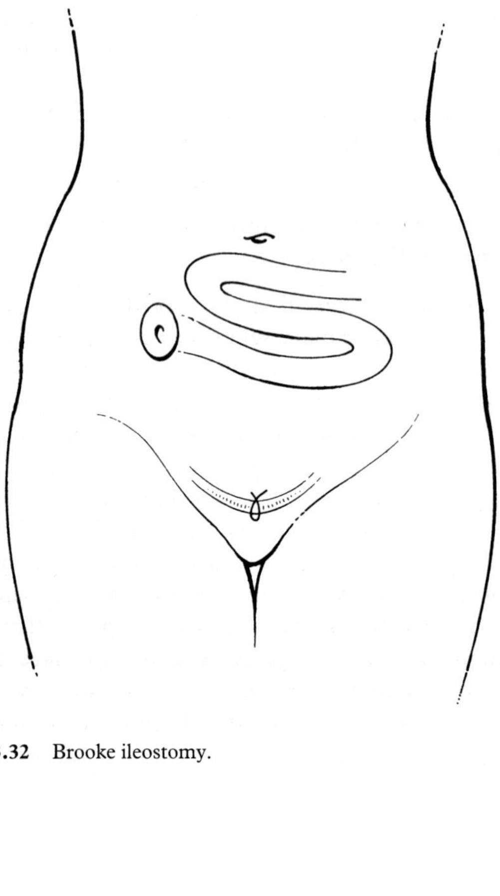

**Fig. 23.32** Brooke ileostomy.

### *Advantages and disadvantages*

The advantages are that the operation is technically simpler than alternative procedures, is associated with fewer complications and, most importantly, removes all of the disease, thus curing the patient. The main disadvantage is that it leaves the patient with a permanent incontinent stoma that requires the constant wearing of an external appliance. Problems with odor, occasional accidents and peristomal skin irritations may interfere with the patient's lifestyle. Also, the perianal wound may occasionally be slow to heal, causing discomfort and the inconvenience of regular dressings. Finally, dissection of the rectum may result in urinary and/or sexual dysfunction.

The operation may be done in one or two stages. The one-stage procedure is suitable in the elective situation when it can be carried out safely with low morbidity and mortality. It obviates the need for a second major operation and avoids the persistent problems of bleeding and inflammation from the residual rectum.

The two-stage procedure is usually reserved for emergency situations when perforation, hemorrhage, severe fulminant disease, toxic megacolon and marked nutritional depletion may increase the morbidity and mortality of a one-stage procedure. It also allows for removal of intraperitoneal colon, improving the patient's general condition and permitting treatment of the residual rectum with topical medication. Occasionally, the rectum may need to be removed as an emergency because of persistent bleeding, toxicity or severe disease. The main disadvantage of the two-stage procedure is offset by its lower morbidity and mortality and the opportunity for a future restorative procedure in those patients who may prove to be suitable candidates. In patients who do not have dysplasia or carcinoma and in whom a one-stage procedure is carried out, dissection of the rectum and anal canal in the intersphincteric plane leaves a smaller perineal wound and a stronger pelvic floor and lessens the chance of delayed healing and injuring pelvic nerves (Lyttle & Parks 1977).

Complications from this operation are infrequent, although not negligible. With careful attention to technical details, infection and hemorrhage should seldom occur. While perineal wound healing may be delayed, eventually most perineal wounds will heal spontaneously within 90 days (Waits et al 1982).

Surgical complications requiring revision affect 5–15% of patients. Stomal skin irritation may occur in up to 40% of patients. Urologic and sexual dysfunction should be mostly avoidable. Impotence occurs in 3–12% of patients and is more likely to occur in older patients. Some women may be troubled by dyspareunia and episodic vaginal discharge as a result of pelvic floor disruption (Metcalf et al 1986b).

In the long term, patients with ileostomies are prone to chronic dehydration and urinary stone formation. Adequate intake of fluids may help prevent these problems. Gallstones are also more common in these patients because of the loss of bile acids through the ileostomy, particularly in those patients who have had a greater portion of their ileum resected.

The quality of life is improved in patients undergoing proctocolectomy and Brooke ileostomy owing to the eradication of the disease and restoration of general health. Social, sexual and sporting activities are, however, somewhat limited because of the incontinent stoma. Eventually, more than 90% of patients adapt to these limitations, have a nearly normal lifestyle and are generally satisfied with their results (Kohler et al 1991).

## Abdominal colectomy and ileorectal anastomosis

Abdominal colectomy and ileorectal anastomosis (Fig. 23.33), mostly popularized by Aylett (1966) in Britain and Loygue in France, has been a useful alternative to proctocolectomy and Brooke ileostomy for many years, especially in selected patients who wish to avoid an ileostomy.

Colectomy with ileorectal anastomosis may be performed as a one-stage procedure in the elective situation or as a two-stage procedure in those requiring emergency surgery. The first stage in the emergency setting is colectomy with ileostomy and either mucus fistula or oversewing of the rectal stump, depending on its quality. The second stage involves restoration of bowel continuity with ileorectal anastomosis.

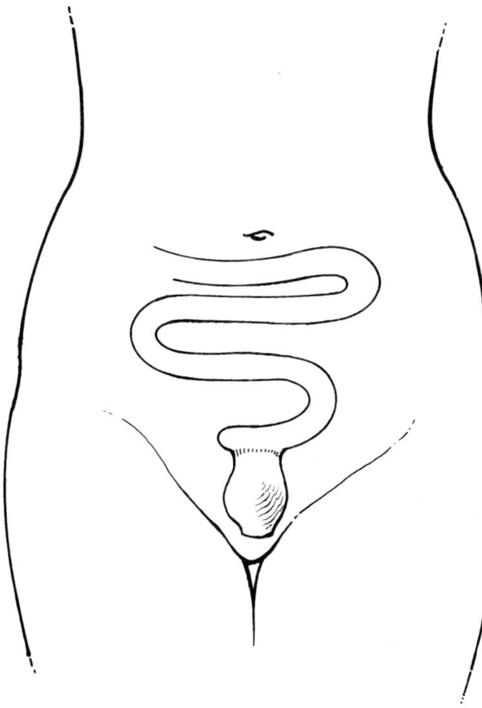

**Fig. 23.33** Ileorectostomy.

### *Indications*

This operation may still be indicated in patients who are not suitable candidates for restorative proctocolectomy and at the same time wish to maintain normal defecation and in those male patients who are particularly concerned with sexual dysfunction. The operation removes the bulk of the disease, usually allowing clinical improvement of symptoms. Also, the diseased rectum must still be pliable so that reservoir capacity is maintained. It is also a suitable operation for patients in whom Crohn's disease cannot be excluded and at times for patients with ulcerative colitis complicated by an advanced malignancy of the proximal colon, provided the rectum is relatively healthy. In this setting, the operation avoids a stoma when life expectancy might be limited. This operation is not suitable for patients with severe rectal disease, especially those with a rigid noncompliant rectum, precancerous changes in the colon or rectum or extraintestinal manifestations, as they are likely to persist due to the residual disease. The procedure should be avoided in the emergency setting under most circumstances because of the increased risk of anastomotic breakdown.

### *Advantages and disadvantages*

The obvious advantage is maintenance of the anal route of defecation. It is also technically safe with minimal immediate complications. There are some significant disadvantages, however, including persistent diarrhea, continuing active disease, the need to be compliant with regard to screening, the need for medication and the cumulative risk of cancer.

### *Results*

In the Mayo Clinic review of patients undergoing ileorectal anastomosis, the procedure was performed in less than 10% of all patients requiring surgery for ulcerative colitis in an era when ileal pouch–anal anastomosis was not yet available (Farnell et al 1985). Of the 63 patients operated, there were two perioperative deaths (3.1%) and one anastomotic leak (1.6%). The follow-up of patients showed that only 55% had satisfactory clinical results. Poor results were due to excessive frequency of bowel motions, continued need for steroid use, incontinence or poor health. More than 30% of patients eventually required proctectomy, all within a few years (Farnell et al 1985). Other studies have shown a spectrum of results with perioperative mortality ranging from 0% to 7%, leakage ranging from 0% to 11% and eventual proctectomy in 4–37% of patients. Satisfactory rectal function has been reported in 32–96% of patients. The results have varied depending on the selection of patients for the procedure, the experience of the surgeon, the varying length of follow-up and the degree of individual enthusiasm for the procedure.

The risk of cancer in the rectal remnant has been reported as 6% after 20 years of disease and 15% after 30 years (Baker et al 1978). The risk is therefore quite significant, considering that most patients are operated in their youth or early adulthood and that these patients need to continue to be surveyed indefinitely. While impotence and urinary dysfunction are not complications expected of this operation because rectal dissection is totally avoided, retrograde ejaculation has been reported (Ambroze et al 1992).

This operation is an acceptable procedure in some patients with ulcerative colitis; however, with the advent of ileal pouch–anal anastomosis, it should be reserved for those who are not suitable candidates for the restorative procedure. Comparative studies have shown no major benefit of colectomy and ileorectostomy over ileal pouch–anal anastomosis in terms of morbidity, mortality, stool frequency and continence (Oakley et al 1985, Parc et al 1989, Ambroze et al 1992).

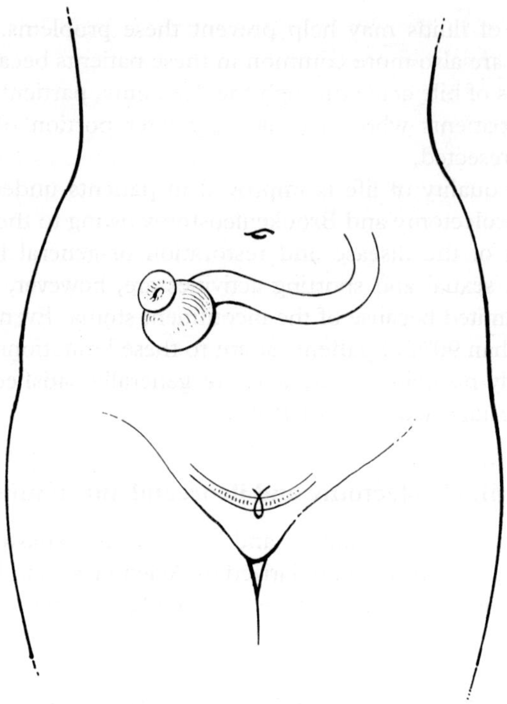

Fig. 23.34 Kock pouch, ileal reservoir, with ileostomy.

## Kock pouch

The continent ileostomy of Kock offers an alternative for those patients who would otherwise need a Brooke ileostomy. The technique, first described by Kock of Sweden (Kock 1976) in 1969, includes an ileal reservoir constructed from a 30 cm segment of terminal ileum and a nipple valve which is interposed between the stoma and reservoir and constructed by intussuscepting a segment of 10 cm of ileum (Fig. 23.34). The early results with the nipple valve were promising, but because of many failed nipple valves the technique was modified through the years to include a longer valve, the use of absorbable sutures, the use of staples and, more recently, stapling the valve to the side wall of the pouch. Because the reservoir is continent, the stoma can be made flush with the abdominal wall and can be located in an inconspicuous place on the abdominal wall. Patients need to intubate the pouch when convenient and between intubations there is no need to wear an appliance.

This operation is suitable for patients who already have had a proctocolectomy but consider their incontinent stoma to be a serious impediment to their lifestyle. Many of these patients are young and feel that the incontinent stoma interferes with personal relationships, sex and participation in sports. Patients who are not suitable for ileal pouch–anal anastomosis because of poor anal sphincter tone are also candidates for this procedure, as are those who have a failed ileal pouch–anal anastomosis. In the latter instance, the existing reservoir can be used and only a nipple valve needs to be constructed from a proximal segment of ileum. The procedure should be avoided in those patients who have had a previous significant resection of small bowel and in the emergency setting. The operation is also best avoided in patients with psychiatric disorders or intellectual or physical disabilities which may make it difficult to manage the pouch or its complications.

### *Advantages and disadvantages*

The major advantage of this operation is that no external appliance need be worn and there is no outward sign that the patient has a stoma. Moreover, the patient can intubate the reservoir at convenient times and places 2–4 times daily. The disadvantage is the excessive need for revisional surgery, most often due to valve malfunction (Dozois et al 1985). Even in the best of hands and despite numerous technical refinements, the risk of valve failure in the long term is about 20%. With better selection of patients, the use of a longer valve, staples and sutures around the base of the pouch and better postoperative management with more prolonged intubation, the early complications of procedures can be minimized.

### *Results*

The results of this operation are quite satisfactory in centers where the operation is performed regularly. Postoperative complications are most often nonpouch-related and include small bowel obstruction and delayed perineal wound healing. Suture line leakage from the reservoir, fistulae and stomal necrosis occur quite infrequently once the surgeon has gained sufficient experience.

Sepsis occurs with the same frequency as with other

abdominal operations. Early suture line leakage may require diversion of the fecal stream. Keeping the reservoir empty and continuously intubated in the immediate postoperative period may help prevent such problems. Bleeding from the suture line is rarely extensive and immediate reoperation has seldom been necessary. It may help at the time of construction of the reservoir to cauterize the incised bowel and to use a full-thickness suturing technique. Stomal necrosis is more likely to occur in obese patients with a thick abdominal wall or if the nipple valve has been revised often. If necrosis is limited to the superficial portion of the bowel traversing the abdominal wall, revision may not be necessary but a stomal stricture may later develop. A late fistula may also develop between the nipple valve and the pouch or the outflow track, resulting in incontinence. Under these circumstances, revisional surgery with construction of a new valve is necessary.

The most frequent problem associated with a Kock pouch is loss of some or all of the surgically constructed intussusception of the distal 10 cm of the ileum used to create the pouch. This reduction of the nipple valve usually occurs within the first year after the surgery and may be precipitated by too early or too infrequent intubations of the pouch and usually results in difficult intubating and ultimately incontinence. Surgery is required to restore continence.

Rarely, the nipple valve will prolapse. This may occur during excessive exercise or pregnancy and is usually easily reducible. Revisional surgery to narrow the size of the site of the outflow tract may be necessary for persistent or recurrent prolapse.

Pouchitis was diagnosed in 7% of Kock pouch patients operated for ulcerative colitis and was associated with diarrhea, discomfort and low-grade fever. Clinical symptoms respond dramatically to antibiotics such as metronidazole or others, suggesting that overgrowth of bacteria plays an important etiologic role. In those patients with recurrent pouchitis that responds poorly to traditional therapy, the possibility of Crohn's disease should be entertained.

Most patients who have had their Brooke ileostomy converted are pleased with the results and have experienced an improved quality of life with less restriction, especially in sexual and sport activities (Kohler et al 1991). Long-term results are excellent in terms of continence and return to normal lifestyle; it is important to remind patients to have their reservoir examined periodically to assess the mucosa.

## Conclusion

Surgical treatment is central in the management of ulcerative colitis because it cures the disease, can be life-saving under urgent and life-threatening circumstances, prevents cancer and restores the patient's health. Several options are currently available and it is important to discuss objectively with patients those best applicable to their own lifestyle, workplace, etc. Surgeons should also clearly emphasize to patients preoperatively the advantages and disadvantages of each of the possible options and have patients participate in the decision-making process. This can be further emphasized by an experienced enterostomal therapist. Although each surgical alternative still has a place, most patients with ulcerative colitis are young and will understandably opt for the ileal pouch–anal anastomosis. The operation is not perfect, but it is curative and does provide patients with a better quality of life than the other options. The impact of the operation may ultimately alter the timing of referral of such patients for surgical consideration. Indeed, if appropriately timed at a stage when the disease is less severe, this newer surgical approach may result in even less morbidity and thus could become even more acceptable to both patients and their treating physicians.

## Surgery for Crohn's disease

Crohn's disease is of unknown etiology, multifocal and incurable. While surgery is limited primarily to the treatment of complications it plays a crucial role since it may be life-saving and most patients will likely require at least one operation during the course of their prolonged illness. The management varies depending on the site(s) of involvement, the nature of the complications and the general status of the patient. The need for surgery relates to the chronicity of the disease and its tendency for obstruction, relapse and recurrence. Less often, an operation may be required for acute and fulminant complications such as hemorrhage, perforation, sepsis or toxic dilatation. Finally, the sole advance in surgery for Crohn's disease in recent years has been the advent of strictureplasty for small bowel obstructive disease, the most common indication for operation in this disease. More emphasis will therefore be placed on this novel technique.

### *Small intestinal disease and strictureplasty*

Bowel obstruction is the most common reason for operating on patients with Crohn's disease and is indicated, by order of decreasing frequency, in patients with small bowel disease, ileocolonic disease and large bowel disease. For isolated distal ileal or ileocolonic disease necessitating surgery, resection remains the procedure of choice. As a rule, resection is preferable to strictureplasty if inflammation is active and multiple strictures are confined to a short segment of bowel (Spencer et al 1994). However, if the disease is multifocal with numerous isolated fibrotic strictures, a conservative yet therapeutic approach would seem most reasonable. The concept of widening the bowel lumen, either by transversely closing a longitudinal inci-

**Table 23.17** Results of strictureplasty in patients with Crohn's disease

| Authors | Number of patients | Number of strictureplasties | % of patients Concomitant resection | Perioperative complications | Recurrent symptoms | Mean follow-up (months) |
|---|---|---|---|---|---|---|
| Alexander-Williams & Haynes (1985) | 57 | 146 | – | 14 | 40 | 6 |
| Silverman et al (1989) | 14 | 36 | 81 | 21 | 26 | 16 |
| Fazio et al (1989) | 50 | 225 | 60 | 16 | 22 | 8 |
| Dehn et al (1989) | 13 | 52 | 31 | 15 | 69 | 24 |
| Spencer et al (1994) | 35 | 71 | 67 | 14 | 20 | 36 |

Modified from Spencer et al (1994)

sion made across the narrowed part if the stricture is short or by approximating the longitudinal incision side-to-side if the stricture is long, as advocated by Lee & Papaioannou (1982) and Alexander-Williams & Haynes (1985), is sound and the results have been most rewarding. In our own experience at the Mayo Clinic with 71 strictureplasties in 35 patients, the operation was safe with no deaths, a low overall complication rate of 14% and no enteric leaks, fistulae or abscesses. The procedure was also effective in that 33 of 35 patients resumed enteral nutrition and discontinued medical treatment (Spencer et al 1994). The symptomatic recurrence rate was 20% at 3 years and six patients required reoperation. Similarly encouraging results have been published by others (Table 23.17). Bypass of a long strictured area is rarely, if ever, indicated because of persistent disease in the diverted segment and its inherent complications, especially cancer.

*Colonic disease*

Crohn's disease may involve most or all of the colon and rectum or the colon alone, either completely or only segmentally. When the disease involves the entire colon and the rectum is spared or minimally involved (15–30% of colitis patients), colectomy with ileorectal anastomosis is reasonable. The surgeon should be concerned with recurrence in the rectum and later proctectomy, anastomotic morbidity and postoperative function and these concerns should be shared with the patient preoperatively. After ileorectostomy, anastomotic breakdown is the most serious complication and may occur in 5–30% of patients (Longo & Ballantyne 1994). Goligher (1979) noted a 70% recurrence rate in the ileum, the rectum or both and 80% required an ileostomy. A 65% recurrence rate was seen at the Cleveland Clinic; however, and most importantly, two-thirds of these patients retained a functional rectum during an average follow-up of nearly 10 years (Longo et al 1992).

The need to conserve functional mucosa is not as imperative in the colon as in the small intestine, although functional derangement may be significant (Longo & Ballantyne 1994). Because of this, some authors advocate segmental resection for segmental colonic disease, further reasoning that the morbidity of colectomy is not negligible and ileostomy should be delayed as long as feasible, especially in younger patients. This is especially true if the right colon can be preserved because of its ability to absorb water and electrolytes. The major disadvantage is the elevated recurrence rate in the remaining large bowel and the need for further surgery, averaging 60–65% at 10 years.

Strictureplasty is rarely indicated to manage colonic strictures except perhaps when preserving the right colon is most important due to previous extensive small bowel resection or for recurrence at the site of a previous ileocolonic anastomosis.

The risk of large bowel cancer complicating Crohn's colitis does not approach that observed with mucosal ulcerative colitis, but it is not negligible and is much greater than in the general population (Weedon et al 1973); one should be suspicious in the presence of extensive disease, bypassed loops or strictured or fistulizing bowel.

Finally, in rare patients with isolated rectal or rectosigmoid disease, proctectomy with end colostomy is reasonable. If later recurrence involves more of the colon, colectomy and ileostomy are indicated. Pouch procedures, such as the continent ileostomy of Kock and the ileal pouch–anal anastomosis, should not be used in definite Crohn's colitis.

In summary, proctocolectomy and ileostomy give the best long-term results in terms of recurrence rates. Colectomy and ileorectal anastomosis may delay or even avoid a stoma and is especially gratifying in young patients in whom it also avoids sexual dysfunction. Segmental resection is reasonable for short segmental colitis as long as the patient understands its limitations.

*Gastroduodenal disease*

Crohn's disease of the distal stomach and duodenum is fortunately uncommon (less than 4%) and is most often associated with obstruction. When necessary, surgery should include gastroenterostomy with proximal gastric or highly selective vagotomy. Total small bowel denervation by truncal ligation should be avoided in the event that diarrhea may complicate it. Strictureplasty of the duodenum is used rarely and only for very short fibrotic strictures. Primary duodenal fistulae are very rare and the duodenal defect can be corrected by simple closure, duodenojejunostomy or serosal onlay patch (Schoetz 1992).

### *Perianal disease*

Anal manifestations of Crohn's disease are common and characteristic, may be the first evidence of the disease and may represent a challenge to the surgeon. Because of the pain it causes and the risk of incontinence that can result from the destructive disease and/or unnecessarily aggressive surgical therapy, conservatism has become of paramount importance; at the same time, however, a tendency to undertreat must be avoided (Abcarian 1994).

Anorectal pain, edema, bleeding and soiling are common manifestations and may result from the disease process and chronic skin irritation by diarrhea, leading to ulceration and excoriation, hemorrhoidal disease, fissures, abscesses and fistulae. Frank incontinence may result not only from the aggressive and destructive nature of the disease with rectovaginal and anoperineal fistulae and loss of rectal compliance, but also from inappropriate surgical therapy. The diagnosis is based on inspection, clinical awareness, digital examination, anoscopy, proctosigmoidoscopy and evaluation of the entire gut. Pain may preclude an adequate examination, which may have to be done under anesthesia. In patients with clinical incontinence in need of surgery, the sphincter mechanism should be assessed carefully with all the modern means at our disposition.

## **Diversion colitis** (Glotzer et al 1981, Lusk et al 1984)

Inflammation may develop in an excluded segment of colon and this has been termed "diversion colitis". The endoscopic and pathological features of the affected mucosa resemble mild ulcerative colitis or there may be aphthous ulcers. The condition occurs in patients with no evidence of previous inflammatory bowel disease and resolves when the fecal stream in restored. However, diversion proctitis has been reported after diversion of the fecal stream in Crohn's disease (Korelitz et al 1984). There is conjecture that the disorder is due to the absence of nutrients, e.g. butyrate, which are normally present in the fecal stream.

## Natural history of inflammatory bowel disease

Among patients with ulcerative colitis, one-quarter present with ulcerative proctitis alone (Hendriksen et al 1985). Among patients with proctitis, the chance of the disease extending into the sigmoid is approximately 30% and the chance of extending to involve the entire colon is between 5% and 10% over 10 years (Ritchie et al 1978). About one-third of patients with ulcerative proctitis have a single attack and the others have a relapsing course (Willoughby 1983). In a population-based study of 783 patients, 9.6% of patients underwent colectomy in the year of diagnosis and the cumulative 10- and 18-year colectomy rates after diagnosis were 23% and 31% (Hendriksen et al 1985). After 3 years from the diagnosis of ulcerative colitis, patients who had undergone surgery and patients who had been treated medically for ulcerative colitis did not differ from the general population in their capacity to work (Hendriksen et al 1985). Among patients with Crohn's disease and ulcerative colitis, the survival at 10 years after diagnosis is 96% of that predicted (Ekbom et al 1992).

About 60–70% of patients with Crohn's disease eventually require at least one surgical treatment (Sales & Kirsner 1983). Following the initial surgical therapy, about 70% of patients will require further surgical therapy. Patients with ileocolitis are more likely to have recurrence following surgery than patients with ileitis alone (Farmer 1981).

REFERENCES


Abcarian H 1994 Perianal Crohn's disease. In: Veidenheimer M (ed) Management of Crohn's disease. Seminars in colon and rectal surgery 5: 204–209

Admans H, Whorwell P J, Wright R 1980 Diagnosis of Crohn's disease. Digestive Diseases and Sciences 25: 911

Alexander-Williams J, Haynes I G 1985 Conservative operations for Crohn's disease of the small bowel. World Journal of Surgery 9: 945–951

Alstead E M, Ritchie J K, Lennard-Jones J E, Farthing M J G, Clark M L 1990 Safety of azathioprine in pregnancy in inflammatory bowel disease. Gastroenterology 99: 443–446

Altman A R, Maltz C, Janowitz H D 1979 Autoimmune hemolytic anemia in ulcerative colitis: report of three cases, review of the literature, and evaluation of modes of therapy. Digestive Diseases and Sciences 24: 282–285

Ambroze W L, Dozois R R, Pemberton J H, Beart R W Jr, Ilstrup D M 1992 Familial adenomatous polyposis: results following ileal pouch–anal anastomosis and ileorectostomy. Diseases of the Colon and Rectum 35: 12–15

Anderson J B, Turner G M, Williamson R C N 1987 Fulminant ulcerative colitis in late pregnancy and the puerperium. Journal of the Royal Society of Medicine 80: 492–449

Anonymous 1987 Reproducibility of colonoscopic findings in Crohn's disease: a prospective, multicenter study of interobserver variation. Groupe d'Etudes Therapeutiques des Affections Inflammatoires du Tude Digestif (GETAID). Digestive Diseases and Sciences 32: 1370–1379

Ariyama J, Wehlin L, Lindstrom C G, Wenkert A, Roberts G M 1980 Gastroduodenal erosions in Crohn's disease. Gastrointestinal Radiology 5: 121–125

Axon A T R, Dickinson R J 1983 Endoscopy in Crohn's disease. In: Allan R N, Keighley M R B, Alexander-Williams J, Hawkins C (eds) Inflammatory bowel diseases. Churchill Livingstone, Edinburgh, p 210

Aylett S O 1966 Three hundred cases of diffuse ulcerative colitis treated by total colectomy and ileorectal anastomosis. British Medical Journal 1: 1001

Aylett S O 1971 Cancer and ulcerative colitis. British Medical Journal 2: 203

Azad Khan A K, Truelove S C 1976 The actions of sulphasalazine. In: Truelove S C, Ritchie J A (eds) Topics in gastroenterology 4. Blackwell, Oxford, p 367

Azad Khan A K, Piris J, Truelove S C 1977 An experiment to determine the active therapeutic moiety of sulphasalazine. Lancet 2: 892–895

Baker W N W, Milton-Thompson G J 1974 Management of anal fistulae in Crohn's disease. Proceedings of the Royal Society of Medicine 67: 58

Baker W N W, Glass R E, Ritchie J K, Aylett S O 1978 Cancer of the rectum following colectomy and ileorectal anastomosis for ulcerative colitis. British Journal of Surgery 65: 862–868

Ball G V, Goldman L N 1976 Chronic ulcerative colitis, skin necrosis, and cryofibrinogenemia. Annals of Internal Medicine 85: 464

Banks B M, Zetzel L, Richter H S 1969 Morbidity and mortality in regional enteritis. Report of 168 cases. American Journal of Digestive Diseases 14: 369

Baron J H, Connell A M, Kanaghinis T G 1962 Outpatient treatment of ulcerative colitis: comparison between three doses of oral prednisolone. British Medical Journal 2: 441–443

Baron J H, Connell A M, Lennard-Jones J E 1964 Variation between observers in describing mucosal appearances in proctocolitis. British Medical Journal 1: 89

Baron T H, Truss C D, Elson C O 1993 Low-dose oral methotrexate in refractory inflammatory bowel disease. Digestive Diseases and Sciences 38: 1851–1856

Bartholomeusz F D L, Shearman D J C 1989 Measurement of activity in Crohn's disease. Journal of Gastroenterology and Hepatology 4: 81–94

Bartram C I 1977 Radiology in the current assessment of ulcerative colitis. Gastrointestinal Radiology 1: 383–392

Beeken W L 1975 Remediable defects in Crohn's disease. A prospective study of 63 patients. Archives of Internal Medicine 135: 686

Behrens R, Devereaux M, Hazleman B, Szaz K, Calvin J, Neale G 1986 Investigation of Auranofin-induced diarrhoea. Gut 27: 59

Bennett R A, Rubin P H, Present D H 1991 Frequency of inflammatory bowel disease in offspring of couples both presenting with inflammatory bowel disease. Gastroenterology 100: 1638–1643

Berger M, Gribetz D, Korelitz B I 1975 Growth retardation in children with ulcerative colitis: the effect of medical and surgical therapy. Pediatrics 55: 459–467

Best W R, Becktel J M, Singleton J W, Kern F Jr 1976 Development of a Crohn's disease activity index. National Cooperative Crohn's Disease Study. Gastroenterology 70: 439–444

Billson F A, de Dombal F T, Watkinson G, Goligher J C 1967 Ocular complications of ulcerative colitis. Gut 8: 102

Binder V, Elsborg L, Greibe J 1981 Disodium cromoglycate in the treatment of ulcerative colitis and Crohn's disease. Gut 22: 55

Blackstone M O, Riddell R H, Rogers B H, Levin B 1981 Dysplasia-associated lesion or mass (DALM) detected by colonoscopy in long-standing ulcerative colitis: an indication for colectomy. Gastroenterology 80: 366–374

Blichfeldt P, Blomhoff J P, Myhre E, Gjone E 1978 Metronidazole in Crohn's disease. A double blind cross-over clinical trial. Scandinavian Journal of Gastroenterology 13: 123

Blomberg B, Rolny P, Jarnerot G 1991 Endoscopic treatment of anastomotic strictures in Crohn's disease. Endoscopy 23: 195–198

Bo-Linn G W, Vendrell D D, Lee E, Fordtran J S 1985 An evaluation of the significance of microscopic colitis in patients with chronic diarrhea. Journal of Clinical Investigation 75: 1559

Borda I T, Southern R F, Brown W F 1973 Cerebral venous thrombosis in ulcerative colitis. Gastroenterology 64: 116

Brant L J, Bernstein L H, Boley S J, Frank M S 1982 Metronidazole therapy for perineal Crohn's disease: a follow-up study. Gastroenterology 83: 383

Brostrom O, Lofberg R, Nordenvall B, Ost A, Hellers G 1987 The risk of colorectal cancer in ulcerative colitis. An epidemiologic study. Scandinavian Journal of Gastroenterology 22: 1193–1199

Brynskov J, Freund L, Rasmussen S N et al 1989 A placebo-controlled, double-blind, randomized trial of cyclosporine therapy in active chronic Crohn's disease. New England Journal of Medicine 321: 845–850

Brynskov J, Freund L, Rasmussen S N et al 1991 Final report on a placebo-controlled, double-blind, randomized, multicentre trial of cyclosporin treatment in active chronic Crohn's disease. Scandinavian Journal of Gastroenterology 26: 689–695

Burul C J, Ritchie J K, Hawley P R, Told I P 1980 Psoas abscess: a complication of Crohn's disease. British Journal of Surgery 67: 355–356

Calkins B M 1989 A meta-analysis of the role of smoking in inflammatory bowel disease. Digestive Disease and Sciences 34: 1841–1854

Camilleri M, Proano M 1989 Advances in the assessment of disease activity in inflammatory bowel disease. Mayo Clinic Proceedings 64: 800–807

Campieri M, Lanfranchi G A, Boschi S et al 1985 Topical administration of 5-aminosalicylic acid enemas in patients with ulcerative colitis. Studies on rectal absorption and excretion. Gut 26: 400

Cangemi J R, Wiesner R H, Beaver S J et al 1989 Effect of proctocolectomy for chronic ulcerative colitis on the natural history of primary sclerosing cholangitis. Gastroenterology 96: 790–794

Carpenter H A, Tremaine W J, Batts K P, Czaja A J 1992 Sequential histologic evaluations in collagenous colitis. Correlations with disease behavior and sampling strategy. Digestive Diseases and Sciences 37: 1903–1909

Cary E R, Tremaine W J, Banks P M, Nagorney D M 1989 Isolated Crohn's disease of the stomach. Mayo Clinic Proceedings 64: 776–779

Chakraborty T K, Bhatia D, Heading R C, Ford M J 1987 Salicylate induced exacerbation of ulcerative colitis. Gut 28: 613

Chan R P, Pope D J, Gilbert A P, Sacra P J, Baron J H, Lennard-Jones J E 1983 Studies of two novel sulfasalazine analogs, ipsalazide and balsalazide. Digestive Diseases and Sciences 28: 609

Chapman N J, Brown M L, Phillips S F et al 1992 Distribution of mesalamine enemas in patients with active distal ulcerative colitis. Mayo Clinic Proceedings 67: 245–248

Chesner I M, Muller S, Newman J 1986 Ulcerative colitis complicated by Budd–Chiari syndrome. Gut 27: 1096

Choen S, Tsunoda A, Nicholls R J 1991 Prospective randomized trial comparing anal function after hand sewn ileoanal anastomosis with mucosectomy versus stapled ileoanal anastomosis without mucosectomy in restorative proctocolectomy. British Journal of Surgery 78: 430–434

Chong S K F, Blackshaw A J, Boyle S, Williams C B, Walker-Smith J A 1985 Histological diagnosis of chronic inflammatory bowel disease in childhood. Gut 26: 55

Chrispin A R, Fry I K 1963 The presacral space shown by barium enema. British Journal of Radiology 36: 319

Collins R H Jr, Feldman M, Fordtran J S 1987 Colon cancer, dysplasia and surveillance in patients with ulcerative colitis: a critical review. New England Journal of Medicine 316: 1654–1658

Cominelli F, Kam L 1993 Inflammatory mediators of inflammatory bowel disease. Current Opinion in Gastroenterology 9: 534–543

Compston J E, Judd D, Crawley E O et al 1987 Osteoporosis in patients with inflammatory bowel disease. Gut 28: 40

Connell W R, Kamm M A, Lennard-Jones J E, Ritchie J K 1992 Twenty seven year experience in 739 patients of bone marrow toxicity from azathioprine in inflammatory bowel disease. Gastroenterology 102 (abstract): A609

Cook M G, Dixon M F 1973 An analysis of the reliability of detection and diagnostic value of various pathological features in Crohn's disease and ulcerative colitis. Gut 14: 255

Cox E V, Meynell M J, Cooke W T, Gaddie R 1958 The folic acid excretion test in the steatorrhea syndrome. Gastroenterology 35: 390

Croft C B, Wilkinson A R 1972 Ulceration of the mouth, pharynx, and larynx in Crohn's disease of the intestine. British Journal of Surgery 59: 249

Crohn B B, Yarnis H 1958 Regional ileitis, 2nd edn. Grune & Stratton, New York

Daly D W, Brooke B N 1967 Ileostomy and excision of the large intestine for ulcerative colitis. Lancet 2: 62

Danielsson A, Hellers G, Lyrenas E et al 1987 A controlled trial of budesonide versus prednisolone retention enemas in active distal ulcerative colitis. Scandinavian Journal of Gastroenterology 22: 987–992
Danzi J T 1988 Extraintestinal manifestations of idiopathic inflammatory bowel disease. Archives of Internal Medicine 148: 297–302
Das K M, Eastwood M A, McManus J P A, Sircus W 1974 The role of the colon in the metabolism of salicylazosulphapyridine. Scandinavian Journal of Gastroenterology 9: 137
Das K M, Sakamaki S, Vecchi M, Diamond B 1987 The production and characterization of monoclonal antibodies to human colonic antigen associated with ulcerative colitis: cellular localization of the antigen by using the monoclonal antibody. Journal of Immunology 139: 77–84
Davidson M 1975 Chronic ulcerative colitis and Crohn's colitis in the pediatric patient. In: Kirsner J B, Shorter R G (eds) Inflammatory bowel disease. Lea & Febiger, Philadelphia, p 154
De Dombal F T, Watts J McK, Watkinson G, Goligher J C 1965 Intraperitoneal perforation of the colon in ulcerative colitis. Proceedings of the Royal Society of Medicine 58: 713
De Dombal F T, Watts J McK, Watkinson G, Goligher J C 1966a Incidence and management of anorectal abscess, fistula and fissure, in patients with ulcerative colitis. Diseases of the Colon and Rectum 9: 201
De Dombal F T, Watts J McK, Watkinson G, Goligher J C 1966b Local complications of ulcerative colitis; stricture, pseudopolyposis and carcinoma of the colon and rectum. British Medical Journal 1: 1442
De Dombal F T, Geffen N, Darnborough A, Watkinson G, Goligher JC 1968 Radiological appearances of ulcerative colitis: an evaluation of their clinical significance. Gut 9: 157
De Dombal F T, Burton I L, Clamp S E, Goligher J C 1974 Short-term course and prognosis of Crohn's disease. Gut 15: 435–443
Dehn T C B, Kettlewell M G W, Mortensen N J M, Lee E C G, Jewell D P 1989 Ten year experience with stricturoplasty for obstructive Crohn's disease. British Journal of Surgery 76: 339–341
Devroede G 1980 Risk of cancer in inflammatory bowel disease. In: Winawer S J, Schottenfeld D, Sherlock P (eds) Colorectal cancer: prevention, epidemiology and screening. Raven Press, New York, p 325–334
Dew M J, Hughes P, Harries A D, Williams G, Evans B K, Rhodes J 1982 Maintenance of remission in ulcerative colitis with oral preparation of 5-aminosalicylic acid. British Medical Journal 285: 1012
Dick A P, Berridge F R, Grayson M J 1959 The pathological basis of the radiological changes in ulcerative colitis. A study of cases treated by colectomy. British Journal of Radiology 32: 432
Dick A P, Holt L P, Dalton E R 1966 Persistence of mucosal abnormality in ulcerative colitis. Gut 7: 355
Diethelm A G, Nickel W F, Wantz G E 1968 Ulcerative colitis in the elderly patient. Surgery, Gynecology and Obstetrics 126: 223
Dixon M F, Brown L J R, Gilmour H M et al 1988 Observer variation in the assessment of dysplasia in ulcerative colitis. Histopathology 13: 385–397
Donaldson R M Jr 1985 Management of medical problems in pregnancy-inflammatory bowel disease. New England Journal of Medicine 312: 1616–1619
Donowitz M 1985 Arachidonic acid metabolites and their role in inflammatory bowel disease. An update requiring addition of a pathway. Gastroenterology 88: 580
Dotevall G, Kock N G 1968 Absorption studies in regional enterocolitis. Scandinavian Journal of Gastroenterology 3: 293
Dozois R R 1988 Pelvis and perianastomotic complications after ileoanal anastomosis. Perspectives in Colon and Rectal Surgery 1: 113–121
Dozois R R, Juhasz E S 1993 Ileal pouch–anal anastomosis: is excision of anal transition zone mucosa essential? Canadian Journal of Gastroenterology 7: 258
Dozois R R, Kelly K A, Beart R WJr, Beahrs O H 1985 Continent ileostomy: the Mayo Clinic experience. In: Dozois R R (ed) Alternatives to conventional ileostomy. Year Book Medical Publishers, Chicago p 180–191
Dozois R R, Nelson H, Metcalf A M 1993 Fonction sexuelle après anastomose iléo-anale. Annales de Chirurgie 47: 1009–1013
Dronfield M W, Fletcher J, Langman M J S 1974 Coincident salmonella infections and ulcerative colitis: problems of recognition and management. British Medical Journal 1: 99
Drossman D A, Patrick, D L, Mitchell C M, Zagami E A, Appelbaum M I 1989 Health-related quality of life in inflammatory bowel disease. Functional status and patient worries and concerns. Digestive Diseases and Sciences 34: 1379–1386
Du Boulay C, Whorwell P J 1982 "Nodular necrobiosis": a new cutaneous manifestation of Crohn's disease? Gut 23: 712
DuBrow R A, Frank P H 1983 Barium evaluation of anal canal in patients with inflammatory bowel disease. American Journal of Roentgenology 140: 1151–1157
Duerr R H, Targan S R, Landers C J, Sutherland L R, Shanahan F 1991a Anti-neutrophil cytoplasmic antibodies in ulcerative colitis. Comparison with other colitides/diarrheal illnesses. Gastroenterology 100: 1590–1596
Duerr R H, Targan S R, Landers C J, LaRusso N F, Wiesner R H 1991b Neutrophil cytoplasmic antibodies: a link between primary sclerosing cholangitis and ulcerative colitis. Gastroenterology: 100: 1385–1391
Duffy L F, Daum F, Fisher S E et al 1985 Peripheral neuropathy in Crohn's disease patients treated with metronidazole. Gastroenterology 88: 681
Dyer N H, Cook P L, Harper R A K 1969 Oesophageal stricture associated with Crohn's disease. Gut 10: 549
Dyer N H, Rutherford C, Visick J H, Dawson A M 1970 The incidence and reliability of individual radiographic signs in the small intestine in Crohn's disease. British Journal of Radiology 43: 401
Edwards F C, Truelove S C 1963 The course and prognosis of ulcerative colitis. Pts I and II. Gut 4: 299
Edwards F C, Truelove S C 1964 The course and prognosis of ulcerative colitis. Pts III and IV. Gut 5: 1
Ekberg O 1977 Double contrast examination of the small bowel. Gastrointestinal Radiology 1: 349–353
Ekberg O, Fork F-Th, Hildell J 1980 Predictive value of small bowel radiography for recurrent Crohn disease. American Journal of Roentgenology 135: 1051
Ekbom A, Helmick C, Zack M, Adami H-O 1990 Ulcerative colitis and colorectal cancer: A population based study. New England Journal of Medicine 323: 1228–1233
Ekbom A, Helmick C G, Zack M, Holmberg L, Adami H-O 1992 Survival and causes of death in patients with inflammatory bowel disease: a population based study. Gastroenterology 103: 954–960
Evans J G, Acheson E D 1965 An epidemiological study of ulcerative colitis and regional enteritis in the Oxford area. Gut 6: 311
Ewen S W B, Anderson J, Galloway J M D, Miller J D B, Kyle J 1971 Crohn's disease initially confined to the appendix. Gastroenterology 60: 853
Fantry G T, James S P 1993 Cellular and molecular immunology and biochemistry of inflammatory bowel disease. Current Opinion in Gastroenterology 9: 544–551
Farmer R G 1981 Factors in the long-term prognosis of patients with inflammatory bowel disease. American Journal of Gastroenterology 75: 97–103
Farmer R G 1989 Study of family history among patients with inflammatory bowel disease. Scandinavian Journal of Gastroenterology. 24 (suppl 170): 64–65
Farmer R G, Brown C H 1967 Ulcerative colitis confined to the rectum and sigmoid flexure. Report of 124 cases. Diseases of the Colon and Rectum 10: 177
Farmer R G, Schumacher O P 1970 Treatment of ulcerative colitis with hydrocortisone enemas: relationship of hydrocortisone absorption, adrenal suppression and clinical response. Diseases of the Colon and Rectum 13: 355
Farmer R G, Hawk W A, Turnbull R B 1972 Crohn's disease of the duodenum (transmural duodenitis): clinical manifestions. American Journal of Digestive Diseases 17: 191
Farmer R G, Hawk W A, Turnbull R B 1975 Clinical patterns in Crohn's disease: a statistical study of 615 cases. Gastroenterology 68: 627
Farnell M B, Adson M A 1985 Ileorectostomy – current results: the

Mayo Clinic experience. In: Dozois R R (ed) Alternatives to conventional ileostomy. Year Book Medical Publishers, Chicago, p 100–121
Farthing M J, Rutland M D, Clark M L 1979 Retrograde spread of hydrocortisone containing foam given intrarectally in ulcerative colitis. British Medical Journal 2: 822–824
Fausa O, Foerster A, Hovig T 1985 Collagenous colitis. A clinical, histological, and ultrastructural study. Scandinavian Journal of Gastroenterology 20 (suppl 107): 8
Fazio V W, Galandiuk S, Jagelman D J, Lavery I C 1989 Stricturoplasty in Crohn's disease. Annals of Surgery 210: 621–625
Feagan B G, McDonald W D, Rochon J et al 1994 Low-dose cyclosporine for the treatment of Crohn's disease. The Canadian Crohn's Relapse Prevention Trial Investigation. New England Journal of Medicine 330: 1846–1851
Ferguson C M, Moncure A C 1985 Benign duodenocolic fistula. Diseases of the Colon and Rectum 28: 852
Fielding J 1972 Crohn's disease of the small intestine and stomach. British Journal of Hospital Medicine 7: 766
Fielding J F 1986 The relative risk of inflammatory bowel disease among parents and siblings of Crohn's disease patients. Journal of Clinical Gastroenterology 8: 655–657
Fielding J F, Cooke W T 1971 Finger clubbing and regional enteritis. Gut 12: 442
Fielding J F, Toye D K M, Beton D C, Cooke W T 1970 Crohn's disease of the stomach and duodenum. Gut 11: 1001–1006
Fiocchi C 1994 Cytokines. In: Targan S R, Shanahan F (eds) Inflammatory bowel disease. From bench to bedside. Williams & Wilkins, Baltimore, p 106–122
Fishman E K, Wolf E J, Jones B, Bayless T M, Siegelman S S 1987 CT evaluation of Crohn's disease. Effect on patient management. American Journal of Radiology 148: 537
Fleckenstein P, Knudsen L, Pedersen E B, Marcussen H, Jarnum S 1977 Obstructive uropathy in chronic inflammatory bowel disease. Scandinavian Journal of Gastroenterology 12: 519–523
Ford G A, Oliver P S, Shephard N A, Wilkinson S P 1992 An Eudragit-coated prednisolone preparation for ulcerative colitis: pharmacokinetics and preliminary therapeutic use. Alimentary Pharmacology and Therapeutics 6: 31–40
Forrest J A H, Shearman D J C 1975 Pulmonary vasculitis and ulcerative colitis. American Journal of Digestive Diseases 20: 482
Francois Y, Dozois RR, Kelly KA et al 1989 Small intestinal obstruction complicating ileal pouch–anal anastomosis. Annals of Surgery 209: 46–50
Frank P H, Riddell R H, Feczko P J, Levin B 1978 Radiological detection of colonic dysplasia (precarcinoma) in chronic ulcerative colitis. Gastrointestinal Radiology 3: 209
Friedman H B, Silver G M, Brown C H 1968 Lymphoma of the colon simulating ulcerative colitis. American Journal of Digestive Diseases 13: 910–917
Froelich J W 1987 Nuclear medicine imaging of inflammatory bowel disease. Radiologic Clinics of North America 25: 133–141
Gabrielsson N, Granqvist S, Sundelin P, Thorgeirsson T 1979 Extent of inflammatory lesions in ulcerative colitis assessed by radiology, colonoscopy, and endoscopic biopsies. Gastrointestinal Radiology 4: 395
Galandiuk S, Scott N A, Dozois R R et al 1990 Ileal pouch–anal anastomosis: reoperation for pouch-related complications. Annals of Surgery 212: 446–454
Galandiuk S, Wolff B G, Dozois R R, Beart R W Jr 1991 Ileal pouch–anal anastomosis without ileostomy. Diseases of the Colon and Rectum 34: 870–873
Gardiner R, Stevenson G W 1982 The colitides. Radiologic Clinics of North America 20: 797
Garrett J M, Sauer W G, Moertel C G 1967 Colonic motility in ulcerative colitis after opiate administration. Gastroenterology 53: 93
Gelfand M D, Tepper M, Katz L A, Binder H J, Yesner R, Floch M H 1968 Acute irradiation proctitis in man. Development of eosinophilic crypt abscesses. Gastroenterology 54: 401
Gemlo B T, Wong W D, Rothenberger D A, Goldberg S M 1992 Ileal pouch–anal anastomosis. Patterns of failure. Archives of Surgery 127: 784–787
Gerson C D, Cohen N, Janowitz H D 1973 Small intestinal absorptive function in regional enteritis. Gastroenterology 64: 907
Gilat T, Lilos P, Zemishlany Z, Ribak J, Benarova Y 1976 Ulcerative colitis in the Jewish population of Tel-Aviv Yafo 111. Clinical course. Gastroenterology 70: 14
Gilat T, Fireman Z, Grossman A et al 1988 Colorectal cancer in patients with ulcerative colitis. A population study in central Israel. Gastroenterology 94: 870–877
Glick S N, Teplick S K 1985 Crohn disease of the small intestine: diffuse mucosal granularity. Radiology 154: 313
Glotzer D J, Glick M E, Goldman H 1981 Proctitis and colitis following diversion of the fecal stream. Gastroenterology 80: 438
Goldberg H I, Jeffrey R B 1980 Recent advances in the radiographic evaluation of inflammatory bowel disease. Medical Clinics of North America 64: 1059
Goldberg H I, Caruthers S B Jr, Nelson J A, Singleton J W 1979 Radiographic findings of the National Cooperative Crohn's Disease Study. Gastroenterology 77: 925
Goldgraber M B, Kirsner J B 1957 "Specific" diseases simulating "nonspecific" ulcerative colitis (lymphopathia venereum, acute vasculitis, scleroderma and secondary amyloidosis). Annals of Internal Medicine 47: 939
Goldgraber M B, Kirsner J B, Palmer W L 1957 The role of ACTH and adrenal steroids in perforation of the colon in ulcerative colitis. A clinical-pathologic study. Gastroenterology 33: 434
Goligher J C 1979 The outcome of excisional operations for primary and recurrent Crohn's disease of the large intestine. Surgery, Gynecology and Obstetrics 148: 1–8
Goligher J C, de Dombal F T, Watts J McK, Watkinson G 1968 Ulcerative colitis. Baillière, Tindall and Cassell, London
Gonzalez-Licea A, Yardley J H 1966 Nature of the tissue reaction in ulcerative colitis. Light and electron microscopic findings. Gastroenterology 51: 825
Goodman M J, Kirsner J B, Riddell R H 1977 Usefulness of rectal biopsy in inflammatory bowel disease. Gastroenterology 72: 952
Gorbach S L 1982 Viral infections and inflammatory bowel disease. Gastroenterology 83: 1318
Gore R M, Cohen M I, Vogelzang R L, Neiman H L, Tsang T-K 1985 Value of computed tomography in the detection of complications of Crohn's disease. Digestive Diseases and Sciences 30: 701
Goulston S J M, McGovern V J 1969 The nature of benign strictures in ulcerative colitis. New England Journal of Medicine 281: 290
Grant C S, Dozois R R 1984 Toxic megacolon: ultimate fate of patients after successful medical management. American Journal of Surgery 147: 106–110
Gravallese E M, Kantrowitz F G 1988 Arthritic manifestations of inflammatory bowel disease. American Journal of Gastroenterology 83: 703–709
Greenstein A J, Aufses A H 1985 Differences in pathogenesis, incidence and outcome of perforation in inflammatory bowel disease. Surgery, Gynecology and Obstetrics 160: 63–69
Greenstein A J, Janowitz H D, Sachar D B 1976 The extra-intestinal complications of Crohn's disease and ulcerative colitis: a study of 700 patients. Medicine 55: 401
Greenstein A J, Sachar D B, Gibas A et al 1985 Outcome of toxic dilatation in ulcerative and Crohn's colitis. Journal of Clinical Gastroenterology 7: 137–144
Grieco M B, Bordan D L, Geiss A C, Beil A R 1980 Toxic megacolon complicating Crohn's colitis. Annals of Surgery 191: 75
Gudmand-Hoyer E, Jarnum S 1970 Incidence and clinical significance of lactose malabsorption in ulcerative colitis and Crohn's disease. Gut 11: 338
Haggitt R C, Meissner W A 1973 Crohn's disease of the upper gastrointestinal tract. American Journal of Clinical Pathology 59: 613
Halls J, Young A 1964 Plain abdominal films in colonic disease. Proceedings of the Royal Society of Medicine 57: 893
Halstensen T S, Mollnes T E, Garred P, Fausa O, Brandtzaeg P 1992 Surface epithelium related activation of complement differs in Crohn's disease and ulcerative colitis. Gut 33: 902–908
Hamilton S R 1985 Colorectal carcinoma in patients with Crohn's disease. Gastroenterology 89: 398
Hanauer S B, Smith M B 1993 Rapid closure of Crohn's disease fistulas

with continuous intravenous cyclosporin A. American Journal of Gastroenterology 88: 646–649
Hanauer S, Schwartz J, Robinson M et al 1993 Mesalamine capsules for treatment of active ulcerative colitis: results of a controlled trial. American Journal of Gastroenterology 88: 1188–1197
Hanngren A, Hansson E, Svartz N, Ullberg S 1963 Distribution and metabolism of salicyl-azo-sulfapyridine. 1. A study with $C^{14}$-salicyl-azo-sulfapyridine and $C^{14}$-5-amino-salicylic acid. 2. A study of $S^{35}$-salicyl-azo-sulfapyridine and $S^{35}$-sulfapyridine. Acta Medica Scandinavica 173: 61, 391
Harries A D, Brown R, Heatley R V, Williams L A, Woodhead S, Rhodes J 1985 Vitamin D status in Crohn's disease: association with nutrition and disease activity. Gut 26: 1197
Harvey R F, Bradshaw J M 1980 A simple index of Crohn's disease activity. Lancet 1: 514
Haslock I, Wright V 1973 The musculo-skeletal complications of Crohn's disease. Medicine 52: 217
Hawley P R 1988 Emergency surgery for ulcerative colitis. World Journal of Surgery 12: 169–173
Hawthorne A B, Hawkey C J 1989 Immunosuppressive drugs in inflammatory bowel disease. A review of their mechanisms of efficacy and place in therapy. Drugs 38: 267–288
Hawthorne A B, Logan R F A, Hawkey C J 1992 Randomized controlled trial of azathioprine withdrawal in ulcerative colitis. British Medical Journal 305: 20–22
Heatley R V 1984 Nutritional implications of inflammatory bowel disease. Scandinavian Journal of Gastroenterology 19: 995
Helgeland L, Tysk C, Janerot G et al 1992 IgG subclass distribution in serum and rectal mucosa of monozygotic twins with or without inflammatory bowel disease. Gut 33: 1358–1364
Helzer J E, Stillings W A, Chammas S, Norland C C, Alpers D H 1982 A controlled study of the association between ulcerative colitis and psychiatric illness. Digestive Diseases and Sciences 27: 513–518
Helzer J E, Chammas S, Norland C C, Stillings W A, Alpers D H 1984 A study of the association between Crohn's disease and psychiatric illness. Gastroenterology 86: 324
Hendriksen C, Kreiner S, Binder V 1985 Long term prognosis in ulcerative colitis – based on results from a regional patient group from the county of Copenhagen. Gut 26: 158–163
Heppell J, Farkouh E, Dube S, Peloquin A, Morgan S, Bernard D 1986 Toxic megacolon: an analysis of 70 cases. Diseases of the Colon and Rectum 29: 789–792
Herlinger H 1982 The small bowel enema and the diagnosis of Crohn's disease. Radiologic Clinics of North America 20: 721–742
Hightower N C Jr, Broders A C Jr, Haines R D, McKenney J F, Sommer A W 1958 Chronic ulcerative colitis. II. Complications. American Journal of Digestive Diseases 3: 861
Holdsworth C D 1981 Sulphasalazine desensitisation. British Medical Journal 282: 110
Hulten L, Kewenter J, Kock N G 1971 The long-term results of partial resection of the large bowel for intestinal carcinomas complicating ulcerative colitis. Scandinavian Journal of Gastroenterology 6: 601
Jackson C W, Haboubi N Y, Whorwell P J, Schofield P F 1986 Gold induced enterocolitis. Gut 27: 452
Jacobson I M, Schapiro R H, Warshaw A L 1985 Gastric and dudoenal fistulas in Crohn's disease. Gastroenterology 89: 1347
Jalan K N, Sircus W, Card W I et al 1969 An experience of ulcerative colitis. 1. Toxic dilation in 55 cases. Gastroenterology 57: 68
Jalan K N, Walker R J, Prescott R J, Butterworth S T G, Smith A N, Sircus W 1970a Faecal stasis and diverticular disease in ulcerative colitis. Gut 11: 688
Jalan K N, Prescott R J, Walker R J, Sircus W, McManus J P A, Card W I 1970b Arthropathy, ankylosing spondylitis and clubbing of fingers in ulcerative colitis. Gut 11: 748
Jalan K N, Prescott R J, Smith A N et al 1970c Influence of corticosteroids on the results of surgical treatment for ulcerative colitis. New England Journal of Medicine 282: 588
Jarnerot G, Rolny P, Sandberg-Gertzen H 1985 Intensive intravenous treatment of ulcerative colitis. Gastroenterology 89: 1005
Jayson M I V, Salmon P R, Harrison W J 1970 Inflammatory bowel disease in ankylosing spondylitis. Gut 11: 506
Johnson M L, Wilson H T H 1969 Skin lesions in ulcerative colitis. Gut 10: 255
Johnson O A, Hoskins D W, Todd J, Thorbjarnarson B 1966 Crohn's disease of the stomach. Gastroenterology 50: 571
Johnson W D, Roth J L A 1975 Diagnosis and differential diagnosis of chronic ulcerative colitis and Crohn's colitis. In: Kirsner J B, Shorter R G (eds) Inflammatory bowel disease. Lea and Febiger, Philadelphia, p 201
Jones B 1985 Double-contrast imaging of inflammatory bowel disease. In: Margulis A R, Gooding C A (eds) Diagnostic radiology. University of California, San Francisco, p 47
Jones H W, Grogono J, Hoare A M 1988 Surveillance in ulcerative colitis: burdens and benefits. Gut 29: 325–331
Jones J H, Chapman M 1969 Definition of megacolon in colitis. Gut 10: 562
Jones J H, Lennard-Jones J E, Young A C 1969 Reversibility of radiological appearances during clinical improvement in colonic Crohn's disease. Gut 10: 738
Juhasz E S, Goudet P, Dozois R R 1995 Surgery in ulcerative colitis. In: Mazier W P, Levien D H, Luchtefeld M A, Senagore A J (eds) Surgery of the colon, rectum, and anus. W B Saunders, Philadelphia
Kantor J L 1934 Regional (terminal) ileitis: its roentgen diagnosis. Journal of the American Medical Association 103: 2016
Kartheuser A H, Dozois R R, LaRusso N F, Wiesner R H, Ilstrup D M, Schleck C D 1993 Complications and risk factors after ileal pouch–anal anastomosis associated with primary sclerosing cholangitis. Annals of Surgery 217: 314–320
Keighley M R B, Eastwood D, Ambrose N S, Allan R N, Burdon D W 1982 Incidence and microbiology of abdominal and pelvic abscess in Crohn's disease. Gastroenterology 83: 1271
Kelly K A, Pemberton J H, Wolff B G, Dozois R R 1992 Ileal pouch–anal anastomosis. Current Problems in Surgery 29: 57–131
Kelvin F M, Oddson T A, Rice R P, Garbutt J T, Bradenham B P 1978 Double contrast barium enema in Crohn's disease and ulcerative colitis. American Journal of Roentgenology 131: 207
Kewenter J, Ahlman H, Hulten L 1978 Cancer risk in extensive colitis. Annals of Surgery 188: 824–828
Kingham J G C, Levison D A, Morson B C, Dawson A M 1986 Collagenous colitis. Gut 27: 570
Kirschner B S, Voinchet O, Rosenberg I H 1978 Growth retardation in inflammatory bowel disease. Gastroenterology 75: 504–511
Kirsner J B 1973 Genetic aspects of inflammatory bowel disease. Clinics in Gastroenterology 2: 557
Kirsner J B 1975 Problems in the differentiation of ulcerative colitis and Crohn's disease of the colon: the need for repeated diagnostic evaluation. Gastroenterology 68: 187
Kirsner J B 1979 The local and systemic complications of inflammatory bowel disease. Journal of the American Medical Association 242: 1177
Kock N G 1976 A new look at ileostomy. Surgery Annual 8: 241–256
Kohler L W, Pemberton J H, Zinsmeister A R, Kelly K A 1991 Quality of life after proctocolectomy. A comparison of Brooke ileostomy, Kock pouch, and ileal pouch–anal anastomosis. Gastroenterology 101: 679–684
Korelitz B I 1977 Colonic-duodenal fistula in Crohn's disease. American Journal of Digestive Diseases 22: 1040
Korelitz B I 1992 Inflammatory bowel disease in pregnancy. Gastroenterology Clinics of North America 21: 827–834
Korelitz B I, Coles R S 1967 Uveitis (iritis) associated with ulcerative and granulomatous colitis. Gastroenterology 52: 78
Korelitz B I, Dyck W P, Klion F M 1969 Fate of the rectum and distal colon after subtotal colectomy for ulcerative colitis. Gut 10: 198–201
Korelitz B I, Cheskin L J, Sohn N, Sommers S C 1984 Proctitis after fecal diversion in Crohn's disease and its elimination with reanastomosis: implications for surgical management. Report of four cases. Gastroenterology 87: 710
Kozarek R A, Patterson D J, Gelfand M D, Botoman V A, Ball T J, Wilske J R 1989 Methotrexate induces clinical and histologic remission in patients with refractory inflammatory bowel disease. Annals of Internal Medicine 110: 353–356
Kristensen E, Mosbech J 1977 Mortality from ulcerative colitis in Denmark 1960–1969. Scandinavian Journal of Gastroenterology 12: 189
Kruis W, Bull U, Eisenburg J, Paumgartner G 1982 Retrograde colonic

spread of sulphasalazine enemas. Scandinavian Journal of Gastroenterology 17: 933

Kunkel J M, Rosenthal D 1986 Management of the ileocecal syndrome. Neutropenic enterocolitis. Diseases of the Colon and Rectum 29: 196

Kyle J 1971 An epidemiological study of Crohn's disease in Northeast Scotland. Gastroenterology 61: 826

Kyle J 1983 Involvement of the urinary tract in Crohn's disease. In: Allan R N, Keighley M R B, Allexander-Williams J, Hawkins C (eds) Inflammatory bowel diseases. Churchill Livingstone, Edinburgh, p 481

Langman M J S 1966 Epidemiology of cancer of the large intestine. Proceedings of the Royal Society of Medicine 59: 132

Laufer I, Costopoulos L 1978 Early lesions of Crohn's disease. American Journal of Roentgenology 130: 307

Laufer I, Mullens J E, Hamilton J 1976 Correlation of endoscopy and double-contrast radiography in the early stages of ulcerative and granulomatous colitis. Radiology 118: 1

Lauritsen K, Hansen J, Ryde M, Rask-Madsen J 1984 Colonic azodisalicylate metabolism determined by in vivo dialysis in healthy volunteers and patients with ulcerative colitis. Gastroenterology 86: 1496

Lee E C G, Papaioannou N 1982 Minimal surgery for chronic obstruction in patients with extensive or universal Crohn's disease. Annals of the Royal College of Surgeons of England 64: 229–233

Lee F I, Costello F T 1985 Crohn's disease in Blackpool – incidence and prevalence 1968–80. Gut 26: 274

Lee J C L, Spittell J A, Sauer W G, Owen C A, Thompson J H 1968 Hypercoagulability associated with chronic ulcerative colitis: changes in blood coagulation factors. Gastroenterology 54: 76

Legge D A, Carlson H C, Judd E S 1970 Roentgenologic features of regional enteritis of the upper gastrointestinal tract. American Journal of Roentgenology 110: 355

Lennard L, van Loon J, Weinshilboum R M 1989 Pharmacogenetics of acute azathioprine toxicity: relationship to thiopurine methyltransferase genetic polymorphism. Clinical Pharmacology and Therapeutics 46: 149–154

Lennard-Jones J E, Powell-Tuck J 1979 Drug treatment of inflammatory bowel disease. Clinics in Gastroenterology 8: 187

Lennard-Jones J E, Baron J H, Connell A M, Jones F A 1962 A double blind controlled trial of prednisolone-21-phosphate suppositories in the treatment of idiopathic proctitis. Gut 3: 207

Lennard-Jones J E, Misiewicz J J, Connell A M, Baron J H, Jones F A 1965 Prednisone as maintenance treatment for ulcerative colitis in remission. Lancet 1: 188

Lennard-Jones J E, Lockhart-Mummery H E, Morson B C 1968 Clinical and pathological differentiation of Crohn's disease and proctocolitis. Gastroenterology 54: 1162

Lennard-Jones J E, Morson B C, Ritchie J K, Williams C B 1983 Cancer surveillance in ulcerative colitis. Experience over 15 years. Lancet 2: 149–152

Levine D S, Rabinovitch P S, Haggitt R C et al 1991 Distribution of aneuploid cell populations in ulcerative colitis with dysplasia or cancer. Gastroenterology 101: 1198–1210

Lichtiger S, Present D H, Kornbluth A et al 1994 Cyclosporine in severe ulcerative colitis refractory to steroid therapy. New England Journal of Medicine 330: 1841–1845

Löfberg R, Danielsson A, Salde L 1993. Oral budesonide in active Crohn's disease. Alimentary Pharmacology and Therapy 7: 611–616

Logan E C M, Williamson L M, Ryrie D R 1986 Sulphasalazine associated pancytopenia may be caused by acute folate deficiency. Gut 27: 868

Lohmuller J L, Pemberton J H, Dozois R R, Ilstrup D, van Heerden J 1990 Pouchitis and extraintestinal manifestations of inflammatory bowel disease after ileal pouch–anal anastomosis. Annals of Surgery 211: 622–629

Longo W E, Ballantyne G H 1994 Segmental Crohn's colitis: options and concerns. In: Veidenheimer M (ed) Management of Crohn's disease. Seminars in colon and rectal surgery: 5: 210–215

Longo W E, Oakley J R, Lavery I C, Church J M, Fazio V W 1992 Outcome of ileorectal anastomosis for Crohn's colitis. Diseases of the Colon and Rectum 35: 1066–1071

Lowdell C P, Shousha S, Parkins R A 1986 The incidence of amyloidosis complicating inflammatory bowel disease. A prospective survey of 177 patients. Diseases of the Colon and Rectum 29: 351

Lumb G, Protheroe R H B, Ramsay G S 1955 Ulcerative colitis with dilatation of the colon. British Journal of Surgery 43: 182

Lusk L B, Reichen J, Levine J S 1984 Aphthous ulceration in diversion colitis. Clinical implications. Gastroenterology 87: 1171

Luukonen P, Jarvinen H J 1992 Hand sutured vs stapled ileoanal anastomosis. ASCRS Annual Meeting. San Francisco, California

Lyttle J A, Parks A G 1977 Intersphincteric excision of the rectum. British Journal of Surgery 64: 413–416

McBride J A, King M J, Baikie A G, Crean G P, Sircus W 1963 Ankylosing spondylitis and chronic inflammatory diseases of the intestines. British Medical Journal 2: 483

MacDougall I P M 1964 The cancer risk in ulcerative colitis. Lancet 2: 655

McGovern V J, Goulston S J M 1968 Crohn's disease of the colon. Gut 9: 164–176

McHugh S M, Diamant N E, McLeod R, Cohen Z 1987 S-pouches versus J-pouches: a comparison of functional outcomes. Diseases of the Colon and Rectum 30: 671–677

McInerney G T, Sauer W G, Baggenstoss A H, Hodgson J R 1962 Fulminating ulcerative colitis with marked colonic dilation: a clinicopathologic study. Gastroenterology 42: 244

McIntyre P B, Macrae F A, Berghouse L, English J, Lennard-Jones J E 1985 Therapeutic benefits from a poorly absorbed prednisolone enema in distal colitis. Gut 26: 822

McIntyre P B, Pemberton J H, Wolff B G, Dozois R R, Beart R W, Kelly K A 1993 Indeterminate colitis: long-term outcome in patients after ileal pouch–anal anastomosis. Diseases of the Colon and Rectum 36 (abstract): 38

McLeod R S, Fazio V W 1984 Quality of life with the continent ileostomy. World Journal of Surgery 8: 90–95

McLeod R S, Lavery I C, Leatherman J R et al 1986 Factors affecting quality of life with a conventional ileostomy. World Journal of Surgery 10: 474–480

McLeod R S, Churchill D N, Lock A M, Vanderburgh S, Cohen Z 1991 Quality of life of patients with ulcerative colitis preoperatively and postoperatively. Gastroenterology 101: 1307–1313

MacPherson B, Pfeiffer C J 1976 Experimental colitis. Digestion 14: 424

Madanagopalan N, Vedachalam S P, Subramaniam R, Murugesan R G 1968 Rectal and colonic mucosal biopsy findings and faeces, sigmoidoscopy and histopathological correlation in amoebiasis and other colitis. Gut 9: 106

Madara J L, Podolsky D K, King N W, Sehgal P K, Moore R, Winter H S 1985 Characterization of spontaneous colitis in cotton-top tamarins (Saguinus oedipus) and its response to sulfasalazine. Gastroenterology 88: 13

Makiyama K, Bennett M K, Jewell D P 1984 Endoscopic appearances of the rectal mucosa of patients with Crohn's disease visualised with a magnifying colonoscope. Gut 25: 337

Margulis A R, Goldberg H I, Lawson T L et al 1971 The overlapping spectrum of ulcerative and granulomatous colitis: a roentgenographic-pathologic study. American Journal of Roentgenology 113: 325

Marshak R H, Lindner A E 1966 Ulcerative and granulomatous colitis. Journal of the Mount Sinai Hospital 33: 444

Marshak R H, Lindner A E 1976 Radiology of the small intestine. W B Saunders, Philadelphia

Marshak R H, Korelitz B I, Klein S H, Wolf B S, Janowitz H D 1960 Toxic dilation of the colon in the course of ulcerative colitis. Gastroenterology 38: 165

Mary J Y, Modigliani R 1989 Development and validation of an endoscopic index of the severity for Crohn's disease: a prospective multicenter study. Gut 30: 983–989

Matts S G F, Gaskell K H 1961 Retrograde colonic spread of enemata in ulcerative colitis. British Medical Journal 2: 614

Max R J, Kelvin F M 1980 Nonspecificity of discrete colonic ulceration on double-contrast barium enema study. American Journal of Roentgenology 134: 1265

Mayberry J F, Rhodes J 1984 Epidemiological aspects of Crohn's disease: a review of the literature. Gut 25: 886

Mayberry J F, Weterman I T 1986 European survey of fertility and

pregnancy in women with Crohn's disease: a case control study by European collaborative group. Gut 27: 821
Mayberry J, Rhodes J, Hughes L E 1979 Incidence of Crohn's disease in Cardiff between 1934 and 1977. Gut 20: 602
Mee A S, McLaughlin J E, Hodgson H J F, Jewell D P 1979 Chronic immune colitis in rabbits. Gut 20: 1
Meiselman M S, Cello J P, Margaretten M 1985 Cytomegalovirus colitis. Report of the clinical, endoscopic, and pathologic findings in two patients with the acquired immune deficiency syndrome. Gastroenterology 88: 171
Mekhjian H S, Switz D M, Melnyk C S, Rankin G B, Brooks R K 1979 Clinical features and natural history of Crohn's disease. Gastroenterology 77: 898
Mellor J A, Chandler G N, Chapman A H, Irving H C 1982 Massive gastrointestinal bleeding in Crohn's disease: successful control by intra-arterial vasopressin infusion. Gut 23: 872
Mendeloff A I, Monk M, Siegel C I, Lilienfeld A 1970 Illness experience and life stresses in patients with irritable colon and with ulcerative colitis. An epidemiologic study of ulcerative colitis and regional enteritis in Baltimore, 1960–1964. New England Journal of Medicine 282: 14
Metcalf A M, Dozois R R, Beart R W Jr, Kelly K A, Wolff B G 1986a Temporary ileostomy for ileal pouch–anal anastomosis: function and complications. Diseases of the Colon and Rectum 29: 300–303
Metcalf A M, Dozois R R, Kelly K A 1986b Sexual function in women after proctocolectomy. Annals of Surgery 204: 624–627
Meyers S, Walfish J S, Sachar D B, Greenstein A J, Hill A G, Janowitz H D 1980 Quality of life after surgery for Crohn's disease: a psychosocial survey. Gastroenterology 78: 1–5
Meyers S, Sachar D B, Goldberg J D, Janowitz H D 1983 Corticotropin vs hydrocortisone in the intravenous treatment of severe ulcerative colitis. A prospective, randomized, double-blind clinical trial. Gastroenterology 85: 351–357
Miller J P 1986 Inflammatory bowel disease in pregnancy: a review. Journal of the Royal Society of Medicine 79: 221–225
Mir-Madjlessi S H, McHenry M C, Farmer R G 1986 Liver abscess in Crohn's disease. Report of four cases and review of the literature. Gastroenterology 91: 987
Misiewicz J J, Lennard-Jones J E, Connell A M, Baron J H, Jones F A 1965 Controlled trial of sulphasalazine in maintenance therapy for ulcerative colitis. Lancet 1: 185
Mitchell A, Guyatt G, Singer J et al 1988 Quality of life in patients with inflammatory bowel disease. Journal of Clinical Gastroenterology 10: 306–310
Miyachi Yoshioka A, Imamura S, Niwa Y 1987 Effect of sulphasalazine and its metabolites on the generation of reactive oxygen species. Gut 28: 190
Monsen U, Brostrom O, Nordenvall B, Sorstad J, Hellers G 1987 Prevalence of inflammatory bowel disease among relatives of patients with ulcerative colitis. Scandinavian Journal of Gastroenterology 22: 214
Morowitz D A, Allen L W, Kirsner J B 1968 Thrombocytosis in chronic inflammatory bowel disease. Annals of Internal Medicine 68: 1013
Morson B C 1972 Pathology of Crohn's disease. Clinics in Gastroenterology 1: 265
Morson B C, Dawson I M P 1979 Gastrointestinal pathology, 2nd edn. Blackwell, Oxford
Mountain J C 1970 Cutaneous ulceration in Crohn's disease. Gut 11: 18
Mower W J, Hawkins J A, Nelson E W 1986 Neutropenic enterocolitis in adults with acute leukemia. Archives of Surgery 121: 571
Mulholland M W, Delaney J P 1983 Neutropenic colitis and aplastic anemia. A new association. Annals of Surgery 197: 84
Naylor A R, Pollet J E 1985 Eosinophilic colitis. Diseases of the Colon and Rectum 28: 615
Nefzger M D, Acheson E D 1963 Ulcerative colitis in the United States Army in 1944. Follow-up with particular reference to mortality in cases and controls. Gut 4: 183
Nelson H, Dozois R R, Kelly K A, Malkasian G D, Wolff B G, Ilstrup D M 1989 The effect of pregnancy and delivery on the ileal pouch–anal anastomosis functions. Diseases of the Colon and Rectum 32: 384–388
Nelson S W 1969 Some interesting and unusual manifestations of Crohn's disease ("regional enteritis") of the stomach, duodenum and small intestine. American Journal of Roentgenology 107: 86–101
Neschis M, Siegelman S S, Parker J G 1968 Diagnosis and management of the megacolon of ulcerative colitis. Gastroenterology 55: 251
Newcomer A D, McGill D B 1967 Incidence of lactase deficiency in ulcerative colitis. Gastroenterology 53: 890
Ni X-Y, Goldberg H I 1986 Aphthoid ulcers in Crohn's disease: radiographic course and relationship to bowel appearance. Radiology 158: 589–596
Nicholls R J, Pezim M E 1985 Restorative proctocolectomy with ileal reservoir for ulcerative colitis and familial adenomatous polyposis: a comparison of three reservoir designs. British Journal of Surgery 72: 470–474
Nicholls R J, Holt S D, Lubowski D Z 1989 Restorative proctocolectomy with ileal reservoir: comparison of two-stage versus three-stage procedures and analysis of factors that might affect outcome. Diseases of the Colon and Rectum 32: 323–326
Nielsen O H, Ahnfelt-Ronne I, Elmgreen J 1987 Abnormal metabolism of arachidonic acid in chronic inflammatory bowel disease: enhanced release of leukotriene $B_4$ from activated neutrophils. Gut 28: 181
Nolan D J 1981 Radiology of Crohn's disease of the small intestine: a review. Journal of the Royal Society of Medicine 74: 294
Nolan D J, Gourtsoyiannis N C 1980 Crohn's disease of the small intestine: a review of the radiological appearances in 100 consecutive patients examined by a barium infusion technique. Clinical Radiology 31: 597
Nostrant T T, Kumar N B, Appelman H D 1987 Histopathology differentiates acute self-limited colitis from ulcerative colitis. Gastroenterology 92: 318
Nyhlin H, Stenling R 1984 The small-intestinal mucosa in patients with Crohn's disease assessed by scanning electron and light microscopy. Scandinavian Journal of Gastroenterology 19: 433
Oakley J R, Jagelman D G, Fazio V W et al 1985 Complications and quality of life after ileorectal anastomosis for ulcerative colitis. American Journal of Surgery 149: 23–30
O'Donoghue D P, Dawson A M, Powell-Tuck J, Bown R L, Lennard Jones J E 1978 Double-blind withdrawal trial of azathioprine as maintenance treatment for Crohn's disease. Lancet 2: 955
O'Duffy J D, Carney J A, Deodhar S 1971 Behcet's disease. Report of 10 cases, 3 with new manifestations. Annals of Internal Medicine 75: 561
O'Morain C, Segal A W, Levi A J 1984a Elemental diet as primary treatment of acute Crohn's disease: a controlled trial. British Medical Journal 288: 1859–1862
O'Morain C, Smethurst P, Dore C J, Levi A J 1984b Reversible male infertility due to sulphasalazine: studies in man and rat. Gut 25: 1078
Ormerod T P 1967 Observations on the incidence and cause of anaemia in ulcerative colitis. Gut 8: 107
Ott D J, Chen Y M, Gelfand D W, Swearingen F V, Munitz H A 1985 Detailed per-oral small bowel examination vs. enteroclysis. Part 1: Expenditures and radiation exposure. Radiology 155: 29
Owyang C, Miller L J, Lie J T, Fleming C R 1979 Takayasu's arteritis in Crohn's disease. Gastroenterology 76: 825
Palmer K R, Groepel J R, Holdsworth C D 1981 Sulphasalazine retention enemas in ulcerative colitis: a double-blind trial. British Medical Journal 1: 1571
Palmer K R, Berry H, Wheeler P J et al 1986 Collagenous colitis – a relapsing and remitting disease. Gut 27: 578
Parc R, Legrand M, Frileux P, Tiret E, Ratelle R 1989 Comparative clinical results of ileal pouch–anal anastomosis and ileorectal anastomosis in ulcerative colitis. Hepatogastroenterology 36: 235–239
Parks A G, Nicholls R J 1978 Proctocolectomy without ileostomy for ulcerative colitis. British Medical Journal 2: 85–88
Parks A G, Nicholls R J, Belliveau P 1980 Proctocolectomy with ileal reservoir and anal anastomosis. British Journal of Surgery 67: 533–538
Pemberton J H 1991 Surgical approaches to proctocolectomy for inflammatory bowel disease. In: Phillips S F, Pemberton J H, Shorter R G (eds) The large intestine: physiology, pathophysiology and diseases. Raven Press, New York, p 629–655
Pemberton J H, Kelly K A, Beart R W Jr, Dozois R R, Wolff B G, Ilstrup D M 1987 Ileal pouch–anal anastomosis for chronic ulcerative colitis: long term results. Annals of Surgery 206: 504–513

Pemberton J H, Phillips S F, Ready R R, Zinsmeister A R, Beahrs O H 1989 Quality of life after Brooke ileostomy and ileal pouch–anal anastomosis: comparison of performance status. Annals of Surgery 209: 620–626
Pena A S, Truelove S C 1973 Hypolactasia and ulcerative colitis. Gastroenterology 64: 400
Penna C, Dozois R R, LaRusso N F, Tremaine W J 1994 Pouchitis after ileal pouch–anal anastomosis for chronic ulcerative colitis occurs with increased frequency in patients with associated primary sclerosing cholangitis. Gastroenterology 106 Part 2 (abstract): A751
Peppercorn M A 1984 Sulfasalazine. Pharmacology, clinical use, toxicity, and related new drug development. Annals of Internal Medicine 3: 377
Pera A, Bellando P, Caldera D et al 1987 Colonoscopy in inflammatory bowel disease. Diagnostic accuracy and proposal of an endoscopic score. Gastroenterology 92: 181
Pezim M E, Pemberton J H, Beart R W Jr et al 1989 Outcome of "indeterminant" colitis following ileal pouch anal anastomosis. Diseases of the Colon and Rectum 32: 653–658
Podolsky D K 1991 Inflammatory bowel disease (1). New England Journal of Medicine 325: 928–937
Poulsen S S, Pedersen N T, Jarnum S 1984 "Microerosions" in rectal biopsies in Crohn's disease. Scandinavian Journal of Gastroenterology 19: 607
Powell F C, Schroeter A L, Su W P D, Perry H O 1985 Pyoderma gangrenosum: a review of 86 patients. Quarterly Journal of Medicine 55: 173
Powell-Tuck J, Lennard-Jones J E, May C S, Wilson C G, Paterson J W 1976 Plasma prednisolone levels after administration of prednisolone-21-phosphate as a retention enema in colitis. British Medical Journal 1: 193
Present D H, Korelitz B I, Wisch N, Glass J L, Sachar D B, Pasternack B S 1980 Treatment of Crohn's disease with 6-mercaptopurine. A long-term, randomized, double-blind study. New England Journal of Medicine 302: 981–987
Present D H, Wolfson D, Gelernt I M, Rubin P H, Bauer J, Chapman M L 1981 The medical management of toxic megacolon: technique of decompression with favorable long term followup. Gastroenterology 80 (abstract): 1255
Present D H, Meltzer S J, Krumholz M P, Wolke A, Korelitz B I 1989 6-mercaptopurine in the management of inflammatory bowel disease: short and long term toxicity. Annals of Internal Medicine 111: 641–649
Price A B 1978 Overlap in the spectrum of non-specific inflammatory bowel disease – "colitis indeterminate". Journal of Clinical Pathology 31: 567
Price W H 1979 A high incidence of chronic inflammatory bowel disease in patients with Turner's syndrome. Journal of Medical Genetics 16: 263–266
Prior P, Gyde S N, Macartney J C, Thompson H, Waterhouse J A H, Allan R N 1982 Cancer morbidity in ulcerative colitis. Gut 23: 490–497
Pullan R D, Ganesh S, Mani V et al 1993 Comparison of bismuth citrate and 5-aminosalicylic acid enemas in distal ulcerative colitis: a controlled trial. Gut 34: 676–679
Pullan R D, Rhodes J, Ganesh S et al 1994 Transdermal nicotine for active ulcerative colitis. New England Journal of Medicine. 330: 811–815
Ransohoff D F, Riddel R H, Levin B 1985 Ulcerative colitis and colonic cancer: problems in assessing the diagnostic usefulness of mucosal dysplasia. Diseases of the Colon and Rectum 28: 383–388
Riddell R H 1983 Dysplasia in inflammatory bowel disease. In: Norris H T (ed) Pathology of colon, small intestine, and anus. Churchill Livingstone, New York, p 77–107
Riddell R H, Goldman H, Ransohoff D F et al 1983 Dysplasia in inflammatory bowel disease: standardized classification with provisional clinical applications. Human Pathology 14: 931
Riley S A, Mani V, Goodman M J, Herd M E, Dutt S, Turnberg L A 1988 Comparison of delayed-release 5-aminosalicylic acid (Mesalazine) and sulfasalazine as maintenance treatment for patients with ulcerative colitis. Gastroenterology 94: 1383
Ritchie J K, Powell-Tuck J, Lennard-Jones J E 1978 Clinical outcome of the first ten years of ulcerative colitis and proctitis. Lancet 1: 1140
Robert J H, Sachar D B, Aufses A H Jr, Greenstein A J 1990 Management of severe hemorrhage in ulcerative colitis. American Journal of Surgery 159: 550–555
Roe T F, Thomas D W, Gilsanz V, Isaacs H Jr, Atkinson J B 1986 Inflammatory bowel disease in glycogen storage disease type Ib. Journal of Pediatrics 109: 55–59
Rosenberg J L, Wall A J, Levin B, Binder H J, Kirsner J B 1975 A controlled trial of azathioprine in the management of chronic ulcerative colitis. Gastroenterology 69: 96–99
Rosenstock E, Farmer R G, Petras R, Sivak M V, Rankin G B, Sullivan B H 1985 Surveillance for colonic carcinoma in ulcerative colitis. Gastroenterology 89: 1342–1346
Rotterdam H Z 1982 The significance of microgranulomas in Crohn's disease. In: Korelitz B I (ed) Inflammatory bowel disease. Experience and controversy. Wright, Bristol, p 91
Rotterdam H, Korelitz B I, Sommers S C 1977 Microgranulomas in grossly normal rectal mucosa in Crohn's disease. American Journal of Clinical Pathology 67: 550
Rowland R, Pounder D J 1982 Crohn's colitis. Pathology Annual 17: 267
Russell A S 1977 Arthritis, inflammatory bowel disease, and histocompatibility antigens. Annals of Internal Medicine 86: 820
Rutgeerts P, Onette E, Vantrappen G, Geboes K, Broeckhaert L, Talloen L 1980 Crohn's disease of the stomach and duodenum: a clinical study with emphasis on the value of endoscopy and endoscopic biopsies. Endoscopy 12: 288
Rutgeerts P, Geboes K, Vantrappen G, Kerremans R, Coenegrachts J L, Coremans G 1984 Natural history of recurrent Crohn's disease at the ileocolonic anastomosis after curative surgery. Gut 25: 665–672
Sales D J, Kirsner J B 1983 Prognosis of inflammatory bowel disease. Archives of Internal Medicine 143: 294–299
Sandberg-Gertzen H, Jarnerot G, Bukhave K, Lauritsen K, Rask-Madsen J 1986a Effect of azodisal sodium and sulphasalazine on ileostomy output of fluid and $PGE_2$, and $PGF_{2a}$ in subjects with a permanent ileostomy. Gut 27: 1306
Sandberg-Gertzen H, Jarnerot G, Kraaz W 1986b Azodisal sodium in the treatment of ulcerative colitis. A study of tolerance and relapse-prevention properties. Gastroenterology 90: 1024–1030
Sandborn W J, Tremaine W J 1992 Cyclosporine treatment of inflammatory bowel disease. Mayo Clinic Proceedings 67: 981–990
Sandborn W J, Landers C J, Tremaine W J, Targan S R 1993 The presence of antineutrophil cytoplasmic antibody correlates with pouchitis after ileal pouch–anal anastomosis for ulcerative colitis. Gastroenterology 104 (abstract): A774
Sandborn W J, Tremaine W J, Schroeder D W et al 1994 A placebo-controlled trial of cyslosporine enemas for mildly to moderately active left-sided ulcerative colitis. Gastroenterology 106: 1429–1435
Sandle G I, Hayslett J P, Binder H J 1986 Effect of glucocorticoids on rectal transport in normal subjects and patients with ulcerative colitis. Gut 27: 309–316
Sandler R S 1994 Epidemiology of inflammatory bowel disease. In: Targan S R, Shanahan F (eds) Inflammatory bowel disease. From bench to bedside. Williams and Wilkins, Baltimore, p 7–9
Sandler R S, Sandler D P, McDonnell C W, Wurzelmann J I 1992 Childhood exposure to environmental tobacco smoke and the risk of ulcerative colitis. American Journal of Epidemiology 135: 603–608
Sartor R B 1994 Cytokines in intestinal inflammation: pathophysiological and clinical considerations. Gastroenterology 106: 533–539
Sartoris D J, Harell G S, Anderson M F, Zboralske F F 1984 Small-bowel lymphoma and regional enteritis: radiographic similarities. Radiology 152: 291
Saxon A, Shanahan F, Landers C, Ganz T, Targan S 1990 A distinct subset of antineutrophil cytoplasmic antibodies is associated with inflammatory bowel disease. Journal of Allergy and Clinical Immunology 86: 202–210
Schinella R A, Greco M A, Cobert B L, Denmark L W, Cox R P 1980 Hermansky–Pudlak syndrome with granulomatous colitis. Annals of Internal Medicine 92: 20
Schmitz-Moormann P, Pittner P M, Malchow H, Brandes J W 1984 The granuloma in Crohn's disease. A bioptical study. Pathology, Research and Practice 178: 467
Schoetz D J 1992 Gastroduodenal Crohn's disease. Perspectives in Colon and Rectal Surgery 2: 145–154

Schofield P F, Staff W G, Moore T 1968 Ureteral involvement in regional ileitis (Crohn's disease). Journal of Urology 99: 412
Schroeder K W, Tremaine W J, Ilstrup D M 1987 Coated oral 5-aminosalicylic acid therapy for mildly to moderately active ulcerative colitis. New England Journal of Medicine 317: 1625–1629
Schuffler M D, Chaffee R G 1979 Small intestinal biopsy in a patient with Crohn's disease of the duodenum. The spectrum of abnormal findings in the absence of granulomas. Gastroenterology 76: 1009
Schwartz A G, Targan S R, Saxon A, Weinstein W M 1982 Sulfasalazine-induced exacerbation of ulcerative colitis. New England Journal of Medicine 306: 409
Shaffer J A, Williams S E, Turnberg L A, Houston J B, Rowland M 1983 Absorption of prednisolone in patients with Crohn's disease. Gut 24: 182
Shanahan F, Duerr R H, Rotter J I et al 1992 Neutrophil autoantibodies in ulcerative colitis: familial aggregation and genetic heterogeneity. Gastroenterology 103: 456–461
Shih W W, Ellison G W, Myers L W, Durkos-Smith D, Fahey J L 1982 Locus of selective depression of human natural killer cells by azathioprine. Clinical Immunology and Immunopathology 23: 672–681
Silverman R E, McLeod R S, Cohen Z 1989 Stricturoplasty in Crohn's disease. Canadian Journal of Surgery 32: 19–22
Sim M, Brooke B N 1958 Ulcerative colitis. A test of psychosomatic hypotheses. Lancet 2: 125
Simon M, Shapiro J H, Parker J G, Schein C J, Weingarten B 1962 The diagnosis and treatment of dilatation of the colon in severe ulcerative colitis. A diagnostic roentgen sign. American Journal of Roentgenology 87: 655
Simpkins K C 1977 Aphthoid ulcers in Crohn's colitis. Clinical Radiology 28: 601
Singleton J W, Law D H, Kelley M L, Mekhjian H S, Sturdevant R A L 1979a National Cooperative Crohn's Disease Study: adverse reactions to study drugs. Gastroenterology 77: 870
Singleton J W, Summers R W, Kern F et al 1979b A trial of sulfasalazine as adjunctive therapy in Crohn's disease. Gastroenterology 77: 887
Sirlin S M, Benkov K J, Kaslow P, Dolgin S, Dische M R, LeLeiko N S 1986 Identical twins concordant for Crohn's disease. Journal of Clinical Gastroenterology 8: 290
Sitrin M D, Rosenberg I H, Chawla K et al 1980 Nutritional and metabolic complications in a patient with Crohn's disease and ileal resection. Gastroenterology 78: 1069–1079
Slaney G, Brooke B N 1959 Cancer in ulcerative colitis. Lancet 2: 694
Slaney G, Muller S, Clay J, Sumathipala A H T, Hillenbrand P, Thompson H 1986 Crohn's disease involving the penis. Gut 27:329
Smith F W, Law D H, Nickel W F, Sleisenger M H 1962 Fulminant ulcerative colitis with toxic dilation of the colon: medical and surgical management of eleven cases with observations regarding etiology. Gastroenterology 42: 233
Snook J A, Lowes J R, Wu K C, Priddle J D, Jewell D P 1991 Serum and tissue autoantibodies to colonic epithelium in ulcerative colitis. Gut 32: 163–166
Sokol R J, Farrell M K, McAdams A J 1984 An unusual presentation of Wegener's granulomatosis mimicking inflammatory bowel disease. Gastroenterology 87: 426
Sommers S C 1985 Dysplasia in inflammatory bowel disease. In: Korelitz B I, Sohn N (eds) Inflammatory bowel disease: experience and controversy. Grune and Stratton, Orlando, p 97
Sonnenberg A, McCarty D J, Jacobsen S J 1991. Geographical variation of inflammatory bowel disease within the United States. Gastroenterology 100: 143–149
Spencer M P, Nelson H, Wolff B G, Dozois R R 1994 Strictureplasty for obstructive Crohn's disease: the Mayo experience. Mayo Clinic Proceedings 69: 33–36
Stack B H R, Smith T, Jones J H, Fletcher J 1969 Measurement of blood and iron loss in colitis with a whole-body counter. Gut 10: 769
Steadman C, Teague C, Kerlin P, Harris O, Hourigan K, Sampson J 1987 Collagenous colitis: clinical and histological spectrum in ten patients. Journal of Gastroenterology and Hepatology 2: 459
Steinberg D M, Cooke W T, Williams J A 1973 Abscess and fistulae in Crohn's disease. Gut 14: 865
Stenson W F 1994 Animal models of inflammatory bowel disease. In: Targan S R, Shanahan F (eds) Inflammatory bowel disease. From bench to bedside. Williams and Wilkins, Baltimore, p 180
Stonnington C M, Phillips S F, Melton I J, Zinsmeister A R 1987 Chronic ulcerative colitis: incidence and prevalence in a community. Gut 28: 402
Streilein J W 1978 Inflammatory bowel disease: T lymphocytes may be the culprits. Gastroenterology 75: 150
Sturniolo G C, Molokhia M M, Shields R, Turnberg L A 1980 Zinc absorption in Crohn's disease. Gut 21: 387
Summers R W, Switz D M, Sessions J T et al 1979 National Cooperative Crohn's Disease Study: results of drug treatment. Gastroenterology 77: 847
Surawicz C M, Belic L 1984 Rectal biopsy helps to distinguish acute self-limited colitis from idiopathic inflammatory bowel disease. Gastroenterology 86: 104
Surawicz C M, Meisel J L, Ylvisaker T, Saunders D R, Rubin C E 1981 Rectal biopsy in the diagnosis of Crohn's disease: value of multiple biopsies and serial sectioning. Gastroenterology 81: 66
Surawicz C M, Goodell S E, Quinn T C et al 1986 Spectrum of rectal biopsy abnormalities in homosexual men with intestinal symptoms. Gastroenterology 91: 651–659
Sutherland L R, Martin F, Greer S et al 1987 5-Aminosalicylic acid enema in the treatment of distal ulcerative colitis, proctosigmoiditis, and proctitis. Gastroenterology 92: 1894
Talbot R W, Heppell J, Dozois R R, Beart R W 1986 Vascular complications of inflammatory bowel disease. Mayo Clinic Proceedings. 61: 140
Talstad I, Rootwelt K, Gjone E 1973 Thrombocytosis in ulcerative colitis and Crohn's disease. Scandinavian Journal of Gastroenterology 8: 135
Tandon H D, Prakash A 1972 Pathology of intestinal tuberculosis and its distinction from Crohn's disease. Gut 13: 260
Teahon K, Pearson M, Levi A J, Bjarnason I 1991 Elemental diet in the management of Crohn's disease during pregnancy. Gut 32: 1079–1081
Teja K, Crum C P, Friedman C 1980 Giant cell arteritis and Crohn's disease. An unreported association. Gastroenterology 78: 796
Tremaine W J 1992 Maintenance of remission in Crohn's disease: is 5-aminosalicylic acid the answer? Gastroenterology 103: 694–696
Truelove S C 1958 Treatment of ulcerative colitis with local hydrocortisone hemisuccinate sodium. A report on a controlled therapeutic trial. British Medical Journal 2: 1072
Truelove S C, Witts L J 1955 Cortisone in ulcerative colitis. Final report on a therapeutic trial. British Medical Journal 2: 1041
Truelove S C, Witts L J 1959 Cortisone and corticotrophin in ulcerative colitis. British Medical Journal 1: 387
Tsunoda A, Talbot I C, Nicholls R J 1990 Incidence of dysplasia in the anorectal mucosa in patients having restorative proctocolectomy. British Journal of Surgery 77: 506–508
Ursing B, Alm T, Barany F et al 1982 A comparative study of metronidazole and sulfasalazine for active Crohn's disease: the Cooperative Crohn's Disease Study in Sweden. II Result. Gastroenterology 83: 550
Utsunomiya J, Iwama T, Imajo M et al 1980 Total colectomy, mucosal proctectomy, and ileoanal anastomosis. Diseases of the Colon and Rectum 23: 459–466
Valero V, Senior J, Watanakunakorn C 1985 Liver abscess complicating Crohn's disease presenting as thoracic empyema. Case report and review of the literature. American Journal of Medicine 79: 659
Van Hees P A M, Bakker J H, van Tongeren J H M 1980 Effect of sulphapyridine, 5-aminosalicylic acid, and placebo in patients with idiopathic proctitis: a study to determine the active therapeutic moiety of sulphasalazine. Gut 21: 632
Waits J O, Dozois R R, Kelly K A 1982 Primary closure and continuous irrigation of the perineal wound after proctectomy. Mayo Clinic Proceedings 57: 185–188
Warwick R R G, Sumerling M D, Gilmour H M, Shearman D J C 1973 Colonoscopy and double contrast barium enema examination in chronic ulcerative colitis. American Journal of Roentgenology 117: 292
Watkinson G 1961 Medical management of ulcerative colitis. British Medical Journal 1: 47
Watkinson G 1967 Cited in Goligher J C, de Dombal F T, Watts J McK,

Watkinson G (eds) 1968 Ulcerative colitis. Baillière, Tindall and Cassell, London, p 208
Watts J McK, de Dombal F T, Goligher J C 1966a Long-term complications and prognosis following major surgery for ulcerative colitis. British Journal of Surgery 53: 1014
Watts J McK, Thompson H, Goligher J C 1966b Sigmoidoscopy and cytology in the detection of microscopic disease of the rectal mucosa in ulcerative colitis. Gut 7: 288
Waye J D 1977 The role of colonoscopy in the differential diagnosis of inflammatory bowel disease. Gastrointestinal Endoscopy 23: 150
Waye J D 1978 Inflammatory bowel disease. Colonoscopic aids in diagnosis and management. New York State Medical Journal 78: 1894
Waye J D 1982 Where has colonoscopy had its greatest value in the management of inflammatory bowel disease? In: Korelitz B I (ed) Inflammatory bowel disease. Experience and controversy. Wright, Massachusetts, p 87
Weber J N, Carmichael D J, Boylston A, Munro A, Whitear W P, Pinching A J 1985 Kaposi's sarcoma of the bowel – presenting as apparent ulcerative colitis. Gut 26: 295
Weedon D D, Shorter R G, Ilstrup D M, Huizenga K A, Taylor W F 1973 Crohn's disease and cancer. New England Journal of Medicine 289: 1099–1103
Werlin S L, Chusid M J, Caya J, Oechler H W 1982 Colitis in chronic granulomatous disease. Gastroenterology 82: 328
Weterman I T 1983 Oral, oesophageal and gastro-duodenal Crohn's disease. In: Allan R N, Keighley M R B, Alexander-Williams J, Hawkins C (eds) Inflammatory bowel diseases. Churchill Livingstone, Edinburgh, p 299
Whitington P F, Friedman A L, Chesney R W 1979 Gastrointestinal disease in the hemolytic-uremic syndrome. Gastroenterology 76: 728
Wiesner R H, LaRusso N F, Dozois R R, Beaver S J 1986 Peristomal varices after proctocolectomy in patients with primary sclerosing cholangitis. Gastroenterology 90: 316–322
Wigley R D, MacLaurin B P 1962 A study of ulcerative colitis in New Zealand, showing a low incidence in Maoris. British Medical Journal 2: 228
Williams C B 1983 Ulcerative colitis: diagnosis and the place of colonoscopy. In: Allan R N, Keighley M R B, Alexander-Williams J, Hawkins C (eds) Inflammatory bowel diseases. Churchill Livingstone, Edinburgh, p 210
Williams C N 1990 Efficacy and tolerance of 5-aminosalicylic acid suppositories in the treatment of ulcerative proctitis: a review of two double-blind, placebo controlled trials. Canadian Journal of Gastroenterology 4: 472
Williams D R, Coller J A, Corman M L, Nugent F W, Veidenheimer M C 1981 Anal complications in Crohn's disease. Diseases of the the Colon and Rectum 24: 22
Williams J A 1972 Surgery and management of Crohn's disease. Clinics in Gastroenterology 1: 469
Willoughby C P 1983 Fertility, pregnancy and ulcerative colitis. In: Allan R N, Keighley M R B, Alexander-Williams J, Hawkins C (eds) Inflammatory bowel diseases. Churchill Livingstone, Edinburgh, p 113
Winthrop J D, Balfe D M, Shackelford G D, McAlister W H, Rosenblum J L, Siegel M J 1985 Ulcerative and granulomatous colitis in children. Comparison of double- and single-contrast studies. Radiology 154: 657
Wright R, Truelove S C 1965 A controlled therapeutic trial of various diets in ulcerative colitis. British Medical Journal 2: 138
Wright R, Truelove S C 1966a Circulating and tissue eosinophils in ulcerative colitis. American Journal of Digestive Diseases 11: 831
Wright R, Truelove S C 1966b Serial rectal biopsy in ulcerative colitis during the course of a controlled therapeutic trial of various diets. American Journal of Digestive Diseases 11: 847
Wright V, Watkinson G 1965 Sacro-iliitis and ulcerative colitis. British Medical Journal 2: 675
Yang H, Rotter J I 1994 Genetics of inflammatory bowel disease. In: Targan S R, Shanahan F (eds) Inflammatory bowel disease. Fom bench to bedside. Williams and Wilkins, Baltimore, p 35–36
Yang J, McElree C, Roth M-P, Shanahan F, Targan S R, Rotter J I 1993 Familial empirical risks for inflammatory bowel disease: differences between Jews and non-Jews. Gut 34: 517–524
Yardley J H, Keren D F 1974 "Precancer" lesions in ulcerative colitis. A retrospective study of rectal biopsy and colectomy specimens. Cancer 34: 835–844
Yates V M, Watkinson G, Kelman A 1982 Further evidence for an association between psoriasis, Crohn's disease and ulcerative colitis. British Journal of Dermatology 106: 323
Young J R 1966 Ulcerative colitis and finger-clubbing. British Medical Journal 1: 278
Zegel H G, Laufer I 1978 Filiform polyposis. Radiology 127: 615

SECTION 5

# Liver structure and function

# 24. The liver: anatomy, physiology, liver biopsy and congenital disorders

*N. D. C. Finlayson*

That the liver has attracted the interest of mankind from time immemorial is not surprising, for it is the largest organ in the body and the bile it produces is impressively dark and bitter. The Babylonians and Assyrians considered it the seat of the soul and used animal livers to foretell the future; Greek and Roman leaders rarely took important decisions without having a priest inspect an animal liver; numerous other peoples have stressed its importance in the balance of human characteristics, particularly in respect of courage or cowardice (lily-livered) and arrogance (gall) or timidity (Mellinkoff 1979).

Modern notions no longer give the liver an important place in determining normal personality, although the effects of hepatic dysfunction on the intellect and emotions can be profound (p. 1045), but the recognition of the enormous diversity of its functions in other directions has more than fulfilled the 18th-century prophecy of Bichat that an organ as large as the liver had to do more than produce a liquid less copious than urine. The history of the development of knowledge about the liver and its diseases in the Western world has been reviewed by Franken (1983) and Arias et al (1994) have produced a comprehensive monograph on current knowledge of its structure and function in health and disease.

## EMBRYOLOGY

The development of the liver begins on about the 18th day of life when the hepatic diverticulum grows ventrally and cranially into the mesenchyme of the septum transversum from that part of the foregut destined to become the duodenal loop (Andres et al 1977). Its origin is associated closely with the pancreatic bud, from which the pancreas develops (p. 1227). As it grows, the hepatic diverticulum divides into a pars hepatica cranially and a pars cystica caudally. The mechanisms of liver development are poorly understood but are probably similar to those of hepatic regeneration during later life (p. 716).

### Parenchyma

The pars hepatica continues to grow cranially and as it does so cords of endodermal cells (hepatoblasts) grow out and anastomose with one another in the mesenchyme. The endodermal cords are solid at first, but at about the eighth week of gestation the intercellular bile canaliculi appear. The liver cells are remarkably uniform in size and shape at birth and the liver cell plates (p. 710) are two cells thick. The transition to liver cell plates one cell thick takes place gradually and is complete by about the age of 6 years. As the endodermal cords extend and anastomose, intercommunicating islands of mesenchymal cells develop between them and form endothelial boundaries peripherally and hemocytoblasts centrally. These hemocytoblasts are an important source of blood cells in fetal life; production reaches a maximum after 6–7 months of intrauterine life, at which point the liver is the main source of blood cells, but little hemopoietic tissue remains in the liver at birth and it disappears within a few weeks. The liver grows uniformly initially, but later the growth of the right lobe exceeds that of the left to give the liver its asymmetric shape.

### Biliary tract

Some of the hepatoblasts in the endodermal cords differentiate to form the intrahepatic bile ducts. These ducts develop from hepatoblasts surrounding the developing portal vein and the ducts develop first in the hilum of the liver and then extend into the hepatic parenchyma. Development of the smallest bile ducts is not complete until a few weeks after birth. The gallbladder, cystic ducts and common bile ducts develop from the pars cystica of the hepatic diverticulum.

### Vasculature

The endodermal cords grow into the septum transversum,

which also contains the anastomosing vessels of the vitelline and umbilical venous system (Fig. 24.1). The spaces between the endodermal cords and these disrupted venous systems become the hepatic sinusoids. At first the sinusoids are lined only with endothelial cells, but other cells such as Kupffer cells and hepatic stellate cells appear in the third month of gestation. The left umbilical vein comes to supply the left lobe of the liver and then divides into the ductus venosus and a branch to the portal vein and the right lobe of the liver. The portal venous blood supplies the right lobe of the liver (Rudolph 1983). The left umbilical vein becomes the round ligament after birth, but its lumen is not completely obliterated (p. 992). The ductus venosus is obliterated completely at birth and becomes the ligamentum venosum. All veins leaving the liver drain to the sinus venosus. Hepatic arterial blood flow is small in fetal life and the closure of the umbilical artery at birth deprives the liver of a considerable supply of arterial blood. Lymphatics appear in the liver in the fourth month of gestation.

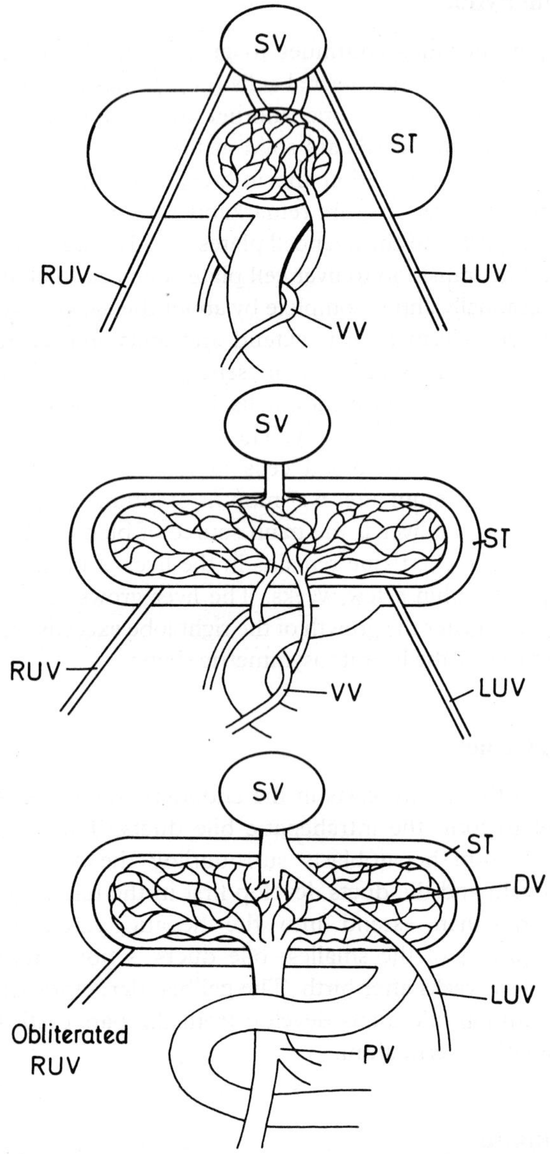


**Fig. 24.1** The development (top to bottom) of the hepatic vasculature from the vitelline and umbilical veins. DV = ductus venosus, LUV = left umbilical vein, RUV = right umbilical vein, PV = portal vein, ST = septum transversum, SV = sinus venosus, VV = vitelline vein.

### Neonatal liver function

The liver begins to function early in fetal life, producing plasma proteins such as alpha-fetoprotein, albumin and $\alpha_1$-antitrypsin within 4 weeks and bile acids within 8 weeks of conception. Unlike the adult liver, it does not show much morphological or functional differentiation within the functional liver acinus (Kanai et al 1984) and the right and left lobes may function differently in relation to blood supply coming from the portal vein or the umbilical vein (Mihaly et al 1982). At birth, many and perhaps most of the liver functions are immature and take weeks or months to reach adult levels. This is exaggerated in premature and lower birth-weight babies. This functional immaturity is best recognized in reduced transport of bilirubin (and other organic anions) from the blood into bile. Uptake of bilirubin from the blood, binding to cytoplasmic proteins such as ligandin and conjugation with glucuronide are all impaired at birth. Impaired conjugation is due to reduced production of the cofactor uridine diphosphate glucuronic acid as well as to reduced activity of glucuronyl transferase. The capacity to secrete conjugated bilirubin into the bile is similarly limited. Bile acid synthesis at birth is also limited (Watkins et al 1973) and secretion of bile acids into bile is low enough to lead to an increase in serum bile acid concentrations after birth, indicating a physiological cholestasis that resolves only gradually over several months (Suchy et al 1981). This increase in serum bile acids occurs in spite of a diminished enterohepatic circulation consequent on limited ileal resorption of bile acids at this time (deBelle et al 1979). Bile acid secretion is important in generating bile flow and impaired bile flow could reduce the clearance into bile of many substances.

Deficient coagulation of the blood is common and there has been disagreement as to whether reduced coagulation factor production or vitamin K deficiency is more important. Vitamin K deficiency is probably more important (Motohara et al 1985), but reduced coagulation factor production can also occur (Corrigan & Krye 1980).

## ANATOMY

### Gross clinical anatomy

The liver is roughly wedge-shaped; it weighs about 1.5 (1.2–1.8) kg and occupies most of the right upper quadrant of the abdomen. In adults its upper border extends from the fifth rib, 2 cm medial to the right mid-clavicular line, to the sixth rib in the left mid-clavicular line (roughly a line just below the nipples) and its oblique inferior border extends inferolaterally from the left extremity of the upper border through the surface marking of the fundus of the gallbladder at the tip of the ninth right costal cartilage to the tip of the tenth rib. The liver at birth is twice as heavy as in the adult relative to body weight, which accounts for the protuberant abdomen of childhood, and this falls gradually to reach adult values in adolescence (Rylance et al 1982).

The liver has a smooth convex superoanterolateral diaphragmatic surface, to which the falciform ligament is attached (Fig. 24.2), and a concave posterolateral visceral surface (Fig. 24.3). The visceral surface contains the porta hepatis, a deep transverse cleft about 5 cm long, from the margins of which descends the lesser omentum containing the bile duct, the hepatic artery and the portal vein. The gallbladder fossa lies anterior and the inferior vena cava posterior to the porta hepatis.

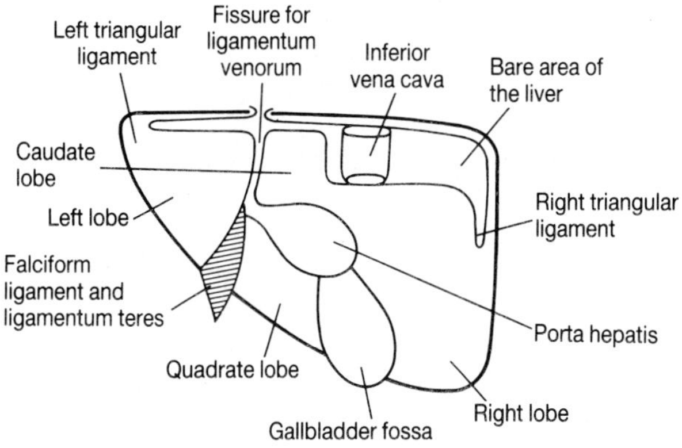


**Fig. 24.3** Posterolateral view of the liver showing its lobes and peritoneal attachments.

*Liver lobes*

The human liver is a single parenchymal mass that was formerly divided arbitrarily into various lobes in accordance with its peritoneal attachments. The insertion of the falciform ligament on the anterior surface and the fissures for the ligamentum teres and the ligamentum venosum on the posterior surface were used to divide the liver into a smaller left and a larger right lobe (Figs 24.2, 24.3). The right lobe contains a quadrate lobe anteriorly between the falciform ligament and the gallbladder and a caudate lobe posteriorly between the inferior vena cava and the ligamentum venosum.

This system does not have much clinical significance and, particularly for the surgeon, a more useful system divides the liver into right and left hemilivers separated by the course of the middle hepatic vein lying roughly on a line between the inferior vena cava and the gallbladder bed and passing through the porta hepatis (Fig. 24.4). The right and left hemilivers are subdivided further into a total of eight segments in accordance with further subdivisions of the hepatic vasculature. The division between the right and left hemilivers lies to the right of the traditional anatomical division and consequently the quadrate lobe and part of the caudate lobe come to lie in the left hemiliver.

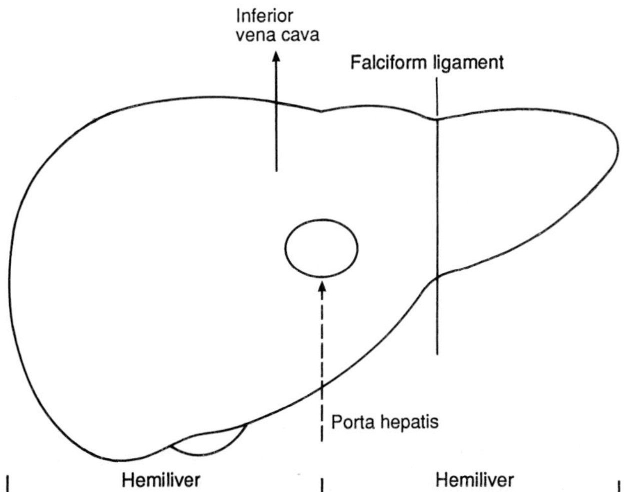

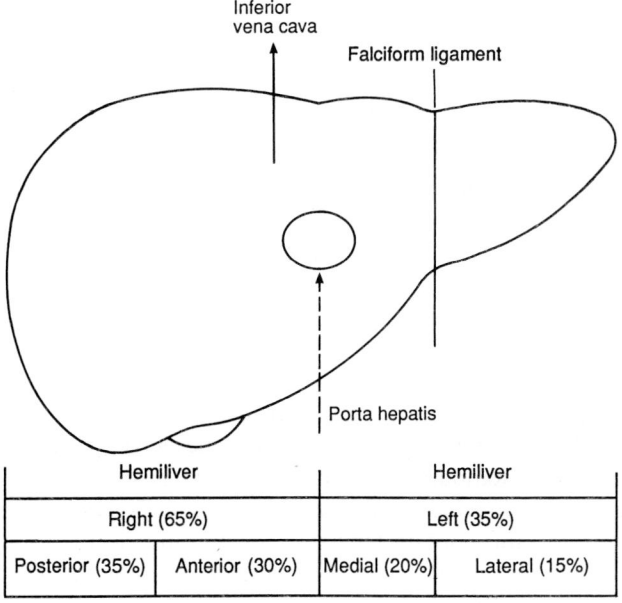

| Hemiliver | | Hemiliver | |
|---|---|---|---|
| Right (65%) | | Left (35%) | |
| Posterior (35%) | Anterior (30%) | Medial (20%) | Lateral (15%) |

**Fig. 24.2** The anterior aspect of the liver showing the traditional division into right and left lobes by the falciform ligament. The sites of the porta hepatis (⇡) and the inferior vena cava (↑) are indicated and the approximate location and relative sizes of the functional lobes of the liver are shown below (Fig. 24.4).

*Clinical examination*

The liver descends 1–3 cm on inspiration and can be felt just below the right costal margin in normal adults; the liver at birth is large relative to the rest of the body and can be felt up to 4.5 cm below the right costal margin in newborns (Ashkenazi et al 1984). Palpation is used to detect hepatomegaly in adults but except in patients with grossly enlarged livers extending below the umbilicus, it is an inaccurate method even when care is taken to define the upper border of the liver by percussion.

The palpability of a liver is determined as much by its consistency as by its size and firm or hard livers are much more easily palpated than soft ones (Castell 1979). Percussion between the upper and lower borders of the liver in the mid-clavicular or mid-sternal lines is a more accurate clinical method, although it tends to underesti-

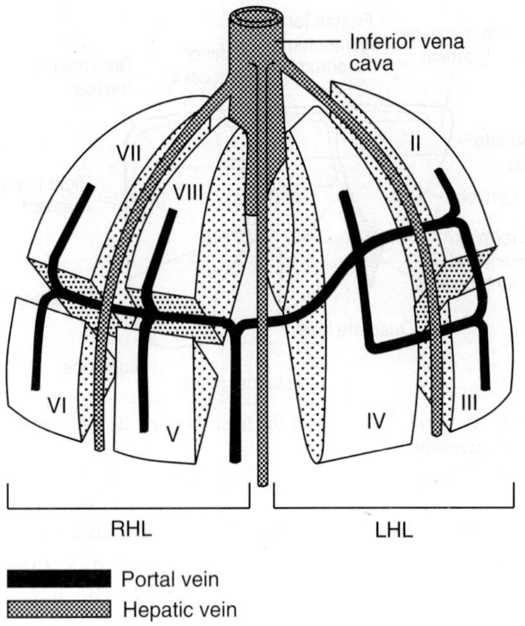


**Fig. 24.4** Schematic representation of the division of the liver into four hepatic sectors by the three main hepatic veins, making up a right hemiliver (RHL) and a left hemiliver (LHL). These sectors are subdivided into eight hepatic segments (I–VIII) by the branches of the portal vein. The caudate lobe (I) is a separate hepatic segment with independent hepatic venous supply and hepatic venous drainage. (Reproduced with permission from Edwards et al 1995 Davidson's Principles and Practice of Medicine, Edinburgh, Churchill Livingstone.)

mate liver size (Castell et al 1969, Sapira & Williamson 1979). Light percussion of both borders gives the best results. Hepatomegaly is unlikely when the mid-clavicular span of the liver is less than 14 cm, and likely when it exceeds 20 cm. In disease, small livers are usually associated with a reduced hepatic blood flow. Auscultation over the liver may reveal an arterial murmur due to a vascular tumor, usually a hepatocellular carcinoma (p. 1119), alcoholic hepatitis (p. 875), a friction rub due to a tumor, a perihepatitis (p. 825) or a recent liver biopsy. A venous hum between the xiphisternum and the umbilicus is characteristic of the Cruveilhier–Baumgarten syndrome (p. 992).

## Microscopic anatomy

The basic histological unit of the liver is the lobule, which comprises a central efferent hepatic vein, with sinusoids and anastomosing columns of liver cells disposed radially around it, and a variable number of portal tracts arranged around the periphery of the sinusoids and liver cell columns. The hepatocyte is the predominant cell in the liver, but other cells constitute a substantial minority (Table 24.1).

*Liver cells (hepatocytes)*

These are large, well-defined, polygonal cells with round nuclei and prominent nucleoli (Fig. 24.5). A few cells are binucleate and mitoses are seen occasionally. Large polyploid nuclei sometimes occur. Some nuclei have vacuoles that contain glycogen. Normal hepatocytes have abundant cytoplasm, which gives a pale stain with hematoxylin and eosin, and fat vacuoles are seen in up to 10% of cells (p. 975). Random hepatocytes die by apoptosis to form acidophilic or Councilman bodies (p. 795) (Searle et al 1987). Fine brownish-yellow lipofuscin granules about 1 μm in diameter are often seen near the biliary canaliculi, particularly in centrilobular cells and in older persons; dark brown hemosiderin granules of about the same size are sometimes seen, particularly in periportal cells. Lipofuscin granules are composed of protein, are found mainly in lysosomes and stain positively with the periodic acid Schiff (PAS) and Ziehl–Neelsen stains. Hemosiderin granules are part of the iron stores in the liver (p. 952) and stain positively with Perl's stain.

**Table 24.1** Cellular composition of the liver

| Cells | % |
|---|---|
| Epithelial cells | 65 |
| Hepatocytes | 60 |
| Biliary cells | 5 |
| Mesenchymal cells | 35 |
| Endothelium | 19 |
| Kupffer cells | 15 |
| Hepatic stellate cells | 1 |

The hepatocytes are disposed in curved plates that separate and surround the sinusoids. They extend from the central veins to the portal tracts and the hepatocyte membranes next to the portal tracts are known collectively as the limiting plate. The hepatocyte plates are only one cell thick in adults, although tangential sectioning sometimes makes them look thicker; tiny bile canaliculi, the walls of which are formed by the hepatocytes themselves, are seen between adjacent liver cells. The bile canaliculi are empty normally. The hepatocytes are separated from the sinusoidal endothelium by the space of Disse.

*Sinusoids*

The sinusoids are the capillary vessels of the liver (Fig. 24.5) and they differ significantly from capillaries elsewhere in the absence of any basement membrane dense enough to be seen on standard electronmicroscopy (below). About a half of the sinusoidal cells are endothelial cells that line the sinusoids and contain fenestrae (below) increasing access to the space of Disse (perisinusoidal space). Their flattened, elongated nuclei can be seen on light microscopy. Other cells found in the sinusoids include the Kupffer cells, which comprise about a third of the sinusoidal cells, hepatic stellate cells, which comprise about a fifth, and rare pit cells (below). Kupffer cells have plumper

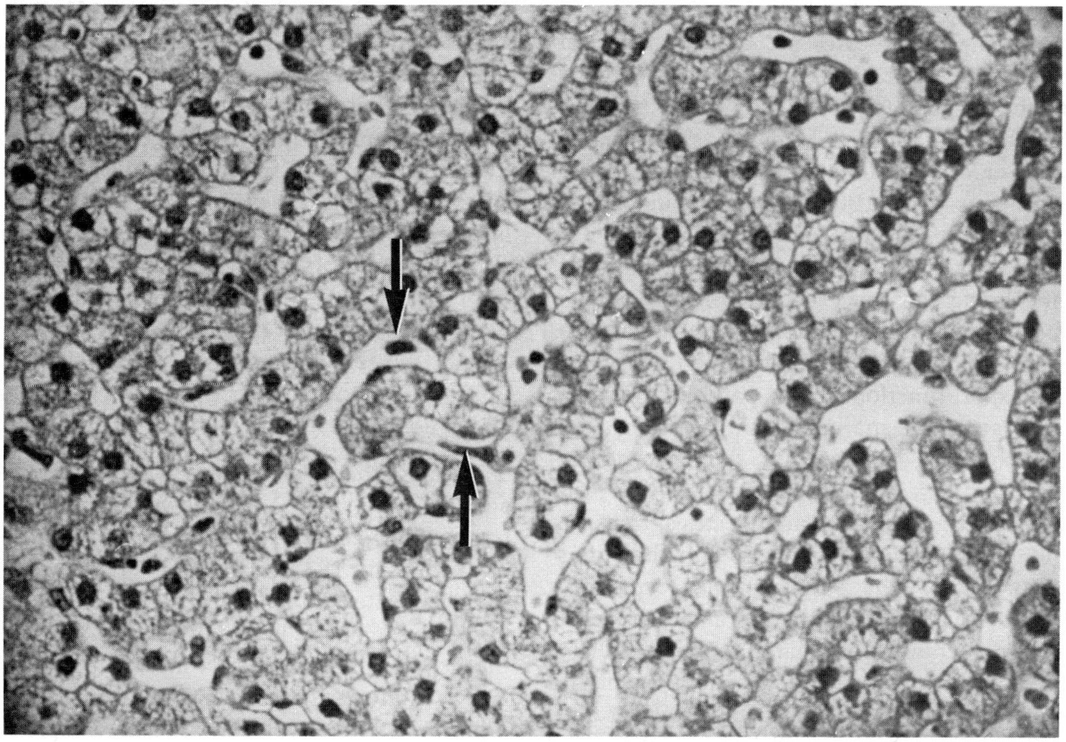

**Fig. 24.5** Normal hepatic parenchyma. Note the single cell plates of hepatocytes and the Kupffer cells (arrowed) in the sinusoids (hematoxylin and eosin, ×25).

nuclei than endothelial cells on light microscopy and can be differentiated from hepatic stellate cells by fat stains, as the latter contain much lipid. The space of Disse contains an extracellular matrix including collagen and other fibrous proteins.

*Portal tracts*

The portal tracts are an integral part of the connective tissue scaffolding of the liver, which is a branching structure extending into the organ from its hilum. They contain branches of the hepatic artery, portal vein and biliary tract as well as nerves and lymphatic vessels and the whole structure is continuous with the liver capsule. The microscopic anatomy varies with the size of the portal tract and that described here relates to the smaller portal tracts seen in needle biopsies of the liver. The smallest portal tracts are round or oval, while larger portal tracts, which give rise to branches, are angulated. The hepatic artery and portal vein branches are usually closely related; the arteries have an intima, a smooth muscle media and an adventitia, with an internal elastic lamina in the larger arteries, while the veins are larger vessels with an endothelial lining and a thin basement membrane and smooth muscle only in quite large veins. The larger septal bile ducts are recognized by their relatively large caliber and their lining of tall columnar epithelial cells with basal nuclei abutting on a basement membrane. These cells stain positively with PAS stain. The smaller interlobular bile ducts are found in the center of small round or oval portal tracts and they have a lining of cuboidal epithelial cells, which do not react positively with the PAS stain, and a basement membrane. These interlobular bile ducts are joined to the hepatocytes by tiny ductules, which are seen occasionally as ducts lined by flattened epithelium in the periphery of the tract. The ductules are joined to the liver cells by the canals of Hering. The lymphatic vessels surround the hepatic artery and portal vein branches and nerves are sometimes seen around larger arterial vessels. The connective tissue of the portal tracts usually contains a variable but moderate number of lymphocytes and large mononuclear cells.

*Hepatic veins*

The centrilobular (hepatic) veins are found at the center of the liver lobule. The smallest branches have very thin walls, but larger branches also have a thin collagen coat, smooth muscle and associated lymphatics.

## Electronmicroscopy

Electronmicroscopy has provided considerable information regarding the structural basis for the functions of liver cells, but it has not proved of particular value in clinical practice.

***Hepatocytes.*** The hepatocytes are large, polyhedral cells arranged in single-cell plates that contain virtually every known subcellular organelle. This reflects the great diversity of hepatocyte functions. Hepatocytes have large nuclei containing at least one nucleolus and mitotic figures are few as only about 1 in 20 000 cells is dividing at any given time.

The plasma membrane shows three different domains. The membrane lining the space of Disse has microvilli occasionally protruding through endothelial fenestrae into the sinusoids. These microvilli reflect the high density of receptor and transport functions of this part of the plasma membrane. The lateral plasma membrane has few or no microvilli but contains desmosomes, which stabilize cell–cell contact, and gap junctions, which allow intercellular communication and chemical and electrical transfer. The canalicular membrane is defined by tight junctions and contains microvilli. The pericanalicular cytoplasm contains numerous vesicles, Golgi bodies and lysosomes, which are involved in transport of material into the biliary canaliculi, and a contractile filamentous system extending into the microvilli, which maintains their structure and may contribute to biliary secretion. The rest of the cytoplasm is also rich in organelles, with the rough endoplasmic reticulum, Golgi bodies and mitochondria more prominent in zone 1 where oxidation and protein synthesis predominate and smooth endoplasmic reticulum more prominent in zone 3 where detoxification reactions related to the cytochrome P-450 enzyme system predominate (p. 837).

***Biliary cells.*** The biliary epithelium is cuboidal in the small intrahepatic bile ducts and becomes columnar as the bile ducts enlarge. There are few microvilli on the plasma membrane and the cytoplasm contains a prominent Golgi apparatus and numerous vesicles. This and a rich peribiliary capillary plexus around the intrahepatic bile ducts support the view that these cells contribute to the composition of bile (p. 757). The gallbladder cells show numerous microvilli and many subcellular organelles reflecting their absorptive function.

***Sinusoidal cells.*** Sinusoidal endothelial cells have prominent nuclei and thin cytoplasmic strands. The cytoplasm contains fenestrae surrounded by microfilaments and bristle-coated membrane invaginations and lysosomes reflecting active endocytosis. The Kupffer cells are most prominent in the periportal area. They are stellate (and are called *sternzellen* in German literature) with pseudopodia extending through endothelial fenestrae and their pseudopodia, pinocytic vesicles and lysosomes reflect their phagocytic functions. Hepatic stellate cells are most prominent in the perivenous area. Many names have been used for these cells (Ito cells, lipocytes, fat-storing cells, perisinusoidal cells, pericytes, parasinusoidal cells) and recently a strong case has been made for the term "hepatic stellate cells" used here (Ahern et al 1996). Quiescent hepatic stellate cells are characterized by numerous vitamin A-containing lipid droplets. Activated hepatic stellate cells develop the features of myofibroblasts and may be related to local production of extracellular fibrous proteins such as collagen. Pit cells have been described in rats. They show the features of large granular lymphocytes and are probably natural killer cells (Bouwens et al 1987). They have not so far been found in humans.

## FUNCTION

### Liver acinus

The classic hepatic lobule was described over 150 years ago in the pig, with a hepatic vein at its center and portal tracts connected by connective tissue septa on its periphery (Kiernan 1833). Few animals, however, show this well-delineated lobular structure and subsequent studies have sought a basic liver unit based on the blood supply to the hepatic parenchyma. None of the units suggested so far is wholly satisfactory and the human liver may be an indivisible whole, but currently the simple liver acinus is favored as the functional unit of the liver (Rappaport 1958). This is defined as a mass of parenchyma dependent on a single blood supply from hepatic arterial and portal venous branches in a small terminal portal tract (Rappaport 1958). The blood from such portal tracts flows into the related sinusoids and drains to several efferent veins supplying the intervening hepatic parenchyma. Each efferent vein drains blood from several different simple acini. The hepatocytes in a simple acinus are divided into zones in accordance with their position relative to the terminal portal tract (Fig. 24.6). Cells in zone 1 are near-

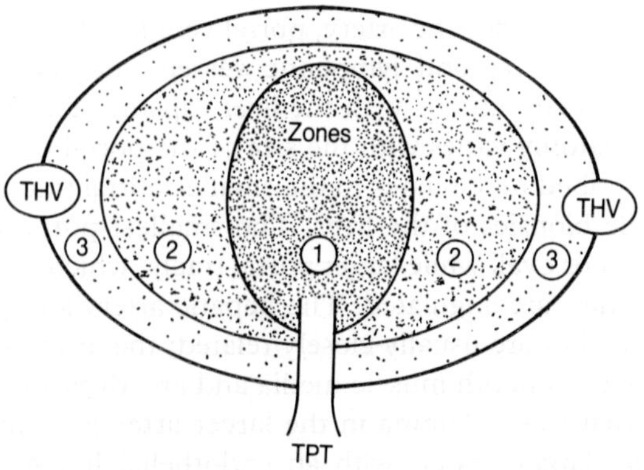


**Fig. 24.6** The zonal subdivisions of the hepatic acinus. Blood enters zone 1 from the portal venule and the hepatic arteriole in a terminal portal tract (TPT) and flows through zone 2 and zone 3 to leave the acinus via the terminal hepatic veins (THV). Stippling represents decreasing vascularity from zone 1 to zone 3.

est and cells in zone 3 are furthest away from the tract. This system of zoning reflects the distribution of blood in the simple acinus and identifies cells at particular risk (zone 3) when blood flow is deficient. Variations also occur in the structure of the sinusoids within the acinus and these variations also determine the extent to which individual hepatocytes have access to blood flowing into the acinus (below).

Complex acini comprise three or more simple acini supplied by a common larger portal tract, the vessels of which divide to enter the terminal portal tracts of each simple acinus. In addition to the simple acini, the complex acinus includes a sheath of hepatocytes surrounding the common larger portal tract that receive their blood supply direct from that tract via small vascular twigs. The hepatocytes supplied by a single vascular twig are known as an acinulus. Acinar agglomerates in turn comprise three or more complex acini with a common blood supply.

## The anatomy of acinar function

The simple acinus looks superficially homogeneous under the light microscope, but it is in fact heterogeneous in respect of the hepatocytes, the sinusoids, the perisinusoidal cells and the extracellular matrix.

***Hepatocytes.*** The hepatocytes constitute a heterogeneous population that has been divided functionally into a predominantly periportal group (zone 1) and a predominantly perivenous group (zone 3) and the localization of material in cells and stuctural and enzymic differences between cells have been used to deduce the predominant functions of cells in different parts of the hepatic acinus (Jungermann & Katz, 1982, 1989). Such functions, however, are not necessarily fixed and depend on metabolic requirements. Immunocytochemical studies have shown that in health only 15–35% of hepatocytes in the human liver contain albumin, whereas all the hepatocytes in the livers of nephrotic animals contain this protein.

All hepatocytes are involved in glucose metabolism, but during absorption the perivenous cells take up glucose and incorporate it into glycogen or convert it to lactate, while the periportal cells convert lactate to glycogen. In the postabsorptive state the periportal cells receive glucose and the perivenous cells release lactate. Thus, the liver acts as the glucostat of the body. All hepatocytes are capable of transporting bile acids from the sinusoids to the biliary canaliculi, but under physiological circumstances this function is probably performed only by periportal hepatocytes, while perivenous hepatocytes may be involved more in the synthesis of new bile acid molecules. Perivenous hepatocytes contain more smooth endoplasmic reticulum and more of the cytochrome P-450 system on which drug metabolism depends, suggesting that centrilobular cells are more active in drug metabolism. The greater susceptibility of these cells to damage by agents such as paracetamol (acetaminophen) has been related to the fact that glutathione, which is conjugated with toxic metabolites of paracetamol metabolism (p. 846), is mainly localized in periportal cells.

Little is known of the determinants of hepatocyte function in different parts of the acinus, but information regarding this is beginning to emerge. Methods for measuring hepatocyte functions directly have shown that the predominant sites of liver functions can be altered by perfusing the liver in a retrograde rather than an anterograde direction (Fig. 24.7). This implies that in normal circumstances the metabolic potential of many hepatocytes is not fully active and that factors in the microenvironment of the cells, including blood flow, oxygen supply and hormone and nutrient substrates in the blood, are likely to be very important. Some hepatocyte functions remain fixed within the acinus, as in the case of the mechanism for ammonia metabolism where conversion of ammonia to urea takes place in the periportal hepatocytes and conversion to glutamine takes place in the perivenous hepatocytes. This constant distribution of function is thought to be due to short-range cell-to-cell information passing from periportal and perivenous endothelium to hepatocytes (Gebhardt 1992).

***Sinusoids.*** Heterogeneity also occurs in the sinusoids. The periportal sinusoids are relatively narrow and tortuous and the perivenous sinusoids wider and more parallel. The periportal endothelial cells have larger fenestrae, but those in the perivenous area have more dense fenestrae and these perivenous sinusoids are probably more permeable. Endothelial cells have many as yet poorly defined functions, reflected in their possession of many cell membrane receptors. These include receptors for connective tissue components such as hyaluronic acid (p. 752) and receptors allowing a variety of scavenger functions. Endothelial cells also produce proteins such as von Willebrand factor, endothelin, fibronectin and cytokines.

***Kupffer cells.*** Kupffer cells are important components

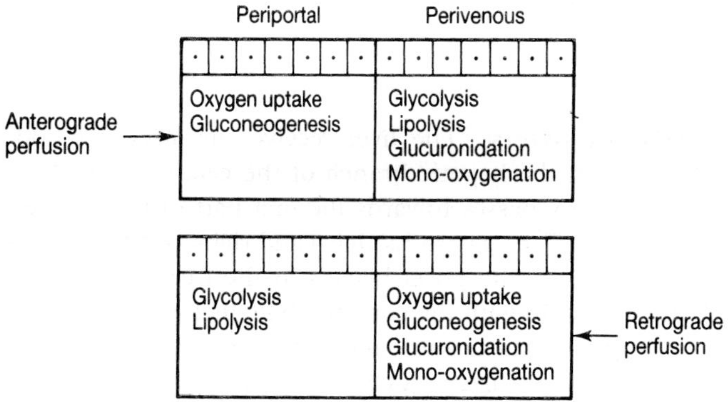


**Fig. 24.7** Predominant metabolic processes in periportal and perivenous regions of the liver acinus related to the direction of perfusion of the acinus (Thurman & Kauffman 1985).

of the reticulo-endothelial system (p. 26.1) and are found in the sinusoids, particularly in the periportal area. They have important phagocytic functions for micro-organisms, effete red blood cells, immune complexes and other substances and this is reflected in the possession of many cell surface receptors including receptors for immune complexes, complement factors, opsonizing agents such as fibronectin and inflammatory mediators such as platelet-activating factor. Kupffer cells also produce cytokines and these affect surrounding cells such as the hepatic stellate cells.

***Hepatic stellate cells.*** Hepatic stellate cells are found in the space of Disse and are most numerous in the perivenous parts of the liver. They possess long interconnecting cytoplasmic filaments and contain characteristic cytoplasmic lipid droplets. They develop features of myofibroblasts on activation. Hepatic stellate cells are now regarded as important in the production of connective tissue components (p. 916) in hepatic repair, and continuing hepatic damage perpetuates this activity leading to increasing fibrosis and cirrhosis (Knittel & Ramadori 1995, Pinzani 1995). Hepatocyte damage due to a variety of factors leads to cytokine production by inflammatory cells, Kupffer cells and platelets and these cytokines activate the hepatic stellate cells. Platelet-derived growth factor is important in hepatic stellate cell proliferation and transforming growth factor β in fibrosis. Hepatic stellate cells are also important in the storage of retinoid (vitamin A). Retinoid is taken up by hepatocytes and transferred to the hepatic stellate cells as retinol bound to retinol-binding protein. Retinol is stored in the hepatic stellate cells and released as required by demand for vitamin A.

## HEPATIC CIRCULATION

The liver has a complex blood supply from the hepatic artery and the portal vein, a unique capillary circulation in the highly permeable sinusoids, a venous drainage through a network of valveless veins and a lymph drainage accounting for half the flow in the thoracic duct (Lautt 1977, Richardson & Withrington 1981a,b).

### Hepatic arteriovenous blood supply

***Hepatic artery.*** The liver receives its arterial blood supply from the hepatic branch of the celiac artery. The hepatic artery passes towards the first part of the duodenum, gives off the gastroduodenal and right gastric arteries and ascends to the porta hepatis in the free edge of the lesser omentum with the common bile duct and the portal vein. In the porta hepatis, the hepatic artery divides into the right hepatic artery, a cystic branch of which supplies the gallbladder, and the left hepatic artery, both of which enter the liver. Hepatic arterial anomalies are fairly common and are important in surgery, in hepatic angiography and when infusing agents such as vasopressin into the splanchnic circulation (p. 503). The hepatic artery may originate from the aorta or from the superior mesenteric artery, accessory hepatic arteries are fairly common and the cystic artery shows frequent variations.

***Portal vein.*** The portal vein drains blood from the gastrointestinal tract, spleen, pancreas and gallbladder. It is formed behind the neck of the pancreas at the level of the second lumbar vertebra by the union of the superior mesenteric vein and the splenic vein, which receives blood from the inferior mesenteric, gastric, gastroepiploic and pancreatic veins. It is about 8 cm long, valveless and passes obliquely to the porta hepatis, initially behind the first part of the duodenum and then in the free edge of the lesser omentum. It receives the right and left gastric veins and the prepyloric vein and in the porta hepatis divides into right and left branches, which enter the liver. The left portal vein is joined by the ligamentum teres and the ligamentum venosum; the remnant of the umbilical vein in the ligamentum teres is not usually obliterated and can be used to catheterize the left portal vein (p. 992). There are communications between tributaries of the portal and systemic veins which become important collateral vessels in portal hypertension. The most important are in the esophagus and stomach (p. 992); others occur in the gastrointestinal tract, especially in the lower rectum and anus, in the anterior abdominal wall, particularly around the umbilicus (p. 992), behind the duodenum and colon and over the bare area of the liver.

***Intrahepatic vessels.*** Within the liver, the hepatic artery and portal vein branches divide in the portal tracts and eventually enter the sinusoids. Most blood enters the sinusoids from the portal venules and afferent or inlet sphincters composed of sinusoidal lining cells are found where these vessels join. Hepatic arterial blood enters only a proportion of the sinusoids, mainly by arteriosinus twigs that enter the sinusoids directly distal to their junction with the portal venules or occasionally via arterioportal anastomoses. The hepatic artery also supplies blood to the biliary tracts via a peribiliar vascular plexus supplied by branches of the hepatic artery and draining mainly to the sinusoids.

***Circulatory control.*** The sinusoids themselves are the main site at which the blood pressure is reduced in the liver and where blood flow into the sinusoids is controlled. This control is exercised mainly by the endothelial and Kupffer cells, which fulfill this function by contracting and swelling to reduce sinusoidal patency. Hepatic arteriolar blood flow is also controlled by the muscular coat of the hepatic arterioles and the portal and hepatic venules also have a small muscular component.

### Sinusoids

The sinusoids are the capillaries of the liver (Fig. 24.5)

and they are in many ways unique (Jones 1983, Bradfield 1984). They are lined completely with endothelial cells but have no underlying basement membrane. On the luminal surface of the endothelium are located the Kupffer cells, which are an important part of the mononuclear phagocyte system (p. 763). Pit cells, containing granules and functioning as natural killer lymphocytes, have been described in some animals but have not been found so far in humans. Hepatic stellate cells are found outside the sinusoids in the space of Disse and are the original *sternzellen* described by von Kupffer in 1876. They probably equate with capillary pericytes elsewhere in the body. They are recognized increasingly as having important functions, especially in relation to fibrosis in the liver (p. 916).

The sinusoids function at a very low pressure (3–5 mmHg) produced by a marked pressure drop at the entrance to the sinusoids and by the relative imperviousness of the sinusoidal system to factors altering capillary pressure elsewhere. This is illustrated in Table 24.2, which compares the effects of vasodilatation on liver sinusoidal and muscle capillary pressures. This feature is related in turn to the high permeability of hepatic sinusoids. Starling (1915) pointed out that the sinusoids were the most permeable capillaries in the body, resulting in the liver interstitial fluid having a similar protein composition to plasma. This is an important factor in the composition of ascites (p. 1018). The high permeability of liver sinusoids results from unique properties of the sinusoidal endothelium and from the absence of a capillary basement membrane (Wisse et al 1985). The endothelial cells have a high endocytotic capacity and in addition possess fenestrae allowing direct access to the space of Disse. The fenestrae are arranged in groups called sieve plates and the majority of fluid, solute and particle exchange between the sinusoids and the space of Disse is thought to take place through the fenestrae. The entrances to and exits from the sinusoids are adjacent to one another and this allows high concentration gradients to be maintained along the sinusoids. Sinusoidal variation occurs within the acinus, as sinusoids in zone 1 anastomose more extensively, have a higher surface/volume ratio and have larger fenestrations than those in zone 3 (Miller et al 1979, Wisse et al 1985).

## Hepatic veins

Blood leaves the liver in the hepatic veins, which constitute a massive venous system. Progressive union of the tributaries draining the hepatic acini leads eventually to the formation of three main valveless hepatic veins draining the left, middle and right thirds of the liver. These vessels join the inferior vena cava at the upper margin of the liver, although frequently the central vein first joins the left vein. Smaller hepatic veins may join the inferior vena cava more distally. A separate vein from the caudate lobe is often present; this separate venous drainage accounts for the frequent sparing of the caudate lobe when the main hepatic veins are obstructed.

**Table 24.2** Variation in rat hepatic and skeletal muscle capillary pressures in response to vasodilatation at a precapillary pressure of 100 mmHg (Lautt 1977)

| State | Liver | Skeletal muscles |
|---|---|---|
| Resting | 2 mmHg | 20 mmHg |
| Maximal vasodilatation | 3.2 mmHg | 37 mmHg |

## Blood flow

The total liver blood flow in humans is about 800–1200 ml/min and constitutes about a quarter of the resting cardiac output. Roughly two-thirds comes via the portal vein and one-third via the hepatic artery. The portal venous system operates at a low pressure (8–10 mmHg), with three-quarters of its blood derived from the mesenteric circulation and one-quarter from the splenic circulation. Controversy continues over the existence of streaming in the portal blood flow, by which mesenteric blood would tend to reach the right hepatic lobe while splenic blood would pass to the left lobe (Groszmann et al 1971, Gates & Dore 1973, Kashiwagi et al 1975). The hepatic artery normally provides only a third of the total liver blood flow, but it is responsible for about half the oxygen supply to that organ. Hepatic oxygen supply is not critical, as the liver extracts only a half of its normal oxygen supply. Hepatic arterial blood flow is maintained provided the systemic arterial pressure remains above 60–80 mmHg.

Liver blood flow is determined mainly by the hepatic arterial vascular resistance and by the intestinal and splenic vascular resistances that control blood flow into the portal venous system. Autoregulation of hepatic arterial flow occurs whereby a rise in arterial pressure results in a rise in arteriolar resistance and vice versa and extrinsic factors such as the neurovascular supply to the hepatic artery and hormonal factors are probably more important in mediating this than intrinsic factors (Richardson & Withrington 1981a,b). The portal venous system, conversely, seems to act mainly as a passive conduit for the splenic and intestinal outflow of blood.

Portal blood flow is governed mainly by factors affecting intestinal and splenic blood flow and consequently increases in response to increased intestinal blood flow postprandially and decreases between meals. There is also a relation between hepatic arterial and portal venous blood flow whereby hepatic arterial flow can increase up to 100% in response to a fall in portal flow. This is not a reciprocal relation, as portal flow does not increase when hepatic arterial flow falls. Entry of hepatic arterial and portal blood into the sinusoids is associated with a major reduction in blood pressure (above).

The hepatic venous system contains no valves and is very sensitive to increases in the central venous pressure. Any increase is transmitted directly to the hepatic sinusoids and causes a marked increase in filtration of fluid across the sinusoids, with a consequent increase in lymphatic drainage. This may lead to the production of ascites (p. 1017). The hepatic venous bed also constitutes a large reservoir of blood; it contains 10–15% of the total blood volume and blood constitutes around a quarter of the total liver volume. About a half of this blood can be expelled rapidly from the liver, which thereby constitutes an important buffering mechanism for blood volume changes. The controlling mechanisms for this function are largely unknown.

### Lymph and lymphatics

The lymphatics deep in the liver run in the portal tracts and in association with the hepatic veins (Comparini 1969). The portal lymphatics are closely related to the branches of the hepatic artery and the portal vein and they carry lymph from the smallest portal tracts to the hepatic lymph nodes in the porta hepatis. The hepatic venous lymphatics follow the course of the hepatic veins and convey lymph to lymph nodes around the inferior vena cava. Superficial lymphatics also emerge directly onto the surface of the liver. Those on the superior and posterior aspects of the liver join the diaphragmatic lymphatic plexuses and the lymphatics emerging with the hepatic veins; the remaining superficial lymphatics converge on the hepatic lymph nodes in the porta hepatis. Lymph leaving the liver may pass through the celiac and para-aortic nodes, posterior mediastinal nodes, internal mammary nodes or the paraesophageal lymphatics before reaching the circulation.

Hepatic lymph is formed in the space of Disse and most passes to the periphery of the hepatic lobule where it enters the lymphatics in the portal tracts (Dumont 1974). Lymph flow to the portal tracts would have to occur against a pressure gradient and the mechanism for this is unknown. Normally, some 80% of the hepatic lymph leaves the liver via the hepatic hilum and the rest via the lymphatics associated with the hepatic veins. About half the thoracic duct lymph derives from the liver and about 40% of the plasma protein pool is returned to the blood in the hepatic lymph daily.

## MAINTENANCE AND REPAIR OF THE LIVER

The size of the liver in relation to the rest of the body remains remarkably constant throughout life and liver transplantation in man and other animals has shown that a transplanted liver grows or shrinks in accordance with the size of the recipient (Kam et al 1987, Kawasaki et al 1992). The mechanisms whereby the liver maintains itself so constantly are poorly understood.

***Maintenance.*** The healthy liver has a slowly renewing cell population with individual hepatocytes living 200–450 days and probably being eliminated by apoptosis. New liver cells originate mainly in the periportal area, possibly from stem cells located at the level of the canals of Hering that are capable of forming hepatocytes or biliary epithelium, and these new hepatocytes stream slowly along the liver cell plate towards the terminal hepatic veins (Zajicek et al 1985). It has been suggested that hepatocytes become more differentiated functionally as they move to the perivenous area, but this seems unlikely in view of the ability of such cells to change function in response to a changing microenvironment (p. 713).

***Repair.*** Liver regeneration has been studied most in animals (mainly rats) subjected to partial hepatectomy and to a lesser extent following toxic liver injury. These experiments show clearly that after injury hepatocytes in any part of the acinus can proliferate and in this circumstance stem cells are not important unless hepatic damage is very severe. Periportal cells proliferate more quickly and more frequently than perivenous cells, but reverse blood flow experiments show that this is not due to intrinsically greater proliferative capacity. The maintenance of adequate liver function during regeneration requires simultaneous hepatic proliferation and the continuance of differentiated hepatocyte functions and this is reflected in the expression of genes related to growth and to liver cell function during this process (Haber et al 1995).

The response to partial hepatectomy relates to the magnitude of the resection and to the age of the animal. Little proliferative activity occurs when less than 40% of the liver is resected, perhaps because of the organ's great functional reserve, but the response then increases as the extent of resection increases. Proliferative activity falls again when resection exceeds 85% of the liver, perhaps because liver function and cell division cannot both then be sustained and death from liver failure is frequent. The proliferative response in older animals is less than in younger animals. Deoxyribonucleic acid (DNA) synthesis begins about 12 h after resection in the rat, peaks at about 24 h, and declines thereafter, sometimes with a second peak at about 36 h in young animals. Even maximum proliferative responses involve DNA synthesis and mitosis in only 30–40% of hepatocytes, even in young animals. Hepatocyte proliferation alone is insufficient for repair of the liver, as new sinusoids must be formed. Hepatocyte proliferation occurs first, leading to formation of hepatocyte clusters without sinusoids, but sinusoidal cells proliferate later with eventual formation of sinusoids in which production of appropriate extracellular matrix is probably very important (Martinez-Hernandez et al 1991).

Liver regeneration in humans is slower. It begins within about 5 days of liver resection in a previously healthy liver and takes up to 6 months to restore the liver mass to normal (Kawasaki et al 1992). There is little or no regeneration in cirrhotic livers following resection, perhaps because a normal reticulin architecture is needed, and resection frequently causes liver failure and death in patients with cirrhosis (Lin et al 1979).

***Mechanisms.*** The mechanisms leading to repair of the liver are poorly understood, although information regarding possibly important factors is becoming available (Knittel & Ramadori 1995). Hepatocytes respond to a complex system of stimulatory and inhibitory signals controlling the regenerative process, although the way in which this is co-ordinated is currently largely unknown. These signals are mediated by growth regulators which stimulate DNA synthesis directly (mitogens), including hepatocyte growth factor (HGF), epidermal growth factor and tumor necrosis factor $\alpha$, which enhance DNA synthesis without stimulating DNA synthesis directly (comitogens), including hormones, neurotransmitters and nutrients, and which inhibit hepatocyte proliferation including transforming growth factor $\beta$ and the interleukins.

HGF is the most potent known inducer of hepatocyte DNA synthesis, although it is not a liver-specific growth factor, and its blood concentration increases during hepatocyte proliferation. It is an important mediator of hepatic regeneration and is essential to normal liver development (Schmidt et al 1995). HGF is synthesized in mesenchymal cells as a promitogen that needs to be activated before it can act as a growth mediator. HGF in the blood is taken up mainly by the liver and is concentrated in the periportal cells. It is probably synthesized in normal liver mainly by hepatic stellate cells, but in regenerating liver the endothelial cells are an important source. The way in which HGF synthesis in nonparenchymal liver cells is regulated is unknown. Major changes in the expression of hepatocyte genes occur during regeneration, but the mechanisms controlling these changes and the means whereby hepatocyte proliferation and differentiation are controlled remains largely unknown.

## LIVER BIOPSY

Liver biopsy has proved invaluable in understanding the liver in health and disease, in substantiating the reliability of other investigations, and in diagnosis. However, it has serious potential complications and should never be done lightly. Needle biopsies can be obtained percutaneously, at laparoscopy or at laparotomy, and wedge biopsies are taken at laparotomy. Percutaneous liver biopsy has been used for over 50 years (Iversen & Roholm 1939), many reviews are available (Hegarty & Williams 1984), and an audit in England and Wales gives an interesting insight into its use in general clinical practice (Gilmore et al 1995). Liver biopsy can be carried out in the fetus for prenatal diagnosis (Rodeck et al 1982).

### *Indications*

***Acute liver disease.*** Most acute liver diseases are self-limiting and are caused by hepatitis viruses or drugs. Viral damage cannot be differentiated readily from drug damage histologically, and liver biopsy is only needed where there is clinical evidence of chronic liver disease. A biopsy is occasionally indicated if alcohol is suspected, if clinical evidence suggests some rare cause such as Wilson's disease, or if the illness fails to resolve. Biopsy can be done in fulminant hepatic failure provided facilities are available for correcting coagulation defects (Scotto et al 1973), but this is hardly ever needed as the diagnosis is made clinically (p. 805) and a biopsy is unlikely to reveal a specific cause or alter the management of the patient.

***Chronic liver disease.*** Liver biopsy is always necessary in the diagnosis of chronic hepatitis and may be needed in the diagnosis of cirrhosis. It confirms their presence, gives some indication of their severity (p. 917), and may reveal causes such as alcohol abuse, hemochromatosis, or $\alpha_1$-antitrypsin deficiency. Laparoscopy increases the diagnostic value of biopsy in cirrhosis (p. 129).

***Jaundice.*** The necessity for liver biopsy depends on the nature of the jaundice. Liver biopsy is most useful when clinical and biochemical evidence points to chronic parenchymal liver disease as the cause of jaundice. Cholestatic jaundice should be investigated first by imaging and by cholangiography (p. 1198), but liver biopsy can be useful when no evidence of mechanical biliary obstruction is found, as an experienced histopathologist may be able to differentiate large bile duct obstruction from parenchymal liver disease (Morris et al 1975, Lance et al 1977). Liver biopsy is not indicated in hemolytic jaundice.

***Abnormal liver function tests.*** Abnormal liver function tests occur in many conditions and are often found on biochemical screening. Minor abnormalities of liver function without clinical evidence of liver disease which cannot be accounted for or which do not disappear after treatment of possible underlying causes require liver biopsy only if they persist for more than 6 months (p. 736).

***Neoplasms.*** Neoplasms are focal lesions and a single percutaneous biopsy often fails to make the diagnosis, as a biopsy represents only 1/50 000 of the liver. It is best, therefore, to localize the neoplasm prior to biopsy by imaging or by laparoscopy. Jori & Peschele (1972) found that a percutaneous biopsy diagnosed liver cancer in 40% of patients, whereas a biopsy at laparoscopy (p. 129) did so in 69% of cases. Conn (1972) found that the best results are obtained when biopsies are directed by a liver scan, when two biopsies are obtained through the same puncture hole, and when cytology is performed on the blood aspirated in the needle. Lymphomas are difficult to diagnose on needle biopsies (p. 1104), and results are better when such biopsies are taken at laparoscopy. Laparotomy to obtain wedge liver biopsies for staging lymphomas is no longer considered important.

***Miscellaneous liver diseases.*** Congenital hepatic fibrosis and nodular transformation of the liver may be associated with portal hypertension; liver function tests are frequently normal, and needle biopsy is often unhelpful. They are diagnosed best from a wedge biopsy. Metabolic diseases involving the liver, such as glycogen storage disease (p. 972) or amyloidosis (p. 979), may be diagnosed by liver biopsy. Biopsy may occasionally be useful in assessing improvement in autoimmune hepatitis prior to stopping therapy, in demonstrating successful treatment of hemochromatosis, and in reassessing liver disease where continuing alcohol abuse is suspected.

***Fever of unknown origin.*** As liver involvement is frequent in systemic illness, liver biopsy may be important in reaching a diagnosis. This is especially so in diseases associated with granuloma formation (p. 829). The biopsy may not reveal the cause of the illness, but findings such as granulomas initiate other appropriate investigations. Fever of unknown origin may also be caused by neoplasms, and in view of their focal nature a biopsy should be preceded by liver imaging and/or done at laparoscopy.

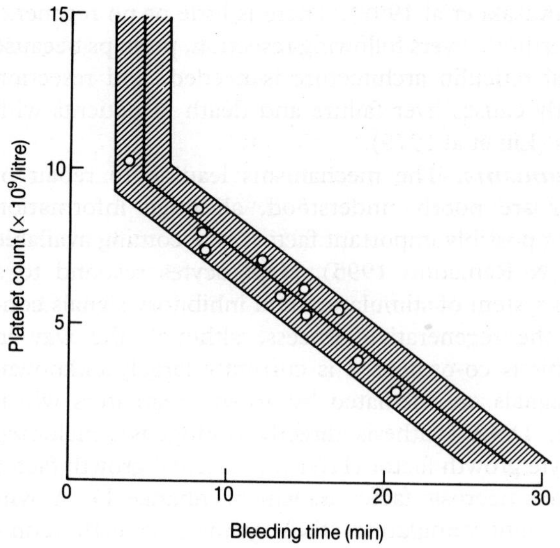


**Fig. 24.8** Relation between platelet count and bleeding time in patients with thrombocytopenia due to splenic pooling (Harker & Slichter 1972). The shaded area represents the expected relation between platelet count and bleeding time for normal platelets. Patients with splenic pooling had hepatic cirrhosis (4), lymphoma (3), myeloid metaplasia (2) and Gaucher's disease (2).

### *Contraindications*

Contraindications to liver biopsy have been discussed by Conn (1975). Many are relative, but in such instances alternative investigations are preferable.

***Unco-operative patients.*** The patient must co-operate in the procedure, as failure may result in laceration of the liver when the biopsy is taken. Unco-operative and psychiatrically disturbed patients require anesthesia for biopsy. Liver biopsy in infancy and childhood can be done safely using general anesthesia or sedation and an assistant to help prevent respiratory movement when the biopsy is taken (Walker et al 1967).

***Defective hemostasis.*** Bleeding is the most common serious complication of liver biopsy, and consequently defective hemostasis is the most important contraindication to the procedure. The prothrombin time is most widely used for checking the adequacy of blood coagulation before biopsy, even though it is a relatively insensitive measure of the function of the coagulation factors produced by the liver (p. 751). A prothrombin time prolonged 3 s or more beyond the control value, or a prothrombin time ratio (patient/control) greater than 1.4 that cannot be corrected by vitamin $K_1$ (phytomenadione) 10 mg given slowly intravenously, is widely held to indicate an increased risk of bleeding. Some laboratories express prothrombin activity as a percentage of normal: activities above 70% are normal, and every reduction of 10% below that corresponds to about a one second prolongation of the prothrombin time. Thrombocytopenia is a relative contraindication depending on its severity and cause. The bleeding time gives a measure of the hemostatic effectiveness of platelets; normal platelets maintain a normal bleeding time down to a count of $100 \times 10^9$/L (100 000/mm$^3$), with a progressive prolongation of the bleeding time as the count falls further, and this relation holds where thrombocytopenia is caused by pooling in a big spleen (Fig. 24.8), as in portal hypertension (Harker & Slichter 1972). In practice, bleeding is unlikely after a liver biopsy when the platelet count exceeds $60 \times 10^9$/L (Sharma et al 1982), and biopsies have been done in patients with platelet counts as low as $20 \times 10^9$/L (20 000/mm$^3$) without complication (Losowsky & Walker 1968). Platelet function is also important and is impaired in uremia prior to dialysis and for about 4 days after therapeutic doses of salicylates. Platelet function may be impaired when the platelet count is high (>$500 \times 10^9$/L, >500 000/mm$^3$), particularly when there is an underlying myeloproliferative disease.

The evidence that measures of hemostasis such as the platelet count and prothrombin time accurately reflect the risk of bleeding at liver biopsy is not good. Indeed, Ewe (1981) found no correlation between the prothrombin time or the platelet count and the immediate duration of bleeding after biopsy at laparoscopy, and Scotto et al (1973) encountered no bleeding after liver biopsy in patients with acute liver failure even when coagulation factors were not used. However, the authors recommend the guidelines given above, and if biopsy is necessary when the prothrombin time is prolonged 3 or more seconds or when the platelet count is below $60 \times 10^9$/L (40 000/mm$^3$), fresh frozen plasma (12–15 ml/kg body weight) and/or platelet concentrate should be given by continuous infusion starting 30 min before biopsy and for 1 h afterwards (Spector et al 1966). Consideration could also be given to plugging the biopsy needle track or performing a transjugular biopsy (below).

***Obstruction of large bile ducts.*** Liver biopsy carries a small risk of biliary peritonitis in this condition (Terry 1952), and septicemia may follow when cholangitis is present. Other investigations are preferable when obstruction of large bile ducts is suspected (p. 1198).

***Infection.*** Biopsy should be avoided when there is active skin disease at the site of needle puncture or infection in the right lower lobe of the lung or in the pleural cavity, as organisms may be carried into the peritoneal cavity or liver. It should also be avoided if a hepatic abscess is suspected; should pus be obtained at liver biopsy, the chance to culture it should not be missed (Lesesne et al 1976). Hydatid disease is an absolute contraindication.

***Pulmonary disease.*** Patients with chronic pulmonary disease and hyperinflated lungs are at risk of pneumothorax. A small pneumothorax in such a patient can precipitate respiratory failure.

***Tumors.*** Very vascular liver tumors, such as hemangiomas or tumors associated with oral contraceptives, should not be biopsied as bleeding may occur.

***Ascites.*** Marked ascites reduces the chance of obtaining an adequate liver biopsy. Biopsy is therefore best deferred until the ascites has been controlled.

***Anemia.*** Severe anemia should be corrected before biopsy.

*Blood*

Usually, 2 units of blood are cross-matched and reserved, but blood transfusion is rarely needed. Edwards (1985) found that only 3.7% of blood reserved for liver biopsy was used, and accordingly the patients's blood can be grouped and an antibody screen done, provided facilities for urgent cross-matching are available.

*Procedure*

Liver biopsy is best carried out in the morning, as most complications occur within about 6 h. This also allows patients who have had no complications to have fewer observations made overnight.

***Patient preparation.*** The written consent of the patient must be obtained before a biopsy is carried out. Nervous patients should be given a mild sedative, such as diazepam (10–20 mg) or temazepam (20 mg), orally 1 h before, and careful instructions are important for obtaining co-operation during the procedure. Prophylactic antibiotics are recommended for patients who are immunosuppressed or at risk of bacterial endocarditis. A lateral puncture site is safest and is preferred unless a specific area of the liver is to be biopsied. The patient should lie supine at the right side of the bed with the right hand behind the head so that the arm does not interfere with the procedure. A point in the midaxillary line is selected which is clearly dull to percussion in expiration, usually in the eight, ninth or tenth intercostal space. The biopsy site should be immediately above the rib below the intercostal space to avoid the intercostal vessels running under the inferior rib margin. The biopsy needle will then enter the upper part of the liver well away from the large structures in the porta hepatis. The skin over and around the selected site is cleaned (thiomersal 0.1%) and surrounded with sterile drapes. Lignocaine is injected into the skin and then into the deeper tissues to ensure that the pleura, diaphragm and liver capsule are anesthetized (Fig. 24.9). A scratchy sensation at the needle tip or pain indicates that the tissue overlying the liver has been reached. Lignocaine is given as a 0.5–1.0% solution, and 5 ml is usually needed; a total dose of 200 mg should never be exceeded (Deacock & Simpson 1964).

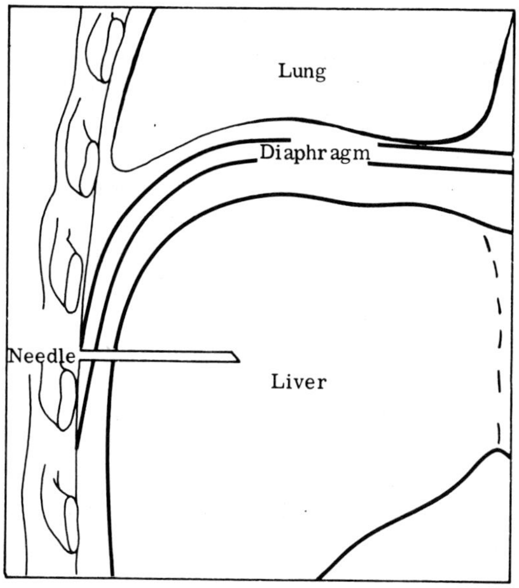


**Fig. 24.9** Diagram showing the tissues traversed during needle biopsy of the liver.

***Biopsy technique.*** The Menghini needle has proved safe and simple. A needle 1.4 mm in diameter and 100 mm in length is recommended, and a guard may be screwed to the needle shaft 35–40 mm from its tip. An obturator is put into the proximal end of the needle to prevent the biopsy being aspirated forcibly into the syringe and fragmented, and the needle is attached to a 5 ml syringe containing approximately 2 ml of sterile physiological saline. The skin is pierced at the biopsy site with an awl or scalpel to allow the needle to be inserted horizontally through the skin. The needle is cleared by injecting 1 ml of saline, the patient is asked to breathe out fully and is then told to stop breathing; negative pressure is applied to the biopsy syringe (1–2 ml) and the needle is plunged into and withdrawn from the liver in less than 1 s while negative pressure is maintained via the syringe (Menghini

1970). Thereafter, the patient can breathe normally. The needle may be inserted a second time in a slightly different direction if an adequate biopsy is not obtained. All equipment used for the biopsy should be regarded as potentially infected, and "sharps" should be put into special disposal units. Modified versions of the Menghini needle include the Klatskin needle, the Hamshidi needle (Kormed, USA), and the Surecut needle (TSK Laboratory, Japan).

The Tru-Cut needle may prevent fragmentation, as the liver biopsy is held in a notch in its inner trocar (Rake et al 1969). The inner trocar is sharply pointed, and when the needle is closed its shaft is covered by a retractable outer cutting sheath. The closed needle is inserted through the skin and is plunged into the liver while the breath is held in expiration. The inner trocar is advanced to allow liver tissue to enter the notch, and the outer sheath is then advanced to cut off the bit of liver held in the notch (Walters & Paton 1980). This relatively complex technique takes 1–2 s to perform even by experienced operators, and small errors can result in failure to obtain tissue. An automatic system for firing the Tru-Cut needle (Radiplast AB, Sweden) quickly and accurately is available (Lindgren 1982).

***Preparation of biopsies.*** The biopsy is removed gently from the needle and is put onto a ground-glass slide or filter paper. A naked-eye examination may be informative (Terry 1954). A normal biopsy has a milk-chocolate color, fragmentation suggests cirrhosis, and a pale yellow and moderately translucent biopsy suggests fatty change. The biopsy may be green in obstructive jaundice, black in the Dubin–Johnson syndrome, deep brown in hemochromatosis, and white in the presence of secondary carcinoma. The biopsy should be put into a fixative, such as 10% formol saline, for light microscopy.

***After-care of patients.*** The patient should be kept in bed for 6–8 h. The pulse and blood pressure are recorded half-hourly for 2 h, hourly for another 6 h, and 3–4 hourly for up to 24 h. The hematocrit should be checked after 24 h. Most complications occur within the first 6 h, and some physicians allow patients to go home after this time (Douds et al 1995).

***Records.*** An adequate entry in the patient's records should include the date and time the biopsy was done, the type and diameter of the needle used, the site of the needle puncture, the number of biopsy attempts, whether a biopsy was obtained, and any complications. It should also include adequate instructions regarding bed rest, pulse and blood pressure recordings, and measures to be taken for pain relief.

### *Complications*

Complications are uncommon in experienced hands but can be serious.

***Pain.*** Little or no pain should be experienced. It is usually transient and is felt either at the puncture site, in the epigastrium, or in the shoulder. It may be pleuritic. An analgesic such as pethidine (50–100 mg) intramuscularly may have to be given. Severe or continuous pain suggests bleeding or biliary peritonitis.

***Hypotension.*** Transient changes of pulse and blood pressure are frequent (Middleton et al 1977). Marked changes within 2 h of biopsy, especially hypotension or an early increase in blood pressure with pain and sweating, suggest hemorrhage. Acute transient hypotension with abdominal or lower chest pain but without tachycardia immediately after biopsy has been described (Sullivan & Watson 1974).

***Hemorrhage.*** This is the commonest serious complication. Terry (1952) reported 16 hemorrhages in 10 600 biopsies (0.15%), but an audit of more general use of liver biopsy reported 26 hemorrhages in 1500 (1.7%) biopsies (Gilmore et al 1995). About half of these patients required blood transfusion and a few needed laparotomy. Hemorrhage usually occurs when the patient breathes during the biopsy and produces laceration of the liver, or occasionally when a hematoma expands progressively and ruptures through the surface of the liver. Hemorrhage can also occur when coagulation is abnormal, as when coagulation factor production is inadequate or in patients with myeloproliferative diseases in which platelet function is poor. It should be treated by blood transfusion and in most cases will stop spontaneously. Angiography is the most appropriate procedure when bleeding continues, as the site of the bleeding can be detected and treated by embolization. Laparotomy may be needed.

***Biliary peritonitis.*** Terry (1952) found seven instances of biliary peritonitis in his review of 10 600 biopsies (0.07%) and added four cases known to himself. Ten had biliary obstruction; one died and three others required laparotomy.

***Bacteremia.*** Bacteremia can follow liver biopsy and has been reported in 13% of cases (McCloskey et al 1973). Patients who are immunosuppressed or at risk of bacterial endocarditis should therefore receive prophylactic antibiotics.

***Other complications.*** Many occasional complications of liver biopsy have been reported, but fortunately they are rare even considered as a whole. Transient febrile episodes sometimes occur and blood culture should be done, as they may result from bacteremia. Pneumothorax or hemothorax can occur, and these are often associated with obvious subcutaneous surgical emphysema, especially in the neck but sometimes extending even to the scrotum (Engelhard et al 1981). Intraheptic hematomas are probably quite common and are usually asymptomatic. Occasionally they may be large and cause pain or biliary obstruction (Forssell et al 1981), and they can rupture through the surface of the liver (Greis et al 1981). Damage to vascular structures can cause arteriovenous fistulae that

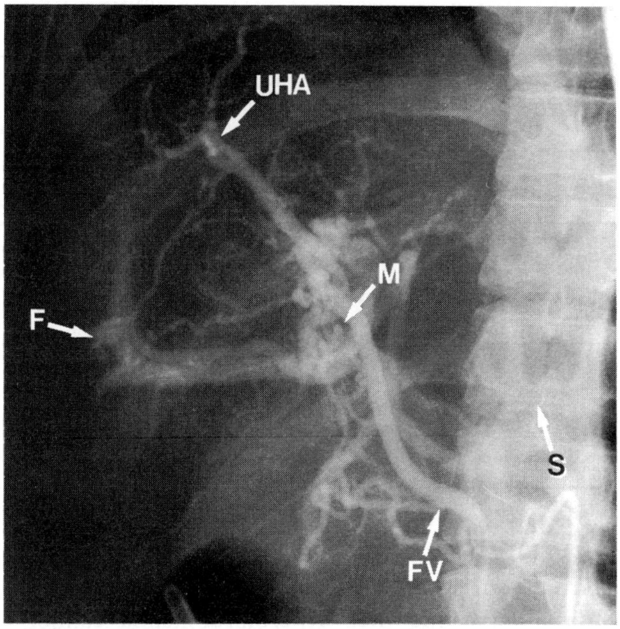


**Fig. 24.10** Hepatic arteriovenous fistula leading to rapidly developing ascites, oesophageal bleeding and a hepatic bruit 2 months after a liver biopsy. Arterial embolization of the fistula led to resolution of all these features. UHA = upper hepatic artery, F= site of fistula, M = mass of vessels, S = spine, FV = feeding vessel.

may occasionally lead to severe portal hypertension with ascites and/or bleeding (Fig. 24.10), and damage to bile ducts can result in hemobilia (p. 493). The site of bleeding can be identified angiographically and treated by embolization (Hultcrantz et al 1983). Bleeding can also cause periumbilical bruising (Tobi et al 1983). Other complications include bile pleuritis or bile embolism; peritonitis; perforation of other organs including the gallbladder, which causes an immediate painful bile peritonitis (Madden 1961); biopsy of other organs such as the kidney, adrenal, pancreas or bowel; tumor seeding in the needle track; and even fracture of the biopsy needle.

***Mortality.*** Terry (1952) recorded a mortality of 0.12% in 10 600 biopsies, Zamchek & Klausenstock (1953) a mortality of 0.17% in 20 016 biopsies using a variety of techniques, and Gilmore et al (1995) a mortality of 0.13–0.33% in 1500 biopsies. Mortality rates of 0.015–0.02% have been achieved using the Menghini method (Menghini 1970).

*Procedures for use in patients with contraindications to liver biopsy*

***Transjugular liver biopsy.*** Transjugular liver biopsy has been used primarily in patients with impaired coagulation or where vascular tumor or hepatic amyloid may predispose to bleeding. The technique and its complications are described elsewhere (p. 34).

***Needle track plugging.*** This technique entails the performance of a percutaneous liver biopsy using a sheathed biopsy needle. The needle is removed from the liver when the biopsy has been obtained, leaving the sheath in place, and the needle tack is then plugged by injecting Sterispon or Gelfoam as the sheath is withdrawn (Riley et al 1984). The method has been advocated for patients with impaired coagulation.

## LIVER ASPIRATION

Localization of focal liver lesions followed by the aspiration of material for cytological and histological examination using fine needles has proved valuable, particularly in the diagnosis of malignant disease (p. 32).

## CONGENITAL DISORDERS

Congenital disorders affecting the liver primarily may be functional or structural. Genetic factors are often important in these disorders but other factors can also be important. The functional disorders considered in this chapter are those related to bilirubin metabolism. Inherited metabolic disorders of the liver are considered in the chapter on metabolic liver disease (p. 951) and in relation to familial intrahepatic cholestasis (p. 945). The liver may be involved in many general metabolic disorders but these are outside the scope of this book (Scriver et al 1995). Genetic factors may also contribute to the development of liver disease, as in alcoholic liver disease (p. 867) or in cholestasis of pregnancy (p. 1091). The main congenital structural disorders are the fibropolycystic diseases and biliary atresia. Hepatic nodules that may be congenital in origin are considered elsewhere (p. 1128). The liver is often involved with other organs in rare syndromes, but these are not considered here (Baraitser & Winter 1991).

## CONGENITAL FUNCTIONAL DISORDERS

### Chronic familial nonhemolytic hyperbilirubinemia

The chronic familial nonhemolytic hyperbilirubinemias (Gilbert's, Crigler–Najjar, Dubin–Johnson and Rotor syndromes) are a group of conditions in which there is fluctuating jaundice of variable severity (Berthelot & Dhumeaux 1978, Billing 1987). Although symptoms may recur, with one rare exception they carry an excellent prognosis. Their clinical importance lies in recognizing them so that patients are not subjected to repeated uncomfortable and potentially dangerous investigations for serious liver disease. These conditions are largely congenital in origin, they are caused by defects in the bilirubin transport mechanisms (p. 737) and they have shed light on the normal mechanism of bilirubin metabolism.

*Gilbert's syndrome*

***Etiology.*** Gilbert's syndrome is the commonest anomaly of bilirubin transport (Gilbert et al 1907). However, its existence, let alone its incidence, has been disputed. This dispute has centered on the nature of the distribution of serum bilirubin concentrations in healthy people (p. 739). Some have held that individuals with high bilirubin concentrations represent a separate population with Gilbert's syndrome and that it affects about 5–10% of healthy people (Owens & Evans 1975), others hold that such a separate population with Gilbert's syndrome does not exist (Bailey et al 1977, Olsson et al 1988). Most accept the existence of Gilbert's syndrome and recent evidence confirms the importance of genetic factors in its development (Schmid 1995). The syndrome is often familial and the single most important pathogenetic factor is impaired production of conjugated bilirubin due to impaired activity of bilirubin uridine diphosphate (UDP)-glucuronosyl transferase (p. 738). The coding and promoter regions of the gene for this enzyme have been sequenced and a consistent abnormality of the promoter region has been found in Gilbert's syndrome, resulting in reduced enzyme production (Bosma et al 1995). Patients with Gilbert's syndrome are homozygous for the abnormal promoter region.

Other factors are probably also important in the pathogenesis of the condition. Gilbert's syndrome occasionally follows viral hepatitis (Arias 1962), but in most such instances viral hepatitis probably only draws attention to pre-existing Gilbert's syndrome. Where there is no evidence of a familial occurrence, the etiology is unknown.

***Pathogenesis.*** Impaired activity of hepatic UDP-glucuronosyl transferase activity resulting in reduced ability to produce bilirubin diglucuronide occurs in all patients with Gilbert's syndrome. Low activities of this enzyme have been found in vitro, bilirubin diglucuronide production following intravenous infusion of bilirubin is diminished and plasma conjugated bilirubin concentrations are low, particularly in relation to unconjugated bilirubin concentrations. However, factors other than deficient enzyme activity must also be important in producing hyperbilirubinemia, as there is no relation between hepatic UDP-glucuronosyl transferase activity and the serum bilirubin concentration and phenobarbitone diminishes the serum bilirubin without increasing enzyme activity (Schmid 1995).

About a third of patients with Gilbert's syndrome have an impaired ability to transport organic anions other than bilirubin from the blood into the bile. This has been shown using organic anions such as bromsulphthalein and indocyanine green, neither of which is conjugated by bilirubin UDP-glucuronosyl transferase. This is consistent with a generalized defect in uptake or intracellular transport of organic anions. About a half of patients with Gilbert's syndrome have a slightly shortened erythrocyte lifespan suggesting mild hemolysis. Increased bilirubin production is therefore probably another factor in the development of jaundice. However, $^{51}$Cr-labeled red blood cell survival tests rarely give values of less than 19 days, indicating that hyperbilirubinemia cannot be attributed primarily to hemolysis (Table 24.3). McColl et al (1987) have described abnormalities of the enzymes of heme synthesis in peripheral blood cells unassociated with any increase of porphyrins or their precursors in Gilbert's syndrome. These abnormalities may have been a consequence of the hyperbilirubinemia. Gilbert's syndrome is probably a heterogeneous condition in which the balance of factors causing hyperbilirubinemia varies, but impaired hepatic UDP-glucuronosyl transferase activity is the most important single factor.

**Table 24.3** Isotopic measurement of red blood cell (RBC) half-life and hyperbilirubinemia (Powell et al 1967a)

| Isotope | RBC half-life (days) | |
|---|---|---|
| | Normal value | Required to produce jaundice |
| Chromium ($^{51}$Cr) | 25–35 | <15 |
| Diisopropylfluorophosphate ($^{32}$P) | 105–130 | <50 |

**Table 24.4** Factors considered to increase the plasma bilirubin concentration in Gilbert's syndrome

| |
|---|
| Fasting |
| Physical exercise |
| Stress |
| Febrile illness |
| Menstruation |

***Clinical features.*** Gilbert's syndrome is often detected fortuitously, usually in adolescence or early adult life. A number of factors have been identified as increasing the serum bilirubin concentration in this condition (Table 24.4) and these can lead to recognition of the syndrome (Schmid 1995). Fasting clearly increases the plasma bilirubin, but normal dietary variations are not important (Gollan et al 1976). The evidence that the other factors actually do induce hyperbilirubinemia is weak (Arias 1962). Malaise, easy fatiguability and nonspecific gastrointestinal symptoms occur episodically in over half the patients, but the relation of these symptoms to the hyperbilirubinemia has been disputed. The symptoms are similar to those of chronic fatigue syndrome and some have thought their relation to hyperbilirubinemia fortuitous (Olsson et al 1988), while others have related them to anxieties caused by fear of chronic liver disease (Foulk et al 1959). However, symptoms often precede jaundice and abdominal pain sufficient to suggest a surgical emergency has been reported (Powell et al 1967b). Examination shows mild jaundice but no other evidence of liver disease.

***Diagnosis.*** Gilbert's syndrome can be diagnosed in a patient who has had constant or intermittent unconjugated hyperbilirubinemia of at least 6 months' duration and who has no clinical or laboratory evidence of liver disease

**Table 24.5** Criteria for the diagnosis of Gilbert's syndrome

*Clinical examination*
Mild icterus. No other evidence of liver disease

*Investigations*
Bilirubin:
  No bilirubinuria
  Hyperbilirubinemia on two occasions over 6 months and conjugated bilirubin <5 μmol/L (0.3 mg/dl) or <20% of total bilirubin
Other liver function tests:
  Plasma transaminase, alkaline phosphatase (liver origin), and γ-glutamyl transferase activities, plasma albumin, globulin and bile acid concentrations and prothrombin time normal
Overt hemolysis:
  Hemoglobin concentration, reticulocyte count, peripheral blood cell morphology and serum haptoglobin concentration normal

*Confirmatory tests*
Liver biopsy normal
Hyperbilirubinemia exacerbated by:
  caloric restriction
  carbohydrate load
  nicotinic acid
Note: these tests are required only in doubtful cases

**Table 24.6** The Crigler–Najjar syndromes

| Feature | Type I | Type II |
|---|---|---|
| Onset | Birth | Birth to adulthood |
| Hyperbilirubinemia | | |
| Type | Unconjugated | Unconjugated |
| Concentration | >350 μmol/L (>20 mg/dl) | 150–300 μmol/L (9–18 mg/dl) |
| Bilirubinuria | Absent | Absent |
| Kernicterus | 75% | Rare |
| Prognosis | Childhood death | Good |
| Liver | | |
| Histology | Normal | Normal |
| Glucuronosyl transferase activity | Absent | Markedly reduced |
| Biliary bilirubin | Absent | Present |
| Phenobarbitone response | None | Reduced serum bilirubin |
| Hemolysis | Absent | Absent |
| Inheritance | Autosomal recessive | Autosomal dominant |

or of overt hemolysis (Table 24.5). About a half of patients with Gilbert's syndrome have a reduced red blood cell lifespan, but reticulocyte counts and plasma haptoglobin concentrations are normal (Powell et al 1967a). Serum bilirubin concentrations can reach about 100 μmol/L (6 mg/dl), but they fluctuate and can be normal intermittently (Foulk et al 1959). Most of the bilirubin is unconjugated and all other biochemical tests of liver function are normal. Hepatic histology is normal on light microscopy (Foulk et al 1959), but increased smooth endoplasmic reticulum has been shown on electronmicroscopy (McGee et al 1975, Dawson et al 1979). However, liver biopsy is not necessary in clinical practice unless there is some reason to suspect chronic liver disease. Unconjugated hyperbilirubinemia without any other clinical evidence of liver disease occurs occasionally in chronic hepatitis, but increased serum transaminase activity is also present (p. 888).

***Specific tests.*** Several tests have been devised to confirm a diagnosis of Gilbert's syndrome based on the ability of dietary manipulation or nicotinic acid to increase the plasma bilirubin or on the normality of measurements of serum bile acids. These tests are only needed in doubtful cases. Restriction of food intake to 400 kcal (1.6 MJ) daily for 3 days increases the plasma unconjugated bilirubin in Gilbert's syndrome but not in other liver diseases (Owens & Sherlock 1973). This is caused by lipid deprivation and the test can be carried out more comfortably for the patient by giving a normal 2500 kcal (10 MJ) diet containing mainly carbohydrate and only 0.6% of energy as lipid (Gollan et al 1976). Nicotinic acid (50 mg over 30 s intravenously) also produces hyperbilirubinemia in Gilbert's syndrome and some have found it a more sensitive test, particularly when the initial plasma bilirubin is normal (Rollinghoff et al 1981).

***Treatment and prognosis.*** Mild jaundice frequently recurs in Gilbert's syndrome, but lifespan is normal and no therapy is needed. Phenobarbitone 60 mg thrice daily can reduce or abolish icterus and may help relieve abdominal symptoms when these are troublesome (Black & Sherlock 1970). The reduction of the serum bilirubin by phenobarbitone may be due to increased uptake and storage of bilirubin by the liver (Ohkubo et al 1981).

### *Crigler–Najjar syndrome*

The Crigler–Najjar syndrome (Crigler & Najjar 1952) is extremely rare and is characterized by severe unconjugated hyperbilirubinemia occurring within hours of birth. There are two distinct forms of this syndrome (Table 24.6), one more severe (type I) and one less severe (type II).

***Etiology.*** Type I and type II Crigler–Najjar syndromes are both the result of markedly diminished hepatic bilirubin UDP-glucuronosyl transferase activity. They are otherwise separate entities and do not coexist in the same families. Two isoforms of bilirubin UDP-glucuronosyl transferase exist in humans and their production is controlled by a single gene. Crigler–Najjar syndrome type I seems to be due to a mutation in the common region of the gene leading to a total failure of enzyme production and a failure of phenobarbitone to reduce the plasma bilirubin (Bosma et al 1992), while Crigler–Najjar syndrome type II seems to be due to a mutation affecting only the more important isoform I (Bosma et al 1993). Both

Crigler–Najjar syndromes may be inherited as recessives. Heterozygotes for Crigler–Najjar syndrome should have normal plasma bilirubin concentrations, but in fact relatives of patients often have hyperbilirubinemia. This may be because of the coexistence of the common genetic abnormality of Gilbert's syndrome (Bosma et al 1995). The chronically jaundiced Gunn rat is a close animal model of the Crigler–Najjar syndrome.

***Type I.*** The plasma bilirubin concentration in Crigler–Najjar syndrome type I exceeds 350 μmol/L (20 mg/dl), kernicterus supervenes in three-quarters of cases and death usually occurs within weeks or months. Patients with kernicterus have occasionally lived to adult life, but survivors are usually mentally retarded and may have epilepsy and other neurological abnormalities (Wolkoff et al 1979). There is no clinical evidence of liver disease and no hemolysis or anemia. Liver function tests and liver histology are normal and there is no bilirubin in the bile and no urobilinogen in the urine. The syndrome is explained by a complete absence of hepatic UDP-glucuronosyl transferase activity that cannot be demonstrated in vitro and cannot be induced by phenobarbitone (Arias et al 1969). There may be deficient conjugation of other substances, such as menthol, and diminished urinary excretion of menthol glucuronide can detect heterozygotes.

Plasmapheresis is the best way of reducing the serum bilirubin rapidly and this should be done to prevent kernicterus. Phototherapy (p. 737) can reduce the serum bilirubin concentration more slowly and phlebotomy can reduce bilirubin production, but both are less effective treatments. Hepatic transplantation has been successful and should be considered when the plasma bilirubin is not controlled by these treatments (p. 1154), as kernicterus then remains a hazard (Kaufman et al 1986).

***Type II.*** Hyperbilirubinemia in Crigler–Najjar syndrome type II is less severe but is still sufficient to cause marked jaundice. It generally develops in childhood, usually during the first year of life, but may not be noted until early adulthood. Kernicterus occurs occasionally, but otherwise the prognosis is excellent. Exercise, fatigue and alcohol excess are said to increase jaundice, although evidence for this is slender (Arias 1962). Fasting increases hyperbilirubinemia and if prolonged, as following surgery, it can be severe and may precipitate kernicterus (Gordon et al 1976). The serum bilirubin varies (150–300 μmol/L; 9–18 mg/dl) and is the only abnormality of liver function. The liver is normal histologically but its hepatic UDP-glucuronosyl transferase activity is reduced. Bilirubin is present in the bile and phenobarbitone can reduce the serum bilirubin to normal for as long as it is given.

*Dubin–Johnson syndrome*

***Etiology.*** This syndrome is a rare, benign condition characterized by chronic fluctuating, predominantly conjugated hyperbilirubinemia (Dubin & Johnson 1954, Sprinz & Nelson 1954). The serum bilirubin is usually less than 100 μmol/L (6 mg/dl) but occasionally reaches 500 μmol/L (30 mg/dl). Hyperbilirubinemia is due to an unexplained inability to excrete conjugated bilirubin into the bile. Hemolysis does not occur. Bromsulphthalein excretion into bile is also impaired and as a result its clearance from the blood follows a characteristic pattern in which clearance is normal at 45 min but the serum bromsulphthalein rises to give higher concentrations 90 min and 120 min after injection. This late rise is characteristic and is due to the regurgitation of conjugated bromsulphthalein into the blood. The hepatic uptake and storage capacity of the liver for bromsulphthalein in the Dubin–Johnson syndrome is normal, but it has virtually no capacity to transport the dye into the bile. Dibromsulphthalein and indocyanine green, which are not conjugated in the liver, do not show secondary rises in plasma concentration, although their clearance into the bile is subnormal. The Dubin–Johnson syndrome is inherited as an autosomal recessive character and it has an animal counterpart in mutant Corriedale sheep.

***Clinical features and diagnosis.*** Jaundice is usually detected first in the second or third decades of life. It fluctuates and exacerbations are sometimes associated with malaise and abdominal discomfort. Pregnancy and oral contraceptive drugs that reduce hepatic excretory function sometimes unmask the condition (Cohen et al 1972). Physical examination reveals only icterus. Investigation confirms hyperbilirubinemia and reveals bilirubinuria and other biochemical tests of liver function are normal.

Liver biopsy is diagnostic. The liver has a dark brown or black appearance, the lobular architecture is normal and the diagnostic feature is a variable amount of dark pigment granules in the hepatocytes and, occasionally, the Kupffer cells. The chemical nature of the pigment is uncertain (Schwartz et al 1979).

***Other features.*** The hepatic excretory defect is not limited to bilirubin. Other organic anions are affected, including bromsulphthalein and biliary contrast media, which explains why the gallbladder cannot be visualized radiologically in this condition. Bile acids are organic anions, but they have received little study in this syndrome. Their transport across the liver may, however, be impaired (Douglas et al 1980). Abnormal porphyrin metabolism, such as has been described in the Rotor syndrome (below), has not been found in the Dubin–Johnson syndrome (Kondo et al 1976).

*Rotor syndrome*

***Etiology.*** This syndrome is a very rare, benign condition characterized by chronic, fluctuating conjugated hyperbilirubinemia (Rotor et al 1948). It has been reported most frequently in the South Pacific islands, Japan, Central and South America and the Mediterranean and is inherited as an autosomal recessive character (Shimizu et al 1981). The cause of the hyperbilirubinemia is related to a reduced hepatic storage capacity for organic anions. Bromsulphthalein is cleared slowly from the blood with increased retention at 45 min and no later increment. This is associated with impaired hepatic bromsulphthalein storage capacity but a normal transport maximum into the bile (Wolpert et al 1977). Mutant Southdown sheep show a defect of bilirubin transport analogous in some respects to that found in Rotor syndrome.

***Clinical features and diagnosis.*** Jaundice is generally mild and is often noted incidentally and physical examination shows no other feature of liver disease. Biochemical liver function tests are normal apart from hyperbilirubinemia and bilirubinuria. Radiological contrast media are transported into the bile normally and consequently the gallbladder can be visualized by cholecystography. Liver biopsy is normal on light microscopic examination, but ultrastructural abnormalities of the mitochondria, lysosomes and microvilli have been reported (Rapaccini et al 1983).

***Other features.*** Individuals with Rotor syndrome show abnormalities of porphyrin metabolism in that there is an increased urinary excretion of coproporphyrins (Shimizu et al 1981). This abnormality has been attributed to a reduced biliary excretion of coproporphyrins and it occurs in otherwise normal first-degree relatives of individuals with Rotor syndrome.

## CONGENITAL STRUCTURAL DISORDERS

### Fibropolycystic disease

Fibropolycystic disease of the hepatobiliary system and often the kidneys comprises a heterogeneous group of rare disorders, some of which are inherited. Their interrelations are poorly understood, owing partly to diagnostic difficulty and partly to their rarity. Patients showing almost every possible combination of lesions have been described. No classification covers all reported cases, but the main groups are shown in Table 24.7.

#### *Adult hepatorenal polycystic disease*

The kidneys are the organs predominantly affected in this condition. Hepatic cysts that do not communicate with the biliary system are present in over half the patients with renal disease (Levine et al 1985); they are lined by cuboidal epithelium and contain fluid that resembles the bile acid-independent fraction (p. 756) of bile (Patterson et al 1982). They vary greatly in number, size and distribution within the liver. Cysts may also be found in other organs, such as the pancreas, spleen and lungs. There may be other associated congenital abnormalities, particularly cerebrovascular aneurysms. The condition usually presents in adult life with palpable renal masses, hyperten-

**Table 24.7** Fibropolycystic diseases of the hepatobiliary system and kidneys

| Type | Inheritance | Lesions | | |
|---|---|---|---|---|
| | | Hepatobiliary | Portal hypertension | Renal |
| Adult hepatorenal polycystic disease | Autosomal dominant | Single or multiple cysts, sometimes with mild fibrosis, in 50% | Very rare | Cysts – usually |
| Isolated polycystic liver disease | Autosomal dominant | Multiple cysts | Unknown | None |
| Childhood hepatorenal micropolycystic disease (congenital hepatic fibrosis) | Autosomal recessive | Hepatic fibrosis, proliferation and ectasia of bile ducts and paucity of portal vein radicals | Common, but only in patients surviving to childhood | Renal tubular ectasia of 10–90% of tubules (medullary sponge kidney) |
| Childhood hepatic micropolycystic disease (congenital hepatic fibrosis) | Autosomal recessive | As above | Usual | None |
| Nonobstructive dilatation of the intrahepatic bile ducts (Caroli's syndrome) | – | Occasional associated congenital hepatic fibrosis or choledochal cyst | None | Occasional renal tubular ectasia or renal cyst |
| Choledochal cyst | – | Occasional associated congenital hepatic fibrosis | None | None |
| Simple (nonparasitic) hepatic cyst | – | None | None | None |

sion, proteinuria, hematuria or renal failure. Lumbar and abdominal pain from very large kidneys is also common. Liver involvement may occur without any evidence of renal cysts.

Complications due to the hepatic cysts are rare and include abdominal pain, jaundice due to enlargement of cysts, hemorrhage into cysts and infection. Occasionally, the liver is enlarged hugely and may cause pressure effects as, for example, in limiting food intake. Portal hypertension and bleeding from esophageal varices occur rarely. In general, treatment is not required, but occasionally a cyst or group of cysts may require drainage or resection. Aspiration of cysts is invariably followed by reaccumulation of the fluid eventually, but instillation of 95% alcohol into the cysts achieves obliteration (Bean & Rodan 1985). Very rarely, cystic involvement has been sufficient to require transplantation. All the various forms of imaging can detect moderate-sized and large cysts (p. 55). Hepatic angiography is not necessary for diagnosis but shows an avascular area without any capillary blush. Multiple congenital cysts may be very small and difficult to demonstrate. Cholangiocarcinoma has been described as a rare complication.

## Isolated polycystic liver disease

Polycystic liver disease in several family members unassociated with renal cysts has been reported. The clinical features associated with these cysts are as in any other form of polycystic liver disease, but there is no associated systemic hypertension, renal failure, or cerebrovascular aneurysms. The condition is inherited as an autosomal dominant.

### *Congenital hepatic fibrosis*

Congenital hepatic fibrosis is a rare condition in which bile ductular proliferation and fibrosis lead eventually to portal hypertension. Liver function is well maintained throughout life. The condition is inherited as an autosomal recessive and the differing presentations found in the literature reflect the severity and distribution of organ involvement (McGonigle et al 1981). Adult autosomal-dominant hepatorenal polycystic disease is a very rare association (Tazelaar et al 1984).

***Pathology.*** Fibrotic linkage of the portal tracts divides the liver into irregular parenchymal masses. The interlobular bile ducts and bile ductules show proliferation and dilatation with the formation of biliary microcysts and there is often a paucity of portal venules, which may be important in the genesis of portal hypertension (Fig. 24.11). In the kidneys a variable proportion of the renal tubules shows general cystic dilatation (medullary sponge kidney). Renal cysts may develop later.

***Clinical features.*** In the perinatal and neonatal forms, renal involvement predominates. The kidneys are large, sometimes massive, and death from renal failure occurs at or soon after birth. The liver shows only mild fibrosis and

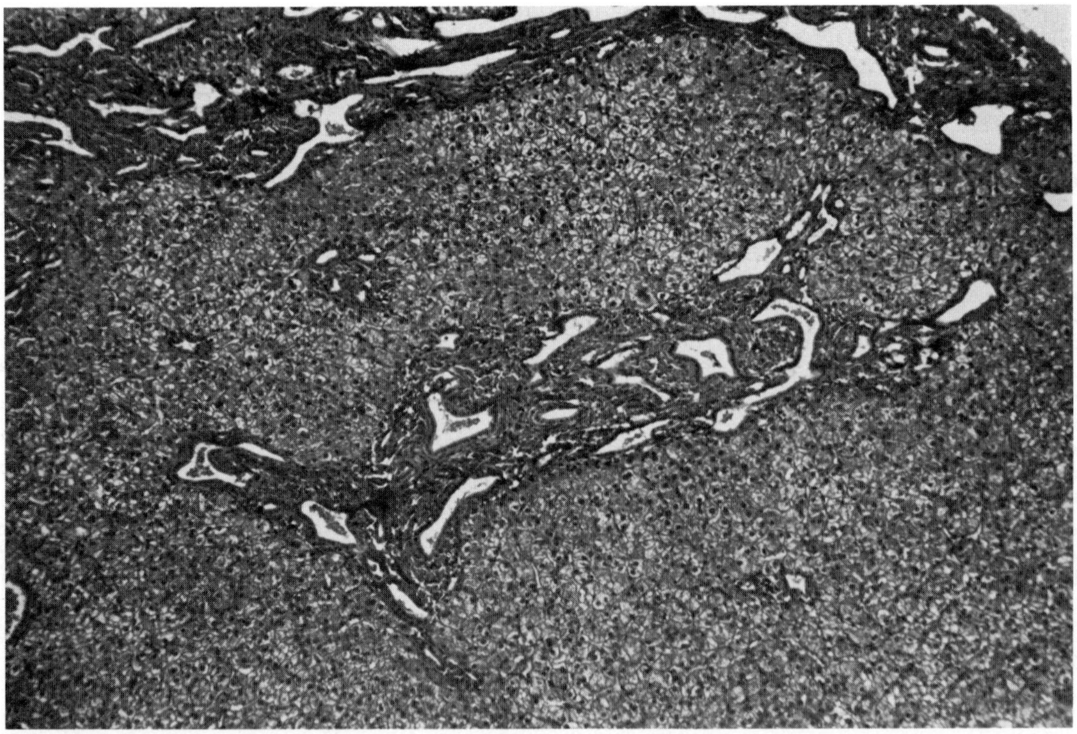

**Fig. 24.11** Congenital hepatic fibrosis. Note the marked fibrosis of portal triads with excess of bile ducts (hematoxylin and eosin ×4)

bile duct dilatation and there is no portal hypertension. In the infantile form, chronic renal failure develops in the first year of life, but if the patient survives long enough, hepatomegaly appears at about the age of 5 years followed by the features of portal hypertension and, in particular, splenomegaly and acute gastrointestinal bleeding from esophageal varices (p. 498). Patients with the juvenile form of the disease do not develop renal failure, as only about 10% of the renal tubules are affected, but portal hypertension develops at about 5 years of age. Finally, when only the liver is involved, patients present with portal hypertension later in childhood or in adolescence and occasionally in adulthood. Hepatocellular function in these patients is good and bleeding is well tolerated. The diagnosis is made ultimately by liver biopsy. Associated renal abnormalities should be sought by intravenous pyelography and ultrasound examination.

Some patients with congenital hepatic fibrosis develop episodes of cholangitis. These arise from infection in dilated intrahepatic biliary radicals. This raises the possibility of Caroli's syndrome (below), to which congenital hepatic fibrosis may be related and with which there is an association.

***Treatment.*** Treatment of congenital hepatic fibrosis includes the treatment of portal hypertension (p. 1005) and chronic renal failure. Portasystemic shunt procedures are tolerated well in view of the good hepatocellular reserve and renal transplantation has been used for childhood renal failure. Cholangitis will require treatment with antibiotics and investigation for associated Caroli's syndrome, which may require treatment in its own right.

### *Caroli's syndrome (nonobstructive intrahepatic biliary dilatation)*

Caroli's syndrome is characterized by multifocal dilatation of the segmental intrahepatic bile ducts and is associated with recurrent bacterial cholangitis (Caroli 1973).

***Pathology.*** Segmental saccular dilatations of the biliary tract occur throughout the liver with normal or dilated intervening bile ducts. Many patients also show the lesions of congenital hepatic fibrosis and they may have associated renal abnormalities (above). The disease in these patients is inherited as an autosomal recessive. Saccular biliary dilatations are restricted to only a part of the liver in a few patients and may be associated with choledochal cysts (Loubeau & Steichen 1976). This localized disease is not associated with congenital hepatic fibrosis and its inheritance is unknown.

***Clinical features.*** Symptoms usually begin in childhood or early adult life, but presentation in middle or old age has been recorded. The symptoms are those of recurring attacks of cholangitis with recurrent fever with or without abdominal pain and jaundice. The liver may be enlarged and tender and hepatic abscesses can occur. Biliary stones form in the dilated bile ducts, thus favoring further attacks of cholangitis or obstructive jaundice. The diagnosis can be made by ultrasonography or computed tomography (Choi et al 1990) and can be confirmed by direct transhepatic or retrograde cholangiography (Fig. 24.12). Invasive biliary investigations should be kept to a minimum, as they can precipitate cholangitis.

***Treatment.*** Treatment of Caroli's syndrome is unsatisfactory. Antibiotics are needed to control episodes of cholangitis, but it is uncertain whether prophylactic antibiotics reduce the frequency of attacks. In the small proportion of patients with disease restricted to one part of the liver, hepatic resection has been claimed to give good results (Nagasue 1984). For the majority of patients, however, such surgery is impossible. Drainage procedures, including choledochoduodenostomy, choledochojejunostomy and hepaticojejunostomy, have been advocated to decompress the biliary system, but cholangitis usually remains a problem and some consider that the only indication for surgery is the presence of biliary stones. The long-term prognosis is poor in patients with recurring cholangitis and transplantation may be needed once infection is controlled. There is an increased risk of the development of cholangiocarcinoma (Dayton et al 1983) and amyloidosis has also been recorded.

### *Choledochal cyst*

Biliary cysts are most frequent in the common bile ducts (choledochus), but the term "choledochal cyst" has come to be applied to cysts in any part of the biliary tree (Flanigan 1975). The majority are probably congenital in origin.

***Pathology.*** Anatomically, choledochal cysts have been subdivided into four types (Fig. 24.13). Type I cysts are the most common; in some instances the dilatation extends outside the common bile duct and occasionally it involves the whole of the extrahepatic and intrahepatic biliary tree. Type II cysts are really biliary diverticula and type III cysts are dilatations or choledochoceles of the intraduodenal bile duct, which may cause duodenal obstruction. Multiple cysts are classified as type IV and this condition merges into Caroli's syndrome (above).

Choledochal cysts are far more common in women (80%) and they are particularly common in Japanese. Almost two-thirds are diagnosed before the age of 10 years, and only 8% after 40 years. They vary greatly in size, some having contained over 5 L of fluid, and they have a fibrotic wall with or without an epithelial lining. Choledochal cysts are liable to the development of carcinomas (Voyles et al 1983). Three-quarters are diagnosed in patients over 20 years of age and 60% are found either at the first operation or within the next 2 years.

***Clinical features.*** Jaundice, an abdominal mass and abdominal pain are the cardinal clinical features and each

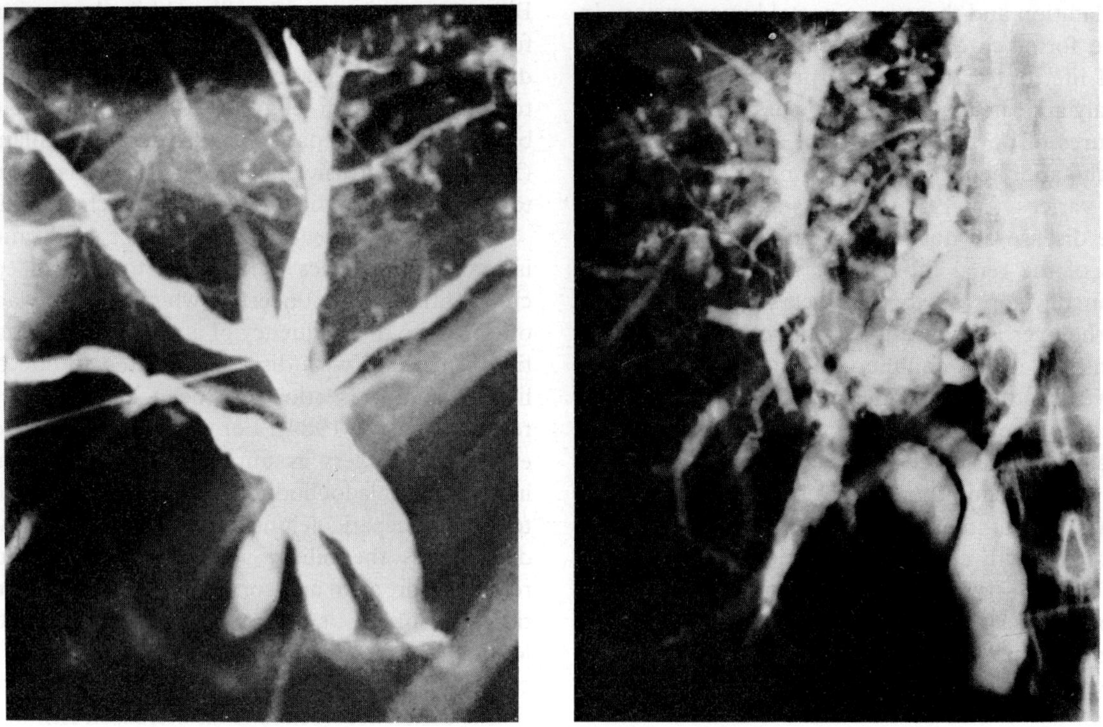

Fig. 24.12 Transhepatic cholangiogram in a patient with Caroli's syndrome showing early (*left*) and late (*right*) filling of the multiple cystic dilatations of the intrahepatic biliary tree.

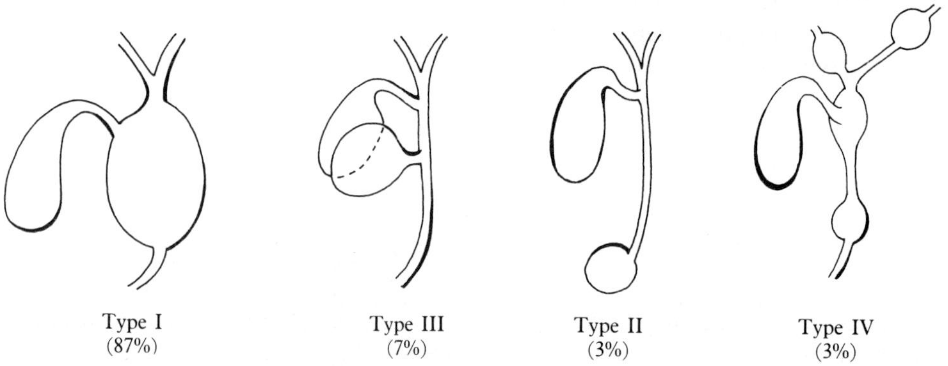


**Fig. 24.13** Classification and frequency of choledochal cysts.

occurs at some time in half to two-thirds of patients. Although the concurrence of all three is recognized as the classic presentation of a choledochal cyst, it occurs in only a third of patients. More often there is a long history of recurrent abdominal pain and jaundice; in a fifth of patients symptoms have been present for over 5 years. Complications of prolonged intermittent or partial biliary obstruction include biliary cirrhosis, cholangitis and occasionally liver abscess. Traumatic or spontaneous rupture may occur and gastrointestinal bleeding, portal vein thrombosis and pancreatitis have been reported. Deterioration in a patient with choledochal cyst may signal the development of carcinoma.

***Diagnosis.*** All the forms of imaging (Fig. 24.14) are accurate ways of making the diagnosis (p. 55), and direct transhepatic (Fig. 24.15) or retrograde cholangiography delineates the anatomy and reveals any associated biliary tract abnormalities.

***Treatment.*** The treatment of choledochal cysts is surgical. The operation of choice for type I cysts is controversial. Excision is the treatment of choice in view of the risk of carcinoma, but its feasibility depends on the anatomy of the cyst, the condition of the patient and the experience of the surgeon. A high-quality cholangiogram and pancreatogram are essential for definition of the duct anatomy. A Roux-en-Y cholecystojejunostomy is performed in many cases with an operative mortality of about 3%. Type II cysts can simply be excised, while type III cysts are treated either by excision and choledochoduodenostomy or by endoscopic sphincterotomy (Venu et al 1984). Type IV

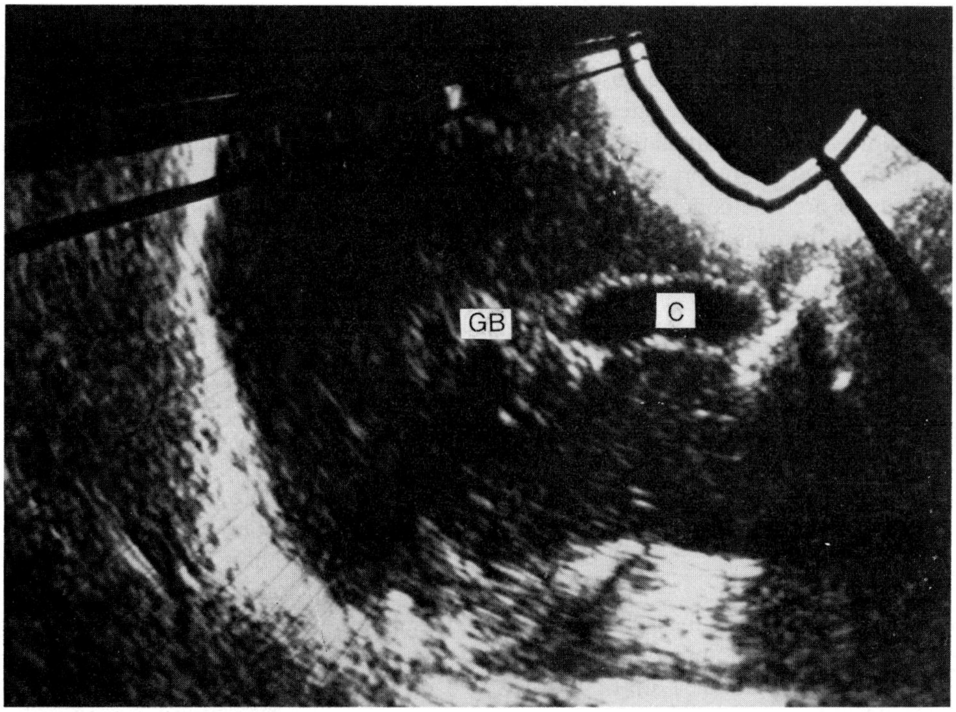


**Fig. 24.14** Ultrasonogram showing choledochal cyst (C) illustrated in Fig. 24.13 Note the gallbladder (GB) and the prominent echoes caused by the anterior abdominal wall above the cyst and by the diaphragm to the left and below it.

cysts are not amenable to surgical therapy and treatment is restricted to antibiotics for attacks of cholangitis.

*Simple (nonparasitic) hepatic cysts* (Hyde et al 1981)

Simple hepatic cysts are usually congenital lesions but are not familial. They have an epithelial lining, are unilocular, contain clear fluid and rarely connect with the biliary tree. Two or more cysts occur in half of patients and occasionally an associated renal cyst is found. Simple cysts are common, occurring in about 1% of the adult population (Larsen 1961), and they are more common in females (1.5:1), particularly when symptomatic (4:1). Larger cysts are usually found in older patients.

Most cysts are found incidentally and are asymptomatic, making it important to exclude alternative causes of symptoms before attributing them to simple cysts. Symptomatic cysts are usually relatively large and occur in otherwise well older patients. Clinical features are usually vague, with nausea and vomiting, acute or chronic abdominal pain and abdominal distention. Hemorrhage causes pain and sudden enlargement of the cyst. Compression of surrounding structures usually causes jaundice and rarely portal hypertension or inferior vena caval obstruction. Rupture into the peritoneum or biliary tract and bacterial infection can occur. Physical examination may reveal an abdominal mass that can extend into the right iliac fossa. Diagnosis is made by imaging (pp. 53 & 55). Angiography

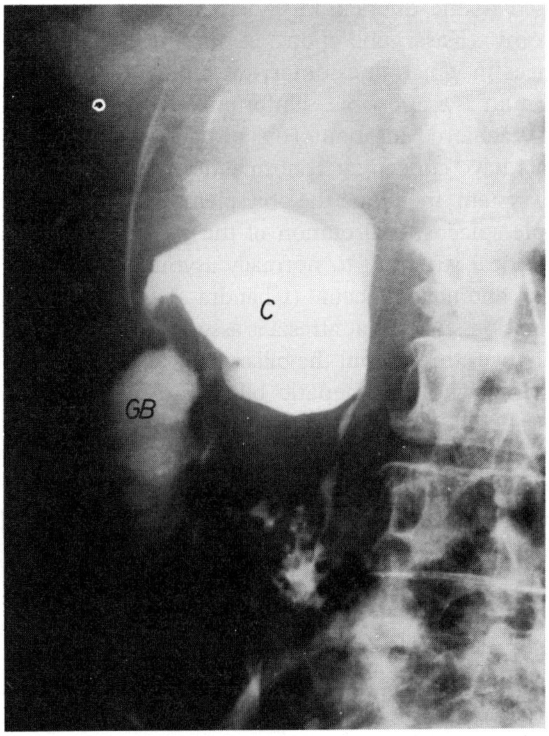


**Fig. 24.15** Transhepatic cholangiogram showing a choledochal cyst (C). Note the common bile duct above the cyst, the attenuated distal common bile duct below it and the gallbladder (GB).

is not necessary for diagnosis but if performed, shows an avascular space-occupying lesion. If the cyst is large enough to produce symptoms, partial excision or injection of sclerosing agents can be carried out (Andersson et al 1989). Drainage is followed by reaccumulation of cystic fluid but excision is rarely needed. The prognosis is good.

Some nonparasitic cysts are not congenital in origin. These include traumatic and neoplastic cysts.

## Biliary atresia

Biliary atresia may affect the extrahepatic or the intrahepatic bile ducts. Affected individuals present early in life and detailed consideration is outside the scope of this book. Atresia is consequently considered in broad outline only here.

### *Extrahepatic atresia*

Extrahepatic biliary atresia is defined as the lack of a biliary lumen in all or part of the extrahepatic biliary tree (Tan & Howard 1989). Atresia occurs in about 1 in 14 000 live births, it is characterized by progressive inflammatory obliteration of the bile ducts and the cause is unknown. Viral infection, failure of vascularization of the biliary tree and toxins such as abnormal bile acids have been suggested but are unproven. Any part of the extrahepatic biliary tree can be affected, but the most useful distinction is between instances in which uninvolved proximal ducts can be anastomosed to the duodenum either directly or by portoenterostomy (Kasai operation) at the hepatic hilum and instances in which anastomosis of remaining ducts to the duodenum is impossible. Unfortunately, anastomosis can only be achieved in about 10% of patients. Some 10% of patients have congenital abnormalities outside the hepatobiliary system, including the polysplenia syndrome in which multiple spleens, malrotation of the gut, situs inversus, a symmetrical structure to normally asymmetric organs and cardiac anomalies occur (Chandra 1974). Histological examination shows that atresia is associated with inflammatory changes throughout the biliary tree.

Patients with extrahepatic biliary atresia present with neonatal cholestatic jaundice and the problem is to differentiate this condition from other causes of neonatal hepatitis. Jaundice is mild at first but becomes more severe, the stools are acholic and hepatomegaly develops after 3–4 weeks. Early diagnosis is important, as patent intrahepatic bile ducts are obliterated progressively over the first 2–3 months of life. Useful investigations include hepatobiliary ultrasonic and scintigraphic imaging and liver biopsy. Cholangiography may become more valuable with the development of appropriate instruments.

The standard treatment for extrahepatic biliary atresia is hepatic portoenterostomy (Kasai operation) in which the dilated bile ducts in the hepatic hilum are anastomosed to the small intestine by a variety of operations. This allows adequate drainage in 90% of patients operated on before the end of the second month of life but in progressively fewer thereafter. Unfortunately, adequate drainage does not equate with cure and continuing intrahepatic inflammation can lead to recurrent cholangitis, cirrhosis, portal hypertension and growth failure. Patients have survived for more than 20 years after successful surgery, but where surgery is not successful few survive beyond 3 years. Liver transplantation can be carried out for patients unsuitable for hepatic portoenterostomy and where this operation is followed by progressive liver disease.

### *Intrahepatic atresia*

Intrahepatic biliary atresia is usually incomplete, showing itself as a reduced ratio of interlobular bile ducts to portal tracts, and hence the alternative names of intrahepatic biliary hypoplasia, ductular hypoplasia and paucity of intrahepatic bile ducts (p. 945). Most patients have associated extrahepatic anomalies (syndromic) known as Alagille's syndrome and have a relatively good long-term prognosis. Some patients have no associated anomalies (nonsyndromic). Nonsyndromic patients probably have a heterogeneous group of diseases and the outlook is worse. A half or more develop hepatic cirrhosis.

### *Combined atresia*

Patients with extrahepatic and intrahepatic bile duct atresia have been described and some of these patients have had features of Alagille's syndrome (p. 945). Microscopic examination has suggested that bile duct hypoplasia and atresia may both be parts of a spectrum of antenatal and perinatal bile duct injury the causes of which are wholly unknown (Kahn et al 1983).

REFERENCES

Ahern M, Hall P, Halliday J et al 1996 Hepatic stellate cell nomenclature. Hepatology 23: 193

Andersson R, Jeppsson B, Lunderquist A, Bengmark S 1989 Alcoholic sclerotherapy of non-parasitic cysts of the liver. British Journal of Surgery 76: 254–255

Andres J M, Mathis R K, Walker W A 1977 Liver disease in infants. I. Developmental hepatology and mechanisms of liver dysfunction. Journal of Pediatrics 90: 686–697

Arias I M 1962 Chronic unconjugated hyperbilirubinemia without overt signs of hemolysis in adolescents and adults. Journal of Clinical Investigation 41: 2233–2245

Arias I M, Gartner L M, Cohen M, Ezzer J B, Levi A J 1969 Chronic nonhemolytic unconjugated hyperbilirubinemia with glucuronyl transferase deficiency. Clinical, biochemical, pharmacologic and genetic evidence for heterogeneity. American Journal of Medicine 47: 395–409

Arias I M, Boyer J L, Fausto N, Jakoby W B, Schachter D, Shafritz D A (eds) 1994 The liver: biology and pathobiology, (3rd edn). Raven Press, New York

Ashkenazi S, Mimouni F, Merlob P, Litmanovitz I, Reisner S H 1984 Size of liver edge in full-term healthy infants. American Journal of Diseases of Children 138: 377–378

Bailey A, Robinson D, Dawson A M 1977 Does Gilbert's disease exist? Lancet 1: 931–933

Baraitser M, Winter R M 1991 Rare diseases with hepatic abnormalities. In: McIntyre N, Benhamou J-P, Bircher J, Rizzetto M, Rodés J (eds) Oxford textbook of clinical hepatology. Oxford Medical Publications, Oxford, p 1489–1520

Bean W J, Rodan B A 1985 Hepatic cysts: treatment with alcohol. American Journal of Roentgenology 144: 237–241

Berthelot P, Dhumeaux D 1978 New insights into the classification and mechanisms of hereditary, chronic, nonhaemolytic hyperbilirubinaemias. Gut 19: 474–480

Billing B H 1987 Familial hyperbilirubinaemia. Journal of Gastroenterology and Hepatology 2: 67

Black M, Sherlock S 1970 Treatment of Gilbert's syndrome with phenobarbitone. Lancet 1: 1359–1362

Bosma P J, Chowdhury N R, Goldhoorn B G et al 1992 Sequence of exons and the flanking regions of human bilirubin-UDP-glucuronosyltransferase gene complex and identification of a genetic mutation in a patient with Crigler–Najjar syndrome type I. Hepatology 15: 941–947

Bosma P J, Goldhoorn B, Oude Elferink R P J, Sinaasappel M, Oostra B A, Jansen P L M 1993 A mutation in bilirubin uridine 5'-diphosphate-glucuronosyltransferase isoform 1 causing Crigler–Najjar syndrome type II. Gastroenterology 105: 216–220

Bosma P J, Chowdhury J R, Bakker C et al 1995 The genetic bases of the reduced expression of bilirubin UDP-glucuronosyltransferase 1 in Gilbert's syndrome. New England Journal of Medicine 333: 1171–1175

Bouwens L, Remels L, Baekeland M, van Bossuyt H, Wisse E 1987 Large granular lymphocytes or "pit cells" from rat liver: isolation, ultrastructural characterization and natural killer activity. European Journal of Immunology 17: 37–42

Bradfield J W B 1984 Liver sinusoidal cells. Journal of Pathology 142: 5–6

Caroli J 1973 Diseases of the intrahepatic biliary tree. Clinics in Gastroenterology 2: 147–161

Castell D 1979 How big is the liver indeed! Archives of Internal Medicine 139: 968–969

Castell D O, O'Brien K D, Muench H, Chalmers T C 1969 Estimation of liver size by percussion in normal individuals. Annals of Internal Medicine 70: 1183–1189

Chandra R S 1974 Biliary atresia and other structural anomalies in the congenital polysplenia syndrome. Journal of Pediatrics 85: 649–655

Choi B I, Yeon K M, Kim S H, Han M C 1990 Caroli disease: central dot sign in CT. Radiology 174: 161–163

Cohen L, Lewis C, Arias I M 1972 Pregnancy, oral contraceptives and chronic familial jaundice with predominantly conjugated hyperbilirubinemia (Dubin–Johnson syndrome). Gastroenterology 62: 1182–1190

Comparini L 1969 Lymph vessels of the liver in man. Microscopic morphology and histotopography. Angiologica 6: 262–274

Conn H O 1972 Rational use of liver biopsy in the diagnosis of hepatic cancer. Gastroenterology 62: 142–146

Conn H O 1975 Liver biopsy in extrahepatic biliary obstruction and in other "contraindicated" disorders. Gastroenterology 68: 817–831

Corrigan J J Jr, Krye J J 1980 Factor II (prothrombin) levels in cord blood: correlation of coagulant activity with immunoreactive protein. Journal of Pediatrics 96: 979–983

Crigler J F Jr, Najjar V A 1952 Congenital familial nonhemolytic jaundice with kernicterus. Pediatrics 10: 169–180

Dawson J, Carr-Locke D L, Talbot I C, Rosenthal F D 1979 Gilbert's syndrome: evidence of morphological heterogeneity. Gut 20: 848–853

Dayton M T, Longmire W P Jr, Tompkins R K 1983 Caroli's disease: a premalignant condition? American Journal of Surgery 145: 41–48

Deacock A R de C, Simpson W T 1964 Fatal reactions to lignocaine. Anaesthesia 19: 217–221

deBelle R C, Vaupshas V, Vitullo B B et al 1979 Intestinal absorption of bile salts: immature development in the neonate. Journal of Pediatrics 94: 472–476

Douds A C, Joseph A E A, Finlayson C, Maxwell J D 1995 Is day case liver biopsy underutilised? Gut 37: 574–575

Douglas J G, Beckett G J, Percy-Robb I W, Finlayson N D C 1980 Bile salt transport in the Dubin–Johnson syndrome. Gut 21: 890–893

Dubin I N, Johnson F B 1954 Chronic idiopathic jaundice with unidentified pigment in liver cells. A new clinicopathologic entity with a report of 12 cases. Medicine 33: 155–196

Dumont A E 1974 Liver lymph. In: Becker F F (ed) The liver: normal and abnormal functions. Part A. Dekker, New York, p 55

Edwards J M 1985 Efficiency of use of blood in surgery. British Medical Journal 291: 1127

Engelhard D, Ornoy A, Deckelbaum R J 1981 Pneumoscrotum complicating percutaneous liver biopsy. Gastroenterology 80: 390–392

Ewe K 1981 Bleeding after liver biopsy does not correlate with indices of peripheral coagulation. Digestive Diseases and Sciences 26: 388–393

Flanigan D P 1975 Biliary cysts. Annals of Surgery 182: 635–643

Forssell P L, Bonkowsky H L, Anderson P B, Howell D A 1981 Intrahepatic hematoma after aspiration liver biopsy. A prospective rendomized trial using two different needles. Digestive Diseases and Sciences 26: 631–635

Foulk W T, Butt H R, Owen C A Jr, Whitcomb F F Jr, Mason H L 1959 Constitutional hepatic dysfunction (Gilbert's disease): its natural history and related symptoms. Medicine 38: 25–46

Franken F H 1983 History of hepatology. In: Csomos G, Thaler H (eds) Clinical hepatology. Springer-Verlag, Berlin pp 1–15

Gates G F, Dore E K 1973 Streamline flow in the human portal vein. Journal of Nuclear Medicine 14: 79–83

Gebhardt R 1992 Metabolic zonation of the liver: regulation and implications for liver function. Pharmacology and Therapeutics 53: 275–354

Gilbert A, Lereboulet P, Hercher M 1907 Les trois cholémies congénitales. Bulletin et Memoires de la Société Médicale des Hôpitaux de Paris 24: 1203–1209

Gilmore I T, Burroughs A, Murray-Lyon I M, Williams R, Jenkins D, Hopkins A 1995 Indications, methods and outcome of percutaneous liver biopsy in England and Wales: an audit by the British Society of Gastroenterology and the Royal College of Physicians of London. Gut 36: 437–441

Gollan J L, Bateman C, Billing B H 1976 Effect of dietary composition on the unconjugated hyperbilirubinaemia of Gilbert's syndrome. Gut 17: 335–340

Gordon E R, Shaffer E A, Sass-Kortsak A 1976 Bilirubin secretion and conjugation in the Crigler–Najjar syndrome Type II. Gastroenterology 70: 761–765

Greis W P, Schulz K A, Giacchino J L, Freeark R J 1981 The fate of unruptured intrahepatic hematomas. Surgery 90: 689–697

Groszmann R J, Kotelanski B, Cohn J N 1971 Hepatic lobar distribution of splenic and mesenteric blood flow in man. Gastroenterology 60: 1047–1052

Haber B, Naji L, Cressman D, Taub R 1995 Coexpression of liver-specific and growth-induced genes in perinatal and regenerating liver; attainment and maintenance of the differentiated state during rapid proliferation. Hepatology 22: 906–914

Harker L A, Slichter S J 1972 The bleeding time as a screening test for evaluation of platelet function. New England Journal of Medicine: 287: 155–159

Hegarty J E, Williams R 1984 Liver biopsy: techniques, clinical applications, and complications. British Medical Journal 288: 1254–1256

Hultcrantz R, Isberg B, Nilsson L H, Thulin L, Tyden G 1983 A case of haemobilia following percutaneous liver biopsy treated by selective arterial embolization. Acta Chirurgical Scandinavica 149: 441–444

Hyde G L, Bertram R L, Schwartz R W 1981 Solitary nonparasitic hepatic cysts. Southern Medical Journal 74: 1357–1360

Iversen P, Roholm K 1939 On aspiration biopsy of the liver with remarks on its diagnostic significance. Acta Medica Scandinavica 102: 1–16

Jones E A 1983 Hepatic sinusoidal cells: new insights and controversies. Hepatology 3: 259–266

Jori G P, Peschele C 1972 Combined peritoneoscopy and liver biopsy in the diagnosis of hepatic neoplasm. Gastroenterology 63: 1016–1019

Jungermann K, Katz N 1982 Functional hepatocellular heterogeneity. Hepatology 2: 385–395
Jungermann K, Katz N 1989 Functional specialization of different hepatocyte populations. Physiological Reviews 69: 708–764
Kahn E I, Daum F, Markowitz J et al 1983 Arteriohepatic dysplasia. II. Hepatobiliary morphology. Hepatology 3: 77–84
Kam I, Lynch S, Svanas G et al 1987 Evidence that host size determines liver size: studies in dogs receiving orthotopic liver transplants. Hepatology 7: 362–366
Kanai K, Kanamura S, Asada-Kubota M, Watanabe J, Oka M 1984 Quantitative analysis of smooth endoplasmic reticulum proliferation in hepatocytes of early postnatal and adult mice treated with phenobarbital. Gastroenterology 87: 1131–1137
Kashiwagi T, Kamada T, Abe H 1975 Dynamic studies on the portal hemodynamics by scintiphotosplenoportography. Streamline flow in the human portal vein. Gastroenterology 69: 1292–1296
Kaufman S S, Wood R P, Shaw B W Jr et al 1986 Orthotopic liver transplantation for Type I Crigler–Najjar syndrome. Hepatology 6: 1259–1262
Kawasaki S, Makuuchi M, Ishizone S, Matsunami H, Terada M, Kawarazaki H 1992 Liver regeneration in recipients and donors after transplantation. Lancet 339: 580–581
Kiernan F 1833 The anatomy and physiology of the liver. Philosophical Transactions of the Royal Society, London 123: 711–770
Knittel T, Ramadori G 1995 Molecular biology. Current Opinion in Gastroenterology 11: 258–266
Kondo T, Kuchiba K, Shimizu Y 1976 Coproporphyrin isomers in Dubin–Johnson syndrome. Gastroenterology 70: 1117–1120
Lance P, Bevan P G, Hoult J G, Paton A 1977 Liver biopsy in "difficult" jaundice. British Medical Journal 2: 236
Larsen K A 1961 Benign lesions affecting the bile ducts in the post-mortem cholangiogram. Acta Pathologica et Microbiologica Scandinavica 51: 47–62
Lautt W W 1977 Hepatic vasculature: a conceptual review. Gastroenterology 73: 1163–1169
Lesesne H R, Holt W, Orringer E 1976 Is hepatic abscess a contraindication to percutaneous liver biopsy? Gasroenterology 70: 297–298
Levine E, Cook L T, Grantham J J 1985 Liver cysts in autosomal-dominant polycystic kidney disease: clinical and computed tomographic study. American Journal of Roentgenology 145: 229–233
Lin T-Y, Lee C-S, Chen C-C, Liau K-Y, Lin W-S-J 1979 Regeneration of human liver after hepatic lobectomy studied by repeated liver scanning and repeated liver biopsy. Annals of Surgery 190: 48–53
Lindgren P G 1982 Percutaenous needle biopsy. Acta Radiologica Diagnosis 23: 653–656
Loubeau J-M, Steichen F M 1976 Dilatation of intrahepatic bile ducts in choledochal cyst: case report with follow-up and review of the literature. Archives of Surgery 111: 1384–1390
Losowsky M S, Walker B E 1968 Liver biopsy and splenoportography in patients with thrombocytopenia. Gastroenterology 54: 241–245
Martinez-Hernandez A, Delgado F M, Amenta P S 1991 The extracellular matrix in hepatic regeneration: localization of collagen types I, III, IV, laminin, and fibronectin. Laboratory Investigation 64: 157–166
McCloskey R V, Gold M, Weser E 1973 Bacteremia after liver biopsy. Archives of Internal Medicine 132: 213–215
McColl K E L, Thompson G G, El Omar E, Moore M R, Goldberg A 1987 Porphyrin metabolism and haem biosynthesis in Gilbert's syndrome. Gut 28: 125–130
McGee J O'D, Allan J G, Russell R I, Patrick R S 1975 Liver ultrastructure in Gilbert's syndrome. Gut 16: 220–224
McGonigle R J S, Mowat A P, Bewick M, Howard E R, Snowden S A, Parsons V 1981 Congenital hepatic fibrosis and polycystic kidney disease: role of porta-caval shunting and transplantation in three patients. Quarterly Journal of Medicine 50: 269–278
Mellinkoff S M 1979 Some meanings of the liver. Gastroenterology 76: 636–638
Menghini G 1970 One-second biopsy of the liver. Problems of its clinical application. New England Journal of Medicine 283: 582–585
Middleton M H III, Griffin J W Jr, Gabilondo J C, Adams H W 1977 Significance of changes in blood pressure and pulse rate after percutaneous liver biopsy. American Journal of Digestive Diseases 22: 989–994
Mihaly G W, Morgan D J, Smallwood R, Hardy K J 1982 The developing liver: the steady-state disposition of propranolol in pregnant sheep. Hepatology 2: 344
Miller D L, Zanolli C S, Gumucio J J 1979 Quantitative morphology of the sinusoids of the hepatic acinus. Quantimet analysis of rat liver. Gastroenterology 76: 965–969
Morris J S, Gallo G A, Scheuer P J, Sherlock S 1975 Percutaneous liver biopsy in patients with large bile duct obstruction. Gastroenterology 68: 750–754
Motohara K, Endo F, Matsuda I 1985 Effect of vitamin K administration on acarboxy prothrombin (PIVKA-II) levels in newborns. Lancet 2: 242–244
Nagasue N 1984 Successful treatment of Caroli's disease by hepatic resection. Annals of Surgery 200: 718–723
Ohkubo M, Okuda K, Iida S 1981 Effects of corticosteroids on bilirubin metabolism in patients with Gilbert's syndrome. Hepatology 1: 168–172
Olsson R, Bliding Å, Jagenburg R et al 1988 Gilbert's syndrome: does it exist? Acta Medica Scandinavica 224: 485–490
Owens D, Evans J 1975 Population studies in Gilbert's syndrome. Journal of Medical Genetics 12: 152–156
Owens D, Sherlock S 1973 Diagnosis of Gilbert's syndrome: role of reduced caloric intake test. British Medical Journal 3: 559–563
Patterson M, Gonzalez-Vitale J C, Fagan C J 1982 Polycystic liver disease: a study of cyst fluid constituents. Hepatology 2: 475–478
Pinzani M 1995 Hepatic stellate (Ito) cells: expanding role for a liver-specific pericyte. Journal of Hepatology 22: 700–706
Pirson Y, Lannoy N, Peters D et al 1996 Isolated polycystic liver disease as a distinct genetic disease, unlinked to polycystic kidney disease 1 and polycystic kidney disease 2. Hepatology 23: 249–252
Powell L W, Billing B H, Williams H S 1967a An assessment of red cell survival in idiopathic unconjugated hyperbilirubinaemia (Gilbert's syndrome) by the use of radioactive diisopropylfluorophosphate and chromium. Australasian Annals of Medicine 16: 221–225
Powell L W, Hemmingway E H, Billing B H, Sherlock S 1967b Idiopathic unconjugated hyperbilirubinemia (Gilbert's syndrome). A study of 42 families. New England Journal of Medicine 277: 1108–1112
Rake M O, Murray-Lyon I M, Ansell I D, Williams R 1969 Improved liver-biopsy needle. Lancet 2: 1283
Rapaccini G L, Anti M, Fedeli G, Vecchio F M, Fabiano A 1983 Porphyrins in Rotor's syndrome. Gastroenterology 84: 667–668
Rappaport A M 1958 The structural and functional unit in the human liver (liver acinus). Anatomical Record 130: 673–687
Richardson P D I, Withrington P G 1981a Liver blood flow. I. Intrinsic and nervous control of liver blood flow. Gastroenterology 81: 159–173
Richardson P D I, Withrington P G 1981b Liver blood flow. II. Effects of drugs and hormones on liver blood flow. Gastroenterology 81: 356–375
Riley S A, Ellis W R, Irving H C, Lintott D J, Axon A T R, Losowsky H S 1984 Percutaneous liver biopsy with plugging of needle track: a safe method for use in patients with impaired coagulation. Lancet 2: 436
Rodeck C H, Patrick A D, Pembrey M E, Tzannatos C, Whitfield A E 1982 Fetal liver biopsy for prenatal diagnosis of ornithine carbamyl tansferase deficiency. Lancet 2: 297–300
Rollinghoff W, Paumgartner G, Preisig R 1981 Nicotinic acid test in the diagnosis of Gilbert's syndrome: correlation with bilirubin clearance. Gut 22: 663–668
Rotor A B, Manahan L, Florentin A 1948 Familial nonhaemolytic hyperbilirubinaemia associated with direct van den Bergh reaction. Acta Medicina Philippina 5: 37–49
Rougier P, Degott C, Rueff B, Benhamou J-P 1978 Nodular regenerative hyperplasia of the liver. Report of six cases and review of the literature. Gastroenterology 75: 169–172
Rudolph A M 1983 Hepatic and ductus venosus blood flows during fetal life. Hepatology 3: 254–258
Rylance G W, Moreland T A, Cowan M D, Clark D C 1982 Liver volume estimation using ultrasound scanning. Archives of Disease in Childhood 57: 283–286

Sapira J D, Williamson D L 1979 How big is the normal liver? Archives of Internal Medicine 139: 971–973
Schmid R 1995 Gilbert's syndrome – a legitimate genetic anomaly? New England Journal of Medicine 333: 1217–1218
Schmidt C, Bladt F, Goedecke S et al 1995 Scatter factor/hepatocyte growth factor is essential for liver development. Nature 373: 699–702
Schwartz C C, Almond H R, Vlahcevic Z R, Swell L 1979 Bile acid metabolism in cirrhosis. V. Determination of biliary lipid secretion rates in patients with advanced cirrhosis. Gastroenterology 77: 1177–1182
Scotto J, Opolon P, Étévé J, Vergoz D, Thomas M, Caroli J 1973 Liver biopsy and prognosis in acute liver failure. Gut 14: 927–933
Scriver C R, Beaudet A L, Sly W S, Valle D (eds) 1995 The metabolic and molecular bases of inherited disease, 7th edn. McGraw-Hill, New York
Searle J, Harmon B V, Bishop C J, Kerr J F R 1987 The significance of cell death by apoptosis in hepatobiliary disease. Journal of Gastroenterology and Hepatology 2: 77
Sharma P, McDonald G B, Banaji M 1982 The risk of bleeding after percutaneous liver biopsy: relation to platelet count. Journal of Clinical Gastroenterology 4: 451–453
Shimizu Y, Naruto H, Ida S, Kohakura M 1981 Urinary coproporphyrin isomers in Rotor's syndrome: a study in eight families. Hepatology 1: 173–178
Spector I, Corn M, Ticktin H E 1966 Effect of plasma transfusions on the prothrombin time and clotting factors in liver disease. New England Journal of Medicine 275: 1032–1037
Sprinz H, Nelson R S 1954 Persistent nonhemolytic hyperbilirubinemia associated with lipochrome-like pigment in liver cells: report of four cases. Annals of Internal Medicine 41: 952–962
Starling E H 1915 Principles of human physiology, 2nd edn. Lea and Febiger, Philadelphia, p 1014
Suchy F J, Balistreri W F, Heubi J E, Searcy J E, Levin R S 1981 Physiological cholestasis: evaluation of the primary serum bile acid concentrations in normal infants. Gastroenterology 80: 1037–1041
Sullivan S, Watson W C 1974 Acute transient hypotension as complication of percutaneous liver biopsy. Lancet 1: 389–390
Tan K C, Howard E R 1989 Biliary atresia. Baillière's Clinical Gastroenterology 3: 211–229
Tazelaar H D, Payne J A, Patel N S 1984 Congenital hepatic fibrosis and asymptomatic familial adult-type polycystic kidney disease in a 19-year-old woman. Gastroenterology 86: 757–760
Terry R 1952 Risks of needle biopsy of the liver. British Medical Journal 1: 1102–1105
Terry R B 1954 Macroscopic diagnosis in liver biopsy. Journal of the American Medical Association 154: 990–992
Thurman R G, Kauffman F C 1985 Sublobular compartmentation of pharmacologic events (SCOPE): metabolic fluxes in periportal and pericentral regions of the liver lobule. Hepatology 5: 144–151
Tobi M, Garretto M, Blackstone M O, Baker A L 1983 Periumbilical hemorrhage complicating percutaneous liver biopsy. New England Journal of Medicine 308: 1541–1542
Venu R P, Geenen J E, Hogan W J et al 1984 Role of endoscopic retrograde cholangiopancreatography in the diagnosis and treatment of choledochocele. Gastroenterology 87: 1144–1149
Voyles C R, Smadja C, Shands C, Blumgart L H 1983 Carcinoma in choledochal cysts: age-related incidence. Archives of Surgery 118: 986–988
Walker W A, Krivit W, Sharp H L 1967 Needle biopsy of the liver in infancy and childhood. A safe diagnostic aid in liver disease. Pediatrics 40: 946–950
Walters J R F, Paton A 1980 Liver biopsy. British Medical Journal 1: 776–778
Watkins J B, Ingall D, Szczepanik P, Klein P D, Lester R 1973 Bile-salt metabolism in the newborn: measurement of pool size and synthesis by stable isotope technic. New England Journal of Medicine 288: 431–434
Wisse E, De Zanger R B, Charels K, Van Der Smissen P, McCuskey R S 1985 The liver sieve: considerations concerning the structure and function of endothelial fenestrae, the sinusoidal wall and the space of Disse. Hepatology 5: 683–692
Wolkoff A W, Chowdury J R, Gartner L A et al 1979 Crigler–Najjar syndrome (Type I) in an adult male. Gastroenterology 76: 840–848
Wolpert E, Pascasio F M, Wilkoff A W, Arias I M 1977 Abnormal sulfobromophthalein metabolism in Rotor's syndrome and obligate heterozygotes. New England Journal of Medicine 296: 1099–1101
Zajicek G, Oren R, Weinreb M Jr 1985 The streaming liver. Liver 5: 293–300
Zamchek N, Klausenstock O 1953 Liver biopsy: II. The risk of needle biopsy. New England Journal of Medicine 249: 1062–1069

# 25. Clinical chemistry of liver disease

*I. W. Percy-Robb N. D. C. Finlayson*

In clinical practice, biochemical investigations are widely used to assess the structural integrity of the liver, its ability to transport substances from the blood into the bile and its ability to synthesize and secrete substances into the blood. While many tests of these functions have been advocated, only a few have proved both informative and feasible to perform on a large scale. In addition, measurements are made of substances such as ceruloplasmin in order to diagnose specific liver diseases.

## LIVER FUNCTION TESTS

These terms refer to a group of blood tests widely used to detect liver disease, to make quantitative assessments of jaundice, to follow the course of an illness and to identify toxic reactions to drugs (Laker 1990). They do not all measure liver functions and they are affected by a number of extrahepatic factors, but the term "liver function tests" or "liver tests" has become hallowed by usage. The tests usually used include the total bilirubin as a measure of hepatic transport, the transaminase activity as a measure of the integrity of the liver cells, the γ-glutamyl transferase as an index of hepatic microsomal induction, the alkaline phosphatase as an index of cholestasis and the albumin concentration as a measure of hepatic synthetic capacity. They should not be regarded as "routine", for they are only useful if there is some reason to suspect hepatic disorder. These liver function tests are used to detect abnormality of the liver and the need for further investigation, but they do not relate to specific liver diseases.

Determining normality for liver function tests is difficult, as values in well people are often not distributed normally and vary with normal factors such as age, sex and body mass. In addition, ethical considerations preclude comparison of such tests in normal people with liver biopsy findings. Plasma bilirubin concentrations in health are skewed to the right (p. 740) so that 5–7% of healthy men have concentrations above 17 μmol/L (0.8 mg/dl), which is widely regarded as the upper limit of normal. Alanine aminotransferase and γ-glutamyl transferase activities are also skewed to the right and vary with age, sex and body mass (Schiele et al 1977, Goldie & McConnell 1990). These considerations emphasize the need for caution in determining normal ranges and laboratories increasingly refer to reference intervals that indicate values covered by a well population without specifying that individual values are necessarily normal or abnormal.

Liver biopsy findings are generally regarded as the "gold standard" by which liver function tests should be judged, but liver biopsies are subject to sampling error and abnormalities are not always distributed uniformly throughout the liver. Accordingly, caution also needs to be applied to such comparisons. Liver function tests accurately reflect active liver diseases such as acute viral or toxic hepatitis or autoimmune hepatitis in relapse, but they may fail to reveal mild or even moderate lesions. Galambos & Wills (1978) compared liver function tests and liver biopsies in obese patients, in whom liver function test abnormalities were generally minor. Patients with steatosis, portal hepatitis, lobular hepatitis or fibrosis had abnormal liver function tests in 60–89% of cases and patients with more marked liver function abnormalities had more severe pathological lesions. However, liver function tests were often normal in spite of more marked lesions on biopsy and abnormalities were often found when pathological lesions were mild or absent. Czaja et al (1981) compared plasma transaminase activity and liver biopsy findings in patients with autoimmune hepatitis receiving corticosteroid therapy and found that activities more than twice normal reliably identified histological abnormality, whereas normal results missed mild periportal hepatitis in 55% of cases during therapy and in 19% of cases after therapy. Liver function tests can also be normal in chronic hepatitis C infection, particularly where the histological lesions are less severe (Fig. 25.1).

Liver function tests should be interpreted in conjunction with other clinical and laboratory information. Normal liver function tests make active or very advanced disease unlikely but do not completely exclude the possibility of liver disease and minor abnormalities, particularly

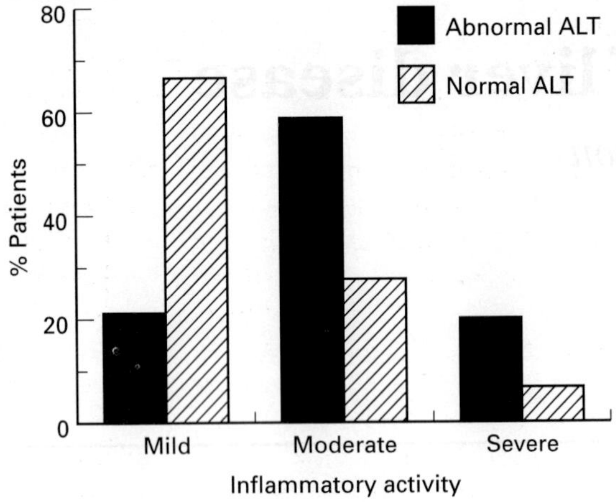


**Fig. 25.1** Plasma alanine aminotransferase (ALT) activity related to inflammatory activity on liver biopsy in chronic hepatitis C virus infection (Stanley et al 1996).

in asymptomatic people, do not necessarily indicate disease likely to be benefited by invasive investigation.

### Quantitative liver function tests

An alternative approach has been to quantitate the ability of the liver to metabolize test substances and to relate the results to the nature or extent of liver pathology (Shiffman et al 1994). A wide range of substances has been used in these studies, including indocyanine green, bromsulphthalein, caffeine, antipyrine, galactose and lignocaine. While these tests can provide quantitative information about the severity of liver disease and about long-term survival of patients, they do not often provide additional information of clinical value once traditional methods (liver function tests and clinical findings) have been taken into account (Villeneuve et al 1986).

### Other liver function tests

The prothrombin time, which requires certain coagulation factors synthesized by the liver, is also used to test hepatic synthetic function (p. 751). The serum globulin concentration is a useful measure of the severity of chronic liver disease; its concentration rises as the albumin concentration falls in chronic liver disease (p. 746). While serum bile acid measurements have been shown to be sensitive indicators of hepatic dysfunction, they have not so far gained wide acceptance in clinical practice. The bromsulphthalein excretion test has been much used in the past but is now obsolete. A quite separate group of biochemical tests is used to detect specific diseases. They include measurements of serum alpha-fetoprotein (p. 749), $\alpha_1$-antitrypsin (p. 748), and ceruloplasmin (p. 751).

### Liver function tests in asymptomatic persons

Liver function tests used for screening purposes identify well persons with abnormal results. This raises the practical and ethical problem of further investigation, particularly in respect of liver biopsy which is invasive and has serious potential complications (Ch 24). Studies in civilian and military blood donors in the United States have identified 0.5% with increased plasma transaminase activity. Three-quarters of the abnormalities in the civilians were attributed to obesity and alcohol (Friedman et al 1987), but only 12% of the abnormalities in the military recruits could be attributed to a specific cause, mainly hepatitis B or hepatitis C infection (Kundrotas & Clement 1993). Gillon et al (1988) found increased transaminase activity in 2.4% of Scottish blood donors and attributed this to obesity and/or alcohol in 82% of cases. Wejstal et al (1988) found raised transaminase activity in 8.8% of Swedish blood donors and increased body weight and fatty liver on biopsy in 10 of 13 with abnormalities for more than a year. The chances of finding a cause increased from 5% where one abnormal transaminase activity was found to 20% where two were found (Kundrotas & Clement 1993). Friedman et al (1987) commented that "few serious liver disorders are found in asymptomatic blood donors with elevated alanine transaminase levels", but the question remains as to whether liver biopsy would have revealed these disorders.

Hultcrantz et al (1986) investigated by liver biopsy 149 asymptomatic patients with moderate elevations of plasma transaminase activity of at least 6 months' duration. Fatty liver was found in 63% and obesity, diabetes mellitus and alcohol excess were prominent associated factors. Hemochromatosis or $\alpha_1$-antitrypsin deficiency was indicated from blood tests and confirmed by biopsy in 7%; chronic hepatitis was found in 20% but was mild (persistent) in a half; cirrhosis was present in 6% and more severe disease was suggested by hypoalbuminemia or hyperglobulinemia in a half; and granulomas were found in 2%. No cause was found on biopsy in 2%. Van Ness & Diehl (1989) investigated 90 asymptomatic patients with increased transaminase activities for 3 months or more and compared the outcome with and without liver biopsy. Treatable liver disease other than that due to alcohol was found in 16 patients (18%) and in 11 the diagnosis was made without biopsy; the remaining patients had granulomas (4) and drug-related disease (1) that should have been recognized from the history.

Clinical evaluation of well patients with mild to moderate abnormalities of liver function tests should include, in particular, alcohol intake, drug therapy, examination for obesity (body mass index), stigmata of chronic liver disease (p. 917) and diabetes mellitus. Investigations should include hepatitis B (p. 785) and C (p. 788), serology, autoantibody tests (p. 887) and ferritin (p. 748), $\alpha_1$-antitrypsin (p. 748) and ceruloplasmin (p. 751) concentrations. An ultrasound examination of the liver and biliary system should also be done. Liver biopsy may be indicated by these further tests, but where all of the further tests are normal, it is recommended that biopsy not be considered unless liver function tests remain abnormal over 3–6 months. The chances of finding severe or treatable liver disease on biopsy are low and patients need to be particularly aware of the hazards of biopsy in these circumstances.

## BILIRUBIN METABOLISM

Bilirubin is a yellow tetrapyrrole derived from heme (Fe-protoporphyrin IX), which is found mainly in hemoglobin. It is also present in myoglobin and in a variety of enzymes such as the cytochromes, peroxidase and catalase. While many tetrapyrroles are water soluble, hydrogen bonding within the bilirubin molecule produces a structure that is lipid soluble (Fig. 25.2). Bilirubin is light sensitive and exposure of bilirubin in the blood to light results in its conversion to substances lacking one or more internal hydrogen bonds, making them more water soluble. These substances can be excreted by the liver without conjugation into the bile where they revert to bilirubin. This property of light sensitivity is used in treating neonatal hyperbilirubinemia and the rare Crigler–Najjar syndrome (p. 723).

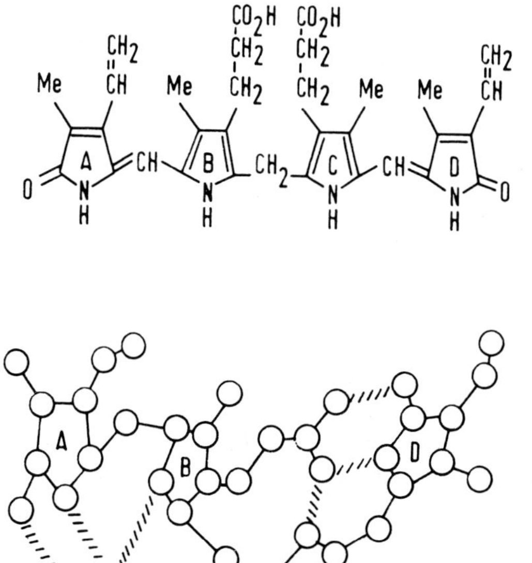

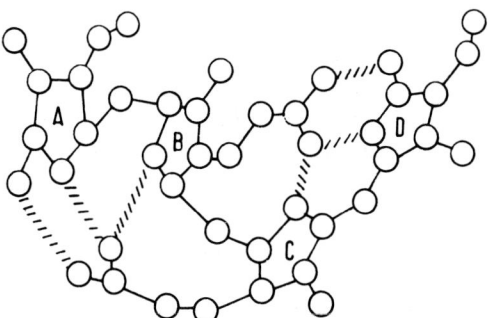

**Fig. 25.2** Structure of bilirubin as written conventionally (*top*) and to show the involuted hydrogen-bonded structure (*bottom*) (Schmid 1978). The hydrogen bonds are shown as discontinuous lines.

### Production

An adult normally produces 425–510 mmol (250–300 mg) of bilirubin daily; 75% comes from the breakdown of effete red blood cells in the spleen, liver and bone marrow while the rest is produced mainly in the liver from the catabolism of proteins containing heme, from heme itself (22%) and from ineffective erythropoiesis in the marrow (3%). Bilirubin metabolism has been studied extensively using heme precursors such as glycine and δ-aminolevulinic acid. This has shown that most bilirubin is produced after 100–140 days from the destruction of red blood cells (Table 25.1). An early phase of bilirubin production (shunt bilirubin), occurring within a few hours and lasting for 2 days, seems to derive mainly from the breakdown of enzymes, particularly microsomal cytochromes, in the liver. The liver contains a high concentration of these enzymes, which have half-lives of only a few hours. A small amount of the bilirubin produced in this early phase is derived from free heme in the liver and some derives from the destruction of immature red blood cells in the marrow. This last source is greatly increased by the "ineffective erythropoiesis" of many blood diseases (p. 740).

The initial rate-limiting step in bilirubin production is the enzyme-mediated oxidation of the α-bridge carbon atom of the heme molecule. The reaction is catalyzed by microsomal heme oxygenase. The α-bridge carbon is eliminated as CO, $Fe^{2+}$ being released and the closed heme molecule being converted into the open tetrapyrrole, biliverdin IXa. Since heme oxidation is the main intrinsic source of CO production, the determination of the CO production rate can be used to quantify bilirubin production and heme degradation (Landaw et al 1970). The iron is conserved (p. 952). Biliverdin is then reduced to free (unconjugated) bilirubin in a reaction catalyzed by cytosolic biliverdin reductase. These two enzymes are present normally only in the reticulo-endothelial cells responsible for heme catabolism, but they can be induced in other tissues by a number of substances, including heme itself.

Heme oxidase and biliverdin reductase appear in the renal tubular cells when intravascular hemolysis produces more heme than can be disposed of by the iron-binding proteins in the blood (p. 747) and by the liver. This

**Table 25.1** Sources of normal bilirubin production (Billing 1978)

| Time of production (days) | Source | Proportion (%) of daily production |
|---|---|---|
| Early (0–2) | Liver enzymes (cytochromes) free heme | 22 |
| | Marrow erythrocyte precursors | 3 |
| Late (100–140) | Effete erythrocytes | 75 |

increases the serum bilirubin rather than the serum heme concentration.

### Transport

Unconjugated bilirubin, which is insoluble in water, is transported in the blood almost wholly bound to albumin. The binding capacity of albumin for unconjugated bilirubin is substantial, amounting to 340–425 μmol/L (20–25 mg/dl), and the degree of binding is high as dialysis does not release appreciable amounts of unconjugated pigment. Nonetheless, there is a small unbound fraction of unconjugated bilirubin in the plasma. Bilirubin is an anion and other endogenous and exogenous anions, such as thyroxin and sulfonamides, can compete with it for the binding sites on albumin. This is sometimes important in neonates because displaced unconjugated bilirubin can enter and damage cells, especially in the brain.

### Hepatic metabolism

Unconjugated bilirubin is lipid soluble and can in principle enter any cell. In fact, it is taken up almost exclusively by the liver, metabolized and excreted in water-soluble form into the bile (Fig. 25.3). It has proved difficult to characterize uptake, metabolism and excretion separately, as these functions are so closely integrated. Entry of bilirubin into the liver is facilitated as the hepatocytes continually lower the intracellular bilirubin concentration by excreting bilirubin into the bile and this maintains a gradient between free plasma and intracellular bilirubin.

### Uptake and storage

Bilirubin dissociates from albumin and is taken up rapidly into the liver. Uptake is facilitated by the size of the liver, by its highly permeable sinusoids that allow easy access of blood to the hepatocyte membrane and possibly by the hepatocyte membrane itself, which may contain a receptor for albumin (Weisiger et al 1981), although this is controversial (Stremmel et al 1981). Albumin and its hepatocyte membrane receptor may ensure a homogeneous distribution of bilirubin between the acinar zones (p. 712), but whether this contributes to bilirubin uptake into the hepatocytes is not known (Gumucio et al 1984). The transport of bilirubin across the hepatocyte membrane is bidirectional and bilirubin may subsequently leave the liver and re-enter the blood.

Hepatocytes contain a series of cytosolic proteins, the glutathione transferases, which have high affinities for bilirubin. One of these was known originally as ligandin (Y protein). These proteins may contribute to the ability of the liver to remove bilirubin from the blood and they bind bilirubin prior to its conjugation in the endoplasmic reticulum. Thus, the return of unconjugated bilirubin from the hepatocytes into the sinusoidal blood is reduced to a minimum and nonspecific diffusion of bilirubin throughout the hepatocyte is prevented.

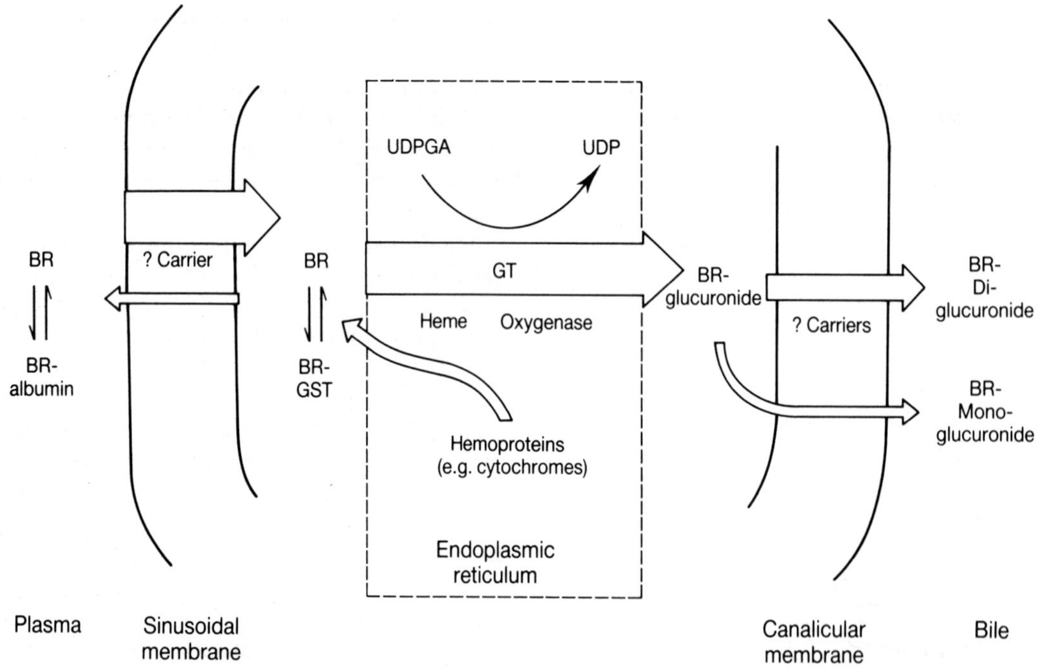


**Fig. 25.3** Bilirubin transport and conjugation in the hepatocyte. BR = bilirubin, GST = glutathione S-transferases, GT = glucuronyl transferase, UDPGA = uridine diphosphate glucuronic acid, UDP = uridine diphosphate (Schmid 1978).

*Conjugation*

Bilirubin is rendered water soluble by conjugation, bilirubin diglucuronide being the main conjugate reaching the bile in humans. The UDP-glucuronosyl transferase enzyme which catalyzes the transfer of glucuronic acid from UDP glucuronic acid to bilirubin and various other aglycone substrates is found in the liver endoplasmic reticulum (Chowdhury & Chowdhury 1983). Both monoconjugated and diconjugated bilirubin are secreted into bile, in a ratio of approximately 1:3. In addition, small amounts (1–2%) of conjugates with other sugars such as glucose and xylose are present as well as similar amounts of the unconjugated form (Fig. 25.4).

***Genetic factors.*** UDP-glucuronosyl transferases occur in several isoforms and in humans UDP-glucuronosyl transferase I contributes most to bilirubin glucuronidation. The isoforms are expressed from a single gene on chromosome 2 containing coding and promoter regions. Mutations in different parts of the gene seem to be responsible for different forms of constitutional hyperbilirubinemia.

*Excretion*

Little is known of the mechanism of the secretion of bilirubin into the bile, but conjugation is a prerequisite, as unconjugated bilirubin is normally present only in trace amounts in bile. Bilirubin is excreted against a concentration gradient, its excretion can be competitively inhibited and the excretion mechanism can be saturated, which suggests that the mechanism requires energy and is mediated by a carrier system. Conjugated bilirubin is secreted across the hepatocyte canalicular membrane by specific mechanisms that are different from those for bile salts. Excretion is the rate-limiting step in the passage of bilirubin from blood to bile. The physical state of bilirubin in bile depends on its solubility in aqueous medium at alkaline pH. Unconjugated bilirubin, which is poorly soluble in water, may exist in bile in association with the bile salt, cholesterol and lecithin micelles (Ostrow & Celic 1984). Bilirubin diconjugate, on the other hand, is present in aqueous solution in bile, the monoconjugate being intermediate between these forms and partly solubilized into the mixed micelles.

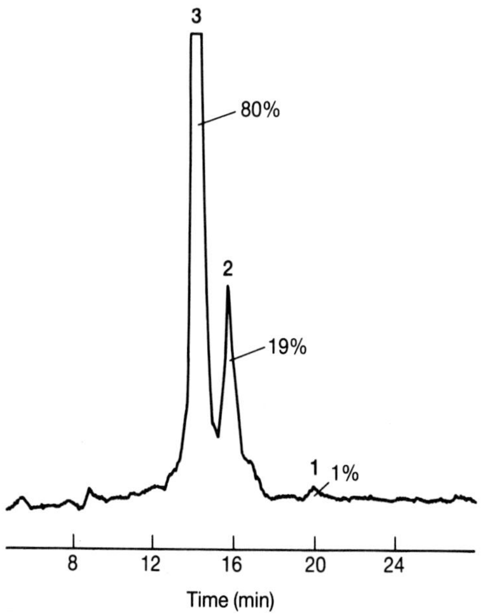


**Fig. 25.4** High pressure liquid chromatograph (HPLC) of normal bile from the gallbladder. Peak 1, unconjugated bilirubin (1%). Peak 2, monoconjugated bilirubin (19%). Peak 3, diconjugated bilirubin (80%).

## Enterohepatic circulation

Conjugated bilirubin is water soluble and is not absorbed from the jejunum or upper ileum. In the terminal ileum and colon, bilirubin is reduced by bacteria to a group of colorless tetrapyrrolic substances, most of which (170–340 μmol/day, 100–200 mg/day) are excreted in the feces (stercobilinogen). Some of these substances are absorbed and most are excreted unchanged into the bile. A small amount (7 μmol/day, 4 mg/day) is excreted into the urine (urobilinogen). Bacterial β-glucuronidase in the colon may partly or wholly deconjugate bilirubin.

## Hyperbilirubinemia

Bilirubin in normal serum is almost entirely unconjugated; both conjugated and unconjugated forms accumulate during hepatobiliary disorders. The normal serum bilirubin concentration is 3–17 μmol/L (0.2–1.0 mg/dl). Concentrations in excess of 17 μmol/L (1.0 mg/dl) therefore constitute hyperbilirubinemia, but it should not be assumed that this necessarily implies disease. Men have higher serum bilirubin concentrations than women and in both sexes concentrations show a distribution skewed to the right (Bailey et al 1977). Thus, 5–7% of apparently normal men have a serum bilirubin exceeding 17 μmol/L and 2% have a serum bilirubin exceeding 25 μmol/L (Fig. 25.5). The nature of the distribution of serum bilirubin concentrations in the normal population is important in the definition of Gilbert's syndrome (p. 722), but the practical implication is that minor increases of serum bilirubin, without other evidence of liver disease, need to be interpreted cautiously. The serum bilirubin concentration can be used to detect liver disease, to confirm that jaundice is present and to follow the progress of a disease or its treatment. Jaundice cannot usually be detected reliably until the serum bilirubin exceeds 45 μmol/L (2.5 mg/dl).

Hyperbilirubinemia may be due to predominantly

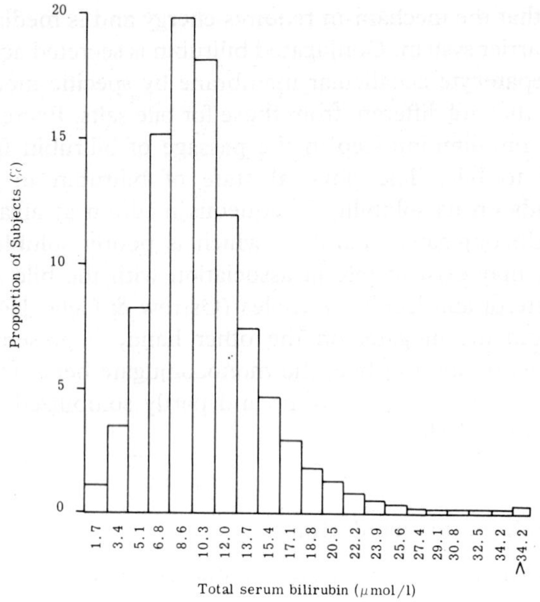


**Fig. 25.5** Distribution of serum bilirubin concentration in 18 454 healthy men (Bailey et al 1977).

unconjugated or conjugated bilirubin and its causes are legion (Table 25.2). Unconjugated hyperbilirubinemia is comparatively uncommon and other than in neonates, it is usually due to hemolysis or to Gilbert's syndrome. Ineffective erythropoiesis occurs in several conditions (Table 25.3) and is occasionally an important factor contributing to hyperbilirubinemia. It is defined as the destruction of developing nucleated red blood cells at the site of their production or the production of abnormal red blood cells that survive for only a few hours in the circulation (Firkin et al 1989). It results in the production of increased amounts of unconjugated bilirubin. Conjugated bilirubin may constitute up to 5 μmol/L (0.3 mg/dl) or up to 20% of the total serum bilirubin in predominantly unconjugated hyperbilirubinemia (Killenberg et al 1980). Conjugated hyperbilirubinemia is most commonly caused by hepatobiliary disease and is accompanied by bilirubinuria. There is usually also a significant increase in the amount of unconjugated bilirubin, but the relative proportions of the different forms of bilirubin are too variable to be of diagnostic value.

Fractionation of the total serum bilirubin into conjugated and unconjugated forms is frequently done to distinguish these two forms of hyperbilirubinemia. However, it needs to be recognized that at total serum bilirubin concentrations below 85 μmol/L (5 mg/dl), many of the current clinical laboratory methods are not capable of performing this fractionation accurately (Killenberg et al 1980). High-performance liquid chromatography, however, provides satisfactory separation into three fractions, namely, unconjugated, monoconjugated and diconjugated forms (Fig. 25.6). Under certain circumstances, a fourth

**Table 25.2** Causes of hyperbilirubinemia and/or cholestasis

**Predominantly unconjugated**
*Increased bilirubin production*
Hemolysis
Ineffective erythropoiesis
Primary shunt hyperbilirubinemia

*Primary failure of bilirubin transport*
Gilbert's syndrome
Crigler–Najjar syndrome (type I and type II)

*Mixed or uncertain pathogenesis*
Neonatal hyperbilirubinemia
Drugs
Altitude-induced
Viral hepatitis
Thyrotoxicosis
Portocaval shunt

**Predominantly conjugated**
*Primary failure of bilirubin transport*
Dubin–Johnson syndrome
Rotor syndrome
Postoperative cholestasis*
Benign familial cholestasis*
Bylers disease*

*Hepatocellular damage**
Viral hepatitis
Drugs
Alcohol
Chronic active hepatitis
Cirrhosis
Neoplasia (1° or 2°)
Neonatal hepatitis
$\alpha_1$-Antitrypsin deficiency

*Biliary obstruction**
Extrahepatic
- Gallstones
- Neoplasia
- Sclerosing cholangitis
- Biliary stricture
- Pancreatitis

Intrahepatic
- Cholestatic viral hepatitis
- Drugs
- Alcohol
- Cirrhosis
- Cholestasis of pregnancy
- Postoperative cholestasis
- Benign recurrent cholestasis
- Primary biliary cirrhosis
- Chronic inflammatory bowel disease
- Biliary atresia
- Parasites

*Conditions causing cholestasis

**Table 25.3** Diseases characterized by increased ineffective erythropoiesis

Megaloblastic anemias, e.g. pernicious anemia
Thalassemia
Myeloproliferative diseases, e.g. myelofibrosis
Sideroblastic anemia
Primary shunt hyperbilirubinemia
Erythropoietic porphyria
Protoporphyria
Lead poisoning

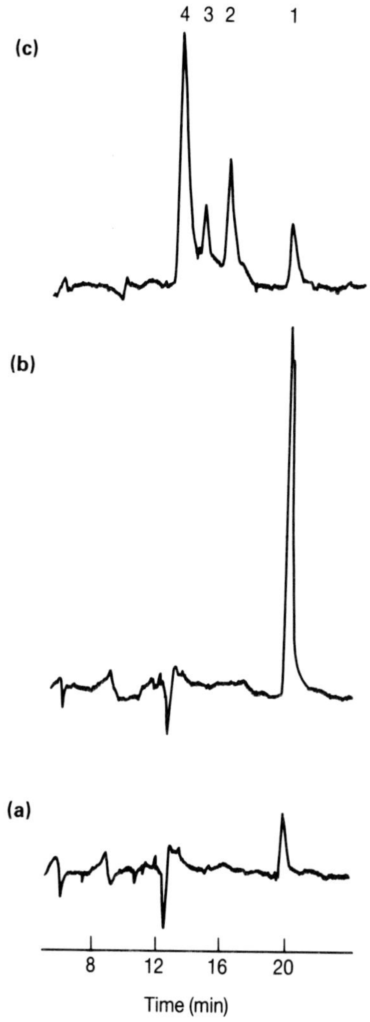


**Fig. 25.6** High pressure liquid chromatograph (HPLC). (a) Normal patient's serum. Total bilirubin 3 μmol/L. (b) Serum from a patient with Gilbert's syndrome. Total bilirubin 25 mmol/L. (c) Serum from a patient with cholestasis caused by gallstones. Total bilirubin 150 μmol/L. Numbered peaks: 1, unconjugated bilirubin; 2, monoconjugated bilirubin; 3, diconjugated bilirubin; 4, protein-bound (δ) bilirubin fraction.

bilirubin fraction becomes detectable in the plasma. This fraction, named δ bilirubin, is firmly (covalently) bound to albumin (Lauff et al 1982, McDonagh et al 1984). δ bilirubin does not pass across the renal glomerular membrane and therefore exhibits a half-life (23 days) that is similar to plasma albumin. As a consequence of this, the total bilirubin concentration in plasma may show a half-life of many days in patients in whom hyperbilirubinemia has been long-standing, such as in biliary obstruction due to gallstones. In these patients, following surgical relief of biliary obstruction, clinicians may be misled into an incorrect assumption that the biliary obstruction has not been successfully relieved. A method for the separation of δ bilirubin has recently been published (Burnett et al 1995).

### Bilirubinuria and urobilinogenuria

Unconjugated bilirubin is almost completely bound to plasma albumin and does not appear in the urine. Conjugated bilirubin, on the other hand, is not protein bound, passes through the glomerulus and is reabsorbed by the renal tubules. It reaches the urine in amounts that can be detected readily only when its concentration in the blood is increased; bilirubinuria therefore indicates the presence of conjugated hyperbilirubinemia. A substantial amount of conjugated bilirubin is excreted in the urine in patients with jaundice due to hepatobiliary disease and this jaundice may be increased by renal failure. An appreciable proportion of urobilinogen in blood (20–30%) is not protein bound, crosses the glomerulus and appears in the urine. It is a weak acid that may be only partly ionized in the tubular fluid, allowing passive back-diffusion into the blood. Ionization increases as the pH rises and consequently more urobilinogen is found in alkaline urine. Urobilinogen in urine is oxidized readily to urobilin on exposure to air. Thus, several factors other than disease affect the results of tests for urobilinogen in the urine and these, and a diurnal variation in urobilinogen excretion, make such tests of little practical value.

## ENZYMES

Enzymes are released when the liver is damaged and measurement of their activity in the blood has proved to have clinical value (Zimmerman & Seeff 1970). However, only those enzymes that have been shown to have clinical value and can be readily measured in large numbers are widely used. Two types are currently important: the transaminases (aminotransferases) which are found inside the liver cells, in both the cytoplasm and mitochondria, and are released by cell damage, and alkaline phosphatase which is bound to cell membranes and is synthesized in increased amounts in cholestasis. Measurements of enzyme activity in serum in liver disease do not give specific diagnoses. Rather, they indicate likely pathologies and therefore help in selecting further investigations. They are also useful in following the progress of diseases and their response to treatment.

### Transaminases

*Nature and distribution*

The activities in serum of two transferase enzymes – aspartate aminotransferase (AST) and alanine aminotransferase (ALT) – are widely used in the diagnosis of hepatic disease. There are two forms of AST in the liver, one in the cell cytoplasm and the other in the mitochondria. ALT is found only in the cytoplasm. Large amounts of AST are present in the liver and heart and lesser amounts in skeletal muscle, erythrocytes, lung, kidney, brain and pancreas. ALT is also widely distributed, but it is more specific in liver disease as its activity is low in organs other than the liver. Both are normally present in serum (5–40 u/L) and in the extracellular fluid. The half-life of ALT (47 ± 10 h) is longer than the half-life of AST (17 ± 5 h) (Price & Alberti 1979).

*Disease*

Increased serum transaminase activity is a sensitive index of liver damage, but it has limited diagnostic or prognostic value (Clermont & Chalmers 1967). Increased activity results principally from the release of enzymes from damaged hepatocytes. Acute liver damage, irrespective of its etiology, usually increases the activity in serum more than 10-fold above the normal reference interval and activities increased over 200-fold can occur. The serum transaminase activity in viral hepatitis is high for up to 2 weeks before the onset of jaundice; it is 10-fold or more above normal in two-thirds of icteric patients (Table 25.4) and about a week after the onset of jaundice it falls rapidly (Strickland et al 1971). Measurement of serum transaminase activity in epidemics of viral hepatitis frequently reveals anicteric and asymptomatic cases. Transaminase activities in anicteric hepatitis are usually lower than in icteric hepatitis (Table 25.5). About 80% of patients with infectious mononucleosis have activities two- to 10-fold above normal; this occurs, albeit less frequently, in other viral illnesses (p. 792). High activities also occur in acute hepatitis due to drugs, particularly in paracetamol poisoning when activities are often increased 200-fold or more.

**Table 25.4** Serum alanine aminotransferase activity in jaundice due to viral hepatitis or to obstructive jaundice (Clermont & Chalmers 1967)

| Alanine aminotransferase activity (fold increase above the normal reference range) | Frequency of alanine aminotransferase activity (%) | |
|---|---|---|
| | Viral hepatitis ($n$ = 177) | Obstructive jaundice* ($n$ = 97) |
| Normal | 1 | 20 |
| Normal to ×5 | 26 | 40 |
| ×5 to ×10 | 12 | 33 |
| ×10 to ×25 | 14 | 7 |
| > ×25 | 47 | 0 |

*Extrahepatic bile duct obstruction

**Table 25.5** Serum aspartate aminotransferase activity in anicteric and icteric viral hepatitis (Clermont & Chalmers 1967)

| Aspartate aminotransferase activity (fold increase above the normal reference range) | Frequency of aspartate aminotransferase activity (%) | |
|---|---|---|
| | Anicteric ($n$ = 35) | Icteric ($n$ = 84) |
| < ×2.5 | 50 | 0 |
| ×2.5 to ×12.5 | 32 | 12 |
| ×12.5 to ×25 | 9 | 31 |
| > ×25 | 9 | 57 |

Acute liver damage due to shock, severe hypoxia, acute cardiac failure and sepsis can cause very high serum transaminase activities and these return to normal rapidly once the underlying cause is rectified. Any other condition damaging the liver can increase the serum transaminase activity, although rarely to such an extent as in the conditions mentioned above. Chronic active hepatitis, in which the serum transaminase is an indication of the activity of the disease, is an exception to this, as serum activity often increases 10-fold or more during exacerbations. In other diseases, such as fatty liver, cirrhosis, secondary carcinoma, granulomatous liver disease, congestive cardiac failure and acute pancreatitis, activity is usually much less than this and has no discriminative value. The raised activity in acute pancreatitis may be caused by biliary obstruction, coincidental cirrhosis or shock and increased AST activity may originate from the pancreas itself. The serum transaminase in alcoholic hepatitis is increased less than fivefold in over 90% of cases (Fulop et al 1971). Biliary obstruction is usually associated with normal or moderately increased activities (Table 25.4), but exceptional activities in excess of 1000 u/L in obstruction of the large bile ducts have been recorded (Shora & Danovitch 1971).

Efforts have been made to increase the usefulness of transaminase measurements by comparing AST and ALT activities. In general, ALT values exceed AST values in acute liver diseases, while AST values exceed ALT values in chronic disorders. Unfortunately, exceptions are so frequent that the AST/ALT ratio is of little clinical value.

Delayed appearance of the mitochondrial form of AST in plasma when compared with the cytosolic form has been shown following myocardial infarction and hepatic injury. It seems that the hepatocyte cell membrane is more vulnerable than the mitochondrial membrane to anoxic injury and, indeed, that leakage of AST across the mitochondrial membrane follows loss of mitochondrial oxidative phosphorylating capacity which probably equates with cell death (Nishimura et al 1986). While there is some evidence that a ratio of the mitochondrial and the total activities improves the sensitivity of these measurements (Nalpas et al 1986), these measurements have not been widely used in clinical practice.

## Alkaline phosphatase

*Nature and distribution*

The alkaline phosphatase enzymes are widely distributed, substantial amounts being present in liver, bone, small intestine, placenta, kidney and white blood cells. They are also found in serum, lymph, urine, intestinal juice, bile, feces and milk. They are the products of three genes each coding for separate isoenzymes. Post-translational modification of the preformed isoenzymes, mainly by the addition of sialic acid residues, leads to the formation of a family of isoforms showing tissue-specific differences of clinical importance. The alkaline phosphatases are found in cell membranes associated with absorptive and secretory functions, and in the liver they are localized in the sinusoidal and canalicular membranes. Bone alkaline phosphatase seems to be important in calcification; intestinal alkaline phosphatase may be involved in the absorption of fat and calcium. It is presumed that elsewhere it is concerned with membrane transport. The functions of alkaline phosphatases in serum, lymph and secretions are unknown. The alkaline phosphatases have been reviewed extensively (Kaplan 1972, Warnes 1972, Fishman 1974).

### *Serum alkaline phosphatase*

The normal serum alkaline phosphatase comes mainly from liver, bone, intestine and the placenta. Electrophoresis, the degree of stability on heating and more recently immunological methods can be used to separate the alkaline phosphatases that are derived from different tissues. This can be valuable in patients who have a raised total alkaline phosphatase activity in serum. On electrophoresis, the liver type migrates fastest, the bone type forms an intermediate zone and the intestinal alkaline phosphatase migrates most slowly. The half-life of alkaline phosphatase in the blood is about 2 days.

***Normal activity.*** Alkaline phosphatase of liver origin usually predominates in normal serum in adults. The intestinal enzyme, which increases after a meal, may account for up to a fifth of the normal serum activity. Skeletal growth in adolescence and up to the age of 20 years increases the total alkaline phosphatase activity by increasing production by bone. Plasma activity may reach two to three times the upper limit of the adult reference interval. Normal activities may also be increased by up to 50% without detectable disease in neonates and in the elderly. Placental alkaline phosphatase becomes detectable after about 8 weeks of pregnancy (Fishman et al 1972), increases the total activity in the third trimester of pregnancy and at term the total serum activity may reach two to two and a half times normal (McMaster et al 1964, Iyengar & Srikantia 1970). Placental alkaline phosphatase constitutes one- to two-thirds of the total serum activity at term. Inherited increases in serum alkaline phosphatase activity due to liver and bone types have been described (Wilson 1979, McEvoy et al 1981).

***Increased activity.*** Increases in alkaline phosphatase activity in serum are the result of increased enzyme production by specific tissues. Increased activity in adults who are not pregnant is most frequently due to liver or bone disease and is usually attributable to liver or bone alkaline phosphatase respectively. Biliary obstruction results in increased production of hepatic alkaline phosphatase leading to increased activity of the liver isoenzyme in serum and in the liver itself. These increases occur irrespective of the site of obstruction in the biliary tract. Increased serum activity of the intestinal alkaline phosphatase isoenzyme can also be caused by hepatic disease, especially alcoholic cirrhosis, but does not occur in bowel disease (Warnes et al 1977). Increased serum activity of bone alkaline phosphatase occurs in diseases causing increased osteoblastic activity such as osteomalacia, Paget's disease and metastatic bone disease.

***Alkaline phosphatase variants.*** Abnormal alkaline phosphatase isoenzymes are sometimes produced by tumors (Fishman 1974). These isoenzymes include the Regan isoenzyme, which has the same properties as placental alkaline phosphatase, the Nagao isoenzyme, which shares certain features with the Regan isoenzyme, and the Regan variant or Kasahara isoenzyme, which has features midway between the other two. The Regan and Nagao isoenzymes are produced occasionally by a variety of tumors; the Regan variant or Kasahara isoenzyme is frequently produced by, and has been considered specific to, hepatocellular carcinomas (p. 1120), although this specificity has been questioned (McKenzie & Henderson 1975). The Regan isoenzyme has also been found in familial polyposis and in ulcerative colitis. Complexes of liver or bone alkaline phosphatase and immunoglobulin sometimes form and are detected as electrophoretically slow forms of alkaline phosphatase. They occur in various diseases and their significance is unknown (Crofton & Smith 1978). These variant forms of alkaline phosphatase are not useful in diagnosis, as they occur in only a minority of patients and often at activities too low to be detected readily.

***Acute jaundice.*** The serum alkaline phosphatase activity in liver disease has been used most widely to differentiate acute hepatitis from biliary obstruction in patients with jaundice of recent onset (Becker & Stauffer 1962, Clermont & Chalmers 1967, Stern et al 1973). Obstruction of larger bile ducts, even of short duration, results in a serum alkaline phosphatase greater than twice the normal activity in over 90% of patients and greater than four times the normal activity in over 75% of patients (Table 25.6). Obstruction of large bile ducts is therefore most unlikely when the serum activity is increased less than twofold and it becomes steadi-

**Table 25.6** Serum alkaline phosphatase activity in jaundice due to viral hepatitis or obstructive jaundice (Becker & Stauffer 1962)

| Alkaline phosphatase activity (fold increase above the normal reference range) | Frequency of alkaline phosphatase activity (%) | |
|---|---|---|
| | Viral hepatitis ($n$ = 81) | Obstructive jaundice* ($n$ = 83) |
| Normal | 1 | 0 |
| Normal to ×2 | 37 | 3 |
| ×2 to ×4 | 41 | 19 |
| ×4 to ×6 | 12 | 27 |
| >×6 | 9 | 51 |

*Extrahepatic bile duct obstruction

ly more likely as the activity rises. A certain differentiation cannot, however, be made even at activities increased more than fourfold, since such activities occur in up to a fifth of patients with viral hepatitis (Table 25.6).

Further help may be obtained by considering the serum alkaline phosphatase and the serum transaminase activities together. Jaundice is due to biliary obstruction in about 90% of patients when the alkaline phosphatase exceeds two and a half times normal and the transaminase is increased less than sixfold; it is due to hepatitis in about 90% of patients when the opposite obtains. These two situations occur in about a half of patients with jaundice and in the rest no sure differentiation can be made. Further differentiation is made best by ultrasonography, which shows dilatation of the large bile ducts increasingly frequently as the duration and severity of obstruction continue (p. 52). This can then be used to decide on the need for cholangiography or liver biopsy. Liver function tests are also useful in following the course of a disease and its response to therapy.

***Parenchymal liver disease.*** Serum alkaline phosphatase activity increases moderately in acute parenchymal liver disease of viral or toxic (drug) origin but reaches four times the reference range in about a fifth of patients with viral hepatitis (Table 25.6). Viral hepatitis of any type can cause a cholestatic illness with high alkaline phosphatase activities, but serum transaminase activities in such cases are usually high (p. 798). Hepatitis due to Epstein–Barr virus (p. 793) and cytomegalovirus (p. 792) is often cholestatic. Hepatotoxic drugs can also cause cholestatic illnesses (p. 850). High alkaline phosphatase activities occur in infiltrative liver diseases such as sarcoidosis (p. 830), when space-occupying lesions are present and in some forms of cirrhosis. High serum alkaline phosphatase activities in chronic liver disease are associated particularly with primary biliary cirrhosis (p. 939), primary sclerosing cholangitis (p. 944) and cholestatic forms of alcoholic liver disease (p. 877). There is often a striking dissociation between serum alkaline phosphatase activity and bilirubin concentration in these conditions and the bilirubin may be normal.

***Systemic disease.*** Increased serum alkaline phosphatase activity of liver origin may occur in diseases that have not involved the liver directly. These include acute and chronic systemic infections (p. 941), collagenoses (p. 1106), neoplasms such as Hodgkin's disease (p. 1104) and renal carcinoma (p. 1110), myelofibrosis, cardiac failure (p. 1097) and inflammatory bowel disease (p. 1101). Liver biopsy shows no abnormality or a nonspecific reactive hepatitis in most of these, centrilobular congestion is seen in cardiac failure and pericholangitis in inflammatory bowel disease.

## γ-Glutamyl transpeptidase

*Nature and distribution*

γ-Glutamyl transpeptidase (GGTP) is a microsomal enzyme that is present in serum and is distributed widely in body tissues. Its activity is highest in the renal tubules and high activities also occur in the liver, pancreas, spleen, brain, breast and small intestine. It is found in the hepatocytes and the epithelium of the small bile ductules in the liver.

*Serum GGTP activity*

GGTP has been used most in the detection of hepatobiliary disease and alcohol abuse (Rosalki & Rau 1972, Goldberg & Martin 1975, Dragosics et al 1976).

***Hepatobiliary disease.*** Increased serum GGTP activity in hepatobiliary disease correlates best with alkaline phosphatase activity, indicating that it reflects mainly alterations in biliary function. The highest activities occur in biliary obstruction, but they give no indication of the site of obstruction; activities are usually increased more than 10-fold and may exceed 40 times the normal upper reference value. Serum GGTP activity is probably a more sensitive index of biliary obstruction than alkaline phosphatase activity because its relative increase is greater, but it is less specific for the liver and it is affected by drugs and alcohol. Serum GGTP activity also increases greatly in acute hepatic damage due to any cause. Increases and decreases in GGTP activity parallel transaminase activity.

Serum GGTP activity in chronic hepatitis is increased when the transaminase activity is increased, but it adds nothing in the diagnosis of the disease or in following its response to treatment. Activities in cirrhosis are highest in patients with alcoholic cirrhosis who are continuing to drink; activities in those who have stopped drinking and in cirrhosis due to other causes are usually increased less than threefold. Space-occupying lesions in the liver, especially metastases, frequently cause increased GGTP activity and this increase may be very marked. The wide distribution of GGTP in the body accounts for the moderate increases in serum GGTP activity in extrahepatic diseases such as pneumonia, pleurisy, pulmonary infarction, pancreatitis, pancreatic cancer, inflammatory bowel disease and diabetes mellitus. Increased activity is uncommon in renal disease in spite of the large amount of GGTP in the renal tubules, but minor increases can occur in chronic renal failure, in the nephrotic syndrome, in renal neoplasms and in rejection reactions after renal transplantation. Increased activity in heart disease is probably due to the effects of cardiac failure on the liver (p. 1097), as the heart contains little GGTP activity.

Serum GGTP activity is a sensitive index of liver damage, but it has not replaced transaminase and alkaline phosphatase measurements in the investigation of hepatobiliary disease. GGTP lacks specificity for liver disease, there is considerable overlap of activities in hepatitis and in biliary obstruction and increased activity can be caused by drugs and alcohol.

***Alcohol abuse and drug use.*** Increased serum GGTP activity is of most value in detecting alcohol abuse (p. 872) and in following the progress of alcoholic patients (Whitehead et al 1978, Chick et al 1981). It is important to realize that the plasma GGTP does not increase in about a third of heavy drinkers and to exclude other causes of increased activity such as liver disease, usually indicated by abnormality of other liver function tests, or drugs, particularly those that are powerful inducing agents (Table 30.3). The distribution of normal plasma GGTP activity is skewed to the right and activities are higher in men, the obese and the elderly (Schiele et al 1977), but increased GGTP activity that cannot be accounted for by such factors, alternative causes or that occurs in otherwise stable liver disease suggests alcohol abuse.

## PLASMA PROTEINS

Plasma contains a wide range of different proteins, many of which are synthesized in the liver. Marked changes in the concentrations of these plasma proteins can occur in liver disease and some of them can be used in the assessment of liver function and in the diagnosis of specific liver diseases. The plasma proteins and the mechanisms whereby proteins are synthesized by liver cells have been reviewed in detail (Putnam 1975, Tavill & Swain 1979).

### Albumin

Albumin is the major secretory protein synthesized by the liver; it accounts for half the protein produced by that organ (Rothschild et al 1988).

#### *Normal metabolism*

The liver synthesizes 8–14 g of albumin daily. Synthesis takes place in the ribosomes of the rough endoplasmic reticulum and the albumin molecules are secreted directly into the sinusoidal blood. Metabolism proceeds rapidly; studies with radio-labeled amino acids show that albumin molecules appear in the blood within half an hour. Two methods have been used to study albumin metabolism in humans. Radio-iodinated albumin has been used to measure albumin distribution and degradation and to calculate the rate of albumin synthesis (p. 349). Radioactive carbon ($^{14}C$) has been used to label intrahepatic arginine, which is then incorporated into albumin, and this allows a direct measure of albumin synthesis.

***Distribution.*** The total exchangeable pool of albumin in an adult male is 280–350 g (Table 25.7). About a third is in the plasma and about two-thirds in the extravascular, extracellular space; the largest single site is the skin, which contains about a fifth of the total exchangeable pool. Albumin given intravenously equilibrates with the intravascular pool in a few minutes, with the extravascular pool in about 10 days and with organs such as the skin even more slowly. Extravascular albumin returns to the circulation via the lymphatics and the thoracic duct. Albumin degradation occurs mainly in the liver, muscle, kidney and skin, although lysosomal proteases present in all cells can degrade albumin (Yedgar et al 1983). Small amounts of albumin are lost in sweat, tears, bile and gastrointestinal secretions. The gut, once considered a major site of loss, accounts for less than 10% of the total amount degraded daily (Fig. 13.6).

**Table 25.7** Normal albumin metabolism (Rothschild et al 1972)

| | Male | Female |
|---|---|---|
| Serum concentration (g/L) | 35–45 | 35–45 |
| Synthesis (mg/kg/day) | 120–200 | 120–150 |
| Degradation (% plasma albumin pool/day) | 6–10 | 6–10 |
| Exchangeable pool (g/kg) | 4–5 | 3.5–4.5 |
| Intravascular pool (% of exchangeable pool) | 38–45 | 38–45 |

***Production.*** The main factors controlling albumin production are nutritional, osmotic and hormonal. Nutrition is the most important factor. A protein-deficient diet in animals rapidly reduces albumin production by about half, the exchangeable albumin pool is reduced to about a third, the plasma albumin concentration falls and the albumin half-life is prolonged. This returns to normal equally rapidly on refeeding. The colloid oncotic pressure in the interstitium of the liver seems also to be important (Rothschild et al 1986). The actual albumin concentration is less important than the total colloid oncotic pressure, as hyperglobulinemia reduces albumin synthesis even when the albumin concentration is low. Albumin synthesis is increased markedly by plasmapheresis during which the intravascular albumin concentration is maintained at the expense of the extravascular pool, which suggests that the site of the controlling mechanism for albumin synthesis is extravascular. Hormones also affect albumin metabolism. Albumin synthesis increases in hyperthyroidism and decreases in hypothyroidism and corticosteroid hormones increase albumin synthesis in health and in patients with cirrhosis. Interaction between hormones is likely to be important.

#### *Function*

Albumin is a water-soluble molecule with a molecular mass of 65 000. It has two main known functions. It is the most important substance in the maintenance of the colloid oncotic pressure of the blood and it serves as a carrier for numerous low molecular mass substances, including bilirubin, bile acids, calcium, fatty acids, urate, hormones such as aldosterone and numerous drugs (Koch-Weser &

Sellers 1976). Analbuminemia (below), however, shows that albumin is not essential to life.

*Liver disease*

Hypoalbuminemia is a feature of advanced chronic liver disease, but it occurs in acute liver damage only if it is severe and of several weeks duration. This can be related to the long biological half-life of albumin (20 days), which ensures that changes in plasma albumin concentration occur slowly and cannot rapidly reflect the effects of acute liver damage. Hypoalbuminemia in chronic liver disease is often taken to indicate reduced hepatic albumin synthesis and this has been supported by indirect measurements of albumin synthesis. However, a normal exchangeable albumin pool, failure of repeated paracenteses to reduce the plasma albumin or its exchangeable pool and direct measurements of albumin synthesis have shown that albumin synthesis can be normal or even increased in cirrhosis despite hypoalbuminemia. Hypoalbuminemia is not, therefore, related simply to a reduced rate of albumin synthesis and other important factors probably include an abnormal distribution of the albumin pool with secretion of albumin directly into ascitic fluid. Impaired albumin synthesis does occur in chronic liver disease, but it need not always be due to the liver alone. The regulation of albumin synthesis by hepatic osmoreceptors could be deranged and hepatic synthetic activity could be limited by nutritional deficiency (p. 922), endocrine abnormalities (p. 920) or alcohol.

The complex relation between the plasma albumin concentration and albumin synthesis does not mean that plasma albumin concentrations are of no clinical value. Post & Patek (1942) showed that patients with cirrhosis but no ascites who had a markedly reduced plasma albumin also had a poor prognosis (Fig. 25.7). The plasma albumin in patients with ascites is not related so clearly to the prognosis and often rises following successful treatment of the ascites. Tygstrup (1973) confirmed the general relation of the plasma albumin to survival, although great individual variations occur. A falling plasma albumin is usually a bad prognostic sign and patients with hypoalbuminemia tolerate operations relatively poorly (p. 1138). A transient fall in plasma albumin frequently follows an operation or gastrointestinal bleed and this does not in itself signify a poor outlook.

*Analbuminemia*

This is a rare condition in which albumin cannot be detected in the blood. No other abnormality of the liver has been found and the condition is compatible with good health. The half-life of infused albumin is very long (Gordon et al 1959). The plasma globulin concentration is high; it falls following albumin infusion, which suggests

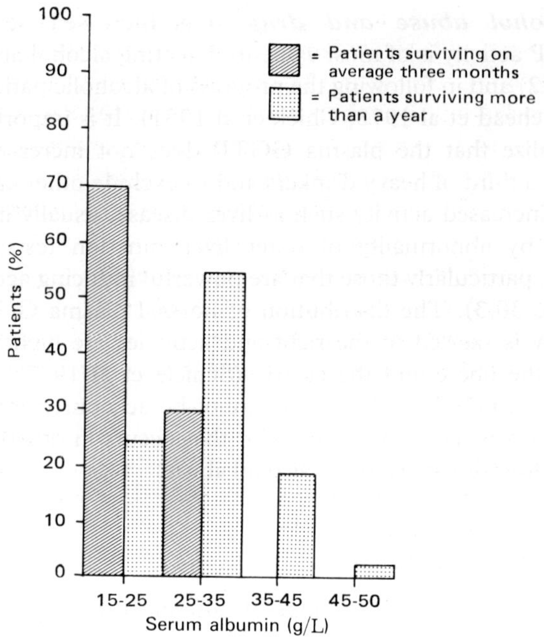


**Fig. 25.7** Serum albumin concentration on admission to hospital related to survival in cirrhosis without ascites (Post & Patek 1942).

that osmotic factors contribute to hyperglobulinemia. Patients are healthy but may suffer mild leg edema.

## Other proteins

While albumin is the predominant protein in plasma, the remaining proteins are a heterogeneous group, many of which are synthesized by the liver, including some of the apolipoproteins, haptoglobin, ceruloplasmin, iron-transport proteins, $\alpha_1$-antitrypsin, $\alpha_2$-macroglobulin and certain components of the complement system. The immunoglobulins are synthesized in the lymphoreticular system. Chronic liver disease is characterized by a fall in the serum albumin concentration and a rise in the concentrations of certain of the other proteins which is related to the severity and duration of the disease (Rothschild et al 1972). The most marked changes occur in chronic active hepatitis, primary biliary cirrhosis and cryptogenic cirrhosis, but overlap with other chronic liver diseases is such that quantitative protein measurements are of no value in differential diagnosis. The measurements give some idea of the severity of liver damage and allow the progress of the disease to be followed. Hyperglobulinemia without hypoalbuminemia can occur in viral hepatitis and in persistent hepatitis.

*Plasma protein electrophoresis*

This technique separates proteins mainly on the basis of their electrical charge. Electrophoresis on cellulose acetate separates the serum proteins into five fractions: albumin and $\alpha_1$-, $\alpha_2$-, β- and γ-globulins. Each of these globulin fractions is heterogeneous. Several abnormalities in the plasma protein electrophoretic pattern occur in liver disease (Hobbs 1967, Larson 1974). None is of great diagnostic value except for an absence of the $\alpha_1$-globulin fraction, which indicates $\alpha_1$-antitrypsin deficiency (p. 966). The most striking changes occur in chronic liver disease, in which a normal pattern is unusual. The typical pattern in cirrhosis is a reduced albumin and a broad (polyclonal) increase in the γ-globulins; analysis of the electrophoretic pattern shows a loss of differentiation between the β- and γ-globulins caused by a particular increase in fast-migrating γ-globulins. The γ-globulins also increase in autoimmune hepatitis but the differentiation between the β- and γ-globulins remains, since the main increase is in the slower moving γ-globulins. The γ-globulins rise in acute hepatitis after the second week and in cholestasis the $\alpha_2$-globulins increase owing to the increased production of lipoproteins. Rarely, a monoclonal increase in γ-globulin occurs and may be associated with a reticulosis or hepatocellular carcinoma (Eliakim et al 1972). Cryoglobulinemia is also a rare occurrence.

### *Immunoglobulins*

Increased concentrations of one or more of the main immunoglobulin (Ig) groups (G, A, M) in serum are found in most patients with chronic liver disease (Feizi 1968). IgG increases are most frequent in autoimmune hepatitis and cryptogenic cirrhosis (65%), IgA increases in alcoholic cirrhosis (60%) and IgM increases in primary biliary cirrhosis (80%). Increases are, however, so variable that Ig levels are of little diagnostic value. In relation to primary biliary cirrhosis, it is notable that 20% of patients with extrahepatic biliary obstruction have a raised serum IgM concentration. In acute viral hepatitis, increased levels of IgM are most typical of type A hepatitis.

Increased serum γ-globulin concentrations in cirrhosis are associated with increased γ-globulin synthesis (Eisenmenger & Slater 1953, Ramsöe et al 1970). This is the result of increased immunoglobulin production by the lymphoreticular system generally and it may be a response to an increased antigenic stimulation (p. 773). It may also be part of a response to maintain the colloid oncotic pressure of the blood.

### *Iron-containing proteins*

The main iron-containing proteins in the blood are transferrin, haptoglobin, hemopexin and ferritin (Grace & Powell 1974, Tavill & Swain 1979).

***Transferrin.*** This is a β-globulin; it is the major iron-containing protein and is responsible for iron transport between the gut, the reticulocytes in the bone marrow and the tissue storage sites (p. 951). Ceruloplasmin (as ferroxidase) may be important in this process (p. 751). Each molecule binds two atoms of iron and 3–4 mg iron are held in the blood in this way. Transferrin is made mainly in the liver and its synthesis is related to the size of the iron stores. Many factors alter its plasma concentration; increases are caused by iron deficiency, pregnancy and oral contraceptive drugs and decreases occur when the iron stores are high, as in hemolysis, aplasia, transfusional siderosis and idiopathic hemochromatosis. Transferrin is also a negative acute-phase reactant and so concentrations fall whenever there is tissue damage or inflammation. Normally, the iron-containing capacity of transferrin is about a third saturated (Table 25.8).

Measurements of serum iron and transferrin concentration made for diagnostic purposes should be done on fasting blood samples. In liver disease, the most characteristic changes occur in idiopathic hemochromatosis (p. 955), in which a raised serum iron concentration and a reduced transferrin concentration result in 60% or more of the iron-binding capacity being saturated. Serum iron concentrations above 36 μmol/L (200 μg/dl) occur in less than 5% of normal people and the serum iron-binding capacity is more than 60% saturated in less than 1% (Card et al 1964, Crosby et al 1974, Edwards et al 1988). This measurement can only be regarded as a screening test for hemochromatosis, since increased saturation of the iron-binding capacity also occurs in acute hepatitis and in alcoholic liver disease. Reduced transferrin concentrations are present in serum from patients with alcoholic liver disease and in about one-third of these there is a raised liver iron content (Chapman et al 1982). In alcoholic cirrhosis it appears that the reduced serum transferrin concentration is due to a reduced hepatic synthesis rate with a normal catabolic rate; in alcoholics with fatty liver, however, the transferrin synthesis rate is increased (Potter et al 1985).

***Carbohydrate-deficient transferrin.*** Transferrin exists as several isoforms varying in respect of their two complex carbohydrate chains. Carbohydrate-deficient transferrin (CDT) isoforms are present at low concentrations in normal serum and concentrations increase after regular intake of alcohol (50–60 g/day) for at least a week and then decrease on abstinence with a half-life of about 15 days. CDT has been advocated as a sensitive means of detecting alcohol abuse which is more specific than other

**Table 25.8** Normal serum iron and transferrin concentrations and transferrin saturation (Card et al 1964)

| Iron | | Transferrin | | |
|---|---|---|---|---|
| μmol/L | μg/dl | μmol/L | μg/dl | Saturation % |
| 10–33 | 55–185 | 45–49 | 250–272 | 14–47 |

Notes: 1. These values refer to fasting morning blood samples. Serum iron concentration varies during the day.
2. <5% normal persons have serum iron concentrations above 36 μmol/L (200 μg/dl).

markers such as the erythrocyte volume (p. 872) or the serum γ-glutamyl transferase activity (Stibler 1991, Bell et al 1993). Sensitivity for detecting continuing alcohol intake of >60 g/day has been reported at about 80% with specificity of about 90%. Moderate increases of CDT occur in about 15% of patients with chronic nonalcoholic liver disease, most of whom have advanced disease with cirrhosis and liver failure. False positive results can also occur in genetic variants of transferrin and in the rare recently described carbohydrate-deficient glycoprotein syndrome. CDT concentrations are not affected by commonly prescribed drugs. Overall, CDT measurement looks to be a useful means for identifying alcohol abuse, although it has not yet become available widely.

***Haptoglobin and hemopexin.*** Haptoglobin is an $\alpha_2$-globulin which complexes with hemoglobin liberated into the circulation by hemolysis. It is synthesized in the liver and is degraded at a constant rate, irrespective of its blood concentration. Its blood level is reduced in parenchymal liver disease and increased in cholestasis, but variable values render it of no diagnostic value (Williams et al 1961). It behaves as a positive acute-phase reactant and is reduced by hemolysis.

Hemopexin is a β-globulin that binds free heme in the blood. It is made in the liver and is removed from the blood by the liver once it is bound to heme.

***Ferritin.*** Ferritin is a large macromolecule of molecular weight 450 000 in which iron is sequestered inside an apoferritin shell. Ferritins differ between tissues in relation to their relative contents of heavier (H) and lighter (L) ferritin subunits. Ferritin provides protection against the toxic effects of iron and provides the main readily accessible storage form of iron. Hemosiderin is an ill-defined degradation product of ferritin. All tissues make ferritin, but ferritin in the blood is cleared by the liver cells which carry ferritin receptors (Adams et al 1988). The plasma ferritin concentration reflects the size of the body's iron stores (Lipschitz et al 1974). It is particularly useful in identifying primary and secondary iron overload and in these conditions the plasma ferritin reflects the iron concentration in the liver (Fig. 25.8). Patients with symptomatic genetic hemochromatosis usually have plasma ferritin concentrations above 1000 μg/L, but this may not be the case in asymptomatic patients with less marked iron overload (p. 956). High plasma ferritin concentrations are not pathognomonic of genetic hemochromatosis or of increased liver iron concentrations, as high plasma concentrations occur in other liver diseases (Prieto et al 1975, Di Bisceglie et al 1992). The highest concentrations are found in acute hepatitis due to drugs or viruses, in which values can reach 30 000 μg/L, but increased values are also found in about a third of patients with chronic hepatitis and alcoholic liver disease and in such patients values above 1000 μg/L are common.

Plasma ferritin concentrations in acute and chronic hepatitis are related to plasma transaminase activity, probably reflecting loss of ferritin from damaged liver cells, and where the plasma transaminase falls rapidly, ferritin concentrations fall within a week or two. Ferritin concentrations fall more slowly in alcoholic liver disease when alcohol intake is reduced or stops (p. 874). It is important to bear in mind that ferritin is an acute-phase reactant (Konijn & Hershko 1977) and that increased ferritin concentrations in plasma occur in inflammatory diseases unrelated to the liver (Fig. 25.9). In these cases, however, plasma concentrations of iron and total iron-binding capacity are usually reduced.

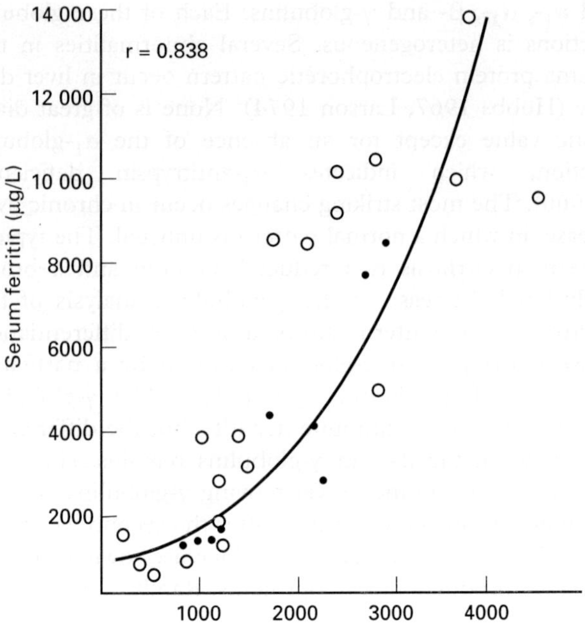

**Fig. 25.8** Relationship between serum ferritin and liver iron concentration in patients with iron overload due to hemochromatosis (●) and to genetic hematological disease (○) (Prieto et al 1975).

*Protease inhibitors*

The protease inhibitor (Pi) system comprises a group of plasma proteins capable of inactivating and eliminating proteolytic enzymes whose uninhibited actions could damage tissues. Its functions are poorly understood, but it seems to act mainly as a protease scavenger system. Major human plasma protease inhibitors include $\alpha_1$-antitrypsin, $\alpha_2$-macroglobulin, antithrombin-3 and an inhibitor of the first component of complement (C-l inactivator). The components of this system can inhibit such varied proteases as trypsin, chymotrypsin, elastases, collagenases, plasmin, thrombin, kallikrein and C-l esterase.

***$\alpha_1$-Antitrypsin.*** $\alpha_1$-Antitrypsin is synthesized wholly in the liver and its synthesis is controlled genetically (p. 966). The normal concentration in serum in individuals with the most common phenotype (PiMM) is 1.5–2.5 g/L, its half-life is about 7 days and it is catabolized largely in the liver. A marked reduction in the serum concentration can be recognized by a reduced or absent

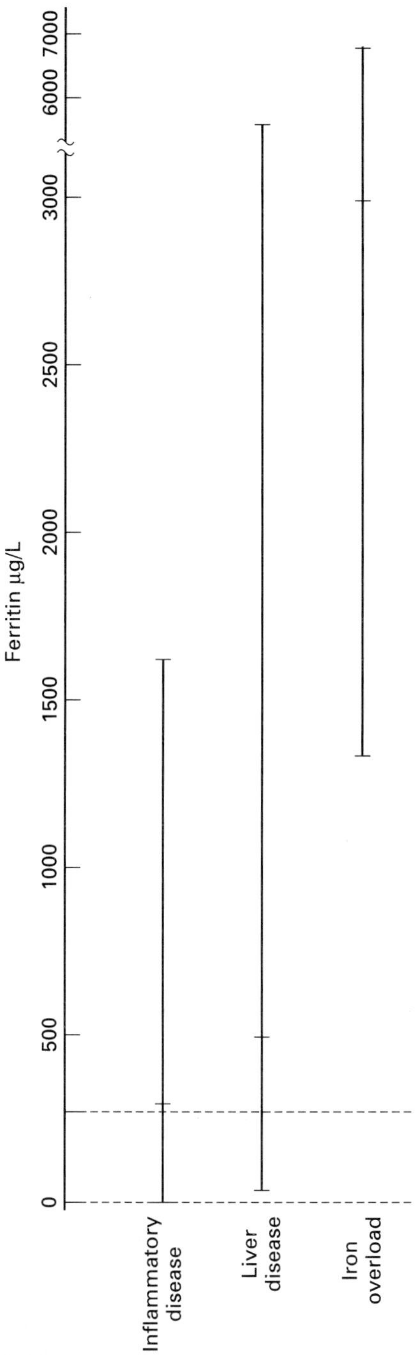


**Fig. 25.9** Plasma ferritin concentrations showing mean values and ranges in nonhepatic inflammatory disease (n = 39), liver disease (alcoholic n = 29, viral hepatitis n = 8), and iron overload (primary n = 3, secondary n= 20) (Lipschitz et al 1974).

α-globulin on serum protein electrophoresis since $\alpha_1$-antitrypsin is the dominant α-globulin in the blood. The actual concentration is measured immunologically. $\alpha_1$-Antitrypsin constitutes 90% of the tryptic inhibitory capacity of the serum and it is the only component of the Pi system related clearly to liver disease (p. 35.15).

$\alpha_1$-Antitrypsin is a relatively small protein of molecular weight 54 000 that passes easily through capillaries. It is distributed widely in the body fluids and accumulates in sites of inflammation and tissue damage where proteolytic enzymes are released. Its production increases in acute and chronic infections, in pregnancy and in response to oral contraceptives, in malignant disease and in cholestasis due to hepatic or biliary disease. In these circumstances, its concentrations in serum may increase two- to threefold. Low concentrations in serum that do not increase in these conditions occur for genetic reasons (p. 966), in severe hepatic necrosis and in protein-losing enteropathy (p. 348). The variation in plasma $\alpha_1$-antitrypsin is such that $\alpha_1$-antitrypsin deficiency can only be diagnosed reliably by determining the phenotype by electrophoresis (p. 966).

### *Alpha-fetoprotein*

Alpha-fetoprotein is a glycoprotein of molecular weight 69 000 showing heterogeneity related mainly to its sialic acid content. It has an electrophoretic mobility between albumin and $\alpha_1$-globulin. Its properties and clinical importance have been reviewed by Taketa (1990).

***Normal occurrence and function.*** Alpha-fetoprotein (AFP) is made during fetal life by the yolk sac, the gastrointestinal epithelium and the liver. The developing liver can make AFP within 4 weeks of conception and by the eighth week it has become its dominant source. Maximum production is reached by the end of the first trimester. AFP is excreted by the fetal kidney into the amniotic fluid. Cord blood contains 10 000–100 000 μg/L of AFP and thereafter the concentration falls with a half-life of 3.5–5 days, reaching its normal adult concentration by the end of a year.

The normal adult serum AFP concentration does not exceed 6 μg/L (or 6 ng/ml). The AFP concentration in maternal serum rises gradually during pregnancy, reaches a maximum of about 500 mg/L at term and falls rapidly to normal after delivery. Rare instances of familial persistence of high serum alpha-fetoprotein concentrations have been reported with concentrations up to about 70 μg/L (Greenberg et al 1990). The functions of AFP are unknown; suggestions have included a role in maintaining the colloid oncotic pressure of fetal blood, control of the entry of fatty acids into cells and the prevention of harmful immune responses.

***Detection.*** Alpha-fetoprotein is now detected routinely by radioimmunoassay which can detect the concentrations in normal blood (<6 μg/L or 6 ng/ml). Electrophoretic methods used previously are much less sensitive and only detect concentrations in excess of 500 μg/L.

***Induction.*** Alpha-fetoprotein is not solely a consequence of liver cell regeneration, as serum concentrations do not rise after partial hepatectomy (Alpert & Feller 1978). Carbon tetrachloride causes a greater increase in serum alpha-fetoprotein than partial hepatectomy in rats, indicating that the nature of the liver damage is also important.

***Hepatocellular carcinoma.*** Serum AFP measurement in adult medical practice is of greatest value in the diagnosis of hepatocellular carcinoma, though increased serum concentrations can occur in other diseases (Table 25.9). Detection of specific forms of alpha-fetoprotein may increase the specificity of diagnosis of hepatocellular carcinoma, but this has not been translated into clinical practice (Burditt et al 1994). Measurements are useful in diagnosis, in following the response to surgical treatment or chemotherapy and in detecting recurrence of tumor several months before symptoms occur. The serum AFP is increased in 70–90% of patients with hepatocellular carcinoma (Fig. 25.10) and in a half or more it is above 400 μg/L and is virtually diagnostic (Chen & Sung 1977). Increased AFP production may be related to chromosomal change occurring in the development of the malignant tumor (Shiou-Hwei et al 1966). The frequency with which the serum alpha-fetoprotein is raised is very variable but is related at least in part to the size of the tumor and to its histological differentiation (Brumm et al 1989, Nomura et al 1989). Larger tumors are more often associated with increased concentrations (Table 25.10) and poorly differentiated tumors more often contain alpha-fetoprotein. These factors are interrelated, as smaller tumors tend to be better differentiated. Alpha-fetoprotein concentrations may also relate to prognosis, as patients with higher concentrations have a shorter survival than those with lower concentrations but similar sized

**Table 25.9** Diseases associated with increased serum alpha-fetoprotein concentration

| | |
|---|---|
| Adults | *Neoplastic* |
| | Hepatocellular carcinoma* |
| | Carcinoma |
| | stomach |
| | pancreas |
| | gallbladder |
| | bile ducts |
| | lungs |
| | *Non-neoplastic* |
| | Viral hepatitis |
| | Chronic hepatitis (esp. chronic active) |
| | Cirrhosis |
| Children | *Neoplastic* |
| | Hepatoblastoma* |
| | Gonadal teratoblastoma* |
| | *Non-neoplastic* |
| | Biliary atresia |
| | Neonatal hepatitis |
| | Indian childhood cirrhosis |
| | Tyrosinosis |
| | Ataxia telangiectasia |
| Pregnancy | Neural tube defects† |
| | Fetal distress |

*Alpha-fetoprotein frequently and greatly increased
†Alpha-fetoprotein also increased in amniotic fluid

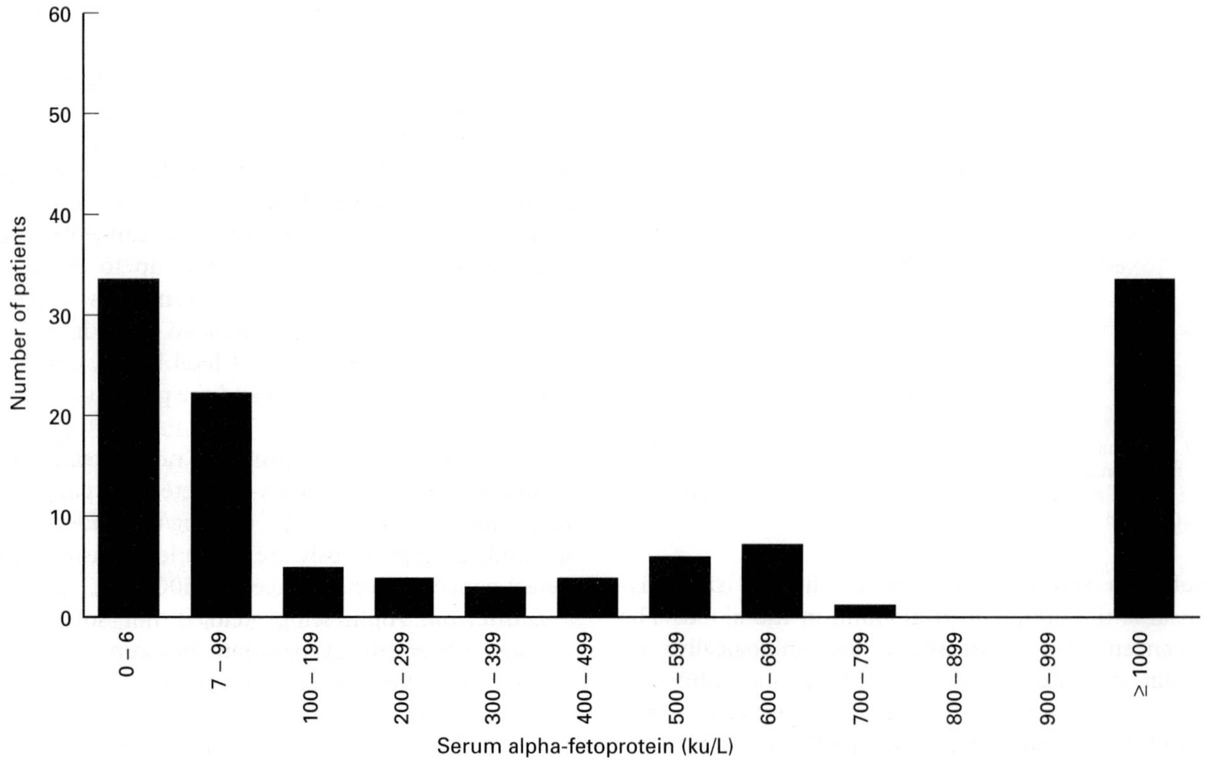


**Fig. 25.10** Serum alpha-fetoprotein (normal 0–6 ku/L) in 115 consecutive patients with hepatocellular carcinoma (Royal Infirmary, Edinburgh).

**Table 25.10** Frequency of increased serum alpha-fetoprotein concentrations related to tumor size (Nomura et al 1989)

| Tumor diameter (cm) | Increased serum alpha-fetoprotein (%) |
|---|---|
| >5 | 77 |
| 3–5 | 72 |
| 2–3 | 76 |
| <2 | 59 |

tumors (Nomura et al 1989). The fibrolamellar variant of hepatocellular carcinoma is not associated with increased serum alpha-fetoprotein (Paradinas et al 1982).

***Other diseases.*** Increased serum AFP concentrations occur in liver diseases other than hepatocellular carcinoma (Table 25.9). They are found in a quarter to a third of patients with acute viral hepatitis or chronic active hepatitis and are related mainly to the biochemical activity of the disease; they are also found occasionally in persistent hepatitis and in quiescent cirrhosis but rarely in other liver diseases (Ruoslahti et al 1974, Silver et al 1974). Increased serum AFP can sometimes be detected in fulminant hepatic failure after the first week of the illness (Alpert & Feller 1978).

***Other carcinomas.*** Cholangiocarcinomas are associated with increased alpha-fetoprotein concentrations occasionally, especially where they show mixed cholangiolar and hepatocellular features histologically. Primary gastrointestinal carcinomas, particularly of the stomach and pancreas, and bronchial carcinomas may give rise to raised serum AFP concentrations, particularly where metastasis to the liver has occurred. The concentrations in these diseases rarely exceed 500 mg/L.

***Childhood.*** Marked increases occur in virtually all hepatoblastomas and in two-thirds of testicular and ovarian teratoblastomas. Serial estimations are useful in assessing the effects of treatment and in detecting recurrence before symptoms develop. Almost any liver injury in the neonatal period may increase the serum AFP, but after the age of 6 months this occurs only in viral hepatitis, ataxia telangiectasia and congenital tyrosinosis. Maternal serum and amniotic fluid alpha-fetoprotein analyses have become important in the antenatal diagnosis of neural tube defects (Brock 1977).

### *Ceruloplasmin*

Ceruloplasmin is an $\alpha_2$-globulin of molecular weight 130 000 produced and catabolized in the liver (Walshe 1995). The gene controlling its production is located on chromosome 3. Each molecule contains six copper atoms that are not exchanged in vivo and it has a 4-day half-life. Ceruloplasmin contains more than 90% of the plasma copper. Most of the rest is bound to albumin (particularly in the portal blood postprandially), and a little is bound to amino acids and may be important in the transport of copper through cell membranes. The functions of ceruloplasmin are poorly understood. Heterozygotes for Wilson's disease may have very low plasma concentrations and yet remain well, while a few patients with Wilson's disease have normal concentrations (p. 962). Patients with hereditary ceruloplasmin deficiency have very low plasma ceruloplasmin concentrations and abnormal iron metabolism (p. 965) and this is because ceruloplasmin (also called ferroxidase) catalyzes the transfer of iron from storage sites in cells to transferrin. Transferrin is the main transporter of iron from storage sites to the bone marrow and consequently ceruloplasmin is important in determining the flow of iron to the marrow. Ceruloplasmin is also a weak oxidase for vasoactive amines in vitro, but this is unlikely to be important in vivo.

***Liver diseases.*** Normal or elevated ceruloplasmin concentrations are frequently found in liver diseases and elevated values are particularly common in cholestasis (Gault et al 1966, Prellwitz et al 1969). A low serum ceruloplasmin concentration is the single most important laboratory feature of Wilson's disease and frequently no ceruloplasmin can be found. Normal values occur in about 5% of patients, usually terminally or during phases of active disease, when they may result from hepatic inflammation or be due to increased circulating estrogen consequent on liver dysfunction (p. 920). Ceruloplasmin concentrations in Wilson's disease which are only moderately reduced may be increased significantly by pregnancy or estrogen therapy (Cartwright et al 1960). No structural abnormality of the ceruloplasmin molecule has been found in these patients. Low ceruloplasmin concentrations may also be found in fulminant hepatic failure and in severe advanced chronic liver diseases other than Wilson's disease (Walshe & Briggs 1962). This is due to failure of synthesis by the grossly damaged liver.

***Other diseases.*** Many factors other than liver disease influence the plasma ceruloplasmin concentration (Table 25.11). Increases in pregnancy and in women taking oral contraceptives (500–1100 mg/L) are attributed to estrogens (Tovey & Lathe 1968, Burrows & Pekala 1971). As ceruloplasmin is a positive acute-phase reactant, its concentration may be elevated in many diseases (Table 25.11). Reduced concentrations occur in malabsorption and when protein is lost from the gastrointestinal tract or from the kidney. Malnutrition rarely reduces the ceruloplasmin concentration unless protein deprivation (kwashiorkor) is severe (Gault et al 1966); low values in malabsorption are probably due to poor copper absorption (Sternlieb & Janowitz 1964).

### *Hemostasis*

The liver has two main functions in hemostasis. It produces inactive proteins of the coagulation and fibrinolytic

**Table 25.11** Abnormal plasma ceruloplasmin concentration in health and disease*

| Increased | Decreased |
|---|---|
| Pregnancy | Neonates |
| Drugs | Malabsorption |
| Estrogen | |
| Oral contraceptives | Protein-losing enteropathy |
| Infections | Nephrotic syndrome |
| Acute | |
| Chronic | Kwashiorkor |
| Myocardial infarction | Liver disease |
| Leukemia | Fulminant hepatic failure |
| Carcinoma† | Severe chronic liver disease |
| Liver disease | Wilson's disease |
| Acute and chronic hepatitis | |
| Cirrhosis | |
| Biliary obstruction | |

*Normal values: 230–440 mg/L
†With or without hepatic metastases

duces inactive proteins of the coagulation and fibrinolytic system, such as fibrinogen, factor VII and plasminogen. During coagulation these proteins are activated in a complex series of interactions with activator molecules in a network involving both positive and negative feedback pathways that result in the orderly formation of a hemostatic plug to limit hemorrhage. To prevent excessive coagulation, the function of the activated proteins is suppressed by specific inhibitors, such as antithrombin-3. In liver disease the clearance of these activated coagulant proteins is reduced. Thus, in patients with liver disease there may be decreased synthesis of coagulant proteins and an increased concentration of activated coagulation factors within the circulation (Mammen 1992, 1994).

The liver synthesizes coagulation factors. The vitamin K-dependent factors II, VII, IX and X are so named because this vitamin is an essential co-factor for γ-carboxy glutamyl transferase, an enzyme that adds a –COOH group to glutamyl residues in each peptide (Table 25.12). This enables each protein to take up a configuration allowing it to participate in the coagulation cascade. Vitamin K deficiency therefore results in a decreased level of function of factors II, VII, IX and X. Vitamin K deficiency is particularly likely to occur in cholestasis because it is fat soluble

**Table 25.12** Coagulation factors, the prothrombin time and changes in liver disease

| Factors affecting prothrombin time | Vitamin K-dependent factors | Changes in plasma factors by degree of liver disease: Moderate | Changes in plasma factors by degree of liver disease: Severe | Plasma half-life (h) |
|---|---|---|---|---|
| | | I ↑ | I ↓ | 96–144 |
| II | II | II ↓ | II ↓ | 55–80 |
| V | | V ↓ | V ↓ | 12 |
| VII | VII | VII ↓ | VII ↓ | 4–6 |
| | | VIII ↑ | VIII ↓ | 12 |
| | IX | IX ↓ | IX ↓ | 18–24 |
| X | X | X ↓ | X ↓ | 52 |

and bile acids are required for efficient absorption from the intestine. The capacity to store vitamin K in the liver is limited and depletion can occur when intake has been impaired for 4 weeks.

In moderately severe liver disease there are often normal or raised concentrations of fibrinogen and factor VIII and reduced concentrations of factors II, V, VII, IX and X. The prothrombin time is particularly sensitive to deficiencies of factors V, VII and X (Table 25.12) and it is therefore a good simple test for assessing the synthetic capacity of the liver (once vitamin K deficiency has been excluded by giving 10 mg intravenously slowly at least 12 h prior to the test). Because factor VII has a short half-life of 5–7 h, the prothrombin time reflects rapid changes in the liver's synthetic capacity in acute hepatitis or fulminant hepatic failure.

In severe liver disease the fibrinogen and factor VIII levels may fall, resulting in a prolonged APTT (activated partial thromboplastin time) and severe thrombocytopenia may also be observed. These changes probably reflect decreased synthesis and a consumptive coagulopathy secondary to increased activation of the coagulation system due to hepatocyte and endothelial cell damage and reduced hepatic clearance of activated clotting factors.

## HYALURONIC ACID (HYALURONATE)

Hyaluronic acid (HYA) is an unbranched high molecular weight polysaccharide that is widely distributed in connective tissue. It is produced mainly by mesenchymal cells, enters the circulation via lymph and is cleared by hepatic endothelial cells that possess a high affinity receptor for HYA (Eriksson et al 1983). The kidneys can excrete low molecular weight HYA, but this accounts for less than 1% of turnover. In the liver, HYA is synthesized primarily by the hepatic stellate cells (p. 714). Conditions such as severe endotoxemia and sepsis increase HYA production by increasing the number of stellate cells, by activation of stellate cells with subsequent increase of HYA production and by activation of the reticuloendothelial cells of the liver with the production of mediators causing proliferation of the stellate cells and increased HYA synthesis. Serum HYA can be measured using a radiometric assay (Pharmacia, Uppsala, Sweden). Its normal half-life in serum is about 2–5 min and this rapid turnover results in a concentration of about 20–40 μg/L at the age of 30–40 years, with an upper limit of 100 μg/L at the age of 60–70 years in normal individuals.

HYA belongs to a group of substances known as acidic glycosaminoglycans, which with collagen are major components of intercellular matrices. Acidic glycosaminoglycans including HYA increase in the liver with advancing cirrhosis in proportion to the hepatic collagen content (Murata et al 1985). Stellate cells are probably largely responsible for this collagen formation and collagenization of the space of Disse leads to capillarization of the hepatic sinusoids (p. 916) including loss of endothelial fenestrae and formation of a basement membrane (Schaffner & Popper 1963). Capillarization is accompanied by increased production of HYA and its release into the blood, as well as by reduced clearance of HYA from the circulation. Capillarization is associated with serum HYA concentrations above 200 μg/L and concentrations above 300 μg/L point strongly to cirrhosis, particularly in primary biliary cirrhosis, chronic hepatitis C infection and alcoholic liver disease (Takato et al 1993). High serum HYA concentrations are not restricted to chronic liver disease. They also occur in rheumatoid arthritis, scleroderma and osteoarthritis, where increased HYA production probably occurs in inflamed synovium, and in fulminant hepatic failure (Fraser et al 1986, Bramley et al 1991).

## LIPIDS

### Plasma lipids

From a chemical standpoint three main types of lipids are important. These are the fatty acids and their esters, cholesterol and its esters and the phospholipids. These lipids act as energy sources, as structural elements in cell membranes and as substrates for a number of important metabolic pathways. In order to fulfill these functions, the lipids must be transported between tissues in the predominantly aqueous bloodstream; this is achieved by physicochemical interactions between the lipids and a series of apoproteins, leading to the formation of lipoproteins that solubilize the insoluble cholesterol, cholesterol esters and fatty acids (triglycerides). In the plasma, fatty acids are also present in unesterified form, being bound to albumin which acts as a carrier.

### Plasma lipoproteins

The lipoproteins and their involvement with liver disease have been reviewed (Kroon & Powell 1992). In plasma the lipoproteins form a complex system that serves both to solubilize and transport lipids and to deliver these lipids to tissues in which they may form structural elements, be stored or be further metabolized. In the lipoproteins a central core of nonpolar lipids is surrounded by a monolayer of amphipathic phospholipid and protein. It is this monolayer that serves to stabilize the core. A schematic diagram of low density lipoprotein (LDL) is shown in Figure 25.11. A single copy of Apo-B is shown with a core of cholesterol esters and triglycerides. Phospholipids form a monolayer over the surface of the core. While a similar arrangement is found in the other classes of lipoproteins, apoproteins other than B are found on their surfaces and these migrate between different classes as metabolism of their lipid content proceeds. The apoproteins not only stabilize the lipid core but also act as cofactors for enzymes such as lecithin cholesterol acyl transferase (LCAT) and lipoprotein lipase and interact with cellular receptors for the lipoproteins.

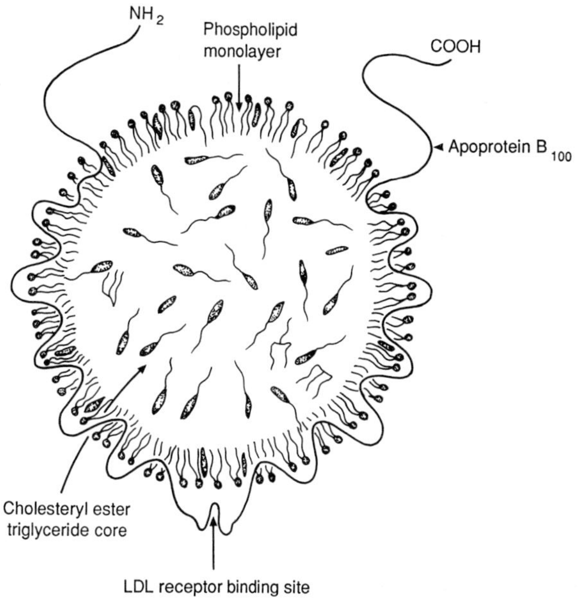


**Fig. 25.11** A schematic model of LDL in which a core of cholesterol esters and triglycerides is surrounded by a monolayer of phospholipid and cholesterol. Apolipoprotein $B_{100}$ is wrapped around the surface and is intimately associated with the phospholipid monolayer. The presence of a binding site for the LDL receptor is indicated (Reproduced with permission from Kroon & Powell 1992).

The lipoproteins have been classified according to their lipid content, their behavior in the ultracentrifuge or in electrophoresis systems and increasingly according to their apoprotein content. Five main classes of lipoproteins are recognized according to their behavior in the ultracentrifuge. It should be recognized that this classification reflects a "snapshot in time" among a series of particles whose lipid and protein content is in a dynamic state, with exchange of lipids and apoproteins between lipoprotein classes as an important feature.

***Chylomicrons.*** The chylomicrons are large particles that originate in the small intestinal mucosa. Their core composition is predominantly tryglycerides (95%) accompanied by small quantities of cholesterol ester. Between 1% and 2% of their mass is formed by apoprotein $B_{48}$, a subgroup of B that is synthesized in the small intestinal mucosa, along with small quantities of $A_1$, $A_{11}$, E and Cs. Chylomicrons act as transport mechanisms for dietary triglycerides, the progressive removal of which, through the action of lipoprotein lipase, leads to the formation of chylomicron remnants in the blood.

***Very low density lipoproteins (VLDL).*** These are synthesized and secreted by the liver. While they are smaller than the chylomicrons, they too have triglycerides (70%) and cholesterol ester (20%) as the main constituents of their core. Approximately 5% of their mass is protein, with apoproteins $B_{100}$, $C_{11}$, and E predominating. The apoprotein $B_{100}$ is synthesized in the liver; $C_1$ and $C_{11}$ are minor constituents. VLDL serve to deliver their load of triglycerides to adipose tissue and muscle (endogenous triglyceride transport) and in doing so lead to the progressive formation of intermediate density lipoproteins and finally low density lipoproteins.

***Intermediate density lipoproteins (IDL).*** These particles arise from the metabolism of VLDL in the blood with the removal of triglyceride and some of the apoproteins C and E. Some of the IDL are taken up by the liver by a receptor-mediated mechanism, thus delivering cholesterol ester to the liver for conversion to bile acids.

***Low density lipoproteins (LDL).*** These particles, which are cholesterol-rich (90%), are formed in the blood from IDL. They retain apoprotein $B_{100}$ as their principal apoprotein along with very small quantities of $C_{111}$ and E. These apoproteins constitute about 20% of the mass of LDL. LDL act as mediators of cholesterol ester transport, being taken up by a receptor-mediated mechanism. LDL receptors are widely distributed, the highest concentrations being found on liver, adrenal and gonadal cells. About 75% of LDL is taken up by the liver.

***High density lipoproteins (HDL).*** About 50% of the mass of HDL consists of apoproteins, principally $A_1$ and $A_{11}$, along with smaller quantities of $B_{100}$, $C_1$, $C_{111}$ and E. The core of this group of lipoproteins consists of about two-thirds cholesterol ester and one-third triglyceride. The cholesterol esters are formed by the action of the enzyme lecithin cholesterol acyl transferase (LCAT), which transfers a fatty acid chain from lecithin to cholesterol that has been accumulated by the HDL through a process of diffusion from cholesterol-rich tissues. HDL serve as a source of cholesterol esters that are, in turn, transferred to other classes of lipoproteins in the plasma. This exchange of cholesterol esters is mediated by cholesterol ester transfer protein (CETP). Cholesterol esters are transferred to VLDL and IDL in exchange for triglycerides that are hydrolyzed by hepatic lipase. The lifecycle of HDL consists of enlargement, due to the influx of cholesterol esters, followed by exchange of these with shrinkage produced by hydrolysis of the imported triglycerides. The sequential actions of LCAT and CETP are believed to mediate the process of transport of cholesterol from peripheral tissues to the liver, via LDL.

***Hepatic metabolism of lipoproteins.*** The liver plays an important role in the metabolism of the lipoproteins, both in their secretion and uptake and in the uptake of unesterified fatty acids that are bound to the surface of albumin. Chylomicron remnants are mainly removed by the liver by a receptor-mediated process that depends on an apo-E receptor. IDL, too, are removed by the liver by a receptor-mediated process that binds to apo-E on its surface. Most of the plasma LDL are removed from the circulation by the liver via the LDL receptor pathway (Brown & Goldstein 1986). Both apo-$B_{100}$ and apo-E are recognized by the LDL receptor. Bound LDL are internalized by the hepatocytes, forming an endocytic vesicle that fuses with the lysosomes with degradation of the LDL; the LDL receptor returns to the cell surface for further use.

Although there has been substantial progress in understanding the molecular basis of lipid metabolism and the role played therein by the liver (Powell & Kroon 1992), these are only now beginning to be translated into advances in understanding of abnormal plasma lipids in liver disease. Alterations in the concentrations of lipids in plasma and in the composition of the lipoproteins that occur in liver disease are further indications of the central role played by the liver in lipoprotein metabolism.

*Cholestasis*

Cholestasis is associated with increased plasma lipid concentrations, particularly marked increases in plasma cholesterol and phospholipids, and with the appearance of a number of unusual lipoproteins including lipoprotein-X (LP-X). LP-X is a bilamellar vesicular structure containing cholesterol and phospholipid along with albumin and apo-C. LP-X in the plasma is characteristic of cholestasis, but LP-X can also appear in LCAT deficiency. The mode of its formation is unclear but may be due to the regurgitation of biliary lipids that subsequently interact with plasma albumin (Manzato et al 1976). LP-X is taken up mainly by the cells of the lymphoreticular system.

While the raised plasma cholesterol concentrations in cholestatic liver disease can be explained, at least in part, by LP-X, the composition of the other lipoproteins is also abnormal. In patients with moderate degrees of primary biliary cirrhosis (PBC), both VLDL and LDL are slightly raised and marked increases in HDL are common. In patients with more advanced PBC, both LDL and LP-X are markedly increased and HDL concentrations are often low. Apoprotein concentrations too are often abnormal in PBC, apo-B and apo-$C_{11}$ being increased, apo-$A_1$ and $A_{11}$ being raised in mild PBC and reduced in more advanced cases (Jahn et al 1985). LP-X has been used in the clinical investigation of patients with cholestasis. Unfortunately, one-quarter of patients with intrahepatic disease also have LP-X in plasma and attempts to improve discrimination by including LCAT measurements have not proved successful (Magnani & Alaupovic 1976).

*Parenchymal liver disease*

Hypercholesterolemia and hypertriglyceridemia are both common in patients with parenchymal liver disease. A reduction in the concentration of cholesterol esters in the plasma is characteristic and is often the result of a reduced activity of LCAT. This is found in severe alcohol-related hepatocellular disease and may be accompanied by a reduction in HDL concentration (Chang et al 1986). It is not certain whether the reduction in LCAT activity is caused by a failure of LCAT synthesis by the liver, loss of the enzyme secondary to hepatic necrosis or the presence of an inhibitor in the blood. Both the lipid (cholesterol ester) and apoprotein content of the lipoproteins may be abnormal. The apo-$A_I$ and $A_{III}$ content of HDL may be reduced and in VLDL apo-E and apo-C may both be raised.

### *LCAT deficiency*

LCAT deficiency may be found secondary to liver disease or as a rare familial condition characterized by absence of LCAT activity in plasma (Gjone 1973). LCAT catalyzes the transfer of fatty acid acyl residues from phospholipids to cholesterol and in LCAT deficiency a reduced concentration of cholesterol esters in plasma is a characteristic abnormality. Patients with LCAT deficiency develop marked arcus senilis, impaired vision and a moderate normochromic anemia. They have proteinuria and death is usually due to uremia. Premature atheroma occurs. While gene therapy may have potential in treating this rare condition, it remains experimental.

## BILE ACID CIRCULATION

Bile acids are important in many physiological processes including the generation of bile flow, the excretion of cholesterol from the body and the absorption of fat-soluble substances from the small intestine. Reviews of the subject include those of Hofmann (1990), Vlahcevic et al (1991), Nathanson & Boyer (1991) and Hayes et al (1992).

### Bile acids

The bile acids are formed in the liver by a series of enzymatic steps that convert cholesterol into cholic and chenodeoxycholic acids. These are known as the primary acids (Fig. 25.12). The rate-limiting step in their synthesis is hydroxylation at the 7-α position, the rate of which depends on the overall flux of bile acids in the enterohepatic circulation, increased fecal losses being compensated for by raised synthesis rates in the liver. Cholic acid synthesis proceeds at a rate twice that of chenodeoxycholic acid, but the latter constitutes about 40% of the total bile acid content as it is more effectively conserved in the intestine (Molino et al 1986). The bile acids are also conjugated in the liver with glycine or taurine. Overall, three times as many glycine conjugates as taurine conjugates are formed.

Conjugation of the bile acids with glycine or taurine causes a reduction in the pKa values (pH at which bile acids are 50% ionized) by about 3 and 5 units respectively. This has important consequences for their solubility in the upper small intestine. At luminal pH the conjugates are essentially fully ionized and therefore more resistant to precipitation or the formation of insoluble calcium salts.

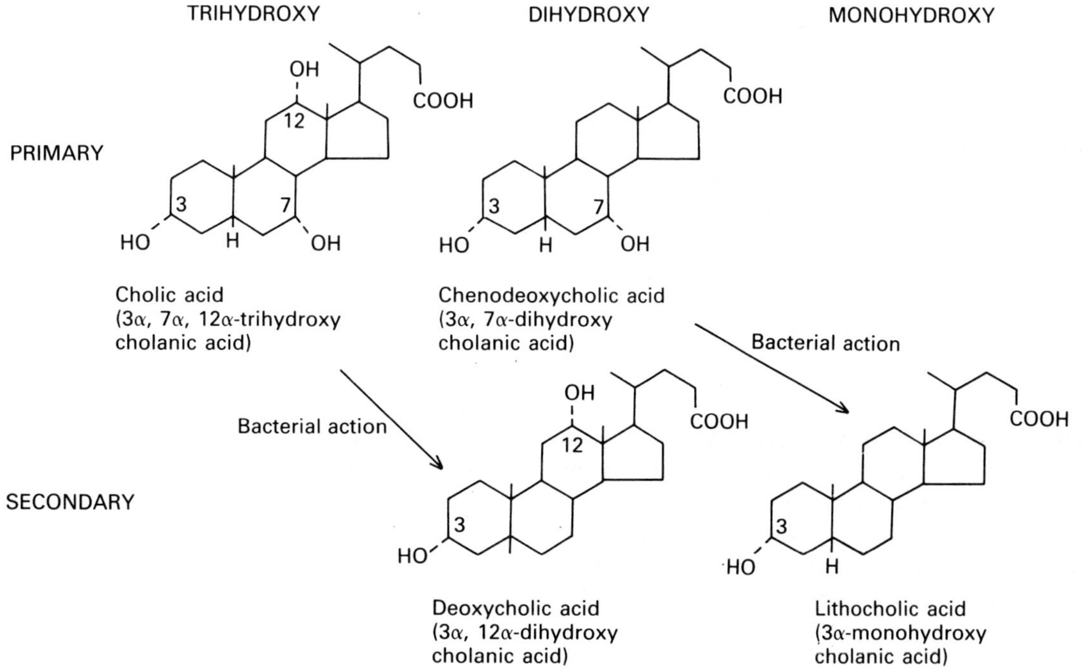


**Fig. 25.12** The important circulating bile acids of man, classified by the number of hydroxyl groups on the ring structure, and into primary and secondary bile acids (Heaton 1972)

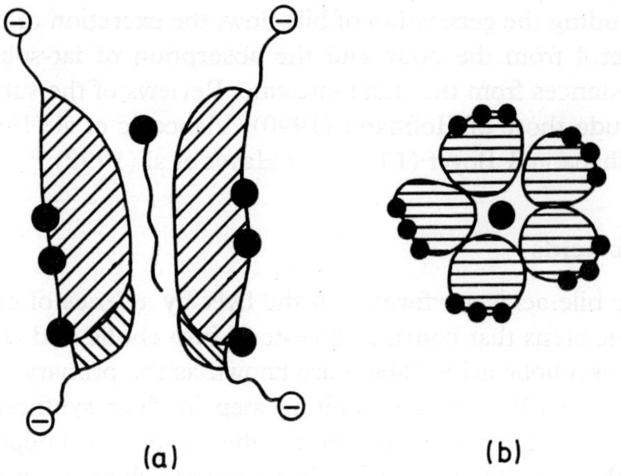


**Fig. 25.13** A bile acid micelle containing a fatty acid molecule — a non-swelling insoluble polar lipid (a) in longitudinal section and (b) in cross-section (Heaton 1972).

In the lower jejunum and ileum about one-quarter of the conjugates are deconjugated by bacterial enzymes. Bacterial action also affects the ring structure with the formation of different products collectively known as the secondary bile acids. The quantitatively more common of these are shown in Figure 25.12.

## Detergent-like properties of conjugated bile acids

The conjugated bile acids are amphipaths as they contain chemical groups (substituents) that are soluble in either water or fat. Given a sufficient concentration in aqueous solution, they can form aggregates called micelles (Fig. 25.13). The hydrophilic or polar parts of the molecule (the hydroxyl substituents on the ring stucture and the carbonyl or sulfonic acid group on the glycine or taurine respectively), which interact with water, form the external surface of the micelle, while the remaining hydrophobic parts that are fat soluble interact inside the micelle. It is implicit in the formation of micellar aggregates that there is a coexistent concentration of unaggregated molecules. This is called the critical micellar concentration and is approximately 4 mmol/L in bile and the small intestine.

## Enterohepatic circulation of bile acids

The bile acids are formed in the liver, secreted as conjugates in bile which passes into the duodenum, reabsorbed from the small intestine mainly at the terminal ileum and hence returned to the liver. This series of processes constitutes the enterohepatic circulation, a mechanism whereby the bile acids are conserved and kept at high concentration in bile, thereby promoting their essential detergent-like effects.

The formation of the bile acids is the main excretory pathway for cholesterol from the body. Conjugation with either glycine or taurine is an essential requirement for their secretion into bile in humans. Secretion of the conjugates takes place across the membrane of the biliary canaliculi against a concentration gradient that is probably as high as 5000:1 and is one of the main driving forces that stimulate bile flow (see below).

The conjugated bile acids are mostly conserved within the jejunal and ileal lumen and active reabsorption by a sodium- and energy-dependent process takes place in the terminal ileum. Some glycine-conjugated chenodeoxycholic acid is reabsorbed across the jejunum (Einarsson et al 1979) and a small quantity of bile acids that have been deconjugated by bacteria in the small intestine is also absorbed in the jejunum and ileum. Following absorption, these bile acids, principally conjugated forms with small amounts of deconjugates, enter the portal bloodstream. In turn they are cleared from portal blood, as it passes through the liver, by a receptor-mediated process, the efficiency of which varies with the type of bile acid being cleared.

The uptake of the bile acids in the terminal ileum is only about 95% efficient and those bile acids that pass through the ileocecal valve are subjected to bacterial action as they pass along the colon. This results in complete deconjugation of the bile acids and degradation with the formation of products that are collectively known as the secondary bile acids. These too are absorbed in part, the unabsorbed compounds being excreted in feces. The absorbed secondary bile acids are passed into the portal blood and are taken up by the liver and secreted into bile after conjugation with glycine or taurine. As a result of these processes conjugates of both the primary and the secondary bile acids appear in bile.

### *Bile formation*

Bile, the exocrine secretion of the liver, is isotonic with plasma. Humans produce about 600 ml daily, three-quarters from the hepatocytes and a quarter from the biliary epithelium.

***Hepatocyte bile formation.*** Hepatocytes make bile by creating osmotic gradients. Hydrostatic pressure is not important, as bile secretory pressure is higher than hepatic sinusoidal pressure. Anions are transported actively by membrane carriers into the biliary canaliculi where negative charges on the tight junctions (p. 712) prevent anion back-diffusion. Cations such as sodium then pass passively across the tight junctions into the canaliculi followed by water passing through or between the liver cells and creating bile and bile flow. Bile acids are the single most important anions generating bile flow (Inoue et al 1984), and there is a good relation between canalicular bile flow rate and biliary bile acid excretion (Fig. 25.14). This is known as bile acid-dependent bile flow. Other mechanisms must exist, as bile flow is maintained at very low bile acid concentrations, and this is known as bile acid-independent

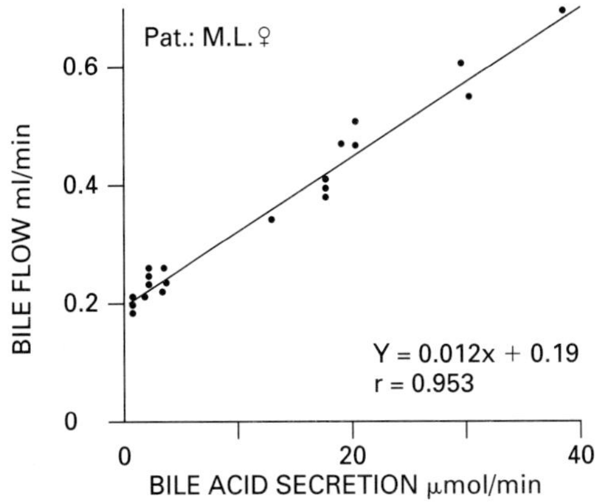


**Fig. 25.14** Relation between bile acid secretion and bile flow (Paumgartner 1977).

bile flow (Boyer & Klatskin 1970). Much less is known of the anions producing bile acid-independent bile flow, but these may include bicarbonate and glutathione. Bile acid-dependent bile flow seems to stem mainly from Zone I of the hepatic acinus (p. 712) and bile acid-independent bile formation from Zone III (Gumucio 1977). The microfilaments in the liver cells (p. 712) are probably important in bile formation, as they are concentrated around the biliary canaliculi and agents causing cholestasis cause canalicular dilatation, loss of canalicular villi, and damage to microfilaments (Phillips et al 1983). Bile acid-dependent and bile acid-independent mechanisms each account for about a half of normal hepatocyte bile formation.

***Biliary bile formation.*** The bile ducts and ductules distal to the biliary canaliculi contribute to bile volume, producing about a quarter of the bile secreted daily. The fluid produced by the biliary epithelium is rich in bicarbonate and its production is stimulated by secretin without any increase of bile acid production by liver cells (Buanes et al 1988). The gallbladder epithelium also influences bile volume but does so by concentrating bile. The mechanism for bile concentration depends on transcellular ion transport (Plevris & Bouchier 1995).

*Bile acids in bile*

The detergent-like properties of the conjugated bile acids are expressed principally in bile, in which phospholipid (principally lecithin) and cholesterol are incorporated into the micelles to form mixed micelles. This increases the solubility of the extremely nonpolar lipids cholesterol and cholesterol ester. In model systems that simulate bile, the solubility of cholesterol is enhanced by as much as 150 000-fold. In addition to these mixed micelles, liquid crystalline phases consisting of phospholipid, bile acid conjugates and cholesterol are present in bile (Patton & Carey 1979). Apoproteins A1, A11 and B are present in bile, but it is unlikely that these play a role in lipid handling therein (Sewell et al 1983).

Hepatic bile, containing the bile acid conjugates, flows down the bile ducts and is partitioned between the gallbladder and the common duct according to pressure changes in the biliary tree (p. 1197). Some bile is secreted continuously into the duodenum even in the fasting state (Mok et al 1980). In the gallbladder, the conjugated bile acids are concentrated by a factor of 5–10 and release of cholecystokinin from the intestinal mucosa in response to ingested food results in contraction of the gallbladder and a rapid rise in the concentrations of conjugated bile acids and lecithin in the duodenum. Bile acids in the intestine initiate a negative feedback inhibiting the release of cholecystokinin (Gomez et al 1988).

*Bile acids in the intestine*

In the intestine, the secretions from the pancreas, intestine and stomach dilute the concentrated bile that has been delivered by contraction of the gallbladder. This in turn dilutes the unaggregated bile acid conjugates, resulting in rearrangement of the lipid-containing micelles into polymolecular disks (Fig. 25.15) (Mazer et al 1980). The products of the hydrolysis of dietary triglyceride become incorporated into these polymolecular disks along with fat-soluble vitamins. In this way, the absorption of dietary fat, cholesterol and fat-soluble vitamins is promoted from the lumen of the jejunum. The following functions take place simultaneously in the intestine but are considered here individually.

***Emulsification.*** Together with monoglycerides, which are themselves the products of lipolysis, the bile acid/phospholipid disks promote the formation of an emulsion of dietary fat that aids lipolysis.

***Lipolysis.*** Hydrolysis of the dietary triglyceride, with the formation of monoglycerides, fatty acids and glycerol, is carried out by pancreatic lipase along with the peptide colipase, which is secreted by the pancreas and promotes the action of the lipase at the surface of the emulsion particles. The bile acid/phospholipid disks are involved in the adhesion of the colipase at the surface of the emulsion particles.

***Solubilization.*** The products of solubilization are further solubilized in the duodenal juice by complex physicochemical interaction with the disk-like particles. These solubilize the products of the hydrolysis, thereby increasing greatly their concentration at the luminal boundary of the unstirred water layer (p. 351) and increasing the concentration gradient and therefore the flux across it (Westergaard & Dietschy 1976).

Having completed their part in the handling of dietary lipid, the conjugated bile acids pass to the terminal ileum, where they are absorbed by an active process. About 20% of the bile acid conjugates are deconjugated during their passage through the small intestine. This is particularly the case in the ileum, in which the numbers of bacteria with deconjugating properties are higher than in the jejunum (p. 459). It is mainly the glycine conjugates that are deconreabsorbed at the terminal ileum by a process that is about 95% efficient. In the colon, the bacterial deconjugation is completed and the formation of the secondary bile acids proceeds. About one-half of the deoxycholic acid and one-fifth of the lithocholic acid are reabsorbed.

*Bile acids in portal blood*

Both conjugated and unconjugated primary and secondary bile acids enter the portal blood. The main source is the sodium- and energy-dependent absorption across the terminal ileum. In portal blood, the bile acids are bound to plasma protein, mainly albumin, and there is a limited association with the lipoproteins, particularly high density lipoprotein (HDL). The extraction of the bile acids from portal blood occurs at the hepatic sinusoids (p. 713) and results in a first-pass clearance (p. 840) of about 80% of chenodeoxycholic acid conjugates and 85% of cholic acid conjugates. Unconjugated acids are taken up less effectively than their corresponding conjugates. There appears to be a constant fractional uptake throughout the day in spite of the dramatic changes in flux rates that occur as a consequence of ingestion of food, contraction of the gallbladder and absorption of the bile acids in the post-prandial period.

*Bile acids in peripheral blood*

Bile acids not removed from the portal blood by the liver can be detected in the peripheral blood. Most are conjugates. In normal individuals, the total bile acid concentration is less than 4 μmol/L in the fasting state, with a rise to 10–12 μmol/L immediately following the ingestion of food. These changes are reflected in the concentrations of both conjugated cholic and deoxycholic acids (Beckett et al 1981). The ratio of cholic acid to chenodeoxycholic acid is about 1:7, reflecting both the short enterohepatic circulation of glycine conjugates of chenodeoxycholic acid and their low first-pass extraction by the liver. Owing to protein binding, little bile acid passes the renal glomerulus and what does is largely reabsorbed by the renal tubules.

***Clinical application.*** Tests of bile acid metabolism have included the serum bile acid concentration fasting and following a test meal when bile acids are returning to the liver in large amounts, the rate at which injected bile acids are removed from the blood and the pattern of bile acids in the blood (Douglas et al 1981). These tests can reveal liver damage when other liver function tests are normal, but in general they increase only slightly the information given by conventional tests (Festi et al 1983). Bile acid measurements have not become part of the routine assessment of patients with liver disease.

REFERENCES


Adams P C, Powell L W, Halliday J W 1988 Isolation of a human hepatic ferritin receptor. Hepatology 8: 719–721

Alpert E, Feller E R 1978 α-Fetoprotein (AFP) in benign liver disease. Evidence that normal liver regeneration does not induce AFP synthesis. Gastroenterology 74: 856–858

Bailey A, Robinson D, Dawson A M 1977 Does Gilbert's disease exist? Lancet 1: 931–933

Becker K L, Stauffer M H 1962 Evaluation of concentrations of serum alkaline phosphatase in hepatitis and obstructive jaundice. American Journal of the Medical Sciences 243: 222–227

Beckett G J, Douglas J G, Finlayson N D C, Percy-Robb I W 1981 Differential timing of maximal postprandial concentrations of plasma chenodeoxycholate and cholate: its variability and implications. Digestion 22: 248–254

Bell H, Tallaksen C, Sjåheim T et al 1993 Serum carbohydrate-deficient transferrin as a marker of alcohol consumption in patients with chronic liver diseases. Alcoholism: Clinical and Experimental Research 17: 246–252

Billing B H 1978 Twenty five years of progress in bilirubin metabolism (1952–77). Gut 19: 481–491

Boyer J L, Klatskin G 1970 Canalicular bile flow and bile secretory pressure. Gastroenterology: 59: 853–859

Bramley P N, Rathbone B J, Forbes M A, Cooper E H, Losowsky M S 1991 Serum hyaluronate as a marker of hepatic derangement in acute liver damage. Journal of Hepatology 13: 8–13

Brock D J H 1977 Prenatal diagnosis of neural tube defects. European Journal of Clinical Investigation 7: 465–472

Brown M S, Goldstein J L 1986 A receptor-mediated pathway for cholesterol homeostasis. Science 232: 34–47

Brumm C, Schulze C, Charels K, Morohoshi T, Klöppel G 1989 The significance of alpha-fetoprotein and other tumour markers in differential immunocytochemistry of primary liver tumours. Histopathology 14: 503–513

Buanes T, Grotmol T, Landsverk T, Raeder M G 1988 Secretin empties bile duct cell cytoplasm of vesicles when it initiates ductular $HCO_3$ secretion in pigs. Gastroenterology 95: 417–424

Burditt L J, Johnson M M, Johnson P J, Williams R 1994 Detection of hepatocellular carcinoma-specific alpha-fetoprotein by isoelectric focussing. Cancer 74: 25–29

Burnett J R, Lim C W, Mahoney G N, Crooke M J 1995 A method for the separation of delta bilirubin using Cibacron Blue affinity chromatography Clinica Chimica Acta 239: 37–46

Burrows S, Pekala B 1971 Serum copper and ceruloplasmin in pregnancy. American Journal of Obstetrics and Gynecology 109: 907–909

Card R T, Brown G M, Valberg L S 1964 Serum iron and iron-binding capacity in normal subjects. Canadian Medical Association Journal 90: 618–622

Cartwright G E, Markowitz H, Shields G S, Wintrobe M M 1960 Studies in copper metabolism XXIX. A critical analysis of serum copper and ceruloplasmin concentrations in normal subjects, patients with Wilson's disease and relatives of patients with Wilson's disease. American Journal of Medicine 28: 555–563

Chang L, Clifton P, Barter P, Mackinnon M 1986 High density lipoprotein subpopulations in chronic liver disease. Hepatology 6: 46–49

Chapman R W, Morgan M Y, Laulicht M, Hoffbrand A V, Sherlock S 1982 Hepatic iron stores and markers of iron overload in alcoholics and patients with idiopathic hemochromatosis. Digestive Diseases and Sciences 27: 909–916

Chen D-S, Sung J-L 1977 Serum alphafetoprotein in hepatocellular carcinoma. Cancer 40: 779–783

Chick J, Kreitman N, Plant M 1981 Mean cell volume and gamma-glutamyl-transpeptidase as markers of drinking in working men. Lancet 1: 1249–1251

Chowdhury J R, Chowdhury N R 1983 Conjugation and excretion of bilirubin. Seminars in Liver Disease 3: 11–23

Clermont R J, Chalmers T C 1967 The transaminase tests in liver disease. Medicine 46: 197–207

Crofton P M, Smith A F 1978 The properties and clinical significance of some electrophoretically slow forms of alkaline phosphatase. Clinica Chimica Acta 83: 235–247
Crosby W H, Likhite V V, O'Brien J E, Forman D 1974 Serum iron levels in ostensibly normal people. Journal of the American Medical Association 227: 310–312
Czaja A J, Wolf A M, Baggenstoss A H 1981 Laboratory assessment of severe chronic active liver disease during and after corticosteroid therapy: correlation of serum transaminase and gamma globulin levels with histologic features. Gastroenterology 80: 687–692
Di Bisceglie A M, Axiotis C A, Hoofnagle J H, Bacon B R 1992 Measurements of iron status in patients with chronic hepatitis Gastroenterology 102: 2108–2113
Douglas J G, Beckett G J, Nimmo I A, Finlayson N D C, Percy-Robb I W 1981 The clinical value of bile salt tests in anicteric liver disease. Gut 22: 141–148
Dragosics B, Ferenci P, Pesendorfer F, Wewalka F G 1976 Gamma-glutamyltranspeptidase (GGTP): its relationship to other enzymes for diagnosis in liver disease. In: Popper H, Schaffner F (eds) Progress in liver diseases, Vol 5. Grune and Stratton, New York, p 436–449
Edwards C Q, Griffen L M, Goldgar D, Drummond C, Skolnick M H, Kushner J P 1988 Prevalence of hemochromatosis among 11,065 presumably healthy blood donors. New England Journal of Medicine 318: 1355–1362
Einarsson K A, Grundy S M, Hardison W G M 1979 Enterohepatic circulation rates of cholic acid and chenodeoxycholic acid in man. Gut 20: 1078–1082
Eisenmenger W J, Slater R J 1953 Distribution and decay of $I^{131}$-tagged albumin and gammaglobulin in patients with cirrhosis. Journal of Clinical Investigation 32: 564
Eliakim M, Zlotnick A, Slavin S 1972 Gammopathy in liver disease. In: Popper H, Schaffner F (eds) Progress in liver diseases, Vol 4. Grune and Stratton, New York, p 403–417
Eriksson S, Fraser J R E, Laurent T C, Pertoft H, Smedsrod B 1983 Endothelial cells are the site of uptake and degradation of hyaluronic acid in the liver. Experimental Cell Research 144: 223–228
Feizi T 1968 Immunoglobulins in chronic liver disease. Gut 9: 193–198
Festi D, Morselli Labate A M, Roda A et al 1983 Diagnostic effectiveness of serum bile acids in liver diseases as evaluated by multivariate statistical methods. Hepatology 3: 707–713
Firkin F, Chesterman C, Penington D, Rush B (eds) 1989 De Gruchy's clinical haematology in medical practice, 5th edn. Blackwell Scientific Publications, Oxford
Fishman W H 1974 Perspectives on alkaline phosphatase isoenzymes. American Journal of Medicine 56: 617–650
Fishman W H, Bardawil W A, Habib H G, Anstiss C L, Green S 1972 The placental isoenzyme of alkaline phosphatase in sera of normal pregnancy. American Journal of Clinical Pathology 57: 65–74
Fraser J R E, Engström-Laurent A, Nyberg A, Laurent T C 1986 Removal of hyaluronic acid from the circulation in rheumatoid disease and primary biliary cirrhosis. Journal of Laboratory and Clinical Medicine 107: 79–85
Friedman L S, Dienstag J L, Watkins E et al 1987 Evaluation of blood donors with elevated serum alanine aminotransferase levels. Annals of Internal Medicine 107: 137–144
Fulop M, Katz S, Lawrence C 1971 Extreme hyperbilirubinemia. Archives of Internal Medicine 127: 254–258
Galambos J T, Wills C E 1978 Relationship between 505 paired liver tests and biopsies in 242 obese patients. Gastroenterology 74: 1191–1195
Gault M H, Stein J, Aronoff A 1966 Serum ceruloplasmin in hepatobiliary and other disorders: significance of abnormal values. Gastroenterology 50: 8–18
Gillon J, Hussey A J, Howe S P, Beckett G J, Prescott R J 1988 Post-transfusion non-A, non-B hepatitis: significance of raised ALT and anti-HBc in blood donors. Vox Sanguinis 54: 148–153
Gjone E 1973 Familial LCAT deficiency. Acta Medica Scandinavica 194: 353–356
Goldberg D M, Martin J V 1975 Role of gamma-glutamyl transpeptidase activity in the diagnosis of hepatobiliary disease. Digestion 12: 232–246
Goldie D J, McConnell A A 1990 Serum alanine transaminase (ALT) reference ranges estimated from blood donors. Journal of Clinical Pathology 43: 929–931
Gomez G, Upp J R, Lluis F et al 1988 Regulation of the release of cholecystokinin by bile salts in dogs and humans. Gastroenterology 94: 1036–1046
Gordon R S, Barrter F C, Waldmann T 1959 Idiopathic hypoalbuminemias. Annals of Internal Medicine 51: 553–576
Grace N D, Powell L W 1974 Iron storage disorders of the liver. Gastroenterology 67: 1257–1283
Greenberg F, Rose E, Alpert E 1990 Hereditary persistence of alpha-fetoprotein. Gastroenterology 98: 1083–1085
Gumucio D L, Gumucio J J, Wilson J A P et al 1984 Albumin influences sulfobromophthalein transport by hepatocytes of each acinar zone. American Journal of Physiology 246: G86–G95
Gumucio J J, Balabaud C, Miller D L et al 1978 Bile secretion and liver cell heterogeneity in the rat. Journal of Laboratory and Clinical Medicine 91: 350–362
Hayes K C, Livingston A, Trautwein E A 1992 Dietary impact on biliary lipids and gallstones. Annual Review of Nutrition 12: 299–326
Hobbs J R 1967 Serum proteins in liver disease. Proceedings of the Royal Society of Medicine 60: 1250–1254
Hofmann A F 1990 Bile acid secretion, bile flow and biliary lipid secretion in humans. Hepatology 12: 517–525
Hultcrantz R, Glaumann H, Linberg G, Nilsson L H 1986 Liver investigation in 149 asymptomatic patients with moderately elevated activities of serum aminotransferases. Scandinavian Journal of Gastroenterology 21: 109–113
Inoue M, Kinne E, Tram T, Arias I M 1984 Taurocholate transport by rat liver canalicular membrane vesicles. Evidence for the presence of a $NA^+$-independent transport system. Journal of Clinical Investigation 73: 659–663
Iyengar L, Srikantia S G 1970 Serum alkaline phosphatase in pregnancy. American Journal of Clinical Nutrition 23: 68–72
Jahn C E, Schaefer E J, Taam L A et al 1985 Lipoprotein abnormalities in primary biliary cirrhosis. Association with hepatic lipase inhibition as well as altered cholesterol esterification. Gastroenterology 89: 1266–1278
Kaplan M M 1972 Alkaline phosphatase. Gastroenterology 62: 452–468
Killenberg P G, Stevens R D, Wildermann R F, Wildermann N M 1980 The laboratory method as a variable in the interpretation of serum bilirubin fractionation. Gastroenterology 78: 1011–1015
Koch-Weser J, Sellers E M 1976 Binding of drugs to serum albumin. New England Journal of Medicine 294: 311–316, 526–531
Konijn A M, Hershko C 1977 Ferritin synthesis in inflammation. 1. Pathogenesis of impaired iron release. British Journal of Haematology 37: 7–16
Kroon P A, Powell E E 1992 Liver, lipoproteins and disease: I. Biochemistry of lipoprotein metabolism. Journal of Gastroenterology and Hepatology 7: 214–224
Kundrotas L W, Clement D J 1993 Serum alanine aminotransferase (ALT) elevation in asymptomatic US Air Force basic trainee blood donors. Digestive Diseases and Sciences 38: 2145–2150
Laker M F 1990 Liver function tests. British Medical Journal 301: 250–251
Landaw S A, Callahan E W Jr, Schmid R 1970 Catabolism of heme in vivo: comparison of the simultaneous production of bilirubin and carbon monoxide. Journal of Clinical Investigation 49: 914–925
Larson P H 1974 Serum proteins: diagnostic significance of electrophoretic patterns. Human Pathology 5: 629–640
Lauff J J, Kasper M E, Wu T-W, Ambrose R T 1982 Isolation and preliminary characterization of a fraction of bilirubin in serum that is firmly bound to protein. Clinical Chemistry 28: 629–637
Lipschitz D A, Cook J D, Finch C A 1974 A clinical evaluation of serum ferritin as an index of iron stores. New England Journal of Medicine 290: 1213–1216
Magnani H N, Alaupovic P 1976 Utilization of the quantitative assay of lipoprotein X in the differential diagnosis of extrahepatic obstructive jaundice and intrahepatic disease. Gastroenterology 71: 87–93
Mammen E F 1992 Coagulation abnormalities in liver disease. Hematology/Oncology Clinics of North America 6: 1247–1257
Mammen E F 1994 Coagulation defects in liver disease. Medical Clinics of North America 78: 545–554

Manzato E, Fellin R, Baggio G, Walch S, Neubeck W, Seidel D 1976 Formation of lipoprotein-X. Its relationship to bile compounds. Journal of Clinical Investigation 57: 1248–1260

Mazer N A, Benedek G B, Carey M C 1980 Quasielastic light-scattering studies of aqueous biliary lipid systems. Mixed micelle formation in bile salt–lecithin solutions. Biochemistry 19: 601–615

McDonagh A F, Palma L A, Lauff J J, Wu T-W 1984 Origin of mammalian biliprotein and rearrangement of bilirubin glucuronides in vivo in the rat. Journal of Clinical Investigation 74: 763–770

McEvoy M, Skrabanek P, Wright E, Powell D, McDonagh B 1981 Family with raised serum alkaline phosphatase activity in the absence of disease. British Medical Journal 282: 1272

McKenzie D, Henderson A R 1975 The occurrence of the Regan variant alkaline phosphatase isoenzyme in the serum of a case of adenocarcinoma of the stomach. Clinica Chimica Acta 62: 447–450

McMaster Y, Tannant R, Clubb J S, Neale F C, Posen S 1964 The mechanism of the elevation of serum alkaline phosphatase in pregnancy. Journal of Obstetrics and Gynaecology of the British Commonwealth 71: 735–739

Mok H Y I, von Bergmann K, Grundy S M 1980 Kinetics of the enterohepatic circulation during fasting: biliary lipid secretion and gallbladder storage. Gastroenterology 78: 1023–1033

Molino G, Hofmann A F, Cravetto C, Belforte G, Bona B 1986 Simulation of the metabolism and enterohepatic circulation of endogenous chenodeoxycholic acid in man using a physiological pharmacokinetic model. European Journal of Clinical Investigation 16: 397–414

Murata K, Ochiai Y, Akashio K 1985 Polydispersity of acidic glycosaminoglycan components in human liver and the changes at different stages in liver cirrhosis. Gastroenterology 89: 1248–1257

Nalpas B, Vassault A, Charpin S, Lacour B, Berthelot P 1986 Serum mitochondrial aspartate aminotransferase as a marker of chronic alcoholism: diagnostic value and interpretation in a liver unit. Hepatology 6: 608–614

Nathanson M H, Boyer J L 1991 Mechanisms and regulation of bile secretion. Hepatology 14: 551–566

Nishimura T, Yoshida Y, Watanabe F et al 1986 Blood level of mitochondrial aspartate aminotransferase as an indicator of the extent of ischemic necrosis of the rat liver. Hepatology 6: 701–707

Nomura F, Ohnishi K, Tanabe Y 1989 Clinical features and prognosis of hepatocellular carcinoma with reference to alpha-fetoprotein levels. Cancer 64: 1700–1707

Ostrow J D, Celic L 1984 Bilirubin chemistry, ionization and solubilization by bile salts. Hepatology 4: 38S–45S

Paradinas F J, Melia W M, Wilkinson M L et al 1982 High serum $B_{12}$ binding capacity as a marker of the fibrolamellar variant of hepatocellular carcinoma. British Medical Journal 285: 840–842

Patton J S, Carey M C 1979 Watching fat digestion. The formation of visible product phases by pancreatic lipase is described. Science 204: 145–148

Paumgartner G 1977 Physiology I. Bile acid-dependent bile flow. In: Bianchi L, Gerok W, Sickinger K (eds) Liver and bile. Lancaster, MTP Press. p 45

Phillips M J, Oshio C, Miyairi M, Watanabe S, Smith C R 1983 What is actin doing in the liver cell? Hepatology 3: 433–436

Plevris J N, Bouchier I A D 1995 Defective acid base regulation by the gallbladder epithelium and its significance for gall stone formation. Gut 37: 127–131

Post J, Patek A J 1942 Serum proteins in cirrhosis of the liver. I. Relation to prognosis and to formation of ascites. Archives of Internal Medicine 69: 67–82

Potter B J, Chapman R W G, Nunes R M, Sorrentino D, Sherlock S 1985 Transferrin metabolism in alcoholic liver disease. Hepatology 5: 714–721

Powell E E, Kroon P A 1992 Liver, lipoproteins and disease: II. Clinical relevance of disordered cholesterol metabolism in liver disease. Journal Gastroenterology and Hepatology 7: 225–231

Prellwitz W, Hammar C-H, Dudeck J 1969 Haptoglobin and caeruloplasmin in diseases of the liver and biliary tract. German Medical Monthly 14: 23

Price C P, Alberti K G M M 1979 Biochemical assessment of liver function. In: Wright R, Alberti K G M M, Karran S, Milward-Sadler G H (eds) Liver and biliary disease. W B Saunders, London, p 381–416

Prieto J, Barry M, Sherlock S 1975 Serum ferritin in patients with iron overload and with acute and chronic liver diseases. Gastroenterology 68: 525–533

Putnam F W (ed) 1975 The plasma proteins, Vols I and II, 2nd edn. Academic Press, London

Ramsöe K, Westergaard H, Jarnum S, Jörgensen M, Schiödt T, Tygstrup N 1970 Albumin and IgG turnover studies in patients with cirrhosis. Scandinavian Journal of Gastroenterology 5 (suppl 7): 25–31

Rosalki S B, Rau D 1972 Serum γ-glutamyltranspeptidase activity in alcoholism. Clinica Chimica Acta 39: 41–47

Rothschild M A, Oratz M, Schreiber S S 1972 Albumin synthesis. New England Journal of Medicine 286: 748–757, 816–823

Rothschild M A, Oratz M, Schreiber S S, Mongelli J 1986 The effects of ethanol and hyperosmotic perfusates on albumin synthesis and release. Hepatology 6: 1382–1385

Rothschild M A, Oratz M, Schreiber S S 1988 Serum albumin. Hepatology 8: 385–401

Ruoslahti E, Salaspuro M, Pihko H, Andersson L, Seppälä M 1974 Serum α-fetoprotein: diagnostic significance in liver disease. British Medical Journal 2: 527–529

Schaffner F, Popper H 1963 Capillarization of hepatic sinusoids in man. Gastroenterology 44: 239–242

Schiele F, Guilmin A-M, Detienne H, Siest G 1977 Gamma-glutamyltransferase activity in plasma: statistical distributions, individual variations and reference intervals. Clinical Chemistry 23: 1023–1028

Schmid R 1978 Bilirubin metabolism: state of the art. Gastroenterology 74: 1307–1312

Sewell R B, Mao S J T, Kawamoto T, LaRusso N F 1983 Apolipoproteins of high, low, and very low density lipoproteins in human bile. Journal of Lipid Research 24: 391–401

Shiffman M L, Luketic V A, Sanyal A J et al 1994 Hepatic lidocaine metabolism and liver histology in patients with chronic hepatitis and cirrhosis. Hepatology 19: 933–940

Shiou-Hwei Y, Chen P-J, Lai M-Y, Chen D-S 1996 Allelic loss on chromosomes 4q and 16q in hepatocellular carcinoma: association with elevated α-fetoprotein production. Gastroenterology 110: 184–192

Shora W, Danovich S H 1971 Marked elevation of serum transaminase activities in extrahepatic biliary tract disease. American Journal of Gastroenterology 55: 575–588

Silver H K B, Gold P, Shuster J, Javitt N B, Freedman S O, Finlayson N D C 1974 $\text{Alpha}_1$-fetoprotein in chronic liver disease. New England Journal of Medicine 291: 506–507

Stanley A J, Haydon G H, Piris J, Jarvis L M, Hayes P C 1996 Asessment of liver histology in patients with hepatitis C and normal transaminase levels. European Journal of Gastroenterology and Hepatology 8: 869–872

Stern R B, Knill-Jones R P, Williams R 1973 Pitfalls in the diagnosis of jaundice due to carcinoma of the pancreas or biliary tree. British Medical Journal 1: 533–534

Sternlieb I, Janowitz H D 1964 Absorption of copper in malabsorption syndromes. Journal of Clinical Investigation 43: 1049–1055

Stibler H 1991 Carbohydrate-deficient transferrin in serum: a new marker of potentially harmful alcohol consumption reviewed. Clinical Chemistry 37: 2029–2037

Stremmel W, Potter B J, Berk P D 1981 Rat liver sinusoidal plasma membranes do not contain a specific albumin receptor. Hepatology 1: 551

Strickland G T, Castell D O, Kronmal R A 1971 Prolonged observation on the liver function tests in infectious hepatitis. American Journal of Gastroenterology 55: 257–264

Takato U, Sadataka I, Takuji T et al 1993 Serum hyaluronate reflects hepatic sinusoidal capillarization. Gastroenterology 105: 475–481

Taketa K 1990 α-Fetoprotein: reevaluation in hepatology. Hepatology 12: 1420–1432

Tavill A S, Swain C P 1979 The protein secretory activities of the liver. In: Duthie H L, Wormsley K G (eds) Scientific basis of gastroenterology. Churchill Livingstone, Edinburgh, p 249–287

Tovey L A D, Lathe G H 1968 Caeruloplasmin and green plasma in

women taking oral contraceptives, in pregnant women, and in patients with rheumatoid arthritis. Lancet 2: 596–603
Tygstrup N 1973 The prognostic value of laboratory tests in liver disease. Scandinavian Journal of Gastroenterology 8 (suppl 19): 47–50
Van Ness M M, Diehl A M 1989 Is liver biopsy useful in the evaluation of patients with chronically elevated liver enzymes? Annals of Internal Medicine 111: 473–478
Villeneuve J-P, Infante-Rivard C, Ampelas M, Pomier-Layrargues G, Huet P-M, Marleau D 1986 Prognostic value of the aminopyrine breath test in cirrhotic patients. Hepatology 6: 928–931
Vlahcevic Z R, Heuman D M, Hylemon P B 1991 Regulation of bile acid synthesis. Hepatology 13: 590–600
Walshe J M 1995 Copper: not too little, not too much, but just right. Journal of the Royal College of Physicians of London 29: 280–288
Walshe J M, Briggs J 1962 Caeruloplasmin in liver disease. A diagnostic pitfall. Lancet 2: 263–265
Warnes T W 1972 Alkaline phosphatase. Gut 13: 926–937
Warnes T W, Hine P, Kay G 1977 Intestinal alkaline phosphatase in the diagnosis of liver disease. Gut 18: 274–278
Weisiger R, Gollan J, Ockner R 1981 Receptor for albumin on the liver cell surface may mediate uptake of fatty acids and other albumin-bound substances. Science 211: 1048–1051
Wejstal R, Hansson G, Lindholm A, Norkrans G 1988 Persistant alanine aminotransferase elevation in healthy Swedish blood donors – mainly caused by obesity. Vox Sanguinis 55: 152–156
Westergaard H, Dietschy J M 1976 The mechanism whereby bile acid micelles increase the rate of fatty acid and cholesterol uptake into the intestinal mucosal cell. Journal of Clinical Investigation 58: 97–108
Whitehead T P, Clarke C A, Whitfield A G W 1978 Biochemical and haematological markers of alcohol intake. Lancet 1: 978–981
Williams R, Speyer B E, Billing B H 1961 Serum haptoglobin in liver disease. Gut 2: 297–303
Wilson J W 1979 Inherited elevation of alkaline phosphatase activity in the absence of disease. New England Journal of Medicine 301: 983–986
Yedgar S, Carew T E, Pittman R C, Beltz W F, Steinberg D 1983 Tissue sites of catabolism of albumin in rabbits. American Journal of Physiology 244: E101–E107
Zimmerman H J, Seeff L B 1970 Enzymes in hepatic disease. In: Coodley E L (ed) Diagnostic enzymology. Lea and Febiger, Philadelphia, p 1–38

# 26. Immunology and infection in liver disease

*Graeme Alexander*

## INTRODUCTION

It is well recognized that the liver is a target for virus infection and immune-mediated diseases, but it is less often appreciated that the liver constitutes an integral part of the body's immune system. This is clearly demonstrated in patients with severe acute liver failure, in whom there is an astonishingly high incidence of bacterial and fungal infections (p. 812). Susceptibility to infection has been attributed to a number of factors, including low levels of complement, reduced opsonization and decreased phagocytosis (p. 773). Kupffer cell function and hepatic transport of immunoglobulin (Ig) A are two features of the liver's role in immune protection that deserve special attention.

***Kupffer cells.*** The Kupffer cells act as an effective barrier between the portal venous system and the systemic system by virtue of their placement among the sinusoidal lining cells, where they are anchored to endothelial cells (p. 713). These cells comprise 70% of the reticuloendothelial system. They are derived from the bone marrow and circulate in blood as monocytes before finally differentiating within the liver. They have the characteristics of peritoneal macrophages with an FC receptor for IgG (Ramadori et al 1986) and a receptor for endotoxin (Wardle 1987). They function as phagocytic cells and are a potential focal point for the initiation of immune responses and induction of tolerance. Kupffer cells have an enormous capacity for phagocytosis which is aided by the opsonin fibronectin synthesized in the liver. Decreased phagocytosis and impaired Kupffer cell function are features of chronic liver disease and of severe acute liver disease (p. 773).

Kupffer cells respond to endotoxin stimulation by the release of a series of cytokines including tumor necrosis factor (Dinarello et al 1986); in addition, they produce interferons and interleukin 1 and almost certainly play a critical role in liver regeneration after injury (Katsumoto et al 1989).

***Immunoglobulin A.*** Secretory IgA is the major immunoglobulin of the mucosal immune system (p. 400). Serum IgA is predominantly monomeric with a ratio of IgA1 to IgA2 of 4 to 1. Secretory IgA is mostly polymeric with equivalent concentrations of IgA1 and IgA2 (Delacroix et al 1982). The two subunits of polymeric IgA are linked by a joining peptide – the J-chain – and one glycoprotein secretory component that is the receptor for the transport of polymeric IgA across the mucosa (Solari & Kraehenbuhl 1985). It is often not appreciated that IgA is the major immunoglobulin of the gastrointestinal system, including the liver.

## IMMUNOGENETICS OF LIVER DISEASE

A major advance in immunology in the last decade has been the clarification of the mechanisms of antigen presentation and processing and the role that the major histocompatibility complex (MHC) class I and MHC class II antigens play. These are also called HLA (human leukocyte antigen) antigens.

### *HLA class I antigens*

The classic HLA class I antigens are cell surface glycoproteins found in greater or lesser density on the surface of virtually all nucleated cells. They are essential for interaction with $CD8^+$ lymphocytes and are therefore critical in the elimination of virus-infected cells. They comprise two polypeptide chains: a 45 kDa $\alpha$ heavy chain (comprising three external domains or regions – $\alpha_1$, $\alpha_2$, and $\alpha_3$) encoded on chromosome 6 and an invariant 12 kDa $\beta_2$-microglobulin molecule encoded on chromosome 15. There are three highly polymorphic class I gene loci that encode class I heavy chains of HLA class I A, B and Cw glycoproteins. Appropriate alignment of a $\beta$-pleated sheet and two $\alpha$-helixes formed from the $\alpha_1$ and $\alpha_2$ domains forms the floor of a groove that is supported by the $\alpha_3$ and $\beta_1$ domains. Recognition that this groove existed and is the site of antigen binding was a critical step in understanding the role of class I antigens.

Bjorkman et al (1987a,b) identified the groove and recognized the locations on HLA A2 critical for peptide binding. Subsequent studies demonstrated that changes in amino acids at specific positions in the groove alter the binding of peptides to class I antigens and thereby the efficiency of their presentation to T-cells (Ajitkumar et al 1988, McMichael et al 1988, Villadangos et al 1992). It is believed now that short peptides comprising fewer than 10 amino acids are presented on the cell surface by class I antigens. These peptides are derived from a complex antigen processing (Villadangos et al 1992). Intracellular antigens are degraded in the cytoplasm following binding to the large multifunctional protosome complex, an intracellular complex responsible for export and degradation of protein. Degraded peptides derived from this process are transported to the endoplasmic reticulum by a protein known as the transporter associated with antigen presentation (TAP). Within the endoplasmic reticulum the newly processed peptide is bound by newly synthesized HLA class I antigens; the HLA class I antigen–peptide complex is then transported via the Golgi to the cell membrane where it can be read by $CD8^+$ cells. It has been shown that different peptide class I complexes vary in immunogenicity and, more importantly, that peptides compete for binding. These features explain why class I antigens play an important role in predisposition to disease.

*HLA class II antigens*

Class II antigens are also heterodimers comprising α and β chains; both are encoded on chromosome 6. Class II antigens, in contrast to class I antigens, are expressed in the membrane of a restricted number of cell types. An antigen-binding cleft, similar to that for class I molecules, has been identified (Villadangos et al 1992). The peptide-binding groove has a different structure and the peptides that can bind within the groove are larger than those that bind to class I antigens. Class II antigens largely recognize peptide antigens derived from extracellular proteins and these are taken into the cell by endocytosis. The antigen is then concentrated in endosomes that fuse with the trans-golgi containing newly synthesized class II antigens transported from the endoplasmic reticulum. This fusion creates an acidic MHC class II compartment in which the protein is cleaved to form peptides that then bind to class II antigens. The resulting class II antigen–peptide complex can then be transported to the plasma membrane where it can interact with CD4-expressing T-cells.

## HLA and autoimmune hepatitis

A haplotype is a number of genes which are inherited as a unit and an association between haplotype HLA 1 B8-DR3 and autoimmune disease in general was recognized many years ago. This association included a link between autoimmune hepatitis and the HLA system (McKay 1972). The new ability to determine HLA class II polymorphism, using molecular techniques of restricted fragment length polymorphism analysis or of analysis of target gene segments amplified by the polymerase chain reaction with sequence-specific oligonucleotide probes, has allowed great progress to be made in autoimmune hepatitis and in other chronic liver diseases not thought previously to have an autoimmune basis.

Donaldson et al (1991a) confirmed that susceptibility to autoimmune hepatitis relates more closely to HLA DR than to either HLA A or HLA B. Although HLA DR3 was the most common association, when $DR3^+$ patients were excluded from analysis, a large proportion of those remaining were HLA $DR4^+$. Patients who were HLA $DR3^+$ were significantly younger at the outset of disease and relapse during treatment was more common. The notion that HLA DR types delineate two subsets of autoimmune hepatitis was supported by the observation that Japanese patients have a high frequency of HLA DR4 (Seki et al 1990). A more recent molecular analysis has shown the greatest risk of autoimmune hepatitis associated with the extended haplotype HLA A1-Ba-DRB1*0301-DRB3*0101-DQA1*0501-DQB1*0201 (Doherty et al 1994). The secondary association with HLA DR4 was confirmed and could be attributed to one particular DR4 allele (DRB1*0401). The most likely alleles related to susceptibility to autoimmune hepatitis are HLA DRB1*0401 and HLA DRB3*0101. It must be stressed that other components of the HLA system may also be relevant. For example, the HLA class III complement C4A and C4B null alleles in children have been associated with autoimmune hepatitis in Europe (Vergani et al 1985) and in North America (Scully et al 1993).

## HLA and primary sclerosing cholangitis

Conventional HLA typing has shown that primary sclerosing cholangitis has an HLA association, suggesting an autoimune basis for the disease, although no classic autoantigen–antibody system has been identified so far. Conventional serological testing has shown an association with HLA B8 and HLA DR3 (Donaldson et al 1991b). As with autoimmune hepatitis, when HLA $DR3^+$ patients were excluded, a secondary association was identified with HLA DR2. Again, as with autoimmune hepatitis, HLA DR3 was associated with an earlier onset of disease. Subsequently, a molecular approach confirmed the association to be with DRB3*0101 and these patients had a reduced survival compared to those without DRB3*0101 (DRB1*0301) (Farrant et al 1992). The two alleles DRB3*0101 and DRB5*0101 (which may also confer susceptibility) encode leucine at position 38 of the DRB polypeptide, whereas all other DRB alleles encode alanine at the same position. Thus, in this particular series susceptibility to and protection from primary sclerosing cholangitis could result from a single amino acid substitution at position 38 on the DRB molecule.

### HLA and primary biliary cirrhosis

Classic serotyping has failed to show any link between HLA and primary biliary cirrhosis, although primary biliary cirrhosis has all the features of an autoimmune disease. More recent studies using a molecular approach show that there is a linkage but that it is not strong. There is an increased frequency of HLA DR8 in studies reported from the United Kingdom even though most patients are HLA DR8$^{-}$ (Underhill et al 1992, Gregory et al 1993). This association has also been found in Japan, where HLA DR8 is more common in the general population (Maeda et al 1992, Seki et al 1993). The HLA DR8 haplotype appears to differ in Japanese and European patients and in the Japanese population DPB1*0501 appears to be the primary susceptibility allele.

## AUTOANTIBODIES IN HEALTHY SUBJECTS

It is important to recognize that autoantibodies occur in apparently healthy people and are not necessarily specific for particular diseases or groups of diseases. Hooper et al (1972) looked for antinuclear (ANA), antithyroid, antiparietal cell, antismooth muscle (SMA) and antimitochondrial antibodies as well as rheumatoid factor in over 90% of the healthy adults in a rural Australian town with a homogeneous Caucasian population. They found at least one autoantibody in 21.6% of subjects (males 13.7%, females 27.5%) and more than one in 3.6% of subjects (males 1.6%, females 5.5%). The frequency of autoantibodies rose with age and reached 48% in those over 85 years old. Antinuclear antibodies were found in 6.4%, the incidence rising with age and reaching 15–20% in persons over 65 years of age, antismooth muscle antibodies occurred in 1.5%, but only one person had antimitochondrial antibodies (0.03%). The antinuclear antibody titers found in this survey were low in over three-quarters of the subjects.

## PRIMARY BILIARY CIRRHOSIS

The diagnosis of primary biliary cirrhosis is generally easy, as a combination of cholestatic liver function tests and the antimitochondrial antibody is diagnostic (p. 940). Several features indicate a likely autoimmune etiology including the association with other diseases thought to have an autoimmune basis (Table 26.1).

**Table 26.1** Disease associations of primary biliary cirrhosis

| |
|---|
| *Common* |
| Sicca syndrome |
| Raynaud's disease |
| Scleroderma |
| CREST syndrome |
| Rheumatoid arthritis |
| Thyroid disease |
| Renal tubular acidosis |
| Pulmonary fibrosis |
| Pancreatic hyposecretion |
| *Uncommon* |
| Polymyositis |
| Systemic lupus erythematosus |
| Pernicious anemia |
| Gluten-sensitive enteropathy |

### Nonspecific abnormalities

A large number of nonspecific immunological abnormalities have been identified in primary biliary cirrhosis. There is a polyclonal elevation of serum immunoglobulin concentrations which is frequently disproportionate with regard to IgM, although that increase may in part be false because the IgM is monomeric. Rarely, there can be oligoclonal immunoglobulin production and in these circumstances the immunoglobulin usually has specificity for mitochondrial antigens (Roux et al 1974). Patients frequently have autoantibodies to smooth muscle, liver membrane, liver-specific protein, nuclear factor, rheumatoid factor and thyroid antigens. They also frequently have immune complex-like material in the serum, increased complement metabolism and decreased Kupffer cell function. Cellular immune abnormalities include skin test anergy, diminished T-cell proliferation, diminished natural killer cell activity and abnormal T-cell regulatory function.

### Autoantibodies

Immunological interest in primary biliary cirrhosis has focused increasingly on autoantibodies (Table 26.2) and particularly on the antimitochondrial antibody which is a specific marker of the disease.

#### *Antimitochondrial antibody*

This was recognized first using immunofluorescence

**Table 26.2** Autoantibodies commonly found in primary biliary cirrhosis

| | |
|---|---|
| Antimitochondrial | Nuclear |
| Rheumatoid factor | DNA |
| Smooth muscle | Histones |
| Thyroid | Ribonucleoprotein (RNP) |
| La | |

(Walker et al 1965) and shortly thereafter the nonorgan-nonspecies-specific staining was localized to mitochondria (Berg et al 1967). It then became apparent that the great majority of patients who had primary biliary cirrhosis had detectable antimitochondrial antibodies. Conversely, although antimitochondrial antibodies do occur in other diseases, including chronic infection, syphilis and myocarditis, the association with primary biliary cirrhosis is such that an asymptomatic individual with normal liver function tests who proves to have antimitochondrial antibody has a high chance of developing primary biliary cirrhosis (p. 938).

Further progress came when an antigen, termed M2, on the inner mitochondrial membrane was identified by sera from patients with primary biliary cirrhosis but not by sera from other patients who were antimitochondrial antibody-positive by immunofluorescence (Berg et al 1982). Two separate groups then showed independently that the 70 kDa M2 antigen (Gershwin et al 1987) was the E2 component of the pyruvate dehydrogenase complex (Van de Water et al 1988, Yeaman et al 1988). Two other major M2 peptides were recognized by Western blotting. These were found to be components of the 2-oxo-acid dehydrogenase multienzyme complex located in mammalian mitochondria (Bassendine & Yeaman 1990). Recognition of the target protein allowed the use of recombinant proteins as antigens in enzyme-linked immunosorbent assays (ELISAs). Combining pyruvate dehydrogenase complex E2 with recombinant E2 of the branched chain 2-oxo-acid dehydrogenase complex gave a sensitivity for antimitochondrial antibody of 96% in ELISAs using sera from patients with primary biliary cirrhosis (Van de Water et al 1989). It is probable that ELISAs using recombinant protein will eventually replace conventional immunofluorescence for the detection of antimitochondrial antibody.

Some of the fluorescence in the immunofluorescence test for antimitochondrial antibody is undoubtedly due to activity against other polypeptides of the outer mitochondrial membrane (i.e. the M4, M8 and M9 polypeptides). Antibodies against these antigens are not found regularly in patients with primary biliary cirrhosis and therefore cannot be used in diagnosis. However, there is evidence that some antibodies to these peptides, particularly to M4 and M8, occur preferentially in patients with progressive disease (Weber et al 1986, Klein et al 1990), whereas antibodies to M9 are associated with a more benign course (Klein et al 1988). Recent data suggest that M9 antibodies recognize an epitope of glycogen phosphorylase (Klein & Berg 1990) and M4 antibodies react with sulfite oxidase (Klein & Berg 1991). Thus, in future a combination of techniques may give sensitive and specific diagnostic and prognostic information.

*Antinuclear antibodies*

Antinuclear antibodies are generally nonspecific and occur in a variety of diseases (Table 26.3). However, two distinct antinuclear antibodies appear to be closely associated with primary biliary cirrhosis. One, found in the sera of up to 40% of patients and particularly associated with the sicca syndrome, is associated with multiple nuclear dots on immunofluorescence. Its polypeptide antigen has a molecular weight of around 100 kDa (Fritzler et al 1985, Szostecki et al 1987, Evans et al 1991, Fusconi et al 1991). A second antinuclear antibody associated with primary biliary cirrhosis shows nuclear ring staining on immunofluorescence (Lozano et al 1988). This antibody appears to react with a nuclear membrane glycoprotein (Lassoued et al 1988, Wozniak et al 1989, Courvalin et al 1990a, Wesierska-Gadek et al 1996) or with the nuclear envelope lamin B receptor (Courvalin et al 1990b). The clinical significance of these more recently identified nuclear antibodies is not yet known, but the observation that some patients with primary biliary cirrhosis have antinuclear antibody with the multiple nuclear dot pattern yet are antimitochondrial antibody-negative suggests that there may be a subgroup of patients recognized by this combination of antibodies (p. 939).

**Table 26.3** Antinuclear antibodies in extrahepatic diseases (Holborow 1978)

| |
|---|
| Systemic lupus erythematosus |
| Progressive systemic sclerosis |
| Rheumatoid arthritis |
| Juvenile chronic polyarthritis |
| Polymyositis/dermatomyositis |
| Sjögren's syndrome |
| Polyarteritis nodosa |
| Chronic discoid lupus erythematosus |
| Hyperglobulinemic purpura |
| Myasthenia gravis |
| Thymoma |
| Hashimoto's thyroiditis |
| Pernicious anemia |
| Ulcerative colitis |
| Chronic membranous glomerulonephritis |
| Cryptogenic fibrosing alveolitis |
| Asbestosis |
| Infectious mononucleosis |
| Dermatitis herpetiformis |

## AUTOIMMUNE CHOLANGITIS

This condition has all the clinical, biochemical and histological features of primary biliary cirrhosis except that antimitochondrial antibody tests are negative (p. 939). Antinuclear antibodies at high titer are usually present and smooth muscle antibodies are often found. Recently, an autoantibody to carbonic anhydrase has been reported in autoimmune cholangitis but not in primary biliary cirrhosis, suggesting that these may be separate diseases.

***Carbonic anhydrase antibody.*** Carbonic anhydrase is widely distributed in tissues and six isoenzymes have been described in humans. It is present in high concentration in the apical cytoplasm of bile duct epithelium, where it may be important in canalicular and ductular choleresis, but in only small amounts in hepatocytes (Buanes et al 1988). Autoantibodies to carbonic anhydrase (anti-CA) have been reported in five of six patients with autoimmune cholangitis one of 12 with primary biliary cirrhosis, none of 12 with primary sclerosing cholangitis and one of 12 with autoimmune hepatitis (Gordon et al 1995). This autoantibody may, therefore, prove a marker of autoimmune cholangitis and show that it is a different disease from primary biliary cirrhosis.

## PRIMARY SCLEROSING CHOLANGITIS

Primary sclerosing cholangitis is a cholestatic disease associated with hypergammaglobulinemia and high concentrations of serum immunoglobulin IgM.

### Autoantibodies

Many patients have smooth muscle antibody and antinuclear antibody, but usually in low titers. Children with primary sclerosing cholangitis typically have high serum IgG concentrations and such patients may have autoantibodies in high titer (Mieli-Vergani et al 1989). Antinuclear antibodies have been found in up to two-thirds of adult women (Zauli et al 1987).

Two other serum autoantibodies have been found that appear to be more specific for primary sclerosing cholangitis and/or ulcerative colitis. One was described originally as associated with portal tract antigens and is now known to be directed against neutrophils and the other is an anticolon antibody (Chapman et al 1986).

***Antineutrophil antibodies.*** Antineutrophil cytoplasmic antibodies (ANCA) have been described in systemic vasculitis and glomerulonephritis and serum antibodies giving a diffuse cytoplasmic staining pattern on immunofluorescence (cANCA) have been found to be very closely associated with Wegener's granulomatosis (Van der Woude et al 1985). Immunofluorescence tests have detected antineutrophil antibodies in patients with ulcerative colitis and primary sclerosing cholangitis, but these differ from cANCA in Wegener's granulomatosis as they give a perinuclear staining pattern and have accordingly been referred to as pANCA (Duerr et al 1991). Antibodies directed against an antigen associated specifically with the nuclei of tissue neutrophils have also been found at high titer in 84% of patients with primary sclerosing cholangitis and titers correlated with disease activity (Snook et al 1989).

A more recent study has analyzed the significance of the specificity of antibodies to neutrophils using Western blotting (Klein et al 1991). Eighty percent of sera from patients with primary sclerosing cholangitis were positive and five antigenic determinants were identified ranging from 30 kDa to 95 kDa. Immunofluorescence tests using neutrophils showed a characteristic perinuclear fluorescence in 87% of patients with primary sclerosing cholangitis. Such fluorescence occurred much less frequently in ulcerative colitis (17%), Crohn's disease (13%), primary biliary cirrhosis (13%), autoimmune hepatitis (16%) and alcoholic liver disease (10%) and was attributable to different antigens. The significance of these antibodies to neutrophil nuclear antigens is not known, but with respect to liver disorders they appear thus far to be relatively specific for primary sclerosing cholangitis. Their full place in diagnosis and prognosis remains to be proved.

***Anticolon antibodies.*** Anticolon antibodies have been found in 63% of patients with ulcerative colitis and primary sclerosing cholangitis but in only 17% with ulcerative colitis alone, in 16% with Crohn's disease alone and in no patient with primary sclerosing cholangitis alone. The anticolon antibodies did not crossreact with human liver. These autoantibodies are not used in clinical diagnosis.

### Other features

Patients with primary sclerosing cholangitis have elevated levels of circulating immune complexes (Bodenheimer et al 1983) and immune complexes can also be found in bile (Alberti-Flor et al 1983). There is no evidence thus far that these immune complexes contain any of the antibodies associated with primary sclerosing cholangitis. It is possible that immune complexes may result from abnormal Kupffer cell function associated with HLA B8 DR3 and chronic liver disease in general. More convincing evidence that circulating antibody may be relevant in patients with primary sclerosing cholangitis is complement activation via the classic pathway (Senaldi et al 1989). A number of studies of T-cell function in this disorder have been carried out. Areas of current research interest include activation markers, HLA DR, interleukin 2 receptors and the phenotype of the infiltrating cells in the liver and circulating cells. None of these experiments has helped in understanding the pathogenesis of the disease so far.

## AUTOIMMUNE HEPATITIS

Autoimmune hepatitis is a multisystem disease characterized by hypergammaglobulinemia, serum autoantibodies (Table 26.4) and in most circumstances a good clinical response to corticosteroids (p. 889). Undoubtedly, there are specific and nonspecific components to the hyperglobulinemia and production of autoantibodies. There is a broad defect of T-cell function in such patients that permits production of antibody in increased quantities (Nouri-Aria et al 1982), although undoubtedly the B-cells have a degree of autonomous function. The humoral responses characteristic of autoimmune hepatitis and their target antigens have been well studied and considerable

**Table 26.4** Autoantibodies associated with autoimmune hepatitis

| | |
|---|---|
| Antinuclear | Antisoluble liver antigens |
| Anti-smooth muscle | Anti-liver–pancreas |
| Antimitochondrial | Anti-liver-specific protein |
| Anti-liver–kidney microsomal | Antiasialoglycoprotein receptor |

progress has been made in this aspect. The T-cell responses, however, have been studied in less detail. Earlier experiments using crude preparations showed specific T-cell responses using a variety of assays for liver-specific protein (LSP) (O'Brien & Eddleston 1987). Many of these experiments are now being repeated using better techniques and more specific antigen preparations. Autoimmune hepatitis was thought initially to be a homogeneous disease, but more recent evidence has identified several subgroups classified in accordance with autoantibodies present (Table 26.5).

## Antinuclear antibodies

Antinuclear antibodies in autoimmune hepatitis are common but nonspecific.

## Anti ds-DNA

The occurrence of anti double-stranded (ds) DNA in autoimmune hepatitis is disputed. These antibodies have been reported as undetectable (Gurian et al 1985) and as common in autoimmune and other forms of chronic hepatitis (Wood et al 1986).

## Smooth muscle antibodies

Smooth muscle antibodies are found characteristically in high titer (>1:40) in autoimmune hepatitis and frequently in association with antinuclear antibodies (Table 26.6). They are identified by immunofluorescence using the smooth muscle in blood vessel walls. The association of smooth muscle antibody and antinuclear antibody in the absence of other antibodies is indicative of type 1 autoimmune hepatitis (p. 917). The target for smooth muscle antibody is F-actin (Lidman et al 1976). F-actin is closely associated with liver plasma cell membrane.

## Liver–kidney microsomal antibodies

Liver–kidney microsomal (LKM) antibodies were identified by their reaction with hepatocyte cytoplasm and proximal renal tubular epithelia and they were found to be directed against microsomes as their reactivity was absorbed by liver microsomal fractions (Rizzetto et al 1973). These antibodies were found to be closely associated with inflammatory liver disease and also occurred in a few patients with nonhepatic autoimmune disease (Smith et al 1974, Manns et al 1989a). The antibodies associated with autoimmune hepatitis have been called liver–kidney microsomal antibody type 1 (LKM1) (Homberg et al 1987). Subsequent studies have shown that they identify a subgroup of patients with autoimmune hepatitis now labeled type 2 (p. 887). A second liver–kidney microsomal antibody (LKM2) has been found to be associated with drug reactions and a third (LKM3) is associated with chronic hepatitis D virus infection (Crivelli et al 1983). Autoantigens for these autoantibodies have been identified (Table 26.7).

### *LKM1*

Molecular identification of microsomal antigens in autoimmune hepatitis has shown that LKM1 recognizes a 50 kDa antigen that is part of human cytochrome P-450 II D6 (Manns et al 1989b). Subsequent experiments have shown specific inhibition of the enzyme function by LKM1 antibody-positive sera. Cytochrome P-450 II D6 is a drug-metabolizing enzyme with an important role in the metabolism in humans of commonly used drugs (Gonzales et al 1988). More recently, the B-cell epitope

**Table 26.5** Classification of autoimmune (nonviral) chronic liver disease in relation to circulating autoantibodies

| | ANA | LKM | SLA | SMA | AMA | Cortico-steroid sensitivity |
|---|---|---|---|---|---|---|
| Classic (autoimmune hepatitis type I) | + | – | – | – | – | + |
| LKM-positive (autoimmune hepatitis type II) | – | + | – | – | – | + |
| SLA-positive autoimmune hepatitis | – | – | + | +/– | +/– | + |
| SMA-positive autoimmune hepatitis (type I) | – | – | – | + | – | + |
| Primary biliary cirrhosis | – | – | – | + | + | – |
| Primary sclerosing cholangitis | + | – | – | +/– | – | – |

Note: ANA = antinuclear antibody; LKM = liver–kidney microsomal; SLA = soluble liver antigen; SMA = smooth muscle antibody; AMA = antimitochondrial antibody

**Table 26.6** Incidence and titer of anti-smooth muscle antibody in chronic active hepatitis and primary biliary cirrhosis (Kurki et al 1980)

| Disease | Number | Anti-smooth muscle antibody Titer | Positive (%) |
|---|---|---|---|
| CAH | 24 | 1:10 | 88 |
| | | 1:50 | 67 |
| | | 1:200 | 54 |
| | | 1:800 | 29 |
| PBC | 15 | 1:10 | 73 |
| | | 1:50 | 33 |
| | | 1:200 | 7 |
| | | 1:800 | – |

Note: CAH = chronic active hepatitis; PBC = primary biliary cirrhosis

**Table 26.7** Autoantigens in autoimmune liver disease

| | Size (kDa) | Character | Association |
|---|---|---|---|
| LKM1 | 50 | Cytochrome p-450 II D6 | Autoimmune hepatitis (type II) |
| LKM2 | 50 | Cytochrome p-450 II C9 | Drug-induced liver disease |
| LKM3 | 55 | UDP glucuronosyl-transferase | Chronic hepatitis D |
| LM | 50 | Cytochrome p-450 I A2 | Autoimmune hepatitis (type II) and drug-induced liver disease |

Note: LKM = liver–kidney microsomal; LM = liver membrane

has been localized on cytochrome P-450 II D6 and comprises a linear sequence of amino acids that are highly conserved among class II D cytochrome P-450s (Manns et al 1990a,b). A small proportion of patients who appear to have autoimmune type 2 hepatitis with LKM1 antibody in their sera have shown no reaction with recombinant P-450 II D6. In these patients, the target appears to be a distinct cytochrome, P-450 IA2 (Manns et al 1989b, Sacher et al 1990). Immunofluorescence has localized this antigen to the perivenous hepatocytes.

### *LKM2*

The antigen recognized by LKM2 has been identified as another cytochrome enzyme, P-450 II C9 (Beaune et al 1987). It has been proposed that a drug metabolized by that particular cytochrome or one of its reactive metabolites could bind to the cytochrome and become antigenic. LKM2 antibodies to this cytochrome have been identified in patients with tienilic acid hepatitis (Homberg et al 1984) and dihydralazine hepatitis (Bourdi et al 1990). By inference, it is possible that a similar process leads to antigen production when cytochrome P-450 II D6 or cytochrome P-450 I A2 is recognized by LKM1 antisera. However, in this instance it is not a drug that has been metabolized but an as yet unidentified environmental antigen.

### *LKM3*

LKM3 antibody has been recognized in about 10% of patients with chronic hepatitis D virus infection. A recent study has shown that these antibodies react with a series of microsomal antigens of molecular weight around 55 kDa and they are probably associated with uridine diphosphate glucuronosyl transferase (Philipp et al 1994). These enzymes are involved in drug metabolism as well as in glucuronidation of endogenous compounds. The functional effect of LKM3 antibody on this enzyme is unknown.

### *Pathogenicity*

It is uncertain whether the target antigens for LKM autoantibodies are involved from the beginning of the disease or whether the autoantibodies develop during the course of the disease (i.e. as a secondary phenomenon). A criticism raised against these antigens being a target for an autoimune response is that they are microsomal and may be inaccessible to the immune system. There is controversy over whether microsomal antigens can be expressed on the liver cell membrane.

## Other autoantibodies

Several autoantibodies have been found in autoimmune hepatitis that are of considerable intrinsic interest, but their clinical significance is unknown.

### *Antisoluble liver antigen*

Autoantibodies against cytosolic components have been recognized in autoimmune hepatitis, including antisoluble liver antigen (anti-SLA) and anti-liver–pancreas (anti-LP).

***Anti-SLA.*** SLA autoantibodies react specifically with cytokeratins 8 and 12 in the cytosol of liver cells, which seem to be the main antigens recognized by these antibodies (Wächter et al 1990). It is not known whether this antigen is expressed in human hepatocyte surface membranes, but it is not specific to the liver as it is also found in lung, pancreas, bowel, brain and thyroid tissue (Manns et al 1987). Three-quarters of patients with anti-SLA also have other autoantibodies, particularly SMA and ANA (Manns et al 1991), and patients with and without anti-SLA cannot be distinguished on clinical, biochemical, histological or prognostic grounds (Czaja et al 1993). Anti-SLA may identify occasional patients with autoimmune hepatitis but no other autoantibodies.

***Anti-LP.*** These autoantibodies react with unknown noncytokeratin cytosolic antigens in liver and pancreatic tissue (Meliconi et al 1987, Stechemesser et al 1993). At least two have been identified and called anti-LP1 and anti-LP2. They occur frequently in type I autoimmune hepatitis in association with SMA and may occasionally identify autoimmune hepatitis in patients without other autoantibodies.

*Anti-liver-specific membrane lipoprotein*

Patients with a variety of liver diseases associated with immune abnormalities have antibodies to a preparation called liver-specific membrane lipoprotein (LSP), which is a crude macromolecular preparation from normal liver containing liver plasma membranes. It contains two liver-specific antigens, one species-specific and one species-nonspecific. Antibodies to this preparation are identified in many liver diseases. The frequency and titers with which this antibody is found in autoimmune hepatitis are the same as in many other forms of liver disease. Long-term immunization with LSP has produced autoimmune hepatitis in rabbits, suggesting that LSP could have a pathogenetic role in the disease (Meyer zum Büschenfelde & Hopf 1974).

***Anti-asialoglycoprotein receptor.*** The hepatic asialoglycoprotein receptor has been identified as a component of LSP (McFarlane et al 1984). This receptor is expressed on the membrane of hepatocytes and is responsible for endocytic removal of galactose-terminating desialyted glycoproteins (McFarlane 1983). It can capture, display and internalize potential antigens, induce T-cell proliferation and activate cytotoxic T-cells (Poralla et al 1991). Antibodies to the asialoglycoprotein (ASGPR) receptor prepared from animal tissue lack disease specificity, but specific antihuman anti-ASGPR occurs in three-quarters of patients with clinically active autoimmune hepatitis compared to frequencies of 7% in chronic hepatitis B, 8% in alcoholic liver disease and 14% in PBC (Treichel et al 1990). Anti-ASGPR was found in 10% of patients with nonhepatic autoimmune disease and malignant disease but not in healthy people. Human anti-ASGPR may prove of value in monitoring the response to treatment, as antibody reactivity correlates with inflammatory reactivity and antibodies disappear during successful therapy and were found in only a third of patients in remission (Treichel et al 1990). Disappearance of antibodies prior to drug withdrawal might identify patients less likely to relapse (McFarlane et al 1984).

## ALCOHOLIC LIVER DISEASE

There is considerable evidence that a variety of immune processes occur in alcoholic liver disease, but the importance of these in producing liver damage remains controversial (p. 867). An individual predisposition to alcoholic liver disease may also be associated with particular MHC class I and II antigens, but this remains contentious. Some patients with alcoholic hepatitis may benefit from corticosteroid therapy (p. 878), and this could reflect the effect of corticosteroids on immune processes.

### Humoral immune responses

Alcoholic liver disease is associated with increased serum immunoglobulin concentration, particularly IgA. Kalsi et al (1983) showed that this increase is due mainly to polymeric IgA but also to monomeric IgA and that the increase is caused primarily by increased production by lymphocytes and not by failure of the liver to transport polymeric IgA into the bile. IgA may also be deposited in the perisinusoidal regions in the liver. This deposition is mainly of IgA2 produced predominantly by mucosal lymphocytes and it may be present as a component of immune complexes (Swerdlow & Chowdhury 1983). The effects of IgA in the liver are not known, but IgA is also deposited in the kidneys and may be responsible for renal damage (p. 1064). Antibodies to ethanol-altered hepatocytes have also been described in patients with alcoholic liver disease (MacSween et al 1981) and the cytotoxicity of these antibodies for liver cells may be closely related to alcohol metabolism, particularly in respect of acetaldehyde (Crossley et al 1986). Indeed, acetaldehyde-modified proteins in the liver may be the antigenic material against which humoral responses are directed (Koskinas et al 1992). Lymphocyte cytotoxicity for human hepatocytes has been shown in alcoholic liver disease and this is probably antibody dependent (Izumi et al 1983).

### Cell-mediated immune responses

T-cell responses to a number of mitogens are impaired in alcoholic liver disease, suggesting a broad defect of T-cell function, and there is a reduced production of interleukin 2 (Devière et al 1988, Bird et al 1989). The number of lymphocytes in peripheral blood is also reduced and there are alterations in the phenotype of circulating $CD4^+$ and $CD8^+$ cells (Alexander et al 1983). However, the circulating lymphocytes appear to be activated with increased expression of interleukin 2 transferrin receptor and HLA DR antigens (Devière et al 1988). The inflammatory infiltration in the liver characteristically includes $CD4^+$ and $CD8^+$ T-cells as well as neutrophils and other mononuclear cells and there is increased HLA class I expression on hepatocytes as well as MHC class II expression on infiltrating cells, indicating that localized cellular activation occurs in areas of tissue damage (Chedid et al 1993). Cytotoxic T-cells appear to be the main cells mediating hepatocyte damage in acute alcoholic hepatitis (Chedid et al 1993). ICAM-1, a cellular adhesion molecule, shows significantly increased expression in areas of tissue damage where the inflammatory cell infiltrate also expresses the ICAM-1 ligand LFA1 (Burra et al 1992). In addition, there are elevated circulating levels of ICAM-1, presumably released from activated T-cells, showing that lymphocyte activation is a feature of alcoholic liver disease.

### Cytokines

The mechanisms involved in cytokine production in alcoholic liver disease are uncertain, but there is no doubt that these mediators and amplifiers of inflammation are detected in high concentrations in alcoholic liver disease. Thus, there are increased serum concentrations and monocyte or hepatocyte production of interleukin 1, tumor necrosis factor α (TNFα), interleukin 6, interleukin 8 and transforming growth factor β (TGFβ) (Bird et al 1989, Khoruts et al 1991, Annoni et al 1992, McClain et al 1993). Interleukin 8 may promote recruitment of neutrophils and T-lymphocytes into the liver in acute alcoholic hepatitis (Thornton et al 1992) and interleukin 6 may be responsible for increased IgA concentrations (Devière et al 1989, 1992) and may enhance the expression of TNFα receptors on hepatocyte membranes (Van Bladel et al 1991). Circulating TNFα and interleukin 6 concentrations correlate with disease severity, including cachexia and muscle wasting (Felver et al 1990, Hill et al 1992), and, particularly in the case of TNFα, are associated with mortality (Bird et al 1990, Sheron et al 1991).

## VIRAL HEPATITIS

Humoral immune responses to hepatitis viruses A (p. 781), B (p. 785), C (p. 788), D (p. 789) and E (p. 791) are important in the diagnosis of infection with these organisms and they are considered elsewhere. Responses possibly related to the pathogenesis of disease due to these viruses are considered briefly here.

### Hepatitis A

The damage mediated by the hepatitis A virus (HAV) is thought to be due to a cytopathic effect. However, T-cells cytotoxic for liver cells circulate in hepatitis A and can be detected early in the disease and for up to 12 weeks after the onset of the illness (Vallbracht et al 1986). It is not known whether the humoral or the cell-mediated response is critical to elimination of the virus in the normal course of events. However, humoral immunity is protective, as shown by the efficacy of immune serum globulin in hepatitis A prophylaxis (p. 782). Circulating immune complexes occur in hepatitis A and these contain virus capsid polypeptides and HAV-RNA (i.e. intact virus) as well as immunoglobulin including specific anti-HAV (Margolis & Nainan 1990). In this regard, it is known that hepatitis A can, rarely, be transmitted by blood.

### Hepatitis B

Liver damage in hepatitis B virus (HBV) infection is thought to be due to the immune response to the virus rather than to the virus itself (p. 783). Elimination of the virus is often, but not always, associated with symptoms of acute hepatitis and where elimination is particularly fast, acute liver failure may develop (Gimson et al 1983, De Cock et al 1986). Cellular immune responses occur in acute hepatitis B and T-cell sensitization to several HBV antigens located on the viral coat, core and polymerase proteins is associated with acute elimination of the virus (Moradpour & Wands 1995). Some patients with hepatitis B virus infection develop polyarteritis nodosa (p. 799), glomerular nephritis (p. 799) or cryoglobulinemia (p. 800) which is associated with immune complexes that may include the HBV. The reasons for the development of chronic HBV infection are poorly understood, but patients with chronic infections show poor or undetectable cellular immune responses pointing to the importance of these responses in eliminating the virus. Impaired T-cell function would explain the increased susceptibility of neonates (p. 784), the elderly, immunodeficient and immunosuppressed individuals to chronic infection (Perrillo et al 1986).

Two clear phases of chronic HBV infection can be delineated (Alexander 1990). The first is characterized by high titers of HBsAg, HBV-DNA and HBeAg in the blood and little HBcAg, HBeAG or HBsAg in the liver. This is compatible with a state of immune tolerance of the virus, which is being exported readily from the liver to the blood. This state is associated with poor expression of HLA class I antigens and cellular adhesion molecules on the hepatocytes (Nagafuchi & Scheuer 1986, Pignatelli et al 1986). Later, and often suddenly, the liver becomes inflamed, hepatocyte necrosis occurs and the serum transaminase activity rises. This is associated with infiltration of T-cell lymphocytes and other mononuclear cells into the liver and the appearance of HLA class I antigens, cell adhesion molecules and viral antigens on the liver cell membranes (Hsu et al 1987). This intermediate phase eventually resolves and leads to the second phase of chronic infection with loss of the HBeAg in the blood, appearance of anti-HBe, reduction or loss of serum HBV-DNA and occasionally elimination of the virus. The reasons for these changes are unknown, but immune factors are clearly important.

Other factors affecting the course of HBV infection include the virus itself and the genetic constitution of the patient and the means whereby these operate probably include the immune system. The HBV genome has a relatively high mutation rate that can lead to mutants less susceptible to the immune defenses or able to escape the effects of prior vaccination (Moradpour & Wands 1995). The activity of the immune system may in its turn facilitate the emergence of such mutants by suppressing the parent virus. One well-recognized mutant, for example, does not produce HBeAg owing to the introduction of a stop codon in the precore region of the genome (Carman et al 1993). Finally, genetic factors in the host determining the immune response may be important in allowing chronic infection. Investigations related to HLA status in determining the outcome of infection have given contradictory findings, but a large recent study points to HLA status as important in determining recovery from HBV infection (Thursz et al 1995).

### Hepatitis C

Humoral responses to the hepatitis C virus (HCV) are well recognized and of considerable diagnostic value (p. 788), but little is known of the mechanisms whereby liver damage occurs or the virus is eliminated. No markers of immunity to the virus are known and viral replication occurs in spite of the presence of currently recognized antibodies. However, rapid progression of liver damage in patients with hypogammaglobulinemia suggests a role for humoral responses at least in controlling viral replication (Bjøro et al 1994). Hypogammaglobulinemic patients also retain a single virus genotype, suggesting that the absence of humoral antibody removes the immune pressure that leads to the appearance of new genotypes (Kurosaki et al 1993, Kumar et al 1994). Liver transplantation in chronic hepatitis C infection followed by infection of the graft is also associated with less antibody to hepatitis C virus and persistence of the original viral genotype (Féray et al 1992, Marzano et al 1994). Cytotoxic T-cell responses have been detected toward several viral components (Koziel et al 1993), but the role of these responses in producing liver damage, viral elimination and immunity is not known.

Autoimmune associations are now well recognized in chronic HCV infection, although the nature of this relation is poorly understood (Lunel 1994, Lunel et al 1994). HCV infection has been associated with immunologic disorders including thyroid diseases, Sjögren's syndrome, glomerulonephritis and polyarteritis nodosa and with an increased frequency of immunologic abnormalities such as cryoglobulinemia and autoantibodies including antinuclear antibody, smooth muscle antibody, LKM antibody, anti-GOR and rheumatoid factors. These associations may all be more frequent when the infection is treated with interferon (p. 895).

Particular interest has centered on LKM antibody and anti-GOR. LKM1 autoantibody, a marker for autoimmune hepatitis type 2, has been reported in chronic HCV infection. However, the LKM1 autoantibodies in these two conditions seem to be different, as a purified recombinant cytochrome P-450 II D6 antigen (p. 768) was recognized by almost all sera from patients with type 2 autoimmune hepatitis but infrequently by sera from patients with chronic HCV infection (Yamamoto et al 1993). Anti-GOR is an antibody found in chronic HCV infections in humans and in primates directed at a host antigen and it is therefore an autoantibody (Löhr et al 1994). This antigen however, shows significant homology with part of the HCV nucleocapsid, which may point to an explanation for induction of autoimmunity by the virus (Hosein et al 1992). Anti-GOR is thought to reflect specific hepatitis C-induced autoimmunity and GOR is therefore a HCV-specific autoantigen (or autoepitope). Patients with LKM1 autoantibodies and HCV infection frequently have anti-GOR, whereas patients with LKM1 autoantibodies and no HCV infection (i.e. autoimmune hepatitis type 2) have anti-GOR infrequently (p. 892).

### Hepatitis D

The hepatitis D virus depends on the hepatitis B virus for its replication (p. 789) and little is known of its pathogenicity. Occasionally, abnormal autoimmune reactions occur, as about 10% of hepatitis D virus infections are associated with the appearance of LKM3 autoantibodies in the blood (p. 769).

### Hepatitis E virus

The hepatitis E antigen has been identified in the cytoplasm of hepatocytes prior to biochemical evidence of liver damage in experimentally infected primates (Krawczynski & Bradley 1989). The means whereby the virus produces liver damage is unknown.

## INFECTION IN LIVER DISEASE

Infection can occur in any patient with liver disease but is particularly common in those with fulminant liver failure or decompensated chronic liver disease (Wyke 1989). Infection in such patients is important, as it may be difficult to detect and is often fatal.

### Etiology

There are many reasons for increased susceptibility to infection in fulminant hepatic failure and in cirrhosis.

***General factors.*** These include malnutrition, which is common in advanced cirrhosis, and other medical complications such as anemia and renal failure. Undernutrition is also a potent cause of immunodeficiency (Dowd & Heatley 1984); malnourished patients with cirrhosis are often anergic and this is associated with an increased mortality (O'Keefe et al 1980). Alcohol abuse is an important factor, partly because of its effects on nutrition and also because it too can impair the ability to combat infection (MacGregor 1986). Factors other than the liver disease itself may also be important. Iron, for example, increases the virulence of *Listeria monocytogenes* which can cause meningitis in patients with cirrhosis and this may be important in hemochromatosis (Van Asbeck et al 1982).

***Immune mechanisms.*** Many mechanisms for preventing and combatting infection are compromised in severe liver disease. Most information relates to chronic liver disease, where impaired cellular defense functions are most important, while in fulminant hepatic failure defects in humoral defense are more important (Rajkovic & Williams 1985). The normal hepatic reticulo-endothelial function of removing bacteria from the blood is diminished by a reduction in hepatic sinusoidal macrophages (Canalese et al 1982, Imawari et al 1985, Mills & Scheuer 1985) and by portasystemic shunts that allow bacteria to bypass the liver (Rimola et al 1984); the normal functions of the leukocytes (DeMeo & Andersen 1972) and the monocytes (Holdstock et al 1982), such as chemotaxis and phagocytosis, are reduced; lymphocyte responsiveness to antigenic challenge is impaired (O'Keefe et al 1980). Serum factors may be important in reducing the function of these cells (Holdstock et al 1982, Wyke et al 1982), the opsonizing capacity of the blood may be reduced by impaired fibronectin production (Gonzales-Calvin et al 1982, Naveau et al 1985) and the concentrations in the blood of complement components made by the liver may be low (Finlayson et al 1972, Wyke et al 1980). Deficient immunoglobulin and antibody production is probably not important in liver disease, but immunoglobulin function may sometimes be impaired (Fierer & Finley 1979).

## Iatrogenic factors

These are frequently important. Ill patients often undergo invasive procedures including intravascular cannulations of various types, bladder catheterization and endoscopy that can allow infective agents to enter the body. They are also given antibiotics that can promote the emergence of resistant organisms or drugs such as corticosteroids that impair immune responses.

## Acute hepatitis

Patients with uncomplicated acute hepatitis who have previously been well are not particularly susceptible to infection. However, infection is very common in fulminant hepatic failure (p. 812), occurring in about 90% of patients and usually within a few days of admission to hospital (Rolando et al 1990). Respiratory infection and bacteremia are most common, but urinary infection and infection of intravascular cannulation sites are also important. Two-thirds of bacterial infections are with Gram-positive organisms and a third of patients acquire a fungal infection.

## Chronic liver disease

Patients with chronic liver disease show an increased susceptibility to infection and the extent of this susceptibility is related to the severity of the liver disease and to alcohol abuse. Studies of bacteremia show that patients with cirrhosis are a significant subgroup. Du Pont & Spink (1969) found that 23 (2.7%) of 860 patients with Gram-negative bacteremia had cirrhosis, no source for the infections could be found and 14 (61%) died. Gransden et al (1985) found that 13 (4%) of 325 with pneumococcal bacteremia had cirrhosis, of whom six had endocarditis and two meningitis, and 10 (77%) died. Many of these patients were also alcoholic.

### *Bacteremia*

Bacteremia is common in patients with cirrhosis, particularly in those with decompensated disease and impaired reticulo-endothelial function where about a fifth develop bacteremia while in hospital (Rimola et al 1984). It is frequently not accompanied by the usual features of fever, rigors and leukocytosis. Often there is only a general deterioration in the patient's condition with a worsening of encephalopathy and it needs to be emphasized that early antibiotic treatment is important in these circumstances, as about half the patients die even when bacteremia is recognized and treated vigorously.

### *Localized infections*

Localized infections usually cause features similar to those seen in patients without liver disease. Sometimes, however, there are no features pointing to the site of the infection and all that is noted is a deterioration of the patient's general condition.

***Pneumonia.*** Pneumonia is common in cirrhosis, particularly associated with alcoholism, and is due frequently to *H. influenzae*, *K. pneumonia* and Gram-negative organisms. Predisposing factors include recumbency, marked ascites with restricted respiratory movement and aspiration during upper gastrointestinal bleeding or consequent on its investigation and treatment by endoscopy or balloon tamponade. Regular pharyngeal suction is important in prevention of pneumonia during gastrointestinal bleeding.

***Urinary infection.*** Urinary tract infection is common and occurs especially in decompensated cirrhosis where up to a quarter of patients acquire infections during hospital admission (Rimola et al 1984). This is often related to catherization of the bladder, which in turn is most frequent in iller patients. Urinary tract infection can occur in any form of cirrhosis but is most frequent in primary biliary cirrhosis for as yet unexplained reasons (Butler et al 1993).

***Fluid collections.*** Fluid collections are very liable to become infected in patients with cirrhosis. This occurs most frequently as spontaneous bacterial peritonitis in ascitic fluid where low ascites protein concentrations, low complement concentrations and poor opsonizing capacity predispose to infection (p. 1033). Infection may also localize in other fluid collections, leading to empyema in pleural effusion and to purulent pericarditis (Flaum 1976, Murray & Marks 1977).

***Other sites.*** Bacterial endocarditis is easily overlooked and carries a high mortality (Gransden et al 1985). It remains unresolved as to whether there is an increased occurrence of bacterial endocarditis in cirrhosis (Snyder et al 1977, McCashland et al 1994). Meningitis can also occur (Pollock et al 1984, Gransden et al 1985) and initially this may suggest only a worsening of encephalopathy (Kibbler et al 1985).

## Prevention and detection

Infection in patients with severe liver disease should be minimized by avoiding invasive procedures wherever possible. Information is not available regarding prophylactic antibiotics, but their use in selected patients undergoing invasive procedures seems reasonable. Such patients would include those with a history of infection, such as bacterial endocarditis or spontaneous bacterial peritonitis, those with severely decompensated disease and those who are immunosuppressed. Prophylactic treatment can be given following spontaneous bacterial peritonitis (p. 812).

Manifestations of infection are often few or absent in ill patients with fulminant hepatic failure or decompensated cirrhosis. Accordingly, culture of blood, urine, ascitic fluid (p. 1034), cannulation sites or drains should be done routinely in fulminant hepatic failure or whenever deterioration occurs in a patient with cirrhosis.

## Treatment

Broad-spectrum antibiotics such as cefotaxime should be given initially to ill or deteriorating patients pending the results of bacterial culture.

REFERENCES


Ajitkumar P, Geier S S, Kesari K V et al 1988 Evidence that multiple residues on both the α helices of the class I MHC molecule are simultaneously recognised by the T cell receptor. Cell 54: 47–56

Alberti-Flor J J, deMedina M, Jeffers L, Schiff E R 1983 Elevated immunoglobulins and immune complexes in the bile of patients with primary sclerosing cholangitis. Hepatology 3: 844

Alexander G J M 1990 Immunology of hepatitis B virus infection. British Medical Bulletin 46: 354–367

Alexander G J M, Nouri-Aria K-T, Eddleston A L W F, Williams R 1983 Contrasting relations between suppressor-cell function and suppressor-cell number in chronic liver disease. Lancet 1: 1291–1293

Annoni G, Weiner F R, Zern M A 1992 Increased transforming growth factor – β1 gene expression in human liver disease. Journal of Hepatology 14: 259–264

Bassendine M F, Yeaman S J 1990 Primary biliary cirrhosis: nature of autoantigens. Springer Seminars in Immunopathology 12: 73–83

Beaune Ph, Dansette P M, Mansuy D et al 1987 Human anti-endoplasmic reticulum autoantibodies appearing in a drug-induced hepatitis are directed against a human liver cytochrome P450 that hydroxylates the drug. Proceedings of the National Academy of Sciences of the United States of America 84: 551–555

Berg P A, Doniach D, Roitt I M 1967 Mitochondrial antibodies in primary biliary cirrhosis. I. Localisation of the antigen to mitochondrial membranes. Journal of Experimental Medicine 126: 277–290

Berg P A, Klein R, Lindenborn-Fotinos J, Kloppel W 1982 ATPase-associated antigen (M2): marker antigen for serological diagnosis of primary biliary cirrhosis. Lancet 2: 1423–1426

Bird G L A, Nouri-Aria K-T, Daniels H, Alexander G J M, Williams R 1989 Contrasts in interleukin-1 and interleukin-2 activity in alcoholic hepatitis and cirrhosis. Alcohol and Alcoholism 24: 541–546

Bird G L A, Sheron N, Goka J, Alexander G J, Williams R S 1990 Increased plasma tumor necrosis factor in severe alcoholic hepatitis. Annals of Internal Medicine 112: 917–920

Bjorkman P J, Saper M A, Samraoui B, Bennett W S, Strominger J L, Wiley D C 1987a Structure of human class I histocompatibility antigen HLA-A2. Nature 329: 506–512

Bjorkman P J, Saper M A, Samraoui B, Bennett W S, Strominger J L, Wiley D C 1987b The foreign antigen binding site and T cell recognition regions of class I histocompatibility antigens. Nature 329: 512–518

Bjøro K, Frøland S S, Yun Z, Samdal H H, Haaland T 1994 Hepatitis C infection in patients with primary hypogammaglobulinemia after treatment with contaminated immune globulin. New England Journal of Medicine 331: 1607–1611

Bodenheimer H C Jr, LaRusso N F, Thayer W R Jr, Charland C, Staples P J, Ludwig J 1983 Elevated circulating immune complexes in primary sclerosing cholangitis. Hepatology 3: 150–154

Bourdi M, Larrey D, Nataf J 1990 Anti-liver endoplasmic reticulum autoantibodies are directed against human cytochrome P4501A2. Journal of Clinical Investigation 85: 1967–1973

Buanes T, Grotmol T, Veel T, Landsverk T, Ridderstrale Y, Raeder M G 1988 Importance of carbonic anhydrase for canalicular and ductular choloresis in the pig. Acta Physiologica Scandinavica 13: 535–544

Burra P, Hubscher S G, Shaw J, Elias E, Adams D H 1992 Is the intercellular adhesion molecule-1/leukocyte function associated antigen 1 pathway of leukocyte adhesion involved in the tissue damage of alcoholic hepatitis? Gut 33: 268–271

Butler P, Valle F, Hamilton-Miller J M T, Brumfitt W, Baum H, Burroughs A K 1993 M2 mitochondrial antibodies and urinary rough mutant bacteria in patients with primary biliary cirrhosis and in patients with recurrent bacteriuria. Journal of Hepatology 17: 408–414

Canalese J, Gove C D, Gimson A E S, Wilkinson S P, Wardle E N, Williams R 1982 Reticuloendothelial system and hepatocyte function in fulminant hepatic failure. Gut 23: 265–269

Carman W, Thomas H, Domingo E 1993 Viral genetic variation: hepatitis B virus as a clinical example. Lancet 341: 349–353

Chapman R W, Cottone M, Selby W S, Shepherd H A, Sherlock S, Jewell D P 1986 Serum auto antibodies, ulcerative colitis and primary sclerosing cholangitis. Gut 27: 86–91

Chedid A, Mendenhall C L, Mortiz T E et al 1993 Cell-mediated hepatic injury in alcoholic liver disease. Gastroenterology 105: 254–266

Courvalin J-C, Lassoued K, Bartnik E, Blobel G, Wozniak R W 1990a The 210-kD nuclear envelope polypeptide recognized by human autoantibodies in primary biliary cirrhosis is the major glycoprotein of the nuclear pore. Journal of Clinical Investigation 86: 279–285

Courvalin J-C, Lassoued K, Worman H J, Blobel G 1990b Identification and characterisation of autoantibodies against the nuclear envelope lamin B receptor from patients with primary biliary cirrhosis. Journal of Experimental Medicine 172: 961–967

Crivelli O, Lavarini C, Chiaberge E et al 1983 Microsomal auto antibodies in chronic infection with the HBsAg associated delta (δ) agent. Clinical and Experimental Immunology 54: 232–238

Crossley I R, Neuberger J, Davis M, Williams R, Eddleston A L W F

1986 Ethanol metabolism in the generation of new antigenic determinants on liver cells. Gut 27: 186–189

Czaja A J, Carpenter H A, Manns M P 1993 Antibodies to soluble liver antigen, P450IID6, and mitochondrial complexes in chronic hepatitis. Gastroenterology 105: 1522–1528

De Cock K M, Govindarajan S, Valinluck B, Redeker A G 1986 Hepatitis B virus DNA in fulminant hepatitis B. Annals of Internal Medicine 105: 546–547

Delacroix D L, Dive C, Rambaud J C, Vaerman J P 1982 IgA subclasses in various secretions and in serum. Immunology 47: 383–385

DeMeo A N, Andersen B R 1972 Defective chemotaxis associated with a serum inhibitor in cirrhotic patients. New England Journal of Medicine 286: 735–740

Devière J, Denys C, Schandene L et al 1988 Decreased proliferative activity associated with activation markers in patients with alcoholic liver cirrhosis. Clinical and Experimental Immunology 72: 377–382

Devière J, Content J, Denys C, Vandenbussche P, Schandene L, Wybran J 1989 High interleukin-6 serum levels and increased production by leucocytes in alcoholic liver cirrhosis. Correlation with IgA serum levels and lymphokines production. Clinical and Experimental Immunology 77: 221–225

Devière J, Content J, Denys C et al 1992 Immunoglobulin A and interleukin 6 form a positive secretory feedback loop: a study of normal subjects and alcoholic cirrhotics. Gastroenterology 103: 1296–1301

Dinarello C A, Cannon J G, Wolff S M et al 1986 Tumor necrosis factor (cachectin) is an endogenous pyrogen and induces production of interleukin-1. Journal of Experimental Medicine 163: 1433–1450

Doherty D G, Donaldson P T, Underhill J A et al 1994 Allelic sequence variation in the HLA class II genes and proteins in patients with autoimmune hepatitis. Hepatology 19: 609–615

Donaldson P T, Doherty D G, Hayllar K M, McFarlane I G, Johnson P J, Williams R 1991a Susceptibility to autoimmune chronic active hepatitis: human leukocyte antigens DR4 and A1-B8-DR3 are independent risk factors. Hepatology 13: 701–706

Donaldson P T, Farrant J M, Wilkinson M L, Hayllar K, Portmann B C, Williams R 1991b Dual association of HLA DR2 and DR3 with primary sclerosing cholangitis. Hepatology 13: 129–133

Dowd P S, Heatley R V 1984 The influence of undernutrition on immunity. Clinical Science 66: 241–248

Duerr R H, Targan S R, Landers C J et al 1991 Neutrophil cytoplasmic antibodies: a link between primary sclerosing cholangitis and ulcerative colitis. Gastroenterology 100: 1385–1391

Du Pont H L, Spink W W 1969 Infections due to Gram-negative organisms: an analysis of 860 patients with bacteremia at the University of Minnesota Medical Center, 1958–1966. Medicine 48: 307–332

Evans J, Reuben A, Craft J 1991 PBC 95K, a 95-kilodalton nuclear autoantigen in primary biliary cirrhosis. Arthritis and Rheumatism 34: 731–736

Farrant J M, Doherty D G, Donaldson P T et al 1992 Amino acid substitutions at position 38 of the DRβ polypeptide confer susceptibility to and protection from primary sclerosing cholangitis. Hepatology 16: 390–395

Felver M E, Mezey E, McGuire M 1990 Plasma tumor necrosis factor alpha predicts decreased long-term survival in severe alcoholic hepatitis. Alcoholism: Clinical and Experimental Research 14: 255–259

Féray C, Samuel D, Thiers V et al 1992 Reinfection of liver graft by hepatitis C virus after liver transplantation. Journal of Clinical Investigation 89: 1361–1365

Fierer J, Finley F 1979 Deficient serum bactericidal activity against *Escherichia coli* in patients with cirrhosis of the liver. Journal of Clinical Investigation 63: 912–921

Finlayson N D C, Krohn K, Fauconnet M H, Anderson K E 1972 Significance of serum complement levels in chronic liver disease. Gastroenterology 63: 653–659

Flaum M A 1976 Spontaneous bacterial empyema in cirrhosis. Gastroenterology 70: 416–417

Fritzler M J, Valencia D W, McCarty G A 1985 Speckled pattern anti-nuclear antibodies resembling anticentromere antibodies. Arthritis and Rheumatism 27: 92–96

Fusconi M, Cassani F, Govoni M et al 1991 Antinuclear antibodies of primary biliary cirrhosis recognise 78-92-kD and 96-100-kD proteins of nuclear bodies. Clinical and Experimental Immunology 83: 291–297

Gershwin M E, Mackay I R, Sturgess A, Coppel R L 1987 Identification and specificity of a cDNA encoding the 70kD mitochondrial antigen recognised in primary biliary cirrhosis. Journal of Immunology 138: 3525–3531

Gimson A E S, Tedder R S, White Y S, Eddleston A L W F, Williams R 1983 Serological markers in fulminant hepatitis B. Gut 24: 615–617

Gonzales F J, Skoda R C, Kimura S et al 1988 Characterisation of the common genetic defect in humans deficient in debrisoquine metabolism. Nature 331: 442–446

Gonzales-Calvin J, Scully M F, Sanger Y et al 1982 Fibronectin in fulminant hepatic failure. British Medical Journal 285: 1231–1232

Gordon S C, Quattrociocchi-Longe T M, Khan B A et al 1995 Antibodies to carbonic anhydrase in patients with immune cholangiopathies. Gastroenterology 108: 1802–1809

Gransden W R, Eykyn S J, Phillips I 1985 Pneumococcal bacteraemia: 325 episodes diagnosed at St. Thomas's Hospital. British Medical Journal 290: 505–508

Gregory W L, Mehal W, Dunn A N et al 1993 Primary biliary cirrhosis: contribution of HLA class II allele DR8. Quarterly Journal of Medicine 86: 393–399

Gurian L E, Rogoff T M, Ware A J, Jordan R E, Combes B, Gillian J N 1985 The immunologic diagnosis of chronic active "autoimmune" hepatitis: distinction from systemic lupus erythematous. Hepatology 5: 397–402

Hill D B, Marsano L, Cohen D, Allen J, Shedlofsky S, McClain C J 1992 Increased plasma interleukin-6 concentrations in alcoholic hepatitis. Journal of Laboratory and Clinical Medicine 119: 547–552

Holborow E J 1978 The serology of connective tissue disorders. British Journal of Hospital Medicine 19: 250 and 257–258

Holdstock G, Leslie B, Hill S, Tanner A R, Wright R 1982 Monocyte function in cirrhosis. Journal of Clinical Pathology 35: 972–979

Homberg J C, Andre C, Abuaf N 1984 A new anti-liver-kidney microsome antibody (anti-LKM2) in tienilic acid-induced hepatitis. Clinical and Experimental Immunology 55: 561–570

Homberg J C, Abuaf N, Bernard O et al 1987 Chronic active hepatitis associated with anti-liver/kidney microsome antibody type I: a second type of "autoimmune hepatitis". Hepatology 7: 1333–1339

Hooper B, Whittingham S, Mathews J D, Mackay I R, Curnow D H 1972 Autoimmunity in a rural community. Clinical and Experimental Immunology 12: 79–87

Hosein B, Fang X, Wang C Y 1992 Anti-HCV, anti-GOR, and autoimmunity. Lancet 339: 871

Hsu H-C, Su I-J, Lai M-Y et al 1987 Biologic and prognostic significance of hepatocyte hepatitis B core antigen expression in the natural course of chronic hepatitis B virus infection. Journal of Hepatology 5: 45–50

Imawari M, Hughes R D, Gove C D 1985 Fibronectin and Kupffer cell function in fulminant hepatic failure. Digestive Diseases and Sciences 30: 1028–1033

Izumi N, Hasumura Y, Takeuchi J 1983 Lymphocyte cytotoxicity for autologous human hepatocytes in alcoholic liver disease. Clinical and Experimental Immunology 53: 219–224

Kalsi J, Delacroix D L, Hodgson H J F 1983 IgA in alcoholic cirrhosis. Clinical and Experimental Immunology 52: 499–504

Katsumoto F, Miyazaki K, Nakayama F 1989 Stimulation of DNA synthesis in hepatocytes of Kupffer cells after partial hepatectomy. Hepatology 9: 405–410

Khoruts A, Stahnke L, McClain C J, Logan G, Allen J I 1991 Circulating tumor necrosis factor, interleukin-1 and interleukin-6 concentrations in chronic alcoholic patients. Hepatology 13: 267–276

Kibbler C C, Jeffrey G P, Epstein O, McIntyre N 1985 Apparent portosystemic encephalopathy in patients with chronic liver disease. British Medical Journal 291: 42–43

Klein R, Berg P A 1990 Anti-M9 antibodies in sera from patients with primary biliary cirrhosis recognise an epitope of glycogen phosphorylase. Clinical and Experimental Immunology 81: 65–71

Klein R, Berg P A 1991 Anti-M4 antibodies in primary biliary cirrhosis react with sulphite oxidase, an enzyme of the mitochondrial inter-membrane space. Clinical and Experimental Immunology 84: 445–448

Klein R, Klöppel G, Fischer R, Fintelmann V, Müting D, Berg P A 1988 The antimitochondrial antibody anti M9: a marker for the diagnosis of early primary biliary cirrhosis. Journal of Hepatology 6: 299–306

Klein R, Klöppel G, Garbe W, Fintelmann V, Berg P A 1990 Antimitochondrial antibody profiles determined at early stages of primary biliary cirrhosis differentiate between a benign and a progressive course of the disease: a retrospective analysis of 76 patients over 6–18 years. Journal of Hepatology 12: 21–27

Klein R, Eisenburg, J, Weber P, Seibold F, Berg P A 1991 Significance and specificity of antibodies to neutrophils detected by western blotting for the serological diagnosis of primary sclerosing cholangitis. Hepatology 14: 1147–1152

Koskinas J, Kenna J G, Bird G L, Alexander G J M, Williams R 1992 Immunoglobulin A antibody to a 200-kilodalton cytosolic acetaldehyde adduct in alcoholic hepatitis. Gastroenterology 103: 1861–1867

Koziel M J, Afdhal N, Dudley D et al 1993 Hepatitis C virus (HCV)-specific cytotoxic T lymphocytes recognize epitopes in the core and envelope proteins of HCV. Journal of Virology 67: 7522–7532

Krawczynski K, Bradley D W 1989 Enterically transmitted non-A, non-B hepatitis: identification of virus-associated antigen in experimentally infected cynomolgus macaques. Journal of Infectious Diseases 159: 1042–1049

Kumar U, Monjardino J, Thomas H C 1994 Hypervariable region of hepatitis C virus envelope glycoprotein (E2/NS1) in an agammaglobulinemic patient. Gastroenterology 106: 1072–1075

Kurki P, Miettinen A, Linder E, Pikkarainen P, Vuoristo M, Salaspuro M P 1980 Different types of smooth muscle antibodies in chronic active hepatitis and primary biliary cirrhosis: their diagnostic and prognostic significance. Gut 21: 878–884

Kurosaki M, Enomoto N, Marumo F, Sato C 1993 Rapid sequence variation of the hypervariable region of hepatitis C virus during the course of chronic infection. Hepatology 18: 1293–1299

Lassoued K, Guilly M N, Andre C et al 1988 Autoantibodies to 200 kD polypeptide(s) of the nuclear envelope: a new serological marker of primary biliary cirrhosis. Clinical and Experimental Immunology 74: 283–288

Lidman K, Biberfeld G, Fragraeus A et al 1976 Anti-actin specificity of human smooth muscle antibodies in chronic active hepatitis. Clinical and Experimental Immunology 24: 266–272

Löhr H F, Gerken G, Michel G, Braun H-B, Meyer zum Büschenfelde K-H 1994 In vitro secretion of anti-GOR protein and anti-hepatitis C virus antibodies in patients with chronic hepatitis C. Gastroenterology 107: 1443–1448

Lozano F, Parés A, Borche L et al 1988 Autoantibodies against nuclear envelope-associated proteins in primary biliary cirrhosis. Hepatology 8: 930–938

Lunel F 1994 Hepatitis C virus and autoimmunity: fortuitous association or reality? Gastroenterology 107: 1550–1555

Lunel F, Musset L, Cacoub P et al 1994 Cryoglobulinemia in chronic liver diseases: role of hepatitis C virus and liver damage. Gastroenterology 106: 1291–1300

MacGregor R R 1986 Alcohol and immune defense. Journal of the American Medical Association 256: 1474–1479

MacSween R N M, Anthony R S, Farquharson M 1981 Antibodies to alcohol-altered hepatocytes in patients with alcoholic liver disease. Lancet 2: 803–804

Maeda T, Onoshi S, Saibara T, Iwasaki S, Yamamoto J 1992 HLA DRw8 and primary biliary cirrhosis. Gastroenterology 103: 1118–1119

Manns M, Gerken G, Kyriatsoulis A, Staritz M, Meyer zum Büschenfelde K H 1987 Characterisation of a new subgroup of autoimmune chronic active hepatitis by autoantibodies against a soluble liver antigen. Lancet 1: 292–294

Manns M, Johnson E F, Griffin K J 1989a Human recombinant LKM (P450 db1) antigen as diagnostic reagent for autoimmune hepatitis. Hepatology 10: 583

Manns M, Johnson E F, Griffin K J 1989b Major antigen of liver kidney microsomal autoantibodies in idiopathic autoimmune hepatitis is cytochrome P450 db1. Journal of Clinical Investigation 83: 1066–1072

Manns M, Griffin K J, Sullivan K F, Meyer zum Büschenfelde K-H, Johnson E F 1990a Molecular mimicry between intermediate early protein (IE175) of herpes simplex virus and cytochrome P450 db1 (IID6), a major autoantigen in autoimmune hepatitis. Hepatology 12: 907

Manns M P, Griffin K J, Quattrochi L C et al 1990b Identification of cytochrome p450 IA2 as a human autoantigen. Archives of Biochemistry and Biophysics 280: 229–232

Manns M P, Griffin K J, Sullivan K F, Johnson E F 1991 LKM-1 autoantibodies recognize a short linear sequence in P450IID6, a cytochrome P-450 monooxygenase. Journal of Clinical Investigation 88: 1370–1378

Margolis H S, Nainan O V 1990 Identification of virus components in circulating immune complexes isolated during hepatitis A virus infection. Hepatology 11: 31–37

Marzano A, Smedile A, Abate M et al 1994 Hepatitis type C after orthotopic liver transplantation: reinfection and disease recurrence. Journal of Hepatology 21: 961–965

McCashland T M, Sorrell M F, Zetterman R K 1994 Bacterial endocarditis in patients with chronic liver disease. American Journal of Gastroenterology 89: 924–927

McClain C, Hill D, Schmidt J, Diehl A M 1993 Cytokines and alcoholic liver disease. Seminars in Liver Disease 13: 170–182

McFarlane I G 1983 Hepatic clearance of serum glycoproteins. Clinical Science 64: 127–135

McFarlane I G, McFarlane B M, Major G N, Tolley P, Williams R 1984 Identification of the hepatic asialoglycoprotein receptor (hepatic lectin) as a component of liver specific membrane lipoprotein (LSP). Clinical and Experimental Immunology 55: 347–354

McKay I 1972 The prognosis of chronic hepatitis. Annals of Internal Medicine 77: 649–651

McMichael A J, Gotch F M, Santos-Aguado J, Strominger J L 1988 Effect of mutations and variations of HLA-A2 on recognition of a virus peptide epitope by cytotoxic T lymphocytes. Proceedings of the National Academy of Sciences of the United States of America 85: 9194–9198

Meliconi R, Facchini A, Miglio F, Gasbarrini G 1987 Antibodies to liver cytoplasmic protein complex in chronic hepatitis disease. Lancet 1: 683–684

Meyer zum Büschenfelde K-H, Hopf U 1974 Studies on the pathogenesis of experimental chronic active hepatitis in rabbits: induction of the disease and protective effect of allogenic liver specific protein. British Journal of Pathology 55: 498–508

Mieli-Vergani G, Lobo-Yeo A, McFarlane B M, McFarlane I G, Mowat A P, Vergani D 1989 Different immune mechanisms leading to autoimmunity in primary sclerosing cholangitis and autoimmune chronic active hepatitis of childhood. Hepatology 9: 198–203

Mills L R, Scheuer P J 1985 Hepatic sinusoidal macrophages in alcoholic liver disease. Journal of Pathology 147: 127–132

Moradpour D, Wands J R 1995 Understanding hepatitis B virus infection. New England Journal of Medicine 332: 1092–1093

Murray H W, Marks S J 1977 Spontaneous bacterial empyema, pericarditis, and peritonitis in cirrhosis. Gastroenterology 72: 772–773

Nagafuchi Y, Scheuer P J 1986 Expression of b2-microglobulin on hepatocytes in acute and chronic type B hepatitis. Hepatology 6: 20–23

Naveau S, Poynard T, Abella A et al 1985 Prognostic value of serum fibronectin concentration in alcoholic cirrhotic patients. Hepatology 5: 819–823

Nouri-Aria K T, Hegarty J E, Alexander G J M, Eddleston A L W F, Williams R 1982 Effect of corticosteroids on suppressor-cell activity in "autoimmune" and viral chronic active hepatitis. New England Journal of Medicine 307: 1301–1304

O'Brien C J, Eddleston A L W F 1987 Immunology of autoimmune and viral chronic active hepatitis. Ballière's Clinical Gastroenterology 1: 647–674

O'Keefe S J, El-Zayadi A R, Carraher T E, Davis M, Williams R 1980 Malnutrition and immunocompetence in patients with liver disease. Lancet 2: 615–617

Perrillo R P, Regenstein F G, Roodman S T 1986 Chronic hepatitis B in asymptomatic homosexual men with antibody to the human immunodeficiency virus. Annals of Internal Medicine 105: 382–383

Philipp T, Durazzo M, Trautwein C et al 1994 Recognition of uridine diphosphate glucuronosyl transferases of LKM-3 antibodies in chronic hepatitis D. Lancet 344: 578–581

Pignatelli M, Water S J, Brown D et al 1986 HLA class I antigens on the hepatocyte membrane during recovery from acute hepatitis B virus infection and during interferon therapy in chronic hepatitis B virus infection. Hepatology 6: 349–353

Pollock S S, Pollock T M, Harrison M J G 1984 Infection of the central nervous system by *Listeria monocytogenes*: a review of 54 adult and juvenile cases. Quarterly Journal of Medicine 53: 331–340

Poralla T, Trichel U, Löhr H, Fleischer B 1991 The asialoglycoprotein receptor as target structure in autoimmune liver diseases. Seminars in Liver Disease 11: 215–222

Rajkovic I A, Williams R 1985 Mechanisms of abnormalities in host defences against bacterial infection in liver disease. Clinical Science 68: 247–253

Ramadori G, Dienes H P, Burger R, Meuer S, Rieder H, Meyer zum Büschenfelde K-H 1986 Expression of Ia-antigens on guinea pig Kupffer cells. Studies with monoclonal antibodies. Journal of Hepatology 2: 208–217

Rimola A, Soto R, Bory F, Arroyo V, Piera C, Rodés J 1984 Reticuloendothelial system phagocytic activity in cirrhosis and its relation to bacterial infections and prognosis. Hepatology 4: 53–58

Rizzetto M, Swana G, Doniach D 1973 Microsomal antibodies in active chronic hepatitis and other disorders. Clinical and Experimental Immunology 15: 331–344

Roux M E B, Florin-Christensen A, Arana R M, Doniach D 1974 Paraproteins with antibody activity in acute viral hepatitis and chronic autoimmune liver diseases. Gut 15: 396–400

Sacher M, Blümel P, Thaler H, Manns M 1990 Chronic active hepatitis associated with vitiligo, nail dystrophy, alopecia and a new variant of LKM antibodies. Journal of Hepatology 10: 364–369

Scully L J, Toze C, Sengar D P S, Goldstein R 1993 Early-onset autoimmune hepatitis is associated with a C4A gene deletion. Gastroenterology 104: 1478–1484

Seki T, Kiyosawa K, Inoko H, Ota M 1990 Association of autoimmune hepatitis with HLA-Bw54 and DR4 in Japanese patients. Hepatology 12: 1300–1304

Seki T, Kiyosawa K, Ota M et al 1993 Association of primary biliary cirrhosis with human leukocyte antigen DPB1*0501 in Japanese patients. Hepatology 18: 73–78

Senaldi G, Donaldson P T, Magrin S et al 1989 Activation of the complement system in primary sclerosing cholangitis. Gastroenterology 97: 1430–1434

Sheron N, Bird G, Goka J, Alexander G, Williams R 1991 Elevated plasma interleukin-6 and increased severity and mortality in alcoholic hepatitis. Clinical and Experimental Immunology 84: 449–453

Smith M G M, Williams R, Walker G, Rizzetto M, Doniach D 1974 Hepatic disorders associated with liver kidney microsomal antibodies. British Medical Journal 2: 80–84

Snook J A, Chapman R W, Fleming K, Jewell D P 1989 Anti-neutrophil nuclear antibody in ulcerative colitis, Crohn's disease and primary sclerosing cholangitis. Clinical and Experimental Immunology 76: 30–33

Snyder N, Atterbury C E, Correia J P, Conn H O 1977 Increased concurrence of cirrhosis and bacterial endocarditis: a clinical and postmortem study. Gastroenterology 73: 1107–1113

Solari R, Kraehenbuhl J-P 1985 The biosynthesis of secretory component and its role in the transepithelial transport of IgA dimer. Immunology Today 6: 17–20

Stechemesser E, Klein R, Berg P A 1993 Characterization and clinical relevance of liver–pancreas antibodies in autoimmune hepatitis. Hepatology 18: 1–9

Swerdlow M A, Chowdhury L N 1983 IgA subclasses in liver tissues in alcoholic liver disease. American Journal of Clinical Pathology 80: 283–289

Szostecki C, Krippner H, Penner E, Bautz F A 1987 Autoimmune sera recognise a 100 kD nuclear protein antigen (sp-100). Clinical and Experimental Immunology 68: 108–116

Thornton A J, Ham J, Kunkel S L 1992 Kupffer cell-derived cytokines induce the synthesis of a leukocyte chemotactic peptide, interleukin-8, in human hepatoma and primary hepatocyte cultures. Hepatology 14: 1112–1122

Thursz M R, Kwiatkowski D, Allsopp C E M, Greenwood B M, Thomas H C, Hill A V S 1995 Association between an MHC class II allele and clearance of hepatitis B virus in the Gambia. New England Journal of Medicine 332: 1065–1069

Treichel U, Poralla T, Hess G, Manns M, Meyer zum Büschenfelde K-H 1990 Autoantibodies to human asialoglycoprotein receptor in autoimmune-type chronic hepatitis. Hepatology 11: 606–612

Underhill J, Donaldson P, Bray G, Doherty D, Portmann B, Williams R 1992 Susceptibility to primary biliary cirrhosis is associated with the HLA-DR8-DQB1*0402 haplotype. Hepatology 16: 1404–1408

Vallbracht A, Gabriel P, Maier K et al 1986 Cell-mediated cytotoxicity in hepatitis A virus infection. Hepatology 6: 1308–1314

Van Asbeck R S, Verbrugh H A, van Oost B A, Marx J J M, Imhof H W, Verhoef J 1982 *Listeria monocytogenes* meningitis and decreased phagocytosis associated with iron overload. British Medical Journal 284: 542–544

Van Bladel S, Libert C, Fiers W 1991 Interleukin-6 enhances the expression of tumor necrosis factor receptors on hepatoma cells and hepatocytes. Cytokine 3: 149–154

Van der Woude F J, Rasmussen N, Lobatto S et al 1985 Autoantibodies against neutrophils and monocytes: tool for diagnosis and marker of disease activity in Wegener's granulomatosis. Lancet 1: 425–429

Van de Water J, Fregeau D, Davis P et al 1988 Autoantibodies of primary biliary cirrhosis recognize dihydrolipoamide acetyltransferase and inhibit enzyme function. Journal of Immunology 141: 2321–2324

Van de Water J, Cooper A, Surh C D et al 1989 Detection of autoantibodies to recombinant mitochondrial proteins in patients with primary biliary cirrhosis. New England Journal of Medicine 320: 1377–1380

Vergani D, Wells L, Larcher V F et al 1985 Genetically determined low C4: a predisposing factor to autoimmune chronic active hepatitis. Lancet 2: 294–298

Villadangos J A, Galocha B, Lopez D, Calvo V, Lopez de Castro J A 1992 Role of binding pockets for amino-terminal peptide residues in HLA-B27 allorecognition. Journal of Immunology 149: 505–510

Wächter B, Kyriatsoulis A, Lohse A W, Gerken G, Meyer zum Büschenfelde K-H, Manns M 1990 Chracterisation of liver cytokeratin as a major target antigen of anti-SLA antibodies. Journal of Hepatology 11: 232–239

Walker J G, Doniach D, Roitt I M, Sherlock S 1965 Serological tests in diagnosis of primary biliary cirrhosis. Lancet 1: 827–831

Wardle E N 1987 Kuppfer cells and their function. Liver 7: 63–75

Weber P, Brenner J, Stechemesser E et al 1986 Characterization and clinical relevance of a new complement-fixing antibody – anti-M8 – in patients with primary biliary cirrhosis. Hepatology 6: 553–559

Wesierska-Gadek J, Hohenauer H, Hitchman E, Penner E 1996 Autoantibodies against nucleoporin p63 constitute a novel marker of primary biliary cirrhosis. Gastroenterology 110: 840–847

Wood J R, Czaja A J, Beaver S J et al 1986 Frequency and significance of double-stranded DNA in chronic active hepatitis. Hepatology 6: 976–980

Wozniak R W, Bartnik E, Blobel G 1989 Primary structure analysis of an integral membrane glycoprotein of the nuclear pore. Journal of Cell Biology 108: 2083–2092

Wyke R J 1989 Bacterial infections complicating liver disease. Ballière's Clinical Gastroenterology 3: 187–210

Wyke R J, Rajkovic I A, Eddleston A L W F, Williams R 1980 Defective opsonisation and complement deficiency in serum from patients with fulminant hepatic failure. Gut 21: 643–649

Wyke R J, Yousif-Kadaru A G M, Rajkovic I A 1982 Serum stimulatory activity and polymorphonuclear leucocyte movement in patients with fulminant hepatic failure. Clinical and Experimental Immunology 50: 442–449

Yamamoto A M, Cresteil D, Homberg J C, Alvarez F 1993 Characterization of anti-liver-kidney microsome antibody (anti-LKM1) from hepatitis C virus-positive and -negative sera. Gastroenterology 104: 1762–1767

Yeaman S J, Fussey S P M, Danner D J, James O F W, Mutimer D J, Bassendine M F 1988 Primary biliary cirrhosis: identification of two major M2 mitochondrial autoantigens. Lancet 1: 1067–1070

Zauli D, Schrumpf E, Crespi C, Cassani F, Fausa O, Aadland E 1987 An autoantibody profile in primary sclerosing cholangitis. Journal of Hepatology 5: 14–18

SECTION 6

# Hepatic infections

# 27. Viral hepatitis

*J. Main*

## INTRODUCTION

Many viruses can cause hepatitis, which can range from an asymptomatic and self-limiting process to life-threatening acute and chronic disease (Zuckerman & Thomas 1993). Advances in molecular biology and virological techniques have enabled us to identify the pathogens responsible for the majority of acute and chronic forms of viral hepatitis. Increased understanding of the virological and immunopathological mechanisms involved has facilitated the development of effective treatments for some patients.

## HEPATITIS A VIRUS

### Virology

Hepatitis A virus (HAV) is a single-stranded RNA virus and is classified as a member of the hepatovirus genus within the picornavirus species (Minor 1991). The virion is a spherical particle about 27 nm in diameter (Feinstone et al 1973). There are three major proteins, VP1–3, which make up the protein shell and the viral genome consists of 7480 nucleotides. In comparison with most picornaviruses, HAV is relatively stable in a range of environmental conditions including heating to 60°C for 60 min. HAV in feces can remain viable for 30 days. Electronmicroscopic detection of viral particles in the feces of hepatitis patients led to the development of diagnostic tests.

### Epidemiology and transmission

HAV is spread principally by the fecal–oral route and is a common virus worldwide. Widespread exposure to HAV occurs early in life in countries with poor levels of sanitation. More than 90% of 5-year-old children in Ethiopia have serological evidence of previous HAV infection compared with fewer than 10% of children in the Western world (Hadler 1991). With improving sanitation, a reduction in HAV infection is noted and this has occurred in the United Kingdom where fewer than 50% of adults now have evidence of previous HAV exposure. Person-to-person spread is particularly common among children, who are not too careful about handwashing, and school outbreaks are a problem in deprived areas. Foodborne outbreaks also occur and are often attributable to poor hygienic practice by foodhandlers. Shellfish are thought to concentrate HAV and are often collected in shallow waters by sewage outfalls. A large outbreak involving 292 301 cases of HAV was reported in Shanghai in 1988–89 due to consumption of hairy clams (Halliday et al 1991). Soft fruits such as strawberries and raspberries have also been implicated as the source of HAV in several small outbreaks and it is thought that the source may have been HAV-infected fruit pickers' urine. Stools from patients with hepatitis A should be regarded as infectious for at least 2 weeks from the time of onset of symptoms and particular care is required when nursing patients with diarrhea, as crossinfection of other patients and health care workers can occur (Centers for Disease Control 1977, Skidmore et al 1985). There have been a few reports of transfused blood and other blood products transmitting HAV. Outbreaks are commonly reported among homosexual men (Corey & Holmes 1980, Coutinho et al 1983).

### Clinical course

The incubation period is 2–7 weeks and HAV infection is usually a mild or subclinical illness (p. 795). There is therefore considerable underdiagnosis of HAV infection. The severity of the illness varies according to the age of the patient. More than 80% of adults are symptomatic and develop jaundice compared with only 5% of children under 5 years (Zachoval & Deinhart 1993). Relapsing hepatitis and cholestasis are occasional complications. The fatality rate is very low and chronic disease does not occur. In severe cases, liver failure and renal failure may develop.

### Diagnosis

The diagnostic test for acute HAV infection is the serum

IgM anti-HAV antibody, which is generally positive at the time of presentation and remains so for 3–4 months. The serum IgG anti-HAV test remains positive for life. HAV vaccine can also cause an initial IgM response followed by an IgG response (Fig. 27.1).

### Antiviral treatments

Generally, HAV is a mild self-limiting infection and no specific therapy is required. In a few cases, a prolonged cholestatic hepatitis may develop and corticosteroid therapy may be helpful (p. 797). Anecdotal reports suggest that interferon may be beneficial in severe HAV infection, but such therapy should not delay transfer to a specialist unit, as liver transplantation may be needed for fulminant hepatic failure (p. 1155).

### Prevention

Careful hygienic measures should help prevent spread of infection and other measures include adequate cooking of shellfish (Giusti & Gaeta 1981). Since the 1940s, passive immunization with normal human immune globulin (NHIG), γ-globulin, has been used for control of outbreaks and for travelers going to areas of high endemicity (Stokes & Neefe 1945, Hadler et al 1983, Winokur & Stapleton 1992). This only offers protection for up to 3 months and the efficacy is dependent on the presence of anti-HAV IgG in the blood donor population. This is declining in Western countries and there have been reports of failed prophylaxis. Immunoglobulin can be given to close contacts in an HAV outbreak and is thought to reduce the severity of the disease, even if given too late to prevent infection (Stokes & Neefe 1945). It seems effective if given within 2 weeks of exposure.

A major advance has been the development of a vaccine for HAV that appears safe and effective (Werzberger et al 1992). HAV is propagated in cell culture and then inactivated by exposure to formaldehyde. Doses are generally administered intramuscularly at 0 and 4 weeks with a booster dose given at 6–12 months. It is thought that this regimen should give at least 5–10 years of protection. Candidates for vaccination include foodhandlers, travelers to areas of poor sanitation and homosexual men. The current relatively high cost of the vaccine is unlikely to encourage mass immunization programs.

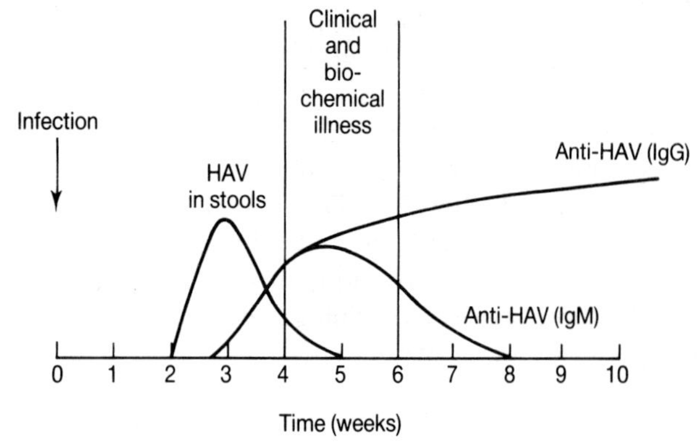


**Fig. 27.1** Occurrence of hepatitis A virus (HAV) in the stools and of antibody to HAV (anti-HAV) in the blood after HAV infection.

## HEPATITIS B VIRUS

### Virology

Hepatitis B virus (HBV) is one of the hepadna group of viruses, which are all small (42–47 nm) viruses. The hepadna viruses are hepatotropic and animal forms of the virus are seen in woodchucks (WHBV), Peking ducks, ground squirrels, herons and snow leopards (Summers et al 1978). HBV has a unique partially double-stranded DNA genome made up of 3182—3221 nucleotides (Robinson & Greenman 1974). HBV particles can be seen on electronmicroscopy of blood and are known as Dane particles after their discoverer (Dane et al 1970). The envelope region of the HBV genome (Fig. 27.2) encodes hepatitis B surface antigen (HBsAg), pre-S1 and pre-S2. The C region encodes hepatitis B core antigen (HBcAg) and e antigen (HBeAg). The P gene product is the viral polymerase, involved in viral replication, and the X gene product is thought to have transactivating activity. Hepatitis B virus is composed, therefore, of three major antigens: HBsAg, HBeAg and HBcAg. All antigens can be detected in an HBV infected liver and the presence of HBsAg and HBeAg in the blood is very useful diagnostically (below).

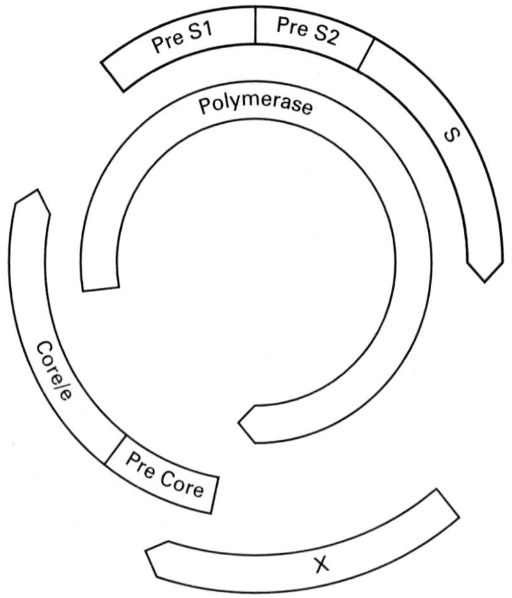


**Fig. 27.2** Diagrammatic representation of the hepatitis B virus genome.

HBsAg was discovered first in the blood of an Australian aborigine and termed Australia antigen (Blumberg et al 1967). The serum hepatitis (SH) antigen described subsequently proved to be the same antigen (Prince 1968). The HBsAg is found in the blood in the coat of complete virions (Dane particles) and as excess coat material seen electronmicroscopically as spheres and filaments (Fig. 27.3). There are three main HBsAg antigenic subtypes, which are mainly of epidemiological interest. All HBV isolates contain a common "a" determinant and "d" or "y" and "w" or "r" determinants. HBcAg is insoluble and can be demonstrated immunohistochemically in infected hepatocytes. It can be detected in the blood only in complete viral particles. HBeAg is not required for the formation of viral particles and its function is not known. It has been postulated that it is secreted by the virus to inhibit host immune response and produce tolerance of the HBV.

***Mutant viruses.*** It has been recognized recently that there are molecular variants or mutants of HBV. Mutation in the gene for HBsAg has been recognized following HBV vaccination or the administration of anti-HBs immune globulin (Carman et al 1990). Despite what would normally be considered protective levels of anti-HBs antibodies, patients have become infected with HBV and in some instances have become chronic carriers. Although only a few cases have been reported worldwide, there is concern that the introduction of mass vaccination programs may lead to further reports. A further molecular variant of clinical significance is associated with mutation in the precore gene of the virus (Carman et al 1989). When this occurs, HBeAg is no longer secreted and the mutant is referred to as a precore or e-minus mutant. The patients remain HBsAg positive and have anti-HBe antibodies. Continuing viral replication is recognized by the presence of HBV-DNA in serum and this is usually associated with continuing liver damage. Patients with fulminant hepatitis B are often HBeAg negative and it has been suggested that the absence of HBeAg and its possible inhibitory effect on the host immune response may allow more severe disease.

***Pathogenicity.*** The HBV does not seem to have any direct pathogenic effect on hepatocytes, and liver damage results from cellular immune responses to viral antigens in infected liver cells. There is a vigorous T-cell response to viral core, envelope and polymerase proteins in acute hepatitis B, but a weak or absent response in chronic infections. Factors determining susceptibility to infection and liability to chronic infection include genetic factors such as HLA types associated with increased likelihood of recovery, age at infection as in vertical infection at an early age leading to immune tolerance of the virus and viral mutation allowing the virus to escape immune recognition (Moradpour & Wands 1995).

### Epidemiology and transmission

It is estimated that there are 300 million chronic carriers of HBV worldwide. In some areas, such as south east Asia, carrier rates are as high as 20% and before the introduction of vaccination programs in countries like Taiwan,

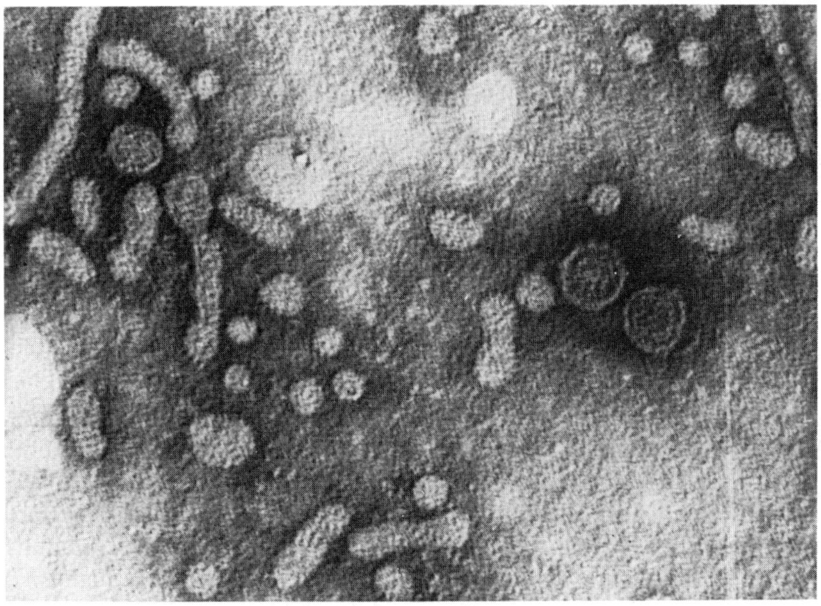

**Fig. 27.3** Electronmicrograph of the types of particles bearing the hepatitis B surface antigen in the blood. Note the small spheres, the filaments and the large spheres with an inner structure (Dane particles), which are the complete virions (phosphotungstic acid stain, ×120 000).

much of the spread was via vertical transmission. Transmission otherwise is by the parenteral route and in the Western world the disease is seen mainly in high-risk individuals such as intravenous drug users and homosexual men.

*Infectious material*

HBV-DNA can be detected in the blood of carriers and at lower levels in saliva, semen and urine (Karayiannis et al 1985).

*Horizontal transmission*

Blood products, before the availability of screening for HBV, were a major source of HBV infection for blood transfusion recipients and hemophiliacs. Sharing of needles and syringes leads to a high incidence in intravenous drug users. Infection has also been reported following tattooing, human bites and dental and surgical procedures. Biting insects remain a hypothetical source of infection.

Sexual transmission, as with HIV, is a major route of infection and HBV appears more easily transmissible than HIV. HBV markers of past or current infection are seen frequently in homosexual men. Blood contamination of toothbrushes and razors has been blamed for transmitting infection. Although HBV-DNA can be detected in saliva, the levels are low and kissing is not thought to be a major cause of transmission. Intact skin serves as an important barrier to infection and breaks in the skin with eczematous or ulcerating lesions may lead to an increased risk of infection. A noteworthy outbreak of hepatitis B in Swedish trackfinders was thought to be caused by contamination of skin abrasions (Ringertz 1967). Close contact in overcrowded situations can lead to spread of infection and this is recognized in prisons and other institutions. In Africa, although some vertical transmission occurs, most HBV infection occurs in the first few years of life and may relate to intrafamilial spread or close contact among young children.

*Vertical transmission*

With the gradual introduction of vaccination programs and antenatal screening, it should now be possible to minimize the risk of mother-to-baby transmission. The main risk is seen with HBeAg-positive mothers and infection appears to occur at the time of birth rather than in utero. Indeed, prior to the availability of effective immunoprophylaxis, the risk of vertical transmission could be reduced by elective cesarean section. Without appropriate immunoprophylaxis, babies born to HBeAg-positive mothers have a more than 90% chance of infection (usually subclinical) and a more than 90% chance of chronic viral infection once infected (Beasley et al 1981a). It is thought that HBeAg crosses the placenta and acts as a tolerogen. The relatively immature neonatal immune system seems unable to mount an effective immune response to HBV and chronic infection occurs.

*Health care workers and patients*

Health care workers who perform invasive procedures are at risk of HBV infection from their patients and are advised to have vaccination. Similarly, patients undergoing procedures can be infected by health care workers who have acute or chronic infections. Surgeons have transmitted HBV, particularly during highly invasive procedures such as thoracic surgery, and the risk is greatest when the surgeon has HBeAg and HBV-DNA in the blood (Harpaz et al 1996). Guidelines to prevent such occurrences are available (Gerberding 1996). Outbreaks have occurred in dialysis units and patients with chronic renal failure should receive HBV vaccination. Infection has also followed upper gastrointestinal endoscopy and poor cleansing of contaminated endoscopes has been blamed. Finger-prick blood sampling devices have also been responsible for HBV transmission. Blood products are now carefully screened for hepatitis B and this has reduced considerably the risk of transmission to recipients of blood products. Vaccination and the development of safer preparations of factor VIII have helped to reduce the incidence of hepatitis B in hemophilic patients. Patients who are given immunoglobulin for hypoglobulinemia are at particular risk of chronic HBV infection, as they are unable to mount an appropriate humoral immune response.

## Clinical course

The incubation period of HBV is 2–6 months and the HBsAg can usually be detected in the blood a few weeks before the onset of the hepatitic illness. The hepatitis appears to coincide with the development of the host immune response, in particular the IgM anti-HBc response, and this has helped establish the hypothesis that the liver damage is caused by the host immune response rather than by the HBV. HBsAg in the blood of a patient with hepatitis may represent acute or chronic infection, but high levels of IgM anti-HBc antibodies are generally diagnostic of acute infection.

Most symptomatic patients have recovered within 6 weeks of onset of the illness, but fatigue can continue for several months (p. 800). Chronic HBV infection occurs in 5–10% of healthy adults and in more than 90% of neonates. Immunodeficient adults, as in those with HIV infection, have a much higher risk of chronic infection. Male children with thalassemia and blood transfusion-acquired HBV infection have shown an increased risk of chronic infection.

***Chronic infection.*** Chronic HBV infection is defined

by the presence of the virus (serum HBsAg positive) for more than 6 months, but in practice chronic infections can be recognized at first testing when the HBsAg and anti-HBc (IgG) tests are both positive. Patients with high levels of viremia have HBV-DNA in the blood and are generally HBeAg positive. Patients with anti-HBe in the blood usually do not have ongoing viral replication, but some do have low levels of replication as evidenced by HBV-DNA in the blood and HBeAg in the liver. Patients who have neither HBeAg nor anti-HBe in the blood may or may not have other evidence of viral replication. Some with chronic HBV infection may clear the virus spontaneously or as a result of interferon treatment. It is also thought that a number of patients recover from the infection but continue to produce HBsAg because of integration of HBV-DNA into the host hepatocyte genome. Chronic HBV infection can occur in patients with normal plasma transaminases and normal liver biopsies ("healthy" carriers) but is associated with chronic liver disease, which may cause cirrhosis (p. 894) and eventually hepatocellular carcinoma (p. 1115).

The natural history of chronic HBV infection has been studied most in people infected either by vertical transmission at birth as in Taiwan (Beasley et al 1981b) or by horizontal transmission in early childhood in Alaska (McMahon et al 1990) or North America (Villeneuve et al 1994). Some 40% of those infected at birth in Taiwan died eventually of complications of HBV infection, mainly cirrhosis and hepatocellular carcinoma, although disease may not become apparent until the fourth or fifth decade of life and many patients have minimal signs of disease. The frequency of death from these causes may be less in other parts of the world, although longer follow-up will be needed to prove this point. Some children and adults have more rapidly progressive disease and cirrhosis caused by HBV has been recognized in a few children under 5 years of age. A variable number of chronic carriers eventually clear the virus themselves and this is often termed "spontaneous seroconversion" (p. 897). Their prognosis depends on the extent of previous liver damage.

### Diagnosis

HBsAg and HBeAg are usually detectable in the blood during the acute illness, but the diagnostic feature of acute HBV infection is the finding of IgM anti-HBc (Fig. 27.4). With resolution of infection, the normal host clears HBsAg and HBeAg and develops antibodies. IgG anti-HBc antibodies denote previous infection with HBV. Anti-HBs antibodies become positive following vaccination (anti-HBc negative) and about 3 months after an acute natural infection (anti-HBc positive).

The persistence of HBsAg for more than 6 months implies chronic viral carriage and some patients may benefit from antiviral therapy (p. 902). Patients with biochemical or histological evidence of hepatitis who are HBsAg positive and anti-HBe positive may have chronic infection with the precore or e-minus mutant virus (p. 894), hepatitis D or other hepatotropic viruses.

### Antiviral therapy

***Acute hepatitis B.*** There is no evidence that interferon is helpful in acute hepatitis B. In theory, an interferon amplification of an activated host immune response to infected hepatocytes could be detrimental, but this has not been demonstrated. The risk of chronic HBV infection in adults is 5–10% and studies so far have been too small to

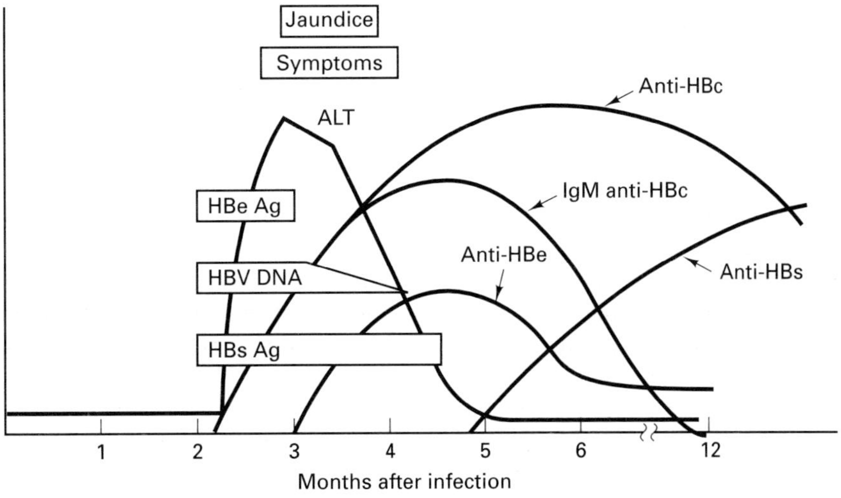


**Fig. 27.4** Serological responses to hepatitis B virus infection (HBsAg = hepatitis B surface antigen; anti-HBs = antibody to HBsAg; HBeAg = hepatitis Be antigen; anti-HBe = antibody to HBeAg; anti-HBc = antibody to hepatitis B core antigen).

show that early administration of interferon in acute disease can prevent chronicity. No benefit has been recorded with interferon given for fulminant hepatitis B (Levin et al 1989). Interferon is not therefore recommended in acute HBV infection.

***Chronic hepatitis B.*** Treatment of chronic hepatitis B virus infection remains suboptimal and the only drug that can be advocated in clinical practice is interferon. This is considered further in relation to chronic hepatitis (p. 902).

## Prevention

### *Active immunization*

The first vaccines were developed from purified 22 nm spherical HBsAg particles derived from the plasma of chronic HBV carriers (Zuckerman et al 1993). The source of the plasma-derived vaccines raised concerns about HIV transmission, but these fears were unfounded (Zuckerman et al 1993). More recent vaccines have been synthesized by recombinant molecular biological techniques in which the gene for HBsAg has been incorporated into a yeast genome and the vaccine derived from cultures. Both types of vaccine are safe and effective. It is still uncertain how long immunity lasts and monitoring anti-HBs levels in large populations is logistically difficult and expensive.

***Use.*** Many countries are considering universal immunization for infants and the USA and Italy instituted their programs in 1992. It is planned that vaccination will be worldwide eventually, but the vaccine is much more expensive than other vaccines used routinely in childhood. This has led to local initiatives to develop cheaper versions. In countries with a low prevalence of hepatitis B, the vaccine is currently given to those in high-risk groups. These include health care workers, patients requiring blood or blood products repeatedly, patients on hemodialysis, homosexual men, intravenous drug users, prostitutes and regular sexual contacts and close family contacts of those with chronic HBV infection. Babies born to carrier mothers are given vaccine in combination with hyperimmune globulin at birth. Vaccine should also be offered to those suffering a medical "sharps" accident involving an infected patient or a patient of unknown HBV status and after sexual intercourse with an infected individual.

***Administration and response.*** The vaccine is given intramuscularly into the deltoid and a typical regimen is 1 ml at 0, 1 and 6 months although accelerated courses have been used successfully. The efficacy of the vaccine can be estimated by measuring the anti-HBs response in serum. Values greater than 10 mi.u./ml are thought to be protective, but individuals require checks of their anti-HBs concentrations every 1–2 years and booster doses may be required every 3–5 years.

The response rate is more than 90% in young immunocompetent individuals but lower in those with concomitant disease or immunodeficiency (Stevens et al 1984, Loke et al 1990). The response rate is lower in males, in obese individuals and in the elderly. It may be that particular MHC haplotypes are associated with a poor response (Kruskall et al 1992). In those who initially fail to respond to vaccine, further booster doses may be successful and alternative experimental strategies to produce a response include the administration of γ-interferon with the vaccine. Those with low or undetectable levels of anti-HBs after vaccination may nevertheless have some cell-mediated immune response, but current practice with nonresponders who are health care workers is to give anti-HBs immune globulin following needlestick injury.

***Vaccine-derived mutants.*** Recently, HBV infection has been diagnosed in patients despite adequate anti-HBs levels (Carman et al 1990). It would seem that some have been infected with the vaccine-derived viral mutant and a mutation can be detected within the gene for HBsAg. Only a few cases have been diagnosed worldwide, but mass vaccination programs may show this to be a more serious problem and accordingly vaccine manufacturers are considering other approaches including the incorporation of pre-S peptides into the vaccine.

***Side-effects.*** Minor skin reactions have been reported following vaccination and there have been occasional case reports of immune-mediated phenomena including polyneuropathy.

### *Passive immunization*

The availability of vaccine has considerably reduced the need for anti-HBs immune globulin (HBIg). It is given in conjunction with vaccine (at the contralateral site) to babies born to carrier mothers and to anyone who has a history of recent exposure to the HBV, no history of vaccination or inadequate levels of anti-HBs. HBIg has also been administered to HBV-infected patients who have undergone liver transplantation to reduce the chance of graft infection (p. 1153). This is very expensive and its long-term efficacy remains to be proved.

# HEPATITIS C VIRUS

## Virology

HAV and HBV testing showed there were many patients with hepatitis, acute and chronic, whose illnesses followed blood transfusion and were associated with negative tests for HAV and HBV. These patients were said to be suffering from non-A, non-B (NANB) hepatitis, also termed PT- (parenterally transmitted/post-transfusion) NANB hepatitis. This was a common problem in intravenous drug users and recipients of blood products. Hemophiliacs who received pooled blood products were especially at risk. Blood products thought to contain the virus were administered to chimpanzees and acute and chronic hepatitis followed. The hepatitis C virus (HCV) was discovered when RNA was extracted from serum from a chimpanzee with NANB hepatitis and was used to establish a library of complementary DNA (cDNA) clones (Choo et al 1989). Gene products were tested for reactivity against a collection of serum samples from patients with NANB hepatitis and eventually clone 5–1–1 (C5–1–1) was recognized to react with patients' sera.

***Virus structure.*** HCV is a single-stranded RNA virus currently regarded as a genus of the flaviviridae which includes insect- and tickborne flaviviruses and pestiviruses (Miller & Purcell 1990). The RNA genome is comprised of approximately 9400 nucleotides (Choo et al 1989) and serves directly as messenger RNA to produce a series of structural and nonstructural proteins (Fig. 27.5). The C region codes for the viral core proteins (nucleocapsid) and is followed by the E1 region that codes for gp33, a 33 kDa envelope glycoprotein. The E2/NS1 gene product is a 70 kDa glycoprotein that is processed by the cell in the same way as gp33, suggesting that it is a second envelope protein as in the pestiviruses. NS2 to NS5 are genes producing nonstructural proteins. The NS3 gene product has protease and/or helicase activity and the NS5 gene product is an RNA-dependent RNA polymerase.

***Virus genotypes.*** The HCV cannot be grown in vitro and accordingly classification of the HCV depends on nucleotide sequencing of its genome or of subgenomic fragments (Simmonds 1995). Sequencing, particularly of hypervariable parts of the genome such as the NS5 and E1/NS1 regions, has revealed different HCV genotypes, but as yet no classification of these has been generally accepted. Simmonds et al (1994) have proposed a classification to include six HCV genotypes (types 1–6) and their subtypes and no doubt others will be added in future. Types 1a, 1b, 2a and 2b have a worldwide distribution, while the others tend to be located more specifically. Types 1a, 1b, 2a, 2b and 3c predominate in western Europe and North America, type 4 is common in the Middle East and Central Africa and type 5a in South Africa. Genotype distribution in the Far East is complex, with types 1a, 2a and 2b predominating in Japan and China, type 3 in Thailand and Singapore and type 6a in Hong Kong. The reasons for these geographic differences in HCV genotype distribution are unknown.

The biological implications of the variations in the HCV genotype are unknown and little is known of the relation of genotypes to viral replication, tendency to damage the liver and susceptibility to interferon therapy. HCV infections frequently become chronic and this has been attributed to the high incidence of variation in parts of the genome determining the viral envelope allowing the virus to escape from the host immune responses by changing viral antigenicity. This is an attractive theory, but evidence that immune pressure drives viral variation has been hard to obtain. All the HCV genotypes seem to damage the liver to some extent, but response to interferon therapy is lowest in type 1 infection (29%) and greater in type 2 (52%) and type 3 (74%) infections (Chemello et al 1994). These differences may be related not solely to the different HCV genotypes but also to other factors related to treatment response. In general, response to therapy is less in

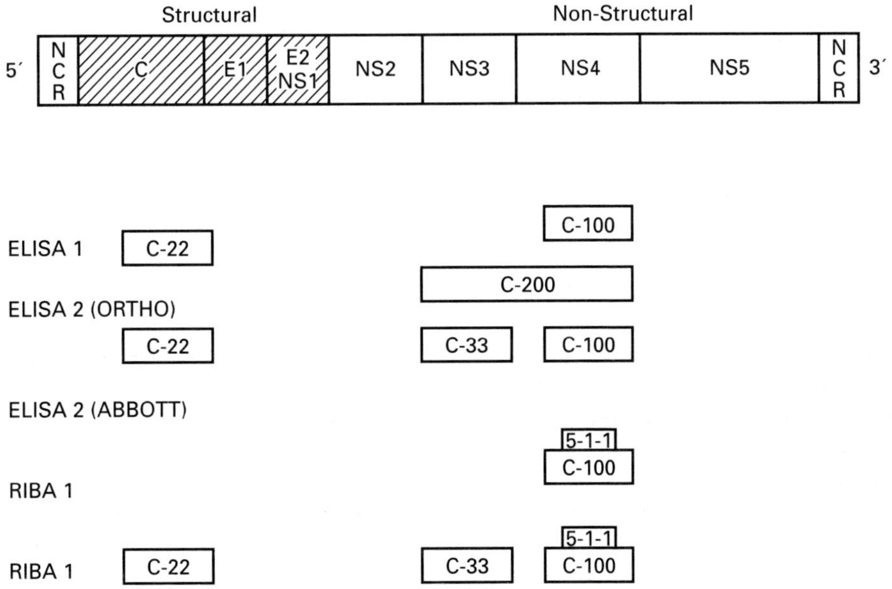


**Fig. 27.5** Diagrammatic representation of the hepatitis C virus and viral antigens important in serodiagnosis.

older patients, in long-standing infections, where cirrhosis is present, and where the pretreatment level of HCV-RNA is high. There have been reports that certain strains are more likely to lead to cirrhosis or hepatocellular carcinoma, but these require confirmation. In view of these unresolved factors, identification of the HCV genotype is not particularly useful in patient management.

## Epidemiology and transmission

HCV infection is frequently associated with the injection of contaminated blood or blood products and is common among hemophiliacs and intravenous drug users, with seroprevalence rates often more than 80% compared with 0.07% in new London blood donors (Ryan et al 1994). Since the introduction of screening of blood products, the incidence of post-transfusion hepatitis has fallen by more than 50% in the USA (Dodd 1992). Inoculation of blood may also be important in sporadic instances of hepatitis C infection. In a detailed study of community-acquired disease (Alter et al 1992), 130 patients with acute community-acquired NANB hepatitis were prospectively followed. Sixty-six (51%) had a history of recent drug use, transfusion or occupational exposure to blood. A study of asymptomatic blood donors found to be infected with HCV showed prior blood transfusion, intranasal and intravenous drug abuse, sexual promiscuity and ear piercing as causative factors in three-quarters (Conry-Cantilena et al 1996). HCV infection is more common in the Mediterranean countries and in Africa and there is a surprisingly high prevalence in Japan where interferon therapy for HCV now accounts for 1.5% of the health budget. Explanations for these higher seroprevalence rates include reuse of needles in mass immunization programs many years ago and the possibility that HCV may be insectborne in tropical climes. Surgical transmission from surgeon to patient can occur (Esteban et al 1996).

Much less is known of transmission routes other than inoculation. Alter et al (1992) attributed eight of 130 (6%) community-acquired infections to household or sexual contact. Studies of the frequency of sexual and household transmission of hepatitis C have given conflicting results, with infection found in 0–30% of sexual partners and 0–20% of children of infected persons (Alter 1994). Sexual transmission seems to occur at a lower rate than in HBV or HIV infection and this may be related to the level of viremia or the genotype (above) involved. Perinatal (vertical) transmission can occur and depends on the level of viremia. Transmission is highly unlikely where HCV-RNA is not found in the mother's blood and occurs in up to a third of infants where maternal titers of HCV-RNA are high (Ohto et al 1994). Associated maternal HIV infection also increases perinatal transmission perhaps for the same reason (Zanetti et al 1995). Breastfeeding does not seem to transmit hepatitis C infection (Zanetti et al 1995). Close contact other than sexual may also be important, as shown by frequent patient-to-patient transfer of hepatitis C unrelated to blood or blood products in a hematology ward (Allander et al 1995). Alter et al (1992) could find no risk factors in only 13 of their 130 (10%) cases of community-acquired hepatitis.

## Clinical course

The incubation period for hepatitis C infection is 6–12 weeks, but much shorter incubation periods have been reported following transfusion of factor VIII (Bamber et al 1981) and this may be because of the high infecting dose. Clinical acute hepatitis (p. 795) develops in only 5–20%, but 60–80% develop chronic infection and it has been estimated that up to 20% will develop cirrhosis eventually with the consequent risk of hepatocellular carcinoma (p. 1116). The risk of chronicity is more in males than in females (Tremolada et al 1992). It is now realized that some patients with chronic infection have normal liver function tests but HCV-RNA can be detected in the blood (Alberti et al 1992, Brillanti et al 1993). Some of these patients have abnormal liver histology, but others have been followed carefully and appear to be "healthy carriers" in that they remain HCV-RNA positive but have normal liver biopsies. The remaining 20–40% of patients who acquire HCV infection appear to clear the virus completely; their liver function tests return to normal and HCV-RNA can no longer be detected in serum. Chronic hepatitis C infection is usually asymptomatic or is associated with mild fatigue only. However, patients can develop chronic hepatitis and cirrhosis, often over 20 years or more, and in such patients hepatocellular carcinoma can develop (p. 898). The frequency with which these sequelae develop has varied in different studies but is generally relatively low.

## Diagnosis

The diagnosis of hepatitis C virus infection requires identification of antibodies to HCV antigens in a patient's blood. The first-generation test identified antibodies against the C100–3 nonstructural antigen, but this test was limited because it only became positive a considerable time after infection and gave false positive results in autoimmune diseases (McFarlane et al 1990). Currently, screening for infection uses a second-generation test identifying antibodies to the C100-3 and C33 nonstructural antigens and the C22 structural nucleocapsid antigen in an enzyme-linked immunosorbent assay (ELISA). The specificity of positive reactions is confirmed using a recombinant immunoblot assay (RIBA) (Van der Poel et al 1991). The RIBA assay checks reactivity against HCV antigens (5-1-1, C100-3, C33a, C22-3) and control human IgG and superoxide dismutase fusion proteins. A

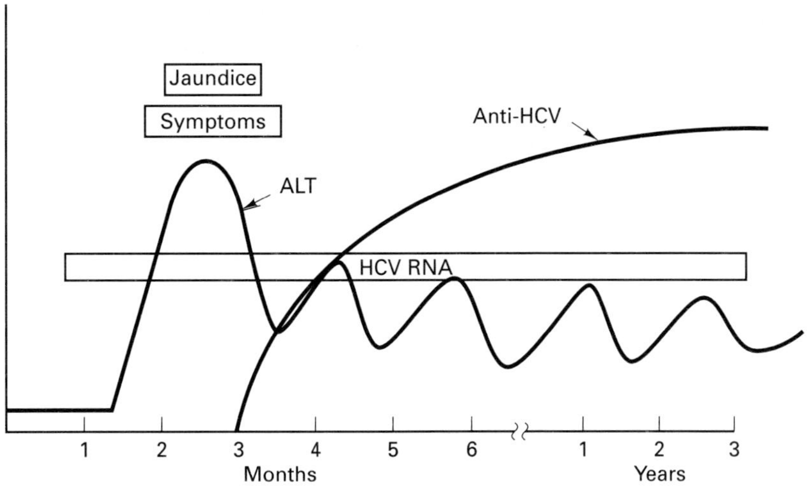


**Fig. 27.6** Development of antibodies of diagnostic importance following hepatitis C virus infection.

third-generation test including a fourth antigen, NS5, is being developed. These antibody tests are usually negative during an acute illness, as antibodies take up to 3 months to develop (Fig. 27.6).

Polymerase chain reaction (PCR) assays can be used to detect HCV-RNA in serum and liver tissue and may become the "gold standard" for diagnosis, but they are not yet widely available. Assays are also being developed in which amplification of the HCV-RNA signal will allow quantification of the HCV-RNA in the blood. However, second-generation ELISA and RIBA tests give a 98% concordance with the results of PCR tests (Nakatsuji et al 1992) unless patients are immunosuppressed, as after transplantation, or have severe autoimmune hepatitis or hypergammaglobulinemia (Poterucha et al 1992). Immunohistochemical methods of detecting HCV antigens in tissue using monoclonal antibodies have shown HCV antigens in hepatocyte cytoplasm, but these methods are still in the developmental stage (Hiramatsu et al 1992).

## Antiviral therapy

### *Acute hepatitis C*

Small trials have reported some benefit from interferon in acute hepatitis C (Alberti et al 1991, Omata et al 1991, Viladomiu et al 1992). Early intervention may be of benefit for the small number of people who recognize that they are at risk of infection, as after a needlestick injury, and where a diagnosis is made early in the disease.

### *Chronic hepatitis C*

Interferon is the only drug advocated in practice for chronic hepatitis C infection. Most patients respond to treatment with a reduction of the plasma transaminase activity and an improvement on liver biopsy, but relapse usually occurs when treatment is stopped and the long-term value of therapy is unknown (p. 900).

## Prevention

Screening of blood and blood products has considerably reduced the incidence of post-transfusion HCV (above). Prior to this, trials suggested that administration of immunoglobulin at the time of blood transfusion reduced the risk of HCV infection (Koretz et al 1976). No vaccine is available and the high mutation rate of the HCV makes it unlikely that a vaccine will be made readily.

# DELTA VIRUS (HEPATITIS D)

## Virology

The delta virus, or agent, is the smallest virus known to infect humans and is similar to plant satellite viruses (Rizzetto et al 1977). Hepatitis D virus (HDV) requires the hepatitis B virus in order to replicate. Viral particles are 35–37 nm in diameter (Bonino et al 1984). The core consists of the delta antigen and the coat consists of the HBsAg (Bonino et al 1986). HDV is a single-stranded RNA virus and the genome consists of 1700 nucleotides. Viral sequencing shows that there are at least three major subtypes of the HDV and these may explain some of the variation in disease outcome and pattern.

## Epidemiology and transmission

HDV is transmitted parenterally and patients can be coinfected with HBV and HDV or an HBV carrier can become superinfected with HDV. Most infections in the Western world relate to intravenous drug use, but sexual transmission can occur. In South American epidemics, the transmission of HDV is not understood. There are three major epidemiological patterns of HDV infection with varying clinical syndromes.

***Epidemic.*** Major epidemics of HDV have been described in various parts of the world, particularly the Amazon basin (Hadler et al 1984) and Kashmir. In South America the clinical syndrome is known as Labrea fever or Santa della Marta fever and has a high mortality rate. The high incidence in children suggests that close contact can transmit the virus.

***Endemic.*** The endemic pattern of infection is seen around the Mediterranean basin, where 10% of HBsAg carriers are also infected with HDV. Romania and other eastern European countries also have high infection levels (Tapalaga et al 1986), but the infection is uncommon in northern Europe. HDV infection is relatively uncommon in Asia.

***High-risk groups.*** This pattern is seen in northern Europe and the USA, where HDV is principally seen in intravenous drug users. Unlike HBV, delta infection is not a major problem in homosexual men, although the seroprevalence rates in this group are higher than in the rest of the population. Screening of blood products for HBsAg has reduced the risks of HDV infection for their recipients, but there are many hemophiliacs who were infected before screening was introduced.

## Clinical course

In coinfection, the patient is infected simultaneously with HBV and HDV. An acute hepatitis can follow, but both agents are generally cleared by the host, with chronic infection occurring in about 77% of patients. In superinfection, a chronic carrier of the HBV is superinfected with HDV. This is a much more serious situation with a high risk of severe clinical hepatitis and very high risk of chronic HDV infection. Progressive liver disease can occur and there are reports of patients developing cirrhosis in 2–3 years (Rizzetto et al 1983). The natural history is very variable, however, and a healthy carrier state can exist (Rizzetto & Durazzo 1991). Immunosuppression is associated with more rapidly progressive disease.

## Diagnosis

In acute coinfection (Fig. 27.7), markers of recent HBV (anti-HBc IgM) and HDV (anti-HDV IgM) infection will be present (Hoofnagle 1989). In superinfection (Fig. 27.8), the patients have evidence of chronic HBV infection (HBsAg positive, anti-HBc IgM negative) and acute HDV infection (anti-HDV IgM positive). In chronic HDV infection, the patients will be anti-HDV IgG positive (IgM negative) and HDV-RNA and antigen can be detected in serum and liver biopsy.

## Antiviral therapy

Interferon may be of benefit. Various regimens have been tried, but there is a high relapse rate (p. 900).

## Prevention

As HDV requires coexistent HBV infection to replicate, a responder to HBV vaccination with adequate anti-HBs levels will be protected from HDV infection. However,

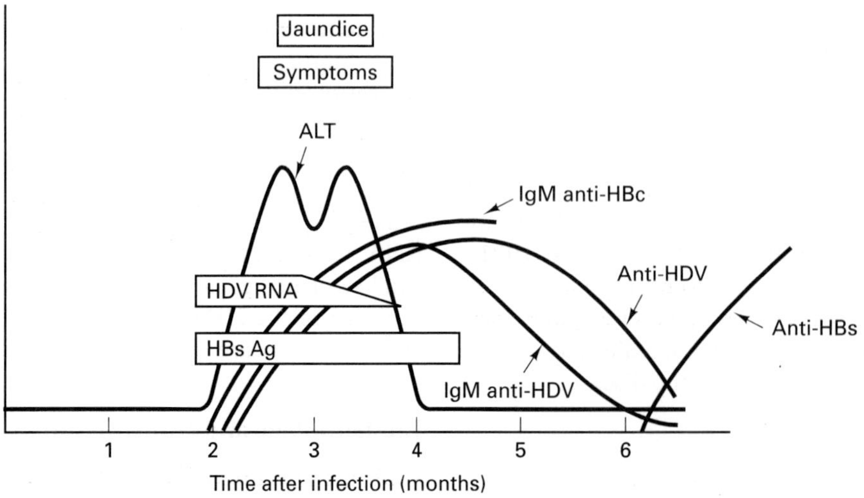


**Fig. 27.7** Serological response to coinfection with hepatitis B virus and hepatitis D virus (HBsAg = hepatitis B surface antigen; anti-HBs = hepatitis B surface antibody; anti-HBc = hepatitis B core antibody (IgM); HDV-RNA = hepatitis D virus RNA; anti-HDV = hepatitis D antibody (IgM)).

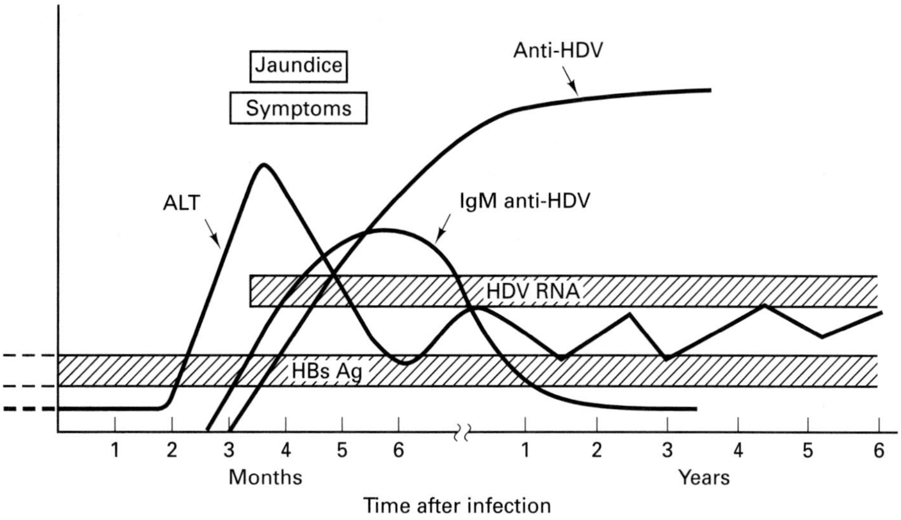


**Fig. 27.8** Serological response to superinfection with hepatitis D virus in chronic hepatitis B virus infection followed by chronic hepatitis D virus infection (HBsAg = hepatitis B surface antigen; HDV-RNA = hepatitis D virus RNA; anti-HDV = hepatitis D antibody (IgM); ALT = alanine aminotransferase).

vaccine will not protect an HBV carrier from HDV superinfection and drug users should be counseled with regard to safer injecting techniques.

## HEPATITIS E VIRUS

Just as it was recognized prior to the discovery of HCV that there were parenterally transmitted cases of hepatitis with no virological evidence of HAV or HBV, so it was recognized that there were outbreaks of hepatitis with a similar epidemiological pattern to HAV with negative tests for HAV and HBV. This was termed enterally transmitted non-A, non-B hepatitis (ET-NANB) and outbreaks were recorded in Asia, Africa and Mexico (Bradley et al 1988). There were clinical similarities, including a peculiarly high mortality rate in pregnancy, not seen with other causes of viral hepatitis. Hepatitis E virus (HEV) proved to be the cause of ET-NANB and it has similarities to caliciviruses. Serological tests are under development. Most patients in Europe and North America with HEV have a history of travel to an area of high endemicity. There are very few secondary cases in an outbreak, suggesting a common source such as an infected water supply. There have been a few cases of HEV in patients with no history of travel to endemic areas and it is unclear how they acquired the infection.

## NON A–E HEPATITIS VIRUSES

Epidemiological and experimental evidence points strongly to causes of hepatitis other than the hepatitis A, B, C, D and E viruses (Simons et al 1995). Further hepatitis viruses are being identified, but evidence about these viruses and the diseases they cause in humans remains scarce. They are likely to become much better defined over the next few years.

### Hepatitis F virus

Hepatitis F virus (HFV) is a DNA virus which was isolated from the stools of French patients with sporadic hepatitis and which has been transmitted to monkeys (Deka et al 1994). Its importance in human disease is not yet well defined but like HAV and HEV, it is transmitted enterically and confers specific immunity on recovery from the illness.

### Hepatitis GB viruses

These are RNA flaviviridae that are quite separate from the HCV. Blood from a surgeon (GB) who had hepatitis was used in transmission experiments and this led to the discovery of two viruses (GB-A and GB-B) in infected tamarins, although it now seems that these viruses are not human viruses (Schlauder et al 1995). However, this discovery led to the finding of a third virus (GB-C) in humans that probably does cause human disease (Simons et al 1995).

### Hepatitis G virus

A further flavivirus different from HCV, GB-A, GB-B and GB-C has been identified in a patient with chronic hepatitis, but further information about it is awaited (Kim et al 1995, James 1996).

### Disease associations of GB-C and HGV

There is little information available on this subject, but GB-C and HGV have been associated with acute hepatitis, including fulminant hepatic failure, chronic liver disease and aplastic anemia (p. 800) (Hadziyannis et al 1995, Kim et al 1995, Yoshiba et al 1995). GB-C and HGV are often associated with HBC and HCV infection and parenteral drug abuse may be an important means of transmission (Aikawa et al 1996).

### Giant cell hepatitis

Phillips et al (1991) have described 10 patients with acute and chronic hepatitis and an unusual and distinctive histological pattern of syncytial giant cell hepatitis. Confusingly, the term "hepatitis G" was suggested for this illness, but there is no evidence that it is due to the HGV (Lancet 1991). Liver biopsy showed that the liver cords were occupied by syncytial giant cells with 3–20 nuclei and a large volume of acidophilic cytoplasm with a ground glass appearance (Fig. 27.9). Cholestasis was prominent. Electronmicroscopy demonstrated large numbers of particles looking like the nucleocapsids of paramyxoviruses. Material derived from infected liver administered to chimpanzees caused no biochemical or histological hepatitis, but one chimpanzee developed a strong serological response to measles virus and parainfluenza 4, which are both paramyxoviruses. Five of the patients required liver transplantation and survived and the remaining patients died.

## OTHER VIRAL CAUSES OF HEPATITIS

Many viral illnesses can cause hepatitis and this often amounts to no more than the finding of abnormal liver function tests that resolve rapidly. Other viruses, particularly in the setting of immunosuppression, can lead to severe and at times fatal disease.

### Cytomegalovirus infection

Infection with cytomegalovirus (CMV) generally requires close contact such as kissing and sexual intercourse. Blood transfusion can also transmit CMV.

#### *Neonatal and childhood infection*

Neonatal cytomegalic inclusion disease is the most dramatic but least common form of the disease. The infection is acquired in utero and presents at or soon after birth with jaundice, thrombocytopenic purpura, hemolytic anemia and frequently cerebral damage. A third of these patients present as neonatal hepatitis. Milder forms of the disease are more common and the prognosis is good if there is no brain damage although hepatomegaly may persist for over a year. Asymptomatic infections in older children may cause hepatomegaly, splenomegaly and abnormal liver function tests, but liver failure is unusual (Hanshaw et al 1965). The histological features in the liver are very variable and include fatty change, focal hepatocellular necro-

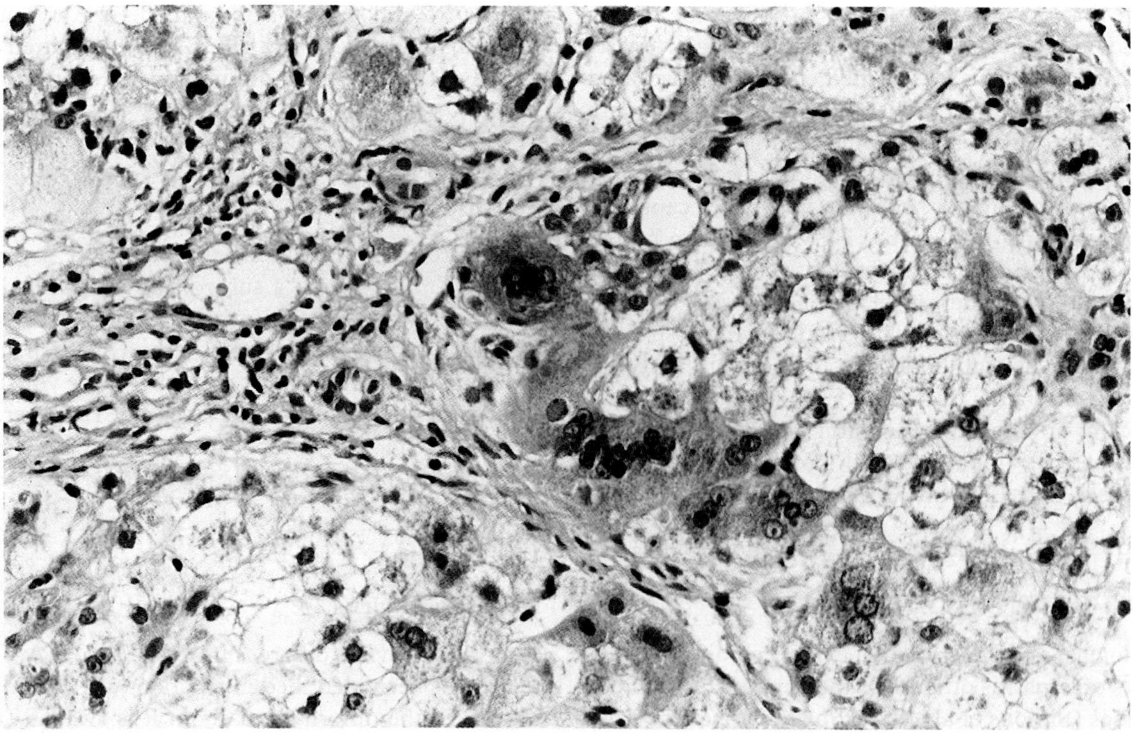

**Fig. 27.9** Giant cell hepatitis of acute onset and following a chronic relapsing course in a young man. Note the prominent multinucleate giant cells (hematoxylin and eosin, ×400).

sis, marked polymorphonuclear and mononuclear cell infiltration of the portal tracts and cholestasis. Giant cells occur and this is one cause of giant cell hepatitis. There may be extensive fibrosis and biliary atresia in fatal cases, but in general the changes are reversible.

### *Adult infection*

Most adult-acquired infections are asymptomatic. However, CMV can cause an illness resembling glandular fever although exudative pharyngitis is unusual. Lymphocytosis with atypical mononuclear cells usually appears in the second week of the illness and liver function tests may be abnormal. Jaundice is rare, but viral hepatitis may be simulated and severe cholestatic jaundice and fulminant hepatic failure have been reported (Lamb & Stern 1966, Toghill et al 1967, Shusterman et al 1978) particularly in immunosuppressed individuals (Evans & Williams 1968). CMV infection is relatively common after liver transplantation (p. 1160). Liver biopsy shows a mononuclear cell infiltrate in the sinusoids with Kupffer cell hyperplasia and inflammation in the portal tracts. Focal hepatocyte necrosis, occasional granuloma formation and sometimes bile duct epithelial damage may be found. Similar appearances can be found in Epstein–Barr infections and certain drug reactions, but if necessary immunohistochemical staining can help confirm the diagnosis. Inclusion bodies are uncommon. Intravenous ganciclovir is the treatment of choice, especially in immunocompromised patients.

### *Diagnosis*

In a primary CMV infection the anti-CMV IgM is positive and IgG negative. In reactivation of disease the patient has evidence of previous infection and is anti-CMV IgG positive. Blood tests for CMV antigens may help to confirm the diagnosis or the liver biopsy may be helpful.

## Epstein–Barr virus

Infectious mononucleosis or glandular fever is caused by the Epstein–Barr virus (EBV). Spread is by close contact such as kissing and this is thought to account for peaks of infection in those under 5 years and then later in the teenage years. In Europe and North America, up to 60% of children under 5 years and 90% of individuals at the age of 20 years have serological evidence of previous infection.

Infectious mononucleosis is an acute illness affecting the reticulo-endothelial system (Hoagland 1967). Pharyngitis, lymphadenopathy, splenomegaly and a fever occur in over three-quarters of teenage patients, but a milder illness is more usual in younger patients. A rash occurs in some patients and jaundice occurs in 5–15%. Fulminant hepatitis (Hart et al 1984) is very rare and in a male suggests Duncan's syndrome, a rare sex-linked condition in which the immune system fails to deal with EBV (Purtilo et al 1975). Fatal disease is the usual outcome. More severe disease may also be seen in older patients with prolonged fever, less peripheral lymphadenopathy and often more abnormal liver function tests (Horwitz et al 1983).

***Diagnosis.*** The diagnosis may be made by a combination of a positive Monospot or Paul Bunnell test and activated (atypical) lymphocytes on the blood film or by a positive anti-EBV IgM antibody test. Serum transaminase activities are elevated in 75% of cases and maximal activities occur between the second and fourth weeks with resolution by the sixth week (Dunnet 1963). The liver shows dense infiltration of the portal tracts and sinusoids with typical and atypical mononuclear cells (Kilpatrick 1966). Small aggregates may be seen in the hepatic parenchyma with focal hepatocyte necrosis and acidophilic bodies. Diffuse hepatic necrosis and cholestasis are not found.

## Human immunodeficiency virus (HIV)

HIV infection can cause an illness like infectious mononucleosis, and liver function tests may show increased serum transaminase activity. Serological tests do not become positive for 1–10 weeks after this acute illness (p. 599), but HIV antigen can be detected in the blood in the acute stage (Molina et al 1992).

## Herpes simplex virus

Herpes simplex virus (HSV)-1 affects mainly the mouth, eyes and central nervous system and HSV-2 mainly causes genital herpes. After the primary infection the viruses lie dormant in the dorsal root sensory ganglia and can reactivate again at any time. Acute hepatitis can occur as part of the primary infection or as a reactivation illness that has been reported mainly in immunosuppressed individuals.

Primary HSV-1 infection generally occurs in very young children and can range from a mild febrile illness to a severe disease with high fever, stomatitis and occasionally hepatitis. Neonatal infection can cause severe disease and generally results from perinatal transmission of HSV-2. The mother may have asymptomatic viral shedding or cervical disease, so there may be none of the classic perineal blisters to alert the obstetrician. Higher levels of virus are seen with primary HSV-2 infection. Severe systemic disease including hepatitis may develop in the neonate. High-dose intravenous acyclovir is the treatment of choice.

Primary HSV infections in adulthood can also cause hepatitis. This is rare but can be life-threatening (Kilpatrick 1966). The features of this disease are nonspecific and include high fever, marked elevation in the plasma transaminase activities, leukopenia in about two-thirds of cases and sometimes disseminated intravascular coagulation. Jaundice is unusual and only half of patients have oropharyngeal or genital lesions suggesting herpes virus infection. Most patients are immunosuppressed due to corticosteroid or other immunosuppressive therapy or are in the third trimester of pregnancy. If there are skin lesions, scrapings or vesicular fluid may be useful for diagnosis. A positive IgM anti-HSV and a negative IgG anti-HSV suggest primary herpetic infection. Liver biopsy may also be useful for diagnosis. A negative IgG anti-HSV and a positive IgM anti-HSV suggest primary herpetic infection. Liver biopsy may also be useful for diagnosis, but coagulopathy may preclude this. High-dose intravenous acyclovir is the treatment of choice.

### Varicella zoster virus

It is not unusual to find an elevated transaminase activity in a child or adult with chickenpox infection. In immunosuppressed individuals and occasionally in immunocompetent adults, chickenpox can be severe with multisystem disease including liver involvement. In such cases there is often significant lung involvement and ventilatory support may be required. Acyclovir in high doses intravenously is the treatment of choice.

### Rubella virus

Rubella, or German measles, is most important when it occurs in the first trimester of pregnancy, when it can cause extensive fetal damage resulting in the congenital rubella syndrome. Immunization programs should reduce this risk in future. Hepatomegaly, with or without splenomegaly, is found at birth in up to three-quarters of cases (Cooper et al 1965) and liver damage varies from mild focal liver cell injury or a few bile thrombi to severe hepatocellular necrosis (Esterly et al 1967). Neonatal giant cell hepatitis or biliary atresia may also occur (Strauss & Bernstein 1968). Mild liver lesions resolve, but in other cases cirrhosis may develop (Stern & Williams 1966). Jaundice and increased serum transaminase activity indicating hepatitis may be present for up to 2 months.

### Measles

Hepatitis in measles is common but asymptomatic and free of chronic complications (Gavish et al 1983, Shalev-Zimels et al 1988). It is revealed by liver function tests that show increased serum transaminase activity in 80% of cases and this tends to be more marked in adults. Liver biopsy is not required but has shown giant cells (Modai et al 1986). Abnormalities have generally disappeared within a month.

### Yellow fever virus

The yellow fever virus may be transmitted from person to person by the mosquito in the urban cycle. More usually, humans may be infected in the forest (sylvatic) cycle, in which the mosquito transmits the virus between primate animals. Yellow fever is now uncommon owing to mosquito control measures and vaccines, but reservoirs of the virus remain in the jungles of Africa and South America and epidemics still occur (Norman 1984).

Lesions in yellow fever are widespread and the most important organs involved are the liver, kidneys and heart. The severity of the disease varies greatly and there are three clinical stages: first, a few days of headache, photophobia and generalized pains, then one or two days of improvement and finally deterioration with vomiting, jaundice, a tender liver, bleeding, hypotension and oliguria with proteinuria. No specific treatment is available. The liver shows hepatic necrosis, usually widespread and severe, involving particularly the mid-zones of the lobules. Many necrotic cells become shrunken, condensed and eosinophilic (Councilman bodies) and fatty change is almost always present. Recovery, when it occurs, is complete. The diagnosis can be confirmed serologically and by culture of the virus from the blood.

### Filovirus (Marburg virus, Ebola virus)

Filoviruses have a filamentous appearance on electronmicroscopy and Marburg virus and Ebola virus both cause hepatitis as part of a generalized hemorrhagic febrile illness (Simpson 1995). The source of the virus is unknown and humans and other primates can be infected. The virus is found in the liver, kidneys, blood and urine in humans. Person-to-person transmission occurs but requires close contact, particularly with blood. Quarantine of known cases effectively contains spread of infection.

Marburg and Ebola viruses cause illnesses that are clinically indistinguishable. The illness described originally occurred in animal handlers and laboratory workers in Europe who had had contact with tissue from African green monkeys, but since then sporadic cases and outbreaks have occurred in sub-Saharan Africa. The illness is severe and about a quarter or more of patients die. The early stage is marked by severe headache, fever, conjunctivitis and generalized aches and pains and the later stage by a skin rash, hepatitis, renal failure, a bleeding tendency, diarrhea and possibly myocarditis. The peripheral blood shows leukopenia and severe thrombocytopenia. The serum transaminase activity is markedly elevated, but the serum bilirubin concentration is usually normal and jaundice is a terminal event. Autopsy shows damage in many organs; the main lesion in the liver is necrosis of hepatocytes. The liver returns to normal in those who survive.

### Adenovirus

Infection with these viruses can be identified pathologically, as they produce large intranuclear inclusions. Hepatitis in adenovirus infection is rare. Indeed, in a volunteer study only one of over 700 infected with adenovirus developed jaundice (Knight 1967).

### Coxsackie viruses; echoviruses

Coxsackie A and B viruses have been isolated from children and from adults with viral hepatitis. Echoviruses have also been thought to have caused hepatitis in infants (Leggiadro et al 1982).

## PATHOLOGY

### Acute hepatitis

Many causes of acute hepatitis give rise to similar histopathological appearances in the liver and it is therefore often difficult or impossible to differentiate between viral and nonviral liver damage. Immunohistochemical techniques and in situ hybridization may sometimes be helpful where serological tests have been nondiagnostic. It is also often difficult to differentiate between acute and chronic disease and full clinical details are required to facilitate histological interpretation.

A detailed description of the histopathology of acute viral hepatitis has been given by MacSween (1980). The main pathological processes in acute viral hepatitis are liver cell death, inflammation and regeneration. Parenchymal damage occurs throughout the lobule but is most marked around the central veins. Hepatocytes become swollen (ballooning degeneration), the uniform pattern of the liver cell plates is disrupted and scattered focal degeneration and death of hepatocytes (spotty necrosis) gives rise to shrunken acidophilic dead cells with pyknotic nuclei (apoptosis) and acidophilic debris (Councilman bodies). Chronic inflammatory cell infiltration occurs at the sites of focal necrosis and multinucleate hepatocytes and mitotic figures are seen as regeneration occurs. More severe hepatitis causes necrosis of large groups of cells (confluent necrosis), sometimes with necrotic cells linking portal tracts and central veins (bridging necrosis or subacute hepatic necrosis), and in fulminant hepatic failure necrosis can affect whole liver lobules (massive necrosis).

Orcein-positive ground glass hepatocytes are not usually evident in acute hepatitis B infection. Fatty change may be evident in acute hepatitis C and acute hepatitis D infection and microvesicular fatty change and often extensive necrosis have been features in South American epidemics. Mild cholestasis is seen in most patients but occurs particularly in hepatitis A. Even when marked, the other features of acute viral hepatitis are also present and prevent confusion with large bile duct obstruction. The portal tracts are expanded and infiltrated with chronic inflammatory cells, mainly lymphocytes, and occasionally the features of periportal hepatitis (piecemeal necrosis) occur but without implying a chronic illness (Fauerholdt et al 1977). Prominent portal tract eosinophilia suggests an acute hepatitis due to drugs. Resolution of these changes occurs with recovery from the illness, but minor changes may persist for 6 months or more and minor residual fibrosis can be permanent.

### Chronic hepatitis

The features of chronic hepatitis are described elsewhere (p. 888).

## CLINICAL FEATURES

Acute viral hepatitis ranges from an asymptomatic process to fatal disease. Most cases are subclinical and there is therefore a considerable underdiagnosis of acute disease. Children generally have mild disease, whereas symptomatic and more severe disease occurs more frequently in adults. The prodromal illness is very nonspecific.

### Prodromal illness

Influenza symptoms are common, with malaise, fever and myalgia. A low-grade fever may occur. Upper respiratory symptoms may predominate and symptoms of pharyngitis, rhinitis and even a cough may cause diagnostic confusion. Anorexia and nausea are common and right hypochondrial discomfort may be present. Smokers develop distaste for cigarettes. Constipation or diarrhea may be present and abdominal discomfort can mimic acute appendicitis (Wewalka 1974). Itching may occur and the patient may notice some darkness of the urine and pallor of the stools.

### Serum sickness syndrome

A few patients can develop a serum sickness-like illness with arthralgia, arthritis, headache and urticaria (Alarcon & Townes 1973). This lasts an average of about 20 days but can persist for up to 6 weeks. Symmetrical polyarthropathy is the usual pattern of joint involvement, but morning stiffness or flitting arthralgia can occur. Skin manifestations include erythema, maculopapular rashes or urticaria. The differential diagnosis includes rheumatic fever, rheumatoid arthritis, systemic lupus erythematosus, polyarteritis nodosa and other viral infections including parvovirus and rubella. The liver function tests may be abnormal and jaundice often follows resolution of the syndrome. Immune complexes are thought to cause the syndrome and hepatitis B virus is more likely than the other hepatotropic viruses to be the trigger factor. HBsAg may not be found during this phase of the disease, but a positive anti-HBc (IgM) test should reveal the diagnosis.

### Icteric phase

The prodromal symptoms usually disappear with the onset of jaundice. The severity and duration of jaundice are very variable. Children usually become anicteric within 2 weeks but more prolonged jaundice occurs in adults, lasting for 2–6 weeks (Wewalka 1974). Severe lethargy, vomiting and drowsiness should alert the physician to impending hepatic failure. The urine remains dark during the icteric phase and pale stools occur in 20–40% of patients. Itching is present in about half the patients but can be troublesome in the minority who develop prolonged cholestasis, particularly in hepatitis A.

### Physical examination

In the prodromal phase, the liver is usually firm, tender and palpable 2–4 cm below the costal margin. Hepatomegaly continues well into convalescence, but tenderness diminishes with recovery. The spleen is palpable in 5–15% of cases and mild posterior cervical lymphadenopathy may be evident. More widespread lymphadenopathy should alert the physician to infectious mononucleosis, cytomegalovirus infection or syphilis (p. 825). Spontaneous rupture of the spleen has occurred but is rare (Van Landingham et al 1984) and would also raise the possibility of Epstein–Barr virus infection.

### Convalescence

The convalescent phase generally begins within 2 weeks of the onset of jaundice. Jaundice fades and the stools and urine return to their normal color. Although by the sixth week of the illness the jaundice has generally resolved and the liver biochemistry may have returned to virtually normal, mental and physical fatigue can persist for several months. A more prolonged course can be seen in those over 60 years of age (Gibinski et al 1973). Most patients have completely recovered from their acute illness within 6 months. Hepatitis B, C and D can lead to chronic disease and persistently deranged liver function tests 6 months after the onset of the acute phase suggest chronic infection.

### Clinical comparison of viral hepatitis

The range and sequence of symptoms and signs are very similar in all the viral hepatides. However, an abrupt onset, prodromal fever and gastrointestinal symptoms are more prominent in hepatitis A infection and the serum sickness syndrome is more typical of hepatitis B. Hepatitis E is more associated with gastrointestinal symptoms in the prodromal illness.

## INVESTIGATIONS

### Urine tests

Bilirubin appears in the urine in the prodromal phase and may lead to the diagnosis. Bilirubinuria gradually disappears in the convalescent phase. Occasionally mild proteinuria and a few red blood cells may be detected in the urine in serum sickness illness or in hepatitis-associated renal disease (Conrad et al 1964).

### Peripheral blood

The white cell count in viral hepatitis is usually normal although leukopenia sometimes occurs in the prodromal phase or in the first week of jaundice. Granulocytopenia increases the proportion of lymphocytes in the blood and atypical lymphocytes similar to those seen in acute Epstein–Barr virus infection are evident in 5–20% of cases (Penington et al 1978). Leukocytosis is unusual in uncomplicated viral hepatitis and alternative diagnoses or fulminant hepatic failure should be considered. Anemia is unusual in viral hepatitis, although a mild reduction in red blood survival can occur (Katz et al 1964, Conrad et al 1964). A hepatitic illness in combination with hemolysis suggests Wilson's disease (p. 807) or autoimmune disease.

### Liver function tests

Liver function tests have to be interpreted in relation to the clinical severity and duration of the illness. A greatly increased serum transaminase activity is the best indication of acute hepatitis and alanine aminotransferase is more specific for liver disease than aspartate aminotransferase (p. 741). Activities greater than 500 u/L generally support the diagnosis and above 1000 u/L usually indicate acute hepatitis. Elevation of the transaminase activity is present in the prodromal phase and activity usually starts to fall with the onset of the icteric phase Transaminase activities reflect the severity of the illness (Zimmerman 1964) and are useful in following progress, but they have no prognostic value (p. 741). Patients with persisting high transaminase activities 6 months after the onset of HBV, HCV or HDV infection most likely have developed chronic infection. Plasma transaminase activity may not reflect the severity of hepatitis in patients with pre-existing chronic liver disease where severe damage may be associated with only moderate enzyme activity. The serum bilirubin concentration is often increased in the prodromal phase and peaks after about 7–10 days. Values have generally returned to normal within 8 weeks (Strickland et al 1971). Most patients with acute viral hepatitis have a moderate (less than twice normal) elevation in the alkaline phosphatase activity that settles rapidly unless the patient develops prolonged cholestasis, which is seen occasionally in acute hepatitis A.

### Serum proteins

The serum albumin and globulin concentrations are of limited value in acute hepatitis. Albumin has a long half-life and is consequently an insensitive reflection of changes of hepatic synthetic function in acute diseases (p. 745). More prolonged disease can be associated with a fall in the albumin concentration and this has been noted in older patients over 60 years of age (Gibinski et al 1973). A low initial serum albumin suggests pre-existing liver disease. After 2–3 weeks the γ-globulin levels rise as a consequence of the immune response.

### Glucose

Hypoglycemia can occur in any severe acute liver disease and the blood glucose should be checked in patients who are clearly unwell. Hypoglycemia occurs most often in fulminant hepatic failure (p. 811).

### Coagulation

Most coagulation factors are made in the liver and have short half-lives (p. 751). Measurements of coagulation are therefore useful reflections of short-term hepatic synthetic function. A steadily increasing prothrombin time is the best readily available indication of a poor prognosis and warns of the development of fulminant hepatic failure (p. 811).

### Serology

Currently available serological tests allow confident diagnoses of hepatitis A, B and D to be made. The hepatitis C antibody test may be negative at the time of the acute illness, but newer tests should facilitate earlier diagnosis and, if available, detection of HCV-RNA helps with the diagnosis if other viral causes of hepatitis have been excluded.

Low autoantibody titers occur during acute viral hepatitis, but high antibody titers in a more prolonged illness suggest an autoimmune chronic hepatitis rather than an acute viral hepatitis.

## MANAGEMENT

### Bed rest

Strict bed rest was routinely prescribed in the past for acute viral hepatitis. Several studies, mainly within the armed forces, have failed to demonstrate any deleterious effect of strenuous exercise on the illness (Repsher & Freebern 1969). However, the recuperative powers of young, previously fit men are likely to be very different from those of older patients. Patients with more severe liver damage feel unwell and know they need rest, including bed rest, whereas younger patients may wish to resume normal activities more quickly.

### Diet

A high-calorie, high-protein diet has been shown to reduce the length of time in hospital for soldiers (Chalmers et al 1955), but civilian patients often find that the anorexia associated with acute hepatitis limits their food intake and this is often associated with weight loss. Low-fat diets are frequently advised, although there is no evidence that dietary fat impairs recovery (Hoagland et al 1946). Patients with severe anorexia, nausea or vomiting occasionally need nutritional support. Felig et al (1970) found that hypoglycemia is common in acute hepatitis, as half their patients had a blood glucose below 3.2 mmol/L (60 mg/dl). Accordingly, hypoglycemia should be sought in those with more severe disease, as a glucose infusion may be needed. Avoidance of alcohol is generally recommended for some months after acute infection, but this is unnecessary and alcohol intake within generally accepted levels (p. 872) is safe once anorexia has resolved (Tözün 1991).

### Corticosteroids

There is no evidence that corticosteroid therapy is of benefit in acute viral hepatitis (Gregory 1981). Indeed, in spite of the view that much of the liver damage in acute hepatitis B is immune mediated, the risk of chronicity is higher in immunocompromised patients with acute hepatitis B and corticosteroid therapy should be avoided. Corticosteroid therapy may benefit a small number of patients with hepatitis A who develop prolonged cholestasis.

### Antiviral therapy

The role of antiviral therapy for viral hepatitis is discussed above in relation to individual hepatitis viruses.

## COMPLICATIONS AND SEQUELAE

Most patients make a full recovery from acute viral hepatitis, but complications and long-term sequelae can occur (Table 27.1).

**Table 27.1** Complications and sequelae of viral hepatitis

| |
|---|
| Relapsing hepatitis |
| Fulminant (acute) hepatic failure |
| Cholestatic hepatitis |
| Connective tissue disease |
| Renal failure |
| Aplastic anemia |
| Posthepatitis syndrome |
| Chronic hyperbilirubinemia |
| Subacute hepatic necrosis |
| Chronic liver disease |
| Chronic hepatitis |
| Cirrhosis |
| Hepatocellular carcinoma |

### Morbidity and mortality

Underdiagnosis limits the collection of accurate data regarding the morbidity and mortality of acute hepatitis. Most data relate to the more severely ill patients who require hospitalization. Gibinski et al (1973) detailed 1335 Polish patients with acute hepatitis. There was no mortality in those under 40 years and 3% in those over 60 years. The Copenhagen Hepatitis Acuta Programme (1982) studied 985 patients admitted to hospital with acute viral hepatitis and followed them for up to 10 years with autopsies in 78% of deaths. Five patients (0.5%) died from fulminant hepatic failure and a further nine patients (0.9%) had hepatitis (2) or cirrhosis (7) at death, although in only four (0.4%) of the nine was death due to liver disease or its treatment with prednisolone. All patients with liver disease at death had HBV or NANB (probably HCV) hepatitis. None of the patients with hepatitis A died with liver disease. As five patients had cryptogenic liver disease at death and as 5–10% of adults with acute HBV and at least 50% of those with acute HCV develop chronic infection, longer follow-up would likely have demonstrated a larger number of deaths due to liver disease. However, from the clinician's viewpoint, clinically apparent acute viral hepatitis in otherwise healthy people has a low mortality rate with the main complications seen in older patients and particularly those with hepatitis B or C. Older people also suffer greater morbidity in that they often have severe and prolonged illness.

### Unusual manifestations

The prodrome in acute viral hepatitis is a generalized nonspecific febrile illness and this may account for occasional unusual manifestations. Neurological complications including encephalitis and meningoencephalitis have occurred (Bromberg et al 1982, Hammond et al 1982). The lymphocytes in the cerebrospinal fluid and a normal prothrombin time and blood glucose help to differentiate these cases from hepatic encephalopathy in fulminant hepatic failure. Guillain–Barré syndrome (Niermeijer & Gips 1975) and various forms of mononeuritis affecting cranial or peripheral nerves (Pelletier et al 1985) have been described. A prodrome with a serum sickness syndrome can delay the diagnosis. Myocardial involvement may cause myocarditis and electrocardiographic changes have been reported (Bell 1971). Pancreatitis should be considered if severe abdominal pain is a feature (Achord 1968). Pleural effusions and ascites characterized by marked lymphocytosis and a high protein concentration in the pleural or ascitic fluid have been reported (Viola et al 1983). These resolve as the patient recovers and have to be differentiated from the ascites and pleural effusions that can occur in liver failure, where the effusions and ascites are transudates with low cell counts.

### Fulminant (acute) hepatic failure

This is a rare and often fatal complication of acute hepatitis (p. 805).

### Relapsing hepatitis

The incidence of clinical relapse has been reported as 1.5–18%, but the reasons for relapse are not understood (Havens 1962). Biochemical relapses are more frequent, but most probably reflect fluctuating serum transaminase activity such as is seen commonly with hepatitis C. Precipitating factors including excessive physical activity, poor nutrition, pregnancy, alcohol and corticosteroid therapy have been cited but often with little evidence.

Relapse occurs particularly in hepatitis A with an incidence quoted variously as 3–20% (Glikson et al 1992). The relapse usually occurs within 3 weeks, subsequent relapses are very rare and the course is generally self-limiting. Persisting infection occurs in some of these patients and the occurrence in others during relapse of rashes, purpura, arthralgia and occasionally nephritis suggests an immune mechanism. Relapse can also occur in other forms of viral hepatitis, but coinfection with more than one hepatitis virus, such as hepatitis B and hepatitis D (Govindarajan et al 1986), needs to be sought serologically, especially where relapse occurs some time after the original episode.

### Cholestatic hepatitis

The term "cholestatic viral hepatitis" has been used in two different contexts. First, it may be used to refer to the histological appearances in the liver. Dubin et al (1960) examined liver biopsies taken within 21 days of the onset of viral hepatitis and classified the appearances as those of acute hepatitis with and without cholestasis, cholestasis with mild hepatitis and isolated cholestasis. The serum bilirubin concentrations were higher in those with histological cholestasis (mean 200 μmol/L, 12 mg/dl) than in those without (mean 100 μmol/L, 6 mg/dl), but there were no other clinical differences between the groups. Second, cholestatic hepatitis may be used to refer to patients in whom acute viral hepatitis causes marked and prolonged cholestatic jaundice (Gall & Braunstein 1955, Shaldon & Sherlock 1957).

***Clinical features.*** The illness starts with the usual prodrome but when jaundice develops, it deepens progressively and the serum bilirubin can reach 300 μmol/L (18 mg/dl) by about the eighth week (range 100–600 μmol/L or 6–36 mg/dl). Pruritus appears after 3–4 weeks, although the patient feels otherwise well. Examination reveals a palpable liver, the spleen is occasionally felt and there may be a nonspecific maculopapular rash. Jaundice persists for 2–6 months after which complete clinical, biochemical and histological recovery almost always occurs.

***Investigations.*** Liver function tests show an obstructive pattern with greatly increased serum bilirubin and alkaline phosphatase and only a moderately increased transaminase activity. Liver biopsy reveals the features of acute hepatitis with centrilobular bile plugs and intracellular cholestasis. Occasionally submassive hepatic necrosis is evident (Schmid & Cueni 1972). It is important to differentiate cholestatic viral hepatitis from obstruction of a large bile duct, as surgical intervention should be avoided in acute viral hepatitis (p. 1138). An acute onset with typical prodromal symptoms suggests a viral cause, whereas fever, rigors and abdominal pain suggest obstruction of a larger bile duct. Ultrasound imaging should be used to exclude biliary obstruction (p. 52). Primary biliary cirrhosis is recognized by its longer clinical course and the presence of high titer antimitochondrial antibody (p. 939). In difficult cases further visualization of the biliary tree with transhepatic or endoscopic retrograde cholangiography may be required.

### Connective tissue disease

Characteristic features of connective tissue disease may arise in patients infected with hepatitis B virus either during the acute illness or in the course of chronic disease. Acute polyarthritis or multisystem disease due to widespread vasculitis are the usual manifestations (Duffy et al 1976, Sergent et al 1976). Many of these patients do not have jaundice and are indistinguishable from patients with other forms of connective tissue disease. They are recognized when abnormal liver function tests are found and/or the HBsAg is identified in the blood.

There are two main syndromes. Acute polyarthritis may last for several weeks but usually responds to bed rest and simple analgesic drugs and settles with the development of jaundice due to acute viral hepatitis. Any joint may be affected, either simultaneously or in a migratory pattern, and a maculopapular, urticarial or occasionally purpuric rash may develop. Patients with widespread vasculitis leading to multisystem disease are often very ill, febrile and have a leukocytosis. Their illness may become chronic and they may die. Many organs may be involved, but particularly common have been the joints, kidneys, heart, gut, nervous system and skin. Arthritis can affect any joint; renal damage is usually indicated by proteinuria (occasionally causing a nephrotic syndrome) and hematuria; cardiac involvement can cause cardiomegaly, cardiac failure or pericarditis; gastrointestinal vasculitis causes abdominal pain and may lead to bowel infarction; nervous system damage may cause peripheral neuropathy or signs of central nervous damage. Hypertension may develop. Treatment with immunosuppressive agents such as corticosteroids and cyclophosphamide and immunomodulatory/antiviral agents such as interferon has given varying results.

### Henoch–Schönlein purpura

There have been a few case reports linking Henoch–Schönlein purpura in children with acute hepatitis B virus infection. The classic IgA deposits and renal involvement have been described and recovery usually occurs (Maggiore et al 1984).

### Renal failure

Renal failure is common in fulminant hepatic failure but rare in uncomplicated viral hepatitis. Chronic hepatitis B virus infection has been associated with glomerulonephritis, particularly in children, and the association is based on finding HBsAg in the blood and in the glomeruli (Levy & Kleinknecht 1980). This condition has been reported mainly from central Europe and Japan and is less common in the United Kingdom and North America. It can cause self-limiting disease or occasionally chronic renal failure and interferon may be beneficial in some cases (Lisker-Melman et al 1989).

Eight patients with membranoproliferative glomerulonephritis in association with chronic HCV have been described (Johnson et al 1993). All had proteinuria (>3.5 g/day in five) and hypocomplementemia and renal biopsies showed membranoproliferative glomerulonephritis with the deposition of IgG, IgM and C3 on capillary walls. Electronmicroscopy was performed on four biopsies and the appearances in three suggested the presence of cryoglobulins. Interferon in four patients reduced protein loss but had a variable response on the serum creatinine. Membranous nephropathy (Rollino et al 1991) and immunoglobulin A nephropathy (Francisco et al 1992) have also been described in association with HCV infection. Spontaneous remission of minimal change nephropathy has been reported following hepatitis A virus infection (Kron & Hedger 1984).

### Aplastic anemia

A variety of hematological abnormalities can occur in acute viral hepatitis (Table 27.2). Aplastic anemia is rare but is the most serious of these complications. The hepatitis is usually uncomplicated and pancytopenia occurs at any time from the early convalescent phase of the illness for a period of about a year. Aplasia is recognized by marrow examination. There is a high mortality rate, but spontaneous recovery has occurred. Posthepatitic aplasia has not been linked to any single hepatitis virus and may be due to an as yet unrecognized hepatotropic virus (Hibbs et al 1992).

**Table 27.2** Hematological changes in viral hepatitis

| Common | Uncommon | Rare |
|---|---|---|
| Moderate anemia | Hemolytic anemia | Aplastic anemia |
| Low reticulocyte count | Agranulocytosis | |
| Shortened red cell survival | Pancytopenia | |
| Macrocytosis | Thrombocytopenia | |
| Leukopenia | | |
| Atypical lymphocytosis | | |
| Megaloblastic changes | | |
| Moderate thrombocytopenia | | |

## Posthepatitis syndrome

This syndrome develops occasionally after acute viral hepatitis when the liver function tests have returned to normal (Sherlock & Walshe 1946). Complaints include malaise, fatigue, anorexia, fat intolerance and upper abdominal discomfort. Myalgia and altered sleeping pattern may occur and the symptoms resemble those of chronic fatigue syndrome. A similar illness can follow other viral infections such as infectious mononucleosis (glandular fever), but the mechanisms are not understood. The peripheral blood count, creatinine and liver function tests are normal and viral serology shows no current hepatitis virus, EBV or CMV infection. Ultrasound examination and liver biopsy may be required in a minority of cases to exclude continuing liver inflammation and other causes of liver disease.

## Sjögren's syndrome

Sjögren's syndrome has been associated with chronic HCV infection (Haddad et al 1992), but there may also be a focal sialadenitis associated with chronic HCV (Aceti et al 1992).

## Porphyria cutanea tarda

A high prevalence of anti-HCV antibodies is seen in patients with porphyria cutanea tarda (DeCastro et al 1993).

## Cryoglobulinemia

Type II cryoglobulinemia appears strongly associated with HCV infection (Agnello et al 1992).

## Chronic liver disease

Chronic hepatitis can follow hepatitis B, C and D and is defined as an increased transaminase activity persisting for more than 6 months following the acute attack (p. 888). Chronic viral hepatitis is generally asymptomatic and the diagnosis may therefore be made by chance when liver function tests are checked incidentally or as part of a screening procedure, as by a blood transfusion center. Patients with chronic HBV infection are generally HBeAg positive, but patients infected with the precore mutant are HBeAg negative and anti-HBe antibody positive but have ongoing viral replication with HBV-DNA in the blood and HBcAg detectable within the liver (Carman et al 1989). Patients with chronic HCV infection are anti-HCV positive and have HCV-RNA detectable in blood. Those with chronic HDV infection are HBsAg positive and HDV antigen or HDV-RNA can be detected in blood or liver samples.

## Cirrhosis

Patients with cirrhosis may have no history of a hepatitic illness. The risk of developing cirrhosis and the time required to do so in chronic hepatitis virus infection is very variable. Most patients with chronic hepatitis B eventually develop cirrhosis, often within 10 years of diagnosis (p. 897), and those with chronic hepatitis D infections usually progress to cirrhosis more quickly, sometimes within 2–3 years (p. 899). Chronic hepatitis C is usually an indolent disease with few or no symptoms, but cirrhosis can eventually develop although it may take 10–20 years to do so (p. 898).

## Hepatocellular carcinoma

Hepatitis B, C and D are all associated with the development of hepatocellular carcinoma (p. 1115). This almost always occurs in patients with established cirrhosis, suggesting that increased cell turnover may predispose to malignant transformation. Occasionally, hepatocellular carcinoma has developed in viral carriers with minimal liver disease, but this is unusual. It is suggested that patients with cirrhosis be screened regularly by imaging and serum alpha-fetoprotein estimation to detect hepatocellular carcinomas at a potentially resectable stage (p. 1125).

## REFERENCES

Aceti A, Taliani G, Sorice M, Amendolea M A 1992 HCV and Sjögren's syndrome. Lancet 339: 1425–1426
Achord J L 1968 Acute pancreatitis with infectious hepatitis. Journal of the American Medical Association 205: 837–840
Agnello V, Chung R T, Kaplan L M 1992 A role for hepatitis C virus infection in type II cryoglobulinemia. New England Journal of Medicine 327: 1490–1495
Aikawa T, Sugai Y, Okamoto H 1996 Hepatitis G infection in drug abusers with chronic hepatitis C. New England Journal of Medicine: 334: 195–196
Alarcon G S, Townes A S 1973 Arthritis in viral hepatitis: report of two cases and review of the literature. Johns Hopkins Medical Journal 132: 1–15
Alberti A, Chemello L, Benvegnu L et al 1991 Pilot study of α-2a

interferon therapy in preventing chronic evolution of acute hepatitis C. In: Hollinger F B, Lemon S M, Margolis H (eds) Viral hepatitis and liver disease. Williams and Wilkins, Baltimore, p 636–658
Alberti A, Morsica G, Chemello L et al 1992 Hepatitis C viraemia and liver disease in symptom-free individuals with anti-HCV. Lancet 340: 697–698
Allander T, Gruber A, Naghavi M et al 1995 Frequent patient-to-patient transfer of hepatitis C in a haematology ward. Lancet 345: 603–607
Alter M J 1994 Transmission of hepatitis C virus – route, dose, and titer. New England Journal of Medicine 330: 784–786
Alter M J, Margolis H S, Krawczynski K et al 1992 The natural history of community-acquired hepatitis C in the United States. New England Journal of Medicine 327: 1899–1905
Bamber M, Murray A, Arborgh B A et al 1981 Short incubation non-A, non-B hepatitis transmitted by factor VIII concentrates in patients with congenital coagulation disorders. Gut 22: 854–859
Beasley R P, Hwang L-Y, Lin C-C et al 1981a Hepatitis B immune globulin (HBIG) efficacy in the interruption of perinatal transmission of hepatitis B virus carrier state. Initial report of a randomised double-blind placebo-controlled trial. Lancet 2: 388–392
Beasley R P, Hwang L-Y, Lin C-C, Chien C-S 1981b Hepatocellular carcinoma and hepatitis B virus: a prospective study of 22,700 men in Taiwan. Lancet 2: 1129–1133
Bell H 1971 Cardiac manifestations of viral hepatitis. Journal of the American Medical Association 218: 387–391
Blumberg B S, Gerstley B J S, Hungerford D A, London W T, Sutnick A I 1967 A serum antigen (Australia antigen) in Down's syndrome, leukemia and hepatitis. Annals of Internal Medicine 66: 924–931
Bonino F, Hoyer B, Shih J W, Rizzetto M, Purcell R H, Gerin J L 1984 Delta hepatitis agent: structural and antigenic properties of the delta-associated particle. Infection and Immunity 43: 1000–1005
Bonino F, Heermann K H, Rizzetto M, Gerlich W H 1986 Hepatitis delta virus: protein composition of delta antigen and its hepatitis B virus-derived envelope. Journal of Virology 58: 945–950
Bradley D W, Andjaparidze A, Cook E H Jr et al 1988 Aetiological agent of enterically transmitted non-A, non-B hepatitis. Journal of General Virology 69: 731–738
Brillanti S, Foli M, Gaiani S, Masci C, Miglioli M, Barbara L 1993 Persistent hepatitis C viraemia without liver disease. Lancet 341: 464–465
Bromberg K, Newhall D N, Peter G 1982 Hepatitis A and meningoencephalitis. Journal of the American Medical Association 247: 815
Carman W F, Jacyna M R, Hadziyannis S et al 1989 Mutation preventing formation of hepatitis $HB_e$ antigen in chronic hepatitis B virus infection. Lancet 2: 588–591
Carman W F, Zanetti A R, Karayiannis P et al 1990 Vaccine-induced escape mutant of hepatitis B virus. Lancet 336: 325–329
Centers for Disease Control 1977 Outbreak of viral hepatitis in the staff of a pediatric ward – California. Morbidity and Mortality Weekly 26: 77
Chalmers T C, Eckhardt R D, Reynolds W E et al 1955 The treatment of acute infectious hepatitis: controlled studies of the effect of diet, rest and physical reconditioning on the acute course of the disease and on the incidence of relapses and residual abnormalities. Journal of Clinical Investigation 34: 1163–1235
Chemello L, Alberti A, Rose K, Simmonds P 1994 Hepatitis C serotype and response to interferon therapy. New England Journal of Medicine 330: 143
Choo Q-L, Kuo G, Weiner A J, Overby L R, Bradley D W, Houghton M 1989 Isolation of a cDNA clone derived from a blood-borne non-A, non-B viral hepatitis genome. Science 244: 359–362
Conrad M E, Schwartz F D, Young A A 1964 Infectious hepatitis: a generalized disease. A study of renal, gastrointestinal and hematologic abnormalities. American Journal of Medicine 37: 789–801
Conry-Cantilena C, Van Raden M, Gibble J et al 1996 Routes of infection, viremia, and liver disease in blood donors found to have hepatitis C virus infection. New England Journal of Medicine 334: 1691–1696
Cooper L Z, Green R H, Krugman S, Giles J P, Mirick G S 1965 Neonatal thrombocytopenic purpura and other manifestations of rubella contracted in utero. American Journal of Diseases of Children 110: 416–421
Copenhagen Hepatitis Acuta Programme 1982 Mortality after acute hepatitis type A, B, and non-A non-B in 981 patients followed up for up to 10 years. Scandinavian Journal of Gastroenterology 17: 193–198
Corey L, Holmes K K 1980 Sexual transmission of hepatitis A in homosexual men: incidence and mechanisms. New England Journal of Medicine 302: 435–438
Coutinho R A, Albrecht-van Lent P, Lelie N, Nagelkerke N, Kuipers H, Rijsdijk T 1983 Prevalence and incidence of hepatitis A among male homosexuals. British Medical Journal 287: 1743–1745
Dane D S, Cameron C H, Briggs M 1970 Virus-like particles in serum of patients with Australia-antigen-associated hepatitis. Lancet 1: 695–698
DeCastro M, Sánchez J, Herrera J F et al 1993 Hepatitis C virus antibodies and liver disease in patients with porphyria cutanea tarda. Hepatology 17: 551–557
Deka N, Sharma M D, MukerjeeR 1994 Isolation of the novel agent from human stool samples that is associated with sporadic non-A, non-B hepatitis. Journal of Virology 68: 7810–7815
Dodd R Y 1992 The risk of transfusion-transmitted infection. New England Journal of Medicine 327: 419–421
Dubin I N, Sullivan B H Jr, LeGolvan P C, Murphy L C 1960 The cholestatic form of viral hepatitis: experiences with viral hepatitis at Brooke Army Hospital during the years 1951 to 1953. American Journal of Medicine 29: 55–72
Duffy J, Lidsky M D, Sharp J T et al 1976 Polyarthritis, polyarteritis and hepatitis B. Medicine 55: 19
Dunnet W N 1963 Infectious mononucleosis. British Medical Journal 1: 1187–1191
Esteban J I, Gómez J, Martell M et al 1996 Transmission of hepatitis C virus by a cardiac surgeon. New England Journal of Medicine 334: 555–560
Esterly J R, Slusser R J, Ruebner B H 1967 Hepatic lesions in the congenital rubella syndrome. Journal of Pediatrics 71: 676–685
Evans D J, Williams E D 1968 Cytomegalic inclusion disease in the adult. Journal of Clinical Pathology 21: 311–316
Fauerholdt L, Asnaes S, Ranek L, Schiødt T, Tygstrup N 1977 Significance of suspected "chronic aggressive hepatitis" in acute hepatitis. Gastroenterology 73: 543–548
Feinstone S M, Kapikian A Z, Purcell R H 1973 Hepatitis A: detection by immune electron microscopy of a virus-like antigen associated with acute illness. Science 182: 1026–1028
Felig P, Brown W V, Levine R A, Klatskin G 1970 Glucose homeostasis in viral hepatitis. New England Journal of Medicine 283: 1436–1440
Francisco S, Wall B M, Cooke C R 1992 Immunoglobulin A nephropathy in a renal allograft of a black transplant recipient. American Journal of Nephrology 12: 121–125
Gall E A, Braunstein H 1955 Hepatitis with manifestations simulating bile duct obstruction (so called "cholangiolitic hepatitis"). American Journal of Clinical Pathology 25: 1113–1127
Gavish D, Kleinman Y, Morag A, Chajek-Shaul T 1983 Hepatitis and jaundice associated with measles in young adults. Archives of Internal Medicine 143: 674–677
Gerberding J L 1996 The infected health care provider. New England Journal of Medicine 334: 594–595
Gibinski K, Fojt E, Suchan L 1973 Hepatitis in the aged. Digestion 8: 254–260
Giusti G, Gaeta G B 1981 Doctors in the kitchen. Experiments with cooking bivalve mollusks. New England Journal of Medicine 304: 1371–1372
Glikson M, Galun E, Oren R, Tur-Kaspa R, Shouval D 1992 Relapsing hepatitis A. Review of 14 cases and literature survey. Medicine 71: 14–23
Govindarajan S, De Cock K M, Rediker A G 1986 Natural course of delta superinfection in chronic hepatitis B virus-infected patients: histopathologic studies with multiple liver biopsies. Hepatology 6: 640–644
Gregory P B 1981 The demise of corticosteroid therapy for acute viral hepatitis. Gastroenterology 80: 404–409
Haddad J, Deny P, Munz-Gotheil C et al 1992 Lymphocytic sialadenitis of Sjögren's syndrome associated with chronic hepatitis C virus liver disease. Lancet 339: 321–323
Hadler S C 1991 Global impact of hepatitis A virus infection changing

patterns. In: Hollinger F B, Lemon S M, Margolis H (eds) Viral hepatitis and liver disease. Williams and Wilkins, Baltimore, p 14–20
Hadler S C, Erben J J, Matthews D, Starko K, Francis D P, Maynard J E 1983 The effect of immunoglobulin on hepatitis A in day-care centers. Journal of the American Medical Association 249: 48–53
Hadler S C, de Monzon M, Ponzetto A et al 1984 Delta virus infection and severe hepatitis. An epidemic in the Yupca Indians of Venezuela. Annals of Internal Medicine 100: 339–344
Hadziyannis S, Wages J, Kim J P et al 1995 Frequency of viraemia with a new hepatitis virus (HGV) in patients with liver disease and in groups at high risk of exposure to blood and blood products. Journal of Hepatology 23 (suppl 1): 78
Halliday M L, Kang L-Y, Zhou T-K et al 1991 An epidemic of hepatitis A attributable to the ingestion of raw clams in Shanghai, China. Journal of Infectious Diseases 164: 852–859
Hammond G W, MacDougall B K, Plummer F, Sekla L H 1982 Encephalitis during the prodromal stage of acute hepatitis A. Canadian Medical Association Journal 126: 269–270
Hanshaw J B, Betts R F, Simon G, Boynton R C 1965 Acquired cytomegalovirus infection: association with hepatomegaly and abnormal liver function tests. New England Journal of Medicine 272: 602–609
Harpaz R, Von Seidlein L, Averhoff F M et al 1966 Transmission of hepatitis B virus to multiple patients from a surgeon without evidence of inadequate infection control. New England Journal of Medicine 334:549–554
Hart G K, Thompson W R, Schneider J, Davis N J, Oh T E 1984 Fulminant hepatic failure and fatal encephalopathy associated with Epstein–Barr virus infection. Medical Journal of Australia 141: 112–113
Havens W P Jr 1962 Viral hepatitis: clinical patterns and diagnosis. American Journal of Medicine 32: 665–678
Hibbs J R, Frickhofen N, Rosenfeld S J et al 1992 Aplastic anemia and viral hepatitis non-A, non-B, non-C? Journal of the American Medical Association 267: 2051–2054
Hiramatsu N, Hayashi N, Haruna Y et al 1992 Immunohistochemical detection of hepatitis C virus-infected hepatocytes in chronic liver disease with monoclonal antibodies to core, envelope and NS3 regions of the hepatitis C virus genome. Hepatology 16: 306–311
Hoagland C L, Labby D H, Kunkel H G, Shank R E 1946 An analysis of the effect of fat in the diet on recovery in infectious hepatitis. American Journal of Public Health and the Nation's Health 36: 1287–1292
Hoagland R J 1967 Infectious mononucleosis. Grune and Stratton, New York
Hoofnagle J H 1989 Type D (delta) hepatitis. Journal of the American Medical Association 261: 1321–1325
Horwitz C A, Henle W, Henle G, Schapiro R, Borken S, Bundtzen R 1983 Infectious mononucleosis in patients aged 40 to 72 years: report of 27 cases including 3 without heterophil-antibody responses. Medicine 62: 256–262
James D G 1996 Viral hepatitis' G string. Quarterly Journal of Medicine 89: 159–160
Johnson R J, Gretch D R, Yamabe H et al 1993 Membranoproliferative glomerulonephritis associated with hepatitis C virus infection. New England Journal of Medicine 328: 465–470
Karayiannis P, Novick D M, Lok A S F, Fowler M J F, Monjardino J, Thomas H C 1985 Hepatitis B virus DNA in saliva, urine and seminal fluid of carriers of hepatitis B e antigen. British Medical Journal 290: 1853–1855
Katz R, Valesco M, Guzman C, Alessandri H 1964 Red cell survival estimated by radioactive chromium in hepatobiliary disease. Gastroenterology 46: 399–404
Kilpatrick Z M 1966 Structural and functional abnormalities of liver in infectious mononucleosis. Archives of Internal Medicine 117: 47–53
Kim J P, Linnen J, Wages J et al 1995 Hepatitis G virus (HGV), a new hepatitis virus associated with human hepatitis. Journal of Hepatology 23 (suppl 1): 78
Knight 1967 Cited in Mosley J W The search for human hepatic viruses. Archiv für die Gesente Virusforschung 22: 252
Koretz R L, Suffin S C, Gitnick G L 1976 Post-transfusion chronic liver disease. Gastroenterology 71: 796–803
Kron M A, Hedger R 1984 Hepatitis A-induced remission of minimal change nephropathy. Archives of Internal Medicine 144: 2279–2280
Kruskall M S, Alper C A, Awdeh Z, Yunis E J, Marcus-Bagley D 1992 The immune response to hepatitis B in humans: inheritance patterns in families. Journal of Experimental Medicine 175: 495–502
Lamb S G, Stern H 1966 Cytomegalovirus mononucleosis with jaundice as presenting sign. Lancet 2: 1003–1006
Lancet 1991 Editorial: hepatitis G? Lancet 337: 1070
Leggiadro R J, Chwatsky D N, Zucker S W 1982 Echovirus 3 infection associated with anicteric hepatitis. American Journal of Diseases of Children 136: 744–745
Levin S, Leibowitz E, Torten J, Hahn T 1989 Interferon treatment in acute progressive and fulminant hepatitis. Israel Journal of Medical Science 25: 364–372
Levy M, Kleinknecht C 1980 Membranous glomerulonephritis and hepatitis B virus infection. Nephron 26: 259–265
Lisker-Melman M, Webb D, Di Bisceglie A M et al 1989 Glomerulonephritis caused by chronic hepatitis B virus infection: treatment with recombinant human alpha interferon. Annals of Internal Medicine 111: 479–483
Loke R H, Murray-Lyon I M, Coleman J C, Evans B A, Zuckerman A J 1990 Diminished response to recombinant hepatitis B vaccine in homosexual men with HIV antibody: an indicator of poor prognosis. Journal of Medical Virology 31: 109–111
MacSween R N M 1980 Pathology of viral hepatitis and its sequelae. Clinics in Gastroenterology 9: 23–45
Maggiore G, Martini A, Grifeo S, de Giacomo C, Scotta M S 1984 Hepatitis B virus infection and Schönlein–Henoch purpura. American Journal of Diseases of Children 138: 681–682
McFarlane I G, Smith H M, Johnson P J, Bray G P, Vergani D, Williams R 1990 Hepatitis C virus antibodies in chronic active hepatitis: pathogenetic factor or false-positive result? Lancet 335: 754–757
McMahon B J, Alberts S R, Wainwright R B, Bulkow L, Lanier A P 1990 Hepatitis B-related sequelae: prospective study of 1400 hepatitis B surface antigen-positive Alaska native carriers. Archives of Internal Medicine 150: 1051–1054
Miller R H, Purcell R H 1990 Hepatitis C virus shares amino acid sequence similarity with pestiviruses and flaviviruses as well as members of two plant virus supergroups. Proceedings of the National Academy of Sciences of the United States of America 87: 2057–2061
Minor P D 1991 Picornaviridae. Springer Verlag, Vienna
Modai D, Pik A, Marmor Z et al 1986 Liver dysfunction in measles, liver biopsy findings. Digestive Diseases and Sciences 31: 333
Molina J-M, Welker Y, Ferchal F, Decazes J-M, Shenmetzler C, Modaï J 1992 Hepatitis associated with primary HIV infection. Gastroenterology 102: 739
Moradpour D, Wands J R 1995 Understanding hepatitis B virus infection. New England Journal of Medicine 332: 1092–1093
Nakatsuji Y, Matsumoto A, Tanaka E, Ogata H, Kiyosawa K 1992 Detection of chronic hepatitis C virus infection by four diagnostic systems: first-generation and second-generation enzyme-linked immunosorbent assay, second-generation recombinant immunoblot assay and nested polymerase chain reaction analysis. Hepatology 16: 300–305
Niermeijer P, Gips C M 1975 Guillain–Barré syndrome in acute HBsAg positive hepatitis. British Medical Journal 2: 732–733
Norman C 1984 The unsung hero of yellow fever. Science 223: 1370–1372
Ohto H, Terazawa S, Sasaki N et al 1994 Transmission of hepatitis C virus from mothers to infants. New England Journal of Medicine 330: 744–750
Omata M, Yokosuka O, Takani S et al 1991 Resolution of acute hepatitis C after therapy with natural beta interferon. Lancet 338: 914–915
Pelletier G, Elghozi D, Trépo C, Laverdant C, Benhamou J-P 1985 Mononeuritis in acute viral hepatitis. Digestion 32: 53–56
Penington D, Rush B, Castaldi P (eds) 1978 De Gruchy's clinical haematology in medical practice, 4th edn. Blackwell, Oxford
Phillips M J, Blendis L M, Poucell S et al 1991 Syncytial giant cell hepatitis – sporadic hepatitis with distinctive pathological features, a severe clinical course, and paramyxoviral features. New England Journal of Medicine 324: 455–460
Poterucha J J, Rakela J, Lumeng L, Lee C-H, Taswell H F, Wiesner R H 1992 Diagnosis of chronic hepatitis C after liver transplantation by the detection of viral sequences with polymerase chain reaction. Hepatology 15: 42–45

Prince A M 1968 An antigen detected in the blood during the incubation period of serum hepatitis. Proceedings of the National Academy of Sciences of the United States of America 60: 814–821

Purtilo D T, Cassel C K, Yang J P S et al 1975 X-linked recessive progressive combined variable immunodeficiency (Duncan's disease). Lancet 1: 935–940

Repsher L H, Freebern R K 1969 Effects of early and vigorous exercise on recovery from infectious hepatitis. New England Journal of Medicine 281: 1393–1396

Ringertz O 1967 Serum hepatitis among Swedish track finders. An epidemiological study. New England Journal of Medicine 276: 540

Rizzetto M, Durazzo M 1991 Hepatitis delta virus (HDV) infections. Epidemiological and clinical heterogeneity. Journal of Hepatology 13 (suppl 4): S116–S118

Rizzetto M, Canese M G, Aricò S et al 1977 Immunofluorescence detection of new antigen–antibody system (∂/anti-∂) associated with hepatitis B virus in liver and in serum of HBsAg carriers. Gut 18: 997–1003

Rizzetto M, Verme G, Recchia S et al 1983 Chronic hepatitis in carriers of hepatitis B surface antigen, with intrahepatic expression of the delta antigen. Annals of Internal Medicine 98: 437–441

Robinson W S, Greenman R L 1974 DNA polymerase in the core of the human hepatitis B virus candidate. Journal of Virology 13: 1231–1236

Rollino C, Roccatello D, Giachino O, Basolo B, Piccoli G 1991 Hepatitis C virus infection and membranous glomerulonephritis. Nephron 59: 319–320

Ryan K W, MacLennan S, Barbara J A J, Hewitt P E 1994 Follow-up of blood donors positive for antibodies to hepatitis C virus. British Medical Journal 308: 696–697

Schlauder G G, Dawson G J, Simons J N et al 1995 Molecular and serologic analysis in the transmission of the GB hepatitis agents. Journal of Medical Virology 46: 81–90

Schmid M, Cueni B 1972 Portal lesions in viral hepatitis with submassive hepatic necrosis. Human Pathology 3: 209–216

Sergent J S, Lockshin H D, Christian C L, Gocke D J 1976 Vasculitis with hepatitis B antigenemia. Medicine 55: 1–18

Shaldon S, Sherlock S 1957 Virus hepatitis with features of prolonged bile retention. British Medical Journal 2: 734–738

Shalev-Zimels H, Weizman Z, Lotan C, Gavish D, Ackerman Z, Morag A 1988 Extent of measles hepatitis in various ages. Hepatology 8: 1338–1339

Sherlock S, Walshe V 1946 The post-hepatitis syndrome. Lancet 2: 482

Shusterman N H, Frauenhoffer C, Kinsey M D 1978 Fatal massive hepatic necrosis in cytomegalovirus mononucleosis. Annals of Internal Medicine 88: 810–812

Simmonds P 1995 Variability of hepatitis C virus. Hepatology 21: 570–583

Simmonds P, Alberti A, Alter H J et al 1994 A proposed system for the nomenclature of hepatitis C viral genotypes. Hepatology 19: 1321–1324

Simons J N, Leary T P, Dawson G J et al 1995 Isolation of novel virus-like sequences associated with human hepatitis. Nature Medicine 1: 564–569

Simpson D I H 1995 The filovirus enigma. Lancet 345: 1252–1253

Skidmore S J, Gully P R, Middleton J D, Hassam Z A, Singal G M 1985 An outbreak of hepatitis A on a hospital ward. Journal of Medical Virology 17: 175–177

Stern H, Williams B M 1966 Isolation of rubella virus in a case of neonatal giant cell hepatitis. Lancet 1: 293–295

Stevens C E, Alter H J, Taylor P E, Zang E A, Harley E J, Szmuness W 1984 Hepatitis B vaccine in patients receiving hemodialysis: immunogenicity and efficacy. New England Journal of Medicine 311: 496–501

Stokes J Jr, Neefe J R 1945 The prevention and attenuation of infectious hepatitis by gamma globulin. Journal of the American Medical Association 127: 144–145

Strauss L, Bernstein J 1968 Neonatal hepatitis in congenital rubella. Archives of Pathology 86: 317–322

Strickland G T, Castell D O, Kronmal R A 1971 Prolonged observation of the liver function tests in infectious hepatitis. American Journal of Gastroenterology 55: 257–264

Summers J, Smolec J M, Snyder F 1978 A virus similar to human hepatitis B virus associated with hepatitis and hepatoma in woodchucks. Proceedings of the National Academy of Sciences of the United States of America 75: 4533–4537

Tapalaga D, Forzani B, Hele C, Paravacini O, Ponzetto A, Theilmann L 1986 Prevalence of the hepatitis delta virus in Rumania. Hepato-Gastroenterology 33: 238–239

Toghill P J, Bailey M E, Williams R, Zeegan R, Bown R 1967 Cytomegalovirus hepatitis in the adult. Lancet 1: 1351–1354

Tözün N, Forbes A, Anderson M G, Murray-Lyon I M 1991 Safety of alcohol after viral hepatitis. Lancet 337: 1079–1080

Tremolada F, Casarin C, Alberti A et al 1992 Long-term follow-up of non-A, non-B (type C) post-transfusion hepatitis. Journal of Hepatology 16: 273–281

Van der Poel C L, Cuypers H T M, Reesnik H W et al 1991 Confirmation of hepatitis C virus infection by new four-antigen recombinant immunoblot assay. Lancet 337: 317–319

Van Landingham S B, Rawls D E, Roberts J W 1984 Pathological rupture of the spleen associated with hepatitis A. Archives of Surgery 119: 224–225

Viladomiu L, Genescà J, Esteban J I et al 1992 Interferon-α in acute posttransfusion hepatitis C: a randomized, controlled trial. Hepatology 15: 767–769

Villeneuve J-P, Desrochers M, Infante-Rivard C et al 1994 A long-term follow-up study of asymptomatic hepatitis B surface antigen-positive carriers in Montreal. Gastroenterology 106: 1000–1005

Viola C, Viñeta L, Bosch J, Rodés J 1983 Exudative ascites in the course of acute type B hepatitis. Hepatology 3: 1013–1015

Werzberger A, Bensch B, Kuter B et al 1992 A controlled trial of a formalin-inactivated hepatitis A vaccine in healthy children. New England Journal of Medicine 327: 453–457

Wewalka F 1974 Clinical course of viral hepatitis. Clinics in Gastroenterology 3: 355–376

Winokur P L, Stapleton J T 1992 Immunoglobulin prophylaxis for hepatitis A. Clinical Infectious Diseases 14: 580–586

Yoshiba M, Okamoto H, Mishiro S 1995 Detection of the GBV-C hepatitis virus genome in serum from patients with fulminant hepatitis of unknown aetiology. Lancet 346: 1131–1132

Zachoval R, Deinhart F 1993 Hepatitis A virus. Natural history and experimental models. In: Zuckerman A J, Thomas H C (eds) Viral hepatitis. Scientific basis and clinical management. Churchill Livingstone, Edinburgh, p 35–53

Zanetti A R, Tanzi E, Paccagnini S et al 1995 Mother-to-infant transmission of hepatitis C virus. Lancet 345: 289–291

Zimmerman H J 1964 Serum enzymes in the diagnosis of hepatic disease. Gastroenterology 46: 613–617

Zuckerman A J, Thomas H C (eds) 1993 Viral hepatitis. Scientific basis and clinical management. Churchill Livingstone, Edinburgh

Zuckerman A J, Zuckerman J L, Harrison T J 1993 Viral hepatitis. Prevention. In: Zuckerman A J, Thomas H C (eds) Viral hepatitis. Scientific basis and clinical management. Churchill Livingstone, Edinburgh, p 217–226

# 28. Fulminant and late-onset hepatic failure

*A. Gimson*

## INTRODUCTION AND DEFINITIONS

Fulminant hepatic failure is a clinical syndrome characterized by sudden massive hepatocyte dysfunction, in the absence of prior chronic liver disease, resulting in hepatic encephalopathy (Trey & Davidson 1970). These neurological changes can progress from minimal confusion to profound coma associated with cerebral edema. Although hepatocellular dysfunction is often very severe, functional and structural regeneration occur on recovery without the development of chronic liver disease (Horney & Galambos 1977, Milandri et al 1980). Recent reviews of fulminant hepatic failure include those of Lee (1993) and Caraceni & van Thiel (1995).

Considerable debate has arisen as to the definition of fulminant hepatic failure (Bernuau et al 1986a, Bernuau & Benhamou 1993). Most have used the definition of the Fulminant Hepatic Failure Surveillance Study where encephalopathy has to develop within 8 weeks of the onset of symptoms (Trey & Davidson 1970), with those cases presenting between 8 and 24 weeks defined as late-onset hepatic failure (Gimson et al 1986). Not all have agreed with this time limitation, restricting the diagnosis to 3, 4 or 6 weeks from onset (Benhamou et al 1972, European Association for the Study of the Liver 1979, Mathiesen et al 1980) and some have even suggested that encephalopathy is not a requirement (Bernuau & Benhamou 1993). The Kings College Hospital group in London, who have a large experience, have recently recommended a new terminology around the core term "acute liver failure" (O'Grady et al 1993). Patients presenting within 7 days of the onset of jaundice were termed hyperacute liver failure and had a high incidence of cerebral edema (69%) and relatively good prognosis with medical management (36% survival), in contrast to acute liver failure presenting within 8–28 days of jaundice with a similar incidence of cerebral edema (56%) but a very poor prognosis (7% survival). Subacute liver failure was defined as a presentation between 29 and 72 days, where cerebral edema was less common (14%) and the prothrombin time was less prolonged, but the survival was again very poor (14%). It is clear that, irrespective of etiology, time to encephalopathy is an independent parameter defining groups of patients with similar clinical features and prognosis, but more comparative studies from different geographical areas are required before these changes will be accepted.

## DIAGNOSIS

The diagnosis of fulminant hepatic failure depends on the recognition of hepatic encephalopathy soon after the onset of an acute hepatic illness and in the absence of any clinical feature of chronic liver disease (p. 917). Liver function tests show particularly a high serum transaminase activity indicating active hepatic damage and in the early stages the serum albumin concentration is normal. Tests of coagulation such as the prothrombin time, however, are abnormal, reflecting severe hepatic damage. Ultrasound imaging is useful in identifying underlying chronic liver disease and in showing unusual causes of fulminant hepatic failure such as the Budd–Chiari syndrome or metastatic liver disease (p. 54). Hepatitis A (p. 781), hepatitis B (p. 785), hepatitis D (p. 790) and less usual viral causes of acute hepatitis (p. 792) are diagnosed serologically. Serological tests often fail to identify hepatitis C owing to delayed appearance of anti-HCV antibodies (p. 788) and serological tests for hepatitis E are not yet available generally. Fulminant hepatic failure due to drugs is diagnosed mainly from the history, but early blood measurements are important in paracetamol overdosage (p. 846).

## ETIOLOGY

Fulminant hepatic failure is uncommon and most cases are due to viral hepatitis or drug hepatotoxicity (Table 28.1). Whether the many patients with negative viral serology, diagnosed as indeterminate viral hepatitis, should be considered as having a viral illness at all is controversial. Other rarer causes account for less than 5% of cases.

**Table 28.1** Etiology of fulminant hepatic failure

| | | |
|---|---|---|
| *Viral* | | |
| Hepatitis A | | |
| Hepatitis B | – acute | |
| | – chronic | – reactivation |
| | | – superinfection (hepatitis D) |
| Hepatitis C | | |
| Hepatitis D | – coinfection (hepatitis B) | |
| Hepatitis E | | |
| Indeterminate hepatitis | | |
| Other viruses | – Epstein–Barr | |
| | – Cytomegalovirus | |
| | – Herpes simplex | |
| | – Herpesvirus-6 | |
| *Drugs* | | |
| Paracetamol overdose | | |
| Halothane, isoflurane, enflurane | | |
| Carbon tetrachloride | | |
| Rare idiosyncratic drug reactions: e.g. isoniazid, rifampicin, sodium valproate, ketoconazole, tricyclic antidepressants, propylthiouracil | | |
| *Rare* | | |
| Pregnancy | – acute fatty liver | |
| | – pre-eclamptic syndromes | |
| Wilson's disease | | |
| Autoimmune hepatitis | | |
| Budd–Chiari syndrome | | |
| Malignant disease | – metastases | |
| | – lymphoma | |
| Heat stroke | | |
| Amanita poisoning | | |
| Circulatory shock | | |
| Reye's syndrome | | |
| Sepsis | | |

## Viral hepatitis

In most series, viral hepatitis is the most common cause of liver failure, accounting for up to 70% of cases. The reasons for the development of liver failure in less than 1% of cases of viral hepatitis are unclear and include host factors as well as the size of innoculum and virus-related factors (Forbes & Williams 1988).

In approximately 0.4% of patients with acute hepatitis A virus (HAV) infection, a fulminant course develops (Fagan & Williams 1990), being more common in the elderly and in intravenous drug abusers (Forbes & Williams 1988, Akriviadis & Redeker 1989). HAV accounts for up to 20% of cases of fulminant hepatic failure in some countries. Although HAV has been considered cytopathic, cell-mediated cytotoxicity has been recorded (Vallbracht et al 1986). In such cases the prognosis is relatively good, with survival rates of over 50% without transplantation (Fagan & Williams 1990).

In many countries hepatitis B virus (HBV) infection is the commonest cause of acute liver failure (Papaevangelou et al 1984). The risk of a fulminant course is higher than with HAV (McNeil et al 1984) and is more common in women and after termination of chemotherapy or immunosuppression in HBV carriers (Bird et al 1989). It is possibly less common in homosexuals (Bernuau et al 1986b). Fulminant hepatic failure is also associated with HBV reactivation, HBe antigen/HBe antibody seroconversion (p. 785), coinfection with HBV and hepatitis D virus (HDV) (p. 789) and superinfection of HBV carriers with HDV (Papaevangelou et al 1984). Coinfection or superinfection occurs in up to 40% of cases of fulminant hepatic failure who are HBsAg positive, with the majority (65%) being superinfection of HBV carriers (Smedile et al 1982, Govindarajan et al 1984), compared to only 4–19% of cases without a fulminant course. Recent reports have also suggested that infections with HBV precore mutants (p. 783), which are unable to secrete HBeAg, are more often associated with a fulminant course (Liang et al 1991, Omata et al 1991).

In contrast to patients with an uncomplicated course, the duration of hepatitis B surface antigenemia and HBV-DNA detection is shorter, the appearance of anti-HBe antibody quicker and the magnitude of the IgM anti-HBc response greater in those with a fulminant course, suggesting an exaggerated immune response to the virus (Trepo et al 1976, Gimson et al 1983, Brechot et al 1984).

The risk of developing fulminant hepatic failure after HCV infection remains unclear but is certainly low (Wright et al 1991, Feray et al 1993) and a fulminant course after post-transfusion hepatitis is exceptional (Farci et al 1996). In many series, up to 50% of patients with fulminant hepatic failure are of indeterminate viral etiology (Liang et al 1993), having no markers of HAV (IgM anti-HAV), HBV (IgM anti-HBc) or HCV infection, and over 80% of patients with late-onset hepatic failure are also negative for all viral markers (Gimson et al 1986).

Hepatitis E virus infection in the Indian subcontinent (Khuroo 1980) and in Africa is associated with a fulminant course predominantly in pregnant women (up to 22%) and may be detectable by specific serological assays (Asher et al 1990, Liang et al 1993).

Rarely, fulminant hepatic failure is associated with other viral infections including Epstein–Barr virus (Davies et al 1980a, Hart et al 1984), cytomegalovirus (Henson et al 1974), herpes simplex (Connor et al 1979), varicella zoster (Morishita et al 1985) and herpes virus-6 (Sobue et al 1991, Asano et al 1991), often in immunocompromised individuals.

## Drug hepatotoxicity

Drugs are common causes of liver damage and should always be suspected in fulminant hepatic failure. Some are directly hepatotoxic, but most damage the liver on an idiosyncratic basis (see Table 30.9).

***Paracetamol.*** Paracetamol (acetaminophen) hepatotoxicity occurs predominantly in the United Kingdom, usually after consumption of more than 12 g of the drug. Paracetamol metabolism produces an unstable nucleophilic intermediate, *N*-acetyl-*p*-benzoquinone imine, which damages cells when produced in amounts greater than can be detoxified by hepatic protective substances such as glutathione (p. 847). Paracetamol hepatotoxicity is more common in alcoholics and in those taking enzyme-inducing drugs (Licht et al 1980, Wootton & Lee 1990, Kumar & Rex 1991), due to induction of the cytochrome system and consequent increased production of the toxic metabolite. Prior depletion of tissue glutathione stores may also be important in alcoholics. In such cases, it is important to appreciate that hepatotoxicity may occur at serum levels of paracetamol substantially below the usually accepted treatment range.

The antidote *N*-acetylcysteine (NAC) (p. 848) given within 20 h of the overdose acts as a sulfhydryl donor (p. 847) to neutralize this toxic metabolite (Prescott et al 1979). Because it is often difficult to identify patients with enzyme induction, it is recommended that NAC should be given to any patient who has consumed more than 7 g. Recent evidence from a retrospective analysis and a randomized controlled trial suggests that patients with significant paracetamol hepatotoxicity who develop liver failure also benefit from NAC infusion even given more than 20 h after the event, with reduced organ dysfunction and significantly improved survival (Harrison et al 1990, Keays et al 1991a). The mechanism of action of NAC at that late stage is likely to be different.

***Halogenated anesthetics.*** Halothane hepatotoxicity usually occurs up to 21 days after exposure and is more common in females (p. 849). It is most common after multiple exposures but can occur after a single anesthetic. Rarely, there are other features of drug hypersensitivity including a rash, liver–kidney microsomal antibodies are found in 25% and a specific antibody against a component of halothane-altered hepatocyte membranes may be of diagnostic use. Hepatotoxicity after enflurane and isoflurane exposure is also recorded but not after desflurane or sevoflurane (p. 850).

### Other causes

These account for fewer than 5% of cases, but their recognition is important, particularly in respect of their management and especially where liver transplantation is being considered.

***Wilson's disease*** (p. 959). Fulminant hepatic failure due to Wilson's disease can be difficult to diagnose, as no single investigation gives consistently reliable diagnostic information (McCullough et al 1983, Da Costa et al 1992, Sallie et al 1992, Schilsky et al 1994). The clinical features may not be helpful. Jaundice is often more marked than in other causes of fulminant hepatic failure but is nonspecific and diagnostic Kayser–Fleischer rings are found in only half of patients and may need slit-lamp examination, which is not always practicable in an ill patient. Associated hemolytic anemia with a negative Coombs test is a very strong indicator of fulminant Wilson's disease and is present in most patients. The liver function tests often show a high plasma bilirubin due to a combination of hemolysis and liver dysfunction, plasma transaminase activity less than in other forms of fulminant hepatic failure and occasionally normal, and plasma alkaline phosphatase little increased or normal. An alkaline phosphatase (units/L) to bilirubin (mg/dl) ratio of less than 2 suggests the diagnosis but is not diagnostic (Berman et al 1991, Sallie et al 1992, Schilsky et al 1994). The plasma ceruloplasmin (p. 751) is low in over 90% of cases, but occasionally it is in the low normal range (p. 962) and sometimes other causes of severe liver failure may cause low concentrations (McCullough et al 1983). The plasma copper, particularly the plasma free copper, and the urine copper are usually high and the urine copper excretion is probably the most useful measurement (Da Costa et al 1992). The diagnosis can almost always be made from a combination of the clinical and laboratory features and measurement of the liver copper is rarely needed and is usually impracticable. The liver copper is high but varies considerably in different parts of the liver and may even be normal in occasional samples in fulminant Wilson's disease (Sallie et al 1992). Liver transplantation is often required, as liver function improves only slowly with medical therapy.

***Reye's syndrome.*** Reye's syndrome is characterized by an acute encephalopathy associated with cerebral edema and fatty change in the viscera (Mowat 1983). It usually occurs between the ages of 5 and 15 years, but cases aged over 20 years have been reported (Ede & Williams 1988). Although considered rare, with an incidence of 0.3–0.5 per 100 000 children, less severe forms of the disease may be more common (Heubi et al 1984). The causes are unknown, but many cases develop a few days after a febrile illness and numerous viruses, including influenza A and B, varicella zoster, Coxsackie, measles and adenoviruses, have been implicated. Interest has also centered on the role of salicylates in precipitating Reye's syndrome. Case-control studies pointed to a strong association, a prospective study supported the association (Hurwitz et al 1987) and avoidance of salicylates in childhood febrile illnesses has reduced the occurrence of Reye's syndrome (Barrett et al 1986). The primary lesions are in the liver and brain, with hepatocytes showing intense, diffuse microvesicular fatty change (p. 977) that can be easily overlooked unless special fat stains are performed. Inflammatory changes and hepatocyte necrosis are not seen, but mitochondrial damage is prominent on electron-microscopy. There is a 40–50% mortality in patients developing coma, but this is reduced to 10% in centers specializing in its management and in patients who do not develop coma (Heubi et al 1984).

***Miscellaneous.*** Liver failure associated with pregnancy (p. 1091) may be due to acute fatty liver of pregnancy or the eclamptic syndrome (Davies et al 1980b, Rolfes &

Ishak 1985, Riely et al 1987) and carries a relatively good prognosis. Budd–Chiari syndrome (p. 1077) can present acutely with fulminant hepatic failure and clinical features suggesting the diagnosis include hepatomegaly, splenomegaly and ascites which may not be marked (Powell-Jackson et al 1986). Ultrasound and Doppler imaging of the hepatic vasculature and the inferior vena cava are particularly important in these patients. Disseminated hepatic malignancy, particularly non-Hodgkin's lymphoma, may cause liver failure in association with splenomegaly (Zafrani et al 1983). Severe circulatory failure can cause fulminant liver failure (Nouel et al 1980) and *Amanita phalloides* mushroom poisoning and exertional heatstroke are also rare causes (Klein et al 1989, Pinson et al 1990, Hassanein et al 1991).

## PATHOLOGY

The commonest histological finding in fulminant hepatic failure, irrespective of etiology, is severe and widespread hepatocyte necrosis (Fig. 28.1). In paracetamol hepatotoxicity, a panacinar eosinophilic necrosis is observed 2–3 days after the injury (Portmann et al 1975). A wide range of less severe changes may be observed. Most damage occurs in the centrizonal regions and the periportal areas are preferentially preserved (Boyer & Klatskin 1970, Goertz & Williams 1973). Cholangiolar proliferation may be prominent in areas related to liver damage. An inflammatory component is often lacking and is more prominent with longer duration of disease. Cholestasis is restricted to surviving hepatocytes and may be most severe when there has been significant sepsis. Previous investigations have reported poor hepatocyte regeneration in patients with fulminant hepatic failure and late-onset hepatic failure. More recently, significant liver cell regeneration has been found, even in fatal cases, and this has been confirmed by immunostaining of proliferating cell nuclear antigen (PCNA) (Gerber et al 1983, Koukoulis et al 1992). There is little correlation between pathological appearances and the etiology of the hepatocyte necrosis.

Microvesicular fatty change is observed characteristically in acute fatty liver of pregnancy, Reye's syndrome, tetracycline hepatotoxicity, sodium valproate toxicity and Jamaican vomiting sickness. In Wilson's disease, established cirrhosis is usually present, but fulminant hepatic failure without cirrhosis has been recorded (p. 961).

## CLINICAL FEATURES

The hallmark of fulminant hepatic failure is hepatic encephalopathy and the most commonly used grading system was developed by Trey & Davidson (1970) (Table 28.2). In patients who deteriorate rapidly, grade 1 encephalopathy may be associated with anxiety and aggres-

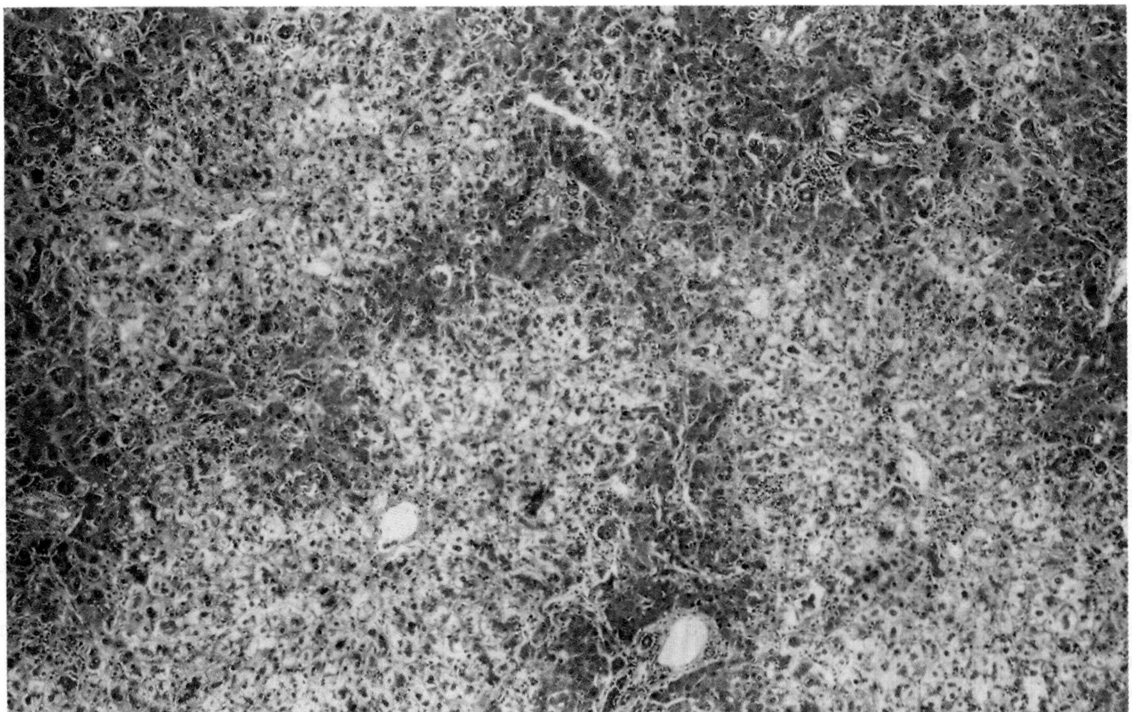

**Fig. 28.1** Submassive hepatic necrosis in fulminant hepatic failure due to acetaminophen (paracetamol). Hepatocyte necrosis is predominantly centrilobular (zone 3) and surviving hepatocytes are predominantly periportal (zone 1) (haematoxylin and eosin ×10).

**Table 28.2** Classification of grades of hepatic encephalopathy

| | |
|---|---|
| Grade 1 | Mild confusion, poor concentration, occasionally dysphoria. Reversed sleep pattern. When roused, fully coherent. |
| Grade 2 | Increasing confusion and disorientation but still rousable and rational. |
| Grade 3 | Sleeping most of the time but can be roused to commands. May be markedly agitated or occasionally aggressive. |
| Grade 4 | Not rousable to commands but may or may not be responsive to painful stimuli. Clinical features of cerebral edema may be apparent during this stage, including hyperventilation, pupillary abnormalities, opisthotonus and extensor plantar response. Abnormal respiratory patterns. |

sive behavior before the development of confusion and coma. Vomiting and abdominal pain are symptoms that may cause confusion in diagnosis. Jaundice and a hepatic fetor are found commonly on examination and as the disease progresses significant reduction in liver size, detected clinically, is also noted. Subconjunctival hemorrhages are particularly common in paracetamol hepatotoxicity. Ascites develops subsequently in up to 10% of patients, but splenomegaly is very unusual and points to some rarer cause of fulminant hepatic failure such as HBV reactivation, HDV superinfection of an HBV carrier, Wilson's disease, the Budd–Chiari syndrome or malignancy presenting as acute liver failure.

## MANAGEMENT AND COMPLICATIONS

Accurate assessment of the etiology and complications of fulminant hepatic failure is central to the general management of these patients. For many years, conservative therapy has concentrated on the prevention and treatment of its numerous complications and detecting the development of these complications at an early stage is of paramount importance (Table 28.3). This is done best in an intensive care unit. Systemic treatment, including corticosteroids, heparin, insulin and glucagon therapy (Woolf & Redeker 1991) and exchange transfusion (Desmet et al 1972), have not been of any therapeutic benefit. Measures specific to the etiology of the liver failure have also been tried and include interferon (Sánchez-Tapias et al 1987) and prostaglandin analogs (Abecassis et al 1987, Sinclair et al 1989), but initial enthusiasm has always evaporated in the face of controlled trials showing no value (Bernuau et al 1989, Sheiner et al 1992).

### Encephalopathy and cerebral edema

For many years the grading of encephalopathy has been that devised by Trey et al (1966). In some patients, progression through the grades is extremely rapid and associated with agitation and aggression, whereas in others it has a slower tempo. Those who remain in grades 1 or 2 have a significantly better prognosis than those progressing to grade 4, where further complications, including cerebral edema, occur in approximately 80% of cases.

**Table 28.3** Investigations in patients with fulminant hepatic failure

| | |
|---|---|
| Hematology | – full blood count<br>– prothrombin time/ratio |
| Biochemistry | – creatinine<br>– sodium, potassium, bicarbonate, phosphate<br>– bilirubin, transaminases, alkaline phosphatase<br>– total protein, albumin, immunoglobulins |
| Virology | – as above |
| Toxicology | – paracetamol (acetaminophen) |
| Autoantibodies | – antinuclear<br>– smooth muscle<br>– antimitochondrial<br>– liver–kidney microsomal |
| Wilson's disease | – serum : ceruloplasmin, copper<br>– urine : copper (± penicillamine) |
| Imaging | – chest radiograph<br>– ultrasound – liver<br>– hepatic vasculature<br>– spleen |

Note: HCV-RNA and HBV-DNA detectable by PCR but not available widely. Tests for HEV (anti-HEV) likely soon to be available generally.

*Encephalopathy*

The pathogenesis of hepatic encephalopathy in acute liver failure, as in those with chronic liver disease (p. 1039), remains unclear. Hyperammonemia, proportionate changes in branched chain and aromatic amino acids and elevation of synergistic toxins, including mercaptans, and short chain fatty acids have all been proposed but have not given consistent results either in animal models of fulminant hepatic failure or in humans (Jones & Schafer 1990). Recent evidence has pointed to the $\gamma$-amino butyric acid (GABA) pathway as the cause of the neuronal depression. Although plasma GABA concentrations are not elevated, it has been hypothesized that benzodiazepine-like substances, acting via a receptor closely linked to the GABA receptor, might be involved (Mullen et al 1988). Increased concentrations of 1,4-benzodiazepines have been detected in brain tissue in both animals and patients with acute liver failure (Basile et al 1990, 1991). Benzodiazepine receptor antagonists such as flumazenil have been reported to improve coma grade at least temporarily (Grimm et al 1988), but they are of no clinical importance.

*Cerebral edema*

Cerebral edema occurs in up to 80% of patients with fulminant hepatic failure (Ware et al 1971). It is one of the major causes of death and has been demonstrated in numerous animal models of acute liver failure. It is associated with elevation of intracranial pressure, reduction of cerebral blood flow and reduction of cerebral oxygen metabolism leading ultimately to cerebral ischemia (Almdal et al 1989, Blei 1991). Tentorial herniation develops in about 25%. Cerebral perfusion pressure, defined as the difference between the mean arterial blood pressure and the intracranial pressure, is critical as cerebral hypoxia occurs when the cerebral perfusion pressure falls below 50 mmHg.

***Pathogenesis.*** Cerebral edema has been divided into cytotoxic and vasogenic types, although recent hypotheses suggest that both share similar pathogenetic mechanisms at the endothelial level (Joo 1987). Studies in fulminant hepatic failure have suggested that cerebral edema is predominantly cytotoxic in nature (Kato et al 1992). This may be related to inhibitors of neuronal $Na^+K^+$-ATPase (Seda et al 1984), although some have not confirmed these findings (Pappas et al 1983). An alteration in the blood–brain barrier has also been proposed in some experimental models (McClung et al 1990). A further possibility is that glial swelling is the primary event, accounting for the localization of cerebral edema to cortical gray matter but not to subcortical white matter (Traber et al 1987). These several hypotheses are not mutually exclusive and increased brain water content may be initially cytotoxic and subsequently associated with altered permeability of the blood–brain barrier (Blei 1991, Kato et al 1992).

***Detection.*** Early detection of cerebral edema is critical and reliance on clinical features such as systemic hypertension, bradycardia, opisthotonus, decerebrate posturing and abnormal pupillary reflexes is unsatisfactory, as these signs occur late and at a time when intervention is often ineffective (Donovan et al 1992). Similarly, computed tomography of the brain has poor sensitivity for detecting cerebral edema (Muñoz et al 1991). The most accurate assessment of brain water has been the use of intracranial pressure monitoring by the subdural or epidural route (Blei 1991, Lidofsky et al 1992, Donovan et al 1992) and the complication rate has been acceptably low (Blei et al 1993). Significant cerebral edema is indicated by a rise in intracranial pressure to >20 mmHg.

***Treatment.*** Stimuli such as pain, movement, bright light and pyrexia can increase intracranial pressure and should be avoided as far as possible. Patients should be nursed in a head-up position approximately 20° to the horizontal, as this reduces cerebral blood flow and limits intracranial pressure (Davenport et al 1990). Osmotic therapy using mannitol is the most effective treatment for cerebral edema and 1 g/kg body weight in a 20% solution is given rapidly over about 30 min. Further doses can be given for recurrent increases of intracranial pressure. When given for an intracranial pressure of >30 mmHg or for clinical signs of cerebral edema, it significantly improves survival (Canalese et al 1982a). Prophylactic mannitol is not indicated. Osmotic therapy is not effective in reducing cerebral edema in the presence of renal failure unless combined with ultrafiltration of twice the infused volume. By reducing brain water, mannitol causes an increase in cerebral blood flow accompanied by an increase in cerebral oxygen extraction.

Barbiturates can lower intracranial pressure significantly, but this therapy may be complicated by significant systemic side-effects (Forbes et al 1989) and an effect on hospital mortality has not been demonstrated. Thiopentone can be infused to a maximum of 250 mg over 5 min followed by a continuous infusion of 50–500 mg hourly. The dose required is determined by the amount needed to control the intracranial pressure and is limited by the occurrence of hypotension. Hypothermia may also occur. The infusion should be stopped when intracranial pressure has been controlled for 4 h. Hyperventilation does not control intracranial pressure (Ede et al 1986) and, in contrast to mannitol, causes a fall in cerebral blood flow (Wendon et al 1992). Dexamethasone has no effect on the raised intracranial pressure of fulminant hepatic failure (Canalese et al 1982a).

### Hemodynamic abnormalities

Acute liver failure is associated with a marked reduction in systemic and pulmonary vascular resistance accompanied by a significant increase in cardiac output. These profound hemodynamic changes are commonly associated with significant hypotension and the magnitude of the changes is of prognostic importance (Wendon et al 1989). This high output/low vascular resistance state is associated with impaired tissue perfusion and an increased blood lactate (Bihari et al 1985, 1986). Moreover, increasing arterial oxygen delivery with a microcirculatory vasodilator is associated with an increase in peripheral oxygen extraction, suggesting the presence of a tissue oxygen debt. Critically ill patients such as these have been considered to show a close relationship between oxygen delivery to the tissues (cardiac output × arterial oxygen content) and oxygen extraction by the tissues over a larger range of oxygen delivery than normal, and this relationship has been observed within organ systems. Cerebral metabolic rate for oxygen rises in parallel with increases in cerebral blood flow that result from either a prostacyclin or *N*-acetylcysteine infusion (Wendon et al 1994). However, although maintenance of adequate delivery is considered important in treatment, it should be realised that technical considerations and the results of clinical studies have cast doubt on this relationship (Gasman et al 1996).

***Treatment.*** Oxygen delivery and oxygen extraction are important and all patients with fulminant hepatic failure need careful intravascular monitoring via systemic and pulmonary arterial lines. Hemodynamic aims are similar to those in other critically ill patients with high output/low vascular resistance states (Shoemaker et al 1990): maintaining pulmonary capillary wedge pressure at 8–12 mmHg with colloid infusions, hemoglobin above 10 g/dl with packed red blood cells and giving oxygen to keep arterial oxygen delivery above 600 ml/min/m$^2$. Inotropes such as adrenaline and dobutamine are of little value in patients with fulminant hepatic failure where the cardiac output is high, but pressor agents such as noradrenaline may be useful in maintaining the mean arterial pressure and improving tissue perfusion. All interventions should be monitored for their effect on oxygen delivery and extraction.

### Respiratory complications

With increasing encephalopathy, central hyperventilation and an associated respiratory alkalosis occur. In the later stages of cerebral edema this hyperventilation is dramatic and may herald sudden apnea as tentorial herniation of the midbrain develops. Arterial hypoxemia may be due to several causes (Bihari et al 1986). Aspiration of gastric contents occurs readily as encephalopathy deepens and pulmonary infection is common although organisms are not found in up to 45% of patients (Rolando et al 1990). Hypoxemia occurs in the absence of sepsis as in chronic liver disease, due in part to a fall in pulmonary vascular resistance and ventilation/perfusion mismatch (p. 1070). Noncardiogenic pulmonary edema is also well recognized and may be related to a widespread increase in endothelial permeability (Trewby et al 1978). Endotracheal intubation is usually undertaken in patients when grade 3 or 4 encephalopathy develops and care must be taken to ensure that changes in ventilation, including positive end expiratory pressure and high minute volumes, do not compromise systemic and cerebral hemodynamics.

### Renal failure

Oliguric renal failure occurs in nearly half of all patients irrespective of etiology (Wilkinson et al 1974). Acute tubular necrosis, with an isotonic urine and high urine sodium, and functional renal failure, with a urine/plasma osmotic ratio >1.2 and a urinary sodium <10 mmol/L, may be found (p. 1061). Renal blood flow is reduced and renin and angiotensin levels are increased (Wilkinson et al 1977). In toxic hepatocellular necrosis due to paracetamol, carbon tetrachloride or solvent abuse, the renal impairment may be out of proportion to the liver cell dysfunction (Baerg & Kimberg 1970, Cobden et al 1982).

***Treatment.*** Management is with regular hemodialysis and care must be taken not to cause too rapid changes in solute or osmolality, as cerebral edema may result. Continuous venovenous or high flow hemofiltration is often used, as initial solute changes are less marked.

### Electrolyte and metabolic abnormalities

Hyponatremia is common and is associated with a shift in sodium to intracellular compartments and inhibition of leukocyte $Na^+/K^+$-ATPase (Wilkinson et al 1974). Saline should not be administered, as urine sodium excretion is usually low (Wilkinson et al 1974). Hypokalemia, associated with respiratory alkalosis, may be profound and requires urgent correction. Hypophosphatemia can occur in patients with normal renal function but correction should be cautious as levels rise rapidly if renal failure develops (Dawson et al 1987).

Hypoglycemia is a hallmark of fulminant hepatic failure and may occur early in paracetamol hepatotoxicity, before the appearance of deep encephalopathy. Low plasma glucose concentrations result from reduced hepatic glycogen stores and hyperinsulinemia due to impaired hepatic insulin clearance. Thus, the routine administration of 10% glucose is necessary.

Hyperlactatemia and metabolic acidosis are found in 30% of cases and have a very poor prognosis, as only 10% of such patients survive (O'Grady et al 1989). They occur predominantly on the second and third day in paracetamol-induced liver failure and have no relation to renal failure or encephalopathy. There is an inverse relation between serum lactate and systemic vascular resistance, suggesting that hyperlactatemia is due not only to stimulation of glycolysis but also to poor tissue perfusion (Bihari & Wendon 1991).

### Abnormalities of coagulation and fibrinolysis

Low concentrations of all the coagulation factors (except factor VIII) are observed. Factor VIII is synthesized in liver and endothelial cells and its concentrations are elevated (Kelly et al 1985). Reduced hepatic synthesis of coagulation factors (p. 751) is important and has been used as a measure of prognosis (see below), but increased intravascular consumption of clotting factors due to disseminated intravascular coagulation is also present. Thrombin–antithrombin complexes are elevated, indicating activation of coagulation, and are associated with high plasma levels of D-dimer, the split product of crosslinked fibrinogen (Langley et al 1990). Activated fibrinolysis is unlikely to be a major cause of significant bleeding, as inhibitors of fibrinolysis are also present (Pernambuco et al 1993). Concentrations of inhibitors of coagulation such as antithrombin-3 are also low. This prolongs the biological half-life of heparin (Sette et al 1985) and a randomized trial of antithrombin-3 replacement demonstrated reduced heparin requirements and preservation of platelet numbers during hemodialysis (Langley et al 1991). Platelet counts commonly fall during fulminant hepatic failure, with selective loss of the larger, more hemostatically active platelets (Rubin et al 1977). Platelets show reduced aggregation to ADP and other agents but enhanced stickiness.

***Treatment.*** Clinically significant hemorrhage from gastric erosions used to be an important cause of morbidity in these patients, but with the use of $H_2$ antagonists the frequency is now low (Macdougall & Williams 1978). As in other critically ill patients, similar reductions in gastrointestinal bleeding risk occur using sucralfate without any risk of colonization of the upper gastrointestinal tract by Gram-negative organisms. However, patients with fulminant hepatic failure often cannot swallow tablets and infusion of an $H_2$ receptor antagonist is appropriate. Hemorrhage is most common in patients with thrombocytopenia and a coagulation defect, but prophylactic administration of fresh frozen plasma is of no benefit. Fresh frozen plasma and platelets should be used as soon as bleeding occurs.

## Sepsis

All patients with significant hepatocellular dysfunction, irrespective of etiology, are susceptible to infection (p. 772) and this is particularly important in fulminant hepatic failure. Complement concentrations, bacterial opsonization, white cell chemoattraction and bacterial killing and Kupffer cell function are all impaired (Wyke et al 1981, Canalese et al 1982b). Bacteremia is common and, in a prospective survey of 50 patients, was observed in 80% of cases (Rolando et al 1990). The sensitivity and specificity of markers for sepsis such as fever and leukocytosis are poor, indicating that daily antimicrobial surveillance is of crucial importance. Surveillance should include a chest radiograph and culture of blood, urine and any other material indicating infection, such as sputum. The majority of infective episodes are caused by Gram-positive organisms, in contrast to the situation in other critically ill patients. Prophylactic antibiotic therapy has only a limited place in preventing these septic episodes (Rolando et al 1993), as many patients become infected early in the illness. Furthermore, regimens of parenteral and enteral decontamination may take up to 5 days to take effect.

Fungal infection, predominantly with *Candida* species, occurs in up to 30% of patients and is associated with leukopenia, renal failure and previous antibiotic therapy. A fever that does not respond to antibiotics for more than 2 days suggests fungal infection and should be treated with fluconazole.

## Hypothermia

Hypothermia is common, especially terminally, and may worsen the cerebral state (Saunders et al 1972). It results from poor central temperature control in a comatose patient.

## Pancreatitis

Pancreatitis is found at postmortem in approximately a third of cases, but clinically significant pancreatitis is rare. The plasma amylase activity should be measured whenever unexplained deterioration occurs.

## Temporary liver support

The studies of prognosis in these patients has confirmed the very poor survival rates in some groups despite the best intensive care therapies. As hepatic regeneration may occur eventually (Milandri et al 1980), a wide range of systems for temporary liver support have been developed. Early devices using highly permeable membranes, charcoal hemoperfusion (Gimson et al 1982) and Amberlite XAD-7 resins (Hughes & Williams 1986) were not found to improve survival significantly over intensive care measures alone (O'Grady et al 1988b). The use of encapsulated hepatocytes in a bioartificial liver is currently undergoing clinical trials (Nyberg et al 1993).

Auxiliary heterotopic liver transplantation has been performed in emergency situations with some success and the native liver may be allowed to regenerate (Moritz & Jarrell 1990, Metselaar et al 1990). Such therapy may have more relevance in paracetamol-induced liver failure than in viral hepatitis. Attempts to promote hepatic regeneration have not been forthcoming and as hepatocyte growth factor levels in this setting are already high, this is unlikely to be a clinically useful therapy (Gohda et al 1991).

## Orthotopic liver transplantation

In those patients with the worst prognosis, orthotopic liver transplantation gives the best chance of long-term survival (p. 1155) and should be considered in all such cases (Table 28.4). Contraindications to transplantation include active sepsis, a cerebral perfusion pressure below 40 mmHg for more than 4 h and treatment-resistant hypotension. As in elective liver transplantation, other factors including age and coexisting diseases need to be taken into account. Intraoperative problems in managing blood pressure and cerebral edema are common and may continue for some hours after the transplant procedure (Keays et al 1991b).

In most centers the overall 1-year survival rate is between 40% and 80%, depending on the severity of the illness at the time of transplantation (Table 28.4). Survival is significantly worse in those with grade 4 encephalopathy and prior cerebral edema (48%) than in those with grades 1 and 2 encephalopathy at operation (71%) (Williams & Wendon 1994). Results in patients transplanted for para-

**Table 28.4** Results of orthotopic liver transplantation for fulminant and late-onset hepatic failure

| Reference | Patients | FHF/LOHF | Encephalopathy (Grade 3/4 (%)) | Survival (%) |
|---|---|---|---|---|
| O'Grady et al 1988a | 31 | 16/15 | 35 | 61 |
| Vickers et al 1988 | 16 | 16/0 | 100 | 56 |
| Schafer & Shaw 1989 | 24 | 24/0 | 50 | 58 |
| Emond et al 1989 | 19 | 19/0 | 84 | 58 |
| Iwatsuki et al 1989 | 42 | 42/0 | 64 | 50 |
| Gallinger et al 1989 | 21 | 9/12 | 81 | 72 |
| Rakela et al 1989 | 8 | 8/0 | 88 | 63 |

Note: FHF = fulminant hepatic failure; LOHF = late-onset hepatic failure cetamol hepatotoxicity are similar to those obtained for other etiologies (O'Grady et al 1991). Although orthotopic liver transplantation remains the only hope of significant improvement in survival for patients with the worst prognosis and the reported results are impressive, only a few patients with fulminant hepatic failure can benefit from such therapy, as many deteriorate too quickly or have contraindications or donor organs cannot be found quickly enough.

## PROGNOSIS

Numerous studies have shown that the prognosis in fulminant hepatic failure depends on the etiology and severity of liver dysfunction, the development of particular complications and various host factors (O'Grady 1988a,b). Fulminant hepatic failure evolves rapidly, so that early assessment of prognosis is important in order that therapeutic interventions, including orthotopic liver transplantation, can be planned. Some prognostic indicants are of limited value as they are difficult to obtain or only available retrospectively and others, such as the volume of viable hepatocytes which is of some discriminative value, are of little practical help as biopsy, even by the transjugular route, carries some risk.

O'Grady et al (1989) have developed a prognostic score based on retrospective analysis of a large cohort of medically treated cases. This system has the advantage of using clinical observations and readily available laboratory tests and is used widely. In cases not attributable to paracetamol, five factors including age, etiology, the duration of jaundice from onset to encephalopathy, peak serum bilirubin and peak prothrombin time were important and a combination of any three or a prothrombin time >100 s was associated with a very poor prognosis (Table 28.5). A recent study in Japan did not confirm the value of this system and accordingly, further evidence of its accuracy will be needed (Takahashi et al 1994). An alternative system, derived from a study of fulminant hepatic failure due to hepatitis B virus infection and using the patient's age and the plasma factor V concentration, has been proposed (Bernuau et al 1986b).

**Table 28.5** Criteria for orthotopic liver transplantation (O'Grady et al 1989)

| |
|---|
| *Paracetamol overdose* |
| Arterial pH <7.3 |
| or |
| All the following: |
| Grade 3 or 4 encephalopathy |
| Creatinine >300 μmol/L |
| Prothrombin time >100 s |
| Prothrombin time rising on day 4 |
| *Nonparacetamol* |
| Any 3 of the following: |
| Prothrombin time >50 s |
| Age <10 years or >40 years |
| Jaundice to encephalopathy >7 days |
| Serum bilirubin >300 μmol/L |
| Etiology non-A, non-B hepatitis, halothane or drug reaction |
| or |
| Prothrombin time >100 s |

In fulminant hepatic failure due to paracetamol the data are more conclusive, as acidosis at any level of encephalopathy and coagulation measurements offer accurate prognostication. A prothrombin time of >100 s in a patient with a serum creatinine >300 μmol/L and grade 3 or 4 encephalopathy and a factor VIII/factor V ratio >30 have had a strong predictive value and high specificity (O'Grady et al 1989, Pereira et al 1992).

Late-onset hepatic failure also carries a poor prognosis and any patient with a duration of illness of more than 8 weeks who develops grade 3 or 4 encephalopathy has an expected survival of only 20% (Gimson et al 1986).

## CONCLUSION

Management of fulminant hepatic failure requires a careful search for an etiology, early detection of complications, the rapid assessment of prognosis and referral for transplantation where appropriate. In those who do not require liver grafting, full regeneration of liver function and structure will occur (Horney & Galambos 1977). In those who do, continuing improvement in organ procurement and postoperative therapy offer the best hope for the future.

## REFERENCES


Abecassis M, Falk J, Makowka L, Dinzans V J, Falk R E, Levy G A 1987 16,16, dimethyl prostaglandin E2 prevents the development of fulminant hepatitis and blocks the induction of monocyte/macrophage procoagulant activity after murine hepatitis virus strain B infection. Journal of Clinical Investigation 80: 881–889

Akriviadis E A, Redeker A G 1989 Fulminant hepatitis A in intravenous drug users with chronic liver disease. Annals of Internal Medicine 110: 838–839

Almdal T, Schroeder T, Ranek L 1989 Cerebral blood flow and liver function in patients with encephalopathy due to acute and chronic liver diseases. Scandinavian Journal of Gastroenterology 24: 299–303

Asano Y, Yoshikawa T, Suga S, Yazaki T, Kondo K, Yamanishi K 1991 Fatal fulminant hepatitis in an infant with human herpesvirus-6 infection. Lancet 335: 862–863

Asher L V S, Innis B L, Shrestha M P, Ticehurst J, Baze W B 1990 Virus-like particles in the liver of a patient with fulminant hepatitis and antibody to hepatitis E virus. Journal of Medical Virology 31: 229–233

Baerg R D, Kimberg D V 1970 Centrilobular hepatic necrosis and acute renal failure "solvent sniffers". Annals of Internal Medicine 73: 713–720

Barrett M J, Hurwitz E S, Schonberger L B, Rogers M F 1986 Changing epidemiology of Reye syndrome in the United States. Pediatrics 77: 598–602

Basile A S, Pannell L, Jaouni T et al 1990 Brain concentrations of benzodiazepines are elevated in an animal model of hepatic encephalopathy. Proceedings of the National Academy of Sciences of the United States of America 87: 5263–5267

Basile A S, Hughes R D, Harrison P M et al 1991 Elevated brain concentrations of 1,4-benzodiazepines in fulminant hepatic failure. New England Journal of Medicine 325: 473–478

Benhamou J-P, Rueff B, Sicot L 1972 Severe hepatic failure: a critical study of current therapy. In: Orlandi F, Jezequel A M (eds) Liver and drugs. Academic Press, London, p 213–228

Berman D H, Leventhal R I, Gavaler J S, Cadoff E M, van Thiel D H 1991 Clinical differentiation of fulminant Wilsonian hepatitis from other causes of hepatic failure. Gastroenterology 100: 1129–1134

Bernuau J, Benhamou J-P 1993 Classifying acute liver failure. Lancet 342: 252

Bernuau J, Rueff B, Benhamou J-P 1986a Fulminant and subfulminant liver failure: definitions and causes. Seminars in Liver Disease 6: 97–106

Bernuau J, Goudeau A, Poynard T et al 1986b Multivariate analysis of prognostic factors in fulminant hepatitis B. Hepatology 6: 648–651

Bernuau J, Babany G, Bezeaud A et al 1989 Does prostaglandin E1 (PGE1) prevent further aggravation in severe, or early fulminant, hepatitis? A preliminary open trial (abstract). Journal of Hepatology 9: S114

Bihari D, Wendon J 1991 Tissue hypoxia in fulminant hepatic failure. In: Williams R, Hughes R D (eds) Acute liver failure: improved understanding and better therapy. London, Mitre Press, p 42–44

Bihari D, Gimson A E S, Waterson M, Williams R 1985 Tissue hypoxia during fulminant hepatic failure. Critical Care Medicine 13: 1034–1039

Bihari D J, Gimson A E S, Williams R 1986 Cardiovascular, pulmonary and renal complications of fulminant hepatic failure. Seminars in Liver Disease 6: 119–128

Bird G L A, Smith H, Portmann B, Alexander G J M, Williams R 1989 Acute liver decompensation on withdrawal of cytotoxic chemotherapy and immunosuppressive therapy in hepatitis B carriers. Quarterly Journal of Medicine 73: 895–902

Blei A T 1991 Cerebral edema and intracranial hypertension in acute liver failure: distinct aspects of the same problem. Hepatology 13: 376–379

Blei A T, Olafsson S, Webster S, Levy R 1993 Complications of intracranial pressure monitoring in fulminant hepatic failure. Lancet 341: 157–158

Boyer J L, Klatskin G 1970 Pattern of necrosis in acute viral hepatitis. Prognostic value of bridging (subacute hepatic necrosis). New England Journal of Medicine 283: 1063–1071

Brechot C, Bernuau J, Thiers V et al 1984 Multiplication of hepatitis B virus in fulminant hepatitis B. British Medical Journal 288: 270–271

Canalese J, Gimson A E S, Davis C, Mellon P J, Davis M, Williams R 1982a Controlled trial of dexamethasone and mannitol for the cerebral oedema of fulminant hepatic failure. Gut 23: 625–629

Canalese J, Gove C D, Gimson A E S, Wilkinson S P, Wardle E N, Williams R 1982b Reticuloendothelial system and hepatocyte function in fulminant hepatic failure. Gut 23: 265–269

Caraceni P, van Thiel D H 1995 Acute liver failure. Lancet 345: 163–169

Cobden I, Record C O, Ward M K, Kerr D N S 1982 Paracetamol-induced acute renal failure in the absence of fulminant liver damage. British Medical Journal 284: 21–22

Connor R W, Lorts G, Gilbert D N 1979 Lethal herpes simplex virus type 1 hepatitis in a normal adult. Gastroenterology 76: 590–594

Da Costa C M, Baldwin D, Portmann B, Lolin Y, Mowat A P, Miele-Vergani G 1992 Value of urinary copper excretion after penicillamine challenge in the diagnosis of Wilson's disease. Hepatology 15: 609–615

Davenport A, Will E J, Davison A M 1990 Effect of posture on intracranial pressure and cerebral perfusion pressure in patients with fulminant hepatic and renal failure after acetaminophen self-poisoning. Critical Care Medicine 18: 286–289

Davies M H, Morgan-Capner P, Portmann B, Wilkinson S P, Williams R 1980a A fatal case of Epstein–Barr virus infection with jaundice and renal failure. Postgraduate Medical Journal 56: 794–795

Davies M H, Wilkinson S P, Hanid M A et al 1980b Acute liver disease with encephalopathy and renal failure in late pregnancy and the early puerperium. A study of fourteen patients. British Journal of Obstetrics and Gynaecology 87: 1005–1014

Dawson D J, Babbs C, Warnes T W, Neary R H 1987 Hypophosphataemia in acute liver failure. British Medical Journal 295: 1312–1313

Desmet V J, de Groote J, van Damme B 1972 Acute hepatocellular failure. A study of 17 patients treated with exchange transfusion. Human Pathology 3: 167–182

Donovan J P, Shaw B W Jr, Langnas A N, Sorrell M F 1992 Brain water and acute liver failure: the emerging role of intracranial pressure monitoring. Hepatology 16: 267–268

Ede R J, Williams R 1988 Reye's syndrome in adults. British Medical Journal 296: 517–518

Ede R J, Gimson A E S, Bihari D, Williams R 1986 Controlled hyperventilation in the prevention of cerebral oedema in fulminant hepatic failure. Journal of Hepatology 2: 43–51

Emond J C, Aran P P, Whitington P F, Broelsch C E, Baker A L 1989 Liver transplantation in the management of fulminant hepatic failure. Gastroenterology 96: 1583–1588

European Association for the Study of the Liver 1979 Randomised trial of steroid therapy in acute liver failure. Gut 20: 620–623

Fagan E A, Williams R 1990 Fulminant viral hepatitis. British Medical Bulletin 46: 462–480

Farci P, Alter H J, Shimoda A et al 1996 Hepatitis C virus-associated fulminant liver failure. New England Journal of Medicine 335: 631–634

Feray C, Gigou M, Samuel D et al 1993 Hepatitis C virus RNA and hepatitis B virus DNA in serum and liver of patients with fulminant hepatitis. Gastroenterology 104: 549–555

Forbes A, Williams R 1988 Increasing age – an important adverse prognostic factor in hepatitis A virus infection. Journal of the Royal College of Physicians of London 22: 237–239

Forbes A, Alexander G J M, O'Grady J G et al 1989 Thiopental infusion in the treatment of intracranial hypertension complicating fulminant hepatic failure. Hepatology 10: 306–310

Gallinger S, Greig P D, Levy G et al 1989 Liver transplantation for acute and subacute fulminant hepatic failure. Transplantation Proceedings 21: 2435–2438

Gasman J D, Ruoss S J, Fishman R S, Rizk N W, Raffin T A 1996 Hazards with both determining and utilizing oxygen consumption measurements in the management of critically ill patients. Critical Care Medicine 24: 6–9

Gerber M A, Thung S N, Shen S, Stromeyer F W, Ishak K G 1983 Phenotypic characterization of hepatic proliferation. Antigenic expression of proliferating epithelial cells in fetal liver, massive hepatic necrosis and nodular transformation of the liver. American Journal of Pathology 110: 70–74

Gimson A E S, Braude S, Mellon P J, Canalese J, Williams R 1982 Earlier charcoal haemoperfusion in fulminant hepatic failure. Lancet 2: 681–683

Gimson A E S, Tedder R S, White Y S, Eddleston A L W F, Williams R 1983 Serological markers in fulminant hepatitis B. Gut 24: 615–617

Gimson A E S, O'Grady J, Ede R J, Portmann B, Williams R 1986 Late onset hepatic failure: clinical, serological and histological features. Hepatology 6: 288–294

Goertz J, Williams R 1973 Histological appearances in fulminant hepatic failure with reference to aetiology, time of survival and role of immunological processes. Digestion 8: 68–79

Gohda E, Tsubouchi H, Nakayama H et al 1991 Human hepatocyte growth factor in blood of patients with fulminant hepatic failure: basic aspects. Digestive Diseases and Sciences 36: 785–790

Govindarajan S, Chin K P, Redeker A G, Peters R L 1984 Fulminant B viral hepatitis: role of delta agent. Gastroenterology 86: 1417–1420

Grimm G, Ferenci P, Katzenschlager R et al 1988 Improvement of hepatic encephalopathy treated with flumazenil. Lancet 2: 1392–1394

Harrison P M, Keays R, Bray G P, Alexander G J M, Williams R 1990 Improved outcome of paracetamol-induced fulminant hepatic failure by late administration of acetylcysteine. Lancet 335: 1572–1573

Hart G K, Thompson W R, Schneider J, Davis N J, Oh T E 1984 Fulminant hepatic failure and fatal encephalopathy associated with Epstein–Barr virus infection. Medical Journal of Australia 141: 112–113

Hassanein T, Perper J A, Tepperman L, Starzl T E, van Thiel D H 1991 Liver failure occurring as a component of exertional heatstroke. Gastroenterology 100: 1442–1447

Henson D E, Grimley P M, Strano A J 1974 Postnatal cytomegalovirus hepatitis: an autopsy and liver biopsy study. Human Pathology 5: 93–103

Heubi J E, Daugherty C C, Partin J S, Partin J C, Schubert W K 1984 Grade I Reye's syndrome – outcome and predictors of progression to deeper coma grades. New England Journal of Medicine 311: 1539–1542

Horney J T, Galambos J T 1977 The liver during and after fulminant hepatitis. Gastroenterology 73: 639–645

Hughes R, Williams R 1986 Clinical experience with charcoal and resin hemoperfusion. Seminars in Liver Disease 6: 164–173

Hurwitz E S, Barrett M J, Bregman D et al 1987 Public Health Service study of Reye's syndrome and medications. Report of the Main Study. Journal of the American Medical Association 257: 1905–1911

Iwatsuki S, Stieber A C, Marsh J W et al 1989 Liver transplantation for fulminant hepatic failure. Transplantation Proceedings 21: 2431–2434

Jones E A, Schafer D F 1990 Fulminant hepatic failure. In: Zakim D, Boyer T D (eds) Hepatology: a textbook of liver disease, Vol 1, 2nd edn. W B Saunders, Philadelphia, p 460–492

Joo F 1987 A unifying concept on the pathogenesis of brain oedemas. Neuropathology and Applied Neurobiology 13: 161–176

Kato M, Hughes R D, Keays R T, Williams R 1992 Electron microscopic study of brain capillaries in cerebral edema from fulminant hepatic failure. Hepatology 15: 1060–1066

Keays R, Harrison P M, Wendon J A et al 1991a Intravenous acetylcysteine in paracetamol induced fulminant hepatic failure: a prospective controlled trial. British Medical Journal 303: 1026–1029

Keays R, Potter D, O'Grady J, Peachey T, Alexander G, Williams R 1991b Intracranial and cerebral perfusion pressure changes before, during and immediately after orthotopic liver transplantation for fulminant hepatic failure. Quarterly Journal of Medicine 79: 425–433

Kelly D A, O'Brien F J, Hutton R A, Tuddenham E G, Summerfield J A, Sherlock S 1985 The effect of liver disease on factors V, VIII and protein C. British Journal of Haematology 61: 541–548

Khuroo M S 1980 Study of an epidemic of non-A, non-B hepatitis; possibility of another human hepatitis virus distinct from post-transfusion non-A, non-B type. American Journal of Medicine 68: 818–824

Klein A S, Hart J, Brems J J, Goldstein L, Lewin K, Busiettel R W 1989 Amanita poisoning: treatment and the role of liver transplantation. American Journal of Medicine 86: 187–193

Koukoulis G, Rayner A, Tan K-C, Williams R, Portmann B 1992 Immunolocalization of regenerating cells after submassive liver necroses using PCNA staining. Journal of Pathology 166: 359–368

Kumar S, Rex D K 1991 Failure of physicians to recognize acetaminophen hepatotoxicity in chronic alcoholics. Archives of Internal Medicine 151: 1189–1191

Langley P G, Forbes A, Hughes R D, Williams R 1990 Thrombin–antithrombin III complex in fulminant hepatic failure: evidence for disseminated intravascular coagulation and relationship to outcome. European Journal of Clinical Investigation 20: 627–631

Langley P G, Keays R, Hughes R D, Forbes A, Delvos U, Williams R 1991 Antithrombin III supplementation reduces heparin requirement and platelet loss during hemodialysis of patients with fulminant hepatic failure. Hepatology 14: 251–256

Lee W M 1993 Acute liver failure. New England Journal of Medicine 329: 1862–1872

Liang T J, Hasegawa K, Rimon N, Wands J R, Ben-Porath E 1991 A hepatitis B virus mutant associated with an epidemic of fulminant hepatitis. New England Journal of Medicine 324: 1705–1709

Liang T J, Jeffers L, Reddy R K et al 1993 Fulminant or subfulminant non-A, non-B virus hepatitis: the role of hepatitis C and E viruses. Gastroenterology 104: 556–562

Licht H, Seeff L B, Zimmerman H J 1980 Apparent potentiation of acetaminophen hepatotoxicity by alcohol. Annals of Internal Medicine 92: 511

Lidofsky S D, Bass N M, Prager M C et al 1992 Intracranial pressure monitoring and liver transplantation for fulminant hepatic failure. Hepatology 16: 1–7

Macdougall B R D, Williams R 1978 $H_2$-receptor antagonist in the prevention of acute upper gastrointestinal hemorrhage in fulminant hepatic failure: a controlled trial. Gastroenterology 74: 464–465

Mathiesen L R, Skinoj P, Nielsen J O, Purcell R H, Wong D, Ranek L 1980 Hepatitis type A, B, and non-A non-B in fulminant hepatitis. Gut 21: 72–77

McClung H J, Sloan H R, Powers P et al 1990 Early changes in the permeability of the blood–brain barrier produced by toxins associated with liver failure. Pediatric Research 28: 227–231

McCullough A J, Fleming C R, Thistle J L et al 1983 Diagnosis of Wilson's disease presenting as fulminant hepatic failure. Gastroenterology 84: 161–167

McNeil M, Hoy J F, Richards M J et al 1984 Aetiology of fatal viral hepatitis in Melbourne: a retrospective study. Medical Journal of Australia 141: 637–640

Metselaar H J, Hesselink E J, de Rave S et al 1990 Recovery of failing liver after auxiliary heterotopic liver transplantation. Lancet 335: 1156–1157

Milandri M, Gaub J, Ranek L 1980 Evidence for liver cell proliferation during fatal acute liver failure. Gut 21: 423–427

Morishita K, Kodo H, Asano S, Fujii H, Miwa S, The Tokyo University Bone Marrow Transplantation Team 1985 Fulminant varicella hepatitis following bone marrow transplantation. Journal of the American Medical Association 253: 511

Moritz M J, Jarrell B E 1990 Heterotopic liver transplantation for fulminant hepatic failure – a bridge to recovery. Transplantation 50: 524–526

Mowat A P 1983 Reye's syndrome: 20 years on. British Medical Journal 286: 1999

Mullen K D, Martin J V, Mendelson W B, Bassett M L, Jones E A 1988 Could an endogenous benzodiazepine ligand contribute to hepatic encephalopathy? Lancet 1: 457–459

Muñoz S J, Robinson M, Northrup B et al 1991 Elevated intracranial pressure and computed tomography of the brain in fulminant hepatocellular failure. Hepatology 13: 209–212

Nouel O, Henrion J, Bernuau J, Degott C, Rueff B, Benhamou J-P 1980 Fulminant hepatic failure due to transient circulatory failure in patients with chronic heart disease. Digestive Diseases and Sciences 25: 49–52

Nyberg S L, Peshwa M V, Payne W D, Hu W-S, Cerra F B 1993 Evolution of the bioartificial liver: the need for randomized clinical trials. American Journal of Surgery 166: 512–521

O'Grady J G, Alexander G J M, Thick M, Potter D, Calne R Y, Williams R 1988a Outcome of orthotopic liver transplantation in the aetiological and clinical variants of acute liver failure. Quarterly Journal of Medicine 69: 817–824

O'Grady J G, Gimson A E S, O'Brien C J, Pucknell A, Hughes R D, Williams R 1988b Controlled trials of charcoal hemoperfusion and prognostic factors in fulminant hepatic failure. Gastroenterology 94: 1186–1192

O'Grady J G, Alexander G J M, Hallyar K M, Williams R 1989 Early indicators of prognosis in fulminant hepatic failure. Gastroenterology 97: 439–445

O'Grady J G, Wendon J, Tan K C et al 1991 Liver transplantation after paracetamol overdose. British Medical Journal 303: 221–223

O'Grady J G, Schalm S W, Williams R 1993 Acute liver failure: redefining the syndromes. Lancet 342: 273–275

Omata M, Ehata T, Yokosuka O, Hosoda K, Ohto M 1991 Mutations in the precore region of hepatitis B virus DNA in patients with fulminant and severe hepatitis. New England Journal of Medicine 324: 1699–1704

Papaevangelou G, Tassopoulos N, Roumeliotou-Karayannis A, Richardson C 1984 Etiology of fulminant virus hepatitis in Greece. Hepatology 4: 369–372

Pappas S, Ferenci P, Jones E A 1983 Evidence against the hypothesis that cerebral oedema in fulminant hepatic failure is due to decreased neural Na–K–ATPase activity (abstract). Hepatology 3: 848

Pereira L M M B, Langley P G, Hayllar K M, Tredger J M, Williams R 1992 Coagulation factor V and VIII/V ratio as predictors of outcome in paracetamol induced fulminant hepatic failure: relation to other prognostic indicators. Gut 33: 98–102

Pernambuco J R B, Langley P G, Hughes R D, Izumi S, Williams R 1993 Activation of the fibrinolytic system in patients with fulminant liver failure. Hepatology 18: 1350–1356

Pinson C W, Daya M R, Benner K G et al 1990 Liver transplantation for severe *Amanita phalloides* mushroom poisoning. American Journal

of Surgery 159: 493–499
Portmann B, Talbot I C, Day D W, Davidson A R, Murray-Lyon I M, Williams R 1975 Histopathological changes in the liver following a paracetamol overdose: correlation with clinical and biochemical parameters. Journal of Pathology 117: 169–181
Powell-Jackson P R, Ede R J, Williams R 1986 Budd–Chiari syndrome presenting as fulminant hepatic failure. Gut 27: 1101–1105
Prescott L F, Illingworth R N, Critchley J A J H, Stewart M J, Adam R D, Proudfoot A T 1979 Intravenous N-acetylcysteine: the treatment of choice for paracetamol poisoning. British Medical Journal 2: 1097–1100
Rakela J, Perkins J D, Gross J B et al 1989 Acute hepatic failure: the emerging role of orthotopic liver transplantation. Mayo Clinic Proceedings 64: 424–428
Riely C A, Latham P S, Romero R, Duffy T P 1987 Acute fatty liver of pregnancy: a reassessment based on observations in nine patients. Annals of Internal Medicine 106: 703–706
Rolando N, Harvey F, Brahm J et al 1990 Prospective study of bacterial infection in acute liver failure: an analysis of fifty patients. Hepatology 11: 49–53
Rolando N, Gimson A, Wade J, Philpott-Howard J, Casewell M, Williams R 1993 Prospective controlled trial of selective parenteral and enteral antimicrobial regimen in fulminant liver failure. Hepatology 17: 196–201
Rolfes D B, Ishak K G 1985 Acute fatty liver of pregnancy: a clinicopathologic study of 35 cases. Hepatology 5: 1149–1158
Rubin M H, Weston M J, Bullock G et al 1977 Abnormal platelet function and ultrastructure in fulminant hepatic failure. Quarterly Journal of Medicine 183: 339–352
Sallie R, Katsiyiannakis L, Baldwin D et al 1992 Failure of simple biochemical indexes to reliably differentiate fulminant Wilson's disease from other causes of fulminant liver failure. Hepatology 16: 1206–1211
Sánchez-Tapias J M, Mas A, Costa J et al 1987 Recombinant $\alpha_{2c}$-interferon therapy in fulminant viral hepatitis. Journal of Hepatology 5: 205–210
Saunders S J, Hickman R, McDonald R, Terblanche J 1972 The treatment of acute liver failure. In: Popper H, Schaffner F (eds) Progress in liver disease, Vol 4. Grune & Stratton, New York, p 333
Schafer D F, Shaw B W Jr 1989 Fulminant hepatic failure and orthotopic liver transplantation. Seminars in Liver Disease 9: 189–194
Schilsky M L, Scheinberg I H, Sternlieb I 1994 Liver transplantation for Wilson's disease: indications and outcome. Hepatology 19: 583–587
Seda H M W, Hughes R D, Gove C D, Williams R 1984 Inhibition of rat brain $Na^+$, $K^+$–ATPase activity by serum from patients with fulminant hepatic failure. Hepatology 4: 74–79
Sette H, Hughes R D, Langley P G, Gimson A E S, Williams R 1985 Heparin response and clearance in acute and chronic liver disease. Thrombosis and Haemostasis 54: 591–594
Sheiner P, Sinclair S, Greig P, Logan A, Blandis L M, Levy G 1992 A randomized control trial of prostaglandin $E_2$ ($PGE_2$) in the treatment of fulminant hepatic failure (FHF) (abstract). Hepatology 16 (suppl): 174
Shoemaker W C, Kram H B, Appel P L 1990 Therapy of shock based on pathophysiology, monitoring, and outcome prediction. Critical Care Medicine 18 (suppl): S19–S25
Sinclair S B, Greig P D, Blendis L M et al 1989 Biochemical and clinical response of fulminant viral hepatitis to administration of prostaglandin E: a preliminary report. Journal of Clinical Investigation 84: 1063–1069
Smedile A, Farci P, Verme G et al 1982 Influence of delta infection on severity of hepatitis B. Lancet 2: 945–947
Sobue R, Miyazaki H, Okamoto M et al 1991 Fulminant hepatitis in primary human herpesvirus-6 infection. New England Journal of Medicine 324: 1290
Takahashi Y, Kumada H, Shimizu M et al 1994 A multicenter study on the prognosis of fulminant viral hepatitis: early prediction for liver transplantation. Hepatology 19: 1065–1071
Traber P G, Dal Canto M, Ganger D R, Blei A T 1987 Electron microscopic evaluation of brain edema in rabbits with galactosamine-induced fulminant hepatic failure: ultrastructure and integrity of the blood–brain barrier. Hepatology 7: 1272–1277
Trepo C G, Robert D, Motin J, Trepo D, Sepetjian M, Prince A M 1976 Hepatitis B antigen (HBsAg) and/or antibodies (anti-HBs and anti-HBc) in fulminant hepatitis: pathogenic and prognostic significance. Gut 17: 10–13
Trewby P N, Warren R, Contini S et al 1978 Incidence and pathophysiology of pulmonary edema in fulminant hepatic failure. Gastroenterology 74: 859–865
Trey C, Davidson C S 1970 The management of fulminant hepatic failure. In: Popper H, Schaffner F (eds) Progress in liver diseases, Vol 3. Grune and Stratton, New York, p 282–298
Trey C, Burns D G, Saunders S J 1966 Treatment of hepatic coma by exchange blood transfusion. New England Journal of Medicine 274: 473–481
Vallbracht A, Gabriel P, Maier K et al 1986 Cell-mediated cytotoxicity in hepatitis A virus infection. Hepatology 6: 1308–1314
Vickers C, Neuberger J, Buckels J, McMaster P, Elias E 1988 Transplantation of the liver in adults and children with fulminant hepatic failure. Journal of Hepatology 7: 143–150
Ware A J, D'Agostino A N, Combes B 1971 Cerebral edema: a major complication of massive hepatic necrosis. Gastroenterology 61: 877–884
Wendon J, Gimson A E, Potter D 1989 Oxygen uptake and delivery in fulminant hepatic failure. Care of the Critically Ill 5: 55–59
Wendon J A, Harrison P M, Keays R, Gimson A E, Alexander G J M, Williams R 1992 Effects of vasopressor agents and epoprostenol on systemic hemodynamics and oxygen transport in fulminant hepatic failure. Hepatology 15: 1067–1071
Wendon J A, Harrison P M, Keays R, Williams R 1994 Cerebral blood flow and metabolism in fulminant liver failure. Hepatology 19: 1407–1413
Wilkinson S P, Blendis L M, Williams R 1974 Frequency and type of renal and electrolyte disorders in fulminant hepatic failure. British Medical Journal 1: 186–189
Wilkinson S P, Weston M J, Parsons V, Williams R 1977 Dialysis in the treatment of renal failure in patients with liver disease. Clinical Nephrology 8: 287–292
Williams R, Wendon J 1994 Indications for orthotopic liver transplantation in fulminant liver failure. Hepatology 20: 5S–10S
Woolf G M, Redeker A G 1991 Treatment of fulminant hepatic failure with insulin and glucagon: a randomized controlled trial. Digestive Diseases and Sciences 36: 92–96
Wootton F T, Lee W M 1990 Acetaminophen hepatotoxicity in the alcoholic. Southern Medical Journal 83: 1047–1049
Wright T L, Hsu H, Donegan E et al 1991 Hepatitis C virus not found in fulminant non-A, non-B hepatitis. Annals of Internal Medicine

# 29. Nonviral infections and granulomatous diseases of the liver

*N. D. C. Finlayson*

Nonviral infections occur remarkably infrequently in the liver in spite of its size and rich blood supply, perhaps because its reticulo-endothelial function makes the liver the main organ responsible for clearing bacteria from the blood (p. 773). Nonviral infections can, however, cause abscesses or more diffuse hepatic involvement; these and the numerous causes of liver granulomas will be considered here. There are many causes of granulomas other than infections, but all these conditions are most conveniently considered together. Hepatic dysfunction, and sometimes jaundice, may occur in systemic infections not involving the liver directly, and these are considered elsewhere (p. 1110).

## PYOGENIC LIVER ABSCESS

Pyogenic liver abscesses are not common but they are important, as they are potentially curable, invariably fatal if untreated and often difficult to diagnose. Their overall incidence may not have changed during this century, but there have been considerable changes in the contexts in which they occur. Recent reviews include those of Frey et al (1989) and Rustgi & Richter (1989).

### *Etiology*

Many conditions can cause a liver abscess (Table 29.1). Infection may reach the liver via the obstructed biliary tree, via the portal vein or the hepatic artery, by direct spread from contiguous structures, from hepatic trauma or by infection of a primary liver lesion. The frequency with which these mechanisms of infection occur varies considerably (Table 29.2).

Biliary obstruction with ascending cholangitis is now the most important single cause of liver abscesses and cholelithiasis, as might be expected, is the most frequent underlying cause (Table 29.2). Cholecystitis may give rise to a hepatic abscess by lymphatic spread of infection or by the direct rupture of the gallbladder into the liver. Appendicitis has diminished greatly as a cause of liver abscess and other intestinal conditions such as diverticular disease, carcinoma of the colon and inflammatory bowel disease (Manjunatha et al 1992) have become more important as causes of spread of infection by the portal vein (Table 29.2). Chronic gastric and duodenal ulcers can cause local intrahepatic suppuration by direct penetra-

**Table 29.1** Causes of pyogenic liver abscess

| Etiological group | |
|---|---|
| Biliary obstruction (cholangitis) | Cholecystolithiasis, choledocholithiasis<br>Neoplasia<br>  bile duct<br>  pancreas<br>  papilla of Vater<br>Stricture<br>Pancreatitis<br>Postoperative<br>Parasites (*Ascaris lumbricoides*) |
| Portal vein infection | Appendicitis<br>Diverticulitis<br>Gastrointestinal neoplasms<br>Inflammatory bowel disease<br>Pancreatitis<br>Gastrointestinal perforation<br>Intra-abdominal abscesses (any site)<br>Umbilical infection, umbilical vein catheterization<br>Hemorrhoids<br>Epididymitis<br>Pelvic inflammatory disease<br>Enteric infections (e.g. *Yersinia*) |
| Hepatic artery infection | Bacteremia (any source) |
| Direct extension | Cholecystitis (empyema)<br>Pancreatic abscess<br>Gastric ulcer<br>Duodenal ulcer<br>Carcinoma (e.g. stomach, colon)<br>Perihepatic abscess<br>Perinephric abscess |
| Primary liver lesion | Malignancy<br>Cysts |
| Trauma | Penetrating (including liver biopsy)<br>Nonpenetrating |

**Table 29.2** Incidence (%) of etiological factors in pyogenic liver abscess

| Etiological factor | Oschner et al 1938 (pre-1940) | Lazarchick et al 1973 (1960–70) | Northover et al 1982 (1967–78) | Farges et al 1988 (1966–86) | Bissada & Bateman 1991 (1982–89) | Robert et al 1992 (1978–88) |
|---|---|---|---|---|---|---|
| Biliary disease | 13 | 39 | 10 | 46 | 33 | 35 |
| Intraperitoneal sepsis | 42 | 20 | 13 | 13 | 33 | 7 |
| (Appendicitis) | (32) | (1) | (3) | (–) | (7) | (3) |
| Generalized sepsis | 12 | 4 | 0 | 24 | 0 | 3 |
| Direction extension | 0 | 10 | 0 | 2 | 0 | 7 |
| Trauma | 4 | 2 | 10 | 0 | 7 | 3 |
| Miscellaneous | 9 | 7 | 3 | 0 | 7 | 10 |
| Unknown cause | 20 | 19 | 63 | 15 | 20 | 38 |
| Total cases (number) | 622 | 75 | 30 | 46 | 27 | 29 |

Note: Oschner et al 1938 includes personal cases (47) and a literature review (575 cases). Dates in parentheses show period during which patients were treated

tion, which is rarely of clinical importance, or may do so as the result of abscess formation following intraperitoneal perforation. Chronic pancreatitis occasionally underlies a liver abscess even in the absence of biliary obstruction, especially in calcific pancreatitis associated with alcohol abuse (Ammann et al 1992). Liver abscess may also result from infection of a pre-existing lesion such as a hepatic cyst or tumor deposit. Hepatic metastases may be especially susceptible to infection with anaerobic bacteria (Trump et al 1978). Abscesses may result from infection in damaged liver tissue or in extravasated blood and bile following liver trauma; this is recognized readily when a penetrating injury has occurred but may be overlooked when it follows a nonpenetrating injury, as the clinical features of the abscess may not arise for 2–4 weeks (Rubin et al 1974). Abscesses have followed arterial embolization or ethanol injection of hepatocellular carcinomas (Hanazaki et al 1993, Okada et al 1993) and have occurred in association with ventriculoperitoneal shunts (Farrell et al 1994). Organisms may spread to the liver from a systemic source and this may not be obvious, as in the case of dental sepsis (Crippin & Wang 1982). No cause can be found for a liver abscess in about 20% of cases and this has remained true over many years (Table 29.2).

The fall in the incidence of liver abscess due to appendicitis and the rise in that due to biliary obstruction have been accompanied by a change in the age distribution of patients with this disease (Fig. 29.1). Previously, 70% of patients were under 40 years old, but now 70% are over 50 and 20% are over 70. Liver abscesses in older adults are usually due to biliary disease and in older children and young adults they are usually a consequence of trauma (Rubin et al 1974). Liver abscesses are uncommon in children.

## Predisposing factors

Predisposing factors include diabetes mellitus, alcoholism, malignant disease, cirrhosis and treatment with immunosuppressive drugs (Rustgi & Richter 1989).

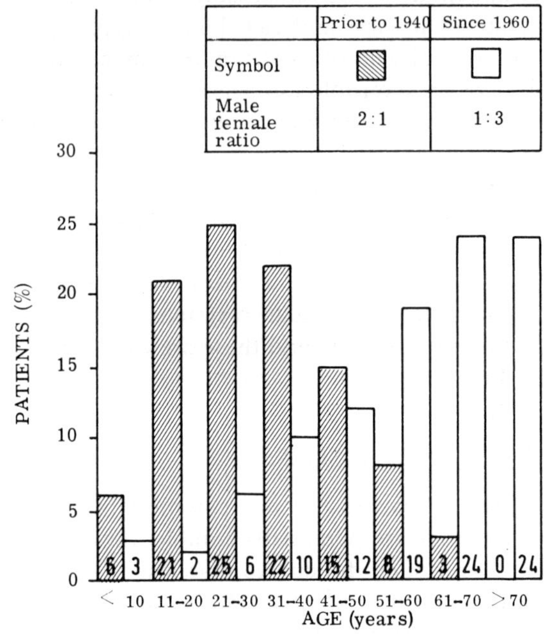


**Fig. 29.1** Age distribution and sex ratio in pyogenic hepatic abscess prior to 1940 and since 1960.

## Bacteriology

Bacteriological investigations in patients with liver abscesses generally reveal a wide range of organisms. This is probably a consequence of the heterogeneous nature of the patients studied, for example in relation to the underlying causes of the abscesses and to the difficulty of growing some organisms such as anaerobes and classifying others such as the streptococci. The predominance of biliary and other intra-abdominal diseases underlying liver abscesses accounts for the frequent isolation of Gram-negative aerobes and anaerobes and these diseases are associated frequently with the isolation of multiple organisms. Gram-positive organisms are more common where liver abscesses originate from systemic infections and single organisms are isolated more often. Lazarchick et al

(1973) isolated organisms from 57 of 65 patients (88%); 59% were Gram-negative bacilli, usually *E. coli* which was overall the organism isolated most often, and 41% were Gram-positive cocci or bacilli, usually a streptococcus. Anaerobic organisms were found in 23% of cases and anaerobes alone were found in 18%.

Similar results have been repeated in more recent series, although anaerobic organisms and isolation of more than one organism are now more frequent (Farges et al 1988, Robert et al 1992). *E. coli* is the most frequently isolated Gram-negative aerobe and others include *Klebsiella*, *Proteus*, *Enterobacter*, and *Pseudomonas* species. Gram-positive organisms include *Enterococcus faecalis*, α- and β-hemolytic streptococci, *Staph. aureus and Staph. epidermidis. Strep. milleri* has been associated increasingly with liver abscesses and its discovery in the blood should lead to a search for a liver abscess.

Anaerobic and microaerophilic organisms, including anaerobic cocci *Bacteroides, Clostridia* and *Fusobacterium* species, have been recognized increasingly as important causes of liver abscesses. Gas in the abscess cavity, foul-smelling pus, unusual bacterial morphology on Gram staining, and failure to grow aerobic organisms all suggest anaerobic infection. No bacteria are isolated from about 20% of liver abscesses and it is likely that most of these are due to anaerobic organisms. Indeed, Sabbaj (1984) considers that anaerobic bacteria are the most numerous and important pathogens in liver abscess and he indicates how frequently these infections involve several organisms.

Almost any organism can cause a hepatic abscess and there are several reports of abscesses caused by unusual organisms. These include abscesses in actinomycosis (Meade 1980), *Yersinia* infection (Capron et al 1981), nocardia (Robinson 1983) and brucellosis (Naveau et al 1983).

***Culture material.*** Blood culture should be carried out in all patients, as the organisms isolated correlate well with those found in the abscess. Sabbaj et al (1972) reviewed 12 series (249 patients) and found that blood culture failed to reveal bacteria in 22% of cases overall, with individual failure rates up to 35%. In practice, it is probably more realistic to expect to isolate organisms in about a half of patients (Table 29.3) and blood culture may be more successful in multiple abscesses (61%) than in single abscesses (24%) in the liver (Lazarchick et al 1973). Culture of abscess material should always be carried out at aspiration or surgery, as this allows identification of organism in about three-quarters of patients (Table 29.3). Previous antibiotic therapy should not be a deterrent to blood and abscess culture, for isolation of organisms is often still successful (Farges et al 1988, Bissada & Bateman 1991). Culture from wounds or drains at a later stage may be misleading owing to secondary invaders.

**Table 29.3** Frequency of isolation of organisms by blood culture and culture of abscess material

| Authors | Positive cultures (%) | |
|---|---|---|
| | Blood | Abscess content |
| Lazarchick et al (1973) | 43 | 88 |
| Farges et al (1988) | 56 | 72 |
| Bissada & Bateman (1991) | 44 | 63 |

## Pathology

Liver abscesses vary from the microscopic to those that occupy a whole liver lobe and they may be single or multiple. Large chronic abscesses have a thick fibrous capsule surrounding an inner wall of granulation tissue that contains acute and chronic inflammatory cells and the cavity itself contains pus and sometimes gas. Enlargement of an abscess may lead to involvement of surrounding structures. Extension into the subphrenic space, pleura or lung may lead to a subphrenic abscess, a pleural effusion or empyema or even infection of the lung itself. Less commonly, the abscess penetrates the peritoneum, leading to generalized peritonitis, or ruptures externally through the skin. Expansion within the liver can lead to obstruction of bile ducts. Metastatic abscesses occur particularly in the lungs and brain (Butler & McCarthy 1969).

The distribution of abscesses within the liver is related to the source of infection (Table 29.4). Biliary obstruction frequently gives rise to multiple abscesses that are found in the distribution of the biliary tree. The pus within them may be bile stained. Other sources of infection usually give rise to a single abscess. Those originating from a source in the portal venous system are more often in the right lobe of the liver and are associated with the portal tracts, which may show evidence of pylephlebitis. The tributaries of the portal vein contain pus and thrombus, the vein walls are infiltrated with inflammatory cells and some veins may have ruptured into the surrounding tissues.

## Clinical features

The patient may show features of the abscess itself, the features of an underlying cause for the abscess and a generalized reaction to infection. Initially, the illness may be due to the underlying cause and evidence of the liver

**Table 29.4** Single and multiple liver abscesses related to the source of infection in 75 patients (Lazarchick et al 1973)

| Source of infection | Number of patients | Abscesses | |
|---|---|---|---|
| | | Single | Multiple |
| Biliary tree | 29 | 5 | 24 |
| Portal system | 15 | 12 | 3 |
| Local spread | 8 | 8 | 0 |
| Miscellaneous | 9 | 5 | 4 |
| Unknown | 14 | 9 | 5 |

abscess may only supervene later. The systemic reaction ranges from fever to bacteremic shock.

The main symptom is pain. More than 80% of patients have variable dull, aching upper abdominal pain, which is usually central or in the right upper quadrant. It may be felt in the left upper quadrant, particularly when there is an abscess in the left lobe. Generalized abdominal pain suggests that peritonitis has developed. Abdominal pain is not invariable and in one report it was absent in half the patients (Rubin et al 1974). The absence of pain does not, therefore, exclude the diagnosis. Diaphragmatic involvement may result in right shoulder pain and pleural involvement causes pleuritic pain in 10–20% of cases, usually on the right. Patients appear ill, have a damp, clammy skin and fetid breath and almost always have lost weight. Half will have lost 5 kg or more and some seem to melt before one's eyes. Anorexia, nausea and vomiting are common and diarrhea occurs in up to a third of patients (Sabbaj et al 1972, Lazarchick et al 1973). Fever is almost always present, often with rigors or night sweats; it can be intermittent, remittent or continuous and is usually above 38°C (100°F). Respiratory symptoms other than pleuritic pain occur in around 10% of patients and include cough and dyspnea.

Hepatomegaly, the commonest positive physical finding, is present in more than half the patients and some have reported it in almost all cases (Sabbaj et al 1972). The enlarged liver is usually tender, especially if there are multiple abscesses (Lazarchick et al 1973), and this may be elicited by gentle percussion over the lower part of the chest on the right side. Mild jaundice is present in a third of cases, splenomegaly is uncommon and ascites is rare. An abdominal mass can sometimes be palpated and generalized abdominal distention may be found. Erythema and edema of the skin due to direct extension of the abscess can occur but is uncommon. Abnormalities are found at the right lung base posteriorly in a quarter of cases and include crepitations, pleural friction and signs of consolidation or pleural effusion. Atypical presentations have become increasingly frequent and are easily mistaken for other diseases (below).

## Investigations

### *Blood*

Two-thirds of patients have a polymorphonuclear leukocytosis and counts over $15 \times 10^9$/L (15 000/mm$^3$) are common. Absence of leukocytosis may actually be a bad prognostic sign (Butler & McCarthy 1969). Anemia occurs in 50% or more and the erythrocyte sedimentation rate is usually over 100 mm in the first hour. The serum alkaline phosphatase activity is the most frequently abnormal liver function test and when more than one test is abnormal, it is generally the most markedly deranged. Rubin et al (1974) found it increased in 95% of cases and in 55% it was markedly abnormal. Normal values may be found with a large solitary abscess. The serum bilirubin exceeds 35 μmol/L (2 mg/dl) in about half the cases, usually in patients with biliary disease, and the serum transaminase activity is raised up to threefold. Hypoalbuminemia, hyperglobulinemia and prolongation of the prothrombin time reflect severe underlying liver disease or a prolonged illness.

### *Radiology and imaging*

Radiological investigations, particularly imaging of the liver, are the most important diagnostic procedures. The chest radiograph shows an elevated or fixed right hemidiaphragm, pleural effusion, basal atelectasis or consolidation in half the patients and occasionally gives the diagnosis by showing gas in an abscess cavity below the diaphragm. Liver imaging must be done in all suspected cases, for it combines a high detection rate with the capacity to locate the lesion in the liver at no risk or discomfort to an ill patient.

Ultrasonography is the initial method of choice for detecting liver abscesses (p. 55). It should detect almost all abscesses greater than 2 cm in diameter and it can often differentiate abscesses from other focal lesions, although neoplastic lesions that have undergone liquefaction may give difficulty (Fig. 2.9). Intraoperative ultrasonography should also be used at laparotomy, as visual examination of the liver alone may not identify a deepseated lesion. Ultrasonography can also be used to guide percutaneous aspiration and drainage of liver abscesses and repeated examination is useful in showing resolution of lesions.

Computed tomography is also very effective in identifying liver abscesses (Fig. 29.2). Radionuclide imaging was previously the best means of identifying liver abscesses but it is much less used now and magnetic resonance imaging is much less available and less well established for this purpose (p. 75).

More than one imaging method should be used where suspicion of an abscess is high and the initial method shows no abnormality. Endoscopic retrograde cholangiography is valuable in identifying biliary disease underlying hepatic abscesses and papillotomy and stone removal or the placement of a stent across a stricture relieves biliary obstruction. Arteriography can be used to localize an abscess but is rarely needed and although indirect evidence of a liver abscess can be found on a barium meal, this method is obsolete.

### *Bacteriology*

Blood cultures and culture of any material removed from liver abscesses should be done in all cases.

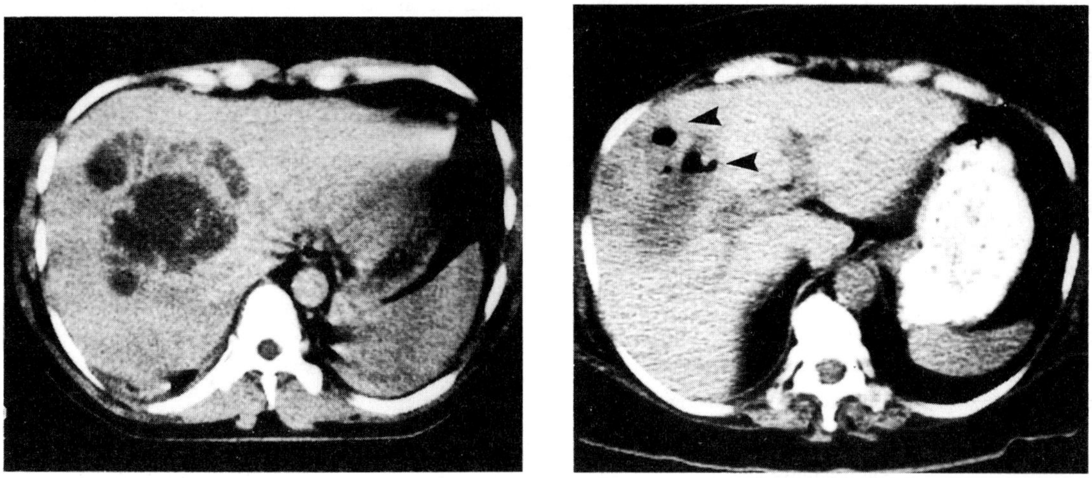

A B

**Fig. 29.2** Liver abscess. (**A**) Large multilocular abscess in right lobe. The low-density areas represent pus. (**B**) Large abscess in right lobe showing gas (arrow) within the abscess cavity.

## Diagnosis

The most important step is to consider the possibility of liver abscesses, which can then almost always be revealed by imaging, for otherwise the diagnosis is made only at autopsy. Altemeier et al (1970) showed that the introduction of radionuclide imaging increased the diagnosis of liver abscess from 20% to 78% and commensurately reduced mortality, although later series still showed up to a third of diagnoses made at autopsy (Northover et al 1982). Farges et al (1988) reported more recently that the use of ultrasound rather than radionuclide imaging was associated with a further reduction of autopsy diagnoses. A rapidly progressive illness with upper abdominal pain, tender hepatomegaly and fever with or without rigors, particularly in a patient with predisposing illnesses such as biliary tract obstruction or appendicitis, will indicate the diagnosis. Cholangitis may be diagnosed correctly, but the fact that hepatic abscesses have developed may be overlooked (Fischer & Beaton 1983).

Other causes of upper abdominal pain, especially pancreatitis, may be mimicked. Unfortunately, cardinal features may not be present and this is increasingly the case (BMJ 1980). Pain may be limited to the lower chest and when this is associated with pleurisy, local tenderness and abnormalities at the right lung base on the chest radiography, pulmonary diseases such as pneumonia or infarction may be diagnosed. A tender, palpable liver with an elevated and fixed right hemidiaphragm should always raise the suspicion of a liver abscess. Pyogenic abscess should be differentiated from amebic abscess (p. 574), and a source for an abscess should always be sought.

***Chronic abscess.*** Major diagnostic difficulties arise where the illness is gradually progressive, as occurs particularly with a solitary abscess. Butler & McCarthy (1969) reported 31 such patients, who constituted two-thirds of all their patients with pyogenic liver abscesses. The clinical presentations were varied (Table 29.5) and the illnesses extended from 3 months to 3 years. Malaise was the commonest symptom and for prolonged periods was the only clinical feature. Two-thirds were febrile, but rigors were uncommon and infrequent. Only half the patients had abdominal pain. Jaundice was uncommon and late. Hepatomegaly occurred in three-quarters, but liver tenderness was a late feature. Anemia and hypoalbuminemic edema were also late features but could be present by the time the patient reached hospital. Radiographs showed hepatomegaly in all patients and liver biopsy gave or suggested the diagnosis in 10 of 12. Some patients even had a laparotomy at which no abscess could be found. Thus, when the diagnosis is suspected, ultrasonography and/or computed tomography should be carried out.

***Other presentations.*** The frequency with which a liver abscess may present as pyrexia of unknown cause should be emphasized. Rarely, an abscess may cause fulminant hepatic failure (Saltzman et al 1978) or a Budd–Chiari syndrome (Mehrota et al 1992).

## Treatment

Successful treatment depends on giving appropriate antibiotic therapy at an early stage and on adequate drainage of the abscess.

### *Antibiotics*

Antibiotics are best given once the responsible organism(s) has been isolated from the blood or the abscess and antibiotic sensitivities are known. They may have to be given to an ill patient before the responsible bacteria have been isolated, but aerobic and anaerobic blood cultures must always be done first and pus should be aspirated from the abscess and cultured if possible.

**Table 29.5** Clinical presentations and sources in 31 patients with chronic pyogenic liver abscesses (Butler & McCarthy 1969)

| Clinical presentation | Source | Metastatic abscesses |
|---|---|---|
| PUO(11) | Diverticulitis(2), lung(1), cholangitis(1), postoperative(1), unknown(6) | Lung(4), brain(1), lung and brain(1) |
| Coma(4) | Pancreas(1), postoperative(1), unknown(2) | Lung(2), brain(1), lung and brain(1) |
| Abdominal pain(3) | Cholangitis(2), unknown(1) | |
| Abdominal mass(3) | Actinomycosis(2), Crohn's disease(1) | Lung(2) |
| Unsuspected(3) | Cholangitis(2), unknown(1) | Lung(1) |
| Lung abscess(2) | Lung(1), unknown(1) | Lung(1) |
| Cardiac failure(2) | Diverticulitis(1), unknown(1) | |
| Collapse(2) | Cholangitis(1), unknown(1) | |
| Diarrhea(1) | Diverticulitis(1) | |

Note: Number of patients shown in parentheses. PUO = pyrexia of unknown origin

The antibiotics used should have an antibacterial spectrum suitable for a polymicrobial infection including aerobes and anaerobes. Suitable combinations would include a third-generation cephalosporin such as cefotaxime or gentamicin, amoxycillin and metronidazole; co-amoxyclav and metronidazole; or ciprofloxacin and metronidazole. Treatment should be given parenterally initially, but the oral route should be used once improvement has occurred. Ciprofloxacin given orally and metronidazole given as suppositories rectally give blood levels equal to those achieved intravenously at much less cost. Patients with decompensated liver disease eliminate metronidazole slowly and may need a reduced dose (Farrell et al 1983). Gentamicin is inexpensive but has to be given parenterally, has considerably renal toxicity and requires blood measurements to ensure peak concentrations less than 10 mg/ml and doses adjusted to renal function (Table 29.6). Imipenem can be used for very ill patients. Subsequent alterations in therapy should be based on a knowledge of the antibiotic sensitivities of the causative bacteria. Prolonged therapy for a period of 2 months or more may be needed.

### *Drainage*

Adequate early drainage of the abscess has always been regarded as of paramount importance (Table 29.7) and liver imaging has greatly improved the achievement of good drainage by localizing the site(s) of disease. Multiple abscesses pose a difficult problem, but large ones at least should be drained. Antibiotic treatment without drainage can be successful, particularly with smaller abscesses, but this treatment should not be continued alone unless the patient is clearly improving (Maher et al 1979, Watanakunakorn 1982). Surgical drainage has previously been regarded as the best treatment for pyogenic abscesses, and some authors still favor this approach (Miedema & Dineen 1984, McCorkell & Niles 1985). Surgical drainage, however, has a high mortality, especially in ill patients, the preferred extraperitoneal approach often cannot be achieved, drains can be difficult to site and intra-abdominal abscesses may develop.

McFadzean et al (1953) showed that solitary liver abscesses could be treated successfully by closed aspiration and local and systemic antibiotics, but this therapy did not find favor at that time. With the advent of imaging, percutaneous drainage (p. 34) and systemic antibiotics have become accepted treatment (Berger & Osborne 1982, Herbert et al 1982, Gerzof et al 1985). Ultrasound and computed tomography are both used to guide aspiration and the siting of drainage catheters. Samples should always be cultured for bacteria to ensure optimal antibiotic therapy. The authors consider that treatment should now begin with closed (nonsurgical) drainage and

**Table 29.6** Gentamicin dosage related to body weight and renal function

| Renal function | | Drug dose | | |
|---|---|---|---|---|
| Blood urea mmol/L (mg/dl) | Creatinine clearance ml/min | Weight >60 kg | Weight <60 kg | Frequency |
| <6 (<40) | >70 | 80 mg | 60 mg | 8-hourly |
| 6–17 (40–100) | 30–70 | 80 mg | 60 mg | 12-hourly |
| 17–34 (100–200) | 10–30 | 80 mg | 60 mg | 24-hourly |
| >34 (>200) | 5–10 | 80 mg | 60 mg | 48-hourly |

**Table 29.7** Drainage of liver abscess and mortality

| Source | Number of cases | Mortality (%) Drainage | Mortality (%) No drainage |
|---|---|---|---|
| Butler & McCarthy (1969) | 31 | 37 | 100 |
| Satiani & Davidson (1978) | 38 | 13 | 100 |

should proceed to surgical drainage only if the patient's condition fails to improve or deteriorates. Solitary abscesses should be aspirated as completely as possible, the largest abscesses should be aspirated where many are present and imaging should be used to follow the resolution of the abscess cavity.

Abdominal disease that has caused a liver abscess may also require surgical treatment. Biliary obstruction should be relieved and drainage instituted, preferably endoscopically (p. 115) or if necessary surgically.

### Complications

Complications occur by extension or rupture into adjacent tissues or spaces or from septic embolization. They develop in about a half of all patients. Most abscesses occur high in the right lobe of the liver and hence a subphrenic abscess or extension to the pleura and lung is most frequent. Pleural or pulmonary involvement may result in fistulas, empyema or a lung abscess. Generalized peritonitis or a perihepatic abscess may result from rupture into the peritoneum. Rarely, rupture into the biliary tree with hemobilia, into other organs such as the pericardium, hepatic vein, vena cava or thoracic duct, or rupture to the exterior may occur. De Bakey & Jordan (1975) considered that antibiotics had reduced the incidence of metastatic abscesses, but Butler & McCarthy (1969) reported brain and/or lung abscesses in 14 of 31 (45%) patients who had had a prolonged illness (Table 29.5).

### Prognosis

Pyogenic liver abscess continues to carry a high mortality. Lazarchick et al (1973) reported a mortality of 40% and Northover et al (1982) a mortality of 43% with many diagnoses made at autopsy. Series describing patients treated more recently have reported lower mortalities of 24% (Farges et al 1988), 11% (Bissada & Bateman 1991) and 24% (Robert et al 1992), suggesting some improvement may have occurred. Farges et al (1988) found that no patients died after the introduction of ultrasound imaging, emphasizing the importance of early diagnosis. However, in spite of diagnostic and therapeutic improvements, mortality is likely to remain significant in those whose illness is severe, indicated by jaundice, multiple abscesses or culture of several organisms, who have serious underlying disease such as malignant disease or who are elderly.

### Prevention

Liver abscess is prevented by early treatment of acute infections within the abdomen, by adequate treatment of biliary disease, by early drainage of intra-abdominal abscesses and by appropriate antibiotics.

## AMEBIC LIVER ABSCESS

Amebic abscesses occur mainly in tropical countries and are considered elsewhere (p. 574). It is important that amebiasis occurs in nonendemic areas (Istre et al 1982) and can cause hepatic abscesses even in patients who have not visited endemic areas (Price 1981).

## LEPTOSPIROSIS

Leptospirosis occurs all over the world and is caused by *Leptospira (L.) interrogans* organisms. More than 170 serotypes affect humans, and those found in most parts of the world are shown in Table 29.8. Public health measures have made it a rare disease in Western countries but it is much more common in less developed countries (Turner 1973, Sanford 1984, Waitkins 1985). Leptospirosis varies from a mild febrile illness with or without meningism and mild proteinuria to a severe and often fatal icteric illness. Jaundice is an uncommon manifestation and has been referred to as Weil's disease. Weil's disease is almost always caused by *L. icterohaemorrhagiae* and most reserve the term for icteric leptospirosis caused by this organism. Unless stated otherwise, the discussion below refers to infection with *L. icterohaemorrhagiae*.

### Epidemiology

Leptospirae survive by proliferating in the renal tubules of their hosts. Rats are the best recognized hosts, but many other wild or domestic animals can be infected, including mice, voles, hedgehogs, oxen, livestock and dogs. Shedding of the leptospirae into the urine occurs transiently in some hosts but permanently in others. Survival of the organism outside the host depends on the urine becoming diluted, as urine contains substances capable of lysing the organism, on the avoidance of drying and on an environment with a neutral pH and a temperature around 30°C. Stagnant water fulfills these criteria well.

Infection in humans occurs sporadically. Previously susceptible groups, such as sewer workers, fish cleaners and miners, now seldom get the disease in the UK or North America owing to better personal and environmental

**Table 29.8** *L. interrogans* organisms commonly causing leptospirosis

| Groups | UK cases (%) |
|---|---|
| Hardjo | 40–50 |
| Icterohaemorrhagiae | 35–55 |
| Hebdomadis | 25–50 |
| Canicola | 5–10 |
| Ballum | Rare |
| Javanica | Rare |
| Autumnalis | Rare |
| Australis | Rare |
| Pomona | Rare |

hygiene. Water-associated leptospirosis in these countries now usually occurs in young people participating in water sports and cattle-associated leptospirosis caused by *L. hebdomadis (hardjo)* has become increasingly important in the UK in farmers, especially cowmen and dairy workers (Hart et al 1984). Infection generally results from indirect contamination with infected urine, blood or tissue. Direct spread by an animal bite, from person to person and by accidental inoculation in the laboratory has occurred but is rare. Asymptomatic leptospirosis, at least in adults, is uncommon (Takafuji et al 1984), but serological evidence of past infection without any history of jaundice is frequent, showing that severe liver involvement is uncommon (Davidson & Smith 1939).

## Pathology

*L. icterohaemorrhagiae* enters the body through the mucous membrane of the eyes, nose, mouth and throat or through abraded skin. The illness begins after an incubation period of 1–2 weeks (2–17 days) with a bacteremic phase that lasts for about a week. All body tissues are invaded during this phase, but especially the kidneys, liver, brain, muscles and capillaries. Thereafter, organisms can be found mainly in the kidneys and liver and in the skin vasculature, giving the skin an erythematous appearance. The disappearance of the organisms from the blood probably results from host immune reactions, as specific serum agglutinins and lysins, important in diagnosis, can be detected first at this time. Titers are low at first and rise rapidly to reach diagnostic levels by the end of the second week. A fourfold increase in titer is diagnostic.

***Liver.*** Most descriptions of the pathological changes in the liver are based on autopsy material, but liver biopsy descriptions are available (Alves et al 1987). The liver is enlarged due to congestion and cholestasis, but a striking feature is the lack of liver cell necrosis despite severe jaundice. This implies that subcellular damage prevents adequate bilirubin excretion and electronmicroscopy has shown loss of microvilli on the sinusoidal and canalicular hepatocyte membranes, which could be related to impaired bilirubin transport. Most abnormalities occur in the centrilobular zones, where hepatocyte swelling, marked mitotic activity, cholestasis and prominent Kupffer cells are seen. Occasional acidophilic bodies indicate focal hepatocyte necrosis and focal fatty change occurs rarely. The portal tracts show mild mononuclear cell infiltration.

***Other organs.*** Lesions may be found in a variety of other tissues, although leptospiral organisms are found only in the kidney, if at all. The renal lesions are more impressive than those in the liver and occur in the convoluted tubules. The tubular cells are swollen, degenerate or dead, casts and cell debris are present in the lumen and the interstitium is infiltrated with mononuclear cells and a few polymorphonuclear leukocytes. Degenerative and inflammatory lesions are also found in the skeletal muscles, myocardium, meninges, lungs and the gastrointestinal tract.

## Clinical features

Leptospirosis manifests itself clinically in two phases: an initial febrile phase that lasts about a week and is related to blood spread of the organism and a subsequent icteric phase that lasts, if the patient survives, for 2–4 weeks. The febrile phase starts suddenly with fever exceeding 38°C (100°F), shivering, anorexia, nausea and perhaps vomiting. Generalized stiffness, arthralgia and especially muscle pain become progressively more severe over the next few days. Most patients have a severe headache from the outset and some develop marked neck stiffness. Conjunctival suffusion is virtually constant and often intense; it usually occurs early, persists throughout the illness and is an important clue to the diagnosis. Additional findings include a sore throat, herpes labialis and a skin rash. The patient either recovers after about a week or develops the icteric phase.

Jaundice usually appears towards the end of the first week (3–10 days), deepens rapidly over a few days and continues for about 2 weeks before subsiding. It develops in about two-thirds of *L. icterohaemorrhagiae* infections but is uncommon in other leptospiral infections. The liver becomes enlarged and tender, the urine dark and sometimes pale stools and pruritus develop. Splenomegaly occurs in fewer than 10% of patients. The fever disappears and muscle pains diminish, but the patient's general condition deteriorates. Anorexia, nausea and vomiting worsen, tachycardia and hypotension develop, the urine output falls and anuria occurs in severe cases. Previously mild proteinuria increases, casts, leukocytes and red blood cells appear in the urine and uremia develops. The blood urea may reach 40 mmol/L (250 mg/dl) in the absence of treatment. Bleeding is common owing to capillary damage. Petechiae and ecchymoses almost always occur, bleeding from the nose and into the conjunctivae is common and occasionally there is severe bleeding from the gastrointestinal tract or into internal organs such as the brain. Cardiac abnormalities include arrhythmias, conduction defects, cardiac failure and sometimes pericarditis.

Improvement begins between the second and fourth week. Full recovery is slow and mild relapses may occur.

## Investigations

***Hematology.*** A polymorphonuclear leukocytosis ($12–35 \times 10^9$/L, 12 000–35 000/$mm^3$) occurs early and bleeding may lead to anemia later. Thrombocytopenia may occur, but other tests of coagulation are normal.

***Renal.*** The urine findings are described above. The blood urea concentration reflects the degree of renal failure due to renal tubular necrosis (Winearls et al 1984).

***Cerebrospinal fluid.*** Lumbar puncture is performed frequently on account of meningism. The cell content of the cerebrospinal fluid is increased to about $100/mm^3$ (Cargill & Beeson 1947). Xanthochromia occurs occasionally.

***Muscles.*** Creatinine phosphokinase activity in the blood is increased in about a third of patients and occasionally very high activities may occur (Farkas et al 1981). Such increases do not occur in viral hepatitis.

***Liver function tests.*** Conjugated hyperbilirubinemia and bilirubinuria are the most prominent findings. The serum alkaline phosphatase activity and γ-glutamyl transferase activity are variably increased and the transaminase activity is normal or only moderately increased, reflecting the absence of hepatocyte necrosis.

***Liver biopsy.*** This can be done in spite of the bleeding tendency (Alves et al 1987), but it is rarely necessary.

***Bacteriology.*** A specific diagnosis depends on isolating the organism or on demonstrating serological responses to it. Organisms may be demonstrated in the blood and cerebrospinal fluid in the first phase of the illness. Microscopy is rapid but unreliable, while blood culture and guinea pig inoculation take a week to yield results. These methods depend on the diagnosis being suspected within a week of the onset of disease, as organisms cannot be found in the blood thereafter. They are excreted in the urine for up to a month, but they are often not viable.

Tests for specific antileptospiral antibodies are the best methods of diagnosing this disease. A test with a compound antigen is used to identify leptospiral antibodies initially and further tests are needed for the precise serotype. Antibodies appear in the second week of the illness and increase rapidly to diagnostic levels over 2–3 weeks before diminishing gradually. They may be detected for years thereafter. A fourfold rise in antibody titer is diagnostic of leptospiral infection.

### Treatment

*Specific*

There is no therapy of proven value. Penicillin kills leptospirae and may help if given within a few days of onset of the illness. It can cause a febrile reaction with headache, myalgia and fever (Winearls et al 1984). Penicillin (600 mg 6-hourly) should be given for 7 days and larger doses are needed if treatment is started after the third day. Alternatively, amoxycillin may be given by mouth. Doxycycline 100 mg twice daily by mouth for 7 days may also be useful provided it is started at an early stage (McClain et al 1984).

*Supportive*

The limitations of specific treatment increase the importance of supportive management. This includes careful fluid balance to avoid dehydration of an anorectic and febrile patient or overhydration of an increasingly oliguric patient. The blood urea and electrolyte concentrations should be measured frequently to guide fluid and electrolyte therapy and to indicate the need for hemodialysis for renal failure. Nutrition should be maintained as far as possible. The hemoglobin should be measured regularly, as minor hemorrhages may gradually lead to anemia. This and overt bleeding should be treated by red blood cell transfusions. Muscle pain may require morphine for relief.

### Prognosis

The prognosis is worse in older patients and in those who develop jaundice. Few anicteric patients die, but about 20% of those with jaundice (Heath et al 1965). Most deaths occur during the second week and renal failure is the main cause. Other causes of death include hemorrhage, cardiac failure and secondary infections. Hepatic failure is uncommon. Recovery, when it occurs, is complete.

### Prevention

This centers on the control of the rodent population and the removal of stagnant water. Individuals in high-risk occupations need protective clothing, especially rubber boots and gloves, and it is inadvisable to swim in stagnant water. Doxycycline 200 mg orally once weekly provides good protection for individuals during periods of particular exposure to leptospirosis (Takafuji et al 1984). Immune serum may protect those known to have been exposed to infection, as in a laboratory accident. Effective vaccines are not available.

## SYPHILIS

Liver damage can occur in all forms of syphilis, although it is a rare cause of liver disease. Congenital syphilis is a widespread disease in which there is a heavy infection of spirochetes in the liver, marked hepatomegaly and diffuse interstitial hepatitis with fibrosis (McIntosh 1909). Granulomatous inflammation in tertiary syphilis gives rise to gummata in which few if any treponemes can be found. These heal with dense fibrosis to give a markedly knobbly liver (hepar lobatum) that is usually asymptomatic. Progressive fibrosis can cause liver failure with jaundice or ascites or portal hypertension with bleeding from esophageal varices (Symmers & Spain 1946).

Secondary syphilis is now recognized as a cause of hepatitis, but it is uncommon and difficult to diagnose, even on liver biopsy (Veeravahu 1985). Concomitant causes of hepatitis, such as viral hepatitis, need to be excluded. The clinical features are variable and include mild jaundice, tender hepatomegaly and the signs of secondary syphilis. Tests of liver function show mild to moderate abnormalities and a markedly increased serum alkaline phosphatase activity is usually a feature. Liver biopsy generally reveals nonspecific abnormalities and granulomas are sometimes seen. Spirochetes are seen in the liver only rarely and they do not prove that hepatitis is caused by syphilis.

## CURTIS–FITZ-HUGH SYNDROME

The Curtis–Fitz-Hugh syndrome is a condition in which urogenital or pelvic inflammatory disease is associated with right upper quadrant abdominal pain due to perihepatitis (Bolton & Darougar 1983). There is usually a sudden onset of pain, suggesting biliary colic or sometimes pleurisy, which is often severe and which may radiate to the right shoulder. Abdominal tenderness and guarding are present and occasionally a rub can be heard over the liver. There may be a leukocytosis and minor abnormalities of liver function tests, but a chest radiograph and ultrasonography or cholecystography show no pulmonary or biliary disease. Cultures from the cervix, urethra and rectum and serological tests reveal either gonorrheal or chlamydial infection.

This disease occurs almost exclusively in women and the upper abdominal pain is caused by a perihepatitis that can give rise to fine "violin string" adhesions between the liver and the abdominal wall. The route of spread of the infection is unknown, but transcelomic spread has been generally favored over lymphatic or blood spread. The condition has been reported rarely in men, which might bring this notion into question, but one male patient was noted to be homosexual and the infection probably originated in the rectum (Fung & Silpa 1981).

Most cases have been caused by *N. gonorrhoea* in the past and these respond well to benzyl penicillin 600 mg intramuscularly 6-hourly for 48 h followed by ampicillin 250 mg four times daily for 12 days. Patients sensitive to penicillin can be given a single dose of co-trimoxazole 3.84 g (eight tablets) or three doses of 2.4 g (five tablets) at 12-hourly intervals. Specialist advice is required for patients with resistant organisms. This syndrome can also be caused by *C. trachomatis* and it is important to look for this organism in all cases (Wood et al 1982). Treatment is with doxycycline 100 mg or erythromycin 500 mg twice daily for seven days.

## MYCOBACTERIA

### Tuberculosis

It has been known for a long time that hepatic involvement at autopsy is common in tuberculosis (Ullom 1909), but it is only rarely that such involvement is manifest clinically. Tuberculosis, however, can present as a primarily hepatic illness and does so in about 1% of patients in countries where the disease is common (Alvarez & Carpio 1983).

#### *Pathology*

The granuloma is the basic lesion and it may be found anywhere in the liver. These lesions are almost always found in miliary tuberculosis and in other forms of tuberculosis the incidence varies from 25% to 80% (Korn et al 1959, Bowry et al 1970, Alvarez & McCabe 1984). Caseation in granulomas is also common, especially where granulomas have coalesced, and can be found in about 80% of patients with hepatic symptoms (Essop et al 1984). Acid-fast bacilli are much less common, occurring in only a third of granulomas in untreated patients at autopsy (Ullom 1909) and in only about 10% of patients during life (Alvarez & McCabe 1984, Essop et al 1984). Freund's adjuvant can produce hepatic granulomas in guinea pigs, suggesting that organisms may not be needed for granuloma production (Jahiel & Koffler 1961). In the absence of caseation or acid-fast bacilli, the granulomas of tuberculosis cannot be identified specifically. The finding of occasional acid-fast rods in granulomas without caseation is not enough for a diagnosis of tuberculosis, as such structures occur in sarcoidosis (Israel & Goldstein 1971). Organisms are hardly ever grown on liver culture, emphasizing the need for guinea pig inoculation (Alvarez & McCabe 1984).

Larger lesions called tuberculomas can develop and show central caseation. They may be single or multiple and, rarely, reach several centimeters in diameter, when they may form a macroscopic "pseudotumor" or develop into a tuberculous abscess. Nonspecific changes are also common and include mononuclear cell infiltration of the portal tracts and sinusoids, periportal fibrosis, fatty change, focal liver cell necrosis and focal Kupffer cell hyperplasia, sometimes forming "microgranulomas". Hepatic amyloid is found occasionally.

#### *Clinical features*

Patients with tuberculous liver disease have usually had a prolonged illness and half have been unwell for more than a year. The main abdominal symptom is right upper quadrant abdominal pain, which occurs in about two-thirds of patients; three-quarters also have respiratory symptoms and many have fever, night sweats and weight loss. Hepatomegaly occurs in almost all patients; it may be marked and in half the liver feels nodular. The spleen is palpable in about a third of patients, usually owing to splenic tuberculosis. Jaundice of hepatocellular or cholestatic type and ascites occur in 10–30%.

#### *Investigations*

Liver function tests are often abnormal in patients who

have no symptoms of liver involvement and are always abnormal in those who do. Increased alkaline phosphatase activity is the most prominent abnormality. Hypoalbuminemia and hyperglobulinemia resulting from systemic infection may be present. Liver imaging can show diffuse or focal abnormalities in severely affected patients, but these findings are nonspecific. Liver biopsy is the most important investigation and gives the diagnosis in more than 90% of patients with symptoms of liver involvement. Laparoscopy is also valuable and in symptomatic patients a correct macroscopic diagnosis can be made. Transhepatic or retrograde cholangiography in patients with cholestatic jaundice may show a normal biliary tree, indicating a hepatocellular cause of cholestasis or a biliary obstruction usually attributed to tuberculous lymphadenopathy in the porta hepatis or sometimes in the common bile duct. Three-quarters of patients with symptomatic hepatic tuberculosis have evidence of tuberculosis on a chest radiograph, but more important for the clinician is that a quarter do not. A negative tuberculin skin test with 10 units of Old Tuberculin (Mantoux 1:1000) virtually excludes tuberculosis in all but moribund patients.

*Treatment*

Antituberculosis chemotherapy is most important. Rifampicin, isoniazid and pyrazinamide (available as Rifater in Europe) should be given for 2 months followed by rifampicin and isoniazid for a further 4 months. Ethambutol is a rather more hepatotoxic drug, but it should also be given where bovine tuberculosis or an atypical mycobacterium is suspected or in areas where resistant organisms are common. Drainage of abscesses by surgical or nonsurgical means is rarely needed. Biliary obstruction may have to be relieved but is not usually necessary. The efficacy of corticosteroids in the very ill is unproven.

### Leprosy

Hepatic granulomas may be found in any form of leprosy but are most frequent in lepromatous leprosy, occurring in two-thirds of cases (Karat et al 1971). Acid-fast bacilli (*M. leprae*) may be seen histologically, but leprosy organisms have not been cultured from liver biopsy material. Liver function tests show minor abnormalities, particularly in patients with granulomas, but clinical evidence of liver involvement does not occur. Diagnosis is based on finding leprosy elsewhere and on a positive lepromin skin test.

### Other mycobacteria

Several mycobacteria other than *M. tuberculosis* and *M. leprae* can cause hepatic granulomas, including *M. bovis*, *M. avium-intracellulare*, *M. serofulaceum*, and other atypical mycobacteria (Guckian & Perry 1966, Patel 1981). *M. avium-intracellulare* has emerged as an important infection causing hepatic involvement in the acquired immunodeficiency syndrome (p. 605). BCG inoculation may also cause an illness associated with hepatic granulomas, particularly when used as immunotherapy in patients with cancer who are particularly susceptible to infection (Hunt et al 1973).

## OTHER INFECTIONS INVOLVING THE LIVER

### Typhoid and paratyphoid

Patients with typhoid fever may develop tender hepatomegaly and splenomegaly, usually during the second week of the illness (p. 563). Jaundice due to a hepatitis-like syndrome occurs in about 0.5–4% of patients admitted to hospital (Dan et al 1982, Pais 1984). These patients have a fever and are very ill clinically and liver function tests show the features of a hepatitis or cholestatic hepatitis. Liver biospy shows chronic inflammatory cell infiltration, focal necroses and sometimes granulomas. Immunoglobulin and complement have been reported in the canaliculi, suggesting the presence of immune complexes (Dan et al 1982). Liver biopsy should not be carried out if the nature of the disease is recognized. Similar changes can occur in paratyphoid fever (Meals 1976).

### Brucellosis

Brucellosis spreads to humans from cattle (*Br. abortus*), sheep or goats (*Br. melitensis*) and pigs (*Br. suis*) and enters the body via the skin or oropharynx. It usually causes an acute, nonspecific illness with malaise, fever, chills, sweating, weight loss, arthralgia and general aches and pains that resolve spontaneously, but it can also follow a subacute relapsing or chronic course. Histological liver involvement is common and biochemical liver function tests are abnormal in about a half of cases, but clinical features of liver disease are not striking (Cervantes et al 1982). Upper abdominal discomfort can occur in acute infection, but jaundice is rare and mild. Minor hepatomegaly and/or palpable splenomegaly occurs in up to a quarter of cases. Biochemical liver function tests show increased plasma transaminase and alkaline phosphatase activity. Liver biopsy shows patchy nonspecific inflammation and necrosis and granulomas occur, particularly in the first 3 months of the illness. Brucellosis rarely causes suppurative disease, but suppurative cholecystitis and liver abscess have been reported (Naveau et al 1983). Calcification may occur in affected organs. Progression to cirrhosis has been reported but is exceedingly rare (McCullough & Eisele 1951). Blood culture and serological tests are used in diagnosis and organisms can be grown from the liver. Brucellosis is usually self-limited but can be treated with tetracycline or trimethoprim-sulphamethoxazole.

### Q-fever

*Coxiella burnetii* causes an acute febrile illness, usually in farm workers or abattoir workers, in which pulmonary symptoms usually predominate. Hepatomegaly occurs in about a half of patients and liver function tests are abnormal in over three-quarters (Spelman 1982). An illness indistinguishable from viral hepatitis clinically occurs occasionally (DuPont et al 1971). Liver biopsy often shows granulomas, but the fibrin-ring granuloma is no longer considered diagnostic of Q-fever (p. 831). Chronic hepatitis may also develop and may occasionally lead to cirrhosis (Turck et al 1976).

### Yersiniosis

*Y. enterocolitica* infection is acquired by ingesting infected food and the commonest symptoms are diarrhea, fever and abdominal pain that may be sufficiently severe to lead to laparotomy. The diagnosis is made by isolating the organism from the stools or by serological tests. Systemic illness is common and hepatic involvement in the acute illness occurs in about 10% of patients, evidenced by a twofold or greater increase of plasma bilirubin, transaminase or alkaline phosphatase (Saebø & Lassen 1992). Occasionally a cholestatic jaundice develops. Liver biopsy usually shows nonspecific changes such as cholestasis, focal necrosis of hepatocytes and fatty change. Subsequent chronic liver damage has been reported in about 5% of patients, only half of whom show hepatic abnormality in the acute illness (Saebø & Lassen 1992). Most show nonspecific abnormalities of liver function and histology, but some show chronic granulomatous hepatitis and portal hypertension and esophageal varices occur occasionally. These patients often show, and may die of, multisystem disease, sometimes with immune abnormalities such as antinuclear factor and rheumatoid factor.

*Y. enterocolitica* is sensitive to tetracycline and third-generation cephalosporins. Corticosteroid therapy improves liver function tests in the acute illness, but relapse is common when treatment is stopped.

### Rickettsial infections

These diseases occur worldwide and are caused by a variety of rickettsia transmitted to humans by ticks, mites or fleas. Lesions occur throughout the body, but clinical manifestations of liver involvement are uncommon. Abnormal liver function tests are common in Rocky Mountain spotted fever (*R. rickettsii*) and in murine typhus (*R. typhi*), with plasma transaminases increased more than five-fold in about a quarter of patients, and the liver shows neutrophil and monocyte infiltration of the liver sinusoids and portal tracts in which the organism can be found (Adams & Walker 1981, Silpapojakul et al 1996). Boutonneuse fever (*R. conori*) can cause granulomas in the liver (Guardia et al 1974), including fibrin-ring granulomas (p. 831). The diagnosis of rickettsial infection is made serologically and the organisms are susceptible to tetracycline and chloramphenicol.

### Listeriosis

*L. monocytogenes* causes foodborne human infection and usually affects the very young or the elderly and those predisposed by immunosuppression, pregnancy or underlying conditions such as diabetes mellitus, renal failure, alcoholism, cirrhosis or malignant disease. It usually causes meningoencephalitis and bacteremia, but other organs can show widespread granulomas or abscesses. Occasional patients can present with the clinical and biochemical features of an acute hepatitis or with hepatic abscess (Braun et al 1993). The organisms can be isolated by blood culture or from an abscess and treatment is with antibiotics such as ampicillin or a cephalosporin.

### Actinomycosis

*A. israelii* and *A. bovis* usually infect the cervicofacial region. Intra-abdominal disease accounts for less than a quarter of cases and in about 15% of these patients there is liver involvement with irregular abscesses (Putman et al 1950). Infection usually spreads to the liver directly or via the portal vein. Occasionally, isolated hepatic abscesses occur and can mimic metastatic disease. Some of these patients have oral actinomycosis and most have had no detectable disease elsewhere (Miyamoto & Fang 1993). The organism is difficult to grow, but pus may contain "sulfur granules" and branching filamentous elements can be seen on microscopy. Treatment is by large doses of penicillin and drainage or resection of abscesses.

### Fungal infections

Fungal infections vary greatly in their geographical distribution. They can occur in otherwise normal people but in practice are most likely to be encountered in patients with diminished immune responses due to myeloproliferative or lymphoproliferative diseases, to the acquired immune deficiency syndrome (p. 605), to the chemotherapy of these diseases or to transplantation. Diagnosis is often unclear, as the organisms can be difficult to isolate and serological tests are not always reliable.

#### *Candidosis*

*Candida albicans* is the most important cause of disseminated fungal infection in immunocompromised patients and the liver is involved in a half or more of cases (Lewis et al 1982). There is often no clinical evidence of infection in the liver, but liver function tests are almost always abnormal, particularly in respect of increased serum alkaline phosphatase or transaminase activity. Jaundice and a clinical syndrome of acute hepatitis are unusual but can occur (Moseley et al 1982). Hepatic imaging can reveal focal defects and liver biopsy, especially guided by imaging or at laparoscopy, is important in giving the diagnosis. Granulomas and microabscesses are the usual liver lesions and large abscesses can occur. Multiorgan involvement is the rule in patients coming to autopsy. Blood cultures reveal the organism in only half the cases and serological tests are not always reliable. Amphotericin and fluconazole are the drugs of choice and neither has major hepatic side-effects.

*Cryptococcosis*

*Cryptococcus neoformans* usually affects immunocompromised individuals and hepatic disease in otherwise normal patients is exceptional (Das et al 1983). The portal of entry is usually the lungs and hepatic involvement can cause a syndrome of hepatitis with transient pulmonary infiltrates on chest radiographs (Howard & Smith 1983). Liver function tests are abnormal, especially with increased serum alkaline phosphatase activity, and there may be an eosinophilia. Liver biopsy shows granulomas and may reveal the organism. Treatment is as for candidiasis.

*Other fungi*

Many other fungi can infect the liver. Some are restricted geographically, as in the case of histoplasmosis, coccidioidomycosis and blastomycosis, which are found in the Americas; others, such as *Aspergillus*, are uncommon causes of liver disease.

## Parasitic infections

These are common worldwide and many affect the liver or biliary tract. Amebiasis (p. 572), giardiasis (p. 575), *Balantidium coli* infection (p. 579), ascariasis (p. 580), enterobiasis (p. 584), visceral larval migrans (p. 585), hydatid disease, schistosomiasis (p. 589), liver flukes (p. 591) and toxocariasis (p. 585) are all considered elsewhere.

## Malaria

The liver is the organ in which malarial sporozoites injected by an infected *Anopheles* mosquito undergo development (schizogony) into merozoites (Hollingdale 1985). The merozoites rupture and destroy the host liver cells as they are liberated into the blood, but this rarely produces clinical features of liver dysfunction, presumably because too few liver cells are destroyed. The clinical features are those of a generalized infection, tissue damage is caused by sequestration of infected red blood cells in vascular beds, but signs of liver involvement are few (Deller et al 1967, Patwari et al 1979). Hepatosplenomegaly is common, especially in children, but is in large part due to involvement of the reticulo-endothelial system. Some patients have abdominal pain and about a half have percussion tenderness over the liver. Jaundice occurs in fewer than 10% of cases and may be caused by hemolysis, hepatocellular damage or cholestasis. Less marked hepatic damage is common, as evidenced by increased transaminase or alkaline phosphatase activity in a half to two-thirds of cases, but liver failure does not occur. Transaminase activity rises more than fivefold in about a fifth of cases and can reach values seen in acute viral hepatitis. These abnormalities disappear following successful treatment.

Liver biopsy is not needed in malaria, but investigations have shown nonspecific mononuclear cell infiltration of the portal tracts and parenchyma, occasional areas of focal hepatocyte necrosis, granulomas, Kupffer cell hyperplasia and brown malarial pigment (Deller et al 1967).

***Tropical splenomegaly syndrome.*** Recurrent malaria can give rise to production of IgM aggregates, phagocytosed in the reticulo-endothelial system, and marked splenomegaly. The liver shows dense sinusoidal lymphocyte infiltration, Kupffer cell hyperplasia, malarial pigment and variable portal tract infiltration.

## Toxoplasmosis

*Toxoplasma gondii* infection can cause a syndrome resembling infectious mononucleosis in adults, but occasional patients present with clinical and biochemical features of an acute hepatitis with jaundice (Vischer et al 1967). The liver shows hepatic cell necrosis, inflammatory cell infiltration and sometimes granulomas and *T. gondii* can be found in these lesions.

# GRANULOMATOUS HEPATITIS

This is a nonspecific condition defined by the presence of granulomas within the liver. The finding of hepatic granulomas should initiate a search for one of their numerous known causes (Tables 29.9, 29.10) and many of these are described in this chapter or elsewhere. The clinical features range from acute self-limiting illnesses to chronic illnesses often causing fever of unknown cause. These features determine what should be sought initially, but a fuller investigation will be needed if the initial search proves fruitless.

## Sarcoidosis

*Definition and pathology*

Sarcoidosis is one of the two commonest causes of hepatic

**Table 29.9** Causes of granulomatous hepatitis (adapted from Fauci & Wolff 1976)

| |
|---|
| Infections (Table 29.10) |
| Drugs (Table 29.12) |
| Primary hepatic disease (Table 29.13) |
| Immune defects |
| Acquired immunodeficiency syndrome (AIDS) |
| Chronic granulomatous disease of childhood |
| Hypogammaglobulinemia |
| Neoplasms |
| Lymphomas |
| Carcinomas |
| Beryliosis |
| Diseases of unknown cause* |
| Sarcoidosis |
| Ulcerative colitis |
| Crohn's disease |
| Allergic granulomatosis (Chung–Strauss syndrome) |
| Connective tissue diseases |
| Chronic idiopathic granulomatous hepatitis |
| Jejunal bypass surgery (Kalat & Martin 1981) |

*Erythema nodosum of unknown cause can be associated with hepatic granulomas

**Table 29.10** Infections causing granulomatous hepatitis (adapted from Fauci & Wolff 1976)

| |
|---|
| *Bacterial* |
| Mycobacterial (typical/atypical) |
| Leprosy |
| Brucellosis |
| Tularemia |
| Listeriosis |
| Granuloma inguinale |
| Melioidosis |
| Typhoid, paratyphoid |
| Whipple's disease |
| Yersiniosis |
| *Fungal* |
| Histoplasmosis |
| Coccidioidomycosis |
| *Viral* |
| Cytomegalovirus |
| Infectious mononucleosis |
| Hepatitis A |
| *Rickettsial* |
| Coxiella burnetii |
| Rickettsia conori |
| Rickettsia typhi |
| *Spirochetal* |
| Syphilis |
| *Parasitic* |
| Schistosomiasis |
| Leishmaniasis |
| Toxocara |
| Giardiasis |
| Others (p. 572) |

granulomas (Table 29.11). Its cause is unknown and its definition has occasioned considerable controversy. It has been defined as:

. . . a disease characterized by the formation in all of several affected organs or tissues of epithelioid-cell tubercles, without caseation though fibrinoid necrosis may be present at the centers of a few, proceeding either to resolution or to conversion into hyaline fibrous tissue (Scadding & Mitchell 1985).

**Table 29.11** Diagnosis in granulomatous liver disease

| Diagnosis | % (range) |
|---|---|
| Sarcoidosis | 28 (0–47) |
| Mycobacterial infection | 21 (7–54) |
| Other | 27 (3–49) |
| No diagnosis | 17 (6–36) |

Notes: (1) Total 711 patients from Klatskin & Yesner 1950, Wagoner et al 1953, Bunim et al 1962, Guckian & Perry 1966, Terplan 1971, Mir-Madjlessi et al 1973, McMaster & Hennigar 1981, Cunningham et al 1982, Anderson et al 1988, Zoutman et al 1991.
(2) Commonest other diagnoses were chronic liver disease 12%, drugs 10%, fungal infections 7%, viral and bacterial infections 5% (brucella, Q-fever, cytomegalovirus), lymphomas 4%, parasites 3%.

Clinicoradiographic findings supported by the presence of such granulomas in more than one organ are sufficient to make the diagnosis (James et al 1976). Virtually every organ and tissue can be involved, although the most common include the lymph nodes, lungs, liver, spleen, skin, eyes, skeleton and salivary glands. When disease occurs in other sites, these commonly involved organs are frequently also affected.

The Kveim test uses a splenic antigen and is highly specific for sarcoidosis, although its basis is not understood (Siltzbach 1961). Eighty percent of typical cases of recent onset are positive, 60% of typical cases of over 2 years' duration are positive and only 40% of cases are positive where extrathoracic tissues only are affected (Israel & Goldstein 1971). The test is no longer used as the splenic antigen cannot be guaranteed free of human immunodeficiency virus.

### *Clinical features*

Clinical evidence of liver involvement is exceptional and is usually limited to hepatomegaly, which is found in about a fifth of patients. Rarely, sarcoidosis may present as a predominantly hepatic illness. Jaundice may occur and can show obstructive clinical and biochemical features. Cholestasis usually develops slowly and can mimic disorders such as primary biliary cirrhosis (p. 940). Acute cholestasis is exceptionally rare (Williams & Cooper 1985). Ascites is very rare and may be associated with jaundice and other evidence of hepatic failure or may be caused by peritoneal involvement (Wong & Rosen 1962). Portal hypertension may result from cirrhosis or from granulomatous inflammation in the portal tracts, leading to presinusoidal portal hypertension, and may result in splenomegaly and bleeding esophageal varices (Vilinskas et al 1970, Berger & Katz 1973).

*Investigations*

Minor abnormalities of liver function are common (Maddrey et al 1970). The most frequent is a raised serum alkaline phosphatase activity. The serum transaminase activity is increased less frequently and hyperbilirubinemia is rarely sufficient to cause jaundice. Biochemical abnormalities are generally associated with more extensive granulomatous liver involvement, although granulomas may occur in the absence of biochemical liver dysfunction. Hypergammaglobulinemia and sometimes hypoalbuminemia may also be present. Serum angiotensin-converting enzyme activity is increased in sarcoidosis but is of no value in patients with hepatic involvement, as activities up to twice normal occur frequently in many liver diseases (Matsuki & Sakata 1982). Liver biopsy in sarcoidosis reveals granulomas in 65–97% of cases (Guckian & Perry 1966). Scadding & Mitchell (1985) found hepatic granulomas in 66% of 73 patients; the incidence was highest in early disease with hilar lymph node enlargement only (87%), lower in those who also had pulmonary infiltration (67%) and lowest in those with pulmonary infiltration alone (59%). Sarcoidosis is, however, usually diagnosed without recourse to liver biopsy; occasionally a biopsy in a patient without specific features may reveal granulomas and lead to the diagnosis.

*Diagnosis*

Sarcoidosis is readily diagnosed when typical clinical features and pulmonary and mediastinal lesions are present. When typical clinical features are not present and when no other cause for granulomatous hepatitis is found, sarcoidosis should be diagnosed only when granulomas are found in hepatic and in extra-abdominal tissues (Israel et al 1984). Granulomas in other abdominal organs make sarcoidosis possible but not certain.

*Treatment*

Therapy in severe hepatic sarcoidosis is based on case reports, as its rarity has precluded any formal therapeutic trial (Maddrey et al 1970, Israel et al 1984). Corticosteroid drugs may reduce or abolish hepatomegaly, splenomegaly and abnormalities of liver function and liver biopsy may show a reduction in granulomas. It is uncertain whether hepatic fibrosis can be prevented. The indications for corticosteroid therapy have varied. Progressive liver disease is a clear indication, but it also seems reasonable to treat in the absence of symptoms when abnormal liver function tests and histological inflammatory changes coexist. Prednisolone 30 mg daily by mouth should be given until liver function tests have returned substantially to normal. A favorable response from continued treatment is unlikely if improvement has not occurred within a month and thereafter the dose should be reduced at 2-weekly intervals by 5 mg/day to 20 mg/day and by 2.5 mg/day thereafter until the minimum dose to maintain remission is reached. After a year in remission, gradual withdrawal of prednisolone over 3–4 months may be tried. Antituberculous chemotherapy should be given when the tuberculin test is positive (Scadding & Mitchell 1985). Treatment for hepatic encephalopathy (p. 1051), for portal hypertension with gastrointestinal bleeding (p. 499), or for ascites (p. 1023) is discussed elsewhere.

## Other causes of granulomatous hepatitis

Other causes of granulomatous hepatitis are legion (Table 29.9) and they may cause either acute or chronic illnesses.

*Drugs*

Drugs are well-established causes of granulomatous hepatitis and they should be considered particularly in acute granulomatous hepatitis. McMaster & Hennigar (1981) incriminated drugs in 29 (30%) of their 95 cases of granulomatous hepatitis, but others have implicated drugs less frequently and an overall frequency may be about 10% (Table 29.11). Drugs associated with hepatic granulomas are shown in Table 29.12.

Granulomatous hepatitis associated with drugs is often asymptomatic and recognized from abnormal liver function tests. Symptomatic acute granulomatous hepatitis is frequently associated with features suggesting hypersensitivity including fever, skin rash, arthralgia and eosinophilia. Histologically, there are no specific features related to drugs although prominent eosinophilia in early granulomas has been emphasized (McMaster & Hennigar 1981).

*Viruses*

Numerous viral infections have been thought to cause liver granulomas, but this is well established only in

**Table 29.12** Drugs reported as causing granulomatous hepatitis (Fauci & Wolff 1976, Bruckstein & Attia 1978, Medline et al 1978, Rotmensch et al 1978, Levy et al 1981, McMaster & Hennigar 1981)

| | |
|---|---|
| Allopurinol | Methyldopa |
| Aspirin | Metozalone |
| Carbamazepine | Mineral oils |
| Cephalexin | Oxacillin |
| Chlorothiazide | Penicillins |
| Chlorpropamide | Phenytoin |
| Dapsone | Phenylbutazone |
| Diazepam | Procarbazine |
| Diltiazem | Procainamide |
| Gold | Quinidine |
| Halothane | Sulfonamides |
| Hydralazine | Sulfonylureas |
| Isoniazid | Tolbutamide |

cytomegalovirus infection and in infectious mononucleosis (Fauci & Wolff 1976).

*Lymphomas*

Hodgkin's disease and non-Hodgkin's lymphomas frequently involve the liver and liver biopsy may reveal neoplastic tissue. Sometimes, however, only nonspecific abnormalities, including granulomas, are found (Kadin et al 1970, Bagley et al 1972). Granulomas occur in 5–15% of cases, they may include giant cells and they do not imply that neoplastic tissue is present elsewhere in the liver. Similar granulomas ("local sarcoid tissue reaction") occur in other tissues, such as lymph nodes, marrow and spleen (Kadin et al 1970).

**Table 29.13** Frequency of granulomas in liver disease (Klatskin 1976)

| | % |
|---|---|
| Hepatitis | |
| Viral | 2 |
| Infectious mononucleosis | 15 |
| Cytomegalovirus* | 100 |
| Drug-induced | 70 |
| Chronic active hepatitis | 12 |
| Fatty liver | 2 |
| Malignant disease | |
| Primary | <1 |
| Secondary | <1 |
| Lymphoma | 2 |
| Cirrhosis | |
| Primary biliary cirrhosis | 40 |
| Alcoholic | 5 |
| Cryptogenic | 3 |

*Two patients only

*Fibrin-ring granulomas*

Fibrin-ring or doughnut granulomas are characterized by a central fat vacuole surrounded by fibrin and were considered previously as pathognomonic of Q-fever. Many other conditions, including infectious mononucleosis, cytomegalovirus infection, hepatitis A virus, leishmaniasis, rickettsial infection, Hodgkin's disease, non-Hodgkin's lymphoma, allopurinol and giant cell arteritis, are now known to cause this type of granuloma (Marazuela et al 1991, De Bayser et al 1993).

*Miscellaneous*

Liver granulomas can occur in the connective tissue diseases (p. 1106) and are well recognized in ulcerative colitis and Crohn's disease (Dordal et al 1967, Eade 1970, Eade et al 1971). They also occur in association with erythema nodosum irrespective of its cause (Table 29.9).

### Granulomas in primary hepatic disease

Granulomas unassociated with systemic granulomatous disease are sometimes found in liver disease (Table 29.13). Primary biliary cirrhosis (p. 936) is most associated with such lesions. They usually occur early in the disease and are almost exclusively within the portal tracts and there is little or no necrosis. They are uncommon in other forms of cirrhosis. Granulomas in which the epithelioid cells contain fat (lipogranulomas) may occur in fatty livers (Iversen et al 1970) and portal tract extravasation of bile in large-duct biliary obstruction occasionally causes granulomas with or without giant cells (Scheuer 1973). Granulomas are rare in viral hepatitis and in cryptogenic cirrhosis (Iversen et al 1970).

### Acute idiopathic granulomatous hepatitis

Self-limited illnesses of unknown cause associated with liver granulomas have been described (Eliakim et al 1968, Gelb et al 1970). Fever and malaise start suddenly and last for 3–6 weeks, sometimes accompanied by cough and headache. Examination may be normal or may reveal local or general lymphadenopathy, hepatomegaly or splenomegaly. There is no jaundice. The leukocyte count is normal or moderately raised, with a lymphocytosis (50–70%), liver function tests show moderate increases in serum transaminase and/or alkaline phosphatase activity and liver biopsy reveals multiple granulomas. Antibiotics are of no value and the granulomas disappear following recovery.

### Chronic idiopathic granulomatous liver disease

*Definition*

Investigation fails to reveal any cause for hepatic granulomas in about 6–36% of cases (Table 29.11). These patients are diagnosed as having chronic idiopathic granulomatous hepatitis. Some turn out to have a self-limiting disorder, while others go on to suffer a prolonged illness that may last for many years. They should be reviewed regularly and should be reinvestigated from time to time, as an underlying cause for the disease may reveal itself.

Cunningham et al (1982) followed up 17 such patients three recovered completely over 1–7 years, four developed diseases known to cause granulomas (sarcoid, tuberculosis, primary biliary cirrhosis and inflammatory bowel disease), six developed other significant diseases and only four continued to have illness of unknown cause. Zoutman et al (1991) followed up seven patients for 4 years and found a good response to corticosteroid therapy, although relapse could occur on withdrawal. Simon & Wolff (1973) reported one patient who responded well to corticosteroids but who was found to have Hodgkin's disease 5 years after his illness started.

*Clinical features and investigations*

Most patients have been unwell for a long time before the diagnosis is made. Guckian & Perry (1966) found that their patients had been unwell for a mean of 16 months before diagnosis and a patient with a 20-year history of illness has been reported (Simon & Wolff 1973). The clinical features are usually nonspecific and include malaise, fatigue, weight loss, abdominal pain and nonspecific musculoskeletal pain (Table 29.14). The illness may also present as a fever of unknown cause (Terplan 1971, Simon & Wolff 1973, Zoutman et al 1991). Hepatomegaly is the usual indicator of liver involvement, but features of advanced liver disease, such as jaundice, spider telangiectasias, palmar erythema, gynecomastia, ascites or encephalopathy, are rare. Only one of 13 patients reported by Simon & Wolff (1973) developed liver failure and portal hypertension. Lymphadenopathy and splenomegaly may be found. Systemic disease with involvement of other organs such as the heart and brain occurs occasionally (Slavutin 1981). Liver function tests show mild to moderate abnormalities in most patients (Table 29.15). Anemia, leukocytosis and eosinophilia are found in up to a third of cases (Guckian & Perry 1966). The erythrocyte sedimentation rate is usually high and may exceed 100 mm in the first hour (Simon & Wolff 1973).

**Table 29.14** Frequency (%) of clinical features in chronic idiopathic granulomatous liver disease

| Clinical feature | Simon & Wolff (1973) | Mir-Madjlessi et al (1973) |
|---|---|---|
| Malaise | 69 | 51 |
| Fatigue | 77 | – |
| Fever | 100 | 16 |
| Weight loss | 62 | – |
| Abdominal pain | 46 | – |
| Hepatomegaly | 54 | 33 |
| Hepatic failure | 8 | – |
| Splenomegaly | 54 | 22 |
| Fever of unknown origin | – | 16 |
| Number of patients | 13 | 18 |

**Table 29.15** Frequency (%) of abnormal liver function tests in chronic idiopathic granulomatous hepatitis

| Clinical feature | Simon & Wolff (1973) | Mir-Madjlessi et al (1973) |
|---|---|---|
| Bilirubin | 8 | 43 |
| Transaminase | 39 | 76 |
| Alkaline phosphatase | 62 | 41 |
| Albumin | 39 | 59 |
| $\gamma$-globulin | 39 | 70 |
| Prothrombin time | – | 6 |
| Number of patients | 13 | 18 |

*Treatment*

The illness may remit spontaneously but only in a minority of patients. Ill health and/or clearly abnormal liver function tests generally respond well to corticosteroid drugs, which usually have to be given on a long-term basis. Corticosteroids may also lead to the disappearance of the hepatic granulomas. Prednisolone 40 mg daily initially results in increased well-being and a return of the laboratory abnormalities towards normal. Sometimes large doses (60–120 mg/day) may be needed to obtain improvement. The dose should be reduced at 2-weekly intervals once the liver function tests are approaching normal, or after 4 weeks of treatment, by 5 mg/day to a level of 15 mg/day and then by 2.5 mg/day until a minimum maintenance dose is reached. This should be 15 mg/day or less if side-effects are to be avoided. Unfortunately, complete remission is not always achieved, although improvement usually occurs, and untoward effects of corticosteroid therapy may occur (p. 901).

Antituberculous treatment is successful only in granulomatous hepatitis due to tuberculosis, but there is always the possibility that the diagnosis has been missed in idiopathic cases. Indeed, corticosteroids can cause an initial improvement in a patient with tuberculosis and subsequent deterioration may not occur for many months (Cunningham et al 1982). Antituberculous treatment should therefore be given initially for 3 months and corticosteroids used thereafter if there is no improvement (Fauci & Wolff 1976). Antituberculous drugs should be continued in patients with a positive tuberculin skin test.

*Prognosis*

As in any condition of unknown cause in which an underlying disease may declare itself later, the prognosis is uncertain. However, where liver damage is not severe and the response to treatment is favorable, survival for many years is usual (Simon & Wolff 1973, Cunningham et al 1982, Zoutman et al 1991). When the duration of the illness prior to diagnosis is considered, survival for 20 years has been recorded.

REFERENCES

Adams J S, Walker D H 1981 The liver in Rocky Mountain spotted fever. American Journal of Clinical Pathology 75: 156–161

Altemeier W A, Schowengerdt C G, Whiteley D H 1970 Abscesses of the liver: surgical considerations. Archives of Surgery 101: 258–266

Alvarez S Z, Carpio R 1983 Hepatobiliary tuberculosis. Digestive Diseases and Sciences 28: 193–200

Alvarez S, McCabe W R 1984 Extrapulmonary tuberculosis revisited: a review of experience at Boston City and other hospitals. Medicine 63: 25–55

Alves V A F, Vianna M R, Yasuda P H, de Brito T 1987 Detection of leptospiral antigen in the human liver and kidney using an immunoperoxidase staining procedure. Journal of Pathology 151: 125–131

Ammann R, Münch R, Largiader F, Akovbiantz A, Marincek B 1992

Pancreatic and hepatic abscesses: a late complication in 10 patients with chronic pancreatitis. Gastroenterology 103: 560–565
Anderson C S, Nicholls J, Rowland R, La Brooy J T 1988 Hepatic granulomas: a 15-year experience in the Royal Adelaide Hospital. Medical Journal of Australia 148: 71–74
Bagley C M Jr, Roth J A, Thomas L B, Divita V T Jr 1972 Liver biopsy in Hodgkin's disease. Clinicopathologic correlations in 127 patients. Annals of Internal Medicine 76: 219–225
Berger I, Katz M 1973 Portal hypertension due to hepatic sarcoidosis. American Journal of Gastroenterology 59: 147–151
Berger I A, Osborne D R 1982 Treatment of pyogenic liver abscesses by percutaneous needle aspiration. Lancet 1: 132–134
Bissada A A, Bateman J 1991 Pyogenic liver abscess: a 7-year experience in a large community hospital. Hepato-Gastroenterology 38: 317–320
BMJ 1980 Leading article: pyogenic liver abscess. British Medical Journal 1: 1155
Bolton J P, Darougar S 1983 Perihepatitis. British Medical Bulletin 39: 159–162
Bowry S, Chan C H, Weiss H, Katz S, Zimmerman H J 1970 Hepatic involvement in pulmonary tuberculosis. Histologic and functional characteristics. American Review of Respiratory Disease 101: 941–948
Braun T I, Travis D, Dee R R, Nieman R E 1993 Liver abscess due to *Listeria monocytogenes*: a case report and review. Clinical Infectious Diseases 17: 267–269
Bruckstein A H, Attia A A 1978 Oxacillin hepatitis. Two patients with liver biopsy, and review of the literature. American Journal of Medicine 64: 519–522
Bunim J J, Kimberg D V, Thomas L B, Van Scott E J, Klatskin G 1962 The syndrome of sarcoidosis, psoriasis, and gout. Annals of Internal Medicine 57: 1018–1040
Butler T J, McCarthy C F 1969 Pyogenic liver abscess. Gut 10: 389–399
Capron J P, Delamarre J, Delcenserie R, Gineston J L, Dupas J L, Lorriaux A 1981 Liver abscess complicating *Yersinia pseudotuberculosis* ileitis. Gastroenterology 81: 150–152
Cargill W H Jr, Beeson P B 1947 The value of spinal fluid examination as a diagnostic procedure in Weil's disease. Annals of Internal Medicine 27: 396–400
Cervantes F, Bruguera M, Carbonell J, Force L, Webb S 1982 Liver disease in brucellosis: a clinical and pathological study of 40 cases. Postgraduate Medical Journal 58: 346–350
Crippin J S, Wang K K 1982 An unrecognized etiology for pyogenic hepatic abscesses in normal hosts: dental disease. American Journal of Gastroenterology 87: 1740–1743
Cunningham D, Mills P R, Quigley E M M et al 1982 Hepatic granulomas: experience over a 10-year period in the west of Scotland. Quarterly Journal of Medicine 51: 162–170
Dan M, Bar-Meir S, Jedwab M, Shibolet S 1982 Typhoid hepatitis with immunoglobulins and complement deposits in bile canaliculi. Archives of Internal Medicine 142: 148–149
Das B C, Haynes I, Weaver R M, Acland P R 1983 Primary hepatic cryptococcosis. British Medical Journal 287: 464
Davidson L S P, Smith J 1939 Weil's disease in the North-East of Scotland: an account of 104 cases. British Medical Journal 2: 753–757
De Bakey M E, Jordan G I Jr 1975 Surgery of the liver. In: Schiff L (ed) Diseases of the liver, 4th edn. J B Lippincott, Philadelphia, p 1089
de Bayser L, Roblot P, Ramassamy A, Silvain C, Levillain P, Becq-Giraudon B 1993 Hepatic fibrin-ring granulomas in giant cell arteritis. Gastroenterology 105: 272–273
Deller J J, Cifarelli P S, Berque S, Buchanan R 1967 Malaria hepatitis. Military Medicine 132: 614–620
Dordal E, Glagov S, Kirsner J B 1967 Hepatic lesions in chronic inflammatory bowel disease. 1. Clinical correlations with liver biopsy diagnoses in 103 patients. Gastroenterology 52: 239–253
DuPont H L, Hornick R B, Levin H S, Rapaport M I, Woodward T E 1971 Q fever hepatitis. Annals of Internal Medicine 74: 198–206
Eade M N 1970 Liver disease in ulcerative colitis. 1. Analysis of operative liver biopsy in 138 consecutive patients having colectomy. Annals of Internal Medicine 72: 475–487
Eade M N, Cooke W T, Brooke B N, Thompson H 1971 Liver disease in Crohn's colitis: a study of 21 consecutive patients having colectomy. Annals of Internal Medicine 74: 518–528
Eliakim M, Eisenberg S, Levij I S, Sacks T G 1968 Granulomatous hepatitis accompanying a self-limited febrile disease. Lancet 1: 1348–1352
Essop A R, Posen J A, Hodkinson J H, Segal I 1984 Tuberculosis hepatitis: a clinical review of 96 cases. Quarterly Journal of Medicine 53: 465–477
Farges O, Lisse T, Bismuth H 1988 Pyogenic liver abscess: an improvement in prognosis. British Journal of Surgery 75: 862–865
Farkas P S, Knapp A B, Lieberman H, Guttman I, Mayan S, Bloom A A 1981 Markedly elevated creatinine phosphokinase, cotton wool spots, and pericarditis in a patient with leptospirosis. Gastroenterology 80: 587–589
Farrell G, Zaluzny L, Baird-Lambert J, Cvejic M, Buchanan N 1983 Impaired elimination of metronidazole in decompensated liver disease. British Medical Journal 287: 1845
Farrell R J, Krige J E, Beningfield S J, Terblanche J 1994 Pyogenic liver abscess following infection of a ventriculo-peritoneal shunt. American Journal of Gastroenterology 89: 140
Fauci A S, Wolff S M 1976 Granulomatus hepatitis. In: Popper H, Schaffner F (eds) Progress in liver diseases, Vol 5. Grune and Stratton, New York, p 609–621
Fischer M G, Beaton H L 1983 Unsuspected hepatic abscess associated with biliary tract disease. American Journal of Surgery 146: 658–662
Frey C F, Zhu Y, Suzuki M, Isaji S 1989 Liver abscesses. Surgical Clinics of North America 69: 259–271
Fung G L, Silpa M 1981 Fitz-Hugh and Curtis syndrome in a man. Journal of the American Medical Association 245: 128
Gelb A M, Brazenas N, Sussman H, Wallach R 1970 Acute granulomatous disease of the liver. American Journal of Digestive Diseases 15: 842–847
Gerzof S G, Johnson W C, Robbins A H, Nabseth D C 1985 Intrahepatic pyogenic abscesses: treatment by percutaneous drainage. American Journal of Surgery 149: 487–494
Guardia J, Martínez-Vázques J M, Moragas A et al 1974 The liver in boutonneuse fever. Gut 15: 549–551
Guckian J C, Perry J E 1966 Granulomatous hepatitis: an analysis of 63 cases and review of the literature. Annals of Internal Medicine 65: 1081–1100
Hanazaki K, Kajikawa S, Horigome N et al 1993 Gas-forming liver abscess after transcatheter arterial embolization for hepatocellular carcinoma: report of a case. Surgery Today 23: 474–479
Hart R J C, Gallagher J, Waitkins S 1984 An outbreak of leptospirosis in cattle and man. British Medical Journal 288: 1983–1984
Heath C W Jr, Alexander A D, Galton M M 1965 Leptospirosis in the United States. Analysis of 483 cases in man, 1949–1961. New England Journal of Medicine 273: 915–922
Herbert D A, Fogel D A, Rothman J, Wilson S, Simmons F, Ruskin J 1982 Pyogenic liver abscesses: successful non-surgical therapy. Lancet 1: 134–136
Hollingdale M R 1985 Malaria and the liver. Hepatology 5: 327–335
Howard P F, Smith J W 1983 Diagnosis of disseminated coccidioidomycosis by liver biopsy. Archives of Internal Medicine 143: 1335–1338
Hunt J S, Silverstein M J, Sparks F C, Haskell C M, Pilch Y H, Morton D L 1973 Granulomatous hepatitis: a complication of B.C.G. immunotherapy. Lancet 2: 820–821
Israel H L, Goldstein R A 1971 Relation of Kveim-antigen reaction to lymphadenopathy. Study of sarcoidosis and other diseases. New England Journal of Medicine 284: 345–349
Israel H L, Margolis M L, Rose L J 1984 Hepatic granulomatosis and sarcoidosis. Further observations. Digestive Diseases and Sciences 29: 353–356
Istre G R, Kreiss K, Hopkins R S et al 1982 An outbreak of amebiasis spread by colonic irrigation at a chiropractice clinic. New England Journal of Medicine 307: 339–342
Iversen K, Christoffersen P, Poulsen H 1970 Epithelioid cell granulomas in liver biopsies. Scandinavian Journal of Gastroenterology 5 (suppl 7): 61–67
Jahiel R I, Koffler D 1961 Hepatic granulomas induced in guinea pigs by Freund's adjuvant with and without homologous liver. British Journal of Experimental Pathology 42: 338–342

James D G, Turiaf J, Hosoda Y et al 1976 Description of sarcoidosis: report of the Subcommittee on Classification and Definition. Annals of the New York Academy of Sciences 278: 742

Kadin M E, Donaldson S S, Dorfman R F 1970 Isolated granulomas in Hodgkin's disease. New England Journal of Medicine 283: 859–861

Kalat E D, Martin D B 1981 Granulomatous hepatitis associated with jejunoileal bypass surgery. Journal of the American Medical Association 246: 982

Karat A B A, Job C K, Rao P S S 1971 Liver in leprosy: histological and biochemical findings. British Medical Journal 1: 307–310

Klatskin G 1976 Hepatic granulomata: problems in interpretation. Annals of the New York Academy of Sciences 278: 427–432

Klatskin G, Yesner R 1950 Hepatic manifestations of sarcoidosis and other granulomatous diseases. A study based on histological examination of tissue obtained by needle biopsy of the liver. Yale Journal of Biology and Medicine 23: 207–248

Korn R J, Kellow W F, Heller P, Chomet B, Zimmerman H J 1959 Hepatic involvement in extrapulmonary tuberculosis: histologic and functional characteristics. American Journal of Medicine 27: 60–71

Lazarchick J, De Souza e Silva N A, Nichols D R, Washington J A 1973 Pyogenic liver abscess. Mayo Clinic Proceedings 48: 349–355

Levy M, Goodman M W, Van Dyne B J, Sumner H W 1981 Granulomatous hepatitis secondary to carbamazine. Annals of Internal Medicine 95: 64–65

Lewis J H, Patel H R, Zimmerman H J 1982 The spectrum of hepatic candidiasis. Hepatology 2: 479–487

Maddrey W C, Johns C J, Boitnott J K, Ibert F L 1970 Sarcoidosis and chronic hepatic disease: a clinical and pathologic study of 20 patients. Medicine 49: 375–395

Maher J A Jr, Reynolds T B, Yellin A E 1979 Successful medical treatment of pyogenic liver abcess. Gastroenterology 77: 618–622

Manjunatha S, McIntyre P B, Lynn A 1992 Multiple liver abscesses in Crohn's disease. British Journal of Hospital Medicine 47: 375–376

Marazuela M, Moreno A, Yebra M, Cerezo E, Goméz-Gesto C, Vargas J A 1991 Hepatic fibrin-ring granulomas: a clinicopathologic study of 23 patients. Human Pathology 22: 607–613

Matsuki K, Sakata T 1982 Angiotensin-converting enzyme in diseases of the liver. American Journal of Medicine 73: 549–551

McClain J B, Ballou W R, Harrison S M, Steinweg D L 1984 Doxycycline therapy for leptospirosis. Annals of Internal Medicine 100: 696–698

McCorkell S J, Niles N L 1985 Pyogenic liver abscesses: another look at medical management. Lancet 1: 803–806

McCullough N B, Eisele C W 1951 Brucella hepatitis leading to cirrhosis of the liver. Archives of Internal Medicine 88: 793–802

McFadzean A J S, Chang K P S, Wong C C 1953 Solitary pyogenic abscess of the liver treated by closed aspiration and antibiotics. A report of 14 consecutive cases with recovery. British Journal of Surgery 41: 141–152

McIntosh J 1909 The occurrence and distribution of spirochaeta pallida in congenital syphilis. Journal of Pathology and Bacteriology 13: 239

McMaster K R III, Hennigar G R 1981 Drug-induced granulomatous hepatitis. Laboratory Investigation 44: 61–73

Meade R H III 1980 Primary hepatic actinomycosis. Gastroenterology 78: 355–359

Meals R A 1976 Paratyphoid fever. A report of 62 cases with several clinical findings and a review of the literature. Archives of Internal Medicine 136: 1422–1428

Mehrota G, Singh R P, Krishna A, Singh B K 1992 Pyogenic liver abcess causing acute Budd-Chiari syndrome. Annals of Tropical Paediatrics 12: 451–453

Medline A, Cohen L B, Tobe B A, Sellers E M 1978 Liver granulomas and allopurinol. British Medical Journal 1: 1320–1321

Miedema B W, Dineen P 1984 The diagnosis and treatment of pyogenic liver abscesses. Annals of Surgery 200: 328–335

Mir-Madjlessi S H, Farmer R G, Hawk W A 1973 Granulomatous hepatitis. A review of 50 cases. American Journal of Gastroenterology 60: 122–134

Miyamoto M I, Fang F C 1993 Pyogenic liver abscess involving Actinomyces: case report and review. Clinical Infectious Diseases 16: 303–309

Moseley R H, Kris M G, Einzig A, West R, Gee T S, Armstrong D 1982 Respiratory alkalosis and abdominal pain heralding candida hepatitis. Occurrence in patients with acute leukemia in remission. Archives of Internal Medicine 142: 1495–1497

Naveau S, Poitrine A, Delfraissy J F, Brivet F, Dormont J 1983 Brucellosis hepatic abscesses and pregnancy. Gastroenterology 84: 1643

Northover J M A, Jones B J M, Dawson J L, Williams R 1982 Difficulties in the diagnosis and management of pyogenic liver abscess. British Journal of Surgery 69: 48–51

Okada S, Aoki K, Okazaki N et al 1993 Liver abscess after percutaneous ethanol injection (PEI) therapy for hepatocellular carcinoma. A case report. Hepato-Gastroenterology 40: 496–498

Oschner A, de Bakey M, Murray S 1938 Pyogenic abscess of liver, II. An analysis of forty seven cases with review of the literature. American Journal of Surgery 40: 292–319

Pais P 1984 A hepatitis like picture in typhoid fever. British Medical Journal 289: 225–226

Patel K M 1981 Granulomatous hepatitis due to mycobacterium scrofulaceum: report of a case. Gastroenterology 81: 156–158

Patwari A, Aneja S, Berry A M, Ghosh S 1979 Hepatic dysfunction in childhood malaria. Archives of Diseases in Childhood 54: 139–144

Price M E 1981 Amoebic liver abscess in a Norfolk factory worker. British Medical Journal 283: 1175

Putman H C Jr, Dockerty M B, Waugh J M 1950 Abdominal actinomycosis: an analysis of 122 cases. Surgery 28: 781–800

Robert J H, Mirescu D, Ambrosette P, Khoury G, Greenstein A J, Rohner A 1992 Critical review of the treatment of pyogenic hepatic abscess. Surgery, Gynecology and Obstetrics 174: 97–102

Robinson P J 1983 Computed tomographic appearance of Nocardia abscesses. British Journal of Radiology 56: 578–580

Rotmensch H H, Yust I, Siegman-Igra Y, Liron M, Ilie B, Vardinon N 1978 Granulomatous hepatitis: a hypersensitivity response to procainamide. Annals of Internal Medicine 89: 646–647

Rubin R H, Swartz M N, Malt R 1974 Hepatic abscess: changes in clinical, bacteriologic and therapeutic aspects. American Journal of Medicine 57: 601–610

Rustgi A K, Richter J M 1989 Pyogenic and amebic liver abscess. Medical Clinics of North America 73: 847–858

Sabbaj J 1984 Anaerobes in liver abscess. Review of Infectious Disease 6: S152

Sabbaj J, Sutter V L, Finegold S M 1972 Anaerobic pyogenic liver abscess. Annals of Internal Medicine 77: 627–638

Saebø A, Lassen J 1992 Acute and chronic liver disease associated with *Yersinia enterocolitica* infection: a Norwegian 10-year follow-up study of 458 hospitalized patients. Journal of Internal Medicine 231: 531–535

Saltzman D A, Smithline N, Davis J R 1978 Fulminant hepatic failure secondary to amebic abscesses. American Journal of Digestive Diseases 23: 561–567

Sanford J P 1984 Leptospirosis – time for a booster. New England Journal of Medicine 310: 524–525

Satiani B, Davidson E D 1978 Hepatic abscesses: improvement in mortality with early diagnosis and treatment. American Journal of Surgery 135: 647–650

Scadding J G, Mitchell D N 1985 Sarcoidosis, 2nd edn. Chapman and Hall, London.

Scheuer P J 1973 The liver in systemic disease, pregnancy and organ transplantation. In: Liver biopsy interpretation, 2nd edn. Baillière Tindall, London, p 128–150

Silpapojakul K, Mitarnun W, Ovartlarnporn P, Chamroonkul N, Khow-Ean U 1996 Liver involvement in murine typhus. Quarterly Journal of Medicine 89: 623–629

Siltzbach L E 1961 The Kveim test in sarcoidosis. American Journal of Medicine 30: 495–501

Simon H B, Wolff S M 1973 Granulomatous hepatitis and prolonged fever of unknown origin: a study of 13 patients. Medicine 52: 1–21

Slavutin L 1981 Chronic granulomatous hepatitis with myocarditis and meningitis. New York State Journal of Medicine 81: 782–786

Spelman D W 1982 Q fever. A study of 111 consecutive cases. Medical Journal of Australia 1: 547–549

Symmers D, Spain D M 1946 Hepar lobatum. Clinical significance of anatomic changes. Archives of Pathology 42: 64–68

Takafuji E T, Kirkpatrick J W, Miller R N et al 1984 An efficacy trial of doxycycline chemoprophylaxis against leptospirosis. New England Journal of Medicine 310: 497–500

Terplan M 1971 Hepatic granulomas of unknown cause presenting with fever. American Journal of Gastroenterology 55: 43–49
Trump D L, Fahnestock R, Cloutier C T, Dickman M D 1978 Anaerobic liver abscess and intrahepatic metastases. A case report and review of the literature. Cancer 41: 682–686
Turck W P G, Howitt G, Turnberg L A et al 1976 Chronic Q fever. Quarterly Journal of Medicine 45: 193–217
Turner L H 1973 Leptospirosis. British Medical Journal 1: 537–540
Ullom J T 1909 The liver in tuberculosis. American Journal of the Medical Sciences 137: 694
Veeravahu M 1985 Diagnosis of liver involvement in early syphilis. A critical review. Archives of Internal Medicine 145: 132–134
Vilinskas J, Joyeuse R, Serlin O 1970 Hepatic sarcoidosis with portal hypertension. American Journal of Surgery 120: 393–396
Vischer T L, Bernheim C, Engelbrecht E 1967 Two cases of hepatitis due to *Toxoplasma gondii.* Lancet 2: 919–921
Wagoner G P, Anton A T, Gall E A, Schiff L 1953 Needle biopsy of the liver. VIII Experiences with hepatic granulomas. Gastroenterology 25: 487–494
Waitkins S A 1985 Update on leptospirosis. British Medical Journal 290: 1502–1503
Watanakunakorn C 1982 *Peptococcus asaccharolyticus* bacteremia with liver involvement cured with oral metronidazole. Gastroenterology 83: 1132–1135
Williams A, Cooper B 1985 Sarcoidosis presenting with acute cholestasis. British Medical Journal 290: 1394
Winearls C G, Chan L, Coghlan J D, Ledingham J G G, Oliver D O 1984 Acute renal failure due to leptospirosis: clinical features and outcome in six cases. Quarterly Journal of Medicine 53: 487–495
Wong M, Rosen S W 1962 Ascites in sarcoidosis due to peritoneal involvement. Annals of Internal Medicine 57: 277–280
Wood J J, Bolton J P, Cannon S R, Allan A, O'Connor B H, Darougar S 1982 Biliary-type pain as a manifestation of genital tract infection: the Curtis–Fitz-Hugh syndrome. British Journal of Surgery 69: 251–253
Zoutman D E, Ralph E D, Frei J V 1991 Granulomatous hepatitis and fever of unknown origin. An 11-year experience of 23 cases with three years' follow-up. Journal of Clinical Gastroenterology 13: 69–75

SECTION 7

# Toxic liver diseases

# 30. Drugs and toxins

*J. Neuberger N. D. C. Finlayson*

## INTRODUCTION

It is not possible to evaluate accurately either the incidence or the prevalence of drug-associated liver damage. Nonetheless, there is a significant morbidity and even mortality associated with drug-induced liver injury. Data from Europe and North America suggest that up to 2% of all cases of jaundice admitted to hospital are drug-induced (Koff et al 1970, Bjornaboe 1980). Studies of adverse drug reaction reports in the United Kingdom and in Denmark show that hepatic reactions account for 3–6% of all reports and are fatal in 5–7% of cases (Bem et al 1988, Friis & Andreasen 1992). In the West Midlands region of the United Kingdom between 1973 and 1987, there were nearly 6500 reports of adverse drug reactions, of which those affecting the liver accounted for 3.6%. The major reactions were jaundice (55%), hepatitis (12.5%) and abnormal liver function tests (23%). The drugs most commonly implicated in liver damage include halothane, antibiotics such as fusidic acid, co-trimoxazole and erythromycin, phenothiazines, nonsteroidal anti-inflammatory drugs and contraceptive drugs.

However, reported drug reactions probably represent a limited view of drug toxicity. Drug reactions of current medical (or media) interest are more likely to be reported, well-recognized reactions are less likely to be reported and poorly recognized reactions are likely to be overlooked. Sadly, doctors are not always very reliable at reporting even recognized reactions. The number of drugs reported as possibly causing hepatotoxic reactions is very great and individual drugs will not be considered in any detail in this chapter other than as illustrations of mechanisms of liver damage. An extensive list of hepatotoxic drugs is given at the end of the chapter and these are considered in detail in the comprehensive monograph of Farrell (1994).

## HEPATIC DRUG METABOLISM

Biotransformation in the body is carried out by enzymes of the smooth endoplasmic reticulum which metabolize a large variety of substances of exogenous and endogenous origin, including most drugs (Benet et al 1990, DeLeve & Kaplowitz 1995). These enzymes are found mainly in the liver, which is more active in drug metabolism than other organs. They are also present in the gastrointestinal epithelium. The gastrointestinal tract and liver act together in their responsibility for the first-pass metabolism of drugs (below). The skin, lungs and kidneys also contain small amounts of these enzymes. Metabolism of the drug usually leads to a relative loss of pharmacological activity and conversion to easily excreted products, but some drugs (prodrugs) only become active when they are metabolized. Drug metabolism can also lead to the production of hepatotoxic intermediates.

Hepatic drug metabolism is classically divided into type I and type II reactions. Type I reactions introduce polar groups into the drug molecule and involve primarily oxidation, reduction and hydrolysis. Type II reactions involve conjugation with water-soluble ligands such as glucuronide, sulfate or glutathione, or acetylation (Jakoby 1994). Type I reactions usually make drugs more polar (water-soluble) and type II reactions result in the production of highly polar acidic metabolites that are usually pharmacologically inactive, less toxic and readily excreted in urine or bile.

### Type I reactions

Drug oxidation, the extraction of an electron from the substrate, accounts for the majority of drug biotransformation reactions (Ziegler 1994). These reactions include O-dealkylation, N-dealkylation, aromatic ring or sidechain hydroxylation, sulfoxide formation, deamination, dehalogenation, N-oxidation and N-hydroxylation. The enzymes catalyzing type I oxidative reactions are the mixed function oxidase enzymes located in the smooth endoplasmic reticulum membranes as associations of cytochrome P-450, cytochrome P-450 reductase and NADPH (Fig. 30.1). The means whereby type I reactions take place are shown in Figure 30.2. Oxidation in the hepatocyte takes place in

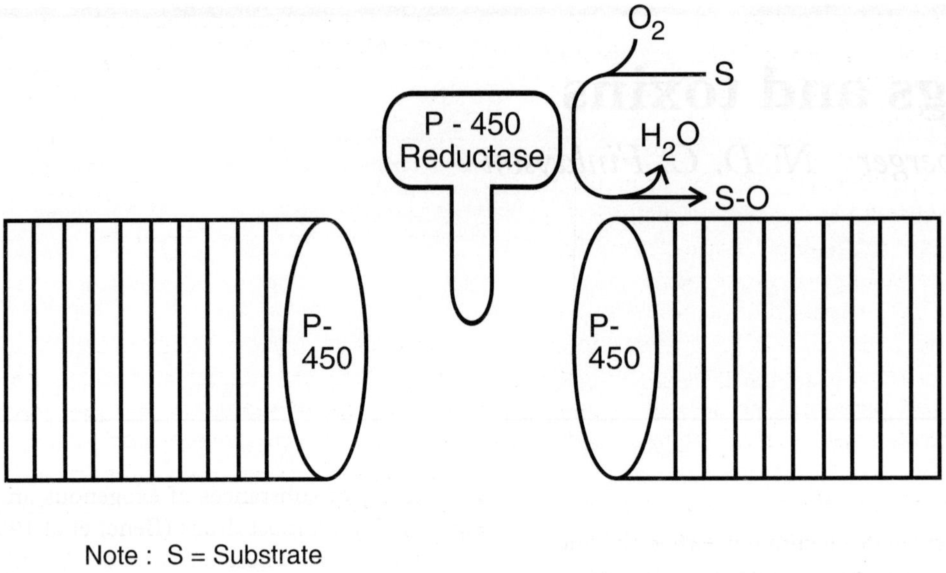


**Fig. 30.1** Site and function of the mixed function oxidase enzyme system in the membranes of the smooth endoplasmic reticulum (after Peterson et al 1976).

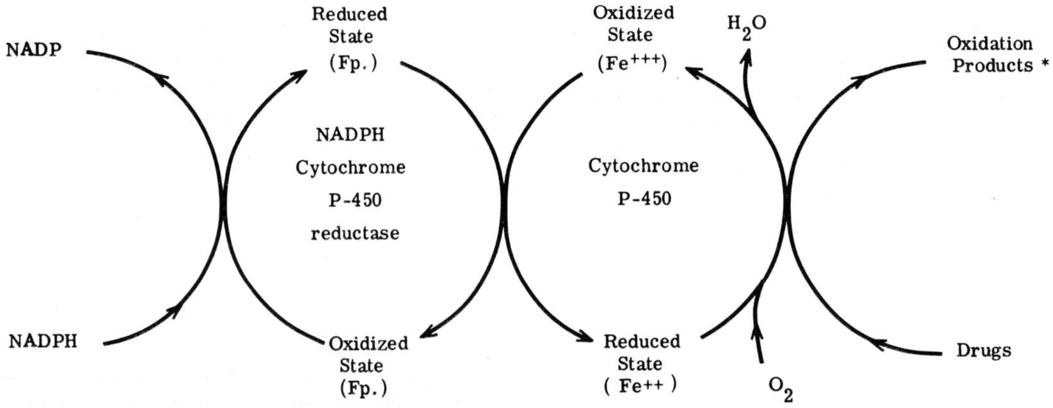


**Fig. 30.2** Principal components of the mixed function oxidase system in the liver endoplasmic reticulum. NADP = nicotinamide adenine dinucleotide phosphate, Fp = flavoprotein.
*Several different drug (R) oxidation products may be formed, e.g.: $R—CH_3 \rightarrow R—CH_2—OH$; $R—S \rightarrow R—S=O$; $R—NH—CH_3 \rightarrow R—NH_2 + CH_2O$

the endoplasmic reticulum and is catalyzed by the cytochrome B5 and cytochrome P-450 enzymes, each of which is associated with cytochrome B5 reductase and cytochrome P-450 reductase. These systems are NADH dependent. Type I reactions generally increase the water solubility of a drug, but their effects on pharmacological activity are very variable. Drugs may be activated or inactivated or their activity may remain unchanged.

***Cytochrome P-450 families.*** Cytochrome P-450 was thought originally to be a single enzyme with broad substrate specificity, but it is now known to constitute a supergene family of enzymes responsible for oxidative metabolism of endogenous and xenobiotic compounds (Nebert & Gonzalez 1987, Watkins 1990). These enzymes have been divided into groups or families according to amino acid sequence homology. At least 10 families with 21 isoenzymes are now recognized. The prefix P-450 can be used to identify individual isoenzymes, but increasingly the supergene family symbol CYP is used for each human P-450, followed by a number to denote the family, a letter to denote the subfamily and a further number to identify an individual P-450 isoenzyme.

Three gene families are important in human drug metabolism and five isoenzymes have been implicated in drug hepatotoxicity. CYP1A2 (P-450 1A2) has been implicated in paracetamol and dihydralazine metabolism and hepatotoxicity. The CYP2 (P-450 2) family is the largest identified so far and contains several subfamilies. CYP2C9 (P-450 2C9) is involved in phenytoin and diclofenac metabolism, CYP2D6 (P-450 2D6) is involved in perhexilene and metoprolol metabolism and CYP2E1 (P450 2E1) is involved in alcohol, paracetamol and halothane metabolism and hepatotoxicity. CYP3A4 (P-450 3A4) is involved in paracetamol metabolism and hepatotoxicity and in the metabolism of many other drugs including amiodarone, carbamazepine, cyclosporin, erythromycin, lovastatin and valproate. These enzymes can all be induced or inhibited selectively by foreign substances (below).

***Toxicity of intermediates.*** Many drugs are converted by type I reactions to reactive metabolites that are potentially toxic and bind to cellular macromolecules. Thus, cytochrome P-450s may oxidize a drug to a reactive electrophile, catalyze the reductive dehalogenation of haloalkanes to the corresponding free radical (such as carbon trichloride from carbon tetrachloride) or cytochrome P-450 reductase may reduce some drugs to free radicals which in the presence of oxygen react with molecular oxygen to regenerate the parent compound and form a superoxide anion. Protection against these processes may occur in a number of ways, including inactivation of cytochrome P-450. Subsequent transformation of metabolites may occur by epoxide hydrolases, superoxide dismutase and glutathione peroxidase. As indicated elsewhere, the reactive metabolites may, if not rapidly removed, bind to cellular macromolecules and disrupt calcium homeostasis within the cell, so leading to cell death.

### *Variation in P-450 enzyme activity*

Cytochrome P-450 activity varies considerably between individuals. This is due partly to genetic factors and partly to drugs or environmental factors such as dietary constituents. These variations in activity can be important in determining hepatotoxic reactions to drugs.

***Genetic factors.*** Genetic polymorphism refers to the occurrence in a population of multiple genetically determined phenotypes, each affecting more than 1% of the population. Much variation in drug metabolism is related to such heterogeneity in genetic factors (Jacqz et al 1986, Meyer 1994). For example, the polymorphism in debrisoquine metabolism is related to several defects in splicing of the CYP2D (P-450 2D) enzyme. Thus, some of the variation in response to drugs, both in clinical effects and in toxicity, may be due to genetic effects on the expression of cytochrome P-450 activity and the effect of drugs and other environmental agents on enzyme induction or inhibition. Other examples of genetic variations in cytochrome P-450 activities resulting in liver damage include variations in CYP3A (P-450 3A) affecting cyclosporin-associated cholestasis and deficiency of thiopurine methyl transferase resulting in azathioprine hepatoxicity due to the accumulation of 6-thioguanine nucleotides.

**Table 30.1** Drugs causing induction of cytochrome P-450 enzymes (Prescott 1980, Fontana & Watkins 1995)

| | |
|---|---|
| Barbiturates | Griseofulvin |
| Carbamazepine | Isoniazid |
| Diphenylhydantoin | Meprobamate |
| General anesthesia | Omeprazole |
| Glucocorticoids | Phenytoin |
| Glutethimide | Rifampicin |

***Enzyme induction.*** Many substances metabolized by the microsomal enzyme system increase the production of the enzymes responsible for their metabolism. This phenomenon is known as enzyme induction and the agents responsible are known as inducing agents. Several drugs are inducing agents (Table 30.1). Environmental factors can also lead to enzyme induction, including dietary constituents such as Brussels sprouts, cabbage and charcoal-broiled meats, alcohol, benzpyrene in tobacco smoke and dichlorodiphenyltrichloroethane (DDT). Enzyme induction leads to an increase in the size of the liver, in the amount of endoplasmic reticulum and in the amount and activity of specific cytochrome P-450 enzymes. Enzyme induction can be detected within 24 h of giving a drug and the response reaches a maximum in 1–3 weeks. Reversion to normal usually occurs within 1–4 weeks once drug therapy has been stopped. As age increases, larger drug doses are needed for induction and the response is less marked. Enzyme induction results in increased tolerance for the inducing agents and for other drugs metabolized by the same enzyme system. It results in diminished activity of the drug when the drug itself is the therapeutic agent and a reduced drug half-life in the blood. Its effects on drug toxicity depend on whether the drug itself or its metabolites are the toxic agents. The extent of enzyme induction in humans varies widely. It is likely to contribute to the phenomenon of tolerance to some drugs, but this may also involve an adjustment in the response of target tissues to the drug (Conney 1967).

***Enzyme inhibition.*** Drugs and other chemicals can inhibit cytochrome P-450 enzymes and reduce the metabolism of drugs (Table 30.2). Dietary factors such as grapefruit juice can also cause inhibition. This can lead to important drug interactions, particularly where the margin between therapeutic and toxic amounts of a drug is small, as with anticoagulants, anticonvulsants and cyclosporin. Immaturity of the enzymes in the neonatal period also results in diminished enzyme activity. Protein deprivation sometimes diminishes enzyme activity and reduces the ability of the liver to metabolize certain drugs (Kato et al

**Table 30.2** Drugs causing inhibition of cytochrome P-450 enzymes

| | |
|---|---|
| Allopurinol | Metronidazole |
| Amiodarone | Neuroleptics |
| Cimetidine | Paroxetine |
| Diltiazem | Propoxyphene |
| Disulfiram | Quinidine |
| Erythromycin | Sertraline |
| Fluoxetine | Sulphinpyrazone |
| Imidazole antifungals | Verapamil |
| Ketoconazole | |

1965). This may explain the sensitivity of undernourished persons to many drugs.

### Type II reactions

Type II reactions involve conjugation of drugs or their type I reaction products to produce water-soluble metabolites that are biologically inactive and excreted readily in urine or bile (Jakoby 1994). Drugs or their metabolites undergoing conjugation require chemical groupings suitable for conjugation with an endogenous substrate in the presence of a transferase enzyme. Type II reactions involve glucuronidation, acetylation, ethylation, sulfation and conjugation with amino acids such as glycine and with transferase enzymes such as uridine diphosphate glucuronosyl transferase, N-acetyl transferase and glutathione-5-transferase found in the endoplasmic reticulum, cytosol and mitochondria.

Uridine diphosphate glucuronosyl transferases are best known as the enzymes catalyzing the conversion of bilirubin to bilirubin diglucuronide (p. 737) and enzyme deficiency can cause jaundice (p. 710). Other endogenous substances metabolized by these enzymes include bile acids and steroid hormones, and drugs metabolized include morphine, chlorpromazine and amitriptyline. Glutathione S-transferases are important in catalyzing the conjugation of many drugs with endogenous intracellular glutathione. Drugs undergoing biotransformation by glutathione S-transferases include epoxides, nitroalkanes, alkenes and nitro compounds. The glutathione conjugate can then be excreted directly into urine or bile but more often undergoes further biotransformation to mercapturic acid conjugates. Glutathione transferases can also bind to drugs or their intermediates within the cell without metabolizing them, thereby limiting their toxicity. Glutathione S-transferases are inducible by barbiturates and other drugs. N-acetyl transferases metabolize drugs such as hydralazine, isoniazid, procainamide and salazopyrine. Genetic factors determine whether individuals are slow or fast acetylators. Sulfotransferases catalyze phase II reactions by sulfating a variety of endogenous and exogenous compounds including drugs.

## DRUG DISPOSITION AND CLEARANCE

The disposition of a drug in the body is dependent on its route of administration, its absorption, distribution and elimination. The physical properties of the drug are also important, including its molecular size, charge, p$K_a$ and lipid solubility. Thus, lipid-soluble drugs cross cell membranes readily, have a large volume of distribution and are metabolized to more hydrophilic compounds for excretion. In contrast, water-soluble drugs have a smaller volume of distribution and may be excreted by the kidneys. Large molecular weight drugs are more often excreted in the bile and smaller molecular weight drugs in the urine after they have been metabolized. The many changes associated with liver disease may alter the pattern of drug disposition in patients with liver disease.

### First-pass metabolism and systemic availability

First-pass metabolism refers to the metabolism of drugs before they reach the systemic circulation and it is an important determinant of their systemic availability (Pond & Tozer 1984). Drugs taken by mouth are absorbed into the mesenteric circulation which passes almost exclusively to the liver via the portal vein (p. 991). Such drugs undergo presystemic metabolism in the gut and liver and the extent of this metabolism is an important determinant of the systemic availability of any drug. The liver is by far the most important site of this metabolism.

The hepatic removal from the blood of drugs with a high clearance depends primarily on the total hepatic blood flow, as the liver is capable of removing any amount of drug reaching it in the blood (below). Toxicity due to such high clearance drugs occurs readily when liver blood flow is reduced, as in shock, or where there is marked portasystemic shunting, as in portal hypertension. Removal of drugs with a low clearance by the liver depends on the amount of drug presented to hepatic clearance sites and this depends on the amount of free drug in the blood and in turn on the extent of drug binding to the plasma proteins.

### Volume of drug distribution

The volume of distribution is defined as the volume into which a drug is distributed in the body when a state of equilibrium has been reached. This volume of distribution (Vd) is defined as the fraction of the dose absorbed into the body (D) divided by $C_{pl}$ ($Vd = D/C_{pl}$), which is the drug concentration in the plasma at equilibrium but before drug elimination. Thus, this is a theoretical concept reflecting the partition of the drug between the plasma, interstitial fluid and intracellular fluid within the body. In liver disease, ascites increases the total fluid compartment within the body and increases the potential volume of distribution for a drug.

### Drug half-life

The clearance of a drug from the body is usually measured

as the elimination half-life, which is the time taken for the concentration and amount in the body to fall by a half. The half-life of a drug ($T_{1/2}$) can be defined from the formula $T_{1/2} = 0.693 \times Vd/CL$ where Vd is the volume of distribution of the drug and CL is the clearance of the drug from the blood. Thus, it can be seen that for a given dose of a drug, if clearance remains unchanged, an increase in the volume of distribution will be associated with an increase in the half-life of the drug. In contrast, changes in the volume of distribution will not alter the steady-state concentrations of the drug once equilibrium has been reached.

### Protein binding of drugs

In general, the activity of a drug is dependent on its free concentration. However, most drugs are bound reversibly to circulating components in the blood including proteins such as albumin, $\alpha_1$-glycoproteins, lipoproteins, ceruloplasmin, transferrins and transcortins. In patients with chronic liver disease, there is often a reduction in these proteins as they are synthesized in the liver. There may also be reduced binding of drugs to binding sites on proteins, since binding sites may be occupied by compounds such as bilirubin retained in liver disease.

There are two possible consequences of changes in protein binding. The first is that for a given blood level of a drug the amount of free drug may be greater. This increase in free drug can lead to an increased pharmacological effect. However, it also leads to an increase in the amount of drug available for metabolism and there may be an increase in the amount of drug metabolized over time. Thus, while free drug clearance remains unchanged, the total clearance of drug will increase, which may result in a decrease in the half-life of the drug.

### Clearance of drugs

The rate of elimination of a drug from the body usually follows first-order kinetics, which means that the amount of drug eliminated with time is independent of the plasma concentration or the dose of drug given. This elimination is usually determined primarily by the liver, but drugs are also cleared from the body by the kidneys and gastrointestinal tract. Within the liver, drugs may be excreted into the biliary system or metabolized to hydrophilic compounds and excreted through the kidneys. The situation is often complex in patients with liver disease owing to changes in hepatic function, biliary excretory capacity, liver blood flow and portasystemic shunting due to portal hypertension. In addition, many patients have impaired renal function (the hepatorenal syndrome).

#### *Hepatic clearance*

The clearance of a drug is defined as the efficiency of removal of the drug across an organ. The hepatic clearance of drug ($CL_H$) defines the efficiency with which a drug is removed from the blood. The amount of drug cleared is determined both by the proportion of the drug extracted from the blood (E) during passage through the liver and by the amount of blood flowing through the liver ($Q_H$). The clearance of a drug through the liver is, therefore, determined by the equation $CL_H = Q_H \times E$. Normally, drugs given orally pass through the portal system to the liver before reaching the systemic circulation. Thus, if a substantial proportion of the drug is removed as it passes through the liver, the fraction of the total dose of drug entering the systemic circulation (F) is reduced. This so-called first-pass effect results in a reduced systemic bioavailability. The fraction of a drug removed is, therefore, determined by the drug's extraction (E) according to the principle $F = 1 - E$. Thus, the greater the hepatic clearance, the lower the systemic availability of the drug. If there is a reduction in the drug clearance due, for example, to liver disease, a greater proportion of drug would reach the systemic circulation and after a single dose the peak plasma concentration would be higher and drug elimination slower (Fig. 30.3). At steady-state concentration, the levels would be higher. For a low-clearance drug, peak plasma concentrations would not be much different from normal but drug elimination would be impaired, resulting in a longer half-life after single administration, and high plasma concentrations would be achieved with chronic administration.

### Classification of drugs by disposition

Drugs may be classified as flow limited, enzyme limited or flow and enzyme limited. When the total intrinsic clear-

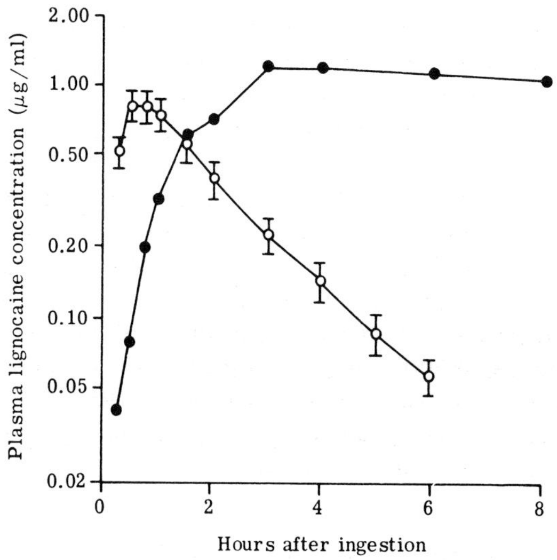


**Fig. 30.3** Plasma concentrations of lignocaine in four healthy subjects (open circles) and in a patient with chronic active hepatitis (closed circles) after 400 mg orally (Adjepon-Yamoah et al 1974).

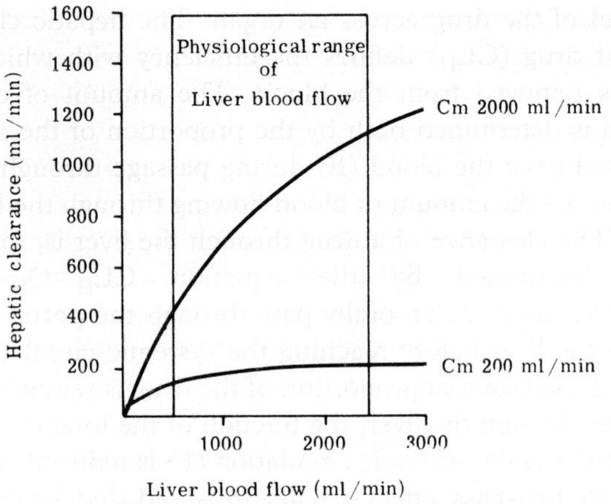


**Fig. 30.4** Theoretical effects of altering hepatic blood flow for a drug with a low intrinsic hepatic clearance (200 ml/min) and a drug with high intrinsic hepatic clearance (2000 ml/min). Cm = maximum drug clearance (Branch et al 1975).

ance of a drug by the liver is high, the overall hepatic clearance of the drug is dependent upon the liver blood flow (i.e. flow limited). These drugs usually have an E >0.6 and only changes in liver blood flow have a significant clinical effect on their clearance (Fig. 30.4). Enzyme-limited drugs are those where the total intrinsic clearance of the drug is small compared with liver blood flow and most have an E <0.2. Thus, hepatic clearance is dependent largely on the intrinsic activity of the liver enzymes and is not affected greatly by changes in liver blood flow (Fig. 30.4). In patients with liver disease, enzyme activity may be reduced by impaired hepatocellular function or may be altered by coadministration of other drugs (p. 839). Many drugs are moderately extracted by the liver and are partially dependent on enzyme metabolism and usually have an E of 0.2–0.6. These drugs are classified as flow and enzyme limited. Examples of drugs with high and low clearance by the liver are shown in Table 30.3.

**Table 30.3** Examples of drugs with high and low clearances by the liver

| High clearance | Low clearance |
|---|---|
| Amitriptyline | Ampicillin |
| Chlormethiazole | Atenolol |
| Chlorpromazine | Carbenicillin |
| Dextropropoxyphene | Chlordiazepoxide |
| Domperidone | Cimetidine |
| Doxepin | Diazepam |
| Labetalol | Digoxin |
| Lignocaine | Frusemide |
| Methadone | Lorazepam |
| Metoprolol | Naproxen |
| Midazolam | Oxazepam |
| Morphine | Prednisolone |
| Nifedipine | Spironolactone |
| Oxprenolol | Theophylline |
| Pentazocine | Tolbutamide |
| Pethidine | Valproic acid |
| Prazosin | Warfarin |
| Propranolol | |
| Verapamil | |

## DRUGS IN LIVER DISEASE

The pharmacokinetics of any drug given to a patient with liver disease can be predicted only from thorough knowledge of the characteristics of the drug and the state of the patient. Thus, to prescribe rationally, not only would the physical characteristics of the drug have to be known but also such factors as the volume of distribution, the degree of shunting in and around the liver and the occurrence of enzyme induction or inhibition. In reality, this never occurs. However, patients with liver disease may require a wide range of drugs and certain principles need to be followed to minimize toxic side-effects (Table 30.4).

**Table 30.4** Principles for prescribing drugs in patients with liver disease

- Drugs should be prescribed only when necessary
- Always start with a low dose, increase gradually if there is no toxicity and achieve therapeutic objectives with the minimum dose
- Consider drug toxicity when unexpected complications occur
- Beware of drug interactions, as patients with liver disease are often treated with several drugs
- If in doubt, stop therapy and consult the textbooks

### Drug metabolism in hepatic disease

Many factors affect hepatic drug metabolism in liver disease and as they occur to a different degree from patient to patient, it is not surprising that the effects of liver disease on drug metabolism are variable (McLean & Morgan 1991). Important factors related to the liver disease include loss of the hepatocyte mass, impaired metabolic capacity of remaining hepatocytes, capillarization of sinusoids (p. 916) reducing access of drugs to remaining hepatocytes, reduced blood flow to the liver (p. 990) and shunting of blood away from the liver by the extrahepatic collateral vessels in portal hypertension (p. 991) and by intrahepatic shunts in cirrhosis (p. 916). Metabolic processes in the hepatocytes are affected to a variable extent. Type I reactions are more affected than type II reactions and among the former, oxidation reactions are most affected, especially where sinusoidal capillarization is present. In contrast, conjugation reactions tend to be preserved.

*Types of hepatic disease*

Impaired drug elimination can occur in acute hepatic damage due to viral hepatitis or to drugs such as paracetamol (Forrest et al 1974, Burnett et al 1976). This is more likely to occur in patients with greatly increased plasma transaminase activity who tend to have more severe liver damage (p. 741) and where fulminant liver failure occurs. Impaired hepatic elimination of drugs is the likely mechanism, as liver blood flow in acute hepatitis is normal (Preisig et al 1966). Impaired elimination also occurs in chronic liver disease, although this is usually common and important only in patients with advanced disease recognized clinically from poor nutritional state, jaundice, ascites and encephalopathy (p. 1007) and biochemically from hypoalbuminemia (p. 745) and prolongation of the prothrombin time (p. 751). Reduced hepatic blood flow and portasystemic shunting make patients with cirrhosis particularly sensitive to drugs that are highly extracted by the liver (below). This is particularly true where a portasystemic shunt operation or a transjugular intrahepatic portasystemic stent shunt (TIPSS) has been carried out, as shunting of blood past the liver in excess of 10% significantly reduces the elimination of these drugs (Huet & Villeneuve 1983). Clinically important impairment of drug elimination does not occur in cholestatic states unless the cholestasis is associated with significant parenchymal liver disease (Miguet et al 1981).

*Types of drug*

Drug toxicity in liver disease is related to the way in which the liver eliminates a drug from the blood. Highly extracted drugs (Table 30.3) depend primarily on hepatic blood flow for their elimination (Fig. 30.4) and reduced liver blood flow is common in chronic liver disease (p. 990). Accordingly, highly cleared drugs should always be used cautiously in patients with chronic liver disease, particularly where the drugs are given orally, as decreased first-pass metabolism (above) and reduced elimination can lead to very high systemic availability of the drug (Fig. 30.5). Drugs with lower extraction (Table 30.3) are, in general, much less likely to cause toxicity. Those that are also poorly bound to plasma proteins are usually only affected to a great extent in advanced cirrhosis, where there is extensive sinusoidal capillarization and loss of activity of drug-metabolizing enzymes. Exceptions to this generalization occur, particularly where drugs are metabolized by oxidation, as in the case of theophylline, as the metabolic pathway for the methylxanthines appears particularly susceptible to damage in cirrhosis. Drugs metabolized by conjugation are much less affected. The elimination of drugs that are poorly extracted but highly bound to plasma proteins is usually impaired only in advanced cirrhosis. However, considerable variation occurs with these drugs, as reduction in protein binding increases the unbound drug fraction and can increase elimination, while impaired hepatocyte enzyme activity can reduce elimination. The outcome for any particular drug depends on the balance between these two factors and drug elimination can be normal, increased or decreased.

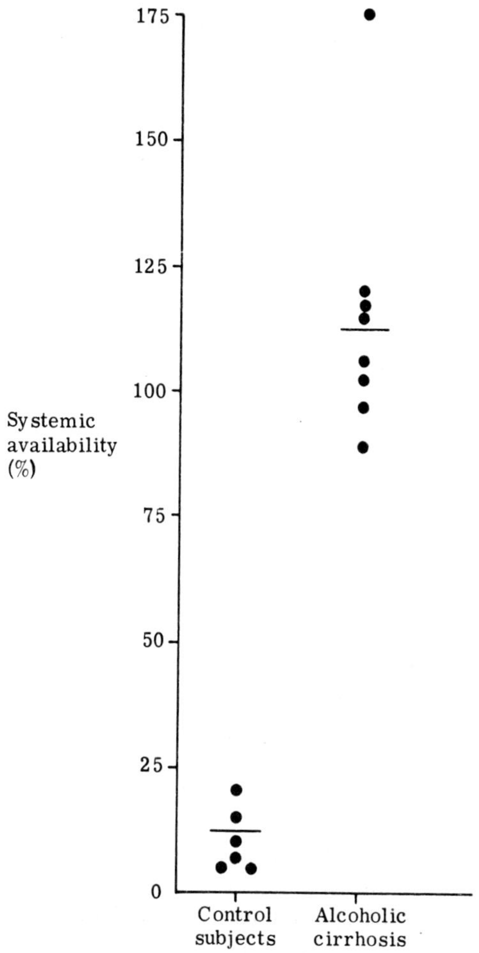


**Fig. 30.5** Systemic availability of chlormethiazole after a single oral dose (192 mg) in normal subjects and in patients with alcoholic cirrhosis (Pentikäinen et al 1980).

*Biliary excretion*

Little information is available regarding the biliary excretion of drugs in chronic liver disease, but such excretion may be normal or impaired (McLean & Morgan 1991).

*Hepatorenal syndrome*

Hepatorenal syndrome occurs in advanced liver disease (p. 81) and may impair the renal excretion of drugs or their metabolites. This does not generally have clinical implications for drug therapy until renal failure is present, as reflected in an increased plasma creatinine concentration.

## Drug receptor responses in liver disease

Altered responsiveness to drugs in patients with liver disease may be due to changes in drug receptors as well as to changes in drug metabolism (McLean & Morgan 1991). There is little information on this subject, but altered receptor responses may account for increased cerebral sensitivity to opiates and benzodiazepines and reduced circulatory responses to catecholamines. Impaired responses to diuretics such as frusemide and bumetanide may be due to a reduction in the number of functional nephrons as well as a reduction in the response of individual nephrons.

## Prescribing in liver disease

Patients with liver disease may require a wide range of drugs. Details of drugs for which precautions may be needed have been reviewed (Bass & Williams 1988) and only a few commonly needed drugs are considered here.

### *Analgesics*

Analgesia may be required for a variety of reasons and patients with chronic liver disease are very likely to undergo invasive procedures. Paracetamol can be used safely in normal therapeutic doses for mild pain (Forrest et al 1979, Benson 1983). Salicylate and nonsteroidal anti-inflammatory drugs should be avoided, since they can exacerbate bleeding from gastritis, precipitate variceal hemorrhage (p. 498) and cause renal sodium retention by interfering with the prostaglandin homeostatic control (p. 1028).

Potent analgesics should be used with caution, but patients should not be deprived of adequate pain relief because of an undue fear of side-effects. Opioid analgesics such as morphine, pethidine, pentazocine, codeine and dextropropoxyphene can all precipitate hepatic encephalopathy, partly because there may be increased cerebral sensitivity to these drugs in liver disease (above) and partly because they have a constipating effect. In addition, they are all highly extracted by the liver and their systemic availability is increased in chronic liver disease, especially when they are given orally. Pethidine is usually well tolerated and a dose of 50 mg intramuscularly can be given initially and increased if this proves inadequate. Pethidine and other opiates have the advantage that the specific antagonist naloxone is available if accidental overdose occurs. Codeine and dextropropoxyphene are not advised, as their effectiveness as analgesics is hardly greater than paracetamol.

Ergotamine for migraine should be avoided since the drug has a high extraction by the liver, leading to the possibility of ergotism.

### *Diuretics*

Many patients require diuretics for the treatment of ascites (p. 1026) or sodium retention from cardiac or other causes. Patients with ascites usually have advanced liver disease with impaired renal function (p. 1057) and diuretics can cause prerenal failure. Potent loop diuretics such as frusemide are particularly liable to precipitate prerenal failure in those without peripheral edema. Spironolactone is widely regarded as the drug of choice for the initial treatment of ascites due to cirrhosis (p. 1027), but the dose of diuretics should always be increased gradually and should be reduced if the serum urea or creatinine starts to rise. A loop diuretic can be added when spironolactone is insufficient.

### *Sedative and psychotropic drugs*

Sedative and psychotropic drugs are potent causes of encephalopathy in patients with severe acute or chronic liver disease. Benzodiazepines are used widely and most have low extraction rates. Those eliminated by glucuronidation (lorazepam, oxazepam) are less affected in liver disease than those eliminated by type I reactions (diazepam, chlordiazepoxide). In practice, diazepam is well tolerated, but care is needed when repeated doses are given since the metabolites themselves cause sedative effects. Midazolam is the most useful benzodiazepine for intravenous use, as its metabolites do not cause sedation. However, it is more highly extracted than most other benzodiazepines and its metabolism is impaired in those with advanced cirrhosis (MacGilchrist et al 1986). Patients with encephalopathy precipitated by benzodiazepines may be treated with the specific antagonist flumazanil.

Chlormethiazole (Heminevrin) is still used extensively in patients with alcohol problems, particularly in the prevention and treatment of delirium tremens. However, it is normally highly extracted by the liver and bioavailability is greatly increased in cirrhosis (Fig. 30.5). Patients have died from respiratory depression and accordingly this drug is not recommended. Chlordiazepoxide is recommended for delirium tremens (p. 1050).

Depression is best treated with a tricyclic drug (e.g. amitriptyline) or a selective serotonin re-uptake inhibitor (e.g. fluoxetine). Amitriptyline is highly extracted by the normal liver and a low starting dose should be used particularly where there is marked portasystemic shunting (Hrdina et al 1985). Fluoxetine is less sedating and is lowly extracted but may be eliminated slowly, and half the normal starting dose should be used (Shenker et al 1988). Phenothiozines often produce prolonged sleepiness, and monoamine oxidase inhibitors should not be used.

### *Antidiarrheals*

Loperamide, which acts locally in the bowel, can be used as an antidiarrheal. Constipation may precipitate hepatic encephalopathy (p. 1039) and drugs such as codeine phosphate should therefore be given with caution.

### *Hypotensives*

Diltiazem, verapamil and nifedipine have high extraction rates, so patients with significant portasystemic shunting are at increased risk of hypotension when standard doses are given. Captopril may induce renal failure, particularly where the plasma creatinine concentration is increased.

## DRUG REACTIONS AND PATTERNS OF DAMAGE

Drug reactions affecting the liver are relatively rare but extremely important causes of liver disease. It is important to remember that significant liver damage may be caused not only by conventional medications but also by recreational drugs (cocaine and ecstasy), by herbal remedies and other agents used in complementary medicine and by environmental and industrial substances.

### General principles

General principles are important in relation to adverse hepatic drug reactions.

- The true incidence and spectrum of liver damage from drugs is not fully known. Adverse drug reactions are often not appreciated by medical attendants or are not reported to the appropriate authorities.
- Reporting of adverse drug reactions does not prove causality. Patients are often taking more than one drug and other factors, either external or due to intrinsic medical problems, may account for the liver reaction.
- Virtually all types of liver injury may be produced by drugs.
- Some drugs are associated with more than one type of liver damage.
- With the possible exception of halothane hepatitis and tienilic acid hepatitis, there are no absolute markers of drug reactions.

Thus, when a patient presents with liver disease or suffers an exacerbation of pre-existing liver disease, the possible contribution of drugs, prescribed or self-administered, must be considered. The use of a challenge test has been advocated, but the specificity and sensitivity of tests are uncertain and in idiosyncratic reactions there is the potential for a fatal reaction, although, to the authors' knowledge, this has not occurred following a controlled challenge. In the case of halothane hepatitis, repeat exposure may well be fatal. The need to confirm that the reaction was due to the drug must be weighed against the possible consequences to the patient and in general, challenge tests are not advocated.

### Diagnostic criteria

Assessment of causality has been discussed by an International Consensus Meeting (Benichou 1990). The diagnosis of drug-induced liver injury should include the following considerations:

- When the drug was being given with special emphasis on the interval between the start of administration of the drug and the onset of the hepatotoxic reaction: hepatocellular injury within 5–90 days (or within 1–15 days of re-exposure) or cholestatic liver injury within 5–90 days (or 1–90 days of re-exposure) of starting drug therapy strongly suggests drug-related injury.
- The course of the reaction when the suspected drug has been discontinued: substantial resolution of abnormal liver function tests following drug withdrawal within 15 days for hepatocellular injury or within a month for cholestatic injury strongly suggests drug-related injury.
- The role of any underlying disease in the etiology of the reaction.
- Laboratory tests.
- Recorded examples of toxicity for any drug under suspicion.
- Response to readministration in rare instances where the use of the suspected drug is essential.

It was also suggested that the term "liver injury" should be used rather than pathological terms such as hepatic necrosis, hepatitis or cirrhosis unless liver tissue had been studied histologically. The criteria for attributing liver injury to drug therapy are shown in Table 30.5, and for defining acute hepatocellular, cholestatic or mixed liver injury in Table 30.6. It is clearly important to exclude other potential causes of liver disease such as pre-existing chronic liver disease, viral infections such as hepatitis A, B or C, Epstein–Barr and cytomegalovirus, underlying nonhepatic

**Table 30.5** The diagnosis of acute drug-induced liver disease

| | |
|---|---|
| Consider the possibility of a drug | |
| Tabulate drugs taken | |
| Prescribed by doctor | |
| Self-administered | |
| Relate drugs to the onset of the illness | |
| Look for pre-existing liver disease | |
| Clinical examination | |
| Previous liver investigations | |
| Consider alternative causes | |
| Viral hepatitis | – serological tests |
| Biliary disease | – cholecystogram |
| | – ultrasound |
| Observe the effects of stopping the suspected drugs | |
| Liver biopsy | |
| Suspected pre-existing liver disease | |
| Failure to improve | |
| Challenge tests with drugs – never (hardly ever) | |

**Table 30.6** Biochemical definition of acute drug-induced hepatocellular injury, cholestatic injury and mixed injury (Benichou 1990)

| Biochemical measurement | Liver injury: Hepatocellular | Cholestatic | Mixed |
|---|---|---|---|
| ALT | >×2 | | >×2 |
| ALP | | >×2 | >×2 |
| ALT/ALP | ≥5 | ≤2 | 2–5 |

Note: ALT = alanine aminotransferase.
ALP = alkaline phosphatase.
Numbers refer to multiples of the upper end of the reference range.

disease such as lymphoma, sepsis and malignancy, and other toxins such as alcohol.

### Acute hepatitis and cholestatic hepatitis

Conventionally, acute drug-induced liver injury is classified into acute hepatitis, cholestasis and mixed forms (cholestatic hepatitis). Although this is logical, in practice differentiating these can be difficult. Acute hepatitis is the commonest adverse hepatic drug reaction. Clinical presentations vary from mild asymptomatic disturbance of liver function tests to fulminant hepatic failure. Most cases present with acute hepatitis clinically and biochemically resembling viral hepatitis and some authors have divided acute hepatitis into hepatocellular hepatitis and cholestatic or mixed hepatitis with features of cellular hepatitis and cholestasis. Drugs causing acute hepatotoxicity may give rise to predictable and idiosyncratic reactions.

***Predictable hepatotoxicity.*** Predictable hepatotoxins (also called true or intrinsic hepatotoxins) destroy the hepatocyte, usually by direct physicochemical methods such as peroxidation or denaturation of cell membranes. One example of this is carbon tetrachloride, which is metabolized to the reactive metabolite $CCl_3$ that results in zonal necrosis with or without steatosis. The incidence of liver damage on exposure to the drug is relatively high. The response is dose-dependent and experimental reproducibility is high.

In contrast, the indirect hepatotoxins require metabolism to generate toxic metabolites. These may result in either cytotoxic or cholestatic effects. Again, indirect hepatotoxins have a relatively high incidence of liver damage, are easy to reproduce experimentally and show a dose-dependent effect. The classic example of an indirect cytotoxin reaction is paracetamol, which is described in detail below. Because the lesion is relatively easy to produce in experimental animals, the pathways of metabolism and toxicity have been defined and in some cases it is possible to generate specific antidotes. It must be remembered, however, that as shown below for paracetamol, external factors such as concomitant use of enzyme inducers or inhibitors may alter individual susceptibility to hepatotoxicity.

***Idiosyncratic hepatotoxicity.*** In contrast to the intrinsic hepatotoxins are the idiosyncratic hepatotoxins. Liver damage may occur as a result of metabolic abnormality or hypersensitivity, the incidence is low, there is no dose dependence and experimental reproducibility is difficult. In the case of metabolic abnormality, the drug is usually metabolized through a minor pathway leading to the generation of hepatotoxic metabolites that result in liver cell necrosis, while immune mechanisms are implicated in hypersensitivity reactions. Liver injury due to toxic metabolites and to immune reactions do not necessarily represent entirely separate mechanisms, for toxic metabolites may bind to cell membrane proteins and give rise to new antigens (neoantigens) recognized by the immune system as foreign (Fontana & Watkins 1995). Immune hepatotoxicity may be associated with features such as pyrexia, rash and an increase in circulating eosinophils, immune complexes and autoantibodies. Autoantibodies may be specific for the drug or nonspecific. Nonspecific reactions include antinuclear antibodies, which occur frequently in patients given procainamide (with liver injury in only a minority), an antimitochondrial antibody in iproniazid liver damage and antiactin antibodies in clometacine liver damage. Hepatitis due to the uricosuric diuretic tienilic acid (not now commercially available in the UK or North America) is associated with autoantibodies to the cytochrome P-450 isoenzymes that metabolize the drug, termed anti-liver/kidney microsomal antibodies type II (p. 769), and halothane hepatitis is associated with an anticarboxylesterase antibody (Zimmerman & Ishak 1995).

#### *Mechanisms*

The mechanisms of hepatotoxicity are illustrated best by individual drugs. Paracetamol is a direct hepatotoxin, halothane causes an idiosyncratic immunoallergic reaction and jaundice resulting from chlorpromazine exhibits metabolism through a minor pathway. These examples of drug hepatotoxicity are considered in some detail below.

#### *Paracetamol*

Paracetamol is an effective analgesic which is safe when taken in therapeutic doses (0.5–1.5 g). However, it is used commonly for self-poisoning and can then cause severe liver necrosis and death (Black 1980). Overdoses taken with therapeutic intent can also cause liver damage and in these cases doses have generally been about 4–15 g over 24 h (Whitcomb & Block 1994). Paracetamol damages the liver in a predictable dose-related manner and the essential lesion is centrilobular necrosis progressing to massive necrosis in those dying of fulminant hepatic failure. Single doses in excess of 7 g (14 tablets) can produce significant liver necrosis in humans if the drug is not removed at an early stage by vomiting or gastric lavage. It is difficult to predict severe liver damage in these patients, but the plasma paracetamol concentration related to the time since the drug was taken and a prolonged plasma half-life are useful pointers (Prescott et al 1971).

***Mechanisms of damage.*** Paracetamol is metabolized by conjugation with sulfate and glucuronic acid leading to excretion of metabolites in the urine (Fig. 30.6). Sulfation is a high-affinity low-capacity pathway, whereas glucuronidation is a high-capacity low-affinity pathway. A small proportion of paracetamol is metabolized by the cytochrome P-450 system to a highly reactive metabolite,

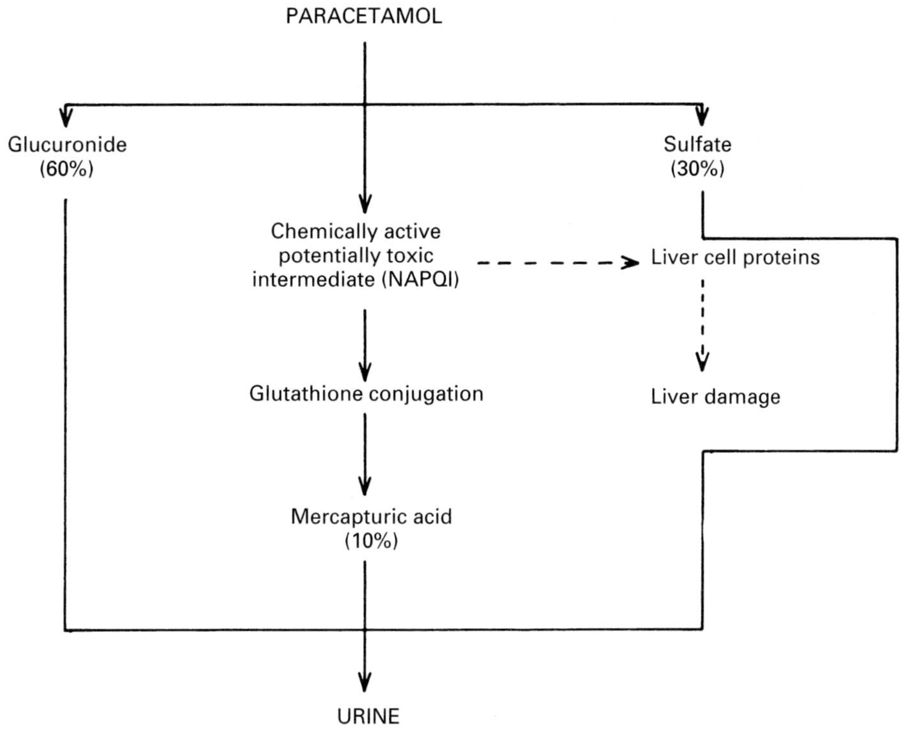


**Fig. 30.6** Metabolism of paracetamol in the liver (NAPQI is *N*-acetyl-*p*-benzoquinoneimine).

*N*-acetyl-*p*-benzoquinone-imine (NAPQI). This reactive metabolite is conjugated with glutathione and excreted as mercapturic acid as a cysteine conjugate. NAPQI oxidizes glutathione to glutathione disulfide and also forms a conjugate with paracetamol. In overdose, the amount of NAPQI is increased and the other metabolic pathways become saturated. It is thought that NAPQI subsequently binds to other major tissue proteins, especially thiol enzymes, which results in alteration of cellular calcium fluxes and disturbance of calcium homeostasis causing loss of mitochondrial calcium and elevation of cytosolic calcium, leading to cell death. These mechanisms have been well studied in laboratory animals and there is good evidence that similar mechanisms occur in humans. In particular, there is a close correlation between binding of paracetamol metabolites and the development of toxicity.

Central to paracetamol toxicity is the development of increased amounts of NAPQI and this can be prevented by replacement of intracellular glutathione. Glutathione itself does not cross cell membranes readily, but methionine or *N*-acetylcysteine can be given. Provided this is done before the generation of toxic amounts of NAPQI, *N*-acetylcysteine or methionine is effective in protecting the liver against damage (below).

***Clinical features.*** Persistent vomiting and right upper quadrant abdominal pain and tenderness usually provide clinical evidence of hepatic necrosis within 24 h, by which time the serum bilirubin, transaminase activity and prothrombin time are all abnormal. These laboratory abnormalities are maximal between 3 and 5 days and return to normal over 10–14 days in those who recover. Transaminase activities often exceed 20 times the normal limit and may reach 15 000 u/L.

The clinical features associated with these abnormalities are very varied: some patients are asymptomatic, almost all with a serum transaminase above 800 u/L suffer anorexia, vomiting and right upper quadrant abdominal pain and a few develop fulminant hepatic failure (p. 805). The prothrombin time is the best guide to the severity of liver damage (p. 751). A prolonging prothrombin time warns of the development of fulminant hepatic failure and in these circumstances should be measured twice daily. Recovery from liver damage of any severity is essentially complete. Some patients also develop acute renal tubular necrosis with renal failure. Rarely, renal failure occurs in the absence of fulminant liver failure (Cobden et al 1982). Plasma creatinine estimations should be used to assess renal function, as the plasma urea concentration may be unreliably low as a consequence of liver damage.

***Treatment.*** This consists of removing paracetamol from the stomach by gastric lavage if the patient is seen within 6 h of drug ingestion, giving a specific antidote for the toxic paracetamol metabolites and providing supportive care for fulminant hepatic failure (p. 809) and acute renal failure. The antidotes provide sulfhydryl groups that can combine with the toxic metabolites produced in the liver when the reserves of glutathione have been exhausted (Proudfoot 1993). The most effective is *N*-acetylcysteine

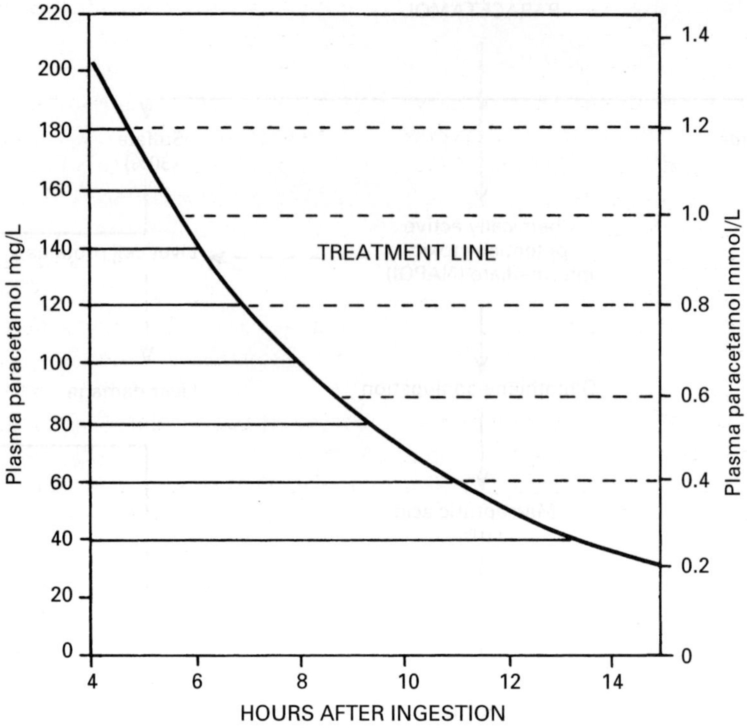


**Fig. 30.7** Plasma paracetamol concentrations in relation to time after overdosage as a guide to prognosis. *N*-acetylcysteine (Parvolex) is indicated in patients with values on or above the treatment line. Two-thirds of patients above the treatment line have serum aminotransferase activities >1000 u/L (Prescott et al 1979).

given intravenously; it provides almost complete protection if given within 8 h of ingestion, but its efficacy diminishes rapidly after 10 h and it is likely that it ceases to be effective after 20 h. Charts relating the plasma paracetamol concentration and time from ingestion to the need for treatment are available (Fig. 30.7) and the mode of administration is shown in Table 30.7. *N*-acetylcysteine causes side-effects in about 10% of patients (Mant et al 1984, Proudfoot 1993). These usually occur within about an hour of starting the infusion, they are dose related and may be more common in asthmatic patients. They are anaphylactoid in nature; flushing, urticaria and pruritus are most common, nausea, vomiting, angioedema and wheezing are much less common and hypertension and hypotension are uncommon. Stopping the infusion usually results in resolution of symptoms and the infusion can then be restarted within about 30 min at a dose of 100 mg/kg body weight given over 16 h. The more serious

**Table 30.7** Dose regimen for *N*-acetylcysteine (Parvolex) in paracetamol poisoning (Prescott et al 1979)

1. 150 mg/kg body weight intravenously in 200 ml 5% dextrose over 15 min
2. 50 mg/kg body weight intravenously in 500 ml 5% dextrose over 4 h
3. Two sequential doses of 50 mg/kg body weight intravenously in 500 ml 5% detrose over 8 h

features may require treatment with antihistamines, but corticosteroids are seldom needed. Methionine 2.5 g by mouth followed by three further doses at 4-hourly intervals is also effective therapy, but inadequate absorption associated with nausea and vomiting may reduce efficacy (Vale et al 1981).

***Other factors.*** Better understanding of the mechanism of paracetamol toxicity allows more insight into factors that increase or decrease paracetamol toxicity. For example, hepatic glutathione concentration is decreased by starvation, making malnourished people more susceptible to paracetamol toxicity. In contrast, children metabolize paracetamol less efficiently and are less susceptible to poisoning. Enzyme-inducing compounds such as phenytoin increase paracetamol metabolism and thereby its toxicity, whereas enzyme inhibitors such as cimetidine reduce paracetamol metabolism and consequently its toxicity. Long-term alcohol ingestion induces enzyme activity, increasing paracetamol metabolism and toxicity, but simultaneous ingestion of alcohol and paracetamol reduces toxicity as alcohol in this circumstance competes for enzyme-binding sites.

### *Chlorpromazine*

Jaundice occurs in up to 2% of patients taking chlorpromazine. The drug is metabolized by sulfoxidation, Nmethylation and hydroxylation. Watson et al (1988) have suggested that since hydroxylated derivatives are more toxic than the parent compound or sulfoxidated metabolites, those who are poor sulfoxidizers but extensive hydroxylaters should be more susceptible to chlorpromazine-induced jaundice. Using debrisoquine and S-carboxymethyl-L-cysteine as probes, sulfoxidation rates were studied in 12 patients with chlorpromazine-induced jaundice. All those with chlorpromazine jaundice were poor sulfoxidizers, compared with 23% of normal subjects. Furthermore, all 11 patients studied for debrisoquine polymorphism were extensive hydroxylaters. Thus, impaired sulfoxidation and increased hydroxylation may result in increased production of toxic chlorpromazine metabolites, causing biliary canalicular damage resulting in jaundice. Metabolic idiosyncrasy may accordingly lead to the appearance of hepatotoxic reactions.

### *Halothane*

Halothane hepatitis is defined as an otherwise unexplained jaundice occurring within 28 days of halothane exposure in patients with previously normal liver function tests (Ray & Drummond 1991). The frequency of halothane hepatitis is unknown. The National Halothane Study in the United States suggested a frequency of clinical hepatitis of 1 in 2500 anesthetics and of fatal fulminant hepatic failure of 1 in 11 000 anesthetics (Subcommittee on the National Halothane Study 1966). Cirrhosis may follow repeated exposures (Klatskin & Kimberg 1969). The likelihood of developing halothane hepatitis is not related to the underlying disease or to the nature or extent of surgery, as would be expected in an idiosyncratic drug reaction. Minor hepatic dysfunction, usually manifest by increased plasma aminotransferase activity, occurs in up to 50% of patients after halothane anesthesia and is unrelated to halothane hepatitis.

***Etiological factors.*** Clinical observations point to several factors associated with an increased likelihood of halothane hepatitis. Most important is previous exposure to halothane. It is rare to encounter halothane hepatitis in a patient with no previous exposure to the agent; most patients have been exposed to halothane on at least one previous occasion and many have had adverse reactions such as fever or jaundice on such occasions (Walton et al 1976, Inman & Mushin 1978). Repeated occupational exposure can lead to halothane hepatitis in operating theater staff, proved by rechallenge (Belfrage et al 1966, Klatskin & Kimberg 1969), and recreational halothane sniffing has also led to hepatitis (Kaplan et al 1979). Other associations include female sex, obesity and older age: two-thirds of patients are females, a high proportion are obese and almost all are older adults although instances in children have been recorded (Lewis & Blair 1982). The importance of associated drug therapy, particularly with microsomal enzyme-inducing agents, is unclear. Genetic factors may be important, as halothane hepatitis has been described in closely related members of three families (Hoft et al 1981). The means whereby halothane might produce liver injury have included immunological and metabolic mechanisms.

***Halothane metabolism.*** About 20% of halothane is metabolized in humans and oxidative and reductive pathways catalyzed by the cytochrome P-450 enzymes have been identified. The oxidative pathway is the predominant route of metabolism and involves hydroxylation followed by debromination to produce trifluoroacetylchloride. This reactive metabolite may be metabolized to trifluoroacetate or may bind covalently to amino acid groups on hepatic macromolecules to produce modified cell proteins and phospholipids that can act as neoantigens. Oxidative metabolism of halothane is probably catalyzed by the enzyme isoform CYP2E1 (P-450 2E1), as it can be inhibited in humans by disulfiram (Kharasch et al 1996). Reductive metabolism is favored by anaerobic conditions and occurs only to a limited extent during surgical anesthesia. Reductive metabolism of halothane is initiated by insertion of an electron to produce a free radical. This undergoes defluorination to produce a compound that is conjugated to glutathione or debrominated. The debrominated compound may be able to initiate lipid peroxidation.

Animal models of halothane toxicity have concentrated on the reductive pathway of halothane metabolism. Guinea pigs pretreated with enzyme inducers such as phenobarbitone will reliably produce centrilobular necrosis and liver failure, which has been attributed to the production of toxic metabolites (Lind et al 1987). However, the clinical relevance of these models to halothane hepatitis in humans is doubtful.

***Immune factors.*** About a half of patients with halothane hepatitis have fever and an eosinophilia and many have immune complexes and a variety of antibodies to normal tissue components and to halothane metabolites, suggesting that immune factors may be important in producing halothane hepatitis. Vergani et al (1980) found that white blood cells from patients with halothane hepatitis showed migration inhibition when cultured with liver antigens isolated from rabbits exposed previously to halothane, indicating the development of a cellular immune reaction to halothane-altered liver components. They subsequently showed that serum from patients with halothane hepatitis contained IgG antibodies recognizing antigens on rabbit hepatocytes exposed to halothane but not on control hepatocytes. This antibody was specific to patients with halothane hepatitis (Neuberger et al 1983). Other antigens have been identified which are recognized by antibodies in the serum of patients with halothane hepatitis. These include protein disulfide isomerase and microsomal carboxylesterase, which have been detected on the surface of hepatocytes, suggesting a possible mechanism of immune liver damage (Kenna et al 1988, Satoh et al 1989).

***Pathogenesis.*** Halothane hepatitis is probably an immune-mediated disease initiated by halothane metabolism. Oxidative metabolism produces trifluoroacetylchloride, which can react with liver cell proteins to produce neoantigens, and halothane hepatitis may result in individuals who react immunologically to these neoantigens. The susceptibility of obese patients may be explained by the increased activity of the CYP2E1 (P-450 2E1) isoform in their livers, but this does not explain female or genetic susceptibility (Kharasch et al 1996). Minor hepatic dysfunction may be associated with reductive metabolism, but this is unproven.

***Prevention.*** Inhibition of CYP2E1 (P-450 2E1) might prevent halothane hepatitis and such inhibition can be achieved using disulfiram (Kharasch et al 1996). Such prevention has not yet been demonstrated on a large scale. It would require the performance of large clinical trials and this has been rendered unnecessary by the introduction of less toxic agents such as isoflurane, enflurane and, most recently, sevoflurane.

### *Other halogenated anesthetics*

Halogenated anesthetics other than halothane have been introduced that cause severe hepatotoxicity less frequently (Eger 1994), perhaps because they undergo less metabolism in the liver (Table 30.8). Enflurane is recognized as being capable of causing severe hepatotoxicity, but only following about 1 in 800 000 exposures (Brown & Gandolfi 1987). Evidence for isoflurane hepatotoxicity is weak (Stoelting et al 1987) and desflurane and sevoflurane have not so far proved hepatotoxic.

## Cholestatic syndromes

Cholestasis is defined as a reduction in bile secretory capacity and its causes lie anywhere in the biliary tract from the hepatocyte canalicular membrane to the ampulla of Vater (p. 931). Cholestasis caused by drugs may be due to effects in the hepatocytes or in the bile ducts. Hepatocyte damage can occur at several sites including individual enzymes, the endoplasmic reticulum, the cellular cytoskeleton, the tight junctions or the plasma membrane. Most cholestatic illnesses due to drugs are self-limiting once the drug is stopped, but sometimes chronic cholestatic illnesses occur.

**Table 30.8** Hepatic metabolism and hepatotoxicity of halogenated anesthetics

| Agent | Hepatic metabolism (%) | Hepatotoxicity |
|---|---|---|
| Desflurane | 0.02 | – |
| Enflurane | 2.4 | 1:800 000 |
| Halothane | 15–20 | 1:11 000 |
| Isoflurane | 0.2 | +/– |
| Sevoflurane | 3.0 | – |

Note: Hepatotoxicity refers to the frequency of severe (fulminant) reactions, +/– indicates uncertain severe hepatotoxicity and – indicates no severe hepatotoxicity reported so far.

### *Acute cholestasis*

Many drugs can cause acute cholestasis. Clinically, the illness may present with nonspecific symptoms of fever, nausea and malaise. Pruritus is usually present before the onset of jaundice. Abdominal pain in the right upper quadrant may be so severe that the diagnosis of acute cholecystitis is made and the patient subjected to laparotomy. In some cases there are features suggestive of hypersensitivity, including circulating eosinophilia and nonorgan-specific autoantibodies. Liver function tests show the features of cholestasis (p. 743) with increases of plasma bilirubin, alkaline phosphatase and γ-glutamyl transferase. As with other forms of drug-induced liver damage, the diagnosis is one of exclusion and considerations of particular importance are shown in Table 30.5. Acute episodes of drug-induced cholestasis usually resolve rapidly once the drug is withdrawn and liver function tests are usually normal within 3 months.

***Bland cholestasis.*** These reactions are characterized by cholestasis without significant hepatocellular damage. The clinical features are jaundice and pruritus and the liver function tests show increased serum alkaline phosphatase and γ-glutamyl transferase activity but little or no increased transaminase activity. Liver biopsy shows only cholestasis. This reaction is generated typically by compounds such as the oral contraceptives, anabolic steroids and cyclosporin which affect the hepatocyte canalicular membrane. Transport of material out of the liver cells across the biliary canalicular membrane is dependent on at least three ATP-dependent transporters and the compounds listed above interfere with one or more of these transporters (DeLeve & Kaplowitz 1995).

***Cholestatic hepatitis.*** These reactions are characterized by a variable amount of hepatocyte damage (hepatitis) and are referred to above (p. 846). The clinical features often include systemic symptoms in addition to cholestasis and more severe forms with fever and abdominal pain are easily mistaken for cholecystitis or bacterial cholangitis. Liver function tests show significantly increased transaminase activity as well as cholestasis. Liver biopsy shows variable hepatocyte damage and more severe illnesses may show damage to bile ducts (cholangiolitis) and follow a more prolonged course.

*Chronic cholestasis*

Chronic cholestasis related to drugs is much less common than acute cholestasis and in some cases jaundice may persist for a year or more. The outlook is good for most patients, although progression to cirrhosis can occur. Some patients develop syndromes closely resembling primary biliary cirrhosis, vanishing bile duct syndrome and sclerosing cholangitis. Death may occur and has been associated with carbutamide, tolbutamide, chlorpromazine, thiobendazole and methyl testosterone. Drugs associated with chronic cholestasis are shown in Table 30.7.

***Primary biliary cirrhosis.*** There have been reports of chronic cholestasis related to drugs leading to a syndrome resembling primary biliary cirrhosis. Drugs implicated include chlorpromazine, imipramine, ajmaline and benoxoprofen (Horst et al 1980). These patients usually do not have the antimitochondrial antibody in the blood and where this antibody is found, it is not known whether the drug has induced primary biliary cirrhosis or merely unmasked pre-existing disease (p. 938).

***Vanishing bile duct syndrome.*** A number of drugs have been associated with chronic progressive cholestasis persisting after the drug is withdrawn and associated with progressive bile duct loss from the portal tracts and increasing fibrosis (Table 30.9). This illness is otherwise indistinguishable from the vanishing bile duct syndrome (p. 945).

***Sclerosing cholangitis.*** Damage to the large bile ducts and gallbladder leading to a syndrome of sclerosing cholangitis has been described in association with a number of drugs. The best recognized is that following intra-arterial administration of fluorouracil and floxuridine. This leads to the characteristic clinical and cholangiographic features of sclerosing cholangitis with histological features of cholestasis and pericholangitis but little hepatocellular damage (p. 943). A major feature differentiating this from primary sclerosing cholangitis is that the distal common bile duct is often spared and occlusion of the small peribiliary arteries may be diagnostic. Sclerosing cholangitis can also occur if scolicidal agents (formaldehyde and saline) are injected accidentally into the biliary tract at operation (Belghiti et al 1986).

## Granulomatous hepatitis

Drugs are recognized as one of the many causes of granulomatous hepatitis (Table 30.9) and this is discussed elsewhere (p. 831).

## Steatosis and steatohepatitis

Hepatic steatosis may be of the microvesicular or macrovesicular type (p. 975). They can be differentiated histologically and there are important clinical differences with respect to mechanisms and prognosis. Steatohepatitis can also occur. Drugs associated with steatosis are listed in Table 30.9.

*Macrovesicular steatosis*

In macrovesicular steatosis, the liver cell contains a single large fat droplet that displaces the nucleus to the periphery of the cell. The principal mechanism underlying macrovesicular steatosis is impaired transport of lipids out of the hepatocyte (p. 975). Triglycerides are incorporated into lipoproteins for transport out of the liver cells and the protein components (apoproteins) of the lipoproteins are synthesized in the rough endoplasmic reticulum and the Golgi apparatus. Decreased lipoprotein synthesis may occur as a consequence of structural damage to the endoplasmic reticulum, the Golgi apparatus or plasma membranes or as a consequence of a specific lesion in one of these sites. Macrovesicular steatosis also occurs in starvation, diabetes and obesity (p. 976). The prognosis is usually excellent, as the liver lesion resolves once the offending drug is withdrawn (Table 35.8).

*Microvesicular steatosis*

In microvesicular steatosis, the hepatocytes are filled with numerous small lipid droplets and the nucleus usually remains in the center of the cell (p. 977). Liver cell necrosis may or may not be present. Microvesicular steatosis is caused by inhibition of mitochondrial oxidation of fatty acids. Fatty acids that are not metabolized by the mitochondria accumulate in the liver in the form of triglycerides. Microvesicular steatosis is usually associated with a serious illness characterized by liver and renal failure that often progresses to coma and death. Valproate is probably the commonest drug causing this condition (Table 35.11).

## Phospholipidosis

Phospholipidosis occurs with the antianginal drugs amiodarone and perhexilene (now obsolete). The drugs enter the lysosomes where they form complexes with phospholipids (Blohm 1978). These complexes inhibit the action of intralysosomal phospholipases and consequently phospholipids accumulate progressively. The drug is removed slowly from the lysosomes once administration is stopped and continues to be detectable in the blood for many months. Perhexilene is hydroxylated by a cytochrome P-450 isoenzyme that is deficient in 5–10% of Caucasians and most patients with perhexilene liver damage have had deficiency of this enzyme, pointing to a genetically determined metabolic basis for perhexilene hepatotoxicity (Morgan et al 1984). Phospholipidosis with no other sign of liver damage occurs frequently when these drugs are given, but in some patients liver function tests become abnormal and in a few overt liver disease develops associated with histological features identical to those of alcoholic liver disease (nonalcoholic steatohepatitis or NASH) (p. 975). Toxicity may be recognized from extrahepatic side-effects such as skin discoloration caused by amiodarone.

## Vascular lesions

Vascular lesions associated with drug administration have been described affecting the portal veins, hepatic veins and sinusoids (Table 30.9).

### *Portal vein*

Thrombosis of the portal vein and its branches has been reported after administration of arsenical derivatives, oral contraceptives and steroids.

### *Hepatic artery*

Arterial intimal hyperplasia may occur following oral contraceptive use. This is usually part of a more general reaction and liver involvement is usually asymptomatic. However, rarely, there may be multifocal hemorrhagic necrosis or even spontaneous rupture of the liver. Necrotizing arterial angiitis has been reported in amphetamine addiction.

### *Perisinusoidal fibrosis*

This is characterized by accumulation of collagen within the space of Disse and it may be asymptomatic or lead to portal hypertension. The most common cause is excessive ingestion of vitamin A, taken often for its effect on skin tanning. There is hyperplasia of the hepatic stellate cells (p. 714) and fibrosis in the space of Disse and, in addition, sinusoidal dilatation and sometimes features resembling veno-occlusive disease. Other drugs are associated with perisinusoidal fibrosis, but the mechanism for the damage is unknown.

### *Sinusoidal damage*

Striking sinusoidal dilatation can occur with some drugs such as oral contraceptives and in the early stages of damage due to azathioprine. Peliosis hepatis has also been attributed to drugs. This condition is characterized by blood-filled cavities distributed randomly within the liver (p. 1086).

### *Veno-occlusive disease*

Veno-occlusive disease is characterized by nonthrombotic concentric narrowing of the small hepatic vein branches. This results in hepatic congestion and centrilobular liver cell necrosis. The clinical features are those of a Budd–Chiari syndrome and presentations may be acute or chronic (p. 1079). Veno-occlusive disease is seen most commonly in bone marrow recipients after irradiation and chemotherapy (p. 1167). Drugs associated with veno-occlusive disease are shown in Table 30.7. Veno-occlusive disease also results from the ingestion of pyrrolizidine alkaloids present in some plants.

### *Budd–Chiari syndrome*

Budd–Chiari syndrome is characterized by obstruction of the large hepatic veins (p. 1079).

### *Other vascular lesions*

Other vascular lesions associated with drugs include hepatoportal sclerosis and nodular hyperplasia. In particular, vitamin A, anabolic steroids, contraceptives and corticosteroids have been associated with nodular hyperplasia of the liver. Azathioprine, methotrexate and arsenicals are associated with hepatoportal sclerosis.

## Chronic hepatitis and cirrhosis

Some drugs have been associated with chronic active hepatitis and cirrhosis and when the drug has been recognized and withdrawn, inflammatory activity within the liver almost always resolves (p. 896). In some cases there are features to suggest autoimmunity, with increased serum IgG concentrations and nonspecific autoantibodies such as antinuclear antibody. Histologically, the liver shows inflammatory features and piecemeal necrosis virtually identical with that of autoimmune hepatitis. Drugs associated with chronic hepatitis and cirrhosis are shown in Table 30.9.

## Hepatic tumors

Both benign and malignant tumors of the liver may be associated with drug ingestion (Table 30.9).

### *Adenoma*

Hepatic adenomas are benign tumors of the liver. In particular, oral contraceptives are associated with an increased risk of hepatocellular adenoma, but this risk is relatively small (p. 1127). Danazol has also been associated with benign hepatic adenomas. The tumors often remain asymptomatic and are discovered incidentally. More rarely, hepatomegaly, abdominal pain or intraperitoneal hemorrhage leads to the diagnosis. For many, discontinuation of the oral contraceptive is associated with slow reduction in tumor size. Clinically, it is difficult to differentiate benign from malignant tumors.

*Hepatocellular carcinoma*

Hepatocellular carcinomas due to drugs usually arise in noncirrhotic liver. Some have been reported to arise within hepatic adenomas. The risk of developing hepatocellular carcinoma from oral contraceptives is very low and is related to the amount and duration of estrogen ingestion (p. 1118).

*Hemangioma*

Hepatic hemangiomas are probably not caused by drug ingestion, but administration of contraceptive steroids may lead to enlargement and occasionally rupture of preexisting hemangiomas.

*Angiosarcoma*

Angiosarcoma is a rare malignant tumor of endothelial cells. It has been associated with drugs and environmental chemicals. There may be a particularly long interval between the ingestion and the development of tumors after thorium and arsenicals administration (p. 1125).

*Cholangiocarcinoma*

Cholangiocarcinoma is a malignant tumor of biliary epithelium. As with angiosarcomas, drugs associated with its development include thorium dioxide, long-term anabolic and androgenic therapy and oral contraceptive pills, but the association remains uncertain.

## HEPATOTOXIC SUBSTANCES

The number of hepatotoxic substances is for practical purposes endless and it is neither possible nor profitable to try to remember them. More important is to remember that hepatotoxic substances are likely explanations for otherwise obscure liver disease and that these substances are encountered not only as the drugs of conventional medicine but as unconventional or alternative medicines, in the recreational use or abuse of drugs, in industrial chemicals and in the environment generally. An appreciation of the many ways in which hepatotoxic substances can damage the liver (above) makes it likely that unusual forms of liver disease will more often be recognized as caused by hepatotoxins and an ordered approach to identifying such diseases (p. 845) will ensure that hepatotoxic liver damage is not identified wrongly and other treatable liver disease overlooked.

Tables of drugs, constituents of herbal medicines, and industrial agents causing liver damage are given here to help the reader in relation to individual patients (Tables 30.9, 30.10, 30.11). These have been adapted with permission from the monograph by Farrell (1994), which is current, extensive, detailed and gives original references. The tables abbreviate different forms of liver damage as jaundice (J), acute hepatitis of all degrees of severity (AH), cholestatic hepatitis (CH), granulomatous hepatitis (GH), fatty liver (FL), nonalcoholic steatohepatitis (NASH), phospholipidosis (PL), nonspecific liver damage (NSLD), acute cholestasis (AC), chronic cholestasis (CC), chronic active hepatitis (CAH), hepatic fibrosis (HF), cirrhosis (Cirr), noncirrhotic portal hypertension (NCPH), peliosis hepatitis or sinusoidal dilatation (PH), veno-occlusive disease (VOD), Budd–Chiari syndrome (BCS), vanishing bile duct syndrome (VBDS), nodular regenerative hyperplasia (NRH), porphyria cutanea tarda (PCT) and tumors of any type (T). The evidence for causality refers to the best evidence available, usually for the most common form of hepatotoxicity, and is listed as recurrence of toxicity on rechallenge with the drug (R) or circumstantial evidence (C) based on the temporal relation between drug usage and toxicity. Other evidence for toxicity may be epidemiological (Ep) or experimental (Ex). Some drug toxicity is dose dependent (DD). Evidence for uncommon forms of hepatotoxicity is often weak. Clearly, the strength of evidence for causality in hepatotoxicity varies. Recurrence of liver injury on rechallenge (R) is very strong evidence of hepatotoxicity, experimental evidence (Ex) in animals is highly suggestive but may be limited by species variability, epidemiological evidence (Ep) does not apply to individual cases and circumstantial evidence (C) varies from many well worked-out cases to sporadic anecdotes. Where doubt exists or circumstantial evidence is mainly anecdotal, a question mark (?) is shown. To help when looking up entries in Tables 30.9, 30.10 and 30.11, these abbreviations have been tabulated (p. 856).

### Drugs

Just as it is impossible to remember all hepatotoxic agents, so too is it impossible to consider every hepatotoxic drug in this chapter. Particular drugs have been considered already as examples of specific hepatotoxic mechanisms and also drugs often giving particular patterns of liver damage have been listed. Most often, doctors wish to know whether a particular drug has been recognized as causing liver damage and in this regard, drug references are useful. The *British Pharmacopoeia* and the *United States Pharmacopeia* are major reference works, Martindale is an excellent single-volume source and the *British National Formulary* and the *Physician's Desk Handbook* in North America are very useful. There are also several reviews and monographs on hepatotoxic substances from which details on individual drugs can be obtained (Ludwig & Axelson 1983, Stricker & Spoelstra 1985, Zimmerman 1990, Stricker 1992, Farrell 1994, Lewis 1995). Most drugs in relatively common use are shown in Table 30.9.

**Table 30.9** Listing of hepatotoxic drugs

| Drug | Liver injury | Causality |
|---|---|---|
| Acebutolol | AH | R |
| Acetohexamide | CH | C |
| *N*-acetylcysteine | NSLD | R |
| Acitretin | AC | C |
| Albendazole | AH | R |
| Allopurinol | AH, GH, AC | R |
| Alprazolam | NSLD, J | R |
| Amineptine | AH, CH, CC, FL | R |
| Aminoglutethimide | CH | R |
| Amiodarone | NASH, PL, FL, CH, GH | C |
| Amitriptyline | CH, AH, VBDS | R |
| Amodiaquine | AH | DD |
| Amoxicillin | GH | C? |
| Amoxicillin/clavulanic acid | CH, AC, AH, GH, VBDS | R |
| Amphotericin B | NSLD | C, DD? |
| Ampicillin | AH, GH, VBDS | C? |
| Androgenic/anabolic steroids | AC, CC, PH, T | C |
| Aprindine | AH, CH | R |
| L-asparaginase | FL | C |
| Aspirin | AH, GH, CH, Reye's syndrome | C, Ep, DD |
| Atenolol | AC | C |
| Azapropazone | CH, GH | C |
| Azathioprine | AH, CH, AC, NCPH, NRH, VOD, PH | R |
| Barbiturates | AH, CH, VBDS | R |
| BCG vaccine | GH | C |
| BCNU | NSLD, AC, VOD | C, Ex |
| Benorylate | AH | C?, DD? |
| Benzarone | AH, CAH | R |
| Bindazac | NSLD | R |
| Bisantrene | NSLD, AC | DD |
| Bleomycin | NSLD | DD |
| Bromocryptine | NSLD, AH | R |
| Busulphan | NRH, VOD, PCT | C |
| Calcium carbimide | AC, CH, Fib, Cirr | C |
| Captopril | CH, AH, AC | C |
| Carbamazepine | GH, AH, CH, VBDS | R |
| Carbenicillin | NSLD | DD? |
| Carbimazole | CH, AH | R |
| Carboplatin | NSLD, VOD | C |
| Carbutamide | GH, CC | C? |
| Carprofen | NSLD | C |
| CCNU | NSLD | R |
| Ceftriaxone | Biliary sludge | C, Ex |
| Cephalosporins | NSLD, AH, CH | C? |
| Chenodeoxycholic acid | NSLD | R |
| Chlorambucil | NSLD | R |
| Chlordiazepoxide | CH, AH | ? |
| Chlormezanone | AH | C |
| Chloroquine | PL | C |
| Chlorothiazide | CH, GH, CC | C |
| Chlorozotocin | AC | C? |
| Chlorpromazine | CH, AH, GH, CAH, VBDS | R |
| Chlorpropamide | CH, GH, VBDS | R |
| Chlorthalidone | CH | C? |
| Chlorzoxazone | NSLD, AH, CH | R |
| Cimetidine | AH, CH, CAH | R |
| Ciprofloxacin | NSLD | C? |
| Cisplatin | FL, AC | R, DD |
| Clindamycin | AH | C |
| Clofibrate | AC, GH, AH, NRH, Stones | C? |
| Clometacin | AH, GH, CAH, Cirr | R |
| Clomipramine | AH | C |
| Clonazepam | AH | R |
| Clorazepate | NSLD | C |
| Clotriazepam | AH | C |

**Table 30.9** (*cont'd*)

| Drug | Liver injury | Causality |
|---|---|---|
| Cloxacillin | CH | C |
| Clozapine | CH, NSLD | R |
| Colchicine | NSLD | DD |
| Corticosteroids | FL | C? |
| Cotrimoxazole | AH, CH, GH, AC, VBDS | R |
| Cromoglycate | CH | C |
| Cyclophosphamide | AH, VOD, PCT | C |
| Cyclosporin A | J, AC, Stones | C, DD? |
| Cyproheptadine | J, AC, VBDS | C |
| Cyproterone acetate | AH, AC, FL | C |
| Cysteamine | VOD | C? |
| Cytosine arabinoside | NSLD, AC, VOD | R |
| Dacarbazine | VOD, BCS | C |
| Dactinomycin | VOD, PH, NC, PH, NRH | C |
| Danazol | PH,T | C |
| Dantrolene | AH, AC, CAH | R |
| Dapsone | CH, GH | C |
| Daunorubicin | VOD | C |
| Desimipramine | AC | C? |
| Dextropropoxyphene | CH | R |
| Diazepam | AH, CH, GH | C? |
| Diclofenac | AH, CH, CAH | R |
| Dicloxacillin | CH | C |
| Didanosine | AH, FL | R, DD? |
| Diethylstilboestrol | AC, PH, T | C? |
| Difenamizole | CAH | C? |
| Diflusinal | NSLD, AH, CH | C |
| Digoxin | NSLD | C? |
| Diltiazem | AH, GH, Mallory bodies | C |
| Disopyramide | CH | C |
| Disulfiram | AH | R |
| Dothiepin | AH | C |
| Doxorubicin | CAH, VOD | C? |
| Enalapril | AH, CH | C |
| Enflurane | AH | R |
| Epipodophyllotoxins | NSLD | C |
| Erythromycin | CH, VBDS | R |
| Ethambutol | CH | R |
| Ethionamide | AH | DD |
| Etretinate | AH, CH, CAH | R |
| Exifone | AH, CH | C |
| Fenamates | NSLD | C? |
| Fenbufen | NSLD, AH | R |
| Fenfibrate | AH, CAH | C? |
| Fenfluramine | GH | C? |
| Fenoprofen | CH | R |
| Fipexidine | AH | R |
| Floxuridine | AH, CC, SclerChol, Cholecystitis | C |
| Flucloxacillin | CH, AC, GH, VBDS | R |
| Fluconazole | CH | R, DD |
| Flucytosine | AH | DD |
| 5-fluorouracil | NSLD | C? |
| Fluphenazine | J | C? |
| Flurazepam | AC | C? |
| Flutamide | AH, AC | R |
| Frentizole | NSLD | Ex, DD |
| Fusidic acid | AC | C, DD |
| Glafenine | AH | R |
| Glibenclamide | AC, AH, GH | C |
| Gold salts | AH, CH, GH | C |
| Griseofulvin | AC | C? |
| Haloperidol | CH, VBDS | C |
| Halothane | AH, GH, CAH | R |
| Heparin | NSLD | C |
| Hycanthone | AH, FL | DD |
| Hydralazine | AH, GH, AC | R |
| Hydroxyurea | NSLD, PH | C? |

**Table 30.9** *(cont'd)*

| Drug | Liver injury | Causality |
|---|---|---|
| Hydroxyzine | NSLD | C? |
| Ibuprofen | AH, CH, AC, FL | R |
| Idarubicin | AH, NSLD | C |
| Imipenem | NSLD | C |
| Imipramine | CH, VBDS | R |
| Indocine N-oxide | AH, VOD | C |
| Indomethacin | AH, CH, FL | C? |
| Interferons | NSLD | C?* |
| Interleukin-2 | NSLD, AC | R |
| Iodipamide meglumine | AH | C |
| Iprindole | AC | R |
| Iproclozide | AH | C |
| Iron | AH, FL | DD |
| Isocarboxazide | AH | C |
| Isoflurane | AH | ? |
| Isoniazid | AH, GH, CAH, Cirr | R |
| Isoxicam | CH | C? |
| Itraconazole | CH | C |
| Kanamycin | CAH | C? |
| Ketoconazole | AH, AC | R |
| Labetalol | AH, CAH, Cirr | R |
| Lergotrile | AH | C |
| Levamisole | NSLD | R |
| Lisinopril | AH | C |
| Lovastatin | NSLD | R |
| Maprotiline | NSLD, CH | C? |
| Mebendazole | NSLD, AH | R |
| Medroxyprogesterone | BCS, PH | C? |
| 6-Mercaptopurine | AH, FL, VOD | R, DD |
| Mesalazine | AH | C |
| Metahexamide | AH, CH | R |
| Metaprine | NLSD, AC | C? |
| Methazolamide | CH | C |
| Methimazole | CH, AH | R |
| Methotrexate | AH, HF, NCPH, Cirr, T | C, DD |
| Methoxsalen | NSLD | R |
| Methoxyflurane | AH | R |
| *N*-methylcarbamate | CAH | C? |
| Methyldopa | AH, CH, GH, CAH | R |
| Metolazone | GH | C? |
| Metoprolol | AH | C |
| Mianserin | NSLD, AH | C |
| Minocycline | AH, FL, CAH | C |
| Mitane | NSLD | C |
| Mithramycin | AH, FL | DD |
| Mitomycin C | NSLD, VOD | C |
| Moxisylyte | AH, CH | R |
| Naficillin | NSLD | C? |
| Naproxen | AH,CH | R |
| Nialamide | NSLD | C? |
| Niclofan | CH | C |
| Nicotinamide | AH, AC | DD |
| Nifedipine | AH, NASH, FL | C |
| Niflumic acid | AH | R |
| Nilutamide | NSLD, AH | C |
| Nitrofurantoin | AH, CH, CAH, GH | R |
| Nitrogen mustard | VOD | C |
| Nizatidine | NSLD | C |
| Norandrostenolone | CC | C |
| Norethandrolone | AC | C |
| Norfloxacin | AH | C |
| Novobiocin | J | C? |
| Octreotide | Stones, NSLD | C |
| Olsalazine | NSLD | C |
| Omeprazole | AH | C? |
| Oral contraceptives | AC, CC, GH, T, PH, BCS, NRH | C |
| Oxacillin | AH, CH, GH | C |
| Oxaprozin | NSLD | C |

**Table 30.9** *(cont'd)*

| Drug | Liver injury | Causality |
|---|---|---|
| Oxyphenbutazone | AH, GH | C? |
| Papaverine | NSLD, GH, CAH, Cirr | R |
| Para-aminosalicylic acid | AH, CAH | DD |
| Paracetamol | AH, CH | DD |
| Pecazine | J | C? |
| Pemoline | AH | C |
| Penicillamine | CH | C |
| Penicillin G and V | AH, GH | C? |
| Pentamidine | NSLD | C? |
| Pentazocine | J | C? |
| Pentostatin | NSLD, FL | DD |
| Perhexiline | NASH, NSLD, FL, GH | C |
| Perphenazine | CH | C? |
| Phencyclidine | AH | C? |
| Phenelzine | AH, Cirr, T | C? |
| Pheniprazine | AH | C? |
| Phenoxyproperazine | AH | C? |
| Phenylbutazone | GH, AH, CH | R |
| Phenytoin | AH, CH, GH, VBDS | R |
| Piperazine | AH | R |
| Piroxicam | AH, CH, AC, FL | C |
| Pirprofen | AH | C |
| Pizotifen | AC | C |
| Prajmalium | CH,VBDS | R |
| Probenecid | J, AH | C |
| Procainamide | GH, AC | R |
| Procarbazine | NSLD, GH | C |
| Prochlorperazine | CH, AH, VBDS | C |
| Progabide | NSLD, AH | C |
| Promazine | AC | C? |
| Propafenone | CH | C |
| Propylthiouracil | AH, CH, CAH | R |
| Pyrazinamide | AC, CAH | C |
| Pyricarbate | AH | R |
| Pyritinol | CH, CAH | R |
| Quinidine | GH, AC | R |
| Quinine | GH | R |
| Ranitidine | AH, CH, GH | C |
| Rifampicin | AH | C? |
| Saramycin | J | |
| Simvastatin | NSLD, AH | C |
| Spiramycin | CH | C |
| Spironolactone | AH | R |
| Stibocaptate | NSLD | DD |
| Stilboestrol | Mallory bodies, T | C? |
| Streptokinase | NSLD | R |
| Streptozotocin | NSLD | C |
| Sulindac | AH,CH | R |
| Sulfonamides | AH, CH, GH, AC, CAH, VBDS | R |
| Tamoxifen | AC, PH | R |
| Terfenidine | NSLD | R |
| Testosterone | PH, T | C |
| Tetracyclines | FL | C |
| Tetrahydroaminoacridine | NSLD | R |
| Thiabendazole | CH, VBDS | R |
| 6-Thioguanine | NCPH, VOD, PH, AC | C |
| Thioridazine | CH | C |
| Tiaprofenic acid | CH | R |
| Ticarcillin-clavulanate | CH | C |
| Ticlopidine | NSLD, AC | C |
| Tocainide | AH, GH | C? |
| Tolazamide | CH, CC | C |
| Tolbutamide | CH, GH, VBDS, T | R |
| Tolmetin | NSLD, FL | C |
| Toloxatone | AH | C |
| Tolrestat | NSLD, AH | C |
| Tranylcypromine | AH, CH | C? |
| Trazodone | AH, AC, CAH | T |

**Table 30.9** *(cont'd)*

| Drug | Liver injury | Causality |
|---|---|---|
| Triamterene | NSLD | R |
| Triazolam | AC | T |
| Trichlormethiazide | GH | C? |
| Triethylene thiophophoramide | AH | C? |
| Trifluoperazine | J | C? |
| Trimethobenzamide | AH | C |
| Trimethoprim | AH | R |
| Troleandomycin | CH, VBDS | R |
| Tumor necrosis factor α | NSLD | T |
| Valproic acid | AH, FL | C |
| Verapamil | AH | R |
| Vincristine | VOD | ? |
| Vitamin A | NSLD, NCPH, Cirr, PH | DD |
| Warfarin | NSLD, AC, FL | C |
| Xenalamine | CH, CC | C |
| Zidovudine | NSLD, FL | R |
| Zimelidine | AH, CH, GH | R |

* Exacerbations of autoimmune hepatitis (p. 32.19).

| Abbreviations used in Tables 30.9, 30.10 and 30.11 | |
|---|---|
| ? | Doubt exists or evidence is mainly anecdotal |
| AC | Acute cholestasis |
| AH | Acute hepatitis |
| BCS | Budd–Chiari syndrome |
| C | Circumstantial evidence |
| CAH | Chronic active hepatitis |
| CC | Chronic cholestasis |
| CH | Cholestatic hepatitis |
| Cirr | Cirrhosis |
| DD | Dose-dependent toxicity |
| Ep | Epidemiological evidence |
| Ex | Expermental evidence |
| FL | Fatty liver |
| GH | Granulomatous hepatitis |
| HF | Hepatic fibrosis |
| J | Jaundice |
| NASH | Nonalcoholic steatohepatitis |
| NCPH | Noncirrhotic portal hypertension |
| NRH | Nodular regenerative hyperplasia |
| NSLD | Nonspecific liver damage |
| PCT | Porphyria cutanea tarda |
| PH | Peliosis hepatitis or sinusoidal dilatation |
| PL | Phospholipidosis |
| R | Rechallenge with the drug |
| T | Tumors of any type |
| VBDS | Vanishing bile duct syndrome |
| VOD | Veno-occlusive disease |

### *Multiple drug therapy*

Difficulty arises in identifying drug hepatotoxicity when patients are taking several drugs and sometimes toxic effects may result from such therapy as drugs interact or exert effects as inducers or inhibitors (p. 839) of the activity of drug-metabolizing enzymes. There is no simple solution to this problem in clinical practice. Fortunately, particular drugs being taken are usually the more likely hepatotoxins and these should be withdrawn first. When this is not the case, it is obviously safest to withdraw all drugs, but this is usually impractical and if possible, one drug should be withdrawn at a time depending on clinical need and the severity of the hepatotoxicity.

### *Recreational drugs*

The use and abuse of drugs for reasons other than medical therapy have increased markedly and should always be considered as possible causes of liver damage. Those taking so-called recreational drugs are frequently using several different drugs of varying degrees of purity and often contaminated by substances that may be hepatotoxic. Histories of drug use are often unreliable (Kothur et al 1991, Conry-Cantilena et al 1996). Furthermore, drugs taken parenterally may lead to infection with identifiable and unidentifiable hepatitis viruses that contribute to liver damage.

***Cocaine.*** Cocaine may produce several medical complications including hyperpyrexia, marked hypertension, renal failure, subarachnoid hemorrhage, disseminated intravascular coagulation and severe liver damage (Silva et al 1991). Animal studies have documented the hepatotoxicity of cocaine administered either acutely or long term. Elevations of serum transaminase activity are time and dose dependent and liver histology shows lobular necrosis, often with fatty change. Susceptibility is dependent on strain, species and enzyme induction.

Liver damage due to cocaine in humans may relate in part to factors such as hyperpyrexia, hypertension and occasionally hypotension (Silva et al 1991), but it is likely that the toxic effect of cocaine is also due to an active metabolite (Roth et al 1992). Cocaine is metabolized to the nontoxic metabolites benzoyl ecgonine, ecgonine methyl ester and ecgonine following hydrolysis by esterases and pseudocholinesterases. However, approximately 10% is demethylated by the cytochrome P-450 enzyme system to norcocaine with further oxidation to *N*-hydroxynorcocaine. Both norcocaine and *N*-hydroxynorcocaine are more potent than cocaine in inducing liver damage. Cocaine toxicity is indicated by early elevation of serum transaminase activity and pathological change characterized by marked coagulative necrosis, predominantly in the pericentral zone, associated with micro- and macrovesicular fat. Inflammatory activity is low.

***Ecstasy (methylenedioxymethylamphetamine).*** The use of ecstasy seems to have increased substantially and upwards of 500 000 people in the UK are said to use the drug at least weekly (Milroy et al 1996). Toxicity causes cardiac arrhythmias, hyperpyrexia, rhabdomyolysis, disseminated intravascular coagulation and renal, liver and brain damage (Henry et al 1992, Milroy et al 1996). Tissue damage may in part be due to hyperpyrexia (p. 1109), but this is not the sole cause. Patients with ecstasy hepatotoxicity present with severe acute hepatitis or with prolonged cholestasis. Fatal fulminant hepatic failure has been reported and one patient has been treated by liver transplantation (Henry et al 1992). Cholestatic hepatitis may resolve slowly over 3 months.

## Traditional or herbal remedies

Unconventional or complementary medicine is used by a significant proportion of the population in many countries. There is an impression that such use has been increasing in the West. A survey in the United States found that a third of the population studied had used at least one unconventional treatment in the previous year and that such treatments were used much more often by younger, better educated and wealthier people. Annual expenditure on such treatments in the United States was estimated at $13.7 billion (Eisenberg et al 1993). People using unconventional treatment for serious illness almost always used conventional treatment as well (83%), but in three-quarters of such cases the doctors providing the conventional treatment were unaware that their patients were also using unconventional remedies.

Herbal medicine or vitamin therapy was used by 5% of patients studied. They are used as general tonics and for a variety of symptoms including headache, pains, skin rashes, rheumatic symptoms, dyspepsia and cough and they are usually taken as tablets or teas. The reasons for this extensive use of unconventional therapy are largely speculative but are likely to include hope for relief from affliction, belief that unconventional therapies are at least harmless, fashion, disappointment with the benefits of conventional therapies and unsatisfactory or unsympathetic encounters with conventional medical practitioners (Cousins 1985, Salmon & Quine 1989).

It is important for doctors to realize that patients will probably not tell them spontaneously about the use of alternative medicines and doctors should inquire specifically about their use, consider them in any explanation for illness and advise patients about their toxic potential. Evidence that herbal medicines can cause liver damage is now good (Table 30.10) and includes the recrudescence of disease on re-exposure to the medicine and reduction of the activity of liver damage on reduction of the dose (Woolf et al 1994). The toxicity of pyrrolizidine alkaloids is thought to result from the binding of active metabolites to hepatocytes, and plants such as comfrey (*Symphytum officinale*) that contain pyrrolizidine alkaloids cause hepatocyte membrane injury in animals (Mattocks 1968, Yeong et al 1993). Liver injury due to the wall germander (*Teucrium chamaedrys*) is probably caused by furano neo-clerodane diterpenoids (Loeper et al 1994). These substances are metabolized by the cytochrome P-450 enzyme system to reactive metabolites that are normally inactivated by glutathione and epoxide hydrolase, but large amounts can be shown to cause liver damage in mice. Accumulating evidence of toxicity has led to the introduction of restrictions on the use of these substances in some countries (Loeper et al 1994, Woolf et al 1994). Herbal remedies often contain many components and the cause of liver damage may be uncertain (DeSmet et al 1996).

**Table 30.10** Listing of hepatotoxic agents used in herbal or folk remedies (From: Farrell 1994. For abbreviations see separate table)

| Agent | Liver injury | Causality |
|---|---|---|
| Arsenic | NCPH, PH, VOD, Cirr, T | Ep, DD |
| *Atractylis gummifera* | AC | C |
| Chaparral leaf (*Lilium rubescens*) | AH | DD |
| Chinese herbs* | NSLD | R |
| Flavaspidic acid | J | C |
| Germander[†] (*Teucrium chamaedrys*) | AH | R |
| *Glycyrrhiza* (liquorice) | NSLD | C |
| Herbal remedies[‡] | NSLD, AH, CAH | R |
| Asafetida (*Ferula foetida*) | | |
| Gentian (*Gentiana*) | | |
| Hops (*Humulus lupulus*) | | |
| Mistletoe (*Viscum album*) | | |
| Motherwort (*Leonurus cardiaca*) | | |
| Skullcap (*Scutellaria*) | | |
| Valerian (*Valeriana*) | | |
| Jin Bu Huan[§] | AH, FL | R |
| Laxatives – natural | NSLD (minor) | C |
| Aloin | | |
| Podophylloxin | | |
| Senna | | |
| Margosa oil | FL | C? |
| Pennyroyal oil (terpenes) | AH | C, DD |
| Pyrrolizidine alkaloids[¶] | VOD, Cirr, T | Ep, C |
| Comfrey (*Symphytum officinale*) | | |
| Crotalaria (*Leguminosae*) | | |
| Heliotropium (*Boraginaceae*) | | |
| Sennecioneae (*Compositae*) | | |
| Seatone (green-lipped mussel) | GH | C |
| *Shohakuhi, shusaikoto* (Japan) | NSLD | C |

* Hepatotoxic component unknown.
[†] Furano neo-clerodane diterpenoids are active metabolites of germander, hepatotoxic in mice (Loeper et al 1994).
[‡] Preparations often contain several ingredients and these do not always remain constant. Suspected hepatotoxins listed.
[§] Chinese herbal containing one active ingredient of the plant genera *Stephania* and *Corydalin*. Structure of l-tetrahydropalmatine similar to pyrrolizidine alkaloids (Woolf et al 1994).
[¶] Usually ingested as herbal teas in many countries.

## Environmental and industrial toxins

There are many potential environmental and industrial toxins (Table 30.11). Alcohol is the most important environmental hepatotoxin. Its effects on the liver are well known and generally disregarded (p. 861). Other environmental hepatotoxins causing serious liver damage are much less common. Mushroom poisoning is common in some countries and is usually due to inexperienced people eating wild mushrooms. *A. phalloides* is the most common cause of liver damage and *A. verna* causes serious poisoning in the United States. Mushroom poisoning causes abdominal pain, nausea, vomiting and diarrhea within 6–18 h followed by improvement for 3–4 days, after which

**Table 30.11** List of environmental and industrial hepatotoxins (From: Farrell 1994. For abbreviations see separate table)

| Agent | Liver injury | Causality |
|---|---|---|
| Aflatoxin | AH, FL, Cirr, VOD, T | C, Ep |
| *Amanita phalloides* (mushrooms) | AH, FL, CAH | C, DD |
| Cadmium | Cirr | Ex |
| Carbon tetrachloride | AH, FL, Cirr, T | DD, Ex |
| Cooking oil – contaminated | | |
| *Yusho* (polychlorinated biphenyls) | AH, T | C |
| Toxic oil syndrome (anilides?) | CH, AH, FL, NASH, NRH, T | C |
| Copper (Bordeaux mixture) | AC, GH, NCPH, T | C, DD |
| Dichlorodiphenyl-trichloroethane (DDT) | NSLD | C |
| Dichloroethane | AH | C |
| Dichloromethane | NSLD | C, Ex |
| Dimethylformamide | NSLD, FL | C, DD |
| Dimethylnitrosamine | Cirr, VOD, T | Ex |
| Dioxins | PCT | Ex, DD |
| Ethanol | FL, Cirr, T | C, Ex, Ep |
| Glyphosate | NSLD | Self-poisoning |
| Methylbromide | NSLD | C |
| Methylenedianiline (Epping jaundice) | CH | C, Ex |
| Methylethylketone peroxide | AH | Poisoning |
| Monochlorobenzene | AH | DD |
| 2-nitropropane | AH, FL, AC | C |
| Organochlorines | NSHD, AH, PCT | DD |
| Paint solvents* | NSLD, FL, Cirr | C? |
| Paraquat | AH, CH, FL | DD |
| Polychlorinated biphenyls | AH, NSLD, Cirr | C, Ex |
| Tetrachloroethane | AH, FL, Cirr | DD |
| Tetrachloroethylene | NSLD | C? |
| Thallium | FL | DD |
| Trichloroethane | FL, Cirr | Ex |
| Trinitrotoluene | AH, Cirr | R |

* E.g. acetone, methylethylketones, styrene, toluene, xylene.

hepatic failure and uremia occur (p. 807). Liver function tests are abnormal in the initial illness, fatal liver failure is associated with severe fatty changes in the liver and the liver returns to normal in those who survive, although recovery may take up to 6 months after a severe illness (Bartoloni St Omer et al 1985). Heavy intake of aflatoxins can cause jaundice, which may be fatal (Ngindu et al 1982), and in the long term may produce hepatocellular carcinomas (p. 1117).

Legislation has done much to prevent disease due to industrial toxins and liver disease due to industrial causes is considered uncommon (Døssing & Skinhøj 1985). However, detection of industrial liver damage is difficult owing to nonspecific symptoms, nonspecific liver function tests and limitations on investigations due to the invasiveness of liver biopsy. An open mind should therefore be kept on this subject.

## PREVENTION OF HEPATOTOXICITY (SURVEILLANCE)

Opportunities for the prevention of drug hepatotoxicity are limited, as overt toxicity is uncommon in drugs accepted into medical practice and virtually all toxicity is idiosyncratic. Repetition or continuance of drug hepatotoxicity can be prevented by investigating the relation of previous hepatic illness to drug administration (p. 845), by asking about intake of unconventional or recreational medicines and by considering drugs as possible causes of otherwise unexplained hepatic abnormality. Exposure to environmental and industrial toxins should also be considered (above).

Surveillance for hepatotoxicity during drug therapy usually utilizes liver function tests, but it is important to recognize the limitations of this undertaking. First, minor liver function test abnormalities are relatively frequent in well people and may be intermittent (p. 736). Accordingly, liver function tests need to be checked before treatment starts and alternative causes for abnormalities need to be considered even when these arise during treatment. Second, asymptomatic abnormal tests during drug therapy do not necessarily identify serious drug hepatotoxicity or signify the development of more severe overt toxicity. Transient minor liver function test abnormalities occur with many drugs and the frequency of such abnormalities varies from less than 5% with some drugs to 20–50% with others (Lewis & Zimmerman 1989). Isoniazid causes asymptomatic abnormality, which is usually self-limiting in spite of continued therapy, in up to 20% of patients, while unrelated serious hepatotoxicity occurs in fewer than 1% of patients (Mitchell & Jollows 1975).

Generally speaking, surveillance is only worthwhile during long-term therapy with newer drugs or with drugs having a known hepatotoxic potential. Watkins et al (1994) checked plasma alanine aminotransferase activity weekly in 2446 patients with Alzheimer's disease given tetrahydroaminoacridine (Tacrine) and found asymptomatic increased activity in 49% at some time. Three-quarters of activities were increased less than twice the upper normal limit, 90% occurred within 12 weeks of starting therapy and increases occurred suddenly. This study illustrated the early occurrence of most hepatotoxicity and the consequent need for frequent liver function tests during this period. Liver function abnormalities after 12 weeks are increasingly likely to be due to other causes. Drug withdrawal only needs to be considered where therapy is not absolutely essential and when asymptomatic increases of serum enzyme activity exceed three to four times the normal upper limit (Zimmerman & Ishak 1995). The limits of surveillance in identifying hepatotoxicity also need to be remembered, as some drugs such as methotrexate and amiodarone can cause severe liver damage without producing abnormal liver function tests.

REFERENCES


Adjepon-Yamoah K K, Nimmo J, Prescott L F 1974 Gross impairment of hepatic drug metabolism in a patient with chronic liver disease. British Medical Journal 4: 387–388

Bartoloni St Omer F, Giannini A, Botti P et al 1985 Amanita poisoning: a clinical–histopathological study of 64 cases of intoxication. Hepato-gastroenterology 32: 229–231

Bass N M, Williams R L 1988 Guide to drug dosage in hepatic disease. Clinical Pharmacokinetics 15: 396–420

Belfrage S, Ahlgren I, Axelson S 1966 Halothane hepatitis in an anaesthetist. Lancet 2: 1466–1467

Belghiti J, Benhamou J-P, Houry H, Grenier P, Huguier M, Fékété F 1986 Caustic sclerosing cholangitis. A complication of the surgical treatment of hydatid disease of the liver. Archives of Surgery 121: 1162–1165

Bem J L, Mann R D, Rawlins M D 1988 Review of yellow cards – 1986 and 1987. British Medical Journal 296: 1319

Benet L Z, Mitchell J R, Sheiner L B 1990 Pharmacokinetics: the dynamics of drug absorption, distribution, and elimination. In: Gilman A G, Rall T W, Nies A S, Taylor P (eds) Goodman and Gilman's the pharmacological basis of therapeutics, 8th edn. Pergamon Press, New York, ch 1, pp 3–32

Benichou C 1990 Criteria for drug-induced liver disorders. Report of an International Consensus Meeting. Jounal of Hepatology 11: 272–276

Benson G D 1983 Acetaminophen in chronic liver disease. Clinical Pharmacology and Therpeutics 33: 95–101

Black M 1980 Acetaminaphen hepatotoxicity. Gastroenterology 78: 382–392

Blohm, T R 1978 Drug-induced lysosomal lipidosis: biochemical interpretations. Pharmacological Reviews 30: 593–603

Branch R A, Nies A S, Read A E 1975 The liver and drugs. In: Read A E (ed) Modern trends in gastroenterology 5. Butterworths, London. Ch 14 p 289

Brown B R Jr, Gandolfi A J 1987 Adverse effects of volatile anaesthetics. British Journal of Anaesthesia 59: 14–23

Burnett D A, Barak A J, Tuma D J, Sorrell M F 1976 Altered elimination of antipyrine in patients with acute viral hepatitis. Gut 17: 341–344

Cobden I, Record C O, Ward M K, Kerr D N S 1982 Paracetamol-induced acute renal failure in the absence of fulminant liver damage. British Medical Journal 284: 21–22

Conney A H 1967 Pharmacological implications of microsomal enzyme induction. Pharmacological Reviews 19: 317–366

Conry-Cantilena C, Van Raden M, Gibble J et al 1996 Routes of infection, viremia, and liver disease in blood donors found to have hepatitis C virus infection. New England Journal of Medicine 334: 1691–1696

Cousins N 1985 How patients appraise physicians. New England Journal of Medicine 313: 1422–1424

DeLeve L D, Kaplowitz N 1995 Mechanisms of drug-induced liver disease. Gastroenterology Clinics of North America 24: 787–810

De Smet P A G M, Van Den Eertwegh A J M, Lesterhuis W, Stricker B H Ch 1996 Hepatotoxicity associated with herbal tablets. British Medical Journal 313: 92

Døssing M, Skinhøj P 1985 Occupational liver injury: present state of knowledge and future perspective. International Archives of Occupational and Environmental Health 56: 1–21

Eger E I 1994 New inhaled anesthetics. Anesthesiology 80: 906–922

Eisenberg D M, Kessler R C, Foster C, Norlock F E, Calkins D R, Delbanco T L 1993 Unconventional medicine in the United States. Prevalence, costs, and patterns of use. New England Journal of Medicine 328: 246–252

Farrell G C 1994 Drug-induced liver disease. Churchill Livingstone, Edinburgh

Fontana R J, Watkins P B 1995 Genetic predisposition to drug-induced liver disease. Gastroenterology Clinics of North America 24: 811–838

Forrest J A H, Roscoe P, Prescott L F, Stevenson I H 1974 Abnormal drug metabolism after barbiturate and paracetamol overdose. British Medical Journal 4: 499–502

Forrest J A H, Adriaenssens P, Finlayson N D C, Prescott L F 1979 Paracetamol metabolism in chronic liver disease. European Journal of Clinical Pharmacology 15: 427–431

Friis H, Andreasen P B 1992 Drug-induced hepatic injury: an analysis of 1100 cases reported to The Danish Committee on Adverse Drug Reactions between 1978 and 1987. Journal of Internal Medicine 232: 133–138

Henry J A, Jeffreys K J, Dawling S 1992 Toxicity and deaths from 3,4-methylenedioxymethamphetamine ("ecstasy"). Lancet 340: 384–387

Hoft R H, Bunker J P, Goodman H I, Gregory P B 1981 Halothane hepatitis in three pairs of closely related women. New England Journal of Medicine 304: 1023–1024

Horst D A, Grace N D, LeCompte P H 1980 Prolonged cholestasis and progressive hepatic fibrosis following imipramine therapy. Gastroenterology 79: 550–554

Hrdina P D, Lapierre Y D, Koranyi E K 1985 Altered amitriptyline kinetics in a depressed patient with portocaval anastomosis. Canadian Journal of Psychiatry 30: 111–113

Huet P-M, Villeneuve J-P 1983 Determinants of drug disposition in patients with cirrhosis. Hepatology 3: 913–918

Inman W H W, Mushin W W 1978 Jaundice after repeated exposure to halothane: a further analysis of reports to the Committee on Safety of Medicines. British Medical Journal 2: 1455–1456

Jacqz E, Hall S D, Branch R A 1986 Genetically determined polymorphisms in drug oxidation. Hepatology 6: 1020–1032

Jakoby W B 1994 Detoxication: conjugation and hydrolysis. In: Arias I M, Boyer J L, Fausto N, Jakoby W B, Schachter D, Shafritz D A (eds) The liver. Biology and pathology, 3rd edn. Raven Press, New York, ch 25, p 429–442

Kaplan H G, Bakken J, Quadracci L, Schubach W 1979 Hepatitis caused by halothane sniffing. Annals of Internal Medicine 90: 797–798

Kato R, Vassanelli P, Frontino G, Chiesari E 1965 Variation in the activity of liver microsomal drug-metabolizing enzymes in rats in relation to the age. Biochemical Pharmacology 13: 1037–1051

Kenna J G, Satoh H, Christ D D, Pohl L R 1988 Metabolic basis for a drug hypersensitivity: antibodies in sera from patients with halothane hepatitis recognize liver neoantigens that contain the trifluoroacetyl group derived from halothane. Journal of Pharmacology and Experimental Therapeutics 245: 1103–1109

Kharasch E D, Hankins D, Mautz D, Thummel K E 1996 Identification of the enzyme responsible for oxidative halothane metabolism: implications for prevention of halothane hepatitis. Lancet 347: 1367–1371

Klatskin G, Kimberg D V 1969 Recurrent hepatitis attributable to halothane sensitization in an anesthetist. New England Journal of Medicine 280: 515–522

Koff R S, Gardner R C, Harinasuta U, Pihl C O 1970 Profile of hyperbilirubinemia in three hospital populations. Clinical Research 18: 680

Kothur R, Marsh F, Posner G 1991 Liver function tests in nonparenteral cocaine users. Archives of Internal Medicine 151: 1126–1128

Lewis J H (ed) 1995 Drug-induced liver disease. Gastroenterology Clinics of North America 24: 739–1094

Lewis J H, Zimmerman H J 1989 Drug-induced liver disease. Medical Clinics of North America 73: 775–792

Lewis R B, Blair M 1982 Halothane hepatitis in a young child. British Journal of Anaesthesia 54: 349–354

Lind R C, Gandolfi A J, Brown B R, Hall P de la M 1987 Halothane hepatotoxicity in guinea pigs. Anesthesia and Analgesia 66: 222–228

Loeper J, Descatoire V, Letteron P et al 1994 Hepatotoxicity of germander in mice. Gastroenterology 106: 464–472

Ludwig J, Axelsen R 1983 Drug effects on the liver. An updated tabular compilation of drugs and drug-related hepatic diseases. Digestive Diseases and Sciences 28: 651–666

MacGilchrist A J, Birnie G G, Cook A et al 1986 Pharmacokinetic and pharmacodynamics of intravenous midazolam in patients with severe alcoholic cirrhosis. Gut 27: 190–195

Mant T G K, Tempowski J H, Volans G N, Talbot J C C 1984 Adverse reactions to acetylcysteine and effects of overdose. British Medical Journal 289: 217–219

Mattocks A R 1968 Toxicity of pyrrolizidine alkaloids. Nature 217: 723–728

McLean A J, Morgan D J 1991 Clinical pharmacokinetics in patients with liver disease. Clinical Pharmacokinetics 21: 42–69
Meyer U A 1994 The molecular basis of genetic polymorphisms of drug metabolism. Journal of Pharmacy and Pharmacology 46 (suppl 1): 409–415
Miguet J-P, Vuitton D, Deschamps J-P et al 1981 Cholestasis and hepatic drug metabolism. Comparison of metabolic clearance rate of antipyrine in patients with intrahepatic or extrahepatic cholestasis. Digestive Diseases and Sciences 26: 718–722
Milroy C M, Clark J C, Forrest A R W 1996 Pathology of deaths associated with "ecstasy" and "eve" misuse. Journal of Clinical Pathology 49: 149–153
Mitchell J R, Jollows D J 1975 Metabolic activation of drugs to toxic substances. Gastroenterology 68: 392–410
Morgan M Y, Reshef R, Shah R R, Oates N S, Smith R L, Sherlock S 1984 Impaired oxidation of debrisoquine in patients with perhexiline liver injury. Gut 25: 1057–1064
Nebert D W, Gonzalez F J 1987 P450 genes: structure, evolution and regulation. Annual Review of Biochemistry 56: 945–993
Neuberger J, Gimson A E S, Davis M, Williams R 1983 Specific serological markers in the diagnosis of fulminant hepatic failure associated with halothane anaesthesia. British Journal of Anaesthesia 55: 15–19
Ngindu A, Johnson B K, Kenya P R et al 1982 Outbreak of acute hepatitis caused by aflatoxin poisoning in Kenya. Lancet 1: 1346–1348
Pentikäinen P J, Neuvonen P J, Jostell K-G 1980 Pharmacokinetics of chlormethiazole in healthy volunteers and patients with cirrhosis of the liver. European Journal of Clinical Pharmacology 17: 275–284
Peterson J A, Ebel R E, O'Keeffe D H, Matsubara T, Estabrook R W 1976 Temperature dependence of cytochrome P-450 reduction. A model of NADPH-cytochrome P-450 reductase: cytochrome P-450 interaction. Journal of Biological Chemistry 251: 4010–4016
Pond S M, Tozer T N 1984 First-pass elimination: basic concepts and clinical consequences. Clinical Pharmacokinetics 9: 1–25
Preisig R, Rankin J G, Sweeting J, Bradley S E 1966 Hepatic hemodynamics during viral hepatitis in man. Circulation 34: 188–197
Prescott L F 1980 Clinically important drug interactions. In: Avery G S (ed) Drug treatment. Principles and practice of clinical pharmacology and therapeutics. Addis Press, Sydney, ch 8, p 236–262
Prescott L F, Wright N, Roscoe P, Brown S S 1971 Plasma-paracetamol half-life and hepatic necrosis in patients with paracetamol overdosage. Lancet 1: 519–522
Prescott L F, Illingworth R N, Critchley J A J H, Stewart M J, Adam R D, Proudfoot A T 1979 Intravenous *N*-acetylcysteine: the treatment of choice for paracetamol poisoning. British Medical Journal 2: 1097–1100
Proudfoot A T 1993 Acute poisoning: diagnosis and management, 2nd edn. Butterworth-Heinemann, Oxford, p 177–179
Ray D C, Drummond G B 1991 Halothane hepatitis. British Journal of Anaesthesia 67: 84–99
Roth L, Harbison R D, James R C, Tobin T, Roberts S M 1992 Cocaine hepatotoxicity: influence of hepatic enzyme inducing and inhibiting agents on the site of necrosis. Hepatology 15: 934–940
Salmon P, Quine J 1989 Patients' intentions in primary care: measurement and preliminary investigation. Psychology and Health 3: 63–110
Satoh H, Martin B M, Schulick A H, Christ D D, Kenna J G, Pohl L R 1989 Human anti-endoplasmic reticulum antibodies in sera of patients with halothane-induced hepatitis are directed against a trifluoroacetylated carboxylesterase. Proceedings of the National Academy of Sciences of the United States of America 86: 322–326
Shenker S, Bergstrom R F, Wolen R L, Lemberger L 1988 Fluoxetine disposition and elimination in cirrhosis. Clinical Pharmacology and Therapeutics 44: 353–359
Silva M O, Roth D, Reddy K R, Fernandez J A, Albores-Saavedra J, Schiff E R 1991 Hepatic dysfunction accompanying acute cocaine intoxication. Journal of Hepatology 12: 312–315
Stoelting R K, Blitt C D, Cohen P J, Merin R G 1987 Hepatic dysfunction after isoflurane anesthesia. Anesthesia and Analgesia 66: 147–153
Stricker B H Ch 1992 Drug-induced hepatic injury. In: Dukes M N G (ed) Drug-induced disorders, vol 5, 2nd edn. Elsevier, Amsterdam, p 1–550
Stricker B H Ch, Spoelstra P 1985 Drug-induced hepatic injury. In: Dukes M N G (ed) Drug-induced disorders, vol 1. Elsevier, Amsterdam
Subcommittee on the National Halothane Study of the Committee on Anesthesia, National Academy of Sciences–National Research Council 1966 Summary of the national halothane study. Possible association between halothane anesthesia and postoperative hepatic necrosis. Journal of the American Medical Association 197: 775–788
Vale J A, Meredith T J, Goulding R 1981 Treatment of acetaminophen poisoning. The use of oral methionine. Archives of Internal Medicine 141: 394–396
Vergani D, Mieli-Vergani G, Alberti A et al 1980 Antibodies to the surface of halothane-altered rabbit hepatocytes in patients with severe halothane-associated hepatitis. New England Journal of Medicine 303: 66–71
Walton B, Simpson B R, Strunin L, Doniach D, Perrin J, Appleyard A J 1976 Unexplained hepatitis following halothane. British Medical Journal 1: 1171–1176
Watkins P B 1990 Role of cytochromes P-450 in drug metabolism and hepatotoxicity. Seminars in Liver Disease 10: 235–250
Watkins P B, Zimmerman H J, Knapp M J, Gracon S I, Lewis K W 1994 Hepatotoxic effects of Tecrine administration in patients with Alzheimer's disease. Journal of the American Medical Association 271: 992–998
Watson R G P, Olomu A, Clements D, Waring R H, Mitchell S, Elias E 1988 A proposed mechanism for chlorpromazine jaundice – defective hepatic sulfoxidation combined with rapid hydroxylation. Journal of Hepatology 7: 72–78
Whitcomb D C, Block G D 1994 Association of acetaminophen hepatotoxicity with fasting and ethanol use. Journal of the American Medical Association 272: 1845–1850
Woolf G M, Petrovic L M, Rojter S E et al 1994 Acute hepatitis associated with the Chinese herbal product Jin Bu Huan. Annals of Internal Medicine 121: 729–735
Yeong M L, Wakefield S J, Ford H C 1993 Hepatocyte membrane injury and bleb formation following low dose comfrey toxicity in rats. International Journal of Experimental Pathology 74: 211–217
Ziegler D M 1994 Detoxication: oxidation and reduction. In: Arias I M, Boyer J L, Fausto N, Jakoby W B, Schachter D, Shafritz D A (eds) The liver. Biology and pathology, 3rd edn. Raven Press, New York, ch 24, p 415–427
Zimmerman H J 1990 Update of hepatotoxicity due to classes of drugs in common clinical use: non-steroidal drugs, anti-inflammatory drugs, antibiotics, antihypertensives, and cardiac and psychotropic agents. Seminars in Liver Disease 10: 322–338
Zimmerman H J, Ishak K G 1995 General aspects of drug-induced liver disease. Gastroenterology Clinics of North America 24: 739–757

# 31. Alcohol and the liver

*K. J. Simpson   Peter W. Brunt*

## INTRODUCTION

The use and misuse of alcohol is worldwide and dates from the origins of civilization. Damage by alcohol was recognized by both the ancient Chinese and the Egyptians, although the first good description of alcoholic cirrhosis was recorded by John Brown, a Norfolk surgeon, in 1685. The association between alcohol and cirrhosis is now well recognized but has done little to promote moderation. Alcohol consumption has been rising steadily in most Western countries since World War II and is second only to viral hepatitis as a cause of liver disease worldwide. In the United States, alcoholism cost $60 billion annually, consumed 12% of the total cost of health care and was a factor in one in 10 deaths (West et al 1984). The problems of alcohol abuse and alcoholic liver disease have been extensively reviewed (Hall 1985, Dufour et al 1993, Hayes 1993, Edwards & Peters 1994, Lieber 1994). Alcohol and the more specific term "ethanol" have been used interchangeably as seems appropriate in this chapter.

## EPIDEMIOLOGY (Lelbach 1976, Pequignot et al 1978, Hall 1985)

Epidemiological studies have shown repeatedly the close relation between national alcohol consumption and mortality from cirrhosis (Fig. 31.1). Deaths from cirrhosis fell during prohibition in the United States and when wine was rationed in France during World War II but rose again when alcohol once more became available (Fig. 31.2). The recent increase in alcohol consumption in many countries has been accompanied by an increase in cirrhosis. Studies in many countries have shown that mortality from cirrhosis is 7–14 times higher in heavy drinkers than in the general population. The prevalence of liver disease in heavy drinkers is more difficult to determine and has varied greatly in different studies. Christoffersen & Nielsen (1972) found a high incidence of damage in liver biopsies from 330 chronic alcoholics admitted to hospital consecutively who had drunk in excess of 50 g of alcohol daily for

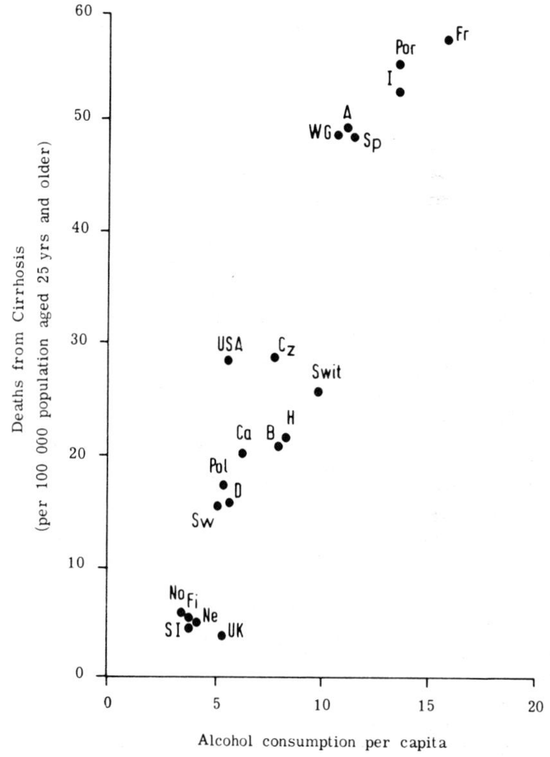


**Fig. 31.1** Relation between death from cirrhosis and alcohol consumption in Europe and North America. A = Austria, B = Belgium, Ca = Canada, Cz = Czechoslovakia, D = Denmark, Fr = France, Fi = Finland, H = Hungary, I = Italy, Ne = Netherlands, No = Norway, Pol = Poland, Por = Portugal, SI = Southern Ireland, Sp = Spain, Sw = Sweden, Swit = Switzerland, UK = United Kingdom, USA = United States of America, WG = West Germany (Schmidt 1977). Alcohol consumption per capita = liters/year of absolute alcohol.

more than a year previously; 64% had a fatty liver, 18% had cirrhosis and 10% had nonspecific abnormalities or hemosiderosis. Only 8% had a normal liver.

Liver disease is much underestimated if investigations are limited to biochemical tests of liver function. Underreporting of alcoholic liver disease also occurs in many countries. Until legislation was changed in 1984, doctors in England were reticent to report a death as due to "alco-

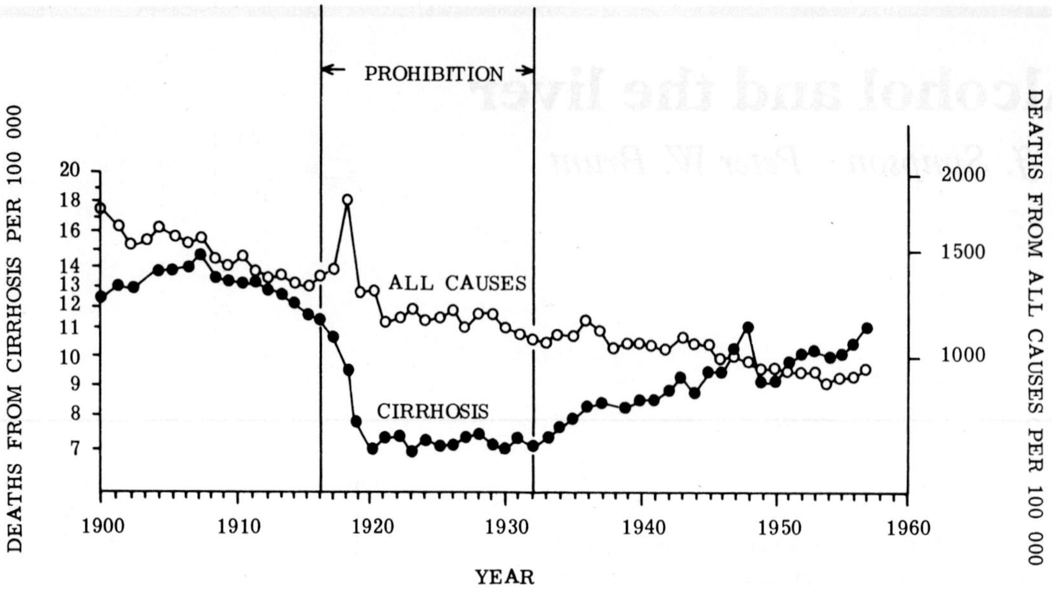


**Fig. 31.2** General mortality and deaths from cirrhosis in the USA from 1900 to 1959. Note the fall in deaths from cirrhosis when the sale of alcohol was forbidden (Prohibition 1916–32) (Klatskin 1961).

holic liver disease" because this would have led to automatic reporting to the coroner with its attendant distress to bereaved families (Maxwell & Knapman 1985, Maxwell 1986).

Many factors influence the intake of alcohol and hence the incidence of alcoholic liver damage. Those engaged in the manufacture, distribution and sale of alcohol, those who have ready access to alcohol and those in the higher income brackets who can afford alcohol have a relatively high mortality from cirrhosis (Table 31.1). Indeed, the availability of alcohol and its cost in relation to income are closely related to alcohol consumption and hence to the likelihood of liver damage (Fig. 31.3).

## ALCOHOL METABOLISM

Ethanol is rapidly absorbed from the stomach and upper small intestine. Absorption from the stomach is slower than from the intestine and normally about 25% is absorbed from the former and 75% from the latter. Absorption tends to be slower and peak blood alcohol concentrations lower when alcohol is taken with food and factors such as drugs or gastric surgery that decrease or increase the rate of gastric emptying decrease or increase peak blood concentrations respectively (Holt 1981). A small proportion is metabolized in the gastric mucosa, oxidized in extrahepatic tissues or excreted unchanged by the kidneys, lungs and sweat glands. However, the majority (80%) of ingested ethanol is catabolized in the liver (Peters 1982). There are three pathways for ethanol metabolism in hepatocytes: the dehydrogenase pathway, the microsomal ethanol oxidizing system (MEOS) and catalase (Fig. 31.4).

**Table 31.1** Standard mortality ratios (SMR) for hepatic cirrhosis for men in the UK, 1959–63 (Morgan 1985)

| Occupation | SMR |
|---|---|
| Publicans | 773 |
| Actors, musicians | 550 |
| Hoteliers | 450 |
| Armed forces | 350 |
| Medical practitioners | 350 |
| Insurance brokers | 330 |
| Waiters | 241 |
| Laborers | 166 |
| Commercial travelers | 150 |
| Teachers | 44 |
| Cleaners | 25 |

Note: Average SMR = 100

### The dehydrogenase pathway

Ethanol is oxidized to acetaldehyde and then to acetate by the sequential action of nicotinamide adenine dinucleotide (NAD)-linked alcohol dehydrogenase (ADH) and acetaldehyde dehydrogenase (ALDH). Less than 30% of the acetate produced by this pathway is metabolized further in the liver, the remainder being released into the circulation, transported to peripheral tissues and oxidized to $CO_2$ and water. NAD is regenerated from the NADH produced during ethanol oxidation by the transfer of hydrogen ions into the mitochondria via aspartate-malate and glycerol 3-phosphate shuttles.

Human liver contains many ADH isoenzymes. Class 1 isoenzymes of ADH are the predominant forms and consist of homodimers or heterodimers of $\alpha$, $\beta$ and $\gamma$ protein chains (e.g. $\alpha$–$\alpha$, $\alpha$–$\beta$, $\gamma$–$\gamma$) (Smith et al 1971). These

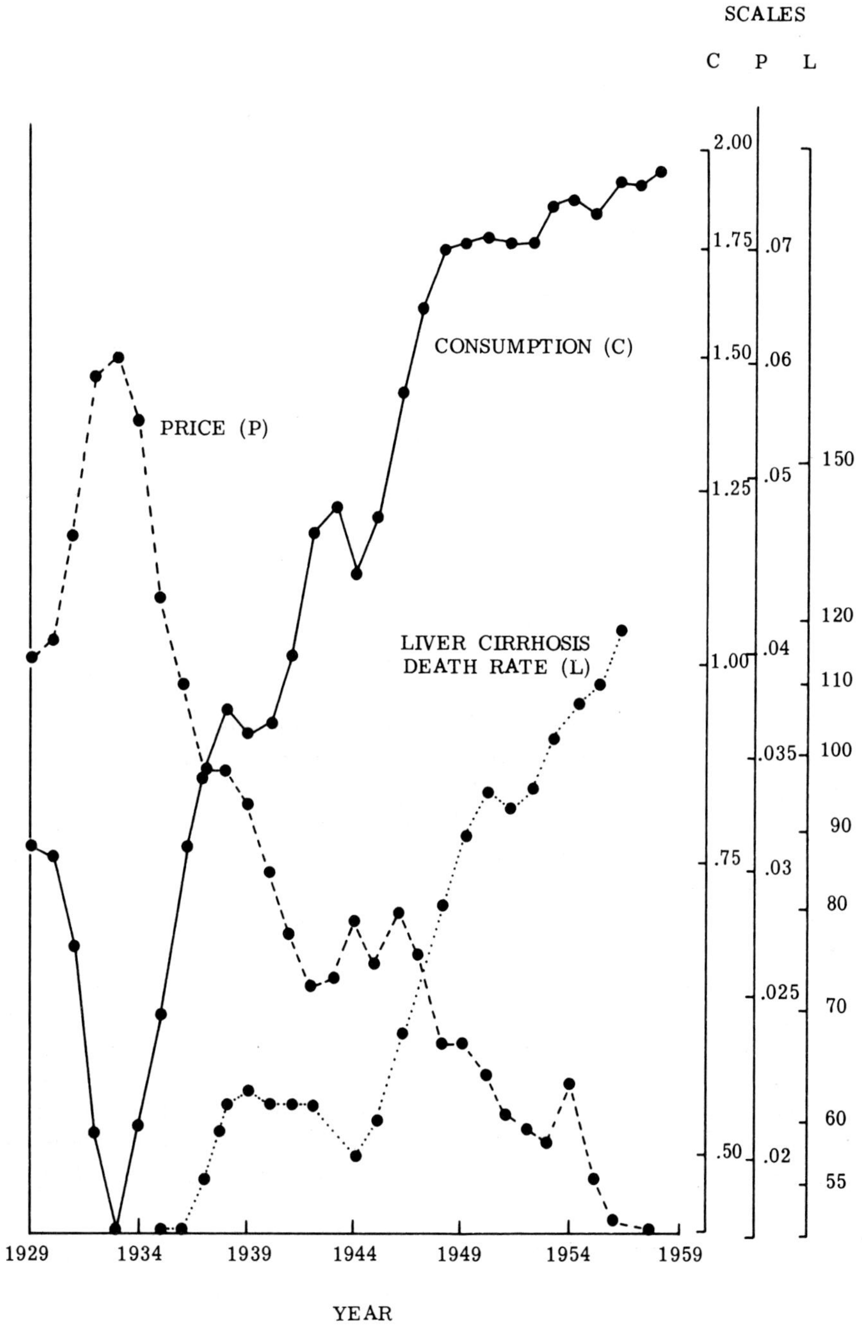


**Fig. 31.3** The relation of the price of alcohol to alcohol consumption and death from cirrhosis of the liver in Ontario, Canada, from 1929 to 1958. P = price of average gallon of absolute alcohol as a fraction of an average disposable income for persons of 20 years of age and over. C = number of gallons of absolute alcohol consumed per person of 20 years and over per year. L = number of deaths from cirrhosis of the liver per 100 000 adults (Seeley 1960).

zinc-binding proteins have a high degree of homology in their protein and DNA sequences but are encoded by three different genes on the long arm of chromosome 4. The ADH genes demonstrate developmental and tissue-specific regulation (Smith et al 1972, 1973); the ADH1 gene codes for the α chain and is the predominant form in fetal and infant liver, the adult stomach and kidney express mainly the ADH3 gene that codes for the γ protein chain and adult lung expresses only the ADH2 gene that codes for the β protein chain. Genetic variation of the ADH2 gene results in the production of $\beta_1$ and $\beta_2$ proteins; the $\beta_2$ homodimer has a 100-fold greater activity than the $\beta_1$ homodimer and is found more commonly in Orientals (Yoshida et al 1988). Genetic variation of the ADH3 gene encodes the $\gamma_1$ and $\gamma_2$ proteins, both of which are common in Caucasians, whereas $\gamma_2$ is rarely found in

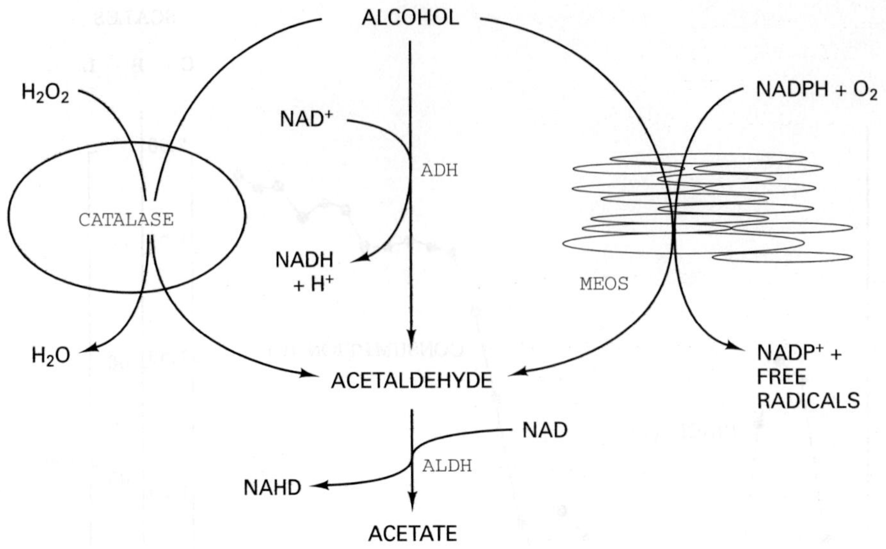


**Fig. 31.4** Pathways for alcohol metabolism in hepatocytes.

Orientals (Yoshida et al 1988). The $\gamma_1$ homodimer is more active in alcohol catabolism than the $\gamma_2$ homodimer.

ALDH is located in both the cytoplasm and the mitochondria of hepatocytes. The gene for cytosolic ALDH (ALDH1) is located on the long arm of chromosome 9, whereas the gene for the mitochondrial form (ALDH2) is located on the long arm of chromosome 12 (Hsu et al 1986). A single nucleic acid base substitution in ALDH2, producing a glutamine to lysine substitution, results in a catalytically inactive form of acetaldehyde dehydrogenase. This mutation occurs in approximately 50% of Orientals and is responsible for the flushing reaction produced by alcohol in this ethnic group (Yoshida et al 1988). The relative importance of cytosolic and mitochondrial ALDH in the metabolism of acetaldehyde is still debated, although the balance would favor the high-affinity mitochondrial form.

Within the gastric mucosa at least three different forms of ADH exist with varying activities in ethanol catabolism. The activity of gastric ADH may reduce the systemic bioavailability of ethanol and hence its harmful systemic effects (Lieber 1994). There is ethnic variation in the expression of the different gastric isoenzymes and inhibition of ADH in the stomach can occur following chronic alcohol consumption and ingestion of aspirin or $H_2$ receptor antagonists such as cimetidine and ranitidine (Seitz et al 1993). Interestingly, *Helicobacter pylori* expresses ADH but not ALDH, suggesting acetaldehyde could perhaps play a pathogenic role in the mucosal damage induced by this organism (Salmela et al 1993).

**The microsomal ethanol oxidizing system** (Lieber 1987, 1988a, 1994)

Proliferation of the endoplasmic reticulum following chronic ethanol consumption in man and experimental animals suggested a microsomal pathway for ethanol metabolism (p. 839). This microsomal ethanol oxidizing system (MEOS) was characterized further by reconstitution of its activity in vitro using NADPH-cytochrome P-450 reductase, phospholipids and purified microsomal P-450 from rats. Although several cytochrome P-450 isoenzymes are capable of ethanol oxidation, cytochrome P-450IIE1 (CYPIIE1) is most specifically induced by ethanol consumption. Human CYPIIE1 has been purified in a catalytically active form; it has a high turnover rate for ethanol, but its Km (Michaelis constant: the substrate concentration at which an enzyme is working at half maximum velocity for any given substrate concentration) is higher (10–15 mM) than that of many ADH isoenzymes (0.2–2 mM), implying that the latter pathway is quantitatively most important at low blood ethanol concentrations. The MEOS utilizes NADPH and oxygen with the production of acetaldehyde, NADP and free radicals during ethanol catabolism. CYPIIE1 is also capable of metabolizing other higher aliphatic alcohols (e.g. acetone), carbon tetrachloride, paracetamol and other drugs, dimethylnitrosamine and other carcinogens, androgenic steroids and certain fat-soluble vitamins. The gene for CYPIIE1 is located on chromosome 10 and demonstrates developmental and tissue-specific expression. Induction of CYPIIE1 by ethanol occurs after short-term light alcohol consumption and in humans is associated with increased CYPIIE1 mRNA levels (Takahashi et al 1993).

**Catalase**

Catalase is located primarily in the peroxisomes and mitochondria of cells. In the presence of hydrogen peroxide catalase oxidizes ethanol, producing acetaldehyde and water. Because of low endogenous production of hydrogen peroxide, the catalase pathway does not contribute to the overall rate of ethanol metabolism under physiological conditions (Peters 1982).

### Nonoxidative pathways

A nonoxidative pathway of ethanol catabolism that produces fatty acid ethyl esters has been identified in the pancreas, liver, heart and adipose tissue (Laposata & Lange 1986). This pathway is of minor importance in the liver because of the large metabolic capacity of the dehydrogenases and MEOS. However, other tissues such as the heart lack the ADH and MEOS pathways and the disruptive effects of fatty acid ethyl esters on membrane function may contribute to the development of alcoholic cardiomyopathy.

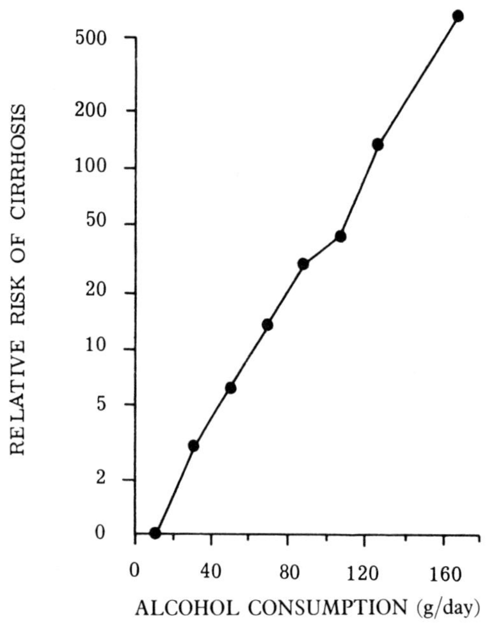


**Fig. 31.5** The relative risk of developing cirrhosis of the liver with increasing daily alcohol consumption (Pequignot et al 1978).

## PATHOGENESIS OF ALCOHOLIC LIVER DISEASE

Studies in experimental animals and in man have proven conclusively that ethanol per se is hepatotoxic (Rubin & Lieber 1968). The mechanisms mediating the hepatotoxicity are not understood fully, but there are several potential pathogenetic mechanisms that could account for the spectrum of liver pathology including fatty liver, hepatitis and cirrhosis (Lieber 1988b, 1993, Sherman & Williams 1994).

**Table 31.2** Frequency (%) of development of cirrhosis over 10–13 years in 258 men drinking more than 50 g alcohol daily related to initial liver biopsy findings (Sørensen et al 1984)

| Normal | Fatty change | | | Alcoholic hepatitis |
|---|---|---|---|---|
| | Slight | Moderate | Severe | |
| 5.6 | 11 | 19 | 28 | 50 |

### Alcohol

The form in which alcohol is taken is not important, as liver damage may result from beer, wines or spirits. Congeners and other additives play at most a very limited part. The amount and duration of alcohol ingestion are the most important factors in animal experiments and man. Cirrhosis can be produced in chronic (up to 7 years) ethanol-fed baboons and bridging fibrosis and hepatitis occur in rats fed ethanol and a high-fat diet for 16 weeks. In humans, increased risk of hepatic cirrhosis can be detected at a daily alcohol intake above 40 g/day (Fig. 31.5) and the risk of cirrhosis is increased 25 times when consumption exceeds 100 g/day (a third of a bottle of spirits). In women, an increased risk of cirrhosis can be detected at lower daily alcohol intakes of between 20 and 40 g/day. The duration and pattern of drinking is also important in humans. It may take 10–25 years to produce symptomatic cirrhosis and continuous alcohol ingestion seems more likely to produce cirrhosis than episodic bouts of drinking.

The amount and duration of drinking may not, however, be the only factors involved. Sørensen et al (1984) have reported a 10–13-year follow-up of liver histology in men who consumed alcohol to excess. Cirrhosis developed in about 2% of their patients annually and this was related to the findings on initial liver biopsy rather than to the degree or duration of drinking (Table 31.2). They concluded that alcohol does not cause cumulative effects as such but rather establishes conditions favorable to the development of cirrhosis. It has long been recognized that only a small proportion of heavy drinkers develop cirrhosis and this study has emphasized the importance of factors other than alcohol in the development of cirrhosis.

### Acetaldehyde

Acetaldehyde is generated by the metabolism of ethanol via the dehydrogenase, MEOS and catalase pathways. It can also be produced by other endogenous metabolic pathways and by micro-organisms within the gut that produce acetaldehyde from dietary sugars. Further catabolism in the liver is dependent on the action of two different aldehyde dehydrogenases, as discussed above.

Acetaldehyde is a very reactive molecule with a high affinity for sulfhydryl groups, allowing it to bind to a variety of intracellular proteins (Lieber 1994). It can impair enzyme function by forming Schiff bases with sulfhydryl groups in the active sites of several enzymes. Acetaldehyde can also reduce enzymatic activity by displacement of the cofactor pyridoxal phosphatase or by enhanced enzyme degradation. Similarly, binding of acetaldehyde to intracellular and plasma membranes interferes with mitochondrial and Golgi function, disrupting hepatocyte energy production and the export of proteins and lipids.

Acetaldehyde also enhances lipid peroxidation and interferes with protective mechanisms in cells, including interfering with glutathione synthesis and reducing the activity of free radical scavenging enzymes such as superoxide dismutase. Hepatic iron accumulation, often associated with chronic ethanol abuse, also serves to enhance free radical production (Kawase et al 1989, Kamimura et al 1992). Binding to cell membrane proteins can result in the formation of neoantigens, seen as foreign by the immune system, which may generate an autoimmune response (Koskinas et al 1992, Holstege et al 1994). Acetaldehyde can also directly interfere with cellular and humoral immune mechanisms. Interaction between acetaldehyde and nuclear histones can result in transcriptional activation of hepatocyte collagen genes and the production of fibrosis (Parés et al 1994).

## NADH generation

During ethanol catabolism via the dehydrogenase pathway, NAD is converted to NADH. This results in an increased intracellular NADH/NAD ratio, or redox (reduction-oxidation) potential, which has been implicated in the lactic acidosis, hyperuricemia and ketonemia that can occur following ethanol consumption. It has also been implicated in impaired gluconeogenesis, with the risk of subsequent hypoglycemia, reduced protein synthesis and reduced metabolism of galactose, serotonin and other vasoactive amines (Lieber 1994).

It has been suggested that the increased NADH/NAD ratio is also implicated in the pathogenesis of alcoholic fatty liver, the excess NADH directly stimulating endogenous hepatic fatty acid synthesis and increasing the concentration of $\alpha$-glycerophosphate, which is a precursor for triglyceride synthesis. However, recent studies have shown clearly that changes in the hepatocyte redox potential are attenuated with continued alcohol consumption and are not responsible for the production of hepatic steatosis. Alcoholic fatty liver arises primarily from enhanced triglyceride synthesis (Day et al 1993, Simpson et al 1994) and impaired secretion of triglyceride-rich very low density lipoproteins (VLDL) secondary to defective microtubular function (Venkatesan et al 1988, Simpson et al 1990). Although fatty acid oxidation is depressed in alcoholics and alcohol-fed animals, this is quantitatively only a minor pathway in the metabolism of fatty acids.

## Malnutrition

Although ethanol can be regarded as a dietary component, its contribution to nutrition is solely as a source of energy (1 g = 7.1 kcal) and therefore in excess it tends to produce obesity. Alcoholics may obtain 50% of their total calorie intake from alcohol, often at the expense of other dietary components. The intake of calories from sources other than alcohol is often lowest in those with the most severe liver disease (Mendenhall et al 1984).

Alcoholism and malnutrition often coexist, the latter being multifactorial (Table 31.3). This has led to a debate on the relative contributions of malnutrition and hepatotoxic effects of ethanol in the pathogenesis of liver disease. Early work showed that alcoholic liver damage in humans could improve in spite of continued alcohol intake provided that an adequate diet was taken simultaneously (Morgan 1982) and experimental work showed that alcohol could produce cirrhosis in rats if a diet deficient in such factors as choline was given and that correcting these deficiencies could reverse the cirrhosis in spite of continuing alcohol intake (Hartroft & Porta 1973). However, the particular nutritional circumstances causing cirrhosis in rats do not pertain to humans. Furthermore, nutritional deficiencies are not inevitable in alcoholic cirrhosis and they may develop more as a consequence than a cause of chronic liver disease.

Recently more emphasis has been placed on the direct hepatotoxic effects of alcohol on the liver. Isocaloric substitution of alcohol for dietary carbohydrate, while maintaining a normal protein intake, causes fat accumulation and typical electronmicroscopic changes in the mitochondria and endoplasmic reticulum in the livers of normal humans within a few days. These changes occur at blood alcohol concentrations below 16 mmol/L (80 mg/dl) and cannot be prevented by a high-protein diet (Lieber & Rubin 1968). Similar long-term experiments in well-fed baboons have led to the production of fatty liver, fibrosis and cirrhosis (Lieber et al 1985). While others have found these results difficult to reproduce, most workers now believe that in humans alcohol is itself hepatotoxic and does not act by inducing nutritional deficiency. This does not, of course, imply that nutritional deficiency in alcoholic cirrhosis is of no importance.

**Table 31.3** Causes of malnutrition in alcohol abuse

| |
|---|
| Social disintegration |
| Anorexia |
| Malabsorption |
|    Small intestinal damage |
|    Pancreatic dysfunction |
|    Biliary dysfunction |
|    Motility disturbances |
| Impairment of nutrient storage and metabolism |
| Increased nutrient losses |

### Immune-mediated injury

A number of abnormalities of humoral and cellular immunity have been described in patients with alcoholic liver disease (p. 770), but it is not yet known to what extent they are causative or simply epiphenomena (Paronetto 1993). Increased production, rather than reduced clearance, is involved in the increased IgA and IgG concentrations often observed (p. 747). Increased circulating tumor necrosis factor (TNF) α, interleukin 1, interleukin 6 and other cytokines have been identified in alcoholic hepatitis and may be involved in hepatic and extrahepatic tissue damage (Bird et al 1990a, Khoruts et al 1991). Increased circulating and hepatic levels of chemotactic cytokines (e.g. interleukin 8) also occur in alcoholic hepatitis (Sheron et al 1993). Adhesion molecules, important in directing circulating white cells to sites of inflammation, are expressed in infiltrating leukocytes and hepatocytes in patients with alcoholic hepatitis (Chedid et al 1993). Immunohistochemical studies have also revealed increased hepatic expression of HLA antigens on cytotoxic T-lymphocytes mediating cellular injury. There is continuing debate regarding the stimulus for these abnormalities and the formation of acetaldehyde–protein adducts and Mallory's hyaline seems the most likely explanation at present (Koskinas et al 1992, Yokoyama et al 1993, Holstege et al 1994).

### Coexistent hepatotrophic virus infection

Several studies have identified increased frequency of serological markers of present or previous hepatitis B virus infection in patients with alcoholic liver disease, although this is not by any means a universal finding (Villa et al 1982, Saunders et al 1983). More recently, it has been recognized that, depending upon the country of origin of the study, a proportion of patients with alcoholic liver disease have coexistent hepatitis C virus infection (Zignego et al 1994). It is not yet clear from epidemiological data to what extent these viral infections are important in the development of irreversible alcoholic liver disease, but it is clear that for the individual the concurrence of hepatitis B or hepatitis C virus infection and heavy drinking has a synergistic effect in accelerating disease (Parés et al 1990, Fong et al 1994). It may also be critically relevant to the development of hepatocellular carcinoma in some patients.

### Disordered collagen metabolism

During alcohol consumption, the balance between synthesis and degradation of extracellular matrix components is altered to favor fibrogenesis. This results in accumulation of fibril-forming collagens and fibronectin in the subendothelial space of Disse which, with continued damage, progresses to cirrhosis.

The hepatic stellate cell (p. 714) has been recognized as the major source of extracellular matrix during chronic liver injury, with smaller contributions from endothelial cells and hepatocytes (Friedman 1993, Clément et al 1993, Gressner 1994). Many different forms of liver injury activate these cells, transforming them from their resting phenotype into myofibroblast-like (or transitional) cells. This activation occurs in at least two steps called initiation and perpetuation. During initiation, the cells enlarge, lose vitamin A, synthesize rough endoplasmic reticulum and express smooth muscle actin. They then express a variety of cytokine and growth factor receptors on their surfaces and therefore are more responsive to stimulation. The mechanisms of stellate cell initiation remain unclear but may involve a variety of stimuli including Kupffer cell, hepatocyte, lymphocyte and platelet-derived factors, lipid peroxidation, platelet-derived growth factor and transforming growth factor β1. Acetaldehyde and the lipid peroxides produced during ethanol metabolism also stimulate activated stellate cells to synthesize and secrete collagen (Lieber 1994). In addition, impaired release of proteinases and increased release of proteinase inhibitors leading to increased production and reduced degradation of collagen may contribute to fibrogenesis (Li et al 1994).

Collagen deposition in the space of Disse contributes to portal hypertension and helps to perpetuate injury by diminishing hepatocyte nutrient supply. Necrosis in the most hypoxic area of the lobule around the central vein (p. 712) leads to fibrosis (sclerosing hyaline necrosis) and portal hypertension. Bridging fibrosis between the portal tracts and central veins following alcoholic hepatitis disrupts the normal cellular and vascular structure of the liver so that hepatocyte regeneration takes a nodular form leading to the end-stage disease (cirrhosis). Recent studies by Worner & Lieber (1985) in baboons have suggested that collagen deposition around central veins may herald cirrhosis even in the absence of a frank "alcoholic hepatitis".

### Genetic susceptibility

Genetic predisposition to alcoholic liver disease must involve multiple genes that increase or reduce susceptibility to ethanol-induced damage. In most instances these genes become clinically important only when patients also have a genetic predisposition to alcoholism. Familial and adoption studies have shown a concordance for alcoholic cirrhosis in monozygotic and dizygotic twins (Ball & Murray 1994). Certain ethnic groups, such as those from the Indo-Pakistan subcontinent, also have an increased genetic susceptibility to alcoholic liver disease (Mendenhall et al 1989).

Recent studies have focused on the different isoenzymes of alcohol dehydrogenase and acetaldehyde dehydrogenase, ADH and ALDH (Day et al 1991, Poupon et al 1992, Chao et al 1994, Lumeng & Crabb 1994, Tanaka et al 1996). Although studies to date have included only small numbers of patients, there is evidence that the more active forms of ADH, such as ADH $\beta_2$ homodimer (encoded by the gene ADH 2*2) and ADH $\gamma_1$ homodimer (encoded by the gene ADH 3*1), are protective with regard to the development of alcoholic liver disease in Chinese patients. In Caucasian alcoholics, the gene ADH 3*1 may actually increase the risk of developing alcoholic cirrhosis. Certainly, patients homozygous for the inactive form of ALDH (ALDH 2*2) experience an intense flushing reaction on drinking alcohol and are presumably "protected" from alcoholism by this adverse reaction. However, ALDH heterozygotes (ALDH 2*1/2*2) may be at higher risk of developing alcoholic liver disease.

Other studies of genetic susceptibility have examined the association (linkage) of certain restriction fragment polymorphisms within the alcohol metabolizing genes and alcoholic liver disease. Such polymorphisms arise when the specific DNA sequence (usually five nucleotide zones long) recognized by a restriction endonuclease enzyme is mutated or deleted. Alteration of the DNA sequence within the ADH2 gene, recognized by the restriction enzyme Pvu II, results in a change of the DNA fragments identified by an ADH2 probe from 5.1 kilobases (kb) to 3.1 and 2.9 kb. The latter restriction fragment polymorphism is significantly associated with alcoholic cirrhosis. Studies on HLA status and susceptibility have on the whole been disappointing and confusing. Earlier reports implicated HLA-B8 (Saunders et al 1982), but a recent meta-analysis has shown no correlation between alcoholic liver disease and HLA status.

### Sex and susceptibility

Women are more susceptible than men to the hepatotoxic effects of alcohol, developing cirrhosis at a younger age, following a shorter period of alcohol excess and at lower levels of alcohol consumption (Morgan & Sherlock 1977). This effect may be related to differences in body size and composition resulting in a lower volume of distribution for alcohol. There is evidence that the hormonal status of women may influence blood alcohol levels. Also, gastric ADH activity is reduced in women, which will result in increased systemic bioavailability of ethanol (Frezza et al 1990).

## PATHOLOGY

Alcohol abuse is associated with a remarkably diverse spectrum of pathological changes in the liver (MacSween & Burt 1986, Harrison & Burt 1993), ranging from minor subcellular abnormalities visible only on electronmicroscopy to fatty change, spotty necrosis, chronic hepatitis, active (micronodular) cirrhosis and end-stage (macronodular) cirrhosis. Hepatocellular carcinoma may complicate alcoholic cirrhosis.

There is a striking lack of correlation between the lesions seen on liver biopsy and the clinical features and laboratory indices. Patients may present for the first time with end-stage disease, cirrhosis can be present despite normal liver function tests and a significant proportion of heavy drinkers have no detectable liver pathology on light microscopy.

### Minimal change disease

Many heavy drinkers have no light microscopic abnormality in the liver but show organelle changes on electronmicroscopy, notably mitochondrial swelling with distortion of the cristae, increased bulk of smooth endoplasmic reticulum (reflecting the inducing property of alcohol) and a paucity of rough endoplasmic reticulum. These abnormalities do not necessarily imply damage to the liver cells but may be an adaptation to alcohol, as in the case of increased smooth endoplasmic reticulum which results from enzyme induction (p. 839).

### Steatosis

Alcohol abuse, obesity and diabetes mellitus are the three commonest causes of fatty change (p. 975) in the liver (Fig. 31.6). The liver can be grossly enlarged with up to 50% of its weight as fat. Fatty change is not usually regarded as precirrhotic, but deposition of fibrous tissue is sometimes seen around central veins and hepatocytes (Fig. 31.6) and there is evidence that this may progress to cirrhosis although less frequently than alcoholic hepatitis (Sørensen et al 1984).

The major accumulating lipids are triacylglycerol and esterified cholesterol (Cairns & Peters 1983) and accumulation occurs because of enhanced synthesis and reduced hepatic release of triacylglycerol-rich VLDLs (Lieber 1994). Characteristically, the fat accumulates as large droplets (macrovesicular steatosis) mainly around the central veins, this being relatively the most hypoxic area of the lobule (p. 712). Occasionally the fat accumulation is microvesicular (p. 977). Small foci of inflammatory cells surrounding fat-laden hepatocytes are called lipogranulomas (Fig. 31.7).

### Alcoholic hepatitis

Hepatitis may occur as a distinctive pathological picture in association with steatosis or established cirrhosis (Figs 31.8, 31.9). The principal features, which are predominantly centrilobular, comprise neutrophil infiltration around foci of hepatocyte necrosis (Fig. 31.8), changes in the hepatocyte cytoskeleton which may be seen as Mallory's hyaline (Fig. 31.9) and pericellular and perivenular fibrosis. Cholestasis is also common. Thrombosis and sclerosis of the central veins are characteristic features and, when

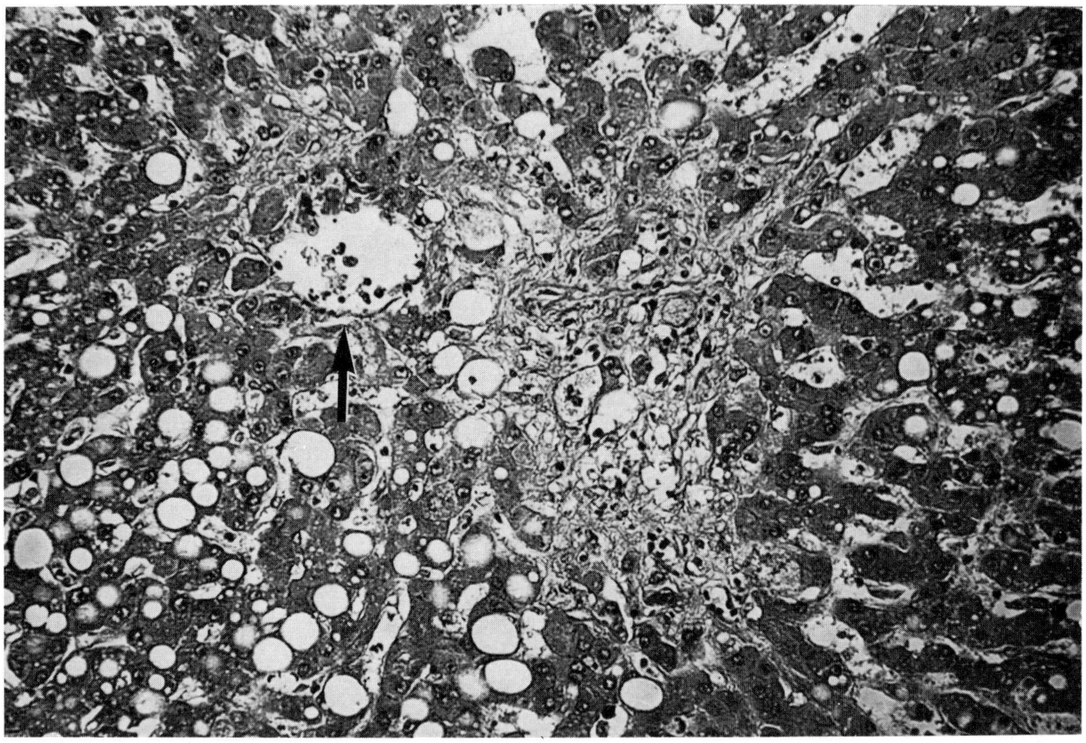

**Fig. 31.6** Central hyaline sclerosis and fatty change. Note the central vein (arrow) and an area of diffuse sclerosis containing neutrophils on its right and hepatocyte cytoplasm displaced by fat droplets (hematoxylin and eosin, ×10).

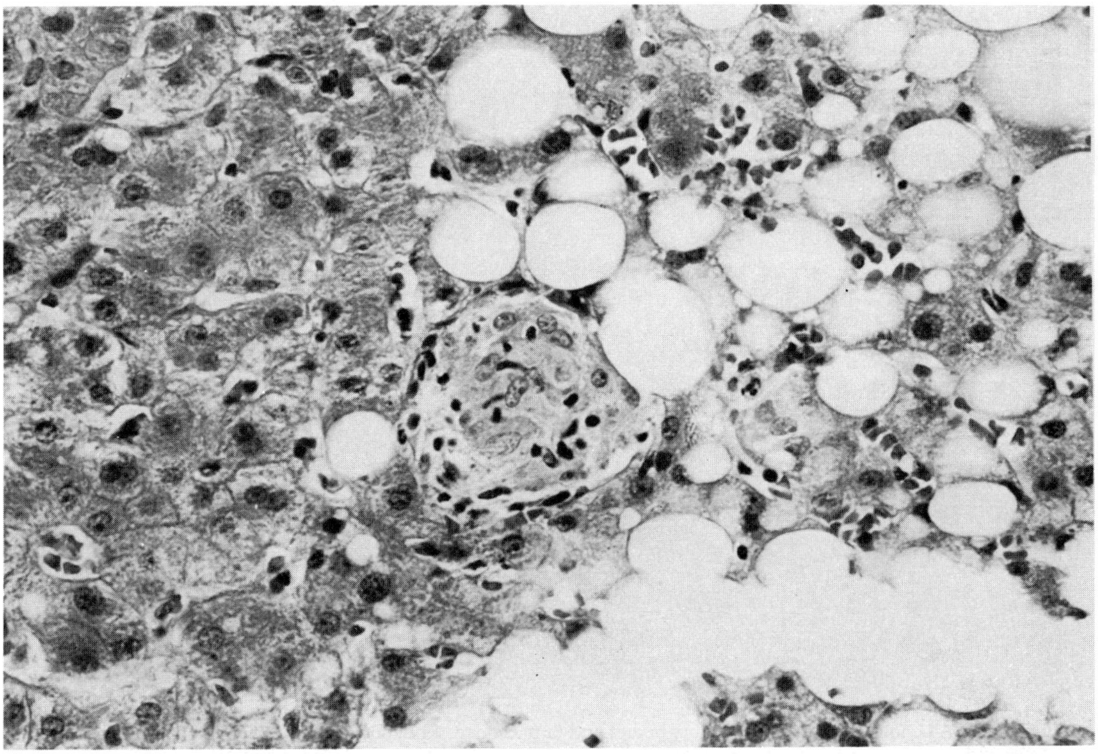

**Fig. 31.7** Granuloma formation (lipogranuloma) in a liver showing fatty change (hematoxylin and eosin, ×25).

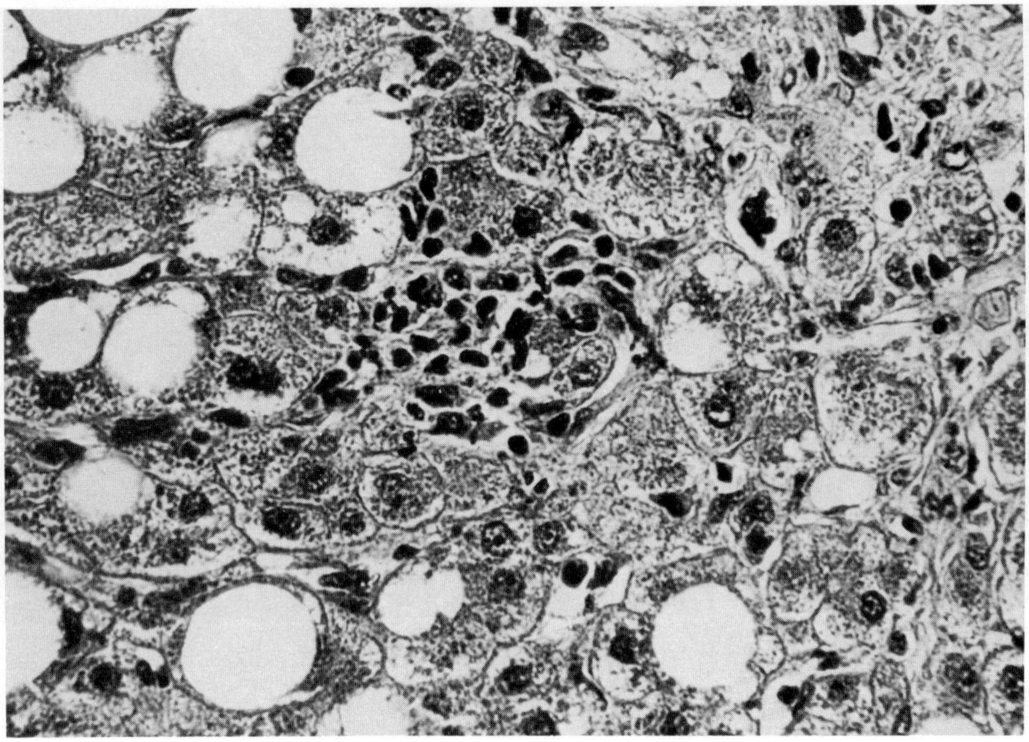

**Fig. 31.8** Alcoholic hepatitis and fatty change. Note central focus of "spotty" focal hepatocyte necrosis with a neutrophil reaction and hepatocyte cytoplasm displaced by fat droplets (hematoxylin and eosin, ×10).

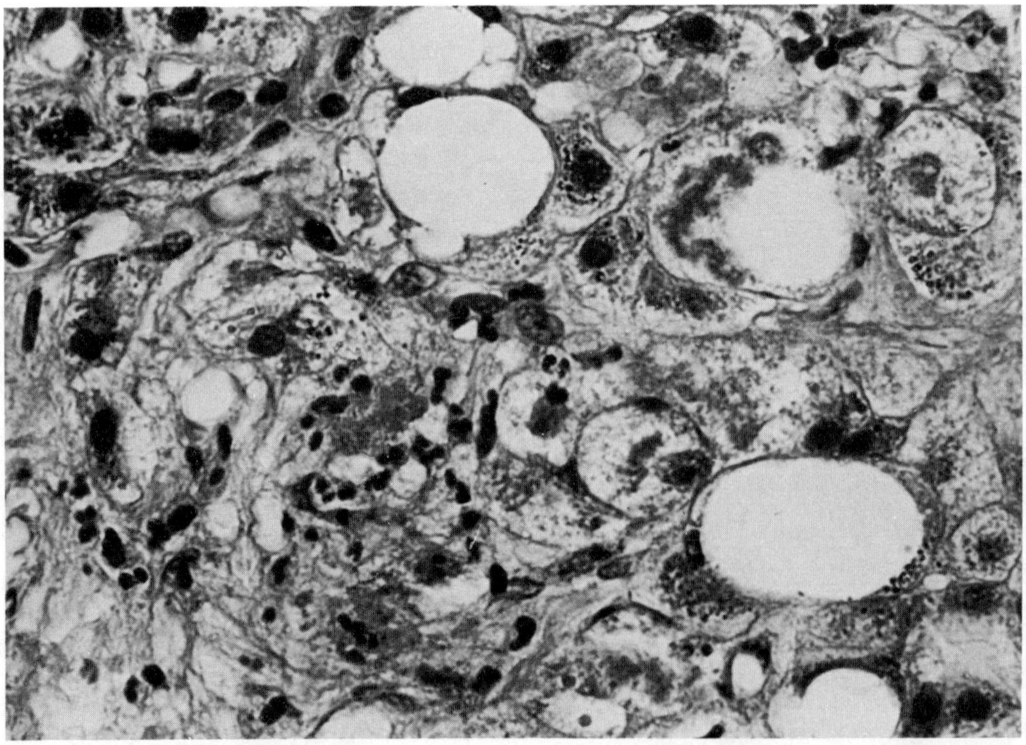

**Fig. 31.9** Alcoholic hepatitis with Mallory bodies and fatty change. Note flocculent intracellular deposits of Mallory's hyaline with a related neutrophil reaction and hepatocyte cytoplasm displaced by fat droplets (hematoxylin and eosin, ×25).

prominent, are termed sclerosing hyaline necrosis or central hyaline sclerosis (Fig. 31.6). They can cause portal hypertension, which may disappear if the lesions resolve, and accordingly can give rise to transient esophagogastric varices. Hyaline bodies or Mallory's hyaline (Fig. 31.9) are characteristic but not pathognomonic features of alcoholic hepatitis, as they may also be seen in drug-associated liver disease (e.g. griseofulvin, perhexiline maleate) and after jejunoileal bypass. The pathological lesions of alcoholic hepatitis occur much more frequently than the florid clinical picture and histological severity bears little correlation to clinical and biochemical features.

### Chronic hepatitis

Occasionally, chronic aggressive (interface) hepatitis with piecemeal necrosis and lobular hepatitis resembling autoimmune hepatitis is seen in alcohol abusers. A high proportion of these patients have serological markers of hepatitis B or C infection (Takase et al 1991).

### Cirrhosis

The gradual development of fibrous bridging between the central veins and portal tracts in a liver damaged by alcohol signals the onset of cirrhosis characterized by fibrous destruction of the lobular architecture and the formation of regenerating hepatocyte nodules with distorted vascular anatomy. Initially, and while drinking continues, the nodules are small ("micronodular cirrhosis") and usually readily recognizable on biopsy (p. 916). The liver is usually large with associated steatosis and other features such as Mallory's hyaline strongly suggest an alcoholic etiology. Deposition of iron in hepatocytes and Kupffer cells is common and may be so heavy as to make distinction from genetic hemochromatosis difficult (p. 958). With progression to a more inactive cirrhosis, especially if drinking lessens or ceases, development of a coarse, irregular pattern ("macronodular cirrhosis") occurs when the alcoholic etiology and even the diagnosis of cirrhosis itself may not be obvious on needle biopsy (Gluud et al 1987).

### Hepatocellular carcinoma

Hepatocellular carcinoma (HCC) develops in about 10% of patients with alcoholic cirrhosis (MacSween & Burt 1986), usually in those with a macronodular pattern. This parallels HCC developing in other forms of cirrhosis and reflects change resulting from the necroinflammatory state. However, some HCC in alcoholic cirrhosis has been shown to be associated with markers of previous hepatitis B virus infection and integration of hepatitis B virus DNA into the host genome. Recently, evidence has suggested that hepatitis C virus infection may be an even more significant precursor. Very occasionally, HCC has been reported in noncirrhotic liver and it has been suggested that this may arise from induction by alcohol of cytochrome P-450-CYPI-IE1 (p. 838), leading to altered metabolism of some as yet unrecognized carcinogen (Guengerich & Shimada 1993).

## DETECTION OF ALCOHOL ABUSE

It is now well known that a substantial proportion (up to 90%) of very heavy drinkers, both in the community and in hospital, remain unrecognized for a variety of reasons. The cost of this in preventable physical or psychiatric complications, wasted investigations and social and economic disaster is incalculable. The three principles of successful detection are a high index of suspicion, an awareness of situations, occupations and people at special risk, and the application of suitable and effective screening systems. Information obtained from patients, relatives and friends is generally most useful (Bernadt et al 1982).

### Clinical features

Many of the clinical features of alcohol abuse are nonspecific and may be detected in the history or the physical examination.

***History.*** Patients may present complaining of a variety of nonspecific symptoms such as nausea, anorexia, retching or vomiting (most commonly in the morning), vague abdominal pain or tenderness and diarrhea. The alcohol history is the single most important element in the detection of alcohol abusers but is frequently poorly performed or omitted, even by doctors with training in psychiatry (Barrison et al 1980, Farrell & David 1988). Doctors and nurses need training in obtaining an alcohol history, which can be difficult especially in patients who are reticent, guilty or frankly deceptive. The true situation often emerges only after a period of time during which the patient's confidence in the medical attendant increases.

Alcohol intake over a prolonged period of time should be assessed, as fluctuating intake can allow a patient to concentrate on periods of lesser intake. Apart from direct questioning on alcohol intake, specific alcohol questionnaires have been devised that may be "disguised" within general health/lifestyle questions (Bloor 1992). These include the rather unsatisfactory four questions of CAGE and the much more comprehensive Michigan questionnaire MAST (Selzer 1971, Mayfield et al 1974). Recently, a World Health Organization questionnaire has been devised, primarily for community use, called AUDIT (Alcohol Use Disorders Test) that gets over some of the inherent problems of such instruments (Babor et al 1989). Good patient rapport is essential for any successful history. Information gleaned from relatives and friends and the communication of information between medical attendants is often most revealing.

An attempt should be made to quantify intake (Table 31.4), but the pattern of drinking (continuous or

**Table 31.4** Average alcohol content of alcoholic drinks

| Form of alcohol | Alcohol concentration (%) | Volume per drink | Total alcohol content |
|---|---|---|---|
| Beers | | | |
| Ordinary | 3–5 | 500* | 20 |
| Special | 7–10 | 250* | 18 |
| Wine | | | |
| Table | 10 | 150 | 15 |
| Fortified | 20 | 60 | 12 |
| Spirits | 40 | 30† | 12 |

*Pint = 560 ml; can = 440 ml
†Equivalent to 1/5 gill

"binges") is almost as important as total intake in determining the harmful effects of alcohol. Prolonged, regular heavy drinking is more likely to be associated with alcoholic cirrhosis and pancreatitis, whereas heavy bout drinking is more characteristically associated with accidents, acute alimentary problems and stroke. It is widespread practice to assess quantity in units – somewhat arbitrarily defined as approximately 10 g of pure ethanol (Paton & Saunders 1981). Unit calculations have their limitations and there is still much debate on so-called "safe limits", an unfortunate term that implies safety up to an arbitrary level but takes no account of individual variation and susceptibility.†

***Physical examination.*** Apart from the obvious signs of liver disease and its complications, the careful observer may notice other pointers to alcohol abuse. These include evidence of personal neglect, suffused conjunctivae, plethoric facies with telangiectasia or acne rosaceae, breath smelling of alcohol (and acetaldehyde) or disguised by peppermint or scent, tachycardia with mild hypertension, tremulousness, excessive sweating and right upper quadrant tenderness on abdominal palpation.

## Laboratory investigation

Laboratory markers indicating hazardous levels of drinking have long been sought, because obtaining a history of alcohol abuse is often time consuming and can be misleading (Johnson & Williams 1985, Sharpe et al 1996). The alcohol history remains the most important single way of detecting alcohol abuse, but some useful laboratory aids have emerged.

### *Alcohol*

Alcohol can be measured directly most readily in the breath or blood. Unfortunately, random measurements in the clinic are of limited value in detecting alcohol abuse, as alcohol is found in the blood in only about a third of patients giving a history of heavy drinking (Hamlyn et al 1975). However, blood alcohol measurements are valuable in patients who deny drinking alcohol, as positive results establish that drinking is occurring and concentrations above 22 mmol/L (100 mg/dl) are highly suspicious of alcohol abuse (Criteria Committee 1972). Alcohol measurements should always be used to confirm a clinical impression that a patient is smelling of alcohol.

### *Macrocytosis and γ-glutamyl transferase*

The two most widely used markers of alcohol abuse are erythrocyte macrocytosis and increased serum γ-glutamyl transferase (GGT) activity. Both supplement the alcohol history, as neither is specific for alcohol abuse.

Macrocytosis is frequent in chronic alcoholism but can also occur in any form of chronic liver disease (Wu et al 1974). It is, however, more frequent and generally more marked in alcoholism than in chronic liver disease not caused by alcohol (Fig. 31.10). About a third of alcoholics with macrocytosis are folate deficient, but the macrocytosis cannot be corrected by giving folate and disappears only when drinking ceases.

Serum GGT activity is increased because of enzyme induction in up to three-quarters of heavy drinkers but can also be increased in many other forms of liver disease, by certain drugs, in hyperlipidemia and in some otherwise apparently normal people (p. 745). Enzyme activity is not increased by isolated episodes of heavy drinking (Dunbar et al 1982); increases generally require an intake above about 60 g daily (Chick et al 1981) and serum activities take some 1–2 months to fall when drinking ceases (Wadstein & Skude 1979). The GGT activity is usually increased two- to

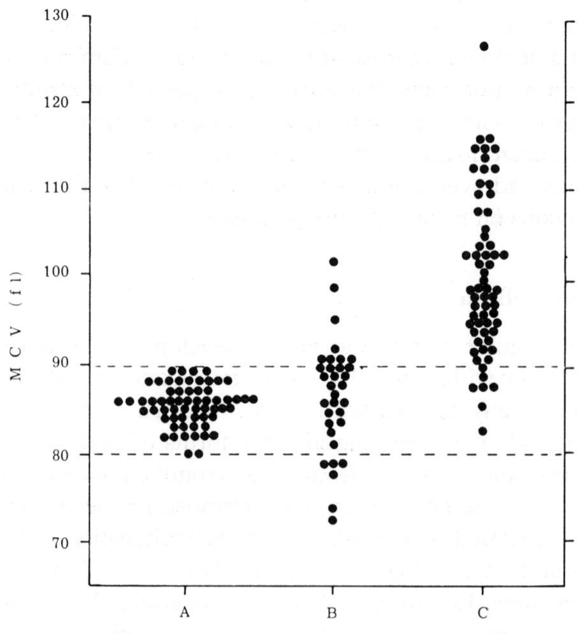


**Fig. 31.10** The erythrocyte mean corpuscular volume (MCV) in control subjects (A), in chronic liver disease not due to alcohol (B) and in alcoholic patients (C) (Wu et al 1974).

†The authors recommend the safe maximum weekly alcohol intake as 21 units for men and 14 units for women.

fourfold, but activities 20 times the upper normal value can occur. Elevated GGT is not predictive of significant liver damage, irrespective of the extent of the increase.

***Use in practice.*** The practical value of these two markers depends on the circumstances in which they are used and on the availability of information about the patient. Sensitivity is generally lowest when "low-risk" individuals are tested, as in health screening. "Higher risk" individuals such as general medical or psychiatric patients are more likely to have abnormal tests and sensitivities are higher. Several investigations have shown that discriminant function analysis using several measurements increases the capacity to detect heavy drinkers. Chalmers et al (1981) showed that a combination of the MCV, serum GGT and alkaline phosphatase activities could identify 80% of patients who had been drinking more than 80 g daily for over a year from those with a low alcohol intake or with liver disease not caused by alcohol. Discrimination resulted from the higher MCV and GGT activities in drinkers compared to the normal or slightly increased MCV and higher alkaline phosphatase activities in patients with nonalcoholic liver disease.

Overall, laboratory markers are useful in detecting alcohol abuse in patients but are relatively insensitive when used to screen otherwise well individuals. Skinner et al (1986) emphasized this point by finding that the medical history and clinical findings are more useful than laboratory findings in detecting alcohol abuse.

*Ferritin*

Plasma ferritin concentrations are increased in about a third of patients with alcoholic liver disease, especially alcoholic hepatitis and cirrhosis (p. 748). This is probably due partly to release of ferritin from damaged liver cells and to ferritin being an acute-phase protein. Ferritin concentrations can exceed 1000 μg/L, leading to confusion with genetic hemochromatosis, and sometimes alcoholic liver disease and hemochromatosis may coexist as hemochromatosis is relatively common (p. 953). The iron saturation of the plasma iron-binding capacity is usually less than 60% in alcoholic liver disease, but where serious doubt exists a liver biopsy and histological, or preferably biochemical, assessment of iron content and calculation of the quantitative iron index are needed (p. 956).

Noninvasive methods of assessing liver iron content such as imaging are not sufficiently sensitive to differentiate these two diseases (p. 67). The plasma ferritin concentration in alcoholic liver disease falls gradually on abstinence, usually with improvement of other markers of alcohol abuse, and may become normal, thereby excluding genetic hemochromatosis (Fig. 31.11).

*Other investigations*

The limitations of existing methods of detecting alcohol abuse have led to a search for more sensitive and specific laboratory markers (Bird 1993). Chronic alcohol misuse alters the sialic acid content of transferrin and isoelectric focusing has shown that the appearance of desialylated transferrin in the blood has a high sensitivity and specificity for detecting alcohol abuse in high-risk populations. Studies using different detection methods such as radioimmunoassay have suggested that elevated desialylated transferrin is a marker of alcoholic liver disease rather than simply of alcohol abuse (p. 747). Measurement of low molecular weight forms of plasma alanine aminotransferase (ALT) and the mitochondrial isoenzyme of aspartate aminotransferase (AST) is no more sensitive or specific than more commonly available tests in identifying heavy drinkers. However, the AST/ALT ratio may be helpful, for a ratio greater than one, particularly when combined with macrocytosis, is a sensitive indicator of alcoholic liver disease. Elevated serum apolipoprotein A1 (apo-A1) in heavy drinkers is suggestive of alcoholic steatosis and incorporation of apo-A1 measurements into a biological index with the prothrombin time and serum γ-glutamyl transferase may be useful in identifying cirrhosis in a group of patients who are heavy drinkers (Teare et al 1993). The finding of fractures of the ribs or clavicles on chest radiographs is associated with unsuspected alcoholism or alcoholic liver disease, but this is not a practicable screening test for alcohol abuse (Lindsell et al 1982, Johnson et al 1984).

## CLINICAL FEATURES AND PROGNOSIS

The clinical features of alcoholic liver disease are diverse and include nonspecific symptoms of alcohol abuse (p. 871) as well as features of liver damage (Brunt et al 1974, Levi & Chalmers 1978, Hislop et al 1983, Finlayson 1993). The relative frequency of individual clinical and biochemical features and their relation to particular pathological changes vary and the pathological changes of alcoholic liver damage can occur in various combinations. In general, women suffer more florid features of liver disease and clinical features of liver disease, such as spider telangiectasia, gynecomastia or liver failure, are seen more often in older patients and in those with advanced liver damage (Table 31.5).

Alcoholic liver disease can be divided for descriptive purposes into four main clinical syndromes – alcoholic fatty liver, alcoholic hepatitis, alcoholic cholestasis and alcoholic cirrhosis – but as with the histological features, these overlap with one another. Alcohol can also cause chronic hepatitis and alcoholic cirrhosis predisposes to hepatocellular carcinoma.

### General

Many patients with alcoholic liver disease are detected coincidentally at routine health checks, insurance exami-

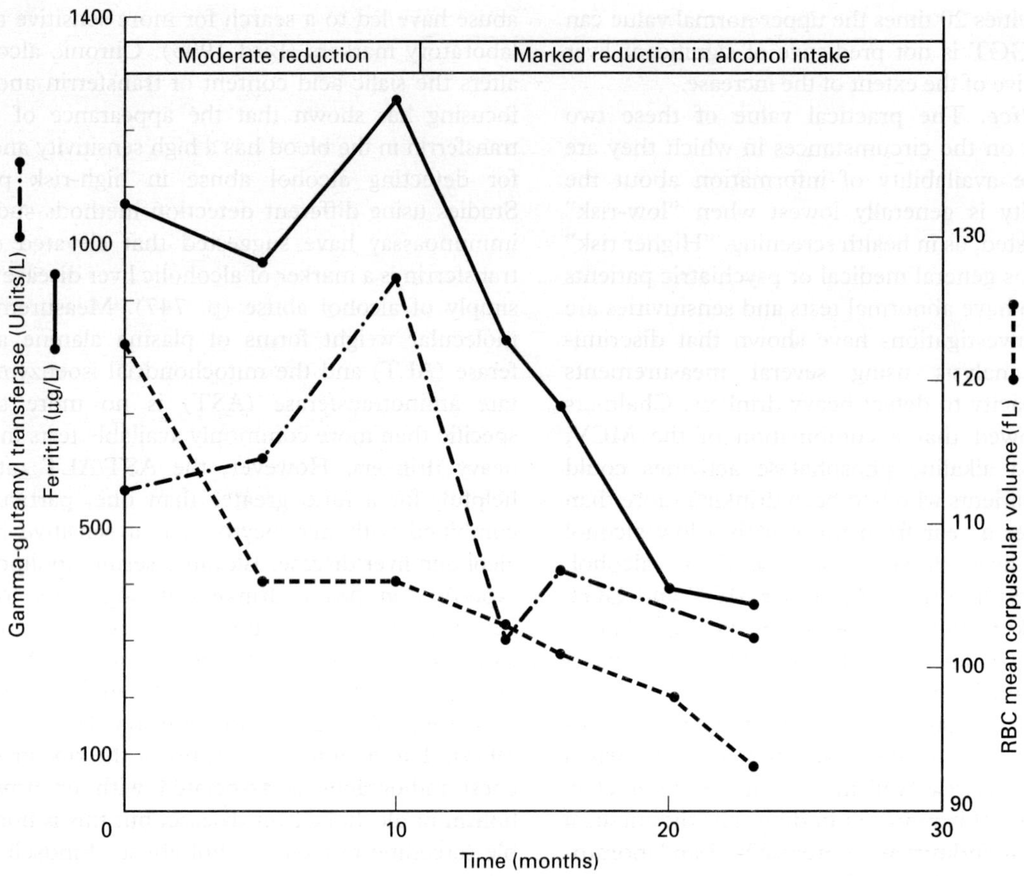


**Fig. 31.11** Changes in plasma ferritin, γ-glutamyl transferase and mean red blood cell volume in a patient with alcholic cirrhosis following marked reduction in alcohol intake (Royal Infirmary, Edinburgh).

**Table 31.5** Frequency of clinical and biochemical features at presentation in alcoholic liver disease related to initial liver histology. Statistical significance is related to the overall prevalence (Hislop et al 1983)

| Feature | Overall ($n$=510) | Fatty liver ($n$=222) | | Hepatitis ($n$=73) | | Active cirrhosis ($n$=3) | | Inactive cirrhosis ($n$=118) | |
|---|---|---|---|---|---|---|---|---|---|
| | % | % | *P* | % | *P* | % | *P* | % | *P* |
| Jaundice | 32 | 29 | <0.001 | 33 | — | 59 | <0.001 | 36 | <0.05 |
| Palmar erythema | 38 | 18 | <0.001 | 26 | — | 41 | <0.001 | 31 | — |
| Spider telangiectasia | 32 | 16 | <0.001 | 36 | — | 55 | <0.001 | 42 | <0.001 |
| Gynecomastia | 5 | 2 | <0.01 | 3 | — | 12 | <0.001 | 8 | — |
| Hepatomegaly | 83 | 71 | <0.001 | 86 | — | 98 | <0.001 | 91 | <0.01 |
| Splenomegaly | 9 | 5 | <0.01 | 7 | — | 13 | — | 16 | <0.01 |
| Ascites | 21 | 8 | <0.001 | 28 | — | 40 | <0.001 | 31 | — |
| Encephalopathy | 12 | 8 | <0.05 | 5 | — | 25 | <0.001 | 13 | — |
| Hyperbilirubinemia | 53 | 34 | — | 65 | <0.05 | 83 | <0.001 | 62 | <0.05 |
| Increased transaminase | 82 | 76 | <0.001 | 85 | — | 96 | <0.001 | 83 | — |
| Increased alkaline phosphatase | 56 | 44 | <0.001 | 64 | — | 77 | <0.001 | 58 | — |
| Hypoalbuminemia | 43 | 28 | <0.001 | 48 | — | 66 | <0.001 | 51 | <0.05 |
| Leukocytosis | 18 | 11 | <0.001 | 29 | — | 30 | <0.05 | 16 | — |

nations or assessments of unrelated problems when the most likely finding is hepatomegaly and subcostal tenderness. Even more common is the finding of an unexplained raised plasma aminotransferase or γ-glutamyl transferase activity or macrocytosis. Some patients present with another alcohol-related problem and alcoholic liver disease is then detected. These problems are many and varied, but the more frequent are given in Table 31.6. Nonspecific features of alcohol abuse (p. 871) are common and easily overlooked. Occasionally, alcoholic

**Table 31.6** Nonhepatic disorders induced by alcohol

| |
|---|
| Intoxication/withdrawal |
| Injury |
| Burns |
| Fractures |
| Subdural hematoma (p. 1051) |
| Epileptic fits |
| Encephalopathy |
| Delirium tremens (p. 1050) |
| Wernicke's encephalopathy (p. 1050) |
| Stroke |
| Peripheral neuropathy |
| Hematemesis – Mallery–Weiss tears (p. 490) |
| Hypertension |
| Cardiomyopathy |
| Atrial fibrillation |
| Cardiac failure |
| Pancreatitis |
| Opportunistic infection – tuberculosis |

liver disease presents acutely with alcoholic hepatitis or cholestasis following an alcohol binge. Finally, a patient with established but hitherto unrecognized liver disease can present with a complication such as jaundice, ascites, peripheral edema, hematemesis from varices, encephalopathy or an opportunistic infection, sometimes associated with a bout of drinking.

***Prognosis.*** It is important to see the prognosis of alcoholic liver disease in the wider context of alcoholism and to recognize that alcohol carries implications for health and survival well beyond the liver. Alcohol, perhaps particularly wine, consumed within so-called safe limits (p. 872) may have a beneficial effect on survival by reducing deaths from vascular disease (Grønbaek et al 1995), but heavier intake undoubtedly increases mortality. The 10-year mortality in those drinking more than 40 units of alcohol weekly is twice that of those drinking less than 20 units weekly and those drinking 20–40 units weekly show a 50% increased mortality by comparison with those drinking less than 20 units weekly (Klatsky et al 1981). The major causes of increased mortality are accidents, cancer, hepatic cirrhosis and respiratory disease.

Controversy has surrounded the value of abstinence in altering the prognosis of alcoholic liver disease. Most have found that abstinence improves survival (Borowsky et al 1981, Saunders et al 1981), but others have not (Pande et al 1978). The present authors have found that few patients who continue to drink heavily do well and consider that abstinence is the best advice for patients.

## Alcoholic steatosis

Fatty change is the commonest form of alcoholic liver disease and is characterized by hepatomegaly, which is sometimes massive and may be accompanied by tenderness. It is commonly symptomless and not usually associated with signs of chronic liver disease, liver failure or portal hypertension. Liver function tests show mild or moderate elevation of transaminase or γ-glutamyl transferase activity, but indices of synthetic function (albumin, prothrombin time) are normal.

***Prognosis.*** Alcoholic steatosis usually resolves within a few months of becoming abstinent and consequently alcoholic steatosis is regarded generally as a benign condition. This is not entirely the case. Progressive liver failure and cholestasis leading to death may occur, usually in generally ill and malnourished patients (Morgan et al 1978), and some less ill patients show signs of significant liver dysfunction such as ascites or hypoalbuminemia (Table 31.5). Long-term follow-up has shown that alcohol abuse carries 2–5 times the risk of developing cirrhosis over 10 years where fatty liver is present as compared to a normal liver (Table 31.2) and survival over 10 years in alcoholic fatty liver is about 70%, which represents a mortality about twice that in the general population (Bouchier et al 1992). Sudden and unexpected death associated only with severe steatosis has long been recognized by forensic scientists but is less well known to clinicians (Randall 1980, Clark 1988). Alcohol abuse is the most common background factor in such cases, but the immediate causes of death are speculative and may include such factors as hypoglycemia, hypomagnesemia and fat embolism. Only a minority of such individuals have had prior contact with medical services.

## Alcoholic hepatitis

This is a much more serious condition than alcoholic steatosis and carries a substantial mortality, particularly in females, of up to 40%. It usually follows heavy drinking, especially when nutrition is impaired, and presents with anorexia, vomiting, upper abdominal pain, jaundice, hepatomegaly and clinical signs of liver failure. A hemorrhagic diathesis is common, ascites is often present and splenomegaly may point to portal hypertension. The liver is often tender. An audible systolic bruit may be heard over the liver, which needs to be distinguished from a transmitted cardiac bruit (Fig. 31.12). The only other likely cause of a hepatic bruit is a hepatocellular carcinoma. Encephalopathy may supervene and create a difficult clinical problem, since other causes of clouding of consciousness and disturbed behavior occurring in such patients include alcohol withdrawal, delirium tremens, subdural hematoma, Wernicke–Korsakoff syndrome and hypoglycemia (p. 1050). Marked jaundice due to cholestasis can be severe and may be prolonged in spite of abstinence. Marked ascites without peripheral edema may be due to severe central venous damage (p. 868) causing clinical features suggesting veno-occlusive disease (p. 1081).

***Investigations.*** Fever is common and may be accompanied by neutrophil leukocytosis, sometimes of leukemoid proportions. This may reflect hepatic necrosis, but as

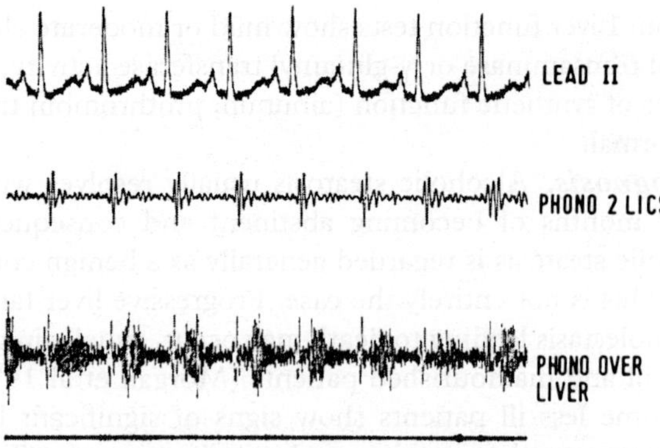


**Fig. 31.12** Phonographic recording of a bruit heard over the liver of a patient with acute alcoholic hepatitis. Simultanaeous electrocardiographic (lead II) and phonocardiographic (2 LICS = second left intercostal space) recordings show that the bruit did not originate from the heart (Royal Infirmary, Edinburgh).

opportunistic infections are important and easily overlooked in alcoholic hepatitis, it is essential to culture blood, ascitic fluid and urine (and, if necessary, cerebrospinal fluid) and to obtain a chest radiograph at the slightest suspicion of sepsis. A mild macrocytic anemia is common and occasionally an acquired sideroblastic anemia is found. Hemolysis can also occur, usually causing a mild anemia with reticulocytes of about 5% but occasionally causing severe anemia with spur cells and cell fragments in the blood. Thrombocytopenia is common and is due to a toxic effect of alcohol on the marrow that reverses on abstinence and to the hypersplenism of portal hypertension. The plasma bilirubin reflects the degree of jaundice and may exceed 100 mmol/L (6 mg/dl) in cholestatic patients. The plasma aminotransferase activities are rarely increased more than fourfold and alkaline phosphatase activity is moderately elevated (Fulop et al 1971). The plasma albumin is usually low, reflecting poor hepatic synthesis and hemodilution where fluid retention is present. Coagulopathy is due largely to synthetic failure of the liver-associated coagulation factors and the prolonged prothrombin time does not respond to vitamin K therapy. Hyponatremia is common but should not be corrected with saline since total body sodium is increased and ascites may be precipitated (p. 1025). The combination of a falling serum sodium concentration, oliguria and increasing uremia is a sign of very serious hepatic dysfunction and is rarely associated with survival. Hypokalemia, hypocalcemia and hypomagnesemia also occur and are due mainly to urinary electrolyte losses (De Marchi et al 1993). Hyperlipidemia with lipemic serum occurs but is uncommon (Zieve 1958). The plasma ferritin may be high and can exceed 1000 µg/L, but it falls with abstinence (Fig. 31.11). Occasionally hemochromatosis needs to be excluded (p. 956).

Imaging techniques, such as ultrasound and computed tomography, are mainly helpful in excluding alternative causes of liver disease or biliary obstruction, but claims that liver histology can be predicated from imaging are exaggerated (p. 54). Liver biopsy is diagnostic and can be carried out unless precluded by coagulopathy (p. 718).

***Prognosis.*** The prognosis for a particular episode of alcoholic hepatitis depends on its severity. Malnutrition, jaundice, fluid retention and encephalopathy are therefore all associated with a poor outlook. Laboratory investigations can also be a guide to prognosis. Mortality does not exceed a few percent when the prothrombin time remains normal, lengthening of the prothrombin time in the acute illness is associated with a mortality of around 20% and a third to a half of patients in whom the prothrombin time precludes biopsy without the aid of coagulation factors at any time die in the acute illness (Galambos 1972). More recently, it was found that a coagulation factor V below 15% of normal on admission to hospital was associated with an 87% mortality over the next 4 weeks (Pereira et al 1992). Alcoholic hyaline in the liver biopsy is associated with more severe hepatitis and in some series it has been related to an increased mortality (Harrison & Burt 1993). Maddrey has combined clinical and laboratory features to produce a prognostic discriminant function (discriminant function = 4.6 [prothrombin time-control] + [serum bilirubin in µmol/L/17.1]) and a value greater than 32 is associated with a 2-month mortality of 50% (Maddrey et al 1978, Carithers et al 1989).

The annual mortality for patients who recover from alcoholic hepatitis exceeds that of the general population. About a half of patients die within 10 years, which is 3–4 times the mortality of the general population (Bouchier et al 1992). More than half of this mortality is caused by liver failure or gastrointestinal hemorrhage. Ascites is associated with a particularly poor prognosis, but other factors, including the histological severity of the hepatitis, the extent of hepatic fibrosis and whether or not the patient stops or significantly moderates alcohol intake, also affect the outlook (Table 31.7). Conventional liver function tests are of little prognostic help.

## Cholestasis

Cholestasis is common in alcoholic hepatitis and may not

**Table 31.7** Factors related to long-term survival after acute alcoholic hepatitis (Galambos 1972)

| Factors | | Survival (%) 1 year | 5 years |
|---|---|---|---|
| Ascites | Absent | 98 | 66 |
| | Present | 62 | 38 |
| Hepatitis* | Mild | 81 | 67 |
| | Moderate | 76 | 48 |
| Fibrosis | Absent | 87 | 69 |
| | Moderate | 83 | 52 |
| Drinking | Moderate or stopped | 98 | 78 |
| | Unchanged | 84 | 50 |

*Judged from liver biopsy

resolve for weeks or months and in cirrhotic patients it signifies serious liver dysfunction and is not a good prognostic sign. Sometimes a cholestatic syndrome (p. 931) dominates the clinical picture in alcoholic liver disease and in this situation two conditions are important.

***Alcoholic pancreatitis.*** Advanced calcific pancreatitis can cause common bile duct obstruction either by compression or by stricture formation. Cholangitis with pain, fever and rigors is often recurrent (Scott et al 1977, Littenberg et al 1979). Anorexia, vomiting and malabsorption lead to considerable weight loss. The alkaline phosphatase is high and features of pancreatic dysfunction, such as glucose intolerance, may occur (p. 1271). Diagnosis is confirmed by endoscopic retrograde cholangiopancreatography or by percutaneous cholangiography (Fig. 31.13).

***Alcoholic cholestasis.*** This may occur occasionally, independently of alcoholic hepatitis, and is similar to drug-induced cholestasis (Fig. 31.14). It may be due to a direct toxic effect on hepatocytes. The diagnosis should be established by liver biopsy and, where doubt exists, by excluding obstruction of the large bile ducts at direct cholangiography. Laparotomy should be avoided as it may be fatal (p. 1138). Recovery usually occurs with abstinence.

### Alcoholic cirrhosis

The clinical features of alcoholic cirrhosis are similar to those of cirrhosis from other causes (p. 917). Dupytren's contracture, palmar erythema, spider telangiectasia and bilateral parotid enlargement are said to be more common in alcoholic cirrhosis, but this is unhelpful in individual patients.

***Prognosis.*** The prognosis in cirrhosis generally is poor, but patients often present with severe complications and those who survive this stage have a much better outlook (p. 925). The importance of abstinence has been questioned, but in general abstinence brings improved health and improvement in the clinical and biochemical features of liver disease (above). Sudden deterioration in a previously stable abstinent patient with alcoholic cirrhosis should raise the suspicion of hepatocellular carcinoma.

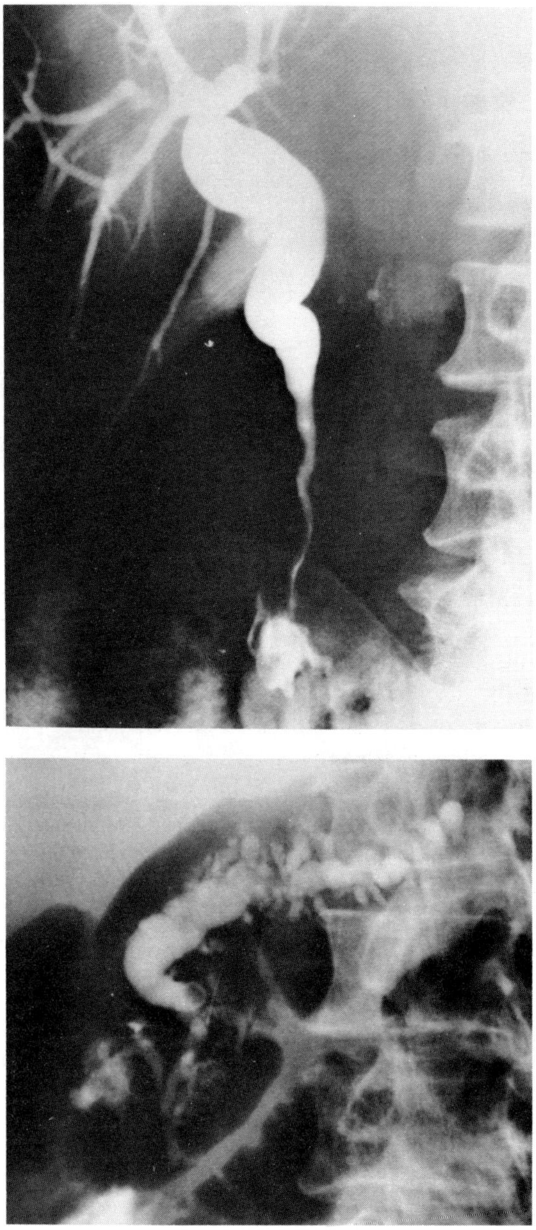

**Fig. 31.13** Transhepatic cholangiogram (*above*) in a patient with alcoholic pancreatitis and cholestatic jaundice showing a long, tapering biliary stricture due to the pancreatitis. Note the pancreatic calcification. Retrograde pancreatography (*below*) showed stricturing of the pancreatic duct, but the bile duct could not be cannulated. Findings confirmed at operation (Royal Infirmary, Edinburgh).

## TREATMENT

### Alcohol abuse

Treatment of alcohol abuse is the most important aspect of the therapy of alcoholic liver disease. Some patients show little alcohol dependence and stop drinking readily, but most have more difficulty and come to realize that they need help. Such help includes the continued encouragement and supervision provided by a follow-up clinic and any available support group for patients with liver disease as well as more specialized agencies for alcohol abuse. Psychiatric help is expensive and time consuming and limited counseling about drinking habits may be equally effective (Chick et al 1985). Help also needs to be extended to patients' families, as they are essential supports for the patients themselves. Abstinence rather than reduction of alcohol intake should be advised even though the latter will often be all that is achieved, as patients need to appreciate the central role of alcohol in liver damage. Abstinence is associated with improved general and social health as well as longer survival (Borowsky et al 1981, Saunders et al 1981).

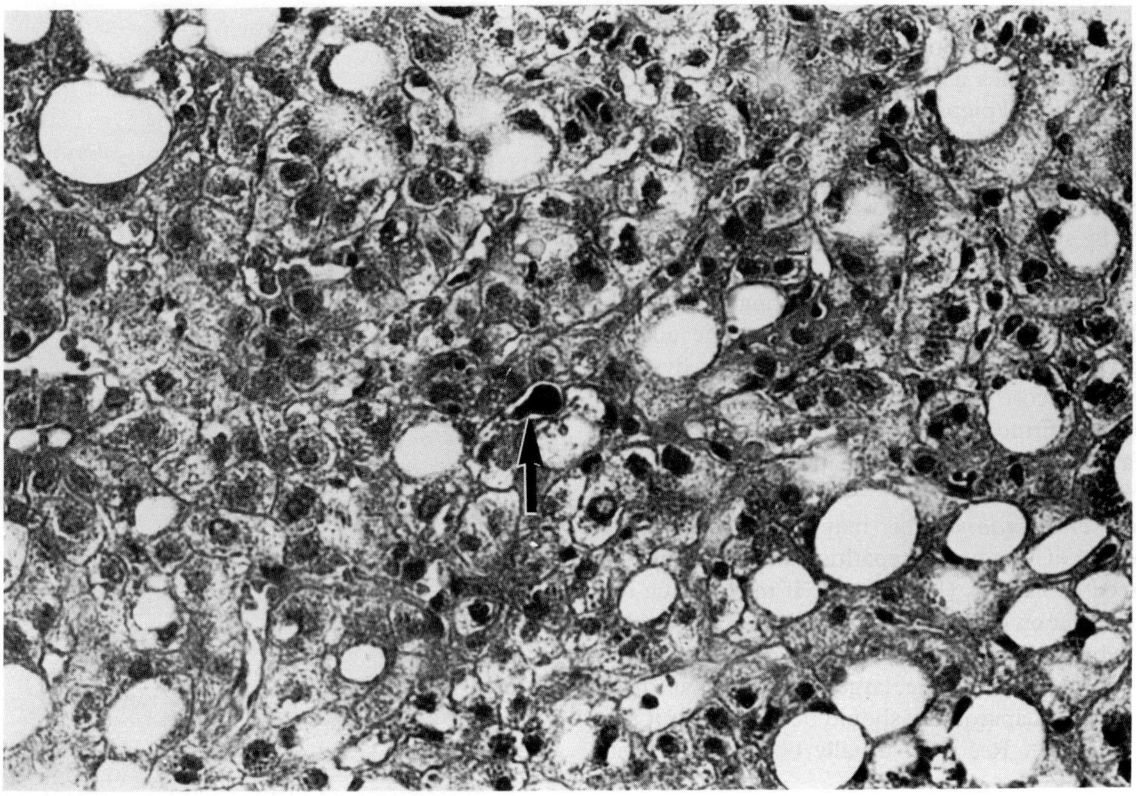

**Fig. 31.14** Alcoholic cholestasis and fatty change. Note intracanalicular bile plug (arrow) and hepatocyte cytoplasm displaced by fat droplets (hematoxylin and eosin, ×25).

## Alcoholic fatty liver

Abstinence from alcohol is the only effective treatment for alcoholic steatosis. Any nutritional deficiencies should be corrected. Following abstinence there is usually but not invariably a rapid clinical, biochemical and histological resolution.

## Hepatitis

Patients with less severe alcoholic hepatitis will respond to withdrawal of alcohol and correction of nutritional deficiencies, as in alcoholic steatosis. However, severe alcoholic hepatitis marked by spontaneous encephalopathy, jaundice or marked disturbance of hepatic synthetic function indicated by prolongation of the prothrombin time has a mortality of over 50% within 3 months and this has prompted a search for specific treatments. Unfortunately, except for the re-emergence of corticosteroids, no other medical therapy has proved useful. Treatment for alcohol withdrawal may also be needed (p. 1050).

### *Corticosteroids*

Despite initial encouraging reports of the use of corticosteroids in alcoholic hepatitis, subsequent publication of negative results, most persuasively the multicenter Veterans Administration Co-operative Study (Mendenhall et al 1984), led to waning interest in the use of corticosteroids in the 1980s. However, Carithers et al (1989) showed that 66 patients randomized to receive methyl prednisolone (32 mg daily for 28 days and then withdrawn over 14 days) in a double-blind study showed a significant improvement of mortality at 1 month compared with controls. Subsequently, a French multicenter randomized study of 61 patients treated with prednisolone 40 mg daily for 28 days showed a reduction in mortality at 66 days, with 16/29 dead (55%) in the placebo group and 4/32 (13%) dead in the prednisolone-treated group (Ramond et al 1992). This study included only patients with alcoholic hepatitis and severe disease established by liver biopsy and a discriminant function using the plasma bilirubin and prothrombin time and/or spontaneous hepatic encephalopathy.

These studies show there is a small group of patients with severe alcoholic hepatitis in whom short-term mortality is improved with corticosteroid treatment. However, such treatment is contraindicated in patients with concomitant viral hepatitis. In addition, complications of alcoholic hepatitis, such as gastrointestinal hemorrhage and local or generalized bacterial infection, must be adequately treated before the introduction of corticosteroid therapy.

*Nutritional therapy*

Many patients with alcoholic hepatitis are malnourished and feeding with as high a protein intake as can be tolerated seems reasonable. However, in the studies to date on the effect of intensive nutritional replacement, early mortality has not been reduced (Ramond et al 1993). However, there may be some long-term benefit from hyperalimentation (Schenker & Halff 1993).

*Other therapies*

Many other therapies have been used, but studies of their efficacy have not shown any reduction in mortality (Table 31.8). However, several of these studies, as with previous studies of corticosteroids, have not confirmed the diagnosis of alcoholic hepatitis histologically. This is important, as up to 20% of patients with clinical and biochemical indices suggestive of the diagnosis of hepatitis have coexistent cirrhosis. In addition, a proportion of patients with suspected alcoholic liver disease may on subsequent examination have disease due to other etiologies.

### Cirrhosis

Nutritional and vitamin deficiency should be corrected and a diet with an adequate caloric intake encouraged. Protein intake is particularly important in malnourished patients and intakes of 1.5 g/kg body weight can be achieved in the absence of encephalopathy with subsequent improvement in serum albumin and other indices of nutritional status. Oral branched chain amino acids do not confer any nutritional value over that provided by other sources of protein. Treatment of encephalopathy (p. 1051), gastrointestinal hemorrhage (p. 499) and ascites (p. 1023) is the same as in patients with other forms of cirrhosis.

Studies of medical therapy in alcoholic cirrhosis are scanty compared with those in alcoholic hepatitis. Several treatments have been tried and some have given promising results, but none can be recommended yet as standard. Colchicine inhibits the synthesis of collagen and increases its breakdown (p. 925). One controlled trial of 100 patients, of whom 45% had alcoholic cirrhosis, found that colchicine (1 mg daily for 5 days per week for a minimum of 3 years) was associated with significant improvement in survival (Kershenobich et al 1988). However, this trial has been criticized for the poor matching of control and treated patients, a high drop-out rate and failure to monitor abstinence. Trials of propylthiouracil (300 mg/day for 3 out of every 4 months over an average of 45 weeks) and silymarin (420 mg daily for periods up to 2 years) have shown improved mortality in the treatment groups compared with placebo (Orrego et al 1987, Ferenci et al 1989). Treatment with anabolic steroids such as testosterone have not shown any survival advantages and long-term treatment with prednisolone 10–15 mg/day was associated with an increased mortality in women (Juhl & Christensen 1985). More recently, treatment with polyunsaturated phosphatidylcholine reduced the development of fibrosis in alcohol-fed baboons (Lieber 1994). This treatment has not improved survival in alcoholic hepatitis (Panos et al 1990), but its effects in cirrhosis are awaited with interest. Ursodeoxycholic acid reportedly reduces circulating free radicals and improves liver function tests in patients with alcoholic cirrhosis (Plevris et al 1991). Clinical trials with 5-adenosyl L-methionine, a methyl donor and precursor of glutathione, are in progress.

Liver transplantation is now used for selected patients with alcoholic cirrhosis (Starzl et al 1988, Bird et al 1990b, Lucey 1993, Krom 1994), as survival rates compare favorably with liver transplantation undertaken for other causes of cirrhosis (p. 1153). Reversion to drinking postoperatively appears less common than might be expected and is in the order of 7–10%.

**Table 31.8** Other therapies used in the treatment of alcoholic hepatitis

| Therapy | References | Efficacy* |
|---|---|---|
| Insulin and glucagon | Baker et al 1981 | No difference |
| | Fehér et al 1987 | Significant difference |
| | Bird et al 1991 | No difference |
| Colchinine | Akriviadis et al 1990 | No difference |
| Propylthiouracil | Orrego et al 1979 | No difference |
| | Hallé et al 1982 | No difference |
| Silymarin | Trinchet et al 1989 | No difference |
| Penicillamine | Resnick et al 1974 | No difference |

*No difference = no significant differences in death rates between placebo and treatment groups

## PREVENTION

Alcohol abuse is a major burden on almost all "Western" societies and alcoholic liver disease is a significant part of this. Cirrhosis, much of it alcoholic, is now the third or fourth commonest cause of death in adult males in the United States. Hence, prevention presents a major challenge.

### Primary prevention

There is no doubt that reduction in alcohol intake is the cornerstone of preventive action. There is evidence that reducing overall consumption in society reduces the problems, including liver disease. Means to this end include tighter legal constraints, improved education, firmer controls on media portrayal and, perhaps most effective, increased fiscal (price) control. Attempts to prevent onset of liver damage by hepatoprotective agents have thus far proved disappointing, although as knowledge of the mechanisms of liver damage increases there are hopes for improved methods.

Identification of those at special risk is an important

opportunity for prevention. Pre-existing nonalcoholic liver disease, genetic susceptibility, including those at risk from hemochromatosis, and infection with the hepatitis B and C viruses all represent added hazards for those who consume alcohol.

## Secondary prevention

This involves the early recognition of dangerous drinking, followed by effective intervention. There is growing evidence that "minimal intervention" in the form of simple, structured advice that can be given by doctors, nurses or counselors is effective in many patients. In some, especially those with features of alcohol dependence, more formal and sustained support is necessary. This may involve alcohol problems clinics, alcohol councils, Alcoholics Anonymous and other agencies.

## Tertiary prevention

Much can be achieved by the early recognition and control of complications of alcoholic liver disease, including variceal hemorrhage, fluid retention and infection. Care in the prescribing of drugs and avoidance where possible of invasive investigation or treatment, such as surgery, are clearly important.

REFERENCES


Akriviadis E A, Steindel H, Pinto P C et al 1990 Failure of colchicine to improve short term survival in patients with alcoholic hepatitis. Gastroenterology 99: 811–818

Babor T F, La Fuente J R, Saunders J, Grant M 1989 Audit – the alcohol use disorders test. WHO MNH/DAT 89 4, World Health Organization, Geneva

Baker A L, Jaspan J B, Haines N W et al 1981 A randomized clinical trial of insulin and glucagan infusion for treatment of alcoholic hepatitis: progress report in 50 patients. Gastroenterology 80: 1410

Ball D M, Murray R M 1994 Genetics of alcohol abuse. British Medical Bulletin 50: 18–35

Barrison I G, Viola L, Murray-Lyon I M 1980 Do housemen take an adequate drinking history? British Medical Journal 281: 1040

Bernadt M W, Taylor C, Mumford J, Smith B, Murray R M 1982 Comparison of questionnaire and laboratory tests in the detection of excessive drinking and alcoholism. Lancet 1: 325–328

Bird G, Lau J Y N, Koskinas J, Wicks C, Williams R 1991 Insulin and glucagon infusion in acute alcoholic hepatitis: A prospective randomized controlled trial. Hepatology 14: 1097–1101

Bird G L A 1993 Investigation of alcoholic liver disease. Clinical Gastroenterology 7: 663–682

Bird G L A, Sheron N, Goka A K J, Alexander G J, Williams R 1990a Increased plasma tumor necrosis factor in severe alcoholic hepatitis. Annals of Internal Medicine 112: 917–920

Bird G L A, O'Grady J G, Harvey F A H, Calne R Y, Williams R 1990b Liver transplantation in patients with alcoholic cirrhosis: selection criteria and rates of survival and relapse. British Medical Journal 301: 15–17

Bloor R N 1992 Social drinker? Detecting and assessing alcohol problems. Hospital Update 18: 607–611

Borowsky S A, Strome S, Lott E 1981 Continued heavy drinking and survival in alcoholic cirrhotics. Gastroenterology 80: 1405–1409

Bouchier I A D, Hislop W S, Prescott R J 1992 A prospective study of alcoholic liver disease and mortality. Journal of Hepatology 16: 290–297

Brunt P W, Kew M C, Scheuer P J, Sherlock S 1974 Studies in alcoholic liver disease in Britain. I. Clinical and pathological patterns related to natural history. Gut 15: 52–58

Cairns S R, Peters T J 1983 Biochemical analysis of hepatic lipid in alcoholic and diabetic and control subjects. Clinical Science 65: 645–652

Carithers R L Jr, Herlong H F, Diehl A M et al 1989 Methylprednisolone therapy in patients with severe alcoholic hepatitis: a randomized multicenter trial. Annals of Internal Medicine 110: 685–690

Chalmers D M, Rinsler M G, MacDermott S, Spicer C C, Levi A J 1981 Biochemical and haematological indicators of excessive alcohol consumption. Gut 22: 992–996

Chao Y-C, Liou S-R, Chung Y-Y et al 1994 Polymorphism of alcohol and aldehyde dehydrogenase genes and alcoholic cirrhosis in Chinese patients. Hepatology 19: 360–366

Chedid A, Mendenhall C L, Moritz T E et al 1993 Expression of the β1 chain (CD29) of integrins and CD45 in alcoholic liver disease. American Journal of Gastroenterology 88: 1920–1927

Chick J, Kreitman N, Plant M 1981 Mean cell volume and gamma-glutamyl-transpeptidase as markers of drinking in working men. Lancet 1: 1249–1251

Chick J, Lloyd G, Crombie E 1985 Counselling problem drinkers in medical wards: a controlled study. British Medical Journal 290: 965–967

Christoffersen P, Nielsen K 1972 Histological changes in human liver biopsies from chronic alcoholics. Acta Pathologica et Microbiologica Scandinavica 80A: 557–565

Clark J 1988 Sudden death in the chronic alcoholic. Forensic Science International 36: 105–111

Clément B, Loréal O, Lavavasseur F, Guillouzo A 1993 New challenges in hepatic fibrosis. Journal of Hepatology 18: 1–4

Criteria Committee, National Council on Alcoholism, New York 1972 Criteria for the diagnosis of alcoholism. Annals of Internal Medicine 77: 249–258

Day C P, Bashir R, James O F W et al 1991 Investigation of the role of polymorphisms at the alcohol and aldehyde dehydrogenase loci in genetic predisposition to alcohol-related end-organ damage. Hepatology 14: 798–801

Day C P, James O F W, Brown A St J M, Bennett M K, Fleming I N, Yeaman S J 1993 The activity of the metabolic form of hepatic phosphatidate phosphohydrolase correlates with the severity of alcoholic fatty liver in human beings. Hepatology 18: 832–838

De Marchi S, Cecchin E, Basile A, Bertotti A, Nardini R, Bartoli E 1993 Renal tubular dysfunction in chronic alcohol abuse – effects of abstinence. New England Journal of Medicine 329: 1927–1934

Dufour M C, Stinson F S, Caces M F 1993 Trends in cirrhosis morbidity and mortality: United States 1979–1988. Seminars in Liver Disease 13: 109–125

Dunbar J A, Hagart J, Martin B, Ogston S, Devgun M S 1982 Drivers, binge drinking and gammaglutamyltranspeptidase. British Medical Journal 285: 1083

Edwards G, Peters T J (eds) 1994 Alcohol and alcohol problems. British Medical Bulletin 50: 1–234

Farrell M P, David A S 1988 Do psychiatric registrars take a proper drinking history? British Medical Journal 296: 395–396

Fehér J, Cornides A, Romány A et al 1987 A prospective multicenter study of insulin and glucagon infusion therapy in acute alcoholic hepatitis. Journal of Hepatology 5: 224–231

Ferenci P, Dragosics B, Dittrich H et al 1989 Randomized controlled trial of silymarin treatment in patients with cirrhosis of the liver. Journal of Hepatology 9: 105–113

Finlayson N D C 1993 Clinical features of alcoholic liver disease. Clinical Gastroenterology 7: 627–640

Fong T-L, Kanel G C, Conrad A, Valinluck B, Charboneau F, Adkins R H 1994 Clinical significance of concomitant hepatitis C infection in patients with alcoholic liver disease. Hepatology 19: 554–557

Frezza M, di Padova C, Pozzato G, Terpin M, Baraona E, Lieber C S 1990 High blood alcohol levels in women: role of decreased gastric alcohol dehydrogenase activity and first-pass metabolism. New England Journal of Medicine 322: 95–99
Friedman S L 1993 Seminars in medicine of the Beth Israel Hospital, Boston. The cellular basis of hepatic fibrosis: mechanisms and treatment strategies. New England Journal of Medicine 328: 1828–1835
Fulop M, Katz S, Lawrence C 1971 Extreme hyperbilirubinemia. Archives of Internal Medicine 127: 254–258
Galambos J T 1972 Alcoholic hepatitis: its therapy and prognosis. In: Popper H, Schaffner F (eds) Progress in liver diseases, Vol 4. Grune and Stratton, New York, p 567–588
Gluud C, Christoffersen P, Eriksen J, Wantzin P, Knudson B B and Copenhagen Study Group for Liver Diseases 1987 Influence of ethanol on development of hyperplastic nodules in alcoholic liver with micronodular cirrhosis. Gastroenterology 93: 256–260
Gressner A M 1994 Perisinusoidal lipocytes and fibrogenesis. Gut 35: 1331–1333
Grønbaek M, Deis A, Sørensen T I A, Becker U, Schnohr P, Jensen G 1995 Mortality associated with moderate intakes of wine, beer, or spirits. British Medical Journal 310: 1165–1169
Guengerich F P, Shimada T 1993 Human cytochrome P450 enzymes and chemical carcinogens. In: Jeffrey E H (ed) Human drug metabolism from molecular biology to man. CRC Press, Florida, p 5–12
Hall P D 1985 The pathological spectrum of alcoholic liver disease. Pathology 17: 209–218
Hallé P, Paré P, Kaptein E, Kanel G, Redeker A G , Reynolds T B 1982 Double-blind, controlled trial of propylthiouracil in patients with severe acute alcoholic hepatitis. Gastroenterology 82: 925–931
Hamlyn A N, Brown A J, Sherlock S, Baron D N 1975 Casual blood-ethanol estimations in patients with chronic liver diseases. Lancet 2: 345–347
Harrison D J, Burt A D 1993 Pathology of alcoholic liver disease. Clinical Gastroenterology 7: 641–662
Hartroft W S, Porta E A 1973 Alcohol, food factors and liver disease. Gastroenterology 64: 350–351
Hayes P C (ed) 1993 Alcoholic liver disease. Baillières Clinical Gastroenterology 7: 555–755
Hislop W S, Bouchier I A D, Allan J G et al 1983 Alcoholic liver disease in Scotland and northeastern England: presenting features in 510 patients. Quarterly Journal of Medicine 52: 232
Holstege A, Bedossa P, Poynard T et al 1994 Acetaldehyde-modified epitopes in liver biopsy specimens of alcoholic and nonalcoholic patients: localization and association with progression of liver fibrosis. Hepatology 19: 367–374
Holt S 1981 Observations on the relation between alcohol absorption and the rate of gastric emptying. Canadian Medical Association Journal 124: 267–271, 297
Hsu L C, Yoshida A, Mohandas T 1986 Chromosomal assignment of the genes for human aldehyde dehydrogenase-1 and aldehyde dehydrogenase-2. American Journal of Human Genetics 38: 641–648
Johnson R D, Williams R 1985 Prevention of hazardous drinking: the value of laboratory tests. British Medical Journal 290: 1849–1850
Johnson R D, Davidson S, Saunders J B, Williams R 1984 Fractures on chest radiographs as indicators of alcoholism in patients with liver disease. British Medical Journal 288: 365–366
Juhl E, Christensen E 1985 Anti-inflammatory and immunosuppressive treatment of alcoholic liver disease. Acta Medica Scandinavica 703 (suppl): 195–199
Kamimura S, Gaal K, Britton R S, Bacon B R, Triadafilopoulos G, Tsukamoto H 1992 Increased 4-hydroxynonenal levels in experimental alcoholic liver disease: association of lipid peroxidation with liver fibrogenesis. Hepatology 16: 448–453
Kawase T, Kato S, Lieber C S 1989 Lipid peroxidation and antioxidant defense systems in rat liver after chronic ethanol feeding. Hepatology 10: 815–821
Kershenobich D, Vargas F, Garcia-Tsao G et al 1988 Colchicine in the treatment of cirrhosis of the liver. New England Journal of Medicine 318: 1709–1713
Khoruts A, Stahnke L, McClain C J, Logan G, Allen J I 1991 Circulating tumor necrosis factor, interleukin-1 and interleukin-6 concentrations in chronic alcoholic patients. Hepatology 13: 267–276
Klatskin G 1961 Alcohol and its relation to liver damage. Gastroenterology 41: 443–451
Klatsky A L, Friedman G D, Siegelaub A B 1981 Alcohol and mortality. A ten-year Kaiser-Permanente experience. Annals of Internal Medicine 95: 139–145
Koskinas J, Kenna J G, Bird G L, Alexander G J M, Williams R 1992 Immunoglobulin A antibody to a 200 kilodalton cytosolic acetaldehyde adduct in alcoholic hepatitis. Gastroenterology 103: 1860–1867
Krom R A F 1994 Liver transplantation and alcohol: who should get transplants? Hepatology 20: 28S–32S
Laposata E A, Lange L G 1986 Presence of nonoxidative ethanol metabolism in human organs commonly damaged by ethanol abuse. Science 231: 497–499
Lelbach W K 1976 Epidemiology of alcoholic liver disease. In: Popper H, Schafner F (eds) Progress in liver diseases, Vol 5. Grune and Stratton, New York, p 494–515
Levi A J, Chalmers D M 1978 Recognition of alcoholic liver disease in a district general hospital. Gut 19: 521–525
Li J, Rosman A S, Leo M A, Nagai Y, Lieber C S 1994 Tissue inhibitor of metalloproteinase is increased in the serum of precirrhotic and cirrhotic alcoholic patients and can serve as a marker of fibrosis. Hepatology 19: 1418–1423
Lieber C S 1987 Microsomal ethanol-oxidizing system. Enzyme 37: 45–56
Lieber C S 1988a The microsomal ethanol oxidizing system: its role in ethanol and xenobiotic metabolism. Biochemical Society Transactions 16: 232–239
Lieber C S 1988b Biochemical and molecular basis of alcohol-induced injury to liver and other tissues. New England Journal of Medicine 319: 1639–1650
Lieber C S 1993 Aetiology and pathogenesis of alcoholic liver disease. Baillières Clinical Gastroenterology 7: 581–608
Lieber C S 1994 Alcohol and the liver: 1994 update. Gastroenterology 106: 1085–1105
Lieber C S, Rubin E 1968 Alcoholic fatty liver in man on a high protein and low fat diet. American Journal of Medicine 44: 200–206
Lieber C S, Leo M A, Mak K M, DeCarli L M, Sato S 1985 Choline fails to prevent liver fibrosis in ethanol-fed baboons but causes toxicity. Hepatology 5: 561–572
Lindsell D R M, Wilson A G, Maxwell J D 1982 Fractures on the chest radiograph in detection of alcoholic liver disease. British Medical Journal 285: 597
Littenberg G, Afroudakis A, Kaplowitz N 1979 Common bile duct stenosis from chronic pancreatitis: a clinical and pathologic spectrum. Medicine 58: 385–412
Lucey M R 1993 Liver transplantation for alcoholic liver disease. Clinical Gastroenterology 7: 717–727
Lumeng L, Crabb D W 1994 Genetic aspects and risk factors in alcoholism and alcoholic liver disease. Gastroenterology 107: 572–578
MacSween R N M, Burt A D 1986 Histologic spectrum of alcoholic liver disease. Seminars in Liver Disease 6: 221–232
Maddrey W C, Boitnott J K, Bedine M S, Weber F L Jr, Mezey E, White R I Jr 1978 Corticosteroid therapy of alcoholic hepatitis. Gastroenterology 75: 193–199
Maxwell J D 1986 Accuracy of death certification for alcoholic liver disease. British Journal of Addiction 81: 168
Maxwell J D, Knapman P 1985 Effect of coroners' rules on death certification for alcoholic liver disease. British Medical Journal 291: 708
Mayfield D, McLeod G, Hall P 1974 The CAGE questionnaire; validation of a new alcoholism screening instrument. American Journal of Psychiatry 131: 1121–1123
Mendenhall C L, Anderson S, Garcia-Pont P et al and the Veterans Administration Co-operative Study on Alcoholic Hepatitis 1984 Short-term and long-term survival in patients with alcoholic hepatitis treated with oxandrolone and prednisolone. New England Journal of Medicine 311: 1464–1470
Mendenhall C L, Gartside P S, Roselle G A et al 1989 Longevity among ethnic groups in alcoholic liver disease. Alcohol and Alcoholism 24: 11–19

Morgan M Y 1982 Alcohol and nutrition. British Medical Bulletin 38: 21–29
Morgan M Y 1985 Epidemiology of alcoholic liver disease: United Kingdom. In: Hall P (ed) Alcoholic liver disease: pathobiology, epidemiology and clinical aspects. Arnold, London, p 193
Morgan M Y, Sherlock S 1977 Sex related differences among 100 patients with alcoholic liver disease. British Medical Journal 1: 939–941
Morgan M Y, Sherlock S, Scheuer P J 1978 Acute cholestasis, hepatic failure and fatty liver in the alcoholic. Scandinavian Journal of Gastroenterology 13: 299–303
Orrego H, Blake J E, Blendis L M, Campton K V, Israel Y 1987 Long term treatment of alcoholic liver disease with propylthiouracil. New England Journal of Medicine 317: 1421–1427
Orrego H, Kalant H, Israel Y et al 1979 Effect of short term therapy with prophylthiouracil in patients with alcoholic liver disease. Gastroenterology 76: 105–115
Pande N V, Resnick R H, Yee W, Eckardt V F, Shurberg J L 1978 Cirrhotic portal hypertension: morbidity of continued alcoholism. Gastroenterology 74: 64–69
Panos M Z, Polson R, Johnson R, Portmann B, Williams R 1990 Polyunsaturated phosphatidyl choline for acute alcoholic hepatitis: a double-blind randomised placebo-controlled trial. European Journal of Gastroenterology and Hepatology 2: 351–355
Parés A, Barrera J M, Caballería J et al 1990 Hepatitis C virus antibodies in chronic alcoholic patients: association with severity of liver injury. Hepatology 12: 1295–1299
Parés A, Potter J J, Rennie L, Mezey E 1994 Aldehyde activates the promoter of the mouse $a_2$(I) collagen gene. Hepatology 19: 498–503
Paronetto F 1993 Immunologic reactions in alcoholic liver disease. Seminars in Liver Disease 13: 183–195
Paton A, Saunders J B 1981 ABC of alcohol: definitions. British Medical Journal 283: 1248–1250
Pequignot G, Tuyns A J, Berta J L 1978 Ascitic cirrhosis in relation to alcohol consumption. International Journal of Epidemiology 7: 113–120
Pereira L M M B, Langley P G, Bird G L D, Hayllar K M, Tredger J M, Williams R 1992 Coagulation factors V and VIII in relation to severity and outcome in acute alcoholic hepatitis. Alcohol and Alcoholism 27: 55–61
Peters T J 1982 Ethanol metabolism. British Medical Bulletin 38: 17–20
Plevris J N, Hayes P C, Bouchier I A D 1991 Ursodeoxycholic acid in the treatment of alcoholic liver disease. European Journal of Gastroenterology and Hepatology 3: 653–656
Poupon R E, Nalpas B, Coutelle C et al 1992 Polymorphism of alcohol dehydrogenase, alcohol and aldehyde dehydrogenase activities: implications in alcoholic cirrhosis in white patients. The French Group for Research on Alcohol and Liver. Hepatology 15: 1017–1022
Ramond M-J, Poynard T, Rueff B et al 1992 A randomized trial of prednisolone in patients with severe alcoholic hepatitis. New England Journal of Medicine 326: 507–512
Ramond M J, Rueff B, Benhamou J-P 1993 Medical treatment of alcoholic liver disease. Clinical Gastroenterology 7: 697–716
Randall B 1980 Fatty liver and sudden death. A review. Human Pathology 11: 147–153
Resnick R H, Boitnott J, Iber F L et al 1974 Preliminary observations of d-penicillamine therapy in acute alcoholic liver disease. Digestion 11: 257–265
Rubin E, Lieber C S 1968 Alcohol-induced hepatic injury in nonalcoholic volunteers. New England Journal of Medicine 278: 869–876
Salmela K S, Roine R P, Koivisto T et al 1993 Characteristics of *Helicobacter pylori* alcohol dehydrogenase. Gastroenterology 105: 325–330
Saunders J B, Walters J R F, Davies P, Paton A 1981 A 20-year prospective study of cirrhosis. British Medical Journal 282: 263–266
Saunders J B, Wodak A D, Haines A 1982 Accelerated development of alcoholic cirrhosis in patients with HLA-B8. Lancet 1: 1381–1384
Saunders J B, Wodak A D, Morgan-Capner P et al 1983 Importance of markers of hepatitis B virus in alcoholic liver disease. British Medical Journal 286: 1851–1854
Schenker S, Halff G A 1993 Nutritional therapy in alcoholic liver disease. Seminars in Liver Disease 13: 196–209
Schmidt W 1977 The epidemiology of cirrhosis of the liver: a statistical analysis of mortality data with special reference to Canada. In: Fisher M M, Rankin J G (eds) Alcohol and the liver. Plenum Press, New York, p 1–26
Scott J, Summerfield J A, Elias E, Dick R, Sherlock S 1977 Chronic pancreatitis: a cause of cholestasis. Gut 18: 196–201
Seeley J R 1960 Death by liver cirrhosis and the price of beverage alcohol. Canadian Medical Association Journal 83: 1361–1366
Seitz H K, Egerer G, Simanowski U A et al 1993 Human gastric alcohol dehydrogenase activity: effect of age, sex, and alcoholism. Gut 34: 1433–1437
Selzer M L 1971 The Michigan Alcoholism Screening Test: the quest for a new diagnostic instrument. American Journal of Psychiatry 127: 1653–1658
Sharpe P C, McBride, Archbold G P R 1996 Biochemical markers of alcohol abuse. Quarterly Journal of Medicine 89: 137–144
Sherman D I, Williams R 1994 Liver damage: mechanisms and management. British Medical Bulletin 50: 124–138
Sheron N, Bird G, Koskinas J et al 1993 Circulating and tissue levels of the neutrophil chemotaxin interleukin-8 are elevated in severe acute alcoholic hepatitis, and tissue levels correlate with neutrophil infiltration. Hepatology 18: 41–46
Simpson K J, Venkatesan S, Smith G D, Peters T J 1990 Very low density lipoprotein–triacylgycerol (VLDL–TG) turnover in alcoholic subjects. Biochemical Society Transactions 18: 1189–1191
Simpson K J, Venkatesan S, Martin A, Brindley D N, Peters T J 1994 Effect of alcohol on the activity and subcellular distributions of phosphatidate phosphohydrolase in rat liver. Biochimica et Biophysica Acta 1201: 411–414
Skinner H A, Holt S, Sheu W J, Israel Y 1986 Clinical versus laboratory detection of alcohol abuse: the alcohol clinical index. British Medical Journal 292: 1703–1708
Smith M, Hopkinson D A, Harris H 1971 Developmental changes and polymorphism in human alcohol dehydrogenases. Annals of Human Genetics 34: 251–271
Smith M, Hopkinson D A, Harris H 1972 Alcohol dehydrogenase isoenzymes in adult human stomach and liver, evidence for activity of the $ADH_3$ locus. Annals of Human Genetics 35: 243–253
Smith M, Hopkinson D A, Harris H 1973 Studies on the properties of the human alcohol dehydrogenase isozymes determined by the different loci $ADH_1$, $ADH_2$, $ADH_3$. Annals of Human Genetics 37: 49–67
Sørensen T I A, Orholm M, Bentsen K D, Høybye G, Eghøje K, Christoffersen P 1984 Prospective evaluation of alcohol abuse and alcoholic liver injury in men as predictors of development of cirrhosis. Lancet 2: 241–244
Starzl T E, van Thiel D, Tzakis A G et al 1988 Orthotopic liver transplantation for alcoholic cirrhosis. Journal of the American Medical Association 260: 2542–2544
Takahashi T, Lasker J M, Rosman A S, Lieber C S 1993 Induction of cytochrome P-4502E1 in the human liver by ethanol is caused by a corresponding increase in encoding messenger RNA. Hepatology 17: 236–245
Takase S, Takada N, Enomoto N, Yasuhara M, Takada A 1991 Different types of chronic hepatitis in alcoholic patients: does chronic hepatitis induced by alcohol exist? Hepatology 13: 876–881
Tanaka F, Shiratori Y, Yokosuka O, Imazeki F, Tsukada Y, Omata M 1996 High incidence of ADH2*1/ALDH2*1 genes among Japanese alcohol dependents and patients with alcoholic liver disease. Hepatology 23: 234–239
Teare J P, Sherman D, Greenfield S M et al 1993 Comparison of serum procollagen III peptide concentrations and PGA index for assessment of hepatic fibrosis. Lancet 342: 895–898
Trinchet J C, Coste T, Lévy V G et al 1989 Traitement de l'hépatite alcoolique par la silymarine. Gastroenterologie Clinique et Biologique 13: 120–124
Venkatesan S, Ward R J, Peters T J 1988 Effect of chronic ethanol feeding on the hepatic secretion of very low density lipoproteins. Biochimica et Biophysica Acta 960: 61–66
Villa E, Barchi T, Grisendi A et al 1982 Susceptibility of chronic symptomless HBsAg carriers to ethanol-induced hepatic damage. Lancet 2: 1243–1244

Wadstein J, Skude G 1979 Changes in amylase, hepatic enzymes, and bilirubin in serum upon initiation of alcohol abstinence. Acta Medica Scandinavica 205: 313–316
West L J, Maxwell D S, Noble E P, Solomon D H 1984 Alcoholism. Annals of Internal Medicine 100: 405–416
Worner T M, Lieber C S 1985 Perivenular fibrosis as precursor lesion of cirrhosis. Journal of the American Medical Association 254: 627–630
Wu A, Chanarin I, Levi A J 1974 Macrocytosis of chronic alcoholism. Lancet 1: 829–831
Yokoyama H, Ishii H, Nagata S, Kato S, Kamegaya K, Tsuchiya M 1993 Experimental hepatitis induced by ethanol after immunization with acetaldehyde adducts. Hepatology 17: 14–19
Yoshida A, Hsu L C, Ikuta T, Kikuchi I, Shibuya A, Mohandas T K 1988 Molecular genetics of alcohol-metabolising enzymes. Biochemical Society Transactions 16: 230–232
Zieve L 1958 Jaundice, hyperlipemia and hemolytic anemia: a heretofore unrecognized syndrome associated with alcoholic fatty liver and cirrhosis. Annals of Internal Medicine 48: 471–496
Zignego A L, Foschi M, Laffi G et al 1994 "Inapparent" hepatitis B virus infection and hepatitis C virus replication in alcoholic subjects with and without liver disease. Hepatology 19: 577–582

SECTION 8

# Chronic liver diseases

# 32. Chronic hepatitis

*Albert J. Czaja*

## INTRODUCTION

Chronic hepatitis is a general term referring to hepatocellular inflammation of at least 6 months' duration (Czaja 1981). Temporal criteria for chronicity are no longer needed in autoimmune hepatitis, since the disease may present acutely and the diagnosis can be made at presentation from clinical, laboratory and histological features (Johnson & McFarlane 1993).

There are many forms of chronic hepatitis and their names reflect etiologic or pathogenic factors (Table 32.1). Terms such as "chronic persistent hepatitis", "chronic active hepatitis", "chronic lobular hepatitis" and "chronic aggressive hepatitis" have been discarded, since they refer to the clinical disease as well as to the histological findings, do not reflect pathogenic mechanisms and may wrongly imply prognosis and need for treatment (Czaja 1993). Additionally, transitions may occur spontaneously between the histological patterns of "chronic persistent hepatitis" and "chronic active hepatitis", thereby confounding the clinical diagnosis and the assessments of prognosis (Schalm et al 1977).

Autoimmune hepatitis, chronic hepatitis B, C and D, indeterminate chronic viral hepatitis cryptogenic chronic hepatitis and drug-related chronic hepatitis are the main currently accepted diagnostic groups (Czaja 1993) (Table 32.1). Within each of these, subtypes may be defined based on pathogenic distinctions such as autoimmune hepatitis type 1 or type 2, precore mutant chronic hepatitis B or methyldopa hepatitis (Czaja 1993). Designations for the subtypes reflect jargon rather than official nomenclature, since in many instances it is uncertain that the subtypes are valid clinical entities.

Unfortunately, not all patients with chronic hepatitis can be classified confidently, since they may simultaneously have features characteristic of different diagnostic categories (Czaja 1993). Some patients with viral infections may have autoimmune markers (Czaja et al 1993a). Other patients with autoimmune hepatitis have concurrent findings of primary biliary cirrhosis (PBC) or primary sclerosing cholangitis (PSC), referred to as "overlap syndromes" (p. 939), and some patients with smooth muscle antibodies" (SMA) or antinuclear antibodies (ANA) have findings suggesting PBC although antimitochondrial antibodies

**Table 32.1** Classification of chronic hepatitis

| Groups | Subgroups |
|---|---|
| Autoimmune hepatitis | Type 1<br>• $ANA^+$<br>• $SMA^+$<br>• $Actin^+$ |
| | Type 2a<br>• Anti-$LKM1^+$<br>• Anti-$HCV^-$<br>• Anti-$LC1^+$ |
| | Type 2b<br>• Anti-$LKM1^+$<br>• Anti-$HCV^+$ |
| | Type 3<br>• Anti-$SLA^+$<br>• Anti-$LP^+$ |
| | Autoantibody-negative |
| Chronic hepatitis B | $HBeAg^+$<br>(Replicative) |
| | $HBeAg^-$/HBV-$DNA^+$<br>(Precore mutant) |
| | $HBeAg^-$/HBV-$DNA^-$<br>(Integrative) |
| Chronic hepatitis C | Genotypes I–IV |
| Chronic hepatitis D | $HBsAg^+$/Anti-$HDV^+$ |
| Indeterminate chronic viral hepatitis | |
| Cryptogenic chronic hepatitis | |
| Drug-related chronic hepatitis | Drug type |
| Chronic hepatitis with mixed features | Autoimmune/viral<br>Autoimmune/PSC<br>Autoimmune/PBC<br>"Autoimmune cholangitis" |

SMA = smooth muscle antibodies, ANA = antinuclear antibodies, LKM1 = liver-kidney microsome type 1, LC1 = liver cytosol type 1, SLA = soluble liver antigen, LP = liver–pancreas, PSC = primary sclerosing cholangitis, PBC = primary biliary cirrhosis.

(AMA) are not present. These findings are incompatible with diagnoses of either autoimmune hepatitis or PBC and they necessitate the creation of a diagnostic pigeonhole, "autoimmune cholangitis" (p. 939), that differentiates these entities from the classic conditions.

The nomenclature of chronic hepatitis is in evolution as newer immunoserologic and virologic assays improve the precision of diagnosis and as advances in molecular biology clarify pathogenic mechanisms. Terms based on clinical features ("lupoid hepatitis", "juvenile cirrhosis"), histological features ("plasma cell hepatitis", "submassive chronic hepatitis", "chronic lobular hepatitis", "chronic persistent hepatitis", "chronic active hepatitis") and serologic findings ("HBsAg-positive chronic hepatitis", "chronic active hepatitis non-A, non-B") are being replaced by terms based on etiologic or pathogenic factors (Desmet et al 1994, International Working Party Report 1995). The new nomenclature must define homogeneous populations so that descriptions of natural history, treatment and investigations of disease mechanisms can be precise. However, temporary categories for conditions with mixed or incompatible features are essential to preserve the integrity of the established syndromes and facilitate understanding of atypical disorders.

## DIAGNOSTIC CRITERIA

The diagnosis of chronic hepatitis requires the presence of certain clinical, laboratory and histological findings and the exclusion of conditions of a similar but different nature (Czaja 1981).

### Clinical

Six months of continuous inflammatory activity, as reflected in the clinical history, abnormal liver function tests or histological findings are sufficient to exclude most self-limited, slowly resolving acute disorders and this is the temporal criterion for chronicity. Autoimmune hepatitis is the only form of chronic hepatitis that does not require 6 months of disease activity, since the diagnosis itself implies chronicity and acute, even fulminant, presentations of the disease are now recognized (Johnson & McFarlane 1993).

### Biochemical

The biochemical features of chronic hepatitis are persistent, although often fluctuating, abnormalities of serum alanine and aspartate aminotransferase activities that predominate over serum alkaline phosphatase elevations. The diagnosis implies a "hepatitic" rather than a "cholestatic" illness (p. 741), although hyperbilirubinemia and increased alkaline phosphatase activity may be present. Hypergammaglobulinemia is a manifestation of disease severity and chronicity rather than etiology (p. 917). It is an important feature of autoimmune hepatitis, however, and the diagnosis is suspect without this finding. In autoimmune hepatitis, the hypergammaglobulinemia is polyclonal in nature, but increased immunoglobulin G concentrations characterize the disorder (Czaja 1984a).

### Pathology

*Portal tracts*

Mononuclear cell infiltration of the portal tracts is the histological hallmark of chronic hepatitis. Preservation of the limiting plate characterizes portal hepatitis (Fig. 32.1). Disruption of the limiting plate (p. 710) characterizes periportal hepatitis and piecemeal necrosis (Fig. 32.2). "Interface hepatitis" is the term now used for piecemeal necrosis because the main liver cell injury is apoptosis rather than lytic necrosis (Ishak et al 1995). Extension of the necroinflammatory process between portal tracts or

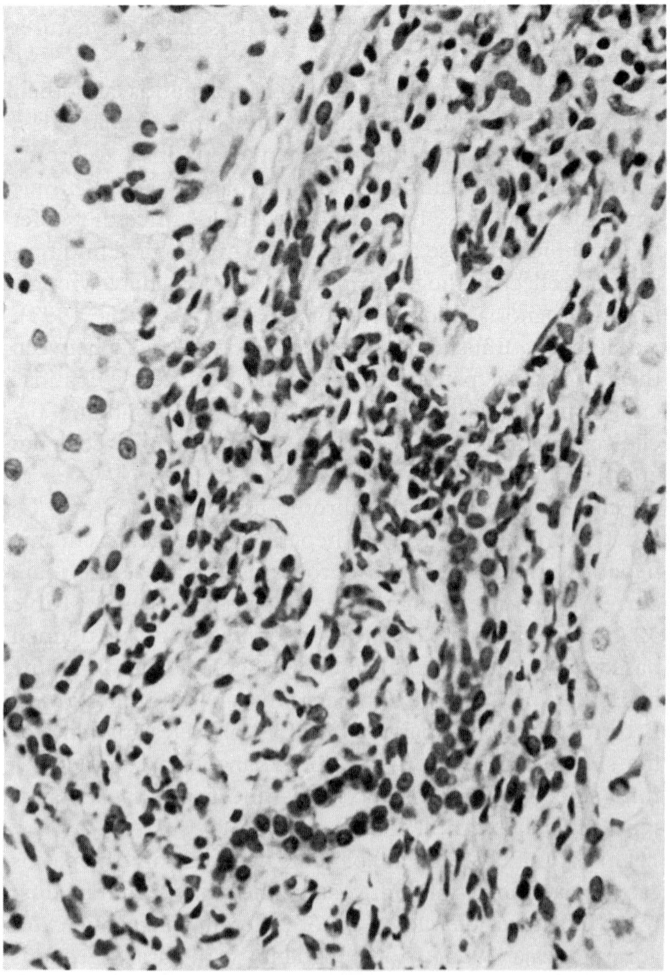

**Fig. 32.1** Portal hepatitis. The lymphocytic infiltrate is confined to the portal tract and the limiting plate is preserved (hematoxylin and eosin, ×200).

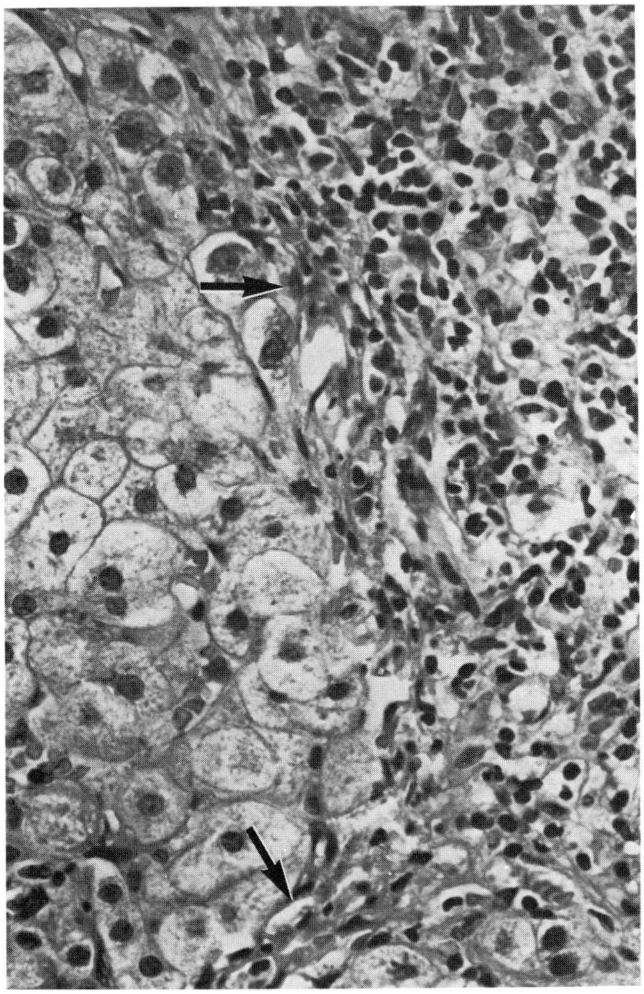

**Fig. 32.2** Periportal hepatitis (piecemeal necrosis or interface hepatitis). The lymphocytic infiltrate disrupts the limiting plate (arrowed) resulting in piecemeal necrosis. A spur of fibrosis extends into the parenchyma (arrowed) (hematoxylin and eosin, ×400).

between portal tracts and central veins (bridging necrosis) or destruction of contiguous lobules (multilobular necrosis) represents more severe manifestations of the same condition (Baggenstoss et al 1972, Cooksley et al 1986).

*Parenchyma*

Sinusoidal mononuclear cell infiltration, lobular disarray, Kupffer cell hyperplasia and dead hepatocytes (acidophilic or Councilman bodies) are manifestations of lobular hepatitis (Fig. 32.3) and they are part of the histological spectrum of chronic hepatitis (Popper & Schaffner 1971, Johnson & McFarlane 1993). Typically, the inflammatory activity in and around the portal tracts predominates over the lobular changes, although in certain stages of chronic hepatitis, such as autoimmune hepatitis in relapse or chronic hepatitis B in transition from a stage of active viral replication to an inactive stage, the reverse may be true.

*Etiological correlates*

Bile duct destruction and loss (ductopenia) do not occur in autoimmune hepatitis (Johnson & McFarlane 1993), but they may be features of chronic hepatitis C (Bach et al 1992, Scheuer et al 1992, Czaja & Carpenter 1993). Steatosis and portal lymphoid aggregates are histological features also suggesting chronic hepatitis C (Fig. 32.4) (Bach et al 1992, Scheuer et al 1992, Czaja & Carpenter 1993). Moderate to severe periportal hepatitis, lobular hepatitis and plasma cell infiltration of the portal tracts support a diagnosis of autoimmune hepatitis (Bach et al 1992, Czaja & Carpenter 1993), while ground-glass hepatocytes indicate chronic hepatitis B (Czaja & Carpenter 1993, Lefkowitch et al 1993). Multinucleated giant cells can be found in autoimmune hepatitis as well as in chronic hepatitis B (Bach et al 1992, Czaja & Carpenter 1993).

It is important that individual histological features lack sensitivity and are not pathognomonic of specific etiologies for chronic hepatitis. This is illustrated in Table 32.2, which shows the reliability of liver biopsy in each of the main clinical forms of chronic hepatitis (Czaja & Carpenter 1993).

*Differential diagnosis*

Hereditary conditions such as Wilson's disease (p. 959), hemochromatosis (p. 953), $\alpha_1$-antitrypsin deficiency (p. 966), alcoholic (p. 875) and nonalcoholic steatohepatitis (p. 975), drug-induced liver disease (p. 845), primary biliary cirrhosis (p. 935) and primary sclerosing cholangitis (p. 943) may have features similar to those of chronic hepatitis, but they are separate conditions and must be excluded. Fortunately, this is usually done easily from the clinical history, other laboratory tests and histological examination (Czaja 1984b). Slit-lamp examination for Kayser–Fleischer rings, serum ceruloplasmin, iron concentration and saturation of the serum iron-binding capacity, ferritin concentrations, $\alpha_1$-antitrypsin concentration and phenotype, liver biopsy assessment and observation after discontinuation of potentially hepatotoxic drugs are important in differential diagnosis.

## CLASSIFICATION OF CHRONIC HEPATITIS

### Autoimmune hepatitis

Autoimmune hepatitis is a disease of unknown cause characterized by periportal hepatitis in the liver and autoantibodies in serum (Czaja 1984a). It constitutes 34% of cases of chronic hepatitis in Germany and 62% of cases in Australia, but only 1% of cases in Hong Kong. Its incidence in the United Kingdom is estimated as 0.69 cases per 100 000 persons per year (Hodges et al 1982). Three subtypes have been proposed based on immunoserologic markers (Maddrey 1987), although they have not been

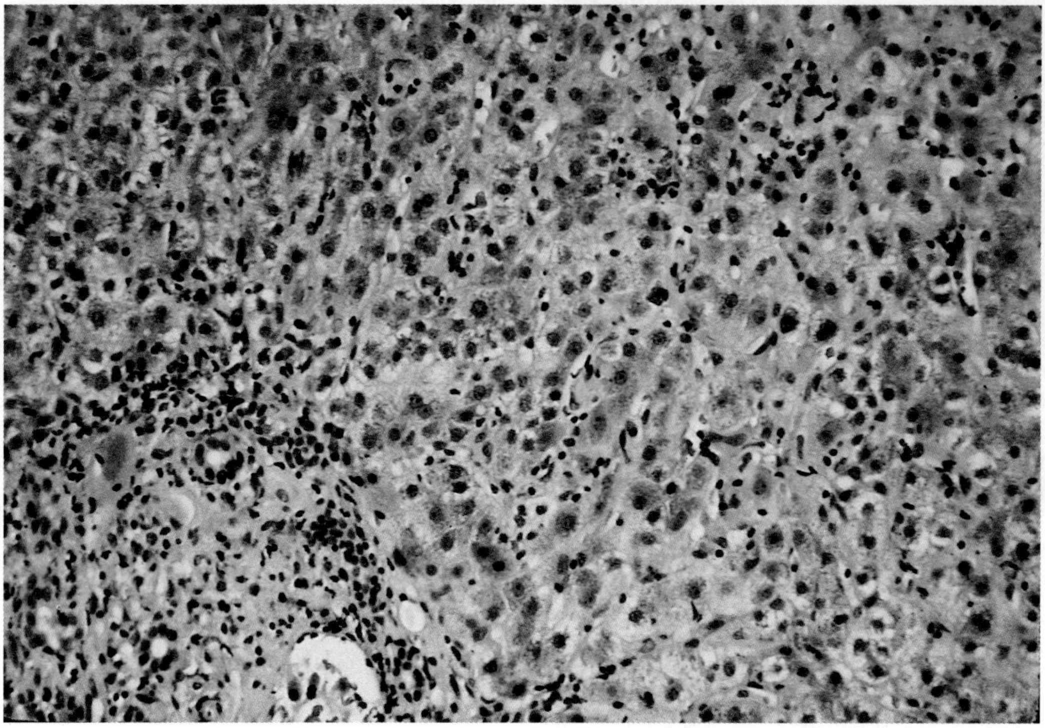

**Fig. 32.3** Lobular hepatitis. Sinusoidal mononuclear cell infiltration, Kupffer cell hyperplasia and lobular disarray are present (hematoxylin and eosin, ×200).

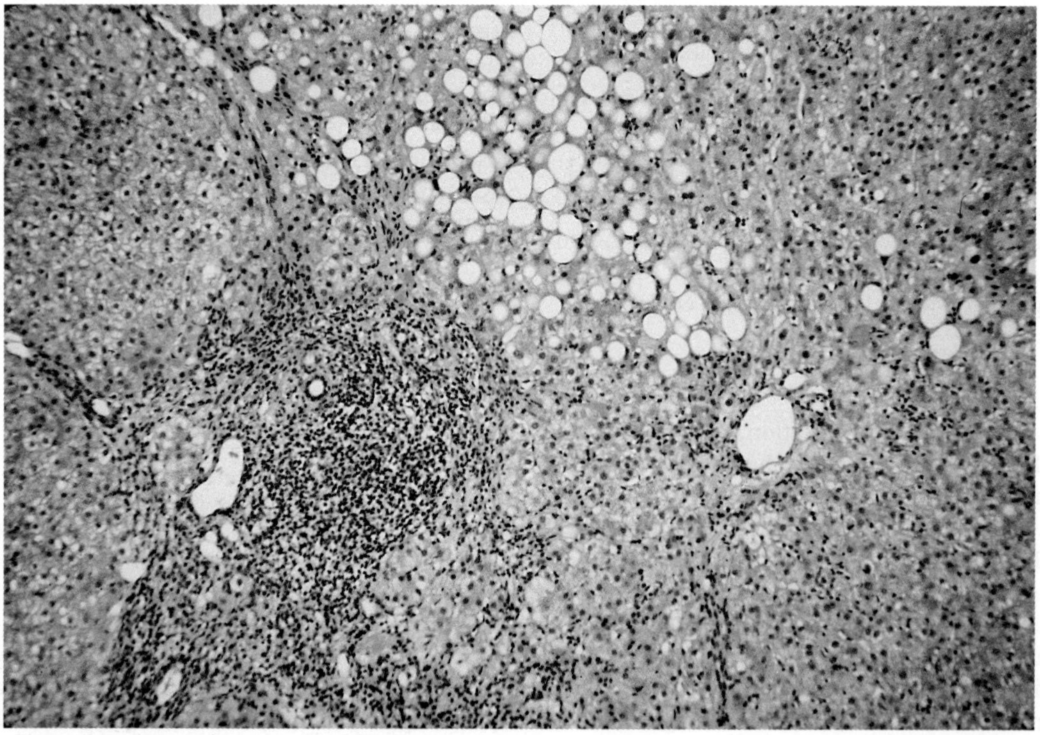

**Fig. 32.4** Portal lymphoid aggregates, steatosis and lobular hepatitis. The constellation of findings suggests the diagnosis of chronic hepatitis C (hematoxylin and eosin, ×100).

**Table 32.2** Sensitivity, specificity and predictability of histological interpretations for the most common forms of chronic hepatitis

| Biopsy performance | Clinical diagnoses (%) | | |
|---|---|---|---|
| | Autoimmune hepatitis | Chronic hepatitis B | Chronic hepatitis C |
| Sensitivity | 40 | 36 | 57 |
| Specificity | 81 | 99 | 91 |
| Positive predictability | 68 | 80 | 67 |
| Negative predictability | 57 | 91 | 87 |
| Overall predictability | 62 | 91 | 82 |

shown to be independent entities (Johnson & McFarlane 1993).

### *Type 1 autoimmune hepatitis*

Type 1 autoimmune hepatitis is characterized by smooth muscle antibodies (SMA) and/or antinuclear antibodies (ANA) (p. 765). Previous, and now obsolete, terms for this condition include lupoid hepatitis, idiopathic autoimmune chronic active hepatitis and classic autoimmune hepatitis. Antibodies to actin, especially polymerized F-actin, are specific markers for the condition (Lidman et al 1976) and some already call the disease "anti-actin hepatitis" (Homberg et al 1987).

Type 1 autoimmune hepatitis is the commonest form of autoimmune hepatitis in adults (80%), most patients are women who are usually less than 40 years old (70%) and concurrent immunologic diseases, such as autoimmune thyroiditis, Graves' disease, ulcerative colitis and rheumatoid arthritis, occur in 17% (Czaja et al 1983). Ulcerative colitis can coexist with autoimmune hepatitis, but cholangiograms and histological examinations are essential to exclude primary sclerosing cholangitis (PSC). Indeed, 42% of patients with autoimmune hepatitis and ulcerative colitis will have features of PSC and these patients typically do not respond to corticosteroid therapy (Perdigoto et al 1992).

Twenty-five percent of patients with type 1 autoimmune hepatitis have cirrhosis at presentation, indicating that the disease has an indolent but progressive subclinical stage (Czaja et al 1983). Forty percent of patients have an acute onset of symptoms easily mistaken for acute viral hepatitis (Czaja et al 1983). This error can delay potentially life-saving therapy, but fortunately most patients have features such as ascites, hypoalbuminemia, hypergammaglobulinemia or thrombocytopenia suggesting chronic liver disease and allowing appropriate therapy to be undertaken promptly (Davis et al 1982). The "acute" onset of the illness in these cases probably represents an exacerbation of long-standing subclinical disease (Nikias et al 1994).

***Pathogenesis.*** The pathogenesis of type 1 autoimmune hepatitis is unknown. None of the associated autoantibodies have been shown to be cytotoxic and a target autoantigen has not been identified (Czaja 1990a). An early hypothesis attributed the disease to antibody-dependent cell-mediated cytotoxicity whereby impairment of suppressor T-cell function allows the production of immunoglobulin G, which binds to normal hepatocyte membrane protein. The antigen–antibody complex so formed on the hepatocyte surface allows lymphocytes (natural killer cells) with receptors for the Fc portion of the antibody molecule to destroy the hepatocytes through a cell-mediated cytolysis (Eddleston 1985, Czaja 1995).

A more recent alternative hypothesis attributes the disease to an antigen-sensitized cell-mediated immunoreaction. The triggering event may be the aberrant expression of major histocompatibility antigens on the hepatocyte surface (p. 763), possibly as a result of viral, genetic or environmental factors (Czaja 1995). This facilitates recognition of normal hepatocyte proteins and leads to production of a lymphocyte clone causing autoimmune cytodestruction (Czaja 1995).

***Hepatitis C virus.*** Initial surveys using first-generation immunoassays (p. 788) for the detection of antibodies to hepatitis C virus (anti-HCV) in type 1 autoimmune hepatitis gave positive reactions in 44% of patients (Esteban et al 1989). Subsequent studies showed frequent false positive reactions with these assays related to hypergammaglobulinemia in autoimmune hepatitis (McFarlane et al 1990). HCV-RNA has been detected by polymerase chain reaction (PCR) in no more than 11% of patients with type 1 autoimmune hepatitis and it appears that HCV is either an infrequent and unimportant etiologic factor or a coincidental finding in some patients with type 1 disease (Mitchel et al 1993, Silva et al 1993, Czaja et al 1995a). Importantly, second- and third-generation immunoassays for anti-HCV in type 1 autoimmune hepatitis also show frequent false positivity (20–60%) and low sensitivities (57%), so that confident diagnosis (or exclusion) of HCV infection in such patients requires detection of HCV-RNA in serum by PCR (Czaja et al 1995a).

### *Type 2 autoimmune hepatitis*

Type 2 autoimmune hepatitis is characterized by serum antibodies to liver–kidney microsome type 1 (anti-LKM1). Patients are typically children (2–14 years); a bimodal age distribution has been described and in Europe about 20% of patients are adults (Homberg et al 1987) whereas in the United States only 4% of patients are adults (Czaja et al 1992a).

Type 2 autoimmune hepatitis differs from type 1 disease in several respects. Patients lack ANA and SMA; they have lower serum concentrations of γ-globulin (especially immunoglobulin A); they more commonly have extrahepatic immunologic diseases such as vitiligo, insulin-dependent diabetes and autoimmune thyroiditis; they more frequently have autoantibodies to parietal cells, islets of Langerhans and thyroid; and they more frequently progress to cirrhosis despite corticosteroid therapy (Homberg et al 1987, Czaja & Manns 1995). As in type 1 autoimmune hepatitis, a fulminant presentation is possible and patients with acute liver failure should be screened for anti-LKM1 (Porta et al 1990).

***Pathogenesis.*** Unlike type 1 autoimmune hepatitis, the target autoantigen of type 2 autoimmune hepatitis has been identified. Antibodies to LKM1 recognize a linear 33 amino acid epitope on the cytochrome mono-oxygenase P-450 IID6 and they are able to inhibit its activity in vitro (Manns et al 1990, 1991). P-450 IID6 is expressed on the human hepatocyte membrane surface and its expression can be modulated by interleukins and tumor necrosis factor (Loeper et al 1993). It shows genetic polymorphism and it is deficient in 10% of individuals who presumably are not susceptible to the disease.

***Autoantibody detection.*** Anti-LKM1 in serum is detected by indirect immunofluorescence against the proximal tubules of the murine kidney. A strong pattern of renal tubular immunofluorescence may make it difficult to distinguish anti-LKM1 from antimitochondrial antibody (AMA) which produces distal tubular immunofluorescence (Czaja et al 1992a). Consequently, patients with autoimmune hepatitis and inexplicably high titers of AMA may actually be anti-LKM1 positive (Czaja et al 1992a).

Recombinant P-450 IID6 has been used in an immunoassay to detect antibodies (anti-P-450 IID6) and this assay has facilitated the diagnosis of type 2 autoimmune hepatitis. Antibodies to P-450 IID6 are directed against a core amino acid motif on the recombinant antigen, which is the 254-271 amino acid sequence, and this reactivity is specific for type 2 disease (Yamamoto et al 1993). Patients with anti-LKM1 and true HCV infection either lack anti-P-450 IID6 or their antibodies react against different epitopes.

***Hepatitis C virus.*** As many as 86% of patients with anti-LKM1 are seropositive for anti-HCV and unlike those with type 1 autoimmune hepatitis, many have true HCV infection (Lenzi et al 1990, Garson et al 1991). This has led to a proposal that type 2 disease be subdivided into type 2a, in which HCV does not occur, and type 2b, in which HCV does occur (Lunel et al 1992).

Patients with type 2a disease are usually young women with clinical features of an autoimmune hepatitis, high titers of anti-LKM1, high plasma aminotransferase activity indicating severe inflammatory activity and a good response to corticosteroid therapy (Lunel et al 1992, Michel et al 1992). Antibodies to liver cytosol type 1 have been proposed as a second marker for type 2a disease (Martini et al 1988, Abuaf et al 1992). These antibodies are present in 67% of patients with anti-LKM1 and they are absent in patients with concurrent HCV infection.

Patients with type 2b disease have HCV infection and the clinical features of a chronic viral hepatitis. Men are commonly afflicted, onset can be late in life, titers of anti-LKM1 are low, serum aminotransferase abnormalities are mild, corticosteroid treatment is ineffective and interferon therapy may be beneficial (Lunel et al 1992, Michel et al 1992). Anti-GOR antibodies are also present. These antibodies are directed against the host-derived GOR-47 antigen and they may reflect an autoimmune reaction induced by the HCV (Löhr et al 1994). The International Autoimmune Hepatitis Group, the World Congress of Gastroenterology and the International Association for the Study of the Liver have recently reaffirmed the nonviral nature of autoimmune hepatitis and have advised that active viral infection precludes its diagnosis (Johnson & McFarlane 1993, Desmet al al 1994, International Working Party Report 1995). They have reclassified patients with anti-LKM1 and true HCV infection as having "chronic hepatitis C with autoimmune features" and they have preserved the homogeneity of type 2 autoimmune hepatitis, obviating the need for type 2a and type 2b designations.

Patients with chronic hepatitis C virus infections rarely have anti-LKM1 (Czaja et al 1992a), while patients with anti-LKM1 are commonly seropositive for anti-HCV (Lenzi et al 1990). This suggests that the HCV in patients with anti-LKM1 may be mutants or variant genotypes. Unfortunately, attempts to define a virus-specific genotype or mutant associated with anti-LKM1 production have been unsuccessful (Gerotto et al 1994, Michitaka et al 1994). Molecular mimicry could explain the concurrence of anti-LKM1 and anti-HCV, as homologies have been described between cytochrome mono-oxygenase P-450 IID6, the HCV genome and the GOR-47 antigen (Manns et al 1991). Consequently, it is possible that antigens such as these generate crossreacting antibodies and possibly cause the induction of autoimmune reactions (Löhr et al 1994).

### *Other autoantibodies*

Several autoantibodies have been found in autoimmune hepatitis that are of considerable intrinsic interest, but as yet their clinical importance in defining subgroups of patients with chronic hepatitis remains uncertain. These include antisoluble liver antigen, anti-liver-specific membrane lipoprotein and anti-liver–pancreas antibodies (p. 769).

### *Autoimmune cholangitis*

This condition is characterized by clinical and biochemical cholestasis associated with ANA and/or SMA but not AMA and it may improve with corticosteroid therapy (Ben-Ari et al 1993). As its histological hallmark is nonsuppurative destructive cholangitis, it has been classified as AMA-negative PBC. However, the recent description of carbonic anhydrase antibodies in this condition but not in PBC suggests that autoimmune cholangitis and

PBC may be separate entities (p. 939). Bile duct destruction is not a feature of autoimmune hepatitis and diagnoses of "cholestatic autoimmune hepatitis" should be regarded with suspicion (Johnson & McFarlane 1993). Corticosteroids may improve the clinical and biochemical manifestations of autoimmune cholangitis, but they do not improve the histological lesions and ursodeoxycholic acid can be used for corticosteroid-resistant patients (p. 941).

*Genetic aspects*

The study of human leukocyte antigens (HLA) has shown particular associations in autoimmune hepatitis. This has important implications for susceptibility to and development of the disease and also relates to the course and evolution of the illness. However, determination of HLA status is not currently important in diagnosis or management of individual patients (p. 763).

***Associations.*** The human leukocyte antigens (HLA) DR3 and DR4 have been recognized as independent risk factors in autoimmune hepatitis (Donaldson et al 1990) and recent studies have shown that these phenotypes are associated with different disease manifestations and prognoses (Opelz et al 1977, Czaja et al 1990a, 1993b, Sanchez-Urdazpal et al 1992). Fifty-two percent of patients with type 1 autoimmune hepatitis have HLA DR3 and 42% have HLA DR4 (Czaja et al 1993c). HLA B8 is closely associated with HLA DR3 (94% co-occurrence) and is present in 47% of patients. The HLA phenotype A1-B8-DR3 is found in 37% of patients and 11% of individuals are heterozygous for HLA DR3 and HLA DR4 (Czaja et al 1993c).

Further dissection of the genotypes of autoimmune hepatitis shows that the alleles DRB3*0101, which encodes DR52a, and the DR4 subtype DRB1*0401 are also strongly associated with autoimmune hepatitis (Doherty et al 1994a). Indeed, 81% of patients with autoimmune hepatitis possess either allele and each is associated with a clinically distinct disease pattern. Additionally, these alleles encode specific amino acid sequences in the DR $\beta$ polypeptide that determine the ability of each class II molecule to bind and present antigens to T-cells (Doherty et al 1994a). The implications are that these residues influence the immunoreactivities of the effector cells and in turn the clinical manifestations and behavior of the disease. Clearly, many genetic loci, including genes outside the major histocompatibility complex (MHC), may affect susceptibility to and severity of autoimmune hepatitis. The possibility of a susceptibility gene (or genes) located within the MHC, however, cannot as yet be discounted and this hypothesis requires demonstration of a linkage between the HLA DR3 and HLA DR4 loci (Donaldson et al 1990, 1994). The predominant phenotype of type 2 autoimmune hepatitis (or other subtypes) has not yet been fully defined, but preliminary studies have implicated HLA B14, DR3 and C4A-QO with type 2 disease (Manns & Kruger 1994).

***Disease manifestations.*** Patients with HLA B8 are younger and have more active disease, as reflected in higher serum aminotransferase activities and histological findings of confluent necrosis and cirrhosis, than those without HLA B8 (Czaja et al 1990a). Similarly, patients who are HLA A1 negative and B8 positive relapse more frequently after treatment is stopped than patients with other phenotypes (Czaja et al 1990a). Patients with HLA DR3 enter remission less frequently and deteriorate more often during corticosteroid therapy than those with other phenotypes and they more frequently require liver transplantation (Sanchez-Urdazpal et al 1992, Czaja et al 1993b). In contrast, older female patients have HLA DR4 more often than patients with HLA DR3, they also have higher serum $\gamma$-globulin concentrations and more frequent concurrent immunologic diseases and they more often remit in response to therapy (Czaja et al 1993b). SMA and high-titer ANA have also been associated with the HLA DR4 phenotype (Czaja et al 1993b). Patients with DRB1*0401 have less severe disease at presentation, develop the disease later in life and relapse less frequently when treatment is stopped than those with DRB3*0101 (Doherty et al 1994a).

Early onset type 1 autoimmune hepatitis has been associated with a C4A gene deletion that is manifested by low serum complement levels and a possible inability to clear immune complexes, viruses or other antigens (Scully et al 1993, Donaldson et al 1994, Manns & Kruger 1994). Ninety percent of patients with childhood-onset type 1 autoimmune hepatitis have null allotypes at the C4A and C4B locus (Scully et al 1993) and in adult patients the C4A deletions have been associated with a greater mortality and relapse frequency (Doherty et al 1994b).

***Viral hepatitis.*** Patients with chronic viral hepatitis have a frequency of HLA DR4 positivity similar to that in autoimmune hepatitis (39% vs 42%) and concurrent extrahepatic immunologic diseases in chronic viral hepatitis are also associated with HLA DR4 (Czaja et al 1993c, 1995b,c). This suggests that patients with chronic viral hepatitis and autoimmune hepatitis share a genetic predisposition to immunologic diseases. The expression of concurrent immunologic diseases, such as autoimmune thyroiditis, rheumatoid arthritis and ulcerative colitis, in patients with chronic viral hepatitis and HLA DR4 may be coincidental with or facilitated by the viral infection (Czaja et al 1995b,c).

## Cryptogenic chronic hepatitis

Cryptogenic chronic hepatitis implies a continuing hepatocellular inflammation that defies etiologic classification. Patients with cryptogenic chronic hepatitis have the clinical, laboratory and histological features of chronic hepatitis (p. 888), but they lack serological markers of chronic hepatitis B and hepatitis C, immunoserological markers of autoimmune hepatitis (ANA, SMA, anti-LKM1) and epidemiological features that suggest a hepatic viral infection including contact with infected persons, high-risk sexual activity, parenteral drug abuse and blood or blood product transfusion (Czaja et al 1990b). About 13% of adults with nonviral chronic hepatitis are assigned to this cryptogenic category. Cryptogenic chronic hepatitis can progress to cryptogenic cirrhosis, a term referring to inactive end-stage cirrhosis, but cryptogenic cirrhosis should be distinguished from cryptogenic chronic hepatitis, as the former may present without a hepatitic phase. Many patients considered previously to have cryptogenic cirrhosis are now recognized to have chronic hepatitis C infection (Czaja et al 1990c, Brown et al 1992, Jeffers et al 1992).

Recent studies have shown that some patients with cryptogenic chronic hepatitis have autoimmune hepatitis that has escaped detection because tests have looked only for autoantibodies well established in clinical practice (Czaja et al 1993d). These patients may show the age, gender and laboratory and histological features of autoimmune hepatitis and share the same HLA types as patients with autoimmune hepatitis. Most important, they also respond to corticosteroid therapy. Patients with chronic viral hepatitis have different clinical and histological features and HLA phenotypes (Czaja et al 1993d). "Autoantibody-negative autoimmune hepatitis" is a fitting designation for these patients who lack only a conventional autoantibody to secure their diagnosis. Antibodies to SLA and LP reveal autoimmune hepatitis in some patients with cryptogenic chronic hepatitis and undoubtedly new markers will diminish further this cryptogenic category (Czaja et al 1993e, Stechemesser et al 1993). Interestingly, patients with cryptogenic chronic hepatitis may develop SMA and/or ANA later in their disease, showing that the expression of autoantibodies is variable in some patients (Czaja 1990a).

## Chronic hepatitis B

Chronic hepatitis B constitutes 20% of the cases of chronic hepatitis in the United Kingdom (Hodges et al 1982), 25% in the United States and 90% in Asia (Davis & Czaja 1981). It is caused by the hepatitis B virus (HBV) (p. 782), which is transmitted mainly by blood inoculation (blood transfusion, needlestick injury) or sexual contact (p. 783). Perinatal transmission is important, especially where the virus is endemic, and infected infants typically develop an asymptomatic chronic carrier state (p. 784).

### *Clinical and biochemical*

Patients with chronic hepatitis B are commonly men who are older than 30 years (Hoofnagle 1981, Perrillo & Aach 1981). The disease is usually insidious in onset and only 50% of individuals have symptoms, such as easy fatiguability and myalgias, at presentation. Most patients are anicteric and show few clinical stigmata of chronic liver disease. Serum aminotransferase activities exceed fivefold normal in only 25% of cases and hypergammaglobulinemia occurs in only 10%. Cryoglobulinemia may be present in patients who manifest arthralgias, purpura and nephritis (Levo et al 1977) and, rarely, a polyarteritis syndrome may occur with pancreatitis, membranous glomerulonephritis and pericarditis (Gocke et al 1970).

### *Diagnosis*

The diagnosis of chronic hepatitis B is based on finding HBsAg and anti-HBc (IgG) in serum in association with the other diagnostic features of chronic hepatitis (Czaja 1979, Hoofnagle 1981). The activity of HBV replication, the risk of infectivity and candidacy for antiviral therapy can be assessed by looking for HBeAg and HBV-DNA in serum. HBeAg and HBV-DNA indicate viral replication and their absence indicates the nonreplicative (integrative) stage of the disease and is confirmed by the presence of anti-HBe (p. 784).

Immunohistochemical techniques can demonstrate HBsAg and HBcAg in liver tissue and support the diagnosis. Concurrent infection with the human immunodeficiency virus or the hepatitis δ agent can each independently worsen chronic hepatitis B and these viruses as well as the hepatitis C virus must be sought in every patient (Housset et al 1992).

***Mutant HBV.*** A mutant strain of HBV has been described that has clinical and therapeutic significance. The precore or e-minus mutant is incapable of producing HBeAg (Carman et al 1989). A single substitution of adenosine for guanosine in the viral genome results in a stop codon that prevents the cleavage of HBeAg from the precore/core peptide (Omata et al 1991). Consequently, patients infected with this mutant have active HBV replication but are HBeAg seronegative. Preliminary studies have suggested that the precore mutant may produce a more severe hepatitis than the wild type and there has been concern that it is less responsive to interferon therapy (Carman et al 1991, Omata et al 1991). The diagnosis is suggested by the presence of HBV-DNA in serum, the demonstration of hepatitis B core antigen (HBcAg) in liver tissue and the exclusion of other concurrent infections or toxicities.

***Subclassification.*** Patients with chronic hepatitis B can be subclassified into three groups based on the serum HBeAg and aminotransferase activity (Schalm 1994). Patients with the HBeAg have active viral replication and they may or may not have symptoms or laboratory features of inflammatory activity. Included in this group are asymptomatic carriers of HBV. Patients who do not have the HBeAg but who have increased serum aminotransferase activity may be infected with a mutant strain of HBV incapable of producing HBeAg ("precore mutant"/ "e-minus mutant") or they may have a coincidental viral or toxic hepatitis, including infection with the hepatitis δ virus (HDV). Patients who do not have the HBeAg and who have normal serum aminotransferase activity have entered the integrative stage of their disease and they are asymptomatic HBsAg carriers whose long-term risks relate to reactivation of the virus or the development of hepatocellular carcinoma. Individual patients may move from one classification to another, but the status at any particular time is useful in decisions regarding treatment.

### Chronic hepatitis C

Chronic hepatitis C is caused by a single-stranded RNA virus (flavivirus) that is transmitted mainly by blood transfusion or needlestick injury. Sexual transmission is possible but uncertain, the risk of perinatal transmission correlates with the titer of HCV-RNA in the mother and sporadic disease within communities is well recognized (Alter et al 1992). Low socioeconomic status is an important risk factor for HCV infection in the community and this may be related to poor sanitation, crowding, sexual promiscuity and drug abuse (Alter et al 1992). Asymptomatic chronic infection undoubtedly contributes to an unrecognized reservoir of virus (p. 788).

#### *Clinical and biochemical*

The clinical features of chronic hepatitis C are similar to those of chronic hepatitis B. The disease is mild, anicteric and commonly asymptomatic (Czaja et al 1992b). Nonspecific symptoms such as tiredness occur and physical examination is often normal as features of chronic liver disease (p. 917) are uncommon. The development of cirrhosis leads eventually to features such as jaundice, ascites, encephalopathy and malnutrition. Liver function tests in the earlier stages show mild to moderate abnormality, particularly of serum transaminase activity, and in the later stages hyperbilirubinemia and hypoalbuminemia reflect deteriorating liver function.

***Associated conditions.*** In contrast to chronic hepatitis B, serum sickness-like manifestations are unusual, although urticaria and purpura can occur (Czaja & Davis 1982). Autoimmune thyroiditis (Pateron et al 1992, Tran et al 1993, Marcellin et al 1995) and Sjögren's syndrome (Haddad et al 1992, Pawlotsky et al 1994) have been reported and there has been speculation that the virus may trigger autoimmune manifestations (Czaja et al 1993a,c). Autoimmune disease may occur before and after interferon therapy (p. 903) and autoantibodies that are typically of low serum titer are common at presentation (Czaja et al 1995b, Clifford et al 1995). Mixed cryoglobulinemia has been described in association with the disease and acquired porphyria cutanea tarda (p. 975) may occur (Misiani et al 1994, Pawlotsky et al 1994).

#### *Diagnosis*

The diagnosis of chronic hepatitis C requires satisfaction of the criteria for chronic hepatitis given above and demonstration of antibodies in serum that react specifically against HCV-encoded antigens (p. 772). Demonstration of HCV-RNA in the blood is the "gold standard" for diagnosis, but it is not often needed and is not generally available.

### Chronic hepatitis D

Chronic hepatitis D is caused by the hepatitis δ virus (HDV), a unique virus ("viroid") that requires the hepatitis B virus for its expression (p. 773). Consequently, it is present only in patients with HBV infection. Transmission is mainly by parenteral inoculation and the disease is most common among intravenous drug users, hemodialysis patients and hemophiliacs (Rizzetto et al 1980). In the United States, 5% of HBsAg-positive patients are seropositive for anti-HDV (Shiels et al 1985). Hepatitis δ virus has direct cytotoxicity and it produces an aggressive hepatocellular injury (Smedile et al 1982). Patients have more active histological features than uninfected counterparts and they are more commonly symptomatic (Shiels et al 1985). Superinfection of an asymptomatic HBV carrier can present as a fulminant hepatitis or a rapidly progressive cirrhosis (Colombo et al 1983, Govindarajan et al 1984). Hepatocellular carcinoma is unusual in chronic hepatitis D, possibly because patients do not survive long enough to develop this complication.

The diagnosis is made by detecting antibodies to HDV in serum by enzyme immunoassay (p. 790). Only patients with serologic evidence of HBV infection need be screened. Immunoglobulin M antibodies to HDV imply a recent HDV infection (acute superinfection), while their absence implies a chronic coincidental infection. HDV-RNA can be detected in serum, but this is not usually necessary for diagnosis and is not available generally. Hepatitis δ antigen can also be sought in liver tissue and this is another method of detecting HDV infection and active replication (Schalm 1994).

### Indeterminate chronic viral hepatitis

About 18% of patients with epidemiologic risk factors for chronic viral hepatitis lack markers for HBV or HCV infection (Alter et al 1992). Such patients have been designated as having "chronic hepatitis non-A, non-B, non-C", but they are more appropriately classified as "indeterminate chronic viral hepatitis" (Czaja 1993). They are distinguished from patients with cryptogenic chronic hepatitis by the presence of viral risk factors including transfusion of blood or blood products, parenteral drug abuse, occupational exposure (health care) and sexual or household contact. Patients with indeterminate chronic viral hepatitis have been studied best in the community (Alter et al 1992). They tend to be older than those with chronic hepatitis C and they are more commonly of a lower socioeconomic class. They have less inflammatory activity, as reflected by serum alanine aminotransferase activity, than patients with chronic hepatitis C.

Indeterminate chronic viral hepatitis could be due to the HCV and reflect insensitivity of currently available diagnostic assays, including PCR, for HCV infection. It could be due to an unknown virus or to a form of autoantibody-negative autoimmune hepatitis.

### Chronic hepatitis with mixed viral and autoimmune features

Patients with chronic hepatitis may have autoantibodies in serum and serologic evidence of viral infection (Sánchez-Tapias et al 1990, Magrin et al 1991a,b, Cassani et al 1992, Nishiguchi et al 1992). Predominance of viral or autoimmune disease needs to be determined, as corticosteroid therapy in viral infection can increase the virus burden and cause clinical deterioration (Magrin et al 1994), while interferon can exacerbate autoimmune hepatitis (Vento et al 1989, Papo et al 1992, Shindo et al 1992a).

Patients with clinical features of autoimmune hepatitis and antibodies to HCV that are nonreactive by RIBA tests (p. 772) should be regarded as having false positive HCV results (Nishiguchi et al 1992). False positive reactions for anti-HCV by second-generation enzyme immunoassay occur in 60% and by third-generation assays in 20% of patients with autoimmune hepatitis (Czaja et al 1995a). These patients usually have borderline anti-HCV seropositivity and they commonly become seronegative for anti-HCV during corticosteroid therapy (Schrumpf et al 1990, Czaja et al 1992c). They have autoimmune hepatitis with false positive viral markers and should be treated as autoimmune hepatitis.

Patients with indeterminate reactions by RIBA tests frequently have true HCV infections, but in the absence of a confirmatory test such as PCR for the detection of HCV-RNA in serum, they should be considered to have autoimmune hepatitis with false positive viral markers (Czaja 1994). A closely monitored corticosteroid regimen can be administered if the disease is severe unless there are strong epidemiologic risk factors indicating viral infection.

Patients with true viral infection and low titers of autoantibodies should be considered as having true viral infection. Nonspecific low-titer autoantibodies occur in 38% of patients with chronic viral hepatitis and they should not confuse a diagnosis based on major clinical and laboratory evidence of viral disease (Abuaf et al 1993, Czaja et al 1993a,c, Pawlotsky et al 1994, Clifford et al 1995). Titers of SMA and ANA exceed 1:160 in only 11% of patients with chronic hepatitis C and only 23% of patients with chronic hepatitis B or C and immunoserologic markers have titers of 1:320 or greater (Czaja et al 1993a,c). In contrast, patients with autoimmune hepatitis without viral features have median titers of SMA of 1:160 and ANA of 1:320 (Czaja et al 1993c). Indeed, only 6% of patients with autoimmune hepatitis have an isolated immunoserologic marker in a titer of less than 1:80. Accordingly, patients with unequivocal serological evidence of viral infection and titers of SMA or ANA of 1:160 or less should be regarded as having HCV infection. The presence of concurrent SMA and ANA regardless of titer is unusual in chronic viral hepatitis and this combination strongly supports a diagnosis of autoimmune hepatitis (Cassani et al 1992, Czaja et al 1995a).

Rarely, true chronic viral hepatitis can be associated with ANA or SMA titers of 1:320 or greater (Czaja et al 1993a,c). These patients probably have both diseases and usually the manifestations of autoimmune hepatitis predominate. Patients in whom a confident diagnosis of autoimmune hepatitis would have been made if viral markers had not been present should be treated as having autoimmune hepatitis. Corticosteroid therapy for 3–6 months would be appropriate followed by interferon if there is no improvement or predominant viral features emerge (Bellary et al 1995). About 57% of patients with severe autoimmune hepatitis and HCV-RNA in serum respond to corticosteroid therapy (Czaja et al 1995a). The nonresponders do not deteriorate during treatment and this tolerance has been a justification for administering corticosteroids first rather than interferon.

### Drug-related chronic hepatitis

Drugs are important causes of chronic hepatitis and must be excluded in all patients (p. 845). Few drugs are free of risk. Drugs have been reported as causing 67% of chronic hepatitis in Australia (Goldstein et al 1973), 48% in Denmark (Dietrichson 1975) and 28% in Sweden (Lindberg et al 1975). Drug-induced disease may be cholestatic, hepatocellular or mixed. Discontinuation of the drug is usually followed by a slow recovery, especially in cholestatic reactions, but all drug-induced injuries are self-limited. Continuation of the liver disease after drug withdrawal should lead to consideration of alternative diagnoses.

The drugs most commonly associated with chronic hepatitis and their typical patterns of injury are shown in Table 32.3. Oxyphenisatin, α-methyldopa, nitrofurantoin and propylthiouracil may be associated with immunoserologic markers that mimic autoimmune hepatitis (Seeff 1981). Dantrolene, isoniazid, sulfonamides, acetaminophen, aspirin and chlorpromazine may produce

**Table 32.3** Drugs associated with chronic hepatitis

| Histological patterns of injury | |
|---|---|
| *Hepatocellular* | *Cholestatic* |
| Oxyphenisatin* | Azathioprine |
| α-Methyldopa* | Chlorpromazine |
| Nitrofurantoin* | Erythromycin |
| Propylthiouracil* | Ethinyl estradiol |
| Dantrolene | Flurazepam |
| Isoniazid | Griseofulvin |
| Sulfonamides | Imipramine |
| Acetaminophen | Indomethacin |
| Chlorpromazine | Meprobamate |
| Halothane | Phenytoin sodium |
| Aspirin | Propoxyphene |
| | Rifampicin |
| | Tolbutamide |

* Associated with autoantibodies

chronic hepatitis and/or cirrhosis, but this is not usually associated with serum autoantibodies (Seeff 1981).

## NATURAL HISTORY

The natural history of chronic hepatitis relates mainly to its cause, the degree of inflammatory activity and the presence or absence of cirrhosis.

### Autoimmune hepatitis

Autoimmune hepatitis is a chronic condition that is subject to remission and relapse. Unfortunately, there is no way of predicting mortality or response to treatment at presentation. Even hepatic encephalopathy, which is usually associated with a dismal prognosis, can respond well to treatment. Spontaneous resolution can occur and patients with mild disease improve as frequently as those with severe disease (13% vs 20%). There is no way of predicting this outcome (Czaja 1984a). Patients who survive an initial severe stage of disease show spontaneous resolution of inflammatory activity in 41% (Mistilis et al 1968), but they typically have inactive cirrhosis as a consequence of their illness.

#### *Inflammatory activity*

Patients with severe inflammatory activity reflected by serum aminotranferase sustained above tenfold, or above fivefold with hypergammaglobulinemia of at least twice normal, have a 3-year survival of 50% and a 10-year survival of 10% if no treatment is given (Czaja 1984a). Prospective studies in patients with disease of similar severity have indicated a mortality as high as 40% within 6 months (Czaja 1984a). Patients with less severe inflammatory activity have a better prognosis. In such patients, cirrhosis develops in only 49% within 15 years and the 10-year mortality is only 10% (Czaja 1984a). In asymptomatic patients with mild disease, 5- and 10-year survivals of 91% and 81%, respectively, have been reported (Czaja 1984a). Patients with type 2 autoimmune hepatitis may progress to cirrhosis more commonly than those with type 1 disease, but differences in natural history between the various subtypes of autoimmune hepatitis have not been established (Homberg et al 1987).

Bridging necrosis or multilobular necrosis on liver biopsy indicates severe inflammatory disease and in such patients cirrhosis develops in 82% within 5 years and death from liver failure in 45% (Schalm et al 1977). Bridging necrosis between portal tract and central vein progresses to cirrhosis more commonly than bridging necrosis between portal tracts (Cooksley et al 1986). In contrast, periportal hepatitis progresses to cirrhosis in only 17% of patients within 5 years and it is associated with a normal 5-year survival (Schalm et al 1977).

#### *Cirrhosis*

Cirrhosis at presentation is associated with a 5-year mortality of 58% (Schalm et al 1977). Esophageal varices develop in 54% of such patients within 2 years and death from hemorrhage occurs in 20% (Murray-Lyon et al 1973).

#### *Hepatocellular carcinoma*

Primary hepatocellular carcinoma does occur in autoimmune hepatitis but is rare, possibly because untreated patients succumb before they can develop this complication (Burroughs et al 1981, Jakobovits et al 1981).

### Chronic hepatitis B

Chronic HBV infection may not be associated with abnormal liver function tests or abnormal liver histology ("healthy" carrier) (p. 784), but cirrhosis develops when chronic hepatitis is present in up to 70% of patients within 10 years and the mortality during this period is 30% (Czaja 1988). Survival relates to the degree of histological inflammatory activity at presentation. Five-year survival is 97% in patients with portal hepatitis, 86% in patients with periportal hepatitis and 55% is patients with cirrhosis (Weissberg et al 1984). Interestingly, stratification based on histological activity shows that life expectancy in chronic hepatitis B is similar to that in autoimmune hepatitis where the histology is similar (Czaja 1990a). Factors associated with a poor survival by multivariate analysis are age of 40 years or greater, serum bilirubin of 27 μmol/L (1.5 mg/dl) or greater, ascites and spider nevi (Weissberg et al 1984).

Clinical and biochemical remission can occur spontaneously and in Asia remission occurs in 90% of patients (Lam et al 1981). Prospective trials in the United States show that biochemical resolution occurs in 19% and loss of HBV-DNA and HBeAg in 7% of patients within 1 year of observation (Perrillo et al 1990). The frequency of seroconversion from HBeAg to anti-HBe is 2.6–20.8% of patients per year and the median time to seroconversion is 28 months (range 7–75 months) (Czaja 1988). Spontaneous disappearance of HBsAg is very uncommon and is associated with reduction of plasma aminotransferase activity and improvement of inflammation on liver biopsy. However, minor increases of plasma aminotransferase activity and mild inflammatory change in the liver can persist and recent reports have shown that HBV-DNA may be found in the liver (Fong et al 1993). Accordingly, such patients may remain at risk of cirrhosis and hepatocellular carcinoma.

Hepatocellular carcinoma can occur in patients who are asymptomatic chronic carriers of the virus as well as in those with chronic hepatitis (Omata et al 1979). The risk of hepatocellular cancer is 20- to 390-fold greater than that in uninfected patients and surveillance based on hepatic ultrasonography and serum alpha-fetoprotein determinations may not enhance survival (Colombo et al 1991).

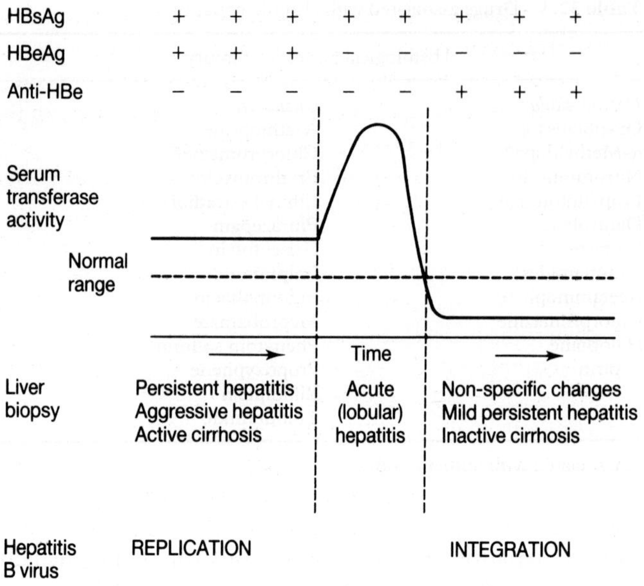


**Fig. 32.5** Seroconversion and histological transitions in chronic hepatitis B.

### *Natural history stages*

Two stages in the natural history of chronic hepatitis B have been described.

***Replication.*** The replicative stage is associated with active hepatitis B virus (HBV) replication and viremia and is characterized by HBeAg and HBV-DNA in serum. Patients are infectious and they have active hepatocellular inflammation reflected in increased serum aminotransferase activity and histological findings of periportal hepatitis (piecemeal necrosis) or active cirrhosis (Fig. 32.5).

***Integration.*** The integrative stage evolves from the replicative stage either spontaneously or during treatment with interferon. It is characterized by the disappearance of HBeAg and HBV-DNA from serum, the appearance of anti-HBe and improvement in the inflammatory manifestations of the disease (Fig. 32.5) (Realdi et al 1980, Wood et al 1987). Patients have a low level of infectivity during this stage, since viremia is absent or minimal. The histological findings are those of portal hepatitis, nonspecific hepatitis or inactive cirrhosis, the last finding being most common in individuals undergoing natural seroconversion (Hoofnagle et al 1981, Liaw et al 1983, 1987, Fattovich et al 1986). The integrative stage is associated with incorporation of the HBV genome into the genome of host hepatocytes (Shafritz et al 1981). The HBV-altered host hepatocytes are capable of producing HBsAg indefinitely in the absence of intact virions. Such cells may be susceptible to subsequent malignant transformation and they have been demonstrated in hepatocellular carcinomas (Shafritz et al 1981, Popper et al 1987, Okuda 1992).

***Transition.*** The transition period between the replicative and integrative stages is heralded by loss of HBV-DNA from serum and seroconversion from HBeAg to anti-HBe (Liaw et al 1983, 1987, Fattovich et al 1986). Clearance of the infected hepatocytes usually produces a hepatitic reaction characterized by an abrupt increase of serum aminotransferase activity. Fatigue and malaise may develop during seroconversion and, rarely, jaundice and other features of hepatic decompensation may ensue. Histological assessment at this time shows a lobular hepatitis (Fig. 32.5). Importantly, the seroconversion period is self-limited and, as integration evolves, inflammatory activity subsides. Seroconversion occurs naturally in 2–20% of patients per year. Patients do not usually lose the HBsAg, although it may disappear in 1–2% of individuals per year.

***Reactivation.*** Unfortunately, reactivation of HBV replication is possible and spontaneous transition from the integrative to the replicative stage can occur (Davis et al 1984a). Reactivation is usually self-limited, but it can have serious clinical consequences including progression to cirrhosis, appearance of ascites or encephalopathy and occasionally even fulminant hepatic failure (Meyer & Duffy 1993). Immunosuppressive agents may precipitate reactivation and they should be used with caution in such patients.

## Chronic hepatitis C

Long-term follow-up studies show that chronic hepatitis C is usually asymptomatic or associated with fatigue. It seems to be less aggressive than chronic hepatitis B and has a relatively good immediate prognosis. Follow-up studies have been of post-transfusion non-A, non-B hepatitis, but retrospective serological tests show that almost all these patients have chronic hepatitis C infection.

Koretz et al (1993) found that only a third of patients developed symptomatic acute hepatitis following transfusion, that chronic hepatitis was asymptomatic and that 18% of patients had some evidence of liver disease after 16 years. The main sign of liver disease was hypersplenism and only one patient each had variceal bleeding or decompensated cirrhosis. Seeff et al (1992) followed patients over 18 years and found that the incidence of death, cirrhosis (1.4%) and hepatocellular carcinoma (0.2%) was the same as in control patients. Tong et al (1995) found a much higher incidence of fatigue (67%), chronic hepatitis (43%), cirrhosis (51%) and hepatocellular carcinoma (5%) at presentation and 15% died of liver disease during a mean follow-up of 4 years. This, however, may reflect selection factors leading to referral to a specialist liver center. Kiyosawa et al (1990) studied patients with chronic hepatitis, cirrhosis or hepatocellular carcinoma following non-A, non-B post-transfusion hepatitis. Almost all patients had chronic hepatitis C virus infection and retrospective serological tests showed persistence of the virus since transfusion. Evolution of chronic hepatitis took about 10 years, cirrhosis about 21 years and hepatocellular carcinoma about 29 years. The evolution of chronic hepatitis C acquired other than by transfusion is not well known. Thus, although cirrhosis, liver failure and hepatocellular carcinoma are well-recognized outcomes of chronic hepatitis C, they do not occur frequently within 20 years of infection and are slow to develop.

The natural history of chronic hepatitis C is characterized by unpredictable spontaneous fluctuations in serum aminotransferase activity (Alter et al 1992). Intervals of biochemical normality can be interspersed with periods of inflammatory activity and viremia may be dissociated completely from clinical and biochemical expression of the disease. Patients with chronic hepatitis C infection can recover spontaneously and lose the markers of HCV infection, but this is infrequent and the rate of loss of anti-HCV does not exceed 0.6 per 100 person-years of observation (Alter et al 1992, Lok et al 1992). Evidence of persistent HCV viremia has been found uniformly during surveillance periods of 42–48 months following return of liver function tests to normal (Alter et al 1992). This implies that HCV viremia can persist indefinitely without clinical expression, that clinical and biochemical resolution does not mean recovery from HCV infection, that spontaneous exacerbation of disease may occur unpredictably and that the risk of developing cirrhosis cannot be discounted in a viremic patient (Czaja 1992). Thus, future treatments need to focus on eliminating the virus if patients are to enjoy clear therapeutic benefit.

Factors predicting the outcome of chronic hepatitis C are few, because the disease is variable in activity and slow in evolution. Retrospective studies show that the duration from onset to cirrhosis in post-transfusion hepatitis is 21 ± 10 years and the mean interval to hepatocellular carcinoma is 29 ± 13 years (Kiyosawa et al 1990). Duration of disease, level of viremia, HCV genotype or variant and cirrhosis may affect response to interferon therapy and hence these factors may be the most important determinants of ultimate outcome (Pagliaro et al 1994).

### Chronic hepatitis D

Chronic coinfection with hepatitis B virus and hepatitis D virus is widely thought to cause more rapidly progressive liver disease than hepatitis B virus alone. However, the development of liver disease in chronic hepatitis D virus infection has been found to be very variable geographically and although cirrhosis can develop within 1–2 years of an acute infection, less severe and less rapidly progressive chronic hepatitis also occurs (Rizzetto & Durazzo 1991).

## INDICATIONS FOR TREATMENT

The decision to institute therapy is a highly individualized judgement and it must balance the possibility of spontaneous improvement and the risks of the untreated disease against the desirable and undesirable consequences of the treatment. Patients with symptomatic disease, severe inflammatory activity or evidence of disease progression are candidates for drug therapy, while patients with few or no symptoms, mild or minimal inflammatory activity, no evidence of disease progression, or advanced decompensated disease have an uncertain benefit–risk ratio from therapy (Table 32.4). The etiologic diagnosis itself does not compel treatment.

### *Autoimmune hepatitis*

Controlled treatment trials have demonstrated a favorable benefit–risk ratio only for patients with sustained severe

**Table 32.4** Indications for treatment in chronic hepatitis

| Absolute | Relative | None |
|---|---|---|
| Incapacitating symptoms | Mild symptoms | Asymptomatic |
| Severe biochemical changes | Mild–moderate biochemical changes | Minimal changes |
| Aminotransferase ≥×10 | | |
| Aminotransferase ≥×5 and γ-globulin ≥×2 | Periportal hepatitis | Portal hepatitis |
| | Disease progression | Inactive cirrhosis |
| Severe histological activity | Decompensation | Advanced decompensation |
| Bridging necrosis | Encephalopathy | |
| Multilobular necrosis | Ascites | |

biochemical abnormalities and/or histological features of confluent (bridging or multilobular) necrosis (Table 32.4). Patients with severe symptoms, such as marked fatigue, or with evidence of progressive disease are also candidates for treatment. Individuals with minimal or no symptoms and mild biochemical and histological activity (periportal hepatitis or mildly active cirrhosis) are best observed (Table 32.4).

*Chronic hepatitis B*

In patients with chronic hepatitis B, active viral replication manifested by sustained presence of HBeAg and/or HBV-DNA in the blood is required before considering antiviral therapy. Individuals most likely to respond to antiviral treatment are women, those with short-duration disease and those who do not have coincident hepatitis D virus or HIV infection, those with serum alanine aminotransferase activity above 200 units/L and those with low levels of HBV viremia (HBV-DNA 99 pg/ml in serum) (Perrillo et al 1990). Failure to manifest any of these findings does not preclude treatment, but it does indicate a low benefit–risk ratio. Patients who have had perinatal infection rarely respond to treatment. Patients with cirrhosis and hypersplenism tolerate medication poorly and are also unlikely to benefit from treatment.

*Chronic hepatitis C*

In patients with chronic hepatitis C, mild asymptomatic disease is common and the value of antiviral therapy is controversial (Terrault & Wright 1995). Mild disease, good health and therefore presumed better tolerance for the drug and greater likelihood of treatment success must be weighed against lack of symptomatic improvement, frequent drug side-effects, unknown long-term benefit and uncertain cost effectiveness. Until clinical trials resolve these issues, the treatment in individual patients with mild disease is a personal one. Patients with chronic hepatitis who are more likely to respond to antiviral therapy are symptomatic, have short-duration disease and low levels of viremia and do not have cirrhosis (Pagliaro et al 1994). Recent reports that interferon therapy may prevent subsequent hepatocellular carcinoma may modify considerations regarding treatment (p. 1125).

***Genotypes.*** Several genotypes of HCV have now been recognized although their classification has not yet been agreed generally (p. 787). Laboratory tests to identify individual genotypes are restricted to a few laboratories, but it already looks likely that the number and nature of genotypes a patient carries will be important in determining response to interferon therapy. In Japan HCV III (HCV-K2) has been found to respond more frequently to interferon therapy than HCV I (HCV prototype) and HCV II (HCV-J) subtypes and another as yet unclassified genotype has been described that responds well to interferon (Yoshioka et al 1992). In Western Europe and the United States, the HCV genotype 1, especially the subtype 1b (Simmonds 1995), has been associated with severe inflammatory activity, a high frequency of cirrhosis, a poor response to interferon therapy and aggressive recurrent liver disease following transplantation (Dusheiko et al 1994, Feray et al 1995). Similarly, the level of viremia is an important but not absolute predictor of outcome (Kobayashi et al 1993, Magrin et al 1994), as are the degree and complexity of quasispecies of HCV that develop as a result of errors in viral replication (Kanazawa et al 1994).

Serum HCV-RNA concentrations are significantly lower in complete responders to interferon than in partial responders or nonresponders and it is possible that the susceptibility of certain HCV subtypes to interferon reflects their lower replicative capacities (Yoshioka et al 1992). The diversity of the HCV strains in an individual patient may also influence the response to treatment. Individuals infected with multiple viral subtypes, as may occur with blood transfusions, respond less well to interferon than those with a single virus subtype, as may occur after a needlestick inoculation (Okada et al 1992). Individuals who fail to respond to interferon can develop an increasingly heterogeneous virus infection under the selective immune pressures of the treatment and of the host. This development of "escape mutants" may in turn impair the response to additional antiviral therapy (Okada et al 1992).

*Chronic hepatitis D*

HDV infection has a significantly worse prognosis than HBV infection and accordingly antiviral treatment is often given. However, response to treatment is poor.

*Other chronic hepatitis*

Patients with cryptogenic chronic hepatitis ("autoantibody-negative autoimmune hepatitis") and chronic indeterminate viral hepatitis should be selected for treatment by the same criteria that govern the therapy of autoimmune hepatitis or chronic hepatitis C respectively. Patients with mixed viral and autoimmune features must be classified according to their predominant etiologic features (p. 896) and then treated according to disease severity (Czaja 1994).

## TREATMENT REGIMENS

### Autoimmune hepatitis

Anti-inflammatory immunosuppressive drugs are used to treat autoimmune hepatitis and corticosteroids such as prednisone or prednisolone in equal doses and azathioprine are the drugs of choice. Prednisone or prednisolone in conjunction with azathioprine (50 mg daily) has been shown to ameliorate symptoms, resolve biochemical abnormalities, improve histological features and enhance survival in patients with severe autoimmune hepatitis (Czaja 1991). Each corticosteroid regimen is comparable in efficacy and each is superior to azathioprine alone or prednisone in alternate day doses (Table 32.5). Postmenopausal patients and individuals with brittle diabetes, hypertension, obesity or emotional lability are ideal candidates for therapy with prednisone and azathioprine. Patients who are cytopenic, pregnant or contemplating pregnancy, with concurrent nonhepatic malignancy or where a short trial of treatment is proposed are best managed with prednisone alone (Czaja 1991). Postmenopausal patients respond as well to corticosteroid therapy as premenopausal patients and they have a similar frequency of drug-related complications during initial treatment (Wang & Czaja 1989). Consequently, these patients should be treated vigorously initially to induce remission. Therapy after relapse is poorly tolerated and postmenopausal patients become candidates for a long-term low-dose maintenance regimen with either prednisone or azathioprine alone.

Treatment is continued until remission is achieved, intolerance to the medication develops, deterioration despite therapy occurs or protracted therapy incurs side-effects (Czaja 1991). There is no evidence that subgroups of autoimmune hepatitis require different treatments. All the subgroups, including cryptogenic chronic hepatitis (autoantibody-negative chronic hepatitis), respond to the treatment regimens given here. Failure to respond to treatment should lead to a review of the original diagnosis.

**Table 32.5** Treatment regimens

| Diagnosis | Treatment | |
|---|---|---|
| Autoimmune hepatitis | Prednisone or prednisolone | + azathioprine: |
| | 30 mg daily × 1 week | + 50 mg daily |
| | 20 mg daily × 1 week | + 50 mg daily |
| | 15 mg daily × 2 weeks | + 50 mg daily |
| | 10 mg daily maintenance | + 50 mg daily |
| | Prednisone alone: | |
| | 60 mg daily × 1 week | |
| | 40 mg daily × 1 week | |
| | 30 mg daily × 2 weeks | |
| | 20 mg daily maintenance | |
| Chronic hepatitis B | α-Interferon (subcutaneously): | |
| | 5 mu daily × 4 months or | |
| | 10 mu alternate days × 4 months | |
| Precore mutant | 9 mu thrice weekly × 4 months | |
| Drug intolerance | 5 mu thrice weekly × 26 weeks | |
| Chronic hepatitis C | α-Interferon (subcutaneously): | |
| | 3 mu thrice weekly × 6 months | |
| Drug intolerance | 1 mu thrice weekly × 6 months | |
| Relapse | 3 mu thrice weekly × 6 months | |
| Chronic hepatitis D | α-Interferon (subcutaneously): | |
| | 5 mu thrice weekly followed by | |
| | 3 mu weekly × 8 months or | |
| | 10 mu thrice weekly × 12 months | |

Note: mu = million units

*Complications*

A combination of prednisone and azathioprine is generally preferred to prednisone alone because it has a lower frequency of severe drug-related complications (10% vs 44%). Each regimen, however, if administered long enough, will induce cosmetic changes with comparable frequency. Indeed, 80% of patients treated with either schedule for at least 2 years will manifest truncal obesity, facial rounding, dorsal hump formation, acne or hirsutism (Czaja 1991). Fortunately, only 13% of patients develop complications that necessitate the premature discontinuation of medication and patients with cirrhosis are affected most commonly (25% vs 8%) (Czaja et al 1984).

Severe complications such as osteoporosis with vertebral collapse, aseptic necrosis, diabetes mellitus, hypertension, cataracts and psychosis usually develop only after 18 months of continuous therapy and at doses of prednisone exceeding 10 mg daily. Since complications of prednisone relate to the concentration of unbound prednisolone in the blood and this in turn is affected by hypoalbuminemia (reduced carrier availability) and/or hyperbilirubinemia (enhanced competition for carrier sites), patients with jaundice and/or hypoalbuminemia are at the greatest risk of corticosteroid-induced complications (Lewis et al 1971, Czaja 1991). It is important to be aware that the consequences of liver disease can resemble the side-effects of drugs and consequently medication may be wrongly incriminated and withdrawn prematurely.

The side-effects of azathioprine are cholestatic hepatitis, skin rash, nausea, vomiting and leukopenia or thrombocytopenia (Czaja 1991). These reactions occur in fewer than 10% of patients receiving the 50 mg daily dose and they improve following dose reduction or drug withdrawal. In pregnant mice, azathioprine has been associated with skeletal anomalies, cleft palate, reduced thymic size, hydrops fetalis, anemia and hematopoietic depression in the fetus. These have not been observed in humans but animal experiments discourage the use of azathioprine in pregnant patients.

Unfortunately, long-term immunosuppression has been associated with an increased risk of malignancy and this must be considered in the treatment decision. The incidence of nonhepatic neoplasms in treated autoimmune hepatitis is 1 per 194 patient-years of surveillance and the probability of cancer is 3% after 10 years (Wang et al 1989). The risk of malignancy cannot be predicted by age, sex, treatment regimen, cumulative duration of treatment or stage of the liver disease. The risk is only 1.4-fold greater than that in the general population, but it does emphasize the importance of treatment only where there are good indications (Table 32.4).

## Chronic hepatitis B

Interferon is currently the only drug used in clinical practice. It has antiviral and antiproliferative actions that affect the HBV directly and in addition it induces HLA expression on hepatocyte membrane surfaces and stimulates immune effector cells to enhance the elimination of infected hepatocytes. Recombinant α-interferon has been shown by controlled clinical trials to induce resolution of biochemical abnormalities (44% vs 19%), seroconversion from HBeAg to antiHBe (37% vs 7%), loss of HBV-DNA from serum (37% vs 7%) and disappearance of HBsAg from serum (12% vs 0%) in patients with replicative chronic hepatitis B (Perrillo et al 1990). Additionally, histological improvement in the liver after therapy occurs more commonly than in untreated patients (64% vs 16%) (Perrillo et al 1990). Reactivation, as evidenced by reappearance of HBeAg or HBV-DNA, after seroconversion occurs in only 2%. Patients with the precore or e-minus mutant should be treated in the same fashion as individuals with the wild type virus. Hadziyannis et al (1990) showed that disappearance of serum HBV-DNA and normalization of the serum alanine aminotransferase activity occurred in 42% of patients treated with 9 million units thrice weekly and prolongation of the treatment period increased the frequency of response to 67% (Table 32.5). Unfortunately, biochemical relapse is more frequent in patients with the precore or e-minus mutant and a sustained biochemical remission can be anticipated in only 15% of patients. Retreatment giving corticosteroids over 4–6 weeks before interferon has been tried on the grounds that corticosteroid-induced immunosuppression may be followed by an immune rebound, improving the chances of success with interferon, but most trials have not found this successful or superior to interferon alone (Perrillo et al 1990). Patients with high serum aminotransferase activity or active hepatitis on biopsy before treatment are more likely to respond to interferon than those with normal aminotransferase activity or minimal abnormality on biopsy (Brook et al 1989). Treatment is unlikely to succeed in patients with coincident HIV infection (Brook et al 1989) or in patients with HBV infection acquired at birth (Lai et al 1987).

***Regimens.*** Two regimens, designed to deliver 30–35 million units of interferon per week are equally effective. Depending on drug tolerance and pre-existent cytopenia, interferon can be administered as a 5 million unit dose subcutaneously each day for 4 months or as a 10 million unit dose subcutaneously on alternate days for 4 months (Table 32.5) (Schalm 1994). Therapy with prednisone followed by interferon has also been effective but offers no advantage (Perrillo et al 1990). A lower dose regimen of 5 million units of interferon thrice weekly for 26 weeks can be administered to individuals intolerant of the recommended schedules (Schalm 1994).

***Response to therapy.*** Within days of starting interferon a reduction is noted in the serum HBV-DNA (Fig. 32.6). Responders show an increase of serum aminotransferase activity after 6–8 weeks, which is thought to represent immune recognition and lysis of infected hepatocytes, followed by the disappearance of HBeAg and the development of anti-HBe antibodies (seroconversion). HBsAg continues to be detected in the blood for some time, but long-term follow-up may show its eventual disappearance. Korenman et al (1991) found that 36% of their patients responded to interferon with loss of HBeAg and reduction

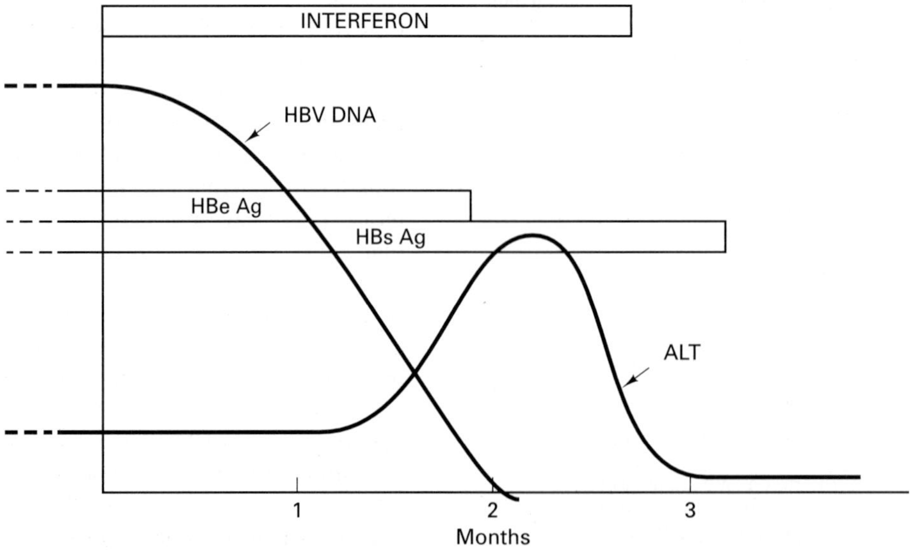


**Fig. 32.6** Serological and biochemical response of chronic hepatitis B virus infection to interferon therapy.

of plasma aminotransferase activity, that relapse occurred in 13% of responders within a year of therapy and that 56% of responders lost the HBsAg within 6 years of therapy. The seroconversion response is associated with an increase of inflammatory activity in the liver, but liver histology returns to normal when this subsides provided cirrhosis was not present before treatment began. Immune lysis of infected hepatocytes in cirrhotic patients may precipitate liver failure, so more cautious, highly supervised regimens of interferon are advised.

***Toxicity.*** Almost all patients experience side-effects from interferon (Davis et al 1989). The most common are fatigue, myalgias, headaches, fever and nausea and these usually improve spontaneously over about 6 weeks as therapy is continued. Taking interferon with acetaminophen (1 g) in the evening before going to bed can minimize the symptoms. More severe side-effects include depression, neutropenia and thrombocytopenia and each may limit the course of treatment. Reduction in the neutrophil count below $0.7 \times 10^9$/L (750/mm$^3$) and/or platelet count below $50 \times 10^9$/L (50 000/mm$^3$) requires reduction in the dose of interferon by 50%. Interferon should be stopped if the neutrophil count falls below $0.5 \times 10^9$/L (500/mm$^3$) and/or the platelet count falls below $30 \times 10^9$/L (30 000/mm$^3$). The peripheral blood count, creatinine, liver function tests and plasma thyroid-stimulating hormone and thyroxine should be checked monthly and in response to new symptoms during treatment.

Interferon therapy can enhance the expression of autoimmune manifestations, possibly because it induces HLA display on surface membranes and impairs suppressor T-cell function (Vento et al 1989). A plethora of autoantibodies have been found in patients after interferon treatment (Mayet et al 1989, Fattovich et al 1991) and there have been reports of interferon-induced autoimmune thyroiditis (Chung & Shong 1993), conversion of chronic hepatitis B to autoimmune hepatitis after therapy (Silva et al 1991) and exacerbation of autoimmune diseases, such as autoimmune hepatitis (Vento et al 1989) or ulcerative colitis (Mitoro et al 1993), after administration of the drug. The autoantibodies induced by interferon do not seem to be cytotoxic and there is no need to stop treatment (Mayet et al 1989, Saracco et al 1990). The drug should be used with caution, however, in individuals with concurrent autoimmune diseases.

## Chronic hepatitis C

Clinical trials have shown that recombinant α-interferon is effective in patients with chronic hepatitis C (Table 32.5) (Davis et al 1989, Di Bisceglie et al 1989). Interferon 3 million units subcutaneously thrice weekly for 6 months induces biochemical resolution more often than 1 million units thrice weekly (46% vs 28%) or no therapy (46% vs 8%) (Davis et al 1989). Eighty-five percent of patients who respond do so within 3 months of treatment and the drug can be discontinued in nonresponders after 4 months. Histological improvement occurs in 52% of patients given 3 million units thrice weekly and improvement may occur even without biochemical resolution (Davis et al 1989). Recent studies have shown that patients with increased hepatic iron concentrations have a diminished response to interferon and phlebotomy in such patients enhances drug efficacy. Relapse after drug withdrawal may be prevented by a gradual reduction in the dose of interferon rather than an abrupt cessation. These observations need to be corroborated, but checking the serum ferritin to detect patients needing phlebotomy and withdrawing interferon gradually may be beneficial. Several HCV genotypes have been identified and some are more susceptible to therapy than others (p. 787).

Interferon therapy can eliminate HCV-RNA from serum, but the disappearance of viremia is frequently temporary (Shindo et al 1991). Biochemical relapse of chronic hepatitis C occurs in 50% of the individuals who respond fully to therapy and these individuals typically have reappearance of HCV-RNA in serum (Davis et al 1989, Shindo et al 1991). Most patients fail to respond to interferon or relapse after drug withdrawal (Davis et al 1989). Only about 25% of treated patients achieve a sustained biochemical remission and HCV-RNA may reappear in the liver within 6 months of stopping treatment (Balart et al 1993). Since biochemical exacerbations after interferon withdrawal may be transient, repeat administration of the drug should be deferred for at least 6 months unless hepatic decompensation has occurred.

Exacerbations of inflammatory activity during interferon treatment suggest the development of a separate viral infection, a toxic reaction, the emergence of an autoimmune disease or interferon "breakthrough" (Roffi et al 1995). Each instance must be evaluated comprehensively. Interferon therapy should be stopped while these are being investigated. Interferon "breakthrough" occurs in 12% of treated patients, half have neutralizing interferon antibodies and they do not respond to higher doses of α-interferon. The reasons for the "breakthrough" are unclear; interferon antibodies are an insufficient explanation, but patients may respond to natural lymphoblastoid interferon (Roffi et al 1995).

## Chronic hepatitis D

Patients with chronic hepatitis D respond less well to interferon than those with chronic hepatitis B or C (Schalm 1994). Higher doses for longer periods of time can reduce disease activity and HDV replication, but biochemical resolution and sustained improvement are infrequent. Since the disease is aggressive, there are compelling clinical reasons to treat but expectations should be limited. The poor response to treatment in chronic hepatitis D may be due in part to factors other than the HDV. Patients are commonly drug addicts and may be infected with other viruses, especially HCV or human immunodeficiency virus, or they may have superimposed toxic liver injury (Schalm 1994). However, poor response rates occur in trials where patients' risk factors have been excluded.

Recombinant interferon 5 million units subcutaneously thrice weekly for 4 months, followed by 3 million units thrice weekly for 8 months, has resulted in a decrease in serum alanine aminotransferase activity in 58% of patients (Table 32.5) (Rosina et al 1991). Unfortunately, liver function tests returned to normal in only one of 48 patients and serum aminotransferase activities increased to pretreatment levels in the majority when the dose of interferon was reduced. Higher response rates occur if interferon 10 million units thrice weekly is given for 12 months, but liver function tests returned to normal in only 33% of patients (Table 32.5) (Hadziyannis 1991). Trials indicate that the best results require high-dose medication for prolonged, possibly indefinite, periods.

## TREATMENT RESULTS

### Autoimmune hepatitis

Remission, defined as resolution of symptoms, biochemical abnormality limited to a serum aminotransferase level of less than twofold normal and minimal or no histological activity, is achieved in 65% of patients within 2 years of instituting therapy (Czaja 1991). "Cure", defined as reversion to normal hepatic architecture and absence of disease for at least 5 years, eventuates in only 10% (Czaja et al 1984). Individuals who do not have cirrhosis at presentation have 5- and 10-year survivals after treatment exceeding 90%, while patients with cirrhosis have 5- and 10-year survivals of 80% and 65% respectively (Czaja 1984a). Thirteen percent of patients improve but fail to enter remission in spite of 3 years' continuous therapy (incomplete responders) and serious drug toxicity that compels premature discontinuation of therapy develops in 13% (Czaja 1991). Intolerable obesity or cosmetic changes (47%), osteoporosis with vertebral compression (27%), brittle diabetes (20%) and peptic ulceration (6%) are the most common reasons for termination of therapy (Czaja et al 1984). Treatment failure, defined by clinical, biochemical and/or histological deterioration, occurs in 9% of patients (Czaja 1991).

#### *Relapse*

Relapse is defined as recrudescence of symptoms after drug withdrawal, elevation of the serum aminotransferase activity to more than threefold normal, hypergammaglobulinemia of greater than 20 g/L and/or histological features of periportal hepatitis. This occurs in as many as 87% of patients within 1 year (Czaja et al 1980, 1981, Hegarty et al 1983). Reinstitution of the original treatment typically re-establishes remission, but later drug withdrawal is commonly followed by further relapse (Czaja et al 1980). Patients who relapse more often progress to cirrhosis (38% vs 10%) and death from liver failure (14% vs 4%) than those who sustain remission after drug withdrawal (Czaja et al 1987). The major consequences of relapse and retreatment, however, are drug-induced complications. Indeed, more than 70% of individuals who have been retreated after multiple relapses have drug-related complications (Czaja et al 1987).

#### *Cirrhosis*

Cirrhosis occurs in 47% of patients with autoimmune hepatitis within 10 years despite corticosteroid therapy (Davis et al 1984b). It develops most commonly during the initial course of treatment when the disease is most active, especially if the duration of treatment required for remission exceeds 2 years (frequency of cirrhosis 56%). If remission can be attained without cirrhosis, it develops subsequently in only 5% of patients. In those who relapse, however, the frequency of cirrhosis is 23% and the mean annual incidence is 2.6% for up to 10 years (Davis et al 1984b).

The development of cirrhosis during or after treatment has not diminished immediate life expectancy. The 5-year survival of such patients is 93% and comparable to that of patients without cirrhosis (Davis et al 1984b). Similarly, esophageal varices develop infrequently in treated patients (13%) and hemorrhage from varices is unusual (5%) (Czaja et al 1979). Recent studies have indicated that hepatic fibrosis may actually diminish during corticosteroid treatment and this improvement may account for the prolonged and uncomplicated survival of patients with early cirrhosis (Schvarcz et al 1993).

#### *Malignant disease*

Hepatocellular carcinoma develops in 7% of patients with cirrhosis of at least 5 years' duration (Wang & Czaja 1988). The incidence of hepatocellular cancer in these patients is 1 per 182 patient-years of follow-up and the probability of neoplasm is 29% after 13 years. There is also the possibility of malignant disease arising as a consequence of immunosuppressive therapy and this is considered elsewhere (p. 901).

### Chronic viral hepatitis

The immediate consequences of interferon therapy in chronic viral hepatitis are well described and include complete response, incomplete response, nonresponse, drug toxicity, sustained remission and relapse after drug withdrawal. The long-term consequences of such treatment are ill defined and it is unknown whether improvements achieved during therapy can be maintained indefinitely or whether progression to cirrhosis, liver failure and hepatocellular carcinoma can be prevented (p. 1125). In a retrospective analysis of patients with chronic hepatitis C in whom serum aminotransferase activities remained normal after therapy, HCV-RNA disappeared in all patients and there was no evidence of recurrent infection or hepatitis after 3–6 years (Shindo et al 1992b). These studies suggest that a complete response to interferon therapy may be long-lasting, but "long-term" studies are still relatively "short-term" in relation to the total duration of chronic HCV infections and the critical issue of eventual outcome has not yet been resolved. Even patients with normal serum aminotransferase and no HCV-RNA detectable in the liver at the end of treatment may relapse within 6 months (Balart et al 1993).

**Table 32.6** Treatment of suboptimal responses

| Diagnosis | Treatment |
|---|---|
| Autoimmune hepatitis | |
| Relapse | Retreatment (original regimen) |
| Multiple (≥2) relapses | Low-dose prednisone or azathioprine (2 mg/kg) |
| Treatment failure | High-dose prednisone 60 mg daily or prednisone 30 mg + azathioprine 150 mg daily × 1 month, then dose reduction every month of improvement |
| | Liver transplantation |
| Incomplete response | Low-dose prednisone |
| Chronic viral hepatitis | |
| Drug intolerance | α-Interferon |
| | Half-dose regimen or discontinuation |
| Relapse | α-Interferon<br>Retreatment (original regimen) |
| Treatment failure | Liver transplantation |

## TREATMENT OF SUBOPTIMAL RESPONSES

### Autoimmune hepatitis

*Relapse after drug withdrawal*

This is the most common problem in autoimmune hepatitis. The causes of relapse are uncertain, but they include premature withdrawal of medication, failure to control pathogenic mechanisms and complicating factors such as viral infection. The frequency of relapse can be reduced if liver function tests and liver histology are normal prior to drug withdrawal (Czaja et al 1984). This may not be attainable, however, and relentless pursuit of these goals may be at the cost of serious side-effects.

Cessation of treatment once hepatic architecture has become normal is followed by relapse in only 20% (Czaja et al 1984), whereas cessation of therapy when portal hepatitis is still present is associated with relapse in at least 50%. Patients who develop cirrhosis during treatment or who still have periportal hepatitis at the time of drug withdrawal invariably relapse. Unfortunately, the possibility of relapse can never be eliminated, but histological assessment prior to termination of treatment is valuable in ensuring the best opportunity for a sustained remission.

Reinstitution of the original treatment after relapse consistently induces another remission, but the likelihood of further relapse after drug withdrawal is 60% and this increases to 86% after a third treatment and subsequent drug withdrawal (Czaja et al 1980). Patients who relapse after two courses of treatment require long-term therapy, as shown in Table 32.6 (Czaja 1990b). Prednisone or prednisolone should be used in the lowest dose found to prevent symptoms and maintain the serum aminotransferase activity below fivefold normal. Side-effects acquired during conventional treatment subside, the development of new side-effects is minimized and mortality can be as low as with conventional regimens (9% vs 10%). Indeed, 87% of patients have been managed on 10 mg or less of prednisone daily (median dose 7.5 mg daily) for up to 149 months (mean duration of follow-up 44 ± 7 months) (Czaja 1990b). Treatment with high-dose prednisone (90 mg daily) for 5 consecutive days each month ("pulse therapy") does not control the disease and alternate-day corticosteroid therapy, which is not effective in managing the disease at presentation, is untested in managing the disease after relapse (Czaja et al 1993f). These two regimens are not recommended.

Long-term maintenance therapy with azathioprine (2 mg/kg daily) can be used for patients who are prone to relapse (Table 32.6) (Stellon et al 1988). Myelosuppression is uncommon (8%) and malignancy has not been reported during relatively short periods of observation. Unfortunately, most patients (75%) experience arthralgias and myalgias as corticosteroid is withdrawn and these may last for up to 12 months. Nonsteroidal anti-inflammatory drugs may be helpful, but patients with esophageal varices should only be given acetaminophen (paracetamol) (p. 844). Additionally, the teratogenic and oncogenic risks of indefinite azathioprine therapy remain uncertain in these patients.

*Treatment failure*

This can occur at any time after institution of corticosteroid therapy, but it typically develops within 2 months. High doses of prednisone (60 mg daily) or prednisone (30 mg daily) in conjunction with azathioprine (150 mg daily) for at least a month bring about a remission in 75%

of cases (Table 32.6) (Schalm et al 1976). Treatment can then be reduced each month in the hope of achieving a conventional maintenance regimen. Prednisolone is an alternative to prednisone.

Patients in whom conventional therapy fails occasionally remit spontaneously (20%), but usually they require long-term corticosteroid treatment with or without azathioprine. Drug-related side-effects are common, as are manifestations of liver failure. Cyclosporin has been used in patients who have not responded to conventional therapy or who have had incapacitating side-effects (Mistilis et al 1985, Hyams et al 1987). Favorable results have been reported using 5–6 mg/kg daily for 1 year, but the drug has not been tested in controlled clinical trials and its value remains to be established. Severe side-effects are possible (p. 1157), and all patients who have responded to the drug have relapsed after termination of therapy.

Liver transplantation is an effective treatment for patients who develop liver failure in spite of medical therapy (p. 1151). Recurrence of the disease after transplantation is rare, but it has been described in patients who are inadequately immunosuppressed and in HLA DR3-positive recipients of HLA DR3-negative grafts (Neuberger et al 1984, Wright et al 1992a). The optimal timing for liver transplantation is uncertain, since there are no findings at presentation that reliably predict response to corticosteroid therapy. Consequently, the decision for transplantation must be based on an assessment of the response to treatment. In most instances, this requires deferment of the transplant decision for no more than 2 weeks. Failure to demonstrate clinical or laboratory improvement (especially reduction in the serum bilirubin level) during this interval justifies liver transplantation (Czaja et al 1988).

*Incomplete response*

An incomplete response to therapy does not mean that clinical deterioration will occur. However, such patients are unlikely to achieve remission even with protracted treatment and limitation of hepatic damage rather than induction of remission becomes the treatment priority (Table 32.6) (Czaja 1991). The proper course of action has not been defined, but reduction in the dose of medications to the lowest level possible to maintain a stable clinical and biochemical state is logical. The first manifestation of liver decompensation justifies consideration of liver transplantation (Sanchez-Urdazpal et al 1992).

### Chronic viral hepatitis

Treatment for patients who fail to respond to interferon is empiric or investigational. The dose of interferon can be halved for patients who are intolerant of the drug or where side-effects occur but are not severe. Regimens as low as 1 million units subcutaneously thrice weekly for 6 months have proved more effective than no therapy in returning liver function tests to normal in chronic hepatitis (Davis et al 1989). Relapse of chronic hepatitis C more than 6 months after interferon withdrawal or reactivation of chronic hepatitis B can be managed by reinstituting the original treatment regimen (Table 32.6). A slow, tapered withdrawal from interferon rather than an abrupt cessation may diminish the likelihood of relapse in patients with chronic hepatitis C. High-dose regimens (5 million units thrice weekly for 6 months), combination regimens (interferon and ursodeoxycholic acid) and long-term indefinite treatment schedules are possible approaches to relapse, but none has yet been proven in clinical trials.

Liver transplantation should be considered for decompensated patients with chronic viral hepatitis, but reinfection is almost invariable (p. 1153). Infection of the allograft can jeopardize the immediate and long-term success of the procedure and in patients with chronic hepatitis B the frequency and seriousness of these consequences have dampened enthusiasm for the procedure. In patients with chronic hepatitis C, viremia after liver transplantation occurs in 95% but 56% of infected recipients have no evidence of allograft injury after 1 year of observation (Wright et al 1992b). Of those with post-transplant hepatitis, 58% have histological features of periportal hepatitis but only 16% have severe histological disease. Other studies have indicated a low frequency of histological progression over a 1–5-year period (1.6%) and low occurrence of severe graft dysfunction (Martin et al 1991, Shah et al 1992). Clearly, HCV infection is an important cause of post-transplant graft dysfunction and has the potential for eventual progression to cirrhosis (Poterucha et al 1992). However, the natural history of chronic HCV infection in transplant recipients has not been defined long-term and although there is skepticism about the eventual outcome, chronic liver disease due to HCV infection remains an indication for liver transplantation.

## OTHER THERAPIES

### Autoimmune hepatitis

Unsubstantiated therapies for autoimmune hepatitis include immunosuppressive drugs, cytoprotective drugs and drugs with a putative immunomodulatory action.

*Tacrolimus (FK-506)*

This is an immunosuppressive agent derived from a soil fungus *(Streptomyces tsukubaenis)*. Its actions are similar to cyclosporin, but it is less toxic and is used most in organ transplantation (p. 1158). Its immunosuppressive actions could be useful in autoimmune hepatitis and an open-labeled trial in a small group of patients with autoimmune hepatitis showed that tacrolimus can decrease serum aminotransferase activities and bilirubin concentrations at an oral dose of 4 mg twice daily (Van Thiel et al 1992, Thomson et al 1993). However, treatment was not continued into remission, liver biopsies were not performed to show any drug-related improvements and most patients showed renal impairment. Furthermore, experimental studies suggest tacrolimus may enhance fibrosis (Frizell et al 1994). This drug requires further evaluation.

*Thymic hormone extracts*

These stimulate suppressor T-cell activity and inhibit immunoglobulin production. Consequently, there is a rationale for their use in autoimmune hepatitis. Unfortunately, an early controlled trial failed to demonstrate that thymic hormone extract could prevent relapse of disease after remission had been achieved by conventional therapy (Hegarty et al 1984). Optimal doses, duration of treatment and mode of administration remain undefined and benefit may yet be shown by further trials.

*Polyunsaturated phosphatidylcholine*

This has been used successfully in conjunction with prednisone in the initial management of autoimmune hepatitis, but its value has not been established. A double-blind controlled trial has shown that this combination reduces histological activity better than prednisone alone, presumably by modifying the hepatocyte membrane and blocking or altering the cytotoxic attack on the liver cell (Jenkins et al 1982). This success has not been confirmed and the combination cannot be recommended as an initial therapy (Neuberger et al 1983). Similar preliminary results have been reported using arginine thiazolidinecarboxylate (Miracco et al 1984).

*Ursodeoxycholic acid*

Administered daily for 2 months in doses of 250 mg, 500 mg, and 750 mg, this reduces serum aminotransferase and γ-glutamyl transferase activities in patients with chronic hepatitis (Crosignani et al 1991). Most of the patients treated have had viral disease, but the drug has actions that may be of benefit to patients with autoimmune hepatitis, including displacement of hydrophobic (highly detergent) bile acids from hepatocytes, prevention of their ileal absorption, protection of the hepatocyte membrane from noxious insults and alteration of class I HLA expression on hepatocyte membranes (Calmus et al 1990). Clinical trials are needed to define the potential of ursodeoxycholic acid in autoimmune hepatitis.

*Budesonide*

This is a potent corticosteroid with a high first-pass clearance by the liver and a low systemic availability (Danielsson & Prytz 1994). Ninety percent of an oral dose is metabolized during the first pass through the liver, its metabolites lack glucocorticoid activity and its affinity for the glucocorticoid receptor is 15-fold greater than that of prednisolone. Theoretically, budesonide could deliver high concentrations of drug to the liver with a low risk of systemic side-effects. A limited trial in 13 patients treated for up to 9 months showed significant reduction in serum alanine aminotransferase and immunoglobulin while plasma cortisol levels remained normal or slightly below normal (Danielsson & Prytz 1994). These encouraging findings justify further assessment.

## Chronic hepatitis B

*Acyclovir*

Acyclovir has an inhibitory effect on HBV replication (Weller et al 1982), but low oral bioavailability has limited its use. Famciclovir has greater oral bioavailability and is under trial (Vere Hodge et al 1989).

*Fialuridine and lamivudine*

Trials with fialuridine, a nucleoside analog, were discontinued when some patients developed fatal multisystem failure and lactic acidosis, suggesting drug-related mitochondrial toxicity. Trials continue with lamivudine, another nucleoside analog, which has an inhibitory effect on HBV replication (Tyrrell et al 1993).

*Bovine thymus extract* (thymosin)

This agent enhances T-cell function, promotes endogenous production of α- and γ-interferon and increases the expression of interleukin 2 receptors on lymphocytes. In a small trial comparing thymosin to placebo in 12 patients with chronic hepatitis B, individuals receiving thymosin lost HBV-DNA from serum and HBcAg from liver tissue more frequently than those receiving placebo (Mutchnick et al 1991). Additionally, liver biopsy showed significant improvement after therapy in patients treated with thymosin in comparison with placebo-treated patients. Thymosin is currently being assessed in a multicenter treatment trial.

## Chronic hepatitis C

*Interferons*

There are three classes of interferons (α, β, and γ), which are divided into two types based on cell of origin, methods of induction and physical properties. Type I interferons include α- and β-interferon and type II interferon implies γ-interferon. α-Interferon is derived from leukocytes and β-interferon from fibroblasts. Each of these heat- and pH-resistant molecules is induced by viruses or polynucleotides. γ-Interferon is derived from T-lymphocytes, is heat and pH labile and is induced by mitogens and antigens. Recombinant α-interferon is the drug currently used to treat chronic hepatitis C. Other interferons are under investigation.

β-Interferon has more rapid antiviral activity in vitro than either the α or γ varieties and it has a greater binding affinity to type I interferon receptors than α-interferon (Kiyosawa et al 1989). Indeed, it may have its own receptor, It is also less toxic than α-interferon. Clinical trials evaluating its efficacy in chronic hepatitis C are in progress.

Recombinant methionyl interferon consensus ("consensus interferon") is a synthetic type I interferon that was derived by scanning the amino acid sequences of the 11 known subtypes of α-interferon and determining the most common amino acid at each position (Ozes et al 1992). A synthetic DNA coding sequence was then constructed based on the consensus sequence and the molecule was expressed in *Escherichia coli*. "Consensus interferon" has 30% homology with β-interferon and has specific antiviral activity that is greater than that of either α-interferon 2a or interferon 2b (Ozes et al 1992). Lower concentrations give equal biologic activity with other interferons and may equate with fewer side-effects at comparable doses or a greater response without increased side-effects at higher doses. This product of molecular engineering needs to be tested in clinical trials.

### *Ribavirin*

This is an antiviral agent quite separate from the interferons that has potent antiviral actions and can be given orally. A small uncontrolled study of 13 patients given ribavirin 600 mg daily increasing to 1200 mg daily for 6 months showed improvement in serum alanine aminotransferase activity in all patients and a return to normal liver function tests in 31% (Di Bisceglie et al 1992). HCV-RNA titers in serum decreased, but viremia was not eradicated and there was no evidence of histological improvement. Not surprisingly, 12 of 13 patients relapsed within 6 months of drug withdrawal. Similar results were reported in a Japanese study in which patients were randomly assigned to ribavirin, β-interferon or a combination therapy (Kakumu et al 1993). Each regimen reduced serum aminotransferase activity and HCV-RNA, but elimination of HCV-RNA occurred in only six of 27 patients (22%). Relapse followed cessation of treatment. Combination therapy with ribavirin and interferon requires further study (Kakumu et al 1993).

The search for better treatment of chronic hepatitis C is intense and at the last count 24 different drugs had been evaluated in some fashion. High-dose interferon regimens tapered to low-dose regimens, indefinite long-term interferon schedules and combination or sequential therapies are all being tested. It is certain that current treatment strategies for chronic viral hepatitis will change.

## REFERENCES


Abuaf N, Johanet C, Chretien P, Martini E, Soulier E, Laperche S, Homberg J C 1992 Characterization of the liver cytosol antigen type 1 reacting with autoantibodies in chronic active hepatitis. Hepatology 16: 892–898

Abuaf N, Lunel F, Giral P et al 1993 Non-organ specific autoantibodies associated with chronic C virus hepatitis. Journal of Hepatology 18: 359–364

Alter M J, Margolis H S, Krawczynski K et al for the Sentinal Counties Chronic Non-A Non-B Hepatitis Study Team 1992 The natural history of community-acquired hepatitis C in the United States. New England Journal of Medicine 327: 1899–1905

Bach N, Thung S N, Schaffner F 1992 The histological features of chronic hepatitis C and autoimmune chronic hepatitis: a comparative analysis. Hepatology 15: 572–577

Baggenstoss A H, Soloway R D, Summerskill W H J, Elveback L R, Schoenfield L J 1972 Chronic active liver disease. The range of histological lesions, their response to treatment, and evolution. Human Pathology 3: 183–198

Balart L A, Perrillo R, Roddenberry J et al 1993 Hepatitis C RNA in liver of chronic hepatitis C patients before and after interferon alpha treatment. Gastroenterology 104: 1472–1477

Bellary S, Schiano T, Hartman G, Black M 1995 Chronic hepatitis with combined features of autoimmune chronic hepatitis and chronic hepatitis C: favorable response to prednisone and azathioprine. Annals of Internal Medicine 123: 32–34

Ben-Ari Z, Dhillon A P, Sherlock S 1993 Autoimmune cholangiopathy: part of the spectrum of autoimmune chronic active hepatitis. Hepatology 18: 10–15

Brook M G, Karayiannis P, Thomas H C 1989 Which patients with chronic hepatitis B virus infection will respond to α-interferon therapy? A statistical analysis of predictive factors. Hepatology 10: 761–763

Brown J, Dourakis S, Karayiannis P et al 1992 Seroprevalence of hepatitis C virus nucleocapsid antibodies in patients with cryptogenic chronic liver disease. Hepatology 15: 175–179

Burroughs A K, Bassendine M F, Thomas H C, Sherlock S 1981 Primary liver cell cancer in autoimmune chronic liver disease. British Medical Journal 282: 273

Calmus Y, Gane P, Rouger P, Poupon R 1990 Hepatic expression of class I and class II major histocompatibility complex molecules in primary biliary cirrhosis: effect of ursodeoxycholic acid. Hepatology 11: 12–15

Carman W F, Jacyna M R, Hadziyannis S et al 1989 Mutation preventing formation of hepatitis B e antigen in patients with chronic hepatitis B infection. Lancet 2: 588–591

Carman W F, Fagan E A, Hadziyannis S et al 1991 Association of a precore genomic variant of hepatitis B virus with fulminant hepatitis. Hepatology 14: 219–222

Cassani F, Muratori L, Manotti P et al 1992 Serum autoantibodies and the diagnosis of type-1 autoimmune hepatitis in Italy: a reappraisal at the light of hepatitis C virus infection. Gut 33: 1260–1263

Chung Y-H, Shong Y K 1993 Development of thyroid autoimmunity after administration of recombinant human interferon-α 2b for chronic viral hepatitis. American Journal of Gastroenterology 88: 244–247

Clifford B D, Donahue D, Smith L et al 1995 High prevalence of serological markers of autoimmunity in patients with chronic hepatitis C. Hepatology 21: 613–619

Colombo M, Cambieri R, Rumi M G, Ronchi G, Del Ninno E, de Franchis R 1983 Long-term delta superinfection in hepatitis B surface antigen carriers and its relationship to the course of chronic hepatitis. Gastroenterology 85: 235–239

Colombo M, de Franchis R, Del Ninno E et al 1991 Hepatocellular carcinoma in Italian patients with cirrhosis. New England Journal of Medicine 325: 675–680

Cooksley W G E, Bradbear R A, Robinson W et al 1986 The prognosis of chronic active hepatitis without cirrhosis in relation to bridging necrosis. Hepatology 6: 345–348

Crosignani A, Battezzati P M, Setchell K D R et al 1991 Effects of ursodeoxycholic acid on serum liver enzymes and bile acid metabolism in chronic active hepatitis: a dose-response study. Hepatology 13: 339–344

Czaja A J 1979 Serologic markers of hepatitis A and B in acute and chronic liver disease. Mayo Clinic Proceedings 54: 721–732

Czaja A J 1981 Current problems in the diagnosis and management of chronic active hepatitis. Mayo Clinic Proceedings 56: 311–323

Czaja A J 1984a Natural history, clinical features, and treatment of autoimmune hepatitis. Seminars in Liver Diseases 4: 1–12

Czaja A J 1984b Diagnosis and treatment of chronic hepatitis. Comprehensive Therapy 10: 58–63

Czaja A J 1988 Diagnosis and management of chronic active hepatitis B. Comprehensive Therapy 14: 46–53

Czaja A J 1990a Autoimmune chronic active hepatitis: a specific entity? The negative argument. Journal of Gastroenterology and Hepatology 5: 343–351

Czaja A J 1990b Low-dose corticosteroid therapy after multiple relapses of severe HBsAg-negative chronic active hepatitis. Hepatology 11: 1044–1049

Czaja A J 1991 Diagnosis, prognosis, and treatment of classical autoimmune chronic active hepatitis. In: Krawitt E L, Weisner R H (eds) Autoimmune liver diseases. Raven Press, New York, p 143–166

Czaja A J 1992 Chronic hepatitis C virus infection: a disease in waiting? New England Journal of Medicine 327: 1949–1950

Czaja A J 1993 Chronic active hepatitis: the challenge for a new nomenclature. Annals of Internal Medicine 119: 510–517

Czaja A J 1994 Autoimmune hepatitis and viral infections. Gastroenterology Clinics of North America 3: 547–566

Czaja A J 1995 Autoimmune hepatitis: evolving concepts and treatment strategies. Digestive Diseases and Sciences 40: 435–456

Czaja A J, Carpenter H A 1993 Sensitivity, specificity and predictability of biopsy interpretations in chronic hepatitis. Gastroenterology 105: 1824–1832

Czaja A J, Davis G L 1982 Hepatitis non A, non B. Manifestations and implications of acute and chronic disease. Mayo Clinic Proceedings 57: 639–652

Czaja A J, Manns M P 1995 The validity and importance of subtypes in autoimmune hepatitis: a point of view. American Journal of Gastroenterology 90: 1206–1211

Czaja A J, Wolf A M, Summerskill W H J 1979 Development and early prognosis of esophageal varices in severe chronic active liver disease (CALD) treated with prednisone. Gastroenterology 77: 629–633

Czaja A J, Ammon H V, Summerskill W H J 1980 Clinical features and prognosis of severe chronic active liver disease (CALD) after corticosteroid-induced remission. Gastroenterology 78: 518–523

Czaja A J, Ludwig J, Baggenstoss A H, Wolf A 1981 Corticosteroid-treated chronic active hepatitis in remission: uncertain prognosis of chronic persistent hepatitis. New England Journal of Medicine 304: 5–9

Czaja A J, Davis G L, Ludwig J, Baggenstoss A H, Taswell H F 1983 Autoimmune features as determinants of prognosis in steroid-treated chronic active hepatitis of uncertain etiology. Gastroenterology 85: 713–717

Czaja A J, Davis G L, Ludwig J, Taswell H F 1984 Complete resolution of inflammatory activity following corticosteroid treatment of HBsAg-negative chronic active hepatitis. Hepatology 4: 622–627

Czaja A J, Beaver S J, Shiels M T 1987 Sustained remission after corticosteroid therapy of severe hepatitis B surface antigen-negative chronic active hepatitis. Gastroenterology 92: 215–219

Czaja A J, Rakela J, Ludwig J 1988 Features reflective of early prognosis in corticosteroid-treated severe autoimmune chronic active hepatitis. Gastroenterology 95: 448–453

Czaja A J, Rakela J, Hay J E, Moore S B 1990a Clinical and prognostic implications of HLA B8 in corticosteroid-treated severe autoimmune chronic active hepatitis. Gastroenterology 98: 1587–1593

Czaja A J, Hay J E, Rakela J 1990b Clinical features and prognostic implications of severe corticosteroid-treated cryptogenic chronic active hepatitis. Mayo Clinic Proceedings 65: 23–30

Czaja A J, Taswell H F, Rakela J, Schimek C M 1990c Frequency and significance of antibody to hepatitis C virus in severe corticosteroid-treated cryptogenic chronic active hepatitis. Mayo Clinic Proceedings 65: 1303–1313

Czaja A J, Manns M P, Homburger H A 1992a Frequency and significance of antibodies to liver/kidney microsome type 1 in adults with chronic active hepatitis. Gastroenterology 103: 1290–1295

Czaja A J, Taswell H F, Rakela J, Schimek C 1992b Frequency of antibody to hepatitis C virus in asymptomatic HBsAg-negative chronic active hepatitis. Journal of Hepatology 14: 88–93

Czaja A J, Taswell H F, Rakela J, Rabe D 1992c Duration and specificity of antibodies to hepatitis C virus in chronic active hepatitis. Gastroenterology 102: 1675–1679

Czaja A J, Carpenter H A, Santrach P J, Moore S B, Taswell H F, Homburger H A 1993a Evidence against hepatitis viruses as important causes of severe autoimmune hepatitis in the United States. Journal of Hepatology 18: 342–352

Czaja A J, Carpenter H A, Santrach P J, Moore S B 1993b Significance of HLA DR4 in type 1 autoimmune hepatitis. Gastroenterology 105: 1502–1507

Czaja A J, Carpenter H A, Santrach P J, Moore S B 1993c Genetic predispositions for the immunological features of chronic active hepatitis. Hepatology 18: 816–822

Czaja A J, Carpenter H A, Santrach P J, Moore S B, Homburger H A 1993d The nature and prognosis of severe cryptogenic chronic active hepatitis. Gastroenterology 104: 1755–1761

Czaja A J, Carpenter H A, Manns M P 1993e Antibodies to soluble liver antigen, P450IID6, and mitochondrial complexes in chronic hepatitis. Gastroenterology 105: 1522–1528

Czaja A J, Wang K K, Shiels M T, Katzmann J A 1993f Oral pulse prednisone therapy after relapse of severe autoimmune chronic active hepatitis. A prospective randomized treatment trial evaluating clinical, biochemical, and lymphocyte subset responses. Journal of Hepatology 17: 180–186

Czaja A J, Magrin S, Fabiano C, Fiorentino G, Diquattro O, Craxi A, Pagliaro L 1995a Hepatitis C virus infection as a determinant of behavior in type 1 autoimmune hepatitis. Digestive Diseases and Sciences 40: 33–40

Czaja A J, Carpenter H A, Santrach P J, Moore S B 1995b Immunologic features and HLA associations in chronic viral hepatitis. Gastroenterology 108: 157–164

Czaja A J, Carpenter H A, Santrach P J, Moore S B 1995c Significance of human leukocyte antigens DR3 and DR4 in chronic viral hepatitis. Digestive Diseases and Sciences 40: 2098–2106

Czaja et al 1995c: the journal details should be as follows: Digestive Diseases and Sciences 40: 2098–2106

Danielsson A, Prytz H 1994 Oral budesonide for treatment of autoimmune chronic active hepatitis. Alimentary Pharmacology and Therapeutics 8: 585–590

Davis G L, Czaja A J 1981 Current concepts in the diagnosis and management of hepatitis B surface antigen-positive chronic active hepatitis. Journal of Clinical Gastroenterology 3: 381–388

Davis G L, Czaja A J, Baggenstoss A H, Taswell H F 1982 Prognostic and therapeutic implications of extreme serum aminotransferase elevation in chronic active hepatitis. Mayo Clinic Proceedings 57: 303–309

Davis G L, Hoofnagle J H, Waggoner J G 1984a Spontaneous reactivation of chronic hepatitis B virus infection. Gastroenterology 86: 230–235

Davis G L, Czaja A J, Ludwig J 1984b Development and prognosis of histologic cirrhosis in corticosteroid-treated hepatitis B surface antigen-negative chronic active hepatitis. Gastroenterology 87: 1222–1227

Davis G L, Balart L A, Schiff E R et al 1989 Treatment of chronic hepatitis C with recombinant interferon alfa. A multicenter randomized, controlled trial. New England Journal of Medicine 321: 1501–1506

Desmet V J, Gerber M, Hoofnagle J H, Manns M, Scheuer P J 1994 Classification of chronic hepatitis: diagnosis, grading and staging. Hepatology 19: 1513–1520

Di Bisceglie A M, Martin P, Kassianides C et al 1989 Recombinant interferon alfa therapy for chronic hepatitis C: a randomized double-blind, placebo-controlled trial. New England Journal of Medicine 321: 1506–1510

Di Bisceglie A M, Shindo M, Fong T-L et al 1992 A pilot study of ribavirin therapy for chronic hepatitis C. Hepatology 16: 649–654
Dietrichson O 1975 Chronic active hepatitis. Aetiological considerations based on clinical and serological studies. Scandinavian Journal of Gastroenterology 10: 617–624
Doherty D G, Donaldson P T, Underhill J A et al 1994a Allelic sequence variation in the HLA class II genes and proteins in patients with autoimmune hepatitis. Hepatology 19: 609–615
Doherty D G, Underhill J A, Donaldson P T et al 1994b Polymorphisms in the human complement C4 genes and genetic susceptibility to autoimmune hepatitis. Autoimmunity 18: 243–249
Donaldson P T, Doherty D G, Hayllar K M, McFarlane I G, Johnson P J, Williams R 1990 Susceptibility to autoimmune chronic active hepatitis: human leukocyte antigens DR4 and A1-B8-DR3 are independent risk factors. Hepatology 13: 701–706
Donaldson P, Doherty D, Underhill J, Williams R 1994 The molecular genetics of autoimmune liver disease. Hepatology 20: 225–239
Dusheiko G, Schmilovitz-Weiss H, Brown D et al 1994 Hepatitis C virus genotypes: an investigation of type-specific differences in geographic origin and disease. Hepatology 19: 13–18
Eddleston A L W F 1985 Immunology of chronic active hepatitis. Quarterly Journal of Medicine 55: 191–198
Esteban J I, Esteban R, Viladomiu L et al 1989 Hepatitis C virus antibodies among risk groups in Spain. Lancet 2: 294–297
Fattovich G, Rugge M, Brollo L et al 1986 Clinical, virologic and histologic outcome following seroconversion from HBeAg to anti-HBe in chronic hepatitis type B. Hepatology 6: 167–172
Fattovich G, Betterle C, Brollo L et al 1991 Autoantibodies during α-interferon therapy for chronic hepatitis B. Journal of Medical Virology 34: 132–135
Feray C, Gigou M, Samuel D et al 1995 Influence of the genotypes of hepatitis C virus on the severity of recurrent liver disease after liver transplantation. Gastroenterology 108: 1088–1096
Fong T-L, Di Bisceglie A M, Gerber M A, Waggoner J G, Hoofnagle J H 1993 Persistence of hepatitis B virus DNA in the liver after loss of HBsAg in chronic hepatitis B. Hepatology 18: 1313–1318
Frizell E, Abraham A, Doolittle M et al 1994 FK506 enhances fibrogenesis in in vitro and in vivo models of liver fibrosis in rats. Gastroenterology 107: 492–498
Garson J A, Lenzi M, Ring C et al 1991 Hepatitis C viraemia in adults with type 2 autoimmune hepatitis. Journal of Medical Virology 34: 223–226
Gerotto M, Pontisso P, Giostra F et al 1994 Analysis of the hepatitis C virus genome in patients with anti-LKM-1 autoantibodies. Journal of Hepatology 21: 273–276
Gocke D J, Morgan C, Lockshin M, Hsu K, Bombardieri S, Christian C L 1970 Association between polyarteritis and Australia antigen. Lancet 2: 1149–1153
Goldstein G B, Lam K C, Mistilis S P 1973 Drug-induced active chronic hepatitis. American Journal of Digestive Diseases 18: 177–184
Govindarajan S, Chin K P, Redeker A G, Peters R L 1984 Fulminant B viral hepatitis: role of delta agent. Gastroenterology 86: 1417–1420
Haddad J, Deny P, Munz-Gotheil C et al 1992 Lymphocytic sialadenitis of Sjögren's syndrome associated with chronic hepatitis C virus liver disease. Lancet 339: 321–323
Hadziyannis S J 1991 Use of alpha-interferon in the treatment of chronic delta hepatitis. Journal of Hepatology 13: S21–S26
Hadziyannis S, Bramou T, Makris A, Moussoulis G, Zignego L, Papaioannou C 1990 Interferon alfa-2b treatment of HBeAg negative/serum HBV DNA positive chronic active hepatitis type B. Hepatology 11: S133–S136
Hegarty J E, Nouri Aria K T, Portmann B, Eddleston A L W F, Williams R 1983 Relapse following treatment withdrawal in patients with autoimmune chronic active hepatitis. Hepatology 3: 685–689
Hegarty J E, Nouri-Aria K T, Eddleston A L W F, Williams R 1984 Controlled trial of a thymic hormone extract (Thymostimulin) in "autoimmune" chronic active hepatitis. Gut 25: 279–283
Hodges J R, Millward-Sadler G H, Wright R 1982 Chronic active hepatitis: the spectrum of disease. Lancet 1: 550–552
Homberg J-C, Abuaf N, Bernard O et al 1987 Chronic active hepatitis associated with antiliver/kidney microsome antibody type 1: a second type of "autoimmune" hepatitis. Hepatology 7: 1333–1339
Hoofnagle J H 1981 Type B hepatitis: virology, serology and clinical course. Seminars in Liver Disease 1: 7–14
Hoofnagle J H, Dusheiko G M, Seeff L B, Jones E A, Waggoner J G, Bales Z B 1981 Seroconversion from hepatitis B e antigen to antibody in chronic type B hepatitis. Annals of Internal Medicine 94: 744–748
Housset C, Pol S, Carnot F et al 1992 Interactions between human immunodeficiency virus-1, hepatitis delta virus and hepatitis B virus infections in 260 chronic carriers of hepatitis B virus. Hepatology 15: 578–583
Hyams J S, Ballow M, Leichtner A M 1987 Cyclosporine treatment of autoimmune chronic active hepatitis. Gastroenterology 93: 890–893
International Working Party Report 1995 Terminology of chronic hepatitis. American Journal of Gastroenterology 90: 181–189
Ishak K, Baptista A, Bianchi L et al 1995 Histological grading and staging of chronic hepatitis. Journal of Hepatology 22: 696–699
Jakobovits A W, Gibson P R, Dudley F J 1981 Primary liver cell carcinoma complicating autoimmune chronic active hepatitis. Digestive Diseases and Sciences 26: 694–699
Jeffers L J, Hasan F, de Medina M et al 1992 Prevalence of antibodies to hepatitis C virus among patients with cryptogenic chronic hepatitis and cirrhosis. Hepatology 15: 187–190
Jenkins P J, Portmann B P, Eddleston A L W F, Williams R 1982 Use of polyunsaturated phosphatidyl choline in HBsAg negative chronic active hepatitis: results of prospective double-blind controlled trial. Liver 2: 77–81
Johnson P J, McFarlane I G 1993 Meeting report: International Autoimmune Hepatitis Group. Hepatology 18: 998–1005
Kakumu S, Yoshioka K, Wakita T, Ishikawa T, Takayanagi M, Higashi Y 1993 A pilot study of ribavirin and interferon beta for the treatment of chronic hepatitis C. Gastroenterology 105: 507–512
Kanazawa Y, Hayashi N, Mita E et al 1994 Influence of viral quasispecies on effectiveness of interferon therapy in chronic hepatitis C patients. Hepatology 20: 1121–1130
Kiyosawa K, Sodeyama T, Nakano Y et al 1989 Treatment of chronic non-A, non-B hepatitis with human interferon beta: a preliminary study. Antiviral Research 12: 151–161
Kiyosawa K, Sodeyama T, Tanaka E et al 1990 Interrelationship of blood transfusion, non-A, non-B hepatitis and hepatocellular carcinoma: analysis by detection of antibody to hepatitis C virus. Hepatology 12: 671–675
Kobayashi Y, Watanabe S, Konishi M et al 1993 Quantitation and typing of hepatitis C virus RNA in patients with chronic hepatitis C treated with interferon-β. Hepatology 18: 1319–1325
Korenman J, Baker B, Waggoner J, Everhart J E, Di Bisceglie A M, Hoofnagle J H 1991 Long-term remission of chronic hepatitis B after alpha interferon therapy. Annals of Internal Medicine 114: 629–634
Koretz R L, Abbey H, Coleman E, Gitnick G 1993 Non-A, non-B post-transfusion hepatitis. Looking back in the second decade. Annals of Internal Medicine 119: 110–115
Lai C-L, Lok A S-F, Lin H-J, Wu P-C, Yeoh E-K, Yeung C-Y 1987 Placebo-controlled trial of recombinant $\alpha_2$-interferon in Chinese HBsAg-carrier children. Lancet 2: 877–880
Lam K C, Lai C L, Ng R P, Trepo C, Wu P C 1981 Deleterious effect of prednisolone in HBsAg-positive chronic active hepatitis. New England Journal of Medicine 304: 380–386
Lefkowitch J H, Schiff E R, Davis G L et al 1993 Pathologic diagnosis of chronic hepatitis C: a multicenter comparative study with chronic hepatitis B. Gastroenterology 104: 595–603
Lenzi M, Ballardini G, Fusconi M et al 1990 Type 2 autoimmune hepatitis and hepatitis C virus infection. Lancet 335: 258–259
Levo Y, Gorevic P D, Kassab H J, Zucker-Franklin D, Franklin E C 1977 Association between hepatitis B virus and essential mixed cryoglobulinemia. New England Journal of Medicine 296: 1501–1502
Lewis G P, Jusko W J, Burke C W, Graves L 1971 Boston Collaborative Drug Surveillance Program. Prednisone side-effects and serum-protein levels. Lancet 2: 778
Liaw Y-F, Chu C-M, Su I-J, Huang M-J, Lin D-Y, Chang-Chien C-S 1983 Clinical and histological events preceding hepatitis B e antigen seroconversion in chronic type B hepatitis. Gastroenterology 84: 216–219
Liaw Y-F, Pao C C, Chu C-M, Sheen I-S, Huang M-J 1987 Changes of serum hepatitis B virus DNA in two types of clinical events preceding

spontaneous hepatitis Be antigen seroconversion in chronic type B hepatitis. Hepatology 7: 1–3
Lidman K, Biberfield G, Fagraeus A et al 1976 Anti-actin specificity of human smooth muscle antibodies in chronic active hepatitis. Clinical and Experimental Immunology 24: 266–272
Lindberg J, Lindholm A, Lundin P, Iwarson S 1975 Trigger factors and HL-A antigens in chronic active hepatitis. British Medical Journal 4: 77–79
Loeper J, Descatoire V, Maurice M et al 1993 Cytochromes P-450 in human hepatocyte plasma membrane: recognition by several autoantibodies. Gastroenterology 104: 203–216
Löhr H F, Gerken G, Michel G, Braun H-B, Meyer zum Büschenfelde K-H 1994 In vitro secretion of anti-GOR protein and anti-hepatitis C virus antibodies in patients with chronic hepatitis C. Gastroenterology 107: 1443–1448
Lok A S F, Cheung R, Chan R, Liu V 1992 Hepatitis C viremia in patients with hepatitis C virus infection. Hepatology 15: 1007–1012
Lunel F, Abuaf N, Frangeul L et al 1992 Liver/kidney microsome antibody type 1 and hepatitis C virus infection. Hepatology 16: 630–636
Maddrey W C 1987 Subdivisions of idiopathic autoimmune chronic active hepatitis. Hepatology 7: 1372–1375
Magrin S, Craxi A, Fabiano C et al 1991a Hepatitis C virus replication in "autoimmune" chronic hepatitis. Journal of Hepatology 13: 364–367
Magrin S, Craxi A, Fiorentino G et al 1991b Is autoimmune chronic active hepatitis a HCV-related disease? Journal of Hepatology 13: 56–60
Magrin S, Craxi A, Fabiano C et al 1994 Hepatitis C viremia in chronic liver disease: relationship to interferon-α or corticosteroid treatment. Hepatology 19: 273–279
Manns M P, Kruger M 1994 Immunogenetics of chronic liver diseases. Gastroenterology 106: 1676–1697
Manns M, Zanger U, Gerken G et al 1990 Patients with type II autoimmune hepatitis express functionally intact cytochrome P-450 db 1 that is inhibited by LKM-1 autoantibodies *in vitro* but not *in vivo*. Hepatology 12: 127–132
Manns M P, Griffin K J, Sullivan K F, Johnson E F 1991 LKM-1 autoantibodies recognize a short linear sequence in P450IID6, a cytochrome P-450 monooxygenase. Journal of Clinical Investigation 88: 1370–1378
Marcellin P, Pouteau M, Benhamou J-P 1995 Hepatitis C virus infection, alpha interferon therapy and thyroid dysfunction. Journal of Hepatology 22: 364–369
Martin P, Muñoz S J, Di Bisceglie A M et al 1991 Recurrence of hepatitis C virus infection after orthotopic liver transplantation. Hepatology 13: 719–721
Martini E, Abuaf N, Cavalli F, Durand V, Johanet C, Homberg J-C 1988 Antibody to liver cytosol (anti-LC1) in patients with autoimmune chronic active hepatitis type 2. Hepatology 8: 1662–1666
Mayet W-J, Hess G, Gerken G, Rossol S, Voth R, Manns M, Meyer zum Büschenfelde K-H 1989 Treatment of chronic type B hepatitis with recombinant α interferon induces autoantibodies not specific for autoimmune chronic hepatitis. Hepatology 10: 24–28
McFarlane I G, Smith H M, Johnson P J, Bray G P, Vergani D, Williams R 1990 Hepatitis C virus antibodies in chronic active hepatitis: pathogenetic factor or false-positive result? Lancet 335: 754–757
Meyer R A, Duffy M C 1993 Spontaneous reactivation of chronic hepatitis B infection leading to fulminant hepatic failure. Report of two cases and review of the literature. Journal of Clinical Gastroenterology 17: 231–234
Michel G, Ritter A, Gerken G, Meyer zum Büschenfelde K-H, Decker R, Manns M P 1992 Anti-GOR and hepatitis C virus in autoimmune liver diseases. Lancet 339: 267–269
Michitaka K, Durazzo M, Tillman H L, Walker D, Philipp T, Manns M P 1994 Analysis of hepatitis C virus genome in patients with autoimmune hepatitis type 2. Gastroenterology 106: 1603–1610
Miracco A, Iodice G, Peluso C et al 1984 Arginine thiazolidinecarboxylate in the treatment of chronic active hepatitis: double-blind comparison with placebo. Journal of Internal Medical Research 12: 35–39
Misiani R, Bellavita P, Fenili D et al 1994 Interferon alfa-2a therapy in cryoglobulinemia associated with hepatitis C virus. New England Journal of Medicine 330: 751–756
Mistilis S P, Skyring A P, Blackburn C R B 1968 Natural history of active chronic hepatitis. I. Clinical features, course, diagnostic criteria, morbidity, mortality, and survival. Australasian Annals of Medicine 17: 214–223
Mistilis S P, Vickers C R, Darroch M H, McCarthy S W 1985 Cyclosporin, a new treatment for autoimmune chronic active hepatitis. Medical Journal of Australia 143: 463–465
Mitchel L S, Jeffers L J, Reddy K R et al 1993 Detection of hepatitis C virus antibody by first and second generation assays and polymerase chain reaction in patients with autoimmune chronic active hepatitis types I, II, and III. American Journal of Gastroenterology 88: 1027–1034
Mitoro A, Yoshikawa M, Yamamoto K et al 1993 Exacerbation of ulcerative colitis during alpha-interferon therapy for chronic hepatitis C. Internal Medicine 32: 327–331
Murray-Lyon I M, Stern R B, Williams R 1973 Controlled trial of prednisone and azathioprine in active chronic hepatitis. Lancet 1: 735–737
Mutchnick M G, Appelman H D, Chung H T et al 1991 Thymosin treatment of chronic hepatitis B: a placebo-controlled pilot trial. Hepatology 14: 409–415
Neuberger J, Hegarty J E, Eddleston A L W F, Williams R 1983 Effect of polyunsaturated phosphatidylcholine on immune mediated hepatocyte damage. Gut 24: 751–755
Neuberger J, Portmann B, Calne R, Williams R 1984 Recurrence of autoimmune chronic active hepatitis following orthotopic liver grafting. Transplantation 37: 363–365
Nikias G A, Batts K P, Czaja A J 1994 The nature and prognostic implications of autoimmune hepatitis with an acute presentation. Journal of Hepatology 21: 866–871
Nishiguchi S, Kuroki T, Ueda T et al 1992 Detection of hepatitis C virus antibody in the absence of viral RNA in patients with autoimmune hepatitis. Annals of Internal Medicine 116: 21–25
Okada S, Akahane Y, Suzuki H, Okamoto H, Mishiro S 1992 The degree of variability in the amino terminal region of the E2/NS1 protein of hepatitis C virus correlates with responsiveness to interferon therapy in viremic patients. Hepatology 16: 619–624
Okuda K 1992 Hepatocellular carcinoma: recent progress. Hepatology 15: 948–963
Omata M, Ashcavai M, Liew C-T, Peters R L 1979 Hepatocellular carcinoma in the U.S.A., etiologic considerations. Localization of hepatitis B antigens. Gastroenterology 76: 279–287
Omata M, Ehata T, Yokosuka O, Hosoda K, Ohto M 1991 Mutations in the precore region of hepatitis B virus DNA in patients with fulminant and severe hepatitis. New England Journal of Medicine 324: 1699–1704
Opelz G, Vogten A J M, Summerskill W H J, Schalm S W, Terasaki P I 1977 HLA determinants in chronic active liver disease: possible relation of HLA-Dw3 to prognosis. Tissue Antigens 9: 36–40
Ozes O N, Reiter Z, Klein S, Blatt L M, Taylor M W 1992 A comparison of interferon-con$_1$ with natural recombinant-interferon-alfa: antiviral, antiproliferative, and natural killer-inducing activities. Journal of Interferon Research 12: 55–59
Pagliaro L, Craxi A, Cammaá C, Tiné F, Di Marco V, Iacono O L, Almasio P 1994 Interferon-α for chronic hepatitis C: an analysis of pretreatment clinical predictors of response. Hepatology 19: 820–828
Papo T, Marcellin P, Bernuau J, Durand F, Poynard T, Benhamou J-P 1992 Autoimmune chronic hepatitis exacerbated by alpha-interferon. Annals of Internal Medicine 116: 51–53
Pateron D, Hartmann D J, Duclos-Vallee J C, Jouanolle H, Beaugrand M 1992 Latent autoimmune thyroid disease in patients with chronic HCV hepatitis. Journal of Hepatology 16: 244–245
Pawlotsky J-M, Ben Yahia M, Andre C et al 1994 Immunological disorders in C virus chronic active hepatitis: a prospective case-control study. Hepatology 19: 841–848
Perdigoto R, Carpenter H A, Czaja A J 1992 Frequency and significance of chronic ulcerative colitis in severe corticosteroid-treated autoimmune hepatitis. Journal of Hepatology 14: 325–331
Perrillo R P, Aach R D 1981 The clinical course and chronic sequelae of hepatitis B virus infection. Seminars in Liver Diseases 1: 15–25

Perrillo R P, Schiff E R, Davis G L et al and the Interventional Therapy Group 1990 A randomized, controlled trial of interferon alfa-2b alone and after prednisone withdrawal for the treatment of chronic hepatitis B. New England Journal of Medicine 323: 295–301
Popper H, Schaffner F 1971 The vocabulary of chronic hepatitis. New England Journal of Medicine 284: 1154–1156
Popper H, Shafritz D A, Hoofnagle J H 1987 Relation of the hepatitis B carrier state to hepatocellular carcinoma. Hepatology 7: 764–772
Porta G, da Costa Gayotto L C, Alvarez F 1990 Anti-liver-kidney microsome antibody-positive autoimmune hepatitis presenting as fulminant liver failure. Journal of Pediatric Gastroenterology and Nutrition 11: 138–140
Poterucha J J, Rakela J, Lumeng L, Lee C-H, Taswell H F, Wiesner R H 1992 Diagnosis of chronic hepatitis C after liver transplantation by the detection of viral sequences with polymerase chain reaction. Hepatology 15: 42–45
Realdi G, Alberti A, Rugge M et al 1980 Seroconversion from hepatitis B e antigen to anti-HBe in chronic hepatitis B virus infection. Gastroenterology 79: 195–199
Rizzetto M, Durazzo M 1991 Hepatitis delta virus (HDV) infections. Epidemiological and clinical heterogeneity. Journal of Hepatology 13 (suppl 4): S116–S118
Rizzetto M, Purcell R H, Gerin J L 1980 Epidemiology of HBV-associated delta agent: geographical distribution of anti-delta and prevalence in polytransfused HBsAg carriers. Lancet 1: 1215–1218
Roffi L, Mels G C, Antonelli G et al 1995 Breakthrough during recombinant interferon alfa therapy in patients with chronic hepatitis C virus infection: prevalence, etiology, and management. Hepatology 21: 645–649
Rosina F, Pintus C, Meschievitz C, Rizzetto M 1991 A randomized controlled trial of a 12-month course of recombinant human interferon-α in chronic delta (type D) hepatitis: a multicenter Italian study. Hepatology 13: 1052–1056
Sánchez-Tapias J M, Barrera J M, Costa J et al 1990 Hepatitis C virus infection in patients with nonalcoholic chronic liver disease. Annals of Internal Medicine 112: 921–924
Sanchez-Urdazpal L, Czaja A J, van Hoek B, Krom R A F, Wiesner R H 1992 Prognostic features and role of liver transplantation in severe corticosteroid-treated autoimmune chronic active hepatitis. Hepatology 15: 215–221
Saracco G, Touscoz A, Durazzo M et al 1990 Antibodies and response to α-interferon in patients with chronic viral hepatitis. Journal of Hepatology 11: 339–343
Schalm S 1994 Treatment of chronic hepatitis B. Netherlands Journal of Medicine 44: 103–109
Schalm S W, Ammon H V, Summerskill W H J 1976 Failure of customary treatment in chronic active liver disease: causes and management. Annals of Clinical Research 8: 221–227
Schalm S W, Korman M G, Summerskill W H J, Czaja A J, Baggenstoss A H 1977 Severe chronic active liver disease. Prognostic significance of initial morphologic patterns. American Journal of Digestive Diseases 22: 973–980
Scheuer P J, Ashrafzadeh P, Sherlock S, Brown D, Dusheiko G M 1992 The pathology of hepatitis C. Hepatology 15: 567–571
Schrumpf E, Elgjo K, Fausa O, Haukenes G, Kvale D, Rollag H 1990 The significance of anti-hepatitis C virus antibodies measured in chronic liver disease. Scandinavian Journal of Gastroenterology 25: 1169–1174
Schvarcz R, Glaumann H, Weiland O 1993 Survival and histological resolution of fibrosis in patients with autoimmune chronic active hepatitis. Journal of Hepatology 18: 15–23
Scully L J, Toze C, Sengar D P S, Goldstein R 1993 Early-onset autoimmune hepatitis is associated with a C4A gene deletion. Gastroenterology 104: 1478–1484
Seeff L B 1981 Drug-induced chronic liver disease, with emphasis on chronic active hepatitis. Seminars in Liver Diseases 1: 104–115
Seeff L B, Buskell-Bales Z, Wright E C et al and the National Heart, Lung and Blood Institute 1992 Long-term mortality after transfusion-associated non-A, non-B hepatitis. New England Journal of Medicine 327: 1906–1911
Shafritz D A, Shouval D, Sherman H I, Hadziyannis S J, Kew M C 1981 Integration of hepatitis B virus DNA into the genome of liver cells in chronic liver disease and hepatocellular carcinoma. New England Journal of Medicine 305: 1067–1073
Shah G, Demetris A J, Gavaler J S, Lewis J H, Todo S, Starzl T E, Van Thiel D H 1992 Incidence, prevalence, and clinical course of hepatitis C following liver transplantation. Gastroenterology 103: 323–329
Shiels M T, Czaja A J, Taswell H F et al 1985 Frequency and significance of delta antibody in acute and chronic hepatitis B. A United States experience. Gastroenterology 89: 1230–1234
Shindo M, Di Bisceglie A M, Cheung L, Shih W-K, Cristiano K, Feinstone S M, Hoofnagle J H 1991 Decrease in serum hepatitis C viral RNA during alpha-interferon therapy for chronic hepatitis C. Annals of Internal Medicine 115: 700–704
Shindo M, Di Bisceglie A M, Hoofnagle J H 1992a Acute exacerbation of liver disease during interferon alfa therapy for chronic hepatitis C. Gastroenterology 102: 1406–1408
Shindo M, Di Bisceglie A M, Hoofnagle J H 1992b Long-term follow-up of patients with chronic hepatitis C treated with α-interferon. Hepatology 15: 1013–1016
Silva E, Sallie R, Tibbs C, McFarlane I, Johnson P, Williams R 1993 Absence of hepatitis C virus in British patients with type 1 autoimmune chronic active hepatitis – a polymerase chain reaction and serological study. Journal of Hepatology 19: 211–215
Silva M O, Reddy K R, Jeffers L J, Hill M, Schiff E R 1991 Interferon-induced chronic active hepatitis? Gastroenterology 101: 840–842
Simmonds P 1995 Variability of hepatitis C virus. Hepatology 21: 570–583
Smedile A, Farci P, Verme G et al 1982 Influence of delta infection on severity of hepatitis B. Lancet 2: 945–947
Stechemesser E, Klein R, Berg P A 1993 Characterization and clinical relevance of liver–pancreas antibodies in autoimmune hepatitis. Hepatology 18: 1–9
Stellon A J, Keating J J, Johnson P J, McFarlane I G, Williams R 1988 Maintenance of remission in autoimmune chronic active hepatitis with azathioprine after corticosteroid withdrawal. Hepatology 8: 781–784
Terrault N, Wright T 1995 Interferon and hepatitis C. New England Journal of Medicine 332: 1509–1511
Thomson A W, Carroll P B, McCauley J et al 1993 FK 506: a novel immunosuppressant for treatment of autoimmune disease. Rationale and preliminary clinical experience at the University of Pittsburgh. Springer Seminars in Immunopathology 14: 323–344
Tong M J, El-Farra N S, Reikes A R, Co R L 1995 Clinical outcomes after transfusion-associated hepatitis C. New England Journal of Medicine 332: 1463–1466
Tran A, Quaranta J-F, Benzaken S et al 1993 High prevalence of thyroid autoantibodies in a prospective series of patients with chronic hepatitis C before interferon therapy. Hepatology 18: 253–257
Tyrrell D L J, Mitchell M C, De Man R A et al 1993 Phase II trial of lamivudine for chronic hepatitis B. Hepatology 18 (suppl): 112A
Van Thiel D H, Wright H, Carroll P, Abu-Elmagd K, Rodriguez-Rilo H, McMichael J, Starzl T E 1992 FK 506 in the treatment of autoimmune chronic active hepatitis: preliminary results. American Journal of Gastroenterology 87: 1309
Vento S, DiPerri G, Garofano T et al 1989 Hazards of interferon therapy for HBV-seronegative chronic hepatitis. Lancet 2: 926
Vere Hodge R A, Sutton D, Boyd M R, Harnden M R, Jarvest K L 1989 Selection of an oral prodrug (BRL42810; famciclovir) for the antiherpesvirus agent BRL 39123 [9-(4-hydroxy-3-hydroxymethylbut-1-yl) guanine; penciclovir]. Antimicrobial Agents and Chemotherapy 33: 1765–1773
Wang K K, Czaja A J 1988 Hepatocellular carcinoma in corticosteroid-treated severe autoimmune chronic active hepatitis. Hepatology 8: 1679–1683
Wang K K, Czaja A J 1989 Prognosis of corticosteroid-treated hepatitis B surface antigen-negative chronic active hepatitis in postmenopausal women: a retrospective analysis. Gastroenterology 97: 1288–1293
Wang K K, Czaja A J, Beaver S J, Go V L W 1989 Extrahepatic malignancy following long-term immunosuppressive therapy of severe hepatitis B surface antigen-negative chronic active hepatitis. Hepatology 10: 39–43
Weissberg J I, Andres L L, Smith C I et al 1984 Survival in chronic hepatitis B. An analysis of 379 patients. Annals of Internal Medicine 101: 613–616

Weller I V D, Carreno V, Fowler M J F et al 1982 Acyclovir inhibits hepatitis B virus replication in man. Lancet 1: 273

Wood J R, Czaja A J, Taswell H F, Ludwig J, Rakela J, Chase R 1987 Hepatitis B virus deoxyribonucleic acid in serum during hepatitis B e antigen clearance in corticosteroid-treated severe chronic active hepatitis B. Gastroenterology 93: 1225–1230

Wright H L, Bou-Abboud C F, Hassanein T, Block G D, Demetris A J, Starzl T E, Van Thiel D H 1992a Disease recurrence and rejection following liver transplantation for autoimmune chronic active liver disease. Transplantation 53: 136–139

Wright T L, Donegan E, Hsu H H et al 1992b Recurrent and acquired hepatitis C viral infection in liver transplant recipients. Gastroenterology 103: 317–322

Yamamoto A M, Cresteil D, Homberg J C, Alvarez F 1993 Characterization of anti-liver–kidney microsome antibody (anti-LKM1) from hepatitis C virus-positive and -negative sera. Gastroenterology 104: 1762–1767

Yoshioka K, Kakumu S, Wakita T et al 1992 Detection of hepatitis C virus by polymerase chain reaction and response to interferon-α therapy: relationship to genotypes of hepatitis C virus. Hepatology 16:

# 33. Cirrhosis

*Peter C. Hayes*

Cirrhosis, a combination of hepatic fibrosis and regenerative nodule formation, is generally considered to be irreversible and is the final common pathway of many chronic hepatic injuries. The clinical manifestations of cirrhosis are protean and vary with the duration and severity of the liver disease rather than the underlying diagnosis. Many individuals remain asymptomatic. This chapter considers the features of cirrhosis in general, while those related to specific causes are considered elsewhere.

## ETIOLOGY

The prerequisite for cirrhosis is chronic injury, the causes of which are legion (Table 33.1). Most cases, however, are due to a relatively small number of causes. In the developed world alcohol remains the single most important cause and much of the variation in frequency relates to reporting accuracy. For this reason there is generally an inverse relationship between the prevalence of alcoholic and cryptogenic cirrhosis. In the Far East and Africa hepatitis B virus infection is an important cause and more recently hepatitis C virus has been recognized as being of major etiological significance. Apparently autoimmune chronic liver diseases, such as primary biliary cirrhosis and autoimmune hepatitis, are less frequent but important causes of cirrhosis, as they make up a significant proportion of the candidates for liver transplantation. Metabolic causes of cirrhosis are also important, since early recognition can lead to effective treatment as in hemochromatosis and Wilson's disease. There is no treatment for others such as $\alpha_1$-antitrypsin deficiency. Drug toxicity is an unusual cause for cirrhosis but should be excluded since drug withdrawal prevents progression. Other factors such as malnutrition and diabetes are rarely, if ever, causes of cirrhosis alone but may play a constitutive role. Despite increased understanding of the pathogenesis of cirrhosis and the recognition of many etiological factors (Table 33.1), the cause in a significant minority of cases remains unknown (cryptogenic).

**Table 33.1** Causes of cirrhosis (frequency %)

| | |
|---|---|
| Alcoholic | 50–60 |
| Hepatitis B & C | 10–20* |
| Primary biliary cirrhosis | 5–10 |
| Cryptogenic | 5–10 |
| Autoimmune hepatitis | 5 |
| Hemochromatosis | 1–5 |
| *Others* | |
| Metabolic (adults) | – $\alpha_1$-antitrypsin deficiency<br>– Wilson's disease<br>– Cystic fibrosis |
| Metabolic (children) | – Galactosemia<br>– Tyrosinosis<br>– Fructose intolerance<br>– Glucagon storage disease |
| Biliary (adults) | – Strictures<br>– Stones<br>– Neoplasms |
| Biliary (children) | – Biliary atresia<br>– Caroli's syndrome<br>– Choledochal cyst |
| Drugs | – Methotrexate |
| Vascular | – Budd–Chiari syndrome<br>– Veno-occlusive disease<br>– Cardiac failure or tamponade<br>– Hereditary hemorrhagic telangiectasia |
| Miscellaneous | – Sarcoidosis<br>– Indian childhood cirrhosis<br>– Intestinal bypass for obesity |

*Note: 5–30% of alcoholic cirrhotics have chronic HCV infection

## INCIDENCE

The occurrence of cirrhosis in most communities is not well known and must vary considerably geographically. The incidence of cirrhosis in Western countries is probably around 15–25 per 100 000 population. The incidence in the UK was 5.6 per 100 000 in 1959 and rose to 15.3 per 100 000 in 1974, mainly due to an increasing incidence of alcoholic liver disease (Saunders et al 1981). The incidence was 23.3 per 100 000 population from 1981 to 1985 in Denmark, with peak incidence rates for alcoholic cirrhosis in the fifth and sixth decades of life and for nonalcoholic nonbiliary cirrhosis and primary biliary cirrhosis in the seventh and eighth decades of life (Almdal et al 1991).

Incidence information based on diagnoses made during life do not take into account that cirrhosis is often asymptomatic during life. Powell et al (1971) found that 9.7% of their 414 patients were diagnosed incidentally at autopsy with an overall frequency of cirrhosis at autopsy of 1.9%. Saunders et al (1981) found that 11.3% of their patients were diagnosed incidentally at autopsy. Incidences of individual liver diseases may also be subject to diagnostic errors, particularly in relation to underdiagnosis of alcoholic cirrhosis (Prytz & Anderson 1988).

## PATHOGENESIS

The prerequisite for the development of cirrhosis is chronic hepatic injury leading to cell death and fibrosis. The mechanisms resulting in hepatocellular necrosis are complex. In alcoholic liver disease, for example, cytotoxic effects of alcohol and/or acetaldehyde, the production of damaging free radicals, genetic factors and immunological mechanisms with the formation of neoantigens have all been implicated (p. 865). Hypoxia and cholestasis secondary to the hepatic injury may also contribute to ongoing liver cell damage.

It is believed that hepatic stellate cells (p. 714) play a critical role in the process of fibrosis. These cells are situated in the space of Disse and are activated, possibly by Kupffer cell and hepatocyte factors including cytokines such as transforming growth factor $\beta_1$ (TGF$\beta_1$), leading to proliferation, loss of vitamin A and synthesis of collagen types I, III, IV and laminin (Friedman 1993). This in turn leads to the production of high density matrix in the subendothelial space, resulting in "capillarization" of the hepatic sinusoids. Simultaneously, the hepatocytes lose their microvilli and the sinusoidal fenestrations are obliterated (p. 714). The net result of this is reduced hepatic uptake of water and solute from the splanchnic circulation which interferes progressively with liver function as cirrhosis advances (Villeneuve et al 1996). At the same time significant microvascular changes occur, notably a dilated and increased peribiliary plexus, venous branches around cirrhotic nodules and increased arterioportal anastomoses as well as flattening of hepatic veins. These microvascular changes are important in the development of intrahepatic shunting and portal hypertension (Haratake et al 1991).

As fibrosis progresses, increases in all types of collagen occur but not equally. The ratio of type III to type I collagen is significantly lower in cirrhotic livers than in normal livers and type IV collagen increases, particularly in the early stage of alcoholic liver disease (Tsutsumi et al 1993). It is generally held that cirrhosis is an irreversible process, but in occasional reports in the literature (Rojkind & Dunn 1979) and more recently in a study from Scandinavia (Schvarcz et al 1993) apparent reversal has been documented. The significance of these observations, if true, cannot be overestimated.

Active fibrogenesis and the formation of passive septa as a result of liver cell necrosis and collapse cause disruption of the liver framework and hepatocyte regeneration occurring in this situation causes nodule formation. The humoral and/or paracrine factors responsible for regeneration are still obscure (p. 716) and a better understanding of this process may provide insights into hepatocellular carcinoma development in the cirrhotic liver.

## PATHOLOGY

The histological diagnosis of cirrhosis requires that the whole liver, although not necessarily every lobule, is involved with both fibrosis and nodular regeneration. Conditions that involve fibrosis alone occur in schistosomiasis and congenital hepatic fibrosis, while nodule formation without fibrosis occurs in nodular transformation and atypical adenomatous hyperplasia. In cirrhosis the nodules are surrounded by connective tissue and may or may not contain portal tracts and central veins. The liver architecture in the nodules may be apparently normal, making diagnosis from small biopsies difficult. Other abnormalities, such as variation in the size of hepatocytes, increase in the thickness of the liver cell plates, abnormal vascular channels and an excess of hepatic venous tributaries, may be identified.

Cirrhosis is the final common pathway for many causes of chronic hepatic injury and in itself seldom provides etiological information. Identification of the cause from liver biopsy lies primarily in the recognition of other features such as fatty change and Mallory's hyaline in alcoholic liver disease, biliary duplication and copper accumulation in primary biliary cirrhosis, lymphoid aggregates in chronic hepatitis C virus infection, antigen detection by immunohistochemistry or orcein staining in hepatitis B virus infection, PAS-positive diastase-resistant cytoplasmic granules in perinodular hepatocytes in $\alpha_1$-antitrypsin deficiency and heavy hepatocellular iron staining in hemochromatosis.

Traditionally, cirrhosis has been divided into two main categories depending on nodule size. Micronodular cirrhosis is typified by nodules of less than 3 mm in diameter (Fig. 33.1), whereas in macronodular cirrhosis the nodules are larger than 3 mm (Fig. 33.2). When nodules of both sizes are present, this is either described as mixed type or, because of the presence of some larger nodules, as macronodular (Fogarty International Center Proceedings 1976, Anthony et al 1977). The synonyms for the two main subtypes of cirrhosis are shown in Table 33.2. Histological confirmation of cirrhosis is usually made by needle biopsy. This is reliable in micronodular cirrhosis, but in macronodular cirrhosis the needle core can be composed entirely of tissue from within a nodule, making the diagnosis difficult or impossible. Thus, percutaneous biopsy underestimates cirrhosis by approximately 5–10% when compared with laparoscopy (p. 129).

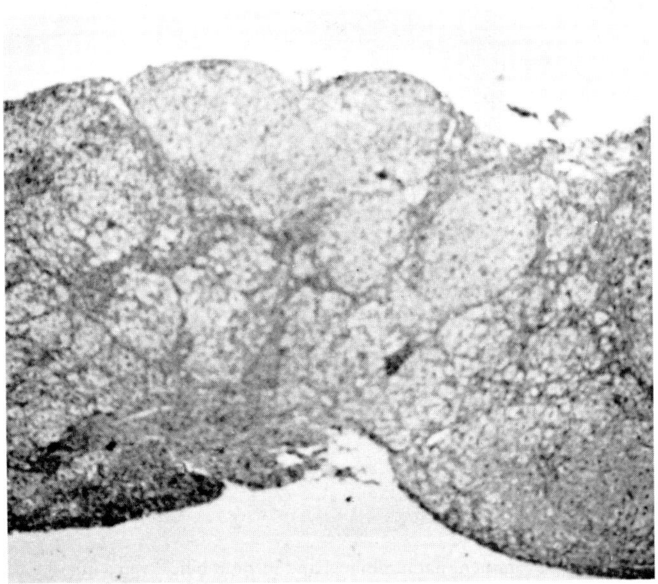

**Fig. 33.1** Micronodular cirrhosis showing small nodules less than 3 mm in diameter.

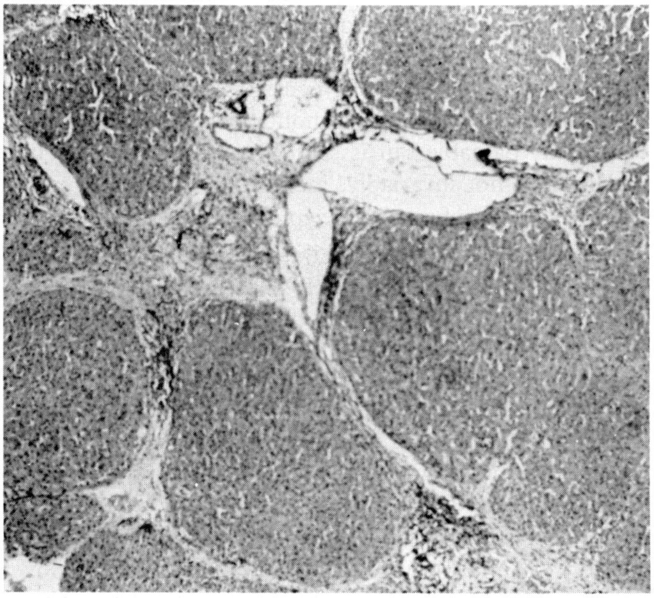

**Fig. 33.2** Macronodular cirrhosis showing nodules greater than 3 mm in diameter.

## ACTIVITY AND SEVERITY

The activity of liver disease is generally best reflected in the plasma transaminase activity. However, this is less true in cirrhosis, because ongoing hepatocellular necrosis may take place in the reduced parenchymal cell mass of cirrhosis with minimal or even no transaminase abnormality. Thus, disease activity in patients suspected of having cirrhosis is best judged histologically by the severity of the inflammatory cell infiltrate and the amount of hepatocellular damage at the interface of parenchymal and connective tissue (interface hepatitis) (p. 888).

**Table 33.2** Synonyms for micronodular and macronodular cirrhosis

| Micronodular* | Macronodular† |
|---|---|
| Laennec | Postnecrotic |
| Portal | Posthepatitic |
| Regular | Irregular |
| Monolobular | |
| Septal | |
| Uniform | |

* Relatively uniform nodules not >3 mm diameter, usually without portal tracts or central veins, and regular, relatively fine septa
† Irregular nodules, frequently multilobular, up to 5 cm diameter with irregular and often broad septa

On the other hand, disease severity in patients with cirrhosis is generally better determined biochemically from the plasma albumin (p. 745) and from coagulopathy (p. 751) than histologically. Although it is accepted generally that there is an evolution in alcoholic liver disease from micro- to macronodular cirrhosis, this is not a good guide to the severity of liver failure. For example, it has been observed that the change from micro- to macronodular cirrhosis is more frequent in abstainers from alcohol than in those who continue to drink (Gluud et al 1987). Laparoscopic assessment may be useful in assessing disease severity, as well-formed nodules, right lobe atrophy and left lobe hypertrophy represent more advanced disease (Tameda et al 1990) and laparoscopy also allows recognition of ascites and portal hypertension.

## CLINICAL FEATURES

Many symptoms and signs occur in cirrhosis and their frequency increases with the duration of disease and extent of liver damage (Martini 1975, Galambos 1979). The sensitivity and specificity of these clinical features is poor, as many patients with cirrhosis have no clinical abnormalities and some signs occur in precirrhotic patients and in conditions other than liver disease. Some of the features correlate more with disease activity than severity. General health and nutrition are usually good in patients with early cirrhosis but these deteriorate as the disease progresses. The major complications of cirrhosis result from portal hypertension, portasystemic shunting and hepatocellular failure and include variceal hemorrhage (p. 998), hepatic encephalopathy (p. 1039), ascites (p. 1017) and renal dysfunction (p. 1057). Rapid deterioration should suggest the possibility of hepatocellular carcinoma (p. 1118).

The clinical features of cirrhosis can be divided into those related to the liver and portal venous system and those that are extrahepatic. The common signs associated with cirrhosis vary in different liver diseases (Fig. 33.3) but are generally unhelpful in determining the underlying cause.

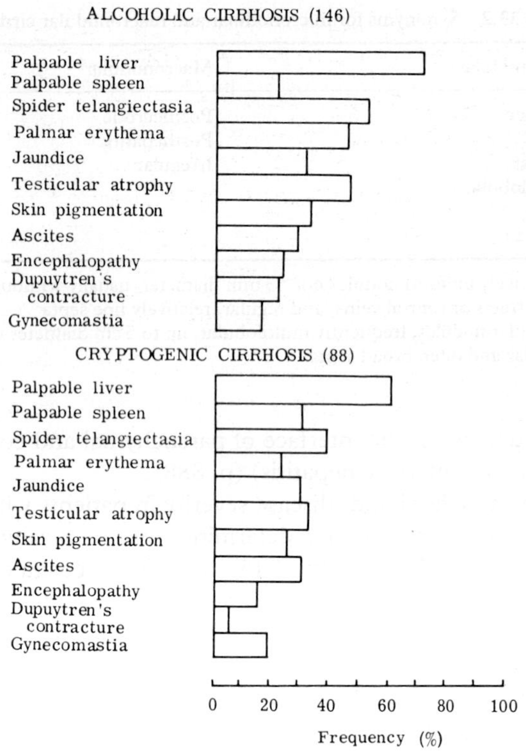


**Fig. 33.3** The frequency of various clinical features in alcoholic cirrhosis and in cryptogenic cirrhosis. The numbers of patients in each group are in parentheses (Powell et al 1971).

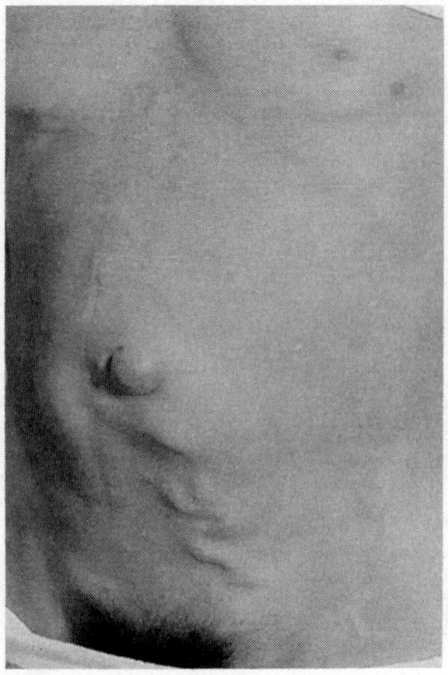

**Fig. 33.4** Prominent paraumbilical and infraumbilical veins in a patient with primary biliary cirrhosis and portal hypertension (Royal Infirmary, Edinburgh).

## Hepatic and portal venous features

### *Symptoms*

Abdominal pain is not uncommon in patients with cirrhosis. Although the cause may be due to peptic ulceration, gallstones or pancreatitis, in the majority its origin is unknown (Table 33.3). The pain may be constant, intermittent or colicky and is more common in patients with hemochromatosis.

### *Signs*

The liver is palpable in most patients with cirrhosis, but this does not necessarily indicate hepatomegaly (Rosenfield et al 1974). Generally, the right lobe is more easily palpable, but in more advanced disease disproportionate enlargement of the left lobe may occur. The liver is not usually tender in cirrhosis, in contrast to hepatitis (p. 796), and irregularity may be detected in patients with macronodular cirrhosis. A hepatic bruit may be heard in patients with primary and occasionally secondary liver cancer and in those with alcoholic hepatitis. The spleen is commonly palpable but is seldom grossly enlarged. This usually, but not invariably, indicates portal hypertension but the absence of a palpable spleen does not exclude this complication (p. 991). There is no correlation between the spleen size and the severity in portal hypertension.

Dilated superficial collateral vessels reflecting portal hypertension may be seen on the abdomen and chest (Fig. 33.4). They may be large and radiate from the umbilicus, a caput Medusae, but this is relatively uncommon. The direction of flow is away from the umbilicus, allowing differentiation from the collaterals that develop in inferior vena caval obstruction. These vessels reflect portal hypertension and indicate patency of the portal vein. Occasionally a venous hum may be detectable over them and this is the hallmark of the rare Cruveilhier–Baumgarten syndrome (p. 992). Hemorrhoids are probably no more common than in the general population and they should not be confused with anorectal varices (p. 993).

**Table 33.3** Abdominal pain in chronic liver disease (Powell et al 1971)

| Causes | Alcoholic cirrhosis | | Cyptogenic cirrhosis | | Chronic active hepatitis | | Hemochromatosis | |
|---|---|---|---|---|---|---|---|---|
| | Number | % | Number | % | Number | % | Number | % |
| Unknown | 32 | 70 | 17 | 59 | 10 | 90 | 14 | 78 |
| Peptic ulcer | 5 | 11 | 2 | 7 | 1 | 10 | 0 | 0 |
| Gallstones | 2 | 4 | 3 | 10 | 0 | 0 | 1 | 6 |
| Pancreatitis | 3 | 6 | 0 | 0 | 0 | 0 | 0 | 0 |
| Other | 4 | 9 | 7 | 24 | 0 | 0 | 3 | 17 |

Ascites may be obvious and confirmed by eliciting shifting dullness or a fluid thrill (p. 1019).

## Extrahepatic features

### *Skin*

Jaundice is usually relatively mild in hepatic cirrhosis compared with biliary cirrhosis. It is present in about a half of patients at presentation, although this may be an overestimate as the presence of jaundice is commonly the primary indication for investigation. Generalized pigmentation due to increased melanin deposition in the skin may occur in cirrhosis but is particularly pronounced in some cases of hemochromatosis and primary biliary cirrhosis. Mild finger clubbing similarly is common when looked for specifically and can, rarely, be associated with periostitis of the tibia and fibula, which may result in tenderness of the affected bones (Epstein et al 1981). Leukonychia may occur in patients with cirrhosis but has low specificity, as it is primarily related to hypoalbuminemia (BMJ 1974). Terry's nails, characterized by a distal pink to brown transverse band 0.5–3 mm wide associated with underlying telangiectatic vessels and pale light nails proximally, is associated with cirrhosis but also with chronic cardiac failure and diabetes mellitus (Holzberg & Walker 1984). In patients with chronic pruritus the nails may be noticeably smooth and shiny. Dupuytren's contracture has been associated with liver disease but is probably no commoner in patients with cirrhosis than in the rest of the population. Xanthomas and xanthelasmas are common in patients with primary biliary cirrhosis. Acne vulgaris is common in patients with underlying autoimmune hepatitis, and porphyria cutanea tarda (p. 975), characterized by skin that is excessively fragile and blisters with minor trauma and with ultraviolet light exposure, is associated strongly with chronic hepatitis C infection (p. 895) (Fargion et al 1992). Bruising is common in patients with coagulopathy, while purpura, especially on the legs, is associated with thrombocytopenia.

### *Vascular abnormalities*

The commonest and most characteristic vascular abnormality in cirrhosis is spider telangiectasia (spider nevus), which occurs in approximately three-quarters of patients (Martini 1975). This lesion comprises a central spiral arteriole with numerous radiating precapillary vessels (Fig. 33.5). The central arteriole may occasionally be both palpable and pulsatile. Pressure on the central arteriole causes blanching with a rapid return of blood flow from the center when the pressure is released. Spider telangiectasias occur almost exclusively on the upper half of the body and are most common on exposed areas. They vary in size from 1 mm (which can be easily overlooked) to 2–3 cm in diameter. When large and/or numerous they are highly suggestive of cirrhosis, but they are not pathognomonic as they occur in the third trimester of pregnancy, disappearing after delivery, in rheumatoid arthritis and occasionally in normal people (Table 33.4). The cause of spider telangiectasias is unknown and although endocrine changes have been implicated, they may regress without resolution of the hormonal abnormalities (Sherlock 1989). Cutaneous white spots also mark the sites of spiral arterioles in chronic liver disease and they are most easily seen over the buttocks and proximal limbs on exposure to cold. Ectasia of cutaneous venules, especially on the face, is common particularly in alcoholic liver disease. Palmar erythema, a blotchy distribution over the thenar and hypothenar eminences, is common, particularly in alcoholic cirrhosis, but also occurs in fever, in thyrotoxicosis and in otherwise well people. Thermographic studies have shown that in cirrhotic patients reduction in the temperature of the fingers relative to the palms is present and is probably due to arteriovenous shunting (Plevris et al 1991).

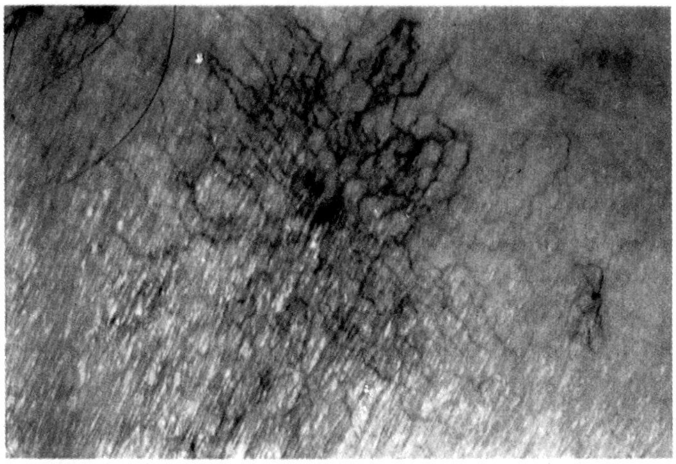

**Fig. 33.5** Large spider telangiectasias with central arterioles and radiating capillaries in a patient with hepatic cirrhosis (Royal Infirmary, Edinburgh).

**Table 33.4** Frequency of spider telangiectasias (Martini 1975)

| Group | Frequency (%) |
|---|---|
| Cirrhosis | 75 |
| Pregnancy | 40* |
| Healthy adults | 2.5 |

* Telangiectasias disappear soon after delivery

### *Epistaxis*

Epistaxis, particularly from the anterior nares, is common in cirrhosis, especially in association with alcohol abuse where trauma, thrombocytopenia and coagulopathy are associated risk factors. Indeed, it has been reported that most epistaxes associated with coagulation deficiencies occur in patients with cirrhosis (Hara 1962). Bleeding from the posterior nares may occur and blood may be swallowed, resulting in hematemesis or melena, which may be severe and which can cause diagnostic difficulties with regard to the site of bleeding (Hutchison & Finlayson 1987). Insertion of a Sengstaken tube through the nose should be discouraged, as it can cause this complication.

### *Cardiorespiratory abnormalities*

A hyperdynamic circulation develops in cirrhosis, becoming more pronounced as liver failure increases (Siegel et al 1974, Braillon et al 1986). The circulatory abnormality is characterized by tachycardia, an increase in cardiac output and a reduction in mean arterial pressure and peripheral vascular resistance (Table 33.5). Hypertension, which may occur with alcohol abuse, is unusual in cirrhosis (Schwartz 1967, Powell et al 1971). The hemodynamic changes affect not only the systemic but also the splanchnic circulation characterized by increased splanchnic blood flow, portal venous hypertension and an increase in portasystemic collateral flow as measured by azygos venous blood flow. Evidence suggests that these circulatory changes are due to humoral factors, including possibly glucagon, catecholamines and bile acids (Grose & Hayes 1992), but the precise etiology remains obscure. The most recent agent to be implicated is the potent vasodilator nitric oxide. Levels of nitric oxide appear to be increased in patients with cirrhosis and the nitric oxide antagonist LNMMA reverses some of the hemodynamic abnormalities (Pizcueta et al 1992, Forrest et al 1995).

Hypoxia is common in cirrhosis but is usually mild. Occasionally, however, it may be severe enough to cause central cyanosis. Numerous factors have been implicated in its development and of these pulmonary ventilation–perfusion imbalance is probably most important (p. 1071). Pulmonary hypertension is an uncommon but serious complication, particularly if liver transplantation is being considered (p. 1072). Hyperventilation characterized by respiratory alkalosis is not uncommon but the cause is unknown (p. 1069).

**Table 33.5** Hemodynamic measurements in hepatic cirrhosis related to liver failure (Braillon et al 1986)

| Measurement | Liver function* | | |
|---|---|---|---|
| | A($n$=16) | B($n$=18) | C($n$=16) |
| Mean arterial pressure (mmHg) | 88±16 | 87±10 | 80±12 |
| Heart rate (beats/min) | 74±13 | 87±12 | 96±12 |
| Cardiac index (L/min/m) | 3.5±0.5 | 4.0±1.1 | 4.7±1.6 |
| Systemic vascular resistance (dynes/s/cm$^{-5}$) | 1252±419 | 1085±341 | 951±307 |
| Wedged hepatic venous pressure (mmHg) | 26±5 | 30±8 | 32±6 |
| Azygos blood flow (ml/min) | 477±242 | 642±224 | 1061±476 |
| Azygos blood flow/cardiac output (%) | 7.6±3.5 | 10.2±4.4 | 14.6±6.9 |

* Assessed by Child (Pugh) grading (Table 36.7)

### *Hypogonadism and feminization*

Hypogonadism and feminization are the commonest endocrine abnormalities in cirrhosis (Baker et al 1976, Green 1977). In males, loss of libido, impotence and seminal fluid abnormalities are common, up to three-quarters have clinical and histological testicular atrophy and benign prostatic hypertrophy is rare. Loss of body hair and gynecomastia are evidence of feminization and have been attributed to imbalance in estrogenic/androgenic activity (Carlson 1980). Gynecomastia defined as an increase in the quantity of breast tissue occurs in approximately 20% of males with cirrhosis (Martini 1975) and is associated with a number of other diseases (Table 33.6) and drugs (Table 33.7). Although progesterone and prolactin are involved in breast growth and lactation, blood concentrations do not correlate with gynecomastia in cirrhosis (Farthing et al 1982). Hypogonadism in women with cirrhosis is characterized by amenorrhea or dysmenorrhea, infertility, benign cystic breast disease and acne vulgaris.

The pathogenesis of hypogonadism in cirrhosis is poorly understood. For example, the correlation between estrogen and androgen activity in the blood and the severity of liver disease and hypogonadism does not support a simple causal relationship. It is not surprising that, since patients show greater abnormalities in the hypothalamo–

**Table 33.6** Causes of gynecomastia (Carlson 1980)

| |
|---|
| Puberty |
| Old age |
| Hypogonadism (primary or secondary) |
| Neoplasia (adrenal, testis, liver) |
| Malnutrition (during refeeding) |
| Renal failure (during haemodialysis) |
| Hepatic cirrhosis |
| Hyperthyroidism |
| Cystic fibrosis |
| Drugs (Table 33.7) |

**Table 33.7** Drugs causing gynaecomastia (Carlson 1980)

| |
|---|
| Antihypertensives (methyldopa, reserpine) |
| Cimetidine |
| Cytotoxics (busulphan, nitrosoureas, vincristine) |
| Digoxin |
| Hormones (oestrogens, androgens, human chorionic gonadotrophin) |
| Isoniazid |
| Psychotrophics (amphetamines, diazepam, marijuana, phenothiazines, tricyclics) |
| Spironolactone |

pituitary–gonadal axis, impotence is commoner in those with alcoholic cirrhosis (70%) than in those with nonalcoholic liver disease (25%) (Cornely et al 1984). Alcohol abuse, even in the absence of liver disease, may cause testicular atrophy and influence the hypothalamo–pituitary–gonadal axis (Van Thiel et al 1975, Van Thiel & Lester 1976). In hemochromatosis, hypothalamo-pituitary injury occurs and hypogonadism is common.

*Parotid enlargement*

Parotid enlargement occurs in patients with alcoholic cirrhosis. It may also be associated occasionally with Sjögren's syndrome in primary biliary cirrhosis, with autoimmune hepatitis and with chronic hepatitis C virus infection. Other causes of parotid enlargement include diabetes mellitus and malnutrition.

## ASSOCIATED CONDITIONS

### Multisystem disease

Multisystem disease is common in autoimmune liver disease, principally type I autoimmune hepatitis, and in primary biliary cirrhosis. Features include arthralgia and arthritis, Raynaud's phenomenon, thyroid disease, inflammatory bowel disease, renal tubular acidosis and Sjögren's syndrome (Table 33.8).

### Diabetes mellitus

Impaired glucose tolerance occurs in approximately 60–80% of patients with cirrhosis, and diabetes mellitus in approximately 10–30%. Diabetes mellitus is insulin-independent (type II) and responds to carbohydrate restriction and oral hypoglycemic drugs. Impaired glucose tolerance is related to the severity of liver disease and there is no evidence that diabetes mellitus predisposes to cirrhosis (p. 1105).

Glucose intolerance in cirrhosis is caused by the simultaneous occurrence of insulin resistance in the muscles and inadequate secretion of insulin by the β-cells of the islets of Langerhans to overcome the insulin resistance (Petrides et al 1994). Diabetes mellitus then develops if insulin secretion decreases and as hepatic insulin resistance increases. Portasystemic shunting may play some part, but glucose tolerance is normal in patients with portal hypertension due to portal vein thrombosis (Smith-Laing et al 1979) and does not deteriorate after portasystemic shunt surgery (Cavallo-Perin et al 1985). The importance of hepatocellular function is supported by the observation that insulin resistance is more pronounced in alcoholic and cryptogenic cirrhosis than in primary biliary cirrhosis, where liver cell function is preserved until late in the disease (Taylor et al 1985).

**Table 33.8** Multisystem disease in 63 patients with cryptogenic cirrhosis (Golding et al 1973)

| Manifestation | Frequency (%) Method of detection | |
|---|---|---|
| | Clinical examination | Specific investigation |
| Arthropathy | 4 | — |
| Skin lesions | 5 | — |
| Thyroid disease | 6 | — |
| Ulcerative colitis | 8 | — |
| Sjögren's syndrome | 0 | 25 |
| Renal tubular acidosis | 0 | 22 |
| Pulmonary diffusion defects | 0 | 24 |
| Neuropathy/myopathy | 0 | 26 |

### Thyroid dysfunction

Abnormal thyroid function tests are common in cirrhosis, but clinical thyroid disease is unusual.

***Thyroid function tests.*** The commonest pattern of abnormality is a reduction in total and free serum thyroxine ($T_3$ and $T_4$) and a reduction in $T_3$ concentration has been related to the severity of cirrhosis (Borzio et al 1983). An increase in reverse $T_3$ occurs in patients with severe liver disease and the $T_3/T_4$ ratio has also been related to prognosis (Rees et al 1977, Griffin 1985). Serum thyroid stimulating hormone concentrations are usually normal, but the thyroid releasing hormone stimulation test is impaired in a third of patients.

***Clinical thyroid disease.*** Thyroid disease is most common in primary biliary cirrhosis and includes Hashimoto's thyroiditis, hyperthyroidism and particularly hypothyroidism (p. 937). Autoimmune thyroid disease with thyroid autoantibodies in the blood has also been reported in patients with chronic hepatitis C virus infection (Tran et al 1993) and irreversible changes in thyroid function may be associated with interferon treatment in this condition (p. 903).

### Cholelithiasis

Autopsy studies have shown an increased frequency of gallstones in cirrhosis (Bouchier 1969, Nicholas et al 1972). Normally, the incidence of gallstones increases with age and is higher in women; in cirrhosis there are no sex differences and the incidence of gallstones is high at all ages. This is due mainly to a high incidence of small pigment stones that may result from frequent mild hemolysis in cirrhosis. The failure to find an increase in cholesterol gallstones in cirrhosis in spite of a low bile salt pool may be due to the fact that bile is undersaturated with cholesterol in cirrhotic patients (Vlahcevic et al 1973). Biliary obstruction by gallstones is uncommon, perhaps because pigment stones are usually small enough to pass through the biliary tree (Nicholas et al 1972).

## Peptic ulcer

The prevalence of duodenal ulcer disease in patients with cirrhosis is increased, principally in those with alcoholic liver disease, primary sclerosing cholangitis and chronic active hepatitis due to hepatitis B virus infection, and an association with large esophageal varices and ascites has been suggested (Rabinowitz et al 1990). This increase in duodenal ulcer disease may be related to the high prevalence of *Helicobacter pylori* infection in cirrhosis and could explain the earlier observation of hypergastrinemia and impaired gastric acid secretion in cirrhosis (Lam 1976).

## Abdominal hernias

Abdominal hernias of all types are frequent in cirrhosis, especially in patients with ascites owing to the frequency with which this causes umbilical herniation (Pescovitz 1984). Umbilical hernias constitute about half of all hernias in such patients. Hernia repair can be performed in patients with good liver function who have no ascites or well-controlled ascites. Pescovitz (1984) reported a 10% mortality in 96 patients in the literature, but no mortality in 26 patients where a prophylactic operation had been done in such low-risk patients. Operations in patients with cirrhosis and poorly controlled ascites are hazardous (p. 1138) and hernia repair should not be considered other than for pressing symptoms or emergencies such as incarceration, strangulation, ulceration or leakage until ascites has been controlled and the nutritional state improved as far as possible. Fears that umbilical hernia repair might often lead to variceal bleeding have not been realized, although such bleeding has been associated with about a half of the postoperative deaths.

## Pleural effusion

Pleural effusion usually occurs in association with ascites, but effusions sometimes occur when ascites cannot be detected clinically (p. 1072).

## Malnutrition

Malnutrition is commonest in alcoholic patients (p. 866) but occurs frequently in all forms of cirrhosis (Mezey 1978). It involves not only deficient total caloric intake and deficiency of the main calorie sources, especially protein, but also deficiency of vitamins, particularly folate, thiamine, ascorbic acid, pyridoxine and all the fat-soluble vitamins, and deficiency of minerals. A body weight record is useful, as 20–30% weight loss indicates moderate calorie deficiency while loss of over 30% indicates severe protein calorie deficiency. Weight loses its value as a nutritional measure when fluid retention occurs. Examination of important muscle groups (temporal muscles, limb girdle, buttocks, thighs) is valuable, supplemented if possible by triceps skinfold (fat reserves) and mid-arm circumference (muscle) measures (Nompleggi & Bonkovsky 1994). Several factors contribute to its development.

***Food intake.*** Inadequate intake is the main cause for malnutrition. It results from the anorexia of liver disease and from the restricted and unpalatable diets prescribed for patients with encephalopathy and ascites. Alcoholics eat particularly badly, because they frequently suffer from abdominal discomfort, their finances are diverted into the purchase of alcohol and orderly family life is often destroyed. Other factors, however, have been recognized increasingly as contributing to malnutrition.

***Malabsorption.*** Malabsorption is common and is most frequently detected as steatorrhea, which occurs in about a half of patients. It is usually mild and fecal fat excretion rarely exceeds 10 g/day. Other nutrients, particularly the fat-soluble vitamins, are also malabsorbed. Many factors contribute to steatorrhea, including deficient pancreatic secretion (Van Goidseahoven et al 1963), reduced intestinal bile salt concentrations (p. 934), and the effects of alcohol (p. 866) and of drugs such as neomycin (p. 1052) and cholestyramine on absorption (p. 933). Small intestinal mucosal abnormalities are slight and are probably unimportant. Protein-losing enteropathy occurs but is mild and does not contribute significantly to hypoalbuminemia (Davcev et al 1969).

***Metabolic abnormalities.*** Liver damage causes widespread metabolic abnormality reflected in impaired carbohydrate tolerance and hyperinsulinism (above), altered blood lipids (p. 754) and increased blood concentrations of amino acids metabolized by the liver (p. 1041). This is associated with a low resting respiratory quotient indicating reduced carbohydrate utilization and increased fat utilization (Müller et al 1992). Glucose production by the cirrhotic liver is impaired and plasma free fatty acid concentrations and turnover are increased, indicating increased energy production from lipolysis (Owen et al 1981). Energy utilization in cirrhosis is very variable by comparison with the norm of 30–35 kcal/kg/24 h. About 20% of patients show increased energy utilization (hypermetabolic) associated with more advanced disease, loss of muscle mass and normal body fat, while about 30% show reduced energy utilization associated with increased fat and fat-free body mass. Hypermetabolism in cirrhosis is probably due mainly to extrahepatic factors and may be important in the development of malnutrition (Müller et al 1992). Increased muscle catabolism is common in cirrhosis and loss of muscle mass is striking in advanced disease (Marchesini et al 1981). In alcoholic liver disease, ethanol-induced abnormalities in mitochondria and induced microsomal enzymes lead to energy wastage (Lieber 1991, Coleman & Cunningham 1991). Indeed, even in the absence of liver disease a moderate to high alcohol intake in women is associated with weight loss despite increased calorie intake (Colditz et al 1991).

### Bone disease

Hepatic osteodystrophy is the term used to encompass the spectrum of bone abnormalities in cirrhosis (p. 932). The commonest abnormality is reduced bone formation and reduced bone mineral content similar but not identical to the osteoporosis observed in postmenopausal women (Diamond et al 1989, Resch et al 1990). Chronic cholestasis may cause vitamin D malabsorption and osteomalacia, but this is uncommon.

Hepatic osteodystrophy leads to an increased prevalence of spinal and peripheral fractures in patients with both cholestatic and noncholestatic liver disorders (Diamond et al 1990). Effective treatment of hepatic osteodystrophy remains elusive (p. 934). Liver transplantation eventually reverses the process, but in the early postoperative phase fractures are common.

### Neuropathy

Autonomic dysfunction occurs commonly in all forms of cirrhosis and is associated with increasing severity of liver disease (Thuluvath & Triger 1989, Dillon et al 1994). Symptoms associated with autonomic dysfunction are unusual. The parasympathetic system appears to be more affected than the sympathetic system and it is unclear whether the abnormality is neuronal or postsynaptic. Peripheral neuropathy occurs in patients with alcoholic liver disease and is associated with alcohol abuse rather than hepatic impairment. Central nervous system abnormalities occur and some must be differentiated from hepatic encephalopathy. These include Wernicke's encephalopathy, vitamin E deficiency in chronic cholestasis and chronic forms of encephalopathy (p. 1050).

### Kidney disease

The kidney plays an important role in the development of ascites and hepatorenal failure often occurs during complications of cirrhosis and as a terminal event (p. 1057). Patients with chronic liver disease may also show pathological abnormalities in the kidneys and the relation of these to the liver disease is uncertain (p. 1064). However, primary renal disease rarely presents clinically in cirrhosis.

## INVESTIGATIONS

### Liver function tests

Liver function tests are neither sensitive nor specific for cirrhosis. The serum transaminase activities accurately reflect disease activity in patients without cirrhosis but are less sensitive in cirrhosis, presumably because of the reduced hepatocellular mass. Hypoalbuminemia reflects disease severity but is normal in many patients with cirrhosis. Serum bilirubin in hepatic cirrhosis increases late in the disease compared with biliary cirrhosis. Serum alkaline phosphatase activity is often moderately increased, but activities above 300 units/L are unusual except in cholestatic diseases. Although serum bile acid concentrations are a sensitive index for liver dysfunction, they are not widely available. Dynamic liver function tests such as indocyanine green, galactose, antipyrine and caffeine clearance are more sensitive than static tests and are valuable research tools, but they are cumbersome and are not commonly used in clinical practice. A number of new tests such as serum procollagen III peptide and hyaluronic acid have been proposed for identifying cirrhosis, but their specificity remains unproven.

### Hematology

Peripheral blood abnormalities are common in cirrhosis and involve all the main cell types (Friedman & Schwartz 1961, Martini 1975, Chanarin 1982). Mild hypochromic or normochromic anemia occurs at some time in almost all patients, macrocytes and target cells are often present and occasionally red cells with spur-like projections (spur cells) are seen. The causes of these morphological abnormalities are uncertain, but they are associated with marked changes in the lipid composition of the red blood cell membrane and are most florid in patients with severe liver damage (Salvioli et al 1978). Mild hemolysis is common but in rare instances, and usually in alcoholic patients, more severe hemolysis occurs and numerous spur cells appear in the blood (Smith et al 1964). Many factors contribute to anemia in cirrhosis, including dilution due to an increased plasma volume (p. 1019), blood loss, mild hemolysis, hypersplenism, depressed marrow function and nutritional deficiency. The marrow is almost always normoblastic or macronormoblastic and megaloblastic changes usually result from folate deficiency.

Leukopenia, especially neutropenia, is also common and is usually due to hypersplenism. This is not always so, as some patients have neutropenia without splenomegaly and sometimes neutropenia is not corrected fully by splenectomy. Thrombocytopenia is more frequent than leukopenia and occurs in a half of patients, although counts below $50 \times 10^9$/L ($50\,000/mm^3$) are rare. Several factors contribute to thrombocytopenia, including a reduced platelet lifespan, an increased splenic platelet pool size, intrinsic and extrinsic platelet abnormalities and alcohol (p. 1190). Bleeding attributable directly to thrombocytopenia is rare, but variceal bleeding is rare in primary biliary cirrhosis when the count is greater than $150 \times 10^9$/L and common when the count is below $100 \times 10^9$/L (Plevris et al 1995).

There is a strong association between essential mixed cryoglobulinemia and hepatitis C virus infection with hepatitis C virions and HCV antigen–antibody complexes found in the cryoprecipitate (Agnello et al 1992).

### Hemostasis

Hemostatic abnormalities are found in a half or more of patients and are complex and multifactorial (p. 751). The severity of coagulopathy is a valuable prognostic marker. Investigation of hemostasis is important before invasive procedures and in revealing deficient hemostasis in bleeding from sites such as esophageal varices. The most useful laboratory investigations are the prothrombin time, the partial thromboplastin time and the platelet count. A prolonged prothrombin time in cholestatic cirrhosis may be caused by vitamin K deficiency, while inability to correct the prothrombin time after intravenous vitamin K 10 mg is administered slowly indicates severe hepatocellular dysfunction.

### Imaging

Ultrasonic imaging is noninvasive and provides accurate information about liver and spleen size and ascites. However, its sensitivity and specificity for cirrhosis is poor. Computed tomography is more accurate and nuclear magnetic resonance may be of value in detecting large amounts of iron or fat. Imaging cannot exclude cirrhosis but is valuable in detecting hepatic tumors, principally hepatocellular carcinoma. Radionuclide imaging is now little used in diagnosis, but it shows an abnormal pattern of uptake by the liver with increased uptake by the bone marrow and spleen in cirrhosis.

### Angiography

Hepatic angiography is not important in the diagnosis of cirrhosis, although characteristic appearances may be seen when it is undertaken for other reasons such as the identification of sites of gastrointestinal bleeding or surgical or transhepatic portasystemic shunt construction. The most characteristic abnormalities are a corkscrew appearance of the intrahepatic arteries in small shrunken livers (Fig. 36.2) and stretched and separated arteries in enlarged livers. The venous phase of a mesenteric angiogram provides imaging of the portal vein and portasystemic collaterals.

### Liver biopsy

Traditionally, ultimate proof of cirrhosis is obtained only by liver biopsy, although this may result in underdiagnosis (p. 717). Diagnostic accuracy can be improved by performing the biopsy laparoscopically (p. 129). Indeed, in certain cases, particularly where the etiology is known, laparoscopy alone without histological confirmation may be sufficient. Laparoscopy also allows the biopsy to be undertaken under direct vision and any bleeding can be controlled by pressure or heater probe application. The necessity for liver biopsy in the diagnosis of cirrhosis is discussed below.

### Other investigations

In most instances the etiology of cirrhosis can be determined by noninvasive techniques. These include the detection of the hepatitis B, C and D viruses, $\alpha_1$-antitrypsin deficiency, hemochromatosis, Wilson's disease and inflammatory bowel disease. Autoantibodies against nuclei, smooth muscle, mitochondria and liver and kidney microsomal antigens are important in the diagnosis of autoimmune liver disease. Serum hyaluronic acid may prove useful in the noninvasive diagnosis of cirrhosis (p. 752).

## DIAGNOSIS

### Differential diagnosis

The conditions from which cirrhosis must be differentiated depend on what causes the patient to consult the doctor. A half to two-thirds of patients present with jaundice or ascites with or without edema and another quarter present with abdominal pain, acute gastrointestinal bleeding or features of encephalopathy. Patients with jaundice usually have some other feature pointing to parenchymal liver disease, most often spider telangiectasias and bilirubinuria indicating hepatobiliary disease (p. 741). Mild jaundice, pallor and a palpable spleen suggest hemolytic anemia, but there are no associated features of cirrhosis and no bilirubinuria in that condition. Abdominal pain occurs in about a third of patients with cirrhosis and usually suggests peptic ulceration, biliary disease or pancreatitis. The diagnosis of ascites (p. 1019), encephalopathy (p. 1045) or gastrointestinal bleeding (p. 499) is considered elsewhere.

Sometimes patients present with nonspecific symptoms, particularly weakness, lassitude, anorexia, nausea or vomiting, and up to a third complain of diarrhea at some time. The absence of an alternative cause for the symptoms, clinical evidence of liver disease and abnormal liver function tests are the main pointers to cirrhosis. Loss of libido or impotence may suggest psychiatric or endocrine disease, but cirrhosis should always be considered in older males. Increasingly, cirrhosis is being diagnosed incidentally when patients present with other diseases or for a routine examination. Prolonged heavy alcohol intake is the most valuable clinical clue to the diagnosis in these patients.

### Investigations

The question arises regarding the investigations needed to make a diagnosis of cirrhosis, especially the need for laparoscopy and/or liver biopsy.

Liver biopsy is an invasive procedure with a small but real mortality (p. 721) and it should not be used automatically in the diagnosis of cirrhosis. Patients with clinical features of cirrhosis, such as multiple spider telangiectasias, clearly abnormal liver function tests and imaging appearances of cirrhosis, do not need a biopsy for cirrhosis to be recognized, especially if a complication of cirrhosis such as ascites, varices or encephalopathy is also present. Biopsy is more useful and better justified where features such as jaundice, ascites, varices and encephalopathy are not associated with other features of parenchymal liver disease. Causes of liver disease can often be determined from blood examination as in autoimmune hepatitis, Wilson's disease and $\alpha_1$-antitrypsin deficiency, but biopsy may also be needed to identify the cause of liver disease, as when a high plasma ferritin suggests hemochromatosis, or to know whether cirrhosis is present before deciding on interferon therapy for chronic hepatic virus infection (p. 902). Ultimately, the decision is a clinical one, but the potential hazards of liver biopsy need to be recognized. Biopsy in the face of blood coagulation abnormalities always demands a very clear indication.

## TREATMENT

Specific treatment is indicated for many causes of cirrhosis, including corticosteroids for autoimmune hepatitis (p. 900), venesection for hemochromatosis (p. 956), α-interferon for hepatitis B and C virus (p. 902), penicillamine for Wilson's disease (p. 964) and alcohol withdrawal for alcoholic cirrhosis (p. 877). In many patients, however, no specific treatment is available and therapy is directed at maintaining nutrition and at controlling encephalopathy (p. 1051), ascites (p. 1023), gastrointestinal bleeding due to portal hypertension (p. 499) and renal failure (p. 1061).

### Nutrition

Patients should be specifically encouraged to take an adequate diet. The nutritional state of malnourished patients who show no signs of encephalopathy can be improved by increasing normal food intake and in those with encephalopathy or ascites it needs to be remembered that adequate nutrition cannot be maintained on a protein intake of less than 30 g/day. It is important to maintain an adequate caloric intake of about 30–35 kcal/kg/day containing 1 g protein/kg ideal body weight, fat not in excess of 35% of calories, and carbohydrate. Supplements, including vitamins and minerals, can be given and this should be done orally whenever possible. Such supplements are expensive but can be valuable (Nompleggi & Bonkovsky 1994).

Malabsorption is only occasionally a major factor impairing nutrition, but in such cases the main causes should be determined. Steatorrhea of undetermined cause is best treated by restricting fat intake to 40 g daily and increasing calorie intake from other sources. Treatment with pancreatic extracts may be beneficial (p. 1273). Anorexia is a feature in many patients with advanced liver disease and where it is important to improve nutrition, as before liver transplantation, nutritional intake can be improved by enteral feeding using a fine-bore nasogastric tube (Nompleggi & Bonkovsky 1994).

### Cramps

Painful leg cramps are common in patients with cirrhosis. They usually occur at night and are occasionally prolonged. The causes are poorly understood but may include electrolyte losses due to diuretic therapy and a reduced circulating blood volume (Angeli et al 1996). Electrolyte deficiencies should be corrected. Quinine salts 200–300 mg by mouth at bedtime usually relieve the cramps where no cause can be found. Weekly infusions of 100 ml 25% albumin may also be helpful (Angeli et al 1996).

### Drugs

No treatment can reverse cirrhosis, but as continuing inflammation and fibrosis are presumably responsible for the progressive death of hepatocytes and for destruction of the hepatic architecture, the value of anti-inflammatory and antifibrotic drugs has been investigated. Corticosteroids are of proven value in autoimmune hepatitis and there is some evidence that in this condition even cirrhosis may be improved (Schvarcz et al 1993). The question therefore arises as to whether corticosteroids might benefit patients with chronic liver disease, including cirrhosis, who do not have serum autoantibodies related to liver disease but who do have other autoantibodies or autoimmune diseases (Shindo et al 1992). The treatment of these patients and those with cryptogenic chronic hepatitis and cirrhosis includes treatment with corticosteroid drugs and is discussed elsewhere (p. 899). Antifibrotic drugs such as colchicine have been tried in alcoholic cirrhosis (Kershenobich et al 1988) and colchicine, penicillamine and ursodeoxycholic acid have been tried in primary biliary cirrhosis (p. 941) but they have not yet been accepted as standard therapy.

## COMPLICATIONS

The main complications of cirrhosis are due either to portal hypertension, such as bleeding from esophageal varices, or to hepatocellular failure, such as ascites, encephalopathy and renal failure. Patients with cirrhosis are also susceptible to infection, particularly bacteremia (p. 772) and spontaneous bacterial peritonitis (p. 1033), and these are considered elsewhere.

## PROGNOSIS

The overall prognosis in cirrhosis is poor and depends largely on the severity of liver failure at presentation and on the underlying etiology. The prognosis is obviously bet-

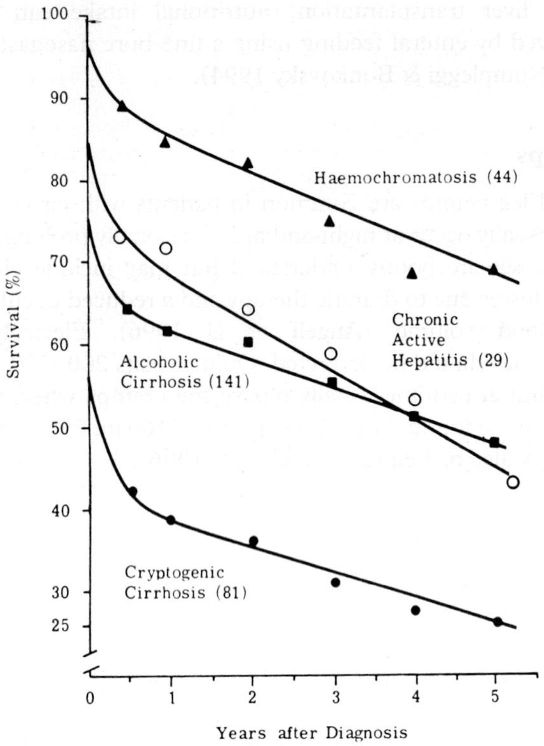


**Fig. 33.6** Cumulative 5-year survival of patients with different forms of cirrhosis (Powell et al 1971).

**Table 33.9** Age at death and main causes of death in different forms of cirrhosis (Powell et al 1971)

| Child (Pugh) grade | Survival (%) 1 year | 5 years | 10 years | Hepatic deaths (%) |
|---|---|---|---|---|
| A | 82 | 45 | 25 | 43 |
| B | 62 | 20 | 7 | 72 |
| C | 42 | 20 | 0 | 85 |

Note: For Child (Pugh) grading see Table 36.7.
Hepatic deaths included hepatic failure, gastrointestinal bleeding, and hepatocellular carcinoma

ter for patients with forms of cirrhosis for which treatment is available, such as autoimmune hepatitis and hemochromatosis (Fig. 33.6, Table 33.9). The prognosis in alcoholic cirrhosis has generally been found to be better in those who stop drinking, but this is not a universal finding (p. 877).

**Table 33.10** Survival and liability to death from hepatic causes related to hepatocellular function (Child Grade) in 231 patients admitted as controls to a clinical trial (Christensen et al 1984)

| Cause of cirrhosis | Mean age at death (years) | Frequency (%) of causes of death: Cirrhosis related* | Infection | Vascular |
|---|---|---|---|---|
| Alcoholic | 54 | 70 | 8 | 1 |
| Cryptogenic | 62 | 61 | 8 | 17 |
| Autoimmune hepatitis | 49 | 92 | 0 | 0 |
| Hemochromatosis | 56 | 55 | 14 | 9 |

* Liver failure, gastrointestinal bleeding and hepatocellular carcinoma

The Child–Pugh classification of severity of liver disease (Pugh et al 1973), which combines biochemical and clinical features, is an imperfect prognostic index but the best generally available (Table 33.10). It should be remembered, however, that patients frequently present during exacerbations of liver disease that are caused by treatable factors or may be followed by spontaneous improvement and accordingly decisions regarding prognosis are best postponed until the patient has been observed for a few months. The question of prognosis is of vital importance in considering the timing for liver transplantation and this remains a problem (p. 1152). Fairly accurate scoring systems have been identified for primary biliary cirrhosis, but for other conditions the unpredictability of disease progression has rendered scoring systems of limited value. Features other than those in the Child–Pugh scoring system that are relevant to prognosis include nutritional status and quality of life and these are taken into account in assessment of transplantation.

## PREVENTION

Since cirrhosis is an irreversible condition, every effort should be made to identify and treat patients before it develops. Improved education regarding the risks of alcohol abuse and the wider application of hepatitis B vaccines as well as specific treatments for chronic liver disease should have some impact. Unfortunately, a large number of patients present for the first time with complications of cirrhosis, limiting effectiveness of preventive measures.

## REFERENCES

Agnello V, Chung R T, Kaplan L M 1992 A role of hepatitis C virus infection in Type II cryoglobulinemia. New England Journal of Medicine 327: 1490–1495

Almdal T P, Sørensen T I A and the Danish Association for the Study of the Liver 1991 Incidence of parenchymal liver disease in Denmark, 1981 to 1985: analysis of hospitalization registry data. Hepatology 13: 650–655

Angeli P, Albino G, Carroro P et al 1996 Cirrhosis and muscle cramps: evidence of a causal relationship. Hepatology 23: 264–273

Anthony P P, Ishak K G, Nayak N C, Poulsen H E, Scheuer P J, Sobin L H 1977 The morphology of cirrhosis. Recommendation on definition, nomenclature and classification by a working group sponsored by the World Health Organization. Journal of Clinical Pathology 31: 395–414

Baker H W G, Burger H G, de Kretser D M et al 1976 A study of the

endocrine manifestations of hepatic cirrhosis. Quarterly Journal of Medicine 45: 154–178
BMJ 1974 Leading article: white marks on nails. British Medical Journal 1: 257–258
Borzio M, Caldara R, Borzio F, Piepoli V, Rampini P, Ferrari C 1983 Thyroid function tests in chronic liver disease: evidence for multiple abnormalities despite clinical euthyroidism. Gut 24: 631–636
Bouchier I A D 1969 Postmortem study of the frequency of gallstones in patients with cirrhosis of the liver. Gut 10: 705–710
Braillon A, Cales P, Valla D, Gaudy D, Geoffroy P, Lebrec D 1986 Influence of the degree of liver failure on systemic and splanchnic haemodynamics and of the response to propranolol in patients with cirrhosis. Gut 27: 1204–1209
Carlson H E 1980 Gynecomastia. New England Journal of Medicine 303: 795–799
Cavallo-Perin P, Cassader M, Bozzo C et al 1985 Mechanism of insulin resistance in human liver cirrhosis. Evidence of a combined receptor and post-receptor defect. Journal of Clinical Investigation 75: 1659–1665
Chanarin I 1982 Haemopoiesis and alcohol. British Medical Bulletin 38: 81–86
Christensen E, Schlichting P, Fauerholdt L et al 1984 Prognostic value of Child–Turcotte criteria in medically treated cirrhosis. Hepatology 4: 430–435
Colditz G A, Giovannucci E, Rim E B et al 1991 Alcohol intake in relation to diet and obesity in women and men. American Journal of Clinical Nutrition 54: 49–55
Coleman W B, Cunningham C C 1991 Effect of chronic ethanol consumption on hepatic mitochondrial transcription and translation. Biochemica et Biophysica Acta 1058: 178–186
Cornely C M, Schade R R, Van Thiel D H, Gavaler J S 1984 Chronic advanced liver disease and impotence: cause and effect? Hepatology 4: 1227–1230
Davcev P, Vanovski B, Sestakov D, Tadze R 1969 Protein-losing enteropathy in patients with liver cirrhosis. Digestion 2: 17–22
Diamond T H, Stiel D, Lunzer M, McDowall D, Eckstein R P, Posen S 1989 Hepatic osteodystrophy. Static and dynamic bone histomorphometry and serum bone Gla-protein in 80 patients with chronic liver disease. Gastroenterology 96: 213–221
Diamond T, Stiel D, Lunzer M, Wilkinson M, Roche J, Posen S 1990 Osteoporosis and skeletal fractures in chronic liver disease. Gut 31: 82–87
Dillon J F, Plevris J N, Nolan J et al 1994 Autonomic function in cirrhosis assessed by cardiovascular reflex tests and 24-hour heart rate variability. American Journal of Gastroenterology 89: 1544–1547
Epstein O, Dick R, Sherlock S 1981 Prospective study of periostitis and finger clubbing in primary biliary cirrhosis and other forms of chronic liver disease. Gut 22: 203–206
Fargion S, Piperno A, Cappellini M D et al 1992 Hepatitis C virus and porphyria cutanea tarda: evidence of a strong association. Hepatology 16: 1322–1326
Farthing M J G, Green J R B, Edwards C R W, Dawson A M 1982 Progesterone, prolactin and gynaecomastia in men with liver disease. Gut 23: 276–279
Fogarty International Center Proceedings No. 22 1976 Diseases of the liver and biliary tract. Standardization of nomenclature, diagnostic criteria and diagnostic methodology. DHEW Publication No. (NIH) 76–725, Ch 3, p 17
Forrest E H, Jones A L, Dillon J F, Walker J, Hayes P C 1995 The cffect of nitric oxide synthase inhibition on portal pressure and azygos blood flow in patients with cirrhosis. Journal of Hepatology 23: 254–258
Friedman I A, Schwartz S O 1961 The relation between the liver and the hemopoietic system. In: Popper H, Schaffner F (eds) Progress in liver diseases, Vol 1. Grune and Stratton, New York, p 134–144
Friedman S L 1993 The cellular basis of hepatic fibrosis. The mechanisms and treatment strategies. New England Journal of Medicine 328: 1828–1835
Galambos J T 1979 Cirrhosis. Major problems in internal medicine, Vol 17. W B Saunders, Philadelphia
Gluud C, Christoffersen P, Eriksen J, Wantzin P, Knudsen B B and the Copenhagen Study Group for Liver Diseases 1987 Influence of ethanol on development of hyperplastic nodules in alcoholic men with micronodular cirrhosis. Gastroenterology 93: 256–260
Golding P L, Smith M, Williams R 1973 Multisystem involvement in chronic liver disease. Studies on the incidence and pathogenesis. American Journal of Medicine 55: 772–782
Green J R B 1977 Mechanism of hypogonadism in cirrhotic males. Gut 18: 843
Griffin J E 1985 Southwestern Internal Medicine Conference: the dilemma of abnormal thyroid function tests – is thyroid disease present or not? American Journal of the Medical Sciences 289: 76–88
Grose R D, Hayes P C 1992 Review article: the pathophysiology and pharmacological treatment of portal hypertension. Alimentary Pharmacology and Therapeutics 6: 521–540
Hara H J 1962 Severe epistaxis. Archives of Otolaryngology 72: 258–269
Haratake J, Hisaoko M, Yamamoto O, Horie A 1991 Morphological changes of hepatic microcirculation in experimental rat cirrhosis: a scanning electron microscopic study. Hepatology 13: 952–956
Holzberg M, Walker H K 1984 Terry's nails: revised definition and new correlations. Lancet 1: 896–899
Hutchison S M W, Finlayson N D C 1987 Epistaxis as a cause of hematemesis and melena. Journal of Clinical Gastroenterology 9: 283–285
Kershenobich D, Vargas F, Garcia-Tsao G, Tamayo R P, Gent M, Rojkind M 1988 Colchicine in the treatment of cirrhosis of the liver. New England Journal of Medicine 318: 1709–1713
Lam S K 1976 Hypergastrinaemia in cirrhosis of the liver. Gut 17: 700–708
Lieber C S 1991 Perspectives: do alcohol calories count? American Journal of Clinical Nutrition 54: 976–982
Marchesini G, Zoli M, Angiolini A, Dondi C, Bianchi F B, Pisi E 1981 Muscle protein breakdown in liver cirrhosis and the role of altered carbohydrate metabolism. Hepatology 1: 294–299
Martini G A 1975 Extrahepatic manifestations of cirrhosis. Clinics in Gastroenterology 4: 439–460
Mezey E 1978 Liver disease and nutrition. Gastroenterology 74: 770–783
Müller M J, Lautz H U, Plogmann B, Bürger M, Körber J, Schmidt F N 1992 Energy expenditure and substrate oxidation in patients with cirrhosis: the impact of cause, clinical staging and nutritional state. Hepatology 15: 782–794
Nicholas P, Rinaudo P A, Conn H O 1972 Increased incidence of cholelithiasis in Laennec's cirrhosis. A postmortem evaluation of pathogenesis. Gastroenterology 63: 112–121
Nompleggi D J, Bonkovsky H L 1994 Nutritional supplementation in chronic liver disease: an analytical review. Hepatology 19: 518–533
Owen O E, Reichle F A, Mozzoli M A et al 1981 Hepatic, gut, and renal substrate flux rates in patients with hepatic cirrhosis. Journal of Clinical Investigation 68: 240–252
Pesçovitz M D 1984 Umbilical hernia repair in patients with cirrhosis. No evidence for increased incidence of variceal bleeding. Annals of Surgery 199: 325–327
Petrides A S, Vogt C, Schulze-Berge D, Matthews D, Strohmeyer G 1994 Pathogenesis of glucose intolerance and diabetes mellitus in cirrhosis. Hepatology 19: 616–627
Pizcueta P, Piqué J M, Fernández M et al 1992 Modulation of the hyperdynamic circulation of cirrhotic rats by nitric oxide inhibition. Gastroenterology 103: 1909–1915
Plevris J N, Hauer J L, Hayes P C, Bouchier I A 1991 The hands in alcoholic liver disease. American Journal of Gastroenterology 86 467–471
Plevris J N, Dhariwal A, Elton R A, Finlayson N D C, Bouchier I A D, Hayes P C 1995 The platelet count as a predictor of variceal hemorrhage in primary biliary cirrhosis. American Journal of Gastroenterology 90: 959–961
Powell L W, Mortimer R, Harris O D 1971 Cirrhosis of the liver: a comparative study of the four major aetiological groups. Medical Journal of Australia 1: 941–950
Prytz H, Anderson H 1988 Underreporting of alcohol-related mortality from cirrhosis is declining in Sweden and Denmark. Scandinavian Journal of Gastroenterology 23: 1035–1043
Pugh R N H, Murray-Lyon I M, Dawson J L, Pietroni M C, Williams R 1973 Transection of the oesophagus for bleeding oesophageal varices. British Journal of Surgery 60: 646–649
Rabinowitz M, Schade R R, Dindzans V, Van Thiel D H, Gavaler J S

1990 Prevalence of duodenal ulcer in cirrhotic males referred for liver transplantation. Does the etiology of the cirrhosis make a difference? Digestive Diseases and Sciences 35: 321–326

Rees L H, Bessar G M, Jeffcoat W J, Goldie D J, Marks V 1977 Alcohol-induced pseudo-Cushing's syndrome. Lancet 1: 726–728

Resch H, Pietschmann P, Krexner E, Woloszczuk W, Willvonseder R 1990 Peripheral bone mineral content in patients with fatty liver and hepatic cirrhosis. Scandinavian Journal of Gastroenterology 25: 412–416

Rojkind M, Dunn M A 1979 Hepatic fibrosis. Gastroenterology 76: 849–863

Rosenfield A T, Laufer I, Schneider P B 1974 The significance of a palpable liver. A correlation of clinical and radioisotope studies. American Journal of Roentgenology, Radium Therapy and Nuclear Medicine 122: 313–317

Salvioli G, Rioli G, Lugli R, Salati R 1978 Membrane lipid composition of red blood cells in liver disease: regression of spur cell anaemia after infusion of polyunsaturated phosphatidylcholine. Gut 19: 844–850

Saunders J B, Walters J R F, Davies P, Paton A 1981 A 20-year prospective study of cirrhosis. British Medical Journal 282: 263–266

Schvarcz R, Glaumann H, Weiland O 1993 Survival and histological resolution of fibrosis in patients with autoimmune chronic active hepatitis. Journal of Hepatology 18: 15–23

Schwartz D T 1967 The relation of cirrhosis of the liver to renal hypertension: a review of 639 autopsied cases. Annals of Internal Medicine 66: 862–869

Sherlock S 1989 Spiders and capillaries. Hepatology 10: 388–389

Shindo M, Di Bisceglie A M, Hoofnagle J H 1992 Acute exacerbation of liver disease during interferon alpha therapy for chronic hepatitis C. Gastroenterology 102: 1406–1408

Siegel J H, Goldwyn R M, Farrell E J, Gallin P, Herman P, Friedman M A 1974 Hyperdynamic states and the physiologic determinants of survival in patients with cirrhosis and portal hypertension. Archives of Surgery 108: 282–292

Smith J A, Lonergan E T, Sterling K 1964 Spur-cell anemia: hemolytic anemia with red cells resembling acanthocytes in alcoholic cirrhosis. New England Journal of Medicine 271: 396–398

Smith-Laing G, Sherlock S, Faber O K 1979 Effects of spontaneous portal-systemic shunting on insulin metabolism. Gastroenterology 76: 685–690

Tameda Y, Yoshizawa N, Takase K, Nakano T, Kosaka Y 1990 Prognostic value of peritoneoscopic findings in cirrhosis of the liver. Gastrointestinal Endoscopy 36: 34–38

Taylor R, Heine R J, James O F W, Alberti K G M M 1985 Insulin action in cirrhosis. Hepatology 5: 64–71

Thuluvath P J, Triger D R 1989 Autonomic neuropathy and chronic liver disease. Quarterly Journal of Medicine 72: 737–747

Tran A, Quaranta J-F, Benzaken S et al 1993 High prevalence of thyroid autoantibodies in a prospective series of patients with chronic hepatitis C before interferon therapy. Hepatology 18: 253–257

Tsutsumi M, Urashima S, Matsuda Y, Takase S, Takada A 1993 Changes in type IV collagen content in livers of patients with alcoholic liver disease. Hepatology 17: 820–827

Van Goidsenhoven G E, Henke W J, Vacca J B, Knight W A Jr 1963 Pancreatic function in cirrhosis of the liver. American Journal of Digestive Diseases 8: 160–173

Van Thiel D H, Lester R 1976 Sex and alcohol: a second peak. New England Journal of Medicine 295: 835–836

Van Thiel D H, Gavaler J S, Lester R, Goodman M D 1975 Alcohol-induced testicular atrophy. An experimental model for hypogonadism occurring in chronic alcoholic men. Gastroenterology 69: 326–332

Villeneuve J-P, Dagenais M, Huet P-M, Roy A, Lapointe R, Marleau D 1996 The hepatic microcirculation in the isolated perfused human liver. Hepatology 23: 24–31

Vlahcevic Z R, Yoshida T, Jutti J U, Data P, Bell C C, Swell L 1973 Bile acid metabolism in cirrhosis III. Biliary lipid secretion in patients with cirrhosis and its relevance to gallstone formation. Gastroenterology 64: 298

# 34. Jaundice and cholestasis

*Keith D. Lindor*

## INTRODUCTION

Jaundice and cholestasis are common clinical problems and they are often thought of synonymously as they frequently occur together. However, patients with jaundice may or may not have cholestasis and patients with cholestasis may or may not be jaundiced.

Jaundice is a discoloration of the tissues due to hyperbilirubinemia, which can result from excessive bilirubin production, failure of bilirubin transport across the liver or biliary obstruction; cholestasis is a failure of normal bile flow, which gives rise to a typical clinical and biochemical syndrome. The two conditions meet in the biliary canaliculus, where bilirubin is excreted into the bile (p. 739) and where bile flow is generated (p. 756). The mechanisms for transporting bilirubin and bile acids across the liver are different. A patient with an isolated inability to transport bilirubin, as in Gilbert's syndrome (p. 717), does not have cholestasis and this is reflected in a normal serum bile acid concentration (Douglas et al 1981), while a patient with an inability to excrete conjugated bile acids, as in Byler's syndrome (p. 946), develops cholestasis but not necessarily jaundice (Linarelli et al 1972). Frequently, however, jaundice and cholestasis (cholestatic jaundice) occur together, either because both transport mechanisms are affected by the same disorder or because severe cholestasis results in such a low bile flow that bilirubin cannot be excreted even though its transport mechanism may be intact.

## JAUNDICE (HYPERBILIRUBINEMIA)

Jaundice is a clinical phenomenon that develops when the bilirubin concentration in the body fluids increases sufficiently to give the skin and mucous membranes a yellow discoloration. Hyperbilirubinemia occurs when the plasma bilirubin concentration exceeds the normal range (2–17 μmol/L; 0.2–0.8 mg/dl) and jaundice can usually be seen once the plasma bilirubin exceeds 40–50 μmol/L (2.5–3.0 mg/dl). There are numerous causes of hyperbilirubinemia and they can be divided into those in which the increased plasma bilirubin is predominantly of the unconjugated type and those in which the plasma conjugated and unconjugated bilirubin are both increased (Table 34.1). Normal plasma contains unconjugated and conjugated bilirubin, but the latter constitutes not more than 10% of the total bilirubin concentration (Muraca & Blanckaert 1983). Unconjugated hyperbilirubinemias are those in which the proportion of conjugated bilirubin remains normal even though the actual conjugated bilirubin concentration is increased, as in hemolysis (Muraca et al 1987); mixed hyperbilirubinemias are those in which the conjugated bilirubin constitutes more than 10% of the total bilirubin. The most widely used methods for differentiating unconjugated ("indirect-reacting") and conjugated ("direct-reacting") bilirubin are relatively inaccurate and in practice mixed hyperbilirubinemias can be regarded as those in which conjugated bilirubin constitutes more than 20% of the total bilirubin. Conditions causing isolated hyperbilirubinemias will be considered in this section and conditions causing cholestasis will be considered later in this chapter. The metabolism of bilirubin is described elsewhere (p. 737).

### Increased bilirubin production

Hemolysis leads to increased bilirubin production and unconjugated hyperbilirubinemia occurs once the rate of hemolysis exceeds the capacity of the liver to excrete bilirubin. This capacity is normally very great; intravenous infusion of bilirubin has shown that red blood cell destruction has to increase more than threefold before the capacity of the liver to excrete bilirubin is exceeded (Powell 1967). Measurements of red blood cell survival using labeled cells have shown that there has to be a considerable reduction in red blood cell half-life before jaundice occurs (Table 34.2) and consequently serum bilirubin concentrations rarely exceed 100 μmol/L (6 mg/dl), even in severe hemolysis. Minor degrees of hemolysis cannot, therefore, explain hyperbilirubinemia when the liver is normal. The plasma unconjugated and conjugated biliru-

**Table 34.1** Causes of hyperbilirubinemia and/or cholestasis

*Unconjugated hyperbilirubinemia*
Increased bilirubin production
- Hemolysis
- Ineffective erythropoiesis
- Primary shunt hyperbilirubinemia

Primary failure of bilirubin transport
- Gilbert's syndrome
- Crigler–Najjar syndrome (type I and II)

Mixed or uncertain pathogenesis
- Neonatal hyperbilirubinemia
- Drugs
- Altitude-induced
- Viral hepatitis
- Thyrotoxicosis
- Portacaval shunt

*Mixed (conjugated) hyperbilirubinemia*
Primary failure of bilirubin transport
- Dubin–Johnson syndrome
- Rotor syndrome
- Postoperative cholestasis*
- Byler's disease*

Hepatocellular damage*
- Viral hepatitis
- Drugs
- Alcohol
- Chronic active hepatitis
- Cirrhosis
- Neoplasia (1° or 2°)
- Neonatal hepatitis
- $\alpha_1$-antitrypsin deficiency

Biliary obstruction*
- Extrahepatic
  - Gallstones
  - Neoplasia
  - Sclerosing cholangitis
  - Biliary stricture
  - Pancreatitis
  - Parasites
- Intrahepatic
  - Cholestatic viral hepatitis
  - Drugs
  - Alcohol
  - Cirrhosis
  - Cholestasis of pregnancy
  - Postoperative cholestasis
  - Benign recurrent cholestasis
  - Primary biliary cirrhosis
  - Chronic inflammatory bowel disease
  - Biliary atresia
  - Parasites

*Causes of cholestasis

**Table 34.2** Isotopic measurement of red blood cell (RBC) half-life and hyperbilirubinemia (Powell et al 1967)

| Isotope | RBC half-life (days) | |
|---|---|---|
| | Normal value | Required to produce jaundice |
| Chromium ($^{51}$Cr) | 25–35 | <15 |
| Diisopropylfluorophosphate ($^{32}$P) | 105–130 | <50 |

bin both increase in hemolytic jaundice, but they increase in proportion to their normal plasma concentrations, probably because both forms of bilirubin can normally cross the hepatocyte sinusoidal membrane in either direction (Muraca et al 1987). However, a plasma conjugated bilirubin exceeding 5 μmol/L (0.3 mg/dl) or 20% of the total plasma bilirubin would strongly suggest that impaired liver function was also present (p. 739).

Unconjugated hyperbilirubinemia may also result from increased bilirubin production without a significant increase in the hemolysis of red blood cells in the peripheral blood. This occurs when there is excessive destruction of red blood cell precursors in the marrow, which is known as ineffective erythropoiesis (below). Sometimes, as in pernicious anemia, ineffective erythropoiesis and peripheral hemolysis both contribute to hyperbilirubinemia.

## Primary shunt hyperbilirubinemia

This is a rare condition, affecting men and women, in which increased shunt (p. 737) bilirubin production is caused by ineffective erythropoiesis of unknown cause (Israels 1970). It usually manifests itself as mild jaundice in the second decade of life and splenomegaly is found in half the patients; it carries an excellent prognosis, although patients are liable to develop gallstones (p. 107). It may be familial. Chronic unconjugated hyperbilirubinemia up to 150 μmol/L (9 mg/dl) occurs with otherwise normal liver function tests. The marrow shows erythroid hyperplasia, there is usually a mild to moderate reticulocytosis and the red blood cell survival time is normal. Ineffective erythropoiesis results in a high serum iron concentration, a highly saturated serum iron-binding capacity and increased fecal and urinary excretion of urobilinogen. Increased deposition of iron in the liver occurs, but marked iron overload is exceptional (Frank et al 1979).

## Secondary shunt hyperbilirubinemia

This term refers to the situation in which an increase in the production of shunt bilirubin (p. 737) due to some known cause of ineffective erythropoiesis (Table 34.3) produces or contributes significantly to hyperbilirubinemia.

## Hepatocellular jaundice

Any disease of the hepatic parenchyma can cause jaundice

**Table 34.3** Diseases characterized by increased ineffective erythropoiesis

Megaloblastic anemias, e.g. pernicious anemia
Thalassemia
Myeloproliferative diseases, e.g. myelofibrosis
Sideroblastic anemia
Primary shunt hyperbilirubinemia
Erythropoietic porphyria
Protoporphyria
Lead poisoning

once it has reduced bilirubin transport sufficiently. These diseases (Table 34.1) are discussed elsewhere.

### Cholestatic jaundice

This is discussed in detail below.

## CHOLESTASIS

The term "cholestasis" means a reduction of bile flow (p. 757) and its many causes can affect the biliary tree anywhere from the tiny biliary canaliculi to the sphincter of Oddi in the duodenum. Cholestasis cannot be defined strictly in clinical practice, as there are no readily available methods of measuring bile flow directly in patients, and consequently it has to be recognized from the clinical and biochemical results of failure of bile flow. These features are used to define the cholestatic syndrome, which is described below.

### Cholestatic syndrome

This syndrome comprises features that are characteristic of a failure of bile flow. They are not related directly to the causes of cholestasis, although individual causes may affect the balance of symptoms and signs and add clinical features of their own, as when a pancreatic carcinoma results in a distended gallbladder. The particular features of extrahepatic causes of cholestasis are considered elsewhere (p. 1197).

*Clinical features* (Table 34.4)

Jaundice is a cardinal but not a necessary feature of the cholestatic syndrome and its severity varies greatly. When the underlying cause is a progressive extrahepatic biliary obstruction, as in pancreatic carcinoma, jaundice can become so intense that the skin may acquire a greenish hue. Dark urine is caused by the excretion of retained conjugated bilirubin by the kidneys and renal excretion of bile acids can make the urine noticeably frothy. Failure of sufficient bile pigment to reach the intestine causes pale stools and the stools may also show the characteristics of steatorrhea. Steatorrhea results from the failure of bile acids to reach the small intestine where they are necessary for micellar solubilization of fats (p. 756). Pruritus is another cardinal feature and, like jaundice, it may or may not be present. It is usually generalized although often felt more in some parts of the body than others and it is usually worst at night. There are no local skin lesions apart from scratch marks. Pruritus can be the presenting and only feature in cholestasis and it then needs to be differentiated from other causes of pruritus unassociated with local skin lesions (Table 34.5). Pruritus in cholestasis is usually attributed to retained bile acids, but the evidence for this is weak (Garden et al 1985). Endogenous opiods have also been suggested as mediators of pruritus (Jones & Bergasa 1992).

Less common complaints include bone pain, particularly backache, from hepatic osteodystrophy (below) and tingling, numbness and pain, especially in the hands and feet, from xanthomatous neuropathy (see below). Recurring flitting arthralgia and arthritis attributed to hyperlipidemia have been described (Mills et al 1979). These complaints are generally seen only in patients with more severe and prolonged cholestasis.

Physical examination usually reveals an enlarged liver, but splenomegaly is unusual and evidence of liver failure and portasystemic collateral circulation such as ascites, encephalopathy and esophagogastric varices occurs only in long-standing cases when cirrhosis has developed. Many patients become pigmented due to an increased deposition of melanin in the skin. A few develop lipid deposits (xanthelasmas/xanthomas) in the skin (Fig. 34.1). Xanthelasmas are most common around the eyes, particularly under the skin of the medial part of the upper eyelid, but they also occur in the palmar creases, in the neck and below the breasts. Tuberous xanthomas are rare and occur in tendon sheaths and over pressure points on the elbows, knees, buttocks and extensor surfaces of the wrists. Lipid deposits occur in patients with long-standing cholestasis and marked hyperlipidemia. Kyphosis from vertebral collapse and other spontaneous fractures can occur.

**Table 34.4** Clinical features of cholestasis

| |
|---|
| Jaundice |
| Pale stools |
| Dark frothy urine |
| Pruritus |
| Pigmentation |
| Hepatomegaly |
| Less common or late features: |
| Xanthomas |
| Hepatic osteodystrophy |
| Neuropathy |
| Arthropathy |
| Abnormal coagulation |
| Splenomegaly |
| Esophagogastric varices |
| Ascites |
| Encephalopathy |

**Table 34.5** Internal causes of pruritus unassociated with skin lesions other than scratch marks

| | |
|---|---|
| Liver disease (especially cholestatic) | Mastocytosis |
| Cholestasis of pregnancy | Polycythemia vera |
| Hemochromatosis | Thyroid disease |
| Iron deficiency | Diabetes mellitus |
| Chronic renal failure | Carcinoid syndrome |
| Lymphomas | Aquagenic |
| Leukemias | Psychogenic |
| Multiple myeloma | Senile |

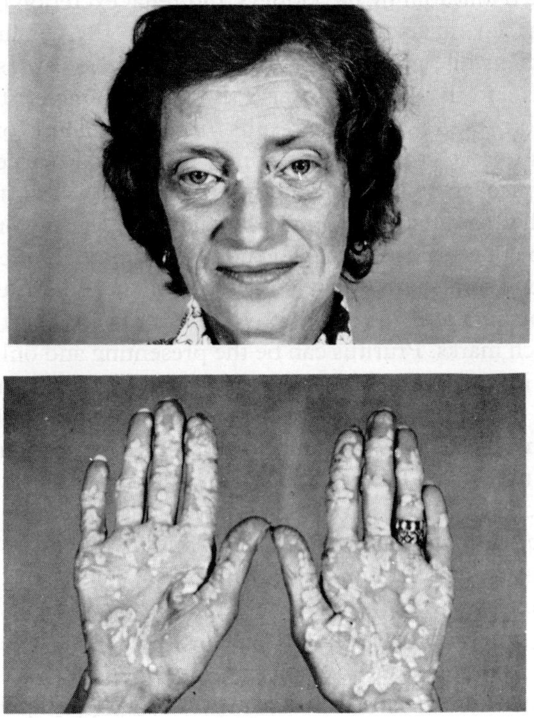

**Fig. 34.1** Xanthelasmas around the eyes and xanthomas on the hands of a patient with primary biliary cirrhosis (Royal Infirmary, Edinburgh).

Nutritional deficiencies occur when cholestasis is prolonged, as in primary biliary cirrhosis (p. 936). This probably results mainly from a poor appetite and malabsorption and it leads to weight loss and to complications due to deficiencies of fat-soluble vitamins. Deficiency of vitamin K causes prolongation of the prothrombin time, which is readily corrected by vitamin $K_1$ (p. 751) provided that severe liver damage has not occurred. Spontaneous bleeding from vitamin K deficiency is uncommon. Deficiencies of vitamin D and of calcium contribute to bone disease (below), which is a particular feature of chronic cholestasis. Plasma concentrations of vitamin A tend to be low, but deficiencies severe enough to cause clinical symptoms such as impaired night vision are uncommon (Shepherd et al 1984). Vitamin E deficiency can cause neurological syndromes including peripheral neuropathy, cerebellar dysfunction, abnormal eye movement and retinal degeneration in children with chronic cholestasis (Elias et al 1981, Alvarez et al 1983), but these are exceptional in adults (Knight et al 1986).

### *Hepatic osteodystrophy*

A combination of osteoporosis and osteomalacia can occur in any chronic liver disease and is known as hepatic osteodystrophy (Heaf 1985, Compston 1986). It develops most frequently in the course of long-standing cholestasis and is consequently particularly common in primary biliary cirrhosis. It is infrequent in primary biliary cirrhosis at presentation (Mitchison et al 1988) but develops as the disease progresses (Christensen et al 1980). It also occurs in other diseases causing chronic cholestasis such as primary sclerosing cholangitis (Hay et al 1991). Hepatic osteodystrophy is frequently asymptomatic, but it can cause considerable pain and deformity and it predisposes to fractures.

***Osteoporosis.*** Osteoporosis is characterized by overall bone loss and is the predominant form of bone disease in hepatic osteodystrophy. Its main clinical manifestations are back pain, kyphosis and vertebral collapse. Its prevalence has been reported variously, depending on the investigative methods used and the populations studied, but radiological evidence of osteoporosis can be found in about a half of patients with symptomatic primary biliary cirrhosis, particularly in the spine. Christensen et al (1980) found that vertebral collapse occurred in 20% of patients with primary biliary cirrhosis followed for 5 years. The main factor contributing to osteoporosis in chronic cholestasis is reduced osteoblastic activity. Osteoblasts are responsible for the synthesis of bone matrix, the maturation of bone and its mineralization and impairment of the first of these is thought currently to be the most important. The possibility of increased osteoclastic activity increasing bone resorption is unresolved. It is possible that different mechanisms operate in chronic liver disease not associated with cholestasis.

***Osteomalacia.*** Osteomalacia is characterized by defective mineralization of bone and is much less common than osteoporosis in hepatic osteodystrophy. It can occur in any chronic liver disease but is most common in the more severe forms of chronic cholestasis. Bone pain is the most common feature and later manifestations include bone tenderness, proximal muscle weakness and fractures. The typical biochemical features of hypocalcemia, hypophosphatemia and increased plasma alkaline phosphatase activity are of limited value in chronic liver disease, as these estimations are altered by the liver disease itself, and radiological features such as pseudofractures and pathological fractures (Fig. 34.2) are late findings. The diagnosis is therefore best made by iliac crest biopsy. Osteomalacia is due primarily to deficiency of vitamin D.

***Vitamin D.*** Vitamin D is derived mainly from the action of sunlight (ultraviolet light) on the skin, leading to the conversion of 7-dehydrocholesterol to cholecalciferol (vitamin $D_3$). Dietary sources of cholecalciferol include fatty fish, fish liver oils, dairy products such as butter and eggs (but not milk) and vitaminized margarine, and as vitamin D is fat-soluble, its absorption is bile acid dependent (p. 357).

Vitamin $D_3$ is hydroxylated by the microsomal enzymes in the liver to 25-hydroxy vitamin D (25(OH)D3) and is then hydroxylated further in the renal tubules to 1,25(OH)D3 and to 24,25(OH)D3. These metabolites are important in promoting the absorption of calcium and the formation of bone. 25(OH)D3 is the main form of vit-

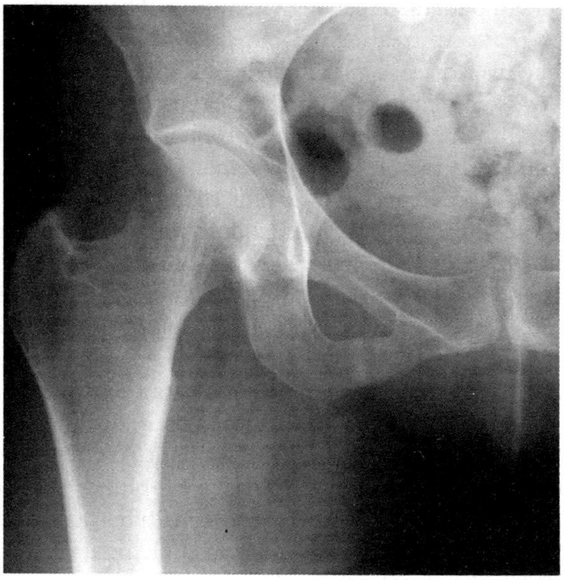

**Fig. 34.2** Pseudofracture of the right inferior pubic ramus due to osteomalacia in primary biliary cirrhosis (Royal Infirmary, Edinburgh).

amin D in the blood and it is carried on a specific globulin produced by the liver. This carrier protein is normally only about 2–3% saturated by 25(OH)D3.

Several factors could therefore contribute to vitamin D deficiency in chronic liver disease, but the main factors are dietary inadequacy and insufficient exposure to sunlight. Malabsorption can occur and may be made worse by cholestyramine, hepatic 25-hydroxylation of cholecalciferol is usually normal even in patients with advanced liver disease and saturation of the plasma-binding protein is normally so low that impaired production of the protein is not important. Dermal synthesis of cholecalciferol seems to be normal in jaundiced patients. Vitamin D metabolites may be lost in the urine, but this is not important in causing deficiency.

*Biochemical features of cholestasis*

Liver function tests substantiate the presence of cholestasis but do not differentiate one cause from another. The cardinal feature is a serum alkaline phosphatase activity more than two and a half times the upper limit of the reference range (>250 u/L). Increased serum alkaline phosphatase due to cholestasis is for practical purposes always associated with increased serum γ-glutamyl transferase, but the hepatic origin of the alkaline phosphatase can be confirmed electrophoretically (p. 742). The serum alkaline phosphatase activity remains high for as long as cholestasis continues and falls to normal when cholestasis is relieved. The serum bilirubin concentration may be normal, as in the early stages of primary biliary cirrhosis, or increased. Hyperbilirubinemia is of the conjugated type (p. 739) and bilirubinuria is present. Serum transaminase activity is usually normal or only slightly increased (p. 742). Serum albumin and globulin concentrations are normal until chronic liver disease develops, when the changes seen in cirrhosis (p. 745) occur. Hyperlipidemia is common but is not of diagnostic value unless lipoprotein X, which is characteristic of cholestasis (p. 754), is sought; this is rarely done. Serum bile acid concentrations are also high, but they are not usually measured in the investigation of cholestasis. There is no urobilinogen in the urine when biliary obstruction is complete and the findings in partial obstruction are so variable that tests for urine urobilinogen are of little value (p. 741). Liver copper concentrations are high in long-standing cholestasis irrespective of cause, but this is not useful in diagnosis (Salaspuro & Sipponen 1976).

*Other investigations*

These are described elsewhere (p. 1198).

*Treatment*

Treatment should be directed to the underlying cause, wherever possible, and to the symptomatic relief of cholestasis. Symptomatic treatment is described here and it applies especially to chronic forms of cholestasis. The most important treatments are those that relieve pruritus and those that prevent or alleviate the effects of malabsorption, especially on the skeleton. Rarely, hyperlipidemia may cause neuropathy that can be relieved.

***Pruritus.*** Garden et al (1985) have reviewed the treatment of this troublesome and frequently disabling symptom. Cholestyramine, an anion-binding resin, gives most effective relief where cholestasis is due to partial biliary obstruction and this action is attributed to its ability to bind bile acids. Relief from itching usually occurs in 1–2 weeks and continues for as long as the agent is given (Schaffner et al 1965, Datta & Sherlock 1966). Cholestyramine powder 4 g daily by mouth is given initially and the dose is increased by 4 g every fifth day until pruritus is relieved or a daily dose of 16 g is reached. It is best taken with breakfast, as bile acid concentrations in the small intestine are likely to be highest at that time (Javitt 1974). A total of 8 g should be taken at breakfast and subsequent doses taken at lunch. The main disadvantage of cholestyramine is that many patients find its taste intolerable. This may be overcome by disguising it with, for example, fruit juice and there is a somewhat more palatable alternative available (cholestipol). Otherwise, side-effects are few and include hyperchloremic acidosis in patients with renal failure (p. 1057), constipation or diarrhea and abdominal discomfort may occur. Prolongation of the prothrombin time has been reported but is not usually sufficient to cause bleeding and can be prevented by vitamin K 10 mg intramuscularly every month. Cholestyramine can interfere with absorption and other drugs should be taken about 3 h after it.

Patients who fail to respond adequately to cholestyramine pose a considerable therapeutic problem. Possible drug therapies for the pruritus itself include antihistamines, phenobarbitone, rifampicin and anabolic steroids. Antihistamines have not proved successful generally, but benefit has been recorded with terfenadin 60 mg twice daily (Duncan et al 1984). Unfortunately, this drug has been associated with cardiac arrhythmias in patients with liver disease and should be avoided when liver function is poor. Cetirizine 5 mg twice daily has similar properties and could be tried as an alternative. Phenobarbitone 3–4 mg/kg body weight daily can improve pruritus, perhaps related to its action as an enzyme inducer (p. 839), but may cause excessive sedation (Bloomer & Boyer 1975); rifampicin 10 mg/kg body weight daily, which is also an enzyme inducer, relieves pruritus and can be given long term (Bachs et al 1992). Anabolic steroids such as methyltestosterone in men and nandrolone in women can reduce pruritus, but they increase jaundice and in practice are hardly ever used. Stanozolol, a C17-substituted derivative of testosterone, 5 mg/day has been found effective in pruritus within about a week, although it too may worsen jaundice (Walt et al 1988). Drugs that improve liver function, such as corticosteroids and azathioprine in autoimmune hepatitis or perhaps ursodeoxycholic acid in primary biliary cirrhosis (p. 941), also help relieve pruritus.

Physical treatment may also be helpful in some patients. Many notice that pruritus improves during sunny weather and phototherapy can give effective relief. The simplest method is to give ultraviolet irradiation and to repeat the therapy as needed if it is successful. Repeat treatment will usually be needed every 1–2 weeks (Hanid & Levi 1980). A tepid bath containing 1–2 cups of sodium bicarbonate can give quite prolonged relief from itching and is particularly helpful before going to bed. Plasmapheresis has improved itching temporarily in patients with intractable pruritus (Cohen et al 1985) and some perfusions have been carried out over charcoal-coated beads to try to remove substances causing pruritus (Lauterburg et al 1980), but this is expensive and unproven.

***Bone disease.*** Vitamin D and its metabolites are effective in the treatment of osteomalacia in chronic liver disease, especially in patients with chronic cholestasis (Heaf 1985, Compston 1986). Calciferol (vitamin $D_2$) 100 000 units intramuscularly weekly has been effective, but smaller doses of 400–4000 units (10–100 µg) orally daily have also been found to be effective (Davies et al 1983). Parenteral treatment is probably preferable in patients with steatorrhea. Vitamin D metabolites are effective but expensive; they have short half-lives (2–4 days) compared with calciferol (30 days) and this provides some protection against vitamin D toxicity. Effective regimens include 25-hydroxycholecalciferol (25(OH)D3) 50–200 µg daily orally, calcitriol (1,25(OH)2D3) 15 µg daily orally and alfacalcidol (IA(OH)D3) 2 µg daily orally. Serum calcium and phosphate concentrations should be measured regularly in all patients receiving vitamin D. There is little evidence that any treatment is effective for osteoporosis in chronic liver disease and evidence in respect of vitamin D therapy is conflicting (Compston 1986).

Recommendations regarding prophylactic treatment are difficult, as it is not known whether hepatic osteodystrophy can be prevented. Some think that all patients, including those without symptoms, should be offered treatment (Heaf 1985), but others consider that the lower prevalence of osteomalacia makes routine vitamin D prophylaxis unnecessary (Compston 1986). The author does not think that patients who are asymptomatic or generally well and free of jaundice need prophylactic treatment, although, like all patients, they should be advised to take a good diet and get good exposure to sunlight. Deficiencies of vitamin D can be sought by measuring blood levels with replacement prescribed if needed (50 000–150 000 units orally/week in divided doses). Supplemental calcium (1000 mg elemental calcium/day) should be recommended as well.

Bone disease may progress in spite of vitamin D and calcium therapy. Some patients suffer considerable pain, which may be relieved by intravenous calcium infusions (Ajdukiewicz et al 1974). Daily infusions of calcium gluconate (1 mg calcium/kg body weight in 500 ml of 5% dextrose) are given over 4 h on 12 successive days. Relief of pain occurs in 3–12 days and lasts for 2–3 months, when treatment may be repeated.

***Malabsorption.*** Patients with primary biliary cirrhosis have a limited ability to absorb fat and fat-soluble vitamins. This is usually attributed to deficient bile acid concentrations in the small intestine, but other factors probably also contribute to malabsorption (Beckett et al 1980, Ros et al 1984, Lanspa et al 1985). Dietary fat should be restricted to 40 g daily and vitamin A (50 000–150 000 units/week) and vitamin K (5 mg/day) can be given as water-soluble forms of the vitamins. Vitamin D is discussed above.

***Neuropathy.*** Peripheral neuropathy due to infiltration of nerves by fat occurs rarely and may be relieved by plasmapheresis (Turnberg et al 1972, Cohen et al 1985). Neuropathy, cerebellar dysfunction, abnormal eye movements and retinal degeneration can occur in children and very rarely in adults and can be treated with vitamin E 500 mg intramuscularly or 100–200 mg/day twice daily by mouth.

## Investigations in jaundice and cholestasis

### *Clinical considerations*

Investigation is based on a thorough history and clinical examination that frequently suggest the likely cause of the illness. It is particularly important to discover all drugs the patient has taken, including those not prescribed by doctors which the patient may forget to mention (857), and to inquire about alcohol consumption. The latter may entail questioning a relative, especially a spouse, if the true situation is to be revealed. Increased bilirubin production is usually identified readily by mild jaundice, the absence of clinical signs of liver disease, associated anemia and the absence of bilirubinuria. The spleen may be palpable. Hemolytic anemia is indicated by the peripheral blood count, reticulocyte count, erythrocyte morphology and serum haptoglobin concentrations; the cause of the hemolysis must be sought. Ineffective erythropoiesis is usually due to a disease (Table 34.3) with clinical features more obvious than mild jaundice. Isolated hyperbilirubinemia in an otherwise well person without evidence of hemolysis or hepatic dysfunction is likely to be due to a constitutional hyperbilirubinemia (p. 721), of which Gilbert's syndrome is much the most common.

*Laboratory investigations*

Most patients with jaundice have hepatobiliary disease. The next step is to ensure that liver function tests confirm cholestasis and to determine with ultrasonography whether the cause of this lies within the liver parenchyma or in the major bile ducts (p. 52). Autoantibodies (p. 765) should be sought as an indication of parenchymal liver disease, particularly the antimitochondrial antibody that identifies primary biliary cirrhosis, and the hepatitis B surface antigen (HBsAg) and hepatitis C antibodies (anti-HCV) should be sought in the blood to identify hepatitis B or C virus infection before invasive investigations are performed. Blood in the stools indicates the need for endoscopic examination of the stomach and duodenum.

*Imaging*

Hepatic imaging is a safe means for investigating cholestasis initially. Most important is ultrasonography (p. 52), which can identify dilatation of the bile ducts and enlargement of the gallbladder caused by biliary obstruction. It is less effective for identifying the cause of biliary obstruction. Gallstones and defects in the liver parenchyma due to neoplasia can also be detected. Computed tomography may complement ultrasonography, especially when malignant obstruction is of concern (p. 66). Magnetic resonance imaging may become more important, as recent reports show it to have a diagnostic capacity similar to endoscopic retrograde cholangiography (Soto et al 1996).

*Further investigations*

The selection of further investigations depends on the results of imaging. Gallstones may be seen occasionally on a plain abdominal radiography (p. 5), but this is not sufficient for a confident diagnosis in cholestatic jaundice. If ultrasonic examination shows dilated bile ducts, retrograde cholangiography (p. 117) or transhepatic cholangiography are the best investigations. The choice depends on local availability but the retrograde approach, while more complex, is usually preferred by patients and can show the pancreatic ducts as well as the bile ducts. Sometimes both methods are needed. When imaging does not show dilated bile ducts, attention should focus on the liver. Needle aspiration (p. 721) or biopsy (p. 717) of any focal intrahepatic lesion seen at imaging should be done (p. 55). Liver biopsy is needed where no lesion has been seen and most information is obtained where this is done at laparoscopy (p. 129). Liver biopsy is no longer used in the diagnosis of obstruction of the large biliary ducts (p. 719).

It should be emphasized that not all the above investigations are needed for every patient. The clinical features may point strongly to a particular cause and in this case the investigations needed to substantiate the likely diagnosis should be done first. Most diseases causing cholestasis are considered elsewhere; others are described below.

## Primary biliary cirrhosis

Primary biliary cirrhosis is characterized by chronic cholestasis with an insidious onset and a steadily progressive course resulting from damage to the intrahepatic biliary tree. The disease was first recognized over a century ago; current clinical concepts and the name "primary biliary cirrhosis", however, date from the report of Ahrens et al (1950) and there have been reports of substantial numbers of patients since then (Foulk et al 1964, Sherlock & Scheuer 1973, Schaffner 1975, Christensen et al 1980). The condition has also been called "chronic nonsuppurative destructive cholangitis", as true cirrhosis is a late development; this clumsy term has never been accepted widely. Primary biliary cirrhosis was previously considered rare, but increased awareness and the wider availability of diagnostic tests have shown that it is relatively common, with a prevalence of 50–150 per million (Triger 1980, Almdal et al 1991).

*Etiology*

The etiology of primary biliary cirrhosis is unknown. The almost constant occurrence of serum autoantibodies, especially the antimitochondrial antibody, lymphocyte infiltrates and granulomas in the liver, circulating immune complexes and abnormal cellular immune responses have all suggested that immunological abnormalities might be important, but so far no immunological mechanism for the liver damage has been conclusively demonstrated.

The disease is not usually familial, but there are reports of its occurrence in siblings and in successive generations (Feizi et al 1972, Chohan 1973, Galbraith et al 1974, Brown et al 1975, Douglas & Finlayson 1979). Feizi et al (1972) found the antimitochondrial antibody in 7% of 125 close relatives of 27 patients and an additional relative also had cirrhosis. This high frequency suggests a familial immune abnormality that might increase susceptibility to whatever causes primary biliary cirrhosis. A previous study found no relation between primary biliary cirrhosis and the HLA-DR antigens that are important in immune responses (Bassendine et al 1985) and a more recent finding that an association with HLA-DR8-DBQ1*0402 was relatively weak suggests that factors other than immunogenetic factors are more important in the etiology of the disease (Underhill et al 1992).

Other factors have been considered as possible causes for primary biliary cirrhosis, but none has emerged as important. The heavy female preponderance among patients has suggested that hormonal factors could be important, but no evidence of this has emerged. Some studies have reported clustering as pointing to environmental causes (Triger 1980), but others have failed to find clusters (Hamlyn et al 1983). Drugs have also been considered as causes. Chronic cholestasis similar to primary biliary cirrhosis can be caused by drugs (p. 851) and primary biliary cirrhosis has been described in patients who had taken neoarsphenamine (Foulk et al 1964), practolol (Brown et al 1978) or benoxaprophen (Babbs & Warnes 1986). Impaired sulfoxidation has been reported recently in most patients with primary biliary cirrhosis and as impaired sulfoxidation is also involved in the cholestatic hepatitis caused by chlorpromazine (p. 848), there is the interesting possibility that an idiosyncratic response to some exogenous toxin could be important in primary biliary cirrhosis (Olomu et al 1988).

The role of the hepatitis B and C viruses in chronic liver diseases is discussed elsewhere (p. 894); there is no evidence that these viruses are responsible for primary biliary cirrhosis. Prolonged cholestatic viral hepatitis (p. 798) can cause a similar syndrome, but it eventually resolves.

### *Pathology*

The pathology of primary biliary cirrhosis changes with progression of the disease and the most widely accepted classification describes four overlapping stages characterized sequentially by cholangiolytic bile duct lesions, ductular proliferation, precirrhotic scarring and cirrhosis (Scheuer 1980, MacSween 1987). The correlation between the clinical features and these pathological stages is poor, partly at least because the pathological changes do not develop uniformly throughout the liver and in some patients cirrhosis may already be present when the clinical features first appear. Portmann et al (1985) have suggested a new pathological classification based on four types of piecemeal necrosis (biliary, lymphocytic, ductular and fibrotic), but the value of this classification will need to be confirmed.

***Stage one.*** Initially, bile duct lesions occur segmentally in the medium-sized and small (<80 μm diameter) bile ducts (Nakanuma & Ohta 1979). The duct epithelium may be swollen, ruptured, necrotic or hyperplastic and there is periductal edema and fibrosis. Normal bile ducts are also seen, as the lesions are segmental, and the bile ductules are normal. The portal tracts are expanded and densely infiltrated with lymphocytes, plasma cells and sometimes eosinophils that surround both normal and damaged bile ducts. Lymphocyte follicles, sometimes with germinal centers, and granulomas without central necrosis usually develop. Granulomas may also occasionally be seen in the parenchyma. The inflammatory cells are confined to the portal tracts, the limiting plates are intact and the parenchyma is normal or shows only nonspecific changes, often with little cholestasis at this stage.

***Stage two.*** The second stage is characterized by disappearance of the characteristic focal ductal lesions, diminution in the number of bile ducts and proliferation of small atypical ductules. The portal tract infiltrate contains more leukocytes and the inflammatory cells erode the limiting plate to give the features of chronic aggressive (interface) hepatitis. Granulomata can still be seen, cholestasis is more prominent and occasional liver cells may contain Mallory's hyaline.

***Stage three.*** The florid inflammatory features of the second stage then subside, leading to a third stage of increasing portal fibrosis and periportal cholestasis.

***Stage four.*** Finally a cirrhosis develops that is characterized by a paucity of bile ducts and an absence of marked fibrosis. Frequently, however, the origin of the cirrhosis cannot be recognized once this stage has been reached.

***Differential diagnosis.*** The diagnosis of primary biliary cirrhosis can be difficult, as only the focal bile duct lesions seen mainly in stage one are pathognomonic of the disease. Confusion occurs most often with autoimmune hepatitis (p. 889) and sclerosing cholangitis (p. 943) and misdiagnosis may well account for instances of autoimmune hepatitis with a positive antimitochondrial antibody test or liver function tests showing cholestasis (Williamson et al 1985).

***Prognosis.*** Attempts to relate liver biopsy findings to prognosis have not proved useful in clinical practice. Patients with cirrhosis have a generally worse outlook than those who do not, as would be expected, and marked cholestasis, severity of fibrosis and piecemeal necrosis, and Mallory's hyaline have all been associated with a worse outlook (Roll et al 1983, Portmann et al 1985). Granulomas have been associated with a better prognosis (Lee et al 1981, Portmann et al 1985).

### *Clinical features*

The disease usually has an insidious onset and 90% or more of the patients are women. Three-quarters are diagnosed in the fifth and sixth decades of life, with an overall range from the third to the ninth decade. The disease has been found in all races but has been described most often in Caucasians, which probably reflects at least in part the uneven distribution of medical facilities in the world.

Pruritus is the first feature to develop in half of cases (Table 34.6). Hepatic features develop first in a fifth of cases. Jaundice is the commonest of these and others include intestinal bleeding and ascites; they indicate more advanced disease. Other early complaints are frequently nonspecific and consequently liver disease may not be suspected. Foulk et al (1964) found that such symptoms had been present for a year or more in three-quarters of their patients. Fatigue, arthralgia, abdominal pain and dyspepsia are the commonest nonspecific complaints. Diarrhea may result from malabsorption and be associated with steatorrhea. Symptoms occur first during pregnancy in 5–10% of patients. Peripheral neuritis occasionally causes pain, tingling and tenderness, especially in the hands and feet; this results from lipid infiltration of peripheral nerves (Thomas & Walker 1965). Sensory neurological abnormalities are absent or slight. Increased awareness, greater use of automated biochemical liver function tests and more widespread availability of tests for antimitochondrial antibodies have led to primary biliary cirrhosis being diagnosed much more frequently in patients with associated conditions (below) or in asymptomatic people (p. 938).

At presentation, the general health and nutrition are often good. Jaundice may be present but is usually mild; almost half the patients have a serum bilirubin below 35 μmol/L (5 mg/dl). Other features of chronic liver disease, such as palmar erythema and spider telangiectasias, are infrequent. Dusky pigmentation, especially of the exposed skin, is common and increases as the disease progresses. Scratch marks are common and lichenification of the skin occasionally occurs. Lipid deposits may be seen in the skin, but they are late features and are not now often seen at presentation (Fig. 34.1). Ahrens et al (1950) found them in most of their patients, Foulk et al (1964) reported them in about half of their patients and Christensen et al (1980) reported them in about a quarter at presentation and about a half after 5 years. Xanthelasmas are the commonest lipid deposits; they are usually found on the eyelids and are unrelated to the serum lipid concentrations. Xanthomas are rare and usually appear late in the disease; they usually develop in the palmar creases, over pressure points, on tendons, especially over the knuckles and elbows, and on the trunk and they occur in patients with marked hyperlipidemia (Schaffner 1975). Examination of the abdomen often reveals hepatomegaly and the liver is generally smooth, firm and painless. The spleen is palpable in fewer than half the patients at presentation.

**Table 34.6** The frequency of presenting feaures in primary biliary cirrhosis

| Presenting features | Frequency (%) | |
|---|---|---|
| | Sherlock & Scheuer (1973) (100 patients) | Christensen et al (1980) (236 patients) |
| Pruritus | 57 | 46 |
| Liver disease | 35 | 20 |
| Jaundice | (28) | (12) |
| Intestinal bleeding | (3) | (6) |
| Ascites | (1) | (2) |
| Hepatosplenomegaly | (3) | – |
| Nonspecific | – | 22 |
| Fatigue, abdominal pain or dyspepsia, arthralgia | | (18) |
| Associated disease | 4 | 5 |
| Incidental diagnosis | 4 | 7 |

The course of the disease is relentlessly though often slowly progressive. Portal hypertension is usually a late development, but some two-thirds of patients have a palpable spleen and about a half have some gastrointestinal bleeding within 5 years of diagnosis (Christensen et al 1980). Kew et al (1971) found portal hypertension in 46% of their patients, but in only 4% did the illness present as gastrointestinal bleeding. Portal hypertension developed 1–10 years after the onset of symptoms (Fig. 34.3) and nodular regeneration in the liver was a frequent though not a constant association. Liver failure develops as the disease progresses and causes increasing jaundice, ascites and encephalopathy. Bone disease is a frequent development (p. 934). Vertebral collapse is particularly common. Hepatocellular carcinoma is exceedingly rare in primary biliary cirrhosis (Krasner et al 1979).

*Associated conditions*

Associated conditions, particularly connective tissue and autoimmune disease, occur frequently in primary biliary cirrhosis. Clinical evidence of extrahepatic disease occurs in 15–25% of patients (Sherlock & Scheuer 1973, Christensen et al 1980) and the frequency of asymptomatic extrahepatic disease is even higher. Golding et al (1973) tested 47 patients for Sjögren's syndrome, renal tubular acidosis, pulmonary diffusion defects and peripheral neuropathy and two-thirds had one or more of these conditions.

Sjögren's syndrome and scleroderma are the connective tissue diseases most prominently associated with primary biliary cirrhosis. Christensen et al (1980) found the former in 5% and the latter in 6% of their 236 patients. Sjögren's syndrome is usually mild and its clinical presence may be revealed only by inquiring about dry mouth and gritty eyes. The diagnosis is confirmed most simply by measuring the capacity to secrete tears with Schirmer test tapes. Scleroderma is frequently associated with the CRST (calcinosis cutis, Raynaud's phenomenon, sclerodactyly, telangiectasia) syndrome in primary biliary cirrhosis (Murray-Lyon et al 1970, Reynolds et al 1971, O'Brien

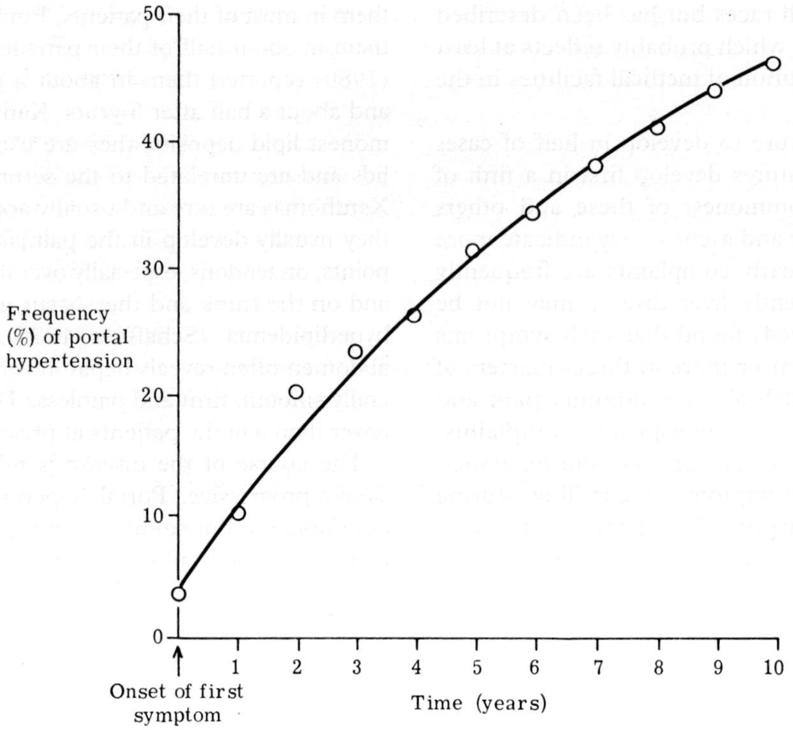


**Fig. 34.3** Frequency of portal hypertension in primary biliary cirhosis related to the onset of symptoms (Kew et al 1971).

et al 1972). Other connective tissue diseases have been reported occasionally, but except for nonspecific arthralgia and an arthropathy involving many large and small joints, they are rare (Child et al 1977, Clarke et al 1978). Thyroid diseases are also frequent and include Hashimoto's disease, thyrotoxicosis and primary hypothyroidism. Hypothyroidism is the most frequent manifestation of thyroid disease and a prevalence of 22% was found in one large series (Crowe et al 1980). Thyrotoxicosis is much less frequent. Several other extrahepatic diseases have been reported in individual patients, including renal tubular acidosis (p. 1046), fibrosing alveolitis, autoimmune hemolytic anemia, glomerulonephritis, ulcerative colitis and a variety of skin rashes (Golding et al 1973, Rai et al 1977, Orlin et al 1980, Bush et al 1987).

Conditions other than connective tissue and autoimmune diseases also occur more frequently in primary biliary cirrhosis than in the general population. Gallstones are common in all forms of cirrhosis (p. 1203) and are present in 30–40% of patients with primary biliary cirrhosis, although they do not often cause symptoms (Summerfield et al 1976). Urinary tract infection is also more common than in women of comparable age and is associated with advanced liver disease. Burroughs et al (1984) found that a fifth of their patients developed bacteriuria over a 1-year period and that a third of these became reinfected subsequently. An increased frequency of breast carcinoma has also been reported (Goudie et al 1985). An increased incidence of ischemic heart disease might be expected in primary biliary cirrhosis, as prolonged hyperlipidemia is frequent; however, it is not a common complication (Crippin et al 1992).

## Variant syndromes

### *Asymptomatic disease*

Asymptomatic primary biliary cirrhosis is usually discovered by finding a high serum alkaline phosphatase activity of liver origin or a positive antimitochondrial antibody test. This often occurs during the investigation of diseases associated with primary biliary cirrhosis (Long et al 1977, James et al 1981, Roll et al 1983, Nyberg & Lööf 1989, Balasubramaniam et al 1990). Such patients may remain asymptomatic in respect of liver disease for up to 10 years and fatigue, musculoskeletal aches and pains and pruritus are usually the first symptoms to appear. Physical examination is usually normal, but hepatomegaly is found in about half and splenomegaly is occasionally present. Liver function tests show cholestasis but, as would be expected, the plasma bilirubin is lower than in symptomatic patients and hypoalbuminemia is rare. The frequency of the antimitochondrial antibody is the same as in symptomatic patients. Liver biopsy usually shows less advanced hepatic disease, but cirrhosis can be present in spite of a complete lack of symptoms.

*Primary biliary cirrhosis in men*

Rubel et al (1984) compared 30 male and 30 female patients with primary biliary cirrhosis and found no difference related to sex. Lucey et al (1986), in a larger series of 39 male and 191 female patients, found that the age at onset and survival were the same, but men had less pruritus, less skin pigmentation and fewer associated autoimmune conditions, especially sicca syndrome. Hepatocellular carcinoma developed more often in men (10.3%) than in women (1.6%).

*Autoimmune cholangitis (antimitochondrial antibody-negative PBC)*

Patients with all the clinical, biochemical and histological features of primary biliary cirrhosis but who lack the antimitochondrial antibody constitute 1–6% of most large series (Goodman et al 1995, Lacerda et al 1995). This may be due occasionally to autoantibody concentrations too low for detection by immunofluorescence, but in most instances antimitochondrial antibody cannot be found even with more sensitive methods (Michieletti et al 1994). These patients have antinuclear antibodies and smooth muscle antibody more frequently and at higher titers than patients with antimitochondrial antibody. They also have lower serum IgM concentrations. They do not have clinical or biochemical features of autoimmune hepatitis and diagnoses of cholestatic autoimmune hepatitis should be regarded with scepticism (p. 892). This condition may be a variant of, or may be distinct from, primary biliary cirrhosis and the term "autoimmune cholangitis" has been suggested. That they may be distinct has been supported by a recent report that an autoantibody to carbonic anhydrase is usually found in autoimmune cholangitis but is uncommon in primary biliary cirrhosis and autoimmune hepatitis (p. 892). Irrespective of these considerations, this condition should be managed in the same way as primary biliary cirrhosis (Michieletti et al 1994).

*Overlap syndromes*

Occasional patients show clinical, biochemical, serological or histological features of autoimmune hepatitis and primary biliary cirrhosis either simultaneously or at different times in the evolution of their disease (Okuno et al 1987, Ben-Ari et al 1993). They have antismooth muscle and antinuclear antibodies and may or may not have antimitochondrial antibodies. Liver function tests usually show cholestasis with high serum transaminase activity during active disease and liver biopsy shows a combination of interlobular bile duct damage and piecemeal necrosis (interface hepatitis). Active disease responds well to prednisolone as used in autoimmune hepatitis and the antimitochondrial antibody may diminish in titer or disappear during such therapy (Okuno et al 1987).

## Investigations

*Biochemistry*

A high serum alkaline phosphatase activity is the most striking biochemical abnormality. Only about 5% of patients have activities less than twice the upper normal limit and where lower values are found a diagnosis of primary biliary cirrhosis should not be made without other excellent evidence (Roll et al 1983). Asymptomatic patients with serological and histological evidence of primary biliary cirrhosis may have normal alkaline phosphatase activity, but this usually increases on follow-up if symptoms arise (Mitchison et al 1986). The plasma bilirubin concentration varies widely in symptomatic patients; at presentation it is less than 35 μmol/L (2 mg/dl) in half and less than 85 μmol/L (5 mg/dl) in three-quarters and only 5% have a bilirubin above 170 μmol/L (10 mg/dl). Increased serum transaminase activity is frequent but rarely exceeds 150 u/L. The serum albumin concentration and the prothrombin time remain normal until liver failure occurs and there is a polyclonal hyperglobulinemia. Hypercholesterolemia is common at all stages of the disease and increases as disease advances, but it is not of diagnostic importance (Crippin et al 1992). Lipoprotein X is present as in other cholestatic conditions (p. 754). Serum lipid concentrations may eventually fall as liver failure progresses.

*Serology*

Serological investigation is important, as 95% or more of patients have the antimitochondrial antibody in the blood (p. 765). The antigen recognized by this specific antibody (termed $M_2$) has been cloned and well characterized as belonging to an enzyme complex in the inner mitochondrial membrane (Leung et al 1992). It is strongly associated with the hepatic lesions of primary biliary cirrhosis, may be specific for the disease and the diagnosis should be made in its absence only if the other evidence is very strong (James et al 1981, Caldwell et al 1992). The serum immunoglobulin M concentration is raised in 80% of cases but is not of any diagnostic value.

*Liver biopsy*

A liver biopsy is diagnostic in primary biliary cirrhosis only if it reveals focal damage to septal or interlobular ducts. These focal lesions are seen much more frequently in wedge biopsies taken at laparotomy than in needle biopsies (Table 34.7). Needle biopsies, however, usually show lesions compatible with primary biliary cirrhosis, such as a biliary pattern of fibrosis, granulomas, heavy portal lymphocytic infiltration and proliferation of biliary ductules. These findings, together with the clinical features and a positive antimitochondrial antibody test, are sufficient for a confident diagnosis.

**Table 34.7** Surgical biopsies and needle biopsies in the diagnosis of primary biliary cirrhosis (Sherlock & Scheuer 1973)

| Type of biopsy | Number | Results | |
|---|---|---|---|
| | | Diagnostic (%) | Compatible (%) |
| Surgical | 41 | 70 | 30 |
| Needle | 59 | 29 | 71 |

*Imaging*

Ultrasonographic imaging is desirable, as failure to show dilatation of the biliary tract makes mechanical obstruction of the large bile ducts very unlikely (p. 52). Ultrasonography can also reveal gallstones and may show diffuse abnormality of the liver. Splenomegaly and collateral vessels signify portal hypertension.

*Cholangiography*

Direct cholangiography is necessary only when the diagnosis of primary biliary cirrhosis is in doubt or when features suggesting obstruction of a large duct develop in the course of the disease. Retrograde cholangiography is the method of choice, as the diseased intrahepatic bile ducts make transhepatic cholangiography more difficult. The large biliary ducts are of normal caliber in primary biliary cirrhosis. The intrahepatic ducts may be normal or they may be tortuous and show irregularities of caliber. Abnormal intrahepatic ducts suggest that cirrhosis has developed (Summerfield et al 1976).

## Diagnosis

The cardinal features of primary biliary cirrhosis are a painless cholestatic syndrome of gradual onset in a middle-aged woman, with pruritus as the dominant symptom and jaundice either mild or absent. A plasma alkaline phosphatase activity more than twice the upper normal limit, a positive antimitochondrial antibody test, ultrasonography showing a normal biliary tract and a compatible liver biopsy complete the diagnosis in such a patient. Atypical features such as abdominal pain, prominent jaundice (bilirubin >85 µmol/L, 5 mg/dl), a male patient or absence of the antimitochondrial antibody indicate the need for direct cholangiography and/or liver biopsy. Cholangiography is also indicated where unexplained abdominal pain, worsening of cholestasis or deterioration of general health develops in the course of the disease.

***Differential diagnosis.*** Primary biliary cirrhosis can be confused with cholestasis due to drugs, cholestasis of pregnancy, primary sclerosing cholangitis (PSC), intrahepatic lesions in inflammatory bowel disease previously referred to as pericholangitis but now as small-duct PSC, adult ductopenia or any cause of obstruction of a large bile duct. The history is crucial in cholestasis due to drugs in which the antimitochondrial antibody is absent or found only transiently and at low titer and the liver biopsy usually does not suggest primary biliary cirrhosis. Cholestasis resolves on withdrawal of the drug, although recovery sometimes takes several months (p. 850). In cholestasis of pregnancy the antimitochondrial antibody is absent and cholestasis remits after delivery (p. 1091). Primary sclerosing cholangitis may be associated with inflammatory bowel disease and the antimitochondrial antibody is not found (p. 943). Sometimes inflammatory bowel disease is revealed only by investigation. Sclerosing cholangitis is diagnosed most accurately by retrograde cholangiography and lesions such as pericholangitis can be revealed by liver biopsy. The antimitochondrial antibody test is negative in idiopathic adult biliary ductopenia (p. 945). Obstruction of a large biliary duct is usually associated with a relatively short history, jaundice, abdominal pain and fever. Pruritus is less prominent than in primary biliary cirrhosis. However, a carcinoma at the junction of the main hepatic ducts (p. 1219) can cause prolonged cholestasis and the finding of an unobstructed extrahepatic biliary tree at laparotomy adds to the confusion. This is obviated by obtaining a transhepatic or retrograde cholangiogram that demonstrates the intrahepatic and the extrahepatic biliary tree. The antimitochondrial antibody is probably never present in uncomplicated obstruction of the large bile ducts (p. 765).

Prominent granulomas in the liver may suggest some other granulomatous disease (p. 829), particularly sarcoidosis. The clinical and biochemical syndrome usually distinguishes clearly between sarcoidosis and primary biliary cirrhosis (Stanley et al 1972). Primary biliary cirrhosis occurs in patients over 40 years old who have pruritus, jaundice, finger clubbing, skin pigmentation, xanthomas or hepatomegaly, none of which are features of sarcoidosis. Sarcoidosis is uncommon over the age of 40 years and is characterized by erythema nodosum, respiratory symptoms, hilar adenopathy on the chest radiograph and uveitis, none of which occur in primary biliary cirrhosis. The antimitochondrial antibody is present in primary biliary cirrhosis and the Kveim test is positive in sarcoidosis (Stanley et al 1972). Rarely, the antimitochondrial antibody test and the Kveim test are positive when both diseases are present (Karlish et al 1969).

Differentiation between primary biliary cirrhosis and autoimmune hepatitis or cryptogenic cirrhosis can be difficult and depends on the degree of cholestasis, the presence of antimitochondrial antibody and careful consideration of the liver biopsy findings (Williamson et al 1985). Sometimes the two conditions seem to occur in the same patient (above).

## Treatment

*Symptomatic*

Treatment includes measures to alleviate the symptoms

and complications of chronic cholestasis (p. 933) and to treat ascites (p. 1023), encephalopathy (p. 1051) and gastrointestinal bleeding resulting from liver failure and portal hypertension (p. 499).

*Specific*

Several drugs have been used to try to prevent or delay the progression of primary biliary cirrhosis, but none can be recommended fully at present. Corticosteroids are beneficial in autoimmune hepatitis (p. 900) and equal efficacy might be expected in primary biliary cirrhosis with its autoimmune associations. Some benefit has been shown in a long-term trial but treatment was associated with worsening of hepatic osteodystrophy (Mitchison et al 1992). Azathioprine (50–100 mg/day) did not prove beneficial in early trials. Late follow-up of one trial of 248 patients showed that, after a statistical adjustment for higher plasma bilirubin in the treated patients, treated patients lived about 20 months longer than untreated patients, suffered fewer complications of the disease and did not experience serious drug toxicity (Christensen et al 1985). Unfortunately, about a quarter of the patients were lost to follow-up.

Other immunosuppressant drugs tried have included chlorambucil and cyclosporin A. Chlorambucil improved liver function tests and liver histology but did not reduce mortality (Hoofnagle et al 1986), while cyclosporin A improved liver function but only after adjusting for imbalances between the trial groups at entry (Lombard et al 1993). There have been several trials of D-penicillamine, as the hepatic copper concentration is high in primary biliary cirrhosis and it was hoped that removal of this would be beneficial, as in Wilson's disease (p. 964). Furthermore, D-penicillamine reduces the deposition of immune complexes and impairs collagen formation. Unfortunately, the results have been conflicting and disappointing and up to a third of patients have suffered serious side-effects (James 1985). Colchicine (1 mg/day), an anti-inflammatory agent, has improved liver function tests in three controlled trials without producing serious side-effects, but long-term follow-up of one trial showed no improvement in survival (Zifroni & Shaffner 1991). Ursodeoxycholic acid (10–15 mg/kg/day) is currently the drug most used in primary biliary cirrhosis. Four trials have shown improvement in symptoms, liver function tests and some aspects of liver histology and either improvement in survival or survival to the point of liver transplantation (Lim et al 1995). The drug is expensive but is virtually free of serious side-effects and is probably the drug of choice if any specific treatment is given.

*Liver transplantation*

Patients with primary biliary cirrhosis are often relatively young and usually have no extrahepatic disease. They are therefore often suitable for liver transplantation, which gives a 1-year survival of about 90%, with 5-year survival around 75% (p. 1162).

**Prognosis**

Primary biliary cirrhosis is a steadily progressive disease, although its rate of progression is slow. Earlier studies reported an average survival of 5–6 years with a wide range of 1–13 years in symptomatic patients and death was due to hepatic failure, bleeding from esophageal varices or a combination of these in 90% of patients (Sherlock 1959, Foulk et al 1964). Hepatocellular carcinoma rarely develops and is more likely in male patients (p. 939). Subsequent reports have shown a more favorable outlook even in symptomatic patients, with 50% surviving about 10 years (Nyberg & Lööf 1989). Asymptomatic patients have been reported to have an average life expectancy of 11–12 years and 80% of patients survive beyond 5 years (Roll et al 1983). A more recent report was less optimistic, with 90% of patients becoming symptomatic and 23% dying or coming to transplantation within about 10 years, but 60% had fibrosis or cirrhosis at diagnosis (Balasubramaniam et al 1990). Nyberg & Lööf (1989) found that asymptomatic patients do have an increased mortality but that this occurs 10 years or more after diagnosis and is more common in those with fibrosis or cirrhosis.

The survival of individual patients is impossible to predict, but certain features suggest a relatively poor outlook. Anicteric patients usually survive for several years, but any sustained rise in the plasma bilirubin is an ominous sign and survival is related to the extent of such increases (Table 34.8). Occasionally, however, the plasma bilirubin can remain above 200 μmol/L (12 mg/dl) for 2–3 years before death (Foulk et al 1964). Other signs of impaired liver function are also associated with a worse prognosis. These include a plasma albumin below 30 g/L, a prolonged prothrombin time and fluid retention, which are features of more severe liver failure (Roll et al 1983). The development of portal hypertension is also a bad prognostic sign owing to the increased mortality from bleeding esophageal varices (Table 34.9). Kew et al (1971) found that patients survived a mean of 15 months after

**Table 34.8** The relation of increases of plasma bilirubin concentration to survival in primary biliary cirrhosis (Shapiro et al 1979)

| Plasma bilirubin increase over 6 months (μmol/L [mg/dl]) | Geometric mean survival (months) | 95% confidence limits on survival (months) |
|---|---|---|
| >34 (2.0) | 49 | 32–74 |
| >102 (6.0) | 25 | 19–32 |
| >170 (10) | 17 | 13–22 |

**Table 34.9** Mortality in primary biliary cirrhosis related to the presence of esophageal varices (Kew et al 1971)

| Esophageal varices | Number of patients | Number of deaths | Mortality (%) | Cause of death | | |
|---|---|---|---|---|---|---|
| | | | | Hepatic failure | Variceal bleeding | Unrelated to liver disease |
| Present | 50 | 27 | 54 | 13 | 13 | 1 |
| Absent | 59 | 14 | 24 | 12 | 0 | 2 |

the discovery of varices, although the range of survival (0–71 months) was wide. A fall in the serum cholesterol concentration or alkaline phosphatase activity and the diminution or disappearance of pruritus or lipid deposits in the skin are very late features and indicate an early fatal end. Survival models have been developed and validated to aid in the timing of liver transplantation (p. 1152).

### Prevention

No preventive measures are possible.

## SECONDARY BILIARY CIRRHOSIS

Secondary biliary cirrhosis results from prolonged obstruction of the extrahepatic biliary tree. It is rare in adults because obstruction due to gallstones can almost always be relieved, other benign causes of obstruction are uncommon and obstruction due to malignant disease causes death before secondary biliary cirrhosis develops. There are consequently few descriptions based on a large number of patients (Scobie & Summerskill 1965).

### Etiology

Biliary stricture is the commonest cause of secondary biliary cirrhosis in adults (Table 34.10). Most strictures result from operations on the biliary ducts (p. 1215) and some are due to sclerosing cholangitis (below) or chronic pancreatitis (p. 1270). Choledocholithiasis or carcinomas originating in the bile ducts, in the head of the pancreas or at the papilla of Vater are also causes, but biliary cirrhosis due to the former can almost always be prevented by removal of the stones and carcinomas usually cause death before cirrhosis can develop. Secondary biliary cirrhosis in children usually results from atresia of the bile ducts (p. 730).

**Table 34.10** Causes of secondary biliary cirrhosis (Scobie & Summerskill 1965)

| Causes | Number | Frequency (%) |
|---|---|---|
| Common duct stricture | 40 | 67 |
| Postoperative | (40) | (67) |
| Other | (0) | (0) |
| Choledocholithiasis | 13 | 22 |
| Carcinoma | 7 | 12 |
| Hepatic ducts | (3) | (5) |
| Pancreas | (2) | (3.5) |
| Papilla of Vater | (2) | (3.5) |
| Total | 60 | 100 |

**Table 34.11** Duration of obstruction in the development of secondary biliary cirrhosis (Scobie & Summerskill 1965)

| Cause | Duration of obstruction (years) | |
|---|---|---|
| | Mean | Range |
| Common duct stricture | 7.1 | 0.5–26 |
| Choledocholithiasis | 4.6 | 0.3–17 |
| Carcinoma | 0.8* | 0.2–1.5 |

*Significantly less than for the other two causes ($P < 0.05$)

Biliary obstruction and cholangitis are thought to be the main factors leading to cirrhosis; obstruction is probably the more important, as it can cause cirrhosis in biliary atresia and following ligation of the common bile duct in animals without associated infection. The time required for the development of secondary biliary cirrhosis is variable, but in general it develops slowly (Table 34.11). It has been found within 3 months of a bile duct injury, but only a third of patients develop cirrhosis within a year. Cirrhosis develops relatively rapidly in biliary atresia and in biliary obstruction due to carcinoma, perhaps because obstruction is more complete in these cases.

### Pathology

Biliary obstruction quickly leads to enlargement of the portal tracts due to edema and an inflammatory infiltrate, including substantial numbers of polymorphonuclear leukocytes, and to a proliferation of small bile ductules. Bile infarcts in the hepatic parenchyma and extravasation of bile in the portal tracts are rare but pathognomonic signs of large bile duct obstruction. Continuing obstruction causes portal fibrosis, which eventually links the portal tracts and accentuates the hepatic lobules. Fibrosis may be particularly marked around the interlobular and septal bile ducts. Nodular regeneration eventually arises in single lobules or in groups of lobules and results in true cirrhosis with irregular nodules separated by broad serpiginous bands of fibrous tissue. This gives the jigsaw pattern of biliary cirrhosis. Occasionally, liver cells containing material indistinguishable from Mallory's hyaline may be found.

## Clinical features

Jaundice is almost invariably present and is more marked than in patients with primary biliary cirrhosis. It often fluctuates, particularly in patients with strictures or stones. Severe abdominal pain occurs in three-quarters of patients with stones but is much less common in those with strictures or carcinomas; recurrent cholangitis occurs in three-quarters of patients with strictures or stones but in only a few with carcinomas; pruritus occurs in most patients but is least severe in those with stones. Weight loss is common and diarrhea is an occasional feature. Hepatomegaly, splenomegaly and scratch marks are the most frequent physical findings, but other features of cirrhosis are relatively uncommon. Liver failure and portal hypertension can cause ascites and gastrointestinal bleeding in advanced disease.

## Investigations

Investigations are those needed to determine a cause for obstructive jaundice (p. 1198) or to confirm a likely cause, such as a biliary stricture. Liver function tests almost always show cholestasis. Three-quarters of patients have a serum bilirubin above 100 μmol/L (6 mg/dl) and a third above 200 μmol/L (12 mg/dl), in contrast to those with primary biliary cirrhosis (above). A half have an alkaline phosphatase activity increased more than threefold and three-quarters more than twofold. Hypoalbuminemia, hyperglobulinemia and prolongation of the prothrombin time are common signs of advanced disease. Antimitochondrial antibodies are not found in the blood.

## Treatment

Treatment is directed whenever possible to the relief of biliary obstruction by surgical means or by the use of stents (p. 119). Otherwise, the treatment is that of chronic cholestasis (p. 933) and antibiotics are used to treat episodes of cholangitis (p. 1212).

## Prognosis

The prognosis is related to the cause of biliary obstruction and to whether or not that obstruction can be relieved. Patients with carcinomas have a poor outlook and most do not live long enough to develop a true cirrhosis. The prognosis is also poor in patients without malignant disease if obstruction cannot be relieved and it improves to the extent that relief of obstruction is achieved (Table 34.12). Unfortunately, relief of obstruction does not necessarily prevent progressive liver damage and the development of liver failure and portal hypertension once secondary biliary cirrhosis is present, but the prime importance of relieving obstruction is emphasized by the symptomatic relief and prolongation of life this achieves. Reversible biliary cirrhosis has been described in children where relief of obstruction has been achieved, but this is a rare occurrence (Yeong et al 1982). Hepatocellular carcinoma is a rarity in secondary biliary cirrhosis, perhaps because most do not survive long enough for this to occur. Hepatocellular carcinoma has been described in a patient 28 years after a common bile duct injury (Jakobovits et al 1984).

**Table 34.12** Outcome of surgery for biliary obstruction due to stones or strictures related to survival (Scobie & Summerskill 1965)

| Result of surgery | Patients | | Survival (years) | |
|---|---|---|---|---|
| | Alive | Dead | Mean | Range |
| Obstruction relieved | 12 | 8 | 10.8 | 3–26 |
| Recurrent obstruction | 4 | 22 | 10.3 | 3–26 |
| Persistent obstruction | 0 | 6 | 3 | 0.5–7 |

## Prevention

Secondary biliary cirrhosis becomes rare when choledocholithiasis is treated promptly and when biliary surgery is performed only by skilled surgeons.

# PRIMARY SCLEROSING CHOLANGITIS

## Etiology

Primary sclerosing cholangitis (PSC) is a rare disease, the cause of which is unknown (Wiesner & LaRusso 1980). Its most important association is with ulcerative colitis, which is present in about 70% of the patients. It is occasionally associated with Crohn's disease, but this is much less common. Thyroid diseases such as thyroiditis, hypothyroidism and Riedel's struma, retroperitoneal fibrosis and pancreatitis have also been reported in PSC, but their relation to it is obscure. An autoimmune basis for the disease has been proposed, but compelling evidence for this is not available. Antinuclear and other autoantibodies have been found in a high proportion of patients by some (Zauli et al 1987) but not by others (Chapman et al 1980). Antineutrophil cytoplasmic autoantibodies (ANCA) have been reported recently in inflammatory bowel disease, particularly ulcerative colitis, and in primary sclerosing cholangitis (p. 767). Two major subclasses of ANCA have been defined by indirect immunofluorescence, one giving diffuse cytoplasmic fluorescence (c-ANCA) and associated with Wegener's granulomatosis and one giving perinuclear fluorescence (p-ANCA) and associated with ulcerative colitis and sclerosing cholangitis. p-ANCA is found in 70–80% of patients with sclerosing cholangitis and in 15–20% of their unaffected relatives. p-ANCA is not related to the extent or activity of ulcerative colitis or sclerosing cholangitis and is probably not important in causing tissue damage, but it may be a genetic marker of the diseases. Sclerosing cholangitis with identical radiological appearances to primary sclerosing cholangitis has occurred after intra-arterial floxuridine (FUDR) for hepatic metastases from colorectal carcinoma (Shea et al 1986), after accidental intrabiliary injection of scolicidal agents (Belghiti et al 1986), following bone marrow transplantation (Geubel et al 1990) and in AIDS (Dowsett et al 1988).

### Pathology

Sclerosing cholangitis is a progressive obliterative fibrosis of the extrahepatic and often the intrahepatic biliary tree. Segmental lesions have also been described. The ducts show widespread irregular narrowing, sometimes with beaded dilatation between the narrowed segments. At surgery, the porta hepatis is typically edematous, the serosal vessels congested and the local lymph nodes enlarged. The affected bile duct may resemble a beaded cord. The histological features of involved bile ducts are similar irrespective of whether the disease is diffuse or segmental. The major ducts show luminal narrowing, epithelial atrophy and in places loss of epithelium. The duct wall is fibrotic and there is a transmural, mainly mononuclear, inflammatory cell infiltration. The liver biopsy shows a range of changes including a reduced number of bile ducts, portal fibrosis, inflammation of the portal tracts and lobules, cholestasis, increased deposition of copper and cirrhosis. In some instances, the appearances may resemble large duct obstruction or sometimes primary biliary cirrhosis (Chapman et al 1980). Hepatic damage is the most important determinant of the prognosis in an individual case.

### Clinical features

The clinical features are those of chronic cholestasis with fluctuating jaundice, pruritus, abdominal pain and recurring cholangitis. Examination often shows hepatomegaly and sometimes splenomegaly. The features and complications of cirrhosis eventually develop. Rapid clinical deterioration suggests the development of a cholangiocarcinoma (Rosen et al 1991).

### Investigations

Liver function tests reflect cholestasis; the serum bilirubin is usually high and fluctuates with progression of the disease and the alkaline phosphatase activity is usually very high. Normal alkaline phosphatase activity has been found in about 3% of patients and this may remain normal on follow-up or become abnormal intermittently. Such patients may be symptomatic and may have well established disease on cholangiography and liver biopsy (Balasubramaniam et al 1988). The antimitochondrial antibody test is negative, but antinuclear and smooth muscle antibodies are occasionally present in adults (Helzberg et al 1987) and more often in children (El-Shabrawi et al 1987). Several other autoantibodies may be found, including p-ANCA, but they are not important in diagnosis (p. 767). The peripheral blood count may show an eosinophilia. Cholangiography is usually diagnostic and shows diffuse or, rarely, a localized smooth narrowing of the bile ducts. Endoscopic retrograde cholangiopancreatography is preferred because the intrahepatic bile ducts are usually attenuated. Bile duct dilatation occurs proximal to the stenotic portion when the lesion is segmental. Liver biopsy shows features consistent with PSC but is often not diagnostic (Helzberg et al 1987).

The definitive diagnosis can be made at operation by operative cholangiography and choledochoscopic biopsy, but this is not often necessary. Biopsy of peridochal lymph nodes is helpful only if it reveals cancer.

### Diagnosis

The diagnosis of PSC includes consideration of causes of chronic cholestasis. The essential diagnostic criteria are a diffuse or segmental inflammatory thickening and stenosis involving mainly the extrahepatic bile ducts in the absence of previous biliary surgery, gallstones or other local intra-abdominal sepsis (Table 34.13).

### Treatment

Treatment is unsatisfactory, as no specific measures are available and results are unpredictable.

#### *Medical treatment*

Broad-spectrum antibiotics are useful in controlling episodes of cholangitis. They should not be given on a long-term basis unless there is continuing liver pain and fever, when a rotation of antibiotics, each given for about 2 weeks, may be used. Corticosteroids, penicillamine, colchicine, methotrexate and azathioprine are of no proven value. Ursodeoxycholic acid treatment has been associated with biochemical and histological hepatic improvement in a small trial extending over a year and is the most promising drug available currently (Beuers et al 1992). Treatment for chronic cholestasis is required (p. 933). There is no evidence to advocate total colectomy for patients who also have ulcerative colitis (p. 684).

**Table 34.13** Criteria for the diagnosis of primary sclerosing cholangitis

| |
|---|
| Diffuse thickening and stenosis of the extrahepatic bile ducts |
| No previous biliary surgery |
| No biliary tract calculi |
| Exclusion of sclerosing carcinoma of the bile ducts by long follow-up (5 years) |

*Surgical treatment*

Surgical treatment should only be undertaken in specialist centers, as it can compromise subsequent management. In a few patients, biliary drainage can be improved by hepatico-jejunostomy for isolated extrahepatic strictures, but the role of prolonged T-tube drainage or transhepatic biliary stenting is unproven (Wood & Cuschieri 1980, Krige et al 1987). For patients with primary involvement of the extrahepatic ducts or a major extrahepatic obstruction, an overall 5-year survival of 82% has been reported following hepatico-jejunal anastomosis (Pitt et al 1982). Despite these encouraging results in selected patients, sclerosing cholangitis remains a difficult disease to treat surgically. Liver transplantation should be considered for patients with severe pruritus and is undertaken when medical measures fail and cirrhosis or portal hypertension has supervened (p. 1152).

### Prognosis

The overall outlook in diffuse primary sclerosing cholangitis has been considered to be poor, although the course of the illness in individual patients is unpredictable. Previously reported survival from diagnosis has been about 5–7 years. However, Helzberg et al (1987) found that 75% of patients were alive 9 years after the diagnosis, partly due to the increasing recognition of asymptomatic disease. Hepatomegaly and a serum bilirubin of more than 30 μmol/L (>1.5 mg/dl) at the time of diagnosis indicated a poor prognosis. Death is usually due to liver failure or to bleeding varices, which can best be avoided by liver transplantation as the disease reaches the end stage. The prognosis of the less common localized type is better and can be improved by adequate surgical decompression of the biliary tract. Cholangiocarcinoma complicates up to 10% of PSC cases, especially with more advanced disease. Surgery is rarely successful and liver transplantation for cholangiocarcinoma is usually followed by recurrent tumor (Rosen et al 1991).

## BILIARY DUCTOPENIA

Damage to small interlobular bile ducts ("vanishing bile duct syndrome") occurs in many diseases (Table 34.14), causing cholestasis and sometimes eventually biliary cirrhosis (Sherlock 1987). These diseases include the familial intrahepatic cholestasis syndromes and a recently described progressive loss of interlobular bile ducts leading to biliary cirrhosis in young adults.

**Table 34.14** Causes of interlobular bile duct damage

| |
|---|
| Primary biliary cirrhosis (above) |
| Primary sclerosing cholangitis (above) |
| Sarcoidosis (p. 830) |
| Drugs (p. 851) |
| Lymphoma (p. 1104) |
| Liver transplant rejection (p. 1159) |
| Graft-versus-host disease (p. 1167) |
| Histiocytosis X (p. 1105) |
| Familial intrahepatic cholestasis syndromes |
| Idiopathic adult ductopenia |

### Idiopathic adult biliary ductopenia

This rare condition usually occurs in young men and women with no previous history of liver disease (Ludwig et al 1988, Zafrani et al 1990). It presents with pruritus and cholestatic jaundice, which may remit and relapse spontaneously. Some patients experience abdominal pain and development of cirrhosis can lead to portal hypertension and ascites or variceal bleeding. Physical examination shows jaundice and often hepatomegaly, and splenomegaly becomes more common as the disease progresses. Liver function tests show a cholestatic pattern (p. 743) and hypoalbuminemia occurs with the development of liver failure. The antimitochondrial antibody test is negative. Cholangiography shows normal intrahepatic and extrahepatic bile ducts. Liver biopsy shows marked portal inflammation with cholangiolar proliferation and sometimes damage to interlobular bile ducts, cholestasis and sometimes hepatocyte necrosis and eventually fibrosis and cirrhosis.

The main alternative diagnoses are drug-induced cholestasis and primary sclerosing cholangitis. The former is detected from the history of drug ingestion, especially of drugs recognized as causing chronic cholestasis. The latter is identified at cholangiography and by features of ulcerative colitis, exclusion of which may require endoscopy and biopsy. Sarcoidosis is a very rare cause of cholestatic jaundice and there is always granulomatous involvement of organs other than the liver (p. 830). The antimitochondrial antibody is positive in primary biliary cirrhosis and lymphoma is diagnosed from findings outside the liver. The disease follows a remitting and relapsing but progressive course. No specific treatment is available and liver transplantation may be needed for liver failure.

### Familial intrahepatic cholestasis syndromes

The familial intrahepatic cholestasis syndromes comprise a group of poorly understood inherited disorders giving rise to cholestasis, which usually presents first early in life (Riely 1979, Alagille et al 1987). They occasionally present in adolescence (Haratake et al 1985) and long-term survivors have developed hepatocellular carcinoma (Ugarte & Gonzalez-Crussi 1981, Kaufman et al 1987).

The mechanisms of cholestasis in these conditions remain unknown but may include the production of abnormal bile acids (Hanson et al 1975), malfunction of the hepatocyte microfilament system (Weber et al 1981) and abnormality of peroxisomes (Goldfischer et al 1973). The various cholestatic syndromes cannot always be readily differentiated from one another and several forms have been described. The most common of these conditions is intrahepatic biliary atresia or intrahepatic bile duct hypoplasia (p. 730), which may be associated with other extrahepatic anomalies (syndromic) or occur as an isolated defect (nonsyndromic). Syndromic intrahepatic bile duct hypoplasia (Alagille's syndrome) is characterized by neonatal cholestatic jaundice and a number of extrahepatic features including a prominent forehead, deep wide-set eyes, a straight nose and a small pointed chin, pulmonary artery stenosis or aortic coarctation, vertebral arch defects (butterfly vertebrae), growth retardation and sometimes renal failure. Posterior embryotoxon, an asymptomatic embryologic remnant, is present in the eye in almost all patients but requires slit-lamp examination for its identification. Familial occurrence is common and an autosomal dominant inheritance has been suggested. The jaundice usually disappears by the age of 4 years, but cholestasis persists permanently. Liver biopsy shows a paucity of intrahepatic bile ducts, but in most cases progressive liver disease does not occur, so that patients survive at least beyond the first decade. Autosomal dominant and recessive inheritance has been suggested. Nonsyndromic intrahepatic bile duct hypoplasia, in which there are no extrahepatic features, is less common. The long-term outlook in this condition is much worse and a half of patients have cirrhosis and liver failure by adolescence.

Several other syndromes have been described, all presenting in infancy or childhood. Byler's disease was described originally in Amish families, where jaundice and steatorrhea occur in the first year of life, sometimes associated with mental and growth retardation, and progress to death from cirrhosis in adolescence. Norwegian familial intrahepatic cholestasis (Aagenaes' syndrome) is characterized by recurrent cholestasis starting in infancy and progressing to cirrhosis associated with lymphedema due to lymphatic hypoplasia. North American Indian cholestasis shows cholestasis progressing to cirrhosis with associated facial telangiectasias. Zellweger's syndrome (cerebrohepatorenal syndrome) presents in the first year of life with a characteristic facial appearance, mental retardation and other congenital abnormalities including renal cysts, hepatomegaly and cholestasis. Occasional instances of bile acid synthesis defects have been described in which the bile acids produced may lack choleretic activity, and a familial chronic cholestasis associated with pigmentation, hypertrichosis, facial telangiectasias and hypothyroidism.

## BENIGN RECURRENT INTRAHEPATIC CHOLESTASIS

This is a rare condition in which recurrent episodes of cholestasis resolve spontaneously. There are usually repeated attacks over many years but patients remain healthy, the structure and function of the liver is normal during remission and chronic liver disease does not develop (Putterman et al 1987). Males are affected more often than females. The first episode of cholestasis develops before the age of 20 years in three-quarters of the patients, but this can vary from as early as the second week of life to the age of 59 years. Individual episodes of cholestasis usually last from 1 to 6 months, although occasional attacks may continue for over 2 years and 20 or more episodes have been reported in the same patient. Most episodes begin with an anicteric phase lasting for up to a month during which pruritus is the main feature. Malaise and anorexia are also often present, jaundice then develops and may be associated with tender hepatomegaly, but there is no abdominal pain or fever and the spleen is not palpable. Liver function tests in the anicteric phase show a much increased plasma alkaline phosphatase activity and bile acid concentrations are high (Van Berge Henegouwen et al 1974). Later, the plasma bilirubin rises, but albumin and globulin concentrations remain normal.

**Table 34.15** Criteria for the diagnosis of benign recurrent intrahepatic cholestasis

| |
|---|
| Recurrent pruritus and jaundice |
| No clinical evidence of chronic liver disease |
| No known cause of cholestasis, especially: |
| drugs |
| pregnancy/oral contraceptives |
| Liver function tests show cholestasis |
| Liver biopsy shows cholestasis |
| Biliary tree normal radiologically |
| No hepatic abnormality during remission |

Benign recurrent intrahepatic cholestasis can be diagnosed in a patient who has had spontaneously resolving cholestasis previously and in whom other causes of cholestasis, especially drugs, have been excluded (Table 34.15). It needs to be differentiated from cholestasis of pregnancy and from cholestasis in women taking oral contraceptive drugs (p. 1091). Liver biopsy shows cholestasis only during relapse and is normal during remission. Cholangiography is necessary to ensure that the biliary tree is normal. There is no specific therapy; treatment during exacerbations is that of the cholestatic syndrome (p. 933).

The cause of this syndrome, which may not be a single entity, is unknown. Sometimes more than one family member is affected and this points to a genetic factor (De Pagter et al 1976). There may also be a relation to cholestasis of pregnancy, as some patients with benign recurrent intrahepatic cholestasis have also developed cholestasis in pregnancy or while taking oral contraceptive drugs. There is a familial factor in the cholestasis of pregnancy and a family has been described in which these two conditions and cholestasis due to oral contraceptives have all occurred (De Pagter et al 1976). It is likely that the cause of the cholestasis operates in the hepatocyte itself, perhaps at the biliary canalicular membrane, but the mechanism of its action is unknown.

## REFERENCES


Ahrens E H Jr, Payne M A, Kunkel H G, Eisenmenger W J, Blondheim S H 1950 Primary biliary cirrhosis. Medicine 29: 299–364

Ajdukiewicz A B, Agnew J E, Byers P D, Wills M R, Sherlock S 1974 The relief of bone pain in primary biliary cirrhosis with calcium infusions. Gut 15: 788–793

Alagille D, Estrada A, Hadchouel M, Gautier M, Odièvre M, Dommergues J P 1987 Syndromic paucity of interlobular bile ducts (Alagille syndrome or arteriohepatic dysplasia): review of 80 cases. Journal of Pediatrics 110: 195–200

Almdal T P, Sørensen T I A and the Danish Association for the Study of the Liver 1991 Incidence of parenchymal liver disease in Denmark, 1981 to 1985: analysis of hospitalization registry data. Hepatology 13: 650–655

Alvarez F, Landrieu P, Laget P, Lemonnier F, Odièvre M, Alagille D 1983 Nervous and ocular disorders in children with cholestasis and vitamin A and E deficiencies. Hepatology 3: 410–414

Babbs C, Warnes T W 1986 Primary biliary cirrhosis after benoxaprophen. British Medical Journal 293: 241

Bachs L, Pares A, Elena M, Piera C, Rodés J 1992 Effects of long-term Rifampicin administration in primary biliary cirrhosis. Gastroenterology 102: 2077–2080

Balasubramaniam K, Wiesner R H, LaRusso N F 1988 Primary sclerosing cholangitis with normal serum alkaline phosphatase activity. Gastroenterology 95: 1395–1398

Balasubramaniam K, Grambsch P M, Wiesner R H, Lindor K D, Dickson E R 1990 Diminished survival in asymptomatic primary biliary cirrhosis. A prospective study. Gastroenterology 98: 1567–1571

Bassendine M F, Dewar P J, James O F W 1985 HLA-DR antigens in primary biliary cirrhosis: lack of association. Gut 26: 625–628

Beckett G J, Dewhurst N, Finlayson N D C, Percy-Robb I W 1980 Weight loss in primary biliary cirrhosis. Gut 21: 734–737

Belghiti J, Benhamou J-P, Houry H, Grenier P, Huguier M, Fekete F 1986 Caustic sclerosing cholangitis. A complication of the surgical treatment of hydatid disease of the liver. Archives of Surgery 121: 1162–1165

Ben-Ari Z, Dhillon A P, Sherlock S 1993 Autoimmune cholangiopathy: part of the spectrum of autoimmune chronic active hepatitis. Hepatology 18: 10–15

Beuers U, Spengler U, Kruis W et al 1992 Ursodeoxycholic acid for treatment of primary sclerosing cholangitis: a placebo-controlled trial. Hepatology 16: 707–714

Bloomer J R, Boyer J L 1975 Phenobarbital effects in cholestatic liver disease. Annals of Internal Medicine 82: 310–317

Bown R, Clark M L, Doniach D 1975 Primary biliary cirrhosis in brothers. Postgraduate Medical Journal 51: 110–115

Brown P J E, Lesna M, Hamlyn A N, Record C O 1978 Primary biliary cirrhosis after long-term practolol administration. British Medical Journal 1: 1591

Burroughs A K, Rosenstein I J, Epstein O, Hamilton-Miller J M T, Brumfitt W, Sherlock S 1984 Bacteriuria and primary biliary cirrhosis. Gut 25: 133–137

Bush A, Mitchison H, Walt R, Baron J H, Boylston A W, Summerfield J A 1987 Primary biliary cirrhosis and ulcerative colitis. Gastroenterology 92: 2009–2113

Caldwell S H, Leung P S C, Spivey J R et al 1992 Antimitochondrial antibodies in kindreds of patients with primary biliary cirrhosis: antimitochondrial antibodies are unique to clinical disease and are absent in asymptomatic family members. Hepatology 16: 899–905

Chapman R W G, Arborgh B A M, Rhodes J M et al 1980 Primary sclerosing cholangitis: a review of its clinical features, cholangiography, and hepatic histology. Gut 21: 870–877

Child D L, Mathews J A, Thompson R P H 1977 Arthritis and primary biliary cirrhosis. British Medical Journal 2: 557

Chohan M R 1973 Primary biliary cirrhosis in twin sisters. Gut 14: 213–214

Christensen E, Crowe J, Doniach D et al 1980 Clinical pattern and course of disease in primary biliary cirrhosis based on an analysis of 236 patients. Gastroenterology 78: 236–246

Christensen E, Neuberger J, Crowe J et al 1985 Beneficial effect of azathioprine and prediction of prognosis in primary biliary cirrhosis. Final results of an international trial. Gastroenterology 89: 1084–1091

Clarke A K, Galbraith R M, Hamilton E B D, Williams R 1978 Rheumatic disorders in primary biliary cirrhosis. Annals of Rheumatic Diseases 37: 42–47

Cohen L B, Ambinder E P, Wolke A M, Field S P, Schaffner F 1985 Role of plasmapheresis in primary biliary cirrhosis. Gut 26: 291–294

Compston J E 1986 Hepatic osteodystrophy: vitamin D metabolism in patients with liver disease. Gut 27: 1073–1090

Crippin J S, Lindor K D, Jorgensen R et al 1992 Hypercholesterolemia and atherosclerosis in primary biliary cirrhosis: what is the risk? Hepatology 15: 858–862

Crowe J P, Christensen E, Butler J et al 1980 Primary biliary cirrhosis: the prevalence of hypothyroidism and its relationship to thyroid autoantibodies and sicca syndrome. Gastroenterology 78: 1437–1441

Datta D V, Sherlock S 1966 Cholestyramine for long term relief of the pruritus complicating intrahepatic cholestasis. Gastroenterology 50: 323

Davies M, Mawer E B, Klass H J, Lumb G A, Berry J L, Warnes T W 1983 Vitamin deficiency, osteomalacia, and primary biliary cirrhosis. Response to orally administered vitamin $D_3$. Digestive Diseases and Sciences 28: 145–153

De Pagter A G F, van Berge Henegouwen G P, ten Bokkel Huinink J A, Brandt K-H 1976 Familial benign recurrent intrahepatic cholestasis. Interrelation with intrahepatic cholestasis of pregnancy and from oral contraceptives? Gastroenterology 71: 202–207

Douglas J G, Finlayson N D C 1979 Are increased individual susceptibility and environmental factors both necessary for the development of primary biliary cirrhosis? British Medical Journal 2: 419–420

Douglas J G, Beckett G J, Nimmo I A, Finlayson N D C, Percy-Robb I W 1981 Bile salt measurement in Gilbert's syndrome. European Journal of Clinical Investigation 11: 421–423

Dowsett J F, Miller R, Davidson R et al 1988 Sclerosing cholangitis in acquired immunodeficiency syndrome. Case reports and review of the literature. Scandinavian Journal of Gastroenterology 23: 1267–1274

Duncan J S, Kennedy H J, Triger D R 1984 Treatment of pruritus due to chronic obstructive liver disease. British Medical Journal 289: 22

Elias E, Muller D P R, Scott J 1981 Association of spinocerebellar disorders with cystic fibrosis or chronic childhood cholestasis and very low serum vitamin E. Lancet 2: 1319–1321

El-Shabrawi M, Wilkinson M L, Portman B et al 1987 Primary sclerosing cholangitis in childhood. Gastroenterology 92: 1226–1235

Feizi T, Naccarato R, Sherlock S, Doniach D 1972 Mitochondrial and other tissue antibodies in relatives of patients with primary biliary cirrhosis. Clinical and Experimental Immunology 10: 609–622

Foulk W T, Baggenstoss A H, Butt H R 1964 Primary biliary cirrhosis. Reevaluation by clinical and histologic study of 49 cases. Gastroenterology 47: 354–374

Frank D J, Dusol M Jr, Schiff E R 1979 Primary shunt hyperbilirubinemia with secondary iron overload: a case report. Gastroenterology 77: 754–757

Galbraith R M, Smith M, Mackenzie R M, Tee D E, Doniach D, Williams R 1974 High prevalence of seroimmunologic abnormalities in relatives of patients with active chronic hepatitis or primary biliary cirrhosis. New England Journal of Medicine 290: 63–69

Garden J M, Ostrow J D, Roenigk H H Jr 1985 Pruritus in hepatic cholestasis. Pathogenesis and therapy. Archives of Dermatology 121: 1415–1420

Geubel A P, Cnudde A, Ferrant A, Latinne D, Rahier J 1990 Diffuse biliary tract involvement mimicking primary sclerosing cholangitis after bone marrow transplantation. Journal of Hepatology 10: 23–28

Goldfischer S, Moore C L, Johnson A B et al 1973 Peroxisomal and mitochondrial defects in the cerebro-hepato-renal syndrome. Science 182: 62–64

Golding P L, Smith M, Williams R 1973 Multisystem involvement in chronic liver disease. Studies in incidence and pathogenesis. American Journal of Medicine 55: 772–782

Goodman Z D, McNally P R, Davis D R, Ishak K G 1995 Autoimmune cholangitis: a variant of primary biliary cirrhosis. Clinico pathologic and serologic correlations in 200 cases. Digestive Diseases and Sciences 40: 1232–1242

Goudie B M, Burt A D, Boyle P et al 1985 Breast cancer in women with primary biliary cirrhosis. British Medical Journal 291: 1597–1598

Hamlyn A N, Macklon A F, James O 1983 Primary biliary cirrhosis: geographical clustering and symptomatic onset seasonality. Gut 24: 940–945

Hanid M A, Levi A J 1980 Phototherapy for pruritus in primary biliary cirrhosis. Lancet 2: 530

Hanson R F, Isenberg J N, Williams G C et al 1975 The metabolism of 3α, 7α, 12α-trihydroxy-5β cholestan-26-oic acid in two siblings with cholestasis due to intrahepatic bile duct anomalies. An apparent inborn error of cholic acid synthesis. Journal of Clinical Investigation 56: 577–587

Haratake J, Horie A, Ishii N, Okuno F 1985 Familial intrahepatic cholestatic cirrhosis in young adults. Gastroenterology 89: 202–209

Hay J E, Lindor K D, Weisner R H, Dickson E R, Krom R A F, LaRusso N F 1991 The metabolic bone disease of primary sclerosing cholangitis. Hepatology 14: 257–261

Heaf J G 1985 Hepatic osteodystrophy. Scandinavian Journal of Gastroenterology 20: 1035–1040

Helzberg J H, Petersen J M, Boyer J L 1987 Improved survival with primary sclerosing cholangitis. A review of clinicopathologic features and comparison of symptomatic and asymptomatic patients. Gastroenterology 92: 1869–1875

Hoofnagle J H, Davis G L, Schafer D F et al 1986 Randomized trial of chlorambucil for primary biliary cirrhosis. Gastroenterology 91: 1327–1334

Israels L G 1970 The bilirubin shunt and shunt hyperbilirubinemia. In: Popper H, Schaffner F (eds) Progress in liver diseases, Vol 3. Grune and Stratton, New York, p 1–12

Jakobovits A, Dudley F J, Allen P 1984 Primary liver cell carcinoma complicating secondary biliary cirrhosis. British Medical Journal 289: 227

James O, Macklon A F, Watson A J 1981 Primary biliary cirrhosis – a revised clinical spectrum. Lancet 1: 1278–1281

James S P 1985 Primary biliary cirrhosis. New England Journal of Medicine 312: 1055–1056

Javitt N B 1974 Timing of cholestyramine doses in cholestatic liver disease. New England Journal of Medicine 290: 1328–1329

Jones E A, Bergasa N A 1992 The pruritus of cholestasis and the opioid system. Journal of the American Medical Association 268: 3359–3362

Karlish A J, Thompson R P H, Williams R 1969 A case of sarcoidosis and primary biliary cirrhosis. Lancet 2: 599

Kaufman S S, Wood R P, Shaw B W Jr, Markin R S, Gridelli B, Vanderhoof J A 1987 Hepatocarcinoma in a child with Alagille syndrome. American Journal of Diseases of Children 141: 698–700

Kew M C, Varma R R, Dos Santos H A, Scheuer P J, Sherlock S 1971 Portal hypertension in primary biliary cirrhosis. Gut 12: 830–834

Knight R E, Bourne A J, Newton M, Black A, Wilson P, Lawson M J 1986 Neurologic syndrome associated with low levels of vitamin E in primary biliary cirrhosis. Gastroenterology 91: 209–211

Krasner N, Johnson P J, Portmann B, Wilkinson G, MacSween R N M, Williams R 1979 Hepatocellular carcinoma in primary biliary cirrhosis: report of four cases. Gut 20: 255–258

Krige J E J, Terblanche J, Harries-Jones E P, Bornman P C 1987 Primary sclerosing cholangitis: biliary drainage and duct dilatation. British Journal of Surgery 74: 54–57

Lacerda M A, Ludwig J, Dickson E R, Jorgensen R A, Lindor K D 1995 Autimitochondrial antibody-negative primary biliary cirrhosis. American Journal of Gastroenterology 90: 247–249

Lanspa S J, Chan A T H, Bell J S III, Go V L W, Dickson E R, DiMagno E P 1985 Pathogenesis of steatorrhea in primary biliary cirrhosis. Hepatology 5: 837–842

Lauterburg B H, Taswell H F, Pineda A A, Dickson E R, Burgstaler E A, Carlson G L 1980 Treatment of pruritus of cholestasis by plasma perfusion through USP-charcoal-coated glass beads. Lancet 2: 53–55

Lee R G, Epstein O, Jauregui H, Sherlock S, Scheuer P J 1981 Granulomas in primary biliary cirrhosis: a prognostic feature. Gastroenterology 81: 983–986

Leung P S C, Krams S, Munoz S et al 1992 Characterization and epitope mapping of human monoclonal antibodies to PDC-E2, the immunodominant autoantigen of primary biliary cirrhosis. Journal of Autoimmunity 5: 703–718

Lim A G, Jazrawi R P, Northfield T C 1995 The ursodeoxycholic acid story in primary biliary cirrhosis. Gut 37: 301–304

Linarelli L G, Williams C N, Phillips M J 1972 Byler's disease: fatal intrahepatic cholestasis. Journal of Pediatrics 81: 484–492

Lombard M, Portmann B, Neuberger J et al 1993 Cyclosporin A treatment in primary biliary cirrhosis: results of a long-term placebo controlled trial. Gastroenterology 104: 519–526

Long R G, Scheuer P J, Sherlock S 1977 Presentation and course of asymptomatic primary biliary cirrhosis. Gastroenterology 72: 1204–1207

Lucey M R, Neuberger J M, Williams R 1986 Primary biliary cirrhosis in men. Gut 27: 1373–1376

Ludwig J, Wiesner R H, LaRusso N F 1988 Idiopathic adulthood ductopenia. A cause of cholestatic liver disease and biliary cirrhosis. Journal of Hepatology 7: 193–199

MacSween R N M 1987 Diseases of the intrahepatic bile ducts. In: MacSween R N M, Anthony P P, Scheuer P J (eds) Pathology of the liver, 2nd edn. Churchill Livingstone, Edinburgh, p 424

Michieletti P, Wanless I R, Katz A et al 1994 Antimitochondrial antibody negative primary biliary cirrhosis: a distinct syndrome of autoimmune cholangitis. Gut 35: 260–265

Mills P R, Rooney P J, Watkinson G, MacSween R N M 1979 Hypercholesterolaemic arthropathy in primary biliary cirrhosis. Annals of Rheumatic Diseases 38: 179–180

Mitchison H C, Bassendine M F, Hendrick A et al 1986 Positive antimitochondrial antibody but normal alkaline phosphatase: is this primary biliary cirrhosis? Hepatology 6: 1279–1284

Mitchison H C, Malcolm A J, Bassendine M F, James O F W 1988 Metabolic bone disease in primary biliary cirrhosis at presentation. Gastroenterology 94: 463–470

Mitchison H C, Palmer J M, Bassendine M F, Watson A J, Record C O, James O F W 1992 A controlled trial of prednisolone treatment in primary biliary cirrhosis. Three-year results. Journal of Hepatology 15: 336–344

Muraca M, Blanckaert N 1983 Liquid-chromatographic assay and identification of mono- and diester conjugates of bilirubin in normal serum. Clinical Chemistry 29: 1767–1771

Muraca M, Fevery J, Blanckaert N 1987 Relationships between serum bilirubins and production and conjugation of bilirubin. Studies in Gilbert's syndrome, Crigler–Najjar disease, hemolytic disorders, and rat models. Gastroenterology 92: 309–317

Murray-Lyon I M, Thompson R P H, Ansell I D, Williams R 1970 Scleroderma and primary biliary cirrhosis. British Medical Journal 3: 258–259

Nakanuma Y, Ohta G 1979 Histometric and serial section observations of the intrahepatic bile ducts in primary biliary cirrhosis. Gastroenterology 76: 1326–1332

Nyberg A, Lööf L 1989 Primary biliary cirrhosis: clinical features and outcome, with special reference to asymptomatic disease. Scandinavian Journal of Gastroenterology 24: 57–64

O'Brien S T, Eddy W M, Krawitt E L 1972 Primary biliary cirrhosis associated with scleroderma. Gastroenterology 62: 118–121

Okuno T, Seto Y, Okanoue T, Takino T 1987 Chronic active hepatitis with histological features of primary biliary cirrhosis. Digestive Diseases and Sciences 32: 775–779

Olomu A B, Vickers C R, Waring R H et al 1988 High incidence of poor sulfoxidation in patients with primary biliary cirrhosis. New England Journal of Medicine 318: 1089

Orlin J B, Berkman E M, Matloff D S, Kaplan M M 1980 Primary biliary cirrhosis and cold autoimmune hemolytic anemia: effect of partial plasma exchange. Gastroenterology 78: 576–578

Pitt H A, Thompson H H, Tompkins R K, Longmire W P Jr 1982 Primary sclerosing cholangitis. Results of an aggressive surgical approach. Annals of Surgery 196: 259–268

Portmann B, Popper H, Neuberger J, Williams R 1985 Sequential and diagnostic features in primary biliary cirrhosis based on serial histologic study in 209 patients. Gastroenterology 88: 1777–1790

Powell L W 1967 Bilirubin metabolism and jaundice with special reference to unconjugated hyperbilirubinaemia. Australasian Annals of Medicine 16: 343

Powell L W, Billing B H, Williams H S 1967 An assessment of red cell survival in idiopathic unconjugated hyperbilirubinaemia (Gilbert's

syndrome) by the use of radioactive diisopropylfluorophosphate and chromium. Australasian Annals of Medicine 16: 221
Putterman C, Keidar S, Brook J G 1987 Benign recurrent intrahepatic cholestasis – 25 years of follow-up. Postgraduate Medical Journal 63: 295–296
Rai G S, Hamlyn A N, Dahl M G C, Morley A R, Wilkinson R 1977 Primary biliary cirrhosis, cutaneous capillaritis, and IgM-associated membranous glomerulonephritis. British Medical Journal 1: 817
Reynolds T B, Denison E K, Frankl H D, Lieberman F L, Peters R L 1971 Primary biliary cirrhosis with scleroderma, Reynaud's phenomenon and telangiectasia. American Journal of Medicine 50: 302–312
Riely C A 1979 Familial intrahepatic cholestasis: an update. Yale Journal of Biology and Medicine 52: 89–98
Roll J, Boyer J L, Barry D, Klatskin G 1983 The prognostic importance of clinical and histologic features in asymptomatic and symptomatic primary biliary cirrhosis. New England Journal of Medicine 308: 1
Ros E, García-Pugés A, Reixach M, Cusó E, Rodés J 1984 Fat digestion and exocrine pancreatic function in primary biliary cirrhosis. Gastroenterology 87: 180–187
Rosen C B, Nagorney D M, Wiesner R H, Coffey R J Jr, LaRusso N F 1991 Cholangiocarcinoma complicating primary sclerosing cholangitis. Annals of Surgery 213: 21–25
Rubel L R, Rabin L, Seeff L B, Licht H, Cuccherini B A 1984 Does primary biliary cirrhosis in men differ from primary biliary cirrhosis in women? Hepatology 4: 671–677
Salaspuro M, Sipponen P 1976 Demonstration of an intracellular copper-binding protein by orcein staining in long-standing cholestatic liver diseases. Gut 17: 787–790
Schaffner F 1975 Primary biliary cirrhosis. Clinics in Gastroenterology 4: 351–366
Schaffner F, Klion F M, Latuff A J 1965 The long term use of cholestyramine in the treatment of primary biliary cirrhosis. Gastroenterology 48: 293–298
Scheuer P J 1980 Liver biopsy interpretation, 3rd edn. Baillière Tindall & Cassell, London
Scobie B A, Summerskill W H J 1965 Hepatic cirrhosis secondary to obstruction of the biliary system. American Journal of Digestive Diseases 10: 135–146
Shapiro J M, Smith H, Schaffner F 1979 Serum bilirubin: a prognostic factor in primary biliary cirrhosis. Gut 20: 137–140
Shea W J Jr, Demas B E, Goldberg H I, Hone D C, Ferrell L D, Kerlan R K 1986 Sclerosing cholangitis associated with hepatic arterial FUDR chemotherapy: radiographic-histologic correlation. American Journal of Roentgenology 146: 717–721
Shepherd A N, Bedford G I, Hill A, Bouchier I A D 1984 Primary biliary cirrhosis, dark adoptometry, electro-oculography, and vitamin A state. British Medical Journal 289: 1484–1485
Sherlock S 1959 Primary biliary cirrhosis (chronic intrahepatic obstructive jaundice). Gastroenterology 37: 574–586
Sherlock S 1987 The syndrome of disappearing intrahepatic bile ducts. Lancet 2: 493–496
Sherlock S, Scheuer P J 1973 The presentation and diagnosis of 100 patients with primary biliary cirrhosis. New England Journal of Medicine 289: 674–678
Soto J A, Barish M A, Yucel E K, Siegenberg D, Ferrucci J T, Chuttani R 1996 Magnetic resonance cholangiography: comparison with endoscopic retrograde cholangiopancreatography. Gastroenterology 110: 589–597
Stanley N N, Fox R A, Whimster W F, Sherlock S, James D G 1972 Primary biliary cirrhosis or sarcoidosis – or both. New England Journal of Medicine 287: 1282–1284
Summerfield J A, Elias E, Hungerford G D, Nikapota V L B, Dick R, Sherlock S 1976 The biliary system in primary biliary cirrhosis. A study by endoscopic retrograde cholangiopancreatography. Gastroenterology 70: 240–243
Thomas P K, Walker J G 1965 Xanthomatous neuropathy in primary biliary cirrhosis. Brain 88: 1079–1088
Triger D R 1980 Primary biliary cirrhosis: an epidemiological study. British Medical Journal 281: 772–775
Turnberg L A, Mahoney M P, Gleeson M H, Freedman C B, Gowanlock A H 1972 Plasmapheresis and plasma exchange in the treatment of hyperlipaemia and xanthomatous neuropathy in patients with primary biliary cirrhosis. Gut 13: 976–981
Ugarte N, Gonzalez-Crussi F 1981 Hepatoma in siblings with progressive familial cholestatic cirrhosis of childhood. American Journal of Clinical Pathology 76: 173–177
Underhill J, Donaldson P, Bray G, Doherty D, Portmann B, Williams R 1992 Susceptibility to primary biliary cirrhosis is associated with the HLA-DR8-DQB1* 0402 haplotype. Hepatology 16: 1404–1408
Van Berge Henegouwen G P, Brandt K-H, de Pagter A G F 1974 Is an acute disturbance in hepatic transport of bile-acids the primary cause of cholestasis in benign recurrent intrahepatic cholestasis? Lancet 1: 1249
Walt R P, Daneshmend T K, Fellows I W, Toghill P J 1988 Effect of stanozolol on itching in primary biliary cirrhosis. British Medical Journal 296: 607
Weber A M, Tuchweber B, Yousef I et al 1981 Severe familial cholestasis in North American Indian children: a clinical model of microfilament dysfunction? Gastroenterology 81: 653–662
Wiesner R H, LaRusso N F 1980 Clinicopathologic features of the syndrome of primary sclerosing cholangitis. Gastroenterology 79: 200–206
Williamson J M S, Chalmers D M, Clayden A D, Dixon M F, Ruddell W S J, Losowsky M S 1985 Primary biliary cirrhosis and chronic active hepatitis: an examination of clinical, biochemical and histopathological features in differential diagnosis. Journal of Clinical Pathology 38: 1007–1012
Wood R A B, Cuschieri A 1980 Is sclerosing cholangitis complicating ulcerative colitis a reversible condition? Lancet 2: 716–718
Yeong M L, Nicholson G I, Lee S P 1982 Regression of biliary cirrhosis following choledochal cyst drainage. Gastroenterology 82: 332–335
Zafrani E S, Metreau J-M, Douvin C et al 1990 Idiopathic biliary ductopenia in adults. A report of five cases. Gastroenterology 99: 1823–1828
Zauli D, Schrumpf E, Crespi C, Cassani F, Fausa O, Aadland E 1987 An autoantibody profile in primary sclerosing cholangitis. Journal of Hepatology 5: 14–18
Zifroni A, Schaffner F 1991 Long-term follow-up of patients with primary biliary cirrhosis on colchicine therapy. Hepatology 14: 990–993

# 35. Metabolic diseases of the liver

*John B. Gross*

Metabolic liver diseases continue to provide among the best opportunities for effective prevention and medical therapy in hepatology. Phlebotomy has transformed the outlook for patients with genetic hemochromatosis and treatment in the prefibrotic phase prevents the development of cirrhosis and hepatocellular carcinoma. Long-term survival in Wilson's disease treated with penicillamine is excellent and alternative medical therapy is available for patients sensitive to penicillamine. Treatment of asymptomatic relatives of patients with genetic hemochromatosis and Wilson's disease prevents the development of disease. The long-term outlook for patients with homozygous $\alpha_1$-antitrypsin deficiency now appears better than was thought previously.

Considerable advances have been made in understanding the genetics of these disorders. The gene for genetic hemochromatosis has been traced to chromosome 6; that for Wilson's disease is located on chromosome 13 and the gene product shows 60–70% homology with the gene product of Menkes' disease (p. 965) where the gene is on the X chromosome; and the gene for ceruloplasmin is located on chromosome 3. The complexity of the codominant inheritance of $\alpha_1$-antitrypsin is now much better appreciated. The genes for a number of rarer metabolic disorders have been isolated. Unfortunately, mutations among affected individuals are often multiple and heterogeneous. Nonalcoholic steatohepatitis is common and usually associated with obesity or diabetes mellitus but is rarely a cause of liver failure. Diseases associated with microvesicular steatosis, such as acute fatty liver of pregnancy or Reye's syndrome, are potentially more serious and have been found in some patients to be associated with underlying mitochondrial enzyme defects.

## IRON AND THE LIVER (HEMOCHROMATOSIS)

The term "hemochromatosis" refers to a group of conditions in which the amount of iron in the body is increased and in which iron is deposited in and damages various organs. It is caused by an inappropriately increased absorption of iron from the intestine and/or the excessive administration of iron. The primary form of the disease and its genetic nature were recognized first by Sheldon (1935). In secondary hemochromatosis, a nonhereditary condition is present that leads to an excessive accumulation of iron in the body. The three major consequences of hepatic iron overload are hepatic fibrosis leading eventually to cirrhosis, porphyria cutanea tarda and hepatocellular carcinoma (Bonkovsky 1991). The terms "siderosis" and "hemosiderosis" cause confusion and are best avoided. A number of excellent reviews of iron metabolism and hemochromatosis are available (Finch & Huebers 1982, Smith 1990, Tavill & Bacon 1990, Bonkovsky 1991).

### Iron metabolism

The body of a normal adult contains 3–4 g of iron (Table 35.1). Most is within cells as hemoglobin, as ferritin or as part of the cell structure and 3–4 mg is present in plasma (Finch & Huebers 1982).

#### *Absorption and excretion*

The daily loss of iron varies little, as the ability to excrete

**Table 35.1** Distribution of iron in the adult human

| Site | Amount | % |
|---|---|---|
| Total body iron | 3–4 g | 100 |
| Hemoglobin iron | 1.5–3 g | 60–70 |
| Plasma iron | 3–4 mg | <1 |
| Tissue iron | | |
| Cellular (essential) | 300 mg | 6–8 |
| Storage* | 600–800 mg | 20–30 |

*Mainly in the liver, muscle and reticuloendothelial system.

iron is limited. Adult males lose about 1 mg daily, mainly in the stools but also from the skin and in the urine. This loss falls to about 0.5 mg daily in iron deficiency and may reach 3 mg daily in iron overload. In women, menstruation adds 0.5–1.5 mg to the average daily loss and each pregnancy calls for about 1 g iron. As the average intake of iron in Western countries is 15 mg/day and the ability to excrete iron is limited, the body avoids accumulating an excessive amount of iron by strictly limiting iron absorption. The factors that influence iron absorption and the way in which iron absorption is controlled are detailed elsewhere (p. 359).

*Iron transport*

Transferrin is the main protein concerned in the transport of iron from its site of absorption in the small intestine to other body tissues (Bomford & Munro 1985). It is made mainly in the liver (molecular weight of 80 000), and each molecule has two iron-binding sites that are normally 20–50% saturated. All cells possess surface membrane transferrin receptors that allow them to remove iron from transferrin and return the apotransferrin to the interstitial fluid otherwise unchanged. Hepatic transferrin synthesis does not change greatly in relation to iron deficiency or excess, but the synthesis of transferrin receptors on cells is increased markedly in iron deficiency and decreased in iron excess. Two other proteins, haptoglobin and hemopexin, bind iron in the blood. Haptoglobin binds heme iron and hemopexin binds heme; much less is known of their functions.

Ferritin is found mainly inside cells but is also present normally in serum where its concentration reflects the total iron stores in health and disease (Jacobs & Worwood 1975). In iron deficiency anemia its concentration may be nearly immeasurable, while in iron overload due to transfusion or hemochromatosis, levels may reach 10 000 μg/L (p. 748). Serum concentrations that are inappropriately high relative to iron stores occur in leukemia due to ferritin synthesis by leukemic cells. Increased concentrations also occur for unknown reasons in other neoplastic diseases, especially Hodgkin's disease.

*Tissue iron*

Most of the body iron is in the hemoglobin of the circulating red blood cells and it is retained and reutilized when red blood cells are destroyed by the macrophages of the reticuloendothelial system (Fig. 35.1). Every milliliter of normal blood (hemoglobin 150 g/L) contains about 0.5 mg iron. Iron in other tissues is either an integral part of the cell or is in a storage form. It is a constituent of myoglobin and of certain cell enzymes, including cytochromes, catalases and peroxidases. This iron is not available for hemoglobin formation, even in severe iron deficiency anemia. The storage forms of iron are ferritin and hemosiderin, which are found in appreciable amounts only in the liver and in the macrophages of the spleen and bone marrow (Valberg 1978). The iron in the macrophages is intimately related to the generation and destruction of red blood cells while iron enters or leaves the liver in relation to the plasma iron concentration. Ferritin is a large water-soluble protein (molecular weight 450 000) with a hollow core in which iron is sequestered. Each tissue produces characteristic isoferritins that are immunologically and electrophoretically distinct; the functions and interrelations of these various ferritins are as yet unknown. Hemosiderin consists mainly of aggregated ferritin molecules, is less soluble and is probably a more stable form of storage iron. The largest iron stores are in the liver, the marrow and the muscles (Valberg 1978).

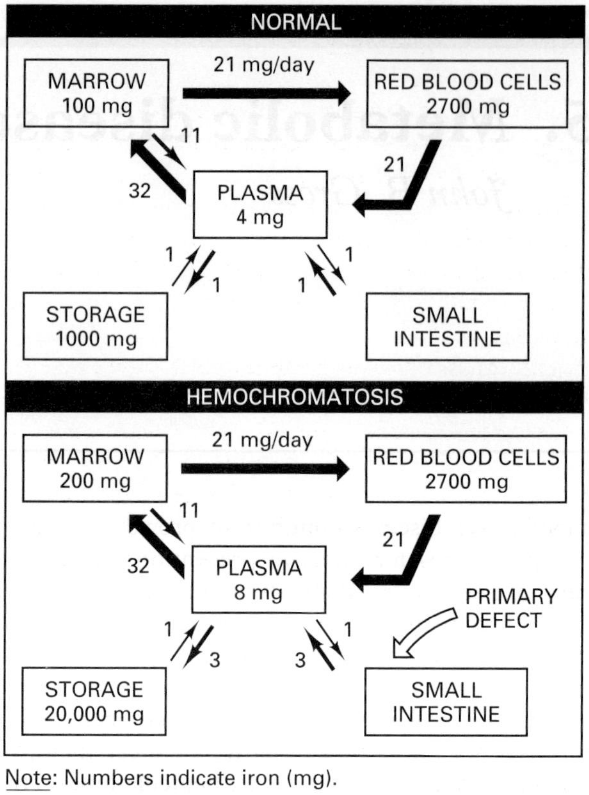


**Fig. 35.1** Iron metabolism in the normal adult and in hemochromatosis (Smith 1990).

## Genetic (idiopathic) hemochromatosis

*Etiology*

The mechanisms whereby iron accumulates in the body

and the nature of the defect in the control of body iron are gradually becoming clearer.

***Inheritance.*** Genetic hemochromatosis is the most common hereditary disease. Confusion in the past regarding the genetic basis of the disease reflected the fact that hemochromatosis presents clinically at a late stage and that methods for identifying asymptomatic patients and potential carriers of any defect were not available. The demonstration of an association with the histocompatibility antigen in patients with hemochromatosis has clarified the situation.

The disease is inherited as an autosomal recessive trait determined by a gene on chromosome 6 that is in close proximity to the A locus of the HLA complex (Simon et al 1980, Simon & Brissot 1988). The HLA-A3 phenotype is found in about 70% of patients with genetic hemochromatosis (Edwards et al 1982). Family studies using HLA typing and linkage analysis allow homozygotes and heterozygotes to be identified (Bassett et al 1981, Edwards et al 1981). Despite its close proximity to the HLA-A locus, the gene has not yet been isolated and the gene product is unknown. Increased serum transferrin saturation or ferritin concentrations occur in about a quarter of heterozygotes and they have increased amounts of iron in the liver but do not develop clinical or biochemical evidence of liver damage. LeSage et al (1983) have found that hepatic iron overload in genetic hemochromatosis develops regardless of alcohol consumption but that affected individuals present with advanced disease at lower iron concentrations if they also happen to drink. In Western countries and Australia the gene frequency is about 5%, which means that roughly 1 in 10 persons is heterozygous and 1 in 200 has the disease (Edwards et al 1988). The discrepancy between the expected and observed prevalences of the disease is probably due partly to lack of recognition and partly to incomplete phenotypic expression (Bacon 1992).

***Pathophysiology.*** The basic defect lies in the failure of the intestinal mucosal cells to limit iron absorption and early in the development of the disease the amount of iron absorbed is several times normal. Later, iron absorption falls as the condition progresses and is usually normal by the time the disease is diagnosed. Normal absorption, however, is inappropriately high when the total body iron is greatly increased. Mean absorption after iron removal therapy reaches four times normal and increased absorption continues for 5 years or more after the completion of therapy. The uptake of iron into the intestinal mucosal cell is normal, but an increased proportion of that iron is then transported into the body (McLaren et al 1988). The intestinal cells, particularly the duodenal absorptive epithelial cells, contain little or no ferritin, which may limit their ability to retain iron and make it available for loss into the gut (Fracanzani et al 1989). In secondary hemochromatosis there is downregulation of transferrin-receptor gene expression and an increase in ferritin mRNA content in duodenal epithelial cells. By contrast, downregulation of the transferrin-receptor gene is absent and intestinal cell ferritin mRNA levels are abnormally low in patients with genetic hemochromatosis (Lombard et al 1990, Pietrangelo et al 1992).

Defects have also been proposed in the liver and in the reticuloendothelial system in genetic hemochromatosis. Liver abnormality is unlikely to be important. Transferrin receptors are appropriately absent in genetic hemochromatosis when the hepatic iron content is high and reappear as iron is removed (Lombard et al 1989) and iron overload disappeared spontaneously after a liver from a donor with genetic hemochromatosis was transplanted into a patient with fulminant hepatic failure (Adams et al 1991a). A generalized defect in the ability of macrophages to retain iron has been described in genetic hemochromatosis, but the importance of this is unknown (Fillet et al 1989).

*Pathology*

***Liver.*** (Powell & Kerr 1975). The main features are a heavy deposition of iron, fibrosis and eventually cirrhosis, which is usually micronodular (Fig. 35.2). Inflammatory changes are characteristically absent or minimal. The iron is deposited mainly in the hepatocytes but also in Kupffer cells, portal tracts and areas of fibrosis. Histologically, the amount of iron in the liver may be graded semiquantitatively. Fibrosis is mild or absent early in the disease, when the patient is asymptomatic. By the time the iron concentration reaches 400 μmol/g (23 000 μg/g) dry weight, fibrosis and/or cirrhosis occurs (Bassett et al 1986). The portal tracts become expanded and fine fibrous septa radiate into the parenchyma giving a "holly leaf" pattern that progresses to cirrhosis. The junction between fibrous tissue and parenchyma is well defined and piecemeal necrosis is not seen. The parenchymal cells may contain fat and much lipofuscin is present.

The pathological similarities in genetic and secondary hemochromatosis and the correlation of hepatic fibrosis with the iron load in idiopathic and secondary hemochromatosis support the view that iron is important in causing fibrosis. Animal experiments show that iron overload has to be present for a long time to produce serious liver damage.

***Other organs.*** Excess iron deposition occurs mainly in the pancreas, heart and joint synovia and in the anterior pituitary, thyroid, parathyroid and adrenal glands. Fibrosis is an almost constant finding in the pancreas but does not occur in the other endocrine organs. In the heart, iron is deposited mainly in the myocardium, which

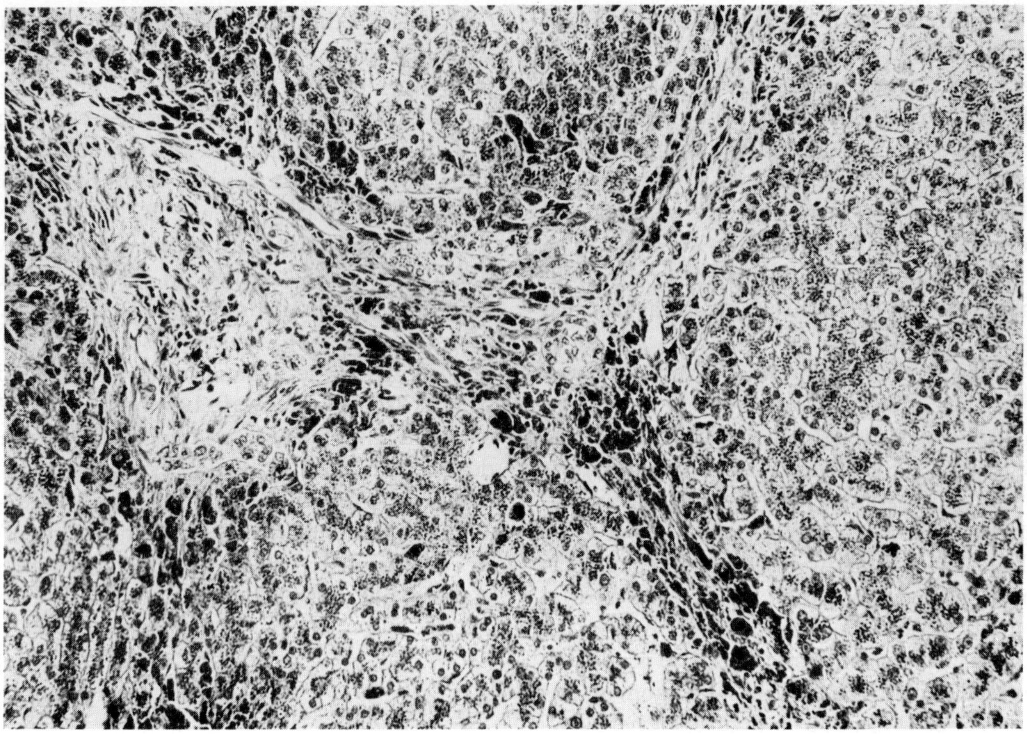

**Fig. 35.2** Hemochromatosis. Note the stellate fibrosis. Heavy iron deposits are present in the hepatocytes and in macrophages in the fibrous tissue (hematoxylin and eosin, ×10).

may show muscle degeneration and fibrosis. There are heavy iron deposits in synovial tissue and degenerative changes occur in the related cartilaginous tissue. The skin in genetic hemochromatosis has a characteristic pigmentation due to increased melanin deposition, although iron deposition may also occur there. Testicular atrophy occurs in about a quarter of cases, but iron deposition is usually scanty. In contrast to secondary iron overload, relatively little iron is found in the spleen, marrow and small bowel mucosa.

### *Clinical features*

Genetic hemochromatosis is about 10 times more common in men than in women and usually presents between the ages of 40 and 60 years (Fig. 35.3). Instances have been reported in childhood (Finch & Finch 1955, Perkins et al 1965) and in women who were still menstruating even though menstruation and pregnancy are thought to protect women by providing a source of blood loss (Lloyd et al 1964). Table 35.2 shows the main features at presentation in a large series of patients (Niederau et al 1985). Historically, most patients have presented with skin pigmentation, diabetes mellitus, cardiac failure or impotence. Patients in the precirrhotic stage of the disease have less florid features and may present with fatigue or arthralgia in the absence of signs of liver disease. Clinical evidence of advanced liver disease at presentation is unusual, as increasing numbers of patients are being diagnosed at an

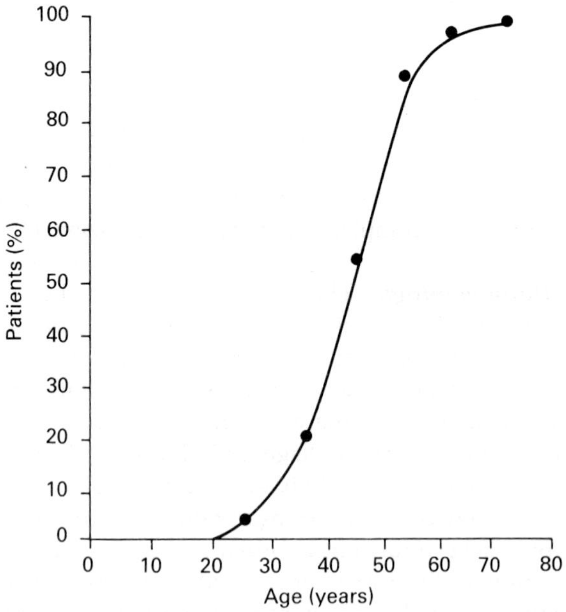


**Fig. 35.3** Age at onset of symptoms of idiopathic hemochromatosis in 787 patients (Finch & Finch 1955).

**Table 35.2** Clinical features at the time of diagnosis in genetic hemochromatosis (Niederau et al 1985)

| Features | Patients (number = 163; cirrhosis = 112) | | |
|---|---|---|---|
| | All patients (%) | Cirrhosis (%) | Precirrhosis (%) |
| *Symptoms* | | | |
| Weakness, lethargy | 83 | 88 | 73 |
| Abdominal pain | 58 | 67 | 39 |
| Arthralgia | 43 | 44 | 41 |
| Loss of libido, impotence | 38 | 43 | 25 |
| Amenorrhea | 22 | 18 | 29 |
| Dyspnea | 15 | 15 | 16 |
| Psychoneurotic symptoms | 6 | 7 | 2 |
| *Signs* | | | |
| Hepatomegaly | 83 | 90 | 69 |
| Pigmentation | 75 | 79 | 69 |
| Loss of body hair | 20 | 23 | 12 |
| Splenomegaly | 13 | 17 | 4 |
| Edema | 12 | 14 | 6 |
| Jaundice | 10 | 13 | 2 |
| Gynecomastia | 8 | 9 | 7 |
| Ascites | 6 | 9 | 0 |
| Esophageal varices | 9 | 13 | 0 |
| *Diabetes mellitus* | | | |
| Non-insulin-dependent | 22 | 27 | 12 |
| Insulin-dependent | 33 | 44 | 8 |
| Impaired glucose tolerance | 10 | 9 | 14 |

asymptomatic stage, primarily due to the inclusion of serum iron indices in many routine biochemical analyses.

***Liver disease.*** Hepatomegaly is a common feature and peripheral evidence of chronic liver disease may be present, but jaundice and ascites are infrequent. Iron removal therapy regularly leads to a reduction in the size of the liver and to improvement in the liver tests. Histologically, iron disappears from the liver and whatever inflammation was present is reduced. Fibrosis occasionally regresses but is usually unchanged (Williams 1971).

***Pigmentation.*** Dusky brown skin pigmentation is more prominent on the exposed parts of the body, especially the forehead and cheeks, and in the body creases. Pigment may also be found in the lips, gums, buccal mucosa, tongue and around the optic disc. It is caused by an excess production of melanin, the cause of which is unknown. There may also be an increase of iron in the skin, especially related to the sweat glands, but it is rarely marked. Iron removal therapy usually leads to lessening of pigmentation (Cawley et al 1969).

***Diabetes mellitus.*** This is common, particularly in patients with cirrhosis (Table 35.2). Dymock et al (1972) studied 115 patients and found impaired glucose tolerance in 11% in addition to the 63% with overt diabetes mellitus. Diabetes mellitus may improve when the hemochromatosis is treated, leading to a reduction in the therapy needed for the diabetes.

***Cardiomyopathy.*** Cardiac dysfunction is rare at presentation but is an important cause of death. The usual manifestations are cardiomyopathy or cardiac arrhythmias. Cardiac dysfunction sometimes begins suddenly and progresses rapidly (Borsey & Lawson 1982). Response to conventional therapy for cardiac failure is poor, but iron removal may be effective and has reduced the frequency of cardiac complications (Easley et al 1972).

***Arthropathy.*** Any joint can be affected, but the second and third metacarpophalangeal joints are most commonly involved. The remaining joints of the hands may become involved along with the wrists, shoulders, knees and hips. The distribution of the changes resembles rheumatoid arthritis. Pain, stiffness, bony swelling and limitation of movement are common in the joints of the hands but are much less common in the larger joints. Radiological changes in the hand joints include loss of cartilage, sclerosis of the metacarpal heads and thinning of the bony cortex; in larger joints, loss of cartilage and chondrocalcinosis are the main changes. Chondrocalcinosis is caused by the deposition of calcium pyrophosphate dehydrate crystals and this can occasionally cause acute attacks of pseudogout. Arthropathy occurs in both primary and secondary iron overload and is not improved by iron removal treatment.

***Endocrine abnormalities.*** Hypogonadism leading to loss of libido, testicular atrophy and loss of body hair (Table 35.2) is the most frequent abnormality (Kley et al 1985). It is commonly attributed to deficient function of the anterior pituitary gland, in which marked iron deposits are usually found. Clinical hypogonadism is usually hypogonadotrophic in origin and does not often improve after iron removal treatment.

***Infection.*** Patients with genetic hemochromatosis are susceptible to infection because of excess tissue iron. Iron overload impairs phagocytosis (van Asbeck et al 1982) and may favor the growth of iron-limited organisms such as *Listeria monocytogenes* (van Asbeck et al 1982) and *Yersinia enterocolitica* (Capron et al 1984).

### *Laboratory tests*

Tests are directed at demonstrating excessive iron stores, excluding secondary causes, and assessing the extent of liver disease. Table 35.3 shows the results of investigations in one large study of idiopathic hemochromatosis.

***Iron and transferrin (iron-binding capacity).*** These are the most widely available measurements for detecting the possibility of excess iron stores, although they are not very specific (p. 747). The serum iron almost always exceeds 36 μmol/L (200 mg/dl) in hemochromatosis and is rarely above 28 μmol/L when the liver iron is below 10 μmol/100 mg of liver tissue (Brissot et al 1981). A transferrin saturation greater than 60% accurately predicted the homozygous genotype in two large studies (Dadone et al 1982, Milman 1991). However, in a large Red Cross screening study involving over 11 000 healthy donors, a

**Table 35.3** Laboratory features of iron overload in 163 patients with genetic hemochromatosis (Niederau et al 1985)

| Measurement | With cirrhosis (mean ± SE) | Without cirrhosis (mean ± SE) |
|---|---|---|
| Plasma iron (μmol/L; μg/dl) | 38±1; 230±7 | 35±1; 210±8 |
| Transferrin saturation (%) | 95±2 | 87±3 |
| Serum ferritin (μg/L) | 3376±325 | 2280±332 |
| Iron removed by venesection (g) | 27.8±1.1 | 20.3±1.3 |

transferrin saturation of 62% detected only 60% of the expected number of female homozygotes (Edwards et al 1988), leading to the suggestion that a threshold of 50% be used to screen women (Edwards & Kushner 1993). The transferrin saturation exceeds 60% in more than two-thirds of patients presenting with genetic hemochromatosis and constitutes strong evidence of iron overload. The increased saturation is a result of both increased serum iron and decreased serum transferrin. A high serum iron concentration and a high transferrin saturation are not, however, diagnostic of genetic hemochromatosis, as they also occur in secondary iron overload, hemolysis and ineffective erythropoiesis. Furthermore, there is no relationship between these measurements and the degree of iron overload. They indicate only that excess iron stores may be present.

***Ferritin.*** The serum ferritin concentration is related quantitatively to the total body iron and increased concentrations are good evidence of excess iron stores (p. 748). In genetic hemochromatosis, the serum ferritin reflects the iron content of the liver rather than a homozygous genotype for the disease. Thus, the serum ferritin usually exceeds 1000 μg/L in symptomatic patients (Chapman et al 1982) but is normal in asymptomatic homozygotes who do not yet have significant hepatic iron overload (Wands et al 1976). The serum ferritin is only about 70% accurate in predicting the homozygous genotype (Dadone et al 1982). Furthermore, a high serum ferritin is not diagnostic of genetic hemochromatosis, as high concentrations occur in alcoholic liver disease, falling when alcohol abuse ceases (p. 873), and in acute and chronic hepatitis where the disease is active. The plasma ferritin can also be increased in inflammatory disease unrelated to the liver, as it is an acute-phase reactant (p. 748).

The serum ferritin is now regarded as a good screening test for excess body iron in the relatives of patients with genetic hemochromatosis who have not yet developed cirrhosis.

***Liver biopsy.*** Liver biopsy establishes the extent of liver damage and the presence of excess iron. Perl's stain (Prussian blue) is used to demonstrate hemosiderin and the amount in the liver cells can be graded (Scheuer et al 1962). Histologic estimates of iron content correlate well with direct measurements of tissue iron and patients with genetic hemochromatosis can usually be distinguished by the grade of parenchymal iron staining (Barry 1974, Brissot et al 1981). The normal liver iron is 500–900 μg/g (10–16 μmol/g) dry liver and in symptomatic genetic hemochromatosis the concentration reaches 21 000 ± 2300 μg/g (375 ± 41 μmol/g) (Chapman et al 1982). Direct measurement of iron in liver biopsy tissue allows calculation of the hepatic iron index (the hepatic iron concentration divided by the age of the patient), which is based upon the fact that individuals with genetic hemochromatosis accumulate hepatic iron progressively with time. Values ≥1.9 μmol/g dry liver/year (100 μg/g dry liver/year) are characteristic of the homozygous genotype, while heterozygotes rarely have an index greater than 1.5 μmol/g dry liver/year (88 μg/g dry liver/year) (Summers et al 1990). If the hepatic iron determination is not possible, an analogous index expressing the degree of histological iron staining per year of age may help separate homozygotes from heterozygotes (Deugnier et al 1993).

***Imaging.*** Hepatic iron concentrations above about 170 μmol/g dry liver (10 000 μg/g dry liver) are detectable by computed tomography or magnetic resonance imaging and are relatively specific for iron overload (Guyader et al 1989, 1992, Harada et al 1992). However, both techniques are insensitive in detecting iron concentrations below this level and cannot therefore be used to diagnose homozygous patients in earlier stages of iron accumulation.

***Iron removal.*** Phlebotomy, in addition to being therapeutic, confirms that excess iron has been present if removal of 500 ml blood at weekly intervals does not reduce the serum iron concentration or produce a 25% fall in the hemoglobin concentration within 8 weeks. Most patients require the removal of 20 g iron (80 units of blood) or more before becoming depleted of iron.

***Diagnostic approach.*** Patients presenting with chronic liver disease should have the serum ferritin and/or the transferrin saturation measured. A serum ferritin above 1000 μg/L or a transferrin saturation above 60% strongly suggests iron overload but is not specific enough for diagnosis and in such cases a liver biopsy should be done. Histological evidence of clear iron excess (Grades 3 and 4) is sufficient for diagnosis, but the liver iron should be measured chemically where possible. Venesection therapy can be carried out where the diagnosis is in doubt or where other factors such as impaired blood coagulation preclude liver biopsy. The serum ferritin and the transferrin saturation should be used in screening asymptomatic relatives (above), even if they are apparently healthy, and suggestive results require that a liver biopsy be done for determination of the tissue iron and calculation of the hepatic iron index.

*Treatment*

The treatment of idiopathic hemochromatosis is to

remove the excess body iron. This is done by weekly phlebotomy of 500 ml blood containing about 250 mg iron. As the total body iron varies from 10 to 40 g, this regimen may have to be continued for 1–3 years. The amount of iron removed by venesection is closely related to the amount of iron removed from the liver (Brissot et al 1981). The hemoglobin concentration is measured before each phlebotomy and the serum ferritin is measured monthly (Garry & Saiki 1982). The former may fall initially, but thereafter increased erythropoiesis maintains it within 10% of the initial values until the iron stores are depleted. The serum ferritin falls gradually.

Once the iron stores have been removed, reaccumulation is prevented by phlebotomy every 1–3 months. Patients with coincidental thalassemia trait or other mild chronic anemias can usually be depleted of iron successfully without further aggravation of anemia. Desferrioxamine given by infusion may induce marked urinary iron excretion (below), but it is only important when iron must be removed quickly, as in those with cardiac failure (Volkholz et al 1984, De Bont et al 1987). An iron-free diet is unnecessary, as the amount of iron absorbed from a normal diet is small relative to that lost by phlebotomy. Iron removal therapy leads to increased well-being and improvement in skin pigmentation, cardiac failure and diabetes mellitus. Hypogonadism may benefit from testosterone therapy.

### *Prognosis*

Williams et al (1969) studied patients treated before and soon after the introduction of venesection and showed that this therapy clearly improved survival. Eighteen untreated patients survived a mean of 4.9 years, whereas 40 treated patients survived 8.2 years and showed regression of their disease. Niederau et al (1985) analyzed a group of patients diagnosed between 1959 and 1983 and found that the prognosis for most patients was excellent. Patients without cirrhosis had the same life expectancy as the normal population. Positive prognostic indicators included absence of cirrhosis, absence of diabetes and depletion of iron within 18 months of beginning phlebotomy (Table 35.4). Adams et al (1991b) reviewed patients diagnosed between 1953 and 1989 and found that cirrhosis was the main determinant of survival. Patients with cirrhosis were 5.5 times more likely to die and accounted for deaths due to liver failure and hepatocellular carcinoma. The main causes of death related to genetic hemochromatosis are hepatocellular carcinoma, liver failure, variceal bleeding, cardiac failure and the consequences of diabetes mellitus (Table 35.5).

Hepatocellular carcinoma has become the most common cause of death in genetic hemochromatosis. Finch & Finch (1955) reported that it caused about 15% of deaths in their series, whereas later series have reported frequencies of 37% (Powell et al 1971), 29% (Bomford & Williams 1976) and 30% (Niederau et al 1985). Hepatocellular carcinoma in hemochromatosis rarely occurs before the age of 40 years and increases in frequency in linear fashion thereafter. Patients with precirrhotic hemochromatosis do not have an increased risk of hepatocellular carcinoma after adequate iron removal, but patients with cirrhosis remain at risk indefinitely and should be put on a regular surveillance program. One such regimen would consist of annual imaging with determination of the serum alpha-fetoprotein.

**Table 35.4** Cumulative survival in genetic hemochromatosis and in an age- and sex-matched normal population (Niederau et al 1985)

| Group | Cumulative survival (%) | | | |
|---|---|---|---|---|
| | 5 yrs | 10 yrs | 15 yrs | 20 yrs |
| Hemochromatosis | | | | |
| Without cirrhosis | 98 | 80 | 69 | 69 |
| With cirrhosis | 89 | 72 | 55 | 42 |
| Without diabetes mellitus | 98 | 90 | 75 | 75 |
| With diabetes mellitus | 88 | 65 | 45 | 37 |
| Iron depleted ≤ 18 months | 98 | 90 | 75 | 75 |
| Not iron depleted ≤ 18 months | 85 | 63 | 50 | 35 |
| Normal population | 96 | 88 | 78 | 65 |

**Table 35.5** Causes of death in 163 patients with genetic hemochromatosis (from Niederau et al 1985)

| Cause | Number | % | Mortality ratio (observed/expected)* |
|---|---|---|---|
| Hepatocellular carcinoma | 16 | 30 | 219.4 |
| Hepatic cirrhosis | 10 | 19 | 12.8 |
| Cardiomyopathy | 3 | 5.7 | 306.3 |
| Diabetes mellitus | 3 | 5.7 | 7.1 |
| All causes | 53 | 100 | 3.0 |

*Note: Significantly more deaths in all categories than expected.

### *Prevention*

Siblings of a patient with genetic hemochromatosis have an approximately 25% chance of having the disease and a 50% chance of being a heterozygote carrier. Parents are almost always carriers but may occasionally be undiagnosed homozygotes and should therefore also be screened. In Western countries, assuming random association of sexual partners, children of an index patient have an approximately 5% chance of being affected with the disease (10% chance that the patient's partner is a heterozygote and 50% chance of passing the abnormal gene). Edwards & Kushner (1993) have recommended routine measurement of the transferrin saturation as a screening measure in the medical population at large, with subsequent measurement of the serum ferritin if the transferrin saturation is over 50% and a liver biopsy for iron determination if both blood test results are elevated. In screening first-degree relatives of an index case, they believe the transferrin saturation is a reliable marker and would add the serum ferritin only in doubtful cases. It should be remembered that body iron stores increase with age, so in cases under 40 where the screening tests are normal, the tests should be repeated every 4–5 years. If any one test is abnormal, then a liver biopsy should be carried out.

Once the diagnosis is established in an index case by liver biopsy, HLA phenotyping may be used in that family to find others with the disease, with about 97% accuracy (Powell et al 1990). However, the method is expensive and does not necessarily indicate the presence of iron overload, so does not relieve the physician of the necessity of doing a liver biopsy (Beaumont et al 1979, Bassett et al 1981).

## Secondary hemochromatosis

There are several causes of secondary hemochromatosis (Table 35.6). Differentiation from genetic hemochromatosis is not usually difficult except where hepatic iron accumulation has occurred as a result of cirrhosis from another cause.

### *Anemia, ineffective erythropoiesis and blood transfusion*

Iron overload is frequent in anemia in which blood transfusions are required over a number of years (Schafer et al 1981). The main conditions in which this occurs are shown in Table 35.6. Much of the iron is derived from the transfused blood, but increased iron absorption can also occur when there is increased marrow activity resulting from increased but ineffective erythropoiesis. Barron et al (1989) studied the family of a patient with refractory sideroblastic anemia and concluded that patients with refractory anemia and significant iron overload probably have at least one allele for genetic hemochromatosis. Ineffective erythropoiesis on its own can occasionally be associated with iron overload, as in primary shunt hyperbilirubinemia (Frank et al 1979). Extensive tissue iron deposition occurs in all who have received over 100 units (50 L) of blood. Hepatic damage may be due to a combination of excess iron in the liver (Risdon et al 1975) and transfusion-related chronic hepatitis C (p. 788). Children with these conditions have often developed cirrhosis by the end of the second decade of life. Phlebotomy therapy is not usually possible. Desferrioxamine does not mobilize much iron and needs to be injected daily, but it is most effective given by infusion in large amounts and with ascorbic acid to increase the amount of iron available for chelation (Lancet 1984). Urinary iron excretion can reach 3700 mg/month in heavily iron overloaded patients (Propper et al 1977).

**Table 35.6** Causes of secondary hemochromatosis

| |
|---|
| Chronic anemia, ineffective erythropoiesis, multiple blood transfusions |
| Thalassemia major |
| Sickle cell anemia |
| Hereditary spherocytosis |
| Sideroblastic anemia |
| Idiopathic hypoplastic anemia |
| Primary shunt hyperbilirubinemia |
| Excess iron ingestion |
| Iron therapy |
| Dietary (e.g. Bantu) |
| Cirrhosis |
| Portacaval shunt |
| Porphyria cutanea tarda |
| Xanthinuria |
| Congenital transferrin deficiency |

### *Oral iron*

Iron overload may be due to a diet rich in iron. This occurs in the South African Bantu, who drink beer rich in iron from having been brewed in iron pots (Gordeuk et al 1986). The daily iron intake in Bantu males may reach 50–100 mg and at autopsy over a third of adult Bantu males have grossly increased iron stores (Brink et al 1976). Relatively few develop clinical features of iron overload and a recent family study suggests that it may be caused by an interaction between the amount of dietary iron and a gene distinct from the HLA-linked gene (Gordeuk et al 1992). Red wine may be a source of excess iron for alcoholics in Western countries, containing as much as 12 mg/L (Barry et al 1970). Prolonged oral iron therapy only rarely leads to a gross increase in body iron (Johnson 1968).

### *Cirrhosis*

For reasons that remain unclear, body iron stores are increased in a third to a half of patients with cirrhosis, although rarely to the extent seen in genetic hemochromatosis (Barry et al 1970). This occurs most often in alcoholic cirrhosis. Some patients with cirrhosis gradually accumulate hepatic iron until the distinction from hemochromatosis is difficult clinically. Measurement of iron in the liver, however, shows amounts much less than in hemochromatosis and the hepatic iron index is less than 1.9. Iron removal in such patients shows that the total body iron rarely exceeds 10 g and therapy does not bring the benefits seen in idiopathic hemochromatosis. Greater iron overload in an alcoholic patient should be regarded as due to the coexistence of genetic hemochromatosis.

### *Portasystemic shunt surgery*

Conn (1972) reported that portacaval anastomosis resulted in an increase in the frequency and amount of hepatic iron deposition. Adams et al (1994) more recently studied 26 consecutive nonalcoholic cirrhotic patients who had previously had portacaval shunts and then liver transplantation and compared them with 37 transplanted patients who had cirrhosis but no shunt. Although many of the shunted patients had increased iron staining, only six of 26 actually had elevated hepatic iron concentrations, versus three of 37 controls. The two highest iron measurements were in patients with liver iron stores of 2.6 g and 3.3 g. This compares with values of up to 1.5 g in normal people and 25–30 g or more in hemochromatosis.

### *Other causes*

Excess iron in the liver occurs in porphyria cutanea tarda, congenital transferrin deficiency and xanthinuria. Increased amounts of iron in the liver also occur in patients on long-term hemodialysis (Kothari et al 1980).

## WILSON'S DISEASE

Wilson's disease (Wilson 1912), or hepatolenticular degeneration, is a hereditary condition resulting in the accumulation of excess body copper that causes a variety of hepatic, neurologic and/or psychiatric manifestations. It is caused by a defect in the gene on chromosome 13 that codes a membrane-bound ATPase copper transport protein (Bull et al 1993, Tanzi et al 1993).

The accumulation of tissue copper is considered the cause of organ damage and some of the effects of the disease can be reversed by copper reduction therapy. The liver is the site of the main metabolic defect, which is therefore cured by liver transplantation (Groth et al 1973). Subsequent reviews have made only minor improvements on the comprehensive and now classic monograph by Scheinberg & Sternlieb (1984).

### *Inheritance and prevalence*

Wilson's disease is transmitted in an autosomal recessive manner and consequently men and women are affected approximately equally. Heterozygotes do not develop the disease. Current estimations of the prevalence and the gene frequency suggest that the disease is significantly underdiagnosed (Walshe 1984). In western Caucasian populations, the gene frequency is approximately 0.5%, the carrier rate is about 1 in 100 and the disease prevalence is about 1 in 30 000. Once the diagnosis is established in an index case, siblings have a 25% chance of having the disease and a 50% chance of being heterozygous. Offspring have roughly a 0.5% chance of having the disease (1% chance of the patient's spouse being a heterozygote and a 50% chance of passing the gene). The gene for Wilson's disease has been cloned recently and shows a 60% homology with the gene for Menkes' disease (p. 965), an inherited disorder of copper deficiency (Bull et al 1993, Tanzi et al 1993). Four mutations have been reported thus far, but they have accounted for only one-third of 50 American patients tested (Tanzi et al 1993). Accordingly, the gene defects are probably heterogeneous and unlikely to lead to a specific diagnostic test.

### *Normal copper metabolism* (Dowdy 1969, Sternlieb 1980, Walshe 1995)

The human body contains 100–150 mg of copper and the normal daily intake is about 2–5 mg matched in health by an equal excretion in the stools and urine (Fig. 35.4). Copper is absorbed rapidly from the stomach and upper small bowel into the portal blood, where it is bound mainly to albumin. It is then taken up avidly by the hepatocytes, where it is bound to two cytosolic copper-binding proteins of low molecular weight. From the cytosolic pool, copper is incorporated into ceruloplasmin, other copper-containing proteins such as cytochrome c oxidase and superoxide dismutase, or is taken up by the lysosomes. Copper is stored in the liver and leaves it either by passing into the blood incorporated into ceruloplasmin or by passing into the bile. It enters the bile in a protein-bound form that is not reabsorbed from the intestine. Copper has several functions in the body, acting most frequently as a catalyst. Its most vital function is in energy metabolism as the prosthetic group in cytochrome c oxidase. It is also important for collagen and elastin synthesis, normal erythropoiesis, conversion of tyrosine to melanin and perhaps myelin synthesis.

### *Copper metabolism in Wilson's disease*

In Wilson's disease there is a high copper concentration in several tissues, especially in the liver, brain, cornea and kidneys. The liver concentration may be up to 100 times normal and the brain concentration up to 10 times normal. Normal newborns have a high copper concentration in the liver and the concentrations of copper and ceruloplasmin in the blood are low. The liver copper falls to normal adult levels over the first 3 months of life and this is accompanied by a steady increase of the ceruloplasmin in the blood. These changes do not occur in Wilson's disease, in which impaired biliary copper excretion and poor incorporation of copper into ceruloplasmin result in hepatic copper accumulation. Once the storage capacity of the liver is surpassed, copper begins to accumulate elsewhere and this may account for

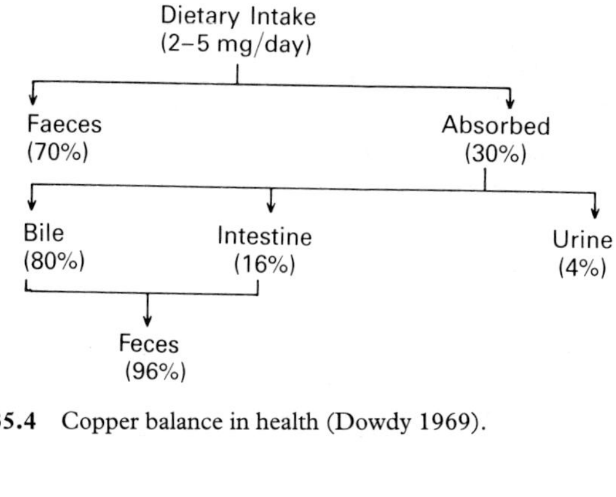


**Fig. 35.4** Copper balance in health (Dowdy 1969).

the frequent occurrence of liver disease in childhood while neurological features rarely occur before the age of 10 years. The mechanisms of copper accumulation should be elucidated by a better understanding of the normal role of the membrane-bound copper-transporting ATPase that is defective in Wilson's disease. It is likely that the defect is present in the canalicular membrane of the hepatocyte.

When radioactive copper is given to normal persons, it is rapidly taken up by the liver and later re-enters the blood incorporated into ceruloplasmin. In Wilson's disease the incorporation of copper into ceruloplasmin occurs very slowly or not at all, despite the liver's ability to synthesize normal apoceruloplasmin (Matsuda et al 1974). The plasma ceruloplasmin may be low in heterozygotes without any excess tissue copper. Conversely, occasional patients with Wilson's disease have normal ceruloplasmin concentrations (Scheinberg & Sternlieb 1963) due to the fact that ceruloplasmin is an acute-phase reactant during inflammation and its induction may occur in Wilson's disease despite the low basal synthesis rate.

## Pathogenesis

Copper accumulation in the liver precedes the development of tissue damage and appears to be its main cause, as removal of copper by treatment prevents further tissue damage. Copper may damage liver cells in a variety of ways. Possible mechanisms include alteration of lysosomal and plasma membranes, interference with sulfhydryl-rich proteins such as tubulin and depletion of glutathione (Sternlieb 1994).

## Pathology

### *Liver*

Histological changes occur long before clinical evidence of liver disease. The earliest change is the deposition of triglyceride, giving rise to a fatty liver. Chronic portal and periportal hepatitis may develop, leading to periportal fibrosis and eventually to cirrhosis. This, together with fatty change and sometimes prominent glycogen vacuolation of liver cell nuclei, gives a characteristic but not pathognomonic appearance. In some patients with extensive hepatocyte necrosis, acidophilic bodies and Mallory's hyalin occur. Excess hepatic copper can be identified histochemically by rubeanic acid or rhodanine staining. Unfortunately, negative reactions occur in half or more of patients with Wilson's disease, in contrast to iron staining in hemochromatosis. Electronmicroscopy shows characteristic mitochondrial damage (Sternlieb 1993).

### *Central nervous system*

The main gross changes are seen in the corpus striatum, which is shrunken (Blackwood & Corsellis 1976). Cavitation often occurs in the putamen but rarely in the other nuclei. Occasionally, the cerebral and cerebellar white matter show softening or cavitation with atrophy of the overlying cortex. The putamen is also most affected histologically with a marked increase in Alzheimer cells and a decrease in the number of neurones. Lesser changes occur in the other thalamic and brainstem nuclei. Degeneration of neurones occurs in the cerebral cortex, especially the frontal lobes, and in the cerebellar cortex, but the brainstem and cord are virtually never affected.

### *Eye*

Microscopic examination of the cornea shows brown granules in Descemet's membrane near the limbus (Blackwood & Corsellis 1976). These granules, which are mainly on the inner surface of the membrane, contain copper. Occasionally, copper deposition in the lens causes a "sunflower cataract" that resembles the changes occurring when copper fragments enter the eye (Cairns et al 1969).

## Clinical features

Symptoms usually start between the ages of 5 and 25 years (Fig. 35.5). It is exceptional for the condition to occur earlier than 5 years of age, but about 10% of patients present after 25 years. Presentation after the age of 20 years is seen in 5% of patients with a hepatic syndrome and 40% of those with neuropsychiatric symptoms (Scheinberg & Sternlieb 1984). Rarely, patients remain asymptomatic until the fifth decade of life and a few patients have been diagnosed after age 50. The main manifestations are due to hepatic and neurological damage and to the deposition of copper in the cornea, leading to Kayser–Fleischer rings; other features include hemolysis, renal and skeletal damage and fever (Cartwright 1978). Although hepatic disease occurs predominantly in children and neurological disease in adolescents and adults, there is a considerable overlap

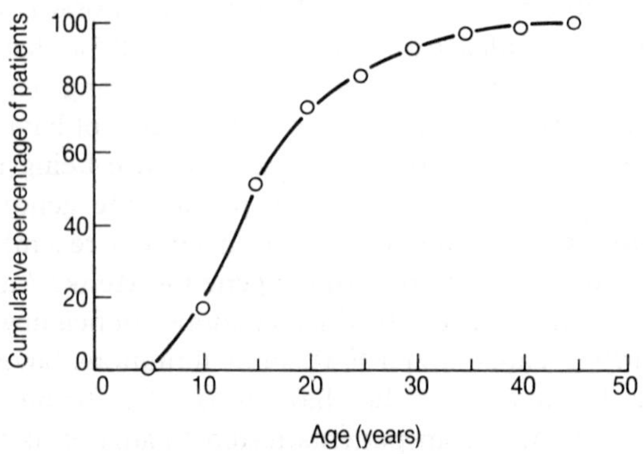


**Fig. 35.5** Age at development of symptoms in 121 patients with Wilson's disease (Sternlieb & Scheinberg 1968).

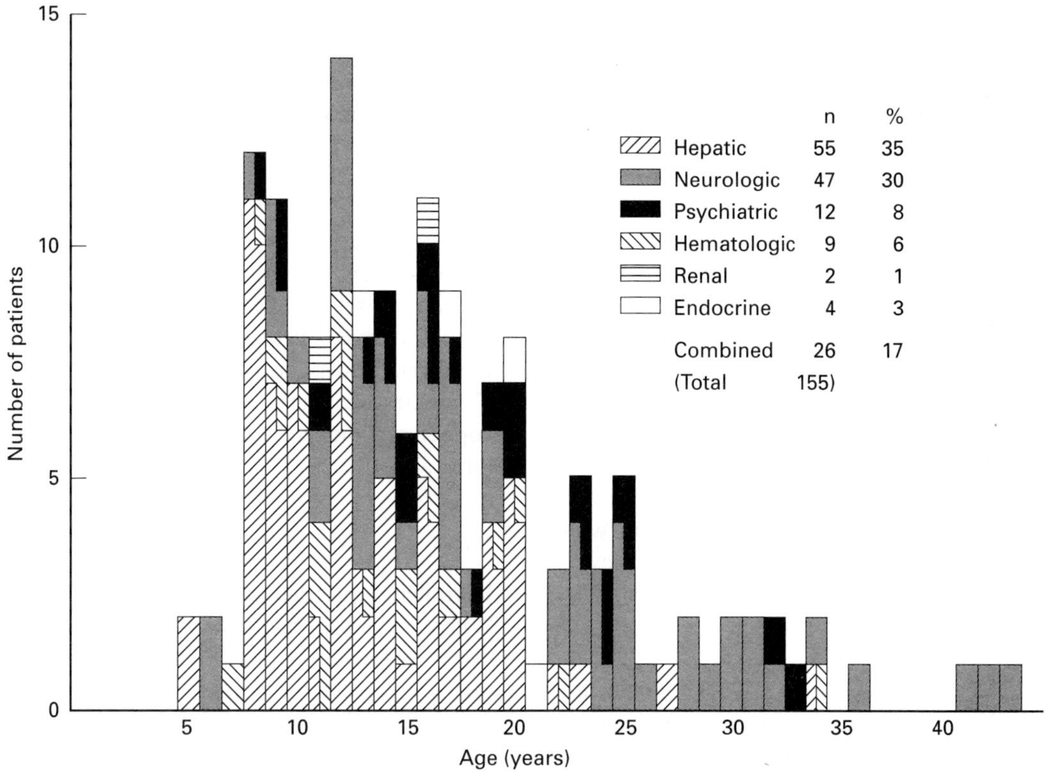


**Fig. 35.6** Presenting features in Wilson's disease related to age. Combined presentations are shown as vertically divided bars (Scheinberg & Sternlieb 1984).

leading to various combined clinical presentations in about 15% of patients (Fig. 35.6).

*Liver*

Liver damage in Wilson's disease may mimic any acute or chronic liver disease. The two most important clues to the diagnosis are a family history of hepatic or neurological disease and Kayser–Fleischer rings, but the family history is usually negative and hepatic disease may occur in the absence of Kayser–Fleischer rings. Acute hepatitis may be the first manifestation and recurrent acute hepatitis for which no cause can be found in a young person should always lead to a search for Wilson's disease, particularly if accompanied by hemolysis. Fulminant hepatic failure is a rare manifestation of Wilson's disease that is difficult to diagnose and almost uniformly fatal unless treated by liver transplantation (p. 807). Most patients with fulminant presentation already have cirrhosis, but acute necrosis without cirrhosis has been recorded (Enomoto et al 1989).

Chronic hepatitis may also be caused by Wilson's disease (Sternlieb & Scheinberg 1972, Scott et al 1978). Patients with chronic hepatitis of unknown cause who are under 40 years old should therefore be investigated fully to exclude Wilson's disease, as prompt treatment with penicillamine is life saving. Patients often present with the clinical features and complications of cirrhosis and portal hypertension, with minimal or no evidence of active hepatitis. Progression to hepatocellular carcinoma is rare (p. 965).

Spontaneous resolution of acute or chronic hepatitis cannot be taken as excluding Wilson's disease, as this may occur for unknown reasons only to be followed by neurological damage. Diagnosis in patients with liver disease can be difficult, as there may be no associated neurological abnormality, Kayser–Fleischer rings may not be seen and the plasma ceruloplasmin may be in the lower part of the normal range. This is particularly the case in children, as Kayser–Fleischer rings do not develop before the age of about 7 years and may not be found in older children with liver disease even with a slit-lamp examination (Sass-Kortsak 1975).

*Brain*

Most patients present with neuropsychiatric symptoms and many are referred initially to psychiatrists. Many patients are labeled as having behavioral or thought disorders for years prior to the correct diagnosis and many probably remain undiagnosed. Deterioration of performance at school is a frequent initial sign of the onset of this aspect of the illness. The psychiatric features are caused partly by the disease itself and partly by an emotional reaction to its distressing nature. They include bizarre behavior, anxiety, mania, depression, hysteria and occasionally schizophrenia.

The neurological features are usually mild at first, but they become progressively more severe. Inco-ordination and tremor are common initial features. Inco-ordination affects fine or complex movements and leads to deterioration in such activities as writing, sports and the playing of musical instruments. The tremor may be fine, coarse or occasionally choreoathetoid, localized or generalized and made worse by activity and emotion. Dysarthria becomes progressively worse with the development of microphasia and eventually aphasia and there may be a peculiar inspiratory laugh. Excessive salivation may be an early and especially distressing feature. Late manifestations include spasticity, rigidity, dystonia and dysphagia, any of which may be incapacitating.

*Eye*

The Kayser–Fleischer ring (Fig. 35.7) is the single most important clinical sign in Wilson's disease. It is present in nearly all adult symptomatic patients and in patients with neuropsychiatric symptoms. It may be difficult to see and should be sought by slit-lamp examination. It is seen first as a green-brown or golden-brown crescent of discoloration at the upper periphery of the cornea and should be viewed obliquely from above with a magnifying glass. The discoloration then appears at the lower margin of the cornea and later at the sides. During treatment, these deposits disappear gradually in the reverse order of their appearance.

Kayser–Fleischer rings visible to the naked eye are pathognomonic of Wilson's disease. Kayser–Fleischer rings found by slit-lamp examination have been reported in primary biliary cirrhosis, long-standing biliary atresia, chronic active hepatitis and cryptogenic cirrhosis (Fleming et al 1975, Frommer et al 1977). These patients generally have increased liver copper concentrations but few of the other biochemical features of Wilson's disease. False Kayser–Fleischer rings have been ascribed to bilirubin in severe jaundice (Weinberg et al 1981) and to carotene in vitamin A intoxication (Giorgio et al 1964).

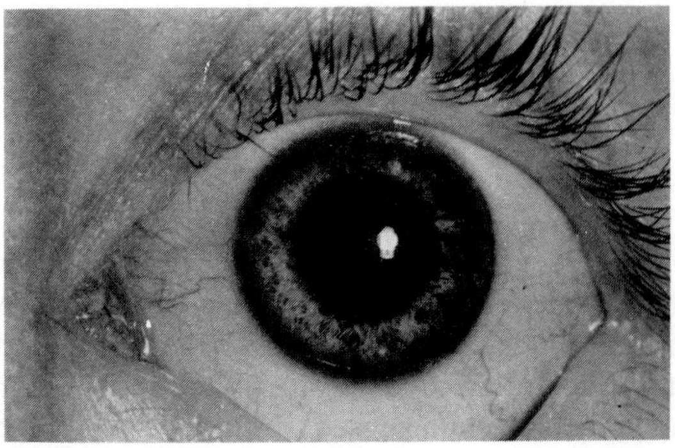

**Fig. 35.7** Kayser–Fleischer rings at the junction of the cornea and sclera in a patient with Wilson's disease.

*Kidney*

Clinical evidence of renal damage is usually minor and almost always occurs in patients already known to have Wilson's disease. Most of the abnormalities reflect renal tubular damage: proteinuria, glycosuria, uricosuria, hypercalciuria, phosphaturia, amino aciduria and hematuria. Hypercupriuria also occurs and results from abnormal copper metabolism. Renal rickets has been reported but is rare.

*Blood*

Hemolytic episodes are a well-recognized complication in Wilson's disease (Iser et al 1974). They are self-limited and show the usual laboratory features of hemolysis but may be very severe, leading to hemoglobin concentrations as low as 5 g/dl. The Coombs test is negative. A hemolytic episode may be the first sign of the disease and when associated with hepatic decompensation it may be rapidly fatal (above). Kayser–Fleischer rings are usually present. The hemolysis is thought to be caused by red blood cell damage due to the sudden release of a large amount of ionic copper into the blood. Serum copper concentrations are high and urinary copper excretion far exceeds that usually found in Wilson's disease. The hemolysis may be analogous to that seen in copper intoxication during hemodialysis (Manzler & Schreiner 1970). The source of the copper is probably the liver, although what causes its sudden release is unknown. Treatment with penicillamine prevents recurrence.

## Laboratory tests

Until diagnostic tests can be developed based on direct genetic analysis, the diagnosis of Wilson's disease continues to require the demonstration of coincident poor ceruloplasmin synthesis and excess body copper. This ordinarily requires a liver biopsy. Confirmation is desirable even when grossly observable Kayser–Fleischer rings are present, as they disappear during treatment and the original diagnosis may be questioned later.

*Ceruloplasmin*

The serum ceruloplasmin concentration is less than 20 mg/dl in almost all cases (Fig. 35.8). It is the most reliable of the routine biochemical tests for Wilson's disease (p. 751). It is normal or only slightly reduced in about 5% of patients, but concentrations above 30 mg/dl effectively exclude Wilson's disease (Sternlieb & Scheinberg 1979).

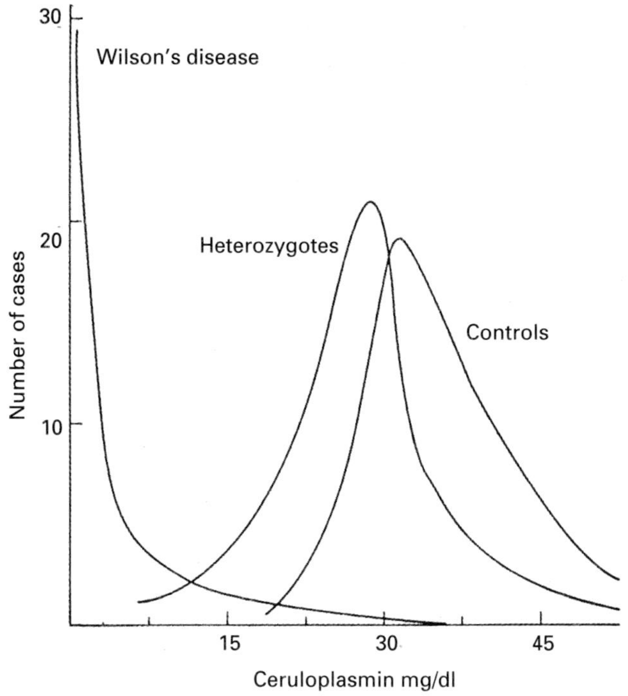


**Fig. 35.8** Distribution of plasma ceruloplasmin concentrations in normal persons ($n$ = 144), heterozygotes ($n$ = 150) and untreated patients with Wilson's disease ($n$ = 70) (Reprinted with permission from Walshe 1995).

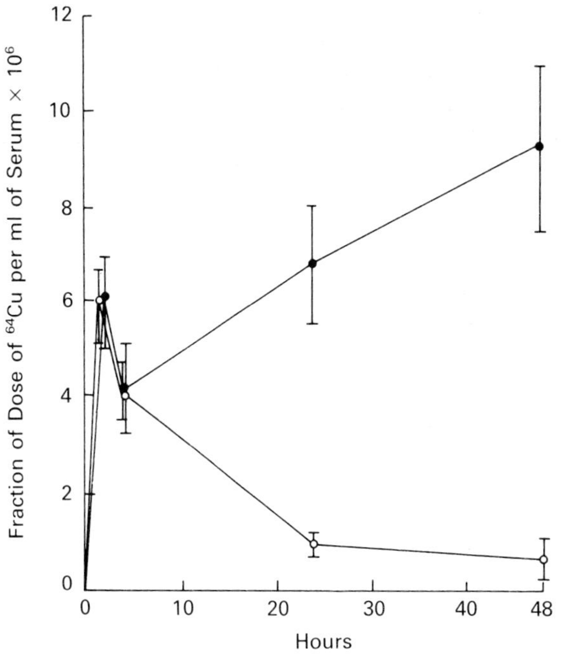


**Fig. 35.9** The concentration (mean ± standard error of mean) of radioactive copper ($^{64}$Cu) in the serum after an oral dose of $^{64}$Cu in health (•) and in Wilson's disease (◦) (Sternlieb & Scheinberg 1979).

Conditions other than Wilson's disease can reduce the ceruloplasmin concentration, including the nephrotic syndrome, protein-losing enteropathy and severe liver failure of any cause. Healthy individuals rarely have a plasma ceruloplasmin concentration below 25 mg/dl.

The main confusion comes from heterozygotes, 20% of whom have ceruloplasmin concentrations below 20 mg/dl (Fig. 35.8) in association with other mild abnormalities of copper metabolism (Scheinberg & Sternlieb 1984). When this occurs, usually in an asymptomatic sibling of an index case, a liver biopsy is required for determination of the tissue copper concentration.

*Copper*

The serum copper concentration parallels the ceruloplasmin, which contains 0.3% copper (33 mg/dl ceruloplasmin carries 1000 μg/L copper). As there is usually an increased plasma nonceruloplasmin ("free") copper, the total serum copper may be reduced slightly or not at all. The urinary copper is rarely less than 1.6 μmol/24 h (100 μg/24 h), but increased copper excretion also occurs in other liver diseases (Gross et al 1985). Penicillamine produces a particularly marked increase in urinary copper excretion in Wilson's disease and most patients excrete more than 16 μmol/24 h (1000 μg/24 h) after starting therapy. Falsely high urine copper estimations are a frequent cause of misdiagnosis, probably because of inaccurate urine collection or use of containers contaminated with copper (Walshe & Yealland 1995). Wide-necked copper-free containers allowing urine to be passed directly into the container should be used.

The hepatic copper content in Wilson's disease is always high and usually exceeds 250 μg/g dry liver. It is the best single test to establish total body copper excess and should be performed in most cases. Liver copper concentrations are also high in any form of chronic cholestasis, especially primary biliary cirrhosis, but this is readily differentiated on other grounds. Autoimmune hepatitis can pose greater difficulty, as about half of patients have increased hepatic copper and 10% may have concentrations similar to those in Wilson's disease (LaRusso et al 1976). The plasma ceruloplasmin in these patients is usually elevated and they rarely have Kayser–Fleischer rings.

*Tests of copper metabolism*

Serum ceruloplasmin and copper measurements in serum, urine and liver will almost always establish the diagnosis of Wilson's disease. Occasionally, the diagnosis remains unclear and in this situation a test may be employed that measures the ability of the liver to incorporate radioactive copper into ceruloplasmin (Sternlieb & Scheinberg 1979). Radioactive copper is normally taken up rapidly from the blood by the liver, incorporated into ceruloplasmin and subsequently released again into the blood. The efficiency with which this is done can be estimated by determining the plasma radioactivity at intervals after the copper is given (Fig. 35.9). This test clearly separates homozygous patients from normals, but heterozygotes may have intermediate values, so not all test results are clearly positive or negative. Unfortunately, the confusion arises most commonly among the heterozygotes with low serum ceruloplasmin concentrations, which probably accounts for the fact that these tests are seldom used.

*Genetic studies*

Family linkage studies after establishing the diagnosis in an index case can correctly classify family members as heterozygotes or homozygotes with 95% accuracy (Farrer et al 1991), but these are not widely available. Gene sequencing is not likely to be useful clinically, as multiple mutations occur (p. 959).

## Treatment

Wilson's disease was untreatable only a few decades ago, but now a variety of effective therapies are available (Walshe 1996).

*Penicillamine*

Among the several copper-reducing agents that have been used for the treatment of Wilson's disease, penicillamine remains the drug of choice (Scheinberg & Sternlieb 1984). It is absorbed readily from the intestine and is excreted rapidly in the urine. The drug should be taken between meals to avoid chelation of metallic substances in the diet. Most patients require 1.0–1.5 g daily. Penicillamine 500 mg four times a day should be started as soon as possible, because patients with Wilson's disease can deteriorate abruptly. This dose will almost always produce an adequate cupriuresis, but may need to be increased if the urine copper does not exceed 2000 μg/24 h. The urinary excretion of copper gradually falls to around 500 μg/day over 6–12 months and should be measured periodically during follow-up. The nonceruloplasmin copper in the serum drops to <0.50 μg/ml and should remain in that range. Kayser–Fleischer rings gradually disappear, but this can take years. Once the disease is in remission, care must be taken that copper reaccumulation does not occur. It is vital for patients to understand that treatment must be continued for life, that stopping treatment will result inevitably in death and that deterioration after stopping treatment does not occur immediately.

Some patients develop neurologic symptoms for the first time and others experience worsening of neurologic symptoms after starting D-penicillamine. These symptoms usually improve subsequently, but this is not invariable (Scheinberg & Sternlieb 1984, Glass et al 1990). About half of patients on D-penicillamine have some side-effect and about one in 10 cannot tolerate the drug. Acute sensitivity reactions include fever, skin rashes, leukopenia, eosinophilia and thrombocytopenia. A nephrotic syndrome may occur and also seems to be a sensitivity reaction. When these reactions occur, the drug must be stopped but can often be restarted in slowly increasing doses, with or without corticosteroid cover. A chronic syndrome resembling systemic lupus erythematosus is a rare development. Penicillamine inhibits pyridoxal-dependent enzymes, but this is not important with the D-isomer and in practice it is not necessary to give pyridoxine supplements.

Young women with Wilson's disease may wish to have children and will naturally worry about the effects of the drug on the fetus, but experience with penicillamine in humans has not revealed any adverse effect in pregnancy (Scheinberg & Sternlieb 1975, Walshe 1977). Conversely, stopping penicillamine during pregnancy leads to the risk, even if small, of an exacerbation of Wilson's disease.

*Trientine*

Triethylene tetramine dihydrochloride (trientene) is a nonsulfhydryl chelating agent that is the drug of choice for patients intolerant of penicillamine. The cupriuresis produced is slightly less than that of penicillamine, but the drug is capable of removing excess copper from the body and of effecting improvement in patients (Walshe 1982). It is also effective in preventing long-term deterioration and has occasionally been used as initial therapy (Scheinberg et al 1987). It is given orally 3–4 times daily before meals (1–2 g daily). Part of its effect may be due to interference with gastrointestinal copper absorption. Iron deficiency is the most common side-effect and is prevented with iron supplementation. Sideroblastic anemia has been reported in a few cases. Experience with the drug in pregnancy is limited.

*Other drugs*

Zinc given by mouth reduces copper absorption and has been used successfully to induce negative copper balance and to treat Wilson's disease (Hoogenraad et al 1979, Brewer et al 1983). Hoogenraad et al (1984) reported good results over 2–20 years in eight patients given oral zinc sulfate as initial therapy in doses from 600 to 1200 mg/day. Not all patients necessarily achieve negative copper balance (Hill et al 1987), so the limited experience thus far would suggest that zinc might best be used for maintenance of copper balance after initial decoppering therapy. In one case, zinc appeared to reverse acute neurological deterioration occurring during penicillamine treatment but this might have been due to withdrawing penicillamine and neurological deterioration recurred eventually after 20 months of zinc (Veen et al 1991). Newer chelating agents such as tetrathiomolybdate are under investigation (Brewer et al 1991). Patients who cannot tolerate penicillamine should be referred if possible to those with special expertise in Wilson's disease.

*Diet*

The efficacy of penicillamine in reducing body copper is such that it is not necessary to recommend special diets to reduce copper intake. Indeed, copper is so ubiquitous that its elimination from the diet is hardly compatible with good general nutrition. Certain foods, however, do contain large amounts of copper and are best avoided: liver, nuts, shellfish, dried fruit, chocolate and mushrooms.

*Transplantation*

Transplantation cures the metabolic defect in Wilson's disease. The main indications for transplantation are deteriorating liver function in spite of adequate medical therapy (p. 1154) and fulminant hepatic failure (p. 1155). Transplantation for crippling neurologic symptoms remains controversial.

### Prognosis

The prognosis in Wilson's disease is excellent except for those presenting with fulminant hepatic failure. One study of 51 patients concluded that long-term survival in treated patients is normal (Stremmel et al 1991), while another report of 85 treated patients found that treatment improved survival two- to threefold but did not return it to normal (Balan et al 1994). No population-based data are available. No hepatocellular carcinomas were found in a long-term follow-up of 117 patients at the Mayo Clinic (Balan et al 1994) and only a handful of such cases are reported in the literature (Polio et al 1989). Clearly, Wilson's disease is not an intrinsically premalignant condition and differs from hemochromatosis in this regard.

### Prevention

Relatives of patients may include healthy individuals who are either heterozygotes or homozygotes for the Wilson's disease gene. Heterozygotes remain healthy, but all homozygotes eventually develop the disease. All siblings and offspring of patients with Wilson's disease should be investigated to detect homozygotes. About 20% of heterozygotes have reduced serum ceruloplasmin and copper concentrations and because of the prevalences of heterozygotes and asymptomatic homozygotes, diagnosis of Wilson's disease on these tests alone would lead to lifetime treatment of 99 heterozygotes for each homozygote (Sternlieb & Scheinberg 1968). Therefore, screening tests should include the serum ceruloplasmin, serum copper, 24-h urinary copper excretion and slit-lamp examination of the eyes. Final diagnosis requires measurement of the liver copper concentration (p. 963) or demonstration of an inability to incorporate radioactive copper into ceruloplasmin (p. 963).

### Other abnormalities of copper metabolism

Diseases of copper metabolism other than Wilson's disease are rare, and they are not associated with liver disease. However, they are of interest in relation to Wilson's disease, as they are associated with low plasma ceruloplasmin concentrations unrelated to copper overload.

***Menkes' disease.*** Menkes's disease is caused by a gene located on the X chromosome (Walshe 1995). It is inherited as a sex-linked recessive and is found only in males. It presents a few months after birth with failure to thrive, kinky hair, micrognathia, and cerebral and cerebellar degeneration leading to mental degeneration, fits, and spastic paraplegia. Death occurs within a few years. This disease is caused by copper deficiency and is associated with low plasma copper and ceruloplasmin concentrations. The primary defect may be deficiency of a zinc-binding protein causing an excess of ionic zinc and leading in turn to excess metallothionine production by cells. This causes copper malabsorption in the small intestine. There is no satisfactory treatment for this condition.

***Occipital horn syndrome.*** This very rare condition is related closely to Menkes' disease and is due to copper deficiency (Danks 1989).

***Hereditary ceruloplasmin deficiency.*** This rare condition is inherited as an autosomal recessive and is due to a mutation of the ceruloplasmin gene on chromosome 3 (Harris et al 1996). Homozygotes develop the disease in adult life and heterozygotes are normal. Some patients have dementia and diabetes mellitus and some have other neurological abnormalities, but all have abnormal iron metabolism characterized by a low plasma iron, a high liver iron, and mild iron-deficiency anemia. Plasma ceruloplasmin concentrations are very low, but there is no copper overload. The abnormalities of iron metabolism are probably the result of ceruloplasmin deficiency (p. 751).

## INDIAN CHILDHOOD CIRRHOSIS

This condition occurs primarily in children in the Indian subcontinent (Joshi 1987), but a similar condition has also been described in 11 non-Indian cases, including two American families (Adamson et al 1992). It accounts for more than half of the chronic liver disease in children in India. Three-quarters of patients are 1–3 years old and a quarter have a positive family history (Joshi 1987).

Three clinical stages are described, progressing from disturbance of appetite and bowel movements to hepatosplenomegaly, portal hypertension and hepatocellular failure (Joshi 1987). About 25% of cases present with an illness resembling acute hepatitis that fails to resolve and progresses to death within a few months.

The liver histology is characterized by liver cell necrosis and mild to moderate inflammation, in association with Mallory's hyaline. There is no fatty change. Hepatocytes show orcein-staining granules that contain copper-associated protein (Adamson et al 1992). "Creeping" fibrosis occurs and progresses to a micronodular cirrhosis (Joshi 1987).

Hepatic copper is markedly increased and is largely cytoplasmic (Tanner et al 1983). Livers of unaffected siblings do not show an excess of copper (Nayak et al 1981). In contrast to Wilson's disease, copper accumulation in the eye is absent and ceruloplasmin levels are normal.

The cause of the disease remains unknown (Joshi 1987). It is not clear whether the high hepatic copper concentration results from an inherited metabolic defect, from excessive oral intake of copper in infancy, or both. Tanner et al (1983) provided evidence that the Indian custom of boiling animal milk in brass and copper household utensils resulted in a significant increase in copper concentration. Fatal nutritional copper intoxication associated with a high concentration of copper in the liver and micronodular cirrhosis has been described in infants from two separate German families whose drinking water was found to be contaminated with high levels of copper (Schramel et al 1988). Penicillamine is of no benefit in advanced cases but was shown to lower the mortality from 93% to 52% in preicteric patients (Tanner et al 1987).

## $\alpha_1$-ANTITRYPSIN DEFICIENCY

$\alpha_1$-Antitrypsin is the protease inhibitor responsible for inhibiting neutrophil elastase. Inherited deficiency of $\alpha_1$-antitrypsin is associated with pulmonary and hepatic disease (Schwarzenberg & Sharp 1990, Birrer et al 1991). Van Steenbergen (1993) has written a useful general review and there are several reviews of the molecular and genetic aspects (Crystal 1990, Perlmutter 1991, Sifers et al 1992).

### Etiology

#### *Genetics*

The concentration of $\alpha_1$-antitrypsin in the blood is determined by two codominant alleles, one from each parent. At least 75 different alleles have been described, but only four variants account for approximately 95% of those encountered in persons with normal serum levels of $\alpha_1$-antitrypsin. The Pi (protease inhibitor) alleles are named by letter according to the electrophoretic mobility of the corresponding $\alpha_1$-antitrypsin protein. The most common is PiM (medium) which occurs in 86–99% of individuals. The PiS (slow) and PiZ (ultra-slow) are the most frequent variations. Full deletion of an allele occurs only rarely (Pi null). The phenotype PiMM produces a normal serum $\alpha_1$-antitrypsin concentration and the presence of other alleles results in lower concentrations (Table 35.7). There are distinct population differences; blacks rarely have alleles other than PiM, while the highest frequency of the PiZ variant is in Scandinavian populations.

**Table 35.7** Human Pi phenotypes and their corresponding plasma $\alpha_1$-antitrypsin concentrations

| Phenotype | Approximate plasma concentration (% of normal) |
|---|---|
| MM | 100 |
| MS | 80 |
| MZ | 60 |
| SS | 60 |
| M null | 50 |
| SZ | 40 |
| ZZ | 15 |
| Null null | 0 |

#### *Pathogenesis*

Liver disease in $\alpha_1$-antitrypsin deficiency is believed to be related to accumulation of $\alpha_1$-antitrypsin in the endoplasmic reticulum of the hepatocytes (Schwarzenberg & Sharp 1990, Perlmutter 1991). Patients who have one or two Z alleles produce an $\alpha_1$-antitrypsin protein with a single amino acid substitution that leads to a change in the conformation of the newly formed polypeptide, resulting in retention and accumulation of most of the protein within the hepatocyte endoplasmic reticulum. In contrast, the protein produced by the S allele is degraded intracellularly and is neither accumulated within the cell nor secreted into the blood. In the case of the null phenotype, no protein is produced at all. The significance of these differences is that liver disease develops only in phenotypes associated with intracellular accumulation of $\alpha_1$-antitrypsin within the hepatocytes (ZZ, MZ, or SZ) and seems not to correlate with the amount of $\alpha_1$-antitrypsin in the blood.

The occurrence of panlobular emphysema is thought to be related to a reduced serum concentration of $\alpha_1$-antitrypsin (Van Steenbergen 1993). Patients with serum concentrations less than 80 mg/dl develop progressive loss of lung elasticity secondary to the unopposed action of neutrophil elastase on elastin in the extracellular matrix of the lung.

#### *Liver disease*

The association of liver disease, plasma $\alpha_1$-antitrypsin deficiency and the phenotype PiZZ was first noted in children (Sharp et al 1969) but was subsequently recognized as a cause of chronic liver disease in adults (Berg & Eriksson 1972). Sveger (1988) carried out a prospective study of 127 consecutive PiZZ individuals found by systematic screening of 200 000 Swedish infants from 1972 to 1974. Most of these patients escaped serious liver injury, but about 25% had a rapidly progressive course leading to cirrhosis and death (or transplantation) in early childhood. After 12 years of follow-up, only two patients (1.5%) had died of liver cirrhosis and a third was found to have cirrhosis incidentally at autopsy after dying of aplastic anemia. No other child had clinical evidence of liver disease and only 15% had abnormal serum aminotransferase activities. Ten to 15% of infants with the PiZZ phenotype present with neonatal hepatitis (Schwarzenberg & Sharp 1990, Birrer et al 1991, Hussain et al 1991), and, as might be expected, studies of smaller or more selected groups of patients at pediatric referral centers suggest that serious liver disease is more likely to develop in patients who present with neonatal jaundice (Alagille 1984, Ghishan & Greene 1988).

The spectrum of liver disease associated with the PiZZ phenotype in adults ranges from mild or insignificant involvement to end-stage liver disease with death due to cirrhosis or hepatocellular carcinoma (Eriksson et al 1986a, Birrer et al 1991). A case-control autopsy study over 20 years in Malmö, Sweden, estimated that individuals with the PiZZ phenotype had an eightfold increased risk of developing cirrhosis and a 20-fold increased risk of developing primary liver cancer, particularly in men. These results were confirmed in a later study of all Swedish patients dying with PiZZ phenotype during the same period (Eriksson 1987). Ninety-four such patients were identified, 35 had cirrhosis and 27 were male. Most presented with signs or symptoms of portal hypertension and the mean survival following diagnosis was only 2 years. Fourteen of the 35 (40%) cirrhotic patients had primary liver cancer at autopsy.

Following reports of cirrhosis in individuals heterozygous for the Z allele (Campra et al 1973), investigators have tried to establish whether this is a significant association. Phenotypes heterozygous for the Z allele are found with greater than expected frequency in patients with otherwise unexplained chronic liver disease (Hodges et al 1981, Carlson & Eriksson 1985). That this may be a "dose-related" phenomenon is suggested by the observation that the age at presentation among heterozygous individuals with chronic liver disease is approximately 15 years later than that of patients who are homozygous for the Z allele (Rakela et al 1987). However, a recent study of 164 consecutive patients either homozygous (9) or heterozygous (155) for the Z allele found that approximately 90% with cirrhosis and 80% with chronic active hepatitis had at least one other identifiable possible cause for chronic liver disease (Propst et al 1992). This raises the possibility that a partial deficiency increases the risk of developing liver disease from other causes.

## Pathology

The histology is characterized by intracytoplasmic globules of retained $\alpha_1$-antitrypsin protein in the hepatocytes (Fig. 35.10). They are more prominent in homozygous

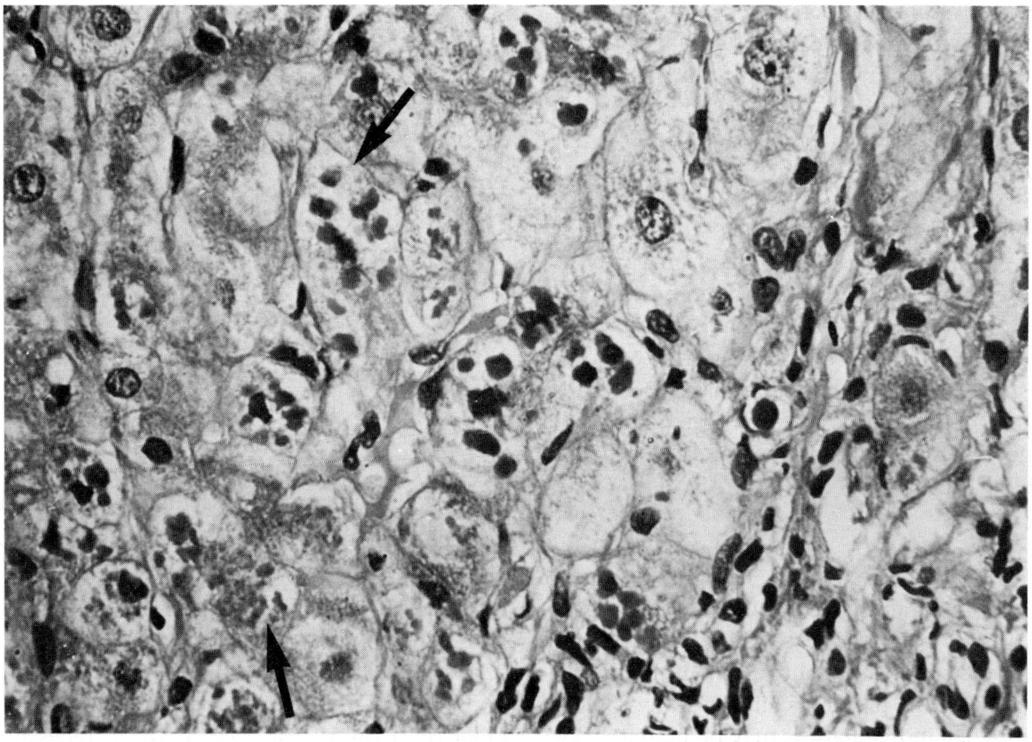

**Fig. 35.10** $\alpha_1$-Antitrypsin bodies. Note the rounded hyaline bodies (arrowed) within the hepatocytes (PAS, ×25).

than in heterozygous individuals and are easily overlooked in sections stained with hematoxylin and eosin; they are strongly PAS-positive and diastase-resistant, varying in size between 1 and 40 μm (Ludwig 1992). The inclusions are found primarily in periportal hepatocytes and at the periphery of regenerating nodules. Intracytoplasmic inclusions may occasionally be found in bile duct epithelial cells (Callea et al 1985).

Patients with neonatal jaundice usually show marked cholestasis with bile retention in the liver cells and canaliculi. PAS-positive globules are not always obvious in the first few months of life but may be identified by immunostains or electronmicroscopy. Children with PiZZ-related neonatal liver disease may show a pattern indistinguishable from giant cell neonatal hepatitis or simply a pattern of periportal fibrosis. A third group shows paucity of intralobular bile ducts (Dorney et al 1987, Van Steenbergen 1993).

Cirrhosis results from irregular expansion of the portal tracts with fibrosis and is usually of the macronodular type.

### Clinical features

*Childhood*

Liver disease usually presents within the first few weeks of life as jaundice and nonspecific abnormalities of serum transaminase and alkaline phosphatase activities. This almost always subsides spontaneously within 6 months, but liver dysfunction may persist and become associated with hepatomegaly or splenomegaly. Early death is rare and children usually develop normally once jaundice subsides. Where liver dysfunction persists, progressive liver disease may ensue, with the clinical features of cirrhosis and complications of portal hypertension occurring in late childhood or adolescence.

*Adults*

The majority of homozygous individuals survive childhood and significant liver disease usually presents later as cirrhosis or chronic hepatitis. These may often be "cryptogenic" and only a search for the abnormal $\alpha_1$-antitrypsin phenotype will reveal a cause. Only a minority of adult patients have simultaneous pulmonary disease. Homozygous individuals present with liver disease at age 50–60, while heterozygotes for the Z allele are often age 65 or above (Rakela et al 1987).

### Laboratory tests

The only sure way to establish or exclude $\alpha_1$-antitrypsin deficiency as a cause of liver disease is to determine the $\alpha_1$-antitrypsin phenotype by electrophoresis. Although the serum concentration of the protein is almost always below normal in homozygous individuals, it may be increased or decreased by associated inflammation or drugs and is therefore unreliable for making the diagnosis (Cox 1989). Appropriate investigations would include tests to exclude other causes of jaundice in infancy or other causes of chronic liver disease in adults.

It is possible to detect $\alpha_1$-antitrypsin variants by direct analysis of DNA using the polymerase chain reaction (Cox & Mansfield 1987, Abbott et al 1992, Andresen et al 1992). These techniques allow the prenatal diagnosis of $\alpha_1$-antitrypsin deficiency and may be performed on minute quantities of tissue such as dried blood spots (Andresen et al 1992).

### Treatment

Augmentation therapy with purified human plasma $\alpha_1$-antitrypsin may prevent pulmonary damage (Van Steenbergen 1993) but is of no avail in liver disease. Indeed, elastase–$\alpha_1$-antitrypsin complexes might increase the tendency to liver cell injury by inducing further $\alpha_1$-antitrypsin synthesis in the liver. No medical therapy has been found effective for the liver disease associated with $\alpha_1$-antitrypsin deficiency (Hussain et al 1991) and liver transplantation remains the only treatment for end-stage liver disease (p. 1151). Gene replacement therapy in the future will have to use hepatocyte-targeted strategies, as Birrer et al (1991) have pointed out that increasing the serum $\alpha_1$-antitrypsin level without changing liver secretion or synthesis is not likely to help the liver disease.

### Prognosis

Impressions of the prognosis in $\alpha_1$-antitrypsin deficiency based upon reports from referral centers were gloomy (Nebbia et al 1983, Ghishan & Greene 1988), but the Swedish study described above suggests a benign course for the majority of PiZZ individuals at least through childhood (Sveger 1988). A small proportion will develop neonatal liver disease, with a fraction of these going on to an accelerated course with early death from cirrhosis (Fig. 35.11). The vast majority of patients, however, survive to adulthood and, if they do not die of respiratory failure from emphysema, have perhaps a 20% chance of developing cirrhosis by the time they are 50–60 years old. The chance of developing hepatocellular carcinoma is many times that of the general population. The prognosis in adults with cirrhosis is relatively poor, perhaps because most are fairly old at the time of presentation and the risk of hepatocellular carcinoma is high (Rakela et al 1987).

## METABOLIC DISEASES OF THE LIVER IN INFANCY AND CHILDHOOD

### Galactosemia

Galactosemia is the result of a recessively inherited deficiency of one of the three main enzymes in the galac-

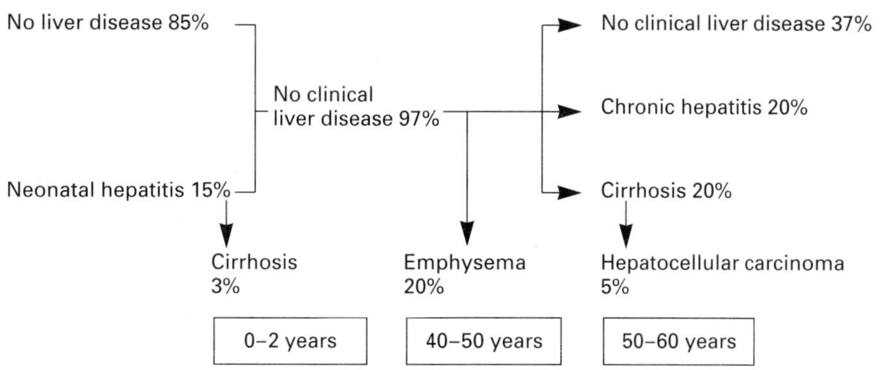


**Fig. 35.11** Natural history of homozygous (PIZZ) $\alpha_1$-antitrypsin deficiency.

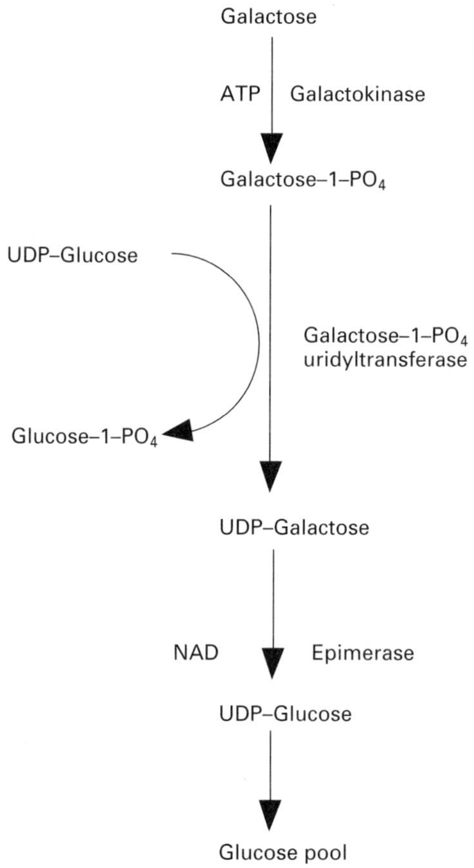


**Fig. 35.12** Metabolic pathway for galactose. ATP = adenosine triphosphate; NAD = nicotinamide adenine dinucleotide; UDP = uridine diphosphate.

tose metabolism pathway (Fig. 35.12) (Beutler 1991). Deficiency of galactose-1-phosphate uridyl transferase is the most common defect and is associated with neonatal liver disease and eventual cirrhosis. A variety of mutations in the gene have been discovered and the disorder is therefore heterogeneous at the molecular level (Reichardt 1992). A similar illness may be caused by a deficiency of the epimerase enzyme, but this is much more rare (Landing et al 1993). Children with galactokinase deficiency may develop cataracts but do not develop liver disease.

The toxic effects of galactosemia are thought to result from the accumulation of galactose and its metabolites, galactose-1-phosphate and galactitol, in blood and body tissues, although the mechanism of action remains unknown. The discovery that UDP-galactose concentrations in the red blood cells of galactosemic patients were lower than normal has led to suggestions that uridine replacement might be helpful, but the value of this treatment is unproven (Lehotay 1993).

### *Pathology*

Liver histology is similar to that in other metabolic disorders, with diffuse macrovesicular fatty change and periportal ductular proliferation in the newborn. This evolves within a few weeks to pseudoglandular change with bile plugs within the liver acini (Ludwig 1992). Giant cell transformation and liver cell adenomas have also been observed. Cirrhosis develops within 3–6 months.

### *Clinical features*

The main source of galactose in the diet is lactose, so symptoms and signs of galactosemia appear during the first week of life with anorexia, vomiting, jaundice, hepatomegaly, lethargy, hypotonia and susceptibility to infection, particularly with Gram-negative organisms (Levy et al 1977). Despite initial response to dietary restriction, surviving individuals may show ataxia, intention tremor, microcephaly, speech abnormalities, low intelligence, ovarian failure or growth retardation (Waggoner et al 1990, Schweitzer et al 1993). Cataract formation appears to be related to poor dietary control but does not correlate with erythrocyte galactose-1-phosphate levels (Beigi et al 1993).

### *Diagnosis*

Galactosuria suggests the diagnosis, but absence of galactosuria does not exclude the diagnosis. The diagnostic test for galactose-1-phosphate uridyl transferase deficiency is assay of the enzyme and its substrate galactose-1-phosphate in red blood cells (Beutler 1991, Kirkman 1992, Lehotay 1993).

*Treatment and prognosis*

Treatment with a galactose-free diet usually leads to rapid improvement with regression of jaundice, hepatomegaly and cataracts. Unfortunately, brain damage is irreversible. Komrower & Lee (1970) reported a 40% mortality at 6 months and persistent hepatomegaly in 18% of survivors. Even with lifelong maintenance of a galactose-free diet, the long-term results in surveys of large patient groups have not been as good as expected (Waggoner et al 1990, Schweitzer et al 1993). Liver transplantation corrects the metabolic defect (p. 1154).

## Hereditary fructose intolerance

Illness from ingestion of fructose, sucrose or sorbitol results from a deficiency of aldolase B, which catalyzes the reversible splitting of fructose-1-phosphate to form dihydroxyacetone phosphate and D-glyceraldehyde. The other two aldolase isoenzymes (A and C) show greater activity toward fructose-1-6-diphosphate and fructose intolerance may, rarely, be due to a deficiency of one of these isoenzymes (Fig. 35.13). The disease results from one of several mutations in the gene on chromosome 9 coding the aldolase B protein and causing catalytic deficiency despite normal amounts of protein (Cox 1990, Cross & Cox 1990). As a result of the deficiency, fructose-1-phosphate accumulates, glycolysis and gluconeogenesis are impaired and hypoglycemia, lactic acidosis and hypophosphatemia result. These abnormalities appear only when the system is challenged with one of the above sugars and affected individuals remain healthy during prolonged fasting. Essential fructosuria results from a deficiency of fructokinase and does not cause liver disease.

*Genetics*

Inheritance is autosomal recessive and the incidence is approximately one in 20 000 in Europe and the United States. At least seven different mutations have been documented and patients are either homozygotes or compound heterozygotes (Cox 1991).

*Clinical features*

Infants develop vomiting, diarrhea and failure to thrive following weaning from breast milk or after administration of sugar-containing medications or sweetened formulas. Hypoglycemia, acidosis, jaundice, seizures and coma occur and death may result from hepatic failure. Children who survive show selective aversions to fruits, sweets, certain vegetables and syrup preparations of vitamins and medicine. Inadvertent ingestion of offending sugars causes abdominal distress and sometimes impaired consciousness. Adults with fructose intolerance may remain undiagnosed due to self-selected restrictive diet (Burmeister et al 1991).

*Diagnosis*

Diagnosis is confirmed by assay of fructose-1-phosphate aldolase activity in the liver or intestinal mucosa. Some specialist laboratories can detect the genetic defect directly in peripheral blood leukocytes or buccal epithelial cells, using the polymerase chain reaction technique.

*Pathology*

Histologic changes resemble those found in galactosemia (Ludwig 1992).

*Treatment*

Complete exclusion of fructose, sucrose and sorbitol is the only treatment available. Death has resulted from intravenous administration of sorbitol solutions to anesthetized patients (Cox 1990). Hepatomegaly and fibrosis are reversible on withdrawal of offending sugars from the diet.

## Hereditary tyrosinemia

This is a rare, recessively inherited disorder that, in its

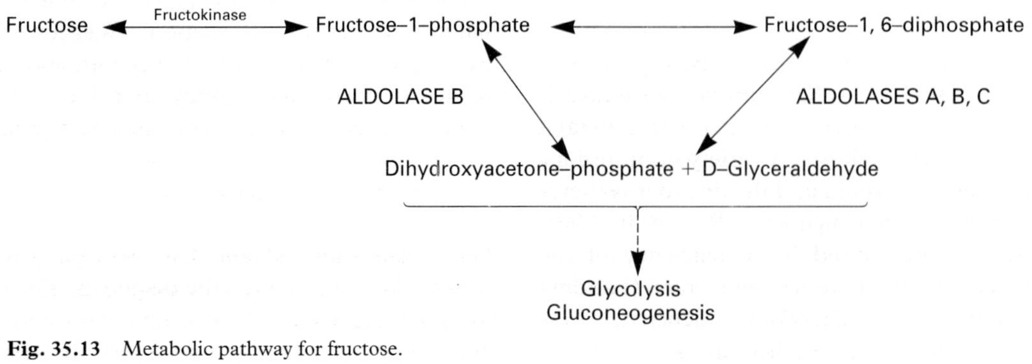


**Fig. 35.13** Metabolic pathway for fructose.

most common form (type I), is caused by deficiency of fumarylacetoacetase, the final enzyme in the tyrosine degradation pathway. Affected individuals accumulate malyl and fumaryl acetoacetate, which are metabolized to succinylacetone, an inhibitor of ALA-dehydrase, and this leads to accumulation of δ-aminolevulinic acid. The liver and kidney are the major target organs and there is a high frequency of neurologic crises similar to those seen in the acute porphyrias (Mitchell et al 1990). The gene for the enzyme is located on chromosome 15 and affected individuals show molecular heterogeneity with regard to the defect (Phaneuf et al 1992).

*Clinical features*

Acute and chronic forms of the disease have been described. The acute form presents during the first few months of life with vomiting, diarrhea, failure to thrive, jaundice and hepatosplenomegaly. Most affected infants die in the first year. The chronic form presents in older infants and young children with cirrhosis, renal tubular dysfunction, renal failure and episodic crises of peripheral neuropathy characterized by pain, extensor hypertonia, vomiting or ileus, muscle weakness and even self-mutilation. Eight of 20 patients seen with neurologic symptoms at one center required mechanical ventilation and 14 died (Mitchell et al 1990).

The liver disease often progresses rapidly to cirrhosis and hepatocellular carcinoma and individuals who survive infancy almost invariably have high serum levels of alpha-fetoprotein (Weinberg et al 1976). Even among young children who have undergone transplantation without evidence of hepatocellular carcinoma, studies of liver tissue show hepatocellular dysplasia and strong staining for alpha-fetoprotein (Manowski et al 1990).

*Diagnosis*

Any child with liver disease or rickets of unknown cause should be considered as having hereditary tyrosinemia type I. Marked abnormality of liver function tests is usual in the acute form, but these tests can be normal in the chronic form and even serum tyrosine and alpha-fetoprotein concentrations can be normal (Kvittingen 1991). Serum levels of tyrosine, methionine and alpha-fetoprotein are elevated. Renal acidosis may be present and there is phosphaturia, glucosuria, aminoaciduria and excretion of δ-aminolevulinic acid.

The most characteristic biochemical abnormality is an elevation of succinylacetone in the blood or urine. Fumarylacetoacetase activity can be assayed directly in lymphocytes or fibroblasts and has been used for prenatal diagnosis in amniotic fluid, but the existence of a "pseudodeficiency" gene means that demonstration of deficient tissue enzyme activity may not be conclusive (Kvittingen 1991). The gene coding the enzyme has been isolated and characterized and direct sequencing of the gene in individual patients is now possible. Single amino acid substitutions have been identified and patients may be compound heterozygotes (Labelle et al 1993).

*Treatment*

Standard treatment is to restrict phenylalanine and tyrosine in the diet. This improves the renal tubular disease but does not necessarily affect the liver disease. Liver transplantation has been successful and inability to predict or prevent complications such as hepatocellular carcinoma has led to the suggestion that liver transplantation be done within the first year of life (p. 1154). An inhibitor of 4-hydroxyphenylpyruvate dioxygenase has been reported to reduce substantially the excretion of succinylacetoacetate, succinylacetone and 5-aminolevulinic acid and the serum concentration of alpha-fetoprotein, but it remains to be seen whether this will be a realistic alternative to transplantation (Lindstedt et al 1992).

## Urea cycle disorders

These result from an inherited mutation in the gene controlling any one of the five enzymes of the urea cycle: carbamylphosphate synthetase, ornithine transcarbamylase (OTC), argininosuccinic acid synthetase (AS), argininosuccinate lyase (AL) and arginase. Deficiencies in the first four of these enzymes produce hyperammonemia. OTC deficiency is the commonest, accounting for about 40% of patients (Bachmann 1987). It is inherited as an X-linked recessive trait, while the other four are autosomal recessive disorders. As with many of the inherited metabolic disorders, a variety of mutations in the OTC gene have been documented (Tuchman 1993). The liver is the site of metabolic failure in these syndromes but normal otherwise. Liver biopsy sometimes shows fatty change and rarely fibrosis (Zimmerman et al 1987).

***Clinical features.*** Most patients present as neonatal lethargy with vomiting, seizures and coma. Death occurs if the condition is not recognized and survivors may suffer permanent brain damage (Brusilow 1985). Late-onset symptoms may arise any time after the first year of life and occasionally first presentation occurs as an adult. Precipitating factors include any intercurrent illness and treatment with total parenteral nutrition. Late-onset illness symptoms include poor appetite with avoidance of protein, impaired growth, mental retardation and sometimes psychiatric syndromes (DiMagno et al 1986, Finkelstein et al 1990). Hyperammonemic coma has also occurred in heterozygous women following valproic acid treatment (Felig et al 1995).

***Diagnosis.*** Patients show increased blood concentrations of ammonia and glutamine and increased urinary orotic acid (Bachmann 1987). Allopurinol-induced increased urinary excretion of orotic acid can also be used, but protein challenge tests can be dangerous. OTC activity in the liver can be measured directly.

***Management.*** Urgent treatment of marked hyperammonemia (>500 μmol/L) requires peritoneal dialysis or hemodialysis. Long-term therapy includes a nitrogen-restricted diet, citrulline or arginine supplements depending on the specific metabolic defect and sodium benzoate or sodium phenylacetate to promote alternative routes of nitrogen dispersal (Brusilow 1984, Batshaw & Monahan 1987). Long-term mortality is considerable, particularly in late-onset patients (Finkelstein et al 1990), and liver transplantation has been carried out (p. 1154).

### Glycogen storage diseases

These diseases include at least 10 separate genetic defects of impaired glycogen breakdown (Ghishan & Greene 1990, Talente et al 1994). Types I and III are the commonest, but still rare (one per 100 000).

***Glycogen storage disease (GSD) type Ia.*** This is due to a deficiency of glucose-6-phosphatase in liver, kidney and intestine and results in an inability to form glucose from glucose-6-phosphate, leading to dependence on dietary carbohydrate to avoid hypoglycemia. In response to low plasma insulin concentrations, a large amount of fatty acid is released from fat and delivered to the liver where it accumulates. Hepatomegaly appears anywhere from several days to several months after birth. Hypoglycemia results in chronic hypercortisolism and consequently poor growth with delayed puberty. The chronic stimulus for glycogenolysis without formation of glucose results in increased production of lactate, uric acid, triglycerides and cholesterol. Common problems in adult patients include hepatic adenomas, anemia of chronic disease, proteinuria and nephrocalcinosis.

***GSD type Ib.*** This is due to a deficiency of the enzyme necessary to translocate glucose-6-phosphate into the endoplasmic reticulum. It is therefore indistinguishable clinically from type Ia, except that patients have a high incidence of neutropenia and recurrent bacterial infections.

***GSD type III.*** This is due to a deficiency of the glycogen debranching enzyme. Hypoglycemia and poor growth are common in childhood, but growth increases around the time of puberty and height is normal in adulthood, by which time hypoglycemia is also uncommon. Serum aminotransferase activities are usually elevated and patients may develop hepatic fibrosis and cirrhosis. Most patients also lack the enzyme in muscle and muscle weakness may occur in childhood or adulthood; cardiomyopathy appears after the age of 30.

***Diagnosis.*** The diagnosis can be confirmed by demonstration of enzyme deficiency in liver (type I) or in peripheral blood leukocytes (other types).

***Treatment.*** Most patients can be treated successfully with cornstarch 2 g/kg orally four times a day or continuous nocturnal nasogastric glucose feedings providing one-third of the daily calories (Chen et al 1993). For patients with GSD type Ib, granulocyte colony-stimulating factor may prevent bacterial infections. It is not clear whether the myopathy associated with GSD type III can be avoided.

Liver transplantation should be considered for patients with GSD type IV (branching enzyme deficiency), as most patients die of liver failure by 4 years of age (p. 1154).

**Cholesterol ester storage disease** (Beaudet et al 1977, Ghishan & Greene 1990)

This is a recessively inherited deficiency of the lysosomal enzyme cholesterol ester hydrolase (lysosomal acid lipase). Most patients develop progressive hepatomegaly in childhood and this may progress to portal hypertension and hepatic fibrosis. In the more severe form of the disorder (Wolman's disease), patients fail to thrive and die in infancy. Otherwise, patients survive into adulthood but develop accelerated atherosclerosis. The liver is markedly enlarged and has a distinctive orange color. The inability to release cholesterol from lysosomal cholesterol ester results in elevated production of endogenous cholesterol. There are anecdotal reports that treatment with lovastatin may produce biochemical improvement (Ginsberg et al 1987).

## CYSTIC FIBROSIS

Improvement in survival of patients with cystic fibrosis has led to increasing numbers surviving into adulthood and developing the hepatic complications of the disease. Cystic fibrosis is the commonest fatal autosomal recessive disorder, affecting one in 2 000 in northern European populations. It results from one or more of 100 mutations in the gene on chromosome 7 coding the transmembrane conductance regulator protein (Mulherin & FitzGerald 1992). The prevalence of overt liver disease in a large referral population of cystic fibrosis patients in England was 4% (Scott-Jupp et al 1991), but characteristic pathological changes have been found in the liver at autopsy in 70% of patients over 24 years of age (Williams et al 1992). Although a familial concordance for clinical liver disease of 20% was found in one study, there were no significant differences in the frequencies of the three most common genetic mutations in subgroups with severe or mild liver disease or without liver disease (Duthie et al 1992).

### Pathology

Focal biliary fibrosis is the characteristic histological lesion and it progresses eventually to biliary cirrhosis. The small intrahepatic bile ducts contain inspissated eosinophilic material that produces partial biliary obstruction characterized by portal edema and fibrosis in association with bile duct proliferation (Ludwig 1992, Williams et al 1992). Electronmicroscopy has shown collagen deposition around bile ducts and ductules with an increase in hepatic stellate cells (p. 714) but no evidence of dilated canaliculi (Lindblad et al 1992). Thus, cholestasis may not be the main pathogenetic factor. A minority of cases show extensive hepatic steatosis, probably related to malnutrition resulting from malabsorption (Colombo et al 1992).

### Clinical features

Neonatal cholestasis may be the first manifestation of cystic fibrosis. More commonly, clinical features of biliary cirrhosis appear in childhood or in adulthood, often in patients with pancreatic and respiratory involvement. Asymptomatic hepatosplenomegaly may be discovered incidentally. Occasionally, complications of portal hypertension such as variceal hemorrhage may be the first indication of liver disease (Williams et al 1992). Biliary complications include abdominal pain and fever due to cholecystitis associated with pigment gallstones or cholangitis associated with intrahepatic ductal strictures or intrahepatic stones.

### Diagnosis

Nonspecific liver function test abnormalities are common. Imaging may show hepatomegaly, echogenic features of fibrosis and steatosis or cirrhosis. Radionuclide biliary scans may be abnormal irrespective of extrahepatic obstruction (Colombo et al 1992). Cholangiography shows features similar to those of primary sclerosing cholangitis, with radiologic abnormalities usually confined to the intrahepatic bile ducts (O'Brien et al 1992). It may be needed to show the cause of abdominal pain or worsening cholestasis. Liver biopsy demonstrates the extent of disease in the liver but is not often needed.

### Treatment

Recent studies have shown that benefit may accrue from ursodeoxycholic acid (Colombo et al 1990, Cotting et al 1990) which may exert a beneficial effect by replacing toxic hydrophobic bile acids in the bile acid pool and by inducing a bicarbonate-rich choleresis. Six months of therapy produced significant improvement in standard liver function tests, BSP retention and the aminopyrine breath test (Cotting et al 1990). Excretory hepatobiliary scans were improved after 1 year of treatment in 13 patients (Colombo et al 1992). The management of cirrhosis (p. 925) and portal hypertension (p. 1005) are described elsewhere.

Liver transplantation can be carried out, but because of the multisystem nature of the disease its place is not as clear as in other inherited metabolic disorders of the liver (p. 1154). Transfer of the human cystic fibrosis transmembrane conductance regulator gene to rat biliary epithelial cells has been successfully accomplished in vivo, suggesting that it may ultimately be feasible to prevent liver involvement by restoring expression of the protein in the biliary tract (Yang et al 1993).

## PORPHYRIA

Porphyrins are tetrapyrrole molecules that form complexes with metals and are the intermediates in heme synthesis. The porphyrias are a group of diseases in which inherited partial enzyme deficiencies lead to accumulation of porphyrins and porphyrin precursors that appear in the urine and stools. The liver is the main site in which the defect is expressed in five of the porphyrias: acute intermittent porphyria (AIP), variegate porphyria (VP), hereditary coproporphyria (HCP), aminolevulinic acid (ALA) dehydrase deficiency and porphyria cutanea tarda (PCT). The sites of expression are the bone marrow and the liver in protoporphyria and hepatoerythropoietic porphyria.

The pattern of inheritance is autosomal dominant in most of the porphyrias except for hepatoerythropoietic porphyria and ALA dehydrase deficiency, which are autosomal recessive. The sporadic form of PCT is expressed only in the liver and is commonly associated with alcohol, estrogens and chronic hepatitis C virus infection (below). The familial form of PCT is expressed in all tissues. PCT is the commonest form generally, VP is relatively common in South Africa (about three per 1000), and the prevalence of AIP is estimated at 5–10/100 000 in the US (Bloomer & Straka 1988).

The three major clinical effects of the porphyrias are neurologic symptoms, skin lesions and liver damage. Skin manifestations are found in the porphyrias in which there is increased porphyrin excretion (Fig. 35.14). Neurologic symptoms do not occur in PCT, hepatoerythropoietic porphyria and protoporphyria, in which liver damage occurs.

Several recent reviews are available (Billett 1988, Bloomer & Straka 1988, Bloomer & Bonkovsky 1989, Bonkovsky 1990, Rank et al 1990). Only the porphyrias affecting the liver are considered further.

### Hepatic porphyrias with acute neurologic symptoms

AIP, HCP and VP all cause episodes of acute abdominal pain severe enough to lead to consideration of surgical exploration. Initial attacks rarely occur before puberty, but thereafter abdominal pain is the most common presentation. Skin involvement does not occur in AIP, but otherwise the three types cannot readily be differentiated clinically.

***Clinical features.*** Acute episodes are characterized by abdominal pain (95%), tachycardia (80%), hypertension (50%), constipation (50%) and vomiting (40%). The pain is attributed to autonomic neuropathy, is usually colicky and lasts from a few hours to several days. Palpation often shows tenderness and bowel sounds may be diminished,

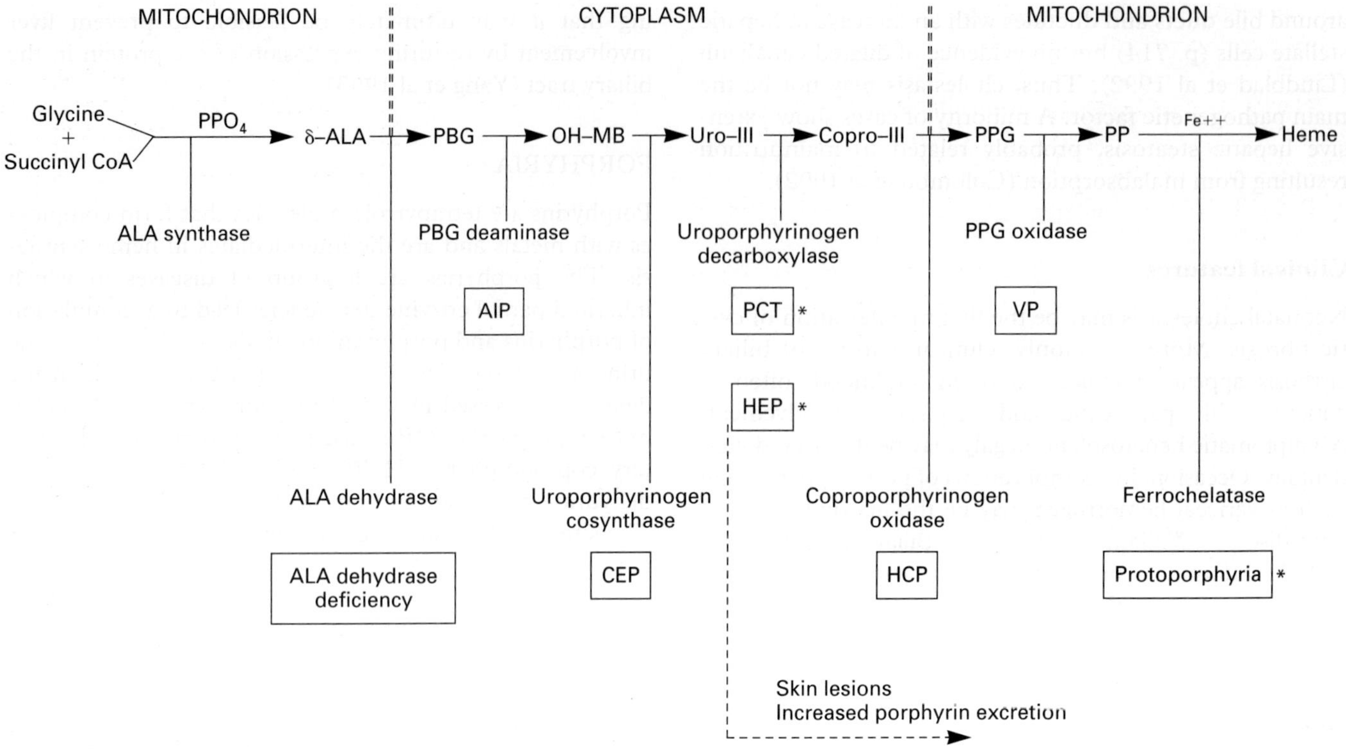


Note: *Structural liver damage but no neurological symptoms. Individual porphyrias shown in boxes (ALA = aminolevulinic acid; AIP = acute intermittent porphyria; CEP = congenital erythropoietic porphyria; PCT = porphyria cutanea tarda; HEP = hepatoerythropoietic porphyria; HCP = hereditary coproporphyria; VP = variegate porphyria).

**Fig. 35.14** Metabolic pathway for porphyrins and associated deficiency syndromes.

but rebound tenderness is unusual and suggests peritonitis from some other cause. Modest hepatomegaly is an occasional finding and serum aminotransferase activity may be moderately increased, but there are no other clinical features of liver disease. Peripheral or cranial neuropathy, manifested as pain or paresis, occurs in 50–60%. Deaths have occasionally occurred from respiratory paralysis. Central nervous system dysfunction is frequent and may appear as confusion (40%), seizures (20%) or coma (10%) (Bloomer & Straka 1988).

***Diagnosis.*** Freshly passed urine looks normal but becomes dark on standing owing to the formation of uroporphyrin from porphobilinogen. Virtually all patients excrete an excess of porphobilinogen in the urine in an acute attack, which gives a pink color with Ehrlich's reagent that cannot be extracted by organic solvents (Watson–Schwartz test). Positive tests should be confirmed by direct measurement of urine porphobilinogen. Subsequent measurement of coproporphyrin and protoporphyrin in the stools usually differentiates acute intermittent porphyria (both normal) from coproporphyria (coproporphyrins greatly increased and protoporphyrins moderated increased) and variegate porphyria (protoporphyrins greatly increased and coproporphyrins moderately increased). Direct measurement of enzyme activity in red cells or liver tissue is the most definitive diagnostic method. The differential diagnosis includes lead poisoning and tyrosinemia, both of which inhibit ALA dehydrase and can produce attacks of abdominal pain.

***Treatment.*** A correct diagnosis is important, as drugs, anesthetics and operations may worsen an attack and cause respiratory failure. Environmental and endogenous factors are both important in producing attacks, as evidenced by the fact that latent enzyme defects are found in asymptomatic patients. Conditions increasing the demand for heme, such as induction of cytochrome P-450 by drugs, or increasing hepatic iron are to be avoided.

The management of an acute attack involves recognizing, removing or treating precipitating factors such as drugs, alcohol, fasting, infections, trauma (including surgery), menstruation and pregnancy and giving supportive therapy until the attack subsides spontaneously. Drugs most frequently reported to exacerbate acute porphyria include barbiturates, estrogens, alcohol, phenytoin, sulfonamides, meprobamate and griseofulvin, but any drug known to induce cytochrome P-450 may be risky (Bonkovsky 1990). The production of porphyrins should be minimized by suppressing ALA synthase activity. Hematin is the mainstay of treatment, given in a dose of 3–4 mg/kg intravenously every 12 h for 3 days and repeated as needed. By exerting a negative feedback effect on ALA synthase (Fig. 35.14), hematin reduces the demand for heme in acute porphyria and produces clinical improvement in most cases (McColl et al 1981, Bissell 1988).

Coagulopathy may occur rarely as an adverse effect. Glucose (400–500 g daily intravenously) may also be helpful.

Narcotics may be required for pain relief. Nausea and vomiting can be treated with promazine or chlorpromazine. Seizures pose a particular problem and are probably best treated with diazepam or possibly sodium valproate. Anesthesia requires specialist anesthetic advice.

***Prevention.*** The relatives of porphyric patients need to be screened, as porphyria is latent in three-quarters of cases, and they may need advice on avoiding factors that precipitate attacks.

### Protoporphyria

Protoporphyria usually begins in childhood and is generally a benign disease characterized by mild skin photosensitivity. Sunlight produces itching, erythema and eczema but not blistering. Some patients complain of upper abdominal pain, but neuropsychiatric dysfunction does not occur. Excess protoporphyrin is detected in red cells and stool. The ferrochelatase deficiency can be detected by direct measurement in red cells. Porphobilinogen excretion in the urine is normal.

Occasional patients develop severe liver disease and die from liver failure (Mooyaart et al 1986, Rank et al 1990). Most are over 30 years old, but fatal liver disease in childhood has been described. Cirrhosis is present in patients who have died of liver disease and the liver is black owing to the presence of crystalline protoporphyrin. The main source of excess protoporphyrin is the bone marrow and the main route of excretion is into the bile. However, excess protoporphyrin causes cholestasis and subsequent precipitation in the liver can lead to hepatocellular damage (Bloomer & Enriquez 1982). Patients with very high red blood cell and plasma protoporphyrin concentrations may be particularly liable to liver damage.

Treatment should be directed at limiting protoporphyrin overproduction by correcting any iron deficiency and giving a high carbohydrate diet. Blood transfusions and hematin given intravenously reduce protoporphyrin production and are theoretically beneficial and cholestyramine has been given to interrupt the enterohepatic circulation of protoporphyrin. Liver transplantation has been used for those with advanced liver disease, but it does not correct the metabolic defect (p. 1154).

### Porphyria cutanea tarda

PCT results from a deficiency of uroporphyrinogen decarboxylase. The clinical symptoms are usually limited to the skin (Billett 1988). There is excess uroporphyrin in the urine and some increased excretion of coproporphyrin in the urine and occasionally in the stools. The sporadic form of PCT is the most common and is associated with iron overload, alcohol abuse, estrogen therapy and chronic hepatitis C virus infection (p. 895). Some centers have reported prevalences of chronic hepatitis C virus infection as high as 60–80% among patients with PCT, particularly in patients with more advanced liver disease (Fargion et al 1992, DeCastro et al 1993, Herrero et al 1993). PCT can be precipitated by hexachlorobenzene in persons who have no enzyme deficiency.

The skin lesions occur in areas exposed to the sun and begin as mild erythema that may progress to blisters; eventually these become crusted erosions that heal slowly with scarring. Excessive facial hair, alopecia, hyperpigmentation and hypopigmentation, milia and indurated plaques in the skin can also occur. Most patients have mild increases of serum aminotransferase activity and more than half have an increased serum transferrin saturation. Five to 20% of patients have cirrhosis, usually associated with alcohol abuse. It has been suggested that PCT may predispose to hepatocellular carcinoma, particularly in males with cirrhosis (Rank et al 1990). Almost all patients have increased amounts of iron in the liver, but the total iron stores usually do not exceed 2–3 g (p. 951). Fatty change, focal hepatocellular necrosis and chronic portal hepatitis may be seen.

PCT may be confused with variegate porphyria or coproporphyria, but acute visceral and neurological attacks do not occur. PCT should be distinguished from photosensitization due to drugs. Urine and fecal porphyrin estimations differentiate these conditions. The condition can usually be kept in remission by eliminating precipitating causes and by removing 500 ml blood every 1–2 weeks until the urine uroporphyrin excretion falls substantially or the hemoglobin falls below 11 g/dl.

## NONALCOHOLIC STEATOSIS AND STEATOHEPATITIS

Fatty change is common in the liver, it becomes visible histologically when hepatic lipid exceeds about 5% and involvement of up to 10% of hepatocytes is regarded as normal. Above this level, fatty change may be mild (to 20%), moderate (to 50%) or severe (above 50%) (Braillon et al 1985). Necroinflammatory damage is not a feature of fatty change and, when present, has always suggested alcohol abuse (p. 868). However, it is now recognized that nonalcoholic conditions can produce this combination and mimic alcoholic hepatitis and cirrhosis. This is now called "nonalcoholic steatohepatitis" (NASH) (Ludwig et al 1980).

### Etiology

The common causes of steatosis and NASH relate to lipid metabolism (Table 35.8). The lipid that accumulates in liver cells under most circumstances is triglyceride. The pathogenesis is probably multifactorial and related to varying combinations of increased fatty acid uptake, increased

**Table 35.8** Causes of steatosis and nonalcoholic steatohepatitis (NASH)

| Common | Uncommon |
|---|---|
| Diabetes mellitus | Chronic viral hepatitis |
| Obesity | Malabsorptive disorders |
| Jejunoileal bypass | Total parenteral nutrition |
| Rapid weight reduction | Wilson's disease |
| Starvation (kwashiorkor) | Abetalipoproteinemia |
| Drugs (Table 35.9) | Weber–Christian disease |
| | Gastric bypass operations |
| | Familial hepatic steatosis |

Note: Steatosis is often incidental.

synthesis of fatty acids by the liver, increased synthesis of triglycerides and impaired secretion of triglycerides into the blood as lipoprotein.

***Starvation.*** Chronic starvation as in kwashiorkor is often associated with hepatomegaly and steatohepatitis. The severity of fatty change in the liver is related to the severity and duration of starvation and the liver returns to normal if recovery occurs (Cook & Hutt 1967). Steatohepatitis after jejunoilcal bypass operations occurs during the period of most rapid weight loss and is most severe in those losing most weight (Haines et al 1981). However, obese patients losing equal amounts of weight without surgery show improvement of liver histology and accordingly weight loss alone cannot be the only factor (Drenick et al 1970). Dietary factors during weight loss may be important and in this regard glucose feeding during weight loss prior to death was associated with more steatohepatitis in an autopsy study (Wanless & Lentz 1990). Such dietary factors may also be important during total parenteral nutrition. Very little information is available in patients with eating disorders, but abnormal liver function tests occur in anorexia nervosa and severe steatohepatitis has been reported in a patient with anorexia nervosa and bulimia (Cuellar et al 1987).

***Obesity and diabetes mellitus.*** Ten to 15% of obese patients have fatty liver on biopsy, 20–30% of morbidly obese patients have histologic evidence of portal hepatitis and up to 5% have cirrhosis (McGill 1994). An autopsy study found steatohepatitis in 18% of grossly obese persons (>40% above ideal weight) as opposed to only 3% of those who were lean; steatohepatitis became more frequent as the severity of obesity and hepatic steatosis increased (Wanless & Lentz 1990). Obesity and adult-onset diabetes mellitus often occur together and steatohepatitis is more common when this is the case, but diabetes mellitus is associated statistically with steatohepatitis in its own right and may also be associated with cirrhosis (p. 921).

***Jejunoileal bypass.*** This operation was performed commonly for morbid obesity until the high incidence of adverse effects was realized. Clinical and hepatic histologic changes are most marked in the first 6 months after operation and are usually reversible, but about 10% of patients develop progressive fibrosis and cirrhosis, leading eventually to hepatic failure (Hocking et al 1983). The relative importance of weight loss, malnutrition and bacterial overgrowth in the bypassed intestinal loop in causing the hepatic damage is unclear.

***Total parenteral nutrition (TPN).*** TPN has been associated with hepatic steatosis, steatohepatitis and occasionally cholestasis (p. 979). These changes are frequent in TPN given for more than a week and chronic liver damage including cirrhosis develops occasionally when long-term TPN is necessary (Bowyer et al 1985).

***Drugs.*** Several drugs may cause steatohepatitis (Table 35.9) and amiodarone, diltiazem, nicardipine and nifedipine can cause a histologic picture resembling alcoholic hepatitis, including Mallory bodies (Ludwig 1992).

***Unknown cause.*** Steatohepatitis can occur in patients who are not obese and who do not have diabetes mellitus. Bacon et al (1994) found that most of their patients were neither obese nor diabetic and Wanless & Lentz (1990) found that 2.5% of nonobese subjects in their autopsy study had steatohepatitis.

***Familial fatty liver.*** This rare condition causes death in infancy and childhood and siblings are often affected (Suprun & Freundlich 1981). The main finding at autopsy is marked macrovesicular steatosis in the liver, kidneys and heart.

## Pathology

Fatty change in steatohepatitis should be prominent and of macrovesicular or mixed macrovesicular and microvesicular type. Macrovesicular fatty change is characterized by a single large cytoplasmic fat vacuole with the cell nucleus pushed to the periphery of the hepatocyte, while microvesicular fatty change is characterized by many small fat vacuoles with the nucleus remaining in the center of the hepatocyte (Fig. 35.15). It is now commonly accepted that microvesicular changes can occur in practically any condition in which macrovesicular steatosis occurs, but the opposite is not necessarily true (see below).

Two cautions are worth noting. First, fatty change and portal hepatitis may be the result of two different causes and steatohepatitis does not include this situation. Second, it may be difficult to distinguish mild steatohepatitis from fatty change with minimal inflammation. Furthermore,

**Table 35.9** Drugs causing steatohepatitis (Ludwig 1992)

| | |
|---|---|
| Amiodarone | Nifedipine |
| Diltiazem | Oxacillin |
| Dimethylaminoethoxyhexestrol | Perhexiline |
| Methotrexate | Spironolactone |
| Naproxen | Sulfasalazine |
| Nicardipine | |

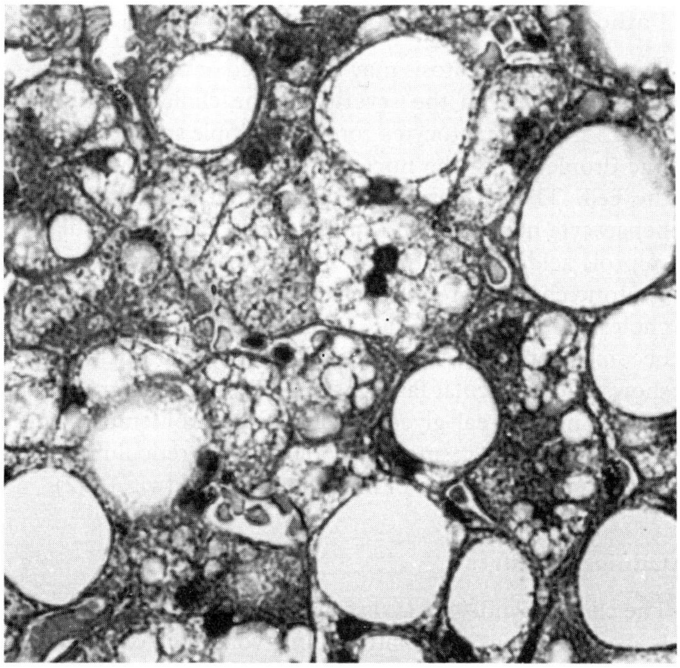

**Fig. 35.15** Macrovesicular steatosis (hepatocytes with single large cytoplasmic fat globules and peripheral nuclei) and microvesicular steatosis (hepatocytes with multiple small cytoplasmic fat globules and central nuclei) of the liver (hematoxylin and eosin, ×680).

inflammatory changes may be spotty and not readily apparent on a given biopsy specimen (Ludwig 1992).

NASH does not differ substantially from alcoholic hepatitis in appearance (p. 868), although NASH tends to produce more fat in proportion to the amount of hepatocellular damage and inflammation (Diehl et al 1988). Prominent nuclear vacuolization of hepatocytes may be seen in steatohepatitis associated with diabetes mellitus. The steatohepatitic changes associated with malabsorptive disorders and total parenteral nutrition tend to be spotty and cholestatic changes and pigment deposition may be important clues to these causes (Bowyer et al 1985). Mallory bodies are associated with the steatohepatitis seen in Wilson's disease, jejunoileal bypass and rapid weight loss after previous morbid obesity. They have also been observed in amiodarone toxicity, Weber–Christian disease and abetalipoproteinemia (Ludwig 1992).

### Clinical features

Most patients with NASH are asymptomatic, the diagnosis being made incidentally after discovery of abnormal liver function tests. Although the condition can occur at any age, patients are usually middle aged and there is a female predominance. Upper abdominal pain may occur, hepatomegaly is common and the liver may be tender on palpation. Signs and symptoms of advanced chronic liver disease are rare.

### Investigations

Serum aminotransferase activities are mildly elevated, usually less than three times normal. Autoantibodies are not found or show only low titers and are incidental. Diffuse fatty change in the liver can be suspected noninvasively by a hyperechoic appearance on ultrasound (p. 54) and a decrease in density relative to the spleen on a computed tomogram (p. 67). Fat cannot usually be distinguished from fibrosis by ultrasound imaging. Occasionally, fatty change occurs focally and presents a pseudotumor appearance. Radiological methods for detecting fat are insensitive and only become positive when more than 30% of liver cells are affected (McGill 1994).

### Treatment

Gradual weight reduction in obese patients results in return of serum aminotransferase activities to normal and in disappearance of fat from the liver (Eriksson et al 1986b). Rapid weight loss may precipitate steatohepatitis and should be avoided. Patients who have had a jejunoileal bypass should seek alternate methods of weight loss after reversal of the operation. Possibly offending drugs should be discontinued. Modifications of parenteral nutrition solutions may be helpful. It is not clear whether close control of diabetes is helpful, as most patients are obese as well. A study of ursodeoxycholic acid therapy in 24 patients with NASH showed modest improvement in liver enzyme results and an improvement in the histologic grading of steatosis in a third of patients (Laurin et al 1994).

## MICROVESICULAR STEATOSIS

Microvesicular steatosis may occur to some extent in any cause of fatty change, including nonalcoholic steatohepatitis, but there is a group of more serious liver diseases in which microvesicular steatosis is the chief histologic finding. The common metabolic denominator is probably an inherited or acquired mitochondrial enzyme defect. In macrovesicular steatosis many patients with excessive alcohol use, obesity and/or diabetes mellitus develop the histologic lesion, but only a small minority of patients exposed to factors causing microvesicular steatosis become ill, suggesting the possibility of an underlying metabolic defect. Urea cycle enzymopathies (p. 971) and defects in β-oxidation of fatty acids have been found to be the sole cause in some patients, but it is also suspected that they are underlying defects uncovered by environmental factors in other cases (Hautekeet et al 1990).

### Etiology

The conditions associated with microvesicular steatosis

**Table 35.10** Causes of microvesicular steatohepatitis

| |
|---|
| Acute fatty liver of pregnancy |
| Reye's syndrome |
| Drugs (Table 35.11) |
| Alcohol |
| Jamaican vomiting sickness (hypoglycin A) |
| Viral hepatitis (δ) |
| Inherited metabolic disorders* |

*Urea cycle defects, fatty acid β-oxidation defects, cholesterol ester storage disease, Wolman disease, Alper's syndrome.

**Table 35.11** Drugs causing microvesicular steatosis (Hautekeete et al 1990, Ludwig 1992)

| | |
|---|---|
| Amineptine | Ketoprofen |
| Amiodarone | Pirprofen |
| Aspirin | Salicylate* |
| Chlortetracycline | Tetracycline* |
| Didanosine (DDI) | Valproic acid |
| Hopantenate | Warfarin* |

*At high doses only.

form a heterogeneous group (Table 35.10). Acute fatty liver of pregnancy occurs in the third trimester and appears to be more common in primiparous women (p. 1091). Reye's syndrome occurs mainly under the age of 18 years and a preceding viral illness and/or aspirin use is virtually universal (p. 807). Several drugs have been associated with microvesicular steatosis (Table 35.11). Sodium valproate is probably now the drug most often responsible. A number of patients taking the drug show increased serum aminotransferase activity, but rare individuals develop an illness like Reye's syndrome associated with extensive necrosis, suggesting an idiosyncratic reaction. Jamaican vomiting sickness is caused by ingestion of unripe akee fruit, which contains a hepatotoxin called hypoglycin A that can reproduce the disease in animals (Tanaka et al 1976). Hypoglycin A is an amino acid metabolized to the mitochondrial poison methylenecyclopropylacetic acid, which is in turn structurally similar to 4-pentanoic acid, a substance capable of reproducing Reye's syndrome in rats and related to metabolites of sodium valproate (Hautekeet et al 1990). Alcohol can induce microvesicular steatosis and produce a clinical syndrome similar to alcoholic hepatitis except that serum aminotransferase activities are higher.

Microvesicular steatosis occurs in inherited metabolic defects such as the urea cycle enzymopathies (p. 971) and disorders of fatty acid oxidation including deficiencies in carnitine metabolism and of acetylcoenzyme A dehydrogenases (Vockley 1994). Microvesicular steatosis may also be associated with cholesterol ester storage disease (acid cholesterol ester hydrolase deficiency), Wolman's disease (lysosomal acid esterase deficiency) (above) and Alper's syndrome, which is associated with progressive neuronal degeneration, microvesicular steatosis and cirrhosis.

### Pathology

Microvesicular steatosis may be marked or mild and correlates roughly with the severity of the clinical syndrome (Fig. 35.15). Hepatocytes contain multiple small cytoplasmic droplets with the nucleus remaining in the center of the cell. The fat vesicles stain with oil red-O. Massive hepatocyte necrosis can occur in severe cases, particularly valproic acid toxicity. In acute fatty liver of pregnancy, the steatotic changes are diffuse early in the disease, but later cholestasis, centrilobular endotheliitis and necrosis become prominent. In Reye's syndrome, light microscopy shows microvesicular fatty change only, but ultrastructural studies may reveal glycogen depletion, proliferation and dilatation of the smooth endoplasmic reticulum and swelling and distortion of mitochondria (Ludwig 1992).

### Clinical features

The clinical syndrome is similar regardless of age or cause. It usually begins with fatigue and vomiting followed by lethargy, impairment of consciousness and coma. Jaundice is characteristic of acute fatty liver of pregnancy, alcoholic liver disease and viral infections but is rare in Reye's syndrome, Jamaican vomiting sickness and the inherited metabolic disorders. It is unpredictable in drug reactions.

### Investigations

Liver function tests show increased serum aminotransferase activities, often very marked, and variable increases of alkaline phosphatase and γ-glutamyl transferase. Prolongation of the prothrombin time reflects the severity of liver damage. Other biochemical abnormalities include hypoglycemia, hyperammonemia, hyperuricemia, acidosis and occasionally myoglobinuria.

### Treatment

The mainstay of treatment in acute fatty liver of pregnancy is prompt interruption of pregnancy. In other cases, possibly toxic drugs should be discontinued. Otherwise, treatment is supportive with correction of metabolic abnormalities. Patients with defects in fatty acid oxidation should avoid fasting. Patients with defects of long-chain fat metabolism may take cornstarch as an alternative source of glucose and administration of fat as medium-chain triglycerides has been reported to be of value (Vockley 1994). Carnitine replacement is effective in patients with carnitine metabolism deficiencies. Emergency liver transplantation should be considered for progressive fulminant hepatic failure (p. 1155).

## HEPATOBILIARY DYSFUNCTION AND PARENTERAL NUTRITION

Total parenteral nutrition (TPN) (p. 634) is commonly

associated with hepatobiliary abnormalities (Quigley et al 1993). Most of these abnormalities are reversible, but in a few patients hepatic cirrhosis can develop. Short-term abnormalities in adults are usually revealed by abnormal liver function tests reflecting underlying steatosis and steatohepatitis, while in infants cholestatic liver function tests reflect histological changes of cholestasis in the liver. Biliary sludge and gallstones can occur at any age and long-term TPN can cause irreversible hepatic cirrhosis.

### Etiology

Many factors contribute to the development of hepatobiliary abnormalities during TPN and these may be related to the TPN itself or to other patient abnormalities. It has been difficult to separate these factors, but the finding of abnormal liver function tests in 61.5% of patients with inflammatory bowel disease receiving TPN and in 6.2% of matched patients receiving enteral nutrition points to the importance of TPN itself (Abad-Lacruz et al 1990). Factors related to TPN include an excess calorie input over requirement, an excess of calories given as carbohydrate and an imbalance between carbohydrate and nitrogen provision. Other less important factors may also contribute (Quigley et al 1993). Cholestasis during TPN is more related to the duration of the TPN therapy. The development of biliary sludge and gallstones is associated with diminished bile secretion. Patient factors contributing to hepatobiliary abnormality include malnutrition, glucose intolerance, sepsis, lack of oral food intake leading to poor enteric stimulation of biliary secretion and intestinal disease and its consequences for which TPN is given. Immaturity of the biliary secretory system leading to low bile flow is important in premature infants.

### Manifestations and pathology

TPN-related hepatic dysfunction is usually recognized from the development of abnormal liver function tests. These develop some 1–4 weeks after starting TPN in anything from a quarter to all patients, perhaps related to their underlying diseases. Increased plasma enzyme activities are usually mild to moderate and may resolve even if TPN is continued. Increased transaminase activity usually reflects hepatic steatosis or steatohepatitis, increased alkaline phosphatase activity usually reflects cholestasis and increased $\gamma$-glutamyl transferase activity is nonspecific. Hyperbilirubinemia is much less common and jaundice is uncommon. The most frequent finding on liver biopsy in adults is steatosis, steatohepatitis is less common and cholestasis is seen mainly after prolonged TPN. Cholestasis is the most frequent finding in infants and the histological features may mimic neonatal hepatitis or biliary atresia.

### Diagnosis and management

TPN-related hepatic dysfunction is recognized from its relation to the administration of TPN (above) and it needs to be differentiated from abnormality related to the disease for which TPN is being given, sepsis (p. 1109), drug toxicity (p. 845) and viral hepatitis. Liver biopsy shows the features described above but is required only if liver function tests deteriorate or fail to improve spontaneously or on moderation of TPN. TPN-related liver damage can be minimized by avoiding giving excess calories, by including lipid as a caloric source, by cycling calorie intake during the day, by giving some oral food intake as soon as possible and by omitting copper from TPN in patients with cholestasis (Bowyer et al 1985). TPN may need to be withdrawn temporarily when liver function tests do not improve.

### Chronic liver disease

Patients receiving long-term TPN may develop persistent liver function test abnormality. This occurs in about 15% of patients, liver biopsy shows steatohepatitis, fibrosis and cholestasis and death from cirrhosis can occur (Bowyer et al 1985). Patients on long-term treatment can also develop hepatic phospholipidosis (Degott et al 1988). Infants may be even more liable to develop chronic liver disease, including hepatocellular carcinoma.

### Biliary disease

Impaired bile flow and gallbladder stasis occur during TPN and predispose to biliary disease. Biliary sludge develops rapidly in patients on TPN and may be present in most or all patients within 3–4 months (Messing et al 1983). Gallstones develop in about a third of patients within about 2 years (Pitt et al 1983). The liability to gallstones is increased where the terminal ileum has been resected. Consequently, these patients are liable to biliary colic and calculous or acalculous cholecystitis and may require cholecystectomy.

## AMYLOIDOSIS

Amyloidosis results from tissue deposition of an insoluble fibrillar protein called amyloid that interferes with normal organ function. The kidneys, heart and peripheral nervous system are most commonly affected. Hepatic infiltration is found at autopsy in the majority of patients, but hepatic involvement was found during life in only 16% in one large series and it is uncommon for liver disease to cause the dominant clinical features (Gertz & Kyle 1988).

Amyloid was formerly classified by its anatomic distribution but is now classified by the biochemical composition of its subunit protein (Gertz & Kyle 1989). Amyloid AL

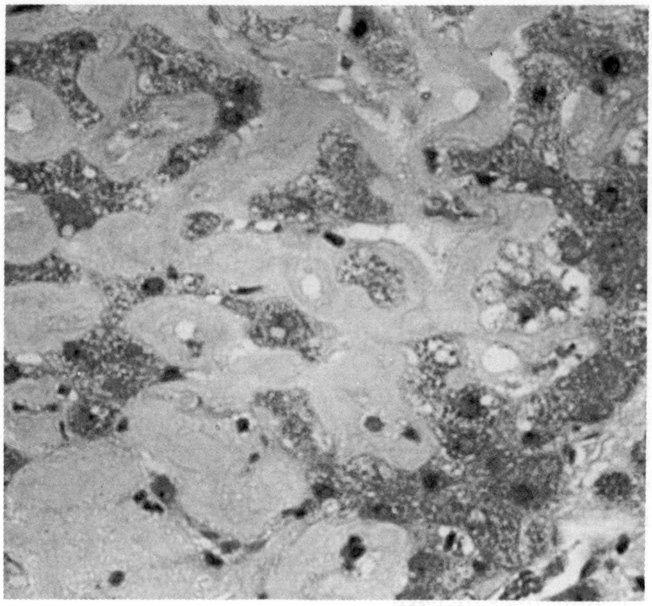

**Fig. 35.16** Extensive amyloidosis (pale staining material) deposited diffusely in the hepatic parenchyma with atrophy of the hepatocytes (hematoxylin and eosin, ×425).

(composed of immunoglobulin light chain) is associated with primary amyloidosis and multiple myeloma. Amyloid AA is composed of a unique protein ("protein A") and is found in chronic inflammatory disorders and familial Mediterranean fever. Other specific types of amyloid are found in familial (AF), senile (SSA), cerebral angiopathic (CAA), isolated atrial (IAA) and other forms of the disease.

### Pathology

The involved liver is enlarged and firm, with a pale, waxy appearance at autopsy. Microscopically there is characteristic deposition of amorphous eosinophilic and hyaline material in the sinusoids, which eventually compresses the liver cell plates (Fig. 35.16). The pathologic changes are usually diffuse and easily seen with routine staining, but Congo red may be used to demonstrate the characteristic green birefringence with polarized light. The homogeneous fibrillar structure of the material can be demonstrated by electronmicroscopy.

### Clinical features

Gertz & Kyle (1988) have reviewed the findings in 80 patients with dominant hepatic involvement associated with light-chain (AL) protein. Most complained of fatigue and two-thirds had abdominal bloating, early satiety or weight loss. Occasionally, hepatic amyloidosis presents with severe intrahepatic cholestasis (Rubinow et al 1978). The main physical finding was hepatomegaly, present in 90% of patients with liver involvement. Liver biopsy was usually diagnostic and the indications for biopsy included hepatomegaly of unknown cause (60%), suspected hepatic metastatic malignancy (25%) and cholestasis of unknown cause (7%). Three-quarters of patients had extrahepatic involvement: nephrotic syndrome (36%), congestive heart failure (20%), orthostatic hypotension (13%) and/or peripheral neuropathy (8%). Fourteen percent had associated myeloma on bone marrow biopsy, but this proved of no clinical importance. Proteinuria, a serum monoclonal protein or hypogammaglobulinemia, hyposplenism on the peripheral blood smear indicating splenic involvement and hepatomegaly out of proportion to liver enzyme abnormalities were all useful pointers to hepatic disease.

### Investigations

Liver function tests are normal in two-thirds of patients or show only minor abnormalities in spite of obvious hepatomegaly. Hypoalbuminemia is common but most often a consequence of proteinuria. Liver biopsy confirms the diagnosis, but as there may be an increased risk of hepatic bleeding in amyloidosis, examination of a rectal biopsy or fat aspirate should be tried first (Gertz & Kyle 1988).

### Treatment

There is no effective treatment for amyloidosis. Melphalan and prednisone have been tried with some success and could be used given the poor prognosis in patients with liver involvement.

### Prognosis

The median survival in patients with primary hepatic amyloidosis is around 9 months, with a 5-year survival of 13% (Gertz & Kyle 1988). Patients do not die of hepatic failure but rather of progressive heart failure, sudden death (presumably cardiac) or progressive renal failure. Complications of portal hypertension are rare (Itescu 1984). About 10% of patients have a slowly progressive form of the disease and prolonged survival (Gertz & Kyle 1988).

REFERENCES

Abad-Lacruz A, Gonzáles-Huix F, Esteve M et al 1990 Liver function tests abnormalities in patients with inflammatory bowel disease receiving artificial nutrition: a prospective randomized study of total enteral nutrition vs. total parenteral nutrition. Journal of Parenteral and Enteral Nutrition 14: 618–621

Abbott C M, Lovegrove J U, Whitehouse D B, Hopkinson D A, Povey S

1992 Prenatal diagnosis of alpha-1-antitrypsin deficiency by PCR of linked polymorphisms: a study of 17 cases. Prenatal Diagnosis 12: 235–240

Adams P C, Ghent C N, Grant D R, Frei J V, Wall W J 1991a Transplantation of a donor liver with haemochromatosis: evidence against an inherited intrahepatic defect. Gut 32: 1082–1083

Adams P C, Speechley M, Kertesz A E 1991b Long-term survival analysis in hereditary hemochromatosis. Gastroenterology 101: 368–372

Adams P C, Bradley C, Frei J V 1994 Hepatic iron and zinc concentrations after portacaval shunting for nonalcoholic cirrhosis. Hepatology 19: 101–105

Adamson M, Reiner B, Olson J L et al 1992 Indian childhood cirrhosis in an American child. Gastroenterology 102: 1771–1777

Alagille D 1984 Alpha-1-antitrypsin deficiency. Hepatology 4: 11S–14S

Andresen B S, Knudsen I, Jensen P K A, Rasmussen K, Gregersen N 1992 Two novel nonradioactive polymerase chain reaction-based assays of dried blood spots, genomic DNA, or whole cells for fast, reliable detection of Z and S mutations in the alpha-1-antitrypsin gene. Clinical Chemistry 38: 2100–2107

Bachmann C 1987 Diagnosis of urea cycle disorders. Enzyme 38: 233–241

Bacon B R 1992 Causes of iron overload. New England Journal of Medicine 326: 126–127

Bacon B R, Farahvash M J, Janney J G, Neuschwander-Tetri B A 1994 Nonalcoholic steatohepatitis: an expanded clinical entity. Gastroenterology 107: 1103–1109

Balan V, Scolapio J S, Harrison J M, Mahoney D W, Zinsmeister A R, Gross J B 1994 Survival in Wilson's disease is less than expected: an analysis of 127 patients followed long-term. Gastroenterology 106: A863

Barron R, Grace N D, Sherwood G et al 1989 Iron overload complicating sideroblastic anemia – is the gene for hemochromatosis responsible? Gastroenterology 96: 1204–1206

Barry M 1974 Liver iron concentration, stainable iron, and total body storage iron. Gut 15: 324–334

Barry M, Cartei G, Sherlock S 1970 Differential ferrioxamine test in haemochromatosis and liver diseases. Gut 10: 697–704

Bassett M L, Halliday J W, Powell L W 1981 HLA typing in idiopathic hemochromatosis: distinction between homozygotes and heterozygotes with biochemical expression. Hepatology 1: 120–126

Bassett M L, Halliday J W, Powell L W 1986 Value of hepatic iron measurements in early hemochromatosis and determination of the critical iron level associated with fibrosis. Hepatology 6: 24–29

Batshaw M L, Monahan P S 1987 Treatment of urea cycle disorders. Enzyme 38: 242–250

Beaudet A L, Ferry G D, Nichols B L, Rosenberg H S 1977 Cholesterol ester storage disease: clinical, biochemical, and pathological studies. Journal of Pediatrics 90: 910–914

Beaumont C, Simon M, Fauchet R et al 1979 Serum ferritin as a possible marker of the hemochromatosis allele. New England Journal of Medicine 301: 169–174

Beigi B, O'Keefe M, Bowell R, Naughton E, Badawi N, Lanigan B 1993 Ophthalmic findings in classical galactosaemia – prospective study. British Journal of Ophthalmology 77: 162–164

Berg N O, Eriksson S 1972 Liver disease in adults with $alpha_1$ antitrypsin deficiency. New England Journal of Medicine 287: 1264–1267

Beutler E 1991 Galactosemia: screening and diagnosis. Clinical Biochemistry 24: 293–300

Billett H H 1988 Porphyrias: inborn errors in heme production. Hospital Practice (Office edn) 23: 40–42

Birrer P, McElvaney N G, Chang-Stroman L M, Crystal R G 1991 Alpha-1-antitrypsin deficiency and liver disease. Journal of Inherited Metabolic Disease 14: 512–525

Bissell D M 1988 Treatment of acute hepatic porphyria with hematin. Journal of Hepatology 6: 1–7

Blackwood W, Corsellis J A N (eds) 1976 Greenfield's neuropathology, 3rd edn. Arnold, London, p 172–177

Bloomer J R, Bonkovsky H L 1989 The porphyrias. Disease a Month 35: 1–54

Bloomer J R, Enriquez R 1982 Evidence that hepatic crystalline deposits in a patient with protoporphyria are composed of protoporphyrin. Gastroenterology 82: 569–572

Bloomer J R, Straka J G 1988 Porphyrin metabolism. In: Arias I M, Jakoby W B, Popper H, Schachter D, Schafritz D A (eds) The liver: biology and pathobiology, 2nd edn. Raven Press, New York, p 451

Bomford A, Williams R 1976 Long term results of venesection therapy in idiopathic haemochromatosis. Quarterly Journal of Medicine 45: 611–623

Bomford A B, Munro H N 1985 Transferrin and its receptor: their roles in cell function. Hepatology 5: 870–875

Bonkovsky H L 1990 Porphyrin and heme metabolism and the porphyrias. In: Zakim D, Boyer T D (eds) Hepatology: a textbook of liver disease, 2nd edn. W B Saunders, Philadelphia, p 378–424

Bonkovsky H L 1991 Iron and the liver. American Journal of Medical Science 301: 32–43

Borsey D Q, Lawson A A H 1982 Idiopathic haemochromatosis presenting as cardiac failure in a young male. British Journal of Clinical Practice 36: 409–411

Bowyer B A, Fleming C R, Ludwig J, Petz J, McGill D B 1985 Does long-term home parenteral nutrition in adult patients cause chronic liver disease? Journal of Parenteral and Enteral Nutrition 9: 11–17

Braillon A, Capron J P, Herve M A, Degott C, Quenum C 1985 Liver in obesity. Gut 26: 133–139

Brewer G J, Hill G M, Prasad A S, Cossack Z T, Rabbani P 1983 Oral zinc therapy for Wilson's disease. Annals of Internal Medicine 99: 314–319

Brewer G J, Dick R D, Yuzhasiyan-Gurkin V, Tankanow R, Young A B, Kluin K J 1991 Initial therapy of patients with Wilson's disease with tetrathiomolybdate. Archives of Neurology 48: 42–47

Brink B, Disler P, Lynch S, Jacobs P, Charlton R, Bothwell T 1976 Patterns of iron storage in dietary iron overload and idiopathic hemochromatosis. Journal of Laboratory and Clinical Medicine 88: 725–731

Brissot P, Bourel M, Herry D et al 1981 Assessment of liver iron content in 271 patients: a reevaluation of direct and indirect methods. Gastroenterology 80: 557–565

Brusilow S W 1984 Arginine, an indispensable amino acid for patients with inborn errors of urea synthesis. Journal of Clinical Investigation 74: 2144–2148

Brusilow S W 1985 Disorders of the urea cycle. Hospital Practice (Office edn) 20: 65–72

Bull P C, Thomas G R, Rommens J M, Forbes J R, Cox D W 1993 The Wilson disease gene is a putative copper transporting P-type ATPase similar to the Menkes gene. Nature Genetics 5: 327–337

Burmeister L A, Valdivia T, Nuttall F Q 1991 Adult hereditary fructose intolerance. Archives of Internal Medicine 151: 773–776

Cairns J E, Williams H P, Walshe J M 1969 "Sunflower cataract" in Wilson's disease. British Medical Journal 3: 95–96

Callea F, Fevery J, Massi G, de Groote J, Desmet V J 1985 Storage of alpha-1-antitrypsin in intrahepatic bile duct cells in alpha-1-antitrypsin deficiency (PiZ phenotype). Histopathology 9: 99–108

Campra J L, Craig J R, Peters R L, Reynolds T B 1973 Cirrhosis associated with partial deficiency of alpha-1-antitrypsin in an adult. Annals of Internal Medicine 78: 233–238

Capron J-P, Capron-Chivrac D, Tossou H, Delamarre J, Eb F 1984 Spontaneous *Yersinia enterocolitica* peritonitis in idiopathic hemochromatosis. Gastroenterology 87: 1372–1375

Carlson J, Eriksson S 1985 Chronic "cryptogenic" liver disease and malignant hepatoma in intermediate alpha-1-antitrypsin deficiency identified by a PiZ-specific monoclonal antibody. Scandinavian Journal of Gastroenterology 20: 835–842

Cartwright G E 1978 Diagnosis of treatable Wilson's disease. New England Journal of Medicine 298: 1347–1350

Cawley E P, Hsu Y T, Wood B T, Weary P E 1969 Hemochromatosis and the skin. Archives of Dermatology 100: 1–6

Chapman R W G, Hussain M A M, Gorman A et al 1982 Effect of ascorbic acid deficiency on serum ferritin concentration in patients with β-thalassaemia major and iron overload. Journal of Clinical Pathology 35: 487–491

Chen Y T, Bazzarre C H, Lee M M, Sidbur J B, Coleman R A 1993 Type I glycogen storage disease: nine years of management with cornstarch. European Journal of Pediatrics 152 (suppl 1): S56–S59

Colombo C, Setchell K D R, Podda M et al 1990 The effects of

ursodeoxycholic acid therapy in liver disease associated with cystic fibrosis. Journal of Pediatrics 117: 482–489
Colombo C, Apostolo M G, Assaisso M, Roman B, Bottani P 1992 Liver disease in cystic fibrosis. Netherlands Journal of Medicine 41: 119–122
Conn H O 1972 Portacaval anastomosis and hepatic hemosiderin deposition: a prospective, controlled investigation. Gastroenterology 62: 61–72
Cook G C, Hutt M S R 1967 The liver after kwashiorkor. British Medical Journal 3: 454–457
Cotting J, Lentze M J, Reichen J 1990 Effects of ursodeoxycholic acid treatment on nutrition and liver function in patients with cystic fibrosis and long-standing cholestasis. Gut 31: 918–921
Cox D W 1989 Alpha-1-antitrypsin deficiency. In: Scriver C R, Beaudet A L, Sly W S et al (eds) The metabolic basis of inherited disease, 6th edn. McGraw-Hill, New York, p 2409–2437
Cox D W, Mansfield T 1987 Prenatal diagnosis of alpha-1-antitrypsin deficiency and estimates of fetal risk for disease. Journal of Medical Genetics 24: 52–59
Cox T M 1990 Hereditary fructose intolerance. Ballière's Clinical Gastroenterology 4: 61–78
Cox T M 1991 Fructose intolerance: diet and inheritance. Proceedings of the Nutrition Society 50: 305–309
Cross N C P, Cox T M 1990 Hereditary fructose intolerance. International Journal of Biochemistry 22: 685–689
Crystal R G 1990 Alpha-1-antitrypsin deficiency, emphysema, and liver disease: genetic basis and strategies for therapy. Journal of Clinical Investigation 85: 1343–1352
Cuellar R E, Tarter R, Hays A, Van Thiel D H 1987 The possible occurrence of "alcoholic hepatitis" in a patient with bulimia in the absence of diagnosable alcoholism. Hepatology 7: 878–883
Dadone M M, Kushner J P, Edwards C Q, Bishop D T, Skolnick M H 1982 Hereditary hemochromatosis: analysis of laboratory expression of the disease by genotype in 18 pedigrees. American Journal of Clinical Pathology 78: 196–207
Danks D M 1989 Disorders of copper transport. In: Scrivner C R, Beaudet A L, Sly W S, Valle D (eds) The metabolic basis of inherited disease, 6th edn. McGraw-Hill, New York. Ch 54, pp. 1411–1431
De Bont B, Walker A C, Carter R F, Oldfield R K, Davidson G P 1987 Idiopathic hemochromatosis presenting as acute hepatitis. Journal of Pediatrics 110: 431–434
Degott C, Messing B, Moreau D et al 1988 Liver phospholipidosis induced by parenteral nutrition: histologic, histochemical, and ultrastructural investigations. Gastroenterology 95: 183–191
DeCastro M, Sánchez J, Herrera J F et al 1993 Hepatitis C virus antibodies and liver disease in patients with porphyria cutanea tarda. Hepatology 17: 551–557
Deugnier Y M, Turlin B, Powell L W et al 1993 Differentiation between heterozygotes and homozygotes in genetic hemochromatosis by means of a histological hepatic iron index: a study of 192 cases. Hepatology 17: 30–34
Diehl A M, Goodman Z, Ishak K G 1988 Alcohollike liver disease in nonalcoholics: a clinical and histologic comparison with alcohol-induced liver injury. Gastroenterology 95: 1056–1062
DiMagno E P, Lowe J E, Snodgrass P J, Jones J D 1986 Ornithine transcarbamylase deficiency – a cause of bizarre behavior in a man. New England Journal of Medicine 315: 744–747
Dorney S F A, Hassall E G, Arbuckle S M, Vargas J H, Berquist W E 1987 SZ phenotype alpha-1-antitrypsin deficiency with paucity of the intralobular bile ducts. Australian Pediatric Journal 23: 55–56
Dowdy R P 1969 Copper metabolism. American Journal of Clinical Nutrition 22: 887–892
Drenick E J, Simmons F, Murphy J F 1970 Effect on hepatic morphology of treatment of obesity by fasting, reducing diets and small-bowel bypass. New England Journal of Medicine 282: 829–834
Duthie A, Doherty D G, Williams C et al 1992 Genotype analysis for ΔF508, G551D, and R553X mutations in children and young adults with cystic fibrosis with and without chronic liver disease. Hepatology 15: 660–664
Dymock I W, Casser J, Pyke D A, Oakley W G, Williams R 1972 Observations on the pathogenesis, complications and treatment of diabetes in 115 cases of hemochromatosis. American Journal of Medicine 52: 203–210
Easley R M Jr, Schreiner B J Jr, Yu P N 1972 Reversible cardiomyopathy associated with hemochromatosis. New England Journal of Medicine 287: 866–867
Edwards C Q, Kushner J P 1993 Screening for hemochromatosis. New England Journal of Medicine 328: 1616–1620
Edwards C Q, Skolnick M H, Kushner J P 1981 Hereditary hemochromatosis: contributions of genetic analyses. Progress in Hematology 12: 43–73
Edwards C Q, Dadone M M, Skolnick M H, Kushner J P 1982 Hereditary haemochromatosis. Clinics in Haematology 11: 411–435
Edwards C Q, Griffen L M, Goldgar D, Drummond C, Skolnick M H, Kushner J P 1988 Prevalence of hemochromatosis among 11,065 presumably healthy blood donors. New England Journal of Medicine 318: 1355–1362
Enomoto K, Ishibashi H, Irie K et al 1989 Fulminant hepatic failure without evidence of cirrhosis in a case of Wilson's disease. Japan Journal of Medicine 28: 80–84
Eriksson S 1987 Alpha-1-antitrypsin deficiency and liver cirrhosis in adults: an analysis of 35 Swedish autopsied cases. Acta Medica Scandinavica 22: 461–467
Eriksson S, Carlson J, Velez R 1986a Risk of cirrhosis and primary liver cancer in alpha-1-antitrypsin deficiency. New England Journal of Medicine 314: 736–739
Eriksson S, Eriksson K F, Bondesson L 1986b Nonalcoholic steatohepatitis in obesity: a reversible condition. Acta Medica Scandinavica 220: 83–88
Fargion S, Piperno A, Cappellini M D et al 1992 Hepatitis C virus and porphyria cutanea tarda: evidence of a strong association. Hepatology 16: 1322–1326
Farrer L A, Bowcock A M, Hebert J M et al 1991 Predictive testing for Wilson's disease using tightly linked and flanking DNA markers. Neurology 41: 992–999
Felig D M, Brusilow S W, Boyer J L 1995 Hyperammonemic coma due to parenteral nutrition in a woman with heterozygous ornithine transcarbamylase deficiency. Gastroenterology 109: 282–284
Fillet G, Beguin Y, Baldelli L 1989 Model of reticuloendothelial iron metabolism in humans: abnormal behavior in idiopathic hemochromatosis and in inflammation. Blood 74: 844–851
Finch C A, Huebers H 1982 Perspectives in iron metabolism. New England Journal of Medicine 306: 1520–1528
Finch S C, Finch C A 1955 Idiopathic hemochromatosis and iron storage disease, A. Iron metabolism in hemochromatosis. Medicine 34: 381–430
Finkelstein J E, Hauser E R, Leonard C O, Brusilow S W 1990 Late-onset ornithine transcarbamylase deficiency in male patients. Journal of Pediatrics 117: 897–902
Fleming C R, Dickson E R, Hollenhorst R W, Goldstein N P, McCall J T, Baggenstoss A H 1975 Pigmented corneal rings in a patient with primary biliary cirrhosis. Gastroenterology 69: 220–225
Fracanzani A L, Fargion S, Romano R et al 1989 Immunohistochemical evidence for a lack of ferritin in duodenal absorptive epithelial cells in idiopathic hemochromatosis. Gastroenterology 96: 1071–1078
Frank D J, Dusol M, Schiff E R 1979 Primary shunt hyperbilirubinemia with secondary iron overload: a case report. Gastroenterology 77: 754–757
Frommer D, Morris J, Sherlock S, Abrams J, Newman S 1977 Kayser–Fleischer-like rings in patients without Wilson's disease. Gastroenterology 72: 1331–1335
Garry P J, Saiki J H 1982 Idiopathic hemochromatosis: serum ferritin concentrations during therapy by phlebotomy. Clinical Chemistry 28: 1806–1808
Gertz M A, Kyle R A 1988 Hepatic amyloidosis (primary [AL], immunoglobulin light chain): the natural history in 80 patients. American Journal of Medicine 85: 73–80
Gertz M A, Kyle R A 1989 Primary systemic amyloidosis – a diagnostic primer. Mayo Clinic Proceedings 64: 1505–1519
Ghishan F K, Greene H L 1988 Liver disease in children with PiZZ alpha-1-antitrypsin deficiency. Hepatology 8: 307–310
Ghishan F K, Greene H L 1990 Inborn errors of metabolism that lead to permanent liver injury. In: Zakim D, Boyer T D (eds) Hepatology: a textbook of liver disease, 2nd edn. W B Saunders, Philadelphia, p 1300–1348
Ginsberg H N, Le N-A, Short M P, Ramakrishnan R, Desnick R J 1987

Suppression of apolipoprotein B production during treatment of cholesteryl ester storage disease with lovastatin. Journal of Clinical Investigation 80: 1692–1697

Giorgio A J, Cartwright G E, Wintrobe M M 1964 Pseudo-Kayser–Fleischer rings. Archives of Internal Medicine 113: 817–818

Glass J D, Reich S G, DeLong M R 1990 Wilson's disease. Development of neurological disease after beginning penicillamine therapy. Archives of Neurology 47: 595–596

Gordeuk V R, Boyd R D, Brittenham G M 1986 Dietary iron overload persists in rural sub-Saharan Africa. Lancet 1: 1310–1313

Gordeuk V, Mukiibi J, Hasstedt S J et al 1992 Iron overload in Africa. Interaction between a gene and dietary iron content. New England Journal of Medicine 326: 95–100

Gross J B Jr, Ludwig J, Wiesner R H, McCall J T, LaRusso N F 1985 Abnormalities in tests of copper metabolism in primary sclerosing cholangitis. Gastroenterology 89: 272–278

Groth C G, Dubois R S, Corman J et al 1973 Metabolic effects of hepatic replacement in Wilson's disease. Transplantation Proceedings 5: 829–833

Guyader D, Gandon Y, Deugnier Y et al 1989 Evaluation of computed tomography in the assessment of liver iron overload. A study of 46 cases of idiopathic hemochromatosis. Gastroenterology 97: 737–743

Guyader D, Gandon Y, Robert J Y et al 1992 Magnetic resonance imaging and assessment of liver iron content in genetic hemochromatosis. Journal of Hepatology 15: 304–308

Haines N W, Baker A L, Boyer J L et al 1981 Prognostic indicators of hepatic injury following jejunoileal bypass performed for refractory obesity: a prospective study. Hepatology 1: 161–167

Harada M, Hirai K, Sakisaka S, Ueno T, Abe H, Tanikawa K 1992 Comparative study of magnetic resonance imaging, computed tomography and histology in the assessment of liver iron overload. Internal Medicine 31: 180–184

Harris Z L, Migas M C, Hughes A E, Logan J I, Gitlin J D 1996 Familial dementia due to a frameshift mutation in the caeruloplasmin gene. Quarterly Journal of Medicine 89: 355–359

Hautekeet M L, Degott C, Benhamou J-P 1990 Microvesicular steatosis of the liver. Acta Clinica Belgica 45: 311–326

Herrero C, Vicente A, Bruguera M et al 1993 Is hepatitis C virus infection a trigger of porphyria cutanea tarda? Lancet 341: 788–789

Hill G M, Brewer G J, Prasad A S, Hydrick C A, Hartmann D E 1987 Treatment of Wilson's disease with zinc. I. Oral zinc therapy regimens. Hepatology 7: 522–528

Hocking M P, Duerson M C, O'Leary J P, Woodward E R 1983 Jejunoileal bypass for morbid obesity. Late follow-up in 100 cases. New England Journal of Medicine 308: 995–999

Hodges J R, Millward-Sadler G H, Barbatis C, Wright R 1981 Heterozygous MZ alpha$_1$-antitrypsin deficiency in adults with chronic active hepatitis and cryptogenic cirrhosis. New England Journal of Medicine 304: 557–560

Hoogenraad T U, Koevoet R, de Ruyter-Korver E G W M 1979 Oral zinc sulphate as long-term treatment in Wilson's disease (hepatocellular degeneration). European Neurology 18: 205–211

Hoogenraad T U, Van den Hamer C J A, Van Hattum J 1984 Effective treatment of Wilson's disease with oral zinc sulphate: two case reports. British Medical Journal 289: 273–276

Hussain M, Miele-Vergani G, Mowat A P 1991 Alpha-1-antitrypsin deficiency and liver disease: clinical presentation, diagnosis and treatment. Journal of Inherited Metabolic Disease 14: 497–511

Iser J H, Stevens B J, Stening G F, Hurley T H, Smallwood R A 1974 Hemolytic anemia of Wilson's disease. Gastroenterology 67: 290–293

Itescu S 1984 Hepatic amyloidosis. An unusual cause of ascites and portal hypertension. Archives of Internal Medicine 144: 2257–2259

Jacobs A, Worwood M 1975 Ferritin in serum: clinical and biochemical implications. New England Journal of Medicine 292: 951–956

Johnson B F 1968 Hemochromatosis resulting from prolonged oral iron therapy. New England Journal of Medicine 278: 1100–1101

Joshi V V 1987 Indian childhood cirrhosis. Perspectives in Pediatric Pathology 11: 175–192

Kirkman H N Jr 1992 Erythrocytic uridine diphosphate galactose in galactosaemia. Journal of Inherited Metabolic Disease 15: 4–16

Kley H K, Stremmel W, Niederau C et al 1985 Androgen and estrogen response to adrenal and gonadal stimulation in idiopathic hemochromatosis: evidence for decreased estrogen formation. Hepatology 5: 251–256

Komrower G M, Lee D H 1970 Long-term follow-up of galactosaemia. Archives of Disease in Childhood 45: 367–373

Kothari T, Swamy A P, Lee J C K, Mangla J C, Cestero R V M 1980 Hepatic hemosiderosis in maintenance hemodialysis (MHD) patients. Digestive Diseases and Sciences 25: 363–368

Kvittingen E A 1991 Tyrosinaemia type I – an update. Journal of Inherited Metabolic Disease 14: 554–562

Labelle Y, Phaneuf D, Laclerc B, Tanguay R M 1993 Characterization of the human fumarylacetoacetate hydrolase gene and identification of a missense mutation abolishing enzymatic activity. Human Molecular Genetics 2: 941–946

Lancet 1984 Leading article: high-dose chelation therapy in thalassaemia. Lancet 1: 373–374

Landing B H, Ang S M, Villarreal-Engelhardt G, Donnell G N 1993 Galactosemia: clinical and pathologic features, tissue staining patterns with labeled galactose- and galactosamine-binding lectins, and possible loci of nonenzymatic galactosylation. Perspectives in Pediatric Pathology: 17: 99–124

LaRusso N F, Summerskill W H J, McCall J T 1976 Abnormalities of chemical tests for copper metabolism in chronic active liver disease: differentiation from Wilson's disease. Gastroenterology 70: 653–655

Laurin J M, Crippin J S, Gossard A et al 1994 Ursodeoxycholic acid improves indices of liver injury in nonalcoholic steatohepatitis. Gastroenterology 106: A926

Lehotay D C 1993 Current controversies about galactosemia. Clinical Biochemistry 26: 69–74

LeSage G D, Baldus W P, Fairbanks V F et al 1983 Hemochromatosis: genetic or alcohol-induced? Gastroenterology 84: 1471–1477

Levy H L, Sepe S J, Shih V E, Vawter G F, Klein J O 1977 Sepsis due to *Escherichia coli* in neonates with galactosemia. New England Journal of Medicine 297: 823–825

Lindblad A, Hultcrantz R, Strandvik B 1992 Bile-duct destruction and collagen deposition: a prominent ultrastructural feature of the liver in cystic fibrosis. Hepatology 16: 372–381

Lindstedt S, Holme E, Lock E A, Hjalmarson O, Strandvik B 1992 Treatment of hereditary tyrosinaemia type I by inhibition of 4-hydroxy-phenylpyruvate dioxygenase. Lancet 340: 813–817

Lloyd H M, Powell L W, Thomas M J 1964 Idiopathic haemochromatosis in menstruating women. Lancet 2: 555–557

Lombard M, Bomford A, Hynes M et al 1989 Regulation of the hepatic transferrin receptor in hereditary hemochromatosis. Hepatology 9: 1–5

Lombard M, Bomford A B, Polson R J, Bellingham A J, Williams R 1990 Differential expression of transferrin receptor in duodenal mucosa in iron overload. Evidence for a site-specific defect in genetic hemochromatosis. Gastroenterology 98: 976–984

Ludwig J 1992 Practical liver biopsy interpretation: diagnostic algorithms. ASCP Press, Chicago

Ludwig J R, Viggiano T R, McGill D B, Ott B J 1980 Nonalcoholic steatohepatitis; Mayo Clinic experience with a hitherto unnamed disease. Mayo Clinic Proceedings 55: 434–438

Manowski Z, Silver M M, Roberts E A, Superina R A, Phillips M L 1990 Liver cell dysplasia and early liver transplantation in hereditary tyrosinemia. Modern Pathology 3: 694–701

Manzler A D, Schreiner A W 1970 Copper-induced acute hemolytic anemia: a new complication of hemodialysis. Annals of Internal Medicine 73: 409–412

Matsuda I, Pearson T, Holtzman N A 1974 Determination of apoceruloplasmin by radioimmunoassay in nutritional copper deficiency, Menke's kinky hair syndrome, Wilson's disease and umbilical cord blood. Pediatric Research 8: 821–824

McColl K E L, Moore M R, Thompson G G, Goldberg A 1981 Treatment with haematin in acute hepatic porphyria. Quarterly Journal of Medicine 50: 161–174

McGill D B 1994 Nonalcoholic steatohepatitis. In: Yoshida Y (ed) Recent advances in hepatology. Churchill Livingstone, London

McLaren G D, Nathanson M H, Jacobs A, Trevett D, Thomson W 1988 Control of iron absorption in hemochromatosis. Mucosal iron kinetics in vivo. Annals of the New York Academy of Sciences 526: 185–198

Messing B, Bories C, Kunstlinger F, Bernier J-J 1983 Does total

parenteral nutrition induce gallbladder sludge formation and lithiasis? Gastroenterology 84: 1012–1019
Milman N 1991 Hereditary haemochromatosis in Denmark 1950–1985: clinical, biochemical, and histological features in 179 patients and 13 preclinical cases. Danish Medical Bulletin 38: 385–393
Mitchell G, Larochelle J, Lambert M et al 1990 Neurologic crises in hereditary tyrosinemia. New England Journal of Medicine 322: 432–437
Mooyaart B R, de Jong G M, van der Veen S et al 1986 Hepatic disease in erythropoietic protoporphyria. Dermatologia 173: 120
Mulherin D, FitzGerald M 1992 Cystic fibrosis in adolescents and adults. Digestive Disease 10: 29–37
Nayak N C, Marwaha N, Kalra V, Roy S, Ghai O P 1981 The liver in siblings of patients with Indian childhood cirrhosis: a light and electron microscopic study. Gut 22: 295–300
Nebbia G, Hadchouel M, Odièvre M, Alagille D 1983 Early assessment of liver disease associated with $\alpha_1$-antitrypsin deficiency in childhood. Journal of Pediatrics 102: 661–665
Niederau C, Fischer R, Sonnenberg A, Stremmel W, Trampisch H J, Strohmeyer G 1985 Survival and causes of death in cirrhotic and in noncirrhotic patients with primary hemochromatosis. New England Journal of Medicine 313: 1256–1262
O'Brien S, Keogan M, Casey M et al 1992 Biliary complications of cystic fibrosis. Gut 33: 387–391
Perkins K W, McInnes I W S, Blackburn C R B, Beal R W 1965 Idiopathic hemochromatosis in children: report of a family. American Journal of Medicine 39: 118–126
Perlmutter D H 1991 The cellular basis for liver injury in alpha-1-antitrypsin deficiency. Hepatology 13: 172–185
Phaneuf D, Lambert M, Laframboise R, Mitchell G, Lettre F, Tanguay R M 1992 Type I hereditary tyrosinemia; evidence for molecular heterogeneity and identification of a causal mutation in a French Canadian patient. Journal of Clinical Investigation 90: 1185–1192
Pietrangelo A, Rocchi E, Casalgrandi G et al 1992 Regulation of transferrin, transferrin receptor, and ferritin genes in human duodenum. Gastroenterology 102: 802–809
Pitt H A, King W III, Mann L L et al 1983 Increased risk of cholelithiasis with prolonged total parenteral nutrition. American Journal of Surgery 145: 106–112
Polio J, Enriquez R E, Chow A, Wood W M, Atterbury C E 1989 Hepatocellular carcinoma in Wilson's disease. Case report and review of the literature. Journal of Clinical Gastroenterology 11: 220–224
Powell L W, Kerr J F R 1975 The pathology of the liver in hemochromatosis. Pathobiology Annual 5: 317–337
Powell L W, Mortimer R, Harris O D 1971 Cirrhosis of the liver: a comparative study of the four major aetiological groups. Medical Journal of Australia 1: 941–950
Powell L W, Summers K M, Board P G, Axelsen E, Webb S, Halliday J W 1990 Expression of hemochromatosis in homozygous subjects. Implications for early diagnosis and prevention. Gastroenterology 98: 1625–1632
Propper R D, Cooper B, Rufo R R et al 1977 Continuous subcutaneous administration of deferoxamine in patients with iron overload. New England Journal of Medicine 297: 418–423
Propst T, Propst A, Dietze O, Judmaier G, Braunsteiner H, Vogel W 1992 High prevalence of viral infection in adults with homozygous and heterozygous alpha-1-antitrypsin deficiency and chronic liver disease. Annals of Internal Medicine 117: 641–645
Quigley E M M, Marsh M N, Shaffer J L, Markin R S 1993 Hepatobiliary complications of total parenteral nutrition. Gastroenterology 104: 286–301
Rakela J, Goldschmiedt M, Ludwig J 1987 Late manifestation of chronic liver disease in adults with alpha-1-antitrypsin deficiency. Digestive Diseases and Sciences 32: 1358–1362
Rank J M, Straka J G, Bloomer J R 1990 Liver in disorders of porphyrin metabolism. Journal of Gastroenterology and Hepatology 5: 573–585
Reichardt J K V 1992 Genetic basis of galactosemia. Human Mutation 1: 190–196
Risdon R A, Barry M, Flynn D M 1975 Transfusional iron overload: the relationship between tissue iron concentration and hepatic fibrosis in thalassaemia. Journal of Pathology 116: 83–95
Rubinow A, Koff R S, Cohen A S 1978 Severe intrahepatic cholestasis in primary amyloidosis. A report of four cases and a review of the literature. American Journal of Medicine 64: 937–946
Sass-Kortsak A 1975 Wilson's disease. A treatable liver disease in children. Pediatric Clinics of North America 22: 963–984
Schafer A I, Cheron R G, Dluhy R et al 1981 Clinical consequences of acquired transfusional iron overload in adults. New England Journal of Medicine 304: 319–324
Scheinberg I H, Sternlieb I 1963 Wilson's disease and the concentration of caeruolplasmin in serum. Lancet 1: 1420–1421
Scheinberg I H, Sternlieb I 1975 Pregnancy in penicillamine-treated patients with Wilson's disease. New England Journal of Medicine 293: 1300–1302
Scheinberg I H, Sternlieb I 1984 Wilson's disease. W B Saunders, Philadelphia
Scheinberg I H, Jaffe M E, Sternlieb I 1987 The use of trientine in preventing the effects of interrupting penicillamine therapy in Wilson's disease. New England Journal of Medicine 317: 209–213
Scheuer P J, Williams R, Muir A R 1962 Hepatic pathology in relatives of patients with haemochromatosis. Journal of Pathology and Bacteriology 84: 53–64
Schramel P, Müller-Höcker J, Meyer U et al 1988 Nutritional copper intoxication in three German infants with severe liver cell damage (features of Indian childhood cirrhosis). Journal of Trace Elements, Electrolytes, Health, and Disease 2: 85–89
Schwarzenberg S J, Sharp H L 1990 Pathogenesis of alpha-1-antitrypsin deficiency-associated liver disease, 1990. Journal of Pediatric Gastroenterology and Nutrition 10: 5–12
Schweitzer S, Shin Y, Jakobs C, Brodehl J 1993 Long-term outcome in 134 patients with galactosaemia. European Journal of Pediatrics 152: 36–43
Scott J, Gollan J L, Samourian S, Sherlock S 1978 Wilson's disease, presenting as chronic active hepatitis. Gastroenterology 74: 645–651
Scott-Jupp R, Lamaw M, Tanner M S 1991 Prevalence of liver disease in cystic fibrosis. Archives of Disease in Childhood 66: 698–701
Sharp H L, Bridges R A, Krivit W, Freier E F 1969 Cirrhosis associated with alpha-1-antitrypsin deficiency: a previously unrecognized inherited disorder. Journal of Laboratory and Clinical Medicine 73: 934–939
Sheldon J H 1935 Haemochromatosis. Oxford University Press, London
Sifers R N, Finegold M J, Woo S L C 1992 Molecular biology and genetics of alpha-1-antitrypsin deficiency. Seminars in Liver Disease 12: 301–310
Simon M, Brissot P 1988 The genetics of haemochromatosis. Journal of Hepatology 6: 116–124
Simon M, Fauchet R, Hespel J P et al 1980 Idiopathic hemochromatosis: a study of biochemical expression in 247 heterozygous members of 63 families: evidence for a single major HLA-linked gene. Gastroenterology 78: 703–708
Smith L H, Jr 1990 Overview of hemochromatosis. Western Journal of Medicine 153: 296–308
Sternlieb I 1980 Copper and the liver. Gastroenterology 78: 1615–1628
Sternlieb I 1993 The outlook for the diagnosis of Wilson's disease. Journal of Hepatology 17: 263–264
Sternlieb I 1994 Copper and zinc. In: Arias I M, Boyer J L, Fausto N, Jacoby W B, Schachter D, Shafritz D A (eds) The liver: biology and pathobiology, 3rd edn. Raven Press, New York, p 585–596
Sternlieb I, Scheinberg I H 1968 Prevention of Wilson's disease in asymptomatic patients. New England Journal of Medicine 278: 352–359
Sternlieb I, Scheinberg I H 1972 Chronic hepatitis as a first manifestation of Wilson's disease. Annals of Internal Medicine 76: 59–64
Sternlieb I, Scheinberg I H 1979 The role of radiocopper in the diagnosis of Wilson's disease. Gastroenterology 77: 138–142
Stremmel W, Meyerrose K-W, Niederau C, Hefter H, Kreuzpaintner G, Strohmeyer G 1991 Wilson disease: clinical presentation, treatment, and survival. Annals of Internal Medicine 115: 720–726
Summers K M, Halliday J W, Powell L W 1990 Identification of homozygous hemochromatosis subjects by measurement of hepatic iron index. Hepatology 12: 20–25
Suprun H, Freundlich E 1981 Fatal familial steatosis of myocardium, liver and kidneys in three siblings. Acta Paediatrica Scandinavica 70: 247–252

Sveger T 1988 The natural history of liver disease in alpha-1-antitrypsin deficiency. Acta Paediatrica Scandinavica 77: 847–851

Talente G M, Coleman R A, Alter C et al 1994 Glycogen storage disease in adults. Annals of Internal Medicine 120: 218–226

Tanaka K, Kean E A, Johnson B 1976 Jamaican vomiting sickness: biochemical investigation of two cases. New England Journal of Medicine 295: 461–467

Tanner M S, Kantarjian A H, Bhave S A, Pandit A N 1983 Early introduction of copper-contaminated animal milk feeds as a possible cause of Indian childhood cirrhosis. Lancet 2: 992–995

Tanner M S, Bhave S A, Pradhan A M et al 1987 Clinical trials of penicillamine in Indian childhood cirrhosis. Archives of Disease in Childhood 62: 1118–1124

Tanzi R E, Petrukhin K, Chernov I et al 1993 The Wilson disease gene is a copper transporting ATPase with homology to the Menke's disease gene. Nature Genetics 5: 344–350

Tavill A S, Bacon B R 1990 Hemochromatosis: iron metabolism and the iron overload syndromes. In: Zakim D, Boyer T D (eds) Hepatology: a textbook of liver disease, 2nd edn. W B Saunders, Philadelphia, p 1273–1299

Tuchman M 1993 Mutations and polymorphisms in the human ornithine transcarbamylase gene. Human Mutation 2: 174–178

Valberg L S 1978 Tissue iron distribution in idiopathic hemochromatosis. Gastroenterology 75: 915–916

van Asbeck B S, Verbrugh H A, van Oost B A, Marx J O J M, Imhof H W, Verhoef J 1982 *Listeria monocytogenes* meningitis and decreased phagocytosis associated with iron overload. British Medical Journal 284: 542–544

Van Steenbergen W 1993 Alpha-1-antitrypsin deficiency: an overview. Acta Clinica Belgica 48: 171–189

Veen C, Van den Hamer C J A, de Leeuw P W 1991 Zinc sulphate therapy for Wilson's disease after acute deterioration during treatment with low-dose D-penicillamine. Journal of Internal Medicine 229: 549–552

Vockley J 1994 The changing face of disorders of fatty acid oxidation. Mayo Clinic Proceedings 69: 249–257

Volkholz H-J, Sailer D, Rödl W 1984 New diagnostic and therapeutic possibilities in manifest idiopathic hemochromatosis. Hepato-Gastroenterology 31: 289–294

Waggoner D D, Buist N R M, Donnell G N 1990 Long-term prognosis in galactosemia: results of a survey of 350 cases. Journal of Inherited Metabolic Disease 13: 802–818

Walshe J M 1977 Pregnancy in Wilson's disease. Quarterly Journal of Medicine 46: 73–83

Walshe J M 1982 Treatment of Wilson's disease with trientine (triethylene tetramine) dihydrochloride. Lancet 1: 643–647

Walshe J M 1984 Wilson's disease. British Medical Journal 288: 1689

Walshe J M 1995 Copper: not too little, not too much, but just right. Journal of the Royal College of Physicians of London 29: 280–288

Walshe J M 1996 Treatment of Wilson's disease: the historical background. Quarterly Journal of Medicine 89: 553–555

Walshe J M, Yealland M 1995 Not Wilson's disease: a review of misdiagnosed cases. Quarterly Journal of Medicine 88: 55–59

Wands J R, Rowe J A, Mezey S E et al 1976 Normal serum ferritin concentrations in precirrhotic hemochromatosis. New England Journal of Medicine 294: 302–305

Wanless I R, Lentz J S 1990 Fatty liver hepatitis (steatohepatitis) and obesity: an autopsy study with analysis of risk factors. Hepatology 12: 1106–1110

Weinberg A G, Mize C E, Worthen H G 1976 The occurrence of hepatoma in the chronic form of hereditary tyrosinemia. Journal of Pediatrics 88: 434–438

Weinberg L M, Brasitus T A, Lefkowitch J H 1981 Fluctuating Kayser–Fleischer-like rings in a jaundiced patient. Archives of Internal Medicine 141: 246–249

Williams R 1971 Haemochromatosis. In: Bouchier I A D (ed) Seventh symposium on advanced medicine. Pitman, London, p 199–209

Williams R, Smith P M, Spicer E J F, Barry M, Sherlock S 1969 Venesection therapy in idiopathic haemochromatosis. An analysis of 40 treated and 18 untreated patients. Quarterly Journal of Medicine 38: 1–16

Williams S G J, Westaby D, Tanner M S, Mowat A P 1992 Liver and biliary problems in cystic fibrosis. British Medical Bulletin 48: 877–892

Wilson S A K 1912 Progressive lenticular degeneration: a familial nervous disease associated with cirrhosis of the liver. Brain 34: 295–509

Yang Y, Raper S E, Cohn J A, Engelhardt J F, Wilson J M 1993 An approach for treating the hepatobiliary disease of cystic fibrosis by somatic gene transfer. Proceedings of the National Academy of Sciences 90: 4601–4605

Zimmermann A, Moll C, Bachmann C 1987 Liver fibrosis in carbamoylphosphate synthetase deficiency. Pediatric Pathology 7: 191–200

SECTION 9

# Complications of chronic liver disease

# 36. Portal hypertension

*Peter C. Hayes*

Portal hypertension is defined as a portal venous pressure greater than 7 mmHg. The portal venous pressure, however, cannot be measured easily and the term "portal hypertension" is also applied to the syndrome associated with increased portal venous pressure characterized by abnormal portasystemic venous anastomoses usually with splenomegaly. It arises because of a combination of increased portal venous resistance and increased portal blood flow.

## CLASSIFICATION

The site of increased portal venous resistance is used to classify portal hypertension into extrahepatic and intrahepatic types and the latter into presinusoidal, mixed and postsinusoidal forms (Table 36.1).

### Extrahepatic portal hypertension

This results from obstruction in the main portal vein and accounts for about 10% of patients with portal hypertension in Europe and North America. Regional extrahepatic portal hypertension is caused by splenic vein occlusion and does not affect the portal vein itself but is conveniently considered with portal vein occlusion. These conditions are described in detail in relation to vascular liver diseases (p. 1083), but their investigation and treatment are very similar to the more common intrahepatic form of portal hypertension reviewed in this chapter.

**Table 36.1** Classification of portal hypertension

| Type | Site of obstruction | Venous pressures | | Commonest cause |
|---|---|---|---|---|
| | | Hepatic | Portal | |
| Extrahepatic | Portal vein | Normal | Increased | Portal vein thrombosis |
| | Splenic vein* | Normal | Normal | Splenic vein thrombosis |
| Intrahepatic | Presinusoidal | Normal | Increased | Schistosomiasis |
| | Mixed | Increased | Increased | Hepatic cirrhosis |
| | Postsinusoidal | Unmeasurable | Increased | Budd–Chiari syndrome |
| | | Normal | Increased | Veno-occlusive disease |

*Not strictly a cause of increased pressure in the portal vein, but usefully considered with portal hypertension.

### Intrahepatic portal hypertension

Obstruction in intrahepatic portal hypertension may be limited to the presinusoidal blood vessels (intrahepatic presinusoidal portal hypertension) or may involve presinusoidal, sinusoidal and postsinusoidal vessels (mixed intrahepatic portal hypertension). Postsinusoidal obstruction alone is rare and occurs in veno-occlusive disease (p. 1081) and in the Budd–Chiari syndrome (p. 1077).

#### *Intrahepatic presinusoidal portal hypertension*

***Schistosomiasis.*** Schistosomiasis due to *S. mansoni* or *S. japonicum* causes liver disease affecting more than 200 million humans (p. 589) and is the commonest cause of portal hypertension in the world. Schistosome eggs find their way into the portal venous radicals in the portal tracts of the liver, where they elicit an inflammatory response (p. 590). An antibody-mediated cellular immune reaction involving eosinophils leads to the destruction of the eggs and antigens released from the eggs then elicit a granulomatous inflammation in the portal tracts (Warren 1984). This inflammation destroys the small portal vessels, particularly in the periphery of the liver, causing presinusoidal portal hypertension, but the liver parenchyma is not affected and total liver blood flow is maintained by an increase in hepatic arterial vessels in the liver, allowing increased hepatic arterial flow (Coutinho 1968, Andrade & Cheever 1971). Portal hypertension leads to the development of esophagogastric varices from which recurrent bleeding can occur, but by contrast with patients who have hepatic cirrhosis, mortality from bleeding is low and hepatic encephalopathy and ascites only occur transiently when bleeding occurs.

***Other causes.*** Myeloproliferative and lymphoproliferative diseases, such as myelofibrosis, chronic myeloid leukemia and Hodgkin's disease, can cause portal hypertension by infiltrating the portal tracts and destroying the portal venous radicals. Drug treatment of these diseases occasionally produces the same effect (p. 852). Other causes include congenital hepatic fibrosis and, rarely, sarcoidosis, arsenic and polyvinyl chloride.

***Diagnosis.*** Esophageal varices establish the presence of portal hypertension, ultrasonography confirms its presence and shows no obstruction in the portal venous system (p. 56), and arterial portography (p. 29) shows the features of portal hypertension with no portal vein obstruction. The wedged hepatic venous pressure is normal, showing that the portal hypertension is presinusoidal in origin. Liver biopsy is required to help establish the underlying cause.

#### *Mixed intrahepatic portal hypertension*

Hepatic cirrhosis is responsible for about 90% of portal hypertension in Europe and North America. Patients with cirrhosis do not always have portal hypertension. There is a poor correlation between the severity of liver disease and portal pressure and the portal pressure may fall during follow-up in spite of progression of disease. However, it should also be noted that wedged hepatic venous pressure, the most commonly used measure of portal pressure, may underestimate true portal pressure, particularly in patients with macronodular cirrhosis where a significant presinusoidal component exists (p. 996). Conditions other than cirrhosis can also cause mixed intrahepatic portal hypertension. These include obstruction of the hepatic venous outflow (p. 1077), partial nodular transformation of the liver (p. 1129) and cystic liver disease (p. 725). Portal hypertension occasionally results from secondary neoplasm in the liver (Kurtz et al 1974) or from congestive cardiac failure (Luna et al 1968), but this is rarely of clinical significance. Chronic vitamin A intoxication has been reported to cause portal hypertension leading to ascites, with recovery following withdrawal of vitamin A (p. 852). Enlargement of sinusoidal lipocytes may be a factor causing the increased portal pressure.

Despite considerable investigation in humans and in animal models, the precise cause of portal hypertension in patients with cirrhosis remains unclear. Two components are probably involved in most patients: increased intrahepatic or outflow resistance and increased portal blood inflow. Increased resistance to blood flow is probably more important in most patients, as reduction of portal blood flow in portal hypertension in cirrhosis leads to only a modest fall in portal pressure (Witte et al 1976).

Intrahepatic resistance has a fixed component and a dynamic component. The fixed component is caused by destruction and distortion of the hepatic vasculature due to fibrosis and nodular regeneration. The dynamic component has been demonstrated experimentally in the isolated perfused cirrhotic rat liver where nitrates have been found to decrease intrahepatic resistance (Bhathal & Grossman 1985), probably by relaxing perisinusoidal myofibroblasts (Bhathal & Grossman 1982). Increased portal blood inflow is the result of increased splanchnic blood flow consequent on the generalized hyperdynamic circulation and high cardiac output in cirrhosis (p. 920). There is probably also selective splanchnic vasodilatation (Vorobioff et al 1984, Benoit et al 1985). Potential mediators of increased portal blood flow include glucagon, bile acids, prostacyclin, 5-hydroxytryptamine and adrenaline (Grose & Hayes 1992). Recently, it has been postulated that high circulating endotoxin concentrations in patients with cirrhosis induce nitric oxide synthetase, leading to the production of nitric oxide and consequently systemic vasodilatation. N-monomethyl-L-arginine (L-NMMA), an inhibitor of vascular nitric oxide synthesis, reduces cardiac output and increases systemic blood pressure in cirrhotic rats, but this has little effect on portal hypertension (Pizcueta et al 1992).

### Idiopathic portal hypertension

This rare condition is caused by damage to the terminal tributaries of the portal vein in the liver. It is described in relation to vascular diseases of the liver (p. 105).

## PORTAL BLOOD FLOW

For many years it was thought that portal blood flow was reduced in patients with cirrhosis (Moreno et al 1975a). Indeed, flow in the portal vein itself is often reduced (Fig. 36.1), but if flow in portacollateral vessels such as the azygos vein that drains esophageal varices is included, flow within the portal vascular bed is increased, supporting the forward flow theory. This is supported further by finding that blood flow in transjugular intrahepatic portasystemic stent shunts (TIPSS) that have reduced portal pressure to normal is around 2 L/min.

### Retrograde portal blood flow

Some controversy exists regarding retrograde (hepatofugal) blood flow away from the liver in the portal vein. Indirect measurements of flow made from pressure gradients across a portal vein clamp at operation suggested that retrograde flow occurred in 5–10% of patients and in up to a third undergoing emergency portasystemic shunt surgery (Charters et al 1974). By contrast, direct measurement of portal blood flow at operation has shown absence of portal flow but not retrograde flow and experimental models and correlation of blood flow and pressure mea-

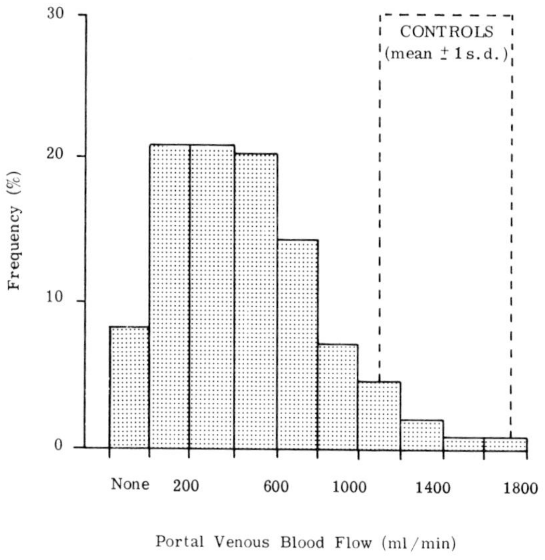


**Fig. 36.1** Portal blood flow in 153 patients with cirrhosis and portal hypertension requiring a portacaval shunt (Moreno et al 1975a).

surements have shown that pressure measurements cannot be related simply to blood flow (Moreno et al 1975b, Archie 1977).

Radiological studies of portal blood flow have their limitations, but direct introduction of contrast material into the portal circulation shows that retrograde blood flow can occur, usually in patients with large collateral vessels, but only in about 1–3% of patients (Takayasu et al 1982, Rector et al 1988). Pollard & Nebesar (1967) found retrograde flow in the Budd–Chiari syndrome. More recently, Doppler studies have demonstrated retrograde flow in intrahepatic portal vessels in 20% of patients with cirrhosis (Rössle et al 1994) and hepatofugal flow has been shown to be commoner in patients with advanced liver disease and encephalopathy after distal splenorenal shunt surgery (Lacy et al 1992).

### Portasystemic shunts

Virtually all of the portal venous blood normally flows to the liver, but in portal hypertension a variable proportion is shunted directly from the portal to the systemic circulation. This may occur via collateral blood vessels or via blood vessels in the diseased liver that bypass the sinusoids and join the hepatic veins. The proportion of the portal blood that passes through such shunts varies greatly and may reach 100%; the proportion traversing intrahepatic or extrahepatic shunts and the proportion of splenic vein and superior mesenteric vein blood passing into shunts are equally variable (Lebrec et al 1976, Okuda et al 1977). The extent to which shunting occurs seems to increase with time and presumably therefore with the progression of liver disease and may be especially marked in patients who suffer bleeding from esophagogastric varices (Groszmann et al 1972, Lebrec et al 1976). Blood flow through the azygos vein reflects the degree of shunting through gastroesophageal collaterals and the flow in patients who have bled from varices reaches about 600 ml/min (Bosch & Groszmann 1984).

### Splenic blood flow in portal hypertension

In Western countries portal hypertension principally due to increased splenic blood flow is unusual. It usually occurs in association with massive splenomegaly and splenic blood flow accounting for 10–50% of cardiac output (Garnett et al 1969). Such conditions include tropical splenomegaly, Felty's syndrome, myelofibrosis, chronic lymphatic leukemia, systemic mastocytosis, polycythemia rubra vera and vascular disorders of the spleen and all of these can be associated with portal hypertension and bleeding from esophageal varices. Investigation does not reveal any obstruction in the portal venous system and splenectomy may entirely alleviate the portal hypertension.

## CLINICAL FEATURES

An increased portal venous pressure does not itself give rise to clinical features and its presence is often not suspected.

### Splenomegaly

This most important sign of portal hypertension is found in almost all patients. The spleen may not be palpable, but enlargement can usually be detected by abdominal radiography or by imaging (p. 1184). Portal hypertension can occur in the absence of splenomegaly, as Liebowitz (1963) found spleens weighing 250 g or less at autopsy in 20% of patients with cirrhosis and esophageal varices, but even so portal hypertension should not be diagnosed when splenomegaly cannot be demonstrated unless other clear evidence is obtained. Splenic congestion in portal hypertension is one factor causing splenomegaly in cirrhosis (Fig. 36.2), but there is no relation between the size of the spleen and the portal pressure and factors such as reticuloendothelial hyperplasia consequent on liver dysfunction, possibly related to impaired Kupffer cell function (p. 763), may also be important (Dumont et al 1974). Splenomegaly on its own, therefore, suggests but is not sufficient for a diagnosis of portal hypertension in cirrhosis. Massive splenomegaly can occur in children and in adolescents with portal hypertension, but in adults it should raise the possibility of causes other than portal hypertension.

A palpable spleen is an important indication that varices may be the source of an acute gastrointestinal bleed and some have felt that failure to feel the spleen is good evidence that such bleeding is not coming from varices (Bull

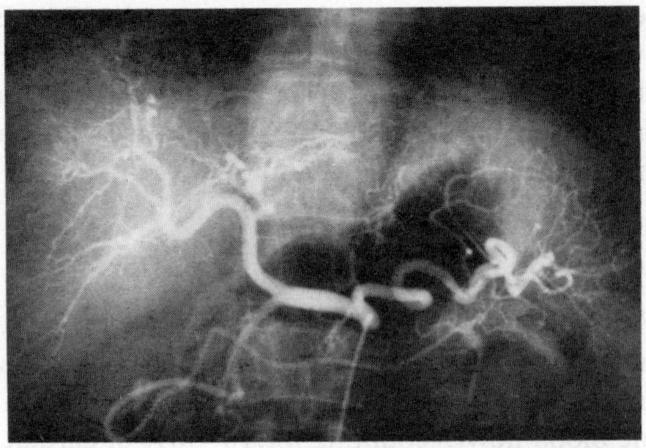

**Fig. 36.2** Arteriogram in a patient with cirrhosis of the liver and portal hypertension showing diminished intrahepatic arterial branches ("tree in winter") with an irregular or corkscrew appearance and a greatly enlarged spleen.

et al 1979). The author has found this unreliable and others have had a similar experience (Harries 1980). The spleen may diminish in size temporarily after a massive hemorrhage from varices (Tumen 1970), but this usually occurs only in children.

## Collateral vessels

Collateral blood vessels are an important sign of raised portal pressure. The sites for their development have been described (p. 714), but those of clinical importance are mainly in the anterior abdominal wall, in the esophagus and stomach, on stomas or in the rectum and anus. Bleeding can also occur from unusual varices that cannot be identified readily (p. 1000).

### *Anterior abdominal wall collateral vessels*

These derive from the left branch of the portal vein via the umbilical and paraumbilical veins. Usually only one or two can be seen in the abdomen (Fig. 36.3) and the direction of blood flow is away from the umbilicus. Rarely, many prominent veins radiate from the umbilicus to form a "caput medusae", so-called because the vessels are deemed to resemble writhing snakes. Collateral vessels radiating from the umbilicus must be differentiated from those due to inferior vena caval obstruction, which originate in the groin, are most prominent in the flanks and carry blood towards the superior vena cava. Differentiation may be difficult, especially when ascites is present.

***Cruveilhier–Baumgarten syndrome.*** This is a rare condition in which portal hypertension is associated with blood flow through a patent umbilical vein and a murmur heard between the xiphisternum and the umbilicus (Armstrong et al 1942). The murmur is usually continuous, often loud, may be accompanied by a thrill and can be obliterated by pressure above the umbilicus (Hardison 1977). Blood flow through a patent umbilical vein is relatively common in intrahepatic portal hypertension, but a murmur occurs in only about 5% of such cases, perhaps because it depends on the nature of the collateral vessels (Salmi et al 1990). The syndrome is always associated with intrahepatic portal hypertension, as the umbilical vein derives from the left branch of the portal vein. It is almost always caused by cirrhosis. Rarely, the liver is not cirrhotic but is small and shows periportal fibrosis. The spleen is often very large.

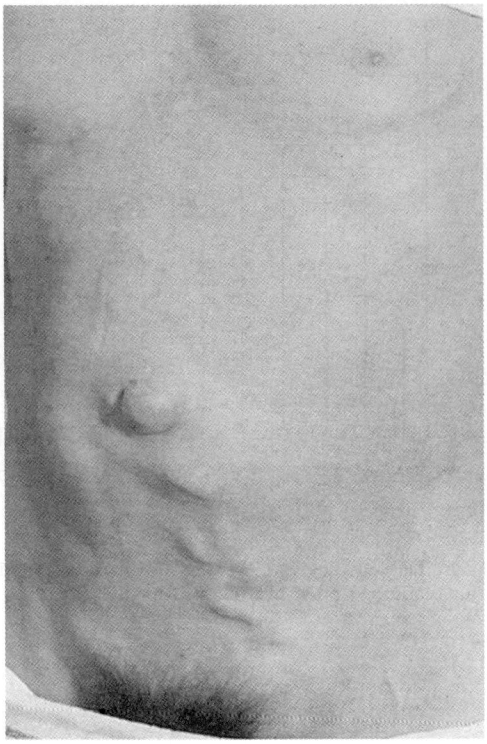

**Fig. 36.3** Prominent abdominal varix in primary biliary cirrhosis with portal hypertension. (Reprinted with permission from Hayes & Simpson 1995 Colour guide to Gastroenterology and Liver Disease, Edinburgh, Churchill Livingstone).

### *Esophagogastric varices*

Although not accessible to clinical examination, esophagogastric varices give such unequivocal evidence of portal hypertension that they should always be sought (p. 105). They indicate portal hypertension without identifying its cause. The identification of esophagogastric varices is described below.

***"Uphill" and "downhill" varices.*** The esophageal veins normally drain to the inferior thyroid, azygos and hemiazygos and left gastric veins. The terms "uphill" and "downhill" have been used to indicate the direction of flow of blood in the varices. Esophageal varices in portal hypertension relieve portal pressure by allowing portal blood to flow "uphill" and reach the heart via the azygos veins and superior vena cava. Such varices occur in the

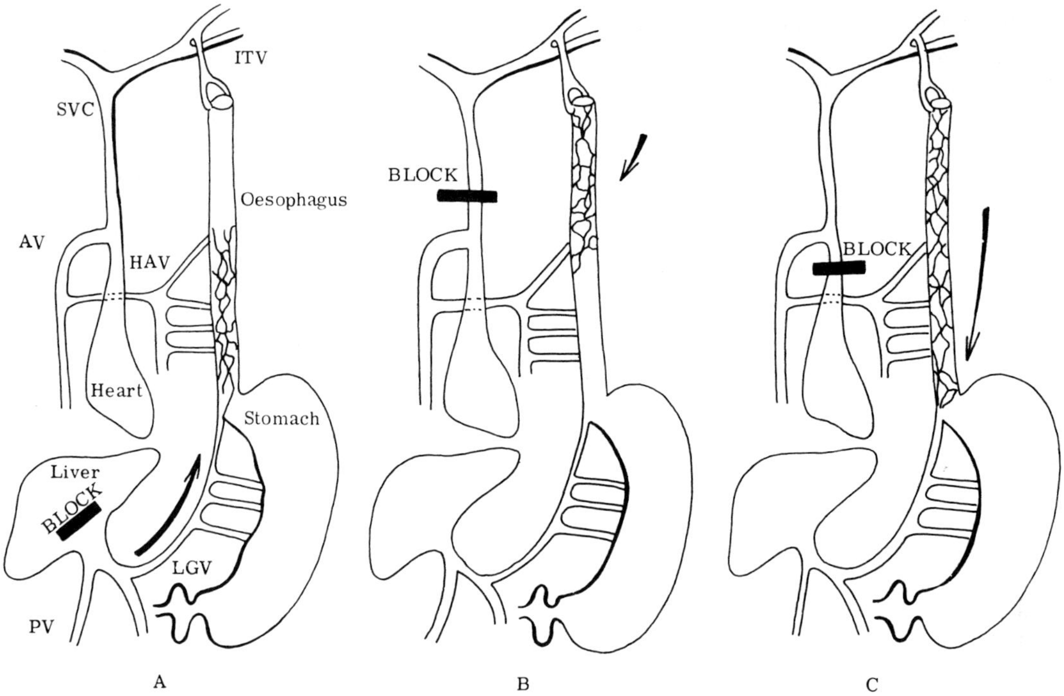


**Fig. 36.4** Schematic diagram of "uphill" esophageal varices in portal hypertension (A), "downhill" varices of the upper esophagus with obstruction of the superior vena cava proximal to the azygos vein (B), and "downhill" varices of the entire esophagus with obstruction of the superior vena cava and azygos vein. Arrows indicate the direction of blood flow in the varices. AV = azygos vein; HAV = hemiazygos vein; ITV = inferior thyroid veins; LGV = left gastric vein; PV = portal vein; SVC = superior vena cava (Sorokin et al 1977)

lower esophagus (Fig. 36.4). Rarely, esophageal varices develop in the absence of portal hypertension. This occurs when the superior vena cava and/or the azygos venous system is obstructed, usually by thyroid masses, after thyroid surgery or by mediastinal masses or fibrosis. Varices occur only in the upper esophagus when the superior vena cava alone is obstructed; they occur throughout the esophagus when the superior vena cava and the azygos veins are obstructed (Sorokin et al 1977, Fleig et al 1982).

***Local varices.*** Local varices have been reported in diseases of the esophagus such as achalasia (Kraft et al 1973).

### *Stomal varices*

Varices can be seen on and around ileostomies and colostomies following bowel resection in patients who have or who develop portal hypertension. They can also develop in the stoma of an ileal conduit (Hollands 1982). Most patients have undergone proctocolectomy for ulcerative colitis and have associated chronic liver disease or sclerosing cholangitis (Cooper et al 1981, Wiesner et al 1986), but varices have been reported at a colostomy consequent on the development of portal hypertension due to hepatic metastases from a rectal carcinoma (Watkins 1981). Stomal varices develop some 1–10 years after proctocolectomy and hepatosplenomegaly, thrombocytopenia, esophageal varices and hypoalbuminemia are frequently also present as most patients have advanced liver disease. Manipulation of the stoma often causes oozing of blood, but overt bleeding is also common and can be severe. The source of the bleeding is recognized easily if the patient or the doctor examines the stoma during bleeding, but bleeding is often attributed to associated esophageal varices if the stoma is not examined carefully.

### *Hemorrhoids and anorectal varices*

Hemorrhoids have been regarded as particularly common in portal hypertension, but in fact they are no more frequent than in the general population (Jacobs et al 1980). This is in keeping with the observation that hemorrhoids are vascular cushions within the hemorrhoidal plexus (p. 1451) that do not communicate with the portal system (Bernstein 1983). They can, however, bleed severely, particularly when coagulation defects are also present.

Anorectal varices are dilated and often tortuous submucosal veins in the rectum and anal canal joining the superior hemorrhoidal veins with the middle and inferior hemorrhoidal veins and often emerging subcutaneously at the anal margin (Hosking & Johnson 1988). They are usually situated in the same position as hemorrhoids (left lateral, right anterior, right posterior) but are easily compressed and refill rapidly when pressure is released. Bleeding from anorectal varices (p. 1000) and its treatment (p. 1010) are considered below.

*Portal gastropathy and colopathy*

Portal hypertension can cause vascular abnormalities in the stomach (p. 1000) and colon (p. 1001) leading to occult and occasionally acute blood loss, iron deficiency and anemia.

### Fetor hepaticus

Fetor hepaticus, in the absence of severe liver failure, suggests an extensive collateral circulation (p. 1046).

### Ascites

Portal hypertension contributes to the formation of ascites (p. 1017).

## INVESTIGATIONS

### Endoscopy

Endoscopy is generally considered the standard method for identifying esophageal varices and for assessing the risk of variceal hemorrhage (see below). The observations are subjective with considerable interobserver variation, particularly for small varices that may be difficult to differentiate from prominent esophageal folds. Varices are virtually diagnostic of portal hypertension and develop only rarely for other reasons. The size of varices is important in determining the risk of bleeding and they are usually classified as small or grade I when they flatten with air insufflation; medium or grade II when they remain despite air insufflation, but where an individual variceal cord does not extend up to the mid-point of the lumen; and large or grade III where individual cords reach the mid-point of the lumen and collectively often occlude the lumen. Endoscopy will also identify the presence of red color signs such as red spots (p. 999) and red wale signs, which are associated with an increased risk of bleeding (North Italian Endoscopic Club 1988, Kleber et al 1991). A combination of the severity of liver disease, the size of varices and the presence or absence of red color signs may be used to identify patients who are particularly at risk of hemorrhage (Fig. 36.5).

New endoscopic techniques such as endoscopic ultrasonography and the electronic endoscope using near-infrared light have been advocated as having certain advantages over straightforward endoscopy, for example in identifying gastric varices and portal hypertensive gastropathy (Caletti et al 1992) and predicting bleeding (Ohta et al 1992), but they require further study.

### Radiology

Esophageal varices may also be identified by barium swallow examination which, although probably less sen-

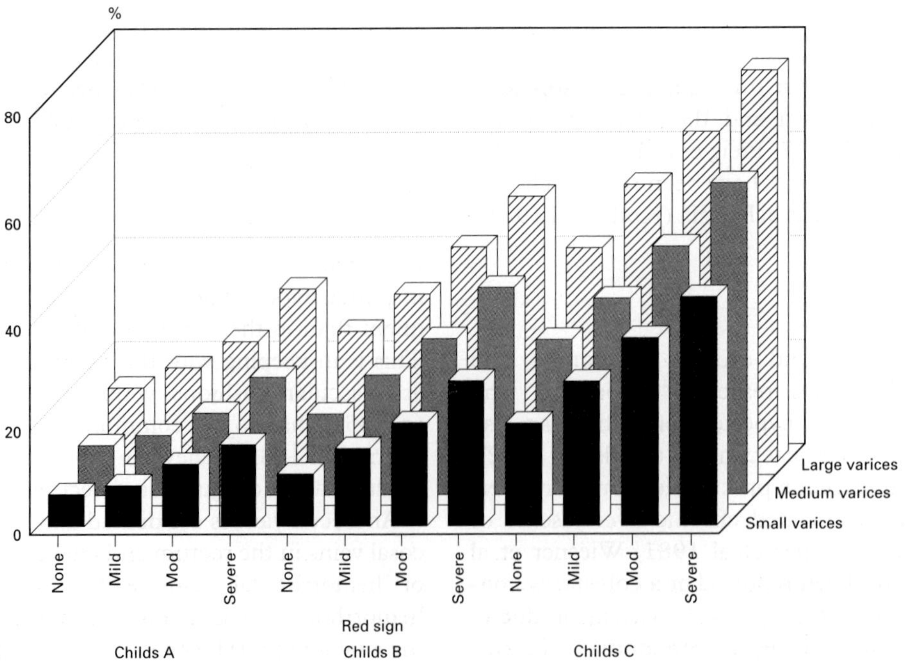


**Fig. 36.5** Probability (%) of variceal bleeding within 1 year of identification of varices (North Italian Endoscopic Club 1988).

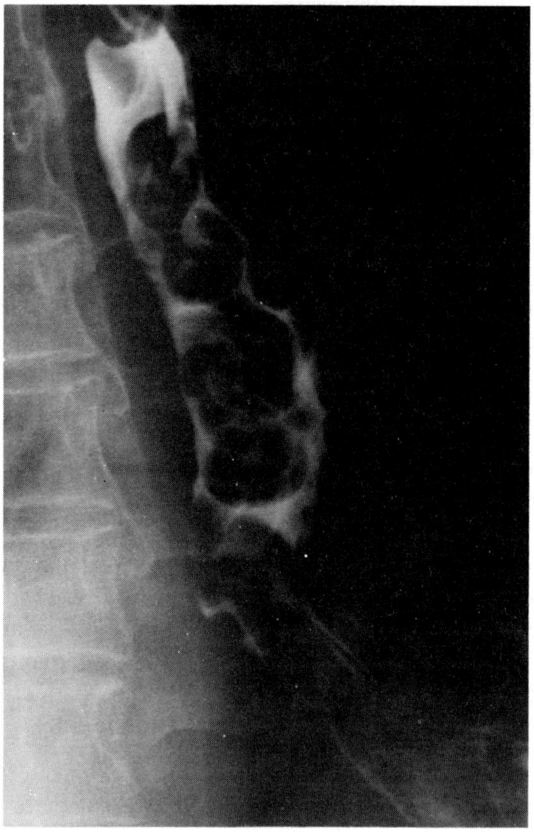

Fig. 36.6 Barium swallow showing large varices in the lower esophagus.

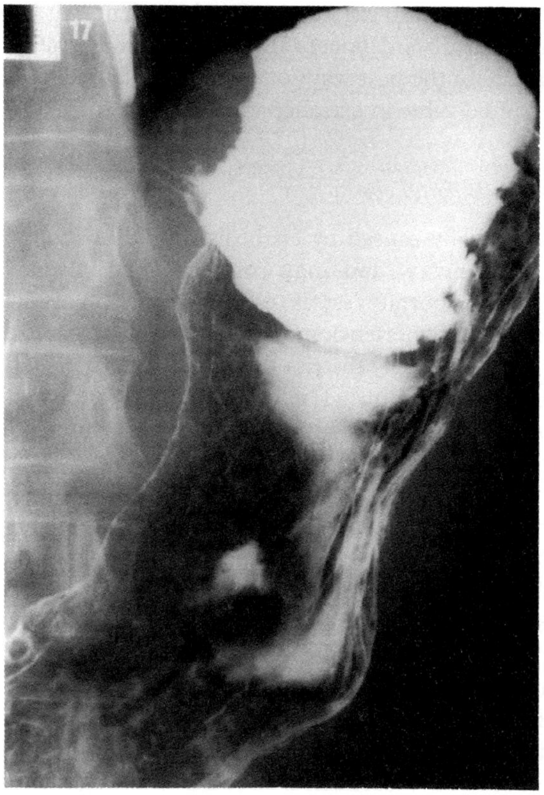


Fig. 36.7 Barium meal showing a gastric varix large enough to simulate a gastric carcinoma in a patient with splenic vein thrombosis.

sitive than endoscopy, remains a reliable investigation (Fig. 36.6). The accuracy of barium swallow may be improved by videoradiology or by giving dextran or anticholinergic drugs to accentuate varices (Dalinka et al 1972, Waldram et al 1977). Gastric varices are more difficult to identify radiologically and if large, may mimic a mass lesion (Fig. 36.7). Paraesophageal varices can sometimes be seen on a chest radiograph as a retrocardiac mass in the low mediastinum.

## Imaging

Ultrasound, computed tomography and nuclear magnetic resonance are all noninvasive methods of detecting the vascular changes of portal hypertension. Ultrasound (p. 56) is the most useful and most generally available method, provided an experienced operator is available and repeated examinations can be done easily (Kane & Katz 1982). Important ultrasonographic signs of portal hypertension include enlargement of the portal vein to a diameter greater than 1.3 cm, seen in a half or more of patients, with loss of variation in the caliber of the mesenteric vessels during respiration, splenomegaly with dilated hilar collateral vessels in almost all patients and dilated umbilical veins and other collateral vessels in some patients (Bolondi et al 1984). Occasionally, very large collateral vessels can be seen (Takayasu et al 1984). They usually run between the splenic vein and the left renal vein and may be responsible for recurring episodes of encephalopathy. Cottone et al (1983) have shown that esophagogastric varices increase in frequency as the diameter of the veins in the portal venous system increases.

Duplex–Doppler ultrasonography is now widely available and can be used as a noninvasive method for quantitating portal vein flow velocity, which may be particularly useful in assessing the influence of pharmacological treatment of portal hypertension (Cioni et al 1992). Computed tomography (McCain et al 1985) and nuclear magnetic resonance (Williams et al 1985) can both detect portal hypertension and varices but are much less generally available and unnecessarily complicated.

## Portal venography

Portal venography (p. 75) is important in identifying the nature and the site of portal venous obstruction in portal hypertension of unknown cause and in defining suitable veins prior to portasystemic shunt surgery. Arterial portography (p. 75) is being used increasingly because of its safety and simplicity, while umbilical portography is not widely available because of its complexity. Transhepatic portography (p. 76) is a relatively invasive technique that carries a significant risk of bleeding in patients with coagulopathy but does delineate the portal venous system well and is one of the best ways of showing collateral vessels. It is of limited value in extrahepatic portal obstruction.

*Intrahepatic portal obstruction*

This is usually caused by cirrhosis (p. 990). Venographic appearances vary and may sometimes be normal. The intrahepatic portal vessels can become abnormal even before portal hypertension develops, becoming sparse, distorted and unevenly distributed to give the so-called "tree in winter" appearance. The liver does not become diffusely opacified as contrast enters the sinusoids but acquires a mottled appearance (Fig. 36.2). The portal vein widens to reach a diameter of 2–3 cm as portal hypertension develops and it loses its tapered shape. Collateral venous channels, which vary greatly from patient to patient, become visible as blood flow reverses in tributary veins and as previously rudimentary embryonic veins develop. Most of the collateral circulation is through tributary vessels, over 90% occurring in the left gastric (coronary) and short gastric veins. An inferior mesenteric collateral system occurs in a third of patients and a superior mesenteric collateral system in about 5%. Collateral circulation through embryonic vessels occurs in a quarter to a third of patients, usually via the paraumbilical and deep epigastric veins to the iliac veins and vena cava or via a spleno–adreno–renal system. Occasionally, very large collateral vessels occur (Fig. 36.8); they rarely decompress the portal venous system sufficiently to prevent bleeding, but they can cause recurrent encephalopathy.

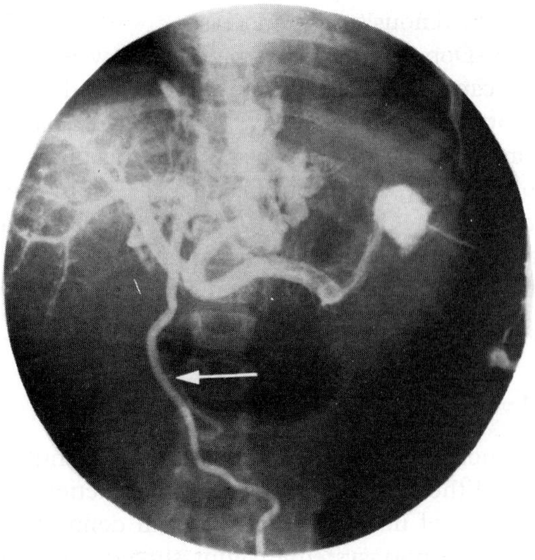

**Fig. 36.8** Splenoportogram in a patient with cirrhosis of the liver, portal hypertension and bleeding esophageal varices, showing a large left gastric vein supplying esophageal collateral vessels (arrowed). Note the paucity of intrahepatic portal venous radicals. Injected contrast material is seen in the spleen.

*Extrahepatic portal obstruction*

Collateral vessels arise from the spleen and from the splenic vein in extrahepatic portal venous obstruction. Their distribution depends on the site of obstruction in the splenic and portal veins. No collateral pathway occurs via the umbilical vein. The hallmarks of extrahepatic portal obstruction are collateral vessels bridging the point of obstruction (p. 1083). The intrahepatic portal venous branches either do not fill or show delayed filling from the collateral vessels. Incomplete obstruction may cause an irregularity of the vein wall or radiolucent areas within the vein.

*Portacaval shunt and TIPSS patency*

Portography can be used to investigate the patency of portasystemic anastomoses when recurrent gastrointestinal bleeding occurs or ascites reaccumulates after shunt surgery or TIPSS insertion (Fig. 36.9). Although patency can be assessed noninvasively by Doppler ultrasound techniques, direct selective catheterization through the anastomosis itself allows both portography, which may reveal shunt narrowing or intimal hyperplasia in patients with TIPSS, and direct portal pressure measurement.

## Portal venous pressure measurements

The extent to which portal pressure is raised can be established only by measuring the portal venous pressure. This

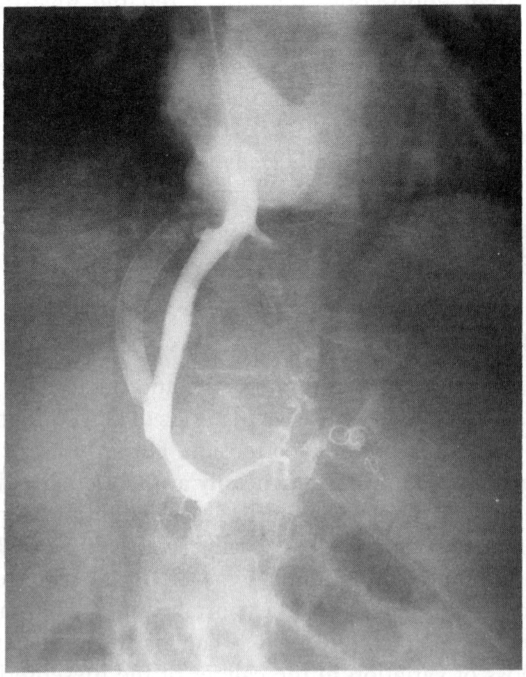

**Fig. 36.9** Portogram showing patent (opacified) and occluded (unopacified) TIPSS shunts, and radio-opaque springs in variceal vessels in portal hypertension due to primary sclerosing cholangitis leading to bleeding from ileostomy varices after colectomy for ulcerative colitis.

can be done directly by passing a catheter into the portal vein through the liver or via the umbilical vein, or indirectly by measuring the wedged hepatic venous pressure or the pressure in the splenic or hepatic parenchyma. All these measurements are invasive, uncomfortable and time consuming and they should be done only for specific reasons. The normal portal venous pressure is about 3–5 mmHg and the pressure in portal hypertension is usually between 15 and 30 mmHg but can exceed 40 mmHg. Radiological assessment of the portal hepatic venous system is frequently done at the same time (p. 75).

*Wedged hepatic venous pressure (WHVP)*

***Procedure.*** The WHVP can be measured safely and relatively simply. A curved-tip cardiac catheter is passed under radiological control via the basilic, external jugular or external iliac vein into a hepatic vein. The catheter is advanced until it is wedged, contrast medium is injected to confirm its position in a small hepatic vein and the wedged pressure is then recorded. An alternative approach is to use a balloon catheter to obtain occluded hepatic venous pressure measurements, as it can be difficult to ensure that a catheter has been fully wedged in a small hepatic vein. Several measurements should be made in different positions to ensure an accurate reading (Reynolds 1974, Groszmann et al 1979). Thereafter, the free hepatic venous pressure (FHVP) in a large hepatic vein or the inferior vena cava pressure (IVCP) is measured as a zero-reference pressure. These internally measured zero references are an important advantage of the WHVP; other methods use arbitrary and approximate external references that do not allow for the effects of ascites or gaseous abdominal distention on intra-abdominal venous pressure (Iwatsuki & Reynolds 1973). The superior vena cava and right atrial pressures should be measured whenever the IVCP is raised, especially when the procedure is being done in a patient with ascites. This ensures that conditions such as cardiac failure, cardiac tamponade and tricuspid valve disease are not overlooked.

***Interpretation.*** The portal pressure gradient (PPG) is the difference between the WHVP and the FHVP or IVCP. It reflects the free portal venous pressure and increases in parallel with the portal venous pressure. Most investigations have been carried out in alcoholic cirrhosis, in which the PPG accurately reflects the true portal venous pressure (Fig. 36.10), but where there is a significant presinusoidal component to the portal hypertension, the PPG underestimates portal pressure (Fig. 36.11) (Pomier-Layrargues et al 1985). The PPG is not raised in presinusoidal portal hypertension and a normal PPG in a patient with portal hypertension implies presinusoidal portal venous obstruction.

*Splenic pulp pressure*

This procedure carries a significant risk of bleeding and is no longer recommended. The range of normal intrasplenic pressure (3–17 mmHg) is higher than for PPG because arbitrary external zero-pressure reference points do not allow for alterations in intra-abdominal pressure unrelated to portal pressure (Reynolds et al 1970). Spuriously high pressures are sometimes found, which may be due to penetration of an artery or to the pathological changes in the spleen in portal hypertension.

*Hepatic parenchymal pressure*

Hepatic sinusoidal pressure can be measured via a needle or a plastic catheter passed into the liver parenchyma. The method is not recommended, as its reproducibility and its relation to the portal venous pressure is poor (Fenyves et al 1988).

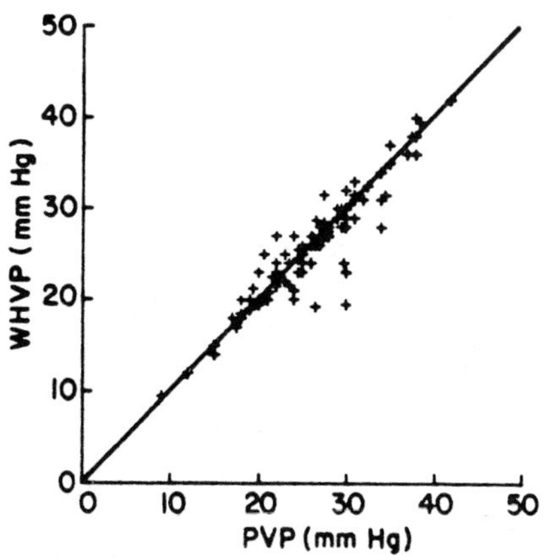


**Fig. 36.10** Simultaneous measurements of wedged hepatic venous pressure (WHVP) and portal venous pressure (PVP) in 110 patients with alcoholic cirrhosis (Pomier-Layrargues et al 1985).

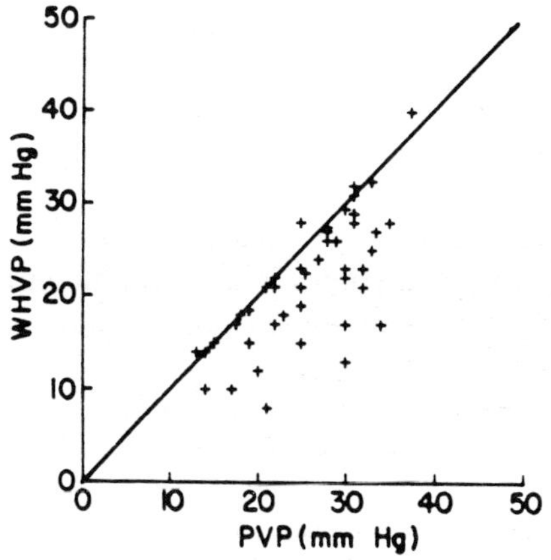


**Fig. 36.11** Simultaneous measurements of wedged hepatic venous pressure (WHVP) and portal venous pressure (PVP) in 46 patients with nonalcoholic cirrhosis (Pomier-Layrargues et al 1985).

*Direct measurements of portal pressure*

Portal venous pressure can be measured directly by passing a catheter through the liver and into the portal vein. This is done during transjugular intrahepatic portasystemic shunt insertion but is rarely required otherwise. Portal pressure can also be measured directly at operation by puncturing the portal vein or one of its mesenteric or omental tributaries. In either case, the FHVP or IVCP pressure should be measured to determine the PPG.

*Indications for measurement of portal venous pressure*

Portal venous pressure measurements are not often needed for diagnosis, but they can be valuable when uncertainty arises.

***Splenomegaly.*** Portal pressure measurements may be useful in patients with splenomegaly for which no cause can be found. If the WHVP is high, portal hypertension due to liver disease, usually well-compensated cirrhosis, is present. If the WHVP is normal, arterial portography can then show the features of presinusodal portal hypertension and usually establishes its cause.

***Esophagogastric varices.*** Varices are virtually always due to portal hypertension, but when there is no other evidence of liver disease, portal pressure measurements and portography are needed to determine the cause of the portal hypertension.

***Ascites.*** Portal pressure measurements are valuable when no cause can be found for ascites (p. 1020). The WHVP is the measurement of choice, as intra-abdominal venous pressures are raised in ascites and this is taken into account by using the IVCP as the zero-reference pressure. A WHVP more than 5 mmHg above the IVCP establishes portal hypertension and indicates chronic liver disease as the likely cause of the ascites. A normal PPG excludes chronic liver disease as the cause of ascites. Where ascites is due to cardiac failure, constrictive pericarditis or tricuspid valve disease, the superior and inferior vena cava pressures and the WHVP are all raised equally.

***Gastrointestinal bleeding.*** The source of gastrointestinal bleeding in a patient with varices may remain questionable, particularly where the varices are relatively small (p. 105). In these circumstances, a portal venous pressure of 12 mmHg or less makes a variceal source of bleeding unlikely. Sometimes it can be difficult to decide whether or not varices are present and this question can be answered best by portography.

***Budd–Chiari syndrome.*** Hepatic vein catheterization is usually diagnostic, as the WHVP usually cannot be measured and the hepatic venogram is abnormal (p. 1079).

***Pharmacological treatment of portal hypertension.*** Pharmacological treatment of portal hypertension, especially with propranolol, can now be used to prevent variceal bleeding (p. 1009). In practice, measurement of portal pressure before and after treatment is not indicated and may even be misleading. Propranolol, for example, reduces the risk of primary and secondary variceal bleeding but does not lower the portal pressure in approximately 40% of patients. It does, however, invariably reduce azygos venous blood flow (p. 1006).

## Esophageal variceal pressure measurement

Esophageal variceal pressure can be measured by puncturing varices with a sclerotherapy needle. The meaning of such pressures remains unclear in view of the structure of esophageal varices (below). Staritz et al (1985) found that pressures in large varices (22.7 ± 2.5 mmHg) were higher than in moderate varices (15.7 ± 0.6 mmHg) and variceal pressure during Valsalva maneuvers could reach 40 mmHg, suggesting that sudden increases of intra-abdominal pressure might precipitate bleeding. Intravariceal pressure has also been found to be an independent risk factor for first variceal bleeding (Feu et al 1990). Doppler ultrasound has shown an increased blood flow in esophageal varices during inspiration and a reduction with expiration (McCormack et al 1983) and Valsalva maneuvers affect variceal flow as measured by azygos venous blood flow, showing a rapid increase at the start of the maneuver followed by profound reduction, resulting in virtual cessation of flow in some patients after 3–5 s (Hayes et al 1992).

## Tolerance tests

These tests were devised to quantitate collateral flow, but they are now obsolete (Grace et al 1969).

## Peripheral blood count

Splenomegaly in portal hypertension often causes hypersplenism and mild to moderate thrombocytopenia is the commonest finding (p. 1187). A relationship between variceal bleeding and a platelet count below $100 \times 10^9$/L has been reported in primary biliary cirrhosis but not in other forms of liver disease (Pleuris et al 1995). Mild leukopenia can also occur, and anemia may be present but is often caused by factors other than hypersplenism (p. 1187). Macrocytosis associated with underlying cirrhosis and alcoholism is frequent (p. 872).

# COMPLICATIONS

## Esophageal variceal bleeding

Acute gastrointestinal bleeding is the most important complication of portal hypertension and it may be due to varices or to portal gastropathy (p. 1000). Bleeding from varices is frequently profuse. In cirrhosis, it may occur in patients who have so little clinical evidence of portal hypertension that the diagnosis is easily missed in an emergency when conditions for a thorough clinical examination are usually inadequate. Conversely, patients with obvious chronic liver disease and gastrointestinal bleeding may be bleeding from erosions or peptic ulceration rather than varices.

*Precipitating factors and variceal structure*

The factors predisposing to and initiating bleeding from esophageal varices remain largely unknown. Attention has centered on variceal structure, the site of bleeding, the size of varices, the degree of portal hypertension, the occurrence of erosive esophagitis and the severity of liver disease.

***Structure of varices.*** The term "varices" implies the presence of venous varicosities at the lower end of the esophagus. Recent studies, notably those of Vianna et al (1987), have shown using cast corrosion methods and radiology that the structure of varices, particularly in the lower 2–3 cm of the esophagus, is complicated (Fig. 36.12). Veins within the gastric wall, as they approach the gastroesophageal junction, arborize extensively and run together as small dilated vessels within the mucosal folds of the esophagus, often so close to the epithelial surface that they are seen as red marks on the varices at endoscopy (below). There is then a 2–3 cm "palisade" zone of straight vessels that subsequently interconnect, frequently forming a "treble clef" arrangement before passing more deeply into the mucosa and joining perforating vessels that communicate with the paraesophageal vasculature. Branches that do not connect with the perforating vessels run proximally in the "truncal" zone within the mucosal folds but deeper than their tributaries just above the gastroesophageal junction. This complex arrangement appears to produce a zone of low vascular resistance in the 2–3 cm above the gastroesophageal junction in which bidirectional flow occurs and in which changes in pressure from positive to negative occur during respiration (McCormack et al 1983).

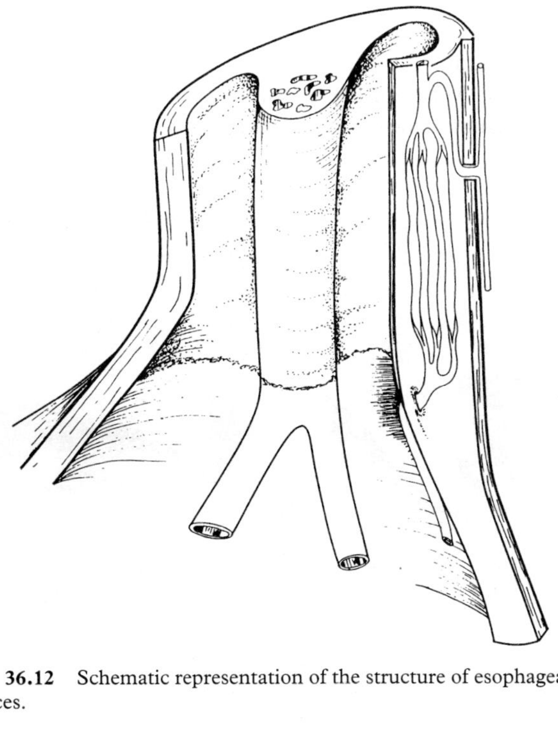

Fig. 36.12 Schematic representation of the structure of esophageal varices.

***Site of bleeding.*** Variceal bleeding almost always occurs within 2–5 cm of the gastroesophageal junction. This may be attributable to the structure of the varices at this site (above), their superficial position, changing blood flow and the possibility of marked pressure changes in the varices. The venous anatomy in this area may also account for the efficacy of endoscopic sclerotherapy in controlling acute bleeding from this site, its effectiveness in eradicating varices and perhaps also its susceptibility to ulceration. Certainly a not uncommon cause of failure to obliterate varices by endoscopic sclerotherapy is injection too proximal in the esophagus into the larger vessels that exist there, resulting in rapid removal of the sclerosant away from the injection site.

***Appearance of varices.*** The mechanisms involved in variceal hemorrhage are incompletely understood, but risk factors for bleeding include the size of varices (Table 36.2) (Lebrec et al 1980), the presence on the varices of cherry red spots or red stripes or ridges (wales) (Beppu et al 1981) and the severity of liver disease. The North Italian Endoscopic Club devised an index using these variables which reasonably predicted bleeding (North Italian Endoscopic Club 1988, De Franchis et al 1990). The risk of bleeding in patients with Child grade A liver disease with small varices and no red markings was 6% over 12 months compared to 76% in Child grade C patients with large varices and severe red markings (Fig. 36.5). These red signs on varices may be related to superficial intraepithelial vessels in the esophageal mucosa (Spence et al 1983).

***Portal pressure.*** It would seem logical to assume a relationship between portal venous pressure and the size and liability to bleeding of esophageal varices, but there is little evidence for this. Some have found that portal pressure is related to variceal size (Willoughby et al 1964, Joly et al 1971), but others have shown that this relation disap-

**Table 36.2** Size of esophageal varices related to source of bleeding at endoscopy in patients presenting with acute upper gastrointestinal bleeding (Royal Infirmary, Edinburgh)

| Variceal size | Source of bleeding | | | |
|---|---|---|---|---|
| | Varices | | Nonvariceal bleeding | |
| | Number | % | Number | % |
| Large | 45 | 78 | 10 | 53 |
| Moderate | 11 | 19 | 6 | 31 |
| Small | 2 | 3 | 3 | 16 |

pears at higher portal pressures (Lebrec et al 1980). It is generally agreed that varices are uncommon and bleeding unusual at portal pressures below 12 mmHg, but the risk of bleeding does not relate to portal pressure above that level (Viallet et al 1975, Lebrec et al 1980, Garcia-Tsao et al 1985). A more important measurement may, of course, be the pressure in the varices themselves (above).

***Drugs.*** Salicylates may precipitate bleeding from varices and should not be used (Franco et al 1977). Other drugs known to produce esophageal ulceration should also be avoided (p. 485) and there is anecdotal evidence that bleeding may follow the use of high-dose corticosteroid therapy.

***Esophagitis.*** Simpson & Conn (1968) found that raised intragastric pressure and gastroesophageal reflux were associated with ascites in cirrhotic patients and they suggested that erosive esophagitis from reflux might precipitate bleeding. However, more recent studies make it unlikely that reflux esophagitis is a common precipitant of bleeding, as studies of the lower esophagus removed at stapling transection have not shown much evidence of esophagitis (Ponce et al 1981, Spence et al 1983) and a normal lower esophageal sphincter pressure has been reported in cirrhotic patients irrespective of esophageal varices, recent variceal bleeding or ascites (Eckhardt et al 1976). Furthermore, variceal bleeding can occur in achlorhydric patients and after total gastrectomy. The observation that $H_2$ receptor antagonists do little to affect the incidence of rebleeding following an index bleed would support a minimal influence of acid reflux on variceal bleeding.

***Hepatic failure.*** As detailed above, the severity of liver disease is an important risk factor of variceal bleeding. Gastrointestinal bleeding is common in hepatic failure and is often a terminal event. Bleeding from varices, however, occurs frequently in patients without marked hepatic failure and as might be expected, this is most common in younger patients (Terés et al 1976, Franco et al 1977).

***Paracentesis.*** Variceal hemorrhage occasionally follows paracentesis. One explanation for this may be hemodynamic changes that include an acute increase in cardiac output following this procedure (Panos et al 1990).

## Bleeding from other varices

Bleeding from varices other than esophageal varices is rare but can occur from a variety of sites. Most patients also have esophageal varices, but those with regional portal hypertension may not (p. 1085). It has been suggested that bleeding from varices in these unusual sites may be particularly common after successful injection sclerotherapy of esophageal varices. Bleeding from gastric varices can be difficult to identify endoscopically and may occur more often than is recognized; it is particularly likely to occur after splenic vein thrombosis where the varices are usually mainly in the stomach (p. 1085). Bleeding from intestinal varices has been reported in the duodenum (Spence & Roy 1984), in the small intestine (Case Records of the Massachusetts General Hospital 1976) and in the colon (Mills et al 1980, Gudjonsson et al 1986). Bleeding from small intestinal varices in the absence of varices elsewhere has been reported in regional superior mesenteric venous hypertension (p. 1085) and bleeding from the colon has occurred with varices throughout the colon (Weingart et al 1982) and in association with intestinal hemangiomas (Lieberman et al 1983). Anorectal varices account for about 5% of bleeds due to portal hypertension (Hosking & Johnson 1988), can cause profuse bleeding and are often mistaken for hemorrhoids (p. 993). Bleeding usually occurs from the squamous part of the anal canal and anoscopy often shows the site of bleeding with or without active bleeding. Varices form at the site of previous operations and bleeding from such varices has occurred at stomas of various types (p. 993). External bleeding can occur from vaginal varices (Eriksson et al 1982) and from umbilical varices (Fig. 36.13) and intraperitoneal bleeding can occur from paraumbilical, mesenteric or even retroperitoneal varices (Rothschild et al 1968, Ross 1970).

## Portal hypertensive gastropathy

Endoscopy in patients with portal hypertension reveals appearances often described as gastritis (McCormack et al 1985). Small pink to red spots a millimeter or two in diameter are seen most often and with increasing severity the spots coalesce to form larger red areas that may show central clot or even bleeding. Other appearances include linear erythematous areas, usually on the surface of rugae, or a white reticular pattern surrounding areas of red edematous-looking mucosa ("snake skin mucosa"). The extent and severity of these lesions vary considerably, but they are usually most severe distally in the stomach and

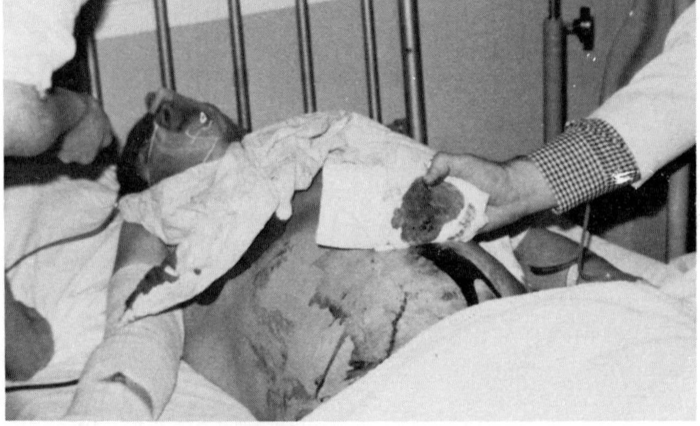

**Fig. 36.13** Profuse bleeding from an umbilical vessel in a patient with cirrhosis and portal hypertension. Bleeding began suddenly during a fit of coughing. Esophagogastric varices were also present.

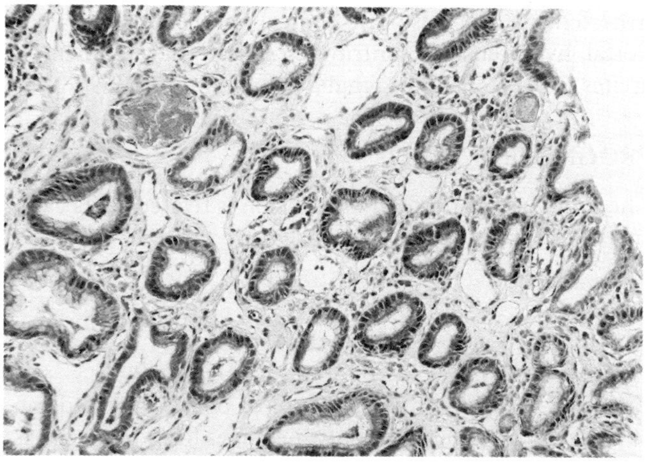

**Fig. 36.14** Congestive gastropathy in the antrum of a patient with cirrhosis, portal hypertension and recurring iron-deficient anemia. Note the numerous dilated blood vessels, some containing fibrin, in the submucosa (hematoxylin and eosin, ×125).

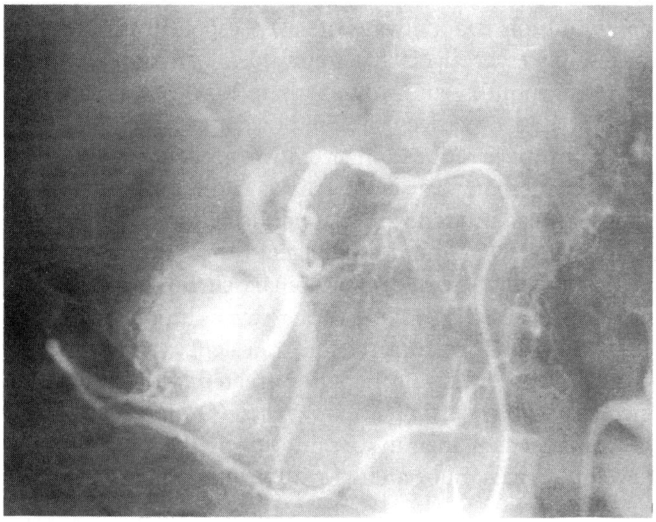

**Fig. 36.15** Angiogram in congestive gastropathy (same patient as in Fig. 36.13) showing a very vascular stomach.

they stop abruptly at the pylorus. Mucosal biopsy shows vascular ectasia rather than inflammation (Fig. 36.14), and angiography may reveal dense gastric collateral vessels in severe cases (Fig. 36.15). McCormack et al (1985) found these lesions at endoscopy in 65 of 127 (51%) patients with portal hypertension and the appearances were classified as mild in 37 (57%). The endoscopic appearances probably represent the most marked instances of vascular changes occurring generally in the stomach in all patients with portal hypertension (Hashizume et al 1983). Cirrhotic patients with portal hypertensive gastropathy have an increase in gastric blood flow (Panés et al 1992) and sclerotherapy of esophageal varices may well exacerbate portal hypertensive gastropathy and promote the development of gastric varices (Tanoue et al 1992).

Patients with congestive gastropathy do not suffer dyspeptic symptoms. Bleeding is the most important complication. It usually causes recurring iron-deficient anemia, sometimes needing repeated blood transfusion, but it can occasionally give rise to more acute bleeding with melena. Reduction in portal pressure and collateral flow with propranolol (p. 1006) is the best initial treatment for active bleeding and for prevention of bleeding (Hosking et al 1987, Perez-Ayuso et al 1991) and a TIPSS procedure (p. 1007) may be valuable although experience remains limited. Operations such as portasystemic shunts, gastric devascularization and distal gastrectomy can prevent recurrent bleeding but are too hazardous and $H_2$ receptor antagonists, bismuth and sucralfate are ineffective.

### Portal hypertensive colopathy

Lesions similar to those of portal gastropathy occur in the colon and are associated microscopically with dilated capillaries (Kozarek et al 1991). Colonoscopic appearances include cherry red spots, ectatic vessels, lesions identical to those of angiodysplasia and occasionally diffuse friable mucosa resembling colitis. The frequency of these lesions in portal hypertension is unknown, but they are often associated with esophagogastric varices, portal gastropathy and sometimes rectal varices.

### Portal venous thrombosis

Portal venous thrombosis can occur in any form of portal hypertension but is seen most often in patients with cirrhosis. This is considered in more detail in relation to vascular diseases of the liver (p. 1083).

### Hypersplenism

This is defined as the association of anemia, leukopenia ($<5 \times 10^9$ cells/L or <5000 cells/$mm^3$) or thrombocytopenia ($<150 \times 10^9$ cells/L or <150 000 cells/$mm^3$) with hyperplasia of the bone marrow and splenomegaly detected by palpitation, radiology or imaging. It is common in cirrhosis and is most frequent in patients with portal hypertension of sufficient duration and severity to have produced esophagogastric varices (Tumen 1970). Hypersplenism in cirrhosis is generally mild (p. 1187); platelet counts below $50 \times 10^9$/L (50 000/$mm^3$) are exceptional and leukopenia rarely gives counts below $2 \times 10^9$/L (2000/$mm^3$). Anemia alone should not be attributed to hypersplenism in cirrhosis with portal hypertension until special investigations have shown a reduced red blood cell lifespan and increased pooling of red blood cells in the spleen. These are not usually prominent features in the hypersplenism of cirrhosis and there are many other causes of anemia in these patients.

The mechanisms producing hypersplenism in portal hypertension have not been well defined and most work has related to thrombocytopenia. Platelets normally survive for about 9 days in the circulation and this survival is reduced in most patients with chronic liver disease. The splenic platelet pool is usually increased, as would be expected in patients with splenomegaly, but there is a poor relation between the platelet count, the splenic platelet pool and spleen size in chronic liver disease, unlike other disease associated with hypersplenism, and consequently other factors must be operating (Toghill & Green 1983). These may include intrinsic platelet abnormalities (Rubin et al 1979) and platelet-associated immunoglobulin (Barrison et al 1981, Bassendine et al 1985) promoting platelet destruction.

Complications of hypersplenism are uncommon in cirrhosis and are not important factors in the prognosis of the disease. Spontaneous bleeding due to thrombocytopenia is rare even when the platelet count is below $50 \times 10^9$/L (50 000/mm$^3$), but platelet depletion may become important during bleeding. Leukopenia severe enough to cause recurrent infection is exceptional. The leukocyte count usually fails to rise after acute gastrointestinal bleeding and this is a clue to underlying hypersplenism. The effects of portasystemic shunts are variable: hypersplenism hardly ever improves (Fig. 36.16), but it rarely develops or gets worse after surgery (Macpherson 1979, Toghill & Green 1979). Splenectomy abolishes hypersplenism and embolization of the spleen can alleviate it (p. 1011). Hypersplenism has also disappeared after spontaneous massive splenic infarction in portal hypertension (Capron et al 1976). The TIPSS procedure reduces splenic congestion, but the increase in platelet count following this procedure is modest.

## Other complications

Portal vein aneurysm is a rare development in portal hypertension, but it is of no clinical significance (p. 1085). Portal hypertension contributes to the development of ascites (p. 1017) and to renal dysfunction (p. 1059).

## PROGNOSIS

The prognosis in portal hypertension is related to its cause and to the presence of esophagogastric varices.

### Cirrhosis

*Development of varices*

Cirrhosis is the commonest cause of portal hypertension, but portal hypertension only becomes important in its prognosis once esophageal varices, from which bleeding can occur, have developed. Christensen et al (1981) found that about a quarter of patients with various forms of cirrhosis had varices at presentation and about two-thirds of the rest developed varices over the next 10 years (Fig. 36.17). Once present, varices tend to enlarge gradually, but this is not always the case, especially in the early stages. Cales et al (1990) followed 84 cirrhotic patients over 16 months and found that 20% developed new varices, 42% of varices already present enlarged and 16% of small varices reduced in size during follow-up.

The underlying cause of cirrhosis and its rate of progression may also influence the rate of development of varices. Kew et al (1971) found esophageal varices at presentation in 4% of patients with primary biliary cirrhosis and about a half of the rest developed varices over the next 10 years (Fig. 36.17). By contrast, the prevalence of esophageal varices in autoimmune hepatitis treated with prednisone increased by only 5% over 5 years (Czaja et al 1979). Bleeding occurs in only a minority of the patients who develop varices, but patients with primary biliary cirrhosis

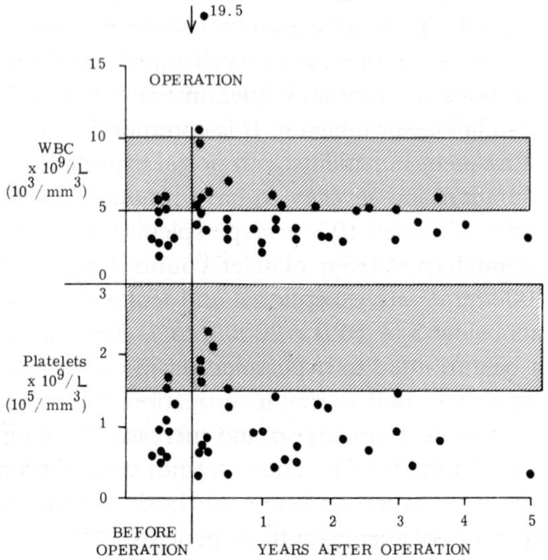


**Fig. 36.16** Leukocyte and platelet counts before and after portacaval anastomosis. Shaded areas represent normal values. The vertical arrow represents the time of operation (Macpherson 1979).

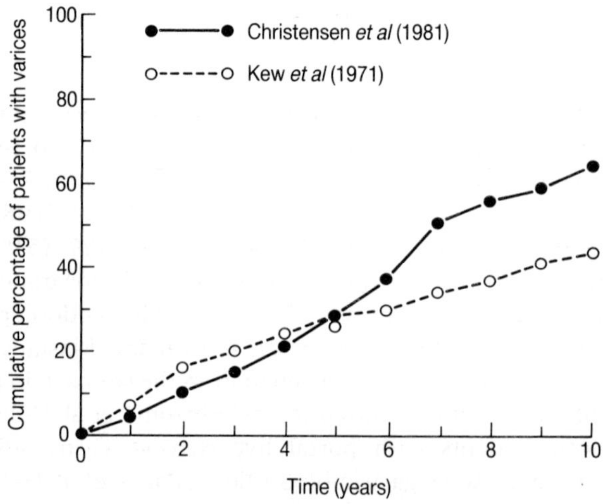


**Fig. 36.17** The development of esophageal varices with time in patients presenting with cirrhosis of various types (Christensen et al 1981) or with primary biliary cirrhosis (Kew et al 1971).

**Table 36.3** Causes of death in 115 patients with cirrhosis and esophageal varices followed for 2–6 years (mean 3.3 years) (Baker et al 1959)

| Cause of death | Number of deaths | Proportion (%) | |
|---|---|---|---|
| | | All patients | All deaths |
| Gastrointestinal bleeding | 20 | 17 | 27 |
| Hepatic failure | 31 | 27 | 42 |
| Other related to the liver | 2 | 2 | 3 |
| Nonhepatic disease | 21 | 18 | 28 |
| Total deaths | 74 | 64 | 100 |

**Table 36.4** Variceal bleeding and survival in the combined control and shunt-refusal groups in prophylactic trials of portasystemic shunt operations

| Trial | Year | No. of patients | Bleeding (%) | Survival (%) | Deaths due to variceal bleeding (%) | Follow-up period (years) |
|---|---|---|---|---|---|---|
| Jackson et al | 1968 | 75 | 19 | 72 | 43 | 5 |
| Resnick et al | 1969 | 45 | 27 | 58 | 26 | 8 |
| Conn et al | 1972 | 35 | 40 | 43 | 40 | 12 |
| Conn et al | 1972 | 24 | 29 | 46 | 45 | 6 |

with varices have twice the mortality of those without varices and this is attributable to acute gastrointestinal bleeding. The development of esophageal varices in a patient with cirrhosis clearly has serious prognostic implications.

### *Varices without previous bleeding*

Kew et al (1971) showed that the development of varices increased mortality in primary biliary cirrhosis because of bleeding. However, hepatic failure is the other major cause of death in cirrhosis (Table 36.3) and liver function has to be taken into account in assessing the prognostic importance of esophageal varices.

***Good liver function.*** Patients who took part in trials of portasystemic shunt surgery for preventing variceal bleeding are likely to have had relatively good liver function and those who did not undergo surgery have been followed for up to 12 years (Jackson et al 1968, Resnick et al 1969, Conn et al 1972). A half to two-thirds of these patients survived 5 years, variceal bleeding occurred in approximately one-third, half of the bleeds were fatal and bleeding accounted for a quarter to a half of all deaths (Tablc 36.4). Similar data regarding the frequency of variceal bleeding in patients with cirrhosis and varices during follow-up can be obtained from the control groups in trials of propranolol in the prophylaxis of variceal bleeding (Pascal et al 1987, Italian Multicenter Project for Propranolol 1989, Conn et al 1991). Over 2 years 25–60% of patients bled, the frequency being higher where there were more patients with decompensated liver disease. Baker et al (1959) found that survival was better when patients with cirrhosis and esophageal varices had less advanced liver disease. About half the deaths in their patients were due to the hepatic disease, a quarter to gastrointestinal bleeding and a further quarter to unrelated causes (Table 36.3). The overall mortality from gastrointestinal bleeding was only 17%, but when bleeding did occur, the outlook became much worse (Fig. 36.18). Thus, only a minority of patients with relatively good liver function die of bleeding within about 5 years of the discovery of varices, but bleeding has a serious prognosis when it does occur.

***Poor liver function.*** The situation is very different when liver function is poor. Garceau & Chalmers (1963) studied a large group of patients with advanced cirrhosis and found that the survival of those with varices that had not bled was about the same as the survival of the group as a whole (Table 36.5). Most of their patients had advanced disease; almost half had jaundice, ascites and hepatic precoma and 96% had one or more of these. Their findings therefore indicate that hepatic failure rather than portal hypertension determines the prognosis in patients with advanced disease. Indeed, Olsson (1972) found that survival was somewhat better in cirrhotic patients who developed bleeding varices than in those who developed other complications, such as liver failure or hepatocellular carcinoma.

### *Variceal bleeding*

Once bleeding from varices occurs, the immediate prognosis is related to the severity of the bleeding and to the degree of hepatic dysfunction (p. 505). Graham & Smith (1981) found that one-third of patients, most with fairly advanced alcoholic cirrhosis, died from their initial bleed, a third rebled within 6 weeks and only a third survived 1 year. Longer term survival is determined largely by the state of liver function (Fig. 36.19), although renewed bleeding continues to occur and causes 40% of late deaths in patients surviving an initial bleed, including those with good liver function (Graham & Smith 1981). The effects of treatment on survival are much debated, but there are grounds for thinking that we have traveled a long way in the last 50 years without getting very far (Fig. 36.20). New treatments, such as variceal banding and the TIPSS procedure, are probably effective in reducing recurrent variceal bleeding, but they do not improve liver function and are unlikely therefore to affect survival significantly. Liver transplantation is the only treatment that corrects hepatocellular function and should improve prognosis, but it is very expensive and of limited availability (p. 1151).

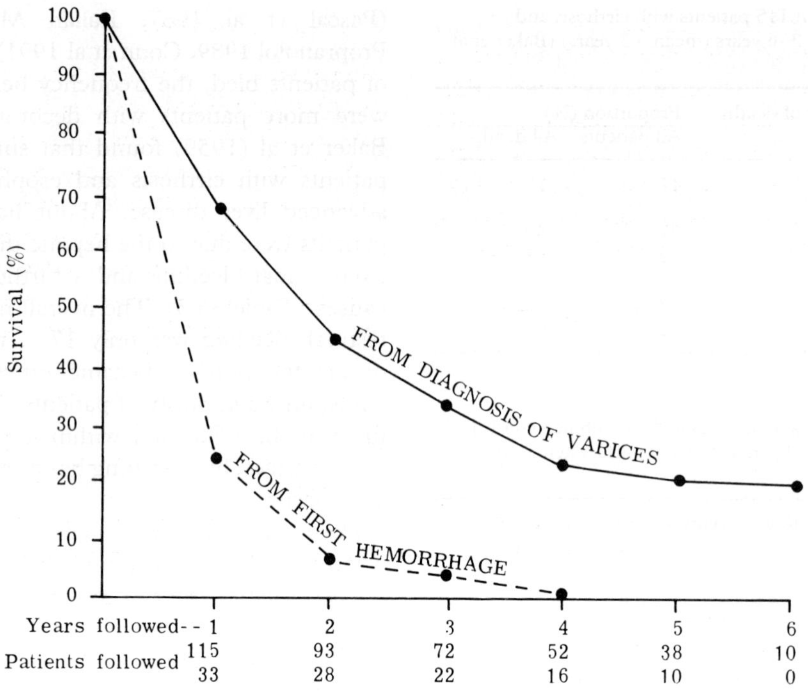


**Fig. 36.18** Survival of patients with varices with and without gastrointestinal hemorrhage (Baker et al 1959).

**Table 36.5** Survival of patients with advanced cirrhosis and esophageal varices (Garceau & Chalmers 1963)

| Time (years) | Survival (%) | |
|---|---|---|
| | Varices, no prior bleeding (288) | Whole group (467) |
| 1 | 42.8 | 34.3 |
| 2 | 24.8 | 20.6 |
| 5 | 8.3 | 5.5 |

Number of patients in parentheses.

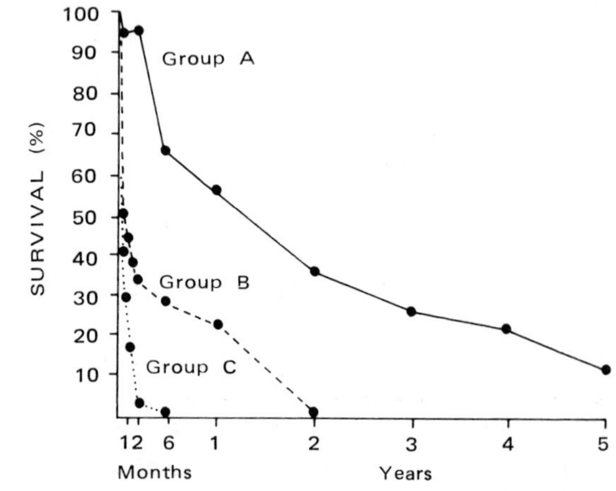


**Fig. 36.19** Survival after first bleed from varices related to hepatic function (see Table 36.7) (Olsson 1972).

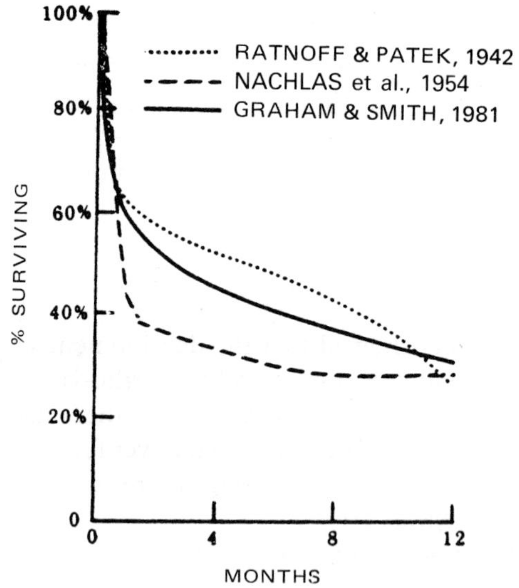


**Fig. 36.20** Comparison of survival curves for patients with variceal bleeding obtained over four decades (Graham & Smith 1981).

## Presinusoidal portal hypertension

The prognosis in presinusoidal forms of portal hypertension is generally better than in portal hypertension due to cirrhosis, as liver function is usually good.

***Extrahepatic portal hypertension.*** This is considered in relation to vascular diseases of the liver (p. 1084).

***Intrahepatic presinusoidal portal hypertension.*** Younger patients usually have conditions such as congenital hepatic fibrosis (p. 726) and their prognosis is much better than patients of similar age with cirrhosis, as liver function is usually well maintained over a long period of time. Older patients do less well because portal obstruction is usually caused by a progressive disease such as carcinoma, lymphoma (p. 1104) or a myeloproliferative disorder (p. 1103) or by diseases such as paroxysmal nocturnal hemoglobinuria (p. 1079) that are associated with recurrent thromboses.

***Primary portal hypertension.*** The prognosis is much better than in cirrhosis (p. 1085).

## TREATMENT

### Esophagogastric variceal bleeding

This is the most important complication of portal hypertension. Management can be divided into three components: emergency treatment of acute bleeding (p. 499), prevention of rebleeding and prophylaxis of bleeding in patients who have never bled. Many treatments have been advocated, implying that there is debate about which are the most effective or appropriate. They can be divided into two main groups: those that aim to obstruct or obliterate varices and those designed to reduce portal pressure. As a general rule, since many of the treatments are probably of similar efficacy, it seems sensible that individual practitioners and centers should develop experience and expertise in a limited number that will cover the range of clinical problems rather than seek to provide all treatments. This is particularly relevant with regard to surgical techniques and such interventions as TIPSS.

*Prevention of rebleeding*

After control of acute bleeding (p. 499), without further intervention rebleeding will recur in approximately 70% of patients within 6 months (Westaby et al 1985).

***Injection sclerotherapy.*** Seven randomized clinical trials over the last 10 years have been undertaken to assess the efficacy of sclerotherapy in reducing rebleeding (Hayes & Bouchier 1990). All seven demonstrated a reduction in rebleeding, but no effect on survival was seen in three. A meta-analysis pooling the results demonstrated an improvement in survival, but as the trials differed in design, patient selection and follow-up, some doubt about the validity of pooling must exist (Infante-Rivard et al 1989). In general, gastric varices respond less well to sclerotherapy than esophageal varices. This is particularly true for varices confined to the fundus of the stomach, which are generally resistant to treatment with conventional sclerosants. However, gastric varices that extend across the gastroesophageal junction from esophageal varices can more readily be treated by sclerotherapy (Gimson et al 1991, Korula et al 1991). Tissue adhesives such as bucrylate may be more effective than conventional sclerosants in this setting (Feretis et al 1990). Injection of thrombin into gastric varices has recently been reported as being valuable (Williams et al 1994). Fifty percent of patients rebleed while variceal obliteration is being undertaken (Fig. 36.21), but rebleeding after eradication of varices is unusual even though varices may recur. Thus, most advocate rapid obliteration by weekly or fortnightly injections followed by 6- or 12-monthly endoscopic review.

As approximately 50% of rebleeding during injec-

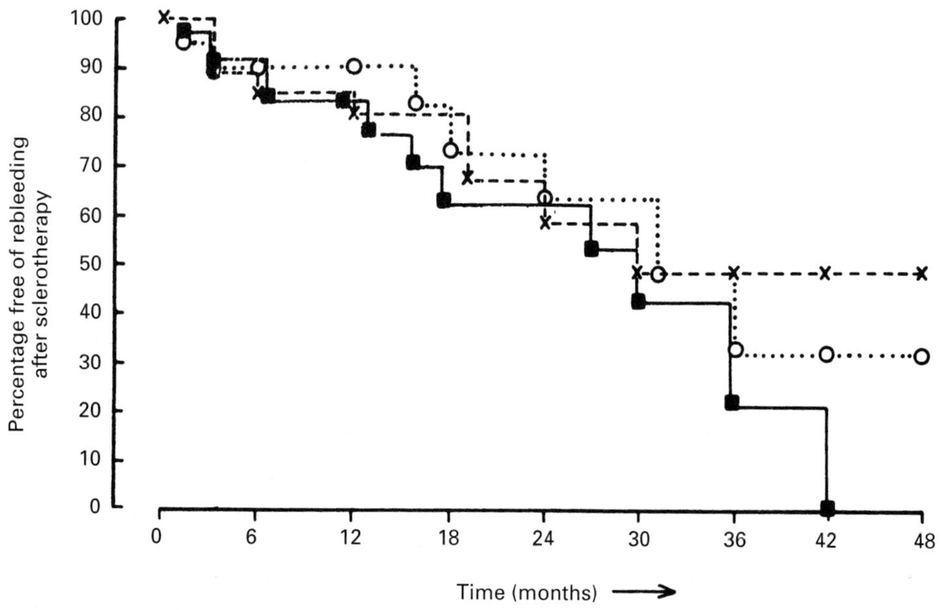


**Fig. 36.21** Cumulative proportion of freedom from rebleeding related to hepatic function in 100 patients with bleeding from esophageal varices treated by sclerotherapy (Royal Infirmary, Edinburgh). Note: hepatic function assessed by Child grade (Table 36.7). ×–× = A; ○–○ = B; ■–■ = C.

tion sclerotherapy is due to sclerotherapy-related ulcers (Westaby et al 1986), it would seem best to balance over-aggressive sclerotherapy to achieve rapid variceal obliteration by a more gradual approach leaving patent varices in place for longer. However, the frequency with which sclerotherapy-related ulcers are found seems to depend on how soon endoscopy is repeated and there is controversy as to whether the frequency of sclerotherapy influences the risk of sclerotherapy-related ulcer bleeding. Sucralfate has been demonstrated to reduce the risk of variceal rebleeding, but the effect is minor and it appears to have little to do with reducing the incidence of ulceration (Polson et al 1989). The major benefit of sclerotherapy in reducing variceal rebleeding occurs over the initial injection sessions and overzealous attempts at complete variceal obliteration may produce more harm than good.

Few doubt that injection sclerotherapy reduces the risk of variceal rebleeding, but it is far from ideal. The treatment is prolonged, is associated with complications such as ulceration, stricture formation and even esophageal perforation and has financial implications for patients and hospitals involved. The value of long-term surveillance has recently been called into question in a trial comparing sclerotherapy and surveillance with sclerotherapy only after each bleed (Burroughs et al 1989). At present injection sclerotherapy, aimed at achieving variceal obliteration, is the most popular treatment, but alternatives such as esophageal variceal band ligation, propranolol, surgical intervention and TIPSS deserve consideration.

***Band ligation of esophageal varices.*** Three recent studies have compared variceal band ligation with injection sclerotherapy after bleeding from esophageal varices (Stiegmann et al 1992, Gimson et al 1993, Laine et al 1993). All three reported advantages of banding, including fewer complications, less rebleeding and more rapid obliteration of varices. Previously, the endoscope had to be withdrawn for reloading after each band was in place, but devices (albeit expensive) that discharge bands sequentially are now available. Many now believe that band ligation should replace injection sclerotherapy at least in nonemergency situations (Hayes 1996). In active bleeding, the restricted view caused by the outer cylinder at the tip of the endoscope is a disadvantage and the suction required to prolapse the varix into the banding device commonly results in obliteration of the field of vision by blood. A combination of injection of small volumes of sclerosant to obtain hemostasis followed by banding may be a practical solution in this situation.

***Propranolol.*** It is over 10 years since Lebrec and colleagues in France first reported that propranolol could reduce portal pressure in patients with cirrhosis and portal hypertension and reduce recurrent gastrointestinal bleeding (Lebrec et al 1981). Over the intervening period there have been numerous trials of the efficacy of propranolol in reducing rebleeding from esophageal varices, some confirming and some refuting this original observation. On balance, however, the evidence favors a beneficial effect (Table 36.6) and this view has been confirmed using meta-analysis (Hayes et al 1990). Some have adjusted the dose of propranolol to reduce the resting heart rate by 25%, while others have used fixed doses; there appears to be little difference in the results and a fixed dose has the merit of simplicity.

**Table 36.6** Results of meta-analysis of 19 trials of β blockade for the prevention of rebleeding from esophageal varices (Hayes et al 1990)

| | Total patients | Patients who rebled | Deaths from rebleeding | Total mortality |
|---|---|---|---|---|
| Treated | 565 | 210 | 49 | 121 |
| Controls | 515 | 299 | 76 | 149 |
| % reduction | – | 39 | 40 | 25 |
| Treatment effect ($p$) | – | <0.0001 | 0.002 | 0.009 |

Note: $p$ = probability.

The mechanism whereby propranolol reduces variceal bleeding remains controversial. Although its use was prompted initially by the observation that it could reduce portal hypertension, it achieves this in only 60% of patients, while a reduction in collateral blood flow, as measured by azygos venous flow, always occurs (Bosch et al 1984). Studies of variables predicting rebleeding in patients receiving propranolol have identified failure of the pulse rate to fall as being important (Poynard et al 1987). This could indicate lack of compliance, also a risk factor for rebleeding, or an unresponsive patient rather than inadequate dose, as there is no correlation between the dose of propranolol and the risk of rebleeding (Westaby et al 1990). This study also identified a high resting heart rate before treatment as a correlate of poor response to therapy. Garcia-Pagán et al (1990) showed recently that a combination of propranolol and isosorbide mononitrate reduced portal pressure more than propranolol alone, but studies of the clinical efficacy of this are not available.

Studies of the relative merits of propranolol and injection sclerotherapy in preventing rebleeding have shown the two treatments to be similar (Alexandrino et al 1988, Westaby et al 1990). In practice, sclerotherapy is the more popular treatment principally because propranolol is poorly tolerated in 20–30% of patients and it depends upon patient compliance. Trials of the effects of combining propranolol and sclerotherapy have given conflicting results. Early studies showed no benefit from adding propranolol (Westaby et al 1986, Vickers et al 1987), whereas two more recent trials of combination therapy did show a reduction in rebleeding (Jenson & Krarup 1989, O'Connor et al 1989). The evidence is therefore unconvincing, but it would seem reasonable at least in the early weeks of sclerotherapy or banding to add propranolol where β-receptor blockade is not contraindicated.

***Portalazygos disconnection operations.*** These oper-

**Table 36.7** Hepatic functional reserve in cirrhosis (Pugh et al 1973)

| Assessment criteria | Points scored for abnormality 1 | 2 | 3 | Grade | Scores |
|---|---|---|---|---|---|
| Encephalopathy grade* | None | 1–2 | 3–4 | A | 5–6 |
| Ascites | None | Slight | Moderate | | |
| Bilirubin µmol/L | <35 | 35–50 | >50 | | |
| Biliary cirrhosis | <70 | 70–170 | >170 | B | 7–9 |
| Albumin g/L | >35 | 28–35 | <28 | | |
| Prothrombin time ratio | <1.4 | 1.4–2.0 | >2.0 | C | 10–15 |
| Seconds prolonged | 1–4 | 4–10 | >10 | | |

*See Table 38.3

**Table 36.8** Mortality of portasystemic shunt surgery in cirrhosis related to hepatic functional reserve

| Series | Number of patients | Postoperative mortality (%) Hepatic reserve A | B | C |
|---|---|---|---|---|
| Wantz & Payne (1961) | 131 | 2 | 13 | 29 |
| Turcotte et al (1969) | 102 | 10 | 16 | 54 |
| Macpherson (1979) | 96 | 0 | 4 | 33 |

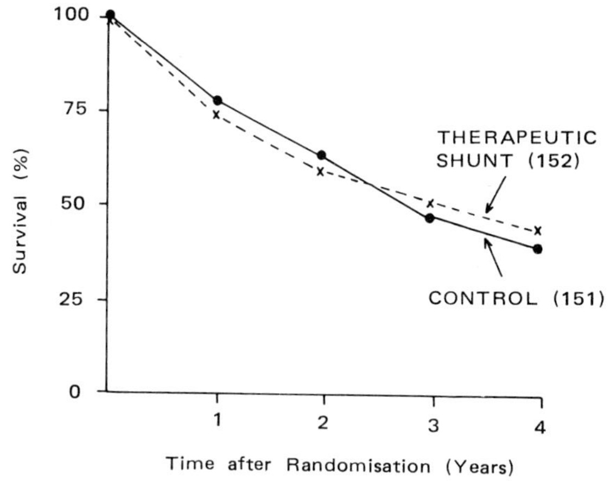


**Fig. 36.22** Cumulative survival after a portacaval shunt operation calculated from the combined results of the Veterans Administration Co-operative Study, the Boston Inter-Hospital Liver Group Study and the Hôpital Beaujon Study (Conn 1974).

ations, the most popular of which is esophageal staple transection, are designed to arrest bleeding from esophageal varices and to prevent rebleeding by interrupting the blood flow to esophageal varices without impairing portal blood flow to the liver. They are used to stop variceal bleeding that has failed to respond to other treatments (p. 504), but they are not used much otherwise in Europe or North America. Portalazygos disconnection operations are frequently favored for variceal bleeding caused by schistosomiasis.

***Portasystemic shunt operations.*** The portacaval shunt was introduced over 50 years ago and quickly became a standard treatment (Blakemore & Lord 1945). Clinical and biochemical assessment in the form of Child grading gave a good indication of the risk of surgery (Table 36.7) and operative mortalities were low in patients with good liver function (Table 36.8). However, where liver function was poor (grade C), the mortality was 30–55%. Eventually, controlled trials of portacaval shunting and of several other portasystemic shunts revealed that they did not prolong life (Figs 36.22, 36.23) and as a result there has been a considerable reduction in the use of these operations (Conn 1974). Liver failure is the main cause of death after portasystemic shunt surgery (Table 36.9) and although survival after surgery is not reduced, patients may experience severe hepatic encephalopathy that mars their quality of life (Table 36.10).

The portacaval shunt and its derivative shunts divert virtually all the portal blood away from the liver (unselective or total shunts) and the liability of patients to hepatic encephalopathy and liver failure has been attributed to this diversion of blood away from the liver. Accordingly, considerable efforts have gone into developing selective portasystemic shunts that decompress the esophageal varices while maintaining as much portal blood flow to the liver as possible. The best known of these shunts is the distal splenorenal shunt, which reduces postoperative encephalopathy at least initially (Table 36.11), although with the passage of time blood flow to the liver falls and encephalopathy can appear (Rikkers et al 1978, Warren et al 1982). Trials comparing the distal splenorenal shunt with unselective shunts have given conflicting results, but it is probably now the portasystemic shunt of choice (Harley et al 1986). The distal splenorenal shunt is not suitable for patients with centrifugal portal blood flow, as in the Budd–Chiari syndrome (p. 1079), but it is not so strongly contraindicated in patients with ascites as was thought previously (Warren et al 1982). A selective left gastric vein to inferior vena cava shunt has also been developed but is used almost exclusively in Japan.

Esophagogastric varices diminish in size over about a year after portasystemic shunt surgery and recurrent bleeding is almost always due to occlusion or stenosis of the shunt, which occurs in 5–10% of patients after portacaval shunt and in 5–20% after splenorenal shunts. However, the lack of suitability of shunt surgery for patients with poor liver function, the significant postoperative mortality and morbidity and the lack of effect on long-term mortality has meant that shunt surgery has gradually become less used and outside certain centers in the United States is now performed infrequently. It may well be that portasystemic shunt surgery in patients with cirrhosis will be reduced even further by the TIPSS procedure where a shunt can be created without recourse to surgery. Shunt surgery still has an important place in patients with presinusoidal portal hypertension, particularly portal vein thrombosis, but since few surgeons are experienced in the technique it is likely to be undertaken only in specialist units.

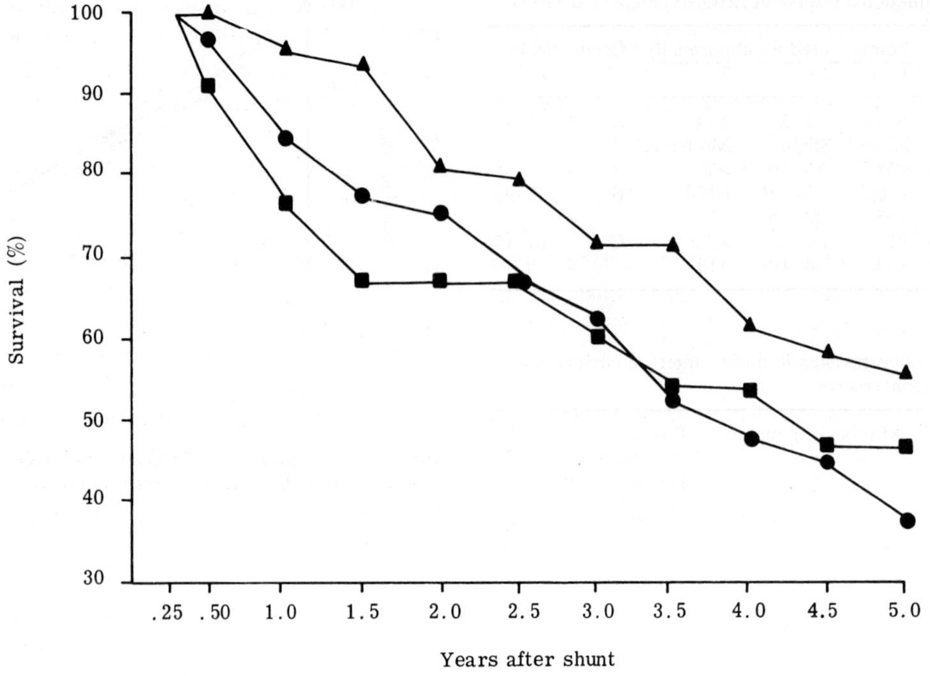


**Fig. 36.23** Life table survival of patients with hepatic cirrhosis who lived at least 3 months after a portacaval shunt operation. ▲ = grade A (48 patients), ● = grade B (61 patients), ■ grade C (22 patients) (Turcotte 1974).

**Table 36.9** Causes of death in a controlled study of the therapeutic portacaval shunt (Resnick et al 1974)

| Cause of death | Portacaval shunt Yes | No |
|---|---|---|
| Gastrointestinal bleeding* | 2 (4) | 10 (44) |
| Hepatic failure* | 13 (28) | 2 (9) |
| Nonhepatic | 5 (11) | 0 |
| Patients at risk | 46 | 23 |

Note: Percentage values shown in parentheses.
*$p < 0.05$

**Table 36.10** The frequency of portasystemic encephalopathy before and for 4 years after random selection for surgery in patients with cirrhosis and varices. Relation to portacaval anastomosis (PCA) (Mutchnick et al 1974)

| Encephalopathy | No PCA (60) Number | % | PCA (40) Number | % | $p$* |
|---|---|---|---|---|---|
| Mild | 21 | 35 | 13 | 33 | >0.05 |
| Severe | 2 | 3 | 8 | 20 | <0.01 |

*$p$ = probability that differences are due to chance.
Number of patients in each group in parentheses.

***Transjugular intrahepatic portasystemic stent shunts.*** Transjugular intrahepatic portasystemic stent shunting (TIPSS) is a new treatment for portal hypertension in which portal decompression is achieved by the creation of an intrahepatic fistulous track between the hepatic and portal veins. Colapinto and colleagues (1982) used balloon dilatation to produce the fistulous track, but early reports were disappointing because of thrombosis of the track and it was only with the development of expandable vascular stents (Palmaz et al 1985) that shunt patency could be maintained (Fig. 36.9). Two stents are available currently: the Palmaz stent, which has the advantage of a diameter that can be varied to produce adequate reduction of the portal pressure with the minimum diameter shunt, and the longer and more flexible Wallstent, which we find associated with fewer complications (Jalan et al 1994).

An explosion of interest in this technique has taken place, but only now are trials of large numbers of patients with reasonable follow-up becoming available (LaBerge et al 1993, Rössle et al 1994). These studies have shown that the procedure is highly effective in reducing rebleeding from esophagogastric varices in the short and medium term and has a low morbidity and mortality (Hayes et al 1994). The procedure can be undertaken successfully in

**Table 36.11** Frequency of hepatic encephalopathy after selective and nonselective portasystemic shunts (Warren et al 1982)

| Shunt | % | 3 years (%) | 7 years* |
|---|---|---|---|
| Selective | 11 | 12 | 3/10 |
| Nonselective | 55 | 52 | 6/6 |

*Encephalopathy subclinical in 3/6 nonselective shunt patients and in 3/10 selective shunt patients.
Restoration of hepatic portal blood flow in 6 selective shunt patients abolished encephalopathy.

around 90% of patients and rebleeding is almost invariably due to shunt obstruction, particularly by neointimal hyperplasia or hepatic vein stenosis. Encephalopathy occurs in 15–20% of patients, which appears to be less frequent than in nonselective surgical shunts, perhaps because of the relatively small diameter of the fistulous connection and continued centripetal portal blood flow. Whether encephalopathy will remain relatively infrequent compared to surgical shunts in the long run remains uncertain, but it should not be forgotten that patients in whom TIPSS is undertaken may have advanced liver disease and would not have been candidates for surgical therapy.

Long-term follow-up and assessment of shunt function is very important, because 20–30% of patients develop intimal hyperplasia and hepatic vein stenosis. We have found that Doppler ultrasound examination, although reliable in detecting shunt patency, is of limited value in detecting narrowing and transjugular portography with pressure measurements are required. The frequency with which this should be undertaken remains unclear. An alternative approach would be to undertake regular endoscopy to ensure that collapse of varices is maintained and to assess further those in whom varices become prominent. In the majority of cases of intimal hyperplasia, balloon dilatation can reduce portal pressure to below 12 mmHg, which appears to be the threshold below which variceal bleeding is unusual. In the case of hepatic vein stenosis, extension of the stent into the hepatic vein is required.

Although most experience with the TIPSS procedure has been in preventing recurrent esophagogastric variceal bleeding, it has also been effective in arresting acute bleeding (p. 504), in bleeding from portal hypertensive gastropathy (p. 990) and in the treatment of intractable ascites (p. 1032). TIPSS insertion has also been used to reduce the risk of bleeding while liver transplantation is considered. Fuller evaluation of TIPSS in these settings is awaited and comparison of TIPSS with injection sclerotherapy and band ligation will be required before this new approach can be recommended unreservedly. Early results suggest that rebleeding is less following TIPSS than after endoscopic therapies. The main influence on survival following variceal hemorrhage is the severity of liver dysfunction and it is unlikely therefore that the TIPSS procedure will have a major impact in prolonging life.

***Splenectomy.*** Splenectomy is an effective means of preventing recurrent variceal bleeding in patients with regional portal hypertension due to splenic vein thrombosis (Røder 1984). It is ineffective in other forms of portal hypertension (Macpherson & Goddard 1977).

### *Prophylaxis of initial variceal bleeding*

As bleeding from esophagogastric varices is unpredictable and carries a high mortality, the possibility of preventing bleeding in patients who have never bled is attractive. However, varices do not bleed inevitably (p. 1002) and none of the treatments available is free of hazard. The problems have therefore been to identify patients at particular risk of bleeding (p. 999) and to find an effective treatment with sufficiently few hazards.

***Injection sclerotherapy.*** Although two original studies by Paquet (1982) and Witzel et al (1985) held out a promise that injection sclerotherapy could be used in primary prophylaxis of variceal hemorrhage, subsequent studies have not confirmed these findings. Sauerbruch et al (1988) in Germany showed no significant reduction in initial variceal bleeding despite obliterating varices in 70% of patients treated by sclerotherapy and Santangelo et al (1988) in the United States found more bleeding in patients treated by sclerotherapy than in control patients. Some have suggested that better selection of patients, such as those with large varices and multiple red signs who are known to be at high risk of bleeding, may allow benefit from sclerotherapy, but trials on this point are not available and ethically would require comparison with propranolol rather than no treatment (see below). Only about 30% of patients with varices ever bleed, many patients present for the first time with bleeding (Hayes et al 1988), and injection sclerotherapy itself may cause bleeding from sclerotherapy-related ulceration, perhaps making it overoptimistic to look to sclerotherapy as an effective prophylactic treatment. Whether band ligation of varices will prove more effective awaits the results of ongoing trials.

***Propranolol.*** Although debate continues on the role of propranolol in reducing rebleeding from varices, a recent meta-analysis of the prophylactic use of β blockers, principally propranolol, showed a marked reduction in bleeding and a reduction in death from bleeding (Hayes et al 1990), although overall mortality was at the boundary of statistical significance (Table 36.12). The main disadvantage of propranolol is the significant number of patients unable to tolerate it owing to side-effects. At present oral nitrates appear the most promising alternative candidates (Angelico et al 1993).

**Table 36.12** Results of meta-analysis of seven studies of β blockade for the prophylaxis of a first variceal bleed (Hayes et al 1990)

| | Total patients | Patients who bled | Deaths from bleeding | Total mortality |
|---|---|---|---|---|
| β blocker | 402* | 50 | 21 | 86 |
| Control | 395 | 92 | 38 | 107 |
| Bleeding reduction % | | 47 | 45 | 22 |
| Treatment effect ($p$) | – | <0.0001 | 0.017 | 0.052 |

*Propranolol
Note: $p$ = probability.

*Choice of treatment*

Injection sclerotherapy or band ligation, propranolol and TIPSS are the main treatments for patients who have bled from esophageal varices. It is not yet clear which of these is best, but many would consider band ligation the treatment of choice. The author favors TIPSS, since we have found it particularly effective in reducing rebleeding (Jalan et al 1996). Injection sclerotherapy and band ligation are not effective for gastric varices and alternative sclerosants such as acrylamide glue and thrombin have not yet proved of any advantage. Propranolol can be used for patients who are compliant and who tolerate the drug, but in general TIPSS is the most appropriate therapy. Propranolol is the only treatment worth considering for prophylaxis in patients whose varices have never bled and the author recommends this for patients with large varices or with varices showing red signs (p. 999).

## Extrahepatic portal hypertension

The choice of treatment in extrahepatic portal hypertension is considered in relation to vascular diseases of the liver (p. 1084).

## Intrahepatic presinusoidal portal hypertension

***Schistosomiasis.*** Treatment of the schistosomiasis itself is an essential preliminary (p. 590). A portasystemic shunt would seem the ideal treatment for portal hypertension in this condition, as the extrahepatic portal venous system is patent, liver function is excellent and liver blood flow is mainly by the hepatic artery. Indeed, good results from unselective portasystemic shunts have been reported in small series of patients (Obeid et al 1983), but most surgeons have found that these operations give rise to liver failure and a high incidence of hepatic encephalopathy (Warren et al 1965). Surgeons in endemic areas have made considerable use of devascularization operations and splenectomy, which can be done electively with a mortality of 5–10% after control of acute bleeding by conservative methods; later rebleeding occurs in about a fifth of patients, but the mortality of rebleeding is relatively low (Hassab 1967, El-Masri & Hassan 1982). Sclerotherapy and propranolol can and perhaps should be used more widely in these patients, but evidence about efficacy, particularly of propranolol, is limited (Küre 1989).

***Other causes.*** The principles of management in young patients with conditions such as a congenital hepatic fibrosis or cysts (p. 726) are as in the extrahepatic forms of presinusoidal portal hypertension, except that a greater variety of shunts may be done as the extrahepatic portal venous system is intact. In general, however, shunt surgery has been undertaken less frequently in recent years, as many patients can be managed effectively with sclerotherapy or band ligation.

## Nonesophagogastric variceal bleeding

Bleeding from varices other than those in the esophagus or stomach is uncommon, but such bleeding can occur from a variety of sites (p. 1000).

***Anorectal varices.*** Anorectal varices occasionally cause rectal bleeding in patients with portal hypertension and such bleeding can be severe (Hosking & Johnson 1988). Proctoscopy is important to differentiate bleeding from anorectal varices (p. 993) and bleeding hemorrhoids in order to avoid useless and sometimes disastrous treatments such as injection or banding of supposed hemorrhoids (McCormack et al 1984). Emergency control of heavy bleeding can be effected by passing a large Foley catheter into the rectum, inflating its balloon fully and then exerting traction on the catheter manually or with a weight (Bark 1981). There is no generally accepted definitive treatment for bleeding rectal varices, but underrunning sutures of the variceal columns is probably the best initial therapy, although it does cause quite a lot of postoperative pain. Hosking & Johnson (1988) treated 13 patients with early rebleeding in only two and late rebleeding in only one. Portasystemic shunt surgery has been tried, but a TIPSS procedure would seem an attractive option where bleeding recurs, particularly in those with compensated liver disease and no encephalopathy.

***Stomal varices.*** Varices can develop at a variety of stomas (p. 993) and can cause severe bleeding. Local treatment with pressure dressings and materials such as Gelfoam or by ligation of the bleeding vessel stops individual episodes of bleeding, but recurrent bleeding is the rule. Frequent or severe recurrences can be prevented by a portasystemic shunt and subsequent hepatic encephalopathy should not be a major problem in those with an ileostomy who have had a proctocolectomy. The TIPSS procedure can also be applied in this setting and has the advantage of avoiding further surgery (Fig. 36.9). However, experience is limited at present. Hepatic transplantation also leads to resolution of the varices and portasystemic shunt procedures should not be done if transplantation is being considered (Wiesner et al 1986). Wiesner et al (1986) have suggested that ileoanal anastomosis may be less likely to give rise to varices, but few patients with portal hypertension have been observed after this operation.

***Intestinal varices.*** The site of bleeding from intestinal varices can be difficult to identify and methods that may prove useful include endoscopy, imaging with $^{99m}$Tc-tagged red blood cells (p. 87) and angiography (p. 27). Treatments for bleeding intestinal varices include lysis of associated adhesions, resection of involved intestine and portasystemic shunt operations. TIPSS is likely to prove most useful in future.

### Portal hypertensive gastropathy

Many patients with this condition do not require treatment or need only long-term oral iron if anemia or iron deficiency has developed. Propranolol is probably the treatment of choice when anemia needing repeated blood transfusion occurs. In a recent Spanish study of patients with severe portal hypertensive gastropathy, propranolol reduced the risk of chronic or acute rebleeding so that after 30 months over 50% of patients receiving propranolol remained free of rebleeding as compared with 7% in the control group. The number of rebleeding episodes was also significantly reduced, but survival was not affected (Perez-Ayuso et al 1991). The author has used TIPSS successfully to treat bleeding from portal hypertensive gastropathy refractory to propranolol.

### Portal hypertensive colopathy

Lesions of portal hypertensive colopathy oozing blood have been treated by heater probe coagulation (Kozarek et al 1991). The same treatment as for portal hypertensive gastropathy can be used, although currently there is no information regarding the efficacy of such therapy.

### Hypersplenism

Hypersplenism sufficient to require treatment is rare (p. 1187). Splenectomy abolishes hypersplenism but leaves portal hypertension unrelieved and may make subsequent surgery in the upper abdomen more difficult. It should not therefore be performed. A proximal splenorenal shunt, which includes splenectomy, or a distal splenorenal shunt can relieve hypersplenism (Macpherson & Goddard 1977, Warren et al 1984). There is disagreement regarding the effect of portacaval anastomosis on hypersplenism, but it cannot be used reliably to relieve this complication (p. 1001) and the same probably also applies to the TIPSS procedure. Splenic embolization sufficient to reduce splenic blood flow by a half relieves hypersplenism (Sangro et al 1993). Platelet and leukocyte counts usually return to normal within a week and are maintained for up to 2 years. Postembolization pain, vomiting and fever are common and transient ascites, pleural effusion and atelectasis may occur. Embolization can therefore be considered where hypersplenism merits treatment, particularly in patients with poor liver function.

### Ascites

Ascites resistant to medical therapy has been relieved by certain portasystemic shunts. The mortality of these operations is such as to prohibit this approach to ascites. More recently, the TIPSS procedure has been used and although it is effective in relieving ascites, its value remains to be confirmed. Since most patients with refractory ascites have a poor prognosis, it is unlikely that TIPSS will have a major effect on survival (p. 1032).

REFERENCES


Alexandrino P T, Alves M M, Correia J P 1988 Propranolol or endoscopic sclerotherapy in the prevention of recurrence of variceal bleeding. A prospective randomised controlled trial. Journal of Hepatology 7: 175–185

Andrade Z A, Cheever A W 1971 Alterations of the intrahepatic vasculature in hepatosplenic schistosomiasis mansoni. American Journal of Tropical Medicine and Hygiene 20: 425

Angelico M, Carli L, Piat C et al 1993 Isosorbide-5-mononitrate versus propranolol in the prevention of first bleeding in cirrhosis. Gastroenterology 104: 1460–1465

Archie J P Jr 1977 Hemodynamic analysis of the portal circulation during temporary portal vein occlusion and after portal-systemic shunt surgery. Surgery 82: 674–679

Armstrong E L, Adams W L Jr, Tragerman L J, Townsend E W 1942 The Cruveilhier–Baumgarten syndrome; a review of the literature and report of two additional cases. Annals of Internal Medicine 16: 113–151

Baker L A, Smith C, Lieberman G 1959 The natural history of esophageal varices. A study of 115 cirrhotic patients in whom varices were diagnosed prior to bleeding. American Journal of Medicine 26: 228–237

Bark C J 1981 Control of massive bleeding from hemorrhoidal veins. Journal of the American Medical Association 245: 921

Barrison I G, Knight I D, Viola L, Boots M A, Murray-Lyon I M, Mitchell T R 1981 Platelet associated immunoglobulins in chronic liver disease. British Journal of Haematology 48: 347–350

Bassendine M F, Collins J D, Stephenson J, Saunders P, James O F W 1985 Platelet associated immunoglobulins in primary biliary cirrhosis: a cause of thrombocytopenia? Gut 26: 1074–1079

Benoit J N, Womack W A, Hernandez L, Granger D M 1985 "Forward" and "backward" flow mechanisms of portal hypertension: relative contributions in the rat model of portal vein stenosis. Gastroenterology 89: 1092–1096

Beppu K, Inokuchi K, Koyanagi N et al 1981 Prediction of variceal hemorrhage by esophageal endoscopy. Gastrointestinal Endoscopy 27: 213–218

Bernstein W C 1983 What are hemorrhoids and what is their relationship to the portal system? Diseases of the Colon and Rectum 26: 829–834

Bhathal P S, Grossman H J 1982 Contractile fibroblasts in the pathogenesis of cirrhotic portal hypertension. Hepatology 2: 155

Bhathal P S, Grossman H J 1985 Reduction of the increased portal vascular resistance of the isolated perfused cirrhotic rat liver by vasodilators. Journal of Hepatology 1: 325–327

Blakemore A H, Lord J W Jr 1945 The technic of using vitallium tubes in establishing portacaval shunts for portal hypertension. Annals of Surgery 122: 476–489

Bolondi L, Mazziotti A, Arienti V et al 1984 Ultrasonography study of portal venous system in portal hypertension and after portosystemic shunt operations. Surgery 95: 261–269

Bosch J, Groszmann R J 1984 Measurement of azygos venous blood flow by a continuous thermal dilution technique: an index of blood flow through gastroesophageal collaterals in cirrhosis. Hepatology 4: 424–429

Bosch J, Masti R, Kravetz D et al 1984 Effects of propranolol on azygos venous blood flow and hepatic and systemic hemodynamics in cirrhosis. Hepatology 4: 1200–1205

Bull J, Keeling P W N, Thompson R P M 1979 Palpable spleen and bleeding oesophageal varices. British Medical Journal 2: 1328–1329

Burroughs A K, McCormick P A, Siringo S, Phillips A, Sprengers D, McIntyre N 1989 Randomized trial of long term sclerotherapy for variceal rebleeding using the same protocol to treat rebleeding in all patients. Final report. Gut 30: A1506

Cales P, Desmorat H, Vinel J P et al 1990 Incidence of large oesophageal varices in patients with cirrhosis: application to prophylaxis of first bleeding. Gut 31: 1298–1302

Caletti G C, Brocchi E, Ferrari A, Fiorino S, Barbara L 1992 Value of endoscopic ultrasonography in the management of portal hypertension. Endoscopy 24 (suppl 1): 342–346

Capron J-P, Chivrac D, Dupas J-L, Rémond A, Ossart J-L, Lorriaux A 1976 Massive splenic infarction in cirrhosis: report of a case with spontaneous disappearance of hypersplenism. Gastroenterology 71: 308–310

Case Records of the Massachusetts General Hospital 1976 Anatomical diagnoses. Ileal varices, involving submucosa and postoperative fibrous adhesions to right pelvic wall. Right oophorectomy, remote Laennec's cirrhosis, with portal hypertension. New England Journal of Medicine 294: 385–391

Charters A C, Chandler J G, Condon J K et al 1974 Spontaneous reversal of portal flow in patients with bleeding varices treated by emergency portacaval shunt. American Journal of Surgery 127: 25–29

Christensen E, Fauerholdt L, Schlichting P et al and CSL 1981 Aspects of the natural history of gastrointestinal bleeding in cirrhosis and the effect of prednisone. Gastroenterology 81: 944–952

Cioni G, d'Alimonte P, Zerbinati F et al 1992 Duplex–Doppler ultrasonography in the evaluation of cirrhotic patients with portal hypertension and in the analysis of their response to drugs. Journal of Gastroenterology and Hepatology 7: 388–392

Colapinto R F, Stronell R D, Birch S J et al 1982 Creation of an intrahepatic portosystemic shunt with a Grüntzig balloon catheter. Canadian Medical Association Journal 126: 267–268

Conn H O 1974 Therapeutic portacaval anastomosis: to shunt or not to shunt. Gastroenterology 67: 1065–1070

Conn H O, Lindenmuth W W, May C J, Ramsby G R 1972 Prophylactic portacaval anastomosis. A tale of two studies. Medicine 51: 27–40

Conn H O, Grace N D, Bosch J et al 1991 Propranolol in the prevention of the first hemorrhage from esophagogastric varices: a multicenter, randomized clinical trial. Hepatology 13: 902–912

Cooper M J, Mackie C R, Dhorajiwala J, Baker A L, Moossa A R 1981 Hemorrhage from ileal varices after total proctocolectomy. American Journal of Surgery 141: 178–179

Cottone M, Sciarrino E, Marcenò M P et al 1983 Ultrasound in the screening of patients with cirrhosis with large varices. British Medical Journal 287: 533

Coutinho A 1968 Hemodynamic studies of portal hypertension in schistosomiasis. American Journal of Medicine 44: 547–556

Czaja A J, Wolf A M, Summerskill W H 1979 Development and early prognosis of esophageal varices in severe chronic active liver disease (CALD) treated with prednisone. Gastroenterology 77: 629–633

Dalinka M K, Smith E H, Wolfe R D, Goldenberg D, Langdon D E 1972 Pharmacologically enhanced visualization of esophageal varices by probanthine. Radiology 102: 281–282

De Franchis R, Arcidiacono P, Nolte A, Primignani M, Vazzoler C, Vitagliano P 1990 Development of a simplified prognostic index to predict the first esophageal bleed in cirrhotics. Journal of Hepatology 11 (suppl 2): S18

Dumont A E, Becker F F, Jacob H S 1974 Regulation of spleen growth in hepatic dysfunction. Annals of Surgery 179: 465

Eckhardt V F, Grace N D, Kantrowitz P A 1976 Does lower esophageal sphincter incompetency contribute to esophageal variceal bleeding? Gastroenterology 71: 185–189

El-Masri S H, Hassan M A 1982 Splenectomy and vasoligation for patients with haematemesis secondary to bilharzial hepatic fibrosis. British Journal of Surgery 69: 314

Eriksson L S, Hårdstedt C, Law D H, Thulin L 1982 Massive haemorrhage from vaginal varicose veins in patient with liver cirrhosis. Lancet 1: 1180

Fenyves D, Pomier-Layrargues G, Willems B, Côté J 1988 Intrahepatic pressure measurements: not an accurate reflection of portal venous pressure. Hepatology 8: 211–216

Feretis C, Tabakopoulous D, Benakis P, Xenofontos M, Golimatis B 1990 Endoscopic hemostasis of esophageal and gastric variceal bleeding with histoacryl. Endoscopy 22: 282–284

Feu F, Bordes J M, García-Pagan J C, Bosch J, Rodés J 1990 Endoscopic measurement of variceal pressure (VP) in patients with cirrhosis. Correlation with the NIEC Index (NI) and with the risk of variceal haemorrhage. Journal of Hepatology 11 (suppl 2): S22

Fleig W E, Stange E F, Ditschuneit H 1982 Upper gastrointestinal hemorrhage from downhill esophageal varices. Digestive Diseases and Sciences 27: 23–27

Forrest E H, Jones A L, Dillon J F, Walker J, Hayes P C 1995 The effect of nitric oxide synthase inhibition on portal pressure and azygos blood flow in patients with cirrhosis. Journal of Hepatology 23: 254–258

Franco D, Durandy Y, Deporte A, Bismuth H 1977 Upper gastrointestinal haemorrhage in hepatic cirrhosis: causes and relation to hepatic failure and stress. Lancet 1: 218–220

Garceau A J, Chalmers T C 1963 The natural history of cirrhosis I. Survival with esophageal varices. New England Journal of Medicine 268: 469–473

Garcia-Pagán J C, Navasa M, Bosch J, Bru C, Pizcueta P, Rodés J 1990 Enhancement of portal pressure reduction by the association of isosorbide-5-mononitrate to propranolol administration in patients with cirrhosis. Hepatology 11: 230–238

Garcia-Tsao G, Groszmann R J, Fisher R L, Conn H O, Atterbury C E, Glickman M 1985 Portal pressure, presence of gastroesophageal varices and variceal bleeding. Hepatology 5: 419–424

Garnett E S, Goddard B A, Markby D, Webber C E 1969 The spleen as an arteriovenous shunt. Lancet 1: 386–388

Gimson A E S, Westaby D, Williams R 1991 Endoscopic sclerotherapy in the management of gastric variceal haemorrhage. Journal of Hepatology 13: 274–278

Gimson A E S, Ramage J K, Panos M Z et al 1993 Randomized trial of variceal banding ligation versus injection sclerotherapy for bleeding oesophageal varices. Lancet 342: 391–394

Grace N D, Castell D O, Wennar M H 1969 A comparison of the oral fructose and ammonia tolerance tests in cirrhosis. Archives of Internal Medicine 124: 330–335

Graham D Y, Smith J L 1981 The course of patients after variceal hemorrhage. Gastroenterology 80: 800–809

Grose R D, Hayes P C 1992 Review article: the pathophysiology and pharmacological treatment of portal hypertension. Alimentary Pharmacology and Therapeutics 6: 521–540

Groszmann R J, Kotelanski B, Cohn J N, Khatri I M 1972 Quantitation of portasystemic shunting from the splenic and mesenteric beds in alcoholic liver disease. American Journal of Medicine 53: 715–722

Groszmann R J, Glickman M, Blei A T, Storer E, Conn H O 1979 Wedged and free hepatic venous pressure measured with a balloon catheter. Gastroenterology 76: 253–258

Gudjonsson H, Zeiler D, Gamelli R L, Kaye M D 1986 Colonic varices. Report of an unusual case diagnosed by radionuclide scanning with review of the literature. Gastroenterology 91: 1543–1547

Hardison J E 1977 Venous hum of the Cruveilhier–Baumgarten syndrome. Response to the Valsalva maneuver. Archives of Internal Medicine 137: 1623–1624

Harley H A J, Morgan T, Redeker A G et al 1986 Results of a randomized trial of end-to-side portacaval shunt and distal splenorenal shunt in alcoholic liver disease and variceal bleeding. Gastroenterology 91: 802–809

Harries A D 1980 Palpable spleen and bleeding oesophageal varices. British Medical Journal 281: 1568

Hashizume M, Tanaka K, Inokuchi K 1983 Morphology of gastric microcirculation in cirrhosis. Hepatology 3: 1008–1012

Hassab M A 1967 Gastroesophageal decongestion and splenectomy in the treatment of esophageal varices in bilharzial cirrhosis: further studies with a report on 355 operations. Surgery 61: 169–176

Hayes P C 1996 The coming of age of band ligation for oesophageal varices. British Medical Journal 312: 1111–1112

Hayes P C, Bouchier I A D 1990 Injection sclerotherapy in the treatment of variceal haemorrhage. European Journal of Gastroenterology and Hepatology 2: 334–337

Hayes P C, Westaby D, Williams R 1988 Prophylactic injection sclerotherapy for esophageal varices: a critical appraisal. Gastrointestinal Endoscopy 34: 359–360

Hayes P C, Davis J M, Lewis J A, Bouchier I A D 1990 Meta-analysis of value of propranolol in prevention of variceal haemorrhage. Lancet 336: 153–156

Hayes P C, Terrace D, Peaston I, Bouchier I A D, Redhead D,

Brash H M 1992 Computerised system for the continuous measurement of azygos venous blood flow. Gut 33: 372–374
Hayes P C, Redhead D N, Finlayson N D C 1994 Transjugular intrahepatic portasystemic stent shunt. Gut 35: 445–446
Hollands M J 1982 Parastomal haemorrhage from an ileal conduit secondary to portal hypertension. British Journal of Surgery 69: 675
Hosking S W, Johnson A G 1988 Bleeding anorectal varices – a misunderstood condition. Surgery 104: 70–73
Hosking S W, Kennedy H J, Seddon I, Triger D R 1987 The role of propranolol in congestive gastropathy of portal hypertension. Hepatology 7: 437–441
Infante-Rivard C, Esnaola S, Villeneuve J P 1989 Role of endoscopic variceal sclerotherapy in the long-term management of variceal bleeding. A meta-analysis. Gastroenterology 96: 1087–1092
Italian Multicenter Project for Propranolol in Prevention of Bleeding 1989 Propranolol prevents first gastrointestinal bleeding in non-ascitic cirrhotic patients. Final report of a multicenter randomized trial. Journal of Hepatology 9: 75–83
Iwatsuki S, Reynolds T B 1973 Effect of increased intraabdominal pressure on hepatic hemodynamics in patients with chronic liver disease and portal hypertension. Gastroenterology 65: 294–299
Jackson F C, Perrin E B, Smith A G, Degradi A E, Nadal H M 1968 A clinical investigation of the portacaval shunt. II. Survival analysis of the prophylactic operation. American Journal of Surgery 115: 22–42
Jacobs D M, Bubrick M P, Onstad G R, Hitchcock C R 1980 The relationship of hemorrhoids to portal hypertension. Diseases of the Colon and Rectum 23: 567–569
Jalan R, Redhead D N, Ferguson J, Simpson K J, Elton R A, Hayes P C 1994 Wall stents or Palmaz stents for the transjugular intrahepatic portasystemic stent-shunt. Journal of Investigational Radiology 9: 147–152
Jalan R, Forrest E H, Stanley A J et al 1996 TIPSS vs variceal band ligation for prevention of variceal rebleeding in cirrhosis: a randomized controlled trial. Gut 38 (Suppl 1): S24
Jenson L S, Krarup N 1989 Propranolol in prevention of rebleeding from oesophageal varices during the course of endoscopic sclerotherapy. Scandinavian Journal of Gastroenterology 24: 339–345
Joly J G, Marbleau D, Legare A, Lavoie P, Bernier J, Viallet A 1971 Bleeding from esophageal varices in cirrhosis of the liver: hemodynamic and radiological criteria for the selection of potential bleeders through hepatic and umbilicoportal catheterization studies. Canadian Medical Association Journal 104: 576–580
Kane R A, Katz S G 1982 The spectrum of sonographic findings in portal hypertension: a subject review and new observations. Radiology 142: 453–455
Kew M C, Varma R R, Dos Santos H A, Scheuer P J, Sherlock S 1971 Portal hypertension in primary biliary cirrhosis. Gut 12: 830–834
Kleber G, Sauerbruch T, Ansari H, Paumgartner G 1991 Prediction of variceal hemorrhage in cirrhosis: a prospective follow-up study. Gastroenterology 100: 1332–1337
Korula J, Chin K, Ko Y, Yamada S 1991 Demonstration of two distinct subsets of gastric varices. Observations during a seven year study of endoscopic sclerotherapy. Digestive Diseases and Sciences 36: 303–309
Kozarek R A, Botoman V A, Predfeldt J E, Roach J M, Patterson D J, Ball T J 1991 Portal colonopathy: prospective study of colonoscopy in patients with portal hypertension. Gastroenterology 101: 1192–1197
Kraft A R, Frank H A, Glotzer D J 1973 Achalasia of the esophagus complicated by varices and massive hemorrhage. New England Journal of Medicine 288: 405–406
Küre C F 1989 Controlled trial of propranolol to prevent recurrent variceal bleeding in patients with non-cirrhotic portal fibrosis. British Medical Journal 298: 1363–1365
Kurtz R C, Sherlock P, Winawer S J 1974 Esophageal varices. Development secondary to primary and metastatic liver tumors. Archives of Internal Medicine 134: 50–51
LaBerge J M, Ring E J, Gordon R L et al 1993 Creation of transjugular intrahepatic portosystemic shunts with the Wallstent endoprosthesis: results in 100 patients. Radiology 187: 413–420
Lacy A M, Navasa M, Gilabert R et al 1992 Long-term effects of distal splenorenal shunt on hepatic hemodynamics and liver function in patients with cirrhosis: importance of reversal of portal blood flow. Hepatology 15: 616–622
Laine L, Hussein M, El-Newihi M, Migikovsky B, Sloane R, Carcia F 1993 Endoscopic ligation compared with sclerotherapy for the treatment of bleeding esophageal varices. Annals of Internal Medicine 119: 1–7
Lebrec D, Kotelanski B, Cohn J N 1976 Splanchnic hemodynamics in cirrhotic patients with esophageal varices and gastrointestinal bleeding. Gastroenterology 70: 1108–1111
Lebrec D, de Fleury P, Rueff B, Nahum H, Benhamou J-P 1980 Portal hypertension, size of esophageal varices, and risk of gastrointestinal bleeding in alcoholic cirrhosis. Gastroenterology 79: 1139–1144
Lebrec D, Nouel O, Bernuau J, Bouygues M, Rueff B, Benhamou J-P 1981 Propranolol in prevention of recurrent gastrointestinal bleeding in cirrhotic patients. Lancet 1: 920–921
Lieberman D A, Krippaehne W W, Melnyk C S 1983 Colonic varices due to intestinal cavernous haemangiomas. Digestive Diseases and Sciences 28: 852–858
Liebowitz H R 1963 Splenomegaly and hypersplenism pre- and post-portacaval shunt. New York State Journal of Medicine 63: 2631–2638
Luna A, Meister H P, Szanto P B 1968 Esophageal varices in the absence of cirrhosis. Incidence and characteristics in congestive heart failure and neoplasms of the liver. American Journal of Clinical Pathology 49: 710–717
Macpherson A I S 1979 Portal hypertension: a pilgrim's progress. Journal of the Royal College of Surgeons of Edinburgh 24: 317–335
Macpherson A I S, Goddard M J 1977 Comparison of splenectomy alone and with lieno-renal anastomosis in the treatment of portal hypertension. Journal of the Royal College of Surgeons of Edinburgh 22: 255–259
McCain A H, Bernardino M E, Sones P J Jr, Berkman W A, Casarella W J 1985 Varices from portal hypertension: correlation of CT and angiography. Radiology 154: 63–69
McCormack T, Martin T, Smallwood R H, Robinson P, Walton L, Johnson A G 1983 Doppler ultrasound probe for assessment of blood-flow in oesophageal varices. Lancet 1: 677–678
McCormack T T, Bailey H R, Simms J M, Johnson A G 1984 Rectal varices are not piles. British Journal of Surgery 71: 163–165
McCormack T T, Sims J, Eyre-Brook I et al 1985 Gastric lesions in portal hypertension: inflammatory gastritis or congestive gastropathy? Gut 26: 1226–1232
Mills P R, Behan W M H, Watkinson G 1980 Haemorrhage from colonic varices associated with portal hypertension. British Journal of Clinical Practice 34: 347–351
Moreno A H, Burchell A R, Reddy R V, Panke W F, Nealon T F Jr 1975a The hemodynamics of portal hypertension revisited: determinants and significance of occluded portal pressures. Surgery 77: 167–179
Moreno A H, Burchell A R, Reddy R V, Steen J A, Panke W F, Nealon T F Jr 1975b Spontaneous reversal of portal blood flow: the case for and against its occurrence in patients with cirrhosis of the liver. Annals of Surgery 181: 346–358
Mutchnick M G, Lerner E, Conn H O 1974 Portalsystemic encephalopathy and portacaval anastomosis: a prospective, controlled investigation. Gastroenterology 66: 1005–1019
North Italian Endoscopic Club for the Study and Treatment of Esophageal Varices 1988 Prediction of the first variceal hemorrhage in patients with cirrhosis of the liver and esophageal varices. A prospective multicenter study. New England Journal of Medicine 319: 983–989
Obeid F N, Smith R F, Elliott J P Jr, Reddy D J, Hageman J H 1983 Bilharzial portal hypertension. Archives of Surgery 118: 702–708
O'Connor K W, Lehman G, Yune H et al 1989 Comparison of three nonsurgical treatments for bleeding esophageal varices. Gastroenterology 96: 899–906
Ohta H, Kohgo Y, Goto Y et al 1992 The near-infra-red electronic endoscope for diagnosis of esophageal varices. Gastrointestinal Endoscopy 38: 330–335
Okuda K, Suzuki K, Musha H, Arimizu N 1977 Percutaneous transhepatic catheterization of the portal vein for the study of portal hemodynamics and shunts. A preliminary report. Gastroenterology 73: 279–284
Olsson R 1972 The natural history of esophageal varices. A retrospective study of 224 cases with liver cirrhosis. Digestion 6: 65–74
Palmaz J C, Sibbitt R R, Reuter S R, Garcia F, Tio F O 1985 Expandable intrahepatic portacaval shunt stents: early experience in the dog. American Journal of Roentgenology 145: 821–825

Panés J, Bordas J, Piqué J et al 1992 Increased gastric mucosal perfusion in cirrhotic patients with portal hypertensive gastropathy. Gastroenterology 103: 1875–1882
Panos M Z, Moore K, Vlavianos P et al 1990 Single, total paracentesis for tense ascites: sequential hemodynamic changes and right atrial size. Hepatology 11: 662–667
Paquet K J 1982 Prophylactic endoscopic sclerosing treatment of the esophageal wall in varices – a prospective controlled randomized trial. Endoscopy 14: 4–5
Pascal J P, Calès P and Multicenter Study Group 1987 Propranolol in the prevention of first upper gastrointestinal tract hemorrhage in patients with cirrhosis of the liver and esophageal varices. New England Journal of Medicine 317: 856–861
Perez-Ayuso R M, Piqué J M, Bosch J et al 1991 Propranolol in prevention of recurrent rebleeding from severe portal hypertensive gastropathy in cirrhosis. Lancet 337: 431–434
Pizcueta P, Piqué J M, Fernández M et al 1992 Modulation of the hyperdynamic circulation of cirrhotic rats by nitric oxide inhibition. Gastroenterology 103: 1909–1915
Plevris J N, Dhariwal A, Elton R A, Finlayson N D C, Bouchier I A D, Hayes P C 1995 The platelet count as a predictor of variceal hemorrhage in primary biliary cirrhosis. American Journal of Gastroenterology 90: 959–961
Pollard J J, Nebesar R A 1967 Altered hemodynamics in the Budd–Chiari syndrome demonstrated by selective hepatic and selective splenic arteriography. Radiology 89: 236–243
Polson R J, Westaby D, Gimson A E S et al 1989 Sucralfate for the prevention of early rebleeding following injection sclerotherapy for esophageal varices. Hepatology 10: 279–282
Pomier-Layrargues G, Kusielewicz D, Willems B, Villeneuve J-P, Marleau D, Côté J, Huet P-M 1985 Presinusoidal portal hypertension in nonalcoholic cirrhosis. Hepatology 5: 415–418
Ponce J, Froufe A, de la Morena E et al 1981 Morphometric study of the esophageal mucosa in cirrhotic patients with variceal bleeding. Hepatology 1: 641–646
Poynard T, Lebrec D, Hillon P et al 1987 Propranolol for prevention of recurrent gastrointestinal bleeding in patients with cirrhosis. A prospective study of factors associated with rebleeding. Hepatology 7: 447–451
Pugh R M H, Murray-Lyon I M, Dawson J L, Pietroni M C, Williams R 1973 Transection of the oesophagus for bleeding oesophageal varices. British Journal of Surgery 60: 646–649
Rector W G Jr, Hoefs J C, Hossak K F, Everson G T 1988 Hepatofugal portal flow in cirrhosis: observations on hepatic hemodynamics and the nature of the arterioportal communications. Hepatology 8: 16–20
Resnick R H, Chalmers T C, Ishihara A M et al 1969 A controlled study of the prophylactic portacaval shunt. Annals of Internal Medicine 70: 675–688
Resnick R H, Iber F L, Ishihara A M, Chalmers T C, Zimmerman H and The Boston Inter-Hospital Liver Group 1974 A controlled study of therapeutic portacaval shunt. Gastroenterology 67: 843–857
Reynolds T B 1974 The role of hemodynamic measurements in portosystemic shunt surgery. Archives of Surgery 108: 276–281
Reynolds T B, Ito S, Iwatsuki S 1970 Measurement of portal pressure and its clinical application. American Journal of Medicine 49: 649–667
Rikkers L F, Rudman D, Galambos J T et al 1978 A randomized controlled trial of the distal splenorenal shunt. Annals of Surgery 188: 271–282
Røder O Chr 1984 Splenic vein thrombosis with bleeding gastroesophageal varices. Reports of two splenectomized cases and review of the literature. Acta Chirurgica Scandinavica 150: 265–268
Ross A P 1970 Portal hypertension presenting with haemoperitoneum. British Medical Journal 1: 544
Rössle M, Haag K, Ochs A et al 1994 The transjugular intrahepatic portasystemic stent-shunt procedure for variceal bleeding. New England Journal of Medicine 330: 165–171
Rothschild J J, Gelernt I, Sloan W 1968 Ruptured mesenteric vein in cirrhosis – unusual cause for hemoperitoneum. New England Journal of Medicine 278: 97–98
Rubin M H, Weston J M, Langley P G, White Y, Williams R 1979 Platelet function in chronic liver disease: relationship to disease severity. Digestive Diseases and Sciences 24: 197–202
Salmi A, de Cotiis R, Rusconi C 1990 On the rarity of Cruveilhier–Baumgarten's venous hum. Journal of Hepatology 11: 279–280
Sangro B, Bilbao I, Herrero I et al 1993 Partial splenic embolization for the treatment of hypersplenism in cirrhosis. Hepatology 18: 309–314
Santangelo W C, Dueno M I, Estes B L, Krejs G J 1988 Prophylactic sclerotherapy of large esophageal varices. New England Journal of Medicine 318: 814–818
Sauerbruch T, Wotzka R, Köpcke W et al 1988 Prophylactic sclerotherapy before the first episode of variceal hemorrhage in patients with cirrhosis. New England Journal of Medicine 319: 8–15
Simpson J A, Conn H O 1968 The role of ascites in gastroesophageal reflux with comments on the pathogenesis of bleeding esophageal varices. Gastroenterology 55: 17–25
Sorokin J J, Levine S M, Moss E G, Biddle C M 1977 Downhill varices: report of a case 29 years after resection of a substernal thyroid gland. Gastroenterology 73: 345–348
Spence R A J, Roy A D 1984 Bleeding duodenal varices. British Journal of Surgery 71: 588
Spence R A J, Sloan J M, Johnston G W 1983 Oesophagitis in patients undergoing transection for varices – a histological study. British Journal of Surgery 70: 332–334
Staritz M, Poralla T, Meyer zum Buschenfelde K-H 1985 Intravascular oesophageal variceal pressure (IOVP) assessed by endoscopic fine needle puncture under basal conditions, Valsalva's manoeuvre and after glyceryl trinitrate application. Gut 26: 525–530
Stiegmann G V, Goff J S, Michaletz-Onody P A et al 1992 Endoscopic sclerotherapy as compared with endoscopic ligation for bleeding esophageal varices. New England Journal of Medicine 326: 1527–1532
Takayasu K, Takashi M, Musha H et al 1982 Spontaneous reversal of portal blood flow demonstrated by percutaneous transhepatic catheterization: report of two cases. Gastroenterology 82: 753–757
Takayasu K, Moriyama N, Shima Y et al 1984 Sonographic detection of large spontaneous spleno-renal shunts and its clinical significance. British Journal of Radiology 57: 565–570
Tanoue K, Hashizume M, Wada H, Ohta M, Kitano S, Sugimachi K 1992 Effects of endoscopic injection sclerotherapy on portal hypertensive gastropathy: a prospective study. Gastrointestinal Endoscopy 38: 582–585
Terés J, Bordas J M, Bru C, Diaz F, Bruguera M, Rodés J 1976 Upper gastrointestinal bleeding in cirrhosis: clinical and endoscopic correlation. Gut 17: 37–40
Toghill P J, Green S 1979 Splenic influences on the blood in chronic liver disease. Quarterly Journal of Medicine 48: 613
Toghill P J, Green S 1983 Platelet dynamics in chronic liver disease using the $^{111}$Indium oxine label. Gut 24: 49–52
Tumen H T 1970 Hypersplenism and portal hypertension. Annals of the New York Academy of Science 170: 332
Turcotte J G 1974 Portal hypertension as I see it. In: Child C G 3rd (ed) Portal hypertension. W B Saunders, Philadelphia, p 78
Turcotte J G, Wallin V W, Child C G 3rd 1969 End-to-side versus side-to-side portacaval shunts in patients with hepatic cirrhosis. American Journal of Surgery 117: 108–116
Viallet A, Marleau D, Huet M et al 1975 Hemodynamic evaluation of patients with intrahepatic portal hypertension. Relationship between bleeding varices and the portohepatic gradient. Gastroenterology 69: 1297–1300
Vianna A, Hayes P C, Moscoso G, Driver M, Portmann B, Westaby D, Williams R 1987 Normal venous circulation of the gastroesophagus junction. A route to understanding varices. Gastroenterology 93: 876–889
Vickers C, Rhodes J, Hillenbrand P et al 1987 Prospective controlled trial of propranolol and sclerotherapy for prevention of rebleeding from oesophageal varices. Gut 28: A1359
Vorobioff J, Bredfeldt J E, Groszmann R J 1984 Increased blood flow through the portal system in cirrhotic rats. Gastroenterology 87: 1120–1126
Waldram R, Nunnerley H, Davis M, Laws J W, Williams R 1977 Detecting and grading of oesophageal varices by fibre-optic endoscopy and barium swallow with and without buscopan. Clinical Radiology 28: 137–145
Wantz G E, Payne M A 1961 Experience with portacaval shunt for portal hyeprtension. New England Journal of Medicine 265: 721–728

Warren K S 1984 "Schistosomiasis". Hepatology 4: 979
Warren K S, Rebouças G, Baptista A G 1965 Ammonia metabolism and hepatic coma in hepatosplenic schistosomiasis. Patients studied before and after portacaval shunt. Annals of Internal Medicine 62: 1113–1133
Warren W D, Millikan W J Jr, Henderson J M et al 1982 Ten years portal hypertensive surgery at Emory. Results and new perspectives. Annals of Surgery 195: 530–542
Warren W D, Millikan W J Jr, Henderson J M, Rasheed M E, Salam A A 1984 Selective variceal decompression after splenectomy or splenic vein thrombosis with a note on splenopancreatic disconnection. Annals of Surgery 199: 694–702
Watkins R M 1981 Variceal haemorrhage from a colostomy due to portal hypertension secondary to intrahepatic metastases from rectal carcinoma. British Medical Journal 282: 189–190
Weingart J, Höchter W, Ottenjann R 1982 Varices of the entire colon – an unusual cause of recurrent intestinal bleeding. Endoscopy 14: 69–70
Westaby D, Macdougall B R D, Williams R 1985 Improved survival following injection sclerotherapy for esophageal varices: final analysis of a controlled trial. Hepatology 5: 827–830
Westaby D, Melia W, Hegarty J, Gimson A E S, Stellon A J, Williams R 1986 Use of propranolol to reduce the rebleeding rate during injection sclerotherapy prior to variceal obliteration. Hepatology 6: 673–675
Westaby D, Polson R J, Gimson A E S, Hayes P C, Hayllar K, Williams R 1990 A controlled trial of oral propranolol compared with injection sclerotherapy for the long-term management of variceal bleeding. Hepatology 11: 353–359
Wiesner R H, LaRusso N F, Dozois R R, Beaver S J 1986 Peristomal varices after proctocolectomy in patients with primary sclerosing cholangitis. Gastroenterology 90: 316–322
Williams D M, Cho K J, Aisen A M, Eckhauser F E 1985 Portal hypertension "evaluated" by MR imaging. Radiology 157: 703–706
Williams S G J, Peters R A, Westaby D 1994 Thrombin — an effective treatment for gastric variceal haemorrhage. Gut 35: 1287–1289
Willoughby E O, David D, Smith C W, Fruin R C, Baker L A 1964 The significance of small esophageal varices in portal cirrhosis. Gastroenterology 47: 375–381
Witte C L, Witte M H, Renert W, O'Mara R E, Lilien D L 1976 Splenic artery ligation in selected patients with hepatic cirrhosis and in Sprague–Dawley rats. Surgery, Gynecology and Obstetrics 142: 1–12
Witzel L, Wolbergs E, Merki H 1985 Prophylactic endoscopic sclerotherapy of oesophageal varices: a prospective controlled study. Lancet 1: 773–775

# 37. Ascites

*H. Ring-Larsen   N. D. C. Finlayson*

Ascites refers to the accumulation of free fluid in the peritoneal cavity. Cirrhosis is one of its commonest causes and the appearance of ascites has serious prognostic implications for the cirrhotic patient (p. 1032).

## PATHOGENESIS

Two main groups of factors underlie the development of ascites in cirrhosis: those leading to a general increase in total body fluid, and those leading to a localization of fluid in the peritoneal cavity (Arroyo et al 1988).

### Generalized fluid retention

Patients with cirrhosis and ascites have a greatly increased total body sodium and water. The main reason for this is a marked retention of sodium and water by the kidneys and three theories have been advanced to explain this occurrence (Ring-Larsen & Henriksen 1986). One suggests that portal hypertension causes increased hepatic and splanchnic interstitial fluid formation, leading to ascites and depletion of the intravascular volume when interstitial fluid formation exceeds the capacity to return the fluid to the circulation (the underfilling theory). This results in a reduction of the "effective" plasma volume and a consequent retention of sodium by the kidneys. A second theory suggests that renal retention of sodium and water, with a consequent expansion of the plasma volume, is the initial event, caused by the liver disease via a hepatorenal reflex. Portal hypertension then determines the development of ascites (the overflow theory).

Recently, a third hypothesis has been advocated. It stresses the importance of a systemic circulatory derangement in which there is a decreased effective arterial plasma volume as an integral part of renal sodium and water retention and ascites formation (the peripheral arterial vasodilatation theory). According to this theory, the size of the arterial circulation is the major determinant of sodium and water retention in cirrhosis rather than the total plasma volume and thus arterial vasodilatation, mainly in the splanchnic circulation, is a consequence of portal hypertension leading to underfilling of the arterial vascular compartment (Schrier et al 1988). The recent demonstration of central vascular and arterial underfilling in patients with cirrhosis supports this latest theory of ascites formation (Henriksen et al 1989) and is consistent with animal experiments (Colombato et al 1996).

The investigation of these theories has been hampered by inability to define and measure precisely "effective" plasma volume or arterial volume and by the difficulty of making sequential measurements of factors leading to sodium retention before, during and after the development of ascites. Experimental work in animals with cirrhosis has shown that end-to-side portacaval shunts do not prevent sodium retention (Levy & Wexler 1978), whereas side-to-side shunts and transjugular intrahepatic portasystemic stent shunts (TIPSS), which decompress both the hepatic and the splanchnic circulation, do prevent sodium retention (Unikowsky et al 1983). This emphasizes the importance of sinusoidal hypertension or other intrahepatic factors in ascites formation (p. 990). The neuroendocrine mechanisms determining the renal sodium–water retention are discussed elsewhere (p. 1059).

### Ascites formation

Ascites forms when fluid enters the peritoneal cavity more quickly than it can be returned to the circulation by the capillaries and lymphatics (Witte et al 1971).

***Portal circulation and lymphatic drainage.*** The portal vasculature is a low pressure system with a portal venous pressure of approximately 8–10 mmHg and a small pressure gradient across the liver sinusoids of 3–5 mmHg (p. 714). The microcirculation in the gut has capillaries that are relatively impermeable to macromolecules but permeable to smaller molecules such as water and crystalloids. Consequently, normal mesenteric lymph has a protein content only about 60% that of plasma (Witte et al 1971). In contrast, normal liver sinusoids have large endothelial fenestrae occupying approximately 10%

of the microvascular wall without any basement membrane (p. 714). These large fenestrae allow almost unrestricted passage of large and small molecules, limiting only the passage of very large proteins. Thus, hepatic lymph has a protein concentration approximately 90% that of plasma (Witte et al 1971). This protein-rich filtrate drains via the liver lymphatics to the thoracic duct. The peritoneal space is drained mainly through diaphragmatic lymphatics to the right lymphatic duct, which has a more limited transport capacity than the thoracic duct.

***Portal hypertension.*** Hepatoportal hypertension is an essential element in ascites formation in cirrhosis. The important pressure gradient, probably due to hepatic fibrosis and regeneration nodules, is located postsinusoidally although an additional minor presinusoidal augmentation of vascular resistance may exist. Therefore, in this condition the hydrostatic pressure in the liver sinusoids is increased and is almost identical to the pressure in the portal vein (p. 996). The location of the pressure gradient according to the nature of the portal hypertension is important. Splanchnic venous hypertension, produced in experimental animals by ligation of the portal vein, does not cause ascites. This is analogous to presinusoidal portal hypertension in man, in which ascites occurs only if the liver function has deteriorated or has been stressed by factors such as gastrointestinal bleeding. In this situation, ascites is produced solely by a greatly increased electrolyte and water flux through the splanchnic capillaries (Witte et al 1981). By contrast, hepatic venous obstruction in man (p. 1077) and in experimental animals rapidly produces marked ascites, since in this instance the hydrostatic pressure is increased in the liver sinusoids as well as in the splanchnic capillaries.

***Hepatic sinusoids in liver disease.*** Due to the large size of fenestrae in the normal sinusoidal endothelium, no oncotic (colloid osmotic) pressure gradient exists across the sinudoids. In cirrhosis, a certain degree of "capillarization" of the sinusoidal wall with appearance of a basal membrane and collagenization of the perisinusoidal space takes place (Schaffner & Popper 1963). However, protein kinetics and scanning electronmicroscopic studies indicate that the fenestrae are decreased in number rather than in size (Henriksen et al 1984, Horn et al 1986). This implies that the oncotic pressure gradient is still small in cirrhosis and that the morphological changes represent a limited counterweight to the increased hydrostatic pressure in the sinusoids (Witte et al 1981).

Ascites formation in cirrhosis and in hepatic vein obstruction probably shares the same pathogenesis although the decreased plasma oncotic pressure in cirrhosis due to hypoalbuminemia may play a role in the flux of water and electrolytes through the splanchnic capillaries. The relation between portal hypertension and hypoalbuminemia has previously been overemphasized and it is not possible to predict the likelihood of ascites from these two factors alone (Witte et al 1971).

***Lymphatics.*** A large amount of fluid exudes from the highly permeable hepatic sinusoids (p. 716) into the perisinusoidal space and enters the hepatic lymphatics. This lymph is rich in protein even in patients with cirrhosis and is removed via the thoracic duct. Lymph also exudes from the mesenteric capillaries, which are relatively impermeable to proteins (Witte et al 1981), and as portal hypertension leads to a disproportionate increase in filtration of water and electrolytes, mesenteric lymph in this condition has a very low protein content (Witte et al 1971). As long as the lymph drainage keeps pace with the enhanced trans-sinusoidal lymph production, the spillover of fluid (water, crystalloids and proteins) into the peritoneal space is minimal and the patient remains free of ascites. When the lymph production in the sinusoids as well as in the splanchnic capillaries exceeds the lymphatic transport capacity, surplus fluid will pass into the peritoneal space. The rate of transport into the peritoneal space is, however, relatively small compared with that of lymph going directly into the thoracic duct, often less than 5% (Henriksen & Ring-Larsen 1984). The transport capacity of the thoracic duct in this situation is increased five- to tenfold from its normal 60–120 ml/h.

***Ascites composition.*** Ascites is composed of lymph derived from the liver and from the mesentry (Witte et al 1981). Prolonged portal hypertension in cirrhosis leads to a marked increase in the passage of water out of the mesenteric capillaries, but there is no similar loss of plasma protein. Consequently, mesenteric lymph in cirrhotic ascites has a low protein content that is only about 20% of the plasma protein and may sometimes be undetectable. Mesenteric lymph composition can return to normal when portal hypertension is relieved, emphasizing the importance of capillary pressure in portal hypertension. Hepatic lymph in cirrhosis has a much greater protein content than mesenteric lymph, but the content is lower than for normal hepatic lymph or for hepatic lymph in acute congestive cardiac failure (Witte et al 1969a), being about 65% of the plasma concentration. This probably reflects fibrosis (capillarization) of the sinusoids as cirrhosis progresses. The protein concentration of ascitic fluid reflects the balance between these two sources of ascites and the concentration may change with time, reflecting changes in the degree of mesenteric portal hypertension and increasing capillarization of the hepatic sinusoids as cirrhosis progresses. This accounts for the wide variation in ascites protein concentrations in cirrhosis (Witte et al 1969b), although most concentrations are in the transudate range (p. 1021).

The transport rates to and from the peritoneal space are important in therapy. Thus, mobilization of fluid by diuretic treatment should not exceed the rate of influx into the peritoneal cavity, since the mechanism of diuretics is in the main to decrease the influx rate (Hoefs 1981a).

### Hemodynamic changes

Cirrhosis with ascites is associated with striking circulatory changes that are probably closely related to the process of sodium and water retention leading to cirrhosis (p. 920). The plasma and blood volumes are usually expanded, the cardiac output is increased, the arterial blood pressure is lower than normal and the systemic vascular resistance is reduced considerably. The etiology of this hyperkinetic circulatory state is still obscure and the regions of the circulation responsible for the reduced systemic resistance are not yet known, but the circulatory abnormalities have important functional effects in the kidneys (p. 1058) and in the lungs (p. 1071).

## CLINICAL FEATURES

Ascites must be differentiated from abdominal distention due to obesity, pregnancy, gaseous distention of the bowel, bladder distention and various cysts and tumors. The cardinal signs are fullness in the flanks, dullness on percussion in the flanks with the patient lying supine, redistribution of dullness when the patient lies on one side so that dullness remains only in the dependent flank (shifting dullness) and the ability to elicit a fluid wave or thrill. These signs appear once more than a liter of ascites is present, but it is important to realize that they are difficult to elicit when ascites is not marked or in obese patients even when it is marked.

Auscultatory methods have been devised that have been claimed to identify as little as 200 ml of ascites in experimental studies. These include eliciting a "puddle" sign in prone patients in the "all fours" position (Lawson & Weissbein 1959) or a change in percussion note in the erect patient (Guarino 1986). Cattau et al (1982) have illustrated the limitations of physical examination in patients with up to about a liter of ascites identified by ultrasonography and paracentesis. Flank dullness proved the most sensitive but least specific sign, while a fluid thrill was most specific but least sensitive (Table 37.1). Auscultation for an ascitic "puddle" is probably useful only if skill in eliciting this sign is developed. The presence or absence of ascites in this difficult group of patients was determined correctly in only a half of examinations, emphasizing the need for clinical humility when ascites is not obvious or the patient is obese. One useful negative point is that resonance in the flanks gives a 90% chance that there is no ascites.

**Table 37.1** Sensitivity and specificity of physical signs in the detection of equivocal ascites (Cattau et al 1982)

| Sign | Sensitivity (%) | Specificity (%) |
|---|---|---|
| Bulging flanks | 78 | 44 |
| Flank dullness | 94 | 29 |
| Shifting dullness | 83 | 56 |
| Fluid wave | 50 | 82 |
| Puddle sign | 55 | 51 |

Note: Sensitivity = true positive/total with ascites × 100.
Specificity = true negative/total with ascites × 100.

***Associated findings.*** Abdominal findings resulting from ascites include distortion or eversion of the umbilicus, herniae, pale abdominal striae and scrotal edema. Abdominal herniae occur in about 10% of patients with cirrhosis who do not have ascites and in about 40% with ascites and half of these herniae are of the umbilical type (p. 922). When ascites is gross, intra-abdominal organs (p. 1182) and masses cease to be palpable and can be detected only by ballottement, the diaphragms are elevated and divarication of the recti may occur. The high intra-abdominal pressure that results is transmitted to the chest, where it has deleterious effects on cardiorespiratory function. Limitation of pulmonary expansion may lead to dyspnea and an increased right atrial pressure and superior vena caval pressure may be seen clinically as a high jugular venous pressure. These changes are discussed further in relation to paracentesis (p. 1029). Gross ascites can also cause meralgia paresthetica from entrapment of the lateral cutaneous nerve of the thigh by the distended abdomen, as can also happen in obesity and pregnancy (Radvan & Vidikan 1982). Such patients may get temporary relief by lying down (Deal & Canoso 1982).

***Pleural effusion.*** Pleural effusions, usually on the right, unrelated to pulmonary or cardiac disease occur in 10% of patients with cirrhosis and ascites (Johnston & Loo 1964). Most are small and are noted on chest radiographs in patients with obvious ascites. Occasionally, large or massive pleural effusions occur and this is referred to as hepatic hydrothorax. These large effusions result from the passage of ascitic fluid through defects in the tendinous part of the diaphragm and they are usually associated with marked ascites (Johnston & Loo 1964, Lieberman & Peters 1970). Rarely, they occur in the absence of clinically detectable ascites, but in such cases the origin of the pleural fluid from the peritoneum can be shown by pleural accumulation of $^{99m}$Tc-sulfur colloid injected into the peritoneal cavity (Rubinstein et al 1985). Presumably, passage of ascitic fluid to the pleural space and clearance of ascites from the peritoneum are sufficient to prevent clinical ascites in these patients.

Left-sided pleural effusions in patients with cirrhosis and ascites should be investigated carefully before they are attributed to ascites. Mirouze et al (1981) found that left-sided effusions accounted for only 18% of all effusions in patients with ascites and four of 22 (18%) were tuberculous. Analysis of cytology and culture of such pleural fluid and perhaps pleural biopsy are required.

***Development.*** Ascites may develop slowly over weeks or months. This is usually due to gradually deteriorating liver function, as a precipitating cause can rarely be found, and the prognosis is poor (p. 1032). Rapid onset of ascites may be due to gastrointestinal hemorrhage, infection, the trauma of surgery, portal venous thrombosis or the development of a hepatocellular carcinoma. It may also develop suddenly during a period of severe alcohol abuse or excessive sodium intake in food or drugs.

## INVESTIGATIONS

### Paracentesis

Paracentesis is a simple and safe procedure that is used to confirm the presence of ascites, to investigate its cause and to identify ascitic infection (Ryan & Neale 1980). Small amounts of ascites or loculated ascites may not be identified. Paracentesis can also be used to relieve the discomfort of massive ascites or to administer drugs.

The patient should empty the bladder and then lie comfortably in the supine position. The iliac fossae away from the inferior epigastric blood vessels or the midline (linea alba) can be used for the puncture. The skin is cleaned and 3–6 ml of lidocaine (1–2%) is infiltrated into the anterior abdominal wall down to the peritoneum. A fine-bore needle (19–23 gauge) attached to a large syringe is used to minimize the chances of subsequent leakage of ascites and the needle is inserted into the peritoneal cavity. Fluid can usually be aspirated easily, but if none comes the needle should be repositioned or the patient rolled slightly to the side of the puncture. At least 50 ml should be taken for biochemical and bacteriological investigation and at least 100 ml for cytology. The scars of previous operations should be avoided as puncture sites; they may have caused adhesions that can be vascular, they may be the site of varices or they may be adherent to loops of bowel. Bleeding or infection are rare complications, even when the bowel has been punctured, and leakage is minimized by using a small-bore needle.

### Appearance

Ascitic fluid due to liver disease is usually clear and straw or light green in color. It can be differentiated from urine in a patient who does not have diabetes mellitus by its glucose content. Bloody ascites, in the absence of trauma, is usually due to malignancy. Pronounced bile staining indicates a communication with the biliary system, usually due to gallstones, neoplasm or trauma. Infection may cause the fluid to be cloudy (p. 1033).

***Chylous ascites.*** Chylous ascites is rare (Nix et al 1957) and has a milky white appearance due to chylomicrons that pass into the supernatant on centrifugation (Press et al 1982). It is usually due to malignant disease, often a lymphoma, or trauma, including surgery, in adults, but there are other causes (Table 37.2). Fat droplets are seen on ascites microscopy, the ascites triglyceride concentration exceeds the serum concentration, and no

**Table 37.2** Causes of ascites

| |
|---|
| *Transudates* |
| Hypoalbuminemia |
|   Nephrotic syndrome |
|   Protein-losing enteropathy |
|   Malnutrition |
| High central venous pressure |
|   Congestive cardiac failure |
|   Tricuspid insufficiency |
|   Constrictive pericarditis/cardiomyopathy |
| Hepatic venous obstruction |
|   Inferior vena cava obstruction |
|   Hepatic vein obstruction (Budd–Chiari syndrome) |
|   Veno-occlusive disease |
| Chronic liver disease with portal hypertension |
| Hepatic infiltration |
|   Malignant disease |
|   Granulomatous disease |
| Portal vein obstruction (rare) |
| *Exudates* |
| Intestinal perforation |
| Inflammatory diseases |
|   Tuberculosis |
|   Spontaneous bacterial peritonitis |
|   Fungi |
|   Parasites |
|   Pancreatitis |
|   Biliary peritonitis |
| Malignant diseases |
|   Metastatic (liver or peritoneum) |
|   Lymphomas/leukemias |
|   Hepatic |
|     Hepatocellular carcinoma |
|     Cholangiocarcinoma |
|     Mesothelioma |
| *Chylous* |
| Trauma to cisterna chyli/thoracic duct |
| Tumors |
| Radiotherapy |
| Pancreatitis |
| Portal vein thrombosis |
| Congenital lymphatic diseases |
| Filariasis, tuberculosis, sarcoidosis |
| Cirrhosis (rare) |
| *Miscellaneous* |
| Meig's syndrome |
| Vasculitis |
|   DLE and other collagenoses |
|   Henoch–Schönlein purpura |
| Eosinophilic ascites |
| Whipple's disease |
| Granulomatous disease |
|   Sarcoid/Crohn's disease |
| Psychotropic drugs |
| Hypothyroidism |
| Chronic dialysis/renal transplantation |
| Familial paroxysmal peritonitis |
| Gynecological — endometriosis, fibroma |
| Pseudomyxoma peritonei |
| Peritoneal mastocytosis |
| POEMS syndrome |
| *Mimics* |
| Pregnancy |
| Obesity |
| Urinary bladder retention |
| Cysts |
|   Ovarian |
|   Pancreatic |
|   Mesenteric |

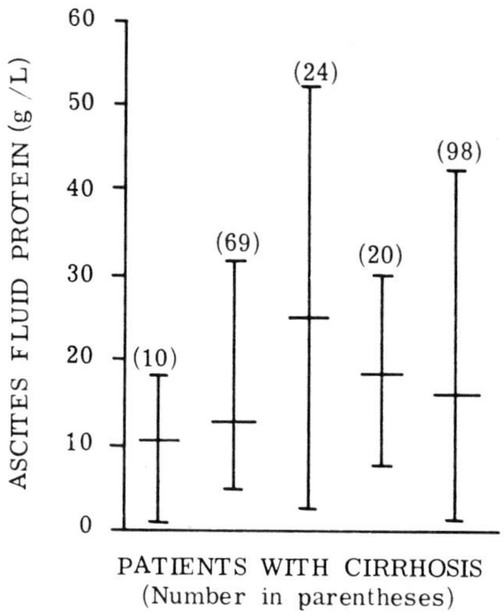


**Fig. 37.1** Ascites fluid protein concentrations (ranges and means) in five series of patients with hepatic cirrhosis (Sampliner & Iber 1974).

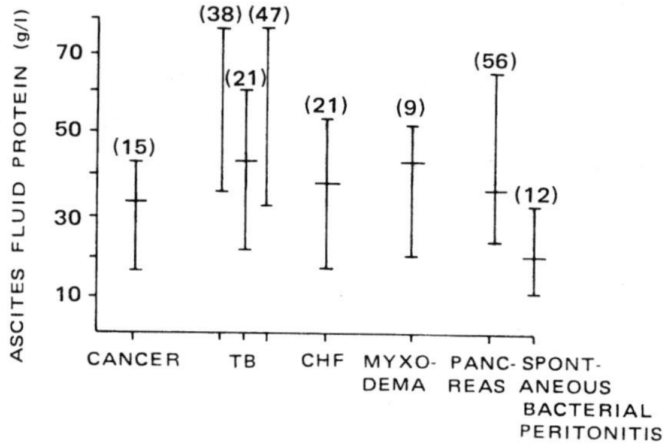


**Fig. 37.2** Ascites fluid protein concentrations (ranges and means) in diseases other than hepatic cirrhosis (Sampliner & Iber 1974).

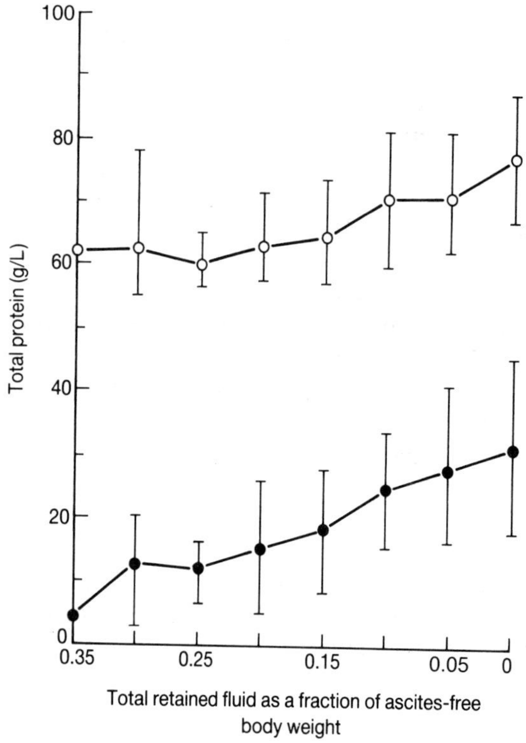


**Fig. 37.3** Total protein concentration in serum (○) and ascitic fluid (●) during diuresis (Hoefs 1981b).

organisms grow on culture. The ascites protein usually exceeds 30 g/L and hypoproteinemia and lymphopenia may be present. Chylous ascites occasionally occurs in cirrhosis; even clear ascites contains small chylomicrons, probably due to intestinal lymphatic hypertension, but where there is chylous ascites, the number and size of the chylomicrons entering the ascites from the lymphatics is increased greatly (Malagelada et al 1974). Whether this results from increased permeability or from rupture of the lymphatics is unknown.

## Biochemistry

Biochemical measurements on ascitic fluid usually include its protein concentration, amylase activity and glucose concentration. The differential diagnosis of ascites concerns mainly cirrhosis, malignancy, cardiac failure and tuberculosis, since other causes of ascites account for less than 1% of cases.

***Protein.*** The ascites protein concentration has been used to determine whether ascitic fluid is a transudate (<25 g/L) or an exudate (>25 g/L). Previously, a transudate was considered as indicating cirrhosis or decompensated heart failure, while an exudate was considered most frequently as due to malignancy. This division has limited diagnostic value, as protein concentrations in different diseases overlap considerably (Figs 37.1, 37.2) and neither the sensitivity nor the specificity is high enough for practical clinical purposes.

The ascites protein in cirrhosis is usually less than 25 g/L, but concentrations above this have been found in up to 20% of cases and concentrations as high as 52 g/L occur (Sampliner & Iber 1974). Hoefs (1981a) has shown that the ascites protein concentration in cirrhosis depends on when it is measured, as the concentration and the ratio of ascites to serum protein rise during diuresis (Fig. 37.3).

Attempts have been made to improve the diagnostic discrimination of ascites protein measurements, particularly in differentiating patients with or without portal hypertension. Rector & Reynolds (1984) showed that the serum/ascites albumin gradient (i.e. the difference between the serum albumin concentration and the ascites albumin concentration) was more reliable in this respect than the ascites protein concentration. The gradient in ascites associated with portal hypertension is usually <11 g/L and by setting the discrimination value at this level the analysis has a sensitivity of 80–93% and a specificity of 97–98% (Paré et al 1983, Prieto et al 1988).

***Amylase.*** The ascites amylase activity is always above 1000 u/L in pancreatic ascites (p. 1270), frequently exceeds 10 000 u/L and is almost always greater than the serum amylase activity. This analysis is important in intra-abdominal inflammatory disease, since other causes of ascites do not increase amylase activity.

***Glucose.*** A low ascites glucose concentration, unrelated to the blood glucose, may be found in malignant disease when the number of malignant cells in the ascitic fluid is high, exceeding about 300/mm$^3$ (Clarkson 1964) and in tuberculous peritonitis (Brown & Dac An 1976).

***pH lactate.*** The acidity of ascitic fluid has been used as an indication of the presence of infection (p. 1035), but pH and ascitic fluid lactate concentrations have proved worthless in most studies (Crossley & Williams 1985).

### Other biochemical analyses

Several analyses on ascitic fluid have been carried out to improve the differential diagnosis of benign or malignant ascites. However, by and large these attempts have been disappointing. A suggestion that a high γ-glutamyl transpeptidase activity is indicative of hepatocellular carcinoma has not been confirmed (Olsson & Waldenström 1979). Likewise, lactate dehydrogenase activity (Schölmerich et al 1984), cholesterol concentration (Mortensen et al 1988) and carcinoembryonic antigen (CEA) (Loewenstein et al 1978) are generally not sensitive or specific enough. The only analysis that seems of some value is the ascitic fluid fibronectin concentration which may be a supplement to cytology (Schölmerich et al 1984).

### Bacteriology

Bacteriological examination usually yields organisms in only about a quarter of patients with tuberculous ascites (Palmer et al 1985), although examination of a liter of fluid may increase the yield to three-quarters or more (Singh et al 1969). Spontaneous bacterial peritonitis can occur in cirrhosis with ascites and bacteriological examination of ascitic fluid in such patients is most likely to reveal the infecting organisms if blood culture bottles are inoculated at the bedside (p. 1034).

### Cytology

Cytological examination should always be carried out immediately ascites is withdrawn, as cells degenerate rapidly. Examination for inflammatory cells can indicate the presence of infection (p. 1034). Examination of the sediment after centrifugation may reveal malignant cells and this is of great diagnostic value because of the specificity of the observation. Unfortunately, the analysis is not very sensitive, as there is a high frequency of false negative observations. In malignancy, "abnormal" cells are found in ascites in approximately 65% of cases, while the frequency in peritoneal carcinomatosis with or without liver metastases is approximately 95%, with certain malignant cytology in 83% (Runyon et al 1988b).

### Peritoneal biopsy

Peritoneal biopsy can be useful when other investigations have failed to reveal the cause of ascites. The biopsy may be obtained with an Abrams punch and the best results are obtained in tuberculous peritonitis (Jenkins & Ward 1980). However, laparoscopy, which allows inspection and biopsies from areas of suspicion on the peritoneum as well as the liver, improves the investigation (p. 120).

### Ultrasonography

Ultrasonography is the best means of identifying ascites where the clinical evidence is equivocal (p. 59), as it can detect as little as 100 ml of intraperitoneal fluid whether it is free or loculated (Goldberg et al 1970). In addition, it may provide evidence as to the cause of the ascites.

### Radiology

Plain abdominal radiographs are widely used to identify ascites, but they are both insensitive and nonspecific in this regard (Bundrick et al 1984).

### Other investigations

These are directed to determining the cause of the ascites and are indicated by the associated clinical features. Liver imaging (p. 53), liver biopsy (p. 717) and measurements of portal hypertension are of greatest value in differentiating two of the more common causes: cirrhosis and malignant disease.

## DIAGNOSIS

The detection of ascites may be difficult when the volume is small, when another disease, such as an ovarian cyst, simulates ascites or when the patient is obese. Ultrasonography is the best means of identifying ascites in these circumstances. Once it is detected, the cause of the ascites (Table 37.2) can usually be discovered from its associated clinical features and their investigation and from an examination of the ascitic fluid itself.

Cirrhosis, malignant disease and congestive cardiac failure are the causes accounting for 90% or more of patients who present with ascites in Europe and North America (Berner et al 1964). Carcinomas involving the peritoneum or, occasionally, restricted to the liver are the usual causes in malignant ascites and the common primary sites include the female genital organs, especially the ovaries, the gastrointestinal tract, especially the stomach and colon, the pancreas, the liver and extra-abdominal sites such as the breast and bronchus. The diagnosis of ascites due to peritoneal mesothelioma is usually a puzzle unless the patient suffers from asbestosis with concurrent clinical signs in the lungs or pleura. Ascites in patients with cirrhosis should not be attributed automatically to the liver disease, particularly when liver function is good or when there is no evidence of portal hypertension; some complicating condition, such as a hepatocellular carcinoma, portal venous thrombosis, infection or an independent cause, should then be sought. Berner et al (1964) found that 13 of 73 (18%) patients with cirrhosis and ascites also had a hepatocellular carcinoma at autopsy.

The circulation should be examined carefully, as right ventricular failure is an easily overlooked cause of ascites. Ascites disproportionate to peripheral edema may be misleading in constrictive pericarditis and giant jugular venous waves in the neck and a pulsating liver are important signs in tricuspid incompetence. Ascites may also be due to marked hypoalbuminemia (<25 g/dl) and when there is no evidence of liver disease the nephrotic syndrome should be sought. Such patients have edema elsewhere and the urine generally contains >5 g of protein daily. Marked hypoalbuminemia without proteinuria or liver disease may be due to protein-losing enteropathy (p. 348). When the protein concentration in the ascitic fluid is high (>25 g/dl), infection – especially tuberculosis (p. 568), hepatic venous obstruction (p. 1081), hypothyroidism and pancreatic ascites (p. 1270) – should always be considered. In older patients clinical evidence of hypothyroidism may not be obvious and a pleural effusion is often also present (Brown et al 1983). The serum thyroxine concentration is always very low, but it is best to confirm the diagnosis by showing that the serum thyroid-stimulating hormone concentration is high, as the serum thyroxine can also be low in liver disease (p. 921). Chylous ascites usually results from malignant lymphatic obstruction but can rarely be due to cirrhosis (p. 1020). Gynecological causes of ascites include small benign ovarian tumors, usually fibromas, which give rise to the rare Meig's syndrome (Pollock 1975, Hurlow et al 1976). Most patients with this condition have a pleural effusion as well as ascites. Endometriosis can also cause ascites of any degree (Naraynsingh et al 1985).

Rare causes of ascites include collagen disorders (Jones et al 1977, Barcells-Gorina et al 1981, McAleer et al 1986), drugs (Goonewardene & Toghill 1977, Witz et al 1987), unusual peritoneal infections with organisms such as *Chlamydia trachomatis* (Cawdell 1986), long-term hemodialysis (Arismendi et al 1976), eosinophilic ascites (Adams & Mainz 1977), peritoneal involvement in systemic mastocytosis (Capron et al 1978) and the POEMS syndrome (Loeb et al 1989).

## TREATMENT

### General principles

The treatment of ascites due to cirrhosis includes bed rest, the restriction of sodium and, sometimes, water intake, the promotion of sodium and water excretion by diuretic drugs and the correction, where possible, of precipitating factors (below). Most patients will respond to these measures, but other treatments (p. 1028) are available for those who do not (Forns et al 1994). Treatment does not necessarily improve the prognosis for patients with cirrhosis (p. 1032) and may even cause serious complications (p. 1028). It is not necessary, therefore, to treat minor amounts of ascites that are not causing the patient any trouble.

Admission to hospital is advisable when ascites is severe, as it reduces the chances of continued alcohol abuse, facilitates the investigation of causes for the ascites and allows the institution of sodium restriction. Treatment is limited initially to bed rest, a sodium-restricted diet and the correction of any potassium deficiency. The patient should be weighed daily and the plasma urea, creatinine, sodium, potassium and bicarbonate concentrations should be measured thrice weekly initially. Unfortunately, there are no good studies of the effect of sodium restriction during diuretic therapy, but there is good evidence that a sodium intake of 20 mmol/24 h alone, without any diuretics, creates a negative sodium balance in nearly 20% of patients with cirrhosis and ascites (Gregory et al 1977). It is not possible to predict in which patients this will occur, but it is most frequent when the glomerular filtration rate (GFR) is above 90 ml/min, the urinary sodium excretion above 10 mmol/day and the serum sodium concentration above 130 mmol/L (Gabuzda 1970). Such patients always have relatively good liver function. Occasionally ascites follows an excessive intake of salty food (Table 37.3) or sodium-containing drugs (Tables 37.4 and 37.5), cessation of

**Table 37.3** Foods containing sufficient sodium* to require elimination from a severely salt-restricted diet

| |
|---|
| *Cereals*: Bread, biscuits, cakes, pastries, breakfast cereals (except those in Table 37.8) |
| *Vegetables*: All tinned, packet or frozen savory vegetables or vegetable salads; spinach, celery, beets, radishes, carrots, turnips, salted potato chips, salted nuts |
| *Fruit*: Crystallized or glazed fruit, maraschino cherries, dried fruit (except dates) |
| *Meat/fish*: All tinned, smoked or prepared products; meat pies, sausage rolls, bridies, hamburgers, pasties; luncheon meat, kosher meat, sausages, ham, bacon, salami, haggis, scrapple; meat or fish pastes or spreads; shellfish, cod roe, duck, goose, turkey, kidney, heart, brains; meat or yeast extracts (Bovril, Marmite, stock cubes) |
| *Dairy*: Salted butter or margarine; cheese (except unsalted cream cheese) |
| *Other*: Tinned and packet soups; bottled and prepared sauces (tomato sauce, salad cream, mayonnaise, barbecue sauce; olives, pickles, mustards, chutneys, horseradish; ice cream, chocolate, toffee, cocoa, syrup |

*Sodium content of these foods >45 mg/oz (2 mmol/28.4 g).

**Table 37.4** Drugs containing relatively large amounts of sodium or causing sodium retention

| High sodium content | Sodium retention |
|---|---|
| Antacids | Carbenoxolone |
| Alginates | Caved-S |
| Antibiotics (Table 37.5) | Corticosteroids |
| Aspirin | Diazoxide |
| Effervescent (Seltzer) preparations | Metoclopramide |
| e.g. Aspirin | Nonsteroidal anti-inflammatory drugs |
| Alka-Seltzer | Estrogens |
| Calcium | |
| Paracetamol | |
| Fybogel | |
| Phenytoin | |
| Valproate | |

**Table 37.5** Sodium and injectable antibacterial agents (Baron et al 1984)

| | |
|---|---|
| Amoxycillin | Cefuroxime |
| Ampicillin | Cephradine |
| Azlocillin | Chloramphenicol |
| Benzylpenicillin | Cloxacillin |
| Cefoperazone | Flucloxacillin |
| Cefotaxime | Mezlocillin |
| Cefoxitin | Piperacillin |
| Ceftazidime | Ticarcillin |

Note: Significant increases of sodium intake due to antibacterial therapy usually occur only during parenteral therapy when large (gram) amounts of drug are used. Maximum parenteral doses of the above drugs increase daily sodium intake by about 20–50 mmol. Drugs that do not themselves contain sodium increase sodium intake if they are infused in sodium-containing fluids. Oral antibacterial therapy rarely increases sodium intake but can occur with fucidin and para-aminosalicylate.

which is followed by diuresis. More often a diuretic will be required.

Diuretic drugs are given if 2 kg of weight have not been lost within 4 days. The author starts with spironolactone 100 mg daily by mouth and simultaneously reduces any potassium being given (p. 1026) by half. The dose of spironolactone is increased by 100 mg/day every 3 or 4 days to 400 mg/day if a daily weight loss of 0.5–1 kg is not achieved. Potassium supplements can be stopped once the plasma potassium has risen into the normal range. A further diuretic is added if daily weight loss remains unsatisfactory. Powerful diuretics are most useful, as their short duration of action gives great therapeutic flexibility (p. 1027). Therapy thereafter depends on the diuretic response and on the development of complications; weight loss exceeding 1.0 kg/day, an increase in the plasma urea or creatinine concentration, abnormalities of serum electrolyte concentrations or increasing alkalosis indicates that therapy should be reduced or stopped for a few days, while failure to respond is an indication to increase the dose of the diuretics or change to another drug. The aim is a moderate steady diuresis and when this is well established treatment can be reduced. In this respect, diuretic drugs are so powerful that the first change can be an increased sodium intake to allow a more palatable diet and so improve food intake. Indeed, some have questioned the need for severe sodium restriction in patients who are not uremic and who have reasonably good liver function (Reynolds et al 1978). The author's experience accords with those who find sodium restriction improves removal of ascites at least initially (Gauthier et al 1986), but once diuresis is established it can then soon be relaxed. Control of ascites is achieved once the patient looks and feels comfortable.

Some patients (20%) will not require diuretics once ascites has been controlled, provided that moderate sodium restriction is continued (Sherlock et al 1966). More often, however, diuretics continue to be needed. They are particularly valuable in outpatients, most of whom cannot reasonably be expected to master the intricacies of low-sodium diets that are frequently only poorly comprehended by their medical advisers. Patients on long-term diuretics should be seen every few months and their plasma urea and electrolyte concentrations should be measured. Patients maintained on spironolactone seem less likely to develop potassium deficiency (Wheeler et al 1977).

## Bed rest

Bed rest in hospital is usually recommended for marked ascites. Such patients often feel most comfortable propped up in bed, elevation of the legs may facilitate the mobilization of peripheral edema and being in bed in hospital at least reduces the likelihood of continued alcohol intake. In addition, it has been shown that the urinary excretion of sodium and water and the GFR increase in the supine position (Table 37.6). An initial period of bed rest while diuresis is being established is therefore reasonable and a supine position for a few hours after diuretics are given is probably desirable. The dangers of bed rest need to be remembered, however, and patients should be mobilized as soon as diuresis is under way (Asher 1972).

**Table 37.6** Effect of posture on the response to diuretic therapy in hepatic cirrhosis with ascites and in congestive cardiac failure (Ring-Larsen et al 1986)

| Observation | Supine | Erect |
|---|---|---|
| Urine volume (ml) | 1133 | 626 |
| Urine sodium (mmol) | 96 | 45 |
| Glomerular filtration rate (ml/min) | 100 | 66 |
| Heart rate (per min) | 76 | 83 |
| Mean arterial pressure (mmHg) | 86 | 85 |

Note: Six patients with cirrhosis and six with cardiac failure studied over 6 h after bumetanide 1 mg intravenously. Differences in urine volume and sodium, glomerular filtration rate and heart rate all significant ($p$ <0.01).

## Sodium and water

As would be expected from the importance of sodium retention in the development of ascites (p. 1017), restriction of sodium intake is a cornerstone of therapy. The daily urinary sodium in patients with cirrhosis and ascites who are eating a normal diet rarely exceeds 10 mmol (230 mg) and sodium losses from other sources amount to only about 1 mmol (23 mg). The maximum sodium intake to avoid positive sodium balance is therefore only about 11 mmol (250 mg). In practice, successful treatment of marked ascites requires restriction of daily sodium intake to about 20–40 mmol (460–920 mg) in addition to diuretic drugs.

***Hyponatremia.*** Hyponatremia is common in cirrhosis with ascites and becomes more frequent and more severe as liver function deteriorates. Mild hyponatremia does not require treatment if the serum sodium is stable and an increased sodium intake should not be allowed, as patients with ascites always have a high total body sodium (normal 30–35 mmol/kg body weight). Moderate hyponatremia (115–124 mmol/L) is not a serious sign if the patient is not uremic and there are no other electrolyte abnormalities and restriction of water intake (0.5–1.0 L/day) is all that is required. Severe hyponatremia (<115 mmol/L) occurs occasionally and results from a combination of excessive water intake (sometimes given as treatment intravenously) and a limited free water clearance due to increased antidiuretic hormone production (p. 1063). Since hyponatremia in ascites usually develops over a period of time, a certain degree of adaptation by the brain takes place and even very low serum sodium concentrations in these patients are rarely accompanied by symptoms. However, when symptoms do occur, hyponatremic encephalopathy may be difficult or impossible to distinguish from hepatic encephalopathy and in such cases hyponatremia should be treated.

Asymptomatic patients, those with less severe symptoms such as anorexia, nausea and headache and those with a serum sodium above 110 mmol/L should be treated by water restriction. Water intake is reduced to 500 ml/day. If treatment is unsuccessful or if patients are not compliant, slow correction of the serum sodium combined with paracentesis and an albumin infusion may be tried. In patients with more severe symptoms such as vomiting, confusion and ataxia or who have had a fit and who are at risk of respiratory arrest, more active treatment is obligatory. The objective in such patients is to reduce brain edema by increasing the serum sodium concentration such that the patient becomes asymptomatic with adequate ventilation (Arieff 1993). The best place for correction of symptomatic hyponatremia is the intensive care unit, where the patient can be monitored adequately and intubated in case of respiratory insufficiency. The target is to achieve a serum sodium of 130 mmol/L slowly with a maximum increase of 25 mmol/L over 24–48 h. This is achieved best by hypertonic sodium chloride administered via a constant infusion pump. It is important to ensure that the serum sodium does not rise more than 1 mmol/L/h in order to avoid damage to the nervous system (Nairns 1986). The risk of central nervous system damage in the form of central pontine myelinolysis (p. 1046) due to rapid correction of symptomatic hyponatremia in cirrhosis with ascites has probably been overestimated and the use of this term in patients with hyponatremia and brain damage seems unwarranted (Arieff 1993).

Sometimes patients lose their ascites and edema and then develop hyponatremia in association with a mixed sodium and water depletion. This is uncommon and usually follows large paracentesis, a major diuresis due to potent diuretics or enteric fluid and electrolyte losses. These patients show the clinical features of dehydration, tachycardia, hypotension and uremia. It then becomes necessary to give sodium and water parenterally to replace their water and electrolyte losses.

## Diet

It is important that doctors should be aware of the difficulties involved in sodium-restricted diets, even when the details are being supervised by a dietitian. Daily sodium intake varies widely throughout the world and in northern Europe amounts to about 350–450 mmol (8–10 g). Even mild sodium restriction involves a substantial reduction of normal intake, for as little as a level teaspoonful of salt (sodium chloride) contains about 100 mmol (2 g) of sodium (Table 37.7). Furthermore, food itself accounts for only 10% of sodium intake and salt added to food during cooking and at the table (discretionary salt) accounts for only a further 15%, while salt added to processed foods, including bread, scones, biscuits, sauces and food produced by manufacturers, accounts for 75% of salt intake (James et al 1987). Labels on containers stating that a food contains "no added salt" may also be misleading, as some foods contain much sodium. In short, anything containing more than 40 mg (2 mmol) of sodium per ounce (0.07 mmol/g) must be avoided or greatly restricted in a low-sodium diet (Table 37.3). Foods that need not be restricted are shown in Table 37.8. A diet limited to 25 mmol (600 mg) of sodium and containing about 2000 kcal (8400 kJ) and 50 g of protein can readily be

**Table 37.7** Sodium content of salt-restricted diets

| Diet | Sodium (mmol) | (g) |
|---|---|---|
| Low | 25 | 0.6 |
| Moderate | 50 | 1.2 |
| Mild ("no-added-salt diet") | 100 | 2.3 |

Level teaspoon of table salt contains 100 mmol (2.3 g)

**Table 37.8** Foods not requiring restriction for a salt-restricted diet

*Cereals*: Shredded wheat, oatmeal, puffed wheat, puffed rice (not rice crispies), plain flour, rice, macaroni, spaghetti, matzo meal, sago, tapioca, semolina, cornflour, custard powder
*Vegetables*: Fresh or frozen vegetables (except those in Table 37.3), unsalted potato chips, unsalted shelled nuts
*Fruit*: All fresh or tinned fruit, fruit juices except bought tomato juice, fruit squashes, lemonade
*Meat/fish*: Unsalted fresh meat, poultry, fish, sweetbreads, tripe (6–8 oz/day if salt allowance >44 mmol)
*Dairy*: Cream and unsalted cream cheese; milk (1 pint = 12 mmol or 280 mg)
*Fats*: Vegetable oils (olive, corn, groundnut); cooking oil, dripping, lard, suet
*Confections*: Jam, jelly, marmalade, boilings, fruit drops, barley sugar, peppermints, sugar, honey
*Other*: Tea and coffee
Salt substitutes (Selora, Ruthmol) both contain 12.6 mmol or 494 mg potassium/g

**Table 37.9** The "no-added-salt" diet

Foods containing little sodium (Table 37.8) can be taken freely. A little salt may be used in cooking but not added later or a little may be sprinkled on food not cooked in salt (e.g. boiled egg)
Food with a moderate sodium content allowed in limited amounts:
*Eggs*: 1–2/day
*Milk*: 600 ml (1 pint)/day (12 mmol or 280 mg sodium); milk pudding portion or a yoghurt = 150 ml ($^1/_4$ pint)
*Bread*: 1–3 large (5 small) slices/day; 1 large slice = 1 roll or 2 small scones
*Biscuits*: 1–6 plain biscuits/day
*Chocolate/toffee*: 1 chocolate biscuit or chocolate/toffee sweet/day
*Cake*: 1 slice = 1 small slice of bread
*Malted milk or chocolate drinks*: 1/day
*Breakfast cereals*: 1 portion/day (of those listed in Table 37.8)

devised but requires supervision by a dietitian. A wide variety of drugs also contain sodium, sometimes in large amounts, and these will need to be restricted if the purpose of the diet is not to be negated (Tables 37.4 and 37.5); some are available to the public and may be taken without the doctor's knowledge. Patients requiring only moderate sodium restriction can be recommended a diet without added salt (Table 37.9).

## Potassium

Potassium depletion is generally regarded as common in hepatic cirrhosis, especially in alcoholics and when ascites is present (Soler et al 1976). However, measurement of the potassium content of tissues such as muscle (Maschio et al 1971), red blood cells (Astrup et al 1980) and leukocytes (Mas et al 1981) has not always confirmed potassium deficiency. Mas et al (1981) concluded that potassium depletion did not occur in cirrhotic patients who had not been given diuretics and that potassium depletion was usually apparent rather than real and due to an expansion of the extracellular fluid volume (ascites and edema) and consequent reduction of the potassium concentration. Unfortunately, there are no simple clinical or laboratory indicators of potassium depletion, as about 99% of the total body potassium (about 55–60 mmol/kg body weight) is inside cells. In practice, a clearly low plasma potassium (<3.0 mmol/L) can be taken as making potassium depletion likely, especially if the patient has been taking diuretic drugs, and potassium replacement should be given. Potassium 50 mmol/day can be given as potassium chloride or potassium bicarbonate if the blood urea or creatinine concentration is normal; potassium chloride slow-release or effervescent tablets, each containing 6–12 mmol of potassium, are suitable preparations. Patients, however, often prefer potassium in the form of fruit or fruit juice. A plasma potassium of 3.0 mmol/L or more can be observed, especially if spironolactone is being used, and replacement given only if the concentration falls.

## Diuretic drugs (Weiner 1990)

Diuretic drugs are so effective that they have made intractable ascites uncommon. Many drugs are available and the diuresis each produces in normal persons varies (Table 37.10). However, as they do not prolong life in cirrhotic patients (Steigmann & Mejicano 1969) and as they may lead to serious side-effects (below), they have to be used carefully.

Fluid enters the peritoneal cavity more readily than it can leave and diuretics act in the main to decrease the rate of influx (Hoefs 1981b). However, even with diuretic drugs the amount of ascites that can be removed daily does not exceed 900 ml (Shear et al 1970). Thus, if a diuresis of 4 L/day is produced with diuretic drugs, more than 3 L/day have come from other sources than ascitic fluid. Patients with cirrhosis and ascites already have poor renal perfusion (p. 1059) and if such diuretic therapy is continued the blood volume available for renal perfusion will be reduced further, leading to oliguria, uremia and hyponatremia (the hepatorenal syndrome), from which the patient may die. Patients with peripheral edema as well as ascites have a greater extracellular fluid volume and are at less risk of this complication (Shear et al 1970). In order to avoid these complications, therapy should produce a daily

**Table 37.10** Relative potency of diuretics and their effect on urinary electrolyte excretion (Weiner 1990)

| Diuretics | Urine volume (ml/min) | Urine electrolytes (mmol/L) | | | |
|---|---|---|---|---|---|
| | | $Na^+$ | $K^+$ | $Cl^-$ | $HCO_3^-$ |
| Normal | 1 | 50 | 15 | 60 | 1 |
| Potassium-sparing | 2 | 130 | 5 | 110 | 15 |
| Loop | 8 | 140 | 10 | 155 | 1 |
| Thiazides | 3 | 150 | 25 | 150 | 25 |
| Mannitol | 10 | 90 | 15 | 110 | 4 |

Note: A single mean value is given, but individual values vary widely.

weight loss of about 1 kg in patients with peripheral edema and 0.5 kg in those without. This implies 4–6 weeks of therapy, as 20–40 L of excess fluid is usually present in more severe cases. A modest amount of ascites is of no consequence once the patient is comfortable and the temptation to get a good cosmetic result by getting rid of all ascites and edema must be resisted.

## Potassium-sparing drugs

*Aldosterone antagonists*

Spironolactone is a safe and specific inhibitor of the action of aldosterone on the distal renal tubules. It produces a diuresis after 3–4 days by competitive antagonism of the action of aldosterone on the distal renal tubules. This reduces sodium reabsorption and allows more sodium to pass into the urine. Spironolactone 100 mg daily is given initially and the dose is increased by 100 mg/day every 4 days to 400 mg/day if the diuretic response is inadequate (above). A previous study showing that 90% of patients with cirrhosis and ascites can be treated successfully with spironolactone alone is probably too optimistic (Pérez-Ayuso et al 1983). A more recent, and perhaps more realistic, study has shown that about 45% of patients do not respond to spironolactone alone in doses up to 500 mg daily (Gatta et al 1991). After the treatment has been supplemented with a loop diuretic, only 4% of patients remain refractory to treatment. Another diuretic can be added if the diuretic response remains inadequate, although larger doses of spironolactone may be effective (Eggert 1970).

Spironolactone does not cause increased urinary potassium loss. Indeed, hyperkalemia may occur in patients who are uremic or who are receiving potassium supplements and it should be remembered that the salt substitutes used to make sodium-restricted diets more palatable contain much potassium (Table 37.8). Spironolactone can reduce the potassium loss caused by more powerful diuretics although the extent of this is unpredictable. Gynecomastia often develops and seems to be related to the dose and duration of treatment. It may be painful, but it disappears when the drug is stopped. Potassium canrenoate, which has a similar diuretic action, causes less gynecomastia and can be used when the complication occurs (Bellati & Idéo 1986). Other side-effects include gastrointestinal symptoms, headache, drowsiness, skin rashes, impotence and a single case of agranulocytosis, but they are all uncommon.

*Other potassium-sparing diuretics*

The main other potassium-sparing diuretics are triamterene and amiloride. Both produce a moderate increase in urinary sodium and only a slight increase, or even a decrease, in urinary potassium. They are not aldosterone antagonists but act directly on the distal renal tubules to reduce sodium reabsorption and thereby to inhibit potassium excretion. Given orally, the maximum diuretic activity occurs within 6 h and ceases within 24 h. These drugs are usually used in combination with a more powerful diuretic (below), when they may potentiate the diuresis and be useful in limiting urinary potassium loss. Both can produce hyperkalemia and need to be used cautiously in patients with renal dysfunction. More than one potassium-sparing diuretic should not be given simultaneously, as this increases the risk of hyperkalemia.

Triamterene, which is now rarely used, is given orally in a dose of 100–250 mg daily. Side-effects are few and include gastrointestinal symptoms, headache, weakness and skin rashes. Combination of triamterene with a thiazide drug may predispose to renal stone formation and this combination should be avoided (Lancet 1986). Amiloride is given orally in a dose of 10–20 mg daily. Side-effects are few and include gastrointestinal symptoms, weakness and headache.

## Loop diuretics

The main drugs in this group are frusemide and bumetanide. The diuresis they produce exceeds that of all other diuretics; it occurs within an hour of an oral dose and within 10 min of an intravenous dose and lasts about 8 h. All act primarily on the ascending limb of the loop of Henle by inhibiting sodium and chloride reabsorption; a similar effect is probably exerted on the proximal tubules but is quantitatively less important. Urinary potassium loss increases because potassium is secreted by the distal tubules in reabsorbing the increased sodium load presented to them. The excretion of calcium and magnesium is also increased and metabolic alkalosis may occur. These drugs increase the diuresis obtained from other diuretics, but they do not augment one another. Toxicity usually results from fluid and electrolyte imbalance, but other side-effects are unusual. Gastrointestinal symptoms, blood dyscrasias, skin rashes, paresthesia and hepatic or renal dysfunction can occur. Hyperuricemia and hyperglycemia develop but are rarely significant.

Frusemide is the drug most often used in ascites and large doses may be needed to produce an adequate diuresis. This may be a consequence of hyperaldosteronism or a reduced renal sensitivity to the drug, but it is not due to any change in the disposition of frusemide in patients with cirrhosis (Sawhney et al 1981). An initial dose of 40 mg is given and the dose increased by 40 mg increments to a maximum of 250 mg/day. Bumetanide (1–5 mg/day) is also suitable and may cause less potassium loss. Frusemide (40–80 mg) and bumetanide (1–2 mg over 5 min) can also be given intravenously, but this is rarely necessary.

## Thiazides

The thiazides are diuretics of intermediate potency that are not greatly used in liver disease. Many are available; the most commonly used in the UK is bendrofluazide. They are readily absorbed from the gut and diuresis starts within an hour. The duration of action varies, that of bendrofluazide being about 24 h. Diuretic action is due mainly to inhibition of sodium and chloride reabsorption in the distal tubules. All thiazides increase potassium secretion by the distal renal tubules. Other renal effects include a reduction in the GFR, important only in renal failure, a reduction of calcium and urate excretion and an increase of magnesium excretion. Toxic side-effects are uncommon and include purpura, photosensitive dermatitis, blood dyscrasias, vasculitis and pancreatitis. Hyperglycemia may occur and cholestatic hepatitis has been reported. Sometimes thiazides seem to worsen renal or hepatic insufficiency; in the case of the liver, this has been associated with hypokalemia, alkalosis and a raised blood ammonia. Hypokalemia occurs particularly when potassium supplements have not been given. Bendrofluazide is given orally in a dose of 5–10 mg daily.

Probably the only indication for treatment with thiazides in cirrhosis with ascites is the patient refractory to treatment with potassium-sparing drugs and loop diuretics. In this situation, supplementation with a thiazide may result in natriuresis due to the fact that these drugs have a site of action more distal in the nephron than the loop diuretics (Olesen & Sigurd 1971).

## Complications

The intrinsic toxicity of diuretic drugs is low. The common complications in cirrhotic ascites are uremia and abnormalities of plasma electrolyte concentrations, which result directly from the therapeutic actions of the drugs. These complications are frequent (Sherlock et al 1966); up to three-quarters of patients develop abnormal plasma urea or electrolyte concentrations and multiple abnormalities occur in a quarter of these (Table 37.11). Mild hyponatremia is commonest and is not in itself a serious complication. Multiple abnormalities are much more serious and even minor increases of blood urea concentration can be associated with rapidly worsening hepatic encephalopathy. Oliguric renal failure heralds the onset of the hepatorenal syndrome and if treatment is not stopped promptly, this may become irreversible. Patients with cirrhotic ascites have serious liver disease and may develop any of these abnormalities from the liver disease itself (Gregory et al 1977); there seems no doubt, however, that they are more frequent and more severe when diuretic drugs, particularly powerful ones, are used (Conn 1977).

**Table 37.11** Frequency of abnormal plasma urea and electrolyte concentrations in 112 patients with cirrhosis and ascites receiving diuretic drugs (Sherlock et al 1966)

| Abnormalities | Abnormal (%) |
|---|---|
| Urea >6.6 mmol/L (40 mg/dl) | 34 |
| Sodium <130 mmol/L (mEq/L) | 41 |
| Potassium <3.1 mmol/L (mEq/L) | 38 |
| Hypochloremic alkalosis | 13 |
| Chloride <90 mmol/L (mEq/L) | |
| Bicarbonate >35 mmol/L (mEq/L) | |
| Frequency of abnormality | |
| ≥1 | 75 |
| ≥3 | 26 |

*Prevention and treatment*

Complications are prevented by recognizing that there are no short cuts to relieving ascites. Weight loss should not be allowed to exceed 1 kg/day (p. 1024), powerful diuretics should be used only if necessary and their dose should only be increased slowly.

## Interactions

Several drugs may influence the effect of diuretic treatment (Henriksen & Ring-Larsen 1993). This is especially true for nonsteroidal anti-inflammatory drugs, which reduce prostaglandin synthesis in the kidneys and thereby decrease the renal blood flow and the GFR, resulting in diminished natriuresis (Gentilini 1993). ACE-inhibitors, even in doses that do not reduce arterial blood pressure, reduce glomerular filtration and natriuresis in patients with decompensated cirrhosis (Gentilini et al 1993). The angiotensin II reduction caused by these drugs involves primarily the efferent arteriole of the glomerulus, which results in an increased renal blood flow but a reduced GFR, filtration fraction and urinary sodium excretion. The use of vasoactive drugs to reduce portal pressure as a prophylaxis against variceal bleeding may simultaneously decrease the arterial blood pressure and influence renal perfusion, glomerular filtration and secondarily the effect of diuretics. The increasing use of such treatment may be a future problem. β-Adrenergic blockade, which is currently a standard treatment of portal hypertension, simultaneously reduces the activity of the renin–angiotensin–aldosterone system. However, recent studies show that the GFR is by and large unchanged during β-adrenergic blockade in patients with decompensated cirrhosis (Bernardi et al 1989), which is in accordance with clinical experience that propranolol per se does not seem to influence sodium excretion during diuretic treatment in cirrhosis.

## Refractory ascites

Refractory ascites is defined as ascites that cannot be

controlled by restriction of sodium intake and by giving diuretic drugs (Arroyo et al 1996). Between 5% and 10% of patients admitted to hospital with ascites belong to this category. The definition of refractory ascites usually used is a patient who does not mobilize ascites despite sodium restriction of 50 mol/day, spironolactone 400 mg/day and frusemide 160 mg/day or who develops progressive uremia, hepatic encephalopathy or serious electrolyte disturbances during the treatment. Patients with refractory ascites usually have a very low GFR, which prevents access of diuretics to their receptors (Brater 1985) and which is also responsible for a reduced delivery of sodium to the loop of Henle and the distal tubules, the site of action for the diuretics. Moreover, in this situation sodium reabsorption in the proximal tubules is greatly enhanced (Chiandussi et al 1978).

The degree of resistance to diuretic therapy is best determined during hospitalization to ensure compliance with diet and drug therapy and quite frequently the treatment turns out to be only apparently ineffective. Most often the patient is still taking too much salt; occasionally the hospital diet is inadequate, sometimes a drug containing sodium is being given (Table 37.4) and frequently the patient is obtaining extraneous salt-containing food or drink. The patient may also be taking a sodium-retaining drug such as a nonsteroidal anti-inflammatory drug (Mirouze et al 1983) or metoclopramide (D'Arienzo et al 1985) which can reduce diuretic-induced natriuresis by some 30–80%. Rarely, the diuretic drugs are not being given or not being taken. These patients often appear generally well and do not develop complications of diuretic therapy. It is worth measuring the 24-h urinary sodium excretion, as a good output implies that the patient must be ingesting an excess of sodium. The treatment of this group of patients is obvious, while the treatment of patients with true refractory ascites, who usually have advanced disease, often with multiple electrolyte disturbances, functional renal failure and severe circulatory changes, can be considered as follows if it is felt that any further therapy is at all justified. Refractory ascites signals a very poor prognosis.

### *Paracentesis*

During the past decade large-volume paracentesis in patients with refractory ascites has been carried out with increasing frequency and is now a well-established treatment. The procedure used in performing a large-volume paracentesis is similar to that of the diagnostic tap, but a larger 16 or 18 gauge needle should be used. A modified Kuss needle, a sharp-pointed blind-ended metal needle inside a 7 cm long metal blunt-edged cannula with side-holes, is also widely used. The procedure is performed under local analgesia and strict aseptic conditions. Attachment to a vacuum bottle or suction pump is advisable, so that the procedure may be carried out in about an hour. Albumin is usually administered intravenously, either 40 g irrespective of the amount of ascites removed or, less frequently, 6 g/L of ascites removed.

Former fear that large-volume paracentesis might lead to hemoconcentration and oliguria (Gabuzda et al 1954), especially in patients without peripheral edema to compensate for the hemodynamic hazards of ascites loss (Shear et al 1970), has apparently been overemphasized. A single paracentesis of 5 L of ascites over about 30 min has not proved dangerous in cirrhotic patients with considerable ascites whether peripheral edema is present (Kao et al 1985) or not (Pinto et al 1988). Furthermore, the removal of this amount of ascites usually relieves respiratory distress, reduces central venous pressure and increases cardiac output (Table 37.12) in patients with gross ascites. Total paracentesis, followed by an infusion of albumin 6 g/L of ascites removed, in patients with tense, refractory ascites likewise caused marked reduction of intra-abdominal, intrathoracic, right atrial and pulmonary pressures. Heart rate did not change, while cardiac output increased. Although systemic vascular resistance and mean arterial pressure decreased slightly, markedly increased baseline plasma renin and aldosterone values decreased during paracentesis even before albumin infusion and only regained baseline levels 6 days later (Pozzi et al 1994). Apparently, ascitic fluid does not reaccumulate as rapidly as previously presumed (Shear et al 1970). In one study this happened at a rate of about 40% within 1 week (Gentile et al 1989).

***Therapeutic paracentesis.*** Quintero et al (1985), in a preliminary study, found that the removal of 4–6 L of ascites with replacement of 40 g albumin intravenously daily in patients with tense ascites was as effective as and no more hazardous than spironolactone and frusemide. Furthermore, the time in hospital in those treated with

**Table 37.12** Hemodynamic effects of the removal of up to 5 L of ascitic fluid in patients with hepatic cirrhosis (Guazzi et al 1975)

| Observation | Paracentesis | | |
|---|---|---|---|
| | Before | 3 L | 5 L |
| Heart rate (per min) | 84 ± 14 | 79 ± 13 | 81 ± 14 |
| Mean arterial pressure (mmHg) | 105 ± 21 | 104 ± 24 | 102 ± 19 |
| Cardiac output (L/min)* | 4.7 ± 0.5 | 5.4 ± 0.9 | 5.9 ± 0.2 |
| Mean right atrial pressure (mmHg)* | 10 ± 4.5 | 6 ± 3.9 | 5 ± 2.2 |
| Inferior caval pressure (mmHg)* | 16 ± 0.7 | 12 ± 2.1 | 10 ± 3.2 |
| Intra-abdominal pressure (mmHg)* | 18 ± 3.8 | 13 ± 5 | 10 ± 4.2 |
| Total peripheral resistance (dynes/s/$cm^{-5}$)* | 1716 ± 340 | 1458 ± 434 | 1388 ± 339 |

Note: No deleterious effects in 21 patients studied.
*Each change significantly different from preceding value ($p$ <0.01).

paracentesis was 12 days as compared with 34 days in those given diuretics. With a similar regimen, Ginès et al (1987) treated 117 patients with tense ascites, the majority of whom had peripheral edema, and found that paracentesis proved quicker, safer and more effective than therapy with spironolactone and frusemide. These studies have been confirmed (Salerno et al 1987) and even total paracentesis (complete removal of ascites by a single paracentesis) and intravenous albumin infusion (6–8 g/L removed) in a 1-day regimen has proved effective and safe (Titó et al 1990).

These studies show that paracentesis with intravenous albumin replacement does not impair systemic hemodynamics or renal function. The procedure is effective, is associated with a low incidence of complications and may be carried out during a 1-day hospital stay. However, patients with refractory ascites often require longer hospitalization and to avoid reaccumulation of ascites, patients require sodium restriction and diuretics after the procedure. Most patients respond well to sodium restriction and diuretics and paracentesis is most useful for those 10% of patients who do not respond to this treatment. Where tense ascites is compromising respiration and causing abdominal pain and discomfort, paracentesis is a useful initial step before starting or adjusting diuretic therapy (Angueira & Kakadia 1994).

***Colloid replacement.*** Several trials have been carried out to determine whether less expensive plasma expanders than albumin (dextran 70, dextran 40, hemacel 5%, isotonic saline) could be used during paracentesis. Dextran 70 does not cause more hyponatremia, renal impairment or encephalopathy compared with albumin, but patients have a significant increase in plasma renin activity and aldosterone concentration signifying systemic hemodynamic changes (Planas et al 1990, Fassio et al 1992). Hemacel has been found as effective as albumin and plasma renin, aldosterone and atrial natriuretic factor measurements were the same with the two plasma expanders (Salerno et al 1991). Cabrera et al (1991) have suggested that isotonic saline is a safe alternative to albumin, but these results have not been confirmed.

Finally, some investigators have looked into the need for any plasma expansion after large-volume paracentesis. One study showed that paracentesis without albumin infusion was followed by a significant increase in blood urea nitrogen, hyponatremia and marked elevation in plasma renin activity and plasma aldosterone in patients who did not receive a plasma expander (Ginès et al 1988). Large-volume paracentesis without plasma expansion results in an increased cardiac output within an hour, followed some hours later by a decreased cardiac output, central venous pressure and pulmonary wedge capillary pressure, with an increased plasma renin activity (Simon et al 1988, Panos et al 1990). Thus, large-volume paracentesis cannot be done safely without plasma expansion.

*Ascites reinfusion*

Ascites may be reinfused as an inexpensive substitute for albumin either directly or after concentration of colloids two to three times by passage through hemodialysis membrane (Rhodiascit). It has been found as effective as large-volume paracentesis (Bruno et al 1992). The method is not widely used partly because it is time consuming and partly because of the problem of keeping the hemodialysis filters free from clotting (Wilkinson et al 1975).

*Peritoneovenous shunts*

Peritoneovenous shunts were developed by LeVeen et al (1976) to drain ascites from the peritoneum directly into the systemic circulation via the superior vena cava.

***Shunt procedure.*** The shunt comprises a long perforated tube that is put into the peritoneal cavity, a one-way valve that is placed extraperitoneally and deep to the abdominal muscles and a silicone rubber tube that passes subcutaneously to the neck where it enters the internal jugular vein and ends in the superior vena cava (Fig. 37.4). Modified peritoneovenous shunts such as the Denver and Hakim–Cordis shunts incorporate a subcutaneous pump over the lower ribs which can be operated by the patient. The advantage of this modification is uncertain

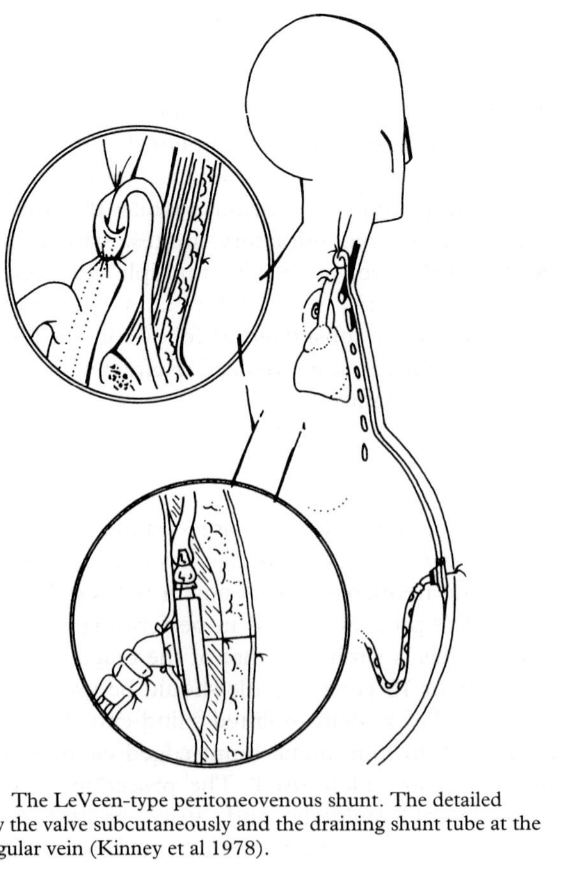

**Fig. 37.4** The LeVeen-type peritoneovenous shunt. The detailed views show the valve subcutaneously and the draining shunt tube at the internal jugular vein (Kinney et al 1978).

(Fulenwider et al 1986). The ascitic fluid should always be cultured first to prevent systemic dissemination of infection in the ascites. Most patients requiring this form of therapy have marked ascites and it is advisable to evacuate a half or more at operation to avoid an excess of fluid entering the circulation after the shunt is in place. The peritoneum must be closed around the tubing meticulously to avoid leakage which predisposes to infection (Smadja & Franco 1985).

Fluid balance in the immediate postoperative period is important and a diuretic such as frusemide given intravenously may be needed to maintain a good diuresis and avoid pulmonary edema or congestive cardiac failure (Greenlee et al 1981). Respiration provides the driving force to carry the ascitic fluid into the central veins, for during inspiration rising intraperitoneal pressure and falling intrathoracic pressure produce a differential of about 5 $cmH_2O$, which is sufficient to open the one-way valve. Respiratory exercises and an abdominal binder can be used to promote ascites flow after operation. The need for such a pressure differential to open the valve helps to prevent the circulation becoming overloaded with ascitic fluid and the one-way valve prevents reflux of blood into the shunt.

***Results.*** Successful treatment with the peritoneovenous shunt results in a marked diuresis associated with a reduction of ascites, an increased renal blood flow and an increased creatinine clearance (Epstein 1982). However, patients often continue to need diuretics. Despite a high rate of complications, some patients get excellent results from peritoneovenous shunting (Fulenwider et al 1984) and their general health and nutrition may improve (Blendis et al 1986).

Only a few prospective randomized controlled trials estimating the efficacy of the peritoneovenous shunt have been carried out, the largest including 299 patients with cirrhosis and ascites (Stanley et al 1989). The peritoneovenous shunt resulted in a significantly faster resolution of ascites (3 weeks) compared with medically treated patients (5.4 weeks). The peritoneovenous shunt also resulted in significant delay in the recurrence of ascites. There was an improvement in the quality of life in shunted patients, but the procedure did not change survival. The prevalence of gastrointestinal bleeding, encephalopathy and infections was similar in the surgically and medically treated groups and although the initial duration of hospitalization was halved in the surgical patients, they were admitted more often and the total number of days in hospital was the same.

Studies in cirrhotic patients with refractory ascites, comparing the peritoneovenous shunt treatment with repeated paracentesis and albumin infusion, have shown that the rate of mobilization of ascites was similar in the two treatments (Ginès et al 1991). However, while the initial admission was shorter in the paracentesis group, these patients were admitted four times more frequently for recurrence of ascites. The probability of shunt obstruction was 40% at 1 year. The rate of complications and survival was similar in the two groups. Similar frequency of obstruction has been found in other studies (Ring-Larsen 1991) and the hope of a beneficial effect from a titanium tip at the venous end of the shunt (Franco et al 1987) has not been confirmed in a multicenter controlled study.

***Complications.*** These are frequent (Table 37.13) and they occur in about a half of patients (Rubinstein et al 1985). Some 10–20% of patients die within 2 months of operation and a third to a half are dead within a year (LeVeen et al 1976, Greenlee et al 1981, Fulenwider et al 1984, Smadja & Franco 1985). This cannot be attributed solely to the operation, as patients treated by peritoneovenous shunts usually have cirrhosis with resistant ascites, which itself has a poor prognosis (Fig. 37.5), and it is notable that mortality is related to liver function at operation. Smadja & Franco (1985) assessed their 140 patients as having good, moderate or poor liver function and noted operative mortalities of 6%, 8% and 25% and 1-year mortalities of 22%, 39% and 75% respectively.

Early complications include particularly pulmonary edema which can be minimized by releasing the ascites at

**Table 37.13** Complications associated with peritoneovenous shunting for ascites

| |
|---|
| *Technical* |
| Shunt failure (occlusion or malposition) |
| Hematoma |
| Migration of shunt out of vein |
| Shunt fracture |
| Skin necrosis over shunt |
| Superior caval thrombosis |
| Ascites leak |
| Bowel obstruction |
| Air embolism |
| Pneumothorax |
| Recurrent laryngeal nerve palsy |
| *Infection* |
| Peritonitis |
| Shunt infection |
| Bacterial endocarditis |
| Septicemia |
| *Cardiorespiratory* |
| Pulmonary edema |
| Hypotension |
| Congestive cardiac failure |
| *Hepatic* |
| Gastrointestinal bleeding |
| Varices |
| Erosions |
| Liver failure |
| *Coagulopathy* |
| Asymptomatic |
| Disseminated intravascular coagulopathy |
| *Renal* |
| Hypokalemia |
| Fever |

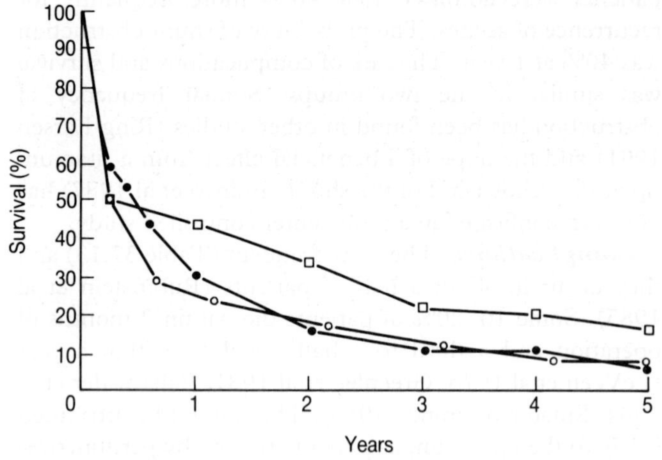


**Fig. 37.5** The survival of three groups of patients with ascites due to hepatic cirrhosis (Ratnoff & Patek 1942 [●], Stone et al 1968 [○], Saunders et al 1981 [□]).

operation and using diuretics after operation, hypotension which may occur for no known cause, and sepsis, while later complications include gastrointestinal bleeding from varices or erosions and sepsis. Shunt failure can occur at any stage. Early on it is usually due to technical errors in placement, thrombosis or cardiac failure and later to fibrin deposition, thrombosis or fibrosis. Suspicion of shunt failure should be investigated early by radiological assessment of the great veins and the shunt, as thrombosis should be treated as soon as possible (LeVeen et al 1984). Venous occlusion, usually of the superior vena cava, is generally due to thrombosis, which may cause fatal pulmonary embolism. It can be relieved by early treatment with a fibrinolytic agent such as streptokinase. Consumption coagulopathy, which occurs in up to a third of patients, is usually asymptomatic and the risk of its occurring may be reduced by evacuating the ascites, but when bleeding occurs the shunt should be interrupted (LeVeen et al 1984). Cardiac failure may occur and be due to overloading of the circulation by ascitic fluid. Examination for previously unrecognized heart lesions revealed by the increased load on the heart should be undertaken (Gur et al 1983). The overall complication rate is approximately 50%, nearly half of which proves to be fatal (Greig et al 1980, Lund & Mortiz 1982).

***Indications.*** Peritoneovenous shunts are associated with considerable risk and should be used only in patients who fail to respond to medical treatment of their ascites, including paracentesis, or if diuretic treatment is accompanied by serious side-effects (p. 1028). Only about 5% of patients with cirrhosis and ascites meet this criterion (Greenlee et al 1981). Shunts can, however, be particularly useful for patients with hydrothorax associated with ascites (below). Patients with Budd–Chiari syndrome often fail to respond to medical therapy for ascites, but they usually respond well to the insertion of a peritoneovenous shunt (p. 1080), perhaps because they have relatively good liver function.

Peritoneovenous shunts have been advocated for the hepatorenal syndrome but evidence is lacking that this syndrome can be reversed, let alone life prolonged, where the diagnosis has been based on appropriate criteria (p. 1061). A peritoneovenous shunt is a prolongation of misery for most patients meeting these criteria. Finally, peritoneovenous shunts can be used to alleviate ascites due to malignant disease. These patients almost all die within 6 months, but they usually get good relief and seem to suffer fewer complications than patients with liver disease (Kostroff et al 1985).

*Transjugular intrahepatic portasystemic stent shunt*

TIPSS has been used to relieve resistant ascites. Ochs et al (1995) treated 50 such patients with grade B (18) or grade C (32) cirrhosis (p. 1007) in an uncontrolled study and obtained a full response in 74% and a partial response in 18%. All patients continued to need diuretic therapy to maintain the response and 16% developed hepatic encephalopathy for the first time after the TIPSS was in place. Long-term shunt occlusion or insufficiency occurred in two-thirds of patients and only a half survived for 2 years. The place of TIPSS in treating resistant ascites requires further investigation.

*Portasystemic shunts*

Surgical portacaval anastomosis can relieve refractory ascites and in general a side-to-side shunt is preferable since it also reduces the sinusoidal pressure (Talman et al 1983). However, patients with refractory ascites usually have poor liver function and are therefore poor candidates for major surgery. Moreover, portasystemic shunts are complicated by hepatic encephalopathy in nearly one-fourth of patients (p. 1007), making this procedure less attractive. Today such patients are more likely to be candidates for orthotopic liver transplantation unless contraindications are present.

### Hydrothorax

Hydrothorax (p. 1019) should be treated initially with sodium restriction and diuretic drugs as for ascites, but in most cases this will not be successful. The insertion of a peritoneovenous shunt (above) may lead to resolution of the hydrothorax or allow it to be aspirated and the pleura sealed with sclerosing agents such as tetracycline or nitrogen mustard (LeVeen et al 1984). TIPSS can also relieve hepatic hydrothorax (Strauss et al 1992).

## PROGNOSIS

The long-term prognosis for patients with cirrhosis who

develop ascites is generally poor. A treatable cause may sometimes be found, usually when the ascites has been of sudden onset, and in such patients the outlook is better. More often, no immediate cause other than increasing and irreversible hepatic failure can be found. Mortality is particularly high initially, as almost a half of patients die within 6 months of diagnosis and in the longer term only 10–20% survive 5 years (Fig. 37.5). Saunders et al (1981) found no improvement in prognosis over the 18 years of their survey (1959–76) and Stone et al (1968) found no difference in the prognosis of their patients and those of Ratnoff & Patek (1942). This supports the view that diuretic drugs have allowed ascites to be controlled without increasing life expectancy (Steigmann & Mejicano 1969).

Some patients have a better outlook than others and this is largely related to liver function, which is also the most important determinant of response to therapy. Sherlock et al (1966) showed that patients who respond readily to diuretic drugs have a better prognosis than those who do not (Table 37.14). Llach et al (1988) investigated 193 patients admitted to hospital with tense ascites uncomplicated by recent gastrointestinal bleeding, infection, encephalopathy, severe renal failure or hepatocellular carcinoma to identify prognostic factors. One-year survival from diagnosis was 56% overall and seven variables reflecting the condition of the liver, the circulation, renal function and nutritional status had independent prognostic value (Table 37.15). Patients without hepatomegaly, with a serum albumin ≤ 28 g/L, with a mean arterial pressure ≤82 mmHg, a urine sodium <1.5 mmol/day, a glomerular filtration rate ≤50 ml/min or poor nutritional state had a 1-year survival of only about 20–40%.

**Table 37.14** Survival of patients with cirrhosis and ascites in relation to response to diuretic therapy (Sherlock et al 1966)

| Group | Number of patients | One-year survival (%) |
|---|---|---|
| Diuretics unnecessary after diuresis | 22 | 85 |
| Diuretics necessary after diuresis | 84 | 71 |
| No diuresis | 6 | 0 |

**Table 37.15** Independent prognostic variables in patients with hepatic cirrhosis and ascites (Llach et al 1988)

| Variables | *p* |
|---|---|
| Mean arterial pressure* | 0.0001 |
| Plasma noradrenaline | 0.0001 |
| Nutrition | 0.004 |
| Hepatomegaly | 0.007 |
| Serum albumin | 0.016 |
| Urine sodium excretion | 0.002 |
| Glomerular filtration rate | 0.04 |

*Diastolic pressure + 1/3(systolic pressure − diastolic pressure).

## SPONTANEOUS BACTERIAL PERITONITIS

Spontaneous bacterial peritonitis (SBP) is a well-recognized complication of cirrhosis with ascites (Crossley & Williams 1985, Runyon 1988). Conn & Fessel (1971) concluded that the incidence of SBP was about 18%, but a more recent prospective investigation reported that the incidence can reach 24% (Pinzello et al 1983). It is not known whether this increase is due to greater awareness of SBP or to an increased occurrence of the condition, but it emphasizes the need to consider SBP whenever deterioration occurs in a patient with ascites.

### Etiology

No source of infection can be found in most patients with SBP. Most infections are thought to be enteric in origin, as enteric organisms are most often found in the ascites. However, the infrequency of anaerobic infection indicates that other sources of infection are probably also important. The most likely pathogenesis of SBP is that bacteria from the gut flora gain access to ascites via the systemic circulation due to an impaired Kupffer cell filter in the liver or directly from the lymphatics in the gut mucosa (Hoefs et al 1982). SBP has followed the use of vasopressin, suggesting that ischemia may increase gut permeability to bacteria (Bar-Meir & Conn 1976), and SBP has also been reported as more frequent after gastrointestinal bleeding and preventable by nonabsorbable antibiotics (Rimola et al 1985).

Rarely, a local source, such as cholangitis, appendicitis or a bowel perforation, is present and occasionally an organism from an infection outside the abdomen, such as pneumonia or pyelonephritis, may reach the peritoneum (Hoefs et al 1982, Pinzello et al 1983). Dental infection has been reported as a source of recurrent infection (Borowsky et al 1979) and the Fallopian tubes are occasional routes of access in sexually transmitted diseases (Stassen et al 1985) or in patients with intrauterine contraceptive devices (Gruer et al 1983). The general increased susceptibility of patients with cirrhosis to infection is doubtless also important (p. 772).

***Organisms.*** SBP is usually caused by a single organism and in at least two-thirds of cases it is of enteric origin (Table 37.16). *Escherichia coli* is responsible for a half or more of cases. Streptococci are found in a quarter or more of cases, including *Diplococcus pneumonia*, which also causes peritonitis in the nephrotic syndrome and in children. Unusual organisms isolated occasionally include *Aeromonas* organisms, *Pasteurella multocida*, *Campylobacter jejuni* and *Yersinia enterocolitica*. Anaerobic organisms are uncommon and are often found with other organisms. The isolation of several enteric organisms should arouse suspicion of perforation of a viscus (Runyon & Hoefs 1984a).

***Recurrence.*** Recurrence of SBP is common and is

**Table 37.16** Organisms isolated from ascitic fluid in 43 patients with spontaneous bacterial peritonitis (Hoefs et al 1982)

| Bacteria | Isolates Single | Multiple |
|---|---|---|
| *Aerobes* | | |
| Gram-negative bacilli | 27 (71%) | |
| *E. coli* | 21 (55%) | 2 (40%) |
| *Citrobacter freundii* | 2 (5%) | 1 (20%) |
| *Klebsiella* | 2 (5%) | 1 (20%) |
| *Proteus morganii* | 1 (2.6%) | – |
| *Enterobacter* | 1 (2.6%) | 1 (20%) |
| Gram-positive cocci | | |
| *Streptococcus* | 11 (29%) | |
| Group D | 5 (13%) | 2 (40%) |
| *viridans* | 4 (11%) | 1 (20%) |
| *pneumoniae* | 1 (2.6%) | |
| others | 1 (2.6%) | |
| *S. aureus* | – | 1 (20%) |
| *Anaerobes* | | |
| *Bacteroides* | – | 1 (20%) |
| Clostridia | – | 1 (20%) |
| *Lactobacillus* | – | 1 (20%) |

Note: Single organisms were isolated from 38 of 43 (88%) patients. Multiple organisms were isolated from 5 of 43 (12%) patients (2 organisms in 4 patients and 4 organisms in 1 patient).

particularly liable to occur in patients with ascites protein concentrations ≤10 g/L (Runyon 1986, Titó et al 1988). The opsonic activity of ascitic fluid is correlated closely with the total protein and complement $C_3$ and $C_4$ concentrations in ascitic fluid. The ascites $C_3$ concentration may be a particularly important marker of susceptibility to SBP. Mal et al (1991) showed in 35 consecutive patients with cirrhosis and ascites without previous SBP that 14 (40%) developed SBP and that these patients had significantly lower chemoattractant activity, $C_3$ and total protein concentrations in the ascitic fluid. In a multivariant analysis, only the $C_3$ concentration in ascitic fluid had independent predictive value for SBP development. Likewise, the probability of SBP recurrence within 4 months was related to the ascites $C_3$ concentration.

## Clinical features

SBP is characterized by fever, abdominal pain and tenderness, nausea, vomiting and frequently encephalopathy and impairment of renal function. Abdominal rigidity is uncommon and does not occur in patients with gross ascites. Clinical features of cirrhosis are usually obvious. The temperature exceeds 38°C (>100°F) in over three-quarters of patients, rigors may occur and hypotension may develop. The clinical features are mild initially in about a third of patients and include mild abdominal pain without rebound tenderness, fever and worsening encephalopathy. SBP can be asymptomatic (bacterascites), even when associated with bacteremia, but this occurs in only about 5% of patients. Thus, the absence of signs of peritonitis in a patient who is unwell does not mean that the ascites need not be examined. It should also be appreciated that bacteria may not be found in the ascites in spite of clinical signs of peritonitis (below).

**Table 37.17** Ascites polymorphonuclear leukocyte (PMN) counts in patients with spontaneous bacterial peritonitis, bacterascites and sterile ascites cultures (Pinzello et al 1983)

| Ascites PMN count ($mm^3$) | SBP $n = 27$ | % | BA $n = 18$ | % | SA $n = 145$ | % |
|---|---|---|---|---|---|---|
| <100 | 2 | 7 | 13 | 72 | 136 | 94 |
| 100–249 | 1 | 4 | 5 | 18 | 5 | 3.5 |
| 250–500 | 3 | 11 | – | – | 3 | 2 |
| >500 | 21 | 78 | – | – | 1 | 0.5 |

Note: Three patients with spontaneous bacterial peritonitis (SBP) and cell counts <250/$mm^3$ had clinical features of SBP. Bacterascites (BA) was defined as the isolation of organisms from ascites in the absence of clinical features of peritonitis and a cell count <250/$mm^3$. Four patients with sterile ascites (SA) had organisms on an ascites Gram stain, but 4 were asymptomatic, 1 had fever and all had cell counts <250/$mm^3$.

## Investigations

### *Ascitic fluid*

The most important step is to examine the ascitic fluid. Ultimately, bacterial culture is most important and this allows the antibiotic sensitivities of any organism to be determined. As the results of culture take time, the total and differential white cell count of the ascitic fluid has been used widely as an indication of infection.

***Leukocyte counts.*** The total and differential white cell count in the ascitic fluid has been used. However, it is known that the cell content of ascitic fluid changes with time in the absence of infection and that diuresis in particular increases the ascites total white cell count due to an increase in the concentration of the long-lived lymphocytes even though there is a decrease in the short-lived polymorphonuclear leukocytes (Hoefs 1981a). Accordingly, decisions should be made on the basis of the ascites polymorphonuclear leukocyte count and infection should be regarded as present when this exceeds 250 cells/$mm^3$ (Table 37.17). A cell count below this level does not exclude SBP. Some patients have a high ascitic fluid cell count but no organisms can be isolated from the ascitic fluid (Runyon & Hoefs 1984b). This may be due to suboptimal culture techniques.

***Culture.*** "Conventional" cultures detect bacterial growth in about 40% of ascites samples with polymorphonuclear leukocyte counts ≥250 cells/$mm^3$, whereas inoculation of blood culture bottles with ascitic fluid can detect growth in 91–93% of cases (Runyon et al 1988a).

### *Blood*

Peripheral blood leukocyte counts are of no value in differentiating patients with or without SBP. Blood culture should always be carried out, as the organism causing SBP can be found in a half to three-quarters of cases (Conn & Fessel 1971, Hoefs et al 1982).

### *Radiology*

Erect and supine abdominal radiographs should be obtained. Free gas in the peritoneum usually indicates perforation but can rarely be caused by a gas-forming organism.

### *Other investigations*

A low ascites pH and an increased ascites lactate have been advocated as indicating SBP, but these tests have not proved superior to the ascites polymorphonuclear leukocyte count (Reynolds 1986). The ascites protein and glucose concentrations are of no diagnostic value in SBP (Runyon & Hoefs 1985).

## Treatment

Treatment with broad-spectrum antibiotics should be given to all patients with clinical evidence of peritonitis, an ascites polymorphonuclear leukocyte count above 250/mm$^3$ or the finding of bacteria in the ascitic fluid. Cefotaxime administered intravenously in a dose of 2 g/8-hourly provides the highest rate of SBP resolution (86%) with minimal nephrotoxicity or superinfection (Felisart et al 1985). Treatment should start as soon as possible and can be adjusted in accordance with bacterial sensitivity tests. Change of antibiotics in patients unresponsive to initial treatment may have to be done empirically if organisms cannot be isolated (e.g. to amoxicillin-clavulanic acid). Antibiotics should never be given before removing blood and ascites for culture. The optimal duration of therapy for SBP has recently been shown to be 5 days (Runyon et al 1991).

***Prophylaxis.*** Aerobic enteric bacteria are the usual cause of SBP and attempts have been made to prevent SBP occurring. Rimola et al (1985) showed that a combination of poorly absorbed antibiotics could prevent SBP, bacteremia and urinary tract infection in cirrhotic patients following gastrointestinal hemorrhage, but the treatment regimen was complex. More recently, Soriano et al (1991) have shown that norfloxacin, which is active against aerobic enteric organisms but not anaerobic organisms, can prevent SBP in at-risk (above) ascitic patients admitted to hospital. Prophylactic therapy for all cirrhotic patients with ascites is not recommended, but oral norfloxacin 400 mg daily can be considered for patients in hospital who have a low ascites protein (<15 g/L) or who have had gastrointestinal bleeding.

REFERENCES


Adams H W, Mainz D L 1977 Eosinophilic ascites: a case report and review of the literature. American Journal of Digestive Diseases 22: 40–42

Angueira C E, Kakadia S C 1994 Effects of large-volume paracentesis on pulmonary function in patients with tense cirrhotic ascites. Hepatology 20: 825–828

Arieff A I 1993 Management of hyponatraemia. British Medical Journal 307: 305–308

Arismendi G S, Izard M W, Hampton W R, Maher J F 1976 The clinical spectrum of ascites associated with maintenance dialysis. American Journal of Medicine 60: 46–51

Arroyo V, Bernardi M, Epstein M, Henriksen J H, Schrier R W, Rodés J 1988 Pathophysiology of ascites and functional renal failure in cirrhosis. Journal of Hepatology 6: 239–257

Arroyo V, Ginés P, Gerbes A L et al 1996 Definition and diagnostic criteria of refractory ascites and hepatorenal syndrome in cirrhosis. Hepatology 23: 164–176

Asher R 1972 The dangers of going to bed. In: Sir Francis Avery Jones (ed) Richard Asher talking sense. Pitman, London, p 199

Astrup J, Prytz H, Thomsen Å C, Westrup M 1980 Red cell sodium and potassium contents in liver cirrhosis. Gastroenterology 78: 530–534

Barcells-Gorina A, Villalta J, Martinez-Orozco F, Ingelmo M 1981 Ascites from polyserositis in periarteritis nodosa. Journal of the American Medical Association 246: 1659–1660

Bar-Meir S, Conn H O 1976 Spontaneous bacterial peritonitis induced by intraarterial vasopressin therapy. Gastroenterology 70: 418–421

Baron D N, Hamilton-Miller J M T, Brumfitt W 1984 Sodium content of injectable β-lactam antibiotics. Lancet 1: 1113–1114

Bellati G, Idéo G 1986 Gynaecomastia after spironolactone and potassium canrenoate. Lancet 1: 626

Bernardi M, DePalma R, Trevisani F et al 1989 Renal function and effective β-blockade in cirrhosis with ascites. Relationship with baseline sympathoadrenergic tone. Journal of Hepatology 8: 279–286

Berner C, Fred H L, Riggs S, Davis J S 1964 Diagnostic probabilities in patients with conspicuous ascites. Archives of Internal Medicine 113: 687–690

Blendis L M, Harrison J E, Russell D M et al 1986 Effects of peritoneovenous shunting on body composition. Gastroenterology 90: 127–134

Borowsky S A, Hasse A, Wiedlin R, Lott E 1979 Dental infection in a cirrhotic patient. Source of recurrent sepsis. Gastroenterology 76: 836–839

Brater D C 1985 Resistance to loop diuretics. Why it happens and what to do about it. Drugs 30: 427–443

Brown J D, Dac An N 1976 Tuberculous peritonitis. Low ascitic fluid glucose concentration as a diagnostic aid. American Journal of Gastroenterology 66: 277–282

Brown J D, Brashear R E, Schnute R B 1983 Pleural effusion in a young woman with myxedema. Archives of Internal Medicine 143: 1458–1460

Bruno S, Borzio M, Romagnoni M et al 1992 Comparison of spontaneous ascites filtration and reinfusion with total paracentesis with intravenous albumin infusion in cirrhotic patients with tense ascites. British Medical Journal 304: 1655–1658

Bundrick T J, Cho S-R, Brewer W H, Beachley M C 1984 Ascites: comparison of plain film radiographs with ultrasonograms. Radiology 152: 503–506

Cabrera J, Inglada L, Quintero E et al 1991 Large-volume paracentesis and intravenous saline: effects on the renin-angiotensin system. Hepatology 14: 1025–1028

Capron J-P, Lebrec D, Degott C, Chivrac D, Coevoet B, Delobel J 1978 Portal hypertension in systemic mastocytosis. Gastroenterology 74: 595–597

Cattau E L Jr, Benjamin S B, Knuff T E, Castell D O 1982 The accuracy of the physical examination in the diagnosis of suspected ascites. Journal of the American Medical Association 247: 1164–1166

Cawdell G M 1986 Diffuse peritonitis and chronic ascites due to infection with *Chlamydia trachomatis*. British Medical Journal 293: 393

Chiandussi L, Bartoli E, Arras S 1978 Reabsorption of sodium in the proximal renal tubule in cirrhosis of the liver. Gut 19: 497–503

Clarkson B 1964 Relationship between cell type, glucose concentration, and response to treatment in neoplastic effusions. Cancer 17: 914–928

Colombato L A, Albillos A, Groszmann R J 1996 The role of central blood volume in the development of sodium retention in portal hypertensive rats. Gastroenterology 110: 193–198

Conn H O 1977 Diuresis of ascites: fraught with or free from hazard. Gastroenterology 73: 619–621

Conn H O, Fessel J M 1971 Spontaneous bacterial peritonitis in cirrhosis: variations on a theme. Medicine 50: 161–197

Crossley I R, Williams R 1985 Spontaneous bacterial peritonitis. Gut 26: 325–331

D'Arienzo A, Ambrogio G, di Siervi P, Perna E, Squame G, Mazzacca G 1985 A randomized comparison of metoclopramide and domperidone on plasma aldosterone concentration and on spironolactone-induced diuresis in ascitic cirrhotic patients. Hepatology 5: 854–857

Deal C L, Canoso J J 1982 Meralgia paresthetica and large abdomens. Annals of Internal Medicine 96: 787–788

Eggert R C 1970 Spironolactone diuresis in patients with cirrhosis and ascites. British Medical Journal 4: 401–403

Epstein M 1982 Peritoneovenous shunt in the management of ascites and the hepatorenal syndrome. Gastroenterology 82: 790–799

Fassio E, Terg R, Landeire G et al 1992 Paracentesis with Dextran-70 vs paracentesis with albumin in cirrhosis with tense ascites. Results of a randomized study. Journal of Hepatology 14: 310–316

Felisart J, Rimola A, Arroyo V et al 1985 Cefotaxime is more effective than is ampicillin–tobramycin in cirrhosis with severe infections. Hepatology 5: 457–462

Forns X, Ginès A, Ginès P, Arroyo V 1994 Pathogenesis and management of the hepatorenal syndrome. Seminars in Liver Disease 14: 71

Franco D, Labianca M, Smadja C, Fragoso J, Halabi S 1987 Titanium catheter tip for peritoneovenous shunts. Artificial Organs 12: 81–82

Fulenwider J T, Smith R B III, Redd S C et al 1984 Peritoneovenous shunts. Lessons learned from an eight-year experience with 70 patients. Archives of Surgery 119: 1133–1137

Fulenwider J T, Galambos J D, Smith R B III, Henderson J M, Warren W D 1986 LeVeen vs Denver peritoneovenous shunts for intractable ascites in cirrhosis. A randomized, prospective trial. Archives of Surgery 121: 351–355

Gabuzda G J 1970 Cirrhosis, ascites and edema. Gastroenterology 58: 546–553

Gabuzda G J, Traeger H S, Davidson C S 1954 Hepatic cirrhosis: effects of sodium chloride administration and restriction and of abdominal paracentesis on electrolyte and water balance. Journal of Clinical Investigation 33: 780–789

Gatta A, Angeli P, Caregaro L, Menon F, Sacerdoti D, Merkel C 1991 A pathophysiological interpretation of unresponsiveness to spironolactone in a stepped-care approach to the diuretic treatment of ascites in nonazotemic cirrhotic patients. Hepatology 14: 231–236

Gauthier A, Levy V G, Quinton A et al 1986 Salt or no salt in the treatment of cirrhotic ascites: a randomized study. Gut 27: 705–709

Gentile S, Angelico M, Bologna E, Capocaccia L 1989 Clinical, biochemical, and hormonal changes after a single, large-volume paracentesis in cirrhosis with ascites. American Journal of Gastroenterology 84: 279–284

Gentilini P 1993 Cirrhosis, renal function and NSAIDs. Journal of Hepatology 19: 200–203

Gentilini P, Romanelli R G, LaVilla G et al 1993 Effects of low-dose captopril on renal hemodynamics and function in patients with cirrhosis of the liver. Gastroenterology 104: 588–594

Ginès P, Arroyo V, Quintero E et al 1987 Comparison of paracentesis and diuretics in the treatment of cirrhotics with tense ascites. Results of a randomized study. Gastroenterology 93: 234–241

Ginès P, Titó L, Arroyo V et al 1988 Randomized comparative study of therapeutic paracentesis with and without intravenous albumin in cirrhosis. Gastroenterology 94: 1493–1502

Ginès P, Arroyo V, Vargas V et al 1991 Paracentesis with intravenous infusion of albumin as compared with peritoneovenous shunting in cirrhosis with refractory ascites. New England Journal of Medicine 325: 829–835

Goldberg B B, Goodman G A, Clearfield H R 1970 Evaluation of ascites by ultrasound. Radiology 96: 15–22

Goonewardene A, Toghill P J 1977 Gross oedema occurring during treatment for depression. British Medical Journal 1: 879–880

Greenlee H B, Stanley M M, Reinhardt G F 1981 Intractable ascites treated with peritoneovenous shunts (LeVeen). A 24- to 64-month follow-up of results in 52 alcoholic cirrhotics. Archives of Surgery 116: 518–524

Gregory P B, Broekelschen P H, Hill M D et al 1977 Complications of diuresis in the alcoholic patient with ascites: a controlled trial. Gastroenterology 73: 534–535

Greig P D, Langer B, Blendis L M, Taylor B R, Glynn M F X 1980 Complications after peritoneovenous shunting for ascites. American Journal of Surgery 139: 125–131

Gruer L D, Collingham K E, Edwards C W 1983 Pneumococcal peritonitis associated with an IUCD. Lancet 2: 677

Guarino J R 1986 Auscultatory percussion to detect ascites. New England Journal of Medicine 315: 1555–1556

Guazzi M, Polese A, Magrini F, Fiorentini C, Olivari M T 1975 Negative influences of ascites on the cardiac function of cirrhosis patients. American Journal of Medicine 59: 165–170

Gur H, Shalit M, Shouval D 1983 Aortic insufficiency unmasked by a peritoneovenous shunt. Annals of Internal Medicine 99: 129

Henriksen J H, Ring-Larsen H 1984 Determination of albumin transport rate between plasma and peritoneal space in decompensated cirrhosis. Scandinavian Journal of Clinical and Laboratory Investigation 44: 143–149

Henriksen J H, Ring-Larsen H 1993 Renal effects of drugs used in the treatment of portal hypertension. Hepatology 18: 688–695

Henriksen J H, Horn T, Christoffersen P 1984 The blood–lymph barrier in the liver. A review based on morphological and functional concepts of normal and cirrhotic liver. Liver 4: 221–232

Henriksen J H, Bendtsen F, Sørensen T I A, Stadeager C, Ring-Larsen H 1989 Reduced central blood volume in cirrhosis. Gastroenterology 97: 1506–1513

Hoefs J C 1981a Increase in ascites white blood cell and protein concentrations during diuresis in patients with chronic liver disease. Hepatology 1: 249–254

Hoefs J C 1981b The mechanism of ascitic fluid protein concentration during diuresis in patients with chronic liver disease. American Journal of Gastroenterology 76: 423–431

Hoefs J C, Canawati H N, Sapico F L, Hopkins R R, Weiner J, Montgomerie J Z 1982 Spontaneous bacterial peritonitis. Hepatology 2: 399–407

Horn T, Henriksen J H, Christoffersen P 1986 The sinusoidal lining cell in "normal" human liver. A scanning electron microscopic investigation. Liver 6: 98–110

Hurlow R A, Greening W P, Krantz E 1976 Ascites and hydrothorax in association with struma ovarii. British Journal of Surgery 63: 110–112

James W P T, Ralph A, Sanchez-Castillo C P 1987 The dominance of salt in manufactured food in the sodium intake of affluent societies. Lancet 1: 426–428

Jenkins P F, Ward M J 1980 The role of peritoneal biopsy in the diagnosis of ascites. Postgraduate Medical Journal 56: 702—703

Johnston R F, Loo R V 1964 Hepatic hydrothorax. Studies to determine the source of the fluid and report of thirteen cases. Annals of Internal Medicine 61: 385–401

Jones P E, Rawcliff P, White N, Segal A W 1977 Painless ascites in systemic lupus erythematosus. British Medical Journal 1: 1513

Kao H W, Rakov N E, Savage E, Reynolds T B 1985 The effect of large volume paracentesis on plasma volume – a cause of hypovolemia? Hepatology 5: 403–407

Kinney M J, Wapnick S, Ahmed N, Ip M, Grosberg S, LeVeen H H 1978 Cirrhosis, ascites, and impaired renal function: treatment with the LeVeen-type chronic peritoneal–venous shunt. In: Epstein M (ed) The kidney in liver disease. Elsevier, New York, p 363

Kostroff K M, Ross D W, Davis J M 1985 Peritoneovenous shunting for cirrhotic versus malignant ascites. Surgery, Gynecology and Obstetrics 161: 204–208

Lancet 1986 Leading article: triamterene and the kidney. Lancet 1: 424

Lawson J D, Weissbein A S 1959 The Puddle Sign – an aid in the diagnosis of minimal ascites. New England Journal of Medicine 260: 652–654

LeVeen H H, Wapnick S, Grosberg S, Kinney M J 1976 Further experience with peritoneo-venous shunt for ascites. Annals of Surgery 184: 574–581

LeVeen H H, Vujic I, d'Ovidio N G, Hutto R B 1984 Peritoneovenous shunt occlusion. Etiology, diagnosis, therapy. Annals of Surgery 200: 212–223

Levy M, Wexler M J 1978 Renal sodium retention and ascites formation in dogs with experimental cirrhosis but without portal hypertension or increased splanchnic vascular capacity. Journal of Laboratory and Clinical Medicine 91: 520–536

Lieberman F L, Peters R L 1970 Cirrhotic hydrothorax. Further evidence that an acquired diaphragmatic defect is at fault. Archives of Internal Medicine 125: 114–117

Llach J, Ginès P, Arroyo V et al 1988 Prognostic value of arterial pressure, endogenous vasoactive systems, and renal function in cirrhotic patients admitted to the hospital for the treatment of ascites. Gastroenterology 94: 482–487

Loeb J M, Hauger P H, Carney J D, Cooper A D 1989 Refractory ascites due to POEMS syndrome. Gastroenterology 96: 247–249

Loewenstein M S, Rittgers R A, Feinerman A E et al 1978 Carcinoembryonic antigen assay of ascites and detection of malignancy. Annals of Internal Medicine 88: 635–638

Lund R H, Mortiz M W 1982 Complications of Denver peritoneovenous shunting. Archives of Surgery 117: 924–928

Mal F, Pham Huu T, Bendahou M, Trinchet J C, Garnier M, Hakim J, Beaugrand M 1991 Chemoattractant and opsonic activity in ascitic fluid: a study in 47 patients with cirrhosis or malignant peritonitis. Journal of Hepatology 12: 45–49

Malagelada J R, Iber F L, Linscheer W G 1974 Origin of fat in chylous ascites of patients with liver cirrhosis. Gastroenterology 67: 878–886

Mas A, Bosch J, Piera C, Arroyo V, Setoain J, Rodés J 1981 Intracellular and exchangeable potassium in cirrhosis. Evidence against the occurrence of potassium depletion in cirrhosis with ascites. Digestive Diseases and Sciences 26: 723–727

Maschio G, d'Angelo A, Sirigu F et al 1971 Muscle biopsy studies in liver cirrhosis. Scandinavian Journal of Gastroenterology 6: 363–368

McAleer J J A, Cunningham S R, Dickey W, Burrows D, Callender M E 1986 Transient ascites in progressive systemic sclerosis. British Medical Journal 293: 1211–1212

Mirouze D, Juttner H-U, Reynolds T B 1981 Left pleural effusion in patients with chronic liver disease and ascites. Prospective study of 22 cases. Digestive Diseases and Sciences 26: 984–988

Mirouze D, Zipser R D, Reynolds T B 1983 Effect of inhibitors of prostaglandin synthesis on induced diuresis in cirrhosis. Hepatology 3: 50–55

Mortensen P B, Kristensen S D, Bloch A, Jacobsen B A, Rasmussen S N 1988 Diagnostic value of ascitic fluid cholesterol levels in the prediction of malignancy. Scandinavian Journal of Gastroenterology 23: 1085–1088

Nairns R G 1986 Therapy of hyponatraemia: does haste make waste? New England Journal of Medicine 314: 1573–1574

Naraynsingh V, Raju G C, Ratan P, Wong J 1985 Massive ascites due to omental endometriosis. Postgraduate Medical Journal 61: 539–540

Nix J T, Albert M, Dugas J E, Wendt D L 1957 Chylothorax and chylous ascites: a study of 302 selected cases. American Journal of Gastroenterology 28: 40–55

Ochs A, Rössle M, Haag K et al 1995 The transjugular intrahepatic portosystemic stent-shunt procedure for refractory ascites. New England Journal of Medicine 332: 1192–1197

Olesen K H, Sigurd B 1971 The supra-additive natriuretic effect addition of quinethazone or bendroflumethiazide during long-term treatment with furosemide and spironolactone. Acta Medica Scandinavica 190: 233–240

Olsson R, Waldenström J 1979 Gamma-glutamyltransferase activity in ascitic fluid in diagnosis of hepatocellular carcinoma. British Medical Journal 2: 830–831

Palmer K R, Patil D H, Basran G S, Riordan J F, Silk D B A 1985 Abdominal tuberculosis in urban Britain – a common disease. Gut 26: 1296–1305

Panos M Z, Moore K, Vlavianos P et al 1990 Single, total paracentesis for tense ascites: sequential hemodynamic changes and right atrial size. Hepatology 11: 662–667

Paré P, Talbot J, Hoefs J C 1983 Serum-ascites albumin concentration gradient: a physiologic approach to the differential diagnosis of ascites. Gastroenterology 85: 240–244

Pérez-Ayuso R M, Arroyo V, Planas R et al 1983 Randomized comparative study of efficacy of furosemide versus spironolactone in nonazotemic cirrhosis with ascites. Relationship between the diuretic response and the activity of the renin–aldosterone system. Gastroenterology 84: 961–968

Pinto P C, Amerian J, Reynolds T B 1988 Large-volume paracentesis in nonedematous patients with tense ascites: its effect on intravascular volume. Hepatology 8: 207–210

Pinzello G, Simonetti R G, Craxi A, Di Piazza S, Spanò C, Pagliaro L 1983 Spontaneous bacterial peritonitis: a prospective investigation in predominantly nonalcoholic cirrhotic patients. Hepatology 3: 545–549

Planas R, Ginès P, Arroyo V et al 1990 Dextran-70 versus albumin as plasma expanders in cirrhotic patients with tense ascites treated with total paracentesis: results of a randomized study. Gastroenterology 99: 1736–1744

Pollock A V 1975 The treatment of resistant malignant ascites by insertion of a peritoneo–atrial Holter valve. British Journal of Surgery 62: 104–107

Pozzi M, Osculati G, Boari G et al 1994 Time course of circulatory and humoral effects of rapid total paracentesis in cirrhotic patients with tense, refractory ascites. Gastroenterology 106: 709–719

Press O W, Press N O, Kaufman S D 1982 Evaluation and management of chylous ascites. Annals of Internal Medicine 96: 358–364

Prieto M, Gómez-Lechón M J, Hoyes M, Castell J V, Carrasco D, Berenguer J 1988 Diagnosis of malignant ascites. Comparison of ascitic fibronectin, cholesterol and serum-ascites albumin difference. Digestive Diseases and Sciences 33: 833–838

Quintero E, Ginès P, Arroyo V et al 1985 Paracentesis versus diuretics in the treatment of cirrhotics with tense ascites. Lancet 1: 611–612

Radvan G H, Vidikan P 1982 Meralgia paresthetica and liver disease. Annals of Internal Medicine 96: 252–253

Ratnoff O D, Patek A J Jr 1942 The natural history of Laennec's cirrhosis of liver. An analysis of 386 cases. Medicine 21: 207–268

Rector W G Jr, Reynolds T B 1984 Superiority of the serum-ascites albumin difference over the ascites total protein concentration in separation of "transudative" and "exudative" ascites. American Journal of Medicine 77: 83–85

Reynolds T B 1986 Rapid presumptive diagnosis of spontaneous bacterial peritonitis. Gastroenterology 90: 1294–1297

Reynolds T B, Lieberman F L, Goodman A R 1978 Advantages of treatment of ascites without sodium restriction and without complete removal of excess fluid. Gut 19: 549–553

Rimola A, Bory F, Teres J, Peréz-Ayuso R M, Arroyo V, Rodés J 1985 Oral, nonabsorbable antibiotics prevent infection in cirrhotics with gastrointestinal hemorrhage. Hepatology 5: 463–467

Ring-Larsen H 1991 Surgical treatment of ascites. European Journal of Gastroenterology and Hepatology 3: 735–740

Ring-Larsen H, Henriksen J H 1986 Pathogenesis of ascites formation and hepatorenal syndrome: humoral and hemodynamic factors. Seminars in Liver Disease 6: 341–352

Ring-Larsen H, Henriksen J H, Wilken C, Clausen J, Pals H, Christensen N J 1986 Diuretic treatment in decompensated cirrhosis and congestive heart failure: effect of posture. British Medical Journal 292: 1351–1353

Rubinstein D, McInnes I E, Dudley F J 1985 Hepatic hydrothorax in the absence of clinical ascites: diagnosis and management. Gastroenterology 88: 188–191

Runyon B A 1986 Low-protein-concentration ascitic fluid is predisposed to spontaneous bacterial peritonitis. Gastroenterology 91: 1343–1346

Runyon B A 1988 Spontaneous bacterial peritonitis: an explosion of information. Hepatology 8: 171–175

Runyon B A, Hoefs J C 1984a Ascitic fluid analysis in the differentiation of spontaneous bacterial peritonitis from gastrointestinal tract perforation into ascitic fluid. Hepatology 4: 447–450

Runyon B A, Hoefs J C 1984b Culture-negative neutrocytic ascites: a variant of spontaneous bacterial peritonitis. Hepatology 4: 1209–1211

Runyon B A, Hoefs J C 1985 Ascitic fluid chemical analysis before, during and after spontaneous bacterial peritonitis. Hepatology 5: 257–259

Runyon B A, Canawati H N, Akriviadis E A 1988a Optimization of ascitic fluid culture technique. Gastroenterology 95: 1351–1355
Runyon B A, Hoefs J C, Morgan T R 1988b Ascites fluid analysis in malignancy-related ascites. Hepatology 8: 1104–1109
Runyon B A, McHutchison J G, Antillon M R, Akriviadis E A, Montano A A 1991 Short-course versus long-course antibiotic treatment of spontaneous bacterial peritonitis: a randomized controlled study of 100 patients. Gastroenterology 100: 1737–1742
Ryan E, Neale G 1980 Tapping ascites. British Medical Journal 281: 499–500, 550–551
Salerno F, Badalamenti S, Incerti P et al 1987 Repeated paracentesis and i.v. albumin infusion to treat "tense" ascites in cirrhotic patients: a safe alternative therapy. Journal of Hepatology 5: 102–108
Salerno F, Badalamenti S, Lorenzano E, Moser P, Incerti P 1991 Randomized comparative study of hemacel vs. albumin infusion after total paracentesis in cirrhotic patients with refractory ascites. Hepatology 13: 707–713
Sampliner R E, Iber F L 1974 High protein ascites in patients with uncomplicated hepatic cirrhosis. American Journal of the Medical Sciences 267: 275–279
Saunders J B, Walters J R F, Davies P, Paton A 1981 A 20-year prospective study of cirrhosis. British Medical Journal 282: 263–266
Sawhney V K, Gregory P B, Swezey S E, Blaschke T F 1981 Furosemide disposition in cirrhotic patients. Gastroenterology 81: 1012–1016
Schaffner F, Popper H 1963 Capillarization of hepatic sinusoids in man. Gastroenterology 44: 239–242
Schölmerich J, Volk B A, Köttgen E, Ehlers S, Gerok W 1984 Fibronectin concentration in ascites differentiates between malignant and nonmalignant ascites. Gastroenterology 87: 1160–1164
Schrier R W, Arroyo V, Bernardi M, Epstein M, Henriksen J H, Rodés J 1988 Peripheral arterial vasodilation hypothesis: a proposal for the initiation of renal sodium and water retention in cirrhosis. Hepatology 8: 1151–1157
Shear L, Ching S, Gabuzda G J 1970 Compartmentalization of ascites and edema in patients with hepatic cirrhosis. New England Journal of Medicine 282: 1391–1396
Sherlock S, Senewiratne B, Scott A, Walker J G 1966 Complications of diuretic therapy in hepatic cirrhosis. Lancet 1: 1049–1053
Simon D M, McCain J R, Bonkovsky H L, Wells J O, Hartle D K, Galambos J T 1988 Effects of therapeutic paracentesis on systemic and hepatic hemodynamics and on renal and hormonal function. Hepatology 7: 423–429
Singh M M, Bhargava A N, Jain K P 1969 Tuberculous peritonitis – an evaluation of pathogenetic mechanisms, diagnostic procedures and therapeutic measures. New England Journal of Medicine 281: 1091–1094
Smadja C, Franco D 1985 The LeVeen shunt in the elective treatment of intractable ascites in cirrhosis. A prospective study on 140 patients. Annals of Surgery 201: 488–493
Soler N G, Jain S, James H, Paton A 1976 Potassium status of patients with cirrhosis. Gut 17: 152–157
Soriano G, Guarner C, Teixidó M, Such J, Barrios J, Enríquez J, Vilardell J 1991 Selective intestinal decontamination prevents spontaneous bacterial peritonitis. Gastroenterology 100: 477–481
Stanley M M, Ochi S, Lee K K et al 1989 Peritoneovenous shunting as compared with medical treatment in patients with alcoholic cirrhosis and massive ascites. New England Journal of Medicine 321: 1632–1638
Stassen W N, McCullough A J, Hilton P K 1985 Spontaneous bacterial peritonitis caused by *Neisseria gonorrhoeae*. Evidence for a transfallopian route of infection. Gastroenterology 88: 804–807
Steigmann F, Mejicano R 1969 The impact of diuretics on chronic liver disease. American Journal of Gastroenterology 52: 37–44
Stone W D, Islam N R K, Paton A 1968 The natural history of cirrhosis. Experience of an unselected group of patients. Quarterly Journal of Medicine 37: 119–132
Strauss R M, Martin L G, Kaufman S L, Galloway J R, Waring J P, Boyer T D 1992 Role of transjugular intrahepatic portosystemic shunt (TIPS) in the primary management of refractory cirrhotic hydrothorax. Hepatology 16: 85A
Talman E A, Johns T N P, Regan W W 1983 A 25-year experience with total portosystemic shunts and reappraisal of colon exclusion. Annals of Surgery 197: 566–573
Tító L, Rimola A, Ginès P, Llach J, Arroyo V, Rodés J 1988 Recurrence of spontaneous bacterial peritonitis in cirrhosis: frequency and predictive factors. Hepatology 8: 27–31
Tító L, Ginès P, Arroyo V et al 1990 Total paracentesis associated with intravenous albumin management of patients with cirrhosis and ascites. Gastroenterology 98: 146–151
Unikowsky B, Wexler M J, Levy M 1983 Dogs with experimental cirrhosis of the liver but without intrahepatic hypertension do not retain sodium or form ascites. Journal of Clinical Investigation 72: 1594–1604
Weiner I M 1990 Diuretics and other agents employed in the mobilization of edema fluid. In: Gilman A G, Rall T W, Nies A S, Taylor P (eds) Goodman and Gilman's The pharmacological basis of therapeutics, 8th edn. Pergamon Press, New York, p 713–731
Wheeler P G, Smith T, Golindano C et al 1977 Potassium and magnesium depletion in patients with cirrhosis on maintenance diuretic regimes. Gut 18: 683–687
Wilkinson S P, Davidson A R, Henderson J, Williams R 1975 Ascites reinfusion using the Rhodiascit apparatus – clinical experience and coagulation abnormalities. Postgraduate Medical Journal 51: 583–587
Witte C L, Witte M H, Dumont A E, Cole W R, Smith J R 1969a Protein content in lymph and edema fluids in congestive heart failure. Circulation 40: 623–630
Witte M H, Witte C L, Cole W R, Kochler P R 1969b Contrasting patterns of ascites formation in hepatic cirrhosis. Journal of the American Medical Association 208: 1661–1666
Witte M H, Witte C L, Dumont A E 1971 Progress in liver disease: physiological factors involved in the causation of cirrhotic ascites. Gastroenterology 61: 742–750
Witte M H, Witte C L, Dumont A E 1981 Estimated net transcapillary water and protein flux in the liver and intestine of patients with portal

# 38. Hepatic encephalopathy

*N. D. C. Finlayson*

A syndrome of neuropsychiatric symptoms and signs, including coma, may develop in severe liver disease. It is referred to as hepatic encephalopathy or hepatic precoma or coma and reviews of it include those of Zieve (1981), Crossley et al (1983), Jones et al (1984), Fraser & Arieff (1985) and Jalan et al (1996).

## ETIOLOGY

Hepatic encephalopathy may be acute, as in fulminant hepatic failure, or chronic and recurrent, as in cirrhosis, or it may manifest itself as acquired hepatocerebral degeneration. Most believe that all these manifestations are due to neurotoxins that interfere with normal brain function without necessarily producing structural damage. Many potential neurotoxins have been suggested, more than one may be important and they could act synergistically (James et al 1979). Furthermore, different mechanisms could predominate in different forms of encephalopathy. Cerebral edema is more important in the encephalopathy of fulminant hepatic failure, while certain chemical neurotoxins could contribute more to some forms of encephalopathy than others. The duration of exposure to the factors causing encephalopathy may also be important, especially in determining the development of irreversible cerebral changes (Prensky 1984).

### *Origin of neurotoxins*

Most of the important neurotoxins are probably produced in the gut and they reach the peripheral circulation, and hence the brain, because the diseased liver fails to metabolize them or because they are carried past or through it in portasystemic shunts. These neurotoxins are likely to be nitrogenous substances because ingested protein and other nitrogenous material readily provoke hepatic encephalopathy and they are probably produced largely by bacterial metabolism since antibiotic therapy alleviates encephalopathy (Schafer et al 1981). Small bowel bacterial overgrowth in cirrhosis could increase neurotoxin production (Shindo et al 1993) and could be related to impaired intestinal motility in cirrhosis particularly in patients with encephalopathy (Chesta et al 1993, Van Thiel et al 1994). There is evidence, however, that bacterial action in the gut may not be the source of all such neurotoxins. Germ-free dogs with a portacaval shunt develop encephalopathy (Nance & Kline 1971) and germ-free rats develop encephalopathy after hepatectomy (Schalm & van der May 1979). Important neurotoxins may also come from sites outside the bowel, as portacaval shunts produce exactly the same electroencephalographic changes irrespective of whether the bowel is left in situ or removed (Degos et al 1974).

### *Precipitants of encephalopathy*

The brain in liver disease may be especially sensitive to anything disturbing cerebral function, as conditions that rarely produce encephalopathy in normal people do so when liver disease is present (Table 38.1). This sensitivity could result from simultaneous exposure to concentra-

**Table 38.1** Precipitating factors in 100 consecutive episodes of hepatic encephalopathy (Fessel & Conn 1972)

| Factors | Frequency (%) |
|---|---|
| Uremia | 29 |
| Spontaneous (50%) | |
| Induced by diuretic drugs (50%) | |
| Drugs* | 24 |
| Gastrointestinal bleeding | 18 |
| Hypokalemic alkalosis | 11 |
| Excess nitrogen intake | 10 |
| Constipation | 3 |
| Infection | 3 |
| Liver failure | 2 |
| Others | |
| Trauma (surgery) | – |
| Shock | – |
| Hypoxia | – |
| Paracentesis abdominis | – |
| Portasystemic shunts | |
| Surgical | – |
| Spontaneous | – |

*Tranquilizers, sedatives, anesthetics, analgesics, alcohol.

tions of neurotoxins insufficient in themselves to produce overt encephalopathy or from changes in the brain cells themselves, as in the case of increased sensitivity to benzodiazepines or benzodiazepine-like substances (p. 1043).

### Cerebral blood flow and energy metabolism

Overall cerebral blood flow and cerebral energy metabolism in humans with overt hepatic encephalopathy are reduced. Measurements in patients without encephalopathy and following successful therapy have generally been normal (Lockwood 1987). These factors may contribute to symptomatic hepatic encephalopathy, but they are probably not important in early or latent encephalopathy.

### Regional cerebral effects

Cerebral functions are not affected equally in hepatic encephalopathy. This is seen most clearly in early or latent encephalopathy, where performance may be affected sufficiently to impair motor skills such as driving or performance of mechanical or skilled occupations, while verbal or learning functions are preserved (Gitlin et al 1986). This shows that some parts of the brain are more affected than others by hepatic encephalopathy and emphasizes the difficulty of interpreting abnormalities found in blood or cerebrospinal fluid in terms of their roles in producing encephalopathy.

O'Carroll et al (1991) have shown increased basal ganglia blood flow and decreased limbic blood flow with associated psychomotor abnormalities in patients with latent encephalopathy and Lockwood et al (1993) found significant reduction of glucose uptake in the cingulate gyrus, which subserves attention, target analysis and response formulation, and concluded that different parts of the brain differ in their sensitivity to whatever causes hepatic encephalopathy. Lavoie et al (1987) found reduced amounts of glutamate, an important excitatory neurotransmitter, in the prefrontal cortex, caudate nucleus and cerebellar vermis and Al Mardini et al (1993) found increased amounts of serotonin, an important inhibitory neurotransmitter, particularly in the thalamus. Abnormalities such as these could produce disordered neurotransmission leading to alterations of consciousness. These findings emphasize that regional brain factors such as blood flow, energy metabolism and neurotransmitter amounts or sensitivity are likely to be important in producing encephalopathy.

### Ammonia

Ammonia has long been considered important in hepatic encephalopathy. It enters the central nervous system readily and its activity and metabolism there have the potential to interfere with cerebral function.

***Normal metabolism.*** The metabolism of ammonia is complex (Dawson 1978, Onstad & Zieve 1979). Digestion of protein and conversion of glutamine to glutamate and ammonia in the small intestine accounts for about a half to two-thirds of ammonia reaching the blood (Klimberg & Souba 1990), bacterial metabolism of protein, products of digestion and urea in the colon account for about a third to a half and some ammonia is produced by tissues such as the liver and the kidneys. Ammonia is removed from the blood mainly by the liver, which metabolizes it mainly to urea and also to glutamine, and by muscles (Häussinger 1989). About a quarter of the urea produced is excreted into the colon to become a major contributor to colonic ammonia production.

***Ammonia and encephalopathy.*** Ammonia precipitates encephalopathy in patients with cirrhosis and can also produce encephalopathy in patients who do not have liver disease (below). Furthermore, feeding nitrogenous substances other than ammonia increases the blood ammonia and worsens encephalopathy in patients with cirrhosis and withdrawal of nitrogenous substances and antibiotic treatment reduces blood ammonia and improves encephalopathy. However, blood ammonia concentrations are not related quantitatively to the degree of encephalopathy, as they may be raised equally in patients with and without cirrhosis whether or not encephalopathy is present and about 10% of patients with cirrhosis and encephalopathy have normal blood ammonia concentrations (Stahl 1963). This does not exclude ammonia as a cause of encephalopathy, for ammonia crosses the blood–brain barrier readily and can be present in increased amounts in the brain at normal or near-normal blood concentrations (Lockwood et al 1991). Ammonia in the brain can interfere with neurotransmission directly or could do so as a consequence of its further metabolism (Szerb & Butterworth 1992). Ammonia in the brain is removed by combining it with glutamate to produce glutamine in the glutamate–glutamine cycle, a metabolic process shared by the astrocytes and the neurones (Fig. 38.1), and this leads to increased glutamine production.

There is a close relation between the cerebrospinal fluid glutamine and the degree of encephalopathy (Hourani & Reynolds 1971). Increased glutamine production may reduce the amount of glutamate available for neurotransmission in the brain and this could produce the neuroinhibition of hepatic encephalopathy, as glutamate is an important excitatory neurotransmitter. Excess glutamine might itself act as a false neurotransmitter and the active removal of glutamine from the brain by the cerebral capillaries could facilitate the entry into the brain of other amino acids that are substrates for neurotransmitter substances (Goldstein 1984).

Animal experiments exploring the role of ammonia in hepatic encephalopathy have shown that large amounts of ammonia are needed to produce stupor, but these studies

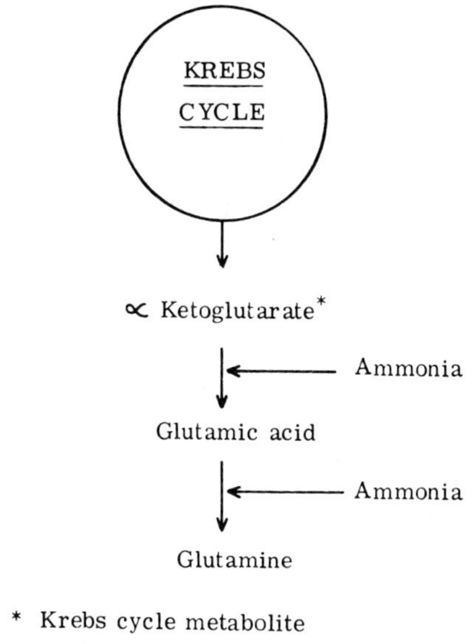


**Fig. 38.1** Ammonia metabolism in the brain.

can be criticized for their short duration and for the presence of a normal liver. Slow infusion of ammonia into Rhesus monkeys has produced gradually decreasing consciousness ending in coma (Voorhies et al 1983). However, it may also be significant that hepatectomy alone and hepatectomy and evisceration in rats with end-to-side portacaval shunts produce exactly the same electroencephalographic signs of encephalopathy, although the eviscerated animals have much lower blood ammonia concentrations (Degos et al 1974). Furthermore, it has been noted that changes in visually evoked potential wave form (p. 1047) and in cerebral neurotransmitter receptors due to hyperammonemia are different from those in hepatic encephalopathy (Ferenci et al 1984).

***Noncirrhotic hyperammonemic encephalopathy.*** Evidence for the ability of ammonia to produce encephalopathy directly or indirectly comes from other conditions in which hyperammonemia occurs. Breakdown of nitrogenous material produces ammonia and its accumulation in the body is prevented by incorporating it into urea in the hepatic urea cycle. Inborn metabolic errors occur at each step of the urea cycle and these give rise to marked hyperammonemia associated with encephalopathy, which improves if hyperammonemia is controlled (p. 971). Hyperammonemic coma has also occurred during treatment of leukemia due to impaired urea formation (Watson et al 1985), during hyperalimentation with essential amino acids (Grazer et al 1984) and from excessive ammonia production in an infected neurologic bladder with increased cerebrospinal fluid glutamine concentrations (Drayna et al 1981).

## Amino acids

***Plasma amino acids.*** The liver is a major site of amino acid metabolism and marked changes in plasma amino acid concentrations occur in liver disease. The most consistent changes in cirrhosis are an increase in the concentration of the aromatic amino acids (phenylalanine, tyrosine, tryptophan and methionine) and a decrease in the concentrations of the branched chain amino acids (valine, leucine and isoleucine); the most consistent changes in fulminant hepatic failure are a great increase in the concentrations of the aromatic amino acids while the concentrations of the branched chain amino acids remain normal (Record et al 1976, Ono et al 1978, Morgan et al 1982b). The reasons for these changes are uncertain. In cirrhosis, the increase in the aromatic amino acids probably results from failure of the liver to metabolize them. The reduction in the branched chain amino acids, which are not metabolized to any great extent by the liver, may be due to increased utilization by other tissues, especially the muscles, possibly as the result of hyperinsulinemia and hyperglucagonemia consequent on failure of the damaged liver to extract insulin from the blood. In fulminant hepatic failure, the increased amino acids probably derive mainly from hepatic necrosis and the general catabolic state.

***Amino acids and encephalopathy.*** It has been suggested that these amino acid abnormalities may be responsible for hepatic encephalopathy, as the aromatic amino acids are precursors of several cerebral neurotransmitters. Plasma amino acid concentrations are the same in cirrhosis with or without hepatic encephalopathy (Morgan et al 1978), but infusions of amino acid mixtures deficient in arginine, which increases ammonia production and impairs the synthesis of urea from ammonia, produce lethargy and coma in normal individuals (Fahey 1957). Experiments in dogs with normal livers have shown that the simultaneous intravenous infusion of tryptophan and phenylalanine causes coma associated with increased concentrations of phenylalanine, tyrosine, octopamine and phenylethanolamine but not of ammonia in the cerebrospinal fluid (Rossi-Fanelli et al 1982).

Less is known about amino acid concentrations in the cerebrospinal fluid and brain in humans; Record et al (1976) found that concentrations of all the aromatic and branched chain amino acids were increased in the brain in fulminant hepatic failure and Ono et al (1978) found that the concentrations of the aromatic amino acids were increased and the concentrations of the branched chain amino acids were normal in the cerebrospinal fluid in cirrhosis. Ono et al (1978) also found that the only difference between patients with and without hepatic encephalopathy was a high cerebrospinal fluid tryptophan concentration in the former. These findings show that the plasma amino acid abnormalities extend to the cerebrospinal fluid and brain but that any effect they have in encephalopathy is likely to be indirect or mediated only by certain amino acids. It seems more likely that amino acids would produce any effects by altering the production of normal neurotransmitters or by leading to the production of false neurotransmitters.

## Neurotransmitters

Over 50 transmitter substances have been recognized in the brain and most of those most recently discovered are peptides (Perry 1991). The "classic" neurotransmitters are shown in Table 38.2. Several of these are derived from amino acids: dopamine and noradrenaline are synthesized from tyrosine and to a lesser extent from phenylalanine (Fig. 38.2), serotonin (5-hydroxytryptamine) is synthesized from tryptophan and γ-aminobutyric acid (GABA) is synthesized from glutamate. Individual neurotransmitters produce either excitation (glutamate, dopamine and noradrenaline) or inhibition (GABA and serotonin) and cerebral activity depends on the balance between these actions. The synthesis of neurotransmitters is thought to be controlled by the availability of their amino acid precursors and this is controlled in turn by the relative concentrations of amino acids in the blood and by the function of the blood–brain barrier where various amino acids compete with one another for transport into the brain. Alteration in particular transmitters or in sensitivity to them could be important in producing hepatic encephalopathy (Record 1991).

**Table 38.2** Neurotransmitters in the brain (Kreiger 1983)

| Neurotransmitters | Central nervous system synapses (%) |
|---|---|
| Acetylcholine | 5–10 |
| Monoamines | |
| Adrenaline | 5–10 |
| Noradrenaline | 0.5 |
| Dopamine | 0.5 |
| Serotonin | 0.5 |
| Amino acids | 25–40 |
| Aspartate | |
| Glycine | |
| Glutamate | |
| γ-aminobutyric acid (GABA) | |
| Neuropeptides | |

***Glutamate.*** Glutamate is an important excitatory neurotransmitter, the metabolism of which is controlled by neurones and astrocytes in the glutamate–glutamine cycle (above). Hyperammonemia increases the synthesis of glutamine by astrocytes and may reduce the amount of glutamate available for neurotransmission. In this regard, measurement of glutamate, glutamine and GABA in the brain at autopsy has shown reduced amounts of glutamate in the prefrontal cortex, caudate nucleus and cerebellar vermis in chronic hepatic encephalopathy (Lavoie et al 1987). Alteration of glutamate receptors on neurones may also occur in hepatic encephalopathy, but this has not yet been shown in humans. Changes in brain glutamate and possibly glutamate receptors, especially in the cortex and caudate nucleus, could explain many features of hepatic encephalopathy and would explain the importance of ammonia in this condition.

***Serotonin.*** Serotonin (5-hydroxytryptamine) is an important inhibitory transmitter involved in the control of sleep. Tryptophan, the precursor of serotonin, is present in increased concentration in the cerebrospinal fluid in hepatic encephalopathy (Ono et al 1978) and recent measurements of tryptophan, serotonin and its metabolite 5-hydroxyindoleacetic acid in the brains of patients dying with hepatic encephalopathy showed increased amounts particularly in the frontal cortex, globus pallidus and putamen (Al Mardini et al 1993). This is likely a result of increased passage of tryptophan from the blood to the brain and could be closely related to hyperammonemia and consequent increased glutamine production (above). These changes could account for the drowsiness characteristic of hepatic encephalopathy.

***γ-Aminobutyric acid (GABA).*** GABA is an impor-

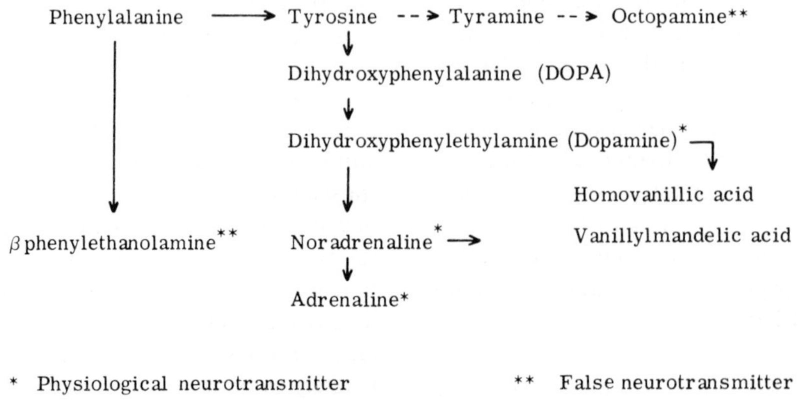


**Fig. 38.2** Catecholamine metabolism and the production of neurotransmitters and false neurotransmitters (Fischer & Baldessarini 1976).

tant inhibitory neurotransmitter and it has been thought that excess activity in the brain might be the cause of drowsiness in hepatic encephalopathy (Schafer & Jones 1982, Hoyumpa 1986). GABA is thought to originate from the gut by bacterial action and reaches the systemic circulation in liver disease as a result of defective liver function. It could then gain access to the brain across the blood–brain barrier. GABA is increased in the blood in hepatic encephalopathy and increased GABA receptors have been found in the brain in animal models of acute liver failure, but human investigations have shown normal cerebrospinal fluid and brain GABA concentrations and GABA receptors in the brain have proved to be normal (Record 1991). It may be, however, that the effect of normal GABA activity in the brain in hepatic encephalopathy is increased by the presence of other substances binding to the related benzodiazepine receptor (below).

***False neurotransmitters.*** Adrenergic neurones in the brain can take up and store compounds structurally similar to the true neurotransmitters, noradrenaline and dopamine, and release them when stimulated. These compounds, however, have little or no physiological function as neurotransmitters and consequently interfere with normal neurotransmission. They are therefore known as false neurotransmitters (Fischer & Baldessarini 1976). A number of aromatic amines found in patients with encephalopathy can act as false neurotransmitters and could be important in the production of encephalopathy. They include octopamine and β-phenylethanolamine (Fig. 38.2), which could be produced by metabolic abnormalities resulting from the marked changes in plasma amino acid concentrations in liver disease. Glutamine could also act as a false neurotransmitter. Much effort has gone into looking for a role for false neurotransmitters in hepatic encephalopathy, but so far none has been established.

### Benzodiazepine-receptor ligands

The GABA receptor subtype A ($GABA_A$) is a complex transmembrane receptor controlling entry of chloride ions into neurones. The binding of GABA to its binding site increases the passage of chloride into the cell and inhibits depolarization of the neurone. The $GABA_A$ complex has several other binding sites that allow other substances – agonists and antagonists – to modulate GABA activity. One of these sites is the benzodiazepine receptor and ligands binding at this site increase the inhibitory effect of GABA on neurones. This has raised the possibility that the benzodiazepine receptor or benzodiazepine receptor ligands could be important in hepatic encephalopathy (Record 1991, Mullen & Basile 1993, Rothstein 1994). The observation that the benzodiazepine antagonist flumazenil could improve hepatic encephalopathy provided strong support for this idea, but although occasional patients show a striking response, this is not often the case (p. 1054). Abnormalities of the benzodiazepine receptor site have not been found in animal models or in humans and interest has centered on the nature and source of benzodiazepine ligands. Human investigations have been difficult, as it is hard to exclude intake of synthetic benzodiazepines that are readily available and can persist for a long time. Nevertheless, patients have been found who have not taken benzodiazepines and who have responded to flumazenil (Pomier-Layrargues et al 1994). Improvements in cognitive rather than motor function have been found (Gooday et al 1995). The origin and nature of the benzodiazepine receptor ligands in these patients are unknown, but they may contribute to encephalopathy in some patients although it is unlikely that they will emerge as sole causes in any instance.

### Other possible toxins

Numerous other substances have been suggested as cerebral toxins in hepatic encephalopathy (Zieve 1981). They include short chain fatty acids and mercaptans which can produce reversible coma in animals, albeit only in large quantities. Their role in hepatic encephalopathy in humans is unknown.

### Intracranial hypertension

Intracranial hypertension is common and is an important cause of death (p. 809) in the encephalopathy of fulminant hepatic failure (Blei 1991). It can occur in hepatic encephalopathy in chronic liver disease but is rare (Crippin et al 1992). Cerebral edema has emerged as the main cause of the increase in intracranial pressure, cerebral blood flow in acute and in chronic liver failure is generally reduced and there does not seem to be any increase in cerebrospinal fluid production. The mechanism for cerebral edema remains uncertain. Normally the passage of water and solutes into and out of the brain is controlled by the capillaries of the central nervous system. All materials entering and leaving the central nervous system have to pass through endothelial cells of the cerebral capillaries, which are wholly bound to one another by tight junctions, and they do this in proportion to their lipid solubility. The endothelial cells transport essential hydrophilic solutes such as glucose and neutral amino acids into the brain by specific carrier-mediated systems, but they resist the transfer of other molecules and large amounts of water and electrolytes such as sodium, potassium, chloride and bicarbonate. This blood–brain barrier maintains homeostasis in the cerebral fluids and damage to this function would obviously impair cerebral function (Bradbury 1979, Goldstein 1984).

Evidence has been obtained in animal models of blood–brain barrier dysfunction with increased water and solute uptake into the brain and electronmicroscopic abnormalities of cerebral capillaries in fulminant hepatic failure in humans have been reported (Kato et al 1992). However, methodological difficulties make interpretation of these findings controversial and some have failed to find evidence of blood–brain barrier dysfunction (Knudsen et al 1993). Other potential mechanisms include inhibition of brain ATPase in fulminant hepatic failure, astrocyte injury, the osmotic effect of a variety of solutes such as glutamine or a complex of several mechanisms.

### Summary

In spite of much research, no definitive neurotoxins have been found to explain hepatic encephalopathy and explanations of the actions of currently suspected neurotoxins are incomplete. This reflects the difficulty of prolonged investigations on humans and the currently limited ability to study different parts of the brain separately. Furthermore, several neurotoxins may be important, other mechanisms such as modulation of the actions of normal neurotransmitters may operate and several mechanisms may be operating in any one patient (James et al 1979). Many neurotoxins potentiate one another in experimental studies (Zieve 1981). Recently, the older hyperammonemia theories have attracted renewed interest and the coming decade should see further evidence emerging regarding benzodiazepine receptor ligands.

## PATHOLOGY

The pathological findings in the brain in patients who have suffered hepatic encephalopathy can be divided roughly into three groups: those related to acute encephalopathy of short duration as occurs in fulminant hepatic failure, those occurring in patients with chronic liver disease who have suffered chronic or recurrent encephalopathy and those occurring in the rare conditions of acquired hepatocerebral degeneration and central pontine myelinolysis.

***Acute encephalopathy.*** No histological abnormality may be found in patients dying after a short period of hepatic encephalopathy, but varying degrees of cerebral edema are found in 25–50% of patients who have died of fulminant hepatic failure (p. 809).

***Chronic encephalopathy.*** Patients dying after chronic or recurrent encephalopathy show marked hypertrophy and hyperplasia of astrocytes, which are greatest in the cerebral cortex and in the basal ganglia. The severity of these changes is broadly proportional to the severity of the hepatic encephalopathy (Adams & Foley 1953) and it is of interest that similar changes occur in hyperammonemic conditions other than chronic liver disease (Perry 1991). The astrocyte is responsible for ammonia metabolism in the brain (p. 1040) and this could be related to the pathological changes observed. Brain imaging has revealed that structural brain damage is probably more common in chronic liver disease than was realized previously. Investigations are complicated by the fact that alcohol produces cerebral damage in its own right (Thomas 1986), but cerebral abnormalities have been detected by computed tomography in nonalcoholic cirrhosis and they are related significantly to measurements of hepatic dysfunction (Tarter et al 1986).

***Acquired hepatocerebral degeneration.*** This is a rare occurrence in chronic liver disease (p. 1046) and is a consequence of irreversible degenerative changes in the central nervous system. There is diffuse but variable necrosis with microcavity formation in the cortex and the corpus striatum. Neuronal degeneration occurs in the cortex, basal ganglia and cerebellum and demyelination occurs in the spinal cord. Chronic hepatic encephalopathy and acquired hepatocerebral degeneration are closely related clinically and acquired hepatocerebral degeneration may simply result from prolonged action of the same factors causing other forms of hepatic encephalopathy, which would explain why such changes are absent in the encephalopathy of fulminant hepatic failure.

***Central pontine myelinolysis.*** This rare condition is characterized by the development of a symmetrical central area of demyelination (myelinolysis) with preservation of the axis cylinders of variable size in the pons (Adams et al 1959). Lesions have also been found in the thalamus, putamen, internal capsule, cerebral cortex and cerebellum in about 10% of patients (Laureno & Karp 1988).

## CLINICAL FEATURES

### Latent hepatic encephalopathy

The effects of liver disease on cerebral function are obvious in patients with overt hepatic encephalopathy, but impaired cerebral function unlikely to be detected in a routine clinical assessment is also common even in patients with well-compensated chronic liver disease. Psychometric tests in such patients show that they perform well in tests of intellect, language, memory and attention capacity but poorly in tests requiring visual, motor and constructional skills (Tarter et al 1984, Gitlin et al 1986). Psychometric tests were abnormal in 70% of cirrhotic patients who were free of clinical encephalopathy compared to the blood ammonia or electroencephalogram, which was abnormal in 46% and 8% respectively (Gitlin et al 1986). Chronic alcoholism may contribute to psychometric abnormalities in some patients, but abnormalities are also common in nonalcoholic cirrhosis (Tarter et al 1984). This may partly explain earlier findings that patients with jobs requiring intellectual function did better in terms of continued employment than patients with jobs requiring manual skills (Kardel et al 1970) and is emphasized by the finding that 60% of a group of cirrhotic patients failed tests of fitness to drive a car and a further 25% did poorly enough to make driving inadvisable (Schomerus et al 1981). These investigations also found that the outcome of psychomotor tests is not related to the cause of the liver disease but to the degree of liver dysfunction. These findings emphasize the clinical importance of making inquiries of relatives and professional colleagues, who are more likely than the doctor to notice functional deterioration, and of asking patients to perform simple drawing or trailmaking tests before concluding that encephalopathy is not present.

## Hepatic encephalopathy

***Symptoms.*** The features of hepatic encephalopathy include changes in intellect, personality, emotions and consciousness, with the development of typical but not pathognomonic neurological signs. The earliest changes are very mild and may be detected only by careful testing (above). Inability to concentrate, apathy, untidiness and reduced alertness all occur later. Behavior is often abnormal and includes irritability, childishness, euphoria, inappropriate laughing or crying, variable restlessness and maniacal outbursts. Emotional responses seem superficial and anxiety or depression occurs. The memory is impaired and intellectual functions such as the ability to add and subtract deteriorate. Drawing, which involves several neurological functions, is also impaired.

Confusion leading to disorientation in time and space is frequent and progression of encephalopathy leads to drowsiness, sleep inversion, stupor and eventually coma. Assessment of the severity of these changes gives a useful indication of the progression or regression of encephalopathy and clinical grading should be based on relatively simple criteria (Table 38.3). Other features are slurring of speech, repetition of inappropriate phrases or sentences (perseveration), convulsions and evidence of brainstem dysfunction such as hypothermia, hyperventilation and sweating (Schenker et al 1974). Decerebrate rigidity is seen rarely and is due to hypoglycemia. It is not necessarily a sign of irreversible cerebral damage.

***Examination.*** Examination usually reveals an asynchronous jerky tremor (asterixis) and sometimes hyperreflexia, extensor plantar responses or, rarely, neck stiffness. Grasping and sucking reflexes may be present in comatose patients. Asterixis is the most characteristic of these neurological signs and is elicited best with outstretched arms, hyperextension of the wrists and separation of the fingers. It occurs with the hands supinated or pronated. Irregular, flapping, bilateral flexion/extension movements at the metacarpophalangeal joints, sometimes with lateral movements of the fingers, are seen. Similar movements can also be seen in tightly closed eyelids and in the protruded tongue or can be felt by having the patient squeeze two of the examiner's fingers steadily (Conn 1977). Asterixis can be elicited in a comatose patients if the hand is dorsiflexed by pressing on the fingertips. Unilateral asterixis occurs but is very rare and has been described with focal lesions of the thalamus and parietal cortex (Stell et al 1994). Electromyography has shown that the tremor is closely related to electrical lapses in the contracting muscles, which may result from inadequate cerebral co-ordination of afferent sensory information important in the maintenance of posture (Schenker et al 1974). Although asterixis is characteristic of hepatic encephalopathy, it also occurs in other conditions (Table 38.4). Reflex activity and asterixis diminish and disappear as coma deepens.

Lateralizing neurological features, such as signs of a unilateral upper motor neurone lesion, are very uncommon but occasionally occur and they resolve on treatment. They should not be accepted as due to hepatic encephalopathy until other causes have been sought. Hypoventilation and apnea are terminal events.

***Variations in presentation.*** Although these features can occur in any liver disease, the encephalopathic

**Table 38.3** Stages in the onset and development of hepatic coma (Trey et al 1966)

| Grade or stage | Mental state | Tremor | Electroencephalographic changes |
|---|---|---|---|
| Prodrome or stage 1 (often diagnosed in retrospect) | Euphoria; occasionally depression; fluctuant, mild confusion; slowness of mentation and affect; untidy; slurred speech; disorder in sleep rhythm | Slight | Usually absent |
| Impending coma or stage 2 | Accentuation of stage 1; drowsiness; inappropriate behavior; sphincter control maintained | Present (easily elicited) | Abnormal; generalized slowing |
| Stupor or stage 3 | Somnolent most of the time but rousable; speech incoherent; confusion marked | Usually present (if patient can co-operate) | Always abnormal |
| Deep coma or stage 4* | Patient may or may not respond to painful stimuli | Usually absent | Always abnormal |

*When patient not responsive to pain, this is regarded as stage 5 in some classifications.

**Table 38.4** Causes of asterixis

| |
|---|
| Liver failure |
| Uremia |
| Cardiac failure |
| Hypercapnia |
| Hypokalemia |
| Sedative drug overdosage |
| Recovery from anesthesia |

**Table 38.5** The differential diagnosis of hepatic coma

| |
|---|
| *Cerebral diseases* |
| Head injury – bilateral subdural hematoma |
| Chronic meningitis (e.g. tuberculosis) |
| Encephalitis |
| Polioclastic |
| Demyelinating |
| Wernicke's encephalopathy |
| *Metabolic disorders* |
| Uremia |
| Diabetic ketoacidosis |
| Hypoglycemia |
| Hypothermia |
| Hyperammonemia (other than hepatic) |
| Hypercapnia (respiratory failure) |
| Anoxia |
| *Endocrine disorders* |
| Hypopituitarism |
| Hypothyroidism |
| Adrenal failure |
| *Narcotic and sedative drugs* |

syndromes in fulminant hepatic failure (p. 808) and in cirrhosis differ. In fulminant hepatic failure, encephalopathy is rapid in onset and progression, with confusion, noisy delirium, convulsions and decerebrate rigidity as prominent features. The response to treatment is often poor and death is frequent. In cirrhosis, encephalopathy is more insidious, frequently responds to treatment and tends to recur. An exogenous factor may precipitate encephalopathy acutely in cirrhosis and produce an encephalopathy resembling that of fulminant hepatic failure (Table 38.1).

### Acquired hepatocerebral degeneration

Occasionally, patients with chronic liver disease and extensive portasystemic shunting of blood develop largely irreversible encephalopathic syndromes referred to as acquired hepatocerebral degeneration (Victor et al 1965, Mendoza et al 1994). The blood may be shunted through a marked collateral circulation or through a surgical portasystemic shunt. Rarely, extensive portasystemic shunts have allowed this syndrome to develop in the absence of histological abnormality of the liver. The most frequent clinical features are those of damage to the basal ganglia and the cerebellar system and the development of spastic paraplegia. Cerebral damage sometimes leads to varying degrees of dementia or the neuropsychiatric features of paranoia or thought disorder. Epilepsy may occur. These several syndromes are not mutually exclusive and may appear together. Sometimes they mimic Wilson's disease, but abnormalities of copper metabolism are absent (p. 961).

Rosenblum et al (1981) have described a gradually progressive neurological syndrome in children with chronic cholestatic liver disease characterized by areflexia, gait disturbance, loss of proprioception and vibration sense and paresis of gaze. There is degeneration of the posterior columns, the gracile and cuneate nuclei and the peripheral nerves. It was suggested that these changes were the result of lack of vitamin E consequent on malabsorption.

### Pontine and extrapontine myelinolysis

This rare condition usually occurs in severe alcoholism, in malnutrition even in the absence of alcoholism, in chronic liver disease and in association with severe systemic illness (Adams et al 1959). The clinical features vary widely in severity, but the cardinal signs are a progressive upper motor neurone flaccid quadriparesis, lower cranial nerve paralyses and behavioral changes in a patient who is often mentally alert. It is caused by an over-rapid increase of the plasma sodium concentration in hyponatremic patients (Laureno & Karp 1988). This may include treatment that has produced hypernatremia. The underlying pathology is myelinolysis mainly in the central pontine region (p. 1044). The lesions can be identified by imaging (p. 1049).

### Associated features

Associated clinical features of underlying liver disease make it unlikely that the hepatic origin of an encephalopathy will be overlooked, but sometimes there may be no such evidence. The encephalopathy of fulminant hepatic failure may then be mistaken for other causes of coma (Table 38.5) and that of chronic liver disease may be attributed to psychiatric or neurological disease (p. 1050).

***Fetor hepaticus.*** Fetor hepaticus, which gives a sweet, musty odor to the breath, is usually present in patients with hepatic encephalopathy but is easily overlooked. It is caused by varying degrees of hepatocellular failure and portasystemic shunting of blood and is more an indication of these factors than of hepatic encephalopathy. It does, however, point to the cause of the encephalopathy. Fetor hepaticus has been attributed to indoles and mercaptans; Chen et al (1970) studied the breath in cirrhosis and concluded that the odor is due to dimethylsulfide. Mercaptans are formed in the intestine from methionine by the action of bacteria and in the liver from the metabolism of sulfur-containing amino acids. They are metabolized rapidly by the normal liver, but in liver disease significant amounts reach the systemic circulation and hence the breath. They have been suggested as contributing to the encephalopathy itself (p. 1043).

## INVESTIGATIONS

Investigations are used to detect encephalopathy, to assess its severity, to exclude alternative causes and to determine any precipitating factor (Table 38.1).

### Clinical tests

Simple tests of mental function assess the ability to draw or construct objects, such as stars and clocks, fluently (Figs 38.3, 38.4). The speed with which numbered circles can be joined in sequence is a similar test that has the advantage of measuring the degree of abnormality (Conn 1977). Twenty-five numbered circles can normally be joined within about half a minute and serial observations can be made provided that the position of individual numbers is changed to allow for learning. Assessment of the ability to perform simple addition and subtraction and of the quality of the handwriting is also useful. A general assessment of the state of consciousness should be made (Table 38.3). Such tests can be repeated easily to follow the progress of encephalopathy and its response to therapy (Figs 38.3, 38.4). It is important to recognize that only relatively marked encephalopathy will be made apparent by such clinical examination and that psychometric testing frequently reveals marked intellectual impairment in superficially normal patients with cirrhosis (above). This emphasizes the clinical importance of speaking to a close relative or colleague who is more likely to have noticed deterioration of a patient's abilities.

### Electroencephalography (EEG)

This is a sensitive means of detecting hepatic encephalopathy that is safe and easily repeated if the facilities are available (Hawkes & Brunt 1974). A normal EEG shows a dominant α rhythm (8–13 c/s), the amplitude of which is altered by altering stimuli such as opening the eyes (Fig. 38.5). The reduction in α rhythm amplitude that follows such stimuli is reduced or lost in the earliest stages of hepatic encephalopathy and thereafter a progressive slowing of the dominant rhythm into the θ range (4–7 c/s) and eventually the δ range (0–3 c/s) occurs (Fig. 38.5). These changes start in the frontal or central cerebral areas in paroxysms and with increasing severity, they extend posteriorly and become continuous. Eventually, electrical activity becomes grossly diminished and asynchronous. These electroencephalographic changes are not specific to hepatic encephalopathy (Table 38.6), which cannot therefore be diagnosed from the EEG alone, and they are not related to any particular liver disease. The appropriate changes in a patient known to have liver disease are, however, virtually diagnostic.

The main uses of the EEG are to support a clinical diagnosis of hepatic encephalopathy if there is doubt, to follow the effects of therapy and to give early warning of encephalopathy in the first 2 weeks or so after portasystemic shunt operations. This last depends on the fact that EEG changes occur before clinical features develop and persist for longer after successful therapy has dispelled them. Attempts have been made to develop "provocative tests" for the detection of latent hepatic encephalopathy in patients with a normal EEG. EEGs are performed before and after stresses such as morphine or a high-protein diet. These tests are not recommended, as they have not been very reliable and may not always be safe.

### Sensory evoked potentials

The function of specific sensory pathways in the nervous system can be investigated in a noninvasive manner by stimulating the pathway and then recording the central electrical potentials elicited by the stimulus as a series of positive and negative waves. Such sensory evoked potentials have been used to investigate the visual pathways, the brainstem auditory pathways and the somatosensory pathways in peripheral nerves (Aminoff 1986). Sensory evoked potentials have also been applied to the assessment of hepatic encephalopathy. Zeneroli et al (1984) found reductions in the peaks and delays in the latencies of the peaks of visual evoked potentials in patients with cirrhosis and hepatic encephalopathy and the extent of these changes related to the severity of the encephalopathy. Abnormalities were found in 10 of 16 patients without clinical or electroencephalographic evidence of encephalopathy, corresponding to preclinical encephalopathy. Yang et al (1985) reported similar results from a study of somatosensory evoked potentials. Visual evoked potentials can therefore be used to detect preclinical encephalopathy and to follow the course of overt encephalopathy, but in clinical practice this can be done more easily using trailmaking and construction tests.

### Ammonia

The arterial ammonia concentration (normal 11–35 μmol/L; 20–63 μg/dl) is raised in most patients with hepatic encephalopathy, but it does not correlate with the degree of encephalopathy and raised concentrations also occur in patients with portasystemic shunts who do not have encephalopathy. It is not, therefore, of great value.

### Cerebrospinal fluid

Lumbar puncture is of no value in the investigation of hepatic encephalopathy, as the cerebrospinal fluid shows no important diagnostic features. The protein concentra-

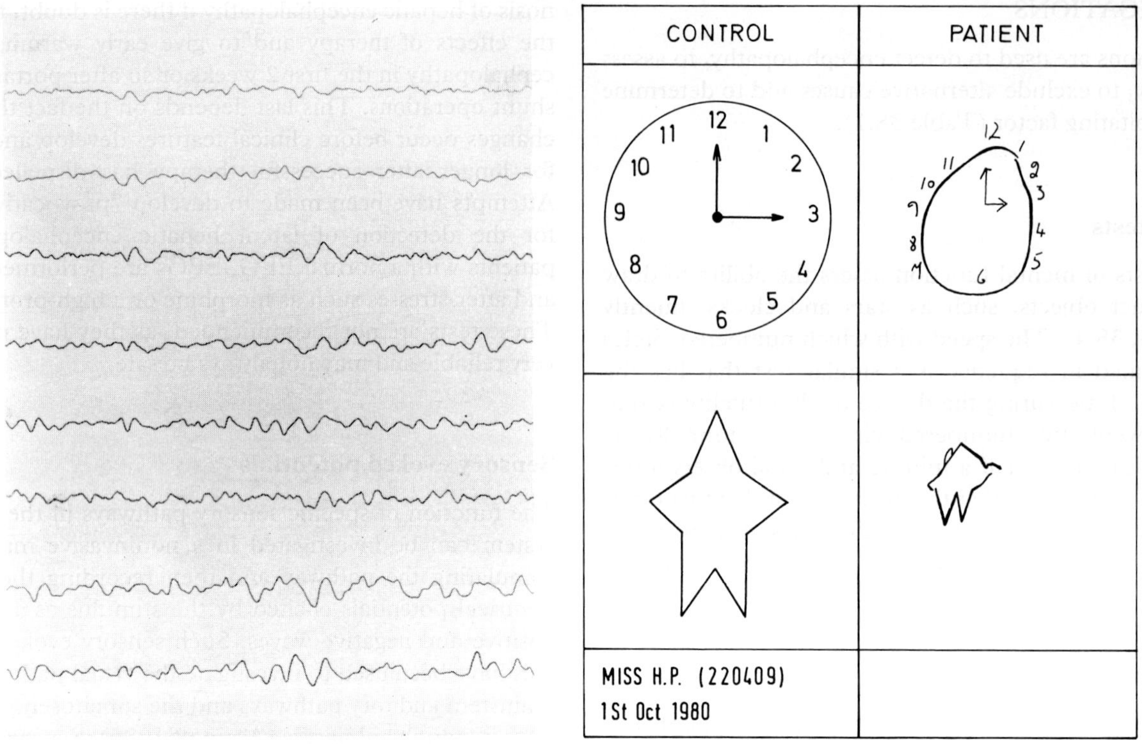


**Fig. 38.3** Construction tests in a patient with hepatic cirrhosis and encephalopathy. Note the impaired ability to draw and the abnormal electroencephalogram (cf. Fig. 38.4).*

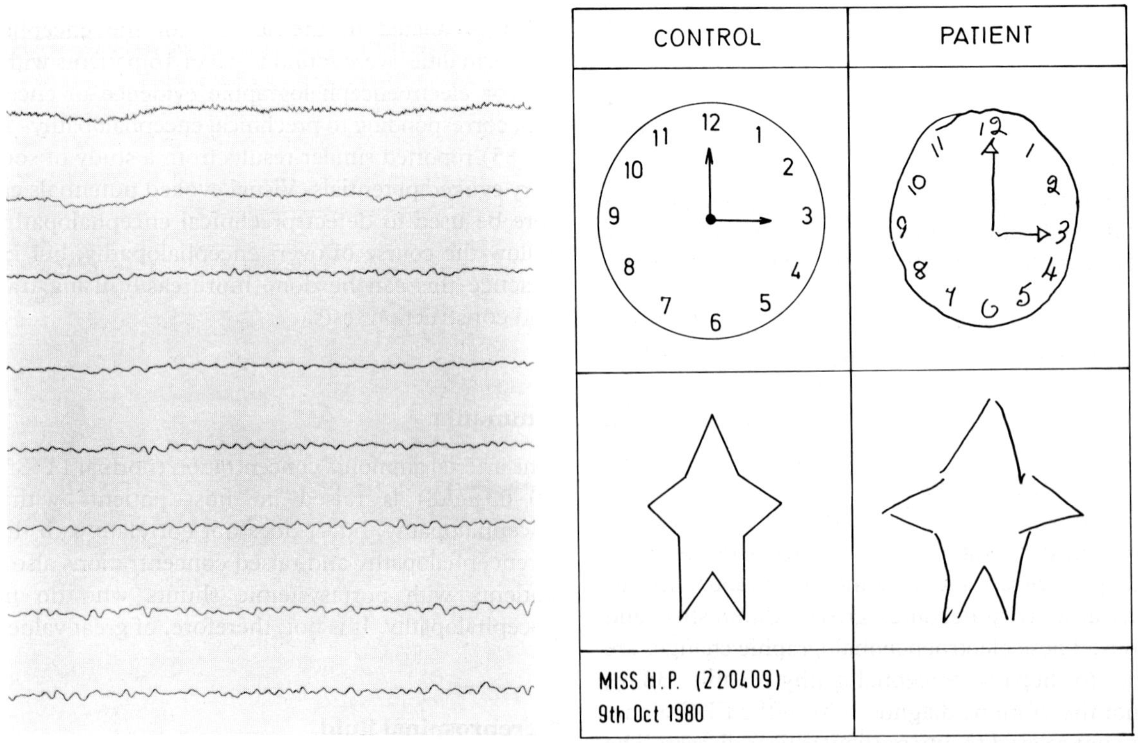


**Fig. 38.4** Improved construction tests and electroencephalogram after treatment in the patient with hepatic cirrhosis and encephalopathy shown in Fig. 38.3.*

*The electroencephalogram uses the 10–20 international electrode placement system and is of a longitudinal temporal montage alternating right and left.

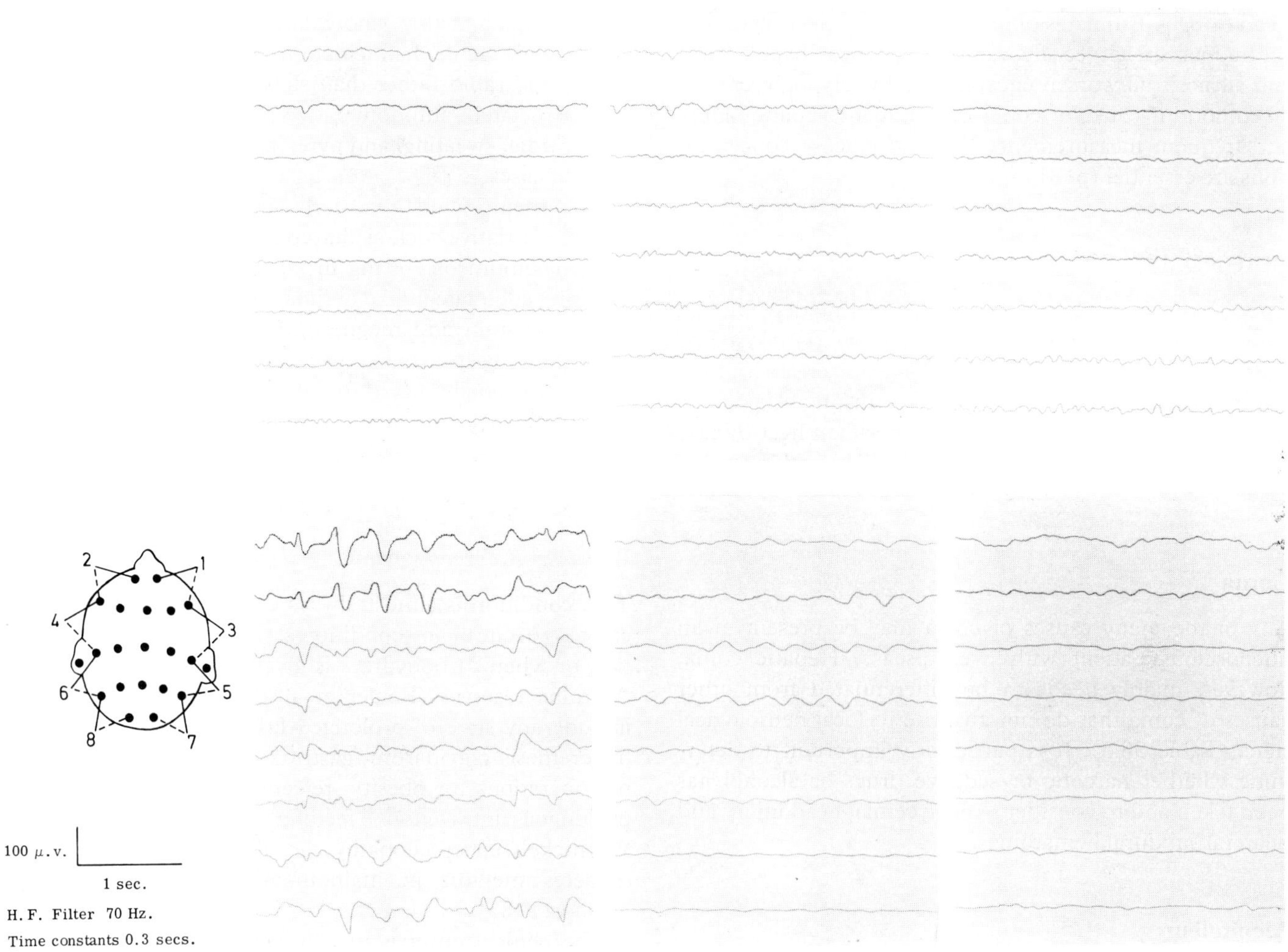


**Fig. 38.5** Electroencephalograms showing the normal appearances and the changes that occur with increasingly severe hepatic encephalopathy. All electroencephalograms use the 10–20 international electrode placement system and are of a longitudinal temporal montage alternating right and left.

**Table 38.6** Alternative causes of electroencephalographic changes typically seen in hepatic encephalopathy

| |
|---|
| Uremia |
| Hypercapnia |
| Hypoglycemia |
| Vitamin $B_{12}$ deficiency |

tion may be increased to about 1.3 g/L, but this occurs in only 6% of cases and an alternative explanation, such as infection or a tumor, should therefore be sought before such an increase is attributed to encephalopathy (Dillon & Schenker 1972). Bilirubin may cause xanthochromia but can be distinguished from other causes of this by spectrophotometry. Ammonia and glutamine concentrations are increased and the latter has been reported to differentiate patients with liver disease who do and do not have encephalopathy (p. 1040). In fulminant hepatic failure, the cerebrospinal fluid pressure may be increased due to cerebral edema (p. 809) and consequently very good reasons are needed to justify lumbar puncture in this condition.

*Acquired hepatocerebral degeneration*

A myelogram may be needed to exclude a space-occupying lesion in the spinal cord if this condition causes spastic paraplegia, although the absence of a sensory level may obviate the need. Myelography is normal in acquired hepatocerebral degeneration.

*Central pontine myelinolysis*

Computed tomography (Thompson et al 1981) or magnetic resonance imaging (DeWitt et al 1984) shows symmetrical pontine lesions and can also reveal lesions in other areas of the brain (p. 1044).

## Other investigations

These are used to differentiate hepatic encephalopathy from other causes of encephalopathy (below). They may also reveal factors precipitating or exacerbating encephalopathy

(Table 38.1). Estimates of plasma urea and electrolyte concentrations are especially valuable. Uremia, hypokalemia and alkalosis all worsen encephalopathy. Hypoglycemia is an important cause of coma in fulminant hepatic failure and frequent measurements of blood glucose concentrations are essential (p. 811).

## DIAGNOSIS

The diagnosis of hepatic encephalopathy depends on demonstrating hepatic disease and/or portasystemic shunting of blood in patients who have one or other of the syndromes described above. It must be distinguished from encephalopathy due to conditions other than liver disease and such conditions may coexist in patients with liver disease.

### Coma

Any of the many causes of coma may be present in an unconscious patient with liver disease. Hepatic coma, however, mainly needs to be differentiated from other causes of coma that do not give rise to focal neurological signs (Table 38.5). It is particularly important to determine whether narcotic or sedative drugs or alcohol has been taken and to consider hypoglycemia, head injury and bilateral subdural hematomas.

### Alcoholism

#### *Drunkenness*

Any patient with cirrhosis, and particularly those with alcoholic cirrhosis, can get drunk. This may be difficult to differentiate from encephalopathy and the blood ethanol concentration may have to be measured. It usually exceeds 30 mmol/L (150 mg/dl) in the drunk and 50 mmol/L (250 mg/dl) in the very drunk or comatose.

#### *Delirium tremens*

Delirium tremens often causes difficulty in alcoholic patients and it may prove impossible to differentiate from hepatic encephalopathy. Indeed, the two may coexist. Delirium tremens may develop during a drinking spree or after 3 or 4 days' abstinence, as following admission to hospital for an unrelated infection, operation or accident. The onset may be acute, but it is more often gradual with nervousness, anorexia and insomnia. The cardinal features are tremor, confusion and hallucination. In contrast to hepatic encephalopathy, the patient with delirium tremens is not drowsy, although inattention, incoherence and misrepresentation of the surroundings attest to altered consciousness. In addition, restlessness, anxiety, insomnia, incessant talking, anorexia and unpleasant auditory, visual and tactile hallucinations occur. The tremor is coarse and rapid rather than slow, irregular and flapping and associated autonomic overactivity causes flushing, tachycardia, sweating, and pyrexia. Convulsions occur in a third of cases.

Treatment includes the early and adequate administration of a sedative such as diazepam 20 mg orally every 2 h to a maximum of 160 mg in 24 h to control symptoms, ensuring adequate intake of fluid and electrolytes (particularly potassium and magnesium) and nursing with adequate lighting to avoid sensory deprivation. The sedative may occasionally need to be given intravenously and chlormethiazole should be avoided as its safety margins are narrow. It is also advisable to give these patients thiamine, as in Wernicke's encephalopathy (below).

#### *Wernicke–Korsakoff syndrome*

This condition is almost always due to alcoholism, but it can also occur in any condition associated with poor nutrition or when carbohydrate is given to patients with poor thiamine reserves (Reuler et al 1985). Such conditions include any state of prolonged fasting, anorexia nervosa, hyperemesis gravidarum, gastric carcinoma, gastrointestinal operations for obesity, refeeding after starvation and prolonged intravenous feeding or hyperalimentation. Wernicke's encephalopathy can also follow treatment of diabetes mellitus in malnourished patients (Kwee & Nakada 1983).

The clinical onset is usually gradual, with inability to concentrate, insomnia, vomiting and nystagmus. The patient is disorientated, has a marked loss of recent memory and compensates for the latter by confabulating. The cardinal feature is ophthalmoplegia, especially affecting the lateral rectus muscle, with horizontal, vertical or ataxic nystagmus and various defects of conjugate gaze. Ataxia of the limbs is frequent, retinal hemorrhages may be seen and peripheral neuropathy may be present coincidentally. Hypotension and hypothermia can also occur. Pontine myelinolysis may occur in Wernicke's encephalopathy and bulbar dysfunction or pyramidal signs should alert to this occurrence (Bergin & Harvey 1992).

Wernicke's encephalopathy should be suspected and treated whenever a few of these features occur in any of the clinical settings described, as classic features such as the triad of disorientation, ophthalmoplegia and ataxia occur in only a minority. This condition constitutes a medical emergency and requires immediate therapy to ensure the best chance of recovery. Thiamine 250 mg intravenously should be given at once and then daily for at least a week. Thereafter thiamine 50 mg daily should be given orally, preferably in a multivitamin preparation as multiple vitamin deficiencies are common in patients with liver disease (p. 922).

*Other*

Alcoholic dementia and alcoholic cerebellar degeneration may need to be differentiated from acquired hepatocerebral degeneration.

### Wilson's disease

This (p. 961) should always be considered in young patients. Confusion is most likely in patients with acquired hepatocerebral degeneration in which the cerebral features do not fluctuate. Patients with Wilson's disease are identified by the disordered copper metabolism.

### Cerebral diseases

Patients with liver disease are as liable to such cerebral disorders as cerebrovascular accidents, neoplasms, meningitis and subarachnoid hemorrhage as are persons who are otherwise well. When these develop, headache, meningism and focal or lateralizing neurological signs will usually suggest the diagnosis. Impaired coagulation in liver disease, however, increases the possibility of a subdural hematoma following injury to the head and alcoholic patients are obviously at particular risk. The injury is often trivial, may be forgotten and may have occurred several weeks before. Headache and disturbance of consciousness are prominent and frequently fluctuate, while focal or lateralizing signs often develop only at a late stage. Papilledema is not usually found. In doubtful cases, a space-occupying lesion should be sought and computed axial tomography is the method of choice. Lumbar puncture is contraindicated.

### Psychiatric disease

Hepatic encephalopathy may mimic or precipitate psychiatric illness. Such illnesses should be treated in their own right.

### Uremia

Some patients with advanced liver disease develop uremia (hepatorenal syndrome, p. 1057), which itself may cause cerebral symptoms. Such patients frequently also have hepatic encephalopathy, but the contributions of renal and hepatic dysfunction to the encephalopathy are usually impossible to separate.

## TREATMENT

Treatment of the hepatic encephalopathy of chronic liver disease depends on the removal of precipitating factors and on measures to alleviate the syndrome itself. The most important measures are to reduce the availability of nitrogenous material from which cerebral toxins can be produced and to reduce the production of such toxins by intestinal bacteria. Drugs that may alter the activity of cerebral neurotransmitters have been advocated, but they have not yet proved particularly effective. Encephalopathy in fulminant hepatic failure is due more to cerebral edema and does not respond to these measures (p. 809).

### General

Patients with clinical evidence of encephalopathy clearly require treatment, but those with latent encephalopathy can also benefit and this may be important in relation to employment or to driving motor vehicles (Plauth et al 1993). Long-term treatment with a protein-restricted diet is likely to exacerbate malnutrition in chronic liver disease and accordingly protein restrictions should be relaxed as far as possible when improvement occurs. Vegetable protein supplements can be used if they are tolerated by the patient and branched chain amino acid supplements can be considered although their nutritional value has not been established (Morgan 1990). Lactulose is the best single agent for long-term therapy, but lactitol may be needed for patients who cannot tolerate the sweet taste of lactulose or its side-effects. Antibiotics are best reserved for short-term use, particularly neomycin which may cause serious side-effects when given long term. Neomycin should never be used in established or developing renal failure. Patients may need advice in relation to their jobs and those with clinical evidence of encephalopathy should be advised not to drive motor vehicles.

### Precipitating factors

Several factor predispose to the development of encephalopathy (Table 38.1).

***Uremia.*** Uremia is the commonest of the precipitating factors and in about a half of cases it is precipitated by diuretic drugs. About a quarter of the normal production of urea enters the gut and is the source of some 80% of the ammonia produced there (Wolpert et al 1970). This ammonia is absorbed, enters the portal blood and is converted to urea by the normal liver. Uremia increases the availability of urea and the diseased liver is unable to metabolize the increased ammonia produced.

***Drugs.*** Diuretic drugs produce hypokalemic alkalosis, which increases ammonia production by the kidneys and facilitates the passage of amines and ammonia into cells (Fischer & Baldessarini 1976). Uremia precipitated by diuretic drugs is especially likely after a marked diuresis and in these cases, reduction of the blood volume may also diminish liver perfusion. Sedative drugs, tranquilizers and opiate analgesics precipitate encephalopathy readily and should be used cautiously in patients with clinical or biochemical evidence of poor liver function (p. 844). Propranolol (Tarver et al 1983) and cimetidine (Grahnén et al 1982) can also cause encephalopathy occasionally. Increased susceptibility to these drugs results mainly from increased cerebral sensitivity to their actions and in the case of the benzodiazepines, this may be related to an increased uptake of the drug into the brain and/or an increased number of benzodiazepine receptors on brain cells in chronic liver disease (Samson et al 1987). The ability of the liver to metabolize many of these drugs is also impaired in chronic liver disease and this allows accumulation of the drug in the blood (p. 842).

***Gastrointestinal bleeding.*** Gastrointestinal bleeding increases the amount of protein entering the gut and may impair liver function by reducing hepatic perfusion. Transfused blood may contain increased concentrations of ammonia.

***Other factors.*** Infection may worsen encephalopathy by inducing a catabolic state and increasing the availability of amino acids. Excess nitrogen intake and constipation, which increases amine production in the bowel, also worsen encephalopathy and are readily treated.

### Nitrogen intake

The relation between nitrogen intake and hepatic encephalopathy is now so well established that it is standard practice to reduce nitrogen intake when patients develop hepatic encephalopathy (Lancet 1983). It is usually sufficient to reduce protein intake to 20–40 g/day in patients with Grade 1 or 2 encephalopathy (Table 38.3) and protein intake is then increased by 10 g/day every third day as encephalopathy improves until a normal intake (60–80 g/day) is reached. If deterioration occurs, intake is reduced to the previously tolerated level. Patients with chronic liver disease need protein and in the long term adequate nutrition requires a protein intake of at least 40 g/day. Acute or severe encephalopathy (Grade 3 or 4 encephalopathy; Table 38.3) should be treated initially by withdrawal of all dietary protein until the encephalopathy improves. Glucose is given to provide 1500 kcal or more daily and a 20% solution can be administered into the superior vena cava to avoid water overloading if the intravenous route has to be used.

The view that abnormalities of amino acid metabolism and altered plasma concentrations of amino acids in cirrhosis may be important in the development of hepatic encephalopathy (p. 1041) has led to attempts to influence nutrition and encephalopathy by altering the type of protein and amino acids ingested.

***Vegetable protein.*** Diets that provide protein from vegetable sources rather than from animal sources reduce urea production and increase fecal nitrogen excretion but do not change plasma amino acid concentrations in patients with stable cirrhosis and no clinical evidence of hepatic encephalopathy (Weber et al 1985). Clinical trials have shown that diets substituting vegetable protein for animal protein can improve nitrogen balance in patients with encephalopathy but improvements in encephalopathy are marginal (Uribe et al 1982, Bianchi et al 1993). Vegetable protein diets are therefore only an adjunct to the treatment of hepatic encephalopathy, but their use in the long term might improve nutritional status. Unfortunately, most patients find exclusively vegetable protein diets bulky and unpalatable once protein intake reaches about 0.5–0.8 g/kg body weight per day and many complain of feeling bloated and of passing an excessive volume of flatus, so that compliance is poor. It seems reasonable to increase the vegetable component of dietary protein in these patients, but exclusively vegetable protein diets should be reserved for patients with chronic debilitating encephalopathy.

***Branched chain amino acids.*** Chronic liver disease is associated with an increase in the plasma concentrations of straight chain amino acids and a decrease in the concentrations of branched chain amino acids (p. 1041). Fischer et al (1976) found that amino acid infusions containing relatively large amounts of branched chain amino acids designed to correct the plasma amino acid imbalance improved hepatic encephalopathy and the electroencephalographic findings and reduced the blood ammonia even though the intake of nitrogen was increased. Unfortunately, controlled trials have given no more than equivocal support to these promising initial findings. Morgan (1990) has reviewed information on the use of branched chain amino acids given intravenously in acute episodes of hepatic encephalopathy and orally in chronic hepatic encephalopathy and concluded that there is no good evidence that they are effective. Branched chain amino acids can probably improve the nutritional condition of patients, but they are very expensive and may be no better than other sources of protein in nutritional terms.

### Antibiotics

Broad-spectrum antibiotics are established in the treatment of hepatic encephalopathy. They probably act by destroying enteric bacteria capable of producing ammonia and toxic amines from nitrogenous substrates (p. 1039). The most important of these are probably the urease-producing bacteria in the colon that can metabolize urea to ammonia. *Helicobacter pylori* in the stomach may also be important in patients infected with this organism (Gubbins et al 1993).

***Neomycin.*** This aminoglycoside, which is poorly absorbed from the bowel, remains the antibiotic of choice for treating hepatic encephalopathy. It is active mainly against aerobic Gram-negative bacilli and staphylococci and has little action against streptococci and anaerobes. Neomycin (1–2 g) is given orally every 6 h and neomycin elixir (100 mg/5 ml) may be used orally or rectally when patients cannot swallow. This treatment improves the electroencephalogram, reduces the blood ammonia concentration and can eliminate fetor hepaticus. Neomycin is not without serious side-effects, but these are uncommon. About 3% of an oral dose is absorbed and is excreted rapidly by the kidneys, so that blood concentrations remain low (Weinstein 1975). However, neomycin should not be used in uremia as the renal excretion is reduced, blood concentrations may reach potentially toxic levels (>10 μg/ml) and nerve deafness and renal damage can occur (Kunin et al 1960). Neomycin is also less desirable for long-term treatment, as patients can occasionally develop irreversible deafness despite normal blood urea and creatinine concentrations and low serum levels of neomycin (Berk & Chalmers 1970). Other side-effects include malabsorption (Dobbins et al 1968) and enteric superinfection (Bolton 1979).

***Metronidazole.*** Metronidazole is active against Bacteroides and other anaerobes now known to contribute significantly to colonic ammonia production and to produce potentially toxic amines. It has been shown to be effective in hepatic encephalopathy in a dose of 200 mg four times daily (Morgan et al 1982a).

***Tetracycline.*** Tetracyclines have also been used in treatment, but enteric superinfection is more likely and hepatic damage is possible when uremia is present (p. 977).

### Lactulose

Lactulose, a synthetic disaccharide composed of fructose and galactose, is effective in the treatment of hepatic encephalopathy and treatment is accompanied by improvement in the electroencephalogram and a fall in the blood ammonia concentration (Bircher et al 1971, Conn et al 1977, Conn & Lieberthal 1979). Lactulose is neither absorbed nor metabolized in the small intestine, but bacteria in the colon hydrolyze it to its components, fructose and galactose. These are then metabolized further to lactic and acetic acids, which cause a catharsis directly and by osmotic means, as well as a reduction of the stool pH. The mechanism of action of lactulose in alleviating encephalopathy is uncertain, but lactulose alters colonic bacterial metabolism so that less ammonia is produced and increased nitrogen excretion in the stools occurs probably in the form of ammonia precursors (Weber 1979, Weber & Fresard 1981). Lactulose may reduce colonic ammonia formation as it reduces colonic transit time and it also reduces ammonium ion absorption from the colon by reducing colonic pH.

Lactulose, which is contaminated with other sugars such as galactose and lactose, is given as a syrup (67 g/dl) in an initial dose of 20 ml thrice daily with meals. Thereafter, the dose must be adjusted, as the needs of individual patients vary greatly (20–200 ml/day). The aim is to produce two or three soft but solid stools daily, although it has been recommended that once the stool pH is consistently below 5.5, the actual habit is not important (Bircher et al 1971). Side-effects are few; diarrhea is eliminated by reducing the dose, urgency of bowel action can occur and can be unpredictable and abdominal cramps usually abate within a week. Some patients find the sweet taste intolerable, although it can be disguised by fruit juices. Diarrhea should be avoided, as it can cause serious fluid and electrolyte losses, sometimes with serious hypernatremia (Nelson et al 1983). Lactulose may also be given as an enema.

### Other carbohydrates

***Lactitol.*** Lactitol is a disaccharide composed of galactose and sorbitol that is effective in treating hepatic encephalopathy (Morgan & Hawley 1987). It acts in a manner similar to lactulose and is given in a dose of 0.5–0.75 g/kg body weight/day to produce two soft stools daily. It is less sweet and therefore more palatable than lactulose and is said to produce a less urgent bowel action.

***Lactose.*** Lactose is an effective substitute for lactulose in encephalopathic patients who are known to be lactase deficient. Lactose enemas (1000 ml of 10% solution thrice daily) are also effective in acute hepatic encephalopathy (Uribe et al 1981). Lactulose and lactose presumably act in a similar way in the colon.

***Sorbitol.*** Sorbitol is a food sweetener and cathartic that is metabolized in the colon in a manner similar to lactulose. It has been used as a placebo in hepatic encephalopathy, but it is probably effective in its own right as 30 ml of 20% three times daily has improved psychomotor function in patients with cirrhosis (McClain et al 1981).

### Other laxatives

Lactulose and the other carbohydrates discussed above are all laxatives and catharsis may be one way in which they alleviate hepatic encephalopathy. Magnesium sulfate 5–15 g/day is a laxative that is often used with benefit in hepatic encephalopathy. It increases stool weight, stool solids and stool nitrogen to the same extent as lactulose, but it does not reduce urea production or reduce the fecal pH (Weber & Fresard 1981).

### Combined treatment

Lactulose and neomycin are often given simultaneously, although it is not certain that their effects in alleviating encephalopathy are additive. They do, however, seem to have an additive effect in reducing ammonia production (Weber et al 1982).

## Surgery

When encephalopathy persists despite medical therapy, surgery has been advocated to exclude colonic bacteria from continuity with the intestinal tract. Ileosigmoidostomy has been used most often and can improve encephalopathy, reduce the need for medical therapy and increase protein tolerance (Resnick et al 1968, Talman et al 1983). The operative mortality, even in patients who are considered reasonable operative risks, is about 25% and growth of a colonic flora in the terminal ileum after operation may lead to recurrence of encephalopathy. Loop ileostomy has been suggested as a simpler operation applicable and effective even in patients with advanced disease (Hebbard et al 1993).

## Other treatments

Several treatments have been proposed for patients who fail to respond to protein restriction, lactulose and neomycin.

### *Benzodiazepine inhibitors*

The benzodiazepine receptor in the brain and benzodiazepine receptor ligands have been implicated in hepatic encephalopathy (p. 1043) and consequently the benzodiazepine inhibitor flumazenil has been used to treat this condition. Rapid improvement occurred when flumazenil (2 mg in 20 ml saline) was given by intravenous infusion over 5 min in about a half of patients and was unrelated to finding benzodiazepine in the blood (Pomier-Layrargues et al 1994). Flumazenil is then beneficial, at least transiently, in some patients, but its place in the longer term treatment of hepatic encephalopathy remains to be determined.

### *Others*

Levodopa and bromocriptine, which act on the dopamine neurotransmitter system, have been used without any consistent success. Measures designed to reduce ammonia production have been tried, but none has proved effective. They include feeding lactobacilli, which do not produce urease, to displace urease-producing bacteria from the bowel, the use of acetohydroxamic acid, which is an inhibitor of urease and injections of jackbean urease to produce antiurease antibodies.

## Summary

Most patients respond well to the removal of factors precipitating encephalopathy, restriction of protein intake, the prevention of constipation and the use of lactulose and/or antibiotics. The minimum therapy needed should be used and patients who recover from an episode of encephalopathy may not require continuous treatment. Therapy should allow the patient as good a protein intake as possible once the more severe features have been controlled. Few remain incapacitated and where liver transplantation is not appropriate, a vegetable protein diet or branched chain amino acid supplements could be considered. Colonic surgery is rarely needed.

## REFERENCES

Adams R D, Foley J M 1953 Neurological disorder associated with liver disease. Association for Research in Nervous and Mental Disease, Proceedings 32: 198–237

Adams R D, Victor M, Mancall E L 1959 Central pontine myelinolysis. A hitherto undescribed disease occurring in alcoholic and malnourished patients. Archives of Neurology and Psychiatry 81: 154–172

Al Mardini H, Harrison E J, Ince P G, Bartlett K, Record C O 1993 Brain indoles in human hepatic encephalopathy. Hepatology 17: 1033–1040

Aminoff M J 1986 Evoked potentials in clinical medicine. Quarterly Journal of Medicine 59: 345–362

Bergin P S, Harvey P 1992 Wernicke's encephalopathy and central pontine myelinolysis associated with hyperemesis gravidarum. British Medical Journal 305: 517–518

Berk D P, Chalmers T 1970 Deafness complicating antibiotic therapy of hepatic encephalopathy. Annals of Internal Medicine 73: 393–396

Bianchi G P, Marchesini G, Fabbri A et al 1993 Vegetable versus animal protein diet in cirrhotic patients with chronic encephalopathy. A randomized cross-over comparison. Journal of Internal Medicine 233: 385–392

Bircher J, Haemmerli U P, Scollo-Lavizzari G, Hoffmann K 1971 Treatment of chronic portal-systemic encephalopathy with lactulose. Report of six patients and review of the literature. American Journal of Medicine 51: 148–169

Blei A T 1991 Cerebral edema and intracranial hypertension in acute liver failure: distinct aspects of the same problem. Hepatology 13: 376–379

Bolton R P 1979 *Clostridium difficile*-associated colitis after neomycin treated with metronidazole. British Medical Journal 2: 1479–1480

Bradbury M W B 1979 The concept of a blood–brain barrier. Wiley, Chichester

Chen S, Zieve L, Mahadevan V 1970 Mercaptans and dimethylsulfide in the breath of patients with cirrhosis of the liver. Journal of Laboratory and Clinical Medicine 75: 628–635

Chesta J, Defilippi C, Defilippi C 1993 Abnormalities in proximal bowel motility in patients with cirrhosis. Hepatology 17: 828–832

Conn H O 1977 Trailmaking and number-connection tests in the assessment of mental state in portal-systemic encephalopathy. American Journal of Digestive Diseases 22: 541–550

Conn H O, Lieberthal M M 1979 The hepatic coma syndromes and lactulose. Williams and Wilkins, Baltimore

Conn H O, Leevy C M, Vlahcevic Z R et al 1977 Comparison of lactulose and neomycin in the treatment of chronic portal-systemic encephalopathy: a double blind controlled trial. Gastroenterology 72: 573–583

Crippin J S, Gross J B, Lindor K D 1992 Increased intracranial pressure and hepatic encephalopathy in chronic liver disease. American Journal of Gastroenterology 87: 879–882

Crossley I R, Wardle E N, Williams R 1983 Biochemical mechanisms of hepatic encephalopathy. Clinical Science 64: 247–252

Dawson A M 1978 Regulation of blood ammonia. Gut 19: 504–509

Degos F, Degos J-D, Bourdiau D et al 1974 Experimental acute hepatic encephalopathy: comparison of the electroencephalographic changes in the liverless and in the eviscerated rat. Clinical Science and Molecular Medicine 47: 599–608

DeWitt L D, Buonanno F S, Kistler J P et al 1984 Central pontine myelinolysis: demonstration by nuclear magnetic resonance. Neurology 34: 570–576

Dillon D, Schenker S 1972 Cerebrospinal fluid protein concentration in hepatic coma. Journal of the American Medical Association 221: 507

Dobbins W O III, Herrero B A, Mansbach C M 1968 Morphologic alterations associated with neomycin induced malabsorption. American Journal of the Medical Sciences 255: 63–77

Drayna C J, Titcomb C P, Varma R R, Soergel K H 1981 Hyperammonemic encephalopathy caused by infection in a neurogenic bladder. New England Journal of Medicine 304: 766–768

Fahey J L 1957 Toxicity and blood ammonia rise resulting from intravenous amino acid administration in man: the protective effect of L-arginine. Journal of Clinical Investigation 36: 1647–1655

Ferenci P, Pappas S C, Munson P J, Jones E A 1984 Changes in glutamate receptors on synaptic membranes associated with hepatic encephalopathy or hyperammonemia in the rabbit. Hepatology 4: 25–29

Fessel J M, Conn H O 1972 An analysis of the causes and prevention of hepatic coma. Gastroenterology 62: 191

Fischer J E, Baldessarini R J 1976 Pathogenesis and therapy of hepatic coma. In: Popper H, Schaffner F (eds) Progress in liver diseases (Vol 5). Grune & Stratton, New York. p 363–397

Fischer J E, Rosen H M, Ebeid A M, James J H, Keane J M, Soeters P B 1976. The effect of normalization of plasma amino acids on hepatic encephalopathy in man. Surgery 80: 77–91

Fraser C L, Arieff A I 1985 Hepatic encephalopathy. New England Journal of Medicine 313: 865–873

Gitlin N, Lewis D C, Hinkley L 1986 The diagnosis and prevalence of subclinical hepatic encephalopathy in apparently healthy, ambulant, non-shunted patients with cirrhosis. Journal of Hepatology 3: 75–82

Goldstein G W 1984 The role of brain capillaries in the pathogenesis of hepatic encephalopathy. Hepatology 4: 565–567

Gooday R, Bezizi K, O'Carroll R, Hayes P C 1995 Benzodiazepine receptor antagonism improves reaction time in latent hepatic encephalopathy. Psychopharmacology 19: 295–298

Grahnén A, Tyllström J, Tyllström B, Jameson S, Lööf L 1982 Cimetidine accumulation and mental confusion in cirrhosis. New England Journal of Medicine 307: 187

Grazer R E, Sutton J M, Friedstrom S, McBarron F D 1984 Hyperammonemic encephalopathy due to essential amino acid hyperalimentation. Archives of Internal Medicine 144: 2278–2279

Gubbins G P, Moritz T E, Marsano L S et al 1993 *Helicobacter pylori* is a risk factor for hepatic encephalopathy in acute alcoholic hepatitis: the ammonia hypothesis revisited. American Journal of Gastroenterology 88: 1906–1910

Häussinger D 1989 Glutamine metabolism in the liver: overview and current concepts. Metabolism 38 (suppl 1): 14–17

Hawkes C H, Brunt P W 1974 The current status of the EEG in liver disease. American Journal of Digestive Diseases 19: 75–80

Hebbard G S, Jenney A W J, Gibson P R, Jacobs R, Penfold J C B 1993 Chronic hepatic encephalopathy following portacaval shunt: management by loop ileostomy. Australian and New Zealand Journal of Surgery 63: 231–234

Hourani B T, Reynolds T B 1971 Cerebrospinal fluid glutamine as a measure of hepatic encephalopathy. Archives of Internal Medicine 127: 1033–1036

Hoyumpa A M 1986 The unfolding GABA story. Hepatology 6: 1042–1044

Jalan R, Seery J P, Taylor-Robinson S D 1996 Review article: pathogenesis and treatment of chronic hepatic encephalopathy 10: 681–697

James J H, Ziparo V, Jeppsson B, Fischer J E 1979 Hyperammonaemia, plasma aminoacid imbalance, and blood–brain amino acid transport: a unified theory of portal-systemic encephalopathy. Lancet 2: 772–775

Jones E A, Schafer D F, Ferenci P. Pappas S C 1984 The neurobiology of hepatic encephalopathy. Hepatology 4: 1235–1242

Kardel T, Lund Y, Zander Olsen P, Möllgaard V, Gammeltoft A 1970 Encephalopathy and portacaval anastomosis. Scandinavian Journal of Gastroenterology 5: 681–685

Kato M, Hughes R D, Keays R T, Williams R 1992 Electronmicroscopic study of brain capillaries in cerebral edema from fulminant hepatic failure. Hepatology 15: 1060–1066

Klimberg V S, Souba W W 1990 The importance of intestinal glutamine metabolism in maintaining a healthy gastrointestinal tract and supporting the body's response to injury and illness. Annals of Surgery 20: 61–76

Knudsen G M, Schmidt J, Almdal P, Paulson O B, Vilstrup H 1993 Passage of amino acids and glucose across the blood–brain barrier in patients with hepatic encephalopathy. Hepatology 17: 987–992

Kreiger D T 1983 Brain peptides: what, where and why? Science 222: 975–985

Kunin C M, Chalmers T C, Leevy C M, Sebastyen S C, Lieber C S, Finland M 1960 Absorption of orally administered neomycin and kanamycin with special reference to patients with severe hepatic and renal disease. New England Journal of Medicine 262: 380–385

Kwee I L, Nakada T 1983 Wernicke's encephalopathy induced by tolazamide. New England Journal of Medicine 309: 599–600

Lancet 1983 Leading article: diet and hepatic encephalopathy. Lancet 1: 625–626

Laureno R, Karp B I 1988 Pontine and extrapontine myelinolysis following rapid correction of hyponatraemia. Lancet 1: 1439–1441

Lavoie J, Giguère J-F, Pomier-Layrargues G, Butterworth R F 1987 Amino acid changes in autopsied brain tissue from cirrhotic patients with hepatic encephalopathy. Journal of Neurochemistry 49: 692–697

Lockwood A H 1987 Hepatic encephalopathy: experimental approaches to human metabolic encephalopathy. CRC Critical Reviews in Neurobiology 3: 105–133

Lockwood A H, Yap E W H, Wong W-H 1991 Cerebral ammonia metabolism in patients with severe liver disease and minimal hepatic encephalopathy. Journal of Cerebral Blood Flow and Metabolism 11: 337–341

Lockwood A H, Murphy B W, Donnelly K Z, Mahl T C, Perini S 1993 Positron-emission tomographic localization of abnormalities of brain metabolism in patient with minimal hepatic encephalopathy. Hepatology 18: 1061–1068

McClain C J, Kromhout J P, Zieve L, Duane W C 1981 Effect of sorbitol on psychomotor function. Its use in alcoholic cirrhosis. Archives of Internal Medicine 141: 901–903

Mendoza G, Marti-Fàbregas J, Kulisevsky J, Escartín A 1994 Hepatic myelopathy: a rare complication of portacaval shunt. European Neurology 34: 209–212

Morgan M H, Read A E, Speller D C E 1982a Treatment of hepatic encephalopathy with metronidazole. Gut 23: 1–7

Morgan M Y 1990 Branched chain amino acids in the management of chronic liver disease. Facts and fantasies. Journal of Hepatology 11: 133–141

Morgan M Y, Hawley K E 1987 Lactitol vs. lactulose in the treatment of acute hepatic encephalopathy in cirrhotic patients: a double-blind, randomized trial. Hepatology 7: 1278–1284

Morgan M Y, Milsom J P, Sherlock S 1978 Plasma ratio of valine, leucine and isoleucine to phenylalanine and tyrosine in liver disease. Gut 19: 1068–1073

Morgan M Y, Marshall A W, Milsom J P, Sherlock S 1982b Plasma amino-acid patterns in liver disease. Gut 23: 362–370

Mullen K D, Basile A S 1993 Benzodiazepine-receptor antagonists and hepatic encephalopathy: where do we stand? Gastroenterology 105: 937–940

Nance F C, Kline D G 1971 Eck's fistula encephalopathy in germfree dogs. Annals of Surgery 174: 856–862

Nelson D C, McGrew W R G, Hoyumpa A M 1983 Hypernatremia and lactulose therapy. Journal of the American Medical Association 249: 1295–1298

O'Carroll R E, Hayes P C, Ebmeier K P et al 1991 Regional cerebral blood flow and cognitive function in patients with chronic liver disease. Lancet 337: 1250–1253

Ono J, Hutson D G, Dombro R S, Levi J U, Livingstone A, Zeppa R 1978 Tryptophan and hepatic coma. Gastroenterology 74: 196–200

Onstad G R, Zieve L 1979 What determines blood ammonia? Gastroenterology 77: 803–805

Perry E K 1991 Neurotransmitters and diseases of the brain. British Journal of Hospital Medicine 45: 73–83

Plauth M, Egberts E-H, Hamster W et al 1993 Long-term treatment of latent portosystemic encephalopathy with branched-chain amino acids. Journal of Hepatology 17: 308–314

Pomier-Layrargues G, Giguère J F, Lavoie J et al 1994 Flumazenil in cirrhotic patients in hepatic coma: a randomized double-blind placebo-controlled crossover trial. Hepatology 19: 32–37

Prensky A L 1984 Time – a fourth dimension for encephalopathies. New England Journal of Medicine 310: 1527–1529

Record C O 1991 Neurochemistry of hepatic encephalopathy. Gut 32: 1261–1263

Record C O, Buxton B, Chase R A, Curzon G, Murray-Lyon I M, Williams R 1976 Plasma and brain amino acids in fulminant hepatic failure and their relationship to hepatic encephalopathy. European Journal of Clinical Investigation 6: 387–394

Resnick R H, Ishihara A, Chalmers T C, Schimmel E M and The Boston Inter-Hospital Liver Group 1968 A controlled trial of colon bypass in chronic hepatic encephalopathy. Gastroenterology 54: 1057–1069

Reuler J B, Girard D E, Cooney T G 1985 Current concepts: Wernicke's encephalopathy. New England Journal of Medicine 312: 1035–1039

Rosenblum J L, Keating J P, Prensky A L, Nelson J S 1981 A progressive neurologic syndrome in children with chronic liver disease. New England Journal of Medicine 304: 503–508

Rossi-Fanelli F, Riggio O, Cangiano C et al 1982 Branched-chain amino acids vs lactulose in the treatment of hepatic coma. A controlled study. Digestive Diseases and Sciences 27: 929–935

Rothstein J D 1994 Benzodiazepine-receptor ligands and hepatic encephalopathy: a causal relationship? Hepatology 19: 248–250

Samson Y, Bernuau J, Pappata S, Chavoix C, Baron J C, Magiere M A 1987 Cerebral uptake of benzodiazepine measured by positron emission tomography in hepatic encephalopathy. New England Journal of Medicine 316: 414

Schafer D F, Fowler J M, Jones E A 1981 Colonic bacteria: a source of γ-aminobutyric acid in blood. Proceedings of the Society of Experimental Biology and Medicine 167: 301–303

Schafer D F, Jones E A 1982 Hepatic encephalopathy and the γ-aminobutyric acid neurotransmitter system. Lancet 1: 18–20

Schalm S W, Van Der May T 1979 Hyperammonemic coma after hepatectomy in germ-free rats. Gastroenterology 77: 231–234

Schenker S, Breen K J, Hoyumpa A M Jr 1974 Hepatic encephalopathy: current status. Gastroenterology 66: 121–151

Schomerus H, Hamster W, Blunck H, Reinhard U, Mayer K, Dölle W 1981 Latent portasystemic encephalopathy I. Nature of cerebral functional defects and their effect on fitness to drive. Digestive Diseases and Sciences 26: 622–630

Shindo K, Machida M, Miyakawa K, Fukumura M 1993 A syndrome of cirrhosis, achlorohydria, small intestinal bacterial overgrowth, and fat malabsorption. American Journal of Gastroenterology 88: 2084–2091

Stahl J 1963 Studies of the blood ammonia in liver disease. Its diagnostic, prognostic and therapeutic significance. Annals of Internal Medicine 58: 1–24

Stell R, Davis S, Carroll W M 1994 Unilateral asterixis due to a lesion of the ventrolateral thalamus. Journal of Neurology, Neurosurgery and Psychiatry 57: 116–118

Szerb J C, Butterworth R F 1992 Effect of ammonium ions on synaptic transmission in the mammalian central nervous system. Progress in Neurobiology 39: 135–153

Talman E A, Johns T N P, Regan W W 1983 A 25-year experience with total portosystemic shunts with reappraisal of colon exclusion. Annals of Surgery 197: 566–573

Tarter R E, Hegedus A M, Van Thiel D H, Schade R R, Gavaler J S, Starzl T E 1984 Nonalcoholic cirrhosis associated with neuropsychological dysfunction in the absence of overt evidence of hepatic encephalopathy. Gastroenterology 86: 1421–1427

Tarter R E, Hays A L, Sandford S S, Van Thiel D H 1986 Cerebral morphological abnormalities associated with non-alcoholic cirrhosis. Lancet 2: 893–895

Tarver D, Walt R P, Dunk A A, Jenkins W J, Sherlock S 1983 Precipitation of hepatic encephalopathy of propranolol in cirrhosis. British Medical Journal 287: 585

Thomas P K 1986 Brain atrophy and alcoholism. British Medical Journal 292: 787

Thompson D S, Hutton J T, Stears J C, Sung J H, Norenberg M 1981 Computerized tomography in the diagnosis of central and extra pontine myelinolysis. Archives of Neurology 38: 243–246

Trey C, Burns D G, Saunders S J 1966 Treatment of hepatic coma by exchange blood transfusions. New England Journal of Medicine 274: 473–481

Uribe M, Berthier J M, Lewis H et al 1981 Lactose enemas plus placebo tablets vs. neomycin tablets plus starch enemas in acute portal systemic encephalopathy. Gastroenterology 81: 101–106

Uribe M, Ramos-Uribe M H, Vargas F, Villalobos A, Ramos C 1982 The treatment of chronic portal-systemic encephalopathy with vegetable and animal protein diets. A controlled cross-over study. Digestive Diseases and Sciences 27: 1109–1116

Van Thiel D H, Fagiuoli S, Wright H I, Chien M-C, Gavaler J S 1994 Gastrointestinal transit in cirrhotic patients: effect of hepatic encephalopathy and its treatment. Hepatology 19: 67–71

Victor M, Adams R D, Cole M 1965 The acquired (non-Wilsonian) type of chronic hepatocerebral degeneration. Medicine 44: 345–396

Voorhies T M, Ehrlich M E, Duffy T E, Petito C K, Plum F 1983 Acute hyperammonemia in the young primate: physiologic and neuropathologic correlates. Pediatric Research 17: 970–975

Watson A J, Karp J E, Walker W G, Chalmers T, Risch V R, Brusilow S W 1985 Transient idiopathic hyperamonaemia in adults. Lancet 2: 1271–1274

Weber F L Jr 1979 The effect of lactulose on urea metabolism and nitrogen excretion in cirrhotic patients. Gastroenterology 77: 518–523

Weber F L Jr, Fresard K M 1981 Comparative effects of lactulose and magnesium sulfate on urea metabolism and nitrogen excretion in cirrhotic subjects. Gastroenterology 80: 994–998

Weber F L Jr, Fresard K M, Lally B R 1982 Effects of lactulose and neomycin on urea metabolism in cirrhotic subjects. Gastroenterology 82: 213–219

Weber F L Jr, Minco D, Fresard K M, Banwell J G 1985 Effects of vegetable diets on nitrogen metabolism in cirrhotic subjects. Gastroenterology 89: 538–544

Weinstein L 1975 Antimicrobial agents. In: Goodman L S, Gilman A (eds) The pharmacological basis of therapeutics, 5th edn. Macmillan, New York, p 1167–1247

Wolpert E, Phillips S F, Summerskill W H J 1970 Ammonia production in the human colon. Effects of cleansing, neomycin and acetohydroxamic acid. New England Journal of Medicine 283: 159–164

Yang S-S, Chu N-S, Liaw Y-F 1985 Somatosensory evoked potentials in hepatic encephalopathy. Gastroenterology 89: 625–630

Zeneroli M L, Pinelli G, Gollini G et al 1984 Visual evoked potential: a diagnostic tool for the assessment of hepatic encephalopathy. Gut 25: 291–299

Zieve L 1981 The mechanism of hepatic coma. Hepatology 1: 360–365

# 39. Renal dysfunction in hepatobiliary disease

*Charles P. Swainson*

The liver and the kidneys are the major excretory organs of the body and failure of either leads to serious risks of fluid overload, sepsis and bleeding. Such failure may be caused by related or unrelated conditions. Renal failure in liver disease may be due to factors that damage both organs simultaneously, such as infections, circulatory disorders and toxins, to diseases affecting both organs independently such as polycystic disease or to chronic renal disease that may or may not be related to chronic liver disease (Table 39.1). Renal failure can also occur in the absence of any other identifiable cause in patients with chronic parenchymal liver disease or biliary tract obstruction. This last form of renal failure, which is usually a functional result of hepatobiliary disease, has been called the hepatorenal syndrome and has been reviewed extensively (Arroyo et al 1988, Epstein 1988, Sherlock 1993). In addition, end-stage renal failure due to structural damage to the kidneys in chronic liver disease can occur and renal tubular dysfunction consequent on poor liver function causes sodium retention, water retention and occasionally renal tubular acidosis.

This chapter considers functional renal failure and renal tubular dysfunction in chronic liver disease, renal failure in biliary disease and end-stage renal failure which may be a consequence of liver disease. Renal dysfunction in acute liver disease is considered elsewhere (p. 811).

**Table 39.1** Causes of coincident renal and hepatic disease (Conn 1973)

| |
|---|
| *Generalized disorders* |
| Infectious |
| Gram-negative septicemia |
| Leptospirosis |
| Yellow fever |
| Circulatory |
| Shock |
| Congestive heart failure |
| Genetic |
| Sickle cell anemia |
| Vasculitis |
| Systemic lupus erythematosus |
| Polyarteritis nodosa |
| Unknown etiology |
| Toxemia of pregnancy |
| Amyloidosis |
| Sarcoidosis |
| Waterhouse–Friedrichson syndrome |
| Hyperthermia |
| Reye's syndrome |
| *Toxins* |
| Direct |
| Carbon tetrachloride |
| Paracetamol |
| Paraquat |
| Chromium |
| Mushroom toxins |
| Idiosyncratic or mixed |
| Methoxyflurane |
| Tetracyclines |
| Streptomycin |
| Sulfonamides |
| Iproniazid |
| *Neoplasms* |
| Metastatic |
| Hypernephroma |
| *Chronic renal and hepatic disease* |
| Related |
| Polycystic disease |
| Amyloid |
| Cirrhotic glomerulonephritis |
| Unrelated |
| *The hepatorenal syndrome* (functional renal failure) |

## RENAL DYSFUNCTION IN CIRRHOSIS

Oliguric renal failure in cirrhosis has been recognized since 1863 (Papper 1983). It is usually attributed to functional renal failure, but it can also be caused by acute tubular necrosis or by associated end-stage renal disease.

### Functional renal failure

The term "hepatorenal syndrome" was introduced in 1932 to denote a form of renal failure occurring after biliary tract surgery, but it was applied subsequently to such a wide range of conditions characterized by hepatic and renal dysfunction (Table 39.1) that it ceased to have any precise meaning (Papper 1983). Later, attention became focused on renal failure developing for no identifiable cause in patients with liver disease (Hecker & Sherlock 1956). These patients almost always have advanced cirrhosis. This is the form of renal dysfunction in liver disease to which the term "hepatorenal syndrome" should now be applied. A number of alternative names for the syndrome have been suggested; of these, "functional renal failure" avoids the confusion surrounding the original term, does not imply any particular hepatorenal mechanism and conforms to current conceptions of the development of renal dysfunction.

Renal hemodynamic abnormalities are thought to underlie functional renal failure, but no unifying explanation of these changes has been agreed. It may be that they are caused by several mechanisms operating in a related way. Evidence exists that both primary sodium retention and a decrease in "effective" blood volume contribute to circulatory changes in the same patients and at different times and there is also substantial evidence for a central role of abnormal activation of the sympathetic nervous system (below). It seems likely that many of the hormonal changes observed are secondary and are mainly important in maintaining glomerular filtration in the face of markedly reduced renal blood flow.

*Occurrence*

Renal dysfunction in cirrhosis is common. Three-quarters or more of patients with advanced cirrhosis have a raised blood urea concentration not associated with primary renal or cardiac disease and in a half of these uremia is severe (Shear et al 1965). The features of renal dysfunction are not specific to functional renal failure and include diminished renal blood flow, diminished glomerular filtration rate, oliguria and an altered diurnal rhythm of urine excretion (Shear et al 1965, Kew et al 1971). It seems likely that most patients with advanced cirrhosis have a characteristic circulatory disturbance (p. 920), consisting of a tendency to arterial hypotension, reduced renal blood flow and avid renal sodium retention. Patients with functional renal failure represent the extreme of a spectrum of disturbances in salt and water homeostasis.

*Recognition*

Functional renal failure can be diagnosed from the criteria outlined in Table 39.2. This combination of features is typical of a reduction in renal cortical perfusion. It is important to exclude reversible, prerenal acute renal failure defined as an abrupt decrease in glomerular filtration caused by hypoperfusion (Arroyo et al 1996). This is often the result of volume depletion, acute cardiac disease or sepsis.

**Table 39.2** Diagnostic criteria for functional renal failure in cirrhosis (Papper 1983)

| |
|---|
| *General* |
| Cirrhosis of the liver |
| No primary cause of renal disease |
| No other known cause of acute/chronic renal failure |
| Acute or subacute onset of progressive renal failure |
| No sustained improvement after volume expansion (p. 1062) |
| *Renal* |
| Reduced glomerular filtration rate |
| Urine sodium concentration $<10$ mmol/L |
| Urine/plasma osmolality ratio $>1.2$ |
| Fractional sodium excretion $<1\%$* |

*Fractional sodium excretion can be calculated on a random urine as $(U[Na]/P[Na]) \times (P[creatinine]/U[creatinine]) \times 100$ when urinary (U) and plasma (P) concentrations of sodium and creatinine are all in mmol/L.

*Pathology*

Renal lesions are common at autopsy in patients with cirrhosis irrespective of uremia during life (p. 1065). These lesions may sometimes cause renal failure, but in most cases they are insufficient to account for renal failure. Indeed, transplant operations have demonstrated normal intrinsic renal functional capacity in most patients with cirrhosis. Koppel et al (1969) transplanted kidneys from patients who had died of cirrhosis with functional renal failure into seven patients with terminal renal disease; in five recipients, diuresis began within 6–14 days, creatinine clearance values of 52 ml/min were achieved and no recipient died of renal failure. Conversely, Iwatsuki et al (1973) found that liver transplantation in three patients with cirrhosis and functional renal failure led to immediate restoration of liver function followed by improvement in renal function over about 2 weeks. These findings indicate that normal renal function depends in some unknown way on normal liver function and experiments in rats have shown that the function of an isolated perfused kidney is significantly prolonged when the liver is included in the perfusion circuit (Mondon et al 1969).

*Circulatory disturbances*

The extrarenal circulation in patients with cirrhosis is abnormal (p. 920) and two main theories have been advanced to account for this. The "underfilling" theory suggests that peripheral vasodilatation combined with the formation of ascites occurs at the expense of the systemic circulation, which is thereby depleted (Schrier et al 1988). Greatly increased splanchnic and pulmonary circulations, a general reduction in systemic vascular resistance, elevated plasma concentrations of catecholamines and of other vasoactive hormones, such as renin, and impaired pressor responses to vasoconstrictors provide evidence of chronic underfilling of the circulation. Numerous observations demonstrate that circulatory improvement can occur in these patients after volume replacement. A brisk natriuresis ensues after volume expansion, reinfusion of ascitic fluid or surgical diversion of the thoracic duct drainage into the venous system, which increases lymphatic return. However, these maneuvers do not work in all patients and improvement is always temporary (Tristani & Cohn 1967). Thus, effective volume depletion, whether absolute or relative, cannot be the only explanation for renal dysfunction.

A second theory, called the "overflow" theory, suggests that renal sodium retention is a primary event causing plasma volume expansion and later ascites (Lieberman et al 1969). Support has come from observations of spontaneous natriuresis in some patients, which may be independent of measurable changes in circulating volume, and of failure to demonstrate a normal "escape" from the sodium-retaining effects of mineralocorticoids. Experimental studies in cirrhotic dogs have shown that renal sodium retention can precede the formation of ascites and that nonportal blood volume increases markedly in this experimental preparation (Levy 1983). The overflow theory does not explain how natriuresis occurs after volume expansion and neither can it account for the changes in vasoactive hormones observed in many of these patients.

A third theory points to the size of the arterial circulation rather than the plasma volume as the main determinant of renal sodium retention (p. 1017).

*Renal blood flow*

Patients with cirrhosis have a hyperdynamic circulation with diminished peripheral vascular resistance that becomes more pronounced as the disease progresses (p. 920). In the early stages of the disease, when general health and liver function is good and before ascites or hypoalbuminemia has developed, renal vascular resistance is reduced and renal blood flow and glomerular filtration rate are increased (Wong et al 1993). Renal blood flow falls as liver disease progresses, even in patients whose disease remains well compensated and where the glomerular filtration rate is normal (Kew et al 1971, Epstein 1988), and renal blood flow and glomerular filtration rate are both considerably reduced once oliguria is present (Tristani & Cohn 1967). In general, total renal blood flow falls progressively, renal hemodynamics become more unstable and renal function deteriorates with increasingly severe cirrhosis.

Investigations have also shown that reduction in renal blood flow does not affect the kidney uniformly but is particularly marked in the outer renal cortex. This maldistribution becomes more severe in advanced disease and, as in any form of acute renal failure, poor outer cortical perfusion is associated with low glomerular filtration rates. Angiography in patients with terminal disease has revealed severe underperfusion of the renal cortex and a high renal vascular resistance that disappears at autopsy. Abnormal renal blood flow is therefore common in cirrhosis; it occurs before the development of oliguria and becomes more marked as renal failure progresses. The fall in renal blood flow is due to a diversion of blood away from the kidneys, associated with a high renal vascular resistance caused by renal vasoconstriction in the presence of a normal or low peripheral vascular resistance. These abnormalities are not due to a fall in cardiac output (Baldus et al 1964a,b, Tristani & Cohn 1967) or to a reduction in the plasma volume (Lieberman & Reynolds 1967) and they explain why the fraction of the cardiac output going to the kidneys is low even in subjects with a normal cardiac output (Baldus et al 1964a,b).

*Renal vasoconstriction*

Abnormal renal arteriolar vasoconstriction, the causes of which remain unknown, is increasingly being considered as the primary factor in reducing renal blood flow. Numerous causes for renal arteriolar vasoconstriction have been proposed and several could be important at any one time. This complex field has been reviewed in detail (Epstein 1992, 1994).

***Sympathetic nervous system.*** There is good evidence that sympathetic control of blood volume and of circulatory reflexes is abnormal in patients with cirrhosis. A complete reflex arc linking the liver and the kidneys has been described by Kostreva et al (1980), who have demonstrated experimentally that an increase in intrahepatic sinusoidal wedged pressure causes a simultaneous increase in hepatic efferent and renal afferent sympathetic nerve activity causing renal vasoconstriction. This reflex arc could be abolished by local anesthetics or by hepatic nerve section. There is evidence also for increased renal afferent sympathetic nerve activity in cirrhosis in humans. Renal venous noradrenaline concentrations are higher than in arterial blood and correlate with increased wedged hepatic venous pressures and infusion of adrenergic antagonists causes an increase in renal blood flow in some cirrhotic patients. Renal noradrenaline release is much higher in cirrhotic than in normal subjects in response to maneuvers such as head-up tilt and natriuresis after a water load in head-out water immersion studies correlates inversely with plasma noradrenaline concentrations in patients with cirrhosis and functional renal failure. Radiolabeled tracer kinetic studies have shown that elevated noradrenaline concentrations are due to increased release and not to reduced clearance (Esler et al 1992).

***Renin–angiotensin–aldosterone.*** Functional renal failure is characterized by a high plasma renin activity that leads to the production of increased amounts of angiotensin II and this in turn could cause efferent glomerular arteriolar vasoconstriction and a reduced blood flow to the renal glomeruli. There is a deficiency of plasma renin substrate, which is produced by the liver, but this is not a limiting factor in angiotensin II production. Infusion of renin substrate can improve glomerular filtration rate and sodium excretion. Several stimuli could be responsible for an elevated plasma renin concentration, including arterial hypotension, increased sympathetic nerve activity to the kidney, decreased hepatic clearance of aldosterone and diminished delivery of sodium to the macula densa in the kidney. The administration of an angiotensin-converting enzyme inhibitor may produce arterial hypotension, suggesting that angiotensin II is activated to compensate for a decreased blood volume. Glomerular filtration may decrease even further in these circumstances because constriction of the efferent arteriole induced by angiotensin II is an important mechanism for the maintenance of glomerular filtration in the face of reduced renal blood flow. There is evidence also for increased sensitivity of the renal tubule to aldosterone; however, during head-out immersion renin and aldosterone are both suppressed independent of whether a natriuresis or diuresis subsequently occurs. The aldosterone antagonist, spironolactone, is effective in the majority of patients and becomes less so only when renal failure supervenes. These data suggest that the renin–angiotensin–aldosterone system is activated principally in a defensive role and is not a primary cause of renal vasoconstriction.

***Atrial natriuretic peptide (ANP).*** ANP is released by maneuvers that increase right atrial pressure, such as rapid volume expansion or head-out immersion, and it may be that an increase in plasma ANP concentrations is responsible for the natriuresis and diuresis observed in these experiments. Most studies have found normal or elevated plasma concentrations in cirrhotic patients, so deficiency of ANP does not contribute to functional renal failure.

***Kallikrein–kinin.*** Plasma prekallikrein concentrations are reduced because the protein is synthesized by the liver. Urinary kallikrein may be reduced in cirrhosis in patients with good renal function but who have elevated plasma renin and urinary prostaglandin E (Zipser et al 1981). Limited measurements have been made in patients with renal dysfunction and MacGilchrist et al (1994) have demonstrated improvements in systemic vascular resistance and renal function after infusion with the kallikrein inhibitor, aprotinin.

***Prostaglandins.*** The renin–angiotensin and kallikrein–kinin systems can increase the renal production of prostaglandins and renal prostaglandin $E_2$ is a potent vasodilator agent. Deficient prostaglandin $E_2$ production in the kidney could contribute to vasoconstriction. The urinary excretion of prostaglandin $E_2$ is controversial, seems to be elevated in most studies of patients with cirrhosis and ascites with normal renal function and is usually low in patients with functional renal failure. This is consistent with the observation that the prostaglandin inhibitor indomethacin can reduce effective renal plasma flow, glomerular filtration rate and urinary sodium excretion even in well-compensated cirrhosis (Wong et al 1993). The potent vasoconstrictor prostaglandin, thromboxane $A_2$, may also be important in the pathogenesis of functional renal failure in cirrhosis. The urinary excretion of thromboxane $B_2$, the stable urinary metabolite of thromboxane $A_2$, is normal in cirrhotic patients with normal renal function but is markedly elevated in those with functional renal failure (Zipser et al 1983).

***Endotoxin.*** Endotoxinemia is a feature of functional renal failure that probably results from the inability of the liver to remove endotoxin from the portal blood. It too may be important in producing renal dysfunction, for it has powerful renal vasoconstrictor activity, by activating thromboxane $A_2$ release, and in addition can lead to nitric oxide release and fibrin deposition in the glomeruli.

***Nitric oxide (NO) and endothelins.*** NO is a powerful vasodilator released from endothelial cells and the enzyme catalyzing its production is inducible by endotoxin. NO causes peripheral vasodilatation and hypotension. A preliminary report suggests that nitrite and nitrate concentrations are elevated in cirrhotic patients and are higher in those with ascites and there was a direct correlation with endotoxinemia. Endothelin concentrations are elevated in patients with hepatorenal syndrome and have been correlated with plasma creatinine concentrations. Further studies of kinetics and with antagonists will be required.

***Other natriuretic factors.*** Vasoactive intestinal peptide, vasopressin and false neurotransmitters have all been implicated in this syndrome. Little evidence for a direct role exists for any of these and indeed, false neurotransmitters would be expected to result in renal vasodilatation.

*Clinical features* (Baldus et al 1964a,b)

Functional renal failure usually occurs in patients with advanced cirrhosis and ascites. The onset may be abrupt or gradual. Frequently, no immediate cause can be found, but possible precipitating factors include infection, gastrointestinal hemorrhage, the removal of large amounts of ascitic fluid (p. 1029), diuretic therapy (p. 1026), nephrotoxic drugs (e.g. NSAIDS, tetracyclines) and surgical procedures. It is impossible to ascribe symptoms specifically to renal rather than hepatic failure; apathy, weakness, fatigue and anorexia are the rule and as renal failure progresses, nausea, vomiting, thirst, drowsiness and a nonspecific tremor lead to clinical features indistinguishable from hepatic encephalopathy (p. 1045).

Examination shows advanced cirrhosis; ascites is usually marked and has often become resistant to medical therapy (p. 1028), bruising is common and fatal gastrointestinal bleeding may occur. The systolic blood pressure is commonly below 100 mmHg and falls further terminally. Pericarditis has been noted occasionally and may contribute to hypotension (Wise et al 1980). Encephalopathy usually worsens as uremia increases (p. 1051) and oliguria is present although it may only be marked terminally.

Rarely, functional renal failure occurs without jaundice or ascites (Conn 1973).

### *Investigations*

***Blood.*** Hypoalbuminemia, often below 30 g/L, and a prolonged prothrombin time confirm very poor liver function. The results of other tests of liver function are variable. The blood urea is increased and terminally may exceed 30 mmol/L (180 mg/dl). The serum creatinine concentration is increased proportionately less than the blood urea and may be normal early in uremia (Baldus et al 1964a,b). This may reflect the reduced muscle mass in advanced cirrhosis (Shear et al 1965). Hyponatremia is the rule, even early in uremia, and it becomes more severe as uremia advances, so that serum sodium concentrations below 120 mmol/L are common terminally. The high serum potassium concentrations seen in other causes of renal failure are unusual in functional renal failure even in patients who have had potassium therapy. In the early stages, hypokalemia is common, the concentration rises as uremia advances and high concentrations with acidosis may occur terminally. Hyperkalemia also occurs in patients receiving spironolactone (p. 1027).

***Urine.*** Functional renal failure should be differentiated from acute tubular necrosis and from pre-existing chronic renal disease coincident with cirrhosis (Table 39.3). The diagnosis is suggested by a gradual onset of oliguria and by the absence of protein, blood, casts and leukocytes from the urine. The osmolality of the urine exceeds the osmolality of the plasma, the urine specific gravity is above 1.015 and the sodium excretion in the urine is less than 10 mmol/day. Kidney size is normal. The glomerular filtration rate in uremia due to functional renal failure or chronic renal disease is reduced. Acute tubular necrosis (Table 39.3) supervenes occasionally in the functional renal failure of cirrhosis.

***Imaging.*** Ultrasound imaging of the kidneys and the lower urinary tract is useful in excluding chronic renal disease with small kidneys and urinary tract obstruction.

### *Treatment*

The outlook for a patient with cirrhosis who develops functional renal failure depends ultimately on the liver. The first step, therefore, is to look for complications that have impaired hepatic function and that could be treated. These include infection, fluid and electrolyte disorders following vigorous treatment of ascites (p. 1028) and gastrointestinal bleeding. A chest radiograph should be taken, the blood, ascitic fluid, urine and any sputum should be cultured, the stools tested for blood and the development of renal failure studied in relation to previous drug therapy. Separate disease that may have compromised both hepatic and renal function, such as cardiac failure, should be sought and the possibility of renal failure being due to intrinsic renal tract disease, such as urinary tract obstruction or nephritis, should be considered. Such diseases should be treated in their own right.

Otherwise, the aim of treatment in functional renal failure is to keep the patient alive in the hope that a spontaneous improvement in liver function will occur (Table 39.4) or the patient is suitable for liver transplantation (p. 1149). It needs to be recognized that the chances of survival are poor and the extent to which treatment, other than that

**Table 39.3** Differential diagnosis of renal failure in cirrhosis

| Factor | Functional renal failure | Acute tubular necrosis | Pre-existing renal disease |
|---|---|---|---|
| Liver disease | Advanced | Variable | Variable |
| Ascites | Present | Variable | Variable |
| Encephalopathy | Present | Variable | Variable |
| Hypotension | Late | Early | Not present |
| Course | Slow | Rapid | Slow |
| Oliguria | Late | Early | Variable |
| Urine protein | < 0.5 g/L | Present | Present |
| Urine sediment* | Normal | Abnormal | Abnormal |
| Urine/plasma osmolality** | > 1.2 | Low | Low |
| Urine sodium | < 10 mmol/L | Moderate | Moderate |
| Glomerular filtration rate | Low | Very low | Low |
| Renal size | Normal | Normal | Reduced |
| Renal pathology | None | Present | Present |

*Fresh centrifuged normal urine examined microscopically contains an occasional red blood cell and white blood cell every few high power fields. A few transitional epithelial cells, and in women vaginal squames, are also seen.
**See Table 39.2.

**Table 39.4** Treatment of functional renal failure

1. Minimize uremia
   - Reduce or eliminate protein intake (<20 g/day)
   - High carbohydrate intake
   - Avoid drugs that increase catabolism
   - Avoid nephrotoxic drugs
2. Increase renal excretory function
   - Expand plasma volume, e.g. salt-poor albumin
   - Diuretic therapy
   - Dopamine 1–2 μg/kg/min intravenously
3. Body fluids and electrolytes
   - Water: occasional depletion due to gastrointestinal, renal or ascitic fluid loss
   - Sodium: occasional depletion due to gastrointestinal, renal or ascitic fluid loss
   - Potassium: give potassium when plasma concentration <3.5 mmol/L
   - Magnesium: depletion may prevent potassium repletion
4. General therapy
   - Hepatic encephalopathy (avoid neomycin)
   - Gastrointestinal bleeding
   - Infection
5. Other therapy
   - LeVeen shunt (p. 1030)
   - TIPSS (p. 1032)
   - Portacaval shunt (p. 1032)

required for the comfort of the patient, is justified should be considered. This applies particularly to the elderly, to those who have had a gradual deterioration of liver function for which no cause can be found and to those with serious associated diseases. Many forms of treatment have been tried, but none is of proven value.

***General measures.*** Hepatic encephalopathy should be treated by protein restriction and with lactulose (p. 1053). Neomycin should not be given, but a less toxic antibiotic can be used if necessary (p. 1052). Almost all patients are overhydrated, as evidenced by ascites and edema, and they often have a dilutional hyponatremia that may require treatment by restriction of water intake (p. 1025). Occasionally, a patient can become sodium and water depleted, in which case replacement therapy may lead to a marked improvement in renal and hepatic function (Galambos & Wilkinson 1962). Such patients are recognized from a history of fluid loss by vomiting, aspiration, diarrhea, paracentesis or vigorous diuretic therapy and by the absence of ascites or edema on examination. A review of records will often show that uremia has accompanied or followed such events.

Volume depletion is best assessed and corrected using a central venous catheter inserted percutaneously by the internal jugular route. This can be done safely by experienced personnel even when the prothrombin time is grossly prolonged. Volume expansion may be started with 0.5–1.0 L of fresh frozen plasma, plasma protein or albumin solution until the central venous pressure is between 2–5 $cmH_2O$. Potassium depletion may be present in these patients in spite of uremia. The plasma potassium concentration does not reflect the total body potassium, but it is the best available guide to therapy; hypokalemia affects renal function adversely and worsens encephalopathy (p. 1039). Treatment should be given when the plasma potassium is below 3.5 mmol/L. Some patients have large potassium deficits (>200 mmol) and large amounts of potassium may have to be given intravenously but at rates not exceeding 25 mmol/h and in concentrations not exceeding 40 mmol/L, with frequent checks of the serum potassium concentration. Magnesium deficiency is also common (Lim & Jacob 1972) and may account for an inability to correct hypokalemia. Magnesium may be administered as magnesium chloride at a rate between 25 and 100 mmol/day depending on the plasma magnesium concentration.

***Renal function.*** The most important measures are to limit uremia and ensure an adequate renal blood flow. The former is achieved by restricting protein intake to 20 g/day and by providing at least 200 g carbohydrate/day to minimize endogenous protein breakdown. Hemodialysis or peritoneal dialysis are of limited value and may be complicated by gastrointestinal bleeding or hypotension (Perez & Oster 1978). However, some reports suggest that intermittent or continuous venovenous hemofiltration is a well-tolerated, safer therapy allowing recovery of hepatic and renal function after an acute insult. Renal blood flow is maximized by infusing colloidal fluid as described above until the central venous pressure is about 2–5 $cmH_2O$.

**Table 39.5** Drugs used without proven success in the treatment of functional renal failure

| | |
|---|---|
| Metaraminol | Papaverine |
| Octapressin | Angiotensin |
| Isoproterenol | Prostaglandin A |
| Phenoxybenzamine | Dopamine |
| Phentolamine | L-dopa |
| Acetylcholine | Propranolol |
| Aminophylline | |

Numerous drugs have been used to improve renal function (Table 39.5), but only dopamine has proved successful enough to recommend its use in practice. It should be administered continuously through a central line at a dose of 1–2 μg/kg/min, which is sufficient to provide a maximal stimulus to the kidney. Diuretic drugs such as frusemide or bumetanide (p. 1027) can be given along with this treatment once vascular volume depletion has been corrected to improve urine output. The urine output and its sodium content, the plasma urea and the plasma creatinine are measured daily during this therapy. The creatinine clearance is also a useful measurement.

Improvement in renal function is often only temporary, and within a few days a decision has to be taken as to whether the treatment should be repeated. When improvement is maintained and the patient remains reasonably well, it may be worth considering the insertion of a transjugular intrahepatic portasystemic stent shunt (TIPSS) (p. 1032) or a peritoneovenous shunt (p. 1030).

***Other treatments.*** A portacaval shunt can relieve functional renal failure in cirrhosis (Schroeder et al 1970), but hardly any of the patients are fit for such surgery. The value of TIPSS in functional renal failure is not known. The possibility of hepatic transplantation (p. 1149) should be considered in younger, fitter patients, as it restores liver function and relieves renal failure (Iwatsuki et al 1973).

*Prognosis*

The prognosis in functional renal failure is very bad. Many patients die within days and few survive beyond 3 months (Conn 1973). Death usually results from progressive hepatic failure; recovery from renal failure is preceded by improving liver function. Death is usually due to hepatic failure or gastrointestinal bleeding or, less commonly, to intercurrent infection or renal failure.

## Acute tubular necrosis

Acute tubular necrosis is uncommon in cirrhosis. It may supervene in patients who have had prolonged functional renal failure (Table 39.3). Plasma urea and creatinine concentrations rise further and the urinary sodium increases. Careful hemodialysis, or preferably hemofiltration, is justified to allow time for recovery from an acute insult, e.g. infection, hypotension or a nephrotoxic drug.

## Renal tubular dysfunction

Several types of renal tubular dysfunction occur in cirrhosis.

### *Increased sodium retention*

Patients with cirrhosis and ascites have a greatly increased total body sodium and water. Marked retention of sodium by the kidneys is central to this and little or no sodium is found in the urine (p. 1025). The reasons for sodium and water retention are poorly understood (Epstein 1994). Alterations in renal blood flow and hyperaldosteronism are the two known abnormalities that are likely to be important; they could be inter-related, as diminished renal cortical blood flow increases plasma renin activity, which is a stimulus to aldosterone secretion. However, it is certain that other unknown factors are also important.

***Renal blood flow.*** Altered renal blood flow in cirrhosis (p. 1059) could itself be an important reason for increased sodium retention by the kidney. Total renal blood flow is diminished, even in the absence of ascites, and once this becomes severe enough the glomerular filtration rate is reduced. Diminished glomerular filtration itself is associated with increased proximal tubular sodium retention. This, however, is not an important factor, as the glomerular filtration rate is diminished only slightly, if at all, in most patients. The redistribution of blood flow within the kidney may also be important, as a greater proportion of the total blood flow passes to the juxtamedullary nephrons. These nephrons are capable of greater sodium retention than those in the outer cortex. Finally, changes in the hydrostatic and oncotic pressure in the peritubular capillaries, resulting from the altered blood flow and hypoalbuminemia, may be important, but this remains unproved. Increased renal sympathetic nerve activity is also important. A reflex arc exists between the liver and the kidney, so that increases in intrahepatic sinusoidal pressure cause an increase in efferent hepatic nerve activity and a simultaneous increase in renal afferent sympathetic nerve activity. An increase in renal afferent sympathetic nerve activity causes avid sodium retention in animals and is thought to be a direct tubular effect. Further increases in nerve activity cause vasoconstriction within the kidney, particularly in the outer cortex, as shown by xenon washout and angiography studies.

***Hyperaldosteronism.*** Increased plasma aldosterone concentrations and increased aldosterone excretion in the urine is a marked and constant feature in patients with cirrhosis and ascites and it is most intense in patients with the most severe ascites. This results principally from an increased secretion of aldosterone; impaired aldosterone metabolism by the liver is probably only a contributory factor (Rosoff et al 1975). The reasons for the increased production of aldosterone are uncertain. Aldosterone secretion is controlled normally by the renin–angiotensin–aldosterone system, but opinions on the importance of this controlling system in cirrhosis with ascites have varied and other unknown factors may become important (Wilkinson et al 1977, Arroyo et al 1979).

Aldosterone, a mineralocorticoid with powerful sodium-retaining properties, and other mineralocorticoids have been shown to increase the blood volume and to produce or worsen ascites in cirrhotic patients (Denison et al 1971). In addition, a close relationship exists between the urinary excretion of sodium and aldosterone in cirrhotic ascites (Wilkinson et al 1977). Hyperaldosteronism has therefore come to be regarded as an important cause of sodium and water retention in cirrhotic ascites. Other evidence, however, has questioned its importance or has at least indicated that other factors must be equally important. Healthy individuals given mineralocorticoids cease to retain sodium and in primary hyperaldosteronism edema does not occur and urinary sodium excretion is normal (Denison et al 1971). Furthermore, some investigators have failed to find a relation between the serum aldosterone concentration and the intake or urinary excretion of sodium (Chonko et al 1977), spontaneous diuresis has been reported in cirrhotic ascites in spite of continuing high serum aldosterone concentrations and reduction of the serum aldosterone concentration by aminoglutethamide, which blocks aldosterone synthesis, produces only a modest diuresis (Rosoff et al 1975). Finally, immersion, which causes a redistribution of the blood volume and a natriuresis in normal people, produces a natriuresis in cirrhosis with ascites in spite of pharmacological doses of mineralocorticoid (Epstein 1979). Other factors must also be responsible for continued sodium retention in cirrhosis.

***Other factors.*** Other factors have been proposed as causes of avid sodium retention in cirrhosis, but they are still poorly understood. They include failure to elaborate natriuretic factors that normally increase sodium excretion when the blood volume is increased and failure to elaborate renal prostaglandins and kinins produced by the kallikrein–kinin system, which directly or indirectly produce natriuresis (Epstein 1983). Increased antidiuretic hormone production could contribute to water retention in patients with ascites, but its role is probably limited (Conn 1972).

### *Impaired water excretion*

Patients with cirrhosis and ascites vary greatly in their abil-

**Table 39.6** Free water clearance, hyponatremia and prognosis in cirrhosis and ascites (Arroyo & Rodés 1975)

| Free water clearance (ml/min) | Patients (number) | Hyponatremia (<130 mmol/L) | Died in hospital | *p* |
|---|---|---|---|---|
| <1 | 17 | 13 | 11(65%) | <0.05 |
| >1 | 38 | 3 | 4(11%) | |

ity to excrete a water load. In some this ability is normal, while in others it is markedly impaired (Arroyo et al 1976, Vaamonde 1983). Patients with a limited ability to excrete water generally have advanced liver disease with renal failure, as evidenced by a significant decrease in their glomerular filtration rates. Inability to excrete water eventually contributes significantly to hyponatremia, which becomes common in patients with free water clearance rates reduced to less than 1 ml/min (Table 39.6). Such patients respond poorly to diuretic therapy and have a particularly poor prognosis (Table 39.6).

Apart from the impaired glomerular filtration rate, three mechanisms have been put forward to explain impaired water excretion. A significant decrease in the delivery of filtrate to the distal parts of the nephron and an increased back-diffusion of water in its terminal segments, consequent on a low flow of fluid in the tubules, are probably the most important factors. Increased concentrations of antidiuretic hormone also contribute to this increased retention of water, but the overall importance of this hormone remains unclear. Patients with cirrhosis who do not have ascites excrete water normally.

Patients with cirrhosis also have a minor impairment in their ability to concentrate urine irrespective of whether they have ascites. This is related to their inability to produce enough urea for concentration within the medulla and is not in itself of any clinical importance.

*Renal tubular acidosis*

Although metabolic acidosis is very uncommon in chronic liver disease, it is now recognized that renal tubular acidosis is quite common (Oster 1983). This paradox is explained by the fact that the renal tubular acidosis is almost always incomplete. There are two types of renal tubular acidosis: in one (type I or classic) the distal tubules cannot maintain the normal steep hydrogen ion gradient between the tubular lumen and the peritubular fluid, and in the other (type II) an acidification defect in the proximal tubules results in a failure to absorb bicarbonate filtered by the glomeruli. Type I renal tubular acidosis in liver disease occurs most frequently in primary biliary cirrhosis, chronic active hepatitis and cryptogenic cirrhosis and has been described in alcoholic cirrhosis (Fig. 39.1).

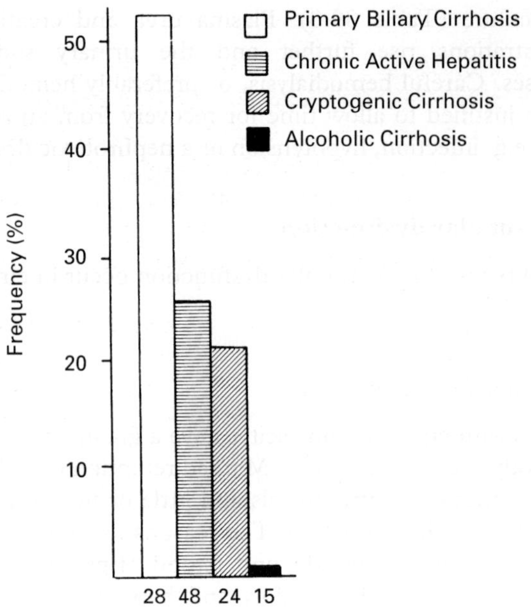


**Fig. 39.1** The frequency of renal tubular acidosis in chronic liver diseases. The figures under each column refer to the number of patients investigated (Golding et al 1973).

Both types of renal tubular acidosis can occur in Wilson's disease in which defects of urine-concentrating capacity, glycosuria, hypercalciuria, phosphaturia and aminoaciduria also occur (p. 962).

The causes of renal tubular acidosis in liver disease are unknown, but immune-mediated tubulointerstitial nephritis has been suggested in primary biliary cirrhosis, chronic active hepatitis and cryptogenic cirrhosis (Golding et al 1973, Tsantoulas et al 1974). Copper deposition in the renal tubules is probably the cause in Wilson's disease. Chronic cholestasis leads to the accumulation of large amounts of copper in the liver (p. 933) and to increased amounts of copper in the blood and urine. Copper depositions in the kidneys have been put forward as an alternative explanation for tubular damage in primary biliary cirrhosis, as renal tubular acidosis in that disease is associated with more prolonged and severe cholestasis leading to especially large amounts of copper in the blood and urine (Parés et al 1981).

Renal tubular acidosis can occasionally have important clinical implications in that hypercalciuria and an alkaline urine may predispose to nephrocalcinosis and nephrolithiasis and potassium loss and an impaired ability to excrete ammonia may increase susceptibility to and aggravate hepatic encephalopathy (Shear et al 1969).

## End-stage renal failure (acute glomerulonephritis)

Renal failure in chronic liver disease is usually due to functional renal failure, but the possibility of end-stage (chronic) renal failure is easily overlooked.

*Clinical features*

Patients with chronic liver disease and end-stage renal failure may present with renal disease, for example with hematuria, but most present because of their liver disease (Nochy et al 1976). End-stage renal failure should be suspected where microscopic hematuria or proteinuria is found, where liver function is relatively good and where renal failure reflected in increased plasma urea and creatinine concentrations has not followed deterioration of liver function, treatment with diuretics or paracentesis or complications such as sepsis. Nakamoto et al (1981) found microscopic hematuria and/or proteinuria in 9.1% and proteinuria >3 g/day in 1.6% of 752 consecutive patients.

*Pathology*

Renal lesions are found at autopsy in cirrhosis irrespective of cause in a half or more of patients (Newell 1987). These lesions include thickening and splitting of the glomerular basement membrane, widening of the mesangeal matrix, tubular dilatation and patchy interstitial nephritis. An early autopsy study of 100 patients with cirrhosis and 100 noncirrhotic controls showed chronic changes in the glomerular basement membranes in 28% of cirrhotic patients compared with 10% of controls, but there were no cases of chronic nephritis (Jones et al 1961). Mesangiocapillary (membranoproliferative) nephritis appears to be the next most common condition, followed by membranous nephropathy, glomerulosclerosis and necrotizing and rapidly progressive (crescentic) nephritis. The frequency of nephritis in unselected cirrhotic patients generally is unknown.

Proliferative forms of glomerulonephritis in which immunoglobulins and complement are deposited in the mesangium have been reported in cirrhosis (Fisher & Perez-Stable 1968). Numerous reports have described changes typical of IgA nephropathy in cirrhotic patients investigated for microscopic hematuria and/or proteinuria with or without raised plasma creatinine concentrations (Nochy et al 1976) and these patients may show a combination of increased plasma IgA, reduced plasma complement (C3) and circulating immune complex containing IgA (Woodruffe et al 1980). There are no comparative studies in cirrhotic patients without nephritis. Defective antigen processing and/or immunoglobulin synthesis by the gut mucosa in cirrhosis are possible pathogenetic mechanisms leading to the renal lesions, but this needs to be explored further.

*Investigations*

The urine should be tested for blood and protein and positive results followed by more definitive tests including urine microscopy for casts and a 24-h urine collection for creatinine clearance and protein excretion. The size of the kidneys should be measured by ultrasonography, which can also be used to exclude an obstructive uropathy. Renal biopsy is rarely needed and may be contraindicated by impaired blood coagulation in liver disease.

*Treatment*

The treatment is that of end-stage renal failure, which may require dialysis or renal transplantation. Renal assessment of patients being considered for liver transplantation who have renal failure is particularly important.

## RENAL FAILURE IN BILIARY DISEASE

Renal failure is usually associated with biliary obstruction, but it can also occur in conditions affecting both the biliary system and the kidneys.

### Biliary obstruction

Acute renal failure is a common cause of death following surgery for biliary obstruction and it is often associated with other fatal complications such as pneumonia and gastrointestinal bleeding. It can also occur in patients undergoing endoscopic retrograde cholangiopancreatography for biliary obstruction (p. 119). The frequency of acute renal failure is greatest in patients with high serum bilirubin concentrations (>170 μmol/L; >10 mg/dl) and the most important precipitating factor is a period of hypotension (systolic pressure <90 mmHg for over 2 h) (Williams et al 1960, Dawson 1965).

***Mechanisms.*** The underlying lesion in the kidney is acute tubular necrosis, but the mechanism whereby it is produced is uncertain. Animal experiments have shown that renal cortical perfusion is reduced after bile duct ligation and that susceptibility to hypotensive renal damage is increased by obstructive jaundice (Williams et al 1960, Bomzon & Kew 1983). Experimentally, obstructive jaundice is associated with hypotension and decreased sensitivity of vascular smooth muscle to catecholamines. Infusion of bile salts causes a brisk natriuresis and kaliuresis, although glomerular filtration rate and renal blood flow are usually maintained in the short term. This may be because of activation of intrarenal angiotensin II. Endotoxinemia, from infection with Gram-negative bacteria, is also important in humans (Wardle 1975, Wilkinson et al 1976). Both mannitol and saline can protect the kidneys from the effects of hypotension in obstructive jaundice (Dawson & Stirling 1964).

***Prevention.*** The implications of these findings for preventing acute renal failure are that the patient should be given appropriate antibiotics (below) and should come to operation well hydrated. Antibiotics and intravenous saline (1–2 L) should begin no later than the evening before surgery. Mannitol 10% (200 ml) can be given during the operation and further mannitol should be given after the operation if the urine output falls below 60 ml/h despite adequate fluid therapy. Similar precautions should also be taken when patients undergo retrograde transhepatic cholangiography, as septicemia and hypotension may occur. Antibiotics such as ciprofloxacin 75 mg orally or cefotaxime 1 g intravenously should be given parenterally before the procedure and if obstruction of a large biliary duct is found, this treatment should be continued and surgical or endoscopic relief of any obstruction carried out as quickly as is practicable.

## Fibropolycystic diseases

The fibropolycystic diseases are a heterogeneous group of hepatobiliary disorders affecting the liver and the kidney. The renal lesions include renal cysts and renal tubular ectasia, including medullary sponge kidney, and renal failure can occur.

## REFERENCES


Arroyo V, Rodés J 1975 A rational approach to the treatment of ascites. Postgraduate Medical Journal 51: 558–562

Arroyo V, Rodés J, Gutierrez-Lizárraga M A, Revert L 1976 Prognostic value of spontaneous hyponatremia in cirrhosis with ascites. American Journal of Digestive Diseases 21: 249–256

Arroyo V, Bosch J, Mauri M et al 1979 Renin, aldosterone and renal haemodynamics in cirrhosis with ascites. European Journal of Clinical Investigation 9: 69–73

Arroyo V, Bernardi M, Epstein M, Henriksen J H, Schrier R W, Rodés J 1988 Pathophysiology of ascites and functional renal failure in cirrhosis. Journal of Hepatology 6: 239–257

Arroyo V, Ginès P, Gerbes A L et al 1996 Definition and diagnostic criteria of refractory ascites and hepatorenal syndrome in cirrhosis. Hepatology 23: 164–176

Baldus W P, Feichter R N, Summerskill W H J, Hunt J C, Wakim K G 1964a The kidney in cirrhosis. II. Disorders of renal function. Annals of Internal Medicine 60: 353–365

Baldus W P, Summerskill W H J, Hunt J C, Maher F T 1964b Renal circulation in cirrhosis: observations based on catheterization of the renal vein. Journal of Clinical Investigation 43: 1090–1097

Bomzon L, Kew M C 1983 Renal blood flow in experimental obstructive jaundice. In: Epstein M (ed) The kidney in liver disease. Elsevier, New York, p 313

Chonko A M, Bay W H, Stein J H, Ferris T F 1977 The role of renin and aldosterone in the salt retention of edema. American Journal of Medicine 63: 881–889

Conn H O 1972 The rational management of ascites. In: Popper H, Schaffner F (eds) Progress in liver diseases, Vol 4. Grune and Stratton, New York, p 269–288

Conn H O 1973 A rational approach to the hepato-renal syndrome. Gastroenterology 65: 321–340

Dawson J L 1965 The incidence of postoperative renal failure in obstructive jaundice. British Journal of Surgery 52: 663–665

Dawson J L, Stirling G A 1964 Protective effect of mannitol on anoxic jaundiced kidneys: a histological study. Archives of Pathology 78: 254–259

Denison E K, Lieberman F L, Reynolds T B 1971 9-α- fluoro-hydrocortisone induced ascites in alcoholic liver disease. Gastroenterology 61: 497–503

Epstein M 1979 Deranged sodium homeostasis in cirrhosis. Gastroenterology 76: 622–635

Epstein M 1983 Renal sodium handling in cirrhosis. In: Epstein M (ed) The kidney in liver disease. Elsevier, New York, p 25

Epstein M 1988 The kidney in liver disease, 3rd edn. Williams and Wilkins, Baltimore

Epstein M 1992 The hepatorenal syndrome – new perspectives. New England Journal of Medicine 327: 1810–1811

Epstein M 1994 Hepatorenal syndrome: emerging perspectives of pathophysiology and therapy. Journal of the American Society of Nephrology 4: 1735–1753

Esler M, Dudley F, Jennings G 1992 Increased sympathetic nervous activity and the effects of its inhibition with clonidine in alcoholic cirrhosis. Annals of Internal Medicine 116: 446–455

Fisher E R, Perez-Stable E 1968 Cirrhotic (hepatic) lobular glomerulonephritis. Correlation of ultrastructural and clinical features. American Journal of Pathology 52: 869–889

Galambos J T, Wilkinson H A III 1962 Reversible hyponatremia and azotemia in a patient with cirrhosis and ascites. American Journal of Digestive Diseases 7: 642–647

Golding P L, Smith M, Williams R 1973 Multisystem involvement in chronic liver disease. Studies on the incidence and pathogenesis. American Journal of Medicine 55: 772–782

Hecker R, Sherlock S 1956 Electrolyte and circulatory changes in terminal liver failure. Lancet 2: 1121–1125

Iwatsuki S, Popovtzer M M, Corman J L, Ishikawa M, Putnam C W, Katz F H 1973 Recovery from "hepatorenal syndrome" after orthotopic liver transplantation. New England Journal of Medicine 289: 1155–1159

Jones W T, Rao D R G, Braunstein H 1961 The renal glomerulus in cirrhosis of the liver. American Journal of Pathology 39: 393–404

Kew M C, Varma R R, Williams H S, Brunt P W, Hourigan K J, Sherlock H 1971 Renal and intrarenal blood flow in cirrhosis of the liver. Lancet 2: 504–510

Koppel M H, Coburn J W, Mims M M, Goldstein H, Boyle J D, Rubini M E 1969 Transplantation of cadaveric kidneys from patients with hepatorenal syndrome. Evidence for the functional nature of renal failure in advanced liver disease. New England Journal of Medicine 280: 1367–1371

Kostreva D R, Castaner A, Kampine J P 1980 Reflex effects of hepatic baroreceptors on renal and cardiac sympathetic nerve activity. American Journal of Physiology 238: R390–394

Levy M 1983 Pathophysiology of ascites formation. In: Epstein M (ed) The kidney in liver disease. Elsevier, New York, p 245

Lieberman F L, Reynolds T B 1967 Plasma volume in cirrhosis of the liver: its relation to portal hypertension, ascites and renal failure. Journal of Clinical Investigation 46: 1297–1308

Lieberman F L, Ito S, Reynolds T B 1969 Effective plasma volume in cirrhosis with ascites. Evidence that a decreased value does not account for renal sodium retention, a spontaneous reduction in glomerular filtration rate (GFR) and a fall in GFR during drug-induced diuresis. Journal of Clinical Investigation 48: 975–981

Lim P, Jacob E 1972 Magnesium deficiency in liver cirrhosis. Quarterly Journal of Medicine 41: 291–300

MacGilchrist A, Craig K J, Hayes P C, Cumming A D 1994 Effect of the serine protease inhibitor, aprotinin, on systemic haemodynamics and renal function in patients with hepatic cirrhosis and ascites. Clinical Science 87: 329–335

Mondon C E, Burton S D, Ishida T 1969 Functional status of isolated rat kidney perfused in combination with isolated liver. Clinical Research 17: 168

Nakamoto Y, Iida H, Kobayashi K 1981 Hepatic glomerulonephritis. Characteristics of hepatic IgA glomerulonephritis as the major part. Virhaus Archiv (Pathology und Anatomie) 392: 4S–54

Newell G C 1987 Cirrhotic glomerulonephritis: incidence, morphology, clinical features and pathogenesis. American Journal of Kidney Disease 9: 183–190

Nochy D, Callard P, Bellon P 1976 Association of overt glomerulonephritis and liver disease: a study of 34 patients. Clinical Nephrology 6: 422–427

Oster J 1983 Acid base homeostasis and liver disease. In: Epstein M (ed)

The kidney in liver disease. Elsevier, New York, p 60
Papper S 1983 Hepatorenal syndrome. In: Epstein M (ed) The kidney in liver disease. Elsevier, New York, p 87
Parés A, Rimola A, Bruguera M, Mas E, Rodés J 1981 Renal tubular acidosis in primary biliary cirrhosis. Gastroenterology 80: 681–686
Perez G O, Oster J R 1978 A critical review of the role of dialysis in the treatment of liver disease. In: Epstein M (ed) The kidney in liver disease. Elsevier, New York, p 325–336
Rosoff L Jr, Williams J, Moult P, Williams H, Sherlock S 1975 Renal hemodynamics and the renin angiotensin system in cirrhosis: the effects of portacaval anastomosis. Gastroenterology 69: A-58/858
Schrier R W, Arroyo V, Bernardi M, Epstein M, Henriksen J H, Rodés J 1988 Peripheral arterial vasodilation hypothesis: a proposal for the initiation of renal sodium and water retention in cirrhosis. Hepatology 8: 1151–1157
Schroeder E J, Numann P J, Chamberlain B E 1970 Functional renal failure in cirrhosis. Recovery after portacaval shunt. Annals of Internal Medicine 72: 923–928
Shear L, Kleinerman J, Gabuzda G J 1965 Renal failure in patients with cirrhosis of the liver. I. Clinical and pathologic characteristics. American Journal of Medicine 39: 184–198
Shear L, Bonkowsky M, Gabuzda G 1969 Renal tubular acidosis in cirrhosis. A determinant of recurrent hepatic precoma. New England Journal of Medicine 280: 1–7
Sherlock S 1993 The kidneys in hepatic cirrhosis: victims of portal-systemic venous shunting (portal-systemic nephropathy). Gastroenterology 104: 931–933
Tristani F E, Cohn J N 1967 Systemic and renal hemodynamics in oliguric hepatic failure: effect of volume expansion. Journal of Clinical Investigation 46: 1894–1906
Tsantoulas D C, McFarlane I G, Portmann B, Eddleston A L W F, Williams R 1974 Cell-mediated immunity to Tamm–Horsfall glycoprotein in autoimmune liver disease with renal tubular acidosis. British Medical Journal 4: 491–494
Vaamonde C A 1983 Renal water handling in liver disease. In: Epstein M (ed) The kidney in liver disease. Elsevier, New York, p 55
Wardle E N 1975 Renal failure in obstructive jaundice – pathogenic factors. Postgraduate Medical Journal 51: 512–614
Wilkinson S P, Moodie H, Stamatakis J D, Kakker V V, Williams R 1976 Endotoxaemia and renal failure in cirrhosis and obstructive jaundice. British Medical Journal 2: 1415–1418
Wilkinson S P, Bernardi M, Smith I K, Jowett T P, Slater J D H, Williams R 1977 Effect of β-adrenergic blocking drugs on the renin–aldosterone system, sodium excretion and renal hemodynamics in cirrhosis with ascites. Gastroenterology 73: 659–663
Williams R D, Elliott D W, Zollinger R M 1960 Surgery for malignant jaundice. Archives of Surgery 80: 992–997
Wise W J, Mamdani B M, Bakir A A, Dunea G 1980 Fibrinous pericarditis in hepatorenal failure. Lancet 2: 1336–1337
Wong F, Massie D, Hsu P, Dudley F 1993 Indomethacin-induced renal dysfunction in patients with well-compensated cirrhosis. Gastroenterology 104: 869–876
Woodruffe A J, Gormley A A, McKenzie P 1980 Immunologic studies in IgA nephropathy. Kidney International 18: 366–374
Zipser R D, Kerlin P, Hoefs J C, Zia P, Barg A 1981 Renal kallikrein excretion in alcoholic cirrhosis: relationship to other vasoactive systems. American Journal of Gastroenterology 75: 183–187
Zipser R D, Radvan G H, Kronborg I J, Duke R, Little T E 1983 Urinary thromboxane B2 and prostaglandin $E_2$ in the hepatorenal syndrome: evidence for increased vasoconstrictor and decreased vasodilator factors. Gastroenterology 84: 697–703

# 40. Pulmonary dysfunction in liver disease

*Michael J. Krowka*

## INTRODUCTION

Pulmonary dysfunction is common in liver disease, and dyspnea is the predominant clinical presentation (Agusti et al 1990). The differential diagnosis of pulmonary dysfunction in liver disease includes abnormalities of the pulmonary parenchyma, pleural space and pulmonary arterial circulation (Krowka & Cortese 1989). This chapter will consider pulmonary dysfunction in specific hepatic disorders and their most frequent pulmonary associations (Table 40.1) and particular attention will be given to pulmonary problems that may compromise liver transplantation (Rodriguez-Roisin & Krowka 1994).

## ASSESSMENT OF PULMONARY FUNCTION IN LIVER DISEASE

The most important physiological measurement in evaluating respiratory dysfunction in patients with liver disease is the identification of arterial oxygenation. Impaired arterial oxygenation leading to hypoxemia ($PaO_2$ <70 mmHg [9.3 kPa] or hemoglobin saturation <90%) in liver disease has been reviewed extensively (Krowka & Cortese 1989). Hypoxemia is common and in selected series ranges from 16% (Rodman et al 1960) to 45% (Hourani et al 1991).

### Arterial gas analysis

Hypoxemia can be quantitated by pulse oximetry, which determines hemoglobin saturation, or by blood gas analysis. Screening for hypoxemia with pulse oximetry using either the ear or fingertip technique may be misleading in patients with significant hyperbilirubinemia (>2.5 mg/dl; 43 mmol/L). These individuals may give falsely low hemoglobin saturations (<90%) in spite of normal oxygenation, due to the circulating bile pigments. Accordingly, the best way to determine arterial oxygenation in patients with liver disease, particularly where jaundice is present, is by blood gas analysis. The measured $PaO_2$ or the calculated alveolar-arterial (a-A) gradient can be used to determine the degree of abnormality of oxygenation. The measured

**Table 40.1** Pulmonary abnormalities associated with specific chronic liver diseases

| | Cirrhosis* | Primary biliary cirrhosis | Chronic active hepatitis | Primary sclerosing cholangitis | $\alpha_1$-antitrypsin deficiency | Noncirrhotic portal hypertension |
|---|---|---|---|---|---|---|
| Interstitial lung disease | | | | | | |
| Subclinical alveolitis | | x | | | | |
| Lymphocytic alveolitis | | x | x | | | |
| Organizing pneumonitis | | x | | | | |
| Fibrosing alveolitis | | x | x | | | |
| Obstructive airways disease | | | | | | |
| Bronchitis/bronchiectasis/emphysema | | x | | x | | |
| Emphysema | | | | | x | |
| Hepatopulmonary syndrome | x | x | x | | x | x |
| Pulmonary hypertension | x | x | | | x | x |
| ARDS | x | | | | | |
| Pulmonary hemorrhage | | x | | | | |
| Pleural effusions | x | x | x | | | |

*Cryptogenic, alcoholic and/or postnecrotic.

$PaO_2$ is the most practical assessment, but the a-A gradient is more sensitive because it considers the fact that the $PaCO_2$ is reduced in these patients. Accordingly, oximetry can be used to screen for hypoxemia, but patients with central cyanosis or finger clubbing should be evaluated with a $PaO_2$ determination breathing room air.

Patients with liver disease generally hyperventilate, resulting in reductions in $PaCO_2$ and increased arterial pH. This respiratory alkalosis occurs in the absence of intrinsic pulmonary abnormality and has no clinically important effect from a pulmonary perspective.

### Pulmonary function tests

Selected pulmonary function tests (PFTs) measuring the $FEV_1/FVC$ ratio (forced expiratory volume in 1 second/forced vital capacity) and DLCO (single breath diffusing capacity for carbon monoxide) aid in the assessment of dyspnea. $FEV_1/FVC$ (normal >70%) quantifies expiratory airflow obstruction which occurs variably in $\alpha_1$-antitrypsin deficiency, primary biliary cirrhosis and primary sclerosing cholangitis. DLCO (normal >80% predicted) measures the efficiency of gas exchange within the lung and is most helpful in detecting interstitial lung disease and pulmonary circulatory abnormalities. Abnormal DLCO is common in end-stage liver disease, occurring in up to 45% of patients (Hourani et al 1991). Reductions in lung volumes, as measured by the FVC, are found frequently in patients with interstitial lung disorders and with massive ascites and/or pleural effusions due to liver disease (Turner-Warwick 1968, Stanley & Woodgate 1972). Improvement in FVC occurs frequently following large volume paracentesis or thoracentesis with subsequent improvement in dyspnea (Berkowitz et al 1993, Krowka & Cortese 1989).

### Chest imaging

Chest imaging (standard chest radiograph or high-resolution computed tomography) combined with pulmonary function assessment is required for a full assessment of the pulmonary dysfunction in liver disease (Table 40.2).

## PULMONARY DYSFUNCTION IN SPECIFIC HEPATIC DISORDERS

### Acute respiratory failure

Acute respiratory failure in liver disease occurs most often in acute liver failure, but it can also develop in any sudden deterioration in chronic liver disease.

#### *Acute (fulminant) liver failure*

The major pulmonary concern in patients with acute (fulminant) liver disease is the development of hypoxemic respiratory failure due to noncardiogenic pulmonary edema (adult respiratory distress syndrome – ARDS). This occurred in 37 of 100 consecutive patients with acute hepatic failure, accounting for a mortality of approximately 80% (Trewby et al 1978). Liver disease was due to acute viral hepatitis, paracetamol or halothane hepatitis and respiratory deterioration occurred within 4 days of stage 4 coma. Aspiration pneumonitis and cerebral edema have both been implicated as causes for noncardiogenic

**Table 40.2** Pulmonary evaluation in patients with chronic liver disease

| | Suspected pulmonary abnormality | | | | |
|---|---|---|---|---|---|
| | Pleural effusion | Expiratory airflow obstruction | Interstitial lung disease | Pulmonary hypertension | Hepatopulmonary syndrome |
| Physiologic studies | | | | | |
| ABGs ($PaO_2\downarrow$) | x | | x | x | x (D) |
| PFTs ($FEV_1/FVC\downarrow$) | | x (D) | | | |
| (DLCO↓) | | | x | x | x |
| Imaging studies | | | | | |
| Chest radiograph | x (D) | | x | | |
| Chest CT (high resolution) | x (D) | | x (D) | | |
| Echocardiography | | | | x (D) | x (D) |
| $^{99Tc}$MAA lung scanning | | | | | x (D) |
| Pulmonary angiography | | | | | x (D) |

x = usually abnormal (see text)
D = abnormality is essentially diagnostic (see text)
$PaO_2$ = partial pressure of oxygen
$FEV_1/FVC$ = forced expiratory flow in 1 second/forced vital capacity
DLCO = diffusing capacity
PVR = pulmonary vascular resistance
MAA = macroaggregated albumin

pulmonary edema. Pathologic studies of the lungs from patients dying of acute hepatic failure showed the development of diffuse pulmonary arterial dilatation within 4 days of the onset of illness and coma (Williams et al 1979). These vascular dilatations were functionally important in causing hypoxemia, as up to 39% of blood was shunted across the lungs (normal <5%), implying that substantial amounts of venous blood were not oxygenated during passage through the dilated pulmonary vessels (see hepatopulmonary syndrome below).

*Chronic liver disease*

Acute respiratory failure can also develop in patients with chronic liver disease who deteriorate, primarily as a consequence of extrapulmonary infection (Matuschak et al 1987). A retrospective study of 100 patients with deteriorating hepatic function admitted to an intensive care unit found that 91% of those requiring mechanical ventilation died (Shellman et al 1988). The usual reasons for intubation and mechanical ventilation in these patients are progressive hypoxemia, the need for airway protection and cardiac arrest. Only 2% of patients with jaundice (bilirubin >3.5 mg/dl or 60 mmol/L), poorly controlled ascites, encephalopathy, a serum albumin <20 g/L or a serum creatinine above 1.3 mg/dl or 115 mmol/L survived where mechanical ventilation was needed.

## Cirrhosis and portal hypertension

Impaired arterial oxygenation sufficient to cause cyanosis has long been recognized as a complication of cirrhosis or portal hypertension (Rodman et al 1960, Berthelot et al 1966). The pulmonary pathophysiology is multifactorial (Table 40.3) even in a particular patient and has been reviewed extensively (Krowka & Cortese 1989, Agusti et al 1990). The degree of respiratory impairment (dyspnea) may be the dominating clinical complaint if hypoxemia is severe ($PaO_2$ <50 mmHg, 6.7 kPa), overshadowing other manifestations of liver disease. Hypoxia improves in most patients if they are given supplemental inspired oxygen. Three particular pulmonary problems deserve special mention in patients with cirrhosis: hepatopulmonary syndrome, pulmonary hypertension and pleural effusions.

**Table 40.3** Mechanisms of hypoxemia in liver disease

| | |
|---|---|
| Ventilation–perfusion mismatch | |
| Impaired hypoxic pulmonary vasoconstriction | |
| Pulmonary vascular dilatations/shunting | Profound hypoxemia |
| Pulmonary vascular leak | |
| Pulmonary vascular constriction | |
| Portopulmonary vein anastomosis | Minimal contribution |
| Pleural "spiders" | |
| Right shift of hemoglobin dissociation curve | |

*Hepatopulmonary syndrome*

***Clinical features.*** The hepatopulmonary syndrome is characterized by a triad of reduced arterial oxygenation and intrapulmonary vascular dilatation in a patient with chronic liver disease (Krowka & Cortese 1994). Patients present with the features of hepatic disease in 80% of cases and the liver disorders are usually chronic (cirrhotic and noncirrhotic portal hypertension) and associated with clubbing, cyanosis and spider telangiectasias (Rodriguez-Roisin et al 1987, Krowka & Cortese 1994). The syndrome can result in severe hypoxemia causing cyanosis (Rydell & Hoffbauer 1956), associated with an excellent response to 100% inspired oxygen and a reduction of $PaO_2$ when moving from the supine to the standing position (orthodeoxia) (Krowka et al 1993). Hypoxia may worsen in spite of clinically stable liver disease.

The natural history of the syndrome is still poorly defined, but in the largest series published to date approximately 40% of patients died within 4 years of diagnosis (Krowka et al 1993). Medical therapy and interventional radiologic procedures (coil embolotherapy) have resulted in occasional improvements in this syndrome (Krowka & Cortese 1994). Hepatopulmonary syndrome can resolve after liver transplantation and may occasionally be an indication for transplantation (p. 1074).

***Pulmonary pathophysiology.*** The hepatopulmonary syndrome is thought to be due to a "diffusion-perfusion defect" with essentially normal ventilation (Edell et al 1989). Arterial vasodilatation has been demonstrated by contrast echocardiography (Hind & Wong 1981), perfusion lung scanning using technetium-99m labeled macroaggregated albumin ($^{99Tc}$MAA) (Stanley et al 1972, Genovesi et al 1976, Wolfe et al 1977) and pulmonary angiography. Angiograms may be normal in spite of substantial arterial oxygen abnormalities in this syndrome. Two angiographic appearances have been described, characterized by diffuse (type I) and discrete (type II) dilatations (Krowka et al 1993).

The pulmonary hemodynamics in this syndrome are similar to those found in chronic liver disease generally and include an elevated cardiac index, normal or reduced mean pulmonary artery pressure and normal to substantially reduced pulmonary vascular resistance (Groszmann 1993). This syndrome is not to be confused with hypoxemia caused by pulmonary hypertension in which the hemodynamics are substantially different and include elevated pulmonary vascular resistance and perhaps a reduced cardiac index. A spectrum of arterial oxygenation abnormalities occurs in the hepatopulmonary syndrome and due to the near-normal response to 100% inspired oxygen in some patients, it is inappropriate to characterize this syndrome as intrapulmonary "shunting" in all patients.

Most patients with hepatopulmonary syndrome probably have impaired hypoxic vasoconstriction (Rodriguez-Roisin et al 1992). The reason for this is unclear, but it most likely relates to a vasodilator substance that is not cleared by the liver and which is present in increased amount because of the liver disease or perhaps because an inhibitor of a normal vasoconstrictor substance is present (Krowka & Cortese 1994). The leading candidate as the mediator of this hyperdynamic and subsequent vasodilatory state is currently nitric oxide (endothelial-derived relaxing factor) (Whittle & Moncada 1992).

### *Pulmonary hypertension*

The association between pulmonary hypertension (mean pulmonary artery pressure greater than 25 mmHg at rest or pulmonary vascular resistance greater than 120 dynes/s/cm$^{-5}$) and portal hypertension is well documented but uncommon (Hadengue et al 1991, Plevak et al 1993).

***Clinical features.*** Cirrhosis is the usual cause and the diagnosis of cirrhosis and portal hypertension has usually preceded that of pulmonary hypertension by years (Lebrec et al 1979, Lockhart 1985, Shah et al 1995). Approximately 40% of these patients have had previous portasystemic shunt surgery (Lockhart 1985). Patients with portal hypertension due to portal vein thrombosis and nodular regenerative hyperplasia have also been documented to have pulmonary hypertension. Children and young adults rarely get pulmonary hypertension and if it does occur, it usually complicates noncirrhotic portal hypertension (Portmann et al 1993). There is no consistent relation between measurements of hepatic dysfunction (biochemical parameters) and the development of pulmonary hypertension (Robalino & Moodie 1991).

The natural history of pulmonary hypertension in patients with portal hypertension is not favorable. A mean survival of 15 months and mortality of nearly 50% within 6 months of diagnosis in patients with severe pulmonary hypertension have been reported (Robalino & Moodie 1991). Many feel that cardiac function and reserve is probably the single most important prognostic factor indicated by a reduced cardiac index (<2 L/min/m$^2$) (Hadengue et al 1991).

***Pulmonary pathophysiology.*** The diagnosis of pulmonary hypertension certainly requires a high degree of suspicion, as many patients do not have clinical problems due to hypoxemia. Transthoracic or transesophageal echocardiography is very helpful in suggesting the diagnosis, but confirmation requires measurement of pulmonary artery hemodynamics using pulmonary artery catheterization. It is important to distinguish elevated pulmonary artery pressures caused by increased vascular resistance from pulmonary artery pressures that are high due to the hyperdynamic circulation associated with liver disease.

The etiology of pulmonary hypertension in these clinical situations is complex and probably represents a combination of factors including a hyperdynamic systemic circulation with high pulmonary artery blood flow, vasoactive substances that are not cleared because of the dysfunctional liver and absence of critical factors preventing vasoconstriction due to hepatic dysfunction and perhaps other unknown physiologic mechanisms (Robalino & Moodie 1991). Although thrombi have been documented in pathologic specimens, thromboembolic disease is not thought to be a major factor in these patients (Lockhart 1985).

### *Pleural effusion*

Pleural effusion occurs in about 6% of patients with cirrhosis complicated by ascites (Krowka & Cortese 1989). Most are small and are noted on chest radiographs, but some are massive and are referred to as hepatic hydrothorax (Fig. 40.1). Hepatic hydrothorax usually occurs in patients with obvious ascites (p. 1019) and the ascitic fluid is thought to pass from the abdomen to the pleural space via diaphragmatic defects or blebs that have been well documented at autopsy (Lieberman & Peters 1970). However, due to negative intrathoracic pressure generated on inspiration, effusions can occur without clinical evidence of ascites in patients with liver disease, as the fluid is transferred into the pleural space from the abdomen as it is produced (Singer et al 1977, Rubinstein et al 1985). The peritoneal origin of the pleural fluid in such cases can be demonstrated by injecting $^{99m}$Tc sulfur colloid into the

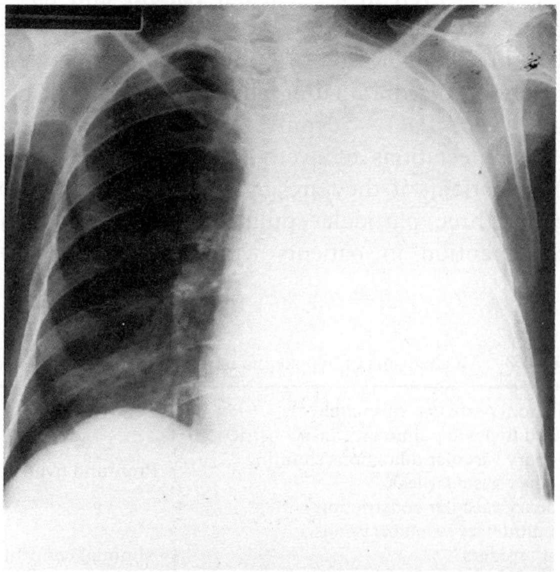

**Fig. 40.1** Hepatic hydrothorax in a patient with alcoholic cirrhosis and gross ascites. Investigations and autopsy revealed no alternative cause.

peritoneal cavity and noting its rapid subsequent accumulation in the pleural fluid (Rubinstein et al 1985).

Most effusions are in the right hemithorax, but about a fifth are on the left side and these are more often due to a cause other than cirrhosis such as tuberculosis (Mirouze et al 1981). They may be massive and associated with reduced lung volumes and substantial hypoxemia. Diagnostic thoracentesis should be carried out, especially if there is fever or any recent change in the effusion. The fluid is usually a clear transudate with a serum/effusion total protein ratio <0.5 and a serum/effusion LDH ratio <0.6. It should be examined cytologically for malignant cells and neutrophil counts, cultures and pH assessment should be done to rule out infection (below). Therapeutic thoracentesis can be attempted but is not usually satisfactory due to rapid recurrence. However, removal of up to 2 L can effectively relieve dyspnea rapidly. In general, the insertion of a chest tube for drainage or pleurodesis is not helpful because of the inability permanently to sclerose the pleural space (Krowka & Cortese 1989). Recently, transjugular intrahepatic portal stent shunts (p. 1007) have been reported to improve hepatic hydrothorax substantially (Strauss et al 1994).

***Spontaneous bacterial empyema (SBEM).*** This condition is characterized by infection in a pleural effusion that cannot be attributed to any local cause (Xiol et al 1990). Most patients have ascites and it is likely that infection reaches the pleural space directly from the abdomen or via the blood. *E. coli, K. pneumonia* and *Cl. perfringens* are the organisms most commonly isolated from the pleural fluid and may also be found in the ascitic fluid or blood. Pleural fluid containing >500 polymorphonuclear leukocytes/min$^3$ should be regarded as infected even though organisms are not grown (culture-negative SBEM). The pleural fluid is usually a transudate but may become an exudate during the infection.

SBEM should be suspected in any patient with a pleural effusion who becomes febrile or who develops cough, dyspnea or chest pain. Sometimes the clinical features are those of associated spontaneous bacterial peritonitis (p. 1033) or a general deterioration in the patient's condition. Occasionally, there are no clinical features and SBEM is found incidentally. SBEM needs to be differentiated from infection due to underlying lung disease, usually a pneumonia, and this can be done from the chest radiograph appearances of pneumonia and by finding organisms more typical of spontaneous bacterial peritonitis than of pneumonia in the pleural fluid. Patients should be treated with a broad-spectrum antibiotic such as cefotaxime 1 g 6-hourly intravenously pending results of microbiological sensitivity tests. Patients with SBEM usually have advanced liver disease and the mortality of SBEM is around 20%. Recurrence is common, but it is not yet known whether the chances of recurrence can be predicted from analysis of the pleural fluid, as is the case for peritoneal fluid and spontaneous bacterial peritonitis (p. 1033). The value of prophylactic therapy is unknown but is recommended by analogy with spontaneous bacterial peritonitis (p. 1035).

### **Primary biliary cirrhosis** (PBC)

A spectrum of pulmonary abnormalities (Table 40.1) has been documented in PBC (Rodriguez-Roisin et al 1981). Early PBC has been associated with subclinical lymphocytic alveolitis (Wallaert et al 1986) and late PBC can be complicated by progressive fibrosing alveolitis (Wallace et al 1987), expiratory airflow obstruction, intrapulmonary granulomas (Stanley & Woodgate 1972) and pulmonary hemorrhage (Bissuel et al 1992). These relationships underscore the possible autoimmune aspects of PBC (sicca complex and Sjögren's syndrome) as they relate to the lung (Culp et al 1982). In addition, similarities between PBC and sarcoidosis have been proposed (p. 940). Studies reporting bronchoalveolar lavage findings or T-lymphocytosis in patients with PBC suggest a probable clinical and immunologic overlap (Krowka & Cortese 1989, Spiteri et al 1990).

A recent study of 67 PBC patients who had never smoked showed a good correlation between deteriorating pulmonary diffusing capacity for carbon monoxide (DLCO) and severity of PBC as defined by the Mayo model risk score for PBC (p. 1152). Reduced DLCO (<80% predicted) occurred in 26 patients (39%) and was not related to the presence of sicca complex or Sjögren's syndrome, suggesting a subclinical alveolitis or even hepatopulmonary syndrome (Krowka et al 1991). Pulmonary hypertension and the hepatopulmonary syndrome have been well documented in advanced PBC (Krowka & Cortese 1989, Stoller et al 1990) and severe pulmonary hypertension has been reported in PBC in the absence of portal hypertension (Yoshida et al 1994).

### $\alpha_1$-Antitrypsin deficiency

Most patients with PiZZ homozygote $\alpha_1$-antitrypsin deficiency have pulmonary dysfunction as a clinical manifestation of this type of liver disease (Crystal 1990). In a study of 124 adults with homozygous PiZZ $\alpha_1$-antitrypsin deficiency referred to a single pulmonary center because of respiratory complaints, 5% had severe expiratory airflow obstruction ($FEV_1$/FVC <40%) but fewer than 10% had abnormal liver function tests (Brantley et al 1988). The National Institutes of Health Registry of patients with $\alpha_1$-antitrypsin deficiency records 1129 patients, of whom 90% had severe expiratory airflow obstruction (mean $FEV_1$/FVC = 42.5%) and 16% had a self-reported history of pulmonary disease (unpublished data). In contrast, a study of 19 adult patients referred to a single center for evaluation of cirrhosis caused by $\alpha_1$-antitrypsin deficiency showed that 53% had only moderate expiratory airflow obstruction (Rakela et al 1987). The predominant clinical manifestation in children with $\alpha_1$-antitrypsin deficiency is hepatic dysfunction (10–20%), whereas clinically important pulmonary abnormalities are rare irrespective of the severity of liver disease (Crystal 1990).

### Hepatic veno-occlusive disease (HVOD)

HVOD is frequently associated with pulmonary and renal dysfunction. In a study of 355 consecutive bone marrow transplant patients, 56% developed HVOD; pulmonary abnormalities appeared approximately 5–12 days after the onset of liver dysfunction (McDonald et al 1993). Pulmonary infiltrates, pleural effusions and the need for mechanical ventilation developed in 48%, 28% and 15% of patients respectively. Mortality was greater than 90% for those requiring mechanical ventilation.

### Chronic hepatitis

Interstitial lung disease (fibrosing alveolitis) with reduced DLCO has been well documented in autoimmune hepatitis (Turner-Warwick 1968, Stanley & Woodgate 1972, Golding et al 1973, Krowka & Cortese 1989). A relation between hepatitis C virus infection and interstitial lung disease has been described, but the nature of the relation is controversial (Ueda et al 1992, Irving et al 1993). Some have attributed the lung disease to an adverse effect of natural and recombinant α-interferon on the lung during the treatment of hepatitis C virus infection (Chin et al 1994).

### Primary sclerosing cholangitis

Expiratory airflow obstruction associated with bronchitis and/or bronchiectasis in patients with primary sclerosing cholangitis and inflammatory bowel disease has been reported (Butland et al 1981). Pulmonary function abnormalities have been noted in primary sclerosing cholangitis patients prior to liver transplantation, but their clinical significance is unknown (Krowka & Cortese 1989).

## PULMONARY CONSIDERATIONS IN LIVER TRANSPLANTATION

Pulmonary dysfunction and pulmonary disease are important factors in the assessment of patients for liver transplantation (p. 1155). In practice, pulmonary infection and identification of pulmonary vascular dysfunction are the two main pretransplant pulmonary issues. Pulmonary indications and contraindications for liver transplantation are in a state of evolution and will change as knowledge of the effects of liver disease on the pulmonary circulation increases (Krowka & Cortese 1990, Rodriguez-Roisin & Krowka 1994), but clinically significant pulmonary dysfunction will be revealed by a chest radiograph, measurement of arterial oxygenation and appropriate echocardiography (Krowka & Cortese 1994).

***Infection.*** It is essential to identify infection when pleural effusions or pulmonary infiltrates are present, as infection has potentially devastating consequences after an otherwise successful liver transplantation due to the need for immunosuppressive drugs (Afessa et al 1993). Pleural fluid should be cultured and its pH determined, as pH <7.1 strongly suggests empyema. Bronchoscopy with bronchoalveolar lavage or even a limited thoracoscopy is appropriate to determine the etiology of pulmonary infiltrates (alveolar or interstitial) in selected clinical settings.

***Adult respiratory distress syndrome (ARDS).*** Acute respiratory failure requiring mechanical ventilation can develop in fulminant hepatic failure or decompensated chronic liver diseases. The severe hypoxemia associated with ARDS can resolve entirely after liver transplantation provided that infection is not present (Doyle et al 1993). Without transplantation, the mortality in these patients is extremely high (Matuschak et al 1987).

***Hepatopulmonary syndrome.*** This remains a clinical problem in that a favorable response to liver transplantation is usual (Stoller et al 1990, Laberge et al 1992, Scott et al 1993b, Van Obbergh et al 1993) but not universal (Hobeika et al 1994). Complete resolution of the pulmonary vascular dilatations with normalization of arterial oxygenation has been well documented in children and adults (Krowka & Cortese 1990). Indicators associated with a poor post-transplant outcome have yet to be defined but may include the response to 100% oxygen administration, at least in adults (Krowka & Cortese 1994). Deteriorating arterial oxygenation in patients with stable hepatic dysfunction has been proposed as an indication for liver transplantation due to the poor prognosis of this pulmonary complication (Rodriguez-Roisin & Krowka 1994).

***Pulmonary hypertension.*** Pulmonary hypertension can be missed if clinicians rely only on arterial oxygen assessment to define the need for further study. Severe pulmonary hypertension can result in sudden death after transplantation due to acute right heart failure if the pulmonary vascular resistance or cardiac reserve is substantially abnormal (Cheng & Woehlck 1992, Prager et al 1992, Scott et al 1993a). It is important that substantial pulmonary hypertension (pulmonary vascular resistance [PVR] above 400 units [dynes/s/cm$^{-5}$]) can occur in the setting of only mild hypoxemia. Reversibility of pulmonary hypertension has been documented if PVR is not excessive (<120 dynes/s/cm$^{-5}$) or if cardiac reserve is acceptable (Plevak et al 1993, Yoshida et al 1993). Echocardiography with Doppler estimates of pulmonary artery pressure is the screening method of choice for detecting pulmonary hypertension prior to liver transplantation, but findings should be confirmed with pulmonary arterial catheterization measurements.

REFERENCES

Afessa B, Guy P C, Plevak D J, Swenson S J, Patel H G, Krowka M J 1993 Pulmonary complications of orthotopic liver transplantation. Mayo Clinic Proceedings 68: 427–434

Agusti A G N, Roca J, Bosch J, Rodriguez-Roisin R 1990 The lung in patients with cirrhosis. Journal of Hepatology 10: 251–257

Berkowitz K A, Butensky M S, Smith R L 1993 Pulmonary function changes after large volume paracentesis. American Journal of Gastroenterology 88: 905–907

Berthelot P, Walker J G, Sherlock S, Reid L 1966 Arterial changes in the lungs in cirrhosis of the liver: lung spider nevi. New England Journal of Medicine 274: 291–298

Bissuel F, Bizollon T, Dijoud F et al 1992 Pulmonary hemorrhage and glomerulonephritis in primary biliary cirrhosis. Hepatology 16: 1357–1361

Brantley M L, Paul L D, Miller B H, Falk R T, Wu M, Crystal R G 1988 Clinical features and history of the destructive lung disease associated with alpha$_1$-antitrypsin deficiency of adults with pulmonary symptoms. American Review of Respiratory Disease 138: 327–336

Butland R J A, Cole P, Citron K M, Turner-Warwick M 1981 Chronic bronchial suppuration and inflammatory bowel disease. Quarterly Journal of Medicine 50: 63–75

Cheng E Y, Woehlck H J 1992 Pulmonary artery hypertension complicating anesthesia for liver transplantation. Anesthesiology 77: 389–392

Chin K, Tabata C, Satake N, Nagai S, Moriyasu F, Kuno K 1994 Pneumonitis associated with natural and recombinant interferon alfa therapy for hepatitis C. Chest 105: 939–941

Crystal R G 1990 $\alpha_1$ Antitrypsin deficiency, emphysema and liver disease. Journal of Clinical Investigation 85: 1343–1352

Culp K S, Fleming C R, Duffy J, Baldus W P, Dickson E R 1982 Autoimmune associations in primary biliary cirrhosis. Mayo Clinic Proceedings 57: 365–370

Doyle H R, Marino I R, Miro A et al 1993 Adult respiratory distress syndrome secondary to end-stage liver disease – successful outcome following liver transplantation. Transplantation 55: 292–296

Edell E S, Cortese D A, Krowka M J, Rehder K 1989 Severe hypoxemia in liver disease. American Review of Respiratory Disease 140: 1631–1635

Genovesi M G, Tierney D F, Taplin G V, Eisenberg H 1976 An intravenous radionuclide method to evaluate hypoxemia caused by abnormal alveolar vessels. Limitation of conventional techniques. American Review of Respiratory Diseases 114: 59–65

Golding P L, Smith M, Williams R 1973 Multisystem involvement in chronic liver disease. Studies on the incidence and pathogenesis. American Journal of Medicine 55: 772–782

Groszmann R J 1993 Hyperdynamic state in chronic liver diseases. Journal of Hepatology 17 (suppl 2): S38–S40

Hadengue A, Benhayoun M K, Lebrec D, Benhamou J-P 1991 Pulmonary hypertension complicating portal hypertension: prevalence and relation to splanchnic hemodynamics. Gastroenterology 100: 520–528

Hind C R K, Wong C M 1981 Detection of pulmonary arteriovenous fistulae in patients with cirrhosis by contrast 2-D echocardiography. Gut 22: 1042–1045

Hobeika J, Houssin D, Bernard O, Devictor D, Grimon G, Chapuis Y 1994 Orthotopic liver transplantation in children with chronic liver disease and severe hypoxemia. Transplantation 57: 224–228

Hourani J M, Bellamy P E, Tashkin D P, Batra P, Simmons M S 1991 Pulmonary dysfunction in advanced liver disease: frequent occurrence of an abnormal diffusing capacity. American Journal of Medicine 90: 693–700

Irving W L, Day S, Johnston I 1993 Idiopathic pulmonary fibrosis and hepatitis C virus infection. American Review of Respiratory Diseases 148: 1683–1684

Krowka M J, Cortese D A 1989 Pulmonary aspects of liver disease and liver transplantation. Clinics in Chest Medicine 10: 593–616

Krowka M J, Cortese D A 1990 Hepatopulmonary syndrome: an evolving perspective in the era of liver transplantation. Hepatology 11: 138–142

Krowka M J, Cortese D A 1994 Hepatopulmonary syndrome: current concepts in diagnostic and therapeutic considerations. Chest 105: 1528–1537

Krowka M J, Grambsch P M, Edell E S, Cortese D A, Dickson E R 1991 Primary biliary cirrhosis: relation between hepatic function and pulmonary function in patients who never smoked. Hepatology 13: 1095–1100

Krowka M J, Dickson E R, Cortese D A 1993 Hepatopulmonary syndrome. Clinical observations and lack of therapeutic response to somatostatin analogue. Chest 104: 515–521

Laberge J-M, Brandt M L, Lebecque P et al 1992 Reversal of cirrhosis-related pulmonary shunting in two children by orthotopic liver transplantation. Transplantation 53: 1135–1165

Lebrec D, Capron J P, Dhumeaux D, Benhamou J-P 1979 Pulmonary hypertension complicating portal hypertension. American Review of Respiratory Diseases 120: 849–856

Lieberman F L, Peters R L 1970 Cirrhotic hydrothorax: further evidence that an acquired diaphragmatic defect is at fault. Archives of Internal Medicine 125: 114–117

Lockhart A 1985 Pulmonary arterial hypertension in portal hypertension. Clinics in Gastroenterology 14: 123–138

McDonald G B, Hinds M S, Fisher L D et al 1993 Veno-occlusive disease of the liver and multiorgan failure after bone marrow transplantation: a cohort of 355 patients. Annals of Internal Medicine 118: 255–267

Matuschak G M, Rinaldo J E, Pinsky M R, Gaveler J S, van Thiel D H 1987 Effect of end-stage liver failure on the incidence and resolution of adult respiratory distress syndrome. Journal of Critical Care 2: 162–173

Mirouze D, Juttner H-U, Reynolds T B 1981 Left pleural effusion in patients with chronic liver disease and ascites. Prospective study of 22 cases. Digestive Diseases and Sciences 26: 984–988

Plevak D, Krowka M, Rettke S, Dunn W, Southorn P 1993 Successful liver transplantation in patients with mild to moderate pulmonary hypertension. Transplantation Proceedings 25: 1840

Portmann B, Stewart S, Higenbottam T W, Clayton P T, Lloyd J K, Williams R 1993 Nodular transformation of the liver associated with portal and pulmonary arterial hypertension. Gastroenterology 104: 616–621

Prager M C, Cauldwell C A, Ascher N L, Roberts J P, Wolfe C L 1992 Pulmonary hypertension associated with liver disease is not reversible after liver transplantation. Anesthesiology 77: 375–378

Rakela J, Goldschmier M, Ludwig J 1987 Late manifestation of chronic liver disease in adults with alpha$_1$-antitrypsin deficiency. Digestive Diseases and Sciences 32: 1358–1362

Robalino B D, Moodie D S 1991 Association between primary pulmonary hypertension and portal hypertension: analysis of its pathophysiology and clinical, laboratory and hemodynamic manifestations. Journal of the American College of Cardiology 17: 492–498

Rodman T, Sobel M, Close H P 1960 Arterial oxygen unsaturation and the ventilation-perfusion defect of Laënnec's cirrhosis. New England Journal of Medicine 263: 73–77

Rodriguez-Roisin R, Krowka M J 1994 Is severe arterial hypoxaemia due to hepatic disease an indication for liver transplantation? A new therapeutic approach. European Respiratory Journal 7: 839–842

Rodriguez-Roisin R, Parés A, Bruguera M et al 1981 Pulmonary involvement in primary biliary cirrhosis. Thorax 36: 208–212

Rodriguez-Roisin R, Roca J, Agusti A G N, Mastai R, Wagner P D, Bosch J 1987 Gas exchange and pulmonary vascular reactivity in patients with liver cirrhosis. American Review of Respiratory Diseases 135: 1085–1092

Rodriguez-Roisin R, Agusti A G N, Roca J 1992 The hepatopulmonary syndrome: new name, old complexities. Thorax 47: 897–902

Rubinstein D, McInnes I E, Dudley F J 1985 Hepatic hydrothorax in the absence of clinical ascites: diagnosis and management. Gastroenterology 88: 188–191

Rydell R, Hoffbauer F W 1956 Multiple pulmonary arteriovenous fistulas in juvenile cirrhosis. American Journal of Medicine 21: 450–460

Scott V, DeWolf A, Kang Y et al 1993a Reversibility of pulmonary hypertension after liver transplantation: a case report. Transplantation Proceedings 25: 1789–1790

Scott V, Miro A, Kang Y et al 1993b Reversibility of the hepatopulmonary syndrome by orthotopic liver transplantation. Transplantation Proceedings 25: 1787–1788

Shah H A, Piris J, Finlayson N D C 1995 Primary pulmonary hypertension developing 11 years after a splenorenal shunt for portal hypertension in hepatic cirrhosis. European Journal of Gastroenterology and Hepatology 7: 283–286
Shellman R G, Fulkerson W J, de Long E, Piantadosi C A 1988 Prognosis of patients with cirrhosis and chronic liver disease admitted to the medical intensive care unit. Critical Care Medicine 16: 671–678
Singer J A, Kaplan M M, Katz R L 1977 Cirrhotic pleural effusion in the absence of ascites. Gastroenterology 73: 575–577
Spiteri M A, Johnson M, Epstein O, Sherlock S, Clarke S W, Poulter L W 1990 Immunological features of lung lavage cells from patients with primary biliary cirrhosis may reflect those seen in pulmonary sarcoidosis. Gut 31: 208–212
Stanley N N, Woodgate D J 1972 Mottled chest radiograph and gas transfer defect in chronic liver disease. Thorax 27: 315–323
Stanley N N, Ackrill P, Wood J 1972 Lung perfusion scanning in hepatic cirrhosis. British Medical Journal 4: 639–643
Stoller J K, Moodie D, Schiavone W A et al 1990 Reduction of intrapulmonary shunt and resolution of digital clubbing associated with primary biliary cirrhosis after liver transplantation. Hepatology 11: 54–58
Strauss R M, Martin L G, Kaufman S L, Boyer T D 1994 Transjugular intrahepatic portal systemic shunt for the management of symptomatic cirrhotic hydrothorax. American Journal of Gastroenterology 89: 1520–1522
Trewby P N, Warren R, Contini S, Crosbie W A, Wilkinson S P, Laws J W 1978 Incidence and pathophysiology of pulmonary edema in fulminant hepatic failure. Gastroenterology 74: 859–865
Turner-Warwick M 1968 Fibrosing alveolitis and chronic liver disease. Quarterly Journal of Medicine 37: 133–149
Ueda T, Ohta K, Suzuki N et al 1992 Idiopathic pulmonary fibrosis and high prevalence of serum antibodies to hepatitis C virus. American Review of Respiratory Diseases 146: 266–268
Van Obbergh L, Carlier M, de Clety S C et al 1993 Liver transplantation and pulmonary gas exchanges in hypoxemic children. American Review of Respiratory Medicine 148: 1408–1410
Wallace J G, Tong M J, Ueki B N, Quismorio F P 1987 Pulmonary involvement in primary biliary cirrhosis. Journal of Clinical Gastroenterology 9: 431–435
Wallaert B, Bonniere P, Prin L, Cortot A, Tonnel A B, Voisin C 1986 Primary biliary cirrhosis. Subclinical inflammatory alveolitis in patients with normal chest radiographs. Chest 90: 842–848
Whittle B J R, Moncada S 1992 Nitric oxide: the elusive mediator of the hyperdynamic circulation of cirrhosis. Hepatology 16: 1089–1092
Williams A, Trewby P, Williams R, Reid L 1979 Structural alterations to the pulmonary circulation in fulminant hepatic failure. Thorax 34: 447–453
Wolfe J D, Tashkin D P, Holly F E, Brachman M B, Genovesi M G 1977 Hypoxemia of cirrhosis: detection of abnormal small pulmonary vascular channels by a quantitative radionuclide method. American Journal of Medicine 63: 746–754
Xiol X, Castellote J, Baliellas C et al 1990 Spontaneous bacterial empyema in cirrhotic patients: analysis of eleven cases. Hepatology 11: 365–370
Yoshida E M, Erb S R, Pflugfelder P W et al 1993 Single-lung versus liver transplantation for the treatment of portopulmonary hypertension – a comparison of two patients. Transplantation 55: 688–690

SECTION 10

# Miscellaneous liver diseases

# 41. Vascular disorders of the liver

*A. J. MacGilchrist Peter C. Hayes*

## INTRODUCTION

Liver damage can result from impaired supply of blood to the liver due to hepatic artery or portal vein occlusion or from impaired venous drainage from the liver due to obstruction of the hepatic veins. The dual blood supply provides considerable protection for the normal liver against occlusion of either hepatic artery or portal vein and vascular liver damage is consequently rare. Problems can arise within the vascular bed of the liver itself, namely sinusoidal dilatation, perisinusoidal fibrosis and peliosis hepatis. Liver damage can also result from systemic circulatory changes in shock (p. 1099) and cardiac failure (p. 1097) and these are considered elsewhere.

## HEPATIC VENOUS DISEASE

### Budd–Chiari syndrome

Obstruction of the larger hepatic veins, with or without involvement of the vena cava, gives rise to the Budd–Chiari syndrome (Tavill et al 1975, Powell-Jackson et al 1982, Dilawari et al 1994, Mahmoud et al 1996).

#### *Etiology*

Budd–Chiari syndrome is more common in females. An underlying thrombotic tendency is present in up to a half of patients, especially where there has been an acute onset, and causes include pregnancy, oral contraceptive drugs, abdominal trauma, Behçet's disease, systemic lupus erythematosus and a number of hematological diseases including paroxysmal nocturnal hemoglobinuria, other myeloproliferative disorders and thrombophilic states such as deficiencies of protein C and protein S or a circulating antiphospholipid antibody. Recent bone marrow culture studies suggest that more subtle thrombotic tendencies are common in patients without overt causes of thrombosis (Pagliuca et al 1990). Rarely, local obstruction by hepatic tumors, abscesses or liver cysts may occur and there is a particular association with renal carcinoma. Intravascular webs in the hepatic veins or inferior vena cava are particularly common in Asia, India and South Africa but also occur occasionally elsewhere (Simson 1982, Benbow 1986). Frequently, no cause for the Budd–Chiari syndrome can be found.

#### *Pathology*

Acute severe occlusion causes marked centrilobular congestion with survival of periportal hepatocytes (Fig. 41.1). Less severe occlusion causes only sinusoidal dilatation. Long-standing occlusion leads to fibrosis with central linkage leading eventually to cirrhosis.

#### *Clinical features*

The cardinal features are abdominal pain, ascites and hepatomegaly. Fulminant hepatic failure with rapidly progressive severe abdominal pain, ascites and jaundice leading to encephalopathy occurs in about 10% of patients (p. 808). This is an urgent and important diagnosis because rapid surgical decompression is effective in restoring hepatic function. More commonly, the onset is less acute with a prodrome of general malaise and vague abdominal pain lasting from a week to several months followed by abdominal pain and ascites with absent or only mild jaundice. Increasingly, the condition presents with ascites or variceal bleeding once cirrhosis and portal hypertension are established. Leg edema suggests obstruction of the inferior vena cava. Jaundice, hepatomegaly and ascites also occur in right heart failure and it is critical to seek elevation of the jugular venous pulse on clinical examination.

#### *Investigations*

Liver function tests are not usually helpful, the degree of elevation of the transaminases reflecting the acuteness of the presentation. The protein content of ascitic fluid may be high, indicating an exudative ascites, but this is only common in acute presentations. Ultrasound imaging is

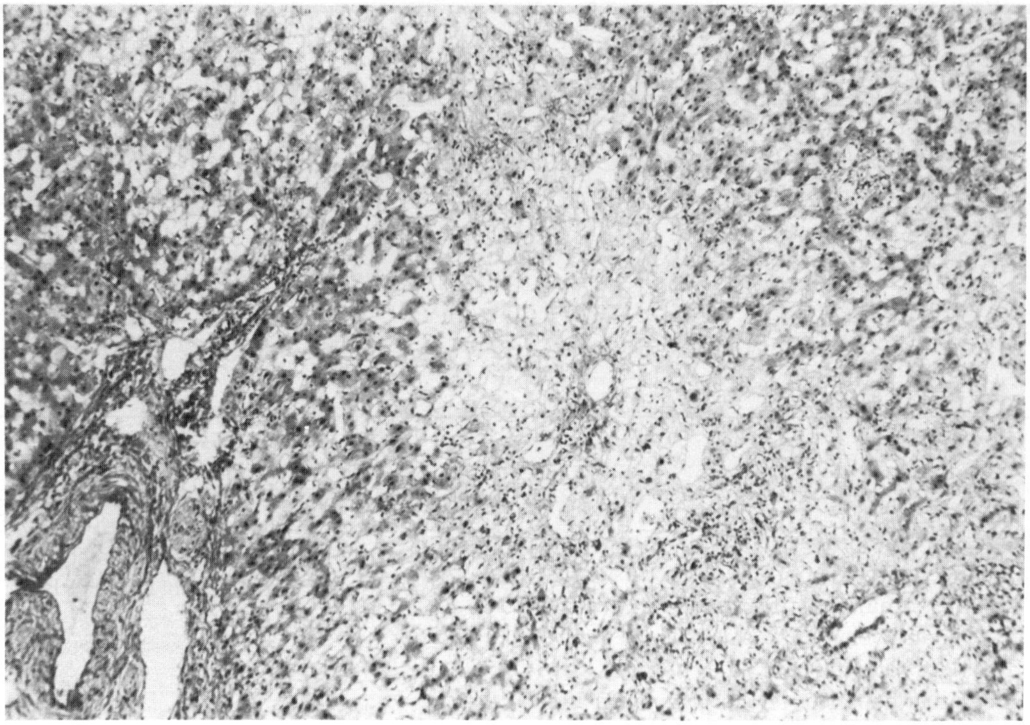

**Fig. 41.1** Budd–Chiari syndrome. Note the thickened central vein with loss of hepatocytes and fibrosis in the surrounding lobule (hematoxylin and eosin, ×4).

helpful, as Doppler signals can identify the patency or occlusion of the hepatic veins (p. 51). Computed tomography (p. 66) and magnetic resonance (p. 76) scanning may visualize hepatic veins and demonstrate sparing of the caudate lobe that drains directly to the inferior vena cava. Hepatic venography remains the best method for demonstrating patency or otherwise of the hepatic veins (Fig. 41.2). The inferior vena cava is often compressed by the enlarged caudate lobe. In these circumstances it is important to measure pressures within the inferior vena cava, as the functional obstruction is often less than it would appear radiologically. Radioisotope scanning, which yielded indirect evidence of the Budd–Chiari syndrome by highlighting the caudate lobe, is no longer employed. Liver biopsy is useful in chronic disease to assess the reversibility of the lesion, although surgical decompression may still be beneficial even when fibrosis is present. A careful search for an underlying thrombotic tendency is essential.

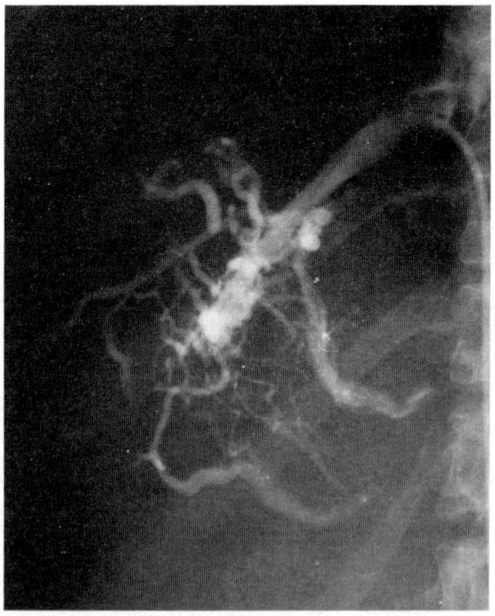

**Fig. 41.2** Budd–Chiari syndrome. Hepatic venography. Abnormal venous channels secondary to obstruction of the hepatic vein.

*Treatment*

Treatment in Budd–Chiari syndrome includes hepatic decompression, medical therapy for thrombosis and the complications of cirrhosis and occasionally liver transplantation.

***Hepatic decompression.*** This is the key to successful treatment in patients with more acute disease. In the past, this has been achieved by surgical mesocaval or portacaval shunts, although such shunts may be made difficult or impossible if the inferior vena cava is obstructed by thrombosis or if an enlarged caudate lobe impairs access to vascular structures. The use of synthetic grafts should be avoided if possible because of the continuing thrombotic tendency. Recently, nonsurgical approaches to decompression have been employed. A patent hepatic vein may be cannulated percutaneously and a route to the inferior vena cava opened by balloon dilatation (Vickers et al 1989, Fock et al 1993). Transjugular intrahepatic portasystemic stent shunting (TIPSS) may also be possible if the hepatic vein can be cannulated. However, these procedures require highly skilled invasive radiology and are not universally available.

***Medical therapy.*** Specific treatment of the underlying thrombotic tendency is rarely possible and most patients require lifelong anticoagulation. Thrombolytic therapy has been used in a few patients and can be successful even after several weeks of illness. The agent of choice is probably recombinant tissue plasminogen activator (Kwan & Hansard 1992, McMullin et al 1994). This therapy is unlikely to replace decompression but may prevent extension of the thrombus into the inferior vena cava and render surgery possible. Treatment of chronic Budd–Chiari syndrome includes the treatment of ascites (p. 1023), where care must be taken to avoid hypovolemia from diuretics or from paracentesis, as this can acutely compromise hepatic function. It also includes treatment of gastrointestinal bleeding from varices (p. 499) and of encephalopathy (p. 1051).

***Liver transplantation.*** Liver transplantation may be indicated occasionally, either in severe acute damage leading to fulminant hepatic failure or in chronic disease with liver failure due to irreversible cirrhosis.

### Veno-occlusive disease

Veno-occlusive disease (VOD) is a condition in which there is widespread occlusion of the small central hepatic veins.

#### *Etiology*

VOD was described originally in Jamaica following ingestion of bush teas containing pyrollizidine alkaloids (Stuart & Bras 1957). It is now principally caused by chemotherapeutic agents and is seen particularly following bone marrow transplantation for hematological malignancies where it is a consequence of the cytoreductive regime of radiotherapy and chemotherapy (McDonald et al 1986). Alcohol can cause the VOD syndrome when severe central hyaline sclerosis of the hepatic veins is present (p. 875).

#### *Pathology*

Sinusoidal blood flow is obstructed by concentric narrowing of the terminal hepatic venules, initially by subintimal edema and later by partial or complete fibrosis. This results in sinusoidal congestion and hepatocellular degeneration, most marked in the centrilobular zones (Shulman et al 1980). The process is usually self-limiting, but occasionally progressive central fibrosis leads to a cirrhosis similar to that in the Budd–Chiari syndrome.

#### *Clinical features*

The presentation is usually acute with abdominal pain, hepatomegaly and ascites. Jaundice is not marked. VOD following bone marrow transplantation usually develops within 2 weeks of the transplant. The condition is usually self-limiting but can lead to a fatal fulminant hepatic failure.

***Treatment.*** Treatment is limited to withdrawal of the causative agent and symptomatic treatment for the ascites.

## HEPATIC ARTERIAL DISEASE

### Hepatic artery occlusion

Hepatic artery occlusion is rare and is usually diagnosed at autopsy. It may be caused by neoplasms, emboli, polyarteritis nodosa, surgical trauma, blunt abdominal trauma or spontaneous thrombosis (O'Connor et al 1976). It may also complicate liver transplantation (p. 1161). Hepatic artery embolization or chemoembolization can be used to treat hepatic tumors (p. 1124), although this usually involves occluding arterial branches close to the tumor itself. Occlusion does not necessarily lead to hepatic infarction, as there is a good collateral circulation, and permanent hepatic damage is rare provided the liver is otherwise normal and the portal blood supply intact. Thrombosis of the hepatic artery and the portal vein is invariably fatal. Hepatic infarction is characterized clinically by sudden severe right upper quadrant abdominal pain with tenderness and guarding and by variable tachycardia, hypotension and peripheral circulatory failure. The features of the underlying causative condition may also be found.

Fever and leukocytosis are usually prominent and liver function tests show hepatocellular damage with the serum transaminase activity increased to levels seen in other causes of acute hepatitis (p. 742). The prothrombin time is prolonged if liver damage is severe enough. Radionuclide liver imaging may show multiple "cold" areas and a liver biopsy may show hepatic necrosis. Patients should be kept well oxygenated (6 L/min or more) and the circulation and fluid and electrolyte balance should be maintained by appropriate intravenous infusion.

### Hepatic artery aneurysm

The hepatic artery is the second most common site of splanchnic arterial aneurysms after the splenic artery, but they are rarely diagnosed. They are an important cause of bleeding into the biliary tract, the liver and the peritoneal cavity (Shaw 1982, Blue & Burney 1990). Three-quarters occur in the extrahepatic course of the artery and a quarter are within the liver; they may be saccular or fusiform in shape and a few are dissecting aneurysms. Extrahepatic aneurysms are usually caused by atheroma and occur in older patients, while intrahepatic aneurysms usually result from trauma, including liver biopsy and biliary surgery. Less common causes include vasculitis, especially polyarteritis nodosa, bacterial endocarditis, portal pyemia, liver abscess and inherent weakness of the arterial wall as in Marfan's syndrome. Some aneurysms occur in otherwise healthy people for no known cause.

Bleeding, the most important complication, is often recurrent and usually occurs into the biliary tract (hemobilia) (p. 493), the peritoneal cavity or directly into the gastrointestinal tract in some 10% of cases. The bleeding can be very severe, especially when it occurs into the peritoneal cavity or gastrointestinal tract, and it is usually accompanied by severe abdominal pain. Abdominal pain that is persistent and unrelated to meals can also be a presenting feature and occasionally compression of the biliary tract leads to the development of obstructive jaundice (Lewis et al 1982). Jaundice is usually the only abnormality on physical examination, but abdominal examination occasionally reveals an upper abdominal mass or a bruit and the gallbladder may become palpable during hemobilia.

The diagnosis is often missed, as it is frequently not considered. An abdominal radiograph shows calcification in the aneurysm in less than a half of cases and the lesion is revealed better by ultrasonography or computed tomography (Kibbler et al 1985). Arteriography is the definitive diagnostic method. Cholangiography may show a smooth tapering stricture in patients with obstructive jaundice (Lewis et al 1982). Surgical treatment is required unless medical contraindications are present. Extrahepatic aneurysms are usually ligated if they are proximal to the gastroduodenal artery and revascularization is required for those distal to or involving the gastroduodenal artery. Intrahepatic aneurysms are treated by ligation of the involved artery, hepatic resection of the involved area or percutaneous angiographic embolization.

### Systemic vasculitis

Vasculitides such as polyarteritis nodosa, Wegener's granulomatosis, rheumatoid arthritis and certain connective tissue disorders are associated with hepatomegaly in up to 30% of cases and with abnormal liver function tests in up to 60%, but they rarely cause major hepatic disease (p. 1106). Needle liver biopsy is generally unhelpful in the diagnosis of the various vasculitides (p. 1106). There is a strong association between polyarteritis nodosa (PAN) and hepatitis B (p. 799). Hepatitis B virus-associated PAN is a serious complication occurring early in the course of hepatitis B infection. It is ameliorated by immunosuppressive therapy (cyclophosphamide and corticosteroids) (McMahon et al 1989) and more recently α-interferon (p. 799) and plasma exchange have been effective (Guillevin et al 1994).

### Hemangioma

These are the most common hepatic tumors. They are usually small and asymptomatic, but larger tumors can be symptomatic (Yamamoto et al 1991). Symptomatic tumors cause abdominal pain, fullness and intraperitoneal bleeding. Jaundice and consumption coagulopathy are occasional occurrences. Treatment of large or symptomatic tumors is by resection or by transcatheter arterial embolization in patients unfit for surgery.

## PORTAL VENOUS DISEASE

Portal venous disease may affect the portal vascular system anywhere from the mesenteric veins to the terminal portal radicals in the liver.

### Portal venous thrombosis

Portamesenteric venous thrombosis is rare, but it can cause infarction of the bowel and death (p. 543). More often the manifestations are less severe and are difficult to diagnose. Thrombosis can occur in an otherwise normal venous system, particularly where a thrombophilic condition is present (p. 1077), in association with inflammatory or neoplastic intra-abdominal disease or as a consequence of portal hypertension (Witte et al 1985). Portal hypertension may be a long-term consequence of portal thrombosis.

***Investigations.*** Ultrasound imaging and computed tomography are noninvasive means of showing portal venous occlusion (p. 51). Portal angiography gives more definitive information (Stringer et al 1994). Patients with hypercoagulable states often show widespread mesenteric occlusion, those with idiopathic portal hypertension usually show only intrahepatic portal venous occlusion and most other patients show occlusion of the main portal vein with or without superior mesenteric venous occlusion.

#### *Acute thrombosis*

Thrombosis in an otherwise normal portal venous system is unusual and is often associated with underlying conditions predisposing to thrombosis. These are the conditions predisposing to hepatic vein thrombosis and hepatic vein thrombosis and portal vein thrombosis can occur together (p. 1077). Symptoms usually start suddenly with severe abdominal pain and often diarrhea. Clinical examination may or may not show peritonism and abdominal radiographs often show segmental small intestinal dilatation. Imaging and portal angiography are usually diagnostic.

**Table 41.1** Causes of portal venous obstruction in extrahepatic portal hypertension

| | |
|---|---|
| *Thrombosis* | |
| Sepsis | |
| | Umbilical |
| | Portal pyemia |
| | Systemic infection |
| Exchange transfusion via the umbilical vein | |
| Thrombotic disease | |
| | Polycythemia rubra vera |
| | Myeloproliferative diseases |
| | Paroxysmal nocturnal hemoglobinuria |
| | Hereditary protein C deficiency |
| Oral contraceptive drugs | |
| Pregnancy | |
| Abdominal trauma | |
| Biliary surgery | |
| Secondary | |
| | Cirrhosis |
| | Budd–Chiari syndrome |
| *Neoplasm* | |
| Extrinsic: pancreatic carcinoma | |
| Intrinsic: hepatocellular carcinoma | |
| *Inflammation* | |
| Pancreatitis | |
| *Congenital abnormality* | |
| *No identifiable cause* (50–75%) | |

There is often extensive thrombosis in the portal and mesenteric veins. Survival depends on early diagnosis and operation to remove infarcted bowel. Factors predisposing to thrombosis include those leading to more chronic portal vein thrombosis with portal hypertension (Table 41.1).

### *Thrombosis and intra-abdominal disease*

Patients who develop portal vein thrombosis in the course of intra-abdominal inflammatory disease show the features of an acute portal thrombosis, but in addition they have the features of such underlying conditions as suppurative or perforated diverticular disease, suppurative appendicitis or necrotizing pancreatitis. It is frequently difficult to differentiate the two conditions and the high mortality is due to sepsis and to bowel infarction consequent on the portal thrombosis. Patients who develop portal vein thrombosis in association with intra-abdominal carcinoma more often develop new or worsening abdominal pain and progressive ascites. These patients have advanced disease and generally deteriorate and die rapidly.

### *Thrombosis in portal hypertension*

Portal hypertension is associated with portal venous obstruction and altered portal blood flow (p. 990) and this in itself predisposes to portal venous thrombosis.

***Cirrhosis.*** Cirrhosis is the commonest cause of portal hypertension and the frequency with which it gives rise to portal thrombosis has been variously estimated. Early reports of an incidence of 10% or more are probably too high and may reflect selection factors or the inclusion of agonal thrombi in autopsy studies. Okuda et al (1985) used angiography to study 708 Japanese patients with cirrhosis and found portal thromboses in only four of 698 (0.6%) who had not had a previous abdominal operation. Portal thrombosis is therefore probably rare in cirrhosis and several factors, including the severity of the liver disease and associated surgical operations, are likely predisposing causes. Okuda et al (1985) found portal thrombosis only in advanced disease (Child grade C), giving an incidence of 1.3% in such patients, and four of 18 (22%) patients who had undergone splenectomy had portal thromboses. It is likely that all operations, especially abdominal operations, predispose to portal thrombosis, but splenectomy may be a particular hazard owing to consequent increases in the number of circulating platelets. The development of a hepatocellular carcinoma is also an important factor and should always be sought. Portal venous thrombosis in cirrhosis is usually characterized by the appearance or worsening of ascites and/or severe esophageal variceal bleeding. Ascites is often progressive or resistant to treatment and spontaneous bacterial peritonitis may occur.

***Noncirrhotic portal hypertension.*** Portal thrombosis in portal hypertension is not linked specifically to cirrhosis and can occur irrespective of the cause. Okuda et al (1985) found portal thrombosis in two of 70 (2.9%) patients with idiopathic portal hypertension and Terayama et al (1995) reported its occurrence in partial nodular transformation of the liver. These conditions are associated with excellent liver function and other factors must be important in thrombosis.

***Extrahepatic portal hypertension.*** This is usually the long-term consequence of portal venous thrombosis. It most often presents with variceal hemorrhage or the discovery of splenomegaly and is considered in detail below.

## Extrahepatic presinusoidal portal hypertension

This results from obstruction in the main portal vein and it accounts for about 10% of cases of portal hypertension in Europe and North America (Webb & Sherlock 1979, Macpherson 1984). In a half or more no etiological factors can be found (Table 41.1), but in many of these thrombotic factors may be important (p. 1179).

### *Childhood and adolescence*

Extrahepatic portal hypertension in these patients is usually due to thrombosis of the portal vein in early life. Neonatal infection is the most common cause. Umbilical infections (omphalitis) are most frequent, although infections outside the portal venous system are also important, perhaps because associated hemoconcentration due to dehydration predisposes to thrombosis. Neonatal infections are in fact rarely complicated by portal thrombosis and portal hypertension (Thompson & Sherlock 1964) and some have questioned their importance as causes of this condition (Mikkelsen 1966). Umbilical catheterization may also lead to portal vein thrombosis and portal hypertension, but this too is a rare event as few such cases have been reported (Junker et al 1976). Congenital portal vein anomalies, once considered the main cause of portal obstruction in the young, are very rare (p. 1085).

Bleeding is uncommon before the age of 3 and most frequent between the ages of 10 and 15 years. These patients usually present with gastrointestinal bleeding or with splenomegaly. They have no clinical evidence of liver disease, ascites is uncommon but may occur transiently soon after bleeding and biochemical tests of liver function are usually normal. Encephalopathy is rare. Evidence of hepatic dysfunction may develop when patients reach adulthood and hyperbilirubinemia, hypoalbuminemia and a raised serum alkaline phosphatase activity are then the commonest abnormalities (Thompson et al 1964). The liver biopsy is normal initially, but irregular atrophy, chronic inflammatory cell infiltration and portal tract fibrosis often develop later (Thompson et al 1964, Stathers et al 1968).

*Adults*

The causes of extrahepatic portal hypertension in adults include conditions predisposing to thrombosis, trauma, portal vein invasion by neoplasms and involvement in inflammatory processes as well as infections (Table 41.1). Splenic arteriovenous fistulas or hepatic artery–portal vein aneurysms are exceptional causes of portal hypertension (Johnston & Gibson 1965). Gastrointestinal bleeding is the usual presenting feature and splenomegaly is less common than in younger patients. Ascites may develop in those with associated hepatocellular disease. Encephalopathy and ascites may follow a gastrointestinal hemorrhage, intercurrent infection or surgery and are associated with a poor prognosis.

*Diagnosis*

The diagnosis of extrahepatic portal hypertension depends on demonstrating the site of obstruction in the portal venous system, showing that portal hypertension is confined to the extrahepatic part of that system and excluding primary liver disease. Portal hypertension is usually obvious from the finding of esophageal varices and Doppler ultrasound can be used to identify the site of venous obstruction. Visualization of the portal and venous system at mesenteric angiography is generally diagnostic and direct measurement of the portal pressure is unnecessary (Fig. 36.8). The wedged hepatic venous pressure is normal in those with pure extrahepatic portal hypertension. Lack of stigmata of chronic liver disease, normal liver function tests and a normal liver on imaging are generally sufficient to exclude liver disease and a liver biopsy, if undertaken, is generally normal although it may provide evidence of the underlying etiology (Table 41.1).

*Investigations*

The investigations used in portal hypertension are described elsewhere (p. 994).

*Prognosis*

The prognosis in presinusoidal portal hypertension is generally much better than in portal hypertension due to cirrhosis, but it is much less common and information regarding prognosis is limited by the relatively small number of patients in most studies (Webb & Sherlock 1979, Fonkalsrud 1980, Macpherson 1984). The important prognostic factors are age, the site of the portal venous obstruction, the cause of the obstruction and the hepatic function. Patients who present as children or adolescents usually have a good prognosis, as most have excellent liver function and extrahepatic portal obstruction due to an intrinsically benign condition. These patients grow and develop normally and three-quarters or more are alive 10 years after diagnosis. Variceal bleeding can begin early in childhood and recurrent bleeding often occurs, but exsanguinating hemorrhage is uncommon and recurrent bleeding tends to become less frequent with time. Liver function is excellent but can deteriorate in the long term, usually in patients over 30 years of age, and sudden fatal bleeding can occur.

*Treatment*

The methods available for treating extrahepatic portal hypertension are discussed elsewhere (p. 1005). The choice of treatment is considered here.

***Children.*** Varices due to extrahepatic presinusoidal portal hypertension are most common in young people and bleeding usually occurs first in childhood or adolescence. Three factors determine the management in these patients: they have good hepatic and cardiovascular reserve and so tolerate bleeding well, the natural history is often towards improvement with cessation of bleeding in up to a fifth and the portal vessels in young children are so small that portasystemic shunts often become occluded (Keighley et al 1973, Macpherson 1984, Spence & Roy 1984). Bleeding is treated by sclerotherapy or band ligation until patients are over 10 years old, with devascularizing operations to stop acute bleeding that fails to respond to such therapy (Stamatakis et al 1982). Sclerotherapy alone is often effective in preventing rebleeding and beyond adolescence bleeding is unusual. Recurrent bleeding, often from gastric rather than esophageal varices, beyond this age can be treated by a portasystemic shunt, as anastomoses at least 10 mm in diameter should be possible. The operation of choice will depend on the availability of suitable veins and includes the selective distal splenorenal shunt (Warren et al 1984). A few surgeons advocate early portasystemic shunt surgery (Alvarez et al 1983), but few support this view (Fonkalsrud 1983, Starzl 1983).

***Adults.*** This form of portal hypertension in adults is usually due to thrombosis or to neoplastic invasion or compression of the portal venous system (Table 41.1). Treatment is the same as in childhood. Portal venous angioplasty has been undertaken occasionally with some success (Uflacker et al 1985) and where thrombosis is confined to the splenic vein, portal hypertension can be eliminated by splenectomy (below). Patients with malignant disease do not live long enough to justify surgical treatment.

### Regional extrahepatic portal hypertension

***Splenic vein.*** Splenic vein thrombosis causes splenomegaly and the formation of gastric varices. Esophageal varices are rarely prominent. The commonest causes of splenic vein thrombosis are pancreatitis, pancreatic pseudocysts, pancreatic neoplasia and, less often, gastric surgery or hepatic cirrhosis (Lankisch 1990). Occlusion of the splenic vein results in the formation of collateral vessels that may be portoportal (from the spleen to the portal vein via the stomach and left gastric vein) or portosystemic (from the spleen to the vena cava via the left renal and retroperitoneal veins, or to the azygos vein via stomach veins when the left gastric vein is occluded). Three-quarters of patients present with variceal bleeding. The diagnosis should be confirmed by ultrasonography with Doppler studies and/or venous phase mesenteric angiography. Computed tomography may help reveal the underlying cause of the splenic vein thrombosis. Control of active bleeding may be achieved by treatments used for other causes of varices (p. 493), but splenectomy is the definitive treatment. Because of the risk of bleeding and the fact that gastric varices are less responsive to endoscopic injection sclerotherapy than their esophageal counterparts, prophylactic splenectomy is recommended.

***Mesenteric veins.*** Regional portal hypertension restricted to the mesenteric circulation with cavernous transformation of the superior mesenteric vein has occurred but is rare. This condition caused recurring gastrointestinal bleeding in a patient who had isolated duodenojejunal varices without splenomegaly or esophageal varices. Bleeding ceased during a year of follow-up after an ileocolic to vena cava anastomosis (Rosen et al 1967). Portal hypertension restricted to the inferior mesenteric vein has occurred in stenosis or absence of the portal vein (below).

### Idiopathic portal hypertension

This condition is diagnosed in a patient with portal hypertension when no obstruction can be demonstrated radiographically in the portal venous system and no primary liver disease can be detected (Mikkelsen et al 1965, Boyer et al 1974, Kingham et al 1981). The hypertension is of the intrahepatic presinusoidal type. Postmortem casts have shown widespread obliteration of the terminal intrahepatic portal tributaries by thrombus and there is often marked perivenous fibrosis. This may be reflected in a paucity of small intrahepatic portal vessels on portography. Histologically, the liver shows a deranged lobular structure with portal tract fibrosis despite the lack of clinical and biochemical evidence of liver disease. The disease progresses very slowly (Levison et al 1982). Cirrhosis does not occur, but ascites, encephalopathy and hypoalbuminemia develop eventually. In the late stages there may be a moderate rise in the wedged hepatic venous pressure.

### Portal venous aneurysm

Portal vein aneurysms are rare (Hagiwara et al 1991). They can occur anywhere in the portal vein, but the commonest sites are at the junction of the superior mesenteric and splenic veins and in the main branches of the portal vein. Aneurysms have also been described in the superior mesenteric vein and splenic vein, but they are very rare (Ohhira et al 1994). About half have occurred in patients with portal hypertension, but in other patients the aneurysms may have been congenital in origin. Most aneurysms are asymptomatic but abdominal pain, rupture with bleeding, including into the biliary tree, and common bile duct compression have been reported. They are best demonstrated by ultrasonography and confirmed by angiography and they are usually found incidentally.

### Congenital portal vein anomalies

Congenital abnormalities of the portal vein are rare but are occasional causes of extrahepatic portal hypertension (Webb & Sherlock 1979). Stenosis of the portal vein and absence of the portal vein have both been reported and in these patients portal hypertension affects primarily the inferior mesenteric vein, leading to recurrent rectal bleeding from colorectal varices (Bell 1970, Lee et al 1994). Treatment of portal hypertensive bleeding in these patients depends on the mesenteric vascular anatomy, but a lienorenal shunt is potentially most useful.

## HEPATIC SINUSOIDAL DISEASE

### Perisinusoidal fibrosis

Perisinusoidal fibrosis is recognized from an accumulation of collagen in the space of Disse. It can be recognized on light microscopy but is best demonstrated by electron-microscopy. Perisinusoidal fibrosis can contribute to the production of portal hypertension and can be caused by inorganic arsenicals, vinyl chloride, vitamin A and several chemotherapeutic drugs (Zafrani et al 1983). The diagnosis should be considered in patients who present with portal hypertension but have neither hepatic cirrhosis nor thrombosis within the portal venous system.

### Sinusoidal dilatation

Sinusoidal dilatation can occur in the absence of hepatic venous outflow obstruction. The histological appearance is of patchy ectasia of the sinusoids and atrophy of the related hepatocytes. It can be idiopathic or associated with certain drugs (p. 852), including oral contraceptives and anabolic steroids. It is generally asymptomatic and a coincidental finding, although abdominal pain, hepatomegaly and raised transaminase and alkaline phosphatase activity have been reported.

### Peliosis hepatis

Peliosis hepatis refers to intrahepatic blood-filled spaces that are not lined by sinusoidal cells. Previously regarded as of little significance, it has, as with sinusoidal dilatation, been associated with oral contraceptive and anabolic steroid ingestion. More recently, it has been reported in patients who are immunosuppressed, for example following liver transplantation (Scheuer et al 1990) and renal transplantation (Cavalcanti et al 1994) and in patients with the acquired immune deficiency syndrome (AIDS) (Perkocha et al 1990). In patients with AIDS, it occurs in conjunction with a skin condition called bacillary angiomatosis; both conditions have been shown to be due to a previously unrecognized rickettsial organism called *Rochalimaea henselae* (Slater et al 1992).

Peliosis hepatis can be asymptomatic or can cause painful hepatomegaly or, rarely, liver failure (Bagheri & Boyer 1974, Zafrani et al 1983). Rupture can lead to severe intraperitoneal bleeding. Diagnosis of peliosis hepatis is best made by laparoscopy, where superficial lesions are visible as blue-black blebs (Ito 1982). Computed tomography and magnetic resonance imaging may also demonstrate the focal lesions. Prompt treatment of the bacillary form in AIDS with erythromycin can be effective.

## VASCULAR FISTULAE

Symptomatic hepatic vascular fistulae are rare and most are arterioportal fistulae. They are usually caused by trauma, including iatrogenic trauma, but others are associated with tumors or ruptured aneurysms. Some are congenital or occur in hereditary hemorrhagic telangiectasia.

### Hereditary hemorrhagic telangiectasia

Telangiectasias, aneurysms and arteriovenous shunts occur frequently in several internal organs in hereditary hemorrhagic telangiectasia (Guttmacher et al 1995). These organs include the liver, gastrointestinal tract, lungs, spleen, brain, kidneys and genital tract. The gastrointestinal features are discussed on p. 492. Liver involvement occurs in older patients; hepatomegaly is common, a liver bruit may be present, a half have upper abdominal pain and another half have splenomegaly (Martini 1978). Liver function tests may show minor abnormalities, but overall liver function is generally good. There may be hepatic artery aneurysms, cavernous hemangiomas and hepatoportal or hepatic artery–hepatic venous fistulae and there may also be an associated coarse nodular cirrhosis with irregular fibrous bands containing telangiectasias and blood-filled cavities lined with endothelium. Portal hypertension can occur and variceal bleeding may be treated best by hepatic artery ligation (Zentler-Munro et al 1989).

### Arterioportal fistulae

Arterioportal fistulae are rare, they may be intrahepatic or extrahepatic in position and they can cause severe portal hypertension. Portal hypertension is probably due mainly to high blood flow and the transmission of arterial pressure but increased vascular resistance may become important, as closure of a fistula does not always correct the portal pressure fully (Van Way et al 1971). Trauma, blunt or penetrating, is the commonest cause and most fistulae related to trauma are in the mesenteric veins. Liver biopsy is the usual cause of intrahepatic fistulae due to penetrating injury. Congenital fistulae or fistulae due to ruptured aneurysms usually occur between the hepatic artery and portal vein or between the splenic artery and vein. They may be multiple and may be associated with other congenital abnormalities (Heaton et al 1995). Other causes include hepatocellular carcinoma and hereditary hemorrhagic telangiectasia (above).

Fistulae can cause abdominal pain, variceal bleeding, which may be severe, or ascites and a bruit may be heard over the liver. Congenital fistulae can cause failure to thrive, diarrhea, hepatosplenomegaly, ascites and bleeding within a year of birth. Extrahepatic fistulae can be closed surgically. Intrahepatic fistulae can be occluded by embolization, but this may only bring temporary improvement where there are multiple fistulae and in such cases hepatic artery ligation is preferable (Zentler-Munro et al 1989, Heaton et al 1995).

### Portasystemic fistulae

Intrahepatic portasystemic shunts unassociated with hepatic cirrhosis or hepatocellular carcinoma are very rare. They may be congenital or acquired and occasionally an aneurysm of the portal vein may rupture into a hepatic vein (Park et al 1990). Most patients with such shunts have presented with hepatic encephalopathy in later life, possibly because hepatic function diminishes with age (p. 1111). Diagnosis is made by Doppler ultrasonography and mesenteric angiography.

REFERENCES


Alvarez F, Bernard O, Brunelle F, Hadchouel P, Odièvre M, Alagille D 1983 Portal obstruction in children. II. Results of surgical portosystemic shunts. Journal of Pediatrics 103: 703–707

Bagheri S A, Boyer J L 1974 Peliosis hepatis associated with androgenic-anabolic steroid therapy. A severe form of liver injury. Annals of Internal Medicine 81: 610–618

Bell J W 1970 Portal-vein hypoplasia with inferior mesenteric hypertension. New England Journal of Medicine 283: 1149–1150

Benbow E W 1986 Idiopathic obstruction of the inferior vena cava: a review. Journal of the Royal Society of Medicine 79: 105–108

Blue J M, Burney D P 1990 Current trends in the diagnosis and treatment of hepatic artery aneurysms. Southern Medical Journal 83: 966–969

Boyer J L, Hales M R, Klatskin G 1974 “Idiopathic” portal hypertension due to occlusion of intrahepatic portal veins by organized thrombi. Medicine 53: 77–91

Cavalcanti R, Pol S, Carnot F et al 1994 Impact and evolution of peliosis hepatis in renal transplant recipients. Transplantation 58: 315–316

Dilawari J B, Bambery P, Chawla Y et al 1994 Hepatic outflow obstruction (Budd–Chiari syndrome). Experience with 177 patients and a review of the literature. Medicine (Baltimore) 73: 21–36

Fock K M, Chan C C, Khoo T K 1993 Budd–Chiari syndrome: successful treatment by percutaneous transluminal angioplasty. Australasian Radiology 37: 108–110

Fonkalsrud E W 1980 Surgical management of portal hypertension in childhood: long-term results. Archives of Surgery 115: 1042–1045

Fonkalsrud E W 1983 Shunt operations for portal hypertension in children. Journal of Pediatrics 103: 742–743

Guillevin L, Lhote F, Sauvaget F et al 1994 Treatment of polyarteritis nodosa related to hepatitis B virus with interferon-alpha and plasma exchanges. Annals of Rheumatic Diseases 53: 334–337

Guttmacher A E, Marchuk D A, White R I Jr 1995 Hereditary hemorrhagic telangiectasia. New England Journal of Medicine 333: 918–924

Hagiwara H, Kasahara A, Kono M et al 1991 Extrahepatic portal vein aneurysm associated with a tortuous portal vein. Gastroenterology 100: 818–821

Heaton N D, Davenport M, Karani J, Mowat A P, Howard E R 1995 Congenital hepatoportal arteriovenous fistula. Surgery 117: 170–174

Ito T 1982 Peritoneoscopy in peliosis hepatis. Endoscopy 14: 14–18

Johnston G W, Gibson J B 1965 Portal hypertension resulting from splenic arteriovenous fistulae. Gut 6: 500–502

Junker P, Egeblad M, Nielsen O, Kamper J 1976 Umbilical vein catheterization and portal hypertension. Acta Paediatrica Scandinavica 65: 499–504

Keighley M R B, Girdwood R W, Wooler G H, Ionescu M I 1973 Long-term results of surgical treatment for bleeding oesophageal varices in children with portal hypertension. British Journal of Surgery 60: 641–646

Kibbler C C, Cohen D L, Cruicshank J K, Kushwaha S S, Morgan M Y, Dick R D 1985 Use of CAT scanning in the diagnosis and management of hepatic artery aneurysm. Gut 26: 752–756

Kingham J G C, Levison D A, Stansfeld A G, Dawson A M 1981 Non-cirrhotic intrahepatic portal hypertension: a long term follow-up study. Quarterly Journal of Medicine 50: 259–268

Kwan T, Hansard P 1992 Recombinant tissue-plasminogen activator for acute Budd–Chiari syndrome secondary to paroxysmal nocturnal hemoglobinuria. New York State Journal of Medicine 92: 109–110

Lankisch P G 1990 The spleen in inflammatory pancreatic disease. Gastroenterology 98: 509–516

Lee J S Y, Yeong K Y, Soo K C 1994 Absent portal vein presenting as rectal bleeding: a case report. Journal of the Royal College of Surgeons of Edinburgh 39: 118–119

Levison D A, Kingham J G C, Dawson A M, Stansfeld A G 1982 Slow cirrhosis – or no cirrhosis? A lesion causing benign intrahepatic portal hypertension. Journal of Pathology 137: 253–272

Lewis D R Jr, Kung H, Connon J J 1982 Biliary obstruction secondary to hepatic artery aneurysm: cholangiographic appearance and diagnostic considerations. Gastroenterology 82: 1446–1451

Macpherson A I S 1984 Portal hypertension due to extrahepatic portal venous obstruction. A review of 40 cases. Journal of the Royal College of Surgeons of Edinburgh 29: 4–10

Mahmoud A E A, Mendoza A, Meshikhes S et al 1996 Clinical spectrum, investigations and treatment of Budd–Chiari syndrome. Quarterly Journal of Medicine 89: 37–43

Martini G A 1978 The liver in hereditary haemorrhagic telangiectasia: an inborn error of vascular structure with multiple manifestations: a reappraisal. Gut 19: 531–537

McDonald G B, Shulman H M, Sullivan K M, Spencer G D 1986 Intestinal and hepatic complications of human bone marrow transplantation. Part I. Gastroenterology 90: 460–477

McMahon B J, Heyward W L, Templin D W, Clement D, Lanier A P 1989 Hepatitis B-associated polyarteritis nodosa in Alaskan Eskimos: clinical and epidemiologic features and long-term follow-up. Hepatology 9: 97–101

McMullin M F, Hillmen P, Jackson J, Ganly P, Luzzatto L 1994 Tissue plasminogen activator for hepatic vein thrombosis in paroxysmal nocturnal haemoglobinuria. Journal of Internal Medicine 235: 85–89

Mikkelsen W P 1966 Extrahepatic portal hypertension in children. American Journal of Surgery 111: 333–340

Mikkelsen W P, Edmondson H A, Peters R L, Redeker A G, Reynolds T B 1965 Extra- and intrahepatic portal hypertension without cirrhosis (hepatoportal sclerosis). Annals of Surgery 162: 602–620

O'Connor P J, Buhac I, Balint J A 1976 Spontaneous hepatic artery thrombosis with infarction of the liver. Gastroenterology 70: 599–601

Ohhira Mo, Ono M, Ohhira Ma, Matsumoto A, Ohta H, Namiki M 1994 Case report: splenic vein aneurysm – report of a lesion that progressively expanded. British Journal of Radiology 67: 656–658

Okuda K, Ohnishi K, Kimura K et al 1985 Incidence of portal vein thrombosis in liver cirrhosis. An angiographic study in 708 patients. Gastroenterology 89: 279–286

Pagliuca A, Mufti G J, Janossa-Tahernia M et al 1990 In vitro colony culture and chromosomal studies in hepatic and portal vein thrombosis – possible evidence of an occult myeloproliferative state. Quarterly Journal of Medicine 76: 981–989

Park J H, Cha S H, Han J K, Han M C 1990 Intrahepatic portosystemic venous shunt. American Journal of Roentgenology 155: 527–528

Perkocha L A, Geaghan S M, Yen T S B et al 1990 Clinical and pathologic features of bacillary peliosis hepatis in association with human immunodeficiency virus infection. New England Journal of Medicine 323: 1581–1586

Powell-Jackson P, Greenway B, Williams R 1982 Adverse effects of exploratory laparotomy in patients with unsuspected liver disease. British Journal of Surgery 69: 449–451

Rosen H, Silen W, Simon M 1967 Selective portal hypertension with isolated duodenojejunal varices. New England Journal of Medicine 277: 1188–1190

Scheuer P J, Schachter L A, Mathur S, Burroughs A K, Rolles K 1990 Peliosis hepatis after liver transplantation. Journal of Clinical Pathology 43: 1036–1037

Shaw J F L 1982 Hepatic artery aneurysms. British Journal of Hospital Medicine 28: 404–409

Shulman H M, McDonald G B, Matthews D et al 1980 An analysis of hepatic venocclusive disease and centrilobular hepatic degeneration following bone marrow transplantation. Gastroenterology 79: 1178–1191

Simson I W 1982 Membranous obstruction of the inferior vena cava and hepatocellular carcinoma in South Africa. Gastroenterology 82: 171–178

Slater L N, Welch D F, Min K-W 1992 Rochalimaea henselae causes bacillary angiomatosis and peliosis hepatis. Archives of Internal Medicine 152: 602–606

Spence R A J, Roy A D 1984 Bleeding duodenal varices. British Journal of Surgery 71: 588

Stamatakis J D, Howard E R, Psacharopoulos H T, Mowat A P 1982 Injection sclerotherapy for oesophageal varices in children. British Journal of Surgery 69: 74–75

Starzl T E 1983 Portal vein thrombosis and portal diversion. Journal of Pediatrics 103: 741–742

Stathers G M, Ma M H, Blackburn C R B 1968 Extrahepatic portal hypertension: the clinical evaluation, investigation and results of treatment of 28 patients. Australasian Annals of Medicine 17: 12

Stringer M D, Heaton N D, Karani J, Olliff S, Howard E R 1994 Patterns of portal vein occlusion and their aetiological significance. British Journal of Surgery 81: 1328–1331

Stuart K L, Bras G 1957 Veno-occlusive disease of the liver. Quarterly Journal of Medicine 26: 291–315

Tavill A S, Wood E J, Kreel L, Jones E A, Gregory M, Sherlock S 1975 The Budd–Chiari syndrome: correlation between hepatic scintigraphy and the clinical, radiological, and pathological findings in nineteen cases of hepatic venous outflow obstruction. Gastroenterology 68: 509–518

Terayama N, Terada T, Hoso M, Nakanuma Y 1995 Partial nodular transformation of the liver with portal vein thrombosis. A report of two autopsy cases. Journal of Clinical Gastroenterology 20: 71–76

Thompson E N, Sherlock S 1964 The aetiology of portal vein thrombosis with particular reference to the role of infection and exchange transfusion. Quarterly Journal of Medicine 33: 465–480

Thompson E N, Williams R, Sherlock S 1964 Liver function in extrahepatic portal hypertension. Lancet 2: 1352–1356

Uflacker R, Alves M A, Cantisani G G, Souza H P, Wagner J, Moraes L F 1985 Treatment of portal vein obstruction by percutaneous transhepatic angioplasty. Gastroenterology 88: 176–180

Van Way C W III, Crane J M, Riddell D H, Foster J H 1971 Arteriovenous fistula in the portal circulation. Surgery 70: 876–890

Vickers C R, West R J, Hubscher S G, Elias E 1989 Hepatic venous webs and resistant ascites: diagnosis, management and implications. Journal of Hepatology 8: 287–293

Warren W D, Millikan W J Jr, Henderson J M, Rasheed M E, Salam A A 1984 Selective variceal decompression after splenectomy or splenic vein thrombosis with a note on splenopancreatic disconnection. Annals of Surgery 199: 694–702

Webb L J, Sherlock S 1979 The aetiology, presentation and natural history of extra-hepatic portal venous obstruction. Quarterly Journal of Medicine 48: 627–639

Witte C L, Brewer M L, Witte M H, Pond G B 1985 Protean manifestations of pylethrombosis: a review of 34 patients. Annals of Surgery 202: 191–202

Yamamoto T, Kawarada Y, Yano T, Noguchi T, Mizumoto R 1991 Spontaneous rupture of hemangioma of the liver: treatment with transcatheter hepatic arterial embolization. American Journal of Gastroenterology 86: 1645–1649

Zafrani E S, Pinaudeau Y, Le Cudonnec B, Larde D, Dhumeaux D 1983 Computed tomography abnormalities in hepatic infarction. Digestive Diseases and Sciences 28: 285

Zentler-Munro P L, Howard E R, Karani J, Williams R 1989 Variceal haemorrhage in hereditary haemorrhagic telangiectasia. Gut 30: 1293–1297

# 42. The liver in pregnancy

*Ian A. D. Bouchier*

Liver disease is uncommon in pregnancy and, conversely, pregnancy is uncommon in chronic liver disease, as such patients are usually infertile. When the two occur together, any of three situations may confront the physician: a liver disease may have occurred in a pregnant woman with a previously normal liver; a liver disease specific for pregnancy may have developed; or pregnancy may have occurred in a woman with pre-existing chronic liver disease (Knox & Olans 1996). Furthermore, results of liver function tests that would be abnormal in women who are not pregnant are encountered and may cause anxiety.

## THE NORMAL LIVER IN PREGNANCY

There is no clinically significant impairment of liver function in normal pregnancy and the histological appearances of the liver are normal (Ingerslev & Teilum 1946). Palmar erythema and small spider telangiectasias may develop, especially in the third trimester, but they do not indicate liver disease and they disappear after delivery (p. 919). Biochemical liver function tests are normal until the third trimester, when an increase in plasma alkaline phosphatase activity occurs in about a third of women (Kreek & Sleisenger 1970). This increase becomes more marked towards term, but in only about 5% of women does the activity exceed twice the normal maximum. It returns to normal within 2 months of delivery. The increased activity is almost all due to placental alkaline phosphatase. A mild physiological cholestasis occurs in the third trimester as plasma bile acid concentrations are increased at this time (Fulton et al 1983). The plasma bilirubin concentration and the transaminase and $\gamma$-glutamyl transferase activities remain normal. The plasma albumin concentration is often slightly reduced (30–35 g/L), owing to an increased plasma volume, and the globulin concentration may be a little increased. There is a two- to fourfold increase in triglycerides and a 50% increase in cholesterol (Freund & Arvan 1990).

## LIVER DISEASE IN PREGNANCY

### Viral hepatitis

Acute viral hepatitis is the commonest liver disease causing jaundice in pregnancy (Snydman 1985). Pregnancy does not increase susceptibility to viral hepatitis, but the frequent close contact of young mothers with children who may already have the disease would increase their exposure to it (Hadler et al 1980). The clinical features and the results of liver function tests in viral hepatitis are the same in otherwise healthy pregnant women and in women who are not pregnant (p. 795). Liver biopsy can be performed in pregnancy but is hardly ever needed.

The course and outcome of viral hepatitis in Europe and North America are not altered by pregnancy, but in many other parts of the world there is a substantially increased mortality, especially during the last trimester. Christie et al (1976), for example, reported a mortality of 13% in pregnant women with hepatitis in Libya. This increased mortality has been attributed to malnutrition, but malnutrition did not account for the increased severity of acute non-A, non-B hepatitis during pregnancy in Kashmir (Khuroo et al 1981). It may be that a virus such as the hepatitis E virus (p. 791) accounts for the greater severity of the disease in these countries. Viral hepatitis can cause fulminant hepatic failure, as in patients who are not pregnant. It has to be differentiated from acute fatty liver of pregnancy, eclampsia and septicemia, which may also be associated with severe liver dysfunction (Davies et al 1980).

There have been conflicting reports regarding the effect of hepatitis on pregnancy itself. Some have found no adverse effects, while others have reported a greatly increased frequency of abortion and of premature delivery. Adverse effects seem mainly related to the severity of the hepatitis. There is no evidence yet that the hepatitis viruses cause congenital abnormality. The treatment of viral hepatitis (p. 797) in pregnancy does not differ from that advised for patients who are not pregnant save that the authors empirically advise a greater degree of rest. Liver transplantation has been carried out where fulminant hepatic failure has developed (p. 1155).

*Hepatitis B virus*

Type B hepatitis is especially important in pregnancy, as it may cause vertical transmission of the virus from mother to child (Snydman 1985). Risk factors increasing the chances of chronic hepatitis B include women of Asian or African origin, previous hepatitis exposure, intravenous drug abuse and multiple episodes of sexually transmitted diseases. Women with acute type B hepatitis in the first and second trimesters are unlikely to transmit the virus to their offspring, but transmission occurs in a half to two-thirds when the infection occurs in the third trimester. Women who are chronic carriers of the hepatitis B virus and who show evidence that viral replication is occurring (p. 784) transmit the virus to their offspring in 80–90% of cases and about 90% of the offspring themselves become chronic carriers of the virus. When women do not have evidence of active viral replication, only one in four or fewer of the offspring is infected and the chances of a chronic infection are less.

It is likely that transmission occurs most frequently at delivery, presumably because of infection of the child by contaminated maternal blood and other body fluids. The hepatitis B surface antigen can be found in the umbilical cord blood in a half of cases, in the amniotic fluid in a third of cases and in the breast milk in about three-quarters of cases when mothers are infected with the hepatitis B virus. Newborns could be infected by swallowing one or other of these fluids, as the hepatitis B surface antigen is found in the gastric contents of most infants. Transplacental infection in utero can occur but is probably unusual (Wong et al 1980). Infection in the child may result in acute hepatitis, which is frequently severe and perhaps fatal, and subsequent development of a chronic carrier state occurs in some 90% of cases. Most children remain asymptomatic but become chronic carriers with or without abnormal liver function tests. Liver biopsy usually shows persistent hepatitis. The ultimate prognosis for children who are chronic carriers is variable, but about a half of male children eventually develop cirrhosis or hepatocellular carcinoma or both.

Prophylactic treatment to prevent transmission of the virus to neonates and in particular to prevent chronic infection is very important. Some consider that such treatment is not necessary when the mother does not show signs of active viral replication, but it is recommended strongly that the neonates of all infected women should be treated. Suitable therapy would include administration of hepatitis B immune globulin (0.5 ml [110–150 units] intramuscularly) within 12 h of birth along with hepatitis B vaccine (0.5 ml; 10 mg) at birth and 1 and 6 months later.

*Other hepatitis viruses*

Other hepatitis viruses can cause maternal infection in pregnancy and can be transmitted to the offspring.

***Hepatitis A virus.*** The hepatitis A virus does not seem to be transmitted from mother to infant even when maternal infection is present in the third trimester or at delivery.

***Hepatitis C virus.*** The hepatitis C virus can be transmitted from mother to infant but less readily than the hepatitis B virus. Transmission occurs only when there is marked maternal viremia as evidenced by HCV-DNA in the blood. Prevention can be attempted by giving 0.5 ml immune serum globulin within 24 h of birth and 26 days later (Seef & Hoofnagle 1979).

***Hepatitis D virus.*** Infection with the hepatitis D (δ) virus can occur in pregnancy and transmission to the offspring can occur along with the hepatitis B virus. Prevention of transmission is as for the hepatitis B virus.

***Hepatitis E virus.*** The hepatitis E virus does not seem to be transmitted from mother to infant.

### Other liver diseases

Acute liver diseases other than viral hepatitis are very rare in pregnancy. Budd–Chiari syndrome occurs occasionally as an expression of an increased occurrence of hypercoagulability (p. 1079).

### Gallstones

The gallbladder empties incompletely during the second and third trimesters, possibly a progesterone effect. Sludge is frequent, but only 3–5% of obstetric patients have gallstones (Gray & Bouchier 1992). The clinical features, course and management are the same as in the absence of pregnancy.

## LIVER DISEASES OF PREGNANCY

Recurrent cholestatis of pregnancy is the only common disease associated specifically with pregnancy. The others are all rare. These conditions have been reviewed (Haemmerli & Wyss 1967, BMJ 1975).

### Hyperemesis gravidarum

Nausea and vomiting are common in early pregnancy but rarely affect the pregnancy. If symptoms are severe, malnutrition, dehydration and liver dysfunction may occur. It is well known that jaundice can occur in hyperemesis gravidarum, but the relationship between the two has been questioned. Larrey et al (1984) have provided good clinical evidence that hyperemesis gravidarum can cause hepatic damage and jaundice. Jaundice should not be attributed to mild hyperemesis gravidarum; hepatitis due to drugs should be considered, hepatitis virus infection should be sought serologically and ultrasonography of the liver and biliary tract should be normal before the diagnosis is made. Treatment includes the relief of vomiting by an antihistamine or phenothiazine drug given parenterally and fluid replacement.

## Intrahepatic cholestasis of pregnancy

This is a condition in which cholestasis appears during pregnancy and remits spontaneously after delivery, often within a few days and generally within 2 weeks. It is the second most common cause of jaundice during pregnancy. Symptoms start in the third trimester in at least two-thirds of cases and in the second trimester in practically all the rest.

***Etiology.*** The incidence of this condition varies widely. Most cases have been reported from Scandinavia and from Chile and half the patients have a close relative who is also affected, suggesting that genetic factors are important (Furhoff & Hellström 1973, Reyes et al 1978). Estrogens reduce the capacity of the biliary canalicular membrane to transport substances into the bile and they are the likely cause of the mild cholestasis that occurs normally in the third trimester of pregnancy and that is characterized by reduced biliary excretion of bromsulphthalein (Simcock & Forster 1967) and increased plasma bile acid concentrations (Fulton et al 1983). Estrogens sometimes produce overt cholestasis in women taking oral contraceptives and this occurs especially frequently in those who have had cholestasis of pregnancy. Patients with recurrent cholestasis of pregnancy seem to develop overt cholestasis because of a marked sensitivity of their livers to estrogens. The abnormalities of estrogen metabolism in these patients are probably the result and not the cause of the cholestasis (Adlercreutz et al 1974).

***Clinical and laboratory features.*** Pruritus is the first and dominant symptom. It is usually worst at night and may lead to lack of sleep. Mild jaundice occurs after 3 or 4 weeks in about half the patients and the serum bilirubin rarely exceeds 100 μmol/L (6 mg/dl). The urine darkens with the onset of jaundice, but the stools often retain their normal color. Sometimes there may be malaise, anorexia or even vomiting, but usually the patient feels well. Abdominal pain is extremely unusual and fever does not occur. Mild jaundice and scratch marks are the only abnormalities. Liver function tests are abnormal, but the changes are rarely marked; the alkaline phosphatase activity is always high and the transaminase activity may be elevated to a maximum of about fivefold. Serum bile acids increase up to 100-fold (Schorr-Lesnick et al 1991). The prothrombin time may be prolonged but can be corrected by vitamin $K_1$ (p. 751) and the plasma albumin is no more reduced than would be expected in any normal pregnancy. Liver biopsy is needed only when there is doubt about the diagnosis, which is rare; it shows only patchy cholestasis. The antimitochondrial antibody is not found in the blood.

***Differential diagnosis.*** Differentiation from viral hepatitis in patients with jaundice is the most common difficulty (Piccinino et al 1975). Viral hepatitis usually starts with prodromal symptoms (p. 795), pruritus is rarely severe or prolonged, hepatic tenderness may be found and the serum transaminase activity is usually much greater (p. 741). Serological tests may show infection with the hepatitis A, B or C virus. Biliary colic or cholecystitis is accompanied by abdominal pain and often fever or leukocytosis. Gallstones are best identified by ultrasound during pregnancy. Occasionally, primary biliary cirrhosis starts during pregnancy (p. 935), which may be misleading. However, the antimitochondrial antibody test is positive and failure of the illness to resolve after delivery leads to further investigation.

***Treatment.*** Treatment consists of assuring the patient that the symptoms will remit after delivery. Cholestyramine (p. 933) can be used to reduce pruritus if it is severe.

***Prognosis.*** Cholestasis of pregnancy carries an increased risk of prematurity and stillbirth but not of congenital abnormality (Fisk & Storey 1988). It almost always recurs in successive pregnancies and can be precipitated by oral contraceptives. There are no deleterious long-term effects on the liver, but the patients have an increased frequency of gallstones (Dalén & Westerholm 1974).

## Acute fatty liver of pregnancy

This condition usually develops between the 35th and 40th week of pregnancy and toxemia of pregnancy is often also present (Kaplan 1985, Reyes et al 1994). It occasionally develops as early as the 30th week or shortly after delivery. It is an uncommon condition, occurring in about one in 13 000 deliveries. The cause is unknown.

***Clinical features.*** The initial features are nonspecific and include fatigue, malaise, nausea and vomiting. Abdominal pain is common but not invariable, is situated in the upper abdomen and particularly in the epigastrium and right upper quadrant, and may be burning or aching and of any degree of severity. Pain sometimes radiates through to the back and this may be due to associated pancreatitis. The disease usually progresses quickly over hours or a few days, with the appearance of jaundice, bruising and bleeding from puncture sites due to coagulopathy and the development of encephalopathy. Encephalopathy may be due to profound hypoglycemia or to hepatic failure. Gastrointestinal bleeding can occur and is usually caused by acute mucosal erosions aggravated by coagulation defects and eventually renal failure develops.

General physical examination usually shows an afebrile

patient and small spider telangiectasias that are generally attributable to the pregnancy itself (p. 919). About 40% of patients have proteinuria, hypertension and edema, which point to associated pre-eclampsia. Abdominal examination is often difficult because of the large uterus and tenderness and guarding, but neither the liver nor the spleen is palpable.

***Investigations.*** Liver function tests invariably show an increased plasma aminotransferase activity, which is usually increased about five- to sevenfold. Activities increased more than tenfold occur in fewer than 20% of patients. The plasma bilirubin may be normal initially but rises as the disease progresses. The plasma alkaline phosphatase activity is usually increased, but this may simply be a reflection of the production of placental isoenzyme (p. 743). The peripheral blood almost always shows a polymorphonuclear leukocytosis that usually exceeds $15 \times 10^9$/L (15 000/mm$^3$) and evidence of microangiopathic hemolysis such as the appearance of burr cells, fragmented erythrocytes, Howell–Jolly bodies and normoblasts is often present. Disseminated intravascular hemolysis is also usually found, giving rise to thrombocytopenia, prolonged prothrombin and partial thromboplastin times, hypofibrinogenemia and fibrin split products. Hypoglycemia, which can be profound, is common.

Liver biopsy is often contraindicated by impaired coagulation, but the characteristic finding is marked microvesicular fatty change (Fig. 35.15), particularly in the pericentral regions. This fatty change can be overlooked in hematoxylin and eosin stains, where the hepatocytes look pale and swollen with central nuclei, and is most readily appreciated when fresh frozen tissue is stained with special fat stains. Patchy hepatocellular necrosis and some lobular inflammation and giant mitochondria may also be seen. Autopsy examination usually shows a small, pale liver and autopsy may also show renal tubular damage.

***Differential diagnosis.*** The main differential diagnosis is from acute viral hepatitis and some of the more helpful points are shown in Table 42.1. The differentiation from fulminant forms of hepatitis is more difficult, but pre-eclampsia, marked leukocytosis and microangiopathic hemolysis or disseminated intravascular coagulation favor fatty liver of pregnancy, while increased plasma transaminase activity progressively favors fulminant hepatitis as it increases more than tenfold above the normal upper limit. Alcoholic hepatitis is very rare late in pregnancy and is difficult to recognize when it occurs, as many of its clinical and biochemical features can mimic fatty liver of pregnancy (p. 875). It is recognized mainly from the history of alcohol abuse. The abdominal pain of fatty liver of pregnancy may be mistaken for cholecystitis, cholangitis or pancreatitis and indeed, pancreatitis can occur in the course of fatty liver of pregnancy. These disorders on their own do not cause liver failure or blood coagulopathy. Ultrasonography is useful in detecting underlying gallstones and dilatation of the bile ducts and the plasma amylase activity should be measured to detect pancreatitis.

**Table 42.1** Features differentiating acute fatty liver of pregnancy and uncomplicated acute viral hepatitis

| Feature | Acute fatty liver of pregnancy | Acute viral hepatitis |
|---|---|---|
| Palpable liver | Rare | Common |
| Transaminases | <×10 (80%) | >×10 (50%) |
| Pre-eclampsia | Present | Absent |
| Leukocytosis | Common | Rare |
| Intravascular coagulopathy | Common | Rare |
| Microangiopathic hemolysis | Common | Rare |
| Hypoglycemia | Common | Rare |
| Uremia | Common | Rare |
| Hepatitis serology | Negative | Positive (type A and type B) |
| Pathology | Fatty change | Necrosis |

***Treatment.*** The management of fatty liver of pregnancy depends on the stage at which it is recognized. The diagnosis is often in doubt at an early stage when there is no hepatic failure and blood coagulation is normal or nearly normal. Liver biopsy should be done at this stage and termination of pregnancy is probably the best course of action if the diagnosis is confirmed, as rapid unexpected deterioration can occur. Liver function usually improves quickly after delivery, so rapid termination by cesarean section or by the vaginal route is best, especially as the patient is usually close to term, so the baby is not endangered. Once liver failure and coagulopathy have occurred, the pregnancy should be terminated, as delivery offers the best chance to mother and baby in fatty liver of pregnancy. Otherwise, the management is that of any cause of fulminant hepatic failure (p. 809), with particular emphasis on the use of platelets and fresh frozen plasma during delivery and on the prevention and treatment of hypoglycemia in the mother and the infant. Liver transplantation may be needed (p. 1155).

***Prognosis.*** Fatty liver of pregnancy was previously a condition with a dismal outlook, as almost all mothers and their infants died. More recent experience shows that mortality can be very low. Series with no maternal mortality are reported (Riely et al 1987, Reyes et al 1994), but fetal mortality can still be high (Reyes et al 1994). This is probably due partly to the recognition of milder cases, but possibly also to better supportive therapy and to early delivery of the baby. The outlook for mothers and infants who recover is excellent. The mother's liver returns to normal and recurrence of fatty liver in a subsequent pregnancy is very rare (Reyes et al 1994).

## Pre-eclampsia–eclampsia

Pre-eclampsia is characterized by hypertension, proteinuria and peripheral edema. Occasionally, there are associated coagulation abnormalities and disseminated intravascular coagulation (DIC). Eclampsia is the additional association of fits and hyperreflexia. Pre-eclampsia–eclampsia occurs in 5% of pregnancies after the 20th week and is more frequent in nulliparas. The liver is damaged as part of the eclamptic process, with hemorrhage and ischemic infarction. The patient has no symptoms referable to the liver and hepatic involvement is diagnosed because of abnormal liver function tests: an increase in transaminases (usually <500 u/L) and modest elevation of the serum bilirubin and alkaline phosphatase.

Severe hepatic involvement in pre-eclampsia–eclampsia is uncommon and takes the form of hepatic infarction, hematomas or rupture of the liver. The clinical features are those of nausea, vomiting, right upper quadrant pain and sudden hypotension in the last trimester of pregnancy. The mortality rate is 50–75% for mothers and 60% for the fetus (Schorr-Lesnick et al 1991).

***Treatment.*** The hepatic complications are best managed by early recognition and treatment of pre-eclampsia. Once hepatic involvement is diagnosed, immediate delivery of the fetus should be undertaken if the fetus is mature. If the condition occurs early in gestation, management with bed rest, antihypertensive therapy and magnesium sulfate is recommended.

***HELLP syndrome.*** A variant of eclampsia is the combination of hemolysis, elevated liver enzymes and low platelets (HELLP). The usual occurrence is around the 32nd week of pregnancy in patients with eclampsia. The symptoms are nausea, vomiting, headache and right upper quadrant or epigastric pain. The diastolic blood pressure is usually above 110 mmHg. Laboratory investigations show evidence of DIC (low platelet count, low fibrinogen levels, raised fibrin degradation products and prolonged prothrombin time). There is evidence of intravascular hemolysis and a moderate elevation of bilirubin and moderate to marked elevation of transaminases (AST 72–1350 u/L) (Freund & Arvan 1990). The maternal mortality rate is about 3%, but the infant perinatal mortality rate is 35%. Early delivery by cesarean section under general anesthesia is recommended. Correction of the clotting abnormalities is necessary (Schorr-Lesnick et al 1991).

### Other conditions

Spontaneous rupture of the liver in pregnancy is a rare condition in which subcapsular hematomas burst into the peritoneum (p. 1110). Primary hepatic pregnancy is an exceptionally rare condition in which the placenta is attached to and invades the liver (Kirby 1969). It causes slow intraperitoneal bleeding leading to pallor, anemia, faintness and upper abdominal pain. Gradually developing oligemic shock indicates the need for blood transfusion and laparotomy. Hepatic venous thrombosis causing the Budd–Chiari syndrome (p. 1079) (Rosenthal et al 1972) may occur in pregnancy or in the puerperium. Mild cases may be managed with diuretics. Most patients require either a portasystemic shunt or liver transplant. The outcome is poor (Gray & Bouchier 1992). Portal venous thrombosis (p. 1082) may also occur (Chambers & Goodbody 1963).

## PREGNANCY IN PATIENTS WITH LIVER DISEASE AND/OR PORTAL HYPERTENSION

Women with liver disease and/or portal hypertension who become pregnant fall into three main groups: those with mild persistent hepatitis, those with chronic active hepatitis or cirrhosis who may or may not have portal hypertension and those who have portal hypertension from extrahepatic portal venous obstruction. Pregnancy in persistent hepatitis has been reported by Infeld et al (1979). The effects of pregnancy in the other two groups have been reviewed by Cheng (1977) and by Varma et al (1977).

### Persistent hepatitis

Persistent hepatitis is a relatively mild condition. These patients usually have a normal menstrual cycle, are normally fertile and do not run any unusual risk from pregnancy.

### Autoimmune hepatitis and cirrhosis

Women with cirrhosis rarely become pregnant, partly because they are often older and partly because amenorrhea or anovulatory menstrual cycles are common in cirrhosis. Consequently, when pregnancy does occur, it is most frequent in patients with cryptogenic cirrhosis or autoimmune hepatitis, who tend to be younger, although it can occur in almost any form of cirrhosis. Pregnancy usually occurs in patients with relatively inactive disease and good liver function.

Spontaneous abortion is no more common than in women without cirrhosis and is not related to the state of liver function. Premature delivery occurs in a fifth of cirrhotic patients and accounts largely for the high perinatal mortality (18%). Premature delivery tends to occur when liver function has deteriorated, as evidenced by jaundice or fluid retention, and when complications such as gastrointestinal bleeding or toxemia of pregnancy have occurred. The only other complication of pregnancy that is more frequent than normal is postpartum hemorrhage and this occurs in a quarter of patients who have had portasystemic shunt surgery. A normal vaginal delivery should be attempted and the second stage should be shortened by forceps delivery if needed. Blood and other facilities for treating gastrointestinal or postpartum bleeding should be immediately available. Cesarean section should be avoided. Surviving babies are not particularly liable to congenital abnormalities or to liver disease provided the mother is not a carrier of the hepatitis B virus (p. 784).

Patients may require treatment for their liver disease during pregnancy. The general rule of avoiding drugs, especially in the first trimester, should be followed but the overriding consideration must be the mother's health. Patients with autoimmune hepatitis (p. 900) must continue treatment with corticosteroids, although fetal and neonatal adrenal suppression can occur when the dose of prednisolone exceeds 10 mg/day, and additional corticosteroids may be needed to cover delivery. Antimetabolites such as azathioprine should be avoided, as they may be teratogenic. Patients with Wilson's disease should continue to receive penicillamine, as it does not cause fetal abnormalities (Scheinberg & Sternlieb 1975, Walshe 1977). Deterioration of liver function may occur during pregnancy but is unpredictable. Bleeding from varices is the most serious complication and carries a high mortality, although whether it is especially liable to occur in pregnancy is unknown. Increased intra-abdominal pressure due to the uterus and the frequency of gastroesophageal reflux might reasonably predispose to it. Bleeding is treated in the usual way (p. 499) and portasystemic shunt surgery can be done without interrupting the pregnancy. Maternal mortality can only be guessed at, but 12 of 92 (13%) reported cases died during pregnancy, at delivery or in the puerperium (Cheng 1977). The main causes have been gastrointestinal bleeding, hepatic coma and postpartum bleeding. Those with biliary cirrhosis may be at less risk.

Advice regarding pregnancy in patients with cirrhosis is difficult. Patients should be aware that pregnancy may not be possible and that, although a surviving baby stands a normal chance of being healthy, there is an increased risk of losing the baby. Patients should also know that deterioration of liver function or gastrointestinal bleeding during pregnancy can occur in any patient and cannot be foretold. The overall maternal mortality of about 10% needs to be kept in mind and it needs to be remembered that the long-term prognosis for the mother is likely to be limited. Faced with these risks, many patients will probably not want to become pregnant and patients who already have a child, who have active or decompensated liver disease, who have esophageal varices or who are over 30 years old should be advised strongly against pregnancy.

### Extrahepatic portal hypertension

Fifty-eight patients with this condition who have become pregnant have been reported and cavernous transformation or thrombosis of the portal vein has been the usual cause of the portal hypertension. Spontaneous abortion is not a hazard, but premature delivery and an increased perinatal mortality (12%) due mainly to prematurity occur. Surviving children are normal. Acute gastrointestinal bleeding is the main complication. It occurs in a third to a half of patients even after successful previous shunt surgery. In contrast to patients with cirrhosis, bleeding is rarely fatal and its treatment should be conservative, as surgery is unsatisfactory (p. 1084). Postpartum hemorrhage is not unduly frequent. Delivery should be the same as for patients with cirrhosis (above). Advice regarding pregnancy in these patients is easier. The only major hazard they face is gastrointestinal bleeding and as their liver function is generally good, their long-term prognosis is much better.

### Contraception

Advice about contraception in patients with extrahepatic portal hypertension does not differ from that given to any healthy woman. Patients with cirrhosis, or their husbands, should consider sterilization. Otherwise, estrogen and progesterone or progesterone-only oral contraceptive drugs may be given and the sheath or an intrauterine device used if these are not tolerated.

## PREGNANCY AND LIVER TRANSPLANTATION

### Pregnancy after liver transplantation

Most major complications occur within a year of liver transplantation and accordingly women are usually advised not to become pregnant during this time (Laifer & Guido 1995). However, menstruation is usually re-established within a year of transplantation, often within 2 months, and consequently contraceptive advice is needed. Oral contraceptives are convenient but can interfere with cyclosporin elimination and increase plasma concentrations and they should not be used by those with Budd–Chiari syndrome who often have thrombotic tendencies. Mechanical contraceptives such as condoms are preferable, but intrauterine devices may best be avoided in patients at risk of infection. Sterilization should be advised if children are not wanted.

Pregnancy does not increase the frequency of hepatic complications such as rejection. Cyclosporin does not seem to have any adverse effect on the fetus, but particular care is needed over blood levels as the dose required may increase as pregnancy progresses and decrease rapidly after delivery (Roberts et al 1995). Tacrolimus has been used without ill effects on the newborn child (Jain et al 1993). Azathioprine should be stopped owing to its teratogenic potential. Pregnancy after liver transplantation has a higher rate of complications due mainly to hypertension, pre-eclampsia and premature delivery, but the long-term outlook for babies normal at delivery is good.

Cytomegalovirus infection of the fetus is a serious complication in maternal carriers of this virus (Laifer et al 1995). Breastfeeding is not advised, as cyclosporin is excreted in breast milk.

## Liver transplantation during pregnancy

Liver transplantation has been carried out only rarely during pregnancy. It is a formidable undertaking and ready availability of a donor liver is required. Transplantation has been carried out for fulminant viral hepatitis (Shanley et al 1995) and fulminant drug-related hepatitis (Bourliere et al 1992), Budd–Chiari syndrome (Valentine et al 1995) and liver disease related to the pregnancy itself (Morrissette & Riely 1991, Hunter et al 1995). Pregnancy is uncommon in patients with chronic liver disease, but transplantation might need consideration where progressive liver failure occurs during pregnancy. Fetal mortality is high and the fetus may suffer injury during transplantation (Finlay et al 1994), but healthy children have survived.

REFERENCES


Adlercreutz H, Tikkanen M J, Wichmann K, Svanborg A, Änberg Ä 1974 Recurrent jaundice in pregnancy. IV. Quantitative determination of urinary and biliary estrogens, including studies in pruritus gravidarum. Journal of Clinical Endocrinology and Metabolism 38: 51–57

BMJ 1975 Leading article: Itching in pregnancy. British Medical Journal 3: 608

Bourliere M, Le Treut Y P, Manelli J C et al 1992 Chlormezanone-induced fulminant hepatitis in a pregnant woman: successful delivery and liver transplantation. Journal of Gastroenterology and Hepatology 7: 339–341

Chambers J S W, Goodbody R A 1963 Portal phlebothrombosis in the puerperium: a report of three cases. British Medical Journal 2: 1104–1106

Cheng S-Y 1977 Pregnancy in liver cirrhosis and/or portal hypertension. American Journal of Obstetrics and Gynecology 128: 812–822

Christie A B, Allam A A, Aref M K, Elmuntasser I H, El-Nageh M 1976 Pregnancy hepatitis in Libya. Lancet 2: 827–829

Dalén E, Westerholm B 1974 Occurrence of hepatic impairment in women jaundiced by oral contraceptives and in their mothers and sisters. Acta Medica Scandinavica 195: 459–463

Davies M H, Wilkinson S P, Hanid M A et al 1980 Acute liver disease with encephalopathy and renal failure in late pregnancy and the early puerperium. A study of fourteen patients. British Journal of Obstetrics and Gynaecology 87: 1005–1014

Finlay D E, Foshager M C, Longley D G, Letourneau J G 1994 Ischemic injury to the fetus after maternal liver transplantation. Journal of Ultrasound in Medicine 13: 145–148

Fisk N M, Storey G N B 1988 Fetal outcome in obstetric cholestasis. British Journal of Obstetrics and Gynaecology 95: 1137–1143

Freund G, Arvan D A 1990 Clinical biochemistry of preeclampsia and related liver diseases of pregnancy: a review. Clinica Chimica Acta 191: 123–152

Fulton I C, Douglas J G, Hutchon D J R, Beckett G J 1983 Is normal pregnancy cholestatic? Clinica Chimica Acta 130: 171–176

Furhoff A-K, Hellström K 1973 Jaundice in pregnancy. A follow-up study of the series of women originally reported by L Thorley. I. The pregnancies. Acta Medica Scandinavica 193: 259–266

Gray J R, Bouchier I A D 1992 Pregnancy and the liver. In: Calder A A, Dunlop W (eds) High-risk pregnancy. Butterworth Heinemann, Oxford, pp 210–232

Hadler S C, Webster H M, Erben J J, Swanson J E, Maynard J E 1980 Hepatitis A in day-care centers. New England Journal of Medicine 302: 1222–1227

Haemmerli U P, Wyss H I 1967 Recurrent intrahepatic cholestasis of pregnancy. Medicine 46: 299–321

Hunter S K, Martin M, Benda J A, Zlatnik F J 1995 Liver transplant after massive spontaneous hepatic rupture in pregnancy complicated by preeclampsia. Obstetrics and Gynecology 85: 819–822

Infeld D S, Borkowf H I, Varma R R 1979 Chronic persistent hepatitis and pregnancy. Gastroenterology 77: 524–527

Ingerslev M, Teilum G 1946 Biopsy studies on the liver in pregnancy. II. Liver biopsy on normal pregnant women. Acta Obstetricia et Gynaecologica Scandinavica 25: 352–360

Jain A, Venkataramanan R, Lever J et al 1993 FK506 and pregnancy in liver transplant patients. Transplantation 56: 1588–1589

Kaplan M M 1985 Acute fatty liver of pregnancy. New England Journal of Medicine 313: 367–370

Khuroo M S, Teli M R, Skidmore S 1981 The incidence and severity of viral hepatitis in pregnancy. American Journal of Medicine 70: 252–255

Kirby N G 1969 Primary hepatic pregnancy. British Medical Journal 1: 296

Knox T A, Olans L B 1996 Liver disease in pregnancy. New England Journal of Medicine 335: 569–576

Kreek M J, Sleisenger M H 1970 Estrogen induced cholestasis due to endogenous hormones. Scandinavian Journal of Gastroenterology 5 (suppl 7): 123–131

Laifer S A, Guido R S 1995 Reproductive function and outcome of pregnancy after liver transplantation in women. Mayo Clinic Proceedings 70: 388–394

Laifer S A, Ehrlich G D, Huff D S, Balsan M J, Scantlebury V P 1995 Congenital cytomegalovirus infection in offspring of liver transplant recipients. Clinical Infectious Diseases 20: 52–55

Larrey D, Rueff B, Feldmann G, Degott C, Danan G, Benhamou J-P 1984 Recurrent jaundice caused by recurrent hyperemesis gravidarum. Gut 25: 1414–1415

Morrissette C T, Riely C A 1991 Acute fatty liver of pregnancy. European Journal of Gastroenterology and Hepatology 3: 869–872

Piccinino F, Manzillo G, Sagnelli E 1975 The differential diagnosis between intrahepatic cholestatic jaundice and viral hepatitis during pregnancy. Acta Hepato-gastroenterologica 22: 144

Reyes H, Gonzales M C, Ribalta J et al 1978 Prevalence of intrahepatic cholestasis of pregnancy in Chile. Annals of Internal Medicine 88: 487–493

Reyes H, Sandoval L, Wainstein A et al 1994 Acute fatty liver of pregnancy: a clinical study of 12 episodes in 11 patients. Gut 35: 101–106

Riely C A, Latham P S, Romero R, Duffy T P 1987 Acute fatty liver of pregnancy. A reassessment based on observations in nine patients. Annals of Internal Medicine 106: 703–706

Roberts M, Brown A St J M, James O F W, Davison J M 1995 Interpretation of cyclosporin A levels in pregnancy following orthotopic liver transplantation. British Journal of Obstetrics and Gynaecology 102: 570–572

Rosenthal T, Shani M, Deutsch V, Samra H 1972 The Budd–Chiari syndrome after pregnancy. American Journal of Obstetrics and Gynecology 113: 789–792

Scheinberg I H, Sternlieb I 1975 Pregnancy in penicillamine-treated patients with Wilson's disease. New England Journal of Medicine 293: 1300–1302

Schorr-Lesnick B, Lebovics E, Dworkin B, Rosenthal W S 1991 Liver diseases unique to pregnancy. American Journal of Gastroenterology 86: 659–670

Seeff L B, Hoofnagle J A 1979 Immunoprophylaxis of viral hepatitis. Gastroenterology 77: 161–182

Shanley C J, Braun D K, Brown K et al 1995 Fulminant hepatic failure secondary to herpes simplex virus hepatitis. Successful outcome after orthotopic liver transplantation. Transplantation 59: 145–149

Simcock M J, Forster F M C 1967 Pregnancy is cholestatic. Medical Journal of Australia 2: 971–973

Snydman D R 1985 Hepatitis in pregnancy. New England Journal of Medicine 313: 1398–1401

Valentine J M J, Parkin G, Pollard S G, Bellamy M C 1995 Combined orthotopic liver transplantation and Caesarean section for the Budd–Chiari syndrome. British Journal of Anaesthesia 75: 105–108

Varma R R, Michelsohn N H, Borkowf H I, Lewis J D 1977 Pregnancy in cirrhotic and non-cirrhotic portal hypertension. Obstetrics and Gynecology 50: 217–222

Walshe J M 1977 Pregnancy in Wilson's disease. Quarterly Journal of Medicine 46: 73–83

Wong D C, Purcell R H, Sreenivasan M A, Prasad S R, Pavri K M 1980 Epidemic and endemic hepatitis in India: evidence for a non-A, non-B virus aetiology. Lancet 2: 876–879

# 43. The liver in systemic disease

*John F. Dillon N. D. C. Finlayson*

## INTRODUCTION

Liver disease sufficient to compromise liver function significantly has serious secondary effects on the function of many other organs in the body. Conversely, diseases of other organs can interfere with liver function either directly or indirectly. This chapter considers the effects a number of extrahepatic diseases can have on the liver itself.

## CARDIOVASCULAR DISEASE

### Heart failure

Hepatic damage always occurs in congestive cardiac failure, although this may be so minor that no clinical evidence of liver damage is found. Frequently, the only sign of hepatic involvement is the finding of abnormal biochemical liver function tests, which may suggest erroneously the presence of intrinsic liver disease. Occasionally the discovery of the abnormal liver function tests may actually lead to the diagnosis of heart failure (Dunn et al 1973, Cohen & Kaplan 1978, Ware 1978).

#### *Etiology*

Any heart disease leading to low-output cardiac failure with right-sided congestion can cause liver damage. It is unclear if the hepatic changes noted in high-output cardiac failure are due to the heart failure itself or to the underlying disease process. Previously, rheumatic heart disease was the commonest cause of hepatic dysfunction due to heart failure, partly because it was the commonest cause of heart failure but also because of its tendency to cause gross right heart failure. Ischemic heart disease and hypertensive heart disease are now the most frequent causes, but the whole disease spectrum has been considerably modified with the introduction of effective diuretics and angiotensin-converting enzyme inhibitors for the treatment of heart failure. Cardiomyopathy can also cause marked hepatic congestion. Four mechanisms contribute to the genesis of hepatic damage in cardiac failure: decreased hepatic blood flow and increased hepatic venous pressure with sinusoidal congestion and dilatation and atrophy of hepatocytes are probably most important, decreased arterial oxygen saturation can occur but is probably not so important in causing hepatocellular hypoxia, and some suggest that endotoxin may have a role.

#### *Pathology*

A large congested liver is the characteristic finding at autopsy. The cut surface has a dark red and yellow mottled appearance (nutmeg liver) due respectively to the contrasting congested hemorrhagic central areas and the paler periportal areas. Fibrosis may be prominent in advanced cases, but nodularity is not usually marked even when cardiac cirrhosis is present. Liver biopsy shows the characteristic features of centrilobular congestion with the central veins and the sinusoids dilated and filled with red blood cells. The centrilobular hepatocytes show degenerative changes including shrinkage, granularity, vacuolation and pyknotic nuclear changes and they often contain brown pigment. The periportal liver cells are relatively normal. The lobular architecture is usually normal, but fibrosis may link central veins and produce a reverse lobulation with portal tracts in the center of the lobules. Cardiac cirrhosis may develop eventually but is rare.

#### *Clinical features*

Most patients with cardiac failure have few symptoms clearly attributable to the liver. Lethargy, confusion, tremor and even coma may occur but are most often due to cardiac failure. Hypoglycemia due to liver failure consequent upon cardiac failure has been reported. Right upper quadrant abdominal discomfort or pain associated with a large, tender liver is common and is attributed to stretching of the liver capsule. In addition to other signs of cardiac failure, examination reveals hepatomegaly in most patients with right ventricular failure. The liver is smooth, often tender and is 5 cm or more below the costal margin in half the patients. When tricuspid incompetence is present, systolic pulsation may be felt over the liver as blood is forced back into the hepatic veins. Pulsation is not found in cardiac cirrhosis. The spleen may be palpable even in the absence of cardiac cirrhosis. Cardiac cirrhosis is rare and not normally associated with peripheral stigmata of chronic liver disease.

***Ischemic hepatitis.*** Occasionally, heart disease can mimic a primary liver disease, particularly viral hepatitis, and rarely fulminant hepatic failure (p. 808) may develop (Cohen & Kaplan 1978, Nouel et al 1980). This occurs most often when there is a sudden change in cardiac output in chronic heart disease or cor pulmonale or in progressive cardiac tamponade. The patient is usually very ill and has obvious tender hepatomegaly with or without jaundice and the biochemical features of an acute hepatitis (p. 741). Constrictive pericarditis may also mimic cirrhosis or the Budd–Chiari syndrome (p. 1079). The single most useful clinical sign in these patients is a raised jugular venous pressure that is easily overlooked if the pressure is very high.

*Investigations*

Liver function tests may be normal in cardiac failure. Abnormalities become more frequent as the severity of the cardiac failure increases or at times of sudden decompensation in the heart failure. The plasma bilirubin is frequently increased, but values are usually below 50 μmol/L and rarely above 100 μmol/L. Hepatic dysfunction or hemolysis is the main contributing factor and the hyperbilirubinemia may be of the conjugated or unconjugated type (p. 739). Apart from hemolysis, cardiac failure is one of the commonest causes of unconjugated hyperbilirubinemia (Levine & Klatskin 1964). Plasma transaminase activity is increased in about a third of cases and usually does not exceed twice the normal upper limit. Occasionally, activities may exceed 1000 μ/L, usually in valvular heart disease and in acute heart failure with a very high central venous pressure, hypotension or shock. Such high transaminase activity may lead to mistaken diagnosis of viral hepatitis (Cohen & Kaplan 1978, Gibson & Dudley 1984). The plasma alkaline phosphatase activity is sometimes increased but rarely exceeds twice the normal upper limit. Hypoalbuminemia is common but values below 25 g/L are exceptional, mild hypergammaglobulinemia may be found, a mild to moderate prolongation of prothrombin time is a very frequent abnormality and occasionally it may be marked and cannot be reversed by vitamin K. These patients are extremely sensitive to anticoagulation treatment.

Ultrasound is useful in showing congested hepatic veins and in excluding other hepatobiliary diseases. Liver biopsy is rarely necessary. Experience has shown no increased risk from liver biopsy in these patients, but they are less able to tolerate any complication when it occurs. If biopsy is necessary, it is best delayed until treatment has improved the patient's condition.

*Diagnosis*

Hepatic dysfunction can be attributed to cardiac failure when the two conditions occur together, when there is no clinical or biochemical evidence of an alternative cause for the liver disease and when successful treatment of cardiac failure leads to improvement or resolution of the hepatic dysfunction. High plasma transaminase activity in cardiac failure is usually associated with a high lactate dehydrogenase activity and these return to normal within 5–10 days of successful treatment of the cardiac failure.

Hepatic congestion and cardiac cirrhosis cannot be differentiated clinically as causes of hepatic dysfunction in cardiac failure. Cardiac cirrhosis may be suspected in patients with prolonged or recurrent cardiac failure, with longstanding tricuspid incompetence or constrictive pericarditis and where the liver is not enlarged in spite of cardiac failure and abnormal liver function tests. A specific diagnosis requires a biopsy, but this is rarely needed. In any patient presenting with both heart disease and liver disease the diagnosis of hemochromatosis should be considered.

*Treatment*

The treatment is that of the underlying heart disease. The congested liver may not metabolize drugs normally and this needs to be considered when planning treatment.

### Myocardial infarction

Many patients with acute myocardial infarction have abnormal liver function tests, even in the absence of congestive cardiac failure or significant hypotension (Das et al 1974). There are, however, usually no signs of clinical liver disease. The plasma bilirubin is elevated in 50% of patients and is mainly due to an increase in unconjugated bilirubin (Cowan et al 1981). The causes of these changes are uncertain. Cardiac output falls significantly in the first few days after uncomplicated myocardial infarction and myocardial ischemia in animals reduces total liver blood flow by 60% at 5 h. However, hepatic clearance of unconjugated bilirubin is relatively independent of hepatic blood flow and accordingly there may be an increase in the amount of bilirubin reaching the liver. One source could be myoglobin released from necrotic myocardium.

### Constrictive pericarditis

Constrictive pericarditis can be confused easily with hepatic cirrhosis, because it causes marked ascites without comparably severe peripheral edema, fatigue rather than breathlessness may be the main complaint and hepatomegaly and sometimes splenomegaly may be found. It can also be mistaken for the Budd–Chiari syndrome (p. 1079) because of the prominent ascites and hepatomegaly and, as in the Budd–Chiari syndrome the ascites may have a high protein concentration (Solano et al 1986). The most important clue to the true diagnosis is a raised jugular venous pressure which may be so high as to be overlooked. Most patients also have a pulsatile liver, best appreciated in mid-inspiration and at end-expiration. This may be felt as a double pulsation with a diastolic dip after the carotid pulse as blood rapidly enters the heart and a pulsation late in diastole as blood refluxes into the hepatic veins once right ventricular filling is complete (Manga et al 1984). The most important investigations in confirming the diagnosis are echocardiography and cardiac catheterization. The treatment is that of the cardiac disease.

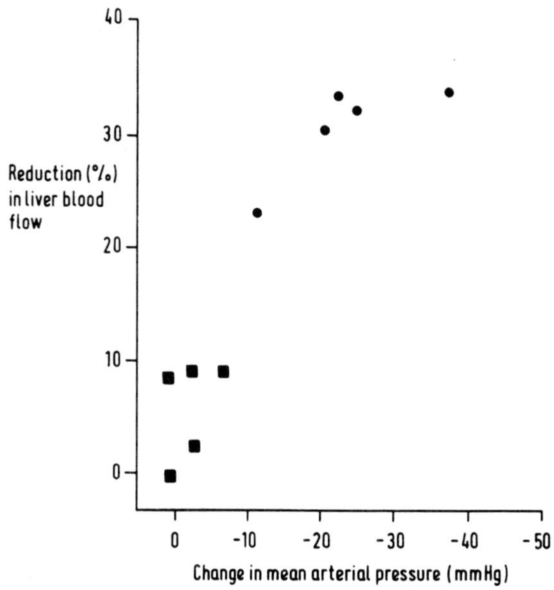


**Fig. 43.1** Relation of hepatic blood flow to change in mean systemic arterial blood pressure in normotensive subjects (■) and in subjects with orthostatic hypotension (●) (Feely et al 1982).

## Cardiomyopathy

Cardiomyopathy can produce hepatic abnormalities either by causing cardiac failure or by causing the syndrome of constrictive pericarditis (above). The combination of cardiomyopathy and hepatic abnormality should also lead to consideration of conditions such as alcohol abuse, hemochromatosis (p. 955), amyloidosis (p. 979) and connective tissue diseases (p. 1106).

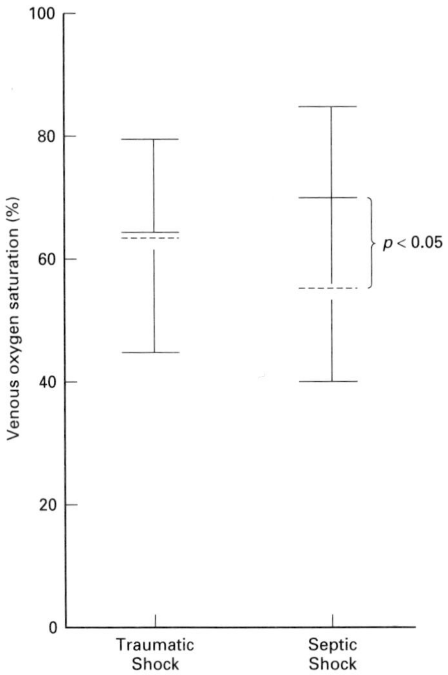


**Fig. 43.2** Central mixed venous oxygen saturation in traumatic and septic shock showing lower mean venous oxygenation in hepatic (– – –) than in central mixed (——) venous blood in septic shock (Dahn et al 1988).

## Shock

Shock liver or ischemic hepatitis is a severe hepatic derangement due to failure of the circulation to the liver (Kantrowitz et al 1967, Nunes et al 1970). It is frequently associated with the syndrome of multiple system organ failure in which the liver, lungs, kidneys and gut are particularly affected (Fry et al 1980). Liver injury is essentially ischemic and is associated with hypotension, which produces an approximately 10% reduction in hepatic blood flow for every 10 mmHg fall in mean arterial pressure (Fig. 43.1). It can be produced by hemorrhage, myocardial infarction, sepsis, postoperative hypotension, pulmonary embolism or major trauma. Hypoxia may be more important in septic shock where tissue oxygen demand is high and hepatic venous oxygenation is low (Fig. 43.2).

### *Clinical features*

The clinical features include those of the cause of the shock, shock itself and the hepatic consequences of the shock. The hepatic consequences often appear sometime after the shock has resolved, but the severity and duration of the shock are important in predicting the likelihood of liver damage. There may be no clinical sign of hepatic dysfunction, even when investigations reveal clear liver damage. Jaundice may appear at any time within 2 weeks of a more severe episode of shock and the serum bilirubin may exceed 200 μmol/L (12 mg/dl) in very ill patients. A serum bilirubin above 50 μmol/L (3 mg/dl) is a bad prognostic sign in traumatic shock. Occasionally, fulminant hepatic failure may be caused by shock (p. 808) and its development is characterized by encephalopathy. Stigmata of chronic liver disease are important only in identifying patients with underlying chronic liver disease who are very sensitive to the hepatic effects of shock.

*Investigations*

Liver function tests show mainly a marked increase of serum transaminase activity that falls rapidly once shock is treated successfully. The bilirubin rises later and a delayed increased alkaline phosphatase and γ-glutamyl transferase may indicate some cholestasis during recovery. Prolongation of the prothrombin time should warn of fulminant hepatic failure. Increased urea and creatinine indicate associated renal damage.

*Pathology*

The main histological findings in patients dying of shock are variable centrilobular congestion, hepatocyte damage and necrosis and cholestasis that includes inspissated bile in the biliary canaliculae and ductules. Liver biopsy is not needed in these patients, but biopsies in fulminant hepatic failure after shock have shown similar findings. The severity and duration of shock are important in the development of these lesions. Congestion and hepatocyte damage occur within about 10 h and progress to necrosis by about 24 h (Table 43.1). Reduced hepatic blood flow and hepatic congestion are probably the main causes of liver damage, but other factors such as hypoxia (Fig. 43.1) may also be important. Animal research suggests that the development of centrilobular necrosis is more severe where there is endotoxemia.

*Treatment*

Treatment is that of the underlying shock and its causes and supportive therapy is necessary for any symptoms of liver failure that develop. Recovery depends upon the underlying disease process and is accompanied by a return to normal liver function. It has been suggested that hepatic calcification may occur following recovery from ischemic hepatitic injuries (Shibuya et al 1985).

## PULMONARY DISEASE

Hepatic abnormalities are quite common in patients with pulmonary disease. The pulmonary abnormalities resulting from liver disease are considered elsewhere (p. 1069).

**Table 43.1** Duration of shock related to development of centrilobular hepatic damage and necrosis (Ellenberg & Osserman 1951)

| Duration of shock (hours) | Centrilobular histology (%) Necrosis | Damage | Normal |
|---|---|---|---|
| 0–10 | 5 | 7 | 88 |
| 10–24 | 22 | 70 | 9 |
| >24 | 92 | 4 | 4 |
| Patient numbers | 32 | 20 | 41 |

### Chronic obstructive airway disease

Liver function tests including bilirubin, aminotransferases, alkaline phosphatase and γ-glutamyl transferase have been found to be abnormal in patients with chronic respiratory insufficiency. The cause of these abnormalities is uncertain. Hypoxemia on its own does not seem a sufficient cause (Whelan et al 1969), unless it is very severe (Refsum 1963), and it may be that in most cases a combination of hypoxemia and cardiac failure is required.

### Asthma

Elevation of serum aspartate and alanine aminotransferases has been reported in severe asthma, particularly during status asthmaticus. The enzyme activities fall rapidly after resolution of the attack and the increase in enzyme activity seems related to the severity of the attack (El-Shaboury et al 1964).

### Pneumonia

It is well recognized that patients with severe pneumococcal pneumonia can become jaundiced. The incidence is reported to be 3–26%. Jaundice usually appears between the third and sixth day of the illness, most often with right lower lobe pneumonias. The liver is frequently tender, but rarely enlarged. Patients with jaundice tend to have had prolonged fever, but they have a similar prognosis to those without jaundice. The serum bilirubin is usually around 70 μmol/L (5 mg/dl) but may reach up to 350 μmol/L (20 mg/dl). Some jaundiced patients show a modest elevation of serum aminotransferase activity and in a few patients there may be a slight rise in alkaline phosphatase activity. The main cause of hyperbilirubinemia is probably hepatocellular dysfunction caused by hypoxia, fever or direct toxicity, but hemolysis due to glucose-6-phosphate dehydrogenase deficiency is a major factor in parts of the world where this condition is common (Tugwell 1973). The atypical pneumonias, particularly legionnaires disease but also mycoplasma, psittacosis and cytomegalovirus pneumonia, are associated with abnormalities of the liver function tests in 50% of reported cases. Jaundice is much less common and is a marker of very severe infection (Kirby et al 1978).

## HEPATIC ANOXIA

Anoxia is a contributory factor in hepatic damage due to shock, especially septic, pulmonary disease and cardiac failure (above). Occasionally, it may be sufficient to cause serious liver damage in its own right (hypoxic hepatitis).

This has been reported in severe hypoxia due to carbon monoxide poisoning (Watson & Williams 1984) and during obstructive sleep apnea (Mathurin et al 1995). The main biochemical finding is a greatly increased serum transaminase activity and a prolonged prothrombin time if liver damage is very severe. Liver biopsy shows severe centrilobular necrosis.

## GASTROINTESTINAL DISEASE

### Inflammatory bowel disease

Ulcerative colitis and Crohn's disease are associated with a number of complications outside the gastrointestinal tract including various disorders of the liver and biliary tree (Cohen et al 1971, Cello et al 1977, Desmet & Geboes 1987). The inflammatory bowel disease usually presents first and causes the predominant clinical features, but occasionally it develops after the extraintestinal complications or remains asymptomatic. The hepatobiliary complications are often asymptomatic but can cause any of the clinical features associated with the underlying hepatobiliary lesion.

The incidence of abnormal liver function tests in unselected ulcerative colitis patients is 11% but nearly half are transient, mainly associated with active bowel disease (Broomé et al 1994).

#### *Fatty liver*

Fatty change has been regarded as the commonest abnormality in the liver in inflammatory bowel disease. This was based on finding fatty change in 90% of liver biopsies taken at surgical resections and fatty change occurring in the liver in 50% of patients dying of inflammatory bowel disease. Clearly such patients have severe inflammatory bowel disease and may be malnourished or suffering nonspecific ill health. Indeed, in one postmortem series the incidence of fatty liver in patients who had died of inflammatory bowel disease was the same as in those dying of other chronic debilitating illness. With better treatment for inflammatory bowel disease and earlier diagnosis in less severely affected individuals, the incidence of fatty change has been shown to be much lower (Broomé et al 1994). The lesion of fatty change causes no clinical feature other than mild hepatomegaly associated with mild abnormalities of the serum transaminase activity. The lesion does not progress and resolves with successful treatment of the underlying bowel disease.

#### *Primary sclerosing cholangitis and small duct primary sclerosing cholangitis* (pericholangitis)

Primary sclerosing cholangitis is an uncommon condition that is associated with ulcerative colitis in about 70% of cases (p. 943). In a series of unselected patients with ulcerative colitis found to have abnormal liver function tests, 11% of the group had some form of hepatobiliary disease and 2.1% had primary sclerosing cholangitis (Broomé et al 1994). Three percent of patients attending a referral center had persistently abnormal liver function tests and most of these had primary sclerosing cholangitis (Shepherd et al 1983). This may be an underestimate, as liver function tests may be normal in sclerosing cholangitis (p. 944). Sclerosing cholangitis can occur in Crohn's disease but with a much lower incidence and largely in patients with colonic disease.

Pericholangitis is a histological term used to describe inflammatory reactions characterized by periductular inflammation and fibrosis in the portal tracts of the liver. The term has also been used to describe a host of nonspecific changes within the liver. Most of these patients have cholangiographic appearances of primary sclerosing cholangitis (Shepherd et al 1983) and they can go on to develop cirrhosis and cholangiocarcinoma. The term "pericholangitis" should probably be abandoned and all patients with periductular inflammation and normal ERCP findings should be regarded as suffering from small duct sclerosing cholangitis (Wee & Ludwig 1985).

#### *Cholangiocarcinoma*

Patients with ulcerative colitis develop bile duct carcinomas 10–30 times more frequently than persons not so affected (Ritchie et al 1974, Mir-Madjlessi et al 1987). This does not seem to occur in Crohn's disease. It usually occurs in patients whose bowel disease is of long duration, up to 15 years or more, and in those in whom most or all of the colon is involved. It has been suggested that primary sclerosing cholangitis may be the precursor of cholangiocarcinoma in patients with ulcerative colitis (Mir-Madjlessi et al 1987).

#### *Cirrhosis*

The incidence of cirrhosis in inflammatory bowel disease is variously reported as being between 1% and 5%. The cirrhosis is normally of the macronodular type and where classification is possible, it is normally of the biliary type. Since sclerosing cholangitis is frequently asymptomatic in ulcerative colitis, it seems likely that most cirrhosis represents end-stage primary sclerosing cholangitis. Patients with ulcerative colitis and cirrhosis develop the usual complications of cirrhosis and in addition, stomal varices and bleeding may develop following colectomy (p. 993). The occasional patient with cirrhosis and ulcerative colitis who suffers severe encephalopathy responding poorly to treatment may benefit from colectomy (p. 1054).

*Autoimmune hepatitis*

Autoimmune hepatitis has been reported in ulcerative colitis. Differentiation from primary sclerosing cholangitis can be difficult and some reported cases have had cholestatic liver function tests (Olsson & Hultén 1975). The pathological lesion of interface hepatitis can occur in primary sclerosing cholangitis, so a diagnosis of autoimmune hepatitis should not be made without an entirely normal cholangiogram and even this would not exclude small duct primary sclerosing cholangitis. Antinuclear antibodies occur in both diseases, but smooth muscle antibody at high titer would favor autoimmune hepatitis (p. 889) and p-ANCA would favor primary sclerosing cholangitis (p. 943). In spite of the difficulties of separating these diseases, there does seem to be an overlap syndrome with the features of both diseases. The importance of recognizing this is that patients with markedly elevated serum transaminase activities may respond to treatment with corticosteroids.

*Other hepatobiliary diseases*

Gallstones occur more frequently in Crohn's disease of the terminal ileum and after resection of the terminal ileum than in the general population. There is no such increase in inflammatory bowel disease restricted to the colon. Rare hepatic lesions in inflammatory bowel disease include granulomatous hepatitis (p. 829), amyloidosis (p. 979) and hepatic abscesses (p. 817). The association of primary biliary cirrhosis with ulcerative colitis remains uncertain (p. 937).

### Jejunoileal diseases

All these disorders are capable of producing severe malnutrition causing gross fatty infiltration in the liver. This lesion normally reverses completely when the underlying malnutrition is alleviated; however, it has been suggested in some conditions at least that this fatty change, if untreated, can develop into fibrosis and lead to cirrhosis.

*Celiac disease*

Clinical evidence of liver disease in celiac disease is rare but asymptomatic liver disease can occur. Hägander et al (1977) found abnormal liver function tests in 39% of 74 consecutive patients and liver biopsies showed chronic aggressive hepatitis or cirrhosis in seven patients. The etiology of this is uncertain. Primary biliary cirrhosis and celiac disease have been reported together (Logan et al 1978) and small intestinal subtotal villus atrophy was found in five of 26 (19%) patients with primary biliary cirrhosis in one report (Olsson et al 1982).

*Tropical sprue*

Abnormalities of the liver function tests are unusual and there are no significant changes on liver histology.

*Whipple's disease*

The liver is commonly involved in Whipple's disease. Periodic acid Schiff-positive macrophages are seen on liver biopsy and occasionally granulomas are also present (Haubrich et al 1960).

*Jejunoileal bypass*

Significant liver disease occurs in 5–50% of patients after jejunoileal bypass (Buchwald et al 1974, Nasrallah et al 1980) and consequently this operation has fallen into disuse (p. 458). Gastroplasty replaced it, but similar abnormalities of liver function have been reported following this operation, suggesting that malnutrition superimposed on obesity may have been responsible for the injury (Hamilton et al 1983). Histological findings range from simple fatty change to fibrosis and cirrhosis and features identical to those of alcoholic hepatitis (nonalcoholic steatohepatitis) can occur (p. 975). Liver disease may present acutely with jaundice and abnormal liver function tests or insidiously with eventual development of hepatic cirrhosis. Changes are most severe during the period of rapid weight loss and persistently abnormal liver function tests 3 months after operation suggest progressive liver disease. This is treated initially by hyperalimentation, but reversal of the ileal bypass is necessary. The response of the existing liver damage to reversal is unclear.

## BLOOD DISEASES

### Hemophilia and Christmas disease

There is no primary liver disease in either of these hemostatic disorders. Unfortunately, however, most of these patients have contracted chronic hepatitis C virus infection (p. 788) from blood products used prior to the availability of serological tests for the hepatitis C virus. Previous reports of abnormal liver function associated with hemophilia are attributable largely to hepatitis C virus infection.

### Hemolytic anemias

Jaundice can occur in any of the hemolytic anemias due to increased production of unconjugated bilirubin (p. 739). This is associated with an increased risk of gallstones (p. 1203). Patients receiving transfusions prior to routine screening of blood for the hepatitis C virus may have been infected with this virus (p. 788) and those needing repeated transfusions are at risk of developing secondary hemochromatosis (p. 958).

### *Sickle cell anemia*

Several hepatobiliary complications can occur in sickle cell anemia and they are generally attributable to aggregations of red blood cells sickling in the hepatic sinusoids or to long-standing hemolysis leading to gallstone formation (Johnson et al 1985). The liver shows sinusoidal sickling, prominence of the Kupffer cells, erythrophagocytosis and increased collagen in the space of Disse and hepatic infarction and abscess formation. Cirrhosis also occurs (Bauer et al 1980).

The commonest complication is the hepatic crisis, which accounts for about 10% of all painful crises in this disease. The clinical features are indistinguishable from acute cholecystitis and individual episodes last about 2–3 weeks. Treatment is the same as in acute cholecystitis and cholecystectomy is advised if gallstones are found. Some patients develop marked jaundice and are found to have thick inspissated bile rather than stones in the gallbladder at operation. Biliary obstruction has been attributed to the inspissated bile and patients may benefit from cholecystectomy. Right upper quadrant abdominal pain, fever and jaundice have also resulted from the development of an intrahepatic bile-filled cyst, a biloma, possibly consequent on hepatic infarction (Middleton & Wolper 1984). Episodes of painless cholestatic jaundice with mild to moderate increases of plasma aminotransferase and alkaline phosphatase activities lasting for up to 2 months can occur. These resolve without producing chronic liver damage and have been attributed to drugs. Rarely, severe and progressive cholestasis occurs with abdominal pain, marked hyperbilirubinemia, greatly increased plasma alkaline phosphatase activity and eventually the development of thrombocytopenia, coagulation defects and renal failure. Death occurs from bleeding or liver failure.

Other uncommon developments in sickle cell disease include hepatic infarction, possibly resulting in bile cysts or abscesses, and cirrhosis. Severe sickling of erythrocytes in the liver can also cause rapid enlargement of the liver with increasingly severe anemia, a "sequestration crisis". This is easily overlooked as the liver enlargement is painless and liver function tests can remain normal (Hatton et al 1985).

### *Thalassemia*

Liver damage in thalassemia is attributable largely to chronic hepatitis C virus infection (p. 895) from repeated blood transfusion. In addition, iron overload leading to secondary hemochromatosis can cause cirrhosis in long-term survivors (p. 958). This is becoming less common with the prophylactic use of desferrioxamine.

## Leukemia

Hepatic involvement is common in acute and chronic leukemias and occurs with increasing frequency as the disease progresses. Hepatomegaly is the commonest clinical evidence of the liver involvement and massive hepatomegaly occurs occasionally. Splenomegaly is also present and is usually due to leukemic involvement rather than portal hypertension due to disruption of portal blood flow within the liver. Some chronic leukemias can cause portal hypertension and varices. Other clinical evidence of liver disease is uncommon. Jaundice may be due to hemolysis or liver damage and ascites can be caused by exudates or transudates. Biochemical tests of liver function are often abnormal and the most frequent abnormality is an increase in plasma alkaline phosphatase activity.

The pattern of liver involvement varies in different forms of leukemia (Rozman et al 1991). Chronic lymphocytic leukemia mainly infiltrates the portal tracts and sometimes the periportal areas. Acute leukemia and granulocytic leukemia mainly infiltrate the sinusoids. Infiltration of both the portal tracts and the sinusoids is unusual and occurs most often in chronic monocytic leukemia, hairy cell leukemia and malignant histiocytosis. Hairy cell leukemia (a rare disease with a proliferation of mononuclear cells with lymphocytic and monocytic features and typically hairy cytoplasmic protrusions) is also characterized by cells with clear perinuclear halos and the development of angiomatous parenchymal cavities lined by hairy cells and containing red blood cells (Roquet et al 1985).

## Multiple myeloma

Hepatic involvement is common in multiple myeloma and hepatomegaly occurs in half to two-thirds of patients coming to autopsy (Thomas et al 1973). Liver function tests are often abnormal. An increased plasma alkaline phosphatase activity is the most common. Plasma cell infiltration of the liver can occur in the portal tracts or in the parenchyma. Parenchymal infiltration can involve the sinusoids diffusely even in the absence of plasma cell leukemia or can produce nodules of plasma cells. Amyloidosis of the liver is an occasional complication of multiple myeloma.

***Osteosclerotic myeloma.*** This is a rare condition in which one or more osteosclerotic skeletal lesions are associated with polyneuropathy and other manifestations include organomegaly (lymph nodes, liver, spleen), endocrinopathy (usually hypothyroidism or hypogonadism), monoclonal gammopathy and skin lesions. Some patients show all these features and are said to have POEMS syndrome (Miralles et al 1992). About a quarter of patients have hepatomegaly and/or splenomegaly and about 10% have ascites. Treatment is with radiotherapy to osteosclerotic lesions and with corticosteroids and 5-year survival is about 60%.

## Light chain disease

This is a rare condition in which immunoglobulin light

chains, usually of κ type, are deposited in multiple organs. A few patients have multiple myeloma, but usually no definite underlying diseases can be found. The material deposited is composed of light chains, appears amorphous and does not react with Congo red dye or polarized light as does amyloid. Kidneys are the organs most often affected and the clinical features are those of renal failure. Hepatic involvement usually also occurs and light chains are deposited in the space of Disse and in the portal tracts with associated fibrosis and peliosis (p. 1086). Clinical features include hepatomegaly, abnormal liver function tests and occasionally ascites, but these are seldom prominent. Cirrhosis has been reported.

### Paroxysmal nocturnal hemoglobinuria

This disease, characterized by intravascular hemolysis with episodes of hemoglobinuria and venous thrombosis, is caused by proliferation of abnormal hematopoietic stem cells (Hillmen et al 1995). Venous thromboses occur in a third or more of patients and may be multiple. Common sites include the hepatic veins and portal venous system, where thrombosis can cause the Budd–Chiari syndrome (p. 1079), portal hypertension (p. 1083) and mesenteric infarction (p. 1082). Thrombosis is also common in the leg veins, leading to pulmonary embolism, and in the cerebral veins. Hemorrhage can occur, including gastrointestinal, subarachnoid and intracerebral. Survival may be prolonged and as venous thromboses account for about a quarter of deaths, prophylactic anticoagulants should be considered.

### Systemic mastocytosis

This is an uncommon and often misdiagnosed condition in which abnormal mast cell proliferation occurs. Some 90% of patients develop a maculopapular rash that shows urticaria on scratching and a proportion have infiltration of organs other than the skin, especially bones, liver, gastrointestinal tract, spleen and lymph nodes. A few patients have no skin lesions and cause particular diagnostic difficulty. Fatigue, weight loss, fever and night sweats are common. Gastrointestinal symptoms are also common and can be the sole features. Hepatic involvement occurs in patients with systemic disease (Yam et al 1986). Hepatomegaly is the most common clinical feature and liver function tests most often show increased plasma alkaline phosphatase activity and hypoalbuminemia. Liver function generally remains good. Liver biopsy shows fibrosis, sometimes with cirrhosis, portal tract and parenchymal infiltration with mononuclear cells in which mast cells are not always prominent, and occasionally granulomas. Portal hypertension may occur and cause esophageal varices and ascites (Sawers et al 1982).

### Extramedullary hemopoiesis

Extramedullary hemopoiesis in the liver is common in neonatal and childhood anemias. It can occur in adults in any of the myeloproliferative disorders and is particularly prominent in myelofibrosis (Silverstein et al 1973). It also occurs in chronic myeloid leukemia and polycythemia rubra vera. Hepatosplenomegaly, which can be massive, is present. Liver function tests show an increased plasma alkaline phosphatase activity in half of the patients and portal hypertension and esophageal varices can occur. Erythroblasts, normoblasts and megakaryocytes are found mainly in sinusoids, while granulocytes and their precursors are found mainly in the portal tracts.

## LYMPHOMAS

### Hodgkin's and non-Hodgkin's lymphomas

Primary lymphoma of the liver is extremely rare, reflecting the fact that lymphoreticular tissue other than Kupffer cells is not normally found in the liver (Zafrani & Gaulard 1993). Secondary lymphomas in the liver are common and are found at autopsy in about half of patients with Hodgkin's and non-Hodgkin's lymphoma (Kim et al 1976, Rozman et al 1991). The recognition of liver involvement in lymphoma is important in patient management, as it implies the need for systemic therapy. Unfortunately, noninvasive measures such as liver function tests, particularly the plasma alkaline phosphatase activity and imaging, are unreliable in detecting liver involvement and liver biopsies are needed for diagnosis. Targeted biopsies taken at laparoscopy are more reliable than percutaneous biopsies and wedge biopsies are more reliable than needle biopsies.

Lymphomatous infiltration of the liver begins in the portal tracts, which then become expanded with eventual invasion of the hepatic parenchyma. Widespread infiltration is the commonest pattern of invasion. Focal deposits can occur and may be single or few in number and sometimes of large size. All deposits may be widely distributed as uniform miliary nodules. The differentiation of lymphomatous infiltrates confined to portal tracts from other nonmalignant diseases can be difficult and depends on recognizing the uniform monomorphic features with atypical cellular characteristics of lymphomas or on recognizing Reed–Sternberg cells in Hodgkin's lymphoma. The diagnostic difficulties are made greater by the nonspecific portal tract infiltrates of lymphocytes, histiocytes and eosinophils that can occur in up to a third of patients with lymphomas and sometimes noncaseating granulomas can be seen in the portal tracts or in the parenchyma, especially in Hodgkin's disease. Focal parenchymal deposits are more easily recognized. The difficulty of diagnosing lymphomas from liver biopsy is such that diagnosis should be confirmed by examination of extrahepatic tissues.

### Malignant histiocytosis

This rare condition is characterized by fever, wasting, lymphadenopathy and hepatosplenomegaly associated with widespread infiltration of organs with malignant histiocytes. Rapid progression in the liver can give rise to clinical and biochemical features of fulminant hepatic failure (Colby & LaBrecque 1982). Intestinal malignancy in histiocytosis associated with jejunal ulceration and malabsorption has also been described (p. 467). The liver is enlarged and diffusely infiltrated with malignant histiocytes, which are often highly pleomorphic and which include giant cells. The infiltrates are found in the portal tracts and in the sinusoids and erythrophagocytosis may be found. Focal hepatocyte necrosis sometimes occurs in relation to infiltrating malignant cells.

### Differential diagnosis of lymphomas

Nonmalignant diseases associated with hepatic infiltrates of inflammatory cells in the portal tracts and hepatic sinusoids need to be kept in mind in the diagnosis of lymphomas. These diseases include infectious mononucleosis, cytomegalovirus infection, angioimmunoblastic lymphadenopathy (in which the typical angiomatous formations found elsewhere are not seen in the liver) and tropical splenomegaly syndrome.

## ENDOCRINE DISEASES

Of the diseases of the endocrine system, only diabetes mellitus and thyroid dysfunction have significant effects upon the liver, although hepatomegaly is a recognized feature of acromegaly. With effective treatments for thyroid disease and diabetes mellitus, changes in liver function are now seen less often and are less severe than in previous times.

### Diabetes mellitus

Clinical evidence of hepatic disease does not occur in established, well-controlled diabetes mellitus. Biochemical tests of liver function, however, are abnormal in about 20% of cases even when the disease is well controlled. These abnormalities are usually slight increases in serum alkaline phosphatase and $\gamma$-glutamyl transferase activities. More marked abnormalities can occur at presentation and in poorly controlled diabetes mellitus and include hepatomegaly and more marked increases of serum transaminase, alkaline phosphatase and $\gamma$-glutamyl transferase activities (Foster et al 1980). This occurs most often in obese adult insulin-independent diabetes mellitus but can also occur in insulin-dependent children (Marble et al 1938). The most common histological abnormality in the liver is fatty change or steatosis (Creutzfeldt et al 1970) but more severe lesions, such as pericentral hepatic fibrosis and intracellular hyalin (Falchuk et al 1980) and steatohepatitis (p. 975), also occur.

The relation of diabetes mellitus to cirrhosis is complex. Cirrhosis itself is associated with impaired glucose tolerance and overt diabetes mellitus (p. 921) and hemochromatosis causes both diseases independently (p. 955). Whether diabetes mellitus predisposes to later development of cirrhosis is controversial and it is difficult to disentangle the relative possible contributions of diabetes mellitus, obesity and alcohol abuse in much available data. The incidence of cirrhosis in various studies has ranged from 0% to 21% (Falchuk et al 1980). Diabetes mellitus is not generally regarded as predisposing to cirrhosis, but the occurrence of lesions such as steatohepatitis (p. 975) makes the development of cirrhosis possible. There may be an increased incidence of gallstones in diabetes mellitus, but this is controversial. The incidence of abnormalities of bile or gallbladder motility that may predispose to gallstones appears to be the same in diabetics as in the general population (Johnson 1991).

### Thyrotoxicosis

Hepatic damage in thyrotoxicosis was common prior to the advent of effective therapy and early autopsy studies reported hepatic inflammation, necrosis and cirrhosis (Sheridan 1983). Clinical signs of liver dysfunction are now uncommon, but nonspecific liver function test abnormalities occur in up to three-quarters of patients at diagnosis (Ashkar et al 1971, Fong et al 1992) and occasionally an increased serum alkaline phosphatase activity is the only clue to thyroid dysfunction (Shetty et al 1987). Jaundice occurs in a minority of patients and is usually mild and of unconjugated type, suggesting Gilbert's syndrome, but more severe jaundice can occur in severe thyrotoxicosis, including thyroid crisis, with superimposed infection and when cardiac failure develops. Rarely, marked jaundice with serum bilirubin as high as 350 μmol/L (20 mg/dl) occurs without any complicating factor (Yao et al 1989, Fong et al 1992).

### Hypothyroidism

Hypothyroidism in adults is not accompanied by clinical evidence of liver disease, although minor abnormalities of liver function tests that disappear on treatment do occur (Gaede 1977). Sensitive tests show that liver function abnormalities are more likely to result from treatment with thyroxine (Beckett et al 1985).

### Addison's disease

Persistent increase of plasma transaminase activity can occur in Addison's disease and resolves on treatment with corticosteroids (Boulton et al 1995). Transaminase abnormality can occur in asymptomatic patients prior to the onset of the features of Addison's disease as well as during the illness itself. Liver biopsy shows no or minor nonspecific abnormality.

## CONNECTIVE TISSUE DISEASES

The connective tissue diseases are characterized by inflammatory lesions in connective tissue anywhere in the body. They include systemic lupus erythematosus, rheumatoid arthritis, systemic sclerosis, Sjögren's syndrome, polyarteritis nodosa and related disorders, and intermediate forms (mixed connective tissue disease). Clinical evidence of hepatic involvement in these diseases is infrequent, but subclinical abnormalities such as abnormal liver function tests and nonspecific histological abnormalities are more common. Hepatic abnormalities may be due to involvement of the liver by the connective tissue disease itself, to associated drug therapy or to consequences of chronic debilitating disease such as amyloidosis.

Many of the connective tissue diseases are associated with autoimmune abnormalities and with a high frequency of the HLA-B8 tissue type; it is not surprising therefore that hepatic abnormalities in connective tissue diseases may also be caused by associated liver diseases such as primary biliary cirrhosis (p. 935) or autoimmune hepatitis (p. 893). Autoantibodies are often found in the blood in connective tissue diseases. Rheumatoid factor occurs frequently in almost all, antinuclear antibodies are virtually universal in systemic lupus erythematosus and common in rheumatoid arthritis but less common in the other disorders and particularly in systemic vasculitis, and antidouble-stranded DNA antibodies are virtually specific to systemic lupus erythematosus. Antismooth muscle antibodies and antimitochondrial antibodies occur in a few patients with rheumatoid arthritis or Sjögren's syndrome (Table 43.2) and may indicate associated autoimmune liver disease (Webb et al 1975). Chronic hepatitis B virus infection can be associated with polyarteritis nodosa.

Liver biopsy is not usually needed in the investigation of patients with connective tissue diseases and should be reserved for those with evidence of severe or active disease. Surgical biopsies are probably preferable for detecting vasculitis, as needle biopsies rarely show this focal lesion.

**Table 43.2** Pattern of clinical and laboratory findings (%) related to liver disease in patients with rheumatoid arthritis (RA)

| Finding | RA ($n$ = 216) (Webb et al 1975) | RA with abnormal liver* ($n$ = 31) (Mills et al 1980) |
|---|---|---|
| Hepatomegaly | 10.6 | 41.9 |
| Palpable spleen | 5.6 | 25.8 |
| Abnormal liver function tests | | |
| Bilirubin | 0 | 3.2 |
| Transaminase | 1.5 | 6.5 |
| Alkaline phosphatase | 18.1 | 64.5 |
| Autoantibodies | | |
| Rheumatoid factor | 76.4 | 96.8 |
| Antinuclear | 34.4 | 44.0 |
| Smooth muscle | 8.8 | 21.7 |
| Antimitochondrial | 3.2 | 33.3 |

*Hepatomegaly, palpable spleen or abnormal liver function tests on two or more occasions.

### Systemic lupus erythematosus (SLE)

There have been conflicting views on the nature and frequency of liver involvement in SLE and in particular, on the relationship between SLE and autoimmune hepatitis. These two conditions are generally regarded as quite separate entities and this view has been supported by several studies that have failed to find clinically significant liver disease in most patients with SLE.

Gibson & Myers (1981) reviewed 81 patients with SLE and found hepatomegaly in 19 (24%) and hepatosplenomegaly in three (3.7%) attributable to SLE. Forty-five (55%) patients had abnormal liver function tests attributable in 19 instances to SLE with up to fivefold elevations of serum transaminase and alkaline phosphatase activity; abnormalities were caused by drugs in 14 (usually aspirin), by cardiac failure in three and by nonhepatic causes in nine cases. Nonspecific histological changes were found in the liver in six of seven cases and interface hepatitis in one only.

Miller et al (1984) studied 260 patients with SLE prospectively and found clinical or biochemical evidence of liver disease in only 63 (24%). Clinical features of liver disease were found in only five patients (2%) and were restricted to hepatomegaly and jaundice; they were attributable to alcohol abuse or malignant disease in three patients and to SLE in only two, in whom they disappeared following corticosteroid therapy. Palmar erythema and leukonychia were encountered, but they occur in SLE per se. Increased serum transaminase and alkaline phosphatase activities were found in 60 patients (23%); two-thirds were attributable to an identifiable cause, including salicylate toxicity in 27 of 60 (45%), alcohol abuse in six of 60 (10%) and hepatitis B virus infection in two of 60 (3%), and one-third were attributed to SLE. Sequential biochemical tests showed that abnormalities attributed to SLE fluctuated in relation to the activity of the disease and liver biopsy in 14 such patients did not show any serious lesion. Hypoalbuminemia and hyperglobulinemia occur in SLE per se and do not in themselves imply liver involvement. SLE is usually therefore a cause of mild subclinical liver damage in which serum transaminase, especially alanine aminotransferase, and alkaline phosphatase activities increase up to about fivefold.

The view that SLE causes only minor liver disease and

is a wholly separate entity from autoimmune chronic active hepatitis has been challenged. Runyon et al (1980) found that 43 of 238 patients (18%) had liver disease evidenced by jaundice (24%), hepatomegaly (39%) and splenomegaly (6%). Liver tissue was available in 33 patients and severe lesions included cirrhosis (4), interface hepatitis (4), granulomatous hepatitis (3) and primary biliary cirrhosis (1). Alternative causes for the liver disease usually could not be found, many patients responded to corticosteroid therapy and three died of progressive liver failure. The authors raise the question whether such patients represent coincident SLE and liver disease, SLE with liver involvement or autoimmune hepatitis with systemic features (p. 891) and point to the fact that such occasional cases show that these two diseases cannot always be readily separated. Indeed, antibody to double-stranded DNA, thought to be specific for SLE, may occur in autoimmune chronic active hepatitis (p. 768). Individual case reports have described granulomatous hepatitis with increased serum alkaline phosphatase activity during exacerbations of SLE responding to treatment with prednisolone and cyclophosphamide (Feurle et al 1982), spontaneous rupture of the liver (Levitin et al 1977) and a possible association of SLE and primary biliary cirrhosis (Iliffe et al 1982). Serious liver disease can therefore occur in SLE but is uncommon.

### **Rheumatoid arthritis** (RA)

Clinical evidence of chronic liver disease in RA is rare, but abnormal liver function tests are more common. Webb et al (1975) studied 216 patients, three-quarters of whom were seropositive, and found hepatomegaly in 10% and a palpable spleen in 5%. Abnormal liver function tests occurred in about a fifth of patients and the most common abnormality was a raised serum alkaline phosphatase in 18% of patients.

Mills et al (1980) have reported the liver biopsy findings in 31 patients with RA who had hepatomegaly, a palpable spleen or abnormal liver function tests on at least two occasions. Most patients (23/31, 74%) had nonspecific abnormalities in the liver, the appearances were normal in a few (4/31, 13%) and individual patients had primary biliary cirrhosis autoimmune hepatitis, alcoholic cirrhosis, and amyloidosis. Autoantibodies occur more often in patients with clinical or biochemical evidence of liver disease (Table 43.2), which may account for the occasional coincidence of "autoimmune" chronic liver diseases (Ellman et al 1974, Mills et al 1980). Rupture of the liver can occur in RA and is probably a consequence of arteritis causing thrombosis, aneurysm formation and vessel rupture (Hocking et al 1981).

***Felty's syndrome.*** Felty's syndrome comprises severe seropositive RA, splenomegaly, and hypersplenism. Blendis et al (1970) described abnormal liver function tests and histological abnormalities in the liver, including lymphocytic infiltration of the sinusoids and portal tracts, portal tract fibrosis, cirrhosis and nodules in the absence of cirrhosis. Thorne et al (1982) subsequently studied 18 patients prospectively and showed that hepatic abnormalities occur frequently; 12 of the patients had histological abnormalities, including five with portal fibrosis, two with lobular abnormalities in the form of double hepatocyte cell plates, and five with nodular regenerative hyperplasia (p. 1129), seven had abnormal liver function tests and four had portal hypertension with bleeding from varices in three.

***Still's disease.*** Acute hepatic dysfunction in Still's disease (juvenile RA) is probably caused mainly by coincident viral infection or by drug therapy (Kornreich et al 1971). Occasional patients develop marked hepatomegaly, fever and systemic features such as skin rash, lymphadenopathy and pleurisy or pericarditis. Liver biopsy in these patients has shown nonspecific periportal infiltration of inflammatory cells and Kupffer cell hyperplasia. The syndrome remits with regression of the underlying juvenile RA (Schaller et al 1970).

### **Sjögren's syndrome**

Patients with Sjögren's syndrome or sicca syndrome have hepatomegaly and/or splenomegaly in about 10% of cases and abnormal liver function tests, almost always with increased plasma alkaline phosphatase activity with or without increased transaminase activity, in a quarter of cases (Webb et al 1975). Liver biopsy usually shows nonspecific changes. Conversely, mild or subclinical features of sicca syndrome are common in patients with autoimmune hepatitis (p. 891), primary biliary cirrhosis (p. 937) and cryptogenic cirrhosis (p. 921).

### **Systemic sclerosis**

Liver disease is uncommon in systemic sclerosis. Bartholomew et al (1964) reviewed 727 patients with systemic sclerosis and found chronic liver disease in only eight (1.1%). The nature of the liver disease in these patients is unknown, but the histological appearances in five were those of an aggressive hepatitis and bile duct lesions and high plasma alkaline phosphatase activity in two strongly suggest primary biliary cirrhosis. More recent case reports have strengthened the association with primary biliary cirrhosis, particularly in the case of the CREST syndrome (p. 937).

***Eosinophilic fasciitis.*** This condition resembles systemic sclerosis and is characterized by fasciitis, myositis, eosinophilia and hypergammaglobulinemia. Liver involvement with focal hepatitis histologically has been reported in a single case (Chan & Lages 1982).

## Dermatomyositis and polymyositis

Hepatomegaly and abnormal liver function tests occur occasionally in primary dermatomyositis (Bitnum et al 1964). Dermatomyositis is associated with carcinomas, usually of the bronchus, breast, stomach or ovary, in about 10% of adult patients (Bohan et al 1977) and liver involvement in such patients is most often due to secondary tumor. Polymyositis has been seen in association with primary biliary cirrhosis (Willson 1981).

## Mixed connective tissue disease

This syndrome shows overlapping features of systemic sclerosis, systemic lupus erythematosus and polymyositis. High titers of antibody to nuclear ribonucleoprotein are found in almost all cases, although the antibody does occur in other connective tissue diseases. Associated autoimmune hepatitis and primary biliary cirrhosis have been reported in individual patients (James et al 1981, Marshall et al 1983).

## Primary systemic vasculitis

The primary systemic vasculitides are a complex group of syndromes with overlapping clinical features that make them difficult to classify (Table 43.3). There are few specific diagnostic tests and consequently diagnoses usually rest on the recognition of patterns of multisystem involvement in patients with general features of systemic disease such as fever, weight loss, anemia, leukocytosis and a high erythrocyte sedimentation rate (each of which occurs in about three-quarters of cases), sometimes eosinophilia and the finding of aneurysms on angiography or vasculitis on biopsy of affected tissue. The presence of a positive antineutrophil cytoplasmic antibody (c-ANCA) (p. 767) can be diagnostic.

***Polyarteritis nodosa.*** Hepatic involvement is common in both the classical form of polyarteritis nodosa affecting medium-sized vessels and the microscopic form affecting small blood vessels (Travers 1979, Scott et al 1982, Camilleri et al 1983, Savage et al 1985). Hepatitis B and hepatitis C virus infection can cause the syndrome of polyarteritis without other clinical features of viral hepatitis and they should be sought serologically in all cases (p. 799). Hepatomegaly occurs in a third to a half of patients, but splenomegaly is rare. Abnormal liver function tests are found in a half or more and these abnormalities usually take the form of increased plasma transaminase and/or alkaline phosphatase activity, reaching a maximum of about five times the upper normal value. Needle biopsies of the liver usually show nonspecific abnormalities but can be normal even when liver function tests are abnormal (Travers 1979); they rarely show vasculitis, perhaps because the focal nature of this lesion predisposes to sampling error, which may be avoided by a surgical biopsy (Ogilvie et al 1981). Visceral angiography should precede liver biopsy, as the finding of multiple aneurysms can establish the diagnosis and avoid the danger of needle puncture of an intrahepatic aneurysm. Vasculitis can lead to arterial occlusion or rupture and bleeding consequent on aneurysm formation and these can cause acute hepatic infarction (Kanter 1965) or hepatic rupture (Li et al 1979).

**Table 43.3** Classification of primary systemic vasculitis (Savage et al 1985)

| Vessels | Granulomas: Present | Granulomas: Absent |
|---|---|---|
| Large | Giant cell arteritis | Takayasu's disease |
| Medium | Churg–Strauss syndrome* | Polyarteritis nodosa |
| Small | Wegener's granulomatosis | Microscopic polyarteritis<br>Henoch–Schönlein purpura<br>Hypersensitivity vasculitis |

*Eosinophilic granulomatosis.

***Churg–Strauss syndrome.*** This rare condition is characterized by severe asthma, fever and eosinophilia with necrotizing granulomas and eosinophils in affected tissue. Coincident primary biliary cirrhosis has been reported in a patient with this syndrome (Conn et al 1982).

***Wegener's granulomatosis.*** Wegener's granulomatosis is a form of systemic granulomatous vasculitis in which the upper and lower respiratory tract and the kidneys are particularly affected. Hepatic involvement manifests itself as hepatomegaly in about a half of patients and by increased plasma alkaline phosphatase activity to 2–4 times the normal upper limit in three-quarters or more. Small increases of serum transaminase activity occur in a minority. Needle biopsies of the liver may be normal or show nonspecific changes (Pinching et al 1983).

***Giant cell (cranial or temporal) arteritis/polymyalgia rheumatica.*** Cranial arteritis and polymyalgia rheumatica occur particularly in elderly women and are associated with granulomatous vasculitis in larger arteries (Long & James 1974, Ogilvie et al 1981). They probably represent aspects of the same disease and the name "polymyalgia arteritica" has been suggested. Liver involvement can cause hepatomegaly and liver function tests usually show a considerable increase of plasma alkaline phosphatase activity with or without minor increases of transaminase activity. Autoantibodies are not usually found in the blood. Autopsy examination has shown arteritis in the hepatic arteries and this can be revealed by larger wedge biopsies of the liver (Ogilvie et al 1981). Needle liver biopsies may be normal or show nonspecific changes and can occasionally reveal granulomas (Long & James 1974).

## HYPERPYREXIA

### Heat stroke

Hyperpyrexia can cause serious damage to many organs including the liver (Simon 1993). Prostration with cerebral symptoms and a temperature above 40°C is the most common presentation, but liver function abnormalities may be prominent with elevation of the serum aminotransferase and alkaline phosphatase activities. Jaundice is relatively rare, normally occurring on about the third day of the illness and reaching a peak within the first week. In one large series of 244 patients, only 10 had jaundice and a further 17 had evidence of hepatic abnormalities (Herman & Sullivan 1959). Kew et al (1970) studied the hepatic effects of heat stroke in 34 Bantu gold miners in South Africa who had rectal temperatures of 40.6–44.2°C. All were confused or comatosed and 14 (41%) were hypotensive (systolic pressure below 100 mmHg). All had increased serum aminotransferase activity of liver origin and in 12 (35%) this was increased more than 10-fold. Half had prolongation of the prothrombin time, but only six had increased alkaline phosphatase activity. Six had hyperbilirubinemia; three of these were jaundiced and two died in hepatorenal failure. Full recovery of the liver occurred in those who survived. Liver biopsies showed relatively mild changes with centrilobular hepatocellular degeneration. Marked necrosis was noted in those who came to autopsy.

### Malignant hyperpyrexia

This is an anesthetic complication related to suxamethonium sensitivity and is considered similar in some respects to heat stroke. Abnormalities of liver function are unusual (Simon 1993).

## MISCELLANEOUS CONDITIONS

### Skin disease

In patients with extensive skin loss due to exfoliative dermatitis, erythroderma or burns, abnormal liver function may be caused by the same mechanisms as operate in the shock liver. Abnormal liver function tests have been reported in patients with psoriasis. These are usually mild. Where liver biopsy has been done, the most common finding has been fatty change and focal necrosis and periportal inflammation and fibrosis have also been reported. Hepatic abnormalities in psoriasis have been related to alcohol abuse rather than to the psoriasis (Poikolainen et al 1990). Systemic sclerosis and lichen planus have also been associated with primary biliary cirrhosis.

### Systemic infection

Systemic bacterial infections not involving the liver directly can cause hepatic dysfunction. Hyperbilirubinemia is usually the most prominent abnormality and jaundice was recognized as a bad prognostic sign in infected patients prior to the advent of antibiotics. Hepatic damage is not severe, however, and does not constitute a threat to the patient; it is more important that hepatic dysfunction may distract attention from serious disease elsewhere (BMJ 1984).

Jaundice due to systemic infection is seen most frequently in infants and young children and it may be severe. It occurs particularly in *Escherichia coli* urinary tract infections and usually within the first 3 months of life (Hamilton & Sass-Kortsak 1963). Jaundice generally appears suddenly and may be the first evidence of a severe infection. The hyperbilirubinemia is usually of the conjugated type (p. 739), the total serum bilirubin may reach 500 μmol/L (30 mg/dl) and other tests of liver function show little or no abnormality. Cholestasis is the main histological finding in the liver.

Hepatic dysfunction can also develop in adults with severe bacterial infections. Hyperbilirubinemia is usually the most prominent abnormality and concentrations of 100–200 μmol/L (6–12 mg/dl) may be reached. Gourley et al (1981) reported abnormal liver function tests in all of 22 women with the toxic shock syndrome. Miller et al (1976) have shown that infections anywhere with a wide variety of Gram-positive and Gram-negative organisms can cause jaundice and they emphasized that conjugated hyperbilirubinemia was the dominant abnormality (Fig. 43.3). Adults with infections severe enough to cause jaundice are generally very ill and most have marked pyrexia, often with rigors, markedly increased leukocyte counts and erythrocyte sedimentation rates, normochro-

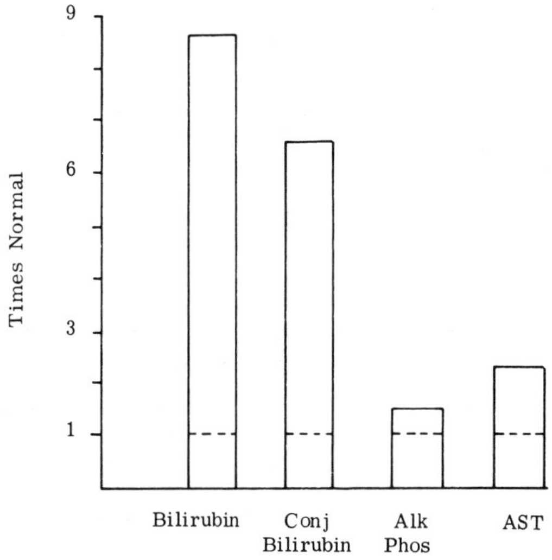


**Fig. 43.3** Mean values for liver function tests in patients with jaundice due to severe bacterial infection. The upper normal limit is shown as a broken line (Miller et al 1976).

mic anemia, hypoalbuminemia and hyperglobulinemia. Increased serum alkaline phosphatase activity may also occur. This usually does not exceed 2–3 times the normal maximal activity, but occasionally activities up to 10 times normal may be found in the absence of jaundice and these remit on successful treatment of the infection (Fang et al 1980). Transaminase activities are generally normal or only a little elevated.

Hepatic dysfunction in infection has been ascribed principally to impaired bilirubin transport by the liver and to cholestasis (Fahrländer et al 1964, Miller et al 1976). Gourley et al (1981) found increased serum bile acid concentrations that would be in keeping with cholestasis and cholestasis is the most common pathological finding, although it is not present invariably. Factors possibly important in producing hepatic dysfunction include fever (above), hypotension (p. 1099) and the effect of bacterial toxins, of which endotoxin is the best recognized (Utili et al 1977). Anorexia and nutritional deficiency may be minor additional factors, but direct bacterial invasion of the liver is not important. Hemolysis is usually also a minor factor except in patients predisposed to hemolysis, as in the case of glucose-6-phosphate dehydrogenase deficiency (Tugwell & Williams 1977).

### Nephrogenic hepatic dysfunction syndrome

This syndrome is a condition in which abnormal biochemical tests of liver function that are not due to secondary deposits occur in association with renal carcinoma (Strickland & Schenker 1977). The incidence is unknown. Patients with this syndrome frequently have hepatomegaly, fever, weight loss and anemia. The serum alkaline phosphatase activity is usually raised and the prothrombin time prolonged, but the serum bilirubin concentration and the transaminase activity are usually normal. Thrombocytosis has been found in two-thirds of patients. Occasional patients with cholestatic jaundice have been reported (Jakobovits et al 1981). Liver biopsy shows nonspecific abnormalities including fatty change and focal hepatocyte necrosis with lymphocytic infiltration. There may be nothing to suggest the presence of renal carcinoma, which is revealed only by investigation. The syndrome is not associated with any particular type of renal carcinoma. The cause of the syndrome is unknown. Patients with renal carcinoma and abnormal liver function tests should not be assumed to have hepatic metastases, as removal of the primary tumor leads to the complete resolution of nephrogenic hepatic dysfunction syndrome.

### Spontaneous rupture of the liver

Spontaneous rupture of the liver is rare and is usually associated with underlying liver disease (BMJ 1976). A vascular primary tumor, usually a hepatocellular carcinoma (p. 1119) but occasionally a benign tumor (p. 1128), is the most common underlying cause. Venous obstruction probably causes hemorrhage into the tumor and the resulting hematoma eventually bursts through the liver capsule and bleeding into the peritoneal cavity occurs. Secondary liver tumors virtually never cause hepatic rupture. Spontaneous hepatic rupture occasionally occurs in patients with collagen diseases, possibly as a consequence of hepatic arteritis leading to thrombosis, hepatic infarction and hematoma formation. Such ruptures have been reported in systemic lupus erythematosus (Levitin et al 1977), polyarteritis nodosa (Li et al 1979) and rheumatoid arthritis (Hocking et al 1981). Late or delayed rupture of a hepatic hematoma into the peritoneum can occur following blunt abdominal trauma (Greis et al 1981). Patients usually present with severe upper abdominal pain of sudden onset sometimes radiating to the shoulder and frequently associated with shock. Abdominal examination reveals tenderness, rebound pain and guarding and an upper abdominal mass can be felt in two-thirds of patients. Imaging can show free fluid in the peritoneal cavity and paracentesis can confirm bleeding by yielding blood. Treatment consists of resuscitation by blood transfusion followed by hepatic resection or hepatic artery ligation.

Spontaneous rupture of a normal liver is exceedingly rare; it usually occurs during the third trimester of pregnancy or soon after delivery and over 80% of cases are associated with vomiting, hypertension or pre-eclampsia (Manas et al 1985). The abrupt onset of severe constant right upper quadrant and epigastric pain with abdominal tenderness and guarding, particularly in a patient with pre-eclampsia, are the cardinal features. Tachycardia, hypotension and a falling hemoglobin or hematocrit point to bleeding. Thrombocytopenia may be present and there may be an increase of fibrin split products in the blood, but other tests of blood coagulation are usually normal. Liver function tests are usually abnormal but do not help in diagnosis. Imaging, particularly by computed tomography with shielding of the abdomen below the liver, is valuable in showing intrahepatic and subcapsular hepatic hematomas and the presence or absence of free intra-abdominal fluid. Resuscitation followed by operation to control the hepatic bleeding by suture, packing or sometimes ligation of the hepatic artery and deliver the fetus by cesarean section has usually been advocated. However, it is now recognized that hepatic hemorrhage is not always associated with rupture and those who remain hemodynamically stable after resuscitation can be treated conservatively and go on to a vaginal delivery. Two-thirds to three-quarters of patients with hepatic rupture die and in these cases only fetuses delivered by cesarean section survive.

### Radiation hepatitis

Liver damage from irradiation was reported first over

70 years ago (Case & Warthin 1924), but subsequent animal experiments led to the view that the liver was relatively resistant to radiation. However, it is now well recognized that radiotherapy can cause liver damage. Wharton et al (1973) found that 14 of 65 (22%) patients receiving whole abdominal radiotherapy (25–30 Gy) for ovarian carcinoma subsequently developed radiation hepatitis and more recently it has been suggested that a combination of radiotherapy and chemotherapy may cause particularly severe and even fatal liver damage (Hansen et al 1982). Radiation hepatitis often occurs in patients who have received over 20 Gy and particularly over 30 Gy in the region of the liver.

Clinical evidence of liver damage does not occur during radiotherapy, but around 2–8 weeks afterwards the patient becomes unwell, with abdominal distention and sometimes abdominal pain, which can be severe. Examination shows ascites and often pleural effusion, the liver is enlarged and tender and mild jaundice and peripheral edema may be present. Liver function tests show mild to moderate abnormalities with particularly an increased serum alkaline phosphatase activity and radionuclide liver imaging usually shows a focal defect in the most damaged area. The liver has been reported as swollen and dusky at laparotomy and liver biopsy shows central vein damage with intimal thickening, occasionally thrombosis and later fibrous obliteration, marked centrilobular congestion and atrophy of the centrilobular hepatocytes. Veno-occlusion of the central veins has been suggested as the primary lesion (Fajardo & Colby 1980) and the term "radiation hepatitis" can be justified only by usage, as inflammation is conspicuous only by its absence histologically. The most important differential diagnoses are recurrence or progression of any underlying neoplastic disease or drug hepatotoxicity.

Spontaneous recovery occurs in most patients, but a few die after a short illness and others may gradually develop liver failure (Lansing et al 1968). Some patients maintain good liver function but develop portal hypertension over a period of years and eventually bleed from esophageal varices. This usually occurs in patients with diseases, such as Wilms' tumor, that have a relatively good prognosis after therapy. Portal hypertension in these cases is a consequence of hepatic vascular damage, usually to the central veins but also possibly to the small portal venous radicals (hepatoportal sclerosis) (p. 1085) and both chemotherapy (p. 852) and radiotherapy probably contribute to the damage (Barnard et al 1986).

## THE LIVER IN OLD AGE

The structure and function of the normal liver changes only gradually in adult life, but by the time an individual has passed their 70th year some appreciable changes have occurred (Mooney et al 1985). The most striking is the reduction in the size of the liver, both absolutely and relative to the rest of the body. The liver constitutes about 4% of the body at birth and about 2% in old age and by the age of 90 years liver volume has fallen from 1475 ml to about 930 ml (Wynne et al 1989). This reduction in size results from a reduction in the number of hepatic parenchymal cells, although individual hepatocytes tend to be larger than in younger people. The cells have more cytoplasm and consequently the nuclei are relatively small and in addition are more often binucleate. Histological changes are slight and include portal tracts containing rather more inflammatory cells than in younger people, some bile ductular proliferation around the peripheries of the portal tracts, occasional foci of necrotic apoptotic hepatocytes and an increased amount of lipofuscin in the cells. Another important change in old age is a reduction in hepatic blood flow of about 35% by the 10th decade of life with a fall in liver perfusion of about 11% (Wynne et al 1989). One factor in this may be the reduction in cardiac output that occurs in old age.

Investigations of liver function in the elderly have given very variable results and reductions in function are in part related to factors such as diet, nutrition, sex and smoking (Vestal 1989). There does, however, seem to be a reduction in oxidative capacity with age, but not of conjugation. Whether this is related to a reported increase in drug hepatotoxicity in the elderly is not known (Nolan & O'Malley 1988a,b). Plasma concentrations of bilirubin and albumin and activities of transaminases and $\gamma$-glutamyl transferase, all of which may be used as tests of liver function, give values very similar to those in younger people. However, alkaline phosphatase activity rises in old age, probably as a consequence of raised bone isoenzyme.

## REFERENCES

Ashkar F S, Miller R, Smoak W M III, Gilson A J 1971 Liver disease in hyperthyroidism. Southern Medical Journal 64: 462–465

Barnard J A, Marshall G S, Neblett W W, Gray G, Ghishan F K 1986 Noncirrhotic portal fibrosis after Wilms' tumor therapy. Gastroenterology 90: 1054–1056

Bartholomew L G, Cain J, Winkelman R K, Baggenstoss A H 1964 Chronic disease of the liver associated with systemic scleroderma. American Journal of Digestive Diseases 9: 43–55

Bauer T W, Moore G W, Hutchins G M 1980 The liver in sickle cell disease: a clinicopathologic study of 70 patients. American Journal of Medicine 69: 833–837

Beckett G J, Kellett H A, Gow S M, Hussey A J, Hayes J D, Toft A D 1985 Raised plasma glutathione S-transferase values in hyperthyroidism and in hypothyroid patients receiving thyroxine replacement: evidence of hepatic damage. British Medical Journal 291: 427–431

Bitnum S, Daeschner C W Jr, Travis L B, Dodge W F, Hopps H C 1964 Dermatomyositis. Journal of Pediatrics 64: 101–131

Blendis L M, Ansell I D, Lloyd-Jones K, Hamilton E, Williams R 1970 Liver in Felty's syndrome. British Medical Journal 1: 131–135
BMJ 1976 Leading article: spontaneous rupture of the liver. British Medical Journal 2: 1278–1279
BMJ 1984 Leading article: Sepsis and cholestasis. British Medical Journal 289: 857
Bohan A, Peter J B, Bowman R L, Pearson C M 1977 A computer-assisted analysis of 153 patients with polymyositis and dermatomyositis. Medicine 56: 255–286
Boulton R, Hamilton M I, Dhillon A P, Kinloch J D, Burroughs A K 1995 Subclinical Addison's disease: a cause of persistent abnormalities in transaminase values. Gastroenterology 109: 1324–1327
Broomé U, Glaumann H, Hellers G, Nilsson B, Sörstad J, Hultcrantz R 1994 Liver disease in ulcerative colitis: an epidemiological and follow up study in the county of Stockholm. Gut 35: 84–89
Buchwald H, Lober P H, Varco R L 1974 Liver biopsy findings in seventy-seven consecutive patients undergoing jejunoileal bypass for morbid obesity. American Journal of Surgery 127: 48–52
Camilleri M, Pusey C D, Chadwick V S, Rees A J 1983 Gastrointestinal manifestations of systemic vasculitis. Quarterly Journal of Medicine 52: 141–149
Case J T, Warthin A S 1924 The occurrence of hepatic lesions in patients treated by intensive deep roentgen irradiation. American Journal of Roentgenology 12: 27–46
Cello J P, Baumgartel E D, Filly R A et al 1977 Cholestasis in ulcerative colitis. Gastroenterology 73: 357–374
Chan M K L, Lages W 1982 Eosinophilic fasciitis. Visceral involvement. Archives of Internal Medicine 142: 2201–2202
Cohen J A, Kaplan M M 1978 Left-sided heart failure presenting as hepatitis. Gastroenterology 74: 583–587
Cohen S, Kaplan M, Gottlieb L, Patterson J 1971 Liver disease and gallstones in regional enteritis. Gastroenterology 60: 237–245
Colby T V, LaBrecque D R 1982 Lymphoreticular malignancy presenting as fulminant hepatic disease. Gastroenterology 82: 339–345
Conn D L, Dickson E R, Carpenter H A 1982 The association of Churg–Strauss vasculitis with temporal artery involvement, primary biliary cirrhosis and polychondritis in a single patient. Journal of Rheumatology 9: 744–748
Cowan R E, Thompson R P H, Kaye J P, Hall R J C 1981 Plasma bilirubin and serum free fatty acids after myocardial infarction. Postgraduate Medical Journal 57: 9–12
Creutzfeldt W, Frerichs H, Sickinger K 1970 Liver diseases and diabetes mellitus. In: Popper H, Schaffner F (eds) Progress in liver diseases, Vol 3. Grune and Stratton, New York, p 371–407
Dahn M S, Lange M P, Jacobs L A 1988 Central mixed and splanchnic venous oxygen saturation monitoring. Intensive Care Medicine 14: 373–378
Das G, Nussbaum H E, Leff W A 1974 Hepatic function in acute myocardial infarction. Journal of the American Medical Association 230: 1558–1560
Desmet V J, Geboes K 1987 Liver lesions in inflammatory bowel disorders. Journal of Pathology 151: 247–255
Dunn G D, Hayes P, Breen K J, Schenker S 1973 The liver in congestive heart failure: a review. American Journal of the Medical Sciences 265: 174–189
Ellenberg M, Osserman K W 1951 Roll of shock in production of central liver cell necrosis. American Journal of Medicine 11: 170–178
Ellman H H, Weis M J, Spellberg M A 1974 Liver disease in rheumatoid arthritis. American Journal of Gastroenterology 62: 46–53
El-Shaboury A H, Thomas A J, Williams D A 1964 Serum transaminase activity in status asthmaticus. British Medical Journal 1: 1220 –1223
Fahrländer H, Huber F, Gloor F 1964 Intrahepatic retention of bile in severe bacterial infections. Gastroenterology 47: 590–599
Fajardo L F, Colby T V 1980 Pathogenesis of veno-occlusive liver disease after radiation. Archives of Pathology and Laboratory Medicine 104: 584–588
Falchuk K R, Fiske S C, Haggitt R C, Federman M, Trey C 1980 Pericentral hepatic fibrosis and intracellular hyalin in diabetes mellitus. Gastroenterology 78: 535–541
Fang M H, Ginsberg A L, Dobbins W O III 1980 Marked elevation in serum alkaline phosphatase activity as a manifestation of systemic infection. Gastroenterology 78: 592–597
Feeley J, Wade D, McAllister C B, Wilkinson G R, Robertson D 1982 Effect of hypotension on liver blood flow and lidocaine disposition. New England Journal of Medicine 307: 866–872
Feurle G E, Bröker H-J, Tschahargane C 1982 Granulomatous hepatitis in systemic lupus erythematosus. Report of a case. Endoscopy 14: 153–154
Fong T L, McHutcheson J G, Reynolds T B 1992 Hyperthyroidism and hepatic dysfunction. A case series analysis. Journal of Clinical Gastroenterology 14: 240–244
Foster K J, Griffith A H, Dewbury K, Price C P, Wright R 1980 Liver disease in patients with diabetes mellitus. Postgraduate Medical Journal 56: 767–772
Fry D E, Pearlstein L, Fulton R L, Polk H C 1980 Multiple system organ failure. Archives of Surgery 115: 136–140
Gaede J T 1977 Serum enzyme alterations in hypothyroidism before and after treatment. Journal of the American Geriatric Society 25: 199–201
Gibson P R, Dudley F J 1984 Ischaemic hepatitis: clinical features, diagnosis and prognosis. Australian and New Zealand Journal of Medicine 14: 822–825
Gibson T, Myers A R 1981 Subclinical liver disease in systemic lupus erythematosus. Journal of Rheumatology 8: 752–759
Gourley G R, Chesney P J, Davis J P, Odell G B 1981 Acute cholestasis in patients with toxic-shock syndrome. Gastroenterology 81: 928–931
Greis W P, Schulz K A, Giacchino J L, Freeark R J 1981 The fate of unruptured intrahepatic hematomas. Surgery 90: 689–697
Hägander B, Berg N O, Brandt L, Nordén Å, Sjölund K, Stenstam M 1977 Hepatic injury in adult coeliac disease. Lancet 2: 270–272
Hamilton D L, Vest T K, Brown B S, Shah A N, Menguy R B, Chey W Y 1983 Liver injury with alcoholic like hyalin after gastroplasty for morbid obesity. Gastroenterology 85: 722–726
Hamilton J R, Sass-Kortsak A 1963 Jaundice associated with severe bacterial infection in young infants. Journal of Pediatrics 63: 121–132
Hansen M M, Ranek L, Walbom S, Nissen N I 1982 Fatal hepatitis following irradiation and vincristine. Acta Medica Scandinavica 212: 171
Hatton C S R, Bunch C, Weatherall D J 1985 Hepatic sequestration in sickle cell anaemia. British Medical Journal 290: 744–745
Haubrich W S, Watson J H L, Sieracki J C 1960 Unique morphologic features of Whipple's disease. A study by light and electron microscopy. Gastroenterology 39: 454–468
Herman R H, Sullivan B H Jr 1959 Heatstroke and jaundice. American Journal of Medicine 27: 154–166
Hillmen P, Lewis S M, Bessler M, Luzzatto L, Dacie J V 1995 Natural history of paroxysmal nocturnal hemoglobinuria. New England Journal of Medicine 333: 1253–1258
Hocking W G, Lasser K, Ungerer R, Bersohn M, Palos M, Spiegel T 1981 Spontaneous hepatic rupture in rheumatoid arthritis. Archives of Internal Medicine 41: 792–794
Iliffe G D, Naidoo S, Hunter T 1982 Primary biliary cirrhosis associated with features of systemic lupus erythematosus. Digestive Diseases and Sciences 27: 274–278
Jakobovits A W, Crimmins F B, Sherlock S, Erlinger S, Rambaud J 1981 Cholestasis as a paraneoplastic manifestation of carcinoma of the kidney. Australian and New Zealand Journal of Medicine 11: 64–67
James O, Macklon A F, Watson A J 1981 Primary biliary cirrhosis – a revised clinical spectrum. Lancet 1: 1278–1281
Johnson C S, Omata M, Tong M J, Simmons J F Jr, Weiner J, Tatter D 1985 Liver involvement in sickle cell disease. Medicine 64: 349–356
Johnson P J 1991 The effect of endocrine diseases on liver function. In: McIntyre N, Benhamou J-P, Bircher J, Rizzetto M, Rodès J (eds) Oxford textbook of clinical hepatology. Oxford University Press, Oxford, p 1194–1196
Kanter D M 1965 Hepatic infarction. Archives of Internal Medicine 115: 479–481
Kantrowitz P A, Jones W A, Greenberger N J, Isselbacher K J 1967 Severe postoperative hyperbilirubinemia simulating obstructive jaundice. New England Journal of Medicine 276: 591–598
Kew M, Bersohn I, Seftel H, Kent G 1970 Liver damage in heatstroke. American Journal of Medicine 49: 192–202
Kim H, Dorfman R F, Rosenberg S A 1976 Pathology of malignant lymphomas in the liver: application in staging. In: Popper H, Schaffner F (eds) Progress in liver diseases, Vol 5. Grune and Stratton, New York, p 683–698

Kirby B D, Snyder K M, Moyer R D, Finegold S M 1978 Legionnaires' disease: clinical features of 24 cases. Annals of Internal Medicine 89: 297–309
Kornreich H, Malouf N N, Hanson V 1971 Acute hepatic dysfunction in juvenile rheumatoid arthritis. Journal of Pediatrics 79: 27–35
Lansing A M, Davis W M, Brizel H E 1968 Radiation hepatitis. Archives of Surgery 96: 878–882
Levine R A, Klatskin G 1964 Unconjugated hyperbilirubinemia in the absence of overt hemolysis (importance of acquired disease as an etiological factor in 366 adolescent and adult subjects). American Journal of Medicine 36: 541–552
Levitin P M, Sweet D, Brunner C M, Katholi R E, Bolton W K 1977 Spontaneous rupture of the liver: an unusual complication of SLE. Arthritis and Rheumatism 20: 748–750
Li A K C, Rhodes J M, Valentine A R 1979 Spontaneous liver rupture in polyarteritis nodosa. British Journal of Surgery 66: 251–252
Logan R F A, Ferguson A, Finlayson N D C, Weir D G 1978 Primary biliary cirrhosis and coeliac disease. An association? Lancet 1: 230–233
Long R, James O 1974 Polymyalgia rheumatica and liver disease. Lancet 1: 77–79
Manas K J, Welsh J D, Rankin R A, Miller D D 1985 Hepatic hemorrhage without rupture in preeclampsia. New England Journal of Medicine 312: 424–426
Manga P, Vythilingum S, Mitha A S 1984 Pulsatile hepatomegaly in constrictive pericarditis. British Heart Journal 52: 465–467
Marble A, White P, Bogan I K, Smith R M 1938 Enlargement of the liver in diabetic children. I. Its incidence, etiology and nature. Archives of Internal Medicine 62: 740–750
Marshall J B, Ravendhran N, Sharp G C 1983 Liver disease in mixed connective tissue disease. Archives of Internal Medicine 143: 181–188
Mathurin P, Durand F, Ganne N et al 1995 Ischemic hepatitis due to obstructive sleep apnea. Gastroenterology 109: 1682–1684
Middleton J P, Wolper J C 1984 Hepatic biloma complicating sickle cell disease. A case report and a review of the literature. Gastroenterology 86: 743–744
Miller D J, Keeton G R, Webber B L, Saunders S J 1976 Jaundice in severe bacterial infection. Gastroenterology 71: 94–97
Miller M H, Urowitz M B, Gladman D D, Blendis L M 1984 The liver in systemic lupus erythematosis. Quarterly Journal of Medicine 53: 401–409
Mills P R, MacSween R N M, Dick W C, More I A, Watkinson C 1980 Liver disease in rheumatoid arthritis. Scottish Medical Journal 25: 18–22
Miralles G D, O'Fallon J R, Talley N J 1992 Plasma-cell dyscrasia with polyneuropathy. The spectrum of POEMS syndrome. New England Journal of Medicine 327: 1919–1923
Mir-Madjlessi S H, Farmer R G, Sivak M V 1987 Bile duct carcinoma in patients with ulcerative colitis. Relationship to sclerosing cholangitis: report of six cases and review of the literature. Digestive Diseases and Sciences 32: 145–154
Mooney H, Roberts R, Cooksley W G E, Halliday J W, Powell L W 1985 Alterations in the liver with ageing. Clinics in Gastroenterology 14: 757–771
Nasrallah S M, Wills C E Jr, Galambos J T 1980 Liver injury following jejunoileal bypass. Annals of Surgery 192: 726–729
Nolan L, O'Malley K 1988a Prescribing for the elderly: Part I. Sensitivity of the elderly to adverse drug reactions. Journal of the American Geriatrics Society 36: 142–149
Nolan L, O'Malley K 1988b Prescribing for the elderly: Part II. Prescribing patterns: differences due to age. Journal of the American Geriatrics Society 63: 245–254
Nouel O, Henrion J, Bernuau J, Degott C, Rueff B, Benhamou J-P 1980 Fulminant hepatic failure due to transient circulatory failure in patients with chronic heart disease. Digestive Diseases and Sciences 25: 49–52
Nunes G, Blaisdell W, Margaretten W 1970 Mechanism of hepatic dysfunction following shock and trauma. Archives of Surgery 100: 546–556
Ogilvie A L, James P D, Toghill P J 1981 Hepatic artery involvement in polymyalgia arteritica. Journal of Clinical Pathology 34: 769–772
Olsson R, Hultén L 1975 Concurrence of ulcerative colitis and chronic active hepatitis. Clinical courses and results of colectomy. Scandinavian Journal of Gastroenterology 10: 331–335
Olsson R, Kagevi I, Rydberg L 1982 On the concurrence of primary biliary cirrhosis and intestinal villous atrophy. Scandinavian Journal of Gastroenterology 17: 625–628
Pinching A J, Lockwood C M, Pussell B A et al 1983 Wegener's granulomatosis: observations on 18 patients with severe renal disease. Quarterly Journal of Medicine 52: 435–460
Poikolainen K, Reunala T, Karvonen J, Lauharanta J, Kärkkäinen P 1990 Alcohol intake: a risk factor for psoriasis in young and middle aged men? British Medical Journal 300: 780–783
Refsum H E 1963 Arterial hypoxaemia, serum activities of GO-T, GP-T and LDH, and centrilobular liver cell necrosis in pulmonary insufficiency. Clinical Science 25: 369–374
Ritchie J K, Allan R N, Macartney J, Thompson H, Hawley R P, Cooke W T 1974 Biliary tract carcinoma associated with ulcerative colitis. Quarterly Journal of Medicine 43: 263–279
Roquet M-L, Zafrani E-S, Farcet J-P, Reyes F, Pinaudeau Y 1985 Histopathological lesions of the liver in hairy cell leukemia: a report of 14 cases. Hepatology 5: 496–500
Rozman C, Cervantes F, Bruguera M 1991 The effect of haematologic and lymphatic diseases on the liver. In: McIntyre N, Benhamou J-P, Bircher J, Rizzetto M, Rodès J (eds) Oxford textbook of clinical hepatology. Oxford University Press, Oxford, p 1188–1194
Runyon B A, LaBrecque D R, Anuras S 1980 The spectrum of liver disease in systemic lupus erythematosus. Report of 33 histologically proved cases and a review of the literature. American Journal of Medicine 69: 187–194
Savage C O S, Winearls C G, Evans D J, Rees A J, Lockwood C M 1985 Microscopic polyarteritis: presentation, pathology and prognosis. Quarterly Journal of Medicine 56: 467–483
Sawers A H, Davson J, Braganza J, Geary C G 1982 Systemic mastocytosis, myelofibrosis and portal hypertension. Journal of Clinical Pathology 35: 617–619
Schaller J, Beckwith B, Wedgewood R J 1970 Hepatic involvement in juvenile rheumatic arthritis. Journal of Pediatrics 77: 202–210
Scott D G I, Bacon P A, Elliott P J, Tribe C R, Wallington T B 1982 Systemic vasculitis in a district general hospital 1972–1980: clinical and laboratory features, classification and prognosis of 80 cases. Quarterly Journal of Medicine 51: 292–311
Shepherd H A, Selby W S, Chapman R W G et al 1983 Ulcerative colitis and persistent liver dysfunction. Quarterly Journal of Medicine 52: 503–513
Sheridan P 1983 Thyroid hormones and the liver. Clinics in Gastroenterology 12: 797–818
Shetty N, Camilleri M, Moss D W, Hodgson H J 1987 Subtle hyperthyroidism presenting as suspected hepatobiliary disease. Journal of Clinical Gastroenterology 9: 186–188
Shibuya A, Unuma T, Sugimoto T et al 1985 Diffuse hepatic calcification as a sequela to shock liver. Gastroenterology 89: 196–201
Silverstein M N, Willaeger E E, Baggenstoss A H 1973 Gastrointestinal and abdominal manifestations of agnogenic myeloid metaplasia. Archives of Internal Medicine 131: 532–537
Simon H B 1993 Current concepts. Hyperthermia. New England Journal of Medicine 329: 483–487
Solano F X, Young E, Talamo T S, Dekker A 1986 Constrictive pericarditis mimicking Budd–Chiari syndrome. American Journal of Medicine 80: 113–115
Strickland R C, Schenker S 1977 The nephrogenic hepatic dysfunction syndrome: a review. American Journal of Digestive Diseases 22: 49–55
Thomas F B, Clausen K P, Greenberger N J 1973 Liver disease in multiple myeloma. Archives of Internal Medicine 132: 195–202
Thorne C, Urowitz M B, Wanless I, Roberts E, Blendis L M 1982 Liver disease in Felty's syndrome. American Journal of Medicine 73: 35–40
Travers R L 1979 Polyarteritis and related disorders. British Journal of Hospital Medicine 22: 38–45
Tugwell P 1973 Glucose-6-phosphate-dehydrogenase deficiency in Nigerians with jaundice associated with lobar pneumonia. Lancet 1: 968–969
Tugwell P, Williams A O 1977 Jaundice associated with lobar pneumonia: a clinical, laboratory and histological study. Quarterly Journal of Medicine 46: 97–118
Utili R, Abernathy C O, Zimmerman H J 1977 Inhibition of $Na^+$, $K^+$-adenosinetriphosphatase by endotoxin: a possible mechanism for

endotoxin-induced cholestasis. Journal of Infections Diseases 136: 583–587

Vestal R E 1989 Aging and determinants of hepatic drug clearance. Hepatology 9: 331–334

Ware A J 1978 The liver when the heart fails. Gastroenterology 74: 627

Watson A, Williams R 1984 Anoxic hepatic and intestinal injury from carbon monoxide poisoning. British Medical Journal 289: 1113

Webb J, Whaley K, MacSween R N M, Nuki G, Dick W C, Buchanan W 1975 Liver disease in rheumatoid arthritis and Sjögren's syndrome. Prospective study using biochemical and serological markers of hepatic dysfunction. Annals of Rheumatic Disease 34: 70–81

Wee A, Ludwig J 1985 Pericholangitis in chronic ulcerative colitis: primary sclerosing cholangitis of small bile ducts? Annals of Internal Medicine 102: 581–587

Wharton J T, Delclos L, Gallager S, Smith J P 1973 Radiation hepatitis induced by abdominal irradiation with the cobalt 60 moving strip technique. American Journal of Roentgenology 117: 73–80

Whelan G, Pierce A K, Schenker S, Combes B 1969 Hepatic function in patients with hypoxaemia due to chronic pulmonary disease. Australasian Annals of Medicine 216: 243–247

Willson R A 1981 Therapeutic quandary. Asymptomatic primary biliary cirrhosis associated with polymyositis. Digestive Diseases and Sciences 26: 372–375

Wynne H A, Cope L H, Mutch E, Rawlins M D, Woodhouse K W, Jares O F W 1989 The effect of age upon liver volume and apparent liver blood flow in healthy man. Hepatology 9: 297–301

Yam L T, Chang C H, Li C Y 1986 Hepatic involvement in systemic mast cell disease. American Journal of Medicine 80: 819–826

Yao J D, Gross J B Jr, Ludwig J, Purnell D C 1989 Cholestatic jaundice in hyperthyroidism. American Journal of Medicine 86: 619–620

Zafrani E S, Gaulard P 1993 Primary lymphoma of the liver. Liver 13: 57–61

# 44. Hepatic tumors and nodules

*Charles B. Rosen David M. Nagorney*

This chapter will discuss primary hepatic tumors (excluding cholangiocarcinoma, which will be considered with the tumors of the biliary system). Malignant primary tumors include hepatocellular carcinoma, fibrolamellar carcinoma, angiosarcoma, epithelial hemangioendothelioma, sarcoma and hepatoblastoma. Benign primary tumors include cavernous hemangioma and hepatocellular adenoma. Focal nodular hyperplasia, nodular regenerative hyperplasia and partial nodular transformation of the liver are nodular hepatic lesions which are not neoplastic. All secondary liver tumors are malignant; the most amenable to treatment are metastatic colonic and rectal carcinoma and carcinoid tumor. Cystic liver disease is discussed elsewhere (Ch 24)

## HEPATOCELLULAR CARCINOMA

Hepatocellular carcinoma is the most common malignant primary liver tumor, accounting for over 90% of primary hepatic malignancies (Okuda 1992). It is also one of the most common malignancies worldwide and accounts for approximately 250 000 deaths per year (Tang et al 1982, Okuda & Okuda 1991).

### Incidence

Although hepatocellular carcinoma occurs throughout the world, its incidence varies widely. The incidence is highest in sub-Saharan Africa and parts of south east Asia, where it exceeds 50 cases per year per 100 000 population, and in the Shangaan tribe in Mozambique. In Europe, North and South America, Australia and northern India the incidence is less than five cases per year per 100 000 population. Racial differences are also seen. A higher incidence is found in the black population compared to the white population in South Africa and North America and in Chinese compared to Indians in Singapore (Waterhouse et al 1976, 1982). Men are affected more often than women, the male : female ratio is 4–8:1 in high incidence areas and approximately 2:1 in low incidence areas (Ken 1990, Okuda & Okuda 1991).

### Etiology

A number of possible etiological agents have been implicated in the genesis of hepatocellular carcinoma. The geographical variation in the incidence suggests that the relative importance of the agents concerned (hepatitis B and C viruses, environmental carcinogens and predisposing liver disease) differ by geographic region.

*Hepatitis B virus* (Arthur et al 1984, Lieberman & Shafritz 1986)

A large and increasing body of epidemiological, biological and animal evidence implicates chronic infection with hepatitis B virus (HBV) as an important cause of hepatocellular carcinoma, particularly in areas with a high incidence of the disease. The cornerstone of the epidemiological evidence is the association between the incidence of hepatocellular carcinoma and the prevalence of persistent HBV infection. Thus, countries with a high prevalence of HBV infection also have a high incidence of hepatocellular carcinoma, while countries with a low prevalence of HBV infection have a correspondingly low incidence. Serological markers of HBV infection are present in 45–90% of patients with hepatocellular carcinoma in areas with a high rate of chronic HBV infection. Hepatitis B surface antigen (HBsAg), antibody to the hepatitis B core antigen (anti-HBc) and antibody to the hepatitis Be antigen (anti-HBe) are commonly present, but the presence of the hepatitis e antigen (HBeAg) itself is uncommon (p. 785). Acute infection followed by clearing of the HBV (as indicated by the presence of antibody to the HBsAg [anti-HBs] as the sole marker of infection) does not appear to confer an increased risk of developing hepatocellular carcinoma. In a prospective study of over 22 000 Taiwanese men, serological markers of chronic

HBV infection were associated with a relative risk of developing hepatocellular carcinoma of 390 (Beasley 1982). Population subgroups, such as the Chinese in Singapore, with a high rate of HBV carriage also have a high incidence of hepatocellular carcinoma when compared with other racial groups in the same area. Vertical transmission of infection may be important in areas of high incidence of hepatocellular carcinoma, as the mothers of patients with hepatocellular carcinoma are frequently carriers of the HBV (Sung & Chen 1980), suggesting that chronic infection for many years may be required before the development of carcinoma. The strength of the epidemiological evidence linking chronic carriage of the HBV to hepatocellular carcinoma can be appreciated from the fact that it is greater than that linking carcinoma of the bronchus to cigarette smoking (Arthur et al 1984).

Molecular biological studies using deoxyribonucleic acid (DNA) hybridization techniques have shown that HBV-DNA can integrate into the genome of the host liver cell (as opposed to existing free in the cytoplasm). HBV-DNA integration has been demonstrated both in cell lines cultured from hepatocellular carcinomas and in the carcinomas themselves. Integration occurs only with prolonged carriage of the virus, probably taking at least 2 years (Shafritz et al 1981).

Animal viruses closely resembling human HBV occur in a variety of animals, of which the woodchuck virus is the most closely studied. In that animal, persistent infection with the woodchuck hepatitis virus results in chronic hepatitis and the development of hepatocellular carcinoma. Integration of the woodchuck hepatitis virus DNA into the host liver cell genome has also been demonstrated.

There are, however, some inconsistencies in the evidence supporting a causal relationship between HBV and hepatocellular carcinoma. The male preponderance of the disease is not explained by the association with HBV infection. In females with hepatocellular carcinoma, the frequency of markers of HBV infection is similar to that in males with the disease (Kew et al 1983). Moreover, not all populations with high HBV infections have a high incidence of hepatocellular carcinoma; for example, it is uncommon in Greenland Eskimos despite endemic chronic HBV infection (Skinhoj et al 1978). Although underreporting of hepatocellular carcinoma in Greenland probably accounts for the finding, a similar association holds true in Alaskan Eskimos (Heyward et al 1981). In South Africa, the rate of hepatocellular carcinoma is greater in blacks born in rural areas than in those born in cities, despite a similar frequency of markers of chronic HBV infection (Kew et al 1986). These findings imply that chronic HBV infection may need an environmental factor as cocarcinogen for the development of hepatocellular carcinoma.

In areas where the incidence of hepatocellular carcinoma is low, HBV infection is a much less common cause of chronic liver disease and its relationship to the development of hepatocellular carcinoma is less clear. Cirrhosis from almost any cause confers an increased risk of hepatocellular carcinoma (see below). It is difficult to accurately distinguish the increased risk due to cirrhosis from that due to chronic HBV infection. In California the rate of hepatocellular carcinoma in noncirrhotic patients is proportional to the frequency of HBV infection in the community (Omata et al 1979). In Britain the frequency of markers of chronic HBV infection is of the order of 40–50% in patients with cirrhosis and hepatocellular carcinoma (Zaman et al 1985, Cobden et al 1986). However, male gender and increasing age are more important as risk factors than HBV infection (Zaman et al 1985). Interestingly, integration of HBV-DNA was demonstrated in the liver cells of 17 of 20 French patients with alcoholic cirrhosis and hepatocellular carcinoma, including seven of nine patients with no serological markers of HBV infection (Brechot et al 1985), a finding which has important implications for the pathogenesis of hepatocellular carcinoma in areas where the prevalence of chronic HBV infection is low.

Superinfection of chronic hepatitis B virus infection with the δ agent is not important in the pathogenesis of hepatocellular carcinoma (Nicholson 1985).

### *Hepatitis C virus*

Hepatitis C virus, although long known to exist, has only recently become identifiable by assay. After the introduction of first-generation enzyme-linked immunosorbent assays for antibody to hepatitis C virus during the late 1980s, multiple studies reported epidemiological data suggesting an association between hepatitis C virus infection and hepatocellular carcinoma (Colombo et al 1989, Hasan et al 1990, Caporaso et al 1991, Di Bisceglie et al 1991, Jeng & Tsai 1991, Kaklamani et al 1991, Levrero et al 1991, Nishioka et al 1991, Tanaka et al 1991, Watanabe et al 1991).

Colombo et al (1989) studied 447 Italian patients with cirrhosis, performing serum alpha-fetoprotein assays and real-time ultrasonography every 3–12 months. Thirty of the 447 patients (7%) were found to have hepatocellular carcinoma at the outset and 29 additional patients (7%) were found to have tumor during follow-up (1–48 months, average 33 months). Hepatitis C virus infection was the most common cause for cirrhosis in the entire group of patients (201 of 447, 45%) and in those with tumor detected at the outset (12 of 30, 40%) or during follow-up (eight of 29, 28%). In comparison, hepatitis B virus infection accounted for cirrhosis in 47 of 447 patients (11%) and was present in one of 30 (3%) with hepatocellular carcinoma at the outset and one of 29 patients (3%) with tumor detected during follow-up.

More evidence has accumulated from studies utilizing second-generation enzyme-linked immunosorbent assays, recombinant immunoblot assay (RIBA) and polymerase chain reaction assay (PCR) (Gerber et al 1992, Liang et al 1993). Liang et al (1993) studied American patients with hepatocellular carcinoma who were hepatitis B surface antigen negative and had no other predisposing factors. Evidence of hepatitis C virus infection was detected in 42 of 91 patients (46%) by RIBA-IL, in 40 of 90 patients (44%) by PCR for hepatitis C virus RNA in serum and in seven of nine patients by PCR for hepatitis C virus RNA in liver and/or tumor tissue. Altogether, 53 of the 91 patients (58%) had evidence of hepatitis C virus infection.

The association between hepatitis C virus and hepatocellular carcinoma varies throughout the world. Areas with a high prevalence of hepatitis B virus infection, such as sub-Saharan Africa and China, have stronger associations between hepatocellular carcinoma and hepatitis B virus infection than with hepatitis C virus infection. In other areas such as Japan, Spain and Italy, the opposite has been found (Bruix et al 1989, Colombo et al 1989, Nishioka et al 1991, Tanaka et al 1991, Ruiz et al 1992). In other countries and in the United States, hepatitis B and C viruses are more equally associated with hepatocellular carcinoma (Di Bisceglie et al 1991, Kaklamani et al 1991, Liang et al 1993). Antibody to hepatitis C virus has been reported in about 20% of French (Zarski et al 1991) and Swiss (Zala et al 1992) patients and 31% of Saudi Arabian patients (Karawi et al 1992) with hepatocellular carcinoma.

The mechanism by which hepatitis C virus infection leads to hepatocellular carcinoma remains unknown. Hepatitis C virus is a single-stranded RNA virus (p. 786). No related viruses such as flaviviruses and pestiviruses have been shown to cause cancer (Houghton et al 1991). Unlike hepatitis B virus, hepatitis C virus does not integrate into host DNA (Shafritz et al 1981, Yoneyama et al 1990). It is noteworthy that all patients with hepatitis C virus related to hepatocellular carcinoma have had advanced chronic liver disease. In the series of 91 hepatitis B surface antigen-negative patients reported by Liang et al (1993), only four without underlying liver disease were negative for both hepatitis B virus and hepatitis C virus markers. Also, patients with hepatitis C virus-related hepatocellular carcinoma tend to be older than patients with hepatitis B virus- or nonviral-related hepatocellular carcinoma. These observations suggest that hepatitis C virus infection may lead to hepatocellular carcinoma through an indirect mechanism mediated by chronic hepatocellular inflammation.

Hepatitis C virus infection may also increase the risk of tumor in patients with cirrhosis from other causes. Simonetti et al (1992) reported that 74% of Italian patients with hepatocellular carcinoma and cirrhosis had anti-hepatitis C virus antibody compared to 62% of those with cirrhosis alone. Farinati et al (1992) also showed a difference in hepatitis C virus infection rates in Italian patients – 60% for those with both alcoholic cirrhosis and hepatocellular carcinoma compared to 38% for those with alcoholic cirrhosis alone. A study of Swiss patients showed similar results (Zala et al 1992), but a Japanese study did not (Yuki et al 1992).

Some patients with hepatocellular carcinoma have evidence of coinfection with both hepatitis B and C viruses – 15% of hepatitis B surface antigen-negative and 29% of hepatitis B surface antigen-positive patients in the American study reported by Liang et al (1993) were also infected with hepatitis C virus. Interestingly, more than half (14 of 26) of the hepatitis B surface antigen-negative patients with positive PCR for hepatitis B virus DNA had hepatitis C virus infection as well (Liang et al 1993). This observation is consistent with other reports which suggest that coinfection with hepatitis B and C viruses suppresses hepatitis B virus replication (Bradley et al 1983, Brotman et al 1983, Fong et al 1991). However, coinfection with hepatitis B and C viruses has not been observed to affect the clinical course of hepatocellular carcinoma.

### *Aflatoxin* (Linsell & Peers 1977)

Aflatoxins are a series of poisonous substances produced by the mold *Aspergillus flavus* which grows readily on peanuts and grain stored in warm, humid conditions. Epidemiologically, a relationship between levels of aflatoxin intake and the incidence of hepatocellular carcinoma is observed in Africa and Thailand, while in Mozambique both aflatoxin intake and the incidence of hepatocellular carcinoma are very high. Experimental administration of aflatoxin to animals produces hepatic necrosis, fibrosis and neoplasia and in rats a single dose may cause hepatocellular carcinoma. Although very high levels of aflatoxin ingestion can cause an acute hepatitis in humans, chronic hepatitis has not been documented. Furthermore, chronic HBV infection is endemic in those areas of Africa and south east Asia where high levels of food contamination by aflatoxin are found. High levels of aflatoxin ingestion are found in India where there is a low incidence of hepatocellular carcinoma. Current evidence supports only a subsidiary or co-carcinogenic role for aflatoxin in the pathogenesis of hepatocellular carcinoma (Enwonwu 1984).

### *Malnutrition*

Little evidence supports malnutrition alone as a cause of chronic liver disease. However, hepatocellular carcinoma is common in areas of the world where malnutrition is rife. The carcinogenic effects of aflatoxin are potentiated by starvation in laboratory rats. Perhaps malnutrition in humans impairs the response of the liver to potential carcinogens.

*Hormones*

Hormonal factors may be important cocarcinogens, as male sex is strongly associated with hepatocellular carcinoma and is an important risk factor for progression of cirrhosis to hepatocellular carcinoma (Zaman et al 1985). This may also be important in the high incidence of hepatocellular carcinoma in hemochromatosis (p. 957) and the low incidence in primary biliary cirrhosis (p. 939). Both androgen and estrogen receptors have been demonstrated in hepatocellular carcinomas, but their significance is unclear. In one study, partial regression of hepatocellular carcinoma was achieved by administering progesterone to two women (Friedman et al 1982). On the other hand, prolonged use of both the combined oral contraceptive steroids (Neuberger et al 1986) and synthetic anabolic steroids has been associated with hepatocellular carcinoma.

*Hemochromatosis*

Hepatocellular carcinoma is particularly common in hemochromatosis and accounted for 30–45% of deaths in several recent series (Bradbear et al 1985, Niederau et al 1985, Fargion et al 1992). The relative risk of hepatocellular carcinoma for patients with hemochromatosis is greater than 200 (Bradbear et al 1985, Niederau et al 1985). Hepatocellular carcinoma related to hemochromatosis has a presentation and clinical course similar to that of hepatocellular carcinoma related to other chronic liver disease. However, unlike hepatitis C virus-related hepatocellular carcinoma, hemochromatosis-related hepatocellular carcinoma may arise rarely in noncirrhotic livers (Deugnier et al 1993).

*Cirrhosis*

More than three-quarters of the patients in most series of hepatocellular carcinoma have an underlying cirrhosis. This frequency of cirrhosis occurs in both high- and low-incidence areas, though in high-incidence areas the cirrhosis is more likely to be subclinical. Hepatocellular carcinoma usually occurs in macronodular cirrhosis but, at least in black South Africans, is now occurring more frequently in micronodular cirrhosis than in the past (Paterson et al 1985). It can occur in virtually any form of chronic liver disease complicated by cirrhosis. Hepatocellular carcinoma is uncommon in autoimmune hepatitis, primary biliary cirrhosis, cirrhosis associated with inflammatory bowel disease and $\alpha_1$-antitrypsin deficiency but is strikingly rare in Wilson's disease.

Large hepatocytes showing nuclear pleomorphism, and sometimes multiple nuclei, occur focally or even throughout whole nodules in some cirrhotic livers. This is known as liver cell dysplasia and is almost exclusively seen in patients with HBV-associated cirrhosis (Ho et al 1981). In Chinese patients it may be a premalignant condition, but this does not appear to be the case in Africans (Cohen et al 1979). It does not lead to alpha-fetoprotein production.

*Miscellaneous associations*

An increased incidence of hepatocellular carcinoma has been claimed in a number of conditions, including diabetes mellitus (Lawson et al 1986), acute intermittent porphyria (Lithner & Wetterberg 1984) and porphyria cutanea tarda (Salata et al 1985). Thorotrast is an obsolete radiological contrast agent associated with the production of hepatic angiosarcomas, cholangiocarcinomas and sometimes hepatocellular carcinomas. Although it was last used more than 30 years ago, patients still present with hepatic tumors attributable to its use.

## Pathology

*Macroscopic features*

Hepatocellular carcinomas occur most frequently in the right lobe of the liver, either as solitary masses or as multiple small nodules. Occasionally, hepatocellular carcinoma may spread diffusely within the liver and may not be immediately obvious to the naked eye. The tumor tissue usually looks white, but there may be areas of necrosis, hemorrhage or bile staining. Invasion of veins is frequent and may lead to portal or hepatic venous obstruction. Arterial invasion is uncommon.

*Microscopic features*

Microscopically, hepatocellular carcinomas usually have a trabecular structure with thick cell plates and are relatively well differentiated so that their origin is easily established (Fig. 44.1). Some have a ductular or papillary pattern and pleomorphic, clear or anaplastic cells occur. Hepatocellular carcinomas with a ductular pattern are not related to cholangiocarcinomas (as suggested by the term "mixed carcinoma" which is often applied to them). Bile secretion by tumor cells into channels resembling canaliculi can occur and is diagnostic when present (Fig. 44.1). Immunoreactive staining techniques may show the presence of alpha-fetoprotein or albumin on the tumor cell surface (Kojiro et al 1981). Hepatocellular carcinomas are usually highly vascular and have little stroma. The vascular channels are lined by epithelial cells, few of which are true Kupffer cells. Venous invasion is common and sometimes widespread invasion of the surrounding sinusoids is seen. Careful examination sometimes shows that a hepatocellular carcinoma has a multifocal origin.

*Metastases* (Nakashima et al 1983)

In patients dying from hepatocellular carcinoma, secondary spread is common (Nakashima et al 1983). The most frequent sites of involvement are the lungs (52%) and the lymphatic system (27%). Infiltration of the diaphragm by direct local extension occurs in 10%, but

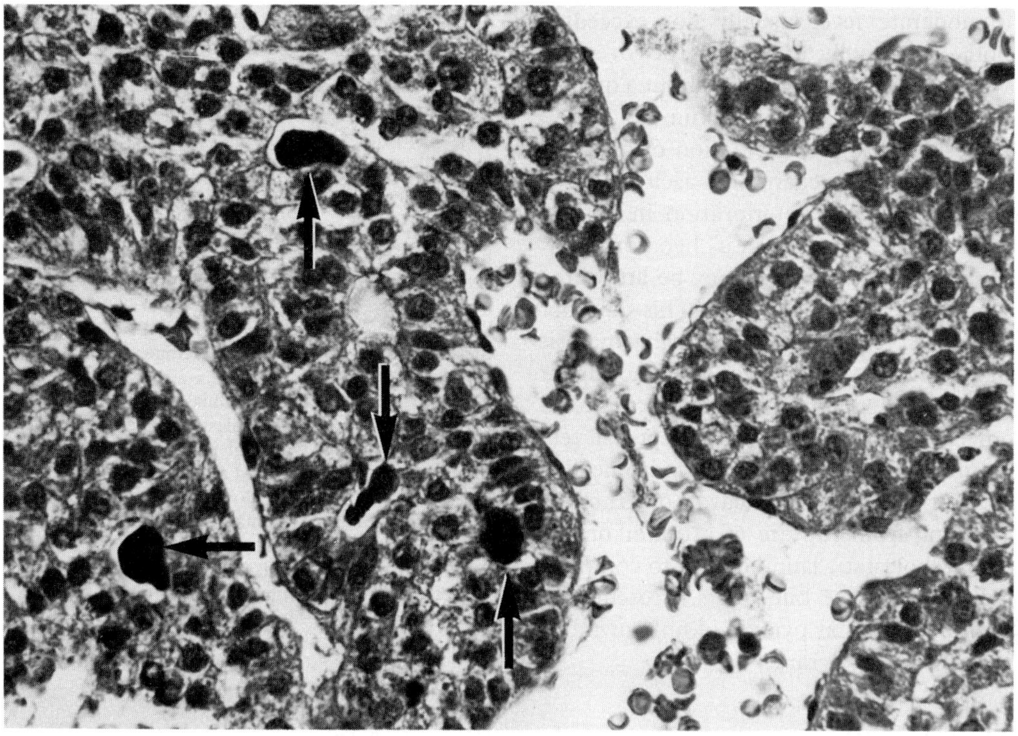

**Fig. 44.1** Hepatocellular carcinoma. This is a well-differentiated carcinoma producing bile (arrow) with well-developed sinusoids lined by epithelium (hematoxylin and eosin ×25).

peritoneal seedlings occur in only 6% of patients. The carcinoma has a particular propensity to invade portal and hepatic veins. Portal vein obstruction may rarely lead to portal hypertension, while involvement of the hepatic veins may produce a secondary Budd–Chiari syndrome and extension of the tumor into the right atrium is well recognized (Kojiro et al 1984). Distant metastases to other sites are rare.

## Clinical features

Most patients present with a general deterioration in health and abdominal symptoms (Table 44.1). Abdominal pain occurs in 50% or more of patients and is usually located in the epigastrium or right hypochondrium. It may be generalized and can radiate through to the back or to the shoulder. Anorexia, nausea and vomiting can be present and weakness, fatigue and weight loss become increasingly common. Diarrhea has also been described. Descriptions of the disease from different parts of the world suggest that there may be geographic variations in the pattern of symptoms.

Physical examination reveals hepatomegaly in almost all patients and ascites and clinical signs of cirrhosis are present in over half (Table 44.2). Mild jaundice may be present, but deep jaundice is rare. The enlarged liver is usually hard and often irregular and a localized mass may be palpable within it. Other physical features include

**Table 44.1** Symptoms in patients with hepatocellular carcinoma

| Symptoms | Frequency (%) | | |
|---|---|---|---|
| Study | Kew et al (1971) | Lai et al (1981) | Kew & Geddes (1982) |
| Country | UK | China | S. Africa |
| Number of patients | 75 | 211 | 548 |
| Weight loss | 71 | 19 | 34 |
| Abdominal pain | 69 | 48 | 95 |
| Anorexia | 28 | 73 | 25 |
| Weakness and fatigue | 23 | ns | 32 |
| Nausea and vomiting | 21 | ns | 2 |
| Pruritus | 8 | ns | ns |
| Diarrhea | ns | 21 | ns |

ns = not stated

**Table 44.2** Physical signs in patients with hepatocellular carcinoma

| Sign | Frequency (%) | | |
|---|---|---|---|
| Study | Kew et al (1971) | Lai et al (1981) | Kew & Geddes (1982) |
| Country | UK | China | S. Africa |
| Number of patients | 75 | 211 | 548 |
| Hepatomegaly | 93 | 93 | 92 |
| Ascites | 61 | 81 | 51 |
| Splenomegaly | 48 | ns | 42 |
| Jaundice | 44 | 5 | 28 |
| Hepatic bruit | 25 | ns | 23 |
| Fever | 24 | most | ns |
| Signs of cirrhosis | 51 | most | 60 |

ns = not stated

splenomegaly, a moderate fever usually not exceeding 38°C (100°F) and occasionally a friction rub over the liver. A bruit may be heard over the liver in about a quarter of patients, reflecting the vascularity of the tumor.

Most patients present with a combination of abdominal pain, weight loss, hepatomegaly and ascites. However, some complain only of a deterioration in general health and other clinical features, such as hepatomegaly, ascites and increasing encephalopathy, may be attributed to decompensation of underlying cirrhosis. This development in a patient with cirrhosis or hemochromatosis should always suggest the development of a hepatocellular carcinoma. Occasional presentations include gastrointestinal bleeding from esophageal varices due to portal vein invasion and thrombosis, a Budd–Chiari syndrome due to hepatic venous or inferior vena caval obstruction, intraperitoneal bleeding from rupture of a tumor on the surface of the liver or cholestatic jaundice due to compression by the tumor of the large bile ducts. Presentation without hepatic features (such as pyrexia of unknown origin or with metastatic disease) is rare.

## **Systemic manifestations** (Cochrane & Williams 1976)

A wide variety of systemic effects due to hepatocellular carcinoma (paraneoplastic syndromes) has been described (Table 44.3). Most of them are rare and some have been described in only one or two cases. The chance of an individual patient having one of these syndromes is approximately 5–10%.

**Table 44.3** Systemic manifestations of hepatocellular carcinoma (Cochrane & Williams 1976)

| | |
|---|---|
| *Endocrine manifestations* | |
| Erythrocytosis | |
| Hypercalçemia | |
| Hypocalcemia | |
| Cushing's syndrome | |
| Hyperthyroidism | |
| Precocious puberty | |
| Feminization | |
| Hypertrophic pulmonary osteoarthropathy | |
| Raised plasma chorionic gonadotrophin | |
| Raised plasma chorionic somatotrophin | |
| Raised plasma human placental lactogen | |
| *Metabolic change* | |
| Glucose | Hypoglycemia |
| Lipids | Hypercholesterolemia |
| | Hypertriglyceridemia |
| Proteins | Increased alpha-fetoprotein |
| | Macroglobulinemia |
| | Myelomatous globulinemia |
| | Increased haptoglobin |
| | Increased ceruloplasmin |
| Others | Porphyria cutanea tarda |
| | Pseudoporphyria |
| | Carcinoid syndrome |
| | Variant alkaline phosphatase |
| | Cystathionuria |
| | Ethanolaminuria |
| *Hematological changes* | |
| Hyperfibrinogenemia | |
| Cryofibrinogenemia | |
| Functional dysfibrinogenemia | |
| Antifibrinolysis | |
| Plasmacytosis | |
| Hemolytic anemia | |
| Leukemoid reaction | |

### *Erythrocytosis*

Erythrocytosis, one of the more common manifestations, occurs in about 10% of Asian patients with hepatocellular carcinoma but is probably less common in other races. It is attributed to increased production of the globulin precursor of erythropoietin by the tumor, which is normally produced by the liver, or to erythropoietin itself. The red cell mass is increased, with erythroid hyperplasia in the marrow, but white cells and platelets are unaffected. The development of erythrocytosis in a patient with cirrhosis is highly suggestive of hepatocellular carcinoma. The erythrocytosis may be masked by concurrent gastrointestinal bleeding and, conversely, the presence of erythrocytosis may prevent the development of anemia despite blood loss into the gut.

### *Disorders of calcium metabolism* (Oldenburg et al 1982)

Although uncommon, hypercalcemia can occur in hepatocellular carcinoma from tumor production of parathormone or a parathormone-like peptide. It is usually associated with hypophosphatemia and the calcium level may be reduced by corticosteroid treatment. Hypercalcemia may also result from bone destruction due to metastatic disease. Hypocalcemia has also been reported due to the production of a calcitonin-like substance by the hepatocellular carcinoma.

### *Hypoglycemia*

Hypoglycemia may affect up to a third of patients. It occurs by two distinct mechanisms. In the first, more common type, the hepatocellular carcinoma is poorly differentiated and contains little glycogen. Hypoglycemia occurs late in the disease in patients with anorexia, weakness and much weight loss and it probably arises because the capacity of the remaining liver is insufficient for the glucose requirements of a massive tumor. It is probably not a true paraneoplastic syndrome but a reflection of the terminal stages of a large tumor. Management is based on oral or intravenous glucose supplementation (300–500 g daily).

The second, much rarer type occurs in well-differentiated hepatocellular carcinomas which contain much glycogen. These patients are often relatively well, but their hypoglycemia may be profound and can constitute a major clinical problem. The hypoglycemia is probably due to abnormalities of the enzymes involved in hepatic glucose metabolism in normal and neoplastic cells, leading to an inability to release glucose from glycogen, and is a true paraneoplastic syndrome. Control of hypoglycemia is difficult and sometimes impossible. A high carbohydrate diet (up to 1500 g/day) may help, but large intravenous infusions of glucose (200–300 g) are usually also necessary.

*Other endocrine manifestations*

The most common endocrinopathy is Cushing's syndrome due to production of an ACTH-like peptide. Although abnormalities of thyroid hormone levels may occur, true hyperthyroidism is rare.

*Miscellaneous systemic disorders*

Rarely, clinical features such as porphyria cutanea tarda, carcinoid syndrome, clubbing of the digits, feminization and hemihypertrophy, or precocious puberty in children, may be associated with hepatocellular carcinoma (Table 44.3).

*Abnormal metabolic products*

Hepatocellular carcinoma is associated with changes in the concentration of many constituents of the blood (Table 34.3). Alpha-fetoprotein has proved valuable diagnostically and, with other tumor products, may be used to follow effects of therapy.

## Diagnosis

Abdominal pain, hepatomegaly, ascites and weight loss are the main symptoms and signs of hepatocellular carcinoma. Their development in a patient with cirrhosis is especially suggestive of hepatocellular carcinoma. For practical purposes, the diagnosis is nearly certain in the setting of an elevation of serum alpha-fetoprotein concentration and the presence of a mass within the liver. Ultrasonography is usually the initial imaging mode when hepatocellular carcinoma is suspected, but computed tomography (CT) and magnetic resonance imaging (MRI) are also quite useful. Histological confirmation of the diagnosis may be obtained by fine-needle aspiration or liver biopsy guided by ultrasonography or CT. Liver biopsy is often not necessary and may be contraindicated in patients with tumors potentially amenable to resection or liver transplantation due to the risk of spreading tumor. Patients who might be suitable for resection or liver transplantation should have abdominal CT to rule out extrahepatic intra-abdominal disease. Chest CT and radionuclide bone imaging are suggested to rule out distant metastases.

*Clinical chemistry*

Liver function tests are abnormal at the time of presentation in most patients. In about 5% of patients they may be normal despite the presence of an obvious mass in the right upper quadrant of the abdomen. As the disease progresses, they become abnormal in virtually all patients. The most common abnormality is an elevation of plasma alkaline phosphatase activity, often in association with increased $\gamma$-glutamyl transpeptidase activity. The plasma bilirubin is normal, or only mildly raised, with levels less than 170 $\mu$mol/L (10 mg/dl). Reduction in plasma albumin, a prolonged prothrombin time and a raised plasma globulin may also be found and become more frequent with progression of the disease. They reflect the degree of hepatocellular impairment and are of no value in differentiating primary hepatocellular carcinoma from other liver tumors or from cirrhosis.

*Ascites*

The ascitic fluid is usually clear with a protein content of less than 25 g/L and does not, therefore, differ from ascitic fluid due to cirrhosis (Tables 37.1 and 37.2). More suggestive findings are blood staining and a higher protein content, but these occur in less than 25% of patients with hepatocellular carcinoma and ascites (Kew et al 1971). Cytological examination of ascitic fluid may show malignant cells but is diagnostic in only a small proportion because of the infrequency of peritoneal seeding.

*Alpha-fetoprotein*

Alpha-fetoprotein was previously identified in serum by counterelectrophoresis, which is relatively insensitive and only capable of detecting concentrations above 250 ng/ml. Thus, detection of an increased serum alpha-fetoprotein concentration was almost diagnostic of hepatocellular carcinoma. However, more sensitive radioimmunoassay techniques now allow the detection of much smaller amounts and consequently this protein is measurable in normal serum in concentrations up to 30 ng/ml (p. 749). Very high concentrations (>400 ng/ml) remain virtually diagnostic of hepatocellular carcinoma, but intermediate values may cause diagnostic confusion. Moderate elevations may occur in acute and chronic hepatitis, cirrhosis and hepatic metastatic carcinoma and in a variety of nonhepatic conditions (pregnancy, embryonal germ cell tumors and sometimes in the neonatal period). The sensitivity for hepatocellular carcinoma may be increased by chromatographic separation of different subgroups of alpha-fetoprotein, but such techniques are still research tools (Buamah et al 1984). Furthermore, not all hepatocellular carcinomas produce alpha-fetoprotein, the proportion of those failing to do so varying from about 10% in high-incidence areas to about 30% in low-incidence areas. Thus, only very high serum alpha-fetoprotein concentrations are diagnostic of hepatocellular carcinoma, lower concentrations are compatible with the diagnosis and normal concentrations do not exclude the tumor. Alpha-fetoprotein measurements are also useful in following the results of therapy and may be capable of detecting small hepatocellular carcinomas in high-risk groups who have normal levels at the start of screening (Heyward et al 1985). They have less value in the detection of early lesions in cirrhosis, due to the frequency with which background levels are moderately raised in these patients and the hepatocellular carcinoma may be large by the time levels have increased to allow detection (Kubo et al 1978).

*Liver imaging*

Imaging methods usually identify hepatocellular carcinomas as space-occupying lesions which cannot be differentiated reliably from other primary and secondary tumors. Difficulty can arise with diffusely invading tumors and from the effects of underlying cirrhosis. Imaging on its own, therefore, is insufficient for a certain diagnosis. Imaging is very useful in localizing the likely site of a hepatocellular carcinoma and directing fine-needle aspiration for a definitive diagnosis.

***Radionuclide imaging.*** The sensitivity and specificity of radionuclide imaging are currently too low to allow its use as a reliable indicator of the presence or absence of a hepatocellular carcinoma, particularly in patients with hepatic cirrhosis (p. 93). Hepatocellular carcinomas appear as areas which lack colloid uptake, but such "cold" areas may also be seen in hepatic cirrhosis. Attempts to improve sensitivity by using delayed scans and tracers concentrated in the tumor (such as $^{75}$Se-selenomethionine or $^{67}$Ga citrate) have only been partially successful, because only about 75% of hepatocellular carcinomas give a positive result. Radionuclide imaging is particularly poor in detecting small lesions (≤2 cm). Other methods of imaging (below) are more effective in diagnosis.

***Ultrasonography.*** In experienced hands, ultrasonography will detect the majority of moderate-sized (>2 cm) hepatocellular carcinomas (p. 55), even in patients with cirrhosis (Cottone et al 1983). The advent of real-time ultrasound has improved resolution so that lesions as small as 1 cm in diameter may be detected (Sheu et al 1984). There are no specific ultrasonographic features of hepatocellular carcinoma which will reliably differentiate it from metastatic liver tumors (Dubbins et al 1981). Ultrasonography is particularly useful for guiding fine-needle aspiration.

***Computed tomography.*** Computed tomography (CT) usually reveals hepatocellular carcinoma as hypodense or isodense compared with the surrounding liver (Fig. 44.2). Accurate definition of the extent of the lesion therefore requires enhancement after injection of intravenous contrast (p. 66). The sensitivity of CT scanning compares well with ultrasonography in that both have a 96% detection rate (La Berge et al 1984). CT scanning is better than ultrasound at detecting parenchymal involvement and extrahepatic spread but less sensitive at detecting vascular invasion (La Berge et al 1984), though Doppler studies coupled with ultrasound improve recognition of vascular abnormalities. With modern machines and studies with contrast, the resolution of the method is such that 70% of lesions less than 2 cm diameter and 86% of lesions between 2 and 5 cm diameter can be detected (Inamoto et al 1983). CT appearances do not differentiate reliably between hepatocellular carcinoma and secondary hepatic tumors.

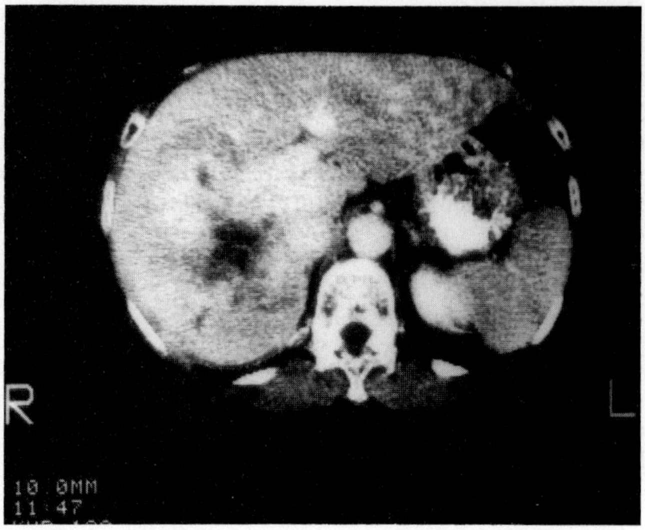


**Fig. 44.2** Computed tomographic imaging of a hepatocellular carcinoma.

***Magnetic resonance imaging.*** MRI (p. 75) is better than CT in detecting tumor margins, portal vein involvement and a tumor pseudocapsule (Itoh et al 1987). It detects 75% of tumors less than 1 cm and over 80% of tumors less than 2 cm in diameter (Hirai et al 1991) and may be better than CT for detection of tumor recurrence after resection or lipiodol embolization (Havard et al 1992). MRI is also better than CT for the detection of hepatocellular carcinoma in hemochromatosis because the high intensity signal from tumor contrasts with the lower intensity signal of the iron-rich liver (Berland et al 1989).

*Angiography*

Angiography is required for diagnosis in only a few patients (p. 26). Hepatocellular carcinoma has characteristic angiographic appearances. The normal intrahepatic arteries are displaced around the tumor, which is supplied by large abnormal vessels emptying into an area of disorderly new vessel formation. The capillaries in the neoplasm give an intense tumor blush, pooling of contrast may occur and there may be extensive arteriovenous shunts. Less vascular tumors, including most cholangiocarcinomas, are characterized mainly by displacement of normal blood vessels. A tumor blush of lower intensity may be seen and there are few arteriovenous shunts. The vascularity of secondary tumors varies considerably and in general reflects that of the primary lesion.

Angiography can detect small lesions and its sensitivity may be increased by injection of iodized oil contrast media into the hepatic artery. This material is taken up and retained by hepatocellular carcinomas and may be detected on plain abdominal X-ray or CT scanning several days later (Yumoto et al 1985). However, the invasiveness, expense and morbidity of angiography, coupled with its uncertainty in distinguishing between primary and secondary tumors, mean that its use as a diagnostic tool is limited. However, it may provide relevant vascular information regarding the resectability of hepatocellular carcinoma.

*Liver biopsy and laparoscopy*

Histological confirmation of hepatocellular carcinoma is usually required when a tumor is not amenable to liver resection or transplantation. Simple "blind" percutaneous liver biopsy is unlikely to be successful unless the tumor is large and located in the right liver. Thus, biopsy is often guided by real-time ultrasound. Simple aspiration cytology is theoretically safer than biopsy because hepatocellular tumors are highly vascular. Although liver biopsy is a relatively safe procedure, the highest risk for bleeding is in patients with hepatocellular carcinoma (McGill et al 1990).

Although laparoscopy is superior to ultrasound or CT for the diagnosis of tumors less than 2 cm in diameter located on the surface of the liver, the procedure is limited by its inability to visualize the posterior and superior aspects of the liver surface (p. 129). Also, tumors deep in the parenchyma or in the hilus cannot be adequately visualized. Laparoscopy does facilitate biopsy of lesions close to the liver surface and laparoscopic ultrasonography may help to overcome the limitations of the procedure. Laparoscopy may also detect extrahepatic disease and thus may avoid unnecessary operations (Bornman & Krige 1995).

*Laparotomy*

Diagnostic or staging laparotomy is now unnecessary in hepatocellular carcinoma and should be reserved for patients in whom surgical resection is contemplated.

*Other investigations*

There are no characteristic changes in the peripheral blood, although erythrocytosis may occur. The leukocyte and platelet count may both be raised. Serology for hepatitis B and C should be obtained as positive serology for past or present infection indicates the need for special care to avoid spreading infection, particularly to medical, nursing and laboratory staff. Autoantibodies are not a feature of hepatocellular carcinoma but reflect the nature of underlying cirrhosis. Plasma protein estimation usually shows a diffuse increase in $\gamma$-globulin and a monoclonal gammopathy may occur.

## Treatment

*Resection*

Liver resection, with complete extirpation of tumor, offers most hope for prolonged survival and the only (albeit small) chance of cure. However, most patients with hepatocellular carcinoma have an underlying chronic disease and impaired hepatocellular function which prohibits major liver resection. Few hepatocellular carcinomas are thus amenable to resection. Resectability rates vary from 6% to 17% depending on the criteria for selection and enthusiasm of the surgeon (Tang et al 1982). Overall survival is poor, but 30–37% 5-year survival rates have been reported for patients able to undergo complete extirpation of tumor (Thompson et al 1983, Sesto et al 1987, Iwatsuki & Starzl 1988, Nagorney et al 1989). Recently, Vauthey et al (1995) reported a 41% 5-year survival rate and 32% 10-year survival rate for 106 patients treated by resection. The prognosis was significantly better in patients with tumors without vascular invasion. Other favorable prognostic factors included absence of symptoms, solitary tumor, negative margin of resection, small (less than or equal to 5 cm) tumor and presence of a pseudocapsule (Vauthey et al 1995).

*Orthotopic liver transplantation*

Liver transplantation at one time seemed an ideal treatment for patients with unresectable hepatocellular carcinoma confined to the liver. Unfortunately, 5-year survival rates were less than 20% (Penn 1991) due to the advanced stage of the disease. However, recent progress has allowed identification of patients with hepatocellular carcinoma who are most likely to have long-term survival after treatment with liver transplantation (p. 1154). A 60–83% 5-year survival rate has been reported after liver transplantation for patients with early-stage (UICC stage II) tumors (Iwatsuki et al 1991, Ringe et al 1991, Gores et al 1992). Recently, several centers have reported encouraging early results with liver transplantation and adjuvant systemic chemotherapy and/or tumor embolization and local chemotherapy for early-stage tumors (Stone et al 1993, Venook 1995, Carr et al 1993, Schnatz 1994). Indeed, some clinicians now feel that patients with early-stage hepatocellular carcinoma and less advanced chronic liver disease (a group previously thought to be best treated by liver resection) are probably best treated by liver transplantation. Underlying chronic liver disease predisposes patients to the development of additional tumors after even potentially curative resection and also inevitably progresses to end-stage liver disease. Since the risk for tumor reappearance after transplantation is low for small tumors, liver transplantation provides excellent treatment for both the carcinoma and the underlying liver disease (Gores 1993, Bismuth et al 1993). Interestingly, the two most common initial sites for tumor reappearance after transplantation are the liver allograft and the lungs (Ringe et al 1989, Yokoyama et al 1990). Also hepatocellular carcinoma has a faster rate of growth after transplantation, presumably due to immunosuppression therapy (Yokoyama et al 1991).

*Hepatic dearterialization and tumor embolization*

Hepatocellular carcinomas derive their blood supply almost entirely from the hepatic artery and in theory, ligation of the hepatic artery might produce worthwhile palliation. However, the tumor soon revascularizes from hepatic capsular vessels. Dearterialization is contraindicated in patients with portal vein obstruction and in those with advanced cirrhosis because massive hepatic necrosis may be precipitated. Surgical dearterialization has not been widely employed because of operative risks and the adverse technical impact on subsequent arterial embolization of the tumor. Arterial embolization involves injection of gelatin sponge, metal coils or autologous blood clot into the branches of the hepatic artery supplying the carcinoma during angiography. Although cure is unlikely, clinical palliation is often worthwhile. In a series of 120 patients, survival at 1 year was 44%, at 2 years 29% and at 3 years 15% (Yamada et al 1983). Portal vein thrombosis is a contraindication but cirrhosis is not. Embolization produces tumor infarction and gas bubbles may be seen on computed tomography. They do not necessarily indicate infection. The procedure is generally well tolerated with low morbidity and mortality and can be repeated. Addition of chemotherapeutic agents to the embolic material may prolong the response.

*Sclerotherapy*

Sclerotherapy of hepatocellular carcinoma by direct tumor injection of ethanol was developed by Sugiura et al (1983). Early results were promising (Livraghi et al 1992), but tumor recurrence was frequent. Survival rates are approximately 60% at 3 years (Livraghi et al 1992) and 34% at 5 years (Okuda 1994). These results are comparable to those obtained with resection in patients with cirrhosis and hepatocellular carcinoma, because the underlying liver disease and propensity to develop additional tumors are the main determinants of life expectancy. However, tumor size (≤5 cm) limits the application of this therapy.

*Chemotherapy*

The results of chemotherapy for hepatocellular carcinoma have been disappointing. A randomized, controlled trial involving over 300 patients examined various treatment protocols using 5-fluorouracil, methyl-CCNU, adriamycin, and streptozotocin as single agents or in combination (Falkson et al 1984). The overall response rate was only 13%, with a median survival time of only 28 weeks and 1-year survival of 20–25%. There was considerable morbidity from drug toxicity. New agents such as mitomycin-C are being evaluated, but early results are similarly disappointing. Interferon has been tried but is of no benefit. Theoretically, intrahepatic arterial infusion of chemotherapeutic agents might deliver a high concentration of antineoplastic drugs to the tumor without systemic side-effects. However, major complications include hemorrhage, infection and thrombosis related to the indwelling arterial catheter and cholestatic jaundice, cholangitis, biliary strictures and gastritis (presumably due to gastroduodenal perfusion of the agent via the right gastric artery). To date, regional infusion chemotherapy for hepatocellular carcinoma has not been associated with either an improved response rate or survival when compared with systemic chemotherapy. Currently the main effect of chemotherapy in most patients with hepatocellular carcinoma has been to diminish the quality of their remaining life without significantly prolonging it.

## Prognosis

Not surprisingly, survival is related to the extent of the disease. A scoring system has been devised which depends on the degree of replacement of normal tissue by the hepatocellular carcinoma and on the severity of hepatocellular dysfunction (Okuda et al 1985). The results of such a staging process on survival are shown in Table 44.4. Only stage I patients (with smaller tumors and no hepatocellular dysfunction) have a median survival of over 3 months. Surgery prolongs survival in stage I and stage II disease, but medical therapy has little or no effect.

**Table 44.4** Median survival in months of 850 patients with hepatocellular carcinoma (Okuda et al 1985)

| Treatment | No. of patients | Stage I | Stage II | Stage III |
|---|---|---|---|---|
| Untreated | 227 | 8.3 | 2.0 | 0.7 |
| Surgery | 157 | 25.6 | 12.2 | – |
| Medical | 464 | 9.4 | 3.6 | 1.6 |

Medical treatment includes transarterial embolization and all forms of chemotherapy.

Death in most patients is due to the local effects of the carcinoma, which causes either liver failure or massive bleeding from the tumor or from esophageal varices. A few patients survive for over a year and there are anecdotal reports of patients surviving for several years despite the presence of tumor.

### Prevention

Chronic HBV infection is the most important cause of hepatocellular carcinoma worldwide and prevention of HBV infection is probably the best way of reducing the incidence of the disease. Vaccination against HBV infection is the best preventive method currently available, but most hepatocellular carcinomas related to chronic HBV infection occur in impoverished countries with limited economic resources for vaccines (p. 786). Improvement of the poor social conditions favoring spread of the virus combined with a selective vaccination program aimed, for example, at preventing vertical spread of infection to newborns would be most beneficial. Current treatments for chronic HBV infection are unlikely to have any effect because they are applicable to only a small proportion of patients and promote viral integration rather than elimination of the virus. Recent reports raise the possibility that treatment of chronic HCV infection with interferon may prevent subsequent development of hepatocellular carcinoma (Nishiguchi et al 1995, Mazella et al 1996). Improved methods of food storage might be valuable in reducing the incidence of hepatocellular carcinoma in parts of the world where aflatoxin contamination of food is high. There are no ready means for preventing hepatocellular carcinoma in low endemic areas because precipitating causes are unknown.

### Screening

The dismal results of treatment of symptomatic hepatocellular carcinoma and the possibility of identifying small tumors prior to metastases with modern ultrasonography and sensitive radioimmunoassay of alpha-fetoprotein have led to attempts to diagnose hepatocellular carcinoma in asymptomatic patients at high risk. Screening programs based on serial alpha-fetoprotein levels and hepatic ultrasonography have been shown to be practical (Liaw et al 1986) and effective (Tang et al 1982). The rate of detection of subclinical hepatocellular carcinomas in such surveys approaches 45%. Moreover, the resection rate of these patients has increased to 33–45%. The 5-year survival rate in such surveys is nearly 30%, a 10-fold improvement over survival in unscreened patients. These programs are most practical in high-incidence areas but can be applicable in low-incidence areas if a population at increased risk is identified, such as the Alaskan Eskimos (Heyward et al 1985), though the yield is considerably lower. Not all programs have given such optimistic results, as new tumors detected may not be operable (Colombo et al 1991). Whether an increased risk of subsequent development of hepatocellular carcinoma persists after resection of an asymptomatic tumor is unresolved. However, the presence of risk factors in such patients with proven hepatocellular carcinoma mandates continued follow-up screening.

## FIBROLAMELLAR HEPATOCELLULAR CARCINOMA (Rosen & Nagorney 1993)

Fibrolamellar hepatocellular carcinoma is a distinct type of hepatocellular carcinoma which has a relatively favorable prognosis. It most often afflicts adolescents and young adults. Unlike hepatocellular carcinoma, an underlying chronic liver disease is unusual. Fibrolamellar carcinomas are often solitary large tumors. Histologically, they have deeply eosinophilic, polygonal, neoplastic cells surrounded by a dense layered fibrous stroma. The mainstay of therapy is surgical resection and resectability rates are higher (75%) than for hepatocellular carcinoma (49%) (Nagorney et al 1985). Overall survival ranges from 25% to 63% at 5 years; patients with resectable tumors fare better with 40–65% survival at 5 years and median survival between 33 and 15 months (Rosen & Nagorney 1993). Patients with unresectable but localized lesions may be candidates for orthotopic liver transplantation. Iwatsuki et al (1991) reported a 37.5% 5-year survival and 3-year median survival after orthotopic liver transplantation, while Ringe et al (1992) reported 28.5 month median survival. Prolonged survival is also possible for patients with unresectable tumors and distant metastases, especially if the tumor responds to chemotherapy (Ihde et al 1985).

## ANGIOSARCOMA (Forbes et al 1987)

This rare, highly malignant tumor has risen to prominence because of its relation to environmental carcinogens. However, no cause can be identified in one-half of the patients. Irrespective of the etiology, the pathological nature of the tumor is that of malignant endothelial cells which line or project into vascular spaces or form solid masses surrounding liver cells. A bruit may be heard over the liver and thrombocytopenia may occur as a result of deposition of platelets within the tumor. Tumor multicentricity and extent almost always preclude resection, therefore survival after diagnosis is brief.

### Thorotrast

The radio-opaque colloidal thorium dioxide (Thorotrast) was widely used as a radiological contrast agent until its causal relationship to liver tumors was recognized. Thorotrast contains radioactive thorium which produces high-energy α, β, and γ emissions and has a biological half-life of 50 years. It is cleared by the reticuloendothelial system and 70% lodges in the liver, 20% in the spleen and 10% in the marrow, lymph nodes and lungs. Thorotrast deposits in the liver are associated with prominent capsular thickening and destruction of hepatocytes and fibrosis may lead to cirrhosis. Angiosarcomas and cholangiocarcinomas occur with about equal frequency, but hepatocellular carcinomas can also develop. A single exposure is sufficient, but most tumors develop 12 to 36 years after exposure. Despite the interest in its relationship with angiosarcoma, an epidemiological study could implicate exposure to Thorotrast in only 7% of patients (Vianni et al 1981).

### Arsenic

Chronic industrial or medicinal exposure to arsenic is implicated in 15% of angiosarcomas (Vianni et al 1981). Unlike Thorotrast, a single exposure is insufficient to promote carcinogenesis.

### Vinyl chloride

Polyvinyl chloride, one of the most commonly used modern plastics, is a polymer made from vinyl chloride monomer. Prolonged repeated exposure to the monomer produces hepatic fibrosis, portal hypertension and splenomegaly. Although workers involved in the manufacture of polyvinyl chloride are at highest risk, people living close to production plants are probably at increased risk. Vinyl chloride has been implicated in 20% of angiosarcomas (Vianni et al 1981). Repeated chronic exposure is necessary for carcinogenesis and the latent period to the development of angiosarcoma is 12 to 30 years.

## EPITHELIOID HEMANGIOENDOTHELIOMA (Ishak et al 1984)

Epithelioid hemangioendothelioma is a slow-growing malignant tumor which arises from endothelial cells. This typically multicentric tumor is composed of dendritic and epithelioid cell elements with a marked sclerotic stroma and extensive infiltration of sinusoids and veins. Sixty percent of the tumors occur in women. The tumor presents with abdominal pain and hepatomegaly or as an incidental finding. These tumors may originate in either the liver or lung and metastases of liver tumors to the lung or lung tumors to the liver are common. Although epithelioid hemangioendothelioma of the liver is slow-growing, the disease inevitably spreads to the lung, bone, spleen and regional lymph nodes. The 5-year survival rate is approximately 30%. Surgical resection provides the only chance for cure, but advanced tumor stage often precludes resection. Several centers have reported favourable results after liver transplantation with a projected 5-year survival rate of 76% (Marino et al 1988, Scoazec et al 1988). Remarkably, favourable results have been obtained even in the presence of extrahepatic disease (Marino et al 1988).

## SARCOMA (Forbes et al 1987)

Sarcomas of the liver are exceptionally rare. They are highly malignant, resistant to treatment and rapidly fatal.

## HEPATOBLASTOMA AND CHILDHOOD TUMORS (Weinberg & Finegold 1983)

### Classification

Hepatic tumors in childhood are rare, comprising between 0.5% and 2% of pediatric malignancies. Their classification is difficult (Table 44.5) and intermediate forms have been described. Most are malignant and present within the first 2 years of life. Hepatoblastomas, hepatocellular carcinomas or hemangiomas are most common. Metastatic liver deposits are exceptionally rare. Most metastases are from adrenal neuroblastomas or nephroblastomas (Wilm's tumor) and they occur in 5–20% of patients who harbor such tumors. Rhabdomyosarcomas and lymphomas are even less common.

### Clinical presentation

Regardless of specific pathology, clinical presentation is similar. Abdominal swelling, a palpable abdominal mass, splenomegaly, abdominal pain, anorexia, vomiting and weight loss are all common features. Hepatoblastoma is the most common of the malignant tumors and usually presents in the first year of life. It is slightly more common in boys and there is no association with either chronic HBV infection or underlying cirrhosis. An association with polyposis coli has been described (Kingston et al 1983). Hepatocellular carcinomas are uncommon below the age of 5 years, though cases are seen occasionally in infancy. They may be associated with hemihypertrophy and virilization. The fibrolamellar variant is more common in the pediatric age group than in adults.

Benign tumors in childhood are rare. Hemangiomas of the liver comprise about 60% of cases (Ehren et al 1983).

**Table 44.5** Primary liver tumors in childhood

| Origin | Benign | Malignant |
|---|---|---|
| Epithelial | Adenoma | Hepatoblastoma<br>Hepatocellular carcinoma<br>Cholangiocarcinoma |
| Mesenchymal | Cavernous hemangioma<br>Hemangioendothelioma<br>Mesenchymal hamartoma | Sarcoma<br>Rhabdomyosarcoma<br>Angiosarcoma<br>Teratocarcinoma |

Cutaneous hemangiomas may also be present. These tumors present as outlined below, but rarely they present with hemorrhagic shock due to rupture of the highly vascular tumor into the peritoneum. Congestive cardiac failure also occurs frequently owing to massive arteriovenous shunting within the tumor. Damage to red cells and platelets within the tumor may cause a microangiopathic anemia, thrombocytopenia and disseminated intravascular coagulation, a combination which has been termed the Kasabach–Merritt syndrome. Adenomas also occur in infancy but are usually associated with other conditions affecting the liver (Chandra et al 1984).

### Investigations

The methods of investigation for liver tumors in infants and children are similar to those used in adults. Serum alphafetoprotein levels are increased in nearly 90% of patients with hepatoblastoma and between 50% and 60% of patients with hepatocellular carcinoma. Calcification is occasionally seen on plain abdominal radiographs in patients with hepatocellular carcinoma or hemangioma. Increased urinary excretion of 4-hydroxy 3-methoxymandelic acid (HMMA) is the single most useful means of detecting neuroblastoma. Liver biopsy may be needed for diagnosis but is contraindicated in hemangiomas because of their vascularity.

### Treatment

The treatment of choice for malignant tumors is surgical resection. Low operative mortality and morbidity rates can be achieved with proper selection of patients and high-quality surgical and postoperative care (Price et al 1982). Resection is possible in about 75% of patients with hepatoblastomas and a cure rate of 30–50% can be expected. Recurrence usually occurs within 3 years but may be delayed for up to 5 years. The histopathological nature of the tumor may have prognostic importance (Weinberg & Finegold 1983). Preoperative chemotherapy with adriamycin may reduce the size of hepatoblastomas and allow subsequent resection (Quinn et al 1985). Adjuvant chemotherapy or radiotherapy after liver regeneration may prolong remission, but recurrence signifies a poor prognosis. Prognosis is best for the fibrolamellar variant of hepatocellular carcinoma.

Benign tumors should be removed only if symptomatic. Hemangiomas may respond to treatment with corticosteroids or radiotherapy, but the response is variable and unpredictable. Recently, α-interferon has proven effective in causing involution of hemangiomas and eliminating life-threatening complications (Ezekowitz et al 1992). If cardiac failure cannot be controlled by medical means, hepatic artery ligation or embolization should be considered (Larcher et al 1981). Hepatic metastases from nephroblastomas are occasionally suitable for resection.

## BENIGN PRIMARY LIVER TUMORS

### Cavernous hemangioma

Cavernous hemangiomas are the most common primary hepatic tumors and are present in up to 1% of autopsies. They may be single or multiple and probably represent congenital ectasia of intrahepatic sinusoidal spaces which gradually dilate. Most are subcapsular, small and asymptomatic. A hepatic bruit may accompany large tumors and thrombocytopenia may follow platelet sequestration within the tumor. Rupture with intraperitoneal hemorrhage is very rare.

Diagnosis is usually made by ultrasound or CT imaging. Radionuclide imaging with $^{99m}$Tc-labeled autologous red cells is specific. Hepatic arteriography is only necessary when there is doubt about the nature of the lesion; the large, orderly sinusoidal spaces of the hemangioma fill and empty slowly so that contrast material remains in the lesion in the venous stage of the angiogram. CT is usually diagnostic. MRI is at least equally diagnostic and both CT and MRI are less invasive than angiography. Arteriovenous shunting does not occur. Although liver biopsy is generally contraindicated because of risk of hemorrhage, fine-needle aspiration is safe provided the liver capsule is not punctured immediately above the hemangioma. Hepatic resection, hepatic artery ligation and irradiation have all been employed. Although most tumors require no treatment, most hemangiomas can be enucleated without major hepatic resection. They grow very slowly and asymptomatic lesions rarely become symptomatic.

### Hepatocellular adenoma

*Etiology*

Hepatocellular adenoma is rare. An association has been reported with oral contraceptive steroids and occasionally with androgenic or anabolic steroids. Less frequently, glycogen storage disease, transfusional hemosiderosis and other forms of hormonal therapy have been implicated in pathogenesis.

*Pathology*

Adenomas are composed of normal hepatocytes without bile ducts but lack lobular organization. They may be difficult to differentiate from focal nodular hyperplasia (below). They are usually single but may be multiple (Flejou et al 1985).

The main clinical features of hepatocellular adenomas are acute abdominal pain with or without shock due to hemorrhage into the tumor or peritoneal cavity, chronic abdominal pain or an upper abdominal mass (Table 44.6). The diagnosis is made incidentally at operation in 20% of patients. Although the general clinical features are the same irrespective of the etiology of the lesion, hemorrhage

**Table 44.6** Presenting complaints due to hepatic adenoma and focal nodular hyperplasia in 106 women taking oral contraceptives (Klatskin 1977)

| Presenting complaint | Patients | |
|---|---|---|
| | Number | Frequency (%) |
| Acute abdominal pain and shock* | 59 | 55 |
| Palpable mass | 21 | 20 |
| Chronic abdominal pain | 5 | 5 |
| Asymptomatic† | 21 | 20 |

*Bleeding into the peritoneum or the tumor.
†Incidental diagnosis at operation.

is more common in adenomas related to oral contraceptive use (66%) (Fig. 44.3); while asymptomatic lesions are more common in those not associated with use (20–50%). Rarely, adenomas may be associated with hepatocellular carcinoma.

*Investigations*

Liver function tests are usually normal although minor increases of serum transaminases or alkaline phosphatase may occur. Serum alpha-fetoprotein levels are normal. Ultrasonography is the initial imaging investigation of choice and can detect nearly 95% of cases. CT and MRI are similarly efficacious and localize a vascular mass in addition to defining anatomic characteristics which will help to plan resection. These investigations will not reliably differentiate an adenoma from focal nodular hyperplasia. Percutaneous liver biopsy should not be performed because of tumor vascularity. However, as with hemangiomas, fine-needle aspiration guided by ultrasound is reasonably safe.

*Treatment*

The treatment of choice is surgical resection and the prognosis is excellent thereafter. Adenomas associated with oral contraceptive use may regress after discontinuation, though response is unpredictable (Buhler et al 1982, Marks et al 1988). Emergency hepatic artery ligation or embolization may be necessary to control bleeding. Rarely, transition to hepatocellular carcinoma has been reported in an adenoma and this potential should prompt resection of most adenomas (Foster & Berman 1994).

## BENIGN LIVER NODULES

The nodular liver lesions constitute a confusing group of conditions for which a multitude of terms has been used (Table 44.7). Focal nodular hyperplasia has often been confused with adenoma or hepatocellular carcinoma and has variously been described as focal cirrhosis, focal nodular cirrhosis, solitary hyperplastic nodule, or isolated nodular regenerative hyperplasia. Nodular regenerative hyperplasia affects the liver generally and has been described as nodular transformation of the liver, miliary hepatocellular adenomatosis, nodular noncirrhotic liver,

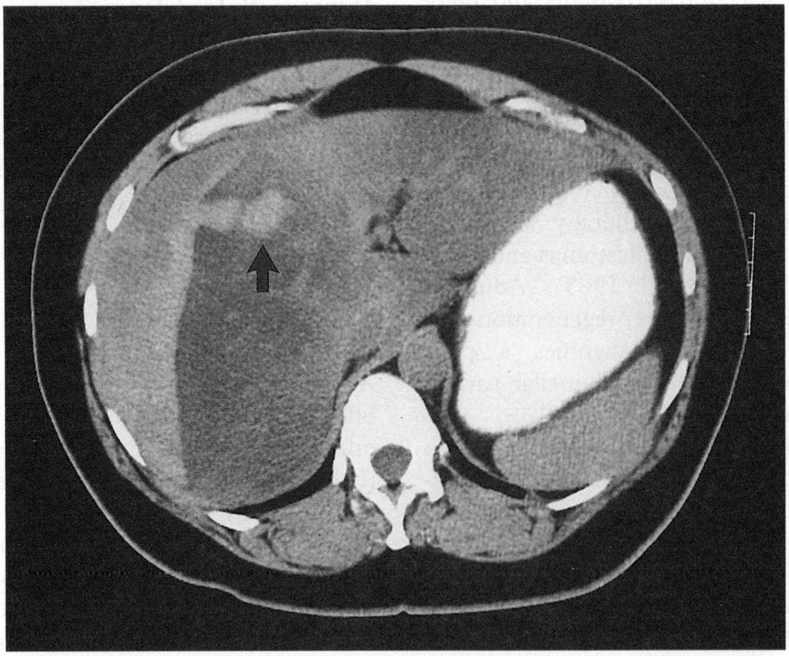

**Fig. 44.3** Hemorrhagic hepatic adenoma. CT of the liver demonstrates subcapsular hematoma from bleeding adenoma in a 38-year-old female on oral contraception. Two additional adenomata were found in resected right liver.

**Table 44.7** Conditions characterized by nodular liver lesions (Rougier et al 1978)

| Characteristics of nodules | Nodular regenerative hyperplasia of the liver | Focul nodular hyperplasia of the liver | Partial nodular transformation of the liver | Adenoma | Cirrhosis |
|---|---|---|---|---|---|
| Distribution | Diffuse | Single | Perihilar | Single (occasionally multiple) | Diffuse |
| Size | Small | Large | Large | Large | Small or large |
| Associated fibrosis | Absent or slight | Limited to lesion | Absent or slight | Absent or slight | Marked |
| Liver cell abnormality | None | None | None | None | Present |

and noncirrhotic portal hypertension. Partial nodular transformation of the liver usually affects the hepatic hilum, but nodules can occur elsewhere in the liver and patients have been described with the lesions of nodular regenerative hyperplasia, partial nodular transformation, and even idiopathic portal hypertension (p. 1085), making it possible that these conditions are part of a spectrum of diseases (Shedlofsky et al 1980, Wanless et al 1985). Hepatocellular adenoma is described above and cirrhosis elsewhere (p. 916).

### **Focal nodular hyperplasia of the liver** (Nichols et al 1990)

Focal nodular hyperplasia of the liver occurs more frequently than hepatocellular adenoma. There is no age predominance, but 80% of patients are female. The condition may be confused with hepatic adenoma, but unlike adenoma there is no causal association with oral contraceptive steroids. The cause is unknown, but it has been postulated that it is an abnormal regenerative response to vascular liver injury. The lesion is usually solitary, round, yellow-brown, 1–7 cm in diameter and situated immediately under the liver capsule. Typically, it has a central scar with fine stellate septa and surface nodularity similar to cirrhosis. Microscopically, it contains all hepatic parenchymal components surrounded by variably vascularized connective tissue stroma and mimics a focus of cirrhosis. The lesion is almost always asymptomatic and requires removal only if its size causes symptoms. Diagnosis is made by ultrasonography, CT, MRI and angiography (which shows a vascular lesion with a focal central scar and an intense capillary blush) (Rogers et al 1981, Welch et al 1985). Technetium-labeled colloid will concentrate within most lesions because of the presence of Kupffer cells. Therefore, the technetium scan should be normal and any filling defects point to the presence of other pathology. Focal nodular hyperplasia has no malignant potential.

### **Nodular regenerative hyperplasia of the liver** (Rougier et al 1978, Stromeyer & Ishak 1981)

Nodular regenerative hyperplasia of the liver is a rare condition in which small hepatocyte nodules are found diffusely throughout the liver. Unlike cirrhosis, fibrosis is slight or absent and does not surround the nodules (Fig. 44.4). It is commonly found in older patients and only rarely in childhood. Frequently this condition is associated with rheumatoid arthritis, Felty's syndrome, renal transplantation, Crohn's disease and hematological diseases. Immunosuppressive drugs and corticosteroids have been implicated etiologically, as has the toxic oil syndrome produced by the ingestion of adulterated cooking oil (Solis-Herruzo et al 1986). The cause is unknown, but an abnormal healing response of the liver to injury has been postulated. The patient usually presents with an abdominal mass. A mixed intrahepatic portal hypertension may be present, presumably as a result of distortion of the hepatic vasculature by the nodules. Liver function remains good and there is no jaundice, ascites, hypoalbuminemia or prolongation of prothrombin time. There is no association with chronic hepatitis B virus infection or with cirrhosis. Serum alpha-fetoprotein concentration is usually normal. Needle biopsies may be normal and a surgical wedge biopsy is preferable for making the diagnosis. The prognosis is good, but liver cell dysplasia may occur and progression to hepatocellular carcinoma has been reported.

### **Partial nodular transformation of the liver**

This is also a rare disease in which nodules are found in the perihilar region. As in nodular regenerative hyperplasia, the nodules may cause portal hypertension while liver function remains good. The diagnosis cannot be made from a needle biopsy, as the rest of the liver is normal or atrophic. The cause is unknown.

## SECONDARY LIVER TUMORS

Metastatic or secondary tumors are the most common malignant tumors of the liver in Western countries and may originate from primary tumors in any part of the body (Table 44.8). The liver is affected by metastatic tumor more frequently than any other organ and is the site of secondary tumor in a third of autopsies involving malignant disease (Willis 1973). Most tumors reach the liver through the

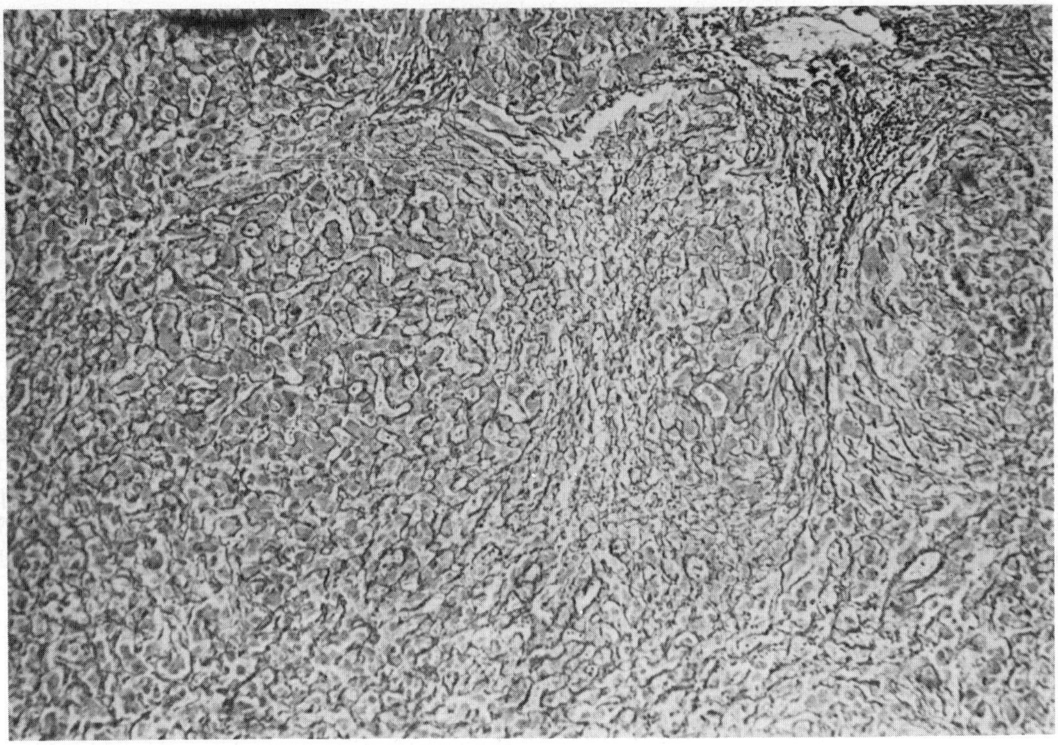

**Fig. 44.4** Nodular regenerative hyperplasia. Note regenerating nodules outlined by compressed reticulin (reticulin, ×4).

**Table 44.8** Frequency of secondary carcinoma in the liver at autopsy (Willis 1973)

| Primary site | Frequency (%) of hepatic metastases Literature survey | Willis |
|---|---|---|
| All sites | – | 36 |
| Portal | – | 48 |
| Extraportal | – | 31 |
| Esophagus | 27 | 41 |
| Stomach | 33 | 46 |
| Pancreas | 60 | 73 |
| Large bowel | 33 | 53 |
| Lung | 39 | 47 |
| Breast | 41 | 49 |
| Uterus | 12 | 20 |

blood. Intra-abdominal malignancies gain access via the portal venous system and extra-abdominal malignancies via the hepatic artery. Tumors arising in organs drained by the portal venous system are particularly prone to metastasize to the liver (Table 44.8). Tumors may also reach the liver via the lymphatic system, by invading and growing along portal or hepatic veins, or (less frequently) by direct invasion.

## **Pathology** (Willis 1973)

Metastatic tumors usually grow as well-defined spheres and are randomly distributed throughout the liver. There are usually multiple deposits. Size varies widely and often the volume of metastatic disease greatly exceeds that of the primary tumor. Most secondary tumors are hard and white and are often umbilicated from central necrosis. Foci of secondary tumors may become hemorrhagic or liquefied. Occasionally, there may be diffuse invasion of the liver, especially in the case of malignant melanoma or breast carcinoma, and rarely a marked scirrhous reaction may mimic cirrhosis. Secondary tumors may reproduce the histological structure of the tissue of origin, indicating the likely primary site, though often the liver deposit is anaplastic and its origin is obscure.

The liver is also frequently involved in the malignant reticuloses (p. 1104). Lymphosarcoma, reticulum cell sarcoma and occasionally myeloma or macroglobulinemia may involve the portal tracts and malignant cells may also be seen in the sinusoids. In particular, Hodgkin's disease frequently involves the liver. The diagnosis may be difficult to make on needle biopsy alone.

## Clinical features

Asymptomatic secondary growths in the liver may be found during the investigation of complaints arising from a primary tumor or its metastases elsewhere. Occasionally, liver metastases are the first or only indication of disease. Clinical features may mimic those of hepatocellular carcinoma except that the clinical stigmata of cirrhosis are present. Abdominal distention and discomfort, pain of varying degrees or a dragging sensation due to hepatic enlargement are the most common complaints. Jaundice may occur, but is usually mild unless there is widespread hepatic invasion or the major bile ducts are obstructed. Pruritus and skin excoriation often accompany jaundice. Peritoneal seedlings may cause ascites and compression of the inferior vena cava may cause edema of the legs. In regions where the incidence of hepatocellular carcinoma is low, a large irregular liver in an adult is usually indicative of hepatic metastases. Auscultation occasionally reveals a friction rub but rarely a bruit, as the common secondary hepatic tumors are generally of low vascularity. Constitutional symptoms of advanced malignancy such as fatigue, malaise, weight loss and fever are common. Flushing, plethora, diarrhea and wheezing suggest a carcinoid tumor.

The liver may be involved in any of the lymphoproliferative disorders. Hepatic involvement indicates an advanced stage of disease. Rarely, however, a malignant lymphoma may present as a primary hepatic disease (Colby & LaBrecque 1982).

## Diagnosis

The diagnosis of secondary liver tumor involves the same imaging strategy as that for hepatocellular carcinoma (pp. 55 & 61). Usually, a diagnostic problem arises only if the primary tumor and other metastases are asymptomatic. If multiple lesions are present on imaging and malignancy is confirmed on liver biopsy or fine-needle aspiration, an extensive, time-consuming search for the primary tumor is inappropriate. Unless potential therapy has significant palliative potential (e.g. in the case of the carcinoid syndrome), prolonged investigation for a primary tumor in a patient with a poor clinical performance status is contraindicated.

## Investigations

Diagnostic laboratory studies are similar to those used for hepatocellular carcinoma. Liver function tests are almost always abnormal, but abnormalities are nonspecific and may be minor in spite of extensive growths. Plasma alkaline phosphatase activity is the test most frequently abnormal. Serum alpha-fetoprotein concentration is usually normal except for some germ cell malignancies. The serum carcinoembryonic antigen (CEA) concentration is often increased in patients with colorectal cancer, but its value is limited as increased concentrations occur in other liver diseases.

Imaging is useful for localizing metastases and may help to differentiate them from hepatocellular carcinoma or hepatic abscess. Final confirmation is dependent on histopathology. Definitive diagnosis is easily accomplished by biopsy or aspiration cytology. Preferably, needle biopsy or aspiration cytology should be guided by ultrasonography, CT or laparoscopy to avoid false negative findings and reduce the risk of complications such as intraperitoneal hemorrhage and viscus perforation.

## Prognosis

The prognosis for patients with untreated secondary carcinoma of the liver is poor (Table 44.9). Half of the patients are dead within 3 months and fewer than 10% survive beyond a year (Bengmark et al 1972). The best prognoses are associated with neuroendocrine and carcinoid tumors, and to a lesser extent with metastatic colonic and rectal carcinoma (see below).

## Treatment

Symptomatic treatment is all that can be offered to most patients with secondary carcinoma of the liver, as their metastases are usually multiple and widely scattered in the organ. The survival of these patients is short, especially where jaundice, ascites, grossly abnormal liver function tests, or a greatly enlarged liver indicate extensive invasion by tumor. Chemotherapy has been used, but its benefits are limited and its potential complications considerable. The most encouraging results have been obtained in patients with hepatic metastases from carcinomas of the colon and rectum and in patients with neuroendocrine tumours. Patients with hepatic lymphomas may benefit from chemotherapy (p. 1104).

*Metastatic colonic and rectal carcinoma* (Rosen et al 1995)

The rationale for operative intervention for metastatic colonic and rectal carcinoma is that the natural history of untreated liver metastases is dismal and that prolonged survival is possible after liver resection. Median survival for patients with untreated metastases is less than 2 years and survival for 5 years is exceedingly rare (Table 44.9). Wagner et al (1984) compared 116 patients treated by potentially curative liver resection with a group of 70 patients with potentially resectable metastases who did not undergo liver resection. Five-year survival was 25% for the resection group but only 2% for the patients who did not undergo resection (Fig. 44.5). Scheele et al (1990) have recently reported similar results from Germany.

**Table 44.9** Survival of patients with hepatic metastases related to the site of the primary carcinoma (Bengmark et al 1972)

| Primary site | Survival | |
|---|---|---|
| | Median (days) | One year (%) |
| Stomach | 90 | 9 |
| Pancreas/biliary | 60 | 3 |
| Colon/rectum | 90 | 21 |
| Breast | 120 | 13 |

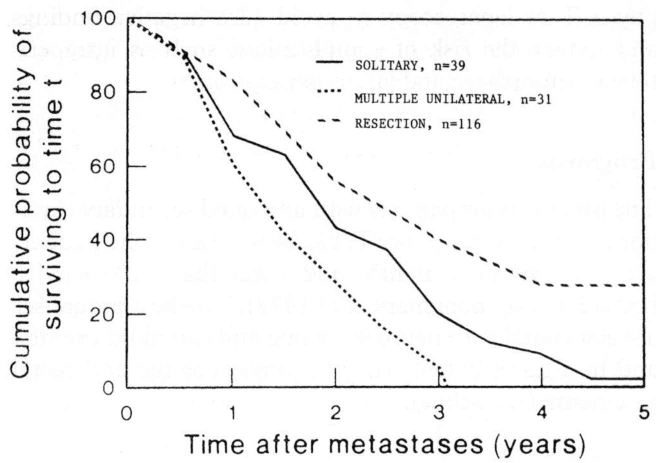


**Fig. 44.5** Comparison of the survival of 116 patients who had solitary and multiple hepatic metastases *resected* without evidence of residual primary tumor or extrahepatic metastases with 70 patients who had *unresected* potentially resectable solitary and multiple hepatic metastases (Wagner et al 1984).

Two large registries (Hughes et al 1988, Nordlinger et al 1992) and many single centers have reported 5-year survival rates of 25–35% for patients with metastatic colonic and rectal carcinoma (Schlag et al 1990, Younes et al 1991, Scheele et al 1991, Doci et al 1991, Rosen et al 1992). Clinical presentation with symptoms or an elevation of serum alkaline phosphatase, extensive liver involvement, multiplicity of lesions, satellite configuration of multiple metastases and extrahepatic or locally recurrent disease all suggest advanced disease and portend a poor prognosis (Rosen et al 1995). Despite complete removal of all known tumor, over 90% of patients in most series eventually succumb to metastatic disease (Rosen et al 1995). The most frequent sites for reappearance of tumor are the liver, lungs and peritoneal cavity. A few highly selected patients have undergone repeat liver resections and surprisingly, the results are similar to those achieved with initial liver resection (Nordlinger et al 1992, Que & Nagorney 1994).

Cryosurgery has been shown to be a safe method of treatment of metastatic liver tumors. Tumor responses have been demonstrated by decreases in serum levels of tumor markers (e.g. carcinoembryonic antigen) and tumor size (demonstrated by cross-sectional imaging studies). However, the ability of cryoablation to prolong life has yet to be demonstrated (Ravikumar 1995) and treatment is reserved for patients with tumors which are not amenable to potentially curative resection (Ravikumar 1995).

Hepatic arterial chemotherapy has also been shown to decrease tumor size and serum levels of tumor markers in patients with metastatic disease not amenable to resection. Several large trials have shown a greater response rate for patients treated with hepatic arterial chemotherapy as opposed to systemic chemotherapy. However, none of the studies show a survival advantage for either group (Kemeny & Seiter 1995).

*Metastatic neuroendocrine tumors*

Neuroendocrine tumors which metastasize to the liver include carcinoid tumor, insulinoma, glucagonoma, polyfunctioning islet-cell carcinoma, gastrinoma and nonfunctioning neuroendocrine tumors. These tumors are rare and have in common a protracted natural history with slow tumor growth.

Incapacitating symptoms often occur due to excessive hormone production. Que et al (1995) reported a series of 74 patients treated by liver resection. Diarrhea and flushing were very common with carcinoid tumors. Other symptoms due to carcinoid tumor included abdominal pain and distention, wheezing, syncope, nausea, vomiting and borborygmi. Glucagonoma caused anorexia, weight loss and necrolytic migratory erythema. Diarrhea was common with gastrinoma. Islet-cell carcinomas caused diarrhea, epigastric pain, fatigue, weight loss and lightheadedness.

The natural history of these rare tumors is not known, but prolonged survival is possible. Thirty to 40% 5-year survival rates and 3- to 4-year median survival have been reported for untreated or unresponsive patients with metastases from carcinoid and islet-cell carcinomas (Moertel et al 1994, Thompson et al 1988).

The goals of therapy for metastatic neuroendocrine tumors are prolongation of life and amelioration of incapacitating symptoms. Therapeutic options include systemic chemotherapy, hepatic artery occlusion or embolization and liver resection. Systemic chemotherapy has afforded tumor regression in less than one-third of patients and relief of symptoms has been brief (Moertel 1989). Octreotide (Sandostatin) effectively lowers hormone levels and affords complete or substantial relief of symptoms in nearly 80% of patients (Kvols et al 1986, 1987) but long-term treatment is very expensive. Symptoms eventually become refractory to treatment and actual tumor regression is uncommon. Tumor regression has been observed in 60% of patients treated by hepatic arterial occlusion and 80% of patients treated with arterial occlusion and chemotherapy (Moertel et al 1994). In a series of 123 patients with hepatic metastases treated by arterial occlusion and subsequent chemotherapy, median survival was 49 months for patients with carcinoid tumor and 35 months for those with islet-cell carcinoma (Moertel et al 1994).

Resection of liver metastases has also been shown to be safe, provide effective palliation and probably prolong survival (Que et al 1995). In a series of 74 patients treated by liver resection, perioperative mortality was 2.7% and 4-year survival rate was 73%. Ninety percent of patients experienced partial or complete amelioration of symptoms for a mean duration of 19.3 months. The clinical response was related directly to the amount of resected tumor and indirectly to the amount of residual disease. Patients were selected for operation if imaging studies (CT and MRI) suggested that the primary and regional tumor and at least

90% of the hepatic tumor volume were resectable. Echocardiography was performed to evaluate the heart and its valves (for patients with carcinoid syndrome) and perioperative somatostatin analog (octreotide) was used to prevent carcinoid crisis.

A few patients with completely controlled local and regional disease and no extrahepatic disease have been treated by orthotopic liver transplantation (Makowka et al 1989, Arnold et al 1989). Although complete relief of symptoms has been achieved, follow-up and overall experience is too limited to advocate widespread use of this approach.

## REFERENCES


Arnold J C, O'Grady J G, Bird G L, Calne R Y, Williams R 1989 Liver transplantation for primary and secondary hepatic apudomas. British Journal of Surgery 76: 248–249

Arthur M J P, Hall A J, Wright R 1984 Hepatitis B, hepatocellular carcinoma, and strategies for prevention. Lancet 1: 607–610

Beasley R P 1982 Hepatitis B virus as the etiologic agent in hepatocellular carcinoma – epidemiologic considerations. Hepatology 2: 21S

Bengmark S, Hafström L, Olsson A 1972 The natural history of primary and secondary liver tumours. V. The prognosis for conventionally treated patients with liver metastases from breast cancer. Digestion 6: 321

Berland L, Lee J K T, Stanley R J 1989 Liver and biliary tract. In: Lee J K T, Sagel S S, Stanley R J (eds) Computed body tomography with MRI correlation, 2nd edn. Raven Press, New York, p 593–659

Bismuth H, Chiche L, Adam R, Castaing D, Diamond T, Dennison A 1993 Liver resection versus transplantation for hepatocellular carcinoma in cirrhotic patients. Annals of Surgery 218: 145–151

Bornman P C, Krige J E J 1994 Liver biopsy and laparoscopy. In: Terblanche J (ed) Hepatobiliary malignancy: its multidisciplinary management. Edward Arnold, London, p 100–105

Bradbear R A, Bain C, Siskind V et al 1985 Cohort study of internal malignancy in genetic hemochromatosis and other chronic nonalcoholic liver diseases. Journal of the National Cancer Institute 75: 81–84

Bradley D W, Maynard J E, McCaustland K A, Murphy B L, Cook E H, Ebert J W 1983 Non-A non-B hepatitis in chimpanzees: interference with acute hepatitis A virus and chronic hepatitis B virus infections. Journal of Medical Virology 11: 207–213

Bréchot C, Degos F, Lugassy C et al 1985 Hepatitis B virus DNA in patients with chronic liver disease and negative tests for hepatitis B surface antigen. New England Journal of Medicine 312: 270–276

Brotman B, Prince A M, Huima T, Richardson L, van den Ende M C, Pfeifer U 1983 Interference between non-A, non-B and hepatitis-B virus infection in chimpanzees. Journal of Madical Virology 11: 191–205

Bruix J, Barrera J M, Calvet X et al 1989 Prevalence of antibodies to hepatitis C virus in Spanish patients with hepatocellular carcinoma and hepatic cirrhosis. Lancet 2: 1004–1006

Buamah P K, Gibb I, Bates G, Ward A M 1984 Serum alpha-fetoprotein heterogeneity as a means of differentiating between primary hepatocellular carcinoma and hepatic secondaries. Clinica Chimica Acta 139: 313–316

Bühler H, Pirovino M, Akovbiantz A et al 1982 Regression of liver cell adenoma. A follow-up study of three consecutive patients after discontinuation of oral contraceptive use. Gastroenterology 82: 775–782

Caporaso N, Romano M, Marmo R, deSio I, Morisco F, Minerva A, Coltorti M 1991 Hepatitis C virus infection is an additive risk factor for development of hepatocellular carcinoma in patients with cirrhosis. Journal of Hepatology 12: 367–371

Carr B I, Selby R, Madariaga J, Iwatsuki S, Starzl T E 1993 Prolonged survival after liver transplantation and cancer chemotherapy for advanced-stage hepatocellular carcinoma. Transplantation Proceedings 25: 1128–1129

Chandra R S, Kapur S P, Kelleher J Jr, Luban N, Patterson K 1984 Benign hepatocellular tumors in the young. A clinicopathologic spectrum. Archives of Pathology and Laboratory Medicine 108: 168–171

Cobden I, Bassendine M F, James O F W 1986 Hepatocellular carcinoma in north-east England: importance of hepatitis B infection and ex-tropical military service. Quarterly Journal of Medicine 60: 855–863

Cochrane M, Williams R 1976 Humoral effects of hepatocellular carcinoma. In: Okuda K, Peters R L (eds) Hepatocellular carcinoma. Wiley, New York, p 333–352

Cohen C, Berson S D, Geddes E W 1979 Liver cell dysplasia. Association with hepatocellular carcinoma, cirrhosis and hepatitis B antigen carrier status. Cancer 44: 1671–1676

Colby T V, LaBrecque D R 1982 Lymphoreticular malignancy presenting as fulminant hepatic disease. Gastroenterology 82: 339–345

Colombo M, De Franchis R, Del Ninno et al 1991 Hepatocellular carcinoma in Italian Patients with cirrhosis. New England Journal of Medicine 325: 675–680

Colombo M, Kuo G, Choo Q L et al 1989 Prevalence of antibodies to hepatitis C virus in Italian patients with hepatocellular carcinoma. Lancet 2: 1006–1008

Cottone M, Marceno M P, Maringhini A et al 1983 Ultrasound in the diagnosis of hepatocellular carcinoma associated with cirrhosis. Radiology 147: 517–519

Deugnier Y M, Guyader D, Crantock L et al 1993 Primary liver cancer in genetic hemochromatosis: a clinical, pathological, and pathogenetic study of 54 cases. Gastroenterology 104: 228–234

Di Bisceglie A M, Order S E, Klein J L et al 1991 The role of chronic viral hepatitis in hepatocellular carcinoma in the United States. American Journal of Gastroenterology 86: 335–338

Doci R, Gennari L, Bignami P, Montalto F, Morabito A, Bozzetti F 1991 One hundred patients with hepatic metastases from colorectal cancer treated by resection: analysis of prognostic determinants. British Journal of Surgery 78: 797–801

Doty J E, Tompkins R K 1989 Management of cystic disease of the liver. Surgical Clinics of North America 69: 285–295

Dubbins P A, O'Riordan D, Melia W M 1981 Ultrasound in hepatoma – can a specific diagnosis be made? British Journal of Radiology 54: 307–311

Ehren H, Mahour G H, Isaacs H Jr 1983 Benign liver tumors in infancy and childhood. Report of 48 cases. American Journal of Surgery 145: 325–329

Enwonwu C O 1984 The role of dietary aflatoxin in the genesis of hepatocellular cancer in developing countries. Lancet 2: 956–958

Ezekowitz R A B, Mulliken J B, Folkman J 1992 Interferon alfa-2a therapy for life-threatening hemangiomas of infancy. New England Journal of Medicine 326: 1456–1463

Falkson G, MacIntyre J M, Moertel C G, Johnson L A, Scherman R C 1984 Primary liver cancer. An Eastern Cooperative Oncology Group trial. Cancer 54: 970–977

Fargion S, Mandelli C, Piperno A et al 1992 Survival and prognostic factors in 212 Italian patients with genetic hemochromatosis. Hepatology 15: 655–659

Farinati F, Fagiuoli S, De Maria N et al 1992 Anti-HCV-positive hepatocellular carcinoma in cirrhosis: prevalence, risk factors, and clinical features. Journal of Hepatology 14: 183–187

Flejou J-F, Barge J, Menu Y et al 1985 Liver adenomatosis. An entity distinct from liver adenoma? Gastroenterology 89: 1132–1136

Fong T-L, Di Bisceglie A M, Waggoner J G, Banks S M, Hoofnagle J H 1991 The significance of antibody to hepatitis-C virus in patients with chronic hepatitis B. Hepatology 14: 64–67

Forbes A, Portmann B, Johnson P, Williams R 1987 Hepatic sarcomas in adults: a review of 25 cases. Gut 28: 668–674

Foster J H, Berman M M 1994 The malignant transformation of liver cell adenomas. Archives of Surgery 129: 712–717

Friedman M A, Demanes D J, Hoffman P G Jr 1982 Hepatomas: hormone receptors and therapy. American Journal of Medicine 73: 362–366

Gerber M A, Shieh Y S C, Shim K-S et al 1992 Detection of replicative hepatitis C virus sequences in hepatocellular carcinoma. American Journal of Pathology 141: 1271–1277
Gores G J 1993 Liver transplantation for malignant disease. Gastroenterology Clinics of North America 22: 285–299
Gores G J, Wahlstrom H E, Sanchez-Urdazpal L et al 1992 Stage II hepatocellular carcinoma: accuracy of preoperative staging and results with orthotopic liver transplantation. Abstract booklet of the International Liver Transplantation Society, p 32
Hasan F, Jeffers L J, DeMedina M et al 1990 Hepatitis C-associated hepatocellular carcinoma. Hepatology 12: 589–591
Havard A C, Collins D J, Guy R L, Husband J E 1992 Magnetic resonance behaviour of Lipiodol. Clinical Radiology 45: 198–200
Heyward W L, Lanier A P, Bender T R et al 1981 Primary hepatocellular carcinoma in Alaskan natives, 1969–1979. International Journal of Cancer 28: 47–50
Heyward W L, Lanier A P, McMahon B J, Fitzgerald M A, Kilkenny S, Paprocki T R 1985 Early detection of primary hepatocellular carcinoma. Screening for primary hepatocellular carcinoma among persons infected with hepatitis B virus. Journal of the American Medical Association 254: 3052–3054
Hirai K, Aoki Y, Majima Y et al 1991 Magnetic resonance imaging of small hepatocellular carcinoma. American Journal of Gastroenterology 86: 205–209
Ho J C I, Wu P-C, Mak T-K 1981 Liver cell dysplasia in association with hepatocellular carcinoma, cirrhosis and hepatitis B surface antigen in Hong Kong. International Journal of Cancer 28: 571–574
Houghton M, Weiner A, Han J, Kuo G, Choo Q-L 1991 Molecular biology of hepatitis C viruses: implications for diagnosis, development, and control of viral disease. Hepatology 14: 381–388
Hughes K S, Simon R, Songhorabodi S et al 1988 Resection of the liver for colorectal carcinoma metastases: a multi-institutional study of indications for resection. Surgery 103: 278–288
Ihde D C, Matthews M J, Makuch R W, McIntire K R, Eddy J L, Seff L B 1985 Prognostic factors in patients with hepatocellular carcinoma receiving systemic chemotherapy. American Journal of Medicine 78: 399–406
Inamoto K, Tanaka S, Yamazaki H, Okamoto E 1983 Computed tomography in the detection of small hepatocellular carcinomas. Gastrointestinal Radiology 8: 321–326
Ishak K G, Sesterhenn I A, Goodman M Z D, Rabin L, Stromeyer F W 1984 Epithelioid hemangioendothelioma of the liver: a clinicopathologic and follow-up study of 32 cases. Human Pathology 15: 839–852
Itoh K, Nishimura K, Togshi K et al 1987 Hepatocellular carcinoma: MR imaging. Radiology 164: 21–25
Iwatsuki S, Starzl T E 1988 Personal experience with 411 hepatic resections. Annals of Surgery 208: 421–434
Iwatsuki S, Starzl T E, Sheahan D G et al 1991 Hepatic resection versus transplantation for hepatocellular carcinoma. Annals of Surgery 214: 221–229
Jeng J-E, Tsai J-F 1991 Hepatitis C virus antibody in hepatocellular carcinoma in Taiwan. Journal of Medical Virology 34: 74–77
Kaklamani E, Trichopoulos D, Tzonou A et al 1991 Hepatitis B and C viruses and their interaction in the origin of hepatocellular carcinoma. Journal of the American Medical Association 265: 1974–1976
Karawi M A, Shariq S, el Sheikh Mohamed A R, Saeed A A, Ahmed A M 1992 Hepatitis-C virus infection in chronic liver disease and hepatocelluar carcinoma in Saudi Arabia. Journal of Gastroenterology and Hepatology 7: 237–239
Kemeny N E, Seiter K 1995 Hepatic bacterial chemotherapy. In: Cohen A M, Winawer S J, Friedman M A, Gunderson L L (eds) Cancer of the colon, rectum, and anus. McGraw-Hill, New York, p 831–843
Ken M D 1990 Tumors of the liver. In: Zakim D, Boyer T D (eds) Hepatology. A textbook of liver diseases, 2nd edn. W B Saunders, Philadelphia, p 1206–1240
Kew M C, Geddes E W 1982 Hepatocellular carcinoma in rural Southern African blacks. Medicine 61: 98–108
Kew M C, Dos Santos H A, Sherlock S 1971 Diagnosis of primary cancer of the liver. British Medical Journal 4: 408–411
Kew M C, Rossouw E, Paterson A, Hodkinson J, Whitcutt M, Dusheiko G 1983 Hepatitis B virus status of black women with hepatocellular carcinoma. Gastroenterology 84: 693–696
Kew M C, Kassianides C, Hodkinson J, Coppin A, Paterson A C 1986 Hepatocellular carcinoma in urban born blacks: frequency and relation to hepatitis B virus infection. British Medical Journal 293: 1339–1341
Kingston J E, Herbert A, Draper G J, Mann J R 1983 Association between hepatoblastoma and polyposis coli. Archives of Disease in Childhood 58: 959–962
Klatskin G 1977 Hepatic tumors: possible relationship to use of oral contraceptives. Gastroenterology 73: 386–394
Kojiro M, Kawano Y, Isomura T, Nakashima T 1981 Distribution of albumin- and/or α-fetoprotein-positive cells in hepatocellular carcinoma. Laboratory Investigation 44: 221–226
Kojiro M, Nakahara H, Sugihara S, Murakami T, Nakashima T, Kawasaki H 1984 Hepatocellular carcinoma with intra-atrial tumor growth. A clinicopathologic study of 18 autopsy cases. Archives of Pathology and Laboratory Medicine 108: 989–992
Kubo Y, Okuda K, Musha H, Nakashima T 1978 Detection of hepatocellular carcinoma during a clinical follow-up of chronic liver disease. Observations in 31 patients. Gastroenterology 74: 578–582
Kvols L K, Moertel C G, O'Connell M J, Schutt A J, Rubin J, Hahn R G 1986 Treatment of the malignant carcinoid syndrome: evaluation of a long-acting somatostatin analogue. New England Journal of Medicine 315: 663–666
Kvols L K, Buck M, Moertel C G et al 1987 Treatment of metastatic islet cell carcinoma with a somatostatin analogue (SMS 201–995). Annals of Internal Medicine 107: 162–168
La Berge J M, Laing F C, Federle M P, Jeffrey R B Jr, Lim R C Jr 1984 Hepatocellular carcinoma: assessment of resectability by computed tomography and ultrasound. Radiology 152: 485–490
Lai C L, Lam K C, Wong K P, Wu P C, Todd D 1981 Clinical features of hepatocellular carcinoma: review of 211 patients in Hong Kong. Cancer 47: 2746–2755
Larcher V F, Howard E R, Mowat A P 1981 Hepatic haemangiomata: diagnosis and management. Archives of Disease in Childhood 56: 7–14
Lawson D H, Gray J M B, McKillop C, Clarke J, Lee F D, Patrick R S 1986 Diabetes mellitus and primary hepatocellular carcinoma. Quarterly Journal of Medicine 61: 945–955
Levrero M, Tagger A, Balsano C et al 1991 Antibodies to hepatitis C virus in patients with hepatocellular carcinoma. Journal of Hepatology 12: 60–63
Liang T J, Jeffers L J, Reddy K R et al 1993 Viral pathogenesis of hepatocellular carcinoma in the United States. Hepatology 18: 1326–1333
Liaw Y-F, Tai D-I, Chu C-M et al 1986 Early detection of hepatocellular carcinoma in patients with chronic type B hepatitis. A prospective study. Gastroenterology 90: 263–267
Lieberman H M, Shafritz D A 1986 Persistent hepatitis B virus infection and hepatocellular carcinoma. In: Popper H, Schaffner F (eds) Progress in liver diseases, Vol 8. Grune and Stratton, New York, pp 395–415
Linsell C A, Peers F G 1977 Aflatoxin and liver cell cancer. Transactions of the Royal Society of Tropical Medicine and Hygiene 71: 471–473
Lithner F, Wetterberg L 1984 Hepatocellular carcinoma in patients with acute intermittent porphyria. Acta Medica Scandinavica 215: 271–274
Livraghi T, Bolondi L, Lazzaroni S et al 1992 Percutaneous ethanol injection in the treatment of hepatocellular carcinoma in cirrhosis: a study of 207 patients. Cancer 69: 925–929
Makowka L, Tzakis A G, Mazzaferro V et al 1989 Transplantation of the liver for metastatic endocrine tumors of the intestine and pancreas. Surgery, Gynecology and Obstetrics 168: 107–111
Marino I R, Todo S, Tzakis A G et al 1988 Treatment of hepatic epithelioid hemangioendothelioma with liver transplantation. Cancer 62: 2079–2084
Marks W H, Thompson N, Appleman H 1988 Failure of hepatic adenomas (HCA) to regress after discontinuance of oral contraceptives. An association with focal nodular hyperplasia (FNH) and uterine leiomyoma. Annals of Surgery 208: 190–195
Mazella G, Accogli E, Sottili et al 1996 Alpha interferon treatment may prevent hepatocellular carcinoma in HIV-related cirrhosis. Journal of Hepatology 24: 141–147
McGill D B, Rakela J, Zinsmeister A R, Ott B J 1990 A 21-year

experience with major hemorrhage after percutaneous liver biopsy. Gastroenterology 99: 1396–1400
Moertel C G 1989 An odyssey in the land of small tumors. Journal of Clinical Oncology 5: 1503–1522
Moertel C G, Johnson C M, McKusick M A et al 1994 The management of patients with advanced carcinoid tumors and islet cell carcinomas. Annals of Internal Medicine 120: 302–309
Nagorney D M, Adson M A, Weiland L H, Knight C D Jr, Smalley S R, Zinsmeister A R 1985 Fibrolamellar hepatoma. American Journal of Surgery 149: 113–119
Nagorney D M, van Heerden J A, Ilstrup D M, Adson M A 1989 Primary hepatic malignancy: surgical management and determinants of survival. Surgery 106: 740–749
Nakashima T, Okuda K, Kojiro M et al 1983 Pathology of hepatocellular carcinoma in Japan. 232 consecutive cases autopsied in ten years. Cancer 51: 863–877
Neuberger J, Forman D, Doll R, Williams R 1986 Oral contraceptives and hepatocellular carcinoma. British Medical Journal 292: 1355–1357
Nichols F C III, van Heerden J A, Weiland L H 1990 Benign liver tumors. Surgical Clinics of North America 69: 297–314
Nicholson K G 1985 Hepatitis delta infections. British Medical Journal 290: 1370–1371
Niederau C, Fischer R, Sonnenberg A, Stremmel W, Trampisch J H, Strohmeyer G 1985 Survival and causes of death in cirrhotic and in noncirrhotic patients with primary hemochromatosis. New England Journal of Medicine 313: 1256–1262
Nishiguchi S, Kuroki A, Nakatani S et al 1995 Randomised trial of effects of interferon-α on incidence of hepatocellular carcinoma in chronic active hepatitis. Lancet 346: 1051–1055
Nishioka K, Watanabe J, Furuta S et al 1991 A high prevalence of antibody to the hepatitis-C virus in patients with hepatocellular carcinoma in Japan. Cancer 67: 429–433
Nordlinger B, Jaeck D, Guiget M et al 1992 Multicentric retrospective study by the French Surgical Association. In: Nordlinger B, Jaaeck D (eds) Treatment of hepatic metastases of colorectal cancer. Springer-Verlag, Paris, p 129–146
Okuda H, Okuda K 1991 Primary liver cell carcinoma. In: McIntyre N, Benhamou J-P, Bircher J, Rizzetto M, Rodes J (eds) Oxford textbook of clinical hepatology. Oxford University Press, Oxford, p 1019–1052
Okuda K 1992 Hepatocellular carcinoma: recent progress. Hepatology 15: 948–963
Okuda K 1994 Other therapies. In: Terblanche J (ed) Hepatobiliary malignancy: its multidisciplinary management. Edward Arnold, London, p 145–157
Okuda K, Ohtsuki T, Obata H et al 1985 Natural history of hepatocellular carcinoma and prognosis in relation to treatment. Study of 850 patients. Cancer 56: 918–928
Oldenburg W A, van Heerden J A, Sizemore G W, Abboud C F, Sheedy P F II 1982 Hypercalcemia and primary hepatic tumors. Archives of Surgery 117: 1363–1366
Omata M, Ashcavai M, Liew C-T, Peters R L 1979 Hepatocellular carcinoma in the U.S.A., etiologic considerations. Localization of hepatitis B antigens. Gastroenterology 76: 279–287
Paterson A C, Kew M C, Herman A A B, Becker P J, Hodkinson J, Isaacson C 1985 Liver morphology in Southern African blacks with hepatocellular carcinoma: a study within the urban environment. Hepatology 5: 72–78
Penn I 1991 Hepatic transplantation for primary and metastatic cancers of the liver. Surgery 110: 726–735
Price J B Jr, Schullinger J N, Santulli T V 1982 Major hepatic resections for neoplasia in children. Archives of Surgery 117: 1139–1141
Que F G, Nagorney D M 1994 Resection of "recurrent" colorectal metastases to the liver. British Journal of Surgery 81: 255–258
Que F G, Nagorney D M, Batts K P, Linz L J, Kvols L K 1995 Hepatic resection for neuroendocrine carcinomas. American Journal of Surgery 169: 36–43
Quinn J J, Altman A J, Robinson H T, Cooke R W, Hight D W, Foster J H 1985 Adriamycin and cisplatin for hepatoblastoma. Cancer 56: 1926–1929
Ravikumar T S 1995 Cryosurgery for hepatic metastases. In: Cohen A M, Winawer S J, Friedman M A, Gunderson L L (eds) Cancer of the colon, rectum, and anus. McGraw-Hill, New York, p 823–829
Ringe B, Wittekind C, Bechstein W O, Bunzendahl H, Pichlmayr R 1989 The role of liver transplantation in hepatobiliary malignancy. Annals of Surgery 209: 88–98
Ringe B, Pichlmayr R, Wittekind C, Tusch G 1991 Surgical treatment of hepatocellular carcinoma: experience with liver resection and transplantation in 198 patients. World Journal of Surgery 15: 270–285
Ringe B, Wittekind C, Weimann A, Tusch G, Pichlmayr R 1992 Results of hepatic resection and transplantation for fibrolamellar carcinoma. Surgery, Gynecology and Obstetrics 175: 299–305
Rogers J V, Mack L A, Freeny P C, Johnson M L, Sones P J 1981 Hepatic focal nodular hyperplasia: angiography, CT, sonography and scintigraphy. American Journal of Roentgenology 137: 983–990
Rosen C B, Nagorney D M 1993 Fibrolamellar and less aggressive hepatocellular carcinomas. In: Terblanche J (ed) Hepatobiliary malignancy: its multidisciplinary management. Edward Arnold, London, p 203–214
Rosen C B, Nagorney D M, Taswell H F et al 1992 Perioperative blood transfusion and determinants of survival after liver resection for metastatic colorectal carcinoma. Annals of Surgery 216: 493–505
Rosen C B, Donohue J H, Nagorney D M 1995 Liver resection for metastatic colonic and rectal carcinoma. In: Cohen A M, Winawer S J, Friedman M A, Gunderson L L (eds) Cancer of the colon, rectum, and anus. McGraw-Hill, New York, p 805–821
Rougier P, Degott C, Rueff B, Benhamou J-P 1978 Nodular regenerative hyperplasia of the liver. Report of six cases and review of the literature. Gastroenterology 75: 169–172
Ruiz J, Sangro B, Cuende J I, Beloqui O, Reizu-Boj J I, Herrero J I, Preito J 1992 Hepatitis B and C viral infections in patients with hepatocellular carcinoma. Hepatology 16: 637–641
Salata H, Cortés J M E, Enriquez de Salamanca R et al 1985 Porphyria cutanea tarda and hepatocellular carcinoma. Frequency of occurrence and related factors. Journal of Hepatology 1: 477–487
Scheele J, Stangl R, Altendorf-Hofmann A et al 1991 Indicators of prognosis after hepatic resection for colorectal secondaries. Surgery 110: 13–29
Scheele J, Stangl R, Altendorf-Hofmann A 1990 Hepatic metastases from colorectal carcinoma: impact of surgical resection on the natural history. British Journal of Surgery 77: 1241–1246
Schilling A, Gewiese B, Berger G et al 1992 Liver tumors: follow-up with P31 MR spectroscopy after local chemotherapy and chemotherapy and chemoembolization. Radiology 182: 887–890
Schlag P, Hohenberger P, Herfarth C 1990 Resection of liver metastases in colorectal cancer: competitive analysis of treatment result in synchronous versus metachronous metastases. European Journal of Surgical Oncology 16: 360–365
Schnatz M E 1994 Primary hepatocellular carcinoma: transplant versus resection. Seminars in Liver Disease 14: 135–139
Scoazec J-Y, Lamy P, Degott C et al 1988 Epithelioid hemangioendothelioma of the liver diagnostic features and role of liver transplantation. Gastroenterology 94: 1447–1453
Sesto M E, Vogt D P, Hermann R E 1987 Hepatic resections in 128 patients: a 24-year experience. Surgery 102: 846–851
Shafritz D A, Shouval D, Sherman H I, Hadziyannis S J, Kew M C 1981 Integration of hepatitis B virus DNA into the genome of liver cells in chronic liver disease and hepatocellular carcinoma. Studies in percutaneous liver biopsies and post-mortem tissue specimens. New England Journal of Medicine 305: 1067–1073
Shedlofsky S, Koehler R E, De Schryver-Kecskemeti K, Alpers D H 1980 Noncirrhotic nodular transformation of the liver with portal hypertension: clinical, angiographic, and pathological correlation. Gastroenterology 79: 938–943
Sheu J-C, Sung J-L, Chen D-S et al 1984 Ultrasonography of small hepatic tumors using high-resolution linear-array real-time instruments. Radiology 150: 797–802
Simonetti R G, Camma C, Fiorello F et al 1992 Hepatitis C virus infection as a risk factor for hepatocellular carcinoma in patients with cirrhosis. A case-control study. Annals of Internal Medicine 116: 97–102
Skinhøj P, Hansen J P H, Nielsen N H, Mikkelsen F 1978 Occurrence of cirrhosis and primary liver cancer in an Eskimo population hyperendemically infected with hepatitis B virus. American Journal of Epidemiology 108: 121–125
Solis-Herruzo J A, Vidal J V, Colina F, Santalla F, Castellano G 1986

Nodular regenerative hyperplasia of the liver associated with the toxic oil syndrome: report of five cases. Hepatology 6: 687–693
Stone M J, Klintmalm G B G, Polter D et al 1993 Neoadjuvant chemotherapy and liver transplantation for hepatocellular carcinoma: a pilot study in 20 patients. Gastroenterology 104: 196–202
Stromeyer F W, Ishak K G 1981 Nodular transformation (nodular regenerative hyperplasia) of the liver. A clinicopathologic study of 30 cases. Human Pathology 12: 60–71
Sugiura N, Takara K, Oho M, Hirooka N, Okuda K 1983 Treatment of small hepatocellular carcinoma by intratumor ethanol injection with the aid of ultrasound. Acta Hepatologica Japonica 24: 920
Sung J-L, Chen D-S 1980 Maternal transmission of hepatitis B surface antigen in patients with hepatocellular carcinoma in Taiwan. Scandinavian Journal of Gastroenterology 15: 321–324
Tanaka K, Hirohata T, Koga S et al 1991 Hepatitis C and hepatitis B in the etiology of hepatocellular carcinoma in the Japanese population. Cancer Research 51: 2842–2847
Tang Z-Y, Ying Y-Y, Gu T-J 1982 Hepatocellular carcinoma: changing concepts in recent years. In: Popper H, Schaffner F (eds) Progress in liver diseases, Vol 7. Grune and Stratton, New York, p 637–647
Tesluk H, Lawrie J 1981 Hepatocellular adenoma. Its transformation to carcinoma in a user of oral contraceptives. Archives of Pathology and Laboratory Medicine 105: 296–299
Thompson G B, van Heerden J A, Grant C S, Carney J A, Ilstrup D M 1988 Islet cell carcinomas of the pancreas: A twenty-year experience. Surgery 104: 1011–1017
Thompson H H, Tompkins R K, Longmire W P Jr 1983 Major hepatic resection. A 25-year experience. Annals of Surgery 197: 375–388
Vauthey J-N, Klimstra D, Franceschi D et al 1995 Factors affecting long-term outcome after hepatic resection for hepatocellular carcinoma. American Journal of Surgery 169: 28–35
Venook A P, Ferrell L D, Roberts J P 1995 Liver transplantation for hepatocellular carcinoma: Results with preoperative chemoembolization. Liver Transplantation and Surgery 1: 242
Vianni N J, Brady J A, Cardamone A T 1981 Epidemiology of angiosarcoma of liver in New York State. New York State Journal of Medicine 81: 895–899
Wagner J S, Adson M A, Van Heerden J A, Adson M H, Ilstrup D M 1984 The natural history of hepatic metastases from colorectal cancer. A comparison with resective treatment. Annals of Surgery 199: 502–508
Wanless I R, Mawdsley C, Adams R 1985 On the pathogenesis of focal nodular hyperplasia of the liver. Hepatology 5: 1194–1200
Watanabe Y, Harada S, Saito I, Miyamura T 1991 Prevalence of antibody against the core protein of hepatitis C virus in patients with hepatocellular carcinoma. International Journal of Cancer 48: 340–343
Waterhouse J, Muir C, Correa P, Powell J (eds) 1976 Cancer incidence in five continents, Vol 3. International Agency for Research into Cancer, Scientific Publications No. 15
Waterhouse J, Muir C, Shanmugaratnam K, Powell J (eds) 1982 Cancer incidence in five continents, Vol 4. International Agency for Research into Cancer, Scientific Publications No. 42
Weinberg A G, Finegold M J 1983 Primary hepatic tumors in childhood. Human Pathology 14: 512–537
Welch T J, Sheedy P F II, Johnson C M et al 1985 Focal nodular hyperplasia and hepatic adenoma: comparison of angiography, CT, US and scintigraphy. Radiology 156: 593–595
Willis R A 1973 Secondary tumours of the liver. In: The spread of tumours in the human body, 3rd edn. Butterworths, London, p 175
Yamada R, Sato M, Kawabata M, Nakatsuka K, Nakamura K, Takashima S 1983 Hepatic artery embolization in 120 patients with unresectable hepatoma. Radiology 148: 397–401
Yokoyama I, Todo S, Iwatsuki S, Starzl T E 1990 Liver transplantation in the treatment of primary liver cancer. Hepato-Gastroenterology 37: 188–193
Yokoyama I, Carr B, Saitsu H, Iwatsuki S, Starzl T E 1991 Accelerated growth rates of recurrent hepatocellular carcinoma after liver transplantation. Cancer 68: 2095–2100
Yoneyama T, Takeuchi K, Watanabe Y et al 1990 Detection of hepatitis-C virus cDNA sequence by the polymerase chain reaction in hepatocellular carcinoma tissues. Japanese Journal of Medical Science and Biology 43: 89–94
Younes R N, Rogatko A, Brennan M F 1991 The influence of intraoperative hypotension and perioperative blood transfusion on disease-free survival in patients with complete resection of colorectal liver metastases. Annals of Surgery 214: 107–113
Yuki N, Hayashi N, Kasahara A et al 1992 Hepatitis B virus markers and antibodies to hepatitis C virus in Japanese patients with hepatocellular carcinoma. Digestive Diseases and Sciences 37: 65–72
Yumoto Y, Jinno K, Tokuyama K et al 1985 Hepatocellular carcinoma detected by iodized oil. Radiology 154: 19–24
Zala G, Havelka J, Altorfer J et al 1992 Hepatitis C virus and hepatoma. Schweizerische Medizinische Wochenschrift 122: 194–197
Zaman S N, Melia W M, Johnson R D, Portmann B C, Johnson P J, Williams R 1985 Risk factors in development of hepatocellular carcinoma in cirrhosis: prospective study of 613 patients. Lancet 1: 1357–1360
Zarski J P, Lunel F, Dardelet D et al 1991 Hepatitis C virus and hepatocellular carcinoma in France: detection of antibodies using two second generation assays. Journal of Hepatology 13: 376–377

# 45. Surgery, anesthesia and the liver

*O. James Garden A. Lee*

## INTRODUCTION

Hepatic surgery is always a major undertaking and has become increasingly common in recent times. Hepatic resection is usually carried out to remove tumors and may be undertaken for the treatment of trauma to the liver. Apart from technical considerations, a major issue in such operations is the amount of liver tissue that can be removed safely. Previously normal livers regenerate vigorously after resection (p. 716), but this does not occur in cirrhotic livers and resections have to be much more limited. Patients with liver disease may need operations that may or may not be related to their liver conditions and these need to be considered carefully as liver disease increases the risks of surgery. Liver disease can also mimic other conditions for which surgery is required, leading to unnecessary operations that carry significant morbidity and mortality, and these need to be avoided. Finally, surgery may be followed by hepatic abnormalities, the causes of which are often multifactorial. These causes need to be identified and their relative importance assessed. Liver transplantation is considered elsewhere (p. 1156).

## HEPATIC OPERATIONS

### Hepatic resection

Hepatic operations are usually performed for the removal of tumors or the treatment of trauma and should be done only on patients with a previously normal liver or, where cirrhosis is present, very good liver function.

***Extent of resection.*** Patients with a previously normal liver can withstand extensive hepatic resections, but there is an increasing danger of postoperative liver failure if the resection exceeds 80% of the liver (Bismuth 1982, Friedman 1993). Preoperative laboratory tests are of value in patients being assessed for hepatic resection, as a plasma bilirubin above 200 μmol/L (12 mg/dl), hypoalbuminemia or a prolonged prothrombin time precludes even a limited liver resection. Patients with tumors and a very high plasma alkaline phosphatase activity have large lesions and a higher risk of postoperative liver failure even when the plasma bilirubin is normal (Didolkar et al 1989). Patients with hepatic cirrhosis are particularly prone to liver failure after hepatic resection. Only patients classified as grade A on the Child–Pugh classification (p. 1007) should be considered and more conservative operations such as segmentectomy should be planned. Postoperative reduction in the plasma bilirubin and increase of alkaline phosphatase activity are indicators of hepatic regeneration that can be seen by computed tomography (Didolkar et al 1989).

***Tumor assessment.*** Preoperative assessment by ultrasonography (p. 55), computed tomography (p. 67) and angiography (p. 26) allows selection of patients for whom hepatic resection may be possible. Laparoscopy (p. 129) also gives valuable information, particularly in respect of spread of tumor outside the liver. Peroperative ultrasonography has become indispensable to hepatic surgery, as direct application of the ultrasound probe onto the liver allows the detection of tumor masses less than a centimeter in diameter, the identification of seedlings around a tumor mass and intravascular invasion (Traynor et al 1988). These all greatly affect the feasibility of surgery. Peroperative ultrasonography is also useful in the examination of cirrhotic livers, which are difficult to assess by conventional imaging methods. Direct ultrasonic examination can now be done at laparoscopy, avoiding the need for laparotomy.

### Hepatic artery occlusion

Hepatic artery ligation can be done for hepatic tumors and is generally well tolerated with no more than transient postoperative increases of transaminase activity. Radiological embolization of the hepatic artery is now generally preferred, as it is less invasive and the tumor circulation alone can often be occluded. The procedure should not be done where the portal vein is occluded or in patients with cirrhosis unless the occlusion can be limited to the tumor circulation.

## OPERATIONS IN PATIENTS WITH HEPATOBILIARY DISEASE

Operations unrelated to the liver in patients with hepatic disease should be considered carefully, as they are associated with a high morbidity and mortality (Powell-Jackson et al 1982). This is related mainly to the severity of the liver disease but also partly to the extent of the operation and to anesthesia.

### Acute hepatitis

Liver function can deteriorate after anesthesia and surgery and liver failure and sometimes death may occur. Harville & Summerskill (1963) reported that four of 42 (9.6%) of their patients with viral hepatitis undergoing laparotomy died of liver failure within 3 weeks of operation and five others (11.9%) suffered major postoperative complications. Hardy & Hughes (1968) reported two deaths in their 30 patients (6.7%) and both patients were considered to have developed chronic hepatitis. Estimates of the risk of operations, particularly laparotomy, in acute viral hepatitis have therefore varied, but most of the evidence points to significantly increased morbidity and mortality. It is obviously important to exclude acute hepatitis as the cause of a hepatobiliary illness prior to operation and only the most urgent surgery should be done in patients with acute hepatitis. Tests for the hepatitis A (p. 779), B (p. 785) and C (p. 788) viruses are important in identifying acute hepatitis and in identifying patients who pose an infectious risk for hospital staff (p. 784).

### Alcoholic liver disease

Patients with alcoholic hepatitis (p. 875) or alcoholic cholestasis (p. 877) can present with features suggesting intra-abdominal malignant disease or biliary obstruction, but about a half of such patients die after laparotomy (Greenwood et al 1972). This high mortality can be reduced by abstinence for about 3 months (Friedman & Maddrey 1987). Patients with fatty liver usually have better liver function (p. 875) and tolerate surgery well. Patients with alcoholic cirrhosis react to surgery similarly to those with other forms of chronic liver disease (see below).

### Chronic liver disease

Patients with chronic liver disease may need surgical treatment related to or independent of their liver disease. However, surgery is a particular hazard for these patients and should be carried out only for clear reasons and as far as possible electively after medical therapy has optimized their general condition. Abdominal herniae are common in cirrhosis, particularly in patients with ascites (p. 922). Herniae should not be repaired until ascites has been controlled and, if possible, the nutritional state improved, unless an emergency such as incarceration, strangulation, ulceration or leakage has occurred. Pescovitz (1984) reported a 14% mortality in 96 patients in the literature but no mortality in 26 patients where a prophylactic operation had been done on relatively well patients.

Abdominal operations are the more major operations required most often. Garrison et al (1984) reviewed 100 such operations, mainly for biliary disease and peptic ulceration, and found a mortality of 30% with 43% of survivors suffering one or more serious complications. Emergency operations had a 57% mortality compared to 10% for elective operations and mortality by Child–Pugh grade was 10% for grade A, 31% for grade B and 76% for grade C. Most patients died of multiorgan failure and/or infection. Adverse prognostic factors in descending order of importance were ascites, intra-abdominal infection, emergency operations, malnutrition, bilirubin >55 μmol/L (3 mg/dl), albumin <30 g/L, a prolonged prothrombin time and a leukocyte count $>10 \times 10^9$/L. The type of operation was not a major factor. Aranha et al (1982) reported a considerable mortality following cholecystectomy in cirrhotic patients (Table 45.1). Mortality related well to prolongation of the prothrombin time and hemorrhage was often the cause of death. These findings are not surprising, as the components of the Child–Pugh grading system are known to relate to the mortality of portasystemic shunt operations (p. 1007), but they emphasize the need for care in recommending surgery for patients with cirrhosis.

Operations on patients with chronic active hepatitis should be postponed whenever possible until active disease, indicated by a high plasma transaminase activity, is controlled by corticosteroid drugs (p. 900). Hydrocortisone hemisuccinate should then be given by intravenous infusion over the operative period. Vitamin $K_1$ (p. 751) should be given preoperatively if the prothrombin time is prolonged and fresh frozen plasma may be needed before and during operation. The hepatitis B and C viruses should always be sought before operation, as their presence requires care to avoid the spread of infection.

### Cholestasis

Adequate investigation is essential to avoid unnecessary operations in patients with cholestasis attributable to

**Table 45.1** Mortality of cholecystectomy in patients with hepatic cirrhosis related to prolongation of the prothrombin time (PT)

| Group | PT prolongation (s) | Number | Deaths | Mortality (%) |
|---|---|---|---|---|
| Normal | 0 | 374 | 4 | 1.1 |
| Cirrhosis | ≤2.5 | 43 | 4 | 9.3 |
| Cirrhosis | >2.5 | 12 | 10 | 83.3 |

wholly intrahepatic causes (below) and less invasive procedures such as endoscopic papillotomy for the removal of common bile duct stones should be considered for patients who have underlying liver disease. The most important medical considerations when operations are carried out for the relief of obstruction to a large bile duct are the correction of vitamin K deficiency by injections of vitamin $K_1$ (p. 751), the control of cholangitis and septicemia (p. 1213) and the prevention of postoperative renal failure (p. 1065).

### Unnecessary operations

Patients sometimes undergo operation before it is realized that they are suffering from parenchymal liver disease and this usually occurs when the liver disease presents in such a way as to suggest a disorder for which laparotomy may be needed (Powell-Jackson et al 1982). Abdominal pain similar to biliary colic, jaundice and fever point to a diagnosis of cholelithiasis, cholangitis or common bile duct obstruction and ascites, especially if it develops quickly or is associated with weight loss, suggests intra-abdominal malignancy or tuberculous peritonitis. However, one or more of these features occurs in many liver diseases, including acute hepatitis due to viruses (p. 781) or drugs (p. 846), alcoholic liver disease, especially alcoholic hepatitis (p. 875) and alcoholic cholestasis (p. 877), chronic active hepatitis (p. 889), hemochromatosis (p. 954), primary biliary cirrhosis (p. 936), sclerosing cholangitis (p. 943) and the Budd–Chiari syndrome (p. 1077). Findings such as a leukocytosis, which can occur in alcoholic hepatitis or in spontaneous bacterial peritonitis (p. 1034), or cholestatic liver function tests, such as occur in primary biliary cirrhosis, may be taken as confirming the clinical diagnosis.

The most important means of avoiding such errors are to obtain an adequate history of contact with jaundice or hepatitis, travel to areas where hepatitis is endemic, homosexuality, transfusion of blood or blood products, alcohol intake (p. 871) and drug ingestion, to examine the patient carefully for stigmata of chronic liver disease, especially spider telangiectasias, and to review the liver function tests. Diagnoses of obstructive biliary disease should be regarded as suspect when the plasma transaminase is elevated more than fivefold and the alkaline phosphatase less than twofold (p. 743) and hypoalbuminemia, hyperglobulinemia and a prolonged prothrombin time that cannot be corrected with vitamin K given parenterally (p. 751) all point to significant damage to the liver itself. Hepatitis A, B and C virus serology is important when clinical and biochemical features are compatible with acute hepatitis and autoantibody tests are important when there are features to suggest chronic liver disease. Imaging is very important, particularly in the detection of biliary obstruction, and laparotomy should not be performed without obtaining retrograde or transhepatic cholangiograms if imaging does not show biliary dilatation.

## ANESTHESIA

Problems for anesthesia may arise prior to, during or after the operation.

### Preoperative evaluation

The preoperative evaluation should include an assessment of the risks of surgery and should identify factors that might be improved preoperatively within an acceptable period to reduce operative risk and improve outcome. Clinical features of poor liver function such as jaundice, ascites and encephalopathy and laboratory features such as hypoalbuminemia and a prolonged prothrombin time all point to patients for whom surgery carries a higher risk.

#### *Nutrition*

Malnutrition is a consistent feature of advanced chronic liver disease that is not easily improved. Weight may be a poor reflection of nutritional status in the presence of ascites (p. 922). Aggressive feeding may precipitate encephalopathy and poor nutritional status may have to be accepted.

#### *Encephalopathy*

Even mild encephalopathy is significant because of the many factors in the perioperative period such as sedative drugs, sepsis and hypoxia that can precipitate encephalopathy with its attendant risks of aspiration and difficulty in patient management. Restriction of protein intake and the administration of enemas and/or lactulose (p. 1053) in the preoperative period may be valuable. Thiamine should be given to alcoholic patients to prevent the development of Wernicke's encephalopathy (p. 1050).

#### *Ascites*

Ascites is an indication of poor liver function and increases the risk of wound dehiscence or herniation. It should be treated wherever possible before surgery (p. 1023). Daily weighing and urinary sodium excretion are useful in controlling the treatment of ascites.

#### *Liver function tests*

Liver function tests should be reviewed in respect of the severity and activity of liver disease. Hyperbilirubinemia, hypoalbuminemia and a prolonged prothrombin time all point to significantly impaired liver function (p. 917) and these are associated with increased mortality from surgery (above). High plasma transaminase activity suggests continuing active liver damage (p. 741) and should prompt consideration of viral hepatitis, drug toxicity, ischemic liver damage or an exacerbation of chronic hepatitis requiring control prior to surgery whenever possible. High alkaline phosphatase activity (p. 743) requires the exclusion of large bile duct obstruction by imaging and consideration of intrahepatic diseases such as tumor or primary biliary cirrhosis.

*Coagulopathy*

Parenteral vitamin K preoperatively will improve coagulation disorders caused by poor nutrition or bile salt deficiency but will not correct coagulopathy due to hepatocellular dysfunction. In this circumstance, fresh frozen plasma should be administered to correct the prothrombin time, if possible, to within 2 seconds of control. Thrombocytopenia is usually secondary to hypersplenism and may not respond well to platelet transfusion, which should be given immediately prior to surgery, but conventionally platelet transfusion is administered when the platelet count is <50 000 u/L. Platelet function may be deranged and a normal platelet count does not preclude difficulties in controlling hemorrhage.

*Renal function*

Prerenal failure should not be mistaken for hepatorenal syndrome, as the former can be improved by appropriate fluid therapy (p. 1061). Central venous pressure monitoring is important in ensuring that the vascular volume is sufficient for normal renal function. Hypoxia, sepsis, fluid imbalance, blood loss and drugs (e.g. aminoglycosides, metoclopramide and nonsteroidal analgesics) can all contribute to renal failure in these patients and these factors need to be sought and treated.

*Obstructive jaundice*

Surgery for obstructive jaundice due to malignancy, particularly in anemic patients, has a high mortality (Dixon et al 1983). Relief of obstructive jaundice by the endoscopic or percutaneous placement of a stent in the preoperative period may reduce operative risk. Such procedures must be weighed against the dangers of introducing infection, especially when percutaneous drainage is used (Blenkharn & Blumgart 1985, Guthrie et al 1993). There is an increased risk of renal failure and this can be minimized by adequate hydration throughout the perioperative period. Mannitol and dopamine (p. 1065) may have a role, but fluid therapy is of prime importance.

*Cardiorespiratory function*

Cardiorespiratory fitness for surgery should be assessed as for any operation. Patients with advanced liver disease often have a hyperdynamic circulation with a resting tachycardia, hypotension and systolic flow murmurs on cardiac auscultation (p. 920). Alcoholic patients may have a cardiomyopathy (p. 875). Alcoholic patients are often also heavy smokers and chronic bronchitis and chronic obstructive airway disease should be sought. Ascites may be associated with pleural effusion, especially on the right side (p. 1072). Hypoxia and sometimes cyanosis occur as part of the portopulmonary syndrome (p. 1071) and occasionally pulmonary hypertension is present (p. 1072). Malnourished patients have poor respiratory musculature and are more likely to need prolonged ventilation after surgery. All patients should have a chest radiograph and an electrocardiogram and any abnormality found may require further investigation.

**Intraoperative management**

The effects of anesthesia and surgery on liver function are often inseparable, but the physiologial changes associated with anesthetic agents and techniques are mostly well defined, as are some of the possible postoperative hepatic consequences such as minor abnormalities of liver function tests (p. 1143).

*Effects of anesthesia*

Anesthetic agents and techniques have many effects outside the liver and there is a balance of risks to consider before adopting a particular method of anesthesia. Intubation and positive pressure ventilation (IPPV), for example, is indicated in an obese patient with the potential for gastroesophageal reflux undergoing surgery in the prone position, but IPPV may contribute to a reduction in liver blood flow. A decrease in liver blood flow could result in hepatic decompensation in a patient with chronic liver failure, but this possibility is theoretical rather than proven (Cowan et al 1991). Studies of total liver blood flow during anesthesia have shown that hepatic blood flow frequently falls by about a third in the half-hour after anesthesia begins, especially in patients over 55 years of age, but these studies have often used anesthetic agents that are now obsolete and have not investigated hepatic oxygen supply or consumption (Cowan et al 1991). Recent evidence that impaired hepatic blood flow can be associated with reduced oxygen supply and that this can have detrimental effects is provided by studies of hepatic venous oxygen saturation intraoperatively. The duration and the degree of oxygen deprivation are both important and correlate with postoperative increases in plasma hepatic enzyme activities, liver failure and death (Kainuma et al 1992).

It is therefore important to use techniques that are least likely to affect liver blood flow, but more research is required to elucidate fully the effects of modern anesthetic agents and surgery on the liver. The effects of anesthesia are probably minor compared with the effects of surgical procedures and, in particular, surgical manipulation of the liver and associated structures (Gelman 1976).

### *Nonanesthetic factors affecting liver blood flow*

Normal total liver blood flow in adults is approximately 1.5 L/min, 25–30% of which is supplied by the hepatic artery, accounting for approximately 50% of the liver oxygen supply (p. 715). An increased oxygen demand can be met by increased oxygen extraction and hepatic arterial flow may increase in response to a decreased portal venous pressure.

***Mechanical factors.*** Poor patient positioning, increased intra-abdominal pressure, surgical retraction and positive pressure ventilation with or without positive end-expiratory pressure (PEEP) can reduce liver blood flow (Sha et al 1987). Mechanical factors can be ameliorated by increasing the circulating blood volume (Matuschak et al 1987).

***Hypotension.*** Hypotension reduces hepatic blood flow (p. 1099), particularly in cardiac failure where there is also an increase in hepatic venous pressure. Portal venous flow is particularly sensitive to decreases in blood pressure and cardiac output. An increase in hepatic arterial flow may compensate for a reduced portal venous flow in the hypotensive patient, maintaining liver oxygenation without a significant increase in oxygen extraction. Spinal and epidural blockade is also associated with a decrease in liver blood flow if hypotension occurs.

***Blood gases.*** Hypocapnia reduces both portal venous and hepatic arterial blood flow (Hughes et al 1979). Hypercapnia reduces hepatic arterial flow, but there is a marked increase in portal venous flow. Profound hypoxemia reduces hepatic arterial flow and can damage the liver in its own right (p. 1100).

***Drugs.*** Some drugs commonly used in liver failure are effective because they reduce portal and consequently total liver blood flow, including propranolol, vasopressin and somatostatin (Lebrec et al 1980, Jenkins et al 1985). Cimetidine reduces liver blood flow by approximately 25%, a fact that does not seem to worry physicians who view with alarm similar reductions in association with surgery. The causes of reduction in liver blood flow, whether any decrease in portal flow is offset by increased arterial flow and whether such decreases require significant increases in oxygen extraction within the liver, are probably all important factors in determining the significance and sequelae of the reduced liver blood flow.

### *Premedication*

This is best omitted in patients with liver disease. A reassuring preoperative visit often provides as effective anxiolysis as drugs and this is generally the only function of premedication in present-day anesthetic practice.

### *Induction*

Any intravenous agent should be used with caution, as it can lead to hypotension. Propofol undergoes hepatic glucuronide conjugation which may be better maintained than the P-450 enzyme systems in late liver disease (p. 842). Although the response to thiopentone may be little altered with liver disease, its long elimination half-life (5 h) makes it less suitable.

### *Maintenance*

Isoflurane is the volatile agent of choice. There is preservation of or an increase in hepatic arterial blood flow, which may be a primary vasodilatory effect of isoflurane or may occur secondary to the reduction in portal vein blood flow that occurs with all volatiles (Hongo 1994). Isoflurane undergoes minimal metabolism and may be safer in respect of postoperative hepatic dysfunction.

Patients undergoing major surgery will usually require opioids for adequate analgesia. Fentanyl elimination is unchanged in cirrhosis and is a suitable drug. Morphine undergoes glucuronidation and may be suitable, but patients with severe liver disease are often sensitive to the cerebral effects of any opioid or sedative and these agents should be titrated cautiously against their effect and given as required.

Regional analgesic techniques are commonly used after major surgery and may have a helpful opioid-sparing effect. Coagulopathy may limit their applicability. Neuromuscular blocking agents that are eliminated in a manner uninfluenced by hepatic and renal failure are now available. Atracurium and more recently rocuronium may be employed without risk of prolonged effect (Khalil et al 1994).

### *Recovery*

A volatile-based general anesthetic will lead to a rapid recovery of consciousness. The risk of liver damage postoperatively from the use of volatile agents is not increased in patients with chronic liver failure. A patient obtunded from opioid and sedative intravenous drugs is at much greater risk in the postoperative period. Reversal of neuromuscular blockade using neostigmine is usually accompanied by the use of atropine to prevent muscarinic side-effects. Glycopyrrolate is preferable in patients with advanced liver disease because, unlike atropine, it does not cross the blood–brain barrier and produce central sedative effects.

*Regional anesthesia*

Regional anesthetic techniques may be employed as the sole form of anesthesia or combined with very light general anesthesia. In either circumstance the risk of precipitating encephalopathy is reduced. There are very few absolute contraindications to regional anesthesia. Most patients accept the techniques if these are carefully explained. Coagulopathy is a contraindication to central (spinal, i.e. subarachnoid or epidural) anesthesia. The risk can be reduced by transfusion of platelet concentrate and fresh frozen plasma preoperatively and most would consider this only a relative contraindication when the risk of hepatic encephalopathy is great; a prothrombin time less than 3 s prolonged and a platelet count above 50 000 may be acceptable in these circumstances, although individual practice varies as central blockade in these circumstances does carry risk (Wildsmith & McClure 1991).

*Fluids*

The use of large quantities of sodium-containing solutions may contribute to general fluid retention and ascites in cirrhotic patients, but operative losses should be replaced appropriately. The maintenance of circulating volume is important to conserve liver and renal blood flow. Patients with blood loss in excess of 1–1.5 liters should have red cell replacement if blood loss is continuing.

*Coagulation*

Careful maintenance of coagulation status may reduce postoperative bleeding complications and wasteful use of blood products after surgery. The postoperative patient with continued blood loss into drains or intra-abdominal bleeding caused by a coagulopathy that has not been adequately addressed earlier is not uncommon. Extrapolation from studies in healthy subjects, suggesting that fresh frozen plasma is not indicated until many units of blood have been transfused or when coagulation tests are relatively normal, is not appropriate in patients with liver disease. Plasma volume is best maintained with fresh frozen plasma at an early stage.

*Temperature*

Maintenance of body temperature is of prime importance in any patient undergoing major surgery, particularly where coagulation is abnormal, as in liver disease. It is achieved by adequate warming of all fluids (water bath blood warmers are inadequate for rapid transfusion), warming of inspired gases, adequate ambient temperature, an effective warming blanket and swaddling of the patient. Coagulopathy becomes worse during hypothermia, as the coagulation cascade and platelet function are adversely affected by even mild reductions in temperature (Valeri et al 1987, Rohrer & Natale 1992).

**Postoperative management**

Postoperative recovery facilities appropriate to the preoperative state of the patient and the magnitude of the surgery should be organized in advance. High dependency or intensive care facilities will often be necessary to provide adequate nursing observation, particularly of consciousness and ongoing blood losses, monitoring of vital functions and frequent laboratory measurements. After major surgery, routine observations include heart rate, blood pressure, oxygen saturation, urine output, central venous pressure, drain losses and consciousness judged using a simple sedative scoring system combined with an assessment of pain control.

*Postoperative liver investigations*

Patients undergoing a major hepatic resection or with poor preoperative liver function are at risk of postoperative decompensation and postoperative monitoring should detect this rapidly. Maintenance of adequate liver function can be judged by regular assessment of consciousness, plasma glucose (BM stick), lactate and prothrombin time. Daily plasma alanine aminotransferase (ALT) activity provides additional information.

*Analgesics and sedatives*

Patients with liver disease need analgesia after surgery and should not have to endure pain because of an inordinate fear of the effects of analgesic drugs (p. 844). Alcoholic patients may develop delirium tremens after operation and in addition to the general features of this condition (p. 1050), they may develop seizures, cardiac arrhythmias or hallucinations leading to self-harm. Alcohol itself can be given to patients preoperatively and postoperatively where they make it clear they have no intention of stopping drinking. All patients undergoing major surgery should receive thiamine to prevent Wernicke's encephalopathy (p. 1050).

## POSTOPERATIVE HEPATIC DYSFUNCTION

Abnormal liver function tests are quite common after surgery, even in patients without liver disease. There are usually no symptoms and the abnormalities resolve in a few days. Occasionally, more severe dysfunction manifests itself as postoperative jaundice.

**Liver function tests before surgery**

Liver function tests found to be abnormal after surgery may reflect an asymptomatic preoperative abnormality and should not be attributed automatically to the operation or anesthetic. The records of personal physicians, medical examinations and previous hospital admissions should be reviewed whenever possible in analyzing postoperative abnormalities. Surveys show that increased liver enzyme activities occur in some 1–5% of the general population (p. 736). Abnormalities in these asymptomatic individuals are usually mild, unassociated with clinical features of chronic liver disease and rarely indicate serious underlying liver disease. The more common causes include alcohol, obesity, diabetes mellitus, drugs and chronic hepatitis B or C infection, but often no cause can be found. Routine liver function tests should be done before any major operation, but they are no substitute for a thorough medical history and clinical examination.

### Liver function tests after surgery

Minor transient abnormalities of liver function tests are common after general anesthesia and surgery. Clarke et al (1976) studied the effects of minor, surface, gastric and biliary surgery on liver function tests over 4 days in patients without preoperative liver dysfunction. Minor surgery produced no abnormality and surface surgery only a minor increase of bilirubin at 24 h. Gastric and especially biliary surgery produced minor increases of bilirubin to about 25 µmol/L (1.3 mg/dl) and alanine aminotransferase activity increased twofold, resolving over 4 days. Evans et al (1974) studied patients undergoing major operations, mainly abdominal, and found that mild jaundice occurred in 16.5% and minor abnormality of other liver function tests in 6.9%. Severe jaundice occurred in 3.7% and was related mainly to sepsis and/or hypotension. Halevy et al (1994) reported the plasma bilirubin increased in 14% and the alanine aminotransferase activity increased 2.2-fold transiently after uncomplicated laparoscopic cholecystectomy.

Overall, these abnormalities are asymptomatic, they occur and resolve within a week of operation and they are usually detected as minor increases of plasma alanine aminotransferase activity. The maximum activity rarely exceeds a fourfold increase and in about three-quarters is less than twice the upper normal limit. The plasma alkaline phosphatase and γ-glutamyl transferase remain normal; abnormalities of these tests and those continuing for more than a week suggest a more significant complication. The cause of these transient and minor abnormalities of liver function is not known but may relate to reductions in liver blood flow, mild systolic hypotension, transient hypoxemia or minor anesthetic toxicity. Liver biopsy is not helpful in revealing a cause (Evans et al 1974).

## POSTOPERATIVE JAUNDICE

Jaundice usually follows only major surgery, is mild in 17% and marked in 4% of patients (Evans et al 1974).

**Table 45.2** Potentially important factors in postoperative hepatic dysfunction

| |
|---|
| *Preoperative factors* |
| Alcohol abuse |
| Drugs |
| Hepatitis exposure |
| Pre-existing hepatic disease |
| Pre-existing extrahepatic disease |
|   Hemolysis |
|   Cardiac failure |
| *Operative and postoperative factors* |
| Operation itself |
|   Nature, duration, findings |
|   Hematomas/hemoperitoneum |
| Drugs |
|   Anesthetic |
|   Other drugs |
| Blood and blood products |
| Parenteral nutrition |
| Complications |
|   Hypotension/shock |
|   Hypoxia |
|   Sepsis |
|   Fever |
| *Biliary obstruction* |
|   Common duct stone |
|   Bile duct injury |
|   Postoperative pancreatitis |

Although postoperative jaundice is usually mild and readily explained, in certain situations its unexpected development may herald serious complications. Several factors usually contribute and this should be borne in mind before individual factors are dismissed because they seem insufficient to be responsible on their own (Table 45.2).

### Pre-existing liver damage

Patients with pre-existing liver disease are at high risk of developing postoperative jaundice and this is particularly true for patients with cirrhosis. Mild to moderate elevations of serum bilirubin, alkaline phosphatase and prothrombin time were noted more frequently in cirrhotic patients following portasystemic shunt surgery than in individuals with normal liver function undergoing cholecystectomy (French et al 1952). Surgery may have a detrimental effect on hepatic function by reducing hepatic blood flow and should be avoided if possible in patients with hepatic disease (Cooperman et al 1977). Unfortunately, liver function tests in patients undergoing elective surgery may not detect underlying liver pathology (Schemel 1976). Particular attention should therefore be paid to a history of high alcohol consumption, recent viral illness, recent contact with jaundiced persons, overseas travel and the findings on clinical examination.

### Increased bilirubin production

Postoperative jaundice due mainly to increased bilirubin

production occurs following multiple trauma and after aortic surgery, but otherwise it is usually a contributing factor. Breakdown of extravasated blood may increase bilirubin production. Blood transfusion may be a factor in that 10% of red blood cells stored for 14 days hemolyze within 24 hours of transfusion. This leads to the production of 425 μmol (250 mg) of bilirubin, equivalent to the normal daily production, from each unit (500 ml) of blood. Patients with normal hepatic function can be given multiple blood transfusion without developing hyperbilirubinemia unless other factors, such as shock or sepsis, are present. Marked hyperbilirubinemia may develop in patients with any form of hemolytic anemia and hemolysis can also be caused by sepsis, drug therapy, the use of extracorporeal circulation or prosthetic heart valves and myoglobin catabolism following muscle injury. These causes of postoperative jaundice do not increase the serum transaminase or alkaline phosphatase activities. A normal blood hemoglobin concentration and a normal reticulocyte count effectively exclude hemolysis as the main cause of postoperative jaundice.

### Postoperative hepatitis

Most major causes of postoperative jaundice impair liver cell function and cause either a hepatitic or a cholestatic syndrome (Table 45.3).

***Anesthetics.*** Anesthetics are the drugs to which postoperative jaundice has been attributed most often. There is good evidence that halothane (p. 849) and possibly other volatile anesthetic agents (p. 850) can cause massive hepatic necrosis and death from liver failure (Ray & Drummond 1991). However, it is important that postoperative hepatitis is attributed to anesthetic agents only after a thorough investigation (p. 845).

Halothane hepatotoxicity is most likely in obese female patients undergoing a second or subsequent halothane anesthetic with a short interval (<28 days) between administrations. Classically, it presents with nausea, fever and upper abdominal tenderness several days after an anesthetic and is associated with eosinophilia and marked increases in plasma transaminase activity. Halothane hepatitis can cause death from fulminant hepatic failure and this has led to questions regarding its use. Halothane is one of the easiest volatile agents to use in the spontaneously breathing patient. It is very potent and its concentration can be increased rapidly with less risk of airway difficulties such as laryngospasm than with other anesthetic agents. Furthermore, a "confidential enquiry into postoperative death" (CEPOD) shows that most anesthetic deaths are not attributable to liver failure and therefore halothane may remain the agent of choice in certain circumstances. Some would consider repeated use reasonable for children, in whom the risk of halothane hepatitis is very low, or for gas induction in children or adults when there is a serious risk of airway obstruction (Buck et al 1987). The introduction of sevoflurane, which is also an excellent induction agent, will likely reduce further the use of halothane.

***Viral hepatitis.*** Viral hepatitis should be considered whenever a hepatic illness follows surgery. Viral hepatitis and hepatitis due to drugs cannot usually be differentiated clinically, biochemically or histologically. It is highly unlikely that a hepatitis virus introduced at operation would cause hepatitis in the postoperative period, but such an illness could result from preoperative exposure to persons with viral hepatitis or from transfusions with blood or blood products. Serological investigations to detect hepatitis A (p. 781), B (p. 785) or C (p. 788) virus infection should be undertaken. The risk of developing post-transfusion viral hepatitis is related to the quantity of blood transfused and the number of donors from whom the blood is harvested (Norrans et al 1981). Post-transfusion hepatitis is now much less common owing to the screening of donor blood for the hepatitis B and C viruses. The incubation time will vary according to which virus is involved, but the incubation period may be as short as 1–4 weeks after transfusion and must be considered in the differential diagnosis of postoperative jaundice.

***Other causes.*** Anesthetics are frequently implicated, probably because they are the drugs most obviously used in relation to operations. Patients who have undergone major surgery have, however, always been given a number of other drugs and these should not be disregarded. Other perioperative factors may be implicated. These include shock or prolonged hypotension that may result in hepatic damage sufficient to cause jaundice (p. 1099). This may follow massive gastrointestinal bleeding, pulmonary embolism or interference with cardiac function by infarction or tamponade as well as major trauma and surgery (Nunes et al 1970, Van Dyke & Gandolfi 1976). Jaundice usually occurs within 10 days of operation and may be marked, plasma transaminase activity rises within days and reaches 500 u/L or more and alkaline phosphatase activity often increases more slowly as recovery occurs. Bacterial infection and fever can also cause jaundice (p. 1109) and infection from *Clostridium welchii*, pneumococci, staphylococci and *Escherichia coli* may be implicated.

**Table 45.3** Postoperative jaundice due to impaired hepatocellular function

| |
|---|
| *Hepatitic syndrome* |
| Drugs (including anesthetics) |
| Shock |
| Viral hepatitis |
| *Cholestatic syndrome* |
| Hypotension |
| Sepsis |
| Drugs |
| Nutritional support |

The causes of abnormal liver function tests in patients receiving parenteral nutrition have not been clearly established, but abnormal liver function tests are common within 1–4 weeks of starting this treatment (p. 978).

### Postoperative intrahepatic cholestasis

Hypotension and multiple blood transfusions may give rise to an unusual but characteristic postoperative cholestatic jaundice. It arises most often following open heart surgery (Sanderson et al 1967). In mild cases, jaundice occurs early in the postoperative period and reaches a peak by the 7th to 10th day before returning to normal rapidly. Prolonged postoperative jaundice is often associated with a high mortality. More often, the jaundice is severe and associated with a marked increase in plasma alkaline phosphatase activity. Liver biopsy shows canalicular bile stasis, centrilobular liver cell degeneration and mild focal fatty change (Kantrowitz et al 1967, LaMont & Isselbacher 1973). In some studies an association with blood transfusion has been emphasized but other factors may contribute to the syndrome, including bleeding, which increases the bilirubin load, sepsis, which causes renal failure and so reduces conjugated bilirubin excretion, and hypotension, which impairs renal function and liver function and in particular liver excretory function (Kantrowitz et al 1967, Nunes et al 1970). The syndrome has been labeled as "benign" but only in the sense that death from liver failure does not occur. Such patients often succumb from extrahepatic disease.

### Impaired bilirubin transport

The hyperbilirubinemia of Gilbert's syndrome (p. 721) is exacerbated by fasting and possibly by infection, trauma and surgery itself. These patients may develop mild jaundice even after minor and uncomplicated surgery. Patients with Gilbert's syndrome are at no increased risk of developing liver failure and the jaundice rapidly resolves with feeding. Jaundice may also develop or increase after surgery in the rare Dubin–Johnson syndrome (p. 724). Patients with Crigler–Najjar syndrome (p. 723) are always obviously jaundiced and this may increase markedly after surgery.

### Surgical factors

Biliary obstruction is a rare cause of postoperative jaundice and is usually due to ligation or transection of the common bile duct (Garden 1991). After cholecystectomy, retention of a common bile duct stone may declare itself as postoperative jaundice. Postoperative jaundice may complicate postoperative pancreatitis and this arises in a third of patients as a consequence of obstruction at the lower end of the bile duct from the associated pancreatic inflammation (Saidi & Donaldson 1963). Postoperative acalculous cholecystitis is an unusual postoperative complication of nonbiliary surgery and also occurs in seriously ill patients who have not undergone operations (Howard & Delaney 1972, Johnson 1987). The pathogenesis of the associated jaundice is unclear and may be similar to other forms of cholecystitis associated with trauma (p. 1206). There is no obstruction of the common bile duct. The diagnosis may be suspected if the patient experiences upper abdominal pain (which may be masked by analgesics), leukocytosis and abnormal liver function tests. At cholecystectomy, gallstones are found in only half the patients and local bacterial infection is common. Most patients have not had previous clinical evidence of gallstones.

### Hepatic resection

This is invariably followed by postoperative jaundice and derangement of liver function tests. These abnormalities are dependent upon the extent of hepatic resection, existing liver disease and operative blood loss (Nagao et al 1985). The serum transaminase activities are at their highest within 48 h of surgery, although the serum bilirubin levels may continue to rise and peak about a week after surgery. The prothrombin time is the most sensitive indicator of hepatic dysfunction.

## INVESTIGATION OF POSTOPERATIVE JAUNDICE

Postoperative jaundice usually develops because of impaired hepatic function with or without increased bilirubin production and many contributory factors are often present. The main cause can usually be identified from the nature of the surgical operation and the development of complications, knowledge of the drugs prescribed, the time of onset of jaundice, clinical examination and the pattern of hepatic injury as assessed by liver function tests. The liver function tests show whether the jaundice is due to hyperbilirubinemia alone or whether there is additional evidence of liver dysfunction. The presence or absence of bilirubin in the urine indicates conjugated and unconjugated hyperbilirubinemia respectively and the pattern of the liver function tests may indicate a hepatitic or cholestatic syndrome.

### Hepatitic syndrome

Hepatocellular damage is most likely to be due to such factors as drug toxicity, sepsis, hypotensive (ischemic) liver injury and viral hepatitis. Patients with halothane hepatitis and a history of previous halothane exposure may develop jaundice earlier, compared with viral hepatitis which usually causes jaundice after some weeks if acquired from blood products at surgery. The time of development of jaundice due to drug toxicity and sepsis is variable. Sepsis should be identified by culture of blood and samples taken from potentially infected sites. Abdominal ultrasound and computed tomography may be useful in identifying intra-abdominal sepsis but liver biopsy is rarely helpful in identifying the cause.

### Cholestatic syndrome

The cholestatic pattern of liver function tests suggests either mechanical biliary obstruction or intrahepatic cholestasis. Ultrasonography should be undertaken to identify biliary obstruction, gallstones and pancreatitis. Pancreatitis should be sought by measuring plasma amylase activity, especially when upper abdominal pain is present. Delineation of the biliary tree may require cholangiography by either the percutaneous or the endoscopic route. The latter approach will allow sphincterotomy and stone removal if required or insertion of a stent to relieve mechanical obstruction. Liver biopsy is not usually helpful in identifying the cause and cannot reliably identify large bile duct obstruction (p. 719).

### Isolated hyperbilirubinemia

The commonest form of hyperbilirubinemia, namely Gilbert's syndrome, is readily differentiated from hemolysis by the normality of liver function tests, reticulocyte counts and haptoglobin levels. The nature of the surgical intervention and the extent of blood loss are important. Drug toxicity may cause hemolysis by either direct or immunological mechanisms and is to be suspected in patients with a reticulocytosis and reduced haptoglobin levels.

### Treatment

Treatment has to be based on a sound diagnosis. The presence of cardiac or renal failure should be excluded, since these may contribute to any hepatic dysfunction. Where sepsis is identified, appropriate antibiotic therapy and drainage of infected collections will be required. Retained gallstones or other mechanical obstruction in the biliary tree should be treated as appropriate.

General supportive measures should be applied to all patients, with maintenance of ventilation and cardiac output. If liver failure or encephalopathy develops, more specific supportive measures may include the use of laxatives, correction of electrolyte, glucose and coagulation abnormalities, early treatment of cerebral edema and antibiotic therapy, if indicated. Consideration should be given to liver transplantation where appropriate.

REFERENCES

Aranha G V, Sontag S J, Greenlee H B 1982 Cholecystectomy in cirrhotic patients: a formidable operation. American Journal of Surgery 143: 55–60

Bismuth H 1982 Postoperative strictures of the bile duct. In: Blumgart L H (ed) The biliary tract. Churchill Livingstone, Edinburgh, p 209–218

Blenkharn J I, Blumgart L H 1985 Streptococcal bacteremia in hepatobiliary operations. Surgery, Gynecology and Obstetrics 160: 139–141

Buck N, Devlin H B, Lunn J N 1987 The report of a confidential enquiry into perioperative deaths. Nuffield Provincial Hospitals Trust, The King's Fund, London

Clarke R S J, Doggert J R, Lavery T 1976 Changes in liver function after different types of surgery. British Journal of Anaesthesia 48: 119–128

Cooperman L H, Wollman H, Marsh M L 1977 Anesthesia and the liver. Surgical Clinics of North America 57: 421–428

Cowan R E, Jackson B T, Grainger S L, Thompson R P H 1991 Effects of anesthetic agents and abdominal surgery on liver blood flow. Hepatology 14: 1161–1166

Didolkar M S, Fitzpatrick J L, Elias E G et al 1989 Risk factors before hepatectomy, hepatic function after hepatectomy and computed tomographic changes as indicators of mortality from hepatic failure. Surgery, Gynecology and Obstetrics 169: 17–26

Dixon J M, Armstrong C P, Duffy S W, Davies G C 1983 Factors affecting morbidity and mortality after surgery for obstructive jaundice: a review of 373 patients. Gut 24: 845–852

Evans C, Evans M, Pollock A V 1974 The incidence and causes of postoperative jaundice. British Journal of Anaesthesia 46: 520–525

French A B, Barss T P, Fairlie C S et al 1952 Metabolic effects of anesthesia in man. V: A comparison of effects of ether and cyclopropane anesthesia on the abnormal liver. Annals of Surgery 135: 145–163

Friedman L S 1993 When patients with liver disease need surgery. Internal Medicine 14: 25–34

Friedman L S, Maddrey W C 1987 Surgery in the patient with liver disease. Medical Clinics of North America 71: 453–476

Garden O J 1991 Iatrogenic injury to the bile duct. British Journal of Surgery 78: 1412–1413

Garrison R N, Cryer H M, Howard D A, Polic H C Jr 1984 Clarification of risk factors for abdominal operations in patients with hepatic cirrhosis. Annals of Surgery 199: 648–655

Gelman S I 1976 Disturbances in hepatic blood flow during anesthesia and surgery. Archives of Surgery 111: 881–883

Greenwood S M, Leffler C T, Minkowitz S 1972 The increased mortality rate of open liver biopsy in alcoholic hepatitis. Surgery, Gynecology and Obstetrics 134: 600–604

Guthrie C M, Haddock G, de Beaux A C, Garden O J, Carter D C 1993 Changing trends in the management of extrahepatic cholangiocarcinoma. British Journal of Surgery 80: 1434–1449

Halevy A, Gold-Deutch R, Negri M et al 1994 Are elevated liver enzymes and bilirubin levels significant after laparoscopic cholecystectomy in the absence of bile duct injury? Annals of Surgery 219: 362–364

Hardy K J, Hughes E S R 1968 Laparotomy in viral hepatitis. Medical Journal of Australia 1: 710–712

Harville D D, Summerskill W H J 1963 Surgery in acute hepatitis. Causes and effects. Journal of the American Medical Association 184: 257–261

Hongo T 1994 Sevoflurane reduced but isoflurane maintained hepatic blood flow during anesthesia in man. Journal of Anesthesia 8: 55–59

Howard R J, Delaney J P 1972 Postoperative cholecystitis. American Journal of Digestive Diseases 17: 213–218

Hughes R L, Mathie R T, Fitch W, Campbell D 1979 Liver blood flow and oxygen consumption during hypocapnia and IPPV in the greyhound. Journal of Applied Physiology 47: 290–295

Jenkins S A, Baxter J N, Corbett W, Devitt P, Ware J, Shields R 1985 A prospective randomised controlled clinical trial comparing somatostatin and vasopressin in controlling acute variceal haemorrhage. British Medical Journal 290: 275–278

Johnson L B 1987 The importance of early diagnosis of acute acalculus cholecystitis. Surgery, Gynecology and Obstetrics 164: 197–203
Kainuma M, Nakashima K, Sakuma I et al 1992 Hepatic venous hemoglobin oxygen saturation predicts liver dysfunction after hepatectomy. Anesthesiology 76: 379–386
Kantrowitz P A, Jones W A, Greenberger N J, Isselbacher K J 1967 Severe postoperative hyperbilirubinemia simulating obstructive jaundice. New England Journal of Medicine 276: 590–598
Khalil M, D'Honneur G, Duvaldestin P, Slavov V, de Hys C, Gomeni R 1994 Pharmacokinetics and pharmacodynamics of rocuronium in patients with cirrhosis. Anesthesiology 80: 1241–1247
LaMont J T, Isselbacher K J 1973 Postoperative jaundice. New England Journal of Medicine 288: 305–307
Lebrec D, Nouel O, Corbic M, Benhamou J-P 1980 Propranolol – a medical treatment for portal hypertension? Lancet 2: 180–182
Matuschak G M, Pinsky M R, Rogers R M 1987 Effects of positive end-expiratory pressure on hepatic blood flow and performance. Journal of Applied Physiology 62: 1377–1383
Nagao T, Inoue S, Mizuta T, Saito H, Kawano N, Morioka Y 1985 One hundred hepatic resections: indications and operative results. Annals of Surgery 202: 42–49
Norrans G, Widell A, Teger-Nilsson A-C, Kiellman H, Frösner G, Iwerson S 1981 Acute hepatitis non-A, non-B following administration of factor VIII concentrates. Vox Sanguinis 41: 129–133
Nunes G, Blaisdell W, Margaretten W 1970 Mechanism of hepatic dysfunction following shock and trauma. Archives of Surgery 100: 546–556
Pescovitz M D 1984 Umbilical hernia repair in patients with cirrhosis. No evidence for increased incidence of variceal bleeding. Annals of Surgery 199: 325–327
Powell-Jackson P, Greenway B, Williams R 1982 Adverse effects of exploratory laparotomy in patients with unsuspected liver disease. British Journal of Surgery 69: 449–451
Ray D C, Drummond G B 1991 Halothane hepatitis. British Journal of Anaesthesia 67: 84–99
Rohrer M J, Natale A M 1992 Effect of hypothermia on the coagulation cascade. Critical Care Medicine 20: 1402–1405
Saidi F, Donaldson G A 1963 Acute pancreatitis following distal gastrectomy for benign ulcer. American Journal of Surgery 105: 87–92
Sanderson R G, Ellison J H, Benson J A Jr, Starr A 1967 Jaundice following open heart surgery. Annals of Surgery 165: 217–224
Schemel W H 1976 Unexpected hepatic dysfunction found by multiple laboratory screening. Anesthesia and Analgesia 55: 810–812
Sha M, Saito Y, Yokoyama K, Sawa T, Amaha K 1987 Effects of continuous positive-pressure ventilation on hepatic blood flow and intrahepatic oxygen delivery in dogs. Critical Care Medicine 15: 1040–1043
Traynor O, Castaing D, Bismuth H 1988 Peroperative ultrasonography in the surgery of hepatic tumours. British Journal of Surgery 75: 197–202
Valeri C R, Feingold H, Cassidy G, Ragno G, Khuri S, Altschule M D 1987 Hypothermia-induced reversible platelet dysfunction. Annals of Surgery 205: 175–181
Van Dyke R A, Gandolfi A J 1976 Anaerobic release of fluoride from halothane. Relationship to the binding of halothane metabolites to hepatic cellular constituents. Drug Metabolism and Disposition 4: 40–44
Wildsmith J A W, McClure J H 1991 Anticoagulant drugs and central nerve blockade. Anaesthesia 46: 613–614

SECTION 11

# Transplantation

# 46. Transplantation

*A. J. MacGilchrist   E. M. M. Quigley*

## INTRODUCTION

This chapter will review general and disease-specific indications, timing of transplantation, the operative process, and both early and late postoperative management in liver transplantation. Pancreatic and small intestinal transplantation and the effects of bone marrow and solid organ transplantation on the gastrointestinal and hepatobility organs will also be considered.

## TRANSPLANTATION OF THE LIVER

Liver transplantation is now established as a successful treatment for acute and chronic liver failure. It is over 30 years since the first human liver transplant (Starzl et al 1963). Progress was slow initially and prior to 1980 fewer than 100 transplants were performed annually worldwide, with a 1-year survival of only 25%. Subsequent improvements have included better immunosuppression, notably the introduction of cyclosporin, and improvements in operative technique, postoperative care and patient selection (NIH Consensus Conference 1984). There has been a dramatic increase in operations and since 1990 the number of transplants being performed annually exceeds 4500 worldwide (Fig. 46.1). Survival following transplantation for cirrhosis is around 80% at 1 year (Health Resources and Service Administration 1991, UNOS releases 1993), with some subsequent fall-off to 70% at 5 years (European Liver Transplant Registry Update 1993). For acute liver failure, the figures are less good: approximately 60% survival at 1 year and 50% at 5 years (Iwatsuki et al 1989, Mutimer & Elias 1992, European Liver Transplant Registry Update 1993).

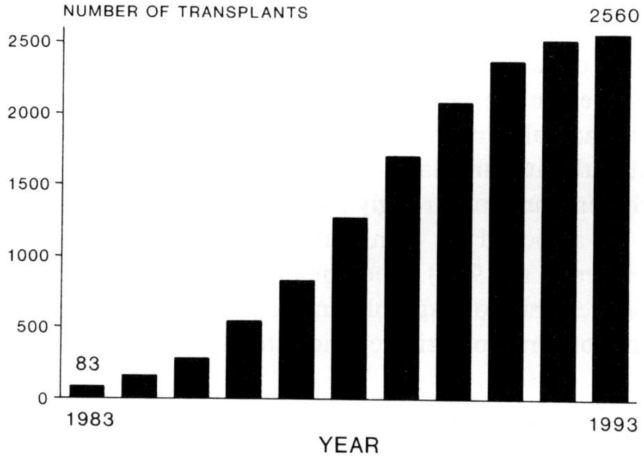


**Fig. 46.1** Liver transplants performed in Europe, 1983–1993 (European Liver Transplant Registry Update 1993).

## INDICATIONS

The indications in adults and children are listed in Table 46.1 and their proportions are illustrated in Figure 46.2. In general, liver transplantation is performed

**Table 46.1** Indications for liver transplantation

| Adults | Children |
|---|---|
| *Chronic liver disease* | *Cholestatic liver disease* |
| Primary biliary cirrhosis | Biliary atresia |
| Primary sclerosing cholangitis | Familial syndromes |
| Chronic hepatitis B | (Alagille's, Byler's) |
| Chronic hepatitis C | *Other chronic liver disease* |
| Alcoholic liver disease | Chronic viral hepatitis |
| Autoimmune hepatitis | Autoimmune hepatitis |
| Cryptogenic cirrhosis | Cryptogenic cirrhosis |
| Budd–Chiari syndrome | Fibrocystic liver disease |
| *Metabolic diseases* | *Fulminant hepatic failure* |
| Wilson's disease | Tyrosinemia type I |
| Hemochromatosis | Reye's syndrome |
| $\alpha_1$-antitrypsin deficiency | As for adults |
| Protoporphyria | |
| *Fulminant hepatic failure* | *Inborn errors of metabolism* |
| Paracetamol poisoning | Tyrosinemia type I |
| Acute viral hepatitis | Familial hypercholesterolemia |
| Drug hepatotoxicity | Crigler–Najjar type I |
| Toxins (amanita phylloides, | Galactosemia |
| "ecstasy") | Urea cycle enzyme deficiency |
| Wilson's disease | Glycogen storage disease |
| *Malignancy* | *Malignancy* |
| Hepatocellular carcinoma | Benign tumors replacing liver |
| Epithelioid hemangioendothelioma | Hepatocellular carcinoma |
| Carcinoid tumor | Hepatoblastoma |

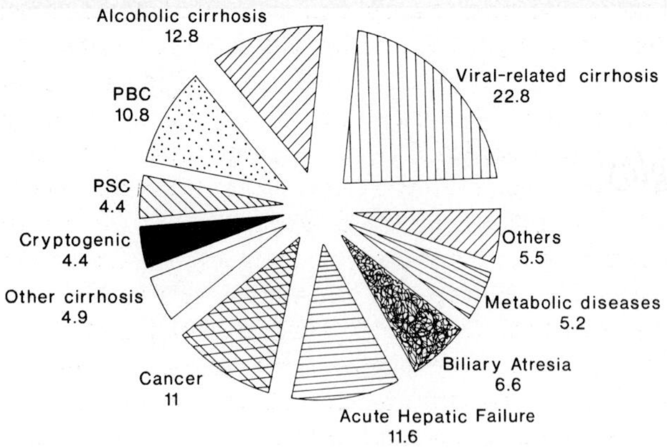


**Fig. 46.2** Indications for liver transplantation in Europe, 1988–1993 (European Transplant Registry Update 1993). Numerical values give the percent frequency of each indication.

for four categories of liver disease: cirrhosis, acute liver failure, hepatic malignancy and metabolic disorders whose defect lies within the liver. Cirrhosis is the largest category, making up three-quarters of all adult cases. Transplantation for acute liver failure is increasing and now exceeds 20% of cases in some programs. Poor results have led to transplantation for malignant disease being performed only rarely, although it is still appropriate in well-selected cases. Transplantation for metabolic disorders is rare unless associated with liver failure, as in hemochromatosis, Wilson's disease or tyrosinosis, but it is occasionally performed in combination with other organ transplants, as in combined heart and liver transplant for cardiac failure associated with hereditary hyperlipidemia or amyloidosis.

## Cirrhosis

Transplantation should be considered for all patients whose progressive liver disease significantly reduces their life expectancy or impairs their quality of life, unless an alternative therapy is available or there are contraindications.

In deciding when to transplant, therefore, it would be valuable to have disease-specific prognostic indications. Unfortunately, with the notable exceptions of the cholestatic cirrhoses primary biliary cirrhosis (PBC) and, to a lesser extent, primary sclerosing cholangitis (PSC), such indications are lacking. There are, however, general pointers to a poor prognosis in cirrhosis. These include ascites, encephalopathy, variceal bleeding, malnutrition and fatigue. Ascites complicated by infection (spontaneous bacterial peritonitis) or renal impairment (functional renal failure or the hepatorenal syndrome) carries a life expectancy of less than 50% at 2 years (Llach et al 1988, Tito et al 1988). Even uncomplicated ascites carries a high mortality when associated with poor nutrition, hypotension (mean arterial pressure <85 mmHg) and hypoalbuminemia (<28 g/L) (p. 1032). Variceal bleeding has alternative therapies but indicates advanced liver disease (p. 1002). Child–Pugh classification, developed over 20 years ago, remains valuable in predicting outcome (p. 925). Thus, survival without transplant in patients with variceal hemorrhage but good liver function (grade A) is 75–100% at 3 years, in contrast to those in grade C with poor liver function, whose 3-year survival is only 20–45% (Di Magno et al 1985, Westaby et al 1985, Garden et al 1990). Similarly, encephalopathy, especially if occurring spontaneously or with minimal precipitating factors, heralds a poor prognosis in addition to greatly impairing quality of life. Malnourished patients and those with renal failure have advanced liver disease and a particularly high operative mortality and it is advisable to transplant patients before that stage is reached. Fatigue can be most disabling and is easily overlooked by the physician. Once nonhepatic causes such as hypothyroidism and depression have been excluded, severe fatigue should prompt a transplant referral even in the absence of other complications.

The laboratory indices of impaired hepatic function used in the Child–Pugh score (p. 1007) are useful in timing transplant. However, only in PBC should the serum bilirubin alone be considered a possible indication for transplant irrespective of the patient's clinical health.

### *Primary biliary cirrhosis*

Results of liver transplantations are good, exceeding 90% at 1 year in some centers. Once the serum bilirubin is consistently greater than 180 µmol/L, the average life expectancy is only 18 months (Shapiro et al 1979) and 1-year mortality approaches 50%. Initial referral to a transplant center should therefore be made once the bilirubin consistently exceeds 100 µmol/L.

Several prognostic models relying on Cox's multiple regression analysis have been validated for PBC (Christensen et al 1985, Dickson et al 1989). Attempts have been made to develop similar models for predicting survival after transplantation (Neuberger 1989), but they are less well validated and become dated as survival continues to improve. These models are too cumbersome for general clinical use, but research application has provided evidence for the benefit of liver transplantation by comparing actual survival post-transplant with predicted survival without transplant (Fig. 46.3) (Markus et al 1989). Such comparisons strongly suggest that improved survival can be achieved by transplanting earlier in the disease (Weisner et al 1992). Poor quality of life should prompt earlier referral, for example, intractable pruritus, disabling fatigue or symptomatic hepatic osteodystrophy (p. 932).

### *Primary sclerosing cholangitis*

As with PBC, several centers have established prognostic models that have the same limitations in clinical practice

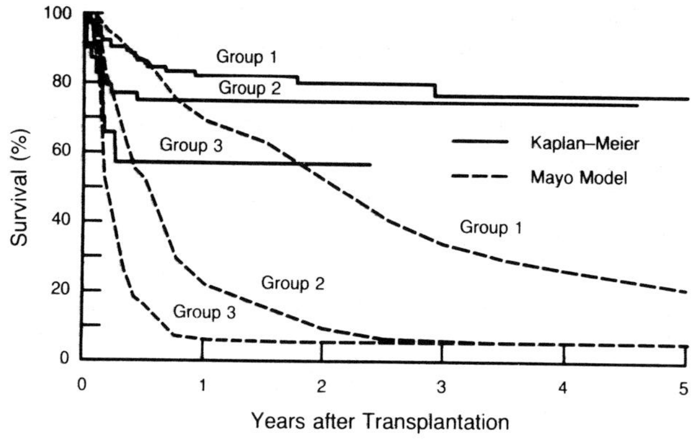


**Fig. 46.3** Actual (Kaplan–Meier) survival after transplantation in three groups of patients with primary biliary cirrhosis and estimated survival without transplantation as predicted by the Mayo model (Markus et al 1989). Group 1 = low risk, Group 2 = medium risk, Group 3 = high risk.

(Farrant et al 1991, Dickson et al 1992). Worsening jaundice in a patient with PSC is not an automatic indication for transplant. Bacterial cholangitis may respond to antibiotics although recurrent attacks may necessitate transplantation. A single, dominant extrahepatic biliary stricture may be treated by dilatation and temporary insertion of a biliary stent, giving lasting relief (Johnson et al 1991). Unfortunately, it is difficult to differentiate a benign stricture from a cholangiocarcinoma and the latter contraindicates transplantation as results are poor (Iwatsuki et al 1985). This is important, as cholangiocarcinoma becomes apparent in life in about 10% of patients and is found at autopsy in 40%.

The diagnosis of cholangiocarcinoma complicating PSC is particularly difficult, as mass lesions demonstrable by imaging techniques are often absent and negative biliary cytology does not exclude the diagnosis. Thus, the patient with PSC and a single dominant biliary stricture poses a difficult management problem. However, with the above exceptions, a patient with persistent jaundice in PSC should be considered for transplantation. Liver failure is a late development and most patients are transplanted because of progressive jaundice, intractable pruritus, recurrent cholangitis, malnutrition or fatigue. Nontransplant biliary surgery should be avoided so as not to compromise the success of later transplant surgery.

### *Alcohol-induced liver disease*

There has been an ethical debate regarding the appropriateness of liver transplantation for alcohol-induced liver disease. This debate has centered on the use of such a scarce resource as a transplant organ for patients with "self-inflicted" disease and the major shortage of donor organs in the United States since 1990 has coincided with alcohol-induced liver disease becoming the most frequent indication for liver transplant in that country. Fears that alcohol abuse after transplantation would damage liver grafts have not yet been realized. Return to drinking has occurred in less than 20% at 2 years (Bird et al 1990, Kumar et al 1990, Lucey et al 1992), but in the longer term a study from London has suggested that most return to regular drinking (Howard et al 1994). Although alcohol can damage other organs such as the heart, pancreas and brain, the 1-year survival following transplant for alcohol-induced liver disease is 70%, similar to that for other forms of cirrhosis (Starzl et al 1988, Bird et al 1990).

Success lies in using social and psychiatric/psychological evaluation to identify patients likely to drink again. Patients with alcohol-induced liver disease are not automatically alcohol-dependent. Most transplant programs prefer a period of abstinence for about 6 months before considering transplantation, as this demonstrates a patient's ability to abstain and allows an opportunity for spontaneous hepatic and general improvement. Improvement happens quite frequently, especially in younger patients, but it occurs over many months after cessation of alcohol intake. Unfortunately, the patient with life-threatening acute alcoholic hepatitis poses a particularly difficult problem and the price of delaying surgery may be death. Few such patients are considered for transplant currently, as their survival is poor and the chances of postoperative relapse of alcohol abuse are high.

### *Chronic viral hepatitis*

***Hepatitis B.*** Hepatitis B almost invariably recurs in the liver graft following transplantation for chronic hepatitis B and recurrence is often particularly aggressive, with progression to cirrhosis within 2 years (Todo et al 1991). Sometimes recurrent disease has a distinct histological pattern termed "fibrosing cholestatic hepatitis" with cholestasis and fibrosis but relatively little cellular infiltrate (Davies et al 1991). It has been speculated that immunosuppression allows the hepatitis B virus (HBV) to become hepatotoxic although this remains unproven. The risk is highest in patients with active viral replication demonstrated by HBeAg or HBV-DNA in serum before transplant. Many centers now regard such findings as a contraindication to transplantation, as the rate of HBV recurrence in HBV-DNA-positive recipients has been 93% as compared to 33% in HBV-DNA-negative recipients (Samuel et al 1991a).

There have been several studies examining the effect of passive immunization by high-dose intravenous hepatitis B immunoglobulin (HBIg) after transplantation. Evidence is accumulating that maintaining the patient's serum anti-HBs titer over 1:100 can delay, perhaps indefinitely, clinically significant recurrent hepatitis B, certainly in patients without evidence of active viral replication before transplantation (Müller et al 1991, Samuel et al 1991b). The results are best in patients transplanted for fulminant hepatitis B (0% HBsAg recurrence), coexisting hepatitis B and hepatitis D infection (13%) and HBV-DNA negative posthepatitis B cirrhosis (30%) and worst in HBV-DNA-positive patients (90% HBsAG recurrence). A multicenter retrospective analysis of all European patients undergoing transplantation for hepatitis B confirmed these findings and emphasized that the HBIg must be continued long-term (Samuel et al 1993). Treatment is costly – £7000 in the UK in the first year – and may have to be continued indefinitely, since cessation of treatment results in recurrent disease. Active immunization with hepatitis B vaccine and interferon is ineffective in the prevention or treatment of recurrent hepatitis B in the graft.

In summary, patients with chronic hepatitis B should be transplanted only if they are HBV-DNA negative and they should receive passive immunization with intravenous HBIg postoperatively.

***Hepatitis C.*** Despite initial reports to the contrary, it is now clear, using sensitive detection techniques such as polymerase chain reaction for HCV-RNA, that reactivation of the hepatitis C virus is inevitable following transplantation for chronic hepatitis C (Wright et al 1992b). However, hepatitis C runs a more benign course than hepatitis B after liver transplantation. Consequently, at least up to 2 years post-transplant, very few patients have clinically significant recurrent hepatitis (Ferrell et al 1992). The long-term outlook is unknown and there are no preventive strategies. At present, liver transplantation is still being undertaken for patients with chronic hepatitis C.

### Metabolic diseases

Patients with metabolic liver diseases constitute only a minority of patients coming to liver transplantation (Fig. 46.2), but transplantation sometimes results in cure of the underlying disease. Genetic hemochromatosis should not often require transplantation, as patients usually present before liver function is seriously impaired and adequate treatment leads to significant improvement (p. 956). Sometimes hemochromatosis is only diagnosed on examination of the explanted liver after transplantation. Unfortunately, the outlook after transplantation may be worse than in other forms of liver disease, with only a half of patients surviving at 1 year. Factors contributing to this poor outlook include postoperative cardiac dysfunction (p. 955), infection (p. 955) and a high incidence of hepatocellular carcinoma (p. 957) in the explanted liver. Iron accumulation occurs in the transplanted liver and phlebotomy may be needed long term (Farrell et al 1994).

Treatment of Wilson's disease usually allows the long-term maintenance of good liver function (p. 963), but transplantation may be required for deteriorating function in spite of medical therapy or for acute liver failure (p. 807). Transplantation cures the metabolic defect, as evidenced by return of the plasma ceruloplasmin and the urine copper excretion to normal, and there is a gradual loss of Kayser–Fleischer rings and resolution of neurologic symptoms (Schilsky et al 1994). The outlook after transplantation is similar to that in other liver diseases. Transplantation for severe neurologic symptoms unresponsive to medical therapy or in the absence of severe liver disease remains controversial.

There is no effective medical treatment for chronic liver disease due to $\alpha_1$-antitrypsin deficiency and progressive liver failure requires liver transplantation (Putnam et al 1977). The plasma $\alpha_1$-antitrypsin concentration returns to normal after transplantation, the phenotype is that of the donor and the patient should be protected from development or worsening of pulmonary disease.

Patients with cystic fibrosis are increasingly surviving into adult life and liver disease has become an important cause of death. Some 35 patients had received liver transplants by 1992 with a good quality of life in the 50% who survived (Williams et al 1992). However, the multisystem nature of cystic fibrosis makes the long-term survival of these patients more problematic and the place of liver transplantation is less clear than in other metabolic diseases.

Protoporphyria occasionally causes liver failure, usually in adult life. Liver transplantation has been used at this stage, but it does not correct the metabolic defect (p. 975). Most other hepatic metabolic diseases for which transplantation can be considered require treatment in childhood. These include urea cycle enzyme deficiencies in which transplantation cures the defect (Todo et al 1992a), although arginine may remain an essential amino acid (Rabier et al 1991); galactosemia in which the metabolic defect is corrected (Otto et al 1989); tyrosinosis in which transplantation has been very successful (Mieles et al 1990, Paradis et al 1990), leading some to recommend operation within the first year of life in view of the high incidence of hepatocellular carcinoma (Freese et al 1991); and glycogen storage disease type IV in which death from liver failure usually occurs by 4 years of age, although it is not yet known if transplantation will prevent later myopathy (Selby et al 1993). Diseases causing microvesicular steatosis (p. 977) may present as fulminant liver failure and need consideration for transplantation (below).

### Malignancy

#### *Hepatocellular carcinoma*

In the early days of liver transplantation, malignant disease, usually primary hepatocellular carcinoma, was a relatively common indication. However, the results were poor with recurrent tumor in the graft or at a distant site leading to a survival at 2 years of only 30% (Bismuth et al 1987a, O'Grady et al 1988c, Penn 1991). This may be associated with a shortening of tumor doubling time in the presence of immunosuppression. Resection rather than transplantation is therefore a more attractive option, but most tumors arise in cirrhotic liver or involve both lobes at presentation, effectively preventing resection (p. 1123). The fibrolamellar variant, which usually arises in a noncirrhotic liver, has a better prognosis with a 5-year survival after transplantation exceeding 50% (Ismail et al 1990). Irresectable lesions may be considered for transplantation as recurrent tumor may not develop for several years.

***Small tumors.*** Liver transplantation for small hepatocellular carcinoma is currently being reconsidered. A number of studies have looked at the outcome for transplant recipients with tumors found only at the time of surgery (Iwatsuki et al 1985, Williams & O'Grady 1990). The prognosis in such patients is the same as for patients transplanted without malignancies. This has led to recognition of the critical importance of tumor size. Most centers now transplant patients with cirrhosis and small single tumors less than 3–5 cm in diameter. Unfortunately, the detection of such tumors by ultrasound, conventional computed tomography (CT) and magnetic resonance imaging (MRI) is low. CT angiography, where CT scanning is combined with venous and arterial phases of selective hepatic angiography, is the most sensitive test but is neither widely available nor a practical screening procedure. Serum alpha-fetoprotein is usually normal when the hepatocellular carcinoma is small (p. 750). Conversely, when referring a patient with malignancy for transplantation with the combination of a mass on imaging and a raised serum alpha-fetoprotein, percutaneous biopsy should not be done to avoid disseminating tumor along the needle tract.

#### *Other tumors*

Cholangiocarcinoma usually recurs rapidly after transplantation, even when found coincidentally, and is therefore a contraindication in most centers. There have, however, been more promising results with up to 60% 2-year survival in highly selected cases (Ringe et al 1989). There is little enthusiasm for transplanting for metastatic disease of the liver. One exception is the slow-growing carcinoid tumor, where transplantation can give prolonged palliation where surgical resection or medical therapy such as octreotide has failed or is not possible. A rare vascular liver tumor that is slow-growing and yields good results with transplantation is the hepatic epithelioid hemangioendothelioma.

### Fulminant hepatic failure

Patients who develop fulminant hepatic failure (p. 805) without pre-existing liver disease may be considered candidates for liver transplantation. If such patients recover with medical management, they do not suffer chronic liver disease and return to full health. However, once encephalopathy has progressed to grade III or IV, the mortality varies from 50% to 90%. If such patients undergo liver transplantation, the 1-year survival is 60–70% (Bismuth et al 1987b, O'Grady et al 1988b). The balance of risks in patients with fulminant hepatic failure and severe encephalopathy would therefore seem to be in favor of transplantation. However, the prognosis is also dependent on the underlying etiology, with more favorable results from medical therapy in hepatitis A, hepatitis B and paracetamol poisoning than in other conditions such as non-A, non-B hepatitis, drug hepatotoxicity and fulminant Wilson's disease. In addition, because of the delay between deciding on a liver transplant and a suitable organ becoming available, it is important to be able to predict as early as possible which patients with fulminant hepatic failure will do badly.

The Liver Unit at King's College Hospital, London, has drawn up a series of prognostic guidelines (Table 28.5) arrived at by retrospective analysis of 310 cases from 1973 to 1985 and tested in a further retrospective analysis of 175 cases from 1986 to 1987 (O'Grady et al 1989). Other centers have used simpler guidelines, including a French group predicting an unfavorable outcome if clotting factor V is less than 20% of normal for patients <30 years or less than 30% for patients >30 years, irrespective of degree of coma (Bernuau et al 1991). The London criteria allow identification of poor prognosis at an early stage for nonparacetamol failure, but neither set of criteria is ideal for predicting which patients with severe encephalopathy will survive (Pauwels et al 1993).

These guidelines are valuable but not foolproof. Referral to a transplant center should take place before these criteria have been reached, as patients may deteriorate on transfer. Patients with severe acute liver disease who have impaired consciousness, a prolonged prothrombin time or impaired renal function should be discussed with a liver transplant center.

## CONTRAINDICATIONS

Absolute contraindications to liver transplantation are few and with medical and surgical advances, certain contraindications that would have been regarded as absolute in the past are now only relative (Table 46.2). Age is a good example. Initial evidence showed that the survival of patients older than 50 years was as good as that of younger patients, but even patients in the eighth decade have been transplanted successfully (Emre et al 1993). As in many other situations, biological age is more relevant than chronological age, although particular attention needs to be paid to cardiovascular disease in older patients.

Portal venous thrombosis, once an absolute contraindication, can be circumvented by recanalization or insertion of a vascular graft, but thrombosis extending into the splenic and superior mesenteric veins renders transplantation impossible. If the portal vein is thrombosed, care should be taken to exclude underlying hepatic malignancy.

**Table 46.2** Contraindications to liver transplantation

| | |
|---|---|
| *Absolute* | |
| Active infection | |
| | Sepsis |
| | HIV infection |
| | Hepatitis B virus (HBeAg+ / HBV−DNA+) |
| Continuing substance abuse | |
| | Alcohol |
| | Other drugs |
| Malignant disease | |
| | Tumor >5 cm diameter |
| | Multicentric |
| | Extrahepatic |
| Extensive portal venous thrombosis | |
| Hyponatremia (<125 mmol/L) | |
| Advanced cardiorespiratory disease | |
| *Relative* | |
| Portal vein thrombosis | |
| Major previous biliary surgery | |
| Psychiatric ilness | |
| Cardiorespiratory disease | |
| Advanced age | |

Previous major upper abdominal surgery renders the operation more difficult, without necessarily worsening survival. It is advisable to avoid major upper abdominal surgery, particularly portacaval or mesocaval shunts or biliary surgery in cirrhotic patients who may require transplant at a later date. Significant cardiac disease increases the anesthetic risk, particularly at the time of reperfusion of the liver graft when major circulatory and metabolic disturbances can occur. Significant respiratory disease may render the patient inoperable or increase the chance of a prolonged period of assisted ventilation postoperatively with the attendant increased risks of sepsis. Hepatopulmonary syndrome causing hypoxia due to arteriovenous shunting consequent on the liver disease itself is no longer regarded as a contraindication and usually reverses after surgery (p. 1071). Pulmonary hypertension consequent on portal hypertension (p. 1072) can also reverse after transplantation, but elevated pulmonary pressures, which may be clinically silent, increase the risk of intraoperative complications.

Alcoholic liver disease per se is not a contraindication to transplantation, but most would not transplant a patient actively abusing alcohol or other drugs. HIV infection is regarded generally as a contraindication, as rapidly progressive AIDS may occur following transplantation. Patients with HIV infection and normal T-lymphocyte counts may prove an exception in this regard. Active replication of the HBV, indicated by the presence in serum of HBeAg or HBV-DNA, is a contraindication, although patients with chronic hepatitis B without such serum markers can be transplanted. Extrahepatic malignancy remains an absolute contraindication.

Temporary contraindications requiring correction prior to transplant are active sepsis and severe hyponatremia. The introduction of immunosuppression when sepsis is present is almost invariably fatal. One exception is where the sepsis is confined within the liver, on the assumption that it will be removed at hepatectomy. The sudden correction of hyponatremia during transplantation may cause central pontine myelinolysis leading to a catatonic state that is irreversible and ultimately fatal. Transplantation is best avoided until serum sodium exceeds 125 mmol/L.

## THE TRANSPLANT PROCESS

The decision on whether or not to transplant will usually be made by a multidisciplinary team including a transplant surgeon, a hepatologist, an anesthetist and various paramedical and support staff.

***Donor organs.*** The supply of suitable organs is limited and patients with chronic liver disease may have to wait weeks or months. Most donors have died while on artificial ventilation, usually as a result of head injury or intracranial hemorrhage, and brain death is confirmed by standard bedside neurological tests. In most countries the consent of the next of kin is required for the use of donor organs. In a few European countries organs may be utilized unless the patient donor had made specific provisions to the contrary. In the United States, 35% of patients listed for transplantation die before an organ becomes available (First 1992). No health care system has unlimited financial resources or organ supplies and patient priority will remain a subject of professional and public controversy.

***Graft matching.*** Donors and recipients are matched for ABO blood group and size. Matching for HLA status is not performed routinely. There is a suggestion that allograft rejection is less common with an HLA class II match and an HLA class I mismatch (O'Grady et al 1988a). Recently, an analysis of almost 500 liver transplants demonstrated an adverse effect on survival of HLA-A+B+DR mismatches, where the 4-year survival was 86% if there were more than two mismatches compared to 62% if there were six mismatches (Nikaein et al 1994).

The main difficulty in size matching is in obtaining small livers for small patients. The difficulty of obtaining suitably small donor livers for children has led to the successful use of reduced grafts, where only a portion of the donor liver, usually segments II and III, is implanted. A more controversial technique is the use of living related donors. In this situation, a relative of the (usually pediatric) patient requiring transplant undergoes a partial hepatectomy, which is then utilized as a reduced graft (Broelsch et al 1991, Ozawa et al 1992). Although technically feasible, this has not yet gained wide acceptance.

***Graft harvesting.*** A hepatectomy is performed by a specialized surgical transplant team. The organ is preserved cold in a suitable medium and transported to the transplant unit, where the potential recipient will have been admitted. Advances have been made in the quality of the preservative, the most widely used being University of Wisconsin solution. Although this maintains the organ

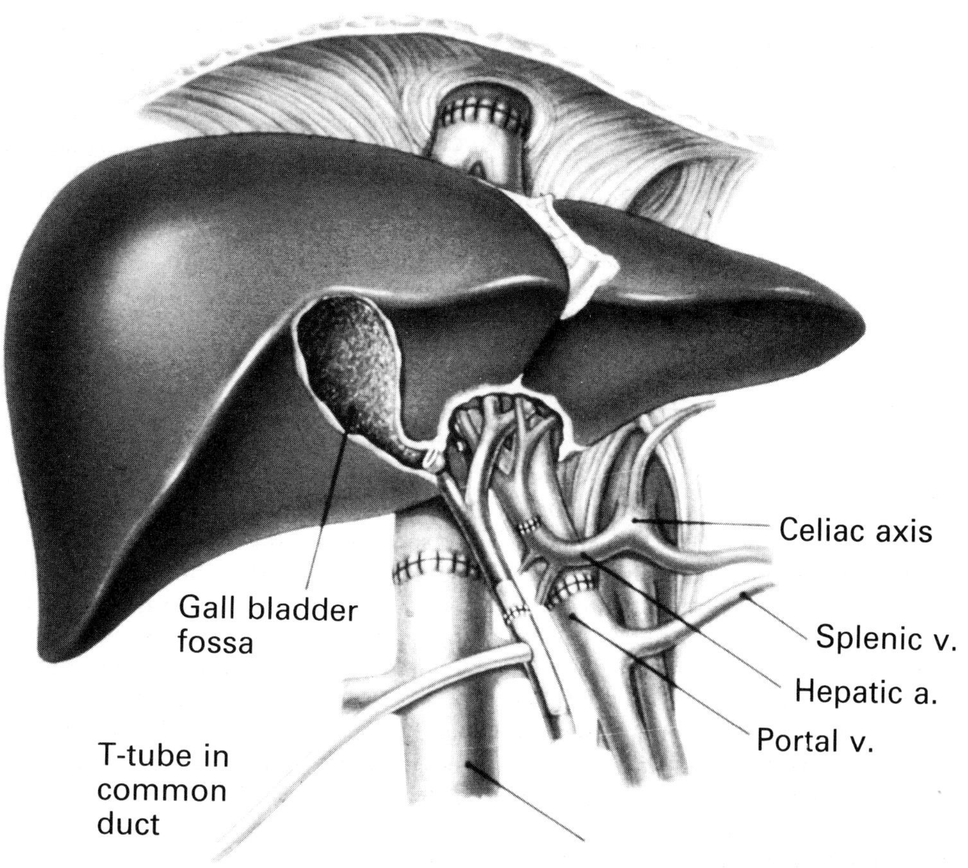


**Fig. 46.4** Diagrammatic representation of transplanted liver showing the five anastomoses (see text).

viable for 24 h, there is a suggestion of increased biliary complications (Sanchez-Urdazpal et al 1992) and poorer graft survival if preservation time exceeds 12 h (Adam et al 1992). Nevertheless, even this period allows most transplant operations to take place during normal working hours with a fresh surgical team.

***Transplant operation.*** The orthotopic transplant operation usually employed comprises the removal of the patient's liver and the insertion of the entire new graft, anastomosing the upper and lower inferior vena cava, the portal vein and the hepatic arteries. The biliary reconstruction will be an end-to-end choledochocholedochostomy or, in the presence of biliary tract disease, as in PSC, biliary atresia or retransplantation, a Roux-en-Y choledochojejunostomy (Fig. 46.4). During the hepatectomy and prior to reperfusion of the liver, some surgeons employ venovenous bypass, redirecting venous blood from the inferior vena cava and portal vein into the superior vena cava via an extracorporeal pump. This lengthens the procedure but reduces blood loss. Reperfusion of the new graft may be accompanied by metabolic disturbances including hyperkalemia and acidosis and by circulatory disturbances including systemic hypotension, myocardial depression and pulmonary hypertension. Transfusion requirements have fallen as surgical techniques have improved. The serine protease inhibitor aprotinin probably reduces transfusion requirements by preventing fibrinolysis, although the studies have all been on small numbers of patients and not all have drawn a positive conclusion.

## Postoperative care

### *Immunosuppression*

Conventional immunosuppression consists of cyclosporin, azathioprine and corticosteroids. No two transplant programs have identical immunosuppressive regimens and there are few, if any, controlled trials comparing such regimens. Prescribing is tailored to the individual, attempting to strike a balance between allograft rejection on the one hand and infection and drug toxicity on the other.

***Cyclosporin.*** The introduction of cyclosporin, a macrolide antibiotic of fungal origin, in 1981 represented a major advance in organ transplantation. The principal immunosuppressive action of cyclosporin is to block T-cell activation by inhibiting production of interleukin 2 and 4 (IL2 and IL4). Cyclosporin concentrations in serum are usually maintained in the range 150–200 nmol/L where the assay measures parent cyclosporin alone by

**Table 46.3** Side-effects of cyclosporin

| |
|---|
| Renal impairment |
| Hypertension |
| Neurotoxicity |
| Headaches |
| Tremor |
| Neuropathy |
| Metabolic disturbance |
| Hyperkalemia |
| Hypomagnesemia |
| Cosmetic |
| Weight gain |
| Hirsutism |
| Gingival hypertrophy |
| Arthralgia |

**Table 46.4** Drugs altering cyclosporin plasma concentration or nephrotoxicity

| *Increased cyclosporin concentration* | *Reduced cyclosporin concentration* |
|---|---|
| Aminoglycosides | Anticonvulsants |
| Calcium channel antagonists | Isoniazid |
| (except nifedipine) | Octreotide |
| Danazol | Rifampicin |
| Erythromycin | *Enhanced cyclosporin* |
| Itraconazole and ketoconazole | *nephrotoxicity* |
| Quinidine | Aminoglycosides |
| | Amphoteracin B |
| | Ketoconazole |
| | NSAIDs |
| | Trimethoprim |
| | Ganciclovir |

HPLC or approximately twice that value where the assay also includes cyclosporin metabolites by radioimmunoassay. The former is the preferred method, as cyclosporin metabolites probably do not contribute significant immunosuppression. Some authorities recommend measurement of both the parent compound and its metabolites to reduce toxicity, but this is not widely practiced.

The major side-effects of cyclosporin, apart from the increased susceptibility to infection (below), are nephrotoxicity, hypertension, neurotoxicity including headaches, tremor, neuropathy and delirium, impaired glucose tolerance, weight gain, hirsutism, gingival hypertrophy, hyperkalemia and hypomagnesemia (Table 46.3). Although such effects are often an indication of toxicity, they can occur at therapeutic blood concentrations. The mechanism of early renal damage is vasoconstriction, principally of the efferent glomerular arteriole, but later tubular damage can occur. As the number of long-term transplant survivors increases, the long-term morbidity of the mild chronic renal impairment seen in the majority of patients will be of increasing importance. Similarly, it is important, particularly in younger patients, to treat hypertension and obesity adequately. Many different antihypertensive agents are employed, including calcium channel antagonists, β-adrenergic antagonists and ACE inhibitors. The last requires careful monitoring of renal function and serum potassium levels. Many drugs interact with cyclosporin (Table 46.4), and it is important to consider this whenever prescribing for a post-transplant patient.

***Azathioprine.*** Azathioprine, whose immunosuppressive action is to inhibit T-cell proliferation by interfering with cell division, is employed by most programs in dosages of 1–2 mg/kg/day. The dose is reduced if myelosuppression occurs and there is anxiety about the long-term risk of malignancy. As with renal transplantation, patients should be screened for skin, anal and cervical tumors.

***Corticosteroids.*** Prednisone or prednisolone are used and dosages vary enormously, commencing at relatively high levels, reducing to low doses or even discontinuing completely over a period of months. At the dosages now employed, major corticosteroid-related side-effects are rare. One important risk is worsening osteoporosis leading to spontaneous fractures. The combined effect of corticosteroid therapy, immobilization and pre-existing hepatic osteodystrophy leads to a reduction in bone density during the first 6 months post-transplant, followed by gradual improvement. Particularly in patients with cholestatic cirrhosis, hepatic osteodystrophy should be taken into consideration in deciding on the timing of transplantation. If bone density is reduced, transplantation should not be delayed and severe bone disease with multiple previous fractures may indicate that it is already too late to transplant.

***Tacrolimus.*** Tacrolimus is another fungus-derived antibiotic with very potent immunosuppressive effects whose mechanism of action is similar to cyclosporin. Two recent multicenter trials have demonstrated a small but significant reduction in the incidence of both acute and chronic rejection when using tacrolimus as compared to cyclosporin and azathioprine. However, the side-effects of tacrolimus, particularly at high doses, showed an increased risk of nephrotoxicity and glucose intolerance (European FK506 Multicentre Liver Study Group 1994, US Multicenter FK506 Liver Study Group 1994). There is some evidence that tacrolimus may be able to reverse early chronic rejection (Todo et al 1990, Shaw et al 1991).

***Other drugs.*** A number of other immunosuppressive agents are undergoing clinical trials. One of the most promising is RS-61443 (mycophenylate mofetil), which has a low toxicity and may be synergistic with cyclosporin. The goal of more effectively targeted immunosuppression with less toxicity may be achieved by the use of monoclonal antibodies directed at specific sites in the rejection cascade such as the T-cell receptor, the IL2 receptor and intercellular adhesion molecules. The options available to clinicians are likely to increase over the next few years.

### *Rejection*

Allograft rejection is common and can be divided into

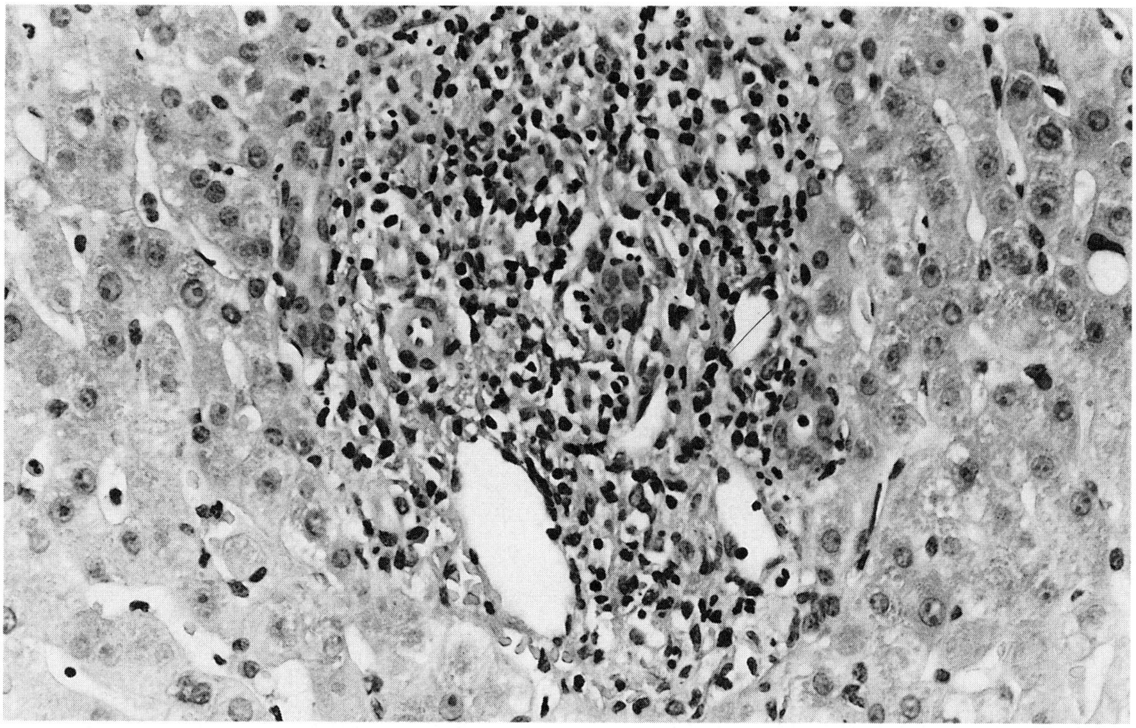

**Fig. 46.5** Acute cellular rejection showing portal triaditis, bile duct damage (center) and portal vein endothelialitis (hematoxylin and eosin × 250).

acute or cellular rejection and chronic or ductopenic rejection, although elements of both can be present simultaneously and whether they represent continuous or separate pathological processes is not known.

***Acute rejection.*** This tends to occur early in the post-transplant period, with a peak incidence at 1 week. It occurs in approximately 70% of liver grafts. The clinical features are jaundice and fever accompanied by elevation of transaminases and white blood cell count. Routine liver biopsies have demonstrated that cellular rejection may be asymptomatic. Rejection should be confirmed histologically by liver biopsy. The classic histological picture of acute rejection is a mixed inflammatory cell infiltrate in the portal tracts, damage to the small bile ductules and endotheliolitis affecting the branch of the portal vein (Fig. 46.5). Mild degrees of rejection often settle spontaneously. More severe degrees usually respond to high-dose corticosteroids such as methylprednisolone 1 g intravenously on three successive days. When so-called "steroid-resistant" rejection occurs, which is rare, an anti-lymphocyte monoclonal antibody such as ALG or OKT3 may be effective. Such agents should be used sparingly because of a possible link with subsequent malignancy, particularly non-Hodgkin's lymphoma, often referred to as PLD (post-transplant lymphoproliferative disorders) (Swinnen et al 1990).

***Chronic rejection.*** This tends to occur later, with a peak onset at 3 months post-transplant. It is less common than acute rejection, affecting 10–15% of transplants. The presentation is usually an insidious onset of cholestasis with jaundice, itching, elevated plasma alkaline phosphatase activity and liver histology showing the "disappearing bile duct syndrome" (DBDS) (p. 945) with a paucity of bile ducts within portal triads and a relative absence of inflammatory cellular infiltrate (Fig. 46.6). There is vascular damage with "foamy cell" degeneration of medium-sized hepatic arterioles, but this is not usually apparent on needle biopsy specimens. No medical treatment is of proven benefit. The suggestion that the early stages of the process can be reversed by tacrolimus has not gained wide acceptance (Todo et al 1990). Once more than 50% of the portal tracts examined have lost their bile ducts, DBDS is regarded as irreversible. Such patients often require a second liver transplant. A link between cytomegalovirus (CMV) infection early post-transplant and the subsequent development of DBDS (O'Grady et al 1988a) has not been confirmed (Paya et al 1992).

Recent evidence has for the first time demonstrated an association between acute and chronic rejection. The Pittsburgh group have suggested that prompt treatment of acute rejection with three 1 g doses of methylprednisolone reduces the subsequent incidence of chronic rejection. This has to be weighed against the increased risk of sepsis associated with such treatment and against the knowledge that moderate degrees of acute rejection often settle spontaneously without high-dose corticosteroids.

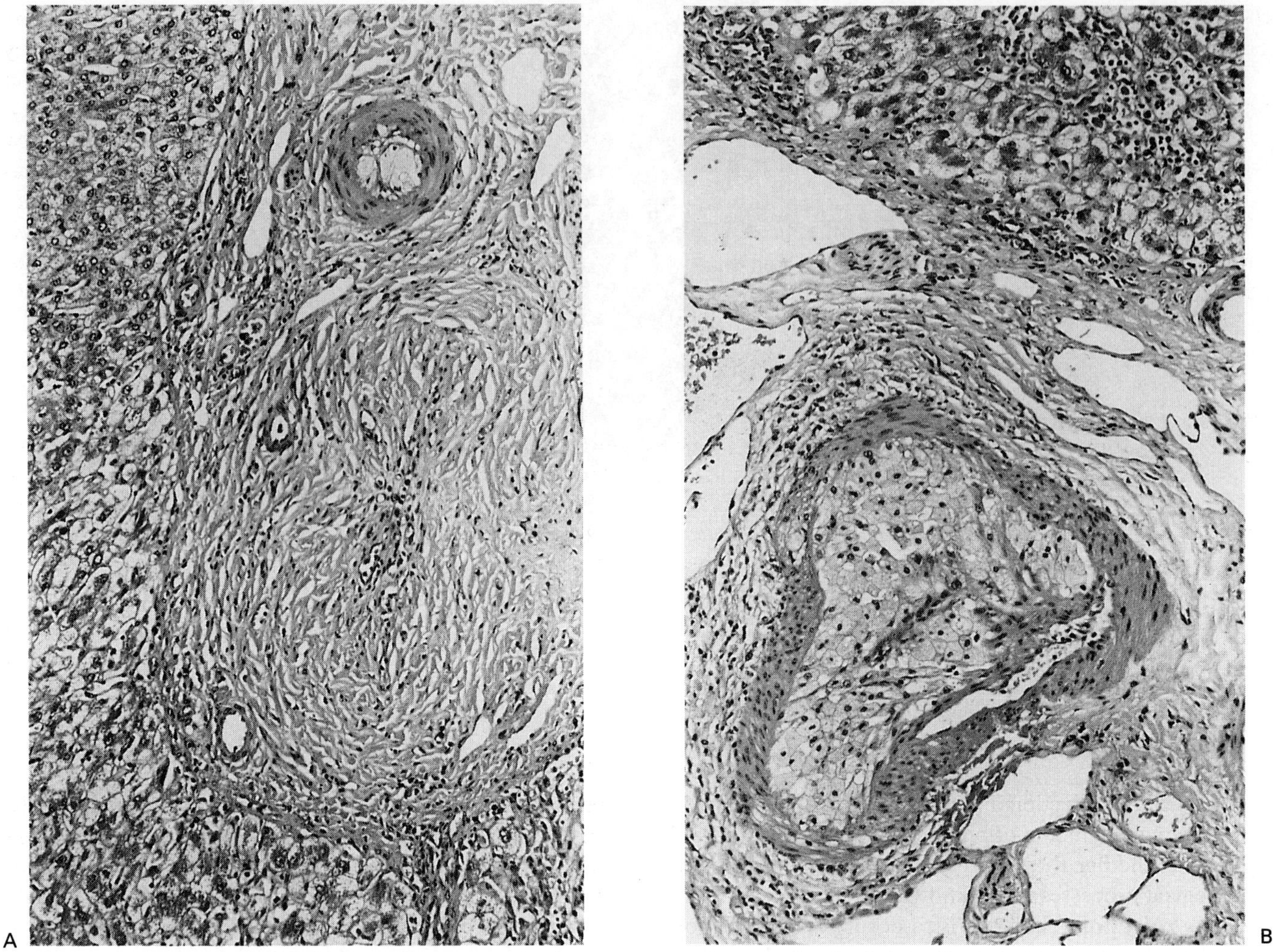


**Fig. 46.6** Chronic rejection showing loss of bile ducts (ductopenia) in a portal tract (**A**) and arterial occlusion with foamy macrophages (**B**).

*Infection*

The commonest cause of death after liver transplantation is infection. The risk is highest in the early postoperative period, especially in patients who were in hospital, malnourished or had renal impairment prior to transplantation. Postoperative risk factors include major intraoperative blood transfusion, high-dose immunosuppression, renal failure and the need for prolonged intensive care. The commonest bacterial pathogens are Gram-negative bacilli and staphylococci.

***Cytomegalovirus.*** The most significant viral infection is cytomegalovirus (CMV), which usually occurs between 3 weeks and 3 months postoperatively. Risk factors include a CMV-positive donor, especially if the recipient was CMV-negative, pre-existing immunosuppression as in retransplantation and high-dose immunosuppression, especially with OKT-3 (Paya et al 1993). A generalized infection with fever and myalgia can occur or specific organs may be affected, especially the liver, the lung and the gastrointestinal tract. CMV hepatitis is one of the differential diagnoses of jaundice and/or disordered liver function tests in the transplanted patient and frequently it causes a cholestatic hepatitis (p. 792). CMV pneumonitis causes variable dyspnea with hypoxia and pulmonary infiltrates. CMV affects the upper gastrointestinal tract with symptoms of delayed gastric emptying and the lower gastrointestinal tract with diarrhea and/or rectal bleeding.

Early diagnosis can be made by detection of CMV antigenemia using a monoclonal antibody detection test or by detection of CMV-DNA by polymerase chain reaction (The et al 1992). Histology of the affected organs may be diagnostic with either conventional or immunocytochemical staining, but false negative results occur. Confirmation of the diagnosis is by cell culture of urine, blood or tissue, but this takes up to 2 weeks. Treatment with ganciclovir is effective in 80% of cases (Stratta et al 1991a). Various regimens, including anti-CMV immunoglobulin, oral acyclovir and intravenous ganciclovir in a variety of combinations, have been assessed as prophylaxis against

CMV, as CMV infection affects up to 50% of patients, with clinical illness in about a half in some series. Intravenous ganciclovir is the most effective, but it is costly.

***Other viruses.*** Infection and/or reactivation of herpes simplex virus is rarely a clinical problem and responds to acyclovir. Epstein–Barr virus (EBV) can be a late cause of post-transplant hepatitis and is associated with post-transplant lymphoproliferative disorders. Treatment is with acyclovir or ganciclovir.

***Fungi.*** Fungal infection may be local or systemic. Oral candidiasis is extremely common. Prophylaxis with oral nystatin, amphoteracin or fluconazole is used. Other local sites for candidiasis include skin, vagina and urine. Systemic fungal infection is less common, usually occurring in a patient already ill, often in intensive care and having required high-dose immunosuppression, prolonged antibiotics or both. Systemic candidiasis may be treated with fluconazole or amphoteracin. Pulmonary or systemic aspergillosis requires amphoteracin but is usually fatal. A liposomal amphoteracin formulation has lower nephrotoxicity but is very expensive.

***Pneumocystis carinii.*** Pneumonia due to *Pneumocystis carinii* has been virtually abolished by the use of prophylactic co-trimoxazole.

***Toxoplasma gondii.*** *T. gondii* infection occasionally reactivates after transplantation.

### *Other complications*

Primary nonfunction of the graft is rare (1–2%) and its etiology remains obscure. Hepatic artery thrombosis is also rare (<5%), but its development in the early postoperative period results in rapid hepatic decompensation usually requiring emergency retransplantation. It is suspected by Doppler ultrasonography and confirmed by selective angiography. Ascitic leakage from drain sites is common and usually diminishes over a few days. Large ascitic fluid losses (>2 L/day) develop in about a quarter of patients and can be associated with hypovolemia, coagulopathy and sometimes thrombotic complications. Ascitic fluid protein concentrations tend to be high (29–54 g/L) and venography and liver biopsy may slow outflow venous obstruction somewhere between the central hepatic veins and the inferior vena cava (Gane et al 1995).

Biliary tract complications develop in 20% of cases (Stratta et al 1989). Biliary leaks, usually at the biliary anastomosis, occur early and usually resolve with conservative treatment involving reopening the T-tube and if necessary draining the extrabiliary collection. Bile duct strictures develop later, presenting with cholangitis and/or cholestasis. A single stricture at the site of the biliary anastomosis is usually due to local factors, but multiple or nonanastomosis strictures usually result from ischemic damage due to late occlusion of the hepatic artery, chronic rejection or, possibly, prolonged cold ischemia during organ preservation. Unlike the hepatic parenchyma, which receives its blood supply from the hepatic artery and the portal vein, the extrahepatic biliary tree is supplied solely by the hepatic artery. Diagnosis of a biliary complication should always lead to assessment of the hepatic artery. Anastomotic strictures can be treated endoscopically or by percutaneous balloon dilatation and insertion of permanent metal or temporary plastic prostheses (Donovan 1993). However, patients often eventually require surgical biliary reconstruction, usually a choledochojejunostomy. Multiple or nonanastomotic strictures often require retransplantation.

## Disease recurrence

Most of the complications affecting the post-transplant patient occur in the first 3 months and new infections, rejection or surgical complications after a year are rare. Thereafter, the major risks to the patient are the long-term consequences of immunosuppression such as malignancy, morbidity associated with renal impairment and recurrence of the original hepatic disease. In most conditions, the risk of disease recurrence is not known, but some short- and medium-term information is available.

### *Chronic liver disease*

PBC can recur and can be distinguished from chronic rejection by experienced histopathologists (Hubscher et al 1993). There are isolated reports of possible recurrence of PSC (Harrison et al 1991) and of autoimmune hepatitis (Wright et al 1992a). To date, however, there are only a few case reports of clinically significant disease recurrence. The genetic defects leading to abnormal copper and iron metabolism reside within the liver and it is therefore not surprising that there are no reports of recurrence of Wilson's disease or hemochromatosis. The risk of recurrence of alcoholic liver disease will depend on the recidivism rate. At 2 years in highly selected cases this is less than 20% (Bird et al 1990, Kumar et al 1990, Lucey et al 1992), but long-term results are not yet available.

The risk of recurrence of hepatitis B relates to active HBV replication at the time of transplant and most have found a high recurrence of clinical hepatitis if active replication was present (Samuel et al 1991a). Recent evidence suggests clinically significant disease can be delayed by the use of intravenous immunoglobulin (HBIg) (Müller et al 1991, Samuel et al 1991b). The most promising long-term results using this approach come from Berlin, where 70% 5-year survival in chronic hepatitis B was found irrespective of HBV-DNA status, markedly higher than earlier reports from other centers. Although hepatitis C recurs following transplant, clinically significant hepatitis is rare up to 2 years (Ferrell et al 1992). Long-term results are not yet available.

*Fulminant hepatic failure*

Disease recurrence following transplantation for fulminant hepatic failure from any cause is not a clinical problem. Acute non-A, non-B hepatitis is sometimes associated with aplastic anemia, which can develop in the post-transplant period. Recurrent hepatitis B is less common than after transplantation for chronic liver disease. Transplantation for paracetamol overdose represents a special case. Most patients have no underlying psychiatric disease and have a good long-term prognosis. Patients with psychiatric disease, particularly if chronic or poorly controlled, and/or patients with a history of multiple previous overdoses or parasuicides and/or patients actively abusing drugs or alcohol are usually excluded from transplantation. Their long-term prognosis is deemed to be poor irrespective of hepatic function and postoperative care is likely to be compromised by poor drug compliance.

*Malignant disease*

The risk of recurrent hepatic malignancy is determined by the tumor pathology and size. Patients with hepatocellular carcinomas less than 3–5 cm in diameter appear to have a good prognosis, while those with larger tumors have a 2-year survival of only 30% (Bismuth et al 1987a, O'Grady et al 1988c). Prolonged survival of up to 10 years is seen occasionally, particularly in fibrolamellar carcinomas. Cholangiocarcinomas usually recur rapidly and are not normally considered for transplantation.

### Psychosocial factors and quality of life

Liver transplantation is a major operation that may have significant postoperative morbidity and requires lifelong medical care. Detailed preoperative preparation and counseling of patients and their relatives are required. Following the operation, the quality of life for the majority of patients is markedly improved. The improved well-being in many individuals is self-evident and studies attempting to quantify the quality of life invariably confirm improvement as compared to pretransplant values, although seldom to the level of "normality", and the timing of the improvement varies from immediate to progressive over the first year (Lowe et al 1990, Commander et al 1992).

However, it must be recognized that problems remain. Liver transplant recipients resemble many patients with chronic stable illnesses in their need to take medication and to attend hospital. Typically, early euphoria gives way to mild depression before the patient achieves full adjustment. These adjustments occur more smoothly where the patient has had full, realistic counseling before surgery. Conversely, patients transplanted for fulminant hepatic failure, who were previously in perfect health, have had no opportunity to adjust and often experience more postoperative psychological problems.

## LIVER TRANSPLANTATION IN CHILDREN

Children undergoing liver transplantation deserve separate consideration. The indications are clearly different from those for adults (Table 46.1). Biliary atresia accounts for half of all pediatric patients and three-quarters of patients under 2 years of age. The commonest familial indication is $\alpha_1$-antitrypsin deficiency. The use of liver transplantation to correct inborn errors of metabolism where the target organ is other than the liver, as in primary oxalosis or familial hypercholesterolemia, reflects the growing confidence in the success of the operation. Rarely, irreversible damage to other organs requires transplantation of a liver and a kidney or a liver and a heart. As children with cystic fibrosis survive longer, the incidence of associated liver disease increases (p. 972), although generally portal hypertension rather than hepatic failure is the clinical problem. Occasionally, these patients are considered for combined heart–lung–liver grafting.

Donor organ availability for children remains a major problem, although the use of reduced grafts has eased the shortage. The use of living, related donors, where the child's parent or other close relation undergoes a partial hepatectomy and the removed segment becomes a reduced graft for the child, is technically feasible and is increasing in popularity, although major ethical controversies remain. Children who receive a liver graft have an excellent chance of survival, with 1-year survival approaching 90% (Salt et al 1992). The surgery remains technically demanding, as reflected by the higher rate of hepatic artery thrombosis in children as compared to adults (Merion et al 1989). End-stage liver disease in children is accompanied by malnutrition and growth retardation. The latter used often to persist post-transplant, but increasing emphasis on nutrition pre- and postoperatively and lower doses of corticosteroids have reduced this problem (Becht et al 1993).

## SUMMARY

Liver transplantation is an established treatment for chronic liver disease, acute liver failure and a minority of primary hepatic malignancies and offers 1-year survival of 80% and 5-year survival of 70% in the most favorable groups. Further improvements in survival will require improved selection by determining disease-specific prognostic indices, new immunosuppressive regimens to reduce the problem of chronic rejection and a means to reduce the problem of biliary tract complications.

## TRANSPLANTATION OF THE PANCREAS

Although the first pancreas transplantation was performed over 25 years ago, this procedure has not yet gained the widespread acceptance enjoyed by transplantation of the heart, liver and kidney (Kelly et al 1967). Recent advances in surgical technique, immunosuppression and perioperative management have, however, led to major improvements in patient and graft survival and 1-year patient and graft survival rates (i.e. independent of exogenous insulin) in excess of 90% for combined pancreas–kidney grafts have been reported (Stratta et al 1991b, 1995, Larsen et al 1994).

### PANCREAS–KIDNEY TRANSPLANTS

Combined pancreas–kidney transplantation is gaining acceptance for patients with insulin-dependent diabetes mellitus and dialysis-dependent diabetic nephropathy. These patients benefit from kidney transplantation and the addition of a pancreas allograft does not appear to increase mortality or morbidity significantly and offers the possibility of independence from insulin. Some data suggest that pancreas transplantation may halt progression of diabetic complications such as retinopathy, neuropathy and atherosclerosis, but only long-term follow-up will show the effect of transplantation on the natural history of diabetes mellitus (Larsen et al 1994, Stratta et al 1995).

Some centers now advocate pancreas–kidney transplantation prior to dialysis on the assumption that improved glucose metabolism resulting from transplantation may prevent the development and progression of complications. The results, in some series at least, are the same as for patients already on dialysis at transplantation. The long-term outcome of this approach remains uncertain and the timing of transplantation in these patients remains to be defined (Larsen et al 1994, Stratta et al 1995).

### PANCREAS TRANSPLANTS

The indications for transplantation of the pancreas alone are less clear. Here, the balance between the disadvantages of long-term insulin therapy and of chronic immunosuppression becomes much more difficult to assess. Given the limited experience with this procedure and the lack of long-term follow-up, it seems reasonable to regard isolated pancreas transplantation as an experimental procedure (Larsen et al 1994, Stratta et al 1995).

### CLINICAL ASPECTS

In many centers the preferred technique is transplantation of the pancreas, with its associated duodenal segment, into the native bladder (Stratta et al 1991b). Immunosuppression is commenced with a four-drug regimen, including either ATGAM (anti-thymocyte globulin) or tacrolimus with cyclosporin, prednisone and azathioprine, and it continues with cyclosporin, prenisolone and azathioprine in the long term. Immediate postoperative complications include rejection, vascular thrombosis, pancreatitis and infection. Early rejection of the pancreas graft is difficult to diagnose and this remains the most important cause of graft loss. Combined pancreas–kidney grafts have the advantage that kidney rejection is easier to detect and parallels or precedes rejection of the pancreatic graft. Asymptomatic hyperamylasemia is common following transplantation and symptomatic pancreatitis may occur, precipitated by inadequate drainage of the graft or by vesicoduodenal reflux in patients with a neurogenic bladder consequent on autonomic neuropathy. These patients are prone to dehydration and metabolic acidosis and may also develop a chemical cystitis or urethritis as a result of the close anatomical relationship between the pancreas and urinary tract (Stratta et al 1991b, 1995, Larsen et al 1994).

## TRANSPLANTATION OF THE SMALL INTESTINE

In the past few years transplantation of the small intestine has become a clinical reality and this technically and immunologically daunting procedure has been performed in children and adults (Vanderhoof et al 1992). While its role in the management of intestinal failure continues to be evaluated, this procedure may soon be an accepted therapeutic option for these unfortunate patients.

### INTESTINAL FAILURE

#### Definition and prognosis

Intestinal failure is best defined as the situation in which the "functioning gut mass has been reduced below the minimum necessary for the adequate digestion and absorption of food" (Scott & Irving 1992). It may arise through loss of intestine as a result of resection, trauma or infarction or through the involvement of the intestine in diseases such as Crohn's disease, radiation enteritis, tumors (such as desmoid tumors and intestinal polyposis), congenital disorders (such as microvillus inclusion disease), diffuse motility disorders and necrotizing enterocolitis. Sometimes, as in Crohn's disease, intestinal failure may be the consequence of resection and disease.

Survival rates for intestinal failure have improved considerably, especially since the advent of total parenteral nutrition (TPN). One study in children showed 5-year survival rates for intestinal failure improved from 65% between 1979 and 1984 to over 94% between 1985 and 1990 (Georgeson & Breaux 1992). Similar survival rates have been reported for adults and most patients with intestinal failure can expect to do well on TPN (Howard et al 1991).

**Table 46.5** Factors influencing adaptation in short-bowel syndrome

| Factor | Favorable | Unfavorable |
|---|---|---|
| Extent of resection | <80% (>40 cm infant, >100 cm adult) | >80% |
| Site of resection | Jejunum | Ileum |
| Intestinal disease | Absent | Present |
| Intestinal anatomy | Ileocolic valve intact | Ileocolic valve resected |
| | Colon in situ | Colon diseased/ resected |
| Age | Child | Elderly |

**Table 46.6** Complications of long-term home parenteral nutrition

| |
|---|
| *Intestinal failure complications* |
| Diarrhea, dehydration, electrolyte imbalance |
| Hypocalcemia, hypomagnesemia |
| Trace element and vitamin deficiencies |
| d-lactic acidosis |
| Calcium oxalate stones |
| Metabolic bone disease |
| Gastric acid hypersecretion |
| *Total parenteral nutrition complications* |
| Hyperglycemia |
| Catheter sepsis |
| Thrombosis |
| Air embolus |
| Catheter breakage |
| Hepatobiliary dysfunction |

Several factors exert a significant impact on prognosis (Table 46.5) (Scott & Irving 1992, Vanderhoof et al 1992). The extent of resection appears to exert the greatest influence, as loss of more than 80% of the small intestine is associated with a poor prognosis. Prognosis is also better following jejunal than ileal resection. Not surprisingly, prognosis is best when the remaining intestine is disease-free. Experimental and clinical studies have shown the beneficial prognostic effects of an intact ileocecal valve and colon. Age also influences outcome, the outlook following extensive resection being best for children and worst for the elderly. The influence of each of these factors is related to its effect on adaptation in the intestinal remnant and the fact that adaptation will occur must be borne in mind in decision making. The potential for adaptation was emphasized in one study in which 88% of infants with a remnant that measured at least 40 cm and 57% of infants with an even smaller remnant were eventually able to dispense with TPN. Adaptation may take 1–2 years to reach a maximum, is greater in an ileal than in a jejunal remnant and is greater in children than in adults. Enteral nutrients are a potent stimulus for adaptation and the importance of continuing enteral nutrition regardless of its caloric contribution cannot be overemphasized. Retention of the ileocolonic junction promotes adaptation.

## Management

All patients with intestinal failure will, at least initially, require nutritional support by TPN with or without some enteral nutrition (Purdom & Kirby 1991, Scott & Irving 1992, Vanderhoof et al 1992). Many will undergo adaptation sufficient to allow resumption of oral nutrition alone. The rest will continue to need TPN and the options then will be to continue home parenteral nutrition (HPN), to use surgical or pharmacological treatments that promote digestive function and permit adequate oral intake or to proceed to intestinal transplantation.

Patients who are left with less than 25 cm of small bowel are unlikely ever to be able to do without HPN, but this is very likely with a remnant in excess of 50 cm. It is in those whose intestinal remnants measure between 25 and 60 cm that factors such as the retention or loss of the colon or ileocecal junction, the presence or absence of disease in the remnant and the presence or absence of a stoma become of greatest importance, as they may tip the balance one way or the other. It is also in this group that surgical or pharmacological interventions may be most effective.

### *Long-term home parenteral nutrition – prognosis and problems*

Most patients do very well on HPN. Actuarial survival in a large multicenter study in the United States showed a 4-year survival on HPN in excess of 80% for patients with Crohn's disease and congenital intestinal diseases and in the region of 70% for those with ischemic, radiation-related and motility disorders (Howard et al 1991). Very few deaths were related directly to HPN but were due to the underlying disease or other medical complications. Thus, in contrast to hemodialysis, complications related to HPN are not a major threat for most patients with intestinal failure.

Morbidity related to HPN appears to be low, but there are several problems that may significantly affect the prognosis and quality of life for patients (Table 46.6).

Some patients with a short remnant and an intestinal stoma suffer large fluid and electrolyte losses requiring repeated hospital admissions for rehydration. Such HPN patients should be considered for transplantation. Problems related directly to HPN that are likely to lead to consideration of transplantation include intravascular complications and hepatobiliary dysfunction. Recurrent catheter sepsis and venous thrombosis may lead to complete loss of venous access. Significant hepatobiliary dysfunction is rare with modern TPN solutions and methods of administration (p. 979). Chronic decompensated liver disease appears most frequently among low birth-weight infants who have required TPN from birth and is often preceded by TPN-related cholestasis. When liver disease leads to consideration of hepatic transplantation, it would seem reasonable to consider combined liver–small bowel transplantation.

Quality of life is an important factor in the treatment of chronic intestinal failure. The United Kingdom HPN Registry shows that most patients enjoy an excellent quality of life with half working full-time and less than 10% housebound or requiring major assistance (Scott & Irving 1992). Cost is a major issue. In the United States, for example, it has been estimated that HPN costs between $75 000 and $150 000 per year; for many individuals health insurance does not cover HPN. HPN also limits independence and may interfere with social and sexual activity.

*Surgical and pharmacological approaches*

Several surgical approaches have been evaluated experimentally and clinically in intestinal failure, but their value remains uncertain (Thompson 1993). The most important "pharmacological" treatment is persistence with some enteral nutrition. The factors in any nutritional formulation that best promote adaptation include essential fatty acids and glutamine. Others have demonstrated beneficial effects on adaptation from growth hormone, prostaglandins and polyamines, but none of these agents has yet gained a place in clinical practice. The current limitations of surgical and pharmacological approaches are such that the choice for most patients with intestinal failure lies between long-term HPN and transplantation.

*Small intestinal transplantation* (Fig. 46.7A&B)

Interest in small intestinal transplantation was first sparked by pioneering animal studies in the late 1950s. Although attempts at small intestinal transplantation were made over the next several years, little progress was made until the arrival of effective immunosuppression with the introduction of cyclosporin. The next landmark came with a report of successful combined transplantation of the liver and small intestine and, as with other organs, it was suggested that grafting the liver with the small intestine conferred a degree of immunological protection on the small intestine (Grant et al 1990). This has led to the performance of combined small intestine–liver grafts at a number of institutions over the past few years (Todo et al 1992b, 1994, Vanderhoof et al 1992). However, while such an approach is ideal for patients with intestinal and liver failure, it poses a considerable dilemma for the individual with intestinal failure but normal liver function.

Recently, the new immunosuppressant agent tacrolimus has rekindled interest in isolated intestinal transplantation. Experience using this agent has been confined almost exclusively to the University of Pittsburgh, where 70 intestinal grafts, 16 of which were isolated intestinal transplants, have been performed using tacrolimus immunosuppression (Todo et al 1994).

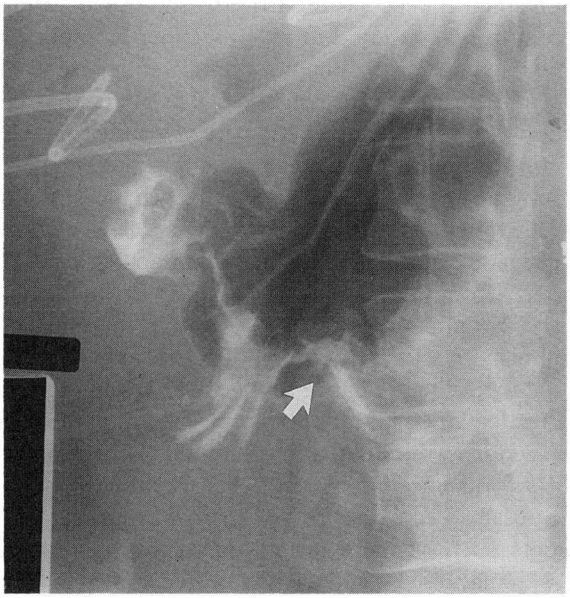

A

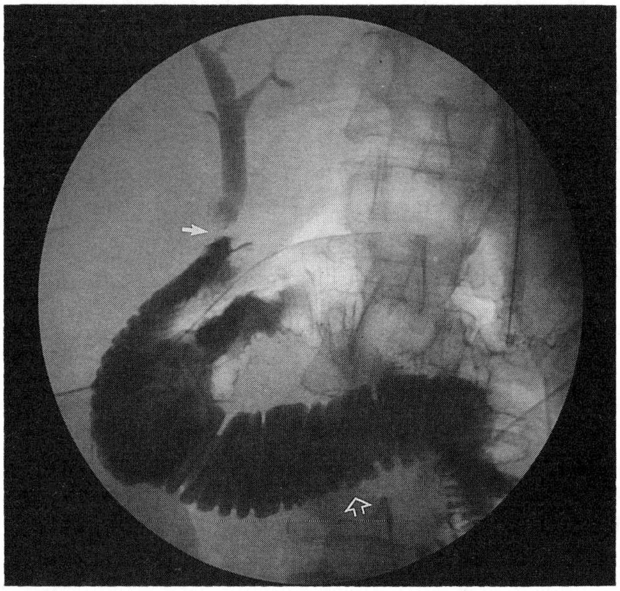

B

**Fig. 46.7** Small intestinal transplantation following intestinal vascular occlusion. The pretransplant radiograph (**A**) shows that only the stomach (gas shadow) and proximal duodenum remain. The latter communicates directly with a duodenostomy tube (arrowed). Post-transplant radiograph (**B**) shows a choledochojejunostomy (closed arrow) and normal-appearing graft (open arrow).

## Transplantation problems

Transplantation of the small intestine remains a formidable procedure and in the largest reported series was accompanied by a mortality of 25–30% (Todo et al 1994). Morbidity among survivors is significant. Rejection is inevitable but because of its patchy nature, it may be difficult to detect and may be missed until irreversible graft damage has occurred. Rejection of the intestinal graft often also leads to infection because of the importance of the intestinal mucosa as a barrier to the translocation of bacteria from the gut lumen. Infectious complications loom large and sepsis is the most important cause of morbidity and death. Transplantation also alters the motor function of the graft muscle and nerve dysfunction may be a prominent manifestation of chronic rejection.

A long-term concern is the development of lymphoma in the grafted intestine (Reyes et al 1994). Several instances, all fatal, of intestinal lymphoma have been reported in long-term survivors. This apparently high incidence of lymphoma is probably related to the intensity of immunosuppression required and to the large amount of immunological tissue native to the gut. Epstein–Barr virus (EBV) infection, as in other transplantation patients, is a major factor in the induction of monoclonal lymphomas. Disease recurrence has not yet been reported but is certainly possible, especially in patients with primary diffuse disorders such as malignancy, inflammatory bowel disease, vascular disease and pseudo-obstruction.

*Selection*

Most patients with chronic intestinal failure do very well on HPN, which carries a relatively low morbidity and mortality and for them intestinal transplantation is an unwarranted risk (Ingham Clark et al 1992). Transplantation should only be considered for HPN patients with major complications related to TPN, such as end-stage liver disease or loss of venous access, or for those who suffer continuing problems of excessive fluid and electrolyte losses or who are not doing well on HPN. Transplantation is certainly not indicated for the well-maintained patient without complications.

## EFFECTS OF ORGAN TRANSPLANTATION ON THE GASTROINTESTINAL TRACT AND LIVER

### GENERAL CONSIDERATIONS

Gastrointestinal, hepatic and biliary complications occur frequently in recipients of bone marrow and solid organ transplants. Several general factors need to be borne in mind to facilitate the diagnosis of symptoms such as gastrointestinal bleeding, abdominal pain and diarrhea in patients who have undergone such transplants.

First, pre-existing gastrointestinal disease may be exacerbated following transplantation. Thus, peptic ulcer disease remains one of the most important causes of gastrointestinal hemorrhage after transplantation, immunosuppression may render previously asymptomatic parasitic infestation invasive and symptomatic and diabetic gastroenteropathy may become symptomatic following pancreas transplantation. The nature of the disease necessitating transplantation and the type of transplantation undertaken are also relevant. Mucositis and veno-occlusive disease (VOD) following bone marrow transplantation are related directly to the intensity of the cytoreductive regimen and graft-versus-host disease (GVHD) is much more frequent following bone marrow allografts than after bone marrow autografts or solid organ transplants. The time from transplantation to the onset of gastrointestinal symptoms may also be important, as bacterial infections tend to occur early and viral infections later. Finally, the effects of various therapies, including the side-effects of antibiotics, immunosuppressives, growth factors and GVHD therapy, and the hepatobiliary effects of parenteral nutrition need to be considered.

Owing to the intensity of pretransplant therapy and the immunological "potency" of the allograft itself, gastrointestinal and hepatobiliary complications are especially prevalent following bone marrow transplantation and will be considered first (see Table 46.8 on p. 1171) (McDonald et al 1986a,b, Wolford & McDonald 1988). The clinical features and evaluation of several of these disorders are common to all transplant patients. Specific comments on gastrointestinal and liver dysfunction following various solid organ transplants will therefore follow.

### GASTROINTESTINAL AND HEPATOBILIARY COMPLICATIONS OF BONE MARROW TRANSPLANTS

#### Intestinal toxicity

This term refers to gastrointestinal symptoms related directly to preoperative therapies, particularly chemotherapy and radiotherapy (Dubois & Walker 1988). The mucosal toxicity (mucositis) induced by these therapies and its related symptoms is a direct consequence of the intensity of the conditioning therapy, occurring in over 80% of patients subjected to some regimens. Abdominal pain and diarrhea (Table 46.7) are prominent symptoms of mucositis and develop within 2 weeks of cytoreductive therapy. Rarely, ileus and peritonism may develop, but perforation is extremely rare and the temptation to proceed to laparotomy should be avoided.

In the early post-transplantation period, previously asymptomatic conditions such as peptic ulcer disease may become symptomatic and must be borne in mind in the differential diagnosis. Furthermore, the clinical features of these disorders may be masked by the effects of chemotherapy and associated neutropenia.

The management of intestinal symptoms related to intestinal toxicity is largely symptomatic. Prophylactic therapy for peptic ulcer disease can be given, as invasive investigations may be relatively contraindicated soon after transplantation. Such therapy should be confined to surface-acting agents such as antacids and sucralfate. $H_2$ receptor antagonists should be avoided given the reported suppressant effects of cimetidine on the bone marrow.

**Table 46.7** Causes of abdominal pain and diarrhea in the bone marrow transplant patient

| |
|---|
| Intestinal toxicity* |
| Graft-versus-host disease* – acute/chronic |
| Infections* |
| Giardia |
| Fungi |
| *C. difficile* |
| Strongyloides |
| *Isospora belli* |
| Cryptosporidium |
| Microsporidium |
| Viral |
| Cytomegalovirus |
| Herpes simplex virus |
| Varicella zoster virus |
| Adenovirus |
| Rotavirus |
| Coxsackie |
| Bacterial translocation |
| Typhlitis |
| Lymphoproliferative disease |
| Hematomas – abdominal wall/intra-abdominal |
| Biliary disease – sludge/stones |
| Pancreatitis - sludge/stones |
| Liver disease |
| Veno-occlusive disease |
| Steatosis |
| Hepatitis |
| Congestion |
| Medications* |
| Jejunal vasculitis |
| Gastric bezoar |

*Indicates cause of diarrhea.

The safety and efficacy of proton pump inhibitors such as omeprazole and lansoprazole have not been evaluated in this patient group.

## Veno-occlusive disease

The two principal hepatic complications of bone marrow transplantation that rarely follow solid organ transplantation are veno-occlusive disease (VOD) and GVHD (McDonald et al 1986a,b, Mieli-Vergani 1993). VOD (p. 1081) is a significant early problem following bone marrow transplantation and has been the subject of several recent reviews (Shulman & Hinterberger 1992, Carreras et al 1993, Baglin 1994). Its cause is probably multifactorial, but it is principally a consequence of concomitant chemotherapy. Other possible risk factors for VOD include female sex, pre-existent liver disease, abnormal liver function tests and metastatic liver disease. The frequency of VOD varies from 2% following transplantation for thalassemia in children (Lucarelli et al 1985) to over 20% following transplantation for hematological malignancies (McDonald et al 1985). Endothelial injury leads to obstruction of small intrahepatic venules and damage to the surrounding centrilobular (zone 3) hepatocytes and sinusoids (p. 712). VOD usually becomes symptomatic within 2 weeks of transplantation.

Abdominal pain is the presenting symptom in 75% of patients. Typical physical findings include right upper quadrant tenderness, hepatomegaly and ascites. These clinical features and characteristic ultrasound findings usually prove diagnostic (Brown et al 1990). The management of VOD is primarily prophylactic and symptomatic. In rare instances, portacaval shunting and liver transplantation have been performed.

## Graft-versus-host disease (GVHD) (Fig. 46.8A,B)

### *Intestinal GVHD*

Acute GVHD develops between 2 and 10 weeks after transplantation, but symptoms usually begin between 3 and 4 weeks (McDonald et al 1986a,b, Wolford & McDonald 1988). The clinical manifestations of gastrointestinal GVHD reflect direct effects on the intestine and infections that develop as a consequence of GVHD. Common secondary infections include viral and fungal enteritis as well as *Cl. difficile* colitis. GVHD promotes bacterial translocation to mesenteric lymph nodes, which can produce abdominal pain. Patients with intestinal GVHD usually also have skin and liver involvement, but this is not always the case.

The most prominent symptoms of intestinal GVHD are abdominal cramps and diarrhea. Diarrhea is typically profuse, secretory in type and the stool contains white blood cells and large amounts of protein. Peritonism may be present, but as with intestinal toxicity perforation is unusual and laparotomy is rarely necessary (McGregor et al 1988). GVHD has a predilection for the distal small intestine and intestinal radiology shows mucosal and submucosal edema and even ulceration of the distal ileum and proximal colon. Pneumatosis cystoides intestinalis has been reported. Intestinal abnormalities usually resolve as symptoms abate, but ileal fibrosis with stricturing and obstruction may develop. GVHD localized to the upper gastrointestinal tract has been reported, causing anorexia, dyspepsia, food intolerance, nausea and vomiting. Endoscopic biopsy may confirm the diagnosis.

Acute GVHD causes necrosis of regenerating mucosal cells and when severe it leads to loss of crypts and sloughing of the mucosa (Galati et al 1993). Upper gastrointestinal biopsies have a greater diagnostic yield for GVHD than biopsies from the colon and lower gastrointestinal endoscopy alone underestimates the incidence of upper gastrointestinal GVHD, which cannot be predicted reliably from symptoms or skin involvement (Roy et al 1991). In one recent study, 25 of 62 (40%) patients with acute upper gastrointestinal GVHD had only limited skin involvement, leading the authors to emphasize that upper gastrointestinal GVHD may be under-recognized. In the same study, 71% of these patients responded to immunosuppressive therapy (Weisdorf et al 1990).

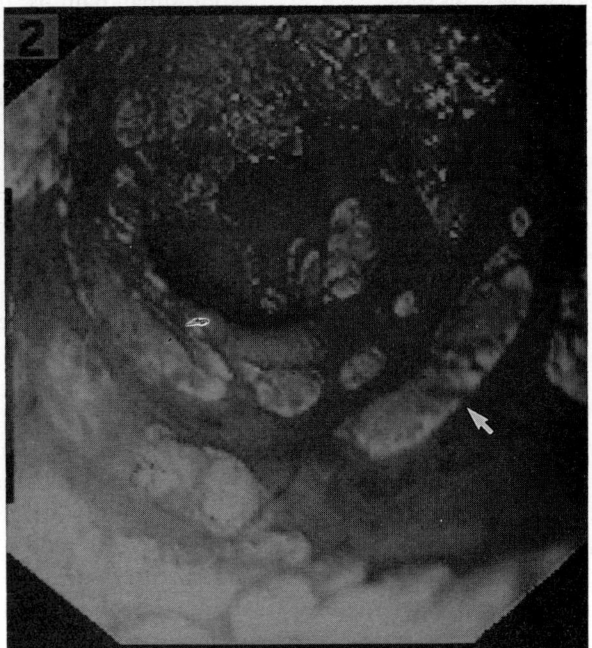


A

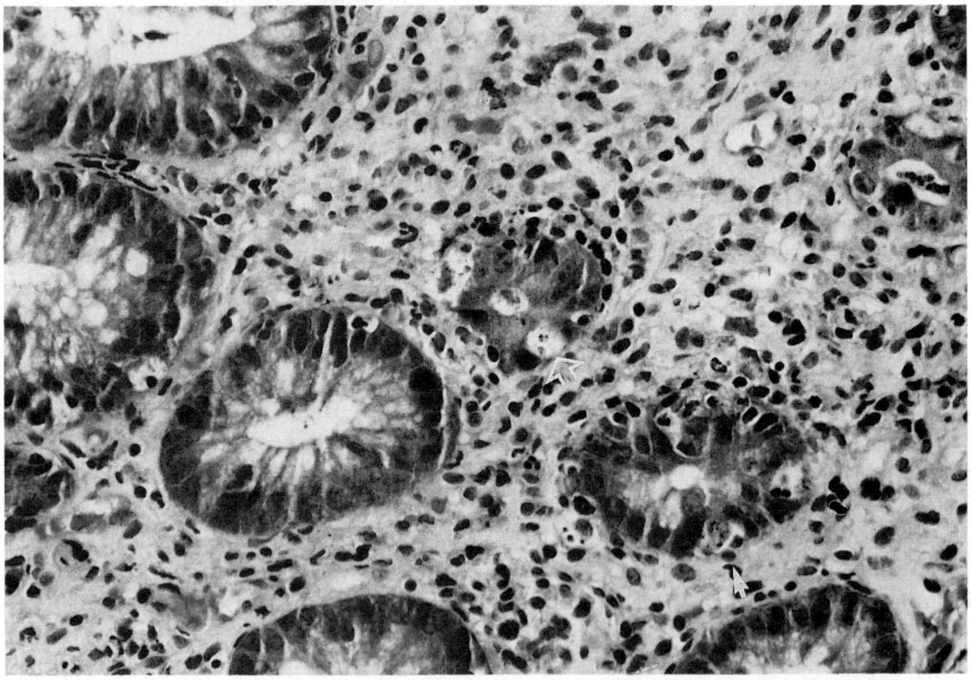

B

**Fig. 46.8** Graft-versus-host disease (GVHD). (**A**) Severe GVHD of the duodenum with extensive sloughing of mucosa with islands (arrowed) of retained mucosa. (**B**) The microscopic features of colonic GVHD with lymphocytic infiltrate and individual cell necrosis of colonic epithelial cells (arrowed) (hematoxylin and eosin, × 200).

The diagnosis of GVHD and several other intestinal complications of bone marrow transplantation frequently depends on examination of mucosal biopsies or luminal fluid at the time of intestinal endoscopy. Unfortunately, pancytopenia increases the risks of hemorrhage and sepsis following gastrointestinal endoscopy, which can only be justified if it provides diagnostic information not available from noninvasive investigations. Macroscopic views of the mucosa are not usually diagnostic and if endoscopy is to be undertaken it should also be safe to obtain brushings for cytology and mucosal biopsies (Galati et al 1993).

Chronic GVHD usually develops more than 100 days

after transplantation and is relatively uncommon in the gastrointestinal tract (Snover 1990). It causes abdominal pain and diarrhea consequent on intestinal obstruction and bacterial overgrowth.

### *Hepatic GVHD*

Acute hepatic GVHD is less common than involvement of the skin and intestine. However, acute hepatic GVHD without skin or intestinal disease can occur and poses a diagnostic dilemma. The presentation with jaundice, hepatomegaly and possibly fever has to be distinguished from VOD and viral hepatitis. GVHD cannot occur until engraftment has taken place and therefore develops later than VOD. The liver function tests are usually markedly cholestatic. Other diagnoses such as viral hepatitis and large duct biliary obstruction can usually be established by viral serology, ultrasonography and measurement of wedged hepatic venous pressure. Liver biopsy may be required but carries some risk in the thrombocytopenic patient. It should be performed laparoscopically after platelet transfusion to minimize the risks of bleeding. Endotheliolitis and bile ductular damage are diagnostic. Treatment with immunosuppression, usually cyclosporin and corticosteroids, is generally successful.

Chronic GVHD, which arises more than 100 days post-bone marrow transplant, is less common but almost invariably involves the liver. Extrahepatic manifestations of chronic GVHD include skin pigmentation, scleroderma, joint contractures, polyserositis and failure of oral and ocular secretions. The hepatic disease resembles chronic rejection after liver transplantation (p. 1159) with progressive cholestasis and pruritus. Histologically, chronic GVHD is one cause of the "vanishing bile duct syndrome". Treatment with cyclosporin is usually successful, but liver transplantation may need to be considered and can be successful (Marks et al 1992).

## Intestinal infections

Intestinal infections are important causes of abdominal pain in bone marrow transplant patients and may occur at any time following transplantation.

### *Nonviral infections*

In the first weeks following transplantation, infections are usually exacerbations of conditions present at the time of conditioning therapy (McDonald et al 1986a,b, Wolford & McDonald 1988). These infections often coexist with or complicate GVHD. Important pathogens include *G. lamblia*, fungi and *Cl. difficile*. Organisms such as *Strongyloides, Cryptosporidium, Microsporidium* and *Isopora belli* may also become invasive and disseminate. Sometimes infection may be detected by stool examination, but direct sampling of duodenal contents and duodenal biopsy will often be necessary to make a definitive diagnosis.

Abdominal pain may also result from invasion of the hepatobiliary system by organisms and bacterial and fungal liver abscesses have been reported (p. 817). Implicated organisms include candida, histoplasma, trichophyton and aspergillus. Splenic microabscesses related to candida and aspergillus and biliary obstruction by aspergillus have also been reported.

An unusual and catastrophic infectious complication of bone marrow transplantation is typhlitis. This syndrome, thought to be caused by *Cl. septicum*, develops in granulocytopenic patients and involves predominantly the cecum and right colon leading to septicemia, perforation and intestinal hemorrhage. Abdominal computed tomography demonstrating a markedly thickened cecum and ascending colon may prove diagnostic. This complication is associated with a high mortality but successful surgical resection has, on occasion, been performed.

### *Viral infections*

Viral infections associated with gastrointestinal symptomatology include cytomegalovirus (CMV), herpes simplex virus (HSV), varicella zoster virus (VZV), adenovirus, rotavirus and coxsackie virus. All may produce a viral enteritis.

***Cytomegalovirus.*** CMV is the most frequent viral pathogen and illness usually occurs more than 2 months following transplant. About 80% of previously CMV-seropositive bone marrow transplant recipients reactivate their infections and 40% of seronegative recipients become seropositive on receiving marrow from seropositive donors (Cicogna & Polsky 1994). About a half of bone marrow transplant patients develop active CMV infection and pneumonitis is the commonest and most serious manifestation. Gastrointestinal involvement may be more common than currently recognized if adequately sought. It has also been suggested that CMV may be important in the pathogenesis of several complications of bone marrow and solid organ transplantations. It may increase the incidence and virulence of other infections by depressing cell-mediated immunity, it may have an influence on the development of rejection and a relationship has been proposed between GVHD and CMV pneumonitis in bone marrow transplant recipients.

The problem, of course, is the ubiquity of CMV infection in the population at large (p. 792). In the United States as many as 50% of adults are seropositive for CMV. Diagnosing CMV as the cause of a particular illness may, therefore, be difficult and investigations have included the demonstration of viral inclusions in biopsy specimens, the detection of CMV antigen or CMV-DNA in tissue specimens and culture of the virus from biopsies. One study compared seven virologic methods for the diagnosis of

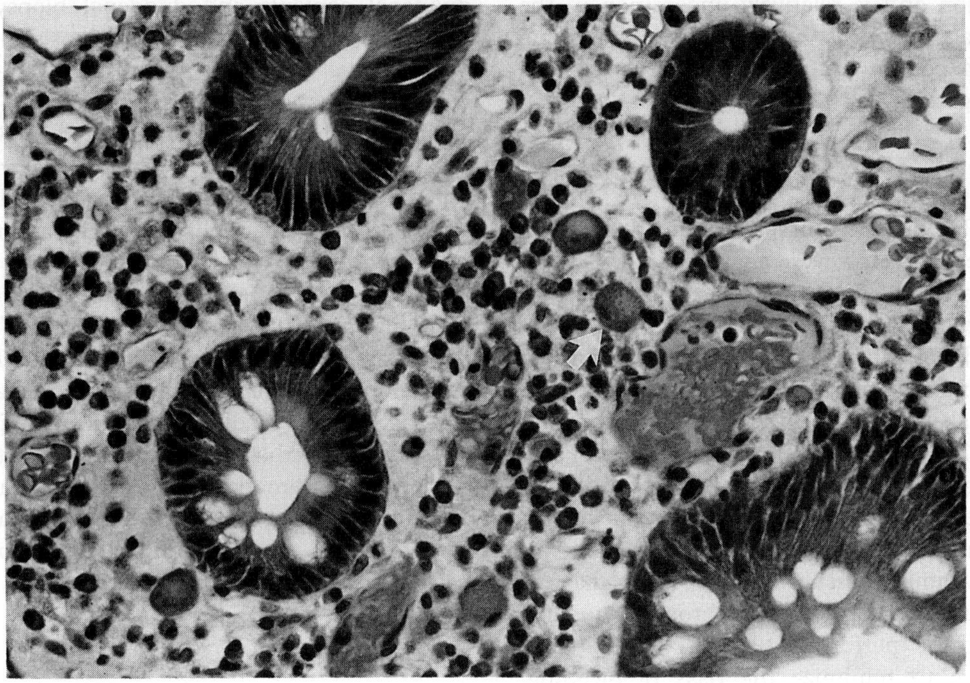

**Fig. 46.9** Cytomegalovirus colitis in a transplant patient showing infected cells bearing typical large intranuclear inclusions (arrowed) (hematoxylin and eosin, × 200).

CMV and found that culture and indirect fluorescent antibody detection of the virus in biopsies gave the greatest diagnostic yield (Hackman et al 1994). CMV inclusions were seen histologically in only 30% of patients and it was concluded that diagnosis should never rely on cytology, histology, immunohistochemistry or DNA hybridization techniques alone.

CMV may be associated with esophagitis, a profound syndrome of gastroparesis, diffuse enteritis, isolated ileitis, colitis, hepatitis and pancreatitis. Discrete ulceration leading to hemorrhage and even perforation of the small intestine and, especially, the colon may occur. The presence of CMV-related gastrointestinal disease may be suggested by systemic manifestations of CMV infection but often relies upon histological examination of endoscopic biopsies (Fig. 46.9). In contrast to HSV, where samples from the ulcer edge are most useful, biopsies obtained from the base of CMV-related ulcers are more likely to prove diagnostic.

***Varicella zoster virus.*** VZV infection may be associated with striking abdominal pain and ileus, hepatitis and pancreatitis. Abdominal pain may precede the appearance of skin lesions, and these lesions may be atypical in transplant patients.

***Epstein–Barr virus.*** An unusual infectious complication that may be associated with the development of abdominal pain is EBV-related lymphoproliferative disease (Davey et al 1989). This malignant B-cell disease usually develops in patients with severe acute GVHD that is being treated with cyclosporin or other immunosuppressive therapy. Intestinal symptoms reflect direct infiltration of the intestinal wall.

*Endoscopy and infection*

Two studies have examined the infectious complications of endoscopic procedures in bone marrow transplant recipients (Bianco et al 1990, Kaw et al 1993). Among patients in whom procedures were performed within 100 days of bone marrow transplant in the Seattle study, 19% developed clinically significant bacteremia. In another series, 67 procedures in 53 patients resulted in fever in one subject and significant sepsis in none, although only 10 of these patients had a neutrophil count of less than 1000. This same study also failed to define any advantage for prophylactic antibiotics. It is our practice to avoid endoscopy whenever possible in the acellular phase and to delay endoscopic procedures, if possible, until the granulocyte count exceeds 500.

### Hematomas

Abdominal pain due to abdominal wall and intra-abdominal hematomas is extremely unusual in the general population, but they should be looked for carefully in bone marrow transplant patients. They are associated with thrombocytopenia, recent biopsy and GVHD. Common sites include the retroperitoneal tissues, the rectus sheath and the intestinal wall. Intramural hematomas of the esophagus and small intestine also occur and are most commonly related to recent endoscopic biopsy but may also occur following retching. Splenic hematomas and infarction have also been described. Therapy includes the correction of any coagulation defect.

### Biliary disease

Almost all bone marrow transplant patients receive TPN at some stage following their transplants and this is associated with hepatic steatosis, cholestasis and gallbladder stasis (Quigley et al 1993). Stasis can lead to the development of sludge and gallstones, which may become symptomatic either by obstruction of the cystic or common bile ducts or by precipitating pancreatitis. In a prospective study, 11 of 18 (61%) patients undergoing bone marrow transplant developed sludge but none was complicated by cholecystitis (Jacobson et al 1993). Acalculous cholecystitis has also been reported in bone marrow transplant patients and this may be more common than calculous cholecystitis (Jardines et al 1993). Possible risk factors for acalculous cholecystitis include multiple blood transfusions, TPN, CMV infections and veno-occlusive disease. Acalculous cholecystitis may present at any time after transplantation and patients develop right upper quadrant abdominal pain and may require cholecystectomy (Jardines et al 1993).

### Pancreatitis

Although several potential causes of pancreatitis occur in bone marrow transplant patients, acute pancreatitis is rare. Causes include biliary sludge, stones, CMV, EBV and HSV infections and the effects of drugs such as methotrexate, cyclophosphamide and prednisone.

### Medication

Iatrogenic gastrointestinal symptoms are common. Medications that can cause abdominal pain include narcotics, anticholinergics, vincristine, granulocyte macrophage colony stimulating factor (GMCSF) and interleukin 2. Narcotic-induced ileus may be a major problem in these patients and can necessitate a change of analgesic or intestinal decompression (Bollinger & Quigley 1994). Medications associated with diarrhea include antibiotics, prokinetics such as metoclopramide and cisapride, antacids and several chemotherapeutic agents.

## GASTROINTESTINAL AND HEPATOBILIARY COMPLICATIONS OF SOLID ORGAN TRANSPLANTS

Gastrointestinal complications are common following transplantation of solid organs (Table 46.8) and occur, for example, in up to 50% of heart transplant recipients (Villar et al 1989, Cates et al 1991, Steck et al 1993). Prominent in these patients are cytomegalovirus, gastroenteritis, upper gastrointestinal hemorrhage, diarrhea, pancreatitis and gallbladder disease. Surgical treatment for gastrointestinal complications has proved necessary in about two-thirds of patients and mortality related to such procedures has been up to 17% (Villar et al 1989). A similar incidence of gastrointestinal complications has been reported in renal transplant recipients (Bardaxoglou et al 1993, Benoit et al 1993). Gastrointestinal perforation occurred in 14 of 416 (3%) kidney transplant recipients and was located in the colon in six, the small bowel in four, the duodenum in two, the stomach in one and the

**Table 46.8** Gastrointestinal and hepatobiliary problems in transplant patients

| Clinical presentation | Causes | Comments |
|---|---|---|
| Dysphagia, odynophagia | Candida<br>Herpes simplex<br>Cytomegalovirus | May not have oropharyngeal symptoms. Endoscopy with cytology/ biopsy essential. |
| Nausea, vomiting | Cytomegalovirus (bone marrow transplant)<br>Gastroparesis | Gastric mucosa may appear normal at endoscopy in cytomegalovirus infection. |
| Upper gastrointestinal hemorrhage | "Stress" ulceration<br>Peptic ulcer disease<br>Esophageal varices<br>Hemobilia<br>Cytomegalovirus | Exacerbation of peptic ulcer disease important. Portal vein thrombosis after liver transplant. |
| Lower gastrointestinal hemorrhage | Cytomegalovirus<br>Ischemia | Multiple, discrete, hemorrhagic ulcers characteristic of cytomegalovirus |
| Diarrhea | Cytomegalovirus<br>*Cl. difficile*<br>GVHD (bone marrow transplant)<br>Giardiasis | Endoscopic biopsy important in GVHD. |
| Abdominal pain | Intestinal toxicity (bone marrow transplant)<br>Cytomegalovirus<br>Pancreatitis<br>Cholecystitis<br>Typhlitis (bone marrow transplant)<br>GVHD<br>Lymphoma | Azathioprine may cause pancreatitis. Gallstones common after kidney and pancreas transplants. |
| Abnormal liver function tests (jaundice) | Veno-occlusive disease<br>GVHD (bone marrow transplant)<br>Viral hepatitis<br>Pre-existing liver disease<br>Drug hepatotoxicity | Acute usually cytomegalovirus. Chronic usually hepatitis C virus. |
| Ascites, hepatomegaly | Veno-occlusive disease<br>GVHD (bone marrow transplant) | |

esophagus in one (Bardaxoglou et al 1993). Other important gastrointestinal complications have included acute pancreatitis, gastrointestinal hemorrhage and cholecystitis. As in other transplant groups, perforation and hemorrhage account for most deaths.

## Graft-versus-host disease

GVHD is much less common following solid organ transplants than bone marrow transplants but has been reported following liver transplantation. Clinical features have included skin rash, fever, pancytopenia and diarrhea (Roberts et al 1991, Collins et al 1992). In contrast to GVHD in bone marrow transplant patients, liver involvement is distinctly uncommon whereas pancytopenia is prominent.

## Infection

Infection is a common occurrence and CMV infection is a particular cause of mortality and morbidity in all organ transplant recipients (Kaplan et al 1989, Cheung & Ng 1993, Goodgame 1993).

### *Cytomegalovirus infection*

The pathological features of CMV infection help to understand the pathophysiology of the clinical manifestations (Goodgame 1993). Epithelial viral inclusions are associated with mild superficial inflammation, whereas endothelial inclusions are associated with severe ulceration and explain the predilection for this infection to cause hemorrhage and perforation. Gastrointestinal bleeding occurred in 11 of 19 (58%) non-AIDS patients with gastrointestinal CMV infection and ulceration was found at endoscopy on 70% of these patients (Cheung & Ng 1993). Important clinical clues to CMV are multiple discrete ulcers in the colon or upper gastrointestinal tract. Ileal CMV has also been described (Lepinski & Hamilton 1990).

CMV esophagitis may lead to dysphagia and odynophagia and may be indistinguishable endoscopically from candida or herpes simplex infection. Gastric involvement was noted in one series in over 80% of all gastrointestinal CMV infections (Sakr et al 1992). Profound gastroparesis related to CMV gastritis and responding to antiviral therapy also occurs. Therapy with ganciclovir has given encouraging results for gastrointestinal CMV in transplant recipients in general (Faulds & Heel 1990). Gastrointestinal CMV has a low incidence of relapse following therapy.

### *Fungal infection*

Fungal infections are potentially devastating complications of any transplantation procedure (Paya 1993). The incidence of fungal infections has varied from 0% to 40% after solid organ transplants and the overall incidence is remarkably similar in heart, heart/lung, lung, pancreas, kidney and liver transplant recipients. *Candida albicans* is the usual organism involved, except in heart transplant recipients where aspergillus infections predominate. Candida esophagitis is perhaps the most common gastrointestinal manifestation and should be suspected in any transplant recipient who develops odynophagia or dysphagia, regardless of the presence or absence of oropharyngeal thrush. Infections with aspergillus are associated with an extremely high mortality and infection may involve the liver and peritoneum.

## Gastrointestinal hemorrhage

Upper and lower gastrointestinal hemorrhage may occur in transplant patients (Alvarez et al 1993). These patients, given the magnitude of the surgical procedure, are at significant risk of developing "stress" ulcers and gastrointestinal hemorrhage in the early postoperative period. Stress ulcer prophylaxis with $H_2$ receptor or proton pump inhibiting drugs has therefore become routine in most centers. Antecedent peptic ulcer disease remains a surprisingly frequent cause of significant upper gastrointestinal hemorrhage in solid organ recipients and symptoms may be masked and presentations obscured by corticosteroid and immunosuppressant therapy. Cytomegalovirus (above) may also lead to gastrointestinal hemorrhage and should be suspected in transplant patients who develop lower gastrointestinal bleeding.

Other causes of gastrointestinal hemorrhage after liver transplantation include esophageal varices consequent upon postoperative portal vein thrombosis and hemobilia related to perianastomatic bleeding. Intestinal ischemia must be considered in the differential diagnosis of gastrointestinal hemorrhage and abdominal pain after any major cardiac surgery, including transplantation.

## Lymphoma

Prolonged survival after transplantation has led to the development of malignancy related to long-term immunosuppression. In renal transplant patients, the risk of cancer generally is estimated to increase 100-fold and that of lymphoma 40-fold (Morrison et al 1994). The rates for lymphoma in renal, heart, liver and pancreas transplant recipients were 1%, 2.4%, 1% and 0.6% respectively (Morrison et al 1994). Lymphomas developed about 18 months after transplantation, B-cell lymphomas predominated and isolated extralymphoreticular disease was common. Among the 38 solid organ recipients in this series who developed lymphoma, most had not received cyclosporin for immunosuppression and 19 of 20 tested for EBV by polymerase chain reaction were positive. The risk of lymphoma appears to be related to the degree of immunosuppression and is more common in patients who have received the monoclonal antilymphocyte agent OKT3.

Several treatments have been recommended. Where possible, immunosuppression should be discontinued or decreased. If disease is localized, surgical excision or local radiation therapy may be attempted; if disease is extensive, antiviral therapy against EBV in the form of high-dose acyclovir has been reported effective in some patients. Conventional chemotherapy for lymphoma has been universally disappointing and interferon therapy remains experimental. The response to treatment has been disappointing, as only 31% of patients achieved remission and 81% died with a median interval of only 14 months (Morrison et al 1994). In some patients with post-transplant lymphoproliferative disorders, gastrointestinal involvement may be predominant. Good results have been reported from decreasing immunosuppression and resection (Nalesnik 1990). Sometimes gastrointestinal involvement becomes obvious only when perforation occurs following the initiation of chemotherapy.

## Diarrhea

Diarrhea is common in transplant patients and while causes such as viral, bacterial or fungal infection and GVHD may be identified in individual patients, a specific cause may not be found. Diarrhea is especially common in liver transplant patients during the first 2–3 weeks following transplantation and tends to improve spontaneously. The cause of the diarrhea is often unknown and although increased fecal fat excretion and altered bile acid metabolism have been demonstrated, it is not certain that they are responsible.

## Hepatobiliary complications

### *Abnormal liver function tests*

Persistently abnormal liver function tests in renal transplant recipients are common, but chronic liver disease is infrequent and occurs in about 7% (Allison et al 1992). About two-thirds of heart transplant recipients have abnormal liver function tests (Cadranel et al 1991). Geographical variation in the incidence of abnormal liver function tests is marked and principally reflects the varying prevalence of viral hepatitis. In addition, most patients with cardiac disease requiring transplantation have abnormal liver function as a result of hepatic congestion and this usually improves after surgery (Gulbis et al 1988).

### *Viral hepatitis*

Chronic hepatitis C (HCV) is the commonest cause of liver dysfunction following renal transplant. The virus has usually been acquired from contaminated blood products prior to transplantation, a problem that should diminish with the introduction of HCV screening of blood donors. Although HCV-infected patients are at increased risk of clinically significant chronic liver disease following renal transplant, most patients have mild disease and HCV infection is not a contraindication to renal transplant (Allison et al 1992, Rohr et al 1993). Chronic hepatitis B, although less common than hepatitis C, has a poor prognosis in renal transplant recipients where the patient shows active viral replication as indicated by HBeAg or HBV-DNA in serum (Fairley et al 1991).

Treatment of viral hepatitis in immunosuppressed transplant recipients is problematic. Theoretical anxieties that the use of the immunomodulatory and antiviral agent interferon would lead to increased graft rejection have not been realized, but it has proved ineffective at eradicating either HBV or HCV.

Infection with CMV, either primary or reactivation due to immunosuppression, can cause an acute hepatitis. This is more frequent following transplantation of the liver than of other solid organs. Treatment with ganciclovir is usually successful. There is no evidence that chronic liver disease can result from CMV infection.

### *Drugs*

Most solid organ transplant recipients receive immunosuppression with a combination of cyclosporin, azathioprine and corticosteroids. Cyclosporin can cause a hepatitic liver disturbance, but this is uncommon. Early reports of a high incidence may have been misdiagnoses or related to much higher doses of the drug. Azathioprine hepatotoxicity is also rare. It can cause veno-occlusive disease and nodular regenerative hyperplasia and both have been reported in renal transplant recipients.

### *Iron overload*

Renal transplant recipients have often received multiple blood transfusions and hepatic siderosis is the second commonest cause of abnormal liver function tests, being present in 12–44% of cases (Allison et al 1992, Rao & Anderson 1992).

## GASTROINTESTINAL AND HEPATOBILIARY PROBLEMS IN THE PANCREAS TRANSPLANT RECIPIENT

Patients who have undergone combined renal and pancreatic transplantation usually have complicated diabetes mellitus and are particularly prone to gastrointestinal and biliary complications. Many patients have autonomic neuropathy and clinical features of diabetic gastroenteropathy. The effects of pancreas transplantation on autonomic neuropathy are uncertain and while symptomatic improvement has been reported, prospective tests of autonomic function have yielded inconclusive results. However, gastroparesis may persist and, indeed, worsen following transplantation and in some patients may lead to considerable nutritional problems. Severe constipation has also caused significant difficulty in the postoperative period, though whether this is also related to pre-existing diabetic autonomic neuropathy remains unclear. Prospective studies on the natural history and management of gastrointestinal manifestation of autonomic neuropathy in pancreas transplantation are not available and current treatment is based on experience with diabetic patients in general. Treatment includes dietary adjustments, prokinetic agents and institution of enteral or even parenteral feeding where indicated.

Recipients of pancreas or pancreas/kidney allografts are prey to the same bacterial, viral and fungal infections as other solid organ recipients. However, the importance of CMV gastritis in the differential diagnosis of gastroparesis needs to be stressed and CMV-induced ulcers have also been implicated in the pathogenesis of leaks from the duodenal segment of the graft (Ozaki et al 1992).

Gallbladder and biliary disease have been recognized as important in pancreas transplant recipients. Acalculous cholecystitis has been reported in patients receiving octreotide to prevent pancreatitis and this complication might be related to the motility-suppressing effects of higher doses of octreotide. Whether octreotide could also contribute to gastroparesis or colonic inertia has not been clarified. Cholelithiasis is especially common in these patients and 30% of pancreas transplant recipients in a prospective study were found to develop gallstones at a mean interval of 13 months following transplantation (Lowell et al 1993). Symptomatic gallbladder disease appears to be infrequent in the short term and these patients appear to tolerate both open and laparoscopic cholecystectomy well. The indications for cholecystectomy and the role of "prophylactic" procedures in management remain to be defined. Two principal factors have been proposed to explain this predisposition to gallstones: gallbladder hypomotility related to diabetic autonomic neuropathy and the effects of cyclosporin on bile composition exacerbated by lack of oral intake in the immediate postoperative period (McCashland et al 1994). The former hypothesis is supported by the higher incidence of cholelithiasis in diabetic than in nondiabetic kidney transplant recipients (Lowell et al 1993) and the latter by reports of an increased risk for gallstones in heart transplant recipients given cyclosporin (Steck et al 1991).

## REFERENCES


Adam R, Bismuth H, Diamond T et al 1992 Effect of extended cold ischaemia with UW solution on graft function after liver transplantation. Lancet 304: 1373–1376

Allison M C, Mowat A, McCruden E A B et al 1992 The spectrum of chronic liver disease in renal transplant recipients. Quarterly Journal of Medicine 83: 355–367

Alvarez L, Puleo J, Balint J A 1993 Investigation of gastrointestinal bleeding in patients with endstage renal disease. American Journal of Gastroenterology 88: 30–33

Baglin T P 1994 Veno-occlusive disease of the liver complicating bone marrow transplantation. Bone Marrow Transplantation 13: 1–4

Bardaxoglou E, Maddern G, Ruso L et al 1993 Gastrointestinal surgical emergencies following kidney transplantation. Transplantation International 6: 148–152

Becht M B, Pedersen S H, Ryckman F C, Balistreri W F 1993 Growth and nutritional management of pediatric patients after orthotopic liver transplantation. Gastroenterology Clinics of North America 22: 367–380

Benoit G, Moukarzel M, Verdelli G et al 1993 Gastrointestinal complications in renal transplantation. Transplantation International 6: 45–49

Bernuau J, Samuel D, Durand F et al 1991 Criteria for emergency liver transplantation in patients with acute viral hepatitis and factor V (FV) below 50% of normal: a prospective study. Hepatology 14: 49A

Bianco J A, Pepe M S, Higano C, Appelbaum F R, McDonald G B, Singer J W 1990 Prevalence of clinically relevant bacteremia after upper gastrointestinal endoscopy in bone marrow transplant recipients. American Journal of Medicine 89: 134–136

Bird G L A, O'Grady J G, Harvey F A H, Calne R Y, Williams R 1990 Liver transplantation in patients with alcoholic cirrhosis: selection criteria and rates of survival and relapse. British Medical Journal 301: 15–17

Bismuth H, Ericzon B G, Rolles K et al 1987a Hepatic transplantation in Europe. First report of the European Transplant Registry. Lancet 2: 674–676

Bismuth H, Samuel D, Gugenheim J et al 1987b Emergency liver transplantation for fulminant hepatitis. Annals of Internal Medicine 107: 337–341

Bollinger S, Quigley E M M 1994 Disordered gastrointestinal motility. In: Quigley E M M, Sorrell M F (eds) Medical care of the gastrointestinal surgical patient. Williams and Wilkins, Baltimore pp 157–174

Broelsch C E, Whitington P F, Emond J C et al 1991 Liver transplantation in children from living related donors: surgical tehniques and results. Annals of Surgery 214: 428–439

Brown B P, Abu-Yousef M, Farner R, LaBrecque D, Gingrick R 1990 Doppler sonography: a non-invasive method for evaluation of hepatic venocclusive disease. American Journal of Roentgenology 154: 721–724

Cadranel J F, Grippon P, Lunel F et al 1991 Chronic liver dysfunction in heart transplant recipients, with special reference to viral B, C and non-A, non-B, non-C hepatitis. A retrospective study in 80 patients with follow-up of 60 months. Transplantation 52: 645–650

Carreras E, Grañema A, Rozman C 1993 Hepatic veno-occlusive disease after bone marrow transplant. Blood Reviews 7: 43–51

Cates J, Chavez M, Laks H et al 1991 Gastrointestinal complications after cardiac transplantation: a spectrum of diseases. American Journal of Gastroenterology 86: 412–416

Cheung A N Y, Ng I O L 1993 Cytomegalovirus infection of the gastrointestinal tract in non-AIDS patients. American Journal of Gastroenterology 88: 1882–1886

Christensen E, Neuberger J, Crowe J et al 1985 Beneficial effect of azathioprine and prediction of prognosis in primary biliary cirrhosis: final result of an international trial. Gastroenterology 89: 1084–1091

Cicogna C, Polsky B 1994 Cytomegalovirus infection in bone marrow transplant patients. Infections in Medicine 11: 258–262

Collins R H, Cooper B, Nikaein A, Klintmalm G, Fay J W 1992 Graft-versus-host disease in a liver transplant recipient. Annals of Internal Medicine 116: 391–392

Commander M, Neuberger J, Dean C 1992 Psychiatric and social

consequences of liver transplantation. Transplantation 53: 1038–1040
Davey D D, Kamat D, Laszewski M et al 1989 Epstein–Barr virus-related lymphoproliferative disorders following bone marrow transplantation: an immunologic and genotypic analysis. Modern Pathology 2: 27–34
Davies S E, Portmann B C, O'Grady J G et al 1991 Hepatic histological findings after transplantation for chronic hepatitis B virus infection, including a unique pattern of fibrosing cholestatic hepatitis. Hepatology 13: 150–157
Dickson E R, Grambasch P M, Fleming T R, Fisher L D, Langworthy A 1989 Prognosis in primary biliary cirrhosis: model for decision making. Hepatology 10: 1–7
Dickson E R, Murtaugh P A, Wiesner R H et al 1992 Primary sclerosing cholangitis: refinement and validation of survival models. Gastroenterology 103: 1893–1901
Di Magno E P, Zinsmeister A R, Larson D E et al 1985 Influence of hepatic reserve and cause of esophageal varices on survival and rebleeding before and after the introduction of sclerotherapy: a retrospective analysis. Mayo Clinic Proceedings 60: 149–157
Donovan J 1993 Non-surgical management of biliary tract disease after liver transplantation. Gastroenterology Clinics of North America 22: 317–336
Dubois A, Walker R I 1988 Prospects for management of gastrointestinal injury associated with the acute radiation syndrome. Gastroenterology 95: 500–507
Emre S, Mor E, Schwartz M E et al 1993 Liver transplantation in patients beyond age 60. Transplant Proceedings 25: 1075–1076
European FK506 Multicentre Liver Study Group 1994 Randomised trial comparing tacrolimus (FK506) and cyclosporin in prevention of liver allograft rejection. Lancet 344: 423–428
European Liver Transplant Registry Update, December 1993. Hôpital Paul Brousse, Villejuif, France
Fairley C K, Mijch A, Gust I D, Nichilson S, Dimitrakakis M, Lucas C R 1991 The increased risk of fatal liver disease in renal transplant patients who are hepatitis B3 antigen and/or HBV DNA positive. Transplantation 52: 497–500
Farrant J M, Hayllar K M, Wilkinson M L et al 1991 Natural history and prognostic variables in primary sclerosing cholangitis. Gastroenterology 100: 1710–1717
Farrell F J, Nguyen M, Woodley S et al 1994 Outcome of liver transplantation in patients with hemochromatosis. Hepatology 20: 404–410
Faulds D, Heel R C 1990 Ganciclovir. A review of its antiviral activity, pharmacokinetic properties and therapeutic efficacy in cytomegalovirus infections. Drugs 39: 597–638
Ferrell L D, Wright T L, Roberts J, Ascher N, Lake J 1992 Hepatitis C viral infection in liver transplant recipients. Hepatology 16: 865–876
First M R 1992 Transplantation in the nineties. Transplantation 53: 1–11
Freese D K, Tuchman M, Schwarzenberg S J et al 1991 Early liver transplantation is indicated for tyrosinemia type I. Journal of Pediatric Gastroenterology and Nutrition 13: 10–15
Galati J S, Wisecarver J L, Quigley E M M 1993 Inflammatory polyps as a manifestation of intestinal graft versus host disease. Gastrointestinal Endoscopy 39: 719–722
Gane E, Langley P, Williams R 1995 Massive ascitic fluid loss and coagulation disturbances after liver transplantation. Gastroenterology 109: 1631–1638
Garden O J, Mills P R, Birnie G G, Murray G D, Carter D C 1990 Propranolol in the prevention of recurrent variceal hemorrhage in cirrhotic patients. A controlled trial. Gastroenterology 98: 185–190
Georgeson K E, Breaux C W Jr 1992 Outcome and intestinal adaptation in neonatal short-bowel syndrome. Journal of Pedriatic Surgery 27: 344–348
Goodgame R W 1993 Gastrointestinal cytomegalovirus disease. Annals of Internal Medicine 119: 924–935
Grant D, Wall W, Mimeault R et al 1990 Successful small bowel/liver transplantation. Lancet 335: 181–184
Gulbis B, Adler M, Ooms H A, Desmet J M, Leclerc J C, Primo G 1988 Liver-function studies in heart-transplant recipients treated with cyclosporin A. Clinical Chemistry 34: 1772–1774
Hackman R C, Wolford J L, Gleaves C A et al 1994 Recognition and rapid diagnosis of upper gastrointestinal cytomegalovirus infection in marrow transplant recipients. A comparison of seven virologic methods. Transplantation 57: 231–237
Harrison R F, Davies M H, Neuberger J M, Hubscher S H 1991 Fibrous and obliterative cholangitis in liver allografts: evidence for recurrent primary sclerosing cholangitis? Hepatology 20: 356–361
Health Resources and Service Administration, Bureau of Health Resources Development 1991 Report of center-specific graft and patient survival rates. US Department of Health and Human Services, Rockville, MD, p 8–10
Howard L, Heaphey L, Fleming C R, Lininger L, Steiger E 1991 Four years of North American registry home parenteral nutrition outcome data and their implications for patient management. Journal of Parenteral and Enteral Nutrition 15: 384–393
Howard L, Fahy T, Wong P, Sherman D, Gane E, Williams R 1994 Psychiatric outcome in alcoholic liver transplant patients. Quarterly Journal of Medicine 87: 731–736
Hubscher S G, Elias E, Buckels J A C, Mayer A D, McMaster P, Neuberger J M 1993 Primary biliary cirrhosis: histological evidence of disease recurrence after liver transplantation. Journal of Hepatology 18: 173–184
Ingham Clark C L, Lear P A, Wood S, Lennard-Jones J E, Wood R F M 1992 Potential candidates for small bowel transplantation. British Journal of Surgery 79: 676–679
Ismail T, Angrisani L, Gunson B K et al 1990 Primary hepatic malignancy: the role of liver transplantation. British Journal of Surgery 77: 983–987
Iwatsuki S, Gordon R D, Shaw B W, Starzl T E 1985 Role of liver transplantation in cancer therapy. Annals of Surgery 202: 401–407
Iwatsuki S, Stieber A C, Marsh J W et al 1989 Liver transplantation for fulminant hepatic failure. Transplantation Proceedings 21: 2431–2434
Jacobson A F, Teefey S A, Lee S P, Holister M S, Higano C A, Bianco J A 1993 Frequent occurrence of new hepatobiliary abnormalities after bone marrow transplantation: results of a prospective study using scintigraphy and sonography. American Journal of Gastroenterology 88: 1044–1049
Jardines L A, O'Donnell M R, Johnson D L, Terz J J, Forman S J 1993 Acalculous cholecystitis in bone marrow transplant patients. Cancer 71: 354–358
Johnson G K, Geenan J E, Venu R P et al 1991 Endoscopic treatment of biliary strictures in sclerosing cholangitis, a larger series and recommendations for treatment. Gastrointestinal Endoscopy 37: 38–43
Kaplan C S, Petersen E A, Icenogle T B et al 1989 Gastrointestinal cytomegalovirus infection in heart and heart–lung transplant recipients. Archives of Internal Medicine 149: 2095–2100
Kaw M, Przepiorka D, Sekas G 1993 Infectious complications of endoscopic procedures in bone marrow transplant recipients. Digestive Diseases and Sciences 38: 71–74
Kelly W D, Lillehei R C, Merkel F K, Idezuki Y, Goetz F C 1967 Allotransplantation of the pancreas and duodenum along with the kidney in diabetic nephropathy. Surgery 61: 827–837
Kumar S, Stauber R E, Gavaler J S et al 1990 Orthotopic liver transplantation for alcoholic liver disease. Hepatology 11: 159–164
Larsen J L, Duckworth W C, Stratta R J 1994 Pancreas transplantation for type I diabetes mellitus. Do the benefits offset the risks and cost? Postgraduate Medicine 96: 105–111
Lepinski S M, Hamilton J W 1990 Isolated cytomegalovirus ileitis detected by colonoscopy. Gastroenterology 98: 1704–1706
Llach J, Ginès P, Arroyo V et al 1988 Prognostic value of arterial pressure, endogenous vasoactive systems and renal function in cirrhotic patients admitted to the hospital for the treatment of ascites. Gastroenterology 94: 482–487
Lowe D, O'Grady J G, McEwen J, Williams R 1990 Quality of life following liver transplantation: a preliminary report. Journal of the Royal College of Physicians of London 24: 43–46
Lowell J A, Stratta R J, Taylor R J, Bynon J S, Larsen J L, Nelson N L 1993 Cholelithiasis in pancreas and kidney transplant recipients with diabetes. Surgery 114: 858–864
Lucarelli G, Polchi P, Galimberti M et al 1985 Marrow transplantation for thalassaemia following busulphan and cyclophosphamide. Lancet 1: 1355–1357

Lucey M R, Merion R M, Henley K S et al 1992 Selection for and outcome of liver transplantation in alcoholic liver disease. Gastroenterology 102: 1736–1741
Marks D I, Dousset B, Robson A et al 1992 Orthotopic liver transplantation for hepatic GVHD following allogeneic BMT for chronic myeloid leukaemia. Bone Marrow Transplantation 10: 463–466
Markus B H, Dickson E R, Grambsch P M et al 1989 Efficacy of liver transplantation in patients with primary biliary cirrhosis. New England Journal of Medicine 320: 1709–1713
McCashland T M, Donovan J P, Amelsberg A et al 1994 Bile acid metabolism and biliary secretion in patients receiving orthotopic liver transplants: differing effects of cyclosporin and FK506. Hepatology 19: 1381–1389
McDonald G B, Sharma P, Matthews D E, Shulman H M, Thomas E D 1985 The clinical course of 53 patients with venocclusive disease of the liver after marrow transplantation. Transplantation 39: 603–608
McDonald G B, Shulman H M, Sullivan K M, Spencer G D 1986a Intestinal and hepatic complications of human bone marrow transplantation. Part I. Gastroenterology 90: 460–477
McDonald G B, Shulman H M, Sullivan K M, Spencer G D 1986b Intestinal and hepatic complications of human bone marrow transplantation. Part II. Gastroenterology 90: 770–784
McGregor G I, Shepherd J D, Phillips G L 1988 Acute graft-versus-host disease of the intestine. A surgical perspective. American Journal of Surgery 155: 680–682
Merion R M, Burtch G D, Ham J M, Turcotte J G, Campbell D A Jr 1989 The hepatic artery in liver transplantation. Transplantation 48: 438–443
Mieles L A, Esquivel C O, Van Thiel D H et al 1990 Liver transplantation for tyrosinemia: a review of 10 cases from the University of Pittsburgh. Digestive Diseases and Sciences 35: 153–157
Mieli-Vergani G 1993 Hepatic complications after bone marrow transplantation. Bone Marrow Transplantation 12 (suppl 1): 96–97
Morrison V A, Dunn D L, Manivel J C, Gajl-Peczalska K J, Peterson B A 1994 Clinical characteristics of post-transplant lymphoproliferative disorders. American Journal of Medicine 97: 14–24
Müller R, Gubernatis G, Farle M et al 1991 Liver transplantation in HBs antigen (HBsAg carriers). Prevention of hepatitis B virus (HBV) recurrence by passive immunization. Journal of Hepatology 13: 90–96
Mutimer D J, Elias E 1992 Liver transplantation for fulminant hepatic failure. In: Boyer J L, Ockner R K (eds) Progress in liver diseases, Vol. 10. W B Saunders, Philadelphia p 349–367
Nalesnik M A 1990 Involvement of the gastrointestinal tract by Epstein–Barr virus-associated posttransplant lymphoproliferative disorders. American Journal of Surgical Pathology 14 (suppl 1): 92–100
National Institutes of Health Consensus Development Conference on Liver Transplantation 1984 Hepatology 4: 1S–110S
Neuberger J, Altman D G, Polson R et al 1989 Prognosis after liver transplantation for primary biliary cirrhosis. Transplantation 48: 444–447
Nikaein A, Backman L, Jennings L et al 1994 HLA compatibility and liver transplant outcome. Transplantation 58: 786–792
O'Grady J G, Alexander G J M, Sutherland S et al 1988a Cytomegalovirus infection and donor/recipient HLA antigens: interdependent co-factors in pathogenesis of vanishing bile duct syndrome after liver transplantation. Lancet 2: 302–305
O'Grady J G, Alexander G J M, Thick M, Potter D, Calne R Y, Williams R 1988b Outcome of orthotopic liver transplantation in the aetiological and clinical variants of acute liver failure. Quarterly Journal of Medicine 69: 817–824
O'Grady J G, Polson R J, Rolles K, Calne R Y, Williams R 1988c Liver transplantation for malignant disease: results in 93 consecutive patients. Annals of Surgery 207: 373–379
O'Grady J G, Alexander G J M, Hayllar K M, Williams R 1989 Early indicators of prognosis in fulminant hepatic failure. Gastroenterology 97: 439–445
Otto G, Herfarth Ch, Senninger N, Fiesk G, Post S, Gmelin K 1989 Hepatic transplantation in galactosemia. Transplantation 47: 902–903
Ozaki C F, Stratta R J, Taylor R J, Langnas A N, Bynon J S, Shaw B W Jr 1992 Surgical complications in solitary pancreas and combined pancreas–kidney transplantations. American Journal of Surgery 164: 546–551
Ozawa K, Uemoto S, Tanaka K et al 1992 An appraisal of pediatric liver transplantation from living relatives. Annals of Surgery 216: 547–553
Paradis K, Weber A, Seidman E G et al 1990 Liver transplantation for hereditary tyrosinemia: the Quebec experience. American Journal of Human Genetics 47: 338–342
Pauwels A, Mostefa-Kara N, Florent C, Levy V G 1993 Emergency liver transplantation for acute liver failure. Evaluation of London and Clichy criteria. Journal of Hepatology 17: 124–127
Paya C V 1993 Fungal infections in solid-organ transplantation. Clinical Infectious Disease 16: 677–688
Paya C V, Wiesner R H, Hermans P E et al 1992 Lack of association between cytomegalovirus infection, HLA matching and the vanishing bile duct syndrome after liver transplantation. Hepatology 16: 66–70
Paya C V, Wiesner R H, Hermans P E et al 1993 Risk factors for cytomegalovirus and severe bacterial infections following liver transplantation: a prospective multivariate time-dependent analysis. Journal of Hepatology 18: 185–195
Penn I 1991 Hepatic transplantation for primary and metastatic cancers of the liver. Surgery 110: 726–735
Purdum P P 3rd, Kirby D F 1991 Short-bowel syndrome: a review of the role of nutrition support. Journal of Parenteral and Enteral Nutrition 15: 93–101
Putnam C W, Porter K A, Peters R L, Ashcavai M, Redeker A G, Starzl T E 1977 Liver replacement for alpha-1-antitrypsin deficiency. Surgery 81: 258–261
Quigley E M M, Marsh M N, Shaffer J L, Markin R S 1993 Hepatobiliary complications of total parenteral nutrition. Gastroenterology 104: 286–301
Rabier D, Narcy C, Bardet J, Parvy P, Saudubray J M, Kamoun P 1991 Arginine remains an essential amino acid after liver transplantation in urea cycle enzyme deficiencies. Journal of Inherited Metabolic Disease 14: 277–280
Rao K V, Anderson W R 1992 Liver disease after renal transplantation. American Journal of Kidney Diseases 19: 496–501
Reyes J, Tzakis A G, Bonet H et al 1994 Lymphoproliferative disease after transplantation under primary FK506 immunosuppression. Transplant Proceedings 26: 1426–1427
Ringe B, Wittekind C, Bechstein W O, Bunzendahl H, Pichlmayer R 1989 The role of liver transplantation in hepatobiliary malignancy. Annals of Surgery 209: 88–98
Roberts J P, Ascher N L, Lake J et al 1991 Graft vs. host disease after liver transplantation in humans: a report of four cases. Hepatology 14: 274–281
Rohr M S, Lesniewski R R, Rubin C A et al 1993 Risk of liver disease in HCV-seropositive kidney transplant recipients. Annals of Surgery 217: 512–517
Roy J, Snover D, Weisdorf S, Mulvahill A, Filipovich A, Weisdorf D 1991 Simultaneous upper and lower endoscopic biopsy in the diagnosis of intestinal graft-versus-host disease. Transplantation 51: 642–646
Sakr M, Hassanein T, Gavaler J et al 1992 Cytomegalovirus infection of the upper gastrointestinal tract following liver transplantation – incidence, location and severity in cyclosporine- and FK506-treated patients. Transplantation 53: 786–791
Salt A, Noble-Jamieson G, Barnes N D et al 1992 Liver transplantation in 100 children: Cambridge and King's College Hospital Series. British Medical Journal 304: 416–421
Samuel D, Bismuth A, Mathieu D et al 1991a Passive immunoprophylaxis after liver transplantation in HBsAg-positive patients. Lancet 337: 813–815
Samuel D, Bismuth A, Serres C et al 1991b HBV infection after liver transplantation in HBsAg positive patients: experience with long-term immunoprophylaxis. Transplantation Proceedings 23: 1492–1494
Samuel D, Muller R, Alexander G et al 1993 Liver transplantation in European patients with the hepatitis B surface antigen. New England Journal of Medicine 329: 1842–1847
Sanchez-Urdazpal L, Gores G J, Ward E M et al 1992 Ischemic-type biliary complications after orthotopic liver transplantation. Hepatology 16: 49–53

Schilsky M L, Scheinberg I H, Sternlieb I 1994 Liver transplantation for Wilson's disease: indications and outcome. Hepatology 19: 583–587
Scott N A, Irving M H 1992 Intestinal failure – the clinical problem. Digestive Diseases 10: 249–257
Selby R, Starzl T E, Yunis E et al 1993 Liver transplantation for type I and type IV glycogen storage disease. European Journal of Pediatrics 152 (suppl 1): S71–S76
Shapiro J M, Smith H, Schaffner F 1979 Serum bilirubin: a prognostic factor in primary biliary cirrhosis. Gut 20: 137–140
Shaw B W Jr, Markin R, Stratta R, Langnas A, Donovan J, Sorrell M 1991 FK506 for rescue treatment of acute and chronic rejection in liver allograft recipients. Transplantation Proceedings 23: 2994–2995
Shulman H M, Hinterberger W 1992 Hepatic veno-occlusive disease – liver toxicity syndrome after bone marrow transplantation. Bone Marrow Transplantation 10: 197–214
Snover D C 1990 Graft-versus-host disease of the gastrointestinal tract. American Journal of Surgical Pathology 14 (suppl 1): 101–108
Starzl T E, Marchioro T L, Von Kaulla K N, Hermann G, Brittain R S, Waddell W R 1963 Homotransplantation of the liver in humans. Surgery, Gynecology and Obstetrics 117: 659–676
Starzl T E, Van Thiel D, Tzakis A G et al 1988 Orthotopic liver transplantation for alcoholic cirrhosis. Journal of the American Medical Association 260: 2542–2544
Steck T B, Costanzo-Nordin M R, Keshavarzian A 1991 Prevalence and management of cholelithiasis in heart transplant patients. Journal of Heart and Lung Transplantation 10: 1029–1032
Steck T B, Durkin M G, Costanzo-Nordin M R, Keshavarzian A 1993 Gastrointestinal complications and endoscopic findings in heart transplant patients. Journal of Heart and Lung Transplantation 12: 244–251
Stratta R J, Wood R P, Langmas A N et al 1989 Diagnosis and treatment of biliary tract complications after orthotopic liver transplantation. Surgery 106: 675–684
Stratta R J, Shaefer M S, Markin R S et al 1991a Ganciclovir therapy for viral disease in liver transplant recipients. Clinical Transplantation 5: 287–293
Stratta R J, Taylor R J, Zorn B H et al 1991b Combined pancreas–kidney transplantation: preliminary results and metabolic effects. American Journal of Gastroenterology 86: 697–703
Stratta R J, Taylor R J, Larsen J L, Cushing K 1995 Pancreas transplantation. International Journal of Pancreatology 17: 1–13
Swinnen L J, Constanzo-Nordin M R, Fisher S G 1990 Increased incidence of lymphoproliferative disorder after immunosuppression with the monoclonal antibody OKT3 in cardiac-transplant recipients. New England Journal of Medicine 323: 1723–1728
The T H, van der Ploeg M, van den Berg A P, Vlieger A M, van der Giessen M, van Son W J 1992 Direct detection of cytomegalovirus in peripheral blood leukocytes – a review of the antigenemia assay and polymerase chain reaction. Transplantation 54: 193–198
Thompson J S 1993 Surgical considerations in the short bowel syndrome. Surgery, Gynecology and Obstetrics 176: 89–101
Tito L, Rimola A, Ginès P, Llach J, Arroyo V, Rodés J 1988 Recurrence of spontaneous bacterial peritonitis in cirrhosis: frequency and predictive factors. Hepatology 8: 27–31
Todo S, Fung J J, Demetris A J, Jain A, Venkataramanan R, Starzl T E 1990 Early trials with FK506 as primary treatment in liver transplantation. Transplant Proceedings 22: 13–16
Todo S, Demetris A J, Van Thiel D, Teperman L, Fung J J, Starzl T E 1991 Orthotopic liver transplantation for patients with hepatitis B virus related liver disease. Hepatology 13: 619–626
Todo S, Starzl T E, Tzakis A et al 1992a Orthotopic liver transplantation for urea cycle enzyme deficiency. Hepatology 15: 419–422
Todo S, Tzakis A G, Abu-Elmagd K et al 1992b Intestinal transplantation in composite visceral grafts or alone. Annals of Surgery 216: 223–234
Todo S, Tzakis A, Reyes J et al 1994 Intestinal transplantation at the University of Pittsburgh. Transplant Proceedings 26: 1409–1410
UNOS releases 1993 1992 transplant statistics. UNOS Update 9: 9
US Multicenter FK506 Liver Study Group 1994 A comparison of tacrolimus for immunosuppression in liver transplantation. New England Journal of Medicine 331: 1110–1115
Vanderhoof J A, Langnas A N, Pinch L W, Thompson J S, Kaufman S S 1992 Short bowel syndrome. Journal of Pediatric Gastroenterology and Nutrition 14: 359–370
Villar H V, Mead D D, Levinson M et al 1989 Gastrointestinal complications after human transplantation and mechanical heart replacement. American Journal of Surgery 157: 168–174
Weisdorf D J, Snover D C, Haake R et al 1990 Acute upper gastrointestinal graft-versus-host disease: clinical significance and response to immunosupressive therapy. Blood 76: 624–629
Weisner R H, Porayko M K, Dickson E R et al 1992 Selection and timing of liver transplantation in primary biliary cirrhosis and primary sclerosing cholangitis. Hepatology 16: 1290–1299
Westaby D, Macdougall B R D, Williams R 1985 Improved survival following injection sclerotherapy for esophageal varices: final analysis of a controlled trial. Hepatology 5: 827–830
Williams R, O'Grady J G 1990 Liver transplantation: results, advances and problems. Journal of Gastroenterology and Hepatology 5 (suppl 1): 110–126
Williams S G J, Westaby D, Tanner M S, Mowat A P 1992 Liver and biliary problems in cystic fibrosis. British Medical Bulletin 48: 877–892
Wolford J L, McDonald G B 1988 A problem-oriented approach to intestinal and liver disease after marrow transplantation. Journal of Clinical Gastroenterology 10: 419–433
Wright H L, Bou-Abboud C F, Hassanein T et al 1992a Disease recurrence and rejection following liver transplantation for autoimmune chronic active liver disease. Transplantation 53: 136–139
Wright T L, Donegan E, Hsu H H et al 1992b Recurrent and acquired hepatitis C viral infection in liver transplant recipients. Gastroenterology 103: 317–322

SECTION 12

# Spleen

# 47. The spleen

*John P. Hanley   Christopher A. Ludlam*

## INTRODUCTION

This chapter gives an overview of the spleen in current clinical practice and describes approaches to the investigation of patients with splenomegaly and functional disorders of the spleen. Enlargement of the spleen is the commonest indicator of a disease process affecting the organ. It should be stressed at the outset that splenomegaly may not be associated with altered splenic function and that hyposplenism may occur in the presence of a normal-sized spleen. The absence of splenic function, either as the result of splenectomy or hyposplenism, is often associated with a normal life expectancy. There are, however, important clinical implications for patients with abnormal splenic function.

## STRUCTURE AND FUNCTION

### Anatomy

The spleen is an encapsulated organ weighing 150–180 g in normal adults. It is at its largest toward the end of puberty and undergoes progressive atrophy through adult life, particularly during the third decade and after the sixth decade of life (DeLand 1970). The normal spleen lies under the left 9th, 10th, and 11th ribs and in an adult its long axis measures up to 12 cm. Its anterior pole reaches the mid-axillary line. It is in close contact with the diaphragm, stomach and pancreas.

Macroscopically, the cut surface reveals two types of parenchyma: the white pulp and the red pulp. The white pulp consists mainly of lymphoid tissue, whereas the red pulp is composed predominantly of vascular tissue including the venous sinuses. Microscopically, a marginal zone can also be identified between the white and the red pulp (Van Krieken et al 1992).

### Circulation

The spleen is extremely vascular, receiving as much as 5% of the cardiac output. The blood supply is derived from the splenic artery, a branch of the celiac axis, which enters the spleen at its hilum and then branches to form trabecular arteries that give rise to central arteries. The central arteries are surrounded by white pulp and ramify before terminating either in the marginal sinus or the marginal zone (Fig. 47.1).

There has been much controversy surrounding the precise nature of the splenic microcirculation. It would appear that there are two distinct routes for blood, a fast and a slow route. The latter provides the opportunity for blood cells to be intimately exposed to phagocytic and immunologically active splenic cells. Due to the anatomical arrangement of the splenic microvasculature, plasma is

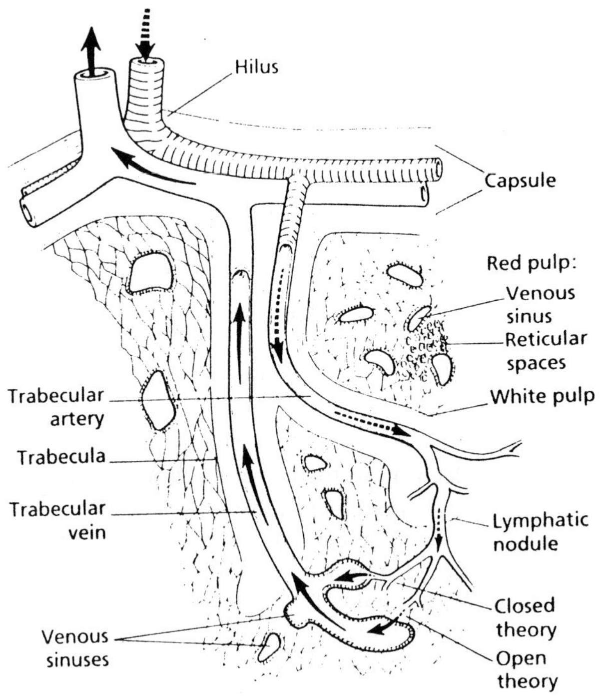


**Fig. 47.1** Schematic diagram of the spleen showing the open and closed forms of the splenic circulation (arterial flow ·····>, venous flow ——>) (Redmond et al 1990).

"skimmed" toward the vessel walls as blood flows through the spleen, enabling immunologically active plasma to be in contact with the parenchyma in the white pulp and the cellular constituents of the blood to be exposed to splenic phagocytes predominantly in the sinusoids.

### Immunological function

The spleen contains the largest collection of lymphoid cells in the body; these are confined mainly to the white pulp. As a result of the high blood flow there is ample opportunity not only for blood filtering but also for the development of immunological responses to foreign antigens. Particulate antigens such as bacteria are trapped initially in the splenic filtration beds. The spleen plays an essential role in protecting the nonimmune individual from infection through its ability to kill bacteria that are not well opsonized (Bohnsack & Brown 1986). Macrophages engulf the particles and subsequently migrate into the lymphoid follicles. The process of killing and disposing of foreign organisms is enhanced by antibody binding and complement activation.

### Reservoir function

The normal spleen contains less than 5% of the total red cells within the body; however, the capacity to pool or sequester erythrocytes is a feature of the diseased spleen. Any cause of splenomegaly may result in up to 40% of the red cell mass being pooled. This may lead to increased red cell transfusion requirements that may be ameliorated by splenectomy. Acute splenic sequestration is a well-recognized life-threatening emergency in infants with sickle cell disease (Harrison & Davies 1992).

## CLINICAL ASSESSMENT

Splenic enlargement occurs into the left hypochondrium and extends diagonally across the abdomen toward the right iliac fossa. The anterior pole of the spleen normally reaches the mid-axillary line and it is widely considered that the spleen has to be enlarged 2–3 times before it becomes palpable. The detection of minor degrees of splenomegaly is very difficult. Zhang & Lewis (1989) related the spleen tip to the costal margin by scintigraphy in patients with hematological disease and found that palpability increased as spleen volume increased (Fig. 47.2). Spleen tips located at or just below the costal margin were palpable in only a half of cases and 31% of spleens of normal volume (<250 $cm^3$) were palpable at this level. Spleen tips located more than 3 cm below the costal margin were always palpable and the spleens were always enlarged and those palpable more than 5 cm below were at least 1000 $cm^3$ or weighed 1 kg or more. Large spleens are occasionally not palpable, often because of obesity, a high diaphragm or other pathology such as ascites (Fig. 47.3).

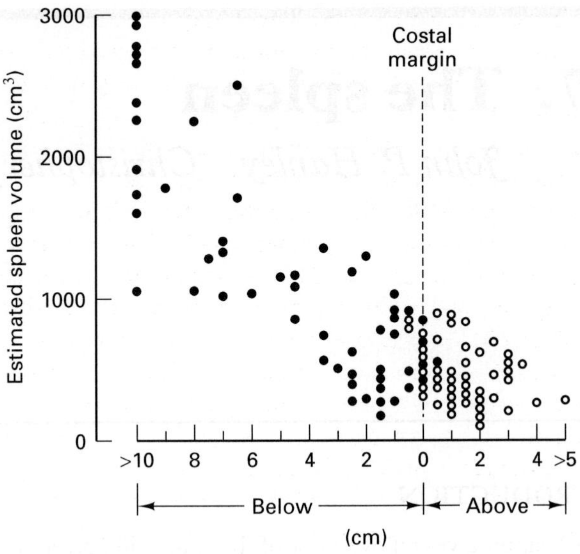


**Fig. 47.2** Palpation of the spleen related to the distance of the spleen tip above or below the costal margin on scintigraphy (Zhang & Lewis 1989). ● = spleen palpable; ○ = spleen not palpable.

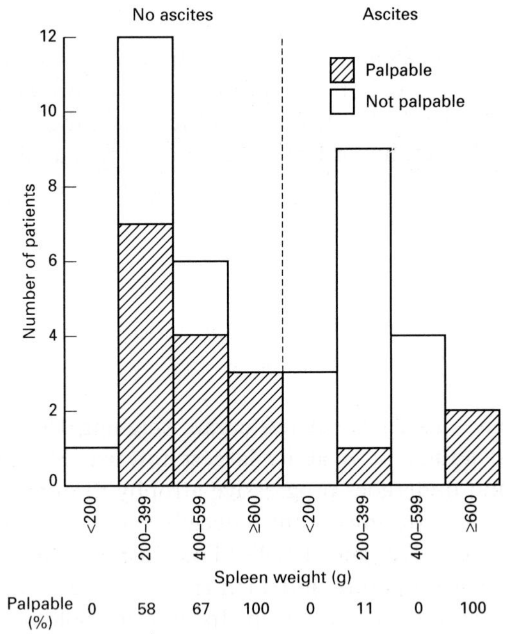


**Fig. 47.3** Spleen weight and palpability related to ascites in 40 patients with hepatic cirrhosis (Royal Infirmary, Edinburgh).

***Clinical examination.*** Examination of the spleen is part of the routine physical examination of the patient (Grover et al 1993). Clues as to the possible underlying cause of splenomegaly should also be sought. Abdominal examination should be performed with the patient supine. Gross splenomegaly may be visible on inspection. The examining hand (the right hand) should be placed flat on the abdomen. Palpation for splenomegaly should start in the right iliac fossa. The patient should be asked to take gentle but deep inspirations. With each inspiration the examining hand should attempt to feel for a descending splenic edge that should then recede toward the left hypochondrium with expiration. If an edge is detected, further palpation should define the extent of the mass. A distinct notch in the right border may be felt in easily palpable spleens. It is not possible to palpate the upper edge of the spleen and percussion techniques may reveal anterior dullness. These features distinguish splenomegaly from other causes of a mass in the left hypochondrium such as an enlarged kidney or a colonic tumor. If no edge is detected the examining hand should be moved 2–3 cm toward the left hypochondrium prior to the next inspiration. This process is repeated with the patient taking deep breaths until the examining hand has reached the left costal margin.

If no splenic enlargement is detected, the patient should be repositioned in the right lateral position. In this position a modestly enlarged spleen may be more easily palpable, although some authors think this maneuver may lead to misdiagnosis of splenomegaly (Barkun et al 1991). Percussion is important in the detection of mild splenomegaly. Dullness to percussion over Traube's space (a triangular area delineated by the sixth rib superiorly, the mid-axillary line laterally and the left costal margin inferiorly) is the earliest detectable sign of splenic enlargement.

***Palpable normal spleens.*** Palpable spleens are almost always enlarged and should be regarded as requiring investigation for a cause. However, it appears that occasionally a normal spleen can be felt, particularly in adolescents and young adults where the size of the spleen is at its greatest (p. 1181). Ebaugh & McIntyre (1979) found a palpable spleen in 2.9% of healthy young American college entrants and follow-up 10 years later did not show any development of serious disease. Berris (1966) found a palpable spleen in 12% of healthy young postpartum Canadian women.

**Table 47.1** Causes of splenomegaly related to spleen size

| |
|---|
| *Massive* |
| Myelofibrosis |
| Chronic myeloid leukemia |
| Hairy cell leukemia |
| Tropical |
| Malaria |
| Leishmaniasis |
| Schistosomiasis |
| Storage diseases |
| Gaucher's disease |
| Niemann–Pick's disease |
| Histiocytosis X |
| *Moderate* |
| Lymphoproliferative disorders |
| Chronic lymphatic leukemia |
| Non-Hodgkin's lymphoma |
| Hodgkin's disease |
| Polycythemia rubra vera |
| Thalassemia major/intermedia |
| Sickle cell anemia (prior to autosplenectomy) |
| Hemolytic anemias |
| Portal hypertension |
| Cirrhosis |
| Hepatic, portal or splenic vein thrombosis |
| *Mild* |
| Sarcoid |
| Amyloid |
| Rheumatoid disease/Felty's syndrome |
| Systemic lupus erythematosus |
| Infections |
| Septicemia |
| Endocarditis |
| Typhoid |
| Infectious mononucleosis |
| Tuberculosis |
| Brucellosis |
| Toxoplasmosis |
| Syphilis |

Note: Massive splenomegaly is palpable below the umbilicus; moderate splenomegaly is easily palpable but not below the umbilicus; mild splenomegaly is palpable below the costal margin or detectable by percussion only.

## INVESTIGATION OF SPLENOMEGALY

Once an enlarged spleen is suspected on clinical grounds, investigations are aimed at confirming splenomegaly and elucidating the underlying cause (Table 47.1). Sometimes the diagnosis is obvious, as in a classic presentation of chronic myeloid leukemia with splenomegaly, a raised white cell count and the presence of the Philadelphia chromosome. In other cases, especially isolated splenomegaly, the diagnosis may not be readily apparent. Approaches to the diagnosis of patients with splenomegaly are outlined in the flow charts (Figs. 47.4, 47.5).

***Splenomegaly of undetermined cause.*** The cause of splenomegaly sometimes remains unknown even after full investigation and diagnostic splenectomy has to be considered. Currently available investigations make this less necessary than previously, but diagnostic splenectomy still accounts for about 10% of splenectomies (Goonewardene et al 1979, Cronin et al 1994). In order to avoid unnecessary operations, investigations for rare causes of isolated splenomegaly should be performed (Table 47.2). This may include ultrasonically guided percutaneous splenic biopsy (Cavanna et al 1992) and with the advent of improved laparoscopic techniques (p. 126), biopsy may become more widely practiced (Carroll et al 1992). Thereafter, a period of observation followed by further investigation is reasonable in asymptomatic patients who do not have marked splenomegaly. However, symptomatic patients or patients with large spleens should be advised to undergo surgery. Cronin et al (1994) reported on 10 such patients where splenectomy revealed lymphoma in seven, all with spleens weighing over 1 kg, and normal histology in only one patient.

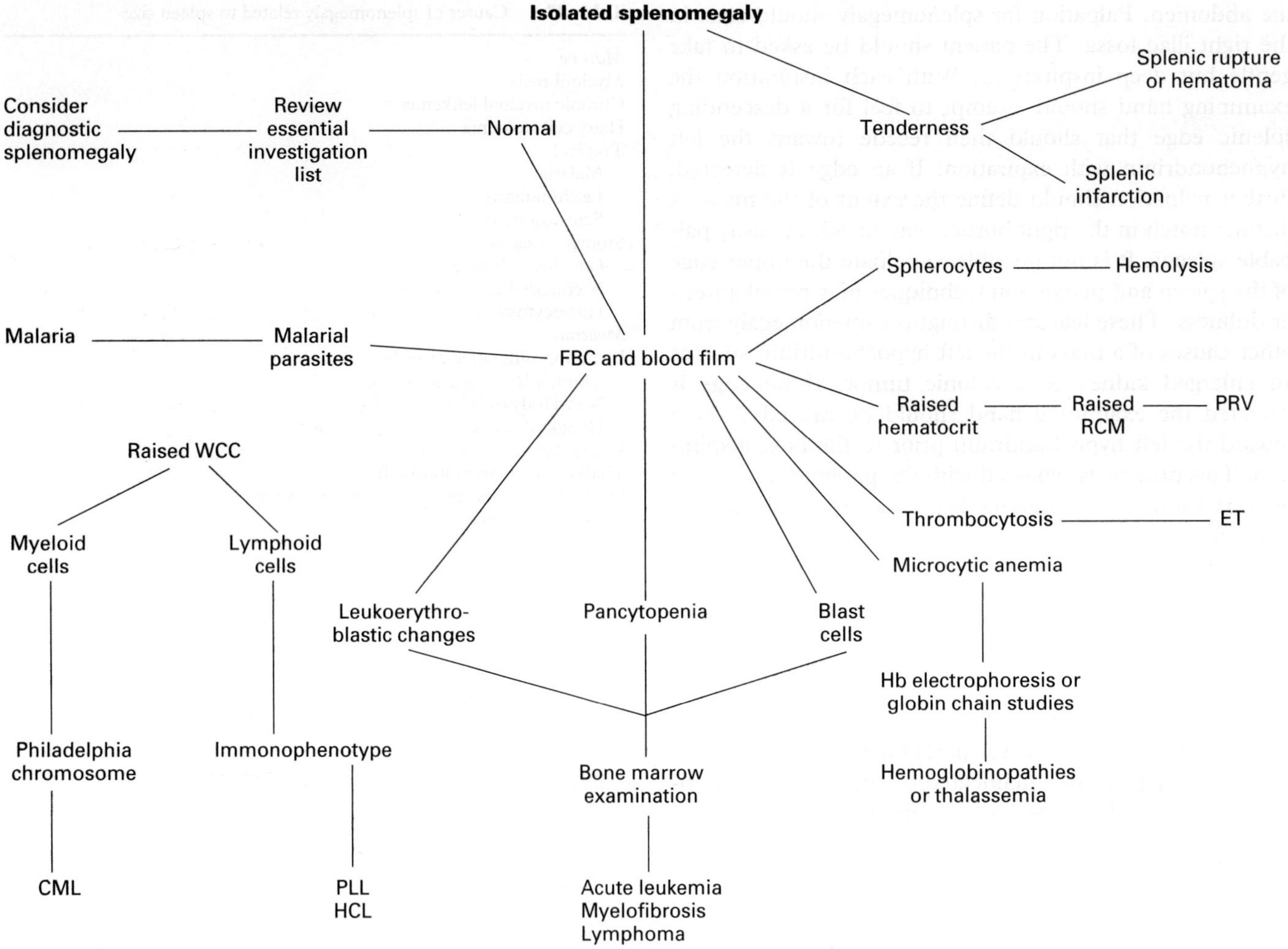


Note: CML = chronic myeloid leukemia; ET = essential thrombocythemia; FBC = full blood count; Hb = hemoglobin; HCL = hairy cell leukemia; PLL = prolymphocytic leukemia; PRV = polycythemia rubra vera; RCM = red cell mass; WCC = white cell count.

**Fig. 47.4** Investigation of isolated splenomegaly.

## IMAGING OF THE SPLEEN

Many methods have been used to measure spleen size including abdominal radiography, ultrasonography, computed tomography, magnetic resonance imaging and radionuclide imaging. Abdominal radiography is relatively insensitive and radionuclide imaging is less used than previously. Relatively few comparative studies have been done, but the main methods for measuring spleen size seem to give comparable results (Meek et al 1984).

### Ultrasound

This is the most useful and generally available investigation to assess splenic size. The splenic volume can be calculated from measurements of splenic length, breadth and thickness, but splenic length alone gives a simple and sufficiently accurate measurement of spleen size (Fig. 47.6). Focal splenic lesions can also be identified. Examination may be hampered by the presence of bowel gas. Ultrasound is often unhelpful in identifying the cause of splenomegaly. However, hepatic abnormalities may point to cirrhosis (p. 917), portal vein abnormalities and collateral vessels indicate portal hypertension (p. 991) and Doppler studies can show portal blood flow and portal or splenic vein thrombosis (p. 56). Patients with lymphoma may show intra-abdominal lymphadenopathy.

### Computed tomography

An accurate assessment of splenic size and volume can be made using computed tomography. Splenic tumors are readily identified, although there are often no specific features that distinguish between benign and malignant lesions. In patients with lymphoma, splenomegaly on computed tomography does not necessarily indicate

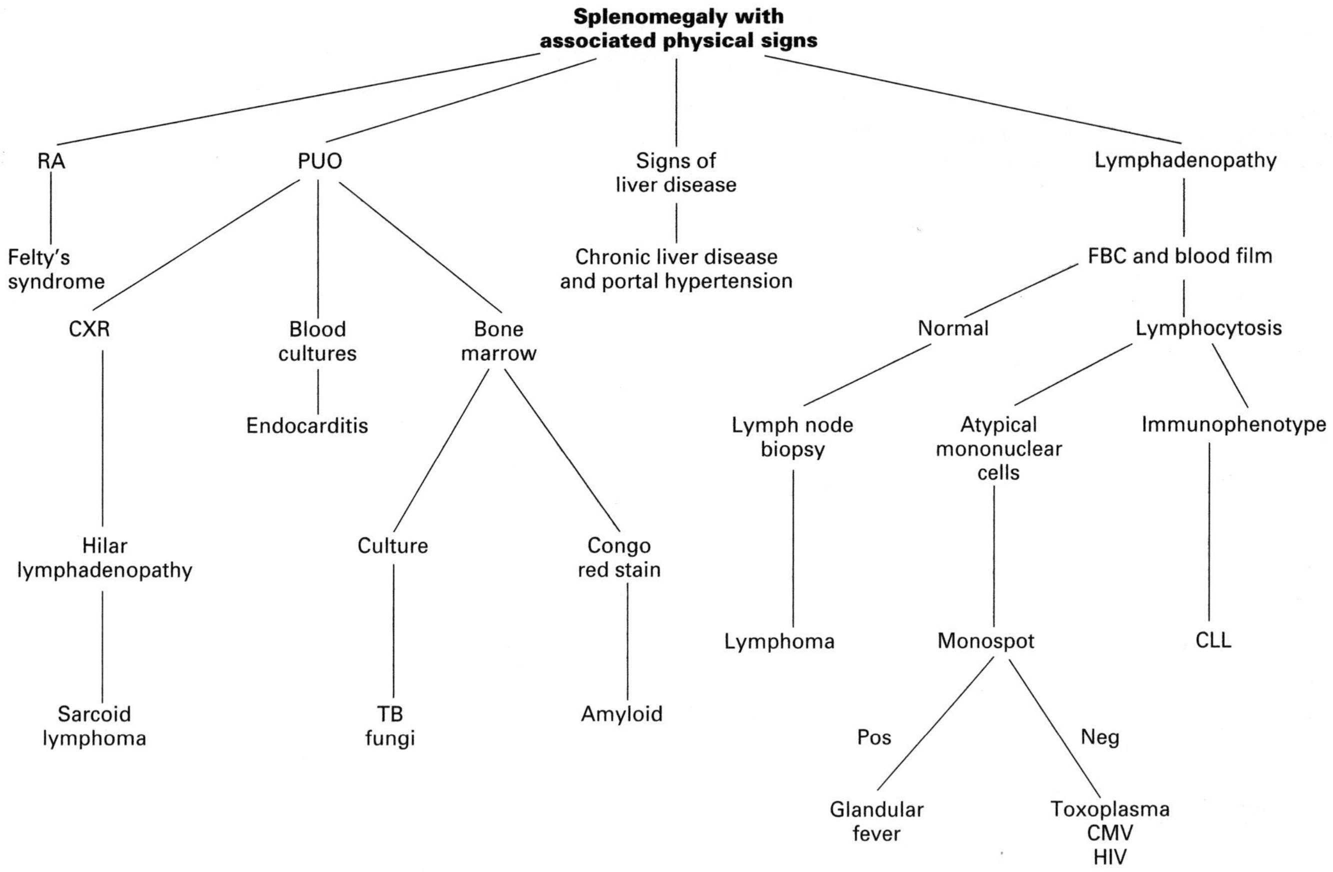


Note: CLL = chronic lymphatic leukemia; CMV = cytomegalovirus; CXR = chest X-ray; FBC = full blood count; HIV = human immunodeficiency virus; PUO = pyrexia of unknown origin; RA = rheumatoid arthritis.

**Fig. 47.5** Investigation of splenomegaly with associated physical signs.

**Table 47.2** Essential investigations in patients with isolated splenomegaly

| |
|---|
| Full blood count and blood film |
| Blood cultures |
| Serology for human immunodeficiency virus, hepatitis B virus, hepatitis C virus |
| Autoantibodies |
| Coomb's test |
| Antinuclear factor |
| Rheumatoid factor |
| Computed tomography of thorax and abdomen |
| Bone marrow aspirate and biopsy |
| Mantoux test |

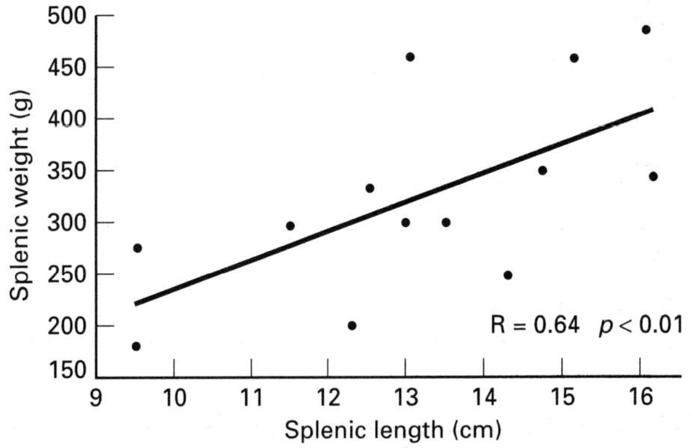


**Fig. 47.6** Relation of splenic weight to splenic length measured by ultrasound (Royal Infirmary, Edinburgh).

involvement but may merely reflect reactive hyperplasia. Equally, small areas of infiltration (<1 cm) may not be detected. Cysts, abscesses and areas of infarction are best identified using computed tomography (Taylor et al 1991).

### Magnetic resonance imaging

Compared to computed tomography and ultrasound, there is no clear role for the use of magnetic resonance imaging in the investigation of abnormal spleens. However, improvements in magnetic resonance imaging and the development of organ-specific contrast agents mean that this investigation is likely to become increasingly useful (Rabushka et al 1994).

### Angiography

Assessment of splenic circulation may be useful, especially to define the vascularity of a focal lesion prior to splenectomy. Therapeutic embolization is also feasible in patients not considered fit for splenectomy (p. 1011).

### Radiology

The spleen can usually be identified on a plain abdominal radiograph. Enlargement results in absent bowel gas shadows in the left hypochondrium. In addition, splenic calcification or fluid levels (e.g. in an abscess) may be detected.

## ASSESSMENT OF SPLENIC FUNCTION

The spleen has numerous functions and it may be useful to assess splenic function in individuals with splenomegaly. Equally, assessment of suspected hyposplenism in patients without splenomegaly (Table 47.3) may be required. There is no single test that gives a "global" assessment of all aspects of splenic function. It is essential, therefore, to approach the investigation of splenic function by deciding which aspects are of particular interest in the individual clinical situation (Table 47.4). For example, when splenomegaly is present in myelofibrosis and in order to assess whether splenectomy is likely to improve anemia, assessment of splenic red cell pooling may be informative. Alternatively, serial assessment of red cell "pit" counts may be useful in patients with potentially reversible functional hyposplenism, as in celiac disease. It should be remembered that splenic function normally declines with age (Markus & Toghill 1991).

**Table 47.3** Causes of hyposplenism

| |
|---|
| Surgical removal |
| Splenic infarction |
|   Sickle cell anemia |
|   Essential thrombocytopenia |
| Splenic atrophy |
| Splenic agenesis |
| Splenic infiltration |
|   Lymphomas |
|   Amyloid |
|   Metastases |
| Postirradiation |

**Table 47.4** Approaches to the assessment of splenic function

| *Question* | *Investigation* |
|---|---|
| Is there functional hyposplenism? | Blood film examination<br>Red cell "pit" counting<br>Damaged red cell clearance<br>Sulfur colloid clearance |
| Is there significant splenic pooling? | $^{51}$Cr-labeled red cell survival |
| Is there significant hypersplenism? | $^{51}$Cr-labeled red cell survival<br>Platelet survival studies |
| Is there extramedullary hemopoiesis? | Ferrokinetic studies |

### Peripheral blood examination

Following splenectomy, characteristic changes are observed in the peripheral blood count and the morphological appearances of the blood film (Fig. 47.7). These changes also occur in functional hyposplenism. Immediately after splenectomy there is usually a neutrophilia and thrombocytosis. The neutrophilia subsides over the following weeks and is replaced by a persistent lymphocytosis and monocytosis. The peak platelet count is usually reached 2 weeks postoperatively and thereafter there is a progressive fall in the platelet count until a steady state is achieved. In some, a moderate thrombocytosis persists; in others, the platelet count returns to normal. Howell–Jolly bodies, intraerythrocyte inclusions that are nuclear remnants usually removed by the spleen, appear on the blood film within hours of splenectomy. In functional hyposplenism and splenic atrophy, increasing numbers of Howell–Jolly bodies correlate with declining splenic function. Acanthocytes and target cells are also seen.

### Erythrocyte "pitting"

In the course of the normal lifespan of a red blood cell, "pits" appear on the red cell membrane (Fig. 47.8). The pits can be visualized under phase-contrast microscopy. Ultrastructural studies have revealed these pits to be vacuoles that contain metabolic waste products. Under normal circumstances and with normal splenic function, these vacuoles are removed from individual cells on pas-

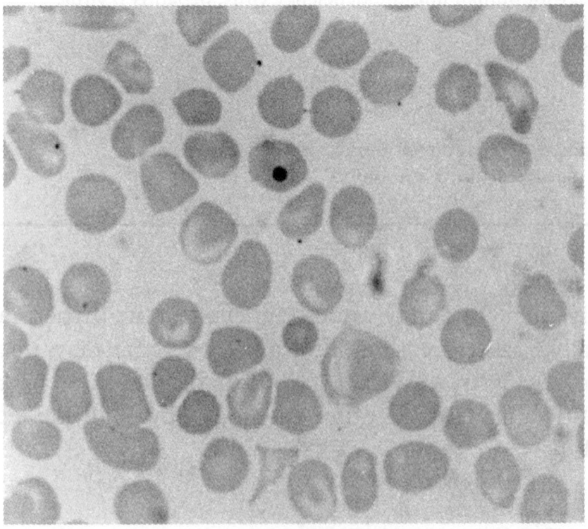

**Fig. 47.7** Peripheral blood film (× 400) following splenectomy showing Howell–Jolley bodies and target cells.

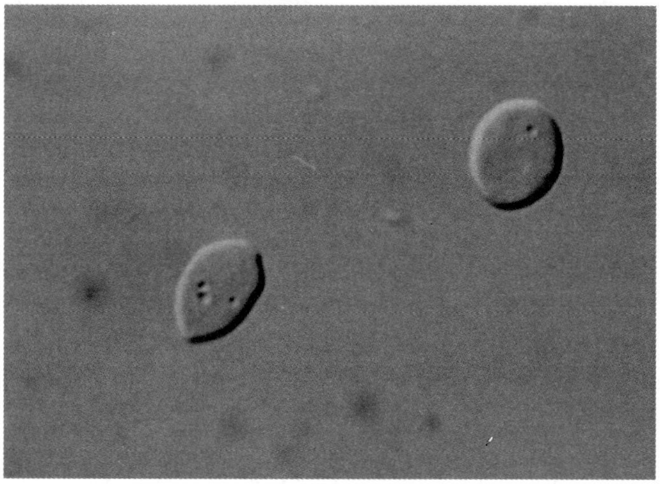

**Fig. 47.8** Pitted red blood cells shown by differential interference microscopy (×1000) (courtesy of Dr A F Muller, The Kent and Canterbury Hospital, England).

sage through the spleen. If splenic function is reduced, the percentage of pitted red cells in the peripheral blood increases. Healthy individuals have 1–4% of circulating red cells with one or more pits visible; after splenectomy, up to 50% of red cells are pitted. Counting pitted red cells is a laborious technique, as up to 2000 individual cells must be counted, but it is very reproducible and there is a good correlation between red cell "pit" counting and other more sophisticated methods of measuring splenic function such as heat-damaged red cell scans (Corazza et al 1981).

### Reservoir function

To assess the ability of the spleen to sequester erythrocytes, autologous red cells are labeled with $^{51}Cr$ and injected into an antecubital vein. Surface counting of radioactivity is performed over the spleen. In splenic sequestration, the counts over the spleen rise slowly over 20 min (the pooling pattern). This contrasts with a maximal reading after 90 s in normal individuals. Further information may be obtained about the sites of red cell destruction by performing differential surface counting over the spleen, liver and heart. This information may be useful to estimate the likely benefits from splenectomy (Patterson & Richards 1992). The degree of extramedullary hemopoiesis may be assessed by ferrokinetic studies.

### Clearance of damaged red blood cells

In health, damaged red cells are removed by the spleen. Consequently, the assessment of damaged autologous red cell clearance from the circulation is a direct measure of the "culling" function of the spleen. For this investigation, red cells can be damaged in vitro by chemical, antibody sensitization or heat methods before being radio-labeled and reinjected into the patient. The rate of isotope disappearance from the circulation can be measured by taking sequential blood samples.

### Clearance of sulfur colloid

Sulfur colloid is taken up selectively by phagocytic cells in the spleen. The rate of clearance of radio-labeled sulfur colloid from the circulation is a method of assessing the phagocytic component of splenic function.

## CONSEQUENCES OF SPLENOMEGALY

Regardless of the cause of splenomegaly, difficulties may arise as a result of splenic enlargement.

### Hypersplenism

The term "hypersplenism" has been employed in a number of different ways. It has been recognized that the presence of splenomegaly, almost regardless of cause, may be associated with certain hematological changes that revert to normal following splenectomy. It is now accepted generally that the term "hypersplenism" should be restricted to individuals with splenomegaly in association with: 1) peripheral blood cytopenias (anemia, leukopenia and thrombocytopenia); 2) a normal or hyperplastic bone marrow; and 3) correction of hematological changes following splenectomy. Patients with hematological malignancies associated with splenomegaly and bone marrow infiltration are particularly difficult to assess, as there is often combined bone marrow failure and hypersplenism leading to peripheral blood cytopenias. The mechanisms leading to the development of hypersplenism are complex. There is increased destruction as well as pooling of blood constituents. For example, the normal spleen contains about 30% of circulating platelets, but with increasing splenomegaly this figure may rise to 90%.

***Chronic liver disease.*** Hypersplenism often accompanies splenomegaly due to chronic liver disease and is associated with portal hypertension (p. 1001). Thrombocytopenia occurs in about 60% of patients with esophagogastric varices, but platelet counts below $70 \times 10^9$/L occur in only about 20% (Fig. 47.9). Thrombocytopenia is not an important direct cause of bleeding from varices, but the chances of bleeding in patients with primary biliary cirrhosis increase as the platelet count falls (p. 923). Leukopenia is less common, occurring in about a quarter of patients with varices, and the total white cell count is below $3 \times 10^9$/L in only 10%. Anemia occurs in about a third of patients with chronic liver disease and splenomegaly, but the hemoglobin is below 100 g/L in only 10%. Anemia in chronic liver disease is usually multifactorial. Factors other than hypersplenism should be considered when the hemoglobin is below 100 g/L, the

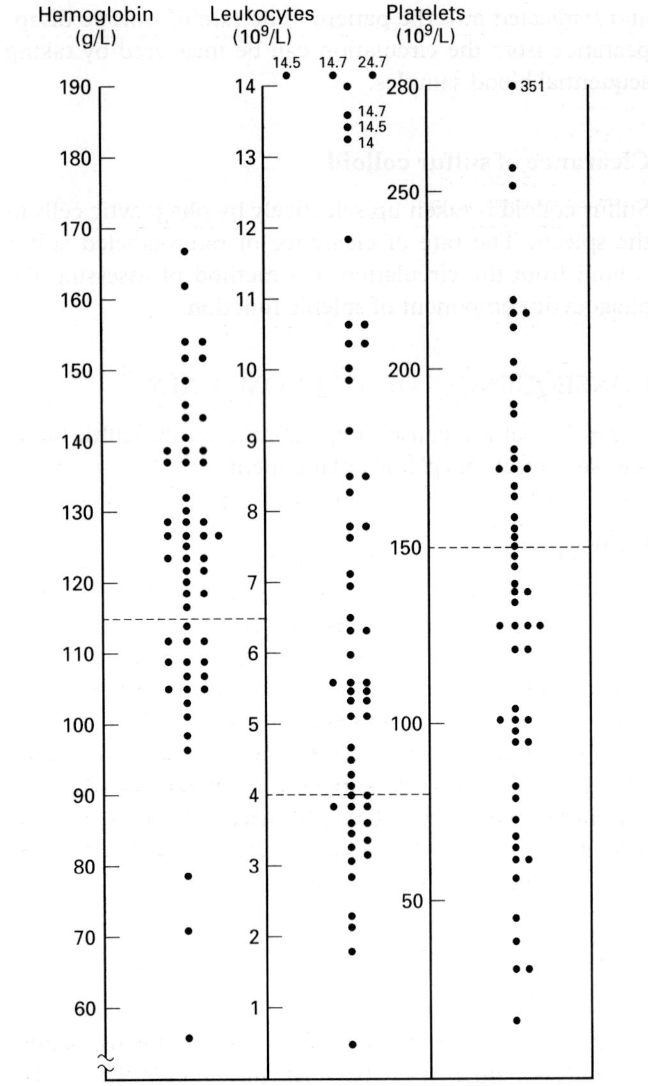


**Fig. 47.9** Peripheral blood counts (lower normal limits ----) in 55 patients with hepatic cirrhosis and esophagogastric varices with no previous or current bleeding (Royal Infirmary, Edinburgh).

leukocytes below 3 × $10^9$/L or the platelets below 70 × $10^9$/L. Decompression of the portal circulation by liver transplantation, portocaval shunt surgery or a transjugular intrahepatic stent shunt (p. 1007) is often followed by a reduction in spleen size and an associated improvement in the peripheral blood count (Jalan et al 1994). Recent studies suggest that granulocyte-macrophage colony-stimulating factor (GM-CSF) may be used to raise the white cell count in patients with cirrhosis and hypersplenism (Gurakar et al 1994). This treatment may be indicated in patients with recurrent infection associated with neutropenia.

## Spontaneous splenic rupture

Nearly all causes of splenomegaly have been implicated as predisposing to spontaneous acute rupture which usually results in severe hemorrhage. This may present abruptly with collapse and severe abdominal pain and necessitates urgent surgical intervention. Chronic presentations of splenic rupture have also been described and controversy remains as to whether a normal spleen may spontaneously rupture (Kumar et al 1992). Splenic rupture has also been reported as a complication of anticoagulant or thrombolytic therapy and may mimic an acute myocardial infarction and cardiogenic shock (Blankenship & Indeck 1993). Peliosis of the spleen may present with splenic rupture.

## Splenic infarction

This usually presents with left upper quadrant pleuritic pain and may be associated with fever and leukocytosis. Management is conservative with analgesia and intravenous fluids.

## Massive spleen syndrome

Portal hypertension with the development of gastric and esophageal varices may occur in patients with massive splenomegaly or with long-standing moderate splenomegaly. This is thought to be due to increased intrahepatic vascular resistance as well as to hemodynamic changes associated with increasing splenic enlargement (p. 990).

# SPLENIC VASCULAR DISEASE

Vascular disease may affect the splenic artery, the intrasplenic vessels or the splenic vein.

### *Splenic artery aneurysm*

Splenic artery aneurysms are uncommon, occurring in about 0.007% of autopsies (Holdsworth & Gunn 1992). Some 80% occur in patients aged over 50 years, but they are more common in women and rupture is associated particularly with pregnancy. They are also strongly associated with portal hypertension. Atherosclerosis accounts for most aneurysms and fibromuscular arterial dysplasia and mycotic aneurysms for a few. The high splenic blood flow of pregnancy and portal hypertension is probably important in the development of the lesion. Most are asymptomatic. Rupture is the commonest complication occurring into any part of the gastrointestinal tract, the pancreatic duct or the peritoneal cavity and causing abdominal pain, shock and hematemesis or melena. Premonitory bleeds can occur and sometimes chronic iron deficiency anemia develops. Abdominal tenderness may be present, an abdominal mass is rare and a bruit is heard in about 10% of cases. Calcification in the aneurysm may be seen on an abdominal radiograph, but urgent arteriography is required when rupture is suspected. Emergency treatment is usually by splenectomy or occasionally by ligation of the aneurysm. Surgical treatment otherwise should be considered for symptomatic lesions, in women of childbearing age and for aneurysms that are greater than 2 cm diameter or increasing in size.

### *Splenic peliosis*

This rare condition, in which blood-filled cystic spaces develop in the red pulp, is invariably found in association with peliosis hepatis and may be linked to the oral contraceptive pill or steroids (p. 1086).

### *Splenic vein thrombosis*

Splenic vein thrombosis is rare but probably underdiagnosed. It is considered further in relation to portal venous thrombosis (p. 1083).

### *Splenic vein aneurysm*

These are exceedingly rare and are considered in relation to aneurysms of the portal and other mesenteric veins (p. 1085).

## THE SPLEEN IN LIVER DISEASE

Splenomegaly is common in chronic liver disease and has been reported in 60–80% of patients with hepatic cirrhosis at autopsy (Tumen 1970). It has usually been attributed to the hemodynamic consequences of portal hypertension and is regarded widely as a consequence of splenic congestion, but reticuloendothelial hyperplasia in the spleen has also been considered important (Merkel et al 1985). Splenomegaly is associated with an increased splenic blood flow and this may make an important contribution to portal hypertension (p. 991). Of further interest is the observation that alcoholic liver disease can be associated with a degree of functional hyposplenism and this may in turn predispose to infection, particularly pneumococcal (Muller & Toghill 1992). This functional hyposplenism may coexist with "hematological" hypersplenism with or without splenomegaly. In 42 patients with alcoholic liver disease, 18 (42%) had functional hyposplenism by measurement of red cell pits, four of these 18 patients had hematological evidence of hypersplenism and only two had splenomegaly. The authors suggested that hyposplenism might be multifactorial and attributable to splenic toxicity of alcohol, liver disease and portal hypertension. The same investigators found no evidence of functional hyposplenism in chronic active hepatitis or primary biliary cirrhosis (Markus et al 1993). There have, however, been occasional reports of reversible hyposplenism following treatment of chronic aggressive hepatitis (Dhawan et al 1979).

**Table 47.5** Gastrointestinal diseases associated with hyposplenism

| |
|---|
| Celiac disease |
| Ulcerative colitis |
| Crohn's disease |
| Whipple's disease |
| Tropical sprue |
| Intestinal lymphangiectasia |
| Idiopathic ulcerative enteritis |

## THE SPLEEN IN GASTROINTESTINAL DISEASE

In recent years there has been increasing evidence of functional hyposplenism in gastrointestinal disease (Muller & Toghill 1995). This has been shown in several disorders (Table 47.5) and has been established best in celiac syndrome. The causative mechanisms are poorly understood. Functional hyposplenism in celiac disease, thought to be due to an autoimmune mechanism, may be reversed by adherence to a gluten-free diet. Splenic atrophy with permanent loss of function occurs in advanced disease (Robinson et al 1980). Hyposplenism has been demonstrated in patients with inflammatory bowel disease using heat-damaged red cell scans (Palmer et al 1981) and "pit" counting methods (Muller et al 1993). The incidence is higher in individuals with extensive colonic disease and there is an increased risk of postoperative infections. In addition, overwhelming infection may occur in patients whose colitis is in remission (Foster et al 1982).

## POSTSPLENECTOMY AND HYPOSPLENIC INFECTION

The spleen plays a crucial role in protecting the body against infecting organisms. Encapsulated bacteria are removed particularly effectively by the spleen, both by phagocytosis and by the rapid development of a specific antibody response. Following splenectomy or in hyposplenic states, these important functions are lost or reduced, resulting in an increased risk of infection which may be sudden, overwhelming and rapidly fatal. The risk of postoperative infection has led to an increasing tendency to limit the indications for splenectomy. Conservative management of the traumatized spleen and the replacement of splenectomy by computed tomography scanning for staging purposes in lymphomas have reduced the number of splenectomies. Previously, the inadvertent seeding of splenic tissue in the peritoneal cavity (splenosis) (Corazza et al 1984) and, more recently, splenic conservation and autotransplantation techniques have almost certainly reduced the risk of postoperative infection (Holdsworth 1991).

The increased risk of serious infection after splenectomy was recognized first in children and subsequently reported in adults. The risk is greatest in the first 2 years after splenectomy but persists throughout life. Recent studies have provided somewhat conflicting estimates of both the incidence and the absolute risk of infection. A consensus view has emerged, however, that the lifelong risk of infection postsplenectomy is increased approximately 12-fold compared to a nonsplenectomized age-matched group. The risk is greater in children (50-fold increase) and in those with coexisting immunosuppression or malignant disease (25-fold increase) (Cullingford et al 1991).

*Overwhelming postsplenectomy infection*

This is the most dramatic form of postsplenectomy sepsis. This syndrome consists of rapidly progressive septicemia associated with circulatory collapse and disseminated intravascular coagulation. *Streptococcus pneumoniae* is the commonest organism to cause postsplenectomy infection, accounting for 90% of cases. Less fulminant episodes of infection may be caused by *E. coli*, *N. meningitidis*, *Pseudomonas* and staphylococci. Once septicemia is established, the mortality is in excess of 50%.

*Other infections*

Malaria, babesiosis and histoplasmosis are also potential hazards (Boone & Watters 1995). The risks associated with travel to endemic areas should be explained to asplenic individuals and the importance of compliance with chemoprophylaxis such as antimalarials should be stressed.

### Prevention

The recommendations for presplenectomy vaccinations and postsplenectomy antibiotic prophylaxis have been reviewed recently (Fielding 1994, Mayon-White 1994). In patients who have functional hyposplenism for reasons other than splenectomy, it is logical to recommend the same program of vaccination and antibiotic prophylaxis (McKay et al 1993). This should be given as soon as the functional hyposplenism has been confirmed by one or more of the methods described above.

Three vaccines are now recommended. Pneumococcal vaccine should be administered at least 2 weeks before an elective splenectomy or 2 weeks after an emergency splenectomy. The response to the vaccine is diminished in the first few postoperative days and to avoid oversights in those who have undergone emergency splenectomy, vaccination should be performed on the day of discharge from hospital even if this is less than 2 weeks postoperatively. A booster dose should be given every 5–10 years. *Haemophilus influenzae* type B (Hib) vaccine is given as a course of three doses at monthly intervals. Meningococcal groups A and C vaccine should be given at the same time as the pneumococcal vaccine and repeated at 5-yearly intervals.

Antibiotic prophylaxis should be recommended for life in addition to vaccinations. This should consist of twice-daily phenoxymethylpenicillin 500 mg for adults, 250 mg for children aged 6–12 years and 125 mg for children under 6 years. Penicillin-allergic individuals should receive erythromycin. If, following full information regarding the risk of infection, the patient declines prophylaxis, a supply of a suitable antibiotic should be given and commenced at the first sign of a pyrexial illness.

## SPLENOSIS

Splenosis is the inadvertent seeding of splenic tissue that can occur after abdominal trauma or splenectomy (Corazza et al 1984). The condition is usually asymptomatic and found incidentally. Symptomatic splenosis usually occurs many years after the causative event. Peritoneal splenosis can cause abdominal pain and intestinal obstruction. Thoracic splenosis is very rare, usually occurs in the pleura and can cause pleuritic pain (Singh et al 1995).

## REFERENCES


Barkun A N, Camus M, Green L et al 1991 The bedside assessment of splenic enlargement. American Journal of Medicine 91: 512–518

Berris B 1966 The incidence of palpable liver and spleen in the postpartum period. Canadian Medical Association Journal 95: 1318–1319

Blankenship J C, Indeck M 1993 Spontaneous splenic rupture complicating anticoagulant or thrombolytic therapy. American Journal of Medicine 94: 433–437

Bohnsack J F, Brown E J 1986 The role of the spleen in resistance to infection. Annual Review of Medicine 37: 49–59

Boone K E, Watters D A K 1995 The incidence of malaria after splenectomy in Papua New Guinea. British Medical Journal 311: 1273

Carroll B J, Phillips E H, Semel C J, Fallas M, Morgenstern L 1992 Laparoscopic splenectomy. Surgical Endoscopy 6: 183–185

Cavanna L, Civardi G, Fornari F et al 1992 Ultrasonically guided percutaneous splenic tissue core biopsy in patients with malignant lymphomas. Cancer 69: 2932–2936

Corazza G R, Bullen A W, Hall R, Robinson P J, Losowsky M S 1981 Simple method of assessing splenic function in coeliac disease. Clinical Science 60: 109–113

Corazza G R, Tarozzi C, Vaira D, Frisoni M, Gasbarrini G 1984 Return of splenic function after splenectomy: how much tissue is needed? British Medical Journal 289: 861–864

Cronin C C, Brady M P, Murphy C, Kenny E, Whelton M J, Hardiman C 1994 Splenectomy in patients with undiagnosed splenomegaly. Postgraduate Medical Journal 70: 288–291

Cullingford G L, Watkins D N, Watts A D J, Mallon D F 1991 Severe late post-splenectomy infection. British Journal of Surgery 78: 716–721

DeLand F H 1970 Normal spleen size. Radiology 97: 589–592

Dhawan V M, Spencer R P, Sziklas J J 1979 Reversible functional asplenia in chronic aggressive hepatitis. Journal of Nuclear Medicine 20: 34–36

Ebaugh F G Jr, McIntyre O R 1979 Palpable spleens: ten year follow-up. Annals of Internal Medicine 90: 130–131

Fielding A K 1994 Prophylaxis against late infection following splenectomy and bone marrow transplant. Blood Reviews 8: 179–191

Foster K J, Devitt N, Gallagher P J, Abbott R M 1982 Overwhelming pneumococcal septicaemia in a patient with ulcerative colitis and splenic atrophy. Gut 23: 630–632
Goonewardene A, Bourke J B, Ferguson R, Toghill P G 1979 Splenectomy for undiagnosed splenomegaly. British Journal of Surgery 66: 62–65
Grover S A, Barkun A N, Sackett D L 1993 Does this patient have splenomegaly? Journal of the American Medical Association 270: 2218–2221
Gurakar A, Fagiuoli S, Gavaler J S et al 1994 The use of granulocyte-macrophage colony-stimulating factor to enhance hematologic parameters of patients with cirrhosis and hypersplenism. Journal of Hepatology 21: 582–586
Harrison J F McK, Davies S C 1992 Acute problems in sickle cell disease. Hospital Update 18: 709–716
Holdsworth R J 1991 Regeneration of the spleen and splenic autotransplantation. British Journal of Surgery 78: 270–278
Holdsworth R J, Gunn A 1992 Ruptured splenic artery aneurysm in pregnancy. A review. British Journal of Obstetrics and Gynaecology 99: 595–597
Jalan R, Redhead D N, Simpson K, Hayes P C 1994 A prospective evaluation of haematological alterations following TIPSS. Gut 35 (suppl): W95
Kumar S, Gupta A, Shrivastava U K, Mathur S B 1992 Spontaneous rupture of normal spleen: an enigma recalled. British Journal of Clinical Practice 46: 67–68
McKay P J, Kennedy D H, Lucie N P 1993 Should hyposplenic patients receive prophylaxis against bacterial infection? Scottish Medical Journal 38: 51–52
Markus H S, Toghill P J 1991 Impaired splenic function in elderly people. Age and Ageing 20: 287–290
Markus H S, Muller A F, Toghill P J 1993 Splenic function, assesssed by quantification of erythrocyte membrane pits, is normal in chronic active hepatitis and primary biliary cirrhosis. Journal of Hepatology 18: 106–111
Mayon-White R 1994 Protection of the asplenic patient. Prescribers' Journal 34: 165–170
Meek D R, Mills P R, Gray H W, Duncan J G, Russell R I, McKillop J H 1984 A comparison of computed tomography, ultrasound and scintigraphy in the diagnosis of alcoholic liver disease. British Journal of Radiology 57: 23–27
Merkel C, Gatta A, Arnaboldi L, Zuin R 1985 Splenic haemodynamics and portal hypertension in patients with liver cirrhosis and spleen enlargement. Clinical Physiology 5: 531–539
Muller A F, Toghill P J 1992 Splenic function in alcoholic liver disease. Gut 33: 1386–1389
Muller A F, Toghill P J 1995 Hyposplenism in gastrointestinal disease. Gut 36: 165–167
Muller A F, Cornford E, Toghill P J 1993 Splenic function in inflammatory bowel disease: assessment by differential interference microscopy and splenic ultrasound. Quarterly Journal of Medicine 86: 333–340
Palmer K R, Sherriff S B, Holdsworth C D, Ryan F P 1981 Further experience of hyposplenism in inflammatory bowel disease. Quarterly Journal of Medicine 50: 463–471
Patterson K G, Richards J D M 1992 The use of radioisotopes in haematology. Blood Reviews 6: 1–9
Rabushka L S, Kawashima A, Fishman E K 1994 Imaging of the spleen: CT with supplemental MR examination. Radiographics 14: 307–332
Redmond H P, Duignan J P, Bouchier-Hayes D 1990 Anatomy of the spleen. In: Cuschieri A, Forbes C D (eds) Anatomy of the spleen. Blackwell Scientific Publications, London, pp 1–24
Robinson P J, Bullen A W, Hall R, Brown R C, Baxter P, Losowsky M S 1980 Splenic size and function in adult coeliac disease. British Journal of Radiology 53: 532–537
Singh P, Munn N J, Patel H K 1995 Thoracic splenosis. New England Journal of Medicine 333: 882
Taylor A J, Dodds W J, Erickson S J, Stewart E T 1991 CT of acquired abnormalities of the spleen. American Journal of Roentgenology 157: 1213–1219
Tumen H J 1970 Hypersplenism and portal hypertension. Annals of the New York Academy of Sciences 170: 332–344
Van Krieken J, Han J M, te Velde J 1992 Spleen. In: Sternberg S S (ed) Histology for pathologists. Raven Press, New York, pp 253–260
Zhang B, Lewis S M 1989 A study of the reliability of clinical palpation of the spleen. Clinical and Laboratory Haematology 11: 7–10

SECTION 13

# Pancreatic-biliary disorders

# 48. Diseases of the biliary tract

*O. James Garden*

ANATOMY AND PHYSIOLOGY

## Normal anatomy

The gallbladder is a pear-shaped sac situated under the right lobe of the liver in the gallbladder fossa between the quadrate lobe (segment IV) of the left hemiliver and segment V of the right hemiliver. It holds approximately 25 ml of fluid. Its fundus lies anteriorly behind the tip of the ninth costal cartilage and its body and neck pass upwards, backwards and medially towards the porta hepatis and the cystic duct. It is covered with peritoneum on its undersurface and is attached to the liver by connective tissue on its upper surface (cystic plate). Its body overhangs the transverse colon and its neck is related to the duodenal cap. The cystic duct follows a variable convoluted course from the neck of the gallbladder to join the common hepatic duct to form the common bile duct. It has a muscular wall and smooth muscle is prolonged into prominent crescentic mucosal folds known as the spiral valves of Heister.

The biliary tract originates in the biliary canaliculi (p. 710) and the intrahepatic ductules derived from them join progressively to form segmental ducts which drain identifiable segments (Fig. 48.1) or compartments of the liver supplied by their own portal venous and arterial blood supply. In the right hemiliver, two posterior segments (segment VI inferiorly and segment VII superiorly) form the posterior sector and two anterior segments (segment V inferior and segment VIII superiorly) form the anterior sector. The two anterior and the two posterior segment ducts join to form the anterior and posterior sectoral ducts respectively, which in the majority of individuals then unite to form the right hepatic duct which emerges from the liver for a distance of less than 1 cm.

The left hemiliver contain three segments. The liver to the left of the falciform ligament, referred to as the left lobe, contains segment III anteriorly and segment II posteriorly. Segment IV lies medial to the falciform ligament and inferiorly is known as the quadrate lobe. The segmental ducts II and III converge at the umbilical fissure and are joined by the segment IV duct at a variable position, but usually to the right of the umbilical fissure. The left

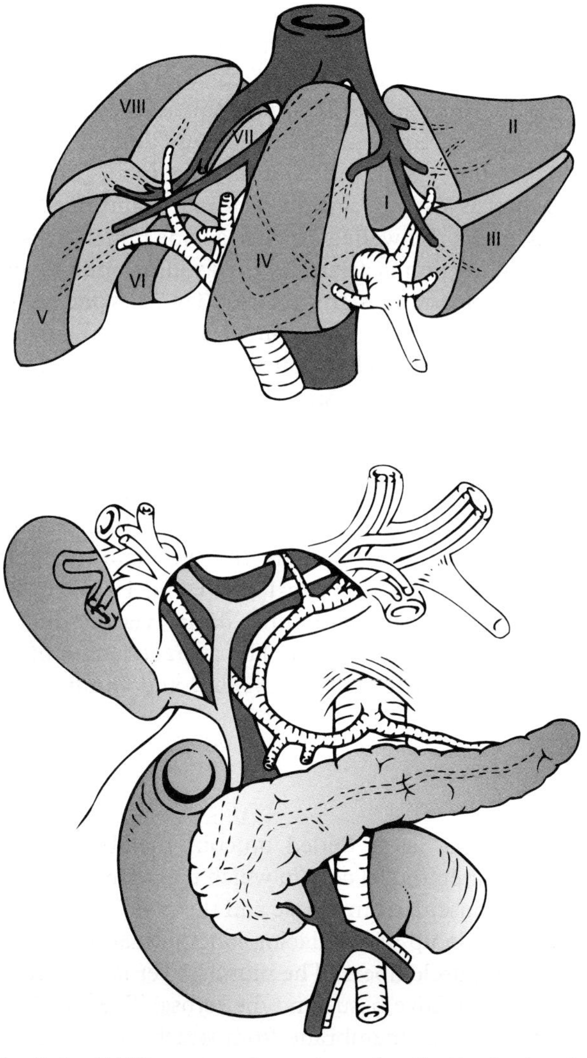

A

B

**Fig. 48.1** (**A**) The segmental anatomy as described by Couinaud with the individual segments labelled (I–VIII). (**B**) The segmental biliary drainage and anatomy of the extrahepatic biliary tree.

hepatic duct is found at the inferior margin of segment IV and pursues a longer and more accessible course than the right hepatic duct with which it unites to form the common hepatic duct. The bile ducts draining segment I (caudate lobe) join both the right and left hepatic ducts.

The common hepatic duct enters the free edge of the lesser omentum and forms the common bile duct following its junction with the cystic duct. At this point, the ducts lie anterior to the portal vein and lateral to the hepatic artery, the right branch of which generally passes posteriorly. The common bile duct passes down behind the duodenal cap, still lying anterolateral to the portal vein and lateral to the gastroduodenal artery. It then passes in a groove on the posterior surface of the head of the pancreas; in some individuals the duct is completely surrounded by pancreatic tissue. The duct then turns laterally towards the second part of the duodenum, passing anterior to the inferior vena cava and between the branches of the pancreaticoduodenal arteries to come into close association with the pancreatic duct. The relative length of the components of the bile duct is variable, but the duct is usually said to be about 5 cm long. The promixal part is thinwalled and has a wide lumen, whereas the distal portion is relatively thickwalled and narrow. Ductal diameter ranges from 4 to 13 mm (Kune 1964) but increases with age (Mahour et al 1967). The duct ends by passing obliquely through the posteromedial wall of the duodenum and its site of entry into the duodenal lumen is marked by the papilla of Vater (major papilla). The main pancreatic duct joins the terminal bile duct to form a common channel in 80% of cases (Fig. 48.2), whereas in 20% of cases there is no common channel and the pancreatic duct enters the duodenum slightly distal to the bile duct (Boyden 1975, Hand 1973). In 2% of cases the main pancreatic duct drains via the duct of Santorini to the minor papilla. The average length of the common channel is usually between 2 and 7 mm (range 1–14 mm).

## Histology

The gallbladder has a folded mucous membrane lined with columnar epithelial cells in which there are no glands. There is no muscularis mucosae and the main thickness of the wall is made up of interlacing longitudinal, transverse and oblique muscle fibers. The muscle layer is covered by subserous connective tissue and the serosa. The bile ducts have a flat mucous membrane from which many mucous glands arise. The proximal bile ducts have thin walls containing collagen and elastic tissue with little muscle, while the distal common bile duct contains the powerful choledochal sphincter muscle which begins about 2 mm outside the duodenal wall and invests the common bile duct and pancreatic duct as far as their opening on the papilla of Vater (Boyden 1957).

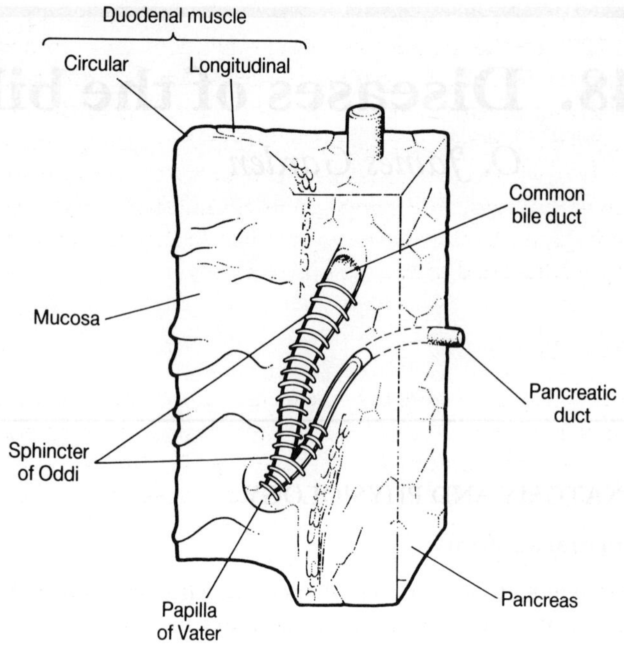


**Fig. 48.2** Schematic representation of the human sphincter of Oddi demonstrating the circular smooth muscle, which surrounds the terminal common bile duct and pancreatic duct. The length of the sphincter along the pancreatic duct is shorter than the length investing the terminal common bile duct. The major part of the sphincter lies within the duodenal wall and enters the duodenum through a slit in the duodenal muscle (Toouli 1984, Toouli et al 1982).

## Anomalies

Variations in biliary anatomy are frequent and important for the biliary surgeon (Kune & Sali 1981). Variations in the sectoral and hepatic ductal anatomy occur in almost 50% of individuals and are important when interpreting radiological studies and when performing hepatic resection, transplantation and operations on the proximal biliary tree. The right anterior or posterior sectoral duct may converge distally to join the rest of the biliary system in up to 25% of individuals and so may be damaged inadvertently during cholecystectomy.

The cystic duct is particularly variable. It may join the right hepatic duct, the retroduodenal or intrapancreatic portion of the common duct or, very rarely, the left hepatic duct. Occasional examples of absence of the cystic duct have been reported, although it is uncertain whether this is a consequence of inflammatory fibrosis. Rare examples of a double cystic duct draining a single gallbladder have been reported (Milroy 1947). The cystic duct may converge on the common hepatic duct at an angle, wind around it or run parallel to it for some distance.

The gallbladder is rarely intrahepatic or attached to the liver by a mesentery, an anomaly which can lead to volvulus (Carter et al 1963). The most frequent gallbladder anomaly is the presence of a Phrygian cap or folded gallbladder, but the gallbladder may also be absent, bilobed or duplicated. Microgallbladder occurs in cystic fibrosis

(p. 1238). Biliary atresia (p. 730) and choledochal cysts (p. 727) are the most important anomalies of the common bile duct. True cholecystohepatic ducts are rare and may arise from severe inflammation. The subvesical or duct of Luschka is a small bile duct which courses in the gallbladder bed within the hilar plate and probably outside the wall of the gallbladder. Such ducts communicate with segment ducts but they have surgical significance in that they may be damaged during cholecystectomy.

### Physiology

The biliary tract conveys bile to the small intestine and stores and concentrates a proportion of it in the gallbladder. Secretion of bile by hepatocytes (p. 713) provides the driving force for bile flow. The muscular activity of the choledochal sphincter, and to a lesser extent the duodenal musculature, determines how much bile enters the duodenum and the gallbladder. Endoscopic retrograde cannulation of the bile duct has allowed study of the choledochal sphincter in health and disease (Carr-Locke & Gregg 1981, Geenen et al 1981, Toouli 1984) (p. 120). Common bile duct pressure is normally some 10 mmHg (140 $mmH_2O$) above duodenal pressure. The choledochal sphincter is 4–6 mm long and its resting pressure exceeds common bile duct pressure by 5–10 mmHg. The pressure in the common bile duct in the fasting state usually exceeds gallbladder pressure so that most, but not all, of the bile enters the gallbladder (Table 48.1).

Resorption of sodium, chloride and bicarbonate by the gallbladder mucosa and the passive diffusion of water and potassium results in concentration of the bile. Phasic high-pressure peristaltic contractions occur within the sphincter at a rate of 4–6 per minute, most moving towards the duodenum and facilitating the flow of bile from the sphincter segment into the duodenum. Cholecystokinin decreases the frequency and amplitude of these contractions, lowers sphincter activity and may affect bile flow. For example, phase III of the migrating motor complex is associated with an increased frequency of phasic contractions (Torsoli et al 1986) while phase II is accompanied by a decrease in gallbladder volume (Toouli et al 1986). The factors which influence the volume of bile secreted by the liver are poorly understood although the rate of secretion of components such as bile acids is influenced by transit time in small bowel (Hardison et al 1979) and by drugs such as chenodeoxycholic acid (Fromm 1988).

The most important cause of gallbladder contraction is food-stimulated cholecystokinin release from the duodenal mucosa (p. 160). The simultaneous relaxation of the choledochal sphincter results in the passage of bile into the duodenum. The gallbladder also receives an autonomic nerve supply derived predominantly from the vagus nerve. Vagal activity in man is probably only important in maintaining gallbladder tone and this may account for the large dilated gallbladders seen after vagotomy (p. 272). The function, if any, of the sympathetic nerves is unknown. Most autonomic fibers are in fact afferents which eventually travel up the splanchnic nerves. Secretin increases the secretion of the biliary epithelium.

**Table 48.1** Pressures (mm bile) in the biliary tract (Hand 1973)

| Secretion pressure of bile | | Common bile duct | Gallbladder | |
|---|---|---|---|---|
| Normal | Maximum | | Resting | Contraction |
| 120–250 | 300 | 60–200* | 10–30 | 200–300 |

*Very variable.

## CHOLESTASIS (OBSTRUCTIVE JAUNDICE)

The principal aims in the management of patients with obstructive jaundice are to establish the cause and to differentiate obstruction of a major bile duct which requires surgical relief from causes of jaundice which cannot be treated surgically (p. 929). Unfortunately, the clinical and biochemical features of jaundice due to biliary obstruction and to hepatic disease overlap and both types of jaundice may coexist. Prolonged obstruction of major bile ducts can produce liver damage, while chronic liver disease may be associated with intrahepatic cholestasis and a high incidence of gallstones (p. 921) which occasionally cause biliary obstruction. However, modern biliary imaging techniques can display precisely the extent and cause of biliary obstruction, even in the absence of jaundice, and allow medical and surgical causes of biliary obstruction to be differentiated with an accuracy of 95% (Zeman et al 1984). Appropriate decisions can then be made regarding the need for surgical or nonsurgical interventional techniques.

### Classification

Jaundice arises when there is an abnormality of bilirubin metabolism (p. 929). It may be due to excessive bilirubin production, defective bilirubin transport or conjugation or impaired bilirubin excretion. Although there are numerous causes of jaundice (see Table 34.1) most cases are due to viral hepatitis, drugs, alcoholic hepatitis, chronic liver disease, choledocholithiasis and malignant disease. In a number of instances no cause can be found.

The word "cholestasis" (p. 931) has replaced the older term "obstructive jaundice" because failure of bile flow is recognized as the underlying reason for the jaundice. Cholestasis may be due to intrahepatic disease, which is rarely amenable to surgical treatment, or to extrahepatic biliary disease which is often amenable to surgical treatment. The latter is often called "surgical jaundice".

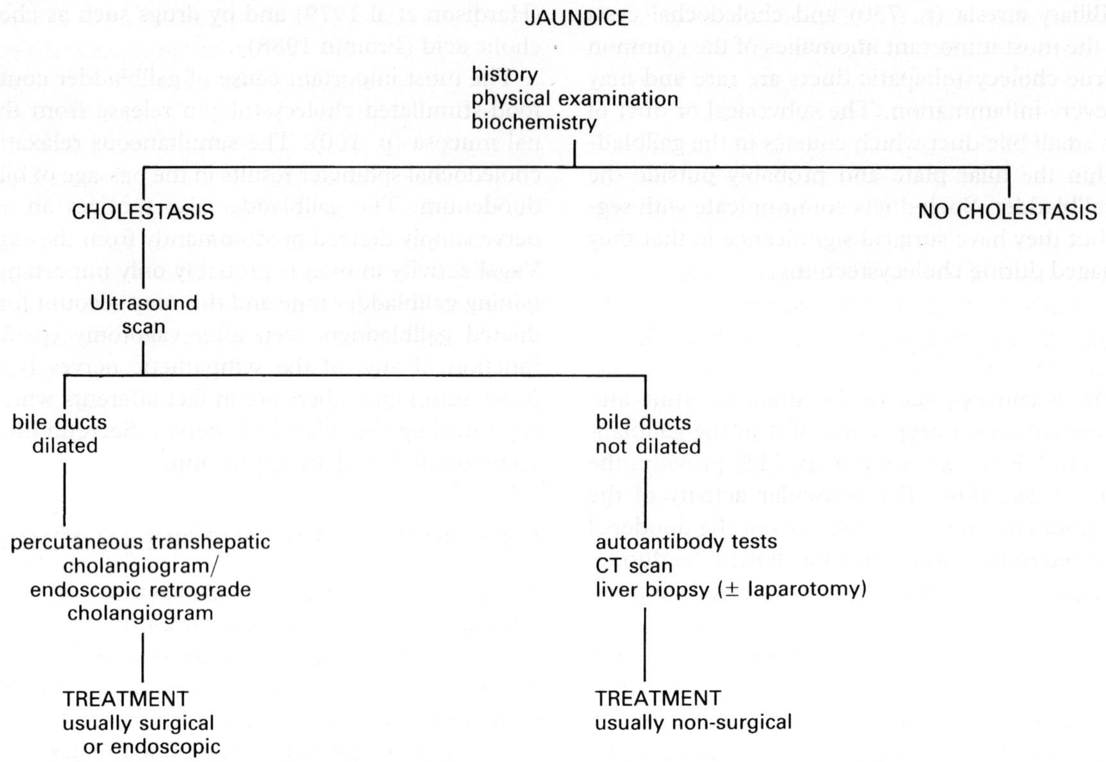


**Fig. 48.3** An algorithm for the diagnostic evaluation of patients with cholestatic jaundice (for biochemical investigation see p. 933; for autoantibody tests see p. 765).

## Diagnosis

This initially involves a careful history, a thorough physical examination, plain radiographs of the chest and abdomen, biochemical liver function tests and ultrasound scans or computed tomography of the liver and biliary tree. It is also advisable in jaundiced patients to test for the hepatitis B surface antigen (HBsAg) in the blood. In many cases, the diagnosis is clear at this stage. If ultrasonography does not show a dilated biliary tree, an intrahepatic cause of jaundice is likely (p. 52). On the other hand, if the biliary tree is dilated, the site and the nature of the obstruction can be further defined by percutaneous transhepatic cholangiography or endoscopic retrograde cholangiography. The diagnostic algorithm outlined in Figure 48.3 may need to be modified according to the availability of investigations and difficulties in their interpretation.

## Clinical features (p. 931)

The important points in the history are the patient's age, family history, contact with hepatitis, recent injections and transfusions, drug and alcohol intake, weight loss, mode of onset of the illness, pruritus, color of the urine and stools, presence of abdominal pain, fever or chills (suggesting cholangitis) and any previous operations on the biliary system or pancreas. Excluding infancy, viral hepatitis is the cause of jaundice in 90% of patients under the age of 30 years and gallstones and malignant disease become progressively more common after the age of 40 years. A family history of jaundice with or without anemia or of gallstones at an early age are also useful clues. Jaundice associated with severe abdominal pain or fever suggests obstruction of the large bile ducts by gallstones and progressive jaundice and weight loss suggest malignant disease.

On physical examination, the important features are depth of the jaundice, peripheral manifestations of chronic liver disease (p. 917), size and shape of the liver, presence of ascites and palpability of the gallbladder or spleen. Deep jaundice favors obstruction of a large bile duct. When the gallbladder is palpable in the presence of obstructive jaundice, calculous obstruction is unlikely (as the gallbladder is usually shrunken and fibrotic) and the common bile duct obstruction is usually due to pancreatic carcinoma (p. 1289). A large irregular liver or ascites suggests malignant disease or cirrhosis and cirrhosis is particularly likely if splenomegaly or other signs of chronic liver disease are found. Splenomegaly and mild jaundice may also suggest hemolysis.

## Investigations

Bilirubinuria (p. 741) reflects the presence of conjugated (water-soluble) bilirubin and supports the diagnosis of cholestasis, while occult blood in the stool (p. 497) suggests a lesion bleeding into the duodenum. A polymorphonuclear leukocytosis suggests choledocholithiasis or a benign stricture and is uncommon in malignant obstruction or viral hepatitis. Eosinophilia occurs occasionally in drug-induced jaundice, particularly that due to chlorpromazine. A high reticulocyte count suggests hemolytic jaundice.

Liver function tests confirm the level of jaundice and may point to a hepatic or cholestatic illness, but never in themselves reveal the precise cause of jaundice. Of the many liver function tests advocated, the serum transaminase and alkaline phosphatase activities, the serum bilirubin, albumin and globulin concentrations and the prothrombin time are of most practical value. The typical results found in hepatitis and cholestasis are described elsewhere (p. 742), but in a proportion of patients the results are not typical and merely show that hepatobiliary disease is present.

*Radiology*

A plain radiograph of the abdomen (p. 5) may show gallstones and the calcification of chronic pancreatitis, while a barium meal examination (p. 8) may show esophageal varices in portal hypertension or duodenal distortion due to pancreatic cancer or chronic pancreatitis. However, the gallstones may not be the cause of cholestasis, while barium meal examination (even when refined by hypotonic duodenography) is a low-yield examination which has been superseded in routine evaluation of cholestasis (Fig. 48.3). Oral cholecystography and intravenous cholangiography are valueless in patients with cholestasis, while radionuclide scanning has been largely superseded by ultrasound and CT scanning as a means of investigating patients with space-occupying lesions and parenchymal liver disease.

*Ultrasound scanning*

Ultrasound scanning is a highly accurate, noninvasive method of detecting bile duct obstruction (p. 52) and can be used as a screening test for biliary disease. While dilatation of intrahepatic ducts is very specific, the detection of extrahepatic bile duct dilatation (Fig. 2.5) is more sensitive and common duct dilatation should be detected in 95% of affected patients (Cooperberg & Golding 1982). Bile duct dilatation is independent of serum bilirubin levels (p. 52), but the absence of dilatation does not exclude extrahepatic biliary obstruction. Additionally, ultrasound scanning can detect gallstones, pancreatic disorders and solid cystic lesions of the liver.

While ultrasound scanning is an extremely accurate method of differentiating between medical and surgical jaundice and the level of obstruction can often be determined, the cause is less often defined (p. 52) and procedures such as direct cholangiography may be required. If, however, gallstones are conclusively demonstrated as the likely cause of bile duct obstruction, further examination is rarely required (Berk et al 1982). Eyre-Brook et al (1983) found that the presence of a dilated extrahepatic duct always reflected obstruction but in 5% of patients the lesion was too proximal for surgical decompression. When extrahepatic obstruction was associated with gallbladder findings typical of calculous obstruction (small gallbladder with multiple stones) or neoplastic obstruction (large empty gallbladder), surgically remediable obstruction was always present.

*Computed tomography* (CT)

While ultrasound followed by cholangiography is the usual combination of investigations for biliary obstruction, some studies have suggested that computed tomography is as sensitive as ultrasound in demonstrating bile duct dilatation (Baron et al 1982) (Fig. 2.20). In addition, the level and cause of obstruction (p. 68) can be defined with greater success than with ultrasound (Pedrosa et al 1981). CT is generally reserved for patients with bile duct dilatation in whom ultrasound has not clearly established the level and cause of obstruction or those in whom the ultrasound findings are equivocal or normal despite clinical or biochemical abnormalities indicating neoplastic cholestasis. CT is a useful method of examining the retroperitoneum and is not limited by overlying bowel gas so that visualization of the pancreas is guaranteed. CT and ultrasound scanning are also used to target fine-needle aspiration of pancreatic lesions.

*Cholangiography*

Percutaneous transhepatic cholangiography (PTC) and endoscopic retrograde cholangiopancreatography (ERCP) can outline the bile ducts clearly and demonstrate the location (and in many cases the nature) of obstruction (Figs 48.4–6, 1.24–28). PTC (p. 22) virtually always outlines the biliary system satisfactorily in the presence of obstruction and will even succeed in outlining it in some 70% of patients who have no biliary dilatation. However, it is invasive and should not be performed when coagulation is impaired or significant ascites is present. In view of the risk of introducing sepsis the procedure should be covered by appropriate prophylactic antibiotic administration and only undertaken following discussion of the patient's subsequent management with a surgical team. ERCP is, if anything, less uncomfortable for the patient and, given its ability to visualize the duodenum and pancreatic duct system, it is preferred when duodenal or pancreatic pathology is suspected. ERCP is also preferred when calculous obstruction is suspected as the cause of cholestasis, since

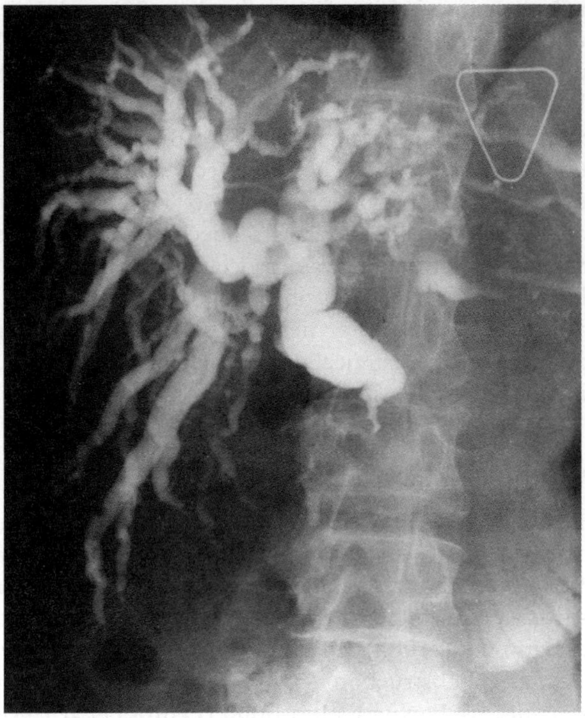

**Fig. 48.4** Percutaneous transhepatic cholangiogram of a patient with cholestatic jaundice caused by a cancer of the head of the pancreas. Note the dilated bile ducts and the complete irregular obstruction at the lower end of the bile duct typical of this type of cancer.

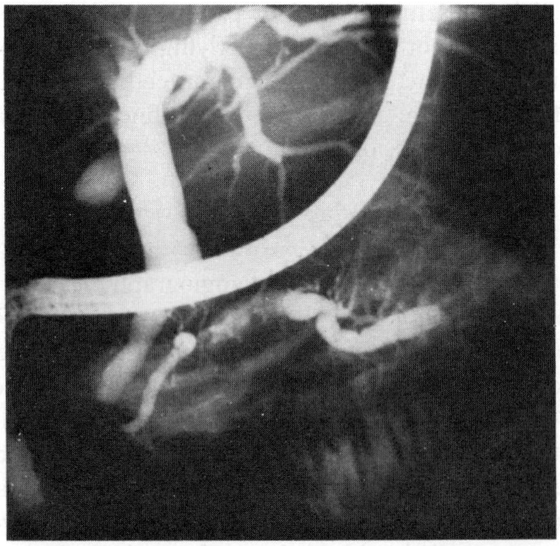

**Fig. 48.5** Endoscopic retrograde cholangiopancreatogram in a patient with cholestasis caused by pancreatic carcinoma. Both the pancreatic and bile ducts are dilated and their distal ends are stenosed.

endoscopic papillotomy can be undertaken. Pancreatitis and cholangitis are the most common serious complications of ERCP. For the individual patient, the choice between these two procedures is determined by the clinician in the light of available radiological and endoscopic expertise.

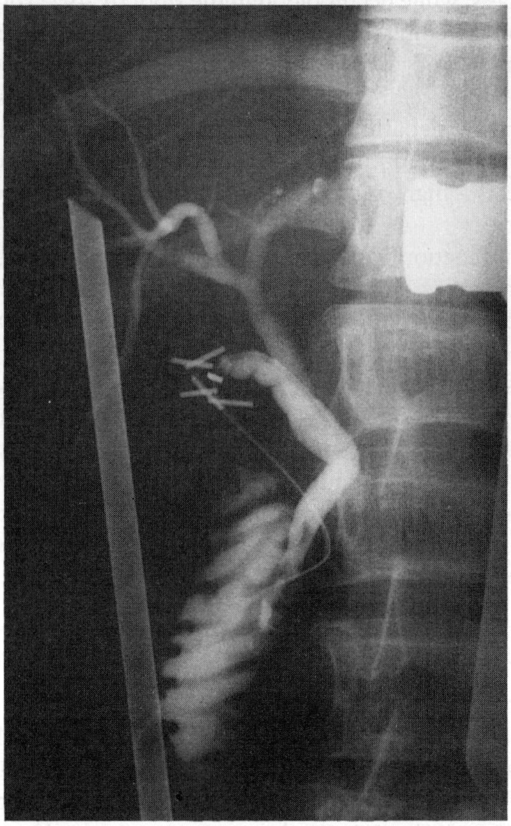

**Fig. 48.6** Operative cholangiogram in a patient with intermittent jaundice confirming the presence of a small stone at the lower end of the bile duct. The patient underwent successful laparoscopic cholecystectomy and transcystic removal of the stone.

*Arteriography*

When resection is contemplated in patients with malignant obstructive jaundice, angiography may be used to detect signs of nonresectability (e.g. portal vein invasion) and display vascular anomalies which may complicate surgery (e.g. origin of hepatic artery from superior mesenteric artery) (Murugiah et al 1993). This investigation is most often employed to assess the resectability of cholangiocarcinoma.

**Surgery**

The role of surgery in the management of obstructive jaundice has changed substantially in recent years. Laparotomy to exclude mechanical bile duct obstruction should never be necessary and can now be avoided in some patients by preoperative demonstration of disseminated malignancy and in others by endoscopic papillotomy with gallstone extraction or insertion of stents (see below). There has been a resurgence of interest in the use of laparoscopy in the assessment and staging of patients with suspected malignant biliary obstruction. The detection of small superficial hepatic metastases and malignant peritoneal seedlings allows unnecessary laparotomy to be avoided in patients with tumors which otherwise appear to be resectable (Warshaw et al 1990). Furthermore, laparoscopic ultrasonography now allows accurate assessment of tumor size and the detection of lymph node and local vascular invasion (John et al 1994).

In patients coming to laparotomy, the abdomen is thoroughly explored to evaluate the gallbladder, bile ducts, pancreas, duodenum and liver. Intraoperative ultrasonography with a high-resolution ultrasound probe can provide additional information which modifies the surgical approach (Garden 1995). Operative cholangiography (Fig. 48.6) may be required and needle biopsy or cytology of any lesion in the pancreas, liver or lymph nodes can be undertaken to stage suspected malignant disease. The distinction between chronic pancreatitis and malignant obstruction may be particularly difficult (p. 1291).

The distinction at operation between benign and malignant conditions such as sclerosing cholangitis and carcinoma of the bile ducts is also problematical. However, it should be stressed that many of the difficulties encountered in the operative diagnosis of the cause of obstructive jaundice can be avoided by appropriate preoperative investigation. The patient should come to surgery with appropriate radiological definition of the cause of obstruction, bearing in mind that some radiological investigations may compromise the surgical approach.

*Procedures to deal with biliary obstruction*

Once obstruction has been confirmed, the procedure depends on its cause and site. Only the principles involved are described here.

Bile duct stones are removed by supraduodenal choledochotomy with removal of the gallbladder, but it is rarely necessary to undertake a further surgical drainage procedure (see below). If there is malignant obstruction in the lower end of the bile duct, biliary bypass can be performed as appropriate. Cholecystjejunostomy is simple and is often preferred, although hepaticojejunostomy may be indicated if a low junction between cystic duct and common bile duct suggests that the cystic duct would soon be blocked by continued tumor growth. If the malignant obstruction is in the head of the pancreas, biliary bypass may be combined with gastrojejunostomy to bypass the duodenum (Sarr & Cameron 1982), as continuing tumor growth otherwise causes duodenal obstruction in some 10–20% of patients (La Ferla & Murray 1987). In some centers, these operations can now be undertaken laparoscopically, but it remains to be seen whether this is advantageous (O'Rourke & Nathanson 1994).

Radical resection of cancer of the head of the pancreas causing jaundice is possible in only a minority of cases and even in this group, long-term survival is rare (p. 1297). If the obstruction is due to cancer at or within 1 cm of the papilla of Vater (periampullary cancer), lower end of bile duct or duodenum, every effort should be made to perform radical resection as these tumors have a lower potential for dissemination than carcinoma of the pancreas (p. 1301). If radical surgery is contemplated for any form of cancer blocking bile flow, preliminary percutaneous transhepatic biliary drainage was once used although it is now generally accepted that the approach failed to influence morbidity and mortality (McPherson et al 1984, Pitt et al 1985). Preoperative endoscopic stenting has also been employed but many surgeons now avoid preliminary biliary drainage and proceed to immediate resection in suitable patients (Lai et al 1992a) .

Proximal bile duct cancer poses considerable management problems (p. 1220). The lesion is rarely resectable and palliative drainage may necessitate an intrahepatic biliary anastomosis or insertion of a prosthesis.

Obstructive jaundice due to less common benign causes is treated according to the circumstances. For example. postcholecystectomy strictures of the bile duct may require hepaticojejunostomy using a Roux limb of jejunum to restore biliary–enteric continuity.

Jaundiced patients are often at high risk when subjected to major surgery. Pitt et al (1981) selected eight factors when assessing risk in patients undergoing cholecystectomy (Table 48.2). Patients with up to two positive factors had no operative mortality, whereas mortality rates rose to 67% in those with six factors and to 100% in those with seven or eight factors. In an analysis of patients undergoing major biliary surgery (i.e. excluding simple cholecystectomy with operative cholangiography), Blamey et al (1983) found that operative mortality was 2% in patients with a serum bilirubin of less than 50 μmol/L, as opposed to 24% in patients with higher serum bilirubin concentrations. Preoperative serum creatinine, serum albumin and serum bilirubin each had independent significance in predicting operative mortality in this study.

Preoperative preparation of jaundiced patients includes correction of anemia and, after measurement of prothrombin time, vitamin K is given (10 mg intravenously/day for 3 days before surgery). Malnutrition is difficult to correct in patients with cholestasis, but endoscopic sphincterotomy with or without stenting can be used in some high-risk patients to buy time with which to improve the general condition. Prophylactic antibiotics are now used routinely

**Table 48.2** Risk factors in biliary surgery (Pitt et al 1982)

| |
|---|
| Malignant obstruction |
| Age > 60 years |
| Albumin < 30g/L |
| Hematocrit < 30% |
| WBC > 10 000/mm$^3$ |
| Bilirubin > 10 mg/ 100 ml |
| Alkaline phosphatase > 100 u/L (normal 0–32) |
| Creatinine > 1.3 mg/100 ml |

in biliary surgery. Whereas a single intravenous dose of a cephalosporin at the time of induction is used to reduce the incidence of wound infection after cholecystectomy, most surgeons prescribe up to 5 days of antibiotics such as cefotaxime or gentamicin combined with ampicillin in high-risk patients with cholestasis and overt sepsis. Bacteria are present in the bile in over 80% of patients with choledocholithiasis and in 30–50% of those with malignant obstruction (Keighley 1982).

Postoperative oliguric renal failure occurs in up to 10% of patients with cholestasis. These patients are often dehydrated and there is evidence that systemic endotoxinemia results from a combination of increased absorption of endotoxin into the portal venous blood and its reduced clearance by the hepatic reticuloendothelial system (Pain & Bailey 1986). It is vital to restore adequate hydration before operation, to monitor hourly urine output during and after surgery and to use a diuretic such as mannitol or frusemide only if hourly output falls in the face of adequate volume replacement.

### Nonsurgical treatment of cholestasis

Endoscopic sphincterotomy (p. 118) now permits clearance of stones from the common bile duct in over 80% of patients, for a complication rate of about 10% and mortality rate of around 1.5% (Cotton 1984, Escourrou et al 1984). The technique is established for the management of retained or recurrent stones after cholecystectomy and is a valuable alternative to surgery in elderly high-risk patients with choledocholithiasis in whom the gallbladder can be left in situ.

Similarly, in patients with malignant biliary obstruction, insertion of an endoprosthesis (p. 119) relieves jaundice with results that are at least as good as those achieved by palliative surgery (Bornman et al 1986). Whereas such prostheses were at one time inserted transhepatically, endoscopic sphincterotomy now allows internal drainage using stents inserted by a transampullary approach (Smith et al 1994).

## GALLSTONE DISEASE

Gallstones are by far the commonest disorder of the biliary system. The metabolic changes which lead to the formation of gallstones, especially cholesterol gallstones, have become much clearer. Important advances have been made in the diagnosis of gallstones by ultrasonography and ERCP. Although the dissolution of gallbladder stones is feasible and nonsurgical methods of treatment are now available, the development of laparoscopic cholecystectomy has restored the role of surgical management (Paterson-Brown et al 1991).

### Composition of gallstones

Gallstones have usually been designated as cholesterol stones, mixed stones or pigment stones (Neoptolemos et al 1986). However, chemical analysis shows a continuous spectrum of stone composition rather than three mutually exclusive stone types. Pure cholesterol and pure pigment stones account for only 20% of gallstones Mixed stones can be considered as variants of cholesterol stones, as they usually contain over 50% cholesterol and account for about 80% of gallstones in Western countries. Ten to 20% of gallstones contain enough calcium to be radio-opaque.

### Gallbladder stones

*Epidemiology*

***Cholesterol gallstones*** (Kaye & Kern 1971, Heaton 1973). The prevalence of gallstones varies considerably from country to country; they are common in Europe, North America and Australasia and rare in Africa and among Eskimos. The extraordinarily high prevalence in American Pima Indians points to the importance of genetic factors. The incidence of gallstones may be increasing. The most striking evidence comes from Japan, whereas evidence in other countries rests principally on increasing cholecystectomy rates, statistics which are difficult to interpret. Increasing cholecystectomy rates in younger people do, however, suggest a real increase.

The predisposing factors have been reviewed by Bennion & Grundy (1978). The two most important determinants of gallstone frequency in any population are age and sex (Fig. 48.7); gallstones become more common with increasing age and are always 2–3 times more common in women. The increased frequency in women becomes manifest at puberty (Fig. 48.8). An increased risk of gallstones is conferred by parity, especially in those under the age of 29, and by oral contraceptives in a susceptible group of young women (Scragg et al 1984a). Obesity is also associated with an increased frequency of

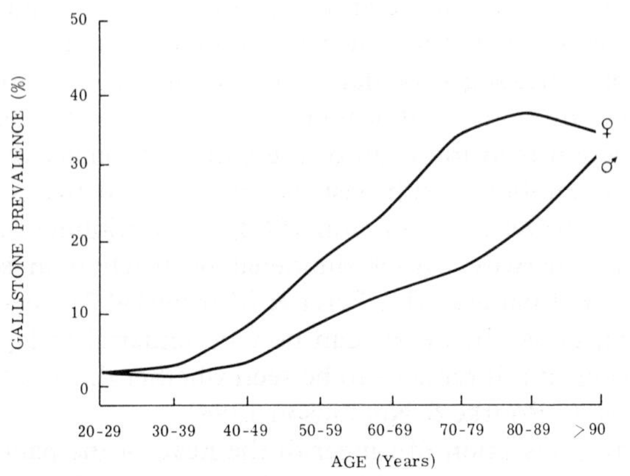


**Fig. 48.7** Autopsy prevalence of gallstones in Oslo showing the steady rise in frequency with increasing age and the approximately twofold incidence in females compared to males (Torvik & Hoivik 1960).

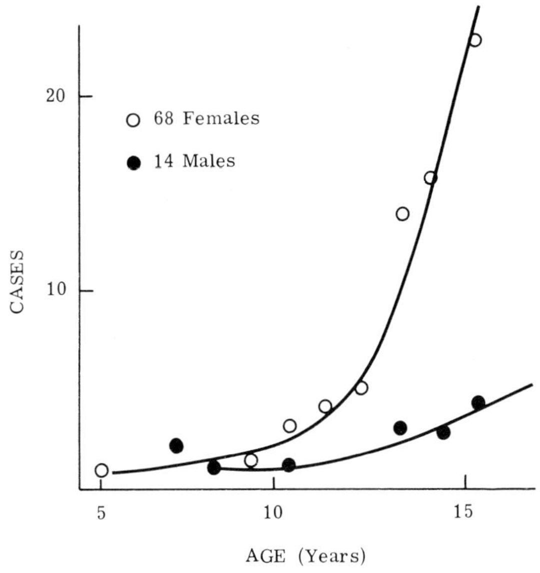


**Fig. 48.8** Cholelithiasis in children in a Swedish community hospital. Note the increase in females at puberty (Nilsson 1966).

gallstones. The precise dietary factors responsible are debatable but may include an increase in animal fat, a decrease in fiber and an increase in total energy intake. Differences related to social class are only found if differences in living standards are marked and they are most likely due to diet. Alcohol appears to be protective (Scragg et al 1984b). The frequency of gallstones is also increased in patients with ileal disease or resection, cirrhosis, cystic fibrosis (p. 1238), diabetes mellitus and in those taking clofibrate or receiving long-term parenteral nutrition (Roslyn et al 1983). Gallstones are found in most patients with gallbladder cancer and in up to 50% of those with acute pancreatitis (p. 1248).

***Pigment stones.*** Much less is known about the epidemiology and cause of bilirubin stones. Black and brown pigment stones arise when excess unconjugated bilirubin leads to precipitation of calcium bilirubinate. The pigment in black pigment stones is a highly crosslinked network polymer; there is considerably less crosslinkage in brown pigment stones (and in the so-called "salt and pepper" pigment stones found in Japan) and this may render them more amenable to dissolution therapy. All forms of stones are especially common in the Far East and they become more frequent with increasing age. Unlike cholesterol stones, pigment stones occur with equal frequency in men and women. They occur particularly in hemolytic anemia, cirrhosis (p. 921), infection of bile with β-glucuronidase-producing bacteria such as *E. coli* and *Bacteroides* spp. and also in primary shunt hyperbilirubinemia (p. 930). However, they often occur in the absence of any known predisposing factor (Soloway et al 1977). The uncommon so-called "primary bile duct stone" is usually also composed mainly of calcium bilirubin.

*Formation*

***Bile.*** Major advances have been made in elucidating the metabolic mechanisms responsible for the formation of cholesterol gallstones (Bennion & Grundy 1978, Smith & LaMont 1986). The three major lipids of bile are the conjugated bile acids, phospholipids (predominantly lecithin) and cholesterol. The bile acid conjugates have detergent-like properties and form micelles in aqueous solution (p. 352). In bile the lecithin is incorporated into bile acid/lecithin mixed micelles and these also incorporate cholesterol, thereby promoting its solubility in the aqueous environment of bile. The capacity of the micellar cholesterol solubilizing system may under certain circumstances be exceeded and the bile is then in a state of cholesterol supersaturation. When this happens the bile is no longer a single-phase system. Dynamic light-scattering experiments have shown that supersaturated human bile is a two-phase system consisting of both cholesterol-containing mixed micelles and cholesterol-containing unilamellar vesicles (radii 400 nm) (Somjen & Gilat 1985). When the concentrations of biliary conjugated bile acids are low, such as in fasting bile secreted by the liver, the cholesterol is solubilized mainly in vesicles and in unsaturated fasting gallbladder bile, micellar solubilization predominates.

Failure of these cholesterol solubilization mechanisms may produce conditions which initiate the nidation of cholesterol microcrystals. These form the basis for the laying down of further cholesterol to form cholesterol gallstones. Gallbladder bile from patients with gallstones has a shorter in vitro cholesterol microcrystal nucleation time than gallbladder bile from control subjects, even when their lipid compositions are similar (Holan et al 1979). This forms the basis for the proposal that both pronucleation and antinucleation factors are present in bile, potential candidates for these being biliary proteins and microproteins respectively (Burnstein et al 1983, Holzbach et al 1984).

Cholesterol gallstones also contain insoluble salts of calcium and this has led to the suggestion that calcium, and possibly other cations, are potential nucleating factors (Williamson & Percy-Robb 1980). A calcium bilirubinate nidus is present at the center of many cholesterol gallstones. However, the mean ionized calcium concentration in bile from patients with gallstones and in controls appears to be similar (Gollish et al 1983) and removal of ionized calcium from supersaturated bile by addition of EDTA has no measurable effect on the rate at which cholesterol microcrystals are produced (Gallinger et al 1986).

Several factors may lead to the production of supersaturated bile and predispose to gallstone formation (LaMorte et al 1979). Some patients secrete large amounts of cholesterol and the bile becomes supersaturated in spite of a normal or even an increased bile acid pool. This occurs in obesity, during rapid weight loss and in patients taking clofibrate. It also occurs in patients taking estrogens and progestogens and may account for the increased frequency of gallstones in women, especially those taking higher dose oral contraceptives and during pregnancy (Pertsemlidis et al 1974). Other patients develop supersaturated bile because of diminished bile acid secretion. This occurs when the ileum is diseased (e.g. Crohn's disease), removed or bypassed or when malabsorption, as in cystic fibrosis (p. 1238), leads to increased loss of bile acid which cannot be compensated for by increased bile acid synthesis. Nonobese patients with gallstones may have a small bile acid pool and a low bile acid secretion rate due to failure to compensate for normal fecal bile acid losses. In American Indians, who have a very high incidence of gallstones, this and a high cholesterol secretion rate may occur. Patients with recurrent cholestasis of pregnancy (p. 1091) have a high incidence of gallstones for unknown reasons.

***Biliary tract.*** Biliary stasis was long regarded as important in the formation of gallstones until attention focused on chemical changes in the bile. However, as such changes have not wholly explained gallstone formation, interest in the biliary tract has reawakened (LaMorte et al 1979). Mechanical biliary obstruction is not important in gallstone formation other than in so-called "primary bile duct stones" (p. 1208), but more subtle aspects of gallbladder and choledochal sphincter function (p. 1197) could be important. The integrated actions of the gallbladder and choledochal sphincter determine the partition of hepatic bile between the gallbladder and the duodenum during fasting and the frequency and vigor of gallbladder contraction largely determines how much bile acid passes around the enterohepatic circulation (Schersten 1973). These factors determine the amount of bile acid reaching the liver and re-entering the bile, which in turn helps to determine the capacity of the bile to solubilize cholesterol. Diminished gallbladder function, as in certain phases of the menstrual cycle, pregnancy and diabetes (Stone et al 1988), after vagotomy and when the diet is rich in refined carbohydrate and poor in fat or when prolonged parenteral nutrition is used, could reduce the cycling of the bile acid pool and contribute to the production of supersaturated bile.

***Bilirubin.*** (Soloway et al 1977, Neoptolemos et al 1986). Pigment stones account for about 40% of stones in the Far East but for only 5–10% in the West. Important factors in their production include hemolysis, with increased amounts of bilirubin in the bile, and the ability to deconjugate bilirubin leading to the production of insoluble unconjugated bilirubin which then precipitates as calcium bilirubinate. Infection is important in the deconjugation of bilirubin and organisms such as *E. coli* contain abundant β-glucuronidase. Other sources of β-glucuronidase may also be present (Boonyapisit et al 1978). Conjugated bilirubin may also be formed by spontaneous hydrolysis and isomerization of bilirubin monoglucuronide in alkaline bile (Spivak et al 1984). Suture material has been identified in almost one-third of patients with ductal stones after cholecystectomy and may be an important nidus for stone formation (Wosiewitz et al 1983).

### *Dissolution*

As most gallstones seem to develop in bile supersaturated with cholesterol, bile acids have been given orally to increase bile acid concentrations so that cholesterol gallstones dissolve (Thistle & Schoenfield 1971, Iser et al 1975, Gerolami et al 1977, Watts et al 1982). Only patients with cholesterol gallstones in a functioning gallbladder are potentially suitable for treatment. While such stones appear radiolucent on oral cholecystography, not all radiolucent stones are cholesterol rich. Smaller stones dissolve more rapidly and, while size is not an absolute contraindication, stones larger than 15 mm in diameter dissolve at best so slowly that dissolution therapy is inadvisable. Gallstone dissolution has only a limited place in management and Watts et al (1982) considered that only some 10% of their gallstone patients would be suitable for such therapy. Dissolution may prove useful in the elderly and patients who are poor surgical risks. If used in women of childbearing age, contraception is mandatory as the teratogenic potential of these drugs is unknown. Dissolution therapy is contraindicated in liver disease and in patients with severe or recurrent biliary colic (p. 1206).

Chenodeoxycholic acid (CDCA) has been used most extensively for the dissolution of gallstones. Complete dissolution rates of 14–38% have been reported following treatment for 6 months to 2 years (Watts et al 1982). The usual dose is 13–15 mg/kg per day but obese patients may require up to 20 mg/kg per day. Cholecystography is performed every 3–6 months to ensure that the stones are decreasing in size. However, small gallstones (under 5 mm) may be undetectable at oral cholecystography and ultrasound scanning has been recommended for follow-up (Shapero et al 1982). CDCA may cause diarrhea which is dose related and usually remits spontaneously. It may be necessary to decrease the dose transiently or add an antidiarrheal agent. Increased serum transaminase activity may occur, but liver biopsies have not shown evidence of significant liver damage. Ursodeoxycholic acid (8–10 mg/kg per day) can be used in the same way as CDCA but with less risk of causing diarrhea (Tokyo Co-operative Society Gallstone Study Group 1980).

Gallstones often recur when dissolution therapy is stopped and recurrence rates of 20–30% within a short period have been recorded (Watts et al 1982). O'Donnell & Heaton (1988) found that recurrence rates increase rapidly in the first few years with rates of 13% at 1 year, 31% at 3 years, 43% at 4 years and 49% at 11 years. Recurrent stones were readily redissolved, but generally recurred again when therapy ceased.

*Asymptomatic gallstones*

There has been debate regarding the need for surgery in patients with asymptomatic gallstones. However, only 10% of the asymptomatic patients followed for a mean of almost 5 years by McSherry et al (1985) developed symptoms and only 7% required operation. While gallstones are undoubtedly associated with an increased risk of gallbladder cancer, only one of 691 gallstone patients followed by McSherry et al (1985) was found eventually to have an incidental carcinoma at operation. Thus patients with asymptomatic gallstones can be followed with reasonable safety without surgery or attempts at dissolution therapy. An exception may be made for diabetics with cholelithiasis, given their increased mortality from acute cholecystitis.

*Complications of gallstones*

Gallstones can cause biliary colic, acute cholecystitis, chronic cholecystitis, biliary obstruction (p. 1197) and cholangitis. They are associated with acute pancreatitis (p. 1248) and carcinoma of the gallbladder (p. 1218) and can fistulate into the gastrointestinal tract (p. 1217), leading to gallstone ileus (p. 1217).

## Biliary colic and chronic cholecystitis

*Pathology*

The condition is due to stones in the gallbladder. There is a poor correlation between the pathological findings in the gallbladder wall and the clinical features. Calculi in the gallbladder may cause only minimal histological abnormality but are often associated with a constellation of changes known together as chronic cholecystitis. In chronic cholecystitis the gallbladder wall is thickened and the organ may be contracted. The mucosa loses its fine honeycomb pattern, becomes flattened and may ulcerate. On microscopy there is fibrosis and a variable chronic inflammatory cell infiltration. The reactive and hyperplastic mucosal changes are sometimes difficult to distinguish from low-grade neoplasm. If lymphocytic infiltration is marked and aggregated, the term "follicular cholecystitis" is applied. Rokitansky–Aschoff sinuses (mucosal diverticula) are usually present. These extend into or through the muscle coat, which may be hypertrophied. When numerous diverticula are present it may be termed "cholecystitis glandularis". By contrast, a focal collection of diverticula with smooth muscle hyperplasia is termed an "adenomyoma" (p. 1211; Fig. 1.22). These are most common at the fundus but may occur elsewhere. Xanthogranulomatous cholecystitis (Goodman & Ishak 1981) is characterized by the development of a soft yellow tumorlike mass of foamy histocytes in the gallbladder wall, probably as a result of breakdown of a Rokitansky–Aschoff sinus with local extravasation of bile. Extensive calcification of the wall, usually associated with outlet obstruction due to calculus, gives rise to so-called "porcelain gallbladder".

*Clinical features*

Biliary colic is the most important symptom and its principal characteristics are that it has sudden onset, rises quickly to a peak, is not colicky (despite its name) and is felt in the upper abdomen. The first attack often occurs a few hours after the main meal and so frequently occurs at night in Western countries. Biliary colic is experienced typically in the epigastrium and along the right costal margin. It commonly radiates to the right subscapular region and only rarely moves to the left costal margin. Retrosternal pain of sudden and dramatic onset may be mistaken for myocardial infarction. When pain is felt only in these less common sites, gallstones may not be suspected and ultrasound examination or cholecystogram may be omitted from the investigation.

Patients with gallstones frequently complain of nonspecific symptoms such as flatulence, fullness and dyspepsia after fatty food. However, these symptoms are as common in patients with a normal cholecystogram and should not be attributed to gallstones. Furthermore, patients commonly find that these symptoms are not relieved by cholecystectomy (Table 48.3).

*Investigations*

***Oral cholecystography*** (p. 19) is a simple, safe and effective means of diagnosing gallbladder stones (Figs. 1.20, 1.21 & 2.1A) but false negative rates for small gallstones of 6–8% are reported (Berk et al 1982). If the gallbladder fails to opacify on cholecystography (nonfunctioning gallbladder), gallbladder disease with cystic duct obstruction is highly likely. Despite its accuracy, cholecystography has now been essentially superseded by ultrasound scanning in the detection of gallstones.

**Table 48.3** Pattern of symptoms recorded by patients with gallstones before and after cholecystectomy and by age- and sex-matched control surgical patients without gallstone disease (Bates et al 1991)

| | Controls | Gallstone patients Preop | | |
|---|---|---|---|---|
| | | | 1 yr postop | 2 yr postop |
| | $n = 278$ % | $n = 218$ % | $n = 278$ % | $n = 274$ % |
| Flatulence | 30 | 66 | 44 | 42 |
| Distention | 33 | 57 | 37 | 40 |
| Indigestion | 38 | 71 | 43 | 42 |
| Nausea | 15 | 62 | 23 | 19 |
| Vomiting | 10 | 54 | 9 | 10 |
| Fever | 4 | 34 | 5 | 4 |
| Rigor | 4 | 30 | 5 | 2 |
| Abdominal pain | 0 | 100 | 34 | 27 |
| Consulted GP for pain | 0 | 100 | 23 | 18 |

***Ultrasound scanning of the gallbladder*** (p. 49) is even more sensitive than oral cholecystography, particularly in the case of small gallstones which are sometimes obscured by contrast material in cholecystography. Gallstones as small as 1–3 mm can be identified with real-time ultrasonography (Cooperberg & Burhenne 1980). Additional advantages include ease of performance, avoidance of irradiation and potentially toxic contrast media (making it the method of choice in pregnancy) and the demonstration of other structures in the upper abdomen.

Gallstones on ultrasound scanning appear typically as mobile, echogenic foci with posterior acoustic shadowing (Figs 2.1 & 2.2). Small calculi do not always produce acoustic shadowing but their intraluminal position and mobility are usually enough to provide the diagnosis. If the gallbladder cannot be identified, the presence of an echogenic focus in the gallbladder area is nearly as specific a finding as that of calculi in a distended gallbladder (Durrell et al 1984). With high-quality ultrasound scanning, gallstones should be detected in at least 95% of cases studied and ultrasonography is the first investigation indicated when gallbladder disease is suspected. If the examination demonstrates gallstones unequivocally, oral cholecystography is unnecessary. When doubt persists or technical artefacts pose problems, repeat ultrasound scanning or oral cholecystography can be performed.

### *Treatment*

Relief of pain is the immediate objective. Severe pain may be relieved by morphine (15–20 mg intramuscularly) and nausea due to morphine can be minimized by cyclizine (50 mg intramuscularly). Morphine occasionally appears to aggravate symptoms and less severe pain can be relieved by pethidine (100–150 mg) or pentazocine (30 mg intramuscularly). It is equally important to ensure continued pain relief by further doses of analgesic at 2–4-hourly intervals until the attack resolves.

***Surgery.*** Patients who have biliary colic should be considered for cholecystectomy. The timing of surgery is not critical but in general, it should be undertaken at the earliest opportunity to avoid further attacks of biliary colic or cholecystitis. The operative mortality for elective cholecystectomy has fallen in recent years and many series have recorded operative mortality rates of less than 1% and in some cases no mortality at all (McSherry & Glenn 1980, Crumplin et al 1985, Clavien et al 1992, Herzog et al 1992). Mortality rates are approximately four times greater for elective cholecystectomy with choledocholithotomy than for elective cholecystectomy alone (Banting & Carter 1994).

The introduction and widespread adoption of laparoscopic cholecystectomy since 1987 has transformed the treatment of gallstones and alternative treatments such as dissolution therapy and lithotripsy are now rarely used. Laparoscopic cholecystectomy has an acceptably low mortality, a shorter hospital stay, a more rapid return to work or normal activity and a better cosmetic result than open operation. These benefits have had to be balanced against concerns that the risk of bile duct injury may be slightly higher than in open cholecystectomy (Cuschieri et al 1991, Paterson-Brown et al 1991, Southern Surgeons Club 1991).

The principles of cholecystectomy remain the same, irrespective of whether a laparoscopic or open technique is used. A thorough examination is made of the other abdominal viscera to exclude conditions which are frequent is patients with gallstones or which can produce similar symptoms (e.g. peptic ulcer, hiatus hernia). The anatomy in the region of the cystic duct and artery must be carefully defined before removing the gallbladder. The introduction of laparoscopic cholecystectomy has fueled the debate regarding the need for routine operative cholangiography to identify stones in the duct system, display the anatomy of the biliary tree and exclude pathology in and around the lower end of the common bile duct. Some surgeons have a selective policy and obtain cholangiograms only in patients already known to have ductal stones and those with obstructive jaundice, common bile duct dilatation and previous cholangitis or pancreatitis (Wilson 1986, Bogokowsky et al 1987, Garden 1991, Paterson-Brown et al 1994). Intraoperative ultrasonography can be employed as an alternative to cholangiography to detect common bile duct stones or select patients for operative cholangiography (Windsor & Garden 1993, Greig et al 1994).

***Nonsurgical treatment.*** Patients who are unfit for or who refuse surgery can he considered for dissolution therapy (p. 1204) or lithotripsy. Lithotripsy is an established treatment for renal stones and has been used for gallbladder stones (Sackmann et al 1988, 1990). It seems to be most successful for single radiolucent stones in a functioning gallbladder where adjuvant dissolution therapy can be given, but calcified stones can be treated with some success.

## Acute cholecystitis

### *Etiology*

The usual cause of acute cholecystitis is occlusion of the cystic duct or Hartmann's pouch by a gallstone. Rarely, a tumor of the bile duct or gallbladder occludes the cystic duct and presents as acute cholecystitis (Thorbjarnarson 1960). Acute acalculous cholecystitis is uncommon but may occur after major trauma, burns or operations (Williamson 1988) and can complicate hemolysis or serious illness in childhood, specific infections such as typhoid fever (p. 562) or brucellosis, acute pancreatitis or diabetes mellitus (Ham 1980). Bacterial infection is probably secondary in most cases (p. 1212). Cholecystitis may also occur in the toxic shock syndrome (Ishak & Rogers 1981).

### *Pathology*

In acute cholecystitis the gallbladder is tense, swollen, edematous and vascular and inflammation extends to the gastrohepatic omentum, involving the region of the common bile duct. The gallbladder wall is thickened and the mucosa is red or gray and may be ulcerated. Mural necrosis appears as areas of thinning and softening of the wall. On microscopy there is transmural edema, congestion, ulceration and a fibroblastic reaction. Lymphocytic infiltration tends to be concentrated in areas of ulceration or necrosis but is often not marked, perhaps because the inflammation is caused by the chemical contents of the gallbladder rather than by infection. Thrombosis of the veins may be present and arteritis is occasionally present as a manifestation of systemic vasculitis. Inflammation resolves spontaneously in about 85% of cases, but in the remainder it may progress to empyema, gangrene or perforation of the gallbladder, usually with the formation of a localized abscess. Free perforation with general biliary peritonitis is uncommon.

### *Clinical features*

The diagnosis of acute cholecystitis can be made on clinical grounds in at least 90% of cases. The illness begins with biliary colic, but the pain continues unabated for one or more days and is associated with variable nausea and vomiting. There is guarding and tenderness in the right upper quadrant of the abdomen and Murphy's sign is usually positive (p. 512). The patient develops pyrexia and sometimes a palpable and tender gallbladder. Mild jaundice is seen in about 15% of cases.

The local complications of empyema, gangrene and pericholecystic abscess can usually be diagnosed from the clinical course; the general condition of the patient deteriorates, pyrexia and tachycardia persist and there is progression of abdominal guarding, rigidity and tenderness. Empyema in the elderly may be particularly difficult to diagnose in that the patient is sometimes remarkably painfree and afebrile.

### *Investigations*

Most patients have a leukocytosis, bilirubinuria may be present and liver function tests may be abnormal. Ultrasound scanning should be used initially to evaluate patients with acute right upper abdominal pain. Gallstones may be detected and signs of acute cholecystitis which may be discerned include gallbladder distention and mural thickening, fluid collections, adjacent liver abscess, intraluminal debris causing nonshadowed echoes and focal tenderness over the gallbladder (Samuels et al 1985) (p. 50). Cholescintigraphy with $^{99m}$Tc-HIDA (p. 91) is claimed to be even more accurate than ultrasound in the diagnosis of acute cholecystitis but it is not employed routinely.

The pain of biliary colic or acute cholecystitis may be mistaken for myocardial infarction. Serum transaminase activities can increase in both diseases (p. 741), but only myocardial infarction produces diagnostic electrocardiographic changes and an increased serum creatinine phosphokinase activity.

### *Treatment*

Initially, the patient requires pain relief (p. 1206), intravenous fluid administration and nil by mouth. A broad-spectrum antibiotic should be given (p. 1212). A few patients with acute cholecystitis require urgent surgical treatment, notably those who develop signs of peritonitis due to abscess formation or perforation and those in whom acute abdominal surgical conditions such as a perforated peptic ulcer cannot be excluded. Patients in whom surgical treatment is contraindicated on medical grounds, usually on account of cardiopulmonary disease, should remain on conservative treatment unless the surgeon's hand is forced by complications such as perforation.

The major area of contention concerns the timing of surgery in patients with a certain diagnosis of uncomplicated acute cholecystitis. In the past, the acute attack was allowed to resolve and surgery was undertaken electively some 2–3 months later. However, there is increasing evidence that there are advantages in operating on such patients during the initial hospital admission. Surgery is not undertaken on an *emergency* basis, but rather as a semi-elective procedure after 2–3 days of medical treatment. The mortality and morbidity, the ease of the operation, the frequency with which the bile duct is explored and the need for cholecystostomy as opposed to cholecystectomy are similar whether the operation is performed during the acute attack or 2–3 months later (McArthur et al 1975, Van der Linden & Edlund 1981). However, the need to convert from laparoscopic to open cholecystectomy is greater in the acute situation than in elective cholecystectomy (Wilson et al 1991, Unger et al 1993). Deferred surgery has the added disadvantages that the number of days spent in hospital is significantly greater and there is the risk that the patient will develop further attacks of acute cholecystitis while awaiting readmission for cholecystectomy.

## Mucocele of the gallbladder

Cystic duct obstruction by a gallstone in Hartmann's

pouch may lead to distention of the gallbladder with mucus (mucocele). The distended gallbladder is not tender and may be felt as a mass in the right upper quadrant, sometimes extending into the right iliac fossa. It is readily confused with colonic carcinoma, hepatic tumors and cysts and omental masses. Plain abdominal X-ray films may show a large soft tissue mass in the right upper quadrant and ultrasound scanning can be diagnostic. Infection in the obstructed gallbladder leads to an empyema and sometimes to septicemia. This causes a severe systemic illness with marked abdominal pain and demands emergency cholecystectomy under antibiotic cover. In the event that cholecystectomy appears unduly hazardous, drainage of the gallbladder after removal of its contained stones (cholecystotomy) may be preferred.

## Emphysematous cholecystitis

Acute emphysematous cholecystitis is a rare condition caused by gas-forming bacteria which presents as a severe episode of acute cholecystitis (p. 1207). Most patients are male and many are diabetic. The patient's condition deteriorates rapidly and a plain abdominal radiograph (Fig. 48.9) shows gas in the gallbladder lumen or concentrically in the gallbladder wall (Blum & Stagg 1963). Treatment consists of immediate parenteral administration of antibiotics to combat aerobic and anaerobic organisms (p. 1212) and urgent cholecystectomy (Pyrtek & Bartus 1967).

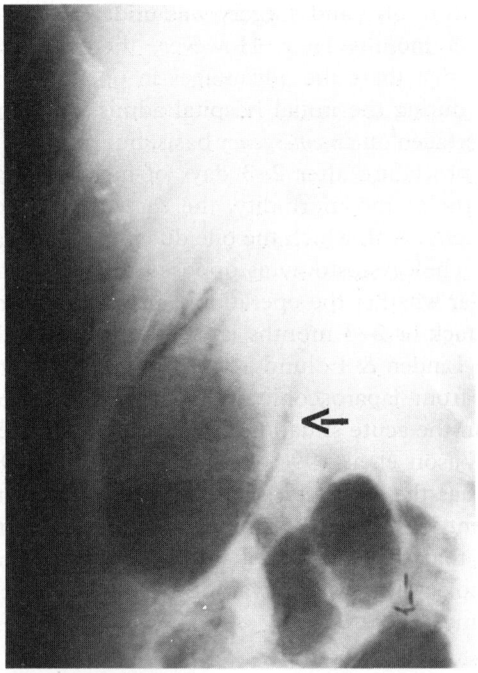

**Fig. 48.9** Plain radiograph of the gallbladder showing acute emphysematous cholecystitis. Note gas in wall of the gallbladder (arrow).

## Choledocholithiasis

*Incidence*

Bile duct stones are found in about 10% of patients with gallbladder stones and their incidence rises with age (Edholm & Jonsson 1962). The incidence of bile duct stones has been declining, probably because patients with gallbladder stones are being operated on sooner than in previous years. This trend may have been accelerated by the introduction of laparoscopic cholecystectomy (Cuschieri et al 1991, Petelin 1991, Southern Surgeons Club 1991, Pace et al 1992).

*Pathology*

The majority of bile duct stones are thought to migrate from the gallbladder into the bile duct, but they probably increase in size in the bile duct with time (Fig. 48.10). There is clinical and experimental evidence that gallstones may also form in the bile duct. Such primary gallstones are usually associated with partial bile duct obstruction and occur in association with iatrogenic biliary strictures or strictures associated with chronic pancreatitis. Occasionally, there is no biliary obstruction; some of these patients have a

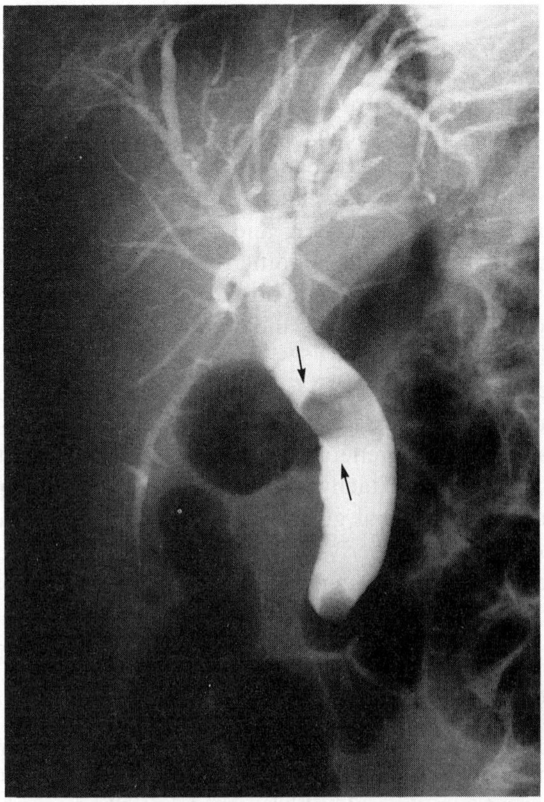

**Fig. 48.10** Cholangiogram showing a large "primary" bile duct stone (arrows). Note the ovoid shape of the stone, the dilated bile duct and the presence of at least one other smaller stone at the lower end of the common bile duct.

thickened bile duct which may impede bile flow, while others may secrete lithogenic bile. Primary bile duct stones are usually single and ovoid and conform to the bile duct in which they are formed. They can be distinguished from secondary stones at operation because they are soft and disintegrate easily.

Secondary pathological changes in the liver vary according to the time the stone(s) has been in the duct, the degree of obstruction and the amount of biliary tract infection that has resulted. Cholangitis may give rise to hepatic abscesses which are often multiple. Secondary biliary cirrhosis may develop but is rare (p. 942).

*Clinical features*

Bile duct stones may give rise to episodes of obstructive jaundice or pancreatitis (p. 1252), cause recurrent symptoms after cholecystectomy (p. 1210) or be discovered at the time of cholecystectomy in patients who have no history of jaundice. The classic Charcot's triad of symptoms produced by bile duct stones consists of pain, obstructive jaundice and fever (with or without rigors) and reflects the development of acute cholangitis. The pain is often identical to that of biliary colic and acute cholecystitis, but may be absent. Jaundice is obstructive with a dark urine and pale stool and be associated with pruritus. It is not usually deep and is characteristically fluctuant, but may occasionally be absent, static or even progressive. Painless jaundice occurs in a few cases.

Acute cholangitis is occasionally associated with rapid development of septicemic shock, a syndrome that has been named acute obstructive suppurative cholangitis (Dow & Lindernauer 1969, Glenn & Moody 1961). Prompt resuscitation (p. 515) and urgent surgical or endoscopic decompression of the bile duct are mandatory.

*Investigations*

Ultrasound scanning is the best screening method with which to detect gallstones and biliary dilatation. However, it often fails to detect stones in the bile ducts and imaging methods such as ERCP should be employed if ultrasonography is negative or equivocal (Einstein et al 1984).

*Treatment*

Endoscopic retrograde cholangiopancreatography (ERCP) is widely accepted as a safe and effective method of evaluating and treating biliary tract disorders and endoscopic treatment of choledocholithiasis has gained similar acceptance. There is general agreement that endoscopic removal of bile duct stones is preferable to surgery in postcholecystectomy patients, high-risk surgical patients when the gallbladder is still present, patients with severe acute cholangitis and selected patients with acute biliary pancreatitis (Varia et al 1982, Cotton 1984, Leese et al 1985). Duct clearance can be expected in 90–95% of patients undergoing successful sphincterotomy and this results in an overall success rate for endoscopic stone clearance of 80–95%, the highest success rates being recorded as experience increases (Varia et al 1982, Leese et al 1985, Lambert et al 1991). Major complications occur in up to 10% of patients and include hemorrhage, acute pancreatitis, cholangitis and retroduodenal perforation, but the overall procedure-related mortality is less than 1% (Varia et al 1982, Leese et al 1985, Lambert et al 1991). However, the 30-day mortality can reach 15%, reflecting the severity of the underlying illness.

Difficulties in removing common bile duct stones endoscopically may be due to unfavorable or abnormal anatomy such as periampullary diverticulum or prior surgery. Stones larger than 15 mm and those situated intrahepatically or proximal to a biliary stricture may be difficult to remove. Adjuvant techniques include mechanical lithotripsy, extracorporeal shockwave lithotripsy and chemical dissolution (Birkett 1992, Webber et al 1992, Shaw et al 1993). Although successful stone fragmentation has been reported in up to 80% of patients, the major drawback is the need for multiple treatment sessions and at least one subsequent ERCP to extract stone fragments. Chemical dissolution of biliary stones has reported success rates of only 26% (Palmer & Hofmann 1986, Neoptolemos et al 1990).

With the introduction of minimal access gallbladder surgery, the traditional surgical treatment of choledocholithiasis by common bile duct exploration and removal of stones has declined. Operative cholangiography (p. 24) is an invaluable aid to define the number and location of stones if exploration is contemplated, while further cholangiograms or choledochoscopy are useful to confirm duct clearance (Carroll et al 1992, Petelin 1994). Preoperative endoscopic sphincterotomy has been suggested as a means of avoiding choledocholithotomy at the time of cholecystectomy, but there is concern that this will result in a large number of unnecessary (and potentially hazardous) ERCP examinations (Paterson-Brown et al 1991). A randomized study had shown no significant differences between patients treated by preoperative sphincterotomy as opposed to open cholecystectomy alone (Neoptolemos et al 1987), but the precise role of ERCP in the era of laparoscopic cholecystectomy has yet to be determined. For surgeons attempting removal of common bile duct stones during laparoscopic surgery, a transcystic approach to the common bile duct is often preferred to supraduodenal choledochotomy (Petelin 1994). A T-tube is left in place for some 10 days to avoid leakage and allow postoperative cholangiography.

The ready availability of endoscopic sphincterotomy has undoubtedly simplified the management of retained biliary duct stones and has undermined the need for routine transduodenal sphincterotomy or choledochoduodenostomy to prevent this problem. Bile duct stones detected in the early postoperative period by T-tube cholangiography which are less than 10 mm in diameter may pass spontaneously or can sometimes be flushed through, with or without the use of glucagon to relax the sphincter of Oddi (Tritapepe et al 1988). If endoscopic extracton is needed it has a success rate of 90% and a morbidity rate of less than 7% (Burhenne 1980, O'Doherty et al 1986, Lambert et al 1988, Tritapepe et al 1988, Cotton 1990, Nussinson et al 1991). Other techniques are also available to avoid the morbidity and mortality of further surgical bile duct exploration; these include T-tube infusion of cholesterol solvents (Palmer & Hofmann 1986), T-tube track choledochoscopy and lithotripsy (Josephs & Birkett 1992) and percutaneous extraction of stones through a mature T-tube track. This last technique (p. 38) involves a delay of some 5 weeks to allow the T-tube track to mature, but succeeds in 77–96% of cases (Burhenne 1980, Tritapepe et al 1988, Cotton 1990, Nussinson et al 1991). However, the small but significant risk of sepsis, biliary trauma and biliary leakage has led many centers to employ early endoscopic sphincterotomy to extract retained stones.

*Results of surgery*

As indicated earlier, choledocholithotomy carries a higher mortality than cholecystectomy alone and the risk is highest in those who are over 60, jaundiced or suffering from cardiorespiratory disease (Banting & Carter 1994). Overlooked or recurrent bile duct stones are the most important cause of persistent or recurrent symptoms after bile duct surgery, but the use of choledochoscopy can reduce the incidence of retained stones. It remains to be seen whether laparoscopic cholecystectomy plus ERCP or laparoscopic exploration of the common bile duct will be able to match the results of open exploration of the common bile duct.

## Postcholecystectomy syndrome, acalculous and functional biliary pain

The term "postcholecystectomy" syndrome has been used to describe residual or recurrent pain or discomfort in the upper abdomen, often indistinguishable from biliary colic, after cholecystectomy. Symptoms occur in 30% of patients, but in only 2–5% are they severe or disabling (Kune & Sali 1981). The cause of the syndrome does not always lie in the biliary tract. Extrabiliary causes include reflux esophagitis, peptic ulceration, chronic pancreatitis, irritable colon and functional pain. The most important biliary causes are overlooked or retained common duct stones, bile stricture and retained gallbladder. Considerable doubt surrounds the significance of a long cystic duct remnant, papillary stenosis, adhesions and painful wound neuromas (Hopkins et al 1979, Moody et al 1983). It is recognized that pain typical of organic biliary disease can arise in the absence of demonstrable biliary calculi. Such patients were often diagnosed as suffering from chronic acalculous cholecystitis and some had fibrotic thickening of the gallbladder, mucosal hypertrophy and Rokitansky–Aschoff sinuses, but the role of these in producing biliary pain remains uncertain.

The mechanism of this pain is poorly understood, but there is increasing evidence that some patients have abnormal motility of the gallbladder and the sphincter of Oddi. The sphincter is not exempt from dysmotility or other functional disorders and a proportion of patients with post-cholecystectomy syndrome fall into this category. It is not uncommon for two or more functional syndromes to coexist in the same individual (p. 1349) and indeed a history of irritable bowel syndrome is often found in patients with post-cholecystectomy syndrome. Altered bowel motility, autonomic dysfunction, particularly sympathetic activation, enhanced visceral nociception together with neuroticism and abnormal illness behavior are present in patients with biliary pain after cholecystectomy. Many patients develop abdominal pain in response to morphine (Roberts-Thomson et al 1990) or CCK-8 (Roberts-Thomson et al 1992). CCK injection or infusion has been used to provoke pain and select patients who may benefit from cholecystectomy (Lennard et al 1984). The test has been refined by combining CCK administration with cholescintigraphy or cholecystography (Griffen et al 1980) but many remain sceptical of its clinical value (Sunderland & Carter 1988).

Abnormalities of sphincter of Oddi motility occur in over 50% of patients. Under normal circumstances, sphincter motility is characterized by phasic contractions superimposed on a basal pressure of about 15 mmHg (p. 120). In patients with biliary pain after cholecystectomy motility abnormalities have been categorized into: (i) dyskinesia, defined as an excess of retrograde contractions, a high frequency of phasic contractions and/or absence of inhibition of phasic contractions when cholecystokinin is given; (ii) high basal pressure (>40 mm Hg) (Roberts-Thomson et al 1989). Theoretically, these abnormalities could result in impaired flow of bile through the sphincter leading to a rise in plasma AST which occurs in about 30% of patients after the administration of morphine.

*Treatment*

Treatment depends on discovering a cause for the cholecystectomy syndrome. The details of the previous cholecystectomy and cholangiograms should be reviewed. ERCP is the investigation of choice (Blumgart 1978). It can detect small overlooked stones and minimal strictures, discriminate between intrahepatic and extrahepatic causes of biliary obstruction and detect pancreatitis (Ruddell et al 1980).

It is difficult to identify objective criteria on which cholecystectomy can be recommended to patients with acalculous biliary type pain. The advent of laparoscopic cholecystectomy should not lead to any relaxation in the indications for cholecystectomy. Only half these patients will benefit from cholecystectomy and the patient must understand that cholecystectomy does not guarantee cure. However, some patients prove to have small biliary calculi which have escaped radiological detection and laparoscopic ultrasonography has been helpful in evaluating the gallbladder during laparotomy for the assessment of abdominal pain (Greig et al 1994a). As experience with ERCP and manometry increases, it may become possible to define with more certainty post-cholecystectomy patients such as those described by Geenen et al (1984a) in whom symptoms can be relieved by endoscopic sphincterotomy without recourse to cholecystectomy. These patients had bile duct dilatation and/or changes in liver enzymes after spontaneous episodes of pain. They underwent sphincterotomy or a sham procedure; 68% with sphincterotomy improved compared to 30% with the sham procedure. Improvement was more frequent in those with a basal pressure >30 mmHg.

If surgical options are rejected, principles of management of functional disorders should be adopted (p. 1360). Further or repeated investigations should be avoided unless new symptoms arise. Frequent explanation and reassurance is given. Some patients may be helped by tricyclic antidepressant drugs, others by sublingual nitrates or calcium channel blocking drugs, but in general medical treatment is disappointing. Some patients can be improved by withdrawal of alcohol, chocolate, fatty foods and analgesics which contain codeine (Toouli & Roberts-Thomson 1987).

## Miscellaneous benign diseases of the gallbladder

*Benign tumors*

Benign biliary tumors are rare (Hossack & Herron 1972). In a series of 180 cases of benign tumors and pseudotumors of the gallbladder, Christensen & Ishak (1970) classified the lesions as polyps (three inflammatory and 21 cholesterol polyps), hyperplasias (18 adenomatous and 73 adenomyomatous), adenomas (22 papillary and 29 nonpapillary), two granular cell tumors, seven gastric heterotopias, seven fibroxanthogranulomatous inflammation, two parasitic inflammation and one traumatic neuroma with suture granuloma.

In general, these conditions are asymptomatic and found coincidentally on ultrasonography or cholecystography. Rarely, they cause abdominal pain due to acute cholecystitis (p. 1206) or pancreatitis from passage of fragments down the biliary tree. On ultrasound scanning, benign biliary tumors are immobile and create echogenic nonshadowing foci in the lumen or attached to the gallbladder wall. They cause filling defects in the gallbladder or the bile ducts on cholecystography or cholangiography.

*Adenomyoma*

The cause of this condition is unknown. It may be diffuse (adenomyomatosis), segmental or localized (Jutras & Jutras 1966). The localized form is almost always found as a nodule measuring up to 12 mm in the fundus of the gallbladder. It may be sessile with a papillary structure, nodular or polypoid with tubular acini lined with epithelium in a stroma of connective tissue and smooth muscle. Gallstones are frequently present and variable epithelial atypia amounts in some instances to carcinoma in situ. On ultrasound scanning, diverticula are seen as small, rounded cystic spaces in the thickened wall and in those with calculi or thickened mucosal projections, the changes are demonstrated by echogenic foci within the lumen or wall, with or without shadowing. On cholecystography, localized fundal lesions are usually best seen after the gallbladder has contracted; annular disease may show as a constricting band dividing the gallbladder and adenomyomatosis or localized disease may produce a corona of contrast material around the gallbladder caused by filling of the Rokitansky–Aschoff sinuses in the lesion (see Fig. 1.22).

It is uncertain whether adenomyomas cause symptoms. However, if a patient continues to have troublesome symptoms compatible with a biliary origin and no other functional or organic alimentary disease is found, cholecystectomy is reasonable. If calculi are present, the decision to proceed to cholecystectomy is more straightforward.

*Cholesterolosis*

Cholesterolosis is a condition in which collections of foamy macrophages in the subepithelial connective tissue of the gallbladder produce yellow streaks on the mucosal folds (strawberry gallbladder). These macrophage collections may become large enough to form polyps. On ultrasonography, polypoid cholesterolosis gives rise to echogenic single or multiple non-shadowing masses fixed to the gallbladder wall which are indistinguishable from polyps and adenomatous tumors. The extent of cholesterolosis varies and it is found in about a fifth of gallbladders removed, irrespective of the presence of gallstones. It is debatable whether cholesterolosis produces symptoms; its management is similar to that of adenomyomatosis.

*Hyperplasia*

Hyperplasia of the gallbladder mucosa may be focal (Sato et al 1985) or widespread and often occurs in association with calculi. Atypia is usually mild but can be difficult to distinguish histologically from adenomyoma or carcinoma in situ.

*Torsion of the gallbladder*

Rarely, the gallbladder has a mesentery which attaches it

to the undersurface of the liver and which may allow torsion to occur (Carter et al 1963, Greenwood 1963, Ashby 1965). The patient usually presents with acute abdominal pain resembling acute cholecystitis, but the progression of symptoms and signs of peritonitis herald the development of necrosis and gangrene. Sometimes, the dilated gallbladder may be felt in an unusual position, such as right iliac fossa, owing to its abnormal mobility.

## BILIARY INFECTION

Biliary tract infection is unusual in the absence of preexisting biliary disease. The only common exception is the primary recurrent pyogenic cholangitis seen in the Orient.

### Bacteriology

Bacteria are not usually found in bile from normal gallbladders unless sophisticated culture methods are used. The frequency with which they are isolated in biliary tract disease is related to the nature of the disease, its site and its duration (Kune & Schutz 1974, Nielsen & Justesen 1976, Dye et al 1978). In gallstone disease, the frequency is low in patients who have a functioning gallbladder and no cystic duct obstruction, high in those with a nonfunctioning gallbladder and highest when gallstones have entered the common bile duct (Table 48.4). Bacteria are cultured more often in elderly patients. In acute cholecystitis, the frequency of positive cultures is low initially but increases sharply after 48 h (Kune & Birks 1970).

The frequency with which bacteria can be isolated from the common bile duct is also related to the cause of the obstruction. Most patients with bile duct obstruction due to stones or benign strictures give positive cultures, while in malignant obstruction less than half of the patients have a positive culture (Keighley 1982).

Organisms isolated from bile are almost always enterobacteria. *E. coli* accounts for up to 50% of isolates and is frequently the only organism found. Numerous other Gram-negative organisms such as *Klebsiella*, *Proteus* and *Pseudomonas* can be found, but they are seldom the sole organism isolated (Dye et al 1978). Mixed growth is obtained in up to one-third of cases. Gram-positive organisms (enterococci, streptococci, staphylococci and diphtheroids) and anaerobic organisms are less common, although the latter are important causes of emphysematous cholecystitis (p. 1208). Clostridia and streptococci are the commonest anaerobes, but bacteroides are rare.

**Table 48.4** Frequency of isolation of bacteria from gallbladder and common bile duct at laparotomy (Dye et al 1978)

| Extrahepatic bile ducts | Gallbladder Functioning | Gallbladder Obstructed | Bacterial isolates (%) GB | Bacterial isolates (%) CBD |
|---|---|---|---|---|
| Normal | Yes | No | 20 | * |
| Cholelithiasis | Yes | No | 30 | 14 |
| Cholelithiasis | No | Yes | 46 | 50 |
| Choledocholithiasis | – | – | 56 | 75 |

* No bacteria were found in the two subjects studied.
GB gallbladder; CBD common bile duct.

### Antibiotic therapy

Controlled studies of antibiotic prophylaxis in biliary surgery have consistently demonstrated a three-to-sixfold reduction in septic complications (Keighley et al 1975, Strachan et al 1977, Morran et al 1978). For routine elective biliary surgery, a single dose of a cephalosporin is given to reduce the incidence of wound infection (Keighley 1982). Local antibiotic sensitivities influence the choice of agent, but the antibiotic is given parenterally before operation so that high blood and tissue concentrations are achieved at the time of surgery. The intravenous route is more convenient. A single dose of prophylactic antibiotics should also be given immediately before interventional techniques such as percutaneous transhepatic cholangiography (p. 22), ERCP (p. 100) or T-tube cholangiography. In patients undergoing more complex biliary surgery, antibiotic resistance can be encountered and avoidance of serious sepsis due to *Streptococcus faecalis* requires the addition of ampicillin or the substitution of a ureidopenicillin such as piperacillin (Blenkharn & Blumgart 1985).

Patients who have jaundice or established infection should be treated over 5 days with gentamicin combined with ampicillin or a broad-spectrum agent such as cefotaxime or ciprofloxacin (Keighley 1982, Keighley et al 1984). Choledocholithiasis, increasing age (over 70 years), recent rigors, emergency operation, obesity, diabetes, concomitant alimentary procedures and previous biliary surgery all increase the risk of infection (Burke 1973, Kune & Burdon 1975, Keighley 1977).

*Acute cholecystitis*

Infection in acute cholecystitis usually results from obstruction of the gallbladder by a stone. It is debatable whether antibiotics affect complications such as empyema and gangrene, but they appear to prevent septicemia, particularly in patients who are especially liable to infection.

### Cholangitis

*Etiology*

Choledocholithiasis and/or benign biliary stricture are the usual predisposing factors in cholangitis. However, the increasing use of diagnostic and therapeutic PTC or ERCP has increased the incidence of cholangitis in patients with malignant obstruction.

*Pathology*

Clinical and experimental evidence indicates that small numbers of bacteria pass intermittently from the gastrointestinal tract via the portal vein to the liver, where most are destroyed by the reticuloendothelial system (Dineen 1964, Kune & Schutz 1974, Nolan 1978). A few return to the gut in the bile, but if there is partial biliary obstruction these organisms can proliferate. They may be present in high concentration without causing symptoms or they may precipitate cholangitis. Progression to cholangitis causes abdominal pain, biliary obstruction leads to jaundice and reflux of organisms into the systemic circulation causes the marked fever and rigors of septicemia. If treatment is witheld, Gram-negative septicemia and shock with renal failure supervene. Cholangitis can spread proximally into the liver and is now the most important single cause of liver abscess in Western countries (p. 817). Obstruction and recurrent cholangitis may lead eventually to biliary cirrhosis and portal hypertension and this is encountered occasionally in patients with neglected traumatic bile duct strictures (Sedgwick et al 1966).

There is debate about the relative importance of bile duct obstruction, foreign bodies and bacterial colonization in the development of cholangitis. Incomplete obstruction is more common than complete obstruction in this disease. Foreign bodies are essential to the pathogenesis and while bacteria are also essential, not all patients with bacteria in their bile develop cholangitis.

There is also debate regarding the mechanism of bacterial colonization of the bile in cholangitis. Potential mechanisms include duodenal reflux (Glenn & Moody 1961), portal bacteremia (Dineen 1964), instrumentation of the biliary tree (Lam et al 1978, Vennes et al 1984) and previous biliary surgery (Goldman et al 1983). Bile stasis secondary to an obstructed biliary-enteric anastomosis is a particular problem in postsurgical cholangitis; Roux-en-Y hepaticojejunostomy is the type of biliary enteric anastomosis with the lowest incidence of cholangitis.

Nonsuppurative (or "ascending") cholangitis due to partial obstruction of the biliary tree is the commonest type of cholangitis seen today. In contrast, suppurative cholangitis accounts for only 15% of cases and is associated with total or near-total obstruction and the rapid accumulation of inflammatory cells, mucus and bacteria contributes to the increase in pressure and the development of hepatic inflammation, septicemia and multiple organ failure.

*Clinical features*

The symptoms of abdominal pain and tenderness are similar to those found in acute cholecystitis but are often more severe. Charcot's triad is present in 90% of patients with suppurative cholangitis and in two-thirds of those with nonsuppurative cholangitis.

*Investigations*

Leukocytosis is usual and although liver function tests show deterioration with the onset of cholangitis, these tests do not discriminate between suppurative and nonsuppurative cholangitis. Deterioration in renal function is a poor prognostic sign. Blood culture may reveal bacteremia.

*Treatment*

The principles of treatment include resuscitation (p. 517), relief of pain (p. 1206), eradication of infection (p. 1212) and relief of biliary obstruction. The commonest cause of suppurative cholangitis is common bile duct obstruction by a stone leading to raised intrabiliary pressure and cholangiovenous reflux (Csendes et al 1988). Most patients respond rapidly to intravenous fluids and antibiotics and further treatment is then based on fitness for surgery. Poor-risk surgical patients should undergo endoscopic sphincterotomy and stone extraction, leaving the gallbladder in situ. Younger low-risk patients should undergo either endoscopic sphincterotomy followed by laparoscopic cholecystectomy or conventional or laparoscopic cholecystectomy with common bile duct exploration.

Urgent ERCP and sphincterotomy is the treatment of choice for patients with acute suppurative cholangitis in whom shock and mental confusion are additional features (Reynolds & Dargan 1959). Temporary percutaneous transhepatic decompression (Nakayama et al 1978) was once used to defer the need for surgery but has been largely superseded by endoscopic sphincterotomy and internal drainage (p. 119). Emergency surgery is reserved for those in whom endoscopic therapy fails, as it is associated with morbidity and a mortality of 10–50% depending upon the severity of illness and the presence of intercurrent disease (Boey & Way 1990). Biliary decompression by a nasobiliary tube or endoprosthesis can buy time if duct stones cannot be removed endoscopically and subsequent attempts at endoscopic stone removal can be performed safely on a semielective rather than emergency basis (Siegel 1981, Kill et al 1989).

In the first retrospective uncontrolled comparison of endoscopic and surgical biliary decompression, Leese and colleagues (1986) found that 30-day mortality was reduced from 21% in patients treated by surgery to 5% in patients managed by endoscopic sphincterotomy. Others have confirmed that mortality is lower in patients managed endoscopically (Leung et al 1989, Lai et al 1992a). In patients with cholangitis due to diseases other than gallstones, the same principles apply but removal of an obstructing foreign body (e.g. blocked stent) or relief of the biliary obstruction (e.g. revision of hepaticojejunostomy) may also be involved.

### Recurrent pyogenic cholangitis

This condition, which is becoming less common in the Far East, is characterized by recurrent attacks of primary bacterial cholangitis with fever, rigors, abdominal pain and jaundice (Lam et al 1978). The cause of the condition is unknown although *Clonorchis sinensis* (p. 591), infestation and ascariasis are reported associations (p. 580). The bile is infected in about 90% of patients, and *E. coli* is the commonest organism recovered. Bile duct proliferation and portal and periportal inflammation and fibrosis are seen in the liver and hepatic abscesses may occur. The large intrahepatic and extrahepatic bile ducts show variable dilatation and stricture formation and frequently contain stones and debris (Choi et al 1982). Episodes of cholangitis usually respond to antibiotic treatment but surgical relief of obstruction is often necessary. Stone removal by choledochotomy and hepatotomy carries a high incidence of recurrence as the strictures remain. Hepaticojejunostomy Roux-en-Y may be used to bypass obstruction but excision of the involved duct system has an acceptably low mortality and gives the best long-term results (Choi et al 1982).

## BILIARY STRICTURES

### Stenosis of the papilla of Vater

*Etiology and pathology*

This rare ill-defined condition accounts for less than 2% of all biliary operations. It seems to result from recurrent or persistent papillitis, the cause of which is unknown (Roberts-Thomson 1980). It is associated with gallstones, but whether this is a causal association is not clear. Histologically, there is an increase in subepithelial fibrous tissue, muscle hypertrophy, glandular proliferation and atrophy of the epithelial elements in the papillary region. In some patients, inflammation is marked. There is associated dilatation and thickening of the common bile duct and some patients have coexisting chronic pancreatitis.

*Definition*

The patient must have had definite biliary symptoms such as pain, jaundice or cholangitis before the diagnosis can be entertained. Indirect evidence of partial biliary obstruction should be present in the form of a dilated common bile duct containing debris and possibly primary bile duct stones. Patients have often had a cholecystectomy and some have had one or more explorations of the bile duct and/or endoscopic sphincterotomy. Ultrasonography or computed tomography shows dilatation of the common bile duct and at endoscopy, cannulation of the biliary and pancreatic ducts is difficult (Roberts-Thomson 1980). Increasing experience suggests that endoscopic manometry is valuable in identifying patients with papillary stenosis and sphincter of Oddi dysfunction (Gregg & Carr-Locke 1984, Toouli et al 1985). In the past, the diagnosis was established at operation by finding narrowing in the region of the sphincter of Oddi and it was impossible to pass anything more than a fine probe through the area. Operative cholangiography usually showed a dilated bile duct. A biopsy of the papillary region and/or brush cytology is advisable to exclude malignancy.

*Treatment*

The most important principle is to provide satisfactory biliary drainage and remove any gallstones and biliary debris. Before the advent of endoscopic sphincterotomy, transduodenal sphincteroplasty was used in younger fitter patients, while in older less fit patients a side-to-side choledochoduodenostomy was used when the common bile duct was distended. Patients thought to have papillary stenosis and sphincter dysfunction can be treated by endoscopic sphincterotomy but careful patient selection is mandatory. Anxieties about re-stenosis after endoscopic sphincterotomy appear misplaced (Geenen et al 1984b, Gregg & Carr-Locke 1984) but further follow-up of larger numbers of patients is needed to establish the definitive value of this approach. If endoscopic sphincterotomy fails, surgical drainage is best effected by means of a hepaticojejunostomy Roux-en-Y.

### Postinflammatory strictures

*Etiology*

Postinflammatory strictures are uncommon and are usually due to choledocholithiasis or chronic pancreatitis. Strictures due to chronic pancreatitis (Fig. 31.13) are usually long and narrow, involve the retropancreatic common bile duct and are thought to be due to peripancreatic sclerosis (Sarles & Sahel 1978). Strictures due to choledocholithiasis may be in any part of the biliary tree and are usually related to the gallstones themselves. Intrahepatic gallstones are quite frequent in advanced cases of recurrent pyogenic cholangitis in the Orient (Choi et al 1982).

*Clinical features*

The clinical features are those of biliary obstruction and cholangitis is common (p. 1212).

*Investigations*

Cholangiography is normally undertaken endoscopically

(p. 114) rather than by the percutaneous transhepatic route. The long distal strictures of chronic pancreatitis can mimic malignant obstruction but contrast usually passes through the narrowed area (Fig. 31.13). In malignant strictures the obstruction is more often complete and the entire biliary system may not be outlined (Fig. 48.4). Strictures due to gallstones are usually short and localized.

*Treatment*

Postinflammatory strictures usually require surgical treatment, although endoscopic or percutaneous stenting may be considered in elderly frail patients. Distal strictures are usually treated by choledochojejunostomy Roux-en-Y, while more proximal strictures are managed by hepaticojejunostomy Roux-en-Y. Intrahepatic strictures are difficult to treat and usually require forcible dilatation and the insertion of a transhepatic splinting tube. Alternatively, partial hepatic resection may be used and is particularly valuable in recurrent pyogenic cholangitis (Choi et al 1982). An access loop of jejunum can be positioned subcutaneously to facilitate subsequent percutaneous dilatation of the biliary tree.

## Bile duct injury and postoperative stricture

Trauma to the extrahepatic biliary tree can result from a number of medical and surgical procedures. Injuries following cholecystectomy have serious consequences and the tragedy is that most occur in young women and that almost all could be prevented by good surgical technique. There is debate about the exact incidence of bile duct injury at cholecystectomy and the few surveys undertaken put the figure at one injury per 300–500 open cholecystectomies (Kune 1979, Bismuth 1982). The early published series of laparoscopic cholecystectomy suggest a slight increase in the incidence of injury to one per 150–200 laparoscopic cholecystectomies (Cuschieri et al 1991, Meyers 1991). Other causes of postoperative jaundice are discussed on page 1143.

*Etiology*

The risk of injury is increased by pathology (such as empyema, cholangitis, portal hypertension and gallstone pancreatitis) which increases vascularity and/or tissue friability. However, most duct injuries occur in patients undergoing otherwise straightforward elective cholecystectomy. In one series of 1554 postcholecystectomy strictures, a junior surgeon was operating on his own in 85% of cases (Smith 1979), while the experience in Sweden showed that 80% of iatrogenic strictures were caused by trainee surgeons with an experience of between 25 and 100 cholecystectomies (Andren-Sandberg et al 1985). Variation in biliary anatomy is often cited as a major factor in such injuries. Potentially dangerous variations include a short cystic duct, a narrow mobile common bile duct which is easily mistaken for the cystic duct and congenital abnormalities of the right hepatic duct. Injury to the common hepatic duct may result from injudicious attempts to control hemorrhage. The value of operative cholangiography in defining abnormal anatomy and preventing inadvertent division of a common bile duct cannot be overemphasized. In one series of 78 iatrogenic strictures, operative cholangiography had been performed in only 29% of cases and the views were often inadequate (Kelley & Blumgart 1985). However, operative cholangiography is no substitute for careful identification of ductal structures.

*Pathology*

The injury is followed by a marked inflammatory reaction leading to fibrosis extending proximally and distally from the site of injury. The arterial supply of the supraduodenal bile duct is axial, with the major supply (60%) coming from below. Northover & Terblanche (1979) have postulated that ischemia creates a vicious cycle whereby bile enters the damaged mucosa causing further inflammation and fibrosis. The fact that most of the blood supply ascends the duct also helps to explain why the final level of the stricture may be much higher in the biliary tree than might have been expected from the site of original injury. In laparoscopic cholecystectomy, the bile duct may be more liable to damage because of the use of diathermy and laparoscopic dissection (Garden 1991); while identification of the junction between gallbladder and cystic duct is essential, dissection of the cystic duct to identify its confluence with the hepatic duct can be both unnecessary and dangerous.

Biliary obstruction results in recurrent cholangitis and late development of biliary cirrhosis may also lead to portal hypertension (p. 942). In some cases, there is also major vessel injury at the time of bile duct damage.

*Clinical features and investigations*

Only some 20% of injuries are appreciated at the time of surgery and most patients present with obstructive jaundice, biliary peritonitis or a biliary fistula within a few days of operation. Jaundice deepens steadily, but recurrent cholangitis may not develop for months or, rarely, years after cholecystectomy. Recurrent stricture after biliary reconstruction may also take years to become manifest.

The diagnosis of bile duct injury is established by ultrasound scanning and PTC (p. 22), supplemented if necessary by ERCP. The stricture is frequently at the level of the confluence or upper common hepatic duct (Fig. 48.11). The frequency of associated vascular injury or portal vein thrombosis means that Doppler ultrasound imaging and/or arteriography is advisable.

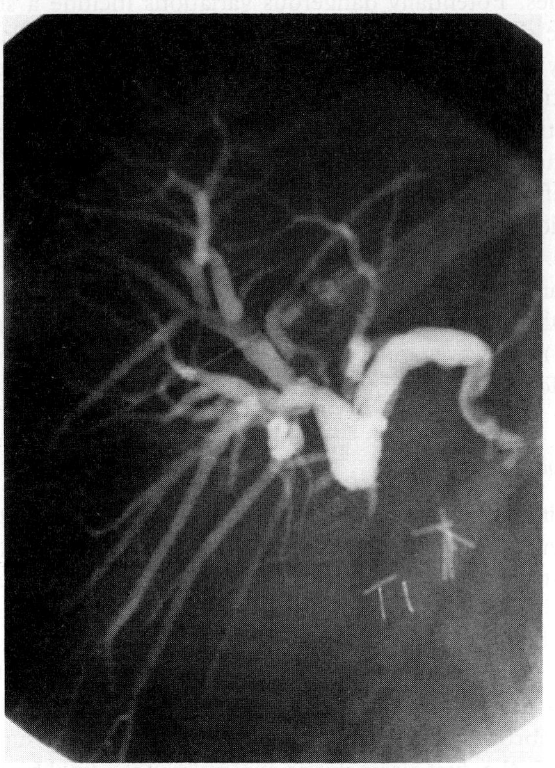


**Fig. 48.11** Percutaneous transhepatic cholangiogram following an operative duct injury during laparoscopic cholecystectomy. Note the typical high injury of the bile duct, which in this case was caused by a metal clip below the confluence of the right and left hepatic ducts. The common hepatic duct and right hepatic artery had been excised.

*Treatment*

If bile duct injury is recognized at surgery and there is no devascularization or duct loss, it may be managed by primary anastomosis constructed without tension over a splinting T-tube. Otherwise, hepaticojejunostomy Roux-en-Y is the most suitable operation. The inexperienced surgeon should not embark on unfamiliar surgery which might aggravate the situation and early referral to a specialist center is indicated.

The outcome of secondary repair in patients with an established biliary fistula is less favorable, because of the small caliber of the hepatic ducts and optimum results are obtained in jaundiced patients with dilated ducts. Control of intra-abdominal sepsis may be necessary in the first instance and percutaneous drainage of the biliary tree may allow a fistula to heal and facilitate delayed repair. The most successful method of reconstruction is direct mucosa-to-mucosa anastomosis of the hepatic duct to a Roux loop of jejunum (Bismuth et al 1978, Bismuth 1982, Blumgart & Kelley 1984) (Fig. 48.11). If the ducts are difficult to define at the confluence, the Roux loop can be anastomosed to the left hepatic duct. There is debate about whether the anastomosis should be protected by a splint and whether this should be kept in place for 6–12 months. Advocates of splinting believe that it lowers the incidence of recurrent stricture formation (Kune 1979), whereas some surgeons do not splint the anastomosis (Bismuth et al 1978). Unilateral duct injury can be managed conservatively in some patients (Hadjis et al 1986) and selected patients may be treated by transhepatic or endoscopic transampullary dilatation or stenting. Such procedures should not be undertaken outside specialist units as inappropriate selection of treatment options can compromise subsequent management and ultimate outcome.

Bleeding varices due to portal hypertension may appear in patients with neglected or recurrent strictures and are difficult to deal with. The mortality of secondary repair increases eightfold once portal hypertension develops (Blumgart & Kelley 1984). Liver transplantation may have to be considered in patients with progressive liver failure (Garden 1991).

*Prognosis*

The difficulty of surgical management is reflected in an average operative mortality of about 8% (Warren et al 1982) and a high morbidity rate after repair. There is a significant risk of re-stenosis (Kune 1979, Smith 1979) and this may occur up to 10 years following repair. The ultimate results are satisfactory in about 85% of patients and the eventual mortality has been reduced beneath 15% in expert centers (Kune 1979, Bismuth et al 1978, Bismuth 1982, Blumgart & Kelley 1984). Death from liver failure or bleeding esophageal varices is uncommon when patients with secondary biliary cirrhosis are considered for liver transplantation at an early stage.

**Primary sclerosing cholangitis**

This rare disease of unknown cause is characterized by progressive obliterative inflammation of the biliary tree. It presents as a chronic fluctuating cholestatic syndrome leading eventually to hepatic cirrhosis and its complications, and it may be complicated by choriocarcinoma. It is considered fully elsewhere (p. 965).

## BILIARY FISTULAE

Biliary fistulae are uncommon. External fistulae communicate between the skin and the biliary tract, while internal biliary fistulae communicate with a part of the gastrointestinal tract, such as the duodenum or the colon, or connect different parts of the biliary tract, such as the gallbladder and the bile duct. Biliary fistulae may develop as a consequence of underlying disease or as a result of surgery. Both internal and external components are occasionally present.

### External fistulae

Surgical external fistulae may be created deliberately (e.g. cholecystostomy) but are usually due to inadequate surgical technique or to an operation which has not relieved biliary obstruction. Spontaneous external biliary fistulae are exceedingly rare. External biliary fistulae lead to fluid and electrolyte depletion and diversion of bile from the gut reduces the absorption of fat and fat-soluble vitamins. A biliary fistula dose not produce excoriation of the skin unless there is associated flow of small intestinal content and pancreatic juice.

Fistulography, PTC or ERCP are used to delineate the bile duct, show whether obstruction is present and detect causes such as division of the common bile duct or overlooked gallstones. Bile leaks from the cystic duct stump or common bile duct following cholecystectomy may heal if the biliary tree is drained temporarily by endoscopic sphincterotomy and/or insertion of a stent.

The principles of treatment are to correct fluid and electrolyte imbalance, treat biliary or intra-abdominal infection and skin digestion (if present) and deal with the underlying cause. This may necessitate temporary biliary drainage by endoscopic or percutaneous means pending further surgical intervention.

### Internal fistulae

These may be created surgically (e.g. cholecystojejunostomy, choledochoduodenostomy and hepaticojejunostomy); unintended postoperative fistulae are rare. Pathological internal fistulae are relatively uncommon; gallstones are usually responsible, but chronic duodenal ulcers and malignancy can be the cause (Pitman & Davies 1963, Dowse 1964, McSherry et al 1969, Collie et al 1994). The fistula usually communicates with the second part of the duodenum, less commonly with the colon, jejunum or stomach.

There are no specific clinical features and most of the symptoms are due to the underlying cause. Plain abdominal radiography may show gas in the biliary tract, particularly following an effervescent drink, and a barium meal may show reflux of barium into the biliary system.

The principles of treatment are to deal with the underlying cause, disconnect the fistula and close the gut and provide satisfactory biliary drainage. Temporary biliary drainage may be required in unfit patients so that definitive surgery can be undertaken under optimal circumstances.

### Gallstone ileus

Gallstone ileus results when a large gallstone perforates into the gastrointestinal tract and obstructs the distal small bowel or, much less commonly, the large bowel. The fistula is usually between the gallbladder and the duodenum. Gallstone ileus accounts for about 1–2% of cases of mechanical intestinal obstructions. This incidence rises with age and most patients are over 60 years of age (Brockis & Gilbert 1957, Cooperman et al 1968). A gallstone has to be at least 2.5 cm in diameter to cause intestinal obstruction. The usual site of impaction is in the lower ileum; large bowel obstruction only occurs if there is a pathological narrowing, as in diverticular disease of the colon.

#### *Clinical features*

The features are those of intestinal obstruction, but the initial symptoms are often intermittent, probably because the gallstone is held up temporarily in several places before it reaches its final site of impaction (Brockis & Gilbert 1957, Collins & Claxton 1966). The diagnosis should be suspected in elderly females known to have gallstones who present with small bowel obstruction in the absence of an obvious cause.

#### *Investigation*

A plain radiograph of the abdomen in the erect and supine positions usually confirms the diagnosis by showing gas in the biliary tract, dilated loops of small bowel with fluid levels suggestive of small bowel obstruction and (sometimes) a radio-opaque gallstone visible in the abdomen.

#### *Treatment*

Treatment consists of nasogastric aspiration and intravenous fluid replacement followed by enterotomy above the site of obstruction to remove the gallstone. The entire small bowel must be examined because recurrent gallstone ileus can be caused by a missed second large gallstone (Claridge 1961, Buetow et al 1963). It is usually unwise to deal with the cholecystoduodenal fistula at the same time since this may have already closed spontaneously and most patients are elderly and poor surgical risks. Attempts at cholecystectomy and repair of the fistula are fraught with difficulty (Cooperman et al 1968) and damage to the main bile duct may occur.

### Mirrizzi's syndrome

This condition usually affects elderly patients who present with obstructive jaundice due to impaction of a gallstone at the cystic duct (type 1) or at the site of an internal fistula between Hartmann's pouch and the common hepatic duct (type 2). Such patients often present with cholangitis and require urgent endoscopic retrograde cholangiography to define the nature of the obstruction and to effect temporary drainage of the biliary tree by endoscopic placement of a stent. The syndrome often mimics the features of gallbladder or bile duct carcinoma, but since the patients are often frail and elderly, definitive surgical intervention is usually not indicated. If surgery becomes necessary, the surgeon should remove the gallbladder in retrograde fashion and avoid leaving a substantial defect of the common hepatic duct. If a portion of Hartmann's pouch is retained, it can be used to repair the defect, although in some patients, it is prudent to drain the biliary tree definitively by means of a hepaticojejunostomy Roux-en-Y.

## CONGENITAL LESIONS

The most important congenital lesions of the biliary tree are choledochal cysts (p. 727) and biliary atresia (p. 730).

## CANCER OF THE GALLBLADDER

### Etiology

Gallstones are found in almost every case, but the risk of gallbladder cancer developing in a patient with untreated gallstones is probably less than 1% (Wenckert & Robertson 1966). This risk may increase the longer the patient has the gallstones. Employees in the automotive, textile, rubber and metal fabricating industries have an increased incidence of gallbladder carcinoma (Krain 1972, Brandt-Rauf et al 1982). Estimates of the incidence of gallbladder cancer range from 0.1 to 0.4% of all gallbladder operations (Perpetuo et al 1978, Welton et al 1979). There is an association between chronic ulcerative colitis and biliary tract malignancy (Almagro 1985).

### Pathology

Carcinoma of the gallbladder are usually adenocarcinomas and are classified as papillary or infiltrative (Edmondson 1967); squamous cell carcinoma and sarcoma are extremely rare (Albores-Saavedra et al 1981). Papillary lesions can be localized or diffuse and form protuberant, nodular and papillary masses which can fill the gallbladder and may resemble empyema. These may become invasive.

Invasive carcinoma is usually characterized macroscopically by a normal-sized or contracted gallbladder. The tumor forms a plaque, ulcer or infiltrating mass in the wall and often spreads directly into the adjacent liver. Less advanced gallbladder cancer may not be obvious macroscopically and can closely mimic the induration of chronic cholecystitis associated with gallstones. In situ carcinoma is usually unrecognizable macroscopically (Albores-Saavedra et al 1984). Evidence is accumulating that the commonest pathway for adenocarcinoma to develop is via dysplasia of metaplastic gallbladder epithelium (Dowling & Kelly 1986, Yamagiwa & Tomiyama 1986). Gallbladder cancer spreads locally via the lymphatics and nerve bundles to involve the liver, lymph nodes and peritoneum. The lungs and other distant sites may become involved (Edmondson 1967).

### Clinical features

Although the condition is encountered in younger individuals, patients are on average in their seventh decade and are six times more likely to be female than male. Obstructive jaundice is a frequent mode of presentation and it almost always implies spread to the bile duct or liver and a very poor prognosis. Other patients present with biliary tract pain and occasionally with acute cholecystitis caused by neoplastic occlusion of the cystic duct. In a substantial number of patients the cancer is reported as an incidental finding at cholecystectomy for cholelithiasis.

### Investigations

Ultrasound scanning (Fig. 2.3) and computed tomography demonstrate a mass filling or replacing the gallbladder in about 50% of patients and in others reveal a mass protruding into the gallbladder or asymmetrical thickening of the wall (Weiner et al 1984). Similar features may be evident if ERCP is undertaken (Fig. 48.12). In many cases, the diagnosis is only made at laparotomy when extensive infiltration into the liver is found or enlarged lymph nodes are identified at cholecystectomy. In other patients the diagnosis is only made on histological examination of a removed gallbladder.

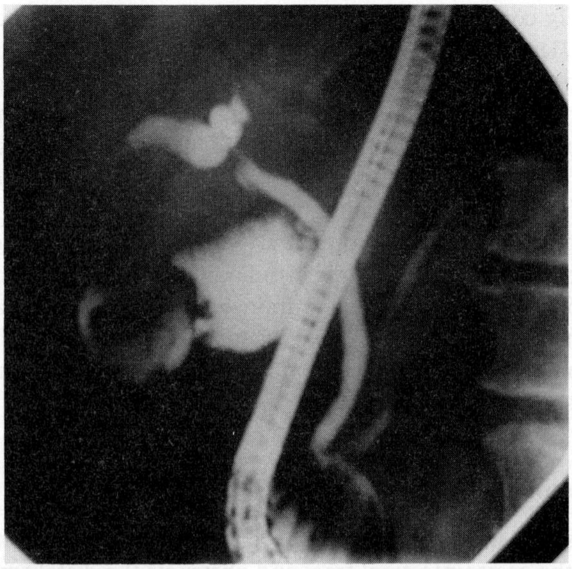

**Fig. 48.12** ERCP showing a polypoidal mass in the fundus of the gallbladder. At operation this proved to be an adenocarcinoma of the gallbladder.

### Treatment

Surgical excision holds the only prospect of cure, but is rarely possible. If the diagnosis has been made before cholecystectomy, radical excision of the gallbladder along with segments IV, V and VI is recommended (Bismuth 1982) rather than atypical resection (Tompkins 1982). Radical lymphadenectomy necessitates excision of the extrahepatic biliary tree and restorative hepaticojejunostomy, but such an aggressive approach or extended right hepatectomy is probably not justified. Excision of the gallbladder bed by trisegmental resection is recommended if the diagnosis has been made subsequent to cholecystectomy and the tumor appears to have breached the gallbladder wall. Unfortunately, in these circumstances, dissemination of the tumor is usually already evident at laparotomy.

In more advanced lesions, palliative decompression of obstructive jaundice may be possible by endoscopic or percutaneous stenting. In younger fitter patients, surgical decompression by segment III cholangiojejunostomy (see below) may be preferable (Fig. 48.13).

The role of chemotherapy and radiotherapy has yet to be established but there is no good evidence that they are beneficial (Tompkins 1982).

### Prognosis

Eighty percent of patients are dead within a year of diagnosis and only 2–5% are alive after 5 years (Warren et al 1968, Vaittinen 1970, Donaldson & Busuttil 1975, Prakash et al 1975). Only a handful of long-term survivors have been reported after radical surgery and most are patients whose gallbladders had been removed for gallstones and have been found incidentally to be the site of cancer.

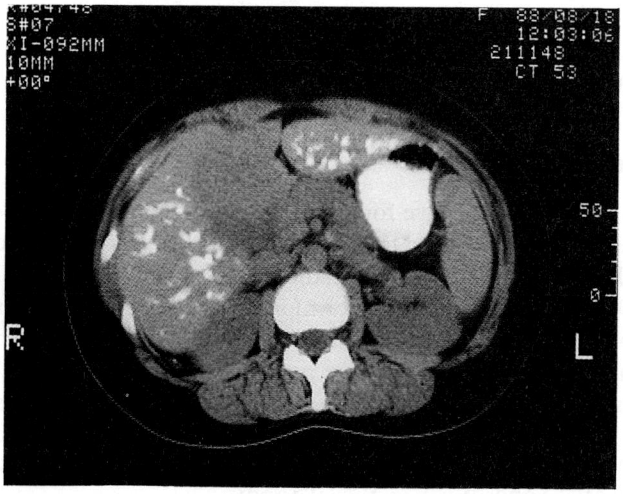


**Fig. 48.13** CT scan demonstrating a tumor mass arising from the gallbladder and infiltrating the right lobe of the liver. The dilated intrahepatic ducts contain contrast from a previous ERCP examination.

### Prevention

Almost all patients with gallbladder cancer have gallstones when their cancers are discovered. The incidence of cancer, however, is very small compared to that of gallstones and as the risk of dying from cholecystectomy is approximately the same as that of developing cancer, it is illogical to recommend cholecystectomy to all gallstone patients as a means of preventing cancer.

## CANCER OF THE BILE DUCTS

### Etiology

Bile duct cancer is less common than gallbladder cancer; it is estimated that it is encountered once in every 100 bile duct operations and once in every 1000 autopsies (Bengmark et al 1986). The cause of bile duct cancer is unknown but the condition may be increasing in frequency. Males are afflicted at least as often as females and the disease is much commoner in the elderly. Gallstones are found in less than a third of cases. Papillomatosis has been recorded as preceding carcinoma, but this is very uncommon. Patients with extensive ulcerative colitis have a high incidence of early onset and aggressive bile duct carcinoma, the course of which is not influenced by successful treatment of the colitis (Akwari et al 1975). Other factors implicated in the pathogenesis of bile duct cancer include *Clonorchis* infestation (p. 591), chronic typhoid infection and cystic dilatation of the biliary system (p. 727) (Tompkins 1982).

### Pathology

No part of the biliary tree is exempt from cancer, but the hepatic duct confluence and the distal common bile duct are the commonest sites. The tumor is usually a solid mass, less commonly it is scirrhous and infiltrating and rarely it is papillary. The cancer is usually an adenocarcinoma or anaplastic carcinoma and is only rarely a papillary carcinoma. Bile duct cancer is frequently multifocal and shows considerable subepithelial spread proximally and distally along the bile duct, which militates against successful surgery. Perineural spread and lymphatic invasion are characteristic. Lymphatic spread occurs first to the regional peridochal nodes and then to the celiac nodes. Direct spread occurs to the portal vein, hepatic artery, pancreas, duodenum and gallbladder. Peritoneal and liver metastases are common but distant metastases are not.

### Clinical features

The usual presentation is with rapidly progressive obstructive jaundice. Upper abdominal pain, pruritus and weight loss are frequent, but cholangitis is uncommon.

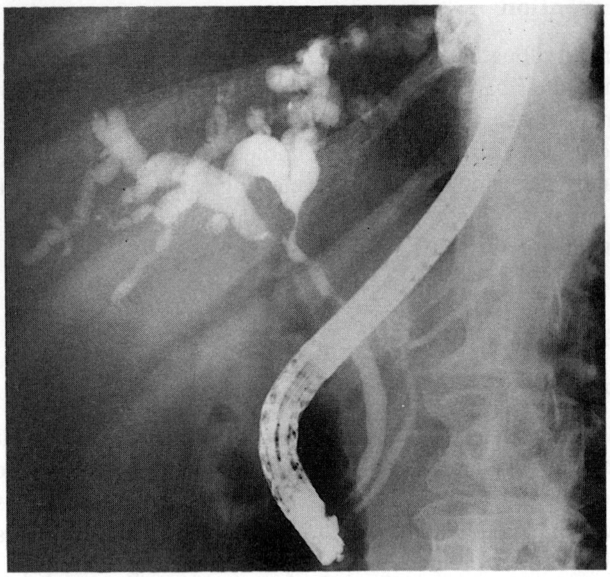

**Fig. 48.14** ERCP showing incomplete bile duct obstruction caused by a cancer of the common hepatic duct. Note the multifocal nature of the tumor which also involves the hepatic duct confluence.

### Investigations

The clue to the diagnosis is intrahepatic duct dilation and a collapsed gallbladder and extrahepatic biliary tree on ultrasonography. CT scanning may demonstrate the level of obstruction and show direct spread to the liver or lymph nodes. Percutaneous transhepatic cholangiography or ERCP may be useful in establishing the level of the obstruction, although it may be difficult to differentiate between a cancer of the bile duct and a benign bile duct stricture due to primary sclerosing cholangitis (Fig. 48.14). Diffusely infiltrating tumors pose particular difficulties and the diagnosis may remain uncertain, even at operation. In patients being considered for radical resection, Doppler ultrasound scanning and/or preoperative angiography is essential to define hepatic arterial and portal venous invasion. In tumors involving the right or left hepatic ducts, contralateral involvement of the branch of the hepatic artery or portal vein constitutes a contraindication to resection.

In patients submitted to operation, the diagnosis may be established by fine-needle aspiration cytology or biopsy of peritoneal, lymph node or liver metastases. Intracholedochoscopic biopsy or brush cytology is often unrewarding, but may differentiate these malignant tumors from benign bile duct strictures.

### Treatment

Cholangiocarcinoma affecting the lower common bile duct is dealt with by Whipple resection if the patient is well enough and the lesion appears potentially curable. Resectability rates of 47–76% and operative mortality rates of 0–8% are now reported for such lesions in the lower third of the biliary tree (Langer et al 1985, Tsunoda et al 1985). Resection rates are lower for middle third tumors and even in specialist centers are usually 20% or less for lesions in the upper third (Blumgart & Kelley 1984, Langer et al 1985, Guthrie et al 1993). Involvement of the biliary tree beyond secondary bifurcations usually indicates the need for hepatic resection (Bismuth et al 1988, Guthrie et al 1993). Resection of the caudate lobe is often advocated (Nimura et al 1990). Hepaticojejunostomy is used to restore intestinal continuity after resection of tumors of the middle and upper third of the extrahepatic biliary tree, but mortality rates of 10–23% reflect the risks of major surgery in these patients (Tompkins et al 1981, Blumgart et al 1984, Bengmark et al 1986, Guthrie et al 1993).

Transhepatic intubation with a U-tube has been advocated as an alternative to resection (Terblanche 1976) or as a means of safeguarding biliary flow following resection of the tumor (Cameron et al 1982). However, anastomosis of a Roux-en-Y limb of jejunum to the segment III duct within the left lobe of the liver (segment III cholangiojejunostomy) is now felt to offer better surgical palliation than surgical intubation or extrahepatic biliary bypass (Bismuth & Corlette 1975, Blumgart & Kelley 1984, Bismuth et al 1988, Guthrie et al 1993). Operative mortality may be as high as 16% following such palliative surgery (Bismuth et al 1988, Guthrie et al 1993) and it should only be contemplated in selected patients. Internal drainage by percutaneous insertion of a prosthesis is preferable to endoscopic stenting in patients unfit for surgery (Gibson et al 1988), although patients are more likely to suffer cholangitis following nonoperative stenting (Guthrie et al 1993). While chemotherapy has little to offer, external irradiation (Langer et al 1985) and irradiation using iridium-192 wire inserted percutaneously or endoscopically (Fletcher et al 1983, Nunnerley & Karani 1990) merit further assessment.

### Prognosis

Most patients survive for about 6 months, but some 10% can survive much longer provided that they have effective biliary decompression or radical surgery (Guthrie et al 1993). Survival of 3 years or more has been reported after palliative decompression alone and is more frequent in patients with a sclerosing or papillary carcinoma. Radical resection of the tumor in the absence of visible metastases is occasionally followed by survival for 5 years or more (Braasch et al 1967, Andersson et al 1977, Inouye & Whelan 1978, Bengmark et al 1988).

## REFERENCES


Akwari O E, van Heerden J A, Foulk W T, Baggenstoss A H 1975 Cancer of the bile ducts associated with ulcerative colitis. Annals of Surgery 181: 303–309

Albores-Saavedra J, Cruz-Oritz H, Alcantara-Vazques A, Henson D E 1981 Unusual types of gallbladder carcinoma. A report of 16 cases. Archives of Pathology and Laboratory Medicine 105: 287–293

Albores-Saavedra J, Manrique J D J, Angeles-Angeles A, Henson D E 1984 Carcinoma in situ of the gallbladder. A clinicopathologic study of 18 cases. American Journal of Surgical Pathology 8: 323–333

Almagro U A 1985 Diffuse papillomatosis of the gallbladder. American Journal of Gastroenterology 80: 274–278

Anderson A, Berdahl L, van der Linden W 1977 Malignant tumors of the extrahepatic bile ducts. Surgery 81: 198–202

Andren-Sandberg A, Alinder G, Bengmark S 1985 Accidental lesions of the common bile duct at cholecystectomy. Pre- and perioperative factors of importance. Annals of Surgery 201: 328–332

Ashby B S 1965 Acute and recurrent torsion of the gallbladder. British Journal of Surgery 52: 182

Banting S W, Carter D C 1994 Expectations of cholecystectomy. In S Paterson-Brown & O J Garden (eds) Principles and practice of laparoscopic surgery. W B Saunders, London, p 53–66

Baron R L, Stanley R J, Lee J K T et al 1982 A prospective comparison of the evaluation of biliary obstruction using computed tomography and ultrasonography. Radiology 145: 91–98

Bates T, Ebbs S R, Harrison M, A'Hern R P 1991 Influence of cholecystectomy on symptoms. British Journal of Surgery 78: 964–967

Bengmark S, Blumgart L H, Launois B 1986 Liver resection in high bile duct tumours. In S Bengmark, L H Blumgart (eds) Liver surgery. Churchill Livingstone, Edinburgh, p 81–87

Bengmark S, Ekberg H, Evander A et al 1988 Major liver resection for hilar cholangiocarcinoma. Annals of Surgery 207: 120–125

Bennion L J, Grundy S M 1978 Risk factors for the development of cholelithiasis in man. New England Journal of Medicine 299: 1161–1221

Berk R N, Cooperberg P L, Gold R P, Rohrmann C A, Ferrucci J T 1982 Radiography of the bile ducts. A symposium on the use of new modalities for diagnosis and treatment. Radiology 145: 1–9

Birkett D H 1992 Biliary laser lithotripsy. Surgical Clinics of North America 72: 641–654

Bismuth H 1982 Postoperative strictures of the bile duct. In L H Blumgart (ed) The biliary tract. Churchill Livingstone, Edinburgh, p 209–218

Bismuth H, Corlette M B 1975 Intrahepatic cholangioenteric anastomosis in carcinoma of the hilus of the liver. Surgery, Gynecology and Obstetrics 140: 170–178

Bismuth H, Franco D, Corlette M B, Hepp J 1978 Long term results of Roux-en-Y hepaticojejunostomy. Surgery, Gynecology and Obstetrics 146: 161–167

Bismuth H, Castaing D, Traynor O 1988 Resection or palliation: priority of surgery in the treatment of hilar cancer. World Journal of Surgery 12: 39–47

Blamey S L, Fearon K C H, Gilmour W H, Osborne D H, Carter D C 1983 Prediction of risk in biliary surgery. British Journal of Surgery 70: 535–538

Blenkharn J I, Blumgart L H 1985 Streptococcal bacteraemia in hepatobiliary surgery: implications for prophylaxis. Surgery, Gynecology and Obstetrics 160: 139–141

Blum L, Stagg A 1963 Emphysematous cholecystitis. American Journal of Roentgenology, Radium Therapy and Nuclear Medicine 89: 840–846

Blumgart L H 1978 Biliary tract obstruction. New approaches to old problems. American Journal of Surgery 135: 19–31

Blumgart L H, Kelley C J 1984 Hepaticojejunostomy in benign and malignant high bile duct stricture: approaches to the left hepatic ducts. British Journal of Surgery 71: 257–261

Blumgart L H, Hadjis N S, Benjamin I S, Beazley R 1984 Surgical approaches to cholangiocarcinoma at confluence of hepatic ducts. Lancet 1: 66–70

Boey J H & Way L W 1990 Acute cholangitis. Annals of Surgery 191: 264–270

Bogokowsky H, Slutzki S, Zaidenstein L, Halpern Z, Negri M, Abramsohn R 1987 Selective operative cholangiography. Surgery, Gynecology and Obstetrics 164: 124–126

Boonyapisit S T, Trotman B W, Ostrow J D 1978 Unconjugated bilirubin, and the hydrolysis of conjugated bilirubin, in gallbladder bile of patients with cholelithiasis. Gastroenterology 74: 70–74

Bornman P C, Harries-Jones E P, Tobias R, van Stiegmann G, Terblanche J 1986 Prospective controlled trial of transhepatic biliary endoprosthesis versus bypass surgery for incurable carcinoma of head of pancreas. Lancet 1: 69–71

Boyden E A 1957 The anatomy of the choledochoduodenal junction. Surgery, Gynecology and Obstetrics 104: 641–652

Braasch J W, Warren K W, Kune G A 1967 Malignant neoplasms of the bile ducts. Surgical Clinics of North America 47: 627–638

Brandt-Rauf P W, Pincus M, Adelson S 1982 Cancer or the gallbladder: a review of forty-three cases. Human Pathology 13: 48–53

Brockis J G, Gilbert M C 1957 Intestinal obstruction by gallstones: a review of 179 cases. British Journal of Surgery 44: 461–466

Buetow G W, Glaubitz J P, Crampton R S 1963 Recurrent gallstone ileus. Surgery 54: 716–718

Burhenne J H 1980 Percutaneous extraction of retained biliary tract stones. American Journal of Radiology 134: 888–898

Burke J F 1973 Preventive antibiotic management in surgery. Annual Review of Medicine 24: 289–294

Burnstein M J, Ilson R G, Petrunka C N, Taylor R D, Strasberg S M 1983 Evidence for a potent nucleating factor in the gallbladder bile of patients with cholesterol gallstones. Gastroenterology 85: 801–807

Cameron J L, Broe P, Zuidema G D 1982 Proximal bile duct tumors. Surgical management with silastic transhepatic biliary stents. Annals of Surgery 196: 412–418

Carr-Locke D L, Gregg J A 1981 Endoscopic manometry of pancreatic and biliary sphincter zones in man. Basal results in healthy volunteers. Digestive Diseases and Sciences 26: 7–15

Carroll J J, Phillips E H, Daykhovsky L et al 1992 Laparoscopic choledochoscopy: an effective approach to the common duct. Journal of Laparoscopic and Endoscopic Surgery 2: 15–21

Carter R, Thompson R J Jr, Brennan L P, Hinshaw D B 1963 Volvulus of the gallbladder. Surgery, Gynecology and Obstetrics 116: 105–108

Choi T K, Wong J, Ong G B 1982 The surgical management of primary intrahepatic stones. British Journal of Surgery 69: 86–90

Christensen A H, Ishak K G 1970 Benign tumors and pseudotumors of the gallbladder. Report of 180 cases. Archives of Pathology 90: 423–432

Claridge M 1961 Recurrent gall stone ileus. British Journal of Surgery 49: 134–135

Clavien P A, Sanabria J R, Mentha G et al 1992 Recent results of elective open cholecystectomy in the North American and the European Centre: comparison of complications and risk factors. Annals of Surgery 216: 618–626

Collie D A, Redhead D N, Garden O J 1994 Cholecystobronchocolic fistula: a late complication of biliary sepsis: diagnosis and management. HPB Surgery 7: 319–326

Collins G M, Claxton R C 1966 Gall stone intestinal obstruction. A review of the literature and presentation of new cases. Medical Journal of Australia 1: 578–581

Cooperberg P, Burhenne H J 1980 Real-time ultrasonography. Diagnostic technique of choice in calculous gallbladder disease. New England Journal of Medicine 302: 1277–1279

Cooperberg P, Golding R H 1982 Advances in ultrasonography of the gallbladder and biliary tract. Radiological Clinics of North America 20: 611–633

Cooperman A M, Dickson E R, ReMine W H 1968 Changing concepts in the surgical treatment of gallstone ileus. Annals of Surgery 166: 377–383

Cotton P B 1984 Endoscopic management of bile duct stones (apples and oranges). Gut 25: 587–597

Cotton P B 1990 Retained bile duct stones, T-tube in place: percutaneous or endoscopic management? American Journal of Gastroenterology 85: 107–108

Crumplin M H K, Jenkinson L R, Kassab J Y, Whitaker C M, Al-Boutiahi F H 1985 Management of gallstones in a district general hospital. British Journal of Surgery 72: 428–432

Csendes A, Sepulveda A, Burdiles P et al 1988 Common bile duct pressure in patients with common bile duct stones with or without acute suppurative cholangitis. Archives of Surgery 123: 697–699
Cuschieri A, Dubois F, Mouiel J et al 1991 The European experience of laparoscopic cholecystectomy. American Journal of Surgery 161: 385–387
Dineen P 1964 The importance of the route of infection in experimental biliary tract obstruction. Surgery, Gynecology and Obstetrics 119: 1001–1008
Donaldson L A, Busuttil A 1975 A clinicopathological review of 68 carcinomas of the gallbladder. British Journal of Surgery 62: 26–32
Dow R W, Lindernauer S M 1969 Acute obstructive suppurative cholangitis. Annals of Surgery 169: 272–276
Dowling G P, Kelly J K 1986 The histogenesis of adenocarcinoma of the gallbladder. Cancer 58: 1702–1708
Dowse J L A 1964 Spontaneous internal biliary fistulae. Gut 429–432
Durrell C A, Vincent L M, Mittelstaedt C A 1984 Gallbladder ultrasonography in clinical context. Seminars on Ultrasonography, Computed Tomography and Magnetic Resonance 5: 315–319
Dye M, McDonald A, Smith G 1978 The bacterial flora of the biliary tract and liver in man. British Journal of Surgery 65: 285–287
Edholm P, Jonsson G 1962 Bile duct stones related to age and duct width. Acta Chirurgica Scandinavica 124: 75–79
Edmondson H A 1967 Tumors of the gallbladder and extrahepatic bile ducts. In: Altas of tumour pathology, Section VII, Fascicle 26. Armed Forces Institute of Pathology, Washington DC
Einstein D M, Lapin S A, Ralls P W, Halls J M 1984 The insensitivity of sonography in the detection of choledocholithiasis. American Journal of Roentgenology 142: 725–728
Escourrou J, Cordova J A, Lazorthes F, Frexinos J, Ribet A 1984 Early and late complications after endoscopic sphincterotomy for biliary lithiasis with and without the gallbladder 'in situ'. Gut 25: 598–602
Eyre-Brook I A, Ross B, Johnson A G 1983 Should surgeons operate on the evidence of ultrasound alone in jaundiced patients? British Journal of Surgery 70: 587–589
Fletcher M S, Brinkley D, Dawson J L, Nunnerley H, Williams R 1983 Treatment of hilar carcinoma by bile drainage combined with internal radiotherapy using $^{192}$iridium wire. British Journal of Surgery 70: 733–735
Fromm H 1986 Gallstone dissolution therapy. Current status and future prospects. Gastroenterology 91: 1560–1567
Gallinger S, Harvey P R C, Petrunka C N, Strasberg S M 1986 Effect of binding of ionised calcium on the *in vitro* nucleation of cholesterol and calcium bilirubinate in human gall bladder bile. Gut 27: 1382–1386
Garden O J 1991 Iatrogenic injury to the bile duct. British Journal of Surgery 78: 1412–1413
Garden O J 1995 The pancreas. In: O J Garden (ed) Intraoperative and laparoscopic ultrasonography. Blackwell, Oxford
Geenen J E, Vennes J A, Silvis S E 1981 Resumé of a seminar on endoscopic retrograde sphincterotomy (ERS). Gastrointestinal Endoscopy 27: 31–38
Geenen J, Hogan W, Toouli J, Dodds W, Venu R 1984a A prospective randomised study of the efficacy of endoscopic sphincterotomy for patients with presumptive sphincter of Oddi dysfunction. Gastroenterology 86: 1086
Geenen J E, Toouli J, Hogan W J et al 1984b Endoscopic sphincterotomy: follow-up evaluation of effects on the sphincter of Oddi. Gastroenterology 87: 754–758
Gerolami A, Sarles H, Brette R et al 1977 Controlled trial of chenodeoxycholic therapy for radiolucent gall stones. A multicentre study. Digestion 16: 299–307
Gibson R N, Yeung E, Hadjis N et al 1988 Percutaneous transhepatic endoprosthesis for hilar cholangiocarcinoma. Journal of Surgery 156: 363–367
Glenn F, Moody F G 1961 Acute obstructive suppurative cholangitis. Surgery, Gynecology and Obstetrics 113: 265–273
Goldman L D, Steer M L, Silen W 1983 Recurrent cholangitis after biliary surgery. American Journal of Surgery 152: 145–150
Gollish S H, Burnstein M J, Ilson R G, Petrunka C N, Strasberg S M 1983 Nucleation of cholesterol monohydrate crystals from hepatic and gall-bladder bile of patients with cholesterol gall stones. Gut 24: 836–844
Goodman Z D, Ishak K G 1981 Xanthogranulomatous cholecystitis. American Journal of Surgical Pathology 5: 653–659
Greenwood R K 1963 Torsion of the gallbladder. Gut 4: 27–29
Greig J D, John T G, Mahadaven M, Garden O J 1994 Laparoscopic ultrasonography in the evaluation of the biliary tree during laparoscopic cholecystectomy. British Journal of Surgery 84: 1202–1206
Greig J D, Mahadaven M, John T G, Garden O J 1996 Comparison of manual and ultrasonographic evaluation of bladder size in patients prior to laparoscopy. Surgical Endoscopy 10: 432–433
Griffen W O, Bivins B A, Rogers E L, Shearer G R, Liebschutz D, Lieber A 1980 Cholecystokinin cholecystography in the diagnosis of gallbladder disease. Annals of Surgery 191: 636–640
Guthrie C M, Haddock G, de Beaux A C, Garden O J, Carter D C 1993 Changing trends in the management of extrahepatic cholangiocarcinoma. British Journal of Surgery 80: 1434–1449
Hadjis N S, Carr D, Blenkharn I, Banks L, Gibson R, Blumgart L H 1986 Expectant management of patients with unilateral hepatic duct stricture and liver atrophy. Gut 27: 1223–1227
Ham J M 1980 Acalculous benign biliary disease. In G A Kune & A Sali (eds) The practice of biliary surgery, 2nd edn. Blackwell, Oxford
Hand B H 1973 Anatomy and function of the extrahepatic biliary system. Clinics in Gastroenterology 2: 3–29
Hardison W G M, Tomaszewski N, Grundy S M 1979 Effect of acute alterations in small bowel transit time upon the biliary excretion rate of bile acids. Gastroenterology 76: 568–574
Heaton K W 1973 The epidemiology of gallstones and suggested aetiology. Clinics in Gastroenterology 2: 67–83
Herzog U, Mesmer P, Sutter M, Tondelli P 1992 Surgical treatment for cholelithiasis. Surgery, Gynecology and Obstetrics 175: 238–242
Holan K R, Holzbach R T, Hermann R E, Cooperman A M, Claffey W J 1979 Nucleation time: a key factor in the pathogenesis of cholesterol gallstone disease. Gastroenterology 77: 611–617
Holzbach R T, Kibe A, Thiel E, Howell J H, Marsh M, Hermann R E 1984 Biliary proteins. Unique inhibitors of cholesterol crystal nucleation in human gallbladder bile. Journal of Clinical Investigations 73: 35–37
Hopkins S F, Bivins B A, Griffen W O Jr 1979 The problem of the cystic duct remnant. Surgery, Gynecology and Obstetrics 148: 531–533
Hossack K F, Herron J J 1972 Benign tumours of the common bile duct. Report of a case and review of literature. Australian and New Zealand Journal of Surgery 42: 22–26
Inouye A A, Whelan T J 1978 Carcinoma of the extrahepatic bile ducts. A ten year experience in Hawaii. American Journal of Surgery 136: 90–95
Iser J H, Dowling R H, Mok H Y I, Bell G D 1975 Chenodeoxycholic acid treatment of gallstones. New England Journal of Medicine 293: 333–378
Ishak K G, Rogers W A 1981 Cryptogenic acute cholangitis – association with toxic shock syndrome. American Journal of Clinical Pathology 76: 619–626
John T G, Greig J D, Crosbie J, Miles W F A, Garden O J 1994 Superior staging of liver tumors with laparoscopy and laparoscopic ultrasound. Annals of Surgery 220: 711–719
Josephs L F, Birkett D H 1992 Laser lithotripsy for the management of retained stones. Archives of Surgery 127: 603–605
Jutras J A, Jutras H P L 1966 Adenomyoma and adenomyomatosis of the gallbladder. Radiological Clinics of North America 4: 483–500
Kaye M D, Kern F 1971 Clinical relationships of gallstones. Lancet 1: 1228–1230
Keighley M R B 1977 Micro-organisms in the bile. A preventable cause of sepsis after biliary surgery. Annals of the Royal College of Surgeons of England 59: 329–334
Keighley M R B 1982 Infection and the biliary tree. In L H Blumgart (ed) The biliary tract. Churchill Livingstone, Edinburgh, p 219
Keighley M R B, Baddeley R M, Burdon D W et al 1975 A controlled trial of parenteral prophylactic gentamicin therapy in biliary surgery. British Journal of Surgery 62: 275–279
Keighley M R B, Razay G, Fitzgerald M 1984 Influence of diabetes on mortality and morbidity following operations for obstructive jaundice. Annals of the Royal College of Surgeons of England 66: 49–51
Kelley C J, Blumgart L H 1985 Per-operative cholangiography and post-

cholecystectomy biliary stricture. Annals of the Royal College of Surgeons of England 67: 93–95
Kill J, Kruse A, Rokkjaer M 1989 Large bile duct stones treated by endoscopic biliary drainage. Surgery 105: 51–56
Krain H S 1972 Gallbladder and extrahepatic bile duct carcinoma. Analysis of 1,808 cases. Geriatrics 27: 111–117
Kune G A 1964 Surgical anatomy of common bile duct. Archives of Surgery 89: 995–1004
Kune G A 1979 Bile duct injury during cholecystectomy: causes, prevention and surgical repair in 1979. Australian and New Zealand Journal of Surgery 49: 35–50
Kune G A, Birks D 1970 Acute cholecystitis. An appraisal of current methods of treatment. Medical Journal of Australia 2: 218–221
Kune G A, Burdon J G W 1975 Are antibiotics necessary in acute cholecystitis? Medical Journal of Australia 2: 627–630
Kune G A, Sali A 1981 Benign biliary strictures. In: L H Blumgart (ed) The practice of biliary surgery. Blackwell, Oxford
Kune G A, Schutz E 1974 Bacteria in the biliary tract. A study of their frequency and type. Medical Journal of Australia 1: 255–258
La Ferla G, Murray W R 1987 Carcinoma of the head of the pancreas: bypass surgery in unresectable disease. British Journal of Surgery 74: 212–213
Lai E C S, Mok F P T, Tan E S Y et al 1992a Endoscopic biliary drainage for severe acute cholangitis. New England Journal of Medicine 326: 1582–1586
Lai E C S, Chu K M, Lo C Y et al 1992b Surgery for malignant obstructive jaundice: analysis of mortality. Surgery 112: 891–896
Lam S K, Wong K P, Chan P K W, Ngan H, Ong G B 1978 Recurrent pyogenic cholangitis as studied by endoscopic retrograde cholangiography. Gastroenterology 74: 1196–1203
Lambert M E, Martin D F, Tweedle D F 1988 Endoscopic removal of retained stones after biliary surgery. British Journal of Surgery 75: 896–898
Lambert M E, Betts C D, Hill J et al 1991 Endoscopic sphincterotomy: the whole truth. British Journal of Surgery 78: 473–476
LaMorte W W, Schoetz D J Jr, Birkett D J, Williams L F Jr 1979 The role of the gallbladder in the pathogenesis of cholesterol gallstones. Gastroenterology 77: 580–592
Langer J C, Langer B, Taylor B R, Zeldin R, Cummings B 1985 Carcinoma of the extrahepatic bile ducts: results of an aggressive surgical approach. Surgery 98: 752–757
Leese T, Neoptolemos J P, Carr-Locke D L 1985 Successes, failures, early complications in their management following endoscopic sphincterotomy: results of 394 consecutive patients from a single centre. British Journal of Surgery 72: 215–219
Leese T, Neoptolemos J P, Baker A R, Carr-Locke D L 1986 Management of acute cholangitis and the impact of endoscopic sphincterotomy. British Journal of Surgery 73: 988–992
Lennard T W J, Farndon J R, Taylor R M R 1984 Acalculous biliary pain: diagnosis and selection for cholecystectomy using the cholecystokinin test for pain reproduction. British Journal of Surgery 71: 368–370
Leung J W, Chung S C S, Sung J J Y, Banez C P, Li A K C 1989 Urgent endoscopic drainage for acute suppurative cholangitis. Lancet 1: 1307–1309
Mahour G R, Wakin K G, Ferris D O 1967 The common bile duct in man: its diameter and circumference. Annals of Surgery 165: 415–419
McArthur P, Cuschieri A, Sells R A, Shields R 1975 Controlled clinical trial comparing early with interval cholecystectomy for acute cholecystitis. British Journal of Surgery 62: 850–852
McPherson G A D, Benjamin I S, Hodgson H J F, Bowley N B, Allison D J, Blumgart L H 1984 Pre-operative percutaneous transhepatic biliary drainage: the results of a controlled trial. British Journal of Surgery 71: 371–375
McSherry C K, Glenn F 1980 The incidence and causes of death following surgery for nonmalignant biliary tract disease. Annals of Surgery 191: 271–275
McSherry C K, Stubenbord W T, Glenn F 1969 The significance of air in the biliary system and liver. Surgery, Gynecology and Obstetrics 128: 49–53
McSherry C K, Ferstenberg H, Calhoun W F, Lahman E, Virshup M 1985 The natural history of diagnosed gallstone disease in symptomatic and asymptomatic patients. Annals of Surgery 202: 59–63
Meyers W C 1991 A prospective analysis of 1,518 laparoscopic cholecystectomies. New England Journal of Medicine 324: 1073–1078
Milroy 1947 An important anomaly of the right hepatic duct and its bearing on the operation of cholecystectomy. British Journal of Surgery 35: 383–385
Moody F G, Becker J M, Potts J R 1983 Transduodenal sphincteroplasty and transampullary septectomy for postcholecystectomy pain. Annals of Surgery 197: 627–636
Morran C G, McNaught W, McArdle C S 1978 Prophylactic cotrimoxazole in biliary surgery. British Medical Journal 2: 462–464
Murugiah M, Windsor J A, Redhead D et al 1993 The role of selective visceral angiography in the management of pancreatic and periampullary cancer. World Journal of Surgery 17: 796–800
Nakayama T, Ideka A, Okuda K 1978 Percutaneous transhepatic drainage of the biliary tract. Technique and results in 104 cases. Gastroenterology 74: 554–559
Neoptolemos J P, Hofmann A F, Moossa A R 1986 Chemical treatment of stones in the biliary tree. British Journal of Surgery 73: 515–524
Neoptolemos J P, Carr-Locke D L, Fossard D P 1987 Prospective randomised study of preoperative endoscopic sphincterotomy versus surgery alone for common bile duct stones. British Medical Journal 294: 470–474
Neoptolemos J P, Hall C, O'Connor D, W R M, Carr-Locke D L 1990 Methyl-tertbutyl-ether for treating bile duct stones: the British experience. British Journal of Surgery 77: 32–35
Nielsen M L, Justesen T 1976 Anaerobic and aerobic bacteriological studies in biliary tract disease. Scandinavian Journal of Gastroenterology 11: 437–446
Nilsson S 1966 Gallbladder disease and sex hormones. A statistical study. Acta Chirurgica Scandinavica 132: 275–279
Nimura Y, Hayakawa N, Kamiya J, Kondo S, Shionoya S 1990 Hepatic segmentectomy with caudate lobe resection for bile duct carcinoma with a hepatic hilus. World Journal of Surgery 14: 535–544
Nolan J P 1978 Bacteria and the liver. New England Journal of Medicine 299: 1069–1071
Northover J M A, Terblanche J 1979 A new look at the arterial supply of the bile duct in man and its surgical implications. British Journal of Surgery 66: 379–384
Nunnerley H B, Karani J B 1990 Interventional radiology of the biliary tract. Introductory Radiation, Radiological Clinics of North America 28: 1237–1240
Nussinson E, Cairns S R, Varia D, Dowsett J F, Mason R R 1991 A ten year single centre experience of percutaneous and endoscopic extraction of bile duct stone with T-tube in situ. Gut 32: 1040–1043
O'Doherty D P, Neoptolemos J P, Carr-Locke D L 1986 Endoscopic sphincterotomy for retained common bile duct stones in patients with T-tube in situ in the early post-operative period. British Journal of Surgery 73: 454 –456
O'Donnell L D J, Heaton K W 1988 Recurrence and re-recurrence of gallstones after medical dissolution: a longterm follow up. Gut 29: 655–658
O'Rourke N, Nathanson L 1994 Laparoscopic biliary-enteric bypass. In: S Paterson-Brown & O J Garden (eds) Principles and practice of surgical laparoscopy. W B Saunders, London, p 179–189
Pace B W, Cosgrove J, Brewer B, Margolis I B 1992 Intraoperative cholangiography revisited. Archives of Surgery 127: 448–450
Pain J A, Bailey M E 1986 Experimental and clinical study of lactulose in obstructive jaundice. British Journal of Surgery 73: 775–778
Palmer K R, Hofmann A F 1986 Intraductal mono-octanoin for the direct dissolution of bile duct stones: experience in 343 patients. Gut 27: 196–202
Paterson-Brown S, Garden O J, Carter D C 1991 Laparoscopic cholecystectomy. British Journal of Surgery 78: 131–132
Paterson-Brown S, de Beaux A, Greig J D, Garden O J 1994 Laparoscopic cholecystectomy. In S Paterson-Brown & O J Garden (eds) Principles and practice of laparoscopic surgery. W B Saunders, London, p 67–77
Pedrosa C S, Casanova R, Rodriguez R 1981 Computed tomography in obstructive jaundice. Part I: The level of obstruction. Radiology 139: 627–634
Perpetuo M D C M O, Valdivieso K, Heilbrun L K, Nelson R S,

Connor T, Bodey G P 1978 Natural history study of gallbladder cancer. A review of 36 years experience at M D Anderson Hospital and Tumor Institute. Cancer 42: 330–335
Pertsemlidis D, Panveliwalla D, Ahrens E H Jr 1974 Effects of clofibrate and of an estrogen-progestin combination of fasting biliary lipids and cholic acid kinetics in man. Gastroenterology 66: 565–573
Petelin J 1991 Laparoscopic approach to common duct pathology. American Journal of Surgery 165: 487–491
Petelin J 1994 Laparoscopic management of choledocholithiasis. In: S Paterson-Brown & O J Garden (eds) Principles and practice of surgical laparoscopy. W B Saunders, London, p 141–156
Pitman R G, Davies A 1963 The clinical and radiological features of spontaneous internal biliary fistulae. British Journal of Surgery 50: 414–416
Pitt H A, Cameron J L, Postier R G, Gadacz T R 1981 Factors affecting mortality in biliary tract surgery. American Journal of Surgery 141: 66–72
Pitt H A, Gomes A S, Lois J F, Mann L L, Deutsch L S, Longmire W P 1985 Does preoperative percutaneous biliary drainage reduce operative risk or increase hospital cost? Annals of Surgery 201: 545–553
Prakash A T M, Sharma L K, Pandit P N 1975 Primary carcinoma of the gallbladder. British Journal of Surgery 62: 33–36
Pyrtek L J, Bartus S A 1967 An evaluation of antibiotics in biliary tract surgery. Surgery, Gynecology and Obstetrics 125: 101–105
Reynolds B M, Dargan E I 1959 Acute obstructive cholangitis – a distinct clinical syndrome. Annals of Surgery 150: 299–303
Roberts-Thomson I C 1980 Stenosis of the papilla of Vater. In: G A Kune & A Sali (eds) The practice of biliary surgery. Blackwell, Oxford
Roberts-Thomson I C, Pannall P R, Toouli J 1989 Relationship between morphine responses and sphincter of Oddi motility in undefined biliary pain after cholecystectomy. Journal of Gastroenterology and Hepatology 4: 317–324
Roberts-Thomson I C, Jonsson J R, Frewin D B, Coates G C 1990 Sympathetic activation: a mechanism for morphine induced pain and rises in liver enzymes after cholecystectomy? Gut 31(2): 217–221
Roberts-Thomson I C, Fettman M J, Jonsson J R, Frewin D B 1992 Responses to cholecystokinin octapeptide in patients with functional abdominal pain syndromes. Journal of Gastroenterology and Hepatology 7: 293–297
Roslyn J J, Pitt H A, Mann L L, Ament M E, DenBesten L 1983 Gallbladder disease in patients on long-term parenteral nutrition. Gastroenterology 84: 148–154
Ruddell W S J, Lintott D J, Ashton M G, Axon A T R 1980 Endoscopic retrograde cholangiography and pancreatography in investigation of post-cholecystectomy patients. Lancet 1: 444–447
Sackmann M, Delius M, Sauerbruch T et al 1988 Shockwave lithotripsy of gallbladder stones: the first 175 patients. New England Journal of Medicine 318: 393–397
Sackmann M, Ippisch E, Sauerbruch T et al 1990 Early gallstone recurrence rate after successful shockwave therapy. Gastroenterology 98: 392–396
Samuels B I, Freitas J E, Gross M D 1985 A pragmatic review of gallbladder imaging. Seminars on Ultrasound, CT and MR 6:156
Sarles H, Sahel J 1978 Cholestasis and lesions of the biliary tract in chronic pancreatitis. Gut 19: 851–857
Sarr M G, Cameron J L 1982 Surgical management of unresectable carcinoma of the pancreas. Surgery 91: 123–133
Sato H, Mizushima M, Ito J, Doi K 1985 Sessile adenoma of the gallbladder. Archives of Pathology and Laboratory Medicine 109: 65–69
Schersten T 1973 Formation of lithogenic bile in man. Digestion 9: 540–553
Scragg R K R, McMichael A J, Seamark R F 1984a Oral contraceptives, pregnancy, and endogenous oestrogen in gall stone disease – a case-control study. British Medical Journal 288: 1795–1799
Scragg R K R, McMichael A J, Paghurst P A 1984b Diet, alcohol, and relative weight in gall stone disease: a case-control study. British Medical Journal 288: 1113
Sedgwick G E, Poulantzas J K, Kune G A 1966 Management of portal hypertension secondary to biliary duct strictures. Annals of Surgery 163: 949–953
Shapero T F, Rosen I E, Wilson S R, Fisher M M 1982 Discrepancy between ultrasound and oral cholecystography in the assessment of gallstone dissolution. Hepatology 2: 587–590
Shaw M J, Mackie R D, Moore J P et al 1993 Results of a multicentre trial using a mechanical lithotriptor for the treatment of large bile duct stones. American Journal of Gastroenterology 88: 730–733
Shea W J, Demas B E, Goldberg H I, Hohn D C, Ferrell L D, Kerlan R K 1985 Sclerosing cholangitis associated with hepatic arterial FUDR chemotherapy: radiographic-histologic correlation. American Journal of Roentgenology 146: 717–721
Siegel J H 1981 Endoscopic papillotomy in the treatment of biliary tract disease: 258 procedures and results. Digestive Diseases and Sciences 26: 1057–1064
Smith B F, LaMont J T 1986 The central issue of cholesterol gallstones. Hepatology 6: 529–531
Smith L O M 1979 Obstructions of the bile duct. British Journal of Surgery 66: 69–79
Smith A C, Dowsett J F, Russell R C G et al 1994 Randomised trial of endoscopic versus percutaneous stent insertion in malignant obstructive jaundice. Lancet 344: 1655–1660
Soloway R D, Trotman B W, Ostrow J D 1977 Pigment gallstones. Gastroenterology 72: 167–182
Somjen G J, Gilat T 1985 Contribution of vesicular and micellar carriers to cholesterol transport in human bile. Journal of Lipid Research 26: 699–704
Southern Surgeons Club 1991 A prospective analysis of 1518 laparoscopic cholecystectomies. New England Journal of Medicine 324: 1073–1078
Spivak W, Hoogerhyde K J, Yuey W 1984 Non-enzymatic alkaline hydrolysis and isomerization of pure bilirubin monoglucuronide (BMG) to unconjugated bilirubin in model bile systems and the coprecipitation of BMG and UCB. Hepatology 4: 1065
Stone B G, Gavaler J S, Belle S H et al 1988 Impairment of gallbladder emptying in diabetes mellitus. Gastroenterology 95: 170–176
Strachan C J, Black J, Powis S J et al 1977 Prophylactic use of cephazolin against wound sepsis after cholecystectomy. British Medical Journal 1: 1245–1256
Sunderland G T, Carter D C 1988 Clinical application of the cholecystokinin provocation test. British Journal of Surgery 75: 444–449
Terblanche J 1976 Is carcinoma of the main hepatic duct junction an indication for liver transplantation or palliative surgery? A plea for the U tube palliative procedure. Surgery 79: 127–128
Thistle J L, Schoenfield L J 1971 Induced alterations in composition of bile of persons having cholelithiasis. Gastroenterology 61: 488–496
Thorbjarnarson B 1960 Carcinoma of the gallbladder and acute cholecystitis. Annals of Surgery 151: 241–244
Tokyo Co-operative Society Gallstone Study Group 1980 Efficacy and indication of ursodeoxycholic acid treatment for dissolving gallstones. A multicenter double-blind trial. Gastroenterology 78: 542
Tompkins R K 1982 Carcinoma of the gallbladder and biliary ducts. In: L H Blumgart (ed) The biliary tract. Churchill Livingstone, Edinburgh, p 183
Tompkins R K, Thomas D, Wile A, Longmore W P 1981 Prognostic factors in bile duct carcinoma. Analysis of 96 cases. Annals of Surgery 194: 447–456
Toouli J 1984 Sphincter of Oddi motility. British Journal of Surgery 71: 251–256
Toouli J, Geenen J E, Hogan W J, Dodds W J, Arndorfer R C 1982 Sphincter of Oddi motor activity: a comparison between patients with common bile duct stones and controls. Gastroenterology 82: 111–117
Toouli J, Bushell M, Stevenson G, Dent J, Wycherley A, Iannos J 1986 Gallbladder emptying in man related to fasting duodenal migrating motor contractions. Australian and New Zealand Journal of Surgery 56: 147–151
Toouli J, Roberts-Thomson I C 1987 Endoscopic manometry of the sphincter of Oddi. Journal of Gastroenterology and Hepatology 2: 431–442
Torsoli A, Corazziari E, Habib F et al 1986 Frequencies and cyclical pattern of the human sphincter of Oddi phasic activity. Gut 27: 363–369
Torvik A, Hoivik B 1960 Gallstones in an autopsy series. Incidence, complications and correlations with carcinoma of the gallbladder. Acta Chirurgica Scandinavica 120: 168

Tritapepe R, di Padova C, di Padova F 1988 Non-invasive treatment for retained common bile duct stones in patients with T-tube in situ: saline wash-out after intravenous ceruletide. British Journal of Surgery 75: 144–146
Tsunoda T, Tsuchiya R, Harada N, Noda T, Yamamoto K 1985 Surgical treatment for carcinoma of the extrahepatic bile duct. Japanese Journal of Surgery 15: 123–129
Unger S W, Rosenbaum G, Unger H M, Edelman D S 1993 A comparison of laparoscopic and open treatment of acute cholecystitis. Surgical Endoscopy 7: 408–411
Vaittinen E 1970 Carcinoma of the gallbladder: a study of 390 cases diagnosed in Finland 1953–1967. Annales Chirurgiae et Gynaecologiae Fenniae 59 (suppl 168): 1–81
Van der Linden W, Edlund G 1981 Early versus delayed cholecystectomy: the effect of a change in management. British Journal of Surgery 68: 753–757
Varia D, Ainley C S W et al 1982 Endoscopic sphincterotomy in 1000 consecutive patients. Lancet 1: 431–433
Vennes J A, Jacobson J R, Silris S E 1984 Endoscopic cholangiography for biliary system diagnosis. Annals of Internal Medicine 80: 61–65
Warren K W, Hardy K J, O'Rourke M G E 1968 Primary neoplasia of the gallbladder. Surgery, Gynecology and Obstetrics 126: 1036–1040
Warren K W, Christophi C, Armendariz R 1982 The evaluation and current perspectives of the treatment of benign bile duct strictures: a review. Surgical Gastroenterology 1: 141–154
Warshaw A L, Zhuo-yun G U, Wittenberg J et al 1990 Preoperative staging and assessment of resectability of pancreatic cancer. Archives of Surgery 125: 230–233
Watts J M, Toouli J, Whiting M J 1982 Gallstone dissolution present and future. In: L H Blumgart (ed) The biliary tract. Churchill Livingstone, Edinburgh, p 17
Webber J, Ademak H E, Riemann J F 1992 Extracorporeal piezoelectric lithotripsy for retained bile duct stones. Endoscopy 24: 239–243
Weiner S N, Koenigsberg M, Morehouse H, Hoffman J 1984 Sonography and computed tomography in diagnosis of carcinoma of the gallbladder. American Journal of Roentgenology 142: 735–739
Welton J C, Marr J S, Friedman S M 1979 Association between hepatobiliary cancer and typhoid carrier state. Lancet 1: 791–794
Wenckert A, Robertson B 1966 The natural course of gallstone disease. Eleven year review of 781 unoperated cases. Gastroenterology 50: 376–381
Williamson B W A, Percy-Robb I W 1980 Contribution of biliary lipids to calcium binding in bile. Gastroenterology 78: 696–702
Williamson R C N 1988 Acalculous disease of the gall bladder. Gut 29: 860–872
Wilson P, Lees E T, Morgan W P, Kelly J F, Brigg J 1991 Elective laparoscopic cholecystectomy for all comers. Lancet 338: 795–797
Wilson T G 1986 Is operative cholangiography always necessary? British Journal of Surgery 73: 637–640
Windsor J A, Garden O J 1993 Laparoscopic ultrasonography. Australian and New Zealand Journal of Surgery 63: 1–2
Wosiewitz U, Schenk J, Sabinski F, Schmack B 1983 Investigations on common bile duct stones. Digestion 26: 43–52
Yamagiwa H, Tomiyama H 1986 Intestinal metaplasia-dysplasia-carcinoma sequence of the gallbladder. Acta Pathologica Japonica 36: 989–997
Zeman R K, Jaffe M H, Grant E G, et al 1984 Imaging of the liver, biliary tract, and pancreas. Medical Clinics of North America 68: 1535–1563

# 49. Physiology of the pancreas, congenital abnormalities and cystic fibrosis

*Randall K. Pearson*

## THE DEVELOPMENT OF THE PANCREATIC DUCT SYSTEM

The pancreas develops from ventral and dorsal outpouchings of the primitive doudenum. The ventral outpouching, which also gives rise to the liver and biliary system, rotates around the gut during development and this allows the eventual fusion of the dorsal pancreas and the ventral pancreas. The dorsal pancreas which forms part of the head, the uncinate process and all of the body and tail empties into the duodenum through the duct of Santorini (Fig. 49.1) and the ventral pancreas is drained by the duct of Wirsung. Once the ventral pancreas has fused with the dorsal pancreas, most of the drainage occurs through the duct of Wirsung. The duct of Santorini remains as a branch of the duct of Wirsung or it may drain directly into the duodenum. The termination of the pancreatic duct is very variable (Berman et al 1960). The common bile duct and the duct of Wirsung share a common opening into the duodenum in 85% of cases. When the duct systems fail to fuse, this is called "pancreas divisum" or "ventral pancreas".

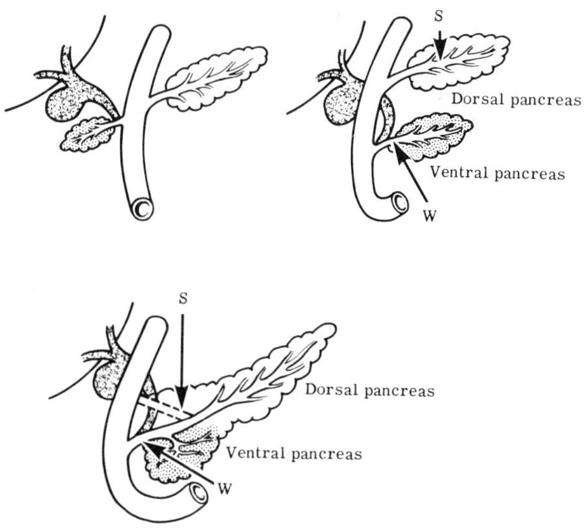


**Fig. 49.1** Development of the pancreatic duct system. The ventral and dorsal pancreas fuse to create an anastomosis between the duct systems. S = duct of Santorini; W = duct of Wirsung (Hadorn 1975).

## CONGENITAL ABNORMALITIES

### Pancreas divisum

Pancreas divisum is present in up to 10% of the population and in the majority is of no clinical significance. The anomaly arises from failure of the dorsal and ventral pancreas to unite, so that most of the pancreas is drained by the duct of Santorini through the accessory papilla.

#### *Pancreatitis in pancreas divisum*

Pancreatitis, whether due to alcohol or other causes, may occur in patients with pancreas divisum as in those with normal fusion. However, it has been suggested that a relative obstruction may occur at the accessory papilla owing to the fact that it is normally smaller than the major papilla. Some workers have suggested that the anomaly may result in an increased incidence of idiopathic recurrent pancreatitis (Cotton 1980, Warshaw et al 1983) and may account for some patients with obscure abdominal pain (Warshaw et al 1983). In practice there is little objective evidence to support this hypothesis (Rosch et al 1976, Mitchell et al 1979, Delhaye et al 1985, Sugawa et al 1987) and figures may have been biased by the referral of these patients to centers with particular interest in the condition. Attempts to treat pancreatitis in these patients by accessory sphincterotomy, either endoscopic or surgical, have not been successful in the long term (Russell et al 1984). It is possible that a small proportion of patients with pancreas divisum have stenosis of the accessory papilla leading to pancreatitis, just as patients with normal fusion of the pancreas may develop pancreatitis as a result of stenosis of the main papilla, but this probably accounts for only a very small minority of cases (p. 1248).

*Clinical features and diagnosis of pancreas divisum* (Warshaw et al 1983)

The majority of individuals with pancreas divisum are asymptomatic. A minority present with idiopathic recurrent pancreatitis or with obscure abdominal pain suggesting pancreatitis. The diagnosis is made at endoscopic retrograde pancreatography. The accessory (minor) papilla can be cannulated in no more than 70% of cases. Cannulation demonstrates that this is the major drainage system and indicates whether stenosis is present. By contrast the duct of Wirsung is foreshortened and ends with fine arborizations; this is in contrast to the abrupt termination seen in cancer of the pancreas.

*Treatment*

Endoscopic papillotomy or surgical sphincteroplasty has been used when no other cause has been found for recurrent pancreatitis in patients with pancreas divisum (Warshaw et al 1983, Ressell et al 1984). However, results have been disappointing and pancreatic resection may be more effective.

## Annular pancreas

This arises from abnormal development of the ventral pancreas which leaves the duodenum surrounded by pancreatic tissue. Half of the cases develop vomiting in the first year of life, mostly during the first week. The other half present in adult life. The condition may be associated with other congenital abnormalities including duodenal atresia (p. 330), malrotation and Down's syndrome. In adults, the symptoms suggest pyloric stenosis. Barium studies show constriction in the second part of the duodenum, usually proximal to the papilla of Vater. The mucosal folds remain intact and the constriction should be differentiated from other causes of duodenal stenosis such as peptic ulcer, pancreatitis and pancreatic cancer. The diagnosis can be confirmed by ERCP (Dharmsathaphorn et al 1979). The treatment is surgical; the pancreatic tissue cannot be resected because of its intimate relationship with the duodenum and so duodenoduodenostomy or duodenojejunostomy is performed.

## Left-sided pancreas (Dunn & Gibson 1986)

The head of the pancreas is not anterior to the aorta and inferior vena cava but is displaced to the left of the midline together with the superior mesenteric artery and vein. This condition may be responsible for a failed ultrasound examination because of failure to locate the organ.

## Ectopic pancreatic tissue

Nodules of ectopic pancreatic tissue occur in the upper gastrointestinal tract in approximately one in 400 persons (Nickels & Laasonen 1976); they may also occur in the lower gastrointestinal tract and possibly elsewhere in the body. Most are found in the submucosa of the stomach or duodenum (Palmer 1951), particularly on the greater curvature of the stomach near to the pylorus.

Nodules may cause symptoms suggesting peptic ulceration and may also cause hematemesis and melena or pyloric obstruction. However, in a large series of cases from the Mayo Clinic it was concluded that ectopic pancreatic tissue was usually unrelated to the patients' symptoms (Dolan et al 1974). The barium meal may show a smooth sessile nodule (1–4 cm diameter) in the stomach or duodenum and barium may occasionally enter the fine duct in the center of the nodule (Kilman & Berk 1977). It is important to differentiate such appearances from those due to neoplasm. Endoscopy confirms that the nodule is submucosal and a central dimple is seen which represents the opening of the duct. Treatment is by local excision.

## Congenital cysts

These are very rare and come to attention as an abdominal mass in an otherwise well patient. Such pancreatic cysts occur occasionally in cystic fibrosis (p. 388) and in polycystic disease of the kidneys and liver. Differentiation of the various cystic conditions affecting the pancreas is considerably aided by computed tomography supplemented where necessary by fine-needle aspiration biopsy.

# THE STRUCTURE OF THE PANCREAS

The pancreas is retroperitoneal and derives its arterial blood supply from branches of the splenic, gastroduodenal and superior mesenteric arteries. The autonomic nerve supply is from the celiac plexus (p. 1233).

The exocrine pancreas consists of epithelial cell acini which synthesize and secrete protein. Many acini make up each lobule (Fig. 49.2). The lumen of the acinus connects with a duct lined by centroacinar cells which, together with the cells lining the other ducts, are responsible for bicarbonate secretion (p. 1229).

The acinar cells are pyramidal in shape with the apex towards the lumen. The basal part of the cell contains the nucleus and basophilic endoplasmic reticulum; the apical part of the cell contains zymogen granules and its surface has microvillous processes; the zymogens are extruded by exocytosis. The Golgi apparatus is situated in the intermediate region of the cell. The centroacinar cells are smaller than acinar cells and have less cytoplasm and no zymogen granules; there are many large mitochondria and a few vesicles. In contrast to the acinar cell, the centroacinar cell contains carbonic anhydrase which is important in fluid and electrolyte secretion. Other morphological features are reviewed by Gorelick & Jamieson (1981). The endocrine cells of the pancreas are grouped in the islets of Langerhans with the A cells outermost (producing

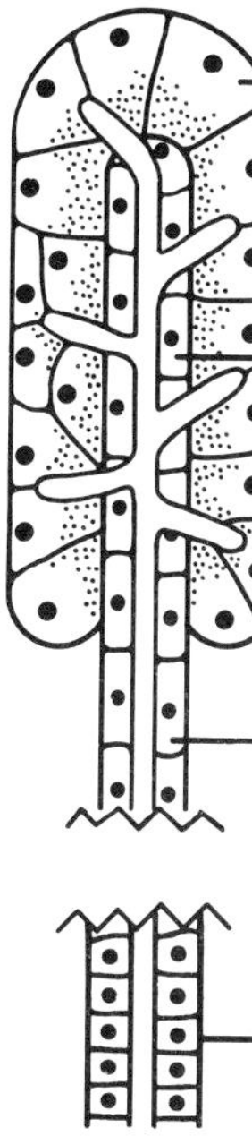


**Fig. 49.2** The cellular structure of the exocrine pancreas (Harper 1967).

glucagon), the B cells innermost (producing insulin) and the D cells in an intermediate position (producing somatostatin, gastrin and pancreatic polypeptide). The islets are surrounded by capillaries which anastomose with capillaries around the acini, implying that islet cell hormones may influence exocrine secretion. Within the pancreas the autonomic nerve fibers are cholinergic (as indicated by the muscarinic receptor on the acinar cell), sympathetic (supplying blood vessels) and peptidergic; these nerve fibers produce somatostatin, vasoactive intestinal polypeptide and enkephalin.

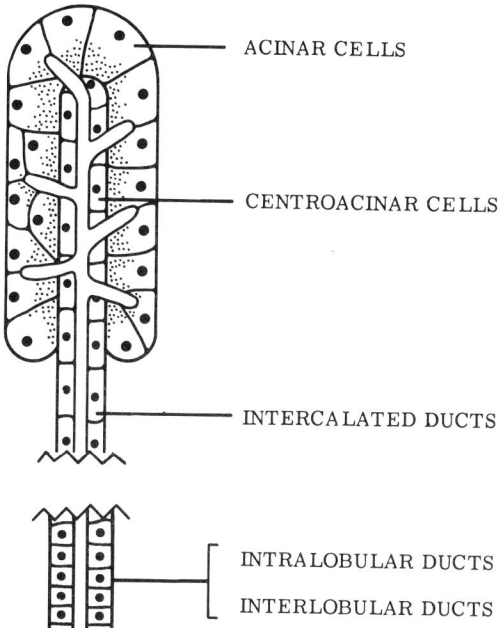

## THE EXOCRINE FUNCTION OF THE PANCREAS

### Secretion of electrolytes

The mechanisms of secretion of electrolytes into pancreatic juice are complex and incompletely understood, with marked species variation (Case & Argent 1993). The most striking features of pancreatic juice are that it is isotonic with plasma under all conditions and that it has a high concentration of bicarbonate which is dependent on flow rate. Hollander and Birnbaum proposed that this bicarbonate secretion originated in the centroacinar and terminal duct cells. Much of the subsequent experimental data has largely supported this proposal. For example, experiments in several animal species in which selective damage to either acinar or ductular elements was induced led to a reduction in enzyme and electrolyte secretion respectively. Carbonic anhydrase has been shown by immunohistochemical techniques to be confined to the ductular and centroacinar cells. The ionic composition of pancreatic juice is shown in Table 49.1.

**Table 49.1** Composition of pancreatic juice (Dreiling 1969)

| | |
|---|---|
| Volume | 1200–3000 ml/24 hours |
| pH | 7.5–8.8 |
| Major cations | |
| $Na^+$ | 148 mmol/l |
| $K^+$ | 4.1–5.6 mmol/l |
| $Ca^{2+}$ | 4.4–6.4 mmol/l (2.2–3.2 mEq/l) |
| $Mg^{2+}$ | 0.6 mmol/l (0.3 mEq/l) |
| Major anions | |
| $HCO_3^-$ | 60–150 mmol/l |
| $Cl^-$ | 60–80 mmol/l |
| $So_4^{2-}$ | 16.8 mmol/l (8.4 mEq/l) |
| Total protein | 1.9–3.4 g/l |

*The cations*

Sodium is secreted at concentrations approximately 10 mmol/L higher than in plasma; potassium concentrations are almost identical in pancreatic juice and plasma. The concentrations of these cations are virtually independent of flow rate. Calcium, on the other hand, is secreted partly in combination with proteins and partly in ionic form. Changes in protein concentration which are produced by infusion of cholecystokinin (CCK) are accompanied by similar changes in calcium concentration and on the basis of regression analysis of these data it is concluded that up to 90% of the calcium is in a protein-associated form. The concentration of both $Ca^{2+}$ and $Mg^{2+}$ shows an inverse relationship to bicarbonate concentration (Nimmo et al 1970).

*The anions*

In contrast to the cations, the concentrations of bicarbonate and chloride are dependent on flow rate, increased flow rates being associated with high bicarbonate and low chloride. The relationship between these anions is reciprocal, their combined concentrations being constant under all conditions of flow. The basis for this reciprocal relationship appears to be an exchange between chloride and bicarbonate ions in the pancreatic duct system. Bicarbonate secretion takes place against an electrochemical gradient and is $Na^+$ dependent. This is balanced by active $H^+$ transport from the lumen to the interstitium of the gland, which can be measured as an acid tide (Anderton et al 1968).

*Mechanisms of secretion*

Secretin and VIP are the main stimuli for provoking water and electrolyte secretion (Chey 1993). There is convincing evidence in experimental animals that cyclic AMP has a role in secretion and in man, cyclic AMP appears in pancreatic juice in concentrations which are correlated with bicarbonate output. This rise in secretin occurs with delivery of scidic chyme to the doudenum. However, infusions of physiological doses of secretin evoke less bicarbonate secretion than does a meat meal in the dog, implying the influence of other factors. While CCK has little or no effect on bicarbonate secretion alone in humans, it potentiates the action of secretin to produce bicarbonate-rich secretion. Thus, large quantities of bicarbonate secretion in humans require the actions of both secretin and CCK. CCK acts via release of intracellular calcium. The site of this important potentiation remains to be clarified.

## Synthesis and secretion of enzymes

### *Synthesis of enzymes*

The pancreas has an extraordinary capacity for synthesis and secretion, delivering between 6 and 20 g of digestive enzymes or zymogen daily in an average volume of 2.5 L of bicarbonate-rich fluid. Thus, the pancreas secretes more protein per gram of tissue than any other organ, reflected by the highest uptake of amino acids per gram of tissue. In malnutrition, it is common to find reduced enzyme secretion as well as diseases producing altered pancreatic architecture (e.g. chronic pancreatitis).

### *Secretion of enzymes*

The receptors for secretagogues present on the acinar cell (Gardner & Jensen 1993) can be divided into those which activate phospholipase C and cAMP. CCK (and structurally related peptides gastrin and cerulein), muscarinic cholinergic agents, gastrin-releasing peptide (bombesin-like) and substance P act through phospholipase C which acts on membrane-bound lipids to release the second messengers inositol triphosphate, which releases intracellular $Ca^{2+}$, and diacylglycerol, which activates protein kinase C. Secretin, VIP and calcitonin gene-related peptide act through receptors linked to adenylate cyclase which raise intracellular cAMP levels, activating cAMP-dependent protein kinase. Both receptor types belong to the superfamily known as G protein coupled receptors. These receptors are integral plasma membrane glycoproteins which when occupied by an agonist, interact to promote the binding of GTP to a specific class of G proteins located on the cytoplasmic plasma membrane. GTP binding activates the G protein which then regulates the ion channel or enzyme responsible for second messenger generation, e.g. adenylate cyclase or phospholipase C. Both pathways result in an activation of protein kinase, which through protein phosphorylation stimulates enzyme secretion. While the two pathways begin functionally distinct, they clearly interact because potentiation of acinar cell secretion occurs when there is simultaneous activation.

The intracellular compartments involved in the secretory pathway were first established in the exocrine pancreas, earning a Nobel Prize for the investigators. The pancreatic acinar cell was a useful model because of its high rate of protein synthesis, such that more than 90% of synthesized proteins are targeted for the secretory pathway. This pathway begins with synthesis of the proenzymes in the rough endoplasmic reticulum, sorting in the Golgi apparatus where condensing vacuoles mature into zymogen granules. Zymogen granules accumulate in the apex of the acinar cell and fuse with their membranes with the apical plasmalemma with the appropriate stimulus and are discharged into the lumen. When the pancreas is stimulated by CCK there is simultaneous reduction in the zymogen granules in the acinar cells (Davies et al 1949). Some enzyme also enters the general circulation directly from the acinar cell; its fate is not known (Rothman & Grendell 1983).

Lysosomal hydrolases are also synthesized by ribosomes attached to the rough endoplasmic reticulum and transported to the Golgi complex and are passed into lysosomes. The lysosomal hydrolases are separated from digestive enzymes because they are phosphorylated at the 6-position of their mannose residues; they are thus recognized by specific phosphorylmannose receptors on the inner surface of the Golgi membranes. The separation of lysosomal and digestive enzymes is perturbed in animal models of pancreatitis and this colocalization of digestive proenzymes and active lysosomal enzymes has been proposed to be of pathogenic importance (Steers & Saluja 1993).

The duodenal fluid of neonates and infants contains no amylase and negligible amounts of lipase (Lebenthal & Lee 1980). By contrast, the levels of proteolytic enzymes are near to those in older children. The secretory response to secretagogues is absent or minimal at birth and is acquired during the postnatal period.

Some studies have shown that the various pancreatic enzymes are secreted in "parallel" (i.e. there is a constant ratio of proteolytic enzyme to lipase and amylase), while others show variations in the ratio between enzymes when the stimulus to secretion is varied (Sommer et al 1985). Enzyme secretion adapts slowly to the predominant component of the diet (Wormsley & Goldberg 1972).

Pancreatic enzymes are hydrolases which digest proteins, carbohydrates and fats. All of the proteolytic enzymes of the pancreas are synthesized in the form of zymogens which are activated in the duodenum by a process of limited proteolysis leading to conformational changes in the molecule. This process is a cascade phenomenon (Rinderknecht 1986) in which the first step is the activation of trypsinogen to form trypsin by enteropeptidase (enterokinase) released from the duodenal mucosa. Released trypsin ensures the activation of other zymogens such as proelastase, chymotrypsinogen, procarboxypeptidase and prophospholipase. Enterokinase deficiency and trypsinogen deficiency have been described (Townes et al

1967, Tarlow et al 1970). The α-amylase present in pancreatic juice hydrolyzes internal glucosidic bonds, producing mainly dextrins with different degrees of branching. Pancreatic juice contains a lipase which hydrolyzes triglycerides and a type A2 phospholipase which hydrolyzes phospholipids.

Among the proteins synthesized by the pancreas there are two which have profound effects on the activities of the enzymes described above. These are pancreatic trypsin inhibitor and pancreatic colipase. Human pancreatic juice contains relatively large concentrations of the trypsin inhibitor which acts to inhibit activated trypsin formed in pancreatic juice (Figarella et al 1980). Pancreatic colipase protein plays an essential role in the hydrolysis of dietary triglyceride by pancreatic lipase. It acts by fixing the lipase enzyme at the lipid–water interface which forms at the surface of the triglyceride emulsion in the duodenum and jejunum (Morgan et al 1969, Sari et al 1975) (p. 342).

## Pancreatic exocrine secretion

The human pancreas is able to secrete at a maximal rate of 4 ml/min with a bicarbonate concentration of 135–150 mmol/L but under physiological conditions it probably secretes just sufficient bicarbonate to neutralize the gastric acid entering the duodenum (DiMagno & Layer 1993). For example, in the dog there is a submaximal response to a solid meal (Henriksen & Worning 1969) and both bicarbonate and enzyme secretion reach only 75% of maximal and in the case of bicarbonate this response is brief, so that the pancreas secretes at 10% of maximal throughout most of the meal.

Pancreatic secretion is regulated by hormonal and neurogenic mechanisms. The important hormones which regulate the flow and composition of the juice are secretin and CCK. They are synthesized in the mucosa of the duodenum and upper jejunum and are released by hydrochloric acid (secretin) and certain nutrients (especially fat > protein) into the portal system whence they reach the general circulation and exert their effects on the pancreas, liver, gallbladder and small intestine, contributing to the co-ordination of pancreatic secretion with other physiological responses to a meal. Other regulatory peptides stimulate bicarbonate (VIP and PHI) and enzyme (bombesin/GRP, motilin, gastrin and substance P) secretion or inhibit secretion (PP, PYY and somatostatin). These peptides may be found in the enteropancreatic nerves. The autonomic nervous system has a major influence on pancreatic secretion through the release of acetylcholine by cholinergic postganglionic vagal neurones. Local nerve reflexes involving the enteric nervous system make important contributions to the regulation of secretion in both the fasting and fed state.

An intestinal feedback mechanism has been proposed whereby the presence of trypsin in the intestinal lumen suppresses the release of CCK. CCK-releasing peptides sensitive to inactivation by trypsin have been isolated from both the proximal small intestine and pancreatic juice. This mechanism is present in the rat and there is some evidence for it in humans (Slaff et al 1985). The regulation of pancreatic secretion is extremely complex. It is designed to respond to the need for a neutral environment in the duodenum and for digestion in the upper small intestine. It is co-ordinated closely with the activities of the stomach, gallbladder, liver and small intestine.

**Table 49.2** Effects of stimulants on pancreatic secretion

| Stimulant | Effect on Flow | Effect on Proenzyme output |
|---|---|---|
| Acetylcholine | + | ++++ |
| Secretin | ++++ | +? |
| Cholecystokinin | + | ++++ |
| Gastrin | +? | +? |

## Phases of pancreatic secretion

The effects of the main stimulants to pancreatic secretion are shown in Table 49.2 (Grossman 1971). The responses to secretin and to CCK, gastrin and acetylcholine are complementary and these main stimulants are involved to varying degrees in the phases of pancreatic secretion.

Grossman (1971) suggested the terms cephalic, gastric and intestinal phases of pancreatic secretion to denote the origin of the stimuli leading to release of the pancreatic stimulant. This is useful for explanatory purposes, but it is artificial since the phases are not sequential but proceed simultaneously. There is also an interdigestive phase.

### *Interdigestive phase*

In the human, the basal secretory rate is low but every 1–2 h secretion of bicarbonate and enzyme occurs for 10–15 min (Vantrappen et al 1979) in concert with increases in bile and gastric acid secretion and the interdigestive myoelectric complex.

### *Cephalic phase* (Fig. 49.3)

This is mediated by the vagus nerves, the stimuli being the thought, smell, taste or chewing of food. Vagal activity releases acetylcholine, which stimulates pancreatic proenzyme secretion and potentiates bicarbonate secretion (Defilippi et al 1982, Anagnostides et al 1984). The flow of proenzyme-rich secretion is perpetuated by other vagally mediated mechanisms, gastrin release from the antrum and gastrin-stimulated acid production which liberates secretin in the duodenum.

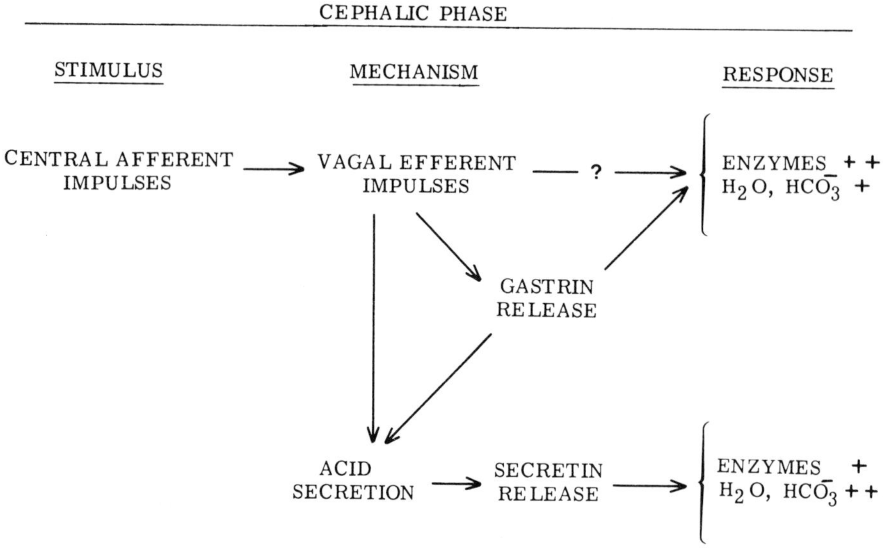


**Fig. 49.3** The cephalic phase of pancreatic secretion (Solomon & Grossman 1977).

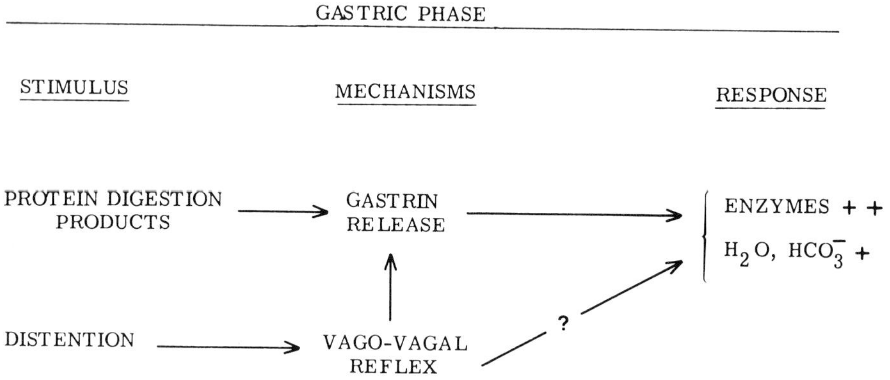


**Fig. 49.4** The gastric phase of pancreatic secretion (Solomon & Grossman 1977).

*Gastric phase* (Fig. 49.4)

Gastric distention causes vagovagal reflexes which activate pancreatic secretion. Although gastrin is also released, it has at most a minor role in these events.

*Intestinal phase* (Fig. 49.5)

This is quantitatively the most important phase. It is mediated by acid, amino acids, peptides, fatty acids, monoglycerides and calcium ions acting on the intestinal mucosa to release CCK, secretin and other hormones, the effects of which are described on page 159. The presence of bile acids in the duodenum will also stimulate the secretion of pancreatic enzymes (Wormsley 1970) and this may be important in co-ordinating fat digestion. These events are also mediated by enteropancreatic, vagovagal reflexes, some of which may be activated by receptors for volume and osmolality in the duodenum (Dooley & Valenzuela 1984). Vagotomy interrupts these reflexes, thereby reducing proenzyme secretion in response to intestinal stimulation (Fried et al 1985). These neural mechanisms likely account for 50% of the pancreatic secretory response to intraluminal nutrients with hormonal action of CCK accounting for most of the rest. When the intestinal mucosa is abnormal, as in celiac disease, pancreatic secretion may be impaired, presumably due to blunting of these neurohormonal stimulatory responses to a meal.

## Secretin

Secretin is the primary stimulant of pancreatic bicarbonate secretion but it may also have a small stimulating effect on proenzyme secretion (Gullo et al 1984, Beglinger et al 1985b). It is a basic polypeptide of 27 amino acids which has common amino acid sequences with glucagon, VIP and GIP. It is found in the S cells mainly in the duodenum but also in the upper small intestine. It has been isolated from porcine intestine, its amino acid sequence has been

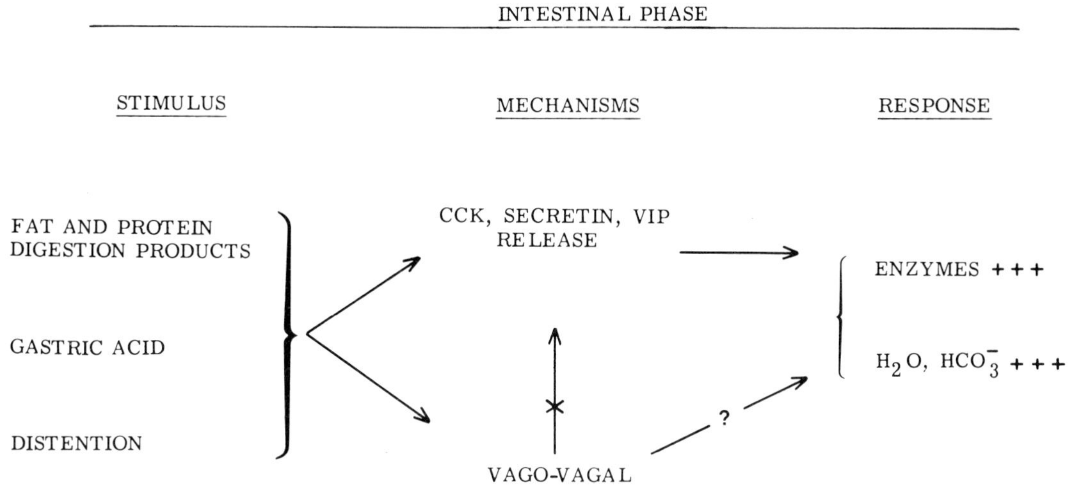


**Fig. 49.5** The intestinal phase of pancreatic secretion (Solomon & Grossman 1977).

determined, it has been synthesized (Mutt & Jorpes 1971) and the gene cloned (Fisher & Klinger 1985). Purified hog secretin and synthetic secretin show equal potency in stimulating pancreatic flow (Grossman 1971).

Secretin may be attached to a protein in the mucosa, from which it is released by bile acid, sodium oleate and by acid (Jorpes 1968) when pH is less than 4.5. Cimetidine abolishes the postprandial increase in secretin, indicating that acid is the most important releasing factor. The release of secretin is inhibited by somatostatin and metencephalin.

The rise in serum secretin in response to acid or food lasts for only 5–10 min (Beglinger et al 1985a) because it is rapidly metabolized in the capillary beds throughout the body. Secretin is also found in duodenal secretions. It stimulates pancreatic bicarbonate secretion in a dose of 0.1 clinical units/kg per hour. Its effect is potentiated by CCK and acetylcholine.

### Cholecystokinin (CCK, cholecystokinin-pancreozymin)

The predominant form of this polypeptide in the gastrointestinal tract has 33 amino acids. CCK 58 and 39 also occur. It is found in the I cells of the duodenum and jejunum, in the nerves of the colon and in the pituitary gland and thyroid. It is one of the most abundant peptides in the central nervous system. It has been isolated from porcine intestine, its amino acid sequence has been determined and the gene cloned. Its structure is similar to gastrin and to the terminal part of the decapeptide cerulein which is present in the skin of the Australian tree toad (*Hyla caerulea*).

CCK is released from the upper small intestine by amino acids, fatty acids and hydrochloric acid (Chen et al 1985). Concentrations of CCK in plasma show a prolonged rise after food. Its most important effect is to promote the output of pancreatic proenzymes (p. 1230), but it also releases enzymes from the small intestinal mucosa (Gotze et al 1972) and may also increase bicarbonate output (p. 1230), particularly via potentiation of the effects of secretin. Many other biological activities are described, some of which may be physiological. It stimulates hepatic bile flow and inhibits the absorption of water and ions from the jejunum and ileum. It stimulates contraction of the gallbladder, relaxes the choledochal sphincter (p. 1197) and stimulates gastric and intestinal motility, these effects being either direct via CCK receptors on smooth muscle or neurally mediated (Grider & Makhlouf 1987). CCK also stimulates pancreatic growth, induces satiety and stimulates the secretion of calcitonin from the thyroid gland and the release of pancreatic polypeptide from the islet cells. CCK antagonizes opiate analgesia and may act physiologically as an antagonist of endogenous opiates (Price et al 1985).

## THE NERVE SUPPLY TO THE PANCREAS

Cancer of the pancreas and acute or chronic pancreatitis cause severe abdominal and back pain. The pain pathways are both sympathetic and parasympathetic. The sympathetic innervation arises from the fifth to the 10th thoracic ganglia and proceeds mainly via the greater splanchnic nerves to the celiac plexus, from which postganglionic fibers accompany the arterial supply to the pancreas. Vagal fibers are also transmitted via the celiac plexus. In intractable pancreatic pain, surgical removal of the celiac plexus or division of the sympathetic trunks at a higher level may bring relief.

Referred pain from the pancreas is felt in the back (p. 1270) or in the upper abdomen. Studies on stimulation of different areas of the pancreas (Bliss et al 1950) show that pain is felt on the side of the stimulus (Fig. 49.6).

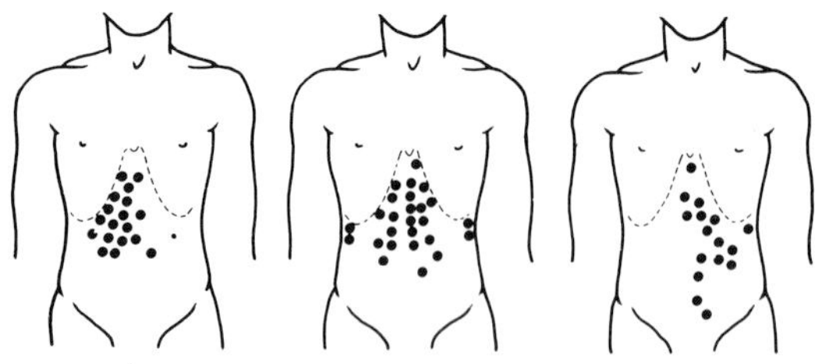


**Fig. 49.6** The site of pain induced by stimulation of the head (A), body (B) and tail (C) of the pancreas (Bliss et al 1950).

## SHWACHMAN SYNDROME (Aggett et al 1980)

This rare multiorgan disease of unknown origin was first delineated as a separate entity in 1964 (Shwachman et al 1964). It is the second most common cause of pancreatic insufficiency in childhood. The major features include exocrine pancreatic insufficiency, growth retardation, metaphyseal chondrodysplasia, neutropenia, thrombocytopenia, elevated fetal hemoglobin levels and increased susceptibility to infection. The familial incidence and analysis of sibship segregation suggest that it is inherited in an autosomal recessive manner.

### Pathology

The pancreas shows extensive fatty infiltration of a normal-sized gland. Most of the acinar cells are replaced by fat but the pancreatic ducts and islet cells appear normal.

### Clinical features

The majority of children present by 4–6 months with symptoms of malabsorption and chronic diarrhea, failure to thrive and recurrent severe infections. Growth failure remains a constant feature despite treatment. Hematological abnormalities include constant or cyclic neutropenia which may be associated with a defect in neutrophil mobility (Aggett et al 1979), thrombocytopenia in 60–70% which may also be cyclical and anemia in about 50%. The bone marrow findings are variable with normal, increased or decreased granulocytic elements being described. Fetal hemoglobin concentration is elevated in 50% of patients (Aggett et al 1980). Bone lesions were not reported initially but have subsequently been well documented, the major lesion being metaphyseal chondrodysplasia. This mainly affects the femoral neck, where it is symmetrical, but can also involve the knees, wrists, ankles and vertebrae. These changes are rare before 1 year of age. Abnormally short ribs with anterior flaring have been described in several infants presenting with neonatal respiratory distress (Danks et al 1976). Abnor-malities of other organ systems have been described, including skin, liver, central nervous system and teeth (Aggett et al 1980). The diagnosis should be suspected in infants with features of malabsorption and chronic diarrhea, growth failure and recurrent severe infections in whom cystic fibrosis has been excluded. Serial blood tests (at least twice weekly for 1 month) are required to confirm neutropenia and thrombocytopenia. Radiographs of chest and a skeletal survey may reveal abnormal ribs and metaphyseal chondrodysplasia which supports the diagnosis. The majority of patients will have steatorrhea as measured by 3-day fecal fat collection and quantitative pancreatic function studies reveal low to absent activities of lipase, colipase, trypsin, amylase and bicarbonate with a low to normal volume (Hadorn et al 1968, Hill et al 1982, Gaskin et al 1982a).

### Treatment

Therapy is symptomatic. Pancreatic enzyme replacement is required in early childhood to correct steatorrhea. Normal fat absorption occurs in most children over age 7 years despite extreme pancreatic insufficiency (Hill et al 1982). Despite correction of steatorrhea, growth retardation usually persists. Fat-soluble vitamins and calorie supplements are advisable early in life. During periods of neutropenia, febrile episodes require careful assessment and antibiotic therapy if appropriate. The anemia is rarely incapacitating and is often refractory to treatment.

### Prognosis

The prognosis is better than for cystic fibrosis, with a mortality rate of between 15% and 25% (Aggett et al 1980). The main cause of death is overwhelming infection. There is also a risk of hemorrhage and neoplasia. Morbidity is quite high owing to repeated infections. Despite the relatively low mortality very few postpubertal patients have been described, raising the possibility that the diagnosis in adults is frequently missed (Hill et al 1982). Late diagnosis is difficult because of the normal bowel habit despite continuing pancreatic insufficiency (Hill et al 1982). The diagnosis should be considered more frequently in adults with short stature, particularly when a history of childhood diarrhea or infection can be elicited.

## ISOLATED PANCREATIC ENZYME DEFICIENCIES

There are a number of case reports of congenital abnormalities of isolated pancreatic enzyme production and combined deficiences are recognized either alone or in various combinations (Stafford & Grand 1982).

### Amylase deficiency

Low levels of amylase are noted in normal infants in the

first 4–6 months of life (Lebenthal & Lee 1980). A patient with diarrhea and growth failure due to amylase deficiency has been described (Lilibridge & Townes 1973).

### Lipase and colipase deficiency

Isolated lipase deficiency has been described in 12 patients (Muller et al 1975, Figarella et al 1980). Most patients present with severe steatorrhea soon after birth but, unlike cystic fibrosis or Shwachman syndrome, failure to thrive does not occur. Pancreatic lipase activity is low, with normal colipase, amylase, trypsin and bicarbonate secretion and the patient responds to therapy with pancreatic enzymes. Two brothers with isolated colipase deficiency have been reported in the literature (Hildebrand et al 1982).

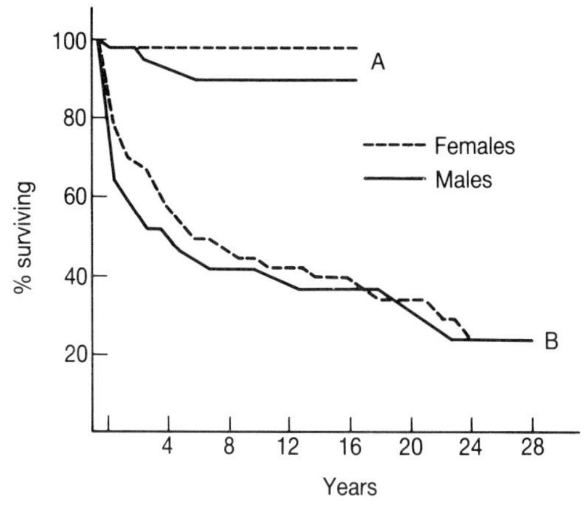


**Fig. 49.7** Cystic fibrosis. Cumulative survival curves by sex for patients diagnosed between 1948 and 1973 (B) and 1973 and 1982 (A) in South Australia (Hill et al 1985).

### Proteolytic enzyme deficiences

Three entities have been defined in patients with steatorrhea, creatorrhea, a normal sweat test and absent trypsin activity in duodenal juice (Lebenthal et al 1976). Shwachman syndrome has been discussed (p. 1234). In congenital enterokinase deficiency the activity of the pancreatic enzymes is normal but mucosal and luminal entero-kinase activity is absent (Tarlow et al 1970, Lebenthal et al 1976). The third group of patients have a deficiency of trypsinogen alone (Townes et al 1967). In all these entities the small intestinal structure and disaccharidase levels were normal.

These patients often present early in life with diarrhea, growth failure and edema due to hypoproteinemia. In order to distinguish enterokinase deficiency, tryptic activity is measured before and after the additon of enterokinase to a sample of duodenal juice. In enterokinase deficiency, addition of the enzyme causes a marked increase in tryptic activity. These patients respond well to pancreatic enzyme replacement therapy and provision of protein hydrolysate formulas.

## CYSTIC FIBROSIS

Cystic fibrosis (CF) is the most common lethal genetic disorder occurring in liveborn Caucasians. It usually presents in the first year of life with failure to thrive, maldigestion and repeated severe respiratory infections. Twenty years ago few children with cystic fibrosis lived beyond 10 years, but now most patients can expect to reach adult life (Fig. 49.7), often with relatively little disability. In developed countries cystic fibrosis is the commonest cause of progressive lung disease or chronic pancreatic insufficiency and cirrhosis of the liver in childhood and young adult life. Until recently pediatricians have managed cystic fibrosis, but now that the majority survive into adult life the physician must be totally familiar with this disease and its management.

In 1989, collaborative investigators led by Dr Frances Collins successfully cloned the gene responsible for cystic fibrosis, culminating one of the most intense and competitive scientific quests in history (Rommens et al 1989, Riordan et al 1989). The cystic fibrosis gene was called the cystic fibrosis transmembrane regulator or CFTR, based on its similarity in the deduced protein structure with other ion-transporting proteins and the chloride conductance defect characteristic of the disease (Quinton 1986).

The identification and cloning of CFTR has ushered in a new era in our understanding of the pathophysiology of cystic fibrosis. Genetic testing for cystic fibrosis is well established in clinical practice and has led to the definitive identification of mild phenotypes. Finally, the advances in molecular genetics have raised the prospects for gene therapy.

### Incidence and genetics

The incidence in Caucasian populations ranges from 1:1500 to 1:15 000 live briths. In Europe, North America and Australia the incidence is approximately one in 2000 live births. As cystic fibrosis is inherited in an autosomal recessive manner the carrier or heterozygote rate in most populations of European extraction is approximately one in 25. Thus, in one of every 400 families there is a risk of producing a child with cystic fibrosis (Romeo 1984). Heterozygotes show no symptoms of cystic fibrosis and at present can only be distinguished from noncarriers through genetic testing for common mutations.

### CFTR cloning and function

The efforts of numerous investigators culminated in the successful cloning of the CF gene in 1989. Remarkably, the CF gene was identified without any structural or functional information of the protein product through a strategy known as positional cloning. The CF gene was initially localized to the long arm of chromosome 7 by restriction fragment length polymorphisms in 1985 (Knowlton et al 1985). Using sophisticated molecular biological techniques (reviewed by Collins 1991), within 5 years the most common mutation in the CF gene was identified, three base pairs amongst 3 billion nucleotide base pairs in the human genome.

The product of the CF gene is a 1480 amino acid protein (168 kDa) which was named the cystic fibrosis transmembrane regulator (CFTR), based on the underlying defect in $Cl^-$ conductance seen in CF epithelia. Transfection of cultured cystic fibrosis cells with normal CFTR cDNA corrects the conductance defect. It was predicted to be an integral membrane protein containing multiple membrane-spanning domains. Consensus sequences for glycosylation, phosphorylation and nucleotide binding were found, consistent with physiological studies in relevant epithelial cells showing regulation of $Cl^-$ conductance by cAMP and ATP. Rather than being merely a regulator of conductance, experimental evidence was quickly collected proving that CFTR is a $Cl^-$ channel itself, reconstituting normal chloride conductance in a number of in vitro systems, including in artificial lipid bilayers. While other functions for CFTR have been proposed, the experimental evidence to date supports the contention that CFTR functions primarily as a cAMP-regulated chloride channel.

The cell biology of CFTR has been extensively characterized in the pancreas. The gene product is localized to the apical region of the epithelial cells lining the proximal pancreatic ducts. As Figure 49.8 illustrates, CFTR supplies the luminal chloride necessary for activation of the apical membrane chloride/bicarbonate exchanger. Responsive to cAMP, CFTR stimulates bicarbonate, water and sodium movement across the apical membrane of the ductular epithelium via its chloride channel (reviewed in Marino & Gorelick 1992).

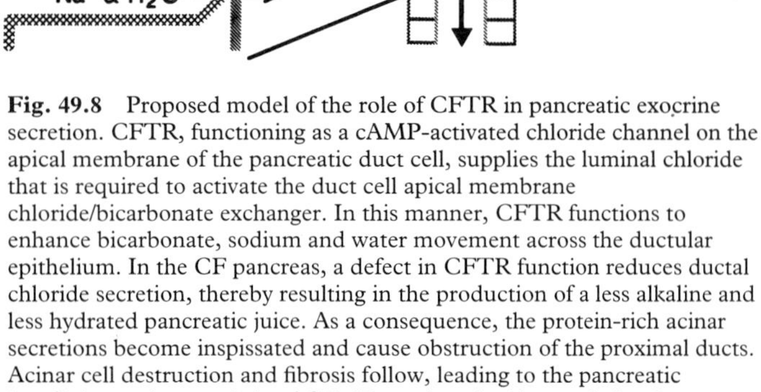

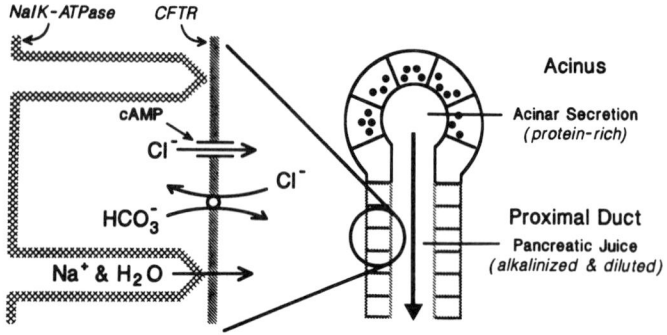


**Fig. 49.8** Proposed model of the role of CFTR in pancreatic exocrine secretion. CFTR, functioning as a cAMP-activated chloride channel on the apical membrane of the pancreatic duct cell, supplies the luminal chloride that is required to activate the duct cell apical membrane chloride/bicarbonate exchanger. In this manner, CFTR functions to enhance bicarbonate, sodium and water movement across the ductular epithelium. In the CF pancreas, a defect in CFTR function reduces ductal chloride secretion, thereby resulting in the production of a less alkaline and less hydrated pancreatic juice. As a consequence, the protein-rich acinar secretions become inspissated and cause obstruction of the proximal ducts. Acinar cell destruction and fibrosis follow, leading to the pancreatic insufficiency characteristic of CF. (Reproduced with permission from Marino et al 1991.)

## CFTR mutations

The CFTR gene on chromosome 7 is large, spanning 250 kilobases with 27 exons. Likewise, the genetics of CF are complex, with over 200 CF-associated mutations identified. The first mutation identified is an unusual one with deletion of an entire 3 bp coding triplet, resulting in loss of a phenylalanine (F) residue at position 508 in the CFTR protein. The *F508 mutation accounts for nearly 70% of CF-associated mutations; the next most common mutation accounting for 3.5%. Many of the mutations described have been found in only a single kindred.

Mutations in CFTR can be categorized by the mechanism of CFTR channel dysfunction which may result from one of several defects in the biosynthesis of the CFTR (Fig. 49.9). As seen in other genetic disorders, nonsense mutations, frameshifts and splice defects lead to loss of protein production by premature truncation of the gene product. By contrast, the common *F508 mutation results in a CFTR protein product which is unable to be appropriately targeted to the apical membrane of epithelial cells under physiological conditions. Degraded intracellularly, *F508 protein is not detected on the cell surface. Other classes of mutations (point mutations; substituting one amino acid for another) result in mutant proteins reaching the plasma membrane with defective function, owing either to defective regulation by stimulating nucleotides (e.g. ATP or cAMP) or to defects in the rate of $Cl^-$ conduction (reviewed by Welsh & Smith 1993).

## Developmental expression of CFTR

CFTR expression has been studied in human fetal tissue using in situ hybridization techniques with a specific CFTR cDNA (Tizzano et al 1993, Trezise et al 1993). CFTR expression was identified at all stage of development with the highest expression found in the developing pancreas, liver, gallbladder, intestine, reproductive tissues, sweat and salivary glands, with lower but significant levels in lung and trachea. This pattern is consistent with the known clinical manifestations and organ dysfunction associated with cystic fibrosis. The expression pattern is similar in adult tissues, with one important exception; much higher levels of mRNA for CFTR were seen in the developing lung than in postnatal respiratory epithelium which contains very little CFTR mRNA.

In the pancreas, CFTR expression is localized to the pancreatic duct epithelium, with the highest levels seen in

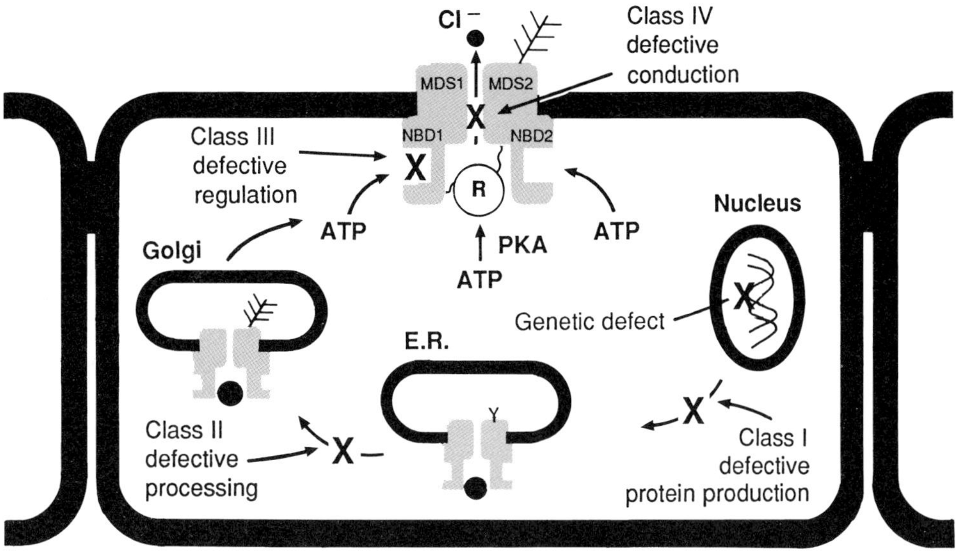


**Fig. 49.9** Biosynthesis and function of CFTR in an epithelial cell. Glycosylation of the protein is indicated by the branched structure. MSD = membrane-spanning domain; NBD = nucleotide-binding domain; R = regulatory domain; ER = endoplasmic reticulum; PKA = protein kinase A. (Reproduced with permission from Welsh & Smith 1993.)

the terminal ducts and centroacinar cells adjacent to the developing acinar cells, which lack CFTR expression. This pattern has also been confirmed in adult pancreas, with CFTR detected in small intralobular and interlobular ducts, but there is no expression in the acinar cells or main pancreatic duct (Marino et al 1991).

## Pathology and pathophysiology

Cystic fibrosis is a generalized exocrinopathy whereby most of the clinical manifestations result from obstruction by abnormal secretions of ducts or passages of the respiratory tract, salivary glands, digestive and biliary tract, pancreas and genitourinary tract (Oppenheimer & Esterly 1975). As outlined, expression of CFTR localizes to epithelia of affected organs; CFTR mRNA or protein is not expressed in organs unaffected in cystic fibrosis. While advances in our understanding of the function and structure of CFTR have been spectacular, the relationship between CFTR dysfunction and the pathophysiology of cystic fibrosis remains poorly understood. Most evidence supports a relationship between diminished electrolyte (and therefore fluid) secretion due to the loss of CFTR conductance resulting in a concentration of macromolecules in the affected duct system. The ensuing obstruction of ducts would result in end organ damage and failure. This hypothesis appears especially pertinent to organs with a high luminal protein concentration such as the exocrine pancreas (Durie 1992).

### *Respiratory system*

Mucopurulent exudates are found in the nasopharynx, sinuses and middle ears in association with congested mucosae and distended acini and ducts of the mucous glands. Nasal polyps are more common in cystic fibrosis.

The lungs are probably normal at birth. The earliest pulmonary lesion is bronchiolar obstruction. As the disease progresses, stagnation of mucus is followed by infection and bronchitis, bronchiolitis, bronchiectasis and abscess formation. Obstruction of the airways with viscid mucopurulent secretion leads to hyperinflation. *Staphylococcus aureus* or *Haemophilus influenzae* are usually cultured early in life, while *Pseudomonas aeruginosa* usually appears in the second decade. Widespread changes eventually occur in both lungs with progressive airway obstruction and peribronchial fibrosis leading to a decrease in gas exchange. Spontaneous pneumothorax, pneumomediastinum and hemoptysis occur mainly in adolescents and adults. With progression of the disease, pulmonary hypertension and right ventricular hypertrophy develop and death is usually due to respiratory failure or to cor pulmonale with right heart failure.

While lung disease accounts for 95% of the premature deaths associated with cystic fibrosis, severity of pulmonary complications correlate poorly with genotype. CFTR expression in the adult lung is low, particularily in the surface epithelium. Higher levels are seen in the submucosal glands of the cartilagenous airways, but it is difficult to attribute the respiratory complications to a malfunction in these glands. This suggests that the respiratory phenotype is heavily dependent on environmental factors (such as exposure to respiratory pathogens) and the host inflammatory response (reviewed by Tizzano & Buchwald 1995). The role of the high fetal expression of CFTR coupled with normal lungs at birth is likely important but remains to be explained.

*Alimentary manifestations*

***Pancreas.*** Structural changes with inspissated eosinophilic mucous secretions in pancreatic ducts are noted from birth. With time, the secretory acini and ducts dilate with flattening of the epithelium, atrophy of exocrine parenchyma and enlargement of acini and ducts to form cysts. Eventually there is fibrosis and replacement by adipose tissue. The islets of Langerhans remain structurally normal, although they are occasionally disorganized by extensive fibrosis and fat. This results in diabetes mellitus in older patients. Recurrent attacks of pancreatitis have been described in older patients and pancreatic insufficiency may develop (Shwachman et al 1975). Pancreatic calcification may follow such episodes.

Pancreatic insufficiency is a prominent clinical manifestation of cystic fibrosis, affecting nearly 85% of patients. A model for the pathogenesis of cystic fibrosis in the pancreas is summarized in Figure 49.8. The state of pancreatic function correlates closely with the genotype. As expected, the common *F508 mutation (and all related mutations resulting in near-complete loss of CFTR function) is associated with pancreatic insufficiency. Some of the point mutations in CFTR, resulting in correctly localized but defective $Cl^-$ conductance, are associated with long-term pancreatic sufficiency. Partial CFTR function is supported by lower sweat sodium studies in these patients. Longitudinal clinical studies confirm that most patients will remain pancreatic sufficient for the long term (Couper et al 1992); however, the pulmonary complications can be mild or severe. Even in pancreatic-sufficient patients, careful pancreatic function studies of bicarbonate secretion will document the secretory defect despite adequate enzyme delivery. It appears that pancreatic-sufficient patients are the subgroup at risk for the development of recurrent attacks of pancreatitis.

***Liver and biliary tract.*** The bile ductules can become blocked by inspissated material with scattered areas of fibrosis (p. 972). Eventually focal biliary cirrhosis becomes multifocal, presenting with severe liver disease in about 2–5% of older patients (Stern et al 1976). Cystic fibrosis is an important cause of hepatic cirrhosis and portal hypertension in adolescents and young adults (p. 972).

Earlier studies reported few biliary abnormalities in cystic fibrosis (Craig et al 1957), but recent investigations show that they are more common in older patients. Microgallbladders, gallbladder cysts and stones in the gallbladder and in the bile ducts all occur. The gallbladder is frequently atrophic or hypoplastic and filled with transparent gray mucus. This is probably due to atresia or obstruction of the cystic duct which can be present at birth. Graham et al (1985) studied 35 adult patients with ultrasonography and found microgallbladders in five (14%), gallstones in three (8.6%), and one patient (2.9%) had already had a cholecystectomy. This incidence of gallstones is clearly high (Newman 1973) as gallstones occur in only 0.25% of children. The reasons for increased stone formation are not known, but lithogenic bile consequent on loss of bile acids in the stools due to malabsorption may be a factor.

Endoscopic retrograde cholangiography has shown that viscid bile, colloquially known as "sludge", may also be important in producing biliary symptoms and obstruction by this material could be important in damaging intrahepatic ducts and in giving rise to a diminished intrahepatic biliary tree with strictures and areas of cystic dilatation (Bass et al 1983). These obstructive lesions cause focal biliary cirrhosis and the cholangiographic and histologic pictures are similar to sclerosing cholangitis (MacSween 1990, O'Brien et al 1992). Biliary obstruction can also result from compression of the common bile duct in the head of a fibrotic pancreas (Lambert et al 1981) and a report of cholangiocarcinoma of the extrahepatic ducts in a young woman with cystic fibrosis raises the possibility that this disease also predisposes to biliary carcinoma (Abdul-Karim et al 1982).

***Intestine.*** Ten to 15% of infants with cystic fibrosis present within 24 h of birth with symptoms of intestinal obstruction. This condition, called meconium ileus, is due to plugging of the intestinal lumen by thick mucus. The lumina of the intestinal crypts are dilated and filled with mucus. In children mucofeculent masses tend to collect in the cecum or terminal ileum. They can become adherent to the wall of the cecum and may calcify. These masses can cause acute or subacute intestinal obstruction, intussusception or appendicitis. This condition, known as meconium ileus equivalent, only presents in patients with steatorrhea and does not occur in any other form of pancreatic malabsorption. Its cause is unknown but it may be due to a combination of slow intestinal transit and the presence of concentrated chyme containing precipitated dietary protein and undigested fat in an intestine lined with densely coagulated mucoprotein (Zentler-Munro 1983).

Recently, the use of microencapsulated formulations of high-strength pancreatic enzyme supplements has been associated with colonic strictures and fibrosis (Smyth et al 1994, McHugh et al 1994). It has been suggested that these fibrotic lesions result from local effects of high potency enzymes that are in contact with proximal colonic mucosa in patients with slow colonic transit.

*Reproductive organs*

In the male reproductive organs, structures derived from the Wolffian duct are obstructed, leading to atrophy and/or atresia of the vas deferens, body and tail of the epididymis and seminal vesicles. Usually there is aspermia. In the female, mucus glands in the cervix may be dilated and vaginal mucus is abnormally viscid.

With the aid of genetic testing for mutations in CFTR, congenital bilateral absence of the vas deferens in the absence of gastrointestinal or pulmonary disease may represent the mild end of the spectrum of cystic fibrosis. This phenotype appears to be related to a specific set of mutations (Anguiano et al 1992).

*Other organs*

In the salivary glands the degree of abnormality is related to the amount of mucus-secreting tissue. Thus, the sublingual glands are most involved and the parotids least. The changes are minor with distention of ducts and acini due to retained secretions. The sweat glands are structurally normal despite the high electrolyte content of sweat and evidence of defective chloride permeability in the ducts (Quinton & Bijman 1983).

## Clinical features

The presentation and severity of the disease is variable. The majority of patients present in early childhood, 55–75% being diagnosed in the first year of life (Hill et al 1985). Occasionally mild disease does not develop until adolescence or early adulthood.

In the neonatal period, 10–15% of babies with cystic fibrosis present with symptoms and signs of intestinal obstruction due to meconium ileus. Occasionally prolonged obstructive neonatal jaundice is the presenting feature. During infancy, respiratory symptoms, failure to thrive and malabsorption with bulky, greasy, offensive stools are the commonest features. Untreated infants may develop severe edema, hypoproteinemia and anemia (Nielsen & Larsen 1982). In late childhood, the presentation may be one of persistent cough and sputum production, rectal prolapse and heat prostration because of excessive sodium loss. Children can present with recurrent abdominal pain which is most frequently due to obstruction by a fecal mass or with features of acute or subacute intestinal obstruction (meconium ileus equivalent) or intussusception. Other important causes of abdominal pain include acute pancreatitis (Shwachman et al 1975), peptic ulcer disease and peptic esophagitis (Bendig et al 1982), cholecystitis usually secondary to cholelithiasis (Isenberg et al 1976) and renal colic due to urate or oxalate stones. Liver disease may become apparent in late childhood (p. 972). Patients presenting for the first time in adult life usually have milder disease. They most commonly present with chest disease. The main features are digital clubbing, chronic bronchitis, bronchiectasis, hemoptysis and spontaneous pneumothorax. Chronic liver disease and cirrhosis may present with jaundice, hepatosplenomegaly and features of portal hypertension (p. 991). Chronic sinusitis and nasal polyps are common. Older male patients may also present via the infertility clinic or the diabetic clinic. Diabetes occurs in 5–10% of patients. Female patients have reduced fertility and pregnancy may cause a deterioration of pulmonary function if this is already poor (Cohen et al 1980).

## Diagnosis and investigations

The diagnosis of cystic fibrosis is based on the clinical features of chronic lung disease and malabsorption together with an elevation of sweat sodium and chloride.

*Sweat test*

The sweat test is the single most important procedure for the diagnosis of cystic fibrosis (Shwachman et al 1981). Most methods are based on the quantitative pilocarpine iontophoresis technique described by Gibson & Cooke (1959). Sweating is stimulated over a small area of skin of the inner forearm by pilocarpine iontophoresis. The sweat is collected on a gauze pad or filter paper of known weight which has been covered with a plastic square and sealed at the edges with waterproof adhesive tape. After 1 h the pad or paper is removed and reweighed, the sweat eluted and chemically analyzed for sodium and chloride. To obtain reliable measurements a minimum of 100 mg sweat is required. In children, chloride values greater than 60 mmol/L are diagnostic for cystic fibrosis whereas values between 50 and 59 mmol are suggestive and require confirmation by genetic testing. As outlined above, pancreatic-sufficient patients will have lower sweat electrolytes. Values for chloride are usually higher than for sodium but by not more than 5–10 mmol/L.

The sweat sodium in normal adults is higher than in normal children and thus a diagnosis of cystic fibrosis in the older patient requires a sweat sodium greater than 70 mmol/L on at least two occasions (McKendrick 1962). Levels below 60 mmol/L exclude the diagnosis. Shwachman et al (1977) have shown the sweat test to be as reliable in the diagnosis of cystic fibrosis in adults as in children. False positive tests have been reported in a variety of illnesses, including untreated adrenal insufficiency, nephrogenic diabetes insipidus, ectodermal dysplasia, congestive heart failure and malnutrition from a variety of causes (Rosenfeld et al 1979).

*Genetic testing* (Hamosh & Corey 1993)

Genetic testing to establish the precise mutations present in an individual suspected of having cystic fibrosis has become routine clinical practice. Despite the large number of different mutations, many are centered on exon 11 of the CFTR gene. Using a combination of polymerase chain reaction and DNA sequencing technology, mutations on both alleles can be defined in >80% of cystic fibrosis homozygotes.

Genetic testing allows for definitive diagnosis and has established mild phenotypes of the disease as described for congenital absence of the vas deferens in men. Knowledge of the precise mutation has some (but limited) prognostic information, particularly regarding pancreatic function as discussed above. Furthermore, genetic testing allows for the possibility of prenatal diagnosis, preimplantation screening (in vitro fertilization) and screening for carrier status in siblings of affected individuals to assess the risk for their future offspring. Screening of the "average risk" population for carrier status is not advocated. The moral, ethical and psychological implications of such testing make formal discussion and informed consent with a medical genetics practitioner mandatory.

*Radiographic features* (Park & Grand 1981)

***Meconium ileus.*** Characteristic changes seen on the plain abdominal radiograph may include uneven distention of small bowel loops with relatively few fluid levels and an empty large bowel. The presence of scattered gas bubbles trapped in the sticky meconium causes a mottled or "soap bubble" appearance and this may be diagnostic. Abdominal calcification may be present, reflecting previous bowel perforation and meconium peritonitis. Occasionally the perforation persists and free gas may be seen in the abdominal cavity and rarely a meconium pseudocyst may cause a soft tissue mass displacing loops of small bowel.

A contrast enema may be needed to differentiate meconium ileus from other causes of intestinal obstruction in infancy, such as Hirschsprung's disease and bowel atresias. Typically the colon is small in meconium ileus and contains only small pellets of feces. Differentiation from long-segment Hirschsprung's disease needs careful examination. While barium may be used as the contrast medium, the use of water-soluble media is also advocated because of its therapeutic potential (Lillie & Chrispin 1972). Gastrografin and similar agents are hypertonic and slightly irritant to the intestine, so that an osmotic diarrhea and intestinal contractions are induced which can cause expulsion of the tenacious meconium with relief of obstruction. A second contrast enema at 24–48 h may be necessary to complete the clearance of meconium. It has been suggested that administration of water-soluble contrast media via a nasogastric tube may dislodge the obstructing meconium if a contrast enema fails (Levick 1972).

A contrast enema is contraindicated in patients in whom perforation is suspected or if other complications such as peritonitis, volvulus or gangrene are thought to be present.

Some precautions are necessary when using water-soluble contrast media. The osmotic diarrhea can produce hypovolemia, which should be treated with intravenous fluid and electrolyte replacement if necessary. If Gastrografin is given through a nasogastric tube, care must be taken to avoid laryngotracheal aspiration.

***Distal intestinal obstruction syndrome*** (meconium ileus equivalent). The plain abdominal radiograph usually show fecal material mixed with bubbles in the proximal colon and distal small bowel. A large fecal mass may develop in the cecum or proximal colon and this is sometimes referred to as an adherent fecolith. This can be visible as a mass which sometimes calcifies. On contrast enema the fecolith similates a large polypoidal filling defect but other features of cystic fibrosis will usually indicate the cause. Occasionally the fecal mass will initiate an intussusception of the ileocolic type and this may be reduced by use of a contrast enema.

***Intestinal mucosal abnormalities.*** Typical radiographic changes may be seen in the duodenum and small intestine. In one series, over 80% of patients showed duodenal abnormalities (Taussig et al 1973), which included markedly thickened mucosal folds, nodular filling defects, distortion, dilatation and redundancy of the duodenal loop. In another series, 12 of 14 patients had similar duodenal abnormalities and one also had a benign duodenal stricture (Phelan et al 1983). Similar radiographic abnormalities have been shown in the small intestine, particularly in the jejunum.

***Other bowel changes.*** The colonic mucosal pattern in older children and young adults may show a coarse, cobblestone appearance usually involving the left side of the colon, but the whole colon may be affected (Berk & Lee 1973). Because of the inability to clear the colon completely of tenacious fecal material and viscid mucus, multiple poorly defined filling defects may be seen along the margins of the colon and may simulate polyposis. Pneumatosis coli may be a complication of cystic fibrosis in older patients.

***Hepatobiliary abnormalities.*** The results of liver function tests are variable and abnormalities can be difficult to interpret, particularly in respect of increased alkaline phosphatase activity, which can be due to coincident liver damage.

The gallbladder and bile ducts are abnormal in one-third to one-half of patients (L'Heureux et al 1977). The gallbladder is frequently small, atrophic and irregular and contains thick, tenacious white bile and mucus and sometimes gallstones. These changes may be demonstrated by ultrasound or oral cholecystography. The latter is not usually successful if the cystic duct is atrophic or occluded, which is not uncommon.

Disorders of the bile ducts such as cholangitis or intraduct stones may be seen at ERCP. Extrinsic compression of the common bile duct by a fibrotic pancreas has been demonstrated to cause biliary tract obstruction, which can present with recurrent abdominal pain or obstructive jaundice (Patrick et al 1986). This can be visualized by percutaneous transhepatic cholangiography.

***Pancreas.*** The pathological changes in the pancreas are best visualized and monitored by ultrasound and computed tomography. Calcification in the pancreas may be seen on an abdominal radiograph in advanced cases. The calcification is generally fine and granular. Ultrasound and computed tomography show a spectrum of abnormalities consistent with the severity of clinical and morphological findings (Daneman et al 1983).

While the findings on ultrasound may be normal, the pancreas is usually smaller than normal and typically is hyperechoic owing to fat replacement. Small anechoic areas may be seen and these are generally due to cystic changes. On computed tomography the pancreas has a variable attenuation density with small areas of calcification and other areas of low attenuation due to cystic change. In some cases the whole pancreas is replaced by fat, the degree of fat replacement appearing to correlate with the patient's age. Daneman et al (1983) advocate the use of ultrasound and computed tomography as non-invasive means of monitoring the progress of pancreatic involvement in cystic fibrosis and other disorders characterized by fat replacement of the pancreas, such as Shwachman syndrome.

As more patients with cystic fibrosis respond satisfactorily to treatment and live into adult life, so the spectrum of radiological abnormalities widens and the differential diagnosis increases. When one or more of the above gastrointestinal, hepatobiliary or pancreatic abnormalities is seen in association with typical abnormalities on the chest radiograph, possibly with evidence of delayed epiphyseal development, the diagnosis of cystic fibrosis is highly likely.

### *Other investigations*

Patients with borderline values for sweat sodium and chloride and those presenting in late adolescence and early adult life with milder disease require careful evaluation, including family history, assessment of respiratory tract with sinus and chest radiographs and lung function tests and analysis of pancreatic secretion. Eighty-five percent of patients with cystic fibrosis have marked steatorrhea and stool microscopy reveals multiple fat globules. In patients without steatorrhea the diagnosis of cystic fibrosis can be confirmed using a test of exocrine pancreatic function with measurements of bicarbonate concentration, lipase, amylase and tryptic activity (Gaskin et al 1982a, 1984). Gaskin et al (1982a, 1984) have also provided a normal range of values for pancreatic secretions. Cystic fibrosis patients without steatorrhea can have low or normal enzyme values but have a depressed water and bicarbonate secretion (Gaskin et al 1982a). Indirect tests of pancreatic function, such as the PABA test, are less reliable, particularly in young infants (Sacher et al 1978) and when pancreatic enzyme secretion is near normal.

Pulmonary function testing does not help in the diagnosis of cystic fibrosis but is a valuable tool in assessing progress and response to treatment.

Celiac disease has been reported in patients with cystic fibrosis (Katz et al 1976), probably as a coincidental finding. The small intestinal biopsy in cystic fibrosis is structurally normal but characteristically shows inspissated eosinophilic secretions in the crypts. Malabsorption of fat-soluble vitamins occurs, although clinical evidence of deficiency is uncommon. An association between low vitamin E levels and spinocerebellar disorders has been described in patients with cystic fibrosis and chronic childhood cholestasis (Muller et al 1983). Measurement of vitamin A and E levels is useful in monitoring vitamin status. Reduced absorption of vitamin $B_{12}$ can be shown in cystic fibrosis patients with steatorrhea but serum $B_{12}$ levels are usually normal and $B_{12}$ absorption is corrected by therapy with pancreatic enzymes (Harms et al 1981).

The results of liver function tests are variable (p. 972) and abnormalities can be difficult to interpret, particularly in respect of increased alkaline phosphatase activity, which can be due to coincident liver damage.

From the time of the diagnosis, management should be multidisciplinary to cover medical, psychological, social, genetic, educational and occupational aspects of the illness. Evidence suggests that optimal therapy is provided by special cystic fibrosis clinics in major pediatric centers (Nielsen & Schiotz 1982, Warwick 1982, Hill et al 1985).

### *Management of gastrointestinal manifestations*

***Pancreatic insufficiency.*** The earliest manifestation of cystic fibrosis is failure to thrive, which correlates closely with survival. To reduce nutrient losses in the face of increased requirements due to chronic lung disease and infection, all patients with pancreatic insufficiency require regular supplementation with pancreatic enzymes. In addition to improving growth and nutrition, enzyme replacement will decrease the number and odor of stools. Primarily because of the sensitivity of lipase to acid and protease inactivation, complete correction of steatorrhea is rarely achieved. Gastric acid secretion in cystic fibrosis is elevated and neutralizing bicarbonate from the CF pancreas diminished, creating a hostile environment. Enterically coated enzyme tablets (designed to release enzyme in the alkaline milieu of the proximal small intestine) are probably more effective than conventional enzyme replacement in improving fat absorption in addition to the ease of administration, particularly in the young infant (Gow et al 1981). The dosage must be varied according to the stool frequency and the degree of malabsorption, as assessed by the amount of fat measured in a 72-h stool collection. Dosages above 30 capsules daily are probably not proportionately more effective. Enzymes should be spread throughout the meal or snack. If a maximal dose of enzyme fails to reduce the frequency of offensive stools and weight gain remains poor, treatment with acid suppression to reduce intragastric enzyme inactivation and intraduodenal bile acid precipitation may be beneficial (Durie et al 1980, Chalmers et al 1985).

***Meconium ileus equivalent.*** In the acute form of the illness, intestinal obstruction is managed conservatively with nasogastric drainage and intravenous therapy followed by the use of the mucolytic agent N-acetyl cysteine given both orally (10–15 ml diluted in cola or orange juice 6- or 8-hourly) and by enemata (Hodson et al 1976). If pain and vomiting continue the possibility of intussusception or appendicitis must be considered.

In the chronic from of meconium ileus equivalent with recurrent abdominal pain and presence of fecal masses, oral therapy with lactulose, bulk agents or N-acetyl cysteine as described above for 7–10 days is often effective. Prevention of this condition is aided by better control of steatorrhea. Enzyme dosage is often inadequate and needs to be increased. Surgery should be avoided if at all possible as it is often unhelpful and may lead to fecal fistula and deterioration in lung function.

***Rectal prolapse.*** This is uncommon after the age of 6 years and is managed by correction of steatorrhea and improvement of nutrition and hence muscle tone. Reduction of coughing by measures to treat recurrent chest infection is also helpful. Operative intervention is rarely if ever indicated.

***Liver and biliary disease*** (Psacharopoulos et al 1981). Biliary colic (p. 1206) and acute cholecystitis (p. 1207) are treated in the usual manner. However, operations are hazardous in cystic fibrosis owing to the high frequency of post-operative pulmonary infection, which may be fatal, and it is probably best to avoid cholecystectomy in patients with poor pulmonary function unless recurrent severe episodes occur. Choledocholithiasis and obstruction due to "sludge" are probably best treated by endoscopic papillotomy, although experience of this is very limited (Bass et al 1983). Biliary strictures can be treated surgically, but the endoscopic insertion of a biliary stent may be more appropriate in patients with advanced pulmonary disease.

## Nutrition

The role of adequate nutrition in improving the clinical status of patients with cystic fibrosis is very important (Chase et al 1979) for those who are underweight tend to have a poorer prognosis (Gaskin et al 1982b). The growth failure is due to an unfavorable energy balance rather than the disease itself (Parsons et al 1983) and an increased intake of protein and energy results in a catch-up of growth (Shepherd et al 1983).

Traditionally, low-fat diets have been used in the treatment of cystic fibrosis (Chase et al 1979). However, since the early 1970s it was shown that a normal to high-fat diet results in improved energy intake and growth (Crozier 1974). Children with cystic fibrosis should be counseled to eat a normal, balanced diet with approximately 40% of the calories from fat with the appropriate pancreatic enzyme replacement rather than diets unusually high in carbohydrate or protein. This strategy also protects against the potential for essential fatty acid deficiency which can complicate cystic fibrosis.

Patients with cystic fibrosis need 120–150% of the recommended daily energy allowance to counteract the increased losses due to residual malabsorption and the energy cost of acute and chronic chest infections. To achieve this, nutritional counseling is required, with promotion of energy-dense foods and increased total energy intake by using high-energy supplements (e.g. glucose polymers, medium-chain triglycerides) and frequent snacks.

Dietary supplements in the form of fat-soluble vitamins in a water-miscible form are required (Chase et al 1979). Essential fatty acid deficiency, a potential problem in those paients with steatorrhea, can be prevented by providing adequate calories (Pencharz 1983). Salt supplements are required during the summer in warm climates to prevent heat prostration (Goodchild & Dodge 1985).

## Prognosis

Improvements in survival in cystic fibrosis in developed countries in the past two decades have brought mean life expectancy from less than 10 years in the early 1960s to 20 years or more (Warwick 1982, Nielsen & Schiotz 1982, Lancet 1984, Hill et al 1985) (Fig. 49.7). The reasons for improved survival are unclear but the influence of specialist cystic fibrosis clinics together with earlier diagnosis are considered major factors (Warwick 1982). A better prognosis is also predicted for those patients without steatorrhea (Gaskin et al 1982b).

## Gene therapy

The cloning of the gene for cystic fibrosis raised hopes for a genetic "cure" for cystic fibrosis but significant challenges remain. However, remarkable progress has been made with research logically centered on delivering a functional CFTR gene to the respiratory epithelium (somatic gene therapy) to ameliorate the morbid lung disease of CF. To date, correction of the electrophysiological defect in CF nasal epithelium has been reported. The search for the appropriate delivery system or vector (viral, liposomes, DNA-ligand complexes) to allow long-term expression in the respiratory epithelium continues. Several Phase 1 clinical trials are underway in the United States and Europe with the realistic hope of further ameliorating the lung disease in cystic fibrosis (reviewed by O'Neal & Beaudet 1994).

## REFERENCES


Abdul-Karim F W, King T A, Dahms B B, Gauderer M W L, Boat T F 1982 Carcinoma of the extrahepatic biliary system in an adult with cystic fibrosis. Gastroenterology 82: 758

Aggett P J, Harries J T, Harvey B A M, Soothill J F 1979 An inherited defect of neutrophil mobility in Shwachman syndrome. Journal of Pediatrics 94: 391

Aggett P J, Cavanagh N P C, Matthew D J, Pincott J R, Sutcliffe J, Harries J T 1980 Shwachman's syndrome. A review of 21 cases. Archives of Disease in Childhood 55: 331

Anagnostides A, Chadwick V S, Selden A C, Maton P N 1984 Sham feeding and pancreatic secretion. Evidence for direct vagal stimulation of enzyme output. Gastroenterology 87: 109

Anguiano A, Oates R D, Amos J A et al 1992 Congential bilateral absence of the vas deferens. A primarily genital form of cystic fibrosis. Journal of the American Medical Association 267: 1794

Anderton J L, Finlayson N D C, Murray-Lyon I M, Smith A F, Shearman D J C 1968 Blood base changes after secretion of bicarbonate by pancreas. British Medical Journal 2: 279

Bass S, Connon J J, Ho C S 1983 Biliary tree in cystic fibrosis. Biliary tract abnormalities in cystic fibrosis demonstrated by endoscopic retrograde cholangiography. Gastroenterology 84: 1592

Beglinger C, Fried M, Whitehouse I, Jansen J B, Lamers C B, Gyr K 1985a Pancreatic enzyme response to a liquid meal and to hormonal stimulation. Correlation with plasma secretin and cholecystokinin levels. Journal of Clinical Investigation 75: 1471

Beglinger C, Kohler E, Whitehouse I, Gyr K 1985b Secretin and pancreatic enzyme secretion. Gut 26: 320

Bendig D W, Seilheimer D K, Wagner M L, Ferry G D, Harrison G M 1982 Complications of gastroesophageal reflux in patients with cystic fibrosis. Journal of Pediatrics 100: 536

Berk R N, Lee F A 1973 The late gastrointestinal manifestations of cystic fibrosis of the pancreas. Radiology 106: 377

Berman L G, Prior J T, Abramow S M, Ziegler D D 1960 A study of the pancreatic duct system in man by the use of vinyl acetate casts of postmortem preparations. Surgery, Gynecology and Obstetrics 110: 391

Bliss W R, Burch B, Martin M M, Zollinger R M 1950 Localization of referred pancreatic pain induced by electric stimulation. Gastroenterology 16: 317

Case R M, Argent B E 1993 Pancreatic duct cell secretion: control and mechanisms of transport. In: Go V L W, DiMagno E P, Gardner J D, Lebenthal E, Reber H A, Scheele G A (eds) The pancreas. Raven Press, New York, p 301

Chalmers D M, Brown R C, Miller M G et al 1985 The influence of long-term cimetidine as an adjuvant to pancreatic enzyme therapy in cystic fibrosis. Acta Paediatrica Scandinavica 74: 114

Chase H P, Long M A, Lavin M H 1979 Cystic fibrosis and malnutrition. Journal of Pediatrics 95: 337

Chen Y F, Chey W Y, Chang T-M, Lee K Y 1985 Duodenal acidification releases cholecystokinin. American Journal of Physiology 249: G29

Chey W Y 1993 Hormonal control of pancreatic exocrine secretion. In: Go V L W, DiMagno E P, Gardner J D, Lebenthal E, Reber H A, Scheele G A (eds) The pancreas. Raven Press, New York

Cohen L F, di Sant'Agnese P A, Friedlander J 1980 Cystic fibrosis and pregnancy. A national survey. Lancet 2: 842

Collins F S 1991 Of needles and pins – finding human disease genes by positional cloning. Clinical Research 39: 615

Cotton P B 1980 Congenital anomaly of pancreas divisum as cause of obstructive pain and pancreatitis. Gut 21: 105

Couper R T L, Corey M, Moore D J, Fisher L F, Forstner G G, Durie P R 1992 Decline of exocrine pancreatic function in cystic fibrosis patients with pancreatic sufficiency. Pediatric Research 32: 179

Craig M, Haddad H, Shwachman H 1957 The pathological changes in the liver in cystic fibrosis of the pancreas. Journal of Diseases of Children 93: 357

Crozier D N 1974 Cystic fibrosis. A not-so-fatal disease. Pediatric Clinics of North America 21: 935

Daneman A, Gaskin K, Martin D J, Cutz E 1983 Pancreatic changes in cystic fibrosis: CT and sonographic appearances. American Journal of Roentgenology 141: 653

Danks D M, Haslam R, Mayne V, Kaufmann H J, Holtzapple P G 1976 Metaphyseal chondrodysplasia, neutropenia, and pancreatic insufficiency presenting with respiratory distress in the neonatal period. Archives of Disease in Childhood 51: 697

Davies R E, Harper A A, Mackay I F S 1949 A comparison of the respiratory activity and histological changes in isolated pancreatic tissue. American Journal of Physiology 157: 278

Defilippi C, Solomon T E, Valenzuela J E 1982 Pancreatic secretory response to sham feeding in humans. Digestion 23: 217

Delhaye M, Engelholm L, Cremer M 1985 Pancreas divisum: congenital anatomic variant or anomaly? Contribution of endoscopic retrograde dorsal pancreatography. Gastroenterology 89: 951

Dharmsathaphorn K, Burrell M, Dobbins J 1979 Diagnosis of annular pancreas with endoscopic retrograde cholangiopancreatography. Gastroenterology 77: 1109

DiMagno E P, Layer P 1993 Human exocrine pancreatic enzyme secretion. In: Go V L W, DiMagno E P, Gardner J D, Lebenthal E, Reber H A, Scheele G A (eds) The pancreas. Raven Press, New York

Dolan R V, ReMine W H, Dockerty M B 1974 The fate of heterotopic pancreatic tissue. Archives of Surgery 109: 762

Dooley C P, Valenzuela J E 1984 Duodenal volume and osmoreceptors in the stimulation of human pancreatic secretion. Gastroenterology 86: 23

Dunn G D, Gibson R N 1986 The left-sided pancreas. Radiology 159: 713

Durie P R 1992 Pathophysiology of the pancreas in cystic fibrosis. 41: 97

Durie P R, Bell L, Linton W, Corey M L, Forstner G G 1980 Effect of cimetidine and sodium bicarbonate on pancreatic replacement therapy in cystic fibrosis. Gut 21: 778

Figarella C, de Caro A, Leupold D, Poley J R 1980 Congenital pancreatic lipase deficiency. Journal of Pediatrics 96: 412

Fisher J H, Klinger K W 1985 Closing in on the cystic fibrosis gene(s). American Review of Respiratory Disease 132: 1149

Fried G M, Ogden W D, Sakamoto T, Greeley G H, Thompson J C 1985 Experimental evidence for a vagally mediated and cholecystokinin-independent enteropancreatic reflex. Annals of Surgery 202: 71

Gardner J D, Jensen R T 1993 Receptors for secretagogues on pancreatic acinar cells In: Go V L W, DiMagno E P, Gardner J D, Lebenthal E, Reber H A, Scheele G A (eds) The pancreas. Raven Press, New York, p 151

Gaskin K J, Durie P R, Corey M, Wei P, Forstner G G 1982a Evidence for a primary defect of pancreatic HCO3-secretion in cystic fibrosis. Pediatric Research 16: 554

Gaskin K J, Gurwitz D, Durie P, Corey M, Levison H, Forstner G G 1982b Improved respiratory prognosis in patients wilh cystic fibrosis with normal fat absorption. Journal of Pediatrics 100: 857

Gaskin K J, Durie P R, Lee L, Hill R, Forstner G G 1984 Colipase and lipase secretion in childhood-onset pancreatic insufficiency. Delineation of patients with steatorrhea secondary to relative colipase deficiency. Gastroenterology 86: 1

Gibson L E, Cooke R E 1959 A test for concentration of electrolytes in sweat in cystic fibrosis of the pancreas utilizing pilocarpine by iontophoresis. Pediatrics 23: 545

Goodchild M C, Dodge J A (eds) 1985 Cystic fibrosis. Manual of diagnosis and management. Baillière Tindall, London

Gorelick F S, Jamieson J D 1981 Structure-function relationships of the pancreas. In: Johnson L R, Christensen J, Grossman M I, Jacobson E D, Schultz S G (eds) Physiology of the gastrointestinal tract, Vol 2. Raven Press, New York, p 773

Gotze H, Adelson J W, Hadorn H B, Portmann R, Troesch V 1972 Hormone-elicited enzyme release by the small intestinal wall. Gut 13: 471

Gow R, Bradbear R, Francis P, Shepherd R 1981 Comparative study of varying regimens to improve steatorrhoea and creatorrhoea in cystic fibrosis: effectiveness of an enteric-coated preparation with and without antacids and cimetidine. Lancet 2: 1071

Graham N, Manhire A R, Stead R J, Lees W R, Hodson M E, Batten J C 1985 Cystic fibrosis: ultrasonographic findings in the pancreas and

hepatobiliary system correlated with clinical data and pathology. Clinical Radiology 36: 199
Grider I R, Makhlouf G M 1987 Regional and cellular heterogeneity of cholecystokinin receptors mediating muscle contraction in the gut. Gastroenterology 92: 175
Grossman M I 1971 Control of pancreatic secretion. In: Beck I T, Sinclair D G (eds) The exocrine pancreas. J & A Churchill, London, p 59
Grossman M I, Jacobson E D, Schultz S G (eds) Physiology of the gastrointestinal tract, Vol 2. Raven Press, New York, p 773
Gullo L, Priori P, Costa P L, Mattioli G, Labo G 1984 Action of secretin on pancreatic enzyme secretion in man. Studies on pure pancreatic juice. Gut 25: 867
Hadorn B 1975 The exocrine pancreas. In: Anderson C M, Burke V (eds) Paediatric gastroenterology. Blackwell, Oxford, p 289
Hadorn B, Zoppi G, Shmerling D H, Prader A, McIntyre I, Anderson C M 1968 Quantitative assessment of exocrine pancreatic function in infants and children. Journal of Pediatrics 73: 39
Hamosh A, Corey M 1993 The cystic fibrosis genotype-phenotype consortium: correlation between genotype and phenotype in patients with cystic fibrosis. New England Journal of Medicine 329: 1308
Harper A A 1967 Hormonal control of pancreatic secretion. In: Code C F, Heidel W (eds) Handbook of physiology, Vol 2, section 6. American Physiological Society, Washington DC, p 969
Harms H K, Kennel O, Bertele R M, Bidlingmeier F, Bohne A 1981 Vitamin B, absorption and exocrine pancreatic insufficiency in childhood. European Journal of Pediatrics 136: 75
Henriksen F W, Worning H 1969 External pancreatic response to food and its relation to the maximal secretory capacity in dogs. Gut 10: 209
Hildebrand H, Borgstrom B, Bekassy A, Erlanson-Albertsson C, Helin I 1982 Isolated co-lipase deficiency in two brothers. Gut 23: 243
Hill D J S, Martin A J, Davidson G P, Smith G S 1985 Survival of cystic fibrosis patients in South Australia. Evidence that cystic fibrosis centre care leads to better survival. Medical Journal of Australia 143: 230
Hill R E, Durie P R, Gaskin K J, Davidson G P, Forstner G G 1982 Steatorrhea and pancreatic insufficiency in Shwachman syndrome. Gastroenterology 83: 22
Hodson M E, Mearns M B, Batten J C 1976 Meconium ileus equivalent in adults with cystic fibrosis of pancreas: a report of six cases. British Medical Journal 2: 790
Isenberg J N, L'Heureux P R, Warwick W J, Sharp H L 1976 Clinical observations on the biliary system in cystic fibrosis. American Journal of Gastroenterology 65: 134
Jorpes J E 1968 Memorial lecture. The isolation and chemistry of secretin and cholecystokinin. Gastroenterology 55: 157
Katz A J, Falchuk Z M, Shwachman H 1976 The coexistence of cystic fibrosis and celiac disease. Pediatrics 57: 715
Kilman W J, Berk R N 1977 The spectrum of radiographic features of aberrant pancreatic rests involving the stomach. Radiology 123: 291
Knowlton R G, Cohen-Haguenauer O, Cong N V et al 1985 A polymorphic DNA marker linked to cystic fibrosis is located on chromosome 7. Nature 318: 380
Lambert J R, Cole M, Crozier D M, Connon J J 1981 Bile duct compression causing jaundice in an adult with cystic fibrosis. Gastroenterology 80: 169
Lancet 1984 Leading article: survival in cystic fibrosis. Lancet 1: 663
Lebenthal E, Lee P C 1980 Development of functional response in human exocrine pancreas. Pediatrics 66: 556
Lebenthal E, Antonowicz I, Shwachman H 1976 Enterokinase and trypsin activities in pancreatic insufficiency and diseases of the small intestine. Gastroenterology 70: 508
Levick R K 1972 The choice of contrast medium in neonatal obstruction. Annales de Radiologie 15: 231
L'Heureux P R, Isenberg J N, Sharp H L, Warwick W J 1977 Gallbladder disease in cystic fibrosis. American Journal of Roentgenology 128: 953
Lilibridge C B, Townes P L 1973 Physiologic deficiency of pancreatic amylase in infancy: a factor in iatrogenic diarrhea. Journal of Pediatrics 82: 279
Lillie J G, Chrispin A R 1972 Investigation and management of neonatal obstruction by gastrograffin enema. Annales de Radiologie 15: 237
MacSween R N 1990 Sclerosing cholangitis and hepatic microvesicular steatosis in cystic fibrosis and chronic pancreatitis. Journal of Clinical Pathology 43: 173
Marino C R, Gorelick F S 1992 Scientific advances in cystic fibrosis. Gastroenterology 103: 681
Marino C R, Matovcik L M, Gorelick F S, Cohn J A 1991 Localization of the cystic fibrosis transmembrane conductance regulator in pancreas. Journal of Clinical Investigation 88: 712
McHugh K, Thomson A, Tam P 1994 Case report: colonic stricture and fibrosis associated with high-strength pancreatic enzymes in a child with cystic fibrosis. British Journal of Radiology 67: 900
McKendrick T 1962 Sweat sodium levels in normal subjects, in fibrocystic patients and their relatives, and in chronic bronchitic patients. Lancet 1: 183
Mitchell C J, Lintott D J, Ruddell W S J, Losowsky M S, Axon A T R 1979 Clinical relevance of an unfused pancreatic duct system. Gut 20: 1066
Morgan R G H, Barrowman J, Borgstrom B 1969 The effect of sodium taurodesoxycholate and pH on the gel filtration behaviour of rat pancreatic protein and lipases. Biochimica et Biophysica Acta 175: 65
Muller D P R, McCollum J P K, Trompeter R S, Harries J T 1975 Studies on the mechanism of fat absorption in congenital isolated lipase deficiency. Gut 16: 838
Muller D P R, Lloyd J K, Wolff O H 1983 Vitamin E and neurological function. Lancet 1: 225
Mutt V, Jorpes J E 1971 The nature of secretin and cholecystokinin-pancreozymin. In: Beck I T, Sinclair D G (eds) The exocrine pancreas. J & A Churchill, London, p 36
Newman D E 1973 Gallstones in children. Pediatric Radiology 1: 100
Nickels J, Laasonen E M 1976 Pancreatic heterotopia. Scandinavian Journal of Gastroenterology 5: 639
Nielsen O H, Larsen B F 1982 The incidence of anemia, hypoproteinemia, and edema in infants as presenting symptoms of cystic fibrosis: a retrospective survey of the frequency of this symptom complex in 130 patients with cystic fibrosis. Journal of Pediatric Gastroenterology and Nutrition 1: 355
Nielsen O H, Schiotz P O 1982 Cystic fibrosis in Denmark in the period 1945–1981. Evaluation of centralized treatment. Acta Paediatrica Scandinavica 301: 107
Nimmo J, Finlayson N D C, Smith A F, Shearman D J C 1970 The production of calcium and magnesium during pancreatic function tests in health and disease. Gut 11: 163
O'Brien S, Keogan M, Casey M, Duffy G, McErlean D, Fitzgerald M X, Hegarty J E 1992 Biliary complications of cystic fibrosis. Gut 33: 387
O'Neal W K, Beaudet A L 1994 Somatic gene therapy for cystic fibrosis. Human Molecular Genetics 3: 1497
Oppenheimer E H, Esterly J R 1975 Pathology of cystic fibrosis. Review of the literature and comparison with 146 autopsied cases. In: Rosenberg H S, Bolande R P (eds) Perspectives in pediatric pathology, Vol 2. Year Book Medical Publishers, Chicago, p 241
Palmer E D 1951 Benign intramural tumors of the stomach. A review with special reference to gross pathology. II. Aberrant pancreatic tumors. Medicine 30: 83
Park R W, Grand R J 1981 Gastrointestinal manifestations of cystic fibrosis: a review. Gastroenterology 81: 1143
Persons H G, Beaudry P, Dumas A, Pencharz P B 1983 Energy needs and growth in children with cystic fibrosis. Journal of Pediatric Gastroenterology and Nutrition 2: 44
Patrick M K, Howman-Giles R, de Silva M, van Asperen P, Pitkin J, Gaskin K J 1986 Common bile duct obstruction causing right upper abdominal pain in cystic fibrosis. Journal of Pediatrics 108: 101
Pencharz P B 1983 Energy intakes and low fat diets in children with cystic fibrosis. Journal of Pediatric Gastroenterology and Nutrition 2: 400
Pencharz P B, Levy L, Durie P R 1984 Nutritional rehabilitation of malnourished cystic fibrosis patients by supplemental nocturnal gastrostomy feeding. In: Lawson D (ed) Cystic fibrosis: horizons. Wiley, Chichester, p 384
Phelan M S, Fine D R, Zentler-Munro P L, Hodson M E, Batten J C, Kerr I H 1983 Radiographic abnormalities of the duodenum in cystic fibrosis. Clinical Radiology 34: 573
Price D D, von der Gruen A, Miller J, Rafii A, Price C 1985 Potentiation of systemic morphine analgesia in humans by

proglumide, a cholecystokinin antagonist. Anesthesia and Analgesia 64: 801
Psacharopoulos H T, Howard E R, Portmann B, Mowat A P, Williams R 1981 Hepatic complications of cystic fibrosis. Lancet 2: 78
Quinton P M 1986 Missing $Cl^-$ conductance in cystic fibrosis. American Journal of Physiology 251: C649
Quinton P M, Bijman J 1983 Higher bioelectric potentials due to decreased chloride absorption in the sweat glands of patients with cystic fibrosis. New England Journal of Medicine 308: 1185
Rinderknecht H 1986 Activation of pancreatic zymogens. Normal activation, premature intrapancreatic activation, protective mechanisms against inappropriate activation. Digestive Diseases and Sciences 31: 314
Riordan J R, Rommens J M, Kerem B et al 1989 Identification of the cystic fibrosis gene: cloning and characterization of complementary DNA. Science 245: 1066
Romeo G 1984 Cystic fibrosis: a single locus disease. In: Lawson D (ed) Cystic fibrosis: horizons. Wiley, Chichester, p 155
Rommens J M, Ianuzzi M C, Kerem B et al 1989 Identification of the cystic fibrosis gene: chromosome walking and jumping. Science 245: 1059
Rosch W, Koch H, Schaffner O, Demling L 1976 The clinical significance of the pancreas divisum. Gastrointestinal Endoscopy 22: 206
Rosenfeld R, Spigelblatt L, Chicoine R 1979 False positive sweat test, malnutrition, and the Mauriac syndrome. Journal of Pediatrics 94: 240
Rothman S S, Grendell J H 1983 The case of the disappearing pancreatic digestive enzymes. Gastroenterology 85: 1438
Russell R C G, Wong N W, Cotton P B 1984 Accessory sphincterotomy (endoscopic and surgical) in patients with pancreas divisum. British Journal of Surgery 71: 954
Sacher M, Kobsa A, Shmerling D H 1978 PABA screening test for exocrine pancreatic function in infants and children. Archives of Disease in Childhood. 53: 639
Sari H, Entressangles B, Desnuelle P 1975 Interactions of colipase with bile salt micelles. 2. Study by dialysis and spectrophotometry. European Journal of Biochemistry 58: 561
Shepherd R W, Thomas B J, Bennett D, Cooksley W G E, Ward L C 1983 Changes in body composition and muscle protein degradation during nutritional supplementation in nutritionally growth-retarded children with cystic fibrosis. Journal of Pediatric Gastroenterology and Nutrition 2: 439
Shwachman H, Diamond L K, Oski F A, Khaw K-T 1964 The syndrome of pancreatic insufficiency and bone marrow dysfunction. Journal of Pediatrics 65: 645
Shwachman H, Lebenthal E, Khaw K-T 1975 Recurrent acute pancreatitis in patients with cystic fibrosis with normal pancreatic enzymes. Pediatrics 55: 86
Shwachman H, Kowalski M, Khaw K-T 1977 Cystic fibrosis: a new outlook. 70 patients above 25 years of age. Medicine 56: 129
Shwachman H, Mahmoodian A, Neff R K 1981 The sweat test: sodium and chloride values. Journal of Pediatrics 98: 576
Slaff J I, Wolfe M M, Toskes P P 1985 Elevated fasting cholecystokinin levels in pancreatic exocrine impairment. Evidence to support feedback regulation. Journal of Laboratory and Clinical Medicine 105: 282
Smyth R L, van Velzen D, Smyth A R, Lloyd D A, Heaf D P 1994 Strictures of ascending colon in cystic fibrosis and high-strength pancreatic enzymes. Lancet 343: 85
Solomon T, Grossman M I 1977 Vagal control of pancreatic exocrine secretion. In: Brooks F P, Evers P W (eds) Nerves and gut. Slack, Thorofare, N J
Sommer H, Schrezenmeir J, Kasper H 1985 Output-dependent nonparallel enzyme secretion of the human pancreas. Hepato-Gastroenterology 32: 246
Soutter V L, Kristidis P, Gruca M A, Gaskin K J 1986 Chronic undernutrition/growth retardation in cystic fibrosis. Clinics in Gastroenterology 15: 137
Stafford R J, Grand R J 1982 Hereditary disease of the exocrine pancreas. Clinics in Gastroenterology 11: 141
Steers M L, Saluja A K 1993 Experimental acute pancreatitis: studies of the early events that lead to cell injury. In: Go V L W, DiMagno E P, Gardner J D, Lebenthal E, Reber H A, Scheele G A (eds) The pancreas. Raven Press, New York
Stern R C, Stevens D P, Boat T F, Doershuk C F, Izant R J, Matthews L W 1976 Symptomatic hepatic disease in cystic fibrosis: incidence, course, and outcome of portal systemic shunting. Gastroenterology 70: 645
Sugawa C, Walt A J, Nunez D C, Masuyama H 1987 Pancreas divisum: is it a normal anatomic variant? American Journal of Surgery 153: 62
Tarlow M L, Hadorn B, Arthurton M W, Lloyd J K 1970 Intestinal enterokinase deficiency. A newly recognized disorder of protein digestion. Archives of Disease in Childhood 45: 651
Taussig L M, Saldino R M, di Sant'Agnese P A 1973 Radiographic abnormalities of the duodenum and small bowel in cystic fibrosis of the pancreas (mucoviscidosis). Radiology 106: 369
Tizzano E, Buchwald M 1995 CFTR expression and organ damage in cystic fibrosis. Annals of Internal Medicine 123: 305
Tizzano E F, Chitayat D, Buchwald M 1993 Cell-specific localization of CFTR mRNA shows developmentally regulated expression in human fetal tissues. Human Molecular Genetics 2: 219
Townes P L, Bryson M F, Miller G 1967 Further observations on trypsinogen deficiency disease. Report of a second case. Journal of Pediatrics 71: 220
Trezise A E O, Chambers J A, Wardle C J, Gould S, Harris A 1993 Expression of the cystic fibrosis gene in human foetal tissues. Human Molecular Genetics 2: 213
Vantrappen G R, Peeters T L, Janssens J 1979 The secretory component of the interdigestive migrating motor complex in man. Scandinavian Journal of Gastroenterology 14: 663
Warshaw A L, Richter J M, Schapiro R H 1983 The cause and treatment of pancreatitis associated with pancreas divisum. Annals of Surgery 198: 443
Warwick W J 1982 Prognosis for survival with cystic fibrosis: the effects of early diagnosis and cystic fibrosis center care. Acta Paediatrica Scandinavica 301: 27
Welsh M J, Smith A E 1993 Molecular mechanisms of CFTR chloride channel dysfunction in cystic fibrosis. Cell 73: 1251
Wormsley K G 1970 Stimulation of pancreatic secretion by intraduodenal infusion of bile salts. Lancet 2: 586
Wormsley K G, Goldberg D M 1972 The interrelationships of the pancreatic enzymes. Gut 13: 398
Zentler-Munro P L 1983 Gastrointestinal disease in adults. In: Hodson M E, Norman A P, Batten J C (eds) Cystic fibrosis. Baillière Tindall, London, p 144

# 50. Acute and chronic pancreatitis — pathophysiology and management

*D. C. Carter*

## CLASSIFICATION OF PANCREATITIS

In 1963 at a symposium in Marseilles, pancreatitis was classified into acute, acute relapsing, chronic relapsing (chronic pancreatitis with acute exacerbations) and chronic pancreatitis. The two chronic forms were characterized by the fact that pancreatic anatomy and/or function did not return to normal once the precipitating cause was removed. This classification was subsequently simplified after meetings in Marseilles and Cambridge (Sarner & Cotton 1984, Sarles 1985) by abolishing the acute relapsing and chronic relapsing categories. Acute pancreatitis is now defined as an acute inflammatory condition typically presenting with abdominal pain and usually associated with raised pancreatic enzyme activity in blood or urine. Chronic pancreatitis is defined as a continuing inflammatory disease of the pancreas, characterized by irreversible morphological change and typically causing pain and/or permanent loss of function.

Within these definitions, it is accepted that acute pancreatitis may cause transient impairment of endocrine and/or exocrine function, that it may recur and that gland destruction in severe necrotizing pancreatitis may leave permanent functional and anatomical derangement. It is also accepted that many patients with chronic pancreatitis have acute exacerbations and that the condition is occasionally completely painless. Pancreatic function can be difficult to assess objectively and there is often little relationship between clinical, morphological, functional and histopathological evidence of pancreatitis.

## ACUTE PANCREATITIS

### Incidence

In Rochester, Minnesota, the incidence of acute pancreatitis was 11 cases per 100 000 population in the period 1940–69 (O'Sullivan et al 1972). In Bristol, England, between 1950 and 1969 the incidence was 5.4 cases per 100 000 (Trapnell & Duncan 1975), but by the next decade it had increased to 9.1 cases per 100 000 (Corfield et al 1985a). In Scotland, the number of patients discharged from hospital with a diagnosis of acute pancreatitis rose 11-fold in males and fourfold in females between 1961 and 1985, the increase being particularly marked in young and middle-aged men and in elderly women (Wilson & Imrie 1990). While this increase may be apparent rather than real, reflecting increasing awareness and improved diagnosis, it may also reflect increasing alcohol abuse. In Finland, a doubling of the incidence of acute pancreatitis in men in the period 1970–89 was correlated with a rising alcohol consumption and incidence of liver cirrhosis (Jaakkola et al 1994). Alcohol is also the predominant cause of acute pancreatitis in Japan where the annual incidence is now 12 cases per 100 000 (Saitoh & Yamamoto 1991).

### Etiology

#### *Alcohol*

In a review of 5019 cases of acute pancreatitis in the decade up to 1980, 55% were attributed to alcohol and 27% to cholelithiasis, while the remainder were idiopathic or attributed to miscellaneous causes (Ranson 1983). Alcohol-associated disease usually predominates in reports from North American inner cities, whereas in most British centers, gallstones are the commonest cause (see Table 50.1), accounting for some 50% of cases (Carter 1989). In Scandinavia, gallstones used to account for two-thirds of cases but in some centers, almost two-thirds of cases are now attributable to alcohol (Svensson et al 1979, Mero 1982).

It is not understood why alcohol causes acute pancreatitis in some individuals and not in others. The amount of alcohol consumed is a determinant of the severity of the first attack of acute pancreatitis but not of recurrent attacks (Jaakkola et al 1994) and it is now appreciated that many patients with so-called acute alcoholic pancreatitis have underlying chronic damage (p. 1270).

**Table 50.1** Etiology of acute pancreatitis in patients admitted to Edinburgh Royal Infirmary 1989–1993

| Etiology | n (%) |
|---|---|
| Gall stones | 116 (42) |
| Alcohol | 97 (35) |
| Idiopathic | 41 (15) |
| Post-ERCP | 11 (4) |
| Pancreatic cancer | 5 (2) |
| After operation | 3 (1) |
| Post-myocardial infarction | 1 (0.4) |
| Trauma | 1 (0.4) |
| Metastatic carcinoma and biliary stent | 1 (0.4) |
| Immunosuppressant therapy post-renal transplant | 1 (0.4) |
| Hyperlipidemia | 1 (0.4) |
| Terminal colon carcinoma | 1 (0.4) |
| Total | 279 |

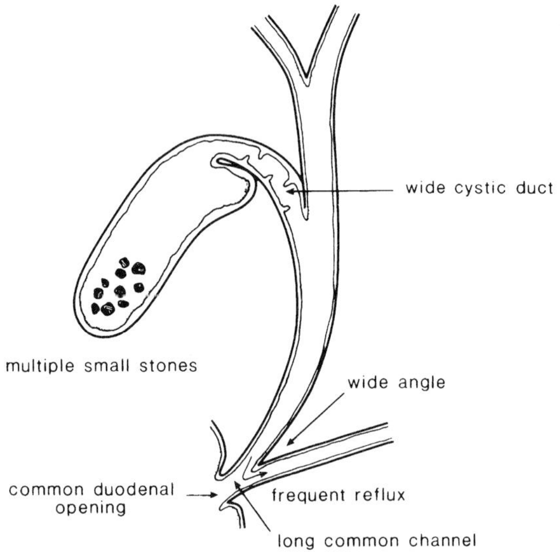


**Fig. 50.1** Summary of anatomical and other abnormalities predisposing to the development of acute gallstone pancreatitis.

*Cholelithiasis*

Some 3–7% of patients with gallstones will develop pancreatitis (Ranson 1979, Moreau et al 1988) and cholelithiasis is the most common cause of acute pancreatitis in patients over the age of 60 years. Factors which predispose to the development of pancreatitis in patients with gallstones include the presence of multiple small stones in the gallbladder, a wide cystic duct, a less acute angle between bile duct and pancreatic duct and a long common channel between them and a greater frequency of reflux into the pancreatic duct on operative cholangiography (McMahon & Shefta 1980, Kelly 1984, Armstrong & Taylor 1985, 1986, Jones et al 1987) (Fig. 50.1). Pregnancy is associated with an increased risk of pancreatitis but this is now attributed to the increased incidence of gallstones during pregnancy.

*Postoperative and postprocedural pancreatitis*

Direct trauma to the pancreas may cause pancreatitis after gastric resection (notably after Polya partial gastrectomy) and biliary tract operations (particularly when there is instrumentation or surgery involving the common bile duct and papilla of Vater). Pancreatitis may also occur after operations unrelated to the pancreas such as cardiac surgery involving cardiopulmonary bypass (see below).

ERCP is now the third commonest defined cause of pancreatitis in some series. The reported incidence of "clinical" as opposed to "biochemical" pancreatitis after ERCP varies from 0.7 to 12% (Roszler & Campbell 1985) although as many as 50% of patients have hyperamylasemia without clinical signs. Excessive manipulation, use of diathermy and high injection pressures with entry of contrast into the acini (acinarization) are all risk factors, although newer nonionic contrast media may reduce some of the risks. Therapeutic maneuvers increase the risk of pancreatitis but in skilled hands the incidence of pancreatitis after endoscopic sphincterotomy for bile duct stones can be less than 1% (Vaira et al 1989). Endoscopic sphincterotomy for sphincter of Oddi dysfunction carries a higher risk, estimated at 3.5% in recent reviews (Sherman et al 1991), and pancreatic duct stricturing in such patients can cause recurrent pancreatitis (Asbun et al 1993) (see also pp. 119 & 120).

Pancreatitis caused by inadvertent injection of contrast at translumbar aortography is no longer seen given the development of other methods of angiography.

*Local obstructive factors* (Warshaw 1989)

Pancreatitis may be caused by chronic duodenal or afferent loop obstruction (Conter et al 1990), duodenal diverticula (Hartley et al 1993), duodenal and periampullary cysts (Holstege et al 1985), stenosis of the papilla of Vater, biliary ascariasis (Khuroo et al 1990) and ductal obstruction by pancreatic and periampullary neoplasms.

*Pancreas divisum*

Pancreas divisum is a congenital abnormality in which the dorsal and ventral pancreatic ducts fail to fuse normally. It has been postulated that pancreatitis arises because secretions from the larger dorsal pancreas have to pass through the small accessory papilla into the duodenum and papillary stenosis may be an important cofactor (Warshaw 1989). However, pancreas divisum is present in about 6% of individuals (Delhaye et al 1985) and there is continuing debate about whether it causes pancreatitis or is merely an incidental finding in patients with idiopathic pancreatitis (Connors & Carr-Locke 1993).

*Trauma*

Pancreatitis may result from penetrating and nonpenetrating abdominal injury, the mortality rate varying according to the severity of trauma and number of organs injured (Imrie et al 1978c).

*Infections and infestations*

Acute pancreatitis may be associated with mumps, Coxsackie, hepatitis A, Epstein–Barr and cytomegalovirus infection, with bacterial infection by *Campylobacter* (Gallagher et al 1981), *Mycoplasma pneumoniae* (Freeman & McMahon 1978) and Legionella, and with infestation by ascariasis (Khuroo et al 1990) and *Clonorchis sinensis* (p. 591).

*Drugs*

Drugs associated with acute pancreatitis include thiazide diuretics, frusemide, sulfonamides, rifampicin, tetracycline, azathioprine and estrogens (Mallory & Kern 1980, Lankisch et al 1995). Drugs with a less certain association include corticosteroids, L-asparaginase, 6-mercaptopurine, chlorthalidone, methyldopa, ethacrynic acid, phenformin, procainamide, agents causing hypercalcemia and cytosine arabinoside.

*Lipid abnormalities* (Toskes 1994)

Acute pancreatitis has a recognized association with types I, IV and V primary hyperlipoproteinemia (Buch et al 1980). It may also occur when there is secondary hyperlipoproteinemia, as in alcohol abuse (Dickson et al 1984), and when there is hyperlipoproteinemia for which no cause can be found. Hyperlipoproteinemia in acute pancreatitis is usually characterized by high serum triglyceride levels with normal cholesterol levels.

The role of hypertriglyceridemia in alcohol-associated pancreatitis remains uncertain. Hypertriglyceridemia is not more common in patients with alcohol-induced pancreatitis than in alcoholics without pancreatitis and plasma triglyceride levels do not account for individual susceptibility to either alcoholic or gallstone pancreatitis (Haber et al 1994). While it is uncertain whether increased serum triglyceride levels can trigger pancreatic inflammation, it is conceivable that pancreatic lipase could hydrolyze triglyceride with release of toxic fatty acids. A high fat intake, with or without alcohol intake, could precipitate pancreatitis through such a mechanism. High triglyceride levels are present in 50% of patients with necrotizing pancreatitis (Dominguez-Muñoz et al 1991) but this hyperlipidemia is almost certainly a pre-existing disorder and not the result of pancreatic necrosis.

Acute pancreatitis may complicate total parenteral nutrition and a high concentration of fat emulsion may be responsible (Lashner et al 1986).

*Ischemia and cardiovascular disease*

Acute pancreatitis is a relatively rare complication of cardiopulmonary bypass (Haas et al 1985); factors implicated include hypotension and hypoperfusion, embolization of cholesterol plaques, nonpulsatile perfusion and hypothermia. Pancreatic cellular injury was evident (i.e. hyperamylasemia of pancreatic origin) in 27% of one series of 300 patients undergoing cardiac surgery, three of whom went on to develop severe pancreatitis (Fernandez-del Castillo et al 1991). Preoperative renal insufficiency, valve surgery, postoperative hypotension and perioperative administration of calcium chloride were significant risk factors for the development of pancreatitis.

Acute pancreatitis is common following fatal rupture of an aortic aneurysm and its association with acute tubular necrosis in this context suggests that prolonged hypotension is important (Warshaw & O'Hara 1978).

Other vascular diseases associated with acute pancreatitis include disseminated lupus erythematosus, polyarteritis nodosa and thrombotic thrombocytopenic purpura. Pancreatitis associated with hypothermia is probably due to impaired vascular perfusion and thrombosis.

*Hypercalcemia*

Acute pancreatitis may complicate hypercalcemia resulting from malignancy (Gafter et al 1976) or total parenteral nutrition (Izsak et al 1980). Its association with hyperparathyroidism is controversial. Between 7% and 19% of patients with hyperparathyroidism once developed acute or chronic pancreatitis (Ludwig & Chaykin 1966) and pancreatitis was sometimes the presenting feature. However, only 1.5% of 1153 patients with hyperparathyroidism in a more recent review had pancreatitis and in two-thirds of them there was an alternative cause (Bess et al 1980). Earlier diagnosis of hyperparathyroidism has undoubtedly reduced the incidence of this form of pancreatitis.

*Miscellaneous causes*

Acute pancreatitis can occur after scorpion stings, in fulminant hepatic failure (Ede et al 1988) and in hypotensive shock. Pancreatitis in relation to organ transplantation (Aziz et al 1985) is probably multifactorial with contributions from altered perfusion, drug therapy, infection and rejection.

*Idiopathic pancreatitis*

With increased understanding of the pathogenesis of pancreatitis and the realization that very small gallstones and biliary debris may cause pancreatitis (Neoptolemos et al 1988b, Lee et al 1992), the proportion of cases without a

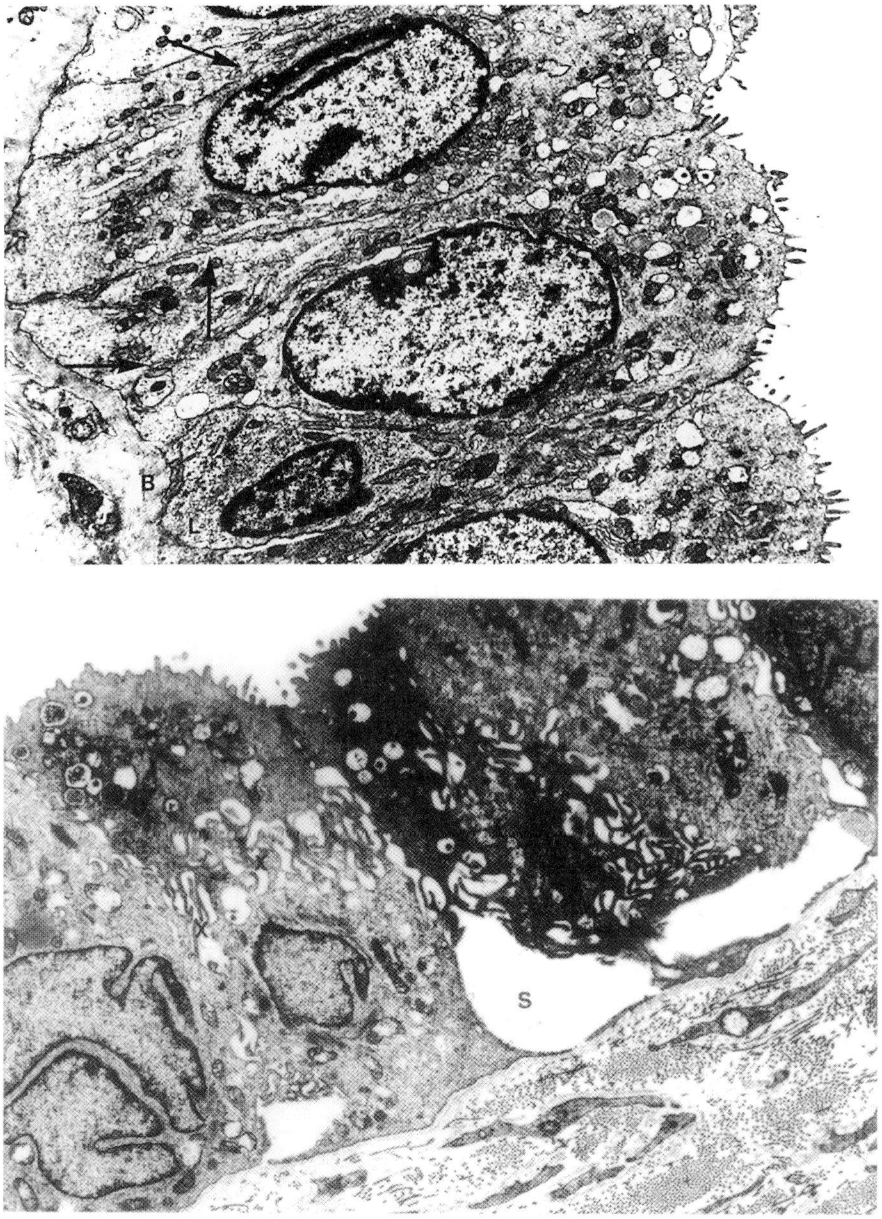


A

B

defined etiological cause has fallen. However, idiopathic pancreatitis still accounts for 30–40% of cases in the elderly and continues to carry a high morbidity and mortality (Browder et al 1993).

## Pathogenesis of acute pancreatitis

Our understanding of the mechanisms which initiate pancreatitis is still imperfect. The disease involves events within the pancreatic acinar cell, inflammation of the pancreas and peripancreatic tissues and a systemic inflammatory response. It has long been held that activated pancreatic proteases such as trypsin and phospholipase A play a role in pancreatic injury, but more recently it has become apparent that release of oxygen-derived free radicals (Sanfey et al 1983) and activation of macrophages and polymorphonuclear leukocytes are also important.

### *Reflux of duodenal juice and bile*

To explain the presence of activated enzymes in the pancreas it is necessary to postulate reflux from the duodenum, mixing of bile and pancreatic juice within the pancreatic duct system or activation of pancreatic enzymes within the acinar cell itself. Normally, the pancreas is protected against its own enzymes by their synthesis as proenzymes. Furthermore, inhibitors in pancreatic tissue and juice inactivate proteases which have been prematurely activated. Mechanisms preventing reflux of activated enzymes from the duodenum include the secretion pres-

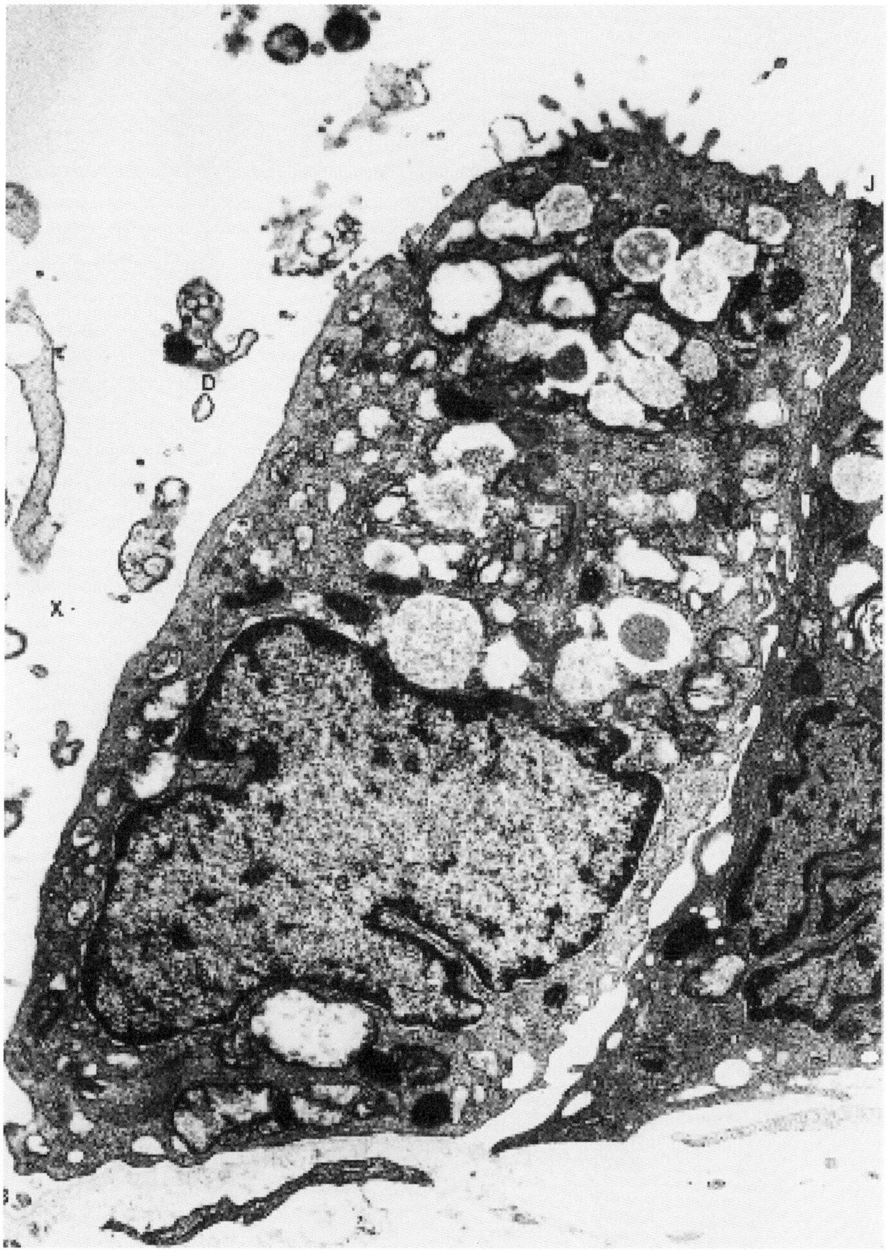


**Fig. 50.2** Transmission electron micrograph of cat pancreatic duct system. (**A**) An intraepithelial lymphocyte (L) is shown just above the basal lamina (B). The arrows point to the intracellular boundaries which are separated by a minimal intracellular space. Note the surface microvilli (× 3500). (**B**) After perfusion with 40 mmol/L sodium taurocholate solution at a pressure of 5 mmHg. No cellular damage is apparent but the lateral contact surfaces (X) are more elaborate than normal and basal intracellular spaces (S) are present (× 4300). (**C**) After perfusion with 40 mmol/L sodium taurocholate solution at a pressure of 30 mmHg. Disintegrated epithelial cells have left debris (D) and wide gaps (X) down to the basal lamina (B). Cells adjacent to the gap show reactive change but are intact and remain firmly attached to their neighbors with normal junctional complexes (J) (× 6000).

sure within the pancreatic duct, the oblique course of the pancreatic duct through the duodenal muscle, the high pressure maintained by the sphincter of Oddi (Carr-Locke & Gregg 1981) and the valvular action of the mucosal folds at the entrance to the pancreatic duct.

Pancreatitis may occur if these protective mechanisms are compromised, for example by sphincterotomy or impaction of a gallstone at the lower end of the common bile duct (McCutcheon 1968). Reflux of duodenal contents into the pancreatic duct could then allow enterokinase to activate trypsinogen, while continued secretion into an obstructed duct could rupture small ducts and allow extravasation of enzymes. Activated proteases have been recovered from pancreatic tissues and juice in human pancreatitis (Geokas & Rinderknecht 1978), but available evidence from animal models suggests that pancreatic secretion, and in particular the secretory response to cholecystokinin, is *reduced* soon after the onset of acute pancreatitis (Niederau et al 1990).

Several enzymes could cause pancreatic inflammation and necrosis in acute pancreatitis, but trypsinogen probably has the central role. This protease is not normally activated until it comes into contact with enterokinase secreted by the duodenal mucosa, but once the molecule has been cleaved to produce the active proteolytic enzyme trypsin, a cascade effect leads to activation of other pancreatic enzymes. Cleavage of trypsinogen also releases trypsinogen activation peptides (TAPs) and the concentration of TAPs in urine and plasma is correlated with the severity of pancreatitis in animals and man (Gudgeon et al 1990, Schmidt et al 1992). Elastase has a key role in the local vascular changes in acute pancreatitis, changes which may be enhanced by the local release of the vasodilator kallikrein. Release of phospholipase A, which damages membranes, may also be important in the production of necrosis.

Bile salts in concentrations normally present in bile disrupt the pancreatic mucosal barrier and produce marked inflammation when injected into the pancreatic duct at physiological pressures (Fig. 50.2) (Farmer et al 1984, Simpson et al 1984). It is possible that bile salts liberate minute amounts of trypsin in the pancreatic cells which in turn activates other pancreatic proenzymes, notably proelastase and prophospholipase A.

Keynes (1988) has argued that necrosis in acute pancreatitis is not the result of autodigestion by proteases but reflux of lysolecithin formed from activation of pancreatic phospholipase by trypsin/bile salts in the duodenum. Infection of refluxing bile could also cause necrosis by triggering a cytotoxic inflammatory response (Keynes 1988). Clinical evidence linking cholangitis and acute pancreatitis (Neoptolemos et al 1987) is supported by experimental evidence that infected bile (particularly *E. coli* infection) readily disrupts the pancreatic duct mucosal barrier (Konok & Thompson 1969).

*Reflux and gallstone pancreatitis*

Patients with gallstone pancreatitis are cured by cholecystectomy, probably because this removes the source of stones passing down the biliary tree (below). Acosta et al (1977) recovered gallstones from the feces in 47 of 51 patients who presented with acute pancreatitis and stones in the gallbladder. In 51 control patients with cholelithiasis but no pancreatitis, stones were recovered in only six patients. Gallstones were present in the ampulla in 75% of patients with gallstone pancreatitis who had surgery within 48 h of the onset of symptoms but in only 25% of those where surgery was delayed for more than 4 days, indicating that most stones pass on spontaneously within days.

Opie's common channel theory (Opie 1901) proposed that obstruction of the papilla allowed bile to reflux from the common bile duct into the pancreatic duct, thus activating pancreatic enzymes. This mechanism is only possible if there is a common channel between the bile duct and pancreatic duct (Fig. 50.1). Despite earlier claims that most individuals lack a common channel (McCutcheon 1968), later anatomical and radiological studies have demonstrated communication in 74–91% of cases (Millbourn 1950, Di Magno et al 1982). Reflux into the pancreatic duct has been found at operative cholangiography in 50–67% of patients who have had gallstone pancreatitis as opposed to 1–18% of patients with cholelithiasis but no history of pancreatitis (Kelly 1976, 1984, Armstrong & Taylor 1986). It is also possible that the passage of a stone into the duodenum renders the pancreatic duct more susceptible to reflux. Acute pancreatitis induced by closed loop obstruction of the duodenum (Pfeffer et al 1957) highlights the potential importance of reflux of duodenal contents since ligation of the pancreatic duct prevents pancreatic inflammation. These experiments may also be relevant to the pancreatitis which may follow Polya partial gastrectomy or chronic duodenal obstruction.

While the ability of gallstones to trigger acute pancreatitis is not in dispute, considerable uncertainty still surrounds the importance of duodenopancreatic or biliary-pancreatic reflux. It is well recognized in experimental models that increasing pancreatic ductal pressure can increase ductal permeability and damage the mucosal barrier (Simpson et al 1984, Harvey et al 1989). Recent studies in the opossum have shown that ligation of the pancreatic duct gives rise to necrotizing pancreatitis which is just as severe as that caused by ligating the bile duct or common pancreaticobiliary channel (Lerch et al 1993); it is clear that duodenal or biliary reflux is not essential for the development of pancreatitis, at least in this experimental model.

*Activation of enzymes within the acinar cell* (Steer et al 1984)

The possibility that enzymes can be activated within the acinar cell itself avoids the need to invoke reflux or a common channel. Under normal circumstances, digestive enzymes and lysosomal hydrolases are both synthesized in the acinar cell by ribosomes attached to the rough endoplasmic reticulum and are then transported to the Golgi complex where secretory proteins accumulate in zymogen granules and lysosomal hydrolases are segregated in lysosomes (p. 1230). Activation of trypsinogen by lysosomal hydrolases is normally prevented by this segregation, by the fact that both are present in low concentrations in the rough endoplasmic reticulum and by the presence of pancreatic trypsin inhibitor in pancreatic tissue. In two forms of experimental pancreatitis, one induced by a choline-deficient diet and the other by infusing cerulein (which stimulates maximal pancreatic secretion), there is evidence of early admixture (colocalization) of digestive and lysosomal enzymes. The fusion of zymogen granules with lysosomes (crinophagy) allows activation of proteases by cathepsin B in the resulting "autophagic vacuoles" (Adler et al 1982, Bettinger & Grendell 1991). Whereas zymogen granules normally discharge into the pancreatic ductules by exocytosis from the apical surface of the acinar cell, disruption of this process may lead to discharge from the basolateral cell surface into the intercellular space (Adler et al 1985). The presence of activated proteases such as trypsin, chymotrypsin and elastase in pancreatic tissues could then lead readily to inflammation, activation of macrophages and polymorphonuclear leukocytes, and pancreatitis.

A unifying concept is that all factors causing pancreatitis act on digestive or lysosomal protein transport within the acinar cell. In this respect, pancreatitis in choline-deficient, ethionine-supplemented mice has an improved mortality when treated with prostaglandin $E_2$ which increases the stability of lysosomal, mitochondrial and cell membranes (Standfield & Kakkar 1983). However, despite the attractions of intracellular activation of proteases as a trigger mechanism, the phenomenon has only been demonstrated in animal models, occurs in mild as well as severe pancreatitis and can occur in ductal obstruction without pancreatitis as well as in normal pancreatic tissue (Warshaw 1993). It follows that its significance in the pathogenesis of acute pancreatitis in man remains uncertain.

### *Alcohol and acute pancreatitis*

Potential mechanisms whereby alcohol exerts its effect on the pancreas include the development of ductal obstruction by precipitates of protein (p. 1269), acetaldehyde toxicity, increased pancreatic duct permeability and alcohol induced hypertriglyceridemia (p. 1249). Ethanol is metabolized to acetaldehyde in the liver (and perhaps to a limited degree in the pancreas itself) by alcohol dehydrogenase and acetaldehyde can induce pancreatitis when given intra-arterially in the isolated perfused canine pancreas (Nordback et al 1991). Acetaldehyde could also serve as a substrate for the generation of oxygen free radicals by the enzyme xanthine oxidase, an enzyme present in high concentrations in the pancreas.

There is little support for the theory that ethanol is directly toxic to the pancreatic acinar cell, causes spasm of the sphincter of Oddi, promotes duodenal reflux by causing incompetence of the sphincter of Oddi or induces pancreatic hypersecretion.

### *Ischemia and pancreatitis*

Ischemia and infarction can cause acute pancreatitis experimentally and clinically (p. 1249). Factors implicated include diffuse small vessel disease as in disseminated lupus, diminished perfusion as in shock (Warshaw & O'Hara 1978) and thrombosis as in hypothermia. Altered blood flow is also important in the pathogenesis of pancreatitis due to other causes. Increased capillary permeability is an early feature of experimental pancreatitis (Sanfey & Cameron 1984) and ultrastructural changes become apparent in the microvasculature within 30 min in cerulein-induced pancreatitis in rats (Kelly et al 1993). Pancreatic necrosis from ischemia may be superimposed on all forms of pancreatitis and there is experimental evidence that α-adrenergic vasoconstrictors (Klar et al 1991) and intravenous contrast agents (Foitzik et al 1994) can accentuate vascular damage.

## Pathology

Acute pancreatitis produces a spectrum of morphological changes which may be patchy or diffuse. In mild, so-called edematous or interstitial pancreatitis, edema predominates with cellular infiltration, fibroblastic proliferation and scattered peripancreatic fat necrosis without parenchymatous or acinar necrosis. To the naked eye the gland appears swollen and pale. In severe or necrotizing pancreatitis, which accounts for some 15% of attacks, there is extensive pancreatic and peripancreatic fat necrosis, parenchymal necrosis and hemorrhage. Liquefaction necrosis is accompanied by thrombosis of small vessels and there may be bleeding in affected areas. Infection may supervene in areas of necrosis.

In both forms of pancreatitis, fat necrosis may be visible as white plaques in surrounding tissues. Histologically, necrotic fat cells are full of granules containing fatty acids to which calcium may bind. Later, the necrotic area is invaded and absorbed by macrophages and giant cells. Pancreatic enzymes can also cause fat necrosis outside the abdomen (p. 1260).

Peripancreatic collections may form which contain pancreatic juice, inflammatory exudate, blood and necrotic tissues. Pseudocysts, infected necrosis and pancreatic abscess are all potential complications of acute pancreatitis. The term "pancreatic phlegmon" was sometimes used to describe an inflamed and indurated pancreatic/peripancreatic mass due to extensive edema, inflammatory exudate and tissue necrosis (Fan et al 1989). When the disease is fully established, the organ may resemble oily mud in which degenerative tissue, fat and hemorrhage coalesce.

## Clinical features

Nearly all patients complain of abdominal pain and the attack is occasionally precipitated by a large meal and/or alcohol. Nausea, vomiting and retching are prominent. The pain is usually epigastric but may radiate to the back or become generalized. Pain is constant and leaning forwards may give some relief whereas vomiting and simple analgesics do not. It is now appreciated that acute pancreatitis can also be painless and that failure to make the diagnosis early increases risk (Lankisch et al 1991). In some cases, acute pancreatitis mimics the presentation of myocardial infarction or uremia and the diagnosis must always be considered in patients who present with unexplained shock or anuria.

Initially, there may be tenderness and guarding in the upper abdomen but these are often minimal, in marked contrast to the severe pain experienced by the patient.

Tenderness and guarding may eventually become generalized and abdominal distention develops with the onset of ileus. Hiccoughs can be troublesome and reflect irritation of the undersurface of the diaphragm. The patient may have low-grade pyrexia and is occasionally jaundiced. Shock is common in severe acute pancreatitis and confusion and toxicity can give rise to "pancreatic encephalopathy". A palpable abdominal mass is rare on admission but may develop if there are complications such as a pseudocyst. Bleeding into fascial planes produces discoloration around the umbilicus (Cullen's sign) or in the flanks (Grey-Turner's sign) in 1–3% of patients (Dickson & Imrie 1984). Neither sign is pathognomonic of acute pancreatitis, but when present they denote severe disease; of the 23 patients reported by Dickson & Imrie, 15 (65%) survived although all but one developed complications. Subcutaneous fat necrosis occasionally produces small red tender nodules in the limbs.

In postoperative pancreatitis, pain, vomiting and abdominal tenderness are often masked by the original operation and diagnosis is difficult. Pancreatitis should be suspected in any patient who develops prolonged hypotension or jaundice within a few days of upper gastrointestinal, pancreatic or biliary surgery.

Acute pancreatitis is seldom absent from the differential diagnosis of the acute abdomen. The clinical findings are seldom sufficiently specific to allow a confident diagnosis of pancreatitis and investigations are always needed. Occasionally the features on examination are such that patients undergo laparotomy because a condition requiring emergency surgical intervention (e.g. perforated peptic ulcer) cannot be excluded.

## Biochemical investigations

*Serum and urinary amylase* (Clavien et al 1989a)

Amylase isoenzymes in the serum can originate from the salivary glands and pancreas. Total amylase activity is measured by its action on synthetic carbohydrate-containing substrates with release of a colored dye (chromogenic method) or glucose (saccharogenic method). The normal range is up to 300 i.u./L although there is no standardized internationally agreed method of measuring serum amylase levels. In acute pancreatitis, the rise in serum amylase activity is confined largely to pancreatic amylase and reflects absorption of enzymes leaking from the acinar cells and duct system. The rise is not proportional to the severity of the pancreatitis and pancreatic necrosis can be associated with activity levels of less than 1000 i.u./L (Winslet et al 1992). Amylase activity is highest during the first 24 h and falls rapidly thereafter following clearance by the kidney, unless there is continuing pancreatitis, pseudocyst or abscess formation. In one recent study, admission amylase activity was diagnostic in 96% of patients with mild pancreatitis and in 87% of those with severe disease, whereas 48 h later these values were 33% and 48% respectively (Winslet et al 1992).

In general, patients with alcohol-associated disease have lower amylase activity than those with gallstone pancreatitis (Blamey et al 1983, Winslet et al 1992) and it is now appreciated that as many as one-third of patients with ultrasonographic or CT scan evidence of acute alcoholic pancreatitis have normoamylasemia (Spechler et al 1983). Hyperlipidemia is found in some 20% of patients with alcoholic pancreatitis and is frequently associated with normal serum and urinary amylase activities (Cameron et al 1973). Gallstone pancreatitis, idiopathic pancreatitis and postoperative pancreatitis occur occasionally in the absence of hyperamylasemia (Clavien et al 1989b).

High amylase activities in serum are found in conditions other than acute pancreatitis (Table 50.2) and isoenzyme determinations (see below) show that up to one-third of patients with hyperamylasemia are not suffering from acute pancreatitis. A serum amylase activity of greater than 1000 or 1200 i.u./L is usually taken as diagnostic for acute pancreatitis and hyperamylasemia of this degree is unusual in the absence of pancreatitis. In some such cases there may be a degree of pancreatic inflammation; for example, ruptured aortic aneurysm is frequently associated with hyperamylasemia (Bagley et al 1994) and Warshaw & O'Hara (1978) found that no less than 29% of patients dying after rupture of an aortic aneurysm had associated pancreatitis, necrosis or abscess. Only about 40% of amylase activity in the serum is normally of pancreatic origin and in some cases of hyperamylasemia, the circulating amylase originates from other organs (notably the salivary glands).

**Table 50.2** Conditions associated with hyperamylasemia

| Abdominal causes | Non-abdominal causes |
|---|---|
| Pancreatitis | Thoracic |
| Pancreatic cancer | Myocardial infarct |
| Biliary tract disease | Pulmonary embolism |
| Perforated peptic ulcer | Pneumonia |
| Acute perforated appendicitis | Metastatic lung cancer |
| Intestinal obstruction | Cardio-pulmonary bypass |
| Mesenteric infarction | Salivary gland |
| Liver disease | Salivary trauma |
| Dissecting aortic aneurysm | Infection (mumps) |
| Ruptured ectopic pregnancy | Salivary duct obstruction |
| Prostatic disease | Irradiation |
| Ovarian neoplasm | Metabolic |
| Recent abdominal operation | Diabetic ketoacidosis |
| Afferent loop syndrome | Drugs |
| | Opiates |
| | Phenylbutazone |
| | Trauma |
| | Cerebral trauma |
| | Burns |
| | Renal disease |
| | Renal insufficiency |
| | Renal transplantation |

A raised serum amylase may also result from impaired renal function or, more rarely, because a macromolecular complex of amylase forms which is too large to be excreted. In most cases, the amylase is bound to an abnormal immunoglycoprotein (usually IgG or IgA) and a raised serum amylase activity in association with a low urinary amylase should lead one to suspect macroamylasemia in a patient with normal renal function. Macroamylasemia is found in up to 3% of cases of acute pancreatitis (Durr et al 1977) and more importantly, in 1–2% of the normal population. Confusion is most simply resolved by measuring serum lipase as an index of pancreatitis.

Urinary levels of amylase frequently remain elevated in acute pancreatitis after serum levels have returned to normal. Amylase can be measured in urine using a rapid colorimetric test (Rapignost-Amylase test) but the test has poor sensitivity and specificity and is not used widely. The amylase:creatinine clearance ratio is raised in acute pancreatitis because of altered renal tubular handling of amylase. Unfortunately, the ratio may be raised in any condition with defective tubular reabsorption of protein and the test is hardly ever used (Clavien et al 1989a).

*Serum lipase*

Lipase and trypsin activity in serum are also increased in acute pancreatitis. The serum lipase is one of the most reliable markers of acute pancreatitis, having a sensitivity and specificity of almost 90% (Ventrucci et al 1989). Lipase activity remains elevated for longer than amylase activity in acute pancreatitis and is not increased when hyperamylasemia is due to salivary amylase or macroamylasemia in the absence of pancreatitis (Kolars et al 1984). Serum lipase activity can now be measured rapidly and reliably by methods such as the lipase latex agglutination test and may yet be used more widely in clinical practice.

## **Radiology and other imaging procedures** (Freeny 1993b)

*Plain radiographs of the abdomen* (Davis et al 1980)

Nonspecific radiological signs associated with acute pancreatitis are seen on the abdominal radiograph in about 50% of cases although the principal value of such films is to exclude other causes of the acute abdomen, notably gastrointestinal perforation and obstruction. Changes in acute pancreatitis include the presence of a soft tissue mass, gas in a pancreatic abscess and soft tissue mottling due to fat necrosis. Gastrointestinal changes include dilatation of the stomach, duodenum, small and large intestine and there may be a "sentinel" loop of jejunum or a colon "cut-off" sign in which gas is seen in the ascending and descending colon but not the transverse colon. Other relevant abnormalities are loss of psoas and renal outlines, opaque gallstones, elevation of the diaphragm, gas in the biliary tract and evidence of ascites.

*Chest radiograph*

Pleuropulmonary complications of acute pancreatitis include pleural effusion, elevation of the diaphragm, widening of the mediastinum, basal atelectasis, lobar consolidation, pulmonary infarction and adult respiratory distress syndrome. Chest radiographs are abnormal in one-third of patients with acute pancreatitis and in over 70% of those with severe pancreatitis, and left-sided pleural effusion is particularly common in patients with severe disease (Millward et al 1983).

*Ultrasound scanning* (Freeny 1993b) (p. 58)

While computed tomography is arguably the best single imaging procedure, ultrasound is useful in the detection of gallstones and biliary obstruction, differentiation between cystic and solid masses and in the detection and serial evaluation of pseudocysts and abscesses. Ultrasonography is also used to establish the diagnosis in an ill patient with normal or marginally increased amylase activity and can be used to guide insertion of a needle for aspiration cytology or percutaneous drainage. Ultrasonography in acute pancreatitis is frequently frustrated because abdominal tenderness prevents good skin contact and because the bowel is often distended with gas as a result of ileus.

Acute pancreatitis produces interstitial edema which alters the size and sonographic texture of the pancreas. The swelling may be generalized or localized (Fig. 50.3), though in recurrent attacks the gland may not be enlarged. Focal swelling always indicates disease regardless of the actual dimensions of the pancreas. As edema increases, the gland becomes relatively echolucent and the pancreatic structures may be indistinguishable from the contiguous portal and splenic veins. Occasionally, in recurrent attacks, the pancreas shows a normal echo pattern. If the disease is particularly severe or associated with hemorrhage or necrosis, the pattern may become hyperechoic.

Dilatation of the pancreatic duct may be seen in acute pancreatitis, though it is more common in chronic disease. As the acute process resolves the duct usually assumes a normal diameter.

*Computed tomography* (Larvin et al 1990, Freeny 1993b)

There is wide variation in the frequency and severity of the manifestations of acute pancreatitis seen on computed tomography and the radiological appearances sometimes conflict with the clinical situation. The morphological changes are similar to those seen on ultrasonography and include changes in size and attenuation of the gland, dilatation and beaded irregularity of the pancreatic duct,

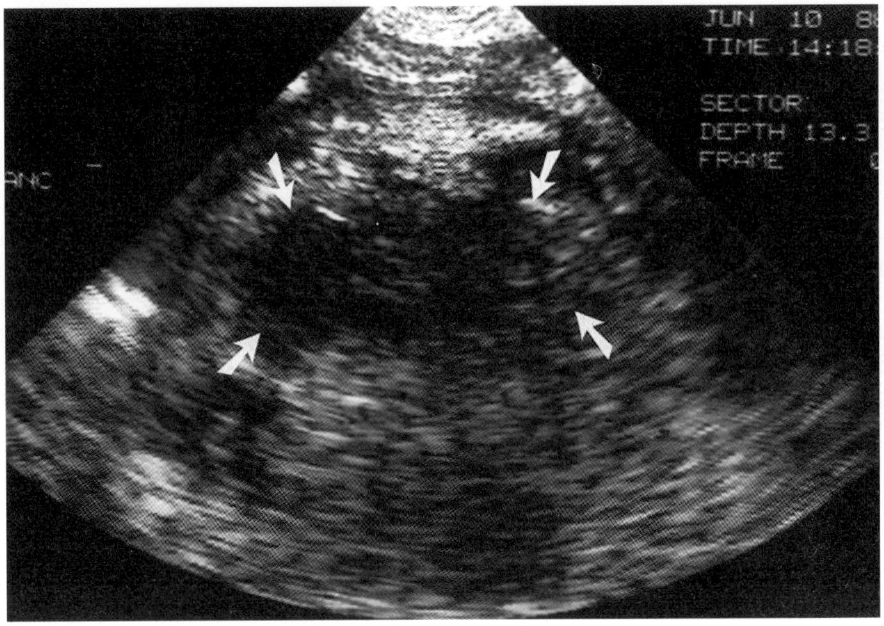


**Fig. 50.3** Acute pancreatitis. Axial ultrasonography shows diffuse enlargement of the pancreas with diminished echo texture (arrows). Normal pancreatic margins and peripancreatic vessels are obscured by the inflammatory process.

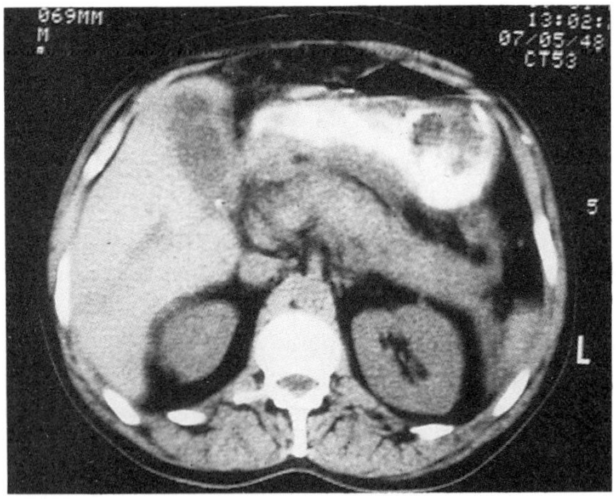


**Fig. 50.4** Non-enhanced CT scan of a patient with mild acute pancreatitis. Contrast is visible in the stomach. The pancreas and surrounding tissues show little inflammation.

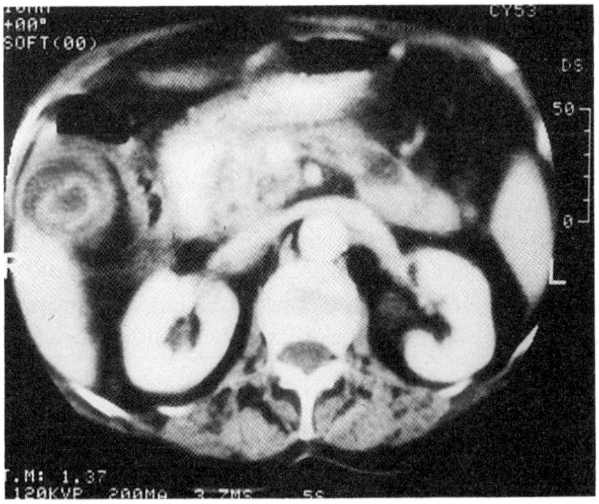


**Fig. 50.5** Dynamic contrast enhanced CT scan in a patient with gall stone pancreatitis. The gall stone (large arrow) is visible in the gallbladder. The pancreas is enhanced with the exception of a few small localized areas of non-enhancement (small arrows).

loss of clarity of the gland margin with abnormal peripancreatic fat planes and pancreatic or peripancreatic fluid collections. The enlargement may be generalized or localized. The contours of the gland usually become indistinct owing to edema in the surrounding soft tissues and a halo of edema may surround the pancreas (Fig. 50.4). The fat around the mesenteric artery is usually preserved, a helpful point in differentiating inflammatory from malignant disease. The pancreatic parenchyma in acute pancreatitis may appear normal or there may be uniform reduction in attenuation or a mixed pattern of attenuation (p. 69).

The pancreas is very vascular and its density on CT scanning can be enhanced considerably following intravenous injection of contrast medium (Figs 50.5, 50.6). Incremental dynamic bolus computed tomography is the best method of detecting the extent and severity of pancreatic and peripancreatic necrosis (Larvin et al 1990, London et al 1991, Freeny 1993a). In the technique used by Freeny (1993a), 5 mm collimated scans are performed

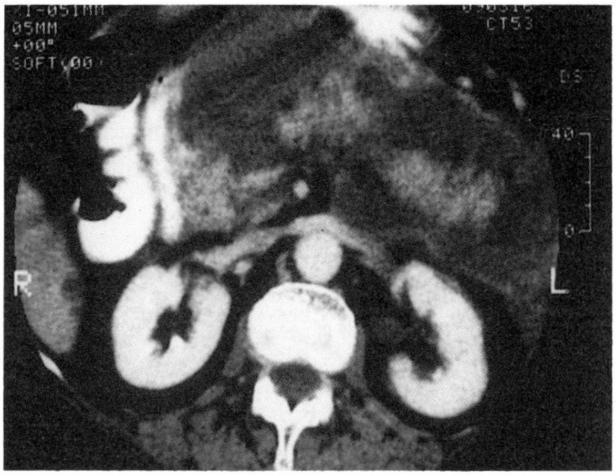


**Fig 50.6** Dynamic contrast enhanced CT scan showing severe pancreatitis with edema and significant areas of non-enhancement. Contrast can be seen in the stomach and duodenum.

at 8 mm intervals using oral contrast to opacify the upper gastrointestinal tract whenever possible. A 150–180 ml bolus of 60% iodinated contrast is given using a monophasic (2–3 ml/s) or biphasic (2–3 ml/s for 20–40 s and then 1–1.5 ml/s) injection sequence. Contraindications to intravenous contrast include a previous severe allergic reaction to iodinated media and severely restricted renal function in a patient not already on renal dialysis. Nonionic contrast media such as iopamidol may carry less risk of renal and cardiovascular complications (Larvin et al 1990), but both ionic and nonionic contrast media can convert borderline ischemia to irreversible necrosis in an experimental model (Foitzik et al 1994). The significance of these findings in human disease remains uncertain but dynamic CT scanning may be best avoided early in the evolution of severe pancreatitis and its routine use is not justified in unselected patients with acute pancreatitis (Lucarotti et al 1993).

Abnormal enhancement in severe pancreatitis may be pancreatic, peripancreatic and a combination of both (Larvin et al 1990). The morphological severity of inflammation on CT scanning can be classified by a five-grade (A–E) system. Stage A denotes a normal CT scan, stage B focal or diffuse pancreatic enlargement, stage C inflammatory change in the peripancreatic fat, stage D single ill-defined fluid collection or phlegmon and stage E two or more fluid collections (Balthazar 1989) or abscess. The score for CT grading (A = zero, E = 4) can be added to a "necrosis score" ( no necrosis = zero, up to one-third = 2, up to one half = 4, more than half = 6) to give a CT Severity Index (CTSI) which shows strong correlation with morbidity and mortality (Balthazar et al 1990).

The presence of necrosis has a strong relationship with morbidity and mortality. Virtually all patients without necrosis survive whereas in the excellent Ulm series, mortality rates of 5%, 7% and 18% respectively have been reported in patients with focal necrosis, extended necrosis and subtotal/total necrosis (Beger et al 1988). Mortality rates are almost twice as high when necrosis becomes infected, as it does in 40–70% of cases (Beger et al 1986a, Gerzof et al 1987, Rattner et al 1992). Fine-needle aspiration of necrotic tissues under CT guidance can be used to detect bacterial contamination (Gerzof et al 1987), while gross infection gives rise to gas in the pancreatic and peripancreatic tissues on CT scanning.

The soft tissues around the lesser sac and anterior pararenal spaces are commonly involved in pancreatitis. The changes are commoner on the left but may be bilateral. Fluid collections may develop in the pancreas, in peritoneal spaces such as the lesser sac and pelvis, in the mediastinum and in the groin. Large peripancreatic collections may be indistinguishable from peripancreatic fat necrosis on CT scanning. Low CT attenuation numbers (<15 Hounsfield units) are more often associated with fluid whereas high attenuation (>25 Hounsfield units) suggests fat necrosis. Other CT findings include vascular complications (e.g. erosion of arteries with bleeding, pseudoaneurysm formation, venous thrombosis and varices), biliary tract involvement (coexisting gallstones, bile duct obstruction [Fig. 2.20]) and gastrointestinal complications (e.g. edema, bleeding, obstruction, necrosis and fistula formation).

The changes seen in acute pancreatitis on computed tomography often persist well beyond the disappearance of clinical symptoms and signs.

### *Barium meal and hypotonic duodenography*

Such studies are not required to diagnose acute pancreatitis but are occasionally performed when excluding other causes of the acute abdomen. Generalized pancreatic enlargement in pancreatitis may displace and indent the stomach and localized inflammation may cause thickening and irregularity of gastric mucosal folds (Fig. 50.7). Similar changes may be seen in the duodenum and can be very marked in the second part where the deformity may assume an "epsilon" shape and mimic pancreatic cancer. The mucosa of the duodenal loop and proximal small bowel may be markedly thickened (Fig. 50.8) and irregular and severe localized inflammation may produce spasm, disturbed motility and displacement of the duodenojejunal flexure.

### *Cholecystography*

Gallbladder opacification by cholecystography is significantly impaired during an attack of acute pancreatitis (Kaden et al 1955), possibly because of poor absorption and/or impaired biliary excretion of contrast medium in the absence of circulating bile salts. The introduction of ultrasound scanning has virtually eliminated the need for cholecystography.

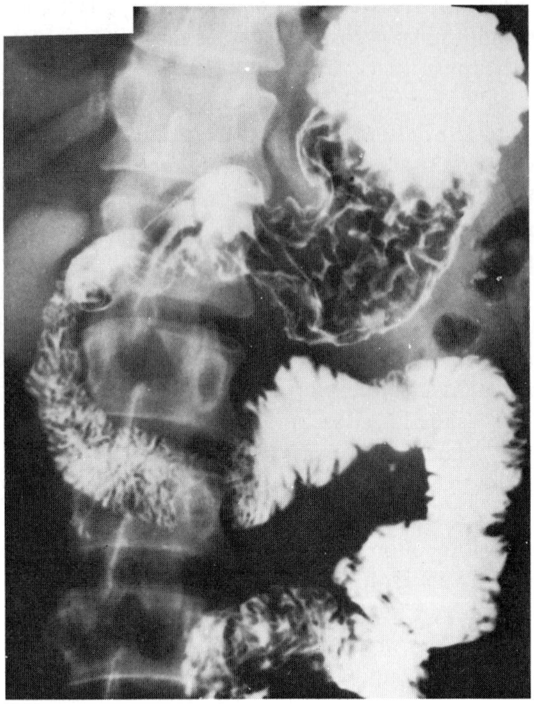

**Fig. 50.7** Barium meal shows edematous gastric folds and enlargement of the duodenal loop with upward displacement of the pyloric antrum due to pseudocyst in the pancreatic head. The gallbladder is opacified as a cholecystogram was performed at the same time.

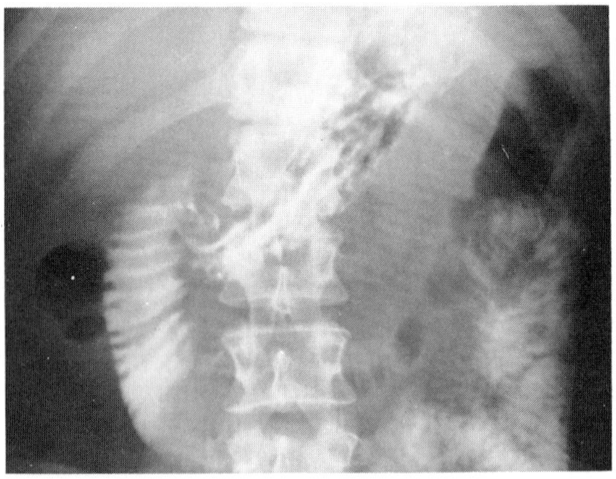

**Fig. 50.8** Acute pancreatitis involving the entire pancreas. Gastrografin meal shows upward displacement of body of stomach and downward displacement of the jejunum. Coarse mucosal pattern in duodenum due to edema with indentation and displacement of its third and fourth parts. Gas in hepatic and splenic flexures but not in transverse colon.

### *Cholescintigraphy*

Failure of the gallbladder to fill during scanning with radionuclides such as $^{99m}$Tc-IDA was once taken to indicate that pancreatitis was likely to be due to gallstones (Glazer et al 1981, Serafini et al 1982). This contention has not been substantiated (Neoptolemos et al 1984) and the test is no longer used.

### *ERCP*

ERCP is not performed to establish the diagnosis of acute pancreatitis. If ERCP is undertaken to treat gallstone pancreatitis (p. 1265), care must be taken to avoid overfilling the pancreatic duct system and so exacerbate existing inflam-mation.

## Other investigations

The hemoglobin concentration commonly rises above 150 g/L as plasma volume falls (see below), but anemia can follow bleeding in necrotizing pancreatitis. Leukocytosis occurs in two-thirds of patients but is usually transient and of little value in differential diagnosis. Persisting leukocytosis suggests necrosis and abscess formation.

Methemalbumin is released in severe pancreatitis as a result of the action of pancreatic enzymes on extravasated red cells. However, methemalbuminemia can occur in other acute abdominal conditions and is not a reliable indicator of severe "hemorrhagic" pancreatitis.

A variety of circulating markers and grading systems have been used to identify patients with severe pancreatitis. High amylase activity in peritoneal lavage fluid has also been used to resolve diagnostic uncertainty and predict the severity of the attack (Mayer & McMahon 1985). These methods of assessment are discussed on page 1262.

## Diagnosis at operation

Laparotomy for diagnosis should be avoided if at all possible in acute pancreatitis. Contrary to earlier contentions that early laparotomy in such circumstances did not increase mortality (Trapnell & Anderson 1964), it is now generally accepted that it significantly increases risk (Imrie & Wilson 1989, Ranson 1990). Increased awareness of acute pancreatitis, recognition of the limitations of the serum amylase in diagnosis and the availability of other methods of diagnosis (peritoneal lavage, ultrasonography and CT scanning) now mean that diagnostic laparotomy is rarely required.

## Complications

Acute pancreatitis may give rise to local or generalized complications. In the first few days, hypovolemic shock is the major threat to life; thereafter sepsis and multiple organ failure are the major dangers.

### *Hypovolemic shock*

Release of enzymes and vasoactive substances increases capillary permeability and results in pancreatic and peripancreatic edema. Hypovolemia is accompanied by tachycardia and hypotension, a raised cardiac index and decreased systemic vascular resistance (Bradley et al 1983), and the hyperdynamic cardiovascular state is significantly more marked in necrotizing pancreatitis (Beger et al 1986b). Kinins may also cause consumptive coagulopathy and reduce renal blood flow, but the existence of a specific "myocardial depressant factor" is now debatable. In necrotizing pancreatitis, there may be bleeding into the pancreas, peritoneal cavity and fascial planes, in rare instances causing discoloration of the flanks (Grey-Turner 1919) or periumbilical tissues.

*Other circulatory changes*

In addition to hypovolemia, the circulation may be impaired by cardiac arrhythmias and myocardial infarction occasionally occurs. Pericarditis or pericardial effusion is a rare consequence of pericardial fat necrosis or hemorrhage. Hypovolemia, disseminated intravascular coagulation and inflammation within the abdominal cavity may predispose to thrombosis and infarction of the small intestine or colon can supervene (Aldridge et al 1989). Sudden blindness caused by microembolization with aggregated granulocytes has even been reported (Jacobs et al 1981).

*Respiratory failure*

Asymptomatic hypoxemia occurs in 50–70% of patients and a $PaO_2$ of less than 60 mmHg indicates severe pancreatitis (Blamey et al 1984). Respiratory failure makes a significant contribution to the mortality of acute pancreatitis in at least one-third of cases.

Neutrophils have been implicated in the pathogenesis of the *adult respiratory distress syndrome* (ARDS) (Willemer et al 1991) and patients destined to progress to ARDS have high concentrations of the neutrophil chemoattractant interleukin 8 (IL8) in bronchoalveolar lavage fluid (Donnelly et al 1993). This cytokine was first isolated from lipopolysaccharide-stimulated monocytes in vitro (Kunkel et al 1991) and its release by lung macrophages could cause neutrophils to migrate into the alveoli, where they become activated with degranulation and the release of histotoxic products such as elastase and collagenase.

The histological features of ARDS have been well described (Lankisch et al 1983). In the first 7 days there is interstitial and intra-alveolar edema, dilatation of lymphatics and capillaries and adhesion of leukocytes. Occasionally, fat droplets are seen in the pulmonary capillaries and fatty deposits are found in the desquamated alveolar epithelium. Between days 3 and 7, hyaline microthrombi in the capillaries and intra-alveolar bleeding are found with increasing frequency. Between 8 and 14 days, hyaline membranes appear and pneumocytes proliferate. After 14 days, there is fibrous organization of hyaline membranes and interstitial fibrosis. These histological features may result from several mechanisms in addition to neutrophil activation, transendothelial migration and degranulation. Circulating enzymes and kinins may contribute in that trypsin can induce disseminated intravascular coagulation, phospholipase A may damage membranes in the lung and increase pulmonary permeability and raised serum triglycerides may be hydrolyzed by pancreatic lipase to form fatty acids which can damage the alveolar capillary membrane. Complement may also cause acute pulmonary injury.

Patients developing ARDS have an increased respiratory rate and hypoxia results from impaired gaseous exchange and right-to-left shunting (Murphy et al 1980). Initially, there are no changes on the chest radiograph but pulmonary edema may develop with hypoxic confusion. Other factors affecting pulmonary function include atelectasis due to abdominal pain, distention and elevation of the diaphragm, pneumonitis secondary to vomiting and aspiration and pleural effusion caused by activated pancreatic enzymes. All of these complications take place against a background of the increased requirement for tissue oxygenation caused by intra-abdominal inflammation.

*Hepatobiliary disorders*

Mild jaundice occurs in about 15% of patients and can be due to impaired bilirubin clearance, biliary tract obstruction or an increased bilirubin load from disseminated intravascular coagulation and intra-abdominal hemorrhage. More severe or increasing jaundice is usually obstructive and reflects compression of the bile duct by pancreatic edema or a pseudocyst or its blockage by a stone. Cholecystitis can occur and portal hypertension due to thrombosis of the portal, splenic or hepatic vein is a rare but recognized complication.

*Gastrointestinal complications*

***Ileus and obstruction.*** Ileus reflects the severity of the attack, lasting 2–3 days in mild cases, up to a week in moderate cases and more than a week in severe cases. Its main causes are local inflammation and the spread of pancreatic enzymes in the mesocolon and mesentery.

Total obstruction may develop when there is mechanical compression of the duodenum by the inflamed pancreas, intramural hematoma, abscess or cyst (Bradley & Clements 1981) or when there is infarction of the bowel due to thrombosis. The colic branches of the superior mesenteric artery, the splenic artery and the gastroduodenal artery are at special risk because of their position. Infarction may also lead to frank necrosis of the colon (Aldridge et al 1989), an enteric fistula or a stricture. The transverse colon and splenic flexure are at particular risk.

Plain radiographs of the abdomen may reveal ileus or obstruction, but barium meal and/or enema may be necessary.

***Hemorrhage.*** Severe acute pancreatitis can be complicated by bleeding into the gastrointestinal tract, retroperitoneum or peritoneal cavity. Severe hemorrhage from the upper gastrointestinal tract occurs in approximately 2% of cases and is a major cause of death (Stroud et al 1981). It may be due to gastric or duodenal erosions, direct involvement of the wall of the duodenum by inflammation or erosion of vessels with pseudoaneurysm formation or frank disruption. Bleeding into the pancreatic duct is uncommon (Brown et al 1985). Gastric or esophageal varices can develop following portal or splenic vein thrombosis and may bleed, while bowel infarction can lead to rectal bleeding.

Initial investigation includes endoscopy. Contrast-enhanced dynamic computed tomography is an excellent method of detecting vascular complications of pancreatitis (Freeny & Lawson 1982). Selective arteriography is occasionally needed and therapeutic embolization may be useful in controlling hemorrhage (Steckman et al 1984).

#### *Renal failure*

Oliguria or anuria are common manifestations of hypovolemia. Cortical or tubular necrosis may develop because of shock, hypoxemia, sepsis, endotoxinemia and disseminated intravascular coagulation.

#### *Role of endotoxin in multiple organ failure*

Endotoxin may play an important role in the pathophysiology of multiple organ failure in severe acute pancreatitis (Foulis et al 1982, Kivilaakso et al 1984b). Translocation of endotoxin from the gut lumen may follow impairment of the gut mucosal barrier and passage through the portal venous system and hepatic reticuloendothelial system can produce bursts of systemic endotoxinemia. Endotoxinemia is known to induce complement and activate coagulation, generate vasoactive kinins and stimulate mononuclear phagocytes to produce cytokines such as IL1, IL6, IL8 and tumor necrosis factor (TNF). Systemic endotoxinemia is difficult to detect because of the need for frequent blood sampling, but recent studies in pancreatitis patients indicate that a fall in serum IgG antiendotoxin antibodies (implying binding of endotoxin and its removal from the circulation) is associated with a high risk of multiple organ failure (Windsor et al 1993).

#### *Metabolic abnormalities*

***Diabetes mellitus.*** Transient hyperglycemia and glycosuria are common in severe pancreatitis and at least one-third of patients have abnormal glucose tolerance in the first few days. Permanent diabetes is unusual unless pancreatic resection is undertaken; 50% of patients with necrotizing pancreatitis treated by pancreatic resection developed diabetes mellitus in a recent Finnish series (Eriksson et al 1992).

***Hypocalcemia.*** Hypocalcemia is a key feature of severity scoring systems (Ranson et al 1974, Imrie et al 1978a, Saitoh & Yamamoto 1991). The mechanism responsible for hypocalcemia is uncertain but frank tetany is exceptionally rare. Calcium is bound in "calcium soaps" when fatty acids are liberated by the action of pancreatic lipase on body fat and this may account for some of the fall in ionized calcium levels in the first 24 h (Croton et al 1981). Patients with hypocalcemic severe pancreatitis have raised parathyroid hormone levels soon after hospitalization, the levels returning to normal within 3 or 4 days (Imrie et al 1978a). This supports the contention that there is indeed a reduction in ionized calcium levels and that parathyroid failure is not the cause of hypocalcemia. Much of the hypocalcemia found in subsequent days reflects reduction in serum albumin concentration and amounts of bound calcium (Allam & Imrie 1977).

#### *Skin and bone lesions*

Subcutaneous fat necrosis can follow release of pancreatic lipase in acute pancreatitis and is seen occasionally in chronic pancreatitis and pancreatic carcinoma. The nodules, which are very similar to those of erythema nodosum, are usually located on the legs but may occur on the arms and trunk (Higgins & Ive 1990). When there is periarticular fat necrosis, polyarthritis may develop and the synovial fluid contains large amounts of hydrolyzed fatty acids (Wilson et al 1983). Intramedullary fat necrosis occasionally causes painful osteolytic bone lesions and intramedullary calcification in pancreatitis and pancreatic carcinoma.

#### *Psychosis and encephalopathy*

These problems are not uncommon in severe pancreatitis and contributory factors include hypoxia, hypovolemia, metabolic abnormalities, alcohol withdrawal, sepsis, opiate administration and cerebral emboli.

### Pancreatic complications

#### *Pseudocysts*

Pseudocysts are localized collections of pancreatic juice which arise from pancreatic inflammation and which are distinguished from other cystic lesions of the pancreas by their lack of epithelial lining. Enzymes within the collection can erode major blood vessels leading to life-threatening hemorrhage. The pseudocyst can compress the common bile duct, leading to obstructive jaundice, and can impair gastric emptying.

In the context of acute pancreatitis, it is important to

stress that most peripancreatic collections of fluid resolve spontaneously as the acute pancreatitis settles. Persistent or recurrent pain, pyrexia and hyperamylasemia should alert the clinician to the possibility of pseudocyst formation. Ultrasonography or CT scanning can then be used to confirm the diagnosis. Collections which persist for more than 4–6 weeks are unlikely to resolve spontaneously, particularly if larger than 5 cms in diameter. Definitive treatment consists of internal drainage into the stomach, Roux loop of jejunum, or (occasionally) duodenum and in some cases this can now be achieved endoscopically without recourse to open surgery. Percutaneous aspiration alone may be worthy of trial in patients unfit for surgery but is followed by recurrence of the pseudocyst in a large proportion of cases. Pseudocysts are discussed further on page 1276.

### *Pancreatic abscess*

A pancreatic abscess is defined as a collection of predominantly liquid purulent material (pus) in the region of the pancreas and enclosed by walls of inflammatory tissue (Frey 1991). The abscess may result from liquefaction of infected necrotic areas or from secondary infection of a pancreatic pseudocyst. The Ulm group (Bittner et al 1987) have emphasized the distinction between pancreatic abscess and infected necrosis, the latter being defined as a diffuse bacterial inflammation of pancreatic and peripancreatic tissue without significant pus formation. Whereas infected necrosis usually becomes evident during the acute phase of acute pancreatitis, abscesses usually become manifest some 4–5 weeks later, often after the acute pancreatitis appears to have subsided. About 85% of all pancreatic infections involve Gram-negative bacteria (particularly *Escherichia coli*), but Gram-positive organisms are found in 10–55% of cases and *Candida* infection has also been reported (Beger 1989). The incidence of abscess has decreased, perhaps reflecting the use of antibiotics, and some 1–4% of patients with acute pancreatitis currently develop this complication.

***Clinical features.*** Some 4 weeks after the onset of the attack of acute pancreatitis the patient's condition deteriorates, with recurrence of abdominal pain, anorexia, nausea, weight loss, fever and abdominal tenderness. A mass is occasionally palpable. Associated cardiorespiratory and renal insufficiency are common (although not as common as in patients with infected necrosis) and the patient looks unwell. There is a leukocytosis, but laboratory findings associated with acute pancreatitis, such as hyperamylasemia, hypocalcemia, hyperglycemia and disturbed liver function, are seldom present (Bittner et al 1987). Factors adversely affecting prognosis are the severity of the precipitating pancreatitis, frank sepsis and positive blood culture, pulmonary dysfunction and persistent postoperative sepsis (Becker et al 1984).

***Radiology.*** The presence of an abscess can be inferred from organ distortion or displacement on a plain radiograph or barium meal, but CT scanning is the investigation of choice (Fig. 50.9). Survival increases dramatically with surgical drainage and early computed tomography is imperative whenever abscess formation is suspected (Ranson et al 1985, Warshaw & Jin 1985). Ranson et al (1985) examined the relationship between CT scan appearances and the risk of abscess formation. No abscesses developed in patients in CT grades A or B, but 57% of patients with CT grade E and predicted severe disease developed abscesses.

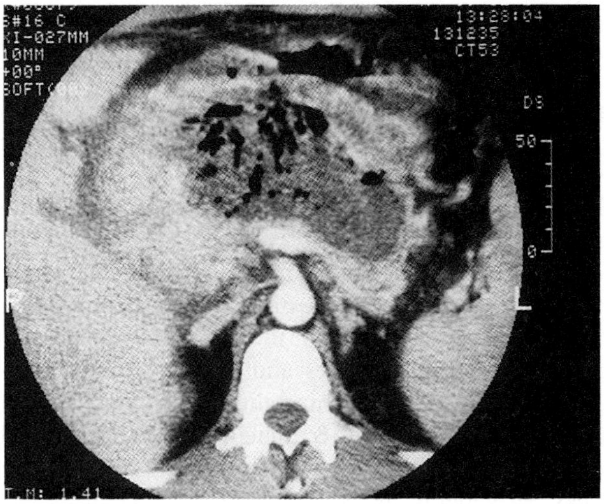

**Fig. 50.9** Dynamic contrast enhanced CT scan of a patient with severe idiopathic pancreatitis. There is a large area of non-enhancement which also contains gas indicating the development of infected necrosis and abscess formation.

The demonstration of gas in the pancreas or peripancreatic tissues (usually due to gas-forming organisms) is a key diagnostic feature. However, gas is seen in only 30–50% of proven abscesses and in some of these it is related to a fistula, a complication which should be excluded in doubtful cases by contrast radiology of the gastrointestinal tract. When gas is not present in an abscess the appearances are indistinguishable from those of a noninfected pancreatic mass or pseudocyst and bacteriological culture following fine-needle aspiration can be invaluable. Abscesses are multiple in up to one-third of cases and may occur at distant sites. Computed tomography is a valuable aid in planning surgical drainage and in some cases, percutaneous aspiration (pp. 34 & 1257).

## Course and prognosis of acute pancreatitis

The mortality rate associated with acute pancreatitis has been of the order of 10–15% and has not changed substantially in 20 years (Mann et al 1994). However, there is some evidence that the situation may be improving. For example, in Scotland mortality rates fell from 17.8% in 1961 to 5.8% in 1985 (Wilson & Imrie 1990) while in

Finland mortality rates fell from 5.9% in 1970 to 2.6% in 1989. Encouraging though these trends may be, it should be borne in mind that in as many as 40% of fatal cases, the diagnosis of acute pancreatitis is not made in life (Wilson et al 1988b) and that the lethality of the disease may still be significantly underestimated.

Edematous pancreatitis nearly always runs a benign course and patients admitted with mild disease on prognostic factor grading have a mortality of 0–3% whereas those with predicted severe disease have a mortality of 25–30% (Mayer et al 1985). Necrotizing pancreatitis develops in 5–15% of cases and has a particularly poor prognosis with reported mortality rates which average some 20–30% (D'Egidio & Schein 1991). Patients who survive a first attack have a low mortality in subsequent attacks. In general, alcohol-associated pancreatitis has a lower mortality than gallstone pancreatitis (Mann et al 1994) (Table 50.3), which in turn has a lower mortality than idiopathic and postoperative pancreatitis (Browder et al 1993, Mann et al 1994). The elderly are at particular risk and mortality rates for those over 60 years of age in Bristol were 28% as opposed to 9% in younger patients (Corfield et al 1985a), while in Hong Kong, mortality rates rose from 6% in those under 50 years to 21% in older patients (Fan et al 1988). Obese patients appear to be at particular risk of developing severe necrotizing pancreatitis and respiratory complications (Porter & Banks 1991, Funnell et al 1993). One large autopsy study involving 405 patients found that 20.5% of deaths occurred in the first 24 h and 60% died within the first week; pulmonary edema and congestion were the prominent findings in deaths during the first week whereas sepsis was the major cause of death thereafter (Renner et al 1985). In a more recent multicenter audit involving 57 deaths, 32% of patients died within the first week, 12% in the second, 19% in the third and 37% died thereafter (Mann et al 1994).

*Assessment of severity* (Williamson 1984)

Prognostic factor grading systems are helpful in predicting disease severity and identifying groups of patients who require monitoring and intensive care. They also provide a useful basis for controlled clinical trials by defining groups of patients with disease that is likely to be severe.

Multiple factor grading systems have been used widely in assessment of severity (Table 50.4). Ranson analyzed 43 early objective measurements in acute pancreatitis and identified 11 factors associated with increased mortality or major complications. When two factors were positive, mortality was about 1%; 3–4 positive, 16%; 5–6 positive, 40%; and 7–8 positive, 100%. These criteria are used in the United States (Ranson et al 1974), whereas the Glasgow system is used in the UK (Imrie et al 1978b). Using an eight-factor modification of the Glasgow system, Blamey et al (1984) found that 39% of 92 attacks classified as severe were associated with death, complications or need for operation as opposed to 9% of the 313 attacks graded as mild. As a rule of thumb, approximately one in four attacks is classified as severe using such systems and approximately one in four of those with severe disease will die. Although useful, these forms of assessment have the disadvantage that 1–2 days elapse before all of the information is available.

The volume and color of free peritoneal fluid also reflect the severity of the attack (MacMahon 1980), although the advantage of immediate assessment is offset by the small risk of visceral puncture. Corfield et al (1985b) assessed the prognostic value of three predictive indices in 436 attacks of acute pancreatitis: clinical assessment identified 34% of patients in whom the attack proved to be severe, multiple laboratory criteria identified 61% and peritoneal lavage identified 53%. Used together, the three indices predicted 82% of the severe attacks.

Serum markers used to predict severity and identify high-risk patients include $\alpha_2$-macroglobulin and $\alpha_1$-antiprotease, complement, C-reactive protein (Wilson

**Table 50.3** Severity and mortality of acute pancreatitis among 279 patients admitted to Edinburgh Royal Infirmary 1989–1993

| Etiology | *n* | Severe disease *n* (%) | Mortality *n* (%) |
|---|---|---|---|
| Gallstones | 116 | 39 (34) | 4 (3) |
| Alcohol | 97 | 16 (16) | 1 (1) |
| Idiopathic | 41 | 12 (29) | 6 (15) |
| Post-ERCP | 11 | 4 (36) | 3 (27) |
| Pancreatic cancer | 5 | 1 | 0 |
| Post-operative | 3 | 3 | 1 |
| Other | 6 | 4 | 2 |
| Total | 279 | 79 (28) | 17 (6) |

**Table 50.4** Basis of factor scoring systems to predict the severity of acute pancreatitis. In both systems disease is classified as severe when three or more factors are present

| Ranson et al (1974) | Imrie et al (1978) |
|---|---|
| On admission<br>Age >55 years<br>White blood cell count 16 × $10^9$/L<br>Blood glucose >10 mmol/L<br>Lactic dehydrogenase >700 u/L<br>Aspartate aminotransferase >250 Sigma Frankel units% | Age >55 years<br>White blood cell count >15 × $10^9$/L<br>Blood glucose >10 mmol/L (no diabetic history)<br>Serum urea >16 mmol/L (no response to i.v. fluids)<br>Arterial oxygen saturation ($PaO_2$) <60 mmHg |
| Within 48 h<br>Blood urea nitrogen rise >5 mg%<br>Arterial oxygen saturation ($PaO_2$) <60 mmHg<br>Serum calcium <2.0 mmol/L<br>Hematocrit fall >10%<br>Base deficit >4 mmol/L<br>Fluid sequestration >6 L | Serum calcium <2.0 mmol/L<br>Serum albumin <32 g/L<br>Lactic dehydrogenase >600 u/L<br>Aspartate aminotransferase/ alanine aminotransferase >100 u/L |

et al 1989), phospholipase A2 (Puolakkainen et al 1987) and ribonuclease (Kemmer et al 1991). These markers have found limited clinical application, although the use of C-reactive protein will be discussed further (p. 1266). As discussed earlier (p. 1251), urinary levels of trypsinogen activation peptides (TAP) are increased in severe pancreatitis, reflecting extensive activation of trypsinogen (Gudgeon et al 1990). It is hoped that an assay will become available for routine use.

The APACHE-II score has also been used to assess and monitor patients with severe acute pancreatitis (Larvin & McMahon 1989).

## Treatment

The falling mortality of acute pancreatitis reflects increased awareness of the disease, improved diagnosis and improved treatment of the disease and its complications.

### *Treatment of circulatory failure*

Hypotension, tachycardia and a raised hemoglobin concentration reflect loss of fluid from the circulation. Treatment is commenced with intravenous isotonic saline but colloid solutions such as albumin are needed in shocked patients. Recent evidence suggests that isovolemic dilution with dextran 60 may improve the pancreatic microcirculation and avoid necrosis (Klar et al 1993). Central venous pressure should be monitored to avoid overloading the cardiopulmonary system. The patient should be catheterized and urine output maintained at 30 ml/h or more. In patients with marked fluid shifts or associated cardiopulmonary disease, monitoring of pulmonary wedge arterial pressures with a Swan–Ganz catheter is of immense value (p. 516).

### *Treatment of pain*

Prompt treatment of pain is essential. Morphine is avoided as it produces spasm of the sphincter of Oddi and while pethidine (75–100 mg given 4-hourly intravenously or by intravenous infusion) is usually preferred, most narcotic drugs produce some degree of sphincter spasm.

### *Fluid and electrolyte balance and nutrition*

Parenteral fluid and electrolyte therapy is usually required for only 3–4 days in mild pancreatitis, but in patients with severe disease it may be needed for much longer. Once the circulation has been restored, the daily fluid intake should equal the output of the previous day plus 1000 ml for insensible losses. Parenteral nutrition is initiated if oral intake cannot be commenced after 3–5 days in patients with severe or complicated disease (Robin et al 1990), but in patients with mild pancreatitis the morbidity of parenteral feeding outweighs any potential benefit (Sax et al 1987).

Treatment of hypocalcemia is necessary only in the rare event that it is symptomatic. When there is severe hypocalcemia, serum magnesium should also be measured and levels below 0.6 mmol/L (1.5 mg/dl) should be corrected by one or more infusions of 10 ml of 50% magnesium sulfate dissolved in at least 200 ml 5% dextrose.

### *Diabetes mellitus* (p. 518)

Persistent hyperglycemia may require insulin therapy, particularly if ketosis develops.

### *Renal failure*

The usual cause of a low urine output is inadequate fluid replacement. If output remains below 30 ml/h despite apparently adequate intravenous therapy, an attempt should be made to induce a diuresis, by giving 25–50 g of mannitol or 400 mg frusemide. If oliguria persists despite adequate volume replacement and dopamine infusion (2–5 μg/kg/min), a program for acute renal failure must be instituted.

### *Respiratory care*

Arterial blood gas concentrations should be measured as soon as pancreatitis is diagnosed and as often as necessary in patients with severe disease. Oxygen is given if the patient is shocked or anoxic and inability to maintain arterial oxygen tension above 8.0 kPa (60 mmHg) is an indication for endotracheal intubation and mechanically assisted ventilation with positive end-expiratory pressure.

### *Measures to suppress pancreatic inflammation* (Ranson 1993)

Agents found to be beneficial in animal models have rarely been beneficial when used in man. The value of most clinical trials is limited by their inclusion of patients with mild disease and lack of sufficient statistical power to give confidence in a negative result (Steinberg & Schlesselman 1987). Agents used to "suppress" pancreatic secretion, such as atropine, glucagon, cimetidine and calcitonin, are of no proven benefit and there is even experimental evidence that cimetidine may be harmful. There is no evidence to support the use of many other agents which have been advocated in the past, including aprotinin, corticosteroids and soya bean trypsin inhibitor. Despite some support for the protease inhibitor gabexate mesilate (Pederzzoli et al 1993), a definitive German study found that it was of no benefit (Buchler et al 1993). Although some reports suggest that somatostatin or its analogs may be of benefit, a recent review concludes that there is insufficient evidence to recommend these agents in prophylaxis or in the treatment of acute pancreatitis (McKay et al 1993). Earlier suggestions that fresh frozen plasma, which contains proteinase inhibitors, might be beneficial (Cuschieri et al 1983) have not been sustained by multicenter study (Leese et al 1987).

Gastric aspiration is often employed in the hope of reducing pancreatic secretion but several studies have shown that it is of no significant benefit, at least in patients with mild disease. However, nasogastric aspiration may relieve persistent vomiting and trials are still needed to assess whether it is beneficial in patients with severe pancreatitis.

There is general agreement that oral feeding should be withheld until pain and tenderness have resolved; persisting fever and leukocytosis may also reflect ongoing pancreatic inflammation.

#### *Antibiotics*

Prophylactic antibiotics do not prevent septic complications and may even promote infection with organisms which are more difficult to treat, such as *Candida albicans*. Some centers use prophylactic broad-spectrum antibiotics in patients with gallstone pancreatitis with the intention of treating cholangitis and some advocate antibiotics in patients with fulminant pancreatitis (Ranson 1993). If water-soluble antibiotics such as the aminoglycoside gentamicin are used, increased endothelial permeability in acute pancreatitis means that normal doses may have to be increased by some 25% to achieve therapeutic peak serum levels (Carr et al 1988).

#### *Other therapeutic agents*

Although anticoagulation is contraindicated in acute pancreatitis, there may be value in giving heparin (750–1000 units/h monitored by partial thromboplastin time) to reduce the danger of disseminated intravascular coagulation in patients with a rising platelet count and serum fibrinogen (Ranson 1993). Attempts to modify pancreatic blood flow by pharmacological means are of uncertain value and are not used clinically. The recent suggestion that the antioxidant vitamin C might be of value in acute pancreatitis (Scott et al 1993) requires evaluation.

#### *Therapeutic peritoneal lavage*

While peritoneal lavage offers a means of confirming the diagnosis of acute pancreatitis and assessing severity (Corfield et al 1985b), the role of therapeutic lavage remains controversial. Animal experiments and uncontrolled studies in man (Ranson & Spencer 1978) initially suggested benefit, but most randomized studies in patients with severe disease have failed to show any benefit in terms of mortality, incidence of major complications or hospital stay (Mayer et al 1985, Ihse et al 1986). However, in a more recent randomized study involving 29 patients with severe disease, lavage for 7 days halved the incidence of pancreatic sepsis (22% versus 40%) and improved mortality (0 versus 20%) when compared to lavage for 2 days (Ranson & Berman 1990). At present, therapeutic peritoneal lavage is used routinely in few centers and lavage with fluid containing proteinase inhibitors (Balldin et al 1983) has also failed to establish a place.

### **Surgical treatment** (Ranson 1990)

As indicated above, laparotomy carried out solely for diagnosis increases risk and is only undertaken when a surgically correctable, potentially lethal disease other than pancreatitis cannot be excluded. Certain complications of acute pancreatitis which can require surgery, namely pancreatic pseudocysts, fistula and ascites, are dealt with for convenience in the section devoted to the complications of chronic pancreatitis (below).

#### *Surgery in gallstone pancreatitis*

It is vitally important to exclude gallstones in all patients with pancreatitis, as their eradication virtually eliminates the risk of further attacks. However, gallstones are not always easy to diagnose in the presence of acute pancreatitis and its associated ileus. Ultrasound is less accurate than normal in detecting gallstones in the first few days; the gallbladder is visualized in only 70–80% of cases and only about two-thirds of patients with gallstone pancreatitis have their gallstones detected at this stage (McKay et al 1982, Neoptolemos et al 1984).

Goodman et al (1985) studied 99 patients discharged from hospital without a defined cause for their attack of acute pancreatitis. While ultrasonography at 6 weeks was of great value, it did not detect all gallstones (sensitivity 87%) and ERCP should be considered in all patients with idiopathic pancreatitis and normal ultrasonography and/or oral cholecystography.

There has been controversy regarding the timing of biliary surgery in gallstone pancreatitis. The classic approach was to allow the pancreatitis to settle on conservative therapy, use radiological investigation to confirm the presence of gallstones and readmit the patient 6–8 weeks later for definitive biliary surgery. This approach had the drawbacks that pancreatitis did not always settle with conservative management and a large number of patients developed further attacks of pancreatitis or cholangitis while awaiting readmission for elective surgery (Osborne et al 1981).

Acosta et al (1978) advocated immediate biliary tract surgery in patients with gallstone pancreatitis, citing a mortality rate of 2% with this policy, as opposed to 16% in historical controls managed by deferred biliary surgery. In a prospective trial, Stone et al (1981) randomized patients to undergo biliary surgery within 73 h of admission or after an interval of 3 months. Biliary tract surgery consisted of cholecystectomy which was always accompanied by transduodenal sphincteroplasty and division of the septum between common bile duct and pancreatic duct. There was one death in the early surgery group and two in the deferred surgery group and there was no significant difference between the groups in terms of major morbidity.

While many surgeons accepted the limitations and risks of the classic deferred surgery approach, few adopted the aggressive policies just outlined. Transduodenal sphincteroplasty is not without risk and exploration of the bile duct increases the morbidity and mortality of biliary surgery. As many of the gallstones responsible for acute pancreatitis impact only transiently at the lower end of the common bile duct, it can be argued that most of them will pass on spontaneously, so obviating the need to explore the duct system if surgery is not undertaken immediately. More recent controlled evaluation has failed to show any benefit from cholecystectomy and bile duct exploration within 48 h of the diagnosis of gallstone pancreatitis in patients with mild disease (Kelly & Wagner 1988); in patients with severe disease, biliary surgery within 48 h had a prohibitive morbidity (83%) and mortality (48%) when compared to the results of surgery after 48 h (18% and 11% respectively).

Osborne et al (1981) have suggested that patients with pancreatitis should be allowed to settle on conservative therapy and undergo cholecystectomy later in the course of the index hospital admission. Operative cholangiography is recommended to detect any stones which remain in the bile duct; if such stones are left in the biliary tree, the reported incidence of further attacks of pancreatitis is as high as 92% (Kelly & Swaney 1982).

Although surgery during the index admission has proved safe and effective in patients who have settled on conservative treatment, it still leaves the real problem of the subgroup of patients with severe disease who fail to settle on such treatment. Rather than subject these patients to immediate surgery with all of its hazards (Kelly & Wagner 1988), ERCP can be used to confirm the presence of gallstones and allow their removal by endoscopic papillotomy (Neoptolemos et al 1988a, Safrany & Cotton 1981). Clinical and biochemical parameters which suggest that gallstones are responsible for an attack of pancreatitis are age over 55, female sex, high alkaline phosphatase and aminotransferase levels and a serum amylase activity of greater than 4000 i.u./L (Blamey et al 1983). If ultrasonography is equivocal in a patient with severe acute pancreatitis, the fact that four or five of these factors are positive means that urgent ERCP should be considered.

Neoptolemos et al (1988a) randomized patients thought to have gallstone pancreatitis to receive conservative management or urgent ERCP (with sphincterotomy if stones were present). In patients with mild disease on Glasgow criteria, urgent ERCP conferred no benefit whereas morbidity was significantly lower in the group of patients with severe disease who underwent urgent ERCP (Table 50.5). None of the patients with mild disease died in this study, but there were fewer deaths in patients with severe disease who received urgent ERCP as opposed to conservative management (although the difference was not statistically significant). In a similar study from Hong Kong, early ERCP (with sphincterotomy if stones were present) reduced the incidence of biliary sepsis but did not affect the mortality or the risk of developing local and systemic complications (Fan et al 1993). It appears that early ERCP is unnecessary in patients with mild pancreatitis and should be avoided if at all possible in patients who do not have gallstones. More data are required to confirm that the approach is beneficial in patients with severe disease. Although the available results are encouraging, some believe that the severity of an attack of pancreatitis (and the risk of necrosis) is determined early and that the amount of activated enzyme may be a more important factor than persisting impaction of a gallstone at the ampulla of Vater (Kelly & Wagner 1988). If there is indeed a "window of opportunity" during which an attack of pancreatitis can be aborted by endoscopic sphincterotomy and stone extraction, the window is likely to be short and may well have passed by the time the patient reaches hospital. On the other hand, necrotizing pancreatitis caused by obstruction of the biliopancreatic duct system by a balloon catheter in the opossum is less severe if the catheter is removed at 1 or 3 days as opposed to 5 days (Runzi et al 1993), lending support to the practice of early endoscopic removal of obstructing stones in gallstone pancreatitis.

If obstructing stones are found and removed at ERCP, the fact that sphincterotomy has been performed may in itself offer some protection against further attacks of pancreatitis. However, unless the patient is unfit for biliary surgery, most surgeons would still advocate early chole-

**Table 50.5** Controlled trial of urgent ERCP (with or without endoscopic sphincterotomy, ±ES) and conventional treatment in patients with acute gallstone pancreatitis (Neoptolems et al 1988)

| | Group A (ERCP ± ES within 72 h) | Group B (conventional treatment) |
|---|---|---|
| Mild acute pancreatitis*(*n*) | 34 | 34 |
| With complications (%) | 4 (12%) | 4 (12%) |
| Deaths | 0 | 0 |
| Severe acute pancreatitis (*n*) | 25 | 28 |
| With complications (%) | 6 (24%) | 17 (61%) |
| Deaths | 1 | 5 |

*Severity assessed by Glasgow criteria (Blamey et al 1984)

cystectomy, an operation which can be carried out laparoscopically where feasible.

The potential importance of "biliary sludge" as a cause of acute pancreatitis has been highlighted recently. Of 31 patients with idiopathic pancreatitis, 23 (74%) had microscopic evidence of sludge (i.e. calcium bilirubinate crystals or cholesterol monohydrate crystals) in duodenal aspirates. Pancreatitis recurred in only one of the 10 patients undergoing cholecystectomy or endoscopic papillotomy, as opposed to eight of the 11 patients having no treatment (Lee et al 1992).

**Table 50.6** Outcome in collected series of patients with necrotizing pancreatitis according to method of surgical treatment (D'Egidio & Schein 1991)

| Treatment | No. of patients | No. of deaths (%) |
|---|---|---|
| Resection or necrosectomy with drainage | | |
| Overall | 516 | 186 (36) |
| Resections excluded | 305 | 89 (29.2) |
| Necrosectomy with local lavage | 216 | 49 (22.7) |
| Necrosectomy with 'open management' | 188 | 46 (24.5) |

### *Surgery for necrotizing pancreatitis*

The development of extensive pancreatic necrosis remains a major cause of death in patients with severe pancreatitis. Although the risk of complications and death can be predicted by clinical and biochemical grading systems (Ranson et al 1974, Blamey et al 1984) or examination of lavage fluid (Corfield et al 1985b), it may still be difficult to identify individual patients who are developing severe necrosis which requires surgical intervention. Multisystem failure is an important marker of fulminant disease and a rising pulse rate, serum creatinine, fever and white cell count in conjunction with difficulty in maintaining arterial blood pressure and $PaO_2$ are ominous signs (Aldridge et al 1985). In some patients it is apparent from the outset that multisystem failure is present and worsening, while others "fail to thrive" or improve temporarily before beginning to deteriorate.

Serum markers which have been advocated for the early detection of pancreatic necrosis include raised levels of ribonuclease (Warshaw & Lee 1979), fibrinogen (Berry et al 1982), $\alpha_1$-antitrypsin (McMahon et al 1984), lactic dehydrogenase and C-reactive protein (Buchler et al 1986) and a falling level of $\alpha_2$-macroglobulin (McMahon et al 1984). Depletion of $\alpha_2$-macroglobulin reflects its consumption during inactivation of circulating proteases and has a sensitivity of 85% in the detection of necrosis (Buchler et al 1986). The acute-phase C-reactive protein (CRP) is a nonspecific index of injury, inflammation, sepsis and ischemia. The level used to signify a high probability of necrosis varies from center to center, but levels greater than 100 mg/L had a sensitivity of 95% in detecting necrosis in the Ulm series (Buchler et al 1986). This is not to say that an elevated CRP level is an indication for surgery, rather that it may be an early indicator of the need for CT scanning to define the presence and extent of necrosis and to determine whether infection is present.

As discussed earlier, incremental dynamic bolus computed tomography is the best method of detecting pancreatic and peripancreatic necrosis, defining its severity and planning surgical intervention (Larvin et al 1990, London et al 1991, Freeny 1993a), while percutaneous fine-needle aspiration under computed tomography guidance may be used to detect infection (Beger et al 1988). It must be emphasized that radiological appearances are not the sole determinant of the need for surgery and that the clinical condition of the patient is also important. However, extensive necrosis and, in particular, the presence of infected necrosis are strong indications for surgery.

Operation is usually undertaken through a bilateral subcostal incision with the lesser sac being opened widely, although some recommend a direct approach to the retroperitoneum through a left lateral subcostal incision (Fagniez et al 1989). Dead and liquefied pancreas is removed and dead retroperitoneal tissue is debrided thoroughly. Blunt (finger dissection) necrosectomy is used and it is now clear that formal pancreatic resection carries unacceptable morbidity and mortality (Table 50.6) (Kivilaakso et al 1984a, Wilson et al 1988a, D'Egidio & Schein 1991, Kiviniemi et al 1993) in addition to removing viable pancreas unnecessarily and incurring a high risk of insulin-dependent diabetes (Eriksson et al 1992). Fortunately, the head of the pancreas usually remains viable but the transverse colon may be affected by necrosis and may have to be resected, with creation of a temporary colostomy. Thorough intraoperative peritoneal lavage is mandatory and the pancreatic bed must be adequately drained. Opinions vary as to whether copious irrigation of the lesser sac is advisable (Beger et al 1988, Larvin et al 1989), or whether the abdominal wound should be packed and left open to facilitate re-exploration, an approach sometimes called "laparostomy" (Bradley 1987, Mughal et al 1987). A recent review has concluded that necrosectomy followed by local lavage or open management with planned re-exploration offers better survival prospects than "conventional" management by resection or necrosectomy followed only by drainage (D'Egidio & Schein 1991). Open management may carry a higher risk of complications such as colonic necrosis, fistula formation and bleeding, but it is clear that specialist units can achieve acceptable results with open management or the lavage method provided that the initial debridement is thorough and re-exploration is undertaken promptly if sepsis persists or recurs. Regardless of the method used, a gastrostomy tube inserted at the time of surgery can avoid the need for prolonged nasogastric intubation in patients liable to protracted duodenal ileus. Insertion of a feeding jejunostomy is also advisable in that enteral nutrition is often practicable and total parenteral nutrition can be avoided. It has been postulated that enteral feeding also reduces the absorption of bacteria and their toxins from the gut by strengthening the intestinal mucosal barrier (Wilmore et al 1988).

*Treatment of pancreatic abscess*

Mortality rates following the conventional treatment of debridement and sump drainage of pancreatic abscess have commonly ranged from 30% to 50% (Bradley & Fulenwider 1984). The recent fall in the mortality of pancreatic abscess to 5–22% reflects early diagnosis by computed tomography and more aggressive surgical intervention with extensive drainage and debridement (Bradley & Fulenwider 1984, Warshaw & Jin 1985, Bittner et al 1987). Warshaw & Jin (1985) counsel against open packing or continuing local peritoneal lavage, although others regard these as valuable innovations (Bradley & Fulenwider 1984, Van Vyve et al 1992) It is essential to provide adequate nutrition following surgery and a feeding jejunostomy established at the time of surgery may be helpful. After drainage, recurrent abscess formation, hemorrhage from the abscess cavity and fistula are common and potentially lethal complications (Warshaw et al 1989), and the importance of eradicating further septic collections cannot be overemphasized. Recurrent abscess may require further surgical treatment, although CT-guided percutaneous drainage may be considered. Bleeding is second only to sepsis as a cause of death in patients with pancreatic abscess and may demand re-exploration, further debridement and packing for its control. Pancreatic fistulae usually close spontaneously but enteric fistulae are more troublesome and may require further surgery if conservative management fails.

## CHRONIC PANCREATITIS

### Incidence

Chronic pancreatitis is often silent or eludes diagnosis but available estimates suggest that its incidence is increasing (Fig. 50.10). A prospective Danish study found an incidence of 8.2 per million with a prevalence of 27.4 cases per million (Copenhagen Pancreatitis Study 1981), figures consistent with those of retrospective studies in Europe and North America. In England and Wales the incidence rose fourfold in men and twofold in women between 1960–64 and 1980–84 and alcohol consumption in the population correlated with the number of patients discharged from hospital with chronic pancreatitis some 6 years later (Johnson & Hosking 1991) (Fig. 50.11).

### Etiology

Chronic pancreatitis may evolve from alcoholic acute pancreatitis (Amman et al 1996)

*Alcohol*

Alcohol accounts for some 60–70% of cases of chronic pancreatitis in Western countries and 85% of those affected are males. Individual sensitivity to the toxic effects of alcohol must vary greatly in that most alcoholics do not develop clinical pancreatitis, although up to 60% have abnormal pancreatic morphology at autopsy (Pichumoni et al 1980, Renner et al 1985). Chronic pancreatitis is unlikely if daily intake is less than 60–80 g, although women may have a lower threshold. The interval between the start of regular alcohol consumption and the clinical manifestations of chronic pancreatitis averages 17–18 years in men but is only 10–12 years in women (Durbec & Sarles 1978). Tobacco smoking may be an additional risk

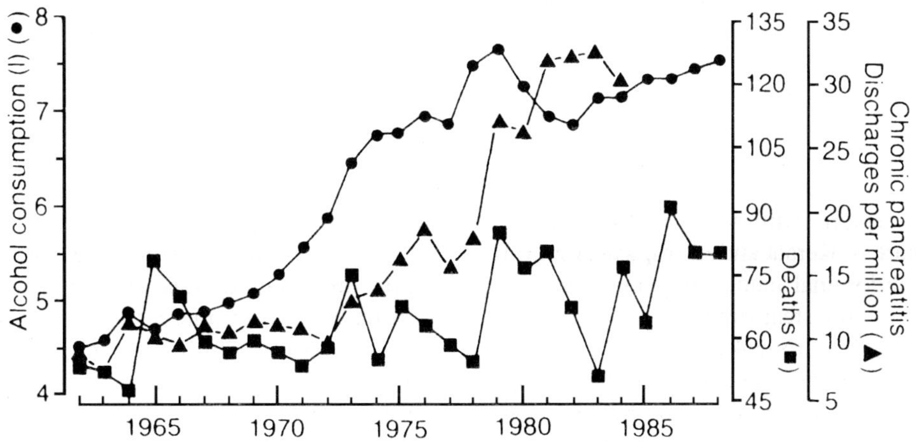


**Fig. 50.10** Changes in annual alcohol consumption (liters per head of population), hospital discharges for chronic pancreatitis per million of population and total number of deaths from chronic pancreatitis in England and Wales 1960–88. (Reproduced with permission from Johnson & Hosking 1991.)

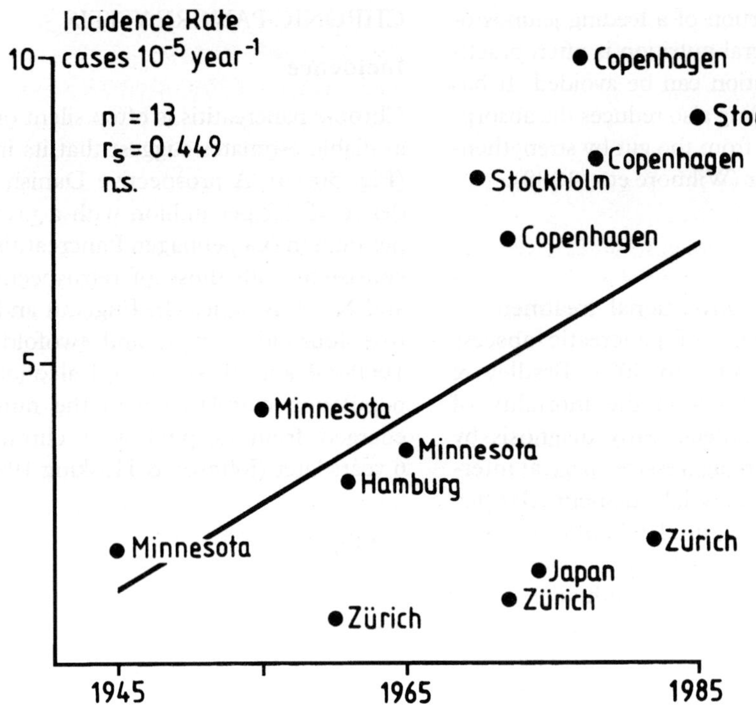


**Fig. 50.11** Incidence of chronic pancreatitis during the years 1945 to 1985. (Reproduced with permission from Worning H 1990 Incidence and prevalence of chronic pancreatitis. In: Beger H G, Buchler M, Ditschuneit H, Malfertheiner P (eds) Chronic pancreatitis. Springer Verlag, Berlin, p 8–14.

factor (Bourliere et al 1991) but its effect is difficult to define given that many heavy drinkers also smoke.

## Nutritional factors

It is uncertain whether alcoholic pancreatitis is associated with nutritional factors. Various studies have implicated a higher than normal, normal or lower than normal intake of calories, fat and protein and an insufficient intake of the trace elements zinc and selenium (see Muller & Singer 1993).

### *Tropical pancreatitis*

Nutritional factors are definitely implicated in tropical pancreatitis, a disease in which alcohol has no role. The condition occurs in regions within 15° of the equator, notably the Indian state of Kerala and in tropical Africa. It is characterized by abdominal pain, pancreatic calcification, diabetes mellitus and steatorrhea and death often occurs "at the prime of life" (Nwokolo & Oli 1980, Gee Varghese 1986). The disease was once thought to be caused by protein-calorie malnutrition or childhood kwashiorkor, but malnutrition is more likely to be the result of the disease. Pancreatic atrophy and insufficiency can be caused by juvenile kwashiorkor but are usually reversible. Epidemiological studies have implicated toxic cyanogenetic glycosides in cassava (*Manihot esculenta*), agents which could theoretically cause pancreatic injury by impairing the action of free radical scavengers such as superoxide dismutase. A cassava-rich diet may also be deficient in methionine and trace elements such as zinc and selenium, leading to impaired detoxification of cyanogens and increased free radical production.

### *Obstructive pancreatitis*

Pancreatic duct obstruction due to congenital strictures, pancreatitis, neoplasia or trauma may cause chronic inflammation. However, obstructive pancreatitis differs from alcoholic pancreatitis in that intraductal protein plugs are less common, calcification is unusual and the inflammatory changes in the obstructed part of the gland are uniform rather than patchy.

*Pancreas divisum*, in which the dorsal and ventral pancreatic ducts fail to fuse, is the commonest congenital abnormality of the pancreas and according to ERCP studies, affects some 7% of the population (see Muller & Singer 1993). It has been suggested that pancreatitis develops because the minor papilla is too small for the free passage of juice from the larger dorsal pancreas. While pressures are indeed abnormally high in the dorsal pancreas in pancreas divisum (Staritz & Meyer zum Buschenfelde 1988), the condition is regarded as a potential cause of recurrent acute pancreatitis rather than chronic pancreatitis (Bernard et al 1990) (see also p. 1227).

### *Hypercalcemia*

Hypercalcemia due to hyperparathyroidism and chronic renal failure can give rise to both acute and chronic pancreatitis. Hyperparathyroidism is now diagnosed early (on the basis of detecting hypercalcemia on routine blood tests) and so accounts for only 1–2% of cases of chronic pancreatitis.

### *Hereditary chronic pancreatitis*

This rare disease is transmitted as an autosomal dominant condition with incomplete penetrance. It does not become manifest until the age of 5–15 years. Associated conditions include hyperlipidemia and aminoaciduria (Dalton-Clarke et al 1980). While hyperlipidemia can be associated with acute pancreatitis, it is not a cause of chronic pancreatitis.

### *Biliary tract disease*

As many as one-half of patients with gallstones have an abnormal pancreatogram and one in six have changes resembling those of chronic pancreatitis (Misra & Dwivedi 1991). However, the significance of these changes is uncertain and while choledocholithiasis is an exceptional cause of chronic pancreatitis, chronic pancreatitis not infrequently causes biliary stasis and the formation of stones in the common bile duct.

### *Idiopathic chronic pancreatitis*

In 20–40% of patients, no etiological factor is identified. Idiopathic chronic pancreatitis affects men and women equally and in the absence of a defined etiology, many of these patients are wrongly labeled as having alcohol-associated disease. *Juvenile idiopathic chronic pancreatitis* has a median age of onset of 19 years and is a painful condition which resembles alcoholic pancreatitis clinically, morphologically and functionally (Layer et al 1994). Late-onset idiopathic chronic pancreatitis is associated with weight loss, functional impairment and pancreatic calcification in the absence of pain (Layer et al 1994). A degree of pancreatic atrophy, functional impairment and morphological change (including calcification) is an accepted feature of aging and it is uncertain whether late-onset chronic pancreatitis is merely an exaggeration of this process.

### *Other factors*

Rare causes of chronic pancreatitis include cystic fibrosis and previous abdominal radiotherapy (Levi et al 1993).

## Pathogenesis

The mechanism by which alcohol damages the pancreas remains controversial (Fig. 50.12). Alcohol diminishes the secretion of bicarbonate and water by duct cells, but increases protein secretion by acinar cells and so produces an abnormally viscous juice. Eosinophilic protein plugs then form within the interlobular and intralobular ducts and subsequently enlarge and calcify with precipitation of calcium carbonate. A 14 000 kDa pancreatic stone protein called lithostatine is the major component of the organic matrix of the resulting stones. Lithostatine is one of the most abundant nonenzyme proteins secreted in pancreatic juice and in vitro evidence supports the contention that it normally prevents the nucleation and growth of calcium carbonate crystals (Sarles et al 1990). Pancreatic juice levels of lithostatine are abnormally low in chronic pancreatitis, particularly when there is calcification (Multinger et al 1985, Mariani et al 1995), and levels of messenger RNA

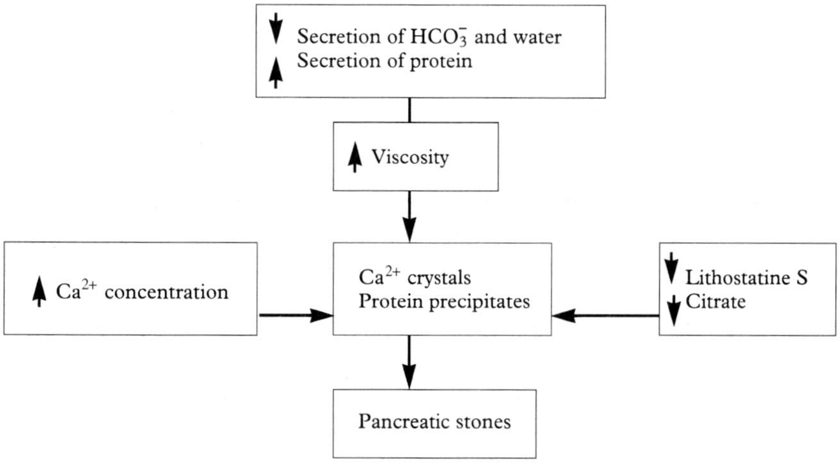


**Fig. 50.12** Factors which contribute to pancreatic calcification.

encoding for lithostatine are lower in all forms of chronic pancreatitis (Giorgi et al 1985, 1989). However, not all accept the central role of lithostatine in the pathogenesis of chronic pancreatitis (Schmiegel et al 1990).

Increased secretion of calcium by acinar cells and a decreased concentration of citrate in pancreatic juice may also be involved in the calcification of chronic pancreatitis (Lohse et al 1983, Lohse & Pfeiffer 1984) and explain the association with hypercalcemia.

In rats, chronic ethanol consumption and protein deficiency increase the capacity of acinar cells to synthesize digestive and lysosomal enzymes (Apte et al 1995). Excessive stimulation of acinar cells by alcohol may also derange intracellular protein transport leading to admixture of digestive enzymes and lysosomal hydrolases and storage of zymogens in acid compartments (Noronha et al 1981, 1984, Bordalo et al 1984). Fatty degeneration of acinar cells rather than ductular obstruction could then lead to periacinar fibrosis.

Alcohol also induces hepatic mixed function oxidases and Braganza (1983) has postulated that disordered hepatic detoxification may generate toxic free radicals and reactive intermediates which are excreted in bile and reflux into the pancreatic duct system. This theory offers an explanation for varied genetic susceptibility to alcohol while emphasizing the potential importance of toxic factors in the pathogenesis of chronic pancreatitis.

## Pathology

The morphological changes in chronic pancreatitis are extremely variable, ranging from minimal morphological and histological change (Walsh et al 1992) to dense fibrosis and destruction of gland architecture. Edema, acute inflammation and necrosis are superimposed on chronic inflammatory change with marked fibrosis, loss of acinar cells and ultimate loss of endocrine cells. The duct system shows variable dilatation and stricture formation with protein plugs and calcification. Perineural disintegration and eosinophilic infiltration and an increase in mean nerve diameter may be related to the painful nature of chronic pancreatitis (Bockman et al 1988). Abnormally large amounts of serotonin and calcitonin gene-related peptide are present and may be related to altered pain thresholds (Walsh et al 1992). Involvement of neighboring organs can produce common bile duct obstruction, splenic vein thrombosis and duodenal stenosis (see below).

It is often difficult to exclude the presence of carcinoma, particularly as chronic pancreatitis may be a premalignant condition. Recent evidence suggests that some 4% of patients develop malignancy within 20 years of diagnosis (Lowenfels et al 1993). Familial chronic pancreatitis carries an even higher risk and as many as 25% of affected individuals develop malignancy.

## Clinical features

Pain is the outstanding symptom and is usually epigastric or subcostal with radiation to the back (p. 1233) and, on occasions, the shoulder tip. It is typically dull, gnawing and severe and is seldom colicky. Some patients lean forwards to relieve the pain, avoid lying supine or on one side or even resort to kneeling on hands and knees to obtain relief. Application of a hot water bottle or a hot bath may ease the pain. The pain is often intermittent, lasting hours, days or weeks, although some patients are rarely free of pain. The need for analgesics is an index of severity, but many patients are already requiring opiates by the time of presentation and fear of addiction is a recurring anxiety in management. Nausea and anorexia are common and vomiting may occur, although it rarely relieves the pain. There are often no identifiable precipitating factors although some patients find that a high fat intake or alcohol consumption may trigger an attack of pain.

Some patients develop constipation because of their consumption of opiate analgesics whereas others develop steatorrhea with the passage of a pale bulky stool which has a particularly offensive smell and is difficult to flush away. The stool can be frankly greasy or oily and many patients are socially incapacitated by their anxiety about using other people's toilets. Steatorrhea indicates that pancreatic exocrine function is less than 10% of normal. Although some have argued that pain diminishes with the onset of marked functional impairment and calcification (Amman et al 1984), this is not generally accepted and the concept that chronic pancreatitis eventually "burns itself out" has been overemphasized.

Diabetes mellitus is a relatively late manifestation and usually develops after overt exocrine insufficiency. The gradual decline in endocrine function is reflected in a transition from diet-controlled diabetes to the use of oral hypoglycemic agents and ultimately to the use of insulin. The risk of developing the complications of diabetes in patients with chronic pancreatitis is no different to that of diabetics in general.

Weight loss is a common result of reduced intake and maldigestion and may be exacerbated by nausea and vomiting. Frank duodenal stenosis due to inflammation in the head of the pancreas is relatively uncommon. Jaundice suggests biliary tract obstruction by inflammation, fibrosis or cyst formation. Gastrointestinal bleeding may occur if gastric and esophageal varices develop as a consequence of splenic vein thrombosis and major bleeding can follow erosion of major vessels by the inflammatory process.

There are no specific findings on examination. Malnutrition and weight loss may be obvious and mottled burn marks (erythema *ab igne*) may reflect the use of heat pads or hot water bottles. Occasional findings include jaundice, a palpable abdominal mass and splenomegaly due to splenic vein thrombosis. Stigmata or chronic liver disease and hepatic decompensation are unusual even in alcohol-related disease. Rupture of a duct or pseudocyst occasionally produces pancreatic ascites or pleural effusion.

## Investigations

### *Biochemical and hematological investigation*

Serum amylase and lipase levels are usually normal or only slightly elevated. Liver function tests may confirm the presence of jaundice and the serum alkaline phosphatase activity is a useful means of excluding or monitoring biliary tract obstruction. Serum electrolyte concentrations are usually normal in the absence of vomiting. Leukopenia and thrombocytopenia suggest that splenic vein thrombosis may have caused splenomegaly. Blood glucose levels are measured to exclude diabetes mellitus.

### *Tests of pancreatic exocrine function* (Lankisch 1993)

Given the accuracy of imaging, few centers now use pancreatic function tests routinely in diagnosis, particularly if there is overt steatorrhea. Function tests are occasionally helpful when chronic pancreatitis is suspected and imaging studies are normal or show minimal change, but none of the available tests are sufficiently sensitive to exclude chronic pancreatitis when negative. Some physicians employ function tests to monitor progression of disease and determine the need for exocrine supplements.

The "gold standard" direct tests involve measuring the concentrations of bicarbonate and enzymes in duodenal juice after stimulating the pancreas by a meal (Lundh test) or by exogenous secretin with or without cholecystokinin or cerulein (secretin-pancreozymin test). These tests are time consuming, expensive, invasive and difficult to standardize and are now used in very few centers. Indirect tests measure digestive capacity, are easier to standardize, noninvasive and easier to perform; some of those available are shown in Table 50.7. At best, function tests are a nonspecific means of diagnosing exocrine insufficiency and they cannot differentiate between chronic pancreatitis and pancreatic cancer.

**Table 50.7** Pancreatic exocrine function tests (Lankisch 1993)

| |
|---|
| *Direct pancreatic function tests* |
| Secretin-pancreozymin test |
| Lundh test |
| *Indirect pancreatic function tests* |
| Measurement of enzymes |
| Serum pancreatitic isoamylase |
| Serum immunoreactive trypsin |
| Fecal trypsin |
| Fecal chymotrypsin |
| Measurement of enzyme actions |
| NBT-PABA (bentiromide) test |
| Pancreolauryl test |
| Fecal fat analysis |

### *Imaging studies*

Pancreatic calcification is apparent in up to one-third of patients with chronic pancreatitis on plain abdominal radiographs but its presence does not exclude pancreatic cancer. Ultrasonography may reveal pancreatic enlargement, duct dilatation, cysts or pseudocysts, splenomegaly and biliary tract obstruction. Computed tomography has a high sensitivity and specificity (approaching 90%) for the diagnosis of chronic pancreatitis, is the best method of detecting calcification (Figs 2.23, 2.24 & 50.13) and may provide useful information about vascular involvement such as splenic vein thrombosis and false aneurysm formation.

Endoscopic retrograde cholangiopancreatography (ERCP) is the single most effective method of detecting chronic pancreatitis (Fig. 50.14), displaying the pancreatic duct system and detecting pancreatic cancer. The combination of ultrasonography, computed tomography and ERCP had a sensitivity of 95–97% and specificity of 100% for the diagnosis of both chronic pancreatitis and

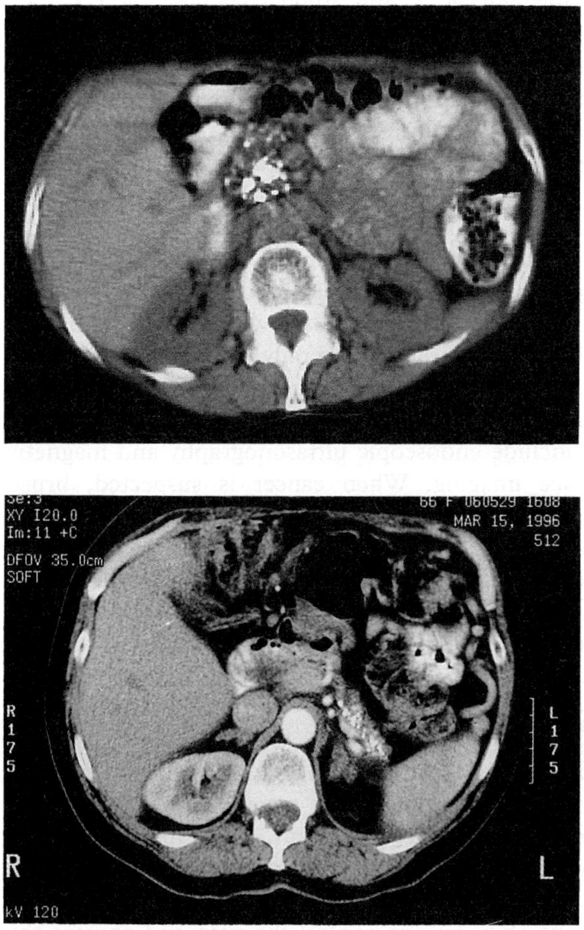


**Fig. 50.13** (**A**) CT scan in a patient with alcohol-associated chronic pancreatitis showing extensive calcification in the head of the pancreas. (**B**) CT scan of a patient with alcoholic chronic pancreatitis showing extensive calcification in the tail of the gland.

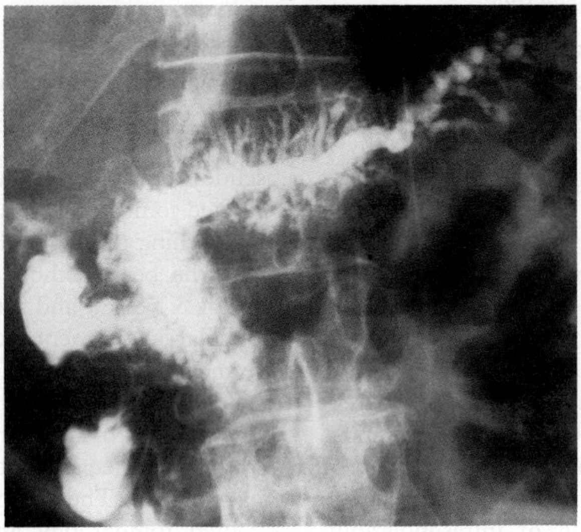

**Fig. 50.14** Endoscopic retrograde pancreatogram in a patient with chronic pancreatitis showing irregular areas of narrowing and dilatation in the pancreatic duct system.

pancreatic cancer in one study (Niederau & Grendell 1985). Ductal changes are classified as mild (normal main duct and three or more abnormal side branches), moderate (abnormal main duct with more than three abnormal side branches) or severe (as in moderate disease but with additional features such as large cavity, filling defect and severe duct dilatation or irregularity). The severity of morphological change frequently does not parallel the degree of functional impairment.

Angiography is now seldom used given that dynamic computed tomography can display vascular abnormality, while barium studies are used only when duodenal stenosis is suspected or in the rare eventuality of colonic obstruction. Investigations which may prove useful in future include endoscopic ultrasonography and magnetic resonance imaging. When cancer is suspected, brush cytology at ERCP, fine-needle aspiration cytology and serum markers such as CA 19-9 may point to the presence of malignancy; in practice it is often extremely difficult to exclude cancer without pathological examination of the resected portion of pancreas (Carter 1992).

## Management

The diagnosis of chronic pancreatitis is not in itself an indication for surgery. Many patients can be managed conservatively for long periods, and in some cases indefinitely, and no surgical procedure can reverse the loss of endocrine and exocrine function. However, medical treatment often fails to control the pain and prevent the development of complications, so that the majority of patients ultimately come to surgical treatment particularly for pain or for pseudocyst.

### *Alcohol*

Abstinence from alcohol is a crucial determinant of long-term prognosis but is often difficult to achieve despite full medical and nursing support, supplemented by counseling, self-help groups and, where necessary, psychiatric help. Abstinence reduces pain in about 50% of patients but many patients continue to have severe pain and serial studies with ERCP have shown that ductal changes may progress despite reduced intake or abstinence (Nagata et al 1981).

### *Pain relief*

Opioid drugs are normally required as nonopioids such as paracetamol and aspirin seldom relieve chronic visceral pain. Dihydrocodeine and codeine (30 mg every 6 h) are suitable for patients with mild to moderate pain but can cause constipation, nausea and dizziness. Sublingual buprenorphine (0.2–0.4 mg every 6–8 h) can be used for more severe pain and has less risk of dependence than morphine, although its combined opioid agonist and antagonist actions can cause withdrawal symptoms in patients who have been taking other opioids. Diconal or pethidine are alternatives for those with severe pain, but the slow-release morphine preparation MST Continus (starting dose 10–20 mg twice daily) is often the best option for long-term relief. Alternatives such as percutaneous celiac plexus blockade have proved disappointing and the early experience with thoracoscopic splanchnicectomy is not encouraging.

In theory, avoidance of a high-fat, high-protein diet should restrict CCK release and physiological stimulation of the pancreas. In practice, patients are advised to avoid foods which cause pain, fat-rich diets and large meals. Elemental diets are no longer employed. There is debate about whether luminal proteases reduce pancreatic exocrine secretion by a negative feedback mechanism and whether oral enzyme supplements reduce pancreatic pain in addition to combating steatorrhoea (Larvin et al 1992, Layer & Holtmann 1994).

### *Diabetes*

Oral hypoglycemic agents are of no value. The patient is managed with diet and insulin, on average 20–30 units/day given as two or three divided doses. This avoids hypoglycemia which is difficult to treat. Because of the danger of hypoglycemia the physician should not aim at normoglycemic control.

### *Pancreatic enzyme replacement*

In chronic pancreatitis, steatorrhoea and protein malabsorption occur only when the secretion of pancreatic lipase and trypsin is reduced to less than 10% of normal

**Table 50.8** Indications for surgery in chronic pancreatitis

| |
|---|
| Intractable pain |
| Pancreatic duct stenosis |
| Cysts and pseudocysts |
| Biliary tract obstruction |
| Splenic vein thrombosis with gastric/esophageal varices |
| Portal vein compression/mesenteric vein thrombosis |
| Pancreatic ascites/pleural effusion |
| Duodenal stenosis |
| Colonic stricture |
| Suspicion of pancreatic carcinoma |

(DiMagno et al 1973). However, a minority of patients have steatorrhoea when pancreatic secretion is reduced to a lesser extent and some others have a normal fat excretion even when pancreatic lipase is extremely low; presumably non-pancreatic lipases are produced which aid absorption in some patients (Lankisch & Creutzfeldt 1984). Pancreatic exocrine insufficiency also occurs in several other conditions (Table 50.8), and while the therapeutic measures listed below apply primarily to chronic pancreatitis they may be of benefit in these situations. In kwashiorkor (Thompson & Trowell 1952) fibrosis of the pancreas may occur; in most children, however, a normal diet results in the restoration of enzyme secretion and recovery of pancreatic cellular structure.

Malabsorption itself may result in an inadequate supply of amino acids to the pancreas, and intestinal disease may result in an inadequate release of secretin and CCK-PZ to stimulate the pancreas (Herskovic 1968). Abnormalities of pancreatic secretion occur occasionally in celiac disease (Dreiling 1957, Worning et al 1967), the characteristic pattern being a normal volume and bicarbonate but a low enzyme output; the pancreas may show acinar atrophy and fibrosis (Adlersberg & Schein 1947). Pancreatic enzyme secretion may also be reduced after small bowel resection, in small-intestinal diverticulosis, in Crohn's disease and in postgastrectomy syndromes (Dreiling 1957).

Pancreatic extracts (Lankisch & Creutzfeldt 1984) are indicated when there is loss of weight, diarrhea or abdominal discomfort from malabsorption. Steatorrhoea of less then 15 g fat per day is not in itself an indication for replacements. The use of extracts may also assist the stabilization of insulin requirements in patients with diabetes. Extracts are also used in cystic fibrosis (p. 1241) to promote normal growth and development. Pancreatic extracts have been used for the treatment of pancreatic pain.

"Pancreatic extracts" are usually prepared from cow or hog pancreas (Saunders & Wormsley 1957) and hypersensitivity to pork protein has been documented. They contain amylase, trypsin and lipase as well as other enzymes, but they are not standardized, and to be effective many have to be given in large doses. Other side-effects are hyperuricosuria in cystic fibrosis and the impairment of folate absorption (Russell et al 1980).

The lipase content of the preparation determines its effectiveness. A large number of tablets, unacceptable to the patient, have to be given to replace the lipase output of the normal pancreas. Therefore a maximum of four capsules are usually given with each meal. The preparations vary in different countries; many are enteric coated or are in granule or microsphere form. These varied forms are intended to prevent the enzyme from being inactivated at pH 4 or below in the stomach and to enhance mixing with food. There is some evidence that more enzyme reaches the small intestine with granulated preparations than with tablets (Ihse et al 1980).

The response to therapy is assessed by fecal fat excretion before and after 3 weeks on therapy. It is best to prescribe a normal fat intake during this period because excessive consumption of fat may obscure improvement brought about by the extract. If there is an inadequate symptomatic response to this treatment then other measures are necessary. The dose of pancreatic extract can be increased but in general this is ineffective and it may result in abdominal cramps. If the response is inadequate, measures should be instituted to reduce gastric acidity with $H_2$ receptor antagonists or preferably a proton pump inhibitor.

*Diet and vitamins*

The diet should be normal and nutritious, with fat restricted to 25% of total calories. Initially the patient may have hyperphagia and under these circumstances fat intake must be monitored. When diarrhea continues despite the administration of pancreatic extracts and a fat intake of 25% of total calories, dietary fat should be reduced further. Under these circumstances medium-chain triglycerides (p. 354) can be given to maintain calorie intake. The absorption of fat-soluble vitamins is reduced even when the steatorrhoea is treated adequately with pancreatic extracts (Dutta et al 1982) and supplements of vitamins A and D are required. Zinc absorption is also impaired. Non-diabetic retinopathy is common in chronic pancreatitis (Toskes et al 1979); patients with steatorrhoea improve with vitamin A supplements while those with a normal fat excretion improve with the administration of zinc sulfate (Toskes & Greenberger 1983).

*Indication for surgery* (Trede & Carter 1993) (Table 50.8)

***Intractable pain.*** This is much the commonest indicator for operation; inability to exclude carcinoma is a factor in some 15% of cases.

***Pseudocysts and cysts*** (p. 1276)

***Pancreatic ascites and pleural effusion*** (1278)

***Obstruction of the common bile duct*** (see also p. 877 and Fig. 31.13). The distal portion of the common bile duct traverses the pancreas in 85% of individuals and is retropancreatic in 15%. When the duct traverses the pancreas it may be involved in dense fibrotic tissue. The complication is present to some degree in 30–65% of cases but is seldom complete and is rarely the sole indication for surgery. In 79 patients with moderate or advanced chronic pancreatitis, ERCP showed narrowing of the common duct in 46% (Wisloff et al 1982). In many cases the patient is symptomatic; however, in some patients the obstruction is an important cause of pain. Jaundice occurs in approximately one-third of patients with chronic pancreatitis (Sarles & Sahel 1978) and in a proportion it is due to obstruction of the common duct. In 51 patients with distal common duct obstruction, serum bilirubin was raised in 44 and serum alkaline phosphatase in 48 (Aranha et al 1984). If the obstructive jaundice is prolonged, complications such as cholangitis, liver abscess, cholestasis and secondary biliary cirrhosis may supervene (p. 942). Obstruction leading to pyogenic liver abscess may occur in the absence of jaundice (Reddy et al 1984).

***Vascular complications.*** About 10% of patients with chronic pancreatitis have portal venous involvement ranging from compression to frank occlusion with thrombosis. Splenic vein thrombosis is the commonest manifestation and the resulting splenomegaly produces hypersplenism and the formation of gastric and esophageal varices. Thrombosis confined to the splenic vein is best dealt with by distal pancreatectomy and splenectomy before bleeding occurs.

Involvement of peripancreatic arteries may cause pseudoaneurysm formation with life-threatening bleeding into a pseudocyst, pancreatic duct, peritoneum or retroperitoneum. Bleeding into a pseudocyst may be apparent from leakage of contrast on dynamic CT scanning and can be confirmed by emergency angiography prior to resection of the affected part of the pancreas. Angiography may also allow embolization and occlusion of the bleeding vessel.

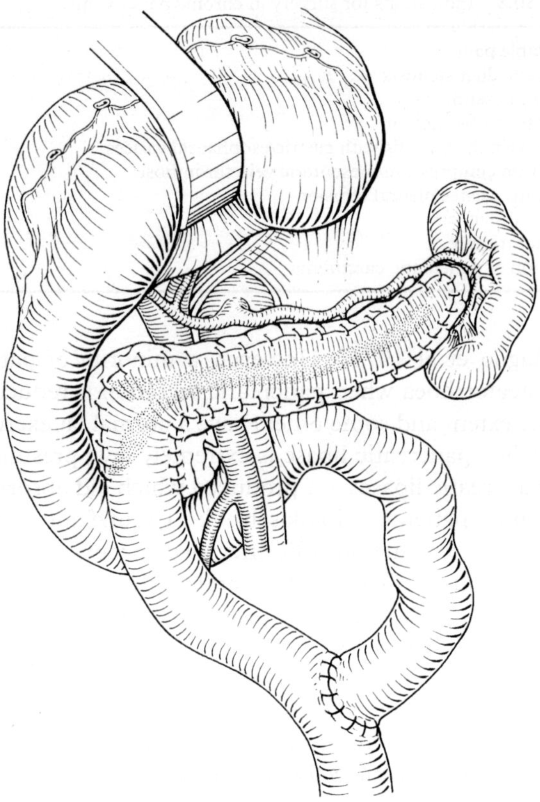

**Fig. 50.15** Longitudinal pancreaticojejunostomy. The pancreatic duct system is opened as widely as possible and anastomosed to a Roux loop of jejunum. Intestinal continuity is restored by an end-to-side jejuno-jejunal anastomosis. The same Roux loop can also be used to drain cystic collections or an obstructed bile duct and to bypass an obstructed duodenum.

### *Surgical options in management*

Chronic pancreatitis causes progressive loss of pancreatic exocrine and endocrine function and no surgical procedure can reverse this process; at best surgical drainage procedures may arrest or slow the rate of decline (Nealon & Thompson 1993), while resection almost invariably leads to further deterioration (partial pancreatectomy) or complete loss of function (total pancreatectomy). Patient selection is all-important, particularly if major resection is complicated, and the decision to undertake surgery must never be made precipitately. The patient must understand the risks and the fact that pain is not always relieved. Operative mortality rates should be close to zero for pancreatic drainage procedures and low single figures for resection. In general, all forms of pancreatic surgery offer complete or substantial pain relief in around 70% of cases when patients are assessed at 5 years (Horn 1993).

Drainage operations such as longitudinal pancreaticojejunostomy (Fig. 50.15) are safer than resection and spare the pancreatic parenchyma and its function. Most surgeons restrict the operation to patients with pancreatic ducts larger than 7–8 mm in diameter, although this restriction is now challenged (Delcore et al 1994). The disadvantages of drainage operations are that they leave diseased pancreas in situ as a source of further pain and complications and the retained pancreas may harbor an unsuspected carcinoma. Some surgeons prefer to overcome some of these limitations by combining excision of most of the head of the pancreas with longitudinal pancreaticojejunostomy (Frey & Amikura 1994). Although the principle of drainage can be extended by using the same Roux loop of jejunum to bypass concurrent obstruction of the bile duct and duodenum, patients requiring "triple drainage" are usually better served by some form of resection.

Chronic pancreatitis generally affects the entire gland and the desire to remove all of the diseased pancreas has to be balanced against the problems posed by brittle insulin-dependent diabetes and total loss of exocrine function which follow total pancreatectomy. A minority of patients have disease confined to the body and tail of the gland and can be dealt with effectively by distal pancreatectomy, but the majority have disease which is maximal in the head of the gland and require some form of Whipple operation or total pancreatectomy. The Whipple operation (Fig. 50.16) removes the head of the gland but conserves function in the remaining pancreas and improves its drainage. The conventional Whipple operation removes the duodenum, gallbladder and common bile duct and antrum of the stomach in addition to the head of the pancreas. Modern variants include pylorus-preserving pancreaticoduodenectomy and duodenum-preserving pancreaticoduodenectomy (Beger & Imaizumi 1995). All forms of resection carry significant operative risk given that tissue planes are often obliterated by dense fibrosis and intraoperative hemorrhage may be problematic.

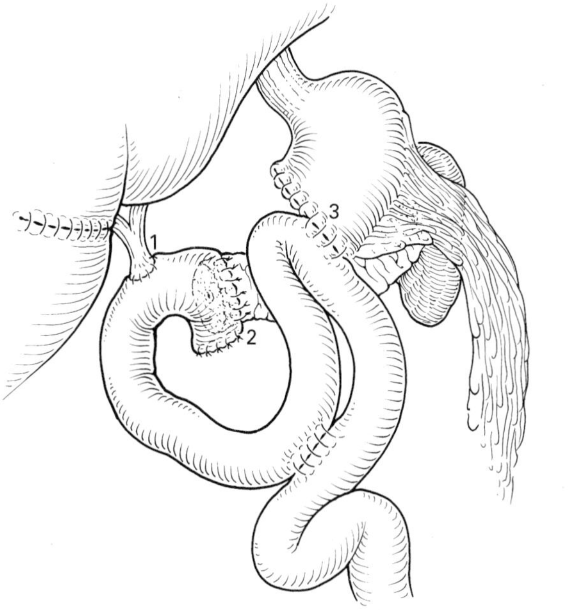


**Fig. 50.16** Reconstruction following resection of the distal stomach, duodenum and head of pancreas by the Whipple operation. The hepaticojejunal (1), pancreaticojejunal (2) and gastrojejunal (3) anastomoses are shown. The side-to-side jejunojejunostomy is performed by some surgeons.

Total pancreatectomy (Fig. 50.17) is occasionally indicated when all else has failed but even after total extirpation of the gland, some 15–30% of patients continue to experience significant discomfort or pain and patients must be selected with extreme care if they are to manage the ensuing brittle diabetes mellitus (Cooper et al 1987). Patients who continue to drink alcohol generally have worse results than those who abstain and the difference is particularly marked in the case of total pancreatectomy.

## Prognosis

Chronic pancreatitis has a mortality rate which approaches 50% over 20–25 years (Horn 1993, Steer et al 1995). Up to 20% of patients die of complications of the disease while the remainder succumb to problems associated with alcohol abuse, tobacco smoking, malnutrition, infection, diabetes mellitus, insulin overdose and suicide. These patients are at greater risk of death from malignancy than the general population and are at particular risk of dying from carcinoma of the pancreas. In patients treated surgically, the long-term results depend more on the drinking habits of the patient than the type of surgery performed.

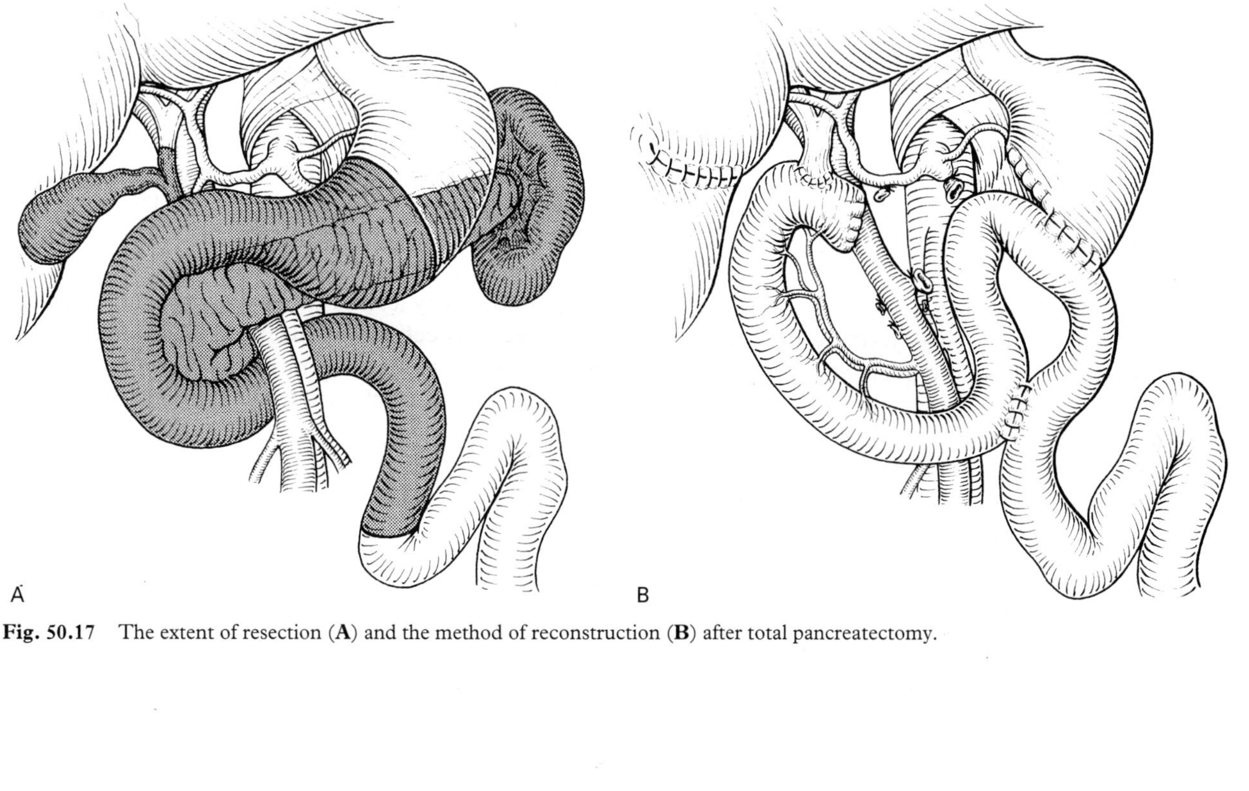


**Fig. 50.17** The extent of resection (**A**) and the method of reconstruction (**B**) after total pancreatectomy.

## PANCREATIC PSEUDOCYSTS

Pseudocysts occur as a complication of acute or chronic pancreatitis, trauma to the pancreas or, rarely, ductal obstruction by cancer. In practice, over 75% arise as a result of pancreatitis (Becker et al 1968, Warren et al 1966). With the advent of ultrasonography, it has become apparent that pseudocysts are multiple in 13% of cases (Goulet et al 1984) and that many resolve spontaneously (Winship et al 1977).

### Pathology

A pseudocyst is a sac which contains fluid, pancreatic enzymes, blood and debris from the pancreas. It is presumed that all pseudocysts connect with a pancreatic duct thus allowing filling with pancreatic secretions, although this is demonstrable by ERCP in only a minority of cases. The pseudocyst develops as a result of autodigestion of the pancreas and has no epithelial lining. It is lined by granulation and fibrous tissue, often with histiocytes, giant cells and blood pigment products, and can be indistinguishable from retention cysts in which the epithelial lining has become eroded. The wall may become calcified (Rowland et al 1985). Pseudocysts may be located within the pancreas or enlarge and involve surrounding structures. Commonly, they occupy the lesser sac and displace the stomach anteriorly and upwards. Several other surrounding organs and structures, such as the colon, may also be displaced or compressed. The cyst tends to spread in the direction of least resistance, and this may lead to unusual abdominal or even intrathoracic localizations (Weidmann et al 1969) (see below).

### Clinical features

In about half of all cases the pseudocyst develops 1–2 weeks after the onset of acute pancreatitis or the acute exacerbation of chronic pancreatitis (Siegleman et al 1980).

Most patients complain of abdominal pain, which is usually epigastric but is located occasionally on the left or right side of the abdomen. Nausea and vomiting are common because a cyst often perpetuates ileus or causes mechanical obstruction. Indeed, the cyst is usually suspected when the patient does not respond to conventional therapy or when the serum amylase and the white count are persistently elevated (pp. 1260–1261). Jaundice may result from obstruction of the common bile duct. Weight loss is marked (Wilson & Costopoulos 1967). Sudden rupture of the cyst into the peritoneal cavity may lead to shock, while a slow leak leads to chronic pancreatic ascites. Secondary infection may lead to the development of an abscess. In patients with chronic pancreatitis, the cyst is occasionally asymptomatic.

On examination, a smooth, round, tender mass is felt in the upper abdomen in half the cases, fever is usual, and there may be jaundice due to compression of the common bile duct. The features of pancreatic abscess are discussed on page 1261. When bleeding into a pseudocyst occurs, there is a sudden increase in the size of the mass, which may become pulsatile, and there may be a bruit. Using ultrasonography, it is now known that approximately 20% of pseudocysts in acute pancreatitis resolve spontaneously and in 90% of cases the resolution occurs in the first 6 weeks after diagnosis (Bradley et al 1979). Resolution is particularly likely with small pseudocysts but in chronic pancreatitis such small cysts are unlikely to resolve.

Since the diagnosis of pseudocyst is usually made by ultrasonography the differential diagnosis consists of those conditions which have a similar ultrasonic appearance (p. 57 and Table 51.6), such as pancreatic abscess, edema of the pancreas, a collection of peripancreatic fluid, cystadenomas (p. 1259), pancreatic retention cysts and loculated ascites.

### Complications

Complications arise in 40% of cases (Bradley et al 1979).

***Rupture.*** Slow rupture results in pancreatic ascites (see below). Sudden rupture into the alimentary canal leads to vomiting or diarrhea and sudden rupture into the peritoneal cavity may simulate a perforation; in both cases there is disappearance of the palpable cyst. Transenteric rupture can be followed by hemorrhage or sepsis, so that up to 50% of such patients die.

***Obstruction.*** Pressure from the cyst can cause obstruction to the common bile duct (Skellenger et al 1983), obstruction of the antrum or duodenum, obstruction or thrombosis of the splenic and portal veins, leading to portal hypertension and varices, and obstruction to the ureter, leading to hydronephrosis.

***Other complications.*** Infection of the cyst converts it into an abscess (p. 1261). Erosion of a major artery, often the splenic, may lead to a pseudoaneurysm which erodes and ruptures into the lumen of the gut, with catastrophic bleeding, or into the peritoneal cavity. Direct involvement of the spleen by the pseudocyst may also lead to severe bleeding (Sitzmann & Imbembo 1984). Splenic vein thrombosis may lead to extrahepatic portal hypertension.

Direct dissection by the pseudocyst may simulate a tumor in the mediastinum, neck or kidney. Dissection to the spleen may result in splenic infarction or rupture.

### Investigations

#### Radiology

Diagnosis is best made by computed tomography and ongoing assessment by ultrasonography. Occasionally a pseudocyst may become apparent when other abdominal radiographic procedures are performed.

***Plain abdominal radiograph.*** This may show a homogeneous mass, usually in the epigastrum or left upper quadrant. Adjacent organs, the stomach and bowel in particular, often show signs of displacement. The psoas or renal shadows may be indistinct or obliterated. The chest radiography may show elevation of the left hemidiaphragm.

***Barium meal or hypotonic duodenogram.*** This may show extrinsic pressure on the stomach and small bowel; a cyst in the head of the pancreas widens the duodenal loop, displaces the antrum upward and flattens the mucosal folds. A cyst in the body displaces the stomach anteriorly and upwards and one in the tail displaces the stomach medially and the proximal jejunum and splenic flexure inferiorly.

***Ultrasound and computerized tomography.*** Ultrasound and computerized tomography may be used to locate pseudocysts, but because of their frequent extrapancreatic location computerized tomography (Fig. 1.39) is more useful in their initial mapping. Ultrasound can then be used to monitor the progress of a particular pseudocyst and the suitability for surgery.

The appearances of a pseudocyst at ultrasound are those of a large sonolucent mass with thick echogenic borders. The appearances on computerized tomography typically show a rounded or oval fluid collection with a thin surrounding capsule. The fluid is usually homogeneous with a low attenuation, though if blood and/or debris are present the attenuation may be non-homogeneous. Initially the margin may be ill-defined, but with time the fibrous capsule matures and may become up to several centimeters thick. Sometimes calcification is visible in the walls of pseudocyst. There is usually no enhancement with intravenous contrast, but if infected there can be faint enhancement of the rim of the pseudocyst. When the pseudocyst is located in the pancreas there may be marked distortion of the gland. About one-half of pseudocysts are located outside the pancreas, most often in lesser sac or pararenal spaces, and in these circumstances the pancreas may be relatively intact. More rarely, fluid collections may occur elsewhere. From time to time a pseudocyst may spontaneously perforate into adjacent bowel and gas can then be seen in the cyst cavity. If such a communication occurs into the colon an abscess frequently follows.

*Analyses of cyst fluid*

Fine needle aspiration of cyst fluid often reveals important diagnostic information. A high carbohydrate antigen 19.9 is common in mucinous tumours, a low CEA in serous cystadenomas and a high amylase level in pseudocysts (Hammel et al 1995).

*ERCP*

Pseudocysts may be demonstrated by endoscopic retrograde pancreatography, either because the cyst fills with contrast medium during the procedure or because it causes obstruction to the pancreatic duct. However, this is not recommended as there is a danger of infection if contaminated contrast medium is introduced into the cyst. However, it is occasionally desirable to perform ERCP in patients with a pseudocyst to obtain information about the duct system prior to surgery (O'Connor et al 1986).

*Surgical, endoscopic or external drainage*

Usually, the cyst is drained internally (p. 1261). It can also be drained externally but with the disadvantage that a pancreatic fistula forms. Drainage can be achieved by percutaneous needle puncture (Fig. 1.39) and insertion of a catheter under ultrasound control, but the pseudocyst is seldom cured in this way and surgery is still recommended. At operation, the cyst should be biopsied to exclude cystadenocarcinoma.

Hemorrhage is the main complication of pseudocysts, and its treatment is difficult. After drainage into the stomach, erosions or ulcerations frequently develop in the gastric mucosa, or bleeding may occur from the cyst wall. Endoscopy should be performed to identify the site and cause of bleeding, and conservative therapy should be pursued if at all possible.

Endoscopic drainage into the duodenum or stomach offers an alternative to surgical drainage into the stomach or Roux loop of jejunum and is used in selected cases where a collection with a relatively thin wall bulges into the gut lumen (Maydeo et al 1993). After puncture with a diathermy needle-knife a pig-tail stent is inserted over a guidewire or the site of puncture can be extended using a conventional papillotome. Complications (bleeding, pancreatitis and abscess) are reported in 5–15% of cases but are rarely fatal.

**Prognosis** (Frey 1978)

When a cyst develops after acute pancreatitis, changes in symptoms or size of the mass, measurements of serum amylase activity or amylase clearance, and ultrasonography indicate progression or resolution of the pseudocyst. As some disappear spontaneously, conservative management should be continued if at all possible for at least 6 weeks. Surgical treatment during this period has a 60% mortality. Conservative treatment allows the wall of the cyst to become well defined, and drainage is easier. However, early operation may become necessary for enlarging pseudocysts which may rupture, for obstructive jaundice, for obstruction of the upper gastrointestinal tract and when a pancreatic abscess is suspected. When a pseudocyst is diagnosed in a patient with chronic pancreatitis when there has been no recent acute attack, it is unnecessary to delay operation (Warshaw & Rattner 1985).

## PANCREATIC ASCITES AND PLEURAL EFFUSION (Cameron 1978)

The term "pancreatic ascites" refers to ascites resulting from duct disruption or from leakage of a pancreatic pseudocyst in patients with chronic pancreatitis. However, these events may also occur in acute pancreatitis. Abdominal trauma is a cause in children.

### Pathogenesis

Damage to the pancreatic ducts can lead to ascites or pleural effusion if the site of duct rupture does not seal off or if a pseudocyst develops and leaks. Anterior duct disruption allows pancreatic secretions to flow into the peritoneal cavity, while posterior disruption allows secretions to track into the mediastinum, where a pseudocyst, pericardial effusion or, more frequently, pleural effusions can develop. Occasionally, the pancreatic-pleural fistula may erode directly through the dome of the diaphragm to cause a pleural effusion. The ascites is maintained by chemical peritonitis and by chronic peritoneal changes which inhibit fluid reabsorption.

### Clinical features

The onset is usually insidious and without any clear episode of acute pancreatitis. There is a slow increase in abdominal girth, abdominal pain, which is severe in one-third of patients, and marked weight loss despite the increase in girth. The ascites is resistant to diuretics. Examination reveals massive ascites, usually without tenderness. Pleural effusions may also be massive, and there may be pleuritic pain. The insidious nature of the disorder may suggest cirrhotic, tuberculous or carcinomatous ascites.

### Investigations

The presence of ascites is easily confirmed by ultrasound or computerized tomography. The diagnosis of pancreatic ascites is made on the serum amylase activity, which is nearly always raised, and the ascitic fluid amylase activity, which is always very high (p. 1021). The ascitic protein concentration usually exceeds 25 g/dl. The ascitic fluid amylase activity often is normal in cirrhosis, and the protein concentration is less than 25 g/dl. Pancreatic pleural effusion fluid also always has a very high amylase activity.

Fistulas to the peritoneum or pleura can be demonstrated by ERCP, but this should only be used to determine the site of the fistula prior to surgery once conservative therapy has failed, because there is a risk of further pancreatitis or the introduction of infection. In some cases the fistula can be demonstrated by computerized tomography (Louie et al 1985).

#### *Treatment*

The initial therapy for pancreatic pleural effusion or panreatic ascites should be conservative. The patient should be treated with nasogastric suction together with parenteral or enteral feeding. *Octreotide* 50–200 μg twice daily by subcutaneous injection is used to minimize pancreatic secretion. Repeated paracentesis or thoracenteses have been advocated (Cameron 1978) but this encourages infection and hypoproteinemia. Conservative measures should be continued for 2 weeks and are successful in one-third of cases. Even if they fail, the patient is usually in better condition for surgery. ERCP or operative pancreatography should be used to locate the site of injury to the pancreatic duct prior to surgical repair. Pancreatic ascites carries a mortality of 20–30% and it is unwise to persist with conservative treatment for more than 2 weeks.

***Surgery.*** If the duct rupture or cyst leakage is localized to the tail of the pancreas and there is no proximal obstruction, a distal pancreatectomy is carried out. If there is proximal obstruction due to stricture or calculi, then a distal pancreatectomy with Roux-en-Y jejunal anastomosis is performed (Bradley & Allen 1993). If the leak cannot be demonstrated or if there are multiple strictures and leaks then a side-to-side pancreaticojejunostomy (Puestow) is performed in patients with dilatation of the pancreatic duct system.

Endoscopic placement of stents across the site of ductal disruption has recently been reported in fistula patients who fail to respond to conservative management. The fistula resolved in all five patients treated by Saeed et al (1993) and none recurred within a follow-up of 14–30 months. It must be emphasized that four of these patients had alcoholic pancreatitis and that in three cases there was evidence of chronic inflammation. The stents were removed after approximately 6 weeks and were thought to have promoted fistula closure by providing a path of least resistance which allowed the fistula tract to collapse. The role of endoscopic stenting in fistulas associated with acute pancreatitis remains uncertain, but stenting may allow surgery to be avoided or deferred in high risk patients, particularly when ERCP has shown a narrowing in the pancreatic duct.

## REFERENCES


Acosta J L, Rossi R, Ledesma C L 1977 The usefulness of stool screening for diagnosing cholelithiasis in acute pancreatitis. A description of the technique. American Journal of Digestive Disease. 22: 168–174

Acosta J M, Rossi R, Galli O M R, Pellegrini C A, Skinner D B 1978 Early surgery for acute gallstone pancreatitis: evaluation of a systematic approach. Surgery 83: 367–380

Adler G, Rohr G, Kern H 1982 Alteration of membrane fusion as a cause of acute pancreatitis in the rat. Digestive Diseases and Sciences 27: 993–1002

Adlersberg D, Schein J 1947 Clinical and pathological studies in sprue. Journal of the American Medical Association 134: 1459

Adler G, Hahn C, Kern H, Rao K 1985 Cerulein-induced pancreatitis in rats: increased lysosomal enzyme activity and autophagocytosis. Digestion 32: 10

Aldridge M C, Ornstein M, Glazer G, Dudley H A F 1985 Pancreatic resection for severe acute pancreatitis. British Journal of Surgery 72: 796–800

Aldridge M C, Francis N D, Glazer G, Dudley H A F 1989 Colonic complications of severe acute pancreatitis. British Journal of Surgery 76: 362–367

Allam B F, Imrie C W 1977 Serum ionized calcium in acute pancreatitis. British Journal of Surgery 64: 665–668

Amman R W, Akovbiantz A, Largadier F, Schueler G 1984 Course and outcome of chronic pancreatitis. Longitudinal study of a mixed medical-surgical series of 245 patients. Gastroenterology 86: 820–828

Amman R W, Heitz P U, Klöpel G 1996 Course of alcoholic chronic pancreatitis: a prospective clinicomorphological long-term study. Gastroenterology 111: 224–231

Apte M, Wilson J S, Korsten M A, McCaughan G W, Haber P S, Pirola R C 1995 Effects of ethanol and protein deficiency on pancreatic digestive and lysosomal enzymes. Gut 36: 287–293

Aranha G V, Prinz R A, Freeark R J, Greenlee H B 1984 The spectrum of biliary tract obstruction from chronic pancreatitis. Archives of Surgery 199: 595

Armstrong C P, Taylor T V 1985 The biliary tract in patients with acute gallstone pancreatitis. British Journal of Surgery 72: 551–556

Armstrong C P, Taylor T V 1986 Pancreatic duct reflux and acute gallstone pancreatitis. Annals of Surgery 204: 59–64

Asbun H J, Rossi R L, Heiss F W, Shea J A 1993 Acute relapsing pancreatitis as a complication of papillary stenosis after endoscopic sphincterotomy. Gastroenterology 104: 1814–1817

Aziz S, Bergdahl L, Baldwin J C, Weiss L M, Jamieson S W, Oyer P E, Stinson E B, Shumway N E 1985 Pancreatitis after cardiac and cardiopulmonary transplantation. Surgery 97: 653–660

Bagley J S, Tyler M P H, Cooper G C 1994 Hyperamylasaemia in ruptured aortic aneurysm: incidence and prognostic implications. British Journal of Surgery 81: 31–32

Balldin G, Borgstrom A, Genell S, Ohlsson K 1983 The effect of peritoneal lavage and aprotinin in the treatment of severe acute pancreatitis. Research in Experimental Medicine 183: 203–212

Balthazar E J 1989 CT diagnosis and staging of acute pancreatitis. Radiologic Clinics of North America 27: 19–37

Balthazar E J, Robinson D L, Megibow A J, Ranson J H C 1990 Acute pancreatitis: value of CT in establishing prognosis. Radiology 174: 331–336

Becker W F, Pratt H S, Ganji H 1968 Psedocysts of the pancreas. Surgery, Gynecology and Obstetrics 127: 744

Becker J M, Pemberton J H, Di Magno E P, Ilstrup D M, McIlrath D C, Dozois R R 1984 Prognostic factors in pancreatic abscess. Surgery 96: 455–460

Beger H G 1989 Management of pancreatic necrosis and pancreatic abscess. In: Carter D C, Warshaw A L (eds) Pancreatitis. Clinical Surgery International 16. Churchill Livingstone, Edinburgh, p 107–119

Beger H G, Bittner R, Block S, Buchler M 1986a Bacterial contamination of pancreatic necrosis. A prospective clinical study. Gastroenterology 91: 433–438

Beger H G, Bittner R, Buchler M, Hess W, Schmitz J E 1986b Hemodynamic data patterns in patients with acute pancreatitis. Gastroenterology 90: 74–79

Beger H G, Buchler M, Bittner R, Block S, Nevalainen T, Roscher R 1988 Necrosectomy and postoperative local lavage in necrotizing pancreatitis. British Journal of Surgery 75: 207–212

Beger H G, Imaizumi T 1995 Duodenum-preserving head resection in chronic pancreatitis. Journal of Hepatobiliary and Pancreatic Surgery 2: 13–18

Bernard J P, Sahel K, Giovanni M, Sarles H 1990 Pancreas divisum is a probable cause of acute pancreatitis: a report of 137 cases. Pancreas 5: 248–254

Berry A R, Taylor T V, Davies G C 1982 Diagnostic tests and prognostic indicators in acute pancreatitis. Journal of the Royal College of Surgeons of Edinburgh 27: 345–352

Bess M, Edis A, van Heerden J A 1980 Hyperparathyroidism and pancreatitis. Chance or a causal association? Journal of the American Medical Association 243: 246

Bettinger J R, Grendell J H 1991 Intracellular events in the pathogenesis of acute pancreatitis. Pancreas 6: S2–S6

Bittner R, Block S, Buchler M, Beger H G 1987 Pancreatic abscess and infected pancreatic necrosis. Different local septic complications in acute pancreatitis. Digestive Diseases and Sciences 32: 1082–1087

Blamey S L, Osborne D H, Gilmour W H, O'Neill J, Carter D C, Imrie C W 1983 The early identification of patients with gallstone pancreatitis using clinical and biochemical factors only. Annals of Surgery 198: 574–578

Blamey S L, Imrie C W, O'Neill J, Gilmour W H, Carter D C 1984 Prognostic factors in acute pancreatitis. Gut 25: 1340–1346

Bockman D, Buchler M, Malfertheiner P, Beger H G 1988 Analysis of nerves in chronic pancreatitis. Gastroenterology 94: 1459–1469

Bordalo O, Bapista, A, Dreiling D, Noronha M 1984 Early pathomorphological pancreatic changes in chronic alcoholism. In: Gyr K E, Singer M V, Sarles H (eds) Pancreatitis – concepts and classification. Excerpta Medica, International Congress Series No 642, Elsevier, Amsterdam

Bourliere M, Barhtet M, Berthezene P, Durbec J P, Sarler H 1991 Is tobacco a risk factor for chronic pancreatitis and alcoholic cirrhosis? Gut 32: 1392–1395

Bradley E L 1987 Management of infected pancreatic necrosis by open drainage. Annals of Surgery 206: 542–550

Bradley E L, Allen K A 1993 Complications of acute pancreatitis and their management. In: Trede M, Carter D C (eds) Surgery of the pancreas. Churchill Livingstone, Edinburgh

Bradley E L, Clements J L 1981 Idiopathic duodenal obstruction. An unappreciated complication of pancreatitis. Annals of Surgery 193: 638–646

Bradley E L, Clements J L, Gonzalez A C 1979 The natural history of pancreatic pseudocoysts: a unified concept of management. American Journal of Surgery 137: 135

Bradley E L, Fulenwider J T 1984 Open treatment of pancreatic abscess. Surgery, Gynecology and Obstetrics 159: 509–513

Bradley E L, Hall J R, Lutz J, Hamner L, Lattouf O 1983 Hemodynamic consequences of severe pancreatitis. Annals of Surgery 198: 130–133

Braganza J M 1983 Pancreatic disease: a casualty of hepatic "detoxification". Lancet 2: 1000–1003

Browder W, Patterson M D, Thompson J L, Walters D N 1993 Acute pancreatitis of unknown etiology in the elderly. Annals of Surgery 217: 469–475

Brown R A, Immelman E J, Harries-Jones E P 1985 Pancreatic duct haemorrhage. British Journal of Surgery 72: 223–224

Buch A, Buch J, Carlsen A, Schmidt A 1980 Hyperlipidaemia and pancreatitis. World Journal of Surgery 4: 307–314

Buchler M, Malfertheiner P, Beger H G 1986 Correlation of imaging procedures, biochemical parameters, and clinical stage in acute pancreatitis. In: Malfertheiner P, Ditschuneit H (eds) Diagnostic procedures in pancreatic disease. Springer-Verlag, Heidelberg, p 123–129

Buchler M, Malfertheiner P, Uhl W et al 1993 Gabexate mesilate in human acute pancreatitis. Gastroenterology 104: 1165–1170

Cameron J L L 1978 Chronic pancreatic ascites and pancreatic pleural effusions. Gastroenterology 74: 134

Cameron J L, Capuzzi D, Zuidema G, Margolis S 1973 Acute

pancreatitis with hyperlipemia: evidence for a persistent defect in lipid metabolism. American Journal of Medicine 56: 482–487
Carr M R, Dick S P, Bordley J, Bertino J S 1988 Gentamicin dosing requirements in patients with acute pancreatitis. Surgery 103: 533–537
Carr-Locke D L, Gregg J A 1981 Endoscopic manometry of pancreatic and biliary sphincter zones in man. Digestive Diseases and Sciences 26: 7
Carter D C 1989 Gallstone pancreatitis. In: Carter D C, Warshaw A L (eds) Pancreatitis. Clinical Surgery International 16. Churchill Livingstone, Edinburgh, p 58–70
Carter D C 1992 Cancer of the head of pancreas or chronic pancreatitis? A diagnostic dilemma. Surgery 111: 602–603
Clavien P-A, Burgan S, Moossa A R 1989a Serum enzymes and other laboratory tests in acute pancreatitis. British Journal of Surgery 76: 1234–1243
Clavien P-A, Robert J, Meyer P 1989b Acute pancreatitis and normoamylasaemia. Annals of Surgery 210: 614–620
Connors P J, Carr-Locke D L 1993 Endoscopic retrograde cholangiopancreatography. In: Trede M, Carter D C (eds) Surgery of the pancreas. Churchill Livingstone, Edinburgh, p 87–110
Conter R L, Converse J O, McGarrity T J, Koch K L 1990 Afferent loop obstruction presenting as acute pancreatitis and pseudocyst: case reports and review of the literature. Surgery 108: 22–27
Cooper M J, Williamson R C N, Benjamin I S et al 1987 Total pancreatectomy for chronic pancreatitis. British Journal of Surgery 74: 912–915
Copenhagen Pancreatitis Study 1981 An interim report from a prospective epidemiological multicenter study. Scandinavian Journal of Gastroenterology 16: 305–312
Corfield A P, Cooper M J, Williamson R C N 1985a Acute pancreatitis: a lethal disease of increasing incidence. Gut 26: 724–729
Corfield A P, Williamson R C N, McMahon M J et al 1985b Prediction of severity in acute pancreatitis: prospective comparison of three prognostic indices. Lancet 2: 403–407
Croton R S, Warren R A, Stott A, Roberts N B 1981 Ionized calcium in acute pancreatitis and its relationships with total calcium and serum lipase. British Journal of Surgery 68: 241–244
Cuschieri A, Wood R A B, Cumming J R G, Meehan S E, Mackie C R 1983 Treatment of acute pancreatitis with fresh frozen plasma. British Journal of Surgery 70: 710–712
D'Egidio A, Schein M 1991 Surgical strategies in the treatment of pancreatic necrosis and infection. British Journal of Surgery 78: 133–137
Dalton-Clarke H J, Lewis M H, Levi A J, Blumgart L H 1980 Familial chronic calcific pancreatitis: a family study. British Journal of Surgery 72: 307–308
Davis S, Parboo S P, Gibson M J 1980 The plain abdominal radiograph in acute pancreatitis. Clinical Radiology 31: 87
Delcore R, Rodriguez F J, Thomas J H, Forster J, Hermreck A S 1994 The role of pancreaticojejunostomy in patients without dilated pancreatic ducts. American Journal of Surgery 168: 598–601
Delhaye M, Engelholm L, Cremer M 1985 Pancreas divisum: congenital anatomic variant or anomaly? Contribution of endoscopic retrograde dorsal pancreatography. Gastroenterology 89: 1431–1435
DiMagno E P, Go V L W, Summerskill W H J 1973 Relations between pancreatic enzyme outputs and malabsorption in severe pancreatic insufficiency. New England Journal of Medicine 288: 813
Di Magno E P, Shorter R G, Taylor W F, Go V L W 1982 Relationships between pancreaticobiliary ductal anatomy and pancreatic ductal and parenchymal histology. Cancer 49: 361
Dickson A P, Imrie C W 1984 The incidence and prognosis of body wall ecchymosis in acute pancreatitis. Surgery, Gynecology and Obstetrics 159: 343–347
Dickson A P, O'Neill J, Imrie C W 1984 Hyperlipidaemia, alcohol abuse and acute pancreatitis. British Journal of Surgery 71: 685–688
Dominguez-Muñoz J E, Malfertheiner P, Ditschuneit H H, Blanco-Chavez J, Uhl W, Buchler M, Ditschuneit H 1991 Hyperlipidaemia in acute pancreatitis. Relationship with etiology, onset and severity of the disease. International Journal of Pancreatology 10: 261–267
Donnelly S C, Strieter R M, Kunkel S L et al 1993 Interleukin-8 and development of adult respiratory distress syndrome in at-risk patient groups. Lancet 341: 643–647
Dreiling D A 1957 The pancreatic secretion in the malabsorption syndrome and related malnutrition states. Journal of the Mount Sinai Hospital 24: 243
Durbec J P, Sarles H 1978 Multicenter survey of the etiology of pancreatic diseases. Relationship between the relative risk of developing chronic pancreatitis and alcohol, protein, and lipid consumption. Digestion 18: 337–350
Durr H K, Bindrich D, Bode J C 1977 The frequency of macroamylasaemia and the diagnostic value of the amylase to creatinine clearance ratio in patients with elevated serum amylase activity. Scandinavian Journal of Gastroenterology 12: 701–705
Dutta S K, Bustin M P, Russell R M, Costa B S 1982 Deficiency of fat-soluble vitamins in treated patients with pancreatic insufficiency. Annals of Internal Medicine 97: 549
Ede R J, Moore K P, Marshall W J, Williams R 1988 Frequency of pancreatitis in fulminant hepatic failure using isoenzyme markers. Gut 29: 778–781
Eriksson J, Doepel M, Widen E, Halme L, Ekstrand A, Groop L, Hockerstedt K 1992 Pancreatic surgery, not pancreatitis, is the primary cause of diabetes after acute fulminant pancreatitis. Gut 33: 843–847
Fagniez P L, Rotman N, Kracht M 1989 Direct retroperitoneal approach to necrosis in severe acute pancreatitis. British Journal of Surgery 76: 264–267
Fan S T, Choi T K, Lai E C S, Wong J 1988 Influence of age on the mortality from acute pancreatitis. British Journal of Surgery 75: 463–466
Fan S T, Choi T K, Chan F L, Lai E C S, Wong J 1989 Pancreatic phlegmon: what is it? American Journal of Surgery 157: 544–547
Fan S T, Lai E C S, Mok F P T, Lo C-M, Zheng S-S, Wong J 1993 Early treatment of acute biliary pancreatitis by endoscopic papillotomy. New England Journal of Medicine 328: 228–232
Farmer R C, Tweedie J, Maslin S, Reber H A, Adler G, Kern H 1984 Effects of bile salts on permeability and morphology of main pancreatic duct in cats. Digestive Diseases and Sciences 29: 740–751
Fernandez-del Castillo C, Harringer W, Warshaw A L, Vlahakes G J, Koski G, Zaslavsky A M, Rattner D W 1991 Risk factors for pancreatic cellular injury after cardiopulmonary bypass. New England Journal of Medicine 325: 382–387
Foitzik T, Bassi D G, Schmidt J, Lewandrowski K B, Fernandez-del Castillo C, Rattner D W, Warshaw A L 1994 Intravenous contrast medium accentuates the severity of acute necrotizing pancreatitis in the rat. Gastroenterology 106: 207–214
Foulis A K, Murray W R, Galloway D 1982 Endotoxaemia and complement activation in acute pancreatitis in man. Gut 23: 656–661
Freeman R, McMahon M J 1978 Acute pancreatitis and serological evidence of infection with *Mycoplasma pneumoniae*. Gut 19: 367–370
Freeny P C 1993a Incremental dynamic bolus computed tomography of acute pancreatitis. International Journal of Pancreatology 13: 147–158
Freeny P C 1993b Pre-operative diagnosis of pancreatic disease. In: Trede M, Carter D C (eds) Surgery of the pancreas. Churchill Livingstone, Edinburgh, p 51–86
Freeny P C, Lawson L (eds) 1982 Radiology of the pancreas. Springer-Verlag, New York
Frey C F 1978 Pancreatic pseudocyst – operative strategy. Annals of Surgery 188: 652
Frey C F 1991 Classification of acute pancreatitis. International Journal of Pancreatology 9: 39–49
Frey C F, Amikura K 1994 Local resection of the head of the pancreas combined with longitudinal pancreaticojejunostomy in the management of patients with chronic pancreatitis. Annals of Surgery 220: 492–507
Funnell I C, Bornman P C, Weakly S P, Terblanche J, Marks I N 1993 Obesity: an important prognostic factor in acute pancreatitis. British Journal of Surgery 80: 484–486
Gafter U, Mandel E, Har-Zahav L, Weiss S 1976 Acute pancreatitis secondary to hypercalcaemia: occurrence in a patient with breast carcinoma. Journal of the American Medical Association 235: 2004
Gallagher P, Chadwick P, Jones D M, Turner L 1981 Acute pancreatitis associated with campylobacter infection. British Journal of Surgery 68: 383
Gee Varghese P J 1986 Calcific pancreatitis. Causes and mechanisms in

the tropics compared with those of the subtropics. St Joseph's Trivandrum. Varghese, Bombay
Geokas M C, Rinderknecht H 1978 Free proteolytic enzymes in pancreatic juice of patients with acute pancreatitis. American Journal of Digestive Diseases 19: 591–598
Gerzof S G, Banks P A, Robbins A H et al 1987 Early diagnosis of pancreatic infection by computed tomography-guided aspiration. Gastroenterology 93: 1315–1320
Giorgi D, Bernard J P, de Caro A, Multinger L, Lapointe R, Sarles H, Dagorn J C 1985 Pancreatic stone protein. I Evidence that it is encoded by a pancreatic messenger ribonucleic acid. Gastroenterology 89: 381–386
Giorgi D, Bernard J P O, Ranquir S, Iovanna J, Sarles H, Dagorn J C 1989 Secretory pancreatic stone protein messenger R N A. Nucleotide sequence and expression in chronic calcifying pancreatitis. Journal of Clinical Investigation 84: 100–106
Glazer G, Murphy F, Clayden G S 1981 Radionuclide biliary scanning in acute pancreatitis. British Journal of Surgery 68: 766–770
Goodman A J, Neoptolemos J P, Carr-Locke D L, Finlay D B, Fossard D P 1985 Detection of gallstones after acute pancreatitis. Gut 26: 125–132
Goulet R J, Goodman J, Schaffer R, Dallemand S, Andersen D K 1984 Multiple pancreatic pseudocyst disease. Annals of surgery 199: 6
Grey-Turner G 1919 Local discolouration of the abdominal wall as a sign of acute pancreatitis. British Journal of Surgery 7: 394–395
Gudgeon A M, Heath D I, Hurley P, Jehanli A et al 1990 Trypsinogen activation peptide assay in the early prediction of severity of acute pancreatitis. Lancet 335: 4–8
Haas G, Warshaw A L, Daggett W, Aretz H 1985 Acute pancreatitis after cardiopulmonary bypass. American Journal of Surgery 149: 508
Haber P S, Wilson J S, Apte M V, Hall W, Goumas K, Pirola R C 1994 Lipid intolerance does not account for susceptibility to alcoholic and gallstone pancreatitis. Gastroenterology 106: 742–748
Hammel P, Levy P, Voitot H et al 1995 Preoperative cyst fluid analysis is useful for the differential diagnosis of cystic lesions of the pancreas. Gastroenterology 108: 1230–1235
Hartley R H, Barlow A P, Kilby J O 1993 Intraluminal duodenal diverticulum: an unusual cause of acute pancreatitis. British Journal of Surgery 80: 488
Harvey M H, Wedgwood K R, Austin J A, Reber H A 1989 Pancreatic duct pressure, duct permeability and acute pancreatitis. British Journal of Surgery 76: 859–862
Herskovic T 1968 The exocrine pancreas in intestinal malabsorption syndromes. American Journal of Clinical Nutrition 21: 520
Higgins E, Ive F A 1990 Subcutaneous fat necrosis in pancreatic disease. British Journal of Surgery 77: 532–533
Holstege A, Barner S, Brambs H J, Wenz W, Gerok W, Farthmann E H 1985 Relapsing pancreatitis associated with duodenal wall cysts. Gastroenterology 88: 814–819
Horn J 1993 Late results of surgical treatment of chronic pancreatitis. In: Trede M, Carter D C (eds) Surgery of the pancreas. Churchill Livingstone, Edinburgh
Ihse I, Lilja P, Lundquist I 1980 Intestinal concentrations of pancreatic enzymes following pancreatic replacement therapy. Scandinavian Journal of Gastroenterology 15: 137
Ihse I, Evander A, Holmberg J T, Gustafson I 1986 Influence of peritoneal lavage on objective prognostic signs in acute pancreatitis. Annals of Surgery 204: 122–127
Imrie C W, Wilson C 1989 Evaluation of severity in acute pancreatitis and the need for early surgery. In: Carter D C, Warshaw A L (eds) Pancreatitis. Clinical Surgery International 16. Churchill Livingstone, Edinburgh, p 31–43
Imrie C W, Beastall G H, Allam B F, O'Neill J, Benjamin I S, McKay A J 1978a Parathyroid hormone and calcium homeostasis in acute pancreatitis. British Journal of Surgery 65: 717–720
Imrie C W, Benjamin I S, Ferguson J C et al 1978b A single centre double blind trial of Trasylol therapy in primary acute pancreatitis. British Journal of Surgery 65: 337–341
Imrie C W, McKay A J, Benjamin I S, Blumgart L H 1978c Secondary acute pancreatitis: aetiology, prevention, diagnosis and management. British Journal of Surgery 65: 399–402
Izsak E, Shike M, Roulet M, Jeejeebhoy K 1980 Pancreatitis in association with hypercalcaemia in patients receiving total parenteral nutrition. Gastroenterology 79: 555
Jaakkola M, Sillanaukee P, Lof K, Koivula T, Nordback I 1994 Amount of alcohol is an important determinant of the severity of acute alcoholic pancreatitis. Surgery 115: 31–38
Jacobs M L, Dagget W M, Civetta J M et al 1981 Acute pancreatitis: analysis of factors influencing survival. Annals of Surgery 185: 43
Johnson C D, Hosking S 1991 National statistics for diet, alcohol consumption and chronic pancreatitis in England and Wales, 1960–1988. Gut 32: 1401–1405
Jones B A, Salsberg B B, Bohnen J M A, Mehta M H 1987 Common pancreatobiliary channels and their relationship to gallstone size in gallstone pancreatitis. Annals of Surgery 205: 123–125
Kaden V G, Howard J M, Doubleday L C 1955 Cholecystographic studies during and immediately following acute pancreatitis. Surgery 38: 1082–1086
Kelly D M, McEntee G P, Delaney C, McGeeney K F, Fitzpatrick J M 1993 Temporal relationship of acinar and microvascular changes in caerulein-induced pancreatitis. British Journal of Surgery 80: 1174–1178
Kelly T R 1976 Gallstone pancreatitis; pathophysiology. Surgery 80: 488–492
Kelly T R 1984 Gallstone pancreatitis. Local predisposing factors. Annals of Surgery 200: 479–484
Kelly T R, Swaney P E 1982 Gallstone pancreatitis: the second time around. Surgery 92: 571–575
Kelly T R, Wagner D S 1988 Gallstone pancreatitis: a prospective randomized trial of the timing of surgery. Surgery 104: 600–605
Kemmer T P, Malfertheiner P, Buchler M, Kemmer M L, Ditschuneit H 1991 Serum ribonuclease activity in the diagnosis of pancreatic disease. International Journal of Pancreatology 8: 23–33
Keynes M 1988 Heretical thoughts on the pathogenesis of acute pancreatitis. Gut 29: 1413–1423
Khuroo M S, Zargar S A, Mahajan R 1990 Hepatobiliary and pancreatic ascariasis in India. Lancet 335: 1503–1506
Kivilaakso E, Lempinen M, Makelainen A, Nikki P, Schroder T 1984a Pancreatic resection versus peritoneal lavation for acute fulminant pancreatitis. A randomized prospective study. Annals of Surgery 199: 426–431
Kivilaakso E, Valtnen V V, Malkamaki M et al 1984b Endotoxaemia and acute pancreatitis: correlation between the severity of the disease and the antienterobacterial common antigen antibody titre. Gut 25: 1065–1070
Kiviniemi H, Makela J, Kairaluoma M 1993 Acute fulminant pancreatitis: debridement or formal resection of the pancreas. HPB Surgery 6: 255–263
Klar E, Rattner D W, Compton C, Stanford G, Chernow B, Warshaw A L 1991 Adverse effect of therapeutic vasoconstrictors in experimental acute pancreatitis. Annals of Surgery 214: 168–174
Klar E, Foitzik T, Buhr H, Messmer K, Herfarth C 1993 Isovolemic hemodilution with dextran 60 as treatment of pancreatic ischemia in acute pancreatitis. Clinical practicability of an experimental concept. Annals of Surgery 217: 369–374
Kolars J C, Ellis C J, Levitt M D 1984 Comparison of serum amylase pancreatic isoamylase and lipase in patients with hyperamylasaemia. Digestive Diseases and Sciences 29: 289–293
Konok G P, Thompson A G 1969 Pancreatic duct mucosa as a protective barrier in the pathogenesis of acute pancreatitis. American Journal of Surgery 117: 18–22
Kunkel S L, Standiford T, Kasahara K, Strieter R M 1991 Interleukin-8: the major neutrophil chemotactic factor in the lung. Experimental Lung Research 17: 17–23
Lankisch P G 1993 Function tests in the diagnosis of chronic pancreatitis. International Journal of Pancreatology 14: 9–20
Lankisch P G, Creutzfeldt W 1984 Therapy of exocrine and endocrine pancreatic insufficiency. Clinics in Gastroenterology 13: 985
Lankisch P G, Dröge M, Gotlesleben F 1995 Drug induced acute pancreatitis: incidence and severity. Gut 37: 565–567
Lankisch P G, Rahlf G, Koop H 1983 Pulmonary complications in fatal acute hemorrhagic pancreatitis. Digestive Diseases and Sciences 28: 111–116
Lankisch P G, Schirren C A, Kunze E 1991 Undetected fatal acute pancreatitis: why is the disease so frequently overlooked? American Journal of Gastroenterology 86: 322–326

Larvin M, McMahon M J 1989 Apache-II score for assessment and monitoring of acute pancreatitis. Lancet 2: 201–205

Larvin M M, McMahon M J, Puntis M C A, Thomas W E G 1992 Marked placebo responses in chronic pancreatitis: final results of a controlled trial of Creon therapy (abstract). British Journal of Surgery 79: 457

Larvin M, Chalmers A G, Robinson P J, McMahon M J 1989 Debridement and closed cavity irrigation for the treatment of pancreatic necrosis. British Journal of Surgery 78: 465–471

Larvin M, Chalmers A G, McMahon M J 1990 Dynamic contrast enhanced computed tomography: a precise technique for identifying and localising pancreatic necrosis. British Medical Journal 300: 1425–1428

Lashner B A, Kirsner J B, Hanauer S B 1986 Acute pancreatitis associated with high-concentration lipid emulsion during total parenteral nutrition therapy for Crohn's disease. Gastroenterology 90: 1039–1041

Layer P, Holtmann G 1994 Pancreatic enzymes in chronic pancreatitis. International Journal of Pancreatology 15: 1–11

Layer P, Yamamoto H, Kalthoff L, Clain J E, Bakken L J, Di Magno E P 1994 The different courses of early- and late-onset idiopathic and alcoholic chronic pancreatitis. Gastroenterology 107: 1481–1487

Lee S P, Nicholls J F, Park H Z 1992 Biliary sludge as a cause of acute pancreatitis. New England Journal of Medicine 326: 589–593

Leese T, Holliday M, Heath D, Hall A W, Bell P F R 1987 Multicentre trial of low volume fresh frozen plasma therapy in acute pancreatitis. British Journal of Surgery 74: 906–911

Lerch M M, Saluja A K, Runzi M, Dawra R, Saluja M, Steer M L 1993 Pancreatic duct obstruction triggers acute necrotizing pancreatitis in the opossum. Gastroenterology 104: 853–861

Levi P, Menzelxhiu A, Palliot B et al 1993 Abdominal radiotherapy is a cause for chronic pancreatitis. Gastroenterology 105: 905–909

Lohse J, Pfeiffer A 1984 Duodenal total and ionised calcium secretion in normal subjects, chronic alcoholics, and patients with various stages of chronic alcoholic pancreatitis. Gut 25: 874–880

Lohse J, Schmid D, Sarles H 1983 Pancreatic citrate and protein secretion of alcoholic dogs in response to graded doses of caerulein. Pflugers Archiv (European Journal of Physiology) 397: 141–143

London N J M, Leese T, Lavelle J M, Miles K, West K P, Watkin D F L, Fossard D P 1991 Rapid-bolus contrast-enhanced dynamic computed tomography in acute pancreatitis: a prospective study. British Journal of Surgery 78: 1452–1456

Louie S, McGrahan J P, Frey C, Cross C E 1985 Pancreatic pleuropericardial effusions. Fistulous tracts demonstrated by computer tomography. Archives of Internal Medicine 145: 1231

Lowenfels A B, Maisonneuve P, Cavallini G et al 1993 Pancreatitis and the risk of pancreatic cancer. New England Journal of Medicine 328: 1433–1437

Lucarotti M E, Virjee J, Alderson D 1993 Patient selection and timing of dynamic computed tomography in acute pancreatitis. British Journal of Surgery 80: 1393–1395

Ludwig G D, Chaykin L B 1966 Pancreatitis associated with primary hyperparathyroidism. Medical Clinics of North America 50: 1403

Mallory A, Kern F 1980 Drug-induced pancreatitis: a critical review. Gastroenterology 78: 813–820

Mann D V, Hershman M J, Hittinger R, Glazer G 1994 Multicentre audit of death from acute pancreatitis. British Journal of Surgery 81: 890–893

Mariani A, Mezzi G, Malesci 1995 Purification and assay of secretory lithostatine in human pancreatic juice by fast protein liquid chromatography. Gut 36: 622–629

Maydeo A, Grimm H, Soehendra N 1993 Endoscopic interventional techniques in chronic pancreatitis In: Trede M, Carter D C (eds) Surgery of the pancreas. Churchill Livingstone, Edinburgh

Mayer A D, McMahon M J 1985 The diagnostic and prognostic value of peritoneal lavage in patients with acute pancreatitis. Surgery, Gynecology and Obstetrics 160: 507–512

Mayer A D, McMahon M J, Corfield A P et al 1985 Controlled clinical trial of peritoneal lavage for the treatment of severe acute pancreatitis. New England Journal of Medicine 312: 399–404

McCutcheon A D 1968 A fresh approach to the pathogenesis of acute pancreatitis. Gut 9: 296

McKay A J, Imrie C W, O'Neill J, Duncan J G 1982 Is an early ultrasound scan of value in acute pancreatitis? British Journal of Surgery 69: 369–372

McKay C J, Imrie C W, Baxter J N 1993 Somatostatin and somatostatin analogues – are they indicated in the management of acute pancreatitis? Gut 34: 1622–1626

McMahon M J, Shefta J R 1980 Physical characteristics of gallstones and the calibre of the cystic duct in patients with acute pancreatitis. British Journal of Surgery 67: 6–9

McMahon M J, Playforth M J, Pickford I R 1980 A comparative study of methods for the prediction of severity of attacks of acute pancreatitis. British Journal of Surgery 67: 22–25

McMahon M J, Bowen M, Mayer A D, Cooper E H 1984 Relationship of alpha-macroglobulin and other antiproteases to the clinical features of acute pancreatitis. American Journal of Surgery 147: 164–170

Mero M 1982 Changing aetiology of acute pancreatitis. Annales Chirurgiae et Gynaecologiae 71: 126–129

Millbourn E 1950 On the excretory ducts of the pancreas in man, with special reference to their relations to each other, to the common bile duct and to the duodenum. A radiological and anatomical study. Acta Anatomica 9: 1

Millward S F, Breatnach E, Simpkins K C, McMahon M J 1983 Do plain films of the chest and abdomen have a role in the diagnosis of acute pancreatitis? Clinical Radiology 34: 133

Misra S P, Dwivedi M 1991 Do gallstones cause chronic pancreatitis? International Journal of Pancreatology 10: 97–102

Moreau J A, Zinsmeister A R, Melton I J, Di Magno E P 1988 Gallstone pancreatitis and the effect of cholecystectomy. Mayo Clinic Proceedings 63: 466–473

Mughal M M, Bancewicz J, Irving M H 1987 The surgical management of pancreatic abscess. Annals of the Royal College of Surgeons of England 69: 64–70

Muller M K, Singer M V 1993 Aetiology and pathogenesis of chronic pancreatitis. In: Trede M, Carter D C (eds) Surgery of the pancreas. Churchill Livingstone, Edinburgh

Multinger I, Sarles H, Lombardo D, de Caro A 1985 Pancreatic stone protein. II Implication in stone formation during the course of chronic calcifying pancreatitis. Gastroenterology 89: 387–391

Murphy D, Pack A I, Imrie C W 1980 The mechanism of arterial hypoxia occurring in acute pancreatitis. Quarterly Journal of Medicine 49: 151–163

Nagata A, Homma T, Tamai K et al 1981 A study of chronic pancreatitis by serial endoscopic pancreatography. Gastroenterology 81: 884–891

Nealon W H, Thompson J C 1993 Progressive loss of pancreatic function in chronic pancreatitis is delayed by main pancreatic duct decompression. Annals of Surgery 217: 458–468

Neoptolemos J P, Hall A W, Finlay D F, Berry J M, Carr-Locke D L, Fossard D P 1984 The urgent diagnosis of gallstones in acute pancreatitis: a prospective study of three methods. British Journal of Surgery 71: 230–233

Neoptolemos J P, Carr-Locke D L, Leese T, James D 1987 Acute cholangitis in association with acute pancreatitis; incidence, clinical features and outcome in relation to ERCP and endoscopic sphincterotomy. British Journal of Surgery 74: 1103–1106

Neoptolemos J P, Carr-Locke D L, London N J M, Bailey I A, James D, Fossard D P 1988a Controlled trial of urgent endoscopic retrograde cholangiopancreatography and endoscopic sphincterotomy versus conservative treatment in patients with acute pancreatitis due to gallstones. Lancet 2: 979–983

Neoptolemos J P, Davidson B R, Winder A F, Vallance D 1988b Role of duodenal bile crystal analysis in the investigation of "idiopathic" pancreatitis. British Journal of Surgery 75: 450–453

Niederau C, Grendell J H 1985 Diagnosis of chronic pancreatitis. Gastroenterology 88: 1973–1975

Niederau C, Niederau M, Luthen R, Strohmeyer G, Ferrell L D, Grendell J H 1990 Pancreatic exocrine secretion in acute experimental pancreatitis. Gastroenterology 99: 1120–1127

Nordback I H, Macgowan S, Potter J I, Cameron J L 1991 The role of acetaldehyde in the pathogenesis of acute alcoholic pancreatitis. Annals of Surgery 214: 671–678

Noronha, M, Bordalo O, Dreiling D A 1981 Alcohol and the pancreas. II Pancreatic morphology of advanced alcoholic pancreatitis. American Journal of Gastroenterology 76: 120–124

Noronha M, Bapista A, Bordalo O 1984 Sequential aspects of pathology in chronic alcoholic disease of the pancreas. In: Gyr K E, Singer M V,

Sarles H (eds) Pancreatitis – concepts and classification. Excerpta Medica, International Congress Series No 642, Elsevier, Amsterdam
Nwokolo C, Oli J 1980 Pathogenesis of juvenile tropical pancreatitis syndrome. Lancet 1: 456–459
O'Connor M, Kolars J, Ansel H, Silvis S, Vennes J 1986 Preoperative endoscopic retrograde cholangiopancreatography in the surgical management of pancreatic pseudocyst. American Journal of Surgery 151: 18
Opie E L 1901 The etiology of acute hemorrhagic pancreatitis. Bulletin of the Johns Hopkins Hospital 12: 182–188
Osborne D H, Imrie C W, Carter D C 1981 Biliary surgery in the same admission for gallstone associated acute pancreatitis. British Journal of Surgery 68: 758–761
O'Sullivan J N, Nobrega F T, Morlock C G, Brown A L, Bartholomew L G 1972 Acute and chronic pancreatitis in Rochester, Minnesota 1940–1969. Gastroenterology 62: 373–379
Pederzzoli P, Cavallini G, Falconi M, Bassi C 1993 Gabexate mesilate vs aprotinin in human acute pancreatitis. International Journal of Pancreatology 14: 117–124
Pfeffer R B, Stasior O, Hinton J W 1957 The clinical picture of sequential development of acute hemorrhagic pancreatitis in the dog. Surgical Forum 8: 248
Pichumoni C S, Sonneshein M, Candido F M, Panchacharam P, Cooperman J M 1980 Nutrition in the pathogenesis of alcoholic pancreatitis. American Journal of Clinical Nutrition 33: 631–636
Porter K A, Banks P A 1991 Obesity as a predictor of severity in acute pancreatitis. International Journal of Pancreatology 10: 247–252
Puolakkainen P, Valtonen V, Paananen A, Schroder T 1987 C-reactive protein (CRP) and phospholipase A2 in the assessment of the severity of acute pancreatitis. Gut 28: 754–761
Ranson J H C 1979 The timing of biliary surgery in acute pancreatitis. Annals of Surgery 189: 654–663
Ranson J H C 1983 Acute pancreatitis. In: Brooks J R (ed) Surgery of the pancreas. W.B. Saunders, Philadelphia, p 146–181
Ranson J H C 1990 The role of surgery in the management of acute pancreatitis. Annals of Surgery 211: 382–393
Ranson J H C 1993 Non-operative management of acute pancreatitis. In: Trede M, Carter D C (eds) Surgery of the pancreas. Churchill Livingstone, Edinburgh, p 209–219
Ranson J H C, Berman R S 1990 Long peritoneal lavage decreases pancreatic sepsis in acute pancreatitis. Annals of Surgery 211: 708–716
Ranson J H C, Spencer F C 1978 The role of peritoneal lavage in severe acute pancreatitis. Annals of Surgery 187: 565–576
Ranson J H, Rifkind K M, Roses D F, Fink S D, Eng K, Spencer J 1974 Prognostic signs and the role of operative management in acute pancreatitis. Surgery, Gynecology and Obstetrics 139: 69–81
Ranson J H C, Balthazar E, Caccavale R, Cooper M 1985 Computed tomography and the prediction of pancreatic abscess in acute pancreatitis. Annals of Surgery 201: 656–663
Rattner D W, Legemate D A, Meuller P R, Warshaw A L 1992 Early surgical debridement of pancreatic necrosis is beneficial irrespective of infection. American Journal of Surgery 163: 105–110
Reddy K R, Jeffers L, Livingstone A S, Gluck C A, Schiff E R 1984 Pyogenic liver abscess complicating common bile duct stenosis secondary to chronic calcific pancreatitis. Gastroenterology 86: 953
Renner I G, Savage W T, Pantoja J L, Renner V J 1985 Death due to acute pancreatitis: a retrospective analysis of 405 cases. Digestive Diseases and Sciences 30: 1005–1018
Robin A P, Campbell R, Palani C K, Liu K, Donahue P E, Nyhus L M 1990 Total parenteral nutrition during acute pancreatitis: clinical experience with 156 patients. World Journal of Surgery 14: 572–579
Roszler M, Campbell W 1985 Post-ERCP pancreatitis: association with urographic visualization during ERCP. Radiology 157: 595
Rowland R, Stevenson G W, Faris I B 1985 Calcified pancreatic pseudocyst – a report of two cases. Australasian Radiology 29: 248
Russell R M, Dutta S K, Oaks E V, Rosenberg I H, Giovetti A C 1980 Impairment of folic acid absorption by oral pancreatic extracts. Digestive Diseases and Sciences 25: 369
Runzi M, Saluja A, Lerch M M, Dawra R, Nishino H, Steer M L 1993 Early ductal decompression prevents the progression of biliary pancreatitis: an experimental study in the opossum. Gastroenterology 105: 157–164
Saeed Z A, Ramirez F C, Hepps K S 1993 Endoscopic stent placement for internal and external pancreatic fistulas. Gastroenterology 105: 1213–1217
Safrany L, Cotton P B 1981 Urgent duodenoscopic sphincterotomy for acute gallstone pancreatitis. Surgery 89: 424–428
Saitoh Y, Yamamoto M 1991 Evaluation of severity of acute pancreatitis. International Journal of Pancreatology 9: 51–58
Sanfey H, Cameron J L 1984 Increased capillary permeability: an early lesion in acute pancreatitis. Surgery 96: 485–491
Sanfey H, Bulkley G B, Cameron J L 1983 Pathogenesis of acute pancreatitis: role of oxygen free radicals. Surgical Forum 34: 222–224
Sarles H 1985 Revised classification of pancreatitis – Marseilles. Digestive Diseases and Sciences 30: 573–574
Sarles H, Sahel J 1978 Cholestases and lesions of the biliary tract in chronic pancreatitis. Gut 19: 851
Sarles H, Bernard J P, Gullo L 1990 Pathogenesis of chronic pancreatitis. Gut 629–632
Sarner M, Cotton P B 1984 Classification of pancreatitis. Gut 25: 756–769
Saunders J H B, Wormsley K G 1975 Pancreatic extracts in the treatment of pancreatic exocrine insufficiency. Gut 16: 157
Sax H C, Warner B W, Talamini M A et al 1987 Early total parenteral nutrition in acute pancreatitis: lack of beneficial effects. American Journal of Surgery 153: 117–124
Schmidt J, Fernandez-del Castillo C, Rattner D W, Lewandrowski K, Compton C C, Warshaw A L 1992 Trypsinogen-activation peptides in experimental rat pancreatitis: prognostic implications and histopathologic correlates. Gastroenterology 103: 1009–1116
Schmiegel W, Buchert M, Kalthoft H et al 1990 Immunochemical characterization and quantitative distribution of pancreatic stone protein in sera and pancreatic secretion in pancreatic disorders. Gastroenterology 99: 1421–1430
Scott P, Bruce C, Schofield D, Shiel N, Braganza J M, McCloy R F 1993 Vitamin C status in patients with acute pancreatitis. British Journal of Surgery 80: 750–754
Serafini A N, Al-Sheikh W, Barkin J S et al 1982 Biliary scintigraphy in acute pancreatitis. Radiology 144: 591–596
Sherman S, Ruffolo T A, Hawes R H, Lehman G A 1991 Complications of endoscopic sphincterotomy. Gastroenterology 101: 1068–1075
Siegleman S S, Copeland B E, Saba G P, Cameron J L, Sanders R C, Zerbouni E A 1980 CT of fluid collections associated with pancreatitis. American Journal of Radiology 134: 1121
Simpson C J, Toner P G, Carr K E, Anderson J D, Carter D C 1984 Effect of bile salt perfusion and intraduct pressure on ionic flux and mucosal ultrastructure in the pancreatic duct of cats. Virchows Archiv fur Cell Pathologie 42: 327–342
Sitzmann J V, Imbembo A L 1984 Splenic complications of a pancreatic pseudocyst. American Jornal of Surgery 147: 191
Skellenger M E, Patterson D, Foley N T, Jordan P H 1983 Cholestasis due to compression of the common bile duct by pancreatic pseudocysts. American Journal of Surgery 145: 343
Spechler S J, Dalton J W, Robbins A H et al 1983 Prevalence of normal serum amylase levels in patients with acute alcoholic pancreatitis. Digestive Diseases and Sciences 28: 865–869
Standfield N J, Kakkar V V 1983 Prostaglandins and acute pancreatitis. British Journal of Surgery 70: 573–576
Staritz M, Meyer zum Buschenfelde K H 1988 Elevated pressure in the dorsal part of the pancreas divisum: the cause of chronic pancreatitis? Pancreas 3: 108–110
Steckman M L, Dooley M C, Jaques P F, Powell D W 1984 Major gastrointestinal hemorrhage from peripancreatic blood vessels in pancreatitis. Treatment by embotherapy. Digestive Diseases and Sciences 29: 486–497
Steer M L, Meldolesi J, Figarella C 1984 Pancreatitis. The role of lysosomes. Digestive Diseases and Sciences 29: 934
Steer M L, Waxman I, Freedman S 1995 Chronic pancreatitis. New England Journal of Medicine 332: 1482–1490
Steinberg W M, Schlesselman S E 1987 Treatment of acute pancreatitis. Comparison of animal and human studies. Gastroenterology 93: 1420–1427
Stone H H, Fabian T C, Dunlop W E 1981 Gallstone pancreatitis.

Biliary tract pathology in relation to time of operation. Annals of Surgery 194: 305–312
Stroud W H, Cullom J W, Anderson M C 1981 Hemorrhagic complications of severe pancreatitis. Surgery 90: 657–663
Svensson J-O, Nordback B, Bokey E L, Edlund Y 1979 Changing pattern in aetiology of pancreatitis in an urban Swedish area. British Journal of Surgery 66: 159–161
Thompson M D, Trowell H C 1952 Pancreatic enzyme activity in duodenal contents of children with a type of kwashiorkor. Lancet 1: 1031
Toskes P P, Dawson W, Curington C, Levy N S, Fitzgerald C 1979 Non-diaetic retinal abnormalities in chronic pancreatitis. New England Journal of Medicine 300: 942
Toskes P P, Greenberger n J 1983 Acute and chronic pancreatitis. Disease-a Month 29: 1
Toskes P P 1994 Is there a relationship between hypertriglyceridemia and development of alcohol- or gallstone-induced pancreatitis? Gastroenterology 106: 810–812
Trapnell J E, Anderson M C 1964 Role of early laparotomy in acute pancreatitis. Annals of Surgery 165: 49–55
Trapnell J E, Duncan E H L 1975 Patterns of incidence in acute pancreatitis. British Medical Journal 2: 179–183
Trede M, Carter D C 1993 Preoperative assessment and indications for operation in chronic pancreatitis. In: Trede M, Carter D C (eds) Surgery of the pancreas. Churchill Livingstone, Edinburgh
Vaira D, d'Anna L, Ainley C et al 1989 Endoscopic sphincterotomy in 1000 consecutive patients. Lancet 2: 431–434
Van Vyve E L, Reynaert M S, Lengele B G, Pringot J T, Otte J B, Kestens P J 1992 Retroperitoneal laparostomy: a surgical treatment of pancreatic abscesses after an acute necrotizing pancreatitis. Surgery 111: 369–375
Ventrucci M, Pezilli R, Gullo L, Plate L, Sprovieri G, Barbara L 1989 Role of serum pancreatic enzyme assays in diagnosis of pancreatic disease. Digestive Diseases and Sciences 34: 39–45
Walsh T N, Rode J, Theis B A, Russell R C G 1992 Minimal change chronic pancreatitis. Gut 33: 1566–1571
Warren K W, Athanassiades S, Frederick P, Kune G A 1966 Surgical treatment of pancreatic cysts. Review of 183 cases. Annals of Surgery 163: 886
Warshaw A L 1989 Obstructive pancreatitis: acute and chronic pancreatitis due to ductal obstruction by causes other than gallstones. In: Carter D C, Warshaw A L (eds) Pancreatitis. Clinical Surgery International 16. Churchill Livingstone, Edinburgh, p 71–89
Warshaw A L 1993 Damage prevention versus damage control in acute pancreatitis. Gastroenterology 104: 1216–1219
Warshaw A L, Jin G 1985 Improved survival in 45 patients with pancreatic abscess. Annals of Surgery 202: 408–415
Warshaw A L, Lee H-L 1979 Serum ribonuclease elevations and pancreatic necrosis in acute pancreatitis. Surgery 86: 227–232
Warshaw A L, O'Hara P J 1978 Susceptibility of the pancreas to ischemic injury in shock. Annals of Surgery 188: 197–201
Warshaw A L, Moncure A C, Rattner D W 1989 Gastrocutaneous fistulas associated with pancreatic abscesses. An aggressive entity. Annals of Surgery 210: 603–607
Warshaw A L, Rattner D W 1985 Timing of surgical drainage for pancreatic pseudocyst. Clinical and chemical criteria. Annals of Surgery 202: 720
Weidmann P, Rutishauser W, Siegenthaler W, Senning A 1969 Mediastinal pseudocyst of the pancreas. Emerican Journal of Medicine 46: 454
Willemer S, Feddersen C O, Karges W, Adler G 1991 Lung injury in acute experimental pancreatitis in rats. I. Morphological studies. International Journal of Pancreatology 8: 305–321
Williamson R C N 1984 Early assessment of severity in acute pancreatitis. Gut 25: 1331–1339
Wilmore D W, Smith R J, O'Dwyer S T et al 1988 The gut: a central organ after surgical stress. Surgery 104: 917–924
Wilson T S, Costopoulos L B 1967 The diagnosis and treatment of pancreatic pseudocysts. Canadian Medical Association Journal 97: 1117
Wilson C, Imrie C W 1990 Changing patterns of incidence and mortality from acute pancreatitis in Scotland, 1961–1985. British Journal of Surgery 77: 731–734
Wilson C, McArdle C S, Carter D C, Imrie C W 1988a Surgical treatment of acute necrotizing pancreatitis. British Journal of Surgery 75: 1119–1123
Wilson C, Imrie C W, Carter D C 1988b Fatal acute pancreatitis. Gut 29: 782–788
Wilson C, Heath D I, Shenkin A, Imrie C W 1989 C-reactive protein, antiproteases and complement factors as objective markers of severity in acute pancreatitis. British Journal of Surgery 76: 177–181
Wilson H A, Askari A D, Neiderhiser D H, Johnson A M, Andrews B S, Hoskins L C 1983 Pancreatitis with arthropathy and subcutaneous fat necrosis. Evidence for the pathogenicity of lipolytic enzymes. Arthritis and Rheumatism 26: 121–126
Windsor J A, Fearon K C H, Ross J A et al 1993 Role of serum endotoxin and antiendotoxin core antibody levels in predicting the development of multiple organ failure in acute pancreatitis. British Journal of Surgery 80: 1042–1046
Winship D, Butt J, Henstorf H et al 1977 Pancreatic pseudocysts and their complications. Gastroenterology 73: 593
Winslet M, Hall C, Londin N J M, Neoptolemos J P 1992 Relation of diagnostic serum amylase levels to aetiology and severity of acute pancreatitis. Gut 33: 982–986
Wisloff F, Jakobsen J, Osnes M 1982 Stenosis of the common bile duct in chronic pancreatitis. British Journal of Surgery 69: 52
Worning H, Mullertz S, Thaysen E H, Bang H O 1967 pH and concentration of pancreatic enzymes in aspirates from the human duodenum during digestion of a standard meal in patients with intestinal disorders. Scandinavian Journal of Gastroenterology 2: 81

# 51. Carcinoma and other tumors of the pancreas

*D. C. Carter*

Most of this chapter is devoted to the common problem of ductal adenocarcinoma of the pancreas. Less common neoplasms of the exocrine pancreas and the separate entity of periampullary cancer are also considered. Neoplasms arising from the endocrine pancreas are also dealt with here with the exception of gastrinoma (see Chapter 9).

## ADENOCARCINOMA OF THE PANCREAS

### Incidence and etiology (Haddock & Carter, 1990)

Ductal adenocarcinoma of the pancreas is a grim disease; 90% of patients are dead within a year of diagnosis and survival beyond 5 years is exceptional. The incidence has risen throughout this century in Western countries such as the United States and United Kingdom and, given the appalling prognosis, incidence and mortality rates are virtually identical. In the United States, pancreatic cancer ranks second only to colorectal cancer as a cause of death from cancer of the digestive system; age-adjusted mortality rates rose from 2.9 to 9 per 100 000 between 1920 and 1970 (American Cancer Society 1977) and have levelled off at approximately 10 per 100 000 (Gordis & Gold 1984). In the United Kingdom, pancreatic cancer is the sixth commonest cause of cancer death, surpassed only by colorectal and gastric cancer as fatal forms of alimentary cancer (Cancer Research Campaign 1989). In Japan, mortality rates rose from 1 to 6 per 100 000 between 1950 and 1974 (Aoki & Ogawa 1978) and are now even higher in men (Table 51.1).

Some of the increased incidence may reflect earlier under-reporting and misdiagnosis, problems which reflect the inaccessibility of the pancreas and ill-founded reluctance to biopsy the gland. Reviews have found that the diagnosis was confirmed histologically in only 38–68% of cases (Gudjonsson et al 1978, Gudjonsson 1987). A review of 78 cases in the Finnish Cancer Registry who survived 5 years after a diagnosis of pancreatic cancer in 1975–84 found that 33 did not have histological confirmation of the diagnosis and that most of the remainder had lesions other than pancreatic adenocarcinoma (Alanen & Joensuu 1993). Targeted cytological or histological sampling under ultrasonographic or radiological control have now improved the accuracy of diagnosis although problems remain (see below).

**Table 51.1** Age-standardized incidence rates of pancreatic cancer in 1978–82 in selected countries (from Muir et al 1987)

| | Age-standardized incidence | |
|---|---|---|
| | Male | Female |
| Canada | 8.6 | 5.5 |
| Colombia, Cali | 5.2 | 3.6 |
| Finland | 10.0 | 6.3 |
| France, Calvados | | |
| Urban | 6.2 | 2.8 |
| Rural | 4.1 | 2.2 |
| Hong Kong | 3.5 | 2.4 |
| India, Madras | 0.9 | 0.4 |
| Israel | | |
| All Jews | 8.9 | 5.9 |
| Non-Jews | 3.1 | 2.1 |
| Japan, Osaka | 7.7 | 4.5 |
| Kuwait | | |
| Kuwaitis | 1.2 | 1.3 |
| Non-Kuwaitis | 2.5 | 3.5 |
| New Zealand | | |
| Maori | 12.1 | 5.0 |
| Non-Maori | 7.5 | 4.7 |
| Puerto Rico | 4.9 | 3.4 |
| Sweden | 8.7 | 6.3 |
| Singapore | | |
| Chinese | 4.5 | 2.8 |
| Indian | 2.6 | 2.4 |
| Malay | 1.9 | 2.2 |
| US, Alameda | | |
| White | 8.4 | 6.2 |
| Black | 16.3 | 9.4 |
| US, New Mexico | | |
| Hispanic | 9.3 | 7.4 |
| Other White | 8.0 | 5.4 |
| American Indian | 5.0 | 3.9 |
| US, New Orleans | | |
| White | 9.8 | 5.3 |
| Black | 12.0 | 7.0 |

The disease is uncommon before the age of 45 years but incidence then rises progressively so that more than 80%

of cases are in the age group 60–80 years. Males are more commonly affected and the overall sex ratio is between 1.5:1 and 2:1 (Aoki & Ogawa 1978, Muir et al 1987). The male preponderance is marked before the age of 50 but diminishes thereafter and virtually disappears after 70 years. Involvement of sex hormones is also suggested by the presence of estrogen receptors (and/or estrogen-binding proteins) in normal and neoplastic pancreas and women with the disease more often have ovarian stromal and endometrial hyperplasia at autopsy and a history of oophorectomy, spontaneous abortion and uterine myomas (Bakkevold et al 1990).

There is a 10-fold difference in incidence between countries with high and low incidences of pancreatic carcinoma (Table 51.1). Rates are generally high in industrialized countries and are particularly high in New Zealand Maoris and native Hawaiians. Mortality rates appear to be increasing in both sexes in all countries.

Japanese migrating to the USA have higher mortality rates than native Americans or those who remain in Japan and their offspring have an intermediate incidence (Haenszel & Kurihara 1968). European migrants to Australia also appear to have a higher incidence (McMichael et al 1980). These findings may reflect dietary change and altered pancreatic exocrine function. However, genetic factors may also be important and contribute to the high incidence reported in Jews, New Zealand Maoris and Hawaiians. Familial aggregations of pancreatic cancer are described (Danes & Lynch 1982) and the disease may occur in "family cancer syndromes".

Pancreatic cancer is approximately twice as common in cigarette smokers but the increased risk does not extend to pipe smoking, snuff inhalation or tobacco chewing. The rising incidence in the USA parallels the increase in cigarette smoking and incidence rises with the number of cigarettes smoked (Ghadirian et al 1991, Weiss & Bernarde 1983). The mechanism is unknown but hyperplastic ductal changes are commoner in smokers and carcinogens excreted in bile could conceivably reflux into the pancreatic duct system; alternatively carcinogens in tobacco smoke could be bloodborne or favor cancer development by an effect on blood lipid levels (Wynder 1975).

Physicochemical agencies have also been implicated in pancreatic cancer (Carter 1993). Employees of coke and gas plants and those exposed to gasoline, dry-cleaning agents and isotopic radiation may have an increased incidence. Nitrosamines are undoubtedly carcinogenic in animal models (Pour et al 1981, Howatson & Carter 1985) but their role in human disease is uncertain; none of the nitrosamines in tobacco smoke appear to be responsible.

There is a correlation between per capita oil and fat consumption and pancreatic cancer mortality in various countries and a controversial association with dietary protein intake (Maruchi 1973, Hirayama 1981, Durbec et al 1983). High intake of fruit, vegetables and vitamins may confer some protection (Gold et al 1985, Norell et al 1986, Mack et al 1986) and micronutrients such as lycopene and selenium could reduce cancer risk by serving as antioxidants (Burney et al 1989). Seventh Day Adventists in California have a lower than expected incidence, but avoidance of smoking rather than diet may be the critical factor (Mills et al 1988). In Norway, incidence was not significantly lower in Seventh Day Adventists (Fonnebo & Helseth 1991), questioning the importance of "cancer lifestyle". Several studies have suggested that coffee consumption is a risk factor but this remains unproven (see Carter 1983). Alcohol is not a risk factor; indeed, modest wine consumption may well be protective (Ghadirian et al 1991).

The incidence of pancreatic cancer (but not other tumors) is 2–3 times greater than expected in diabetes mellitus. Diabetes is almost certainly the result of pancreatic cancer rather than a causal factor; when patients developing cancer within 2 years of the onset of diabetes are excluded, the association disappears (Gullo et al 1994, La Vecchia et al 1994). Pancreatic cancer patients have insulin resistance (with decreased total body glucose use) and a diminished insulin response to glucose because of B-cell dysfunction or deficiency (Cersosimo et al 1991).

The association between chronic pancreatitis and pancreatic cancer is controversial but a recent large cohort study suggests that it is a risk factor (Lowenfels et al 1993). The situation is complicated by the involvement of cigarette smoking in both conditions, by the frequent coexistence of inflammation and cancer and by the ease with which cancer escapes detection in an inflamed pancreas. The rare familial form of chronic pancreatitis is transmitted as an autosomal dominant condition of incomplete penetrance and up to one-third of affected family members develop pancreatic cancer (Miller et al 1992).

Other factors implicated in the etiology of pancreatic cancer include pernicious anemia, cholelithiasis and previous gastric surgery (Haddock & Carter 1990). In each case the evidence is weak and these are still unproven associations.

Overexpression and mutation of oncogenes (such as the K-*ras* oncogene) and alteration or loss of tumor suppressor genes (such as p53) are among the molecular genetic changes described in pancreatic cancer (Simon et al 1994, Kondo et al 1994, Marxsen et al 1994). Involvement of factors controlling cellular growth (e.g. epidermal growth factor, transforming growth factor βs, cholecystokinin, somatostatin) are also being elucidated (Liehr et al 1990, Korc 1991, Friess et al 1993a). The next few years should see further advances in our understanding of the biology of the disease and the realization of the diagnostic, prognostic and therapeutic potential of some of these observations.

*Animal studies* (Longnecker 1983, Longnecker et al 1984)

The two models which have been studied most widely are azaserine-induced acinar cell cancer in rats and N nitrosobis (2-oxopropyl) amine (BOP)-induced ductal adenocarcinoma in hamsters. Azaserine is probably a direct carcinogen whereas nitrosamines are first metabolized. The nitrosamine-hamster model is of particular interest given the importance of ductal adenocarcinoma in man and early intraductal hyperplasia is followed by replacement of acinar tissue by ductules; abnormal ductal and ductular lesions then progress to carcinoma. Carcinogenesis in both models is enhanced by feeding a diet with a high fat content or raw soya or by administering cholecystokinin (Howatson & Carter 1985).

**Pathology** (Cubilla & Fitzgerald 1984, Becker & Stommer 1993)

Ductal adenocarcinoma accounts for at least 80% of all tumors of the exocrine pancreas (Morohoshi et al 1983) (Fig. 51.1). When the cancer-bearing pancreas is examined, a spectrum of ductal dysplastic change extends from papillary hyperplasia and ductal atypia through in situ carcinoma to invasive carcinoma (Klöppel et al 1982, Tsusumi & Konishi 1990). However, it is uncertain whether these are premalignant field changes or intraductal extensions of invasive ductal carcinoma. Diffuse intraductal papillary adenocarcinoma is a rare distinct entity which carries a better prognosis (Morohoshi et al 1989). Duct-ectatic or mucin-secreting carcinoma shares many features with intraductal papillary adenocarcinoma (including a favorable prognosis) and is characterized by extreme duct dilatation and profuse mucin secretion (Rickaert et al 1991). The relationship of mucinous duct-ectatic neoplasms to mucinous cystic neoplasms (see below) is speculative, but the former arise within the duct system rather than outside it and the resulting obstructive pancreatitis frequently results in exocrine (and endocrine) gland failure. Other less common variants of ductal carcinoma include adenosquamous, squamous, giant cell and osteoclastoid giant cell carcinoma (Becker & Stommer 1993). Acinar cell carcinomas account for only 1–2% of pancreatic neoplasms and share the poor prognosis of ductal adenocarcinoma. The patients are often elderly and most tumors have metastasized by presentation (Becker & Stommer 1993). Acinar cells are apparent histologically and contain zymogen granules on electronmicroscopy. Even rarer cystic forms of this neoplasm have been reported (see below).

The common ductal adenocarcinoma is located in the head of the pancreas in 60–80% of cases, the body or tail in 15–20% of cases and a combination of sites in the remainder (Cubilla & Fitzgerald 1978, Becker & Stommer 1993). Macroscopically the tumor usually appears as a poorly delineated, firm, yellow-gray mass. Only about 2% of tumors are less than 2 cm in diameter at diagnosis (Tsuchiya et al 1986). The cancer frequently obstructs the pancreatic duct and ductal dilatation is followed by acinar atrophy or secondary chronic pancreatitis. Up to 5% of patients present with acute pancreatitis and this is an important diagnostic pitfall. Carcinoma of the head of the pancreas frequently occludes the bile duct and dilates the biliary tree. Cancer in the body and tail produces symp-

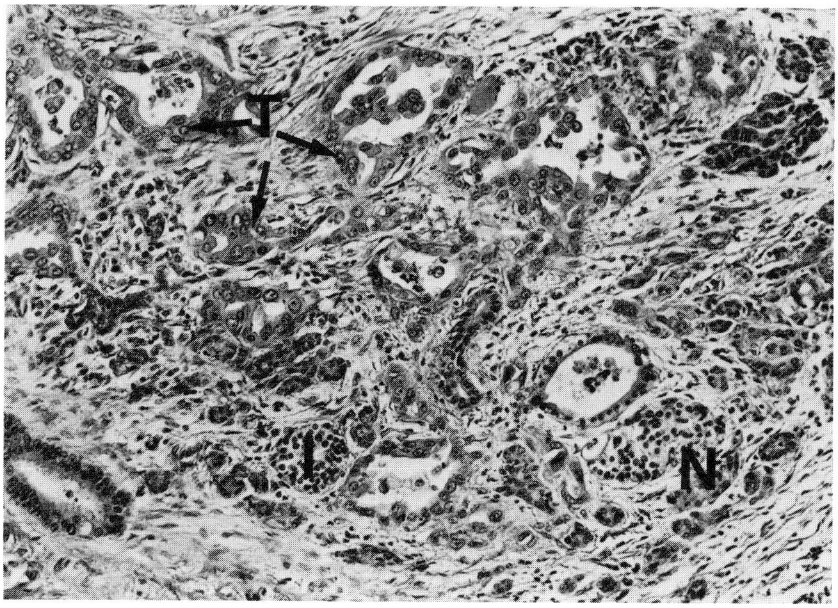


**Fig. 51.1** Pancreatic adenocarcinoma. The tumor (T) is moderately differentiated, infiltrating normal pancreatic tissue (N); islets (I) are also seen (hematoxylin and eosin, ×150).

toms by local extension into the retroperitoneal tissues, mesocolon and portal venous system.

Metastases are detected in about 60% of patients at presentation and commonly involve the liver, abdominal lymph nodes and peritoneum.

Of the various methods of staging, those of the Union Internationale Contre le Cancer (UICC) and the Japanese Pancreas Society (Tables 51.2, 51.3) have been used widely since their introduction in 1987. Whereas the UICC system regards nodal metastasis as the most important prognostic factor, the Japanese classification stresses tumor size and local spread. In the UICC classification, all tumors without lymph node involvement are included in stages I and II regardless of spread to peripancreatic tissues or blood vessels. In the Japanese classification, any invasion of peripancreatic tissue takes the tumor out of stage I. The significance of neural invasion and involvement of peripancreatic plexuses has been emphasized by Japanese studies (Kayahara et al 1991, Nagakawa et al 1992). Neural, plexus and lymph node invasion are related and the risk of nodal metastasis generally increases with tumor size. However, even small cancers may give rise to nodal metastases, particularly to the para-aortic region (Nagakawa et al 1993).

The differences between the two staging systems are highlighted by Tsunoda et al (1991). Using the UICC classification, 6%, 4%, 38% and 51% of their patients were allocated to stages I, II, III and IV respectively while the comparable figures using the Japanese system were 1%, 5%, 13% and 82%. The Japanese system may more accurately reflect prognosis but its complexity will probably inhibit its widespread adoption (Klöppel 1991).

**Table 51.2** UICC classification for staging pancreatic cancer

*Primary tumor (T)*
Tx Primary tumor cannot be assessed
T0 No evidence of primary tumor
T1 Tumor limited to pancreas (T1a 2 cm or less; T1b more than 2 cm)
T2 Tumor extends directly to bile duct, duodenum or peripancreatic tissues
T3 Tumor extends directly to stomach, spleen, colon or large vessels

*Regional lymph nodes (N)*
Nx Regional lymph nodes cannot be assessed
N0 No regional lymph node metastasis
N1 Regional lymph node metastasis

*Distant metastasis (M)*
Mx Presence of distant metastasis cannot be assessed
M0 No distant metastases
M1 Distant metastasis

*Stage grouping*

| | | | |
|---|---|---|---|
| Stage I | T1 | N0 | M0 |
| | T2 | N0 | M0 |
| Stage II | T3 | N0 | M0 |
| Stage III | any T | N1 | M0 |
| Stage IV | any T | any N | M1 |

**Table 51.3** Japanese Pancreas Society staging of pancreatic cancer

| | | | | | |
|---|---|---|---|---|---|
| Stage I | T1 (0–2 cm) | N0 | S0 | Rp0 | V0 |
| Stage II | T2 (2.1–4 cm) | N1 | S1 | Rp1 | V1 |
| Stage III | T3 (4.1–6 cm) | N2 | S2 | Rp2 | V2 |
| Stage IV | T4 (> 6 cm) | N3 | S3 | Rp3 | V3 |

Distant metastasis including hepatic or peritoneal spread is allocated to stage IV.
T = tumor size.
N = lymph node metastasis (N1, nodes close to tumor; N2, secondary nodes between N1 and N3; N3, tertiary or juxtaregional nodes)
S = serosal invasion
Rp = retroperitoneal invasion
V = invasion of portal venous system
S0, Rp0, V0 = no invasion
S1, Rp1, V1 = suspected invasion
S2, Rp2, V2 = definite invasion
S3, Rp3, V3 = severe invasion

*Clinical features* (Table 51.4)

***Pain.*** Pancreatic cancer is rarely painless. In the experience of Warren et al (1983), pain was experienced in 83% of cases and was the first symptom in 58%. It was epigastric in 70% of cases, in the right upper quadrant in 15% and suprapubic in 10%. Radiation to the back occurred in 30% of patients and some experience pain only in the back. The pain is usually difficult to localize, may be exacerbated by meals and is often worse at night and when lying supine. It is sometimes eased by leaning forwards and some patients only find comfort by kneeling on all fours. Initially, pain is intermittent but frequently becomes persistent.

***Jaundice.*** Jaundice is the first symptom in up to one-third of patients and develops at some stage in 90% of cases; it is painless in only 10% of patients (Warren et al 1983). Initially, jaundice may fluctuate but soon becomes progressive. Pruritus is common and can be most distressing.

***Other features.*** Weight loss is common and can be marked even when the tumor is small. Anorexia, nausea and vomiting are major causes (Perez et al 1983) and

**Table 51.4** Frequency of presenting symptoms and signs in 865 cases of carcinoma of the pancreas affecting all parts of the gland (Moldow & Connelly 1968)

| Symptoms | Frequency (%) | Signs | Frequency (%) |
|---|---|---|---|
| Pain | 63 | Hepatomegaly | 41 |
| Weight loss | 48 | Jaundice | 38 |
| Jaundice | 36 | Abdominal mass | 24 |
| Lethargy | 26 | Palpable gallbladder | 7 |
| Dark urine | 26 | Ascites | 5 |
| Pale stool | 25 | | |
| Vomiting | 20 | | |
| Nausea | 18 | | |
| Constipation | 8 | | |
| Diarrhea | 6 | | |

steatorrhea and malabsorption are occasionally the only manifestation of a small resectable tumor. In some patients the cancer triggers an "inappropriate" increase in resting expenditure (Falconer et al 1994a). Such patients have increased production of acute-phase proteins such as C-reactive protein (CRP) and the cytokines interleukin 6 and tumor necrosis factor have been implicated. A raised CRP level is by far the most significant determinant of survival duration in inoperable pancreatic cancer (Falconer et al 1995).

Hematemesis and melena can result from invasion of the duodenum or stomach or from variceal bleeding secondary to portal vein obstruction. Vomiting is usually due to obstruction of the duodenum, pylorus or duodenojejunal flexure and can develop in nonjaundiced patients.

Recurrent acute pancreatitis predated the diagnosis of pancreatic cancer in six of 191 patients reported by Warren et al (1983) and occasionally signals involvement of the pancreas by metastatic disease (Wernecke et al 1986).

Diabetes mellitus is an occasional presenting feature, although rarely the sole feature, and its development in patients over 60 years must always raise suspicions that the patient has pancreatic carcinoma.

Thrombophlebitis and deep venous thrombosis are present in up to 10% of cases, but "classic" migratory thrombophlebitis is uncommon.

Psychiatric upset in the form of depression, anxiety, loss of ambition or premonition of serious illness may precede other manifestations of pancreatic cancer (Fras et al 1968).

***Physical findings.*** Jaundice, hepatomegaly and abdominal tenderness are the commonest physical findings. An abdominal mass is present in one in four cases and is most often epigastric. A dilated gallbladder may be palpable but in many cases is obscured by hepatomegaly. A palpable gallbladder means that gallstones are unlikely to be responsible for the obstructive jaundice (Courvoisier's law) and strongly suggests carcinoma of the head of the pancreas.

***Features specific to carcinoma of the body and tail of the pancreas*** (Bowden & Die Goyanes 1970). Many of the above symptoms occur, but the emphasis is different. Pain, weight loss, anorexia, nausea and vomiting are particulary common and paroxysmal left-sided abdominal pain may be accompanied by constipation (Arlen & Brockunier 1967). Jaundice is much less common and is usually the result of hepatic metastases. Metastases are present at the time of presentation in the liver, supraclavicular lymph nodes, pelvis or peritoneum in 75% of cases. Abdominal distention from ascites can be troublesome. Splenic vein thrombosis is common and the resulting hypersplenism and gastric varices can cause major upper gastrointestinal bleeding. Bleeding can also result from direct invasion of the bowel.

## Investigations

Cancer of the pancreas is a major diagnostic and therapeutic problem. A tumor with a diameter of 2 cm is at the limit of current methods of detection, yet may be three-quarters of the way through its biological life, is usually still asymptomatic and has probably metastasized. At present there is no effective screening test and by the time patients present with symptoms, imaging all too often reveals advanced incurable disease. However, there is evidence that tumor size at operation has fallen (p. 1293) and the importance of appropriate investigation is underlined by the fact that some patients thought clinically to be suffering from pancreatic cancer prove to have benign disease or more favorable neoplasms such as periampullary cancer and cystic pancreatic tumors.

### *Serological markers*

None of the many serum tumor markers available to date have lived up to their early promise and proved suitable for use in screening or routine diagnosis. The list of putative markers includes tumor-associated antigens (e.g. CEA, pancreatic oncofetal antigen, tissue polypeptide antigen, DU-PAN-2 and CA 19-9), enzymes (e.g. ribonuclease, galactosyl-transferase isoenzyme II and elastase) and hormones (e.g. testosterone).

The marker studied most extensively is CA 19-9 (Steinberg 1990) for which an antibody kit is available commercially. The test has a sensitivity of about 80% but CA 19-9 levels are frequently normal in early disease and the test is useless for screening. Furthermore, it is also positive in 14% of cases of benign gastrointestinal disease and in up to two-thirds of cases of nonpancreatic cancer. It may have some value in assessing the completeness of surgical resection and in surveillance for recurrent disease.

Testosterone levels and the ratio of testosterone to dihydrotestosterone are low in men with pancreatic cancer, presumably because of increased conversion of testosterone by the tumor (Greenway et al 1983, Roblez-Diaz et al 1987). However, such measurements are not sufficiently sensitive or specific to be of value in diagnosis.

### *Laboratory investigations*

Liver function tests frequently reflect cholestasis and a raised serum alkaline phosphatase activity is sometimes the sole initial abnormality. Some 50% of cases have mild anemia. Glucose tolerance is impaired in most patients although only about 5% have frank diabetes mellitus.

### *Pancreatic function tests* (Klapdor 1993)

Fecal fat excretion is raised in 25% of patients with pancreatic cancer and the volume of pancreatic enzyme secretion is often reduced despite a normal bicarbonate concentration. However, the pattern is often similar in chronic pancreatitis and function tests have no real diagnostic value. Hopes that pancreatic juice lactoferrin levels or the ratio of lysosomal to digestive enzymes in pancreatic juice would differentiate between pancreatic cancer and chronic pancreatitis have not been fulfilled.

### *Cytology* (Ihse & Isaksson 1984)

Methods for the cytological examination of pancreatic juice include examination of duodenal aspirates following secretin stimulation, aspiration of juice at ERCP and endoscopic brushing of the pancreatic duct. Some two-thirds of cancers can be diagnosed by these methods although Yamada et al (1984) reported an overall accuracy of 80%. As in all cytological techniques, success depends on the skill of the pathologist.

A recent development is the use of the polymerase chain reaction to detect K-*ras* mutations in pancreatic juice. Some 95% of ductal adenocarcinomas contain a mutated K-*ras* oncogene (Almoguera et al 1988) whereas such mutations are rare or nonexistent in chronic pancreatitis, bile duct carcinomas or endocrine tumors (Tada et al 1990). Kondo et al (1994) found K-*ras* mutations in the pancreatic juice of six of nine patients with ductal adenocarcinomas and negative cytology.

Fine-needle aspiration cytology can be performed percutaneously under ultrasound or CT guidance or at operation. The sensitivity of the technique is 49–86% but the specificity is virtually 100% (Ihse & Andren-Sandberg 1993). Sampling difficulty rather than pathologist error is the major cause of false negativity and a negative result does not exclude malignancy. It can be difficult to distinguish between the epithelial atypia of chronic pancreatitis and well-differentiated cancer (Carter 1992), but it is usually possible to tell whether a tumor is of exocrine or endocrine origin. The technique has a complication rate of less than 0.2% and a mortality rate of less than 0.02%. While needle track seeding of tumor is exceptional (see Ihse & Andren-Sandberg 1993), preoperative sampling should be avoided in patients with potentially resectable neoplasms (Di Magno 1994). Intraoperative fine-needle aspiration cytology is if anything more reliable than percutaneous sampling, particularly when guided by ultrasonography, and has a sensitivity of up to 95% (Bodner & Glaser 1993).

### *Biopsy*

Ultrasound-guided percutaneous needle core biopsy is an alternative to aspiration cytology (Jennings et al 1989) but larger needles probably increase the chance of needle track seeding, particularly when multiple passes are made. Operative wedge biopsy has an unacceptably high rate of complications such as pancreatitis, fistula and abscess (Carter & Comis 1975) and is no longer used. However, Tru-cut needle biopsy is still an acceptable method of confirming the diagnosis at laparotomy if cytological facilities are unavailable; whenever possible the transduodenal route is used to minimize the risk of fistula formation.

### *Radiological investigations*

***Plain radiographs.*** Plain radiographs occasionally show displacement of normal structures by a tumor mass but have a very low diagnostic yield and are not used routinely. Calcification is relatively uncommon in pancreatic adenocarcinoma unless there is coexistent chronic pancreatitis and is commoner in cystic neoplasms and neuroendocrine tumors (p. 1297).

***Barium meal and enema.*** Displacement and/or distortion of the stomach, duodenal loop (Fig. 51.2) or proximal small bowel may be visible at barium meal, while barium enema may reveal displacement of the colon. Indentation from an enlarged gallbladder or dilated common bile duct is sometimes apparent. Such barium studies were once used extensively when pancreatic cancer was suspected but their success rate ranged from 30% (Kairaluoma et al 1985) to 62% (Gudjonsson et al 1978). Most of the tumors detected in these series were almost certainly large and incurable. Barium studies are no longer used unless there is a need to assess duodenal obstruction.

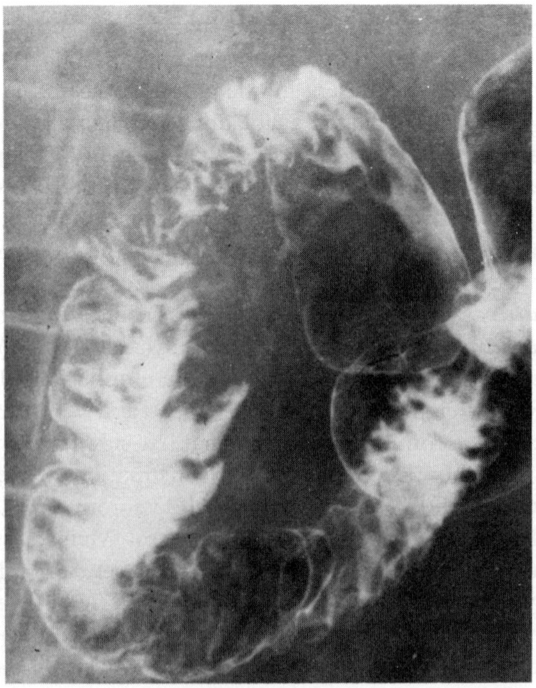

**Fig. 51.2** Barium meal showing carcinoma of head of pancreas causing a constant filling defect on the medial side of the second part of the duodenum.

***Arteriography.*** Most pancreatic adenocarcinomas are hypovascular. The characteristic arteriographic sign is arterial encasement within the tumor mass; neovascularity is uncommon. Neighboring veins may be displaced, invaded or thrombosed. Invasion of larger veins such as the splenic, superior mesenteric and portal veins and/or encasement of larger arteries usually indicates nonresectability. When encasement is marked it may be very difficult to distinguish between malignancy and chronic pancreatitis (Lunderquist 1985).

The availability of imaging methods such as ultrasonography, endoscopic ultrasonography and CT scanning (see below) means that selective visceral arteriography is now seldom used to diagnose pancreatic cancer or assess resectability (Rosch et al 1992a). A recent study of 46 consecutive patients with potentially resectable pancreatic or periampullary cancer showed that angiography had a predictive value for resectability of only 61% (Murugiah et al 1993). Of 27 patients found to have nonresectable disease at operation, only 11 were correctly identified as nonresectable on angiography (sensitivity 41%), while of the 33 patients thought to have resectable disease on angiography, no less than 16 had tumors which could not be resected.

A case is still sometimes made for angiography as a means of detecting vascular anomalies likely to affect the course of resection. Anomalies are found in one-third of patients (Murugiah et al 1993), the most significant being origin of the common hepatic or right hepatic artery from the superior mesenteric artery. However, this anomaly should be suspected at operation if major arterial pulsation is found to the *right* of the common bile duct and even when there is celiac axis stenosis, resection has still been undertaken successfully. The wide availability of intraoperative ultrasonography has further undermined the need for preoperative angiography.

***Ultrasonography.*** Transcutaneous ultrasonography is employed as the initial examination when pancreatic disease is suspected and in jaundiced patients it determines the presence and location of biliary obstruction. The pancreas is imaged satisfactorily in 90% of cases and in cachectic patients, ultrasonography gives better resolution than computed tomography (which relies on peripancreatic fat to outline the pancreas). Most pancreatic carcinomas produce a focal area of hypoechogenicity and alter the contour of the gland. Tumors of the pancreatic head are most easily visualized, but lesions smaller than 2 cm are very difficult to detect, particularly when there are minimal alterations in echogenicity. Dilatation of the pancreatic and/or biliary tree (Fig. 2.11) suggests that a lesion is present even if a mass is not seen. Invasion of large veins points to nonresectability, as does involvement of the origins of the celiac and superior mesenteric arteries. Metastatic spread to the liver and lymph nodes and ascites may be seen.

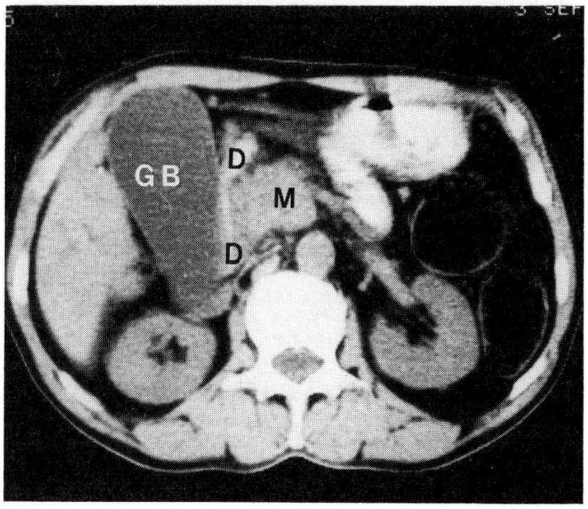


**Fig. 51.3** CT scan showing carcinoma of the head of the pancreas (M), dilated gallbladder (GB) and displaced duodenal loop (D).

Ultrasonography is also used preoperatively or intraoperatively to target needle aspiration or biopsy (see above) and can be used as an adjunct to laparoscopic evaluation (see below). Endoscopic ultrasonography is very useful in detecting small tumors and assessing vascular invasion; it also detects lymph node enlargement although it usually cannot distinguish reactive nodes from those which contain tumor (Di Magno et al 1982, Rosch et al 1992a).

***Computed tomography.*** This is the preferred method of imaging and has an accuracy of 91% in the diagnosis of pancreatic cancer (Freeny 1989), visualizing the entire pancreas, including the tail. The CT signs of pancreatic carcinoma include focal or diffuse pancreatic enlargement (Fig 51.3), changes in the shape or contour of the gland, dilatation of the pancreatic duct (in small tumors this may be the only abnormality) and biliary system (Fig. 2.20) and diminished attenuation of the tumor when intravenous contrast enhancement is used. Tumors smaller than 2 cm can be demonstrated if they show such reduced attenuation (Clark et al 1985). It must be stressed that pancreatitis and other forms of pancreatic neoplasia can produce identical findings, while tumor necrosis can simulate pseudocyst formation.

Computed tomography can spare unnecessary laparatomy by demonstrating inoperability (Freeny & Lawson 1982). For example, direct spread may be seen in areas such as the splenic hilum, root of the mesentery, left adrenal gland, stomach and duodenum. Distant metastases are commonly seen in the liver (47%) and lymph nodes (25%). Tumor invasion of major blood vessels (Fig. 51.4) may be apparent on bolus enhancement as a halo of soft tissue around the celiac and mesenteric arteries or occlusion of major veins with formation of collaterals (Megibow et al 1981, Stephens et al 1983).

Enlargement of pancreaticoduodenal lymph nodes is common but can be mimicked by other forms of neoplasia and benign disease. In one series of 38 patients, the malig-

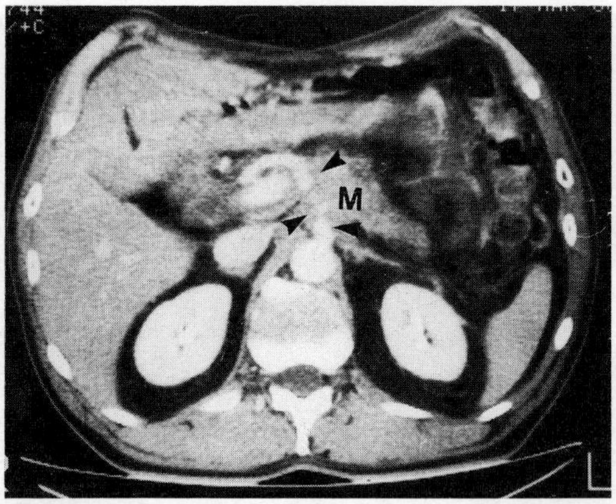


**Fig. 51.4** CT scan showing cancer of the body of the pancreas (M) encasing the celiac axis (arrowed).

nancies responsible for nodal enlargement included lymphoma and tumors of the gastrointestinal tract, breast and lung (Zeman et al 1985). In one-third of patients, biliary obstruction was present. Focally involved posterior pancreaticoduodenal lymph nodes separated by intact fat planes from the anterior border of the pancreas on ultrasonography or computed tomography indicates that the primary problem is extrapancreatic; guided percutaneous fine-needle aspiration biopsy may resolve uncertainty in such cases.

***Magnetic resonance imaging and positron emission tomography.*** Normal pancreas has a low signal intensity compared to peripancreatic fat, while blood vessels are normally void of signal. Magnetic resonance imaging is not used routinely to diagnose pancreatic cancer at present, but technical advances and better contrast media may increase its value. Recent preliminary reports indicate that positron emission tomography using 18-fluoro-deoxy glucose may have a sensitivity as high as 92% in diagnosing pancreatic cancer and differentiate between cancer and chronic pancreatitis (Beger et al 1994).

***Duodenoscopy and ERCP.*** Duodenoscopy shows ulceration or infiltration of the duodenal wall by tumor in 10–20% of patients with pancreatic cancer and allows biopsy or brush cytology to confirm the diagnosis. The case for routine ERCP in the diagnosis of pancreatic cancer can be debated now that less invasive imaging techniques are available. However, it has a sensitivity and specificity of 90% (De Magno 1994) and remains extremely useful where there is diagnostic doubt. The ERCP signs of pancreatic cancer include the double-duct sign, pancreatic duct displacement, stenosis or abrupt cut-off and pooling of contrast in areas of tumor necrosis. Duodenoscopy and ERCP are particularly valuable in jaundiced patients when periampullary cancer is suspected and in patients with inoperable pancreatic cancer, stents can be inserted to relieve jaundice and pruritus.

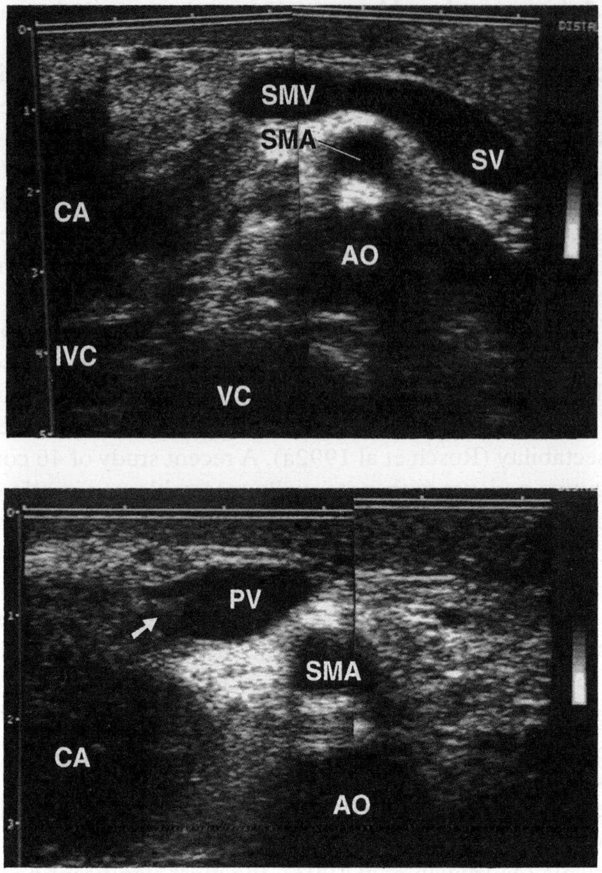


**Fig. 51.5** Laparoscopic ultrasonogram showing (**A**) an infiltrating carcinoma in the head of the pancreas (CA) and (**B**) infiltration of the portal vein (PV). SMV=superior mesenteric vein; SMA=superior mesenteric artery; AO=aorta; SV=splenic vein; IVC=inferior vena cava; VC=vertebral column.

***Laparoscopy and laparoscopic ultrasonography.*** The availability of nonsurgical methods for relieving jaundice and pruritus means that fruitless surgery can now be avoided in patients with nonresectable pancreatic cancer. Warshaw et al (1986) used laparoscopy to evaluate 40 patients with potentially resectable pancreatic cancer; in 14 cases it revealed unsuspected peritoneal or hepatic deposits, thus altering the course of treatment. In three of the 26 patients with "negative" laparoscopy, liver deposits were found at subsequent laparotomy so that laparoscopy detected 82% of the cases where tumor spread precluded resection. In a more recent study of 40 patients also thought to have resectable pancreatic or periampullary cancer after conventional imaging (John et al 1995), laparoscopy showed peritoneal, hilar or hepatic tumor in 14 cases but failed to detect local invasion at the site of the tumor in 12 cases and metastatic tumor in three cases. However, ultrasonography using a 5 mHz contact probe passed down the laparoscope (Fig. 51.5) improved the accuracy of predictability of resection from 65% for laparoscopy alone to 89%. In two cases, laparoscopic ultrasonography wrongly predicted that the disease would be resectable while in one further case it incorrectly predicted that the disease was nonresectable. It appears that laparoscopy, particularly when combined with contact ultrasonography, improves the detection of nonresectable disease and also provides valuable information about vascular invasion.

## Treatment

*Resection* (Carter 1980)

In the past, resection was only undertaken for cancers of the head of the pancreas and cancers arising in the body and tail were regarded as unresectable. However, a recent study showed that resection could be undertaken in 12% of patients with body and tail tumors and that five of these patients survived for more than 2 years (Johnson et al 1993).

The Whipple operation is the conventional curative procedure for cancer of the pancreatic head and consists of en bloc removal of the duodenum with the head, neck and proximal body of the gland. The classic contraindications are the presence of distant metastases, lymph node involvement and involvement of the portal vein or superior mesenteric vessels. However, involvement of regional nodes or major vessels are no longer seen as absolute contraindications (see below). Cholecystectomy and truncal vagotomy with antrectomy are components of the conventional operation. Reconstruction takes the form of gastrojejunostomy, pancreaticojejunostomy and hepaticojejunostomy (Fig. 51.6). Some surgeons now preserve the stomach and pylorus in an attempt to minimize nutritional complications and avoid dumping (Traverso & Longmire 1978). Delayed gastric emptying in the postoperative period, stomal ulceration (McAfee et al 1989) and failure to eradicate intramucosal spread of cancer within the duodenum (Sharp et al 1989) are occasional problems attributed to the pylorus-preserving modification of pancreaticoduodenectomy.

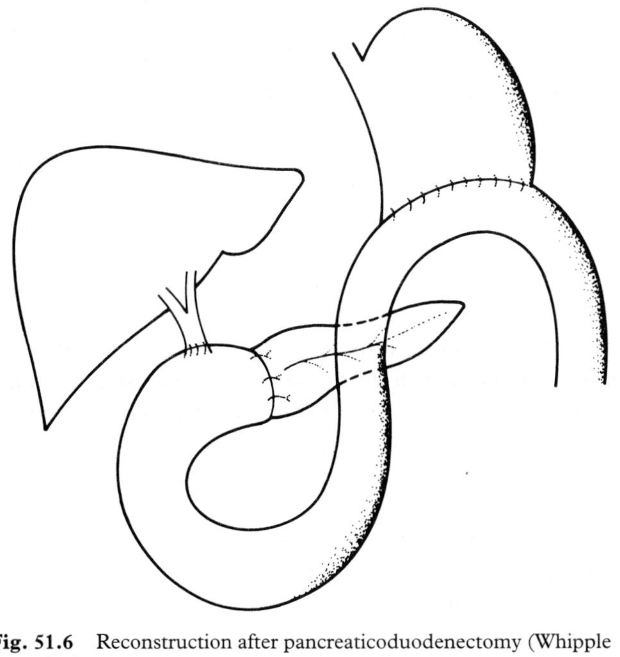

**Fig. 51.6** Reconstruction after pancreaticoduodenectomy (Whipple operation).

Advocates of resection stress that it offers the only prospect of cure and provides better palliation than bypass in incurable disease (Klinkenbijl et al 1993). Resection rates as high as 40% are reported from some surgical centers (Fortner et al 1977, Mackie et al 1979, Klinkenbijl et al 1993) and in Japan, the resection rate was 23% in a multicenter review involving 3315 patients (Tsuchiya et al 1986). A figure of 15% is now representative for Western centers with an interest in pancreatic cancer (Watanapa & Williamson 1992). Tumor size at operation may have fallen while resection rates have risen (Nix et al 1984, Trede 1985), but the great majority of patients still have unresectable disease at the time of diagnosis. Tsuchiya et al (1986) offer a tantalizing glimpse of what might be achieved if pancreatic cancer could be detected before the tumor reaches a diameter of 2 cm. Their 106 patients with small tumors had a resectability rate of 99% and operative mortality of 4%. On examination of the resection specimen, 44% of the patients had stage I disease and the overall cumulative 5-year survival rate of 30% rose to 37% in this subgroup. It must be stressed that small cancer is not necessarily "early" or confined cancer and that such small tumors accounted for only 2.1% of the cases seen by the contributing hospitals.

Returning to the problem of pancreatic cancer in general, an attitude of "surgical pessimism" was fuelled by retrospective analyses showing that comparable groups of patients treated by the Whipple resection fared no better than those having bypass (Shapiro 1975). Critics of resection also highlight the fact that the mean operative mortality in series published in the period 1980–86 was 16%, while the overall 5-year survival rate was only 0.4% (Gudjonsson 1987). Much depends on the denominator used when assessing survival rates and in Gudjonsson's analyses this was the number of patients diagnosed rather than the number undergoing resection. However, there are some recent signs of improvement. Prompt diagnosis and referral mean that patients now being considered for resection are at lower risk than formerly and in jaundiced patients the need for routine preliminary biliary drainage by endoscopically or transhepatically inserted stents is now questioned (McPherson et al 1984, Pitt et al 1985, Lai et al 1994). An exception may still be considered for those at particularly high risk and depth of jaundice, renal function and serum albumin level are important risk markers (Blamey et al 1983). Improvements in patient selection, operative technique and perioperative care now mean that operative mortality can be avoided in specialist centers (Trede et al 1990, Cameron et al 1993). However, results from such centers are not necessarily representative and multicenter studies in the last decade report operative mortalities of 7.8%, 9% and 10% in North America, Norway and France respectively (Edge et al 1993, Bakkevold & Kambestad 1993, Baumel et al 1994). The need to concentrate experience in specialist hands is underlined by the finding that surgeons performing 1–3 pancreatic resections a year in the North American study had significantly more complications (Edge et al 1993).

Recognition that the pancreaticojejunal anastomosis was the major source of morbidity and mortality in the Whipple operation and anxieties about the radicality of cancer resection led many to evaluate the alternative of total pancreatectomy. The argument for total pancreatectomy was strengthened by the frequent finding of tumor cells beyond the Wipple resection line (Ihse et al 1977) and the detection of nodal metastases in areas not normally removed in this operation (Cubilla et al 1978). However, survival is probably more dependent on spread outside the pancreas and total pancreatectomy inevitably causes complete loss of pancreatic exocrine and endocrine function. In fact, the complication rate of total pancreatectomy proved to be up to three times that of Whipple resection (Trede 1985), mortality rates were twice as high (Bakkevold & Kambestad 1993) and survival rates were not improved (Ihse et al 1977, Nakase et al 1977). This led others to use "regional pancreatectomy" in which total pancreatectomy is combined with resection of portal vein and/or major arteries. However, this operation had a prohibitively high operative mortality (25%) and a disappointing long-term survival rate (Fortner 1984) and is no longer recommended.

In Japan, great emphasis has been placed on the need to eradicate involved lymph nodes and retroperitoneal spread by "radical pancreatectomy". Posterior pancreaticoduodenal nodes, retroperitoneal nodes and nodes along the superior border of the pancreas appear particularly important. Manabe et al (1989) found nodal metastases in 21% of patients with stage I and II tumors treated by radical pancreatectomy as opposed to 86% in those treated by nonradical pancreatectomy; for stage III and IV tumors the figures were 50% and 77% respectively. Patients having radical pancreatectomy had a cumulative 5-year survival rate of 33% whereas none of those undergoing nonradical surgery survived beyond 3 years. After macroscopically curative resection, Kayahara et al (1993) detected microscopic tumor in the retroperitoneum in 17 of 45 patients and found local retroperitoneal recurrence in 12 of 15 patients coming to autopsy. Radical retroperitoneal dissection was advocated even when the patient appears to have a small cancer which is not obviously invading the retroperitoneum. Invasion of extrapancreatic neural plexuses such as that surrounding the superior mesenteric artery is also regarded as a critical determinant of survival and the need for radical dissection (Kayahara et al 1991, Nagakawa et al 1992).

Assessment of radical pancreatectomy is limited by the lack of prospective controlled comparisons with nonradical resection, by the frequency with which radical surgery in Japan is combined with adjuvant treatment and by the use of cumulative survival data rather than absolute survival figures. It remains uncertain whether increased radicality of resection will significantly improve overall survival in a disease known to present late and with spread outside the reach of regional surgery. Nevertheless, the Japanese studies highlight the shortcoming of conventional pancreatic resection and help to explain its failure to achieve long-term survival. At present, the best 5-year survival figures following resection in Western medicine are those achieved in Mannhein by Trede (1993) where a cumulative 5-year survival rate of 30% was recorded in 100 patients with $R_0$ disease (i.e. surgeon and pathologist considered that tumor was completely eradicated). Trede found no 5-year survivors in those with $R_1/R_2$ tumors and emphasizes that even survival to 5 years after resection of $R_0$ cancer does not always mean cure; of 17 patients who survived for more than 5 years after resection, nine died subsequently from recurrent disease.

### *Palliative treatment*

***Palliative surgery.*** The great majority of patients with pancreatic cancer have extensive disease or are elderly or so ill that curative resection is not feasible. Biliary bypass effectively relieves jaundice and pruritus and cholecystojejunostomy is the safest and simplest option (Sarr & Cameron 1982). Hepaticojejunostomy is a more complex operation and is often reserved for patients in whom the tumor encroaches on the junction of cystic duct and common hepatic duct. Concomitant gastroenterostomy is usually recommended as 15% of patients otherwise develop duodenal obstruction. Surgical bypass is not without risk and in the days when it was the only means of relieving jaundice, the operative mortality was about 20% with a mean duration of survival of only 5.4 months (Sarr & Cameron 1982). Mortality rates have fallen in the last decade to about 14% (Watanapa & Williamson 1992), although this may reflect the fact that endoscopic stenting now offers a safer alternative to surgery in high-risk patients. There is still debate about whether surgery is the better option in younger, fitter individuals (see below). Minimally invasive techniques mean that cholecystojejunostomy can now be performed without recourse to laparotomy.

***Stenting.*** Biliary drainage can now be achieved by inserting stents (endoprostheses) endoscopically or transhepatically. In the prospective Cape Town study, the 30-day mortality for transhepatic stenting was 8% as opposed to 20% for surgical bypass (Bornman et al 1986). Stented patients spent less time in hospital (although some required readmission to deal with prosthesis blockage) and median survival times were not significantly different (19 versus 15 weeks). Speer et al (1987) found that endoscopic stenting was even more effective than transhepatic stenting and its significantly lower 30-day mortality (15% versus 33%) was attributed to avoiding the bleeding and bile leakage that can complicate hepatic puncture. The transhepatic route is now reserved for when transduodenal stenting fails. In some cases, endoscopic stenting initially proves impossible but can be achieved if the radiologist passes a guidewire transhepatically into the duodenum, the "rendevous technique". If endoscopic stenting fails, some radiologists prefer to establish external transhepatic drainage in the first instance and internalize the stent some days later.

Endoprostheses can be plastic (polyurethane or Teflon) or metallic (Jaschke & Manegold 1993). Plastic stents are relatively inexpensive, but are more prone to bile encrustation and blockage. The risks of migration or perforation are lessened by choosing an appropriate length (usually about 20 cm), placement so that the tips lie in the lumen rather than pressing on the wall of bile duct or duodenum and using small anchoring fins at either end of the stent. Metallic stents such as the Wallstent or Strecker stent are more expensive but are larger and less prone to block (Huibregtse et al 1992), although tumor ingrowth can be problematic. These stents are inserted in a collapsed form and the wire mesh either then expands spontaneously or is dilated by a balloon catheter from a starting diameter of about 2.6 mm to around 8–10 mm. Stent migration does not occur but the stent is virtually impossible to remove and is not used if resection is being considered.

Immediate complications of endoscopic stenting include bleeding, perforation of the bile duct by a guidewire and duodenal perforation. Bleeding, bile leakage and hemobilia may complicate transhepatic drainage, each having an incidence or 1–2% (see Jaschke & Manegold, 1993). Such complications can sometimes be treated non-surgically; for example, biliary peritonitis may be managed by percutaneous drainage while hemobilia can be dealt with by embolization (see also p. 120).

Stent blockage with cholangitis and return of jaundice is a major problem with plastic stents and in one recent study, occurred after a mean period of 113 days (range 4–273 day) (Van den Bosch et al 1994). Although blocked stents can usually be changed, the late morbidity of stenting led Van den Bosch et al (1994) to suggest that patients with favorable prognostic criteria (relative youth, female sex, no liver metastases, large diameter tumors) and a survival expectation exceeding 6 months may be better served by surgical bypass. In the Middlesex Hospital study, patients with malignant low bile duct obstruction were randomized to endoscopic stenting or surgical bypass; stenting had fewer early complications whereas surgery had fewer late complications (Table 51.5) (Smith et al 1994). Both options were regarded as effective forms of palliation and there were no significant differences in median survival, despite the early advantage of stenting.

**Table 51.5** Results of endoscopic stenting versus surgical biliary bypass in patients with malignant low bile duct obstruction (Smith et al 1994)

| | Endoscopic stenting ($n$ = 101) | Surgical bypass ($n$ = 100) |
|---|---|---|
| Technical success rate | 94% | 95% |
| Biliary decompression | 92% | 92% |
| Procedure-related mortality | 3% | 14%* |
| 30-day mortality | 8% | 15% |
| Major complication rate | 11% | 29% |
| Minor complication rate | 29% | 18% |
| Median total hospital stay | 20 days | 26 days* |
| Recurrent jaundice | 36 patients | 2 patients |
| Late gastric outlet obstruction | 17% | 7% |
| Overall median survival (wks) | 21 | 26 |

* = statistically significant difference between the two groups

### *Cytotoxic therapy*

Single agents such as 5-FU and mitomycin C can slow tumor growth and produce a "response", but seldom extend survival in unresectable pancreatic cancer. Combination chemotherapy has also proved disappointingly inconsistent. In the Veterans Administration trial, the combination of 5-FU and CCNU proved no better than supportive care (Frey et al 1981). On the other hand, Mallinson et al (1980) found that combination chemotherapy (5-FU, cyclophosphamide, vincristine, methotrexate and mitomycin C) significantly improved survival (44 weeks versus 9 weeks), whereas Cullinan et al (1990) found that 5-FU alone was just as effective as combination therapy. In Edinburgh, the combination of 5-FU, adriamycin and mitomycin C significantly lengthened median survival (33 weeks versus 15 weeks) when compared to no treatment in patients with unresectable disease (Fig. 51.7) (Palmer et al 1994); side-effects such as nausea and vomiting, leukopenia, oral ulceration and alopecia were common but usually mild. Even in trials where benefit has been demonstrated, survival beyond 2 years is exceptional and doubt still surrounds the use of chemotherapy outside prospective controlled trials in patients with unresectable disease.

Chemotherapy has also been used as an adjunct to surgical resection, but survival and toxicity have been disappointing. The Norwegian Pancreatic Cancer Trial Group randomized 54 patients with pancreatic or periampullary cancer to receive adjuvant chemotherapy (5-FU, doxorubicin and mitomycin C) or no treatment following resection. Median survival in treated patients was significantly

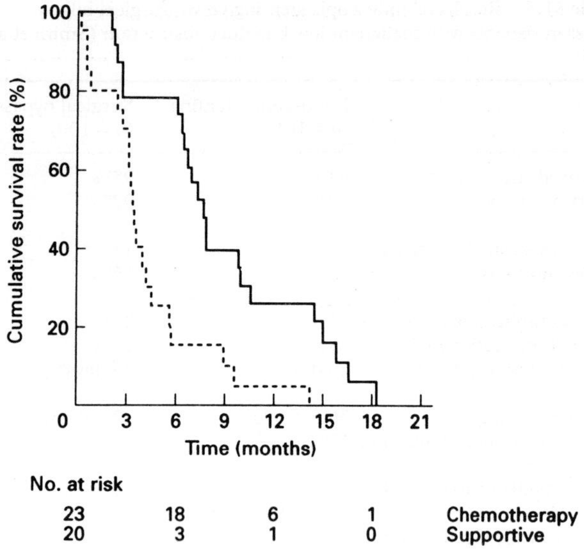


**Fig. 51.7** Kaplan–Meier survival curves in patients receiving combination chemotherapy (continuous line) or supportive therapy (broken line) following diagnosis of inoperable pancreatic cancer (Palmer et al 1994).

better (23 months versus 11 months) but no benefit was observed in terms of actuarial 5-year survival rates (8% versus 4%) (Bakkevold et al 1993).

Recent evidence indicates that certain polyunsaturated fatty acids such as eicosapentaenoic (EPA) and gamma-linolenic (GLA) acid can inhibit growth of pancreatic cancer cell lines in vitro, possibly by enhancing lipid peroxidation (Falconer et al 1994b). Clinical trials of these agents are now underway.

*Radiotherapy*

Radiotherapy has traditionally been regarded as ineffective in pancreatic cancer. However, the combination of radiotherapy and the radiosensitizer 5-FU doubled survival times when compared with radiotherapy alone (10.5 versus 5.5 months) in one early trial (Gastrointestinal Tumor Study Group 1981). Subsequent studies showed that the combination was better than chemotherapy (streptozocin, mitomycin and 5-FU) in 43 patients with locally unresectable disease in terms of median survival (42 weeks versus 32 weeks) and 1-year survival (41% versus 19%) (Gastrointestinal Tumor Study Group 1988).

Adjuvant radiotherapy has also been used after resection. The Gastrointestinal Tumor Study Group (1987) reported 2-year survival rates of 43% in 21 patients randomized to receive radiotherapy and 5-FU as apposed to 18% in 22 patients who were not irradiated. As in all studies of this type, accrual was slow and patient numbers small and the approach has not gained general acceptance. European groups are currently evaluating the use of radiotherapy and chemotherapy following potentially curative resection.

Intraoperative radiotherapy has also been used alone and in combination with external beam therapy and/or chemotherapy in unresectable disease. Survival benefit has not been forthcoming (Tuckson et al 1988, Roldan et al 1988) or unimpressive (Abe et al 1987) and necrotizing pancreatitis and retroperitoneal fibrosis posed problems in earlier series. When used as an adjunct to resection, intraoperative radiotherapy may improve local control of disease but has not improved survival (Zerbi et al 1994). Some consider that intraoperative irradiation combined with external beam therapy offers useful palliation (especially pain relief) when curative resection is not possible (Okamoto et al 1994).

*Hormonal therapy* (Bakkevold et al 1990)

The suggestion that estrogen receptors and/or estrogen-binding proteins might allow pancreatic cancer to respond to antiestrogens, such as tamoxifen, were not confirmed in a controlled Norwegian study in 176 patients with pancreatic or periampullary cancer (Bakkevold et al 1990).

Somatostatin inhibits pancreatic exocrine secretion and the release of trophic hormones such as cholecystokinin and gastrin and it was hoped that it might inhibit the growth of pancreatic cancer. Long-acting analogs inhibited growth of xenografts of human cancer in nude mice (Upp et al 1988), although subsequent studies failed to demonstrate somatostatin receptors in human pancreatic cancer (Reubi et al 1988, Gillespie et al 1992). To date, survival in patients receiving somatostatin analogs has not been improved consistently, despite suggestions of improved performance status (Cannobio et al 1992, Friess et al 1993b).

*Immunotherapy*

Despite encouraging results in animal models, passive immunotherapy with murine monoclonal antibody failed to improve survival in patients after Whipple resection (Buchler et al 1991).

*Pain relief*

Pain due to obstruction of the biliary tree o gastric outlet is usually eliminated by relief of obstruction, while erosion of bony structures can be treated by radiotherapy. However, the pain of pancreatic cancer is more often due to involvement of neural tissues such as the peripancreatic neural plexuses and intercostal nerves. Metastatic involvement of the liver may also cause pain due to stretching of the capsule, infarction and obstruction of hepatic outflow.

Pain due to pancreatic inflammation and/or neural involvement only occasionally responds to nonopioids (e.g. paracetamol) or weaker opioids (e.g. codeine, dextropropoxyphene, buprenorphine) and oral morphine is frequently required. Morphine is best given as modified release tablets (e.g. MST Continus) and the starting dose is 10–20 mg every 12 h. When pain is severe, it may be better to give oral solution of morphine every 4 h to define the dose required and then transfer to the same daily dose given as two doses of MST at 12-h intervals. Nausea and vomiting may be troublesome initially and constipation can be a problem. When swallowing is difficult, diamorphine can be given by subcutaneous injection or infusion; the dose is one-third to one-quarter of the oral dose of morphine.

In patients who are not controlled by opiates, methods which may be used include epidural administration of morphine or local anesthetics (Cherry et al 1985), percutaneous celiac plexus block using 25–50% alcohol injected under CT guidance (Moore et al 1981, Leung et al 1983) and thoracoscopic section of the splanchnic nerves (Cuschieri 1994). Splanchnicectomy and celiac plexus block offer obvious advantages over epidural analgesia, but their efficacy is unpredictable and pain is often only relieved for 6–8 weeks in patients who respond. However, given the appalling prognosis of pancreatic cancer, even this short-lived relief may suffice.

*Nutrition*

When weight loss is associated with malabsorption (Perez et al 1983), pancreatic supplements may be helpful. Elucidation of the mechanism(s) responsible for cachexia (see above) may allow more effective nutritional management.

### Prognosis

Prognostic factors following resection include tumor size (Cubilla & Fitzgerald 1978), serosal and retroperitoneal invasion, nodal involvement and the presence of hepatic metastases (Kayahara et al 1993). In one study, 19% of cases recurring after resection had local failure only (i.e. recurrence in the pancreatic bed, regional nodes, adjacent organs and peritoneum) and 73% had a component of local failure. Extra-abdominal metastases were documented in only 27% of cases but were never the sole site of recurrence; all patients with recurrent disease had recurrence within the abdomen and peritoneal (42%) and hepatic (62%) recurrences were common (Griffin et al 1990).

Gudjonsson (1987) found only 156 5-year survivors among 37 000 or so patients in surgical reports published between 1960 and 1986; the 5-year survival rate was only 0.4%. As a prognostic rule of thumb, patients who undergo apparently curative resection have a median survival of 11–21 months, patients with locally unresectable disease but no hepatic or more distant metastases survive for some 5–11 months, while those with advanced local or disseminated disease have only 2.5–5 months of life.

**Table 51.6** Classification of cystic lesions of the pancreas (after Howard 1989)

| |
|---|
| *Congenital true cysts* |
| Single true cysts |
| Polycystic disease |
| Enterogenous cysts |
| Dermoid cysts |
| *Angiomatous cysts* |
| *Cystic neoplasms* |
| Serous (microcystic) cystadenoma |
| Mucinous (macrocystic) cystic neoplasms |
| Acinar cell cystadenocarcinoma |
| Papillary-cystic epithelial neoplasm |
| Teratomatous cyst |
| Other rare cysts |
| *Aquired (nonproliferative) cysts* |
| Retention cysts |
| Parasitic cysts |
| Pseudocysts |
| *Miscellaneous cysts* |
| Cystic necrosis of exocrine pancreatic cancer |
| Cystic islet cell tumors |
| Cysts of adjacent duodenum |
| Cysts of uncertain nature |

## CYSTIC TUMORS OF THE PANCREAS

Cystic neoplasms account for 10–15% of all pancreatic cysts (Friedman et al 1983, Table 51.6) and 1% of all pancreatic neoplasms. Of 75 cases reported by Compagno & Oertel (1978a, b), 45% were serous microcystic cystadenomas, 29% were benign mucinous cystic neoplasms and 25% were malignant mucinous cystic neoplasms.

*Cystadenoma and cystadenocarcinoma* (Compagno & Oertel 1978a,b) (Fig. 2.25)

***Serous (microcystic) cystadenomas.*** These large tumors arise in any part of the pancreas, predominantly affect middle-aged or elderly women and have an excellent prognosis after complete excision. They are virtually always benign although serous cystadenocarcinomas have been reported (Yoshimi et al 1992). The tumor consists of multiple small cysts (Fig. 51.8) lined by cuboidal glycogen-rich epithelium and presents as a palpable mass or is discovered incidentally on ultrasonography or CT scanning. Late-onset diabetes occurs in 25% of patients and jaundice may complicate lesions of the pancreatic head. Gastrointestinal bleeding is occasionally the presenting symptom. Calcification with a "starburst" patten is seen in approximately 10% of cases. Complete excision of the involved pancreas is indicated although the benign nature of the lesion allows conservative management in elderly or infirm patients.

***Mucinous (macrocystic) cystadenoma and cystadenocarcinoma.*** These tumors have a better prognosis than ductal adenocarcinoma but should be regarded as malignant or potentially malignant and dealt with by

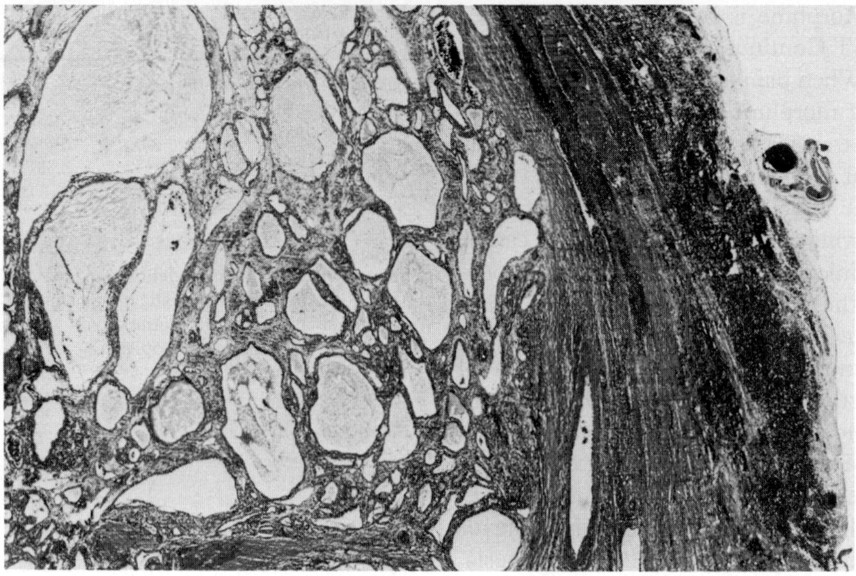

**Fig. 51.8** Serous microcystic cystadenoma of the pancreas showing a multilocular thinwalled cyst with low columnar and cuboidal epithelium (hematoxylin and eosin, ×18).

**Table 51.7** Clinical characteristics in 67 patients with cystic neoplasms of the pancreas (Warshaw et al 1990)

| Type of neoplasm | Mean age (yrs) | Female (%) | Head of pancreas (%) | Mean size (cm) | Symptoms (%) | Wrong diagnosis* (%) |
|---|---|---|---|---|---|---|
| Serous cystadenoma | 64 | 72 | 39 | 5 | 56 | 33 |
| Mucinous cystic tumor | 59 | 81 | 47 | 5 | 60 | 40 |
| Mucinous cystadenocarcinoma | 63 | 74 | 56 | 6 | 85 | 41 |
| Papillary cystic tumor | 44 | 67 | 13 | 8 | 67 | 33 |
| Cystic islet cell tumor | 60 | 50 | 0 | 5 | 50 | 0 |
| Mucinous ductal ectasia | 69 | 0 | 100 | 6 | 100 | 50 |

* Wrongly diagnosed as pancreatic pseudocyst

radical excision whenever feasible. Young and middle-aged women are affected predominantly (Compagno & Oertel 1978b; Table 51.7). The tumor involves any part of the pancreas, is up to 20 cm in diameter and consists of a variable number of cysts lined by columnar mucus-secreting epithelium (Fig. 51.9). The variability of the histological pattern cannot be overemphasized; some areas appear benign, others show marked atypia and others can show frank malignancy. Compagno & Oertel recommend abandoning the terms "mucinous cystadenoma" and "cystadenocarcinoma" in favor of "mucinous cystic neoplasm with latent or overt malignancy". The lesion is thought to originate from duct cells; neuroendocrine cells have the same origin and in one series neuroendocrine elements were found in 87% of mucinous cystic neoplasms and in 47% of those regarded as malignant (Warshaw et al 1990).

The lesion usually presents as an abdominal mass in an otherwise healthy patient. It can cause pain and obstructive jaundice. CT scanning is the investigation of choice and usually reveals solid as well as cystic components. The neoplasm is frequently misdiagnosed as a pseudocyst, but loculation should raise suspicion. Rim (and occasional central) calcification is seen in about 10% of cases and local invasion or nodal and liver metastases are occasionally detected. ERP usually fails to show communication between the neoplasm and the pancreatic duct, but may reveal duct constriction or obstruction. If angiography is undertaken, the solid component of the tumor often appears hypervascular while the cystic areas are hypovascular. Cyst fluid analysis and cytology has been used to aid preoperative diagnosis; high viscosity, high levels of CEA, CA 125 and tumor-asociated glycoprotein-72 (TAG-72) and low amylase levels point to malignancy (Lewandrowski et al 1993, Alles et al 1994).

Treatment consists of surgical excision as this is often a curable tumor, even when malignant. For reasons outlined above, frozen section analysis of an operative biopsy can mislead but the presence of mucus within a cyst

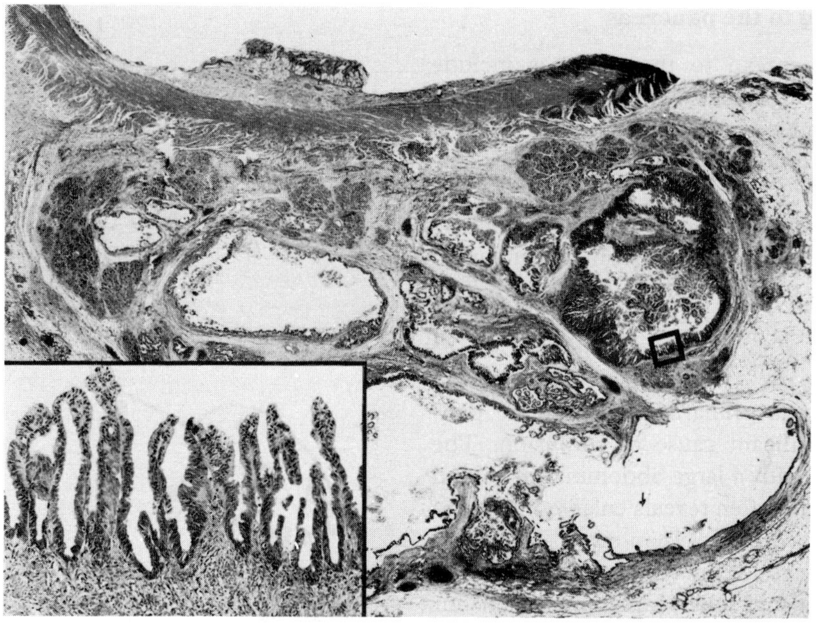

**Fig. 51.9** Mucinous cystic neoplasm of the pancreas, showing fibrosis between locules and pleomorphic proliferative columnar epithelial lining (hematoxylin and eosin, ×5). Insert: papillary pleomorphic epithelium (hematoxylin and eosin, ×75).

should indicate that one is not dealing with a pseudocyst. Lesions thought to be pseudocysts should never be managed by internal drainage without generous biopsy of their wall; the presence of epithelium immediately excludes the diagnosis of pseudocyst (Warshaw & Rutledge 1987).

***Papillary-cystic epithelial neoplasm*** (Frantz 1959). This rare epithelial tumor mainly affects young women. It usually forms a well-circumscribed, even encapsulated mass which on section is soft, necrotic and partly cystic. Histology shows cystic and papillary structures formed by regular polygonal cells with clear cytoplasm and regular round nuclei showing little mitotic activity. The origin is debated but ultrastructural and immunohistochemical studies suggest that the tumor arises from primitive pancreatic epithelial cells exhibiting exocrine and focal endocrine differentiation (Miettinen et al 1987, Stommer et al 1991). Metastases are rare despite local invasion and the neoplasm is often cured by excision (Sanfey et al 1983).

***Acinar cell cystadenocarcinoma.*** The acinar cell origin of this extremely rare multilocular tumor is attested by its high content of zymogen granules on electron-microscopy (Stamm et al 1987). The tumor may be frankly malignant with spread to the peritoneum and liver. Resection is undertaken if feasible.

***Cystic neuroendocrine tumor.*** These rare neuroendocrine tumors are easily mistaken for benign cysts. They account for less than 5% of all pancreatic cystic neoplasms and may be functioning or nonfunctioning (Weissmann et al 1994, Schwartz et al 1994). The tumor commonly presents with abdominal pain and a mass is apparent clinically or on CT scanning. The tumor stains positively for neurone-specific enolase or chromogranin (i.e. neuroendocrine markers) and may stain positively for polypeptide hormones such as pancreatic polypeptide (PP), insulin, gastrin, somatostatin, glucagon and growth hormone. There is little or no correlation between symptoms and immunohistochemical profile.

The value of preoperative aspiration is debated. Weissmann et al (1994) advocate aspiration to allow measurement of tumor markers (e.g. CA 125), amylase, insulin and viscosity and permit cytology, whereas Schwartz et al (1994) argue that aspiration can mislead and disseminate malignancy. As these tumors can be malignant, resection is advocated where possible. Surgical debulking is helpful if extirpation is impossible and streptozotocin and somatostatin analogs may prove useful in adjuvant treatment (see below).

## MISCELLANEOUS PANCREATIC TUMORS AND TUMORS OF CHILDHOOD

### Tumors of childhood

Lack et al (1983) describe eight childhood cases of pancreatic tumor collected over a 30-year period. There were three adenocarcinomas, two acinar carcinomas, two acinar cell adenomas and one papillary cystic neoplasm. Pancreatoblastoma also occurs and may be associated with raised serum alpha-fetoprotein levels (Iseki et al 1986).

### Tumors metastasizing to the pancreas

Neoplasms which can spread to the pancreas include those arising in neighboring organs, lung, breast or kidney, melanoma and lymphoma or sarcoma (Wernecke et al 1986). On computed tomograpy, multiple nodules may deform the surface of the pancreas or a solitary focal mass may simulate a primary pancreatic neoplasm (Rumancik et al 1984). Fine-needle aspiration biopsy may distinguish primary from metastatic tumor.

### Lymphoma

Non-Hodgkin's lymphoma primarily involving the pancreas is a rare but significant cause of confusion. The patient usually presents with a large abdominal mass and confirmatory CT scanning often reveals enlarged peripancreatic nodes. Guided needle biopsy can reveal the correct diagnosis but aspiration cytology may be misinterpreted as showing poorly differentiated adenocarcinoma (Mansour et al 1989). Excellent symptom control and extended remission are usually achieved with chemotherapy and surgery is avoided if possible (Webb et al 1989).

### Miscellaneous tumors

Other rare neoplasms of the pancreas include lipomas, mesenchymal tumors (e.g. Schwannoma), granular cell tumors and plasmacytomas.

## PERIAMPULLARY TUMORS

Periampullary tumors arise at or within 1 cm of the papilla of Vater. They might be more correctly termed "peripapillary" but the term "periampullary" is used widely and is retained here. In some reports, the term "periampullary" is used to include cancers of the head of the pancreas. Given that the two cancers have a different etiology and prognosis, the practice is inappropriate. However, it can sometimes be difficult to be certain that a periampullary tumor has not arisen from the pancreas, terminal bile duct or elsewhere in the duodenum.

Improved diagnosis, and in particular the advent of duodenoscopy and ERCP, may explain the apparent rise in the incidence of periampullary cancer (Levin et al 1981). Conversely, many patients who survive for more than 5 years after resection of a "pancreatic cancer" were undoubtedly suffering from the more favorable periampullary lesion. Only 126 patients with "ampullary cancer" were registered in England and Wales in 1979 whereas 5881 were thought to have pancreatic cancer (Allen-Mersh & Earlam 1986).

Patients with *familial adenomatous polyposis* (FAP) and Gardner's syndrome are at particularly high risk of periampullary or duodenal cancer. Jagelman et al (1988) found 39 such cancers (36 of which were periampullary) in 1225 FAP patients. Endoscopic surveillance of the stomach and duodenum is now advised, bearing in mind that there may be an interval of 20 years between colectomy for FAP and the development of upper gastrointestinal cancer. Spigelman et al (1989) performed gastroduodenoscopy in 102 FAP patients (Fig. 51.10); none had polyps of the duodenal bulb alone, eight had polyps of the first three parts of the duodenum and 80 had polyps of the second and third parts only. Biopsies revealed dysplasia in 94 cases, hyperplasia in six and an abnormal periampullary area in 90%. Nonadenomatous fundic gland polyps were found in 56 patients but were not regarded as premalignant.

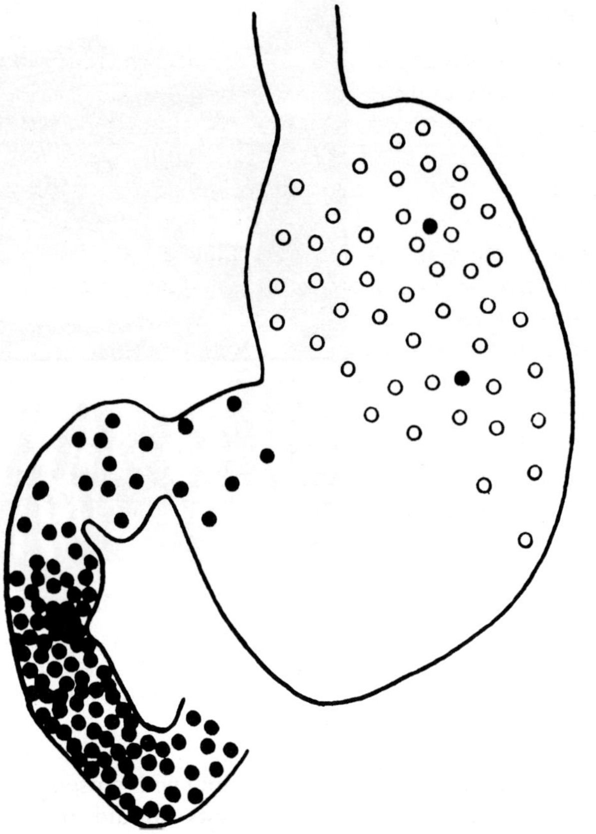

**Fig. 51.10** Gastroduodenal sites affected by polyps in 102 patients with familial adenomatous polyposis undergoing upper gastrointestinal endoscopy. Open circles represent patients with fundic gland polyps; closed circles are patients with adenoma(s). (Reproduced with permission from Spigelman et al 1989.)

*Carcinoids* of the periampullary region are rare but may be associated with Von Recklinghausen's disease (Klein et al 1989), a disease which also increases the risk of developing periampullary neurofibromas, paraganglionomas and ganglioneuromas. Neuroendocrine tumors of the papilla have also been described (Emory et al 1994).

*Primary duodenal carcinomas* are also rare. Although they account for only 0.35% of all gastrointestinal cancers, it should be remembered that up to 50% of all small bowel cancers occur in the duodenum.

### Pathology

The tumor usually appears as a protuberant mass with a papillary surface or as a neoplastic ulcer. Care must be taken when interpreting biopsies as sampling errors are common. This is a particular problem in villous tumors where two-thirds of apparently benign lesions harbor malignancy (Ryan et al 1986). Examination of the entire tumor is the only way to determine if it is malignant. Conversely, inflammatory lesions can easily be mistaken for malignancy (Leese et al 1986). The majority of tumors in surgical series are adenocarcinomas and there is persuasive evidence that adenomas are premalignant lesions (Neoptolemos et al 1988). Protuberant tumors tend to be better differentiated and less aggressive than ulcerated tumors (Blumgart & Kennedy 1973). Local spread and metastasis are less common than in adenocarcinoma of the pancreas.

### Clinical features

The tumor has no sex predilection and a peak incidence in the seventh decade (Schlippert et al 1978, Robertson et al 1987). Over 90% of patients present with obstructive jaundice and almost half report pain (Robertson et al 1987). Nausea and vomiting can occur. Acute pancreatitis is occasionally the first manifestation (Jones et al 1985) and tumor ulceration can lead to iron deficiency anemia. Marked weight loss and inanition are unusual in the absence of metastatic spread, although steatorrhea is troublesome in some cases.

#### *Investigations*

Liver function tests reflect cholestasis. Ultrasonography usually confirms extrahepatic biliary obstruction and may reveal pancreatic duct dilatation. On hypotonic duodenography the lesion appears as a protruding, often irregular, filling defect on the medial wall of the second part of the duodenum (Fig. 4.14). Duodenoscopy is now the preferred investigation in that it allows direct inspection, permits histological confirmation and, where appropriate, allows relief of jaundice by papillotomy and/or stenting. Every attempt should be made to obtain deep biopsies. Resectability is assessed as in pancreatic cancer (p. 1291), and endosonography is particularly helpful in staging (Tio et al 1993).

### Treatment

The choice of curative treatment rests between Whipple resection and transduodenal excision. A review from northwest England favored local excision in that none of the 25 patients dealt with in this way died postoperatively, whereas radical surgery in 24 patients had an operative mortality of 30% (Knox & Kingston 1986). However, no less than 33 surgeons were responsible for the care of these patients and such cases should now be referred to specialist units. A study from Glasgow showed an operative mortality of 8% for Whipple resection, compared to 25% for local excision and 17% for palliative bypass (Robertson et al 1987). Pancreaticoduodenectomy in skilled hands should now have a near-zero operative mortality and is the treatment of choice for otherwise fit patients. Transduodenal excision is reserved for elderly unfit patients, particularly when the lesion appears to be benign. Endoscopic papillotomy can be used as a preliminary maneuver in jaundiced patients before surgery and papillotomy with or without insertion of a stent offers worthwhile palliation in those unfit for laparotomy (Bickerstaff et al 1990).

### Prognosis

Five-year survival rates following resection range from 30% to 57% (Robertson et al 1987, Nordolinger et al 1992, Kawarada et al 1993, Wade et al 1994), emphasizing the importance of distinguishing between periampullary cancer and the much less favorable pancreatic cancer. Periampullary carcinoids are a particularly favorable subgroup with a 5-year survival rate of 90% (Hatzitheoklitos et al 1994). Adenocarcinoma of the duodenum also had a cumulative 5-year survival rate of 45% after resection in a multicenter French report (Rotman et al 1994).

## ISLET CELL TUMORS OF THE PANCREAS

The first operation to deal with a pancreatic neuroendocrine tumor was undertaken by W J Mayo in 1927 in a physician with recurrent hypoglycemia. An extract from a metastasis reproduced the actions of insulin when injected into a rabbit, indicating that the tumor was an insulinoma. At least a dozen syndromes are now known to arise from tumors of pancreatic neuroendocrine cells. With the exception of insulinomas and gastrinomas, most are so rare that single cases rather than series have been report. As shown in Table 51.8, these syndromes can also result from extrapancreatic tumors.

The tumors responsible for a syndrome can be so small that it escapes detection; for example, the Zollinger–Ellison syndrome may be caused by tiny tumors hidden in the pancreas or duodenal well. In rare instances, hyperinsulinemia results from islet hyperplasia rather than tumor formation; this is known as nesidioblastosis and its existence is accepted in children but is still debated in adults.

Multiple endocrine neoplasia type I (MEN-I) or Wermer's syndrome is a hereditary disorder characterized by tumors of the parathyroid (virtually all cases), pancreatic islets (lese than 50% of cases, most often gastrinomas) and pituitary (less than 25% of cases, mostly prolactinomas). Occasionally there are adenomas of the thyroid or adrenal cortex. The MEN-I gene has been assigned to the long arm of chromosome II and allelic deletions have been

**Table 51.8** Endocrine tumors of the pancreas and their clinical syndromes (based on Creutzfeld & Arnold 1993)

| Name (synonym) | Frequency* | Clinical symptoms | Hormone responsible | Other hormones frequently produced |
|---|---|---|---|---|
| Insulinoma | 51% | Fasting hypoglycemia | Insulin | PP, glucagon |
| Gastrinoma | 24% | Gastric hypersecretion, fulminant ulceration, steatorrhea or diarrhea, (Zollinger–Ellison syndrome) | Gastrin | Insulin, PP, glucagon, ACTH |
| VIPoma (Verner–Morrison syndrome, pancreatic cholera, WDHA syndrome, watery diarrhea syndrome) | 1% | Watery diarrhea, hypokalemia, gastric hyposecretion | Vasoactive intestinal peptide | PP, glucagon, calcitonin, peptide histidine, isoleucine (PHI), catecholamine |
| Glucagonoma | 1% | Necrolytic migratory erythema, diabetes mellitus, anemia | Glucagon | PP, somatostatin, insulin |
| Somatostatinoma | Extremely rare | Diabetes mellitus, cholelithiasis, steatorrhea, gastric hyposecretion | Somatostatin | PP, insulin, calcitonin, cortisol, gastrin |

*Frequency refers to frequency distribution of islet cell tumors seen in a series of 322 patients treated at the Mayo Clinic 1960–86 (Van Heerden & Thompson 1993). In this series, nonfunctioning tumors accounted for 18% of cases, while carcinoids and tumors secreting pancreatic polypeptide (PP), CCK, growth hormone, calcitonin, catecholamines, parathyroid hormone-like substance or ACTH collectively accounted for 5% of cases. Somatostatinoma was not seen in this series.

demonstrated in DNA from parathyroid and islet cell tumors (Lairmore & Wells 1993). These deletions affect the chromosome derived from the unaffected parent and this probably allows expression of the germline mutation on the chromosome derived from the affected parent. The tumors are usually benign. Sporadic cases of MEN-I have also been reported.

The widespread use of CT scanning has increased the detection of nonfunctioning islet cell tumors which are not associated with syndromes of hormone production or high circulating hormone levels. Whereas nonfunctioning tumors accounted for 25% of islet cell tumors at the Mayo Clinic in 1970–74, the proportion had risen to 65% by 1980–84 (Van Heerden & Thompson 1993).

Most islet cell tumors consist of uniform cells within a vascular stroma, the cells coalescing into trabecular, acinar or solid patterns. Benign and malignant tumors cannot be distinguished histologically and the diagnosis of malignancy is based on gross invasion or metastases. Immunohistochemistry can establish the nature of stored hormone(s) although there may be little or no stored peptide in undifferentiated tumors. Markers such as chromogranin, neurone-specific enolase and synaptophysin confirm the neuroendocrine nature of a tumor, although not all nonfunctioning tumors show such reactivity. Electronmicroscopy helps to identify secretory granules in some cases but in others, the granules are atypical and nondiagnostic.

The remainder of this chapter discusses the principles of diagnosis, localization and treatment of islet cell tumors and outlines the features of individual syndromes with the exception of the Zollinger–Ellison Syndrome (see p. 252).

## GENERAL PRINCIPLES OF ASSESSMENT AND MANAGEMENT

### Clinical diagnosis

Radioimmunoassay has transformed the diagnosis of functioning islet cell tumors. Pancreatic polypeptide (PP) levels are elevated in some 50% of cases (Polak et al 1976) but there is no useful general marker and preoperative diagnosis rests on demonstrating high circulating hormone levels. In some cases, levels are not particularly high, but are nevertheless inappropriately elevated. For example, plasma insulin levels may be “normal” in insulinoma patients until it is appreciated that there is concurrent hypoglycemia (see below). The rarity of islet cell tumors means that a high index of suspicion is needed if potentially harmful delay in diagnosis is to be avoided.

### Localization

Once an islet cell tumor has been diagnosed, the next step is to locate the tumor(s) and detect any metastases. Nonfunctioning tumors, glucagonomas and somatostatinomas are often large and readily detected on CT scanning.

Small functioning tumors such as insulinomas and gastrinomas can be exceedingly difficult to localize and a recent review of specialist surgical centers found that CT detected only one-third of cases of insulinoma (Rothmund et al 1990). MRI does not yet appear to have any advantages over CT scanning.

Transcutaneous ultrasonography is no better than CT scanning, but *endoscopic ultrasonography* is a highly accurate method of imaging even tumors with a diameter of 0.5–2 cm (Lightdale et al 1991); indeed, Thompson et al (1994) suggest that this is now the only localization study needed for insulinomas. Rosch et al (1992b) found that endoscopic ultrasonography had a sensitivity of 82% in localizing 39 pancreatic endocrine tumors and was negative in all but one of 19 control patients without endocrine tumors (specificity 95%).

Selective visceral arteriography has variable success rates but with magnification, subtraction films, superselective catheterization and additional oblique views, it detected all 30 solitary benign insulinomas in one recent series (Geoghegan et al 1994). Such lesions are usually hypervascular and produce a discrete tumor "blush".

Debate surrounds the use of *percutaneous transhepatic portal venous sampling* to locate occult islet cell tumors. The technique has been used most widely to locate insulinomas (Fig. 51.11) and has an accuracy of 86–100% in recent reports (Vinik et al 1991, Pedrazzoli et al 1994). A variant consists of venous sampling during selective arterial injection of calcium to stimulate insulin release (Doppman et al 1991). These techniques are invasive, need great skill and at best "regionalize" rather than localize the tumor and there is a growing consensus that they are unnecessary if the patient is being dealt with by an experienced surgeon with access to endoscopic and/or intraoperative ultrasonography (Van Heerden et al 1992; see below). However, they still have a valuable place when an insulinoma has not been found at the initial operation (p. 31).

Lamberts et al (1990) visualized tumors in 12 of 13 patients with metastatic carcinoids and seven of nine patients with pancreatic endocrine tumors using $^{123}I$-labeled Tyr$^{3}$-octreotide (a synthetic long-acting analog of somatostatin). Successful localization using $^{111}In$-pentetreotide, a labeled somatostatin analog that is easier to prepare, has also been reported (Scherubl et al 1993, Weinel et al 1993), while Schirmer et al (1993) have used intraoperative somatostatin-receptor scintigraphy. Some 10–20% of islet cell tumors (and carcinoids) do not possess somatostatin receptors (Reubi et al 1990) and cannot be visualized, but useful information is still obtained in that such patients can be spared unnecessary treatment with octreotide.

Radioiodinated VIP has also been used to detect insulinomas and carcinoid tumors, as well as carcinomas of the stomach, exocrine pancreas and colon which express VIP receptors (Virgolini et al 1994).

Laparotomy remains an important method of locating pancreatic endocrine tumors, assessing their resectability or amenability to debulking and detecting metastatic disease. Intraoperative ultrasonography (Sigel et al 1982, Pedrazzoli et al 1994) may prove extremely helpful (Fig. 51.12).

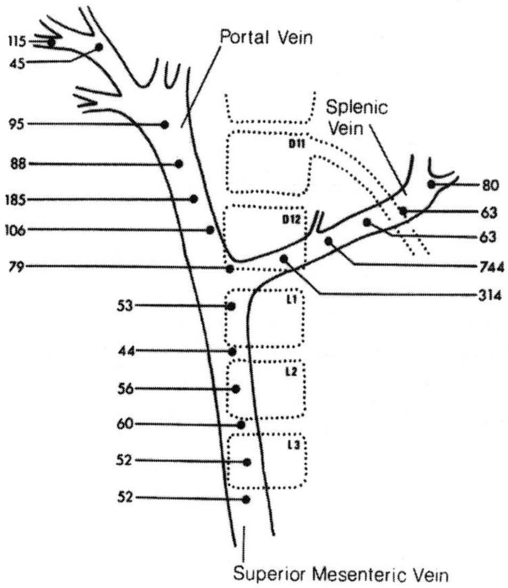


**Fig. 51.11** Concentrations of insulin in samples taken from the portal venous system by transhepatic venous sampling in a patient with an insulinoma subsequently found in the body of pancreas.

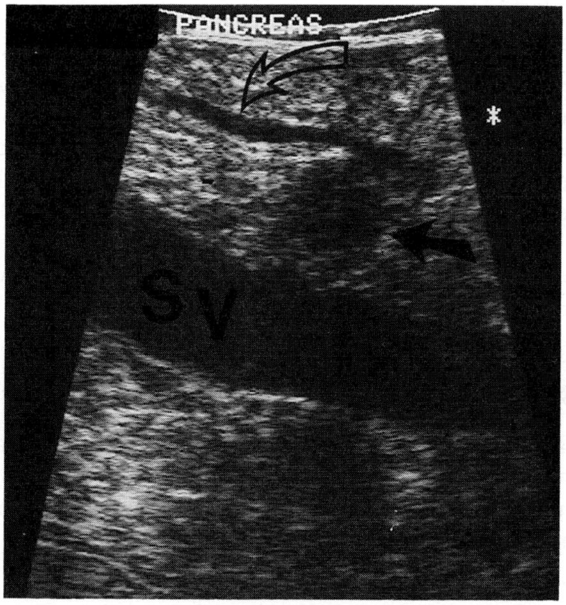


**Fig. 51. 12** Longitudinal ultrasonogram of the pancreas demonstrating a close relationship between the pancreatic duct (open arrow) and islet cell adenoma (solid arrow). SV=splenic vein.

## Treatment

Much depends on whether a tumor is benign or malignant and whether there is locally unresectable disease and/or metastases. Small benign tumors such as insulinomas can usually be enucleated, whereas larger tumors may require formal pancreatic resection.

When there is unresectable or metastatic disease, surgical debulking is usually recommended (McEntee et al 1990), although this is now challenged, at least in nonfunctioning tumors (see below). Streptozotocin (an antibiotic derived from *Streptomyces achromogenes* and closely related to nitrosoureas) is cytotoxic to B-cells and when combined with 5-fluorouracil or doxorubicin, produced an objective response in 45% of 44 patients in one series for a median of 27.5 months (Eriksson et al 1990). Interferon achieved comparable responses in those failing to respond to chemotherapy. In patients with anaplastic neuroendocrine tumors, etoposide plus cisplatin may give worthwhile regression and prolong survival (median 19 months), although well-differentiated islet tumors rarely respond (Moertel et al 1991). Hepatic artery chemoembolization can be considered for symptomatic liver metastases. Perry et al (1994) found that 27 of 30 patients with islet cell tumors or carcinoids experienced subjective improvement after embolization with doxorubicin and iodized oil followed by absorbable gelatin powder of pledgets; hormonal markers and/or tumor size decreased by at least 50% in 79% of cases (see also p. 475).

*Octreotide* is a valuable means of controlling symptoms in patients with unresectable tumors (see p. 475) and experimental and early clinical evidence indicates that it inhibits the growth of somatostatin receptor-positive tumors (Van Eijck et al 1994). Symptoms from specific islet cell tumors may be controlled by specific medication; for example, acid hypersecretion in gastrinomas responds to $H_2$ receptor antagonists or omeprazole, while hypoglycemia in insulinomas can be controlled by diazeoxide (see below).

Whereas nonfunctioning tumors were once thought to have a better prognosis, recent analysis suggests that they have a similar prognosis to functioning tumors when matched for extent of disease (Venkatesh et al 1990). This may reflect earlier diagnosis and treatment of patients with functioning tumors.

# INSULINOMA (Creutzfeldt & Arnold 1993)

This insulin-secreting tumor arises from B-cells and accounts for 70–80% of functioning islet cell tumors. Its annual incidence is about 1 per million, although this may be an underestimate.

## Pathology

Insulinomas are usually solitary benign lesions measuring less than 1–2 cm in diameter and distributed evenly throughout the pancreas. Only 1% are ectopic (Miyazaki et al 1986). Multiple insulinomas are found in about 10% of cases, half of which have the MEN-I syndrome. The tumor is malignant in 10% of patients and one-third of these cases have metastases at the time of diagnosis. Malignant tumors are usually larger and had a mean diameter of 6.2 cm in one review (Danforth et al 1984). Histological differentiation between benign and malignant insulinoma is virtually impossible and follow-up is needed to confirm the absence of metastases.

## Clinical features

Sixty percent of cases occur in women. All age groups can be affected but most patients are between 30 and 50 years old. They often present with episodes of blurred vision, confusion, paresthesiae, difficulties with speech, somnolence or coma. Some present to psychiatrists with personality changes or disturbed behavior, some are misdiagnosed as abusers of alcohol and some are seen by neurosurgeons or neurologists with suspected epilepsy or brain tumor. All of these features are due to neuroglycopenia. Other features such as sweating, tremor, palpitations, pallor and apprehension reflect the adrenergic response to hypoglycemia. Insulinoma patients appear to have reduced awareness of the autonomic and neuroglycopenic symptoms of their hypoglycemia and a decreased response by counter-regulatory hormones (Mitrakou et al 1993). The most important diagnostic feature is that symptoms occur in the night, early morning or before meals, but hardly ever after food. The patients eats to allay hypoglycemia and is often overweight. Diagnosis is frequently delayed for 2–3 years (Auld et al 1988) and prolonged delay can cause permanent mental retardation.

## Diagnosis

The classic *Whipple's triad* is the relationship of symptoms to fasting, their prompt relief by glucose and the demonstration of a low blood glucose during symptoms. The diagnosis is now confirmed by measuring plasma insulin and glucose levels every 3–4 h during a 24–48 h fast in hospital. By 24 h, 75% of insulinoma patients have blood glucose levels lower than 2.2 mmol/L (40 mg/100 ml) with neuroglycopenic and adrenergic symptoms, while by 48 h, 98% have hypoglycemia (Creutzfeldt & Arnold 1993). Insulin levels are inappropriately high for the glucose levels and it is useful to calculate the amended insulin:glucose ratio:

Insulin concentration (pmol/L)/glucose concentration (mmol/L) – 1.7

The figure of 1.7 reflects the fact that B-cells do not

secrete insulin at plasma glucose concentrations beneath 1.7 mmol/L. The upper limit of normal for the amended ratio is a molar ratio of $63\times10^{-6}$, although Creutzfeldt & Arnold (1993) found that a ratio of $39\times10^{-6}$ completely separated patients with and without an insulinoma. The insulin concentration can also be expressed in milliunits/L; a ratio of more than 30 is then strong presumptive evidence of an insulinoma (Auld et al 1988). Tests based on stimulation (tolbutamide, glucagon, calcium) or suppression (exogenous insulin) of endogenous insulin secretion are no longer used, but prolonged fasting to 72 h is occasionally required.

The principal differential diagnosis is factitious hypoglycemia due to insulin or sulfonylurea abuse, a problem which may affect members of the medical/nursing community or relatives of diabetics. The key is to measure glucose, insulin and C-peptide concentrations during an attack (provoked if necessary by a 24–48 h fast). When proinsulin is cleaved, insulin and C-peptide are produced in equimolar amounts. Thus, high levels of endogenous insulin should be accompanied by high levels of circulating C-peptide. Hypoglycemia (blood glucose <2.2 mmol/L) in conjunction with a high insulin concentration (>15 mU/L), but a normal or low C-peptide concentration suggests exogenous insulin administration. Sulfonylurea abuse mimics insulinomas clinically and biochemically and can only be detected by measuring drug levels. Other causes of spontaneous hypoglycemia include alcohol, hypopituitarism, Addison's disease and large retroperitoneal tumors, but these are usually easily discernible on clinical history and examination.

### Localization

Preoperative localization is discussed above. One algorithm would now include CT scanning and the use of endoscopic and/or intraoperative ultrasonography as adjuncts to surgical exploration. Somatostatin-receptor scintigraphy may be used increasingly in localization. Opinions vary about the need for angiography, but most centers avoid transhepatic portal venous sampling prior to the primary operation.

### Treatment

Symptomatic treatment is based on frequent high-calorie snacks and, where necessary, diazoxide (25–200 mg taken orally two or three times a day) can be used to inhibit insulin release (see below).

At surgery, the pancreas is fully exposed and bimanually palpated. Tumors in the head are enucleated, while tumors in the body or tail are enucleated if possible or dealt with by distal pancreatectomy. If tumor is not found, two-thirds distal pancreatectomy was at one time recommended. However, insulinomas are distributed evenly and distal resection fails to cure almost 50% of cases. Most surgeons now avoid blind distal pancreatectomy; the patient can be treated with diazoxide pending further attempts to localize the tumor. In patients with MEN-I syndrome, there are usually multiple adenomas and subtotal pancreatectomy is advised (Rasbach et al 1985).

Once the tumor is removed, transient hyperglycemia is common, particularly if carbohydrate solutions are infused. Postoperative hyperglycemia may be due to a combination of pancreatitis, high levels of counter-regulatory hormones induced by operation, chronic downregulation of insulin receptors and suppression of normal B-cells by long-standing hypoglycemia. However, insulin is rarely required and diabetes does not develop unless large amounts of pancreas have been resected.

When all malignant tumor cannot be removed, debulking (Danforth et al 1984) and cytotoxic therapy may give worthwhile palliation (see above). Hypoglycemia can be controlled with diazoxide although anorexia, nausea, vomiting, water and sodium retention, hypotension, cardiac arrhythmias and hirsutism can be troublesome. Octreotide is considered if diazoxide cannot be tolerated but can worsen hypoglycemia, presumably by suppressing secretion of glucagon and growth hormone.

## VIPOMA (Mozell et al 1990)

This rare syndrome has also been called *pancreatic cholera*, *Verner–Morrison syndrome*, *WDHA syndrome* (watery diarrhea, hypokalemia, achlorhydria) and WDS (*watery diarrhea syndrome*). It was first described by Verner & Morrison (1958) in patients with severe diarrhea, hypokalemia and an islet cell tumor. The tumor secretes vasoactive intestinal peptide (VIP), but it is debated whether this peptide accounts for all of the manifestations of the VIPoma syndrome. Other tumors causing diarrhea are discussed on page 1308.

### Pathology

The tumor is discrete in 80% of cases and most lie in the distal two-thirds of the pancreas. More than 50% are malignant and have metastasized by the time of diagnosis. VIP-producing tumors such as ganglioneuroblastomas and pheochromocytomas (Sackel et al 1985) are also found outside the gastrointestinal tract. The syndrome has also been produced by an argyrophil small cell carcinoma of the esophagus (Watson et al 1985). In childhood, neurogenic tumors such as ganglioneuroblastomas are the commonest VIP-secreting tumors. Previously, diarrhea had been ascribed to catecholamine excess but it is now believed that VIP is the mediator (Kaplan et al 1980).

The tumor is usually poorly differentiated and occasionally has an atypical carcinoid-like appearance. The cells contain granules which may be round and small (Capella et al 1983) or large and irregular and may have both VIP and peptide histidine isoleucine (PHI) immunoreactivity. In one study PHI was found in 22 of 24 VIPomas (Bloom et al 1983).

## Pathophysiology

VIPoma patients have abnormal intestinal absorption, abnormal secretion of sodium, chloride and water into the proximal jejunum, increased pancreatic secretion (especially in response to a meal) and possibly an increase in bile secretion. This causes increased flow at the duodenojejunal flexure, marked increase in net jejunal water, sodium and chloride secretion and increased flow through the distal ileum with reduced ileal absorption. As a result, up to 8 liters of fluid per day are delivered to the colon, exceeding its maximum absorptive capacity (5 liters). While VIP appears to be the central cause, PHI (which has great molecular and biological similarity) may play a role. Hypokalemia results from passive loss of potassium from the small intestine and from active AMP-mediated secretion in the large intestine. Hypochlorhydria occurs in 70% of patients and is probably due to inhibition of acid secretion by VIP. VIP is a vasodilator and this explains the flushing seen in 20% of cases. Calcitonin is also produced by some VIPomas and may enhance intestinal secretion (Booth et al 1983).

## Clinical features (O'Dorisio & Mekhjian 1985)

Middle-aged adults are most often affected but some 10% of tumors occur in children under the age of 10 years. There is severe intermittent diarrhea which later becomes episodic or continuous, with passage of 1–10 liters of thin tea-colored stool each day. Hypokalemia and hyperchloremic metabolic acidosis reflect fecal loss of bicarbonate and potassium. Fluid loss leads to dehydration, profound weakness, uremia and potentially fatal shock. Other features are gastric hypochlorhydria (but rarely achlorhydria), hyperglycemia, hypercalcemia, abnormal glucose tolerance and flushing. Hypercalcemia may be due to both a direct effect of VIP on bone or hyperparathyroidism (MEN-I).

In childhood (Iida et al 1980, Kaplan et al 1980), chronic watery diarrhea is the commonest initial complaint. Hypokalemia may be episodic rather than continuous. Abdominal distention is common, as is growth failure and malnutrition. Hypercalcemia and glucose intolerance are found in 50% of adult patients but not in children. Excess catecholamine excretion is common in childhood VIPomas and may explain the common association with flushing, hyperhidrosis and hypertension.

## Diagnosis (O'Dorisio & Mekhijan 1985)

Plasma VIP concentrations are normally 0–190 pg/ml but range from 225–1850 pg/ml in patients with VIP-secreting tumors. A high VIP concentration is virtually diagnostic but a normal level does not exclude the syndrome and the measurement should be repeated several times. Hypokalemia and acidosis are common and there is occasionally hypercalcemia. The condition is suspected when stool volume exceeds 500 ml/day, when diarrhea persists in the absence of eating and when stool osmolality can be accounted for entirely by its electrolyte content. The stool pH is alkaline and there may be mild steatorrhea.

VIPoma can be differentiated from the Zollinger–Ellison syndrome by nasogastric aspiration and by measuring stool pH, potassium and bicarbonate. In Zollinger–Ellison syndrome the stool is acid and potassium loss is only increased slightly. Differentiation from infectious diarrhea, chronic laxative abuse and diarrhea caused by other tumors is accomplished by measuring plasma VIP levels. However, some patients with secretory diarrhea have no evidence of laxative abuse or endocrine tumor (Read et al 1982).

## Localization

The procedures used are described above (p. 1302), but only a minority of VIPomas are localized before surgery.

## Treatment

Fluid loss, hypokalemia and acidosis are corrected using oral and/or parenteral glucose-electrolyte solutions. Prednisolone (60–80 mg/day) enhances absorption and controls diarrhea initially in most patients. Octreotide (50–200 μg two or three times a day by subcutaneous injection) is used to decrease circulating VIP levels, decrease stool volume and reverse metabolic and electrolyte upsets.

The tumor is removed if at all possible. In childhood, catecholamine levels are measured to determine whether preoperative antiadrenergic therapy is advisable (Kaplan et al 1980). If a tumor cannot be located, blind subtotal pancreatectomy may be considered. In children a search for ganglioneuroma must be carried out. In patients with inoperable tumor, debulking reduces VIP secretion and may facilitate medical management. Streptozotocin relieves diarrhea in some patients (McGill et at 1980) and can induce prolonged remission. Chlorozotocin brings about a response in 60–70% of cases (O'Dorisio & Mekhjian 1985). In patients who have diarrhea despite surgery and cytotoxic therapy, octreotide may be effective (Kraenzlin et al 1985, Wood et al 1985) although escape from control can occur (Koelz et al 1987).

## GLUCAGONOMA (Holst 1985, Van Heerden & Thompson 1993)

The rare glucagonoma syndrome was described by Mallinson et al (1974), although the existence of glucagon-secreting A-cell tumor of the pancreas had been appreciated earlier. The characteristic *necrolytic migratory erythema* means that this is the only islet cell tumor syndrome that can be diagnosed on clinical grounds alone.

### Pathology

The tumors are usually large (3–35 cm), solitary malignant lesions which can be part of the MEN-I syndrome. More than half have metastasized to the liver and regional nodes by diagnosis. Histological examination shows pleomorphism, with immunoreactive cells in strands and ribbons. The granules are often atypical and unrecognizable as A-cell granules. Glucagonomas may contain PP-, insulin-, somatostatin- and gastrin-producing cells.

The skin lesions show marked superficial spongiosis and necrosis. The granular layer is lost and there is a thin parakeratotic layer below the stratum corneum. There is also acanthosis and perivascular leukocyte infiltration of the dermis. The cause of the rash is unknown but it is unlikely to be a direct result of high circulating glucagon levels; low plasma/tissue zinc concentrations, hypoproteinemia, hypoaminoacidemia and the associated catabolic state may be involved.

### Clinical features

Most patients are middle-aged or elderly and the sexes are equally affected. Skin lesions are present in two-thirds of cases and start as annular of figurate erythema at intertriginous sites and around the mouth. The erythema becomes raised and central superficial bullae detach to leave erosions encircled by serous crusts. The lesions become confluent and serpiginous and heal, leaving hyperpigmentation. They are recurrent and migratory and particularly affect the face and the trunk. Secondary *Candida* infection is common, as is stomatitis, glossitis, angular cheilitis, nail dystrophy and vulvovaginitis. Typical necrolytic migratory erythema in the absence of glucagonoma has been termed "pseudoglucagonoma syndrome".

Other features include glucose intolerance (80% of cases), hypoaminoacidemia, weight loss, normochromic normocytic anemia, deep venous thrombosis with pulmonary embolism, psychiatric disturbance, diarrhea and vomiting. Giant intestinal villi have been recorded in a patient with glucagonoma (Stevens et al 1984). Visual scotomas and changes in visual acuity may develop.

### Diagnosis and localization

The diagnosis is confirmed by a raised fasting plasma glucagon concentration (in the absence of pancreatitis, trauma, severe illness, renal insufficiency and advanced liver disease). Normal levels range from 25–250 pg/ml but values above 500–1000 pg/ml are common in glucagonoma syndrome. Localization is as described above (p. 1302), but given the size of the tumor, CT scanning is usually reliable.

### Treatment

The syndrome is treated surgically whenever possible by eradicating the tumor or by debulking. Given the late presentation, cure is only possible in a minority of cases, but worthwhile and extended remission can often be achieved. Dacarbazine (Holst 1985) and streptozotocin may be useful. After apparently curative resection, plasma glucagon levels are monitored to detect recurrence. Recurrence is treated by chemotherapy, but patients who do not respond may obtain remission from their skin lesions by oral zinc and amino acid infusion (Norton et al 1979). Octreotide often relieves symptoms, probably by reducing glucagon levels and changing the responsiveness of target organs.

## SOMATOSTATINOMA (Creutzfeldt & Arnold 1993)

Less than 100 cases of this tumor have been reported.

### Pathology

Only some 30% of reported cases had tumors of the pancreas, elevated plasma somatostatin levels and the "typical" features of the somatostatinoma syndrome (see below). In the remainder, the tumor was in the duodenal mucosa, plasma somatostatin levels were normal and there was often associated Von Recklinghausen syndrome, MEN-II, pheochromocytoma or carcinoid tumor. Somatostatin cell hyperplasia of the stomach and duodenum has also been described in a female with dwarfism, obesity, dry mouth and goiter (Holle et al 1986).

On microscopy, somatostatinomas usually resemble a well-differentiated islet cell or carcinoid tumor. Ultrastructurally, the secretory granules are typical D-cell granules, but most tumors contain other hormones such as calcitonin, VIP, cortisol, PP and gastrin.

### Clinical features

The peak age of presentation is around 50 years and males and females are affected equally. The inhibitory effects of somatostatin explain the common occurrence of diabetes mellitus (usually mild), cholelithiasis, diarrhea and/or steatorrhea (secondary to inhibition of pancreatic secretion) and hypochlorhydria. Epigastric pain, weight loss and anemia are common. Some patients have features such as flushing, tachycardia, hypokalemia and hypoglycemia, which are unlikely to be due to increased somatostatin levels.

### Diagnosis and localization

This is confirmed by finding a raised plasma somatostatin-like immunoreactivity (SLI). Because the tumor is usually large before it produces enough hormone to cause the syndrome, plasma SLI is often measured only after a tumor has already been found at surgery. Other endocrinopathy, especially insulinoma or Cushing's syndrome, may be present. Increased SLI also occurs with medullary carcinoma of the thyroid, small cell lung cancer, pheochromocytomas and catecholamine-producing extra-adrenal paragangliomas. When basal plasma SLI concentrations are normal but somatostatinoma is suspected, the intravenous tolbutamide test and calcium-pentagastrin test can be used to induce a marked increase in plasma SLI (Pipeleers et al 1983). The mechanisms of SLI release probably differ and not all somatostatinomas respond identically to the two tests (Budmiger et al 1987). The value of these tests remains uncertain.

Because the tumors are often large, CT scanning is usually a reliable method of localization.

### Treatment

The surgical and chemotherapeutic management is similar to that of glucagonoma and VIPoma (see above). Twelve of the 20 patients reviewed by Boden & Shimoyama (1985) had surgical treatment, four had chemotherapy and two had surgery plus chemotherapy. At the time of writing, eight of the 20 had died at intervals ranging from 1 week to 14 months from treatment.

## OTHER HORMONE-PRODUCING TUMORS (O'Dorisio & Vinik 1985)

Pancreatic polypeptide is produced in excess by PP-cell tumors of the pancreas, mixed cell tumors and PP-cell hyperplasia. PP-cell tumors may produce abdominal pain and weight loss (Strodel et al 1984) but there are no symptoms specific to pancreatic polypeptide. The tumor is malignant in 50% of cases. PP is also increased in at least 50% of gastrinomas, insulinomas, VIPomas, glucagonomas and carcinoids (Polak et al 1976). Many islet cell tumors contain several different peptides, yet the symptoms are usually characteristic of only one (Larsson 1978). However, the symptoms may change from those produced by one hormone to those caused by another.

Pancreatic tumors occasionally produce extrapituitary growth hormone-releasing factor (GRF) in association with acromegaly. The peptide has also been found in a jejunal gastrinoma (Antonioli et al 1987) and islet cells (Rivier et al 1982) but is mainly confined to the brain.

Diarrhea can be a feature of endocrine tumors other than VIPoma. High circulating prostaglandin levels are found in carcinoid syndrome, medullary carcinoma of the thyroid and some cases of VIPoma (Jaffe & Condon 1976) and may be responsible for the diarrhea. Calcitonin can also produce secretory diarrhea and is produced in excess by medullary carcinomas of the thyroid. This tumor can also contain 5-HT, ACTH, somatostatin, substance P, calcitonin gene-related peptide and gastrin-releasing peptide (Ghatel et al 1985).

## NONFUNCTIONING ISLET CELL TUMORS

Older estimates that nonfunctioning tumors accounted for 15–41% of all islet cell tumors (Cheslyn-Curtis et al 1993) are now replaced by estimates of 55–65% (Venkatesh et al 1990, Van Heerden & Thompson 1993). The tumors are usually solitary and most are in the head of the gland. Some authors regard virtually all nonfunctioning tumors as malignant, as defined by their capacity for uncontrolled local growth and metastasis (Evans et al 1993), and the proportion of patients with distant metastases at presentation ranges from 49% to 91% (Venkatesh et al 1990). As with functioning tumors, histology reveals small uniform cells in cords or nests and the absence of local invasion does not mean that the tumor is benign. Immunoperoxidase staining and ultrastructural examination reveal production or storage of one of more hormones in most cases, despite the lack of symptoms or high circulating hormone levels.

Men and women are equally affected and the mean age of presentation is in the fifth decade (Venkatesh et al 1990). As with adenocarcinoma of the pancreas, patients frequently present with pain, jaundice and an abdominal mass. Gastrointestinal bleeding can occur from erosion of tumor into the stomach or the development of varices following splenic vein thrombosis. In contrast to adenocarcinoma, performance status is usually preserved and weight loss and back pain are less common (Evans et al 1993).

Computed tomography is a reliable means of detecting the tumors and their metastases. The tumor distorts the contour of the gland and on bolus infusion of contrast there is peripheral enhancement. In the 26 patients reviewed by Eelkema et al (1984), the mass was identified in all but one case and was 3–24 cm in diameter. Metastases were present in 15 patients and the biliary or pancreatic ducts were dilated in four. In some patients the findings were indistinguishable from those of pancreatic adenocarcinoma and fine-needle aspiration biopsy was required for differentiation. However, when abdominal computed tomography demonstrates a large, heterogeneous pancreatic mass containing areas of calcification or hyperdensity on contrast enhancement, the diagnosis of islet cell carcinoma should be suspected. If angiography is undertaken, the mass is usually hypervascular.

Resectability rates range from 28% to 73%, but the figure of 44% in the 73 patients reported by Evans et al (1993) is perhaps representative. In this series, median survival following curative resection was 6.8 years. A median survival of 4.7 years in unresected nonmetastatic tumor calls into question the role of heroic and potentially dangerous debulking surgery. Even when distant metastases are present, 5-year survival rates of some 40% have been reported (Evans et al 1993). The role of chemotherapy in management is discussed above (p. 1304).

## REFERENCES


Abe M, Shibamoto Y, Takahashi M et al 1987 Intraoperative radiotherapy in carcinoma of the stomach and pancreas. World Journal of Surgery 11: 459–464

Alanen K A, Joensuu H 1993 Long-term survival after pancreatic adenocarcinoma – often a misdiagnosis? British Journal of Cancer 68: 1004–1005

Allen-Mersh T G, Earlam R J 1986 Pancreatic cancer in England and Wales: surgeons look at epidemiology. Annals of the Royal College of Surgeons of England 68: 154

Alles A J, Warshaw A l, Southern J F, Compton C L, Lewandrowski K B 1994 Expression of CA 72–4 (TAG 72) in the fluid contents of pancreatic cysts. Annals of Surgery 219: 131–134

Almoguera C, Shibata D, Forrester K, Martin J, Arnheim N, Perucho M 1988 Most human carcinomas of the exocrine pancreas contain mutant c-K-*ras* genes. Cell 53: 549–554

American Cancer Society 1977 Cancer facts and figures. American Cancer Society, New York

Antonioli D A, Dayal Y, Dvorak A M, Banks P A 1987 Zollinger–Ellison syndrome. Cure by surgical resection of a jejunal gastrinoma containing growth hormone releasing factor. Gastroenterolgy 92: 814

Aoki K, Ogawa H 1978 Cancer of the pancreas: international mortality trend. World Health Statistics Quarterly 31: 2–26

Arlen M, Brockunier A 1967 Clinical manifestations of carcinoma of tail of the pancreas. Cancer 20: 1920

Auld C D, Beastall G H, Schlinkert R, Carter D C 1988 Surgical treatment of insulinomas of the pancreas. Journal of the Royal College of Surgeons of Edinburgh 33: 132–137

Bakkevold K E, Kambestand B 1993 Morbidity and mortality after radical and palliative pancreatic cancer surgery. Risk factors influencing the short-term results. Annals of Surgery 217: 356–368

Bakkevold K E, Pettersen A, Arnesjø B, Espehaug B 1990 Tamoxifen therapy in unresectable adenocarcinoma of the pancreas and papilla of Vater. British Journal of Surgery 77: 725–730

Bakkevold K E, Arnesjø B, Dahl O, Kambestad B 1993 Adjuvant combination chemotherapy (DMF) following radical resection of carcinoma of the pancreas and papilla of Vater. Results of a controlled prospective randomised multicentre study. European Journal of Cancer 29: 698–703

Baumel H, Huguier M, Manderscheid J C, Fabre J M, Houry S, Fagot H 1994 Results of resection for cancer of the exocrine pancreas: a study from the French Association of Surgery. British Journal of Surgery 81: 102–107

Becker V, Stommer P 1993 Pathology and classification of tumours of the pancreas. In: Trede M, Carter D C (eds) Surgery of the pancreas. Churchill Livingstone, Edinburgh

Beger H D, Schoenberg M H, Birk D 1994 The method of preoperative clinical staging. European experience. International Journal of Pancreatology 16: 109–112

Bickerstaff K I, Berry A R, Chapman R W, Britton B J 1990 Endoscopic sphincterotomy for the palliation of ampullary carcinoma. British Journal of Surgery 77: 160–162

Blamey S L, Fearon K C H, Gilmour W H, Osborne D H, Carter D C 1983 Prediction of risk in biliary surgery. British Journal of Surgery 70: 535–538

Bloom S R, Christofides N D, Yiangou Y, Blank M A, Tatemoto K, Polak J M 1983 Peptide histidine isoleucine (PHI) and Verner–Morrison syndrome. Gut 24: 473

Blumgart L H, Kennedy A 1973 Carcinoma of the ampulla of Vater and duodenum. British Journal of Surgery 60: 33

Boden G, Shimoyama R 1985 Somatostatinoma. In: Cohen S, Soloway R D (eds) Hormone-producing tumors of the gastrointestinal tract. Churchill Livingstone, Edinburgh, p 85

Bodner E, Glaser K 1993 Intraoperative needle aspiration biopsy. In: Trede M, Carter D C (eds) Surgery of the pancreas. Churchill Livingstone, Edinburgh

Booth I W, Fenton T R, Milla P J, Harries J T 1983 A pathophysiological study of the intestinal manifestations of a vasoactive intestinal peptide, calcitonin and catecholamine-secreting tumour. Gut 24: 954

Bornman P C, Harries-Jones E P, Tobias R, van Stiegmann G, Terblanche J 1986 Prospective controlled trial of transhepatic biliary endoprosthesis versus bypass surgery for incurable carcinoma of head of pancreas. Lancet 1: 69

Bowden L, Die Goyanes A 1970 Cancer of the body and tail of the pancreas. In: Glass G B J (ed) Progress in gastroenterology, Vol 2. Grune and Stratton, New York, p 356

Buchler M, Friess H, Schultheiss K-H et al 1991 A randomized controlled trial of adjuvant immunotherapy (murine monoclonal antibody 494/32) in resectable pancreatic cancer. Cancer 68: 1507–1512

Budmiger H, Buhler H, Hacki W, Stamm B, Streuli R, Ammann R 1987 Comparative diagnostic value of the calcium-pentagastrin test versus the tolbutamide test in a patient with a somatostatinoma. Gastroenterology 92: 800

Burney P G J, Comstock G W, Morris J S 1989 Serologic precursors of cancer. Serum micronutrients and the subsequent risk of pancreatic cancer. American Journal of Clinical Nutrition 49: 895–900

Cameron J L, Pitt H A, Yeo C J, Lillemoe K D, Kaufman H S, Coleman J 1993 One hundred and forty-five consecutive pancreaticoduodenectomies without mortality. Annals of Surgery 217: 430–438

Cancer Research Campaign 1989 Facts on cancer. Cancer Research Campaign, London

Cannobio L, Boccardo F, Cannata D, Gallotti P, Epis R 1992 Treatment of advanced pancreatic carcinoma with the somatostatin analogue BIM 23014. Cancer 69: 648–650

Capella C, Polak J M, Buffa R et al 1983 Morphologic patterns and diagnostic criteria of VIP-producing endocrine tumors. A histologic, histochemical, ultrastructural, and biochemical study of 32 cases. Cancer 52: 1860

Carter D C 1980 Surgery for pancreatic cancer. British Medical Journal 280: 744

Carter D C 1992 Cancer of the head of the pancreas or chronic pancreatitis? A diagnostic dilemma. Surgery 111: 602–603

Carter D C 1993 Aetiology and epidemiology of pancreatic and periampullary cancer. In: Trede M, Carter D C (eds) Surgery of the pancreas. Churchill Livingstone, Edinburgh

Carter S K, Comis R L 1975 The integration of chemotherapy into a combined modality approach for cancer treatment. VI. Pancreatic adenocarcinoma. Cancer Treatment Reviews 2: 193

Cersosimo E, Pisters P W T, Pesola G, McDermott K, Bajorunas D, Brennan M F 1991 Insulin secretion and action in patients with pancreatic cancer. Cancer 67: 486–493

Cherry D A, Gourlay G K, Cousins M J, Gannon B J 1985 A technique for the insertion of an implantable portal system for the long-term

epidural administration of opioids in the treatment of cancer pain. Anaesthesia and Intensive Care 13: 145
Cheslyn-Curtis S, Sitaram V, Williamson R C N 1993 Management of non-functioning neuroendocrine tumours of the pancreas. British Journal of Surgery 80: 625–627
Clark L R, Jaffe M H, Choyke P L, Grant E K, Zeman R K 1985 Pancreatic imaging. Radiologic Clinics of North America 23: 489
Compagno J, Oertel J E 1978a Mucinous cystic neoplasms of the pancreas with overt and latent malignancy (cystadenocarcinoma and cystadenoma). A clinicopathologic study of 41 cases. American Journal of Clinical Pathology 69: 573
Compagno J, Oertel J E 1978b Microcystic adenomas of the pancreas (glycogen-rich cystadenomas). American Journal of Clinical Pathology 69: 289
Creutzfeldt W, Arnold R 1993 Endocrine tumours of the pancreas: clinical picture, diagnosis and therapy. In: Trede M, Carter D C (eds) Surgery of the pancreas. Churchill Livingstone, Edinburgh
Cubilla A L, Fitzgerald P J 1978 Pancreas cancer. 1. Duct adenocarcinoma. A clinical-pathologic study of 380 patients. In: Sheldon-Summers C (ed) Pathology annual, Vol 1. Appleton-Century-Crofts, New York, p 241
Cubilla A L, Fitzgerald P J 1984 Tumors of the exocrine pancreas. In: Atlas of tumor pathology, second series. Armed Forces Institute of Pathology, Washington DC
Cubilla A L, Fortner J, Fitzgerald P J 1987 Lymph node involvement in carcinoma of the head of the pancreas. Cancer 41: 880
Cullinan S, Moertel C G, Wieand H S et al 1990 A phase III trial of therapy of advanced pancreatic carcinoma. Evaluations of the Mallinson regimen and combined 5-fluorouracil, doxorubicin and cisplatin. Cancer 65: 2207–2212
Danes B S, Lynch H T 1982 A familial aggregation of pancreatic cancer. An in vitro study. Journal of the American Medical Association 247: 2798
Danforth D N, Gorden P, Brennan M F 1984 Metastatic insulin-secreting carcinoma of the pancreas: clinical course and the role of surgery. Surgery 96: 1027–1035
Di Magno E P 1994 Preoperative staging of pancreatic ductal cancer in the USA. International Journal of Pancreatology 16: 112–114
Di Magno E P, Regan P T, Cain J E, James E M, Buxton J L 1982 Human endoscopic ultrasonography. Gastroenterology 83: 824–829
Doppman J L, Miller D L, Chang R et al 1991 Insulinomas: localization with selective intra-arterial injection of calcium. Radiology 178: 237–241
Durbec J P, Chevillotte G, Bidart J M, Berthezene P, Sarles H 1983 Diet, alcohol, tobacco and the risk of pancreatic cancer: a case-controlled study. British Journal of Cancer 47: 463–470
Edge S B, Scmieg R E, Rosenlof L K, Wilhelm M C 1993 Pancreas cancer resection outcome in American University centers in 1989–1990. Cancer 71: 3502–3508
Eelkema E A, Stephens D H, Ward E M, Sheedy P F 1984 CT features of nonfunctioning islet cell carcinoma. American Journal of Roentgenology 143: 943–948
Emory R E, Emory T S, Goellner J R, Grant C S, Nagorney D M 1994 Neuroendocrine ampullary tumors: spectrum of disease including the first report of a neuroendocrine carcinoma of non-small cell type. Surgery 115: 762–766
Eriksson B, Skogseid B, Lundqvist G et al 1990 Medical treatment and long-term survival in a prospective study of 84 patients with endocrine pancreatic tumors. Cancer 65: 1883–1890
Evans D B, Skibber J M, Lee J E et al 1993 Nonfunctioning islet cell carcinoma of the pancreas. Surgery 114: 1175–1182
Evans W K, Ho C-S, McLaughlin M J, Tao L C 1981 Fatal necrotizing pancreatitis following fine-needle aspiration biopsy of the pancreas. Radiology 141: 61
Falconer J S, Fearon K C H, Plester C E, Ross J A, Carter D C 1994a Cytokines, the acute phase response, and resting energy expenditure in cachectic patients with pancreatic cancer. Annals of Surgery 219: 325–331
Falconer J S, Ross J A, Fearon K C H, Hawkins R A, O'Riordain M G, Carter D C 1994b Effect of eicosapentaenoic acid and other fatty acids on the growth *in vitro* of human pancreatic cancer cell lines. British Journal of Cancer 69: 826–832
Falconer J S, Fearon K C H, Ross J A, Elton R E, Wigmore S J, Garden O J, Carter D C 1995 The acute phase protein response and duration of survival in patients with pancreatic cancer. Cancer 75: 2077–2082
Fønnebø V, Helseth A 1991 Cancer incidence in Norwegian Seventh-day Adventists 1961 to 1986. Cancer 68: 666–671
Fortner J G 1984 Regional pancreatectomy for cancer of the pancreas, ampulla, and other related sites. Tumor staging and results. Annals of Surgery 199: 418
Fortner J G, Kim D K, Cubilla A, Turnbull A, Pahnke L D, Shils M E 1977 Regional pancreatectomy: en bloc pancreatic, portal vein and lymph node resection. Annals of Surgery 186: 42
Frantz V K 1959 Tumors of the pancreas. In: Atlas of tumor pathology, section VII, fascicle 27. Armed Forces Institute of Pathology, Washington DC
Fras I, Litin E M, Bartholomew L G 1968 Mental syndrome as an aid in the early diagnosis of carcinoma of the pancreas. Gastroenterology 55: 191
Freeny P C 1989 Radiologic diagnosis and staging of pancreatic ductal adenocarcinoma. Radiologic Clinics of North America 27: 121–128
Freeny P C, Lawson T C 1982 Radiology of the pancreas. Springer Verlag, New York
Frey C, Twomey P, Keehn R, Elliott D, Higgins G 1981 Randomised study of 5-FU and CCNU in pancreatic cancer: report of the Veterans Administration Surgical Adjuvant Cancer Chemotherapy Study Group. Cancer 47: 27–31
Friedman A C, Lichtenstein J E, Dachman A H 1983 Cystic neoplasms of the pancreas. Radiological-pathological correlation. Radiology 149: 45
Friess H, Yamanaka Y, Buchler M et al 1993a Enhanced expression of transforming growth factor β isoforms in pancreatic cancer correlates with decreased survival. 105: 1846–1856
Friess H, Buchler M, Beglinger Ch, Weber A, Kunz J, Fritsch K, Beger H G 1993b Low dose octreotide treatment is not effective in patients with advanced pancreatic cancer. Pancreas 14: 290–291
Gastrointestinal Tumor Study Group 1981 Therapy of locally resectable pancreatic carcinoma: randomised comparison of high dose (6000 rads) radiation alone, moderate dose (4000 rads) radiation and high dose radiation and 5-fluorouracil. Cancer 48: 1705–1710
Gastrointestinal Tumor Study Group 1987 Further evidence of effective adjuvant combined radiation and chemotherapy following curative resection of pancreatic cancer. Cancer 59: 2006–2010
Gastrointestinal Tumor Study Group 1988 Treatment of locally unresectable carcinoma of the pancreas: comparison of combined-modality therapy (chemotherapy plus radiotherapy) to chemotherapy alone. Journal of the National Cancer Institute 80: 751–755
Geoghegan J G, Jackson J E, Lewis M P N et al 1994 Localization and surgical management of insulinomas. British Journal of Surgery 81: 1025–1028
Ghadirian P, Simard A, Baillargeon J 1991 Tobacco, alcohol and coffee and cancer of the pancreas. A population-based case-control study in Quebec, Canada. Cancer 67: 2664–2670
Ghatel M A, Springall D R, Nicholl C G, Polak J M, Bloom S R 1985 Gastrin-releasing peptide-like immunoreactivity in medullary thyroid carcinoma. American Journal of Clinical Pathology 84: 581
Gillespie J, Poston G J, Schacter M, Guillou P J 1992 Human pancreatic cancer cell lines do not express receptors for somatostatin. British Journal of Cancer 66: 483–487
Gold E B, Gordis L, Diener M D 1985 Diet and other risk factors for cancer of the pancreas. Cancer 55: 460–467
Gordis L, Gold E B 1984 Epidemiology of pancreatic cancer. World Journal of Surgery 8: 808–821
Greenway B, Iqbal M J, Johnson P J, Williams R 1983 Low serum testosterone concentrations in patients with carcinoma of the pancreas. British Medical Journal 286: 93
Griffin J F, Smalley S R, Jewell W, Paradelo J C, Reymond R D, Hassanein R E S, Evans R G 1990 Patterns of failure after curative resection of pancreatic carcinoma. Cancer 66: 56–61
Gudjonsson B 1987 Cancer of the pancreas. 50 years of surgery. Cancer 60: 2284–2303
Gudjonsson B, Livstone E M, Spiro H M 1978 Cancer of the pancreas. Diagnostic accuracy and survival statistics. Cancer 42: 2494
Gullo L, Pezzilli R, Morselli-Labate A M and the Italian Pancreatic

Cancer Study Group 1994 Diabetes and the risk of pancreatic cancer. New England Journal of Medicine 331: 81–84
Haddock G, Carter D C 1990 Aetiology of pancreatic cancer. British Journal of Surgery 77: 1159–1166
Haenszel W, Kurihara M 1968 Studies of Japanese migrants. I. Mortality from cancer and other diseases among Japanese in the United States. Journal of the National Cancer Institute 40: 43–68
Hatzitheoklitos E, Buchler M W, Friess H et al 1994 Carcinoid of the ampulla of Vater: clinical characteristics and morphological features. Cancer 73: 1580–1588
Hirayama T 1981 A large-scale cohort study on the relationship between diet and selected cancer of digestive organs. In: Correa P, Kipkin M, Tannebaums S, Wilkins S (eds) Banbury report no: 7. Gastrointestinal cancer. Endogenous factors. Cold Spring Harbor Laboratory, Cold Spring Harbor
Holle G E, Spann W, Eisenmenger W, Riedel J, Pradayrol L 1986 Diffuse somatostatin-immunoreactive D-cell hyperplasia in the stomach and duodenum. Gastroenterology 91: 733–739
Holst J J 1985 Glucagon-producing tumors. In Cohen S, Soloway R D (eds) Hormone-producing tumors of the gastrointestinal tract. Churchill Livingstone, Edinburgh, p 57
Howard J M 1989 Cystic neoplasms and true cysts of the pancreas. Surgical Clinics of North America 69: 651–665
Howatson A G, Carter D C 1985 Pancreatic carcinogenesis – enhancement by cholecystokinin in the hamster-nitrosamine model. British Journal of Cancer 51: 107
Huibregtse K, Carr-Locke D L, Cremer M et al 1992 Biliary stent occlusion – a problem solved with self-expanding stents? Endoscopy 24: 391–394
Ihse I, Andren-Sandberg A 1993 Percutaneous fine-needle aspiration cytology. In: Trede M, Carter D C (eds) Surgery of the pancreas. Churchill Livingstone, Edinburgh
Ihse I, Isaksson G 1984 Pancreatic carcinoma: diagnosis and treatment. Clinics in Gastroenterology 13: 961
Ihse I, Lilja P, Arnesjo B, Bengmark S 1977 Total pancreatectomy for cancer. An appraisal of 65 cases. Annals of Surgery 186: 675
Iida Y, Nose O, Kai H et al 1980 Watery diarrhoea with a vasoactive intestinal peptide-producing ganglioneuroblastoma. Archives of Disease in Childhood 55: 929
Iseki M, Suzuki T, Koizumi Y et al 1986 Alpha-fetoprotein-producing pancreatoblastoma. A case report. Cancer 57: 1833
Jaffe B M, Condon S 1976 Prostaglandins E and F in endocrine diarrheagenic syndromes. Annals of Surgery 184: 516
Jagelman D G, de Cosse J J, Bussey H J R 1988 Upper gastrointestinal cancer in familial adenomatous polyposis. Lancet 1: 1149–1151
Jaschke W R, Manegold B C 1993 Palliative management with percutaneous and rendezvous techniques. In: Trede M, Carter D C (eds) Surgery of the pancreas. Churchill Livingstone, Edinburgh
Jennings P E, Coral A, Donald J J, Rode J, Lees W R 1989 Ultrasound-guided core biopsy. Lancet 1369–1371
John T G, Greig J D, Carter D C, Garden O J 1995 Carcinoma of the pancreatic head and periampullary region. Tumor staging with laparoscopy and laparoscopic ultrasonography. Annals of Surgery 221: 156–164
Johnson C D, Schwall G, Flechtenmacher J, Trede M 1993 Resection for adenocarcinoma of the body and tail of the pancreas. British Journal of Surgery 80: 1177–1179
Jones B A, Langer B, Taylor B R, Girotti M 1985 Periampullary tumors: which ones should be resected? American Journal of Surgery 149: 46
Kairaluoma M I, Myllyla V, Partio E et al 1985 Impact of new imaging techniques on survival in cancer of the head of the pancreas and the periampullary region. Acta Chirurgica Scandinavica 151: 69
Kaplan S J, Holbrook C T, McDaniel H G, Buntain W L, Crist W M 1980 Vasoactive intestinal peptide secreting tumors of childhood. American Journal of Disease in Childhood 134: 21
Kawarada Y, Takahashi K, Tabata M et al 1993 Surgical treatment for carcinoma of the papilla of Vater. Journal of HBP Surgery 1: 8–13
Kayahara M, Nagakawa T, Konishi I, Ueno K, Ohta T, Miyazaki I 1991 Clinicopathologic study of pancreatic carcinoma with particular reference to the invasion of the extrapancreatic neural plexus. International Journal of Pancreatology 10: 105–111
Kayahara M, Nagakawa T, Ueno K, Ohta T, Takeda T, Miyazaki I 1993 An evaluation of radical resection for pancreatic cancer based on the mode of recurrence as determined by autopsy and diagnostic imaging. Cancer 72: 2118–2123
Klapdor R 1993 Laboratory evaluation of pancreatic function and disease. In: Trede M, Carter D C (eds) Surgery of the pancreas. Churchill Livingstone, Edinburgh
Klein A, Clemens J, Cameron J L 1989 Periampullary neoplasms in von Recklinghausen's disease. Surgery 106: 815–819
Klinkenbijl J H G, Jeekel J, Schmitz P I M et al 1993 Carcinoma of the pancreas and periampullary region: palliation versus cure. British Journal of Surgery 80: 1575–1578
Klöppel G 1991 Editorial. International Journal of Pancreatology 8: 203–204
Klöppel G, Held H, Morohoshi T, Seifert G 1982 Klassification exokriner Pankreastumore. Histologische Untersuchungen an 167 autoptischen und 96 bioptischen Fällen. Pathologe 2: 319–328
Knox R A, Kingston R D 1986 Carcinoma of the ampulla of Vater. British Journal of Surgery 73: 72
Koelz A, Kraenzlin M, Gyr K et al 1987 Escape of the response to a long-acting somatostatin analogue (SMS 201–995) in patients with VIPoma. Gastroenterology 92: 527
Kondo H, Sugano K, Fukayama N et al 1994 Detection of point mutations in the K-*ras* oncogene at codon 12 in pure pancreatic juice for diagnosis of pancreatic carcinoma. Cancer 73: 1589–1594
Korc M 1991 Growth factors and pancreatic cancer. International Journal of Pancreatology 9: 87–91
Kraenzlin M E, Ch'ng J L C, Wood S M, Carr D H, Bloom S R 1985 Long-term treatment of a VIPoma with somatostatin analogue resulting in remission of symptoms and possible shrinkage of metastases. Gastroenterology 88: 185
Lack E E, Cassady J R, Levey R, Vawter G F 1983 Tumors of the exocrine pancreas in children and adolescents. American Journal of Surgical Pathology 7: 319
Lai E C S, Mok F P T, Fan S T, Lo C M, Chu K M, Liu C L, Wong J 1994 Preoperative drainage for malignant obstructive jaundice. British Journal of Surgery 81: 1195–1198
Lairmore T C, Wells S A 1993 Genetic testing for multiple endocrine neoplasia. British Journal of Surgery 80: 1092–1093
Lamberts S W J, Bakker W H, Reubi J-C, Krenning E P 1990 Somatostatin-receptor imaging in the localization of endocrine tumors. New England Journal of Medicine 323: 1246–1249
Larsson L-I 1978 PP-producing and mixed endocrine pancreatic pancreatic tumours. In: Bloom S R (ed) Gut hormones. Churchill Livingstone, Edinburgh, p 605
La Vecchia C, Negri E, Franceschi S, D'Avanzo B, Boyle P 1994 A case-control study of diabetes mellitus and cancer risk. British Journal of Cancer 70: 950–953
Leese T, Neoptolemos J P, West K P, Talbot I C, Carr-Locke D L 1986 Tumours and pseudotumours of the region of the ampulla of Vater: an endoscopic, clinical and pathological study. Gut 27: 1186
Leung J, Bowen-Wright M, Aveling W, Shorvon P, Cotton P B 1983 Coeliac plexus block for pain in pancreatic cancer and chronic pancreatitis. British Journal of Surgery 70: 730–732
Levin D L, Connelly R R, Devesa S S 1981 Demographic characteristics of cancer of the pancreas: mortality, incidence and survival. Cancer 47: 1456
Lewandrowski K B, Southern J F, Pins M R, Compton C L, Warshaw A L 1993 Cyst fluid analysis in the differential diagnosis of pancreatic cysts: a comparison of pseudocysts, serous cystadenomas, mucinous cystic neoplasms, and mucinous cystadenocarcinoma. Annals of Surgery 217: 41–47
Liehr R-M, Melnykovych G, Solomon T 1990 Growth effects of regulatory peptides on human pancreatic cancer lines PANC-1 and MIA PaCa-2. Gastroenterology 98: 1666–1674
Lightdale C J, Botet J F, Woodruff J M, Brennan M F 1991 Localization of endocrine tumors of the pancreas with endoscopic ultrasonography. Cancer 68: 1815–1820
Longnecker D S 1983 Carcinogenesis in the pancreas. Archives of Pathology and Laboratory Medicine 107–154
Longnecker D S, Wiebkin P, Schaeffer B K, Roebuck B D 1984 Experimental carcinogenesis in the pancreas. In: Richter G W, Epstein M A (eds) International review of experimental pathology, Vol 26. Academic Press, New York, p 177

Lowenfels A B, Maisonneuve P, Cavallini G et al 1993 Pancreatitis and the risk of pancreatic cancer. New England Journal of Medicine 328: 1433–1437

Lunderquist A 1985 The pancreas. Clinics in Gastroenterology 14: 355

Mack T M, Yu M C, Hanisch R, Henderson B E N 1986 Pancreas cancer and smoking, beverage consumption, and past medical history. Journal of the National Cancer Institute 76: 49–60

Mackie C R, Cooper M J, Lewis M H, Moossa A R 1979 Nonoperative differentiation between pancreatic cancer and chronic pancreatitis. Annals of Surgery 189: 480

Mallinson C N, Bloom S R, Warin A P et al 1974 A glucagonoma syndrome. Lancet 2: 1

Mallinson C N, Rake M O, Cocking J B et al 1980 Chemotherapy in pancreatic cancer: results of a controlled, prospective, randomised, multicentre trial. British Medical Journal 281: 1589

Manabe T, Ohshio G, Baba N et al 1989 Radical pancreatectomy for ductal cell carcinoma of the head of the pancreas. Cancer 64: 1132–1137

Mansour G M I, Cucchiaro G, Niotis M T et al 1989 Surgical management of pancreatic lymphoma. Archives of Surgery 124: 1287–1289

Maruchi N 1973 An epidemiologic study of pancreatic cancer with special reference to US-Japanese comparison. Japanese Journal of Cancer Clinics 19: 73–82

Marxsen J, Schmiegel W, Roder C et al 1994 Detection of the anti-p53 antibody response in malignant and benign pancreatic tissue. British Journal of Cancer 70: 1031–1034

McAfee M K, van Heerden J A, Adson M A 1989 Is proximal pancreatoduodenectomy with pyloric preservation superior to total pancreatectomy? Surgery 105: 347–351

McEntee G P, Nagorney D M, Kvols L K, Moertel C G, Grant C S 1990 Cytoreductive hepatic surgery for neuroendocrine tumors. Surgery 108: 1091–1096

McGill D B, Miller L J, Carney J A, Phillips S F, Go V L W, Schutt A J 1980 Hormonal diarrhea due to pancreatic tumor. Gastroenterology 79: 571

McMichael A J, McCall M G, Hartshorne J M, Woodings T L 1980 Patterns of gastro-intestinal cancer in European migrants to Australia: the role of dietary change. International Journal of Cancer 25: 431

McPherson G A D, Benjamin I S, Hodgson H J F, Bowley N B, Allison D J, Blumgart L H 1984 Preoperative percutaneous transhepatic biliary drainage: the results of a controlled trial. British Journal of Surgery 71: 371

Megibow A J, Bosniak M A, Ambos M A, Beranbaum E R 1981 Thickening of the celiac axis and/or superior mesenteric artery: a sign of pancreatic carcinoma on computed tomography. Radiology 141: 449

Miettinen M, Partanen S, Fraki O, Kivilaakso E 1987 Papillary cystic tumor of the pancreas: an analysis of cellular differentiation by electron microscopy and immunohistochemistry. American Journal of Surgical Pathology 11: 855–865

Miller A R, Nagorney D M, Sarr M G 1992 The surgical spectrum of hereditary pancreatitis in adults. Annals of Surgery 215: 39–43

Mills P K, Beeson W L, Abbey D E, Fraser G E et al 1988 Dietary habits and past medical history as related to fatal pancreas cancer risk among adventists. Cancer 61: 2578–2585

Mitrakou A, Fanelli C, Veneman T et al 1993 Reversibility of unawareness of hypoglycemia in patients with insulinomas. New England Journal of Medicine 329: 834–839

Miyazaki K, Funakoshi A, Nishihara S, Wasada T, Koga A, Ibayashi H 1986 Aberrant insulinoma in the duodenum. Gastroenterology 90: 1280

Moertel C G, Kvols L K, O'Connell M J, Rubin J 1991 Treatment of neuroendocrine carcinomas with combined etoposide and cisplatin. Cancer 68: 227–232

Moldow R E, Connelly R R 1968 Epidemiology of pancreatic cancer in Connecticut. Gastroenterology 55: 677

Moore D C, Bush W H, Burnett L L 1981 Coeliac axis block: a roentgenographic, anatomic study of technique and spread of solution in humans and corpses. Anaesthesia and Analgesia 60: 3609

Morohoshi T, Held G, Kloppel G 1983 Exocrine pancreatic tumours and their histological classification. A study based on 167 autopsy and 97 surgical cases. Histopathology 7: 645

Morohoshi T, Kanda M, Asanuma K, Klöppel C 1989 Intraductal papillary neoplasms of the pancreas. A clinicopathologic study of six patients. Cancer 64: 1329–1335

Mozell E, Stenzel P, Wolterine E A, Rosch J, O'Dorisio T M 1990 Functional endocrine tumours of the pancreas: clinical presentation, diagnosis and treatment. Current Problems in Surgery 27: 309–326

Muir C, Waterhouse J, Mack T (eds) 1987 Cancer incidence in five continents. Volume V, IARC Scientific Publications No. 88

Murugiah M, Windsor J A, Redhead D N, O'Neill J S, Suc B, Garden O J, Carter D C 1993 The role of selective visceral angiography in the management of pancreatic and periampullary cancer. World Journal of Surgery 17: 796–800

Nagakawa T, Kayahara M, Ueno K, Ohta T, Konishi I, Ueda N, Miyazaki I 1992 A clinicopathologic study on neural invasion in cancer of the pancreatic head. Cancer 69: 930–935

Nagakawa T, Kobayashi H, Ueno K et al 1993 The pattern of lymph node involvement in carcinoma of the head of the pancreas. International Journal of Pancreatology 13: 15–22

Nakase A, Matsumoto Y, Uchida K, Honjo I 1977 Surgical treatment of cancer of the pancreas and the periampullary region: cumulative results in 57 institutions in Japan. Annals of Surgery 185: 52–57

Neoptolemos J P, Talbot I C, Shaw D C, Carr-Locke D L 1988 Long-term survival after resection of ampullary carcinoma is associated independently with tumour grade and a new staging classification that assesses local invasiveness. Cancer 61: 1403–1407

Nix G A J J, Schmitz P I M, Wilson J H P, van Blankenstein M, Groeneveld C F M, Hofwijk R 1984 Carcinoma of the head of the pancreas. Therapeutic implications of endoscopic retrograde cholangiopancreatography findings. Gastroenterology 87: 37

Nordlinger B, Jeppsson B, El-Khoury W et al 1992 Tumours of Oddi: diagnosis and surgical treatment. HPB Surgery 5: 123–133

Norell S E, Ahlborn A, Erwald R 1986 Diet and pancreatic cancer: a case-control study. American Journal of Epidemiology 124: 894–902

Norton J A, Kahn C R, Schiebinger R, Gorschboth C, Brennan M F 1979 Amino acid deficiency and the skin rash associated with glucagonoma. Annals of Internal Medicine 91: 213

O'Dorisio T M, Mekhjian H S 1985 VIPoma syndrome. In: Cohen S, Soloway R D (eds ) Hormone-producing tumors of the gastrointestinal tract. Churchill Livingstone, Edinburgh, p 101

O'Dorisio T M, Vinik A I 1985 Pancreatic polypeptide- and mixed peptide-producing tumors of the gastrointestinal tract. In: Cohen S, Soloway R D (eds) Hormone-producing tumors of the gastrointestinal tract. Churchill Livingstone, Edinburgh, p 117

Okamoto A, Tsuruta K, Isawa T et al 1994 Intraoperative radiation therapy for pancreatic carcinoma. International Journal of Pancreatology 16: 157–164

Palmer K R, Kerr M, Knowles G, Cull A, Carter D C, Lennard R C F 1994 Chemotherapy prolongs survival in inoperable pancreatic carcinoma. British Journal of Surgery 81: 882–885

Pedrazzoli S, Pasquali C, Alfano d'Andrea A 1994 Surgical treatment of insulinoma. British Journal of Surgery 81: 672–676

Perez M M, Newcomer A D, Moertel C G, Go V L W, Di Magno E P 1983 Asseessment of weight loss, food intake, fat metabolism, malabsorption, and treatment of pancreatic insufficiency in pancreatic cancer. Cancer 52: 346

Perry L J, Stuart K, Stokes K R, Clouse M E 1994 Hepatic arterial chemoembolization for metastatic neuroendocrine tumours. Surgery 116: 1111–1117

Pipeleers D, Couturier E, Gepts W, Reynders J, Somers G 1983 Five cases of somatostatinoma: clinical heterogeneity and diagnostic usefulness of basal and tolbutamide-induced hypersomatostatinemia. Journal of Clinical Endocrinology and Metabolism 56: 1236

Pitt H A, Gomes A S, Lois J F, Mann L L, Deutsch L S, Longmire W P 1985 Does preoperative percutaneous biliary drainage reduce operative risk or increase hospital cost? Annals of Surgery 201: 545

Polak I M, Adrian T E, Bryant M G, Bloom S R, Heitz P H, Pearse A G E 1976 Pancreatic polypeptide in insulinomas, gastrinomas, vipomas, and glucagonomas. Lancet 1: 328–330

Pour P M, Runbe R G, Birt D 1981 Current knowledge of pancreatic carcinogenesis in the hamster and its relevance to human disease. Cancer 47: 1573–1587

Rasbach D A, van Heerden J A, Telander R L, Grant C S, Carney J A 1985 Surgical management of hyperinsulinism in the multiple

endocrine neoplasia, type 1 syndrome. Archives of Surgery 120: 584
Read N W, Read M G, Krejs G J, Hendler R S, Davis G, Fordtran J S 1982 A report of five patients with large-volume secretory diarrhea but no evidence of endocrine tumor or laxative abuse. Digestive Diseases and Sciences 27: 193
Reubi J C, Horisberger U, Essed C E, Jeekel J, Klijn J G H, Lamberts S W J 1988 Absence of somatostatin receptors in human exocrine pancreatic adenocarcinomas. Gastroenterology 95: 760–763
Reubi J C, Kvols L K, Nagorney D M et al 1990 Detection of somatostatin receptors in surgical and percutaneous needle biopsy samples of carcinoids and islet cell carcinomas. Cancer Research 50: 5969–5977
Rickaert F, Cremer M, Deviere J et al 1991 Intraductal mucin-hypersecreting neoplasms of the pancreas. A clinicopathologic study of eight patients. Gastroenterology 101: 512–519
Rivier J, Spiess J, Thorner M, Vale W 1982 Characterization of a growth hormone-releasing factor from a human pancreatic islet tumour. Nature 300: 276
Robertson J F R, Imrie C W, Hole D J, Carter D C, Blumgart L H 1987 Management of periampullary carcinoma. British Journal of Surgery 74: 816
Roblez-Diaz G, Diaz-Sanchez V, Mendez J P, Altamirano A, Wolpert E 1987 Low serum testosterone/dihydrotestosterone ratio in patients with pancreatic carcinoma. Pancreas 2: 684–687
Roldan G E, Gunderson L L, Nagorney D M et al 1988 External beam versus intraoperative and external beam irradiation for locally advanced pancreatic cancer. Cancer 61: 1110–1116
Rosch T, Braig C, Gain T et al 1992a Staging of pancreatic and ampullary carcinoma by endoscopic ultrasonography. Gastroenterology 102: 188–199
Rosch T, Lightdale C J, Botet J F et al 1992b Localization of pancreatic endocrine tumors by endoscopic ultrasonography. New England Journal of Medicine 326: 1721–1726
Rothmund M, Angelini L, Brunt M et al 1990 Surgery for benign insulinoma: an international review. World Journal of Surgery 14: 393–399
Rotman N, Pezet D, Fagniez P-L, Cherqui D, Celicout B, Lointier P 1994 Adenocarcinoma of the duodenum: factors influencing survival. British Journal of Surgery 81: 83–85
Rumancik W M, Megibow A J, Bosniak M A, Hilton S 1984 Metastatic disease to the pancreas: evaluation by computed tomography. Journal of Computer Assisted Tomography 8: 829
Ryan D P, Schapiro R H, Warshaw A L 1986 Villous tumors of the duodenum. Annals of Surgery 203: 301
Sackel S G, Manson J E, Harawi S J, Burakoff R 1985 Watery diarrhea syndrome due to an adrenal pheochromocytoma secreting vasoactive intestinal polypeptide. Digestive Diseases and Sciences 30: 1201
Sanfey H, Mendelsohn G, Cameron J L 1983 Solid and papillary neoplasm of the pancreas. Annals of Surgery 197: 272
Sarr M G, Cameron J L 1982 Surgical management of unresectable carcinoma of the pancreas. Surgery 91: 123–133
Scherubl H, Bader M, Fett U et al 1993 Somatostatin-receptor imaging of neuroendocrine gastroenteropancreatic tumors. Gastroenterology 105: 1705–1709
Schirmer W J, O'Dorisio T M, Schirmer T P et al 1993 Intraoperative localization of neuroendocrine tumors with $^{125}$I-TYR(3)-octreotide and a hand-held gamma-detecting probe. Surgery 114: 745–752
Schlippert W, Lucke D, Anuras S, Christensen J 1978 Carcinoma of the papilla of Vater. A review of fifty-seven cases. American Journal of Surgery 135: 763
Schwartz R W, Munfakh N A, Zwent T N et al 1994 Nonfunctioning cystic neuroendocrine neoplasms of the pancreas. Surgery 115: 645–649
Shapiro T M 1975 Adenocarcinoma of the pancreas: a statistical analysis of biliary bypass vs Whipple resection in good risk patients. Annals of Surgery 182: 715
Sharp K W, Ross C B, Halter S A et al 1989 Pancreatoduodenectomy with pyloric preservation for carcinoma of the pancreas: a cautionary note. Surgery 105: 645–653
Sigel B, Coelho J, Nyhus L M et al 1982 Detection of pancreatic tumors by ultrasound during surgery. Archives of Surgery 117: 1058
Simon B, Weinel R, Hohne M, Watz, J, Schmidt J, Kortner G, Arnold R 1994 Frequent alterations of the tumour suppressor genes p53 and DCC in human pancreatic carcinoma. Gastroenterology 106: 1645–1651
Smith A C, Dowsett J F, Russell R C G, Hatfield A R W, Cotton P B 1994 Randomised trial of endoscopic stenting versus surgical bypass in malignant low bile duct obstruction. Lancet 344: 1655–1660
Speer A G, Cotton P B, Russell R C G et al 1987 Randomised trial of endoscopic versus percutaneous stent insertion in malignant obstructive jaundice. Lancet i: 57–62
Spigelman A D, Williams C B, Talbot I C, Domizio P, Phillips R K S 1989 Upper gastrointestinal cancer in patients with familial adenomatous polyposis. Lancet 2: 783–785
Stamm B, Burger H, Hollinger A 1987 Acinar cell cystadenocarcinoma of the pancreas. Cancer 60: 2542–2547
Steinberg W 1990 The utility of the CA 19-9 tumour associated antigen. American Journal of Gastroenterology 85: 350–355
Stephens D H, Sheedy P F, James E M 1983 Neoplastic lesions. In: Margulis A R, Burhenne H J (eds) Alimentary tract radiology, 3rd edn. Part IX, Pancreas. C V Mosby, St Louis, p 1316
Stevens F M, Flanagan R W, O'Gorman D, Buchanan K D 1984 Glucagonoma syndrome demonstrating giant duodenal villi. Gut 25: 784
Stommer P, Kraus J, Stolte M, Giedl J 1991 Solid and cystic pancreatic tumors: clinical, histochemical, and electron microscopic features in ten cases. Cancer 67: 1635–1641
Strodel W E, Vinik A I, Lloyd R V et al 1984 Pancreatic polypeptide-producing tumors. Archives of Surgery 119: 508
Tada M, Yokosuka O, Omata M, Ohto M, Isono K 1990 Analysis of Ras gene mutations in biliary and pancreatic tumors by polymerase chain reaction and direct sequencing. Cancer 66: 930–935
Thompson N W, Czako P F, Fritts L L et al 1994 Role of endoscopic ultrasonography in the localization of insulinomas and gastrinomas. Surgery 116: 1131–1138
Tio T L, Mulder C J J, Eggink W F 1992 Endosonography in staging early carcinoma of the ampulla of Vater. Gastroenterology 102: 1392–1395
Tio T L 1993 Endoscopic ultrasonography. In: Trede M, Carter D C (eds) Surgery of the Pancreas. Churchill Livingstone, London.
Traverso L W, Longmire W P Jr 1978 Preservation of the pylorus in pancreaticoduodenectomy. Surgery, Gynecology and Obstetrics 146: 959
Trede M 1985 The surgical treatment of pancreatic carcinoma. Surgery 97: 28
Trede M 1993 The surgical options. In: Trede M, Carter D C (eds) Surgery of the pancreas. Churchill Livingstone, Edinburgh
Trede M, Schwall G, Saeger H D 1990 Survival after pancreaticoduodenectomy. 118 consecutive resections without an operative mortality. Annals of Surgery 211: 447–458
Tuckson W B, Goldson A L, Ashayeri E, Halyard-Richardson M, DeWitty R L, Leffall L 1988 Intraoperative radiotherapy for patients with carcinoma of the pancreas. Annals of Surgery 207: 648–653
Tsuchiya R, Noda T, Harada N et al 1986 Collective review of small carcinomas of the pancreas. Annals of Surgery 203: 77
Tsunoda T, Ura K, Eto T, Matsumoto T, Tsuchiya R 1991 UICC and Japanese stage classification for carcinoma of the pancreas. International Journal of Pancreatology 8: 205–214
Tsusumi M, Konishi Y 1990 Early pancreatic duct adenocarcinoma. Proceedings of the 4th Meeting of the International Association for Pancreatology, and the 3rd Symposium of the International Pancreatic Cancer Study Group 1: 193
Upp J R, Olson D, Poston G H, Alexander R W, Townsend C M, Thompson J C 1988 Inhibition of growth of two human pancreatic adenocarcinomas in vivo by somatostatin analog SMS 201–995. American Journal of Surgery 155: 29–35
Van den Bosch R P, van der Schelling G P, Klindenbijl J H G et al 1994 Guidelines for the application of surgery and endoprostheses in the palliation of obstructive jaundice in advanced cancer of the pancreas. Annals of Surgery 219: 18–24
Van Eijck C H J, Slooter G D, Hofland L J et al 1994 Somatostatin receptor-dependent growth inhibition of liver metastases by octreotide. British Journal of Surgery 81: 1333–1337
Van Heerden J A, Thompson G B 1993 Islet cell tumours of the pancreas. In: Trede M, Carter D C (eds) Surgery of the pancreas. Churchill Livingstone, Edinburgh

Van Heerden J A, Grant C S, Czako P F, Service J, Charboneau J W 1992 Occult functioning insulinomas: which localizing studies are indicated? Surgery 112: 1010–1015
Venkatesh S, Ordonez N G, Ajani J et al 1990 Islet cell carcinoma of the pancreas. Cancer 65: 354–357
Verner J V, Morrison A B 1958 Islet cell tumor and a syndrome of refractory watery diarrhea and hypokalemia. American Journal of Medicine 25: 374
Vinik A I, Delbridge L, Moattari R, Cho K, Thompson N 1991 Transhepatic portal vein catheterization for localization of insulinomas: a ten-year experience. Surgery 109: 1–11
Virgolini I, Raderer M, Kurtaran A et al 1994 Vasoactive intestinal peptide-receptor imaging for the localization of intestinal adenocarcinomas and endocrine tumors. New England Journal of Medicine 331: 1116–1121
Wade T P, Coplin M A, Virgo K S, Johnson F E 1994 Periampullary cancer treatment in U.S. Department of Veterans Affairs hospitals: 1987–1991. Surgery 116: 819–826
Warren K W, Christophi C, Armendariz R, Basu S 1983 Current trends in the diagnosis and treatment of carcinoma of the pancreas. American Journal of Surgery 145: 813
Warshaw A L, Rutledge P L 1987 Cystic tumors mistaken for pancreatic pseudocysts. Annals of Surgery 205: 393–398
Warshaw A L, Tepper J E, Shipley W U 1986 Laparoscopy in the staging and planning of therapy for pancreatic cancer. American Journal of Surgery 151: 76–79
Warshaw A L, Compton C C, Lewandrowski K, Cardenosa G, Mueller P R 1990 Cystic tumors of the pancreas. Annals of Surgery 212: 432–443
Watanapa P, Williamson R C N 1992 Surgical palliation for pancreatic cancer: developments during the past two decades. British Journal of Surgery 79: 8–20
Watson K J R, Shulkes A, Smallwood R A et al 1985 Watery diarrhea-hypokalemia-achlorhydria syndrome and carcinoma of the esophagus. Gastroenterology 88: 798
Webb T H, Lillemoe K D, Pitt H A, Jones R L, Cameron J L 1989 Pancreatic lymphoma: is surgery mandatory for diagnosis or treatment? Annals of Surgery 209: 25–30
Weinel R J, Neuhaus C, Stapp J et al 1993 Preoperative localization of gastrointestinal endocrine tumors using somatostatin-receptor scintigraphy. Annals of Surgery 218: 640–645
Weiss W, Bernarde M A 1983 The temporal relationship between cigarette smoking and pancreatic cancer. American Journal of Public Health 74: 1403–1404
Weissmann D, Lewandrowski K, Godine J, Centeno B, Warshaw A L 1994 Pancreatic cystic islet-cell tumors. International Journal of Pancreatology 15: 76–79
Wernecke K, Peters P E, Galanski M 1986 Pancreatic metastases: US evaluation. Radiology 160: 399
Wood S M, Kraenzlin M E, Adrian T B, Bloom S R 1985 Treatment of patients with pancreatic endocrine tumours using a new longacting somatostatin analogue: symptomatic and peptide responses. Gut 26: 438
Wynder E L 1975 An epidemiological evaluation of the causes of cancer of the pancreas. Cancer Research 35: 2228–2233
Yamada T, Murohisa B, Muto Y, Okamoto K, Doi K, Tsuchiya R 1984 Cytologic detection of small pancreaticoduodenal and biliary cancers in the early developmental stage. Acta Cytologica 28: 435
Yamamoto R, Tatsuta M, Noguchi S et al 1985 Histocytologic diagnosis of pancreatic cancer by percutaneous aspiration biopsy under ultrasonic guidance. American Journal of Clinical Pathology 83: 409
Yoshimi N, Sugie S, Tanaka T et al 1992 A rare case of serous cystadenocarcinoma of the pancreas. Cancer 69: 2449–2453
Zeman R K, Schiebler M, Clark L R et al 1985 The clinical and imaging spectrum of pancreaticoduodenal lymph node enlargement. American Journal of Roentgenology 144: 1223
Zerbi A, Fossati V, Parolini D et al 1994 Intraoperative radiation therapy adjuvant to resection in the treatment of pancreatic cancer. Cancer 73: 2930–2935

SECTION 14

# Colonic and anorectal disorders

# 52. Colorectal and anorectal motor dysfunctions

*D. C. C. Bartolo   W.-M. Sun*

Healthy intestinal function requires normal transit of gut contents through the small intestine, colon and rectum, followed by efficient and controlled evacuation of rectal contents during defecation. Small intestinal (p. 438) and colonic (p. 1345) physiology is considered elsewhere. Disorders of defecation occur either because control is impaired or lost or because evacuation is delayed or impaired. In this chapter, disorders of continence and evacuation will be considered. The structure of the anorectal region is discussed on page 1449.

## PHYSIOLOGY OF CONTINENCE

Continence depends on the social awareness of the need to control the contents of the rectum until it is appropriate to evacuate in a controlled manner.

### Rectal function

The rectum is a potentially capacious organ with the ability to store feces for variable periods of time. The initial rectal filling induces rectal contraction, followed by a decrease in pressure to a predistension level. This is known as the "accommodation response", a receptive relaxation of the rectal ampulla to accommodate the bowel contents. The rectum can often tolerate more than 300 ml and show no increase in rectal pressure.

### Internal sphincter function

The internal anal sphincter is tonically active at rest, thus keeping the anal canal closed and the perianal skin dry. It contributes to 50–60% of the basal anal pressure. $\alpha$-adrenergic impulses increase resting anal canal pressure, but the tone is primarily dependent on myogenic activity and intramural enteric nerves (Burleigh et al 1979, Bouvier & Gonella 1981, Burleigh 1983, Burleigh & D'Mello 1983, Bouvier et al 1986, 1987).

Fast distension of the rectum with air or liquid in an experimental setting induces relaxation of the internal sphincter via the intrinsic intramural nerves. In the presence of minimal distention, transient relaxation occurs, followed by recovery of internal anal sphincter tone. This latter reflex is known as the rectoanal inhibitory reflex, during which the anal epithelium "samples" the rectal contents. Perception in the anal canal is an important component of defecation and continence (p. 1316). With increasing volume of distention, the amplitude of relaxation becomes larger and its duration longer and, eventually, the amplitude reaches its maximal level. In this situation, the residual anal pressure is maintained by compensatory contraction of the external sphincter. The rectoanal inhibitory reflex is seen most dramatically in gross fecal impaction where, in the presence of weak external sphincter, the anal canal gapes widely.

### External sphincter function

This muscle is also tonically active at rest, contributing to 20–30% of the basal anal pressure (Floyd & Walls 1953, Walls 1959). It contains a high proportion of slow twitch type I muscle fibers which are capable of sustained contraction (Parks et al 1962, 1977, Parks 1975).

Normal skeletal muscle consists of a mosaic of type I and type II fibers. The former are rich in oxidative enzymes, and accordingly are capable of tonic contraction. Type II fibers contain phosphorylating enzymes, accumulate lactate and are prone to fatigue and are therefore useless for continence.

### Anorectal sensation

*Rectal sensation*

Specific sensations are experienced in the rectum with increasing volumes of content (gas, liquid or solid). These are fullness, a desire to defecate, an urgency to defecate, and ultimately pain. However, the rectum is relatively insensitive to pain caused by pinch or cut, temperature and light touch. In the rectal mucosa there are abundant beaded, non-myelinated, nerve fibers, but only one recognizable intraepithelial receptor ending has been identified. Tension at the site of the sensory endings, which may be within or external to the wall of the viscus, provides the stimulus for sensory appreciation. Some sensory endings are present in the walls of the viscera and behave as if they are "in series" with smooth muscle. Others, however, are outside the muscle layers, in the mesentery, and can respond to forces transmitted through mesenteric connections during contraction and distention. Nociceptors are also present in the mucosa and respond to high levels of pressure applied locally to their punctate endings. Rectal sensation can be assessed by the intermittent rectal distension method or the ramp inflation method (p. 1318).

### Anal sensation

The anal canal is extensively innervated with a profusion of sensory nerves. Duthie first demonstrated that the anal canal contained specialized sensory nerve endings, and that these could appreciate light touch, pain and temperature. The canal was more sensitive than the tip of the index finger and the tongue (Duthie & Gairns 1960, Duthie & Bennett 1963, Duthie & Watts 1965, Duthie 1971, 1975). Roe et al (1986) were able to quantitate anal sensation using a specialized probe which delivered minute electrical impulses to the anus. They found the threshold of sensation was of the order of 5 milliamps, whereas the rectum was insensitive to stimuli of over 25 milliamps. Miller et al (1987) demonstrated that temperature could be quantified and the anal canal, but not the rectum, was able to discriminate differences of temperature of 0.5°C. It was concluded that when the anal canal opens progressively in a funnel-like manner, small quantities of rectal contents descend into the anal canal and allow conscious perception of what is in the rectum. The mechanism is sensitive enough to discriminate solid from liquid and gas with virtual certainty. Appropriate action can then occur.

### Anorectal angle

Ambulatory studies and saline continence tests have shown that continence is the result of the anal canal generating a higher pressure than the rectum; incontinence occurs when the sphincter pressures are lower than those generated by the rectum (Bartolo et al 1983a,b, 1986a, Bartolo 1984, Bannister et al 1989). Parks et al (1986) determined that the angle between the rectal axis and the axis of the anal canal in normal subjects was approximately 90°. He observed that some patients with incontinence had obtuse anorectal angles associated with perineal descent. He proposed the flap valve theory of continence and suggested that continence depended not so much on sphincteric action as on the fact that in the presence of an acute anorectal angle, raised intra-abdominal pressure was transmitted to the anterior rectal wall, which was forced into and occluded the anus. Bartolo et al (1986a) studied rectal and anal pressures and external sphincter and puborectalis electromyogram during Valsalva maneuvers. Continence was preserved by sphincteric action with no evidence to substantiate the flap valve theory. Indeed, the anterior rectal wall was displaced away from the anal canal, which remained closed.

### Anal cushions

The anal cushions are three pads of vascular tissue lying underneath the anal epithelium and surrounding the anal canal (Fig. 56.4). They are composed of large blood spaces and are fed by arterioles. Histologically they resemble the erectile tissue of the penis. Analysis of anal wall tension, estimated by using probes of different diameters, indicates that the circular muscle fibers cannot shorten sufficiently enough to close the anal canal completely. The anal cushions could therefore provide an expansile packing which is able to seal the anal canal and maintain the anal pressure despite variation in the tone of the sphincter muscles. The importance of the anal cushions in preserving continence is emphasized by the occurrence of incontinence after more radical types of hemorrhoidectomy which excise the cushions.

## INVESTIGATIONS

Patients with incontinence, constipation, defecatory disorders and prolapse require intensive investigation to aid management. Investigations may be divided into manometric, radiological and neurophysiological. The first measure physical pressures, the second define anatomic variations and the last quantify neurological function.

### Anorectal manometry

*Indications*

Anorectal manometry is indicated in patients with incontinence or constipation not responding to simple measures. Manometry is particularly useful in an incontinent patient who has no evidence of anatomical defect of the anal sphincters. The questions that can be answered by manometric testing are whether the patient has low anal pressures, which sphincter is responsible for the weak anal function, whether the motor and sensory rectal responses to balloon distention are normal, whether the spinal reflex activity is intact, and whether the co-ordination between the rectum and the anal sphincters is normal.

Anorectal manometry is also performed before closing a stoma to ensure that the continence mechanism is preserved. It is also used to assess the success of anorectal surgery.

*Apparatus*

A number of techniques are used to measure anal sphincter pressure. Each technique has particular advantages and disadvantages and influences the pressure recorded.

***Water perfused catheter.*** An assembly that incorporates multiple side-hole sensors is the most commonly used recording device (Read & Sun 1992). This method is inexpensive, versatile and effective. The pressure is recorded in each catheter, which is perfused slowly using a pneumohydraulic pump. The pressure transducers are located outside the body, along the fluid line. Closely spaced sensors can generate a pressure profile along the rectum and anal canal with great accuracy and discriminate between external and internal sphincter activity (Sun et al 1989). They may be combined with a sleeve sensor (see below). This multiple-sidehole manometric technique can be combined with other functional tests — such as rectal distention and dynamic function assessment of anorectal function (see below). However, the disadvantage of the perfused system is that the number of perfusion sideholes may be limited, artifactual contractions may be induced by leakage of fluid in the anal canal, and the method is less useful for recording pressures in large hollow organs, for example rectal ampulla, unless contractions occlude the lumen.

***Sleeve sensor.*** The properties of the sleeve sensor make it ideal for prolonged or ambulatory recordings of anal sphincter pressure due to its relative tolerance of movement of the sphincter (Orkin et al 1991). However, it does not localize the highest pressure point in the anal canal and cannot discriminate between internal and external sphincter activity.

***Solid state probe and microtransducer.*** The microtransducers are mounted on a probe. This system offers high accuracy and fidelity. However, the instrument is fragile and expensive.

***Balloon catheter.*** Anal pressures are measured by two balloons placed in the anal canal, the proximal one measures internal sphincter pressure and the distal one measures external sphincter pressure (Schuster et al 1965). As the two sphincters overlap in the anal canal, the interpretation of the data is limited by the longitudinal arrangement of balloons. A modification using multiple microballoons has been tried (Belliveau et al 1983), but it is not widely used.

*Procedure*

Anorectal manometry is performed by static and ambulatory studies. These are done with concurrent measurement of electrical activity of sphincters (p. 1320) (Fig. 52.1). No bowel preparation is required. However, the patient is encouraged to empty the rectum before the study. If bowel preparation becomes necessary, a small volume enema is used, preferably 3–4 h before the test. Should clean-out of the entire colon be required, a minimum 12 h should be allowed prior to the procedure.

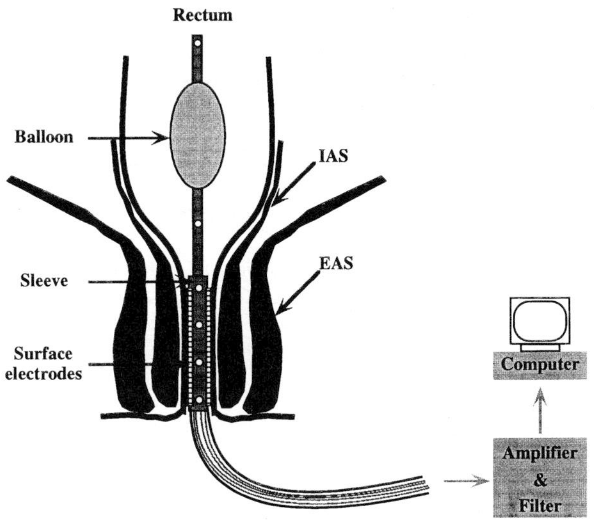


**Fig. 52.1** Diagram of the anal canal showing the different muscle components and the catheter used to measure pressure in multiple sites in the rectum and anal canal. The balloon is used for rectal distension and the intraluminal surface electrodes are used for recording electrical activity. The sleeve sensor situated in the anal canal is particularly useful for ambulatory recordings. IAS = internal anal sphincter, EAS = external anal sphincter.

***Static manometry.*** The study is usually performed in the laboratory. The patient lies in the left lateral position with the hips flexed to 90°. A lubricated catheter is then inserted anally. The internal and external sphincter function, rectal sensation, the rectoanal reflex, spinal reflex and the influence of cerebral control are then assessed.

***Ambulatory manometry.*** An ambulatory study is done using a portable computer while the subject carries out his/her usual daily life (e.g. during sleep and defecation). Event markers allow patients to register their symptoms or any adverse event, so that the correlation between an event and motor abnormality can be made.

*Interpretation* (Fig. 52.2)

***Basal pressure.*** Anal basal pressure has been assessed using three main techniques: station pull-through, rapid pull-through and recording under resting conditions. The latter is now commonly used because the other two methods unavoidably stimulate external sphincter activity.

Basal anorectal pressure is usually recorded for 10–20 min, during which it decreases to a stable level. The pressure recorded immediately after insertion of the catheter is the maximum anal pressure and the pressure recorded at a stable level is the minimum anal pressure. Under resting conditions the high pressure zone is about 2 cm long; this mainly reflects the internal sphincter activity.

The resting pressure in the anal canal undergoes regular fluctuations. These consist of slow waves (amplitude 5–25 mmHg; frequency 6–20 cpm) and much larger

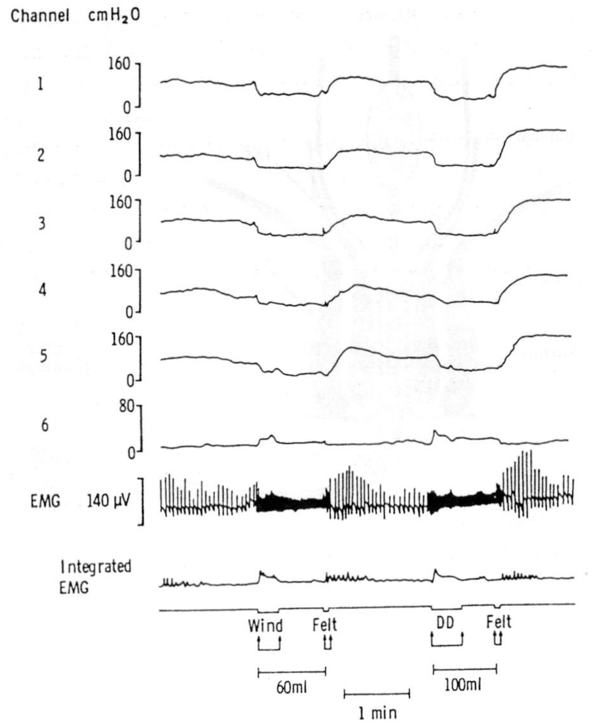


**Fig. 52.2** Recordings of anorectal pressure and the electrical activity of the external and internal sphincters in a normal subject during rectal balloon distension with 60 and 100 ml of air. Channels 1–6 represent ports situated 0.5, 1.0, 1.5, 2.0, 2.5 and 4.5 cm from the anal verge. Note that rectal distension induced increases in rectal pressure (6) and relaxation in sphincter pressure. The reduction in anal pressure was associated with abolition of the electrical oscillations produced by internal sphincter activity, and the residual anal pressure was maintained by an increase in the electrical activity of the external sphincter. Deflation of the balloon produced a rebound increase in pressure which is associated with marked increase in the slow wave oscillations. Rectal sensation of gas in the rectum (wind) and desire to defecate (DD) was elicited during distension. Deflation of the balloon also induced a transient perception of the rectal sensation (Felt). The dips along the horizontal line indicate the duration of each sensation.

amplitude, ultra-slow waves (amplitude 30–100 mmHg; frequency ≤3 cpm). It seems likely that slow and ultra-slow waves are generated by the internal sphincter, since electrical recordings from the internal sphincter show fluctuations at the same frequencies, and rectal distension reduces the tone of the internal sphincter and abolishes both electrical and pressure fluctuations.

The frequency of the internal sphincter slow wave is higher in the distal anal canal than in the proximal anal canal. This inwardly directed contraction gradient may function to encourage small amounts of material in the anal canal to move back into the rectum.

Ultra-slow waves are associated with particularly high resting pressures. They occur in about 40% of normal subjects, but only when the resting pressure is above 100 mmHg. Other workers have reported ultra-slow waves in only 5% of normal subjects, but in 30–45% of patients with hemorrhoids and 67–80% of patients with anal fissures. Resting sphincter pressures are often very high in both of these conditions (Sun et al 1992).

Resting anal pressure is reduced in patients with meningocele, spinal shock, spinal anesthesia and patients who have had a sacral resection with ablation of sacral nerves on one or both sides. It is not, however, lowered in patients with chronic paraplegia.

***Squeeze pressure.*** The squeeze pressure is recorded when the subject contracts the external sphincter maximally — the so-called "squeeze". During this maneuver the high pressure zone lengthens to 2.5–3 cm. Voluntary contraction elevates the pressure throughout the anal canal, but the pressure rise is maximal in the lower canal where the bulk of the external sphincter is situated. Pressures induced by voluntary contraction are higher in males compared with females and are reduced with aging.

The external sphincter contributes 15–20% of the total resting anal pressure. Resting anal pressure is increased in the upright posture and is associated with an increased electrical activity in the external sphincter. Coughing, or increases in intra-abdominal pressure also increase the external sphincter activity, possibly by stimulation of tension receptors in the pelvic floor. This is a spinal reflex activity. Squeeze pressure is reduced with damage to the pudendal nerves, spinal cord or central nervous system and with anal mucosal or spinal anesthesia.

***Rectal pressures.*** The rectum is often quiescent under normal resting conditions with a basal pressure of about 5 mmHg. Arrival of fecal material or gas in the rectum may stimulate rectal contraction. Three major types of rectal contractile activity have been described: runs of contractions occurring at a frequency of 5–10 cpm; sporadic slower contractions, occurring at a frequency of about 3 cpm; and slow contractions of similar characteristics that appear to propagate through the rectum lasting 80–90 min during the day and 50–60 min during the night.

***Rectal activity.*** This is measured by means of rectal distention. Three different methods are routinely used. Intermittent distension is used to mimic the rapid arrival of fecal material into the rectum; this is carried out with a hand-held syringe and the insertion of air at about 40 ml/s. Ramp inflation distends the rectum continuously at a constant rate by means of a peristaltic pump, which is usually much slower than the intermittent distension, at 10–100 ml/min. Rectal distension can also be studied by a barostat technique, with which the rectum is distended either isovolumetrically or isobarically. The compliance of the rectum is derived by calculating the changes in volume over the changes in pressure (dV/dP).

The phasic contractile response to rectal distension is reduced or absent in patients with lesions involving the low spinal cord, suggesting that it is mediated by a spinal reflex. Rectal tone is increased and compliance reduced in patients with a high spinal lesion, while in patients with low spinal lesions rectal tone is reduced and compliance increased (MacDonagh et al 1992). In patients with irritable bowel syndrome both phasic and tonic rectal activity are enhanced.

***Rectal sensation.*** Rectal sensation occurs during rectal distension. The onset and duration of rectal sensation are indicated by the subject pressing an event marker. Abnormal rectal sensations include hypersensitivity, hyposensitivity or delayed sensation (Sun et al 1992).

***Rectoanal inhibitory reflex*** (see p. 1315). This is associated with suppression of internal sphincter electrical oscillations. As the rectal balloon is distended with larger volumes, the amplitude and duration of the relaxation increases.

***External sphincter excitatory response to rectal distension.*** Intermittent distension of a rectal balloon induces a transient increase in anal pressure, which is associated with an increase in the electrical activity of the external sphincter. This reduces to a steady state which increases in amplitude and duration as the rectal volume increases. Very high levels of rectal distension can be associated with an abolition of external sphincter activity causing a profound reduction in anal pressure. This is rare in healthy subjects with rectal volumes of up to 200 ml. The initial external sphincter response to rectal distension is most likely to be a spinal reflex because it is preserved in patients with complete high spinal lesions but diminished after a posterior rhizotomy (Sun et al 1995). It is also absent in patients with low spinal lesions. However, the secondary, prolonged response involves a conscious mechanism because of its close temporal relationship to the conscious perception of the rectal sensation. In patients with complete high spinal lesions this second response is absent (Sun et al 1990).

***Ambulatory studies.*** Ambulatory recordings have allowed a correlation between bowel events and anorectal motor activities. For example, the feeling of gaseous distension or the desire to defecate is associated with reduction of anal pressure (Miller et al 1988a). A disadvantage of the technique is that it may be difficult to determine whether a drop in anal pressure is caused by a shift of the sensor back into the rectum or out of the anal canal. If this technique is combined with measurements of both internal and external anal sphincter electrical activities, the interpretation of the data is much more reliable (Duthie 1990a, b, 1991, Farouk et al 1992, 1993, 1994a, b).

### Laboratory versus ambulatory studies

It is important to introduce a note of caution regarding the interpretation of laboratory studies of anorectal function. In the short period of time that the patient spends in the laboratory, the adverse events may not be detected because they are infrequent. Prolonged recording using the ambulatory technique allows the measurements to be made in the patient's usual environment. On the other hand, the current technology does not permit the use of as many sensors as with laboratory recordings, and the patient sometimes requires after-hours supervision which is not always readily available. Conversely, laboratory studies allow detailed planning and manipulation of the observation parameters. For example, the rate and volume of rectal distension can be changed according to the needs of the investigator. When combined with a dynamic testing technique, it also allows the tests to be conducted in a situation that mimics the life event.

### Dynamic studies

These are done under simulated physiological events, for example, the intrarectal saline infusion test, and the expulsion test in order to test the mechanisms of continence and defecation. Both the saline continence and the expulsion test can be performed at the end of standard anorectal manometry.

### Saline continence test

*Indication*

The saline continence test assesses the overall capacity of the anorectum to maintain continence during conditions that simulate diarrhea. It can detect minor compromises in sphincter function (Penninckx 1995) and can also be used as an indicator of improved anorectal function after treatment (Rao & Read 1990, Miner et al 1990).

*Apparatus and procedure*

A perfusion tube is introduced anally to approximately 10 cm into the rectum. The patient sits on a commode after the intubation. The rectum is then slowly distended with saline which has been pre-warmed to 37°C at a pump rate of 60 ml/min (Haynes & Read 1982, Read et al 1983).

*Interpretation*

The minimum volume at which the first leakage of the infused fluid occurs and the maximum volume of retained fluid is calculated. Abdominal symptoms during the procedure are recorded in relation to the volume of fluid infused. Anorectal manometric recordings can be made at the same time.

### Expulsion test

*Indications*

The expulsion test evaluates the co-ordination of pelvic floor function, spinal control and the modulation of cerebral control. If the patient says they have difficulty in defecation, this test can be used to confirm it.

*Apparatus and procedure*

The test is done by asking the patient to pass simulated sausage or sphere-shaped stools made from silicon rubber or to pass a water-filled balloon. The simulated stools are introduced anally. The patient is transferred to a commode and then allowed to expel the stools in private.

*Interpretation*

Most normal subjects can expel the device within 3 min, whereas patients with obstructed defecation may fail to do so even after staining for 5 min. If the anorectal catheter is left in situ, the pressure patterns and gradient during straining can be recorded. Furthermore, electrical activity of both internal and external sphincter can also be evaluated simultaneously by electromyography.

## Radiological and imaging investigations

*Defecography* (p. 18)

This procedure is used to assess incomplete rectal prolapse and rectoceles, where clinical assessment leaves the clinician in some doubt about the significance of the clinical signs. The rectum is filled with semisolid contrast and the rectum and sigmoid is imaged radiologically during defecation. Abnormalities of rectal morphology including prolapse, perineal descent and rectoceles can then be identified.

*Anal ultrasonography*

Anal ultrasonography is used for the assessment of anal sphincter integrity, sphincter defects and anal fistulae. The results allow patients to be selected for surgical treatment. It is also used for postoperative evaluation, particularly in patients who have a poor outcome of surgery. A recent development of this technique which places the scanner into the vagina has further enhanced the image. This vaginal procedure does not compress the submucosal structure and therefore it may be possible to diagnose submucosal or luminal abnormalities (Sultan et al 1993a, b).

*Magnetic resonance imaging (MRI)*

The muscular structure of anal sphincters can be evaluated by MRI. The quality of the image has been improved by the deployment of an internal coil inserted into an anal canal (deSouza 1995). This technique is still in a development stage and for research purposes only.

*Transit measurements*

In cases of severe constipation, it is important to confirm that stool frequency is abnormal, since some patients deny defecation yet studies show the bowel has emptied. Objective proof of constipation is certainly needed in those patients who require surgery. The simplest test is to give 20 opaque markers and take a plain radiograph of the abdomen 5 days later. Most patients pass 16 markers by 5 days. Those who retain more markers are considered to have slow transit constipation. There are various refinements of this technique which isolate segments of the colon which do not function. This allows more selective surgery if indicated (p. 1347).

Radionuclear methods can be used to measure the transit through the entire gastrointestinal tract (p. 1346). When necessary the rectum can be separated as a region of interest from which information about rectal retention and its volume are derived.

## Neurophysiological investigations

The three commonly used tests are measurement of the latency of the terminal portion of the pudendal nerve, anal sensation and electromyography.

*Pudendal latency*

The pudendal nerve is stimulated at the level of the ischial spine and impulses are recorded from an electrode placed in the anus. The pudendal stimulator is available commercially and testing is well tolerated and reproducible. Prolongation of the latency is seen in severe nerve damage and may herald a poor outcome following sphincter reconstruction after injury.

*Anal sensation*

Tiny electrical currents are delivered to the anal skin until a threshold of sensation is reached. This quantifies sensation and is a moderately useful assessment of sensation in the anal canal. It is the least useful in terms of overall management, but helps to build an overall picture when combined with other investigations.

*Electromyography*

Electromyography can be recorded by two methods and each has its specific indications in the evaluation of sphincter functions.

***Needle electrodes.*** This involves inserting needle electrodes into the anal sphincter and is largely a research procedure. It was used to assess sphincter integrity in patients with suspected sphincter injuries, but has been largely superseded by anal ultrasonography. It requires multiple punctures which are unpleasant for the patient.

Motor unit function can be studied using electromyography to provide evidence of reinnervation. When a motor nerve degenerates, healthy adjacent axons sprout neurofibrils which reinnervate denervated muscle fibers. The resultant motor units are larger and the polyphasic potentials recorded are evidence of previous nerve injury. The technique involves identifying larger motor unit action potentials of increased duration with multiple phases which are generated from the larger motor units. The test is sophisticated, but has largely been superseded by pudendal latency.

***Surface electrodes.*** In a recent development, intraluminal surface electrodes are incorporated into an anorectal catheter. This makes the technique readily acceptable to patients and increasingly used in routine anorectal manometry. It quantitatively measures electrical activity in the external anal sphincter or puborectalis (Kerremans 1969, Jesel et al 1973, Sun et al 1992). This can be facilitated by integration of the raw electrical activity of the external sphincter (Sun 1989). The surface electrodes allow separate recordings of the electromyogram of the internal and external sphincters whereas pressure recording, because of the overlap of the two muscles, produces only one summated estimation (Read 1992, Sun et al 1992).

## INCONTINENCE

Fecal incontinence in the community is much more common than was recognized in the past. In the healthy population aged over 65, 7% wear a pad or experience fecal incontinence at least weekly.

### **Etiology** (Table 52.1)

Incontinence occurs when the sphincter is incapable of sustaining a contraction sufficient to contain rectal contents. Any condition which causes a fall in the pressure gradient between the anus and the rectum may lead to fecal incontinence.

Fecal incontinence is commonly classified as minor or major. Minor incontinence occurs occasionally and is due to inability to control flatus or liquid stool, causing soiling. Major incontinence, by contrast, is defined as the frequent and inadvertent evacuation of stool of normal consistency.

#### *Childbirth*

Childbirth is the most common cause of fecal incontinence in women owing to damage to the anal sphincters and pudendal nerves. Factors which correlate with a reduction in external sphincter function are a prolonged second stage, related to the time spent pushing, the weight of the baby, with increased weight correlating inversely with squeeze pressures, and the circumference of the head of the baby (Sultan et al 1994). Moreover, we know that many women present many years after delivery with a relatively short history of incontinence, so the effects of traumatic delivery are not always apparent immediately.

**Table 52.1** Common causes of fecal incontinence

| |
|---|
| Trauma |
| Obstetric injury |
| Surgery |
| Injury |
| Radiation |
| Pudendal neuropathy |
| Prolonged labor |
| Prolonged straining at stool |
| Perineal descent |
| Injury |
| Neurological and psychological diseases |
| Diabetic autonomic neuropathy |
| Dementia |
| Injury |
| Neoplasms |
| Psychological illness |
| Sleroderma |
| Amyloidosis |
| Multiple sclerosis |
| Irritable bowel syndrome |
| Inflammatory bowel disease |
| Congenital abnormality |
| Spina bifida |
| Myelomeningocele |
| Imperforate anus |
| Prolapse |
| Constiption |
| Faecal impaction |
| Drugs |

Marsh (1994) selected 125 primiparous women for investigations after delivery. They included patients who had had a large number of interventions, so the outcomes were indicative of difficult delivery rather than typical of the whole population. Thirty-seven were delivered without intervention, 37 with forceps, 20 by Ventouse extraction, 10 were breech, six had elective cesarean section and 15 emergency cesarean sections. At 6 months after delivery, 99 returned for follow-up. Thirty-two had urgency of defecation (32%), or 26% of the whole group. However, it should be recognized that those with symptoms were more likely to return for follow-up. Eighteen percent complained of varying degrees of fecal incontinence. Sixteen had both urgency and loss of control. Fourteen of the 22 with fecal incontinence had forceps deliveries, compared with only two following Ventouse extraction. Thus, overall, 14 of 36 delivered with forceps developed varying degrees of incontinence compared with only two of 20 Ventouse deliveries. Whether the latter mode of delivery can replace the former is something obstetricians need to determine, but they do need to be aware of the deleterious consequences of forceps usage. There were 26 perineal tears, 11 were second degree and 15 third degree, out of 104 delivered vaginally. Of the 15 with tears involving the sphincters, seven had had forceps, two Ventouse extraction and six had spontaneous vaginal deliveries.

Further evidence of the adverse effects of forceps was that the outcome of a tear with forceps was worse than a tear associated with a spontaneous vaginal delivery. Thus six of nine patients who sustained a third-degree tear during forceps delivery developed incontinence, whereas only one of six was incontinent after a noninstrumental delivery associated with a similar tear (Marsh 1994). In all these studies it is likely that endoanal ultrasonography would have revealed an even higher incidence of tears (Sultan et al 1993b).

***Pudendal nerve damage.*** The external sphincter is innervated by the pudendal nerve which is relatively fixed as it passes through the pudendal canal. Thus perineal descent will stretch the nerve and may lead to irreversible damage. Childbirth is clearly the most potent cause of neurogenic injury to the external sphincter. Several studies have now shown that immediately following delivery, there is prolongation of the pudendal nerve terminal motor latency but this invariably recovers by 6 months following delivery. Repeated injury during further deliveries or as a result of chronic defecatory straining or simply as a result of aging results in a weakened sphincter, manifesting signs of chronic partial denervation. Biopsies of the sphincter have showed changes consisting of atrophy, hypertrophy and fiber grouping which are characteristic of chronic partial denervation (Parks et al 1977, Beersiek et al 1979). Electromyographic studies are consistent with a neurogenic cause (Buchthal & Pinelli 1953, Stalberg & Trontelj 1979, Henry et al 1980, Neill & Swash 1980, Bartolo et al 1983a,b,c,d, 1986b) and nerve conduction studies have shown delay in the latency of transmission of terminal impulses along the pudendal nerve (Kiff & Swash 1984a,b). These studies support the view that the sphincter mechanism has been denervated. The pudendal latency prolongation is in keeping with denervation in incontinence and suggests nerve entrapment, possibly within the pudendal canal.

The most obvious cause for these neurogenic changes is trauma sustained during delivery. This can result in injury to the pudendal nerve or direct injury to the sphincter musculature (Snooks et al 1984, Cornes et al 1991, Marsh 1994, Sultan et al 1994a).

***Anal sphincter damage.*** Anal ultrasonography (p. 1320) enables accurate definition of defects in the internal and external sphincters and provides a qualitative assessment of the muscle. This has altered the understanding of fecal incontinence, as well as its investigation and management. Such studies have shown a high incidence of structural defects affecting the sphincters. These studies have therefore cast some doubt on the overall importance of neurological factors in the pathogenesis of fecal incontinence (Neilson et al 1992, Deen et al 1993). To determine the incidence of such damage after childbirth, Sultan et al (1993) studied 202 consecutive pregnant women before and after delivery and repeated the study 6 months later if abnormalities were detected. Thirty-five percent of primiparae developed a sphincter defect affecting either the internal or external sphincter or both and this damage persisted at 6 months. Thirteen percent of primiparae developed new symptoms of anal incontinence, mainly of flatus and urgency, after delivery. There was no correlation of bowel symptoms with nerve latency. The same study showed that eight of 10 women who had forceps deliveries sustained a tear compared to none of the five women delivered by vacuum extraction.

***Relative importance of the pudendal nerve and anal sphincter.*** Pudendal nerve denervation has been central to our understanding of the pathophysiology of fecal incontinence, but the advent of anal ultrasound scanning has shown that many more patients have tears than was formerly considered to be the case. This has generated debate over the role of denervation in these patients.

Early postpartum incontinence is usually the result of a direct injury to the anal sphincters. Patients who present with incontinence many years after a traumatic injury almost certainly have a different cause. They have lived and coped with the sphincter injury apparently without ill effects. It is likely that these women present when denervation leads to progressive sphincter weakness. They may also benefit from surgery, but denervation explains why the results of repair are less satisfactory.

### *Neurological and psychological diseases*

All diseases which involve the central nervous system may cause incontinence. Incontinence of feces is a common manifestation of behavioral problems in children, senile dementia and all forms of pyschotic illness.

### *Diabetes mellitus*

Anorectal dysfunction leading to fecal incontinence occurs in up to 20% of unselected patients with diabetes mellitus. In diabetic patients with incontinence there are usually multiple anorectal motor and sensory dysfunctions. Internal and external anal sphincter pressures are reduced, the internal anal sphincter is frequently unstable and rectal sensation may be impaired when compared to healthy subjects. It is usually considered that fecal incontinence in diabetes mellitus is caused by irreversible autonomic neuropathy. Recent studies indicate that the blood glucose concentration may have a major, reversible, effect on motor and sensory function in the anorectum. This suggests that optimization of blood glucose control may be an important component of treatment.

### *Irritable rectum*

Irritable rectum is not confined to the irritable bowel syndrome. The physiological features of irritable rectum are also present in patients with inflammatory bowel diseases, ulcerative colitis and solitary rectal ulcer syndrome.

During physiological tests, such patients feel a desire to defecate, urgency and pain at much lower rectal volumes when compared to normal subjects. The rectal compliance in these patients is also reduced. Furthermore, the rectal contractile response to rectal distension and the rectoanal reflex are abnormally enhanced, making the anal sphincter incapable of maintaining continence under these conditions.

*Constipation*

Fecal impaction (p. 1316) occurs often in elderly and bed-bound patients and accounts for the commonest cause of fecal incontinence in this group of patients. Some drugs may also cause constipation and lead to over-flow incontinence.

## Clinical assessment

A full clinical history and examination is necessary to look for relevant conditions (Table 52.1). In women the history should include information about each delivery, birth weight, use of forceps and the occurrence of tears.

During clinical examination, scars are noted, as are sphincter defects. A digital assessment is made of resting and squeeze tone. The patient is asked to strain and signs of prolapse, either internal or external, are documented. A sigmoidoscopy completes the examination. If necessary, specific tests should be offered to patients in the light of clinical examination in order to identify the cause(s). If trauma to the sphincter is suspected, anal endosonography may localize the sphincter defect and aid surgical reconstruction. A pudendal nerve latency test may provide pathophysiological basis for a weak external sphincter. A saline continence test is a useful objective test and is also valuable for follow-up assessments. Combined measurement of anorectal pressure, sphincter electromyography and rectal sensation may be necessary to elicit the cause of the problem.

## Treatment

*General management*

The initial management of minor incontinence is dietary modification and bowel habit regulation. Bulking agents or a high-fiber diet may increase the stool consistency. Offending agents or drugs should be stopped if possible, otherwise, the dose should be reviewed and adjusted to the minimum effective dose. Fecal impaction is relieved by manual or instrumental disimpaction followed by enemas and laxatives to restore normal bowel habit. Opiate derivatives such as loperamide are the most potent antidiarrheal agents. They reduce intestinal secretion and inhibit propagated motor activity. Opiates also relax the smooth muscles in the proximal colon thereby increasing its capacity. Loperamide is the only opiate that also inhibits rectal sensation in patients with irritable bowel syndrome and increases internal sphincter tone in patients with diarrhea and incontinence.

*Biofeedback*

Biofeedback (p. 1361) aims to increase external sphincter strength, rectal sensation and co-ordination between the rectal activity and the anal response. It is mostly used in improving anorectal function in idiopathic fecal incontinence. The sphincter activity during conscious contraction of the external sphincter is displayed to patients visually. Patients are encouraged to improve the response in both strength and duration. Rectal sensation is improved by reducing the threshold volume of perception of balloon distension. Patient selection is crucial to the success of the retraining. For example, patients with a defect of the external sphincter do not respond to such a treatment.

*Surgical treatment*

Treatment for patients who have sustained a tear of the sphincter muscle is surgical. Several options are available.

***Primary repair.*** It appears that primary repair of the sphincter is often inadequate as half the women who sustained a tear still had symptoms of incontinence and urgency and sonographic defects could be identified in 85% of those who sustained a third-degree tear, compared to 33% of controls who did not (Sultan et al 1993b).

Acute sphincter injuries are best treated by primary repair whenever possible. Direct apposition of the severed sphincter muscles without tension or with slight overlap using prolene sutures may achieve satisfactory results in skilled hands. Where appropriate skills are not available the management depends on the extent of the injury. With a substantial defect of the sphincter the most appropriate course of action is to carry out a loop colostomy to divert the fecal stream until the patient can be referred for elective reconstruction.

***Secondary repair.*** Many incontinent patients have to be treated after the primary repair failed due to sepsis, hematoma, faulty technique or because the injury was simply not recognized.

Secondary repairs should be performed only after all contaminated wounds have healed and inflammation has subsided completely. This generally requires about 3 months following injury. Routine preoperative care includes complete bowel preparation and prophylactic antibiotics. The use of a colostomy is not often necessary. The repair options include a direct overlapping approach which may or may not be combined with a levatorplasty. The purpose of adding this in such injuries is to strengthen and lengthen the anal canal with the theoretical objective of improving continence (Miller et al 1988b, 1989, Orrom et al 1991a).

In a series of 55 women with incontinence, external sphincter damage was delineated preoperatively. Eighty percent became continent postoperatively. Improvement correlated with restoration of normal anatomy (Sultan et al 1994b). In the failures, defects were still present. The above results need to be assessed at 5 years and beyond to ascertain if such improvements are sustained.

***Plication repair.*** In less severe injuries it may be evident that the muscle is not completely divided but rather attenuated anteriorly. In this instance, rather than dividing the splayed out but intact muscle a plication of the intact muscle and scar is achieved using horizontal mattress sutures rather than the conventional overlapping repair. After the sphincters have been reconstructed with one of these three procedures the vaginal wall and perineum is normally repaired with interrupted absorbable sutures. This may require a V-Y plasty or Z-plasty to achieve adequate skin cover. Sometimes, the wounds are left open to heal by secondary intention.

***Postanal repair.*** Postanal repair was based on Park's observation that many incontinent patients have an intact but poorly functioning sphincter with a wide anorectal angle. He proposed direction of the apparent abnormality by performing a posterior levatorplasty to tighten the anorectal angle and lengthen the anal canal. The initial high rate of success (83%) (Parks 1975) has not been reproduced in other centers and the postanal repair may actually lead to progression of neurogenic damage. Lengthening and tightening of the anal canal may be of some value in some patients. Keighley et al (1983) advocated a combined anterior and posterior levatorplasty in selected patients. Analyses of the results from several series suggests the operation is of little help in improving continence to liquid stool, but leads to improvement of control in 77% with incontinence to solid stools.

***Synthetic encirclement procedures.*** Thiersch wiring is now obsolete but Dacron-impregnated silastic sheet have been advocated by some to reinforce weakened sphincters.

***Artificial sphincter.*** The concept of a totally implantable artificial bowel sphincter is particularly attractive for the patient not suited to other options. Indeed, an artificial urinary sphincter has been used in over 4000 patients since 1972. The septic and failure rates are acceptably low with this device. There is limited experience of using a similar device for anal incontinence with reasonable results in the majority of the small series reported.

***Muscle transfer techniques.*** Gracilis muscle transposition has been used to reconstruct the anal sphincter. It is not as effective as expected, because it consists of mostly Type II fibers. Williams et al (1990) developed the concept of using electrical stimulation of the gracilis muscle to transform it from a fast twitch (Type II) to a slow twitch (Type I) muscle, capable of sustained tonic contractility. Stimulating electrodes are sutured to the gracilis muscle before transposition and their leads are connected to a permanent pacemaker device implanted in the chest wall. Once satisfactory function has been obtained, continence rates have been excellent.

## PHYSIOLOGY OF DEFECATION

The basic control mechanism of defecation is present in the newborn. Controlled, conscious defecation which involves control by higher cortical activity develops through 'training'. Stool is propelled into the rectum by propagated colonic contractions. The presence of stool in the rectum elicits sensations which are usually associated with a rectal contraction and a relaxation of the internal sphincter, both of which serve to push the stool down into the proximal anal canal. This increases the defecatory urge, which can only be suppressed by a vigorous contraction of the external sphincter and puborectalis. If conditions are appropriate for defecation, the subject sits or squats, contracts the diaphragm, the abdominal muscles, and the levatores, while relaxing the external sphincter and possibly also the puborectalis. By comparing the findings from patients with complete supraconal spinal lesions and normal subjects, it appears that the relaxation of the external sphincter during defecation requires inhibition from the central nervous system (MacDonagh et al 1992).

## CONSTIPATION

Most people feel they know what constipation is but it is nevertheless hard to define. Some 10% of the population have less than three bowel motions weekly (p. 53.5) and a similar proportion strain at stool (Drossman et al 1982, Dent et al 1986). This is widely regarded as defining constipation, but the form of the stool is also useful as fragmented or lumpy stools are strongly associated with constipation (Table 53.2).

### Etiology

Constipation may be secondary to organic diseases of the anus, rectum or colon including painful anal lesions, stenosis of the anus, stricture of the rectum, neoplasms, diverticular disease, inflammatory bowel disease and some motility disorders. These will be suspected from the history or detected at rectal examination and sigmoidoscopy. The rare disorder of megacolon (p. 66) is characterized by increased rectal or colonic diameter. Megarectum is defined if the rectal width is greater than 6.5 cm at the pelvic brim.

Constipation may also occur secondary to a variety of systemic disorders including hypothyroidism, hypercalcemia, psychiatric and neurological disorders. Drugs causing constipation are analgesics, calcium and aluminium antacids, bismuth, anticholinergics, anticonvulsants, antidepressants and monoamine oxidase inhibitors, diuretics, drugs for Parkinsonism, hypotensives and ganglion-blocking drugs, iron and opiates (Devroede 1985).

Nevertheless, most cases of constipation can be defined as "simple" constipation, i.e. these individuals are simply lacking fiber in their diet. They have normal intestinal transit whilst receiving fiber. Other contributory factors are neglect of the call to stool which can be psychological or due to travel, unfavorable working and living conditions and lack of exercise.

Patients with the most severe constipation are likely to have disordered motility or anal function. Some patients have a slow gastrointestinal transit time. This is termed slow transit constipation (p. 1326) and is usually accompanied by paradoxical contraction of the voluntary anal sphincter during straining. Patients with irritable bowel syndrome may also have constipation but they have a normal transit time. Reynolds et al (1987) studied 25 patients with severe constipation defined as absence of spontaneous bowel movements for periods of 5 days or longer over at least 18 months, absence of mechanical obstruction as defined by radiological and endoscopic studies and absence of systemic disorders known to cause constipation such as scleroderma. Six patients had a generalized motility disturbance of the gastrointestinal tract, six had no rectosigmoid response to a meal and in five there was a failure of relaxation of the internal anal sphincter in response to rectal distension. Of the remaining eight patients, four were thought to have irritable bowel syndrome.

### Diagnosis

The physician must determine whether constipation is real or imagined. Normal subjects pass three or more stools per week and if this is not achieved the patient is constipated (p. 1319). It is difficult to evaluate other complaints, such as stool hardness or difficulty in expelling stool, although the complaint can be taken into account if it fits in with the findings on examination, e.g. hard stool in the rectum. Poor dietary habits, emotional disturbance and ignoring the call to stool may be contributory in the majority of cases where no cause for constipation can be found. There correction is important in treatment. The following questions should be pursued:

1. Is the constipation recent? If it is and the patient is over 30 years old, a full gastrointestinal investigation is indicated.
2. Has the patient taken laxatives regularly for many years? The patient may have a cathartic colon.
3. Is the patient receiving drugs which may cause constipation? Many drugs, including antacids, analgesics, anticholinergics, iron, antidepressants and hypotensives, cause constipation. Even diuretics may contribute to constipation by inducing mild dehydration.
4. Has the patient developed a systemic disorder which could cause constipation, e.g. hypothyroidism, or pregnancy?
5. Is there a neurogenic reason for constipation? This might be Hirschsprung's disease (p. 1333) or meningocele, in which case there will have been a problem since infancy. Constipation may arise with lesions of the lumbosacral cord, including demyelinating diseases, trauma to the lumbosacral region (Devroede et al 1979) and also in cerebral degenerative disorders.

### Investigation

Most patients will have undergone barium enema examination prior to referral to the gastroenterologist. The width of the rectum at the pelvic brim should be reviewed to exclude megacolon. Indeed, constipation with dilatation is seen in Hirschsprung's disease, Chagas' disease and intestinal pseudo-obstruction (Gattuso & Kamm 1993). Sigmoidoscopy should be performed to detect rectal lesions and melanosis coli and it will enable the appearance of the stool to be correlated with the history. Those patients with constipation as part of the irritable bowel syndrome will usually be diagnosed as such on the basis of their symptoms (p. 1357). It is then reasonable to treat the patient as a case of simple constipation and if they do not respond further investigation must be undertaken. A transit study will diagnose slow-transit constipation and other studies may be used to demonstrate paradoxical intestinal sphincter activity in these patients (p. 1356).

### Treatment

*Simple constipation*

Management includes investigation to exclude organic disease if necessary, reassurance, education in the normal functioning of the large bowel and the institution of a high-roughage diet and adequate fluid intake. Fiber should be introduced slowly and if bloating ensues a pharmaceutical bulk-providing agent should be tried. Diet, exercise and living conditions should be reviewed. Initially in severe cases it may be necessary to use laxatives but it should be made clear to the patient that this is a temporary measure.

The treatment of slow-transit constipation and patients with irritable bowel syndrome who are constipated is discussed below and on p. 1362.

## SLOW-TRANSIT CONSTIPATION

This has several possible causes. Many patients have substantial psychological problems, sometimes following sexual abuse during childhood and adolescence. It is possible that some of these patients have profound inhibition of colonic motility at cerebral level. In this regard, recent work has demonstrated the importance of cerebral corticotrophin-releasing hormone in regulating colonic motility, in particular its response to stress (Gue et al 1991). The profound constipation of some of these women may be mediated via similar mechanisms.

In other patients, there is likely to be an abnormality of the enteric nervous system. In some this may be congenital or acquired, perhaps in response to laxatives. Recent studies have failed to confirm the ability of laxatives to cause enteric neural damage (Gattuso & Kamm 1994) but some patients have an identifiable abnormality of the myenteric plexus on silver staining (Krishnamurthy et al 1985). Studies of enteric neurotransmitters have also revealed abnormalities. The total concentration of indoles (serotonin and dopamine b-hydroxylase) have been found to be increased in the mucosa and circular muscle layer of the resected colons from patients with severe idiopathic constipation (Lincoln et al 1990). Vasoactive intestinal peptide appears to be decreased in its colonic wall concentration (Koch et al 1988, Milner et al 1990).

### Clinical features

Slow-transit constipation is predominantly a condition of young and middle-aged women. These patients have no normal call to stool and complain of abdominal pains and bloating. Stool frequency may vary from between weekly and once a month.

### Investigations

The initial assessment should include an evaluation of the patient's psychological state. Transit studies are routinely carried out to measure whole gut transit, using radio-opaque markers or isotopes (p. 1347). These will delineate whether there is a disorder of the whole gut, i.e. a pan-enteric disorder, or possibly one limited to the hindgut, where markers or isotope are held up in the rectum and sigmoid colon.

### Medical treatment

Dietary fiber is rarely helpful and frequently exacerbates pain and bloating. However, in patients who take an inadequate amount of fiber, this option should be tried. The diet should include 14–30 g per day of crude fiber; the type of fiber is not important. Initially it should be a low dose and is gradually increased to minimize possible bloating and distension. Adequate hydration is important in order to facilitate the action of the bulking agents.

The mainstays of treatment are stimulant oral laxatives and stimulant suppositories such as bisacodyl or phosphate enemas and osmotic laxatives. Cisapride, a 5HT4 agonist, accelerates whole gut transit and has been shown to be effective in the treatment of slow-transit constipation. However, it does not act selectively on the colon and is only effective in some patients with a recent onset of constipation.

#### *Surgical treatment*

Surgery should be considered as a last resort in selected patients. The outcome is variable, with some patients having excellent results, while others develop severe diarrhea. A minority will develop recurrent constipation. In 102 patients with severe slow-transit constipation, 32 had colectomy and ileorectal anastomosis. Because early good results may deteriorate with time, these patients were assessed at 5 years after surgery. Bowel frequency was significantly improved from a median of less than one action a week to seven a week. Only 10% of patients were using laxatives. Anismus (see below) did not appear to predict a poor outcome, even at 5 years. Defecatory straining was reduced from over 80% to 40%. Tenesmus or incomplete emptying after defecation reduced from 78% to 41%. Preoperatively, only 20% ever experienced a call to stool. Postoperatively, 80% had normal sensation. Pain and bloating proved the most difficult symptoms to treat. Preoperative rates of 80% were only reduced to 55%, which was particularly disappointing as these symptoms were virtually abolished at 1 year after colectomy. Overall, 67% of patients felt their lives had been significantly improved in the long term and considered their operations had been successful. More importantly, none felt they were worse. Those expressing dissatisfaction were those who either had recurrent constipation, or those with very frequent stools (Duthie & Bartolo 1995).

## OBSTRUCTED DEFECATION

Obstructed defecation is defined as a reported sensation of the desire to defecate when stool is either not passed or the patient is left with a feeling of incomplete evacuation. It may result from failure of sphincter relaxation or ballooning of the pelvic floor because of poor support by the pelvic floor muscles which sag during defecatory straining. In other patients, there is no call to stool, but abdominal discomfort and bloating suggest that defecation is needed and ineffective efforts are made at rectal evacuation. Despite this definition, anismus has been considered to be interchangeable with obstructed defecation. However, others regard anismus as just one category of obstructed defecation. Those clinical entities which fulfil the definition of obstructed defecation (Read & Sun 1992, Sun 1993) are listed in Table 52.2.

**Table 52.2** Causes of obstructed defecation

| |
|---|
| Anismus |
| Hirschsprung's disease |
| Internal sphincter myopathy |
| Levator syndrome |
| Hemorrhoids |
| Intussusception, rectal prolapse and solitary rectal ulcer syndrome |
| Rectocele |
| Fecal impaction |
| Idiopathic megacolon and megarectum |

## Etiology

*Luminal obstruction*

Patients with varying degrees of prolapse or the solitary rectal ulcer syndrome experience fullness in the rectum due to the prolapse intussuscepting towards the anal canal. Strenuous efforts may be made to pass the intussusceptum which can result in rectal bleeding and passage of mucus without evacuating any stool.

Hemorrhoids may act as a plug to obstruct the anal canal during attempts to defecate. A severely impacted rectum associated with hypotonic rectal muscle activity inevitably blocks the outlet of the colon.

*Rectal sensory loss*

Abnormalities in rectal (pelvic) sensation have been found in patients with idiopathic constipation and obstructed defecation. Although some studies have shown a normal threshold of sensation (Read et al 1986, Shouler & Keighley 1986), others have shown a raised threshold as well as a higher volume required to produce the desire to defecate (Farouk et al 1994a). In addition, rectal sensory loss has been observed in patients with defecatory difficulties (Kamm & Lennard-Jones 1990). Whether this sensory loss is a contributing factor is uncertain. It may simply be a reflection of the neuropathic process affecting the pelvic floor muscles (Lubowski et al 1992). This is reinforced by the observation that the rectum in patients with obstructed defecation is often empty at the time of examination, suggesting a failure to fill the rectum rather than a failure to perceive its contents.

*Rectal awareness*

Not all sampling events reach conscious awareness (Miller et al 1988a). Patients with slow-transit constipation rarely have a normal call to stool and it may be that they have fewer sampling events or that these events are abnormal. Similarly patients with obstructed defecation appear to respond (Gowers 1877) to calls to stool far more frequently and are more sensitive to changes in anorectal motility and appreciate significantly more at a conscious level. This explains their frequent calls to stool and possibly why they are often unable to defecate despite the urge to do so. There is no evidence that rectal awareness is impaired in slow-transit constipation.

*Failure of pelvic co-ordinating mechanism*

Normal defecation requires a co-ordinated relaxation of the internal and external sphincters. With impaired function there is inappropriate contraction of the puborectalis and external sphincter, failure of relaxation of the internal sphincter, failure of the levator to lift up the pelvic floor and open the anorectal angle.

## Anismus

The inappropriate contraction of the external anal sphincter is called anismus. This condition was described by Lennard-Jones and colleagues in 1987, in a group of young women with severe constipation. These patients could not expel a simulated stool, and had a paradoxical contraction of the puborectalis and external sphincter during attempts to defecate (Figure 52.3).

These events are attributed to failure of the somatic component of the anal sphincter complex to relax and allow spontaneous defecation. The situation is confused in that similar findings have been reported in the solitary rectal ulcer syndrome, perineal pain and in normal controls (Jones et al 1987, Barnes & Lennard-Jones 1988). Published work

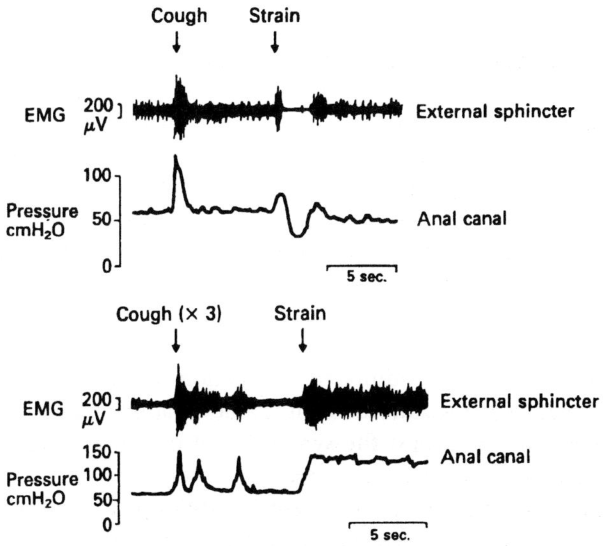


**Fig. 52.3** Recordings of anal pressure and electrical activity of the external sphincter in a normal subject (top) and a constipated patient (below) during attempted defecation. Note that the pressure in the anal canal and the electrical activity of the external sphincter increase during straining in the constipated patient. (From Preston & Lennard-Jones 1985.)

on obstructed defecation and its treatment has emphasized this paradoxical contractility of the pelvic musculature.

However, anismus remains the most common diagnosis in patients with obstructed defecation (Preston & Lennard-Jones 1985, Bleijenberg & Kuijpers 1987, Duthie et al 1989b). As a diagnosis, it has now gained wide acceptance, but is almost certainly overdiagnosed (Duthie & Bartolo 1992) and this has gone largely unchallenged in the literature (Kuijpers & Strijk 1984, Preston & Lennard-Jones 1985, Kamm & Lennard-Jones 1992).

### *Etiology*

Anismus characteristically presents in young or middle-aged females with constipation in whom spontaneous defecation is rare. Laxatives are necessary and digitation is frequently admitted.

***Anismus and constipation.*** Duthie et al (1989a) investigated 132 patients with slow-transit constipation, of whom approximately a half had anismus during defecography. Transit marker studies in these patients failed to demonstrate a correlation between retention of markers in the rectosigmoid segment and outlet obstruction. Indeed, markers were randomly distributed throughout the colon and it was concluded that obstructed defecation per se was not implicated in the genesis of slow-transit constipation. On the other hand, Miller et al (1991) identified a group of constipated subjects with normal transit and symptoms of outlet obstruction who recruited their somatic muscles during evacuation and were able to evacuate completely, whereas others relaxed their sphincters appropriately but were unable to empty their rectums. Thus dynamic proctography in these patients was confusing and casts doubt on the validity of these techniques.

The significance of anismus on laboratory testing has been questioned by Jones et al (1987). Using electromyography it was shown that 76% of patients with constipation, 48% with perineal pain and 50% with solitary ulcer syndrome had anismus and it was concluded that this was a nonspecific finding of questionable significance. A report from the Mayo Clinic (Ambroze et al 1990) described pubococcygeus muscle activity during voluntary straining to defecate in eight normal young patients. A significant increase in puborectalis and external sphincter activity occurred during simulated defecation using a balloon placed in the rectum filled with radio-opaque contrast. All these studies suggest the symptoms of obstructed defecation cannot be simply ascribed to anismus.

***Anismus and physiological behavior patterns.*** When normal subjects were asked to strain (bear down) as if to defecate, four patterns of external sphincter response were observed in the laboratory environment: relaxation of the external sphincter; initial contraction followed by relaxation; relaxation followed by transient contraction; and contraction of the external sphincter. However, when patients with complete supraconal spinal cord lesions were asked to do the same, they demonstrated only one pattern — contraction of the external sphincter. Therefore this pattern has been recognized to be mainly a spinal reflex. These observations confirm the belief that sphincter co-ordination is a learned behavior. Some patients may not have learned this properly during the toilet training period or may have subsequently 'lost' this ability. This may explain its existence in patients with psychological illness or in those who suffered sexual abuse at early age.

***Anismus and neurological diseases.*** An observation of an anismus-type of pelvic floor dysfunction in patients with Parkinson's disease and constipation suggests that a focal dystonic can be the cause of anismus in some patients. It is also quite possible that patients with upper neurone disease may also have anismus as one of their defecational problems.

### *Diagnosis*

True anismus requires physiological studies either during actual defecation, or during the expulsion test. During evacuation, an inappropriate rise in anal canal pressures, accompanied by recruitment of the pelvic floor muscles and failure of rectal emptying should be observed. The diagnosis may require electromyography or combine electromyography, pressure studies and radiology. Recruitment shown by electromyography alone is insufficient to diagnose anismus. Definition should be based on three criteria: demonstration of puborectalis electromyography recruitment of >50%; evidence of an adequate level of intrarectal pressure (>50 $cmH_2O$) on straining; and the presence of defective evacuation. Womack et al (1985) investigated 16 patients with outlet obstruction and compared the findings with those in six control subjects. The controls all exhibited decreased sphincter activity with relaxation of the anorectal angle during defecation. Over half the patients could not evacuate contrast and all patients demonstrated recruitment of puborectalis and external sphincter activity during defecation. Notably, 44% who were able to evacuate showed recruitment and emptied in spite of it. This method had significant advantages over the balloon expulsion tests described by Barnes & Lennard-Jones (1985). Under proctographic examination, patients with anismus demonstrate delayed initiation of evacuation, which is also prolonged and incomplete. Incomplete evacuation after 30 s is highly suggestive of anismus.

An ambulatory technique has provided the most physiological method to date (Duthie & Bartolo 1992). Fifteen female patients who demonstrated anismus in the laboratory with a positive gradient between resting anal and rectal pressures also demonstrated somatic muscle recruitment during defecation on a commode in the laboratory. During home recordings 12 patients relaxed both the puborectalis and external sphincter muscles appropriately. Three of the patients in their home environment continued to have definite evidence of anismus during testing. There seemed no doubt that this inappropriate contractile activity of their sphincters was contributing to their symptoms. It appears, however, on the basis of these findings that all 15 patients would have been considered to have anismus and hence obstructed defecation if they had simply been studied in the laboratory and the incidence of truly obstructed defecation is almost certainly overestimated. This may explain why most therapeutic attempts to treat so-called outlet obstruction constipation have been unsuccessful.

None of the tests used are ideal and the more complex, such as dynamic proctography, are far from physiological. Ambulatory monitoring allows the patient to be studied during spontaneous defecation in their own environment (p. 1319).

### *Treatment*

The choice of treatment in obstructed defecation is difficult and its outcome is often unsatisfactory.

Conservative therapy should always be the first option and the aim of the clinician should be to understand the pathophysiology of the patient's symptoms so that therapy may be addressed to correcting the abnormal physiology.

***Medical treatment.*** Decrease in stool consistency may help. Diet modulation should always be suggested to patients. Laxatives can be useful in some patients (p. 1335). Prokinetic drugs such as cisapride may help those patients who also have slow bowel transit. Paralysis of the sphincter with botulinum toxin has been reported to be successful in a few patients. However, this treatment has to be repeated several times, administrated by a specialist and seems to be associated with a considerable risk of incontinence, and therefore, has not been accepted as an appropriate treatment.

***Surgery.*** Surgery should be considered as a last resort in selected patients. The outcome is variable with some patients having excellent results, when there is associated prolapse and intussusception (Van Tets & Kuijpers 1995), while in others, rectopexy may actually make them worse (Orrom et al 1991b). Attempts have been made to divide the puborectalis either surgically (Wassermann 1964, Barnes et al 1985, Kamm et al 1988) or medically with the injection of botulinum toxin (Hallan et al 1988) and to weaken the internal sphincter (Yoshioka & Keighley 1987a,b, Pinho et al 1989, Binnie et al 1989). Long-term results have been universally disappointing.

***Biofeedback retraining.*** Biofeedback has gained widespread support as a noninvasive and effective treatment. This is usually achieved by concurrent measurement of anorectal pressures and electrical activity of the external sphincter. This information is then fed back to patients via a graphic display and the electrical activity of the external sphincter can also be fed back through a loudspeaker. For biofeedback to achieve its effect, patients with a reversed anal to rectal gradient during defecation must be shown to correct and invert the gradient so that rectal pressures exceed anal pressures during defecation. Moreover, these changes must be shown to correlate with improvement in symptoms as observed by an independent assessor. Bleijenberg and Kuijpers (1987) pioneered this technique in outlet obstruction constipation and reported excellent results. Clearly there may well be a placebo effect of biofeedback which could be profound. Lubowski et al (1992) observed that the outcome following biofeedback was unpredictable. Some patients achieved excellent results, while others were not helped at all.

## Rectal prolapse, intussusception and solitary rectal ulcer syndrome (SRUS)

Rectal prolapse, intussusception and solitary rectal ulcer syndrome are now considered to share a common pathogenesis with prolapse being the unifying pathology. Some patients with SRUS do not have prolapse but strain excessively and ulcerate the anterior rectal wall which is forced into the anus during futile straining efforts. Three-quarters of patients are female and older women are particularly at risk.

### *Etiology and pathology*

Rectal prolapse starts as an intussusception of the upper rectum which passes into the lower part of the viscus (Broden & Snellman 1968). Progression results in its protrusion through the anal canal to emerge as an external prolapse. A mobile sigmoid mesentery and an elongated mesorectum tend to favor prolapse. Constipation and chronic straining at stool are also considered to be important in the etiology (Boulos et al 1984). Conversely, the presence of an intussuscepting rectum will tend to mimic the presence of stool in the rectum and lead to straining efforts to evacuate the prolapse. Since it is uncertain which of these is cause and which effect, the precise etiology remains uncertain. It is likely that both processes are involved to some extent. In some patients, particularly younger ones with normal sphincter function, the presentation is with the solitary rectal ulcer syndrome (Fig. 52.4). In these patients, the intussusception is pushed against a closed sphincter leading to cycles of straining to pass the prolapse which mimics stools in the rectum. Repeated straining leads to traumatic ulceration and mucous discharge.

Solitary ulcers occur most commonly on the anterior wall of the rectum. Ford et al (1983) in a report of 40 cases found all the abnormalities within 13 cm of the anal verge: the majority of ulcers in that series were shallow and approximately 1 cm (range 0.5–4 cm) in diame-

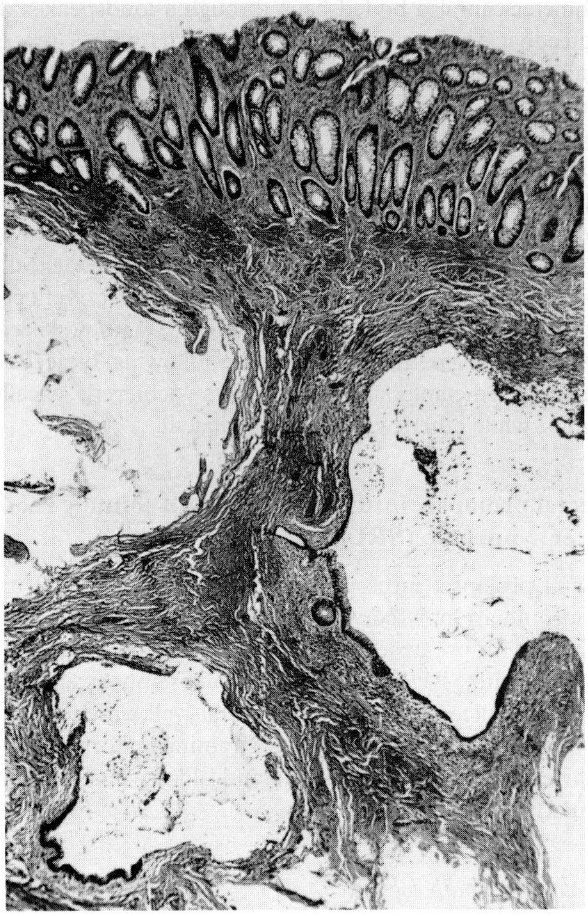

**Fig. 52.4** Solitary ulcer syndrome. Dilated mucus-filled cysts are seen in the submucosa. The overlying mucosa shows increased density of the lamina propria due to fibrosis, and muscle fibers from the muscularis mucosae extending between the crypts (hematoxytin and eosin, ×30).

ter. The ulcers have a white base, are usually irregular but can be well demarcated and are surrounded by a halo of hyperemia. Sometimes there is an inflamed granular hyperemic area without ulceration.

On microscopy, the earliest change is a replacement of the normal lamina propria by fibroblasts arranged at right angles to a thickened muscularis mucosae (Fig. 52.5). The crypt and surface epithelium show regenerative changes and a low villous configuration of the surface may occur. Later the fibers of the muscularis become realigned to point towards the lumen and they occupy the lamina propria between the crypts. The muscularis propria shows marked thickening. The crypts may branch and the epithelium is hyperplastic and shows mucin depletion. Vascular congestion and exudation of fibrin and polymorphs on to the surface of the mucosa are followed by superficial ulceration. A similar histological pattern is seen in mucosal prolapse (Du Boulay et al 1983). The mucosal changes seen in the solitary ulcer syndrome may give rise to misplaced glands in the submucosa (colitis cystica profunda) which may be mistaken for carcinoma.

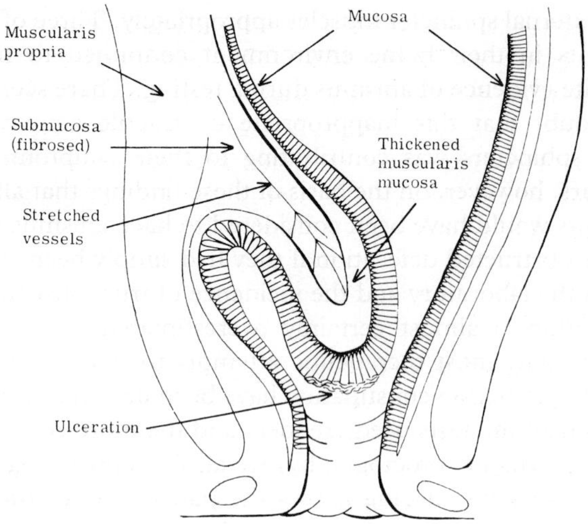


**Fig. 52.5** Mucosal prolapse causing solitary ulcer (Rutter & Riddell 1975).

*Physiology of prolapse*

Farouk and colleagues studied the pathophysiology of prolapse in 54 patients with complete rectal prolapse and fecal incontinence (Farouk et al 1992, 1994b). All the patients reported that fecal leakage occurred without warning which contrasts with patients with sphincter injuries who complain of intense urgency, but are unable to defer defecation and have urge incontinence. Prolapse patients had reduced resting and squeeze pressures, shortened sphincters, prolonged pudendal latencies and relatively noncompliant rectums. The rectoanal inhibitory reflex was only present in five of the 54 patients. Thus, the internal sphincter is fully inhibited in patients with rectal prolapse. Internal anal sphincter ambulatory electromyography measurements showed that the frequency of the electrical response was reduced significantly compared to controls. Resting anal pressures were increased and it was possible to record spontaneous episodes of anal sphincter relaxation, when rectal pressures equalized anal pressures; this did not occur in normal controls. Two patterns of rectal motor activity were observed in the patients with prolapse. The first consisted of sampling reflexes and occurred at a frequency of five times an hour which is similar to controls. The second consisted of rectal motor complexes (Kumar 1989), bursts of rectal motor activity characterized by a rise in rectal pressure with no effect on internal sphincter electromyographic function or anal pressures. They were seen in both normal subjects and patients and occurred sporadically during the day and night, with no obvious periodicity. A second motor complex activity was observed in the prolapse patients which had not previously been described. This consisted of high pressure waves, associated with internal sphincter electromyographic inhibition and falls in anal pressure. Thus rectal pressures grossly exceeded anal pressures favoring leakage of rectal contents. The duration of these episodes varied between 30 and 150 s. They occurred without any periodicity, they did not occur during sleep and were unrelated to meals. Forty-six patients recorded a desire to defecate during these episodes and five were actually incontinent during them. Similar events have never been observed in normal subjects without prolapse.

*Clinical features*

The syndrome is reported in all age groups, but the maximum incidence is between 20 and 40 years of age and it is more common in women.

The patient presents with bleeding and the passage of mucus on defecation, but blood loss is small and may have occurred for several years before the diagnosis is made. Occasionally, there can be severe pain localized to the perineum, sacrum or left iliac fossa. Tenesmus and a sensation of anal obstruction occur. There may be diarrhea and constipation. At digital examination, an indurated area may be felt at the site of the ulcer. The patient is asked to strain to determine if prolapse is present. On sigmoidoscopy, the ulcer or abnormal area may be seen and prolapse of the rectum can often be demonstrated by asking the patient to bear down when the sigmoidoscope is 10–15 cm from the anal verge. The diagnosis is made on the histological features of the biopsy. The differential diagnosis is extensive and includes benign and malignant neoplasms, rectal infections and ulcers produced by drugs and by trauma. In practice, differentiation from Crohn's disease and from traumatic and drug-induced ulcers may present the greatest difficulty. The use of ergotamine suppositories will produce solitary rectal ulcers (Eckardt et al 1986).

*Treatment*

Asymptomatic solitary ulcer syndrome discovered during routine sigmoidoscopy should not be treated. In symptomatic patients, initial management should be directed towards avoiding straining and measures to soften the stool can be employed. If it can be demonstrated that rectal prolapse occurs during defecation, repair of the prolapse should be considered. Most symptomatic patients with rectal prolapse or SRUS require surgical treatment. Many operations have been proposed, but resection rectopexy probably gives the best results.

***Resection rectopexy.*** This operation consists of full rectal mobilization, including lateral ligament division. The splenic flexure is always mobilized and the redundancy is excised. The rectum is fixed by suturing it to the sacrum.

***Recovery of continence.*** Farouk et al (1994c) carried out post-rectopexy studies within 6 months of surgery in 48 patients. Forty-four patients became continent of solid and liquid stool, but one patient complained of constipation despite resection. The so-called prolapse waves were no longer observed and resting pressures rose, mirrored by an increase in internal anal sphincter electromyographic frequency. Furthermore, during rectoanal sampling episodes, rectal pressures no longer exceeded anal pressures. Thus although pressures remained relatively low, they were adequate to cope with the normal rectal events. Moreover, because the anal canal was no longer effaced by the prolapse, the sensitive anal lining was restored to its anatomic position, thereby allowing appropriate perception of rectal contents during sampling, so unconscious soiling and incontinence no longer occurred in the majority. Longitudinal studies showed that pressures and internal sphincter electrical frequency rose progressively over 12 months. Thus, recovery is not immediate and improvement may be expected over this period.

The mechanism of recovery of continence after prolapse surgery has been the subject of considerable debate (Wells 1959, Bearhrs et al 1965, Frykman & Goldberg 1969, Keighley et al 1983, Spencer 1984, Watts et al 1985, Holmstrom et al 1986, Broden et al 1988, Kuijpers & De Moree 1988, Mann & Hoffman 1988, Sainio et al 1991, Duthie & Bartolo 1992a, Deen et al 1994). Fecal incontinence is common in patients with complete rectal prolapse. The exact mechanism of incontinence in such patients appears to be related to profound inhibition of the internal sphincter together with neurogenic damage to the external sphincter (Parks et al 1977, Farouk et al 1994b). Incontinent patients with rectal prolapse have lower resting and squeeze pressures compared to those who retain continence. Moreover, following successful rectopexy a variable proportion of patients recover continence. Reported series for resection rectopexy vary between 40% and 85% (Watts et al 1985, Madoff et al 1992, Duthie & Bartolo 1992a, Deen et al 1994).

Farouk et al (1994c) outlined some of the variables which improve after resection rectopexy and provided an outline for the objectives which should be attained by an operation to treat prolapse. Eliminating the prolapse itself is clearly fundamental, but following this attention to the functional outcome is imperative. Continence depends on a compliant rectal reservoir functioning with an adequate sphincter. Incontinent patients with rectal prolapse have low resting and squeeze pressures and their rectums are less compliant than normal. In part, this test is abnormal because the sphincters are so lax that compliance testing balloons cannot be retained and therefore low maximum tolerable volumes are recorded. It is interesting that continence can be restored in these patients with such poor function, while patients with obstetric injury who often start with better objective measurements do less well.

Resting pressures rise after surgery but remain comparable with other nonprolapse incontinent patients. Squeeze pressures do not change, so this does not explain continence recovery. The explanation for recovery appears to lie in the inverse change following surgery where the high pressure prolapse waves are abolished, resulting in rectal pressures which no longer exceed the weak anal sphincter. An effective operation must therefore be one which allows the sphincter to recover and should not reduce rectal compliance, since this will result in high rectal pressures which will overcome the weak anal canal.

***Alternative operations.*** Operations which involve large implants, particularly polyvinyl alcohol sponges, which induce an intense fibrotic reaction around the rectum, will make the rectum less compliant and so can be expected adversely to affect continence in some patients. Furthermore, a substantial proportion of patients report very severe postoperative constipation (Mann & Hoffman 1988). It appears, therefore, that such implants are ill advised and should probably be abandoned. Nonresection rectopexy may be associated with higher recurrence rates but can be considered in poorer risk patients.

***Perineal procedures.*** Operations which remove the rectal reservoir, such as the perineal rectosigmoidectomy, or which reduce its capacity, like the Delorme procedure, will lead to a noncompliant neorectum, so continence will not be expected to improve to the same extent as an abdominal rectopexy. In the former operation, the rectum is removed and often very narrowed diverticular sigmoid with grossly hypertrophied circular muscle which is used to generate high pressures is anastomosed to the anal canal. In the Delorme procedure, the rectum is plicated and narrowed significantly. These operations are considerably less invasive, so are of benefit in the unfit, but do have high recurrence rates.

***Incomplete prolapse.*** Ihre & Seligson (1975) reported that continence was restored in 75% of patients with rectal intussusception and incontinence treated by surgery. On examination it is important to discriminate between small intussusceptions of very dubious significance and those in whom the prolapse almost emerges from the anal canal with gross bulging of the perineum with circumferential internal incomplete prolapse. Urgency as a symptom is more commonly associated with sphincter injuries and weakness, whereas patients with prolapse frequently report soiling or voiding with no warning. A good squeeze pressure would favor treating the prolapse, especially if ultrasonography confirms the anterior sphincter is intact. This is often a difficult decision but overall, if prolapse predominates, then it is advisable to repair it before considering surgery on the sphincter, as the latter is liable to fail in the presence of prolapse.

### Conclusions

If patients are fit enough, the operation of choice is a resection rectopexy since this has the lowest recurrence rate. A lesser procedure is simply to fix the rectum but this has a higher recurrence rate and may be associated with constipation postoperatively. The perineal operations are best reserved for the elderly patient who may not survive an abdominal procedure. Unfortunately postoperative function is likely to be poor and recurrence rates are high.

## Hemorrhoids

Patients with nonprolapsing or first degree hemorrhoids commonly complain of obstructed defecation. Contrary to popular belief, constipation does not appear to give rise to hemorrhoids, for the prevalence of hemorrhoids was similar in patients with severe slow transit constipation compared with normal subjects. In an epidemiological study, it has also been shown that constipation and hemorrhoids may be unrelated (Johanson 1990). Patients with hemorrhoids strain excessively which exacerbates the obstruction by causing the ‘piles’ to swell. Manometric studies in patients with nonprolapsing hemorrhoids show abnormally high anal pressures (Hancock 1976, Sun 1990). When the rectum is distended with a balloon, the pressures in the distal aspect of the anal canal remain elevated even though the internal sphincter is relaxed and the activity of the external sphincter is not increased. A recent study suggests that the high residual pressure is probably caused by the elevated pressure within the vascular spaces. The treatment is that of hemorrhoids (p. 1452).

## Internal and sphincter myopathy

In this rare autosomal-dominant inherited form, obstructed defecation is caused by smooth muscle myopathy (hypertrophy) (Kamm et al 1991). The hypertrophic muscle is 7–8 mm, 2–4 times thicker than in normal subjects. It does not seem to relax either in vitro or in vivo. These patients also suffer from extreme anal pain, which further inhibits rectal evacuation. Anal manometry demonstrates high pressures with marked ultraslow wave activity. Anal endosonography usually confirms the presence of a grossly thickened internal sphincter. The treatment of choice is sphincterotomy.

## Levator syndrome

During defecation, the levators contract to lift up the pelvic floor while the puborectalis slings open, the net effect being a less acute anorectal angle. Some patients with severe constipation have profound perineal descent and cannot straighten out the anorectal angle. Defecography reveals that they are attempting to pass their rectal contents directly through a bulging perineum. It is usually assumed that the apparently weak and abnormally descended pelvic floor is the result of prolonged straining at stool or obstetric trauma to the pudendal nerve due to prolonged second stage of labor. Biofeedback is the treatment of choice.

## Rectocele

Defecography has revealed that some women appear to attempt to force the rectal contents through the posterior wall of the vagina. The only way that some of these women say they can defecate is to insert their fingers into the vagina and press backwards as they strain. Unfortunately, there is no real evidence that surgical repair of the posterior vaginal wall facilitates defecation. Proctography shows that many of these patients also appear to contract the puborectalis, but fail to contract the bulk of the levators during attempts at defecation.

## Hirschsprung's disease

This is a familial disorder occurring in about one in 5000 births. Most cases present soon after birth or in childhood, but occasionally the diagnosis is not made until later in life. For a review of the disorder in adults see Crocker & Messmer (1991).

### *Etiology and pathology*

In embryonic life, it is thought that the ganglion cells develop in the colon from the proximal to the distal end and in Hirschsprung's disease the process is arrested within a few centimeters of the anus, leaving a short segment of the bowel without normal innervation. Thus, the abnormal area always commences at the anus and extends proximally for a variable distance. However, immunohistochemical localization using neurone-specific enolase suggests that neuronal development proceeds from both ends of the gut to the middle (Tam & Lister 1986). If this is confirmed the pathogenesis of Hirschsprung's disease will need to be reconsidered. About 90% of cases have a short segment of absent innervation varying from 3 to 40 cm and the remaining cases are termed "long segment" forms. On rare occasions, these may extend into the small intestine. The disease is familial, affecting 7% of the siblings of index cases (Kleinhaus et al 1979). In those patients whose disease extended to the cecum or small bowel, the frequency of a family history rose to 21%. Hirschsprung's disease is sometimes associated with other congenital disorders, particularly Down's syndrome, and with megacystis and megaureter. Hirschsprung's disease is not associated with a high incidence of prematurity, most infants being of appropriate weight for gestational age.

The aganglionic segment of bowel remains contracted and shows histological abnormalities of innervation, whilst the bowel proximal to it is normally innervated but becomes dilated and the muscle thickened because of the distal obstruction caused by the aganglionic segment. In addition to the absence of ganglion cells in the plexuses, there is a characteristic abnormality of the nerve fibrils which is clearly recognizable on histological sections. This consists of thick, wavy bundles of nonmyelinated fibers, especially between the circular and longitudinal muscles. There is evidence of a deficiency of peptidergic nerves in the aganglionic segment (Freund et al 1981) (p. 154).

Various studies have shown that the aganglionic segment has neuromuscular activity (Garrett et al 1969) but no propulsive activity and that the internal sphincter fails to relax with distention of the rectum because it has no cholinergic innervation (Lawson & Nixon 1967).

### *Clinical features*

Most cases present in the first 3 days after birth with delay or absence of passage of meconium and with obstruction. Importantly, however, the passage of meconium in the first 48 h of life does not rule out a diagnosis of Hirschsprung's disease (Klein et al 1984). In some instances, particularly when conservative management with enemas has been instituted, severe enterocolitis may supervene. Kleinhaus et al (1979) have shown that in suspected cases conservative management in the first 2 months of life is associated with a high incidence of enterocolitis. In the child, Hirschsprung's disease can occasionally present as severe constipation which has not been present since birth, together with abdominal distention and some rectal bleeding from stercoral ulceration. More rarely, the disorder can present in the young adult with gradually increasing constipation and abdominal distention. Usually the aganglionic segment is short. They recommend against conservative management of unclear cases and strongly support a definitive diagnostic approach as the only way to reduce the very high incidence of enterocolitis with its associated high mortality.

In children and young adults, rectal examination and sigmoidoscopy reveal an empty rectum, the plain radiograph of the abdomen shows colonic but not rectal distention and the barium enema may show the narrowed distal aganglionic segment and a dilated proximal segment; the barium study must be carried out carefully on an unprepared colon (Nixon 1971). A normal barium enema does not exclude the diagnosis. By contrast, in acquired megacolon the rectum is full and a narrowed distal segment is not seen on barium enema. The definitive diagnostic procedure is a suction rectal biopsy carried out 1–2 cm above the internal sphincter. If this shows ganglion cells, it excludes the diagnosis (Dobbins & Bill 1965), but if ganglion cells are absent a full-thickness biopsy is carried out under general anesthesia 2 cm above the dentate line. The staining of suction biopsies for acetylcholinesterase aids the identification of ganglion cells (Barr et al 1985).

Occasionally, it can be difficult to distinguish a very short segment Hirschsprung's disease from an acquired megacolon and in the former there may be feces in the rectum and no narrowed distal segment. Physiological tests are often helpful under these circumstances; for example, distention of the rectum results in failure of relaxation of the internal sphincter, whereas patients with acquired megacolon show relaxation (Lawson & Nixon 1967). This reflex is absent in normal term infants in the first 2 weeks of life. Anomanometry is a technique requiring considerable expertise to obtain reliable results and should not be used as a routine diagnostic test.

*Treatment*

The treatment is surgical after the colon has been decompressed either by colostomy or by repeated enemas. Several definitive surgical procedures are described (Koop 1966, Nixon 1971). All involve the anastomosis of the normally innervated bowel to the region of the internal anal sphincter. The line of demarcation between normal and aganglionic bowel is determined at operation by the use of frozen sections. Kleinhaus et al (1979) have reviewed the procedures used in 1196 patients and shown that the results in terms of operative mortality and postoperative complications are very acceptable. It now seems clear that complete correction should be carried out at about age 1 year or earlier rather than the previously stated 2 years, because it allows more time for normalization of bowel function prior to toilet training (Klein et al 1984). With very short segment disease, it may be possible to carry out an anorectal myotomy or forceful dilatation of the anal canal (Bentley 1971).

### Idiopathic megacolon and megarectum

These terms refer to the increase in the transverse diameter of the colon which occurs secondary to a variety of disorders. However, most commonly, no cause is found and the terms idiopathic acquired megacolon or psychogenic megacolon are used. It has been suggested that idiopathic megacolon may be subdivided into those with onset in childhood and those who present as adults (Barnes 1985, Barnes et al 1986). The former have a megarectum with fecal impaction and soiling. They have a normal rectosphincteric reflex and a paradoxical contraction of the external anal sphincter during straining. The constipation usually arises during the period of training. At this stage, there may be stool withholding due to insecurity and other emotional problems and in some children this may persist into later childhood and present as fecal incontinence and a retained mass of feces which can be felt on examining the abdomen. It is clear that the primary event is a failure to evacuate the bowel which, over a period of time, results in megacolon.

The diagnosis is made on the history, which confirms the absence of bowel problems in the first year or two of life, the fact that the child has the urge to defecate, unlike in Hirschsprung's disease, and examination of the rectum which is found to be full of feces. By contrast, megacolon with onset in later life may have an acquired disorder of the myenteric plexus as the main abnormality. Usually, they do not have impaction or soiling and this makes distinction from adult Hirschsprung's disease difficult. Both conditions have abdominal pain, distention and a palpable abdominal mass. A water-soluble contrast enema examination on unprepared bowel shows a dilated rectum with no evidence of a distal narrow segment. A rectal diameter of more than 6.5 cm at the pelvic brim on the lateral view is diagnostic of megarectum but there is no such agreed diameter for megacolon (Gattuso & Kamm 1993). Rectal biopsy is essential to differentiate megacolon from Hirschsprung's disease.

*Treatment*

The rectum should be disimpacted (see below) and recurrent impaction prevented by the use of laxatives. Daily magnesium sulfate is used to maintain a liquid stool. If it cannot be tolerated, phosphate enemas are used. The patient should be aware that the treatment is usually lifelong. In some patients, colectomy with ileorectal anastomosis is necessary. Despite adequate use of laxatives, some patients may develop recurrent volvulus which can be confirmed with a plain abdominal radiograph or a water-soluble contrast enema.

Acquired megacolon may occur in many other disorders.

***Psychogenic megacolon.*** Patients with schizophrenia or severe depression may develop megacolon, presumably because their mental state allows them to ignore the urge to defecate. Drugs used in the treatment of depression may also contribute to the constipation. Treatment is difficult, but it may be possible to recondition some patients so that they have a regular bowel movement (Haward & Hughes-Roberts 1962). Megacolon also occurs in pseudocyesis, in neurosis and in some cases of prolonged laxative abuse (see below).

***Neurological disorders.*** These include paraplegia, Parkinsonism, diabetic neuropathy, myotonic dystrophy, Chagas' disease, chronic intestinal pseudo-obstruction, diabetes and multiple sclerosis. The radiological appearance in Chagas' disease may mimic Hirschsprung's disease since there is a distal aganglionic segment.

***Smooth muscle disorders.*** Scleroderma is recognized by its effects elsewhere in the body, including other regions of the gastrointestinal tract, such as the esophagus.

***Obstructive lesions or painful rectal lesions.*** These include rectal strictures from tumor, lymphogranuloma venereum or irradiation.

***Metabolic disorders.*** Hypothyroidism, porphyria and amyloidosis are sometimes associated with acquired megacolon.

### Fecal impaction

This can occur in most of the conditions in which

acquired megacolon (p. 1334) is present and also in patients who become bedridden for a variety of causes. The rectum becomes distended by a huge mass of firm feces which the patient cannot expel. The patient complains of rectal fullness and lower abdominal pain and there can be spurious diarrhea. Large bowel obstruction may supervene with nausea and vomiting. Examination of the abdomen reveals a firm mass and the rectal examination demonstrates a large mass of feces in the rectum except in cases where the fecal mass is mainly in the sigmoid colon. Many related problems may develop (Lal & Brown 1967). Elevation of the bladder may lead to angulation of the urethra and retention of urine. In some patients, chronic obstructive problems lead to hydroureter and hydronephrosis. Fecal impaction predisposes to volvulus, rectal prolapse and stercoral ulceration (see below). Spontaneous perforation of the colon is reported.

*Treatment* (Jones & Godding 1972)

On occasions evacuation may be achieved with large doses of oral sennosides (Senokot: X-prep). Usually, 150 ml olive oil is used as a retention enema to soften the fecal mass on 2–4 occasions over 2 days, followed by rectal washouts. An alternative softener is dioctyl sodium sulfhosuccinate given as 40 ml 0.2% solution made up to 120 ml. If symptoms of large bowel obstruction are already present at the time of presentation, manual removal is necessary under general anaesthesia or after anlgesia with 100 mg pethidine.

The treatment of impaction must be followed by a regime to prevent its recurrence. Oral laxatives may be sufficient in the elderly. In severely debilitated patients, it is sometimes necessary to institute regular rectal washouts.

### Stercoral ulceration or the rectum and colon

A stercoral ulcer results from the pressure of a hard mass of feces on the mucosa of the rectum or colon. Such ulcers are usually in the distal bowel, are irregular in outline but well demarcated and are situated in areas of necrotic tissue. On microscopy, the ulcer involves the full thickness of the mucosa and there is marked inflammation in the adjacent muscle layers. Stercoral ulcers can occur at any age in patients with severe constipation. They may be asymptomatic or may present with rectal bleeding or perforation. Treatment is that of their cause – fecal impaction.

## LAXATIVES

**Pharmacology** (Jones & Godding 1972, Cummings 1976)

*Anthracene laxatives*

These include senna, cascara and danthron. Senna and cascara occur as glycosides which pass unchanged into the colon, where they are hydrolyzed at the glycoside bond to produce the active molecule: this stimulates the myenteric plexus and inhibits sodium absorption, thus increasing the amount of water in the stool. These drugs are not excreted into the milk of lactating mothers. Danthron, by contrast, is a free anthraquinone which is partly absorbed from the small intestine and detoxified. Senna and cascara seem to be free from specific side-effects. Danthron may produce skin complaints.

*Phenylmethane laxatives*

These include phenolphthalein, bisacodyl and oxyphenisatin. Oxyphenisatin causes liver damage and is now obsolete. They are substituted methanes which are partly absorbed from the small intestine, conjugated in the liver and excreted in the bile and exert their effect after deconjugation by intestinal bacteria. They act by stimulating the myenteric plexus. By contrast to the anthracenes, they affect small intestinal transport systems as well as colonic water and electrolyte absorption. Bisacodyl is given orally in an enteric-coated form, which is thought to reduce its action on the small intestine. Phenolphthalein has been implicated in skin reactions and hypersensitivity reactions.

*Saline laxatives*

These consist of soluble sulfates, phosphates or tartrates of sodium, potassium or magnesium. They all contain poorly absorbed ions which retain fluid in the intestinal lumen; thus, 15 g magnesium sulfate retains 300–400 ml water in the intestinal lumen. Their mode of action is therefore to stimulate hyperperistalsis. Saline laxatives act rapidly but can result in fluid and electrolyte imbalance; in addition, the absorption of sodium and magnesium ions is undesirable in heart and kidney failure.

*Hydrophilic agents*

These agents exert their effect by producing a substrate for colonic bacteria and by increasing the amount of water in the stool (p. 1345). They are:

1. **Cellulose ethers**, e.g. Celevac, which are prepared from wood or cotton celluloses.
2. **Mucilagenous seeds and gums**, e.g. Normacol, Metamucil and Isogel. Hypersensitivity reactions may occur to sterculia, a constituent of Normacol, which also contains the chemical laxative frangula.

Laxatives in groups 1 and 2 have produced esophageal and intestinal bolus obstruction.

3. **Bran.** This depends upon its fiber content, which is hydrophilic. Because it is consumed together with other foods, it does not cause bolus obstruction.

*Other laxatives*

A detergent-like substance, dioctyl sodium sulfhosuccinate, has laxative properties and is sometimes called a "stool softener". It may act by influencing sodium and water transport in the small intestine and colon.

Lactulose is used as a laxative. In the colon, it is metabolized to short chain fatty acids, which have an osmotic effect (p. 1053).

Castor oil is a hydroxylated fatty acid which impairs water and electrolyte absorption and causes secretion in the jejunum and colon (p. 369 and 462).

Liquid paraffin is a mixture of mineral oil hydrocarbons. It interferes with the absorption of fat-soluble vitamins and causes lipoid pneumonia, it is partly absorbed and deposited in various tissues to form paraffinomas and anal seepage causes pruritus. It should not be used except in children.

## The use of laxatives

Laxatives have very little place in the management of simple constipation (see below) unless all educational and dietary measures have failed. However, they are indicated in some disorders of the large bowel, in chronic psychoses, when there is disease or injury to the spinal cord or when there is painful disease of the anal region. They may have to be used in the elderly and debilitated. If chemical laxatives have to be resorted to, senna and cascara are probably the safest.

## Evacuants and their use

Colonic irrigation with several liters of warm isotonic saline is used to clean the entire colon. To clear the rectum, 150 ml olive oil is used as a retention enema, followed by a washout with 500 ml warm saline. Most often, evacuation is achieved with a disposable enema of 100 ml hypertonic sodium phosphate. These evacuants are used in midwifery, for impaction in the elderly and for preparation of the large bowel prior to endoscopy, radiology or surgery.

*Soap colitis*

Soap is a severe irritant to the large bowel and soap enemas should not be used. On occasions, abdominal pain and severe diarrhea leading to hypovolemia may result. Sigmoidoscopy shows a hyperemic and even hemorrhagic mucosa.

# LAXATIVE ABUSE SYNDROME (Cummings 1976, Morris & Turnberg 1979)

Vast amounts of laxatives are consumed unnecessarily and most patients who take laxatives can be weaned off them by dietary means. The effects of prolonged and often surreptitious laxative abuse are considered here.

## Pathology

The colon may be dilated, often in its entirety but more usually in its proximal part. On microscopy, some studies have shown a reduction in nerve fibers in the myenteric plexus (Smith 1968). These changes were thought to be due to the anthraquinones which stimulate the plexi and ultimately lead to their degeneration. Other studies have failed to show these abnormalities (Müller-Lissner 1993). However, other histological abnormalities are described including damage to microvilli and mitochondria and widening of intracellular spaces.

The pigmentation of melanosis coli is usually maximal in the rectum and can be seen histologically in macrophages in the lamina propria (Fig. 52.6) when it is not visible macroscopically.

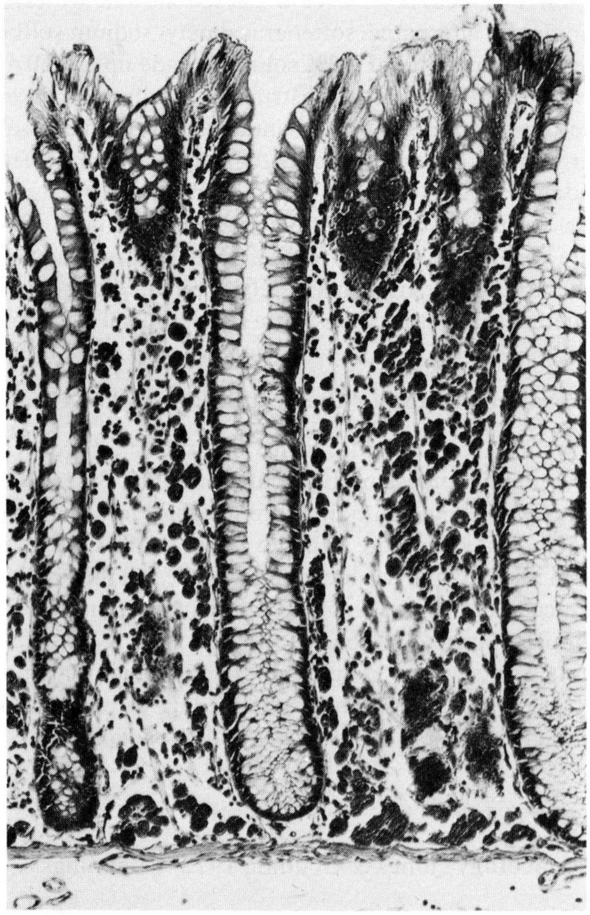

**Fig. 52.6** Melanosis coli. Numerous macrophages containing dark granular pigment within the lamina propria of the colonic mucosa (hematoxytin and eosin, ×120).

## Clinical features

The condition occurs predominantly in women who have taken laxatives regularly for many years. The patient presents with vague abdominal complaints, tiredness, lethargy and constipation or diarrhea. The consumption of laxatives may be denied and laxative abuse may continue during investigation even when the patient is in hospital. Patients with watery diarrhea can develop symptoms of electrolyte imbalance, such as lassitude, weakness, confusion and dementia, cramps, thirst and bone pain. Often a variety of abdominal operations have been performed to no avail. In some patients, anorexia nervosa may be the reason for continued laxative abuse.

## Investigation

*Sigmoidoscopy*

The diagnosis is strongly supported if melanosis coli is seen. The mucosa varies from light brown to black. Often the pigment is not deposited evenly, so that there is a reticular pattern and lymphoid follicles which do not become pigmented appear as tiny dots. Melanosis appears after anthraquinone purgative has been used for 4–13 months and it takes approximately the same time to disappear after the purgative is stopped (Speare 1951).

*Barium enema*

This may assist the diagnosis by demonstrating a cathartic colon. It occurs in about 10% of surreptitious laxative abusers. The featureless mucosa, the loss of haustration and shortening may suggest chronic ulcerative colitis. The changes are more marked on the right side of the colon with shortening of the cecum and loss of patency of the ileocecal valve. The ileum may be tubular and show a loss of mucosal pattern. Characteristic pseudostrictures, which are smooth, tapering and inconstant, and the marked distensibility of the colon suggest cathartic colon (Cummings 1976). In most cases the radiological abnormalities are probably irreversible, but Campbell (1983) reports a case with complete reversion to normal 4 months after stopping laxatives.

*Serum electrolytes*

Frequent laxative consumption results in increased sodium and potassium losses in the stool. Hypokalemia is common. The increased loss of sodium and water leads to secondary hyperaldosteronism, which encourages the retention of sodium and accentuates the loss of potassium in the urine. Hypokalemia damages the renal tubules.

*Other investigations*

Anemia, steatorrhea, malabsorption of xylose, protein-losing enteropathy, hyperglycemia and glycosuria have been described.

*Stool electrolytes*

The stool volume should be measured in patients with diarrhea; if it is over 200 ml/day the stool electrolytes should be measured to distinguish osmotic from secretory diarrhea (p. 369). Investigation in hospital is necessary so that the patient can be observed closely and tests made for purgatives in the stool and urine. Osmotic diuretics can usually be suspected from changes in stool electrolytes (Morris & Turnberg 1979).

## Treatment

Many patients have emotional disturbances requiring treatment. The aim of medical therapy is to withdraw the offending laxative and substitute bulk laxatives and to increase dietary fiber. A long and arduous campaign is required to effect these changes and the patient requires much support. Sometimes, colonic function does not return, presumably because of destruction of the myenteric plexus, and all treatment fails. When constipation is intractable, colectomy can be carried out (Cummings 1976).

## PROCTALGIA FUGAX (Thompson 1981)

This is defined as pain, seemingly arising in the rectum, which recurs at irregular intervals and is unrelated to organic disease (Douthwaite 1962). The pain is usually sudden and severe, lasting a few seconds or minutes and can be localized to just above the anus. There is no disturbance of bowel function. In men the onset is sometimes related to ejaculation and in men and women it may be related to straining at stool. Fainting may occur. Proctalgia is a common phenomenon; it occurred in 14% of 301 individuals and was sometimes related to the irritable bowel syndrome (Thompson & Heaton 1980). Some patients are anxious or neurotic (Schuster 1977).

On examination, the rectum and colon are normal. Examination during an attack of pain has shown a rigid band compressing the rectum in the vicinity of the levator ani and it is postulated that pain is caused by spasm of the pubococcygeus muscle. On the other hand, in two patients, pain was shown to be associated with contraction of the sigmoid colon (Harvey 1979).

## Treatment

Reassurance that there is no organic disease and that the attacks become less frequent with age is important. Each attack may be alleviated by upward pressure on the anus or by a hot bath.

## REFERENCES


Akervall S, Fasth S, Nordgren S, Oresland T, Hulten L 1988 Manovolumetry: a new method for investigation of anorectal function. Gut 29: 614–623

Akervall S, Fasth S, Nordgren S, Oresland T, Hulten L 1989 Rectal reservoir and sensory function studied by graded isobaric distension in normal man. Gut 30: 496–502

Ambroze W I, Pemberton J H, Litchy W J, Hanson R B 1990 The myoelectric activity of the pubococcygeus muscle. Diseases of the Colon and Rectum 33: 29

Bannister J J, Read N W, Donnelly T C, Sun W M 1989 External and internal anal sphincter responses to rectal distension in normal subjects and in patients with idiopathic faecal incontinence. British Journal of Surgery 76: 617–621

Barkel D C, Pemberton J H, Phillips S P, Keely K A, Brown M L 1986 Scintigraphic assessment of the anorectal angle in health and after operation. Surg. Forum 37: 183–186

Barnes P R H 1985 Megacolon in adults. British Journal of Surgery 72: S10

Barnes P R H, Lennard-Jones J E 1985 Balloon expulsion from the rectum in constipation of different types. Gut 26: 1049–1052

Barnes P R H, Lennard-Jones J E 1988 Function of the striated anal sphincter during straining in control subjects and constipated patients with a radiologically normal rectum or idiopathic megacolon. International Journal of Colorectal Disease 3: 207–209

Barnes P R H, Hawley P R, Preston D M, Lennard-Jones J E 1985 Experience of posterior division of the puborectalis muscle in the management of chronic constipation. British Journal of Surgery. 72: 475–477

Barnes P R H, Lennard-Jones J E, Hawley P R, Todd I P 1986 Hirschsprung's disease and idiopathic megacolon in adults and adolescents. Gut 27: 534–541

Barr L C, Booth J, Filipc M I, Lawson J O 1985 Clinical evaluation of the histochemical diagnosis of Hirschsprung's disease. Gut 26: 393–399

Bartolo D C C 1984 A comparative study of the pelvic floor musculature in disorders of defaecation and idiopathic faecal incontinence. MSc thesis, University of London

Bartolo D C C, Read N W, Jarratt J A, Read M G, Donnelly T C, Johnson A G 1983a Differences in anal sphincter function and clinical presentation in patients with pelvic floor descent. Gastroenterology 85: 68–75

Bartolo D C C, Jarratt J A, Read M G, Donnelly T C, Read N W 1983b The role of partial denervation of the puborectalis in idiopathic faecal incontinence. British Journal of Surgery 70: 664–667

Bartolo D C C, Jarratt J A, Read N W 1983c The use of conventional electromyography to assess external sphincter neuropathy in man. Journal of Neurology, Neurosurgery and Psychiatry 46: 1115–1118

Bartolo D C C, Jarratt J A, Read N W 1983d The cutaneo-anal reflex: a useful index of neuropathy? British Journal of Surgery 70: 660–663

Bartolo D C C, Roe A M, Locke-Edmunds J C et al 1986a Flap-valve theory of anorectal continence. British Journal of Surgery 73: 1012–1014

Bartolo D C C, Roe A M, Mortensen N J M 1986b The relationship between perineal descent and denervation of the puborectalis in continent patients. International Journal of Colorectal Disease 1: 91–95

Bearhrs O H, Vandertoll D J, Baker M H 1965 Complete rectal prolapse: an evaluation of surgical treatment. Annals of Surgery 161: 221–226

Beersiek F, Parks A G, Swash M 1979 Pathogenesis of anorectal incontinence: a histometric study of the anal canal musculature. Journal of Neurological Science 42: 111–127

Bell A M, Pemberton J H, Hanson R B, Zinsmeister A R 1991 Variations in muscle tone of the human rectum: recordings with an electromechanical barostat. American Journal of Physiology 260(1 Pt 1): G17–25

Belliveau P, Thomson J P, Parks A G 1983 Fistula-in-ano. A manometric study. Diseases of the Colon and Rectum 26(3): 152–154

Bentley J F R 1971 Constipation in infants and children. Gut 12: 85–90

Binnie N R, Kawimbe B M, Papacrysostomou M, Smith A N 1989 EMG biofeedback as a domicillary treatment of anismus. Gut 30: A714

Bleijenberg G, Kuijpers H C 1987 Treatment of the spastic pelvic floor syndrome with biofeedback. Diseases of the Colon and Rectum 30: 108–111

Boulos P B, Stryker S J, Nicholls R J 1984 The long-term results of polyvinyl alcohol (Ivalon) sponge for rectal prolapse in young patients. British Journal of Surgery 71: 213–214

Bouvier M, Gonella J 1981 Nervous control of the internal anal sphincter of the cat. Journal of Physiology (London) 310: 457–469

Bouvier M, Kirschner G, Gonella J 1986 Action of morphine and enkephalins on the internal anal sphincter of the cat: relevance for the physiological role of opiates. Journal of the Autonomic Nervous System16: 219–232

Bouvier M, Grimaud J C, Naudy B, Salducci J 1987 Effects of morphine on electrical activity of the rectum in man. Journal of Physiology (London) 388: 153–161

Broden B, Snellman B 1968 Procidentia of the rectum studied with cineradiography: a contribution to the discussion of causative mechanism. Diseases of the Colon and Rectum 11: 330–347

Broden G, Dolk A, Holmstrom B 1988 Recovery of the internal anal sphincter following rectopexy: a possible explanation for continence improvement. International Journal of Colorectal Disease 3: 23–28

Buchthal F, Pinelli P 1953 Action potentials in muscular atrophy of neurogenic origin. Neurology 3: 591–603

Burleigh D E 1983 Non-cholinergic, non-adrenergic inhibitory neurons in human internal anal sphincter muscle. Journal of Pharmacy and Pharmacology 35: 258–260

Burleigh D E, d'Mello A 1983 Neural and pharmacologic factors affecting motility of the internal anal sphincter muscle. Gastroenterology 84: 409–417

Burleigh D E, d'Mello A, Parks A G 1979 Responses of isolated human internal anal sphincter to drugs and electrical field stimulation. Gastroenterology 77: 484–490

Campbell W L 1983 Cathartic colon. Reversibility of roentgen changes. Diseases of the Colon and Rectum 26: 445–448

Cornes H, Bartolo D C C, Stirrat G M 1991 Changes in anal sensation after childbirth. British Journal of Surgery 78: 74–77

Crocker N L, Messmer J M 1991 Adult Hirschsprung's disease. Clinical Radiology 44: 257–259

Cummings J H 1976 The use and abuse of laxatives. In: Bouchier IAD (ed) Recent advances in gastroenterology, 3rd edn. Churchill Livingstone, Edinburgh, p 124

Deen K I, Kumar D, Williams J G, Olliff J, Keighley M R B 1993 The prevalence of anal sphincter defects in faecal incontinence: a prospective endosonic study. Gut 34: 685–688

Deen K I, Grant C, Billingham C, Keighley M R B 1994 Abdominal resection rectopexy with pelvic floor repair versus perineal rectosigmoidectomy and pelvic floor repair for full thickness rectal prolapse. British Journal of Surgery 81: 302–304

Dent O F, Goulston K J, Zubrzycki J, Chapuis P H 1986 Bowel symptoms in an apparently well population. Diseases of the Colon and Rectum 29: 243–247

deSouza N M, Puni R, Gilderdale D J, Bydder G M 1995 Magnetic resonance imaging of the anal sphincter using an internal coil. Magnetic Resonance Quarterly 11(1): 45–56

Devroede G 1985 Mechanisms of constipation. In: Read N W (ed) Irritable bowel syndrome. Grune & Stratton, London, p 127

Devroede G, Arhan P, Duguay C, Tetreault L, Akoury H, Perey B 1979 Traumatic constipation. Gastroenterology 77: 1258–1267

Dobbins W O, Bill A H 1965 Diagnosis of Hirschsprung's disease excluded by rectal suction biopsy. New England Journal of Medicine 272: 990

Douthwaite A H 1962 Proctalgia fugax. British Medical Journal 2: 164

Drossman D A, Sandler R S, McKee D C, Lovitz A J 1982 Bowel patterns among subjects not seeking health care. Use of a questionnaire to identify a population with bowel dysfunction. Gastroenterology 83: 529–534

Du Boulay C E H, Fairbrother J, Isaacson P G 1983 Mucosal prolapse syndrome – a unifying concept for solitary ulcer syndrome and related disorders. Journal of Clinical Pathology 36: 1264–1268

Duthie G S, Bartolo D C C 1992a Abdominal rectopexy for rectal prolapse: a comparison of techniques. British Journal of Surgery 79: 107–113
Duthie G S, Bartolo D C C 1992b Anismus: the cause of constipation? Results of investigation and treatment. World Journal of Surgery 16: 831–835
Duthie G S, Bartolo D C C 1995 Slow transit constipation and anismus. In: Wexner S D, Bartolo D C C (eds) Constipation: aetiology, evaluation and management. Butterworths, Landon, p 160–168
Duthie G S, Bartolo D C C, Miller R, Mortensen N J M, Virjee J 1989a Is anismus the result of reduced anorectal sensation in slow transit constipation. Gut 30: A714
Duthie G S, Bartolo D C C, Miller R, Mortensen N J M 1989b Anismus does not adversely affect the outcome of colectomy and ileorectal anastomosis for slow transit constipation. Gut 30: A735
Duthie G S, Miller R, Bartolo D C C 1990a Internal anal sphincter electromyographic frequency is related to anal canal resting pressure. Both are reduced in idiopathic faecal incontinence. Gut 31: A619
Duthie G S, Miller R, Bartolo D C C 1990b Resting anal pressure studies poorly reflect actual pressures recorded during ambulatory monitoring. Diseases of the Colon & Rectum 33: 6–7
Duthie G S, Bartolo D C C, Miller R 1991 Estimation of the incidence of anismus by laboratory tests (abstract). British Journal of Surgery 78: 747
Duthie H L, Bennett R C 1963 The relation of sensation in the anal canal to the functional anal sphincter: a possible factor in anal continence. Gut 4: 179–182
Duthie H L, Gairns F W 1960 Sensory nerve endings and sensation in the anal region of man. British Journal of Surgery 47: 585–595
Duthie H L, Watts J 1965 Contribution of the external anal sphincter to the pressure zone in the anal canal. Gut 6: 64–68
Eckardt V F, Kanzler G, Remmele W 1986 Anorectal ergotism: another cause of solitary rectal ulcers. Gastroenterology 91: 1123–1127
Edwards C A, Brown S, Baxter A J, Bannister J J, Read N W 1989 Effect of bile acid on anorectal function in man. Gut 30(3): 383–386
Farouk R, Duthie G S, Bartolo D C C, MacGregor A B 1992 Restoration of continence following rectopexy for rectal prolapse is associated with recovery of the internal anal sphincter electromyogram. British Journal of Surgery 79: 439–440
Farouk R, Duthie G S, Pryde A, MacGregor A B, Bartolo D C C 1993 Internal anal sphincter dysfunction in neurogenic faecal incontinence. British Journal of Surgery 80: 259–261
Farouk R, Duthie G S, Pryde A, Bartolo D C C 1994a Abnormal transient internal sphincter relaxation in idiopathic pruritus ani: physiological evidence from ambulatory monitoring. British Journal of Surgery 81: 603–606
Farouk R, Duthie G S, MacGregor A B, Bartolo D C C 1994b Rectoanal inhibition and incontinence in patients with rectal prolapse. British Journal of Surgery 81: 743–746
Farouk R, Duthie G S, Bartolo D C C 1994c Recovery of internal anal sphincter and continence after restorative proctocolectomy. British Journal of Surgery 81: 1065–1068
Floyd W, Walls E 1953 Electromyography of the sphincter ani externus in man. Journal of Physiology 16: 638–644
Ford M J, Anderson J R, Gilmour H M, Holt S, Sircus W, Heading R C 1983 Clinical spectrum of "solitary ulcer" of the rectum. Gastroenterology 84: 1533–1540
Freund H R, Humphrey C S, Fischer J E 1981 Reduced tissue content of vasoactive intestinal peptide in aganglionic colon of Hirschsprung's disease. American Journal of Surgery 141: 243–244
Frykman H M, Goldberg S M 1969 The surgical treatment of rectal procidentia. Surgery, Obstetrics & Gynecology 129: 1225–1230
Garrett J R, Howard E R, Nixon H H 1969 Bowel innervation in Hirschsprung's disease. British Medical Journal 3: 718–719
Gattuso J M, Kamm M A 1993 Review article: the management of constipation in adults. Alimentary Pharmacology and Therapeutics 7: 487–500
Gattuso J M, Kamm M A 1994 Adverse effects of drugs used in the management of constipation and diarrhoea. Drug Safety 10: 47–65
Gowers W R 1877 The autonomic action of the sphincter ani. Proceedings of the Royal Society of Medicine London 26: 77–84
Gue M, Junien J L, Bueno L 1991 Conditioned emotional response in rats enhances colonic motility through the central release of corticotrophin-releasing factor. Gastroenterology 100: 964–970
Hallan R I, Williams N S, Melling J 1988 Treatment of anismus in intractable constipation with Botulinum A toxin. Lancet ii: 714–717
Hancock B D 1976 Internal sphincter and the nature of haemorrhoids. Gut 18: 651–656
Harvey R F 1979 Colonic motility in proctalgia fugax. Lancet 2: 713–714
Haward L R C, Hughes-Roberts H E 1962 The treatment of constipation in mental hospitals. Gut 3: 85
Haynes W G, Read N W 1982 Ano-rectal activity in man during rectal infusion of saline: a dynamic assessment of the anal continence mechanism. Journal of Physiology 330: 45–56
Henry M, Parks A G, Swash M 1980 The anal reflex in idiopathic faecal incontinence. An electrophysiological study. British Journal of Surgery 67: 781–783
Holmstrom B, Broden G, Dolk A 1986 Increased anal resting pressure following the Ripstein operation: a contribution to continence? Diseases of the Colon and Rectum 29: 485–487
Ihre T, Seligson U 1975 Intussusception of the rectum – internal procidentia. Treatment and results in 90 patients. Scandinavian Diseases of the Colon and Rectum 18: 391–396
Jesel M, Isch-Treussard C, Isch F 1973 Electromyography of striated muscles of anal and urethral sphincter. New developments in electromyography and clinical neurophysiology. Karger, Basle, pp. 406–420
Johanson J and Sonnenberg A 1990 The prevalence of hemorrhoids and chronic constipation: An epidemiology study. Gastroenterology 98: 380–386
Jones F A, Godding E W 1972 Management of constipation. Blackwell, Oxford
Jones P N, Lubowski D Z, Swash M, Henry M M 1987 Is paradoxical contraction of puborectalis muscle of functional importance? Diseases of the Colon and Rectum 30: 667–670
Kamm M, Hoyle C, Burleigh D et al 1991 Hereditary internal anal sphincter myopathy causing proctalgia fugax and constipation. A newly identified condition. Gastroenterology 100: 805–810
Kamm M A, Lennard-Jones J E, Thompson D G, Sobnack R, Garvie N W, Granowska M 1988 Dynamic scanning defines a colonic defect in severe idiopathic constipation. Gut 29: 1085–1092
Kamm M A, Lennard-Jones J E 1990 Rectal mucosal electrosensory testing – evidence for a rectal sensory neuropathy in idiopathic constipation. Diseases of the Colon and Rectum 33: 419–423
Kamm M A, Lennard-Jones J E 1992 Constipation: pathophysiology. In: Henry M M, Swash M (eds) Coloproctology and the pelvic floor. Butterworth-Heinemann, Oxford, p 411–412
Kamm M A, Hawley P R, Lennard-Jones J E 1988 Lateral division of puborectalis in the management of severe constipation. British Journal of Surgery 75: 661–663
Keighley M R B, Fieldings W L, Alexander-Williams J A 1983 Results of Marlex mesh abdominal rectopexy for rectal prolapse in 100 consecutive patients. British Journal of Surgery 70: 229–232
Kerremans R 1969 Morphological and physiological aspects of anal continence and defaecation. Editions Arscia, Brussels
Kiff E S, Swash M 1984a Slowed conduction in the pudendal nerve in idiopathic (neurogenic) faecal incontinence. British Journal of Surgery 71: 614–616
Kiff E S, Swash M 1984b Normal proximal and delayed distal conduction in the pudendal nerve of patients with idiopathic (neurogenic) faecal incontinence. Journal of Neurology, Neurosurgery and Psychiatry 47: 820–823
Klein M D, Coran A G, Wesley J R, Drongowski R A 1984 Hirschsprung's disease in the newborn. Journal of Pediatric Surgery 19: 370–374
Kleinhaus S, Boley S J, Sheran M, Sieber W K 1979 Hirschsprung's disease. A survey of the members of the Surgical Section of the American Academy of Pediatrics. Journal of Pediatric Surgery 14: 588–597
Koch T R, Carney J A, Go L, Go V L W 1988 Idiopathic chronic constipation is associated with decreased colonic vasoactive intestinal peptide. Gastroenterology 94: 300–310
Koop C E 1966 The choice of surgical procedures in Hirschsprung's disease. Journal of Pediatric Surgery 1: 523
Krevsky B, Malmud L S, D'Ercole F, Maurer A H, Fisher R S 1986

Colonic transit scintigraphy: a physiologic approach to the quantitative measurement of colonic transit in humans. Gastroenterology 91: 1102–1112
Krishnamurthy S, Schuffler M D, Rohrmann C A, Pope C E II 1985 Severe idiopathic constipation is associated with a distinctive abnormality of the colonic myenteric plexus. Gastroenterology 88: 26–34
Kuijpers H C, de Moree H 1988 Towards a selection of the most appropriate procedure in the treatment of complete rectal prolapse. Diseases of the Colon and Rectum 31: 355–357
Kuijpers H C, Strijk S P 1984 Diagnosis of disturbances of continence and defaecation. Diseases of the Colon and Rectum 27: 658–662
Kumar D, Williams N S, Waldron D, Wingate D L 1989 Prolonged manometric recording of anorectal motor activity in ambulant human subjects: evidence of periodic activity. Gut 30: 1007–1011
Lal S, Brown G N 1967 Some unusual complications of fecal impaction. American Journal of Proctology, Gastroenterology and Allied Subjects 18: 226–231
Lawson J O N, Nixon H H 1967 Anal canal pressures in the diagnosis of Hirschsprung's disease. Journal of Pediatric Surgery 2: 544–552
Lincoln J, Crowe R, Kamm M A, Burnstock G, Lennard-Jones J E 1990 Serotonin and 5-hydroxyindoleacetic acid are increased in the sigmoid colon in severe idiopathic constipation. Gastroenterology 98: 1219–1225
Lubowski D Z, King D W, Finlay I G 1992 Electromyography of the pubococcygeus muscles in patients with obstructed defaecation. International Journal of Colorectal Disease 7: 184–187
Lubowski D Z, Meagher A P, Smart R C, Butler S P 1995 Scintigraphic assessment of colonic function during defaecation. International Journal of Colorectal Disease 10(2): 91–93
MacDonagh R, Sun W M, Thomas D G, Smallwood R, Read N W 1992 Anorectal function in patients with complete supraconal spinal cord lesions. Gut 33: 1532–1538
Madoff R D, Williams J G, Wong W D 1992 Long-term functional results of colon resection and rectopexy for overt rectal prolapse. American Journal of Gastroenterology 87: 101–104
Mann C V, Hoffman C 1988 Complete rectal prolapse: the anatomical and functional results of treatment by an extended abdominal rectopexy. British Journal of Surgery 75: 34–37
Marsh H 1994 MD Thesis, University of Bristol
Miller R, Bartolo D C C, Cervero F, Mortensen N J M 1987 Anorectal temperature sensation: a comparison of normal and incontinent patients. British Journal of Surgery 74: 511–515
Miller R, Lewis G T, Bartolo D C C, Cervero F, Mortensen N J M 1988a Sensory discrimination and dynamic activity in the anorectum: evidence using a new ambulatory technique. British Journal of Surgery 75: 1003–1007
Miller R, Bartolo D C C, Locke-Edmunds J C, Mortensen N J M 1988b Prospective study of conservative and operative treatment for faecal incontinence. British Journal of Surgery 75: 101–105
Miller R, Bartolo D C C, Cervero F, Mortensen N J M 1988c Anorectal sampling: a comparison of normal and incontinent patients. British Journal of Surgery 75: 44–47
Miller R, Orrom W J, Cornes H, Duthie G S, Bartolo D C C 1989 Anterior sphincter plication and levatorplasty in the treatment of faecal incontinence. British Journal of Surgery 76: 1058–1060
Miller R, Duthie G S, Bartolo D C C, Roe A M, Locke-Edmunds J, Mortensen N J M 1991 Anismus in patients with normal and slow transit constipation. British Journal of Surgery 78: 690–692
Milner P, Crowe R, Kamm M A, Lennard-Jones J E, Burnstock G 1990 Vasoactive intestinal polypeptide levels in sigmoid colon idiopathic constipation and diverticular disease. Gastroenterology 99: 666–675
Miner P B, Donnelly T C, Read N W 1990 Investigation of mode of action of biofeedback in treatment of fecal incontinence. Digestive Diseases and Sciences 35: 1291–1298
Morris A I, Turnberg L A 1979 Surreptitious laxative abuse. Gastroenterology 77: 780–786
Müller-Lissner S A 1993 Adverse effects of laxatives: fact and fiction. Pharmacology 47(suppl 1): 138–145
Neill M E, Swash M 1980 Increased motor unit fibre density in the external anal sphincter in anorectal incontinence: a single fibre EMG study. Journal of Neurology, Neurosurgery and Psychiatry 43: 343–347
Nielson M B, Hauge C, Rasmussen O O, Pedersen J F, Christensen J 1992 Anal endosonographic findings in the follow-up of primarily sutured sphincteric ruptures. British Journal of Surgery 79: 104–106
Nixon H H 1971 Hirschsprung's disease. British Journal of Hospital Medicine 5: 199
Oresland T, Fasth S, Nordgren S, Akervall S, Hulten L 1990a Pouch size: the important functional determinant after restorative proctocolectomy. British Journal of Surgery 77: 265–269
Oresland T, Fasth S, Akervall S, Nordgren S, Hulten L 1990b Manovolumetric and sensory characteristics of the ileoanal J pouch compared with healthy rectum. British Journal of Surgery 77: 803–806
Orkin B A, Hanson R B, Kelly K A, Phillips S F, Dent J 1991 Human anal motility while fasting, after feeding, and during sleep. Gastroenterology 100(4): 1016–1023
Orrom W J, Miller R, Cornes H, Duthie G S, Mortensen N J M, Bartolo D C C 1991a Comparison of anterior sphincteroplasty and postanal repair in the treatment of idiopathic faecal incontinence. Diseases of the Colon and Rectum 34: 305–310
Orrom W J, Bartolo D C C, Miller R, Mortensen N J M, Roe A M 1991b Rectopexy is an ineffective treatment for obstructive defecation. Diseases of the Colon and Rectum 34: 41–46
Parks A G 1975 Anorectal incontinence. Proceedings of the Royal Society of Medicine 68: 681–690
Parks A G, Porter N H, Melzack J 1962 Experimental study of the reflex mechanism controlling the muscle of the pelvic floor. Diseases of the Colon and Rectum 5: 407–414
Parks A G, Porter N H, Hardcastle J D 1966 The syndrome of the descending perineum. Proceedings of the Royal Society of Medicine 59: 477–482
Parks A G, Swash M, Urich H 1977 Sphincter denervation in anorectal incontinence and rectal prolapse. Gut 18: 656–665
Penninckx F, Lestar B, Kerremans R 1995 Manometric evaluation of incotinent patients. Acta Gastroenterologie Belgique 58(1): 51–59
Pinho M, Yoshioka K, Keighley M R B 1989 Longterm results of anorectal myectomy for chronic constipation. British Journal of Surgery 76: 1163–1164
Preston D M, Lennard Jones J E 1985 Anismus in chronic constipation. Digestive Diseases and Sciences 30: 413–418
Prior A, Fearn U J, Read N W 1991 Intermittent rectal motor activity: a rectal motor complex? Gut 32: 1360–1363
Rao S S and Read N W 1990 Gastrointestinal motility in patients with ulcerative colitis. Scand. J. Gastroenterol. 172(Suppl.): 22–28
Read M G, Read N W 1982 Role of anorectal sensation in preserving continence. Gut 23: 345–347
Read N W, Harford W V, Schmulen A C, Read M G, Santa Ana C, Fordtran J S 1979 A clinical study of patients with faecal incontinence and diarrhoea. Gastroenterology 76: 747–756
Read M G, Read N W, Barber D C, Duthie H L 1982a Effects of loperamide on anal sphincter function in patients complaining of chronic diarrhoea with faecal incontinence and urgency. Digestive Diseases and Sciences 27: 807–814
Read M G, Read N W, Haynes W G, Donnelly T C, Johnson A G 1982b A prospective study of the effect of haemorrhoidectomy on sphincter function and continence. British Journal of Surgery 69: 396–398
Read N W, Haynes W G, Bartolo D C C, Hall J, Read M G, Donnelly T C, Johnson A G 1983a Use of anorectal manometry during rectal infusion of saline to investigate sphincter function in incontinent patients. Gastroenterology 85: 105–113
Read N W, Bartolo D C C, Read M G, Hall J, Haynes W G, Johnson A G 1983b Differences in anorectal manometry between patients with haemorrhoids and patients with descending perineum syndrome: implications for management. British Journal of Surgery 70: 656–659
Read N W, Bartolo D C C, Read M G 1984 Differences in anal function in patients with incontinence to solids and in patients with incontinence to liquids. British Journal of Surgery 71: 39–42
Read N W, Timms J M, Barfield L J, Donnelly T C, Bannister J J 1986 Impairment of defaecation in young women with severe constipation. Gastroenterology 90: 53–60
Read N W, Sun W M 1992 Anorectal manometry. Coloproctology and pelvic floor. London, Butterworths. 2nd edition, pp. 119–145
Reynolds J C, Ouyang A, Lee C A, Baker L, Sunshine A G, Cohen S

1987 Chronic severe constipation. Prospective motility studies in 25 consecutive patients. Gastroenterology 92: 414–420
Roe A M, Bartolo D C C, Mortensen N J M 1986 New method for assessment of anal sensation in various anorectal disorders. British Journal of Surgery 73: 310–312
Rutter K R P, Riddell R H 1975 The solitary ulcer syndrome of the rectum. Clinics in Gastroenterology 4: 505–530
Sainio A P, Voutilainen P E, Husa A I 1991 Recovery of anal sphincter function following transabdominal repair of rectal prolapse: cause of improved continence? Diseases of the Colon and Rectum 34: 816–821
Schuster M M, Hookman P, Hendrix T R 1965 Simultaneous manometric recording of internal and external anal sphincter reflexes. Bulletin of the John Hopkins Hospital 116: 79–88
Schuster M M 1977 Constipation and anorectal disorders. Clinics in Gastroenterology 6: 643–658
Shouler P, Keighley M R B 1986 Changes in colorectal function in severe idiopathic chronic constipation. Gastroenterology 90: 414–420
Smith B 1968 Effect of irritant purgatives on the myenteric plexus in man and the mouse. Gut 9: 139–143
Snooks S J, Setchell M, Swash M, Henry M 1984 Injury to the innervation of the pelvic floor sphincter musculature in childbirth. Lancet 2: 546–550
Speare G S 1951 Melanosis coli. Experimental observations on its production and elimination in twenty-three cases. American Journal of Surgery 82: 631
Spencer R J 1984 Manometric studies in rectal prolapse. Diseases of the Colon and Rectum 27: 523–525
Stalberg E, Trontelj J V 1979 Single fibre electromyography. Miravelle, Woking, UK
Sultan A H, Nicholls R J, Kamm M A, Hudson C N, Beynon J, Bartram C I 1993a Anal endosonography and correlation with in vitro and in vivo anatomy. British Journal of Surgery 80: 508–511
Sultan A H, Kamm M A, Hudson C N, Bartram C I 1993b Anal sphincter disruption during vaginal delivery. New England Journal of Medicine 329: 1905–1911
Sultan A H, Kamm M A, Hudson C N 1994a Pudendal nerve damage during labour: prospective study before and after childbirth. British Journal of Obstetrics and Gynaecology 101: 22–28
Sultan A H, Kamm M A, Bartram C I, Hudson C N 1994b Third degree obstetric anal sphincter tears: risk factors and outcome of primary repair. British Medical Journal 308: 887–891
Sun W M 1993 Obstructed defaecation. Journal of Gastroenterology and Hepatology 8: 383–389
Sun W M, Donnely T C, Read N W 1989 Anorectal function in normal human subjects: effect of gender. International Journal of Colorectal Disease 4: 188–196
Sun W M, Donnelly T C, Read N W 1992 Utility of a combined test of anorectal manometry, electromyography, and sensation in determining the mechanism of 'idiopathic' faecal incontinence. Gut 33: 807–813
Sun W M, MacDonagh R, Forster D, Thomas D G, Smallwood R, Read N W 1995 Anorectal function in patients with complete spinal transection before and after sacral posterior rhizotomy. Gastroenterology 108: 990–998
Sun W M, Peck R J, Shorthouse A J, Read N W 1992 Haemorrhoids are associated not with hypertrophy of the internal anal sphincter, but with hypertension of the anal cushions. British Journal of Surgery 79: 592–594
Sun W M, Read N W, Donnelly T C 1990 Anorectal function in incontinent patients with cerebrospinal disease. Gastroenterology 99: 1372–1379
Sun W M, Read N W, Prior A, Daly J A, Cheah S K, Grundy D 1990 Sensory and motor responses to rectal distention vary according to rate and pattern of balloon inflation. Gastroenterology 99: 1008–1015
Sun W M, Read N W, Shorthouse A J 1990 Hypertensive anal cushions as a cuase of the high anal canal pressure in patients with haemorrhoids. British Journal of Surgery 77: 458–462
Suzuki H, Matsumoto K, Amano S, Fujioka M, Honzumi M 1980 Anorectal pressure and rectal compliance after low anterior resection. British Journal of Surgery 67: 655–657
Tam P K H, Lister J 1986 Development profile of neuron-specific enolase in human gut and its implications in Hirschprung's disease. Gastroenterology 90: 1901–1906
Thompson W G, Heaton K W 1980 Proctalgia fugax. Journal of the Royal College of Physicians of London 14: 247–248
Thompson W G 1981 Proctalgia fugax. Digestive Diseases and Sciences 26: 1121–1124
Van Tets W F, Kuijpers J H C 1995 Internal intussusception: fact or fancy. Diseases of the Colon and Rectum 30: 1080–1083
Wald A, Jafri F, Rehder J, Holeva K 1993 Scintigraphic studies of rectal emptying in patients with constipation and defecatory difficulty. Digestive Diseases and Sciences 38(2): 353–358
Walls E W 1959 Recent observations on the anatomy of the anal canal. Proceedings of the Royal Society of Medicine 52 (suppl): 85–87
Wassermann I F 1964 Puborectalis syndrome (rectal stenosis due to anorectal spasm). Diseases of the Colon and Rectum 7: 87–98
Watts J D, Rothenberger D A, Buls J G, Goldberg S M, Nivatvongs S 1985 The management of procidentia. 30 years experience. Diseases of the Colon and Rectum 28: 96–102
Wells C 1959 New operation for rectal prolapse. Proceedings of the Royal Society of Medicine 52: 602–603
Williams N S, Hallan R I, Koeze T H, Watkins E S 1990 Construction of a neoanal sphincter by transposition of the gracilis muscle and prolonged neuromuscular stimulation for the treatment of faecal incontinence. Annals of the Royal College of Surgeons of England 72: 108–113
Womack N R, Williams N S, Holmfield J H M, Morrison J F B, Simpkins K C 1985 New method for the dynamic assessment of anorectal function in constipation. British Journal of Surgery 72: 994–998
Yoshioka K, Keighley M R B 1987a Anorectal myectomy for outlet obstruction. British Journal of Surgery 74: 373–376
Yoshioka K, Keighley M R B 1987b Randomised trial comparing anorectal myectomy and controlled anal dilatation for outlet obstruction. British Journal of Surgery 74: 1125–1129

# 53. Irritable bowel syndrome

*M. J. Ford*

COLONIC ANATOMY

## The structure of the colon

The colonic muscle consists of an inner meshwork of circular fibers and an outer layer of longitudinal fibers which is largely concentrated into three teniae that fuse in the region of the rectosigmoid junction. Some of the muscle fibers of the teniae penetrate and attach to the circular muscle. The colon is divided by many outpouchings; the indentations between them are known as haustra. The macroscopic and radiological appearance of the colon has not been correlated with findings on dissection. For example, some of the haustrations in the normal colon are permanent, whilst others are not, but the permanent haustrations show no particular organization of the muscle. The mucosal surface shows some folds which are called plicae semilunares.

In the human colon, nerve cells are concentrated in Auerbach's plexus between the circular and longitudinal muscle and in Meissner's plexus in the submucosa (p. 154). The mucosal surface is flat and numerous tubular crypts open into it; the crypts extend to the muscularis mucosae. The lower part of the crypt contains goblet cells, undifferentiated cells and endocrine cells. The luminal part of the crypts and the surface epithelium comprise absorptive cells interspersed with goblet cells. Large lymphoid follicles may be a normal feature of the lamina propria and can extend into the submucosa. The lower two-thirds of the crypt contain the proliferative compartment of relatively undifferentiated cells. Division of these cells gives rise to absorptive and goblet cells which are ultimately extruded from the surface of the colon, a process which takes approximately 3 days. Cell proliferation can be extensively modified by fasting and refeeding, pH, different dietary fibers and the presence of minerals.

Mucus provides lubrication in the rectum for luminal solids and maintains a relatively neutral microclimate at the interface between the lumen and mucosa. Mucus is classified according to its polysaccharide side-chains into neutral and acidic (sialo- or sulfo-) mucins. Mucus becomes more acidic in the distal colon, with the appearance of relatively greater amounts of sialomucins. Studies using monoclonal antibodies to a variety of specific mucus subtypes have demonstrated a relatively even distribution throughout the colon and at various levels in individual crypts, implying sharing of common structures amongst glycoprotein molecules.

## Vascular supply to the colon

The arterial supply to the colon is via the ileocolic, right colic and middle colic branches of the superior mesenteric artery, the left colic, sigmoid and superior rectal branches of the inferior mesenteric artery and the inferior rectal branch of the internal pudendal artery from the internal iliac artery (p. 541). The portal vein receives blood from the superior and inferior mesenteric veins and the internal iliac vein, from the inferior rectal veins. The lymphatic vessels of the appendix and cecum drain via the ileocolic nodes, the ascending and transverse colon via the paracolic nodes to the superior mesenteric set of preaortic nodes and the descending and sigmoid colon and the upper rectum to the inferior mesenteric set of preaortic nodes. The lower 10 cm of rectum drains superiorly via the inferior mesenteric set of preaortic nodes and both laterally and inferiorly via the internal iliac node. Below the pectinate line, i.e. the mucocutaneous junction, lymph drains via the external and common iliac nodes to the superficial inguinal nodes.

## Neural control of the colon

*Extrinsic nervous system* (Furness et al 1990)

The cephalic control of the colon comprises the cerebral cortex and hypothalamus and influences colonic responses to food and stress via neural and hormonal pathways, the latter being mediated in part by β-endorphin and corticotrophin-releasing factor (Rogers et al 1993, Tache et al

1993). The brainstem, spinal cord and prevertebral ganglia control enteroenteric reflexes. The parasympathetic supply to the colon is predominantly via the sacral outflow (S2–S4) and the pelvic nerves (nervi erigentes). The vagus supplies the cecum, ascending and transverse colon and the remainder is supplied by the pelvic nerves. The sympathetic supply comprises the splanchnic, lumbar colonic and hypogastric nerves (T5–L3) via the celiac and mesenteric ganglia. The splanchnic and lumbar colonic sympathetic nerves supply the motor innervation to the proximal colon and the entire colon respectively. The sympathetic hypogastric nerve supplies the motor and sensory innervation of the internal anal sphincter and the parasympathetic nervi erigentes, the sensory innervation of the rectum. Only spinal afferents traveling with the sympathetic fibers supply pain sensation. Parasympathetic stimulation increases muscle and secretory activity and ablation results in colonic inertia and severe constipation, e.g. spinal cord lesions. Sympathetic stimulation decreases smooth muscle contractility and inhibits secretomotor function. When deficient, e.g. in diabetic autonomic neuropathy, the increased and inco-ordinated motor and secretory activity typically results in diarrhea (see also p. 153).

*Enteric nervous system* (p. 154)

The enteric nervous system of the colon is similar in structure and distribution to that of the midgut with myenteric and submucous plexuses. Most of the submucosal ganglia project to the epithelium and facilitate ion transport. Nerve fibers containing norepinephrine or acetylcholine are considered to be extrinsic as their cell bodies are located in the prevertebral ganglia or vagal/spinal cord nuclei respectively. In the submucosal ganglia, the principal neurotransmitters are acetylcholine and VIP; neurones containing 5-HT, enkephalins or GRP are not present, unlike the myenteric ganglia where such neurones synapse with interneurons and help co-ordinate motility patterns with ion transport. In disorders such as Hirschsprung's disease, the enteric nervous system is characteristically involved, often with a predominant loss of VIP or nitrergic neurones, resulting in an impairment of smooth muscle relaxation and severe, intractable constipation (Huizinga et al 1985, Sarna 1991a, b).

## COLONIC PHYSIOLOGY

The major functions of the colon are listed in Table 53.1.

**Table 53.1** Functions of the colon

| |
|---|
| Absorption of water, electrolytes and the products of bacterial fermentation, e.g. short chain fatty acids |
| Reservoir with a slow emptying rate to facilitate bacterial fermentation and absorption |
| Mixing and kneading of intraluminal content to enhance fermentation and absorption |
| Storage of feces until defecation is appropriate |
| Controlled rapid propulsion and expulsion of intraluminal content during mass movements and defecation |
| Detection, discrimination and processing of sensory stimuli |

### Colonic absorption

Colonic absorptive processes are slower than those of the small bowel as the colonic surface area of absorption per unit length is small in the absence of villi. Nonetheless, the absorptive capacity of water by the normal colon, usually 2 liters per day, may increase to 5–6 liters per day. Bacterial fermentation of nonstarch polysaccharides to short chain fatty acids (p. 341), principally acetate, proprionate and butyrate, is a slow process; similarly, the absorption of water, electrolytes and the products of fermentation is slow since it occurs against osmotic and concentration gradients. Degradation of 60–70 g of carbohydrate per day is required in order to maintain colonic bacterial mass, much of which is derived from poorly absorbed, complex polysaccharides. To promote these functions, the motility of the colon ensures extensive mixing and kneading, slow continuous net propulsion and intermittent, forceful sustained contractions to rapidly propel and expel solid or viscous fecal material (Gaginella 1994).

### Intestinal gas production

The volume of gas passed each day by normal subjects is 400–1200 ml and at any time there is 30–200 ml in the bowel. It is possible to make a reasonable estimate of the volume of gas by plain abdominal radiography. Normally, 20–80 ml of gas is present in the stomach, virtually none is in the small intestine and the remainder is in the colon. Nitrogen and carbon dioxide are the predominant gases in flatus; oxygen is present in small amounts and hydrogen and methane vary from undetectable amounts to 30% of the total. Most of the nitrogen is probably swallowed. Carbon dioxide is produced during the process of digestion, e.g. by the interactions of gastric acid with bicarbonate and fatty acids with amino acids. Oxygen is derived from swallowed air; it is rapidly absorbed and some may also be utilized by intestinal bacteria. Most of the hydrogen is produced by the bacterial microflora of the colon and excreted in the breath and flatus. However, substantial quantities are metabolized by methanogenic and sulfate-reducing bacteria. Methane is also produced by bacteria; about one-third of the population are methane producers. Flatus also contains trace amounts of a large number of odoriferous gases, such as hydrogen sulfide, ammonia, volatile amino acids and short chain fatty acids. Thus the composition of the colonic flora determines, in part, the nature and amount of gas production. In normal circumstances it is produced in the colon from malabsorbed simple and complex carbohydrates in the diet. For example, beans contain oligosaccharides which cannot be absorbed in the small intestine and are split by colonic bacteria. In malabsorption syndromes, unabsorbed dietary carbohydrate is fermented in the colon and the absorbed hydrogen forms the basis of the hydrogen breath test (p. 342). In blind loop syndromes, hydrogen can also be produced in the small intestine (Levitt 1980, Christl et al 1992).

## Dietary fiber

Dietary fiber consists of plant cell wall polysaccharides comprising cellulose, hemicellulose, pectin and lignin. Most nonstarch polysaccharides enter the colon undigested. A proportion of dietary starch also enters the colon intact but is not included in the definition of dietary fiber. Some polysaccharides are completely fermented by colonic bacteria in the right colon, resulting in the production of short chain fatty acids (acetate, proprionate and butyrate), hydrogen, methane, carbon dioxide and water (p. 341). Other dietary fiber, for example cellulose, is only partly fermented. The cellulose and other cell wall polysaccharides of wheat bran, because of their lignin content, are relatively resistant to breakdown. Nonstarch polysaccharide is the component of dietary fiber that principally affects bowel habit. This effect is due to its physical and chemical properties particularly the water solubility, extent of digestion, pentose content, viscosity, particle size and lignin content. The method of cooking and the colonic transit time also influence its activity.

Dietary fiber has several important physiological effects. It increases the stool weight, volume and colonic transit rates; the fermented products lead to an increased volume of microflora and the unfermented products trap water within the cellular matrix; both result in increased fecal bulk. Fiber also softens feces, probably owing to an increased content of gas, and the accelerated colonic transit also reduces water reabsorption. Experimental evidence suggests that bran reduces pressures in the sigmoid colon. Other effects of fiber include an increase in the output of fecal bile acids and impairment of mineral absorption from the stool (Cummings 1973, Eastwood & Morris 1992).

## Colonic sensory function (p. 153)

The origin of sensations throughout the gastrointestinal tract is poorly understood. Most visceral sensory information never reaches the level of consciousness and is primarily concerned with the regulation and co-ordination of secretory and motor functions. Visceral afferent neurones are involved both in mediating reflexes which alter motility and in the conscious perception of visceral sensation (Mayer & Raybould 1990).

Conscious, visceral sensation can be grouped into either diffuse, painless sensations (bloating, incomplete rectal evacuation, urgency, desire to pass flatus/feces) or localized, painful sensations concerned with nociceptive stimuli. Visceral sensations from mucosal, muscular or serosal receptors are mediated by spinal afferent fibers running within both the sympathetic and the parasympathetic nerve trunks. Furthermore, parasympathetic afferents may also modulate the sensitivity of spinal afferents via reflex pathways. However, only spinal afferents associated with sympathetic nerve trunks mediate visceral pain (Mayer & Raybould 1990).

In the colon, as in the rest of the gut, there are sensory receptors which exhibit a graded response to both innocuous and noxious levels of stimulation. Such a mechanism may have a role in signaling visceral pain (Ness et al 1990). Though no specific nociceptive receptors have been identified as yet within the gut, nociceptors do exist in other organs. Differences exist in the patterns of perception to colonic distention induced by balloons. Rapid, intermittent distention induces sensations which are quantitatively and qualitatively different from those induced by slower, progressively increasing distention (Sun et al 1990). However, studies have shown a considerable degree of variation in colonic sensitivity between investigators which is attributable to different methodologies. Balloon shape, size, viscoelastic properties, rate and pattern of distention, position in the colon, age and sex, anxiety and arousal ratings may all contribute to these variations (Sun et al 1990). In consequence, the results from different investigators cannot readily be compared.

Gut compliance is usually assessed by analysis of the pressure–volume relationship during balloon-induced distention of the colon. Most viscera are compliant within the physiologic range of distention. Thereafter, even small increases in the distending volume will result in rapid increases in pressure. Colonic compliance, and hence the response of sensory receptors, is dependent upon colonic muscle tone, i.e. activity in efferent nerve fibers.

## Colonic motor function

### *Intrinsic myogenic control*

The stomach and small bowel are programmed by an underlying electrical control activity (ECA). The colon, however, is not programmed in the same manner and exhibits multiple rather than a single contractile pattern. Unlike the stomach and small bowel, colonic ECA is not omnipresent, there is no evidence of colonic pacemaker cells like the interstitial cells of Cajal, there is a near absence of gap junctions and close appositions linking colonic muscle cells and the ECA is phase unlocked, i.e. its frequency, amplitude and intercycle intervals vary considerably in different anatomic sites. Therefore, co-ordination of the ECA between groups of cells in the interdigestive period is poor; when electromechanical coupling does occur, contractions may only involve a small segment of the colonic circumference. Indeed, synchronous, circumferential, propagating contractions are usually only observed following cholinergic stimulation (Sarna 1991a, b).

*The control of motor activity*

Unlike the stomach and small bowel where patterns of phasic and tonic contractility have been well characterized, the motor contractility of the human colon is poorly understood. Though there is a migrating motor complex (MMC) within the rectum in man, no cyclic interdigestive MMC patterns have been shown to extend either distally from the ileum or proximally from the rectum. The ileocecal sphincter controls the entry of ileal contents into the cecum and exhibits short bursts of phasic contractions but basal tone is minimal (Quigley et al 1984). Small bowel MMCs usually fade out before reaching the sphincter. Eating followed by distention of the ileum may relax the sphincter and allow chyme to move into the colon. It is not known to what extent these events are controlled by neural or hormonal mechanisms or how they relate to the ileal brake mechanism. The sphincter may also prevent reflux into the ileum.

The colonic response to eating is influenced by a cephalic phase and though primarily under neural control, humoral influences also contribute to augment the response (Rogers et al 1993). Distention of the stomach or ingestion of a high fat meal leads to an immediate increase in the frequency of both myoelectric and phasic contractile activity in the sigmoid colon. This "gastrocolonic reflex" is predominantly neurally mediated and is diminished by muscarinic or opioid receptor antagonists; it is absent in patients with spinal cord transection or autonomic neuropathy (Holdstock & Misiewicz 1970, Sullivan et al 1978).

Colonic motor contractile activity comprises both propagative and nonpropagative (segmentation) contractions. Studies of the contractile patterns of the colon have shown that colonic motility is sporadic, irregular and nonpropagative for most of the time. Regular propagative contractile activity occurs principally on awakening and postprandially and in toto, represents only 7% of total colonic motility; 87% of regular motility occurs in the sigmoid and descending colon, where the commonest contractile frequency is three per minute (Bassotti et al 1993), but contraction frequencies in the human colon range from one to 13 per minute (Sarna 1991b).

Frequent, relatively low amplitude, nonpropagating, short duration contractions appear to be associated with short spike bursts of myolectric activity. In contrast, infrequent, relatively high amplitude, propagating contractions (HAPC) are associated with long spike bursts and both circular and longitudinal muscle activity. In the human colon, there is anatomic evidence of longitudinal muscle bundles penetrating into the circular muscle coat. The physical coupling of the muscle coats is believed to mediate co-ordination of circular and longitudinal muscle contraction; propagating contractions occur when the slow waves of the circular muscle are synchronous with the onset of long spike bursts of the longitudinal muscle (Sarna 1991a).

High amplitude propagating contractions originate in the ascending colon and occur in health up to six times per day. Half occur on awakening before breakfast and half within 2 h after meals. They are the motility correlate of mass movements and propagate over great distances at speeds of about 1 cm per second. They are usually, but not invariably, antegrade in direction.

*Flow and transit*

Segmentation causes a slow mixing of colonic contents without propulsion. This activity is responsible for the production of some of the haustra. Propulsion or mass movements have been studied using radio-opaque markers with time-lapse cineradiography and radioisotope scanning. Mass movements, which occur three or four times per day, result in feces moving distally for a variable distance; they are preceded by the disappearance of haustra distally. Transit from the cecum to rectum usually takes about 12 h, but in some individuals it can take over 24 h. Segmentation increases when food enters the upper small intestine. Propulsive activity increases after meals, especially if physical activity is also increased (Holdstock et al 1970, Krevsky et al 1986).

Colonic transit and flow patterns are critically dependent on the pattern of contractions which in turn are dependent upon the stimulus of colonic distention produced by the volume and hydraulic properties of the intraluminal contents. However, the contractile frequency and amplitude and the mean regional transit rates appear to be similar in the different colonic regions in the unprepared colon. In the prepared colon, the emptying rate of the ascending colon is considerably more rapid than elsewhere in the colon; emptying is logarithmic rather than linear and the mean $t_{1/2}$ is 1.5 h (Krevsky et al 1986) compared with 5.5 h in the unprepared ascending colon (Proano et al 1990). Fluid loading of the ascending colon increases regional colonic transit rates and the whole colonic transit rate correlates with intraluminal water content (Hammer & Phillips 1993). In addition, dietary fiber may further increase transit rates in a variety of ways depending upon its physicochemical properties.

The functions of the proximal colon are principally those of a reservoir to facilitate mixing, fermentation and reabsorption. Radioscintigraphic studies in the unprepared colon indicate that at 24 h, 40% of the radiolabel is still proximal to the splenic flexure and only 4% proximal to the hepatic flexure. Such data suggest that the transverse colon is the predominant site of mixing, dehydration and storage (Proano et al 1990). The contents of the proximal colon are fluid having different hydraulic properties compared to the more solid contents of the distal colon. The distending stimulus of fluids is different from that of solids; in consequence, it is possible that different colonic sensory receptors will be stimulated, evoking different patterns of contractile activity. Furthermore, competence of the ileocecal sphincter and the incompressibility of fluid ensure that when segmental contractions occur in the proximal colon, the net movement of contents is antegrade, irrespective of whether contractions are isoperistaltic or antiperistaltic.

The motor activity of the proximal colon is predominantly irregular and unco-ordinated. Regular, propulsive contractile activity represents a greater proportion of segmental contractions in the distal than the proximal colon. Most propagative contractility occurs after awakening and after meals and the direction of movement of intraluminal content is determined by the pressure gradient between adjacent colonic segments. In health, the net hourly antegrade movement of colonic contents is approximately 5 cm, i.e. on average, 8 cm caudad and 3 cm cephalad; 71% of colonic contents are defecated by 48 h (using scintigraphic methods) and the mean colonic transit time is about 40 h (using radio-opaque marker methods) (Krevsky et al 1986, Proano et al 1990, Bassotti et al 1993).

## Normal bowel habit

Only 1% of the population has less than three bowel actions per week or more than three per day (Connell et al 1965). The former should be regarded as constipated and the latter as abnormal, particularly if the stools are loose. If the stool is hard and difficult to pass, even persons with one bowel movement per day can be regarded as constipated. Stool consistency is normally highly variable and can best be characterized using standard stool descriptors (Heaton et al 1992a) (Table 53.2). However, only the extremes of stool forms correlate closely with colonic transit rates (Degen & Phillips 1996).

As the intake of dietary fiber increases, colonic transit time decreases and the stools become softer and more frequent. Studies have shown, however, that the variability in stool output in response to increased dietary fiber intake is determined more by psychological factors than by the nature or quantity of the fiber ingested (Tucker et al 1981, Fowlie et al 1992a). In healthy females, colonic transit is slower and stool consistency harder than in males (Heaton et al 1992a). However, no consistent difference in colonic transit between the follicular and luteal phases of the menstrual cycle has been identified and the cause of the gender differences is unknown (Heitkemper & Jarrett 1992, Lampe et al 1993).

**Table 53.2** Stool consistency scale (Heaton et al 1992a)

| | |
|---|---|
| 1. | Separate hard lumps, like nuts |
| 2. | Sausage shaped and lumpy |
| 3. | Sausage shaped, cracked surface |
| 4. | Sausages or "snaky", smooth, soft |
| 5. | Soft blobs, clearcut edges |
| 6. | Fluffy pieces, ragged edges, "mushy" |
| 7. | Watery, no solids |

## Investigation of colonic transit rate

The most popular and appropriate method of estimating transit times in patients with constipation in clinical practice is by abdominal radiography following the ingestion of radio-opaque markers. In this way, mouth-to-anus, whole colon and segmental colonic transit can be assessed. The technique is, however, of limited value in assessing accelerated transit. An alternative strategy is to measure transit using radioisotopic scintigraphic markers and gamma camera imaging. Neither method requires major dietary modification, orocecal intubation or prior bowel preparation. Effective radiation dose equivalents for the two methods are similar (Metcalf et al 1987, Camilleri & Zinsmeister 1992).

### *Radio-opaque marker method*

The modified Hinton technique requires that the bowel is free of any residual barium from previous contrast radiographic studies and that subjects eat a normal diet with a standard 10 g fiber supplementation and avoid the use of laxatives or enemas. At the same hour of the day, the subject ingests 24 radio-opaque markers on days 1, 2 and 3 and a high KV fast-film abdominal X-ray is taken on day 4 (25% of the radiation dose of an ordinary abdominal radiograph). In patients with significant constipation or if transit is delayed, markers are ingested daily for 3 more days and a further radiograph is undertaken on day 7 (Metcalf et al 1987).

The colon is divided into the right, left and rectosigmoid segments by identification of gaseous bowel outlines (if visible) and bony landmarks, i.e. lines drawn on the abdominal X-ray between the lumbar vertebral spines and between the fifth lumbar spine and left anterior superior iliac crest and right pelvic brim. If the bowel outlines clearly show the transverse colon or cecum, markers should be judged to be in the appropriate colonic segment based on the bowel outlines seen. Markers to the right of the lumbar spine above the pelvic brim are assigned to the right colon, markers to the left of the lumbar spine are assigned to the left colon if above the line to the anterior superior iliac crest and to the rectosigmoid colon if below this line (Fig. 53.1).

The mean total colonic transit time (hours) is equivalent to the sum of the total number of markers present on

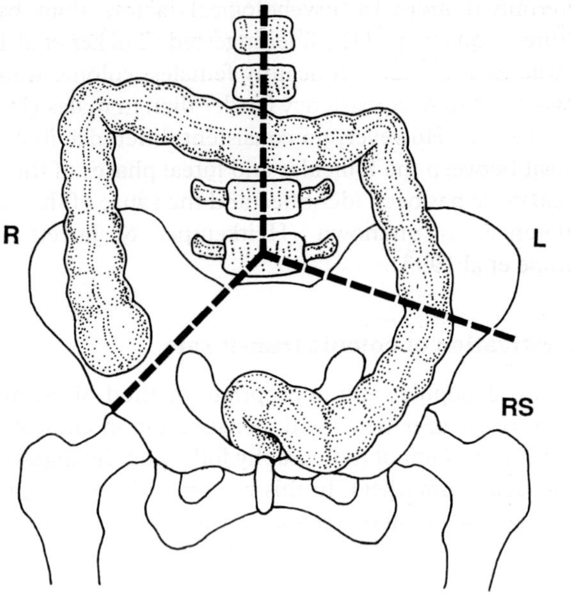


**Fig. 53.1** Ingested radio-opaque markers (24 per capsule, one capsule per day) appearing along the colonic silhouette of an abdominal radiograph taken on day 4 are counted and represent transit time through the regions shown. R = right segment; L = left segment; RS = rectosigmoid segment. Colonic transit time (h) = total number of markers visible.

day 4 (or the sum of the number of markers present on day 4 and day 7). The mean segmental colonic transit times are indicated by the number of markers in each of the three colonic regions. The variability in segmental transit is such that prolongation of the mean segmental transit time should not be considered abnormal unless the mean total colonic transit time is also significantly prolonged. The normal values shown in the example are from a USA population (Table 53.3).

**Table 53.3** Example of a colonic transit study

| Mean colinic transit time (hrs) – normal values (mean : upper limit) | |
|---|---|
| Right colon | 12 markers (day 4) = 12 hours (11.5 : 30.6) |
| Left colon | 22 markers (day 4) = 22 hours (11.2 : 34.6) |
| Rectosigmoid | 38 markers (day 4) = 38 hours (12.4 : 32.0) |
| Total colon | 72 markers (day 4) = >72 hours (35.2 : 72.0) |
| Total colon | 52 markers (day 7) = 124 hours (day 4 + day 7) |

*Combined gastric, small bowel and colonic transit measurements by the radioscintigraphic marker method*

The radioisotope $^{111}$indium (half-life 68 h) is used to label polystyrene ion-exchange pellets which are then placed in a gelatin capsule coated with a single layer of a pH-sensitive polymer, methacrylate. The capsule is designed to release its contents within the pH range 7.2–7.4, i.e. the mean pH observed in the terminal ileum. Concomitant administration of the radioisotope $^{99m}$technetium (adsorbed onto resin pellets) is used if an integrated study of gastric and small intestinal transit times is required. The effective radiation dose equivalent of $^{111}$indium (0.1 mCi) and $^{99m}$technetium (1 mCi) combined is 0.13, an exposure similar to that of a plain abdominal radiograph (80 mrads) (Fig. 53.2).

Scintigraphic, single-plane (anterior and posterior) scanning using a dual gamma camera is undertaken at time 0, 4 and 24 h if only total colonic transit is to be

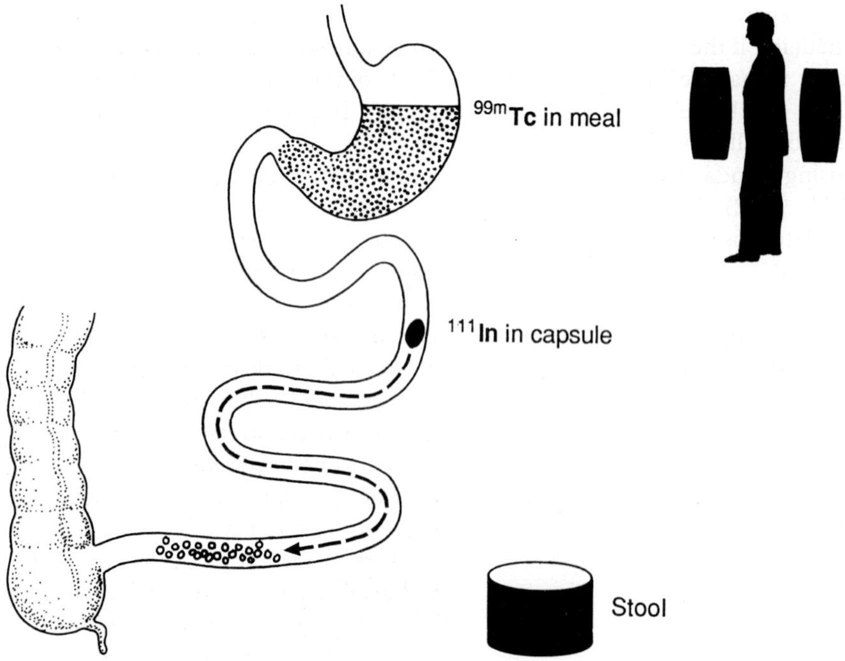


**Fig. 53.2** Scintigraphic transit.

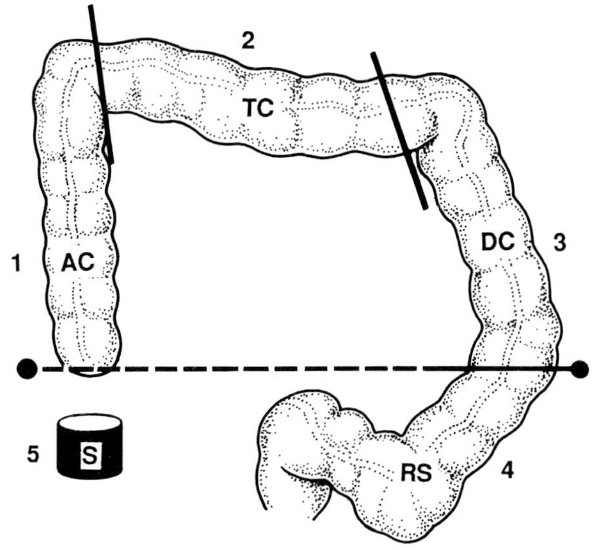


**Fig. 53.3** Colonic scintigraphy. AC = ascending colon; TC = transverse colon; DC = descending colon; RS = rectosigmoid colon; S = stool. The numbers are the weighting factors for each region, used in calculating the geometric center.

**Table 53.4** Geometric center of colonic isotope

| Group | Mean ± SEM (range) 4 h | 24 h |
|---|---|---|
| Healthy subjects | 1.1 ±0.1 (0.8–1.4) | 2.6 ±0.3 (1.6–3.6) |
| Constipation | 1.0 ±0.2 | 1.8 ±0.2 |
| Diarrhea | 2.3 ±0.3 | 3.7 ±0.3 |

assessed. Standard corrections for depth and isotope decay are made, i.e. attenuation and scatter are assessed from the geometric mean of anterior and posterior counts (Camilleri & Zinsmeister 1992). The $^{111}$indium radiolabel is used to identify the colonic regions of interest. The colonic transit time is evaluated as the geometric center (GC), i.e. the weighted mean of the proportion of $^{111}$indium isotope counts in each colonic region at 4, 6 and 24 h, e.g. GC4, GC6, GC24. In practice, the colonic regions – ascending colon, transverse colon, descending colon, rectosigmoid colon and stool – are designated a number from 1–5 respectively as a weighting factor. The proportion of counts in each region is multiplied by the weighting factor and the sum calculated (Fig. 53.3). Thus a low geometric center implies that most of the $^{111}$indium isotope lies within the ascending colon whereas a high geometric center suggests that most of the $^{111}$indium isotope has been evacuated in the stool. Table 53.4 shows ranges of colonic transit rates as measured by scintigraphy.

## FUNCTIONAL GASTROINTESTINAL DISORDERS

### Introduction

Functional disorders can be defined as constellations of symptoms persisting for 3 months or more, associated with altered physiologic function, for which no structural or biochemical cause can be found. Each year, at least one such symptom is experienced by two-thirds of the USA population, of whom one-third will have previously sought medical advice for a functional gastrointestinal disorder (Drossman et al 1993). Functional gastrointestinal disorders are responsible for 50% of outpatient gastroenterological practice in the UK and in the USA, 3.5 million office visits for functional bowel disorders alone per year and 8.7 days missed from work or school per patient per year (Harvey et al 1983, Drossman et al 1993).

Functional disorders affect every site in the alimentary tract from mouth to anus (Tables 53.5, 53.6). The repertoire of symptoms of the alimentary tract is limited and considerable overlap exists between the symptom clusters that define the separate functional syndromes. It is not

**Table 53.5** The functional gastrointestinal disorders (Drossman et al 1993). Classification and point prevalence based on a US householder survey by mailed questionnaire

| Functional disorder | Prevalence (%) | Seen by a doctor (%) |
|---|---|---|
| A. *Functional esophageal disorders* | 42 | 38 |
| A1. Globus | | |
| A2. Rumination syndrome | | |
| A3. Functional chest pain of presumed esophageal origin | | |
| A4. Functional heartburn | | |
| A5. Functional dysphagia | | |
| A6. Unspecified functional esophageal disorder | | |
| B. *Functional gastroduodenal disorders* | 26 | 23 |
| B1. Functional dyspepsia | | |
| B1a. Ulcer-like dyspepsia | | |
| B1b. Dysmotility-like dyspepsia | | |
| B1c. Reflux-like dyspepsia | | |
| B1d. Unspecified functional dyspepsia | | |
| B2. Aerophagia | | |
| C. *Functional bowel disorders* | 44 | 23 |
| C1. Irritable bowel syndrome | | |
| C2. Functional abdominal bloating | | |
| C3. Functional constipation | | |
| C4. Functional diarrhea | | |
| C5. Unspecified functional bowel disorder | | |
| D. *Functional abdominal pain* | 2 | 50 |
| D1. Functional abdominal pain syndrome | | |
| D2. Unspecified functional abdominal pain | | |
| E. *Functional biliary pain* | 1 | 57 |
| E1. Sphincter of Oddi dyskinesia | | |
| F. *Functional anorectal disorders* | 27 | 17 |
| F1. Functional incontinence | | |
| F2. Functional anorectal pain | | |
| F2a. Levator syndrome | | |
| F2b. Proctalgia fugax | | |
| F3. Pelvic floor dyssynergia | | |
| F4. Unspecified functional anorectal disorder | | |

**Table 53.6** Average prevalences of common functional gastrointestinal disorders in surveys conducted in US and UK communities

| Functional disorder | Community prevalence (%) |
|---|---|
| Functional chest pain | 11–14 |
| Functional dyspepsia | 13–18 |
| Irritable bowel syndrome | 14–20 |

(Thompson & Heaton 1980, Drossman et al 1982, Harvey et al 1983, Talley et al 1991b, Talley et al 1992a,c, Jones & Lydeard 1992a,b, Scott et al 1993)

surprising, therefore, that two or more functional syndromes may coexist in the same individual. Symptom patterns in functional disorders are so frequently nonspecific that diagnosis from the clinical history is often not possible without further investigation. For these reasons and to facilitate further research in the field, the symptom criteria used to define the syndromes have become increasingly explicit and restrictive. It seems unlikely, however, that more detailed analyses of symptoms alone will permit identification of specific causation. For clinical purposes, the "lumping" rather than the "splitting" approach makes more sense. However, in this chapter only three of the more common presentations of functional gastrointestinal disorders will be reviewed, the irritable bowel syndrome, functional abdominal pain syndrome and functional dyspepsia.

Table 53.5 shows a breakdown of the point prevalence of the functional gastrointestinal disorders based on a questionnaire mailed to several thousand US householders. While the population surveyed was poorly representative for blacks and low socioeconomic groups, the prevalence figures reflect several other series published to date (Table 53.6; Thompson & Heaton 1980, Drossman et al 1982). It is worth noting that, for the commoner functional bowel disorders, about half the patients will have consulted a physician about the symptoms. There is much overlap of these symptom complexes within the same patient. Thus, one-third to one-half of patients with IBS will have functional dyspepsia and vice versa and two-thirds of patients with functional chest pain have IBS or functional dyspepsia.

## IRRITABLE BOWEL SYNDROME

### Etiological factors

*Alterations in motor function*

Compared with healthy control subjects, patients with irritable bowel syndrome exhibit increased motility in response to a wide variety of stimuli including emotional arousal, food, sympathomimetic and parasympathomimetic drugs, bile acids, cholecystokinin and gut distension (Whitehead & Schuster 1985, Camilleri & Neri 1989). Altered patterns of motility are not limited to the gut. There is evidence of hyper-reactivity of smooth muscle of the urinary bladder and even the bronchial tree in patients with irritable bowel syndrome (Whorwell et al 1986b, White et al 1991).

Changes in proximal gut motility include reduced pressures in the lower esophageal sphincter, increased contractility of the esophageal body, gastric antral hypomotility and increased small bowel motility, particularly in response to stress (Whorwell et al 1981, Kumar & Wingate 1985, Kellow & Phillips 1987, Kellow et al 1992a). Clustered jejunal contractions and ileal propulsive waves are more common than in control subjects and are more likely to be associated with abdominal symptoms (Kellow & Phillips 1987). Significantly, such changes in small bowel motility characteristically disappear during sleep (Kellow et al 1992b, Kumar et al 1992, Gorard et al 1994). Alterations in gastric, small bowel and colonic transit rates have been reported in subsets of patients with irritable bowel syndrome. However, none is consistently or sufficiently pronounced to be of any diagnostic or clinical value.

The predominance of lower bowel symptoms in irritable bowel syndrome and the relative accessibility of the distal colon have resulted in a disproportionately large number of studies of colonic motor function. Most investigators have recorded nonpropagative, phasic contractile activity of the distal colon, where phasic motility is known to be appreciably greater than that of the proximal colon. Distal colonic motility during fasting is greater in patients with irritable bowel syndrome who have pain compared with healthy control subjects, but does not differ significantly in constipation-predominant compared with diarrhea-predominant irritable bowel syndrome. The increase in phasic colonic motility postprandially correlates with the exacerbation of symptoms by meals in irritable bowel syndrome, but is not qualitatively different from that observed in healthy control subjects.

Studies of colonic motility responses to emotional stress have shown only quantitative rather than qualitative differences in irritable bowel syndrome compared with healthy control subjects. In a study using both healthy and psychoneurotic control subjects, no differences were observed in colonic myoelectric activity or phasic motility responses to emotive interviewing compared with patients with irritable bowel syndrome, though baseline phasic contractility was greater in patients (Latimer et al 1981). In health, the dominant frequency of myoelectric activity (electrical control activity or "slow wave") is 3 cpm in the colon and 6 cpm in the rectum. Earlier studies suggested that rectal myoelectric activity was qualitatively different in patients with irritable bowel syndrome in that the proportion of 3 cpm activity was significantly greater in patients than in control subjects. However, this has not been confirmed and the most consistent motor changes in irritable bowel syndrome have been the paradoxical hypomotility in diarrhea and excessive contractility in constipated groups.

The alterations in colonic motility in patients with irritable bowel syndrome in response to numerous stimuli suggest that they differ from healthy control subjects in their susceptibility and sensitivity to stress rather than in the pattern of motility responses. There are no motility responses qualitatively unique to patients with irritable bowel syndrome that are of value in discriminating them from control subjects and few of the alterations in motility that have been described correlate with symptoms. Indeed, the similarities of physiological motility responses are particularly noticeable when individuals are matched for levels of anxiety, suggesting that differences in levels of emotional arousal probably account for the variability.

### *Alterations in sensory function*

In an early study, inflation of a balloon in the distal colon to a standard volume of 60 ml induced pain in 6% of control subjects compared with 56% of patients with irritable bowel syndrome (Ritchie 1973; Fig. 53.4). Many studies have since confirmed that pain thresholds following balloon distention of the colon are significantly lower in patients with irritable bowel syndrome than normal control subjects, which supports the hypothesis of visceral hypersensitivity. However, in studies comparing pain induced by distention in patients with irritable bowel syndrome and in anxious control subjects without bowel symptoms, no significant differences were found with respect to perception or pain thresholds (Latimer et al 1979).

These conflicting results are not easy to reconcile. Only 60% of patients exhibit increased sensitivity to rectal distention and it remains ill understood why some patients experience severe pain. Interestingly, the motility response to distention of the rectosigmoid colon is significantly greater in irritable bowel syndrome compared with control subjects. Furthermore, contractile responses to distention and visceral sensitivity to distention are increased in diarrhea-predominant patients particularly, amongst whom anxiety ratings are significantly greater. Indeed, 75% of patients with irritable bowel syndrome and with elevated anxiety ratings exhibit increased rectal sensitivity. It seems likely therefore that both the increase in visceral sensitivity and the alteration in motility which it induces may represent arousal effects (Prior et al 1993).

Studies using balloon distention illustrate that the somatic referral of pain in irritable bowel syndrome is more widespread and varied than in normal subjects (Swarbrick 1980). Colonic balloon distention at a variety of sites is shown in Figure 53.5. In normal subjects (Fig. 53.5) the pain was mainly hypogastric but occasionally epigastric or periumbilical. In patients with irritable bowel syndrome, the pain was in any segment of the abdomen, especially when the transverse and right side of the colon were inflated (Fig. 53.6). Similar studies in healthy subjects have reproduced such findings when subjects are stressed by frequently repeated balloon distention (Ness et al 1990). In patients with functional abdominal pain, balloon distention in the ileum, proximal jejunum, second part of the duodenum or distal esophagus can also produce pain anywhere in the abdomen (Moriarty & Dawson 1982).

In summary, rather than a normal perception of abnormal motility or an abnormal perception of normal motili-

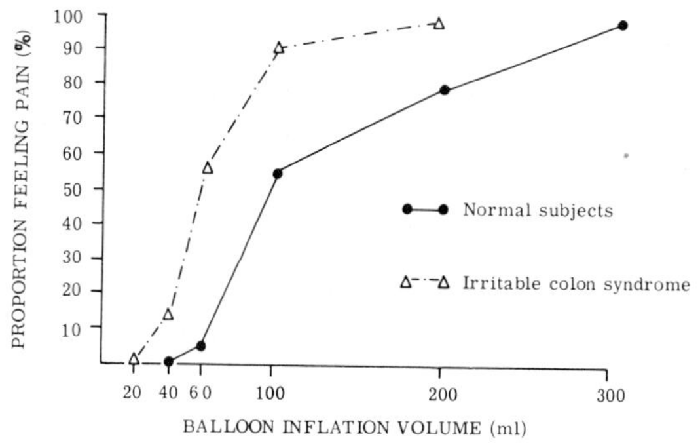


**Fig. 53.4** Onset of pain at different volumes of balloon inflation (Ritchie 1973).

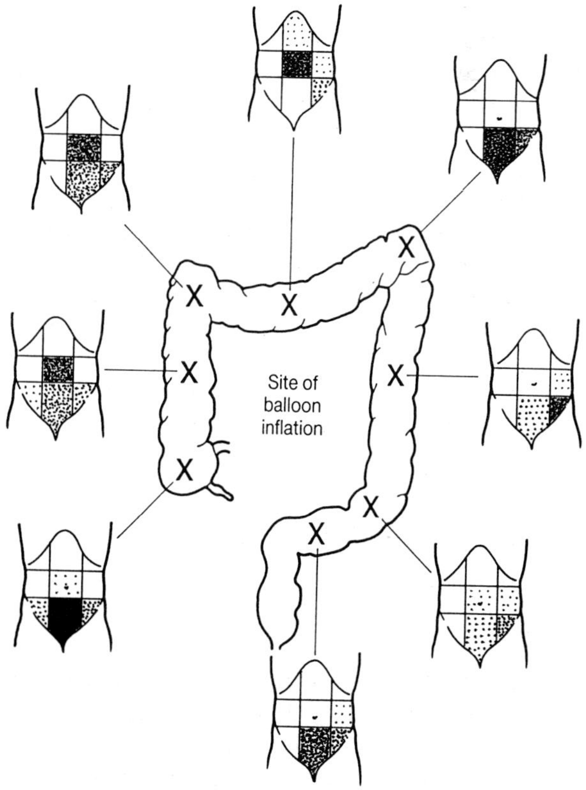


**Fig. 53.5** Distribution of abdominal pain induced by balloon inflation in nine control patients (Swarbrick et al 1980).

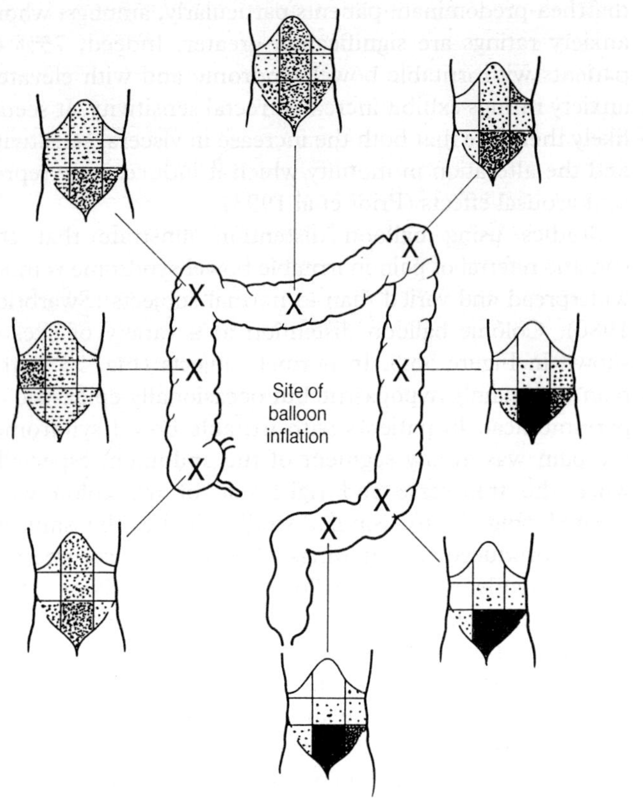


**Fig. 53.6** Distribution of abdominal pain induced by balloon inflation in 48 patients with functional abdominal pain (Swarbrick et al 1980).

ty, irritable bowel syndrome may be the result of visceral hypersensitivity induced by many factors, most notably by an increase in central (autonomic) arousal.

*Alterations in autonomic function*

Patients with functional abdominal pain but without any specific alteration in bowel movement have been shown to have higher basal parasympathetic activity and lower sympathetic neural activity than healthy control subjects (Bharucha et al 1993, Aggarwal et al 1994). Cardiovagal function is impaired in one-third of patients with ulcerative colitis and sympathetic adrenergic function is impaired in half of patients with Crohn's disease (Lindgren et al 1993). Cardiovagal function tests in irritable bowel disease have demonstrated impaired autonomic responses in the diarrhea-predominant group particularly, though similar findings are also found less often in the constipation-predominant group (Aggarwal et al 1994). The sensitivity and specificity of such tests, their etiologic significance with respect to alimentary disorders and the confounding effects of other variables, including the psychologic profile, are all open to question. Assessment of pelvic parasympathetic function would, however, be of more relevance than cardiovagal function given the extrinsic neural control of motility in most of the colon (Camilleri & Ford 1994).

Diarrhea-predominant irritable bowel syndrome is known to be associated with increased levels of anxiety and excretion of free epinephrine in the urine (Esler & Goulston 1973). Increased levels of anxiety confer an increased level of arousal, thereby resetting the sensitivity of the arousal pathways to adrenergic and cholinergic stimulation. Since patients with irritable bowel syndrome have been shown to have increased responsiveness to adrenergic ($\alpha_2$) and cholinergic (muscarinic $M_2$) modulation, it is more likely that the changes in autonomic function described in IBS patients represent alterations in the function of central pathways as a result of the changes in arousal, rather than alterations in the peripheral autonomic function (Dinan et al 1989, Fukudo et al 1993). Before attributing alterations in gastrointestinal function and symptoms of irritable bowel syndrome to the demonstrated changes in extrinsic autonomic function, it is important to control for the potential effects of anxiety and arousal on central autonomic function and hence to include, as a disease control group, those patients with similar levels of anxiety but no gastrointestinal symptoms. Though there are alterations in extrinsic autonomic nervous function in patients with irritable bowel syndrome, their etiologic significance is unknown (Camilleri & Ford 1994).

*Alterations in gastrointestinal hormones*

Given the alterations in motor and sensory function of the gut that have been described in irritable bowel syndrome, many of the gut hormones and neuropeptide transmitters have been studied. The irritable bowel is hypersensitive to many stimuli including hormonal stimuli, a finding exemplified by the increased sensitivity of the gut to cholecystokinin (Kellow et al 1988, Niederau et al 1992). Gastrointestinal hormonal profiles in diarrhea-predominant and constipation-predominant irritable bowel syndrome have shown increased fasting plasma concentrations of motilin and pancreatic polypeptide in the former and decreased fasting concentrations of gastrin and motilin in the latter (Besterman et al 1981, Preston et al 1985). However, since such tests reflect the overflow of peptides into the peripheral circulation, plasma levels may bear little relationship to peptide release. No typical basal or postprandial profiles in the plasma concentrations of gut hormones and neuropeptides have been reported (Sjolund & Ekman 1987).

*Food allergy and food intolerance*

The existence of food intolerance is regarded by many clinicians with cynicism (p. 406). Studies of the putative effects of dietary factors in the irritable bowel syndrome are difficult to reconcile given the contrast between the high frequency of food intolerance reported and the low number documented objectively in clinic populations of patients with irritable bowel syndrome (Jones et al 1982). Most patients experience postprandial exacerbations of symptoms and some consider that their gastrointestinal symptoms are exacerbated by certain foods. In many instances, symptoms cannot be reproduced by double-blinded food challenge and psychiatric studies in patients referred because of suspected food intolerance have established a high prevalence of psychiatric disorders (Rix et al 1984).

Specific food allergy is a difficult diagnosis to establish due to the lack of reliable confirmatory tests. Its diagnosis is best established by the use of an elemental diet with a slow and painstaking introduction of food items, one by one, ideally given as powdered food in a double-blind manner (Nandra et al 1989, Crowe & Perdue 1992). Evidence of food allergy can, however, be established in 2–5% of patients with irritable bowel syndrome, most of whom also have other pre-existing atopic manifestations such as asthma or eczema (Farah et al 1985). The foods most frequently proven to induce allergic manifestations include cow's milk, wheat, eggs, corn, nuts, fish and seafood. Extraintestinal manifestations of food allergy can be dramatic and occasionally life threatening, as with anaphylaxis induced by the ingestion of peanuts.

Even in some nonatopic subjects, however, symptoms can be reproduced by food challenge and relieved by avoidance of the foods concerned. The mechanism for this intolerance is unknown; after food challenge there is no increase in immune complexes, eosinophil counts or plasma histamine and no change in the profile of gastrointestinal hormones (Hunter 1991).

### *Carbohydrate intolerance*

Flatulence and abdominal distention are often considered by patients and clinicians alike to be the result of excessive gas production. However, carefully controlled studies have not shown any significant difference in the composition or rate of accumulation of intestinal gas in patients with irritable bowel syndrome compared with control subjects (Lasser et al 1975, Haderstorfer et al 1989). The flatulence factor associated with certain foods has been shown to be oligosaccharides that cannot be digested in the small bowel and are fermented in the colon, yielding hydrogen, methane and carbon dioxide. The ingestion of wheat products by normal subjects results in hydrogen production due to incomplete carbohydrate absorption. Though this may explain why a gluten-free diet can improve symptoms in some IBS patients, carbohydrate malabsorption occurs as frequently in healthy individuals as it does in the irritable bowel syndrome (Anderson et al 1981).

### *Lactose intolerance* (p. 343)

The importance of lactose intolerance to irritable bowel syndrome clearly depends upon the prevalence of lactase deficiency in the population or ethnic group. Malabsorption of lactose due to intestinal lactase deficiency occurs in 5% of Caucasian adults in the United Kingdom and in 5% of patients with irritable bowel syndrome (Ferguson et al 1984). Such individuals commonly experience abdominal distention and diarrhea following ingestion of lactose. Hence, it should be sought as a contributing factor, particularly in ethnic groups with high prevalence. However, lactase-deficient patients with irritable bowel syndrome do not consistently experience an improvement in symptoms with a lactose-free diet (Gudmand-Hoyer et al 1973).

### *Fructose and sorbitol intolerance* (p. 345)

These simple sugars are natural constituents of many common foodstuffs and are especially abundant in apples, pears and their juices. Most are consumed as artificial additives and sweeteners, particularly in diabetic and low-calorie drinks. The amount of fructose in excess of glucose seems to be the major determinant of fructose malabsorption since glucose stimulates fructose absorption; for this reason, sucrose malabsorption is rare (Rumessen 1993). Fructose or sorbitol malabsorption occurs in approximately 50% of the population, a proportion similar to that in patients with irritable bowel syndrome, and may result in bloating and diarrhea. Ingestion of these sugars has been shown to be more likely to induce troublesome alimentary symptoms in irritable bowel syndrome compared with the ingestion of similar doses of sucrose. It is reasonable, therefore, to consider dietary manipulation to avoid lactose, fructose and sorbitol in diarrhea-predominant patients with irritable bowel syndrome in whom a dietetic history raises suspicion of such possibilities (Rumessen & Gudmand-Hoyer 1988, Nelis et al 1990, Symons et al 1992, Fernandez-Banares et al 1993).

### *Bile acid malabsorption*

In patients with functional diarrhea, abnormalities in fecal bile acid excretion have been demonstrated suggesting primary bile acid malabsorption (Merrick et al 1985, Sciarretta et al 1987, Williams et al 1991, Eusufzai et al 1993). Such patients have impaired ileocecal function. The presence of primary bile acids in the colon stimulates colonic motility and can provoke diarrhea. Furthermore, patients with irritable bowel syndrome have been shown to have increased ileal and colonic sensitivity to perfused bile acids (Oddsson et al 1978, Taylor et al 1980). Impaired absorption of radiolabeled bile acid has been demonstrated in less than 10% of patients, however, and should only be suspected in the patient with painless diarrhea in whom a therapeutic trial of cholestyramine should be considered (Merrick et al 1985).

*Dietary fiber deficiency*

It has been suggested that the symptoms of an irritable bowel reflect the response of a normal bowel coping with an altered environment produced by highly refined carbohydrates and a depletion in dietary fiber (Cummings 1973). Such a concept implies that the irritable bowel would be better termed the "irritated bowel" (Painter 1972). These anecdotal statements are not well supported by fact; there is ample evidence that the irritable bowel syndrome predated the introduction of highly refined carbohydrate diets and little evidence to suggest that irritable bowel patients have a total dietary fiber intake which is significantly different from normal individuals (Hillman et al 1982). Fiber deficiency alone clearly cannot explain why patients develop irritable bowel syndrome or, indeed, constipation. In studies correlating dietary fiber intake with fecal output, there are large variations in fecal output between individuals despite similar dietary fiber intakes (Davies et al 1986). The amount of fiber supplemented in the diet needs to be individualized and comorbidity may also influence the response to this supplementation. Thus, for example, psychoneurotic traits predispose to a reduced fecal output and predetermine the magnitude of the therapeutic response to dietary fiber in patients with the irritable bowel syndrome (Tucker et al 1981, Fowlie ct al 1992a).

*Intestinal infection*

Gastrointestinal infections can trigger prolonged bowel dysfunction (Chaudhary & Truelove 1962, Collins 1992). Similarly acute diarrhea following the use of broad-spectrum antibiotics may result in an irritable bowel which persists for several months. Since infection can be implicated in the onset of less than one-fifth of patients with an irritable bowel, even in patients living in areas where gastroenteritis is endemic, it is unlikely that changes in bowel flora and hence the bile acid pool are of relevance to the majority of such patients (Chaudhary & Truelove 1962, Bordie 1972).

*Altered psychological function*

Surveys of personality traits in patients with irritable bowel syndrome compared with healthy controls, using the Minnesota Multiphasic Personality Inventory (MMPI), indicate elevated subscale scores for hypochondriasis, hysteria and depression, the so-called "psychosomatic triad" (Talley et al 1990, Heymen et al 1993). However, the utility of personality profiles in patients with chronic illness is considerably less than that derived from standard psychometric tests of anxiety and depression ratings. Patients with alternating constipation and diarrhea commonly report changes in bowel function which correlate with changes in mood. Furthermore, patients with irritable bowel syndrome who exhibit visceral hypersensitivity to physical and emotional stress are particularly more likely than those without visceral hypersensitivity to have increased anxiety ratings on psychometric tests (Prior et al 1993).

Most physicians appreciate the inter-relationship between stress, psychological factors and the irritable bowel syndrome; indeed, more than 50% of patients, irrespective of consulting behavior, report that stressful life events exacerbate their symptoms (Whitehead et al 1992). Prospective studies have shown significant life events occurred in 50% of patients followed up for 12 months of whom 75% experienced exacerbation of symptoms at the time of the event (Svedlund et al 1983). Prospective psychiatric studies have shown that anxiety disorders and depression can be diagnosed in 40–50% of patients at presentation and 70–80% have abnormal scores on psychometric tests (Creed & Guthrie 1987, Walker et al 1990, Lydiard et al 1993). Anxiety-provoking life events are strongly associated with the subsequent onset of psychiatric disorder and severe life events or psychiatric illness precede the onset of symptoms of irritable bowel syndrome in two-thirds of patients (Ford et al 1987). Major life events are experienced more often by patients who consult and are perceived as more severe compared to those who are nonconsulters (Hui et al 1991). As with other anxious or depressed patients, those with irritable bowel syndrome exhibit a selective emotional bias when recalling life events and difficulties; for example, such subjects are less likely to recall emotionally charged events, whether joyful or sad, and are more likely to perceive such events as being distressing (Gomborone et al 1993). Life events alone are unlikely to play a major role in the development of symptoms unless associated with significant psychological distress (Ford et al 1987).

If 14–20% of the population have the symptoms of the irritable bowel syndrome, yet only 25% seek medical attention, it must be asked why some seek help and others do not. It has been assumed that psychological factors are predominant in this self-selection given the fact that those with symptoms of irritable bowel syndrome in the community who do not consult doctors (nonconsulters) have apparently normal psychological profiles (Welch et al 1985). Other community studies, however, have shown that the presence of symptoms, particularly abdominal pain, is strongly correlated with psychological factors, especially anxiety states, a correlation which is significant for both nonconsulters and consulters (Drossman et al 1988, Whitehead et al 1988, Smith et al 1990).

Other factors influence consulting behavior, notably sociological factors (Ingham & Miller 1982, 1983). Social learning in relation to illness behavior appears to be important in this regard (Whitehead et al 1982). Individuals with an irritable bowel are more likely than healthy controls to experience multiple somatic complaints of minor severity

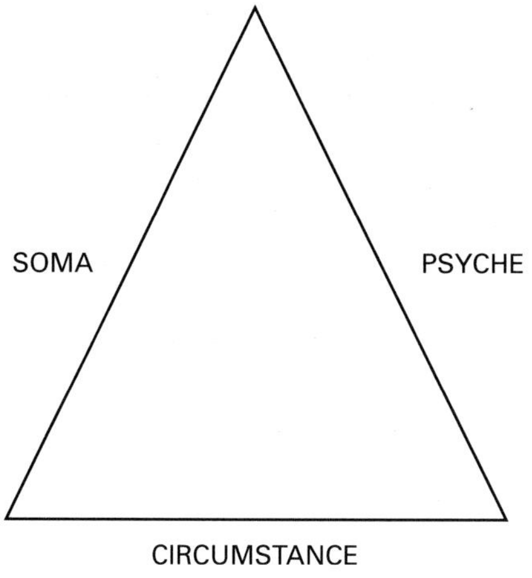


**Fig. 53.7** The triangle of soma, psyche and circumstance (Ford et al 1982).

and for which they consult their physician (Talley et al 1991b). Significantly, more patients with irritable bowel syndrome consult practitioners of alternative medicine than do patients with organic bowel disorders (Smart et al 1986b). The evidence suggests that illness behavior is likely to have been learned in childhood; compared to control subjects, patients with irritable bowel syndrome are more likely to have had recurrent abdominal pain in childhood, experienced sexual abuse in childhood, recall minor childhood illness favorably or had parents with irritable bowel syndrome (Lowman et al 1987, Drossman et al 1990, Walker et al 1993).

It is important to remember that the diagnosis of a functional disorder is not synonymous with the presence of psychiatric illness and that the diagnosis of a psychiatric disorder should be made by a positive assessment of the mental state and not by the exclusion of organic disease. Furthermore, patients with organic diseases are not immune from psychiatric illness. The more appropriate model for illness is, therefore, one which embraces the physical, emotional and situational factors, each of which contributes to the severity of the illness and its responsiveness to therapy (Ford et al 1982, Ford 1986) (Fig. 53.7).

If functional gastrointestinal symptoms are widely prevalent, yet do not give rise to requests for consultation, the implication is that patients seeking advice do so either because symptom severity has become greater or because their tolerance is reduced. However, several factors contribute to the health-seeking behavior of patients (Table 53.7). Studies have shown that the severity of symptoms and the acuteness of their onset are significant predeterminants of self-referral, although often as background factors rather than sole precipitants (Drossman et al 1988, Smith et al 1990, Heaton et al 1992b, Jones & Lydeard 1992a, Kettell et al 1992). The influence of symptom severity upon self-referral is greater when the presenting symptoms are those of anxiety and depression or when symptoms are accompanied by anxiety (Ingham & Miller 1982, 1983). Additional modifying factors include the chronicity and speed of onset of symptoms, the disruption of social function associated with symptoms and pre-existing stressful life events and difficulties (Whitehead & Crowell 1991) (Table 53.7).

**Table 53.7** Determinants of health-seeking behavior

| |
|---|
| Childhood illness experience |
| Learned illness behavior |
| Social support |
| Coping skills |
| Psychological status |
| Life events and difficulties |
| Symptom severity |
| Speed of symptom onset |

There is a social dimension to every illness experience which determines how patients perceive, interpret and react to bodily changes. Some patients have personality traits in which the amplification of physical symptoms is a frequent characteristic, some may be responding to life events and difficulties and others may not have any apparent explanation for their symptoms. Abdominal pain is a common symptom heralding psychiatric illness and, as a subjective experience, is often difficult to assess. Attempts to distinguish between real and imaginary pain are inappropriate. The assessment of pain is influenced by the effects of personality and mood state on the perception of pain, the patient's ability to identify and express feelings of anxiety or depression and the language and imagery used to describe symptoms.

A model that incorporates the biopsychosocial dimensions involved in functional gastrointestinal disorders is shown in Figure 53.8 (Rahe et al 1974). Note the path includes filters that incorporate past experience and developed coping skills, the broadening or exaggeration of symptoms by psychological factors represented by a convex lens and ultimately the illness behavior of the individual that will focus the nature of symptoms with which to present.

### *Stress and gastrointestinal function*

Central to an understanding of functional disorders is the study of stress on physiological functions. Stress can usefully be defined as the physiologic response of an individual to a stimulus perceived as perturbing; the perturbing stimulus provoking physiologic responses is termed the "stressor". Physical and psychological stressors in health influence enteric motor and sensory function via the central nervous system. Stress responses are mediated neurally via the autonomic nervous system and humorally via a number of neuropeptides including corticotrophin-releasing factor and thyrotrophin-releasing hormone from the

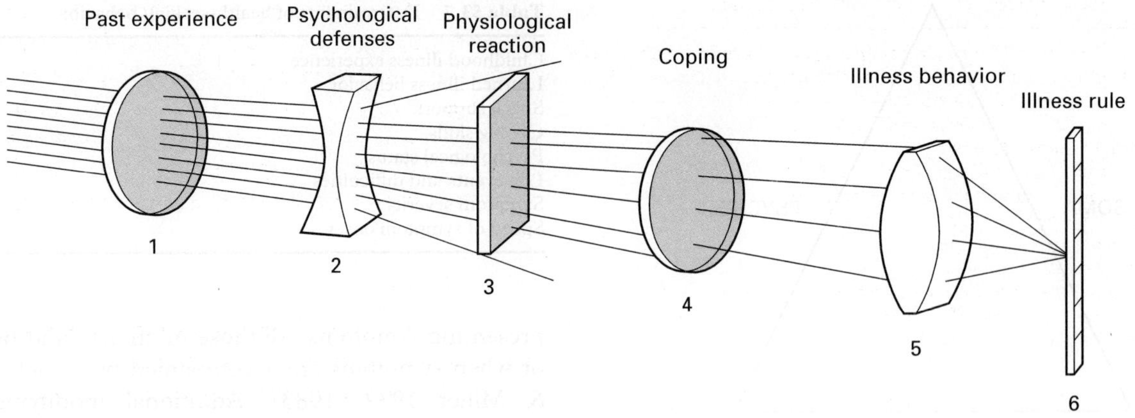


**Fig. 53.8** Life stress and illness model (adapted from Rahe et al 1974).

hypothalamus and β-endorphin from the anterior pituitary. These and other putative mediators of stress such as catecholamines and neuropeptide Y are released both locally and systemically; adrenergic, opiate or corticotrophin-releasing factor (CRF) blockade prevents the effect of stress on gastrointestinal motility (Camilleri & Neri 1989, Dinan et al 1989, Fukudo et al 1993, Tache et al 1993).

Stress affects many of the mechanisms considered to play an etiological role in the evolution or maintenance of irritable bowel symptoms. The measurement and assessment of stress, however, is confounded by many factors. Not all stressors are equivalent qualitatively or quantitatively. Standardization of the potency of a stressor between individuals may be difficult or impossible as the emotional response induced often reflects differences in previous illness experience. Furthermore, the effects of acute stress differ from those of chronic or intermittent stress and the potency of a stressor may be either attenuated or enhanced on repetition (Ness et al 1990).

Physical stressors such as cold pain evoke different physiological responses compared with psychological stressors such as mental performance tasks. Physical stressors can also be psychological stressors if they are associated with anticipatory fear of a distressing stimulus; such responses may decrease with repetition as individuals become habituated. Experimental models of stress bear little resemblance to the chronic stress of everyday life and little is known about the changes in gastrointestinal motility associated with major life events and difficulties.

***Normal gastrointestinal responses to acute stressors.*** Stress-induced alterations in the patterns of smooth muscle contraction are complex; sphincteric and nonsphincteric muscle respond differently and either decreased or increased motor activity can be induced. Stresses such as emotionally charged discussion of personal difficulties (emotive interviewing), dichotomous listening and immersion of the hand in ice-cold water (cold pressor stress) have different effects on different viscera varying with the predominant emotion elicited. For instance, cold pressor stress increases the upper esophageal sphincter pressure and the amplitude of esophageal contractions and stimulates isolated pyloric pressure waves; it also decreases gastric antral contractility and the gastric emptying rate. Similarly, dichotomous listening stress inhibits fasting migrating motor complexes (MMCs) in the jejunum and decreases small bowel transit rate. The induction of anger or anxiety increases colonic motor activity whereas the feeling of hopelessness decreases motility. Cold pressor stress increases the colonic motility response to meals and dichotomous listening stress decreases this response (McRae et al 1982, Camilleri & Neri 1989, Holtmann & Enck 1991).

Stress can increase not only gut contractility but also visceral sensitivity to stimulation. Furthermore, alterations in sensory function influence motor function and vice versa. For example, the increase in colonic motility in response to meals induces an increased sensitivity to colonic distention. Sensory and motor gut function change significantly in healthy subjects during sleep with prolongation of phase 1 and shortening of phase 2 of the MMC (Kellow & Phillips 1987). Similarly, in patients with functional bowel disorders, during sleep, gastrointestinal motor function is normal (Kumar et al 1986). Hypnosis-assisted relaxation also reduces sensitivity to gut distention (Whorwell et al 1992). In healthy subjects, repeated distention of the sigmoid colon with the same intensity produces a progressive increase in both pain ratings and the area of the abdomen over which the stimulus is perceived (Ness et al 1990).

## Clinical manifestations

The irritable bowel syndrome is a constellation of bowel symptoms including abdominal pain or discomfort which is persistent or recurrent for 3 months or more and for which no underlying structural or biochemical cause can be found. Explicit criteria for the diagnosis were agreed by

**Table 53.8** 'Rome criteria' for irritable bowel syndrome

| |
|---|
| *Continuous or recurrent abdominal pain or discomfort*, relieved by defecation or associated with altered stool frequency or consistency, together with either or both of the following features: |
| *Altered pattern of defecation* for at least 25% of the time, i.e. **two** or more of the following: |
| Altered stool frequency (> 3/day or < 3/week) |
| Altered stool form (lumpy, hard, loose, watery) |
| Altered stool passage (straining, fecal urgency, feeling of incomplete emptying) |
| Passage of mucus |
| *Abdominal bloating* or a feeling of abdominal distention |

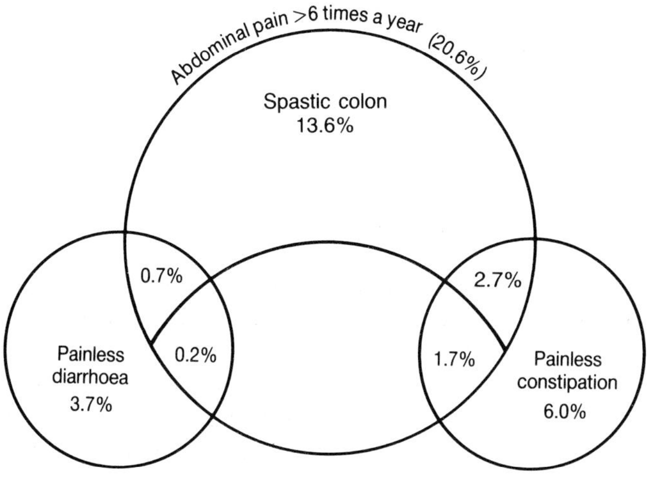


**Fig. 53.9** Prevalence of gut symptoms in healthy adults (Thompson & Heaton 1980).

an international working team in Rome in 1988 (hence the "Rome Criteria") and subsequently further refined (Thompson et al 1992) (Table 53.8).

Symptoms consistent with the diagnosis of irritable bowel syndrome are widely prevalent in the community with prevalence rates of 14–20% and incidence rates of approximately 9% per year; 60% of those with symptoms continued to experience symptoms 1–2 years later (Thompson & Heaton 1980, Drossman et al 1982, Talley et al 1992b) (Fig. 53.9).

The disorder affects most but not all communities throughout the world with a female predominance in the West (3:1) and a male predominance in India (3:1), reflecting cultural and social differences in access to and use of medical services. Indeed, in the Western world, only 25% of individuals with irritable bowel syndrome seek medical advice (consulters). Females are significantly more likely than males to seek medical advice and this is as true for functional bowel disorders as for other nonalimentary disorders. However, among nonconsulters with irritable bowel syndrome, females also predominate.

The majority of patients present before the age of 50 years and presentation for the first time after this age is uncommon. Nonetheless, the prevalence in patients over the age of 65 years is only marginally less than that in a younger population (Talley et al 1992a). Given that the probability of serious ill health increases with advancing age, it is unwise to diagnose the disorder without careful evaluation and investigation in subjects presenting for the first time after the age of 50 years. At presentation, symptoms have been present for an average of at least 5 years.

### *Colonic symptoms*

There are six cardinal symptoms that have been shown to best characterize irritable bowel syndrome (the "Manning criteria"); abdominal pain relieved by defecation, looser and more frequent stools at the onset of abdominal pain, distention, mucus and a feeling of incomplete rectal evacuation (rectal dissatisfaction). Two or more of these symptoms occur in 92% of patients with irritable bowel syndrome compared with 46% of patients with organic abdominal disease (Manning et al 1978). Most studies distinguish at least three clinical forms of the disorder – constipation-predominant, diarrhea-predominant and alternating constipation and diarrhea. All patients undergo relapses and remissions. Diarrhea occurring in the complete absence of abdominal pain is rare and fully justifies extensive further investigations (Bolin et al 1982). Only 50% of the diarrhea-predominant group have a stool volume of greater than 200 g per day. Usually, patients with irritable bowel syndrome have urgency and frequent small motions. The mechanism of the increased stool volume of 50% of diarrhea-predominant patients is thought to relate to faster small bowel and colonic transit rates compared with transit rates associated with constipation-predominant irritable bowel syndrome. There are no major differences in colonic motility and transit rates between constipation-predominant and diarrhea-predominant irritable bowel (Whitehead & Schuster 1985).

In the constipation-predominant variant, there is frequent passage of small, hard rabbit-like stools. When there is alternating constipation and diarrhea, episodes of diarrhea may be accompanied by urgency, tenesmus and rectal dissatisfaction. In the diarrhea-predominant variant, diarrheal episodes occur most commonly in the morning, especially at breakfast time and postprandially, and improve as the day progresses. Symptoms rarely disturb sleep in the absence of significant insomnia, although the patient may arise early in the morning to defecate. The stools are semi-liquid and often small in volume; they may be ribbon or wormlike because of increased anal pressures. An attack is sometimes related to particular foods, for example fresh fruit and salads, excessive coffee or alcoholic drinks, especially beer. Many patients exhibit a heightened defecatory response to meals with an urgent call to stool (Sullivan et al 1978). The passage of mucus is common irrespective of other bowel symptoms; it may be passed with the stool or entirely by itself (Chaudhary & Truelove 1962).

*Abdominal pain*

Abdominal pain is an essential component of the symptomatology of the irritable bowel syndrome. Pain is typically colicky and poorly localized and by convention, has been assumed to be colonic in origin. The evidence suggests, however, that such an attribution is inappropriate. Pain is frequently continuous and a dull ache in character. It is localized to the hypogastric area in only 25% of patients and is experienced in the right side of the abdomen in 18%, the left side of the abdomen in 17% and in the epigastrium in 8% (Chaudhary & Truelove 1962). Balloon distention studies on the esophagus, stomach, small bowel and large bowel clearly reveal that abdominal pain can be perceived anywhere in the abdomen and back and that distention stimuli applied throughout different regions of the gut can both induce and reproduce abdominal pain. Though right iliac fossa abdominal pain can be reproduced by right-sided colonic distention, some patients also experience pain in the right iliac fossa following distention of the pelvic colon (Ritchie 1973, Moriarty & Dawson 1982, Cullingford et al 1992).

Pain may be so distressing as to simulate serious abdominal conditions, such as appendicitis or cholecystitis; when such diagnoses cannot be readily excluded or are made erroneously, abdominal surgery may be undertaken. Some patients with irritable bowel syndrome may experience episodes of pain in the right iliac fossa or right side of the abdomen alone. Approximately 33% of patients have undergone appendicectomy, cholecystectomy or gynecological surgery and often no cause has been found (Chaudhary & Truelove 1962). Operation is particularly likely in patients with right-sided pain. In some patients, pain radiates to the left costal margin and shoulder and to the lower sternum; this has been named the "splenic flexure syndrome" because it can be reproduced by distention of the splenic flexure. The pain may be relieved by passing flatus or defecation.

*Dyspeptic symptoms*

Upper gastrointestinal symptoms are an integral part of irritable bowel syndrome. Dyspeptic symptoms are found in 50% of patients with irritable bowel syndrome and usually include nausea, occasional vomiting, aerophagy and early satiety; heartburn and/or acid reflux are present in 30% and the spectrum merges into that of functional dyspepsia. When the predominant symptoms are reflux-like, the patient either has coexisting, gastroesophageal reflux disease or may have insufficient colonic symptoms to qualify for the diagnosis of irritable bowel syndrome. Some patients complain of abdominal distress not amounting to pain. Usually it takes the form of abdominal distention, belching, borborygmi and passing of a large amount of gas (Smart et al 1986a, Talley 1991b).

*Bloating and abdominal distention*

Characteristically, patients report that abdominal distention and bloating are least troublesome on awaking and progress throughout the day, being exacerbated by food and absent during sleep. The symptom of bloating is a powerful discriminator in favor of the diagnosis and abdominal distention is present in over 90%. Most experience distention affecting the entire abdomen, usually occurring within 10 min of a meal and often within 60 s. The majority do not experience excessive flatus or relief with the passage of flatus or stool. The pathogenesis of distention is unknown but CT scanning of the abdomen has confirmed an increase in intra-abdominal volume and excluded increased intraluminal gas, diaphragmatic descent and lumbar lordosis as possible causes. Its occurrence is likely to reflect alterations in gut smooth muscle tone and visceral perception (Maxton et al 1991).

*Nonalimentary symptoms*

Most patients complain of multiple symptoms often considered to be nonalimentary in origin (Table 53.9). Such symptoms commonly include those characteristic of anxiety, depression and hyperventilation syndromes (Whorwell et al 1986a, b, Nyhlin et al 1993).

Urinary frequency, urgency, nocturia and dysuria may accompany an exacerbation of symptoms together with dysmenorrhea and dyspareunia. Gynecological symptoms are particularly common; indeed, 50% of females attending a gynecological clinic with abdominal pain have symptoms consistent with irritable bowel syndrome (Prior et al 1989). Backache and muscle aches and pains often accompany these symptoms such that patients may present with fibromyalgia; in one series, over 60% of patients with fibromyalgia attending a rheumatological clinic had evidence of irritable bowel syndrome (Triadafilopoulos et al 1991).

Systemic symptoms such as tiredness, lethargy and inability to concentrate, insomnia, palpitation, sweating and flushing are common and should alert the clinician to the possibility that the patient may be seriously anxious or depressed. Patients often rank the severity and distress associated with such symptoms above that attributed to

**Table 53.9** Nonalimentary symptoms in irritable bowel syndrome

| Somatic | Emotional |
|---|---|
| Urinary frequency | Tiredness |
| Backache | Insomnia |
| Dysmenorrhea | Anxiety |
| Dyspareunia | Depression |
| Headaches | Palpitation |
| Dry mouth | Weakness |
| Aches and pains | Dizziness |

alimentary symptoms even though the initial presentation was with the latter (Maxton et al 1989).

## Clinical examination

The patient's demeanor has been summed up as "inappropriate" (Fielding 1983). Many patients appear inappropriately well, the external appearance being at odds with the severity of symptoms and the distress associated with their problem. Smiling may accompany complaints of severe pain or distress and the history is typically vague. Cool clammy hands, the absence of a tachycardia (suggesting increased cardiovagal tone) and brisk knee jerks are characteristic findings. On abdominal palpation, the patient may close their eyes and avoid eye-to-eye contact. Abdominal tenderness may appear to be inappropriately marked; it is present in one or more areas of the colon in 60% of patients. The pelvic colon can often be readily palpated as a firm, "rope-like" tube and a squelching sensation can be elicited on palpation of the right lilac fossa in 30% of instances.

Rectal examination may be experienced as unusually distressing. Sigmoidoscopy may show a hyperemic mucosa with an excess of mucus but not friable. Rectal contractions are frequent and rectal biopsies show a histologically normal mucosa; in the typical patient, however, rectal biopsy is unnecessary unless the clinical picture or the macroscopic appearances of the mucosa raise doubt about the diagnosis. Insufflation of small amounts of air can provoke discomfort or pain and may reproduce the patient's usual pain (Cullingford et al 1992, Kang et al 1994).

## Diagnosis and investigation

In young and otherwise healthy patients in whom the clinical history and physical examination strongly suggest the diagnosis of irritable bowel syndrome, no further investigations are warranted other than hematological and biochemical screening to exclude easily missed diagnoses, e.g. anemia, liver dysfunction, thyroid disease, malabsorption and gluten enteropathy; hence the justification for checking hemoglobin, liver function values, thyroxine, serum iron and folate. In addition, the irritable bowel syndrome may coexist with more sinister disease or even be exacerbated by organic gastrointestinal conditions.

Investigation should therefore be undertaken when doubt exists, especially in the older patient or when symptoms or signs are atypical. Investigation is not, however, an essential part of the process of reassurance nor an alternative to spending time with the patient, listening to and carefully reviewing the history and evolution of the patient's complaints, worries and expectations. Investigations should not be repeated unless there has been a clinically significant change in the symptoms or signs. Depending on the clinical circumstances and judgement, it may occasionally be necessary to perform barium studies of the small or large intestine, upper or lower gastrointestinal endoscopy or ultrasonography of the gallbladder or pelvic organs. Patients with a short history or who have traveled abroad recently should have a rectal biopsy and stool microscopy and culture to exclude enteric pathogens including giardia and amebae. If suspected, the possibility of giardiasis should be excluded by a therapeutic trial of metronidazole as treatment can be quicker and more reliable than laboratory attempts to confirm the diagnosis.

Painless diarrhea requires consideration of an extensive differential diagnosis and should not be readily accepted as functional in origin until proven otherwise by appro-

**Table 53.10** Differential diagnosis of atypical irritable bowel syndrome

| |
|---|
| Drug toxicity or laxative abuse |
| Visceral autonomic neuropathy |
| Inflammatory bowel disease |
| Colonic carcinoma |
| Pancreatic carcinoma |
| Ischemic enterocolitis |
| Food allergy and intolerance |
| Gluten enteropathy |
| Giardiasis or amebiasis |
| Endometriosis |
| Thyrotoxicosis |
| Bile acid malabsorption |
| Carcinoid or gastrinoma |
| Psychiatric disorder |

**Table 53.11** Features suggesting organic bowel disease

| |
|---|
| Absence of psychological features |
| Frequent nocturnal symptoms |
| Watery stools – stool volume > 200 ml/day |
| Urinary sediment or hematuria |
| Persistent weight loss or vomiting |
| Rectal bleeding, anemia or fever |
| Abdominal guarding or mass |
| Proctosigmoidoscopic abnormality |

**Table 53.12** Diagnostic evaluation

| |
|---|
| History and physical examination |
| Proctosigmoidoscopy |
| Fecal occult blood test |
| Urinalysis |
| Hematological profile + ESR |
| Biochemical profile, liver function tests and TSH estimation |
| *Pain predominant* |
| Barium enema |
| Biliary, pancreatic + pelvic ultrasound |
| CT abdominal scan |
| *Diarrhea predominant* |
| Stool weight and culture |
| Malabsorption screen |
| Colonoscopy and biopsies |
| Exclude giardiasis + celiac disease |
| Exclude lactose intolerance |

priate investigation and follow-up (Bolin et al 1982). Disorders such as alcohol abuse, laxative abuse, hyperthyroidism, carbohydrate intolerance, lactose malabsorption and idiopathic bile salt diarrhea should all be considered and excluded (Tables 53.10–12).

### Approach to patients with functional gastrointestinal disorders

Patients need to tell their own story in their own words. It is tempting in a busy practice to lead the questioning. Indeed, in one survey, 70% of clinical consultations were interrupted by the physician within an average of 15 s of the patient beginning to relate their story. In the one-third of patients who were not interrupted, all managed to satisfactorily conclude their opening statement within 2 min, indicating that all but the most loquacious of patients can be allowed sufficient time to tell their story (Beckman & Frankel 1984). Furthermore, the study also showed that the first-named complaint mentioned by the patient was of no more significance than subsequent complaints expressed later in the interview.

The conventional stereotype of the "good doctor" and the "good patient" is unhelpful and should be abandoned. Neither exists and the stereotype is obstructive to the necessary communication required if the consultation is to be helpful. It is important to remember that the patient is also an expert and that the social context, life events and difficulties surrounding illness are never irrelevant or a distraction from the main purpose of the consultation – they are the real "business of medicine". If the consultation is viewed as a meeting of two experts, communication is more likely to be both meaningful and effective. "Listen to the patient, he is telling you the diagnosis" (Osler, 1904). In listening to the history, the physician should have in mind the issues listed in Table 53.13.

Finally, remember too that much of the information communicated during the consultation is conveyed nonverbally. All exchanges between the doctor and the patient transmit clues about the feelings and attitudes of both. Such feelings are often suppressed by both doctor and patient in the belief that they may impair the effectiveness of the consultation. Nonetheless, these feelings invariably "leak" and are usually expressed in "body language". For these reasons, it is important that the process of the consultation is one of listening, observing and feeling.

**Table 53.13** Important considerations in the approach to patients with functional gastrointestinal disorders

| |
|---|
| What are the alternative diagnoses and their possibilities? |
| How appropriate are further investigations? |
| Is there evidence of quantitively abnormal gut function? |
| Are the symptoms or signs potentially amenable to pharmacotherapy? |
| Why is the patient seeking help now? The hidden agenda |
| What is the social context of the illness? |
| Does the patient require specialist psychological assessment? |
| How does the patient perceive the illness, its cause, treatment and outlook? |
| What are the patient's expectations of the consultation and future management? |

Given that 50% of patients referred to gastrointestinal clinics have a functional bowel disorder, of whom 50% have significant and unresolved emotional problems, Alvarez's comment in his book *Nervousness, Indigestion and Pain* (1944) remains just as relevant today:

"The gastroenterologist just has to be a psychiatrist of sorts . . . if he is to help at all".

### Treatment

*General measures*

Since irritable bowel syndrome is common, it can occur coincidentally in patients with serious organic diseases. A complete history and physical examination including proctosigmoidoscopy are therefore essential. Speed in arriving at the diagnosis is counterproductive if by so doing, the patient is left resentful that the clinician did not pay appropriate attention to the details and circumstances of their problems. The necessary investigations should be carried out thoroughly and then the patient can be reassured. These processes are in themselves integral and important components of treatment. Multiple investigations at different times in various clinics and hospitals only serve to increase the patient's anxiety and perpetuate the symptoms. In general, one thorough investigation should be followed by reassurance and treatment. If symptoms continue, anxiety on the part of the inexperienced physician that serious disease may have been overlooked can be the stimulus to unnecessary, fruitless and potentially distressing further investigations. The evidence suggests that the likelihood of overlooking cancer or other serious disorder is remote and every effort should be made to avoid repeated investigation unless there has been a significant change in symptoms (Hawkins & Cockel 1971, Holmes & Salter 1982, Svendsen et al 1985, Harvey et al 1987, Fowlie et al 1992a).

Having reached the diagnosis of an "irritable bowel" an explanation of the condition should be given to the patient to develop a more effective doctor–patient relationship. Though most realize that they do not have carcinoma or colitis, it is as well to emphasize that there is no evidence of these conditions. Even though many patients realize that their symptoms are exacerbated by stress, they commonly experience a sense of disappointment on being told that they do not have any serious underlying disease. Patients often suspect that their physician may not believe or fully appreciate the severity of symptomatology; some may even have doubts themselves in this regard. The physician must be careful to acknowledge their symptoms and to explain where possible the relevant contributory factors; an empathic approach and patient education and reassurance are vital. Other levels of management of patients with irritable bowel syndrome are stress and symptom management.

*Stress management, psychotherapy and biofeedback*

Referral for psychiatric assistance is usually unnecessary, often resented and frequently rejected by patients with the irritable bowel syndrome. In some patients, particularly those exhibiting abnormal illness behavior, even attempted discussion of the possible contribution of psychological factors may provoke hostility or resentment. In such circumstances, it is often more prudent to accept these limitations and work with the patient within the confines of their own frame of reference; for example, behavioral therapy may be promoted as a means to help the patient cope with the stress resulting from their illness (Drossman 1991, Drossman & Thompson 1992).

Some physicians believe they lack the appropriate interactive counseling and psychotherapeutic skills to cope or consider that as bowel specialists, it is not their responsibility to attend to the emotional concerns of their patients. They may feel more comfortable therefore either by avoiding discussion of psychosocial issues or by dealing with the problem by onward referral. However, most patients respond well to firm reassurance and a sensitive exploration of the psychosocial issues contributing to their current level of symptomatic distress. Embracing the basic principles of psychotherapy and behavioral therapy, stress management therapy can help many patients to cope better with their disorder and assists in the control of both symptoms and disability (Shaw et al 1991, Blanchard et al 1992a). Stress management involves teaching the patient to recognize the signs of heightened arousal and anxiety, identify and understand the nature of precipitating factors and then avoid, reduce or control autonomic arousal by a variety of techniques including cognitive restructuring, hypnosis, progressive muscular relaxation, behavioral therapy and biofeedback training (Whorwell et al 1987, Svedlund 1992, Whitehead 1992, Blanchard et al 1993).

Short-term dynamic psychotherapy (10 one-hour sessions over 3 months) has been shown to usefully complement conventional medical therapy in a controlled study of refractory irritable bowel syndrome; the improvement in abdominal pain and bowel habit was significantly greater compared with medical therapy alone and persisted for the 1-year period of follow-up (Svedlund 1983). Similar findings in refractory irritable bowel syndrome have been reported in a controlled study comparing brief, dynamic psychotherapy (seven sessions over 3 months) together with the use of relaxation tape recordings plus standard medical therapy compared with medical therapy alone including follow-up. Despite the absence of any change in constipation, ratings of abdominal pain, diarrhea, anxiety and depression were significantly improved compared to the control group after both 3 months and 12 months (Guthrie et al 1991). Good prognostic factors included the presence of anxiety and/or depression, intermittent pain exacerbated by stress, a short duration of the present symptoms and the absence of constant, unremitting pain, a marker for severe somatization disorders (Creed & Guthrie 1989, Guthrie et al 1991, 1993, Blanchard et al 1992b).

Hypnotherapy, an alternative form of progressive muscular relaxation therapy, has been found to be particularly useful in refractory symptoms, both on an individual basis and in the setting of group therapy (Whorwell et al 1984, 1987, Harvey et al 1989). In a controlled trial comparing hypnotherapy with supportive psychotherapy, hypnotherapy was significantly more effective in improving symptoms and general well-being than psychotherapy over the follow-up period of 1 year (Whorwell et al 1984). Good prognostic factors included the absence of severe psychopathology and age less than 50 years. Progressive muscular relaxation therapy has been shown to significantly reduce levels of autonomic arousal and small bowel phasic contractility and suppress the discrete clustered jejunal contractions. Similarly, hypnotherapy in irritable bowel syndrome significantly reduces distal colonic motility and rectal hypersensitivity, particularly in patients with pre-existing elevated anxiety ratings (Prior et al 1990, 1993).

Biofeedback techniques are of proven value in the treatment of refractory constipation associated with pelvic floor dyssynergy or anismus (Bassotti et al 1993) (p. 1329). Biofeedback has also been used in attempts to control changes in distal colonic motility occurring in response to balloon distention without success. An alternative approach, systematic desensitization, involves the use of relaxation techniques to control elevated levels of autonomic arousal often accompanying stressful situations (Schwarz et al 1986). In a pilot study, prior relaxation training in patients with irritable bowel syndrome has been shown to reduce the frequency and severity of abdominal pain occurring during simulated stressful situations normally associated with symptom exacerbation (Whitehead 1985).

*Symptom management*

Some patients continue to experience refractory symptoms despite a careful explanation of the problem and firm reassurance. Before embarking on detailed and time-consuming therapeutic trials, it is worthwhile asking the patient to keep a diary record of symptoms during a 4-week period and to rank the symptomatology in terms of severity and associated social disruption, noting any possible physical or emotional aggravating or relieving factors. In this way, treatment can be targeted at the most intrusive of troublesome symptoms and its efficacy assessed more objectively. For many patients, nonalimentary symptoms such as tiredness or backache may be their overriding concern (Whorwell et al 1986a, Maxton et al 1989, Nyhlin et al 1993).

*Dietary therapy*

Diarrhea-predominant irritable bowel syndrome raises the possibilities of carbohydrate intolerance (lactose, sucrose, sorbitol or fructose) or true food allergy. No study has shown that carbohydrate intolerance is the sole cause of symptoms in typical irritable bowel syndrome. However, limiting the amount of the appropriate carbohydrates may help diminish the severity of symptoms in some patients in whom both disorders are present (Symons et al 1992). When doubt exists, such patients should avoid beer and other alcoholic drinks and consider elimination of the appropriate carbohydrates from the diet, albeit for a trial period.

The diagnosis of a food allergy involves the use of an elemental diet and the gradual and painstaking introduction of food items, ideally in a powdered form, in a double-blind manner. The clinical efficacy of exclusion diets in management is unproven (McKee et al 1987). In such patients, one open and uncontrolled trial treatment with oral cromoglycate has shown an improvement in the control of diarrhea (Stefanini et al 1992). Patients who remain convinced that they are sensitive to specific foodstuffs in the absence of confirmatory evidence should be encouraged to adopt as balanced a diet as possible.

Patients with constipation may benefit from increased dietary roughage with foods such as wholemeal bread, fruit and vegetables. Constipation may be improved by wheat bran but diarrhea can be exacerbated and the fiber content of the diet is best increased slowly in a stepwise manner. Overall, the response to high-fiber diets is disappointing (Hillman et al 1984, Lambert et al 1991).

*Fiber supplementation*

Supplementation of dietary fiber has traditionally been advocated for constipation-predominant irritable bowel syndrome (Painter 1972). However, studies have shown that the response to bran in terms of daily stool weight, bowel frequency and symptoms is determined more by pre-existing psychometric variables such as anxiety and depression than the amount or nature of the bulking agent administered (Tucker et al 1981, Fowlie et al 1992a). Bran therapy does not influence the pattern or severity of abdominal pain and its effects are no more than those attributable to a placebo effect (Cann et al 1984). The use of bran and other bulking agents in controlled trials has also confirmed the presence of a high placebo response in irritable bowel syndrome (Soltoft et al 1976, Lucey et al 1987). Some patients with constipation do not tolerate bran, often blaming it for "indigestion", bloating or flatulence. In such individuals, dietary modification with the use of wholemeal bread and an increase in other natural fibers may be more acceptable; alternatively, bulking agents such as psyllium or ispaghula may be tried though none is of proven efficacy (Longstreth et al 1981, Prior & Whorwell 1987). As one cynic has stated, bulking agents appear as useful in the treatment of irritable bowel syndrome as they are in depression. Curiously, despite the controversies and the absence of evidence of efficacy, most gastroenterologists continue to advocate a high dietary fiber intake in the treatment of irritable bowel syndrome.

*Drug therapy*

In a busy clinical practice, faced by demanding patients with refractory symptoms, drug therapy can be a tempting means with which to avoid time-consuming discussions or end a difficult consultation. More often, drug therapy is considered in attempts to alleviate distressing symptoms associated with an insoluble problem for which "something must be done". However, there have been few adequately controlled double-blind trials to define the role of drug therapy in the management of irritable bowel syndrome. Symptoms often improve whichever drug is used and placebo responses are usually in the order of 50% (Klein 1988).

Pharmacotherapy should be directed at specific symptoms with the rationale being either to modulate intestinal motility, decrease visceral sensitivity or treat associated psychiatric disorders, particularly anxiety or depression (Pattee & Thompson 1992). In assessing the benefits of drug therapy, it should be appreciated that the placebo response varies for different symptoms; the placebo response of pain may be 50–70% while that for diarrhea about 30% (Klein 1988).

*Psychotropic drugs*

Antidepressant drug therapy has been shown to improve symptoms though whether this effect is attributable to its mood-enhancing, peripheral anticholinergic or central analgesic properties remains controversial (Pilowsky & Barrow 1990). Benzodiazepine anxiolytics also have significant smooth muscle relaxant properties in addition to their central effects on arousal. Their potential for abuse and their association with severe drug dependency states is such that their use for periods of longer than 1 week is contraindicated.

Studies appear to indicate that the central reduction of anxiety is an important ingredient of psychotropic therapy. In a placebo-controlled trial, desipramine hydrochloride (150 mg nocte) was significantly superior to atropine and placebo in improving abdominal pain, diarrhea and depression rating; not surprisingly, constipation was not improved (Greenbaum et al 1987). In a study of trimipramine (50 mg nocte), a low dose unlikely to influence depression, a significant improvement in mood without any improvement in bowel symptoms was observed compared to placebo (Myren et al 1982). A small dose (10–20 mg) of amitriptylene is often of value when there is a sensation of incomplete evacuation.

In summary, antidepressant drug therapy may improve bowel symptoms, especially diarrhea and abdominal pain, and the symptoms of anxiety and depression. Their use, in appropriate dosage, should be considered in patients with the biological markers of depression as an adjunct to cognitive therapy. However, given the placebo response rates and their adverse effects, antidepressants in high dosage should be avoided in the absence of symptoms of depression.

### *Drugs influencing motility*

***Anticholinergic drugs.*** These act by decreasing the abnormal sensitivity of cholinergic (muscarinic $M_2$) receptors in gut smooth muscle in irritable bowel syndrome and have been extensively evaluated (Ivey 1975). They significantly inhibit gut motility in response to food, often without commensurate changes in clinical symptoms (Goyal 1989). *Dicyclomine* or *cimetropium* in adequate dosage usually produces side-effects rendering placebo-controlled, double-blind comparisons difficult. Significant improvements in abdominal pain and rectal urgency compared with placebo have been reported in short-term trials. There is no evidence, however, that anticholinergics are more efficacious than placebo in the longer term (Ivey 1975).

***Smooth muscle relaxants.*** *Mebeverine*, *octylonium*, *nifedipine* and *peppermint oil* are all drugs which have direct relaxant properties on gut smooth muscle mediated in part or in total by their actions on intracellular calcium flux. *Calcium channel blockers* may also inhibit the release of sensory neurotransmitters and so further decrease visceral sensitivity to balloon distention. Placebo-controlled trials, however, have not produced any consensus on their overall efficacy in irritable bowel syndrome and many studies have reported little or no efficacy. As with the anticholinergic agents, though these drugs exert a powerful influence on basal and stimulated gut motility, these effects do not translate into consistently useful, clinical improvements (Gwee & Read 1994).

***Opioid-receptor agonists.*** Opioid receptors are important modulators of gastrointestinal function. At least three different receptor types ($\mu$, $\kappa$ and $\delta$) act at peripheral, spinal and central nervous system sites through a variety of mechanisms including neural stimulation, inhibition of neurotransmitter release and direct smooth muscle effects (Kromer 1988). Opiates that do not cross the blood–brain barrier, like *loperamide* and *trimebutine*, are preferable on the grounds of safety to those which do, e.g. codeine and diphenoxylate. *Loperamide* acts predominantly on peripheral $\mu$ receptors on the myenteric neurone, increasing nonpropulsive contractility and decreasing propulsive contractility. It delays small and large bowel transit, increases the frequency of small bowel phase 3 of the MMC, decreases intestinal secretory activity, colonic myoelectrical activity and rectal sensitivity and increases rectal sphincteric muscle tone. Placebo-controlled studies have confirmed its efficacy in reducing diarrhea, rectal urgency and abdominal pain in irritable bowel syndrome (Lavo et al 1987, Awouters et al 1993).

*Trimebutine*, an opioid that binds equally well to peripheral $\mu$, $\kappa$ and $\delta$ receptors, decreases colonic long spike burst activity and inhibits motility via a naloxone-insensitive pathway. Its clinical efficacy compared with placebo, however, has not been adequately demonstrated in irritable bowel syndrome, though it appears to be superior to placebo in alleviating pain (Schaffstein et al 1990).

*Fedotozine* stimulates peripheral $\kappa$ opioid receptors of the submucosal plexus and gut mucosa, resulting in inhibition of neurotransmitter release by the myenteric neurones. Double-blind, placebo-controlled studies have shown that it is effective in improving abdominal pain and bloating; however, further evaluation of its clinical efficacy is required (Dapoigny et al 1993).

***$\alpha_2$-adrenergic receptor agonists.*** Evidence suggests that enteric smooth muscle is under tonic control by a central "sympathetic brake". Sympathetic stimulation inhibits nonsphincteric gut motility, increases sphincteric muscle tone and reduces gut secretion, most of which effects relate to $\alpha_2$-adrenergic receptor activity (McIntyre & Thompson 1992). *Clonidine*-like $\alpha_2$ agonists have been formally evaluated as an antidiarrheal agent but found to be ineffective in irritable bowel syndrome (Prior et al 1988).

***$\beta_2$-adrenergic receptor antagonists.*** $\beta_2$ and not $\beta_1$-adrenergic receptors mediate an inhibitory influence on colorectal motility (Abrahamsson et al 1983, Lyrenas et al 1985, McIntyre & Thompson 1992). However, placebo-controlled trials of both nonselective and selective $\beta$ blockers have not shown either to be of any value in the management of bowel symptoms in irritable bowel syndrome (Fielding 1981).

***Dopaminergic receptor antagonists.*** Dopamine stimulates colorectal motility, an action that is blocked by domperidone but not metoclopramide. Placebo-controlled trials in irritable bowel syndrome have shown that *domperidone* has no consistent, overall effect on colonic symptoms; however, patients with irritable bowel syndrome with dyspeptic symptoms may represent a subgroup who could benefit (Cann et al 1983).

***Serotonergic 5HT3 receptor antagonists.*** Serotonergic 5HT3 receptors play a central role in visceral sensory function and also possess anxiolytic properties.

They are intimately involved in eating behavior, emesis, peristalsis, diarrhea and abdominal pain (Costall & Naylor 1990, Talley 1992). *Ondansetron* and *granisetron*, 5HT3 receptor antagonists, appear to decrease rectal sensitivity and motility in diarrhea-predominant irritable bowel syndrome; clinical trials are awaited (Prior & Read 1993, Hammer et al 1993).

***Serotonergic 5HT4 receptor agonists.*** *Cisapride* and the substituted benzamides indirectly stimulate cholinergic nerves via 5HT4 receptors on myenteric neurones, in addition to their direct effect on serotonergic transmission. Cisapride increases small and large bowel motility and transit (Talley 1992). The role of cisapride in constipation-predominant irritable bowel syndrome is still controversial.

***Somatostatin analogs.*** The somatostatin analog *octreotide* has been shown to prolong small bowel and colonic transit, reduce secretory function and decrease rectal sensitivity to distention in irritable bowel syndrome (Hasler et al 1994). Its uses await fuller evaluation (Grosman & Simon 1990, Burroughs & Malagelada 1993).

***Gonadotrophin-releasing hormone (GRH) analogs.*** Symptoms of irritable bowel syndrome are commonly exacerbated during the postovulatory phase of the menstrual cycle and in vitro, estrogen facilitates and progesterone inhibits smooth muscle contractility. *Leuprolide* has been shown to improve abdominal pain, nausea, early satiety and bloating in double-blind, placebo-controlled studies of women with the syndrome. However, it is unclear whether its effects are hormonally mediated or due to direct effects of the neuropeptide on brain, spinal or enteric neurones, akin to the effects of thyrotrophin and corticotrophin-releasing hormones (Wood 1994).

### Prognosis

This is a relapsing and remitting disorder; though its prevalence in a community appears stable, the evidence suggests that each year, 10% will develop symptoms and 30% will lose their symptoms (Talley et al 1992b). Most studies have confirmed that over follow-up periods of between 1 and 10 years, 50–70% of individuals become virtually asymptomatic and only one-third will experience persistent, unremitting symptoms. There is disagreement as to whether the prognosis is better in the constipation-predominant or diarrhea-predominant form. The available evidence suggests that a more favorable prognosis is seen in patients whose pain is intermittent rather than continuous, whose symptoms occurred only in response to major stress and in patients without major psychiatric disorders, particularly with no evidence of severe somatization disorders (Hawkins & Cockel 1971, Holmes & Salter 1982, Svendsen et al 1985, Harvey et al 1987, Fowlie et al 1992b).

Why then do symptoms come and go? Given that symptoms disappear during sleep, clearly the central nervous system is a key player. The correlation of symptom severity with psychometric tests in nonconsulters suggests that psychological status and levels of autonomic arousal are among the more important determinants; other factors, however, including previous illness experience, learned illness behavior, degree of social support and concomitant, coexisting illness, may all contribute.

Reassuringly, the diagnosis of irritable bowel syndrome remains a safe one in young patients when established following an appropriate history, examination and investigation. Fewer than 5% of patients develop evidence of missed or misdiagnosed illness during follow-up of 1–5 years duration (Waller & Misiewicz 1969, Harvey et al 1987). Significantly, however, in patients presenting acutely for the first time after the age of 50 years, the likelihood of serious organic disease is greater and may reach 10% or more; in such instances, therefore, detailed investigation and thorough follow-up are mandatory.

## FUNCTIONAL ABDOMINAL PAIN SYNDROME

### Definition

Functional abdominal pain syndrome is characterized by frequently recurrent or continuous, nonspecific, abdominal pain for 6 months or more in the absence of any other gut symptoms and evidence of underlying structural disease despite thorough investigation (Table 53.14; Thompson et al 1992). Functional abdominal pain syndrome is uncommon, with a community prevalence of 2%, but is more common in women than men. It is always associated with abnormal illness behavior, loss of social functioning and significant psychiatric disorder (Drossman 1982).

### Clinical features

*History*

Abdominal pain is either continuous or frequently recurrent, bears little or no relationship with physiological events such as eating, defecation or menstruation and invariably prevents the patient from fulfilling their social

**Table 53.14** Diagnostic criteria of functional abdominal pain syndrome

| |
|---|
| Frequently recurrent or continuous abdominal pain for at least 6 months **and** |
| Incomplete or no relationship of pain with physiological events (e.g. eating, defecation or menses) **and** |
| Some loss of daily social functioning **and** |
| No evidence of organic disease to explain the pain and insufficient criteria to establish the diagnosis of an alternative functional gastrointestinal disorder |

responsibilities and functioning normally. The pattern of abdominal pain does not fit any known disease and its severity is extreme. Unlike organic pain, the severity of pain varies surprisingly little and its onset may coincide with a time of great personal crisis.

Description of the pain usually includes multiple pains with different characteristics, often in multiple sites. The language and imagery used to describe the pain varies and is significantly altered by the prevailing mood and emotional distress. More importantly, there is often considerable disparity between the subjective description of pain severity and the degree of behavioral impairment. Aggravating or relieving factors are characteristically absent but may be inexplicable and even bizarre. For instance, the pain that is constant may not intrude on leisure activities yet makes attendance at work impossible. Analgesic drug therapy is usually characterized by poor efficacy and numerous adverse drug effects. The absence of pain during sleep and the denial of any possibility of emotional factors contributing to the disability are particularly suggestive of a functional pain disorder.

The past history is often especially revealing. Most patients will have previously undergone extensive investigations which may have included abdominal surgery for suspected appendicitis or cholecystitis. Previous episodes of self-harm, attempted suicide and psychiatric illness are clearly important. Dissatisfaction with previous medical care and carers may be openly expressed and is often closely associated with the striking absence of any personal sense of involvement in or responsibility for the management of their illness.

Abnormal illness behavior is an invariable accompaniment. (Table 53.15; Blackwell & Gutman 1986). The patient's family may be as convinced as the patient that serious disease is being overlooked. Often, at the patient's request, a relative is brought into the consulting room to endorse the validity of the illness and its severity.

*Examination*

The physical appearance of the patient is often at odds with the severity of their complaints, especially when pain is apparently present throughout the consultation. Pain behaviors may be remarkable by virtue of their exaggeration or complete absence. Abdominal palpation may reveal shifting sites of pain and tenderness, especially if distracted, disproportionate guarding or rebound tenderness and closure of the eyes throughout the abdominal examination. Objective features of serious disease are by definition absent, e.g. weight loss, anemia and rectal bleeding.

**Table 53.15** Features of abnormal illness behavior

| |
|---|
| Disability disproportionate to the clinical state |
| Relentless search for the validation of disease |
| Adoption and display of the sick role |
| Dissatisfaction with previous care and previous carers |
| Abrogation of responsibility for health to the carers |
| Sense of entitlement to be cared for |
| Avoidance of health promotion activities |

*Psychological evaluation*

Most patients will have clinical features to suggest an anxiety or depressive disorder. Others will exhibit features to suggest a somatoform disorder (Table 53.16; American Psychiatric Association 1987). It can be extremely helpful to enlist the help and support of the patient's primary care physician and, as appropriate, discuss the results of prior investigations with other specialists who may have been previously involved in the patient's care.

*The concept of illness behavior*

Why do some patients present with somatic complaints and minimize the psychological component of their illness? Many of the somatic complaints reported are amplifications of normal physiological sensations experienced by the majority of the population at some time (Mechanic 1986, Pilowsky 1986). It is therefore as important to ask the question "Why is the patient behaving in the way they are?" as it is to ask "What is wrong with them?". This hidden agenda is often central to the request for consultation and is intimately concerned with patterns of illness behavior and the concept of the sick role (Lipowski 1988, Drossman 1991).

The sick role carries with it many privileges. In addition to the exemption from responsibility, there is an unspoken obligation for the carer to be kind and sympathetic to them, as well as to assume some of the patient's responsibilities. The only obligation on the sick patient is to seek and accept appropriate treatment so that the privileges of the sick role are used for as short a time as possible. When patients behave as though they were ill when the demands of everyday life become excessive, they do so because they

**Table 53.16** Somatoform disorders (American Psychiatric Association 1987)

| | |
|---|---|
| Somatisation disorder | Numerous unexplained symptoms<br>Symptom onset aged < 30<br>Multiple specialist referrals |
| Somatoform pain disorder | Onset with life crisis<br>Previous good health |
| Hypochondriasis | Unreasonable fear of disease<br>Unamenable to medical reassurance<br>Repeated demands for investigations |
| Psychotic delusion | Unipolar depression<br>Schizophrenic disorder |

have learned to do so in the past. Such learned illness behavior can best be classified by three overlapping phenomena: overt and covert organic disease, illness motivated by fear of illness and illness rewarded by the advantages of the sick role.

The model of illness behavior and the sick role provides a more convincing explanation of the phenomena of psychosomatic and functional disorders. For most patients, the sick role only becomes attractive when adversity is abnormally great, often at a time of severe stress or exacerbations of chronic psychiatric disorders. However, a small minority of patients may adopt the sick role permanently if they experience the normal demands of life as excessive, either because they lack the ability or the energy to cope or because only when sick do they receive sufficient sympathy and attention.

Since it is usually impossible to separate conscious from unconscious motivation, it is counterproductive to imply either verbally or nonverbally that symptoms are not entirely genuine, particularly as patients may have doubts about this themselves. The wiser approach is to emphasize that symptoms are very familiar, that serious illness can be safely excluded and that a significant improvement can be expected, if necessary confessing ignorance as to the cause of the problem.

### Management

The cornerstone of management is the establishment of an effective doctor–patient relationship and the setting of explicit treatment aims with the patient. The management principles and expectations of both doctor and patient are shown in Table 53.17 (Drossman 1991).

Drug therapy should be carefully planned so as to avoid potentially harmful doses of narcotic agents or drug combinations. Antidepressant therapy may usefully complement analgesic therapy and psychotherapy given their central and peripheral pain-modulating properties (Feinmann 1985, Pilowsky & Barrow 1990). Referral to a psychiatrist should be considered when suicidal ideation, intractable depression or delusional beliefs are apparent. Referral to a pain clinic for behavioral therapy can also be helpful. However, limiting the number of physicians involved in management to a primary care physician supported by one specialist is sensible and, if achieved long term, can be seen as representing a successful outcome.

**Table 53.17** Management of functional abdominal pain syndrome

| |
|---|
| Acknowledgement of the severity of pain and distress |
| Avoidance of inappropriate further investigations |
| Shared responsibility for the management of their illness |
| Focusing on coping better with pain rather than seeking cures |
| Improving disability level and social functioning despite pain |
| Identification and treatment of concomitant emotional illness |

## FUNCTIONAL DYSPEPSIA

### Definition

Although the term "dyspepsia" usually implies upper alimentary symptoms associated with food intake, like the term "indigestion", it is nonspecific and few patients or physicians can agree on an explicit definition. One definition of functional dyspepsia is that of persistent or recurrent upper abdominal pain or discomfort, with or without other upper abdominal symptoms, lasting for 3 months or more and which occurs at least 25% of the time, for which no structural or biochemical cause can be found (Talley et al 1991a). When so defined, 15% of the community will have experienced functional dyspepsia in the previous year, of whom 15–25% will have previously sought medical advice because of symptoms (Talley et al 1992b). The prevalence of all dyspeptic symptoms in the community is 25% and is similar in men and women. The incidence of functional dyspepsia (the number of new cases in the community each year) is approximately 8% each year. One-third of all subjects with functional dyspepsia become asymptomatic within 1 year of the onset of symptoms and one-third remain persistently symptomatic during follow-up (Talley et al 1992b, Jones & Lydeard 1992b).

### Clinical manifestations

The common symptoms of dyspepsia are shown in Table 53.18. Endoscopic review of dyspeptic patients reveals recognizable mucosal lesions in only 20%. In a further 15%, the predominant symptoms are those of reflux dyspepsia, comprising acid reflux, heartburn, odynophagia (pain on swallowing) or dysphagia (Mansi et al 1993, Kay & Jorgensen 1994). When heartburn or acid regurgitation dominates the clinical symptomatology, these symptoms confer a high degree of specificity but lower sensitivity for the diagnosis of gastroesophageal reflux disease. Overall, no underlying structural abnormality of the upper gastrointestinal tract will be found in two-thirds of individuals who regularly experience dyspeptic symptoms in the absence of significant reflux symptomatology (Camilleri et al 1986a, Mansi et al 1993).

**Table 53.18** Dyspeptic symptoms

| |
|---|
| Abdominal pain or discomfort |
| Postprandial fullness |
| Abdominal bloating |
| Belching |
| Early satiety |
| Anorexia |
| Nausea |
| Vomiting |
| Heartburn |
| Acid reflux |

*Ulcer dyspepsia*

This term is used to encompass symptoms characteristic of peptic ulcer disease. Symptoms include episodic upper abdominal pain, pain relieved by food or antacids, pain accurately localized to the epigastrium (the pointing sign), frequent nocturnal pain, a dyspeptic history longer than 4 years, a family history of peptic ulcer disease, water brash (the appearance of clear, tasteless fluid in the mouth), regular vomiting with the relief of pain and the ability to eat immediately after vomiting. Unfortunately, at least 50% of patients with a peptic ulcer do not have the characteristic features. Therefore, the differentiation of peptic ulcer from functional dyspepsia can only be reliably established following an adequate endoscopic examination (Crean et al 1994, Kay & Jorgensen 1994).

Of patients with functional dyspepsia, approximately 17% have the symptom subset of ulcer-like dyspepsia, 9% dysmotility-like dyspepsia and 16% reflux-like dyspepsia; one-third have symptoms from more than one symptom subset and one-third have unspecified functional dyspepsia (Waldron et al 1991, Talley et al 1993) (Table 53.19). It was hoped that these subsets of functional dyspepsia would be of clinical utility; however, other than facilitating identification of patients with heartburn and acid reflux (in whom the diagnosis of gastroesophageal reflux disease is more appropriate) they have not been shown to have discriminant value. At least one-third of patients with functional dyspepsia also have the symptoms of the irritable bowel syndrome. None of the dyspeptic symptom subgroups correlate with the symptoms of irritable bowel syndrome (Talley et al 1993). Furthermore, patients with gastroesophageal reflux or peptic ulcer disease may also have concomitant and unrelated functional dyspepsia. The presence of an organic disorder neither excludes the possibility of a coexistent functional disorder nor alters an individual's susceptibility to functional disorders.

**Table 53.19** Symptom subsets in dyspepsia

| | |
|---|---|
| Ulcer-like dyspepsia: | Symptoms characteristic of peptic ulcer disease, i.e. upper abdominal pain or discomfort with at least two of the following criteria: pain relieved by food or antacids, periodic pain, postprandial pain or nocturnal waking with pain |
| Dysmotility-like dyspepsia: | Upper abdominal pain or discomfort with two or more of the following: anorexia, nausea, vomiting, early satiety, postprandial bloating, belching |
| Reflux-like dyspepsia: | Predominant symptoms of heartburn and acid reflux |
| Unspecified dyspepsia: | Dyspeptic symptoms not clearly aligned with the above groups |

## Functional dyspepsia and the irritable bowel syndrome

Upper alimentary symptoms are present in two-thirds of patients with irritable bowel syndrome, of whom 50% regularly experience dyspepsia. Upper abdominal pain or discomfort occurs in one-third of patients with irritable bowel syndrome. Balloon inflation studies in different parts of the colon indicate that colonic pain from distention is commonly perceived in the upper abdomen (Swarbrick et al 1980). The distinction between functional dyspepsia and irritable bowel syndrome, therefore, is often arbitrary and artificial and represents semantic rather than etiological differences.

## Diagnosis

The diagnosis of functional dyspepsia requires a thorough clinical history and a careful physical examination. The presence of findings favoring alternative diagnoses (Table 53.20) justifies prompt, detailed investigation. Young patients with recent onset of dyspepsia without such factors are unlikely to have underlying disease and usually do not require immediate investigation. Upper gastrointestinal endoscopy, however, is always indicated in those dyspeptic individuals who fail to respond to symptomatic therapy with acid reduction therapy (Mansi et al 1993). When further investigation is required, endoscopy has been found to be superior to barium meal examination. Without endoscopic evidence of disease, additional investigations, including gastric antral biopsies to identify *H. pylori* gastritis, are of little value. Abdominal ultrasonography and endoscopic retrograde cholangiopancreatography have very low diagnostic yields in atypical dyspepsia when a diagnosis of functional dyspepsia is otherwise considered likely. Patients with functional dyspepsia should, however, have a full blood count and biochemical screen to exclude anemia and hepatic dysfunction, as both may escape clinical detection until the underlying disorder is advanced. In some patients, gastric emptying studies are of value (p. 427). In the older patient, lower abdominal symptoms fully justify colonic investigations; carcinoma of the cecum is notoriously difficult to diagnose, especially in the earlier stages when symptoms are characteristically atypical. Conditions which should be considered in the differential diagnosis are listed in Table 53.21.

**Table 53.20** Clinical features favoring organic disease rather than functional dyspepsia

| |
|---|
| Recent onset of dyspepsia for the first time in patients aged 45 years + |
| Frequent vomiting, weight loss, dysphagia, anemia, jaundice, atypical abdominal pain, abdominal mass |
| Heavy consumption of tobacco, alcohol or NSAIDs |
| Previous history or family history of peptic ulceration or gastric cancer |
| Symptoms unresponsive to effective acid reduction therapy |

**Table 53.21** Differential diagnosis of functional dyspepsia

| Disorder | Clinical features |
|---|---|
| Peptic ulcer disease | Ulcer-like dyspepsia<br>Endoscopy essential for diagnosis |
| Gastric carcinoma | Age >45 years<br>Weight loss<br>Frequent vomiting<br>Anemia<br>Endoscopy and biopsy essential for diagnosis |
| Gastroesophageal reflux disease | Acid reflux and heartburn<br>50–66% have a normal endoscopy<br>Response to acid reduction is often diagnostic |
| Gallstones | Characteristic biliary pain lasting > 2 h<br>Vomiting without relief of pain<br>Jaundice; history of cholecystectomy |
| Chronic relapsing pancreatitis | Severe epigastric pain<br>Vomiting without relief of pain<br>Pain lasts > 4 h, often > 8 h<br>Association with high alcohol intake |

## Etiologic factors

### *Gastric acid hypersecretion*

Most studies have confirmed that acid secretion is normal in patients with functional dyspepsia. Controlled trials of gastric acid suppression in functional dyspepsia indicate that, while symptoms may improve, the benefit to be gained is not statistically significantly different from a placebo effect (Nyren et al 1986, Bytzer et al 1994).

### *Chronic gastritis and* Helicobacter pylori *infection*

Histological evidence of *H. pylori* gastritis can be found in 50% of patients with functional dyspepsia. However, up to 40% of the general population may be infected with this organism by the age of 50 and most remain asymptomatic. Symptom profiles in individuals with and without chronic gastritis associated with *H. pylori* are not significantly different and, similarly, gastrointestinal dysmotility is found with the same frequency in functional dyspepsia with and without *H. pylori* infection (Waldron et al 1991, Stanghellini et al 1992, Tucci et al 1992, Talley 1994). Patients with *H. pylori* gastritis and functional dyspepsia show no consistent symptomatic response to antimicrobial therapy. However, one study has shown a significant reduction in the symptomatic relapse rate 1 year after effective antimicrobial therapy (O'Morain & Gilvarry 1993). Confirmatory studies are required. An etiologic relationship between *H. pylori* chronic gastritis and functional dyspepsia remains to be established (Talley 1994).

### *Dietary and other factors*

Food intolerance and food allergy, as established by double-blind challenge testing, is rare in functional dyspepsia in the absence of other atopic manifestations (Young et al 1994). Smoking or the consumption of alcohol, coffee or nonsteroidal anti-inflammatory analgesics are not significantly associated with functional dyspepsia (Talley et al 1994).

### *Altered gastrointestinal motility*

Disordered upper gastrointestinal motility has been implicated in the etiology of functional dyspepsia because of such symptoms as abdominal bloating, early satiety and epigastric fullness. Many studies have confirmed that gastric antral motility is impaired postprandially in functional dyspepsia compared to healthy controls (Mearin et al 1991). Antral hypomotility, however, is a nonspecific motor abnormality which occurs in 50% of patients with functional dyspepsia (Camilleri et al 1986b, Greydanus et al 1991, Camilleri 1993, Hausken et al 1993). Similarly, delayed gastric emptying of solids is found in up to one-third of patients with functional dyspepsia and may be associated with hypochlorhydria (Van Wijk et al 1992, DeVault & Castell 1992). However, the finding of either delayed gastric emptying or antral hypomotility does not correlate with the presence or severity of symptoms (Waldron et al 1991, Galil et al 1993). In some patients with normal gastric emptying, the intragastric distribution of food is different from that of healthy controls. The initial retention of food in the proximal stomach is reduced, consistent with an alteration in gastric receptive relaxation (Scott et al 1993b, Troncon et al 1994).

Small bowel motility studies also indicate altered motility; bursts of nonpropagated, discrete, clustered contractions identical to those recorded in the irritable bowel syndrome have been described in the minority of patients. Indeed, such changes in small bowel motility are rare in functional dyspepsia in the absence of concomitant irritable bowel symptoms (Kellow & Phillips 1989). No consistent changes in gastric tone or gastric antral motility have been found in patients with functional dyspepsia with or without *H. pylori* gastritis compared with patients with ulcer dyspepsia (Waldron et al 1991, Stanghellini et al 1992). However, in a small subset of patients with functional dyspepsia, disordered motility may be of etiological importance. Gastric emptying studies may offer a simple means of screening patients who could benefit from a therapeutic trial of a prokinetic agent; several studies suggest that a prokinetic medication is superior to placebo or $H_2$ receptor antagonist in patients with either documented delay in gastric emptying or dysmotility-like dyspepsia (Corinaldesi et al 1987, Jian et al 1989, Halter et al 1994).

*Gastroduodenal hypersensitivity*

Gastric tone and gastric wall compliance are similar in patients with functional dyspepsia compared with healthy controls (Mearin et al 1991, Lemann et al 1991). However, isobaric gastric distention has been shown to elicit more upper abdominal discomfort in functional dyspeptic patients than in controls with evidence of a lower perception threshold in patients with functional dyspepsia (Mearin et al 1991, Fig. 53.10). Sensory responses to mechanical distention of the duodenum are unaltered in functional dyspepsia. In contrast, gastric emptying of a liquid meal containing fat is significantly prolonged in patients with functional dyspepsia compared with healthy controls, suggesting hypersensitivity of duodenal chemoreceptors (Read & Khan 1992). The fact that upper gastrointestinal symptoms are not significantly different in patients with delayed gastric emptying in response to a fatty liquid meal compared with those patients with normal gastric motility suggests that enhanced gastroduodenal sensitivity is not the predominant physiological factor responsible for symptoms in patients with functional dyspepsia. Interestingly, studies using buspirone, a 5HT1a receptor agonist, have shown that in functional dyspepsia, prolactin release is enhanced, suggesting that central 5HT receptors may be supersensitive. This finding could explain some of the alterations in visceral hypersensitivity recorded in functional dyspepsia (Chua et al 1992).

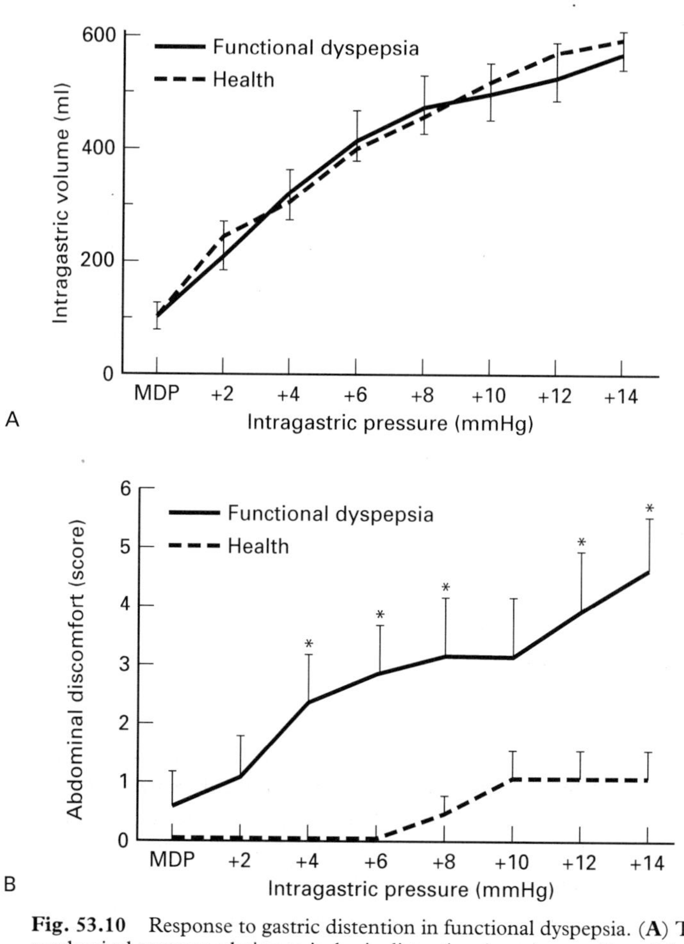


**Fig. 53.10** Response to gastric distention in functional dyspepsia. (**A**) The mechanical accommodation to isobaric distention (gastric compliance) is similar in patients with functional dyspepsia compared with healthy controls. (**B**) However, distention elicited more upper gastrointestinal symptoms in dyspeptics (n = 20) compared with control subjects, suggesting that altered perception may explain the symptomatology in functional dyspepsia (Mearin et al 1991). MDP = minimal distending pressure.

*Psychological factors*

For a psychological factor to be of etiological significance, it must be shown that patients with functional dyspepsia are more vulnerable or more sensitive to major life events and difficulties or that they experience these more often than healthy controls. There is little doubt that psychological stress alters gastrointestinal function and may even induce symptoms in healthy individuals (Richter 1991). Approximately 50% of patients with functional dyspepsia have a psychiatric disorder, usually anxiety or a mixed anxiety and depressive disorder, and in those with psychiatric disorders, abnormal illness behavior is significantly more common (Colgan et al 1988, Langeluddecke et al 1990). In patients with functional dyspepsia without psychiatric disorder, however, illness behavior is similar to that of control subjects. Personality profiles in functional dyspepsia do not help to discriminate functional dyspepsia from ulcer dyspepsia or healthy controls. Nonetheless, the use of the Minnesota Multiphasic Personality Inventory (MMPI) in healthy controls and patients with functional dyspepsia demonstrates that the latter are similar to those with the irritable bowel syndrome in exhibiting significantly elevated subscale scores for hypochondriasis, depression and hysteria, the so-called "psychosomatic triad" (Talley et al 1990). Furthermore, the inability to express feelings of anger or hostility has been shown to be of positive predictive value in identifying patients with functional dyspepsia in whom gastric emptying is delayed (Bennett et al 1992).

Stressful life events and difficulties are more commonly reported by patients presenting to their physician with functional dyspepsia compared with patients with organic dyspepsia and healthy controls. Patients with functional dyspepsia also perceive life events and difficulties as significantly more stressful than matched controls (Hui et al 1991). The association between psychological factors and functional dyspepsia is strongest in patients seeking medical care. It has been argued, therefore, that it is "health-seeking behavior", rather than the underlying condition, which is associated with severe life events and psychiatric illness.

*Summary*

The principal factors in the evolution and maintenance of

functional symptoms are visceral motor and sensory function, both of which may be modulated by central nervous autonomic activity. Symptom severity, psychosocial distress and learned illness behavior determine both the degree of autonomic arousal and health-seeking behavior. It follows that the management of functional dyspepsia should therefore include a careful appraisal of each potential contributory factor (Ford 1986, Jones & Lydeard 1989).

## Treatment

The cornerstone of treatment is a detailed clinical history, physical examination and appropriate further investigations. On this basis, patients can be strongly reassured about the absence of underlying disease. Endoscopic confirmation of the absence of upper gastrointestinal pathology reduces both alimentary- and nonalimentary-related consultation rates and prescription rates in general practice (Jones 1988, Morris et al 1992).

When symptoms are persistent or recurrent, reinvestigation should be avoided unless new symptoms emerge which demand investigation in their own right and which raise the possibility of serious disease, e.g. anemia, weight loss or frequent vomiting. In such instances, upper gastrointestinal endoscopy should be followed by an assessment of gastroduodenal motility and/or gastric emptying rate. The presence of functional dyspepsia associated with psychological distress does not exclude concomitant disorders, specifically gastroesophageal reflux disease or even more serious conditions. When reflux symptoms predominate, a therapeutic trial of a proton pump inhibitor should be considered. However, all patients should not be treated as if they had peptic ulcer disease.

## Principles of management

When symptoms persist and prove troublesome, re-exploration of the social context of illness, the hidden agenda and the reasons why the patient is seeking help at this time can be particularly helpful. A behavioral approach with the appropriate use of stress management techniques such as relaxation therapy, hypnosis, time management and cognitive therapy may all help reduce the level of symptoms and assist the patient to come to terms with their problem (Table 53.22).

**Table 53.22** Principles of therapy

| |
|---|
| Effective doctor–patient relationship |
| Patient education and reassurance |
| Stress management |
| Symptomatic management |

### *Drug therapy*

Many patients expect drug treatment, but few require it. As many as 50% will experience significant improvement with placebo therapy, although this finding does not justify the use of a placebo. When pharmacotherapy is used, it should be directed at controlling specific symptoms. Meta-analysis of randomized, controlled drug trials in functional dyspepsia indicates that in the absence of reflux dyspepsia, only prokinetic therapy is likely to offer any advantage over placebo. There is no convincing evidence, however, to indicate that a symptom-oriented classification is likely to identify responders to prokinetic agents (Waldron et al 1991) and, specifically, prokinetic agents are no more effective in patients with dysmotility-like symptoms compared with ulcer-like symptoms (Dobrilla et al 1989).

***Prokinetic drugs.*** Two classes of prokinetic agents are widely used: dopaminergic $D_2$ receptor blockers (*metoclopramide* and *domperidone*) and serotoninergic receptor agonists (*cisapride* and the substituted benzamides). Dopaminergic $D_2$ receptors are principally located in the proximal gut and their blockade stimulates gastric motility. Serotoninergic neurones comprise 2% of all myenteric neurones and project to the submucosal plexus, thereby facilitating control of motor, sensory, absorptive and secretory functions.

Both metoclopramide and cisapride have been shown to produce a significant improvement in symptoms in patients with functional dyspepsia; cisapride may also reduce gastric hypersensitivity to distention. Metoclopramide is both a dopaminergic $D_2$ receptor antagonist and a 5HT4 receptor agonist; it crosses the blood–brain barrier and induces central adverse drug effects in 20% of patients, i.e. anxiety, drowsiness and extrapyramidal symptoms including tardive dyskinesia. Domperidone is a peripherally acting dopamine antagonist that does not cross the blood–brain barrier. Though it is no more efficacious than metoclopramide, its use avoids the possibility of CNS adverse effects.

Cisapride and the substituted benzamides indirectly stimulate cholinergic nerves via 5HT4 receptors on myenteric neurones, in addition to their direct effects on serotoninergic transmission. Increases in lower esophageal sphincter tone, esophageal motility and gastric and small bowel transit have been reported following its administration. The overall success rate of prokinetic agents is approximately 50% and is most likely for those with impaired gastric emptying (Corinaldesi et al 1987, Jian et al 1989), although clinical trials of efficacy extending beyond the first 4 weeks of treatment are lacking. There is no clearcut evidence that cisapride is superior to metoclopramide or domperidone or that there is any clinical benefit to be obtained by the combined use of both classes of prokinetic agents (Holtmann & Talley 1993).

***Antacids and acid-reducing agents.*** Although the evidence suggests that histamine $H_2$ receptor antagonists (cimetidine and ranitidine) are marginally more effective than placebo in alleviating symptoms of functional dyspepsia, the benefits of antacid therapy appear more obvious in patients whose functional dyspepsia is characterized by reflux-like symptomatology. It remains to be demonstrated by control trials, however, that proton pump inhibitors have any significant role to play in the drug treatment of functional dyspepsia (Bytzer et al 1994).

Sucralfate, an agent which stimulates mucosal prostaglandin synthesis, has been reported as producing a significant symptomatic improvement in patients with functional dyspepsia in placebo-controlled trials. The number of studies reported, however, does not as yet justify its use in functional dyspepsia outside clinical trials.

***Anticholinergic therapy.*** *Pirenzepine*, an antisecretory agent with selective $M_2$ muscarinic receptor antagonist effects, has been evaluated in the treatment of functional dyspepsia. Unfortunately, the initially promising results have not been confirmed by larger placebo-controlled studies. *Dicyclomine* therapy in functional dyspepsia has similarly been found to be no better than placebo in alleviating symptoms (Ivey 1975, Gwee & Read 1994).

***Eradication of* Helicobacter pylori *infection.*** Since 50% of patients with functional dyspepsia have histological evidence of gastritis associated with Helicobacter infection, a number of controlled trials have been undertaken to assess the efficacy of antimicrobial therapy with and without bismuth in functional dyspepsia. One study has suggested that Helicobacter eradication can reduce symptoms for up to 12 months (O'Morain & Gilvarry 1993). However, there is little corroborative evidence that antimicrobial therapy is more effective than placebo in achieving lasting symptomatic improvement or in altering gastric antral hypomotility (Talley 1994).

***Other drugs.*** Serotoninergic 5HT3 receptors have been identified in the central nervous system and on post-ganglionic autonomic and enteric sensory neurones. 5HT3 receptor antagonists (*ondansetron*) are highly effective antiemetics with anxiolytic properties but as yet they have not been fully evaluated in the treatment of functional dyspepsia. The evidence suggests that this class of drugs may have greater effects in reducing visceral hypersensitivity than accelerating gastric and small bowel emptying (Talley 1992); nevertheless there is no current evidence that these drugs are efficacious in dyspepsia.

*Erythromycin* is a macrolide antibiotic with motilin-like properties. In diabetic gastroparesis, it has been shown to improve gastric emptying, though its effects do not last longer than 4 weeks and can only be reliably achieved by intravenous administration. There are no studies reported on its longer term use in functional dyspepsia.

*Octreotide*, a synthetic somatostatin analog, possesses a multiplicity of actions and antagonizes numerous gut hormones and neuropeptides, inhibiting gut secretory, absorptive and motor functions. It can increase the initial phase of gastric emptying and decrease small bowel transit in health. Though it reduces rectal sensitivity to distention, it has little effect on gastric sensory thresholds.

*Fedotozine*, a κ-opioid receptor agonist, increases esophageal contractility and lower esophageal sphincter tone and decreases gastric sensitivity to balloon distention. Its therapeutic role in functional dyspepsia awaits further evaluation.

*Loxiglumide*, a cholecystokinin (CCK-A) receptor antagonist, blocks the effect of intraduodenal fat in delaying gastric emptying. A placebo-controlled trial in functional dyspepsia associated with delayed gastric emptying demonstrated a significant improvement in symptoms unrelated to its effects on gastric emptying; further evaluation is awaited (Gwee & Read 1994).

## Prognosis of functional dyspepsia

The prevalence of functional dyspepsia in the community is approximately 15%, one-third of whom become asymptomatic within 1 year. Each year, 8% of the population experience the onset of functional dyspepsia for the first time or an exacerbation of dyspeptic symptoms. Approximately one-third of individuals with functional dyspepsia have persistent or chronic intermittent symptoms which remain largely unchanged over a course of 3–5 years. In one study, the symptoms of gastroesophageal reflux disease developed for the first time in 9% of patients with functional dyspepsia followed up for a mean period of 18 months. Of the two-thirds of patients still symptomatic at 12 months, 23% underwent repeat endoscopy and of these, 12% were found to have developed peptic ulcer disease, most of whom had a past history of peptic ulcer disease (Jones 1988, Talley et al 1987, Talley et al 1992b, Jones & Lydeard 1992b, Morris et al 1992, Kay & Jorgensen 1994).

REFERENCES

Abrahamsson H, Lyrenas E, Dotevall G 1983 Effects of beta-adrenoreceptor blocking drugs on human sigmoid colonic motility. Digestive Diseases and Sciences 28: 590–594
Aggarwal A, Cutts T F, Abell T L et al 1994 Predominant symptoms in irritable bowel syndrome correlate with specific autonomic nervous system abnormalities. Gastroenterology 106: 945–950
American Psychiatric Association 1987 Somatoform disorders. In: Diagnostic and statistical manual of mental disorders. American Psychiatric Association p 255–267
Anderson I H, Levine A S, Levitt M D 1981 Incomplete absorption of the carbohydrate in all-purpose wheat flour. New England Journal of Medicine 304: 891–892
Awouters F, Megens A, Verlinden M, Schuurkes J, Niemegeers C, Janssen P A J 1993 Loperamide – survey of studies on mechanisms of

its antidiarrheal activity. Digestive Diseases and Sciences 38: 977–995

Bassotti G, Crowell M D, Whitehead W E 1993 Contractile activity of the human colon: lessons from 24 hour studies. Gut 34: 129–133

Beckman H B, Frankel R M 1984 The effect of physician behavior on the collection of data. Annals of Internal Medicine 101: 692–696

Bennett E J, Kellow J E, Cowan H et al 1992 Suppression of anger and gastric emptying in patients with functional dyspepsia. Scandinavian Journal of Gastroenterology 27: 869–874

Besterman H S, Sarson D L, Rambaud J C, Stewart J S, Guerin S, Bloom S R 1981 Gut hormone responses in the irritable bowel syndrome. Digestion 21: 219–224

Bharucha A E, Camilleri M, Low P A, Zinsmeister A R 1993 Autonomic dysfunction in gastrointestinal motility disorders. Gut 34: 397–401

Blackwell B, Gutman M 1986 The management of chronic illness behavior. In: McHugh S, Vallis T M (eds) Illness behavior: a multidisciplinary model. Plenum, New York, p 401–408

Blanchard E B, Schwarz S P, Suls J M et al 1992a Two controlled evaluations of multicomponent psychological treatment of irritable bowel syndrome. Behaviour Research and Therapy 30: 175–189

Blanchard E B, Scharff L, Payne A, Schwarz S P, Suls J M, Malamood H 1992b Prediction of outcome from cognitive-behavioral treatment of irritable bowel syndrome. Behaviour Research and Therapy 30: 647–650

Blanchard E B, Greene B, Scharff L, Schwarz S P 1993 Relaxation training as a treatment for irritable bowel syndrome. Biofeedback and Self Regulation 18: 125–132

Bolin T D, Davis A E, Duncombe V M 1982 A prospective study of persistent diarrhoea. Australian and New Zealand Journal of Medicine 12: 22–26

Bordie A K 1972 Functional disorders of the colon. Journal of the Indian Medical Association 58: 451–456

Burroughs A K, Malagelada R 1993 Potential indications for octreotide in gastroenterology: summary of workshop. Digestion 54 (suppl 1): 59–67

Bytzer P, Hansen J M, Schaffalitzky de Muckadell O B 1994 Empirical H2-blocker therapy or prompt endoscopy in management of dyspepsia. Lancet 343: 811–816

Camilleri M 1993 Study of human gastroduodenojejunal motility – applied physiology in clinical practice. Digestive Diseases and Sciences 38: 785–794

Camilleri M, Ford M J 1994 Functional gastrointestinal disease and the autonomic nervous system: a way ahead? Gastroenterology 106: 1114–1118

Camilleri M, Neri M 1989 Motility disorders and stress. Digestive Diseases and Sciences 34: 1777–1786

Camilleri M, Thompson D G, Malagelada J-R 1986a Functional dyspepsia – symptoms and underlying mechanisms. Journal of Clinical Gastroenterology 8: 424–429

Camilleri M, Malagelada J-R, Kao P C, Zinsmeister A R 1986b Gastric and autonomic responses to stress in functional dyspepsia. Digestive Diseases and Sciences 31: 1169–1177

Camilleri M, Zinsmeister A R 1992 Towards a relatively inexpensive, noninvasive, accurate test for colonic motility disorders. Gastroenterology 103: 36–42

Cann P A, Read N W, Holdsworth C D 1983 Oral domperidone: double-blind comparison with placebo in irritable bowel syndrome. Gut 24: 1135–1140

Cann P A, Read N W, Holdsworth C D 1984 What is the benefit of coarse wheat bran in patients with irritable bowel syndrome? Gut 25: 168–173

Chaudhary N A, Truelove S C 1962 The irritable colon syndrome. A study of the clinical features, predisposing causes, and prognosis in 130 cases. Quarterly Journal of Medicine 31: 307–322

Christl S U, Murgatroyd P R, Gibson G R, Cummings J H 1992 Production, metabolism and excretion of hydrogen in the large intestine. Gastroenterology 102: 1269–1277

Chua A, Keating J, Hamilton D, Keeling P W, Dinan T G 1992 Central serotonin receptors and delayed gastric emptying in non-ulcer dyspepsia. British Medical Journal 305: 280–282

Colgan S, Creed F, Klass H 1988 Symptom complaints, psychiatric disorder and abnormal illness behaviour in patients with upper abdominal pain. Psychological Medicine 18: 887–892

Collins S M 1992 Is the irritable gut an inflamed gut? Scandinavian Journal of Gastroenterology 192 (suppl): 102–115

Connell A M, Hilton C, Irvine G, Lennard-Jones J E, Misiewicz J J 1965 Variation of bowel habit in two population samples. British Medical Journal 2: 1095–1099

Corinaldesi R, Stanghellini V, Raiti C et al 1987 Effect of chronic administration of cisapride on gastric emptying of a solid meal and on dyspeptic symptoms in patients with idiopathic gastroparesis. Gut 28: 300–305

Costall B, Naylor R J 1990 5-hydroxytryptamine: new receptors and novel drugs for gastrointestinal motor disorders. Scandinavian Journal of Gastroenterology 25: 769–787

Crean G P, Holden R J, Knill-Jones R P et al 1994 A database on dyspepsia. Gut 35: 191–202

Creed F, Guthrie E 1987 Psychological factors in the irritable bowel syndrome. Gut 28: 1307–1318

Creed F, Guthrie E 1989 Psychological treatments of the irritable bowel syndrome: a review. Gut 30: 1601–1609

Crowe S E, Perdue M H 1992 Gastrointestinal food hypersensitivity: basic mechanisms of pathophysiology. Gastroenterology 103: 1075–1095

Cullingford G L, Coffey J F, Carr-Locke D L 1992 Irritable bowel syndrome: can the patient's response to colonoscopy help with diagnosis? Digestion 52: 209–213

Cummings J H 1973 Dietary fibre. Gut 14: 69–81

Dapoigny M, Homerin M, Scherrer B, Fraitag B 1993 Efficacy of fedotozine in the irritable bowel syndrome (IBS). A double-blind, placebo-controlled dose-range muticentre study. Gut 34 (suppl 3): S30

Davies G J, Crowder M, Reid B, Dickerson J W T 1986 Bowel function measurements of individuals with different eating patterns. Gut 27: 164–169

Degen L P, Phillips S F 1996 How well does stool form reflect colonic transit? Gut 39: 109–113

DeVault K, Castell D O 1992 The irritable stomach syndrome. American Journal of Gastroenterology 87: 399–400

Dinan T G, Barry S, Ahkion S, Chua A, Keeling P W N 1989 Assessment of central noradrenergic functioning in irritable bowel syndrome using a neuroendocrine challenge test. Journal of Psychosomatic Research 34: 575–580

Dobrilla G, Comberlato M, Steele A, Vallaperta P 1989 Drug treatment of functional dyspepsia. A meta-analysis of randomised controlled clinical trials. Journal of Clinical Gastroenterology 11: 169–177

Drossman D A 1982 Patients with psychogenic abdominal pain: six years' observation in the medical setting. American Journal of Psychiatry 139: 1549–1557

Drossman D A 1991 Illness behavior in the irritable bowel syndrome. Gastroenterology International 4: 77–81

Drossman D A, Thompson W G 1992 The irritable bowel syndrome: review and a graduated multicomponent treatment approach. Annals of Internal Medicine 116: 1009–1016

Drossman D A, Sandler R S, McKee D C, Lovitz A J 1982 Bowel patterns among subjects not seeking health care. Use of a questionnaire to identify a population with bowel dysfunction. Gastroenterology 83: 529–534

Drossman D A, McKee D C, Sandler R S et al 1988 Psychosocial factors in the irritable bowel syndrome. A multivariate study of patients and nonpatients with irritable bowel syndrome. Gastroenterology 95: 701–708

Drossman D A, Leserman J, Nachman G et al 1990 Sexual and physical abuse in women with functional or organic gastrointestinal disorders. Annals of Internal Medicine 113: 828–833

Drossman D A, Li Z, Andruzzi E et al 1993 US householder survey of functional gastrointestinal disorders – prevalence, sociodemography and health impact. Digestive Diseases and Sciences 38: 1569–1580

Eastwood M A, Morris E R 1992 Physical properties of dietary fiber that influence physiological function: a model for polymers along the gastrointestinal tract. American Journal of Clinical Nutrition 55: 436–442

Eisendrath S J, Way L W, Ostroff J W, Johanson C A 1986 Identification of psychogenic abdominal pain. Psychosomatics 27: 705–712

Esler M D, Goulston K J 1973 Levels of anxiety in colonic disorders. New England Journal of Medicine 288: 16–20

Eusufzai S, Axelson M, Angelin B, Einarsson K 1993 Serum 7a-hydroxy-4-cholesten-3-one concentrations in the evaluation of bile acid malabsorption in patients with diarrhoea: correlation with SeHCAT test. Gut 34: 698–701

Farah D A, Calder I, Benson L, Mackenzie J F 1985 Specific food intolerance: its place as a cause of gastrointestinal symptoms. Gut 26: 164–168

Feinmann C 1985 Pain relief by antidepressants. Pain 23: 1–8

Ferguson A, MacDonald D M, Brydon W G 1984 Prevalence of lactase deficiency in British adults. Gut 25: 163–167

Fernandez-Banares F, Esteve-Pardo M, de Leon R et al 1993 Sugar malabsorption in functional bowel disease: clinical implications. American Journal of Gastroenterology 88: 2044–2050

Fielding J F 1981 Timolol treatment in the irritable bowel syndrome. Digestion 22: 155–158

Fielding J F 1983 Detailed history and examination assist positive clinical diagnosis of the irritable bowel syndrome. Journal of Clinical Gastroenterology 5: 495–497

Ford M J 1986 The irritable bowel syndrome. Journal of Psychosomatic Research 30: 399–410

Ford M J, Eastwood J, Eastwood M A 1982 The irritable bowel syndrome: soma and psyche. Psychosomatic Medicine 12: 705–707

Ford M J, Miller P McC, Eastwood J, Eastwood M A 1987 Life events, psychiatric illness and the irritable bowel syndrome. Gut 28: 160–165

Fowlie S, Eastwood M A, Prescott R 1992a Irritable bowel syndrome: assessment of psychological disturbance and its influence on the response to fibre supplementation. Journal of Psychosomatic Research 36: 175–180

Fowlie S, Eastwood M A, Ford M J 1992b Irritable bowel syndrome: the influence of psychological factors on the symptom complex. Journal of Psychosomatic Research 36: 169–173

Fukudo S, Nomura T, Muranaka M, Taguchi F 1993 Brain–gut response to stress and cholinergic stimulation in irritable bowel syndrome. A preliminary study. Journal of Clinical Gastroenterology 17: 133–141

Furness J B, Bornstein J C, Smith T K 1990 The normal structure of gastrointestinal innervation. Journal of Gastroenterology and Hepatology 1: 1–9

Gaginella T S 1994 Absorption and secretion in the colon. Current Opinion in Gastroenterology 10: 5–10

Galil M A, Critchley M, Mackie C R 1993 Isotope gastric emptying tests in clinical practice: expectation, outcome and utility. Gut 34: 916–919

Gomborone J E, Dewsnap P A, Libby G W, Farthing M J 1993 Selective affective biasing in recognition memory in the irritable bowel syndrome. Gut 34: 1230–1233

Gorard D A, Libby G W, Farthing M J 1994 Ambulatory small intestinal motility in "diarrhoea" predominant irritable bowel syndrome. Gut 35: 203–210

Goyal R K 1989 Muscarinic receptor subtypes – physiology and clinical implications. New England Journal of Medicine 321: 1022–1029

Greenbaum D S, Mayle J E, Vanegeran L E, Jerome J A, Mayor J W, Greenbaum R B 1987 The effects of desipramine on irritable bowel syndrome compared with atropine and placebo. Digestive Diseases and Sciences 32: 257–266

Greydanus M P, Vassallo M, Camilleri M, Nelson D K, Hanson R B, Thomforde G M 1991 Neurohormonal factors in functional dyspepsia: insights on pathophysiological mechanisms. Gastroenterology 100: 1311–1318

Grosman I, Simon D 1990 Potential gastrointestinal uses of somatostatin and its synthetic analogue octreotide. American Journal of Gastroenterology 85: 1061–1072

Gudmand-Hoyer E, Riis P, Wulff H R 1973 The significance of lactose malabsorption in the irritable colon syndrome. Scandinavian Journal of Gastroenterology 8: 273–278

Guthrie E, Creed F, Dawson D, Tomenson B 1991 A controlled trial of psychological treatment for the irritable bowel syndrome. Gastroenterology 100: 450–457

Guthrie E, Creed F, Dawson D, Tomenson B 1993 A randomised controlled trial of psychotherapy in patients with refractory irritable bowel syndrome. British Journal of Psychiatry 163: 315–321

Gwee K A, Read N W 1994 Rolling review: disorders of gastrointestinal motility – therapeutic potentials and limitations. Alimentary Pharmacology and Therapeutics 8: 105–118

Haderstorfer B, Whitehead W E, Schuster M M 1989 Intestinal gas production from fermentation of undigested carbohydrate in irritable bowel syndrome. American Journal of Gastroenterology 84: 375–378

Halter F 1993 Clinical use of antacids. Journal of Physiology and Pharmacology 44: 61–74

Halter F, Miazza B, Brignoli R 1994 Cisapride or cimetidine in the treatment of functional dyspepsia. Scandinavian Journal of Gastroenterology 29: 618–623

Hammer J, Phillips S F 1993 Fluid loading of the human colon: effects on segmental transit and stool composition. Gastroenterology 105: 988–998

Hammer J, Phillips S F, Talley N J, Camilleri M 1993 Effect of a 5-HT3-antagonist (ondansetron) on rectal sensitivity and compliance in health and the irritable bowel syndrome. Alimentary Pharmacology and Therapeutics 7: 543–551

Harvey R F, Read A E, Salih S Y 1983 Organic and functional disorders in 2000 gastroenterology outpatients. Lancet 1: 632–634

Harvey R F, Mauad E C, Brown A M 1987 Prognosis in the irritable bowel syndrome: a 5-year prospective study. Lancet 1: 963–965

Harvey R F, Gunary R M, Hinton R A, Barry R E 1989 Individual and group hypnotherapy in treatment of refractory irritable bowel syndrome. Lancet 1: 424–425

Hasler W L, Soudah H C, Owyang C 1994 Somatostatin analog inhibits afferent response to rectal distention in diarrhea-predominant irritable bowel patients. Journal of Pharmacology and Experimental Therapeutics 268: 1206–1211

Hausken T, Svebak S, Wilhelmsen I et al 1993 Low vagal tone and antral dysmotility in patients with functional dyspepsia. Psychosomatic Medicine 55: 12–22

Hawkins C F, Cockel R 1971 The prognosis and risk of missing malignant disease in patients with unexplained and functional diarrhoea. Gut 12: 208–211

Heaton K W, Radvan J, Cripps H, Mountford R A, Braddon F E M, Hughes A O 1992a Defecation frequency and timing, and stool form in the general population: a prospective study. Gut 33: 818–824

Heaton K W, O'Donnell L J, Braddon F E, Mountford R A, Hughes A O, Cripps P J 1992b Symptoms of irritable bowel syndrome in a British urban community: consulters and nonconsulters. Gastroenterology 102: 1962–1967

Heitkemper M M, Jarrett M 1992 Pattern of gastrointestinal and somatic symptoms across the menstrual cycle. Gastroenterology 102: 505–513

Heymen S, Wexner S D, Gulledge A D 1993 MMPI assessment of patients with functional bowel disorders. Diseases of the Colon and Rectum 36: 593–596

Hillman L C, Stace N H, Fisher A, Pomare E W 1982 Dietary intakes and stool characteristics of patients with the irritable bowel syndrome. American Journal of Clinical Nutrition 36: 626–629

Hillman L C, Stace N H, Pomare E W 1984 Irritable bowel patients and their long-term response to a high fiber diet. American Journal of Gastroenterology 79: 1–7

Holdstock D J, Misiewicz J J 1970 Factors controlling colonic motility: colonic pressures and transit after meals in patients with total gastrectomy, pernicous anaemia or duodenal ulcer. Gut 11: 100–110

Holdstock D J, Misiewicz J J, Smith T, Rowlands E N 1970 Propulsion (mass movement) in the human colon and its relationship to meals and somatic activity. Gut 11: 91–99

Holmes K M, Salter R H 1982 Irritable bowel syndrome – a safe diagnosis? British Medical Journal 285: 1533–1534

Holtmann G, Enck P 1991 Stress and gastrointestinal motility in humans: a review of the literature. Journal of Gastrointestinal Motility 3: 245–254

Holtmann G, Talley N J 1993 Functional dyspepsia. Current treatment recommendations. Drugs 45: 918–930

Hui W M, Shiu L P, Lam S K 1991 The perception of life events and daily stress in nonulcer dyspepsia. American Journal of Gastroenterology 86: 292–296

Huizinga J D, Stern H S, Chow E, Diamante N E, El-Sharkawy T Y 1985 Electrophysiologic control of motility in the human colon. Gastroenterology 88: 500–511

Hunter J O 1991 Food allergy – or enterometabolic disorder? Lancet 338: 495–496
Ingham J, Miller P 1982 Consulting with mild symptoms in general practice. Social Psychiatry 17: 77–88
Ingham J G, Miller P McC 1983 Self-referral: social and demographic determinants of consulting behaviour. Journal of Psychosomatic Research 27: 233–242
Ivey K J 1975 Are anti-cholinergics of use in the irritable bowel syndrome? Gastroenterology 68: 1300–1307
Jian R, Ducrot F, Ruskone A et al 1989 Symptomatic, radionuclide and therapeutic assessment of chronic idiopathic dyspepsia: a double-blind, placebo-controlled evaluation of cisapride. Digestive Diseases and Sciences 34: 657–664
Jones R 1988 What happens to patients with non-ulcer dyspepsia after endoscopy? Practitioner 232: 75–78
Jones R, Lydeard S 1989 Factors affecting the decision to consult with dyspepsia: comparison of consulters and non-consulters. Journal of the Royal College of General Practitioners 39: 495–498
Jones R, Lydeard S 1992a Irritable bowel syndrome in the general population. British Medical Journal 304: 87–90
Jones R, Lydeard S 1992b Dyspepsia in the community: a follow-up study. British Journal of Clinical Practice 46: 95–97
Jones V A, McLaughlan P, Shorthouse M, Workman E, Hunter J O 1982 Food intolerance: a major factor in the pathogenesis of irritable bowel syndrome. Lancet 2: 1115–1117
Kang J Y, Gwee K A, Yap I 1994 The colonic air insufflation test indicates a colonic cause of abdominal pain. An aid in the management of irritable bowel syndrome. Journal of Clinical Gastroenterology 18: 19–22
Kay L, Jorgensen T 1994 Epidemiology of upper dyspepsia in a random population. Prevalence, incidence, natural history, and risk factors. Scandinavian Journal of Gastroenterology 29: 2–6
Kellow J E, Phillips S F 1987 Altered small bowel motility in irritable bowel syndrome is correlated with symptoms. Gastroenterology 92: 1885–1893
Kellow J E, Phillips S F 1989 Functional disorders of the small intestine. In: Snape W J (ed) Pathogenesis of functional bowel disease. Plenum, New York
Kellow J E, Phillips S F, Miller L J, Zinsmeister A R 1988 Dysmotility of the small intestine in irritable bowel syndrome. Gut 29: 1236–1243
Kellow J E, Langeluddecke P M, Eckersley G M, Jones M P, Tennant C C 1992a Effects of acute psychologic stress on small-intestinal motility in health and the irritable bowel syndrome. Scandinavian Journal of Gastroenterology 27: 53–58
Kellow J E, Eckersley G M, Jones M 1992b Enteric and central contributions to intestinal dysmotility in irritable bowel syndrome. Digestive Diseases and Sciences 37: 168–174
Kettell J, Jones R, Lydeard S 1992 Reasons for consultation in irritable bowel syndrome: symptoms and patient characteristics. British Journal of General Practice 42: 459–461
Klein K B 1988 Controlled treatment trials in the irritable bowel syndrome: a critique. Gastroenterology 95: 232–241
Krevsky B, Malmud L S, d'Ercole F, Maurer A H, Fisher R S 1986 Colonic transit scintigraphy – a physiologic approach to the quantitative measurement of colonic transit in humans. Gastroenterology 91: 1102–1112
Kromer W 1988 Endogenous and exogenous opioids in the control of gastrointestinal motility and secretion. Pharmacological Reviews 40: 121–162
Kumar D, Wingate D L 1985 The irritable bowel syndrome: a paroxysmal motor disorder. Lancet 2: 973–977
Kumar D, Wingate D, Ruckesbusch Y 1986 Circadian variation in the propagation velocity of the migrating motor complex. Gastroenterology 91: 926–930
Kumar D, Thompson P D, Wingate D L, Vesselinova-Jenkins C K, Libby G 1992 Abnormal REM sleep in the irritable bowel syndrome. Gastroenterology 103: 12–17
Lambert J P, Brunt P W, Mowat N A G et al 1991 The value of prescribed "high fibre" diets for the treatment of the irritable bowel syndrome. European Journal of Clinical Nutrition 45: 601–609
Lampe J W, Fredstrom S B, Slavin J L, Potter J D 1993 Sex differences in colonic function: a randomised trial. Gut 34: 531–536
Langeluddecke P, Goulston K, Tennant C 1990 Psychological factors in dyspepsia of unknown cause: a comparison with peptic ulcer disease. Journal of Psychosomatic Research 34: 215–222
Lasser R B, Bond J H, Levitt M D 1975 The role of intestinal gas in functional abdominal pain. New England Journal of Medicine 293: 524–526
Latimer P, Campbell D, Latimer M, Sarna S, Daniel E E, Waterfall W 1979 Irritable bowel syndrome: a test of colonic hyperalgesia hypothesis. Journal of Behavioral Medicine 2: 285–295
Latimer P, Sarna S, Campbell D, Latimer M, Waterfall W, Daniel E E 1981 Colonic motor and myoelectrical activity: a comparative study of normal subjects, psychoneurotic patients and patients with irritable bowel syndrome. Gastroenterology 80: 893–901
Lavo B, Stenstam M, Nielsen A L 1987 Loperamide in the treatment of irritable bowel syndrome – a double-blind, placebo-controlled study. Scandinavian Journal of Gastroenterology 22 (suppl 130): 77–80
Lemann M, Dederding J P, Flourie B, Franchisseur C, Rambaud J C, Jian R 1991 Abnormal perception of visceral pain in response to gastric distension in chronic idiopathic dyspepsia. The irritable stomach syndrome. Digestive Diseases and Sciences 36: 1249–1254
Levitt M D 1980 Intestinal gas production – recent advances in flatology. New England Journal of Medicine 302: 1474–1475
Lindgren S, Stewenius J, Sjolund K, Lilja B, Sundkvist G 1993 Autonomic vagal nerve dysfunction in patients with ulcerative colitis. Scandinavian Journal of Gastroenterology 28: 638–642
Lipowski Z J 1988 Somatisation: the concept and its clinical application. American Journal of Psychiatry 145: 1358–1368
Longstreth G F, Fox D D, Youkeles L, Forsythe A B, Wolochow D A 1981 Psyllium therapy in the irritable bowel syndrome – a double-blind trial. Annals of Internal Medicine 95: 53–56
Lowman B C, Drossman D A, Cramer E M, McKee D C 1987 Recollection of childhood events in adults with irritable bowel syndrome. Journal of Clinical Gastroenterology 9: 324–330
Lucey M R, Clark M L, Lowndes J O, Dawson A M 1987 Is bran efficacious in irritable bowel syndrome? A double-blind placebo-controlled crossover study. Gut 28: 221–225
Lydiard R B, Fossey M D, Marsh W, Ballenger J C 1993 Prevalence of psychiatric disorders in patients with irritable bowel syndrome. Psychosomatics 34: 229–234
Lyrenas E, Abrahamsson H, Dotevall G 1985 Effects of beta-adrenoreceptor stimulation on rectosigmoid motility in man. Digestive Diseases and Sciences 30: 536–540
Manning A P, Thompson W G, Heaton K W, Morris A F 1978 Towards positive diagnosis of the irritable bowel. British Medical Journal 2: 653–654
Mansi C, Savarino V, Mela G S, Picciotto A, Mele M R, Celle G 1993 Are clinical patterns of dyspepsia a valid guideline for appropriate use of endoscopy? A report on 2253 dyspeptic patients. American Journal of Gastroenterology 88: 1011–1015
Maxton D G, Morris J A, Whorwell P J 1989 Ranking of symptoms by patients with the irritable bowel syndrome. British Medical Journal 299: 1138
Maxton D G, Martin D F, Whorwell P J, Godfrey M 1991 Abdominal distension in female patients with irritable bowel syndrome: exploration of possible mechanisms. Gut 32: 662–664
Mayer E A, Raybould H E 1990 Role of visceral afferent mechanisms in functional bowel disorders. Gastroenterology 99: 1688–1704
McIntyre A S, Thompson D G 1992 Review article: adrenergic control of motor and secretory function in the gastrointestinal tract. Alimentary Pharmacology and Therapeutics 6: 125–142
McKee A M, Prior A, Whorwell P J 1987 Exclusion diets in irritable bowel syndrome: are they worthwhile? Journal of Clinical Gastroenterology 9: 526–528
McRae S, Younger K, Thompson D G, Wingate D L 1982 Sustained mental stress alters human jejunal motor activity. Gut 23: 404–409
Mearin F, Cucala M, Azpiroz F, Malagelada J R 1991 The origin of symptoms on the brain–gut axis in functional dyspepsia. Gastroenterology 101: 999–1006
Mechanic D 1986 The concept of illness behavior: culture, situation and personal predisposition. Psychological Medicine 16: 1–7
Merrick M V, Eastwood M A, Ford M J 1985 Is bile acid malabsorption underdiagnosed? An evaluation of accuracy of diagnosis by measurement of SeHCAT retention. British Medical Journal 290: 665–668

Metcalf A M, Phillips S F, Zinsmeister A R, MacLarty R L, Beart R W, Wolff B G 1987 Simplified assessment of segmental colonic transit. Gastroenterology 92: 40–47
Moriarty K J, Dawson A M 1982 Functional abdominal pain: further evidence that whole gut is affected. British Medical Journal 284: 1670–1672
Morris C, Chapman R, Mayou R 1992 The outcome of unexplained dyspepsia. A questionnaire follow-up study of patients after endoscopy. Journal of Psychosomatic Research 36: 751–757
Myren J, Groth H, Larsen S E, Larsen S 1982 The effect of trimipramine in patients with the irritable bowel syndrome – a double-blind study. Scandinavian Journal of Gastroenterology 17: 871–875
Nandra R, James R, Smith H, Dudley C R K, Jewell D P 1989 Food intolerance and the irritable bowel syndrome. Gut 30: 1099–1104
Nelis G F, Vermeeren M A P, Jansen W 1990 Role of fructose-sorbitol malabsorption in the irritable bowel syndrome. Gastroenterology 99: 1016–1020
Ness T J, Metcalf A M, Gebhart G F 1990 A psychophysiological study in humans using phasic colonic distension as a noxious visceral stimulus. Pain 43: 377–386
Niederau C, Faber S, Karaus M 1992 Cholecystokinin's role in regulation of colonic motility in health and in irritable bowel syndrome. Gastroenterology 102: 1889–1898
Nyhlin H, Ford M J, Eastwood J et al 1993 Non-alimentary aspects of the irritable bowel syndrome. Journal of Psychosomatic Research 37: 155–162
Nyren O, Adami H O, Bates S et al 1986 Absence of therapeutic benefit from antacids or cimetidine in nonulcer dyspepsia. New England of Journal of Medicine 314: 339–343
Oddsson E, Rask-Madsen J, Krag E 1978 A secretory epithelium of the small intestine with increased sensitivity to bile acids in irritable bowel syndrome associated with diarrhoea. Scandinavian Journal of Gastroenterology 13: 409–416
O'Morain C, Gilvarry J 1993 Eradication of *Helicobacter pylori* in patients with non-ulcer dyspepsia. Scandinavian Journal of Gastroenterology 196 (suppl): 30–33
Painter N S 1972 Irritable or irritated bowel. British Medical Journal 2: 46
Pattee P L, Thompson W G 1992 Drug treatment of the irritable bowel syndrome. Drugs 44: 200–226
Pilowsky I 1986 Abnormal illness behaviour (dysnosognosia). Psychotherapy and Psychosomatics 46: 76–84
Pilowsky I, Barrow C G 1990 A controlled study of psychotherapy and amitriptyline used individually and in combination in the treatment of chronic, intractable, "psychogenic" pain. Pain 40: 3–19
Preston D M, Adrian T E, Christofides N D, Lennard-Jones J E, Bloom S R 1985 Positive correlation between symptoms and circulating motilin, pancreatic polypeptide and gastrin concentrations in functional bowel disorders. Gut 26: 1059–1064
Prior A, Read N W 1993 Reduction of rectal sensitivity and postprandial motility by granisetron, a 5-HT3 receptor antagonist, in patients with irritable bowel syndrome. Alimentary Pharmacology and Therapeutics 7: 175–180
Prior A, Whorwell P J 1987 Double-blind study of ispaghula in irritable bowel syndrome. Gut 28: 221–225
Prior A, Wilson K M, Whorwell P J 1988 Double-blind study of an alpha-2 agonist in the treatment of irritable bowel syndrome. Alimentary Pharmacology and Therapeutics 2: 535–539
Prior A, Wilson K, Whorwell P J, Faragher E B 1989 Irritable bowel syndrome in the gynaecological clinic – survey of 798 new referrals. Digestive Diseases and Sciences 34: 1820–1824
Prior A, Colgan S M, Whorwell P J 1990 Changes in rectal sensitivity after hypnotherapy in patients with irritable bowel syndrome. Gut 31: 896–898
Prior A, Sorial E, Sun W M, Read N W 1993 Irritable bowel syndrome: differences between patients who show rectal sensitivity and those who do not. European Journal of Gastroenterology and Hepatology 5: 343–349
Proano M, Camilleri M, Phillips S F, Brown M L, Thomforde G M 1990 Transit of solids through the human colon: regional quantification in the unprepared bowel. American Journal of Physiology 258: G856–862
Quigley E M M, Borody T J, Phillips S F, Wienbeck M, Tucker R L, Haddad A 1984 Motility of the terminal ileum and ileocecal sphincter in healthy humans. Gastroenterology 87: 857–866
Rahe R H, Floistad I, Bergan T et al 1974 A model for life changes and illness research. Archives of General Psychiatry 31: 172–177
Read N W, Khan M I 1992 Gut sensitivity in functional dyspepsia. European Journal of Gastroenterology and Hepatology 4: 622–625
Richter J E 1991 Stress and psychologic and environmental factors in functional dyspepsia. Scandinavian Journal of Gastroenterology 182 (suppl): 40–46
Ritchie J 1973 Pain from distension of the pelvic colon by inflating a balloon in the irritable bowel syndrome. Gut 14: 125–132
Rix K J B, Pearson D J, Bentley S J 1984 A psychiatric study of patients with supposed food allergy. British Journal of Psychiatry 145: 121–126
Rogers J, Raimundo A H, Misiewicz J J 1993 Cephalic phase of colonic pressure response to food. Gut 34: 537–543
Rumessen J J 1993 Functional bowel disease: the role of carbohydrates. European Journal of Gastroenterology and Hepatology 5: 999–1008
Rumessen J J, Gudmand-Hoyer E 1988 Functional bowel disease: malabsorption and abdominal distress after ingestion of fructose, sorbitol, and fructose-sorbitol mixtures. Gastroenterology 95: 694–700
Sarna S K 1991a Physiology and pathophysiology of colonic motor activity (part one of two). Digestive Diseases and Sciences 36: 827–862
Sarna S K 1991b Physiology and pathophysiology of colonic motor activity (part two of two). Digestive Diseases and Sciences 36: 998–1018
Schaffstein W, Panijel M, Luttecke K 1990 Comparative safety and efficacy of trimebutine versus mebeverine in the treatment of irritable bowel syndrome. Current Therapy Research 47: 136–145
Schwarz S P, Blanchard E B, Neff D F 1986 Behavioral treatment of irritable bowel syndrome: a 1-year follow-up study. Biofeedback and Self-Regulation 11: 189–198
Sciarretta G, Fagioli G, Furno A et al 1987 $^{75}$SeHCAT test in the detection of bile acid malabsorption in functional diarrhea and its correlation with small bowel transit. Gut 28: 970–975
Scott A M, Mihailidou A, Smith R R et al 1993a Functional gastrointestinal disorders in unselected patients with non-cardiac chest pain. Scandinavian Journal of Gastroenterology 28: 585–590
Scott A M, Kellow J E, Shuter B et al 1993b Intragastric distribution and gastric emptying of solids and liquids in functional dyspepsia. Lack of influence of symptom subgroups and *H. pylori*-associated gastritis. Digestive Diseases and Sciences 38: 2247–2254
Shaw G, Srivastava E D, Sadlier M, Swann P, James J Y, Rhodes J 1991 Stress management for the irritable bowel syndrome: a controlled trial. Digestion 50: 36–42
Sjolund K, Ekman R 1987 Are gut peptides responsible for the irritable bowel syndrome (IBS)? Scandinavian Journal of Gastroenterology 130 (suppl): 15–19
Smart H L, Nicholson D A, Atkinson M 1986a Gastro-oesophageal reflux in the irritable bowel syndrome. Gut 27: 1127–1133
Smart H L, Mayberry J F, Atkinson M 1986b Alternative medicine consultations and remedies in patients with the irritable bowel syndrome. Gut 27: 826–828
Smith R C, Greenbaum D S, Vancover J B et al 1990 Psychosocial factors are associated with health care seeking rather than diagnosis in irritable bowel syndrome. Gastroenterology 98: 293–301
Soltoft J, Gudmand-Hoyer E, Krag B, Kristensen E, Wulff H R 1976 A double-blind trial of the effect of wheat bran on symptoms of irritable bowel syndrome. Lancet 2: 270–272
Stanghellini V, Ghidini C, Maccarini M R, Paparo G F, Corinaldesi R, Barbara L 1992 Fasting and postprandial gastrointestinal motility in ulcer and non-ulcer dyspepsia. Gut 33: 184–190
Stefanini G F, Prati E, Albini M C et al 1992 Oral disodium cromoglycate treatment on irritable bowel syndrome: an open study on 101 subjects with diarrheic type. American Journal of Gastroenterology 87: 55–57
Sullivan M A, Cohen S, Snape W J 1978 Colonic myoelectrical activity in irritable-bowel syndrome: effect of eating and anticholinergics. New England Journal of Medicine 298: 878–883
Sun W M, Read N W, Prior A, Daly J, Cheah S K, Grundy D 1990

Sensory and motor responses to rectal distention vary according to rate and pattern of balloon inflation. Gastroenterology 99: 1008–1015

Svedlund J 1983 Psychotherapy in irritable bowel syndrome – a controlled outcome study. Acta Psychiatrica Scandinavica 67 (suppl 306): 1–86

Svedlund J 1992 Psychological treatment for the irritable bowel syndrome. Gastroenterology 102: 739–740

Svedlund J, Sjodin I, Ottosson J-O, Dotevall G 1983 Controlled study of psychotherapy in irritable bowel syndrome. Lancet 2: 589–591

Svendsen J H, Munck L K, Andersen J R 1985 Irritable bowel syndrome – prognosis and diagnostic safety. A 5-year follow-up study. Scandinavian Journal of Gastroenterology 20: 415–418

Swarbrick E T, Bat L, Hegarty J E, Williams C B, Dawson A M 1980 Site of pain from the irritable bowel. Lancet 2: 443–446

Symons P, Jones M P, Kellow J E 1992 Symptom provocation in irritable bowel syndrome. Effects of differing doses of fructose-sorbitol. Scandinavian Journal of Gastroenterology 27: 940–944

Tache Y, Monnikes H, Bonaz B, Rivier J 1993 Role of CRF in stress-related alterations of gastric and colonic motor function. Annals of the New York Academy of Sciences 697: 233–243

Talley N J 1991 Spectrum of chronic dyspepsia in the presence of the irritable bowel syndrome. Scandinavian Journal of Gastroenterology 182 (suppl): 7–10

Talley N J 1992 Review article: 5-hydroxytryptamine agonists and antagonists in the modulation of gastrointestinal motility and sensation: clinical implications. Alimentary Pharmacology and Therapeutics 6: 273–289

Talley N J 1994 A critique of therapeutic trials in *Helicobacter pylori*-positive functional dyspepsia. Gastroenterology 106: 1174–1183

Talley N J, McNeil D, Hayden A, Colreavy C, Piper D W 1987 Prognosis of chronic unexplained dyspepsia. A prospective study of potential predictor variables in patients with endoscopically diagnosed nonulcer dyspepsia. Gastroenterology 92: 1060–1066

Talley N J, Phillips S F, Bruce B, Twomey C K, Zinsmeister A R, Melton L J 1990 Relation among personality and symptoms in nonulcer dyspepsia and the irritable bowel syndrome. Gastroenterology 99: 327–333

Talley N J, Colin-Jones D, Koch K L, Nyren O, Stanghellini V 1991a Functional dyspepsia: a classification with guidelines for diagnosis and management. Gastroenterology International 4: 145–160

Talley N J, Phillips S F, Bruce B, Zinsmeister A R, Wiltgen C, Melton L J 1991b Multisystem complaints in patients with the irritable bowel syndrome and functional dyspepsia. European Journal of Gastroenterology and Hepatology 3: 71–77

Talley N J, O'Keefe E A, Zinsmeister A R, Melton L J 1992a Prevalence of gastrointestinal symptoms in the elderly: a population-based study. Gastroenterology 102: 895–901

Talley N J, Weaver A L, Zinsmeister A R, Melton L J 1992b Onset and disappearance of gastrointestinal symptoms and functional gastrointestinal disorders. American Journal of Epidemiology 136: 165–177

Talley N J, Zinsmeister A R, Schleck C D, Melton L J 1992c Dyspepsia and dyspepsia subgroups: a population-based study. Gastroenterology 102: 1259–1268

Talley N J, Weaver A L, Tesmer D L, Zinsmeister A R 1993 Lack of discriminant value of dyspepsia subgroups in patients referred for upper endoscopy. Gastroenterology 105: 1378–1386

Talley N J, Weaver A L, Zinsmeister A R 1994 Smoking, alcohol, and nonsteroidal anti-inflammatory drugs in outpatients with functional dyspepsia and among dyspepsia subgroups. American Journal of Gastroenterology 89: 524–528

Taylor I, Basu P, Hammond P, Darby C, Flynn M 1980 Effect of bile acid perfusion on colonic motor function in patients with the irritable bowel syndrome. Gut 21: 843–847

Thompson W G, Heaton K W 1980 Functional bowel disorders in apparently healthy people. Gastroenterology 79: 283–288

Thompson W G, Creed F, Drossman D A, Heaton K W, Mazzacca G 1992 Working team report. Functional bowel disease and functional abdominal pain. Gastroenterology International 5: 75–91

Triadafilopoulos G, Simms R W, Goldenberg D L 1991 Bowel dysfunction in fibromyalgia syndrome. Digestive Diseases and Sciences 36: 59–64

Troncon L E A, Bennett R J M, Ahluwalia N K, Thompson D G 1994 Abnormal intragastric distribution of food during gastric emptying in functional dyspepsia patients. Gut 35: 327–332

Tucci A, Corinaldesi R, Stanghellini V et al 1992 Helicobacter pylori infection and gastric function in patients with chronic idiopathic dyspepsia. Gastroenterology 103: 768–774

Tucker D M, Sandstead H H, Logan G M et al 1981 Dietary fiber and personality factors as determinants of stool output. Gastroenterology 81: 879–883

Van Wijk H J, Smout A J, Akkermans L M, Roelofs J M, ten Thije O J 1992 Gastric emptying and dyspeptic symptoms in the irritable bowel syndrome. Scandinavian Journal of Gastroenterology 27: 99–102

Waldron B, Cullen P T, Kumar R et al 1991 Evidence for hypomotility in non-ulcer dyspepsia: a prospective mutifactorial study. Gut 32: 246–251

Walker E A, Roy-Byrne P P, Katon W J 1990 Irritable bowel syndrome and psychiatric illness. American Journal of Psychiatry 147: 565–572

Walker E A, Katon W J, Roy-Byrne P P, Jemelka R P, Russo J 1993 Histories of sexual victimization in patients with irritable bowel syndrome or inflammatory bowel disease. American Journal of Psychiatry 150: 1502–1506

Waller S L, Misiewicz J J 1969 Prognosis in the irritable-bowel syndrome. A prospective study. Lancet 2: 753–756

Welch G W, Hillman L C, Pomare E W 1985 Psychoneurotic symptomatology in the irritable bowel syndrome: a study of reporters and non-reporters. British Medical Journal 291: 1382–1384

White A M, Stevens W H, Upton A R, O'Byrne P M, Collins S M 1991 Airways responsiveness to inhaled methacholine in patients with irritable bowel syndrome. Gastroenterology 100: 68–74

Whitehead W E 1985 Psychotherapy and biofeedback in the treatment of irritable bowel syndrome. In: Read N W (ed) Irritable bowel syndrome. Grune and Stratton, London, p 245–266

Whitehead W E 1992 Behavioral medicine approaches to gastrointestinal disorders. Journal of Consulting and Clinical Psychology 60: 605–612

Whitehead W E, Crowell M D 1991 Psychologic considerations in the irritable bowel syndrome. Gastroenterology Clinics of North America 20: 249–267

Whitehead W E, Schuster M M 1985 Irritable bowel syndrome: physiological and psychological mechanisms In: Gastrointestinal disorders. Behavioral and physiological basis for treatment. Academic Press, Orlando, p 179–209

Whitehead W E, Winget C, Fedoravicius A S, Wooley S, Blackwell B 1982 Learned illness behavior in patients with irritable bowel syndrome and peptic ulcer. Digestive Diseases and Sciences 27: 202–208

Whitehead W E, Bosmajian L, Zonderman A B, Costa P T, Schuster M M 1988 Symptoms of psychological distress associated with irritable bowel syndrome. Comparison of community and medical clinic samples. Gastroenterology 95: 709–714

Whitehead W E, Crowell M D, Robinson J C, Heller B R, Schuster M M 1992 Effects of stressful life events on bowel symptoms: subjects with irritable bowel syndrome compared with subjects without bowel dysfunction. Gut 33: 825–830

Whorwell P J, Clouter C, Smith C L 1981 Oesophageal motility in the irritable bowel syndrome. British Medical Journal 1: 1101–1102

Whorwell P J, Prior A, Faragher E B 1984 Controlled trial of hypnotherapy in the treatment of severe refractory irritable bowel syndrome. Lancet 2: 1232–1234

Whorwell P J, McCallum M, Creed F H, Roberts C T 1986a Noncolonic features of irritable bowel syndrome. Gut 27: 37–40

Whorwell P J, Lupton E W, Erduran D, Wilson K 1986b Bladder smooth muscle dysfunction in patients with irritable bowel syndrome. Gut 27: 1014–1017

Whorwell P J, Prior A, Colgan S M 1987 Hypnotherapy in severe irritable bowel syndrome: further experience. Gut 28: 423–425

Whorwell P J, Houghton L A, Taylor E E, Maxton D G 1992

Physiological effects of emotion: assessment via hypnosis. Lancet 340: 69–72
Williams A J K, Merrick M V, Eastwood M A 1991 Idiopathic bile acid malabsorption – a review of clinical presentation, diagnosis and response to treatment. Gut 32: 1004–1006
Wood J D 1994 Efficacy of leuprolide in treatment of the irritable bowel syndrome. Digestive Diseases and Sciences 39: 1153–1154
Young E, Stoneham M D, Petruckevitch A, Barton J, Rona R 1994 A population study of food intolerance. Lancet 343: 1127–1130

# 54. Non-neoplastic structural disease of the colon

*D. C. Carter*

## DIVERTICULAR DISEASE OF THE COLON

### Terminology

In diverticular disease, the colon acquires small outpouchings of the mucosa which herniate through its muscular wall. These occur predominantly in the sigmoid, but can be found anywhere in the colon. The early terminology defined a prediverticular state, diverticulosis and diverticulitis (Spriggs & Marxer 1925) on clinical and radiological grounds but it is now accepted that it may be impossible to determine clinically whether diverticula are uninflamed (diverticulosis) or inflamed (diverticulitis). Morson (1963) examined resection specimens from 173 patients considered to have "diverticulitis" and found that 35% had no pathological evidence of inflammation. Berman et al (1968) argue that the term "diverticulitis" is in any case incorrect since the inflammation is predominantly in the pericolic fat and not in the intestinal wall or diverticula. They use the term "peridiverticulitis" and consider that it arises from the perforation of a single diverticulum. Parks et al (1970) retrospectively examined the symptoms and complications in 461 patients; 230 were considered radiologically to have diverticulosis and 231 diverticulitis. The clinical features and complications were similar in both groups and two radiologists disagreed in their assessment of the barium enema examinations in 15 of 40 (38%) patients.

It is appropriate, therefore, to refer to the condition simply as "diverticular disease" although the terms "diverticulosis" and "diverticulitis" continue to be used widely in clinical practice. In this chapter, the terms "simple (or uncomplicated) diverticular disease" and "diverticulitis" are retained, recognizing that the distinction may be artificial and attempting to reserve the latter term for patients with evidence of local inflammation.

### Incidence

Diverticular disease is common in Western countries but rare in developing countries. In autopsy and barium enema studies, the incidence in most countries is between 5% and 10% (Painter & Burkitt 1975). Approximately one-third of individuals over the age of 60 years have diverticular disease and less than 5% of those affected are under the age of 40 (Eusebio & Eisenberg 1973, Parks 1975); females are affected more often than males. In northern Norway, 25% of males and 43% of females over the age of 20 years have diverticular disease (Eide & Stalsberg 1979) and similar high incidences have been recorded in Northern Ireland and Australia. The disease is rare in Africa, the Middle East, India, Malaysia and Singapore.

### Etiology (Manousos 1989)

The anatomy of the colon facilitates the development of diverticula because the longitudinal muscle is condensed into teniae coli and the circular muscle into fascicles in a way that leaves some areas relatively unprotected by muscle. In addition, the penetration of blood vessels provide weak spots through which mucosa can herniate, although diverticula sometimes have no relationship to vessels (Gennaro & Rosemond 1974). Furthermore, these anatomical factors are present in all colons and some additional factor must be required to produce diverticula; this is generally considered to be raised intraluminal pressure in the sigmoid colon as a result of disordered muscle activity.

#### *Dietary influences*

The disease is only common in countries where the diet is low in fiber. Painter & Burkitt (1971) have pointed out that roller-milling, introduced in 1880, removed most of the fiber from flour and that the disease became common about 40 years later. The death rate for diverticular disease in England and Wales (Fig. 54.1) has shown a steady increase (Cleave et al 1969). Conversely, diverticular disease is rare in countries in which a large amount of fiber is consumed, although its incidence may now be increasing

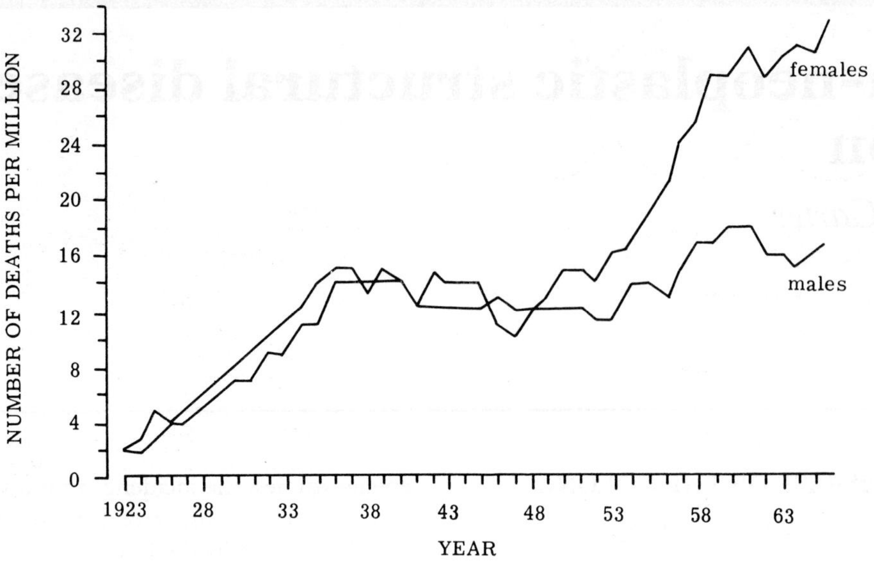


**Fig. 54.1** Crude death rates for diverticular disease: Registrar General's Statistical Review of England and Wales 1923–1966 (Cleave et al 1969).

in parts of Africa where a "Western" type diet has been adopted. The prevalence of diverticular disease increased in Japan during a period in which the consumption of dietary fiber declined (Ohi et al 1983). Diet is further incriminated by the high incidence of diverticular disease in Japanese born in Hawaii compared to the very low incidence in Japan. Furthermore, studies in the UK have shown that diverticular disease is much less frequent in vegetarians, who consume more fiber than nonvegetarians (Gear et al 1979) and a case-control study in Athens showed that patients with the disease consumed significantly less vegetables, brown bread, potatoes and fruit and consumed more meat and milk products (Manousos et al 1985).

Mendeloff (1976) has suggested that the high incidence of diverticular disease in Western societies could relate in part to long life expectancy and to as yet undefined dietary differences. Analysis of changing dietary habits is difficult. For example, the main sources of dietary fiber in the UK have changed in that the relative contribution from cereal has fallen yet overall there may have been little change in total fiber content over the past 100 years (Robertson 1972). However, cereal fiber is probably the most important component of dietary fiber which protects against diverticular disease (Gear et al 1979).

*Colonic intraluminal pressures*

Painter & Truelove (1964) showed that intraluminal pressures in the normal colon and in colons with diverticular disease were similar under basal conditions, but that morphine and neostigmine produced much greater increases in diverticular disease. Morphine increased pressure to 20–40 mmHg in normal subjects, whereas pressures commonly exceeded 50 mmHg in diverticular disease. Subsequent studies employing simultaneous cineradiology and intraluminal pressure measurement showed that pressures in diverticular disease were not high throughout the colon but in localized areas only (Painter et al 1965). Segmentation was responsible for producing localized pressure increases. This process allows the normal colon to move its contents proximally or distally by forming contraction rings (Fig. 54.2). The colon thus functions as a series of "bladders", in which contents are squeezed from one "bladder" to another, rather than as a uniform tube. The formation of two powerful contraction rings occludes a segment of colonic lumen and this, combined with contraction of the muscle between the two rings, generates high intraluminal pressure which could produce diverticula. Those who consider that a low-fiber diet favors formation of diverticula contend that the resulting small fecal volume reduces the diameter of the colonic lumen; under these circumstances, intraluminal pressures increase greatly during segmentation. Conversely, a high-fiber diet produces a high fecal volume which is said to increase the diameter of the colonic lumen and decrease intraluminal pressure (Painter & Burkitt 1971).

It remains an open question whether the ability to generate areas of high intraluminal pressure eventually leads to diverticula. Weinreich & Andersen (1976) suggested that the increased colonic pressure is a chance association. They found an excessive pressure response to neostigmine in patients with a history of lower abdominal colic, irrespective of the presence of diverticular disease, and no such response in patients with asymptomatic diverticular disease.

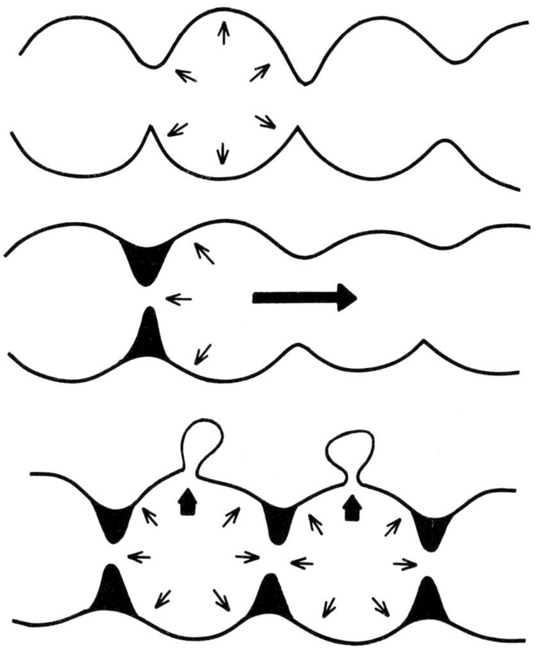

**Fig. 54.2** Segmentation of colon. Contraction rings of thickened circular muscle cause pressure forces which are dissipated either via the unoccluded bowel lumen or by forming diverticula at the point of weakness where arteries pierce the circular muscle layer (Berman & Kirsner 1972).

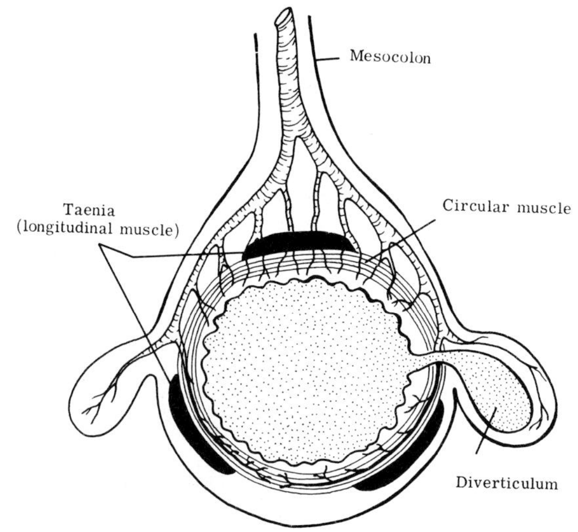


**Fig. 54.3** The human colon in diverticulosis. The colonic wall is weak between the teniae. The blood vessels that supply the colon pierce the circular muscle and weaken it further by forming tunnels. Diverticula usually emerge through these points of least resistance (Painter 1973).

*Muscular abnormalities*

Pathological changes in the muscle of the sigmoid colon (see below) suggest that muscle dysfunction could be the main etiological factor. A primary disorder of the longitudinal muscle would explain the shortening of the sigmoid colon which is often an early feature of the disease. Indeed, muscle thickening without diverticula is found in a few patients undergoing resection for "diverticular disease".

*Relationship to the irritable bowel syndrome*

This relationship is controversial. In both diseases, motility responses in the sigmoid colon are abnormal and the clinical and radiological features of early diverticular disease and spastic colon can be indistinguishable. Fleischner (1971) divided early diverticular disease into two forms, "simple massed diverticulosis" and "spastic colon diverticulosis". In simple massed diverticulosis, there are many diverticula in the descending and sigmoid colon and these areas are shortened and narrow. Fleischner speculated that this type may result from the painless diarrhea variant of the irritable bowel syndrome (p. 437). In spastic colon diverticulosis, the changes are mainly confined to the pelvic colon and consist of marked narrowing with a serrated bowel contour; diverticula are sparse. Williams (1967b) has described this as "diverticular disease without diverticula". Pathological examination shows that the radiological features in these cases are due to shortening of the teniae and thickening of the circular muscle. Fleischner suggested that the spastic colon (p. 1357) is the precursor of spastic colon diverticulosis. Fleischner's classification is seldom used and long-term follow-up of patients with irritable bowel syndrome has so far failed to demonstrate an association with diverticular disease (Parks 1975).

## Pathology

The herniation of mucosa through the muscle wall (Figs 54.3, 54.4) may be reducible at first, but later becomes fixed and the diverticulum loses its thin covering of muscle fibers. On histological examination, the initial reducible stage may be represented by a leash of blood vessels and fibrous tissue passing through the circular muscle (Arfwidsson 1964). In the pelvic, transverse and descending colon, the diverticula appear between the mesenteric and antimesenteric teniae, but small diverticula can be found between the antimesenteric teniae. Diverticula protruding into appendices epiploicae may not be readily apparent on inspection at operation. In the ascending colon, diverticula tend to develop along the branches of the main blood vessels.

The pelvic colon is by far the commonest site involved (Fig. 54.5). Laplace's law states that tension in the wall of a hollow cylinder is inversely proportional to its radius multiplied by the pressure within it; the importance of radius may mean that pulsion diverticula are most likely to form in the sigmoid colon with its relatively narrow lumen. Other sites are almost always involved in association with the sigmoid colon. The incidence of cecal involvement

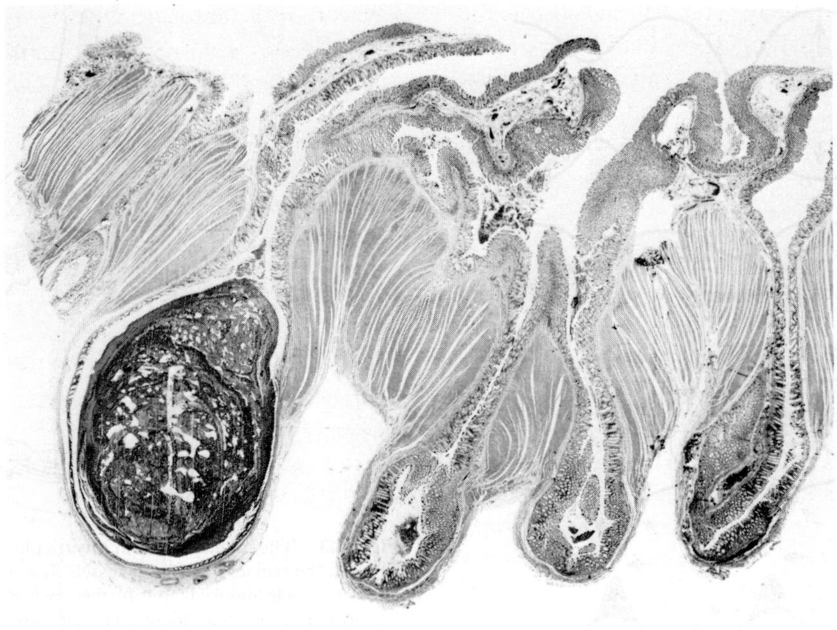

**Fig. 54.4** Diverticular disease of the colon. Several narrow-necked, mucosal-lined diverticula pass through the muscle. The fasciculation of the muscle is striking and the overlying mucosa is thrown into folds (hematoxylin and eosin, ×4).

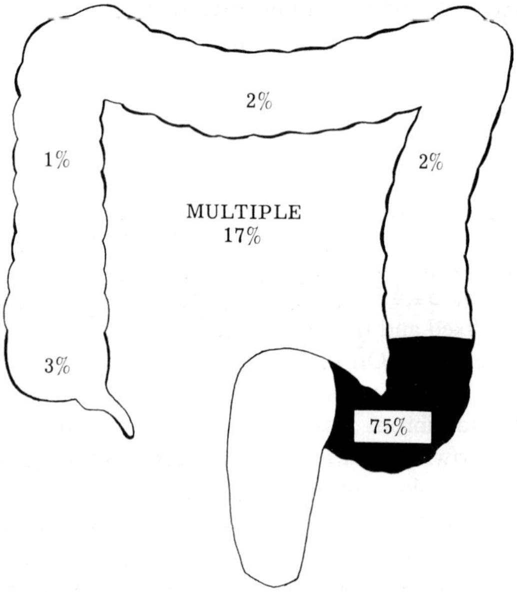


**Fig. 54.5** Areas of colonic involvement in diverticular disease in 374 patients (Zollinger 1968).

varies from 5% (Williams 1960) to as high as 25% (Hughes 1969) in other series and is discussed separately (p. 1392). The rectum is never involved.

*The muscle abnormality* (Morson 1975)

Hughes (1969) defined the muscle changes as shortening and thickening of the teniae, localized thickening of the circular muscle to form bands and, in some cases, uniform thickening of the circular muscle. There is no histological abnormality of the muscle itself, but Hughes believed that it was in a state of "spasm", which can be relaxed at autopsy by perfusing the specimen with propantheline. The mouths of diverticula lie between the bands of circular muscle. It has been maintained that all of the abnormal features in the wall of the sigmoid colon, including the redundant folds of mucosa which add to the narrowing, are due to shortening (Williams 1967b). In fact, the sigmoid colon in diverticular disease is thickened and firm owing to an increase of elastic tissue in the teniae coli which leads to shortening or "contracture" (Whiteway & Morson 1985).

*"Diverticulitis"*

Originally, it was thought that closure of a diverticulum by spasm or inflammation resulted in further inflammation with the possibility of abscess formation, ulceration and perforation. It is now thought that microperforations of diverticula occur during episodes of raised intracolonic pressure (Fleischner & Ming 1965) or that localized inflammation at the apices of diverticula results from abrasion by inspissated fecal material, leading to inflammation in the lymphoid tissue at the apices and then to perforation. In any event, there may be free perforation into the peritoneal cavity or, more usually, there is localized inflammation when perforation has been gradual. Local perforation can cause a pericolic abscess consisting of pus, necrotic tissue and foreign body giant cells and fistula formation may involve the small intestine, bladder or vagina. Extensive localized perforation can result in longitudinal spread of inflammation along the outer aspect of the muscle layer; this causes extramural fibrosis which leads to further narrowing and irregularity of the colon.

*Bleeding*

The pathological findings are discussed on page 1388.

## Clinical features of diverticular disease

Diverticular disease of the colon is common but often remains asymptomatic or causes only insignificant symptoms. Frequent complaints are intermittent pain in the left iliac fossa or suprapubic region and intermittent constipation. The sigmoid colon can be tender to palpation, but in uncomplicated diverticular disease there is no fever or leukocytosis. Minor rectal bleeding or a positive fecal occult blood test are very uncommon (Kewenter et al 1985) and should raise the suspicion of carcinoma. Barium enema in uncomplicated disease demonstrates diverticula with spasm and narrowing of the pelvic colon. Although the symptoms can lead to a diagnosis of "diverticulitis", the resected pelvic colon frequently shows no evidence of inflammation. Symptomatic simple diverticular disease may be difficult to distinguish from the irritable bowel syndrome. Patients with the former often localize pain to the left iliac fossa, while the latter produces generalized abdominal discomfort (Colcock 1971).

Over half the patients admitted with diverticular disease have had symptoms for less than a month (Parks 1969a, MacGregor et al 1970). The main complaints are of abdominal pain and altered bowel habit. In one series, abdominal pain was the presenting feature in 71% of cases and constipation and/or diarrhea occurred in 45% (Zollinger 1968). Nausea, vomiting and fever may be present and occasionally there are urinary symptoms, rectal bleeding, abdominal distention or an abdominal mass.

Parks (1969b) analyzed the pattern of abdominal pain in 521 patients. Pain was most common across the lower abdomen but was often more acute on the left side. Another frequent pattern was pain localized to the left lower quadrant, sometimes spreading to the left upper quadrant. Less frequently, pain was experienced centrally, on the right or even in the epigastrium. "Cramping" pain was more likely to be distributed across the abdomen, while "aching" pain was often more localized. Pain in the lower back is an occasional finding (Botsford & Zollinger 1969). Altered bowel habit takes the form of constant or intermittent constipation or intermittent diarrhea. Alternating constipation and diarrhea are less common and continuous diarrhea is rare. Misdiagnosis is particularly common in patients under 40 years of age despite a similar spectrum of symptoms (Eusebio & Eisenberg 1973) and this reflects the misconception that diverticular disease does not affect younger patients. Immunocompromised patients with severe acute diverticulitis often present with minimal or absent symptoms and few physical findings (Perkins et al 1984).

Complications other than bleeding occur in about one in four patients (Zollinger 1968, Parks 1969b). In a 10-year retrospective study of 673 patients attending hospital with diverticular disease, 14% required operation; the indications were abscess (36 cases), bleeding (18), perforation (10), obstruction (10), suspicion of coexistent carcinoma (8), recurrent symptoms (7) and fistula (5) (Alexander et al 1983). Systemic complications such as arthritis and pyoderma gangrenosum are described in diverticulitis (Klein et al 1988).

The main physical findings in diverticulitis are abdominal tenderness, a painful mass and distention. The sigmoid colon is usually palpable and often thickened. Tenderness and pain are most marked in the left lower quadrant or suprapubic region but can occur in the right lower quadrant. Even gentle palpation of a mass can cause pain and guarding. Parks (1969b) found a mass on abdominal or rectal examination in 20% of patients. Abdominal distention is generalized and is due to obstruction in the sigmoid colon. Fever is common.

## Investigation of diverticular disease

*Blood count and urinalysis*

A leukocytosis may be present although 64% of 130 patients with acute complications of diverticular disease at operation had a white count in the range $5-12 \times 10^9$/L (Hackford et al 1985). If inflammation involves the left ureter or bladder the urine may contain a few red blood cells. Urine culture is indicated if there are urinary symptoms.

*Sigmoidoscopy*

Sigmoidoscopy is carried out to exclude carcinoma of the rectum unless the clinical presentation suggests that complications such as perforation are present. The procedure may cause discomfort. The mucosa of the rectosigmoid may be edematous, but the mouths of diverticula are rarely seen unless fiberoptic sigmoidoscopy is performed, when they are readily visible in association with prominent haustral folds.

*Radiology*

***Plain films and contrast radiology.*** Plain abdominal radiographs are rarely helpful in uncomplicated disease and barium enema is the mainstay of diagnosis (see below). The early radiological features in what Spriggs & Marxer (1925) termed "prediverticular disease" are due to

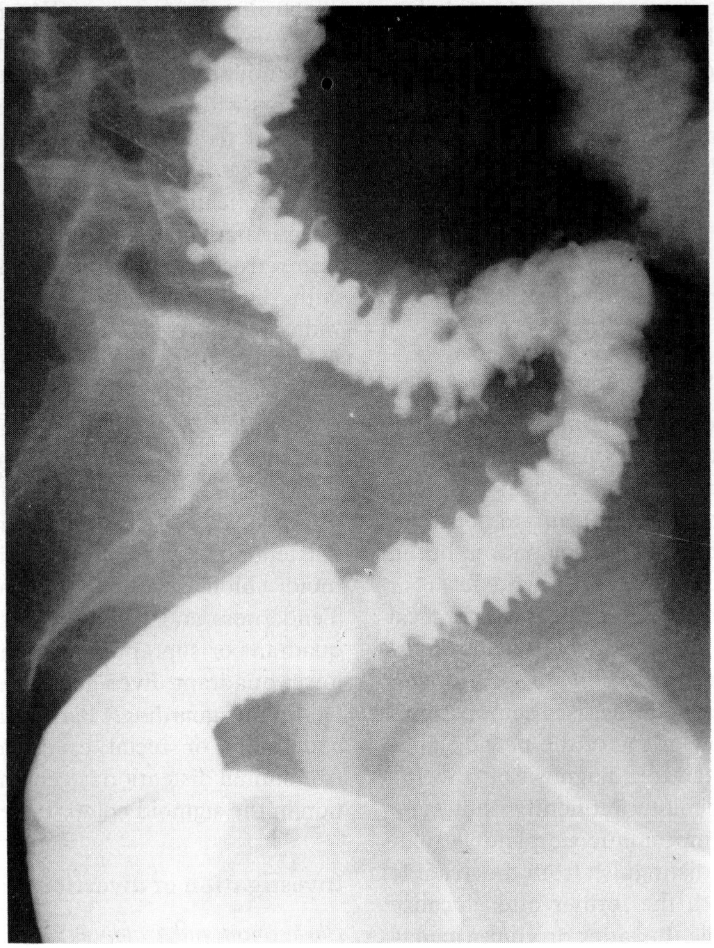

**Fig. 54.6** Diverticular disease of sigmoid colon. The uniformly disposed transverse bars due to thickened circular muscle are clearly demonstrated. The diverticula arise between these bars.

hypertrophy and shortening of the circular muscle in the pelvic colon and much depends on the degree of contraction and the angles from which radiographs are taken (Williams 1967b). Terms such as "palisades", "smooth palisades", "saw-tooth" have been used to describe the appearances of the contour (Fig. 54.6). Unilateral palisades are produced if the infoldings on the walls between the mesenteric and antimesenteric teniae extend slightly into the antimesenteric wall. A lateral radiograph often demonstrates a unilateral palisade opposite the mesenteric attachment. In other cases, close circumferential folds reminiscent of small intestinal folds are seen; they are due to circular folds of mucosa and result from shortening of the sigmoid colon. These changes are evidence of diverticular disease even in the absence of diverticula.

Diverticula may fill with barium. The projection used is important since most diverticula occur between the mesenteric and antimesenteric teniae. Two radiographs taken at right angles can reveal diverticula otherwise hidden by a barium-filled colon. The ease with which barium enters diverticula depends on the degree of contraction of the colonic wall and on whether they are filled with feces. Initially, only "prediverticular" disease of the sigmoid colon may be seen, but radiographs taken a few minutes later will often show diverticula. The openings in the diverticula may be occluded by edema secondary to inflammation and this is illustrated by the apparent disappearance of diverticula in patients who develop ulcerative colitis (Beranbaum & Ring 1968).

The radiological investigation of patients who present clinically with acute diverticulitis deserves special consideration and has been reviewed recently by McKee et al (1993). Abnormalities such as pneumoperitoneum, ileus, complete or partial obstruction or a soft tissue mass are found on abdominal films in 30–50% of such cases but are not specific to diverticular disease. The erect chest X-ray detects coincidental cardiorespiratory disease in up to one-third of patients and detects a pneumoperitoneum in 3–12% of cases of acute diverticulitis. Lateral decubitus films may detect free air if erect films are impractical.

Contrast enema is contraindicated in patients with pneumoperitoneum, those who are hemodynamically unstable and when a deep rectal biopsy has been taken in the preceding 7 days. In other cases, a water-soluble agent such as Gastrografin should be used for contrast enemas during the acute phase (1–7 days) if the clinical diagnosis is in doubt (Simpkins 1984), although the mucosal detail is inferior to that provided by barium. Water-soluble contrast is hyperosmolar and fluid shift into the bowel can compound hypovolemia, although this is seldom a problem in practice in patients receiving adequate resuscitation. The value of contrast radiology is underlined by a recent report in which the clinical diagnosis of diverticular disease was sustained in only 49% of 53 cases after a water-soluble contrast enema (Hiltunen et al 1991). Double-contrast enemas are best avoided in acute diverticulitis.

If the acute attack has subsided, double-contrast barium enema and sigmoidoscopy are advisable to confirm the clinical diagnosis and exclude an underlying or associated carcinoma. It is usually safe to perform a barium enema after 7–14 days of treatment for diverticulitis. Some claim that a conventional enema is safer (Marshak et al 1979), while others believe that double-contrast enema is superior. Whichever technique is adopted, discomfort can be reduced by intravenous antispasmodics such as glucagon (0.5–1 mg) and the abolition of colonic muscle spasm may improve the radiological definition.

The characteristic signs of diverticulitis include a smooth, well-demarcated mass in the colonic wall, an extrinsic impression with distortion of the associated diverticula usually in the sigmoid region, filling of a sinus tract or abscess cavity (Fig. 54.7) and fixed narrowing due to fibrosis (Fleischner 1971). "Double tracking" may be produced if contrast extends longitudinally in the submucosal or subserosal space. Demonstration of diverticula does not necessarily indicate that the patient has complicated diverticulitis; conversely, gross inflammation of the colon may not produce radiological evidence of inflammatory change. Care has to be taken if there is an irregular constricting lesion as both carcinoma and diverticulitis can produce this appearance and error rates of 23% have been recorded when the radiological diagnosis was compared to the final histological diagnosis (Schynder et al 1979). Signs favoring diverticulitis in this context are listed in Table 54.1.

Paracolic abscesses are frequently caused by diverticulitis. Chennells & Simpkins (1981) described five features on double-contrast enema, although it must be emphasized that single water-soluble contrast studies are now preferred in this context. The signs are a soft-tissue mass; extraluminal gas collection; barium-filled cavity; displacement, impression or narrowing of the lumen; and changes in the mucosal pattern. The commonest feature, seen in 95% of cases, was displacement, impression or narrowing of the lumen. A localized perforation often appears as a shallow mound projecting into the lumen (Fleischner 1971). Occasionally, an abscess cavity fistulates to the small intestine (Fig. 54.8), bladder or vagina. Abscesses

**Table 54.1** Radiological features distinguishing diverticular disease from carcinoma of the colon (Rowe & Kollmar 1952, McKee et al 1993)

| |
|---|
| *Diverticular disease* |
| Spastic bowel with 'saw-tooth' appearance |
| Funnel-shaped rather than shouldered margins to the narrow areas |
| Long segments of involved bowel (Fig. 54.9) |
| Preservation of mucosal folds |
| Change in size of the constricted area between examinations |
| Presence of diverticula |
| Relief of spasm by glucagon |
| *Carcinoma* |
| Bowel adjacent to tumor mass is normal |
| Margins of the lesion are sharply defined or shouldered |
| Short segments of involved bowel |
| Destruction of mucosal folds |
| Tendency to increasing obstruction between examinations |
| Absence of diverticula |
| No relief of spasm by glucagon |

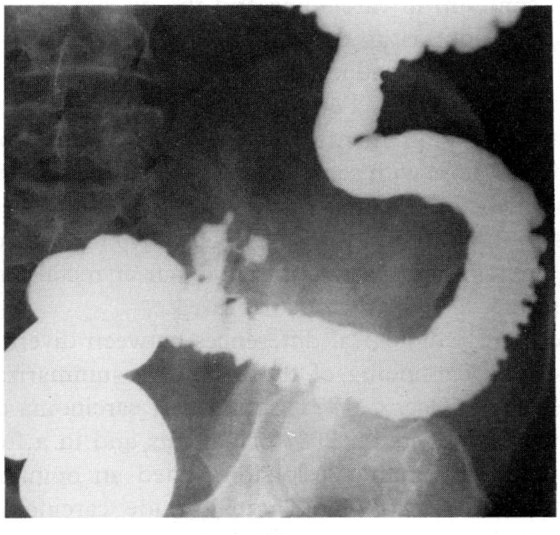

**Fig. 54.7** Short segment of diverticulitis in upper pelvic colon with communication with an abscess cavity.

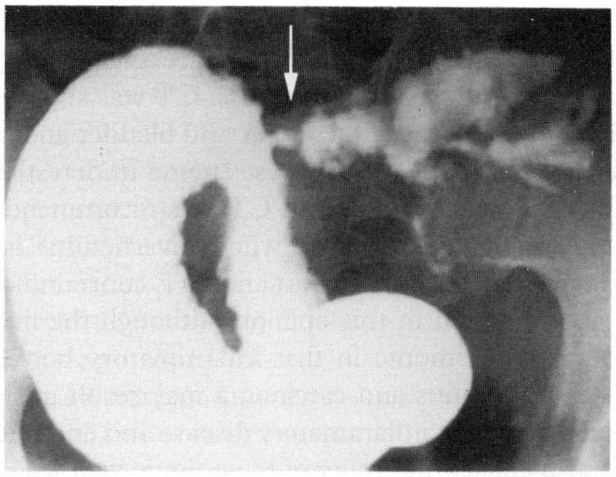

**Fig. 54.8** Short segment of diverticulitis with fistula (arrow) to ileum.

**Table 54.2** Radiological features distinguishing Crohn's colitis from diverticulitis (Marshak et al 1979)

| |
|---|
| *Diverticulitis* |
| Lesion usually short (3–6 cm); usually in sigmoid |
| Diverticula sharply defined; often contain a fecolith |
| Abscess has intramural defect or arcuate configuration of stretched folds |
| No transverse fissures |
| Short pericolonic sinus tract |
| Mucosa normal |
| *Crohn's disease* |
| Lesion usually long (10 cm or more); anywhere in colon |
| Abscess triangular with cap-like configuration; does not contain a fecolith |
| Folds thickened and edematous; increased secretions present |
| Transverse fissures and mucosal edema |
| Long sinus tract which may be intramural or pericolonic |
| Mucosal ulcerations or cobblestoning |

resulting from the perforation of several diverticula can communicate with one another to form a long abscess channel, which results in spasm, irritability, shortening, narrowing, rigidity, distortion and thickening of the folds (Marshak et al 1979). Luminal narrowing is common and fibrosis may produce stenosis. Crohn's disease may be difficult to distinguish from diverticular disease in that both may produce narrowing, fistula and abscess (Table 54.2).

***Ultrasonography*** (McKee et al 1993). Ultrasonography may reveal thickening of the bowel wall, diverticula and abscess cavities and serial scans can be used to monitor resolution. However, bowel wall thickening is far from specific to diverticulitis and in one prospective study, ultrasonography had a sensitivity of 85% and specificity of 80% when compared to the final diagnosis made on contrast radiology or surgical exploration (Verbanck et al 1989).

***Computed tomography*** (Lieberman & Haaga 1983, Hulnick et al 1984). This investigation may be valuable in the assessment of acute diverticulitis and abscess formation. Hulnick et al (1984) studied 43 patients with colonic diverticulitis, 37 of whom also had a contrast enema. Computed tomography showed inflammatory changes in the pericolic fat in 98%, diverticula in 84%, colonic thickening in 70%, pericolic abscess in 35%, peritonitis in 16%, fistula in 14%, colonic obstruction in 12% and intramural sinus tracts in 9%. A distant abscess was revealed in 12% and ureteric obstruction in 7%. CT was superior for revealing involvement of the ureter and bladder and showing distant abscesses and contrast enema underestimated pericolic inflammation in 41%. CT was recommended as the initial imaging procedure when diverticulitis is suspected, especially when contrast enema is contraindicated. Other reports confirm this opinion, although the findings are not pathognomonic in that inflammatory bowel disease, ischemic colitis and carcinoma may result in similar CT findings. Pelvic inflammatory disease and endometriosis can also cause thickening of the colonic wall with pericolic inflammation. Computed tomography and contrast radiology are best regarded as complementary techniques in the evaluation of acute diverticulitis and even when the diagnosis seems certain on CT, subsequent barium enema is still advisable to exclude carcinoma.

*Colonoscopy*

Colonoscopy can be difficult in diverticular disease and there is some danger that the instrument will enter and perforate a diverticulum. The main indication is the need to investigate suspicious areas seen on barium enema. Indeed, barium enema frequently misses cancer when diverticula are present and there is a case for colonoscopy in all patients with sigmoid diverticular disease, particularly in those over the age of 60 years who have evidence of rectal bleeding. Boulos et al (1984, 1985) found cancer on colonoscopy in seven of 105 patients with symptomatic diverticular disease. Radiologically suspicious areas can be visualized in at least 75% of cases (Glerum et al 1977, Max & Knutson 1978, Forde et al 1980) and it may be possible to avoid laparotomy in elderly patients with intercurrent disease. Colonoscopy is also indicated in diverticular disease when there is occult or intermittent bleeding. Its value in patients with overt bleeding falls when bleeding is massive and other methods for identifying the site of bleeding are recommended (p. 27).

## Differential diagnosis

The main problem is the distinction from carcinoma of the colon, although there is occasional difficulty with other diseases, notably Crohn's disease. Diverticular disease and carcinoma of the colon coexisted in 0.4–8.4% of cases in various series (Speer & Bacon 1962) and although their symptoms are similar, there are differences in emphasis. Pain is much less common in carcinoma, but bleeding is more common, tending to be constant and slight. Weight loss is common in carcinoma and the disease progresses steadily, in contrast to the intermittent attacks of diverticular disease. Fever and leukocytosis are uncommon in carcinoma of the colon. Perforation with abscess formation occurs in 40% of patients with diverticular disease but in only 3% of those with carcinoma (p. 1424). Finally, fistula formation occurs in a third of patients with diverticular disease but is rare in cancer (Colcock 1971). Both conditions may cause a mass, but abdominal or rectal tenderness is more likely in diverticular disease.

The main radiological differences between diverticular disease and carcinoma of the colon are summarized in Table 54.1. Colcock (1971) found that carcinoma could not be excluded in 15–20% of patients and in a further 5–10% an obstructing lesion precluded an opinion. In some patients, it is possible to exclude carcinoma by repeating the examination after 2 or 3 weeks of conservative management. Parks et al (1970) found difficulty excluding carcinoma in only 6% of 461 patients. Colonoscopy is definitely indicated in such cases.

Difficulty in diagnosis may affect the prognosis of carcinoma, in that the 5-year survival rate for colon cancer with coexisting diverticulitis was 39%, compared to 53% for cancer of the colon without diverticulitis (Mayo & Delaney 1956).

Crohn's disease localized to the sigmoid region is uncommon, but when it does occur it can be difficult to distinguish from diverticular disease. The distinguishing radiological features are shown in Table 54.2.

## Natural history and prognosis

Analyses of the natural history of diverticular disease are often biased because they deal only with patients referred to hospital. In two large series of hospitalized patients, follow-up for 5 years or more showed that approximately one-third had undergone surgery, one-third were alive and well and one-third were alive but symptomatic (Table 54.3). In some patients the disease is progressive in that more diverticula appear, but prognosis is related mainly to the development of complications rather than the extent of the disease and number of diverticula. It has been estimated that peridiverticular inflammation develops in 10% of patients within 5 years and in 25% within 10 years. In Parks' series (1975), 50% of all patients were in good health until less than 1 month prior to hospital admission and many of the deaths in these patients were due to free perforation. Adhesions may localize a perforation in more chronic cases.

The disease is recurrent; Colcock (1958) estimated that 45% of patients who had one attack would have a recurrence. Symptoms may even recur or continue in patients treated surgically; these symptoms were mild in 20% and severe in 2% of patients in one series (Parks 1969a).

In a UK audit of 300 patients with complicated diverticular disease, complications present on admission were acute phlegmon in 104 cases, pericolic abscess in 34, purulent peritonitis in 40, large bowel obstruction in 31, fecal peritonitis in 23, pericolic abscess complicated by fistula in 28 and bleeding in 40 (Tudor et al 1994). The overall mortality rate was 11.3%. Review of 120 of these patients 5 years later found that 10 had died from recurrent complicated diverticular disease, 29 had died from other disorders and 81 remained alive (Farmakis et al 1994). Excluding those who had died from recurrent complications, 36% of patients were still symptomatic at the time of follow-up or death from unrelated causes. Of the 77 patients initially managed by sigmoid colectomy, only two developed recurrent complications as opposed to 37 of the 43 managed conservatively during their index admission.

**Table 54.3** Features of the natural history of diverticular disease in patients admitted to hospital and then followed up for 5 or more years

| | Parks (1969a) | Zollinger (1968) |
|---|---|---|
| Number of patients | 455 | 374 |
| Initial surgical treatment | 35% | 21% |
| Initial medical treatment | | |
| Alive and well | 41% | 30% |
| Alive but symptomatic | 29% | 35% |
| Died from diverticular disease | 2% | 2% |
| Subsequent surgery | 6% | 4% |

## Treatment

### *Uncomplicated diverticular disease*

Painter et al (1972) studied 70 unselected patients with diverticular disease who were advised to eat highbran cereals, wholemeal bread, fruit and vegetables and reduce their refined sugar intake. Two teaspoons (12–14 g) of unprocessed bran were given three times a day and the dose was increased until one or two normal bowel movements were obtained daily. The patients were followed for an average of 22 months; 62 (89%) obtained relief of symptoms and their bowel habit was restored to normal. Other studies with bran and bulking agents have been reviewed by Dwyer et al (1978) and Thompson & Patel (1986) and the symptomatic relief obtained from a high-fiber diet has been confirmed in a double-blind controlled trial (Brodribb 1977), although this view has been contested (Ornstein et al 1981). It is thought that bran increases the bulk of the stool, which in turn reduces pressures within the sigmoid colon. Bran should also be advised after surgery for diverticular disease.

Antispasmodics such as dicyclomine or propantheline are often prescribed in an attempt to reduce pain and discomfort due to muscle activity, although objective evidence of benefit is lacking. These agents do not cause constipation provided a high-roughage diet is given. Patients should be told not to take laxatives for constipation. Most patients respond to these measures. At one time, surgery was reserved for the treatment of complicated diverticular disease, but there is now growing acceptance that elective surgery can be beneficial in some patients with persistent symptoms (see below).

### *Diverticulitis and complicated diverticular disease*

Patients with diverticulitis and its complications should be admitted to hospital. If the attack is accompanied by nausea and vomiting or abdominal distention, nasogastric suction is instituted and fluid and electrolytes are given intravenously. When these symptoms are absent, nasogastric suction is unnecessary and oral fluids may be given. A broad-spectrum antibiotic such as ampicillin or amoxycillin should be given for 10 days in conjunction with metronidazole. Improvement is manifested by a reduction in leukocytosis and fever and a reduction in the size of any abdominal mass and abdominal tenderness. Improvement can be accompanied by the gradual reintroduction of food. Moderate pain is often relieved by aspirin; severe pain may require pethidine. Deterioration or failure to improve necessitates surgery (below). Barium enema examinations are inadvisable during the acute phase, but water-soluble contrast enemas and computed tomography may be helpful (p. 1386). Even when the acute symptoms have subsided, the barium enema examination should be performed with care.

*Elective surgery*

The decision to recommend elective surgery should take into account the balance between its risks and the danger to life if complications develop during further exacerbations. Only 4–10% of all hospitalized patients treated conservatively during their index admission require subsequent surgery (Zollinger 1968, Parks 1969a, MacGregor et al 1970) and it is conceivable that fibrosis limits the severity of later attacks. Factors influencing the decision are the number and severity of previous attacks of diverticulitis, persistent symptoms and inability to exclude carcinoma (Botsford & Zollinger 1969, Moreaux & Vons 1990). It is often difficult to be certain that persisting symptoms are indeed due to diverticular disease, although colonoscopy has helped to reduce uncertainty about the presence of cancer. Fistulae and suspicion of residual abscess may be additional indications for elective surgery. Transplant patients and others receiving immunosuppressive agents or steroids are at particular risk of developing colonic complications, notably free perforation, and the threshold for elective surgery should be lower in such cases.

***Sigmoid myotomy and its variants.*** (Reilly & Smith 1975, Pescatori & Castiglioni 1978). These procedures were once used in patients with symptomatic but uncomplicated diverticular disease who had failed to respond to medical therapy. The aim of the operation was to reduce intraluminal pressure. In sigmoid myotomy, a longitudinal incision was made through the thickened muscle while in transverse tenia myotomy, multiple transverse incisions were made in the antimesenteric teniae. These operations carried significant morbidity because of perforation of the mucosa and high colonic pressures frequently remained or returned after operation. Daniel (1969a,b) reported perforation in no fewer than 18 of his 30 cases, while Smith et al (1969) reported major abdominal sepsis in three of their 14 cases, with two operative deaths. Sigmoid myotomy and its variants are no longer recommended.

***Primary resection and anastomosis.*** Whereas staged resections were once popular, it is now usually possible to resect the sigmoid colon with immediate end-to-end anastomosis. The main postoperative complication is leakage from the suture line, although given good preoperative bowel preparation, skilled surgery and prophylactic perioperative antibiotics, this is infrequent and mortality rates are low. For example, in a personal series of 156 patients, mostly treated by one-stage operation, Goligher (1984) reported only three deaths due to "medical" causes. More recently, Moreaux & Vons (1990) carried out colonic resection with primary anastomosis in 95% of their 177 patients undergoing elective surgery for diverticular disease (including some with a coexisting extracolonic abscess). There were no postoperative deaths and none of the patients developed clinical evidence of anastomotic leakage. Key technical points were the use of inflammation-free bowel for anastomosis, avoidance of dead space in the pelvis by omental packing and avoidance of transverse colostomy and abdominal drains.

Most surgeons now practice one-stage resection but would not hesitate to exteriorize the bowel ends or perform a Hartmann procedure (see below) if there was gross intraperitoneal sepsis or reservations about the quality of the anastomosis. Generalized debility and age are not in themselves indications for staged resection; elderly patients withstand repeated operations badly and may be best served by primary resection with immediate anastomosis. Inability to prepare the bowel adequately before surgery can now be overcome by on-table intraoperative bowel irrigation (Koruth et al 1985).

## Complications of diverticulitis

*Hemorrhage*

The incidence of this complication varies from 5% to 41% in hospital series (Rigg & Ewing 1966), with an overall incidence of 15% and an incidence of serious bleeding of 3–5% (Zollinger 1968, McGuire & Haynes 1972). McGuire & Haynes (1972) defined serious bleeding as that requiring transfusion because of shock or a fall in the hemoglobin concentration of more than 3 g/dl. Diverticular disease is one of the commonest causes of lower intestinal bleeding in patients over the age of 65 years (Boley et al 1979a).

***Pathology*** (Meyers et al 1976). Bleeding from colonic diverticula is typically acute and massive and may be more commonly right-sided than left-sided. The bleeding is arterial, coming from the vasa recta which lie alongside the diverticula as they emerge at the weak points created where the arteries penetrate the muscle. The ruptured vessels show adjacent intimal thickening, reduplication of the elastic lamina and muscle thinning suggesting an underlying vascular weakness. Bleeding may also arise from granulation tissue at the neck or base of the diverticulum (Hughes 1975). Less commonly, there may be bleeding from a diverticular mass (Salvati et al 1967) or from a diverticulum which becomes inverted or congested. Bleeding can also occur from small vascular mucosal lesions (angiodysplasia) in the cecum or ascending colon (Pounder et al 1982) (p. 495), lesions which can be associated with diverticula (BMJ 1980).

***Clinical features.*** Bleeding tends to occur in older hypertensive patients. Heald & Ray (1971) contrasted a "bleeding group" with a "diverticulitis group". Patients in the latter were admitted because of other symptoms of diverticular disease, while those with bleeding were on average about 10 years older, had a higher diastolic blood pressure and had few symptoms prior to the episode. A previous history of severe pain is rare, as are fever and abdominal tenderness. The paucity of symptoms may reflect the fact that many are bleeding from vascular mucosal lesions (p. 495) rather than diverticular disease.

Bleeding usually starts with a sudden call to stool and the passage of a large quantity of bright or dark red blood, sometimes with clots. The patient feels faint, but shock is rare. There may be a little colic or distention but no marked pain (Heald & Ray 1971). Occasionally, there may be slight intermittent bleeding prior to a major episode. After the major episode, intermittent bleeding for a few days is common with passage of decreasing amounts of altered blood, although as many as one-third of patients may require intervention. A minority of patients suffer recurrence months or years later and frequent recurrence can lead to severe anemia.

The differential diagnosis of bleeding from the lower gastrointestinal tract is discussed on page 494. It should be remembered that duodenal ulceration is the most common cause of severe bleeding per rectum and on occasions the blood may be red; under these circumstances the gastric aspirate contains blood and the patient is shocked to a degree which would be unexpected with a similar rectal blood loss in diverticular disease.

***Conservative management.*** Most patients are elderly and have vascular disease so that a conservative policy is indicated. Transfusion requirements are less than 1 liter in two-thirds of cases and in over half the bleeding stops on arrival at hospital or within the first day (McGuire & Haynes 1972). Up to 30% of patients bleed again in hospital (Taylor & Epstein 1969) and operation for massive or continuous bleeding was necessary in 22–30% of patients in some series (Taylor & Epstein 1969, McGuire & Haynes 1972).

The initial management should be as for any gastrointestinal bleed (p. 482) and it is particularly important to obtain a coagulation screen. Oral intake is limited to fluids. If the patient is shocked, a nasogastric tube is passed to exclude upper gastrointestinal hemorrhage. Sigmoidoscopy is performed to exclude colitis and major hemorrhoids once the patient's condition has become stable. Conservative management should continue for several days provided that less than 1 liter of blood per day is required. If more than a liter is required, operation must be considered and continued blood loss is tolerated particularly badly by the elderly. Olsen (1968) recommends operation before the total blood loss exceeds 3 liters, especially if the bleeding is rapid. Recurrence is not in itself an indication for surgery since bleeding usually stops with conservative measures; it is the rate of bleeding which is important. The plan of management is discussed on page 482.

Selective arteriography of the celiac, superior mesenteric and inferior mesenteric arteries may locate the site of continuous and rapid bleeding, which is often in the right side of the colon. It may reveal extravasation of dye or filling of a diverticulum or may show alternative sources of blood loss, notably vascular ectasia. The bleeding points are often difficult or impossible to locate at operation and the surgeon may not know which part of the colon to resect. Casarella et al (1972) studied 27 patients by angiography, all of whom had a negative gastric aspirate and sigmoidoscopy. The bleeding point was seen in 18 patients and in 13 of them was in a colonic diverticulum. Twelve of the 13 bleeding points were proximal to the splenic flexure.

Angiography also allows embolization or perfusion of adrenaline or pitressin through the catheter and thus avoid surgery even when bleeding is severe (Baum et al 1973; p. 27). Vasodilators and fibrinolytic drugs have been administered to facilitate angiographic diagnosis prior to definitive therapy (Rosch et al 1982).

Colonoscopy and barium enema are difficult to perform in patients with severe bleeding and are seldom helpful. Scintigraphy after administration of technetium-labeled blood cells is an alternative investigation.

***Surgical treatment.*** Surgery carries appreciable morbidity and mortality because of the age of the patient and the decision to undertake laparotomy is often difficult. However, it must be stressed that the elderly withstand repeated hemorrhage badly and may be better served by prompt operation if major bleeding continues or recurs.

A bleeding point localized by extravasation of contrast into the lumen at angiography is treated by segmental resection. A more difficult problem is posed by the patient known to have diverticular disease and shown on angiography to have vascular ectasia but no extravasation of contrast. The inclination at present is to regard the ectasia as the more likely source (Boley et al 1979a,b), although this is controversial. If laparotomy is unavoidable, opinion has now hardened in favor of total colectomy and ileorectal anastomosis as a more certain method of removing the source of bleeding and avoiding recurrent hemorrhage.

Elective surgery is not advised for elderly patients in whom bleeding settles on conservative measures, even though there has been more than one episode. However, fit patients who have had one or more episodes of severe bleeding are advised to undergo elective resection (Olsen 1968).

***Results and prognosis.*** McGuire & Haynes (1972) reviewed the results of treatment in 473 patients in 15 series between 1956 and 1971; 77% were treated conservatively and of these 3% died; 23% were treated by surgery and of these 20% died. The incidence of recurrent bleeding in the survivors was 22% after conservative management and 28% after surgery. However, now that total colectomy and ileorectal anastomosis is accepted as the operation of choice, the incidence of rebleeding approaches zero in modern practice. Wright et al (1980) treated 96 patients with severe lower intestinal bleeding over a 2-year period. The mean age of the patients was 70 years and eight received only supportive treatment before death. Of the remaining 88, 63 stopped bleeding spontaneously with a transfusion volume of less than 1.5 liters. Of the 25 patients who continued to bleed, angiography localized the site of bleeding in 12 of 14 cases. Diverticula were deemed responsible in eight and ectasias in four (all lesions being proximal to the splenic flexure). Twenty-two of these 25 patients came to urgent laparotomy and in 20 the source of bleeding had been determined by angiography, colonoscopy or barium studies; these patients were treated by segmental resection. The two patients without localization were treated by "blind" right hemicolectomy or "blind" total colectomy with ileorectal anastomosis. There was no operative mortality and none of 63 patients who stopped bleeding spontaneously succumbed, although 11 subsequently came to elective colectomy.

### *Perforation and abscess*

Formation of a small abscess is a common cause of an exacerbation of diverticular disease. The abscess may be pericolic, within the leaves of the mesentery or pelvis. Some abscesses resolve or drain back into the bowel, but some fail to subside on conservative management and adherence of small bowel can result in obstruction. Failure to respond to conservative treatment requires drainage, but in some cases this may now be performed percutaneously under radiological or ultrasound control.

Perforation is a very serious complication and often occurs without warning in a patient with only mild symptoms of diverticular disease. Free perforation produces fecal peritonitis or "communicating diverticulitis" (Hughes 1975) and is a devastating condition with a high mortality. Purulent peritonitis or "noncommunicating diverticulitis" develops from rupture of a previously walled off pericolic or pelvic abscess and is still a serious illness although less dangerous than fecal peritonitis.

In acute noncommunicating diverticulitis, there is severe pain of recent onset in the lower abdomen with peritoneal inflammation which is usually maximal in the left iliac fossa; a mass may be felt in the left iliac fossa. Perforating carcinoma of the sigmoid colon or carcinoma of the ovary invading the sigmoid colon can present in the same way. The patient is ill with fever, tachycardia and diminished bowel sounds. Patients with acute communicating diverticulitis are usually profoundly ill with sepsis and hypovolemia and the true diagnosis is immediately apparent at laparotomy.

Perforated diverticulitis can be misdiagnosed as acute appendicitis (Barabas 1971) because the pelvic colon may lie in, or perforate towards, the right iliac fossa. In patients with sudden perforation and no previous history of diverticular disease, generalized abdominal rigidity may lead to a misdiagnosis of perforated duodenal ulcer. Perforation in patients receiving corticosteroids is particularly difficult to recognize and peritonitis often progresses rapidly (Canter & Shorb 1971). An attack of diverticulitis in immunocompromised patients nearly always leads to surgery (Perkins et al 1984); after renal transplantation, the incidence of colonic perforation is 0.7% with a 90% mortality (Archibald et al 1978). The high mortality reflects suppression of symptoms and signs and compromise of the immune response to bacterial infection by azathioprine and corticosteroids. In this respect, patients who perforate while receiving cyclosporin may have better survival prospects than those receiving azathioprine and corticosteroids (Rigotti et al 1986).

***Surgical treatment.*** Krukowski & Matheson (1984) suggest that when the clinical diagnosis is localized sepsis secondary to diverticular disease, management should be conservative in the first instance with systemic antibiotics and supportive therapy. Operation should be reserved for patients with obvious generalized peritonitis or failure of conservative treatment. When operation is necessary, the affected sigmoid loop should be resected with temporary exteriorization of the end of the descending colon and closure of the rectal stump (Hartmann's procedure). If circumstances are favorable and operation is being undertaken by a skilled surgeon, primary anastomosis after on-table bowel irrigation (Koruth et al 1985) may be considered. In their own experience of 57 patients with acute diverticulitis, 37 were managed without operation while 21 had urgent or emergency surgery. None of the conservatively treated patients died whereas three died in the surgical group, although only one death was attributable to peritoneal sepsis (Krukowski et al 1985)

The traditional three-stage approach to perforated diverticular disease is now seldom used. In the first stage a proximal transverse colostomy was created and a drain placed down to the sigmoid colon, elective colectomy with immediate anastomosis was then undertaken after some 2 months and finally the colostomy was closed. It is generally accepted that transverse colostomy does not prevent continued colonic inflammation, peritoneal sepsis and fecal fistula formation and that multiple operations pose a formidable strain on this elderly group of patients. There are few controlled data, but the collected mortality for the conservative approach is 25%, as opposed to 11% for emergency primary resection (Krukowski & Matheson 1984). Despite these considerations, Kronborg (1993) has recently reported a prospective randomized comparison of initial transverse colostomy and suture of the perforation as opposed to immediate resection without anastomosis in perforated diverticulitis. In purulent peritonitis there were no deaths in 21 patients undergoing colostomy and six deaths in 25 patients undergoing immediate resection; mortality rates were not significantly different between the two groups in patients with fecal peritonitis.

Patients younger than 50 years may be more prone to recurrences and complications after conservative treatment of acute diverticulitis, whereas older patients more often require operation during their index admission (Ambrosetti et al 1994).

### *Obstruction*

Thickening of the wall of the sigmoid colon can cause a degree of obstruction and the lumen may be reduced further as a result of peridiverticulitis (Fig. 54.9). The patient may then present with typical features of an acute large bowel obstruction which is of the "closed loop" type if the ileocecal valve is functional. Small bowel obstruction may also occur because of adhesion formation. The traditional approach to obstructed diverticular disease was the three-stage approach outlined above. However, for the same reasons there has been a move towards emergency resection, with a choice thereafter of Hartmann's procedure or immediate end-to-end anastomosis. After a Hartmann's procedure, continuity is restored electively after 2–3 months, although a significant proportion of elderly patients are left with a stoma when it is deemed unwise to attempt restoration of continuity.

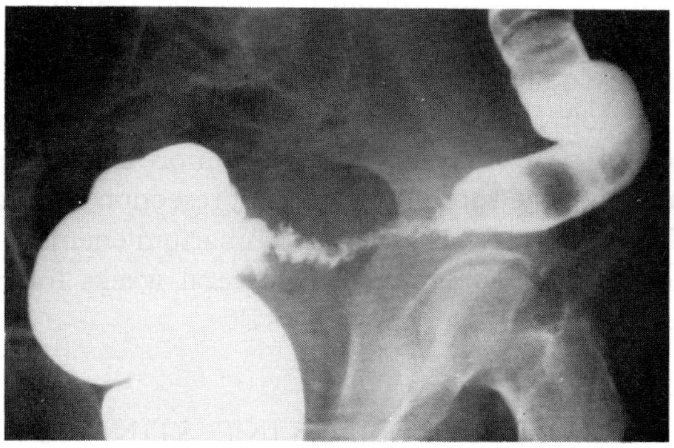

**Fig. 54.9** Obstruction in upper pelvic colon due to markedly active diverticular disease. The colon could be filled with barium only following relaxation with hyoscine butylbromide (Buscopan) 30 mg intravenously.

### *Fistula* (Small & Smith 1975, Woods et al 1988)

Diverticular disease is a commoner cause of fistula formation than Crohn's disease or carcinoma (p. 1424) and its reported incidence varies from 5–33% (Hool et al 1981, Corman 1984). The fistula may be the culmination of an obvious attack of diverticulitis or it may be the first and only clinical evidence of the disease. The commonest variety is the colovesical fistula followed by colocutaneous, colovaginal and coloenteric fistulae. Fistulation to the uterus, fallopian tubes, ureter, perineum and other parts of the colon are exceptionally rare.

***Colovesical fistula.*** Urinary symptoms are common in diverticulitis but the complication of colovesical fistulae develop in a small proportion of cases. The male preponderance reflects the fact that the interposed uterus prevents fistulation in women, a protection that may be lost after hysterectomy. Most colovesical fistulae develop in patients with few or no bowel symptoms; by contrast, colovesical fistulae in Crohn's disease are usually accompanied by bowel symptoms.

The patient complains of frequency, dysuria and hematuria, usually as a consequence of *E. coli* cystitis. Suspicion should be raised if the infection fails to respond to treatment or if the patient is aware of a bubbling sensation at the end of micturition (pneumaturia) or fecaluria. Passage of urine per rectum is very rare. Systemic toxicity and an abdominal mass are present in about one-third of cases.

This fistula is difficult to demonstrate and the diagnosis is often confirmed only at laparotomy. Cystoscopy occasionally reveals the fistulous opening but more usually shows a localized area of cystitis. Cystography is rewarding in only a third of cases in contrast to its helpfulness when there is a fistula from Crohn's disease of the small bowel. A plain abdominal radiograph may show gas in the bladder and a barium enema will demonstrate the fistula in some 50% of cases. Computed tomography may also show the fistula and provide useful information about the extent of pericolic inflammation.

Colovesical fistulae were once treated by staged resection, but with modern methods of bowel preparation and antibiotic cover, primary resection and anastomosis with repair of the bladder is now usually feasible and safe (Rao et al 1987).

***Colovaginal fistula.*** Colovaginal fistula from any cause is rare, but its usual cause is diverticular disease. A persistent foul vaginal discharge develops after an episode of acute diverticulitis. The fistula is treated by resection of the involved colon with primary anastomosis; closure of the vaginal defect is unnecessary.

***Colocutaneous fistula.*** These fistulae may form spontaneously or after an operation for diverticulitis. The clinical diagnosis is obvious and the fistula is demonstrated by barium enema and treated by excision of the diseased segment of colon.

### Right-sided diverticular disease and solitary ulcers of the cecum or ascending colon

*Etiology and pathology*

This disorder differs from the predominantly left-sided disease in its racial distribution, age incidence and pathology. In Japan, 429 of 615 patients with colonic diverticular disease had diverticula confined to the cecum and ascending colon (Sugihara et al 1984). In Hawaii, Caucasians had the usual "Western" distribution of diverticular disease, but the proportion with right-sided disease was 60% in Japanese, 50% in Hawaiians and 30% in Chinese and Filipinos (Peck et al 1968). The average age of these patients was 40 years. Autopsy studies in Hong Kong and Singapore show that the prevalence of diverticular disease was 5% (Coode et al 1985) and 19% (Lee 1986) respectively, but in both studies the right side of the colon was predominantly affected. Perry & Morson (1971) studied the pathology in two cases of right-sided diverticulosis and found no evidence of generalized muscle thickening but rather a mucosal thickening around the mouth of each diverticulum. This thickening was due to lymphoid tissue and the authors speculated that fecoliths found in the diverticula were responsible for the hypertrophy.

The diverticula in right-sided disease are composed of a mucous membrane and a thin layer of longitudinal muscle and it is still debated whether they are congenital or aquired and true or false. Nearly 80% lie within 2 cm of the ileocecal valve (Fischer & Farkas 1984). In a review of right-sided diverticular disease in Caucasians (Wagner & Zollinger 1961), the average age was 41 years compared to 53 years in patients with sigmoid disease. Thus, there is a case for believing that right-sided diverticular disease is a distinct entity in whichever race it occurs. However, abnormal motility may play a role in producing the diverticula (Sugihara et al 1983) by the same mechanisms implicated in sigmoid diverticular disease.

Solitary diverticulum of the cecum is seen in less than 0.1% of barium enema examinations. Greaney & Snyder (1957) classify diverticula of the cecum into "hidden" and "projecting". The former are entirely within the wall of the bowel and appear as a mass rather than as a diverticulum on barium enema. The latter project outwards from the cecum near the ileocecal valve. Solitary ulcer of the cecum and a cecal inflammatory mass may be related to caecal diverticulitis and may progress to perforation. Solitary ulcer is found in the same age group, presents the same clinical features and tends to occur at the same site near the ileocecal valve. Furthermore, ulcer and diverticulum may coexist (Anscombe et al 1967). It is thought that a fecolith in a diverticulum may cause ulceration and inflammation (Williams 1960) and when this occurs in a "hidden" diverticulum, an inflammatory mass may develop.

In a review of 16 Caucasian patients, Pieterse et al (1986) described four distinct groups. Six patients had solitary false diverticula mimicking acute appendicitis, while five patients had diverticula associated with fibrous defects of the muscle coat and typically presented with bleeding similar to angiodysplasia. True diverticula were uncommon and solitary. The fourth category had diverticula similar to those seen on the left side of the colon.

*Clinical features and investigations*

The majority of patients present with the clinical features of acute appendicitis (Fischer & Farkas 1984). Others complain of recurrent pain in the right iliac fossa with localized tenderness and sometimes a mass. Nausea and diarrhea can occur. Obstruction is rare but bleeding may occur, as in the case of right-sided diverticula associated with total colonic diverticular disease. There may be fever and a leukocytosis. Whatever the presentation, a preoperative diagnosis is made in less than 10% of cases (Wagner & Zollinger 1961).

If the patient does not require surgery immediately, the diagnosis may be made by barium enema. A diverticulum may "project" from the cecum or, when the crater does not fill, an excrescence may be seen extending into the bowel lumen (Bahabozorgui et al 1968). Because of the wide lumen of the cecum, abnormalities are easily obscured by the large mass of barium and radiographs in several projections must be taken. The diagnosis is often difficult to establish even at operation since a cecal mass may be misinterpreted as malignant. In their review, Wagner & Zollinger (1961) found that 30% of benign masses had been incorrectly diagnosed as carcinoma.

*Treatment*

In nearly all cases, the diagnosis is only established at operation. Right hemicolectomy is avoided unless there are multiple diverticula or cancer cannot be excluded (Colcock 1971). A diverticulum should be treated by local excision or by inversion, while abscesses are drained. Wagner & Zollinger (1961) found that mortality after right hemicolectomy was five times greater than after simple excision of a diverticulum, although more recent review indicates that the mortality following resection is now less than 2% (Fischer & Farkas 1984). A barium enema is usually advised after an interval of several weeks following treatment.

## PNEUMATOSIS CYSTOIDES INTESTINALIS

This rare disorder has attracted much attention because of its unusual nature and because there is no adequate explanation for the occurrence of gas cysts in the bowel.

**Etiology and pathology** (Koss 1952)

Cysts occur at any level in the bowel and opinions differ as to whether they are most frequent in the large or small bowel. The affected intestine has a nodular mucosal surface with an excess of adherent mucus. On section there are cysts of varying size involving mucosa, submucosa, main muscle coat and subserosa (Fig. 54.10). On microscopy the cysts are lined in part by fibrous tissue and in part by histiocytes, including scattered giant cells. Some surrounding fibrosis may develop. The overlying mucosa is often abnormal, showing the pattern of a chronic colitis which suggests that the gas is entering directly through the mucosa (Pieterse et al 1985).

Several other theories have been postulated to account for the phenomenon. In infancy, pneumatosis develops as a consequence of bacterial invasion of the bowel wall and is frequently associated with enterocolitis (Stone et al 1968). The cysts contain hydrogen, nitrogen and carbon dioxide. Breath hydrogen concentrations are increased in patients with pneumatosis cystoides intestinalis. Under normal circumstances this hydrogen is produced in the colon by bacteria which ferment carbohydrates and proteins. Hydrogen is excreted in the breath and flatus and a large proportion is metabolized by methogenic or sulfate-reducing bacteria. These bacteria are virtually absent in pneumatosis cystoides intestinalis (Christl et al 1993). There is also a "mechanical theory"; in adults, pneumatosis of the small intestine is often associated with obstructive lesions in the pyloric region, whereas pneumatosis of the large bowel is associated with chronic lung or heart disease and may occur after instrumentation of the rectum and lower colon and occasionally in patients with no other disease. It is possible that in chest disease severe coughing causes alveolar rupture and pneumomediastinum and experimental studies have demonstrated that air in the mediastinum eventually tracks into the retroperitoneal tissues and forms cysts in the bowel wall (Keyting et al 1961). In the case of pyloric obstruction, vomiting may force air into the tissues via an ulcer crater.

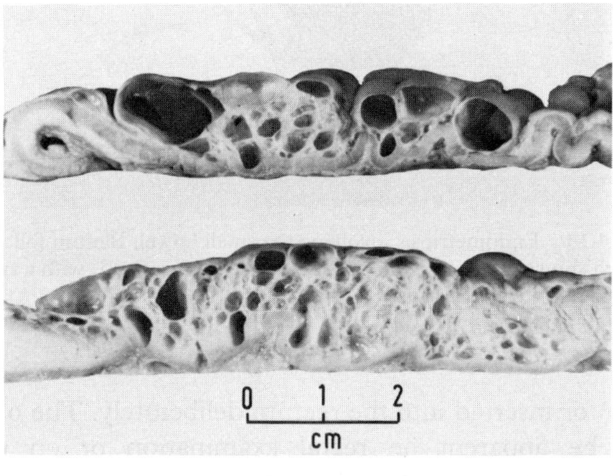


**Fig. 54.10** Pneumatosis coli. Cut sections of the colon showing the cysts, which are mainly in the submucosa and superficial muscle.

**Clinical features**

In adults, the ratio of males to females is 3.5:1 and the disease is commonest between the ages of 30 and 60 years. The patient usually presents with an associated disorder, commonly pyloric stenosis or gastric cancer. Occasionally, the underlying disease may be small intestinal scleroderma, diverticula, a malabsorption syndrome or jejunoileal bypass. Symptoms which can be ascribed to pneumatosis are episodes of constipation or even obstruction, episodes of diarrhea with froth and mucus, rectal bleeding and pneumoperitoneum. When the rectum is involved, the appearance is of multiple sessile polyps (Fig. 4.20) of varying size which puncture and deflate when biopsy is attempted. The condition can be recognized on a plain abdominal radiograph by the small, round, radiolucent shadows along the course of the affected segment. Barium enema shows multiple sessile filling defects which can be mistaken for multiple polyposis (Fig. 54.11).

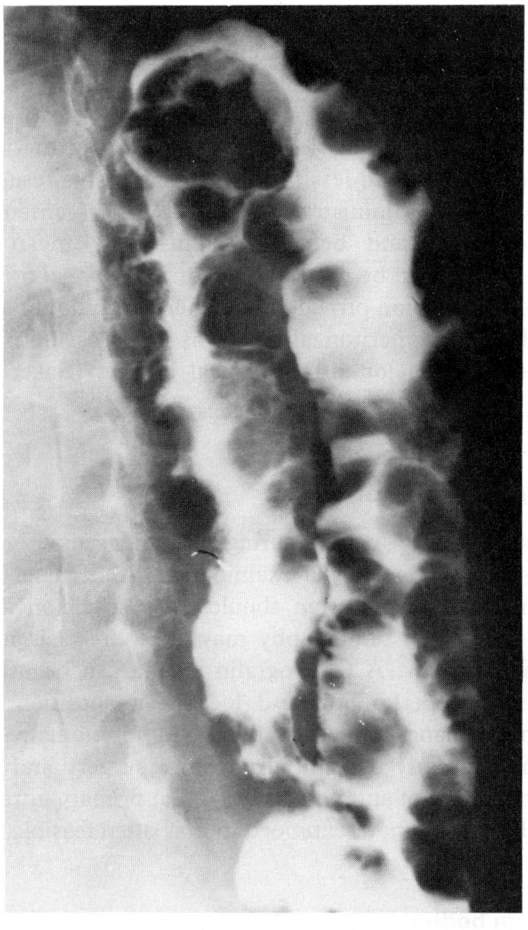

**Fig. 54.11** Pneumatosis coli. Barium enema shows large gas-containing cysts causing a markedly irregular and narrowed lumen.

### Treatment

Underlying gastrointestinal disease should be treated whenever possible. For example, in pneumatosis cystoides secondary to systemic lupus erythematosus, both conditions improved with corticosteroids (Cabrera et al 1994). In patients with obstruction or severe large bowel symptoms, it may be necessary to resect the involved area, but every attempt is usually made to treat such cases conservatively.

Treatment with hyperbaric oxygen produces a symptomatic response and if contained, it often results in a cure (Grieve & Unsworth 1991). Metronidazole 500 mg three times a day for several weeks is also effective in some patients (Tak et al 1992), presumably by reducing the numbers of bacteria which produce hydrogen.

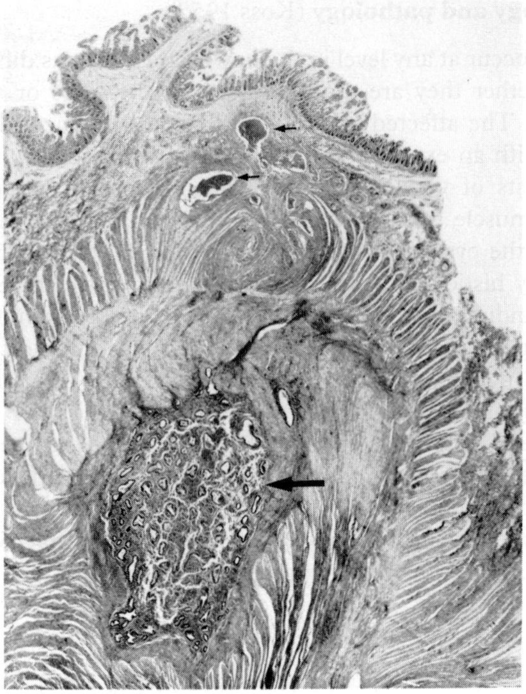

**Fig. 54.12** Endometriosis. Ileum showing occasional blood-filled endometrial glands in the submucosa and muscle (small arrows) with a deeper group of glands and related endometrial stroma (large arrow) (hematoxylin and eosin, ×10).

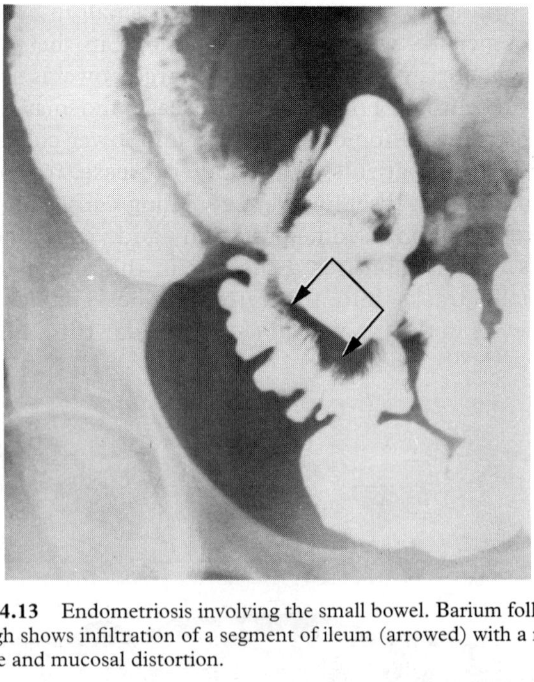

**Fig. 54.13** Endometriosis involving the small bowel. Barium follow-through shows infiltration of a segment of ileum (arrowed) with a ragged outline and mucosal distortion.

## TRAUMA AND FOREIGN BODIES IN THE COLON AND RECTUM

### Colorectal trauma

Colorectal injury in civilian life usually results from penetrating low velocity gunshot wounds or stab injury, whereas in combat settings the injury is caused by high velocity missiles or shrapnel. The injured bowel has been managed traditionally by exteriorization with colostomy formation but where feasible, the bowel has been primarily sutured with early replacement (ca 5–7 days) in the peritoneal cavity if all was well. Reduction of the injury to operation time to less than 12 h, aggressive resuscitation and early administration of antibiotics (gentamicin, metronidazole and benzylpenicillin) now mean that some injuries can be managed by intraperitoneal primary suture of the colon provided that there is no doubt about bowel viability, peritoneal soiling is not gross and there are no other major intraperitoneal injuries (Baker et al 1990).

### Iatrogenic perforation

Perforation may occur during sigmoidoscopy, colonoscopy or barium enema examination. Abdominal pain, tenderness and distention should raise suspicion and a plain abdominal radiography may show free gas in the peritoneal cavity. A Gastrografin enema can be used to confirm the perforation and localize its position. The patient is managed as just described for noniatrogenic trauma but early recognition, prompt surgery and early administration of antibiotics means that primary intraperitoneal suture without exteriorization is often feasible.

### Foreign bodies (Abcarian & Lowe 1978)

These may have been ingested accidentally (e.g. chicken bone) or inserted into the rectum deliberately. The object may be apparent on rectal examination or on plain abdominal radiographs. Most objects can be removed under general anesthesia without the need for laparotomy,

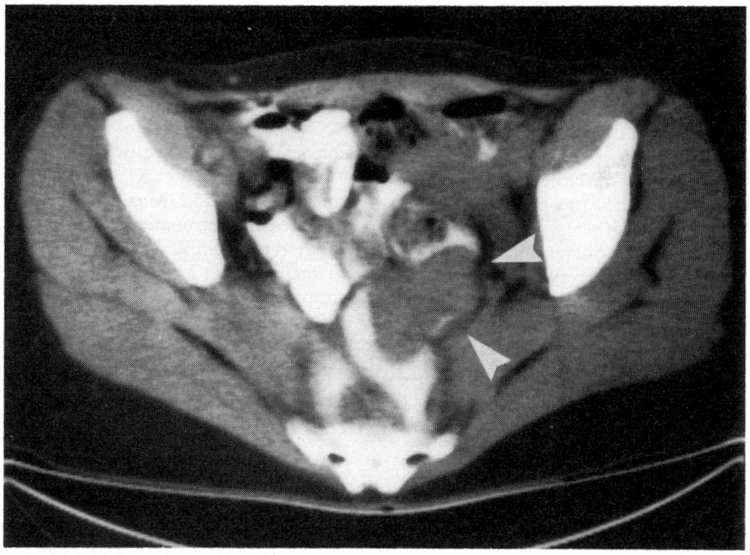

**Fig. 54.14** Endometriosis involving the rectal wall and perirectal tissues (arrows).

but a 24-h period of observation may be advisable to exclude perforation or bleeding.

## ENDOMETRIOSIS

This condition is important to the gastroenterologist because it may give rise to gastrointestinal symptoms and may simulate carcinoma of the lower bowel.

It is not understood how endometrial tissue becomes implanted in the alimentary tract or, indeed, elsewhere; the postulate that it enters the peritoneal cavity via the fallopian tubes has not been seriously challenged (Sampson 1940) and is in keeping with the pathological finding that the serosa is involved initially.

### Pathology

Although endometriosis can occur in the small intestine (Bose & Davson 1969), it involves the sigmoid colon and rectum most frequently. The implant of endometrium initially involves the outer layers of the bowel. Cyclical bleeding from the endometrium creates a cystic mass which gradually expands towards the lumen, but the mucosa of the intestine remains intact even when a polypoid mass projects into the bowel. Sometimes, the entire circumference of the bowel is involved and obstruction ensues. Such obstruction is commonest in the small intestine (McGuff et al 1948) and is partly due to dense adhesions. Histology shows that the mass is composed of hypertrophied muscle, endometrium, inflammatory cells and areas of hemorrhage. An example from the ileum is shown in Figure 54.12. A localized biopsy may be mistaken for adenocarcinoma.

### Clinical features

Most patients never experience bowel symptoms. Symptomatic patients are between 30 and 60 years old and complain of cyclical rectal pain, discomfort and constipation. Occasionally, there may be diarrhea or cyclical rectal bleeding (Miller et al 1994). Other complaints include dysmenorrhea, dyspareunia, pelvic pain and abdominal swelling due to ascites. Endometriosis of the small intestine usually presents as obstruction secondary to fibrosis, adhesions or intussusception (Bose & Davson 1969, Aronchick et al 1983).

The diagnosis is made by palpating a tender nodule on bimanual examination; the size and tenderness may vary during the menstrual cycle. Endoscopic and radiological examination always reveal intact mucosa over the tumor but are frequently not diagnostic. The lesion appears as an intramural tumor or a stenosis. Involvement of a segment of small intestine is shown in Figure 54.13 and of rectum in Figure 54.14.

### Treatment

Lesions causing obstruction are excised and a primary anastomosis is performed. Smaller lesions can be subjected to local dissection without opening the bowel wall. Other lesions can be rendered asymptomatic by progestogen therapy (Williams 1967a).

REFERENCES


Abcarian H, Lowe R 1978 Colon and rectal trauma. Surgical Clinics of North America 58: 519

Alexander J, Karl R C, Skinner D B 1983 Results of changing trends in the surgical management of complications of diverticular disease. Surgery 94: 683

Ambrosetti P, Robert J H, Witzig J-A, Mirescu D, Mathey P, Borst F, Rohner A 1994 Acute left colonic diverticulitis: a prospective analysis of 226 consecutive cases. Surgery 115: 546–550

Anscombe A R, Keddie N C, Schofield P F 1967 Solitary ulcers and diverticulitis of the caecum. British Journal of Surgery 54: 553

Archibald S D, Jirsch D W, Bear R A 1978 Gastrointestinal complications of renal transplantation. 11. The colon. Canadian Medical Association Journal 119: 1301

Arfwidsson S 1964 Pathogenesis of multiple diverticula of the sigmoid colon in diverticular disease. Acta Chirurgica Scandinavica (suppl): 342

Aronchick C A, Brooks F P, Dyson W L, Baron R, Thompson J J 1983 Ileocecal endometriosis presenting with abdominal pain and gastrointestinal bleeding. Digestive Diseases and Sciences 28: 566

Bahabozorgui S, DeMuth W E, Blakemore W S 1968 Diverticulitis of the ascending colon. American Journal of Surgery 115: 295

Baker L W, Thomson S R, Chadwick S J D 1990 Colon wound management and prograde colonic lavage in large bowel trauma. British Journal of Surgery 77: 872–876

Barabas A P 1971 Peritonitis due to diverticular disease of the colon: review of 44 cases. Proceedings of the Royal Society of Medicine 64: 253

Baum S, Rosch J, Dotter C T et al 1973 Selective mesenteric arterial infusions in the management of massive diverticular hemorrhage. New England Journal of Medicine 288: 1269

Beranbaum S L, Ring S M 1968 Ulcerative colitis engrafted upon diverticulitis. An evolutionary case history. American Journal of Roentgenology 104: 551

Berman L G, Burdick D, Heitzman E R, Prior J T 1968 A critical reappraisal of sigmoid peridiverticulitis. Surgery, Gynecology and Obstetrics 127: 481

Berman P M, Kirsner J B 1972 Current knowledge of diverticular disease of the colon. American Journal of Digestive Diseases 17: 741

B M J 1980 Leading article: massive bleeding from the large bowel. British Medical Journal 1: 425

Boley S J, DiBiase A, Brandt L J, Sammartano R J 1979a Lower intestinal bleeding in the elderly. American Journal of Surgery 137: 57

Boley S J, Sammartano R, Brandt L J, Sprayregen S 1979b Vascular ectasias of the colon. Surgery, Gynecology and Obstetrics 149: 353

Bose A, Davson J 1969 Endometriosis of small intestine. British Journal of Surgery 56: 109

Botsford T W, Zollinger R M 1969 Diverticulitis of the colon. Surgery, Gynecology and Obstetrics 128: 1209

Boulos P B, Salmon P R, Karamanolis D G, Clark C G 1984 Is colonoscopy necessary in diverticular disease? Lancet 1: 95

Boulos P B, Cowin A P, Karamanolis D G, Clark C G 1985 Diverticula, neoplasia, or both? Early detection of carcinoma in sigmoid diverticular disease. Annals of Surgery 202: 607

Brodribb A J M 1977 Treatment of symptomatic diverticular disease with a high-fibre diet. Lancet 1: 664

Cabrera G E, Scopelitis E, Cuellar M L et al 1994 Pneumatosis cystoides intestinalis in systemic lupus erythematosus with intestinal vasculitis: treatment with high dose prednisone. Clinical Rheumatology 13: 312–316

Canter J W, Shorb P E 1971 Acute perforation of colonic diverticula associated with prolonged adrenocorticosteroid therapy. American Journal of Surgery 121: 46

Casarella W J, Kanter I E, Seaman W B 1972 Right-sided colonic diverticula as a cause of acute rectal hemorrhage. New England Journal of Medicine 286: 450

Chennells P M, Simpkins K C 1981 The barium enema diagnosis of paracolic abscess. Clinical Radiology 32: 73

Christl S U, Gibson G R, Murgatroyd P R et al 1993 Impaired hydrogen metabolism in pneumatosis cystoides intestinalis. Gastroenterology 104: 392–397

Cleave T L, Campbell G D, Painter N S 1969 Diabetes, coronary thrombosis and the saccharine disease, 2nd edn. Wright, Bristol

Colcock B P 1958 Surgical management of complicated diverticulitis. New England Journal of Medicine 259: 570

Colcock B P 1971 Diverticular disease of the colon. Major problems in clinical surgery, Vol XI. W B Saunders, Philadelphia, p 25

Colcock B P 1975 Diverticular disease: proven surgical management. Clinics in Gastroenterology 4: 99

Coode P E, Chan K W, Chan Y T 1985 Polyps and diverticula of the large intestine: a necropsy survey in Hong Kong. Gut 26: 1045

Corman M L 1984 Colon and rectal surgery. J B Lippincott, Philadelphia

Daniel O 1969a Sigmoid myotomy with peritoneal graft. Proceedings of the Royal Society of Medicine 62: 39

Daniel O 1969b Personal communication

Dwyer J T, Goldin B, Gorbach S, Patterson J 1978 Drug therapy reviews: dietary fiber and fiber supplements in the therapy of gastrointestinal disorders. American Journal of Hospital Pharmacy 35: 278

Eide T J, Stalsberg H 1979 Diverticular disease of the large intestine in Northern Norway. Gut 20: 609

Eusebio E B, Eisenberg M M 1973 Natural history of diverticular disease of the colon in young patients. American Journal of Surgery 125: 308

Farmakis N, Tudor R G, Keighley M R B 1994 The 5-year natural history of complicated diverticular disease. British Journal of Surgery 81: 733–735

Fischer M G, Farkas A M 1984 Diverticulitis of the cecum and ascending colon. Diseases of the Colon and Rectum 27: 454

Fleischner F G 1971 Diverticular disease of the colon. New observations and revised concepts. Gastroenterology 60: 316

Fleischner F G, Ming S C 1965 Revised concepts on diverticular disease of the colon. II. So-called diverticulitis; diverticular sigmoiditis and perisigmoiditis: diverticular abscess, fistula and frank peritonitis. Radiology 84: 599

Forde K A, Lebwohl O, Seaman W B 1980 Colonoscopy as an adjunctive technique in evaluating acquired colonic narrowing. Surgery 87: 243

Gear J S S, Fursdon P, Nolan D J et al 1979 Symptomless diverticular disease and intake of dietary fibre. Lancet 1: 511

Gennaro A R, Rosemond G P 1974 Pathogenesis of diverticulosis of the colon. Diseases of the Colon and Rectum 17: 64

Glerum J, Agenant D, Tytgat G N 1977 Value of colonoscopy in the detection of sigmoid malignancy in patients with diverticular disease. Endoscopy 9: 228

Goligher J C (ed) 1984 Surgery of the anus, rectum and colon. Baillière Tindall, London, p 1103

Greaney E M, Snyder W H 1957 Acute diverticulitis of the cecum encountered at emergency surgery. American Journal of Surgery 94: 270

Grieve D A, Unsworth I P 1991 Pneumatosis cystoides intestinalis: an experience with hyperbaric oxygen treatment. Australian and New Zealand Journal of Surgery 61: 423–426

Hackford A W, Schoetz D J, Coller J A, Veidenheimer M C 1985 Surgical management of complicated diverticulitis. The Lahey Clinic experience, 1967 to 1982. Diseases of the Colon and Rectum 28: 31

Heald R J, Ray J E 1971 Bleeding from diverticula of the colon. Diseases of the Colon and Rectum 14: 420

Hiltunen K M, Kolehmainen H, Vuorinen T, Matikainen M 1991 Early water-soluble contrast enema in the diagnosis of acute colonic diverticulitis. International Journal of Colorectal Disease 6: 190–192

Hool G J, Bokey E L, Pheils M T 1981 Diverticular coloenteric fistulae. Australian and New Zealand Journal of Surgery 51: 358–359

Hughes L E 1969 Postmortem survey of diverticular disease of the colon. Part 1. Diverticulosis and diverticulitis. Gut 10: 336

Hughes L E 1975 Complications of diverticular disease: inflammation, obstruction and bleeding. Clinics in Gastroenterology 4: 147

Hulnick D H, Megibow A J, Balthazar E J, Naidich D P, Bosniak M A 1984 Computed tomography in the evaluation of diverticulitis. Radiology 152: 491

Kewenter J, Hellzen-Ingemarsson A, Kewenter G, Olsson U 1985

Diverticular disease and minor rectal bleeding. Scandinavian Journal of Gastroenterology 20: 922
Keyting W S, McCarver R R, Kovarik J L, Daywitt A L 1961 Pneumatosis intestinalis: a new concept. Radiology 76: 733
Klein S, Mayer L, Present D H, Youner K D, Cerulli M A, Sachar D B 1988 Extraintestinal manifestations in patients with diverticulitis. Annals of Internal Medicine 108: 700
Koruth N M, Krukowski Z H, Youngson G G et al 1985 Intraoperative colonic irrigation in the management of left-sided large bowel emergencies. British Journal of Surgery 72: 708
Koss L G 1952 Abdominal gas cysts (pneumatosis cystoides intestinorum hominis). An analysis with a report of a case and a critical review of the literature. Archives of Pathology 53: 523
Kronborg O 1993 Treatment of perforated sigmoid diverticulitis: a prospective randomized trial. British Journal of Surgery 80: 505–507
Krukowski Z H, Matheson N A 1984 Emergency surgery for diverticular disease complicated by generalized and faecal peritonitis: a review. British Journal of Surgery 71: 921
Krukowski Z N, Koruth N M, Matheson N A 1985 Evolving practice in acute diverticulitis. British Journal of Surgery 72: 684–686
Lee Y S 1986 Diverticular disease of the large bowel in Singapore. An autopsy survey. Diseases of the Colon and Rectum 29: 330
Lieberman J M, Haaga J R 1983 Computed tomography of diverticulitis. Journal of Computer Assisted Tomography 7: 431
MacGregor A B, Abernethy B C, Thomson J W W 1970 The role of surgery in diverticular disease of the colon. Journal of the Royal College of Surgeons of Edinburgh 15: 137
Manousos O N 1989 Diverticular disease of the colon. Diseases of the Colon and Rectum 7: 86
Manousos O, Day N E, Tzonou A et al 1985 Diet and other factors in the aetiology of diverticulosis: an epidemiological study in Greece. Gut 26: 544
Marshak R H, Lindner A E, Maklansky D 1979 Diverticulosis and diverticulitis of the colon. Mount Sinai Journal of Medicine 46: 261
Max M H, Knutson C O 1978 Colonoscopy in patients with inflammatory colonic strictures. Surgery 84: 551
Mayo C W, Delaney L T 1956 Colonic diverticulitis associated with carcinoma. Review of fifty cases. Archives of Surgery 72: 957
McGuff P, Dockerty M B, Waugh J M, Randall L M 1948 Endometriosis as a cause of intestinal obstruction. Surgery, Gynecology and Obstetrics 86: 273
McGuire H H, Haynes B W 1972 Massive hemorrhage from diverticulosis of the colon. Guidelines for therapy based on bleeding patterns observed in fifty cases. Annals of Surgery 175: 847
McKee R F, Deignan R W, Krukowski Z H 1993 Radiological investigation in acute diverticulitis. British Journal of Surgery 80: 560–565
Mendeloff A I 1976 A critique of "Fiber Deficiency". American Journal of Digestive Diseases 21: 10
Meyers M A, Alonso D R, Gray G F, Baer J W 1976 Pathogenesis of bleeding colonic diverticulosis. Gastroenterology 71: 577
Miller L S, Barbarevech C, Friedman L W 1994 Less frequent causes of lower gastrointestinal bleeding. Gastrointestinal Bleeding II 23: 21–52
Moreaux J, Vons C 1990 Elective resection for diverticular disease of the sigmoid colon. British Journal of Surgery 77: 1036–1038
Morson B C 1963 The muscle abnormality in diverticular disease of the sigmoid colon. British Journal of Radiology 36: 385
Morson B C 1975 Pathology of diverticular disease of the colon. Clinics in Gastroenterology 4: 37
Ohi G, Minowa K, Oyama T et al 1983 Changes in dietary fiber intake among Japanese in the 20th century: a relationship to the prevalence of diverticular disease. American Journal of Clinical Nutrition 38: 115
Olsen W R 1968 Hemorrhage from diverticular disease of the colon. The role of emergency subtotal colectomy. American Journal of Surgery 115: 247
Ornstein M H, Littlewood E R, Baird I M, Fowler J, North W R S, Cox A G 1981 Are fibre supplements really necessary in diverticular disease of the colon? A controlled clinical trial. British Medical Journal 1: 1353
Painter N S 1973 Diverticular disease of the colon. In: Truelove S C, Jewell D P (eds) Topics in gastroenterology, Vol 1. Blackwell, Oxford, p 294
Painter N S, Burkitt D P 1971 Diverticular disease of the colon: a deficiency disease of Western civilisation. British Medical Journal 2: 450
Painter N S, Burkitt D P 1975 Diverticular disease of the colon, a 20th century problem. Clinics in Gastroenterology 4: 3
Painter N S, Truelove S C 1964 The intraluminal pressure patterns in diverticulosis of the colon. 1. Resting patterns of pressure. II. The effect of morphine. III. The effect of prostigmine. Gut 5: 201, 207, 365
Painter N S, Truelove S C, Ardran G M, Tuckey M 1965 Segmentation and localization of intraluminal pressures in the human colon, with special reference to the pathogenesis of colonic diverticula. Gastroenterology 49: 169
Painter N S, Almeida A Z, Colebourne K W 1972 Unprocessed bran in treatment of diverticular disease of the colon. British Medical Journal 2: 137
Parks T G 1969a Natural history of diverticular disease of the colon. A review of 521 cases. British Medical Journal 4: 639
Parks T G 1969b Reappraisal of clinical features of diverticular disease of the colon. British Medical Journal 4: 642
Parks T G 1975 Natural history of diverticular disease of the colon. Clinics in Gastroenterology 4: 53
Parks T G, Connell A M, Gough A D, Cole J O Y 1970 Limitations of radiology in the differentiation of diverticulitis and diverticulosis of the colon. British Medical Journal 2: 136
Peck D A, Labat R, Waite V C 1968 Diverticular disease of the right colon. Diseases of the Colon and Rectum 11: 49
Perkins J D, Shield C F, Chang F C, Farha G J 1984 Acute diverticulitis. Comparison of treatment in immunocompromised and nonimmunocompromised patients. American Journal of Surgery 148: 745
Perry P M, Morson B C 1971 Right-sided diverticulosis of the colon. British Journal of Surgery 58: 902
Pescatori M, Castiglioni G C 1978 Sigmoid motility and clinical results after transverse taeniamyotomy for diverticular disease. British Journal of Surgery 65: 666
Pieterse A S, Leong A S-Y, Rowland R 1985 The mucosal changes and pathogenesis of pneumatosis cystoides intestinalis. Human Pathology 16: 683
Pieterse A S, Rowland R, Miliauskas J R, Hoffmann D C 1986 Rightsided diverticular disease of the colon: a morphological analysis of 16 cases. Australian and New Zealand Journal of Surgery 56: 471
Pounder D J, Rowland R, Pieterse A S, Freeman R, Hunter R 1982 Angiodysplasias of the colon. Journal of Clinical Pathology 35: 824
Rao P N, Knox R, Barnard R J, Schofield P F 1987 Management of colovesical fistula. British Journal of Surgery 74: 362–363
Reilly M, Smith A N 1975 Sigmoid myotomy. Clinics in Gastroenterology 4: 121
Rigg B M, Ewing M R 1966 Current attitudes on diverticulitis with particular reference to colonic bleeding. Archives of Surgery 92: 321
Rigotti P, van Buren C T, Payne W D, Peters C, Kahan B D 1986 Gastrointestinal perforations in renal transplant recipients immunosuppressed with cyclosporin. World Journal of Surgery 10: 137
Robertson J 1972 Changes in the fibre content of the British diet. Nature 238: 290
Rosch J, Keller F S, Wawrukiewicz A S, Krippaehne W W, Dotter C T 1982 Pharmacoangiography in the diagnosis of recurrent massive lower gastrointestinal bleeding. Radiology 145: 615
Rowe R J, Kollmar G H 1952 Collective review. Diverticulitis of the colon complicated by carcinoma. Surgery, Gynecology and Obstetrics International Abstracts of Surgery 94: 1
Salvati E, Hak Hyun B, Varga C F 1967 Massive hemorrhage from colonic diverticula caused by arterial erosion: a practical theory of its mechanism and causation: report of two cases. Diseases of the Colon and Rectum 10: 129
Sampson J A 1940 The development of the implantation theory for the origin of peritoneal endometriosis. American Journal of Obstetrics and Gynecology 40: 459
Schynder P, Moss A A, Floeni F R, Margules A R 1979 Double blind study of radiological accuracy in diverticulitis, diverticulosis and carcinoma of sigmoid colon. Clinical Journal of Gastroenterology 1: 55–66

Simpkins K C 1984 Double-contrast examination. Part Ill: colon. Clinics in Gastroenterology 13: 1
Small W P, Smith A N 1975 Fistula and conditions associated with diverticular disease of the colon. Clinics in Gastroenterology 4: 171
Smith A N, Attisha R P, Balfour T 1969 Clinical and manometric results one year after sigmoid myotomy for diverticular disease. British Journal of Surgery 56: 895
Speer C S, Bacon H E 1962 Coexisting diverticular and neoplastic disease of the colon. Surgery 52: 733
Spriggs E I, Marxer O A 1925 Intestinal diverticula. Quarterly Journal of Medicine 19: 1
Stone H H, Allen W B, Smith R B, Haynes C D 1968 Infantile pneumatosis intestinalis. Journal of Surgical Research 8: 301
Sugihara K, Muto T, Morioka Y 1983 Motility study in right sided diverticular disease of the colon. Gut 24: 1130
Sugihara K, Muto T, Morioka Y, Asano A, Yamamoto T 1984 Diverticular disease of the colon in Japan. A review of 615 cases. Diseases of the Colon and Rectum 27: 531
Tak P P, van Duinen C M, Bun P et al 1992 Pneumatosis cystoides intestinalis in intestinal pseudoobstruction. Resolution after therapy with metronidazole. Digestive Diseases and Sciences 37: 949–954
Taylor F W, Epstein L I 1969 Treatment of massive diverticular hemorrhage. Archives of Surgery 98: 505
Thompson W G, Patel D G 1986 Clinical picture of diverticular disease of the colon. Clinical Gastroenterology 15: 903–916
Tudor R G, Farmakis N, Keighley M R B 1994 National audit of complicated diverticular disease: analysis of index cases. British Journal of Surgery 81: 730–732
Verbanck J, Lambrecht S, Rutgeerts L et al 1989 Can sonography diagnose acute colonic diverticulitis in patients with acute colonic inflammation? Journal of Clinical Ultrasound 17: 661–666
Wagner D E, Zollinger R W 1961 Diverticulitis of the cecum and ascending colon. Archives of Surgery 83: 436
Weinreich J, Andersen D 1976 Intraluminal pressure in the sigmoid colon. II. Patients with sigmoid diverticula and related conditions. Scandinavian Journal of Gastroenterology 11: 581
Whiteway J, Morson B C 1985 Elastosis in diverticular disease of the sigmoid colon. Gut 26: 258
Williams B F P 1967a Conservative management of endometriosis: follow-up observations of progestin therapy. Obstetrics and Gynecology 30: 76
Williams I 1967b Diverticular disease of the colon without diverticula. Radiology 89: 401
Williams K L 1960 Acute solitary ulcers and acute diverticulitis of the caecum and ascending colon. British Journal of Surgery 47: 351
Woods R J, Lavery J C, Fazio V W et al 1988 Internal fistulas in diverticular disease. Diseases of the Colon and Rectum 31: 591–596
Wright H K, Pelliccia O, Higgins E F, Sreenivas V, Gupta A 1980 Controlled, semielective, segmental resection for massive colonic hemorrhage. American Journal of Surgery 139: 535
Zollinger R W 1968 The prognosis in diverticulitis of the colon. Archives of Surgery 97: 418

# 55. Polyps and carcinoma

*M. G. Dunlop*

## POLYPS OF THE LARGE INTESTINE

In the large intestine a "polyp" is generally regarded as a benign epithelial tumor, although polyps arising from submucosal lesions can occasionally cause confusion during colonoscopy (see below). The histological classification of polyps of epithelial origin into four groups has clinical relevance (Morson et al 1983; Table 55.1). True neoplastic polyps are classified as tubular adenomas, tubulovillous adenomas and villous adenomas (Morson & Dawson 1979) (Fig. 55.1).

**Table 55.1** Classification of benign intestinal polyps

| Type | Solitary form | Multiple form |
|---|---|---|
| Neoplastic | Adenoma | Familial adenomatous polyposis |
| Hamartomatous | Juvenile<br>Peutz–Jeghers | Juvenile polyposis<br>Peutz–Jeghers syndrome |
| Inflammatory | Benign lymphoid polyp | Benign lymphoid polyposis<br>Inflammatory polyposis in colitis |
| Unclassified | Metaplastic (hyperplastic) | Multiple metaplastic polyps |

## NEOPLASTIC POLYPS

### Evidence that neoplastic polyps are precancerous

Evidence for the adenoma–carcinoma sequence in colorectal malignancy is substantial. The association of benign and malignant lesions could be due to a common etiological agent but the weight of evidence argues strongly that the adenoma is the major precursor of colorectal carcinoma (Morson et al 1983). For obvious reasons, adenomas at high risk of malignant conversion are not left *in situ* and so there are few studies of their natural history. In one study, 49% of adenomas smaller than 5 mm in diameter enlarged over a 2-year period, corresponding to a doubling of adenoma mass (Hoff et al 1986). None of the polyps grew larger than 5 mm but because adenomas larger than 5 mm were excluded, the implication of the study in terms of the larger adenomas is not clear. Another study of untreated polyps larger than 1 cm showed a cumulative risk of cancer at the same site of 2.5%, 8% and 24% at 5, 10 and 20 years respectively (Stryker et al 1987). Over a mean follow-up of some 9 years, 37% of polyps enlarged, 10% of patients developed invasive cancer at the site of the polyp and 5% developed remote cancer.

The adenoma–carcinoma sequence does not exclude the possibility that carcinoma can arise de novo (Jass 1989), a contention supported by the "flat adenoma"

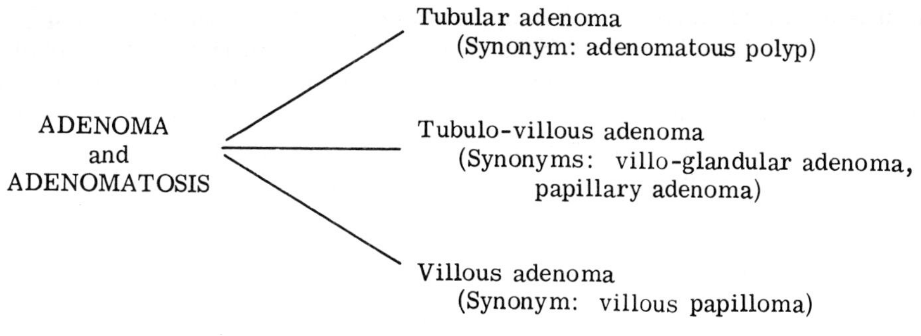


**Fig. 55.1** Classification of neoplastic polyps.

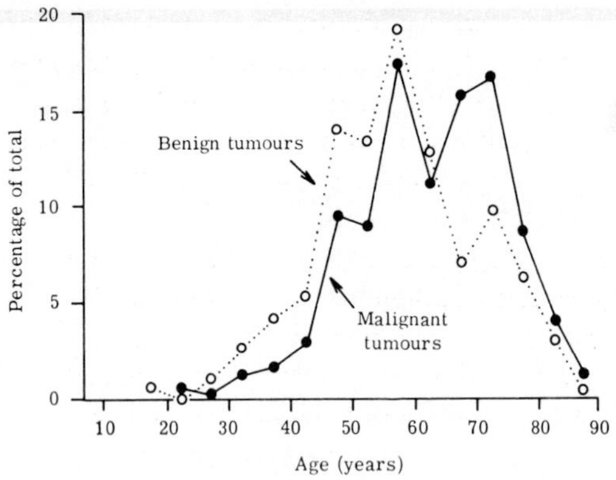


**Fig. 55.2** Age distribution of 188 patients with benign polyps in the large intestine and 98 patients with coexisting polyps and cancer in the large intestine seen at St Mark's Hospital, London (Morson & Dawson 1972).

syndrome (Muto et al 1985; see below). The adenoma–carcinoma sequence has important implications in that population screening and removal of adenomas can only be successful if this is at least the major pathway for the development of colorectal cancer.

*Age distribution studies*

The steep rise in the detection rate of adenomas occurs on average 5 years earlier than the parallel rise in diagnosis of carcinoma (Fig. 55.2). In one study, the average age at detection of single adenomas (58.1 years) predated that of single carcinomas (62.1 years) by 4 years (Muto et al 1975).

*Epidemiological studies* (Weisburger et al 1975, Correa & Haenszel 1978, Restrepo et al 1981)

Demographic variations in incidence of colorectal cancer closely parallel those of adenoma. Areas with a high incidence of large bowel cancer such as Liverpool (Williams et al 1982) have a much higher prevalence of adenomas at autopsy than countries such as Nigeria, where colorectal cancer is uncommon (Williams et al 1975). The prevalence of colorectal adenomas and carcinomas increase in parallel with migration from a low- to a high-incidence area. The prevalence of adenomas in native Japanese over the age of 50 is 27% (Sato et al 1976) whereas in Hawaiian-Japanese in the same age group it is 63% (Stemmerman & Yatani 1973). Adenomas are uncommon in indigenous African populations such as Nigerians and South African Bantus (Bremner & Ackerman 1970), whereas in New Orleans, adenomas (and colorectal cancer) are actually more prevalent in negroes than whites (Correa et al 1977).

*Anatomical distribution of colorectal adenomas and carcinomas*

The segmental distribution of adenomas in autopsy (Clark et al 1985), radiological and colonoscopic studies (Gillespie et al 1979) is similar to that of cancer. Approximately 66–75% of colorectal cancers arise in the rectum and sigmoid colon (Falterman et al 1974, Goligher 1984) and large adenomas are commoner in these regions (Williams et al 1982). In a series of 1187 adenomas, 47% occurred in the sigmoid colon, the distribution decreasing proximally to the right colon (8.2%) (Morson et al 1983). The proportion of adenomas larger than 1 cm was higher in the sigmoid colon whereas adenomas smaller than 5 mm were distributed evenly throughout the colon and rectum.

*Studies on the simultaneous occurrence of polyps and cancer*

Approximately one-third of colorectal cancer resection specimens contain adenomatous polyps (Morson & Dawson 1979). Such patients are twice as likely to develop metachronous large bowel tumors (a tumor which develops subsequently to the primary tumor) as those without polyps (10% versus 5% lifetime risk) (Heald & Bussey 1975, Muto et al 1975, Morson et al 1984). Furthermore, adenomas in patients who develop metachronous tumors show more dysplasia. The risk of metachronous cancer also increases with increasing numbers of polyps, reaching 70% if six or more polyps are present (Muto et al 1975). Fifty percent of colons resected for synchronous cancers (tumors which develop simultaneously) carry incidental polyps (Heald & Bussey 1975) and the incidence of cancer at autopsy is 50% higher in individuals with multiple polyps than in those with a solitary polyp (Ekelund 1963).

*Studies on the pathology of adenomas and cancer*

Muto et al (1975) found that 14% of malignant tumors were partly composed of benign adenomatous tissue. In the experience of Morson (1966), 57% of carcinomas limited to the submucosa had a benign component; when spread was limited to the bowel wall the figure was 18% and when there was transmural involvement, it fell to only 8%. In situ carcinoma virtually always has adjacent benign tissue (Lane 1976). All of this suggests that the development of carcinoma involves replacement of a benign precursor by invasion and/or destruction. Very small cancers are never found (Culp 1967), implying that tumors arise only from polyps. However, the pathological definition of cancer requires invasion of the submucosa and there is clearly a selection bias in favor of larger lesions which have been present for some time.

*The effects of prophylactic polypectomy*

Comparative studies strongly suggest that removing adenomas reduces the risk of colorectal cancer. However, prospective randomized controlled trials with death from colorectal cancer as the endpoint are still needed to determine whether screening and polypectomy are indeed beneficial.

One study concluded that rigid sigmoidoscopy and polypectomy reduced the incidence of rectosigmoid carcinoma in screened patients by 84% (Gilbertsen 1974). However, symptomatic individuals and 27 cases of cancer diagnosed at the first screen were excluded. This, combined with lack of a true control population, makes it likely that the expected and observed numbers of cancers in the study group were similar. Two further studies employing rigid sigmoidoscopy and polypectomy (Hertz et al 1960, Selby et al 1988) also have shortcomings. For example, the Kaiser Permanente study (Selby et al 1988) was randomized and controlled and is frequently cited as showing a 60% reduction in colorectal cancer mortality (Friedman et al 1986). However, the frequency of death from all causes was almost identical in screened and control groups and only subgroup analysis showed reduction in colorectal cancer mortality. In addition, because the controls were also in the Kaiser Permanente health plan, 25% of the controls versus 30% of the screened group underwent sigmoidoscopy. It is difficult to explain the observed mortality benefit given the small difference in access to sigmoidoscopy and polypectomy.

More definitive evidence for benefit in removal of colorectal polyps comes from a recent cohort study of 1418 symptomatic and asymptomatic screened patients who underwent colonoscopic polypectomy (Winawer et al 1993). Although the study has been criticized for lack of a formal control cohort, practical issues in the USA meant that such controls were not possible. However, the polypectomized cohort were compared with historical controls from outside the USA and a 76–90% reduction in expected colorectal cancer risk was noted in the study group compared to each of the three comparative groups.

The evidence for benefit of polypectomy from all of the studies discussed above does seem compelling. However, death from colorectal cancer is the most important endpoint for the individual and recently evidence for a reduction in colorectal cancer mortality in polypectomized patients has been demonstrated in a large randomized study of population screening for colorectal cancer by fecal occult blood testing in which polyps were removed colonoscopically (Mandel et al 1993).

*Study of the molecular genetics of colorectal adenomas and carcinomas*

Molecular genetic evidence supports the adenoma–carcinoma sequence and underlines the increased malignant potential of larger and more villous adenomas. Mutations in the Kirsten *ras* gene can be detected in 40–50% of colorectal cancers (Bos et al 1987, Forrester et al 1987). In small adenomas with low grade dysplasia, *ras* mutations are found in only 13% of tumors but in larger, more histologically aggressive lesions, they are as frequent as in carcinomas (Vogelstein et al 1988). *Ras* mutations can also be demonstrated in both the benign and malignant elements of lesions possessing both these components (Vogelstein et al 1988).

Familial adenomatous polyposis (FAP) is a model for the progression of adenoma to carcinoma. The hundreds or thousands of adenomatous polyps which characterize this disorder render the affected individual at such high risk of cancer that prophylactic colectomy is routinely advised. The cancer risk strongly supports the notion that polyps are the precursors of colorectal cancer. Mutations in the gene responsible for FAP (the APC gene) are ubiquitous in the resulting tumors and are also found in 60% of sporadic colorectal cancers and adenomas (Powell et al 1992, Nagase & Nakamura 1993, Ichii et al 1993). As with other tumor suppressor genes, both copies of APC probably have to be inactivated for neoplastic change. Patients with FAP inherit one mutant APC allele whereas the adenomas in the colon and rectum acquire a somatic mutation in the normal copy of the APC gene as they enlarge and become more dysplastic. Non-FAP cases acquire two inactivated APC alleles by somatic mutation. APC mutations have been detected in 3 mm adenomas (Powell et al 1992, Ichii et al 1993) and the fact that they are as frequent as in late-stage carcinomas indicates that they are involved in initiation of neoplasia.

*Bile acids and progression from adenoma to carcinoma*

Bile acids are not implicated as a cause of adenomas but total fecal bile acid and bile acid profile are correlated with the size of adenomas and possibly with the severity of epithelial dysplasia and villous change (Hill 1985). The contention that bile acids promote the progression of adenoma to carcinoma is supported by evidence from animal studies.

## Etiology and incidence of colorectal adenomas

Adenomas are very common, especially in the elderly. Rickert et al (1979) found one or more in 71% of males in the 65–69 year age group. The rate of sigmoidoscopic detection of polyps in patients over 40 years varies from 4.7% to 9.7% (Rider et al 1954, Winawer et al 1976) although some of these polyps are metaplastic rather than adenomatous. Colonoscopy in asymptomatic individuals over 50 years of age reveals adenomas in around 40% of cases (Foutch et al 1991, DiSario et al 1991), while autopsy studies indicate that the rate of adenoma carriage in developed countries is 37–51% (Morson et al 1983).

*The histological development of adenomas*

This has been studied most extensively in FAP (Bussey

1975, Mughai & Filipe 1978, Maskens 1979). Adenomas develop from an area of epithelial hyperplasia which shows hyperchromatism, decreased mucus production and increased mitotic activity. The glands become irregular and branched. DNA-synthesizing cells accumulate on the mucosal surface and their proliferation results in infolding of the surface epithelium between normal glands, producing the characteristic shape of the tubular adenoma. It is postulated that villous adenomas result from outfolding of the surface epithelium (Maskens 1979).

**Pathology** (Enterline 1976, Morson 1976a,b)

An adenoma is a benign pedunculated or sessile neoplasm of glandular epithelium in which there is cellular atypia of varying degree. The International Histological Classification of Tumours recognizes the following types:

- **Tubular adenomas (adenomatous polyps).** These are composed predominantly of branching tubules embedded in or surrounded by lamina propria (Fig. 55.3). They are usually pedunculated but can be sessile and are occasionally large.
- **Villous adenomas.** These are composed of pointed or blunt finger-like processes of lamina propria and are covered by epithelium which reaches down to the muscularis mucosae (Fig. 55.4). Excess mucus secretion is sometimes seen. The tumor is more often sessile than pedunculated and can cover a large surface area.
- **Tubulovillous adenomas.** These may have both tubular and villous patterns or an intermediate pattern (Fig. 55.5). They are also known as villoglandular adenomas and can be sessile or pedunculated.

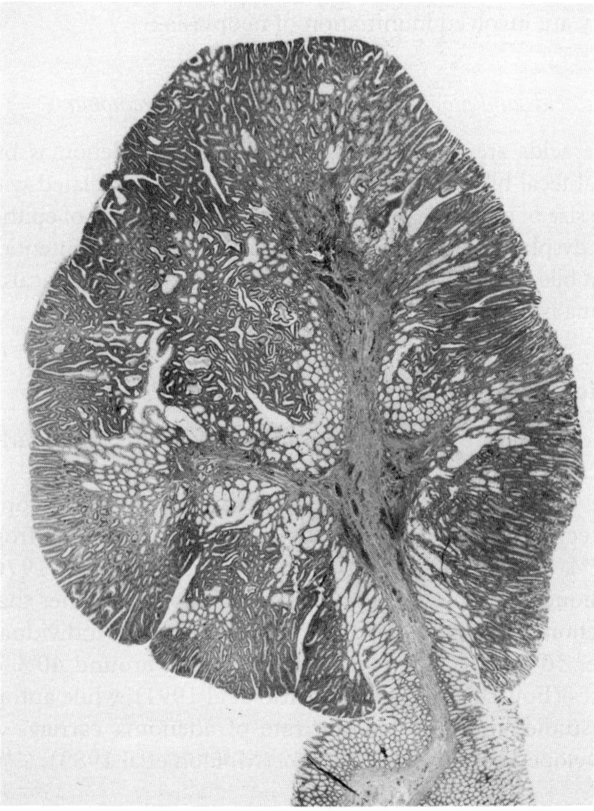

**Fig. 55.3** Tubular adenoma showing tubular glands sectioned both longitudinally and transversely. The adenoma is pedunculated (hematoxylin and eosin, $\times 5\frac{1}{2}$).

The macroscopic appearance of adenomatous and villous polyps led to them being regarded as separate entities. However, the different types result from different growth patterns and a single adenoma can have both tubular and villous architecture. In general, tubular adenomas show mild cellular atypia, whereas villous types show marked atypia. In all of these neoplasms, the columnar epithelium tends to become taller and contain more nuclei which are often large and hyperchromatic. Mitotic figures are increased. Enterochromaffin and Paneth cells are distributed randomly in contrast to their basal location in normal epithelium. Tubular polyps have fewer goblet cells whereas villous tumors continue to produce mucus.

Disordered glandular formation or severe cellular atypia confined to the mucosa is termed noninvasive carcinoma or carcinoma in situ. Invasive carcinoma should be diagnosed only when tumor has penetrated the muscularis mucosae (Fig. 55.6). Difficulties in interpretation may arise when adenomatous tissue is displaced into the submucosa, so-called pseudocarcinomatous invasion.

Tubular adenomas account for 75% of all adenomas, villous adenomas for 10% and intermediate types for 15%. However, villous adenomas account for 60% of lesions larger than 2 cm (Morson 1976a); only 3% of tubular adenomas are larger than 2 cm. Although villous tumors occur throughout the bowel, they are most common in the rectum (Morson 1984).

Adenomas of the colon and rectum are usually small, 48–60% being less than 1 cm in diameter (Morson et al 1976a, Gillespie et al 1979). In the colonoscopic study of Gillespie et al (1979), 65% of patients had one adenoma, 18% had two, 8% had three and only 2.6% had more than five adenomas. With adenomas larger than 1 cm, Morson et al (1983) found that 50% of patients had only one tumor, 24% had two, 14% had three and 12% had four or more. In another large study, 1.4% of patients had six or more adenomatous polyps, the largest number being 48 (Bussey 1975). Studies using sequential flexible sigmoidoscopy and colonoscopy show that 55% of all adenomas arise in the sigmoid colon or rectum (i.e. within approximately 60 cm of the anus) (Dunlop 1992). A radiological study (Bernstein et al 1985) found that 52% of polyps were proximal to the sigmoid colon and that older patients had significantly more right-sided polyps and fewer rectosigmoid polyps.

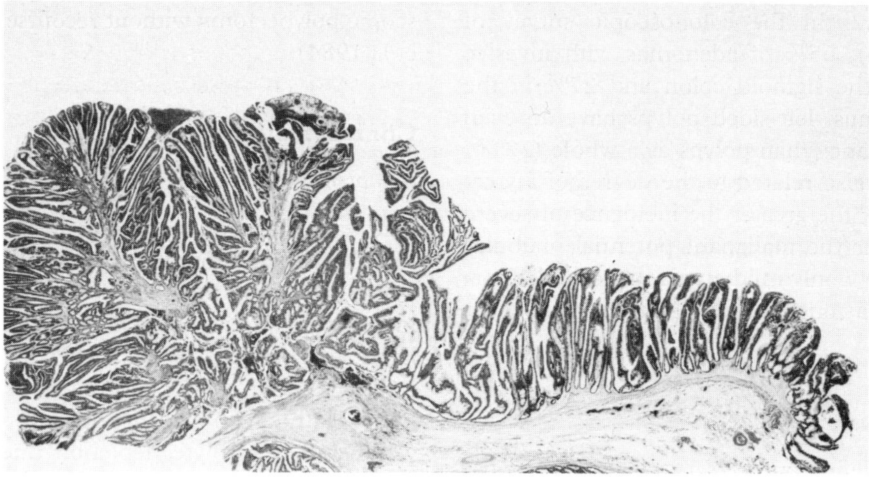

**Fig. 55.4** Villous adenoma. Part of a sessile adenoma composed of long finger-like folds of lamina propria covered by epithelium (hematoxylin and eosin, ×4).

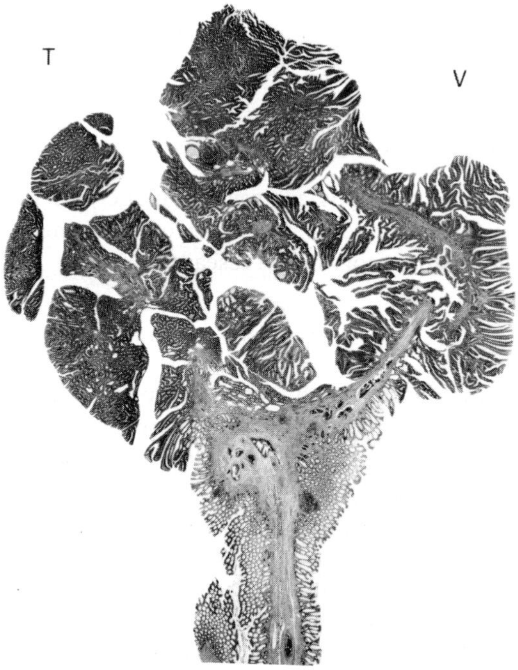


**Fig. 55.5** Tubulovillous adenoma. A large pedunculated adenoma with tubular (T) and villous (V) areas (hematoxylin and eosin, $\times 3\frac{1}{2}$).

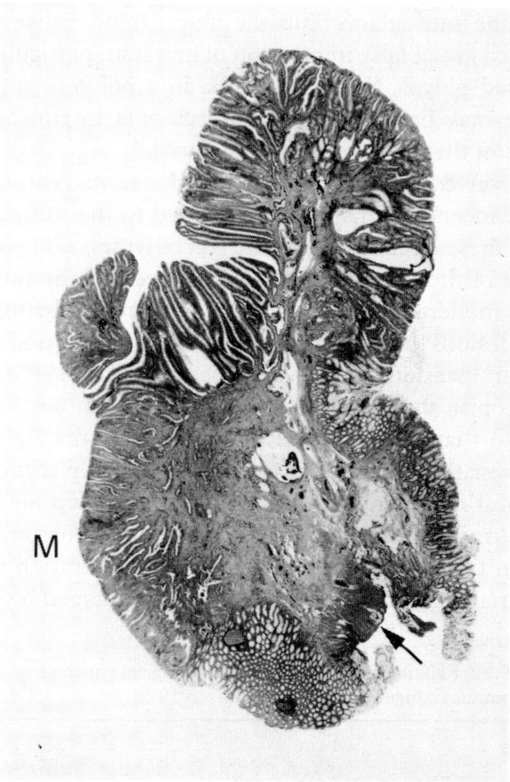


**Fig. 55.6** Cancer in an adenoma. Predominantly villous adenoma showing a focus of malignancy (M) with invasion through the muscularis mucosae. Coagulation diathermy artefact is seen at the base (arrow) (hematoxylin and eosin, ×6).

*The malignant potential of adenomas* (Morson 1976a)

Autopsy studies at St Mark's suggest that around 10% of tubular adenomas larger than 1 cm become malignant (Morson et al 1983), an annual conversion rate of three per 100 adenomas (Eide 1986). The risk of cancer was 1% for adenomas smaller than 1 cm, 10% for those of between 1 and 2 cm and 46% for those larger than 2 cm. Where carcinoma and adenoma were present in the same lesion, the adenoma was tubular in 33%, tubulovillous in 31% and villous in 36% of cases. As only 10% of adenomas are villous, the risk of malignant conversion in a villous adenoma is substantially greater. In an update of this series, the cumulative adenoma risk after removal of one or more adenomas was 50% and the cancer risk was 7% (Morson & Bussey 1985). However, in patients initially presenting with multiple polyps, the cancer risk was 13% at 15 years. The effect of size and histological type on malignancy is shown in Table 55.2. In the colonoscopic survey of Gillespie et al (1979), 65% of adenomas with invasive malignancy were in the sigmoid colon and 27% in the descending colon. Thus, left-sided polyps have an even greater risk of malignancy than polyps as a whole (72%). The risk of cancer is also related to the degree of atypia. The larger the tumor, the greater the incidence of severe atypia and the greater the malignant potential. Tubular adenomas usually show only mild atypia, but when atypia is severe, there is a one in four chance of cancer (Table 55.3).

*The malignant polyp and early cancer*

The pathological definition of a malignant polyp (Fig. 55.6) requires invasion of the pedicle or, in the case of sessile tumors, penetration of the muscularis mucosae. Two problems can arise in interpretation: adenomatous tissue may be displaced into the submucosa and hyperplasia of the muscularis mucosae may extend between the glands to give a false impression of invasion, particularly in left-sided polyps. Severe dysplasia in a polyp or mucosal surface may be classified as a carcinoma in situ and by definition there is no evidence of invasion.

Morson & Dawson (1979) use the term "early colorectal cancer" when spread is confined to the submucosa. Under these circumstances, the risk of lymph node metastases is of the order of only a few percent if the tumor is well or moderately well differentiated, but poorly differentiated lesions have a 66% risk of metastasis and show vascular invasion in 16% of cases (Cooper 1983). The endoscopist should provide an excisional biopsy in one piece so that the pathologist can orientate the specimen and assess the completeness of excision by step sections. It is helpful if the endoscopist impales the polyp on a fine hypodermic needle at the site of resection before immersing it in fixative (Riddell 1985). Such co-operation allows many malignant colorectal polyps to be managed by endoscopic polypectomy without recourse to resection (Morson et al 1984).

**Table 55.2** Relationship between size, histological type and carcinomatous change in adenomas (Morson 1976a)

| Histology | <1 cm | | 1–2 cm | | >2 cm | |
|---|---|---|---|---|---|---|
| | *n* | % cancer | *n* | % cancer | *n* | % cancer |
| Tubular adenoma | 1382 | 1% | 392 | 10% | 101 | 35% |
| Intermediate type | 76 | 4% | 149 | 7% | 155 | 46% |
| Villous adenoma | 21 | 10% | 39 | 10% | 174 | 53% |

## Clinical features

*Symptoms*

The vast majority of polyps are asymptomatic and are found on sigmoidoscopy when abdominal complaints are being investigated or the patient is being checked following colonic surgery. Polyps can cause rectal bleeding or large bowel colic, especially when a large polyp has caused intussusception. Patients with villous adenomas, especially of the rectum, can present with severe watery diarrhea and water and electrolyte depletion due to excessive mucus loss.

*Digital examination of the rectum*

Most adenomas within reach of the examining finger are palpable, but villous tumors are soft and sessile and 26% were missed in one series (Ramirez et al 1965).

## Investigations and diagnosis

Most colorectal polyps are asymptomatic and investigation is usually aimed at excluding or confirming malignancy or inflammatory bowel disease.

*Sigmoidoscopy*

Rigid sigmoidoscopy only detects around 30% of polyps but flexible sigmoidoscopy greatly increases the yield (see above). Although flexible sigmoidoscopy allows negotiation of the rectosigmoid junction, many centers use colonoscopy to inspect even the distal large bowel, given its superior range and the same requirement for instrument cleaning and bowel preparation. The macroscopic appearances of polyps are described on page 1402, but villous tumors often merge into the normal mucosa and can be difficult to identify. Sigmoidoscopy is performed before barium enema as the rectosigmoid junction is a particularly difficult area for the radiologist.

*Double-contrast barium enema and colonoscopy*

Single contrast barium enemas fail to demonstrate a sub-

**Table 55.3** Frequency of carcinoma in relation to the grade of atypia and histological type of adenoma (Morson 1976a)

| Grade of atypia | Tubular adenoma | | Intermediate | | Villous adenoma | |
|---|---|---|---|---|---|---|
| | *n* | (% carcinoma) | *n* | (% carcinoma) | *n* | (% carcinoma) |
| Mild | 1410 | 2% | 208 | 14% | 116 | 36% |
| Moderate | 357 | 9% | 119 | 32% | 73 | 41% |
| Severe | 113 | 27% | 56 | 34% | 54 | 50% |

stantial proportion of polyps (Winawer 1976), while double-contrast studies detect nearly all polyps when carried out by experts (Ott et al 1986). For polyps larger than 5 mm the detection rate should approach 90–95%, but the detection rate for diminutive polyps (under 5 mm) ranges from 26% to 93%, with an average of 61% (Ott et al 1986). In one study, the detection rate was 26% for 2–3 mm polyps, 56% for 4–5 mm polyps, 83% for polyps of 6–9 mm and 100% for polyps larger than 1 cm (Rex et al 1986). Double-contrast barium enema can be less accurate than colonoscopy, particularly when diverticular disease is present (Farrands et al 1983), although the techniques are probably equally accurate when carried out by experts (Thoeni & Petras 1982). Aldridge & Sim (1986) studied 97 patients with persistent large bowel symptoms after double-contrast enemas had been reported as normal or showing diverticular disease and detected four carcinomas and 22 polyps. The frequency of neoplasia in those with a normal barium enema was 32% and in those with diverticular disease, 23%. These data led the authors to suggest that colonoscopy should be the primary investigation for persistent large bowel symptoms.

Polyps appear as filling defects protruding into the barium column or as opacities on the surface of which a thin coat of barium projects into the distended air-filled lumen (p. 18). While a polyp may be suspected on one projection, the diagnosis should only be confirmed when it is seen on two or more radiographs. Adherent fecal residue may mimic polyps; changes in position sometimes show that a fecal lump is mobile and palpation may help differentiation. Air bubbles, mucous streaks, a single small diverticulum, deformities from previous appendicectomy or other operations and prominent lymphoid follicles can also mislead (Kelvin 1982). Errors in interpretation probably account for more than 50% of misdiagnoses. The most common errors are failure to identify a filling defect in the barium pool or recognize a tumor en face in double contrast (Kelvin et al 1981). Careful viewing and double reading all enhance the accuracy of double-contrast barium enema.

### *The detection of malignancy*

Pedunculated polyps are often mobile and move under the influence of gravity; the presence of a long stalk generally signals the absence of invasive cancer. Villous adenomas have a characteristic frond-like appearance, particularly in the rectum, but cannot be characterized as benign or malignant on radiological criteria. The surface of a polyp, whether benign or malignant, tends to be smooth. As size increases, the surface may become lobulated or irregular, but typical malignant changes only become apparent when the polyp reaches 2–3 cm. Retraction of the base of a polyp may indicate bowel wall invasion and malignancy, but was not seen in one series of benign and malignant polyps (Skucas et al 1982). With widespread access to colonoscopy, the subtler aspects of radiological distinction between benign and malignant polyps are largely irrelevant. As discussed above, the only radiological feature of any consequence is size, assuming that the magnification factor of the examination is taken into account.

Colonoscopy is used increasingly in diagnosis since polyps can be removed during the examination. It is indicated when there has been rectal bleeding, when one or more polyps have been detected by sigmoidoscopy and when individuals who have had colonic cancer or multiple polyps are being screened.

### *The differential diagnosis of polyps*

Neoplastic polyps must be differentiated from benign lymphoid polyps, juvenile polyps, submucosal lipomas, leiomyoma and leiomyosarcoma, lymphosarcoma, carcinoid tumor and inflammatory polyps and granulomas (which occur in ulcerative colitis, Crohn's disease, amebiasis and lymphogranuloma venereum). Enlarged anal papillae can be mistaken for polyps on digital examination.

## Treatment

### *Removal of polyps in the lower rectum* (Lawrence 1976)

Pedunculated polyps within reach of the sigmoidoscope can be excised with a cautery snare. If the polyp is benign or if it contains in situ or invasive cancer on microscopy but the pedicle is uninvolved, treatment is regarded as complete. If invasive cancer is identified in the stalk and the excision margins are not clear, resectional surgery appropriate to cancer at that location is indicated. Transanal full thickness excision of lesions close to the anus is a useful means of avoiding low restorative resection with its potential for anastomotic leakage and functional upset (p. 123).

Sessile polyps within reach of the sigmoidoscope should be biopsied or excised. Benign lesions are fulgurated and further treatment is unnecessary. If the lesion is large and a biopsy reveals benign disease or cancer in situ, transanal excision should be attempted. If infiltrating cancer is shown on biopsy, resection must be considered.

Local procedures result in hemorrhage in a small proportion of cases and perforation is a rare complication when the polyp is above the peritoneal reflection.

### *Colonoscopic polypectomy* (p. 125)

Colonoscopic polypectomy has revolutionized the treatment of polyps beyond the reach of the rigid sigmoidoscope. It is possible to remove or ablate over 90% of polyps (Gillespie et al 1979) with mortality and morbidity rates which are lower than those of laparotomy and colotomy (Berci et al 1974). Colonoscopy can usually be carried out on an outpatient basis or with overnight admission. Larger polyps can be removed by electrocautery snare while smaller lesions can be biopsied and destroyed using "hot" biopsy forceps which fulgurate any residual adenoma (p. 125). Every effort should be made to recover polyp tissue for histological examination to confirm the diagnosis and assess malignant potential and completeness of removal. Of 1049 adenomas removed by Gillespie et al (1979), 46 patients had polyp(s) with invasive carcinoma and 30 of them were treated by colonoscopic polypectomy without surgical resection.

Complications of colonoscopic polypectomy are rare; bleeding occurs in 0.7% of cases and perforation in 0.3% (Berci et al 1974).

*Laser treatment of colonic polyps* (Fleischer 1986)

Laser photocoagulation has been used to destroy colorectal adenomas, but is expensive and increases the risk of perforation.

*Resectional surgery for adenomatous polyps of the colon and rectum*

Resection or colotomy with polypectomy are indicated in the rare event that polyps cannot be removed at colonoscopy. Polyps larger than 1 cm or with suspicious irregularities should be removed if the patient is fit enough, but in the elderly and infirm, the risk of malignancy has to be balanced against the risk of surgery.

Subtotal colectomy and ileosigmoid or ileorectal anastomosis is now offered increasingly to patients prone to develop adenomas who would otherwise require frequent colonoscopic surveillance, particularly when there is a strong family history of colorectal cancer. Resection may also be indicated for large villous adenomas, as around one-third of such lesions have a focus of carcinoma which is extremely difficult to detect by biopsy or even by transanal submucosal excision. After resection, patients are followed in the same way as after colonoscopic polypectomy.

*Management after polypectomy*

After removal of a benign polyp, colonoscopy is recommended at 6–12 months and thereafter every 2 years. The same applies when carcinoma in situ is found in the polyp but has been totally excised (Morson et al 1984). When the polyp is sessile, follow-up must be particularly thorough and frequent.

When *invasive carcinoma* is found in the polyp, the situation is controversial (Lancet 1984), in that the risk of death from unexcised malignant disease must be balanced against the risks of segmental resection in patients who are often elderly and have other chronic diseases (Riddell 1985). Advocates of more aggressive treatment cite the fact that lymph node metastases have been found in six of 24 patients with malignant colonic polyps treated by colectomy after apparently complete endoscopic polypectomy (Colacchio et al 1981). However, endoscopic polypectomy is regarded as adequate treatment in many centers, provided careful histopathological studies confirm complete excision. An exception is made for invasive poorly differentiated or anaplastic tumors for which segmental resection is indicated even if removal appears complete. Segmental resection is also indicated when invasive carcinoma extends to the margin of the polypectomy specimen.

## FAMILIAL ADENOMATOUS POLYPOSIS (Bussey 1975, Bulow 1987)

Familial adenomatous polyposis (FAP) is one of the commonest single gene disorders predisposing to cancer. First described in 1881 (Sklifasowski 1881), it was shown to be a heritable disorder in 1882 (Cripps 1882) and the risk of malignant progression was soon appreciated (Smith 1887). An autosomal dominant mode of inheritance was formally documented by Reed & Neel (1955).

In one of the few population studies to achieve complete registration, the annual incidence was 1.8 new patients per million, corresponding to 1/6670 live births/year with a population prevalence of one in 13 528 (Bulow 1987, Bisgaard et al 1994). The incidence around the world appears to be similar although completeness of registration is a logistic problem in developing countries (Reed & Neel 1955, Utsunomiya & Iwama 1978, Hill 1982, Bulow 1987). The syndrome is characterized by the development of 100 or more large bowel adenomas, usually during teenage years and early adulthood, with virtual certainty of colorectal cancer by the third or fourth decade if prophylactic colectomy is not undertaken.

Around 25% of affected individuals have no family history of FAP, the disease arising as a result of a mutation in the APC gene. The new mutation rate is estimated to be nine mutations/million gametes/generation. The incidence of cancer at initial presentation in such patients is the same as for unscreened cases with a positive family history. The offspring of patients with new mutations have a 50% risk of inheriting the mutant gene.

Study of clinical and molecular aspects of FAP has advanced our understanding of the role of tumor suppressor genes in multistage carcinogenesis, in addition to providing a model of the adenoma–carcinoma sequence.

### Pathology

The diagnosis of FAP requires the presence of more than 100 adenomatous polyps of the large bowel. The average

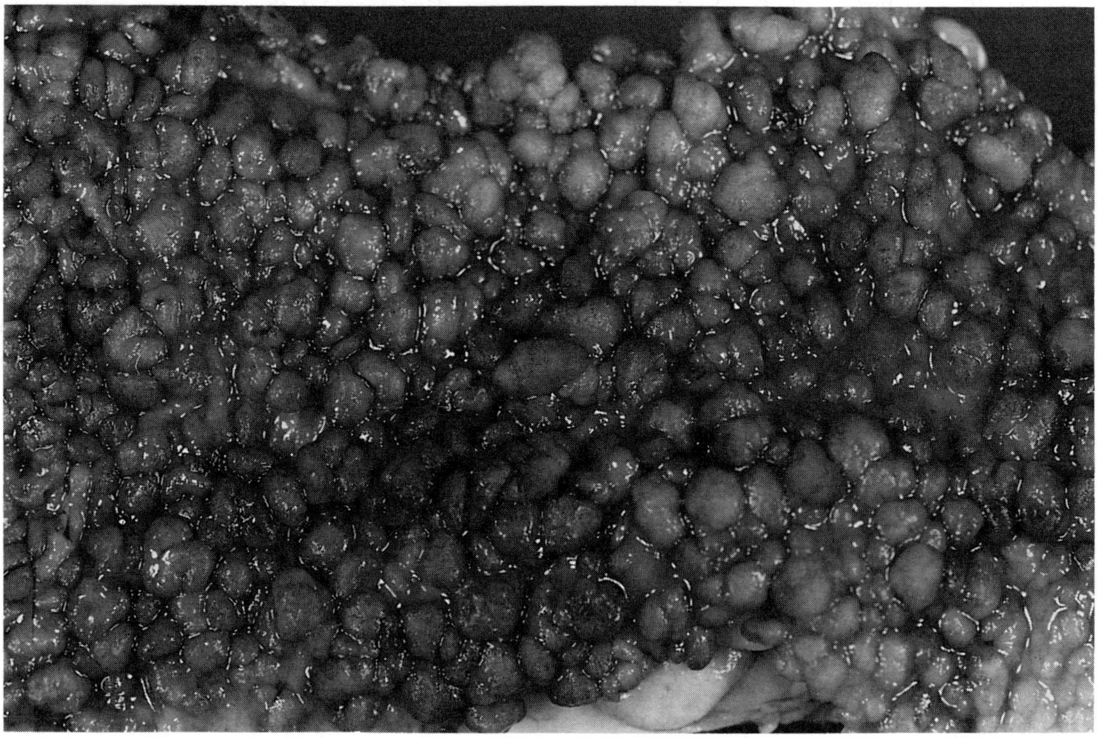

**Fig. 55.7** Colectomy specimen from a patient with familial adenomatous polyposis showing numerous adenomas of varying sizes which were of tubular and tubulovillous architecture.

number is around 1000, but can be 5000 (Bussey 1975). Detailed macroscopic (Fig. 55.7), histological and ultrastructural examination of colectomy specimens has revealed the stages of adenoma development from single crypt lesions to large tubular and villous adenomas (Bussey 1975, Mughai & Filipe 1978, Morson et al 1983). The adenomas and carcinomas show similar pathological features to those found in non-FAP cases and tubular, tubulovillous and villous adenomas are found in similar proportions (Morson et al 1983). The carcinomas are comparable as regards tumor site, stage, degree of differentiation and outcome (Utsunomiya & Iwama 1978). Given the sheer number of adenomas in FAP, the risk of malignant conversion of any one FAP adenoma is actually quite low.

## Clinical aspects

The peak age of detection of the onset of adenomas in screened and nonscreened individuals is 23.7 and 27 years respectively and for the detection of carcinomas, it is 33 and 39.2 years respectively (Bussey 1975, Bulow 1987, Murday & Slack 1989). Polyps do not usually develop before the age of 10 years, although the disorder has been recorded in a 3-year-old infant (Jackman & Beahrs 1968). A few patients have an attenuated form of FAP in which polyps do not appear until after the age of 40 years. The attenuated form is a distinct entity caused by mutations in a particular area of the gene (Spirio et al 1993) (see below) and the change from benign to malignant tumor can be very rapid (Lipkin 1978).

*Symptoms*

Since the aim is to identify affected individuals by screening, most new cases are asymptomatic at diagnosis. Patients with new mutations present with blood in the stool and/or diarrhea; abdominal pain and mucus in the stool are additional features. Two-thirds of patients who present with symptoms already have carcinomas.

*Diagnosis*

Since the rectum is always involved, the diagnosis can usually be established by rigid sigmoidoscopy and biopsy (Bulow 1987). Biopsy is necessary to exclude juvenile polyposis, Peutz–Jeghers syndrome, benign lymphoid polyposis and inflammatory polyposis. In pneumatosis cystoides (p. 1393), the polypoid structure (Fig. 4.20) bursts when biopsy is attempted. Barium enema in FAP shows multiple small filling defects (Marshak et al 1963) with an uneven distribution. In the 27 patients reported by Bartram & Thornton (1984), the predominant polyp size was 2–5 mm although variation was marked. In four cases, most polyps were larger than 5 mm, while in one patient all were less than 2 mm. The largest polyp seen measured

4 cm. In patients identified early (usually family members of index cases), the background nodular pattern was difficult to distinguish from lymphoid hyperplasia.

With the recent introduction of presymptomatic diagnosis by direct APC gene mutation analysis (see below), screening of affected individuals is used increasingly to define the optimal timing of prophylactic surgery relative to important educational or other milestones.

## The value of presymptomatic screening in FAP

Presymptomatic screening of at-risk individuals from polyposis kindreds results in early recognition of gene carriers and reduces the prevalence of colorectal cancer at first screening (Jarvinen 1992). Every effort must be made to identify affected individuals, register them and their relatives with a regional registry or clinical genetics service and screen those at risk. The prevalence of colorectal cancer at diagnosis is 64–69% for symptomatic nonscreened individuals and 3–6% for screened family members (Bussey 1975, Bulow 1987, Morton et al 1993).

## Prophylactic surgery

Early detection of FAP allows prophylactic colectomy before malignancy supervenes. Surgery involves removing all, or most, of the premalignant colorectal mucosa. This can be achieved by proctocolectomy with ileostomy, subtotal colectomy with ileorectal anastomosis or restorative proctocolectomy with formation of an ileal pouch reservoir (Parks et al 1980). Proctocolectomy with ileostomy was the operation of choice in many centers until recently, as it completely removes the premalignant epithelium but at the cost of a permanent ileostomy. A further disadvantage is that at-risk relatives may be so averse to the prospect of a stoma that they avoid surveillance and hence expose themselves to risk of malignancy. Proctocolectomy was carried out in 48% of FAP cases in one series (Bulow 1987) but in only 14% in the St Mark's series (Bussey et al 1985), reflecting the special interest in colectomy with ileorectal anastomosis at that center.

Although there is still a place for proctocolectomy and ileostomy in cases where rectal cancer has already supervened, this operation should not otherwise be performed without first discussing the alternatives. Most patients opt for one of these alternatives (and should be encouraged to do so), although the choice between them is subject to controversy and surgeon preference. The pouch operation is undoubtedly more complex but the best functional results obtained with it are at least as good as those of colectomy with ileorectal anastomosis (Beart 1985, Madden et al 1991). Interference with bladder control, potency or fertility occasionally complicates rectal excision, whereas the main disadvantage of colectomy with ileorectal anastomosis is the risk of cancer in the retained rectum. Estimates of this risk vary widely; Bulow et al (1984) estimated it at 13% at 10 years while Bussey et al (1985) calculated a cumulative risk of death from rectal cancer of 4% at 30 years. DeCosse et al (1992) analyzed data from three population-based registries and found a 13% chance of developing and a 2% chance of dying from rectal cancer after colectomy with ileorectal anastomosis. Long-term follow-up of the St Mark's series suggests that cancer risk increases dramatically with age, the lifetime risk reaching 29% in those who attain the age of 60 (Nugent & Phillips 1992). This led the authors to suggest that, since surveillance of the rectum is inadequate, it may be advisable to offer proctectomy and an ileoanal pouch to patients reaching 60 after colectomy with ileorectal anastomosis. One further consideration is the well-documented regression of polyps after colectomy with ileorectal anastomosis (Hubbard 1957, Williams & Fish 1966, Shepherd 1971, Bussey 1975, Nicholls et al 1988a); such regression does not reduce the need for careful surveillance of the retained rectum but does reduce the need for repeated fulguration.

In conclusion, the optimal treatment for patients who do not have rectal carpeting with polyps or a rectal cancer is now colectomy with ileorectal anastomosis (DeCosse et al 1992). If rectal polyps increase in size or become more dysplastic, proctocolectomy with ileal pouch–anal anastomosis can be performed subsequently.

## Extracolonic features of FAP

FAP is a constitutional genetic defect and its clinical features are not confined to the large bowel.

### *Gastroduodenal polyposis*

Gastric polyps have been found in 70% of FAP patients in some studies (Utsonomiya & Iwama 1978, Jarvinen et al 1983, Bulow 1987). In one prospective study, 55% of patients had gastric polyps although only 8% were adenomas (Spigelman et al 1989). The majority of gastric polyps show cystic enlargement of the fundic glands.

Duodenal adenomas are found in 35–98% of patients (Burt et al 1984, Bulow et al 1985, Sarre et al 1987, Spigelman et al 1989) and the periampullary region is particularly affected. Spigelman et al (1989) attribute this to the high local concentrations of bile. It is estimated that the risk of these tumors is increased 200-fold in FAP patients and the polyps can become malignant (Jones & Nance 1977, Pauli et al 1980, Jagelman et al 1988). The overall lifetime risk of periampullary cancer in patients cured of their colonic disease is 7–12% (Bussey 1972, Harned & Williams 1982, Bulow et al 1985). The prevalence of invasive upper gastrointestinal cancer in one study of 1255 patients was 4.5%, with duodenal and periampullary carcinoma making up 68% of all cases

**Table 55.4** Site of polyps in various polyposis syndromes

| Site | FAP | Turcot's syndrome | Juvenile polyposis | Cronkhite–Canada syndrome | Peutz–Jeghers syndrome |
|---|---|---|---|---|---|
| Esophagus | – | – | | + | – |
| Stomach | + | – | + | +++ | ++ |
| Duodenum | ++ | – | + | ++ | +++ |
| Small intestine | + | – | + | ++ | +++ |
| Colon and rectum | +++ | +++ | ++ | +++ | ++ |

– None; + Rare; ++ Common; +++ Predominant

(Jagelman et al 1988). After colectomy with ileorectal anastomosis, FAP patients are more likely to die of upper gastrointestinal cancer than carcinoma of the retained rectum. There is no clear evidence that screening and intervention have any effect on mortality from upper gastrointestinal malignancy, although this is currently being addressed in a European multicenter trial.

*Ileal polyposis*

Ileal adenomas also occur in FAP (Utsonomiya & Iwama 1978, Bulow 1987) and can develop after colectomy and ileorectal anastomosis (Hamilton et al 1979). The risk of progression to malignancy appears to be very low (Ross & Mara 1974, Jagelman et al 1988). The location of polyps in various syndromes which can be confused with FAP is shown in Table 55.4.

*Craniofacial and long bone osteomata*

The association of bone tumors and FAP was first noted by Gardner (Gardner & Plenk 1952) and the bone lesions were subsequently shown to be osteomas (Ooya et al 1976). The combination of osteomas, FAP and epidermoid cysts was once thought to be the distinct clinical entity of *Gardner's syndrome* but it is now clear that these manifestations are simply part of the spectrum of phenotypic expression of FAP. Osteomas are found in 81–93% of FAP patients (Utsunomiya & Nakamura 1975, Ushio et al 1976), the median number of mandibular osteomas being two, with a range of 1–6 (Bulow et al 1984) Their appearance tends to precede that of polyps by 18–20 years (Duncan et al 1968) and signifies that the patient is affected, even if polyps have yet to appear. Orthopantomography of the mandible as a means of screening at-risk individuals (Bulow 1987) is now irrelevant given the possibility of molecular genetic diagnosis. However, in individuals with multiple osteomas but no family history of FAP, serious consideration should be given to screening the colon as the patient may be a new case of FAP. There are no recorded cases of malignancy developing in an osteoma but local pain may necessitate excision.

*Desmoid tumors*

Intra-abdominal desmoids are a sinister problem in FAP. Their prevalence is variously reported as 4–15% (Smith 1958, Bussey 1975, Bulow 1986, Klemmer et al 1987) and 89% occur in women (Bulow 1986). They can be subdivided into those involving the abdominal wall and those within the abdomen. Most abdominal wall desmoids arise in recent surgical wounds and have a relatively uncomplicated course although they can cause local pain. Intra-abdominal tumors occur in 51% of cases (Bulow 1986) and are a much more capricious problem, frequently compressing and obstructing the ureters and other viscera. Some surgeons recommend rectal excision and ileoanal pouch formation as the primary procedure in FAP because subsequent pelvic desmoid disease can prevent excision of rectal carcinoma if colectomy with ileorectal anastomosis has been undertaken.

The association of desmoid tumors with FAP was first described by Smith (1958). These lesions are classified with other fibromatous conditions such as Dupuytren's contracture and keloid scar, but their nature is not clearly understood. Pain and discomfort can be very difficult to control and the patient may deteriorate progressively as the tumor compresses and obstructs intra-abdominal organs. Although surgical excision can be very effective for abdominal wall tumors, often little can be done for intra-abdominal and retroperitoneal disease. Management consists of surgical palliation as radical excision has unacceptable morbidity and mortality and regrowth is likely even if the patient survives (Lofti et al 1989). Treatment with teromiphene, tamoxifen, sulindac, indomethacin, chemotherapy and radiotherapy has limited value. An understanding of the functional deficit resulting from an inherited mutant APC allele may lead to more effective treatment.

*Epidermoid cysts* (Leppard 1974)

Multiple epidermoid cysts are found in approximately 50% of FAP patients and one-third have had one or more cysts removed in childhood (Leppard & Bussey 1975). The generic term "sebaceous cyst" is too broad and is best avoided in this context. The cysts tend to occur on the face and scalp whereas they are more common on the back in non-FAP cases. The mean number of cysts is around four but up to 20 have been found in one individual. Any epidermoid cyst on the face or scalp of a prepubescent child should be taken seriously as these lesions are very uncommon in this age group when not associated with FAP.

*Retinal pigmented lesions in FAP*

Pigmented lesions of the retina, known as congenital hypertrophy of the retinal pigment epithelium (CHRPE), are well described in association with FAP (Blair & Trempe 1980, Lynch et al 1987, Chapman et al 1989, Iwama et al 1990, Polkinghorne et al 1990) and their number correlates with the age of onset of polyps (Chapman et al 1989). The lesions are multiple, isolated, flat, well-demarcated, hyperpigmented areas and frequently affect both eyes. The hyperpigmented areas are usually surrounded by a hypopigmented halo and patchy depigmentation can occur within the lesion. Histologically, there is hypertrophy of the pigment epithelial cells with enlargement of pigment granules and degeneration of the overlying photoreceptors (Purcell & Shields 1975). The lesions do not appear to cause symptoms or affect visual fields or acuity. They are best visualized by indirect ophthalmoscopy as they are frequently peripheral. One study suggested that three or more pigmented lesions, particularly when occurring in both eyes, is a sensitive (100%) and specific (100%) indication of FAP status (Chapman et al 1989), but others report a sensitivity of 55–97% (Iwama et al 1990, Polkinghorne et al 1990). Clearly CHRPEs are a useful tool for detecting FAP but are of less value in excluding inheritance of the mutant gene. Although most at-risk members of known FAP families are now screened by direct APC gene mutation analysis, ophthalmologists should be aware that CHRPEs in otherwise asymptomatic individuals may indicate that the patient has a new APC mutation and requires colonic screening.

*Thyroid carcinoma*

Women below the age of 35 years with FAP are at 160 times greater risk of thyroid carcinoma than non-FAP counterparts (Alm & Licznerski 1973, Plail et al 1987). Men do not appear to be at increased risk. The carcinomas are predominantly papillary. Careful neck palpation is now part of the follow-up protocol for young women with FAP and fine-needle aspiration and ultrasound screening are used to assess suspicious nodules.

*Other associated conditions*

Other reported associations include hepatoblastoma, carcinoma of the gallbladder, bile duct and pancreas and an increased risk of brain tumors outside the defined Turcot's syndrome (see below).

## Genetics of FAP

*Gene penetrance and polyp formation*

Gene penetrance with regard to polyp formation is age dependent and the peak age incidence for presentation of polyps depends on whether the population was screened (Bussey 1975, Bulow 1987, Murday & Slack 1989). Correct assessment of age-dependent penetrance is important since risk estimations are partly derived from such calculations. The age of onset of polyps is frequently biased upwards as what is measured is the age at which polyps first present clinically. Age-dependent penetrance can only be assessed by calculations based on screened populations, as described by Murday & Slack (1989). Penetrance is close to 100% at 40 years of age (Bulow 1987, Murday & Slack 1989, Bisgaard et al 1994).

*The APC gene: location, function and mutations*

The APC gene was localized by genetic linkage analysis to the long arm of chromosome 5 in the band 21–22 (Bodmer et al 1987, Leppert et al 1987). The gene was then cloned and sequenced and mutations were identified in FAP kindreds (Groden et al 1991, Joslyn et al 1991, Kinzler et al 1991, Nishisho et al 1991). Germline mutations subsequently reported in around 250 FAP families (Nagase et al 1992b, Nagase & Nakamura 1993, Mandl et al 1994) are base substitutions or deletion/insertions which all result in truncation of the APC protein product. The mutations occur along the length of the gene but there are only two which occur in more than 5% of cases. APC gene mutations have also been demonstrated in almost all sporadic (non-FAP) carcinomas and in even the smallest premalignant adenomas (Powell et al 1992, Ichii et al 1993). The causative role of APC mutations in FAP and their detection at the very earliest stages of colorectal neoplasia indicate their crucial role in the genesis of colorectal cancer.

APC protein appears to influence cellular adhesion through cell surface molecules (Rubinfeld et al 1993, Su et al 1993). Antibodies show that the protein is expressed in epithelial cells in the upper portions of the colonic crypts, suggesting that it is functional in mature colonocytes (Smith et al 1993). Subcellular localization has demonstrated that wild type (i.e. normal) APC is closely associated with microtubules and promotes their formation, whereas mutant APC product does not (Munemitsu et al 1994, Smith et al 1994). APC could conceivably afford a direct line of communication from cell surface to microtubule formation.

Mutations in certain regions of the gene predict certain

clinical features. Thus mutations in one region result in an attenuated, usually late onset disease (Spirio et al 1993) whereas mutations in another result in a more extreme phenotype with profuse polyps in the colon and rectum (Nagase et al 1992a). Similarly, patients with mutations upstream of exon 9 do not have CHRPE lesions whereas downstream mutations are associated with a normal retina (Olschwang et al 1993). Other factors must be involved since identical APC mutations can be associated with diverse FAP phenotypes (Paul et al 1993, Groden et al 1993). Environmental interaction can undoubtedly modulate expression of the FAP phenotype since regression of rectal polyps after colectomy and ileorectal anastomosis is well recognized. There is also clear evidence of a modifying gene from a mouse model of FAP (Moser et al 1990) which maps to mouse chromosome 4, corresponding to human chromosomal region 1p35-36 (Dietrich et al 1993). Interestingly, this region is frequently involved in sporadic colorectal tumors. Pharmacological modulation of the FAP phenotype may become possible through manipulation of such a modifier gene. As the number of reported mutations increases and the quality of clinical data improves, elucidation of the clinical effects of different APC mutations may yield clues to the functional significance of various domains of the APC protein.

### *Predictive genetic testing for FAP*

Predictive genetic testing using the relatively crude tool of genetic linkage analysis has had considerable value in identifying affected individuals who had previously been discharged inappropriately from follow-up (Dunlop et al 1991). However, problems such as early death of gene carriers, uncertain paternity within families and the fact that around 25% of FAP patients carry a new mutation and have no family history substantially reduce the value of linkage studies.

Mutation analysis is now the most frequently used technique for presymptomatic testing and linkage analysis is reserved for confirmation of carrier status predictions in individuals where no APC mutation can be detected. Although laborious, identification of every mutation responsible for FAP will elucidate possible genotype-phenotype correlations and provide ultimate diagnostic reliability.

## TURCOT'S SYNDROME

The controversy as to whether Turcot's syndrome (Turcot et al 1959) is distinct from FAP remains unresolved. Adenomatous colorectal polyps occur in Turcot's syndrome but are characteristically less numerous than in FAP (Itoh et al 1979). Although brain tumors do occur rarely in FAP, Turcot's syndrome is characterized by astrocytoma (and medulloblastomas and glioblastomas) of the brain or spinal cord. The condition may well be an autosomal recessive trait, but its molecular basis is not established. Germline mutations in the APC gene have been identified in some Turcot's syndrome patients (Mori et al 1994) but this locus has been excluded in other families (Tops et al 1992). It seems likely that there are two similar syndromes, one which is due to particular APC gene mutations and the other to an unlinked locus.

## HEREDITARY FLAT ADENOMA SYNDROME

Since its description by Muto et al (1985), the flat adenoma has been recognized as an important "fast track" to malignancy (Jass 1989) and a challenge to the concept that all colorectal cancers arise from a pre-existing adenoma. The small flat lesions show varying degrees of dysplasia and more than 40% show focal carcinoma (Muto et al 1985). In lesions 9–10 mm in diameter, the probability of detecting carcinoma is 80%. Small flat carcinomas without any evidence of pre-existing adenomatous tissue are occasionally detected (Jass 1989) and have been termed "de novo carcinomas". It is not clear how often this occurs but it seems likely that the flat adenoma is a stage in the process.

Hereditary aspects of the flat adenoma syndrome have been appreciated in recent years. The lesions have been reported in true hereditary nonpolyposis colorectal cancer (HNPCC) families (Lynch et al 1988) and tend to be right sided. Lynch also found that some families were linked to the APC gene region on chromosome 5q (Lynch et al 1990). This suggests that although the patients did not have FAP, they did have an APC gene mutation which was incapable of inducing the full FAP phenotype.

## JUVENILE POLYPOSIS (Rolles 1987)

Juvenile polyps have an overall prevalence varying from 1% in autopsy series in the United States to around 5% in Colombia (Louw 1968, Correa et al 1977). They are commonest in prepubertal boys and are particularly common in children under 6 years of age. They can be multiple or solitary and multiple polyps are associated with a familial tendency (Veale et al 1966, Grotsky et al 1982). The pathological nature of the lesions is unclear but they are generally thought of as hamartomas.

In some cases there is a mixed juvenile and adenomatous polyposis syndrome (Veale et al 1966, Beacham et al 1978, Mazier et al 1982, Mestre 1986, Jones et al 1987, Sarles et al 1987). Although juvenile polyposis is generally thought not to carry an increased risk of colorectal cancer, it is now clear that there is substantial risk in mixed polyposis, particularly if multiple polyps are present. Several cases of colorectal cancer have arisen in patients with juvenile polyposis (Rozen & Baratz 1982, Jarvinen & Franssila 1984, Baptist & Sabatini 1985). The St Mark's Hospital data indicate that the cumulative risk of developing colorectal cancer is 68% at 60 years of age (Murday & Slack 1989). The risk of malignancy has prompted some to recommend prophylactic colectomy and ileorectal anastomosis if adenomatous polyps are detected in patients with juvenile polyposis (Jarvinen & Franssila 1984).

*Pathology*

Until the advent of routine colonoscopy and double-contrast barium enema, the juvenile polyp was thought to be more often single than multiple and autopsy series suggested a fairly even distribution throughout the colon (Correa & Haenszel 1978). It is now recognized that polyps are multiple in over 50% of cases (Mestre 1986). They are usually confined to the colon but although they are found throughout the gastrointestinal tract, most arise in the colon. The polyps are round, smooth and pedunculated and consist of epithelial tubules which are often cystic (Fig. 55.8), together with a large amount of lamina propria containing many inflammatory cells, particularly eosinophils. The pedicle consists of epithelium and lamina propria; muscularis is usually absent from both the pedicle and the polyp. The polyps frequently undergo volvulus, bleed or become infected. Occasionally, cartilage or bone is found in the stroma.

Some authors classify the polyps as hamartomas (Morson & Dawson 1979), others regard them as inflammatory with blockage of colonic crypts resulting in retention cysts and eventual polyp formation (Roth & Helwig 1963, Franzin et al 1983), while a third school regards the presence of eosinophils as indicating an allergic basis (Alexander et al 1970). Most juvenile polyps are not adenomatous but Mazier et al (1982) found adenomatous lesions in 4% of 258 patients and two were under the age of 5 years. In another series of 144 cases, three showed moderate dysplasia and in one of these a focus of severe dysplasia was also seen (Dajani & Kamal 1984).

*Symptoms*

Intermittent passage of fresh blood or autoamputation of the polyp are the usual modes of presentation. Occasionally children present with rectal prolapse with the polyp as the head of the intussusception. Other symptoms include abdominal pain and constipation. Protein-losing enteropathy can also occur (Gourley et al 1982).

*Diagnosis*

The diagnosis is made at sigmoidoscopy if a smooth, round polyp, often with some superficial ulceration, is seen. In symptomatic patients with negative sigmoidoscopy, colonoscopy or double-contrast barium enema is necessary (Douglas et al 1980). Histological assessment of the polyp confirms the diagnosis.

*Treatment*

Polyps should be removed at sigmoidoscopy or colonoscopy using a cautery snare. All polyps should be removed (Gryboski 1986) and follow-up is mandatory. Recurrence

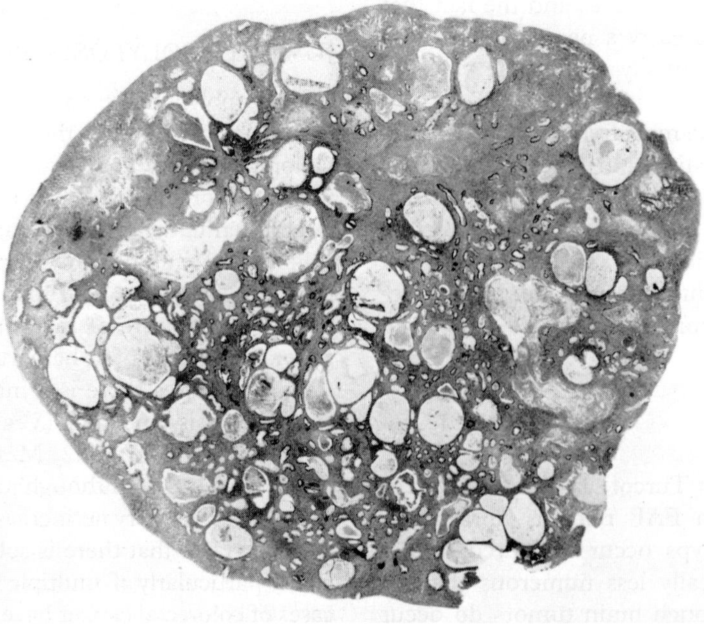

**Fig. 55.8** Juvenile polyp. Rounded polyp with surface erosion, prominent cystic glands and fibrous stroma infiltrated by inflammatory cells (hematoxylin and eosin, ×6).

is common but when single lesions have been removed in early childhood and there is no recurrence after puberty, further screening is unnecessary. However, cases of multiple juvenile polyposis, and particularly those with an adenomatous component, should be screened annually and virtually indefinitely. The question of subtotal colectomy and ileorectal anastomosis should be discussed (Jarvinen & Franssila 1984, Grosfeld & West 1986), given the substantial risk of malignancy.

## CRONKHITE–CANADA SYNDROME (Johnson et al 1972, Daniel et al 1982)

This rare syndrome consists of polyposis throughout the gastrointestinal tract in association with alopecia, atrophy of the nails and brown macular hyperpigmentation. The stomach and colon are involved in almost all cases, the duodenum in 75% and the jejunum and ileum in 50%. There are multiple sessile polyps on a thickened intestinal mucosa. Histological examination shows cystic dilatation of the crypts (Jenkins et al 1985) similar to that seen in juvenile polyposis. Typically the epithelium is orderly, but adenomatous or carcinomatous change may occur (Katayama et al 1985). The primary abnormality is atrophy of the mucosa due to low cellular turnover (Freeman et al 1985) and the condition may remit completely, indicating its non-neoplastic nature (Russell et al 1983). The lamina propria is edematous and secondary acute inflammation may occur. The gastric mucosa may resemble that of Menetrier's disease. The mean age of onset is 60 years. The patient has severe diarrhea with water and electrolyte depletion, steatorrhea and protein-losing enteropathy. The condition does not seem to be inherited.

## PEUTZ–JEGHERS SYNDROME

Peutz–Jeghers syndrome is inherited as an autosomal dominant disorder with high penetrance. The manifestations include gastrointestinal polyps and melanin pigmentation at mucocutaneous junctions and (occasionally) on the dorsum of the hands and feet. Some family members show pigmentation without polyposis and vice versa. There is an overall increased risk of gastrointestinal malignancy (Utsunomiya et al 1974, Giardiello et al 1987). Small intestinal and gastric cancers are relatively common, occurring in 7% of patients in one series (Utsunomiya et al 1974). Analysis of the St Mark's registry revealed a 13-fold increased risk of all gastrointestinal malignancies (Murday & Slack 1989); 15% of patients in this St Mark's series eventually developed cancer.

### *Pathology*

Polyps occur throughout the gastrointestinal tract but are commonest in the jejunum. They usually have a short pedicle and a lobulated surface resembling that of an adenomatous polyp or sometimes a villous tumor. On microscopy, the polyp consists of branches of the muscularis mucosae covered by epithelium and lamina propria. The lesion is classified as a hamartoma but can be distinguished from juvenile polyps histologically (Morson & Dawson 1979). Adenomatous and carcinomatous changes can occur in the stomach, duodenum and small and large intestine (Perzin & Bridge 1982, Tweedie & McCann 1984).

### *Clinical features*

Most cases present in childhood or adolescence. There are usually dark brown or bluish spots on the lips and inside of the mouth and the face, palms, soles, arms and perianal region can also be affected. Patients without pigmentation have been described (Bartholomew et al 1957). The usual presentation is with abdominal pain or obstruction due to intussusception of a polyp. Rectal bleeding and iron deficiency anemia are also common. Gastrointestinal cancer occurs in 2–3% of cases (Bussey 1970) and there may be an increased incidence of gonadal tumors (Wilson et al 1986). Two patients have been reported in whom cancer arose in a jejunal hamartomatous polyp (Matuchansky et al 1979, Cochet et al 1979).

### *Treatment*

Treatment is conservative wherever possible. If surgery is absolutely necessary, enterotomy and polypectomy, rather than resection, is recommended as polyps tend to develop at the anastomosis (Utsunomiya et al 1974). The incidence of cancer is relatively low but continued screening is generally recommended.

## BENIGN LYMPHOID POLYPS

These are round, smooth, sessile tumors, usually in the lower rectum and varying in diameter from a few millimeters to 3 cm. On histological examination, they consist of an aggregate of normal lymphoid tissue (Fig. 55.9) covered by attentuated epithelium. They are most common in the third and fourth decades and usually present with rectal bleeding, anal pain and tenderness or prolapse of the polyp (Cornes et al 1961). Multiple benign lymphoid polyps, sometimes familial, have been described in childhood (Louw 1968, Bussey 1975) and in families with FAP (Venkitachalam et al 1978). In both the single and multiple forms, the follicular pattern of the lymphoid tissue, lack of ulceration and lack of involvement of the muscle layer allow differentiation from lymphosarcoma, but differentiation from giant follicular lymphoma can be difficult (Cornes et al 1961). Treatment consists of local excision and there is no evidence of progression to malignancy if tissue remains.

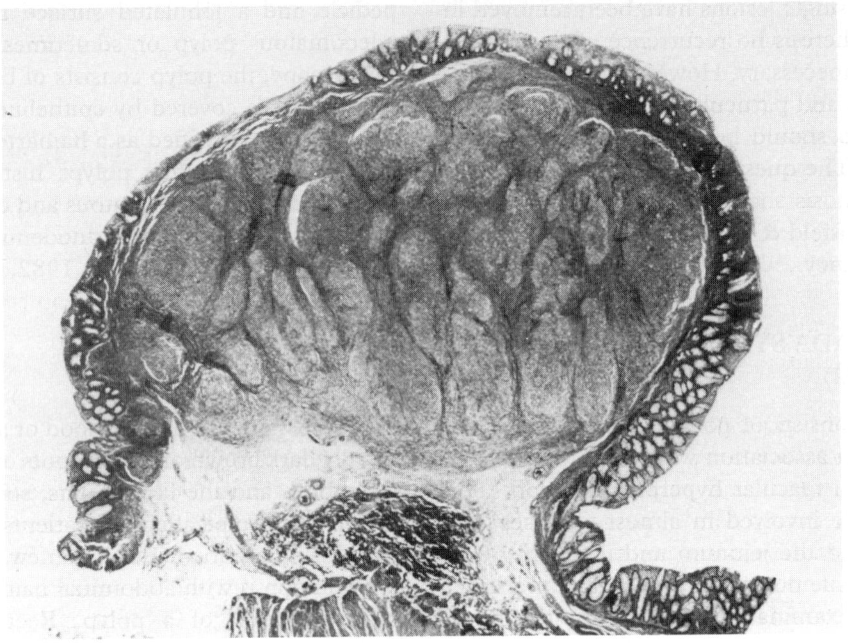

**Fig. 55.9** Benign lymphoid polyp. Polypoid lesion produced by an aggregate of reactive lymphoid follicles in the submucosa of the rectum (hematoxylin and eosin, ×12).

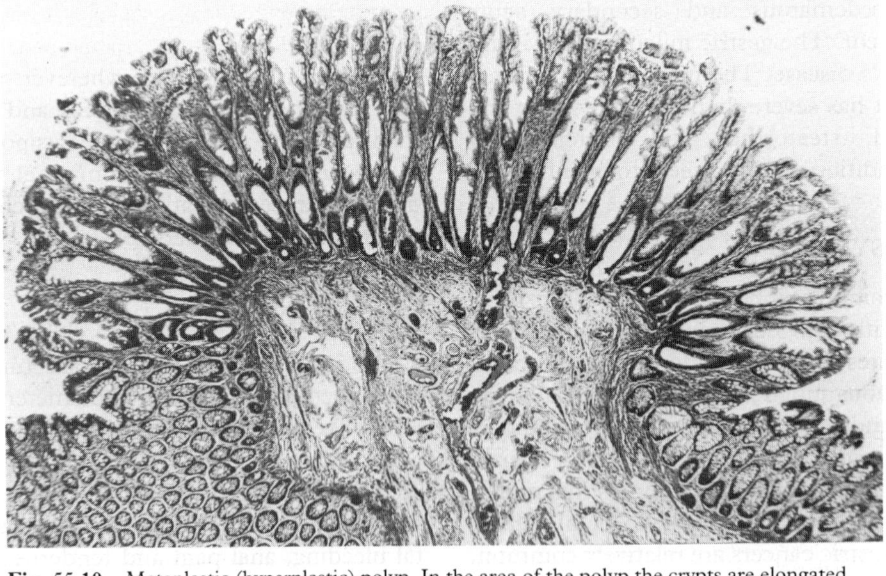

**Fig. 55.10** Metaplastic (hyperplastic) polyp. In the area of the polyp the crypts are elongated and have a prominent serrated or "sawtooth" profile (hematoxylin and eosin, ×30).

## METAPLASTIC (HYPERPLASTIC) POLYPS

Metaplastic polyps occur in the large intestine in increasing numbers with age and are present in some 75% of patients over the age of 40 years. They are commoner in men and are usually less than 5 mm diameter. The polyps tend to be pale, flat-topped, sessile plaques, mainly in the rectum and often on the crest of mucosal folds. Histologically the crypts are elongated, dilated and lined by columnar epithelium which has a sawtooth pattern (Fig. 55.10) due to micropapillary elevations (Williams et al 1980). At the base of the crypts the epithelium is hyperplastic and mitotically active and this can be misinterpreted as invasive tumor and lead to unnecessary resectional surgery.

The epithelium within a metaplastic polyp undergoes maturation, then hypermaturation with apparent delay in migration of the cells to the surface (Hayashi et al 1974). However, the overall cell renewal pattern is normal (Deschner & Lipkin 1976). The more superficial cells are tall and eosinophilic and differ from the normal colonic epithelium in their height, having increased numbers of tall microvilli and a thickened fibroblastic sheath. Larger polyps become pedunculated and may develop a villous surface configuration.

Metaplastic polyps are usually regarded as benign and lacking the premalignant potential of neoplastic polyps (Jass 1983). However, villous adenomas may have metaplastic areas within them and larger metaplastic polyps may contain an adenomatous component (Franzin et al 1984). Carcinoma with adenoma and metaplastic polyp has also been reported (Urbanski et al 1984). Some cases resemble multiple polyposis because the metaplastic polyps are both multiple and large (Williams et al 1980).

## COWDEN'S DISEASE

Cowden's disease (Lloyd & Dennis 1962) is a rare disseminated form of gastrointestinal polyposis with an autosomal dominant pattern of inheritance (Carlson et al 1984). The polyps are hamartomatous, similar to juvenile polyps but fewer in number. Adenomas and colorectal cancer can occur but the greatest risk is for benign and malignant disease of the breast and thyroid (Gentry et al 1974, Burnett et al 1975). Other associated lesions include macrocephaly, fibromas, angiomas, lipomas and sebaceous cysts. All patients have mucocutaneous lesions around the eyes which are warty tricholemmomas (Brownstein et al 1979). The presence of these lesions, oral fibromas and keratoses of the hands and feet are diagnostic. Regular colonoscopic screening is advisable.

## OTHER FORMS OF POLYP

Other polypoid conditions include pseudopolyps in chronic ulcerative colitis, lipomas (Bussey 1975), lymphosarcoma, carcinoid tumor and leiomyoma. Neurofibromatosis rarely results in colonic polyps. Mucosal ganglioneuromatosis has been described in association with multiple adenomatous or juvenile polyps (Weidner et al 1984) and multiple endocrine neoplasia (MEN) type IIb. Neurofibromatosis usually involves the small intestine (Bussey 1975) or stomach (Hochberg et al 1974) and the polyps, which consist of an overgrowth of nerve tissue in the submucosa and muscle layers, may ulcerate. The histology and significance of such polyps is reviewed by Enterline (1976).

Polyposis of the entire gastrointestinal tract has been described (Yonemoto et al 1969) and carries a high incidence of adenocarcinoma.

## COLORECTAL ADENOCARCINOMA

Cancer of the large bowel is the commonest gastrointestinal tract malignancy and second only to lung cancer as a cause of cancer death in Westernized countries. Adenocarcinoma is by far the most common form of invasive large bowel tumor.

### Epidemiology

Colorectal cancer is predominantly a disease of Westernized societies (Burkitt 1971, Haenszel & Correa 1971, Muir et al 1987) and environmental factors are important in its etiology (Correa & Haenszel 1978, Haenszel & Correa 1982). There are approximately 155 000 new cases a year in the USA and 25 000 in the United Kingdom (Muir et al 1987) and less than one-third of patients remain alive 5 years later (Falterman et al 1974, Jass et al 1987). The male:female ratio for cancer of the colon is close to unity (Muir et al 1987) and for cancer of the rectum it reaches 1.7:1 in high-incidence populations. In high-incidence countries, tumors of the sigmoid and descending colon are particularly common, whereas in low-incidence countries, tumors are more evenly distributed (Haenszel & Correa 1982).

The incidence of colorectal cancer in north western Europe and North America is 10-fold higher than in developing countries such as sub-Saharan Africa, India and parts of South America (Table 55.5; Burkitt 1971, Haenszel & Correa 1971, Doll & Peto 1981, Boyle et al 1985, Muir et al 1987). Most European countries are in an intermediate risk category but Scotland has a particularly high risk. Rectal cancer shows a sevenfold variation in risk between high- and low-risk countries. Although incidence may now be falling in high-incidence countries such as the USA and the UK, no other malignancy so closely parallels the affluence of a society.

Within populations there may be wide variation between ethnic groups, such as between Maoris and non-Maoris in New Zealand and Hispanics and whites in New Mexico (Table 55.5). Migrant studies provide strong evidence for environmental factors which operate within two to three decades of immigration (Weisburger et al 1975) so that migrants from low-risk countries take on the risk of their new high-risk country within their lifetime. For example, the risk for native rural Japanese males in Miyagi prefecture is 17.9 per 100 000 compared to 52 per 100 000 in Japanese Hawaiians. Australian immigrants from low-risk countries such as Greece show a marked increase in incidence whereas those from countries with a higher risk than Australia (e.g. Scotland) show a slight reduction (McMichael & Giles 1988).

**Table 55.5** Age standardized rates of colon and rectal cancer combined (Muir et al 1987)

| | | Rates for cancer of colon and rectum combined per 100 000 population (ICD codes 153 and 154) Male | Female |
|---|---|---|---|
| *Developed countries* | | | |
| Australia | | | |
| Victoria | | 46.8 | 37.1 |
| Queensland | | 39.2 | 34.1 |
| Canada | | 39.4 | 32.3 |
| England and Wales | | 30.3 | 22.6 |
| Japan | | | |
| Miyagi | Rural | 17.9 | 14.6 |
| New Zealand | | | |
| Maori | | 22.1 | 16.3 |
| Non-Maori | | 43.6 | 40.1 |
| Scotland | | 33.7 | 27.1 |
| United States | | | |
| Connecticut | White | 52.1 | 37.6 |
| | Black | 45.6 | 34.9 |
| New Orleans | White | 43.9 | 30.0 |
| | Black | 39.4 | 33.1 |
| New Mexico | Hispanic | 22.7 | 17.0 |
| | White | 33.5 | 26.3 |
| Hawaii | White | 41.8 | 28.9 |
| | Japanese | 52.0 | 31.0 |
| *Developing countries* | | | |
| Brazil | | | |
| Recife | | 12.7 | 12.3 |
| São Paulo | | 22.0 | 21.1 |
| Columbia | | | |
| Cali | | 18.6 | 10.0 |
| India | | | |
| Bombay | | 7.9 | 5.4 |
| Madras | | 4.8 | 2.1 |

The high incidence in Western countries is reflected in the contribution of large bowel cancer to the total cancer burden; 18% of all cancer registrations in Connecticut and New Zealand are from colorectal cancer but only 2% in Nigeria. In the USA the risk is higher in the north, within Scandinavia it is greatest in Denmark and diminishes as one moves northwards, while in Europe generally it is higher in northern than in southern or eastern regions. In all countries, urban populations are at greater risk.

In low-risk populations, female cases are preponderant and there is a relatively uniform distribution of cancers throughout the colon (Haenszel & Correa 1982). When a new etiological factor is introduced into a low-risk population, the transition from an "endemic" to an "epidemic" phase is first expressed as an increase in sigmoid cancer in older males followed by a rise in female sigmoid cancer. When the "epidemic" is well established, a rise in cecal and ascending colon cancer is first apparent in males and is accompanied by an increased frequency of cancer of the transverse and descending colon. These findings could be explained by the presence of a carcinogen in intestinal contents which is increasingly concentrated during transit from ileocecal valve to rectum.

## Etiology

### *Dietary factors*

The evidence that the high incidence of colorectal cancer in developed countries is due to factors present in the Western diet comes from observed geographic variation and migrant studies (Burkitt 1971, Weisburger et al 1975, Lipkin 1978, Correa & Haenszel 1978, Doll & Peto 1981, Muir et al 1987, McMichael et al 1988), and from case-control studies of dietary intake (Stubbs 1983). However, it is difficult to dissect out the role of each dietary constituent from that of related dietary factors. Experimental studies of carcinogenesis have also implicated specific dietary factors although few have been sustained by case-control or cohort studies (Bruce 1987). Dietary intervention studies hold great promise as a means of reducing the incidence of colorectal cancer, but as yet few concrete data are available.

***Fiber.*** Burkitt (1971) suggested that a high fiber intake speeds intestinal transit and dilutes potential fecal carcinogens, thereby reducing exposure of the colonic epithelium to carcinogens. While there is virtually no evidence to support this suggestion in man or in laboratory animals (Stubbs 1983), there is undoubtedly a marked inverse correlation between fiber intake and colorectal cancer risk (McKeown & Bright-See 1984) and the risk reduction which could be achieved is estimated to be around 35% (Trock et al 1990). Possible mechanisms to explain risk reduction by dietary fiber include enhanced bacterial fermentation and production of short chain fatty acids with acidification of stool (so reducing the bioavailability of carcinogenic bile acids). However, fiber given to Western subjects does not alter fecal flora (Drasar & Jenkins 1976) and an alternative possibility is that fiber metabolites such as butyrate may have direct antineoplastic effects.

***Fat.*** The epidemiological correlation between fat intake and colorectal cancer is striking (Drasar & Irving 1973). One large cohort study (Willett et al 1990) demonstrated that those taking the most fat (over 65 g/day) were at 1.9 times greater risk than those taking the least fat. A low-fiber and high-fat diet appears to increase fecal pH and this may enhance bile acid toxicity. Bacterial conversion of fecal bile acid to carcinogens related to methylcholanthrene has also been suggested (Stubbs 1983). Bile acids have toxic effects on colonic epithelium in laboratory experiments and high fat intake mobilizes bile acids. However, dietary fat consumption is not a consistent risk factor in case-control studies (Stubbs 1983, Bruce 1987).

Individuals with low serum cholesterol may be at higher risk of colorectal cancer (Doll & Peto 1981), although the association appears to be "U"-shaped with an increased mortality from colorectal cancer at cholesterol concentrations above and below the mean population level (Isles et al 1989).

***Meat.*** It is not clear whether the apparent association between meat ingestion and colorectal cancer is due to the associated intake of animal fat. However, Willet et al (1990) noted an increased risk in women who consumed a greater proportion of red meat relative to fish and chicken, suggesting an effect specific to beef. Cooking of meat, particularly frying, produces carcinogens but epidemiological studies have failed to detect any association with colorectal cancer.

***Energy.*** It is difficult to substantiate a link between total energy intake and colorectal cancer because of the relationship between specific dietary constituents and caloric intake, a problem epitomized by dietary fat with its high caloric content.

***Vegetables and fruit.*** Vegetables contain antioxidants (e.g. carotene) and other potential antineoplastic compounds. Seventh Day Adventists have a high vegetable intake and a low colorectal cancer incidence and a number of case-control studies have found a protective effect for vegetables (Potter 1990), in particular cruciferous vegetables such as broccoli, cabbage and Brussels sprouts. However, as with all dietary constituents, disentangling the effect of vegetables from confounding factors such as dietary fiber is very difficult indeed. The protective effect of fruit is less convincing than that of vegetables (Potter 1990).

***Calcium*** (Sorenson et al 1988). High calcium intake appears to be protective while deficiency of dietary calcium and vitamin D is associated with increased colorectal cancer risk (Garland et al 1985). The beneficial effects of calcium may be due to reduced bioavailability of bile acids.

Failure to repress DNA synthesis in epithelial cells during migration from crypt to lumen is well documented in patients with adenomas and cancer and those with HNPCC (see below). Such cells are not shed normally and form polypoid excrescences (Sherlock et al 1975, Deschner & Lipkin 1976, Lipkin 1978, 1984). Proliferative indices can be normalized by dietary calcium supplements in high-risk patients such as those with multiple polyps and affected members of colon cancer families (Lipkin & Newmark 1985, Rozen et al 1989). Prospective studies of the effect of calcium supplements on adenoma recurrence after polypectomy are in progress.

***Smoking.*** In a prospective study in the United States it was found that smoking in the previous 20 years was associated with an increased prevalence of small adenomas of the colorectum and smoking for more than 20 years was associated with large adenomas. An increased risk of colorectal cancer was noted only after 35 years of smoking. These relationships were apparent for men but in the case of women the associations were not as strong, probably because substantial smoking amongst women occurred later than in men (Giovannucci et al 1994a,b).

***Alcohol.*** Several studies have shown a relationship between high alcohol intake (especially beer) and rectal cancer, whereas others have shown little or no effect. A recent meta-analysis concluded that a small increase in risk with increased beer consumption does not indicate a causal role (Longnecker et al 1990).

***Fecal pH and diet.*** Cellular proliferation is reduced when feces are acidified (Bruce 1987) but few intervention studies have assessed the effect of fecal pH manipulation on colonic epithelial proliferation. McKeown et al (1988) were unable to influence the development of colorectal adenomas or carcinomas following fecal acidification by ingestion of vitamins C and E. However, larger studies with longer follow-up are under way.

*Interaction between diet and intestinal bacteria* (Hill 1978, Lipkin 1978)

The possibility that diet acts by modifying the intestinal flora and providing substrates from which bacteria produce carcinogens has been assessed by studies in populations with different incidences of colon cancer. Suggestions that a Western diet produced a specific type of stool microflora have not been confirmed (Simon & Gorbach 1984), but the metabolic activity of the microflora does appear to be influenced by diet. The concentration of neutral steroids (formed in the large bowel from the degradation of cholesterol) and acid steroids such as dehydroxycholanic acid (derived from bile acids) is increased in high-incidence populations. Furthermore, colon cancer patients have more fecal steroid than controls. The increased degradation is related to increased activity of μ-dehydroxylase and cholesterol dehydrogenase in the fecal flora (Mastromarino et al 1976). Patients with adenomatous polyps also have increased activity and high levels of deoxycholate are found in the colon (Van der Werf et al 1982). High fat intake is an important factor in increasing levels of steroids in the stool and degradation products of bile acids might be carcinogenic.

Bacterial P-glucuronidase activity is also increased by a Western high-meat diet. The enzyme can retoxify compounds previously detoxified by glucuronidation in the liver and it has been postulated that this might apply to some carcinogens.

Rodent models have provided useful information (Rogers & Nauss 1985, Ahnen 1985). The enzymes nitroreductase and azoreductase increase in animals fed a high-beef diet; nitroreductase can produce nitrosamines from nitrogenous compounds while azoreductase can reduce azo food dyes to carcinogens. A high-beef diet also renders animals more susceptible to the effects of a number of carcinogens. Bacteria can also act by activating dietary carcinogens; for example, the glycoside cycasin, which itself is not carcinogenic, is hydrolyzed to the active aglycone by intestinal bacteria. Animal experiments have emphasized the importance of carcinogens contained in and produced by the fecal stream in the development of cancer (Sherlock et al 1975, LaMont & O'Gorman 1978). Cycasin does not produce colonic tumors if the fecal stream is diverted, while the colonic tumors produced by subcutaneous 2,3-dimethyl-4-aminobiphenyl are prevented by proximal colostomy. In man, regression of colonic tumor after proximal colostomy has been described (Dunphy et al 1959).

### *Other etiological factors*

There is a suggestion from epidemiological studies that parity is protective (Zaridze 1983). It has been postulated that endogenous estrogens lower plasma cholesterol and increase bile acid production, while progesterone, pregnancy and high-dose oral contraceptives reduce plasma high-density lipid concentration, hepatic clearance of cholesterol and bile acid production.

Colorectal cancer may develop as a result of a single large dose of radiotherapy (Rotmensch et al 1986) and there is circumstantial evidence that it can follow irradiation for uterine carcinoma. Castro et al (1973) found radiation proctocolitis at the site of the tumor in more than half of a series of 26 patients and 60% of the tumors produced mucin, compared to 10–20% in other series.

An association between lack of physical exercise and colorectal cancer has emerged from case-control and cohort studies (Lee et al 1991). One hypothesis is that colonic transit time is reduced by exercise but other possible mechanisms include alterations in the levels of prostaglandins and antioxidant enzymes.

### *Genetic factors*

The spectrum of predisposition to colorectal cancer ranges from an ill-defined increased risk in individuals with a positive family history to well-defined autosomal dominant genetic traits in which the genes involved have been identified and mutations characterized. About 20–25% of patients with colorectal cancer have a family history of the disease (Dunlop 1992) and there are data to suggest that all cases of colorectal cancer occur on a background of genetic predisposition (Cannon-Albright et al 1988). Familial adenomatous polyposis is discussed above (p. 1406) but the much commoner autosomal dominant condition, hereditary nonpolyposis colorectal cancer (HNPCC), accounts for around 5% of all cases of colorectal cancer (Mecklin et al 1986b, Lynch et al 1993). HNPCC is of major interest because of its prevalence and the potential to identify gene carriers by mutation analysis of blood samples and so target those at risk for colonoscopic screening.

Colorectal cancer in HNPCC gene carriers is associated with only small numbers of adenomas (Lynch et al 1985a) and there is a propensity for both adenomas and carcinomas to develop in the proximal colon. Expression of the HNPCC phenotype is diverse in terms of the age at which cancer occurs and it can be inherited as a site-specific colorectal cancer susceptibility trait or be associated with uterine, gastric, ovarian, upper urinary tract, small intestinal and other malignancies (Mecklin et al 1986b). The HNPCC family shown in Figure 55.11 has a number of cases of colorectal and uterine carcinoma arising at an early age. The pedigree demonstrates the autosomal dominant nature of the syndrome in that almost 50% of each generation are affected but also reveals cases of nonpenetrance in obligate gene carriers. Such large HNPCC fami-

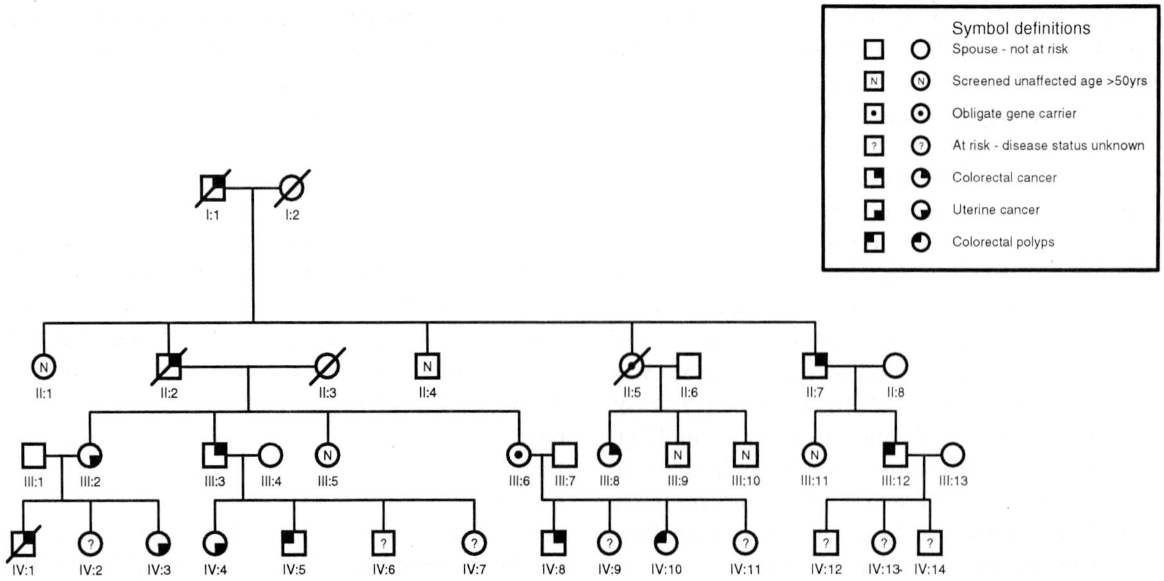


**Fig. 55.11** A large HNPCC family. The autosomal dominant mode of inheritance with a high degree of penetrance is clear but there are two cases (II:5 and III:6) where females are obligate gene carriers who have passed on the defective gene but who are unaffected themselves.

lies are fairly uncommon and the minimum criteria for HNPCC diagnosis are:

1. three or more relatives with histologically proven colorectal cancer, one being a first degree relative of the other two;
2. two or more generations affected;
3. at least one family member affected before the age of 50 years (Vasen et al 1991).

Abnormalities of colonic epithelial cell proliferation have been demonstrated in HNPCC (Lipkin et al 1983, Lynch et al 1985b) and are more pronounced as the strength of family history increases (Gerdes et al 1993). This could be due to shared family environment, but while relatives of colorectal cancer patients are at increased risk, spouses have the same risk as the general population (Jensen et al 1980). Demonstration of a genetic effect in terms of both familial aggregation and alterations in crypt cell turnover does not mean that this is a single gene disorder. A number of genes are now known to be responsible for HNPCC and still more may prove to be involved.

Four human genes have been identified which, when mutated, result in a common functional deficit at the molecular level, a deficit which is responsible for predisposition to colorectal cancer. These genes are human homologs of yeast and bacterial DNA repair genes and are known as hMSH2 on chromosome 2p (Fishel et al 1993, Leach et al 1993), hMLH1 on chromosome 3p (Bronner et al 1994, Papadopoulos et al 1994), hPMS1 on chromosome 2q (Nicolaides et al 1994) and hPMS2 on chromosome 7q (Nicolaides et al 1994). Mutational inactivation of both genes on each chromosome pair in tumors of HNPCC patients is associated with characteristic alterations in tumor DNA, resulting in widespread instability in short repetitive tracts due to defective repair of DNA mismatches (Ionov et al 1993, Aaltonen et al 1993, Thibodeau et al 1993). The proportion of families with mutations in each of the genes is still to be defined but around 40% of families fulfilling the criteria for HNPCC carry mutations in hMSH2 (Liu et al 1994) and some 30% have mutations in hMLH1.

Lynch has calculated that the population gene frequency of an HNPCC allele may be around 0.005 (Lynch et al 1993). Instability in short repetitive DNA tracts (microsatellite instability) has been detected in around 15% of apparently sporadic colorectal cancers (Ionov et al 1993, Aaltonen et al 1993, Thibodeau et al 1993) but it is unlikely that all of these are due to inheritance of HNPCC genes as some individuals could acquire two somatic mutations. However, the fact that virtually every tumor arising in an HNPCC gene carrier exhibits microsatellite instability (Aaltonen et al 1994) offers a potential means of identifying carriers.

Microsatellite instability has been detected in endometrial cancer (Risinger et al 1993) and other cancers in HNPCC gene carriers (Aaltonen et al 1994). It also occurs in tumors from patients with multiple different primary cancers (Horii et al 1994), suggesting that such individuals could carry DNA repair-gene mutations even in the absence of a family history of cancer.

*Inflammatory bowel disease and risk of colorectal cancer*

***Ulcerative colitis.*** The mechanism responsible for the increased risk is not clear but chronic inflammation must be involved. In one population study (Ekbom et al 1990a) the relative risk was 2.8 for patients with left-sided colitis and 14.8 for those with pancolitis. Age at onset was a strong and independent predictor of risk in that the overall risk for patients with pancolitis was 30% at 35 years but 40% after 35 years in those younger than 15 at onset. In another cohort study, the risk was increased eight-fold overall and 19-fold in extensive disease (Gyde et al 1988); the cumulative risk in extensive disease was 7.2% at 20 years and 16.5% at 30 years (see also pp. 672 & 685).

The vexed question is whether colonoscopic surveillance can reduce the occurrence of malignancy. Despite the substantial risk with pancolitis, screening such patients has been of little benefit (Gyde 1990, Jonsson et al 1994); cancer arises in some cases during the screening program and the financial costs are substantial. It therefore seems prudent to discuss the option of proctocolectomy in patients with pancolitis, especially when ulcerative colitis was diagnosed before the age of 15 years.

***Crohn's disease.*** The risk of large bowel malignancy is increased in Crohn's disease but to a lesser extent than in ulcerative colitis. The largest study of a cohort of 1655 patients with colonic Crohn's disease demonstrated an overall relative risk of 2.5 (Ekbom et al 1990b), with a substantially higher risk in those diagnosed under the age of 30. Involvement of the ileum alone does not increase the risk of colorectal cancer but colonic involvement does, even when the ileum is involved (see also p. 674).

## Pathology

Pathological assessment of the resected specimen (despite many shortcomings) remains the most robust prognostic indicator. Pathological staging is not a means of predicting the natural history of a particular tumor, but more a predictor of outcome for the majority of patients with tumors in that staging category.

## Site

Wood (1967) reviewed 7463 cases from five series and noted the following site distribution: rectum 49%, sigmoid colon 14%, rectosigmoid 12%, cecum 6.5%, descending colon 5.5%, transverse colon 4.9%, ascending colon 3.9%, hepatic flexure 2.5% and splenic flexure 1.9%. As in all studies of this type, it is often difficult to determine whether cancers at the rectosigmoid junction are colonic or rectal. Within this limitation, several large studies have shown a tendency for the proportion of right-sided colonic cancers to increase with time. Axtell & Chiazze (1966) found that the increase in proximal cancers over the previous two decades was due to an increase in cancer of the colon without a proportionate rise in rectal cancer. Cady et al (1974) found that between 1928 and 1967, the proportion of right colon cancer rose from 7% to 22% while that of sigmoid, rectosigmoid and rectal carcinoma fell from 80% to 62%. Falterman et al (1974) reported that 10% of tumors in their series were in the cecum and 62% in the rectum and sigmoid and more recently, Stower & Hardcastle (1985) found that 10.4% of tumors were in the cecum. Greene (1983) confirmed the trend for the proportion of proximal tumors to increase, the effect being more marked in women; the proportion of cancers at various sites in 1971–80 was cecum 19%, transverse colon 18%, descending colon 8%, sigmoid colon 29% and rectum 26%.

The elderly have a particularly high proportion of right-sided tumors (Schub & Steinheber 1986). Right colon cancers comprised 8%, 22% and 28% in the age groups 60–69 years, 70–79 years and >80 years respectively compared to 77%, 58% and 49% respectively for rectosigmoid lesions. It is possible that racial differences affect the proportion of right colon tumors (Falterman et al 1974, Johnson & Carstens 1986).

### *Multiplicity of tumors*

Around 3–5% of patients presenting with colorectal cancer have two or more synchronous tumors (Falterman et al 1974, Morson & Dawson 1979, Abrams & Reines 1979, Jarvinen et al 1988). Multiple cancers are more likely when adenomas are present in the resected specimen (Morson 1984). Failure to detect synchronous cancers is a particular problem with rectal cancer where the diagnosis seems clear and histological proof has been obtained from the rectal lesion. It is vital in such patients to assess the entire colon by colonoscopy or barium enema to exclude proximal synchronous lesions. Many apparently metachronous cancers are actually missed synchronous tumors. The true rate of metachronous cancer is clearly affected by the survival of patients following treatment of the primary lesion; estimates of 3–5% are probably underestimates.

### *Macroscopic features*

Tumours may be ulcerating, polypoidal or infiltrative. Two-thirds are ulcerating and a typical malignant ulcer has raised everted edges, slough-covered floor and indurated base. Small tumors, and particularly those in the rectum and cecum, tend to be round or oval but as the tumor enlarges the whole bowel circumference becomes involved. Infiltration causes deformity which is apparent from the serosal aspect and in annular tumors results in an indurated "napkin ring" stricture. Obstruction usually develops slowly and becomes manifest clinically when the luminal diameter is around 6 mm (Messinger et al 1971).

The 10% of tumors which are polypoidal tend to be better differentiated. Infiltrative tumors are uncommon but tend to be poorly differentiated. A substantial proportion of infiltrative tumors are in fact metastases from a distant primary tumor, most commonly arising in stomach and ovary.

Early adenocarcinomas are those which have not spread in continuity beyond the submucosa. As discussed earlier, these have usually arisen in adenomas (Morson 1966) (Fig. 55.12) and the focus of carcinoma may be identifiable as an area of induration or ulceration. As the lesion enlarges the adenomatous component is progressively destroyed until the lesion is diagnosable only as a polypoid carcinoma. Remnants of adenomas were found at the edge of 23% of 169 carcinomas in one series (Eide 1983). Muto et al (1983) studied 155 early cancers and found that the commonest types had a short stalk or broad base.

Tumor size is not a good independent prognostic indicator. Tumors of the right colon and cecum tend to be large exophytic growths, presumably reflecting the capaciousness of the proximal colon. However, this did not affect outcome in some studies (Spratt & Spjut 1967) and larger tumors actually had a more favorable outcome in some series (Osnes 1955).

### *Microscopic features and histological grading*

Almost all colorectal malignancies are adenocarcinomas with a varying degree of differentiation and 10–20% of them are mucinous (Morson 1967). Around 5% of tumors are undifferentiated. Broder's (1925) classification is based on the degree of cellular differentiation but its prognostic value is limited as most tumors are moderately differentiated (Table 55.6). Even with simplified versions of the classification, assignment of grade is wholly subjective and interobserver variation is substantial (Blenkinsopp et al 1981).

Well-differentiated tumors consist of complex or simple tubules lined by epithelium and closely resemble normal colonic mucosa, the cells retaining nuclear polarity. Moderately differentiated lesions have varying degrees of crowding and heaping up of cells within tubules and increasingly aberrant mitotic figures. Poorly differentiated tumors show little or no glandular structure and a loss of nuclear polarity. Colloid tumors have associated lakes of mucin and are usually poorly differentiated. Although many studies have shown that defining the degree of differentiation is useful (Phillips et al 1984a), many others

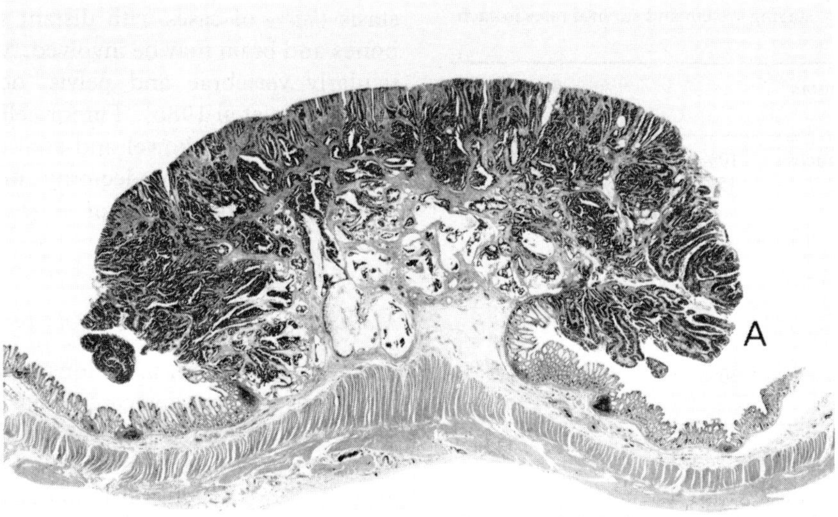


**Fig. 55.12** Polypoidal adenocarcinoma. There is extensive invasion of the core of the polyp and such severe dysplasia of surface glands that there is only one area (A) which could be considered adenomatous (hematoxylin and eosin, ×4).

**Table 55.6** Histological grading and prognosis in colorectal carcinoma

| Degree of differentiation | % of cases | Metastasis to lymph nodes | Crude 5-year survival rate (%) |
|---|---|---|---|
| Well | 20 | 25% | 80% |
| Moderate | 60 | 50% | 60% |
| Poor | 20 | 80% | 25% |

have found that histological grade has no independent prognostic value (Jass et al 1987). However, signet ring tumors do have a very poor prognosis and few patients survive more than 2 years. Mucin-producing undifferentiated tumors are commoner in young patients (Martin et al 1981, Pratt & George 1982) and in HNPCC (Mecklin et al 1986a). A subgroup of undifferentiated tumors with a good prognosis has also been described (Gibbs 1977); these tumors grow large before metastasizing, do not produce mucin, have a solid growth pattern and may show argyrophilia.

*Pathological staging*

Pathological staging has important implications for management. For example, some patients may be given adjuvant chemotherapy on the basis of staging, while in other groups it may be important to avoid chemotherapy. Dukes' stage B patients fared substantially worse than controls when given chemotherapy in one large study which showed benefit from chemotherapy in Dukes' stage C patients (Moertel et al 1990). Staging hinges on the degree of invasion and nodal involvement, but there are subtle variations and no one staging system is in universal use.

In 1932 Dukes modified the classification of rectal tumors first devised by Lockhart-Mummery (1926–27) and later demonstrated its prognostic value (Dukes 1940). Although Dukes' staging was initially applied to rectal cancer, it has since been widely used for colon cancer as well and retains its correlation with survival. Dukes later subdivided stage C into C1 with metastasis to local lymph nodes and C2 with metastasis to apical nodes (Gabriel et al 1935). Kirklin et al (1949) subdivided stage B into B1 (invasion into the muscularis) and stage B2 (invasion through the muscularis to the serosa). Astley & Coller (1954) further subdivided stages B and C, with stage C1 being a stage B1 tumor with lymph node metastases and C2 being a stage B2 tumor with lymph node metastases. Astley–Coller staging is still used extensively in the USA.

The fact that Dukes' staging and its variations remain in use attests its simplicity and reproducibility. A further stage (D) has been added for distant metastases, although this was never proposed by Dukes who based his staging system exclusively on pathological examination of the resection specimen. The generally accepted version of Dukes' staging for colorectal cancer with approximate proportions of tumors in each category and 5-year survival rates (Falterman et al 1974, Gill & Morris 1978, Phillips et al 1984a, Stower & Hardcastle 1985) is shown in Table 55.7.

Due to the number of variations of Dukes' staging system in use, the American Joint Committee on Cancer and the Union Internationale Contre Le Cancer developed the TNM system for colorectal cancer (Hutter & Sobin 1986). The importance of number of involved lymph nodes involved is reflected in this system (Table 55.8) (Phillips et al 1984a, Wolmark et al 1986).

**Table 55.7** Modified Dukes' staging system and survival rates in each group

| Extent of spread | Proportion of tumors | | 5-yr survival |
|---|---|---|---|
| Stage A | Invasion of submucosa | 10% | 82% |
| Stage B1 | Invasion into the muscularis | 35% (Bland 2) | 65% |
| Satge B2 | Invasion through the muscularis to serosa | | |
| Stage C1 | Metastasis to proximal lymph nodes only | 25% (C1 and 2) | 46% |
| Stage C2 | Involvement of apical lymph nodes | | 22% |
| Stage D | Liver or other distant metastases | 30% | 5% |

**Table 55.8** TNM staging for colon and rectal cancer

| | |
|---|---|
| Tx | Primary tumor cannot be assessed |
| Tis | Carcinoma in situ |
| T1 | Cancer invades into the submucosa |
| T2 | Cancer invades into muscularis propria |
| T3 | Cancer invades through muscularis propria and into the subserosa or into nonperitonealized pericolic or perirectal tissues |
| T4 | Cancer perforates the visceral peritoneum or directly invades adjacent organs |
| Nx | The regional lymph nodes cannot be assessed |
| N0 | No regional lymph nodes involved |
| N1 | Metastases in 1–3 pericolic or perirectal lymph nodes |
| N2 | Metastases in 4 or more pericolic or perirectal lymph nodes |
| N3 | Metastases in lymph node along the course of a major named blood vessel |
| Mx | The presence of distant metastases cannot be assessed |
| M0 | No distant metastases |
| M1 | Distant metastases |

*Mode of spread*

Colorectal cancer may extend proximally or distally in the bowel wall, but distal spread beyond 1 cm is unusual and is virtually confined to patients with Dukes' C tumors, patients who die from distant metastases rather than local recurrence (Williams et al 1983). There is increasing evidence that the classic 5 cm margin of distal clearance at surgery is not necessary and a margin of 2 cm is probably adequate. In low rectal tumors, this may allow sphincter-saving resection in patients who would have been treated in the past by abdominoperineal excision of the rectum (Williams 1984b, Williams et al 1985).

Local spread through the bowel wall is resisted initially by the muscularis and later by the peritoneum, but tumor often spreads along blood vessels and nerves. Once the peritoneum is breached, dissemination throughout the abdominal cavity is likely. Invasion of lymphatics results in regional lymph node involvement. Very low rectal tumors may also involve the inguinal nodes. Invasion of veins also allows cells to pass into the portal circulation (Talbot et al 1981, Jass et al 1987). The liver is the main site of metastasis (75% of cases with distant spread) and the lungs, bones and brain may be involved. Metastasis to bone, particularly vertebrae and pelvis, occurs in 4% of cases (Bonnheim et al 1986). Tumor cells may implant in other parts of the large bowel and anal canal implantation can complicate hemorrhoidectomy in the presence of an unsuspected colorectal cancer (Le Quesne & Thomson 1958).

*Molecular pathology of colorectal cancer*

As discussed earlier, mutations in the APC gene occur in sporadic adenomas and carcinomas (p. 1401). Indeed, such mutations appear ubiquitous in colorectal tumors and may be an absolute requirement for initiation of the neoplastic process. Loss of genetic material at markers around the APC gene occurs in around 50% of tumors (Vogelstein et al 1988, Ashton-Rickardt et al 1989), while mutations resulting in truncation of the APC gene product have been identified in 60% of sporadic colorectal cancers and adenomas (Powell et al 1992, Ichii et al 1993). Inactivation of the APC gene by one or other mechanism appears to be implicated in all colorectal cancers.

Mutations in the APC gene have been detected in adenomas as small as 3 mm in diameter (Powell et al 1992, Ichii et al 1993) with the same frequency as in late-stage carcinomas, strengthening the suggestion that they are involved in initiation of the neoplastic process. The spectrum of somatic APC mutations in sporadic colorectal adenomas and carcinomas is remarkably similar to the germline changes in FAP.

Other genetic events observed in DNA from colorectal cancers (Fearon & Vogelstein 1990) include DNA hypomethylation, loss of the DCC gene on chromosome 18 in 85% of cases, inactivation by mutation or large genetic rearrangement of the p53 gene on chromosome 17 in 75% of cases and mutational activation of the K-*ras* oncogene on chromosome 12 in 40% of cases (Vogelstein et al 1988).

## Screening for colon cancer

The good prognosis associated with early tumors has generated great interest in screening apparently healthy asymptomatic populations to reduce the incidence and mortality of colorectal cancer.

*Fecal occult screening for colorectal cancer* (Macrae 1985, Simon 1985, Reasbeck 1987, Hardcastle 1989)

The most extensively studied screening test is the guaiac-impregnated paper test for fecal occult blood (FOB). Sensitivity is reduced if the test paper is dry but can be restored from 50% (Simon 1985, Hardcastle et al 1989) to 90% (Mandel et al 1993) by rehydration before analysis. The predictive value of a nonrehydrated positive FOB test is around 10% for cancer and 50% for adenomas >1 cm and/or cancer (Hardcastle 1989, Hardcastle et al 1989).

Five controlled studies assessing the effect of population-based FOB screening on colorectal cancer mortality are in progress (Hardcastle 1989). Cancers are detected at a more favorable stage (i.e. 50–70% Dukes' stage A) than in nonscreened groups (5–10% Dukes' stage A), but survival benefit is still being determined. Mandel et al (1993) have reported a 33% reduction in mortality from colorectal cancer using an annual rehydrated FOB test, but the increased sensitivity associated with rehydration has to be balanced by a concomitantly increased false positive rate. The overall FOB positive rate was almost 10% and 49% of the entire screened group required colonoscopic assessment during the 13-year study, leading to suggestions that this was more a randomized trial of colonoscopic screening than of FOB testing! It is unlikely that this strategy could be applied to population screening given the need for a massive increase in colonoscopic resources.

Further problems with screening relate to the risks of the investigations triggered by a positive FOB test. Colonoscopy can result in potentially fatal colonic perforation and bleeding after polypectomy (Eddy et al 1987, Ransohoff et al 1991) and it is vital to demonstrate a net benefit from screening in randomized studies. Compliance is also a major factor because it confounds the ability to determine whether there is a true effect in the screened population. Thus if individuals who fail to comply are actually at high risk of colorectal cancer due to diet or genetic factors, there will be an apparent benefit to the group offered screening who do comply. Compliance for biennial FOB test in the UK is around 50% (Hardcastle 1989, Hardcastle et al 1989). Although 75% of individuals completed some of the screens in the study by Mandel et al (1993), only 50% completed all screens.

There is little doubt that FOB screening results in a favorable shift in stage (Hardcastle et al 1989) and survival benefit (Mandel et al 1993). However, it will be important to assess the results of all studies using the 2-yearly nonrehydrated test to determine whether it is a practical and affordable proposition.

*Endoscopic screening*

There is substantial evidence that detection and removal of adenomas reduces the incidence and mortality of colorectal cancer (Winawer et al 1993), but it remains uncertain whether this can be reproduced in an asymptomatic population undergoing screening. As discussed earlier, Gilbertsen's study (Gilbertsen 1974, Gilbertsen & Nelms 1978) is widely cited as proof of the benefit of sigmoidoscopic polypectomy, but does not withstand close scrutiny. Nevertheless screening by rigid (Neugut & Pita 1988) and flexible sigmoidoscopy is widely practiced and has a worthwhile pick-up rate of adenomas and early cancers (Wherry 1981, Reasbeck 1987, Atkin et al 1993). Using assumptions from published studies, it has been calculated that "once only" flexible sigmoidoscopy between the ages of 55 and 60 years would prevent 5500 cases of colorectal cancer and save 3500 lives annually (Atkin et al 1993). The number of screening studies using colonoscopy is relatively small in comparison to the population studies using FOB testing (Hardcastle 1989).

*Screening in high-risk patient groups*

The discussion relating to population screening does not apply to groups at particularly high risk of colorectal cancer. FOB testing is too insensitive (Armitage et al 1986), while flexible sigmoidoscopy will miss a substantial number of tumors in patients with a genetic predisposition who have a high proportion of cancers in the proximal colon (Dunlop 1992). Screening in FAP, other polyp syndromes and ulcerative colitis is discussed above. With the recent identification of genes responsible for HNPCC (see above), blood tests for those at risk will soon be available so that gene carriers can be targeted for colonoscopic follow-up. However, for some time to come, evidence of genetic predisposition will continue to be based on a family history of colorectal cancer. Screening individuals with either a strong family history or a documented mutation in an HNPCC gene should consist of 3-yearly full colonoscopy with polypectomy as appropriate. If multiple polyps are present, prophylactic colectomy should be discussed.

## Clinical features of colon and rectal cancer

*Common symptoms* (Keddie & Hargreaves 1968, Jackman & Beahrs 1968, Falterman et al 1974)

As early tumors rarely produce symptoms and signs, the majority of patients present with established colorectal cancer. There are no specific symptoms or signs and symptoms associated with the disease are also common in healthy individuals. Nevertheless, all such patients must be investigated (Goulston et al 1986).

Rectal bleeding is often the earliest, and in some cases the only, symptom of rectal cancer (Dent et al 1986). Small amounts of blood mixed with mucus are lost; torrential bleeding is rare and more frequently due to diverticular disease or angiodysplasia. Rectal bleeding is reported by 60–90% of patients with rectal cancer, by about 50% with cancer of the left side of the colon and by less than 5% with right-sided lesions. Bleeding occurs with equal frequency in proximal and distal cancers but patients with right-sided tumors are often unaware of blood loss and present with iron deficiency anemia. Patients with left-sided tumors rarely present with iron deficiency anemia in the absence of other symptoms. Hence right-sided tumors are usually discovered later and the patient is more likely to have constitutional symptoms such as weight loss and anorexia. Rarely, patients with proximal cancers present with fresh rectal bleeding (Bacon & Gennaro 1968).

Pain occurs in about two-thirds of cases; its site and character vary and it may amount to no more than abdominal or rectal discomfort. Dull pain may be related to the site of the tumor or referred elsewhere. This is particularly true of cecal tumors which can present with dyspeptic type pain in the epigastrium which is exacerbated by food. Colicky lower abdominal pain is frequently related to bowel movements or the passage of flatus in left-sided lesions. Localized rectal or perineal pain may be the presenting feature in rectal cancer and usually indicates a poor prognosis. Tenesmus occurs in over 50% of patients with low rectal cancers. A relatively short history of fecal incontinence associated with tenesmus is a sinister symptom which must be fully investigated.

Change of bowel habit occurs in over 60% of patients with left-sided and rectal cancer, but as a symptom is more common in non-neoplastic diseases such as infective diarrhea, diverticular disease or irritable bowel syndrome. Increasing constipation or constipation alternating with explosive diarrhea and fecal urgency is commonest in rectal cancer. Altered bowel habit is reported by 40% of patients with tumors in the transverse and descending colon, roughly the same proportion reporting constipation as reporting diarrhea. Only 20% of patients with right-sided lesions have altered bowel habit.

Nausea and vomiting occur in some 10% of patients with right-sided cancer, but are rare with left-sided or rectal tumors. Even when obstruction supervenes, nausea and vomiting affect only 20% of cases (Gennaro & Tyson 1978). Although right-sided cancers produce the greatest absolute number of obstructions (with left-sided tumors in second place), tumors at the splenic flexure are most likely to obstruct. In the study of Phillips et al (1985), the proportion of cancers presenting with obstruction was 22% for right-sided lesions, 23% for left-sided lesions, 6% for rectal and rectosigmoid cancer and 49% for splenic flexure cancers. Goligher & Smiddy (1957) reported that 18% of patients with colorectal cancer had acute obstruction and that 62% of the obstructing tumors were in the splenic flexure, descending colon and sigmoid, 14% in the rectum, 7% in the transverse colon and 17% in the cecum, ascending colon and hepatic flexure. In another series of 1036 patients, 6.5% had acute obstruction; the majority had no symptoms apart from increasing constipation in the several days prior to obstruction (Gennaro & Tyson 1978).

Because colorectal cancer is perceived as a disease of the elderly, sinister symptoms are often ignored by young patients and their doctors. About 3% of patients are under 35 and their symptom pattern is similar to that of older patients, excepting that recurrent abdominal pain and nausea and vomiting may be more common (Miller & Liechty 1967, Pratt & George 1982).

*Presentation with complications*

The clinical presentation is greatly influenced by the development of complications such as obstruction, perforation and peritonitis (with or without associated obstruction), pericolic abscess and bleeding. In one study, obstruction occurred in 16% of the 4583 patients, while perforation occurred in 20% of those with obstruction and in 15% of those without (Phillips et al 1985). Other studies report colonic perforation in 3–8% of patients (Goligher & Smiddy 1957, Donaldson 1958, Crowder & Cohn 1967) and in one large study of colon cancer, 4% of patients had an abscess, 2% had free perforation and 2% had fistulation (Donaldson 1958). As obstruction or perforation significantly worsens prognosis within each tumor stage (Fielding et al 1986), every effort must be made to detect colorectal cancer early. Although the recommendation that all patients with lower gastrointestinal symptoms should undergo investigation may seem somewhat indiscriminant, it is the only way to detect tumors at an early uncomplicated stage without a population screening strategy.

*Other symptoms*

Invasion of the abdominal wall occasionally leads to abscess formation (White et al 1973). Fistulation to other hollow viscera is uncommon in colorectal cancer and much more likely to be due to diverticular disease. Fistulae that do develop are usually due to late diagnosis of a localized perforation.

Cecal carcinoma can mimic acute appendicitis; the appendix may be normal but appendicitis due to obstruction can cause the tumor to be overlooked (Ruderman et al 1967). Occasionally, patients present with hemorrhoids secondary to rectal carcinoma, hence the necessity for a rectal examination and sigmoidoscopy in all patients diagnosed as having piles. However, it is commoner for patients to assume that the symptoms of their rectal cancer are due to hemorrhoids than for them to have hemorrhoids.

More obscure presentations have been reviewed by Hardin (1972). Metastasis to the skin, lungs, bones and brain can cause subcutaneous nodules, unexpected metastasis on a routine chest radiograph, pathological fracture or neurological disorder respectively. Although intussusception is uncommon (Sanders et al 1958, Weilbaecher et al 1971), 60% of large bowel intussusceptions in adults are caused by carcinoma. As with childhood intussusception, there may be rectal bleeding, but the predominant feature is episodic abdominal pain leading to complete obstruction. Rare systemic manifestations (Bartholomew & Schutt 1971) include dermatomyositis, acanthosis nigricans, Cushing's syndrome, hypercalcemia, thrombophlebitis and lymphedema.

### *Clinical examination*

The history is supremely important given that clinical examination is often negative and the clinician must not be dissuaded from investigating the large bowel. General examination may reveal signs of anemia or chronic iron deficiency and occasional evidence of tumor dissemination. Abdominal examination may reveal hepatomegaly and an abdominal mass is palpable in more than 50% of patients (Falterman et al 1974), particularly in patients with right-sided or transverse colon tumors. Such masses are usually hard, painless and irregular and are often fixed to surrounding tissues. By contrast, less than 10% of tumors in the left colon are palpable. Abdominal distention is usually a sign of large bowel obstruction (Gennaro & Tyson 1978) but is occasionally due to ascites.

Digital rectal examination is mandatory to detect low cancers and assess fixity, sphincter involvement and sphincter quality when low rectal anastomosis is planned. Whereas rectal examination once detected 40% of all large bowel tumors (Jackman & Beahrs 1968), the incidence of low rectal cancers may since have fallen. Only 12% of all large bowel cancers and 30% of all rectal cancers extended to within 6 cm of the anal margin in the experience of Berg & Howell (1974), while Halvorsen (1986) found that 21% of 853 colorectal adenocarcinomas had a lower margin within 10 cm of the anal verge.

## Investigations

### *Occult blood testing*

Whereas fecal occult blood testing has a role in population screening, it is not sufficiently sensitive to be used as a diagnostic tool. A negative test is never taken to indicate that a symptomatic patient does not need further investigation.

### *Rigid and flexible sigmoidoscopy*

Although rigid sigmoidoscopy detected over half of all large bowel cancers in the past, more recent studies show that only some 38% of cancers are within reach of the rigid sigmoidoscope and 60% within reach of the flexible sigmoidoscope (Smith 1983). It is essential to inspect the rectosigmoid junction as this site is often poorly visualized at barium enema. Rigid sigmoidoscopy may have a role in assessing the fixity of rectal tumors when carrying out examination under anesthesia to plan resection.

Optimal investigation when large bowel cancer is suspected involves flexible sigmoidoscopy after suitable bowel preparation followed by double-contrast barium enema. However, practical and resource implications may mean that normal practice consists of rigid sigmoidoscopy with inspection of the rectosigmoid junction followed by barium enema at a separate visit.

### *Plain abdominal radiography*

In uncomplicated cases, the plain abdominal radiograph is almost always normal. Occasionally a soft tissue mass or stricture distorts the luminal gas shadow. Mucin-secreting primary cancers occasionally have fine granular calcification and granular "poppyseed" calcification may be present in liver metastases.

Since 8–29% of all colon cancers obstruct (Deans et al 1994a) and colon cancer accounts for approximately 80% of all cases of confirmed large bowel obstruction (Stewart et al 1984), plain radiography has a major role in patients presenting with complications. However, typical features of large bowel obstruction on plain films, even when associated with clinical signs and symptoms, are not necessarily diagnostic of mechanical obstruction. Up to 11% of patients with such features have idiopathic pseudo-obstruction and only 45% have colorectal cancer and many centers regard single contrast enema as mandatory when large bowel obstruction is suspected (Stewart et al 1984, Gilchrist et al 1985).

Obstruction typically produces gaseous distention of the large bowel proximal to the lesion with fluid levels on the erect film. If obstruction is complete and the ileocecal valve incompetent, small bowel obstruction may be superimposed. When the ileocecal valve remains competent, gross distention of the cecum carries a substantial risk of perforation. If perforation occurs, free peritoneal gas, gas in a localized soft tissue abscess or mass or an inflammatory ileus pattern may make diagnosis more difficult. Mucosal edema can result in "thumbprinting" of the bowel outline due to the presence of colitis or acute-on-chronic large bowel obstruction (Whitehouse & Watt 1977, Seaman & Clements 1982). Intussuscepting ileocecal tumors produce diagnostic features on plain films (Weilbaecher et al 1971).

### *Barium enema* (see also p. 481)

As just discussed, urgent contrast radiography is advisable when large bowel obstruction is suspected. Water-soluble media such as Gastrografin should be used although dilute barium can be employed if there is no suspicion of perforation. In pseudo-obstruction, Gastrografin enema can be therapeutic, although care should be taken to avoid dehydration.

In the elective setting, double-contrast barium enema is

a remarkably accurate method of detecting primary colorectal cancer, provided bowel preparation is thorough. Cancer detection rates reach 94–98% in the best hands (Kelvin 1982, Johnson et al 1983, Stevenson 1993) and in one representative study, the error rate was less than 5% (Johnson et al 1983). The four main causes of error were technical problems, radiologist inexperience, misinterpretation and distraction. Distraction accounted for 44% of errors and was due mainly to preoccupation with the first lesion found. The distracting lesion was often a synchronous malignant tumor but lesions such as diverticular disease, fistula, polyps, pelvic masses and ischemic changes can be responsible. Colonic spasm, retained fecal or fluid material and redundant overlapping loops, especially in the sigmoid region, may also cause misdiagnosis. Kelvin et al (1981) also found that the majority of missed diagnoses of colorectal cancer on double-contrast barium enema were due to failure to assess the radiographs rather than fundamental inability of the technique to show the lesion. In around 30% of cases, a combination of assessment and technical factors were responsible. The most common assessment errors were failure to detect a filling defect in the barium pool or a tumor en face in double-contrast films.

Variations in accuracy reflect the operator-dependent nature of double-contrast barium enema (Stevenson 1993). In one study of 2590 patients (Fork 1983), the predictive value of a positive report was 93% but the overall sensitivity was only 84%, whereas Johnson et al (1983) found a sensitivity of 95%. Optimum assessment involves careful viewing by two separate radiologists.

The commonest appearance of colorectal cancer is an annular stricture (Figs 55.13 and 55.14) which is typically abrupt, shouldered, eccentric in outline and up to 5 or 6 cm long. The stricture is fixed and rigid and its mucosal surface often appears ulcerated. This type of cancer appears to arise from one side of the lumen, probably as a plaque-like or saddleshaped lesion which spreads circumferentially (Dreyfuss & Benacerraf 1978). Sigmoid tumors may be difficult to differentiate from diverticular disease.

Polypoidal or fungating tumors produce a large, irregular filling defect in the barium/air contrast column (Fig. 55.15). The deformity may be unilateral owing to irregular involvement of the wall by the base of the tumor and the exophytic soft tissue mass may displace or distort the bowel and neighboring structures. Occasionally, tumor necrosis is apparent as barium and/or air filling of an irregular, ill-defined cavity which projects beyond the colonic lumen. The prognosis in such patients is usually poor (Hunter et al 1983). Sometimes barium outlines a fistula or abscess cavity. Evidence of free perforation (preexisting or iatrogenic as a result of hydrostatic pressure) is rare but necessitates urgent laparotomy.

Progress of barium is occasionally completely arrested by a constricting neoplasm in a patient with no clinical evidence of obstruction. This is most frequently seen in the sigmoid and descending colon. Intravenous antispasmodic agents and careful positioning may allow some contrast to pass through the narrowed area, but excessive pressure must be avoided. Evacuating the barium and introducing a little air sometimes outlines the stricture and allows an estimate of its length and cause. A characteristic appearance is seen in the rare event of intussusception of a polypoid carcinoma of the cecum.

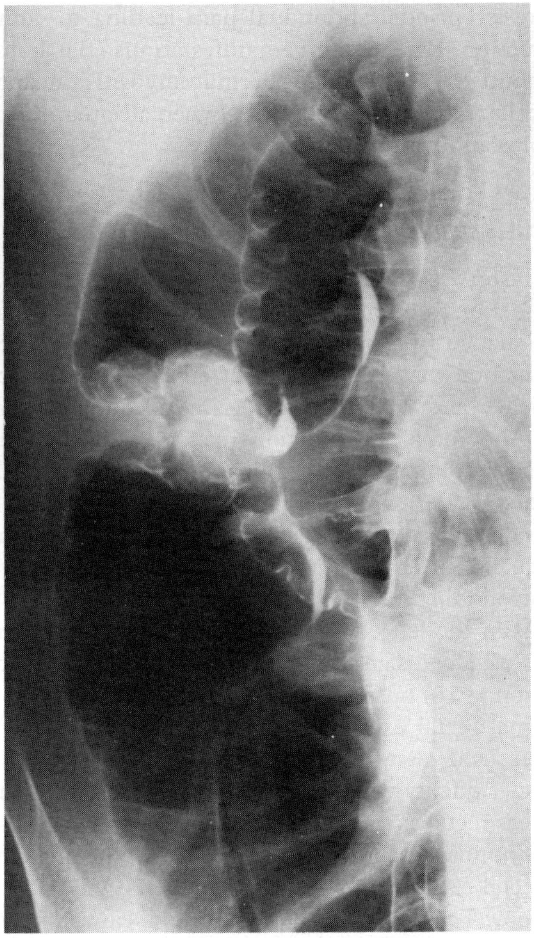

**Fig. 55.13** Large annular carcinoma of the ascending colon demonstrated by double-contrast barium enema.

Other radiological features include a pattern resembling colitis. This can occur proximal to a neoplasm where it is thought to be due to ischemia due to the high intraluminal pressure (Whitehouse & Watt 1977) and the resultant submucosal edema or colonic "urticaria" (Seaman & Clements 1982). Bronen et al (1984) emphasize the need for careful evaluation to exclude neoplasia in patients over 60 years of age with diffuse lymphoid follicles of the colon.

Long neoplastic strictures may simulate inflammatory, granulomatous or ischemic strictures. If the mucosal pattern is preserved, the differential diagnosis includes infiltrating primary adenocarcinoma of the colon, metastases from primary gastric or breast cancer and colonic

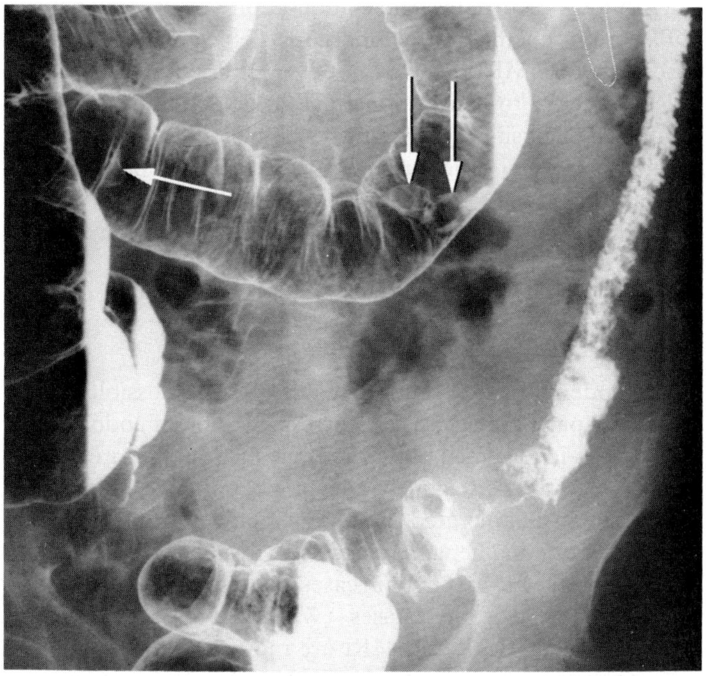

**Fig. 55.14** Carcinoma of sigmoid colon with three polyps (arrows) in the transverse colon, two of which were found to be malignant at histological examination.

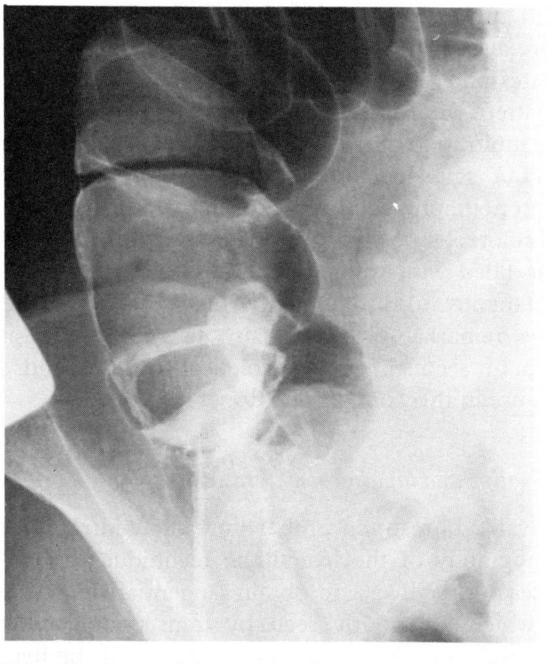

**Fig. 55.15** Carcinoma of the cecum and commencement of ascending colon. Double-contrast barium enema shows characteristic filling defect.

lymphoma (which may present as a bulky intramural mass with extensive infiltration). In chronic ulcerative proctocolitis, any stricture, regardless of length, is highly suspicious of malignancy (Gardiner & Stevenson 1982).

Cecal tumors can present major diagnostic problems. Small tumors can be concealed in the barium pool, indentation can be due to normal structures such as the ileocecal valve and satisfactory bowel preparation can be difficult. However, a major problem is failure to perceive tumors which are visible on subsequent review of the films (Bolin et al 1988). Other causes of cecal abnormality include Crohn's disease, lipoma, appendicitis and appendix mass. Since the cecum is not examined satisfactorily in 6% of colonoscopies (Thoeni & Petras 1982) and as the incidence of cancer of the right colon is increasing (Bernstein et al 1985), double-contrast barium enema of the right side of the colon must be a thorough and complete examination.

*Colonoscopy* (p. 124)

There is a compelling argument for colonoscopy as the primary investigation of all large bowel symptoms. Skilled endoscopists expect to complete the examination in more than 95% of cases (Williams 1984a, Stevenson 1993) and it is at least as well tolerated as barium enema, equally sensitive in detecting cancer and probably more accurate in detecting polyps. However, colonoscopy misses about 10% of polyps 1 cm or larger (Williams 1984a) and a greater proportion of smaller lesions.

One of the main benefits of colonoscopy is the facility to photograph and biopsy lesions and remove polyps. Other therapeutic interventions include sclerotherapy or laser treatment of angiodysplastic lesions. Colonoscopy is the follow-up procedure of choice after colonic resection for cancer and should probably be performed every 2 years. It can also complement double-contrast barium enema by detecting additional lesions which can be removed endoscopically or at the time of surgery (Williams 1984a). As indicated above, adenomatous polyps are present in 30% of cases and synchronous cancers in around 5% of cases of colorectal cancer. In cecal cancer, colonoscopy can confirm the diagnosis prior to surgery when barium enema suggests the presence of cancer.

Colonoscopy is invasive and its particular complications are perforation and bleeding. Mortality rates of 1/2000–1/6000 can be expected (Gilbert et al 1984, Eddy et al 1987) and serious morbidity rates are around 1/300–1/500 and are particularly high after snare polypectomy (Gilbert et al 1984, Ransohoff et al 1991). Although the benefits of colonoscopy far outweigh its drawbacks, serious complication rates must be taken into account when screening otherwise healthy individuals (Eddy et al 1987).

*Computed tomography* (CT) (p. 66)

Computed tomography is of value in diagnosing colorectal cancer, staging rectal tumors, detecting liver metastases and local recurrence. As a primary diagnostic test, it is a useful alternative to barium enema in elderly patients who are unable to retain barium and air (Day et al 1993). Its sensitivity is inferior to that of barium enema although accuracy improves with oral contrast. CT can provide additional information regarding degree of spread (e.g. abdominal wall involvement) and nodal and more distant metastases. However, Freeny et al (1986) found that in local staging it agreed with Dukes' classification of the operative specimen in only 48% of 103 patients. In another study, CT understaged 10 of 25 cases of recto-sigmoid carcinoma (Thompson et al 1986) and it is substantially less accurate than endorectal ultrasonography in the staging of rectal cancer (Hawes 1993).

Due to its noninvasive nature, CT of the abdomen and pelvis is the investigation of first choice when local recurrence is suspected or the patient has a rising postoperative plasma carcinoembryonic antigen (CEA) level. CT of the chest may be of value if pulmonary metastases are suspected. The fact that CT is more sensitive in detecting recurrent disease than CEA levels (Shirkhoda et al 1984, McCarthy et al 1985) has led some to recommend a scan at 2–4 months postoperatively with a follow-up scan 6-monthly for at least 2 years (Thompson et al 1986).

CT is of undoubted value in preoperative detection of unsuspected hepatic metastases and in assessing known hepatic metastases (see below). The sensitivity exceeds 95% with deposits larger than 2 cm but falls beneath 40% with lesions smaller than 1 cm in diameter (p. 67).

### *Arterial portography combined with computed tomography* (CTAP)

Transplenic portography had a high incidence of splenic bleeding and CTAP is now the favored alternative. It involves superior mesenteric angiography and continuous infusion of contrast during CT. Spiral CT during portography has even greater sensitivity in detecting small lesions. CTAP is not part of the routine assessment prior to resection of colorectal cancer. It is reserved for preoperative assessment when resection of liver metastases is being considered and is now the method of choice in this context, having a sensitivity and specificity of around 90% in detecting liver deposits (Karl et al 1993, Howell et al 1993, Small et al 1993, Lindberg et al 1993). McGrath et al (1993) found that 74% of patients referred for resection of liver metastases were deemed unresectable after CTAP.

### *Magnetic resonance imaging* (MRI)

MRI has similar accuracy to CT in detecting liver deposits of 2 cm or larger but is inferior for smaller lesions; in preoperative assessment of such metastases, MRI had a sensitivity of 78% whereas that of CTAP was 94% (Soyer et al 1993a).

With local recurrence, the combination of conventional CT, barium enema and colonoscopy detects 61–88% of cases, whereas MRI detects 80–88%. On the other hand, MRI is inferior to conventional CT in detecting nodal or peritoneal deposits (Charnsangavej 1993). The place of MRI in colorectal cancer remains to be fully explored but its main use may be in assessment of spread in rectal cancer and in deciding between transabdominal resection and peranal excision (p. 75).

### *Transcutaneous abdominal ultrasonography*

With modern, high-definition scanners, it is possible to identify hepatic metastases and assess invasion of abdominal wall or involvement of structures such as the ureter. Ultrasonography is relatively cheap, reproducible, noninvasive and well tolerated, but is a relatively insensitive means of detecting hepatic metastases. Lesions larger than 2 cm are detected in 88% of cases but overall it detects only 53% of liver metastases (Wernecke et al 1991). Although CT, CTAP and MRI are more accurate, ultrasonography has the advantages of availability and cost and can still provide additional information leading to therapeutic benefit (Alderson et al 1983) (p. 55).

Liver metastases appear circumscribed or diffuse and the echoic intensity may be increased, decreased or absent. Diffuse alterations of echogenicity with mixed patterns are also seen. However, increased echogenicity predominates and there is no definite relationship between echo pattern and vascularity or cell type (Lewis 1984). Diffuse infiltration of the liver may give a very bright echo pattern but is nonspecific.

Ultrasonography has been used for the primary detection of colorectal polyps and cancer (Limberg 1990). The colon is filled with water or saline enema and standard transcutaneous ultrasonography performed. The technique is remarkably accurate in detecting even small polyps but it seems likely that practical considerations will limit its use in this context.

### *Intraoperative and laparoscopic ultrasonography*

Autoclavable ultrasound probes now allow intraoperative ultrasonography of the liver. The technique can access most areas of the liver and obtain tangential views of segments which are poorly seen by transcutaneous ultrasonography. In addition, the image quality of the hepatic parenchyma is substantially improved because there is no intervening abdominal wall. The ultrasound probe can be hand-held at open operation or introduced laparoscopically (Miles et al 1992, John & Garden 1994). Intraoperative ultrasonography has proved superior to combinations of all available preoperative investigations, including CTAP (Soyer et al 1993b), but is operator dependent and may not become a routine adjunct to surgery.

*Rectal endosonography* (see also p. 126)

Endorectal ultrasonography is a relatively new method of preoperative staging and follow-up of patients with rectal cancer (Hawes 1993). It is particularly valuable for lesions below the peritoneal reflection. Although 90° array scanners are available, most probes have a rotating transducer which gives a real-time 360° image of the rectal wall and extrarectal tissues. The technique has an overall accuracy of 91% in staging mural spread (Beynon et al 1986) but its accuracy in lymph node assessment is only 78–87% (Beynon et al 1989, Hildebrandt et al 1990, Hawes 1993). Endorectal ultrasonography is substantially more accurate than CT in the staging of rectal cancer (Hawes 1993) and in the detection of local rectal recurrence after apparently curative resection.

*Immunoscintigraphy*

Radiolabeled monoclonal antibodies have been used to target primary or recurrent malignant tissue (Britton & Granowska 1985, Ryan 1993). Although promising results have been reported using antibodies to CEA (Allum et al 1986), the problem to date is lack of specificity of the antibodies.

*Radionuclide scanning*

Radionuclide scanning has been superseded by the methods described above in the detection of hepatic metastases.

## Differential diagnosis of cancer of the colon

Some of the conditions which may simulate colorectal cancer radiologically and clinically are listed below.

*Cecum and ascending colon*

- Ileocecal Crohn's disease
- Appendiceal abnormalities including inverted appendiceal stump after appendicectomy, intussusception of the appendix, mucocele, appendix abscess
- Prominence of the ileocecal valve
- Right-sided diverticular disease resulting in mass or abscess
- Infective conditions resulting in an inflammatory mass or granuloma in the cecal region such as amebiasis, tuberculosis and actinomycosis (Cowgill & Quan 1979)
- Colonic lymphoma

*Transverse colon*

- Extracolonic inflammatory conditions, such as acute pancreatitis and cholecystitis, may simulate tumor radiologically although the correct diagnosis is usually obvious
- Cancer of the pancreas or of the stomach may invade or metastasize to the bowel
- Ischemic colitis, particularly at the splenic flexure (Brandt et al 1985)
- Localized colonic Crohn's disease

*Left colon and rectosigmoid*

- Diverticular disease may be indistinguishable from or coexist with cancer
- Inflammatory lesions, particularly Crohn's disease, may mimic scirrhous cancer (Wolf & Marshak 1963)
- Cancer in adjacent organs (e.g. cancer of ovary, prostate, cecum and stomach). Ovarian cancer typically produces fixed edematous folds of rectal mucosa on sigmoidoscopy which overlie a hard fixed mass
- Cancer of the prostate rarely invades the rectum but can narrow or encircle its lumen and present as a stricture. Although invasion of the rectal mucosa is extremely rare, it may be indistinguishable on inspection from rectal cancer and it is important to review the histology of rectal tumors before radical surgery
- Endometriosis may cause rectal symptoms. On sigmoidoscopy the endometrioma projects into the lumen of the rectum or rectosigmoid junction as a polypoid mass covered by intestinal mucosa
- Rare lesions which can cause diagnostic difficulties include solitary ulcer of the rectum, leiomyoma, leiomyosarcoma, lipoma, carcinoid tumor, lymphoid tumor and hindgut cysts (Hjermstad & Helwig 1988)

## Primary treatment of colorectal cancer

*Primary surgical treatment*

En bloc resection of the primary tumor and locoregional nodes is the principle of radical surgery for large bowel cancer. Locoregional nodes are those nodal groups in the mesentery (including mesorectum), along the course of the feeding blood vessel to its origin. Resection may cure patients with localized disease and palliate those with hepatic or other metastases by preventing such distressing features as obstruction, bleeding, tenesmus and diarrhea. Resectability rates of up to 80% for rectal cancer in specialist centers (Abulafi & Williams 1994) give a false impression of surgical practice as many units achieve a radical resection rate of about 50% (Clarke et al 1980, Phillips et al 1984a). However, rates lower than 75–80% are now unacceptable and referral to specialist surgeons should be encouraged, particularly for rectal cancer.

Radical resection has unquestionable benefit. In combination with extended lymphadenectomy it is popular in Japan and remarkably low local recurrence rates and prolonged survival are reported (Koyama et al 1984). Radical excision of the entire mesorectum in rectal cancer has been advocated by Heald and local recurrence rates are lower than those achieved in adjuvant radiotherapy trials (MacFarlane et al 1993). Crucial aspects of technique may account for large differences between surgeons in terms of local recurrence and survival rates (Phillips et al 1984b, Quirke et al 1986, McArdle & Hole 1991). Thus, survival rates might be improved if techniques employed by surgeons producing the best results were applied universally or if all patients with large bowel cancer were referred to specialist surgeons.

*Segmental and other resectional surgery*

Right hemicolectomy involves excision of the terminal ileum, cecum, right colon and proximal transverse colon, along with the ileocolic, right colic and right branch of the middle colic artery and associated lymphatics. The vessels are taken at their origin to maximize the lymphadenectomy and the ileum is anastomosed to the transverse colon. Extended right hemicolectomy involves ligation of the middle colic artery at its origin and extending the resection to the upper descending colon. Transverse colectomy is now seldom performed as ileocolic anastomosis is superior to colocolic anastomosis. Total colectomy is a further extension of extended right hemicolectomy and includes ligation of the inferior mesenteric vessels and resection of left colon and sigmoid colon followed by an ileorectal anastomosis. Sigmoid colectomy and left hemicolectomy both involve ligation of the inferior mesenteric vessels flush with the aorta to maximize the chance of complete tumor removal.

Surgery for rectal cancer is technically more demanding and local recurrence and survival rates are particularly dependent on surgical skill (Abulafi & Williams 1994). Low anterior resection implies that the tumor is below the pelvic peritoneal reflection and/or is palpable on digital rectal examination. The aim is to excise the tumor-bearing bowel, perirectal fat and lymphatics and preserve the anal sphincters and continence. Distal resection margins of >2 cm are adequate and the recurrence rate is low (Karanjia et al 1990) provided the mesorectum is completely excised (Heald & Ryall 1986, MacFarlane et al 1993) and lateral excision margins are wide and histologically clear (Quirke et al 1986). Stapling devices now facilitate low rectal anastomosis, while endoanal suturing techniques mean that the rectum can be transected just above the anal sphincters. Abdominoperineal resection (APR) of the rectum and anus with formation of an end colostomy is no longer acceptable for mobile rectal lesions which do not invade the sphincter muscle.

Sphincter-saving resections give better quality of life than APR; 75% of patients undergoing low anterior resection are continent and 25% have only occasional incontinence (Williams & Johnston 1983). The functional result can be improved by forming a colonic reservoir before anastomosis to the upper anal canal (Nicholls et al 1988b). APR has significant morbidity related to both the perineal wound and the colostomy. Two-thirds of patients have problems with their colostomy appliance, many use medication or dietary manipulation to aid colostomy function and colostomy hernia is common (Hawley & Ritchie 1979).

There is conflicting evidence about differences between restorative low anterior resection and APR with regards to local recurrence and survival (Abulafi & Williams 1994). There are no controlled studies but the evidence strongly suggests that the most significant variable is the surgeon (McArdle & Hole 1991). Local recurrence rates of 5% have been reported following restorative procedures undertaken by specialists (MacFarlane et al 1993), while a survey involving specialists and nonspecialists found recurrence rates of 18.1% and 11.9% for restorative excision and APR respectively (Phillips et al 1984b).

Invasion of other organs does not preclude radical surgery. Resection of bladder, uterus, small intestine or abdominal wall muscle may be indicated and can provide optimal palliation even if cure is not achieved. En bloc resection is the aim, the area(s) of invasion being excised in continuity with the primary cancer. Adherence to other organs is frequently due to inflammation and even in cases with malignant invasion, 5-year survival rates may not be adversely affected (Eldar et al 1985). On the other hand, attempts to improve survival by extended abdominoiliac lymphadenectomy have proved disappointing in rectal cancer (Glass et al 1985).

*Emergency surgery for obstruction or perforated colorectal cancer*

In cases of perforation or obstruction of right-sided colon cancer, laparotomy is undertaken after appropriate resuscitation. Right hemicolectomy is the operation of choice, although palliative bypass (side-to-side anastomosis of ileum to transverse colon) may be indicated in patients with irresectable and/or disseminated disease. Emergency right hemicolectomy is not a trivial procedure and in the UK Large Bowel Cancer Project had an operative mortality of 14% (Fielding 1981).

Treatment of obstructed left colon cancer has moved away from the classic three-stage procedure to a one-stage resection with anastomosis whenever possible. Measures to reduce the risk of anastomotic leakage in such cases include on-table colonic lavage to remove all fecal residue before anastomosis (Radcliffe & Dudley 1983, Deans et al 1994a) and resection of the entire colon with ileorectal anastomosis. The latter technique avoids a colocolic anastomosis and removes any synchronous tumors (which are present in 5–10% of cases) and any diarrhea and fecal incontinence usually settles with time (Stephenson et al 1990).

Staged resection of obstructing left colon cancer is now rarely used and its overall mortality (almost 20%) is no better than that of primary resection (Fielding 1981, Deans et al 1994a). If staged resection is undertaken, the rectal stump is oversewn and an end colostomy created (Hartmann's procedure) or both ends of bowel are brought out as a colostomy and a mucous fistula. The benefit of the mucous fistula option is that the rectum is easier to find when reconstruction is undertaken. It should be stressed that 30% of patients who undergo Hartmann's resection never have continuity restored (Deans et al 1994a) and primary anastomosis is performed whenever possible.

Patients with peritonitis secondary to perforation of left colon cancer usually require resection with creation of an end colostomy. If contamination is minimal, a specialist surgeon may elect to carry out primary resection and anastomosis.

*Local treatment of rectal cancer*

Rectal cancer can be excised peranally under direct vision or with a resectoscope. Peranal excision gives acceptable results and avoids major abdominal surgery (Savage et al 1994) but should not be used in fit, potentially curable patients. It is particularly applicable to small cancers (< 3 cm) lying low in the rectum (see also p. 125).

Other local techniques include intracavitary irradiation (Papillon 1987), electrocoagulation (Madden & Kandalaft 1983) and Nd:YAG laser therapy (Bown et al 1986). External beam irradiation is sometimes used in palliative local treatment.

*Postoperative morbidity and mortality*

Even in earlier studies, segmental and abdominoperineal resection at the Mayo Clinic had a mortality rate of less than 4% (Judd 1961) and the mortality rate for elective resection should now be no more than 5%. Operative mortalities have fallen from 6.5% to 4.4% in Finland (Jarvinen et al 1988) and from 9% to 5% in north east Scotland (Gordon et al 1993). Even with radical surgery for low rectal cancer, a perioperative mortality of 2% is achievable (Goligher 1984, MacFarlane et al 1993) and the in-hospital mortality of anterior resection is similar to that of APR (Phillips et al 1984b). However, there is wide variation and mortality rates of 15–17% for elective surgery have been reported from district general hospitals (Chester & Britton 1989). Operative mortality is substantially greater following emergency resection and ranges from 16% to 31% (Fielding 1981, Chester & Britton 1989, Deans et al 1994a).

Anastomotic leakage is the major source of morbidity and mortality. Minor leaks can become walled off and pass unnoticed (Goligher et al 1970), while major leaks often lead to a fecal fistula and potentially lethal peritonitis. Bowel preparation and surgical technique have a major influence on leak rates (Fielding et al 1980). Major leaks require urgent reoperation at which the anastomosis is taken down and an end colostomy is created. Continuity can be restored some months later. Anastomotic leakage increases the risk of local recurrence. Akyol et al (1991) found that patients who leaked had a local recurrence rate of 47% compared to 19% in those who did not. However, anastomotic leakage may well reflect inadequate surgery, underlining the critical importance of technique as a determinant of outcome.

After rectal excision, some degree of urinary retention occurs in about 20% of cases and is particularly troublesome in men (Beahrs & Congdon 1957). Impotence occurs in 15–50% of cases and reflects trauma to the autonomic nerve supply (Lapides & Tank 1971, Yeager & Van Heerden 1980).

*Colostomy complications* (Hawley & Ritchie 1979) (p. 1466)

Care is essential when creating a colostomy if stoma-related problems are to be avoided. The end colostomy following rectal excision is usually sited in the left iliac fossa. Early complications are rare but include stomal necrosis if the blood supply is poor. Surgery is sometimes avoidable, but is necessary if necrosis extends to the intraperitoneal colon. Stenosis and/or retraction of the colostomy is usually the result of ischemia and requires surgical treatment.

Paracolostomy herniation is common and some 50% of patients develop some degree of herniation by the sixth postoperative year. The hernia is often asymptomatic and repair can be avoided, but significant prolapse requires excision and refashioning of the colostomy. Some patients have problems with colostomy function and irrigate the colostomy. Perforation of the bowel following irrigation is a rare cause of urgent laparotomy.

A defunctioning transverse colostomy is at less risk of ischemia but prolapse is common. It is usually a temporary procedure designed to protect a low rectal anastomosis and complications can follow its closure. Mortality rates are usually less than 2%, but a fecal fistula occurs in 3–7% of patients (although spontaneous closure is likely unless there is distal obstruction).

## Locally recurrent and metastatic colorectal cancer

*Local recurrence*

Local recurrence implies regrowth of carcinoma in the tumor bed, pericolic fat and local lymph nodes or at the anastomosis after apparently curative resection. The term does not apply to tumor growth after palliative resection. Risk factors are tumor stage, degree of differentiation and, in rectal cancer, the extent of extrarectal spread. Obstruction or perforation at presentation increases the risk of recurrence.

Local recurrence is apparent before the end of the second postoperative year in around two-thirds of patients destined to develop it (Polk & Spratt 1971, Umpleby & Williamson 1987). Most recurrences are asymptomatic and only 20–25% of asymptomatic recurrences can be detected on clinical examination. Therefore, if locally recurrent disease is to be detected at a potentially curable stage, additional means of follow-up are required. Serum CEA levels undoubtedly parallel increases in recurrent tumor bulk (Northover 1985) and can influence the timing of surgery and resectability rate (Abulafi & Williams 1994). However, there is no objective evidence that this improves outcome in terms of further tumor growth or survival. For the present it seems wise to offer serial CEA estimations at least for the first 2 years. Further investigation by CT, MRI and ultrasonography is discussed above.

Symptoms of local recurrence usually imply that the situation is unsalvageable. Perineal discomfort and pain aggravated by sitting after APR is particularly sinister. Other symptoms include weight loss, cramping abdominal pain, change of bowel habit and rectal bleeding. Examination may reveal an abdominal mass, recurrence in the perineal or abdominal scar or recurrence at the anastomosis on rectal or vaginal examination. Inguinal lymph nodes may be palpably involved when low rectal cancer has been resected.

Reported local recurrence rates range from 8.5% to 36% (Wright et al 1969, Umpleby & Williamson 1987) but a rate of 14% in one study of 4228 patients is probably representative. This complication above all depends on the technical skill of the surgeon performing the original operation (Phillips et al 1984b). As discussed above, there has been particular concern about apparently higher rates of pelvic recurrence following anterior resection (18%) than APR (12%) (Phillips et al 1984b). However, no differences were noted in many studies (Abulafi & Williams 1994) and very low recurrence rates are achievable even after restorative resection of high-risk rectal cancers (MacFarlane et al 1993).

Operative technique may minimize the risk of local recurrence. The no-touch technique leaves the tumor undisturbed until high ligation of the vascular pedicle has been performed (Turnbull et al 1967, Jeekel 1986). Seeding of exfoliated cancer cells on raw mucosa is a potential cause of suture line recurrence and may be minimized by isolating the tumor-bearing segment with tapes and irrigating the bowel lumen with cytotoxic agents before anastomosis (Umpleby & Williamson 1987). Local recurrence may be less likely after stapled as opposed to sutured anastomoses (Akyol et al 1991), although some studies report the converse and many have shown no difference (Abulafi & Williams 1994). It is difficult to offer a coherent biological explanation for any such differences.

Surgery for local recurrence usually involves further bowel resection with excision of involved adjacent structures. Excision of ilium and sacrum have been advocated but such radical surgery is usually contraindicated by pulmonary and liver metastases. Some patients who appear to present with recurrent disease may have benign remediable conditions such as adhesive obstruction, diverticular disease, appendicitis and ischemic colitis. In one series of 63 patients coming to further laparotomy with suspected recurrence, nine had benign disease while four had metachronous cancer (Lewi et al 1983).

Local recurrence remains a major cause of morbidity and poor prognosis. Every effort must be made to avoid it, even though the measures discussed above may have no overall effect on mortality.

*Hepatic metastases* (see also p. 1131)

Hepatic metastases may be detected by palpation or by a rising serum CEA level. Further investigation involves ultrasonography, CT, CTAP and MRI, as discussed above. If potentially operable liver metastases are found, intraoperative and laparoscopic ultrasonography help to determine the feasibility and extent of resection. When patients present with jaundice, the situation is usually untreatable.

Around 25% of patients have overt hepatic metastases at the time of primary resection (Stower & Hardcastle 1985, Jarvinen et al 1988, McArdle et al 1990, Ballantyne & Quin 1993) and a further 25% have occult liver metastases which become detectable over the next 2–3 years (Finlay et al 1982). The median survival of patients with overt liver metastases is around 10 months. Metastases are apparently limited to the liver in only 25% of cases and in around 25% of them, only one lobe is involved. It is in this last group of patients (amounting to less than 5% of all patients with colorectal cancer) that liver resection may be worthwhile. Controversy stems from the fact that this highly selected group might have a reasonably good prognosis with several years of survival even without treatment. There have been no prospective randomized studies which compare liver resection with observation and it is now highly unlikely that such studies could be performed for ethical reasons.

While circumstantial and comparative data suggest that resection of liver metastases improves survival (Ballantyne & Quin 1993), few patients actually benefit as most have incurable disease. In one large study of 1209 patients with hepatic metastases, 19% went to resection with a view to cure (Scheele et al 1990). The operative mortality of radical excision was 5.5% and the cumulative survival rate of the remainder was 40% at 5 years and 25% at 10 years.

Other protagonists acknowledge that hepatic resection could only influence outcome in 15–20% of patients with liver metastases (Adson et al 1984). However, there is little doubt that increased survival (and perhaps cure) is possible in a small number of highly selected patients with hepatic metastases from colorectal cancer.

Chemotherapy has been delivered systemically or via hepatic artery perfusion. Response rates are similar and although there are no controlled trials showing conclusive survival advantage (Ballantyne & Quin 1993), arterial perfusion of cytotoxic drugs can palliate severe pain (Priestman 1976). Hepatic artery infusion of 5-FU or 5-fluorodeoxyuridine using implantable pumps is expensive and although response rates of over 50% have been claimed, unequivocal evidence of benefit is lacking (Clark 1986). Complications of hepatic artery infusion include gastrointestinal toxicity, chemical cholecystitis and hepatitis and a form of sclerosing cholangitis (Kemeny et al 1985). Systemic therapy also has significant morbidity including mucositis and diarrhea, especially when high-dose regimens are employed.

Given the absence of proven benefit for regional or systemic chemotherapy in patients with colorectal hepatic metastases, the balance between complications and possible palliation must be assessed on an individual patient basis.

## Adjuvant therapy for colorectal cancer

### *Radiotherapy*

Adjuvant radiotherapy has no place in the management of colon cancer but randomized controlled trials suggest benefit in cancer of the rectum (Duncan 1985, Lancet 1985, Taylor 1987, Buyse et 1988, Gaze 1988, Cummings 1989). It is vital to distinguish between benefit in terms of local recurrence and survival. Local recurrence rate is a function of surgical technique while the predominant arbiter of survival is disease stage and tumor biology.

Radiotherapy in a nonadjuvant setting has a role in palliation of local recurrence and in alleviating bone pain from metastases.

***Effect of adjuvant radiotherapy on survival.*** In a meta-analysis of 3062 patients in all published trials up to 1988, Buyse et al (1988) detected no survival benefit in rectal cancer. More recently, Krook et al (1991) reported a statistically significant 34% and 36% reduction in local recurrence rate and cancer-related deaths respectively in a randomized trial of combination chemoradiotherapy for rectal cancer. Analysis suggests that the benefit is largely due to the addition of chemotherapy. No trial has shown survival benefit for adjuvant radiotherapy alone and this is hardly surprising since the over-riding reason for poor survival is dissemination outside the pelvis at presentation.

In a minority of patients, preoperative radiotherapy may convert an inoperable tumor to an operable, potentially curable lesion. Papillon (1987), in an uncontrolled study, reported that 17% of patients subsequently coming to surgery had tumor-free resection specimens and 32% had Dukes' A tumors. In another series (Taylor et al 1987), complete tumor regression was seen in 38% of radically treated patients and 24% of those treated palliatively; partial regression was seen in 56% and 58% of cases respectively. Pahlman et al (1985) also found that preoperative radiotherapy was more effective in reducing local recurrence rates than postoperative treatment.

***Effect of adjuvant radiotherapy on local recurrence.*** Several trials have shown a statistically significant reduction in the incidence of pelvic recurrence (Gerard et al 1985, Duncan 1985, Pahlman et al 1985, Fisher et al 1988, Gaze 1988, Cummings 1989). The study of patients with Dukes' B2 or C tumors reported by Krook et al (1991) is discussed above and undoubtedly demonstrates a lower local recurrence rate in the combined treatment arm. However, the local recurrence rate was 62.7% and 41.5% with radiotherapy alone and combined treatment respectively. Similar recurrence rates are reported in other US adjuvant radiotherapy trials, rates of 70% being common (Fisher et al 1988). These rates are substantially higher than the rate of 22% achieved by surgery alone (MacFarlane et al 1993, Abulafi & Williams 1994). At best, it appears that radiotherapy converts the results of the poorest surgeons to something approaching those of the best surgeons. Furthermore, adjuvant radiotherapy incurs a cost in terms of radiation proctitis, cystitis and small bowel involvement, in addition to its financial and logistic implications. With increasing specialization and the practice of complete mesorectal excision (Heald et al 1982, Heald & Ryall 1986), many surgeons now feel that routine adjuvant postoperative radiotherapy is inappropriate, even for high-risk rectal cancer (Dukes' B2 and C). However, in patients with large fixed tumors, preoperative radiotherapy may allow surgical excision and the best hope for cure.

### *Chemotherapy* (Buyse et al 1988, Woolley et al 1988, Hunt & Taylor 1989)

Systemic adjuvant chemotherapy using 5-fluorouracil alone or in combination has been studied for over 25 years (Moertel & Reitemeier 1967, Moertel 1976). A meta-analysis of 17 trials involving 6791 patients (Buyse et al 1988) showed no overall benefit or detriment, but when trials involving 5-FU were analyzed separately, there was an overall 10% survival benefit in favor of treatment but this did not reach statistical significance. Only when trials involving treatment for over a year were analyzed did a statistically significant (17%) survival benefit appear. Recently, the American Intergroup study compared 5-FU and levamisole, levamisole alone and no chemotherapy

(Moertel et al 1990) and reported substantial survival benefit for patients with Dukes' C colon cancer. The statistically significant 33% reduction in colon cancer deaths prompted a US government directive that adjuvant chemotherapy was mandatory for patients with Dukes' stage C colon cancer (NIH Consensus Conference 1990). The evidence suggests that the combination of 5-FU and levamisole is no better than 5-FU alone.

The high level of compliance and the intensive regimen have been used to explain the difference between the Intergroup study and the meta-analysis (Buyse et al 1988). However, the Intergroup study also randomized patients with Dukes' B2 tumors and patients in the treatment arm did substantially worse. This could be due to chance misstaging of poor prognosis Dukes' B2 cancers that were actually Dukes' C lesions and were in the treatment arm. Concerns over universal adoption of adjuvant chemotherapy with its side-effects and resource implications are certainly valid. The main side-effect is leukopenia, requiring weekly white blood cell and platelet count. Mucositis, anorexia, occasional vomiting, diarrhea and weakness are all relatively common with intensive regimes. The concerns discussed have resulted in the initiation of a large trial in the United Kingdom (Quasar) which aims to recruit 7500 patients.

A second American Intergroup study has also shown a statistically significant benefit from adjuvant 5-FU plus radiotherapy (4500–5040 cGy) for rectal cancer. The reduction in cancer-related deaths was 36% and in local recurrence was 46%, leading the authors to conclude that radiotherapy and chemotherapy may be synergistic.

In the United States, the position is clear; all patients with lymphatic involvement must have chemotherapy and there is a moratorium on trials including an untreated control arm. Outside the United States there is still substantial doubt about the benefit of adjuvant chemotherapy. Morbidity and financial consequences will be substantial if chemotherapy is used routinely in all patients with Dukes' C tumors. Since many studies and a meta-analysis have shown little or no overall benefit, it seems wiser to await the results of further large trials which do include a "no treatment" arm before concluding that adjuvant chemotherapy is of value. In the meantime, it is likely that patients outside trials will be offered the American Intergroup regimen.

Portal infusion with 5-FU reduced the odds of death by 60% in one trial (Taylor et al 1985). Several trials have shown similar but smaller benefit and the effect may be mainly systemic rather than a specific effect on first pass through the liver (Wolmark et al 1990). The AXIS trial in the United Kingdom was designed to evaluate portal infusion of 5-FU and should soon report its findings.

### Prognosis of colorectal cancer

Prognosis depends on the degree of spread and aggressiveness of the tumor at the time of diagnosis. Cancer-related death rates and local recurrence rates may now be lower than in the 1970s (Jarvinen et al 1988, Gordon et al 1993). It cannot be overemphasized that the technical expertise of the surgeon is a major outcome determinant (Phillips et al 1984b, McArdle & Hole 1991).

Attempts at staging are confounded by the idiosyncratic natural history of some tumors. While Dukes' and other staging systems (Jass et al 1987) remain useful for stratifying patients into prognostic categories for adjuvant trials, outcome cannot be predicted accurately for an individual. The problem is illustrated by the finding that of patients undergoing curative operations with no apparent liver metastases, 30% eventually develop overt liver metastases and clearly had occult disease at the time of surgery (Finlay & McArdle 1986).

Despite these problems, some assessment of prognosis is worthwhile in that it allows tailoring of management. The importance of degree of differentiation and of local venous and lymphatic spread has been discussed above. Dukes' classification gives broad prognostic categories and stages A, B, C and D have approximate 5-year survival rates of 80%, 70%, 30% and 6% respectively. Within each category, the pathologist can provide further information on prognosis (Morson & Dawson 1979); for example, the 5-year survival rate of Dukes' B patients ranges from 90% to 57%, depending upon the degree of spread in continuity. Within the Dukes' C category, 5-year survival rate varies from 60% when only one lymph node is involved to 20% when six or more nodes are affected. In Dukes' B and C stages, more advanced tumors are more likely to have greater local spread and more lymph node involvement.

Prognosis undoubtedly depends on clinicopathological features, including mode of presentation (e.g. obstruction) and tumor mobility, in addition to the purely pathological features discussed above (Fielding et al 1986). Tumor site does not have a major effect and the 5-year survival rates of rectal and colon cancer are not substantially different (Falterman et al 1974, Gill & Morris 1978, Gordon et al 1993). Other factors inter-related with stage and degree of differentiation are spread of tumor into veins outside the bowel wall (Carroll 1963, Talbot et al 1981), perforation and obstruction. Clinical presentation also has a bearing in that discomfort and bleeding for less than 6 months are associated with a much better prognosis than if the symptoms have been present for longer (Thomas et al 1969, Speck et al 1970).

There is conflicting evidence as to whether perioperative blood transfusion reduces survival. Confounding issues are that patients who receive blood do so for a reason and their tumor may be more advanced or their surgeon technically less skilled. One large study in which these variables were controlled to some extent found that transfusion of autologous as opposed to heterologous blood did not affect survival (Busch et al 1993). However, the argument that blood transfusion causes immune depression seems compelling since blood transfusion before renal transplant was used until relatively recently as a means of immunocompromising recipients. The issue may never be resolved but it would seem wise to avoid excessive blood loss by careful surgery and transfuse only when absolutely necessary.

It is important to realize that published survival rates usually refer to patients selected for surgical treatment and that true population survival is much worse. Once there is evidence of distant spread such as liver metastases, the outlook is bleak. In one large study, no patients with liver metastases who did not undergo liver resection survived for 5 years and 3- and 4-year survival rates were 2% and 1% respectively (Scheele et al 1990).

## OTHER MALIGNANT TUMORS OF THE COLON AND RECTUM

### Squamous cancer of the large bowel

Squamous carcinoma which are not simply anal carcinomas which have spread proximally into the rectum are rare. Such tumors frequently arise in the cecum and proximal colon. They can be associated with long-standing ulcerative colitis and are thought to arise in an area of squamous metaplasia secondary to chronic inflammation. In tumors not associated with ulcerative colitis, an adenosquamous pattern may be seen. Tumors with squamous features are very rare and tend to have a very poor prognosis; their etiology is unknown.

### Carcinoid tumors of the large bowel

Large bowel carcinoid tumors are very rare but accounted for 28% of all nonadenomatous or adenocarcinomatous tumors of the colon and rectum in one study (Geboes et al 1978). Rectal carcinoid tumors are the most common and 12–15% of carcinoids arise at that site (Godwin 1975).

Carcinoid tumor of the rectum does not cause the "carcinoid syndrome", but is important in the differential diagnosis of rectal lesions. In reporting 32 rectal neuroendocrine tumors, Shimoda et al (1984) found 27 typical carcinoids and five neuroendocrine carcinomas. Benign carcinoids are usually found incidentally during rectal examination and are solitary, spherical, hard, sessile, yellowish submucosal nodules (Fig. 55.16) which rarely exceed 2 cm in diameter. Ulceration is uncommon (Caldarola et al 1964). Symptoms include rectal pain, bleeding and tenesmus. One-third of patients have other associated malignancy and 10% have synchronous anorectal cancer (Morgan et al 1974). However, this association is almost certainly the result of ascertainment bias due to investigation and surgery for the adenocarcinoma.

Histological features are shown in Figure 55.17. Small rectal carcinoids are treated by local excision. Lesions larger than 1 cm in diameter are often ulcerated, frequently malignant and require segmental resection. Naunheim et al (1983) suggest that radical surgery should be reserved for tumors larger than 2 cm and for smaller tumors which show invasion of the muscularis propria on examination after local excision. This would miss only 6% of aggressive tumors and only 1.2% of individuals would have inappropriately conservative surgery. The 5-year survival rate for

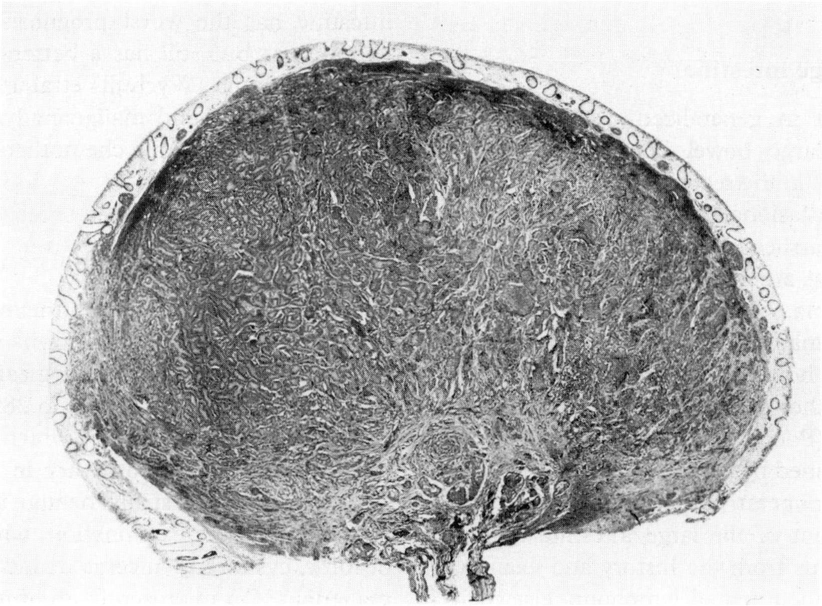

**Fig. 55.16** Benign rectal carcinoid. The lesion is polypoid and has produced attenuation of the overlying mucosa but there is no ulceration.

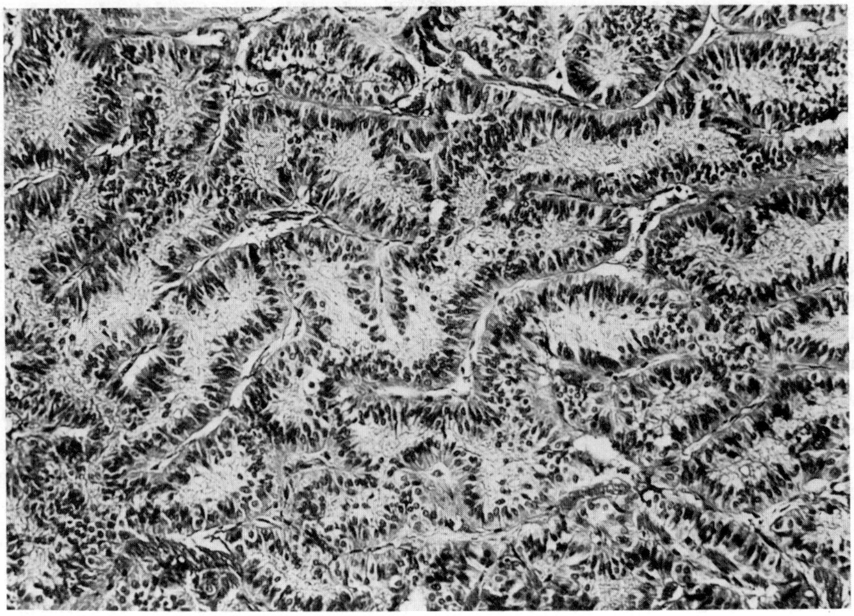

**Fig. 55.17** Benign rectal carcinoid showing the ribbon-like interlacing strands of regular, almost columnar cells typical of hindgut carcinoids (hematoxylin and eosin, ×140).

rectal carcinoids was 76% in one study of 36 patients (Orloff 1971).

Carcinoid tumors of the colon account for 7% of all carcinoid tumors (Godwin 1975). Most arise in the right colon (Rosenberg & Welch 1985) and cause symptoms indistinguishable from those of adenocarcinoma. In contrast to rectal carcinoids, colonic carcinoids can give rise to the carcinoid syndrome (p. 473). They are the most malignant of all carcinoid tumors and 60% have metastasized at diagnosis. Treatment consists of colonic resection and removal or debulking of metastases.

### Lymphoma of the large intestine

Secondary involvement in generalized disease is commoner than primary large bowel lymphoma. Primary lymphomas usually arise in the rectum or cecum (Dawson et al 1961) but are occasionally multicentric (p. 468). Abdominal pain with diarrhea is the usual mode of presentation and the symptoms are often indistinguishable from those of adenocarcinoma. Gastrointestinal bleeding can occur and obstruction may supervene, particularly in the case of ileocecal lymphoma, which may intussuscept. Barium enema often shows a long rigid segment with intramural thickening (Pochaczevsky & Sherman 1962). The diagnosis is established by histological examination of an endoscopic biopsy or operative specimen.

Secondary involvement of the large intestine by lymphoma is usually obvious from the history and examination of a patient with documented lymphoma elsewhere. The colon is involved more often than the rectum, usually with a polypoid mass of tissue. When the rectum is involved, there may be a presacral mass (Culp & Hill 1962) or on sigmoidoscopy the mucosa may appear to have fixed convolutions or a diffuse nodular appearance.

Malignant lymphomatous polyposis is a very rare form of large bowel lymphoma (p. 472). The gastrointestinal tract is primarily involved and multiple tumors may be present (Cornes 1961); lesions can occur elsewhere later. The condition must be differentiated from familial and other forms of polyposis (Table 55.4).

Primary lymphomas are treated by resection followed by chemotherapy and radiotherapy. Lymphoma of the large intestine has the worst prognosis of all gastrointestinal lymphomas but still has a better outlook after resection than carcinoma (Wychulis et al 1966). Secondary malignant lymphoma and malignant lymphomatous polyposis are treated by systemic chemotherapy and targeted radiotherapy (p. 471).

### Leiomyoma and leiomyosarcoma (Nemer et al 1977)

These rare tumors arise from the muscle of the bowel wall. The benign and malignant forms are often impossible to distinguish clinically or histologically. Geboes et al (1978) found that leiomyoma made up 28% and leiomyosarcoma 8% of all colorectal tumors which were not of adenomatous origin. The tumors vary in size from 1 to 20 cm; smaller ones are usually benign and asymptomatic and found on routine examination, while larger tumors often become cystic and ulcerated and are more likely to be malignant. On microscopy, the tumor consists entirely of smooth muscle cells. Metastasis occurs via the bloodstream to the liver and lungs in particular. The patient complains of rectal pain, a rectal mass or bleeding. On sigmoidoscopy, the tumor is usually found in the lower rectum and appears nodular and ulcerated. Tumors should be removed because of the possibility of malignancy. Tumors of up to 3 cm in diameter are usually treated by local excision and larger ones by radical surgery.

### Other tumors in the differential diagnosis of large bowel malignancy

These rare tumors are usually submucosal (Geboes et al 1978). Clinical presentation includes abdominal pain, rectal bleeding and abdominal discomfort. The histological diagnoses include lymphangioma, neurofibroma and granular cell myoblastoma (Kanabe et al 1978) but all are extremely rare. Hemangioma of the rectum may resemble a sessile polyp on sigmoidoscopy, but biopsy causes severe bleeding. Small rectal tumors can be fulgurated, but larger lesions require resection. In patients with vascular rectal lesions, the oral and nasal mucosae should be inspected for hemangiomata and the family history may suggest a diagnosis of hereditary hemorrhagic telangiectasia. Lipomata are usually single, round and soft and have a short pedicle; small ones are asymptomatic, but others cause abdominal pain (Wychulis et al 1964), frequently due to intussusception. Ulceration may cause bleeding. Barium enema usually reveals an intramural filling defect. Rectal tumors can be removed by local excision, more proximal lesions by colonoscopic polypectomy. An excess of adipose tissue in the submucosa of the ileocecal valve may be difficult to distinguish from carcinoma of the cecum on barium enema examination.

Oleoma or oil injection granuloma may follow the use of mineral oil to inject internal hemorrhoids. The tumor in the lower rectum is firm and rubbery. Biopsy reveals oil droplets, fibrous tissue and giant cells. Treatment is unnecessary.

## MALIGNANT TUMORS OF THE ANUS AND PERIANAL REGION

Anal cancer accounts for about 2% of all cancers of the colon, rectum and anus, although its incidence has increased by 70% and 300% in males and females respectively in one population study starting around 1960 (Frisch et al 1993). Anal cancer behaves as two distinct entities depending on its anatomical origin (Morson 1976b). Around 70% of the tumors arise between the anorectal ring and dentate line (Greenall et al 1985a,b). However, the World Health Organization recommends that the anal canal is regarded as extending from the anorectal ring to the junction of the modified squamous anal epithelium (the anal verge) and by this definition, 85% of anal cancers arise in the canal. Hence cancers of the anal margin can be regarded as occurring below the dentate line or distal to the anal verge, depending on classification used. This results in some confusion when assessing the effects of treatment. Most authors regard the dentate line as a convenient landmark and so cancers of the anal verge arise below it and cancers of the anal canal arise above it (Talbot 1988, Deans et al 1994b).

### Etiological factors

The etiology of anal cancer is multifactorial. The high incidence in females in Brazil has been attributed to poor personal hygiene. Smokers have around an eight-fold increase in incidence (Daling et al 1987). Immunosuppression plays a role, as evidenced by the substantially increased incidence in renal transplant recipients (Penn 1986). Anoreceptive intercourse is a risk factor in homosexual men (Leach & Ellis 1981) but the incidence of anal cancer in women indulging in anoreceptive intercourse is much lower (Daling et al 1987). Syphilis and anal warts are associated factors and an increased incidence in homosexual males with AIDS has been noted (Croxson et al 1984, Daling et al 1987). However, the increase in incidence predated recognition of the first AIDS patient in Denmark by 20–25 years (Frisch et al 1993) and so HIV infection could simply be a coinfecting agent rather than a causal factor. There is a strong association between anal and cervical cancer in women and the evidence strongly suggests that human papilloma virus (HPV) is the common etiological factor. HPV can be detected in around 70% of squamous anal carcinomas in males and females (Deans et al 1994b). Homosexual males are particularly prone to HPV infection and around 50% of HIV-positive patients have detectable anal HPV (Palefsky et al 1990). HPV type 16 virus is detected in around 50% of all cases, has been detected in anal warts and correlates with the degree of dysplasia.

### Clinical presentation

The mean age of presentation of anal cancer is 57 years and in population studies, two-thirds of patients are female (Frisch et al 1993). In selected populations with large homosexual communities (e.g. California), the sex ratio is reversed. The most common presenting symptoms are bleeding and anal/perianal pain, usually aggravated by defecation. Pruritis ani and discharge are common and an anal mass may be felt. Presentation is often late and the tumors are usually infiltrative when arising at the anal margin. There may be little ulceration until the disease is advanced. Extension into vagina, bladder or prostate occurs in 15% of patients. Perianal conditions which are frequently present include Paget's disease, leukoplakia, melanoma and lichen sclerosis. It is common practice to send all hemorrhoidectomy specimens for histological examination due to a supposed association with anal cancer. However, only one case of unsuspected anal cancer was noted in over 21 000 hemorrhoidectomy specimens in one study (Cataldo & MacKeigan 1992).

On examination the anal canal may feel thickened and irregular. A distinct mass may be palpable, particularly when cancer arises in the upper anal canal. The diagnosis is confirmed by biopsy under general anesthesia. Biopsy is essential in cases of atypical fissures or pruritis ani, in order to avoid missing early anal cancer.

## Pathology

Anal cancer is classified as epithelial, nonepithelial and malignant melanoma. Tumors with admixture of cell types are classified according to the predominant type. Epithelial tumors are subdivided into squamous carcinoma and adenocarcinoma.

### *Squamous (epidermoid) anal carcinoma*

The two main variants of epidermoid carcinoma of the anus, basaloid and squamous, are distinguished by their histology and area of origin (McConnell 1970, Boman et al 1984). Prognosis is no longer thought to be influenced by cell type (Deans et al 1994b).

Squamous carcinomas account for 80% of all malignant tumors of the anal region. Half of the tumors arising in the anal canal are nonkeratinizing and 80% are poorly differentiated, whereas 80% of anal margin tumors are keratinizing and only 15% are poorly differentiated. Tumors arising from the transitional epithelial zone above the pectinate line often have a basaloid pattern. The cell type may be mixed and a small cell pattern is associated with a very poor prognosis. True squamous lesions usually arise from the anal margin below the pectinate line.

Anal epidermoid carcinomas are usually 2–4 cm in diameter and appear infiltrating, fungating, ulcerating or undermining. Histologically, basaloid carcinomas consist of infiltrating islands of basaloid cells, which have a high nucleocytoplasmic ratio, oval or round nuclei and numerous mitoses. The better differentiated tumors show a peripheral palisade of cells. By contrast, squamous tumors consist of cells with abundant cytoplasm and show pearl formation.

Mucoepidermoid carcinomas are characterized histologically by mucin-producing cells in islands of epidermoid cells which usually show keratinization. These lesions account for some 10% of anal tumors (Berg et al 1960) and may occur in association with Paget's disease (Giltman et al 1985). However, some do not regard mucoepidermoid carcinoma as a distinct entity as its behavior does not differ significantly from that of other anal carcinomas (Dougherty & Evans 1985).

### *Anal adenocarcinoma*

The commonest tumor to involve the anal canal is distal extension of a low rectal adenocarcinoma (Klotz et al 1967). However, true adenocarcinoma of the anal canal does occur and arises from the anal glands. Anal adenocarcinoma accounts for 8–10% of anal cancers and can arise in chronic perianal fistula.

## Spread and staging of anal cancer

Anal epidermoid carcinoma may infiltrate through the anal wall into surrounding structures, including the vagina. Perirectal or inguinal lymph nodes may be involved at an early stage. Inguinal node involvement is particularly common in cancer of the anal margin; 20% of squamous carcinomas already have involvement at presentation and in a quarter of cases this is bilateral (Salmon et al 1984). Pararectal node involvement is detected in 25% of cases involving the upper anal canal, but pelvic lymphatic spread is rare with cancer of the anal margin. Only a small minority of patients have distant metastases at presentation.

Staging classifications used for colorectal adenocarcinoma are not appropriate. Classification involves clinical, radiological and endoscopic assessment (Deans et al 1994b). T1 and T2 tumors are less than 4 cm in diameter, while T3 tumors are 4 cm or greater in diameter and freely mobile. T4a tumors ulcerate the vaginal mucosa and T4b lesions invade the rectum, vagina or perineal skin (Papillon 1982). This classification has substantially better prognostic value than the TNM staging system.

## Treatment

Adenocarcinoma of the anal canal is treated by APR, in the same way as low rectal adenocarcinoma involving the anus. Involvement of the skin of the anal canal and anal margin may signal tumor spread to the inguinal glands.

Small early squamous cancers of the anal margin can be locally excised. Until recently, squamous cancer of the anal canal was usually treated by APR with formation of a permanent colostomy. This was followed by local recurrence in some 40% of cases (Boman et al 1984) and the 5-year survival rate of 71% in those who survived surgery fell to only 60% when patients with inoperable tumors were included. In order to reduce locoregional recurrence, Papillon et al (1983) exploited the extreme radiosensitivity of anal squamous cancer by using radiotherapy with or without operation. They achieved a 5-year survival rate of 65% and most patients retained their anus. Subsequently, concurrent chemotherapy (5-fluorouracil and mitomycin C) and external beam irradiation have been introduced (Nigro 1987) with a projected 5-year survival rate of 83% and with 75% of patients retaining anal function. Radiotherapy with or without chemotherapy is now the treatment of choice for squamous cancer of the anal canal (Deans et al 1994b). A controlled trial administered by the UK Co-ordinating Committee for Cancer Research, which is comparing radiotherapy alone with radiotherapy plus chemotherapy, may determine whether the toxicity of high-dose chemotherapy is justified by material benefit. Radical surgery is now reserved as a salvage procedure when medical treatment fails, although controversy still surrounds the need for inguinal lymph node dissection. Block dissection has substantial morbidity and as prophylactic dissection does not materially affect prognosis, such surgery is reserved for cases with proven nodal involvement which is refractory to chemotherapy.

## OTHER TUMORS OF THE ANAL REGION

### Malignant melanoma

Malignant melanomas arising in the perianal skin, anal canal or rectum are usually advanced at presentation. Most arise from melanocytes in the anal canal but some 70% are nonpigmented. The tumor may invade radially or proximally into the rectum and can present as a "thrombosed hemorrhoid" or as a polypoid mass in the lower rectum. Symptoms include perianal pain, tenesmus and rectal bleeding. On histological examination the tumor is pleomorphic with many mitoses. Spread occurs rapidly to the lymphatics of the pelvis and abdomen and by bloodborne metastasis. Prognosis is dismal with a 5-year survival rate of less than 10% (Chiu et al 1980). There is debate as to whether surgery should take the form of local excision or APR. Many authors regard the latter as the best option for long-term disease-free survival and effective palliation.

Other cell types which may give rise to malignant lesions of the anal region include basal cell carcinoma which presents as an ulcer on the anal verge (Nielsen & Jensen 1981). Paget's disease (Lock et al 1977) and Bowen's disease (Strauss & Fazio 1979) appear as red encrusted lesions in the perianal skin, present with pruritus and are treated by local excision. Neuroendocrine carcinoma (Boman et al 1984) may also occur. Anal intraepithelial neoplasia, possibly related to herpes virus infection, occurs in male homosexuals (Nash et al 1986). Anal tumors which occur in HIV infection are discussed on p. 611.

REFERENCES


Aaltonen L A, Peltomaki P, Leach F S et al 1993 Clues to the pathogenesis of familial colon cancer. Science 260: 812–816

Aaltonen L A, Peltomaki P, Mecklin J-P 1994 Replication errors in benign and malignant tumours from hereditary non-polyposis colorectal cancer patients. Cancer Research 54: 1645–1648

Abulafi A M, Williams N S 1994 Local recurrence of colorectal cancer: the problem, mechanisms, management and adjuvant therapy. British Journal of Surgery 81: 7–19

Abrams J S, Reines H D 1979 Increasing incidence of right-sided lesions in colorectal cancer. American Journal of Surgery 137: 522–526

Adson M A, van Heerden J A, Adson M H, Wagner J S, Ilstrup D M 1984 Resection of hepatic metastases from colorectal cancer. Archives of Surgery 119: 647–651

Ahnen D J 1985 Are animal models of colon cancer relevant to human disease? Digestive Diseases and Sciences 30: 103S–106S

Akyol A M, McGregor J R, Galloway D J, Murray G D, George W D 1991 Anastomotic leaks in colorectal surgery: a risk factor for recurrence? International Journal of Colorectal Disease 6: 179–183

Alderson P O, Adams D F, McNeil B J et al 1983 Computed tomography, ultrasound, and scintigraphy of the liver in patients with colon or breast carcinoma: a prospective comparison. Radiology 149: 225–230

Aldridge M C, Sim A J 1986 Colonoscopy findings in symptomatic patients without X-ray evidence of colonic neoplasms. Lancet 2: 833–834

Alexander R H, Beckwith J B, Morgan A, Bill A H 1970 Juvenile polyps of the colon and their relationship to allergy. American Journal of Surgery 120: 222–225

Allum W H, MacDonald F, Anderson P, Fielding J W L 1986 Localisation of gastrointestinal cancer with a 131 I labelled monoclonal antibody to CEA. British Journal of Cancer 53: 203–210

Alm T, Licznerski G 1973 The intestinal polyposes. Clinics in Gastroenterology 2: 577–602

Armitage N C, Farrands P A, Mangham C M, Hardcastle J D 1986 Faecal occult blood screening of first degree relatives of patients with colorectal cancer. International Journal of Colorectal Disease 1: 248–250

Ashton-Rickardt P G, Dunlop M G, Nakamura Y et al 1989 High frequency of APC loss in sporadic colorectal carcinoma due to breaks clustered in 5q21–22. Oncogene 4: 1169–1174

Astley V B, Coller F A 1954 The prognostic significance of direct extension of carcinoma of the colon and rectum. Annals of Surgery 139: 846–851

Atkin W S, Cuzick J, Northover J M A, Whynes D K 1993 Prevention of colorectal cancer by once-only sigmoidoscopy. Lancet 341: 736–740

Axtell L M, Chiazze L Jr 1966 Changing relative frequency of cancers of the colon and rectum in the United States. Cancer 19: 750–754

Bacon H E, Gennaro A R 1968 Carcinoma of the transverse colon and the splenic flexure. Surgery, Gynecology and Obstetrics 127: 523–527

Ballantyne G H, Quin J 1993 Surgical treatment of liver metastases in patients with colorectal cancer. Cancer 71: 4252–4266

Baptist S J, Sabatini M T 1985 Coexisting juvenile polyps and tubulovillous adenoma of colon with carcinoma in situ. Human Pathology 16: 1061–1063

Bartholomew L G, Schutt A J 1971 Systemic syndromes associated with neoplastic disease including cancer of the colon. Cancer 28: 170–174

Bartholomew L G, Dahlin D C, Waugh J M 1957 Intestinal polyposis associated with mucocutaneous melanin pigmentation (Peutz–Jeghers syndrome). Review of literature and report of 54 cases with special reference to pathologic findings. Gastroenterology 32: 434

Bartram C I, Thornton A 1984 Colonic polyp patterns in familial polyposis. American Journal of Roentgenology 142: 305–308

Beacham C H, Shields H M, Raffensperger E C, Enterline H T 1978 Juvenile and adenomatous gastrointestinal polyposis. American Journal of Digestive Diseases 23: 1137–1143

Beahrs O H, Congdon G H 1957 Morbidity and mortality following combined abdominoperineal resection: with special reference to closure of the posterior wound. Surgical Clinics of North America 37: 999

Beart R W 1985 Familial polyposis. British Journal of Surgery 72: S31–S32

Berci G, Panish J F, Schapiro M, Corlin R 1974 Complications of colonoscopy and polypectomy. Report of the Southern California Society for Gastrointestinal Endoscopy. Gastroenterology 67: 584–585

Berg J W, Howell M A 1974 The geographic pathology of bowel cancer. Cancer 34: 807–814

Berg J W, Lone F, Stearns M W 1960 Mucoepidermoid anal cancer. Cancer 13: 914
Bernstein M A, Feczko P J, Halpert R D, Simms S M, Ackerman L V 1985 Distribution of colonic polyps: increased incidence of proximal lesions in older patients. Radiology 155: 35–38
Beynon J, Mortensen N J M, Foy D M A et al 1986 Endorectal sonography: laboratory and clinical experience in Bristol. International Journal of Colorectal Disease 1: 212–215
Beynon J, Mortensen N J M, Foy D M A et al 1989 Preoperative assessment of mesorectal lymph nodes in rectal cancer. British Journal of Surgery 76: 276–279
Bisgaard M L, Fenger K, Bulow S, Niebuhr E, Mohr J 1994 Familial adenomatous polyposis (FAP): frequency, penetrance and mutation rate. Human Mutation 3: 121–125
Blair N P, Trempe C L 1980 Hypertrophy of the retinal pigment epithelium associated with Gardner's syndrome. American Journal of Ophthalmology 90: 661–667
Blenkinsopp W K, Stewart-Brown S, Blesovsky L et al 1981 Histopathology reporting in large bowel cancer. Journal of Clinical Pathology 34: 509–513
Bodmer W F, Bailey C J, Bodmer J et al 1987 Localisation of the gene for familial polyposis coli on chromosome 5. Nature 328: 614–616
Bolin S, Franzen L, Nilsson E, Sjodahl R 1988 Carcinoma of the colon and rectum: missed tumours in 63 patients. Cancer 61: 1999–2008
Boman B M, Moertel C G, O'Connell M J et al 1984 Carcinoma of the anal canal. A clinical and pathologic study of 188 cases. Cancer 54: 114–125
Bonnheim D C, Petrelli N J, Herrera L, Walsh D, Mittelman A 1986 Osseous metastases from colorectal carcinoma. American Journal of Surgery 151: 457–459
Bos J L, Fearon E R, Hamilton S R et al 1987 Prevalence of ras mutations in human colorectal cancers. Nature 327: 293–297
Bown S G, Barr H, Matthewson K et al 1986 Endoscopic treatment of inoperable colorectal cancers with the Nd YAG laser. British Journal of Surgery 73: 949
Boyle P, Zaridze D G, Smans M 1985 Descriptive epidemiology of colorectal cancer. International Journal of Cancer 36: 9–18
Brandt L J, Katz H J, Wolf E L, Mitsudo S, Boley S J 1985 Simulation of colonic carcinoma by ischemia. Gastroenterology 88: 1137–1142
Bremner C G, Ackerman L V 1970 Polyps and carcinoma of the large bowel in the South African Bantu. Cancer 26: 991–999
Britton K E, Granowska M 1985 Radioimmunoscintigraphy of cancer. British Journal of Surgery 72: S43–S44
Broder A C 1925 The grading of carcinoma. Minnesota Medicine 8: 726
Bronen R A, Glick S N, Teplick S K 1984 Diffuse lymphoid follicles of the colon associated with colonic carcinoma. American Journal of Roentgenology 142: 105–109
Bronner C E, Baker S M, Morrison P T et al 1994 Mutation in the DNA mismatch repair gene homologue hMLH1 is associated with hereditary non-polyposis colon cancer. Nature 368: 258–261
Brownstein M H, Mehregan A H, Bikowski J B et al 1979 The dermatopathology of Cowden's syndrome. British Journal of Dermatology 100: 667–673
Bruce W F 1987 Recent hypotheses for the origin of colon cancer. Cancer Research 47: 4237–4242
Bulow S 1984 The risk of developing rectal cancer after colectomy and ileorectal anastomosis in Danish patients with polyposis coli. Diseases of the Colon and Rectum 27: 726–729
Bulow S 1986 Clinical features of familial polyposis coli. Results of the Danish Polyposis Registry. Diseases of the Colon and Rectum 29: 102–107
Bulow S 1987 Familial polyposis coli. Danish Medical Bulletin 34: 1–15
Bulow S, Sondergaard J O, Witt I N, Larsen E, Tetens G 1984 Mandibular osteomas in familial polyposis coli. Diseases of the Colon and Rectum 27: 105–108
Bulow S, Lauritsen K B, Johansen A, Svendsen L B, Sondergaard J O 1985 Gastroduodenal polyps in familial polyposis coli. Diseases of the Colon and Rectum 28: 90–93
Burkitt D P 1971 Epidemiology of cancer of the colon and rectum. Cancer 28: 3–13
Burnett J W, Goldner R, Calton G J 1975 Cowden disease. Report of two additional cases. British Journal of Dermatology 93: 329–336
Burt R W, Berenson M M, Lee R G, Tolman K G, Freston J W, Gardner E J 1984 Upper gastrointestinal polyps in Gardner's syndrome. Gastroenterology 86: 295–301
Busch O R, Hop W C, Hoynck van Papendrecht M A, Marquet R L, Jeekel J 1993 Blood transfusions and prognosis in colorectal cancer. New England Journal of Medicine 328: 1372–1376
Bussey H J R 1970 Gastrointestinal polyposis. Gut 11: 970–978
Bussey H J R 1972 Extracolonic lesions associated with polyposis coli. Proceedings of the Royal Society of Medicine 65: 294
Bussey H J R 1975 Familial polyposis coli. Family studies, histopathology, differential diagnosis, and results of treatment. Johns Hopkins University Press, Baltimore
Bussey H J R, Eyers A A, Ritchie S M, Thomson J P S 1985 The rectum in adenomatous polyposis: the St. Mark's policy. British Journal of Surgery 72 (suppl): S29–S31
Buyse M, Zeleniuch-Jacquotte A, Chalmers T C 1988 Adjuvant therapy of colorectal cancer. Why we still don't know. Journal of the American Medical Association 259: 3571–3578
Cady B, Persson A V, Monson D O, Maunz D L 1974 Changing patterns of colorectal carcinoma. Cancer 33: 422–426
Caldarola V T, Jackman R J, Moertel C G, Dockerty M B 1964 Carcinoid tumors of the rectum. American Journal of Surgery 107: 844
Cannon-Albright L A, Skolnick M H, Bishop D T, Lee R G, Burt R W 1988 Common inheritance of susceptibility to colonic adenomatous polyps and associated colorectal cancers. New England Journal of Medicine 319: 533–537
Carlson G J, Nivatvongs S, Snover D C 1984 Colorectal polyps in Cowden's disease (multiple hamartoma syndrome). American Journal of Surgical Pathology 8: 763–770
Carroll S E 1963 The prognostic significance of gross venous invasion in carcinoma of the rectum. Canadian Journal of Surgery 6: 281
Castro E B, Rosen P P, Quan S H Q 1973 Carcinoma of the large intestine in patients irradiated for carcinoma of the cervix and uterus. Cancer 31: 45 52
Cataldo P A, MacKeigan J M 1992 The necessity of routine pathologic evaluation of hemorrhoidectomy specimens. Surgery, Gynecology and Obstetrics 174: 302–304
Chapman P D, Church W, Burn J, Gunn A 1989 The detection of congenital hypertrophy of the retinal pigment epithelium (CHRPE) by indirect ophthalmoscopy; a reliable clinical feature of familial adenomatous polyposis. British Medical Journal 298: 353–354
Charnsangavej C 1993 New imaging modalities for follow-up of colorectal carcinoma. Cancer 71: 4236–4240
Chester J, Britton D 1989 Elective and emergency surgery for colorectal cancer in a district general hospital: impact of surgical training on patient survival. Annals of the Royal College of Surgeons of England 71: 370–374
Chiu Y S, Unni K K, Beart R W Jr 1980 Malignant melanoma of the anorectum. Diseases of the Colon and Rectum 23: 122–124
Clark C G 1986 Implantable vascular access devices in the treatment of colorectal liver metastases. British Journal of Surgery 73: 419–421
Clark J C, Collan Y, Eide T J et al 1985 Prevalence of polyps in an autopsy series from areas with varying incidence of large-bowel cancer. International Journal of Cancer 36: 179–186
Clarke D N, Jones P F, Needham C D 1980 Outcome in colorectal carcinoma: seven-year study of a population. British Medical Journal 280: 431–435
Cochet B, Carrel J, Desbaillets L, Widgren S 1979 Peutz–Jeghers syndrome associated with gastrointestinal carcinoma. Report of two cases in a family. Gut 20: 169–175
Colacchio T A, Forde K A, Scantlebury V P 1981 Endoscopic polypectomy: inadequate treatment for invasive colorectal carcinoma. Annals of Surgery 194: 704–707
Cooper H S 1983 Surgical pathology of endoscopically removed malignant polyps of the colon and rectum. American Journal of Surgical Pathology 7: 613–623
Cornes J S 1961 Multiple lymphomatous polyposis of the gastrointestinal tract. Cancer 14: 249
Cornes J S, Wallace M H, Morson B C 1961 Benign lymphomas of the rectum and anal canal: a study of 100 cases. Journal of Pathology and Bacteriology 82: 371
Correa P, Haenszel W 1978 The epidemiology of large bowel cancer. In:

Klein G, Weinhouse S (eds) Advances in cancer research, Vol 26. Academic Press, London, p 2
Correa P, Strong J P, Reif A, Johnson W D 1977 The epidemiology of colorectal polyps. Prevalence in New Orleans and international comparisons. Cancer 39: 2258–2264
Cowgill R, Quan S H Q 1979 Colonic actinomycosis mimicking carcinoma. Diseases of the Colon and Rectum 22: 45–46
Cripps W H 1882 Two cases of disseminated polypus of the rectum. Transactions of the Pathology Society London 33: 165–168
Crowder V H, Cohn I 1967 Perforation in cancer of the colon and rectum. Diseases of the Colon and Rectum 10: 415
Croxson T, Chabon A B, Rorat E, Barash I M 1984 Intraepithelial carcinoma of the anus in homosexual men. Diseases of the Colon and Rectum 27: 325–330
Culp C E 1967 New studies of the colonic polyp and cancer. Surgical Clinics of North America 47: 955
Culp C E, Hill J R 1962 Malignant lymphoma involving the rectum. Diseases of the Colon and Rectum 5: 426
Cummings B J 1989 Influence of radiation therapy on cure and recurrence rates. Cancer Surveys 8: 49–70
Dajani Y F, Kamal M F 1984 Colorectal juvenile polyps: an epidemiological and histopathological study of 144 cases in Jordanians. Histopathology 8: 765–779
Daling J R, Weiss N S, Hislop G T et al 1987 Sexual practices, sexually transmitted diseases, and the incidence of anal cancer. New England Journal of Medicine 317: 973–977
Daniel E S, Ludwig S L, Lewin K J, Ruprecht R M, Rajacich G M, Schwabe A D 1982 The Cronkhite–Canada syndrome. An analysis of clinical and pathologic features and therapy in 55 patients. Medicine 61: 293–309
Dawson I M P, Cornes J S, Morson B C 1961 Primary malignant lymphoid tumours of the intestinal tract. Report of 37 cases with a study of factors influencing prognosis. British Journal of Surgery 49: 80
Day J J, Freeman A H, Coni N K, Dixon A K 1993 Barium enema or computed tomography for the frail elderly patient? Clinical Radiology 48: 48–51
Deans G T, Krukowski Z H, Irwin S T 1994a Malignant obstruction of the left colon. British Journal of Surgery 81: 1270–1276
Deans G T, McAleer J J A, Spence R A J 1994b Malignant anal tumours. British Journal of Surgery 81: 500–508
DeCosse J J, Bulow S, Neale K et al 1992 Rectal cancer risk in patients treated for familial adenomatous polyposis. British Journal of Surgery 79: 1372–1375
Dent O F, Goulston K J, Zubrzycki J, Chapuis P H 1986 Bowel symptoms in an apparently well population. Diseases of the Colon and Rectum 29: 243–247
Deschner E E, Lipkin M 1976 Cell proliferation in normal, preneoplastic and neoplastic gastrointestinal cells. Clinics in Gastroenterology 5: 543
Dietrich W F, Lander E S, Smith J S et al 1993. Genetic identification of Mom-1, a major modifier locus affecting Min-induced intestinal neoplasia in the mouse. Cell 75: 631–639
DiSario J A, Foutch P G, Mai H D, Pardy K, Manne R K 1991 Prevalence and malignant potential of colorectal polyps in asymptomatic, average-risk men. American Journal of Gastroenterology 86: 941–945
Doll R, Peto R 1981 The causes of cancer: quantitative estimates of avoidable risks in the United States. Journal of the National Cancer Institute 66: 1197–1312
Donaldson G A 1958 The management of perforative carcinoma of the colon. New England Journal of Medicine 258: 201
Dougherty B G, Evans H L 1985 Carcinoma of the anal canal: a study of 79 cases. American Journal of Clinical Pathology 83: 159–164
Douglas J R, Campbell C A, Salisbury D M, Walker-Smith J A, Williams C B 1980 Colonoscopic polypectomy in children. British Medical Journal 281: 1386–1387
Drasar B S, Irving D 1973 Environmental factors and cancer of the colon and breast. British Journal of Cancer 27: 167–172
Drasar B S, Jenkins D J A 1976 Bacteria, diet and large bowel cancer. American Journal of Clinical Nutrition 29: 1410–1416
Dreyfuss J R, Benacerraf B 1978 Saddle cancers of the colon and their progression to annular carcinomas. Radiology 129: 289–293
Dukes C E 1932 The classification of cancer of the rectum. Journal of Pathology and Bacteriology 35: 323–332
Dukes C E 1940 Cancer of the rectum: an analysis of 1000 cases. Journal of Pathology and Bacteriology 50: 527
Duncan B R, Dohner V A, Priest J H 1968 The Gardner syndrome: need for early diagnosis. Journal of Pediatrics 72: 479–505
Duncan W 1985 Adjuvant radiotherapy in rectal cancer: the MRC trials. British Journal of Surgery (71) Suppl: S59–S62
Dunlop M G 1992 Screening for large bowel neoplasms in individuals with a family history of colorectal cancer. British Journal of Surgery 79: 488–494
Dunlop M G, Wyllie A H, Steel C M, Piris J, Evans H J 1991 Linked DNA markers for presymptomatic diagnosis of familial adenomatous polyposis. Lancet 337: 313–316
Dunphy J E, Patterson W B, Legg M A 1959 Etiologic factors in polyposis and carcinoma of the colon. Annals of Surgery 150: 488
Eddy D M, Nugent F W, Eddy J F et al 1987 Screening for colorectal cancer in a high risk population. Results of a mathematical model. Gastroenterology 92: 682–692
Eide T J 1983 Remnants of adenomas in colorectal carcinomas. Cancer 51: 1866–1872
Eide T J 1986 Risk of colorectal cancer in adenoma-bearing individuals within a defined population. International Journal of Cancer 38: 173–176
Ekbom A, Helmick C, Zack M, Adami H O 1990a Ulcerative colitis and colorectal cancer. A population based study. New England Journal of Medicine 323: 1228–1233
Ekbom A, Helmick C, Zack M, Adami H O 1990b Increased risk of large-bowel cancer in Crohn's disease with colonic involvement. Lancet 336: 357–359
Ekelund G 1963 On cancer and polyps of colon and rectum. Acta Pathologica et Microbiologica Scandinavica 59: 165
Eldar S, Kemeny M M, Terz J J 1985 Extended resections for carcinoma of the colon and rectum. Surgery, Gynecology and Obstetrics 161: 319–322
Enterline H T 1976 Polyps and cancer of the large bowel. In: Morson B C (ed) Pathology of the gastrointestinal tract. Springer-Verlag, New York, p 97
Falterman K W, Hill C B, Markey J C, Fox J W, Cohn I 1974 Cancer of the colon, rectum and anus: a review of 2313 cases. Cancer 34: 951–959
Farrands P A, Vellacott K D, Amar S S, Balfour T W, Hardcastle J D 1983 Flexible fiberoptic sigmoidoscopy and double-contrast barium enema examination in the identification of adenomas and carcinoma of the colon. Diseases of the Colon and Rectum 26: 725–727
Fearon E R, Vogelstein B 1990 A genetic model for colorectal tumorigenesis. Cell 61: 759–767
Fielding L P 1981 Primary resection for obstructed large bowel cancer. In: DeCosse J J (ed) Large bowel cancer. Churchill Livingstone, Edinburgh, p 128
Fielding L P, Stewart-Brown S, Blesovsky L, Kearney G 1980 Anastomotic integrity after operations for large-bowel cancer: a multicentre study. British Medical Journal 281: 411–414
Fielding L P, Phillips R K S, Fry J S, Hittinger R 1986 Prediction of outcome after curative resection for large bowel cancer. Lancet 2: 904–907
Finlay I G, McArdle C S 1986 Occult hepatic metastases in colorectal carcinoma. British Journal of Surgery 73: 732–735
Finlay I G, Meek D R, Gray H W, Duncan J G, McArdle C S 1982 Incidence and detection of occult hepatic metastases in colorectal carcinoma. British Medical Journal 284: 803–805
Fishel R, Lescoe M K, Rao M R S et al 1993 The human mutator gene homolog MSH2 and its association with hereditary nonpolyposis colon cancer. Cell 75: 1027–1038
Fisher B, Wolmark N, Rockette H et al 1988 Postoperative adjuvant chemotherapy or radiation therapy for rectal cancer: results from the NSABP protocol R-01. Journal of the National Cancer Institute 80: 21–29
Fleischer D 1986 Lasers and colon polyps. Technology and pathology: the courtship continues. Gastroenterology 90: 2024–2025
Fork F-TH 1983 Reliability of routine double contrast examination of the large bowel: a prospective study of 2590 patients. Gut 24: 672
Forrester K, Almonguera C, Han K, Grizzle W E, Perucho M 1987

Detection of high incidence of K-ras oncogenes during human colon tumorigenesis. Nature 327: 298–303
Foutch P G, Mai H, Pardy K, DiSario J A, Manne R K, Kerr D 1991 Flexible sigmoidoscopy may be ineffective for secondary prevention of colorectal cancer in asymptomatic, average-risk men. Digestive Diseases and Sciences 36: 924–928
Franzin G, Zamboni G, Dina R, Scarpa A, Fratton A 1983 Juvenile and inflammatory polyps of the colon – a histological and histochemical study. Histopathology 7: 719
Franzin G, Zamboni G, Scarpa A, Dina R, Iannucci A, Novelli P 1984 Hyperplastic (metaplastic) polyps of the colon. A histologic and histochemical study. American Journal of Surgical Pathology 8: 687–698
Freeman K, Anthony P P, Miller D S, Warin A P 1985 Cronkhite Canada syndrome: a new hypothesis. Gut 26: 531–536
Freeny P C, Marks W M, Ryan J A, Bolen J W 1986 Colorectal carcinoma evaluation with CT: preoperative staging and detection of postoperative recurrence. Radiology 158: 347–353
Friedman G D, Collen M F, Fireman B H 1986 Multiphasic health checkup evaluation: a 16-year follow-up. Journal of Chronic Diseases 39: 453–463
Frisch M, Melbye M, Moller H 1993 Trends in incidence of anal cancer in Denmark. British Medical Journal 306: 419–422
Gabriel W B, Dukes C E, Bussey H J R 1935 Lymphatic spread in cancer of the rectum. British Journal of Surgery 23: 395
Gardiner R, Stevenson G W 1982 The colitides. Radiologic Clinics of North America 20: 797–817
Gardner E J, Plenk H P 1952 Hereditary pattern of multiple osteomas in a family group. American Journal of Human Genetics 4: 31–36
Garland C, Shekelle R B, Barrett-Connor E, Criqui M H, Rossof A H, Paul O 1985 Dietary vitamin D and calcium and risk of colorectal cancer: a 19-year prospective study in men. Lancet 1: 307
Gaze M N 1988 Radiotherapy for rectal carcinoma. Journal of the Royal College of Surgeons of Edinburgh 33: 175–178
Geboes K, de Wolf-Peeters C, Rutgeerts P, Vantrappen G, Desmet B 1978 Submucosal tumors of the colon: experience with twenty-five cases. Diseases of the Colon and Rectum 21: 420–425
Gennaro A R, Tyson R R 1978 Obstructive colonic cancer. Diseases of the Colon and Rectum 21: 346–351
Gentry W C, Eskritt N R, Gorlin R J 1974 Multiple hamartoma syndrome (Cowden disease). Archives of Dermatology 109: 521–525
Gerard A, Berrod J L, Pene F et al 1985 Interim analysis of a phase III study on pre-operative radiation therapy in resectable rectal carcinoma. Cancer 55: 2372–2379
Gerdes H, Gillin J S, Zimbalist E et al 1993 Expansion of the epithelial cell proliferative compartment and frequency of adenomatous polyps in the colon correlate with the strength of family history of colorectal cancer. Cancer Research 53: 279–282
Giardiello F M, Welsh S B, Hamilton S R et al 1987 Increased risk of cancer in the Peutz–Jeghers syndrome. New England Journal of Medicine 316: 1511–1514
Gibbs N M 1977 Undifferentiated carcinoma of the large intestine. Histopathology 1: 77–84
Gilbert D A, Hallstrohm A P, Shaneyfelt S L 1984 The national ASGE complications of colonoscopy survey. Gastrointestinal Endoscopy 30: 156
Gilbertsen V A 1974 Proctosigmoidoscopy and polypectomy in reducing the incidence of rectal cancer. Cancer 34: 936–939
Gilbertsen V A, Nelms J M 1978 The prevention of invasive cancer of the rectum. Cancer 41: 1137–1139
Gilchrist A M, Mills J O M, Russell C G 1985 Acute large-bowel pseudo-obstruction. Clinical Radiology 36: 401–404
Gill P G, Morris P J 1978 The survival of patients with colorectal cancer treated in a regional hospital. British Journal of Surgery 65: 17–20
Gillespie P E, Chambers T J, Chan K W, Doronzo F, Morson B C, Williams C B 1979 Colonic adenomas – a colonoscopy survey. Gut 20: 240–245
Giltman L I, Osborne P T, Coleman S A, Uthman E O 1985 Paget's disease of the anal mucosa in association with carcinoma demonstrating mucoepidermoid features. Journal of Surgical Oncology 28: 277–280
Giovannucci E, Rimm E B, Stampfer M J et al 1994a A prospective study of cigarette smoking and risk of colorectal adenoma and colorectal cancer in U.S. men. Journal of the National Cancer Institute 86: 183–191
Giovannucci E, Colditz G A, Stampfer M J et al 1994b A prospective study of cigarette smoking and risk of colorectal adenoma and colorectal cancer in U.S. women. Journal of the National Cancer Institute 86: 192–199
Glass R E, Ritchie J K, Thompson H R, Mann C V 1985 The results of surgical treatment of cancer of the rectum by radical resection and extended abdomino-iliac lymphadenectomy. British Journal of Surgery 72: 599–601
Godwin J D 2nd 1975 Carcinoid tumors. An analysis of 2837 cases. Cancer 36: 560–569
Goligher J C 1984 Surgery of the anus, rectum and colon, 5th edn. Baillière Tindall, London
Goligher J C, Smiddy F G 1957 The treatment of acute obstruction or perforation with carcinoma of the colon and rectum. British Journal of Surgery 45: 270
Goligher J C, Graham N G, de Dombal F T 1970 Anastomotic dehiscence after anterior resection of rectum and sigmoid. British Journal of Surgery 57: 109–118
Gordon N L M, Dawson A A, Bennett B et al 1993 Outcome in colorectal adenocarcinoma: two seven year studies of a population. British Medical Journal 307: 707–710
Goulston K J, Cook I, Dent O F 1986 How important is rectal bleeding in the diagnosis of bowel cancer and polyps? Lancet 2: 261–265
Gourley G R, Odell G B, Selkurt J, Morrissey J, Gilbert E 1982 Juvenile polyps associated with protein-losing enteropathy. Digestive Diseases and Sciences 27: 941–945
Greenall M J, Quan S H Q, DeCosse J J 1985a Epidermoid cancer of the anus. British Journal of Surgery 72: S97
Greenall M J, Quan S H Q, Stearns M W, Urmacher C, DeCosse J J 1985b Epidermoid cancer of the anal margin. Pathologic features, treatment and clinical results. American Journal of Surgery 149: 95–101
Greene F L 1983 Distribution of colorectal neoplasms. A left to right shift of polyps and cancer. American Surgeon 49: 62–65
Groden J, Thliveris A, Samowitz W et al 1991 Identification and characterization of the Familial Adenomatous Polyposis Coli gene. Cell 66: 589–600
Groden J, Gelbert L, Thliveris A et al 1993 Mutational analysis of patients with adenomatous polyposis: identical inactivating mutations in unrelated individuals. American Journal of Human Genetics 52: 263–272
Grosfeld J L, West K W 1986 Generalized juvenile polyposis coli. Clinical management based on long-term observations. Archives of Surgery 121: 530–534
Grotsky H W, Rickert R R, Smith W D, Newsome J F 1982 Familial juvenile polyposis coli. A clinical and pathologic study of a large kindred. Gastroenterology 82: 494–501
Gryboski J D 1986 All juvenile polyps are not benign. American Journal of Gastroenterology 81: 397
Gyde S N 1990 Screening for colorectal cancer in ulcerative colitis: dubious benefits and high costs. Gut 31: 1089–1092
Gyde S N, Prior P, Allan R N et al 1988 Colorectal cancer in ulcerative colitis: a cohort study of primary referrals from three centres. Gut 29: 206–217
Haenszel W, Correa P 1971 Cancer of the colon and rectum and adenomatous polyps. A review of epidemiologic findings. Cancer 28: 14–24
Haenszel W, Correa P 1982 Epidemiology of large bowel cancer. In: Correa P, Haenszel W (eds) Epidemiology of cancer of the digestive tract. Martinus Nijhoff, The Hague, p 85
Halvorsen T B 1986 Site distribution of colorectal adenocarcinomas. A retrospective study of 853 tumours. Scandinavian Journal of Gastroenterology 21: 973–978
Hamilton S R, Bussey H J R, Mendelsohn G et al 1979 Ileal adenomas after colectomy in nine patients with adenomatous polyposis coli; Gardner's syndrome. Gastroenterology 77: 1252–1257
Hardcastle J D 1989 The prospects for mass population screening in colorectal cancer. Cancer Surveys 8: 123–138
Hardcastle J D, Thomas W M, Chamberlain J et al 1989 Randomised, controlled trial of faecal occult blood screening for colorectal cancer. Results from the first 107,349 subjects. Lancet 1: 1160–1164

Hardin W J 1972 Unusual manifestations of malignant disease of the large intestine. Surgical Clinics of North America 52: 287–298
Harned R K, Williams S M 1982 Familial polyposis coli and periampullary malignancy. Diseases of the Colon and Rectum 25: 227–229
Hawes R H 1993 New staging techniques. Endoscopic ultrasound. Cancer 71: 4207–4213
Hawley P R, Ritchie J K 1979 The colon. Part I. Complications of ileostomy and colostomy following excisional surgery. Clinics in Gastroenterology 8: 403–415
Hayashi T, Yatani R, Apostol J, Stemmermann G N 1974 Pathogenesis of hyperplastic polyps of the colon: a hypothesis based on ultrastructure and in vitro cell kinetics. Gastroenterology 66: 347–356
Heald R J, Bussey H J R 1975 Clinical experiences at St Mark's Hospital with multiple synchronous cancers of the colon and rectum. Diseases of the Colon and Rectum 18: 6–10
Heald R J, Ryall R D H 1986 Recurrence and survival after total mesorectal excision for rectal cancer. Lancet 1: 1479–1482
Heald R J, Husband E M, Ryall R D H 1982 The mesorectum in rectal cancer surgery – the clue to pelvic recurrence? British Journal of Surgery 69: 613–616
Hertz R E, Deddish M R, Day E 1960 Value of periodic examinations in detecting cancer of the rectum and colon. Postgraduate Medicine 27: 290–294
Hildebrandt U, Klein T, Feifel G, Schwarz H P, Koch B, Schmitt R M 1990 Endosonography of pararectal lymph nodes: in vitro and in vivo evaluation. Diseases of the Colon and Rectum 33: 863–868
Hill M J 1978 Some leads to the etiology of cancer of the large bowel. Surgery Annual 10: 135–149
Hill M J 1982 Genetic and environmental factors in human colorectal cancer. In: Malt R A, Williamson R C N (eds) Colonic carcinogenesis. MTP Press, Lancaster, p 73–81
Hill M J 1985 Cancer of the large bowel: human carcinogenesis. British Journal of Surgery 72: S37–S39
Hjermstad B M, Helwig E B 1988 Tailgut cysts. Report of 53 cases. American Journal of Clinical Pathology 89: 139–147
Hochberg F H, Dasilva A B, Gaidabini J, Richardson E P Jr 1974 Gastrointestinal involvement in von Recklinghausen's neurofibromatosis. Neurology 24: 1144–1151
Hoff G, Foerster A, Vatn M H, Sauar J, Larsen S 1986 Epidemiology of polyps in the rectum and colon. Recovery and evaluation of unresected polyps 2 years after detection. Scandinavian Journal of Gastroenterology 21: 853–862
Horii A, Han H-J, Shimada M et al 1994 Frequent replication errors at microsatellite loci in tumours of patients with multiple primary cancers. Cancer Research 54: 3373–3375
Howell J, Facundus D, Kay D, Matthews C, Walker A 1993 Hepatic tumors: role of computed tomographic arterial portography in surgical planning. Southern Medical Journal 86: 1133–1141
Hubbard T B 1957 Familial polyposis of the colon: the fate of the retained rectum after colectomy in children. American Surgeon 23: 577–586
Hunt T M, Taylor I 1989 The role of chemotherapy in the treatment and prophylaxis of colorectal liver metastases. Cancer Surveys 8: 71–90
Hunter G J, Willson S A, Chapman M 1983 Necrotic carcinoma of the colon. Clinical Radiology 34: 297–299
Hutter R V P, Sobin L H 1986 A universal staging system for cancer of the colon and rectum. Let there be light. Archives of Pathology and Laboratory Medicine 110: 367–368
Ichii S, Takeda S, Horii A et al 1993 Detailed analysis of genetic alterations in colorectal tumours from patients with and without familial adenomatous polyposis (FAP). Oncogene 8: 2399–2405
Ionov Y, Peinado M A, Malkhosyan S et al 1993 Ubiquitous somatic mutations in simple repeated sequences reveal a new mechanism for colonic carcinogenesis. Nature 363: 558–561
Isles G G, Hole D J, Gillis C R, Hawthorne V M, Lever A F 1989 Plasma cholesterol, coronary heart disease, and cancer in the Renfrew and Paisley survey. British Medical Journal 298: 920–924
Itoh H, Ohsato K, Yao T, Lida M, Watanabe H 1979 Turcot's syndrome and its mode of inheritance. Gut 20: 414–419
Iwama T, Mishima Y, Okomato N, Inoue J 1990 Association of congenital hypertrophy of the retinal pigment epithelium with familial adenomatous polyposis. British Journal of Surgery 77: 273–276
Jackman R J, Beahrs O H 1968 Tumors of the large bowel. Major problems in clinical surgery, Vol 8. W B Saunders, Philadelphia, p 91
Jagelman D G, DeCosse J J, Bussey H J R 1988 Upper gastrointestinal cancer in familial adenomatous polyposis. Lancet 1: 1149–1151
Jarvinen H J 1992 Epidemiology of familal adenomatous polyposis in Finland: impact of family screening on colorectal cancer rate and survival. Gut 33: 357–360
Jarvinen H, Franssila K O 1984 Familial juvenile polyposis coli: increased risk of colorectal cancer. Gut 25: 792–800
Jarvinen H J, Peltokallio P, Landtman M, Wolf J 1982 Gardner's stigmas in patients with familial adenomatosis coli. British Journal of Surgery 69: 718–721
Jarvinen H, Nyberg M, Peltokallio P 1983 Upper gastrointestinal tract polyps in familial adenomatosis coli. Gut 24: 333–339
Jarvinen H J, Ovaska J, Mecklin J P 1988 Improvements in the treatment and prognosis of colorectal carcinoma. British Journal of Surgery 75: 25–27
Jass J R 1983 Relation between metaplastic polyp and carcinoma of the colorectum. Lancet 1: 28–30
Jass J R 1989 Do all colorectal carcinomas arise in preexisting adenomas? World Journal of Surgery 13: 45–51
Jass J R, Love S B, Northover J M A 1987 A new prognostic classification of rectal cancer. Lancet 2: 1303–1306
Jeekel J 1986 Curative resection of primary colorectal cancer. British Journal of Surgery 73: 687–688
Jenkins D, Stephenson P M, Scott B B 1985 The Cronkhite–Canada syndrome: an ultrastructural study of pathogenesis. Journal of Clinical Pathology 38: 271–276
Jensen O M, Bolander A M, Sigtryggsson P, Vercelli M, Nguyen-Dinh X, MacLennan R 1980 Large-bowel cancer in married couples in Sweden. A follow-up study. Lancet 1: 1161–1163
John T G, Garden O J 1994 Laparosopic ultrasonography: extending the scope of diagnostic laparosopy. British Journal of Surgery 81: 5–6
Johnson C D, Carlson H C, Taylor W F, Wetland L P 1983 Barium enemas of carcinoma of the colon. Sensitivity of double- and single contrast studies. American Journal of Roentgenology 140: 1143–1149
Johnson G K, Soergel K H, Hensley G T, Dodds W J, Hogan W J 1972 Cronkhite–Canada syndrome: gastrointestinal pathophysiology and morphology. Gastroenterology 63: 140–152
Johnson H Jr, Carstens R 1986 Anatomical distribution of colonic carcinomas. Interracial differences in a community hospital population. Cancer 58: 997–1000
Jonsson B, Ahsgren L, Andersson L O, Stenling R, Rutegard J 1994 Colorectal cancer surveillance in patients with ulcerative colitis. British Journal of Surgery 81: 689–691
Jones M A, Hebert J C, Trainer T D 1987 Juvenile polyp with intramucosal carcinoma. Archives of Pathology and Laboratory Medicine 111: 200–201
Jones T R, Nance F C 1977 Periampullary malignancy in Gardner's Syndrome. Annals of Surgery 185: 565–573
Joslyn G, Carlson M, Thliveris A et al 1991 Identification of deletion mutations and three new genes at the Familial Polyposis locus. Cell 66: 601–613
Judd E S 1961 The risk of surgery of the colon: current trends in hospital mortality rates. Proceedings of Staff Meetings of the Mayo Clinic 36: 492
Kanabe S, Watanabe I, Lotuaco L 1978 Multiple granular-cell tumors of the ascending colon: microscopic study. Diseases of the Colon and Rectum 21: 322–328
Karanjia N D, Schache D J, North W R, Heald R J 1990 'Close shave' in anterior resection. British Journal of Surgery 77: 510–512
Karl R C, Morse S S, Halpert R D, Clark R A 1993 Preoperative evaluation of patients for liver resection. Appropriate CT imaging. Annals of Surgery 217: 226–232
Katayama Y, Kimura M, Konn M 1985 Cronkhite–Canada syndrome associated with a rectal cancer and adenomatous changes in colonic polyps. American Journal of Surgical Pathology 9: 65–71
Keddie N, Hargreaves A 1968 Symptoms of carcinoma of the colon and rectum. Lancet 2: 749–750
Kelvin F M 1982 Radiologic approach to the detection of colorectal neoplasia. Radiologic Clinics of North America 20: 743–759

Kelvin F M, Gardiner R, Vas W, Stevenson G W 1981 Colorectal carcinoma missed on double contrast barium enema study: a problem in perception. American Journal of Roentgenology 137: 307–313

Kemeny M M, Battifora H, Blayney D W et al 1985 Sclerosing cholangitis after continuous hepatic artery infusion of FUDR. Annals of Surgery 202: 176–181

Kinzler K W, Nilbert M C, Su L-K et al 1991 Identification of FAP locus genes from chomosome 5q21. Science 253: 661–665

Kirklin J W, Docherty M B, Waugh J M 1949 The role of the peritoneal reflection in the prognosis of carcinoma of the rectum and sigmoid colon. Surgery, Gynecology and Obstetrics 88: 326

Klemmer S, Pascoe L, DeCosse J J 1987 Occurrence of desmoids in patients with familial adenomatous polyposis of the colon. American Journal of Medical Genetics 28: 385–392

Klotz R G, Pamukcoglu T, Souilliard D H 1967 Transitional cloacogenic carcinoma of the anal canal. Clinicopathologic study of three hundred seventy-three cases. Cancer 20: 1727–1745

Koyama Y, Moriya Y, Hojo K 1984 Effects of extended lymphadenectomy for adenocarcinoma of the rectum – significant improvement of survival rate and decrease of local recurrence. Japanese Journal of Clinical Oncology 14: 623–632

Krook J E, Moertel C G, Gunderson L L et al 1991 Effective adjuvant therapy for high risk rectal carcinoma. New England Journal of Medicine 324: 709–715

LaMont J T, O'Gorman T A 1978 Experimental colon cancer. Gastroenterology 75: 1157–1169

Lancet 1984 Editorial: the malignant large-bowel polyp – conservative or radical treatment? Lancet 1: 1387

Lancet 1985 Editorial: adjuvant treatment of carcinoma of the rectum and colon. Lancet 2: 367–368

Lane N 1976 The precursor tissue of ordinary large bowel cancer. Cancer Research 36: 2669–2672

Lapides J, Tank E S 1971 Urinary complications following abdominal perineal resection. Cancer 28: 230–235

Lawrence W Jr 1976 Surgical management of gastrointestinal cancer. Clinics in Gastroenterology 5: 703–742

Leach F S, Nicolaides N C, Papadopolous N et al 1993 Mutations of a MutS homolog in hereditary non-polyposis colorectal cancer. Cell 75: 1215–1225

Leach R D, Ellis H 1981 Carcinoma of the rectum in male homosexuals. Journal of the Royal Society of Medicine 74: 490–491

Lee I M, Paffenbarger R S, Hsieh C C 1991 Physical activity and risk of developing colorectal cancer among college alumni. Journal of the National Cancer Institute 83: 1324–1329

Leppard B J 1974 Epidermoid cysts and polyposis coli. Proceedings of the Royal Society of Medicine 67: 1036–1037

Leppard B J, Bussey H J R 1975 Epidermoid cysts, polyposis coli and Gardner's syndrome. British Journal of Surgery 62: 387–393

Leppert M, Dobbs M, Scambler P et al 1987 The gene for familial polyposis maps to the long arm of chromosome 5. Science 238: 1411–1413

Le Quesne L P, Thomson A D 1958 Implantation recurrence of carcinoma of rectum and colon. New England Journal of Medicine 258: 578

Lewi H J E, Carter D C, Ratcliffe J G, McArdle C S 1983 Second laparotomy following "curative" resection for colorectal cancer. Annals of the Royal College of Surgeons of England 65: 314–315

Lewis E 1984 Screening for diffuse and focal liver disease: the case for hepatic sonography. Journal of Clinical Ultrasound 12: 67–73

Limberg B 1990 Diagnosis of large bowel tumours by colonic sonography. Lancet 335: 144–146

Lindberg C G, Lundstedt C, Stridbeck H, Tranberg K G 1993 Accuracy of CT arterial portography of the liver compared with findings at laparotomy. Acta Radiologica 34: 139–142

Lipkin M 1978 Susceptibility of human population groups to colon cancer. In: Klein G, Weinhouse S (eds) Advances in cancer research, Vol 27. Academic Press, London, p 281

Lipkin M 1984 The identification of high risk populations. Scandinavian Journal of Gastroenterology 19 (suppl 104): 91–97

Lipkin M, Newmark H 1985 Effect of added dietary calcium on colonic epithelial-cell proliferation in subjects at high risk for familial colonic cancer. New England Journal of Medicine 313: 1381–1384

Lipkin M, Blattner W E, Fraumeni J F et al 1983 Tritiated thymidine labelling distribution as a marker for hereditary predisposition to colon cancer. Cancer Research 43: 1899–1904

Liu B, Parsons R E, Hamilton S R et al 1994 hMSH2 mutations in hereditary nonpolyposis colorectal cancer kindreds. Cancer Research 54: 4590–4594

Lloyd K N, Dennis M 1962 Cowden's disease. A possible new symptom complex with multiple system involvement. Annals of Internal Medicine 58: 136

Lock M R, Katz D R, Parks A, Thomson J P S 1977 Perianal Paget's disease. Postgraduate Medical Journal 53: 768–772

Lockhart-Mummery J P 1926–27 Two hundred cases of cancer of the rectum treated by perineal excision. British Journal of Surgery 14: 110–124

Lofti A M, Dozois R R, Gordon H H et al 1989 Mesenteric fibromatosis complicating familial adenomatous polyposis: predisposing factors and results of treatment. International Journal of Colorectal Disease 4: 30–36

Longnecker M P, Orza M J, Adams M E, Vioque J, Chalmers T C 1990 A meta-analysis of alcoholic beverage consumption in relation to risk of colorectal cancer. Cancer Causes Control 1: 59–68

Louw J H 1968 Polypoid lesions of the large bowel in children with particular reference to benign lymphoid polyposis. Journal of Pediatric Surgery 3: 195–209

Lynch H T, Kimberling W J, Albano W A et al 1985a Hereditary nonpolyposis colorectal cancer (Lynch syndromes 1 and 2). 1. Clinical description of resource. Cancer 56: 934–938

Lynch H T, Schuelke G S, Kimberling W J et al 1985b Hereditary nonpolyposis colorectal cancer (Lynch syndromes 1 and 2). 2. Biomarker studies. Cancer 56: 939–951

Lynch H T, Priluck I, Fitzsimmons M L 1987 Congenital hypertrophy of retinal pigment epithelium in non-Gardner's polyposis kindreds. Lancet 2: 333

Lynch H T, Smyrk T C, Lanspa S J et al 1988 Flat adenomas in a colon cancer-prone kindred. Journal of the National Cancer Institute 80: 78–82

Lynch H T, Smyrk T C, Lanspa S J et al 1990 Phenotypic variation in colorectal adenoma/cancer expression in two families. Hereditary flat adenoma syndrome. Cancer 66: 909–915

Lynch H T, Smyrk T C, Watson P et al 1993 Genetics, natural history, tumor spectrum, and pathology of hereditary nonpolyposis colorectal cancer: an updated review. Gastroenterology 104: 1535–1549

MacFarlane J K, Ryall R D H, Heald R J 1993 Mesorectal excision for rectal cancer. Lancet 341: 457–460

Macrae F A 1985 Faecal occult blood testing: sensitivity and specificity. British Journal of Surgery 72: S67–S69

Madden J L, Kandalaft S I 1983 Electrocoagulation as a primary curative method in the treatment of carcinoma of the rectum. Surgery, Gynecology and Obstetrics 157: 164–179

Madden M V, Neale K F, Nicholls R J et al 1991 Comparison of morbidity and function after colectomy with ileorectal anastomosis or restorative proctocolectomy for familial adenomatous polyposis. British Journal of Surgery 78: 788–792

Mandel J S, Bond J H, Church T R et al for the Minnesota Colon Cancer Control Study 1993 Reducing mortality from colorectal cancer by screening for fecal occult blood. New England Journal of Medicine 328: 1365–1371

Mandl M, Paffenholz R, Friedl W, Caspari R, Sengteller M, Propping P 1994 Frequency of common and novel inactivating APC mutations in 202 families with familial adenomatous polyposis. Human Molecular Genetics 3: 181–184

Marshak R H, Moseley J E, Wolf B S 1963 The roentgen findings in familial polyposis with special emphasis on differential diagnosis. Radiology 80: 374–382

Martin E W Jr, Joyce S, Lucas J, Clausen K, Cooperman M 1981 Colorectal carcinoma in patients less than 40 years of age: pathology and prognosis. Diseases of the Colon and Rectum 24: 25–28

Maskens A P 1979 Histogenesis of adenomatous polyps in the human large intestine. Gastroenterology 77: 1245–1251

Mastromarino A, Reddy B S, Wynder E L 1976 Metabolic epidemiology of colon cancer: enzymic activity of fecal flora. American Journal of Clinical Nutrition 29: 1455

Matuchansky C, Babin P, Coutrot S, Druart F, Barbier J, Maire P 1979

Peutz–Jeghers' syndrome with metastasizing carcinoma arising from a jejunal hamartoma. Gastroenterology 77: 1311–1315
Mazier W P, Mackeigan J M, Billingham R P, Dignan R D 1982 Juvenile polyps of the colon and rectum. Surgery, Gynecology and Obstetrics 154: 829–832
McArdle C S, Hole D 1991 Impact of variability among surgeons on postoperative morbidity and mortality and ultimate survival. British Medical Journal 302: 1501–1505
McArdle C S, Hole D, Hansell D, Blumgart L H, Woods C B 1990 Prospective study of colorectal cancer in the West of Scotland: ten year follow-up. British Journal of Surgery 77: 280–282
McCarthy S M, Barnes D, Deveney K, Moss A A, Goldberg H I 1985 Detection of recurrent rectosigmoid carcinoma: prospective evaluation of CT and clinical factors. American Journal of Roentgenology 144: 577–579
McConnell E M 1970 Squamous carcinoma of the anus – a review of 96 cases. British Journal of Surgery 57: 89–92
McGrath F P, Malone D E, Dobranowski J et al 1993 Same-day computed tomography during arterial portography and delayed high-dose iodine computed tomography: an efficient approach to imaging potentially resectable liver tumours. Canadian Association of Radiologists Journal 44: 262–266
McKeown G E, Bright-See 1984 Dietary factors in colon cancer: international relationships. Nutrition and Cancer 6: 160–170
McKeown G E, Holloway C, Jazmaji V, Bright-See E, Dion P, Bruce W R 1988 A randomized trial of vitamins C and E in the prevention of recurrence of colorectal polyps. Cancer Research 48: 4701–4705
McMichael A J, Giles G G 1988 Cancer in migrants to Australia: extending the descriptive epidemiological data. Cancer Research 48: 751–756
Mecklin J-P, Sipponen P, Jarvinen H J 1986a Histopathology of colorectal carcinomas and adenomas in cancer family syndrome. Diseases of the Colon and Rectum 29: 849–853
Mecklin J-P, Jarvinen H J, Peltokallio P 1986b Cancer family syndrome. Genetic analysis of 22 Finnish kindreds. Gastroenterology 90: 328–333
Messinger N H, Beneventano T C, Siegelman S S 1971 Interflexural carcinoma of the colon: clinical-radiologic-pathologic correlations. Diseases of the Colon and Rectum 14: 255–258
Mestre J R 1986 The changing pattern of juvenile polyps. American Journal of Gastroenterology 81: 312–314
Miles W F A, Paterson-Brown S, Garden O J 1992 Laparoscopic contact ultrasonography. British Journal of Surgery 79: 419–420
Miller F E, Liechty R D 1967 Adenocarcinoma of the colon and rectum in persons under thirty years of age. American Journal of Surgery 113: 507–510
Moertel C G 1976 Chemotherapy of gastrointestinal cancer. Clinics in Gastroenterology 5: 777–793
Moertel C G, Reitemeier R J 1967 Chemotherapy of gastrointestinal cancer. Surgical Clinics of North America 47: 929
Moertel C G, Fleming T R, Macdonald J S et al 1990 Levamisole and fluorouracil for adjuvant therapy of resected colon carcinoma. New England Journal of Medicine 322: 352–358
Morgan J G, Marks C, Hearn D 1974 Carcinoid tumors of the gastrointestinal tract. Annals of Surgery 180: 720–727
Mori T, Nagase H, Horii A et al 1994 Germline and somatic mutations of the APC gene in patients with Turcot syndrome and analysis of APC mutations in brain tumours. Genes, Chromosomes and Cancer 9: 168–172
Morson B C 1966 Factors influencing the prognosis of early cancer of the rectum. Proceedings of the Royal Society of Medicine 59: 607–608
Morson B C 1967 Notes on the pathology of carcinoma of the large intestine. National Cancer Institute Monograph 25: 287
Morson B C 1976a Genesis of colorectal cancer. Clinics in Gastroenterology 5: 505
Morson B C 1976b Histological typing of intestinal tumours. In: International Histological Classification of Tumours No. 15. World Health Organization, Geneva, p 65
Morson B C 1984 The evolution of colorectal carcinoma. Clinical Radiology 35: 425–431
Morson B C, Bussey H J R 1985 Magnitude of risk for cancer in patients with colorectal adenomas. British Journal of Surgery 72 (suppl): S23–S25
Morson B C, Dawson I M P 1972 Gastrointestinal pathology. Blackwell, Oxford
Morson B C, Dawson I M P 1979 Gastrointestinal pathology, 2nd edn. Blackwell, Oxford
Morson B C, Bussey H J R, Day D W, Hill M J 1983 Adenomas of large bowel. Cancer Surveys 2: 451
Morson B C, Whiteway J E, Jones E A, Macrae F A, Williams C B 1984 Histopathology and prognosis of malignant colorectal polyps treated by endoscopic polypectomy. Gut 25: 437–444
Morton D G, MacDonald F, Haydon J et al 1993 Screening practice for familial adenomatous polyposis: the potential for regional registers. British Journal of Surgery 80: 255–258
Moser A R, Pitot H C, Dove W F 1990 A dominant mutation that predisposes to multiple intestinal neoplasia in the mouse. Science 247: 322–324
Mughai S, Filipe M I 1978 Ultrastructural study of the normal mucosa-adenoma-cancer sequence in the development of familial polyposis coli. Journal of the National Cancer Institute 60: 753–768
Muir C, Waterhouse J, Mack T, Powell J, Whelan S 1987 (eds) Cancer incidence in five continents. IARC Scientific Publications No 88, Lyon
Munemitsu S, Souza B, Muller O, Albert I, Rubinfeldt B, Polakis P 1994 The APC gene product associates with microtubules in vivo and promotes their assembly in vitro. Cancer Research 54: 3676–3681
Murday V, Slack J 1989 Inherited disorders associated with colorectal cancer. Cancer Surveys 8: 139–157
Muto T, Bussey H J R, Morson B C 1975 The evolution of cancer of the colon and rectum. Cancer 36: 2251–2270
Muto T, Kamiya J, Sawada T, Morioko Y 1983 Morphogenesis of human colonic cancer. Diseases of the Colon and Rectum 26: 257–262
Muto T, Kamiya J, Sawada T et al 1985 Small flat adenoma of the large bowel with special reference to its clinicopathological features. Diseases of the Colon and Rectum 28: 847–851
Nagase H, Nakamura Y 1993 Mutations of the APC (adenomatous polyposis coli) gene. Human Mutation 2: 425–434
Nagase H, Miyoshi Y, Horii A et al 1992a Correlation between the location of germline mutations in the APC gene and the number of colorectal polyps in familial adenomatous polyposis. Cancer Research 52: 4055–4057
Nagase H, Miyoshi Y, Horii A et al 1992b. Screening for germ-line mutations in familial adenomatous polyposis patients: 61 new patients and a summary of 150 unrelated patients. Human Mutation 1: 467–473
Nash G, Allen W, Nash S 1986 Atypical lesions of the anal mucosa in homosexual men. Journal of the American Medical Association 256: 873–876
Naunheim K S, Zeitels J, Kaplan E L et al 1983 Rectal carcinoid tumours – treatment and prognosis. Surgery 94: 670–676
Nemer F D, Stoeckinger J M, Evans O T 1977 Smooth-muscle rectal tumors: a therapeutic dilemma. Diseases of the Colon and Rectum 20: 405–413
Neugut A I, Pita S 1988 Role of sigmoidoscopy in screening for colorectal cancer: a critical review. Gastroenterology 95: 492–499
Nicholls R J, Springall R G, Gallagher P 1988a Regression of rectal adenomas after colectomy and ileorectal anastomosis for familial adenomatous polyposis. British Medical Journal 296: 1707–1708
Nicholls R J, Lubowski D Z, Donaldson D R 1988b Comparison of a colonic reservoir and straight colo-anal reconstruction after rectal excision. British Journal of Surgery 75: 318–320
Nicolaides N C, Papadopoulos B L, Wei Y-F et al 1994 Mutations of two PMS homologues in hereditary nonpolyposis colon cancer. Nature 371: 75–80
Nielsen O V, Jensen S L 1981 Basal cell carcinoma of the anus – a clinical study of 34 cases. British Journal of Surgery 68: 856
Nigro N D 1987 Multidisciplinary management of cancer of the anus. World Journal of Surgery 11: 446–451
NIH Consensus Conference 1990 Adjuvant therapy for patients with colon and rectal cancer. Journal of the American Medical Association 264: 1444–1450
Nishisho I, Nakamura Y, Miyoshi Y et al 1991 Mutations of

chromosome 5q21 genes in FAP and colorectal cancer patients. Science 253: 665–669
Northover J M A 1985 Carcinoembryonic antigen and recurrent colorectal cancer. British Journal of Surgery 72: S44–S46
Nugent K P, Phillips R K S 1992 Rectal cancer risk in older patients with familial adenomatous polyposis and an ileorectal anastomosis: a cause for concern. British Journal of Surgery 79: 1204–1206
Olschwang S, Tiret A, Laurent-Puig P, Muleris M, Parc R, Thomas G 1993 Restriction of ocular fundus lesions to a specific subgroup of APC mutations in adenomatous polyposis coli patients. Cell 75: 959–968
Ooya K, Yamamoto H, Lay K M 1976 Sclerotic masses in the mandible of a patient with familial polyposis of the colon. Journal of Oral Pathology 5: 305–311
Orloff M J 1971 Carcinoid tumors of the rectum. Cancer 28: 175–180
Osnes S 1955 Carcinoma of the colon and rectum: a study of 353 cases with special reference to prognosis. Acta Chirurgica 110: 378
Ott D J, Gelfand D W, Wu W C, Munitz H A, Chen Y M 1986 How important is radiographic detection of diminutive polyps of the colon? American Journal of Roentgenology 146: 875–888
Pahlman L, Glimelius B, Graffmen S 1985 Pre- versus post-operative radiotherapy on rectal carcinoma: an interim report from a randomised multicentre trial. British Journal of Surgery 72: 961–966
Palefsky J M, Gonzales J, Greenblatt R M, Ahn D K, Hollander H 1990 Anal intraepithelial neoplasia and anal papillomavirus infection among homosexual males with group IV HIV disease. Journal of the American Medical Association 263: 2911–2916
Papadopoulos N, Nicolaides N C, Wei Y-F et al 1994 Mutation of a mutL homolog in hereditary colon cancer. Science 263: 1625–1629
Papillon J 1982 Rectal and anal cancers. Springer, Berlin
Papillon J 1987 The future of external beam irradiation as initial treatment of rectal cancer. British Journal of Surgery 74: 449–454
Papillon J, Mayer M, Montbarbon J F et al 1983 A new approach to the management of epidermoid carcinoma of the anal canal. Cancer 51: 1830–1837
Parks A G, Nicholls R J, Belliveau P 1980 Proctocolectomy with ileal reservoir and anal anastomosis. British Journal of Surgery 67: 533–538
Paul P, Letteboer T, Gelbert L, Groden J, White R, Coppes M J 1993 Identical APC exon 15 mutations result in a variable phenotype in familial adenomatous polyposis. Human Molecular Genetics 2: 925–931
Pauli R M, Pauli M E, Hall J G 1980 Gardner syndrome and periampullary malignancy. American Journal of Medical Genetics 6: 205–219
Penn I 1986 Cancers of the anogenital region in renal transplant recipients. Analysis of 65 cases. Cancer 58: 611–616
Perzin K H, Bridge M F 1982 Adenomatous and carcinomatous changes in hamartomatous polyps of the small intestine (Peutz–Jeghers syndrome): report of a case and review of the literature. Cancer 49: 971–983
Phillips R K S, Hittinger R, Blesovsky L et al 1984a Large bowel cancer: surgical pathology and its relationship to survival. British Journal of Surgery 71: 604–610
Phillips R K S, Hittinger R, Blesovsky L, Fry J S, Fielding L P 1984b Local recurrence following "curative" surgery for large bowel cancer: II. The rectum and rectosigmoid. British Journal of Surgery 71: 17–20
Phillips R K S, Hittinger R, Fry J S, Fielding L P 1985 Malignant large bowel obstruction. British Journal of Surgery 72: 296–302
Plail R O, Bussey H J R, Glazer G, Thomson J P S 1987 Adenomatous polyposis: an association with carcinoma of the thyroid. British Journal of Surgery 74: 377–380
Pochaczevsky R, Sherman R S 1962 Diffuse lymphomatous disease of the colon: its roentgen appearance. American Journal of Roentgenology 87: 670
Polk H C Jr, Spratt J S Jr 1971 Recurrent colorectal carcinoma: detection, treatment, and other considerations. Surgery 69: 9–23
Polkinghorne P J, Ritchie S, Neale K, Schoeppner G, Thomson J P S, Jay B S 1990 Pigmented lesions of the retinal pigment epithelium and Familial Adenomatous Polyposis. Eye 4: 216–221
Potter J D 1990 The epidemiology of fiber and colorectal cancer: why don't the analytic epidemiologic data make better sense? In: Kritchevsky D, Boonfield C, Anderson LW (eds) Dietary fiber: chemistry, physiology, and health effects. Plenum Press, New York
Powell S M, Zilz N, Beazer-Barclay Y et al 1992 APC mutations occur early during colorectal tumorigenesis. Nature 359: 235–237
Pratt C B, George S L 1982 Epidemic colon cancer in children and adolescents? In: Correa P, Haenszel W (eds) Epidemiology of cancer of the digestive tract. Martinus Nijhoff, The Hague, p 127
Priestman T J 1976 Cytotoxic therapy for gastrointestinal carcinoma. Gut 17: 313
Purcell J J, Shields J A 1975 Hypertrophy with hyperpigmentation of the retinal pigment epithelium. Archives of Ophthalmology 93: 1122–1126
Quirke P, Durdey P, Dixon M F, Williams N S 1986. Local recurrence of rectal adenocarcinoma due to inadequate surgical resection. Histopathological study of lateral tumour spread and surgical excision. Lancet 2: 996–999
Radcliffe A G, Dudley H A F 1983 Intraoperative antegrade irrigation of the large intestine. Surgery, Gynecology and Obstetrics 156: 721–723
Ramirez R F, Culp C E, Jackman R J, Dockerty M B 1965 Villous tumors of the lower part of the large bowel. Journal of the American Medical Association 194: 863
Ransohoff D F, Lang C A, Kuo H S 1991 Colonoscopic surveillance after polypectomy: considerations of cost effectiveness. Annals of Internal Medicine 114: 177–182
Reasbeck P G 1987 Colorectal cancer: the case for endoscopic screening. British Journal of Surgery 74: 12–17
Reed T E, Neel J V 1955 A genetic study of multiple polyposis of the colon (with an appendix deriving a method of estimating relative fitness). American Journal of Human Genetics 7: 236–263
Restrepo C, Correa P, Duque E, Cuello C 1981 Polyps in a low-risk colonic cancer population in Colombia, South America. Diseases of the Colon and Rectum 24: 29–36
Rex D K, Lehman G A, Lappas J C, Miller R E 1986 Sensitivity of double-contrast barium study for left-colon polyps. Radiology 158: 69–72
Rickert R R, Auerbach O, Garfinkel L, Hammond E C, Frasca J M 1979 Adenomatous lesions of the large bowel. An autopsy survey. Cancer 43: 1847–1857
Riddell R H 1985 Hands off "cancerous" large bowel polyps. Gastroenterology 89: 432–435
Rider J A, Kirsner J B, Moener H C, Palmer W L 1954 Polyps of the colon and rectum. Their incidence and relationship to carcinoma. American Journal of Medicine 16: 555
Risinger J, Berchuck A, Kohler M F et al 1993 Genetic instability of microsatellites in endometrial carcinoma. Cancer Research 53: 5100–5103
Rogers A E, Nauss K M 1985 Rodent models for carcinoma of the colon. Digestive Diseases and Sciences 30: 87S–102S
Rolles C J 1987 Juvenile intestinal polyps – are they always benign? British Medical Journal 294: 529
Rosenberg J M, Welch J P 1985 Carcinoid tumors of the colon. A study of 72 patients. American Journal of Surgery 149: 775–779
Ross J E, Mara J E 1974 Small bowel polyps and carcinoma in multiple intestinal polyposis. Archives of Surgery 108: 736–738
Roth S I, Helwig E B 1963 Juvenile polyps of the colon and rectum. Cancer 16: 468
Rotmensch S, Avigad I, Soffer E E et al 1986 Carcinoma of the large bowel after a single massive dose of radiation in healthy teenagers. Cancer 57: 728–731
Rozen P, Baratz M 1982 Familial juvenile colonic polyposis with associated colon cancer. Cancer 49: 1500–1503
Rozen P, Fireman Z, Fine N, Wax Y, Ron E 1989 Oral calcium suppresses increased rectal epithelial proliferation of persons at risk of colorectal cancer. Gut 30: 650–655
Rubinfeld B, Souza B, Albert I et al 1993 Association of the APC gene product with b-catenin. Science 262: 1731–1734
Ruderman R L, Strawbridge H T G, Bloom H W 1967 Carcinoma of the cecum, presenting as acute appendicitis: case report and review of the literature. Canadian Medical Association Journal 96: 1327
Russell D McR, Bhathal P S, St John D J B 1983 Complete remission in Cronkhite–Canada syndrome. Gastroenterology 85: 180–185
Ryan J W 1993 Immunoscintigraphy in primary colorectal cancer. Cancer 71: 4217–4224

Salmon R J, Fenton J, Asselain B et al 1984 Treatment of epidermoid anal canal cancer. American Journal of Surgery 147: 43–48
Sanders G B, Hagen W H, Kinnaird D W 1958 Adult intussusception and carcinoma of the colon. Annals of Surgery 147: 796
Sarles J C, Consentino B, Leandri R, Dor A M, Navarro P H 1987 Mixed familial polyposis syndromes. International Journal of Colorectal Disease 2: 96–99
Sarre R G, Frost A G, Jagelman D G, Petras R E, Sivak M V, McGannon E 1987 Gastric and duodenal polyps in familial adenomatous polyposis: a prospective study of the nature and prevalence of upper gastrointestinal polyps. Gut 28: 306–314
Sato E, Ouchi A, Sasano N, Ishidate T 1976 Polyps and diverticulosis of the large bowel in an autopsy population of Akita prefecture compared with Miyagi. High risk for colorectal cancer in Japan. Cancer 37: 1316–1321
Savage A P, Reece-Smith H, Faber R G 1994 Survival after peranal and abdominoperineal resection for rectal carcinoma. British Journal of Surgery 81: 1482–1484
Scheele J, Stangl R, Altendorf-Hofman A 1990 Hepatic metastases from colorectal cancer: impact of surgical resection on the natural history. British Journal of Surgery 77: 1241–1246
Schub R, Steinheber F U 1986 Rightward shift of colon cancer. A feature of the ageing gut. Journal of Clinical Gastroenterology 8: 630–834
Seaman W B, Clements J L 1982 Urticaria of the colon: a nonspecific pattern of submucosal edema. American Journal of Roentgenology 138: 545–547
Selby J V, Friedman G D, Collen M F 1988 Sigmoidoscopy and mortality from colorectal cancer: the Kaiser Permanente multiphasic evaluation study. Journal of Clinical Epidemiology 41: 427–434
Shepherd J A 1971 Familial polyposis of the colon with special reference to regression of rectal polyposis after subtotal colectomy. British Journal of Surgery 58: 85
Sherlock P, Lipkin M, Winawer S J 1975 Predisposing factors in carcinoma of the colon. Advances in Internal Medicine 20: 121–150
Shimoda T, Ishikawa E, Sano T, Watanabe K, Ikegami M 1984 Histopathological and immunohistochemical study of neuroendocrine tumors of the rectum. Acta Pathologica Japonica 34: 1059–1077
Shirkhoda A, Staab E V, Bunce L A, Herbst C A, McCartney W H 1984 Computed tomography in recurrent or metastatic colon cancer: relation to rising serum carcinoembryonic antigen. Journal of Computer Assisted Tomography 8: 704–708
Simon G L, Gorbach S L 1984 Intestinal flora in health and disease. Gastroenterology 86: 174–193
Simon J B 1985 Occult blood screening for colorectal carcinoma: a critical review. Gastroenterology 88: 820–837
Sklifasowski N W 1881 Polyadenoma tractus intestinalis. Vrachebnoe Delo (Kiev) 4: 55–57
Skucas J, Spataro R F, Cannucciari D P 1982 The radiographic features of small colon cancers. Radiology 143: 335–340
Small W C, Mehard W B, Langmo L S et al 1993 Preoperative determination of the resectability of hepatic tumors: efficacy of CT during arterial portography. American Journal of Roentgenology 161: 319–322
Smith K J, Johnson K A, Bryan T et al 1993 The APC gene product in normal and tumor cells. Proceedings of the National Academy of Science 90: 2846–2850
Smith K J, Levy D B, Maupin P, Pollard T D, Vogelstein B, Kinzler K W 1994 Wild-type but not mutant APC associates with microtubule cytoskeleton. Cancer Research 54: 3672–3675
Smith L E 1983 Symposium on outpatient anorectal procedures. 4. Flexible fiberoptic sigmoidoscopy: an office procedure. Canadian Journal of Surgery 28: 233
Smith T 1887 Three cases of multiple polypi of the lower colon occurring in one family. St. Bartholomew's Hospital Report 23: 225–229
Smith W G 1958 Multiple polyposis, Gardner's syndrome and desmoid tumours. Diseases of the Colon and Rectum 1: 323–332
Sorenson A W, Slattery M L, Ford M H 1988 Calcium and colon cancer: a review. Nutrition and Cancer 11: 135–145
Soyer P, Levesque M, Caudron C, Elias D, Zeitoun G, Roche A 1993a MRI of liver metastases from colorectal cancer vs CT during arterial portography. Journal of Computer Assisted Tomography 17: 67–74
Soyer P, Elias D, Zeitoun G, Roche A, Levesque M 1993b Surgical treatment of hepatic metastases: impact of intraoperative sonography. American Journal of Roentgenology 160: 511–514
Speck R L, Thomas W H, Larson R A, Wright H K, Cleveland J C 1970 Analysis of 860 patients with carcinoma of the transverse and descending colon. Surgery, Gynecology and Obstetrics 130: 259–262
Spigelman A D, Williams C B, Talbot I C, Domizio P, Phillips R K S 1989 Upper gastrointestinal cancer in patients with familial adenomatous polyposis. Lancet 2: 783–785
Spirio L, Olshwang S, Groden J et al 1993 Alleles of the APC gene: an attenuated form of familial polyposis. Cell 75: 951–957
Spratt J S Jr, Spjut H J 1967 Prevalence and prognosis of indivdual and pathological variables associated with colorectal carcinoma. Cancer 20: 1976–1985
Stemmerman G N, Yatani R 1973 Diverticulosis and polyps of the large intestine. A necropsy study of Hawaii Japanese. Cancer 31: 1260–1270
Stephenson B M, Shandall A A, Farouk R, Griffith G 1990 Malignant left-sided large bowel obstruction managed by subtotal/total colectomy. British Journal of Surgery 77: 1098–1102
Stevenson G W 1993 Radiology and endoscopy in the pretreatment diagnostic management of colorectal cancer. Cancer 71: 4198–4206
Stewart J, Finan P J, Courtney D F, Brennan T G 1984 Does a water soluble contrast enema assist in the management of acute large bowel obstruction: a prospective study of 117 cases. British Journal of Surgery 71: 799–801
Stower M J, Hardcastle J D 1985 The results of 1115 patients with colorectal cancer treated over an 8-year period in a single hospital. European Journal of Surgical Oncology 11: 119–123
Strauss R J, Fazio V W 1979 Bowen's disease of the anal and perianal area. A report and analysis of twelve cases. American Journal of Surgery 137: 231–234
Stryker S J, Wolff B G, Culp C E et al 1987 Natural history of untreated colonic polyps. Gastroenterology 93: 1009–1013
Stubbs R S 1983 The aetiology of colorectal cancer. British Journal of Surgery 70: 313–316
Su L-K, Johnson K A, Smith K J, Hill D E, Vogelstein B, Kinzler K W 1993 Association between wild type and mutant APC gene products. Cancer Research 53: 2728–2731
Talbot I C, Ritchie S, Leighton M H, Hughes A O, Bussey H J R, Morson B C 1981 Spread of rectal cancer within veins: histologic features and clinical significance. American Journal of Surgery 141: 15–17
Talbot R W 1988 Changing nature of anal cancer. British Medical Journal 297: 239–240
Taylor I, Machin D, Mullee M et al 1985 A randomised controlled trial of adjuvant portal vein cytotoxic perfusion in colorectal cancer. British Journal of Surgery 72: 359–363
Taylor R E, Kerr G R, Arnott S J 1987 External beam radiotherapy for rectal adenocarcinoma. British Journal of Surgery 74: 455–459
Thibodeau S N, Bren G, Schaid D 1993 Microsatellite instability in cancer of the proximal colon. Science 260: 816–819
Thoeni R F, Petras A 1982 Double-contrast barium-enema examination and endoscopy in the detection of polypoid lesions in the cecum and ascending colon. Radiology 144: 257–260
Thomas W H, Larson R A, Wright H K, Cleveland J C 1969 Analysis of 830 patients with rectal adenocarcinoma. Surgery, Gynecology and Obstetrics 129: 10–14
Thompson W M, Halvorsen R A, Foster W L, Roberts L, Gibbons R 1986 Preoperative and postoperative CT staging of rectosigmoid carcinoma. American Journal of Roentgenology 146: 703–710
Tops C M J, Vasen H F A, van Berge Henegouwen G et al 1992 Genetic evidence that Turcot syndrome is not allelic to familial adenomatous polyposis. American Journal of Medical Genetics 43: 888–893
Trock B, Lanza E, Greenwald P 1990 Dietary fibre, vegetables, and colon cancer: critical review and metaanalysis of the epidemiological data. Journal of the National Cancer Institute 82: 650–661
Turcot J, Despres J-P, St Pierre F 1959 Malignant tumors of the central nervous system associated with familial polyposis of the colon: report of two cases. Diseases of the Colon and Rectum 2: 465–468
Turnbull R B Jr, Kyle K, Watson F R, Spratt J 1967 Cancer of the

colon: the influence of the no-touch isolation technic on survival rates. Annals of Surgery 166: 420–427
Tweedie J H, McCann B G 1984 Peutz–Jeghers syndrome and metastasising colonic adenocarcinoma. Gut 25: 1118–1123
Umpleby H C, Williamson R C N 1987 Anastomotic recurrence in large bowel cancer. British Journal of Surgery 74: 873–878
Urbanski S J, Kossakowska A E, Marcon N, Bruce W R 1984 Mixed hyperplastic adenomatous polyps – an underdiagnosed entity. American Journal of Surgical Pathology 8: 551–556
Ushio K, Sasagawa M, Doi H et al 1976 Lesions associated with familial polyposis coli: studies of lesions of the stomach, duodenum, bones and teeth. Gastrointestinal Radiology 1: 67–80
Utsunomiya J, Iwama T 1978 Studies of hereditary gastrointestinal polyposes. Asian Medical Journal 21: 12–96
Utsunomiya J, Nakamura T 1975 The occult osteomatous changes in the mandible in patients with familial polyposis coli. British Journal of Surgery 62: 45–51
Utsunomiya J, Gocho H, Miyanaga E et al 1974 Peutz–Jeghers syndrome: its natural course and management. Johns Hopkins Medical Journal 136: 71–82
Van der Werf S D J , Nagengast F M, van Berge Henegouwen G P, Huijbregts A W M, van Tongeren J H M 1982 Colonic absorption of secondary bile acids in patients with adenomatous polyps and in matched controls. Lancet 1: 759–762
Vasen, H F A, Mecklin J-P, Meera-Khan P et al 1991 The International Collaborative Group on Hereditary Non-Polyposis Colorectal Cancer (ICG-HNPCC). Diseases of the Colon and Rectum 34: 424–425
Veale A M, McColl I, Bussey H J R, Morson B C 1966 Juvenile polyposis coli. Journal of Medical Genetics 3: 5–16
Venkitachalam P S, Hirsch E, Elguezabal A, Littman L 1978 Multiple lymphoid polyposis and familial polyposis of the colon. A genetic relationship. Diseases of the Colon and Rectum 21: 336–341
Vogelstein B, Fearon E R, Hamilton S R et al 1988 Genetic alterations during colorectal tumour development. New England Journal of Medicine 319: 525–532
Weidner N, Flanders D J, Mitros F A 1984 Mucosal ganglioneuromatosis associated with multiple colonic polyps. American Journal of Surgical Pathology 8: 779–786
Weilbaecher D, Bolin J A, Hearn D, Ogden W 2nd 1971 Intussusception in adults. Review of 160 cases. American Journal of Surgery 121: 531–535
Weisburger J H, Reddy B S, Joftes D L 1975 Colo-rectal cancer. UICC Technical Report Series No. 19: 7, Geneva
Wernecke K, Rummeny E, Bongartz G et al 1991 Detection of hepatic metastases from colorectal carcinoma: comparative sensitivities of sonography, CT and MR imaging. American Journal of Radiology 157: 731–739
Wherry D C 1981 Screening for colorectal neoplasia in asymptomatic patients using flexible fibreoptic sigmoidoscopy. Diseases of the Colon and Rectum 24: 521–522
White A F, Haskin B J, Jenkins C K, Pfister R C 1973 Abscess of the abdominal wall as the presenting sign in carcinoma of the colon. Cancer 32: 142–146
Whitehouse G H, Watt J 1977 Ischemic colitis associated with carcinoma of the colon. Gastrointestinal Radiology 2: 31–35
Willett W C, Tampfer M J, Colditz G A, Rimm E B, Speizer F E 1990 Relation of meat, fat, and fiber intake to the risk of colon cancer in a prospective study among women. New England Journal of Medicine 323: 1164–1172
Williams A O, Chung E B, Agbata A, Jackson M A 1975 Intestinal polyps in American negroes and Nigerian Africans. British Journal of Cancer 31: 485–491
Williams A R, Balasooriya B A W, Day D W 1982 Polyps and cancer of the large bowel: a necropsy study in Liverpool. Gut 23: 835–842
Williams C B 1984a The clinical yield of colonoscopy. Postgraduate Medical Journal 60: 803
Williams G T, Arthur J F, Bussey H J R, Morson B C 1980 Metaplastic polyps and polyposis of the colorectum. Histopathology 4: 155–170
Williams N S 1984b The rationale for preservation of the anal sphincter in patients with low rectal cancer. British Journal of Surgery 71: 575–581
Williams N S, Johnston D 1983 The quality of life after rectal excision for low rectal cancer. British Journal of Surgery 70: 460–462
Williams N S, Dixon M F, Johnston D 1983 Reappraisal of the 5 centimetre rule of distal excision for carcinoma of the rectum: a study of distal intramural spread and of patients' survival. British Journal of Surgery 70: 150–154
Williams N S, Durdey P, Johnston D 1985 The outcome following sphincter-saving resection and abdomino-perineal resection for low rectal cancer. British Journal of Surgery 72: 595–598
Williams R D, Fish J C 1966 Multiple polyposis, polyp regression and carcinoma of the colon. American Journal of Surgery 112: 846–849
Wilson D M, Pitts W C, Hintz R L, Rosenfeld R G 1986 Testicular tumors with Peutz–Jeghers syndrome. Cancer 57: 2238–2240
Winawer S J 1976 Colon adenomas – to burn or not to burn. Gastroenterology 71: 1101
Winawer S J, Melamed M, Sherlock P 1976 Potential of endoscopy, biopsy and cytology in the diagnosis and management of patients with cancer. Clinics in Gastroenterology 5: 575–595
Winawer S J, Zauber A G, Ho M N et al 1993 Prevention of colorectal cancer by colonoscopic polypectomy. New England Journal of Medicine 329: 1977–1981
Wolf B S, Marshak R H 1963 Linitis plastica or diffusely infiltrating type of carcinoma of the colon. Radiology 81: 502–507
Wolmark N, Fisher B, Wieand H S 1986 The prognostic value of modifications of the Dukes' C class of colorectal cancer. Annals of Surgery 203: 115–122
Wolmark N, Rockette H, Wickerhan D L et al 1990 Adjuvant therapy of Dukes' A, B, and C adenocarcinoma of the colon with portal-vein fluorouracil hepatic infusion: preliminary results of a National Surgical Breast and Bowel Project Protocol C-02. Journal of Clinical Oncology 8: 1466–1475
Wood D A 1967 Atlas of tumor pathology, Section VI, Fascicle 22. Tumors of the intestines. Armed Forces Institute of Pathology, Washington DC
Woolley P V, Treat J, Srivistava S K 1988 Cancers of the large bowel, pancreas and hepatobiliary tract. In: Pinedo H M, Longo D L, Chabner B A (eds) Cancer chemotherapy and biological response modifiers annual, 10. Elsevier, Amsterdam
Wright H K, Thomas W H, Cleveland J C 1969 The low recurrence rate of colonic carcinoma in ileocolic anastomoses. Surgery, Gynecology and Obstetrics 129: 960–962
Wychulis A R, Jackman R J, Mayo C W 1964 Submucous lipomas of the colon and rectum. Surgery, Gynecology and Obstetrics 118: 337
Wychulis A R, Beahrs O H, Woolner L B 1966 Malignant lymphoma of the colon. A study of 69 cases. Archives of Surgery 93: 215–225
Yeager E S, van Heerden J A 1980 Sexual dysfunction following proctocolectomy and abdominoperineal resection. Annals of Surgery 191: 169–170
Yonemoto R H, Slayback J B, Byron R L, Rosen R B 1969 Familial polyposis of the entire gastrointestinal tract. Archives of Surgery 99: 427–434
Zaridze D G 1983 Environmental etiology of large-bowel cancer. Journal of the National Cancer Institute 70: 389–400

# 56. Anorectal conditions

*D. C. Carter*

## ANATOMY OF THE ANORECTAL REGION

The physiology of the anorectum is considered in detail in Chapter 52 but a brief outline of the anatomy will be provided here.

### Musculature of the anorectal region

The anal canal is 3–4 cm long and consists of two muscular tubes. It commences where the rectum narrows at the anorectal ring and ends at the anus (Fig. 56.1).

The internal sphincter makes up the inner tube and is 3 mm thick. It is continuous above with the circular smooth muscle of the rectum, but has a greater number of muscle cells and higher density of nerve fibers. The sphincter is controlled by the autonomic nervous system and has adrenergic, cholinergic and nonadrenergic, noncholinergic nerve fibers (Penninckx et al 1992).

The external sphincter is an outer sheath of striated muscle which is joined in its uppermost part by fibers of the puborectalis portion of the levator ani. These muscles are under voluntary control. The puborectalis fibers originate from the back of the pubic symphysis and form a U-shaped loop which blends with the bowel as it passes through the pelvic floor. This loop helps to maintain the angle of some 80° between the axis of the rectum and anal canal (Fig. 56.2) and compresses the canal into an anteroposterior slit. The anorectal ring is the name given to the condensed ring of muscle formed by puborectalis and upper edges of the two sphincters. The ring can be felt rectally and is vital to continence.

The longitudinal muscle of the anal canal is a continuation of the outer muscle of the rectum which becomes fibrous as it passes between the internal and external anal sphincters, ending as a series of bands which radiate to the perianal skin (Fig. 56.1). The anatomy of this muscle is controversial (Luniss & Phillips 1992). Like the other muscle layers, this coat can be imaged by endoanal ultrasonography.

### The lining of the anal canal

The upper half of the anal canal is plum-colored and lined by epithelium which may be columnar, squamous or transitional. It is thrown into a series of vertical mucosal columns which fuse 2 cm above the anal verge to form crescentic folds (anal valves) which make up the pectinate

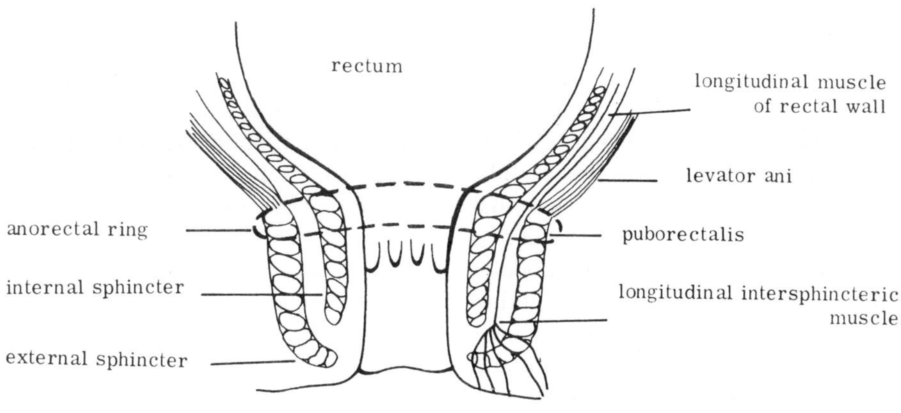


**Fig. 56.1** Transverse section of the anal canal showing disposition of the musculature.

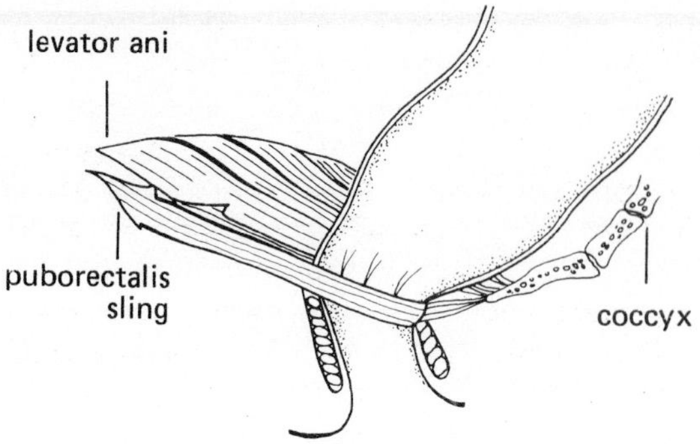


**Fig. 56.2** Sagittal section of the anorectal region to show the disposition of the puborectalis portion of levator ani; forward traction of the puborectalis sling maintains an angle of some 80° between the long axis of the lower rectum and that of the anal canal.

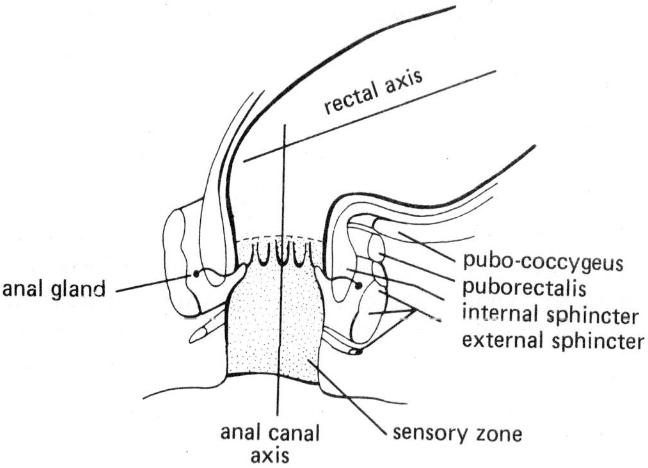


**Fig. 56.3** Transverse section of the anal canal to show the ramification of anal glands and their relationship to the anal sphincters, the angulation at the pelvic floor between the rectum and anal canal (adapted from Duthie 1979).

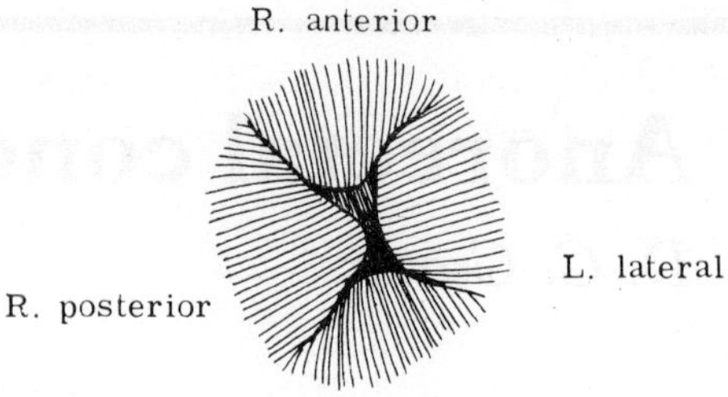


**Fig. 56.4** Configuration of the anal cushions in relation to the lumen of the anal canal.

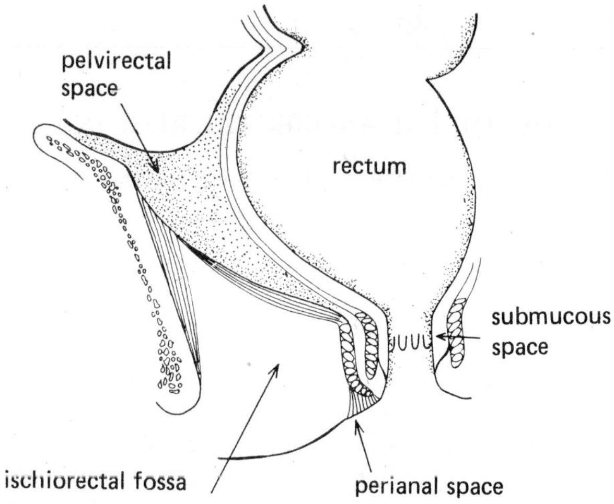


**Fig. 56.5** Transverse section of the rectum and anus showing related tissue spaces.

(dentate) line. Each valve encloses an anal crypt and an anal gland opens into the floor of some of the crypts. These glands ramify in the submucosa to reach the internal sphincter, some of them penetrating to the intersphincteric plane (Fig. 56.3). The glands are important in the spread of anorectal infection. The pectinate line marks the embryological junction of the endodermal cloaca and the ectodermal proctodeum.

For 1.5 cm below the pectinate line the epithelium is pale pink and stratified squamous in type. It is firmly fixed to the underlying muscle by connective tissue. The stratified squamous epithelium gives way to true skin, that is, it becomes keratinized, at the "white line" which is marked by a circumferential groove between the subcutaneous part of the external sphincter and the lower end of the internal sphincter. The term "anal margin" is sometimes applied to the area between the pectinate line and the anal verge (the term applied to the perianal skin).

Above the pectinate line, the anal mucosa is innervated by the autonomic nervous system, whereas distal to the pectinate line the epithelium is innervated by the peripheral nervous system. However, somatic sensation commonly extends slightly above the pectinate line.

The submucosa of the anal canal forms three pads of vascular connective tissue called anal cushions (Thomson 1975). These lie classically in the left lateral, right posterior and right anterior positions and impart a Y-shaped configuration to the lumen (Fig. 56.4).

### Tissue spaces in relation to the anorectal region

The ischiorectal fossa is the pyramidal space bounded laterally by the side wall of the pelvis, medially by the external anal sphincter and superiorly by the levator ani (Fig. 56.5). It contains fatty connective tissue and is crossed by the inferior rectal vessels. The two fossae communicate behind the anal canal.

The perianal space lies below the inferior margins of the anal sphincters and is loculated by fibrous septa.

The submucous space lies between the internal sphincter and the mucocutaneous lining of the upper two-thirds of the anal canal and contains the internal hemorrhoidal venous plexus.

The pelvirectal space is a potential space between the upper surface of the levator ani and the pelvic peritoneum and contains the lateral ligaments of the rectum.

### Blood supply of the anorectal region

The superior rectal artery is the continuation of the inferior mesenteric artery and typically forms three branches which descend through the rectum to the anal canal (Fig. 19.1). However, the arterial anatomy is very variable and does not explain the usual disposition of hemorrhoids (Thomson 1975).

The anal canal is also supplied by branches of the internal iliac artery. The middle rectal artery enters the rectum above the levator ani, while the inferior rectal artery traverses the ischiorectal fossa. There is a profuse anastomosis between the three rectal arteries.

The superior rectal vein drains upwards into the portal vein, while the middle and inferior rectal veins drain laterally into the systemic venous system. Venous anastomoses in the submucosa form the internal hemorrhoidal plexus above the pectinate line and the external hemorrhoidal plexus below.

### Lymphatic drainage of the anorectal region

Carcinoma of the rectum spreads upwards along the superior rectal lymphatic vessels, although lesions in the lower extraperitoneal rectum occasionally spread laterally to the internal iliac nodes. Metastasis to inguinal nodes occurs only when carcinoma involves the skin of the lower anal canal or perianal region.

## HEMORRHOIDS

### **Etiology** (Loder et al 1994)

Hemorrhoids (piles) are one of the commonest ailments of Western society and at least 50% of the over-50 population have some degree of hemorrhoid formation and symptoms (Goligher 1984). Approximately 60% of hospitalized patients with piles are men, although hemorrhoids have equal prevalence in women in the community (Loder et al 1994) and frequently give rise to problems during pregnancy. The etiology of piles remains uncertain and none of the following theories fully explains their development; attenuation of the supporting connective tissue of the anal canal mucosa is the most convincing explanation.

#### *Venous hypertension*

Piles commonly develop or enlarge during pregnancy and are associated with constipation and straining (although most patients have normal bowel frequency). There are no valves in the portal system and it is conceivable that increases in intra-abdominal pressure dilate unsupported anal canal veins. However, the vascular anatomy is unchanged in patients with hemorrhoids and there is normally free communication between the portal and systemic venous systems (Thomson 1975). Burkitt (1972) attributes the increasing incidence of piles in developing countries to a transition to refined low-residue Western diets with consequent straining at stool, but there are no objective data linking prevalence of hemorrhoids and fiber intake.

A number of factors militate against the varicose vein theory. Development of piles in pregnancy may be due to increased laxity and vascularity of the pelvic tissues. Piles are not more common in portal hypertension and if they do develop, they are typically true varices of the anal canal. Rectal cancer may cause piles by obstructing venous drainage, but it must be remembered that these are both common conditions and that they frequently coexist.

#### *The vascular hyperplasia theory*

Stelzner (1963) attributed hemorrhoids to hyperplasia of a submucosal vascular network in which arteries anastomose directly with veins to create a "corpus cavernosum recti". Although high anal pressures in patients with piles are related to high vascular pressures within the anal cushions (see below), the red blood lost from piles probably comes from dilated capillaries rather than arteries (Thomson 1975).

#### *Attenuation of supporting connective tissue*

This theory holds that straining at stool pushes down on the anal cushions so that the supporting framework becomes attenuated, allowing permanent pile prolapse and venous distention (Thomson 1975, Haas et al 1984). Increasing age could exacerbate this attenuation although basal pressure within the anal canal normally falls with advancing age (Hiltunen & Matikainen 1985). Patients with hemorrhoids have higher basal anal pressures than controls but this is probably due to high vascular pressures within the anal cushions (Sun et al 1992, Loder et al 1994).

#### *The pecten band theory*

Lord (1968) introduced anal dilatation as an empirical treatment for piles, suggesting subsequently that constricting fibrous "pecten bands" obstructed the passage of stool and caused venous congestion. This theory for pile formation is not widely accepted.

### Classification of hemorrhoids

Hemorrhoids originate as bulges in the upper anal canal

and lower rectum. The piles contain the internal venous hemorrhoidal plexus, but thickened mucosa and connective tissue contribute to their mass. Progressive enlargement involves the skin-lined lower anal canal with its underlying external hemorrhoidal venous plexus. At this stage, the piles become visible externally.

The piles lie in the left lateral, right anterior and right posterior positions relative to the anal canal. Smaller accessory piles are often present between the three main masses (Fig. 56.4).

Piles which bulge into the lumen without prolapsing through the anus are first degree, those which prolapse on defecation but return spontaneously are second degree, while those which remain prolapsed and have to be pushed back are third-degree piles. Some long-standing piles cannot be returned to the anal canal and are sometimes called fourth-degree piles.

The term "external piles" is sometimes used to describe anal hematomas and skin tags, but is confusing and best avoided.

## Symptoms of uncomplicated hemorrhoids

Bleeding is traditionally regarded as the first symptom. While this is true for first-degree piles, some two-thirds of patients report prolapse as the first manifestation (Thomson 1975). Bleeding is usually first noted as a bright red streak on the stool surface after straining, but can increase in frequency and severity until a steady drip or squirting of blood accompanies defecation. Severe secondary anemia is extremely uncommon, although blood loss can be substantial in patients with portal hypertension.

Prolapse produced symptoms in 114 of 138 patients (83%) requiring hemorrhoidectomy in one series (Bennett et al 1963). It is at first a transient feature on defecation but occurs with increasing frequency and ease until third-degree piles can result. Mucous discharge due to exposure of anal mucosa was troublesome in 22% of Bennett's patients.

Pain is a rare manifestation of uncomplicated piles, but 77% of Bennett's patients experienced discomfort and in 18% it was the main complaint.

Skin tags are found in almost 50% of cases (Steinberg et al 1975) and may cause excoriation and pruritus.

## Assessment and diagnosis

A careful history and abdominal examination must precede anorectal examination. Anal bleeding cannot be attributed to piles until other anorectal pathology has been excluded.

The perianal area is inspected with the patient in the left lateral position. First-degree piles produce no outward abnormality, but separation of the buttocks usually reveals the skin-covered component of second-degree piles and the piles may prolapse when the patient is asked to strain. In third-degree piles, the red anal mucosa is usually visible, separated by a furrow from the skin-lined component.

Digital rectal examination usually reveals no abnormality unless the piles are long-standing and thickened. Proctoscopy is the key investigation, the piles bulging into the lumen as the instrument is withdrawn. The patient is asked to strain during withdrawal to assess vascular engorgement and degree of prolapse. Sigmoidoscopy is essential to exclude coexisting rectal pathology which might mimic bleeding from piles. Barium enema or colonoscopy is indicated when symptoms cannot be explained on proctoscopic and sigmoidoscopic appearances and when hemorrhoidectomy is contemplated (see below).

## Treatment of hemorrhoids

### *Conservative treatment*

Small asymptomatic first-degree piles should be left alone. A high-residue diet or bulk laxative is recommended to combat habitual constipation and straining.

Symptomatic piles merit intervention. While local ointments or suppositories can be used to relieve symptoms such as pruritus or discomfort, they have no long-term role in management.

### *Outpatient and day-patient treatment*

***Manual anal dilatation.*** This technique was popularized by Lord (1968) to treat piles of any degree. Although a number of studies reported long-term symptom relief in 70–80% of patients, incontinence to flatus was troublesome in up to 40% of cases and occasional fecal incontinence was a problem in isolated patients (McCaffrey 1975, Walls & Ruckley 1976). There is no doubt that incontinence is a potentially disastrous complication of manual dilatation (MacDonald et al 1992), particularly when carried out with undue force or in patients with any sphincter weakness, perineal descent or tendency to diarrhea. Most surgeons now avoid dilatation or use gentle dilatation only as a preliminary measure when banding piles under general anesthesia in patients with high sphincter tone (Hancock 1992).

***Injection.*** Injection of 5% phenol in almond oil was once the standard method of treating bleeding hemorrhoids with minimal prolapse. The sclerosant was injected in 2–5 ml quantities into the submucosa above each pile and the subsequent fibrosis tethered the anal cushions at the level of the anorectal junction. Transient deep-seated aching was occasionally noted, but more serious complications such as necrosis, ulceration, abscess and hematuria were rare.

***Infrared coagulation.*** This technique is as effective as injection therapy for piles which have bleeding rather than prolapse as their main manifestation. It is quick, painless and less messy than injection and produces satisfactory results in 85% of patients (Templeton et al 1983). Cryosurgery can also be used to treat second- and third-degree piles (Lloyd-Williams et al 1973) but gives rise to a troublesome discharge for up to 10 days and is now seldom used. Laser therapy has also been used to treat piles but its definitive place remains uncertain.

***Rubber band ligation.*** This is now the standard approach in most clinics to first- and second-degree piles and gives results which are at least as good as those of injection or infrared coagulation (Templeton et al 1983). Each pile is pulled down through the proctoscope and a rubber band is applied by a special applicator to the mucosa-covered pedicle (Barron 1963). Sharp pain indicates that the pile has been banded too low in the anal canal. Although all three piles can be banded at one visit, most surgeons band only one or two piles at a time. Bleeding is the commonest complication and typically occurs 7–14 days after band application. Severe potentially fatal sepsis has been reported on rare occasions after banding (Russell & Donohue 1985) and most cases have occurred in young males. It is uncertain whether immunodeficiency is involved, but all patients should be warned to report to their doctor immediately if they experience marked pain, fever and chills or urinary difficulties.

*Inpatient hemorrhoidectomy*

The standard operation of ligature and excision (Milligan et al 1937) is usually reserved for patients with permanent prolapse and large piles. Formal evaluation of the entire colon and rectum is advisable to exclude bowel pathology and sigmoidoscopy is usually undertaken before commencing hemorrhoidectomy. General anesthesia is employed traditionally but the operation can be performed with sedation and local anesthesia. Each pile mass is dissected free, the plane of dissection passing just within the internal sphincter, which is carefully preserved (Fig. 56.6). Each pedicle is transfixed and ligated and the piles are excised to leave three raw areas separated by bridges of skin and mucosa from which re-epithelialization occurs, so preventing excessive fibrosis and anal narrowing. Some surgeons prefer to reapproximate the edges of each wound by a running suture. Anal dilatation is no longer routine as it fails to reduce postoperative pain and can cause minor defects in anal control (Goligher et al 1969).

Pain is the most troublesome problem and may be extreme during passage of the first bowel motions. The stool is kept soft by hydrophilic agents and analgesics such as buprenorphine can be helpful. Males often have difficulty with micturition but catheterization is rarely needed. Reactionary hemorrhage occurs in less than 2% of patients and secondary bleeding at 7–14 days affects about 1% of cases (Goligher 1984).

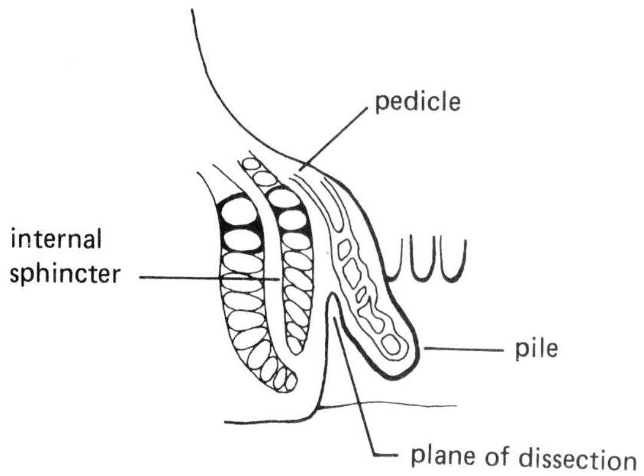


**Fig. 56.6** Section of the anal canal showing the plane of dissection during ligature and excision of hemorrhoids.

Hemorrhoidectomy abolishes pain, discomfort, pruritus and soiling in the majority of patients (Murie et al 1981). Occasional flatus incontinence affected 10% of patients and almost 20% noticed soiling of underclothes despite careful toilet in one study; despite this 93% of patients were satisfied with their long-term result (Bennett et al 1963). First-degree piles are present on proctoscopy in two-thirds of patients after hemorrhoidectomy, but only 5% of patients complain of recurrent symptoms (Bennett et al 1963).

## Thrombosed hemorrhoids

This acute painful condition is often known as "an attack of piles". It occurs when the anal sphincters contract around prolapsed piles, preventing their return to the anal canal and obstructing venous return. Thrombosis and strangulation may be complicated by ulceration and gangrene and the piles become swollen, hard and exquisitely tender. The edematous skin often overhangs and hides the swollen mucosal component.

Immediately after the onset it may be possible to return the piles to the anal canal and allow congestion to settle. By the time patients present to hospital this is seldom feasible. Conservative management (consisting of bed rest, elevation of the foot of the bed, application of dressing soaked in saline, analgesia and mild aperients) is normally recommended in view of the risks said to be associated with emergency surgery (secondary hemorrhage, anal stenosis and portal pyemia).

Recent evidence based on a series of 500 patients undergoing elective hemorrhoidectomy for prolapsed piles and 204 having emergency surgery for thrombosed/gangrenous hemorrhoids in Singapore showed that secondary hemorrhage (5%), anal stenosis (3–6%) and recurrence 7–8%) were no more common after emergency hemorrhoidectomy (Eu et al 1994); portal pyemia was not seen in either group of patients. Lateral internal sphincterotomy (see below) has also been used successfully to provide immediate pain relief and avoid the potential difficulties of emergency surgery in patients with strangulated hemorrhoids (De Roover et al 1994).

### Perianal hematoma

This common condition results from rupture of a vein at the anal verge after straining at stool. The small painful hematoma ("thrombosed external pile") is bluish-black, circumscribed and exquisitely tender. The hematoma is best evacuated by incision under local anesthesia and the wound left to granulate. Alternatively, the hematoma may be left to resolve spontaneously although this takes some days, leaves a skin tag and is occasionally complicated by secondary infection.

## PRURITUS ANI

This common condition of perianal itching occurs more frequently in men, especially between the ages of 30 and 60 years. It may occur in isolation or accompany other anorectal problems such as hemorrhoids.

### Etiology

In more than half of the patients, no cause can be identified and it is assumed that psychogenic problems, chemical irritation by some constituent of feces or food allergy are responsible. In some patients, impaired anal contraction in response to rectal distention may contribute to soiling, which in turn predisposes to pruritus ani (Eyers & Thomson 1979).

Conditions associated with pruritus ani include the following.

***Skin disease.*** Skin lesions may be localized to the perianal area or, as in the case of psoriasis and lichen planus, there may be lesions elsewhere. Contact eczema can be caused by local application of corticosteroid, antibiotic, local anesthetic or lanoline ointment or creams. Bowen's disease is a rare cause of perianal itching.

***Infections.*** Candidiasis must be considered in diabetics and those who have received prolonged courses of corticosteroids or broad-spectrum antibiotics. Fungal infections are occasionally contributory. Threadworms are a cause of nocturnal pruritus ani in children but are uncommon in adults. Anal warts are commonly complicated by pruritus. For anal infections in HIV infection, see p. 611.

***Gastrointestinal diseases.*** Pruritus can be a feature of any anorectal disorder which causes rectal discharge (e.g. piles, fissure, fistula, proctitis, polyps and rectal cancer). Frequent bowel movements in the irritable bowel syndrome, ulcerative colitis or malabsorptive disorders predispose to pruritus.

***Miscellaneous conditions.*** Drugs such as quinidine and colchicine cause pruritus when taken for prolonged periods. Obesity increases the risk of pruritis.

### Clinical features

The itching varies from a minor nuisance to a source of overwhelming misery. The urge to scratch is often irresistible so that the skin is damaged, with local discomfort or pain. Symptoms are worst after defecation and at night, regardless of the cause of pruritus. The perianal skin may show no abnormality on examination, but more often appears raw and excoriated with linear cracks, ulcers and lichenification. Psoriasis and fungal infections often have a well-defined border.

### Investigations

Investigation aims at establishing the underlying cause. The entire skin surface is inspected and proctoscopy and sigmoidoscopy are performed. The urine is examined for glucose. Candidiasis and fungal infection are confirmed on skin scrapings.

### Treatment

Underlying causes such as psoriasis, diabetes and rectal diseases are treated in the usual manner. When no cause can be found, symptomatic measures can be tried. All local applications are discontinued as a first step. Attention to perianal hygiene is essential, as there may be primary or secondary sensitivity to feces or rectal mucus. The region should be washed with lukewarm water in the morning and evening and after defecation. Medicated soaps are avoided to prevent any contained antiseptic from exacerbating inflammation; any excessive use of any form of soap is discouraged. After washing, the area is patted dry with a soft towel; it must not be rubbed vigorously. Application of talcum powder may be useful in warm weather when there is excessive sweating and shaving of the perianal skin may be worthwhile. Woolen and nylon underwear favors sweating and should be replaced by cotton mesh garments. It must also be stressed that some patients become obsessive about hygiene in the mistaken belief that pruritus reflects poor standards of personal cleanliness; excessive washing and use of cleansing agents can make a major contribution to persistent pruritus in such cases and should be discouraged.

It may be possible to identify dietary factors such as beer, red wine, coffee, curries, fruit and milk which exacerbate pruritus. Ingestion of mineral oil may cause anal leakage and advice on laxatives is essential. Bulk laxatives are preferred as a means of achieving a regular soft motion.

Considerable willpower is needed to stop scratching

during waking hours. Involuntary scratching during sleep is also a problem and sedation with phenothiazines can be helpful. Postmenopausal women may benefit from estrogen therapy, particularly if there is also genital pruritus.

The continuing support of the general practitioner is important and regular review ensures that the prescribed measures are being carried out and that remedial causes are detected. Surgical treatment using two curved incisions to produce anesthesia of the perianal skin is no longer advocated as results are far from satisfactory.

## ANORECTAL ABSCESS

### Etiology

Anorectal abscesses are a common cause of admission to hospital. They are 2–3 times commoner in men, the highest incidence being in the third and fourth decades (Buchan & Grace 1973). In general, homosexual men who indulge in penetrative anal sex have a higher incidence of anorectal sepsis (see below).

There is no apparent cause for abscess formation in most patients. Of the 183 cases reported by Buchan & Grace (1973), two had Crohn's disease, three had ulcerative colitis, two had rectal cancer and two had active tuberculosis. Parks (1961) has suggested that infection arises in an anal gland, passes to the intersphincteric space (Fig. 56.3) and then tracks downwards to present as a perianal abscess, outwards to form an ischiorectal abscess or upwards to produce a high intermuscular abscess (Fig. 56.7). Intersphincteric abscesses undoubtedly occur but are less common than this concept suggests (Goligher et al 1967, Buchan & Grace 1973).

It is debated whether anorectal sepsis is commoner in HIV-infected individuals, but when anorectal sepsis does occur in those with persistent generalized lymphadenopathy or AIDS-related complex, there is a higher frequency of intersphincteric, chronic and complex abscesses (Sim 1992).

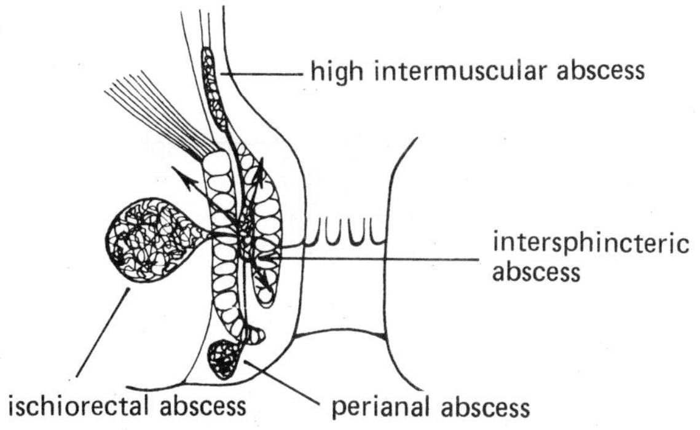


**Fig. 56.7** Transverse section of the anal canal illustrating the manner in which infection could spread from an anal gland.

**Table 56.1** Inciddence of anorectal disease

| Type of abscess | Buchan & Grace (1973) Number | % | Ellis (1958) (as cited by Goligher 1984) Number | % |
|---|---|---|---|---|
| Perianal | 102 | 56 | 109 | 55 |
| Ischiorectal | 77 | 42 | 78 | 39 |
| Submucous (intermuscular intersphincteric) | 1 | – | 0 | |
| Pelvirectal | 0 | | 0 | |
| Uncertain/atypical | 3 | 2 | 3 | 6 |

### Clinical features

***Perianal abscess.*** This common abscess (Table 56.1) presents as an acute painful tender swelling just outside the anal verge. Systemic upset is minimal.

***Ischiorectal abscess.*** This is also common (Table 56.1) and produces a brawny diffuse induration lateral to the anus. The swelling is painful and tender, but fluctuation is a late feature and is associated with marked systemic signs of infection. The swelling may be palpable on digital rectal examination and infection may extend behind the anal canal as a "horseshoe abscess" involving both ischiorectal fossae.

***Intersphincteric abscess.*** This abscess is uncommon or infrequently appreciated, although Parks & Thomson (1973) reported 33 cases. Continuous throbbing anal pain is exacerbated by defecation. There are a few external signs unless the abscess is complicated by perianal or ischiorectal suppuration. Discharge into the anal canal leads to the passage of pus and blood. Digital rectal examination is confirmatory.

***High intermuscular abscess.*** This is rare and resembles an intersphincteric abscess in its presentation.

***Pelvirectal abscess.*** This originates from pelvic sepsis.

***Massive anorectal suppuration.*** Anorectal abscess can become fatally fulminant and obesity and diabetes mellitus are recognized risk factors. Seow-Choen & Nicholls (1992) divide massive anorectal suppuration into anorectal sepsis where infection extends superficially around the perineum causing necrosis of skin, subcutaneous tissue, fascia or muscle, and sepsis which involves the preperitoneal and retroperitoneal spaces. The patient may have subtle signs including abdominal wall induration, tenderness or a vague mass and plain radiographs may show gas in the soft tissues.

### Treatment

Perianal and ischiorectal abscesses are incised and drained under general anesthesia. A specimen of pus is taken for bacteriological examination. The cavity walls are probed gently to detect any communication with the anal lumen.

Fistulous connections were discovered in one-third of the patients reported by Buchan & Grace (1973), but these authors stress that many such "fistulae" may be iatrogenic. Assuming that no communication is detected, the abscess is deroofed by making a cruciate incision and excising the four triangles of skin. The excised skin and a biopsy of the abscess wall are always sent for histological examination. A minority of surgeons perform primary suture of the wound under antibiotic cover (Ellis 1960, Wilson 1964).

Massive anorectal suppuration requires urgent radical debridement and laparotomy may be indicated if intra-abdominal sepsis is suspected. Gram staining of pus is advisable and broad-spectrum antibiotics are started pending the results of culture for anaerobic as well as aerobic organisms.

### Problems in treatment

If an opening into the anal canal is demonstrated below the pectinate line, the fistula should be laid open. This should only be performed by an experienced surgeon and if there is any doubt about the level of the fistula, treatment should be deferred. One-quarter of the patients reviewed by Buchan & Grace (1973) developed recurrent abscess or fistula and ischiorectal abscesses have a particularly high risk of recurrent sepsis. The recurrence rate is similar with primary suture and with incision and drainage (Wilson 1964) and it is now recognized that recurrence may reflect continuing sepsis in offending anal glands and ducts (Seow-Choen & Nicholls 1992).

Anorectal abscess may be the first manifestation of Crohn's disease, ulcerative colitis (p. 662) or, much less commonly, tuberculosis. These abscesses are characteristically indolent and lined by pale gray granulation tissue. They should be incised and drained and bacteriological and histological confirmation of the diagnosis should be obtained. Incision is frequently following by fistula formation, but radical treatment is avoided in the first instance.

## FISSURE-IN-ANO

### Etiology

An anal fissure is a tear in the sensitive skin-lined lower anal canal which produces pain on defecation. The fissure commonly presents in young to middle-aged adults of either sex and can be an isolated primary problem or associated with other gastrointestinal diseases. Its cause is not known. Duthie & Bennett (1964) found no difference between resting internal sphincter pressures in patients with fissure and those in controls, concluding that spasm only occurred in response to defecation. However, Nothmann & Schuster (1974) found higher resting pressures in fissure patients, as well as an abnormal response to rectal distention. Instead of the normal reflex relaxation followed by a gradual return of tone, the internal sphincter relaxed momentarily and then went into marked prolonged contraction.

*Primary fissure-in-ano*

The etiology is uncertain, but some patients first notice symptoms after passing a hard constipated stool. The superficial fibers of the external sphincter are relatively deficient posteriorly and this may explain the frequency with which anal fissures occur in the posterior midline.

*Secondary fissure-in-ano*

Anal fissures are common in Crohn's disease and ulcerative colitis (p. 671). Such secondary fissures are frequently multiple, occur at any point on the canal circumference, are broad-based and characteristically indolent. Fissures are a rare complication of anorectal operations such as hemorrhoidectomy.

### Pathological anatomy

The typical primary fissure is a longitudinal tear extending from the pectinate line to the anal verge in the posterior midline (Fig. 56.8). In 15% of female patients and in 1% of males, the tear is in the midline anteriorly. The tear becomes a canoe-shaped ulcer, the floor of which contains the lower third of the internal sphincter. Inflammation causes swelling of the fissure margins and an edematous skin tag at the anal verge known as a sentinel pile. The swollen anal valve at the upper extent of the fissure is called a hypertrophied anal papilla. Infection may produce a perianal abscess, incision of which results in a lower anal fistula. Anal fissures can heal spontaneously if untreated or become chronic with fibrosis of the spastic internal sphincter.

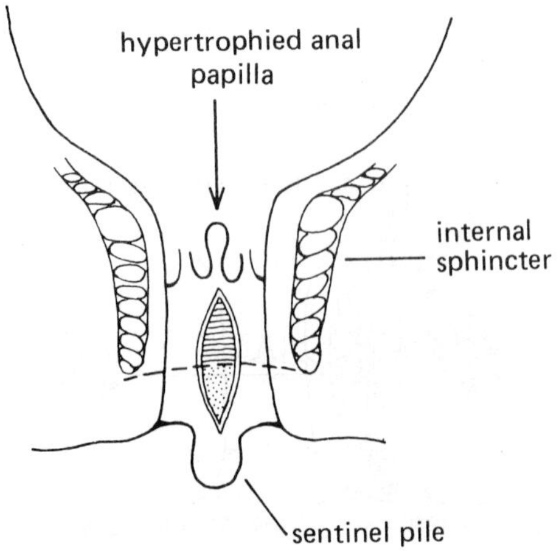


**Fig. 56.8** Transverse section of the anal canal to show the typical features of a primary fissure-in-ano.

### Clinical features

The fissure floor has somatic innervation and excruciating pain on defecation is typical, pain persisting for as long as 6 h and frequently leading to constipation. Pain becomes less troublesome as the fissure heals or becomes chronic. Bleeding sometimes occurs on defecation but is seldom profuse. The sentinel pile and associated serous discharge commonly cause excoriation and pruritus. Perianal abscesses and anal fistulas can complicate the fissure. Recurrent or indolent fissures in unusual sites suggest Crohn's disease or ulcerative colitis.

The diagnosis can usually be made on the history alone. Inspection reveals the sentinel pile and traction on the anal skin may bring the lower part of the fissure into view. Digital rectal examination is painful and often not feasible. If the finger can be inserted, sphincter spasm is confirmed and the indurated margins of the fissure are apparent. Maximal tenderness is elicited when the base of the fissure is palpated. Proctoscopy and sigmoidoscopy are essential to exclude other anorectal disease, but must be performed under anesthesia.

### Treatment

*Conservative treatment*

Anal fissures can heal spontaneously, but conservative treatment with local anesthetic ointments and suppositories has often failed by the time the patient is referred to hospital. Operative treatment allows complete anorectal examination, provides a rapid and more certain cure and is generally advocated. Chronic fissures are unlikely to heal without operation. Whichever method of treatment is selected, a long-term high-fibre diet is advisable to reduce the risk of recurrence.

*Operative treatment*

General anesthesia is essential. The patient is placed in the lithotomy position and the anal canal and rectum are examined thoroughly.

***Anal dilatation.*** Acute fissures frequently respond to gentle dilatation with dramatic relief of pain and spasm and subsequent healing. However, only 50% of patients in one recent review responded to one episode of dilatation (MacDonald et al 1992) and about one in four patients notice some impairment of continence (Watts et al 1964). There is now a greater awareness of the potential consequences of forcible dilatation and the method has lost popularity.

***Lateral subcutaneous internal sphincterotomy.*** This gives a better guarantee of success as a first line of treatment in both acute and chronic fissures. A tenotomy knife is introduced through the perianal skin on one side of the anal canal and the internal sphincter is divided from the pectinate line downwards without entering the lumen (Notaras 1969).

The operation gave immediate relief of pain and was successful in 96 of the 99 patients treated by Hoffmann & Goligher (1970). Minor defects in anal control were noted in 12 patients. Open internal sphincterotomy and excision of the fissure is no longer practiced.

## FISTULA-IN-ANO (Seow-Choen & Nicholls 1992)

### Etiology

Males are more commonly affected and in common with a number of anorectal diseases, the condition has its highest incidence in the age group 30–50 years. Lockhart-Mummery (1929) postulated that infection commences in an anal gland and then spread to produce perirectal abscesses. Parks (1961) extended the cryptoglandular hypothesis by suggesting that infection in perianal glands produces an intersphincteric abscess and infection might then track into the perianal or ischiorectal region. Surgical incision or spontaneous discharge completes the fistula which is kept open by continuing infection from the anal lumen. Not all workers accept this explanation for all cases of anal fistula (see Seow-Choen & Nicholls 1992). Anal fistulae can also be associated with Crohn's disease, ulcerative colitis, tuberculosis, actinomycosis, colloid carcinoma of the rectum and lymphogranuloma venereum.

### Pathological anatomy

Many classifications of anal fistulae exist. Parks et al (1976) divided fistulae into four groups: intersphincteric, trans-sphincteric, suprasphincteric and extrasphincteric. The alternative classification described by Milligan & Morgan and developed by Goligher (1984) will be used here.

*Subcutaneous anal fistula*

These fistulae lie just beneath the perianal skin or skin-lined anal canal.

*Low anal fistula*

This is the commonest anal fistula. The track does not extend higher than the anal crypts and usually enters the bowel at this level. The fistula may traverse both internal and external sphincters as it passes to the exterior or descends in the intersphincteric plane (Fig. 56.9).

*High anal (trans-sphincteric) fistula*

The track extends above the pectinate line but not above the anorectal ring (Fig. 56.9). As with low fistulae, the

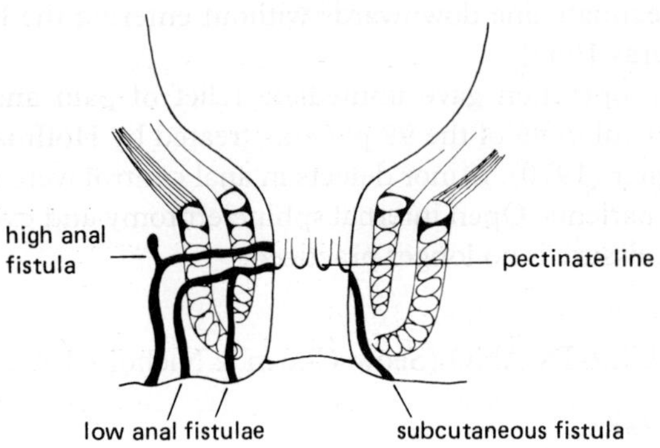


**Fig. 56.9** Transverse section of the anal canal showing the disposition of high and low anal fistulae relative to the pectinate line.

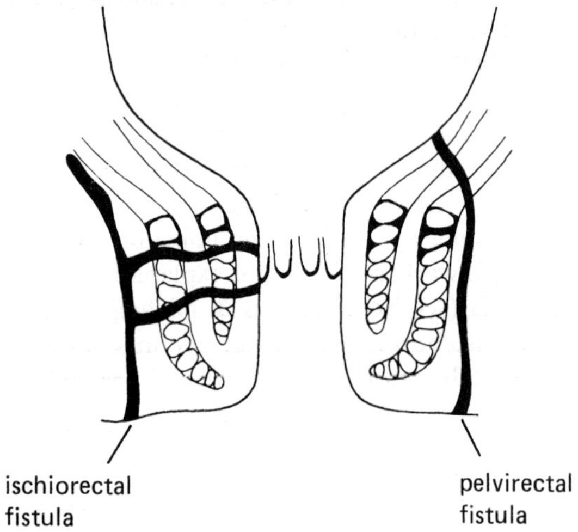


**Fig. 56.10** Transverse section of the anal canal and lower rectum showing the disposition of anorectal fistulae.

track may traverse both sphincters or descend between them.

*Anorectal fistula*

These fistulae are rare. In the ischiorectal variety, the track extends above the anorectal ring but does not pass through the levator ani to enter the rectum (Goligher 1984). The rarer pelvirectal fistula does penetrate the levator, entering the rectum above the anorectal ring (Fig. 56.10).

## Clinical features

Fistulae commonly present as abscesses and are completed when the abscess is incised. In other cases, the patient notices a small discharging sinus with excoriation and pruritus. Once the fistula has formed, it is generally painless unless blockage leads to abscess formation. Malignant transformation is a very rare complication of long-standing fistulae (McAnally & Dockerty 1949), although in some cases the fistula is the result of the cancer rather than its cause.

The purpose of examination is to locate the internal and external opening, define the primary track and any secondary tracks and detect any associated disease. Inspection should reveal the external opening(s). Examination under anesthesia is usually needed but examination without it is also important to assess sphincter tone before any operation.

Digital rectal examination may detect induration along the fistula track, while pressure on the indurated area may express pus from the external opening. The internal opening is occasionally visible on proctoscopy and a malleable probe can be passed carefully along the fistula to define its course without creating false passages. Fistulae with external openings in front of a transverse line passing through the center of the anus generally open into the anal canal at the nearest point on its circumference, whereas fistulae with external openings behind this line tend to open in the posterior midline (and often extend behind the anal canal on both sides to form a horseshoe fistula). This is often known as Goodsall's rule.

Sigmoidoscopy is used to exclude associated rectal disease. Fistulography can mislead and create false passages, whereas endoanal ultrasonography is an accurate method of defining the relation of the tracks to the sphincters and identifying any deep areas of sepsis (Deen et al 1994).

## Treatment

Fistulae associated with other anorectal disease are usually treated conservatively in the first instance. Fistulae arising de novo rarely close spontaneously and operation is generally advised. The course of the fistula must be determined before embarking on surgery and the anorectal ring must be preserved as disastrous permanent incontinence follows its inadvertent division. Approximately 85–95% of fistulae are readily treated by being laid open (fistulotomy) or excised (fistulectomy). Low anal fistulae are usually laid open along their entire length and allowed to heal by granulation and epithelialization. High anal fistulae and the ischiorectal type of anorectal fistulae are treated in the same way, provided that the surgeon is certain that laying open the fistula will not entail division of the anorectal ring.

Management of the 5–15% of difficult fistulae that cannot be laid open without producing incontinence is outside the scope of this text and is reviewed by Goligher (1984) and Seow-Choen & Nicholls (1992). Options include use of a seton (i.e. a nonabsorbable suture passed through the fistula track and tied), formal repair, closure of the internal opening and long-term defunctioning colostomy, or excision of the rectum with permanent iliac colostomy.

## REFERENCES


Alexander-Williams J 1983 Pruritus ani. British Medical Journal 287: 159

Barron J 1963 Office ligation of internal haemorrhoids. American Journal of Surgery 105: 563–570

Bennett R C, Friedman M H W, Goligher J C 1963 Late results of haemorrhoidectomy by ligature and excision. British Medical Journal 2: 216

Buchan R, Grace R H 1973 Anorectal suppuration: the results of treatment and the factors influencing the recurrence rate. British Journal of Surgery 60: 537–540

Burkitt D P 1972 Varicose veins, deep vein thrombosis and haemorrhoids; epidemiology and suggested aetiology. British Medical Journal 2: 556–561

Deen K I, Williams J G, Hutchinson R, Keighley M R B, Kumar D 1994 Fistulas in ano: endoanal ultrasonographic assessment assists decision making for surgery. Gut 35: 391–394

De Roover D M L R, Hoofwijk A G M, van Vroonhoven Th J M V 1989 Lateral internal sphincterotomy in the treatment of fourth degree haemorrhoids. British Journal of Surgery 76: 1181–1183

Duthie H L 1979 Ano-rectal region. In: Duthie H L, Wormsley K G (eds) Scientific basis of gastroenterology. Churchill Livingstone, Edinburgh, p 477

Duthie H L, Bennett R C 1964 Anal sphincter pressure in fissure-in-ano. Surgery, Gynecology and Obstetrics 119: 19

Ellis M 1960 Incision and primary suture of abscesses in the anal region. Proceedings of the Royal Society of Medicine 53: 652

Eu K-W, Seow-Choen F, Goh H S 1994 Comparison of emergency and elective haemorrhoidectomy. British Journal of Surgery 81: 308–310

Eyers A A, Thomson J P S 1979 Pruritus ani: is anal sphincter dysfunction important in aetiology? British Medical Journal 2: 1549

Goligher J C 1984 Surgery of the anus, rectum and colon, 5th edn. Baillière Tindall, London

Goligher J C, Ellis M, Pissides A 1967 A critique of anal glandular infection in the aetiology and treatment of idiopathic anorectal abscesses and fistulas. British Journal of Surgery 54: 977–983

Goligher J C, Graham N C, Clark C G, de Dombal F T, Giles G 1969 The value of stretching the anal sphincters in the relief of posthaemorrhoidectomy pain. British Journal of Surgery 56: 859

Hancock B D 1992 Haemorrhoids. British Medical Journal 304: 1042–1044

Haas P A, Fox T A Jr, Haas G P 1984 The pathogenesis of haemorrhoids. Diseases of the Colon and Rectum 27: 442–450

Hiltunen K M, Matikainen M 1985 Anal manometric findings in symptomatic haemorrhoids. Diseases of the Colon and Rectum 28: 807–809

Hoffmann D C, Goligher J C 1970 Lateral subcutaneous internal sphincterotomy in treatment of anal fissure. British Medical Journal 3: 673

Lockhart-Mummery J P 1929 Discussion on fistula *in ano*. Proceeding of the Royal Society of Medicine 22: 1331–1341

Lloyd-Williams K, Haq I U, Elem B 1973 Cryodestruction of haemorrhoids. British Medical Journal 1: 666–668

Loder P B, Kamm M A, Nicholls R J, Phillips R K S 1994 Haemorrhoids: pathology, pathophysiology and aetiology. British Journal of Surgery 81: 946–954

Lord P H 1968 A new regime for the treatment of haemorrhoids. Proceedings of the Royal Society of Medicine 61: 935–936

Luniss P J, Phillips R K S 1992 Anatomy and function of the anal longitudinal muscle. British Journal of Surgery 70: 882–884

MacDonald A, Smith A, McNeill A D, Finaly I G 1992 Manual dilatation of the anus. British Journal of Surgery 70: 1381–1382

McAnally A K, Dockerty M B 1949 Carcinoma developing in chronic draining cutaneous sinuses and fistulae. Surgery, Gynecology and Obstetrics 88: 87–96

McCaffrey J 1975 Lord treatment of haemorrhoids. Lancet 1: 133–134

Milligan E T C, Morgan C N, Jones L E, Officer R 1937 Surgical anatomy of the anal canal, and the operative treatment of haemorrhoids. Lancet 2: 1119–1124

Murie J A, Sim A J W, Mackenzie I 1981 The importance of pain, pruritus and soiling as symptoms of haemorrhoids and their response to haemorrhoidectomy or rubber band ligation. British Journal of Surgery 68: 247

Notaras M J 1969 Lateral subcutaneous sphincterotomy for anal fissure – a new technique. Proceedings of the Royal Society of Medicine 62: 713

Nothmann B J, Schuster M M 1974 Internal anal sphincter derangement with anal fissures. Gastroenterology 67: 216

Parks A G 1961 The pathogenesis and treatment of fistula-in-ano. British Medical Journal 1: 463–469

Parks A G, Thomson J P S 1973 Intersphincteric abscess. British Medical Journal 2: 537

Parks A G, Gordon P H, Hardcastle J D 1976 A classification of fistula *in ano*. British Journal of Surgery 63: 1–12

Penninckx F, Lestar B, Kerremans R 1992 The internal anal sphincter: mechanisms of control and its role in maintaining anal continence. In: Henry M M (ed) Anorectal disorders. Baillière's Clinical Gastroenterology, vol 6, no 1. Baillière Tindall, London, p 193–214

Russell T R, Donohue J H 1985 Haemorrhoidal banding — a warning. Diseases of the Colon and Rectum 28: 291–293

Sim A 1992 Anorectal HIV infection and AIDS: diagnosis and management. In: Henry M M (ed) Anorectal disorders, Baillière's Clinical Gastroenterology, vol 6, no 1. Baillière Tindall, London, pp. 95–104

Seow-Choen F, Nicholls R J 1992 Anal fistula. British Journal of Surgery 79: 197–205

Steinberg D M, Liegois H, Alexander-Williams J 1975 Long term review of the results of rubber band ligation of haemorrhoids. British Journal of Surgery 62: 144

Stelzner F 1963 Die Hamorrhoiden und andere Krankheiten der Corpus cavernosum recti und dem Analkanals. Deutsche Medizinische Wochenschrift 88: 689

Sun W M, Peck R J, Shorthouse A J, Read N W 1992 Haemorrhoids are not associated with hypertrophy of the internal anal sphincter, but with hypertension of the anal cushions. British Journal of Surgery 79: 592–594

Templeton J L, Spence R A J, Kennedy T L, Parks T G, Mackenzie G, Hanna W A 1983 Comparison of infrared coagulation and rubber band ligation for first and second degree haemorrhoids: a randomised prospective clinical trial. British Medical Journal 286: 1387

Thomson W H F 1975 The nature of haemorrhoids. British Journal of Surgery 62: 542–552

Walls A D F, Ruckley C V 1976 A five-year follow-up of Lord's dilatation for haemorrhoids. Lancet 1: 1212–1213

Watts J M, Bennett R C, Goligher J C 1965 Stretching of the anal sphincters in the treatment of fissure-in-ano. British Medical Journal 2: 342–343

Wilson D H 1964 The late results of anorectal abscess treated by incision, curettage and primary suture under antiobiotic cover. British Journal of Surgery 51: 828–831

# 57. Stoma and pouch care

*Laurie J. Maidl*

In this chapter an overview of issues related to the management of colostomies and ileostomies is presented. A colostomy may result from cancer, diverticular disease, volvulus, incontinence, congenital anomalies or trauma. The most common reasons for an ileostomy are ulcerative colitis, Crohn's disease and familial polyposis.

Preoperative education allows the individual and family the opportunity to ask questions and express concerns. Topics included are the type of ostomy, stoma appearance, usual consistency and quantity of fecal drainage, appliances, gas and odor control, diet, fluids and electrolytes, clothing, sexuality, recreational activities and returning to work.

Postoperatively, the person with an ostomy becomes very experienced in managing their stoma. Health care professionals and the person with the ostomy should work together, maintaining mutual respect for each other's knowledge and experience. If the person's knowledge is inadequate, it can be corrected with the assistance of the enterostomal therapy nurse (ET nurse).

### Role of the enterostomal therapy nurse

Ostomy surgery significantly alters bowel function, necessitating physiological and psychosocial adaptation. An enterostomal therapy nurse (ET nurse) is a specialist who assists the person with an ostomy and their family during the complex process of rehabilitation in collaboration with the person's physician. Equivalent specialists are termed stoma care nurses in the UK and stomal therapists in Australia.

Patients undergoing ostomy surgery benefit from the services of ET nurses across the continuum of care. In the preoperative, outpatient setting the ET nurse discusses the surgical procedure and lifestyle issues with the patient, demonstrates various ostomy appliances and marks the stoma site.

Postoperatively, in the hospital, the ET nurse assists the patient with an ostomy to learn management of the stoma using an appropriate ostomy appliance. Dietary advice, peristomal skin care and resuming daily activities are discussed. Rehabilitation, focusing on body image, sexuality and return to normal life activities such as work or school, are also discussed by the ET nurse.

After hospital discharge, it is important for the person with an ostomy to have regular contact with an ET nurse to assist in the management of changes that may occur. These changes include a decrease in stoma size, changes in body contour, stabilization of weight after surgery and increasing activity with return to normal lifestyle. In the years following ostomy surgery, the ET nurse is available to assist with problem solving of peristomal skin complications, pouching difficulties and psychosocial concerns. Additionally, the person with an ostomy is able to learn about new ostomy equipment (Anonymous 1991a,b, Blackley 1994).

## THE STOMA SITE

Selection and marking of the stoma site preoperatively is important. An ideal stoma site meets the following criteria: within the rectus muscle; visible to the individual; away from the umbilicus, skinfolds, scars, bony prominences and previously irradiated tissue; surrounded by a 4.5–5 cm flat surface. The stoma site should be compatible with other prosthetic devices currently in use, such as corsets or belts (Smith 1992). Siting should be carried out preoperatively with the person lying, sitting and standing. Psychosocial adaptation to a new colostomy or ileostomy is influenced in part by stoma site location and stoma construction. An improperly sited or poorly constructed stoma can result in management problems that adversely affect an individual's lifestyle.

### Colostomy site

Generally, sigmoid and descending colostomies are located in the left lower quadrant (Fig. 57.1). Occasionally, but often temporarily, a colostomy has to be sited elsewhere. For example, a transverse colostomy may be located in an upper quadrant (Fig. 57.2) but sometimes this is impossi-

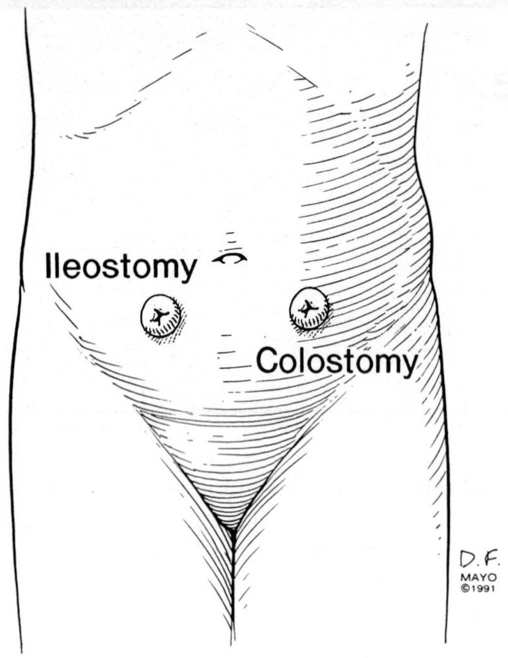


**Fig. 57.1** Preferred stoma sites. (Modified from *Ileostomy: Postoperative Information* by permission of Mayo Foundation for Medical Education and Research).

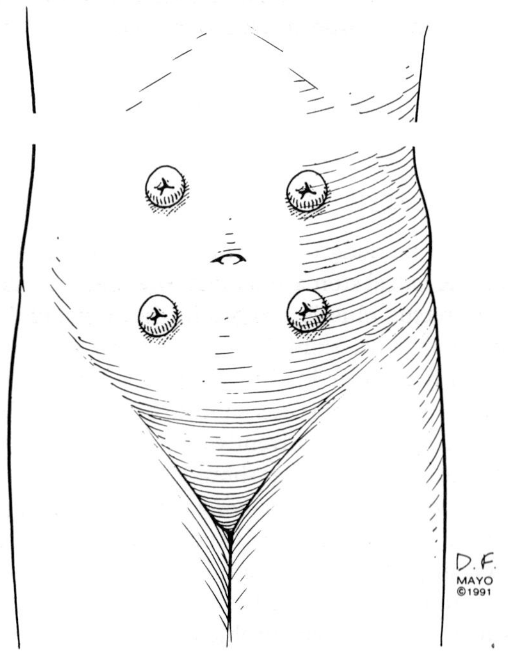


**Fig. 57.2** Alternative sites for transverse colostomy. (Modified from *Ileostomy: Postoperative Information* by permission of Mayo Foundation for Medical Education and Research).

ble because of abdominal contours and it is generally agreed that "no amount of skill can compensate for the poorly sited stoma". The effluent varies from a semi-formed to formed consistency (see also p. 1431).

### Ileostomy site

An ileostomy is most commonly sited in the right lower quadrant (Fig. 57.1). The effluent is initially liquid and although it gradually thickens, it does not become solid. The effluent is discharged intermittently throughout the day.

### Construction of the stoma

A stoma may be constructed as an end, loop or double-barrel stoma. Guidelines regarding the construction of all stoma types include adequate mobilization of the bowel to reduce tension, maturation of the stoma at the time of surgery to reduce risk of stricture, sufficient blood supply and protrusion of 1 cm for colostomy and 2 cm for ileostomy to reduce risk of appliance leakage (Turnbull 1967, McGarity 1992). Initially, the stoma appears red and edematous but gradually decreases in size over 6–8 weeks and develops a shiny pink appearance.

## MANAGEMENT OF THE STOMA

A key factor in optimal management of a stoma is a properly fitting appliance. Certain characteristics are necessary for all ostomy appliances:

- Odor proof
- Protective skin barrier
- Drainable – for ileostomies and some colostomies
- Low profile
- Easy to apply
- Cost effective.

### Appliances

Appliances are available in two types – disposable and reusable. A disposable appliance has an adhesive backing with or without a skin barrier attached. Once this type of appliance has been removed, it cannot be reapplied and is discarded. Disposables are available in a variety of sizes with a cut-to-fit or precut opening. Disposable appliances may be either one piece or two piece, drainable or closed. Some come with flatus filters.

The two-piece type consists of an adhesive base wafer and a pouch which attaches separately. This system allows for changes of the pouch without disturbing the base wafer (Fig. 57.3). In a two-piece system, convexity may be added with the use of a convex insert. Some flanges are available with built-in convexity (Fig. 57.4). A convex appliance may be necessary for the management of a flush or retracted stoma.

With one-piece disposable appliances, the adhesive surface and the pouch are all one piece. These are usually lightweight and very flexible. One-piece appliances are also available with built-in convexity (Fig. 57.5).

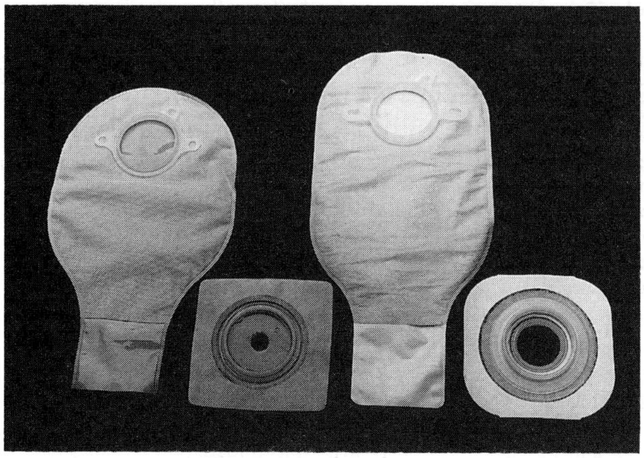

**Fig. 57.3** Two-piece appliance, consisting of adhesive base wafer and pouch.

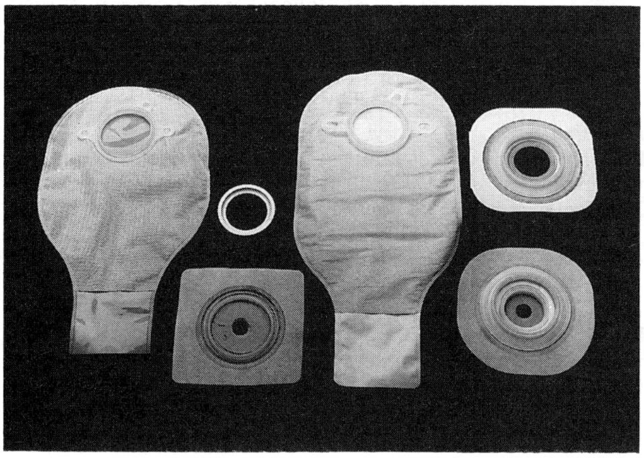

**Fig. 57.4** Convexity may be added to two-piece appliances with use of a convex insert. Wafers are also available with built-in convexity.

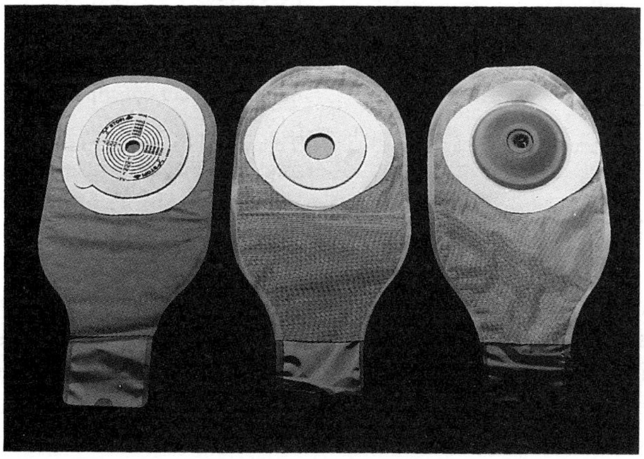

**Fig. 57.5** One-piece appliance, flat and with built-in convexity.

A reusable appliance (rarely used in Australia) is one which may be removed, cleansed and reapplied repeatedly for varying lengths of time. With proper care, some may be reused for 6 months or longer. Reusable appliances are available in one- and two-piece systems, with or without convexity (Fig. 57.6).

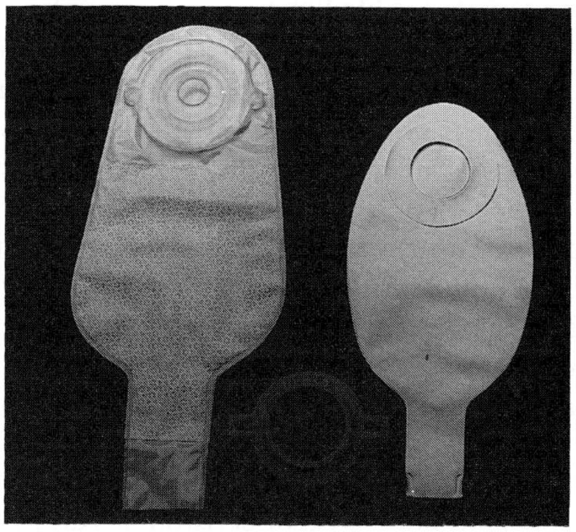

**Fig. 57.6** One and two-piece reusable appliances.

## Special considerations for managing a descending or sigmoid colostomy

Methods for managing a descending or sigmoid colostomy include natural evacuation and colostomy irrigation. The method or combination of methods used will depend on several factors:

- The amount of intestine present above the colostomy
- Bowel habits prior to illness
- Physical ability
- Personal choice.

***Natural evacuation.*** This method allows the bowel to empty naturally. Since the colostomy does not have a sphincter to control the passage of stool, a pouch is worn at all times.

***Colostomy irrigation.*** Irrigation provides stimulation for the colon to empty itself of stool. Special colostomy irrigation equipment is used for this procedure. Colostomy irrigation may allow the individual more control over bowel function. Therefore, a small pouch or gauze covering on the colostomy between irrigations may be all that is needed (Anonymous 1991a).

## Peristomal skin care

The basic principles in the management of peristomal skin are to thoroughly cleanse and dry the skin and to wear a properly fitting appliance.

Peristomal skin should be cleansed with warm water. If soap is used, care should be taken to remove any residual soap film prior to applying the appliance. Products containing alcohol should be avoided due to the dehydrating effect on the skin, which may result in flaking, itching and breakdown of the epithelial layer. Conversely, products with an oil or petroleum base leave an oily residue on the skin, preventing appliance adherence. Better adhesion is obtained if hair is removed either by clipping closely with scissors or by shaving the skin, taking care to avoid damage to the skin and stoma.

The practice of using antacids to treat skin irritation is no longer recommended. Antacids alter the pH level of the skin which may potentiate further skin breakdown.

When removing the appliance, skin trauma is avoided by peeling the appliance gently from the skin. An adhesive remover manufactured specifically for removal of ostomy appliances may also be used.

The most common cause of peristomal skin irritation is stool in contact with the skin. An appliance fitted within 3 mm of the stoma helps eliminate skin irritation due to contact with stool.

A person with a stoma needs to be instructed on methods to reduce the risk of leakage. First, the skin surrounding the stoma should be washed and dried thoroughly before the new appliance is applied. Second, the pouch should be emptied when it is one-third full. Additionally, excessive external pressure on a partially filled pouch has to be avoided. A fourth method to reduce leakage is to evaluate the person's appliance type. If leakage occurs repeatedly in the area of a crease or skinfold, a convex appliance or belt may be necessary. At the first sign of leakage, the entire appliance should be changed.

**Table 57.1** Properties of various foods (from *Ileostomy: Postoperative Information*, by permission of Mayo Foundation for Medical Education and Research)

| | | |
|---|---|---|
| *Gas-forming foods* | *Incompletely digested foods* | |
| Beans | Celery | Coconut |
| Beer | Corn | Dried fruit |
| Broccoli | Green peppers | Lettuce |
| Brussels sprouts | Mushrooms | Nuts |
| Cabbage | Olives | Peas |
| Carbonated beverages | Pickles | Pineapple |
| Cauliflower | Popcorn | Raw vegetables |
| Onions | Seeds | Spinach |
| | Skins of fruits and vegetables | |
| *Thickening foods* | *Thinning foods* | |
| Apple sauce | Alcoholic beverages | |
| Bananas | Grape juice | |
| Breads and starches | Heavily spiced foods | |
| Cheeses | Prune juice | |
| Pastas | | |
| Peanut butter (creamy) | | |
| *Odor-reducing foods* | *Odor-producing foods* | |
| Buttermilk | Asparagus | |
| Parsley | Eggs | |
| Yogurt | Fish | |
| | Garlic | |
| | Onions | |

*Reminders:*
- Eating more than one food from within a list may intensify the effect on the bowel.
- The stool may appear red after eating beets. Broccoli, asparagus and spinach may darken the stool.

**Table 57.2** Dietary guidelines (from *Ileostomy: Postoperative Information*, by permission of Mayo Foundation for Medical Education and Research)

| General guidelines | Rationale |
|---|---|
| 1. Eat meals at regular times, three or more times daily. | 1. Skipping meals may cause more gas production. Bowel function may be more regular. |
| 2. Chew all food thoroughly. | 2. Chewing assists the digestive process and reduces the chance of food blockages. |
| 3. Drink adequate fluids (8–10 glasses per day). | 3. Drinking fluids will help reduce fluids lost through an ileostomy or help prevent constipation with a colostomy. |
| 4. Try new foods one at a time. | 4. This will assist in determining foods that may cause diarrhea, excessive gas or constipation. |

## Flatus

Flatus may make a noise as it passes through the stoma. This sound is decreased when clothing is worn to provide a muffling effect. Factors that may increase the amount of flatus produced include drinking through a straw, chewing gum, eating gas-forming foods, skipping meals and emotional upsets. Medications containing simethicone may be taken to reduce the flatus. Some appliances come with a flatus filter – a vent containing charcoal which allows the gas to escape and be deodorized.

## Odor

Most ostomy appliances are odor proof. Odor may be an indicator of leakage, an appliance left on too long, incorrect fitting of the appliance or failure to cleanse the drainable end of the pouch (Sivly & Todd 1991) Certain foods may also increase the odor of the stool (Table 57.1). Oral preparations, such as chlorophyll tablets (200–400 mg daily) or bismuth subgallate (400 mg), or deodorant drops in the pouch may be used.

## Diet/fluids

There are no special diets for people who have ostomies but some general guidelines are recommended (Anonymous 1991a) (Table 57.2). Some foods have been identified as having certain effects on the bowel. Since individual tolerance to foods will vary, this list may be used as an initial guide (Anonymous 1991b).

## Fluid and electrolyte balance

Initially after surgery, ileostomy effluent is bile green in color and liquid in consistency. As the diet progresses, the effluent changes character quickly and becomes much thicker. In people with well-established ileostomies, the amount of output varies from person to person (Pemberton 1988).

The influence of diet and fluid intake on the consistency and volume of the ileal effluent is well known. If large quantities of water are consumed, no significant increase in the volumes of effluent occurs. Some foods, such as fruit juices, will increase the fluid weight of the effluent (Pemberton 1988).

In general, people with ileostomies excrete more water in their stool than people without ileostomies. Ileostomy effluent also has a relatively high sodium content (38–40 mmol daily) compared to normal daily loss (10 mmol). Despite ileostomy adaptation, there is an 11% reduction in total body water and a 7% reduction in exchangeable sodium present in people with ileostomies (Devlin 1984). They rarely, however, manifest symptoms of sodium or water depletion. This is probably because of enhanced renal conservation of sodium and water. If high output occurs for any reason, volume depletion develops rapidly (Pemberton 1988).

The water and electrolyte loss from the ileostomy results in a decrease in urine output and an increase in urine concentration. People with well-functioning ileostomies have a slightly higher incidence of renal stones than the general population (Pemberton 1988).

Extensive ileal resection reduces the absorptive surface, resulting in less absorption and higher ileostomy output. Management of people with high-volume output is based on its presumed etiology. Hypomotility agents such as loperamide hydrochloride may provide effective treatment for people with high output ileostomies (Pemberton 1988).

### Medications

The absorption and effectiveness of medications may be affected by the type of ostomy. It is helpful for people to inform their pharmacist that they have an ileostomy to insure that they receive medication in a form that is most effectively absorbed. Time-released or enteric-coated medications may be only partially absorbed. Liquids, gelatin capsules, uncoated or chewable tablets may be more effective. Advice should be obtained on specific oral contraceptives.

***Antibiotics.*** Because antibiotics can cause a change in the normal flora of the digestive tract, diarrhea, dehydration and electrolyte losses may result in a person with an ileostomy. Candidiasis may also occur on the peristomal skin. This infection is treated with an antifungal powder.

***Diuretics.*** Diuretics need to be used carefully by a person with an ileostomy because they may cause electrolyte imbalance and dehydration. If diuretics are used, electrolyte supplements may be necessary.

***Potassium supplements.*** The potential for diarrhea from liquid and powder potassium supplements can be reduced by dividing the dosage into smaller amounts. Sustained-released tablets may be only partially absorbed by the person with an ileostomy. Additionally, foods that are a good source of potassium can be suggested to the person.

***Laxatives.*** Laxatives should not be used by the person with an ileostomy as dehydration and electrolyte imbalance may result (Anonymous 1991b). Mild laxatives may be used for managing constipation in a person with a colostomy.

## LIFESTYLE

The person with a stoma has many questions about lifestyle changes following surgery. The usual guidelines of limited weight lifting after surgery should be followed. As strength and endurance increase, the person with an ostomy may return to a normal lifestyle. The time for returning to work will be determined by energy level as well as the physical demands of the job. An ostomy need not be a hindrance to any job or career.

People with new ostomies often express concern about resuming sexual activity and need reassurance that such nervousness is a normal feeling. Good communication between partners about feelings, patience and a sense of humor will decrease the anxiety and promote a positive experience. It is helpful to have a clean, empty, secure appliance in place before initiating any sexual activity.

People who have had surgery in the rectal area or removal of the rectum may experience some changes in sexual function. For women, vaginal penetration may be painful due to incisional pain, decreased lubrication and a change in the angle of the vagina. The pain usually decreases as the rectal area heals. Sensation may be altered and difficulty in reaching orgasm may occur. For men, the ability to achieve or maintain an erection may be a temporary or permanent problem. At first pain from surgery, fatigue and anxiety may be the cause of the dysfunction. If the problem continues, a thorough urologic work-up is indicated to determine the cause and proper treatment options (Anonymous 1991b).

## PSYCHOSOCIAL ISSUES

An individual's ability to cope with an ostomy is directly determined by maturity, educational level, cultural values, self-image, past coping mechanisms, previous experiences with others having an ostomy, current support systems and financial resources. Feelings may include anxiety, depression or hostility. When cancer is newly diagnosed, a person may experience feelings of powerlessness and hopelessness. Conversely, if a disease is ablated, optimism and hopefulness may be felt.

It is important that people facing surgery and their families address the psychosocial issues of life with an ostomy.

Emotional support in the early postoperative phase is essential as the person and family come face to face with the reality of seeing and managing the stoma (Shipes 1987). A person with an ostomy needs to work toward acceptance of a change in body image and an altered pattern of elimination.

As each person's skill level in managing the technical aspects of ostomy care improves, confidence builds toward managing other aspects of their lifestyle. The time it takes for each individual to adjust to a new ostomy is variable. Patience, understanding and support are important to allow the phases of adjustment and acceptance to progress gradually.

## MANAGEMENT OF ALTERED BOWEL FUNCTION

### Colostomy

On occasion, the person with a colostomy may have problems with constipation or diarrhea. The bowel can be affected by certain foods, a virus, medications or emotional factors such as anger or stress.

Constipation may be prevented by drinking 8–10 glasses of fluid in a 24-h period and including fiber in the diet. A stool-bulking agent such as psyllium may be taken 1–3 times daily, to increase fiber. A stool softener taken routinely may help with recurrent problems with constipation. If needed, a mild laxative may be taken.

Foods to help thicken the stool may be helpful if diarrhea occurs. Incompletely digested foods or those that thin the stool should be temporarily avoided (Table 57.1). An over-the-counter antidiarrheal medication may be helpful. It is important to increase intake of liquids to replace the fluid lost from diarrhea and to prevent dehydration (Anonymous 1991a).

### Ileostomy

Normal ileostomy output is about 500–1000 cc of stool per day. Drinking 8–10 glasses of fluid per day will replace the water that is normally lost.

Occasionally problems with high ileostomy output or diarrhea can occur, making it necessary to empty the ileostomy appliance every 1–2 h instead of 5–6 times a day. Diarrhea may begin suddenly and may be accompanied by abdominal cramping (Anonymous 1991b). Salt tablets may be prescribed.

Ileostomy output greater than 1000 cc of liquid stool in 24 h can lead to dehydration. Increasing fluid intake will replace the extra fluids lost and prevent dehydration. Withholding foods and fluids will not decrease ileostomy output. Sodium and potassium lost through high output may need to be replaced. Food sources of sodium are broth, cheese, electrolyte drinks, processed meats and salt used in food preparation. Food sources of potassium include bananas, electrolyte drinks, oranges, potatoes, squash, tomatoes and yogurt (Anonymous 1991b).

### Food blockage

Food blockage is a potential problem for a person with an ileostomy. Incompletely digested foods are the most common cause. A large food mass can become lodged at a kink or narrowing in the intestine. Generally, food blockage occurs close to the opening of the ileostomy, resulting in difficulty or inability to pass stool through the stoma. Symptoms of a food blockage may include abdominal cramping, bloated or distended abdomen, increased odor to the stool, nausea and vomiting, swelling of the stoma, watery diarrhea or no ileostomy output. A food blockage may also cause dehydration because of the watery diarrhea and vomiting that can occur (Anonymous 1991b).

Many food blockages will resolve by themselves. Getting in a knee–chest position, taking a hot shower or bath or drinking a warm liquid may help. Gently massaging the abdomen, especially around the stoma, may resolve a food blockage. During a blockage episode, the stoma may become swollen and appliance resizing may be required. Blockages not resolved in 4–6 h may require further evaluation, such as an ileostomy lavage or endoscopic examination (Anonymous 1991b) or readmission to hospital for investigation.

## STOMAL AND PERISTOMAL SKIN COMPLICATIONS

The primary goal for the person with a stoma is prevention of stomal and peristomal skin complications. Preoperative assessment, postoperative teaching and adequate follow-up visits are all a part of this preventive care. When complications do occur, the first step is to identify the cause. Once the cause has been identified, appropriate interventions are initiated until the problem is resolved. Follow-up is necessary to determine if the intervention has been effective.

### Stomal necrosis

This is the death of mucosal tissue on the surface of the stoma within 5–7 days after surgery. This occurs when there is a compromised blood supply to the stoma.

Clinical features most commonly seen are changes in stoma color from purple to gray to black and a decrease in moisture on the surface of the stoma. Stomal necrosis may involve a portion or the entire stoma surface and is not painful. Sometimes there is a pungent odor to the stoma as the tissue sloughs.

Interventions for a necrotic stoma include documentation of the mucosal color changes, assessment of the depth of necrosis, use of room or pouch deodorizers, debridement of nonviable tissue and psychological support for the person with the stoma. The level of necrosis can be checked by inserting a small test tube gently into the stoma and shining a flashlight into the tube to determine where the mucosa is pink and healthy. The stoma needs to be viable below the fascia or peritonitis can result. As nonviable tissue sloughs or is debrided from the stoma, the appliance will need to be resized. Surgical intervention may be required.

### Mucocutaneous separation

This is a separation of the suture line at the junction between the stomal mucosa and skin. This occurs secondary to inappropriate or insufficient sutures used during surgery, poor stomal construction, suturing under tension and poor tissue healing.

The clinical features are skin irritation around the stoma and separation at the mucocutaneous junction which may be partial or circumferential. Drainage, either serosanguinous or purulent, may be present at the site of the separation. Pain or burning at the separation site may occur from contact with stool.

There is a need to determine the extent of the separation and to rule out fistula formation. Irrigation of the separation with normal saline facilitates removal of any drainage and nonviable tissue. A deep separation may be packed with gauze or a calcium alginate dressing while a superficial separation may be filled with a powder form of skin barrier to promote wound healing. The use of a two-piece appliance is necessary if packing is required. Continued follow-up is needed to evaluate changes needed in the ostomy appliance.

### Stomal retraction

This occurs when the stoma is pulled inward. This is often preceded by stomal necrosis or mucocutaneous separation. Retraction may be caused by the use of insufficient length of bowel to make the stoma, too much tension on the bowel and a significant postoperative weight gain.

The clinical features include the stoma located at or below skin level, a receded or dimpled area around the stoma and difficulty with the pouch adhering to the receded area. A mucocutaneous separation may also occur.

A digital examination is performed to check the stoma for stenosis at the skin or fascial level. Peristomal skin needs to be protected from contact with stool by using an appliance with convexity as well as a belt. Weight loss may also reduce retraction. Surgical intervention may be required should problems persist.

### Stomal stenosis

This occurs when the skin or fascia surrounding the stoma contracts due to scar tissue formation. Insufficient skin excision at the stomal site at the time of surgery and scarring that occurs with stomal necrosis, peristomal abscess or radiation therapy are directly related to stomal stenosis.

Clinical features include stenosis at the skin or fascial level, a small stoma lumen on digital examination and effluent exiting the stoma under pressure. The potential for constipation exists with a colostomy when stenosis is present.

Measures required include short-term dilatation, assessing the volume and ease of evacuation of effluent and refitting the appliance. Dilatation can cause additional scarring with long-term use if the fibrous ring is torn. If problems persist, surgical revision of the stoma may be necessary.

### Peristomal hernia

This is a protrusion of the ileum or colon into the subcutaneous layer of the skin surrounding the stoma. Herniation can occur when the stoma is not placed within the rectus muscle, a defect in abdominal musculature exists or as a result of increased intra-abdominal pressure with lifting or straining. Recently it has been proposed that a stomal hernia occurs in those prone to it, whether or not the stoma is sited within the rectus muscle (Phillips et al, Blackley 1994).

Peristomal hernias vary in size, with progressive bulging that is exaggerated with sitting or increased intra-abdominal pressure. They are usually not painful but obstructive symptoms may be experienced with progression of the hernia (p. 1431).

A supportive undergarment such as a hernia support belt may alleviate the pressure of the hernia. The appliance may need to be refitted due to changes in abdominal contour. Medical assistance is necessary if pain develops or if the stoma changes in color. Surgical revision and possible stoma relocation may be necessary if problems persist.

### Laceration

This is a cut in the stoma mucosa. A laceration can result if the appliance is inappropriate for the size of the stoma, when poor technique is used in applying the ostomy appliance or when there is trauma to the stoma through direct injury.

Notable clinical features include blood in the pouch and bleeding from the stoma with a laceration noted on examination. Stoma lacerations are not painful.

Interventions commonly used include applying direct pressure or the use of topical thrombin to control bleeding and adjusting the appliance to fit the stoma appropriately. Educating the person with a stoma on the cause and treatment of a laceration and providing follow-up to assess healing are also important.

**Irritant dermatitis**

This inflammation of the skin results from contact with a chronic irritant, secondary to poor stoma construction causing effluent to be in contact with the skin or from poor technique in appliance care. Too many products used on the skin may cause increased interaction of product ingredients, resulting in the development of sensitivity to the products.

Irritant dermatitis is manifested by erythema, swelling, denudement, ulceration, bleeding and weeping from involved peristomal skin. Pain, burning and itching are also apparent. Skin manifestations may vary in severity.

Treatment is directed at identifying and eliminating the cause. The goal is to protect damaged skin and avoid other irritants. Patch or skin testing of products may be done to determine the cause in order to eliminate the irritant. Topical steroids may be needed to reduce the inflammation, pain and itching.

**Candidiasis**

This is a fungal infection which may result from moisture around or under the appliance and from systemic antibiotic therapy, immunosuppressive medications or chemotherapy.

Clinical features include erythema of the peristomal skin, extrafollicular lesions, papules and/or pustules, maceration, satellite lesions and lesions that may be seen in other areas of the body, such as the groin or axilla.

The treatment plan involves providing a dry environment and the use of antifungal powders, porous tapes and pouch covers to absorb moisture. The appliance may need to be resized to fit appropriately. Hydrophilic skin barriers which absorb moisture and keep it in contact with the skin may need to be eliminated.

**Mechanical injury**

This term refers to injury to the peristomal skin caused by pressure, friction or stripping of skin during pouch removal. This results from poor technique in appliance changes, improper use of ostomy equipment and fragile skin from steroids or radiation therapy.

Clinical features include erythema, denuded skin, ulceration and pain. The margins of the lesions are irregular.

Management includes the use of skin sealants on intact skin, as well as the use of skin barriers in solid, paste or powder form to promote healing. The technique of appliance application and removal should be evaluated and additional instruction given as needed.

**Radiation injury**

Skin cell destruction and mechanical stripping of the epidermis occur when skin barriers and adhesive are removed from irradiated skin. Small vessel damage after radiation is the underlying cause of tissue damage.

Radiation injury is manifested by dry skin, induration and thinned epithelium which may result in painful ulcerated lesions.

The treatment goals are to protect the damaged skin and promote tissue healing. Avoiding the use of adhesives and irritants such as soaps and solvents, as well as avoiding trauma to the peristomal skin or stoma, are strategies to accomplish this goal. Products containing zinc or mercury should not be used. When the stoma is within the radiation field discussion should take place with the oncologist as to whether the appliance should be removed or folded out of the way. It is totally impractical at times to remove the ostomy appliance for treatment. Frequent removal is in itself a cause of skin stripping. Removal depends on the appliance worn, e.g. a bulky reuseable appliance may have buckles and belt rings, etc. The modern appliance, however, has such a low profile that it can be left in situ provided the planning and measurement of dose of radiation, etc. takes into account the composition and thickness of the appliance and the radiation oncologist and the stoma therapy nurse collaborate on the treatment plan. Marking the stoma site outside of the radiation field when preoperative radiation has been given facilitates postoperative wound healing.

**Hyperplasia**

This is the overgrowth of skin tissue caused by exposure to a chronic irritant, such as stool or an improperly sized appliance.

Clinical features most commonly seen are raised lesions with a wartlike appearance that are hyperpigmented, usually gray. Lesions begin at the stomal base and extend outward and may be partial or circumferential. The lesions may be macerated, hypersensitive and bleed easily. Increased difficulty with pouch adherence may occur due to raised lesions.

The appliance needs to be refitted to cover the hyperplastic area. An acidification program using half-strength vinegar soaks to the hyperplastic area twice a day may be beneficial. Follow-up is necessary to evaluate if the hyperplasia is being reduced and to resize the appliance.

**Folliculitis**

This inflammation of the hair follicles on the peristomal skin is most commonly caused by traumatic removal of peristomal hair when removing the appliance. The most common infecting agent is *Staphylococcus aureus*.

Follicular lesions arise from hair follicles and are erythemic, pinpoint papules or pustules. The lesions may be few or many in number, pruritic and painful if the condition is severe.

The use of nonocclusive adhesives, such as a skin sealant, and removing the peristomal hair with an electric razor or clipping with a scissors should alleviate the problem. Use of straight-edged razors is discouraged. Reinforcement of proper skin care technique is important (Maidl 1990).

### **Pyoderma gangrenosum** (p. 674)

This is an inflammatory skin disease that can be destructive and extensive. It reflects underlying inflammatory processes rather than being a "complication" of ostomy construction. Lesions begin as a pustule and progress to ulcers which may undermine the skin. These ulcers usually have a blue-red border with a red center. These may or may not be covered with necrotic tissue.

Systemic corticosteroids are used to reduce the inflammation and pain. Appliance modification will also need to be addressed. Protecting the skin and facilitating healing remain the treatment goals (Hampton 1992).

## FOLLOW-UP OF PATIENTS

It is important that people with ostomies continue to receive follow-up care after they leave the hospital. Changes will occur during the first few months after surgery which may affect the type of ostomy appliance the person is using. These changes include a decrease in size of stoma, changes in body contour, stabilization of weight and an increase in activity. Follow-up care provides an opportunity to assess the current ostomy appliance and make modifications if necessary. Continued follow-up care also provides an opportunity to assess the person's psychological adjustment to a new ostomy.

## RESOURCES/SUPPORT SERVICES

Nurses who specialize in the care of persons with ostomies are available in many communities. They are an invaluable resource in helping people learn to manage and adjust to their ostomy.

Many communities have ostomy associations or support groups for people with ostomies and their families. These organizations provide psychological support and educational services through meetings, group discussions, newsletters and educational programs.

## ALTERNATIVE PROCEDURES

### **Continent ileostomy** (Kock pouch) (p. 694)

The reservoir is emptied 4–5 times a day by inserting a catheter through the stoma. Individuals with a continent ileostomy are able to wear a small waterproof pad instead of a pouch over the stoma.

Problems with nipple valve dysfunction and the development of the ileal pouch–anal anastomosis procedure have resulted in decreased use of the continent ileostomy as the procedure of choice.

### **Ileal pouch–anal anastomosis (IPAA)** (p. 689)

Management issues for people having IPAA surgery include learning to care for their temporary ileostomy, diet and fluid balance, management of high ostomy output/frequent stools and anal skin care. It is important that individuals with an IPAA are counseled as to what to expect after the surgery with regard to stool frequency and sphincter control. Immediately after ileostomy closure they may have 10–20 bowel movements per day. The internal reservoir will gradually adapt over time and after 6 months to a year they may have only 5–6 bowel movements per day.

Overall, patients undergoing this operation have been satisfied with the outcome, with the elimination of their disease process, avoidance of a permanent stoma and return to an active lifestyle (Kohler et al 1991).

*Acknowledgement*

I recognize the collaborative efforts of the ET nurses at Mayo Medical Center for their contributions in writing this chapter: Karen Brigham, Therese Jacobson, Renee Kromrey, Pam Sivly, Diane Todd and Jean Zuroski.

## REFERENCES

Anonymous 1991a Colostomy: postoperative information, Mayo Foundation for Medical Education and Research, Rochester, Mn

Anonymous 1991b Ileostomy: postoperative information, Mayo Foundation for Medical Education and Research, Rochester, Mn

Blackley P 1994 Professional stomal therapy nursing practice. University of New England Press, Armidale

Devlin H B 1984 Stomas and stoma care. In: Bouchier I A D, Allan R N, Hodgson H J F, Keighley M R B (eds) Textbook of gastroenterology. Baillière Tindall, London, p 1012–1013

Hampton B G 1992 Peristomal and stomal complications. In: Bryant R A, Hampton B G (eds) Ostomies and continent diversions: nursing management. CV Mosby, St Louis, p 107–123

Kohler L W, Pemberton J H, Zinsmeister A R, Kelly K A 1991 Quality of life after proctocolectomy: a comparison of Brooke ileostomy, Koch pouch, ileal pouch–anal anastomosis. Gastroenterology 101: 679–684

McGarity W C 1992 Gastrointestinal surgical procedures. In: Bryant R A, Hampton B G (eds) Ostomies and continent diversions: nursing management. CV Mosby, St Louis, p 354–361

Maidl L 1990 Stomal and peristomal skin complications with urostomies. Urologic Nursing 10: 17–22

Pemberton J H 1988 Management of conventional ileostomies. World Journal of Surgery 12: 203–210

Phillips R, Myers C, Kelly L Principles of stoma siting. Produced with the co-operation of Dansac UK, Pembroke Avenue, Waterbeach, Cambrige, CB5 8BR

Shipes E 1987 Psychological issues: the person with an ostomy. Nursing Clinics of North America 22: 292–302
Sivly P, Todd D 1991 Management of the ileostomy. Practical Gastroenetrology 15: 23–35
Smith D B 1992 Psychosocial adaptation. In: Bryant R A, Hampton B G (eds) Ostomies and continent diversions: nursing management. CV Mosby, St Louis, p 2–8
Turnbull R B 1967 Subtotal colectomy and ileostomy. In: Turnbull R B, Weakley F L (eds) Atlas of intestinal stomas. CV Mosby, St Louis, Missouri, p 24

# Index